Head & Neck Surgery— OTOLARYNGOLOGY

FOURTH EDITION

SECTION EDITORS

Basic Science/General Medicine
Byron J. Bailey
Shawn D. Newlands

Rhinology and Allergy
Matthew W. Ryan
Berrylin J. Ferguson

General Otolaryngology
Byron J. Bailey
Shawn D. Newlands

Airway and Swallowing
David E. Eibling

Voice
Clark A. Rosen

Trauma
Grant S. Gillman
Dean M. Toriumi
Karen H. Calhoun

Pediatric Otolaryngology
Charles M. Myer III
Ronald W. Deskin

Head and Neck Surgery
Jonas T. Johnson
Anna Maria Pou

Otology
Barry E. Hirsch
Arun K. Gadre

Facial Plastic and Reconstructive Surgery
Grant S. Gillman
Dean M. Toriumi
Karen H. Calhoun

Miscellaneous
Byron J. Bailey
Shawn D. Newlands

Consultant (Radiology)
Hugh D. Curtin

Head & Neck Surgery— OTOLARYNGOLOGY

FOURTH EDITION
VOLUME TWO

▬ BYRON J. BAILEY, MD

Chair Emeritus, Department of Otolaryngology
University of Texas Medical Branch at Galveston
Galveston, Texas

▬ JONAS T. JOHNSON, MD

Chair, Department of Otolaryngology
Professor, Departments of Otolaryngology and Radiation Oncology
University of Pittsburgh School of Medicine
Professor, Department of Oral and Maxillofacial Surgery
University of Pittsburgh School of Dental Medicine
Pittsburgh, Pennsylvania

▬ SHAWN D. NEWLANDS, MD, PhD, MBA

Wiess Professor and Chairman
Department of Otolaryngology
University of Texas Medical Branch at Galveston
Galveston, Texas

335 Contributors

Illustrated by Victoria J. Forbes, Anthony Pazos,
and Christine Gralapp

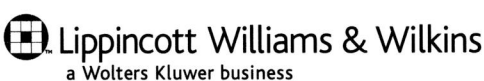
. Lippincott Williams & Wilkins
a Wolters Kluwer business
Philadelphia · Baltimore · New York · London
Buenos Aires · Hong Kong · Sydney · Tokyo

Acquisitions Editor: Robert Hurley
Managing Editor: Michelle LaPlante
Developmental Editor: Molly Connors, Dovetail Content Solutions
Project Manager: Alicia Jackson
Senior Manufacturing Manager: Benjamin Rivera
Marketing Manager: Angela Panetta
Art Director: Risa Clow
Cover Designer: Marie Gardocky Clifton
Production Service: Nesbitt Graphics, Inc.
Printer: Courier-Kendallville

© 2006 by LIPPINCOTT WILLIAMS & WILKINS, a WOLTERS KLUWER BUSINESS
530 Walnut Street
Philadelphia, PA 19106 USA
LWW.com

Third Edition, © 2001 Lippincott Williams & Wilkins
Second Edition, © 1998 Lippincott-Raven Publishers

Library of Congress Cataloging-in-Publication Data

Head and neck surgery--otolaryngology / [edited by] Byron J. Bailey, Jonas T. Johnson, Shawn D. Newlands; illustrated by Victoria J. Forbes, Anthony Pazos, and Christine Gralapp.-- 4th ed.
    p. ; cm.
 Includes bibliographical references and index.
 ISBN-13: 978-0-7817-5561-0   ISBN-10: 0-7817-5561-1 (alk. paper)
 1. Otolaryngology, Operative. 2. Head--Surgery. 3. Neck--Surgery. I. Bailey, Byron J., 1934- II. Johnson, Jonas T. III. Newlands, Shawn D., 1960- . IV. Title.
 [DNLM: 1. Otorhinolaryngologic Diseases--surgery. 2. Head--surgery.
 3. Neck--surgery. WV 168 H432 2006]
 RF51.H43 2006
 617.5'1059--dc22

                                                              2006002393

Care has been taken to confirm the accuracy of the information presented and to describe generally accepted practices. However, the authors, editors, and publisher are not responsible for errors or omissions or for any consequences from application of the information in this book and make no warranty, expressed or implied, with respect to the currency, completeness, or accuracy of the contents of the publication. Application of the information in a particular situation remains the professional responsibility of the practitioner.

The authors, editors, and publisher have exerted every effort to ensure that drug selection and dosage set forth in this text are in accordance with current recommendations and practice at the time of publication. However, in view of ongoing research, changes in government regulations, and the constant flow of information relating to drug therapy and drug reactions, the reader is urged to check the package insert for each drug for any change in indications and dosage and for added warnings and precautions. This is particularly important when the recommended agent is a new or infrequently employed drug.

Some drugs and medical devices presented in the publication have Food and Drug Administration (FDA) clearance for limited use in restricted research settings. It is the responsibility of the health care provider to ascertain the FDA status of each drug or device planned for use in their clinical practice.

To purchase additional copies of this book, call our customer service department at (800) 638-3030 or fax orders to (301) 223-2320. International customers should call (301) 223-2300.

Visit Lippincott Williams & Wilkins on the Internet: at LWW.com. Lippincott Williams & Wilkins customer service representatives are available from 8:30 am to 6 pm, EST.

10 9 8 7 6 5 4 3 2

DEDICATIONS

To our patients and to the vision of improved health for all who inhabit our shrinking world. I am grateful for the opportunity to have led the marvelous efforts of our authors as they assembled and organized this comprehensive collection of important new medical information. May we always keep the needs of our patients foremost in our minds and in our hearts as we study, learn, and practice the science and art of medicine.

Byron J. Bailey, MD, FACS

To my family who indulge my work and my patients who have taught me so much.

Jonas T. Johnson, MD, FACS

To our newest otolaryngologists, our residents, whose probing questions and spirit of inquiry keep alive my interest in learning ever more about our specialty, and to my daughter, Kelsey, whose simple questions keep my life interesting.

Shawn D. Newlands, MD, PhD, MBA, FACS

To Byron J. Bailey, MD, the best friend and mentor an academic otolaryngologist could have had!

Karen H. Calhoun, MD

To all the otolaryngologists that have taken their time to help me learn head and neck radiology over the years. Thank you for your efforts and for your patience.

Hugh D. Curtin, MD

To my good friend and long time mentor, Dr. Byron J. Bailey; to my wife, Nina, and daughters Diane and Jennifer for their lifetime support and encouragement; and to my patients who inspire me to be a better, caring physician.

Ronald W. Deskin, MD, FAAP

To my teachers, especially John Kirchner, Eiji Yanagisawa, Eugene Myers, and Jonas Johnson.

David E. Eibling, MD

To my patients, whose wellbeing and return to health is my primary mission, and to my colleagues and residents who teach and question and advance the primary mission.

Berrylin J. Ferguson, MD

To my parents, Dr. Meena-Ruth and Dr. K. C. Gadre, for their countless sacrifices; to my wife, Dr. Swarupa A. Gadre, for her unwavering support; and to my children Samir-Yitzhak and Sonia, whose smiles make life worthwhile.
Arun K. Gadre, MD

I am forever indebted to Dr. Kris Conrad, Canadian facial plastic surgeon par excellence, without whose inspiration and support I wouldn't be where I am today. And to Drs. Robert Simons, Richard Davis, and Julio Gallo for sharing their expertise with me during my facial plastics fellowship and ever since.
Grant S. Gillman, MD, FRCS(C)

To my wife, Jean, and children David and Peter for their love and support. Many thanks to Eugene Myers, Jonas Johnson, and Mary Lee McAndrew for all the work we have accomplished together.
Barry E. Hirsch, MD

As always, I am appreciative of the support and encouragement of my family and colleagues in the completion of this project.
Charles M. Myer III, MD

To my parents, Jeanette and Frederick Pou, who taught me compassion, kindness, and hard work through example, and to my brother Robert, who in dying taught me courage, dignity, and how to better care for my patients and their families.
Anna Maria Pou, MD

To the first doctor who taught me how to take care of patients, Paul Jack Rosen, MD. I am grateful for the career and personal guidance of the ultimate role model and friend, James I. Cohen, MD, PhD. My involvement and contributions would not be possible without the support, strength, and love from my wife, Monica.
Clark A. Rosen, MD, FACS

To Alex, Ava, Tristan, and August for all your sacrifices made on my behalf.
Matthew W. Ryan, MD

To my family, Colleen, Hannah, and Olivia Toriumi.
Dean M. Toriumi, MD

Contents

Contributing Authors xv
Preface xxix
Acknowledgments xxxi

VOLUME ONE

SECTION 1: BASIC SCIENCE/GENERAL MEDICINE 1

1   Surgical Anatomy of the Head and Neck 3
    Michael D. Maves

2   Understanding Data and Interpreting the Literature 17
    Richard M. Rosenfeld

3   Outcomes and Evidence-Based Medicine 33
    Michael G. Stewart

4   Introduction to Otolaryngic Genetics 41
    Maria J. Worsham, Daniel L. Van Dyke, Bruce R. Korf, and Michael S. Benninger

5   Molecular Otolaryngology 53
    Jessica W. Lim and Michael Friedman

6   Microbiology, Infections, and Antibiotic Therapy 57
    Michael D. Poole and David N. F. Fairbanks

7   Imaging Technology in Otolaryngology 67
    Marvin P. Fried and Richard V. Smith

8   Diagnostic Imaging 85
    Ian J. Witterick, Arnold M. Noyek, Daniel M. Fliss, and Edward E. Kassel

9   Trends in Diagnostic Pathology 99
    Robert L. Reddick and Anne C. Jones

10 Neurology 107
    Frank E. Lucente, Konstantin Tarashansky, and Toby I. Gropen

11 Ophthalmology 125
    Jean Edwards Holt and G. Richard Holt

12 Anesthesiology 141
    Gulshan Doulatram and Shawn D. Newlands

13 Endocrinology 155
    Alfred A. Simental Jr., Lamont Murdoch, and George H. Petti Jr.

14 Degenerative, Idiopathic, and Connective Tissue Diseases 169
    Shawn D. Newlands

15 Dynamics of Wound Healing 197
    Christine G. Gourin and David J. Terris

16 Perioperative Management Issues 215
    David M. Barrs

17 Geriatric Otolaryngology 235
    Byron J. Bailey

18 Headache and Facial Pain 247
    Alan G. Finkel

19 Manifestations of the Acquired Immunodeficiency Syndrome 263
    Mark A. Williams, Thomas A. Tami, and Kelvin C. Lee[†]

20 Tobacco Cessation: How-to Guidance and Resources for Practitioners 277
    Margaret Kuder Hamilton and Nina Markovic

SECTION 2: RHINOLOGY AND ALLERGY 287

21 Olfactory Function and Dysfunction 289
    Richard L. Doty, Steven M. Bromley, and Windolyn D. Panganiban

22 Sinonasal Anatomy, Function, and Evaluation 307
    William E. Walsh and Robert C. Kern

23 Surgical Management of Septal Deformity, Turbinate Hypertrophy, Nasal Valve Collapse, and Choanal Atresia 319
    Michael Friedman and Ramakrishnan Vidyasagar

24 Immunology and Allergy 335
    Paneez Khoury and Robert M. Naclerio

25 Allergic and Nonallergic Rhinitis 351
    John H. Krouse

[†]Deceased.

26   External Approaches in Sinus Surgery 365
     Umamaheswar Duvvuri, Ricardo L. Carrau,
     and Stephen Y. Lai

27   Granulomatous and Autoimmune Diseases of
     the Nose and Sinuses 377
     David M. Poetker, Ricardo Cristobal,
     and Timothy L. Smith

28   Chronic Hypertrophic Rhinosinusitis and Nasal
     Polyposis 393
     Berrylin J. Ferguson and Richard R. Orlandi

29   Nonpolypoid Rhinosinusitis: Classification,
     Diagnosis, and Treatment 405
     José M. Busquets and Peter H. Hwang

30   Fungal Rhinosinusitis 417
     Robert Todd Adelson and Bradley F. Marple

31   Sinus Imaging 429
     Barbara A. Zeifer and Hugh D. Curtin

32   Endoscopic Management of Neoplasms of the
     Nose and Paranasal Sinuses 447
     Lee A. Zimmer, Ricardo L. Carrau,
     Carl H. Snyderman, and Amin B. Kassam

33   Endoscopic Sinus Surgery 459
     Jivianne T. Lee and David W. Kennedy

34   Complications of Sinus Surgery 477
     James A. Stankiewicz

35   Complications of Rhinosinusitis 493
     Carla M. Giannoni and Debra G. Weinberger

36   Epistaxis 505
     Peter-John Wormald

SECTION 3: GENERAL OTOLARYNGOLOGY 515

37   Anatomy and Physiology of the Salivary
     Glands 517
     Benjamin C. Stong, Michael E. Johns,
     and Michael M. Johns III

38   Salivary Gland Imaging 527
     John L. Go, Philip Hoang, and Terry S. Becker

39   Nonneoplastic Diseases of the Salivary
     Glands 545
     Dale H. Rice

40   Controversies in Salivary Gland Disease 555
     Robert J. DeFatta and John M. Truelson

41   Taste 567
     John F. Kveton and Linda M. Bartoshuk

42   Stomatitis 579
     Steven B. Aragon, Bruce W. Jafek, and Steve Johnson

43   Pharyngitis 601
     Lester D. R. Thompson

44   Odontogenic Infections 615
     William Lawson, Anthony J. Reino,
     and Richard W. Westreich

45   Temporomandibular Disorders and Surgery 631
     William C. Donlon

46   Snoring and Obstructive Sleep Apnea 645
     Regina Paloyan Walker

47   Infections of the Deep Spaces of the Neck 665
     Arun K. Gadre and Kamalakar C. Gadre

SECTION 4: AIRWAY AND SWALLOWING 683

48   Upper Digestive Tract Anatomy and
     Physiology 685
     Jeri A. Logemann

49   Upper Airway Anatomy and Function 693
     Gayle E. Woodson

50A Evaluation of Dysphagia 703
     Adrienne L. Perlman and Douglas J. Van Daele

50B Management of Dysphagia 713
     Cathy L. Lazarus

51   Radiographic Examination of the Upper
     Aerodigestive Tract 721
     Barton F. Branstetter IV

52   Management of Intractable Aspiration 733
     David E. Eibling

53   Endoscopic Evaluation of the Upper
     Aerodigestive Tract 745
     Gregory N. Postma, Peter C. Belafsky, Milan R. Amin,
     Stacey L. Halum, and Jamie A. Koufman

54   Esophageal Disorders 755
     William W. Shockley and Subinoy Das

55   Complex Upper Airway Problems 771
     Robert A. Sofferman and Christopher M. Greene

56   Tracheotomy and Intubation 785
     Mark C. Weissler and Marion Everett Couch

57   Controversies in Upper Airway Obstruction 803
     Amelia F. Drake and Michael O. Ferguson

SECTION 5: VOICE 815

58   Voice: Anatomy, Physiology, and Clinical
     Evaluation 817
     Lucian Sulica

59   Laryngitis 829
     *Sumeer K. Gupta, Gregory N. Postma,
     and Jamie A. Koufman*

60   Benign Vocal Fold Lesions and
     Phonomicrosurgery 837
     Clark A. Rosen

61   Treatment of Vocal Fold Paralysis 847
     C. Blake Simpson

62   Neurologic Disorders of the Larynx 867
     Andrew Blitzer and Tanya Meyer

63   Voice Therapy for the Treatment
     of Voice Disorders 883
     Jackie Gartner-Schmidt

64   Care of the Professional Voice 895
     Mark S. Courey

65   Controversies in Laryngology 907
     *Jamie A. Koufman, Stacey L. Halum,
     and Gregory N. Postma*

SECTION 6: TRAUMA 917

66   Principles of Trauma 919
     James Chan and Peter J. Koltai

67   Management of Soft Tissue Trauma
     and Auricular Trauma 935
     J. Randall Jordan and Karen H. Calhoun

68   Laryngeal Trauma 949
     J. Randall Jordan and Scott P. Stringer

69   Mandibular Fractures 961
     Jesse E. Smith and Joseph L. Leach

70   Maxillary and Periorbital Fractures 975
     Brendan C. Stack Jr. and Francis P. Ruggiero

71A Nasal Fractures 995
     Byron J. Bailey

71B Fractures of the Frontal Sinus 1009
     Luke K. S. Tan and Byron J. Bailey

72   Penetrating Face and Neck Trauma 1017
     Michael G. Stewart

73   Complex Facial Trauma with Plating 1027
     Robert M. Kellman and Sherard A. Tatum

SECTION 7: PEDIATRIC OTOLARYNGOLOGY 1045

74   Pediatric Otolaryngology 1047
     Michael J. Cunningham

75   Airway Imaging in Children 1063
     *Susan D. John, J. Alberto Hernandez,
     and Leonard E. Swischuk*

76   Pediatric Sleep-Disordered Breathing 1079
     Liane B. Johnson

77   Neonatal Respiratory Distress 1087
     Mark Boston and Charles M. Myer III

78   Stridor, Aspiration, and Cough 1095
     Cecille G. Sulman and Lauren D. Holinger

79   Congenital Anomalies of the Aerodigestive
     Tract 1119
     Gerald B. Healy

80   Laryngeal Stenosis 1133
     Michael J. Rutter and Robin T. Cotton

81   Pediatric Tracheotomy 1147
     Ronald W. Deskin

82   Caustic Ingestion and Foreign Bodies in the
     Aerodigestive Tract 1157
     Ellen M. Friedman and Gabriel Calzada

83   Recurrent Respiratory Papillomatosis 1167
     Craig S. Derkay

84   Tonsillitis, Tonsillectomy, and
     Adenoidectomy 1183
     Linda Brodsky and Christopher Poje

85   Controversies in Tonsillectomy,
     Adenoidectomy, and Tympanostomy
     Tubes 1199
     Charles D. Bluestone

86   Congenital Neck Masses and Cysts 1209
     Robert L. Pincus

87   Congenital Anomalies of the Nose 1217
     John P. Bent and Roy B. Sessions

88   Pediatric Rhinosinusitis 1229
     Rodney P. Lusk

89   Salivary Gland Disease in Children 1241
     Karen B. Zur and Charles M. Myer III

90   Anatomy and Physiology of the Eustachian Tube
     System 1253
     Charles D. Bluestone

91 Otitis Media with Effusion 1265
    Margaret A. Kenna and Adriane DeWitt Latz

92 Pediatric Audiology 1277
    Deborah L. Carlson and Hilary L. Reeh

93 Sensorineural Hearing Loss 1289
    Patrick E. Brookhouser

94 Genetic Hearing Loss 1303
    Romaine Johnson and John Greinwald

95 Cleft Lip and Palate: Evaluation
    and Treatment of the Primary
    Deformity 1317
    Robin A. Dyleski and Dennis M. Crockett

96 Pediatric Facial Fractures 1337
    Paul R. Krakovitz and Peter J. Koltai

97 Congenital Vascular Lesions 1349
    Norman R. Friedman and Ron Mitchell

98 Pediatric Malignancies 1359
    Mark E. Gerber and Robin T. Cotton

99 The Syndromal Child 1371
    Ted L. Tewfik and John J. Manoukian

VOLUME TWO

SECTION 8: HEAD AND NECK SURGERY 1389

100 Gene Therapy 1391
     Hinrich Staecker, Bert W. O'Malley Jr.,
     and Mark J. Praetorius

101 Tumor Biology and Immunology of Head and
     Neck Cancer 1403
     Peter van der Riet and William J. Richtsmeier

102 Guidelines for Patient Care 1419
     Ara A. Chalian and Sarah H. Kagan

103 Principles of Chemotherapy in the Management
     of Head and Neck Cancer 1427
     Bruce E. Brockstein and Everett E. Vokes

104 Principles of Radiation Oncology 1441
     David H. Hussey

105 Cutaneous Malignancy 1455
     Fred J. Stucker, Cherie-Ann O. Nathan,
     and Timothy S. Lian

106 Malignant Melanoma 1469
     Jeffrey N. Myers and Andrew J. Nemechek

107 Neoplasms of the Nose and Paranasal
     Sinuses 1481
     Lee A. Zimmer and Ricardo L. Carrau

108 Orbital Tumors 1501
     Mark A. Alford and Jeffrey A. Nerad

109 Salivary Gland Neoplasms 1515
     Young S. Oh and David W. Eisele

110 Lip Cancer 1535
     Ramon M. Esclamado and Michael A. Fritz

111 Neoplasms of the Oral Cavity 1551
     Mark J. Jameson and Paul A. Levine

112 Odontogenic Cysts, Tumors, and Related
     Jaw Lesions 1569
     William L. Chung, Darren P. Cox, and Mark W. Ochs

113 Neck Dissection 1585
     Jesus E. Medina

114 Controversies in Management of the N0 Neck
     in Squamous Cell Carcinoma of the Upper
     Aerodigestive Tract 1611
     Karen T. Pitman

115 Lymphomas of the Head and Neck 1621
     Ranjana Advani and Charlotte D. Jacobs

116 Diagnosis and Treatment of Thyroid
     and Parathyroid Disorders 1629
     Cristian M. Slough, Henning Dralle,
     Andreas Machens, and Gregory W. Randolph

117 Nasopharyngeal Cancer 1657
     William I. Wei

118 Oropharyngeal Cancer 1673
     Christopher H. Rassekh and Hadi Seikaly

119 Hypopharyngeal Cancer 1691
     Seungwon Kim and Randal S. Weber

120 Cervical Esophageal Cancer 1711
     Jonas T. Johnson

121A Early Glottic and Supraglottic Carcinoma:
      Endoscopic Techniques 1721
      Steven M. Zeitels

121B Early Glottic and Supraglottic Carcinoma:
      Vertical Partial Laryngectomy and
      Laryngoplasty 1727
      Byron J. Bailey

121C Early Glottic and Supraglottic Carcinoma:
      Open Supraglottic and Supracricoid Partial
      Laryngectomy 1743
      Gregory S. Weinstein, Ollivier Laccourreye,
      and Christopher H. Rassekh

122   Advanced Cancer of the Larynx 1757
      Richard V. Smith and Marvin P. Fried

123   Voice Rehabilitation after Laryngectomy 1779
      Mark. I. Singer and Carla D. Gress

124   Tracheal Tumors 1793
      K. Robert Shen and Douglas J. Mathisen

125   Vascular Tumors of the Head
      and Neck 1811
      Umamaheswar Duvvuri, Ricardo L. Carrau,
      and Amin B. Kassam

126   Cranial-Base Surgery 1827
      Peter D. Costantino, Ahmed S. Ismail,
      and Ivo P. Janecka

127   Surgical Techniques to Enhance Prosthetic
      Rehabilitation 1853
      Mark S. Chambers, James C. Lemon,
      and Jack W. Martin

SECTION 9: OTOLOGY 1867

128   Development of the Ear 1869
      Michael J. Wareing, Anil K. Lalwani,
      and Robert K. Jackler

129   Anatomy and Physiology of Hearing 1883
      John H. Mills, Samir S. Khariwala,
      and Peter C. Weber

130   Vestibular Function and Anatomy 1905
      Shawn D. Newlands and Conrad Wall III

131   Balance Function Tests 1917
      Colin L. W. Driscoll and J. Douglas Green Jr.

132   Assessment of Peripheral and Central Auditory
      Function 1927
      James W. Hall III and Patrick J. Antonelli

133   Neurophysiologic Intraoperative
      Monitoring 1943
      Matthew R. O'Malley, Brian A. Moore,
      and David S. Haynes

134   Imaging Studies of the Temporal Bone 1961
      John A. Butman, Nicholas J. Patronas, and
      Hung Jeffrey Kim

135   Infections of the External Ear 1987
      Christopher J. Linstrom and Frank E. Lucente

136   Neoplasms of the Ear and Lateral Skull
      Base 2003
      Bradley P. Pickett and James P. Kelly

137   Congenital Aural Atresia 2027
      Paul R. Lambert

138   Intratemporal and Intracranial Complications of
      Otitis Media 2041
      J. Gail Neely and H. Alexander Arts

139   Middle Ear and Temporal Bone Trauma 2057
      Rodney Diaz and Hilary A. Brodie

140   Cholesteatoma 2081
      Ted A. Meyer, Chester L. Strunk Jr.,
      and Paul R. Lambert

141   Surgery of the Mastoid and Petrosa 2093
      Richard A. Chole, Hilary A. Brodie,
      and Abraham Jacob

142   Reconstruction of the Tympanic Membrane and
      Ossicular Chain 2113
      Charles M. Luetje II

143   Otosclerosis 2125
      Peter S. Roland and Ravi N. Samy

144   Acute Paralysis of the Facial Nerve 2139
      Jeffrey T. Vrabec and Newton J. Coker

145   Otologic Manifestations of Systemic
      Disease 2155
      Alexander J. Schleuning Jr.,[†]
      Peter E. Andersen, Karen J. Fong, and
      Samuel P. Gubbels

146   Infections of the Labyrinth 2169
      Arun K. Gadre, C. Y. Joseph Chang,
      and Kamalakar C. Gadre

147   Noise-Induced Hearing Loss 2189
      Robert A. Dobie

148   Ototoxicity 2201
      Rita M. Schuman and Gregory J. Matz

149   Cerebellopontine Angle Tumors 2207
      Derald E. Brackmann, James V. Crawford,
      and Douglas Green Jr.

150   Sudden Sensory Hearing Loss 2231
      George T. Hashisaki

151   Tinnitus 2237
      Alexander J. Schleuning Jr.,[†] *"Baker" Y. Shi,*
      and William H. Martin

152   Autoimmune Inner Ear Disease 2247
      Jeffrey P. Harris

153   Aging and the Auditory and Vestibular
      System 2257
      Peter S. Roland and Ravi N. Samy

154   Cochlear Implants and Other Implantable
      Auditory Prostheses 2265
      Richard T. Miyamoto and Karen Iler Kirk

[†]Deceased.

155 Hearing Aids and Assistive Listening
     Devices 2279
     *Todd A Ricketts, Albert R. DeChicchis,
     and Fred H. Bess*

156 Peripheral Vestibular Disorders 2295
     Carol A. Bauer and Horst R. Konrad

157 Central Vestibulopathy 2303
     C. Y. Joseph Chang and Arun K. Gadre

158 Medical Management of Vestibular Disorders
     and Vestibular Rehabilitation 2317
     *P. Ashley Wackym and
     Tammy S. Schumacher-Monfre*

159 Surgical Management of Vestibular
     Disorders 2333
     Jeffrey T. Vrabec

SECTION 10: FACIAL PLASTIC AND RECONSTRUCTIVE SURGERY 2343

160 Grafts and Implants in Facial, Head, and
     Neck Surgery 2345
     G. Richard Holt

161 Local Skin Flaps: Anatomy, Physiology, and
     General Types 2357
     *Kevin A. Shumrick, Jon B. Chadwell,
     and Andrew C. Campbell*

162 Microvascular Free Flaps in Head and Neck
     Reconstruction 2369
     Douglas B. Chepeha and Theodoros N. Teknos

163 Surgical Reconstruction after Mohs Surgery and
     Tissue Expansion 2393
     Karen H. Calhoun and William W. Shockley

164 Scar Camouflage 2411
     Marcelo Hochman and Ricardo A. Beas

165 Nasal Restoration with Flaps
     and Grafts 2421
     Stephen S. Park

166 Surgery for Exophthalmos 2453
     *G. Richard Holt, Jean Edwards Holt,
     and Randal A. Otto*

167 Facial Reanimation 2467
     Steve Parnes and Rami Batniji

168 Facial Analysis and Preoperative
     Evaluation 2481
     Karen H. Calhoun and Kweon I. Stambaugh

169 Pictorial Documentation: Traditional
     Photography and Digital Imaging 2499
     Samuel M. Lam

170 Surgical Anatomy of the Nose 2511
     David W. Kim and Ted Mau

171 Introduction to Rhinoplasty 2533
     Gregory J. Renner

172 Management of the Upper Two Thirds of the
     Nose 2551
     Randolph B. Capone and Ira D. Papel

173 Nasal Tip Surgery 2563
     Grant S. Hamilton III and Dean M. Toriumi

174 Management of the Post-Traumatic Nasal
     Deformity 2579
     Banjamin C. Marcus and Tom D. Wang

175 Secondary Rhinoplasty 2595
     Stephen W. Perkins and Shervin Naderi

176 Blepharoplasty 2611
     Norman J. Pastorek and Andres Bustillo

177 The Aging Face (Rhytidectomy) 2627
     Russell W. H. Kridel and Peyman Soliemanzadeh

178 The Aging Neck 2651
     Edwin F. Williams III and Allison T. Pontius

179 The Aging Forehead 2663
     Peter A. Adamson and Ravi Dahiya

180 Congenital Auricular Malformation 2685
     Eugenio A. Aguilar III

181 Chin and Malar Augmentation 2701
     William E Silver and Anurag Agarwal

182A Chemical Peeling 2717
     J. Gregory Staffel

182B Laser Skin Resurfacing 2725
     Paul J. Carniol

183 Management of Benign Facial Lesions 2731
     *Fred F. Shahan, Karen J. Johnson, John A. Zitelli, and
     Henry H. Roenigk Jr.*

184 Management of Alopecia 2749
     Benjamin A. Bassichis and Raymond J. Konior

185 Cosmetic Uses of Botox and Injectable
     Fillers 2761
     Grant S. Gillman and Julio F. Gallo

186 Rejuvenation of the Midface 2771
     Edwin F. Williams III and Allison J. Pontius

SECTION 11: MISCELLANEOUS 2779

187   **Medical Ethics Rounds** 2781
     Sharen J. Knudsen and Byron J. Bailey

188   **Eponyms in Otolaryngology** 2789
     Kim R. Jones and Harold C. Pillsbury III

189   **Overview of Alternative Medicine** 2797
     Benjamin F. Asher

190   **The Business of Medicine and Planning Your Future** 2805
     Lee D. Eisenberg

191   **Professionalism** 2813
     Byron J. Bailey

192   **Physician Communication Skills: An Essential Competency** 2819
     Byron J. Bailey

Subject Index I-1

Contributing Authors

PETER A. ADAMSON, MD, FRCSC, FACS Professor, Department of Otolaryngology–Head and Neck Surgery, University of Toronto, Toronto; Staff Surgeon, Department of Otolaryngology–Head and Neck Surgery, Toronto General Hospital–University Health Network, Toronto, Ontario, Canada

ROBERT TODD ADELSON, MD Department of Otolaryngology–Head and Neck Surgery, University of Texas Southwestern Medical Center, Dallas, Texas

RANJANA ADVANI, MD Assistant Professor, Department of Medicine, Division of Oncology, Stanford University Medical Center, Stanford, California

ANURAG AGARWAL, MD The Aesthetic Surgery Center, Naples, Florida

EUGENIO A. AGUILAR III, MD, FACS Clinical Assistant Professor, Michael E. Debakey Department of Surgery, Division of Plastic Surgery, Baylor College of Medicine, Houston, Texas

MARK A. ALFORD, MD North Texas Ophthalmic Plastic Surgery, Fort Worth, Texas

MILAN R. AMIN, MD Director, Center for Voice and Swallowing Disorders, Department of Otolaryngology/Head and Neck Surgery, Drexel University College of Medicine, Philadelphia, Pennsylvania

PETER E. ANDERSEN, MD Department of Otolaryngology–Head and Neck Surgery, Oregon Health and Science University, Portland, Oregon

PATRICK J. ANTONELLI, MD Professor and Chair, Department of Otolaryngology, and Assistant Dean for Clinical Informatics, University of Florida School of Medicine, Gainesville; Chief Medical Information Officer, Shands HealthCare, Gainesville, Florida

STEVEN B. ARAGON, MD, DDS Department of Otolaryngology–Head and Neck Surgery, Oral and Maxillofacial Surgery, Sky Ridge Medical Center, Lone Tree, Colorado

H. ALEXANDER ARTS, MD Professor, Department of Otolaryngology and Neurosurgery, University of Michigan School of Medicine, Ann Arbor, Michigan

BENJAMIN F. ASHER, MD Restorative ENT, New York, New York

BYRON J. BAILEY, MD Chairman Emeritus, Department of Otolaryngology, University of Texas Medical Branch, Galveston, Texas

DAVID M. BARRS, MD Otologist and Neurologist, Department of Otolaryngology, Mayo Clinic Arizona, Scottsdale, Arizona

LINDA M. BARTOSHUK, MD, PhD Clinical Professor, Departments of Otolaryngology and Surgery, Yale University School of Medicine, New Haven, Connecticut

BENJAMIN A. BASSICHIS, MD, FACS Clinical Assistant Professor, Department of Otolaryngology–Head and Neck Surgery, University of Texas Southwestern Medical Center, Dallas; Medical Director, Advanced Facial Plastic Surgery Center, Dallas, Texas

RAMI K. BATNIJI, MD Clinical Lecturer, Department of Otolaryngology–Head and Neck Surgery, Indiana University School of Medicine, Indianapolis; Fellow, Facial Plastic and Reconstructive Surgery, Meridian Plastic Surgery Center, Indianapolis, Indiana

CAROL A. BAUER, MD Associate Professor, Department of Surgery, Southern Illinois University School of Medicine, Springfield; Medical Staff, Department of Surgery—Otolaryngology, St. John's Hospital, Springfield, Illinois

RICARDO A. BEAS, MD Visiting International Fellow, The Facial Surgery Center, Charleston, South Carolina; Private practice, Guadalajara, Mexico

TERRY S. BECKER, MD Assistant Professor of Clinical Radiology, Department of Radiology and Otolaryngology, University of Southern California Keck School of Medicine, Los Angeles; Department of Head and Neck Radiology, Los Angeles County/USC Medical Center, Los Angeles, California

PETER C. BELAFSKY, MD, PhD Assistant Professor, Department of Otolaryngology–Head and Neck Surgery, University of California, Davis, School of Medicine, Sacramento, California

MICHAEL S. BENNINGER, MD Chairman, Department of Otolaryngology/Head and Neck Surgery, Henry Ford Hospital, Detroit, Michigan

JOHN P. BENT, MD Assistant Professor, Department of Otolaryngology, Albert Einstein College of Medicine, Bronx; Department of Otolaryngology, Children's Hospital at Montefiore, Bronx, New York

FRED H. BESS, MD   Dan Maddox Hearing Aid Research Laboratory, Vanderbilt Bill Wilkerson Center for Otolaryngology and Communication Sciences, Nashville, Tennessee

ANDREW BLITZER, MD, DDS   Professor of Clinical Otolaryngology, Columbia University College of Physicians and Surgeons, New York; Senior Attending Otolaryngologist, and Director, New York Center for Voice and Swallowing, St. Luke's/Roosevelt Hospital Center, New York, New York

CHARLES D. BLUESTONE, MD   Professor, Department of Otolaryngology, University of Pittsburgh School of Medicine, Pittsburgh; Former Director (1975–2004), Department of Pediatric Otolaryngology, Children's Hospital of Pittsburgh, Pittsburgh, Pennsylvania

MARK BOSTON, MD, MAJ, USAF, MC, FS   56th MDG/SG05L/ENT Clinic, Luke Air Force Base, Arizona

DERALD E. BRACKMANN, MD   Clinical Professor, Department of Otolaryngology–Head and Neck Surgery and Neurosurgery, Los Angeles County/USC Medical Center, Los Angeles; President, House Ear Clinic, Los Angeles, California

BARTON F. BRANSTETTER IV, MD   Assistant Professor, Department of Radiology and Otolaryngology, University of Pittsburgh School of Medicine, Pittsburgh; Director of Head and Neck Imaging, Department of Radiology, University of Pittsburgh Medical Center, Pittsburgh, Pennsylvania

BRUCE E. BROCKSTEIN, MD   Associate Professor, Department of Medicine, Northwestern University Feinberg School of Medicine, Chicago, Illinois; Director, Evanston Kellogg Cancer Cure Center, Department of Oncology and Hematology, Evanston Northwestern Healthcare, Evanston, Illinois

HILARY A. BRODIE, MD, PhD   Professor and Chair, Department of Otolaryngology–Head and Neck Surgery, University of California, Davis, School of Medicine, Sacramento, California

LINDA BRODSKY, MD   Professor, Departments of Otolaryngology and Pediatrics, University of Buffalo School of Medicine and Biomedical Sciences, Buffalo; Director, Department of Pediatric Otolaryngology and Communicative Disorders, Women's and Children's Hospital of Buffalo, Buffalo, New York

STEVEN M. BROMLEY, MD   Assistant Professor, Department of Neurology, University of Medicine and Dentistry of New Jersey–Robert Wood Johnson Medical School, Camden; Attending Neurologist, Department of Medicine, Cooper University Hospital, Camden, New Jersey

PATRICK E. BROOKHOUSER, MD, FACS   Father Flanagan Chair of Otolaryngology, and Director, Boys Town National Research Hospital, Omaha; Chief of Otolaryngology, Creighton University Medical Center, Omaha, Nebraska

JOSÉ M. BUSQUETS, MD   Assistant Professor, Department of Otolaryngology–Head and Neck Surgery, University of Puerto Rico, San Juan; Director, Puerto Rico Nasal and Sinus Institute, San Juan Health Center, San Juan, Puerto Rico

ANDRES BUSTILLO, MD   Department of Facial Plastic and Reconstructive Surgery, Baptist Hospital of Miami, Miami, Florida

JOHN A. BUTMAN, MD, PHD   Senior Staff Neuroradiologist, Diagnostic Radiology Department, Warren G. Magnuson Clinical Center, National Institutes of Health, Bethesda, Maryland

KAREN H. CALHOUN, MD, FACS   William E. Davis Professor and Chair, Department of Otolaryngology–Head and Neck Surgery, University of Missouri–Columbus School of Medicine, Columbia, Missouri

GABRIEL CALZADA, MD   Resident, Bobby R. Alford Department of Otolaryngology–Head and Neck Surgery, Baylor College of Medicine, Houston, Texas

ANDREW C. CAMPBELL, MD   Department of Otolaryngology–Head and Neck Surgery, University of Cincinnati College of Medicine, Cincinnati, Ohio

RANDOLPH B. CAPONE, MD   Director, The Baltimore Center for Facial Plastic Surgery; Co-Director, The Greater Baltimore Cleft Lip and Palate Team; Assistant Professor, The Johns Hopkins Medical Institutions, Baltimore, Maryland

DEBORAH L. CARLSON, PhD   Associate Professor, Department of Otolaryngology, and Director, Center for Audiology and Speech Pathology, University of Texas Medical Branch, Galveston, Texas

PAUL J. CARNIOL, MD, FACS   Clinical Associate Professor, Department of Surgery, Section of Otolaryngology–Head and Neck Surgery, The New Jersey Medical School, Newark, New Jersey; Attending Surgeon, Department of Plastic Surgery and Otolaryngology, Overlook Hospital, Summit, New Jersey

RICARDO L. CARRAU, MD, FACS   Professor, Departments of Otolaryngology and Neurological Surgery, University of Pittsburgh School of Medicine, Pittsburgh; Center for Minimally Invasive Surgery, University of Pittsburgh Medical Center, Eye & Ear Institute, Pittsburgh, Pennsylvania

JON B. CHADWELL, MD   Department of Otolaryngology–Head and Neck Surgery, University of Cincinnati College of Medicine, Cincinnati, Ohio

ARA A. CHALIAN, MD   Associate Professor, Department of Otorhinolaryngology–Head and Neck Surgery, University of Pennsylvania School of Medicine, Philadelphia; Director, Section of Facial Plastic and Reconstructive Surgery, Department of Otorhinolaryngology–Head and Neck Surgery, University of Pennsylvania Health System, Philadelphia, Pennsylvania

MARK S. CHAMBERS, DMD, MS Associate Professor, Department of Head and Neck Surgery, The University of Texas M.D. Anderson Cancer Center, Houston, Texas

JAMES CHAN, MD Department of Otolaryngology, Facial Plastic and Reconstructive Surgery, Stanford University School of Medicine, Stanford, California

C. Y. JOSEPH CHANG, MD, FACS Department of Otolaryngology–Head and Neck Surgery, University of Texas–Houston Medical School, Houston; Chief of Service, Department of Otolaryngology–Head and Neck Surgery, Memorial Hermann Hospital, Houston, Texas

DOUGLAS B. CHEPEHA, MD, MSPH Associate Professor, Department of Otolaryngology–Head and Neck Surgery, University of Michigan Medical School, Ann Arbor, Michigan

RICHARD A. CHOLE, MD, PhD Lindburg Professor and Head, Department of Otolaryngology, Washington University School of Medicine, St. Louis; Chief, Department of Otolaryngology, Barnes-Jewish Hospital, St. Louis, Missouri

WILLIAM L. CHUNG, DDS, MD Assistant Professor, Department of Oral and Maxillofacial Surgery, University of Pittsburgh School of Dental Medicine, Pittsburgh; Staff Surgeon, Department of Oral and Maxillofacial Surgery, University of Pittsburgh Medical Center, Pittsburgh, Pennsylvania

NEWTON J. COKER, MD Professor, Bobby R. Alford Department of Otolaryngology–Head and Neck Surgery, Baylor College of Medicine, Houston, Texas

PETER D. COSTANTINO, MD Associate Professor of Clinical Otolaryngology, Department of Otolaryngology, Columbia University College of Physicians and Surgeons, New York; Vice Chairman, Department of Otolaryngology–Head and Neck Surgery, and Co-Director, Center for Cranial Base Surgery, Department of Otolaryngology and Neuroscience, St. Luke's–Roosevelt Hospital Center, New York, New York

ROBIN T. COTTON, MD Director, Department of Pediatric Otolaryngology, Children's Hospital Medical Center, Cincinnati, Cincinnati, Ohio

MARION EVERETT COUCH, MD, PhD, FACS Assistant Professor, Department of Otolaryngology–Head and Neck Surgery, University of North Carolina at Chapel Hill School of Medicine, Chapel Hill, North Carolina

MARK S. COUREY, MD Clinical Professor of Otolaryngology, Department of Otolaryngology–Head and Neck Surgery, University of California, San Francisco, School of Medicine, San Francisco; Director, Division of Laryngology, The UCSF Voice and Swallowing Center, San Francisco, California

DARREN P. COX, DDS, MBA Assistant Professor of Clinical Oral Pathology, Department of Orofacial Sciences and Pathology, University of California, San Francisco, San Francisco, California

JAMES V. CRAWFORD, MD Associate Professor, Department of Surgery, Uniformed Services University, Bethesda, Maryland; Chief of Neurotology, Department of Surgery, Madigan Army Medical Center, Tacoma, Washington

RICARDO CRISTOBAL, MD Chief Resident, Department of Otolaryngology and Communication Sciences, Medical College of Wisconsin, Milwaukee, Wisconsin

DENNIS M. CROCKETT, MD Associate Professor, Department of Otolaryngology–Head and Neck Surgery, University of Southern California Keck School of Medicine, Los Angeles, California

MICHAEL J. CUNNINGHAM, MD Associate Professor, Department of Otology and Laryngology, Harvard Medical School, Boston; Surgeon, Department of Otolaryngology, Massachusetts Eye and Ear Infirmary, Boston, Massachusetts

HUGH D. CURTIN, MD Professor, Department of Radiology, Harvard Medical School, Boston; Chief, Department of Radiology, Massachusetts Eye and Ear Infirmary, Boston, Massachusetts

RAVI DAHIYA, MD Potomac Facial Plastic Surgery, Chevy Chase, Maryland

SUBINOY DAS, MD Resident, Department of Otolaryngology–Head and Neck Surgery, University of North Carolina at Chapel Hill School of Medicine and University of North Carolina Hospitals, Chapel Hill, North Carolina

ALBERT R. De CHICCHIS, PhD Department of Communication Sciences and Disorders, University of Georgia, Athens, Georgia

ROBERT J. DeFATTA, MD, PhD Resident, Department of Otolaryngology–Head and Neck Surgery, University of Texas Southwestern Medical Center, Dallas, Texas

CARLA DeLASSUS (GRESS), ScD, CCC-SLP Voice Institute Director, International Association of Laryngectomees, Stockton, California

CRAIG S. DERKAY, MD Professor, Departments of Otolaryngology and Pediatrics, Eastern Virginia Medical School, Norfolk; Director, Department of Pediatric Otolaryngology, Children's Hospital of the King's Daughters, Norfolk, Virginia

RONALD W. DESKIN, MD, FAAP Professor, Departments of Otolaryngology and Pediatrics, University of Texas Southwestern Medical Center, Dallas; Attending Otolaryngologist, Department of Otolaryngology, Children's Medical Center of Dallas, Dallas, Texas

RODNEY DIAZ, MD Assistant Professor, Department of Otolaryngology–Head and Neck Surgery, University of California, Davis, School of Medicine, Sacramento, California

ROBERT A. DOBIE, MD Professor, Department of Otolaryngology, University of California, Davis, School of Medicine, Sacramento, California

WILLIAM C. DONLON, DMD, MS Consultant Surgeon, Cherry Blossom Clinical Consulting, Ltd., Ashland, Oregon

RICHARD L. DOTY, PhD Director, Smell and Taste Center, Department of Otorhinolaryngology–Head and Neck Surgery, University of Pennsylvania School of Medicine, Philadelphia, Pennsylvania

GULSHAN DOULATRAM, MD Assistant Professor, Department of Anesthesiology, University of Texas Medical Branch, Galveston, Texas

AMELIA F. DRAKE, MD, FACS Professor, Department of Otolaryngology–Head and Neck Surgery, and Chief, Division of Pediatric Otolaryngology; Newton D. Fischer Distinguished Professor of Surgery, University of North Carolina at Chapel Hill School of Medicine, Chapel Hill, North Carolina

HENNING DRALLE, MD, FRCS Professor of Surgery and Chairman, Department of General, Visceral and Vascular Surgery, University of Halle, Halle, Germany

COLIN L.W. DRISCOLL, MD Associate Professor, Department of Otorhinolaryngology–Head and Neck Surgery, Mayo Clinic College of Medicine, Rochester, Minnesota

UMAMAHESWAR DUVVURI, MD, PhD Resident, Department of Otolaryngology, University of Pittsburgh School of Medicine, Eye & Ear Institute, Pittsburgh, Pennsylvania

ROBIN A. DYLESKI, MD, FACS Director of Pediatric Otolaryngology, Department of Otolaryngology, New York Eye and Ear Infirmary, New York, New York

DAVID E. EIBLING, MD Professor, Department of Otolaryngology–Head and Neck Surgery, University of Pittsburgh School of Medicine, Pittsburgh; Assistant Chief, Department of Surgical Service, Verterans Affairs Pittsburgh, Pittsburgh, Pennsylvania

DAVID W. EISELE, MD Professor, Department of Otolaryngology–Head and Neck Surgery, University of California, San Francisco, School of Medicine, San Francisco; Chairman, Department of Otolaryngology–Head and Neck Surgery, UCSF Comprehensive Cancer Center, San Francisco, California

LEE D. EISENBERG, MD, FACS Associate Clinical Professor, Department of Otolaryngology–Head and Neck Surgery, Columbia University College of Physicians and Surgeons, New York, New York; Chief, Department of Otolaryngology–Head and Neck Surgery, Englewood Hospital, Englewood, New Jersey

RAMON M. ESCLAMADO, MD Professor, Department of Surgery, Duke University School of Medicine, Durham; Chief, Division of Otolaryngology–Head and Neck Surgery, Duke University Medical Center, Durham, North Carolina

DAVID N. F. FAIRBANKS, MD Clinical Professor, Department of Otolaryngology, George Washington University School of Medicine, Washington, DC

BERRYLIN J. FERGUSON, MD, FACS, FAAOA Associate Professor, Department of Otolaryngology, University of Pittsburgh School of Medicine, Pittsburgh; Director, Division of Sino-Nasal Disorders and Allergy, Department of Otolaryngology, University of Pittsburgh Medical Center, Pittsburgh, Pennsylvania

MICHAEL O. FERGUSON, MD Assistant Professor of Otolaryngology–Head and Neck Surgery, University of North Carolina at Chapel Hill School of Medicine, Chapel Hill, North Carolina

ALAN G. FINKEL, MD Associate Professor, Department of Neurology, University of North Carolina at Chapel Hill School of Medicine, Chapel Hill, North Carolina

DANIEL M. FLISS, MD Professor of Otolaryngology, Tel Aviv University, Sackler School of Medicine, Tel-Aviv; Chairman, Department of Otolaryngology–Head and Neck Surgery, The Skull Base Unit, Tel Aviv Sourasky Medical Center, Tel-Aviv, Israel

KAREN J. FONG, MD Assistant Professor, Department of Otolaryngology–Head and Neck Surgery, Oregon Health and Science University, Portland, Oregon

MARVIN P. FRIED, MD, FACS Professor and University Chairman, Department of Otolaryngology, Albert Einstein College of Medicine–Montefiore Medical Center, Bronx; Attending and Chairman, Department of Otolaryngology, Albert Einstein College of Medicine–Montefiore Medical Center, Bronx, New York

ELLEN M. FRIEDMAN, MD Professor, Bobby R. Alford Department of Otolaryngology–Head and Neck Surgery, Baylor College of Medicine, Houston; Chief, Department of Otolaryngology, Texas Children's Hospital, Houston, Texas

MICHAEL FRIEDMAN, MD Professor of Otolaryngology, Chairman of Head/Neck Surgery, Department of Otolaryngology/Head and Neck Surgery, Rush University Medical Center, Chicago; Chairman, Department of Otolaryngology, Advocate Illinois Masonic Medical Center, Chicago, Illinois

NORMAN R. FRIEDMAN, MD, D.ABSM Assistant Professor, Department of Otolaryngology, University of Colorado Health Science Center, Denver; Director of the Rocky Mountain Sleep Disorders Unit, Division of Pediatric Otolaryngology, The Children's Hospital–Denver, Denver, Colorado

MICHAEL A. FRITZ, MD Associate Staff, Head and Neck Institute, Cleveland Clinic Foundation, Cleveland, Ohio

ARUN K. GADRE, MD Associate Professor, Department of Otolaryngology–Head and Neck Surgery, University of Texas School of Medicine at Houston; Department of Otolaryngology, Memorial Hermann Texas Medical Center. Houston, Texas

KAMALAKAR C. GADRE, MS, DLO (LOND), FICS, FACS Chairman and Professor Emeritus, Department of Otolaryngology–Head and Neck Surgery, Lokmanya Tilak Municipal Medical College, Mumbai; Chief, Department of Otolaryngology, Dr. Gadre's Surgical & Maternity Hospital, Mumbai, India

JULIO F. GALLO, MD   Voluntary Clinical Instructor, Division of Facial Plastic Surgery, Department of Otolaryngology, University of Miami School of Medicine, Miami; Medical Director, The Miami Institute for Age Management and Intervention, Miami, Florida

JACQUELINE L. GARTNER-SCHMIDT, PhD   Assistant Professor, Department of Otolaryngology, University of Pittsburgh School of Medicine, Pittsburgh; Associate Director, University of Pittsburgh Voice Center, Department of Otolaryngology, University of Pittsburgh Medical Center, Pittsburgh, Pennsylvania

MARK E. GERBER, MD, FACS, FAAP   Pediatric Otolaryngology–Head and Neck Surgery, Evanston Northwestern Healthcare; Assistant Professor, Department of Otolaryngology, Northwestern University Feinberg School of Medicine, Chicago, Illinois

CARLA GIANNONI, MD   Associate Professor, Pediatric Otolaryngology, Bobby R. Alford Department of Otolaryngology–Head and Neck Surgery, Baylor College of Medicine, Houston; Department of Pediatric Otolaryngology, Texas Children's Hospital, Houston, Texas

GRANT S. GILLMAN, MD, FRCS   Assistant Professor, Director, Division of Facial Plastic Surgery, Department of Otolaryngology, University of Pittsburgh School of Medicine, Pittsburgh, Pennsylvania

JOHN L. GO, MD   Assistant Professor of Clinical Radiology, Departments of Radiology and Otolaryngology, University of Southern California Keck School of Medicine, Los Angeles; Chief, Department of Head and Neck Radiology, Los Angeles County/USC Medical Center, Los Angeles, California

CHRISTINE G. GOURIN, MD, FACS   Assistant Professor, Department of Otolaryngology, Medical College of Georgia, Augusta; Active Staff, Department of Otolaryngology–Head and Neck Surgery Medical College of Georgia Medical Center, Augusta, Georgia

J. DOUGLAS GREEN Jr., MD, MSc, FACS   Active Staff, Department of Otolaryngology–Head and Neck Institute Baptist Medical Center, Jacksonville, Florida

CHRISTOPHER M. GREENE, MD   Associate Professor, Department of Anesthesiology, University of Vermont School of Medicine, Burlington; Attending Anesthesiologist, Department of Anesthesiology, Fletcher Allen Health Care, Burlington, Vermont

JOHN H. GREINWALD Jr., MD   Associate Professor, Department of Otolaryngology–Head and Neck Surgery, University of Cincinnati College of Medicine, Cincinnati; Director of the Auditory Genetics Laboratory at the Center for Hearing and Deafness Research, Division of Otolaryngology–Head and Neck Surgery, Cincinnati Children's Hospital Medical Center, Cincinnati, Ohio

TOBY I. GROPEN, MD   Assistant Professor, Department of Neurology State University of New York–Downstate Medical Center, Brooklyn; Chairman, Department of Neurology, Long Island College Hospital, Brooklyn, New York

SAMUEL P. GUBBELS, MD   Department of Otolaryngology–Head and Neck Surgery, Oregon Health and Science University, Portland, Oregon

SUMEER K. GUPTA, MD   Center for Voice and Swallowing Disorders, Department of Otolaryngology, Wake Forest University School of Medicine, Winston-Salem, North Carolina

JAMES W. HALL III, PhD   Associate Chair and Clinical Professor, Chief of Audiology Division, Department of Communicative Disorders, University of Florida, Gainesville, Florida

STACEY L. HALUM, MD   Center for Voice and Swallowing Disorders, Department of Otolaryngology–Head and Neck Surgery, Wake Forest University School of Medicine, Winston-Salem, North Carolina

GRANT S. HAMILTON III, MD   Assistant Professor, Department of Otolaryngology–Head and Neck Surgery, University of Iowa; Surgeon, Department of Facial Plastic Surgery, University of Iowa Hospitals and Clinics, Iowa City, Iowa

MARGARET KUDER HAMILTON, MHPE, CHES   Research Associate, Department of Dental Public Health, University of Pittsburgh School of Dental Medicine, Pittsburgh, Pennsylvania

JEFFREY P. HARRIS, MD, PhD   Chief of Otolaryngology–Head and Neck Surgery, Professor of Surgery/Otology and Neurological Surgery, University of California, San Diego, School of Medicine, San Diego, California

GEORGE T. HASHISAKI, MD   Associate Professor, Department of Otolaryngology–Head and Neck Surgery, University of Virginia Health Systems, Charlottesville, Virginia

DAVID S. HAYNES, MD   Associate Professor, Department of Otolaryngology, Vanderbilt University Medical Center, Nashville; Director of Otology and Neurotology, The Otology Group of Vanderbilt, Vanderbilt University Medical Center, Nashville, Tennessee

GERALD B. HEALY, MD   Otolaryngologist-in-Chief, Department of Otolaryngology and Communication Disorders, Children's Hospital, Boston; Professor of Otology and Laryngology, Harvard Medical School, Boston, Massachusetts

J. ALBERTO HERNANDEZ, MD   Assistant Professor of Radiology and Pediatrics, Department of Radiology, University of Texas Medical Branch, Galveston; Assistant, Department of Radiology, Children's Hospital, Galveston, Texas

BARRY E. HIRSCH, MD, FACS   Associate Professor, Department of Otolaryngology, University of Pittsburgh School of Medicine, Pittsburgh, Pennsylvania

PHILLIP HOANG, MD   Clinical Instructor, Department of Radiology, University of Southern California Keck School of Medicine, Los Angeles; Clinical Instructor, Department of Radiology, Los Angeles County/USC Medical Center, Los Angeles, California

MARCELO HOCHMAN, MD, FACS   The Facial Surgery Center, Charleston, South Carolina

LAUREN D. HOLINGER, MD   Professor, Department of Otolaryngology–Head and Neck Surgery, Northwestern University Feinberg School of Medicine, Chicago; Head, Department of Pediatric Otolaryngology, Children's Memorial Hospital, Chicago, Illinois

G. RICHARD HOLT, MD   Professor, Department of Otolaryngology-Head and Neck Surgery, The University of Texas Health Science Center, San Antonio, Texas

JEAN EDWARDS HOLT, MD   Clinical Professor, Department of Ophthalmology, The University of Texas Health Science Center, San Antonio, Texas

DAVID H. HUSSEY, MD   Clinical Professor, Radiation Oncology, The University of Texas Health Science Center, San Antonio, Texas

PETER H. HWANG, MD   Associate Professor, Department of Otolaryngology–Head & Neck Surgery, and Director, Stanford Sinus Center, Stanford University School of Medicine, Stanford, California

AHMED S. ISMAIL, MD   Department of Otolaryngology–Head and Neck Surgery, Faculty of Medicine, University of Alexandria, Egypt; Lecturer, Department of Otolaryngology–Head and Neck Surgery, Columbia University College of Physicians and Surgeons, New York, New York

ROBERT K. JACKLER, MD   Sewall Professor and Chair, Department of Otolaryngology, Stanford University School of Medicine, Stanford, California

ABRAHAM JACOB, MD   Otology/Neurotology Fellow, Department of Otolaryngology–Head and Neck Surgery, The Ohio State University Medical Center, Columbus, Ohio

CHARLOTTE D. JACOBS, MD   Professor, Department of Medicine, Division of Oncology, Stanford University School of Medicine, Stanford, California

BRUCE W. JAFEK, MD, FACS, FRSM   Professor, Department of Otolaryngology–Head and Neck Surgery, University of Colorado School of Medicine, Denver; Active Staff, Department of Otolaryngology–Head and Neck Surgery, University of Colorado Hospital, Denver, Colorado

MARK J. JAMESON, MD, PhD   Chief Resident, Department of Otolaryngology–Head and Neck Surgery, University of Virginia Health System, Charlottesville, Virginia

IVO P. JANECKA, MD   Longwood Skull Base Program, Harvard Medical School, Boston, Massachusetts

SUSAN D. JOHN, MD   Professor and Chair, Department of Diagnostic and Interventional Imaging, University of Texas Health Science Center, Houston; Chair, Department of Diagnostic and Interventional Imaging, Memorial Hermann Hospital, Houston, Texas

MICHAEL E. JOHNS, MD   Executive Vice President for Health Affairs, Robert W. Woodruff Health Sciences Center, Emory University, Atlanta; Chairman of the Board, Emory Healthcare, Emory University Hospitals, Atlanta, Georgia

MICHAEL M. JOHNS, III, MD   Assistant Professor, Department of Otolaryngology, Emory University School of Medicine, Atlanta, Georgia

JONAS T. JOHNSON, MD   Chair, Department of Otolaryngology, and Professor, Departments of Otolaryngology and Radiation Oncology, University of Pittsburgh School of Medicine; Professor, Department of Oral and Maxillofacial Surgery, University of Pittsburgh School of Dental Medicine, Pittsburgh, Pennsylvania

KAREN J. JOHNSON, MD   University of Pittsburgh Medical Center–Shadyside Medical Center, Pittsburgh, Pennsylvania

LIANE B. JOHNSON, MDCM, FRCS(C)   Assistant Professor, Department of Surgery, Division of Paediatric Otolaryngology, Dalhousie University, QEII Health Sciences Centre, Halifax; Paediatric Otolaryngologist, Airway Surgeon, Department of Surgery, Division of Paediatric Otolaryngology, IWK Health Centre, Halifax, Nova Scotia, Canada

ROMAINE F. JOHNSON, MD   Pediatric Otolayngology Fellow, Department of Otolaryngology–Head and Neck Surgery, Cincinnati Children's Hospital Medical Center, Cincinnati, Ohio

STEVE JOHNSON, MD   University of Colorado Health Sciences Center, Denver, Colorado

ANNE C. JONES, DDS   Professor, Department of Pathology, University of Texas Health Science Center, San Antonio; Oral Medicine, Oral Pathology, Department of Pathology, University of Texas Health System, San Antonio, Texas

KIM R. JONES, MD, PhD   Department of Otolaryngology–Head and Neck Surgery, University of North Carolina at Chapel Hill School of Medicine, Chapel Hill, North Carolina

J. RANDALL JORDAN, MD, FACS   Associate Professor and Vice Chairman, Department of Otolaryngology and Communication Sciences, University of Mississippi School of Medicine, Jackson, Mississippi

SARAH H. KAGAN, PhD, RN   Associate Professor of Gerantological Nursing, Department of Otolaryngology–Head and Neck Surgery, University of Pennsylvania School of Nursing, Philadelphia; Clinical Nurse Specialist, Department of Nursing, University of Pennsylvania Hospital, Philadelphia, Pennsylvania

AMIN B. KASSAM, MD, FRCS(C)   Associate Professor, Department of Neurological Surgery, University of Pittsburgh School of Medicine, Pittsburgh; Director, Minimally Invasive endoNeurosurgical Center, University of Pittsburgh Medical Center, Pittsburgh, Pennsylvania

EDWARD E. KASSEL, MD, DDS, FRCPC Associate Professor, Department of Medical Imaging, University of Toronto; Department of Medical Imaging, Mount Sinai Hospital, Toronto, Ontario, Canada

ROBERT M. KELLMAN, MD Professor and Chair, Department of Otolaryngology, State University of New York Upstate Medical University, Syracuse, New York

JAMES P. KELLY, MD Director of Research, Department of Surgery, University of New Mexico School of Medicine, Albuquerque, New Mexico

MARGARET A. KENNA, MD, MPH Associate Professor, Department of Otology and Laryngology, Harvard Medical School; Director of Clinical Research, Department of Otolaryngology and Communicative Disorders, Children's Hospital Boston, Boston, Massachusetts

DAVID W. KENNEDY, MD Vice Dean for Professional Services and Senior Vice President, University of Pennsylvania Health System; Director of Rhinology, Department of Otorhinolaryngology–Head and Neck Surgery, Hospital of the University of Pennsylvania, Philadelphia, Pennsylvania

ROBERT KERN, MD Professor, Department of Otolaryngology–Head and Neck Surgery, Northwestern University, Feinberg School of Medicine, Chicago; Chief of Rhinology, Department of Otolaryngology–Head and Neck Surgery, Northwestern Memorial Hospital, Chicago, Illinois

SAMIR S. KHARIWALA, MD Department of Head and Neck Surgery, The Cleveland Clinic Foundation, Cleveland, Ohio

PANEEZ KHOURY, MD Clinical Instructor–Housestaff, Department of Internal Medicine, The Ohio State University, Columbus, Ohio

DAVID W. KIM, MD Assistant Professor, Department of Otolaryngology–Head and Neck Surgery, and Director, Division of Facial Plastic and Reconstructive Surgery, University of California, San Francisco, School of Medicine, San Francisco, California

H. JEFFREY KIM, MD Senior Staff Clinician, Neurology Branch, National Institute on Deafness and Other Communication Disorders, National Institutes of Health, Bethesda, Maryland; Associate Professor, Department of Otolaryngology–Head and Neck Surgery, Georgetown University Medical Center, Washington, DC

SEUNGWON KIM, MD Fellow in Head and Neck Surgical Oncology, Department of Head and Neck Surgery, University of Texas M.D. Anderson Cancer Center, Houston, Texas

KAREN ILER KIRK, PhD Professor, Department of Speech, Language, and Hearing Sciences, Purdue University, West Lafayette, Indiana

SHAREN J. KNUDSEN, MD Private practice, Highland, California

PETER J. KOLTAI, MD, FACS, FAAP Professor and Chief, Division of Pediatric Otolaryngology, Department of Otolaryngology–Head and Neck Surgery, and Professor, Department of Pediatrics, Stanford University School of Medicine, Stanford, California; Service Chief, Pediatric Otolaryngology–Head and Neck, Lucile Packard Children's Hospital, Palo Alto, California

RAYMOND J. KONIOR, MD Oak Brook Aesthetic and Premiere Hair Restoration, Oak Brook, Illinois

HORST R. KONRAD, MD Professor Emeritus, Department of Surgery, Division of Otolaryngology, Southern Illinois University School of Medicine, Springfield; Staff, Department of Surgery and Otolaryngology, St. John's Hospital, Springfield, Illinois

BRUCE R. KORF, MD, PhD Wayne H. and Sara Crews Finley Professor of Medical Genetics, and Chair, Department of Genetics, University of Alabama at Birmingham, Birmingham, Alabama

JAMIE A. KOUFMAN, MD Director, Center for Voice and Swallowing Disorders, Department of Otolaryngology–Head and Neck Surgery, Wake Forest University School of Medicine, Winston-Salem, North Carolina

PAUL R. KRAKOVITZ, MD Associate Staff, Head and Neck Institution, Section of Pediatric Otolaryngology, Cleveland Clinic Foundation, Cleveland, Ohio

RUSSELL W. H. KRIDEL, MD, FACS Clinical Professor, Division of Facial Plastic and Reconstructive Surgery, Department of Otolaryngology–Head and Neck Surgery, University of Texas Health Science Center and Medical School, Houston, Texas

JOHN H. KROUSE, MD, PhD Professor, Department of Otolaryngology–Head and Neck Surgery, Wayne State University School of Medicine, Detroit; Director, Center of Excellence in Sinonasal Diseases, Department of Otolaryngology–Head and Neck Surgery, Harper-Hutzel Hospital, Detroit Medical Center, Detroit, Michigan

JOHN F. KVETON, MD Clinical Professor, Department of Surgery, Division of Otolaryngology, Yale University School of Medicine, New Haven, Connecticut

OLLIVIER LACCOURREYE, MD Professor, Otolaryngology–Head and Neck Surgery, The University of Paris

STEPHEN Y. LAI, MD, PhD Assistant Professor, Department of Otolaryngology, University of Pittsburgh, The Eye & Ear Institute, Pittsburgh, Pennsylvania

ANIL K. LALWANI, MD Mendik Foundation Professor and Chairman, Department of Otolaryngology, and Professor, Department of Physiology and Neuroscience, New York University School of Medicine, New York; Department of Otolaryngology, New York University Medical Center, New York, New York

SAMUEL M. LAM, MD Director, Lam Facial Plastic Surgery Center and Willow Bend Wellness Center, Plano, Texas

PAUL R. LAMBERT, MD, FACS Professor and Chair, Department of Otolaryngology–Head and Neck Surgery, Medical University of South Carolina, Charleston, South Carolina

ADRIANE DEWITT LATZ, MD Assistant Professor, Department of Otolaryngology–Head and Neck Surgery, University of Kansas School of Medicine, Kansas City, Kansas; Children's Mercy Hospital, Kansas City, Missouri

WILLIAM LAWSON, MD, DDS Professor, Department of Otolaryngology, Mount Sinai Medical Center, New York, New York

CATHY L. LAZARUS, PhD Associate Professor, Department of Otolaryngology, New York University School of Medicine, New York; Director, Department of Hearing and Speech, Bellevue Hospital Center, New York, New York

JOSEPH L. LEACH, MD Associate Professor, Department of Otolaryngology, University of Texas Southwestern Medical Center, Dallas; Staff, Department of Otolaryngology, Parkland Hospital, Dallas, Texas

JIVIANNE T. LEE, MD Rhinology Fellow, Department of Otorhinolaryngology–Head and Neck Surgery, University of Pennsylvania School of Medicine, Philadelphia; Clinical Instructor, Department of Otorhinolaryngology–Head and Neck Surgery, Hospital of the University of Pennsylvania, Philadelphia, Pennsylvania

KELVIN C. LEE, MD†

JAMES C. LEMON, DDS Professor (Emeritus), Department of Head and Neck Surgery, The University of Texas M.D. Anderson Cancer Center, Houston, Texas

PAUL A. LEVINE, MD Chairman, Department of Otolaryngology–Head and Neck Surgery, University of Virginia Health System, Charlottesville, Virginia

TIMOTHY S. LIAN, MD Department of Otolaryngology—Head and Neck Surgery, Louisiana State University Health Sciences Center-Shreveport, Louisiana

JESSICA W. LIM, MD Department of Otolaryngology, Long Island College Hospital, Brooklyn, New York

CHRISTOPHER J. LINSTROM, MD Professor, Department of Otolaryngology–Head and Neck Surgery, The New York Medical College, Administration Department, Valhalla, New York; Surgeon Director, Department of Otolaryngology–Head and Neck Surgery, The New York Eye and Ear Infirmary, New York, New York

JERI A. LOGEMANN, MD Professor, Department of Communication Sciences and Disorders, Northwestern University; Professor, Departments of Neurology and Otolaryngology–Head and Neck Surgery, Northwestern University Feinberg School of Medicine, Chicago, Illinois

FRANK E. LUCENTE, MD Professor and Chairman, Department of Otolaryngology, State University of New York–Downstate Medical Center, Brooklyn; Chairman, Department of Otolaryngology, Long Island College Hospital, Brooklyn, New York

CHARLES M. LUETJE III, MD, FACS Otologic Center, Inc., Kansas City, Missouri

RODNEY P. LUSK, MD, FACS, FAAP Boys Town National Research Hospital, Boys Town ENT Institute, Omaha, Nebraska

ANDREAS MACHENS, MD Associate Professor of Surgery, Department of General, Visceral and Vascular Surgery, University of Halle, Klinikum Krollwitz, Halle, Germany

JOHN J. MANOUKIAN, MD, FRCSC Associate Professor, Department of Otolaryngology, McGill University, Montreal; Associate Director, Department of Otolaryngology, Montreal Children's Hospital, Montreal, Quebec, Canada

BENJAMIN C. MARCUS, MD Assistant Professor, Department of Surgery, Division of Otolaryngology–Head and Neck Surgery, University of Wisconsin School of Medicine, Madison, Wisconsin

NINA MARKOVIC, PhD Associate Professor, Department of Dental Public Health, University of Pittsburgh, Pittsburgh, Pennsylvania

BRADLEY F. MARPLE, MD Associate Professor and Vice Chairman, Department of Otolaryngology, University of Texas Southwestern Medical Center, Dallas, Texas

JACK W. MARTIN, DDS, MS Professor, Department of Head and Neck Surgery, The University of Texas M.D. Anderson Cancer Center, Houston, Texas

WILLIAM H. MARTIN, MD Department of Otolaryngology–Head and Neck Surgery, Oregon Health and Science University, Portland, Oregon

DOUGLAS J. MATHISEN, MD Hermes C. Grillo Professor, Department of Thoracic Surgery, Harvard Medical School, Boston; Visiting Surgeon and Chief, Department of General Thoracic Surgery, Massachusetts General Hospital, Boston, Massachusetts

GREGORY J. MATZ, MD Professor, Department of Otolaryngology–Head and Neck Surgery, Loyola University Medical Center, Maywood, Illinois

TED MAU, MD, PhD Chief Resident, Department of Otolaryngology–Head and Neck Surgery, University of California, San Francisco, San Francisco, California

MICHAEL D. MAVES, MD Executive Vice President and Chief Executive Officer, American Medical Association, Chicago, Illinois

JESUS E. MEDINA, MD, FACS Paul and Ruth Jonas Professor, and Chairman, Department of Otorhinolaryngology, University of Oklahoma Health Sciences Center, Oklahoma City, Oklahoma

† Deceased.

TANYA MEYER, MD Assistant Professor, Department of Otorhinolaryngology, University of Maryland School of Medicine, Baltimore; University of Maryland Hospital, Department of Otolaryngology, Baltimore, Maryland

TED A. MEYER, MD, PhD Assistant Professor, Department of Otolaryngology, Medical University of South Carolina, Charleston, South Carolina

JOHN H. MILLS, MD Department of Otolaryngology, Medical University of South Carolina, Charleston, South Carolina

RON B. MITCHELL, MD Associate Professor, Department of Otolaryngology–Head and Neck Surgery, and Director, Pediatric Otolaryngology, Department of Otolaryngology–Head and Neck Surgery, Virginia Commonwealth University School of Medicine, Richmond, Virginia

RICHARD T. MIYAMOTO, MD Professor and Chair, Department of Otolaryngology, Indiana University School of Medicine, Indianapolis, Indiana

BRIAN A. MOORE, MD Clinical Assistant Professor, Department of Otolaryngology–Head and Neck Surgery, Tulane University School of Medicine, New Orleans, Louisiana; Staff Otolaryngologist, Department of ENT Surgery, Eglin Regional Hospital, Eglin Air Force Base, Florida

LAMONT MURDOCH, MD Professor, Department of Internal Medicine, Loma Linda University School of Medicine, Loma Linda; Chief, Division of Endocrinology, Department of Internal Medicine, Loma Linda University Medical Center, Loma Linda, California

CHARLES M. MYER III, MD Vice Chairman of Residency, and Professor, Departments of Pediatrics and of Otolaryngology–Head and Neck Surgery, University of Cincinnati, College of Medicine, Cincinnati; Department of Pediatric Otolaryngology, Cincinnati Children's Hospital Medical Center, Cincinnati, Ohio

JEFFREY N. MYERS, MD, PhD, FACS Associate Professor and Deputy Chair for Academic Programs, Department of Head and Neck Surgery and Cancer Biology, The University of Texas M.D. Anderson Cancer Center, Houston, Texas

ROBERT M. NACLERIO, MD Professor, Department of Surgery, Pritzker School of Medicine, Chicago; Chief, Section of Otolaryngology–Head and Neck Surgery, The University of Chicago Hospitals, Chicago, Illinois

SHERVIN NADERI, MD Clinical Assistant Professor, Department of Otolaryngology, Indiana University School of Medicine, Indianapolis, Indiana; Staff, Division of Plastic Surgery, INOVA Loudoun Hospital, Leesburg, Virginia.

CHERIE-ANN O. NATHAN, MD Department of Otolaryngology–Head and Neck Surgery, Louisiana State University Health Sciences Center–Shreveport, Louisiana

J. GAIL NEELY, MD Professor and Research Director, Department of Otolaryngology–Head and Neck Surgery, Washington University School of Medicine, St. Louis; Director, Otology/Neurotology/Base of Skull Surgery, Department of Otolaryngology–Head and Neck Surgery, Barnes-Jewish Hospital, Center for Advanced Medicine, St. Louis, Missouri

ANDREW J. NEMECHEK, MD, FACS Assistant Clinical Professor, Department of Otolaryngology–Head and Neck Surgery, University of Colorado School of Medicine, Denver, Colorado; Director, Head and Neck Tumor Program, Swedish Medical Center, Englewood, Colorado

JEFFREY A. NERAD, MD, FACS Department of Ophthalmology, University of Iowa Hospitals and Clinics, Iowa City, Iowa

SHAWN D. NEWLANDS, MD, PhD, MBA, FACS Harry Carothers Wiess Professor and Chair, Department of Otolaryngology, University of Texas Medical Branch, Galveston, Texas

ARNOLD M. NOYEK, MD, FRCSC, FACS Professor, Department of Otolaryngology–Head and Neck Surgery, Department of Medical Imaging, Department of Public Health Sciences, University of Toronto; Director, Peter A Silverman Centre for International Health, Department of Otolaryngology–Head and Neck Surgery, Mount Sinai Hospital, Toronto, Ontario, Canada

MARK W. OCHS, DMD, MD Associate Professor and Chairman, Department of Oral and Maxillofacial Surgery, University of Pittsburgh School of Dental Medicine, Pittsburgh; Chairman, Department of Oral and Maxillofacial Surgery, University of Pittsburgh Medical Center, Pittsburgh, Pennsylvania

YOUNG S. OH, MD Clinical Instructor, Department of Otolaryngology–Head and Neck Surgery, University of California, San Francisco, School of Medicine, San Francisco; Clinical Instructor, Department of Otolaryngology, Head and Neck Institute, UCSF Comprehensive Cancer Center, San Francisco, California

BERT W. O'MALLEY Jr., MD Gabriel Tucker Professor and Chairman, Department of Otorhinolaryngology–Head and Neck Surgery, University of Pennsylvania School of Medicine, Philadelphia, Pennsylvania

MATTHEW R. O'MALLEY, MD Department of Otolaryngology–Head and Neck Surgery, Vanderbilt University Medical Center, Nashville, Tennessee

RICHARD R. ORLANDI, MD, FACS Associate Professor, Department of Otolaryngology–Head and Neck Surgery, The University of Utah, Salt Lake City; Attending Physician, Department of Otolaryngology–Head and Neck Surgery, The University of Utah Hospitals and Clinics, Salt Lake City, Utah

RANDAL A. OTTO, MD Thomas W. Folbre Professor, and Chair, Department of Otolaryngology–Head and Neck Surgery, The University of Texas Health Science Center, San Antonio, Texas

WINDOLYN D. PANGANIBAN, MD Clinical Faculty, Department of Otolaryngology–Head and Neck Surgery, St. Luke's College of Medicine, Quezon City; Active Consultant Staff, Department of Otolaryngology–Head and Neck Surgery, St. Luke's Medical Center, Quezon City, Philippines

IRA D. PAPEL, MD Associate Professor, Division of Facial Plastic and Reconstructive Surgery, Department of Otolaryngology–Head and Neck Surgery, The Johns Hopkins University, Baltimore; President, Facial Plastic Surgicenter, Baltimore, Maryland

STEPHEN S. PARK, MD, FACS Professor, Department of Otolaryngology, University of Virginia Health System, Charlottesville, Virginia

STEVEN M. PARNES, MD Professor and Head, Department of Surgery, Division of Otolaryngology, University ENT, Albany; Chief, Division of Otolaryngology, Department of Surgery, Albany Medical Center Hospital, Albany, New York

NORMAN J. PASTOREK, MD Clinical Professor, Department of Otolaryngology, Weill Cornell Medical College, New York; Attending Otolaryngologist, Department of Otolaryngology, New York Presbyterian Hospital, New York, New York

NICHOLAS J. PATRONAS, MD Chief, Neuroradiology Section, Diagnostic Radiology Department, Warren G. Magnuson Clinical Center, National Institutes of Health, Bethesda, Maryland

STEPHEN W. PERKINS, MD Clinical Associate Professor, Department of Otolaryngology–Head and Neck Surgery, Indiana University School of Medicine, Indianapolis; President, Meridian Plastic Surgery Center, Indianapolis, Indiana

ADRIENNE L. PERLMAN, PhD Professor, Department of Speech and Hearing Science, University of Illinois at Urbana-Champaign, Champaign, Illinois

GEORGE H. PETTI Jr., MD Professor, Department of Surgery, Loma Linda University School of Medicine, Loma Linda; Attending Physician, Division of Otolaryngology–Head and Neck Surgery, Jerry L. Pettis Veterans Hospital, Loma Linda, California

BRADLEY P. PICKETT, MD Clinical Assistant Professor, Department of Surgery, University of New Mexico School of Medicine, Albuquerque, New Mexico

HAROLD C. PILLSBURY III, MD Professor, Department of Otolaryngology–Head and Neck Surgery, University of North Carolina at Chapel Hill School of Medicine, Chapel Hill; Chair, Department of Otolaryngology–Head and Neck Surgery, University of North Carolina Hospital, Chapel Hill, North Carolina

ROBERT L. PINCUS, MD Chief, Department of Otolaryngology, New York Otolaryngology Group, New York; and Associate Professor, Department of Otolaryngology–Head and Neck Surgery, New York Medical College, New York, New York

KAREN T. PITMAN, MD Associate Professor, Department of Otolaryngology and Communicative Sciences, University of Mississippi Medical Center, Jackson, Mississippi

DAVID M. POETKER, MD Chief Resident, Department of Otolaryngology and Communication Sciences, Medical College of Wisconsin, Milwaukee, Wisconsin

CHRISTOPHER P. POJE, MD Clinical Assistant Professor, Departments of Otolaryngology and Pediatrics, University at Buffalo School of Medicine & Biomedical Sciences, Buffalo; Attending Physician, Department of Pediatric Otolaryngology and Communicative Disorders, Women's and Children's Hospital of Buffalo, Buffalo, New York

ALLISON T. PONTIUS, MD Attending Staff, The Williams Center, Latham, New York

MICHAEL D. POOLE, MD Georgia Ear Institute and Memorial Health University Physicians, Savannah, Georgia

GREGORY N. POSTMA, MD Director, Voice and Swallowing Center, Department of Otolaryngology, Medical College of Georgia, Augusta, Georgia

ANNA MARIA POU, MD, FACS Associate Professor, Department of Otolaryngology–Head and Neck Surgery, University of Texas Medical Branch, Galveston, Texas

MARK J. PRAETORIUS, MD Assistant Professor, Department of Otolaryngology, University of Heidelberg, Heidelberg, Germany

GREGORY W. RANDOLPH, MD Assistant Professor, Department of Otolaryngology, Harvard Medical School, Boston; Director General and Thyroid Surgical Service, Massachusetts Eye and Ear Infirmary, Boston; Endocrine Surgery Service, Massachusetts General Hospital, Boston, Massachusetts

CHRISTOPHER H. RASSEKH, MD, FACS Associate Professor, Department of Otolaryngology–Head and Neck Surgery; Director, Head and Neck Oncology, and Co-Director, Center for Cranial Base Surgery, West Virginia University, Morgantown; West Virginia University Hospitals, Department of Head and Neck Oncology, Morgantown, West Virginia

ROBERT L. REDDICK, MD Professor and Chair, Department of Pathology, University of Texas Health Science Center, San Antonio; Chief, Department of Pathology, University Of Texas Health System, San Antonio, Texas

HILARY L. REEH, MA Audiologist, Galveston-Brazoria Cooperative for the Hearing Impaired, Webster, Texas

ANTHONY J. REINO, MD, MSc, FACS Assistant Professor, Department of Otolaryngology, Mount Sinai School of Medicine, New York; Attending Physician, Department of Otolaryngology, Mount Sinai Medical Center, New York; Chief, Department of Otolaryngology, Veterans Affairs Medical Center, Bronx, New York

GREGORY J. RENNER, MD Associate Professor, Department of Otolaryngology–Head and Neck Surgery, University of Missouri–Columbia; Attending Physician, Department of Otolaryngology–Head and Neck Surgery, University of Missouri Hospital and Clinics, Columbia, Missouri

DALE H. RICE, MD Tiber/Alpert Professor and Chair, Department of Otolaryngology–Head and Neck Surgery, University of Southern California Keck School of Medicine, Los Angeles, California

WILLIAM J. RICHTSMEIER, MD Department of Otolaryngology–Head and Neck Surgery, Bassett Healthcare, Cooperstown, New York

TODD A. RICKETTS, PhD Director, Dan Maddox Hearing Aid Research Laboratory, Vanderbilt Bill Wilkerson Center for Otolaryngology and Communication Sciences, South, Nashville, Tennessee

HENRY H. ROENIGK Jr., MD Professor, Department of Dermatology, Northwestern University Feinberg School of Medicine, Chicago, Illinois

PETER S. ROLAND, MD Professor and Chairman, Department of Otolaryngology–Head and Neck Surgery, and Neurological Surgery, University of Texas Southwestern Medical Center, Dallas; Chief of Service, Otolaryngology–Head and Neck Surgery, Zale Lipshy University Hospital, Dallas, Texas

CLARK A. ROSEN, MD, FACS Associate Professor, Department of Otolaryngology, University of Pittsburgh School of Medicine, Pittsburgh; Director, University of Pittsburgh Voice Center, Department of Otolaryngology, University of Pittsburgh Medical Center, Pittsburgh, Pennsylvania

RICHARD M. ROSENFELD, MD, MPH Professor, Department of Otolaryngology, State University of New York Downstate Medical Center, Brooklyn; Director of Pediatric Otolaryngology, Department of Otolaryngology, The Long Island College Hospital, Brooklyn, New York

FRANCIS P. RUGGIERO, MD Resident, Division of Otolaryngology, Department of Surgery, Penn State University/Milton S. Hershey Medical Center, Hershey, Pennsylvania

MICHAEL J. RUTTER, MD, FRACS Associate Professor, Director of Clinical Research, Division of Pediatric Otolaryngology, Head and Neck Surgery, Cincinnati Children's Hospital Medical Center, and Department of Otolaryngology, University of Cincinnati College of Medicine, Cincinnati, Ohio

MATTHEW W. RYAN, MD Assistant Professor, Department of Otolaryngology, Division of Pediatric Otolaryngology, University of Texas Medical Branch, Galveston, Texas

RAVI N. SAMY, MD, FACS Assistant Professor, Department of Otolaryngology, University of Cincinnati Medical Center, Cincinnati; Staff, Department of Otolaryngology, Cincinnati Children's Hospital Medical Center, Cincinnati, Ohio

ALEXANDER J. SCHLEUNING Jr., MD†

TAMMY S. SCHUMACHER-MONFRE, MSN, APNP Advanced Practice Nurse Prescriber, Department of Otolaryngology and Communication Sciences, Medical College of Wisconsin, Milwaukee, Wisconsin

RITA M. SCHUMAN, MD Department of Otolaryngology–Head and Neck Surgery, Loyola University Medical Center, Chicago, Illinois

HADI SEIKALY, MD Director, Head and Neck Oncology, and Associate Professor and Chief, Division of Otolaryngology–Head and Neck Surgery, University of Alberta, Edmonton, Alberta, Canada

ROY B. SESSIONS, MD Professor, Department of Otolaryngology, Albert Einstein College of Medicine, New York; Professor, Department of Otolaryngology, Beth Israel Medical Center, New York, New York

FRED F. SHAHAN, MD San Diego Dermatology and Cosmetic Surgery, Inc., San Diego, California

K. ROBERT SHEN, MD Assistant Professor, Department of Surgery, and Surgeon, Department of General Thoracic Surgery, University of Virginia Health System, Charlottesville, Virginia

"BAKER" Y. SHI, MD Department of Otolaryngology–Head and Neck Surgery, Oregon Health and Science University, Portland, Oregon

WILLIAM W. SHOCKLEY, MD Professor, and Vice Chair, Department of Otolaryngology–Head and Neck Surgery, University of North Carolina at Chapel Hill School of Medicine, and Neurosciences Hospital, Chapel Hill; Attending Staff, Department of Otolaryngology–Head and Neck Surgery, University of North Carolina Hospitals, Chapel Hill, North Carolina

KEVIN A. SHUMRICK, MD Clinical Professor, Facial Plastic and Reconstructive Surgery, Department of Otolaryngology–Head and Neck Surgery, University of Cincinnati Medical Center and the University Hospital, Cincinnati, Ohio

WILLIAM E. SILVER, MD, FACS Clinical Assistant Professor, Department of Otolaryngology–Head and Neck Surgery, Emory University School of Medicine, Atlanta; Clinical Assistant Professor, Department of Otolaryngology–Head and Neck Surgery, Medical College of Georgia, Augusta; Medical Director, Facial Plastic Surgery, Northside/Dunwoody Surgery Center, Atlanta, Georgia

ALFRED A. SIMENTAL Jr., MD Associate Professor, Department of Surgery, Loma Linda University School of Medicine, Loma Linda; Chief, Otolaryngology–Head and Neck Surgery, Department of Surgery Loma Linda University Medical Center, Loma Linda, California

C. BLAKE SIMPSON, MD Associate Professor and Deputy Chairman, Department of Otolaryngology–Head and Neck Surgery, University of Texas Health Science Center, San Antonio, Texas

MARK I. SINGER, MD Robert K. Werbe Distinguished Professor of Head and Neck Cancer, Department of Otolaryngology–Head and Neck Surgery, University of California, San Francisco, School of Medicine, San Francisco; Attending Physician, Mt. Zion Cancer Center and Department of Otolaryngology–Head and Neck Surgery, Mt. Zion Hospital, San Francisco, California

† Deceased.

CRISTIAN M. SLOUGH, MD   Thyroid and Parathyroid Surgical Fellow, Department of Otolaryngology, Harvard Medical School, Boston; Massachusetts Eye and Ear Infirmary, Boston, Massachusetts

JESSE E. SMITH, MD   Assistant Professor, Department of Otolaryngology–Head and Neck Surgery, University of Texas Southwestern Medical Center, Dallas; Facial Plastic and Reconstructive Surgeon, Department of Surgery, John Peter Smith Hospital, Fort Worth, Texas

RICHARD V. SMITH, MD   Associate Professor and Vice Chairman, Department of Otolaryngology, Albert Einstein College of Medicine-Montefiore Medical Center, Bronx; Director of Head and Neck Service, Department of Otolaryngology and Surgery, Montefiore Medical Center, Bronx, New York

TIMOTHY L. SMITH, MD, MPH   Chief, Division of Rhinology and Sinus Surgery, Department of Otolaryngology–Head and Neck Surgery and Director, Oregon Sinus Center, Oregon Health and Science University, Portland, Oregon

CARL H. SNYDERMAN, MD   Center for Cranial Base Surgery, Department of Otolaryngology, Head and Neck Surgery and Neurosurgery, University of Pittsburgh Medical Center, Pittsburgh, Pennsylvania

ROBERT A. SOFFERMAN, MD   Professor of Surgery and Chairman, Division of Otolaryngology, University of Vermont School of Medicine, Burlington; Chairman, Department of Surgery, Division of Otolaryngology, Fletcher Allen Health Care, Burlington, Vermont

PEYMAN SOLIEMANZADEH, MD   Staff, Department of Surgery, Aden, Thousand Oaks, California

BRENDAN C. STACK Jr., MD, FACS   Professor and Vice Chairman, Department of Otolaryngology–Head and Neck Surgery, University of Arkansas for Medical Sciences, Little Rock; Chief of Service, Department of Otolaryngology-Head and Neck Surgery, The University Hospital of Arkansas, Little Rock, Arkansas

HINRICH STAECKER, MD, PhD   Associate Professor, Department of Otolaryngology–Head and Neck Surgery, University of Kansas School of Medicine, Kansas City, Kansas

J. GREGORY STAFFEL, MD   Shea Ear Clinic, Memphis, Tennessee

KWEON I. STAMBAUGH, MD   Cabarrus ENT and Facial Surgery Center, Concord, North Carolina

JAMES A. STANKIEWICZ, MD   Chairman and Professor, Department of Otolaryngology–Head and Neck Surgery, Loyola University Medical School, Maywood; Attending Physician, Department of Otolaryngology–Head and Neck Surgery, Loyola University Medical Center, Maywood, Illinois

MICHAEL G. STEWART, MD, MPH   Professor and Chairman, Department of Otorhinolaryngology, Weill Medical College of Cornell University, New York; Otolaryngologist-in-Chief, Department of Otorhinolaryngology, New York Presbyterian Hospital–Weill Cornell Medical Center, New York, New York

BENJAMIN C. STONG, MD   Resident Physician, Department of Otolaryngology–Head and Neck Surgery, Emory University, Atlanta, Georgia

SCOTT P. STRINGER, MD   Professor and Chair, Department of Otolaryngology and Communicative Sciences, University of Mississippi School of Medicine, Jackson; University of Mississippi Medical Center, Jackson, Mississippi

CHESTER L. STRUNK, MD   Clinical Associate Professor, University of Texas Medical Branch, Galveston, Texas; Clear Lake Regional Medical Center, Department of Otolaryngology, Webster, Texas

FRED J. STUCKER, MD   Professor and Chairman, Department of Otolaryngology–Head and Neck Surgery, Louisiana State University Health Sciences Center–Shreveport, Louisiana

LUCIAN SULICA, MD   Assistant Professor, Department of Otorhinolaryngology, Weill Medical College of Cornell University, New York; Attending Physician, Department of Otorhinolaryngology, Beth Israel Medical Center, New York, New York

CECILLE G. SULMAN, MD   Clinical Instructor, Department of Otolaryngology–Head and Neck Surgery, Northwestern University Feinberg School of Medicine, Chicago; Attending Physician, Department of Pediatric Otolaryngology, Children's Memorial Hospital, Chicago, Illinois

LEONARD E. SWISCHUK, MD   Professor, Department of Radiology and Pediatrics; Chairman, Department of Radiology; and Director, Pediatric Radiology, University of Texas Medical Branch, Galveston, Texas

THOMAS A. TAMI, MD   Professor, Department of Otolaryngology–Head and Neck Surgery, University of Cincinnati College of Medicine, Cincinnati, Ohio

LUKE K. S. TAN, MD   Associate Professor and Head, Department of Otolaryngology, National University of Singapore, Singapore; Chief, Department of Otolaryngology–Head and Neck Surgery, National University Hospital, Singapore

KONSTANTIN TARASHANSKY, MD   Clinical Instructor, Department of Otolaryngology, State University of New York–Downstate Medical Center, Brooklyn, New York

SHERARD A. TATUM, MD   Department of Otolaryngology, State University of New York Upstate Medical University, Syracuse, New York

THEODOROS N. TEKNOS, MD   Associate Professor, Department of Otolaryngology–Head and Neck Surgery, University of Michigan School of Medicine, Ann Arbor, Michigan

DAVID J. TERRIS, MD, FACS Porubsky Distinguished Professor and Chairman, Department of Otolaryngology, Medical College of Georgia, Augusta; Chief of Service, Department of Otolaryngology–Head and Neck Surgery, Medical College of Georgia Medical Center, Augusta, Georgia

TED L. TEWFIK, MD Professor, Department of Otolaryngology, McGill University, Montreal; Associate Director, Department of Otolaryngology, Montreal Children's Hospital, Montreal, Quebec, Canada

LESTER D. R. THOMPSON, MD Staff Pathologist, Department of Pathology, Southern California Permanente Medical Group, Woodland Hills, California

DEAN M. TORIUMI, MD Professor, Department of Otolaryngology–Head and Neck Surgery, University of Illinois at Chicago; University of Illinois Medical Center, Chicago, Illinois

JOHN M. TRUELSON, MD Associate Professor, Resident Program Director, Department of Otolaryngology–Head and Neck Surgery, University of Texas Southwestern Medical Center, Dallas, Texas

DOUGLAS J. VAN DAELE, MD Assistant Professor, Department of Otolaryngology–Head and Neck Surgery, University of Iowa Carver College of Medicine, Iowa City; Clinic Physician Director, Department of Otolaryngology–Head and Neck Surgery, University of Iowa Hospitals and Clinics, Iowa City, Iowa

PETER VAN DER RIET, MD Department of Otolaryngology–Head and Neck Surgery, Bassett Healthcare, Cooperstown, New York

DANIEL L. VAN DYKE, PhD Professor, Department of Laboratory Medicine, and Unit Chair, Department of Cytogenetics Laboratory, Mayo Clinic and Foundation, Rochester, Minnesota

RAMAKRISHNAN VIDYASAGAR, MS (ENT), MD Fellow, Department of Otolaryngology–Head and Neck Surgery, Rush University Medical Center, Chicago; Fellow, Department of Surgery, Section ENT, Advocate Illinois Masonic Medical Center, Chicago, Illinois

EVERETT E. VOKES, MD Director, Section of Hematology and Oncology, Department of Medicine, and John E. Ultmann Professor of Medicine, Radiation, and Cellular Oncology, Department of Medicine, University of Chicago Pritzker School of Medicine; University of Chicago Hospitals, Chicago, Illinois

JEFFREY T. VRABEC, MD Associate Professor, Bobby R. Alford Department of Otolaryngology–Head and Neck Surgery, Baylor College of Medicine, Houston, Texas

P. ASHLEY WACKYM, MD, FACS, FAAP John C. Koss Professor and Chairman, Department of Otolaryngology and Communication Sciences, Medical College of Wisconsin, Milwaukee; Surgeon-in-Chief, Department of Otolaryngology–Head and Neck Surgery, Froedtert and Medical College of Wisconsin Hospital, Milwaukee, Wisconsin

REGINA PALOYAN WALKER, MD Clinical Associate Professor, Department of Otolaryngology, Loyola University, Maywood; Department of Surgery, Hinsdale Hospital, Hinsdale, Illinois

CONRAD WALL, III, PhD Associate Professor, Department of Otology and Laryngology, Harvard Medical School, Boston; Director, Jenks Vestibular Laboratory, Department of ENT, Massachusetts Eye and Ear Infirmary, Boston, Massachusetts

WILLIAM E. WALSH, MD, CMI Resident and Certified Medical Illustrator, Department of Otolaryngology–Head and Neck Surgery, Northwestern University Feinberg School of Medicine, Chicago; Resident, Department of Otolaryngology–Head and Neck Surgery, Northwestern Memorial Hospital, Chicago, Illinois

TOM D. WANG, MD Professor, Department of Otolaryngology–Head and Neck Surgery, Division of Facial Plastic and Reconstructive Surgery, Oregon Health and Science University, Portland, Oregon

MICHAEL J. WAREING, MD Consulting Otolaryngologist, Department of Otolaryngology–Head and Neck Surgery, St. Bartholomew's Hospital, West Smithfield, London; Consulting Otolaryngologist, The Lomon Clinic, London, England

PETER C. WEBER, MD Department of Head and Neck Surgery, The Cleveland Clinic Foundation, Cleveland, Ohio

RANDAL S. WEBER, MD Professor and Chairman, Department of Head and Neck Surgery, University of Texas M.D. Anderson Cancer Center, Houston, Texas

WILLIAM I. WEI, MS, FRCS, FRCSE, FRACS(HON), FACS, FHKAM(ORL) (SURG FRCS) Professor, Department of Surgery, The University of Hong Kong, Hong Kong SAR; Chief of Service, Department of ENT, Queen Mary Hospital, Hong Kong SAR, China

DEBRA G. WEINBERGER, MD, FACS Fellow, Pediatric Otolaryngology, Bobby R. Alford Department of Otolaryngology–Head and Neck Surgery, Baylor College of Medicine, Houston, Texas

GREGORY S. WEINSTEIN, MD Professor and Vice Chairman, Otorhinolaryngology–Head and Neck Surgery, University of Pennsylvania School of Medicine, Philadelphia; Director, Division of Head and Neck Surgery, Department of Otorhinolarynoglogy–Head and Neck Surgery, Hospital of the University of Pennsylvania, Philadelphia, Pennsylvania

MARK C. WEISSLER, MD, FACS Joseph P. Riddle Distinguished Professor, Department of Otolaryngology–Head and Neck Surgery, University of North Carolina at Chapel Hill School of Medicine, Chapel Hill, North Carolina

RICHARD W. WESTREICH, MD Assistant Professor, Department of Otolaryngology, State University of New York Downstate Medical Center, Brooklyn; Associate Director, Facial Plastic Surgery, Department of Otolaryngology, Long Island College Hospital, Brooklyn, New York

MARK A. WILLIAMS, MD, PhD Department of Otolaryngology–Head and Neck Surgery, University of Cincinnati Medical Center, Cincinnati, Ohio

EDWIN F. WILLIAMS III, MD, FACS Medical Director, The Williams Center, Latham, New York; Clinical Professor of Surgery, Division of Otolaryngology–Head and Neck Surgery, Albany Medical Center, Albany, New York

IAN J. WITTERICK, MD, MSc, FRCSC Associate Professor, Department of Otolaryngology–Head and Neck Surgery, University of Toronto; Otolaryngologist, Department of Otolaryngology–Head and Neck Surgery, Mount Sinai Hospital and St. Joseph's Health Centre, Toronto, Ontario, Canada

GAYLE E. WOODSON, MD Professor and Chair, Division of Otolaryngology, Southern Illinois University School of Medicine, Springfield, Illinois

PETER-JOHN WORMALD, MD Professor and Chair, Department of Otolaryngology–Head and Neck Surgery, Adelaide and Flinders Universities, Adelaide; Department of Otolaryngology–Head and Neck Surgery, The Queen Elizabeth Hospital, South Australia, Australia

MARIA J. WORSHAM, MD Professor, Department of Pathology, Wayne State School of Medicine, Detroit; Director of Research, Department of Otolaryngology–Head and Neck Research, Henry Ford Health System, Detroit, Michigan

BARBARA A. ZEIFER, MD Associate Professor, Department of Radiology, Albert Einstein College of Medicine, New York; Vice Chair, Department of Radiology, Beth Israel Medical Center, New York, New York

STEVEN M. ZEITELS, MD, FACS Eugene B. Casey Chair of Laryngeal Surgery, and Associate Professor, Department of Surgery, Harvard Medical School, Boston; Director, Center for Laryngeal Surgery & Voice Rehabilitation, Massachusetts General Hospital, Boston, Massachusetts

LEE A. ZIMMER, MD, PhD Assistant Professor, Department of Otolaryngology, University of Cincinnati and University of Cincinnati Medical Center, Cincinnati, Ohio

JOHN A. ZITELLI, MD Adjunct Associate Professor, Departments of Dermatology and Otolaryngology, University of Pittsburgh Medical Center–Shadyside Medical Center, Pittsburgh, Pennsylvania

KAREN B. ZUR, MD Clinical Fellow, Pediatric Otolaryngology, Cincinnati Children's Hospital Medical Center, Cincinnati, Ohio

Preface

The first edition of *Head & Neck Surgery—Otolaryngology*, published in 1993, was developed by an experienced group of teacher-surgeons. Their challenge was to create a comprehensive textbook of head and neck surgery—otolaryngology that could help both residents and practicing otolaryngologists achieve cognitive mastery of the specialty. Rather than itemizing every new finding in otolaryngology, the information was organized around a learning system that made it easier for physicians to achieve clinical competence in a constantly evolving world.

Once this learning system was established, our hope was that otolaryngologists could fit new findings into this system and thereby make it easier to judge the scientific and clinical usefulness of the latest research. The editors of the succeeding editions have used this system as a way of organizing a review of our specialty. For each edition a working group of editors, co-editors, authors, and publisher take more than 2 years to fashion the final product.

The book in your hands today is the result of an intellectual journey by a new team of editors and authors with the goal of producing content relevant to today's practice of head and neck surgery—otolaryngology.

We continue to use a number of features to organize this information in a clinically useful way. There are many new illustrations and the latest relevant references. For emphasis, we have extensively employed summary tables and highlights at the end of each chapter. We take great pride in our illustrious editorial team and the remarkable authors in each subspecialty who have brought you our vision of a learning system. We have enjoyed working with our seasoned international support team at Lippincott Williams & Wilkins, who helped refine our initial ideas and expand our understanding of educational philosophy. We welcome your decision to employ this learning system on your journey toward a higher level of medical understanding.

Byron J. Bailey, MD, FACS
Jonas T. Johnson, MD, FACS

Acknowledgments

This represents the fourth edition of *Head & Neck Surgery—Otolaryngology*. The text has been entirely revised and edited. Even with the experience gained after publishing three editions, the planning and eventual realization of this two-volume text is a remarkable task. Teamwork was essential at every step to complete this project on time and within budget. The efforts of our associate editors and contributing authors have been remarkable. This is truly their book.

Through the leadership of our publisher (Robert Hurley of Lippincott Williams & Wilkins and Molly Connors of Dovetail Content Solutions), we have assembled a production team that has worked efficiently and with great expertise. We are thankful that we were able to employ an all-electronic system for submission and editorial review of these chapters. This facilitated quick turnaround and maximized opportunity for collaborative improvement.

We remain indebted to Victoria Forbes for assistance in developing new illustrations for the fourth edition. We are grateful to Jackie Lynch, our senior editorial coordinator, for her remarkable efficiency, calm demeanor, and consistent advice as we struggled to complete this project on time.

Head and Neck Surgery

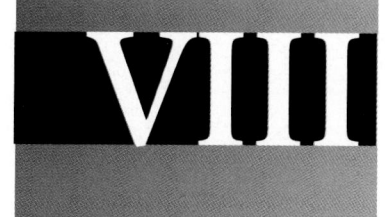

Jonas T. Johnson   *Anna Maria Pou*

Gene Therapy

Hinrich Staecker   Bert W. O'Malley Jr.
Mark J. Praetorius

Despite continued improvements in pharmacotherapy, surgery, chemotherapy, and radiotherapy, these traditional therapeutic modalities remain limited in their efficacy for many common otolaryngologic disorders (1). Dramatic advances in the field of molecular biology and genetics have allowed us to understand cellular pathology at the molecular level. These discoveries have launched the field of molecular medicine of which gene therapy is an important component. Gene therapy is defined as the process of transferring DNA or ribonucleic acid (RNA) to achieve therapeutic goals and alter or cure a disease process (2). Gene therapy has evolved from early attempts at treating inherited monogenic (single gene) diseases such as severe combined immune deficiency (SCID) that is caused by a lack of a single liver enzyme. From there, gene therapy has evolved to deliver exogenous genes and genes producing diffusible substances such as cytokines and growth factors. From these studies, it has become evident that more common illnesses (e.g., cancer, atherosclerosis, autoimmune disorders, and cardiac disease) may also be amenable to gene and molecular therapy approaches whose goal it is to alter the biology and microenvironment of a tissue (3).

Introducing replacement or newly engineered therapeutic genes into body tissues can be accomplished in several different ways. In single gene diseases, transfer of the defective or missing wild type gene into targeted cells, in theory, should correct the disorder. This gene transfer can be achieved through either an *in vivo* strategy whereby genetic vectors are directly injected into the patient or by *ex vivo* strategies whereby selected tissue or cells are removed from the body, manipulated in culture systems, and then reimplanted into the target or patient (Fig. 100.1). For example, in patients with cystic fibrosis, the chloride channels of the respiratory epithelium are dysfunctional. By adding the gene for the chloride channel through gene transfer using viral vectors or nanoparticles (nonviral) vectors to the af-

fected cells or tissues within the body, the ion exchange deficiency can be improved or corrected (*in vivo* strategy) (4). An example for the *ex vivo* strategy is one of the first clinical trials which targeted malignant melanoma (5). Tumors were surgically removed from patients, and tumor-infiltrating lymphocytes (TIL) were harvested and purified from the tumor specimens. The TIL were then amplified in cell culture, and the gene for the tumor necrosis factor (TNF) was delivered into these cells using retroviruses. Subsequently, the "tumor specific" TIL were reintroduced into patients through intravenous injection; they migrated to the tumors and, ultimately, resulted in local production of therapeutic TNF within the melanoma.

Gene therapy can further be divided into somatic and germ cell gene therapy. Somatic gene therapy, which is relatively accepted, is under widespread investigation as it focuses on altering the "mortal" cells of an individual. Germ cell gene therapy, however, is highly controversial because it involves manipulating the "immortal" germ cells that may be passed on to the offspring of an individual. The appeal of germ line gene therapy is the ability, possibly, to cure or even prevent genetic disease in the offspring. Currently, significant ethical and safety concerns with this strategy exist and, thus, the manipulation of germ line DNA is currently banned (6).

Duration of the gene expression can also be used to classify gene therapy. Two general classifications are "permanent" gene therapy and "transient" gene therapy. Permanent gene transfer, which is typically achieved through specially designed viral vectors, may prove most applicable to chronic and single gene diseases (e.g., hemophilia and cystic fibrosis). In other disorders such as juvenile diabetes mellitus, where the secretion of insulin is impaired or missing, the permanent introduction of an insulin gene would be successful only if insulin expression could be tightly controlled and regulated to each patient's need. This controlled

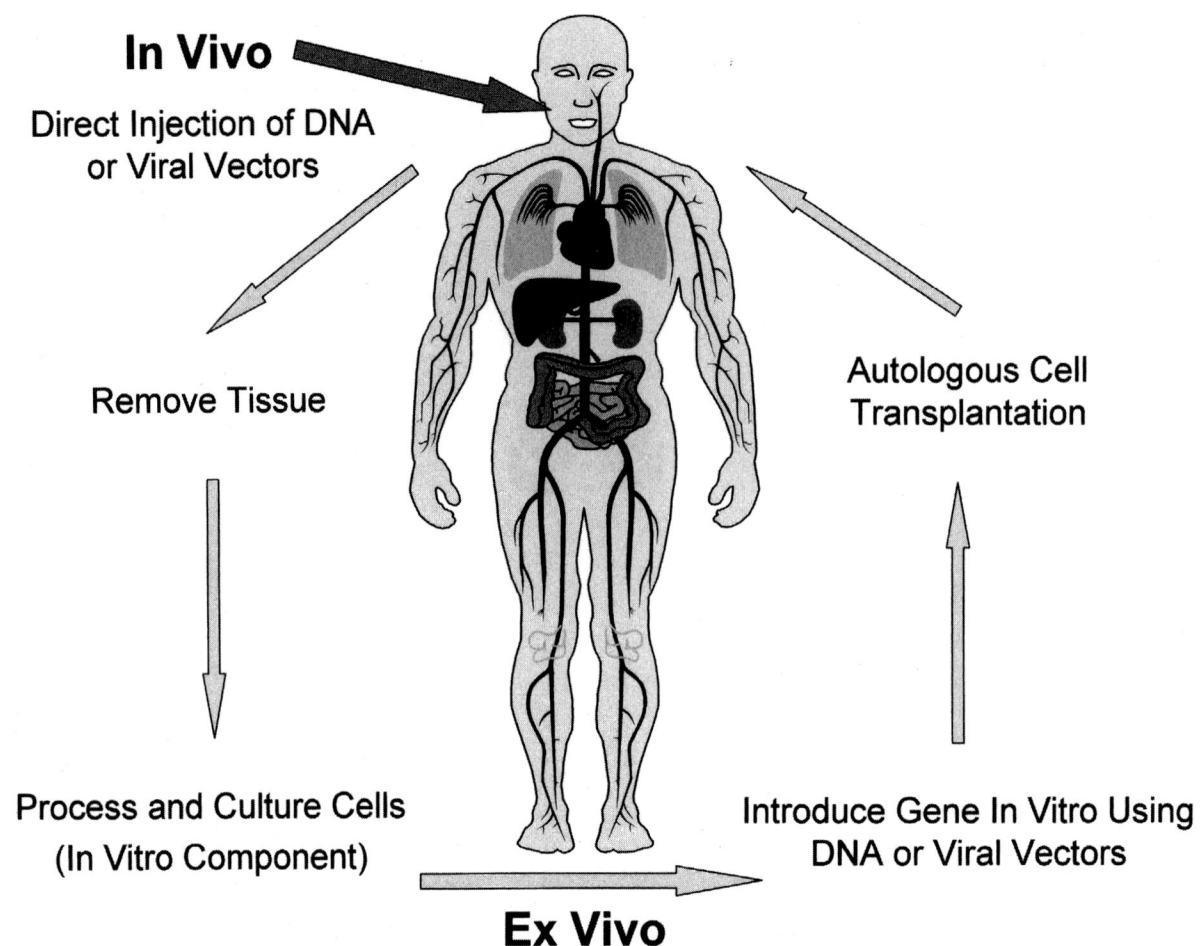

In Vivo

Direct Injection of DNA
or Viral Vectors

Remove Tissue

Autologous Cell
Transplantation

Process and Culture Cells
(In Vitro Component)

Introduce Gene In Vitro Using
DNA or Viral Vectors

Ex Vivo

Figure 100.1   There are two main strategies of gene delivery. *In vivo* therapy involves direct injection of the vector or gene transfer vehicle into the target or patient. *Ex vivo* gene therapy involves biopsy or harvest of designated tissue and then subsequent gene delivery to the cells or tissue in an *in vitro* culture system. The cells are then reintroduced back into a patient through a process of autologous cell transplantation. For tumor vaccine strategies, these harvested tumor cells are typically radiated to prevent growth or metastases of the tumor sample.

or regulated expression of insulin, theoretically, could be achieved using glucose responsive gene regulatory elements engineered into the gene therapy vehicle. Regulated gene transfer for diabetes remains unattainable, however, demonstrating the complexity of molecular medicine. The clinical success of gene therapy will be achieved when the therapeutic agent can be safely targeted to a specific cell type within a tissue and controlled with respect to the time course of therapy. Understanding of disease at a molecular level and the availability to diagnose disease at a molecular level are important adjunctive components of molecular medicine.

TRANSFERRING GENES INTO CELLS: AN OVERVIEW OF COMMON VECTORS

Vectors are vehicles designed to increase the efficiency of gene transfer by delivering genetic material into target cells without degradation. Two main strategies have evolved to accomplish this: viral and nonviral gene transfer (Fig. 100.2).

The viral-mediated approaches take advantage of virus particles that are modified to remove their harmful and toxic components, yet can enter cells and deliver one or multiple genes. Some viruses are also capable of inserting their genes into a targeted cell's genome, thus potentially providing permanent or long-term gene therapy. In contrast, nonviral gene delivery is the administration of therapeutic genes in various degradable envelopes (e.g., liposomes, nanoparticles, polymers, or particles of gold). Nonviral gene transfer predominantly results in short-term expression of the therapeutic gene. Some gene therapy strategies are involved in the application of "naked DNA," which is essentially the gene and its regulatory elements in their most basic form.

ADENOVIRAL VECTORS

Vectors based on the adenoviridae make up 26% of all gene therapy trials (7). Recently, the use of adenoviral vectors came under scrutiny after a patient exposed to high

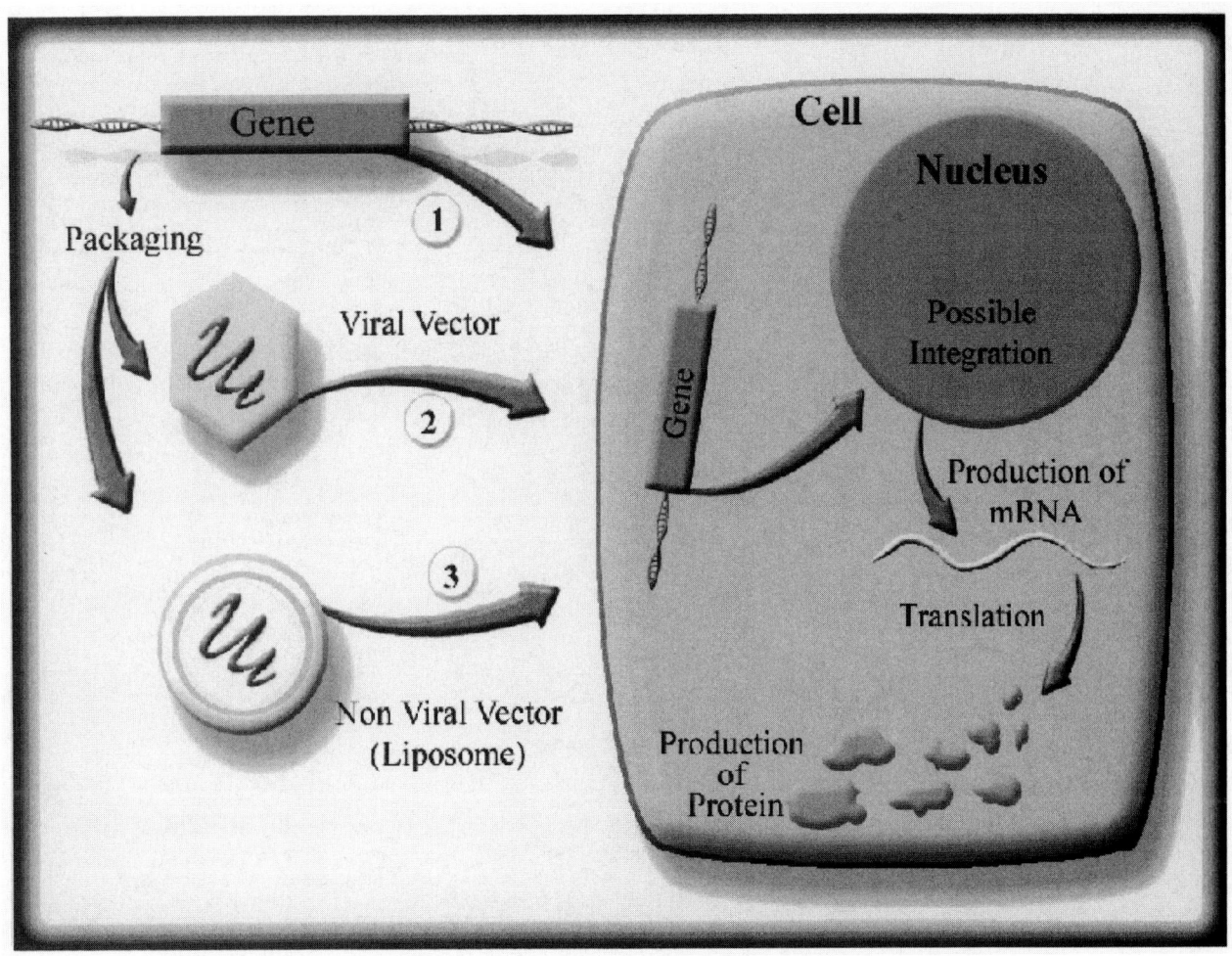

Figure 100.2 Gene therapy involves the delivery of nucleic acids to a cell, resulting in transcription of the delivered gene and expression of a protein. DNA can enter a cell directly or efficiency of delivery can be improved using either viral or nonviral vectors.

titers of intrahepatic delivered recombinant adenovirus died of coagulopathy. This, however, was related to the massive dose of vector delivered, and no other trials have yet shown significant adenoviral vector related toxicity (8). When a cell is infected by an adenovirus vector, the virus particle remains episomal (i.e., the viral genome does not integrate into the cell's chromosome). A major benefit of adenoviral vectors is that they bind to and transfer their genes (transfect) to a wide variety of cells with a high level of efficacy. Transfection takes place via binding to the Coxsackie-adenovirus receptor (CAR), which is expressed on most epithelial cells. On binding to and entering a cell, adenovectors will induce therapeutic gene expression lasting from days to many months, depending on how the vector is designed (9). The genetically engineered vectors of the current generation are replication deficient and stripped of many of the wild type genes, thus reducing or eliminating their native viral toxicities (10). Adenovectors remain capable of expressing some products that can induce immune response and

even cause target cell lysis. It is not yet clear how much of the genome needs to be deleted because some of the viral genes act as modulators of the cellular immune response. The construction of a replication-defective adenoviral vector is shown as an overview in Figure 100.3. Experiments have shown that deleting the E4 region of an adenovirus vector renders it less toxic to its target cells (11). Experience in animal models with attenuated adenoviral vectors such as depicted in Figure 100.3 shows a high margin of safety among the feasible dosing range. One key challenge remains the readministration of adenoviral vectors, because the host or patient's immunity may be mounted against the viral vector after the first administration. This potentially treatment-limiting immune response can be addressed by either administering antiinflammatory drugs as steroids or by altering the serotype of the vector to escape the immune response (12). In local, intralesional adenovirus gene therapy strategies (e.g., used for head and neck cancer), these systemic immune effects are generally dose limiting.

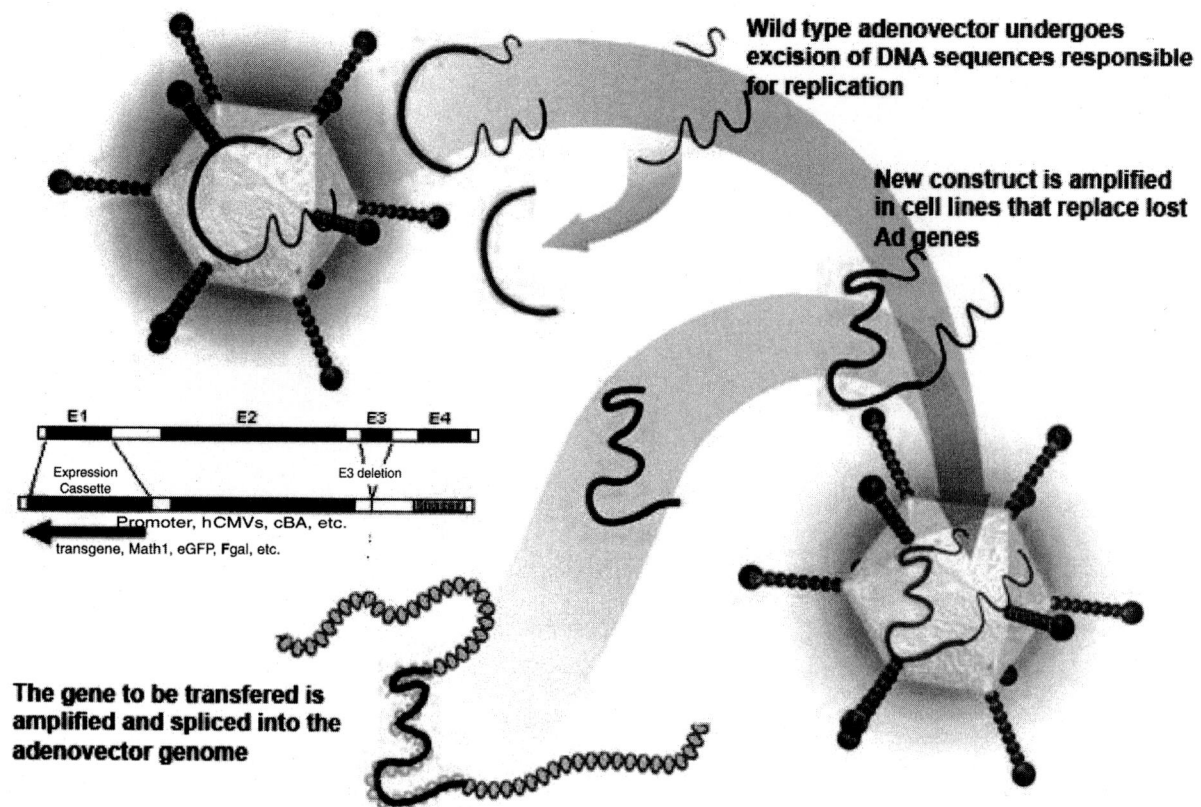

Figure 100.3 Synthesis of a replication-deficient adenovirus initially involves removal of the E1 and E3 regions, which renders the virus incapable of replicating. The targeted gene to be transferred is then annealed into the empty E1 region and the new construct is transfected into a packaging cell line. Vectors can replicate in these designated packaging cell lines, which allows for amplification and then purification of the engineered viral vector.

ADENO-ASSOCIATED VIRUS VECTORS

The adeno-associated virus (AAV) is a nonpathogenic parvovirus composed of single-stranded DNA. Eight AAV serotypes are currently known. Currently, 25 clinical gene therapy trials are underway using AAV vector (7). AAV has the distinct advantage of being capable of infecting a broad range of dividing and nondividing cells. The onset of transgene expression can be as early as 3 days after delivery, and stable gene expression has been seen for as long as 18 months. The AAV genome, however, is small and, thus, this imposes an approximately 14-kb size limit to the possible payload of therapeutic genes. The AAV, which can replicate only in the presence of a helper virus, maintains either a latent infection in the cell or induces target cell lysis. The production of vector is a sophisticated process because three components are necessary: (a) the AAV vector in which the viral genes have been replaced with the therapeutic gene of interest, (b) a plasmid with AAV packaging genes, and (c) a packaging cell line. All of these have to be co-transfected with a helper virus (usually, herpesvirus or adenovirus), which then starts the replication of the AAV vector (13). The helper virus can be difficult to remove completely from

the vector stock, which causes a low risk of enabling wild type vector replication in the target cell or host tissue. Another advantage of AAV vectors is the high titers, up to 10^{10} cfu/mL (colony forming units per milliliter), that can be purified and used for gene therapy applications. High titers of vector translate to higher gene delivery and expression which, in turn, may translate to higher therapeutic efficacy. Another potential disadvantage is that wild type AAV introduces its genome reliably into the 19q13.4 locus of the human genome (13). This locus has a role in the formation of chronic B-cell leukemia, thus raising the concern that AAV could be oncogenic. On the other hand, recombinant AAV vectors do not insert into the 19q13.4 site within the target cell's chromosome, but they insert randomly into the target cell's chromosome. Although this random insertion can result in no untoward effects, it also could alter host cell or tissue biology, causing unwanted side effects. In preclinical studies, treatment of cancer cell lines with "suicide" gene therapy and antisense gene therapy using AAV vectors has been shown to be effective (13). Overall, recombinant AAV represents a versatile vector that can be used for a variety of applications and has promise for use in long-term gene expression.

HERPES VIRUS VECTORS

Most herpes vectors are based on the neurotropic herpes simplex virus type 1 (HSV-1). To date, 30 clinical gene therapy trials using HSV vectors have been registered (7). The HSV is a double-stranded DNA virus that can remain in a latent phase in a broad range of tissues. HSV is highly infectious, does not integrate into the host cell genome, and can be reactivated at the original site of infection. Of the population over 30 years of age, 90% have acquired antibodies to HSV, indicating a prior infection. The native virus has a 152 kb genome, which is almost 15 times bigger than lentivirus and 4 times bigger than adenovirus, which makes the HSV vector unique in its potential therapeutic gene-carrying capacity. In total, 84 genes are nonessential for vector function, resulting in a carrying capacity of up to 40 kb (14). HSV also contains the gene for thymidine kinase (TK), which converts the prodrug acyclovir into its active agent inside the affected cell, thus making this vector useful for suicide therapy. HSV suicide gene therapy using acyclovir has been studied in human brain tumor clinical trials (15). The replication-defective HSV-1 vectors can be prepared to relatively high titers of 10^4 to 10^8 cfu/mL and can be amplified and purified without the need for helper virus. Because helper virus is not needed to produce clinical grade HSV vectors, essentially no risk of contamination exists with wild type pathogenic virus.

RETROVIRUS VECTORS

Retroviruses are small RNA viruses containing two identical single-stranded RNA molecules that induce the reverse transcription process after infecting a cell and then subsequently integrate their genomes into host cell chromosomes in a stable, yet random, fashion. The inserted genes, theoretically, are passed to all subsequent generations of cells which, in turn, raises long-term safety concerns. Because of the small size of the genome (10 kb), the encapsulation capacity is limited, so that large or multiple gene delivery from one vector is often not feasible. Retroviruses can only infect cells that are actively dividing, leaving quiescent (nondividing) cells unaffected. Currently, 263 clinical trials have used retroviral vectors, and these trials have mainly targeted monogenic diseases (7). Retroviruses have been used in cancer vaccine strategies using *ex vivo* techniques such as discussed earlier. In these cases, gene transfer is not the primary curative event, but it is a critical component for altering tissue microenvironment, thereby achieving an indirect therapeutic effect. Cancer vaccine strategies using retroviral vectors for other cancers (e.g., brain, breast, lung, and head and neck) are under investigation (3,5).

Retrovirus-transfected cells generally show no obvious changes in cell biology such as the presence of inclusion bodies. In a recombinant retrovirus, the native retroviral genes are replaced with the therapeutic gene and its promoter, and replication takes place in a packaging cell line, which provides the proteins missing in the altered genome. Relatively high titers of 10^6 to 10^7 cfu/mL can be achieved. These particles, however, are susceptible to rapid degradation by the host's natural systemic complement cascade.

On retroviral binding to a target cell, the vector enters the cell and releases its RNA genome into the cytoplasm. Viral reverse transcriptase then builds a provirus of double-stranded DNA. This provirus integrates into the host cell's chromosomes. The process of integration does not always result in stable or long-term gene expression because cells are able to shut off retroviral vector expression. Another problem with retroviral vector is the possibility of intracellular recombination with human endogenous retroviruses, which could result in replication-competent retrovirus formation within the host.

LENTIVIRUS VECTORS

Lentiviruses are a subgroup of retroviruses. Members of this family include the human and the feline immunodeficiency virus (HIV and FIV). The lentiviruses can infect quiescent nondividing cells with a transfection efficiency that has been reported up to 10 times higher than maximal retroviral vector gene transfer efficiency (16). Although reluctance to use HIV-based vectors in human clinical trials exists because seroconversion can take place and wild type recombination remains a risk, the feline wild type lentivirus is not pathogenic in humans and, therefore, may be developed for human applications.

The general properties of lentiviruses are similar to the retroviruses. The range of possible target cells can be broadened by pseudotyping, where the surface structures of the vector are altered to mimic other viral envelopes. The most well-characterized lentivirus is HIV. Its genome complex contains genes for integrase and a matrix protein which enable the provirus to enter through the nuclear envelope of the infected target cells. FIV is not known to infect humans or to cause disease in humans, although some viral strains can infect human cells in culture (17). The viability of lentivirus vectors for use in gene therapy strategies remains to be tested. The ability to infect nondividing or terminally differentiated cells on a long-term basis, however, make lentivirus vectors good candidates for continued research and evaluation for future gene therapy trials for diseases where long-term stable gene expression is needed.

NONVIRAL GENE TRANSFER

Lingering safety concerns with viral vectors have prompted the search for nonviral gene transfer options. Most nonviral vectors are complex molecules with cationic charges that allow electrostatic interaction with the negatively charged

DNA of the therapeutic gene. This causes formation of a nanoparticle complex consisting of the carrier and nucleic acid. Because these carriers have a surplus of positive charges, they can then interact with the negatively charged outer cell membrane and enter the cell via a process called endocytosis. Liposome-based vectors are positively charged lipid particle emulsions that have been used in 85 clinical gene therapy trials (7). These cationic lipids are amphophilic and have a hydrophilic amino group and one or two fatty acid chains. Their function can be enhanced by constructing multivalent lipids that can condense DNA more effectively and thus deliver higher amounts of the therapeutic gene. Liposomes can also be engineered with protamine, an arginine-rich peptide that can further condense DNA by its electrostatic forces. Other cationic agents include polymers such as polyethylenimine (PEI), poly-L-lysine (PLL), and polyvinyl propamine (PVP). Also, natural polyamines exist as spermidine and spermine that condense the DNA to nanoparticles of a diameter of about 50 to 130 nm (18). These nonviral gene carriers can be categorized into several groups: (a) those to increase the DNA delivery to the nucleus or cytosol by adding the nucleus localizing signal (NLS) (19); (b) those to form condensed complexes to protect the DNA from being degraded by nucleases and other enzymes; (c) those designed to address specific cell types; (d) those that release DNA in the Cytosol; and (e) those to dissociate from the DNA in tissue to provide controlled or continuous gene expression. An example of the latter is a thermosensitive polymer that can be loaded with DNA between 4°C and 20°C and undergo a solution-to-gel transition at 30.3°C, thus remaining at the site of injection over a longer period of time, slowly releasing the DNA into the surrounding cells (19).

Given the inherent inefficiency of nonviral gene transfer, a growing interest is seen in developing adjuvant techniques to enhance efficiency. Ultrasound is one such technique that has been used to increase membrane permeability in target cells, thereby allowing improved nonviral vector uptake and gene delivery (20). Ultrasound increases the intracellular access of dissolved solutes, thus encouraging DNA entry and enhancing endosomal destabilization that results in rapid release of the therapeutic gene (21). Rapid release of the therapeutic gene is of critical importance in preventing endosomal-based degradation of the transferred gene. Also, studies have demonstrated that microbubbles, which are used as ultrasound contrast agents, can bind oligonucleotides, which are short segments of DNA capable of inhibiting gene expression (22). Because ultrasound can destroy these microbubbles, the controlled and directed release of oligonucleotides or therapeutic genes by focused ultrasound may be possible and warrants further investigation (23).

Electroporation, which breaks the electrostatic barrier of the cell membrane with short, high-voltage pulses, can also be used to facilitate gene delivery. By applying an external electric field that just surpasses the capacitance of the cell membrane, a transient and reversible breakdown of the cell membrane is induced. When this technique is used in live tissues *in vivo*, needle electrodes are used that generate fields of 1 kV cm^{-1} (24). To treat a target area or tissue, several applications may be used. This technique also produces a vascular effect composed of reflexive constriction of resistance vessels and interstitial edema, causing a drug or gene to be retained in the area of delivery (25). These effects are more prominent in tumors where the endothelial structures are more vulnerable, which can be an advantage in cancer treatment (26). When designing a potential treatment, the characteristics of each vector type are taken into account. Given the complex factors in human gene therapy and the present technology constraints, it is doubtful that a single gene delivery strategy will meet all our clinical needs. Our current knowledge of vector biology, however, is increasing and is allowing us to pick the vector that is best suited for a particular clinical application.

Ensuring Specificity of Treatment: Targeting Vector to a Tissue or Cell Type

Three different approaches can be used to ensure that a therapeutic gene is targeted into the desired tissue. Most simply, for diseases such as head and neck cancer, the molecular therapeutic can be injected into the site of disease (e.g., a recurrent floor of mouth cancer). Molecular modifications of the vector and the gene construct itself can be used to target the vector only to cells with a specific receptor or surface molecule, whereas modification of promoter can limit gene expression to certain tissues. A promoter is a genetic region involved in binding of the RNA polymerase required for the initiation of messenger RNA (mRNA) transcription. Currently, the majority of vectors use promoters from the cytomegalovirus (CMV) or the simian virus (SV40), which are not tissue specific but allow high levels of gene expression. To reach a higher degree of specific vector expression, tissue-specific promoters that allow gene expression only in tissues capable of binding a specific promoter are being evaluated. Cyclooxygenase-2 (Cox-2) is barely detectable in most tissues, but can be induced by tumor transcription factors, growth factors, and proinflammatory cytokines (27). Linking the Cox-2 promoter to a vector gene has demonstrated specific expression in pathologic tissue while sparing normal cells (28). In cancer cells, the enzyme telomerase prevents apoptosis and promotes uncontrolled proliferation. Vectors under control of the human telomerase reverse transcriptase (hTERT) promoter are restricted to activity in tumor cells, regardless of their tissue's origin (29). Other potential cancer-specific promoters are the carcinoembryonic antigen (CEA) (30), the α-fetoprotein (AFP) (31), and the secretory leukoprotease inhibitor (SLPI) (32). Modification of the gene sequence that controls vector gene expression, thus, can be used specifically to direct gene expression in malignant tissue and will be required to increase the safety of gene therapy that delivers potentially harmful genes.

Gene therapy works best if the vector is targeted to a specific cell type instead of having the vector transfect a broad range of cells. Vectors that are targeted to a specific cell (e.g., a cancer cell) should have less potential toxic effects on normal surrounding or distant cells, organs, or tissues. Retargeting of the vector can be achieved by making modifications in the outer shell and surface of the virus particle (capsid). A sound understanding of the respective viral entry mechanism is necessary to develop a retargeting strategy. The adenovirus is a nonenveloped icosahedral particle with 12 fibers projecting from the surface, of which each tip has a globular region referred to as the knob domain (33). These knobs bind to the Coxsackie-adenovirus receptors (CAR) and the virus enters the cell via endocytosis (Fig. 100.4). The knob domain has been the primary region for retargeting attempts. Several different strategies have been used for retargeting (Fig. 100.5). Immunologic retargeting approaches such as endothelial cell growth factor receptor (EFGR) and fibroblast growth factor receptor (FGFR) retargeting have received the most attention in recent years. In these strategies, FGF or EGF is bound to an antibody fragment that, in turn, covalently binds to the knob fiber of the adenovirus. Thus, no knob fiber is exposed to bind to a target cell's native CAR receptor on its cell surface. Thus, nonspecific binding to any tissue or cell that naturally expresses CAR does not occur. Efficient viral binding and gene transfer, however, will occur on targeted cells that express a high number of EFGR or FGFR, which is the case with many epithelial cancers such as head and neck cancer (34).

Another approach is called indirect targeting, of which three primary strategies are currently under investigation. The first is inverse targeting, which involves the selective inhibition of infectivity on cells expressing the targeted receptor (35). The second is protease targeting, which in contrast, involves the global suppression of infectivity with its selective reactivation on cells expressing a targeted protease (36). A third strategy is based on the interaction of a ligand displayed on the surface of the vector with its specific receptor on the cell. This process is based on the stimulation of target cells and the induction of signaling, which significantly enhances gene transfer (37). These collective retargeting strategies all have the same goal of delivering genetic vectors to specific cell types to

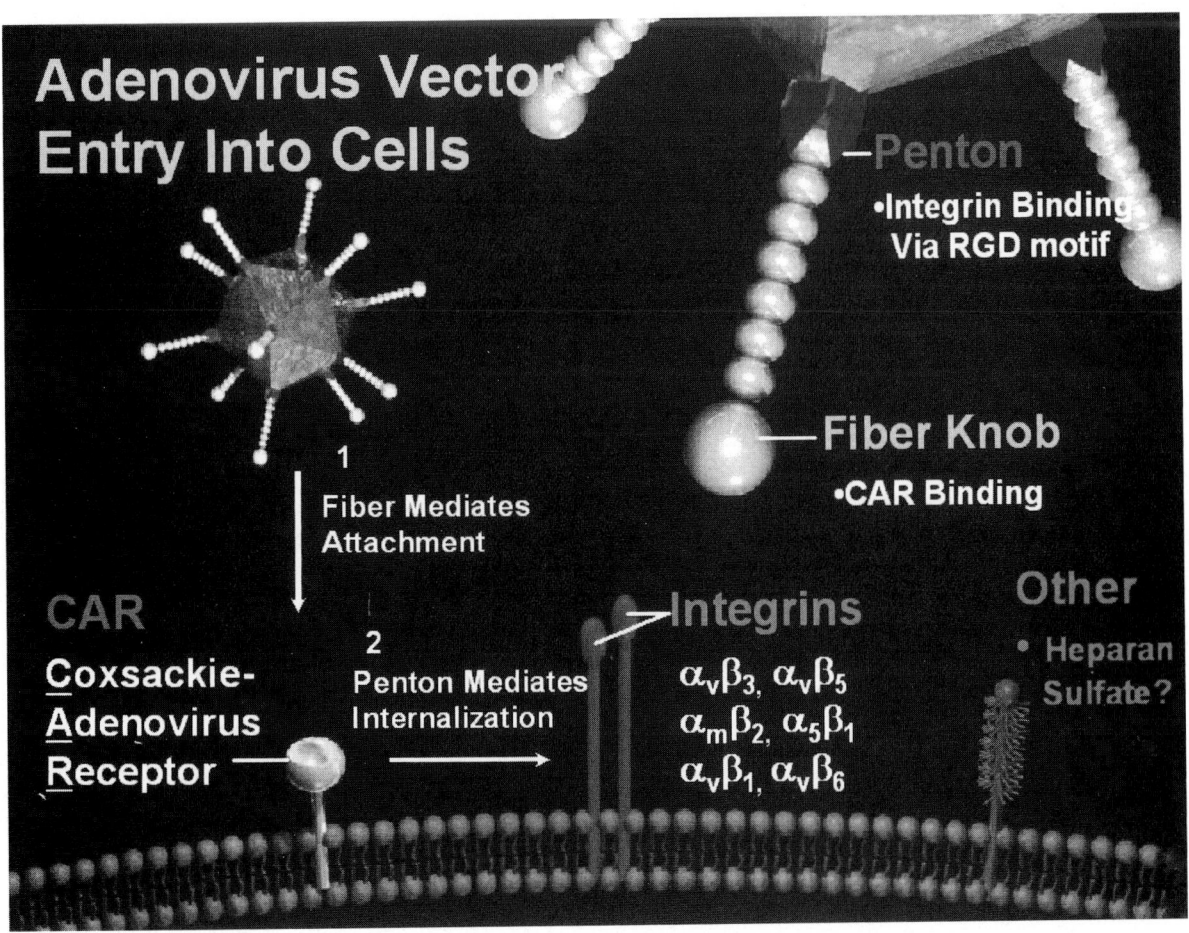

Figure 100.4 Adenovector entry occurs primarily through binding of fiber or knob to cellular Coxsackie-adenovirus receptor (CAR). Integrins and heparin play secondary roles in vector entry.

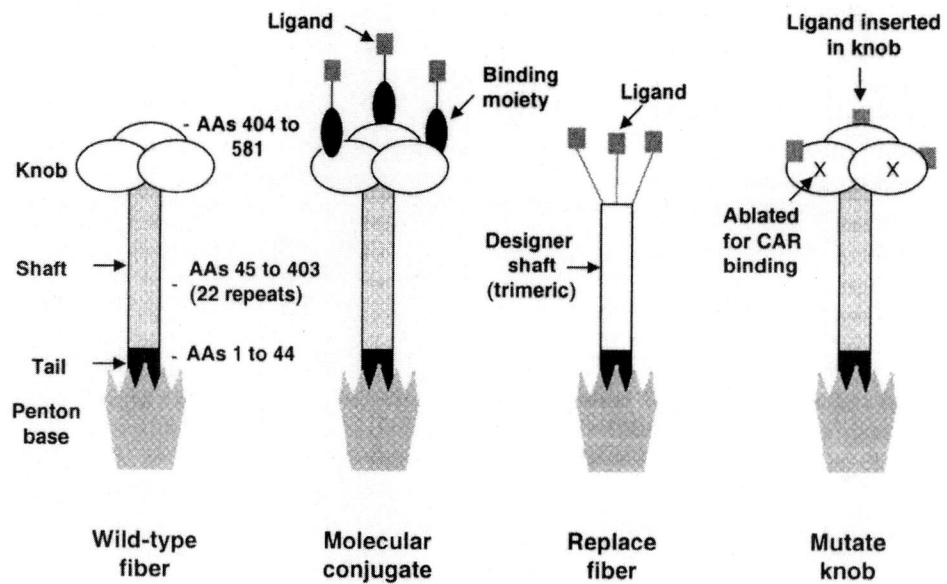

Figure 100.5 To alter tropism of native vectors, chimeric molecules capable of binding vector or target can be used or the vectors binding region can be altered through a variety of strategies.

maintain or enhance therapeutic effect while reducing the potential toxicity caused by nonspecific viral vector binding. In combination with tissue-specific promoters, molecular therapeutics can be targeted to a single cell type within a tissue.

Therapeutic Approaches to Tumor Treatment

Treatment of tumors with gene therapy can take several different forms. Delivery of genes that kill tumor cells is known as suicide gene therapy or gene-directed, enzyme-prodrug therapy. This type of treatment has three components: (a) the prodrug to be activated, (b) the enzyme (usually nonhuman) used for activation, and (c) the delivery system for the corresponding gene (38). The prodrug must be a systemic agent that is metabolically stable and able to diffuse efficiently by paracellular or transcellular routes to the areas in the tumor where the activating enzyme is being generated. The activated drug should be an effective cytotoxin, preferably able to kill cells in all stages of their cycle, and have an ability to diffuse to and kill neighboring tumor cells, a therapeutic benefit called the "bystander effect." Herpes simplex type-1 thymidine kinase enzyme (HSV-Tk)-activated guanosine-based prodrugs, which were originally developed as antiherpes agents, have been widely used. Examples of these prodrugs are ganciclovir, acyclovir, and valcyclovir, which cause cell death by inhibition of incorporation of deoxyguanosine triphosphate (dGTP) into DNA, leading to prevention of chain elongation (39). Another enzyme used in suicide therapy is cytosine deaminase (CD), which catalyzes the conversion of cytosine to uracil, accounting for an impor-

tant biochemical pathway in prokaryotes and fungi, but not in multicellular eukaryotes. The prodrug 5-fluorocytosine efficiently converted within a target cell to the toxic chemotherapy agent 5-fluorouracil (5-FU) by CD. This suicide gene therapy strategy, which has been tested in renal cell carcinoma, was reported as having a stronger therapeutic effect than HSV-Tk gene therapy (40).

Most viral vectors are designed to be replication incompetent or "nonpathogenic." With increasing knowledge and understanding of the details of viral replication and the biology of tumors, replication-selective viruses with oncolytic potential have been developed. These viral vectors are targeted to replicate in cells that show inherent genetic defects such as loss of p53 gene expression (41). Infection of a p53 defective cell allows selective viral replication, killing of the tumor cell, vector spread, and subsequent infection of surrounding tumor cells. Normal noncancerous cells at the tumor margins are spared because they express functional p53 and, thus, are not receptive to virus infection and effect. The ONYX-015 adenovirus is a p53 conditionally replicating vector that has been used in a number of human cancer clinical trials (42). ONYX-015 was shown to be safe and produced limited tumor remissions alone and in combination with standard chemotherapy regimens (43). This treatment approach takes advantage of the fundamental properties of a virus (cell lysis) and an understanding of the molecular basis of disease to produce a novel therapeutic approach. Other types of gene therapy, as discussed earlier, attempt to alter the tumor environment to achieve a therapeutic effect.

The immune system is capable of identifying and destroying target cells and can elicit long-lasting memory of this interaction. Tumor cells, however, express only low levels of key adhesion molecules such as the major histo-compatibility complex (MHC), which allows for the immune system to recognize a cell as foreign or cancerous. Furthermore, tumor cells have a natural defense whereby they secrete immunosuppressive molecules such as interleukin-10 (IL-10) and tumor growth factor-β (TGF-β), which reduces the potential for immune attack. To overcome this shortfall and to make tumor cells more "visible" to the immune system, strategies have been developed to deliver immune-stimulating interleukins to tumor tissues. Local, elevated concentrations of immune-stimulating interleukins (e.g., IL-2) have been shown to promote killer T-cell responses and activate a variety of nonspecific tumor-killing white blood cells (e.g., natural killer cells, lymphokine-activated killer cells, monocytes, and macrophages).

Local delivery of the recombinant interleukin protein requires frequent injections or systemic treatments and can have significant associated systemic toxicity. Thus, the application of gene therapy to enhance immune-stimulating cytokine expression within the tumor site over a prolonged period has many potential therapeutic advantages. The first experimental models and clinical applications of cytokine gene therapy focused on the delivery of the gene for IL-2, which was shown to successfully inhibit tumor growth (44). Transgenes encoding for several other interleukins (IL-1, IL-4, IL-7, IL-7, IL-12, and IL-13), interferons (IFN-γ and IFN-α), hematopoietic growth factors (GC-CSF, G-CSF, and M-CSF), and tumor necrosis factor (TNF) have also shown promise with gene therapy strategies (45).

In addition to delivering genes that replace defective genes or cause direct tumor-killing or immune activation, gene therapy can be used to deliver a variety of constructs that can inhibit gene expression in a therapeutically beneficial manner. RNA that is complementary to the strand of DNA that encodes a specific gene is capable of binding to this DNA and inhibiting its gene expression. This "antisense" RNA can suppress the activity of several oncogenes, including *ras*, *fos*, and *myc* as well as the virus activity of HSV-1, human papilloma virus (HPV), and human T-cell lymphotrophic virus type 1 (HTLV-1) (46). Because the malignant phenotype of tumor cells is dependent on the expression of particular oncogenes, antisense treatment, theoretically, could halt tumor proliferation. Antisense therapy in its present form has been limited by an inability to deliver sufficient antisense molecules to the target (47). Ongoing investigations and clinical trials are focusing on the development of novel gene transfer vectors that are designed to overcome this limitation (48). One such strategy that has potential for the treatment of head and neck cancer is liposome-mediated, intratumoral delivery of antisense to epidermal growth factor receptor (EGFR) and its ligand, transforming growth factor-α (TGF-α) (48).

Gene-specific, double-stranded RNA fragments can trigger the degradation of homologous full-length cellular RNA and, thus, disrupt certain key processes or gene expressions within a cell. The process by which double-stranded RNA degrades homologous RNA is known as RNA interference (RNAi). The degradation is mediated by small, interfering RNA (siRNA), which can be readily custom made (49). In comparative experiments, siRNAs have been shown to be more effective than antisense RNA with one hypothesis being that these short RNA of around 21 base pairs (bp) are more likely to escape intracellular nuclease degradation than the longer antisense RNA molecules (50). RNAi gene therapy is a new concept that is currently evolving under the blanket of RNA-based therapy.

Inhibition of genes that protect tumors from cell death is another potential approach for treatment.

Gene and Molecular Therapy in Head and Neck Surgery

Cancers of the head and neck, which are accessible for locally directed gene therapy, allow close clinical monitoring for both antitumor and toxic effects. For this reason, interest existed in developing gene therapy strategies for head and neck cancer early in the development of the field. Some of the first preclinical investigations focused on using suicide gene therapy strategies alone or in combination with immune-stimulating cytokine gene therapy (51). Whereas data from these preclinical animal studies were encouraging, the limitations of gene therapy alone with standard first generation adenovirus vectors shifted the development and clinical trial focus toward replicating adenovirus therapy or gene therapy in combination with radiation and chemotherapy.

The safety and potential efficacy of replicating viruses that destroy tumor cells has been shown in a phase II trial of a combination of intralesional injection of ONYX-015 vector in combination with cisplatin and 5-FU versus chemotherapy alone in patients with recurrent squamous cell cancer of the head and neck. This study demonstrated substantial objective tumor responses, including a high number of complete responses with no tumor progress in a 6-month follow-up window. All patients who received only chemotherapy experienced disease progression. Biopsies of the tumors from patients who received the replication-competent viral therapy showed tumor-selective viral replication and induction of necrosis; however, no apparent correlation was seen between the mutational tumor status of p53 and the extent of the clinical response (52).

Another evolving combination standard and gene or viral therapy strategy that has entered clinical trials is based on an adenovirus vector that is activated to express an antitumor molecule on exposure to radiation. This adenovirus vector was engineered with a radiation-inducible EGR-1 promoter. When this genetically engineered viral vector infects a tumor cell and then is exposed to radiation, high levels of the antitumor cytokine TNF-α are expressed within the infected tumor cell. This new strategy referred to as "TNFerade" has been studied in phase I clinical trials for patients with breast, lung, rectal, skin, and head and neck cancer (53,54).

A key factor in tumor growth is the vasculature support and blood supply for the tumor. Interference with the protease enzyme function necessary for invasive outgrowth of the tumor vascular endothelium has been shown to inhibit tumor growth (55). Murine preclinical studies using gene transfer of the anti-aniogenic endostatin gene demonstrated significant effects on both primary and metastatic tumor growth (56). Although these anti-angiogenesis strategies are intriguing, there has been little investigation into their application in head and neck cancer. Gene therapy strategies to modulate blood supply have more potential applications than the primary treatment of head and neck cancer and could prove valuable in wound healing and local, regional, or free flap repairs in head and neck and skull base tumor surgery. Various growth factors such as the basic fibroblast growth factor (bFGF) and the heparin-binding factor are known to stimulate new vessel in-growth (57). In general, tissue repair is governed by a plethora of growth factors (e.g., TGF-α and -β, EGF, insulinlike growth factors one and two [IGF-I and II], platelet-derived growth factor [PDGF], and nerve growth factor [NGF]). These factors enhance both blood supply and nerve growth or recovery and are involved in the maintenance of muscle mass, all of which have potential benefit in the field of head and neck reconstructive surgery or in the treatment of laryngeal or facial paralysis.

Gene Therapy Potential Applications in Otology

Inner ear gene therapy is currently purely at the experimental stage. Several vectors have been studied and shown to successfully deliver functional ectopic genes into the mammalian auditory system. Reporter genes, functional markers as green fluorescent protein (gfp), or the β-galactosidase (β-gal) (58) have been used to demonstrate the efficacy of gene delivery to the inner ear (59) (Fig. 100.6). As otologic disease is generally not associated with mortality, the vectors used need to have low immunogenicity and cytotoxicity and no oncogenic potential. Adeno-associated virus-based vectors as well as liposomes as packaging agents have been used to transfect cells of the inner ear (60). Methods for surgical delivery in animal models have been developed (61,62). Transfection of the cochlea of guinea pigs and mice without damaging the hearing threshold has also been demonstrated (63,64).

One of the great challenges of otologic gene therapy is the regeneration of the sensory epithelium, the hair cells. As the Math1 gene is known to be expressed in the inner ear of mice between embryonic days 12.5 and 18.5, and its loss in knock-out mice corresponds with a loss of hair cells, it may prove a key candidate gene for hair cell regen-

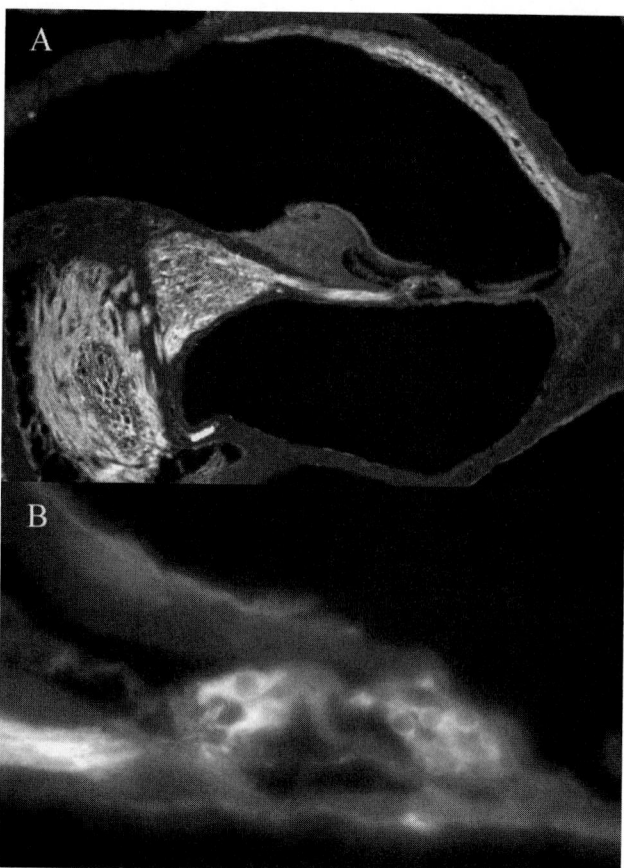

Figure 100.6 Adenovector-mediated delivery of green fluorescent protein (GFP) to the inner ear of mice is shown in low (**A**) and high (**B**) power. Cells in which the gene for GFP has been transduced can be identified by their bright yellow or green staining. Expression of GFP is seen in spiral ganglion cells as well as in inner and outer hair cells.

eration (65,66). In select studies, the regenerative potential of hair cells in mammals after injury has been shown (67,68). Transfer of a plasmid vector expressing Math1 resulted in new hair cell formation in cultures of neonatal cochleae of the rat (69). In recent studies, the application of an adenoviral vector encoding Math1 into the scala media of the cochlea of adult guinea pigs led to ectopic auditory hair cells (70). Hearing loss and vestibular disorders are an emerging area for gene therapy and preclinical data support continued investigation that may lead to human clinical trials.

CONCLUSION

Initial attempts at gene therapy focused on the correction of less-common monogenetic diseases (e.g., severe combined immune disease and hemophilia); however, the field has significantly evolved into the realm of using gene and molecular therapy to treat common afflictions (e.g., cancer, arthritis, and cardiovascular diseases). Over the past 10 years, gene therapy has moved from initial basic science research to active human clinical trials, and the field has broadened to include new viral and nonviral concepts in molecular therapy. Otolaryngology presents the practitioner with a variety of challenging diseases, ranging from malignancies to chronic neurodegenerative disorders. An increased understanding of the molecular basis of otolaryngologic diseases will allow the development of novel molecular-based therapies. Further research with a focus on combining gene and molecular therapy with standard surgery, radiation, and chemotherapy promises to change the course of head and neck cancer care. Ongoing developments in vector design and targeted gene delivery opens possibilities of moving molecular therapy into the fields of reconstruction and hearing and vestibular disorders.

HIGHLIGHTS

- Somatic cell gene therapy is relatively accepted.
- Germ cell gene therapy remains highly controversial. Manipulation of germ line DNA is currently banned.
- Gene transfer vectors can be viral or nonviral.
- Viral vectors have safety concerns.
- Gene therapy works best when properly targeted.
- Understanding the molecular basis for disease offers novel approaches to genetic manipulation.

REFERENCES

1. Schwartz GJ, Mehta RH, Wenig BL, et al. Salvage treatment for recurrent squamous cell carcinoma of the oral cavity. *Head Neck* 2000;22:34–41.
2. Cusack JC Jr, Tanabe KK. Cancer gene therapy. *Surg Oncol Clin N Am* 1998;7:421–469.
3. O'Malley BW Jr, Couch ME. Gene therapy principles and strategies for head and neck cancer. *Adv Otorhinolaryngol* 2000;56:279–288.
4. Griesenbach U, Geddes DM, Alton EW. Advances in cystic fibrosis gene therapy. *Curr Opin Pulmon Med* 2004;10:542–546.
5. Abdel-Wahab Z, Weltz C, Hester D, et al. A phase I clinical trial of immunotherapy with interferon-gamma gene-modified autologous melanoma cells: monitoring the humoral immune response. *Cancer* 1997;80:401–412.
6. Smith KR. Gene therapy: theoretical and bioethical concepts. *Arch Med Res* 2003;34:247–268.
7. Edelstein M. *Gene therapy clinical trials worldwide. 2004.* 2004. Wiley. Ref Type: Electronic Citation.
8. Stephenson J. Studies illuminate cause of fatal reaction in gene-therapy trial. *JAMA* 2001;285:2570.
9. Bergelson JM, Cunningham JA, Droguett G, et al. Isolation of a common receptor for Coxsackie B viruses and adenoviruses 2 and 5. *Science* 1997;275:1320–1323.
10. Lozier JN, Csako G, Mondoro TH, et al. Toxicity of a first-generation adenoviral vector in rhesus macaques. *Hum Gene Ther* 2002;13:113–124.
11. Mizuguchi H, Kay MA. A simple method for constructing E1- and E1/E4-deleted recombinant adenoviral vectors. *Hum Gene Ther* 1999;10:2013–2017.
12. Kolb M, Inman M, Margetts PJ, et al. Budesonide enhances repeated gene transfer and expression in the lung with adenoviral vectors. *Am J Respir Crit Care Med* 2001;164:866–872.
13. Romano G, Michell P, Pacilio C, et al. Latest developments in gene transfer technology: achievements, perspectives, and controversies over therapeutic applications. *Stem Cells* 2000;18:19–39.
14. Latchman DS. Gene delivery and gene therapy with herpes simplex virus-based vectors. *Gene* 2001;264:1–9.
15. Markert JM, Parker JN, Gillespie GY, et al. Genetically engineered human herpes simplex virus in the treatment of brain tumours. *Herpes* 2001;8:17–22.
16. Indraccolo S, Habeler W, Tisato V, et al. Gene transfer in ovarian cancer cells: a comparison between retroviral and lentiviral vectors. *Cancer Res* 2002;62:6099–6107.
17. Johnston MI, Hoth DF. Present status and future prospects for HIV therapies. *Science* 1993;260:1286–1293.
18. Vijayanathan V, Thomas T, Shirahata A, et al. DNA condensation by polyamines: a laser light scattering study of structural effects. *Biochemistry* 2001;40:13644–13651.
19. Cartier R, Reszka R. Utilization of synthetic peptides containing nuclear localization signals for nonviral gene transfer systems. *Gene Ther* 2002;9:157–167.
20. Harvey E. Biological aspects of ultrasonic waves, a general survey. *Biol Bull* 1930;59:306–325.
21. Tata D, Dunn F. Interaction of ultrasound and model membrane systems: analyses and predictions. *J Physical Chem* 1992;96:3548–3555.
22. Porter TR, Iversen PL, Li S, et al. Interaction of diagnostic ultrasound with synthetic oligonucleotide-labeled perfluorocarbon-exposed sonicated dextrose albumin microbubbles. *J Ultrasound Med* 1996;15:577–584.
23. Unger EC, Porter T, Culp W, et al. Therapeutic applications of lipid-coated microbubbles. *Adv Drug Deliv Rev* 2004;56:1291–1314.
24. Gehl J, Sorensen TH, Nielsen K, et al. In vivo electroporation of skeletal muscle: threshold, efficacy and relation to electric field distribution. *Biochim Biophys Acta* 1999;1428:233–240.
25. Gehl J, Skovsgaard T, Mir LM. Vascular reactions to in vivo electroporation: characterization and consequences for drug and gene delivery. *Biochim Biophys Acta* 2002;1569:51–58.
26. Cemazar M, Parkins CS, Holder AL, et al. Electroporation of human microvascular endothelial cells: evidence for an anti-vascular mechanism of electrochemotherapy. *Br J Cancer* 2001;84:565–570.
27. Saukkonen K, Rintahaka J, Sivula A, et al. Cyclooxygenase-2 and gastric carcinogenesis. *APMIS* 2003;111:915–925.
28. Casado E, Gomez-Navarro J, Yamamoto M, et al. Strategies to accomplish targeted expression of transgenes in ovarian cancer for molecular therapeutic applications. *Clin Cancer Res* 2001;7:2496–2504.
29. Huang TG, Savontaus MJ, Shinozaki K, et al. Telomerase-dependent oncolytic adenovirus for cancer treatment. *Gene Ther* 2003;10:1241–1247.
30. Li Y, Chen Y, Dilley J, et al. Carcinoembryonic antigen-producing cell-specific oncolytic adenovirus, OV798, for colorectal cancer therapy. *Mol Cancer Ther* 2003;2:1003–1009.
31. Huang X, Zhang W, Wakimoto H, et al. Adenovirus-mediated tissue-specific cytosine deaminase gene therapy for human hepatocellular carcinoma with different AFP expression levels. *J Exp Ther Oncol* 2002;2:100–106.
32. Barker SD, Coolidge CJ, Kanerva A, et al. The secretory leukoprotease inhibitor (SLPI) promoter for ovarian cancer gene therapy. *J Gene Med* 2003;5:300–310.
33. Shenk T. Adenoviridae: the viruses and their replication. In: Fields BN, Knipe DM, Howley PM, eds. *Fields Virology*, 3rd ed., Philadelphia: Lippincott-Raven, 1996:2118–2148.
34. Barnett BG, Crews CJ, Douglas JT. Targeted adenoviral vectors. *Biochim Biophys Acta* 2002;1575:1–14.
35. Fielding AK, Maurice M, Morling FJ, et al. Inverse targeting of retroviral vectors: selective gene transfer in a mixed population of hematopoietic and nonhematopoietic cells. *Blood* 1998;91:1802–1809.
36. Schneider RM, Medvedovska Y, Hartl I, et al. Directed evolution of retroviruses activatable by tumour-associated matrix metalloproteases. *Gene Ther* 2003;10:1370–1380.
37. Maurice M, Mazur S, Bullough FJ, et al. Efficient gene delivery to quiescent interleukin-2 (IL-2)-dependent cells by murine leukemia virus-derived vectors harboring IL-2 chimeric envelope glycoproteins. *Blood* 1999;94:401–410.
38. Anderson WF. Gene therapy scores against cancer. *Nat Med* 2000;6:862–863.

39. Mesnil M, Yamasaki H. Bystander effect in herpes simplex virus-thymidine kinase/ganciclovir cancer gene therapy: role of gap-junctional intercellular communication. *Cancer Res* 2000;60: 3989–3999.

40. Shirakawa T, Gardner TA, Ko SC, et al. Cytotoxicity of adenoviral-mediated cytosine deaminase plus 5-fluorocytosine gene therapy is superior to thymidine kinase plus acyclovir in a human renal cell carcinoma model. *J Urol* 1999;162:949–954.

41. Zupanska A, Kaminska B. The diversity of p53 mutations among human brain tumors and their functional consequences. *Neurochem Int* 2002;40:637–645.

42. Bischoff JR, Kirn DH, Williams A, et al. An adenovirus mutant that replicates selectively in p53-deficient human tumor cells. *Science* 1996;274:373–376.

43. Nemunaitis J, Khuri F, Ganly I, et al. Phase II trial of intratumoral administration of ONYX-015, a replication-selective adenovirus, in patients with refractory head and neck cancer. *J Clin Oncol* 2001;19:289–298.

44. Bubenik J, Voitenok NN, Kieler J, et al. Local administration of cells containing an inserted IL-2 gene and producing IL-2 inhibits growth of human tumours in nu/nu mice. *Immunol Lett* 1988; 19:279–282.

45. Rosenberg SA, Blaese RM, Brenner MK, et al. Human gene marker/therapy clinical protocols. *Hum Gene Ther* 2000;11: 919–979.

46. Maeda N, Kawamura T, Hoshino H, et al. Inhibition of human T-cell leukemia virus type 1 replication by antisense env oligodeoxynucleotide. *Biochem Biophys Res Commun* 1998;243:109–112.

47. Xi S, Grandis JR. Gene therapy for the treatment of oral squamous cell carcinoma. *J Dent Res* 2003;82:11–16.

48. Thomas SM, Zeng Q, Dyer KF, et al. Tissue distribution of liposome-mediated epidermal growth factor receptor antisense gene therapy. *Cancer Gene Ther* 2003;10:518–528.

49. Cui W, Ning J, Naik UP, et al. OptiRNAi, an RNAi design tool. *Comput Methods Programs Biomed* 2004;75:67–73.

50. Bertrand JR, Pottier M, Vekris A, et al. Comparison of antisense oligonucleotides and siRNAs in cell culture and in vivo. *Biochem Biophys Res Commun* 2002;296:1000–1004.

51. O'Malley BW, Cope KA, Chen SH, et al. Combination gene therapy for oral cancer in a murine model. *Cancer Res* 1996;56: 1737–1741.

52. Khuri FR, Nemunaitis J, Ganly I, et al. A controlled trial of intratumoral ONYX-015, a selectively-replicating adenovirus, in combination with cisplatin and 5-fluorouracil in patients with recurrent head and neck cancer. *Nat Med* 2000;6:879–885.

53. Rasmussen H, Rasmussen C, Lempicki M, et al. TNFerade biologic: preclinical toxicology of a novel adenovector with a radiation-inducible promoter, carrying the human tumor necrosis factor alpha gene. *Cancer Gene Ther* 2002;9:951–957.

54. Kircheis R, Wagner E. Technology evaluation: TNFerade, GenVec. *Curr Opin Mol Ther* 2003;5:437–447.

55. Taniguchi T, Rigg A, Lemoine NR. Targeting angiogenesis: genetic intervention which strikes at the weak link of tumorigenesis. *Gene Ther* 1998;5:1011–1013.

56. Blezinger P, Wang J, Gondo M, et al. Systemic inhibition of tumor growth and tumor metastases by intramuscular administration of the endostatin gene. *Nat Biotechnol* 1999;17:343–348.

57. O'Toole G, MacKenzie D, Buckley MF, et al. A review of therapeutic angiogenesis and consideration of its potential applications to plastic and reconstructive surgery. *Br J Plast Surg* 2001; 54:1–7.

58. Raphael Y, Frisancho JC, Roessler BJ. Adenoviral-mediated gene transfer into guinea pig cochlear cells in vivo. *Neurosci Lett* 1996; 207:137–141.

59. Staecker H, Li D, O'Malley BW Jr, et al. Gene expression in the mammalian cochlea: a study of multiple vector systems. *Acta Otolaryngol* 2001;121:157–163.

60. Wareing M, Mhatre AN, Pettis R, et al. Cationic liposome mediated transgene expression in the guinea pig cochlea. *Hear Res* 1999;128:61–69.

61. Jero J, Tseng CJ, Mhatre AN, et al. A surgical approach appropriate for targeted cochlear gene therapy in the mouse. *Hear Res* 2001; 151:106–114.

62. Praetorius M, Knipper M, Schick B, et al. A novel vestibular approach for gene transfer into the inner ear. *Audiol Neurootol* 2002; 7:324–334.

63. Luebke AE, Foster PK, Muller CD, et al. Cochlear function and transgene expression in the guinea pig cochlea, using adenovirus- and adeno-associated virus-directed gene transfer. *Hum Gene Ther* 2001;12:773–781.

64. Praetorius M, Baker K, Weich CM, et al. Hearing preservation after inner ear gene therapy: the effect of vector and surgical approach. *ORL J Otorhinolaryngol Relat Spec* 2003;65:211–214.

65. Bermingham NA, Hassan BA, Price SD, et al. Math1: an essential gene for the generation of inner ear hair cells. *Science* 1999;284: 1837–1841.

66. Woods C, Montcouquiol M, Kelley MW. Math1 regulates development of the sensory epithelium in the mammalian cochlea. *Nat Neurosci* 2004;7:1310–1318.

67. Lefebvre PP, Malgrange B, Thiry M, et al. Epidermal growth factor upregulates production of supernumerary hair cells in neonatal rat organ of Corti explants. *Acta Otolaryngol* 2000; 120:142–145.

68. Kopke RD, Jackson RL, Li G. Growth factor treatment enhances vestibular hair cell renewal and results in improved vestibular function. *Proc Natl Acad Sci U S A* 2001;98:5886–5891.

69. Zheng JL, Gao WQ. Overexpression of Math1 induces robust production of extra hair cells in postnatal rat inner ears. *Nat Neurosci* 2000;3:580–586.

70. Kawamoto K, Ishimoto S, Minoda R, et al. Math1 gene transfer generates new cochlear hair cells in mature guinea pigs in vivo. *J Neurosci* 2003;23:4395–4400.

Tumor Biology and Immunology of Head and Neck Cancer

Peter van der Riet   *William J. Richtsmeier*

The discussion of tumor biology begins with an overview of genetic events that are known to occur in head and neck cancer. Specific steps in the development and progression of malignant tumors are discussed. It is increasingly important to understand both the molecular mechanisms of neoplastic diseases in the human host, and their environment, so that new diagnostic, prognostic, therapeutic, and preventive strategies can be developed and rationally applied to specific subgroups of patients.

Tumor immunology is the study of the complex interaction between a human host and a neoplasm, which unless adequately treated causes the death of the host. An interest in the relationship between the immune system and tumors goes back to the infancy of immunology and is intimately connected to three areas of study. First, it is related to the studies of infectious diseases and the science of humoral and cellular immunity. Second, are the studies of organ transplantation and the science of rejection and tolerance. Third, are the studies of wound healing and the science of cytokines and cell-growth promoters.

In cancer patients, immune-competent cells kill cancer cells, but some cancer cells escape immune killing. Anergy, the loss of immunologic energy, occurs in many patients with head and neck cancer. Much early work centered on the types of immune effector cells in tumors. This approach, however, provided only a limited understanding of how cancers escape immune killing.

TUMOR BIOLOGY

Most cancers result from a multistep process of accumulated genetic alterations that result in clonal outgrowth of transformed cells (1). These genetic alterations include a variety of changes in the structure and sequence of cellular DNA within this clonal population, resulting in activation of protooncogenes and inactivation of tumor suppressor genes. These DNA changes ultimately arise from a variety of mechanisms, including endogenous mutation and exogenous mutations caused by potent environmental carcinogens. The accumulation of these genetic changes leads to phenotypic expression of different biologic characteristics of any particular neoplasm, including cell growth and death, motility, and invasion. These genetic alterations can also influence the host responses, such as its defense mechanism or immunologic status. To gain full expression of the malignant phenotype, most sporadic solid tumors are thought to require several genetic events. Statistical analysis of age-specific incidence data in patients with head and neck cancer suggests that these cancers arise after six to ten independent genetic events (2), acquired over a 20- to 25-year latency period. During this time, the host is believed to have exposure to carcinogens, particularly tobacco, perhaps augmented by alcohol. The host may also have experienced changes in immune status, exposure both to transforming viruses and to other environmental changes. Circadian rhythms enable humans to adapt to daily environmental changes and serve to synchronize multiple biochemical, physiologic processes with each other. Circadian clocks can interfere with the cell cycle. A circadian system appears important for normal cell growth and cell death. Therefore, deciphering the role of the circadian clock in the cell cycle and the role of these chronobiotic mediators in its tumor microenvironment is important to understand tumorigenesis (3).

The pioneering genetic progression model for colorectal cancer tumorigenesis was proposed by Fearon and Vogelstein 1990 (1). Specific genetic alterations were assigned to each step of the well-established adenoma-carcinoma histopathological sequence in colorectal tumorigenesis. As with colorectal cancer, head and neck squamous cell carcinoma is thought to progress through a series of well-defined clinical histopathologic stages, and recent research has evolved in a genetic progression model for head and neck cancer (4,5) (Fig. 101.1). Allelotypes generated in this fashion have identified several areas of frequent allelic loss and areas of amplification from which some of the responsible tumor suppressor genes and protooncogenes have been cloned or identified (6). The most common areas of loss are at chromosome 9p21; several discrete regions on 3p, 17p21, 13q14; and several discrete regions on 4q, 6p, 7, 8, 14q, and 19q.

Chromosome region 9p21 loss is the most common chromosomal aberation detected not only in head and neck cancer but in most human cancers, occurring in more than 70% of head and neck cancers. Positional cloning strategies led to the identification and characterization of p16 (CDKN2 or MTS1) as a candidate tumor suppressor gene in this area (7). In addition, 9p21 loss, which seems to be one of the earliest detectable events in head and neck cancer, occurs in approximately 20% of benign squamous hyperplastic (leukoplakic) lesions (4). The gene p16 (CDKN2 or MTS1) is a critical inhibitor of cyclin CDK complexes whose inactivation is thought to permit inappropriate progression through critical G1/S cell cycle check points, allowing cell division to occur unchecked (8). Only a few point mutations of the p16 gene have been identified in head and neck cancer, but subsequently two other mechanisms of inactivation of the p16 have been elucidated (9). First, homozygous deletions of p16 have been noted in 50% of head and neck cancers, and methylation of the promotor region has been identified and associated with complete block of transcription of p16 (10,11).

Several discrete regions of deletion have been identified on chromosome 3p (12,13). Loss of chromosome 3p is seen in approximately 60% of head and neck cancers. No conclusive reports of tumor suppressor genes from these regions exist. Mutations and aberrant transcripts of the FHIT gene have been reported in up to 65% of head and neck cancers by several groups (14–16).

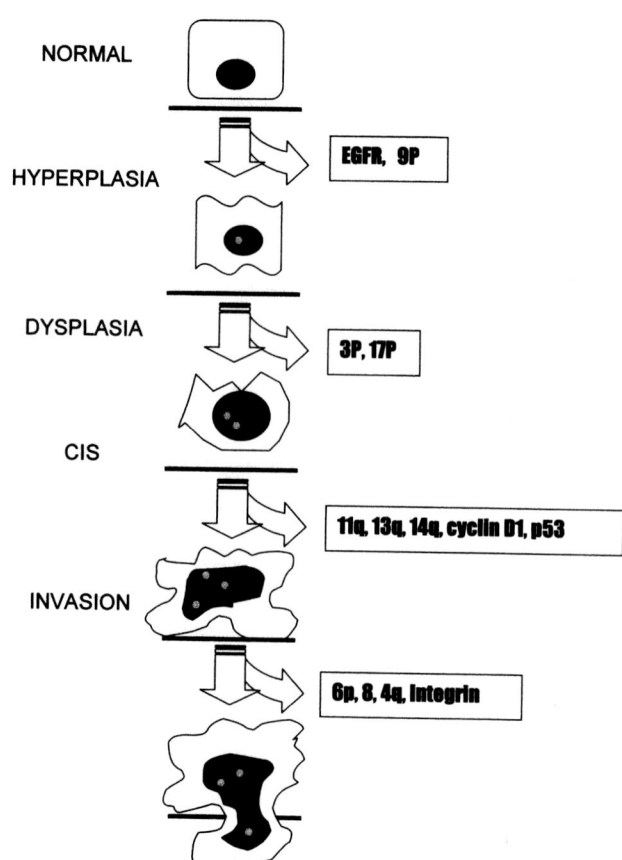

Figure 101.1 Genetic progression model of head and neck squamous cell cancer. Multiple genetic changes are involved in the progression from normal mucosa to dysplasia to carcinoma in situ (CIS) to invasive carcinoma. Genetic alterations have been placed before the lesion at which the frequency of the particular events plateaus. The accumulation, and not necessarily the order, of genetic events determines progression. (Derived from Califano J, van der Riet P, Clayman G, et al. Genetic progression model for head and neck cancer: implications for field cancerization. *Cancer Res* 1996;56:2488–2492, with permission.)

Loss of chromosome 17p has been shown in more than 50% of head and neck cancers and correlates with p53 inactivation. Mutations of p53 increase with tumor progression in head and neck cancer, occurring in approximately 45% of invasive tumors (17). p53 is the most extensively studied of known tumor suppressor genes. The p53 protein has a crucial and complex role in tumor suppression and its function is intimately related to that of other tumor suppressor genes, protooncogenes, and growth factors. It is involved in multiple cellular functions such as inducing the G1 arrest until repair has been effected, or if not possible, directing the cell in a apoptotic pathway (18–22). More than 50% of head and neck cancers arising in the oropharynx contain oncogenic human papilloma virus (HPV) DNA (23). HPV can successfully subvert normal host cellular growth and control regulatory processes to enhance viral survival. The HPV E6 gene product interacts with the p53 protein and promotes its degradation, essentially inactivating p53 and resulting in genomic instability, which promotes neoplastic progression (24–26).

Loss of 13q is another common genetic alteration, displayed in about 60% of head and neck cancers. Further mapping in this region included an excellent candidate at the RB gene locus. Few head and neck cancers showed inactivation of RB, by reliable immunohistochemical analysis (27). Most likely, an alternative target of 13q loss exists. Also, the HPV E7 gene product interacts with the RB gene product, which leads to increased cellular proliferation as the RB gene product negatively modulates the transcription factor E2F (28,29).

Other chromosomal arms in head and neck cancers show loss of chromosomal arms greater than 30% but no candidate genes or loci have been found. These chromosomal arms include 4q, 6p, 7, 8, 14q, and 19q (6).

Consistent amplification of 11q13 implicated cyclin D1 or CCND1 as an important oncogene involved in head and neck cancer pathogenesis (30,31). Cyclin D1 constitutively activates cell-cycle progression (32,33). Transfection of antisense cyclin D1 in head and neck cancer cell lines caused decreased *in vitro* growth rates and decreased tumorigenicity in a nude mouse model (34). Squamous cell carcinoma-related oncogene (SCCRO) and gene-encoding phosphatidyllinositol-3 kinase catalytic alphapolypeptide (PIK3CA) have been identified as targets of 3q26.3 amplification (35).

Growth factors and their receptors mediate signals that stimulate cell division and growth in normal cells under physiologic conditions. Overexpression of these growth factors and their receptors can promote pathologically excessive cell growth and, as such, they could be considered as products of protooncogenes. More than 90% of head and neck cancers overexpress the epidermal growth factor receptor (EGFR), a transmembrane glycoprotein encoded by *c-erb* (36).

The HER-2/*neu* gene encodes for a transmembrane receptor tyrosine kinase that belongs to the EGFR family. The HER-2 gene amplification and extension of HER-2 protein overexpression has been used as a marker for breast cancer and may be a predictor for certain chemotherapy response (37,38). Some patients with non–small-cell lung cancer have specific mutations in the EGFR gene, which appears to correlate with clinical responsiveness to certain small molecules such as gefitinib (Iressa, ZD1839), which is a tyrosine kinase inhibitor (39). Studies have shown direct immortalization of primary human airway epithelial cell through the successive introduction of simian virus 40 early region and the telomerase catalytic subunit hTERT. Cells immortalized in this way are now responsive to malignant transformation by an introduced H-*ras* of K-*ras* oncogene (40).

With the completion of sequencing the entire human genome, it becomes important to understand the relationship between the genes and the proteins. The study of the proteome, includes not only identification of proteins but also the determination of their localization, modifications, interactions, activities, and ultimately, function. Now that a genetic progression model for head and neck cancer has been established, the transcriptional deregulation as a consequence of accumulation of genetic alterations needs to be unraveled to further understand tumorigenesis. Expression microarrays studies for head and neck cancer identify different gene expression in progression from normal tissue to dysplastic epithelium to invasive cancer (41).

CLINICAL APPLICATIONS OF MOLECULAR BIOLOGY

Increasing our understanding of tumor biology is directed at its clinical application in prediction of tumor behavior, improving diagnostic and therapeutic strategies to benefit our patients. More than 50% of head and neck cancers arising from the oropharynx contain oncogenic HPV DNA (23). Recent studies indicate that patients who were HPV-positive were less likely to have tumors that harbor a p53 mutation (42). These patients had better overall survival, suggesting that HPV-positive oropharyngeal tumors comprise a distinct clinical and pathologic disease entity caused at least in part by HPV. Epstein-Barr virus (EBV) has been strongly linked to the development of nasopharyngeal carcinoma (43). EBV DNA has been found in the serum of patients with nasopharyngeal carcinoma and HPV in a subgroup of patients with other head and neck cancers (44–46). The results of quantitative analysis of EBV DNA correlated precisely with disease status and were useful for monitoring and tracking patients during their radiation therapy (47). These findings also raise the possibility of developing vaccines as an approach to protect these patients. A recently reported phase III trial showed that vaccination with HPV-16 L1 VLP in young women can reduce the incidence of both HPV-16 infection and HPV-16 related cervical intraepithelial neoplasia (48). Recently, the antiviral agent cidofovir in combination with irradiation both *in vivo* and in xenografts resulted in marked radiosensitization in HPV-positive cells, which was not observed in virus negative cells. Expression of E6 and E7 were reduced when these cervical and head and neck cancer cells were treated *in vitro* with cidofovir (49).

The concept of molecular staging has also been introduced. Genetic alterations (e.g., p53 mutations) can be used to detect rare cancer cells in samples with normal histologic appearance, including lymph nodes and tissue margins at the periphery of the tumor (50,51). The molecular analysis of tissue from the margins of head and neck cancer has been shown to predict the likelihood of tumor recurrence (52,53).

Strategies have evolved to target p53 mutant tumors. One approach has been to develop an adenovirus with E1b 55 kd gene deleted (ONYX-015), engineered to selectively replicate and lyse p53-deficient cancer cells and spare the normal cells (54). Phase I and II clinical trials have been documented (55,56). Another approach of targeting p53 mutations involves gene replacement using a replication-defective adenoviral vector containing wild-type p53 gene (57). The phase II study is still in progress (58).

Cyclin D1 is commonly overexpressed in head and neck cancer, and p16, endogenous inhibitor of CDK4, is commonly deleted as an early event in head and neck cancer progression. Flavopiridol, a CDK inhibitor, has been shown to repress the transcription of cyclin D, induce cell cycle arrest in G2 and G1 phases, and promote p53 independent apoptosis in preclinical experiments (59). It also enhances chemo- and radiosensitivity of tumor cells *in vitro* and experimental tumor models (60–62). The small molecule modulator, UNC-01, is a protein kinase C inhibitor that can block the cell cycle progression and promote apoptosis. Trials of UNC-01 in combination with standard chemotherapeutic agents are underway (63). Rapamycin (CCI-779) decreases the kinase activity of CDK4-cyclin D complex in a p53-independent fashion, and its role in solid tumors is also being actively investigated (64).

The overexpression of EGFR in head and neck cancer is associated with a poor prognosis (65–67) and, therefore, different EGFR blockers are being investigated in head and neck cancer. These blockers include antibodies, tyrosine kinase small molecule inhibitors, ligand conjugates, immunoconjugates, antisense oligonucleotides, and truncated dominant-negative mutant EGFR. Also, experimental preclinical animal studies have shown promising results with evidence of synergism between EGFR blockade and cytotoxic chemotherapy or radiotherapy (68–71). Potential compensatory up-regulation of downstream pathways can be counteracted with combinations of inhibitors targeting both EGFR and critical downstream molecules [e.g., Stat-3, Ras, or mitogen-activated protein kinase (MAPK)]. A subgroup of patients with non–small-cell lung cancer have specific mutations in the EGFR gene, which correlate with clinical responsiveness of tyrosine kinase inhibitor gefitinib (Iressa, ZD1839) (39). Further molecular markers that identify patients who will benefit from such an approach are desperately needed to optimize the utility of these compounds.

ADVANCES IN BASIC IMMUNOLOGY

Before proceeding further with discussion of the known interactions between tumors and their hosts, it is worth reflecting on basic immune functions that are early events in the immune surveillance system. For many years it was thought that immune competence occurred around the time of birth among mammals and that embryos or the very young did not have competent immune systems. Embryos and newborns were thought fairly immune tolerant. Many of these concepts came from experiments in the 1950s, an example of which is attributed to Billingham et al. (72). The original experiments involved removing hemopoietic stem cells from newborn, inbred (genetically homogeneous) mice and injecting the cells into mice of a different skin color. Scientists already knew that inbred mice tolerate skin grafts from their litter mates but not from mice with a different genetic composition (mice with

a different skin color). In such an experiment, a skin graft from one species to another can be followed easily because of the obvious color difference. Skin grafts from the test animals normally placed on a control animal were rejected within a relatively short period of time. Test animals that had received injections with stem cells in newborn life became tolerant of skin grafts from the stem cell donor species even after they had become otherwise immunologically competent. They rejected grafts from mice different from either of the groups tested.

The concepts of newborn immune competence were revisited by Ridge et al. (73). These investigators used an immunologic difference present in otherwise genetically identical mice. In the test system, the only difference from animal to animal occurred among males that carried an additional antigen on the cell surface. The females lacked this antigen. Such an experiment, with a single different antigen between all the test animals, was a unique circumstance to test various hypotheses. The investigators observed that when spleen cells or B cells from male mice were injected into female mice in the newborn period, the mice became tolerant and lacked specific cellular killing mechanisms to identify the male cells in a controlled test later. If, on the other hand, dendritic cells were harvested from the male mice, concentrated, and injected into the females, the female mice developed specific cellular toxicity for cells displaying the male antigen. These series of experiments showed that the ability to obtain either tolerance or specific immunologic activity can be controlled by the presence or absence of dendritic cells or tolerizing B cells. The opportunity for immunologic activity basically involves an activated dendritic cell coming in contact with a virgin T cell. Any other combination causes no response or tolerization. Because there are many more B cells (and activated T cells) in the donor inoculum than there are dendritic cells, the relative abundance of the tolerizing B cells coming in contact with virgin T cells renders the recipient animal tolerant of any antigens that are on the injected B cells. Activated dendritic cells, which display their own surface antigens the same as they would antigens ingested from another source, can make a killer T cell when they come into contact with the virgin T cell in the proper circumstance.

These activated T cells propagate and allow specific immunologic activity against one antigen. In the newborn period, when dendritic numbers are small, it is much more likely that the donor inoculum causes tolerance than specific immunologic memory. Being able to alter the numbers and activity of dendritic cells displaying any given antigen is an important part of the immune response. The immune system typically is not inclined to respond to antigens of the host, and reasons exist to maintain control of this type of reaction. Otherwise, the individual would quickly die of autoimmune disorders. Therefore, a dendritic cell not activated but expressing some of its own antigens on its surface must have a way of not activating a virgin T cell.

A number of mechanisms have been identified that affect the relation between dendritic cells and lymphocytes and that are important in tumor immunology. The T cell must come into intimate contact with the dendritic cell as part of the antigen recognition process. As shown in Figure 101.2A, dendritic cell–T cell interaction involves, first, presentation of the antigen in the major histocompatibility complex (MHC) and, second, activation of CD28 (T cell) and b7.1 (or b7.2) on the dendritic cell. If both these conditions are not met, the molecule in the antigen MHC is considered nonantigenic or tolerant by the dendritic T-cell system. Tumor cells produce substances (e.g., CTLA-4), which binds more intensely to CD28 than the b7.1 locus and, therefore, confers T cells immunologically tolerant. Although this specific mechanism has not been found present in head and neck cancer, such tolerance has already had power in human transplantation. Preexposing a patient to donor cells in the presence of CTLA-4 has produced what appears to be lifelong graft tolerance that requires no ongoing immunosuppression.

CD8+CD28(−) alloantigen-specific T-suppressor (TS) cells induce the up-regulation of immunoglobinlike transcript 3 (ILT3) and ILT4 on dendritic cells, rendering these antigen presenting cells (APC) tolerogenic through a contact-dependent mechanism (74). This appears to be important in transplant tolerance. Other immunosupressive cytokines may have independent avenues.

Dendritic cells have no specificity in terms of the antigens they present and, therefore, antigens that happen to occur on the surfaces of these cells because of normal biologic characteristics can be presented to T cells. As shown in the lower left portion of Figure 101.2B, internally produced antigens are expressed in the same way as tumor antigens, which undergo pinocytosis and are delivered to the surface for antigen presentation. That is, proteins produced by the dendritic cell endoplasmic reticulum have the same chance of being expressed to a T cell as one that undergoes pinocytosis. In the case of the male mice in the experiments by Ridge et al. (73), the normal male antigen on the transplanted male dendritic cells is constitutive and interacts

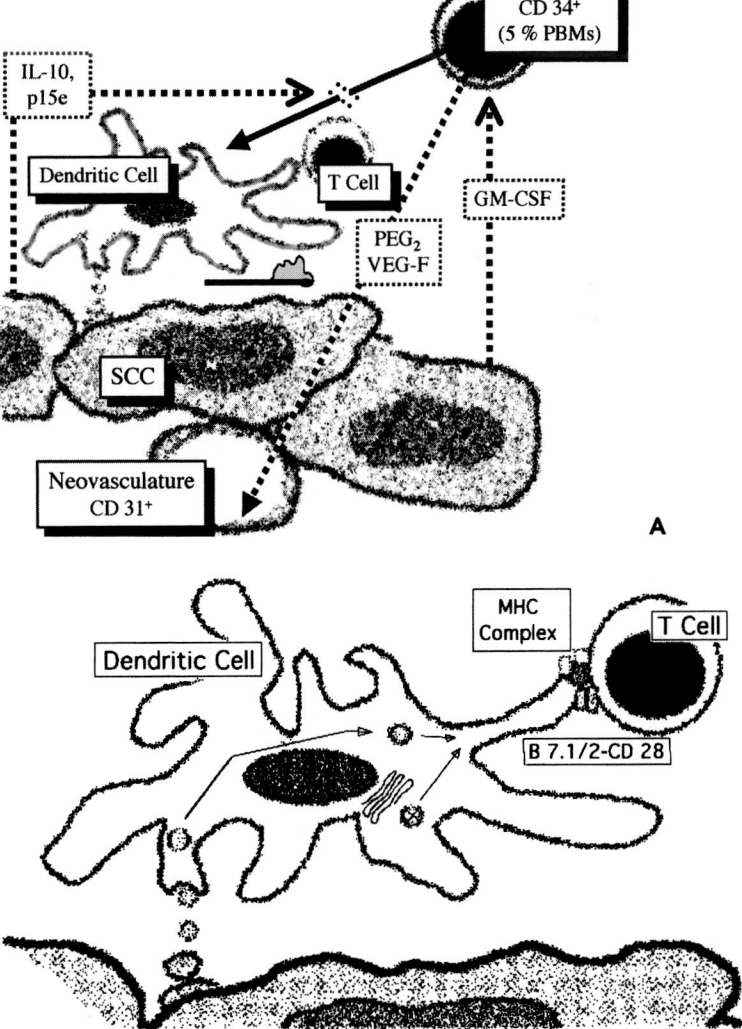

Figure 101.2 A: Near the *bottom*, tumor cells influence the interaction between dendritic cells and lymphocytes and recruitment of predendritic cells, CD34-positive cells, into the tumor environment. Tumor production includes granulocyte-macrocyte colony-stimulating factor and interleukin 1 (IL-1) and other inflammatory mediators. The predendritic, CD34+ cells, however, do not differentiate into active dendritic cells but can be recruited to other activities, which occurs in the presence of squamous cells' condition media. One such substance may be able to induce differentiation of CD34+ cells to CD31 endothelial cells, promoting new blood vessel formation for tumor nutrient supply and growth. **B:** The cancer cell in the *lower portion* of the illustration is shedding antigen, which is processed by the dendritic cell and competes for presentation to T cells and normally produced proteins from its own endoplasmic reticulum. All antigens must be presented in the major histocompatibility antigen complex and the binding of b7.1 or b7.2 on the surface of the dendritic cell and CD28 on the T cell. The dendritic cell must be in an active form, which can be brought about by heat shock protein or other mediators.

with the female virgin T cells to start antimale cytotoxicity. This lack of selectivity caused by dendritic cells requires a number of mechanisms to ensure that an individual does not react inappropriately to a self antigen. Strategies for the use of dendritic cells to manipulate the vaccine approach to cancer therapy has been reviewed (75), but primarily involves exposing competent dendritic cells to tumor antigen in an ideal setting and making the active immune-directing system function in the patient.

TUMOR CELL ANTIGENS

The foundation of the antitumor response rests on the ability of the immune system to differentiate between normal and malignant cells. It has been postulated that tumor cells express distinct antigens that allow the immunologic surveillance mechanisms to discern normal from malignant tissue. Truly unique tumor antigens, those antigens detected only on tumor cells and not the remaining cells of the host, have been difficult to identify in head and neck cancer. Tumor-associated antigens have been found on both normal and malignant cells, and differentiation between the two types of cells is possible because of qualitative and quantitative differences in expression (76). Examples of tumor-associated antigens are the blood group antigens, β_2-microglobulin, and some of the antigens normally found in differentiated squamous epithelium (e.g., keratin) (77,78).

The advent of monoclonal antibody technology has allowed the development of antibodies that bind to a number of types of squamous cell carcinoma, although none has been found completely specific for the malignant cells. Two such monoclonal antibodies are E48, which are used to detect an antigen expressed exclusively by squamous epithelium in the region of the desmosome, and A9, a member of the integrin family that serves as a cell attachment receptor for laminin and may be involved in the development of metastasis. These antibodies may have utility for diagnosis and treatment (79,80). Tumor cells also express other surface antigens that have a direct role in the generation of immunologic signals. The quantity of these immunologically active antigens may be affected by exposure to cytokines. One MHC class II (MHC-II) molecule, HLA-DR antigen, which is involved in the processing of antigenic signals, has been found on the surface of squamous cell carcinoma of the head and neck by means of induction with interferon-γ (IFN-γ) (81). MHC-CII is involved in processing of foreign antigens and may have a similar role in head and neck cancer. Other antigens identified on the surface of squamous cell carcinoma are the intercellular adhesion molecule, which functions as a ligand for cytotoxic T lymphocytes, and other cell adhesion molecules, such as CD44 epithelial cadherin, the integrins α_6 and β_1, and sialyl Lewis X (82,83).

Additional mechanisms that influence this early step in the immune system were identified when it was observed that large numbers of dendritic cell precursors were present in the peripheral blood of patients with a variety of cancers. These cells, which are CD34+, apparently are recruited through the effects of granulocyte-macrophage colony-stimulating factor, which is produced by head and neck tumors (84). In this model, the proportion of CD34+ cells may be as high as 5% of the peripheral blood mononuclear cell population. With such a large number of dendritic cell precursors, why is there such a poor immune response? Multiple methods seem to exist for interfering with maturation of dendritic cells. The mechanisms include tumor production of interleukin-10 (IL-10) and production of a material that interferes with many aspects of immune response, p15e, a retroviral antigen similar to interferon-α (IFN-α).

It also appears that tumors can influence differentiation of CD34 cells to CD31+ endothelial cells. Therefore, tumors recruit predendritic cells but pervert the response by changing them into cells, which only contribute to neovascularization of the tumor and inhibit immune potential. The CD34+ cell derived from patients with squamous cell carcinoma can differentiate into dendritic cells (85). The differentiation could be mediated by 25-hydroxyvitamin D (3,86).

Another tumor-associated immunosuppressive product produced by squamous cell carcinoma of the head and neck is prostaglandin E_2, which inhibits growth of T cells in a system in which specific tumor-associated lymphocytes are harvested and grown in culture. Prostaglandin E_2 influences tumor neovascularization. Experiments with implantation of corneal tumors in rabbits have shown cessation of solid tumors elsewhere than in the head and neck. Neovascularization with cyclooxygenase inhibitors raises the possibility of therapeutic intervention with this class of drugs (87). In an evaluation of immune suppression, Young et al. (84) found a multiplicity of nonmutually exclusive mechanisms of immune suppression that reduced CD8+ cell influx and altered function of intratumor

TABLE 101.1

POSSIBLE MECHANISMS OF IMMUNOSUPPRESSION IN HEAD AND NECK CANCER

Immunoglobulin-A blocking antibody
Circulating immune complexes
Antigenic modulation of the tumor cells
Suppressor T cells
Prostaglandin secretion by tumor, inhibiting interleukin-1
Transforming growth factor-β inhibition of lymphokines
Low levels of exogenous interferon
Exogenous administration of immunosuppressive agents (chemotherapy, radiation)
Histamine activation of suppressor lymphocytes and inhibition of cytokine production
Tumor cell production of p15e
Tumor cell production of vascular endothelial growth factor, granulocyte-macrophage colony stimulating factor, interleukin-1, interleukin-10, and other cytokines

CD4 cells. Other possible mechanisms of tumor immuno-suppression are listed in Table 101.1.

EFFECTOR MECHANISMS AGAINST HEAD AND NECK CANCER

The effector components responsible for surveillance and destruction of malignant disease include the cells of the circulatory and lymphoreticular systems—lymphocytes, monocytes, macrophages, dendritic cells, and endothelial cells, and the secretory products derived from these cellular constituents—the immunoglobulins and cytokines. Although the cellular and humoral parts of the immune system often are considered separately, it is important to recognize that an effective immunologic response depends on the complex interactions and regulatory effects that each exerts on the other. This integrated immune mechanism can behave differently, depending on tumor and host factors; as such, precise delineation of the antitumor response is difficult.

Another old perspective was that newborns were thought to be poor responders to vaccine. Many studies have shown that young animals simply have to have the vaccine dose decreased so that it does not overwhelm the newborn T lymphocytes before the dendritic cells can activate them (88). This perspective also leads to the newer concept that three steps, rather than two, are needed to activate the immune system. It was known that a specific antigen triggered the immune response after being recognized by the T-lymphocyte receptor plus a nonspecific signal provided by dendritic cells, which were co-stimulated. It now appears that the second signal is delivered only after the dendritic cell has been activated by other stressed, damaged, or otherwise injured cells through a danger signal. In this way, graft rejection and cancer are closely linked. Damaged cells that give the danger signal are critical in activating the response to cancer. One candidate group of molecules for the danger signal is heat shock proteins (89).

IMMUNOGLOBULIN STRUCTURE AND FUNCTION

Central to an understanding of the immune response to cancer is recognition of the role of the immunoglobulins in the effector mechanism. The immunoglobulins are serum glycoproteins produced by B lymphocytes in response to foreign antigens. The hallmark of the immunoglobulins is their specificity; they can bind directly to the substance that elicited their production, thus functioning as antibodies. Each immunoglobulin molecule is composed of two heavy (H) and two light (L) chains, each with variable (V) and constant (C) regions. This composition provides a tremendous degree of structural diversity. Classification of the H and L chains based on differences in the constant regions allows differentiation into two types of L chains, κ and λ, and five types of H chains, μ, γ,

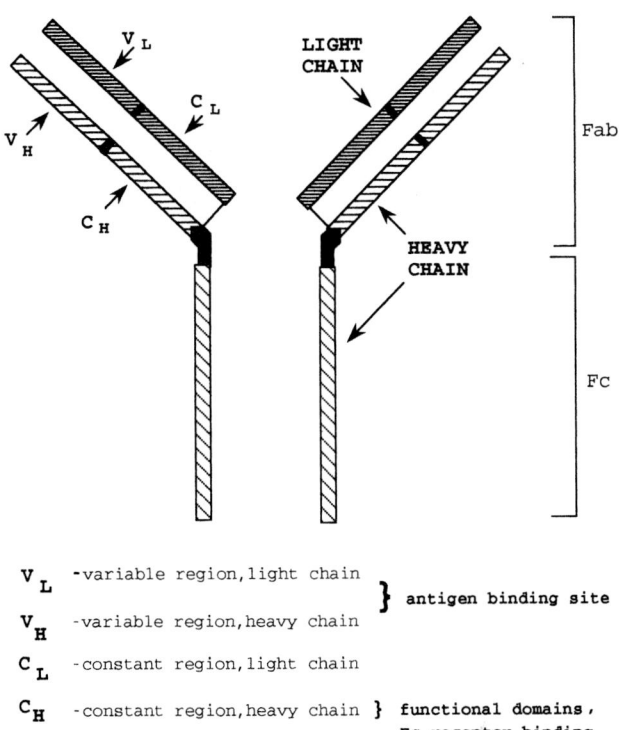

V_L -variable region, light chain

V_H -variable region, heavy chain } antigen binding site

C_L -constant region, light chain

C_H -constant region, heavy chain } functional domains, Fc receptor binding

Figure 101.3 Diagram shows immunoglobulin (Ig) molecule with associated antigen-binding and functional domains. Enzymatic cleavage with papain splits the molecule into Fab and Fc regions. IgG, IgE, and IgD exist as monomers. Secretory IgA is present in a dimeric form joined by one secretory molecule and one J chain. IgM normally exists as a pentamer.

α, ε, and δ. The H-chain classification determines the class of immunoglobulin molecule, hence the five classes: IgG, IgA, IgM, IgE, and IgD. The antigen-binding site is formed by amino acid sequences located in the V regions of the H and L chains. Enzymatic cleavage by papain results in digestion of the immunoglobulin molecule into two Fab (antigen-binding) fragments and an Fc (crystallizable) fragment that can combine with a cell-surface receptor located on certain leukocytes (Fig. 101.3).

Much of the immunologic diversity attributable to immunoglobulins occurs through genetic recombinations that change the antigenic determinants of the variable regions (idiotypes). This provides functional antibody specificity, but further diversity also occurs through variation in the class and subclass of the H and L chains (isotypes) (90). In this way, the immunoglobulins have antigenic specificity as well as differences in secondary biologic activities.

The immunoglobulins primarily involved in the immunologic response to cancer include IgG and IgA. IgG, the predominant immunoglobulin molecule in the serum, appears to have an important role in cytotoxic events directed against malignant cells. Two mechanisms involving IgG are active in this regard. Complement fixation to IgG molecules bound to tumor cells can cause cell death. Molecules in the serum of patients with head and neck cancer can bind C1q, the first component of the complement pathway. These molecules may be circulating immune complexes composed of immunoglobulin bound to tumor antigens. This can have a deleterious effect on the function of complement-mediated cytotoxicity, because elevated levels of C1q binding carry a poor prognosis for patients with advanced-stage disease who are undergoing induction chemotherapy (91).

An alternative and perhaps more efficient mechanism involves antibody-dependent cellular cytotoxicity, in which the immunoglobulin molecule, usually IgG, binds to a specific antigenic target on the tumor cell and attaches to an effector cytotoxic cell through the Fc receptor. A number of immune cells can be effectors, each expressing the Fc receptor on the cell surface. Cells that appear capable of participating in this cytotoxic response include helper T and cytotoxic T lymphocytes, monocytes, macrophages, eosinophils, neutrophils, and platelets. Antibody-dependent cellular cytotoxicity functions *in vitro* in the immune response to squamous cell carcinoma of the head and neck by means of peripheral blood lymphocytes directed against pemphigus antigen present on the malignant cells (78). The previous finding of detectable levels of circulating antitumor antibodies in patients with squamous cell carcinoma of the head and neck supports the role of antibody-dependent cellular cytotoxicity tumor surveillance *in vivo* (92).

The function of IgA in the immunologic response to cancer is less clear. IgA exists in both a monomeric circulatory form and a dimeric secretory form attached to a secretory component. IgA cannot bind complement in either form, although the circulatory form can activate the alternative pathway if aggregation of the immunoglobulins occurs; however, this pathway does not appear to be physiologically active. IgA does not elicit a chemotactic or phagocytic response after binding to antigen. As a result, IgA may confer a protective effect for the benefit of the tumor by isolating malignant cells from cytotoxic mediators.

CELLULAR EFFECTORS

The immune response to cancer centers on the function of the lymphocyte. Lymphocytes, which comprise approximately 20% of the circulating leukocytes, are divisible into three general classes: T cells, B cells, and natural killer (NK) cells. The use of monoclonal antibodies directed against cell-surface antigens has marked heterogeneity among the lymphocytes and allows further differentiation into distinct subsets with differing functions. Characteristic surface markers, designated clusters of differentiation (CD), and the specific antigen receptors present on each cell are used to classify lymphocytes. T cells recognize antigen by means of a specific T-cell antigen receptor complex, designated CD3. Further distinction into two T-cell subsets is possible on the basis of the relation of the T cells to MHC molecules. T cells expressing the CD4 molecule, mainly representing helper T cells, require MHC-II (HLA-DR) for anti-

gen presentation, although lymphocytes expressing the CD8 molecule, cytotoxic T cells, respond to antigen associated with MHC-I (HLA-A, HLA-B, or HLA-C). CD4 T lymphocytes mediate their response by means of stimulating other effector cells, whereas activated CD8 cells cause direct cytolysis. B lymphocytes express surface immunoglobulin that functions as the antigen receptor. Unlike T cells, B lymphocytes can bind directly to antigens without the need for MHC molecules. B cells also have Fc receptors on the cell surface, although the binding affinity for extrinsic immunoglobulin molecules attached to this receptor is much lower than that for the expressed native immunoglobulin.

Activation of B cells can occur by means of T cell–independent or T cell–dependent antigen stimulation. In the first case, clonal proliferation and immunoglobulin production occur without helper T-cell interaction. T cell–dependent activation requires helper T-cell recognition of the antigen and subsequent production of soluble mediators, including IL-2 and IL-4, which stimulate B cells to respond. The third subset of lymphocytes, the NK cells, express neither the T-cell receptor complex nor the B-cell immunoglobulin receptor and appear to represent a distinct lineage. NK cells can be identified through expression of certain differentiation antigens, namely the IgG Fc receptor (CD16) and CD56. Among healthy persons, NK cells comprise 10% to 15% of the circulating lymphocyte pool and are present in the bone marrow and spleen. These cells appear to have marked cytotoxic antitumor activity, which does not depend on prior antigen exposure or MHC restriction. Enhanced cell killing also exists for NK cells activated by the cytokine IL-2 (93). These activated cells, known as *lymphokine-activated killer (LAK) cells,* can lyse fresh tumor cells. Other cytokines (e.g., IFN-α and IFN-γ) also seem to provide NK cells with increased cytotoxic activity (93). In addition to their role as direct cytotoxic effectors, NK cells mediate antibody-dependent cellular cytotoxicity and influence the function of other effector cells by secreting cytokines.

Other cells are recognized as having a role in the immune response to cancer. Most notable are the monocytes and macrophages, constituents of the reticuloendothelial system. Monocytes, present in the circulation, differentiate into macrophages, which function as phagocytic and immunoregulatory cells. Monocytes and macrophages can be differentiated from other lymphoid cells through identification of their cell-surface antigens, including MHC-I and MHC-II molecules, interferon receptor, complement receptors, and Fc receptors CD32 and CD64.

Important in the antitumor response by macrophages is their function as antigen-presenting cells for T lymphocytes. Macrophages can process and present antigen to both CD4 and CD8 T cells, allowing activation of these lymphocytes against malignant cells. Activated lymphocytes, in turn, produce cytokines that enhance the antigen-presenting capabilities of the macrophages and stimulate them to develop direct tumoricidal activity. Other antigen-presenting cells, apparently of leukocytic origin, have been isolated from patients with head and neck cancer. These cells, called *dendritic cells*, may be important in presentation of tumor-specific antigen.

CYTOKINES

The antitumor responses of the immune system depend on a group of immunomodulatory peptides, the cytokines, produced mostly by the mononuclear cells. These cellular products have true hormonelike activity, although in most cases their activity is directed locally in the microenvironment in a paracrine manner. Cytokines produced by lymphocytes are called *lymphokines*. Those produced by monocytes are called *monokines*. These cytokines once were identified and classified according to their *in vitro* functions with such names as T-cell growth factor and macrophage-activating factor.

In the immune response to cancer, the functions of the cytokines are protean. They regulate and activate other cellular effectors, exert growth and differentiation effects on the tumor cells and surrounding tissues, and participate directly as cytotoxic agents. The target cell effects of the cytokines are mediated through specific receptor interactions, presumably located at the cell surface. Technologic advances that allow cloning of the genes for the cytokines enable large-scale production of homologous products that fuel the investigative uses of these agents. Cytokines that have received the most intense investigation in the antitumor response to head and neck cancer are as follows.

INTERFERONS

As a group, the interferons have received a great deal of attention as immunomodulatory, anti-inflammatory, and cytotoxic agents. Interferon was originally recognized as a secretory protein produced in response to viral infection that conferred antiviral protection to cells. Since the initial discovery, three distinct subclasses of interferon have been identified, and a variety of stimuli elicit their production. Two of the subclasses, IFN-α and IFN-β, have been called *type I interferons*. These agents are produced in response to viral infection or exposure to double-stranded RNA and remain stable during exposure to acid. IFN-α was initially thought to be produced by most leukocytes but the major producer is plasmacytoid dendritic cells (94). IFN-β is produced by connective tissue cells. In contrast, IFN-γ, type II interferon, is produced only by T lymphocytes and large granular lymphocytes in response to antigenic stimuli in cooperation with dendritic cells and is labile at acidic pH (77).

In addition to their antiviral effects, interferons mediate a broad range of biologic responses, including antitumor cytotoxicity, inhibition of cell proliferation, gene activation, modulation of cell-surface antigens, immune cell activation, and stimulation of other cytokines and immunomodulators. These effects occur as a result of direct binding of the interferon to specific cell-surface receptors on the target. Different receptors exist for the type I and II interferons, both receptors exhibiting high-affinity binding. After internalization of the interferon-receptor complex, synthesis of specific messenger RNA and proteins occurs that modulates the biologic effect. Some products induced by interferon include the MHC antigens, a protein kinase, and 2858-oligoadenylate synthetase (93). These enzymes have a role in the antiviral effects, although the MHC antigens are intimately involved in the immune response mechanism. The exact events responsible for the cytolytic and cytostatic effects of the interferons are not yet resolved. The expression of a number of protooncogenes, including *myc, ras, mos,* and *abl,* however, is affected by interferon (93).

Interferon-γ has a more potent immunomodulatory effect than the type I interferons. Direct cytotoxic effects have been seen *in vitro* against squamous cell carcinoma of the head and neck, with both cytolytic and cytostatic results (95). These responses depend on the cumulative dose of IFN-γ and the duration of exposure. *In vivo*, IFN-γ can cause cytolysis and increase tumor cell differentiation (96). Interferon-γ also may enhance the cell-mediated response to head and neck cancer. Activation of macrophages and NK cells by IFN-γ, with increased expression of the Fc receptor, enhances the tumoricidal capabilities of these cells and promotes the antigen-presenting function of the macrophages. Interferon-γ also induces expression of the MHC-II antigen and the intercellular adhesion molecule on tumor cells and lymphocytes, which may contribute to the chemotactic and antigen-presenting functions necessary for an effective immune response (81,96). Interferon-γ also can enhance the antitumor effects of other cytokines, such as tumor necrosis factor (TNF).

INTERLEUKINS

The interleukins encompass a group of proteins produced by leukocytes and other cells that exert a wide array of overlapping immunologic and nonimmunologic actions. A number of interleukins have been identified. Many are labeled with numerals, such as IL-1, along with the closely related cytokines TNF-α and TNF-β. Although the complex functions of these cytokines are being intensely investigated, certain effects are clearly important in the immune response to cancer.

Interleukin-1, originally known as lymphocyte-activating factor, has diverse immunologic, inflammatory, and reparative actions. This cytokine is produced by most nucleated cell types, including macrophages, dendritic cells, keratinocytes, lymphocytes, endothelial cells, and fibroblasts. Although a number of agents can stimulate production of IL-1, the immunologically important inducers include antigens presented in conjunction with MHC-II molecules and other cytokines such as IFN-γ and TNF. The main effect of this stimulation is generation of IL-1 by macrophages.

Specific inhibitors of IL-1 production have been identified and appear to have implications for the antitumor response. Corticosteroids and prostaglandins inhibit production of IL-1 by macrophages. The production of prostaglandins by the prostaglandin synthetase enzyme system is specifically inhibited by pharmaceuticals such as the nonsteroidal anti-inflammatory agents. Administration of these agents has reversed inhibition of IL-1 production both *in vitro* and *in vivo* (77). Evidence exists that tumor cells themselves produce prostaglandins and have an inhibitory effect on IL-1 (97). This may be one of the immunosuppressive mechanisms associated with head and neck cancer. It manifests itself as the loss of delayed hypersensitivity skin test response and impaired *in vitro* cytotoxic effects, both of which are mediated in part by IL-1.

Interleukin-1 affects the cells responsible for generating an immune response against tumor. It enhances T-lymphocyte proliferation by inducing production of IL-2 from other lymphocytes. Proliferation of B lymphocytes and antibody production also are augmented. IL-1 also augments the cytotoxic and antigen-presenting capabilities of the macrophages and stimulates these cells to secrete other chemoattractant cytokines (e.g., IL-6 and IL-8). Further chemotactic and lymphoproliferative effects are mediated by induction by IL-1 of the intercellular adhesion molecule on vascular endothelium, cytotoxic T lymphocytes, and tumor cells. Interleukin-1b also generates considerable osteoclast activation with marked bone resorption (98). Such activity is a mechanism of bone invasion by squamous cell carcinoma of the head and neck (99).

Considerable redundancy is present in the actions of IL-1 and TNF. TNF-α was initially described as an inducer of tumor necrosis and later found to be cachectin. TNF-β was originally known as *lymphotoxin*. These substances are produced by lymphocytes and monocytes in response to a number of exogenous and endogenous stimuli, including IL-1, IFN-γ, and TNF itself. In addition to promoting effects similar to those of IL-1, TNF has a more profound *in vivo* and *in vitro* cytotoxic antitumor response (98). IL-1 and TNF enhance one another's effects, providing overlapping pathways for the immune system to mount a response.

Interleukin-2, produced by activated T lymphocytes, has a central role in the immune response. This cytokine is essential for stimulating T-cell, B-cell, and NK-cell proliferation and inducing lymphokine production by these effectors. IL-2 is produced after stimulation of T lymphocytes by MHC-associated antigens in conjunction with IL-1. Secretion of IL-2 by CD4+ helper T cells responding to MHC-II–associated antigens appears to provide the main stimulus for activation of cytotoxic T lymphocytes and NK cells directed against tumor cells. Secretion of IL-2 produced directly by melanoma cells transfected with the IL-2 gene, bypassing the need for helper T cells, has induced greater cytotoxic T-lymphocyte activity against the tumor than that against nontransfected cells (100). Cytotoxic T-lymphocyte function still depended on antigen presentation in conjunction with MHC-I; depletion of CD8 T cells abrogated the antitumor response. This finding suggests that a defect in the helper T-cell arm of the immune

response with ineffective lymphokine production in the region of the tumor may be partly responsible for the absence of an adequate cytotoxic response against malignant cells.

The ability of IL-2 to generate effective cytotoxic cells has been used in the development of strategies for immunotherapy. Lymphoid cells incubated with IL-2 become capable of lysing fresh tumor cells. The cytotoxic effectors generated in this way are known as *LAK cells*, which represent a class of lymphoid cells effective in the antitumor response distinct from cytotoxic T-lymphocytes or NK cells (101,102). In addition to these effects, IL-2–stimulated lymphocytes are induced to secrete a variety of lymphokines, including IFN-γ, transforming growth factor-β (TGF-β), IL-4, and B-cell growth factors, further amplifying and modulating the immune response.

Other lymphokines that participate in the immune response to tumor include IL-4 and TGF-β. IL-4, originally identified as B-cell growth factor, is produced by activated T lymphocytes. Besides stimulating B-cell immunoglobulin production, immunoglobulin isotype switching, and MHC-II and Fc receptor expression, IL-4 serves as a potent activator of macrophages. It enhances tumor-antigen presentation and cytotoxic ability (98). Unlike the previously discussed cytokines, TGF-β is an immunoregulatory peptide that has inhibitory effects on many of the effector mechanisms responsible for the antitumor response. TGF-β can suppress *in vitro* the mitogenic activity of IL-2 on T and B lymphocytes, NK-cell cytotoxic function, and IL-2–induced development of LAK cells (103). The importance of TGF-β to the tumor response *in vivo* is unknown. It is possible that this peptide functions as an endogenously produced immunosuppressive factor. Evidence supports the presence of a soluble factor produced by squamous cell carcinoma of the head and neck that inhibits the cytotoxicity of LAK cells (104). Whether this factor is indeed TGF-β remains to be seen.

Understanding dendritic cells is essential to understanding the response of the immune system. Massard et al. (105) reviewed the activity of these cells. Dendritic cells originate from the bone marrow. Their phenotype of these cells is characterized by high expression of MHC-II molecules and high expression of adhesion molecules. A close relation with alveolar macrophages exists, whereby macrophages down-regulate antigen-presenting function through TNF-α. Gabrilovich et al. (106) showed that peptide-pulsed dendritic cells isolated from tumor-bearing mice had decreased ability to induce specific cytotoxic T lymphocytes in control animals or to restimulate immune T lymphocytes from control mice *in vitro*. This reduction was reversed by means of addition of dendritic cells from control animals. Macrophages did not improve cytotoxic T-lymphocyte function. The dendritic cells from tumor-bearing mice did not respond and process antigens. Gabrilovich et al. (107) achieved further correlation in an investigation of the mechanisms of dendritic cell dysfunction under certain other conditions. Retroviral infection appeared to down-regulate surface MHC-II molecules, which are critical in activating an immune response.

Finkelman et al. (108) found that dendritic cells can present antigens in both a tolerogenic or immunogenic manner. Porgador et al. (109) found that dendritic cells pulsed with peptides outside the body can provide a protective immune response when returned to the host. Dendritic cells harvested from peripheral blood, expanded in culture, and exposed to exogenous agents or tumor-produced substances can elevate the level of secondary immunosuppressive molecules.

EXOGENOUS IMMUNOSUPPRESSION

Exogenous agents given to patients with head and neck cancer (110) include alcohol (shown to be immunosuppressive), chemotherapeutic drugs (intended to be antitumor but may have anti-immune effects), corticosteroids (given for swelling), and the immunosuppressive effects of surgery (which include induction of prostaglandin and histamine, both well-known immunosuppressive agents). Viral effects caused by infection with EBV, human immunodeficiency virus (HIV), or other agents affect both the number and function of immune cells. The third group are immunosuppressive agents made by the immune system in response to other immunologically active processes that can contribute to immunosuppression (e.g., circulating antigen-antibody complexes).

Among the immunologically active peptides produced by tumor cells, p15e, a low–molecular-weight retroviral membrane protein, is of distinct interest. As early as 1984, Snyderman and Cianciolo (111) identified p15e as having an immunosuppressive effect. A synthetic 17-amino-acid peptide homologous to a highly conserved region of several retroviral transmembrane envelope proteins has an immunosuppressive effect similar to that of p15e (112,113). The immunosuppressive activities include inhibition of monocyte chemotactic responses, IL-1–mediated monocyte tumor killing, the respiratory burst of human monocytes, mitogen and alloantigen-stimulated proliferation of human lymphocytes, immunoglobulin synthesis by B lymphocytes, production of IFN-γ, human NK-cell activity, and *in vivo* delayed hypersensitivity to sheep erythrocytes in mice. A region similar to the conserved p15e sequence has been identified in IFN-α, which may explain some of the immunosuppressive effects of IFN-α. In a study with 25 patients, investigators in the Netherlands (112) identified different amounts of activity of p15e-like substance and IFN-α in the tumors. Immunotherapy with monoclonal antibodies against p15e given to tumor-bearing mice in a model other than head and neck cancer markedly improved survival rate (113).

IMMUNOTHERAPY

Methods of therapy directed at augmenting the immune response against cancer can be classified as either active or passive. *Active immunotherapy* involves administration of

agents to the tumor-bearing host that elicited an immune reaction designed to control or eradicate malignant disease. *Passive immunotherapy* is administration of externally stimulated immunologic components initially obtained from the patient being treated. These therapeutic attempts can be specific, as in the use of tumor-cell vaccines for immunization, or nonspecific, in which immune stimulants such as bacille Calmette-Guérin or cytokines are administered to the host. Many of these active therapeutic manipulations were developed after clinicians observed that some patients with cancer and severe postoperative infection had marked tumor regression and improved survival times. The infectious agents, it is now realized, elicited broad immunologic reactions with cytotoxic cell activation. Most of these therapies, however, have been unsuccessful in human treatment trials. Vaccination with tumor cells or tumor cell extracts is limited by the following factors: tumor-specific antigens are difficult to identify; malignant cells have a considerable degree of heterogeneity; tumor cells seem capable of altering their antigenic expression, especially for the MHC antigens; and tumors can produce suppressive factors or augment the function of suppressor T cells, which inhibit the immune response. These problems affect the ability of vaccines to function properly by making it more difficult for the host response mechanisms to consistently and effectively identify and differentiate malignant and normal cells.

Use of cytokines in therapeutic trials designed to augment the immune system has provided a new strategy for affecting the host response to tumor. These agents have been used alone as nonspecific active forms of therapy and in combination with other effectors in passive approaches to tumor immunotherapy. This method of treatment is called *adoptive immunotherapy* when the therapeutic agents being administered include effector cells (114). Initial clinical attention focused on the use of the interferons and IL-2, both as single agents and in combination with tumor-reactive lymphocytes obtained from the patient's circulating cell pool, LAK cells, or the tumor itself, so-called tumor-infiltrating lymphocytes (TIL).

Interferon-α, IFN-γ, and IL-2 have been used as single agents in the management of head and neck cancer. The clinical use of these agents has been complicated by difficulties in establishing the appropriate antitumor and immunomodulatory dosages, routes of administration, and evaluation of the isolated physiologic roles. Only limited antitumor responses have been identified for these individual cytokines. Interferon-γ has a cytolytic and cytostatic effect against squamous cell carcinoma of the head and neck both *in vivo* and *in vitro*, although improvement in survival outcome after IFN-γ therapy has not been found (95,96). Systemic administration has increased tumor cell differentiation and NK-cell activity, suggesting important immunomodulatory and physiologic effects at the local and systemic levels. Similar effects have been observed with IFN-α, although the cytotoxic effect has not been as profound for squamous cell carcinoma of the head and neck as it has been for some of the hematologic malignant diseases. IL-2 has had antitumor and immunomodulatory effects when administered systemically or perilesionally for squamous cell carcinoma of the head and neck (115,116). Activation of peripheral NK cells after systemic infusion of IL-2 combined with IFN-α has been documented, and LAK cells have been generated from tumor-associated nodal lymphocytes after regional injection of the cytokine (117,118). ILO-2 receptors have been identified on some cell lines of squamous cell carcinoma of the head and neck, and *in vitro* IL-2 has a direct growth-inhibitory effect on these cells (119).

Systemic administration of IL-2 as single-agent therapy has been associated with serious morbidity and few clinical responses (120). In an attempt to improve the clinical results obtained with IL-2 therapy, Rosenberg et al. (101), at the National Cancer Institute, used the transfer of IL-2–activated lymphocytes, which they called LAK cells, in adoptive immunotherapy trials. Immunotherapy with LAK cells in combination with high systemic doses of IL-2 led to marked regression of established metastatic disease in both animal and human studies (92,101,102). Most of the experience with this form of therapy has been in the treatment of patients with metastatic renal cell carcinoma, melanoma, and colorectal cancer; however, investigators have evaluated this form of treatment for squamous cell carcinoma of the head and neck. *In vivo* studies with nude mice have shown marked inhibition of tumor growth of squamous cell carcinoma of the head and neck with either local or systemic administration of LAK cells and IL-2 (119). Attempts to generate more homogeneous populations of LAK cells with greater cytotoxic activity are under investigation and may lead to improved clinical outcomes with decreased toxicity (121).

The infiltration of solid tumors by lymphocytic populations has long been recognized. The function of these cells in the control of tumor growth and dissemination is not fully understood, but evidence suggests that the presence of a mononuclear infiltrate may be related to improved prognosis and survival rates among patients with squamous cell carcinoma of the head and neck (122). Methods have been developed for harvesting TIL, and clinical trials have been instituted in which these cells are used for adoptive immunotherapy. Treatment with TIL depends on activation of these cells by IL-2 that results in effectors with cytolytic activity against autologous tumor. Murine studies have shown that TIL expanded in IL-2 and transferred to animals bearing micrometastasis are 50 to 100 times more potent than are LAK cells in eradicating tumor (123,124). A clinical trial with TIL therapy for metastatic melanoma showed marked tumor regression; response rates were higher than those achieved with LAK cells and IL-2 (125). Similar results have been obtained *in vitro* for cultures of squamous cell carcinoma of the head and neck, and isolation and activation of TIL from a patient with head and neck cancer has been accomplished (115,116). The cytolytic specificity exhibited by TIL toward autologous tumor results from MHC restriction. Tumor-specific anti-

gens exposed to dendritic cells harvested from peripheral blood of patients and expanded *in vitro* has been proposed as a form of immunotherapy, but no data are available for patients with head and neck cancer. This specificity makes this form of immunotherapy appealing, but further investigation is needed to determine the effectiveness in the management of head and neck cancer.

An important early report of a study employing biological modifiers to treat active advanced cancers also showed them to prevent metachronos cancers. Shin et al. (126) gave IFN-α, 13-cis-retinoic acid, and α-tocopherol to patients with advanced disease (69% had N2 or N3 disease). They noticed an improvement in control wherein 86% of patients were disease free after 24 months. In addition, they noted a lack of second primary tumors in this population except for one patient who developed acute leukemia but no case of upper aerodigestive tract second primaries.

HIGHLIGHTS

- A cancer progression model specific for head and neck cancer is being developed. This accounts for the multistep process of genetic alterations responsible for the pathogenesis of malignant tumors.
- Mutation of p53 appears to have a central role in the development of cancer by altering the ability of cells to respond to DNA damage.
- Human papillomavirus proteins interact with p53; the result is inactivation of p53 protein.
- Immunoglobulin-associated cytotoxicity directed against malignant cells occur through two mechanisms: complement fixation and antibody-dependent cellular cytotoxicity.
- Interferon-γ may prove useful as an immunotherapeutic agent because of its cytotoxic, immunomodulatory, and cell-differentiating effects.
- Tumor production of immunosuppressive factors may impair the cytotoxic response by inhibiting the immunomodulatory effects of the cytokines.
- Interleukin-1 may have a role in the development of bone invasion by squamous cell carcinoma of the head and neck.
- Defects in the helper T-lymphocyte phase of the immune response may be partly responsible for the impaired cytotoxic response against malignant cells.
- Active immunotherapy for cancer involves administration of agents that can elicit an immune response (e.g., IFN-γ).
- Passive immunotherapy involves administration of externally stimulated immunologic components such as LAK cells, initially obtained from a tumor-bearing patient.
- Systemic and perilesional injection of IL-2 for squamous cell carcinoma of the head and neck has activated NK and LAK cells, but no survival benefit has been shown.
- Adoptive immunotherapy with IL-2–stimulated LAK cells or TIL may improve the rates of tumor regression and control.

REFERENCES

1. Fearon ER, Vogelstein B. A genetic model for colorectal tumorigenesis. *Cell* 1990;61:759–767.
2. Renan MJ. How many mutations are required for tumorigenesis? Implications for human cancer data. *Mol Carcinog* 1993;7:139.
3. Canaple L, Kakizawa T, Laudet V. The days and nights of cancer cells. *Cancer Res* 2003;63:7545–7552.
4. van der Riet P, Nawroz H, Hruban RH, et al. Frequent loss of chromosome 9p21-22 early in head and neck cancer progression. *Cancer Res* 1994;54:1156–1158.
5. Califano J, van der Riet P, Clayman G, et al. A genetic progression model for head and neck cancer; implications for field cancerization. *Cancer Res* 1996;56:2488–2492.
6. Nawroz H, van der Riet P, Hruban RH, et al. Allelotype of head and neck squamous cell carcinoma. *Cancer Res* 1994;54:1152–1155.
7. Kamb A, Gruis NA, Weaver-Feldhaus J, et al. A cell cycle regulator potentially involved in the genesis of many tumor types. *Science* 1994;264:436–440.
8. Hartwell LH, Katan MB. Cell cycle control and cancer. *Science* 1994;266:1821–1828.
9. Cairns P, Mao L, Merlo A, et al. Rates of p16 (MTS1) mutations in primary tumors with 9p loss. *Science* 1994;265:415–416.
10. Merlo A, Herman JG, Mao L, et al. 5′ CpG island methylation is associated with transcriptional silencing of the tumor suppressor p16/CDKN1/MTS1 in human cancers. *Nat Med* 1995;7:686–692.
11. Cairns P, Polascik TJ, Eby Y, et al. Frequency of homozygous deletion at p16/cdkn2 in primary human tumors. *Nat Genet* 1995;11:210–212.
12. Wu CL, Sloan P, Read AP, et al. Deletion mapping on the short arm of chromosome 3 in squamous cell carcinoma of the oral cavity. *Cancer Res* 1994;54:6484–6488.
13. Maestro R, Gasparotto D, Vuksavljevic T, et al. Three discrete regions of deletion in head and neck cancers. *Cancer Res* 1993;53:5775–5779.
14. Mao L, Fan YH, Lotan R, et al. Frequent abnormalities of FHIT, a candidate tumor suppressor gene, in head and neck cancer cell lines. *Cancer Res* 1996;56(22):5128–5131.
15. Gotte K, Hadaczek P, Coy JF, et al. FHIT expression is absent or reduced in a subset of primary head and neck cancer. *Anticancer Res* 2000;20(2A):1057–1060.
16. Ohta M, Inoue H, Cotticelli MG, et al. The FHIT gene, spanning the chromosome 3p14.2 fragile site and renal carcinoma-associated t(3:8) breakpoint, is abnormal in digestive tract cancers. *Cell* 1996;84:587–597.
17. Boyle JO, Hakim J, Koch W, et al. The incidence of p53 mutations increases with progression of head and neck cancer. *Cancer Res* 1993;53:4477–4480.
18. Kastan MB, Onyekere O, Sidransky D, et al. Participation of p53 protein in the cellular response to DNA damage. *Cancer Res* 1991;51:6304–6311.
19. Livingstone LR, White A, Sprouse J, et al. Altered cell cycle arrest and gene amplification potential accompany loss of wild-type p53. *Cell* 1992;70:923–935.
20. Yin Y, Tainsky MA, Bischoff FZ, et al. Wild-type p53 restores cell cycle control and inhibits gene amplification in cells with mutant p53 alleles. *Cell* 1992;70:937–948.
21. Lowe SW, Schmitt EM, Smith SW, et al. p53 is required for radiation induced apoptosis in mouse thymocytes. *Nature* 1993;362:847–849.
22. Yonish-Rouach E, Resnitzky D, Lotem J, et al. Wild-type p53 induces apoptosis of myeloid leukemic cells that are inhibited by interleukin-6. *Nature* 1991;352:345–347.
23. Gillison ML, Koch WM, Capone RB, et al. Evidence for a causal association between human papillomavirus and a subset of head and neck cancers [see comment]. *J Natl Cancer Inst* 2000;92(9):709–720.
24. Steele C, Cowser LM, Shillitoe EJ. Effects of human papilloma virus type 18-specific antisense oligonucleotides on the transformed phenotype of human carcinoma cell lines. *Cancer Res* 1993;53:2330–2337.
25. Werness BA, Levine AJ, Howley PM. Association of human papilloma virus types 16 and 18 E6 proteins with p53. *Science* 1990;248:76–79.
26. Munger K, Phelp WC, Bubb V, et al. The E6 and E7 genes of the human papilloma virus type 16 together are necessary and sufficient for transformation of primary human keratinocytes. *J Virol* 1989;63:4417–4421.
27. Yoo GH, Xu HJ, Brennan JA, et al. Infrequent inactivation of the retinoblastoma gene despite frequent loss of chromosome 13q in head and neck squamous cell carcinoma. *Cancer Res* 1994;54:4603–4606.
28. Munger K, Werness BA, Dyson N, et al. Complex formation of human papillomavirus E7 proteins with the retinoblastoma suppressor gene product. *EMBO J* 1989;8:4099–4105.
29. Martelli F, Livingston DM. Regulation of endogenous E2F1 stability by the retinoblastoma protein. *Proc Natl Acad Sci USA* 1999;96:2858–2863.
30. Barkova J, Lukas J, Muller H, et al. Abnormal patterns of D-type cyclin expression and GI regulation in human head and neck cancer. *Cancer Res* 1995;55:949–956.
31. Jares P, Fernandez PL, Campo E, et al. PRAD-1/cyclin D1 gene amplification correlates with messenger RNA over-expression and tumor progression in human laryngeal carcinomas. *Cancer Res* 1994;54:4813–4817.
32. Peters G. The D-type cyclins and their role in tumorigenesis. *J Cell Sci* 1994;18:89–96.
33. Condon-Cardo C. Mutations of cell cycle regulators: biological and clinical implications for human neoplasia. *Am J Pathol* 1995;147:545–560.
34. Nakashima T, Clayman GL. Antisense inhibition of cyclin D1 in human head and neck squamous cell carcinoma. *Arch Otolaryngol Head Neck Surg* 2000;126(8):957–961.
35. Estilo CL, O-Charoenrat P, Ngai I, et al. The role of novel oncogenes squamous cell carcinoma-related oncogene and phosphatidylinositol 3-kinase p110 alpha in squamous cell carcinoma of the oral tongue. *Clin Cancer Res* 2003;9(6):2300–2306.
36. Dassonville O, Formento JL, Francoual M, et al. Expression of epidermal growth factor receptor and survival in upper aerodigestive tract cancer. *J Clin Oncol* 1993;11:1873–1878.
37. Thor A. Are patterns of HER-2/neu amplification and expression among primary tumors and regional metastases indicative of those in distant metastases and predictive of herceptin response? *J Natl Cancer Inst* 2001;93(15):1120–1121.
38. Xia W, Lau YK, Zhang HZ, et al. Strong correlation between c-erbB-2 over-expression and overall survival of patients with oral squamous cell carcinoma. *Clin Cancer Res* 1997;3(1):3–9.
39. Lynch TJ, Bell DW, Sordella R, et al. Activating mutations in the epidermal growth factor receptor underlying responsiveness of non-small-cell lung cancer to gefitinib. *N Engl J Med* 2004;350(21):2129–2139.
40. Lundberg AS, Randell SH, Stewart SA, et al. Immortalization and transformation of primary human airway epithelial cells by gene transfer. *Oncogene* 2002;21(29):4577–4586.
41. Ha PK, Benoit NE, Yochem R, et al. A transcriptional progression model for head and neck cancer. *Clin Cancer Res* 2003;9(8):3058–3064.
42. Forastiere A, Koch W, Trotti A, et al. Head and neck cancer. *N Engl J Med* 2001;345(26):1890–1900.
43. Chien YC, Chen JY, Liu MY, et al. Serologic markers of Epstein-Barr virus infection and nasopharyngeal carcinoma in Taiwanese men. *N Engl J Med* 2001;345(26):1877–1882.
44. Lo YM, Chan LY, Lo KW, et al. Quantitative analysis of cell-free Epstein-Barr virus DNA in plasma of patients with nasopharyngeal carcinoma. *Cancer Res* 1999;59(6):1188–1191.
45. Shotelersuk K, Khorprasert C, Sakdikul S, et al. Epstein-Barr virus DNA in serum/plasma as a tumor marker for nasopharyngeal cancer. *Clin Cancer Res* 2000;6(3):1046–1051.
46. Capone RB, Pai SI, Koch WM, et al. Detection and quantitation of human papillomavirus (HPV) DNA in the sera of patients with HPV-associated head and neck squamous cell carcinoma. *Clin Cancer Res* 2000;6(11):4171–4175.
47. Lo YM, Chan LY, Chan AT, et al. Quantitative and temporal correlation between circulating cell-free Epstein-Barr virus DNA and tumor recurrence in nasopharyngeal carcinoma. *Cancer Res* 1999;59(21):5452–5455.
48. Koutsky LA, Ault KA, Wheeler CM, et al. Proof of principle study investigators. A controlled trial of a human papillomavirus

type 16 vaccine [see comment]. *N Engl J Med* 2002;347(21): 1645–1651.

49. Abdulkarim B, Sabri S, Deutsch E, et al. Antiviral agent cidofovir restores p53 function and enhances the radiosensitivity in HPV-associated cancers. *Oncogene* 2002;21(15):2334–2346.

50. Leong PP, Rezai B, Koch WM, et al. Distinguishing second primary tumors from lung metastases in patients with head and neck squamous cell carcinoma [see comment]. *J Natl Cancer Inst* 1998;90(13):972–977.

51. Califano J, Leong PL, Koch WM, et al. Second esophageal tumors in patients with head and neck squamous cell carcinoma: an assessment of clonal relationships. *Clin Cancer Res* 1999;5(7): 1862–1867.

52. Brennan JA, Mao L, Hruban RH, et al. Molecular assessment of histopathological staging in squamous-cell carcinoma of the head and neck. *N Engl J Med* 1995;332:429–435.

53. Partridge M, Li SR, Pateromichelakis S, et al. Detection of minimal residual cancer to investigate why oral tumors recur despite seemingly adequate treatment. *Clin Cancer Res* 2000;6(7):2718–2725.

54. Bischoff JR, Kirn DH, Williams A, et al. An adenovirus mutant that replicates selectively in p53-deficient human tumor cells. *Science (Washington, DC)* 1996;274:373–376.

55. Khuri FR, Nemunaitis J, Ganly I, et al. A controlled trial of intratumoral ONYX-015, a selectively-replicating adenovirus, in combination with cisplatin and 5-fluorouracil in patients with recurrent head and neck cancer [see comment]. *Nat Med* 2000;6(8): 879–885.

56. Nemunaitis J, Ganly I, Khuri F, et al. Selective replication and oncolysis in p53 mutant tumors with ONYX-015, an E1B-55kD gene-deleted adenovirus, in patients with advanced head and neck cancer: a phase II trial. *Cancer Res* 2000;60(22):6359–6366.

57. Ishida S, Yamashita T, Nakaya U, et al. Adenovirus-mediated transfer of p53-related genes induces apoptosis of human cancer cells [erratum appears in Jpn J Cancer Res 2000;91(7):767]. *Japn J Cancer Res* 2000;91(2):174–180.

58. Clayman GL, el-Naggar AK, Lippman SM, et al. Adenovirus-mediated p53 gene transfer in patients with advanced recurrent head and neck squamous cell carcinoma [see comment]. *J Clin Oncol* 1998;16(6):2221–2232.

59. Patel V, Senderowicz AM, Pinto D Jr, et al. Flavopiridol, a novel cyclin-dependent kinase inhibitor, suppresses the growth of head and neck squamous cell carcinomas by inducing apoptosis. *J Clin Invest* 1998;102(9):1674–1681.

60. Kortmansky JS, Motwani MV, Jung CP, et al. Flavoperidol potentiates the effect of radiotherapy in HCT-116 colon cancer xenografts (abstract #347). *Proc Am Soc Clin Oncol* 2002;87a.

61. Schwartz GK, Farsi K, Maslak P, et al. Potentiation of apoptosis by flavopiridol in mitomycin-C-treated gastric and breast cancer cells. *Clin Cancer Res* 1997;3(9):1467–1472.

62. Schwartz GK, Ilson D, Saltz L, et al. Phase II study of the cyclin-dependent kinase inhibitor flavopiridol administered to patients with advanced gastric carcinoma. *J Clin Oncol* 2001;19(7): 1985–1992.

63. Senderowicz AM. Small molecule modulators of cyclin-dependent kinases for cancer therapy. *Oncogene* 2000;19(56): 6600–6606.

64. Hashemolhosseini S, Nagamine Y, Morley SJ, et al. Rapamycin inhibition of the G1 to S transition is mediated by effects on cyclin D1 mRNA and protein stability. *J Biol Chem* 1998;273(23): 14424–14429.

65. Dassonville O, Formento JL, Francoual M, et al. Expression of epidermal growth factor receptor and survival in upper aerodigestive tract cancer (abst). *J Clin Oncol* 1993;11:1873–1878.

66. Grandis JR, Melhem MF, Gooding WE, et al. Levels of TGF-alpha and EGFR protein in head and neck squamous cell carcinoma and patient survival. *J Natl Cancer Inst* 1998;90(11):824–832.

67. Ang KK, Berkey BA, Tu X, et al. Impact of epidermal growth factor receptor expression on survival and pattern of relapse in patients with advanced head and neck carcinoma. *Cancer Res* 2002;62(24): 7350–7356.

68. Huang SM, Li J, Armstrong EA, et al. Modulation of radiation response and tumor-induced angiogenesis after epidermal growth factor receptor inhibition by ZD1839 (Iressa). *Cancer Res* 2002; 62(15):4300–4306.

69. Sirotnak FM, Zakowski MF, Miller VA, et al. Efficacy of cytotoxic agents against human tumor xenografts is markedly enhanced by coadministration of ZD1839 (Iressa), an inhibitor of EGFR tyrosine kinase. *Clin Cancer Res* 2000;6(12):4885–4892.

70. Lammering G, Valerie K, Lin PS, et al. Radiosensitization of malignant glioma cells through overexpression of dominant-negative epidermal growth factor receptor. *Clin Cancer Res* 2001;7(3): 682–690.

71. Lammering G, Hewit TH, Hawkins WT, et al. Epidermal growth factor receptor as a genetic therapy target for carcinoma cell radiosensitization [see comment]. *J Natl Cancer Inst* 2001;93(12): 921–929.

72. Billingham RE, Brent L, Medawar PB. Actively acquired tolerance of foreign cells. *Nature* 1953;172:603–606.

73. Ridge JP, Fachs EJ, Matzinger P. Neonatal tolerance revisited: turning on newborn T-cells with dendritic cells. *Science* 1996;271: 1723–1726.

74. Chang CC, Ciubotariu R, Manavalan JS, et al. Tolerization of dendritic cells by T(S) cells: the crucial role of inhibitory receptors ILT3 and ILT4. *Nat Immunol* 2002;3(3):237–243.

75. Blattman JN, Greenberg PD. Cancer immunotherapy: a treatment for the masses. *Science* 2004;305(5681):200–205.

76. Rosenberg SA. Development of cancer immunotherapies based on identification of the genes encoding cancer regression antigens. *J Natl Cancer Inst* 1996;88:1635–1644.

77. Richtsmeier WJ. Basic allergy and immunology. In: Cummings CW, Fredrickson JM, Harker LA, et al., eds. *Otolaryngology head and neck surgery*. Vol 1. St. Louis: Mosby, 1986:115–148.

78. Koch WM, Richtsmeier WJ. Lysis of squamous cell carcinoma via antibody-dependent cellular cytotoxicity. *Arch Otolaryngol Head Neck Surg* 1989;115:669–676.

79. Quak JJ, Balm AJM, Van Dongen GAMS, et al. A 22-kd surface antigen detected by monoclonal antibody E 48 is exclusively expressed in stratified squamous and transitional epithelium. *Am J Pathol* 1990;136:191–197.

80. Wolf GT, Carey TE, Schmaltz SP, et al. Altered antigen expression predicts outcome in squamous cell carcinoma of the head and neck. *J Natl Cancer Inst* 1990;82:1566–1572.

81. Koch WM, Dugan E, Diaz LA, et al. Induction of HLA-DR antigen on human squamous carcinoma by recombinant interferon gamma. *Laryngoscope* 1988;98:511–515.

82. Scher RL, Koch WM, Richtsmeier WJ. Induction of the intercellular adhesion molecule (ICAM-1) on squamous cell carcinoma by interferon gamma. *Arch Otolaryngol Head Neck Surg* 1993;119: 432–438.

83. Wenzel CT, Scher RL, Richtsmeier WJ. Head and neck squamous carcinoma endothelial cell adhesion: the missing link. *Arch Otolaryngol Head Neck Surg* 1995;121:1279–1286.

84. Young MR, Wright MA, Lozano Y, et al. Mechanisms of immune suppression in patients with head and neck cancer: influence on the immune infiltrate of the cancer. *Int J Cancer* 1996;67: 333–338.

85. Lathers DM, Achille N, Kolesiak K, et al. Increased levels of immune inhibitory CD34+ progenitor cells in the peripheral blood of patients with node positive head and neck squamous cell carcinomas and the ability of these CD34+ cells to differentiate into immune stimulatory dendritic cells. *Otolaryngol Head Neck Surg* 2001;125(3):205–212.

86. Lathers DM, Clark JI, Achille NJ, et al. Phase IB study of 25-hydroxyvitamin D(3) treatment to diminish suppressor cells in head and neck cancer patients. *Human Immunol* 2001;62(11): 1282–1293.

87. Masferrer JL, Leahy KM, Koki AT, et al. Antiangiogenic and antitumor activities of cyclooxygenase-2 inhibitors. *Cancer Res* 2000;60: 1306–1311.

88. Sarzotti M, Robbins DS, Hoffman PM. Induction of protective CTL responses in newborn mice by a murine retrovirus. *Science* 1996;271:1726–1728.

89. Pennisi E. Teetering on the brink of danger. *Science* 1996;271: 1665–1667.

90. Schwartz RH. Acquisition of immunologic self-tolerance. *Cell* 1989;57:1073–1081.

91. Schantz SP, Savage HE, Brown BW, et al. Association of levels of circulating C1q binding macromolecules with induction

chemotherapy response in head and neck cancer patients. *Cancer Res* 1988;48:5868–5873.

92. Carey TE, Kimmel KA, Schwartz DR, et al. Antibodies to human squamous cell carcinoma. *Otolaryngol Head Neck Surg* 1983;91:482–491.

93. Rosenberg SA, Lotze MT, Yang JC, et al. Experience with the use of high-dose interleukin-2 in the treatment of 652 cancer patients. *Ann Surg* 1989;210:474–485.

94. Hartmann E, Wollenberg B, Rothenfusser S, et al. Identification and functional analysis of tumor-infiltrating plasmacytoid dendritic cells in head and neck cancer. *Cancer Res* 2003;63(19):6478–6487.

95. Richtsmeier WJ. Interferon gamma induced oncolysis. *Arch Otolaryngol Head Neck Surg* 1988;114:432–437.

96. Richtsmeier WJ, Koch WM, McQuire WP, et al. Phase I-II study of advanced head and neck squamous cell carcinoma patients treated with recombinant human interferon gamma. *Arch Otolaryngol Head Neck Surg* 1990;116:1271–1277.

97. Snyderman C, LeTessier E, Heo DS, et al. Immunosuppressive effects of cultured squamous cell carcinoma (abst). Presented at the Third International Head and Neck Oncology Research Conference. Las Vegas, September 1990.

98. Oppenheim JJ, Ruscetti FW, Faltynek C. Cytokines. In: Stites DP, Terr AI, eds. *Basic and clinical immunology,* 7th ed. Norwalk, CT: Appleton & Lange, 1991:78–100.

99. Meghji S, Sandy JR, Scutt AM, et al. Macromolecular osteolytic factor synthesized by squamous carcinoma cell lines from the head and neck in vitro is interleukin 1. *Br J Cancer* 1988;58:17–21.

100. Fearon ER, Pardoll DM, Toshiuki I, et al. Interleukin-2 production by tumor cells bypasses T helper function in the generation of an antitumor response. *Cell* 1990;60:397–403.

101. Rosenberg SA, Lotze MT, Muul LM, et al. Observations on the systemic administration of autologous lymphokine-activated killer cells and recombinant interleukin-2 to patients with metastatic cancer. *N Engl J Med* 1985;313:485–492.

102. Rosenberg SA, Lotze MT, Muul LM, et al. A progress report on the treatment of 157 patients with advanced cancer using lymphokine-activated killer cells and interleukin-2 or high-dose interleukin-2 alone. *N Engl J Med* 1987;316:889–897.

103. Mule JJ, Schwarz SL, Roberts AB, et al. Transforming growth factor-beta inhibits the in vitro generation of lymphokine-activated killer cells and cytotoxic T cells. *Cancer Immunol Immunother* 1988;26:95–100.

104. Strasnick B, Lagos N, Lichtenstein A, et al. Suppression of lymphokine-activated killer cell cytotoxicity by a soluble factor produced by squamous tumors of the head and neck. *Otolaryngol Head Neck Surg* 1990;103:537–549.

105. Massard G, Tongio MM, Wihlm JM, et al. The dendritic cell lineage: a ubiquitous antigen-presenting organization. *Ann Thorac Surg* 1996;61:252–258.

106. Gabrilovich DI, Patterson S, Timofeev AV, et al. Mechanism of dendritic cell dysfunction in retroviral infection of mice. *Clin Immunol Immunopathol* 1996;80:139–146.

107. Gabrilovich DI, Ciernik IF, Carbone DP. Dendritic cells in antitumor immune responses. *Cell Immunol* 1996;170:101–110.

108. Finkelman FO, Lees A, Birnbaum R, et al. Dendritic cells can present antigen in vivo in a tolerogenic or immunogenic fashion. *J Immunol* 1996;157:1406–1414.

109. Porgador A, Snyder D, Gilboa E. Induction of antitumor immunity using bone marrow-generated dendritic cells. *J Immunol* 1996;156:2918–2926.

110. Wustrow TPU, Mahnke CG. Causes of immunosuppression in squamous cell carcinoma of the head and neck. *Anticancer Res* 1996;16:2433–2468.

111. Snyderman R, Cianciolo GJ. Immunosuppressive activity of the retroviral envelope protein p15E and its possible relationship to neoplasia. *Immunology Today* 1984;5:240–244.

112. Lang MS, Oostendorp AJ, Simons PJ, et al. New monoclonal antibodies against the putative immunosuppressive site of retroviral p15E. *Cancer Res* 1994;54:1831–1836.

113. Lang MS, Hovenkamp E, Savelkoul HFJ, et al. Immunotherapy with monoclonal antibodies directed against the immunosuppressive domain of p15E inhibits tumor growth. *Clin Exp Immunol* 1995;102:468–475.

114. Rosenberg SA, Longo DL, Lotze MT. Principles and applications of biologic therapy. In: DeVita V, Hellman, Rosenberg SA, eds. *Cancer: principles and practice of oncology,* 3rd ed. Vol. 1. Philadelphia: JB Lippincott, 1989:301–347.

115. Heo DS, Whiteside TL, Johnson JT, et al. Long-term interleukin 2-dependent growth and cytotoxic activity of tumor-infiltrating lymphocytes from human squamous cell carcinomas of the head and neck. *Cancer Res* 1987;47:6353–6362.

116. Boscia R, Chen K, Johnson JT, et al. Evaluation of therapeutic potential of interleukin 2, expanded tumor-infiltrating lymphocytes in squamous cell carcinoma of the head and neck. *Ann Otol Rhinol Laryngol* 1988;97:414–421.

117. Schantz SP, Clayman G, Racz T, et al. The in vivo biologic effect of interleukin 2 and interferon alfa on natural immunity in patients with head and neck cancer. *Arch Otolaryngol Head Neck Surg* 1990;116:1302–1308.

118. Rivoltini L, Gambacorti-Passerini C, Squadrelli-Saraceno M, et al. In vivo interleukin-2 induced activation of lymphokine-activated killer cells and tumor cytotoxic T-cells in cervical lymph nodes of patients with head and neck tumors. *Cancer Res* 1990;50: 5551–5557.

119. Sacchi M, Snyderman CH, Heo DS, et al. Local adoptive immunotherapy of human head and neck cancer xenografts in nude mice with lymphokine-activated killer cells and interleukin 2. *Cancer Res* 1990;50:3113–3118.

120. Lotze MT, Custer MC, Rosenberg SA. Intraperitoneal administration of interleukin-2 in patients with cancer. *Arch Surg* 1986;121:373–379.

121. Melder RJ, Whiteside TL, Vujanovic ML, et al. A new approach to generating antitumor effectors for adoptive immunotherapy using human adherent lymphokine-activated killer cells. *Cancer Res* 1988;48:3461–3469.

122. Wolf GT, Hudson JL, Peterson KA, et al. Lymphocyte subpopulations infiltrating squamous carcinomas of the head and neck: correlations with extent of tumor and prognosis. *Otolaryngol Head Neck Surg* 1986;95:142–152.

123. Rosenberg SA, Spiess P, Lafreniere R. A new approach to the adoptive immunotherapy of cancer with tumor-infiltrating lymphocytes. *Science* 1986;233:1318–1321.

124. Spiess PJ, Yang JC, Rosenberg SA. In vivo antitumor activity of tumor-infiltrating lymphocytes expanded in recombinant interleukin-2. *J Natl Cancer Inst* 1987;79:1067–1075.

125. Rosenberg SA, Packard BS, Aebersold PM, et al. Use of tumor-infiltrating lymphocytes and interleukin-2 in the immunotherapy of patients with metastatic melanoma: a preliminary report. *N Engl J Med* 1988;319:1676–1680.

126. Shin DM, Khuri FR, Murphy B, et al. Combined interferon-alfa, 13-cis-retinoic acid, and alpha-tocopherol in locally advanced head and neck squamous cell carcinoma: novel bioadjuvant phase II trial. *J Clin Oncol* 2001;19(12):3010–3017.

Guidelines for Patient Care

Ara A. Chalian   *Sarah H. Kagan*

Care of patients requiring surgical and multimodality treatment for head and neck cancer is increasingly amenable to application of multidisciplinary clinical guidelines and clinical or critical pathways (1). Multidisciplinary care of these patients mandates a coordinated approach from a multispecialty team to ensure best practices, maintenance of standards of care, and meeting individual needs (Table 102.1). Clinical guidelines and critical pathways represent national and institutional efforts, respectively, to affect that coordinated approach and streamline aspects of care that can be standardized within well-defined groups of patients. These clinical tools are aimed at outlining standards of care, specifying targeted outcomes, and improving resource utilization (2). Their structure, basis, and implementation vary across institutions, nationally and cross-nationally (3). Further, data documenting outcomes and other marks of improved practice that result are inconsistent (2,3). The apparent clinical utility of pathways and guidelines juxtaposed against inconsistent data generates debates over their development, application, and true utility.

PURPOSE

This chapter reviews literature on the use of critical pathways in head and neck surgery to identify successful models, findings, and implication for future development. Background on genesis, history, and controversy in pathway and guideline literature begin the discussion. Clinical guidelines are noted primarily as a point of contrast, given limited examples purely within head and neck surgery. The review of pathways centers on clinical care processes to outline and critique outcomes. Implications for practice and suggestions for future research conclude the discussion.

BACKGROUND

History

Guides to establish best practices or codify national standards of care emerged in the United States and gained notoriety beginning in 1990 when the Agency for Healthcare Policy and Research (AHCPR) was established, building on the work of its predecessor agency, the National Center for Health Services Research and Health Care Technology Assessment. The most visible activity of the AHCPR was to convene national expert panels to develop clinical guidelines on topics as diverse as depression in primary care and pressure ulcer prevention. In 1999, this section of the Department of Health and Human Services became the Agency for Healthcare Research and Quality, the federal agency charged with investigating quality, costs, outcomes, and patient safety in American health care (4,5).

Broadly stated, clinical guidelines aim to set national standards in documents developed under governmental or professional organizational auspices. Conversely, clinical pathways—also known as critical pathways—are generally set forth by health care institutions to establish system-level road maps for care delivery (3). Guidelines specify care at a patient level as seen in the AHCPR guidelines, which can be accessed through the National Guideline Clearinghouse (www.guideline.gov). Pathways specify care protocols within systems, often using the strategy of outlining time-sequenced actions for members of the multidisciplinary team and including patient and family educational benchmarks and materials.

Pathways, as generally single institution quality initiatives, are linked to two of the most prominent trends in health care of the past two decades. The movement formally

---

TABLE 102.1

HEAD AND NECK ONCOLOGY TEAM

- Head and neck surgeon
- Subspecialty surgical consultants
- Interventional radiologist
- Radiation oncologist
- Medical oncologist
- Internal medicine physician
- Physiatrist
- Outpatient and inpatient clinical nurses
  - Head and neck surgery clinic
  - Operating room
  - Postanesthesia recovery
  - Intensive care unit
  - Postsurgical unit
  - Rehabilitation, long-term care, and home care settings
- Advanced practice nurses
  - Nurse practitioners in medical and surgical subspecialties
  - Clinical nurse specialists in disease specialties and institutional settings
- Speech-language pathologist
- Audiologist
- Social worker
- Physical therapist
- Occupational therapist
- Behavioral and mental health specialists, including psychiatrist, psychologist, and psychiatric advanced practice nurse
- Religious or spiritual counselor
- Licensed dietician
- Integrative medicine specialists
- Complementary therapy practitioners

---

known as evidence-based medicine (EBM) emerged out of the United Kingdom, marked by development of the Cochrane Collection and other notable repositories for analyses of evidence for practice (6). Pathways and guidelines, in some ways, are tangible products of EBM. Each has a different scope of influence but each emphasizes use of scientific evidence and development of consensus to create a document to guide practice at institutional, regional, or national levels (3,7). Further, they are similar to initiatives that emphasize evidence as the foundation for practice in other disciplines (8).

Disease management protocols arose in the United States somewhat after widespread promulgation of EBM, seemingly to redouble efforts to improve outcomes in common, largely chronic diseases (9–11). Ellrodt et al. (11) defined disease management as necessarily including (a) an integrated health care delivery system; (b) available comprehensive knowledge from prevention through all phases of treatment and including palliation; (c) sophisticated information systems able to analyze practice patterns, resource use, and cost and charge data; and (d) a system of continuous quality improvement. Disease management typically includes use of clinical guidelines and critical pathways to achieve the more global standards for EBM (11). Additionally, ongoing clinician education programs, apart from those necessitated by pathway use, and population or

patient education and behavioral health programming may also be included.

Clinical pathways became widespread in American health care in the early 1990s. The use of a specially designed tool to outline a path to improved outcomes is historical, rooted in Taylor's *Principles of Scientific Management* and resulting critical pathways popularized in the 1950s (12). These critical pathways operationalized ideas akin to those promulgated by Taylor even if they did not directly reference his principles. Taylor's aim was to enhance and refine industrial productivity. Introduction of prospective payment systems triggered interest in, and development of, the original critical pathways in the 1980s. Interest burgeoned with managed care penetration. Both managed care and physician and hospital groups looked to pathways to reduce unnecessary variation in practice patterns that resulted in clinical outcomes seen to be disadvantageous or suboptimal and in cost outcomes that stressed already overburdened systems (2).

Development of Structure and Process

Pathways are fundamentally timed action plans, displayed by time period, action, and actor in an available format with inbuilt mechanisms for data collection and management (2). The format most commonly used is the Gantt chart, which suggests specific actions in a time-task matrix (2). Flow charts (Fig. 102.1) have been offered as an alternate form of time-task matrix, with use of a time line and decision points outlined for critically timed events (e.g., an invasive procedure or operation) (13).

Creation of a pathway requires a team approach, given the needs of broad access to applicable evidence, critical analysis and planned implementation, and structured approaches to documentation and evaluation inherent in the overall aim of pathway use (2). Multidisciplinary teams, most often led by physicians and nurses, are the most common means to successful pathway design, implementation, and evaluation. The lack of physician commitment and involvement is the most significant threat to early failure of pathway initiatives. Physician involvement, particularly in surgical care, connotes value and credibility for other team members (2). In parallel, a lack of a truly multidisciplinary team often unbalances the structure and actions of the pathway. Discrete actions by members of the interdisciplinary team essential to well-coordinated care can be overlooked if representative clinicians are not involved in planning.

The matrix format of pathways proscribes sequences for clinician timing and resource use. Resources generally include, but are not limited to, tests and medications; consultation requests for surgical and medical specialists as well as case managers or discharge nurses or social workers; therapies and treatments, from the most basic (e.g., endotracheal suction) to those administered by consulting therapists such as occupational therapists; and patient and

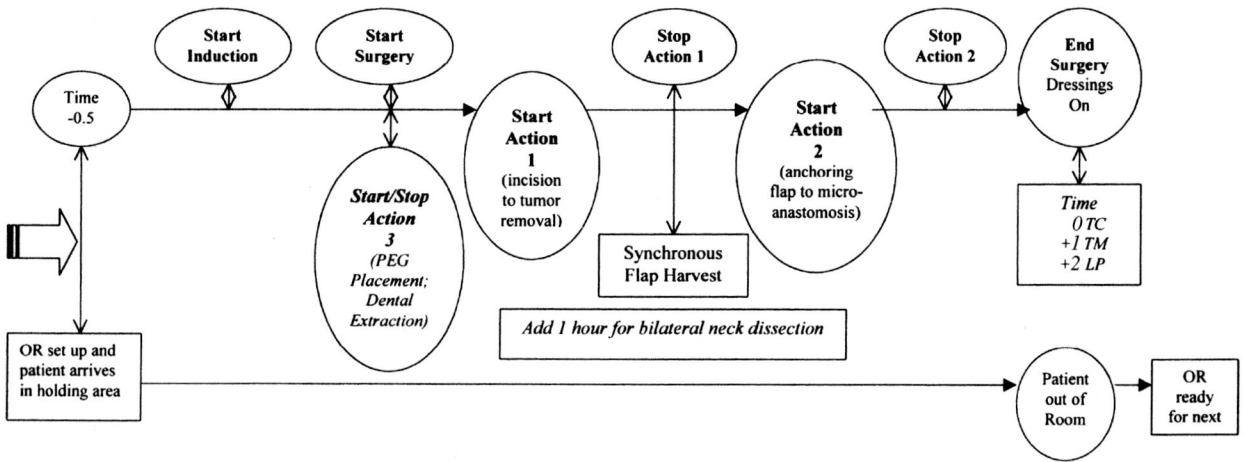

Figure 102.1 Schematic of intraoperative pathway: laryngopharyngectomy (*TLP*) resection, transmandibular (*TM*) resection, transcervical (*TC*) resection.

family education and self-care activities (2). Rarely, if ever, are pathways designed to be interactive, eliciting the input and investment of patients and family members. Sharp et al. (14) offer a singular exception, reporting findings from a patient-held care diary designed to integrate clinical information exchange in a multisetting, multidisciplinary head and neck cancer care center. This project arose in part as a response to clinician concerns over patient and family questions that bespoke confusion about the care process (15). Clinician activities in surveillance and monitoring are generally also specified in pathways when they are viewed as essential, given analysis of available evidence on clinical course and complications. This element of pathway process, in particular, may be undervalued. Surveillance and monitoring likely function to prevent and identify complications as early as possible, thereby triggering appropriate action and, thus, perhaps limiting failure to rescue (16,17).

Consistent and valid documentation, as well as integrated data management and analysis system, have proved critical to pathway use (2,18). With the advent of pathways, mechanisms were developed to ensure completion of the time-task matrix and documentation of variance from the sequence established by the pathway. Placement of pathway materials in the medical record and requirements for physician documentation appear to be associated with greater success in implementation. Pearson et al. (2) note concerns about making the pathway itself the device for nursing documentation. This was a pattern common in the early years of pathway use, which contradicts the contribution to overall success achieved in mandating physician involvement and interdisciplinary collaboration. Team documentation is essential to marking resource over- and underuse as well as individual patient and family data that contribute to pathway maintenance or variance. Analysis of that documentation and upkeep of the pathway database over time ensures fullest ability to gauge outcomes and

overall pathway success. Institutional and departmental or ward electronic infrastructure are generally developing rapidly with widespread use of electronic medical records and efforts to integrate previously noncommunicative data systems. These improvements can facilitate pathway data management considerably beyond early experiences of database introduction and bridging incompatible systems. Nonetheless, despite technologic advances, ensuring access to adequate staff to manage data, query databases, and create reports remains crucial and frequently underestimated in lean organizational climates.

Medicolegal Issues

Pathways, and to a lesser extent guidelines, must be viewed globally as part of a health care system in a litigious context where even the best intended actions may be subject to legal argument. Hart (19), a British barrister, and Tingle (20), writing from a center on law and health in the United Kingdom, offer charged yet practical arguments on the legal aspects of clinical guidelines set within the British system. The lead for Hart's (19) article asserts the double-edged nature of guidelines as they present the threat of poor clinical adherence for which clinicians who use them are then potentially liable and a possibility of inadequately individualized care delivered under the guise of guideline adherence. Taken with Tingle's (20) exhaustive consideration of legal implications and guideline construction, Hart's (19) lead resonates for every clinician who is accountable to a patient and family, a multidisciplinary team, and an institution with every care encounter. Clinician responsibility to evaluate tools with which practice is conducted, the test of adequacy for the new clinician, and redoubled emphasis on teaching and maintaining clinical judgment emerge in consideration of legal implications in design, implementation, and evaluation of both pathways and guidelines.

Outcomes and Gauging Success

Marking success of pathways, as with guidelines, is substantively debated within the health care community (18,21). Measuring outcomes present theoretical and practical challenges. Assessing outcomes requires careful delineation of scope and precise definition. Control of confounders stemming from the field research setting as it were, historical influences in other institutional practices and reimbursement, and other threats to internal validity is invariably limited and threatens internal validity in any given project. Further, most pathways are implemented within a single institution with little opportunity for more than retrospective comparison, immediately implying the threat of history and a Hawthorne-like effect. The Hawthorne effect occurs in "the direction expected but not for the reason expected . . . specifically the effect can be generated by studying the process" (21a). Within head and neck surgery pathway literature for example, only Chen et al. (22) and Yueh et al. (18) transcend the solution of turning to retrospective control groups. Such challenges in design and measurement then lead to findings of pathway outcomes not easily interpreted and for which alternative explanations exist. Institutional or service level indicators (e.g., hospital length of stay, service use per case, and hospital readmission) are commonly included in pathway analysis. Again, the adequacy of judging short- and long-term patient outcomes by these means, the value of institutional outcomes, and the persistence of outcomes (e.g., shortened length of stay) as a virtue of the pathway remains controversial.

Gauging guideline-driven change in practice and regional or national outcomes is similarly bound by analysis of alteration over time and discerning significant changes from confounded effects and spurious coincident findings over a much larger range than is seen with pathways (4,5). Although prescribing or service use patterns are common intermediate variables that are often more easily measured in guideline evaluation, these likely have little direct connection to comprehensive patient outcomes (4,5). Tracking outcomes associated with pathway implementation is less cumbersome, although confounders and spurious findings remain problematic, albeit on a different scale, leading to continued debate around the balance between institutional investment and patient benefit (21).

Various aspects of care for patients having head and neck surgery have been addressed through pathways developed and implemented by a number of health care institutions. With the exception of a single intraoperative pathway, pathways implemented to date have addressed postoperative care for relatively unambiguous procedures (e.g., laryngectomy) (13). The most notable examples of pathways have been published in the otolaryngology and surgical literature, providing a substantive body of literature that shows a progressively sophisticated approach and analysis.

National guidelines for head and neck surgery are less common and less likely to be targeted to surgical care than are pathways. The national guideline for sinus surgery offered by the American Academy of Otolaryngology–Head and Neck Surgery is as relevant a guideline as has been addressed in the literature (23). Most other guidelines obtained through a search of the National Guideline Clearing House (www.guideline.gov), for example, are only tangentially related to head and neck surgery. These guidelines generally address other treatment modalities for diseases such as oral or other head and neck cancers. For instance, guidelines for radiotherapy as well as discrete aspects of general care (e.g., antibiotic prophylaxis) are returned with search terms head+neck+cancer+/-surgery. Table 102.2 offers titles of guidelines returned when the Guidelines.gov collection was queried in March 2005 with the search terms "head and neck cancer" as an example.

PATHWAYS IN HEAD AND NECK CANCER CARE

Outpatient Pathways

Outpatient aspects of head and neck surgery practice have yet to be influenced by pathways and other strategies for clinical management. Outpatient pathways are a clearly minority presence in the pathway and disease management literature. Across specialties, most outpatient pathways focus on pharmacologically driven treatment, as with neutropenia or deep vein thrombosis (24,25). Day surgery units offer an additional opportunity to standardize care. Breast cancer surgery offers the most visible example (26). Pestian et al. (27) report the sole available example within otolaryngology, an outpatient tonsillectomy and adenoidectomy pathway. This pathway showed statistically significant ($\alpha = 0.05$) savings in time, cost, and length of stay for day surgery versus the established practice of postoperative discharge to an outpatient observation short-stay, inpatient unit. The study was limited by its pilot design and small sample. Pestian et al. (27) underscore that a pathway team approach offers advantages in improving outpatient management through shared goals, clear communication, and standard patient and family education. Nonetheless, this strategy, which emphasizes outpatient management, may offer limited utility for head and neck surgery.

Head and neck surgery is sufficiently complex with clear potential of life-threatening complications to warrant the close surveillance of inpatient settings (1). Other surgical subspecialties, however, offer pathways that address the continuum of surgical care that provoke consideration of the intricate nature of best multidisciplinary practice and optimal patient outcomes in head and neck surgery. For example, Reed et al. (28) detail a pathway system to decrease length of stay for patients having vascular surgery. This pathway employs coordinated wound care and rehabilitative services. Although the length of stay and cost savings were not particularly remarkable, with cost savings on the order of $500 per patient day, neither mortality nor

TABLE 102.2

SEARCH RESULTS FROM NATIONAL GUIDELINES CLEARINGHOUSE (WWW.GUIDELINES.GOV)
SEARCH TERM: HEAD AND NECK CANCER

Symptomatic treatment of radiation-induced xerostomia in head and neck cancer patients. Practice Guidelines Initiative—State/Local Government Agency [Non-U.S.]. 1998 October 15 (revised 2004 Mar). 11 pages. NGC:003526

The role of amifostine as a radioprotectant in the management of patients with squamous cell head and neck cancer. Practice Guidelines Initiative—State/Local Government Agency [Non-U.S.]. 2003 April 9 (revised online 2004 March). 22 pages. NGC:003600

American Cancer Society guidelines on nutrition and physical activity for cancer prevention: reducing the risk of cancer with healthy food choices and physical activity. American Cancer Society—Disease Specific Society. 2002 March-April. 28 pages. NGC:002757

Hyperfractionated radiotherapy for locally advanced squamous cell carcinoma of the head and neck. Practice Guidelines Initiative—State/Local Government Agency [Non-U.S.]. 2000 November 27 (revised online 2003 January). 13 pages. NGC:002827

Accelerated radiotherapy for locally advanced squamous cell carcinoma of the head and neck. Practice Guidelines Initiative—State/Local Government Agency [Non-U.S.]. 2000 November 27 (updated online 2002 October). 19 pages. NGC:002990

The role of neoadjuvant chemotherapy in locally advanced squamous cell carcinoma of the head and neck (SCCHN) (excluding nasopharynx). Practice Guidelines Initiative—State/Local Government Agency [Non-U.S.]. 1996 February 15 (updated online 2003 February). 10 pages. NGC:002925

Concomitant chemotherapy and radiotherapy in squamous cell head and neck cancer (excluding nasopharynx). Practice Guidelines Initiative—State/Local Government Agency [Non-U.S.]. 2000 February 23 (updated online 2000 March). Various pages. NGC:002215

The role of chemotherapy with radiotherapy in the management of patients with newly diagnosed locally advanced squamous cell or undifferentiated nasopharyngeal cancer. Practice Guidelines Initiative—State/Local Government Agency [Non-U.S.]. 2003 July 22 (revised 2004 March). 20 pages. NGC:003527

Potassium iodide as a thyroid blocking agent in radiation emergencies. Food and Drug Administration (U.S.) —Federal Government Agency [U.S.]. 2001 November. 12 pages. NGC:002315

Society of Nuclear Medicine procedure guideline for therapy of thyroid disease with iodine-131 (sodium iodide). Society of Nuclear Medicine, Inc.—Medical Specialty Society. 2002 February 10. 11 pages. NGC:002417

Screening for oral cancer: recommendation statement. United States Preventive Services Task Force—Independent Expert Panel. 1996 (revised 2004 February 24). 4 pages. NGC:003454

AACE/AAES medical/surgical guidelines for clinical practice: management of thyroid carcinoma. American Association of Clinical Endocrinologists—Medical Specialty Society. American Association of Endocrine Surgeons; Medical Specialty Society. American College of Endocrinology—Medical Specialty Society. 1997 (updated 2001 May-June). 19 pages. NGC:002074

Thyroid disease in pregnancy. American College of Obstetricians and Gynecologists—Medical Specialty Society. 2001 (revised 2002 August). 10 pages. NGC:003124

Summary of policy recommendations for periodic health examinations. American Academy of Family Physicians—Medical Specialty Society. 1996 November (revised 2004 August). 15 pages. NGC:003954

2002 update of recommendations for the use of chemotherapy and radiotherapy protectants: clinical practice guidelines of the American Society of Clinical Oncology. American Society of Clinical Oncology—Medical Specialty Society. 1999 October (revised 2002 June). 9 pages. NGC:002574

Clinical practice guideline for the management of postoperative pain. Department of Defense—Federal Government Agency [U.S.] Department of Veterans Affairs—Federal Government Agency [U.S.] Veterans Health Administration—Federal Government Agency [U.S.]. 2001 July (revised 2002 May). Various pagings. NGC:002510

Guidelines for preventing health care-associated pneumonia, 2003: recommendations of CDC and the Healthcare Infection Control Practices Advisory Committee. Centers for Disease Control and Prevention—Federal Government Agency [U.S.]. 2004 March 26. 36 pages. NGC:003506

Guidelines for environmental infection control in health care facilities. Recommendations of CDC and the Healthcare Infection Control Practices Advisory Committee. Centers for Disease Control and Prevention—Federal Government Agency [U.S.]. 2003 June 6. 42 pages. NGC:003059

readmission rates were affected (28). This set of neutral findings allays concerns that moving critical elements of physical care and rehabilitation out of the hospital might jeopardize outcomes. Institutional pathway experience coordinating multispecialty, multidisciplinary head and neck surgery care might then be built on this foundational notion of moving care elements to best settings across the continuum (1). Further, important opportunities exist for the American Academy of Otolaryngology–Head and Neck

Surgery to exert national leadership through rigorously developed clinical guidelines that span the continuum of care and cross setting boundaries in a futuristic manner.

Intra- and Perioperative Pathways

Cost and time savings for intraoperative processes and associated aspects of immediate perioperative care have yet to be broadly addressed through a pathways framework.

Strong utility is suggested in the congruence between intraoperative care and Taylor's principles of scientific management and the overriding need for algorithmic precision (12). Postoperative pathways often include particular timed tasks designed to reduce unnecessary intra- or perioperative testing or monitoring (29,30), but few focus exclusively within the operative setting.

Chalian et al. (13) offer the sole example of a pathway designed exclusively to address intraoperative care. Figure 102.1 displays the algorithmic design used, which sequences actions within the operating room from the point at which the room is set up to the point at which the patient leaves and the room is readied for the next procedure and patient. Differences in procedure are accommodated in similar sequences with varying time allotments, wherein the actions timed are expected to increase because of complexity. Time savings across transmandibular resection, total laryngectomy or total pharyngectomy, and bilateral neck dissection were examined through variance on three intraoperative pathways. Patients having laryngopharyngectomy resection, transmandibular resection, or transcervical resection with radial forearm free-flap reconstruction were placed on intraoperative pathways. Time savings of around 20% or 3 to 4 hours, depending on procedure, were sought and achieved (13). The project was limited by relatively small numbers of cases and an inability to analyze cost of labor, equipment, and space. Nonetheless, time savings on the order of hours underscores large opportunities that likely exist within most institutions' intraoperative processes for time, labor, and hence cost savings without threat to patient outcomes in this resource intensive environment.

Both intra- and perioperative care present relatively high risk periods for complications that beget concern about safety and trigger analyses of failure to rescue when untoward events occur. As with intraoperative processes, perioperative care protocols are similarly resource intensive, requiring high staffing levels, sophisticated equipment, and close monitoring. Perioperative care is then likely amenable to time-task analysis inherent in pathways in general and typified by the input-output model useful to intraoperative care (13). Close attention to high risk, high volume conditions, treatments, and procedures has proved amenable to both national guidelines and institutional pathways (31). Given the peril of unexpected complications and the resultant need for rescue, hypothermia, anemia from blood loss, and other predictable events are seemingly ripe for pathway and guideline development as part of an integrated approach. The American Society of Post Anesthesia Nurses, for example, developed a guideline to prevent unplanned perioperative hypothermia that offers a mechanism to enhance an integrated approach to best practice for thermoregulation in the perioperative period (32). Others have focused on transfusion prediction models that could be easily integrated into clinical guidelines or pathways for hemodynamic stability (33).

Postoperative Pathways

Postoperative pathways are prototypical of pathway development in head and neck surgery. In what, by far, is the best literature on pathways and guidelines within the specialty, six major centers report their experience in a series of papers (18,22,34–42), although only one paper uses cross-institutional comparison (18), whereas the others use single institution retrospective designs. Regional and socioeconomic variation are likely well represented as the reporting institutions range from coast to coast, from north to south, and treat patients from a variety of rural, suburban, and urban locations. All, as must be expected, are tertiary institutions of some repute. The findings offered, however, are less homogeneous and evoke discrete questions through review.

Four institutions, those without a comparison, report at least clinically and generally statistically significant improvements in length of hospital stay and associated costs (34,36,38,40,42). Chen et al. (22) used a comparison design having both historical and concomitant institutional controls. They found no significant comparative advantages for pathway patients over nonpathway patients. They concluded that the pathway process had been effective in reducing resources utilization for both groups of contemporaneous patients, offering advantages to all (22). Yueh et al. (18) offer contrast in reporting the sole study using comparison. They found no statistically significant difference in length of stay for patients having laryngectomy at an institution with a pathway in place since 1997 with those treated at a similar tertiary institution that has no pathway and no plans to implement one. Further, when controlling for date of surgery, they found the associated decline in hospital stay at the pathway institution became statistically not significant (18).

Pointed contrast in findings among the papers reporting postoperative pathways in head and neck surgery spurs a more detailed level of analysis and introspection regarding processes to improve care. The benefits of pathway development and implementation are touted by authors both in favor and opposed to their use (13,22,43). These authors question what in the process is most valuable and whether those benefits arise in the pathway itself or in the team that creates and uses it. Those who argue the value of the pathway itself tend to turn to resource analyses, pointing to persistence over time and other benefits. Gendron et al. (41) show persistence of resource savings over time. They argue this persistence supports a sustained impact on resource use in a chronological analysis of intensive care unit (ICU) and ward length of stay in an institution's pathway performance (41). Cohen et al. (36) delved into data from another institution, uncovering the effects of tracheotomy and microvascular reconstruction on resource use. These findings are consistent with common understandings of acuity, risk, and care needs. Kagan et al. (40) turn instead to innate patient characteristics in an examination of age on pathway outcomes. These findings emphasize the complexity of age-associated issues in health care resource use, showing an increase in length of stay for patients more than 65 years of age and for patients who have both a comorbid condition and a complication, although their presence was not associated with age over 65 years (40). These analytically divergent perspectives emerge from a literature insufficient to sustain intensive exploration of these questions without further science (21). Yet, philosophically, the chicken and egg question of process versus product in pathway creation and use remains a compelling debate for a health care environment fraught with constraint and in search of substantive solutions.

CONCLUSIONS

In summary, the egress of pathways and guidelines into head and neck surgery and in health care more broadly is marked by industrial history, resource and productivity concerns, and desires to standardize care. Creating pathways and guidelines is limited by several important factors in the nature of evidence available, systems deficits in information and integration, and human influences on methodology. For example, anecdotal resistance to perceived restriction or prescription of individual practice has often presaged development and implementation of pathways. These human issues commonly require attention rivaling that devoted to analysis of applicable evidence. Conversely, guidelines can be perceived to be primarily educational initiatives that have little "bite" at the patient level. Disease management, in fact, may then be understood in part as a response to this clinical distance in its structured approaches to guideline application at the institutional level. Perhaps most importantly, given the questions of cost-benefit analysis and the scientific limitations of pathway research, the question of whether insufficient data warrant resource investment remains. Future investment in pathways and guidelines must be predicated on thoughtful strategy to maximize human and technological resources needed to make these tools, themselves aimed to curb inefficient resource use, a reality.

Systematic access to, and maintenance of, information and data management, although they are becoming more available in health care, are still often inadequate and must be remedied to optimize analytic ability. The greater questions of whether advantages of institutional pathways outweigh their setup and maintenance costs and disadvantages must be addressed. Research employing tenets of organizational behavioral and other applicable theoretical frames must be implemented with fairly sophisticated multisite design and prospective analyses (44). Further, the question of whether another systematic way exists to gain control in a complex systems over complicated specialty care to achieve optimal patient care has yet to be answered

by those who argue that savings are the byproduct of increased institutional attention and enhanced multidisciplinary communication. Comparative analysis of outcome achieved through various strategies aimed at achieving best practices and optimizing resource use will similarly benefit from carefully designed multisite trials.

HIGHLIGHTS

- Comprehensive care of patients requiring surgical and multimodality treatment for head and neck cancer is well suited to the applicability of multidisciplinary clinical guidelines and clinical or critical pathways.
- Pathways and guidelines have historical roots in evidence-based medicine and the emergence of disease management.
- Few guidelines that directly address head and neck surgery are available and, hence, literature describing implementation and outcomes is thinly developed.
- Development of clinical pathways in head and neck surgery focuses largely on postoperative care. Literature reporting outcomes of these pathways reflects progress in methods and analysis.
- Pathway outcomes for head and neck surgery are subject to increasingly sophisticated analysis and debate.
- Future investigation and clinical improvements in guidelines and pathways, in particular, warrant multisite design and prospective analyses.

REFERENCES

1. Gibson MK, Forastiere AA. Multidisciplinary approaches in the management of advanced head and neck tumors: state of the art. *Curr Opin Oncol* 2004;16(3):220–224.
2. Pearson SD, Kleefield SF, Soukop JR, et al. Critical pathways intervention to reduce length of hospital stay. *Am J Med* 2001;110(3):175–180.
3. Bailey DA, Litaker DG, Mion LC. Developing better critical paths in healthcare: combining 'best practice' and the quantitative approach. *J Nurs Adm* 1998;28(7–8):21–26.
4. Devine EC, Bevsek SA, Brubakken K, et al. AHCPR clinical practice guideline on surgical pain management: adoption and outcomes. *Res Nurs Health* 1999;22(2):119–130.
5. Sebring RH, Herrerias CT. The political anatomy of a guideline: a collaborative effort to develop the AHCPR-sponsored practice guideline on otitis media with effusion. *Jt Comm J Qual Improve* 1996;22(6):403–411.
6. Dickersin K, Manheimer E. The Cochrane Collaboration: evaluation of health care and services using systematic reviews of the results of randomized controlled trials. *Clin Obstet Gynecol* 1998; 41(2):315–331.
7. Butterworth J. Clinical pathways for the high-risk patient. *J Cardiothorac Vasc Anesth* 1997;11(2 Suppl 1):16–18; discussion 24–25.
8. Parry G, Cape J, Pilling S. Clinical practice guidelines in clinical psychology and psychotherapy. *Clin Psychol Psychother* 2003; 10(6):337–351.
9. Fitzner K, Sidorov J, Fetterolf D, et al. Principles for assessing disease management outcomes. *Dis Manag* 2004;7(3):191–201.
10. Ofman JJ, Badamgarav E, Henning JM, et al. Does disease management improve clinical and economic outcomes in patients with chronic diseases? A systematic review. *Am J Med* 2004;117(3): 182–192.

11. Ellrodt G, Cook DJ, Lee J, et al. Evidence-based disease management. *JAMA* 1997;278(20):1687–1692.
12. Freemantle N. Taylorism in a post-modern age? *Health Serv Manag Res* 1995;8(1):3–9.
13. Chalian AA, Kagan SH, Goldberg AN, et al. Design and impact of intraoperative pathways for head and neck resection and reconstruction. *Arch Otolaryngol Head Neck Surg* 2002;128(8):892–896.
14. Sharp L, Laurell G, Tiblom Y, et al. Care diaries: a way of increasing head and neck cancer patient's involvement in their own care and the communication between clinicians. *Cancer Nurs* 2004; 27(2):119–126.
15. Sharp L, Lewin F, Hellborg H, et al. When does my treatment start? The continuum of care for patients with head and neck cancer. *Radiother Oncol* 2002;63(3):293–297.
16. Silber JH, Rosenbaum PR, Schwartz JS, et al. Evaluation of the complication rate as a measure of quality of care in coronary artery bypass graft surgery [see comment]. *JAMA* 1995;274(4):317–323.
17. Clarke SP. Failure to rescue: lessons from missed opportunities in care. *Nursing Inquiry* 2004;11(2):67–71.
18. Yueh B, Weaver EM, Bradley EH, et al. A critical evaluation of critical pathways in head and neck cancer. *Arch Otolaryngol Head Neck Surg* 2003;129(1):89–95.
19. Hart D. Some reflections on how not to get bitten by a clinical guideline. *Heart* 2005;87:501–502.
20. Tingle JH. Do guidelines have legal implications? *Arch Dis Child* 2002;86:387–388.
21. Weingarten S. Critical pathways: what do you do when they do not seem to work? *Am J Med* 2001;110(3):224–225.
21a. Parsons HM. What happened at Hawthorne? *Science* 1974;183:922–932.
22. Chen AY, Callender D, Mansyur C, et al. The impact of clinical pathways on the practice of head and neck oncologic surgery: the University of Texas M. D. Anderson Cancer Center Experience. *Arch Otolaryngol Head Neck Surg* 2000;126(3):322–326.
23. Piccirillo JF, Thawley SE, Haiduk A, et al. Indications for sinus surgery: how appropriate are the guidelines? *Laryngoscope* 1998;108(3):332–338.
24. Vinson DR, Berman DA. Outpatient treatment of deep venous thrombosis: a clinical care pathway managed by the emergency department. *Ann Emerg Med* 2001;37(3):251–258.
25. Escalante CP, Weiser MA, Manzullo E, et al. Outcomes of treatment pathways in outpatient treatment of low risk febrile neutropenic cancer patients. *Support Care Cancer* 2004;12(9):657–662.
26. Sladek ML, Swenson KK, Ritz LJ, et al. A critical pathway for patients undergoing one-day breast cancer surgery. *Clin J Oncol Nurs* 1999;3(3):99–106.
27. Pestian JP, Derkay CS, Ritter C. Outpatient tonsillectomy and adenoidectomy clinical pathways: an evaluative study. *Am J Otolaryngol* 1998;19(1):45–49.
28. Reed J, Taylor, Veith FJ, et al. System to decrease length of stay for vascular surgery. *J Vasc Surg* 2004;39(2):395–399.
29. Correa AJ, Reinisch L, Paty VA, et al. Analysis of a critical pathway in osteoplastic flap for frontal sinus obliteration. *Laryngoscope* 1999;109(8):1212–1216.
30. Brothers TE, Robison JG, Elliott BM. Relevance of quality improvement methods to surgical practice: prospective assessment of carotid endarterectomy. *Am Surg* 1997;63(3):213–219; discussion 219–220.
31. Krizek TJ. Surgical error: ethical issues of adverse events. *Arch Surg* 2000;135(11):1359–1366.
32. Jeran L. Patient temperature: an introduction to the clinical guideline for the prevention of unplanned perioperative hypothermia [see comment]. *J Perianesth Nurs* 2001;16(5):303–304.
33. Krupp NL, Weinstein G, Chalian A, et al. Validation of a transfusion prediction model in head and neck cancer surgery. *Arch Otolaryngol Head Neck Surg* 2003;129(12):1297–1302.
34. Hanna E, Schultz S, Doctor D, et al. Development and implementation of a clinical pathway for patients undergoing total laryngectomy: impact on cost and quality of care. *Arch Otolaryngol Head Neck Surg* 1999;125(12):1247–1251.
35. Husbands JM, Weber RS, Karpati RL, et al. Clinical care pathways: decreasing resource utilization in head and neck surgical patients. *Otolaryngol Head Neck Surg* 1999;121(6):755–759.
36. Cohen J, Stock M, Chan B, et al. Microvascular reconstruction and tracheotomy are significant determinants of resource utilization in head and neck surgery. *Arch Otolaryngol Head Neck Surg* 2000;126(8):947–949.
37. Bhattacharyya N, Fried MP. Benchmarks for mortality, morbidity, and length of stay for head and neck surgical procedures. *Arch Otolaryngol Head Neck Surg* 2001;127(2):127–132.
38. Cohen J, Stock M, Andersen P, et al. Critical pathways for head and neck surgery. Development and implementation. *Arch Otolaryngol Head Neck Surg* 1997;123(1):11–14.
39. Clarke LK. Pathways for head and neck surgery: a patient-education tool. *Clin J Oncol Nurs* 2002;6(2):78–82.
40. Kagan SH, Chalian AA, Goldberg AN, et al. Impact of age on clinical care pathway length of stay after complex head and neck resection. *Head Neck* 2002;24(6):545–548.
41. Gendron KM, Lai SY, Weinstein GS, et al. Clinical care pathway for head and neck cancer: a valuable tool for decreasing resource utilization. *Arch Otolaryngol Head Neck Surg* 2002;128(3): 258–262.
42. Levin RJ, Ferraro RE, Kodosky SR, et al. The effectiveness of a "critical pathway" in the management of laryngectomy patients. *Head Neck* 2000;22(7):694–699.
43. Jacavone JB, Daniels RD, Tyner I. CNS facilitation of a cardiac surgery clinical pathway program. *Clinical Nurse Specialist* 1999; 13(3):126–132.
44. Brief AP, Weiss HM. Organizational behavior: affect in the workplace. *Annu Rev Psychol* 2002;53:279–307.

Principles of Chemotherapy in the Management of Head and Neck Cancer

Bruce E. Brockstein *Everett E. Vokes*

The use of chemotherapy to manage malignant disease is aimed at eradication of systemic cancer, or at an increase in locoregional control when used with surgery or radiation therapy. Patients are treated with chemotherapy for either macroscopic or suspected microscopic metastases, or to help in the management of localized tumors. Patients with macroscopic metastasis have clinical or radiologic evidence of tumor spread. This is commonly called *metastatic disease. Microscopic metastasis* implies that clinically unrecognizable small metastatic tumor deposits are present. If the patient is not treated, the deposits become macroscopic. It is in this setting that adjuvant or neoadjuvant chemotherapy is used.

In practice, cure has been realized for only a few types of metastatic malignant tumors. Most patients with metastatic solid tumors cannot be treated with curative intent. Chemotherapy as a single modality can cure patients with testicular cancer, small-cell lung cancer, ovarian cancer, lymphoma, leukemia, sarcomas of childhood or young adulthood, and occasionally the lymphoepithelioma subtype of nasopharyngeal cancer. In the microscopic or adjuvant setting, chemotherapy is effective for breast cancer, colon cancer, osteosarcoma, and many solid tumors of childhood, as well as head and neck cancer, to an extent. Chemotherapy also is important in combination with radiation therapy (RT) for head and neck cancer and other intermediate-stage solid tumors.

The relative success of chemotherapy depends on the tumor burden, the percentage of tumor cells in a chemotherapy-responsive phase of the cell cycle, and the number of cells with inherent or acquired resistance to chemotherapeutic agents (1). The relative success of targeted therapy drugs such as gefitinab (Iressa), cetuximab (Erbitux C225), or imatinab mesylate (Gleevec) may be dependent on specific mutation subtypes or protein expression (2,3). An effective chemotherapeutic drug must be toxic more to the tumor than to normal tissue. Classic chemotherapeutic drugs can be classified into several broad categories according to chief mechanism of action (1). Alkylating agents cross-link DNA and interfere with DNA replication. Among these are nitrogen mustard, cyclophosphamide, and chlorambucil. Cisplatin and several other drugs, including the antitumor antibiotics doxorubicin, bleomycin, and mitomycin C, also act by binding to DNA. Antimetabolites actively interfere with cellular metabolism, frequently by means of inhibiting one or more target enzymes. Many agents with activity in head and neck cancer fall into this group, including methotrexate, 5-fluorouracil (5-FU), hydroxyurea, and gemcitabine. The naturally occurring vinca alkaloids, including vincristine, vinblastine, and vinorelbine, interfere with mitotic spindle formation. The taxanes include paclitaxel and docetaxol. They are plant derivatives that stabilize microtubules and render them incapable of mitosis. Another class of drugs, topoisomerase I inhibitors, including irinotecan and topotecan, prevent the unwinding and, therefore, replication of DNA. Biologic response modifiers, including interferons and interleukins, and tumor vaccines have a role in renal cell carcinoma, melanoma, and some forms of leukemia and lymphoma. Gene therapy is under active investigation, although progress has been slow. Much of the recent progress and research has focused on molecular or targeted therapies. The first of these were hormonal therapies (e.g., tamoxifen and other drugs) that target the estrogen receptor. Hormonal therapies have had little use in head and neck cancer. Current targets of interest include epidermal growth factor receptor (EGFR) inhibitors, tyrosine kinase inhibitors, and other molecular targets involved in the growth and differentiaition of cancer cells. Successful drugs and targets to date are listed in Table 103.1. Numerous systemic agents with novel mechanisms of action also are under clinical investigation as therapy for solid tumors.

Chemotherapeutic agents often are more effective if used in combination. In selection of appropriate drugs for a combination to manage a given disease, drugs with documented single-agent activity usually are chosen. The ideal drugs have spectra of toxicity that do not overlap. The scheduling of drug administration takes into account possible pharmacologic interactions. Prescribing chemotherapy requires a detailed knowledge of the pharmacology, mechanism of action, general and organ-specific toxicity, and spectrum of activity of a drug.

ROLE OF THE OTOLARYNGOLOGIST

An otolaryngologist frequently is asked to help prevent or manage the side effects of chemotherapy or the complications of cancer. Oral effects are common. Chemotherapy-induced mucositis must be differentiated from infection with bacteria, candida, or viruses such as herpes or cytomegalovirus. Dental caries can cause tooth abscesses in a neutropenic patient. Tonsillar or retropharyngeal abscesses also can occur. Chemotherapy commonly causes dysguesia, which is extremely disturbing to patients. Stridor and airway obstruction can be caused by local tumor, radiation-induced edema, or allergic reactions to chemotherapeutic drugs derived from natural products.

CLINICAL TRIALS

Antitumor drugs and new treatment approaches are tested in several phases of clinical trials before they are accepted or rejected. Whenever possible, chemotherapy is administered as part of a carefully designed clinical trial with clearly stated research goals that follow established guidelines and methods (1).

Phase I Trials

In phase I trials with human participants, tolerance and the pharmacologic properties of newly developed compounds are studied. The endpoint of these studies is determination of the maximally tolerated dose and the spectrum of toxicity among humans for a given schedule of drug administration, although the clinical intent in treating the patient is tumor shrinkage and palliation of symptoms, or prolongation of life. Typically, cohorts of three to six patients are treated with escalating doses of a drug, usually starting with one tenth the dose that was lethal to one tenth of the mice treated in animal experiments. The dose is increased until the maximally tolerated dose, usually defined as the dose at which one third or fewer of the patients have severe toxic reactions, is reached. New drugs or combinations of known drugs not previously used in combination can be studied in this setting. Because the primary endpoint of these trials is the maximally tolerated dose, patients with a variety of tumor types are eligible if no standard therapy with a defined chance for attaining cure or response exists.

TABLE 103.1

ACTIVE CHEMOTHERAPY DRUGS FOR UNCONTROLLED METASTATIC OR RECURRENT HEAD AND NECK CANCER WHEN THE PATIENT HAS HAD NO PRIOR CHEMOTHERAPY

Drug	Response Rate (%)
Cisplatin	20–25
Carboplatin	20–25
Methotrexate	20–25[a]
5-Fluorouracil	15
Paclitaxel	30
Docetaxel	35
Bleomycin	30[a,b]
Ifosfamide	25
Cetuximab	15[c]
Gefitinib	5–10[c]
Erlotinib	5[c]
Hydroxyurea	30[a,b]
Doxorubicin	15[a,b]
Cyclophosphamide	35[a,b]
Gemcitabine	15[b]
Vinorelbine	15[b]
UFT	30[b]

[a]Mostly older studies.
[b]Less rigorously studied.
[c]Patients with prior therapy.

Phase II Trials

In phase II trials, investigators attempt to determine the therapeutic activity, or efficacy, of a new drug in a specific disease and stage at a defined dose or to determine the activity of a combination of drugs at defined doses. Examples include use of a new agent to treat patients with recurrent or metastatic cancer of the head and neck or use of a combination of drugs before surgery or with radiation therapy. The endpoint is definition of activity, usually measured as response rate, at an acceptable rate of toxicity.

In assessing response rates, it is important to follow carefully defined response criteria. Traditional response criteria have been revised recently, replaced by the RECIST criteria (Response Evaluation Criteria in Solid Tumors). A complete response is defined as complete disappearance of all clinically detectable disease. Complete disappearance of microscopic disease at surgery or biopsy is called a *histological complete response*. A partial response is defined as 50% (30% linear reduction by RECIST) or greater reduction in average tumor size, measured by means of multiplying the two largest perpendicular dimensions. Complete or partial responses must last a minimum of 28 days to be considered clinically meaningful. Stable disease is defined as any reduction in average tumor size of less than 50% (30% by RECIST). Progressive disease is defined as appearance of new lesions or a 25% (20% linear increase by RECIST) or greater increase in the size of known lesions. The overall response rate for a new drug or drug combination includes all patients achieving complete or partial responses and is expressed as a percentage of all patients entered in the trial.

A particularly difficult problem is determination of response among patients with cancer of the head and neck having multimodality treatment with chemotherapy, radiation therapy, and surgery. Edema and fibrosis can be difficult to differentiate clinically and radiologically from tumor. Thus, biopsy proof of complete response may be necessary both for clinical decision-making and responsible reporting of the results of clinical trials. Positron emission tomography (PET) scanning may be useful to differentiate residual tumor from changes after radiotherapy or surgery (4).

Phase III Trials

If the information learned in a phase II trial suggests that the new drug or combination has antitumor activity, the drug can be compared with the current standard therapy in a phase III trial. In a phase III trial, two therapies are compared in a randomized manner. Therapeutic activity and toxicity can be endpoints. For example, a new treatment with similar activity but less toxicity is considered superior. Survival is the most commonly and appropriately chosen endpoint for a phase III trial, although other endpoints (e.g., progression-free survival or palliation of defined symptoms) can be used. Because many patients are needed to detect a statistically significant difference in survival rate, these studies are commonly conducted by more than one institution.

Phase III trials are difficult to conduct for head and neck cancer because of the relatively low incidence of these tumors, their anatomic heterogeneity, and differences in standard surgical and radiotherapeutic approaches at different institutions. The use of survival rate as the endpoint is complicated by successful salvage therapies, the older age of many patients at diagnosis, and the high incidence of complicating medical events and second malignant lesions, both of which often are the result of substance abuse. As a result, the endpoints of *disease-free survival* and *disease-specific survival* can be substituted for *overall survival*.

To offset accrual problems caused by the relatively low incidence of disease, most chemotherapy trials of the management of head and neck cancer are not site-specific inquiries, although most limit eligibility to patients who have squamous cell histologic features. This approach is valid, because differences in response rates between most sites in the head and neck (with the exception of nasopharyngeal cancer) have not been consistently demonstrated.

Several prognostic factors affect trial design and results (5,6). In general, the more previous therapy a patient has received, the less likely is the response to another therapy. Extent of disease and size of the largest mass can influence response rates. Pretreatment performance status, a measure of functional activity, is another important prognostic factor. These prognostic factors should be reported in published trials. Multiple molecular markers are also under evaluation for prognositc correlation (7).

ROLES OF CHEMOTHERAPY IN HEAD AND NECK CANCER

Approximately one third of patients with squamous cell carcinoma of the head and neck come to medical attention with highly confined, early-stage lesions. These patients need no chemotherapy. For all other patients, chemotherapy may have a role. For the few patients with metastatic disease and for those with locoregional recurrences that cannot be treated with further surgery or radiation, chemotherapy has a palliative role. Approximately one third of patients in the metastatic setting have tumor shrinkage (a partial or complete response), which lasts an average of 3 to 6 months. For patients with locoregionally advanced stage III and IV cancer, chemotherapy has two main roles: improving survival and organ preservation. Patients with nonresectable head and neck cancer who receive concurrent chemotherapy and RT rather than RT alone have had improved survival rates. For patients with resectable advanced tumors of the larynx and hypopharynx, chemotherapy followed by RT has been associated with laryngeal preservation among two thirds of patients without decreasing survival rate. Concurrent chemoradiation therapy also may allow organ preservation as well or better than induction chemotherapy with a survival rate equivalent to that of surgery.

STANDARD CHEMOTHERAPY FOR RECURRENT OR METASTATIC CANCER

Several drugs have been shown to have reproducible single-agent activity in the management of metastatic or locoregionally recurrent head and neck cancer (6,8) (see Table 103.1). These agents generate response rates of 30% or less, with responses that are almost exclusively partial and of short duration (2 to 6 months). Responding patients have had longer survival times than nonresponding patients, although this may imply selection by chemotherapy response of favorable patients rather than benefit from the chemotherapy. Results of one randomized trial comparing chemotherapy with no chemotherapy (supportive care only) showed a statistically significant increase in survival rate among patients who had chemotherapy (9). Comparison of nonrandomized data suggests an average survival benefit of several months when using the most effective chemotherapy versus best supportive care. Cure is not achieved with chemotherapy alone, with the occasional exception of metastatic nasopharyngeal carcinoma. The primary goal of therapy in this setting is to palliate symptoms, including pain and disfigurement by a mass, or to improve organ function caused by invasive cancer. From the perspective of clinical research, trials with these patients are performed to identify new drugs or combinations of drugs with antitumor activity.

Paclitaxel and Docetaxel

Paclitaxel and docetaxel are among the most active drugs against head and neck cancer (10). Paclitaxel was initially isolated from the bark of the Pacific yew tree, although it is now produced synthetically. The taxanes stabilize tubulin polymers and prevent cell division. A cooperative group phase II study of single-agent paclitaxel given at fairly high doses over 24 hours to 30 patients had a response rate of 40% (11), although the drug usually is given every 3 weeks as a 3-hour outpatient infusion or weekly over an hour. The true response rate is likely slightly less than this, because larger studies of paclitaxel with cisplatin have yielded response rates of only 35% (12). Docetaxel has shown activity approximately equivalent to paclitaxel. These drugs are considered by many to be "first-line" agents for treatment of advanced head and neck cancer.

Cisplatin

Cisplatin, which has been a mainstay in the treatment of head and neck cancer, frequently is used to treat cancer of the head and neck. Its antitumor activity results from intracellular binding of the activated, positively charged form with a nucleophilic site on DNA to form bifunctional covalent links that interfere with normal DNA function (1). Cisplatin usually is administered over 2 to 6 hours in doses of 60 to 120 mg/m^2, with similar efficacy reported for this entire dosage range. Renal toxicity is common and includes mild to moderate azotemia and electrolyte wasting, particularly of magnesium and potassium. Other toxic reactions include nausea and vomiting, peripheral neurotoxicity, ototoxicity, and cumulative myelosuppression if several cycles of the drug are administered. For single-agent doses ranging from 60 to 120 mg/m^2 given every 3 to 4 weeks, partial response rates of approximately 15% to 30% are achieved (10,13).

In three randomized trials, investigators compared single-agent cisplatin with single-agent methotrexate (8). In general, no significant differences in response rates or survival rate were found in any trial, although the overall trend in survival and response favored cisplatin. The improvements may come at the expense of added toxicity; therefore, cisplatin is not necessarily considered superior (8).

Because of the toxicity of cisplatin, in particular its dose-limiting nephrotoxicity and neurotoxicity, analogues of the drug have been developed with the goal of preserving the antitumor activity of the drug and decreasing its toxic effects. Carboplatin has decreased nephrotoxicity and neurotoxicity. Its dose-limiting toxicity is myelosuppression. Another advantage of this compound is a comparable ease of administration. Because nausea and vomiting are reduced, carboplatin can be given easily on an outpatient basis and without vigorous hydration. It is active against cancer of the head and neck, but slightly less so than is cisplatin. Carboplatin is now commonly used, particularly in the palliative setting, in which minimizing side effects and hospital time is essential (14). An additional platinum compound, *oxaliplatin*, is currently in clinical trials for head and neck cancer.

5-Fluorouracil

5-Fluorouracil is an S phase–specific uracil analogue that can be activated with two major intracellular pathways: (a) sequential phosphorylation and incorporation into RNA or (b) activation to 5-fluorodeoxyuridine monophosphate, which blocks both the enzyme thymidylate synthase and the conversion of uridine into thymidine compounds. Cells are depleted of thymidine and cannot synthesize DNA. Many other drugs have been shown to interact with 5-FU, and trials aimed at increasing its activity by means of modulating its intracellular metabolism have been conducted. The most important side effects are myelosuppression, mucositis, diarrhea, dermatitis, and cardiac toxicity. Used as a single-agent intravenous bolus to treat patients with head and neck cancer, 5-FU has limited activity. A response rate of 13% was found in one large, randomized trial (13). 5-Fluorouracil can be substantially more active administered in a 5-day continuous infusion and clearly adds to the response rate of cisplatin.

Methotrexate

Methotrexate is an antimetabolite that interferes with intracellular folate metabolism by binding to the enzyme dihydrofolate reductase. This inhibits conversion of folic acid to tetrahydrofolate. The result is cellular depletion of reduced folates and inhibition of DNA synthesis. This drug is active only during the S phase of the cell cycle. It selectively affects tissues with more rapid cell turnover. The side effects of methotrexate can be minimized by supplying reduced folates in the form of leucovorin within 36 hours after exposure to the drug. As a single agent, methotrexate usually is given in weekly doses of 40 to 50 mg/m^2. Toxic reactions include myelosuppression, mucositis, dermatitis, nausea, vomiting, diarrhea, and hepatic fibrosis. These toxicities are exacerbated with high-dose regimens unless leucovorin rescue is administered. Renal injury occurs with high-dose schedules.

Methotrexate produces a partial response rate of approximately 10% (9,10); the response duration ranges from 1 to 6 months. Improved response and survival rates are not consistently achieved with high-dose methotrexate regimens, but toxicity increases. Therefore, high-dose methotrexate is not used. Although single-agent methotrexate sometimes is used, other drugs or combinations, especially those containing 5-FU, paclitaxel, or cisplatin lead to higher response rates. Survival rate is not clearly improved with these combinations, and toxicity can be greater than that of single-agent therapy. Thus, methotrexate is the minimal standard treatment of patients having chemotherapy (8). Although it is sometimes still used as a control arm in randomized trials, currently it is not generally used as first-line therapy.

OTHER CHEMOTHERAPY DRUGS

Several other drugs have had a moderate degree of activity in the management of head and neck cancer. Bleomycin, a naturally occurring antitumor antibiotic, was often used in combination with cisplatin or methotrexate. The risk of fatal interstitial pneumonitis limits cumulative use of this agent, and the development of other drugs has limited its usefulness. Ifosfamide, an alkylating agent closely related to cyclophosphamide, which has single-agent activity, has been tested in several combination regimens. Other active drugs are listed in Table 103.1.

BIOLOGIC THERAPIES UNDER INVESTIGATION

Most conventional drug therapies for head and neck cancer have used classic cytotoxic drugs whose mechanism involves the disruption of normal mitotic activity, or cell division. Most of the new drugs in development target molecular pathways more specific to malignant than normal cells.

Among the most promising targets for novel therapies are a group of cell-surface receptors called the "growth factor receptors" and "receptor tyrosine kinases" (RTK). RTK activity is tightly controlled in normal cells, but the genes encoding these receptors escape from their usual inhibitory intracellular mechanisms in malignant cells through amplification, mutation, or structural rearrangement. One of these receptors, the EGFR, is dysregulated and overexpressed in most head and neck cancers. Several therapeutic approaches (e.g., monoclonal antibodies [Moab], small molecule tyrosine kinase inhibitors) that specifically target the activated EGFR are in clinical trials for head and neck cancer.

Cetuximab (Erbitux, IMC225)

As noted, most head and neck cancer tumors overexpress EGFR, making it a good target for cetuximab, an anti-EGFR Moab that inhibits receptor activity by blocking the ligand binding site. Cetuximab is currently being investigated as a single agent, in combination with chemotherapy, and as a radiation sensitizer (15–19).

The efficacy of cetuximab monotherapy was shown in a multicenter trial involving 103 patients with recurrent or metastatic cisplatin-refractory head and neck cancer (15). In a preliminary report, cetuximab (400 mg/m^2 initially, followed by 250 mg/m^2 weekly) resulted in 17 responses (5 complete), but the median time to progression and overall survival (OS) were only 2.8 and 5.8 months, respectively.

In a study of 96 patients with recurrent squamous head and neck cancer who failed to respond to a platinum-based regimen, patients were treated with cetuximab plus either cisplatin or carboplatin (16). In a preliminary report, an objective response to therapy was noted in 14 (15%), and 40% maintained disease stabilization. Similar results were noted by others using a similar treatment strategy (17).

In an early report of a phase III study that randomly assigned 121 patients with advanced head and neck cancer to cisplatin with placebo or cetuximab, the median duration of disease-free survival and OS for the entire group of patients were 6.7 and 7.2 months, respectively (18). No significant benefit was seen for the addition of cetuximab to single agent cisplatin, although the response rate to the combination exceeded that of cisplatin alone.

Gefitinib (Iressa, ZD 1839) and Erlotinib (Tarceva, OSI-774)

Gefitinib and erlotinib are the orally active, small molecule tyrosine kinase inhibitors. The efficacy of these agents has been demonstrated in several studies.

Gefitinib was studied as a single agent at 500 mg daily by mouth in a group of 47 assessable patients with recurrent or metastatic head and neck cancer. Of 47, 5 (11%) had a complete or partial response after 8 weeks of therapy, whereas a further 20 had prolonged disease stabilization (20). The main side effects of gefitinib were a characteristic acneiform rash in one half of patients and diarrhea. Notably, the development of skin toxicity predicted for a better outcome from therapy (both in terms of response rate and progression-free survival). Similar results have been noted with gefitinab given at 250 mg daily.

Similar results were noted in a study of erlotinib (150 mg daily) in 115 patients with locally recurrent or metastatic head and neck cancer (21). Five patients had objective disease regression (4.3%), 44 had disease stabilization for a median of 16 weeks, and in subgroup analysis, patients with at least grade 2 skin toxicity had significantly longer survival than those with no skin rash (7.4 vs. 4 months, respectively).

COMBINATION CHEMOTHERAPY

Combinations of drugs are thought to be superior to single agents because cells resistant to one agent may be sensitive to another. In the management of head and neck cancer, most combinations have been based on methotrexate or cisplatin, and most recently on cisplatin or carboplatin, paclitaxel or docetaxel, and 5-FU. Several randomized studies have compared a single agent with a combination regimen. In these studies, investigators attempted to increase response rates by combining drugs with proved single-agent activity, such as cisplatin, carboplatin, 5-FU methotrexate, and bleomycin. In other studies, investigators attempted to use active drugs that might interact synergistically with each other, for which the observed cell destruction would exceed that expected from the sum of the activity of both agents. This may be the case for the combination of cisplatin and 5-FU, which is synergistic *in vitro* (22). One of the "standard" combination regimens has been cisplatin followed by a 4- to 5-day continuous intravenous infusion of 5-FU. In the care of patients with recurrent disease, it has had reproducible response rates ranging from 30% to 40% (13,14). In the neoadjuvant setting of locally advanced, nonmetastatic disease, impressive response rates of about 80%, with 10% to 40% complete responses, have occurred (6,10,23,24). The combination of cisplatin and 5-FU was compared with each of these drugs delivered as single agents in a three-arm randomized trial (13). Although the response rate of the combination (32%) was significantly higher than that of cisplatin alone (17%) or 5-FU alone (13%), no significant difference was seen in the median survival period of 5 to 6 months for all groups. In a three-armed, randomized trial, the Southwestern Oncology Group (14) compared cisplatin and 5-FU with a combination of carboplatin and 5-FU (postulated to be equally active but less toxic) and single-agent methotrexate as standard therapy. Both cisplatin and carboplatin combined with infusion of 5-FU had a better response rate than did methotrexate alone. Both combinations were more toxic, and survival rate was not affected in any of the arms.

The taxanes are commonly used in combination regimens. The Eastern Cooperative Oncology Group (ECOG) directly compared cisplatin (75 mg/m^2) plus paclitaxel (175 mg/m^2) every 21 days to cisplatin (100 mg/m^2) and 5-FU (1,000 mg/m^2 daily infusion, days 1-4) every 21 days as first-line therapy in 194 patients with advanced head and neck cancer (25). In a preliminary report, the cisplatin–paclitaxel combination was associated with similar median (9 vs. 8 months) and 1-year survival rates (30% vs. 41%), but a more favorable toxicity profile. In the palliative setting, carboplatin is often substituted for cisplatin in combination with a taxane. Several other three-drug or four-drug combination regimens containing taxanes have shown high response rates and are under development.

An analysis of the available, appropriately conducted, randomized chemotherapy trials had the following conclusions about combination regimens (8):

- Combinations produce statistically significantly higher response rates than do single agents, including methotrexate.
- In no comparison group (single agent or combinations with taxanes excluded) is survival time meaningfully lengthened.
- The toxicities of cisplatin and infusional 5-FU, especially nausea and vomiting, are significantly greater than those of single agents.
- Clinical research now focuses on identification of new agents and combinations with activity against cancer of the head and neck. In particular, the new drugs with novel mechanisms, such as tyrosine kinase inhibitors, angiogenesis inhibitors, and other inhibitors of invasion and metastasis, are under investigation. The role of retinoids, selenium, and other molecules in the reversal of premalignant lesions and prevention of primary or second malignant tumors also is under investigation (6).

In summary, chemotherapy for recurrent or metastatic cancer of the head and neck is palliative for some patients, although the effect on survival rate is small. Cisplatin, carboplatin, infusional 5-FU, paclitaxel, and docetaxel are the most active single agents. The response rate is 10% to 30% and the response lasts for 1 to 6 months. Combination chemotherapy, particularly cisplatin or carboplatin with 5-FU or paclitaxel or docetaxel, produces higher response rates, although long-term survival rarely is achieved. Because cure with result of any of these drugs or combinations is unlikely among patients previously treated or those with metastatic disease, and in view of the poor outcome with standard single agents and combinations, patients should be treated in a clinical trial whenever possible.

TABLE 103.2

BENEFITS AND MECHANISMS OF CHEMORADIOTHERAPY

Drugs and irradiation can be active against different tumor cell subpopulations based on cell-cycle specificity, pH, and oxygen supply. Cells resistant to one modality of treatment can be eradicated by the other.
Combination therapies can increase tumor cell recruitment from G0 into radiation therapy-responsive cell-cycle phase.
Tumor shrinkage can decrease interstitial pressure and, therefore, increase drug and oxygen delivery.
Early eradication of tumor cells prevents emergence of drug or radiation resistance.
Cell-cycle synchronization increases the effectiveness of both therapies.
Chemotherapy inhibits repair of sublethal radiation damage and inhibits recovery from potentially lethal radiation damage.

OTHER ROLES OF CHEMOTHERAPY

Chemoradiation

In concomitant chemoradiation therapy (CRT), chemotherapy and radiation therapy are used simultaneously or in a rapidly alternating sequence. Chemotherapy can increase the efficacy of radiation therapy within the radiation treatment field. The possible mechanisms underlying this effect are summarized in Table 103.2. Because head and neck cancer manifests predominantly as a locoregional disease, concomitant chemoradiation therapy is valuable because it focuses on the site that determines prognosis. The early use of chemotherapy also can sterilize distant micrometastasis.

Chemoradiation therapy can be used in several settings. For unresectable locoregionally advanced cancer of the head and neck, CRT is clearly better than radiation therapy alone in most settings. In the postoperative setting, results of several studies have shown that CRT in the treatment of patients at high risk for relapse results has a better outcome than RT alone. For patients with resectable disease who are to have RT alone for medical reasons or because they refuse surgical treatment, CRT is generally superior to RT alone. CRT has not been compared directly with surgery and RT for resectable disease. Comparison of results of phase II studies suggests, however, that appropriately administered intensive CRT can be at least equivalent to surgery plus RT for medically fit patients. Representative randomized studies in which cisplatin or carboplatin, with or without 5-FU, was used concomitantly with chemotherapy (and select other studies) are detailed in Table 103.3.

Unresectable Head and Neck Cancer

The definition of *resectability* is variable and is highly dependent on surgical and patient preferences. This is an important factor in interpreting the outcomes of trials involving patients with "unresectable" cancer of the head and

TABLE 103.3

REPRESENTATIVE STUDIES OF CONCOMITANT CHEMOTHERAPY AND RADIATION THERAPY

Investigator	Evaluable Patients	Treatment	OS (%) Chemotherapy/Control
Single-agent 5-FU or cisplatin			
Browman et al. (50)	175	5-FU, RT	63/50 ($P = 0.08$)
Lo et al. (51)	151	5-FU, RT	32/14 ($P < 0.05$)
Jeremic et al. (33)	130	Cisplatin, RT	46/25 ($P = 0.008$)
Bachaud et al. (31)	83	Surgery, then RT + cisplatin	36/13 ($P < 0.01$)[a]
Combination chemotherapy			
Taylor et al. (52)	214	Cisplatin, 5-FU, (neoadjuvant or concomitant), RT	41/36
Merlano et al. (53)	157	Cisplatin, 5-FU, RT	24/10 ($P = 0.01$)
Brizel et al. (29)	116	Cisplatin, 5-FU, RT	55/34 ($P = 0.07$)
Wendt et al. (30)	270	Cisplatin, 5-FU, RT	48/24 ($P < 0.0003$)
Adelstein et al. (32)	100	Cisplatin, 5-FU, RT	50/48[a]
Calais et al. (54)	226	Cisplatin, 5-FU, RT	51/31 ($P = 0.02$)
Adelstein et al. (55)	271	Cisplatin + 5-FU + RT vs. cisplatin + RT vs. RT (with split course for cisplatin + 5-FU + RT)	23/37/27 ($P = 0.014$ for cisplatin + RT vs. RT)
RTOG 91-11	518	CF neoadjuvant vs. cisplatin + RT vs. RT	55/54/56
Bernier et al./EORTC (27)	334	Postoperative RT ± cisplatin	53/40 ($P = 0.02$)[a]
Cooper et al./RTOG (28)	459	Postoperative RT ± cisplatin	47/40 − 9 = 0.19[a]

OS, overall survival; bleo, bleomycin; RT, radiotherapy; 5-FU, 5-fluorouracil[J28]; CF (cisplatin + 5-FU); RTOG, Radiation Therapy Oncology Group; EORTC, European Organization for the Research and Treatment of Cancer.
[a]All patients resectable.

neck. The most current staging system, American Joint Commission on Cancer (AJCC) 6, however, defines resectability. Regardless of definition, the long-term survival rate with RT alone for unresectable cancer of the head and neck historically has been 10% to 30%. Numerous trials have been performed over the last two to three decades in which patients with unresectable cancer of the head and neck have been randomized to undergo RT alone or RT with concomitant chemotherapy. Many drugs have been used alone or in combination with different strategies regarding factors such as timing of chemotherapy and dose of radiation. General conclusions can be drawn from these studies, particularly from three recent, large-scale metaanalyses. In general, with most single-agent chemotherapeutic drugs given concomitantly with chemotherapy, locoregional control and survival are better than with RT alone.

Direct comparisons have not been made between radiosensitizing chemotherapeutic drugs. The most frequently used, and perhaps best single-agent chemotherapeutic drugs, are 5-FU and cisplatin. Although they have not been directly compared with RT alone, paclitaxel and docetaxel also are commonly used. Cetuximab added to RT has recently been shown to be superior to RT alone in a randomized trial (19). Several other drugs are effective but are less commonly used because of concerns about side effects or decreases in efficacy. Many combination regimens have been used with RT, the most well characterized of which is the combination of cisplatin and 5-FU. The combination of carboplatin and taxol is undergoing rigorous study owing to its potential efficacy and relative tolerability. The combination of 5-FU and hydroxyurea has been extensively studied at the University of Chicago, and it appears to be a synergistic regimen that may be as effective or more effective than cisplatin with 5-FU.

The results of several metaanalyses have mostly involved patients with unresectable lesions. In the most comprehensive, the Meta-analysis of Chemotherapy on Head and Neck Cancer Collaborative Group (MACH-NC) performed an individual patient metaanalysis involving more than 10,000 patients in total. The hazard ratio of death among the concomitant group was 0.81 (95% CI, 0.76 to 0.88). This represented an improvement in 5-year survival rate from 32% to 40%. The subset of trials in which multiagent chemotherapy was used showed a hazard ratio of 0.69 (26).

The benefit of CRT must be weighed against the toxicity inherent in its use. The risk of acute mucositis, dermatitis, and chemotherapy-specific side effects is greater than with either mode of therapy alone. Short-term use of gastric feeding devices is needed more frequently. In those studies that have assessed long-term function, no increase in long-term toxicities were noted (27,28). The latest generation of studies continues to show improved survival rates with aggressive CRT. This advantage is maintained even when chemotherapy is added to hyperfractionated RT, so the benefit of chemotherapy is not solely because of the more intensive treatment (hyperfractionation) but to a true radioenhancing effect (17,18).

Postoperative Adjuvant Chemoradiation Therapy

Several studies have specifically assessed postoperative use of CRT versus RT alone. In one study of 83 patients with stage III or IV cancer of the head and neck with extracapsular lymph node spread, patients were treated with RT alone or with weekly administration of cisplatin. The combined modality group had both improved locoregional control and an improved overall survival rate (36% as opposed to 13% 5-year overall survival rate, $P < 0.01$) (31). The results of two larger cooperative group trials have been recently published. Both showed an improvement in outcome for high risk postoperative patients receiving RT plus concomitant cisplatin chemotherapy compared with RT alone (27,28).

One randomized trial sponsored by the European Organization for the Research and Treatment of Cancer (EORTC) studied 334 patients with high-risk resected squamous cell carcinoma (SCC) of the oral cavity, oropharynx, larynx, or hypopharynx who were randomly assigned to RT alone (66 Gy in 33 daily 2 Gy fractions) or the same dose with concomitant cisplatin (100 mg/m², on days 1, 22, and 43 of RT) (27). High-risk disease was defined as a T3 or T4 primary with any nodal stage (excepting T3N0 laryngeal cancer), involved surgical margins, extracapsular extension, perineural invasion, vascular invasion, or oral cavity or oropharyngeal primary sites with involvement of level IV or V lymph nodes. CRT was associated with significantly better 5-year rates of progression-free survival (PFS, 47% vs. 36%) and overall survival (53% vs. 40%), and fewer local-regional relapses (18% vs. 31%). Severe (grade 3 or 4) functional mucosal acute adverse effects were more frequent in the combined therapy group (41% vs. 21%), but the incidence of xerostomia, dysphagia, or late complications did not differ (27).

A similarly designed Radiation Therapy Oncology Group (RTOG) trial randomly assigned 459 patients with resected high-risk (positive resection margins, involvement of two or more lymph nodes, or extracapsular nodal extension) SCC of the oral cavity, oropharynx, larynx, or hypopharynx to RT alone (60 to 66 Gy in 30 to 33 fractions) or with concomitant cisplatin on days 1, 22, and 43 (28). In this study, CRT was associated with a significantly better 4-year disease-free survival (DFS, 40% vs. 30%) and fewer local-regional relapses (19% vs. 30%). The difference in overall survival, however, did not reach the level of statistical significance (hazard ratio 0.84, $P = 0.19$). As with the EORTC study, the incidence of acute severe mucosal toxicity was significantly greater in the chemoradiotherapy group (77% vs. 34%), but long-term toxicity rates were comparable.

Resectable Cancer of the Head and Neck

Until recently, CRT has had a lesser role in the management of resectable cancer of the head and neck. It is becoming evident that at least some intensive CRT programs used to treat patients who are medically fit can yield results that appear to be comparable with and, in some cases, better than those of surgery plus RT. Even when primary-site surgery is not initially used, the head and neck surgeon still has an important role in diagnostic procedures, follow-up evaluation, neck dissection for some patients, and surgical salvage when CRT fails.

No randomized data have been generated to compare the results of CRT with surgery with or without RT. Results of several indirect comparisons suggest CRT can be an alternative to surgery. Adelstein et al. (32) randomized 100 patients, mostly with stage IV disease, to RT alone or RT with concomitant cisplatin and 5-FU administration during weeks 1 and 4 of RT. In the CRT arm, the 5-year survival rate was 50%. Eleven patients needed surgical salvage, and 8 had successful procedures. The overall survival rate with primary site preservation was 42%. Although the survival rate was equivalent in the RT only arm, 27 patients needed surgical salvage, which was successful for 17 patients. Brizel et al. (29) randomized 116 patients to receive hyperfractionated RT alone or to receive chemotherapy (cisplatin and 5-FU) plus hyperfractionated RT. The 3-year survival rate was 55% in the CRT arm. This percentage is comparable with that achieved in most surgical series. Although the survival rate among the patients with resectable disease (47% of patients) was not reported, it was likely as good or better than that for the entire group. In a similar study, 130 patients with mostly stage IV disease had hyperfractionated RT with or without daily administration of cisplatin. Of the patients who had chemoradiation therapy, 47% had resectable lesions and likely had an overall survival rate better than the 46% 5-year survival for the entire group (33). In the RTOG 91-11 study described below, 547 patients received cisplatin and concomitant RT for stage 3 or 4 laryngeal cancer. The overall survival rate at 5 years actuarial follow-up was 54% for the CRT group. The larynx preservation rate was 84% at median follow-up of 3.8 years.

Several phase II trials also have examined the issue of CRT for resectable disease. A Chicago consortium headed by the University of Chicago has published the results of two consecutive trials of induction chemotherapy followed by CRT. In both studies, patients received 6 to 8 weeks of induction chemotherapy with carboplatin and paclitaxel. Patients then received concomitant hyperfractionated split course concomitant chemoradiotherapy. RT was delivered at 150 cGY twice daily every other week with paclitaxel, 5-FU, and hydroxyurea. Although not specifically reported, many patients had potentially resectable disease. In the first 69 patients (96% with stage IV disease) (35), the 3-year PFS and OS rates were 80% and 70%, respectively. The

2-year locoregional control rate was 94% and 2-year distant control rate was 93%. Toxicity included grade 3 or 4 neutropenia in 36%, mucositis in 76%, and dermatitis in 61%. A second trial using lower RT doses (54 vs. 60 Gy to clinically uninvolved sites at risk for microscopic disease and 39 vs. 45 Gy for low-risk sites) showed a more favorable toxicity profile and preserved efficacy (36). The 2-year and 3-year actuarial survival was 77% and 70%, respectively. The 3-year locoregional control rate was 97% and distant control 95%. Notably, in both trials, the rate of distant metastases was lower than expected, based on similar historical control groups, supporting the hypothesis that induction chemotherapy can help to control distant metastases and improve survival when locoregional control rates are high (35–37).

Several other studies have yielded similar results (38). We believe that patients with stage III or IV resectable disease who are likely to have functional or cosmetic sequelae of the surgery and who need postoperative radiation therapy anyway should be offered an aggressive CRT regimen, as primary therapy, if they are medically able.

Induction (Neoadjuvant) Chemotherapy

Neoadjuvant chemotherapy has been an extensively investigated concept in head and neck cancer. The rationale for this mode of therapy is summarized in Table 103.4. Most important among the reasons for using chemotherapy earlier in the course of disease is lowering the systemic tumor cell burden at a time when fewer chemotherapy-resistant cells exist. The regional vasculature is intact, and drug delivery to the tumor may be better. Surgery and RT are more likely to be successful if used against a smaller tumor (downsizing). These theoretic advantages are offset by the disadvantages of increased toxicity, duration, and cost of overall treatment. More importantly, it has been postulated that cells that

TABLE 103.4

ADVANTAGES AND DISADVANTAGES OF INDUCTION CHEMOTHERAPY FOR LOCALLY ADVANCED HEAD AND NECK CANCER

Advantages

Drug delivery to cancer cells is unimpaired.

Macroscopic response may predict for response of microscopic disease. Prompt elimination of micrometastases may aid in cure.

Tumor may be downsized, allowing for more successful surgery or radiation therapy with less radical treatment.

Patient performance status at surgery may be improved.

Disadvantages

Original extent of tumor may be obscured.

Performance status may decline.

Tumor may increase during chemotherapy.

Duration, toxicity, and cost of treatment are increased.

survive chemotherapy may not respond to subsequent RT. In the rare event of disease progression during chemotherapy, a resectable tumor may become unresectable, and the chance for cure is lost. The practical reason to investigate or use neoadjuvant chemotherapy is to attempt to improve the likelihood of organ preservation or cure.

Clinical trials of neoadjuvant chemotherapy have been performed for more than 20 years. In pilot studies, investigators cautiously administered single agents for one or two cycles before administering local therapy. Use of two-drug and three-drug combinations for two to three cycles eventually became a common approach (6,39). The most extensively used and studied combination is a regimen of cisplatin and 5-FU, although other newer regimens have been used with similar but less consistent efficacy. From these phase II and phase III studies (Table 103.5), the following general conclusions can be made:

- Overall response rates exceeding 80% are frequently achieved.
- Complete response rates usually range from 20% to 50%, most trials showing approximately 30%. Some of the clinical complete responses are confirmed histologically at surgery.
- Toxicity usually is moderate to severe, but administration of subsequent standard local therapy is not compromised, although a small percentage of patients with complete responses refuse subsequent planned local therapy.
- Patients achieving complete responses have a better prognosis, particularly if the responses are confirmed histologically.
- Organ preservation is possible, at least in laryngeal and hypopharyngeal carcinoma.
- The rate of distant metastases is decreased.
- Survival, assessed in randomized studies, is not consistently improved.

The last observation was made by analyzing results of randomized trials in which standard local therapy (surgery followed by RT) was compared with the best neoadjuvant chemotherapy (three cycles of an active regimen that produced complete response rates >20% and overall response rates >80%) followed by the same local therapy. Because various anatomic sites and other prognostic factors, including performance status and tumor (T) and node (N) stages of disease, must be accounted for, many patients must be accrued to detect a statistically significant difference in survival rate, such as more than 10% to 20% after 2 to 3 years of follow-up study.

Many randomized trials have been conducted comparing neoadjuvant chemotherapy before local therapy with local therapy alone. Most had too few subjects or were too poorly designed to be conclusive. In approximately 10 studies, however, many patients were enrolled. The most important of these are summarized in Table 103.5 (23,24,40–44), and a complete description has been summarized elsewhere (39). In only 1 of the 10 studies was overall survival time prolonged (44). All eight studies that assessed distant metastasis as a site of first failure showed a decrease among the patients receiving chemotherapy. Most patients died of complications of locoregional disease; therefore, the decreased rate of distant metastasis generally did not translate into a survival benefit. These generally negative results were confirmed in MACH-NC (26). In that individual patient metaanalysis, however, the patients receiving neoadjuvant cisplatin plus 5-FU were shown to have a statistically significant survival benefit (hazard ratio, 0.88; 95% CI, 0.79 to 0.97). Because metastatic lesions decrease with neoadjuvant chemotherapy, it is possible that with improved locoregional treatment, neoadjuvant chemotherapy may improve survival rates (37).

Three studies that pursued organ preservation as a clinical goal deserve special mention. One is the randomized trial conducted by the Department of Veterans Affairs

TABLE 103.5

RANDOMIZED TRIALS OF NEOADJUVANT CHEMOTHERAPY

Investigator	No. of Patients Evaluable	Chemotherapy Drugs	Overall Survival (%) Chemotherapy/Control	Metastases (%) Chemotherapy/Control
HNCP (40)	443	Cisplatin, bleomycin	45/35	9/19 (P = 0.02)
Laramore et al. (41) (Intergroup)	442	Cisplatin, 5-FU	48/44	15/23 (P = 0.03)
VA Laryngeal (23)	325	Cisplatin, 5-FU	68/68	11/17 (P = 0.001)
Paccagnella et al. (24)	237	Cisplatin, 5-FU	37/29	9/32 (P = 0.002)
Lefebvre et al. (42)	197	Cisplatin, 5-FU	NS	NR
Depondt et al. (43)	300	Carboplatin, 5-FU	52/46	14/19
Domenge et al. (44)	318	Cisplatin, 5-FU	53/45	RR 1.36 (control/chemotherapy, P = n.s.)

HNCP, Head and Neck Contracts Program; VA, Veterans Affairs; NS, not stated; NR, not reported; RR, relative risk; n.s., not significant.
Modified from Brockstein BE, Vokes EE. Chemoradiotherapy for head and neck cancer. *PPO Updates* 1996;10:6, with permission.

Laryngeal Cancer Study Group (23). In this study, patients with advanced laryngeal cancer were randomized to standard therapy with surgery and postoperative RT or three cycles of neoadjuvant cisplatin and 5-FU followed by RT. Response was assessed after two cycles of chemotherapy. Patients with partial or complete responses continued with a third cycle of chemotherapy. Only patients who did not respond to the first two cycles of chemotherapy or had residual or recurrent disease after RT proceeded with surgery in the experimental study arm. Two goals were pursued in this study: improved survival and preservation of the larynx. The 2-year actuarial rates of overall survival were identical in the two groups—68%. The most important finding was the high rate of preservation of the larynx. Of patients in the chemotherapy arm, 64% had their larynxes preserved; the median follow-up period was 33 months. Of these, 39% were both free of disease and had an intact larynx. Only two salvage laryngectomies were performed after the first year. A similar rate of disease-free survival with laryngeal preservation (28%) was achieved in another study (41) with a similar design in which the patients had hypopharyngeal cancer. In a follow-up to the VA Larynx study, the RTOG 91-11 study randomized patients with stage 3 or 4 larynx cancer to RT preceeded by three cycles of induction cisplatin and 5-FU versus RT alone or RT concomitant with cisplatin. The survival of all three groups was similar (54% to 56% at 5 years), but the rate of larynx preservation was highest in the concomitant group (84%) versus the induction group (72%) and the RT alone group (67%) (34).

The results of these three studies established that nearly all patients with laryngeal or hypopharyngeal carcinoma who would otherwise have total laryngectomy or pharyngolaryngectomy should be offered organ preservation therapy. The protocol used in the Veterans Affairs larynx trial is acceptable at a minimum, although the addition of concomitant chemotherapy to RT enhances organ preservation and shortens the overall treatment time considerably.

Several new, aggressive, multiagent neoadjuvant chemotherapy regimens administered before RT are showing promise at improving survival (45,46). Neoadjuvant chemotherapy has not conclusively improved survival and, therefore, continues to be investigational therapy for disease of sites other than the larynx and hypopharynx. Ongoing roles include organ preservation in larynx and management of hypopharyngeal cancer. Possibly a role in the management of nasopharyngeal cancer exists. The neoadjuvant setting may be appropriate for testing chemotherapeutic agents and drug combinations. Finally, induction chemotherapy may enhance survival when used before concomitant chemoradiaiton, and several studies are planned to assess this concept.

Nasopharyngeal Cancer

Chemotherapy is important in the treatment of nasopharyngeal cancer. It is now generally considered standard therapy for all but the few early-stage cases. The optimal timing and role of chemotherapy have yet to be determined. Metastatic, undifferentiated carcinoma, or lymphoepithelioma, of the nasopharynx is highly sensitive to chemotherapy. In four consecutive studies involving a total of 165 patients treated with cisplatin-containing regimens for metastatic lymphoepithelioma, 19% achieved a complete response, and 64% had at least a partial response. Of patients, 12% were free of disease 3 years after chemotherapy, and 14 of 165 were disease free after at least 82 months (47).

Chemotherapy also has a role in the management of squamous cell carcinoma and lymphoepithelioma when disease is local. The most compelling results are from an intergroup trial in the United States in which 147 patients were randomized to RT alone or RT with concomitant cisplatin and postradiation therapy with cisplatin and 5-FU. The study was stopped early when a significant difference in 2-year survival rate occurred in favor of the chemotherapy arm. The 3-year survival rate for the patients who had chemotherapy was 78%; the 3-year survival rate was 47% for patients who did not have chemotherapy ($P = 0.005$) (48). Several other studies have shown similar results with the use of concomitant chemotherapy (49).

CHEMOTHERAPY EMERGENCIES

Chemotherapy emergencies can be divided into those characterized by severe symptomatic side effects or organ-specific toxicities (Tables 103.6 and 103.7). Emergencies particularly relevant to cancer of the head and neck drugs

TABLE 103.6   COMPLICATIONS OF CHEMOTHERAPY

Complication	Management
Nausea or vomiting	Antiemetics, fluids, relaxation, support
Diarrhea	Treat infection (*Clostridium difficile*), antidiarrheals
Fatigue	Rest, exercise, corticosteroids, methylphenidate
Alopecia	None versus scarf, turban, prosthesis (wig)
Mucositis	Mouth care, narcotics
Myelosupression	
Neutropenia	Granulocyte colony-stimulating factor, intravenous antibiotics, and hospitalization if febrile
Thrombocytopenia	Platelet transfusion if <10–20, or bleeding at <50
Anemia	Treat bleeding, erythropoietin, transfusions
Nephrotoxicity	Hydration, support, dialysis
Electrolyte wasting	Repletion
Neurotoxicity	Mainly supportive
Allergic reaction	Antihistamine, steroids, epinephrine
Pulmonary toxicity	Support, steroids, treat specific cause
Hepatotoxicity	Mainly supportive

TABLE 103.7	CHEMOTHERAPY-RELATED EMERGENCIES	
Emergency	**Signs and Symptoms**	**Treatment**
Neutropenic fever	Fever, chills, infectious symptoms plus absolute neutrophil count <500	Hospitalization, antibiotics, granulocyte colony-stimulating factor
Thrombocytopenia or bleeding	Platelet count <10–20 petechiae, overt bleeding	Transfuse, find source of bleeding, avoid aspirin and nonsteroidal antiinflammatory drugs
Allergic reaction	Rash, hives, stridor, hypotension	Antihistamine, steroids, epinephrine
Extravasation	Redness, swelling, pain	Subcutaneous epinephrine or hyaluronidase
Overdose	Drug dependent	Supportive, antidote if available

are discussed. Intractable nausea, vomiting, or diarrhea, although less common with modern antiemetic and antidiarrheal agents, still occurs among some patients. Dehydration and electrolyte disturbances can occur, and patients may need hospitalization for administration of antiemetics and intravenous fluids. Severe mucositis can prompt hospitalization for administration of parenteral narcotics and hydration.

With administration of most chemotherapeutic drugs, granulocytopenia and thrombocytopenia regularly occur. Although granulocytopenia itself does not necessitate hospitalization, infection, characterized by fever, chills, or specific signs and symptoms, indicates a need for immediate antibiotic therapy, usually as an inpatient, if the patient has neutropenia. Blood, urine, and other fluids are cultured, and broad-spectrum, antipseudomonal antibiotics are started immediately and empirically. Administration of antibiotics is continued until neutropenia, fever, and infection resolve. Administration of granulocyte colony-stimulating factor has a role in preventing infection among aggressively treated patients but is not as helpful if initiated in the setting of established neutropenic fever.

Thrombocytopenia can be life-threatening, particularly if platelet counts decrease to less than 10,000/L to 20,000/L, in which case spontaneous and fatal hemorrhage can occur. The patient is treated with platelet transfusions until the platelet count returns to a safe range. These patients may need hospitalization because of bleeding or, in some instances, for transfusions of platelets.

Acute renal failure can occur with administration of drugs such as high-dose methotrexate or cisplatin. Patients receiving cisplatin can have severe electrolyte wasting. These conditions necessitate in-hospital evaluation and treatment by a medical oncologist and nephrologist. Allergic reactions, especially to paclitaxel, bleomycin, or cetuximab, can be severe and necessitate treatment with antihistamines, steroids, and other support. Leakage or extravasation of drugs such as vincristine or doxorubicin can cause necrosis of the skin and necessitate immediate treatment.

NEW HORIZONS

Investigational chemotherapy for head and neck cancer has a strong rationale and must be pursued because the results achieved with conventional therapy are not satisfactory. The search for more active systemic therapy for cancer of the head and neck is focused on the development of new active single agents and possible integration of these agents with other drugs and modalities. Drugs with novel mechanisms of action are in various stages of development. Molecular therapies such as monoclonal antibodies and receptor tyrosine kinase inhibitors have begun to demonstrate important activity in head and neck cancer, and these and other targeted therapies will be the focus of future drug development in head and neck cancer. Similarly, integration of chemopreventive agents with the multispecialty treatment of these patients is only just beginning.

Several new approaches are actively being studied for the management of incurable, locoregionally advanced cancer of the head and neck. Photodynamic therapy involves administration of a systemic photosensitizer that becomes preferentially incorporated into tumor cells. An illumination source, which is directed locally or endoscopically near the tumor, induces cell killing. Complete responses have occurred in small tumors, as has shrinkage and palliation of symptoms of larger tumors.

Gene therapy for cancer of the head and neck is being actively studied. In these studies, viral vectors have been used to deliver the p53 tumor suppressor gene to tumor cells by direct intratumoral injection. Both wild-type p53 (AdCMVp53) and genetically altered p53 genes (ONYX-015) have been used; responses have occurred in the tumors treated. Other investigational therapies for locoregionally advanced, incurable tumors include chemotherapy with concomitant repetition of irradiation.

HIGHLIGHTS

■ Standard chemotherapy consists of cisplatin or carboplatin, 5-FU, paclitaxel or docetaxel, and methotrexate. When it is administered to patients with symptomatic recurrent or metastatic cancer of the head and neck, the treatment intent is palliative.

■ Combination chemotherapy for recurrent disease can improve response rates but has little impact on survival rate.

■ Neoadjuvant chemotherapy for locoregionally advanced cancer of the head and neck can produce high overall and complete response rates and decrease the rate of distant metastases, but its effect on survival is minimal.

■ Laryngeal preservation is feasible with induction or concomitant chemotherapy and RT, but administration of neoadjuvant chemotherapy for other cancers of the head and neck is confined to an investigational setting.

■ Concomitant CRT for locoregionally advanced head and neck cancer has a sound rationale. Randomized trials have shown moderately higher disease-free and overall survival rates for many drugs and combinations than obtained with single-modality RT. It is an appropriate treatment option for patients with unresectable disease, for patients with laryngeal or hypopharyngeal carcinoma who would otherwise require laryngectomy or pharyngolaryngectomy, for many patients after surgical treatment, and for some patients with resectable disease in the appropriate treatment setting.

■ Chemotherapy has a role in management of metastatic lymphoepithelioma. Concomitant cisplatin and RT is included in the management of locoregionally advanced nasopharyngeal cancer.

■ Because the outcome with conventional treatment of many patients with advanced head and neck cancer is disappointing, all patients need to be strongly encouraged to participate in clinical trials.

■ New targeted therapies have shown activity in head and neck cancer without typical chemotherapy side effects, and are a major focus of ongoing research.

REFERENCES

1. DeVita VT Jr. Principles of cancer management: chemotherapy. In: DeVita VT Jr, Hellman S, Rosenberg SA, eds. *Cancer: principles and practice of oncology,* 5th ed. Philadelphia: Lippincott-Raven, 1997:333–347.

2. Lynch TJ, Bell DW, Sordella R, et al. Activating mutations in the epidermal growth factor receptor underlying responsiveness of non-small-cell lung cancer to gefitinib. *N Engl J Med* 2004;350:2129–3219.

3. Heinrich MC, Corless CL, Demetri GD, et al. Kinase mutations and imatinib response in patients with metastatic gastrointestinal stromal tumor. *J Clin Oncol* 2003;21:4342–4349.

4. Yao M, Graham MM, Hoffman HT, et al. The role of post-radiation therapy FDG PET in prediction of necessity for post-radiation therapy neck dissection in locally advanced head-and-neck squamous cell carcinoma. *Int J Radiat Oncol Biol Phys* 2004;59:1001–1010.

5. Mick R, Vokes EE, Weichselbaum RR, et al. Prognostic factors in patients with advanced head and neck cancer undergoing multimodality therapy: the University of Chicago experience. *Otolaryngol Head Neck Surg* 1991;105:62–68.

6. Vokes EE, Weichselbaum RR, Lippman S, et al. Head and neck cancer. *N Engl J Med* 1993;328:184–194.

7. Wreesmann VB, Shi W, Thaler HT, et al. Identification of novel prognosticators of outcome in squamous cell carcinoma of the head and neck. *J Clin Oncol* 2004;22:3965–3972.

8. Browman GP, Cronin L. Standard chemotherapy in squamous cell head and neck cancer: what we have learned from randomized trials. *Semin Oncol* 1994;21:311–319.

9. Morton RP, Stell PM. Cytotoxic chemotherapy for patients with terminal squamous carcinoma: does it influence survival? *Clin Otolaryngol* 1984;9:175–183.

10. Brockstein B. Integration of taxanes into primary chemotherapy for squamous cell carcinoma of the head and neck: promise fulfilled? *Curr Opin Oncol* 2000;12:221–228.

11. Forastiere AA, Shank D, Neuberg D, et al. Final report of a phase II evaluation of paclitaxel in patients with advanced squamous cell carcinoma of the head and neck: an Eastern Cooperative Oncology Group Trial (PA390). *Cancer* 1998;82:2270–2274.

12. Forastiere AA, Leong T, Rowinsky E, et al. Phase III comparison paclitaxel + cisplatin + granulocyte colony-stimulating factor versus low-dose paclitaxel + cisplatin in advanced head and neck cancer (HNSCC): an Eastern Cooperative Oncology Group study. *J Clin Oncol* 2001;19:1088–1095.

13. Jacobs C, Lyman G, Velez-Garcia E, et al. A phase III randomized study comparing cisplatin and fluorouracil as single agents and in combination for advanced squamous cell carcinoma of the head and neck. *J Clin Oncol* 1992;10:257–263.

14. Forastiere AA, Metch B, Schuller DE, et al. Randomized comparison of cisplatin plus fluorouracil and carboplatin plus fluorouracil versus methotrexate in advanced squamous cell carcinoma of the head and neck: a Southwest Oncology Group Study. *J Clin Oncol* 1992;10: 1245–1251.

15. Trigo, J, Hitt, R, Koralewski, P, et al. Cetuximab monotherapy is active in patients with platinum-refractory recurrent/metastatic squamous cell carcinoma of the head and neck: results of a phase II study (abst). *Proc Am Soc Clin Oncol* 2004;23:487a.

16. Baselga, J, Trigo, JM, Bourhis, J, et al. Cetuximab (C-225) plus cisplatin/carboplatin is active in patients with recurrent/metastatic squamous cell carcinoma of the head and neck progressing on the same dose/schedule platinum-based regimen (abst). *Proc Am Soc Clin Oncol* 2002;21:226a.

17. Hong WK, Arquette M, Nabell L, et al. Efficacy and safety of the anti-epidermal growth factor antibody (EGFR) IMC-C225, in combination with cisplatin in patients with recurrent squamous cell carcinoma of the head and neck refractory to cisplatin-containing chemotherapy (abst). *Proc Am Soc Clin Oncol* 2001;20:224a.

18. Burtness B, Li Y, Flood W, et al. Phase III trial comparing cisplatin (C) + placebo (P) to C + anti-epidermal growth factor antibody (EGF-R) C225 in patients (pts) with metastatic/recurrent head neck cancer (HNC). *Proc Am Soc Clin Oncol* 2002;21:226a.

19. Bonner JA, Giralt J, Harari PM, et al. Phase III study of high dose radiation with or without cetuximab in the treatment of locoregionally advanced squamous cell cancer of the head and neck (abst). *Proc Am Soc Clin Oncol* 2004;23:489s.

20. Cohen EE, Rosen F, Stadler WM, et al. Phase II trial of ZD1839 in recurrent or metastatic squamous cell carcinoma of the head and neck. *J Clin Oncol* 2003;21:1980.

21. Soulieres D, Senzer NN, Vokes EE, et al. Multicenter phase II study of erlotinib, an oral epidermal growth factor receptor tyrosine kinase inhibitor, in patients with recurrent or metastatic squamous cell cancer of the head and neck. *J Clin Oncol* 2004;22:77.

22. Scanlon KY, Newman EM, Priest DG. Biochemical basis for cisplatin and 5-fluorouracil synergism in human ovarian carcinoma cells. *Proc Natl Acad Sci U S A* 1986;83:8923–8925.

23. Department of Veterans Affairs Laryngeal Cancer Study Group. Induction chemotherapy plus radiation compared with surgery plus radiation in patients with advanced laryngeal cancer. *N Engl J Med* 1991; 324:1685–1690.

24. Paccagnella A, Orlando A, Marchiori C, et al. Phase III trial of initial chemotherapy in stage III or IV head and neck cancers: a study by the Gruppodidi Studio SUI Tumori Della Testa E Del Collo. *J Natl Cancer Inst* 1994;86:265–272.

25. Murphy B, Li Y, Cella D, et al. Phase III study comparing cisplatin 5-fluorouracil versus cisplatin paclitaxel in metastatic/recurrent head neck cancer (abst). *Proc Am Soc Clin Oncol* 2001;20:224a.

26. Pignon JP, Bourhis J, Domenge C, et al. Chemotherapy added to locoregional treatment for head and neck squamous cell carcinoma: three meta-analyses of updated individual patient data. *Lancet* 2000;355:949–955.

27. Bernier J, Domenge C, Ozsahin M, et al. Postoperative irradiation with or without concomitant chemotherapy for locally advanced head and neck cancer. *N Engl J Med* 2004;350:1945.

28. Cooper JS, Pajak TF, Forastiere AA, et al. Postoperative concurrent radiotherapy and chemotherapy for high-risk squamous-cell carcinoma of the head and neck. *N Engl J Med* 2004;350:1937.

29. Brizel DM, Albers ME, Fisher R, et al. Hyperfractionated irradiation with or without concurrent chemotherapy for locally advanced head and neck cancer. *N Engl J Med* 1998;338:1798–1804.

30. Wendt TG, Grabenbauer GG, Rodel CM. Simultaneous radiotherapy versus radiotherapy alone in advanced head and neck cancer: a randomized multicenter study. *J Clin Oncol* 16:1318–1324.

31. Bachaud JM, Cohen-Jonathan E, Alzieu C, et al. Combined postoperative radiotherapy and weekly cisplatin infusion for locally advanced head and neck cancer: final report of a randomized trial. *Int J Radiat Oncol Biol Phys* 1996;36:999–1004.

32. Adelstein DJ, Lavertu P, Saxton JP, et al. Mature results of a phase III randomized trial comparing concurrent chemoradiotherapy with radiation therapy alone in patients with stage III and IV squamous cell carcinoma of the head and neck. *Cancer* 2000; 88:876–883.

33. Jeremic B, Shibamoto Y, Milicic B, et al. Hyperfractionated radiation therapy with or without concurrent low dose cisplatin in locally advanced squamous cell carcinoma of the head and neck: a prospective randomized trial. *J Clin Oncol* 2000;18:1458–1464.

34. Forastiere AA, Goepfert H, Maor M, et al. Concurrent chemotherapy and radiotherapy for organ preservation in advanced laryngeal cancer. *N Engl J Med* 2003; 349:2091–2098.

35. Vokes EE, Stenson K, Rosen FR, et al. Weekly carboplatin and paclitaxel followed by concomitant paclitaxel, fluorouracil, and hydroxyurea chemoradiotherapy: curative and organ-preserving therapy for advanced head and neck cancer. *J Clin Oncol* 2003;21:320.

36. Haraf DJ, Rosen FR, Stenson K, et al. Induction chemotherapy followed by concomitant TFHX chemoradiotherapy with reduced dose radiation in advanced head and neck cancer. *Clin Cancer Res* 2003;9:5936

37. Brockstein B, Haraf DJ, Rademaker AW, et al. Patterns of failure, prognostic factors and survival in locoregionally advanced head and neck cancer treated with concomitant chemoradiotherapy: a 9-year, 337-patient, multi-institutional experience *Ann Oncol* 2004;15:1179–1186.

38. Vokes EE, Kies M, Haraf DJ, et al. Concomitant chemoradiotherapy as primary therapy for locoregionally advanced head and neck carcinoma. *J Clin Oncol* 2000;18:1652–1661.

39. Brockstein BE, Vokes EE. Chemoradiotherapy for head and neck cancer. *PPO Updates* 1996;10:1–19.

40. Final Report of the Head and Neck Contracts Program. Adjuvant chemotherapy for advanced head and neck squamous carcinoma. *Cancer* 1987;60:301–311.

41. Laramore GB, Scott CB, Al-Sarraf M, et al. Adjuvant chemotherapy for resectable squamous cell carcinomas of the head and neck: report on intergroup study 0034. *Int J Radiat Oncol Biol Phys* 1992;23:705–713.

42. Lefebvre JL, Chevalier P, Luboinski B, et al. Larynx preservation in pyriform sinus cancer: preliminary results of a European organization for research and treatment of cancer max III trial. *J Natl Cancer Inst* 1996;88:890.

43. Depondt J, Gehanno P, Martin M, et al. Neoadjuvant chemotherapy with carboplatin/5-fluorouracil in head and neck cancer. *Oncology* 1993;50[Suppl 2]:23.

44. Domenge C, Hill C, Lefebvre JL. Randomized trial of neoadjuvant chemotherapy in oropharyngeal carcinoma. French Groupe d'Etude des Tumeurs de la TÃªte et du Cou (GETTEC). *Br J Cancer* 2000;83:1594–1598.

45. Clark JR, Busse PM, Norris CM, et al. Induction chemotherapy with cisplatin, fluorouracil, and high dose leucovorin for squamous cell carcinoma of the head and neck: long-term results. *J Clin Oncol* 1997;15:3100–3110.

46. Vermorken JB, Remenar E, van Herpen, C, et al. Standard cisplatin/infusional 5FU (PF) vs docetaxel plus PF (TPF) as neoadjuvant chemotherapy for nonresectable locally advanced squamous cell carcinoma of the head and neck (LA-SCCHN): a phase III trial of the EORTC head and neck cancer group (EORTC #24971). *Proc Am Soc Clin Oncol* 2004;22:490S.

47. Fandi A, Bachouchi M, Azli N, et al. Long-term disease free survivors in metastatic undifferentiated carcinoma of the nasopharynx type. *J Clin Oncol* 2000;18:1324–1330.

48. Al-Sarraf M, LeBlanc M, Giri PG, et al. Chemoradiotherapy versus radiotherapy in patients with advanced nasopharyngeal cancer: phase III randomized Intergroup study 0099. *J Clin Oncol* 1998;16:1313–1317.

49. Langendijk JA, Leemans CR, Buter J, et al. The additional value of chemotherapy to radiotherapy in locally advanced nasopharyngeal carcinoma: a meta-analysis of the published literature. *J Clin Oncol* 2004;15(22):4604–4612.

50. Browman GP, Cripps C, Hodson I, et al. Placebo controlled randomized trial of infusional fluorouracil during standard radiotherapy in locally advanced head and neck cancer. *J Clin Oncol* 1994;12:648–653.

51. Lo TC, Wiley AL Jr, Ansfield FJ, et al. Combined radiation therapy and 5-fluorouracil for advanced squamous cell carcinoma of the oral cavity and oropharynx: a randomized study. *Am J Roentgenol* 1976;126:229–235.

52. Taylor S, Murphy AK, Vannetzelj M. Randomized comparison of neoadjuvant cisplatin and fluorouracil infusion followed by radiation versus concomitant treatment in advanced head and neck cancer. *J Clin Oncol* 1994;12:385–395.

53. Merlano M, Benasso M, Corvo R, et al. Five-year update of a randomized trial of alternating radiotherapy and chemotherapy compared with radiotherapy alone in treatment of unresectable squamous cell carcinoma of the head and neck. *J Natl Cancer Inst* 1996;88:583–589.

54. Calais G, Alfonsi M, Bardet E, et al. Randomized trial of radiation versus concomitant chemotherapy and radiation for advanced-stage oropharynx carcinoma. *J Natl Cancer Inst* 1999;15:2081–2086.

55. Adelstein DJ, Li Y, Adams GL. An intergroup phase III comparison of standard radiation therapy and two schedules of concurrent chemoradiotherapy in patients with unresectable squamous cell head and neck cancer. *J Clin Oncol* 2003;21:92–98.

Principles of Radiation Oncology

104

David H. Hussey

Radiation oncology plays a major role in the treatment of cancers of the head and neck. It is often used as the only treatment modality or as an adjuvant treatment in combination with surgery. In recent years, it has been frequently used in combination with chemotherapy to preserve organ function. Radiation oncology requires an understanding of radiation physics and biology, as well as knowledge of the natural history of cancer and its pattern of spread. The fundamental concepts of these fields as they relate to the use of radiation therapy for head and neck cancer are described in this chapter.

RADIATION PHYSICS

Radiation therapy is the treatment of cancer with ionizing radiation. The types of radiation used most commonly for radiation therapy are x-rays, gamma rays, and electrons, although protons and neutrons also are being used in some specialized facilities. In this chapter, the discussion is limited to the beams most commonly used.

Ionizing radiation deposits its energy in biologic material through the production of secondary charged particles. With primary x-rays, gamma rays, and electrons, the secondary particles are electrons, and these secondary particles are ultimately responsible for inflicting the biologic injury (1). The biologic effects of ionizing radiation are the result of its ability to release sufficient energy in a very localized area to break a chemical bond.

Radiation therapy may be delivered with an external beam of radiation (teleradiotherapy), or with a radioactive implant or mold (brachyradiotherapy). With external beam radiotherapy, the tumor is irradiated some distance away from the patient, whereas with brachytherapy, the tumor is irradiated with radioactive sources placed in or near the tumor.

External Beam Irradiation

Most radiation oncology departments today have dual-energy linear accelerators capable of generating low-energy megavoltage x-rays (4 to 6 MV), high-energy megavoltage x-rays (15 to 25 MV), and a range of electron beams (6 to 18 or 25 Mev). Megavoltage x-ray and gamma-ray beams are very penetrating beams that are useful for treating a wide variety of cancers. The characteristics of an x-ray or gamma-ray beam that are important from radiation therapy standpoint are their (a) skin-sparing properties, (b) depth dose (i.e., penetration), and (c) isodose distributions (i.e., beam uniformity). The skin-sparing and depth-dose properties of the photon beams commonly used are shown in Figure 104.1 (2).

The selection of beam energy is usually based on the location of the tumor. Cancers located 12 to 15 cm deep, such as cancer of the prostate or uterine cervix, usually are best managed with 15- to 25-MV x-rays because these beams are more penetrating than are lower-energy beams. Cancers of the head and neck, however, are better managed with 4- to 6-MV x-rays or cobalt 60 gamma rays, at least initially, because these tumors are located no more than 7 to 8 cm deep, and usually regional lymph nodes must be treated, which are located just under the skin. However, 15- to 25-MV x-rays are occasionally used to deliver additional treatment to boost the dose to some head and neck cancers, such as those located in the base of the tongue or nasopharynx.

Electron beams are used for treating cancers that are located superficially. Unlike x-rays, electrons have a finite

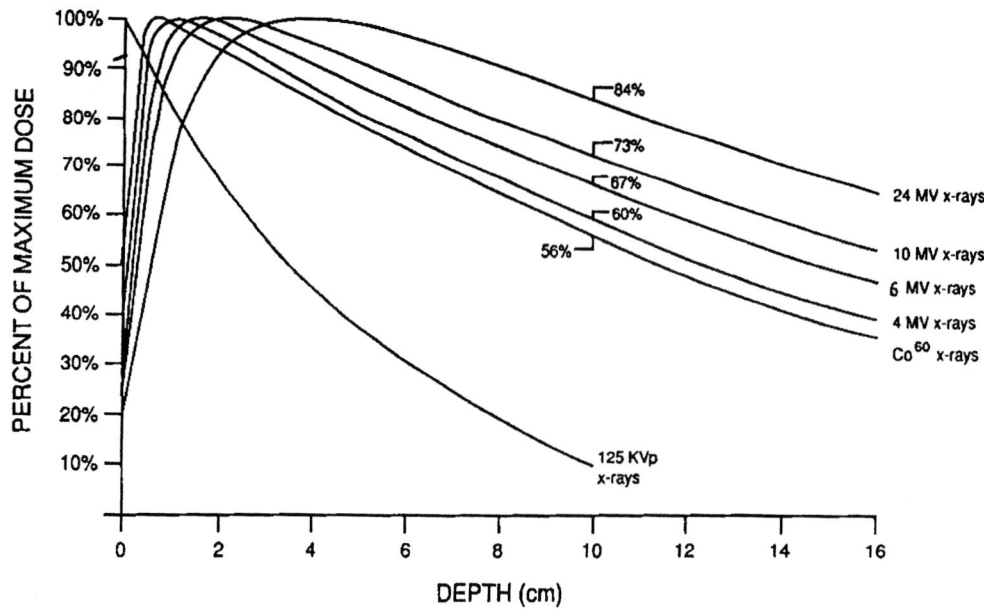

Figure 104.1 Skin-sparing and depth-dose properties of x-ray and gamma-ray beams commonly available in radiation therapy departments.

range and thus are a means of sparing tissues deep to the tumor (Fig. 104.2). The useful range of an electron beam is determined by its energy, and a variety of beam energies are available. Six-MeV electrons are used for cancers of the skin or lip, 6- to 9-MeV electrons for cervical lymph nodes overlying the spinal cord, 9- to 12-MeV electrons for cancers of the buccal mucosa, and 15- to 18-MeV electrons for cancers of the tonsillar fossa or parotid.

Brachyradiotherapy

With brachyradiotherapy, radioactive sources are placed close to the target volume. These sources may be placed directly into the tumor (interstitial therapy), within body cavities (intracavitary therapy), or onto epithelial surfaces (surface molds). Brachytherapy implants may be either temporary or permanent. Temporary implants are usually

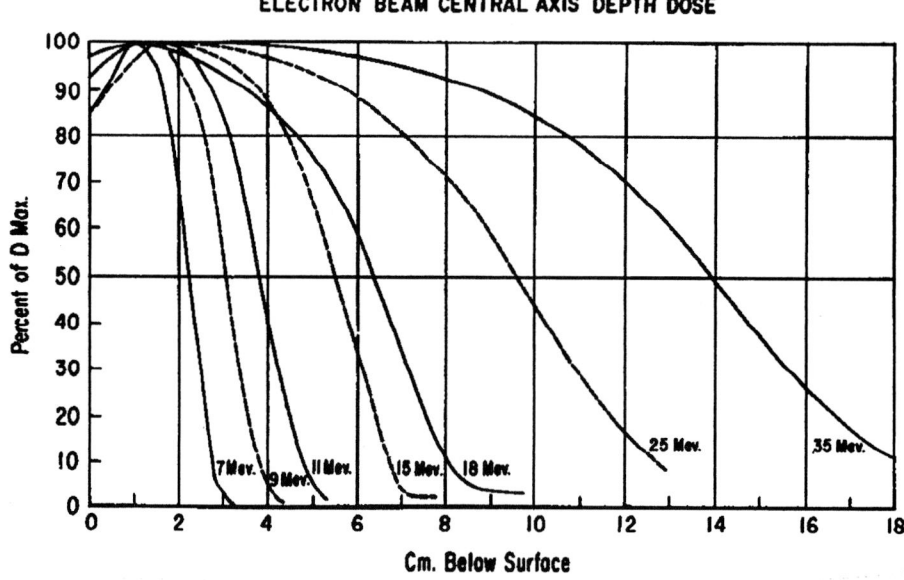

Figure 104.2 Skin-sparing and depth-dose properties of a variety of electron beams. Electron beams have a limited range, so they are useful for sparing tissues deep to the target volume. A rule of thumb is that the useful range of an electron beam in centimeters is equal to the megaelectron volts of the beam divided by three. Electron beams provide less skin sparing than megavoltage x-ray and gamma-ray beams.

TABLE 104.1

PHYSICAL CHARACTERISTICS OF COMMONLY USED BRACHYRADIOTHERAPY SOURCES

Radionuclide	Half-life	X or Gamma ray Energy (keV)	Physical Configuration	Advantages	Disadvantages
Cesium 137	30 y	662	Tubes, needles	Relatively inexpensive	Relatively large sources; limited sizes and strengths
Gold 198	2.7 d	412	Seeds	Small size; higher dose rate; relatively inexpensive	Not usually afterloaded
Iodine 125	60 d	27–35	Seeds	Small size; less exposure to personnel	Low dose rate
Palladium 103	17 d	20–23	Seeds	Small size; higher dose rate; less exposure to personnel	Expensive
Iridium 192	74 d	136–1,060	Wire, seeds, catheters (afterloading)	Wide variety of source strengths and sizes; usually afterloaded	—
Radium 226	1,620 y	47–2,440	Tubes, needles	Relatively large sources; no appreciable decay with time	Limited sizes and strengths; potential for leakage and contamination

performed with long-lived isotopes (e.g., radium 226, cesium 137, or iridium 192). Permanent implants conversely must be performed with short-lived isotopes (e.g., gold 198, iodine 125, or palladium 103) because the activity of the sources must decay to negligible levels in a short time.

The advantages of brachytherapy over external beam irradiation are twofold. First, the irradiation is confined mainly to the implant volume so that a greater dose is delivered to the tumor and a lesser dose is delivered to adjacent normal tissues. This should result in better local tumor control and fewer complications. A second advantage of brachytherapy is that the treatment is delivered continuously at a low dose rate. For several radiobiologic reasons, this should be more effective than intermediate or high dose-rate irradiation in the treatment of hypoxic or slowly proliferating cancers (1,3).

However, implants are effective only if the entire tumor volume can be implanted. The tumor must be accessible and relatively well demarcated. Large or poorly defined tumors are usually not treated with brachytherapy because peripheral extensions of the cancer are difficult to implant effectively.

The isotopes most commonly used for brachytherapy are listed in Table 104.1. If the implant is used as the sole treatment modality, the sources are usually left in place for 5 to 7 days to deliver a total dose of 70 to 80 Gy to the target volume (3). If it is combined with external beam radiation, a dose of 40 to 50 Gy is delivered with external beam irradiation followed by a 2- to 4-day implant to deliver an additional 30 to 40 Gy (total dose, 70–80 Gy).

Conformal Radiation Therapy

Recent improvements in computer technology have led to the development of better techniques for delivering a high dose of radiation to the target volume and a smaller dose

to normal tissues (4). Such techniques are called conformal because the high-dose region is designed to conform to the target volume. At the same time, advancements in diagnostic imaging have made it possible to define better the extent of the cancer. These two advances are complementary, leading to a powerful new tool for the management of many head and neck cancers.

Intensity modulated radiation therapy (IMRT) is one method of delivering conformal radiation therapy. With IMRT, the treatment fields are divided into hundreds of pencil beams, each one contributing radiation to different parts of the target volume. The computer controls the amount of radiation delivered through each of these pencil beams as the treatment machine rotates around the patient.

The radiation oncologist outlines various tumor volumes (e.g., primary tumor, nodal disease, subclinical volumes) on treatment-planning computed tomography (CT) scans, along with critical organs and normal structures (Fig. 104.3). Each is assigned a target dose and an acceptable range of doses. The computer considers these dosage limits as it develops a series of treatment-delivery plans to be evaluated by the radiation oncologist. Once a satisfactory plan has been generated, the patient's computer files are loaded onto the delivery system that is used to administer the treatments.

RADIATION BIOLOGY

Cell Death

The treatment must eradicate every viable cancer cell if the tumor is to be controlled with radiation therapy. Cells are considered to be "viable" from a radiobiologic standpoint if they are capable of unlimited division (1). They are considered to be "dead" if they are unable to proliferate

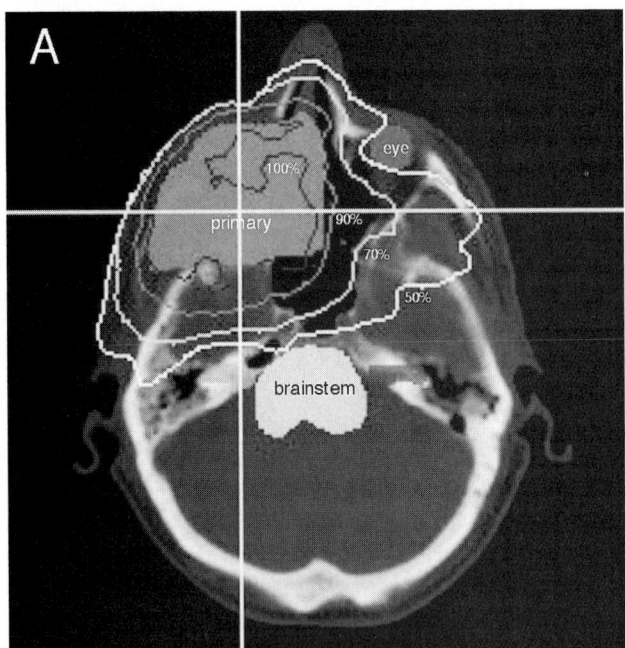

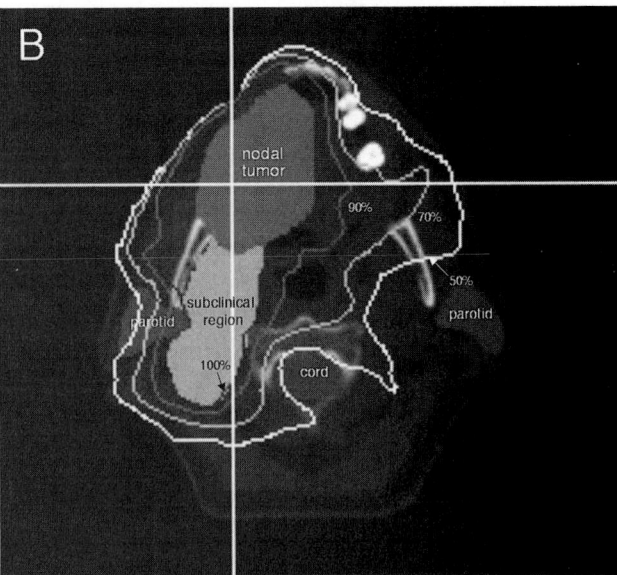

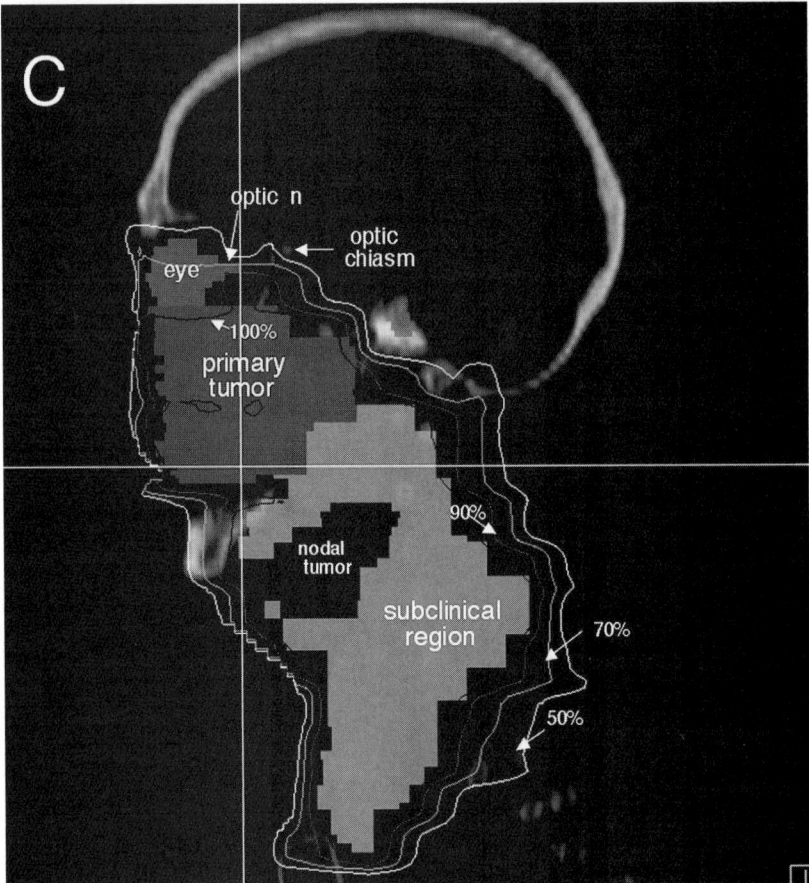

Figure 104.3   Intensity-modulated radiation therapy (IMRT) treatment: 63-year-old man with a T2 squamous carcinoma of the right maxillary antrum was treated initially with a right maxillectomy. The margins were close (0.4 cm). Postoperatively right submandibular lymphadenopathy developed. The patient was treated with IMRT to limit the dose to the visual pathway, salivary glands, and spinal cord. Initially, a dose of 50 Gy was delivered with IMRT to the right maxillary region and upper neck, and 44 Gy was delivered to the right lower neck (see dose distributions). After this, the residual tumor was boosted with an additional 20 Gy, bringing the total tumor dose to 70 Gy in 7 weeks. **A:** Axial dose distribution at the level of the maxilla. **B:** Axial dose distribution at the level of the positive submandibular node. **C:** Sagittal dose distribution.

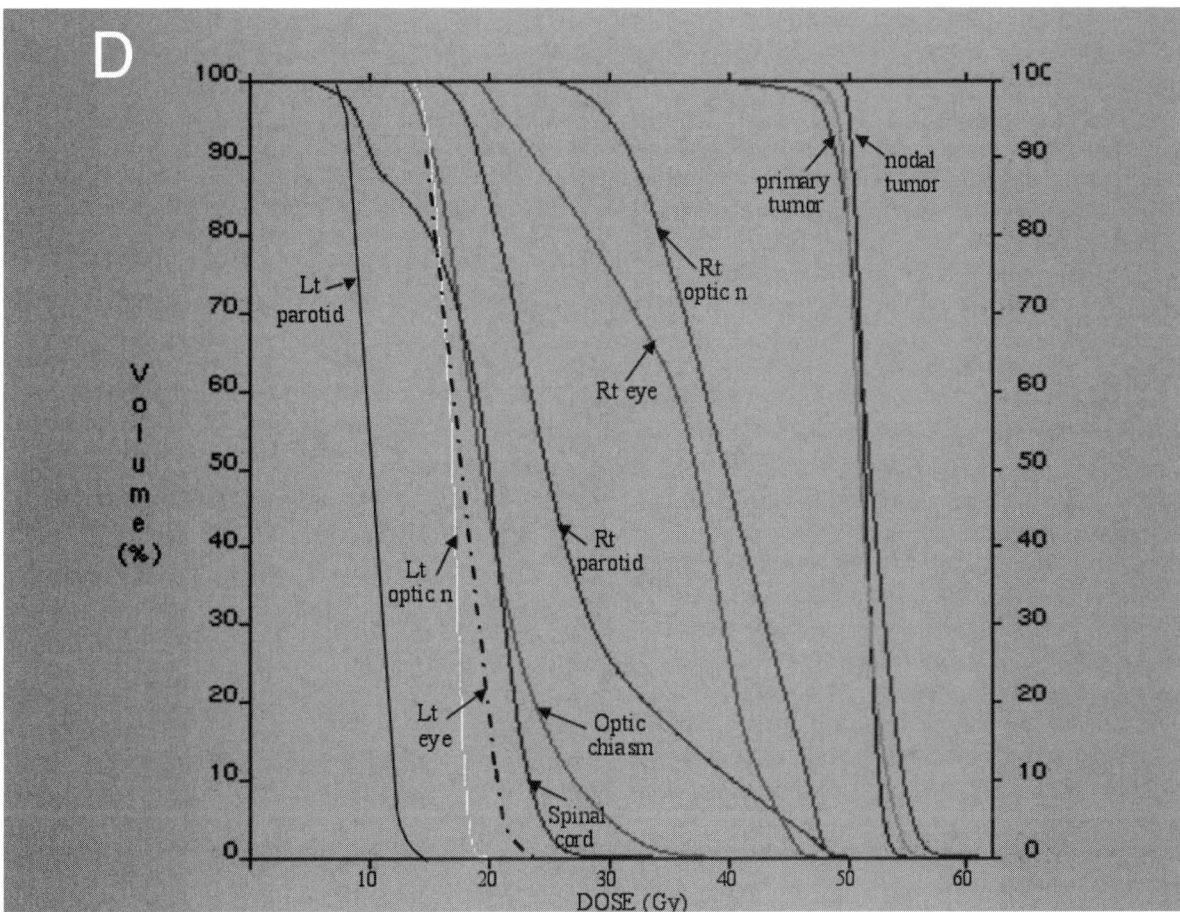

Figure 104.3 *(Continued)* **D:** Dose volume histogram.

indefinitely. It is not necessary that the cells be lysed or morphologically altered to be considered killed.

Several methods of cell death occur after radiation therapy. The most common form of cell death after irradiation is "mitotic death." With mitotic death, cells die while attempting to divide. Cells may undergo four or five divisions before undergoing pyknosis and disintegration. Cell death from radiation is thought to be due to damage to DNA, although other targets also may be important.

A second form of cell death after irradiation is "apoptosis" or programmed cell death (5). Apoptosis also occurs in unirradiated tissues—for example, in the process of organogenesis. It is the mechanism by which tadpoles lose their tails. Apoptosis is identified by a well-defined sequence of morphologic events. Radiation-induced apoptosis occurs in the bone marrow and the salivary glands. It also occurs in tumors, particularly those of lymphoid and hematopoietic origin.

Random Nature of Cell Kill

The deposition of energy from a radiation beam is a random event, and so is the infliction of radiochemical injury. This means that every cell in the tumor has the same chance of being killed by a given dose of radiation. Because of this, other factors being equal, a given dose of radiation kills the same proportion of cells in a tumor, not the same number of cells. It takes the same amount of radiation to reduce the cell population from 100 cells to 10 cells as it does to reduce it from 10 billion to 1 billion cells.

This principle has several important implications for radiation therapy. First, it shows that the amount of radiation needed to eradicate a tumor depends on the total number of viable cells. A greater dose is required to control a 3-cm tumor (which contains $\sim 10^{10}$ cells) than a 1-cm tumor (which contains $\sim 10^{9}$ cells). It also shows the fallacy of using response rates to monitor the effectiveness of treatment. A tumor is no longer palpable when the tumor has been reduced from 10^{10} to 10^{5} cells, yet only half the dose necessary to eradicate that tumor has been delivered.

Repair of Sublethal Injury

When a secondary electron passes through matter, clusters of dense ionization are distributed along an otherwise sparsely ionizing tract. If a sensitive target in a cell is hit by a cluster of dense ionization, it can inflict irreparable damage. However, if the target is hit by an area of sparse ionization, injury may

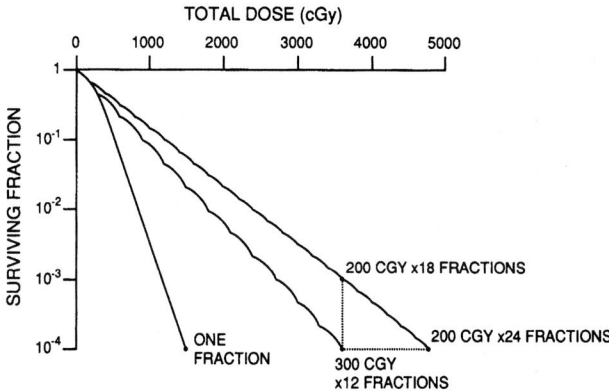

Figure 104.4 Effect of fractionation. Hypothetical model shows that 3,600 cGy in 12 fractions is equivalent to 4,800 cGy in 24 fractions.

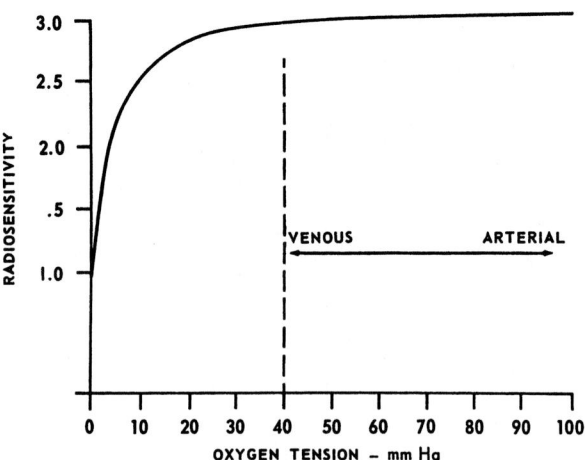

Figure 104.5 Relation between oxygen concentration and radiation sensitivity. Hypoxia is considered a major cause of treatment failure.

be inflicted that is not sufficient to kill the cell. In this situation, additional hits will be required to cause cell death. The cell can repair the sublethal injury if no further hits are incurred. Because of this, a greater dose is required to produce a biologic effect when it is given in several fractions than it is when it is given in only a single fraction. In most tissues, sublethal injury is repaired within 3 hours. However, it can take as long as 24 hours in some tissues (1).

For several reasons, the cells' ability to repair sublethal injury between dose fractions is important. One is that the biologic effect of radiation depends on the fractionation schedule used. The greater the number of fractions, the greater is the opportunity for repair between dose fractions, and the greater is the dose required to produce the same level of biologic effect. For example, a dose of 36 Gy in 12 fractions (3-Gy fractions) over a 2.5-week period produces much more damage than 36 Gy in 18 fractions (2-Gy fractions) over a 3.5-week period (Fig. 104.4). Fractionated irradiation also allows more repair of normal tissue injury, and this should provide a therapeutic advantage because tumor cells are less capable of repair. In general, the sparing effect of fractionation is greater for tissues responsible for late injury than for those responsible for acute reactions or tumor response. This is one reason for fractionating the radiation therapy.

Another reason that sublethal injury is important is that certain tumors have more capacity to repair sublethal injury than do others. For example, some melanomas have a remarkable capacity for repairing sublethal injury. This may be responsible for the belief that melanoma is a radioresistant tumor. Recognition of this biologic characteristic has led some radiation oncologists to treat melanomas with a small number of large fractions (hypofractionation). The fewer the fractions, the smaller is the opportunity for repair between fractions.

Tumor Cell Hypoxia

It has long been known that oxygen significantly increases the effect of ionizing radiation on biologic tissues. The

mechanism by which oxygen radiosensitizes is not completely understood, but it is thought that oxygen combines with an electron in the outer shell of free radicals as they are being formed to make them more stable. Free radicals are otherwise quite labile. They are responsible for the indirect effect of radiation on DNA. In most biologic systems, the dose of radiation necessary to kill hypoxic cells is 2.5 to 3 times more than that required to kill well-oxygenated cells (Fig. 104.5).

Whereas normal tissues are almost always well oxygenated, cancers usually contain hypoxic regions (6). Acute tumor cell hypoxia can occur because capillaries collapse periodically or are compressed, and chronic hypoxia can occur because tumors tend to outgrow their blood supply (7) (Fig. 104.6). Hypoxic tumor cells usually reoxygenate during a course of irradiation. Acute hypoxia improves because collapsed blood vessels periodically open during the course of treatment. Chronic hypoxia improves because the hypoxic cells are brought closer to capillaries as well-oxygenated cells near the capillaries are eradicated, and the requirements for oxygen are diminished as tumor cells are depleted. Reoxygenation is one of the most important reasons for delivering radiation therapy in a fractionated course over a period of time.

Cell-Cycle Effects

Another factor that influences the radiosensitivity of a cell is its position in the cell cycle (1). Cells undergoing DNA synthesis (in the S phase) are more radioresistant than are cells in other phases of the cell cycle (Fig. 104.7). For this reason, a single large dose of radiation is less effective in controlling a tumor than is a fractionated course of radiation. By fractionating the treatment, cells surviving each fraction redistribute themselves into more-sensitive phases of the cell cycle, making them more susceptible to eradication by subsequent fractions. The greater the number of

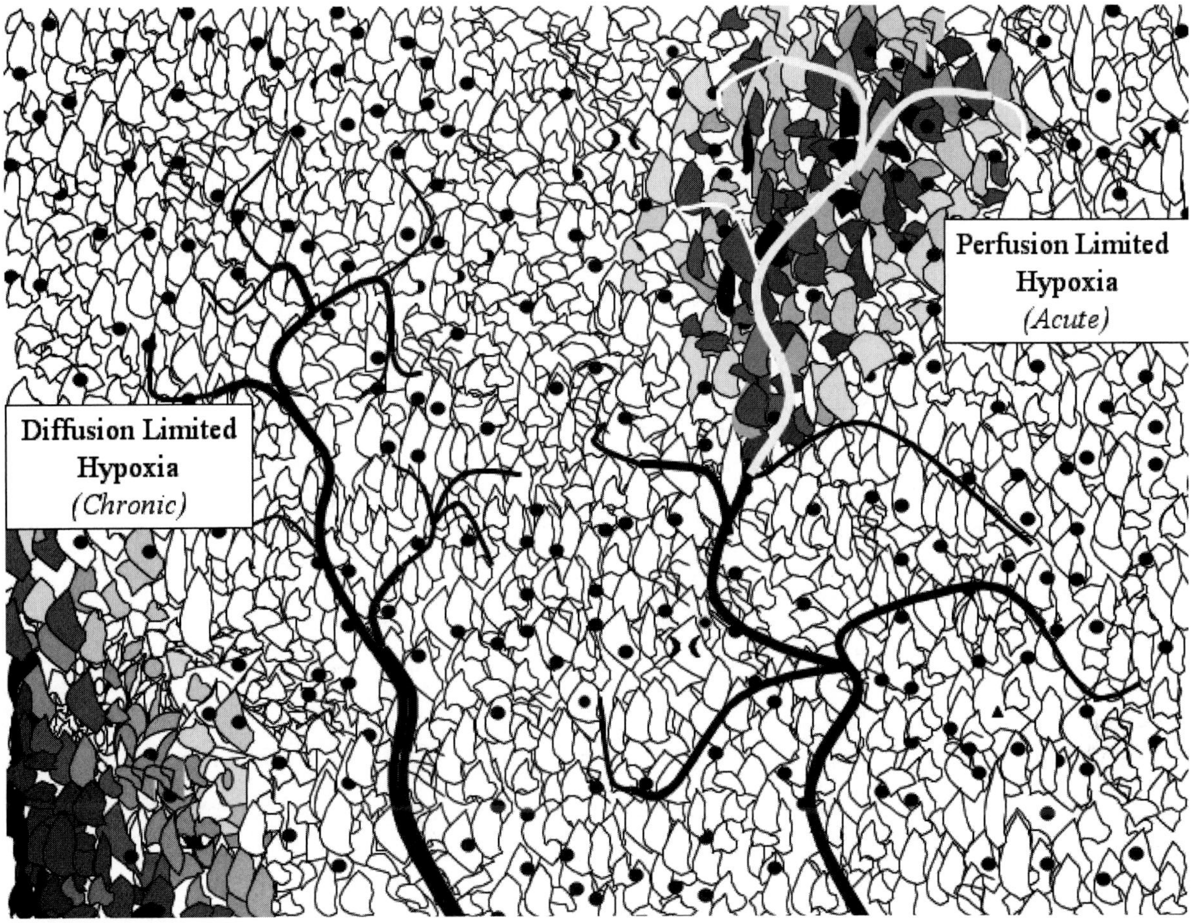

Figure 104.6 Hypoxic cells in lung cancer. Perfusion limited hypoxia (acute). Diffusion limited hypoxia (chronic).

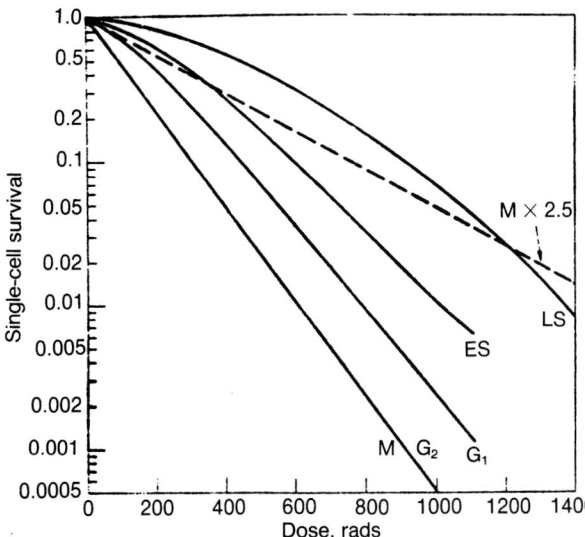

Figure 104.7 Relation between radiosensitivity and the cell cycle. Cells in the late S phase (*LS*) are synthesizing DNA and are most resistant. *M*, mitotic phase; *G1*, presynthetic phase; *G2*, postsynthetic phase. (Modified from Sinclair WK. *Time-dose relationships in radiation biology as applied to radiation therapy.* Report 50203 [C-57]. Berkeley, Calif: Brookhaven National Laboratory, 1969:97, with permission.)

fractions, the greater is the probability of hitting cells in a sensitive phase some time during the course of irradiation. This sensitizing effect of redistribution tends to offset the protective effect of fractionation resulting from the repair of sublethal damage.

Redistribution is greater for cells that are rapidly cycling than for those that are slowly cycling because rapidly cycling cells redistribute better between dose fractions. In general, the cells responsible for acute reactions (e.g., skin, mucosa) are rapidly cycling, and the cells responsible for late effects (e.g., connective tissue, blood vessels) are slowly cycling. The net effect is that tissues responsible for late complications are spared more by fractionation than are tissues responsible for acute reactions.

Repopulation

Tumors are proliferating tissues, and because of this, it is not advisable to protract unnecessarily a course of radiation therapy. Furthermore, if the tumor cell population is reduced, as by surgery or irradiation, the malignant cells respond by accelerated repopulation. Repopulation is a greater problem with rapidly proliferating tumors than it is with slow-growing neoplasms. In recent years, accelerated treatment schedules using twice-daily fractionation have been used to diminish the opportunity for repopulation of rapidly proliferating cancers. Repopulation after incomplete resection is one of the main reasons for not delaying a course of postoperative radiation therapy. It is also a reason for not using split-course radiation therapy.

Radiosensitivity

In the 1960s, radiosensitivity was thought to be related to tumor histology. Squamous carcinomas were thought to be radiosensitive, whereas adenocarcinomas were considered to be radioresistant (8). It also was thought to be related to the location of the cancer. Primary cancers in the oral tongue were considered to be radiosensitive, whereas lymph node metastases from oral tongue cancers were thought to be radioresistant. We now believe that these differences were attributable to other causes (e.g., differences in regression rates, or difficulty delivering adequate doses to these tumors with the equipment then available) rather

than inherent differences in radiosensitivity. In general, squamous carcinomas, adenocarcinomas, mucoepidermoid carcinomas, carcinomas ex pleomorphic adenoma, and soft tissue sarcomas are all thought to be approximately equal in radiosensitivity.

The biologic factors that determine the probability of local tumor control are related mainly to the number of malignant cells and the proportion of cells that are hypoxic. Both of these factors are related to the size of a cancer. Large tumors have more cancer cells, and a greater proportion of these cells are hypoxic.

The clinical appearance of the cancer can often be a clue as to the radiosensitivity of a head-and-neck cancer. In general, superficial exophytic tumors such as many cancers of the faucial arch are well vascularized and respond well to irradiation. Infiltrative and ulcerative cancers are more resistant because they are more extensive than is apparent clinically and have significant hypoxic compartments.

The probability of controlling a cancer with irradiation depends on the size of a neoplasm and the dose of radiation (9) (Table 104.2). A dose of 50 Gy in 5 weeks controls

TABLE 104.2
LOCAL CONTROL AS A FUNCTION OF RADIATION DOSE AND SIZE OF THE TUMOR

Radiation Dose (Gy)	Primary Site and Clinical Stage			Regional Lymph Nodes		
	T1	T2–3	T3–4	Subclinical	1–3 cm	3–5 cm
30–40				~60–70%[a]		
50	60% T1 nasopharynx[b]			~90%[a]	~50%[c]	
55		30% T2–3 supraglottic larynx[d]				
60–65	90% T1 tonsillar fossa[e,f,g]	80% T2 tonsillar fossa[e,f,g]	50% T3–4 tonsillar fossa[e,f]			
	90% T1 RMT, ATP[g]	75% T2–3 supraglottic larynx[d]				
	100% T1 supraglottic larynx[d]	55% glossopharyngeal sulcus[h]				
	88% T1 base of tongue[j]					
70	100% T1 tonsillar fossa[g]	90% T2–3 supraglottic larynx[d]	65% T3–4 tonsillar fossa[g]		90%[j]	70%[j]
	100% T1 glossopharyngeal sulcus[h]	90% T2–3 RMT, ATP[k]				
		80% glossopharyngeal sulcus[h]				
75		80% T2–3 base of tongue[i]	90% T3–4 tonsillar fossa[g]			
		100% T2–3 glossopharyngeal sulcus[h]				

RMT, Retromolar trigone; ATP, anterior tonsillar pillar.
[a]Fletcher. *Cancer* 1972;29:545.
[b]Moench and Phillips. *Am J Surg* 1972;124:515.
[c]Northrup, et al. *Cancer* 1973;29:23.
[d]Shukovsky. *Am J Roentgenol* 1970;108:27.
[e]Fayos and Lampe. *Am J Roentgenol* 1971;111:85.
[f]Perez, et al. *Am J Roentgenol* 1972;114:43.
[g]Shukovsky and Fletcher. *Radiology* 1973;107:621.
[h]Shukovsky, et al. *Radiology* 1976;120:405.
[i]Spanos, et al. *Cancer* 1976;37:2,591.
[j]Schneider, et al. *Am J Roentgenol* 1975;123:42.
[k]Barker and Fletcher. *Int J Radiat Oncol Biol Phys* 1977;2:407.

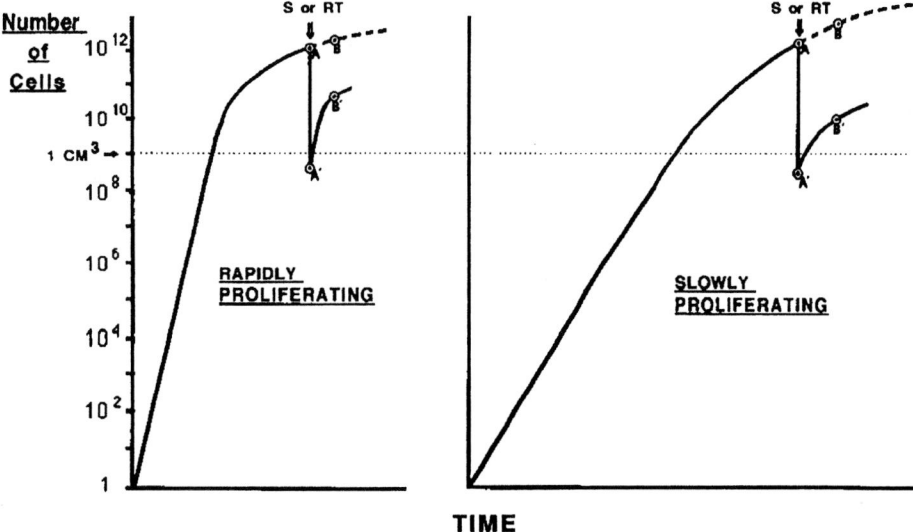

Figure 104.8 Tumor growth curves for a rapidly proliferating tumor and a slowly proliferating tumor. The initial growth of a tumor is exponential. However, growth begins to plateau as the tumor enlarges, presumably because of inadequate blood supply and a lack of nutrients. When the tumor cell population is reduced, as by surgery or irradiation, the malignant cells respond with accelerated repopulation. The difference between the growth rate of unperturbed tumor (*AB*) and the more rapid growth rate after surgery or irradiation (*A8B8*) is evident. Accelerated regrowth is a greater problem with rapidly proliferating tumors than with slowly proliferating tumors.

subclinical disease in >90% of patients, and 1- to 3-cm masses are controlled in ~50% of patients. However, a dose of 60 Gy in 6 weeks controls 1- to 2-cm masses in 80 to 90% of patients, and a dose of 65 Gy in $6^1/_2$ weeks controls 2- to 4-cm tumors in ~70% of patients.

The dose–response relation for small well-vascularized tumors is often quite steep. A modest increase in dose can increase the probability of local tumor control from 25 to 75% (Fig. 104.8). This is because these tumors are relatively homogeneous in size and oxygenation. The dose–response relation for bulky tumors is not as steep as it is for small tumors, however, because large tumors are much more heterogeneous, with considerable variability in the number of cells and the state of oxygenation. The dose–response relation for subclinical disease also is relatively shallow because the tumor burden is heterogeneous, ranging from only a few clonogenic cells to as many as 10^7 cells.

Regression Rates

Cell loss after irradiation is predominantly due to lysis at the time of mitosis, and most cells divide 4 or 5 times before lysis occurs. Regression rates are related to the cycling times of the tumor cells because of this. In general, rapidly proliferating tumors tend to regress quickly after irradiation, whereas slowly proliferating cancers shrink more gradually. Because lethally injured cells and surviving cells are morphologically indistinguishable, biopsies are of little value in the early postirradiation period. For head and neck cancers, a positive biopsy is usually not a reliable indicator of persistent disease until about 3 months after treatment.

TREATMENT

Selection of a Treatment Modality

Selection of a treatment modality for head and neck cancer should be based on the size and location of the primary tumor, the status of the regional lymph nodes, and the general condition of the patient. Early head and neck cancers are usually treated with one modality—either surgery or radiation therapy. The choice between surgery and radiation therapy in these cases is usually determined by the functional deficit that would result from each treatment modality. Larger cancers are usually treated with a combination of surgery and radiation therapy. However, radiation therapy alone may be attempted, reserving surgery for salvage if the tumor persists.

In general, surgery is more effective in salvaging radiation therapy failures than radiation therapy is in salvaging surgical failures. This is because radiation therapy failures usually occur in areas that were grossly involved with cancer initially, often in the center of bulky masses, whereas surgical failures usually occur peripherally, in tissues that are more hypoxic postoperatively because the blood supply has been interrupted.

Patients with massive cancers or with distant metastases are usually treated palliatively. This is usually, but not always, best achieved with radiation therapy. The radiation doses required for palliative treatment of patients with head and neck cancers are similar to those required for definitive treatment. Sometimes palliative surgery, single-agent chemotherapy, or no treatment at all is an appropriate choice for a patient with massive head and neck disease.

INITIAL FIELDS   1ST FIELD REDUCTION†   2ND FIELD REDUCTION*

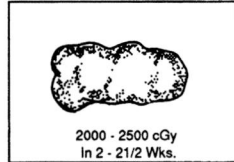

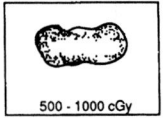

4500 - 5000 cGy
In 41/2 - 51/2 Wks.

2000 - 2500 cGy
In 2 - 21/2 Wks.

500 - 1000 cGy

A   ENCOMPASSES GROSS TUMOR
WITH WIDE MARGINS PLUS
AREAS OF POSSIBLE SPREAD
TO REGIONAL NODES.

B   BOOST FIELD TO GROSS
TUMOR WITH SOME
MARGIN (TOTAL DOSE =
7000 cGy)

C   ADDED BOOST FOR VERY
INFILTRATIVE PRIMARY
TUMORS OR LARGE
NODES (TOTAL DOSE =
7000 - 7500 cGy)

†FOR SMALL TO MODERATE TUMORS

*FOR MASSIVE TUMORS

Figure 104.9   Shrinking-field technique. The total dose is determined according to the size of the tumor. **A:** Initial portals encompass the gross tumor with wide margins, including areas of possible nodal metastasis. **B:** The first field reduction boosts the field to encompass the gross tumor with some margin. The total dose is 6,500 to 7,000 cGy. **C:** The second field reduction is boosted again for highly infiltrative primary tumors or large nodes. The total dose is 7,000 to 7,500 cGy.

Radiation Therapy Alone

If treatment with radiation therapy alone is selected, it can be delivered with external beam irradiation, an interstitial implant, or a combination of the two. The choice is usually based on the site and extent of the disease. Treatment with an implant alone is appropriate only if the tumor is accessible and well circumscribed, with little risk of regional lymph node metastasis. If the disease is more extensive, external beam irradiation or a combination of external beam and an implant is preferred. The neck is usually irradiated if clinically positive nodes are present or if a greater than a 15% risk of subclinical metastasis exists in these areas.

The tumor dose is usually based on the extent of the cancer and the tolerance of normal tissues in the treated area. If the cancer is small, doses of 60 to 65 Gy in 6 to 6.5 weeks may be adequate. Greater doses (e.g., 65 to 70 Gy in 6.5 to 7.5 weeks) are needed for larger tumors, and even larger doses (~70 to 75 Gy and 7.5 to 8 weeks) are required for patients with massive disease (see Table 104.2).

The treatment is usually delivered with a shrinking-field technique (Fig. 104.9). An initial dose of 45 to 50 Gy is delivered in 4 to 5 weeks through large portals covering the clinically involved region and areas of potential regional lymph node metastasis. After this, the fields are reduced to encompass only the gross tumor with a small margin, and an additional 15 to 25 Gy is delivered, bringing the total tumor dose to 60 to 70 Gy in 6 to 7.5 weeks. With massive tumors, often a second field reduction is given at 60 to 65 Gy. An additional 5 to 10 Gy is given with the final boost fields, which cover the residual disease with small or no margins. The total tumor dose is 70 to 75 Gy in 7 to 8 weeks. The spinal cord is limited to a dose of no more than 45 to 50 Gy to avoid the risk of radiation myelitis.

Combined Surgery and Radiation Therapy

The rationale for combining surgery and radiation therapy is based on fundamental surgical and radiobiologic principles (Fig. 104.10). Surgical failures are usually due to microscopic disease beyond the margins of resection, and radiation therapy failures are usually due to an inability to eradicate bulky disease. When combined, these two modalities are complementary. Surgery is used to remove gross masses that are too large to be eradicated by moderate doses

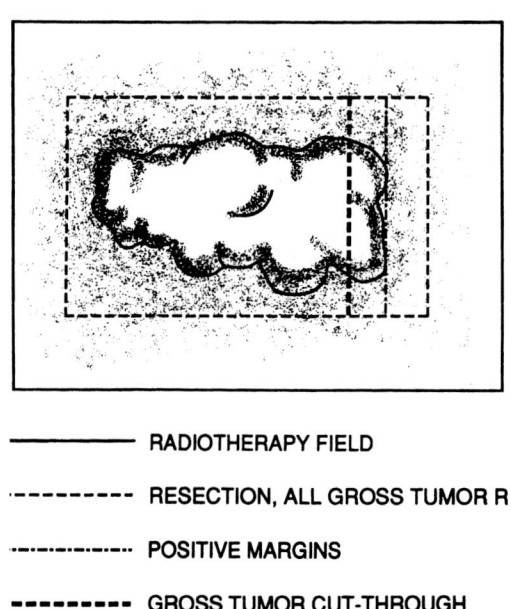

—————   RADIOTHERAPY FIELD

---------   RESECTION, ALL GROSS TUMOR R

-·-·-·-·-   POSITIVE MARGINS

- - - - -   GROSS TUMOR CUT-THROUGH

Figure 104.10   Rationale for combined surgery and radiation therapy. Surgical failures usually are caused by residual microscopic disease, and radiation failures usually are caused by inability to eradicate bulky masses.

of irradiation, and radiation therapy is used to eradicate microscopic extensions of tumors that cannot be excised.

Once a decision to deliver combined radiation therapy and surgery has been made, the management team must decide which treatment modality to use first.

Preoperative Radiation Therapy

The arguments in favor of preoperative radiation therapy are as follows:

1. Unresectable tumors may be made resectable.
2. The extent of the surgical resection may be diminished.
3. The treatment portals preoperatively are usually smaller than would be required postoperatively.
4. Microscopic disease is more radiosensitive preoperatively than it is postoperatively because it has a better blood supply.
5. The viability of tumor cells that may be disseminated by surgical manipulation is diminished, reducing the risk of distant metastasis.

However, wound healing is more difficult after irradiation. Because of this, the dose that can be delivered safely preoperatively is less than that which can be given postoperatively. Furthermore, if a positive margin or gross residual tumor remains after surgery, it is difficult to add a meaningful dose postoperatively when preoperative radiotherapy has already been given. The typical preoperative dose is 45 Gy in 4.5 weeks. This dose is sufficient to eradicate subclinical disease in 85% to 90% of patients. However, it is less than the dose required to control gross disease (8,10).

Postoperative Radiation Therapy

The arguments in favor of postoperative radiation therapy are as follows:

1. The anatomic extent of the tumor can be determined surgically, making it easier to define the treatment portals required.
2. Surgical resection is easier and healing is better in unirradiated tissues.
3. A greater dose of radiation can be given postoperatively than can be given preoperatively.
4. The dose to be given can be adjusted on the basis of the residual tumor burden after surgery.

A theoretic disadvantage of postoperative radiotherapy is that distant metastasis may result from cells that are spread by the surgical procedure. These cells might have been eradicated with preoperative irradiation or rendered less capable of implanting. Another problem with postoperative radiation therapy is that the treatment may have to be postponed if surgical healing is delayed, allowing cancer to repopulate in the interval.

When radiation therapy is given postoperatively, a dose of 60 to 65 Gy is usually delivered in 6 to 7 weeks. Higher doses may be required if gross residual cancer is present.

TABLE 104.3

RECURRENCE RATE AS A FUNCTION OF THE STATUS OF THE SURGICAL MARGINS IN PATIENTS TREATED WITH SURGERY ONLY

Histologic Margins[a]	Recurrence Rate at the Primary Site	
Premalignant change	80% (4/5)	
Carcinoma in situ	84.6% (11/13)	
Close margins (<0.5 cm)	73.7% (14/19)	72.6% (45/62)
Positive margins (invasive microscopically)	64% (16/25)	
Negative margins	31.7% (543/1,713)	

[a]Microscopic findings; patients with gross residual cancer after surgery were excluded.

Positive margins should be regarded as evidence of gross disease because a relatively large number of cells (10^6 to 10^7 cells) must be present to be detectable even microscopically. Looser et al. (11) found that the presence of disease within 0.5 cm of the surgical margins has the same prognostic implication as positive margins (Table 104.3). Postoperative radiation therapy markedly reduces the risk of recurrence in the surgical fields (Fig. 104.11). The results are poorer, however, if the postoperative radiation therapy is delayed beyond 6 weeks (10).

COMPLICATIONS

The effects of irradiation of normal tissues may be classified as acute or late. Acute effects can be a problem during the course of irradiation, but they generally subside several weeks after completion of treatment. Consequently, they are usually not a long-term problem. Late effects are more a concern because the injury is often permanent. The late effects of radiation therapy include xerostomia, damage to the teeth, fibrosis, soft tissue necrosis, bone necrosis, cartilage necrosis, and damage to the eye, ear, and central nervous system (Table 104.4).

Xerostomia occurs when the salivary glands are irradiated to a dose of 35 Gy or more in 3.5 weeks. Even lower doses can have an effect on salivary gland function. Damage to the dentition is usually caused by xerostomia rather than a direct effect on the teeth or surrounding bone. Soft tissue necrosis or osteoradionecrosis may be seen occasionally in head and neck cancer patients. Soft tissue necrosis appears as mucosal ulceration. It is thought to be caused by damage to vascular connective tissue. Most cases of osteoradionecrosis of the head and neck are caused by overlying soft tissue necrosis. Cartilage necrosis also may be secondary to necrosis of overlying soft tissues.

Severe skin damage is relatively uncommon today because modern radiation therapy equipment spares the skin. However, minor skin sequelae are frequent—including epilation

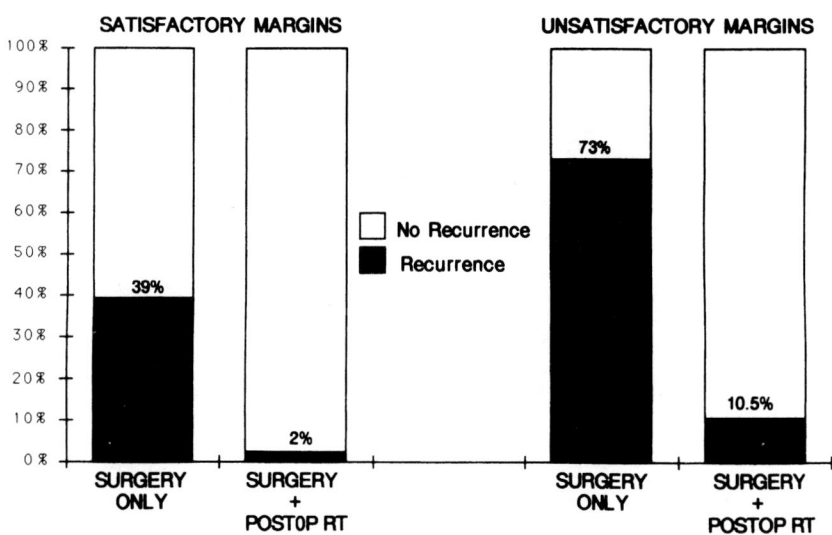

Figure 104.11 Recurrence rates at the primary site with and without postoperative radiation therapy. Unsatisfactory margins include positive margins, close margins (less than 0.5 cm), and margins containing in situ carcinoma. RT, radiation therapy. (From Vikram B, Strong EW, Shah JP, et al. Failure of the primary site following multimodality treatment in advanced head and neck cancer. *Head Neck Surg* 1984;6:720, with permission.)

and dryness due to loss of sweat and sebaceous gland functions, thinning of the epidermis, and telangiectasia.

Fibrosis of the subcutaneous tissues and muscle can be a major problem. It is the principal dose-limiting factor in radiation therapy today. In severe cases, the tissue can develop a woody texture and becomes fixed into a single hard mass. Large daily fractions and massive neck disease increase the severity of subcutaneous fibrosis.

The ocular apparatus is relatively sensitive to radiation, and complications can occur in the form of cataracts, radiation retinopathy, optic nerve injury, and lacrimal gland damage. Cataracts occur with doses as low as 6 Gy, and radiation retinopathy or optic nerve injury can occur with doses in the range of 50 to 55 Gy. The lacrimal glands are similar histopathologically to the salivary glands, and like salivary glands, they are very radiosensitive. The nasolacrimal drainage system, however, is usually quite radioresistant.

Serous otitis media is a frequent complication of radiation therapy for paranasal sinus and nasopharyngeal cancers, but it is usually transient. It is caused by edema of the mucous

membranes lining the eustachian tube. Sensorineural hearing loss is rarely reported, but it is probably more common than generally thought. Radiation damage to the brain or spinal cord is very rare, but it is a major concern to radiation oncologists because the results are devastating. Transient radiation myelopathy can occur with doses as low as 30 Gy in 25 fractions. This is a transitory syndrome characterized by electric shock sensations triggered by flexing the cervical spine (i.e., Lhermitte sign). Transverse myelitis is a rare but permanent complication that may occur after spinal cord doses of 50 to 60 Gy in 5 to 6 weeks.

Radiation effects on the brain also can be transient or permanent. Somnolence syndrome is a transient condition that is self-limited and characterized by lethargy, nausea, headache, cranial nerve palsies, or ataxia. It usually appears 2 to 3 months after treatment and lasts 2 to 4 weeks. Brain necrosis, however, is a permanent injury that can develop after doses in the range of 65 to 70 Gy.

TABLE 104.4 **COMPLICATIONS RADIATION THERAPY FOR HEAD AND NECK CANCER**

Xerostomia
Dental caries
Soft-tissue radionecrosis (mucosa)
Osteoradionecrosis (bone injury)
Cartilage radionecrosis
Fibrosis
Ocular complications (cataracts, retinopathy, optic nerve injury, lacrimal gland injury)
Serous otitis media, sensorineural hearing loss
Spinal cord injury (Lhermitte syndrome, radiation myelopathy, transverse myelitis)
Brain injury (somnolence syndrome, brain necrosis)

HIGHLIGHTS

- Every viable clonogenic cancer cell must be eradicated if the tumor is to be controlled with radiation therapy. Cells are considered to be viable if they are capable of unlimited division.
- The biologic effects of irradiation depend on the fractionation schedules used. The larger the number of fractions, the greater the total dose required to produce a given level of damage.
- Oxygen in the targeted tissues significantly enhances the biologic effects of radiation. Conversely, hypoxia protects tissues from the effects of radiation.
- After a tumor-cell population is reduced by surgery or irradiation, the cells respond by accelerated repopulation. This is one of the main reasons for not delaying postoperative radiation therapy and not delivering radiation therapy in a split course.

- The two biologic factors that determine the probability of local control by irradiation are the number of malignant cells and the proportion of these cells that are hypoxic. Both of these factors are principally related to the size of the cancer.
- Small, well-vascularized, exophytic tumors usually respond well to irradiation, whereas large, infiltrative, or ulcerative cancers are less responsive.
- The probability of controlling a head and neck cancer with radiation therapy is related to the size of the neoplasm. A dose of 50 Gy in 5 weeks controls subclinical disease in 90% to 95% of patients, but 65 to 70 Gy in 6 to 7 weeks is required to control gross masses.
- Because lethally injured cancer cells and surviving cancer cells are morphologically indistinguishable, biopsies are of little value in the early postirradiation period (i.e., within 3 months).
- Radiation therapy for head and neck tumors is usually delivered with a shrinking-field technique. The initial portals are relatively large, encompassing the gross tumor and areas of potential subclinical involvement. The boost fields usually encompass only the gross tumor with a small margin.

REFERENCES

1. Hall EJ. *Radiobiology for the radiologist,* 4th ed. Philadelphia: JB Lippincott, 1994.
2. Khan FM. *The physics of radiation therapy,* 2nd ed. Baltimore: Williams & Wilkins, 1994.
3. Delclos L, Sampier V. Special gamma-ray techniques. In: Fletcher GH, ed. *Textbook of radiotherapy.* Philadelphia: Lea & Febiger, 1980:71.
4. Hevezi JM. Emerging techniques in cancer treatment. *Oncology* 2003;17.10:1445–1464.
5. Dewey WC, Ling CC, Meyn RE. Radiation-induced apoptosis: relevance to radiotherapy. *Int J Radiat Oncol Biol Phys* 1995;33:781.
6. Thomlinson RH, Gray LH. The histological structure of some human lung cancers and the possible implications for radiotherapy. *Br J Cancer* 1955;9:539.
7. Brown JM. Evidence for acutely hypoxic cells in mouse tumours and a possible mechanism for reoxygenation. *Br J Radiol* 1979;52:650.
8. Fletcher GH. The role of irradiation in the treatment of squamous cell carcinomas of the mouth and throat. In: Nahum AM, Bush S, Davidson TM, et al., eds. *Head and neck surgery.* Boston: Houghton Mifflin,1979:1441.
9. Fletcher GH. Basic principles of radiotherapy: basic clinical parameters. In: Fletcher GH, ed. *Textbook of radiotherapy.* Philadelphia: Lea & Febiger, 1980:180.
10. Vikram B, Strong EW, Shah JP, et al. Failure of the primary site following multimodality treatment in advanced head and neck cancer. *Head Neck Surg* 1984;6:720.
11. Looser KG, Shah JP, Strong EW. The significance of "positive" margins in surgically resected epidermoid carcinomas. *Head Neck Surg* 1978;1:107.

Cutaneous Malignancy

Fred J. Stucker   *Cherie-Ann O. Nathan*
Timothy S. Lian

Skin cancer is the most common human malignancy, with more than 1,300,000 cases in the United States annually (1). Most tumors arise on the sun-exposed regions of the head and neck. Basal cell carcinoma is the predominant histologic type and accounts for about 90% of all cutaneous neoplasms in the head and neck region. Second in incidence is squamous cell carcinoma. Less common is melanoma, which accounts for approximately 7,300 deaths each year in the United States, and 2,000 additional deaths are related to other forms of cutaneous cancer (2). Cutaneous malignancies are classically divided into epidermal, dermal, adnexal, and melanocytic. Malignant melanoma has a distinct biologic behavior and is addressed separately in Chapter 106. Many other rare skin malignancies of the dermis and adnexa are not discussed specifically, but some principles of evaluation and treatment of cutaneous cancers are applicable. This chapter is primarily dedicated to a discussion of nonmelanoma cutaneous malignancy, specifically basal cell and squamous cell carcinomas, their precursors, and associated epidermal neoplasms.

RISK FACTORS

Risk factors for basal and squamous cell carcinomas are strikingly similar. These lesions, although seen in younger age groups, are most often encountered in patients aged 60 years or older.

The mechanism by which ultraviolet light causes sundamaged skin has been extensively studied. Laboratory experiments indicate that the wavelengths with the most potential for carcinogenesis are those in the range of 280 to 320 nm, the ultraviolet B band. This ultraviolet B is responsible for the common sunburn. The transition from normal to actinic (i.e., sun damaged) to cancerous skin is usually a progressive process that occurs over a period of several decades.

With the current environmental changes occurring with the earth's protective ozone layer, the concern for skin cancer becomes much more significant. A dramatic ozone depletion above the Antarctic continent has been detected (3). For each 1% reduction in atmospheric ozone concentration, a concomitant 2% increase in ultraviolet B penetration occurs (4).

The carcinogenesis of epidermal tumors parallels the multistep development of other neoplasms. As with other neoplasms, certain characteristics render the host more susceptible to the development of cancer. Traits that are associated with an increased incidence of skin cancer include fair complexion, light hair, blue or green eyes, inability to tan, propensity to sunburn, history of multiple or severe sunburns, and Celtic ancestry (5). Other factors implicated include age, occupation, habits (tanning booths), and residential geography, which are considered indirect causes of increased sun exposure.

The bulbs used in tanning booths are almost exclusively ultraviolet A wavelength and are promoted as providing a safe suntan. However, recent evidence indicates that ultraviolet A (320 to 400 nm) synergistically augments ultraviolet B responses and is independently capable of producing deleterious skin alterations and neoplasias (6).

Other etiologic factors are associated with the development of cutaneous carcinoma (5). Chronic exposure to chemical agents, such as arsenic in patients treated with Fowler solution, has been associated with the development of multiple squamous and basal cell tumors. Patients with chronic radiodermatitis, resulting from superficial radiation therapy, demonstrate a propensity to develop multiple and aggressive lesions. Trauma in the form of burns, ulcers, and scars also is associated with the development of skin cancer (i.e., Marjolin ulcer). Immunosuppression, common in transplant patients and patients with leukemia or lymphoma, can be complicated by an increased incidence or aggressiveness of skin malignancies.

Studies of human papillomavirus offer additional support for the importance of immune dysfunction in the development of skin squamous cell carcinoma. One study showed human papillomavirus presence in 60% of cutaneous squamous cell carcinoma lesions found in renal autograft recipients. Moreover, this human papillomavirus presence was significantly higher than that found in matched transplant recipients without cutaneous malignancy (7). A high incidence of human papillomavirus appears in squamous cell carcinoma lesions of the cervix, penis, and digits (8).

Genetic syndromes, such as xeroderma pigmentosum (autosomal recessive) and nevoid basal cell carcinoma syndrome (autosomal dominant), are associated with a predilection for developing multiple basal cell carcinomas, often at an early age.

BASAL CELL CARCINOMA

Evaluation

Several clinical types of basal cell carcinoma are found. Smith (9) outlined five clinical forms: nodular or noduloulcerative, morphealike or sclerosing, superficial multicentric, pigmented, and fibroepithelioma. Although other less common types exist, subclassification is not clinically useful. The most common type is the nodular or noduloulcerative lesion. This lesion typically is seen as a discrete, raised, circular lesion that appears pink and waxy, with a capillary network that is easily visible. Often an area of central ulceration appears, and the border of the lesion is rolled. This is the type of basal cell carcinoma that is easiest to recognize and treat. A variant of this lesion is cystic basal cell carcinoma, which also is waxy and well demarcated but is more cystic in appearance.

The superficial basal cell carcinoma lesion shows evidence of scarring and atrophy, with a threadlike waxy border. This lesion may consist of one or several red scaling patches. These crusted lesions have irregular borders and gradually increase in size by peripheral extension. They are relatively uncommon in the head and neck and more frequently occur on the trunk or extremities.

The most dangerous clinical form of basal cell carcinoma is the morphea type, also called sclerosing or fibrosing basal cell carcinoma. This variety is typified by its macular, whitish, or yellowish plaque. Some physicians have noticed an increased incidence among women. The margins may be quite indistinct, and the lesion may go unnoticed for years in some patients. Complete excision is difficult because of ill-defined margins. The lesion may look like a scar, may develop telangiectasia, or may ulcerate.

A less common basal cell carcinoma variant is pigmented basal cell carcinoma, which is characterized by its brown pigmentation and may resemble a pigmented nevus or a melanoma. The appearance and behavior of this lesion seems to parallel that of nodular basal cell carcinoma. Pigmented basal cell carcinoma differs from the noduloulcerative type only by the brown pigmentation of the lesion. This type of lesion also may be mistaken for seborrheic keratosis, melanoma, or dermatofibroma.

Fibroepitheliomas, another variant, are seen initially as firm pedunculated lesions that resemble fibromas. It was first described in 1953 by Pinkus (10). These lesions commonly occur on the back.

The nevoid basal cell carcinoma syndrome is an autosomal dominant disease. During childhood, small cutaneous nodules appear, often numbering in the hundreds. These lesions initially have a rather indolent course during the nevoid phase, but as the patient ages, a neoplastic phase may occur in which the lesions show a marked change in aggressiveness. The lesions become invasive, destructive, and mutilating. Abnormalities associated with nevoid basal cell carcinoma syndrome include jaw cysts, bifid ribs, scoliosis, mental retardation, and frontal bossing.

Histopathology

The characteristic cell in basal cell carcinoma has a large, oval, or elongated nucleus with relatively little cytoplasm. These cells may resemble the basal cells of the epidermis, but the neoplastic forms lack intercellular bridges. The nuclei are rather uniform in size and configuration. A connective tissue stroma proliferates with the tumor and is oriented in parallel bundles around the tumor masses, causing peripheral palisading of the cells and stromal retraction. This is commonly referred to as peritumoral lacunae. The stroma is often mucinous. Because mucin shrinks with dehydration and fixation of the specimen, the stroma may show retraction from the tumor islands. This detachment of tumor islands from the stroma is known as *clefting* and is a helpful diagnostic sign.

Lever and Schaumburg-Lever (11) divided basal cell carcinoma into four basic histologic patterns: solid, keratotic, cystic, and adenoid. In the solid pattern, the cells show no differentiation. This type generally displays tumor masses of various sizes and shapes embedded in the dermis (Fig. 105.1). The peripheral cell layer may show a palisading of the nuclei. Basal cell carcinomas that differentiate toward hair structures are referred to as *keratotic*. This lesion is typified by undifferentiated cells in combination with parakeratotic cells and horn cysts (Fig. 105.2). Cystic tumors show differentiation toward sebaceous glands. Histologically, one or several cystic spaces may appear within the tumor lobules. In the adenoid variety of basal cell carcinoma, the tumors display a tubular or glandular formation. The strands of epithelial cells commonly form a lace-like pattern (Fig. 105.3).

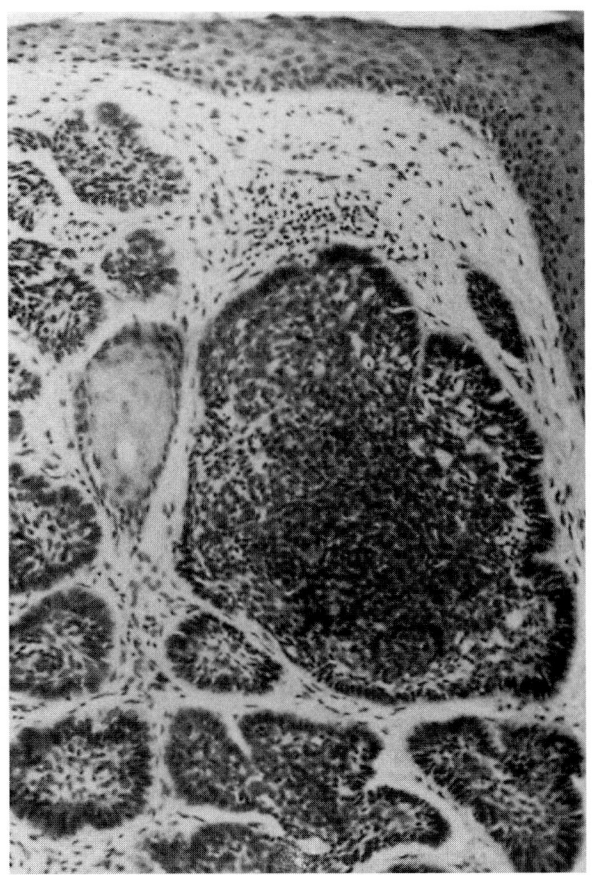

Figure 105.1 Basal cell tumor masses (solid type).

KERATOTIC BASAL CELL CARCINOMA

Keratotic basal cell carcinoma, also known as basosquamous cell carcinoma or metatypical carcinoma, has been the subject of much controversy. The confusion arises because histologically, coexistent features of both basal cell and squamous cell carcinomas occur in the same lesion, frustrating accurate assessment of prognosis and behavior. Most dermatopathologists currently believe that basosquamous tumor is a variant basal cell carcinoma, referred to by many as keratotic basal cell carcinoma (11). Although limited potential exists for metastasis, keratotic basal cell carcinoma is thought to be more biologically aggressive than many of the other types of basal cell carcinomas.

SQUAMOUS CELL CARCINOMA

Evaluation

Far less common than basal cell carcinoma, squamous cell carcinoma accounts for approximately 10% of skin malignancies. As with its counterpart, basal cell carcinoma, squamous cell carcinoma is related to prolonged (i.e., 10 to 20 years) sun exposure. As the equator is approached, the relative incidence of squamous cell carcinoma increases compared with basal cell carcinoma. Cutaneous squamous cell carcinoma, like basal cell carcinoma, is more common in men.

Squamous cell carcinoma of the skin usually is first seen as an erythematous, ulcerated, crusting lesion. The tumor often demonstrates a granular base that may be friable and tends to bleed with minimal trauma. Usually an elevated area of induration is seen at the lesion edge, and an inflammatory response may occur in the adjacent tissues.

These lesions have different patterns. Squamous cell carcinoma can occur as a thickened hyperkeratotic patch or an area of crusting. Under this crust is an ulcerated base with a rolled margin. Other lesions may be recognized as areas of persistent ulceration, possibly in the site of previous trauma, burns, or an old scar (i.e., Marjolin ulcer). Neoplastic change

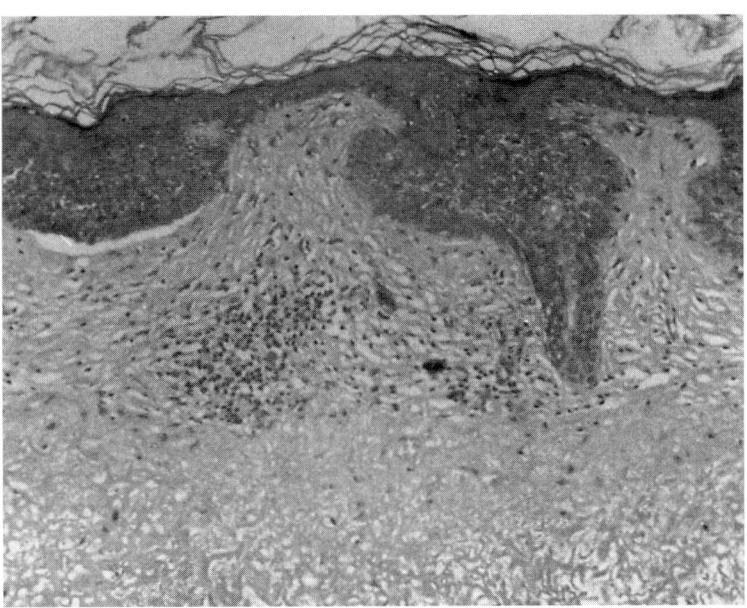

Figure 105.2 Undifferentiated cells with parakeratotic and horn cysts (keratotic type).

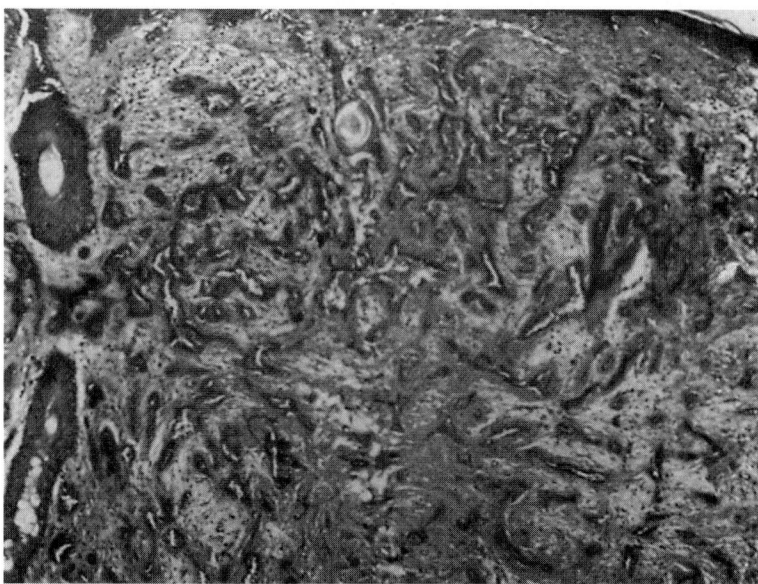

Figure 105.3 Lacelike patterns of epithelial cells (adenoid type).

in a chronic ulcer may result in basal cell or squamous cell carcinoma and is associated with a poorer prognosis and higher rates of metastasis. Superficial multifocal lesions can arise in actinic skin. These lesions are usually accompanied by a scaling patch that bleeds with minimal trauma. Diagnosis and determination of the extent of the lesion can be difficult, and multiple biopsies may be necessary.

Squamous cell carcinoma occasionally appears as a nodular exophytic lesion. Initially cystic, it later tends to become ulcerative and progressively enlarges. These lesions also may demonstrate a sudden growth spurt (13).

Histopathology

Several histologic characteristics are important in analyzing squamous cell carcinoma. The usual histologic picture of squamous cell carcinoma of the skin is that of irregular masses of epidermal cells that proliferate downward and invade the dermis. The tumor masses may be well differentiated or may show atypical or anaplastic cells. The differentiated tumors tend to be associated with evidence of keratinization, such as keratin pearls. Tumors are graded from 1 to 4 by using the Broder classification; grade 1 tumors are well differentiated, and grade 4 tumors are poorly differentiated.

Some squamous cell carcinomas are actinically induced, and some arise de novo. Lesions arising in sun-exposed areas appear to follow a more benign course with a low incidence of metastasis. The de novo lesions are more aggressive in their behavior and exhibit greater potential for metastasis. One researcher estimated that in at least 8% of patients with de novo lesions, regional or distant metastases develop (14). It is often possible to differentiate clinically between the two types of squamous cell carcinoma. Histologically, a determination can usually be made by looking for actinic changes in the skin adjacent to the squamous cell carcinoma.

Squamous cell carcinoma has metastatic potential, and regional metastatic spread is correlated with depth of invasion. Squamous cell carcinoma lesions that penetrate to Clark's level IV or V are associated with a 20% regional metastatic rate.

Histologic variations of squamous cell carcinoma are categorized as generic, adenoid, bowenoid, verrucous, and spindle-pleomorphic types (15). The generic type is characterized by actinic changes. In the adenoid type, a pseudoglandular arrangement is noted. These tubular or alveolar formations result from dyskeratosis and subsequent acantholysis. The lumina are lined with one or several layers of epithelium and are filled with desquamated acantholytic cells. The bowenoid type of squamous cell carcinoma is characterized by evidence of invasion coexistent with the findings of Bowen disease.

Verrucous carcinoma is seldom seen as a skin neoplasm on the head and neck, but it is well known as a tumor of the oral cavity and larynx. It appears as a white cauliflowerlike lesion. The tumor is well differentiated, demonstrating hyperkeratosis, parakeratosis, and acanthosis. Clinical and pathologic correlations are needed to confirm the diagnosis.

In the spindle-pleomorphic type of squamous cell carcinoma, little evidence of differentiation is seen. These tumors are anaplastic, show little or no keratinization, and are usually considered to be a Broder grade 4 tumor. The spindle cells are intermingled with collagen, may be arranged in whorls, and can be associated with pleomorphic giant cells.

PREMALIGNANT LESIONS

Several skin lesions are considered premalignant. This group includes a low-grade malignancy that can be treated as if it were a premalignant lesion. The most common of

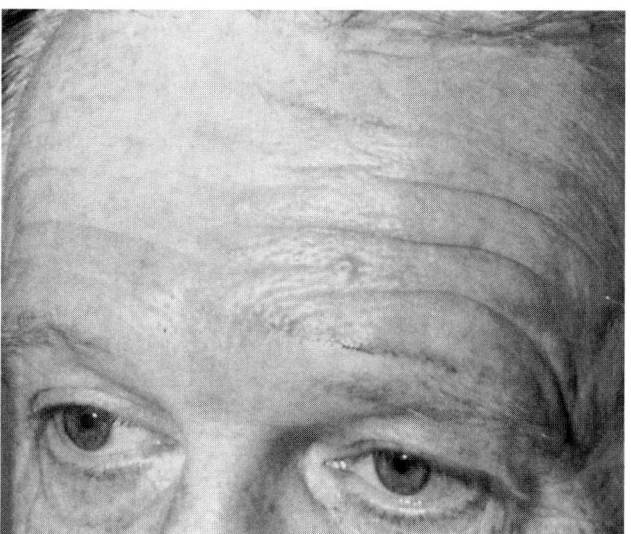

Figure 105.4 Actinic keratosis on forehead.

these are actinic keratosis, Bowen disease, and keratoacanthoma.

Actinic Keratoses

Actinic keratosis (i.e., solar keratoses or senile keratoses) is the most common premalignant lesion of the head and neck and is seen almost exclusively in sun-exposed areas of the skin. The lesions are generally less than 1 cm in diameter and are commonly located on the face, scalp, hands, and forearms (Fig. 105.4). They are considered precancerous. The chance of progression to epidermal cutaneous carcinoma has been estimated to be as great as 20% (11). They usually occur as an erythematous patch, often covered by an adherent scale. Clinically, they show little or no sign of inflammation. Occasionally, a marked hyperkeratosis is seen, giving the appearance of a cutaneous horn. A sandpaper-like scale is the most distinctive feature on clinical examination. Because these lesions have malignant transformation potential, most physicians believe they should be treated. Depending on the clinical setting, superficial shave excision, cryosurgery, topical treatment with 5-fluorouracil, or trichloroacetic acid peel may provide effective treatment. The differential diagnosis includes seborrheic keratosis, benign lentigo, squamous cell carcinoma, and basal cell carcinoma.

Bowen Disease

Bowen disease is considered a preinvasive form of squamous cell carcinoma. It can be considered synonymous with carcinoma in situ of the skin. Histologically, full-thickness dysplasia of the epidermis is noted without evidence of invasion. Clinically, the lesion is a well-circumscribed, erythematous, scaly patch or plaque with an irregular border. As with squamous cell carcinoma, these lesions generally occur in sun-exposed areas. They are particularly common in patients with a history of chronic arsenic ingestion, in whom lesions often occur on nonexposed skin. The lesion may resemble a superficial basal cell carcinoma, but it lacks the fine pearly border.

Keratoacanthoma

Keratoacanthoma is a benign, usually self-limited epithelial tumor that is easily confused clinically and histopathologically with squamous cell carcinoma. It is more common in males and typically is first seen in older patients. A history of rapid growth is reported, usually over a 2- to 6-month period. The lesion begins as a smooth rounded nodule, but with further enlargement, the center becomes ulcerated and filled with keratinous material, taking on a volcano-like appearance. The hallmark of keratoacanthoma is rapid growth over weeks or months.

The most common site affected is the nose. Although histologically the lesion resembles a squamous cell carcinoma (Fig. 105.5), it may involute spontaneously, leaving

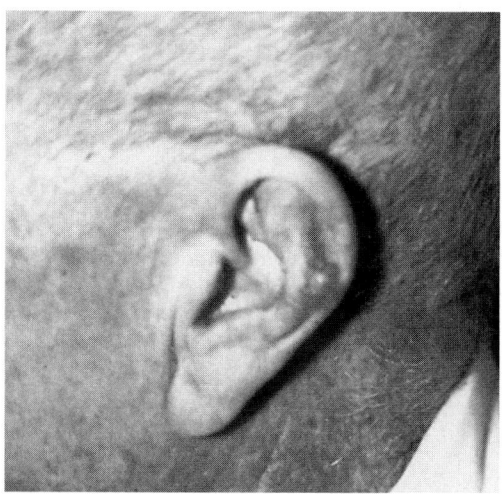

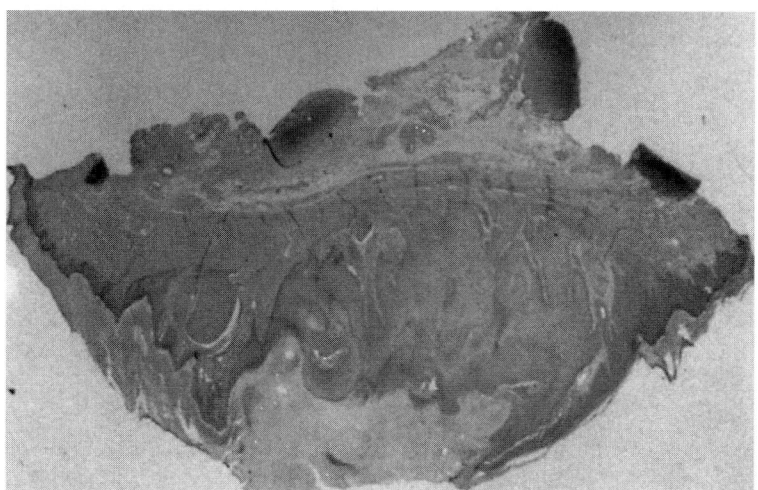

A   B

Figure 105.5 A: Keratoacanthoma of the auricle. **B:** Histologic volcano-like appearance.

only a depressed scar. Because of the lack of predictability, surgical excision is recommended.

PROGNOSIS

Tumor Behavior

Staging for cutaneous basal cell carcinoma and squamous cell carcinoma has been defined by the American Joint Committee on Cancer by using the TNM classification as shown in Table 105.1 (12). Tumor histology, local extent or infiltration, tumor size, anatomic site, associated risk factors (e.g., age, prior irradiation, genetic syndromes), and previous treatment must be considered in determining the risk of recurrence for a given lesion. We consider the risk factors shown in Table 105.2 to be indications for histologic documentation of tumor-free margins.

The clinical and histologic types are significant prognostic variables. The morphea type of basal cell carcinoma is well known for its subversive attitude. This lesion generally spreads centrifugally by way of finger-like projections of tumor. It is deceptive in its behavior and can be difficult to evaluate and control. Keratotic (i.e., basosquamous), recurrent basal cell, and spindle cell variants of squamous cell carcinomas also are associated with worse prognoses.

Squamous cell lesions can be virulent. They have the potential to metastasize to regional nodes and are sometimes

TABLE 105.1

AJCC CLASSIFICATION FOR CUTANEOUS BASAL CELL AND SQUAMOUS CELL CARCINOMA

Primary tumor (T)
TX: Primary tumor cannot be assessed
T0: No evidence of primary tumor
Tis: Carcinoma in situ
T1: Tumor 2 cm or less in greatest dimension
T2: Tumor greater than 2 cm but not more than 5 cm in greatest dimension
T3: Tumor greater than 5 cm in greatest dimension
T4: Tumor invades deep extradermal structures (i.e., cartilage, muscle, bone)

Regional lymph nodes (N)
N0: No regional lymph node metastasis
N1: Regional lymph node metastasis

Distant metastasis (M)
M0: No distant metastasis
M1: Distant metastasis

Stage groupings
Stage 0: Tis, N0, M0
Stage 1: T1, N0, M0
Stage 2: T2, N0, M0; T3, N0, M0
Stage 3: T4, N0, M0; Any T, N1, M0
Stage 4: Any T, any N, M1

TABLE 105.2

FACTORS ASSOCIATED WITH HIGH-RISK CUTANEOUS MALIGNANCIES

Histology
De novo squamous cell carcinoma
Basal cell carcinoma, morphea type
Keratotic basal cell carcinoma (i.e., basosquamous, metatypical)

Location
Nose, nasolabial sulcus, floor of nose, columella
Auricular, postauricular, preauricular
Periorbital region, embryonic fusion planes

Size
Lesions >2 cm

Predisposing factors
Any genetic predisposition or syndrome
History of arsenic use
Tumor arising in burns or scars
Tumors arising in area of radiodermatitis

Other factors
Recurrent tumors
Tumors with significant tissue invasion

associated with distant metastases. Locally, these tumors are more likely to grow in a vertical fashion and less likely to respect the barriers of cartilage and bone than are basal cell carcinomas. It is prudent to evaluate the regional lymphatic drainage when dealing with squamous cell carcinoma.

The anatomic location influences the prognosis because various regions of the head and neck have a propensity for tumor recurrence. Lesions on the nose and ear have higher rates of recurrence, which is probably associated with embryonic fusion planes (16). These embryologic sites of fusion afford greater access for tumors, which use the planes as avenues for spread. The most prominent sites are the preauricular and postauricular regions, the floor of the nose and columella, and the nose–cheek crease. The periorbital region also is at risk for tumors tracking along the bone or periosteum, particularly in the medial canthal region. Mohs (17) speculated that basal cell tumor cells migrate along the periosteum or perichondrium of the nose and the medial canthi because of the close apposition of the skin to the bone and cartilage in these locations.

Swanson (18) determined that the high-risk sites fall within an "H" zone on the face (Fig. 105.6). In highlighting the specific regions at risk, he cited the junction of the ala with the nasolabial fold, the nasal septum, the nasal ala, the inner canthi and lower eyelids of the periorbital region, the periauricular region extending to the temple, and certain scalp lesions.

Recurrent Cutaneous Lesions

A recurrent carcinoma of the skin presents a much more challenging problem than the primary lesion. Recurrent

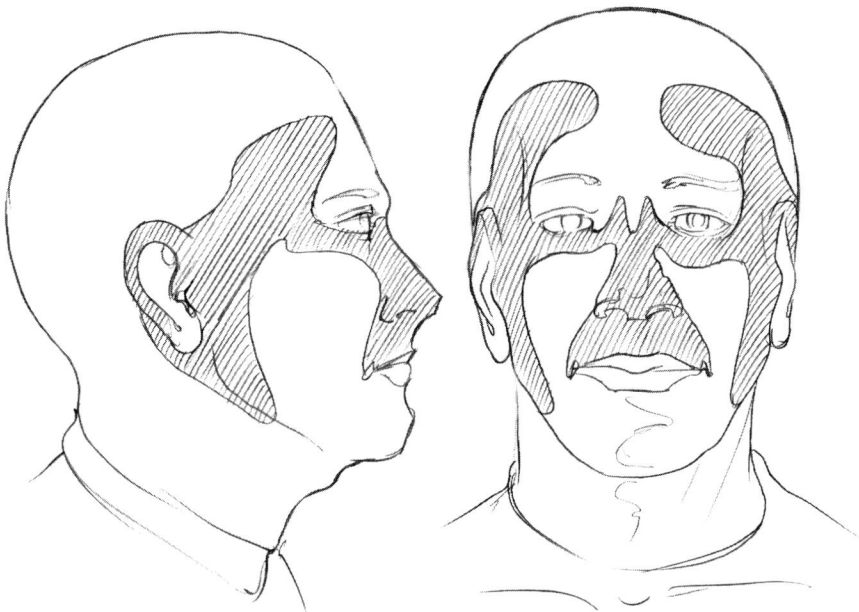

Figure 105.6 H zone: high-risk areas of aggressive cutaneous malignancies. (From Swanson NA. Mohs surgery: technique, indications, applications, and the future. *Arch Dermatol* 1983;119:761, with permission.)

cancer indicates inadequate initial therapy or a persistence of disease in the tissue adjacent to the original lesion. Levine and Bailin (19) evaluated 496 cases of recurrent basal cell carcinoma in an attempt to identify significant risk factors. They found that the midface region was involved in 57.6% of the cases, and the auricular and preauricular areas accounted for 13.4% of the recurrences. The nose is the most common location of recurrence (25.5% to 41%). The relative risk for recurrence was calculated in one study for different locations (19). In order of decreasing magnitude of risk, the locations are the nose (2.38), the ears (1.43), the periorbital areas (1.17), the remainder of the face (1.04), and the neck and scalp (0.55). The distribution of these recurrent tumors is shown in Fig. 105.7.

Jackson and Adams (21) described 33 cases of extensive basal cell carcinoma. These lesions were large (greater than 3 cm), destructive, locally uncontrollable, or metastatic. In defining the predominant characteristic of each lesion, the researchers found that 18 were large, six destructive, five locally uncontrollable, and four metastatic. They concluded that these horrifying tumors usually had an onset before age 40 years and recurred more than twice despite adequate treatment, and that each recurrence appeared sooner and became larger than the preceding tumor. In many patients,

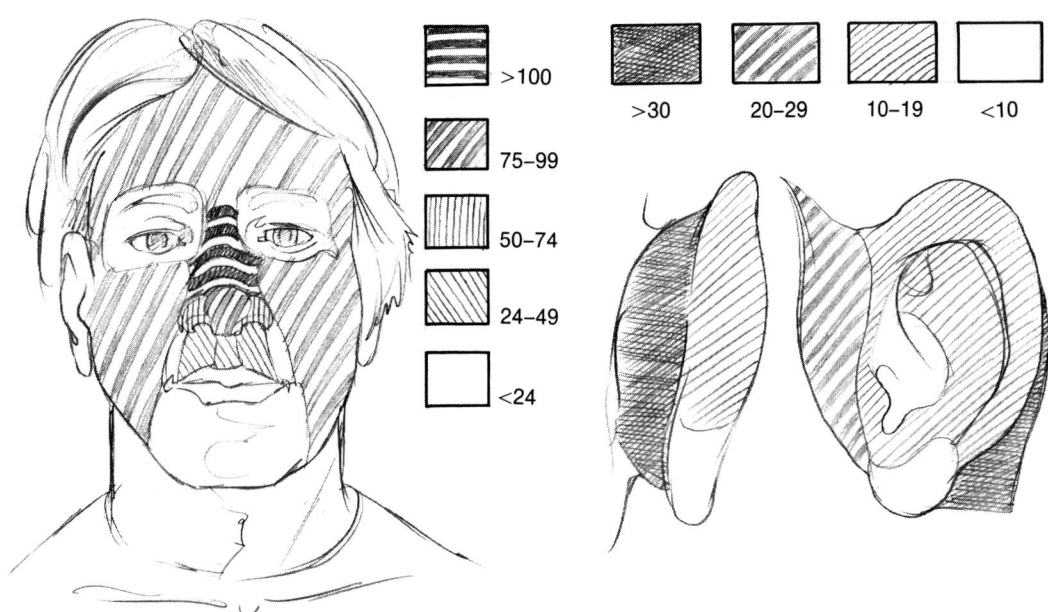

Figure 105.7 Distribution of recurrent cutaneous malignancies.

underlying conditions predisposed them to cutaneous basal cell carcinoma, including arsenic ingestion, nevoid basal cell syndrome, preexisting burns, and radiodermatitis.

Levine (22) studied the pathogenesis and treatment of large recurrent cutaneous neoplasms. The advanced lesions, called massive or previously uncontrolled, met one or more of the following criteria: diameter greater than 3 cm, involvement deeper than skin and subcutaneous fat, four or more previous treatments without control, or proven metastatic disease.

MANAGEMENT

An advantage of nonsurgical management of primary skin malignancies is cure rates reported in excess of 95% for selected skin malignancies. These nonsurgical modalities use field therapy for their mechanism of treatment. Skin cancers grow both radially and vertically in a predictable and proportional manner. Field therapy uses these growth characteristics to treat a defined area containing both tumor and a surrounding layer of normal tissue.

Curettage with Electrodesiccation

One of the most common treatments for basal cell carcinoma is curettage excision combined with electrodesiccation, also known as electrosurgery or electrodesiccation with curettage. It is used primarily by dermatologists, who manage most of these lesions, and is quite successful when used appropriately, yielding cure rates of 92% to 98% (23).

The rationale for using this modality is that basal cell and squamous cell tumors have a soft feel that can be detected as a lesion is curetted. In experienced hands, this allows the removal of all palpable tumor with different sizes of curettes. After normal-feeling tissue is encountered over the entire base of the excision, electrodesiccation or fulguration of the wound is performed. This process is completed from 2 to 6 times, and the wound is treated topically and allowed to heal by second intention.

The advantages of electrosurgery include maximal sparing of normal tissue, ease of performance, and expediency (23). The disadvantages include care of an open wound, depressed or hypertrophic scarring, and delayed bleeding. Electrosurgery should be used only in selected lesions, usually basal cell lesions less than 2 cm in diameter. Contraindications for this treatment modality include lesions with deep invasion, morphea-like and sclerotic basal cell carcinomas, and recurrent tumors (23). If squamous cell tumors are treated with this modality, they should be carefully selected.

Cryosurgery

Cryosurgery is another treatment option that may be appropriate for some basal cell lesions. As with electrosurgery, the skill and experience of the treating physician are critical. The most common cryogen used is liquid nitrogen. A temperature of at least $-30°C$ is considered to be lethal to cutaneous malignant tissue, although some surgeons consider $-50°C$ to be more appropriate. The tumor and an area of surrounding tissue are frozen to ensure the adequacy of the ablation. A thermocouple inserted at the margin of the treatment area ensures that the proper temperature for cell killing is reached. The tissue is allowed to thaw, and after an appropriate period, the freeze–thaw cycle is repeated.

Proponents of this technique cite as advantages its high cure rate, tissue-sparing capabilities, and expedience (24). It is thought to be useful in tumors overlying cartilage that can be frozen without undergoing necrosis. It may be particularly useful in patients with multiple lesions. The disadvantages include a prolonged healing phase and wound care. Hypopigmentation and unsatisfactory scarring can occur. Its use should be limited to lesions with well-defined borders and should not be used for morphea-like tumors or recurrent skin cancers.

Radiation Therapy

Radiation therapy has the capability of curing most skin cancers successfully and has been used extensively in the past (25). As more expedient and less radical methods of treatment have become popular, its use in recent years has waned. The advantages of irradiation include the ability to treat a wide field of tumor and avoidance of surgery. The disadvantages include the protracted treatment course, expense, adjacent tissue effects, limited effectiveness if tumors involve cartilage or bone, and the possibility of radiodermatitis and delayed carcinogenesis. Radiation therapy is currently used in the treatment of poor operative candidates, as an adjuvant to surgery, or for palliation in advanced lesions. It can be curative, but careful selection of lesions and patients is crucial.

Photodynamic Therapy for Cutaneous Malignancy of the Head and Neck

Photodynamic therapy (PDT) is a therapeutic modality using a photosensitizing drug that selectively localizes in tumors and that, on being activated by exposure to light, causes preferential tumor necrosis. Despite its initial promise, PDT now remains an investigational modality. The two components needed for this therapy are a photosensitizer drug and a laser to activate the drug. The most widely used drug in head and neck has been porphyrin. Some of the other drugs that have been used as photosensitizers are tetracyclines, fluorescein, rhodamine, and more recently, sulfonated metallophthalocyanines. The light source consists of a laser either delivered down a fiber for surface illumination (which is the technique of choice for superficial cancer) or implanted into the substance of the tumor (used for bulky tumors). The argon ion dye-pumped laser is most commonly used in North America.

Review of the literature reveals that initially this treatment was used predominantly for palliation of advanced skin cancer. Most series reveal a dramatic initial response in many patients, but long-term follow-up was rarely possible because of the advanced nature of these cancers (26). The response was variable and unpredictable, and severe pain and skin necrosis were common. A major problem in evaluating the literature is the tremendous variability in technique, drug, and light dosage in the reported series.

The advantages of PDT are that multiple lesions can be treated at the same time, it has good cosmetic results, and no anesthesia is required. The disadvantages include lack of predictable response in more advanced lesions and occasional photosensitivity. Once the technique has been further refined, it has great potential in the management of skin cancers.

Interferon-α

Interferon-α (IFN-α) is under investigational use for the treatment of primary skin cancer. Pilot studies demonstrated that basal cell carcinoma of the nodular and superficial types shows excellent responses (27,28). Treatment is initiated with low-dose (1.5 ∞ 106 IU) intralesional IFN-α 3 times per week. Local reactions include pain and persistent erythema. The most common side effect is a flulike illness, the symptoms of which respond to acetaminophen. Hematologic side effects include leukocytopenia and thrombocytopenia.

The mechanism is believed to be due to the antiproliferative and immunomodulating properties of interferon. Through a nonspecific stimulating effect on macrophages and natural killer cells, localized administration of IFN-α focally increases the host response to the neoplastic tissue.

Excisional Surgery

Surgical excision for cutaneous neoplasms is the modality with which most head and neck surgeons have the most experience. The success rate for this method of treatment is 93% to 95% (29). The major advantages of excisional surgery include the ability to obtain tissue for diagnosis and to assess the completeness of excision. By use of frozen sections, the surgeon can evaluate the margins of excision histologically. Another benefit is the excellent cosmesis, particularly if defects are amenable to primary closure. The disadvantages are that excisional surgery can be more time-consuming, inconvenient, and expensive for the patient than other treatments. Most surgeons believe that the histologic confirmation of the adequacy of excision outweighs these relatively minor disadvantages. The carbon dioxide (CO_2) laser also can be used for excision of cutaneous carcinomas.

Mohs Surgery

Mohs pioneered a new technique for removal of cutaneous neoplasms while he was a medical student in the 1930s.

His first results were published in 1941, and the new modality was dubbed *chemosurgery technique* (29). With this method, zinc chloride paste (a chemical fixative) was applied to the cancer, fixing it in situ and permitting careful serial excisions with examination of the entire specimen histologically. This permitted him to map extensions of residual tumor, so that reexcision of these pockets of cancer were possible. The cure rates associated with the technique range from 96% to 99% (30,31). Tromovitch and Stegman (32) revised the original technique and used a fresh-tissue technique that adhered to the same tenets of serial excisions and mapping of residual tumor deposits. The nomenclature for the techniques has now evolved to the point that Mohs chemosurgery implies a fixed-tissue technique, and Mohs micrographic surgery indicates use of the fresh-tissue technique. Most dermatologic surgeons now use the fresh-tissue technique, commonly called Mohs surgery. Details of the technique are published in numerous sources (17,29,31). A schematic of this process is shown in Fig. 105.8.

The advantages of Mohs surgery lie in its ability to examine the resection margins in their entirety, unlike routine or frozen-section margins that evaluate a random sampling of margins. Microscopic foci of tumor can be identified, mapped, and reexcised with this technique. It also allows removal of the neoplasm with maximal preservation of surrounding normal tissue. Another benefit of the Mohs fresh-tissue technique is the ability to reconstruct immediately the defects that have been created. The major advantage is that this technique has the highest cure rate in the management of advanced, high-risk, or recurrent lesions. Mohs surgery is most useful in the high-risk lesions characterized in Table 105.3. The disadvantages of the Mohs technique are the special expertise, time, and expense involved. Someone with this special training may not be available in all communities. These drawbacks are compensated for by achieving a disease-free status.

Carbon Dioxide Laser

Laser excision is appropriate in the management of some skin malignancies. It is indicated instead of standard excision for patients whose cardiac status or other medical conditions render it unwise to use epinephrine in the local anesthesia. Lidocaine without the addition of a vasoconstrictor has a duration of approximately 15 minutes, more than adequate time for the few minutes required to resect most facial lesions in a bloodless fashion with the CO_2 laser. If margins are positive, more anesthesia is infiltrated where required and more tissue removed as needed. After margins are determined to be free of tumor, the area of the local flap is infiltrated, and the reconstruction carried out. We also have found laser excision to be of benefit in patients with bleeding disorders.

Another indication for use of the CO_2 laser is the resection or vaporization of small multiple lesions that then

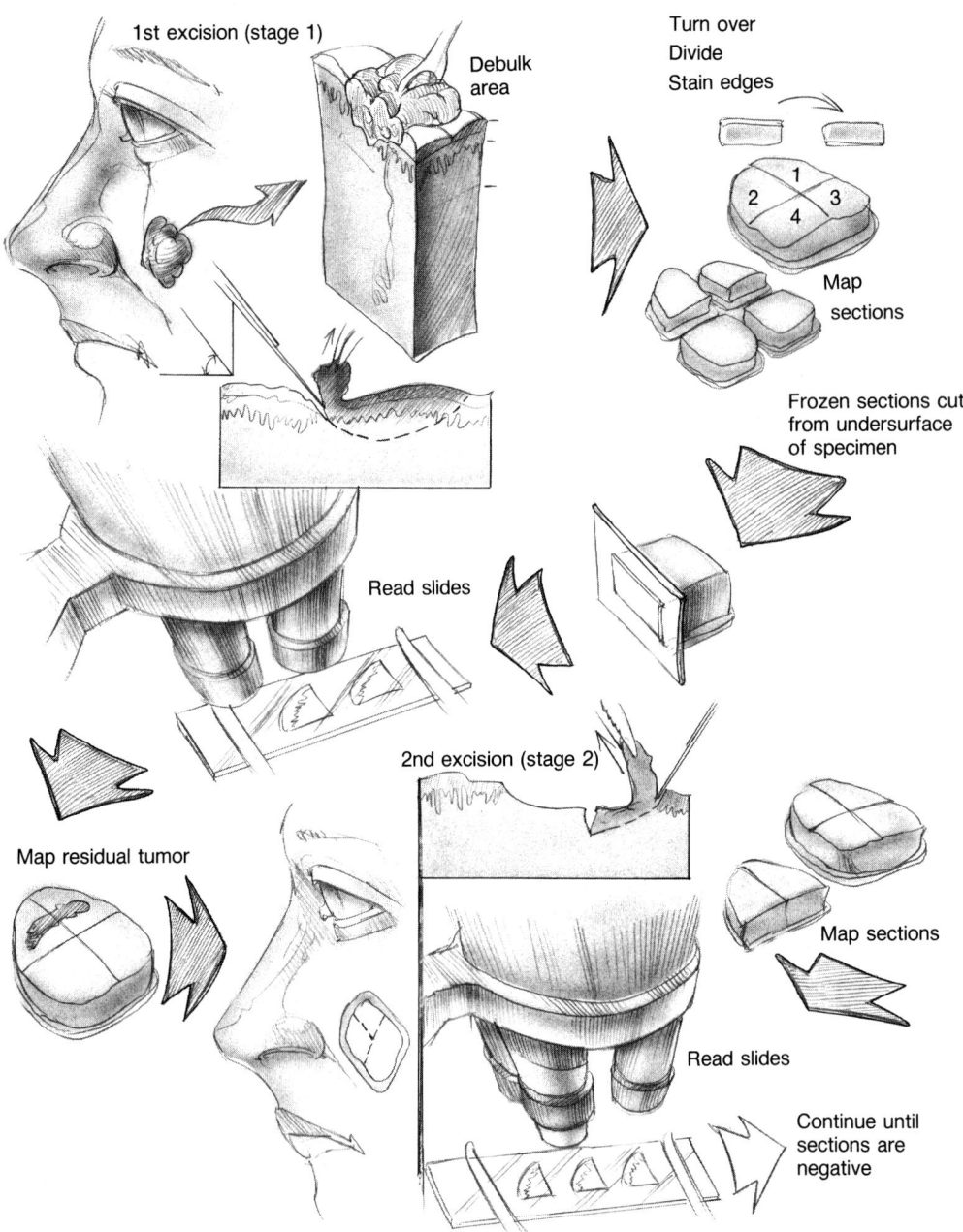

1st excision (stage 1)

Debulk area

Turn over
Divide
Stain edges

Map sections

Frozen sections cut from undersurface of specimen

Read slides

2nd excision (stage 2)

Map sections

Map residual tumor

Read slides

Continue until sections are negative

Figure 105.8 Schema used by micrographic cutaneous tumor excision. (Modified from Mohs FE. Microcontrolled surgery for skin cancer. In: Epstein E, Epstein E, eds. *Skin surgery.* Philadelphia: WB Saunders, 1987:380–381, with permission.)

TABLE 105.3 ℞ **TREATMENT OF BASAL CELL CARCINOMA**

Treatment Method	Success Rate (%)
Electrosurgery	92.6–98.0
Excisional surgery	93.2–95.5
Cryosurgery	94.0–97.0
Radiation surgery	92.1–96.0
Mohs surgery	97.4–99.1

require no reconstruction. Lesions as large as 7 to 8 mm can be resected bloodlessly and are left with a physiologic dressing that heals completely within 10 days, resulting in excellent cosmesis. This method is particularly effective in managing multiple premalignant or potentially malignant lesions in patients with skin cancer.

Palliation of the neglected lesion in the very elderly or debilitated patient whose skin cancer is of less concern than more major health considerations is carried out with alacrity by using the CO_2 laser. These patients often reside in limited-care facilities, and palliation can be directed toward

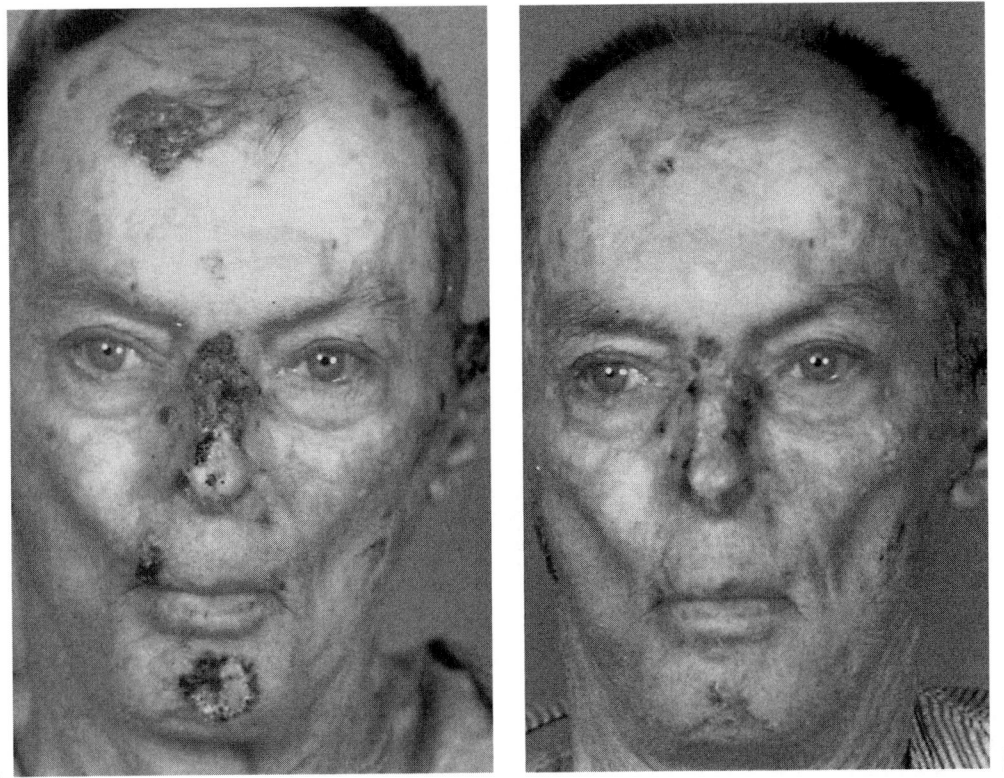

Figure 105.9   A: Multiple basal cell cancers palliated with laser. **B:** Six weeks after laser ablation.

improved nursing care, better patient comfort, and convenience. These goals prompt some type of treatment, although cure may not be realistic or possible (Fig. 105.9). Our approach to management techniques is summarized in Table 105.4.

Surgical Reconstruction

Three fundamental methods exist for managing the defects created by excisional surgery for skin cancer: no reconstruction, immediate repair, or delayed reconstruction. The first alternative is used if the wound is allowed to heal by second intention or is covered by a graft and the subsequent defect not reconstructed. This may be appropriate for patients who are palliated or who for other reasons are not candidates for reconstruction. Other patients may be candidates or better served with a prosthesis. The surgeon's choice is influenced by many factors, such as the general health of the patient and his or her life expectancy. The location and extent of the lesion and the social situation of the patient may play a role in the decisions concerning reconstruction. Large defects are of little concern to some people, but a minimal defect can be devastating to others.

Functional restoration takes precedence over cosmesis if this choice must be made (e.g., reconstruction of the upper lip to ensure a competent oral sphincter before embarking on a nasal reconstruction). Early reconstruction of nasal ala and eyelid defects is of paramount concern because reconstruction after contracture has occurred is rarely satisfactory.

In addition to functional restoration, anatomic, pathologic, and cosmetic considerations influence the surgeon's choice of reconstructive method. Basic to any flap reconstruction is the secondary tissue deficit that, when closed, results in increased tension on the surrounding local tissue. Scar contraction has the potential to distort and create a greater deformity. The use of a skin graft decreases this likelihood by harvesting tissue where an abundance is found, usually some distance from the defect, and substituting this tissue for the resected tumor.

Anatomic considerations control surgical options by imposing constraints such as symmetry, facial landmarks and structures, and the lack of availability of adequate local or adjacent tissue. All flaps create a secondary defect that must be attended to in some manner. This is most often done by primary closure, but the surgeon can use another flap or a graft.

Pathologic considerations influence reconstructive choices. The defects related to certain histologic tumor types might best be covered with a skin graft rather than have potential tumor hidden by a thick flap. Questionable margins are another factor that might prompt a more conservative choice. Tumors located in areas known clinically to be more virulent (e.g., medial canthus, nasal spine, external ear canal) might best not be reconstructed with a

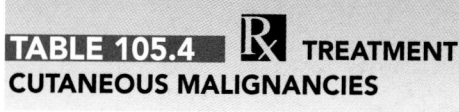

TABLE 105.4 ℞ **TREATMENT**
CUTANEOUS MALIGNANCIES

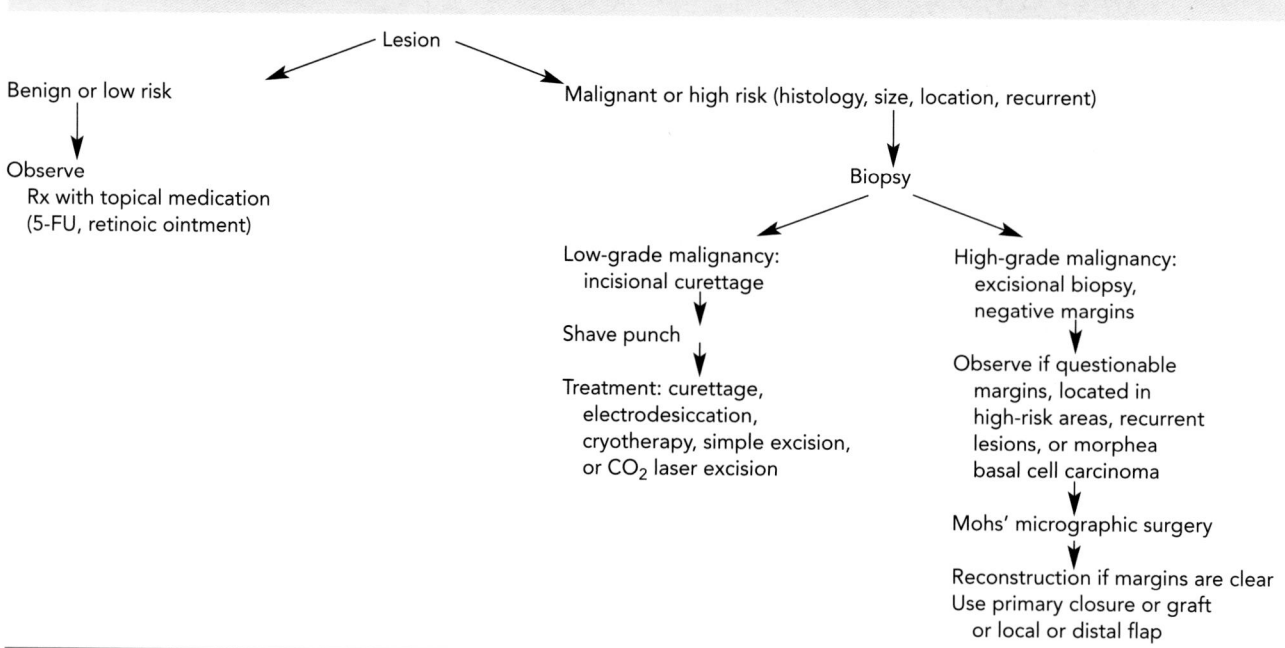

5-FU, 5-fluorouracil.

thick flap. Squamous cell carcinomas of the skin are usually more aggressive and infiltrative than basal cell carcinomas, and this affects their management. An exception to this is the morphea type of basal cell carcinoma, which is infiltrative. Its iceberg-like subdermal extension may make elaborate reconstructive efforts futile and perhaps devastating for the patient. It is wise to defer immediate reconstruction and allow healing by second intention or cover the defect with a skin graft. When the recipient bed has a marginal blood supply, delayed skin grafting is recommended. The wound area is allowed to granulate for 21 days. Then a 1- to 2-mm circumferential strip is removed, followed by cross-hatching of the area. A thick (0.45 to 0.5 mm) split-thickness skin graft is placed. If further reconstruction is needed, it can be undertaken when the patient is confirmed to be tumor free, usually after a period of observation of 1 to 2 years.

Planning Reconstruction

In designing local flap reconstruction, the surgeon must first consider the effects on adjacent tissues and structures. It is essential that the tissue to be moved into the defect is lax and abundant enough to close the surgical void. The donor site also must be closed, usually primarily, without unacceptable consequences to adjacent tissues or structures. Utmost in the surgeon's mind must be the placement of incisions. Closure lines should be in skin creases,

facial structural demarcations, or relaxed skin-tension lines. The tension and direction of maximal pull must not distort, create asymmetry, or result in an unacceptable scar. The ultimate contracture of the resulting scars should not create a deformity.

A review of our surgical cases indicates that the most common management after resection is advancement and primary closure. Obviously, this technique is propitious for most small lesions. For those requiring a more sophisticated form of reconstruction, several reliable reconstructive options exist (Table 105.5). Reconstruction options and techniques are discussed in Chapters 162, 166, and 169.

TABLE 105.5
METHODS OF RECONSTRUCTION

Method	Percentage of Procedures
Midline forehead flap	26
Sliding nasal dorsal flap	24
Perichondrial cutaneous graft	18
Nasolabial flap	15
Other methods	19
Total	100

Data from unpublished series of FJ Stucker.

TABLE 105.6   COMPLICATIONS

CUTANEOUS MALIGNANCIES

Lesion	Diagnosis	Treatment	Closure	Problems or Complications
Superficial basal cell	History of sun exposure, red scaly patches, occasionally central unceration, rolled border	Small: electrodesiccation and curettage, cryosurgery, excisional biopsy	Primary	Lesion recurs; large excision with frozen section or Mohs' surgery
Morphea form basal cell	Macular rough patch, skip lesions, extension down natural facial planes	Resection often to bone, including periosteum, frozen sections of deep layers	Delay reconstruction if margins uncertain	Recurrence common; primary excision should be aggressive; possible role for adjuvant therapy
Squamous cell carinoma	Erythematous and ulcerated patch, usually history of actinic keratosis, friable	Evaluate regional lymph nodes or palpable adenopathy if lesion > 3 cm, perform neck dissection and postoperative irradiation	Local or distant flap or graft	Recurrent and large lesions; requires en bloc excision; may have missed involvement or failure to identify lymph node involvement

COMPLICATIONS

In dealing with facial cutaneous malignancies, the temptation to avoid disfigurement is great (Table 105.6). Unfortunately, this often results in an inadequate excision, dooming the patient to recurrence and quite possibly a much worse prognosis. Perhaps the most important lesson that the Mohs technique has taught us is the insidious behavior of some cutaneous malignancies. Therefore, margins must always be checked and histology confirmed. Questionable margins should not be reconstructed.

What may originally be considered a simple excision is occasionally complicated by positive margins. The surgeon must be flexible. If the patient is under local anesthesia, general anesthesia may be needed. If the patient was not aware of the extent of the resection and subsequent repair, the surgeon should stage the surgery and discuss with the patient what may be involved. In considering reconstruction, function is always more important than cosmesis. The surgeon should avoid designing flaps that adversely affect function (i.e., cheek flap producing ectropion).

Regional nodal metastasis from cutaneous basal cell carinoma is rare, occurring in up to 0.5% of patients (33). Nodal metastasis from cutaneous squamous cell carcinoma occurs in up to 12.5% of patients (34). Thus in dealing with squamous cell carcinoma, regional lymph nodes must be carefully evaluated. Regional nodal metastasis from cutaneous malignancies in the head and neck most frequently involve the parotid nodes, followed by upper cervical nodes. For cutaneous lesions larger than 3 cm, neck dissections or adjuvant therapy should be considered. It is mandatory to monitor all patients with cutaneous malignancies, and biopsies should be performed for suggestive areas. Follow-up of patients with basal cell carcinoma should be every 6 months for 5 years, as in just over one third of patients, a second primary basal cell carcinoma will develop within 5 years. In many patients with skin cancers, constant vigilance is the key to a successful outcome.

> **HIGHLIGHTS**
>
> - Sun exposure is associated with all forms of skin cancer.
> - Unlike other forms of basal cell cancer, the morphea type is particularly difficult to excise because of indistinct margins, skip lesions, and a propensity for deep invasion.
> - De novo squamous cell cancer tends to be far more aggressive locally and metastatically than cancer that develops after actinic changes.
> - Histology, anatomic site, and primary or recurrent status should be considered in managing a cutaneous malignancy.
> - Premalignant and low-grade lesions can be managed with topical chemotherapy (i.e., 5-fluorouracil), electrodesiccation and curettage, or CO_2 laser. All other lesions should be excised with clear margins to maximize success.
> - Consider excising additional tissue to incorporate a complete facial unit if more than one third is involved. This produces a more cosmetic and symmetric repair.
> - If confronted with indistinct deep margins or a high probability of recurrence, consider skin grafting and observation for 6 to 12 months.
> - Planned reconstruction should never limit oncologic resection.
> - If possible, place incisions in a facial crease, hair-bearing areas, junctions of facial units, and parallel to relaxed skin-tension lines.

- Always plan reconstruction from simple to more-complex microvascular patterns: primary closure skin graft > local flap > regional flap > free flap.
- If using a local facial flap, consider the donor site defect and its effect on functional structures (e.g., eyelid, mouth).

REFERENCES

1. Santmyrie BR, Feldman SR, Fleischer AB Jr. Lifestyle high-risk behaviors and demographics may predict the level of participation in sun-protection behaviors and skin cancer primary prevention in the United States: result of the 1998 Nation Health Interview Survey. *Cancer* 2001;92:1315–1324.
2. American Cancer Society. *Cancer facts and figures 2000.* November, 2001; www.cancer.org.
3. Farman J, Gardiner B, Shanklin J. Large losses of total ozone in Antartica reveal seasonal Clx/NOx interaction. *Nature* 1985;315: 207.
4. Cutchis P. Stratospheric ozone depletion and solar ultraviolet radiation on earth. *Science* 1974;184:13.
5. Wagner RF, Casciato DA. Skin cancers. In: Casciato DA, Lowitz BB, eds. *Manual of clinical oncology*, 4th ed. Philadelphia: Lippincott Williams & Wilkins, 2000:336–373.
6. Taylor KS. Unraveling the molecular pathway from sunlight to skin cancer. *Acc Chem Res* 1994;27:76–82.
7. Barr BB, Benton EC, McLaren K, et al. Human papilloma virus infection and skin cancer in renal allograft recipients. *Lancet* 1989;1:124.
8. Eliezri YD, Silverstein SJ, Nuovo GJ. Occurrence of human papillomavirus type 16 DNA in cutaneous squamous and basal cell neoplasms. *J Am Acad Dermatol* 1990;23:836.
9. Smith JL. Pathology of skin tumors of the head and neck. In: Thawley SE, Panje WR, eds. *Comprehensive management of head and neck tumors.* Philadelphia: WB Saunders, 1985:1173.
10. Pinkus H. Premalignant fibroepithelial tumors of the skin. *Arch Dermatol Syph* 1953;67:598–615.
11. Lever WF, Schaumburg-Lever G. *Histopathology of the skin.* Philadelphia: JB Lippincott, 1983.
12. American Joint Committee on Cancer. Carcinoma of the skin (excluding eyelid, vulva, and penis). In: Greene FL, et al., eds. *American Joint Committee on Cancer: staging manual*, 6th ed. New York: Springer, 2002:203–208.
13. Harris TJ. Squamous cell carcinoma. In: Emmett AJJ, O'Rourke MGE, eds. *Malignant skin tumors.* New York: Churchill Livingstone, 1982:67.
14. Jansen GT, Westbrook KC. Cancer of the skin. In: Suen JY, Myers EN, eds. *Cancer of the head and neck.* New York: Churchill Livingstone, 1981:212.
15. Headington JT. Epidermal carcinomas of the integument of the nose and ear. In: Batsakis JG, ed. *Tumors of the head and neck.* Baltimore: Williams & Wilkins, 1979:420.
16. Panje WR, Ceilley RI. The influence of embryology of the midface on the spread of epithelial malignancies. *Laryngoscope* 1979;89: 1914.
17. Mohs FE. Chemosurgery for the microscopically controlled excision of skin cancer. *J Surg Oncol* 1971;3:257–267.
18. Swanson NA. Mohs surgery: technique, indications, applications, and the future. *Arch Dermatol* 1983;119:761.
19. Levine HL, Bailin PL. Basal cell carcinoma of the head and neck: identification of the high risk patient. *Laryngoscope* 1980;90:955.
20. Roenigk RK, Ratz JL, Bailin PL, et al. Trends in the presentation and treatment of basal cell carcinoma. *J Dermatol Surg Oncol* 1986;12:860–865.
21. Jackson R, Adams RH. Horrifying basal cell carcinoma: a study of 33 cases and a comparison with 435 non-horror cases and a report of four metastatic cases. *J Surg Oncol* 1973;5:431.
22. Levine H. Cutaneous carcinoma of the head and neck: management of massive and previously uncontrolled lesions. *Laryngoscope* 1983;93:87.
23. Swanson NA. Basal cell carcinoma: treatment modalities and recommendations. *Prim Care* 1983;10:443.
24. Crissey JT. Curettage and electrodesiccation as a method of treatment for epitheliomas of the skin. *J Surg Oncol* 1971;3:287.
25. Zacarian SA. Cryosurgery of malignant tumors of the skin. In: Epstein E, Epstein E, eds. *Skin surgery.* Philadelphia: WB Saunders, 1987.
26. Carruth JAS, McKenzie AL. Preliminary report of a pilot study of photoradiation therapy for the treatment of superficial malignancies of the skin, head and neck. *Eur J Surg Oncol* 1985;11:47–50.
27. Greenway HT, Cornell RC, Tanner DJ, et al. Treatment of BCC with intralesional interferon. *J Am Acad Dermatol* 1986;15: 437–443.
28. Uede K, Shimakage J, Ohta C, et al. Skin carcinoma successfully treated by interferon (IFN) local injection. In: *Abstracts of the Seventeenth World Congress of Dermatology.* Berlin, 1987;1:358.
29. Swanson NA, Grekin RC, Baker SR. Mohs surgery: techniques, indications, and applications in head and neck surgery. *Head Neck Surg* 1983;6:683.
30. Mohs FE. Chemosurgery: a microscopically uncontrolled method of cancer excision. *Arch Surg* 1941;42:279.
31. Mohs FE. Microcontrolled surgery for skin cancer. In: Epstein E, Epstein E, eds. *Skin surgery.* Philadelphia: WB Saunders, 1987: 280–395.
32. Tromovitch TA, Stegman SJ. Microscopically controlled excision of skin tumors. Chemosurgery (Mohs): fresh tissue technique. *Arch Dermatol* 1974;110:231.
33. Malone JP. Basal cell carcimona metastatic to the parotid: report of a new case and review of the literature. *Ear Nose Throat J* 2000; 79:511.
34. Cherpelis BS, Marcusen C, Lang PG. Prognostic factors for metastasis in squamous cell carcinoma of the skin. *Dermatol Surg* 2002;28:268–273.

Malignant Melanoma 106

Jeffrey N. Myers   *Andrew J. Nemechek*

Community outreach and educational programs have heightened public awareness and resulted in early detection for patients with cutaneous malignant melanoma (CMM). Consequently, 5-year survival rates have improved. However, the incidence of CMM has increased at such an alarming rate that these advances have not translated into lower overall mortality rates. Although traditional staging methods have relied heavily on tumor depth of invasion and size of regional nodes, more recent data on clinicopathologic predictors of treatment outcomes have resulted in the new staging system that incorporates tumor ulceration and depth, the presence of satellitosis and in transit metastases, and the number rather than the size of involved lymph nodes. Work continues that investigates the utility of molecular approaches to staging. Furthermore, results from studies of the various regional staging methods, sentinel lymph node identification, and biopsy have shown the sentinel node status to be the most reliable predictor of treatment outcomes. Surgery with adjuvant postoperative radiation therapy in selected patients has been shown to be extremely effective in achieving locoregional control above the clavicles, but distant failure remains a daunting problem. Systemic adjuvant therapy with high-dose interferon-α has been shown to improve disease-free survival, although it has not been shown to affect overall survival significantly. Data from studies of immunotherapy, chemotherapy, or biochemotherapy for advanced-stage disease are accumulating. However, these have not been proven to increase survival significantly.

We review some of these recent developments in the staging, evaluation, and treatment of CMM and their relevance to the management of CMM of the head and neck region. Mucosal melanomas of the head and neck also are discussed.

EPIDEMIOLOGY

The incidence of melanoma has increased over the past 40-year period and continues to do so at a frightening rate. The number of new cases is increasing approximately 5% annually. Worldwide, more than 50,000 new cases of CMM were diagnosed in 2002. In the United States, the current estimated lifetime risk for developing CMM is 1 in 75 (1). Melanoma is the leading cause of death from malignancies of the skin, accounting for 2% of all cancer deaths in the United States. The number of deaths from CMM has increased 2% annually since 1960. Overall cancer-related survival has increased over the past 20 years. However, survival rates in patients with advanced disease have not changed.

People who are fair in complexion or who have the tendency to sunburn easily, or both, have an increased relative risk of developing malignant melanoma. Head and neck melanomas occur more commonly in men (2:1), with a median age at diagnosis at 55 years, with a range of 12 to 92 years (2). Epidemiologic studies demonstrate higher rates of melanoma in those living in geographic areas that are exposed to intense sunlight (i.e., Australia). This finding and investigations in the laboratory demonstrate that exposure to ultraviolet light plays a major role in the pathogenesis of melanoma, and UV-A and UV-B radiation have both been implicated. This is further supported by the lower rates of melanoma reported in people whose skin natively has more pigmentation. The incidence of melanoma is approximately 10 times higher in whites than in blacks in the same geographic region (3). Although the combined head and neck region accounts for only 9% of body surface area, 15% to 30% of all melanomas arise within the head and neck. Patients with large (larger than 20 cm) congenital nevi at birth, dysplastic nevi, or xeroderma pigmentosa have significantly heightened risk of developing invasive CMM.

CLINICAL PRESENTATION AND DIAGNOSIS

The classic hallmark finding that raises suspicion for malignant melanoma is the presence of a pigmented lesion that changes over a time period of weeks to months. Lesions that change substantially in size or color over time should prompt medical attention. Other features of pigmented lesions, which should alert one to the possibility of a malignant process, include changes in diameter or height, variations in border, color, ulceration, itching, pain, and bleeding (4). Melanomas also may show signs of regression with involution of a primary lesion, which is often manifested by a "halo" lesion with a central area of decreased pigmentation. However, the clinical diagnosis of this disease may not always be straightforward; not all melanomas are pigmented. As many as 10% of melanomas may lack melanin, some may resemble other cutaneous lesions such as basal cell carcinoma, and some tumors may not have a surface component. Patients also may be seen initially with metastasis to cervical lymph nodes with no identifiable primary tumor.

Once a suspicion of melanoma exists, relevant historic factors associated with increased risk of developing this disease should be ascertained. These factors include a history of childhood sun exposure with episodes of severe sunburning and a family history of cutaneous malignancies, including melanomas. Other types of pigmented lesions are important to note as well. These include junctional or acquired nevi that are found in the skin of most adults and are generally smaller than 5 mm. Dysplastic nevi tend to be larger and have irregular borders with variation in color. The identification of a dysplastic nevus should prompt dermatologic evaluation because of an increased risk of developing a malignant melanoma within these lesions.

Melanoma is divided into four distinct clinicopathologic subtypes: lentigo maligna melanoma (LMM), superficial spreading, and nodular and acral lentiginous melanoma. These lesions demonstrate either a radial (intraepithelial) or vertical (intradermal) growth phase or a combination of the two. Radial growth is circumferential in nature and confined to the dermal–epidermal junction. The vertical growth phase (intradermal) demonstrates invasion through the dermal–epidermal junction. The radial growth phase may indicate a lesion's capacity for growth and invasion into the papillary dermis. These lesions may lack metastatic potential. Conversely, cells in the vertical growth phase may represent a clonal change in cells with a growth advantage over neighboring cells, resulting in the clone's ability to invade and metastasize.

Curaneous melanomas may mimic a host of other pathologic cutaneous lesions. Differential diagnosis includes seborrheic keratosis, benign nevi (including junctional, compound, and dermal), hemangioma, blue nevi, pyogenic granuloma, and pigmented basal cell carcinoma. Lentigo maligna, LM, also known as melanoma in situ, is a premalignant pigmented lesion that frequently develops in the head and neck region of elderly patients. Known historically as Hutchinson melanotic freckle, these lesions are associated with solar skin damage and feature atypical melanocytes, which spread radially along the dermal–epidermal junction, exhibit focal nesting, and occasionally extend along skin appendages into the dermis.

Up to 5% of LMs or melanomas in situ progress to invasive LMM. LMM lesions should be excised with 0.5-cm margins, although prediction of tumor margins can prove difficult. This is the least common type of cutaneous melanoma and accounts for between 6% and 10% of melanoma lesions. Its growth is characterized by a slow radial phase that may take up to 10 years to progress. At first, they are quite slow to invade deeply, and affected patients have a better prognosis when compared with those with other forms of melanoma.

Superficial spreading melanoma represents the most common type of melanoma and comprises between 65% and 75% of cases. These lesions may demonstrate a wide variety of colors, including pink, blue–gray, brown, tan, and black. They also may demonstrate radial growth for 5 to 7 years and then become invasive, an event frequently heralded by ulceration and bleeding. High cure rates have been reported when these lesions are clinically detected in the radial growth phase. Spontaneous regression of superficial spreading melanomas also has been reported.

Acral lentiginous is the most common type of melanoma seen in the African-American population. Because these lesions commonly occur on the soles of the feet, surfaces of the hand, and oral/anogenital mucosa, they are less commonly encountered by head and neck surgeons.

Nodular melanoma comprises between 10% and 15% of all melanomas and may affect areas of both exposed and non–sun-exposed areas of the skin. They tend to develop in patients older than 50 years. Nodular melanoma is considered to be the most invasive of the cutaneous melanomas, and affected patients have the poorest prognosis.

When a patient's skin lesion is suggestive of malignant melanoma by both history and physical examination, biopsy is performed. The prognostic importance of lesion ulceration is discussed later. The clinician should document clearly the presence or absence of ulceration *before* biopsy. The technique for obtaining tissue for pathologic analysis has been the subject of considerable debate. A properly performed biopsy not only establishes a diagnosis but also provides critical prognostic data and assists in formulating a specific treatment plan. The type of biopsy is dictated by factors such as the size of the lesion and its anatomic location in relation to vital structures in the head, face, and neck. The site of origin of a primary melanoma in the head and neck also can be of prognostic significance itself, because lesions of the scalp and neck are associated with a worse prognosis than are melanomas of the face. Excisional biopsies are the favored technique to obtain tissue for diagnosis, and several studies have demonstrated an association between decreased survival and incisional or manipulative biopsies (5). Excision is performed with a narrow margin of normal-appearing tissue and should include subcutaneous fat for complete evaluation of the depth.

After excision, the specimen is oriented and discussed with the pathologist. If the lesion's size or other anatomic or cosmetic constraints preclude excision, incisional and punch biopsy techniques are acceptable alternatives. Both should sample the most representative portion of the lesion. Punch biopsy may include sampling the most raised area of the lesion or an area with the most pigmentation. Lesions with variable heights, colors, and borders may require biopsies of multiple areas to be performed for accurate and proper diagnosis. Traditional stains such as hematoxylin–eosin are used. The immunohistochemical stains S-100, HMB-45, and melan-A have helped standardize pathologic evaluataion of cutaneous lesions. Fine-needle aspiration, curettage, and shave techniques have no role in evaluation of suspected invasive melanoma, as they are inadequate in providing precise information regarding the depth of invasion. It should also be clearly stated that the initial excisional biopsy with negative margins is not considered adequate therapy for invasive melanoma but does allow reexcision with the opportunity to perform lymphatic mapping and sentinel lymph node biopsy (SLNB) at the time of reexcision.

MUCOSAL MELANOMA

Noncutaneous mucosal melanomas are relatively rare lesions, representing only 2% of all head and neck melanomas. More than 50% of reported cases arise within the nasal cavity. Other affected areas include the paranasal sinuses, nasopharynx, oral cavity, and oropharynx. Esophageal mucosa also may be affected. Nasal obstruction is the most common presenting symptom for sinonasal lesions. However, a significant number of mucosal melanomas may be asymptomatic until they have progressed to an advanced stage, which contributes to the poor prognosis of patients with this diagnosis. Stern and colleagues (6) at the M.D. Anderson Cancer Center found an average of 9 months between the first onset of symptoms and physician intervention. The differential diagnosis includes vascular lesions, angiomas, and dental amalgam tattoos. Biopsy is confirmatory. Anatomic constraints frequently preclude the use of excisional biopsy techniques in most patients with mucosal melanoma. Immunohistochemistry also can be helpful in making the correct diagnosis, as mucosal melanomas demonstrate staining characteristics similar to those of their cutaneous counterparts. It is not uncommon for the characteristic melanosis to be absent in mucosal melanoma lesions. Ascertaining the depth of invasion is not necessary in mucosal melanomas because it has little or no prognostic impact for these tumors. Desmoplastic variants of mucosal melanoma have been described in the head and neck (7).

Wide excision of mucosal melanoma is the mainstay of therapy. Radiotherapy in the adjuvant setting also is suggested, but its benefits have not been proven, and recent work in mutiple centers has studied its role (8,9). Patients may experience multiple local recurrences and ultimately die of a combination of uncontrolled local and distant disease. Patients with lesions confined to the nasal cavity exhibit improved survival when compared with those with lesions in the oral cavity, and 5-year overall survival rates range between 10% and 45%. The development of distant metastasis is an ominous sign. Most patients in whom distant metastases develop concurrently have local recurrence, and most die of their disease.

DESMOPLASTIC MELANOMA

Desmoplastic melanoma is a histologic variant of melanoma that accounts for fewer than 1% of melanoma cases overall. However, as many as 75% of these tumors occur in the head and neck region. Clinically, desmoplastic melanomas may be amelanotic, a feature that impedes early recognition and leads to significant delays in diagnosis and treatment. Another important characteristic feature of these lesions is their neurotropism. This predisposes them to perineural invasion and spread that often accounts for local recurrence despite histologically "negative margins." Therefore it is suggested that wider resection margins be taken around a desmoplastic tumor and that adjuvant radiation is often recommended after definitive excision. The rates of regional metastasis are lower than those for conventional melanomas of comparable tumor thickness, and the biologic behavior of a particular desmoplastic lesion may be dependent on several histopathologic variations (10). Therefore regional therapy, such as lymph node dissection, is usually not advocated for stage I or II disease (11). The role of sentinel lymph node mapping in the management of desmoplastic melanomas has not yet been determined.

PRIMARY TUMOR STAGING

The staging of malignant melanoma has evolved over the past half century in efforts to determine more reliably a patient's prognosis and to identify the most appropriate treatment schemes. Clark and Breslow made significant contributions to the microscopic staging of melanoma. Clark (12) described five categories known as the Clark levels of invasion. They denote the deepest microscopic anatomic level penetrated by a melanoma. In the Breslow staging system (13), the maximum thickness of melanomas is used as a prognostic indicator.

In the past 25 years, much controversy has surfaced regarding melanoma staging and its importance in clinical decision making. Investigators at the M.D. Anderson Cancer Center studying historical staging parameters correlated clinical outcomes with clinicopathologic criteria and proposed a new staging system. The American Joint Committee on Cancer (AJCC) has incorporated many of these recommendations in the current staging for CMM (14,15). This staging method is based on evaluation of the primary tumor, regional metastasis (satellites, in-transit, and lymph node disease), and presence/location of distant metastasis.

Evaluation of the primary tumor is based on the lesion thickness measured from the granular cell layer to the deepest point of invasion. The importance of ulceration of the primary lesion also is denoted in the new T classification. In addition, the AJCC noted that discrepancies between tumor thickness and Clark level are settled in favor of the least favorable T stage. Approximately 75% of patients with melanoma of the head and neck have intermediate-thickness lesions (0.75 to 4.0 mm). Although cutoff points for T stage have traditionally been 0.75, 1.50, and 4.0 mm, Balch and others found that T stages based on depths of invasion of 1.0, 2.0, and 4.0 mm are easier to use and more accurate, and these are reflected in the latest update of the AJCC staging system (16,17).

REGIONAL NODAL STAGING

Evaluation for regional metastasis relies on both physical examination and complementary imaging studies. In the head and neck, lateralized tumors may drain into the primary echelon nodal basins, including preauricular, parotid, postauricular, suboccipital, posterior cervical, anterior cervical (external or internal jugular), and supraclavicular nodal groups. Nodal drainage basins in the head and neck are less predictable when compared with trunk and extremity sites. Although some areas on the scalp, face, and ears may have predictable lymphatic drainage, bilateral or contralateral metastases are not uncommon, and ambiguous drainage patterns can be seen in up to 55% of patients. Posterior scalp lesions may have lymphatic drainage to the suboccipital and postauricular basins as well. Recent studies using preoperative and intraoperative lymphoscintigraphic methods have helped to define further the patterns of lymphatic drainage in primary melanomas of the head and neck region (18).

The risk of regional metastasis varies directly with tumor thickness. Those measuring less than 0.75 mm demonstrate virtually no risk. Those measuring between 0.76 and 1.49 mm have a 25% risk of regional metastasis. Lesions 1.5 to 3.9 mm in greatest thickness have up to a 60% risk of regional metastasis. Those measuring larger than 4 mm in thickness have a greater than 65% incidence of regional metastasis. When physical examination reveals palpable lymphadenopathy, computed tomography (CT) or magnetic resonance imaging (MRI) is often used to determine the number and extent of cervical metastases. Buzaid et al. (19) showed that the number of lymph nodes involved with regional metastases is more predictive of treatment outcomes than is the size of lymph nodes harboring metastatic disease.

Complete staging for distant metastases is critical in patients with melanoma. Serologic studies, including liver-function tests and CT of the brain, chest, and abdomen, are recommended. Other imaging modalities also are used. These include positron emission tomography (PET) and coregistered PET-CT. [^{18}F]2-Fluoro-2-deoxy-D-glucose (FDG) is used as an analogue of glucose metabolism. Typically, melanoma cells are highyly FDG-avid. To date, PET and PET-CT have not been used to diagnose malanoma. However, their usefulness in detecting regional and distant disease has been demonstrated (20). Their sensitivity is limited by tumor volume (21).

Lymphoscintigraphy may provide an adjunctive method of defining the pathways of regional metastasis. It may be particularly helpful when the primary tumor is located in the midline (scalp, forehead) and has potential bilateral drainage, including one or both parotid glands. As stated, the most important factor in survival in patients with head and neck melanoma is the presence or absence of lymph node metastasis. When palpable lymphadenopathy is present, fine-needle aspiration biopsy can often be used to confirm the metastasis. Once the presence of lymph node involvement by tumor is confirmed, a therapeutic lymph node dissection is recommended.

Detection of Occult Nodal Disease

The evaluation and treatment for occult regional metastasis is perhaps the most controversial aspect of the management of CMM of the head and neck (22). Patients with lesions of less than 1 mm in depth and Clark level less than IV who do not have palpable lymphadenopathy are most often observed. For those patients having lesions more than 1 mm in depth or Clark level IV or V, several options exist to determine the pathologic nodal status.

The rationale for the determination of nodal status is to identify patients who would benefit from regional therapy with surgery or radiation therapy or both to improve local regional control and to identify patients at greater risk for systemic recurrence who could potentially benefit from systemic adjuvant therapy. Imaging methods such as ultrasound, CT, and MRI may slightly increase the sensitivity in detecting regional metastases over palpation alone. They are still not completely reliable in distinguishing regional metastatic disease from reactive adenopathy. The Centers for Medicare and Medicaid Services guidelines approve FDG-PET for the intial staging and restaging of melanoma.

Elective Lymph Node Dissection

Another technique to identify occult regional metastatic disease is elective lymph node dissection (ELND) (22). The use of ELND in the management of patients with CMM of intermediate thickness or thicker lesions has been frequently debated. This debate has largely waned since the prospective, multiinstitutional randomized trial led by The Intergroup Melanoma Surgical Trial that compared ELND with observation for stage I and II melanomas from all regions of the body (23). This study found no survival benefit to ELND except in patients younger than 60 years or those who had lesions 1 to 2 mm in depth. Whether ELND can help improve survival by identifying those with occult disease who might benefit from systemic adjuvant trials has not been resolved (24). The development of SLNB may enhance the sensitivity and specificity of ELND or could replace it in the assessment of regional metastatic disease in patients with CMM of the head and neck region (25).

Sentinel Lymph Node Identification and Biopsy

For patients with CMM below the clavicles, sentinel lymph node mapping and biopsy has been the most important advance in the evaluation and treatment of patients (26). Studies of this method continue. Its ultimate role in head and neck surgical oncology remains to be determined by further investigation (27).

Seminal work by Dr. Donald Morton (28) hypothesized that, within each nodal basin, an orderly progression of lymphatic drainage is found from a first-echelon or sentinel node to nodes of lower echelons. If one can identify the sentinel lymph node in a basin at risk for spread from a melanoma and find it to be free of metastasis, then the remainder of nodes in that basin should also be free of metastatic tumor. This concept has been subsequently supported in a number of trials for non–head and neck CMM, and this has led to the wide practice of this technique as a staging method to determine whether further regional or systemic therapy may be beneficial.

Numerous techniques for intraoperative localization and mapping have been described. These include intraoperative identification of sentinel lymph nodes by their blue color after preexcisional injection of the primary site with isosulfan blue dye or use of a handheld gamma probe to find nodes that take up a radioactive colloid tracer or both. Gershenwald et al. (29) reported the results of a multiinstitutional study using lymphatic mapping for stage I and II melanoma patients. The status of the sentinel nodes was found to be the strongest predictor of disease-free survival. Further, the study concluded that nodal status helps to stratify patients for whom adjuvant therapy is not indicated.

An additional benefit of SLNB is that it can focus a more extensive evaluation of lymph nodes at risk for subclinical metastases. Workers at the M.D. Anderson Cancer Center have shown that analysis of serial sections of a sentinel lymph node can increase the sensitivity in detection of nodal metastases, thereby improving the selection of patients who receive regional and systemic treatment (30). The use of frozen sections for evaluation of a sentinel lymph node is controversial because false negatives have been reported. Additional studies that can be used to evaluate the sentinel node include S-100, HMB-45, melan-AS-100, and more recently, the reverse transcriptase polymerase chain reaction (rt-PCR).

The role of SLNB continues to be refined in the management of CMM of the head and neck region. The complexity of lymphatic drainage patterns and the frequent need to remove sentinel lymph nodes from the parotid gland, placing the facial nerve at risk, have made head and neck surgical oncologists somewhat slow to adapt this method. Multiple centers have reviewed their experience with lymphatic mapping by using preoperative lymphoscintigraphy and intraoperative blue-dye localization and a handheld gamma probe (30,31). The low false-negative rate of lymphatic mapping lends further support for the use of this method for staging the regional lymphatics (32).

Data from these studies suggest that lymphatic mapping by using the combination of blue dye and a handheld gamma probe is an effective method for ruling out regional metastases in patients with melanoma and may be a particularly good method for identifying patients who might benefit from systemic adjuvant therapy. However, several arguments exist against the use of lymphatic mapping for melanoma in the head and neck region.

O'Brien et al. (17), at the Sydney Melanoma Unit, pointed out some limitations of lymphatic mapping in the treatment of head and neck melanoma in a study of 97 patients who underwent lymphoscintigraphy. These authors found a high rate (34%) of disagreement between clinically predicted lymphatic drainage pathways in the head and neck region and the pathways found on the basis of lymphoscintigraphy. Their analysis also revealed a large number of sentinel lymph nodes for each patient—only 13 patients had a single sentinel node. Thirty-three patients had two sentinel nodes, three had three sentinel nodes, 15 had four sentinel nodes, and six had five sentinel nodes, indicating the complexity of lymphatic mapping in the head and neck region. These authors also reported difficulty in the operative identification of all sentinel lymph nodes found on lymphoscintigraphy. In addition, the rate of regional failure was 25% among 16 patients found to have histologically negative sentinel nodes. Furthermore, identification of sentinel lymph nodes may frequently require extensive dissection in multiple areas of the neck and parotid gland. The utility of frozen section at the time of SLNB is dependent on the surgical pathologist (33). Adverse reacctions to isosulfan blue also are reported (34). Despite these concerns, the use of SLNB has continued to expand in the evaluation and treatment of patients with mailgnant melanoma (35,36).

TREATMENT: PRIMARY RESECTION

After a thorough preoperative workup that includes staging of the primary lesion and evaluation for regional and distant metastasis, therapeutic options are discussed with the patient. Surgical resection has been the mainstay of therapy in the treatment of primary cutaneous melanoma in the head and neck. Treatment includes resection of the primary melanoma or previous biopsy site with a rim of normal-appearing tissue surrounding it. The minimal resection margin necessary for adequate resection has been the topic of debate. Historically, 5-cm excision margins were suggested, based on the propensity of melanomas to recur in areas adjacent to the primary site, although no survival advantages could be shown. Based on subsequent retrospective analyses, it was suggested that narrower resection margins might be appropriate for thin or intermediate-thickness lesions (37). Recent randomized trials concluded that local and regional control rates and survival were not different when excisions with large (5-cm) margins and those using more conservative (2-cm) margins were compared (38).

In a collaborative review, investigators at the University of Texas M.D. Anderson Cancer Center and the Moffett Cancer Center found no increase in local recurrence rates or worse survival rates in patients when thick primary melanomas (larger than 4 mm) were excised with a margin of 10 mm or less (39).

The current recommendations for adequate resection margins include the following (each dependent on anatomic and cosmetic constraints):

    in situ, 0.5 cm
    1 to 2 mm, 1.0 cm
    2 to 4 mm, 2.0 cm
    >4 mm, >2 cm

Frequently, in the head and neck, proximity of structures such as the eyes, nose, ears, and circumoral anatomy effectively limits the borders for excision. Excisions are carried out in a full-thickness fashion down to underlying fascia such that all margins, including those that are deeply invaded, may be effectively evaluated. Significant controversy exists regarding the use of frozen section for evaluation and diagnosis. Zitelli et al. (40) and other Mohs surgeons have reported that frozen sections of analysis for surgical margins of melanoma had sensitivity and specificity of 100% and 90%, respectively. However, many dermatopathologists believe that the use of frozen sections is inadequate to distinguish the margins of pigmented lesions. Therefore we recommend control of margins by permanent-section pathologic analysis and often delay reconstruction until margin analysis has been completed. Methods of reconstruction after resection for melanoma are beyond the scope of this chapter. However, most lesions can be enclosed either primarily with the use of local advancement flaps or with the use of skin-grafting techniques. Skin grafting may allow closer surveillance for earlier detection of recurrent disease.

LYMPHADENECTOMY: THERAPEUTIC NECK DISSECTION AND PAROTIDECTOMY

For patients with clinically positive lymph nodes, neck dissection is indicated. However, the extent of neck dissection remains an area of controversy but ranges from removal of gross disease by selective lymphadenectomy to radical neck dissection and its modifications. Studies from Memorial Sloan Kettering Cancer Center, the Melanoma Unit in Sydney, Australia, and Duke University have investigated the effect of neck dissection on outcome for patients with melanoma (17,24). Shah and colleagues (41) concluded that in the presence of clinically positive lymph nodes, a comprehensive neck dissection should be carried out. The type of neck dissection was tailored to the site of the primary tumor. For instance, in patients with melanomas of the face, ear, and anterior scalp, dissection of the parotid gland and lymph node levels I through IV was carried out. Patients with lesions in the postauricular and posterior scalp and neck required dissections of levels II through V. A complete discussion as to type and technique of neck dissection can be found elsewhere in this text.

RADIOTHERAPY

Like many issues important to the treatment of malignant melanoma, radiotherapy, both as the primary modality of therapy and in the adjuvant setting, has sparked much controversy in the past century. Conflicting reports as to its efficacy included investigators unabashedly stating that malignant melanoma cells were radioresistant. However, ground-breaking work by Barranco et al. (42) found that cultured malignant melanoma cells differ from other types of tumor cells in their radiosensitivity. The observed radioresistance of melanoma could be overcome by increasing the individual dose fraction. These studies have helped form the basis for clinical practice, and subsequent studies helped to determine the ideal fraction size and total therapeutic dose that effectively treats melanoma.

Radiotherapy is not generally recommended for the primary treatment of CMM. However, in some exceptional circumstances, its use is advocated. In patients who are poor candidates for surgical resection, radiotherapy may offer an acceptable alternative. For those patients with extensive facial LM melanoma that precludes adequate surgical resection based on cosmetic considerations, radiotherapy can serve as an excellent alternative.

Radiotherapy has been shown to be very effective in the postoperative adjuvant setting in achieving high rates of locoregional control in patients with high-risk CMM of the head and neck region. In prospective nonrandomized clinical trials carried out at The University of Texas M.D. Anderson Cancer, three subgroups of patients were studied (43,44). The first group had primary lesions larger than 1.5 mm or had lesions extending to Clark level IV or V and received elective radiation after a wide local resection. The second group had palpable lymphadenopathy and received radiation in the adjunctive setting after excision of primary lesions coupled with a therapeutic neck dissection (selective or modified radical). The last group of patients underwent radiation after therapeutic neck dissection for regionally recurrent melanoma. Radiotherapy was delivered in five fractions of 6 Gy, twice weekly, to a total dose of 30 Gy. For 174 patients, in only six patients did recurrence develop above the clavicles, whereas in 58 patients, distant metastases developed. The 5-year survival rate was 47%, and the locoregional control rate was 88% for all patients. The 5-year survival rate of the first group of patients was strongly influenced by thickness of the primary lesion. Patients in groups 2 and 3 with fewer than three involved lymph nodes at the time of neck dissection had significantly higher survival rates than did those with three or more involved lymph nodes. Patients with stage I/II melanoma widely excised who received adjuvant radiotherapy had an 89% regional control rate achieved at both 5 and 10 years (45). Additionally, recent studies have confirmed the efficacy of postoperative radiotherapy in controlling regional disease in patients who have undergone therapeutic neck dissection for clinically apparent cervical metastasis (46).

In summary, patients whose primary lesions measure 1.5 mm or greater or are ulcerated should be considered for radiotherapy to the primary site or regional nodal basins or both. Patients with regional metastasis should be offered radiotherapy after excision of primary tumor and neck dissection. Additionally, patients with primary melanomas that demonstrate neurotropism (desmoplastic type) should be considered for radiotherapy after excision. Controversy remains regarding the use of lymphatic mapping and SLNB in an effort to guide the use of regional radiotherapy in the absence of a formal neck dissection.

SYSTEMIC THERAPY

Two major indications exist for systemic therapy in management of patients with CMM. The first indication is the *adjuvant* treatment of patients who have completed locoregional therapy and have no evidence of local, regional, or systemic disease but who are thought to be at high risk for systemic relapse. The second indication for systemic treatment is the presence of distant metastases. A number of systemic therapy options are available to treat patients with either of these indications, including single-agent or multiple-agent chemotherapy, biochemotherapy, or strategies using immune modulation.

A number of clinical studies have been designed to evaluate the role of systemic adjuvant therapies for patients who have completed locoregional treatment and who are believed to be at high risk for the development of distant metastatic disease. Although no universal definition exists for the high-risk patient, a number of studies have accrued patients with primary lesions that are ulcerated lesions, more than 4 mm in depth or Clark level IV, or those patients with satellitosis, in-transit disease, or nodal metastases.

Interferon

Interferon-α is one of the most well-studied agents for the systemic adjuvant therapy of CMM arising from all sites (47,48). However, it has yet to be shown unequivocally to improve overall survival for these patients. The interferons are a family of proteins that have both immunostimulatory and antiangiogenic activity and have excellent preclinical antitumor activity in a number of systems. Interferons enhance phagocytosis and free radical production in macrophages and increase activity of natural killer cells. A prospective, randomized, clinical trial of high-dose interferon-α in the treatment of patients with high-risk melanoma was conducted by the Eastern Cooperative Oncology Group (47). High-risk patients were given high-dose interferon alfa-2b, 20 MU/m^2/day intravenously for 4 weeks. This was followed by 10 MU/m^2/day, administered subcutaneously, 2 days weekly for the remainder of the year. Increases of prolonged survival of 2.8 to 3.8 years were observed, and the recurrence-free survival ranged from 1 month to 1.7 years. The survival advantages were statistically significant in patients with regional lymph node metastasis. Most patients experienced significant toxicity that included chills, fevers, myalgias, and other constitutional symptoms including fatigue and anorexia. A follow-up trial of high- and low-dose interferon alfa-2b in high-risk melanoma, E1690, was recently reported by the Intergroup (48). This study did not confirm the earlier improvement in overall survival but did demonstrate a dose-dependent improvement in 5-year recurrence-free survival rates from 35% to 44%. Finally, Kirkwood and co-workers (49) reported their experience comparing high-dose interferon alfa-2b and GM-2 ganglioside vaccine for patients with resected-melanoma.

Tumor Vaccination

Vaccination is another widely studied strategy for systemic adjuvant therapy of the high-risk melanoma patient, and a variety of different immunization approaches has been used. These studies are predicated on several clinical observations and lines of basic investigation that indicate that the immune system can eradicate melanoma cells and that immune stimulation can overcome immune tolerance to tumor antigens to enhance the immune surveillance of tumor cells. Although a comprehensive review of available vaccine strategies is beyond the scope of this chapter, some of the more encouraging studies are discussed. Ganglioside GM2, an antigen overexpressed by many melanoma cells, given in combination with bacille Calmette-Guérin (BCG) or other immune adjuvants, was developed by Dr. Alan Haughton and colleagues at Memorial Sloan Kettering Cancer Center and has had promising results in clinical trials (50).

Investigators at the John Wayne Cancer Center have developed a polyvalent melanoma cell vaccine capable of inducing humoral and cell-mediated immune responses to melanoma-specific antigens. This is currently undergoing evaluation in a phase III randomized study. Other cancer vaccines have been identified by Dr. Steven Rosenberg and co-investigators at the surgery branch of the National Cancer Institute by using specific peptide antigens recognized by autologous tumor-specific T-cell clone reactivity. These peptide vaccines are most often administered with cytokine or cellular immune adjuvants such as dendritic cells. The results of SWOG trial 9035 using an allogenic vaccine protocol have been reported (51). DiFronzo et al. (52) demonstrated that enhanced humoral responses in patients treated with polyvalent vaccines resulted in limited but improved disease-free survival. It is difficult to advocate any of the current vaccine strategies over another. Therefore, we recommend that patients with high-risk melanoma be enrolled into prospective trials to test these adjuvant therapeutic strategies.

Another approach to adjuvant therapy has been evaluated by the Melanoma Medical Oncology Service at M.D. Anderson. This approach includes the use of biochemotherapy in which conventional chemotherapeutic drugs are combined with the biologically active agents interferon-α and interleukin-2 (IL-2). Currently, biochemotherapy is being compared with high-dose interferon-α alone in a prospective randomized trial at that institution (53).

Systemic Therapy for Metastatic Disease

The prognosis of patients with metastatic melanoma is poor; those with liver, brain, or bone metastasis have a median survival of only 3 to 4 months. Chemotherapy using single-agent dacarbazine (DTIC) or combinations such as bis(2-chloroethyl)nitrosourea (BCNU), cisplatin, lomustine, and hydroxyurea has been reported. The trials comparing DTIC alone or in combination with other agents have shown a significant though brief improvement in survival. The combination of DTIC with cisplatin and vinblastine,

CVD, has been given along with interferon-α and IL-2 either simultaneously or sequentially as biochemotherapy for patients with metastatic melanoma. In 114 patients with stage IV disease who received either sequential or concurrent bichemotherapy, a complete response rate of 21% and a partial response rate of 39% have been obtained, with a prolongation in survival over CVD alone from 9 to 13 months (54).

Based on the immunoresponsiveness of melanoma, Atkins and colleagues (54) treated several hundred patients with metastatic melanoma with high-dose bolus recombinant IL-2 since September 1985 and found a complete response rate of 7% with 10% partial responses. Of the 10 patients who had complete responses, eight had durable responses. The determinants of response to this toxic form of treatment have not been identified at this point, which has made widespread application of this form of treatment impractical. Current studies are focused on the use of IL-2 given with melanoma peptide antigens or melanoma-specific in vitro expanded autologous tumor-infiltrating lymphocytes. A combination of systemic therapies such as interferon alfa-2b, IL-2 cisplatin, dacarbazine, and tamoxifen also has been reported to have activity in patients with metastatic disease (55). Nevertheless, given the overall poor performance of agents in this cohort of patients, continued basic and translational research is warranted to identify active agents for these unfortunate patients. Preemptive strategies are also being developed. Because a majority of patients with CMM have some identifiable risk factor (i.e., sun exposure), chemoprevention using carotenoids and inhibitors of cyclooxygenase-2 (COX-2), vascular endothelial growth factor (VEGF) receptor, and cytochrome P-450 are actively being investigated (56). Outcomes of this work are much anticipated.

SURVEILLANCE

With the rapidly increasing rate of melanoma worldwide, the importance of surveillance of even benign-appearing lesions is understood. The importance of dermatologic evaluation, photo documentation, and close follow-up cannot be overstated. In patients with a diagnosed malignant melanoma, between 55% and 70% of recurrences appear within the first 2 years of therapy, and up to 80% of recurrences will be diagnosed in the first 3 years after treatment. Those with regional metastasis at presentation may have clinically evident tumor recurrences within 24 months. The time to recurrence also correlates with primary tumor thickness, ulcerations, and increasing patient age. Physical examination, liver-function serology, and chest radiography will detect most of these recurrences; therefore, routine screening with CT of the head, chest, and abdomen is not recommended. The utility of PET or PET-CT imaging for the surveillance of affected patients is

TABLE 106.1

RECOMMENDED GUIDELINES FOR THE SURVEILLANCE OF PATIENTS WHO HAVE NO EVIDENCE OF DISEASE AFTER TREATMENT FOR CMM

Stage	Examination	Imaging and Laboratory Tests	Interval
Melanoma in situ	Skin survey		12 mo
Stages I and II			
<4 mm	Skin survey	Chest x-ray, LDH	6 mo for 2 yr; then 12 mo
≥4 mm	Nodes		4 mo for 2 yr; then 12 mo
Stage III	Skin survey Nodes	CXR, LDH, CBC	Every 3 mo for 2 yr; then 6 mo for 5 yr
Stage IV (NED)	Skin survey Nodes	CXR, LDH, CBS	Every 3 mo for 2 yr; then 6 mo for 5 yr

CMM, cutaneous malignant melanoma; LDH; lactase dehydrogenase; CXR, chest x-ray; CBC, complete blood count; NED, no evidence of disease.

being investigated. Additionally, the prospect of using specific serum screening tools such as tyrosinase mRNA detected by rt-PCR is both clinically exciting and ethically challenging (57). The National Cancer Institute has reported a consensus statement on the follow-up evaluation of patients with early melanoma. Most patients without a family history and no atypical nevi should have follow-up evaluations every 6 months for the first 2 years. Thereafter, yearly follow-up is appropriate. Those with a family history or atypical nevi are followed up every 3 months. The guidelines in Table 106.1 have been recommended for the surveillance of patients who have no evidence of disease after treatment for CMM (58).

CONCLUSION

The incidence and mortality rate of CMM are rapidly increasing worldwide. Features of the history and physical examination that are suggestive of malignant melanoma include changes in size or color, sensation of the lesion, and variations in color and margin surface. The presence of ulceration also is quite important. When a suggestive lesion is encountered, excisional biopsy is performed that includes subcutaneous fat for complete evaluation of lesion depth. Biopsy techniques that do not evaluate depth, such as fine-needle aspiration and curettage, have no role in evaluation in suspected melanoma. Once invasive melanoma is diagnosed, histologic type is assessed, and lesion thickness is

established. Tumor thickness (Breslow) and level of invasion (Clark) are prognostically important. Staging in relation to the presence of regional and distant metastasis is established by physical examination, liver-function serology, and chest radiograph in stage I and II disease. Additionally, imaging of the head, chest, and abdomen is recommended for patients with stage III and IV disease.

Lymphoscintigraphy provides an adjunctive method of identifying sentinel lymph nodes and defining routes of lymphatic spread, especially in patients with primary tumors located in the midline that have predicted drainage basins that are ambiguous or include both parotid glands. After staging, a treatment strategy is formulated. For melanomas less than 1 mm in thickness and with no evidence of regional metastasis, surgical excision is carried out with close surveillance thereafter. Current recommendations for adequate resection margins, dependent on anatomic constraints, range from 0.5 to larger than 2 cm, depending on the thickness of the primary lesion. For patients with lesions more than 1 mm thick and for ulcerated lesions without regional metastasis, excision is offered, along with a procedure to assess the status of the regional lymph node, such as SLNB. Once SLNB is performed, serial sectioning of the lymph node(s) with immunohistochemical evaluation is carried out on histologically negative sentinel nodes to increase the sensitivity of pathologic identification of metastases.

In patients with regional lymph nodes that are found to be pathologically positive, radiotherapy is offered. Dosages of 6 Gy are delivered twice weekly over 2.5 weeks to a total of 30 Gy. In addition, patients with ulcerated lesions or those with lesions larger than 1.5 mm or with Clark level IV who do not undergo ELND or SLNB are recommended to receive adjuvant radiotherapy. Patients with clinically positive lymph nodes should undergo excision of the primary lesion and a therapeutic neck dissection that may be modified to preserve neurovascular structures. Parotidectomy is performed if parotid lymph nodes are included in nodal drainage basins. These patients also should be evaluated for systemic adjuvant therapy, as should those who have or develop distant metastasis. The use of systemic therapy includes chemotherapy, bioimmunotherapy, and vaccination, all of which can be used to treat metastatic disease or in the adjuvant setting for patients without evidence of disease who are at high risk for systemic failure. The importance of treating these patients within the confines of thoughtfully designed, preospectve clinical trials cannot be overemphasized.

The number of patients affected with melanoma is increasing. However, survival rates are improving because of early-detection programs and heightened awareness of the general population. It is hoped that this heightened awareness, coupled with progress made in improved pathologic description and staging and the use of systemic therapies, including immune modulation, will result in continued improvement in our ability to cure patients with this disease.

HIGHLIGHTS

- Increased public awareness and early detection have improved survival in patients with CMM, yet the incidence of CMM worldwide is increasing at an alarming rate.
- A skin lesion that changes in size, color, and sensation or one that ulcerates or bleeds requires prompt medical attention.
- Histologic evaluation is carried out via biopsy techniques (i.e., excisional) that include subcutaneous fat for complete evaluation of depth. Fine-needle aspiration and curettage have no role in the evaluation of suspected melanoma.
- Local disease staging involves evaluation of thickness (Breslow) and invasion level (Clark) and the presence or absence of tumor ulceration. In the staging of regional disease, the presence of satellite lesions, in transit disease, and the number (rather than the size of) involved lymph nodes are all of prognostic significance. The type of distant metastasis also is significant.
- For patients with thin, nonulcerated primary tumors without evidence of regional or distant spread on physical examination (stages I and II), chest radiograph and liver-function tests compose the recommended workup. For patients with regional or systemic metastases or both, a comprehensive staging workup should include MRI of the brain and contrast-enhanced CT of the neck, chest, abdomen, and pelvis. PET imaging has been used to aid in detecting regional and distant metastasis. Lymphoscintigraphy and sentinel node mapping may provide an additional means of identifying regional disease for tumors located in areas with ambiguous predicted drainage patterns or that include both parotid glands.
- Nonulcerated melanomas less than 1 mm in thickness without regional metastasis are excised with adequate margins, dictated by anatomic constraints.
- Melanomas more than 1 mm or ulcerated lesions without regional metastasis are excised, and consideration is given to lymphoscintigraphy and SLNB with ELND, followed by pathologic evaluation by serial sectioning.
- Patients with regional metastasis should undergo neck dissection and should be considered for adjuvant hypofractionated radiotherapy, given to a total dose of 30 Gy.
- Patients with high-risk primary tumors or regional metastasis or both should be evaluated for systemic adjuvant therapies, including chemotherapy, bioimmunotherapy, and vaccination given in the context of approved prospective clinical trials.
- Patients with distant metastases should be considered for trials of systemic therapies such as chemotherapy, biochemotherapy, or immunotherapy.
- Vigilant follow-up is mandatory. Recommended follow-up intervals relate to the patient's original staging characteristics.

REFERENCES

1. Greenlee RT, Murray T, Bolders, et al. Cancer statistics. *CA Cancer J Clin* 2001:51:15–36.
2. O'Brien CJ, Coates AS, Petersen-Schaefer K, et al. Experience with 998 cutaneous melanomas of the head and neck over 30 years. *Am J Surg* 1991;162:310.
3. Weinstock MA. Epidemiology of melanoma. *Cancer* 1993;65:29.
4. Abassi NR, Shaw HM, Rigel DS, et al. Early diagnosis of cutaneous melanoma: revisiting the ABCD criterion. *JAMA* 2004; 292:2771–2776.
5. Austin J, Byers RM, Brown WD, et al. Influence of biopsy on the prognosis of cutaneous melanoma of the head and neck. *Head Neck* 1996;18:107–117.
6. Stern SJ, Guillamondegui O. Mucosal melanoma of the head and neck. *Head Neck* 1991;13:22.
7. Prasad ML, Patel SG, Busam KJ. Primary mucosal desmoplastic melanoma of the head and neck. *Head Neck* 2004;26:373–377.
8. Temam S, Mamelle G, Marandas P, et al. Postoperative radiotherapy for primary mucosal melanoma of the head and neck. *Cancer* 2005;103:313–319.
9. Owens JM, Roberts DB, Myers JN. The role of postoperative adjuvant radiation therapy in the treatment of mucosal melanomas of the head and neck region *Arch Otolaryngol Head Neck Surg* 2003; 129:858–864.
10. Busam KJ, Mujumdar U, Hummer AJ, et al. Cutaneous desmoplastic melanoma: reappraisal of morphologic heterogeneity and prognostic factors. *Am J Surg Pathol* 2004;28:1515–1525.
11. Quinn MJ, Crotty KA, Thompson JF, et al. Desmoplastic and desmoplastic neurotropic melanoma: experience with 280 patients. *Cancer* 1998;83:1128–1135.
12. Clark WH, From l, Bernardino LA, et al. The histogenesis and biologic behavior of primary human malignant melanomas of the skin. *Cancer* 1970;29:705.
13. Breslow A. Thickness, cross-sectional areas and depth of invasion in the prognosis of cutaneous melanoma. *Ann Surg* 1970;172:902.
14. Buzaid AC, Ross MI, Balch CM, et al. Critical analysis of the current American Joint Committee on Cancer Staging system for cutaneous melanoma and proposal of a new staging system. *J Clin Oncol* 1997;13:1039.
15. Balch CM, Buzaid AC, Soong SJ, et al. Final version of the American Joint Committee on Cancer Staging System for cutaneous melanoma. *J Clin Oncol* 2001;19:3635–3648.
16. Balch CM, Soong SJ, Gershenwald JE, et al. Prognostic factors analysis of 17,600 melanoma patients: validation of the American Joint Committee on Cancer Melanoma Staging System. *J Clin Oncol* 2001;19:3622–3634.
17. O'Brien CJ, Petersen-Schaefer K, Ruark D, et al. Radical, modified and selective neck dissection for cutaneous malignant melanoma. *Head Neck* 1995;17:232.
18. Cochran AJ, Huang R, Guo J, et al. Current management issues in malignant melanoma. *ASCO;*2003;189–194.
19. Buzaid AC, Tinoca LA, Jendiroba D, et al. Prognostic value of size of lymph node metastases in patients with cutaneous melanoma. *J Clin Oncol* 1997;13:2362.
20. Mihnhout GS, Hoekstra OS, vanTulder MW, et al. Systematic review of the diagnostic accuracy of ^{18}F-fluorodeoxyglucose positron emission tomography in melanoma patients. *Cancer* 2001;91:1530–1542.
21. Wagner JD, Schauwecker D, Davidson, D, et al. FDG-PET sensitivity for melanoma lymph node metastasis is dependent on tumor volume. *J Clin Oncol* 2001;77:237–242.
22. Myers J. A neck dissection is required in the management of patients with cutaneous malignant melanomas of the head and neck (CMMHN) of intermediate thickness. *Arch Otolaryngol Head Neck Surg* 1999;125:110–115.
23. Balch CM, Soong S, Ross MI, et al. Long-term results of a multi-institutional randomized trial comparing prognostic factors and surgical results for intermediate thickness melanoma (1.0 to 4.0mm). *Ann Surg Oncol* 2000;7:87.
24. Fisher SR. Elective, therapeutic, and delayed lymph node dissection for malignant melanoma of the head and neck: analysis

of 1444 patients from 1970 to 1998. *Laryngoscope* 2002;112:99–110.

25. Jansen L, Koops HS, Nieweg OE, et al. Sentinel node biopsy for melanoma in the head and neck region. *Head Neck* 2000;22:27–33.

26. Morton D. Introduction:sentinel lymphadenectomy for patients with clinical stage I melanoma. *J Surg Oncol* 1997;66:267–269.

27. Fincher TR, O'Brien JC, McCarty TM, et al. Patterns of drainage and recurrence following sentinel lymph node biopsy for cutaneous melanoma of the head and neck. *Arch Otolaryngol Head Neck Surg* 2004;130:844–848.

28. Lentsch EJ, Myers JN. Melanoma of the head and neck: current concepts in diagnosis and management. *Laryngoscope* 2001;111:1209–1222.

29. Gershenwald J, Thompson W, Mansfield PF, et al. Multi-institutional melanoma lymphatic mapping experience: the prognostic value of sentinel lymph node status in 612 stage I or II melanoma patients. *J Clin Oncol* 1999;17:976–983.

30. Gershenwald J, Kolome MI, Lee JE, et al. Patterns of recurrence following a negative sentinel lymph node biopsy in 243 patients with stage II or II melanoma. *J Clin Oncol* 1998;16:2253.

31. Patel SG, Coit DG, Shaha AR, et al. Sentinel lymph node biopsy for cutaneous head and neck melanomas. *Arch Otolaryngol Head Neck Surg* 2002;128:285–291.

32. Chao C, Wong SL, Edwards MJ, et al. Sentinel lymph node biopsy for head and neck melanomas. *Ann Surg Oncol* 2003;10:21–26.

33. Tanis PJ, Boomir PA, Koops HS, et al. Frozen section investigation of the sentinel node in malignant melanoma and breast cancer. *Ann Surg Oncol* 2001;8:222–226.

34. Cimmino VM, Brown AL, Szocik JF, et al. Allergic reactions to isosulfan blue during sentinel lynmph node biopsy. *Surgery* 2001;130:439–444.

35. Ariyan S, Ariyan C, Farber LR, et al. Reliability of identification of 655 sentinal lymph nodes in 263 consecutive patients with malignant melanoma. *J Am Coll Surg* 2004;198:924–932.

36. McMasters KM, Reintgen DS, Ross, MI, et al. Sentinel lymph node biopsy for melanoma: controversy despite widespread agreement. *J Clin Oncol* 2001;1:2851–2855.

37. O'Rourke MG, Altmann CR. Melanoma recurrence after excision: is a wide margin justified? *Ann Surg* 1993;217:2.

38. Karakousis CP, Balch CM, Urist MM, et al. Local recurrence in malignant melanoma: long-term results of the multi-institutional randomized surgical trial. *Ann Surg Oncol* 1996;3:446.

39. Heaton K, Sussman J, Gershenwald J, et al. Surgical margins and prognostic factors in thick (>4 mm) primary melanoma patients. *Ann Surg Oncol* 1998;5:322–328.

40. Zitelli JA, Moy RL, Abel E. The reliability of frozen sections in the evaluation of surgical margins for melanoma. *J Am Acad Dermatol* 1991;24:102.

41. Shah JP, Kraus DH, Dubner S, et al. Patterns of regional lymph node metastases from cutaneous melanomas of the head and neck. *Am J Surg* 1991;162:320.

42. Barranco SC, Romsdahl MM, Humphrey RM. The radiation response of human malignant melanoma cell grown in vitro. *Cancer* 1971;31:830.

43. Ang KK, Byers RM, Peters LJ, et al. Regional radiotherapy as adjuvant therapy for head and neck melanoma: preliminary results. *Arch Otolaryngol Head Neck Surg* 1990;116:169–172.

44. Ang KK, Peters LJ, Weber RS, et al. Postoperative radiotherapy for cutaneous melanoma of the head and neck region. *Int J Radiat Oncol Biol Phys* 1994;30:795.

45. Bonner MD, Ballo MT, Myers JN, et al. Elective radiotherapy provides regional control for patients with cutaneous melanoma of the head and neck. *Cancer* 2004;100:283–289.

46. Ballo MT, Bonnen MD, Gaarden AS, et al. Adjunct irradiation for cervical lymph node metastasis from melanoma. *Cancer* 2000:97:1789–1796.

47. Kirkwood JM, Strawderman MH, Ernstoff MS, et al. Interferon alfa-2b adjuvant therapy of high-risk resected cutaneous melanoma: the Eastern Cooperative Oncology Group trial EST 1684. *J Clin Oncol* 1996;14:717.

48. Kirkwood JM, Ibrahim JG, Sundak VK, et al. High- and low-dose interferon alfa-2b in high-risk melanoma: first analysis of Intergroup Trial E1690/S9111/C9190. *J Clin Oncol* 2000;18:2444–2458.

49. Kirkwood JM, Ibrahim JG, Sosman JA, et al. High-dose interferon alfa-2b significantly prolongs relapse-free survival and overall survival compared with the GM2-KLH/QS21 vaccine in patients with resected stage IIB-IV melanoma: results of the intergroup trial 1694/S9512/C509801. *J Clin Oncol* 2001;19:2370–2380.

50. Saleh MN, Khazaeli MB, Wheeler RH, et al. Phase I trial of the murine monoclonal anti-GD2 antibody 1469a in a metastatic melanoma. *Cancer Res* 1992;52:4342.

51. Sondak VK. Adjuvant therapy of T3N0M0 melanoma with allogenic tumor vaccine: results of SWOG 9035. *Melanoma Res* 2001;11:541.

52. DiFronzo AL, Gupta RK, Essner R, et al. Enhanced humoral immune response correlates with improved disease-free survival and overall suvival in American Joint Committee on Cancer stage II melanoma patients receiving adjuvant polyvalent vaccine. *J Clin Oncol* 2002;20:3242–3248.

53. Legha S, Ring S, Eton O, et al. Development of a biochemotherapy regimen with concurrent administration of cisplatin, vinblastine, darcarbazine, interferon alfa, and interleukin-2 for patients with metastatic melanoma. *J Clin Oncol* 1998;16:1752–1759.

54. Atkins MB, Lotze MT, Dutcher JP, et al. High-dose recombinant interleukin 2 therapy for patients with metastatic melanoma: analysis of 270 patients treated between 1985 and 1993. *J Clin Oncol* 1999;17:2105–2116.

55. Rosenberg SA, Yang JC, Schwartzentruber DL, et al. Prospective randomized trial of the therapy of patients with metastatic melanoma using chemotherapy with cisplatin, dacarbazine, and tamoxifen alone or in combination with interleukin-2 and interferon alfa-2b. *J Clin Oncol* 1999;17:968–975.

56. Demierre MF, Nathanson L, et al. Chemoprevention of melanoma: an unexplored strategy. *J Clin Oncol* 2003; 21:158–165.

57. Mellardo B, Velam M, Colomer D, et al. Tyrosinase mRNA in blood of patients with melanoma treated with adjuvant interferon. *J Clin Oncol* 2002;20:4032–4039.

58. Po-Hwu HJ, Ariyan S, Lamb L, et al. Follow-up recommendations for patients with American Joint Committee on Cancer stages I-III malignant melanoma. *Cancer* 1999;86:2252–2258.

Neoplasms of the Nose and Paranasal Sinuses

Lee A. Zimmer   Ricardo L. Carrau

EPIDEMIOLOGY

Malignant tumors of the sinonasal tract constitute about 3% of tumors arising in the upper respiratory tract. They occur most commonly in Caucasians, and the incidence in males is twice the incidence in females (1). Exposure to industrial fumes, wood dust, nickel-refining processes, and leather tanning have been implicated in the carcinogenesis of certain types of sinonasal malignant tumors. Other industrial exposures associated with an increased incidence of sinonasal cancer include mineral oils, chromium and chromium compounds, isopropyl oils, lacquer paint, soldering and welding, and radium dial painting. A recent report demonstrates a higher incidence of nasal cancers in cigarette smokers (1).

EVALUATION

Diagnosis

Tumors of the sinonasal tract commonly appear with symptoms identical to those caused by inflammatory sinus disease, such as nasal airway obstruction, epistaxis, headache, facial pain, and nasal discharge, and are frequently asymptomatic in 9% to 12% of patients, contributing to a delay in the diagnosis and advanced stage of disease. Regional and distant metastases are infrequent despite the advanced stage of the primary tumor. The incidence of cervical metastases on initial presentation varies from1% to 26%, with most large series reporting less than 10%. In only 15% of patients

with malignancies of the paranasal sinuses do cervical metastases develop after treatment of the primary site (2). This number decreased to 11% in patients treated with radiation to the neck. The presence of distant metastasis on initial presentation is even less common, with most series reporting an incidence of less than 7%.

The physical examination should be thorough, with emphasis on the sinonasal region, orbit, and cranial nerves, and should include nasal endoscopy. Although not pathonogmonic, numbness or hypesthesia of the infraorbital (V_2) or supraorbital (V_3) nerve strongly suggests malignant invasion. Other findings such as proptosis; chemosis; extraocular muscle impairment; mass effect in the cheek, gingiva or gingivobuccal sulcus (e.g., ill-fitting dentures); and loose dentition also suggest the presence of a sinonasal tumor. Table 107.1 provides a summary of diagnostic techniques.

Radiologic imaging is essential for staging. Plain films may demonstrate bone destruction; however, a significant number will be interpreted as normal. A screening computed tomography (CT) scan is more accurate than plain films to evaluate the bony framework of the paranasal sinuses and compares favorably with the cost of plain films. High-risk patients with a history of carcinogen exposure, severe persistent pain, cranial neuropathies, exophthalmos, chemosis, sinonasal disease, and those with persistent symptoms after adequate medical treatment should be evaluated with an axial and coronal CT scan with contrast or magnetic resonance imaging (MRI). CT scanning is superior for the evaluation of the bony confines of the sinonasal tract

TABLE 107.1 📖 DIAGNOSIS PARANASAL TUMORS	
History and Physical Exam	**Risk Factors/Cranial Nerve Deficits, Nasal Mass**
Imaging	
Radiograms	Bone erosion, opacification of PNS
CT scanning	Evaluation of bony boundaries of PNS; not cost-effective
MRI	Evaluation of soft-tissue invasion and perineural spread; differentiate retained secretions from tumor
PET	Routine evaluation for recurrent disease after primary treatment and distant metastasis; useful for squamous cell carcinoma; cost-effectiveness unknown
Biopsy	
Sinus lavage/cytology	
Fine-needle aspiration	
Transnasal biopsy	Direct or endoscopic. Preferred modality

PNS, peripheral nerve sheath; CT, computed tomography; MRI, magnetic resonance imaging; PET positron emission tomography.

and skull base. The use of contrast provides an estimate of the tumor vascularity and its relation to the carotid artery.

MRI differentiates adjacent tumor from soft tissue, differentiates secretions in an obstructed sinus from a space-occupying lesion, demonstrates perineural spread, has less artifact effect with dental fillings, offers the advantage of imaging in the sagittal plane, and does not involve exposure to ionizing radiation. Coronal MRI images are superior for the evaluation of the foramen rotundum, vidian canal, foramen ovale, and optic canal. Sagittal images are most useful to demonstrate the replacement of the normal low-intensity signal of Meckel cave and the high-intensity signal of fat in the pterygopalatine fossa by tumor signals similar to brain. MRI, however, is more expensive than CT scan, more prone to motion artifact, and less tolerated because of claustrophobia.

Positron emission tomography (PET) is commonly used for malignancies of the head and neck for staging and surveillance. The combined PET/CT scanner adds anatomic detail that aids in surgical planning by defining the extent of tumor. Although many reports have documented the use of PET in head and neck cancer, none has evaluated the use of this modality for malignant tumors of the nose and paranasal sinuses.

Angiography with carotid-flow study is reserved for surgical candidates with tumors that surround the carotid artery or when sacrifice of the vessel is anticipated to obtain clear margins. Balloon occlusion tests, used with single-photon emission CT (SPECT), xenon CT scan, or transcranial Doppler, offer a reasonable estimate of the risk of ischemic brain infarction if the internal carotid artery is sacrificed. These tests, however, cannot predict ischemia at marginal ("watershed") areas or embolic phenomena.

A CT scan of the chest and abdomen is recommended for patients with tumors that metastasize hematogenously,

such as sarcoma, melanoma, and adenoid cystic carcinoma. Metastatic evaluation is important if an extensive resection is considered. A lumbar puncture and brain and spine imaging are recommended for tumors that invade the meninges or brain.

Pathology

The sinonasal tract pathology, with certain important exceptions, reflects the pathology found in other areas of the head and neck (Table 107.2). We provide a brief description of the most common histologic diagnoses.

Benign Epithelial Tumors

Papillomas arise from squamous or schneiderian epithelium. The keratotic papilloma of the vestibule (vestibular wart) behaves like other cutaneous counterparts. It is easily treated with simple excision or cauterization. Papillomas of the nasal cavity may be classified in three distinct categories (Table 107.3). Fungiform papillomas arise from the nasal septum, whereas inverted and cylindrical papillomas typically arise from the lateral nasal wall. Although they are benign in nature, extension beyond their site of origin can destroy bone, recur when not excised completely, and may be associated with malignant tumors (3,4). They are most commonly diagnosed in white males during the fifth to seventh decades (mean, 50 years). En bloc resection has been the gold standard for the treatment of these lesions (Table 107.4). However, MRI, CT scanning, and nasal endoscopy permit an accurate preoperative mapping of these lesions, allowing a more conservative resection through less-invasive approaches. During the last decade, various endoscopic, transnasal techniques for the resection of inverting papillomas have been reported (4,5). Transnasal techniques avoid the use of incisions and usually require a

TABLE 107.2
TUMORS OF THE SINONASAL TRACT

Epithelial

    Benign

        Exophytic papilloma
        Inverted papilloma
        Columnar papilloma
        Adenoma

    Malignant

        Squamous cell carcinoma
        Transitional cell carcinoma
        Adenocarcinoma
        Adenoid cystic carcinoma
        Melanoma
        Olfactory neuroblastoma
        Undifferentiated carcinoma

Nonepithelial

    Benign

        Fibroma
        Chondroma
        Osteoma
        Neurilemmoma
        Neurofibroma
        Hemangioma

    Malignant

        Soft-tissue sarcoma
        Rhabdomyosarcoma
        Leiomyosarcoma
        Fibrosarcoma
        Liposarcoma
        Angiosarcoma
        Myxosarcoma
        Hemangiopericytoma
        Connective tissue sarcoma
        Chondrosarcoma
        Osteosarcoma

Lymphoreticular tumors

        Lymphoma
        Plasmacytoma
        Giant cell tumor

Metastatic carcinoma

shorter hospital stay than do external approaches. The endoscopic approach provides superior visualization of the posterior ethmoid cells, especially those that extend lateral to the sphenoid sinus or around the optic nerve (Onodi cells). In expert hands, resection with an endonasal, medial maxillectomy approach has recurrence rates equal to those of traditional open, en bloc resections (5).

Adenomas of the sinonasal tract arise more commonly in the nasal septum. Most are found during the fourth to the seventh decades, occurring with an equal sex distribution. The recurrence rate is low after complete removal (10%).

Malignant Epithelial Tumors

Squamous cell carcinoma is the most common tumor of the sinonasal tract. It is most commonly reported in white men in their fifth to sixth decade. The prognosis is related to the extent of the tumor and the site of origin.

Adenocarcinomas make up 4% to 8% of all sinonasal tumors. They originate most commonly in the ethmoid sinuses and nasal cavity and are associated with exposure to hardwood dust. Adenocarcinomas may be divided into low and high grades according to their histologic characteristics and behavior. Low-grade tumors have a uniform glandular architecture and cytologic characteristics, with rare mitoses and seldom perineural invasion or distant metastases. Low-grade adenocarcinomas tend to recur locally. High-grade adenocarcinoma has a solid growth pattern with poorly defined margins, prominent pleomorphism, and large number of mitoses. One third of patients with high-grade adenocarcinomas will initially have distant metastases. Approaches to adenocarcinomas of the paranasal sinuses include anterior craniofacial resection, lateral rhinotomy, and endonasal techniques with or without radiotherapy. The 5-year disease-specific survival for patients with adenocarcinoma of the nose and paranasal sinuses after surgery and radiation therapy is 55% for T1 and T2, 28% for T3, and 25% for T4 lesions (6).

Adenoid cystic carcinomas (ACCs) of the sinonasal tract compose 14% to 20% of all the adenoid cystic carcinomas

TABLE 107.3
PAPILLOMAS OF THE SINONASAL TRACT

	Inverted Papilloma	Fungiform Papilloma	Cylindrical Papilloma
Site of origin	Lateral wall	Septum	Lateral wall
Frequency	47%	50%	3%
Recurrence rate	27%–73%	22%–50%	25%–35%
Associated with malignancy	13%	3%–5%	15%

Adapted from Barnes EL. Surgical pathology of the head and neck. Vol. 1, New York: Marcel Dekker, 1985, with permission.

TABLE 107.4
RECURRENCE RATES FOR INVERTING PAPILLOMA

Authors	Lateral Rhinotomy–Medial Maxillectomy	Conservation Resection[a]
Benninger et al. (1991)	0 (0/20)	36% (5/14)
Myers et al. (1990)	5% (1/22)	0 (0/4)
Pelausa and Fortier (1992)	7% (1/14)	77% (37/48)
Outzen et al. (1991)	7% (3/44)	27% (3/11)
Lawson et al. (1989)	9% (7/77)	10% (1/10)
Segal et al. (1986)	10% (1/10)	70% (10/14)
Kristensen et al. (1985)	12% (7/57)	38% (8/21)
Phillips et al. (1990)	13% (9/72)	44% (4/9)
Smith and Gullane (1987)	27% (3/11)	57% (4/7)
Dolgin et al. (1992)	29% (4/14)	44% (4/9)
Weissler et al. (1986)	29% (37/126)	67% (103/153)
Bielamowicz et al. (1993)	30% (6/20)	74% (17/23)
Averages	16% (79/487)	60% (209/350)

[a]Does not include reports of endoscopic resection.
Adapted from Lawson W, Ho BT, Shaari CM, et al. Inverted papillomas: a report of 112 cases. *Laryngoscope* 1995;105:282–288, with permission.

arising in the head and neck. They are characterized by early spread to neurovascular structures, submucosal spread, and advanced stage at the time of diagnosis. Low-grade tumors are defined by histology with less than 30% solid architecture and include the cribriform and tubular patterns. High-grade tumors correspond to those with a histologic pattern more than 30% solid cellular architecture. The incidence of perineural invasion is similar for both grades, but the incidence of local recurrence and metastases is higher in the solid type. High rates of recurrence (50% to 76%) are likely due to perineural spread and positive microscopic margins not identified at the time of surgery (7,8). The treatment of adenoid cystic carcinoma of the sinonasal tract is primarily surgical, although combined surgery and postoperative radiation therapy appear to yield better local control.

In our experience with 36 patients with ACC of the sinonasal tract, most patients were first seen with locally advanced disease (8). The orbit was invaded in 35% of these patients, and 33% had intradural disease. Only two patients had distant metastasis at the time of diagnosis. Margins are difficult to clear, even with extensive craniofacial resection, because of the proximity to vital structures and the propensity for perineural spread, which in this series was more than 90% of patients. The survival rate at 2 years was 46% after primary treatment and 15% after salvage surgery. Most patients had local recurrences (65%), and in 50%, regional or distant recurrence developed. The median time to death was 44 months.

Melanoma of the sinonasal tract may be primary or metastatic. Although 20% of all melanomas originate in the head and neck, less than 1% arise from the sinonasal tract. They are most commonly found in the nasal cavity, followed by the maxillary sinus, ethmoid sinus, and frontal sinus, in descending order. Most patients initially have disease confined to the site of origin but show a tendency toward early vascular and lymphatic invasion with a high incidence of local recurrence after surgical excision. Postoperative radiation therapy may be beneficial, although its impact on survival and local control has not been addressed in scientific trials. The median survival for patients with sinonasal melanoma is 24 to 36 months. The most common cause of failure is local recurrence, whereas the most important factor in predicting survival is metastatic disease (9,10).

Olfactory neuroblastoma is a rare tumor arising in the olfactory epithelium. Patients often are first seen with nasal obstruction and epistaxis. It has a bimodal frequency at ages 10 to 20 and 50 to 60 years, with a similar incidence in male and female patients. Its prognosis is related to the extent of disease and resectability on initial presentation. Most institutions have adopted combined therapies based on the Kadish staging system (Table 107.5). The UCLA classification (Table 107.6), however, provides better prognostication regarding local recurrences, as factors such as intradural and orbital invasion are not considered in the Kadish staging system. The advent of craniofacial resection with postoperative radiation to the primary site and neck

TABLE 107.5
KADISH STAGING SYSTEM FOR OLFACTORY NEUROBLASTOMA

Stage A	Tumor confined to the nasal cavity
Stage B	Tumor in nasal cavity extending to paranasal sinus
Stage C	Tumor extending to orbit, base of skull, cranial cavity, or with cervical/distant metastasis

TABLE 107.6

UCLA STAGING SYSTEMS FOR OLFACTORY NEUROBLASTOMA

Stage	Description
T1	Tumor involving the nasal cavity or paranasal sinuses (excluding sphenoid) or both, sparing the most superior ethmoidal air cells
T2	Tumor involving the nasal cavity or paranasal sinuses (including the sphenoid) or both with extension to or erosion of the cribriform plate
T3	Tumor extending into the orbit or protruding into the anterior cranial fossa
T4	Tumor involving the brain

has improved the therapeutic results (12). In a recent meta-analysis, the 5-year disease-free survival for all stages is 65% after combined surgery with radiotherapy (12).

Sinonasal undifferentiated carcinomas (SNUCs) are usually composed of small and medium-sized cells and must be differentiated from rhabdomyosarcoma, melanoma, olfactory neuroblastoma, lymphoma, and squamous cell carcinoma. The progression of symptoms is very rapid, and they usually are first seen with a very advanced stage involving multiple sinuses. Treatment includes trimodal therapy using chemotherapy (cyclophosphamide, doxorubicin, and vincristine), radiation therapy, and, in appropriate cases, surgery. Patients with intracranial disease fared poorly despite aggressive combination therapy.

Benign Nonepithelial Tumors

Fibroosseous lesions, including osteomas, fibromas, and chordomas, are the most common benign tumors of the sinonasal tract. Their growth is usually slow and self-limited. Simple surgical excision is recommended when a histologic diagnosis is needed or to relieve obstructive symptoms.

Fewer than 4% of benign peripheral nerve sheath tumors of the head and neck arise in the nose and paranasal sinuses. They are initially seen as polypoid, slow-growing masses, reaching a very large size and often causing facial deformities and local destruction of adjacent structures. Ninety percent of the nerve sheath tumors show a benign histology. Two thirds of these tumors are schwannomas, and one third, neurofibromas. Unlike those in other regions, schwannomas of the nose and paranasal sinuses often lack tumor encapsulation, with neoplastic cells undermining adjacent respiratory mucosa (13). Treatment is by complete surgical excision, or partial removal for massive neurofibromas involving vital areas.

Malignant Nonepithelial Tumors

Neurogenic sarcomas are rare in the head and neck and are commonly associated with neurofibromatosis. Neurogenic sarcomas are locally aggressive and frequently appear with distant metastases. Surgery plays a primary role in their

therapy; radiation and chemotherapy are usually reserved for incomplete removal, inoperable cases, or recurrences (14). The 5-year survival rate is 60%, although sarcomas associated with neurofibromatosis behave more aggressively, yielding a 5-year survival rate of 30% (14).

Rhabdomyosarcomas arise in the head and neck in 35% to 45% of cases. In 10% of patients, they originate in the paranasal sinuses (15). These tumors may assume the morphology of any of the developmental stages of striated muscle, hence the classification into embryonal, alveolar, and pleomorphic types. A bimodal distribution pattern is found in childhood, with the embryonal occurring in the first decade and the alveolar type in adolescents. Rhabdomyosarcomas have a less favorable outcome in adults, with a 5-year survival rate of only 35% (16). The head and neck region is less involved in adults, with the viscera and extremities the most common sites of presentation.

Rhabdomyosarcomas of the sinonasal tract are classified as nonorbital parameningeal and behave more aggressively than those arising in other locations. Systemic and regional metastases are common. In 1987, the Intergroup Rhabdomyosarcoma Study I reported the use of intensive radiation and chemotherapy on patients with nonorbital parameningeal rhabdomyosarcoma, showing an improvement of the survival rate from 51% to 81%. In 2002, Intergroup Rhabdomyosarcoma Study IV reported further improvements in survival for those patients with cranial parameningeal involvement (17). Patients with cranial parameningeal sarcomas, but without meningeal invasion, receive multiagent chemotherapy followed by radiation therapy. High-risk tumors defined as intracranial tumors, tumors that eroded the base of skull, or that caused a cranial neuropathy were treated with triple intrathecal chemotherapy, whole-brain radiation, and spinal radiation. At 5 years, 73% of patients were alive, compared with 45% in IRS I. Overall survival for patients with paranasal sinus involvement was 76% for the low-risk group and 57% for the high-risk group. Failure-free survival was 57% for the low-risk group and 52% for the high-risk group. Aggressive initial surgical therapy was not warranted. These results, however, have never been confirmed in adults. Adult rhabdomyosarcoma is usually treated with wide surgical excision. Radiation is recommended for positive margins or inoperable or recurrent disease. Chemotherapy has a palliative role that must be weighed against its possible morbidity.

Fibrosarcoma is a tumor arising from fibroblasts; thus the term encompasses a spectrum of malignancies that ranges from low-grade fibromatosis to high-grade tumors. Misdiagnosis is very common. Radiation and trauma have been implicated as possible etiologic factors. The treatment of choice is wide surgical excision for previously untreated tumors. Radiation is recommended for involved margins or recurrent or inoperable tumors.

Hemangiopericytoma is a very rare, highly vascular tumor arising from the pericapillary pericytes of Zimmerman. Histologic examination reveals oval and spindle-shaped pericytes. Benign and malignant varieties have been described. Malignant tumors are distinguished by increased mitotic activity, high cell density, and necrotic and hemorrhagic zones. They invade locally and metastasize in 10% to 15% of cases. Hematogenous metastases involve lung, liver, and bone. Sixteen percent are found in the head and neck, with about 50 reported cases arising in the sinonasal tract (18). Their prognosis relates to the size of the lesion, the number of mitoses, and the metastases. The primary treatment is surgical excision.

Osteogenic sarcoma is the most common primary tumor of bone in the United States, with an estimated incidence of one case per 100,000. Those originating within the jaws constitute 7% to 10% of all osteosarcomas. Etiologic factors include ionizing, radiation, fibrous dysplasia, trauma, Paget disease, and the gene associated with retinoblastoma. The most effective therapy is surgical excision. However, during the past decade, several reports have suggested that adjunctive radiation and chemotherapy may improve survival. A multiinstitutional review and meta-analysis demonstrated a 2- and 5-year disease-free survival for maxillary osteosarcomas of 65% and 38%, respectively (19). Adjuvant therapy, including radiation, chemotherapy, or combination therapy, failed to improve outcome. Nonetheless, these authors acknowledge a selection bias, and therefore the role of adjuvant therapy remains unresolved.

Chondrosarcomas are slow-growing tumors that usually arise from cartilaginous structures. These tumors have been graded from I to III on the basis of the rate of mitoses, cellularity, and nuclear size. Size of the tumor and grading correlates with the rate of metastasis, local aggressiveness, and ultimate survival. Surgical removal with wide margins is the treatment of choice. Gross total removal with postoperative radiation is recommended for those involving vital structures.

Although the metastatic potential and oncologic outcome of sarcomas arising in the sinonasal tract is variable among the different histologic types, the local behavior of sarcomas is similar. Sarcomas are infiltrative, usually advancing to areas farther than what is appreciated by the naked eye; thus they are often incompletely resected and therefore recur locally. Wide excision improves the local control, but this is difficult to perform when dealing with the sinonasal tract, which is adjacent to important if not vital structures. Cranial-base surgery may improve the local control of sarcomas of the sinonasal tract.

Lymphoma of the sinonasal tract accounts for only 0.17% of all lymphomas. T-cell lymphomas are more common in Asian populations, whereas B-cell lymphomas are more common in Western populations. The primary sites of occurrence in the sinonasal tract are the maxillary sinus (79%) and nasal cavity (20%) (20). The treatment includes radiation therapy for localized lesions and chemotherapy to prevent systemic recurrence. The biologic behavior is remarkably different in the pediatric and adult populations. Adults have frequent relapses, commonly involving the abdomen, and show a 5-year survival rate of around 45%. Distant metastases is often associated with failure to treat with chemotherapy in the primary setting (20). In children, complete remissions are more common, involvement of the gastrointestinal tract is rare, and the 5-year survival rate is close to 75%.

Of patients with extramedullary plasmacytoma, 80% to 90% have involvement of the head and neck region, and 40% arise in the sinonasal tract. It is more common in the sixth to seventh decades. It tends to spread locally and can be found in the cervical nodes in less than 25% of the cases. The prognosis is unpredictable, and a variable number of the patients will be diagnosed with multiple myeloma. It is of utmost importance to rule out this diagnosis on the initial presentation. Most of these lesions will respond to radiation therapy in doses of 4,000 to 5,000 cGy administered over a 4- to 5-week period.

Metastatic Tumors

Metastatic tumors to the sinonasal tract produce symptoms similar to those of primary tumors. More than 100 cases have been reported, metastasizing to the maxillary, ethmoid, frontal, and sphenoid sinus in descending order. The most common primary sources are the kidneys, breasts, and lungs. The treatment is palliative, using radiation, surgery, or chemotherapy to relieve obstructive and compressive symptoms or pain.

STAGING

A staging system provides a guide to define the extent and prognosis of a tumor and also serves as a communication tool, allowing different institutions to compare their experience with the use of different therapeutic modalities. The American Joint Committee on Cancer (AJCC) TNM staging system of the nose and paranasal sinuses is provided (Table 107.7). The AJCC recommends a different system for soft-tissue sarcomas. This system includes a histologic grading system that differs from the system used for epithelial tumors. Grading is thought to be the most significant prognostic factor in patients with mesenchymal tumors and is based on the number of mitoses, degree of cellularity, amount of stroma, degree of maturation, nuclear pleomorphism, and presence or absence of necrosis.

PRINCIPLES OF TREATMENT

Surgery

Diagnostic (Biopsy)

Tissue sampling may be performed by using endoscopic sinus surgery instruments or through open transcutaneous or transoral procedures (e.g., Caldwell-Luc antrostomy,

TABLE 107.7

MAXILLARY SINUS TNM STAGING FOR PRIMARY TUMOR (T)

TX	Primary tumor cannot be assessed
T0	No evidence of primary tumor
Tis	Carcinoma in situ
T1	Tumor limited to maxillary sinus mucosa with no erosion or destruction of bone
T2	Tumor causing bone erosion or destruction including extension into the hard palate and/or middle nasal meatus, except extension to posterior wall of maxillary sinus and pterygoid plates
T3	Tumor invades any of the following: bone of the posterior wall of the maxillary sinus, subcutaneous tissues, floor or medial wall of orbit, pterygoid fossa, ethmoid sinuses
T4a	Tumor invades anterior orbital contents, skin of cheek, pterygoid plates, infratemporal fossa, cribriform plate, sphenoid or frontal sinuses
T4b	Tumor invades any of the following: orbital apex, dura, brain, middle cranial fossa, cranial nerves other than maxillary division of trigeminal nerve (V_2), nasopharynx, or clivus

From American Joint Committee on Cancer. *Manual for staging of cancer*, 6th ed. New York: Springer-Verlag, 2002, p. 61, with permission.

external ethmoidectomy, rhinotomy). The former is preferred because it provides good access and hemostatic control with less morbidity and does not contaminate other soft tissues.

Drainage/Debridement

An adequate drainage port (e.g., nasoantral window) should be opened in patients with secondary bacterial sinusitis and in patients who will require radiation therapy as primary treatment.

Resection

Surgical resection is usually recommended with curative intent. Palliative excision may be considered to alleviate intractable pain, to provide rapid decompression of vital structures, or to debulk a massive lesion, thus freeing the patient from social embarrassment. Surgery as a single treatment modality for malignant tumors of the sinonasal tract has yielded 5-year survival rates from 19% to 86%. Figures 107.1 through 107.6 demonstrate the most common surgical approaches and techniques.

With recent advances in preoperative imaging, intraoperative image-guidance systems, endoscopic instrumentation, and materials for hemostasis, endonasal techniques for the removal of nasal and paranasal sinus tumors may be a viable alternative to the traditional open techniques. Endoscopic approaches can access and visualize tumors in the nasal cavity, ethmoid, sphenoid, medial frontal, and medial maxillary sinuses (21). Frozen sections must be used, as the tumor is often removed in a piecemeal fashion. Improvements in functional recovery and long-term survival, however, are yet to be described.

Rehabilitation

The main goals of postsurgical rehabilitation are primary wound healing, preservation or reconstruction of the facial contour, and restoration of oronasal separation, thus facilitating speech and swallowing. Functional considerations take precedence over aesthetics. Rehabilitation after surgical resection may be achieved with a dental prosthesis or reconstructive flaps, such as temporalis muscle flaps with and without the inclusion of cranial bone, pedicled or microvascular free myocutaneous flaps (e.g., pectoralis major, latissimus dorsi, trapezius), and cutaneous flaps (e.g., forehead, scalp, deltopectoral). Flaps are recommended to replace resected skin, to provide support for the orbit or brain, or to isolate the cranial cavity from the upper aerodigestive tract.

A total maxillectomy defect should not be obliterated at the initial operation; an open cavity facilitates cleansing and direct visual inspection during the follow-up period. Patients requiring a craniofacial resection, especially those needing an orbital exenteration, deserve special consideration, because a recurrence after an adequate craniofacial resection is uniformly lethal. From the functional standpoint, patients require immediate separation of the cranial cavity from the upper aerodigestive tract and support of the brain. A pericranial flap and transfer of a temporalis muscle flap achieves these goals. The temporalis muscle, however, is often devascularized after an infratemporal fossa dissection, or its bulk may be inadequate to obliterate the dead space. Under these circumstances, the maxillectomy cavity may be obliterated with a free microvascular flap, offering immediate palliation and oronasal separation without the need for a prosthesis.

Radiation Therapy

Radiation may be used as a single modality, as an adjunct to surgery, or as palliative therapy. Recent reports indicate that postoperative radiation improves local control but does not cause specific or absolute survival (2). We and others favor postoperative radiation because there is a smaller volume of tumor cells to kill, the margins of the non-radiated tumor can be better defined during surgery, and the postoperative wound healing is more predictable.

Chemotherapy

The role of chemotherapy for the treatment of tumors of the sinonasal tract is usually palliative, using its cytoreductive effect to relieve pain and obstruction, or to debulk a massive external lesion. Samant et al. (22) in 2004 reported the use of high-dose intraarterial cisplatin with concomitant radiation in patients with carcinoma of the paranasal sinuses. The overall and disease-free survival rates at 5 years were 53% (Table 107.8). Patients who represent a poor sur-

gical risk and those who refuse surgery should be considered for enrollment in protocols that include combinations of radiation and chemotherapy.

MANAGEMENT OF ADVANCED TUMORS

Orbital Invasion

Sinonasal tract tumors may extend to the orbit by invasion or erosion of the bony walls, by perineural or perivascular invasion, or by following preformed pathways (Fig. 107.6). In patients with orbital invasion, ocular symptoms rapidly

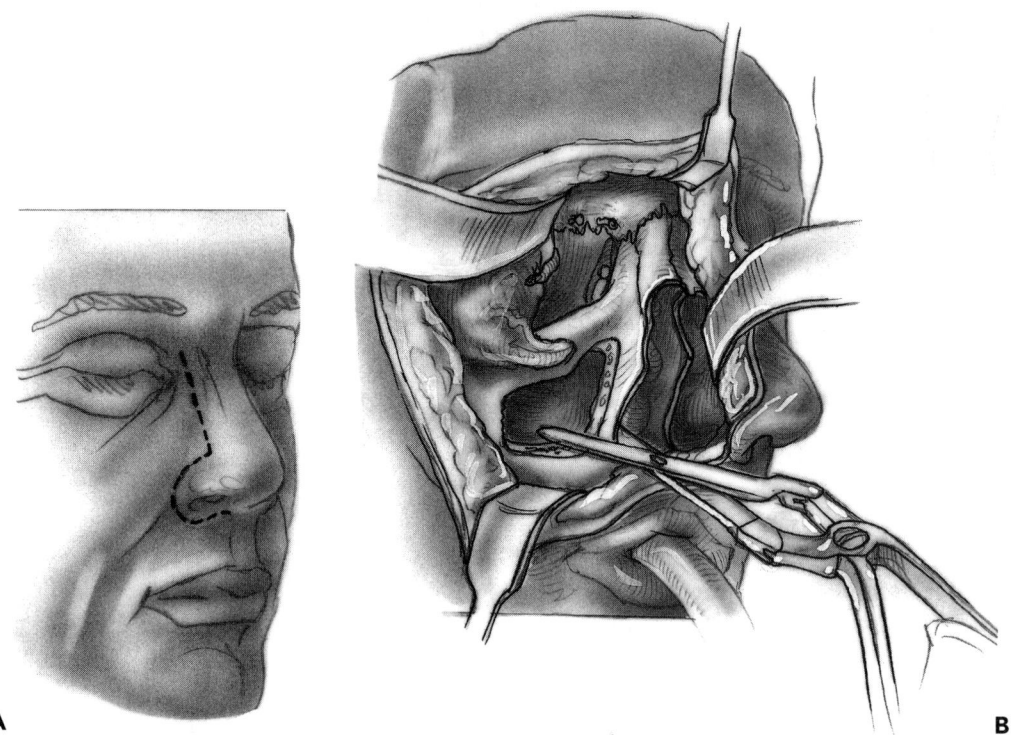

A   **B**

Figure 107.1   Medial maxillectomy. Lateral rhinotomy: **A:** The skin incision begins beneath the medial aspect of the eyebrow and continues 4 to 5 mm anterior to the medial canthus and over the nasal bone along the deepest portion of the nasomaxillary groove and following the alar crease. A lip-splitting extension of the incision is not necessary. To expose the surgical area, the cheek flap is elevated subperiosteally over the maxilla and around the infraorbital nerve. The periorbita is elevated over the lamina papyracea, and the frontoethmoid suture is identified and followed posteriorly until the anterior and posterior ethmoid arteries are identified. The anterior wall of the antrum is penetrated at the canine fossa by using a 4-mm chisel. The antrostomy is enlarged with a Kerrison rongeur around the infraorbital nerve and superiorly toward the inferior orbital rim. **B:** Bone is removed across the orbital rim, including the lacrimal fossa. The nasolacrimal duct is divided, and the lacrimal sac is opened and marsupialized **(C). D:** Osteotomies and removal of the specimen. The first osteotomy involved in the actual removal extends through the piriform aperture at the level of the nasal floor, directed posteriorly until the osteotomy perforates the posterior wall of the antrum. The orbit is retracted laterally, and a second osteotomy is performed at the frontoethmoid suture, extending posteriorly to a point 2 to 3 mm posterior to the posterior ethmoid artery (i.e., anterior to the optic foramen). **E:** The thin bone of the medial floor of the orbit is sawed by following a line that joins the lacrimal fossa with the superior osteotomy. The final bone cut involves three steps. First, a 2-mm osteotome is introduced through the anterior antrostomy and directed through the medial posterior antral wall. The osteotome is advanced superiorly to reach the level of the superior osteotomy and is then pushed medially. Second, a wide osteotome, introduced through the nose, is impacted into the anterior wall of the sphenoid sinus, and then pushed laterally. Heavy right-angle scissors (e.g., upper-lateral-cartilage scissors) are guided through the inferior osteotomy with one blade in the nose and the other in the antrum to start the posterior cut, behind the turbinates. **F:** Heavy curved scissors are then introduced with one blade in the nasal cavity and the other in the superior osteotomy, directed through or along the posterior attachments of the turbinates. The specimen is removed by anterior and inferior traction. Hemostasis is achieved by direct clamping or cautery. The bony edges are smoothed with a rongeur. Residual ethmoid mucosa is removed with ethmoid forceps, and a wide sphenoidotomy is opened with Kerrison rongeurs. The cavity is covered with absorbable gelatin (Gelfoam) for hemostasis. The medial canthal tendon is sutured to the periosteum of the nasal bones. The wound is closed by using a meticulous layered closure.

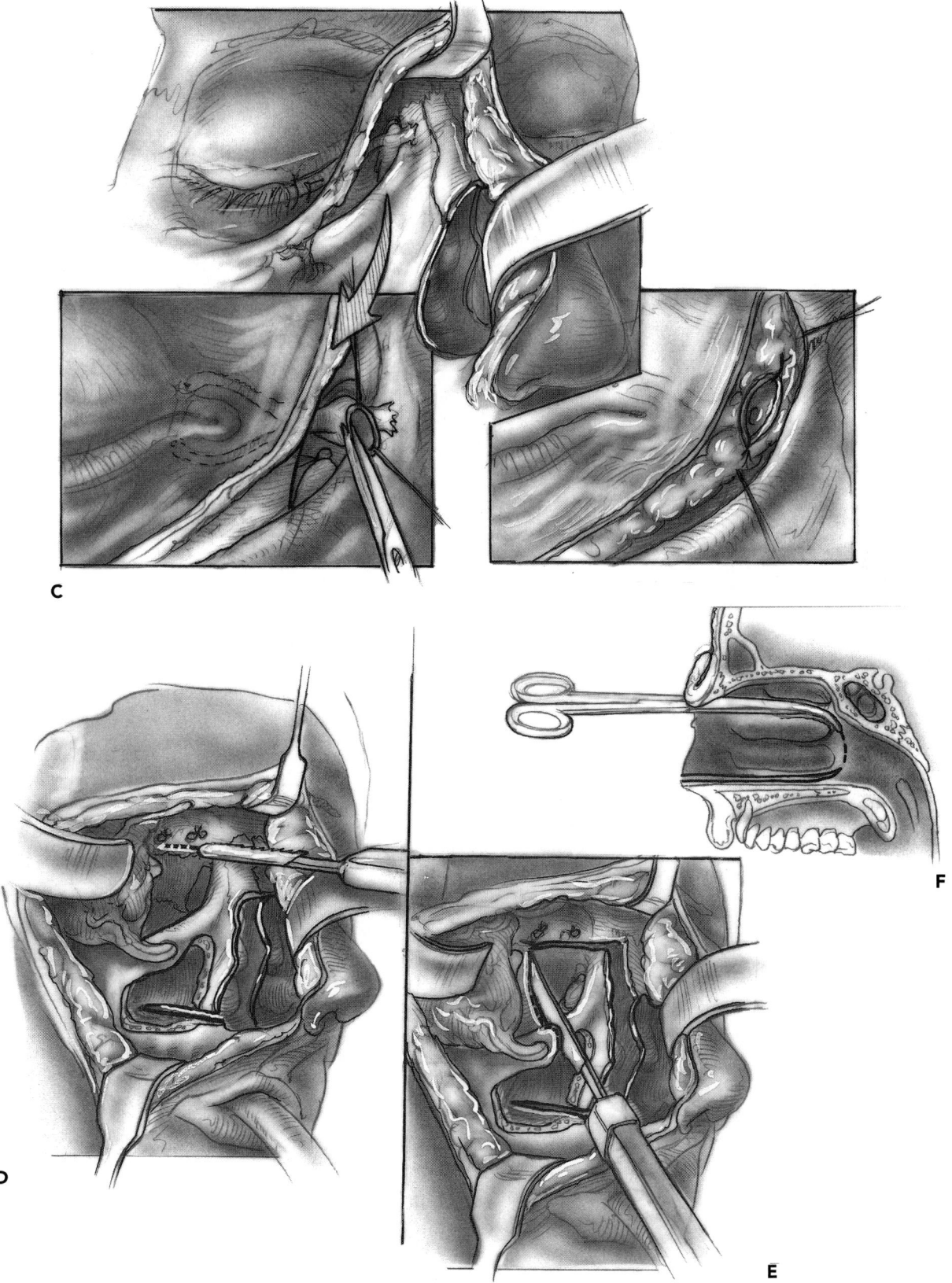

Figure 107.1 *(continued)*

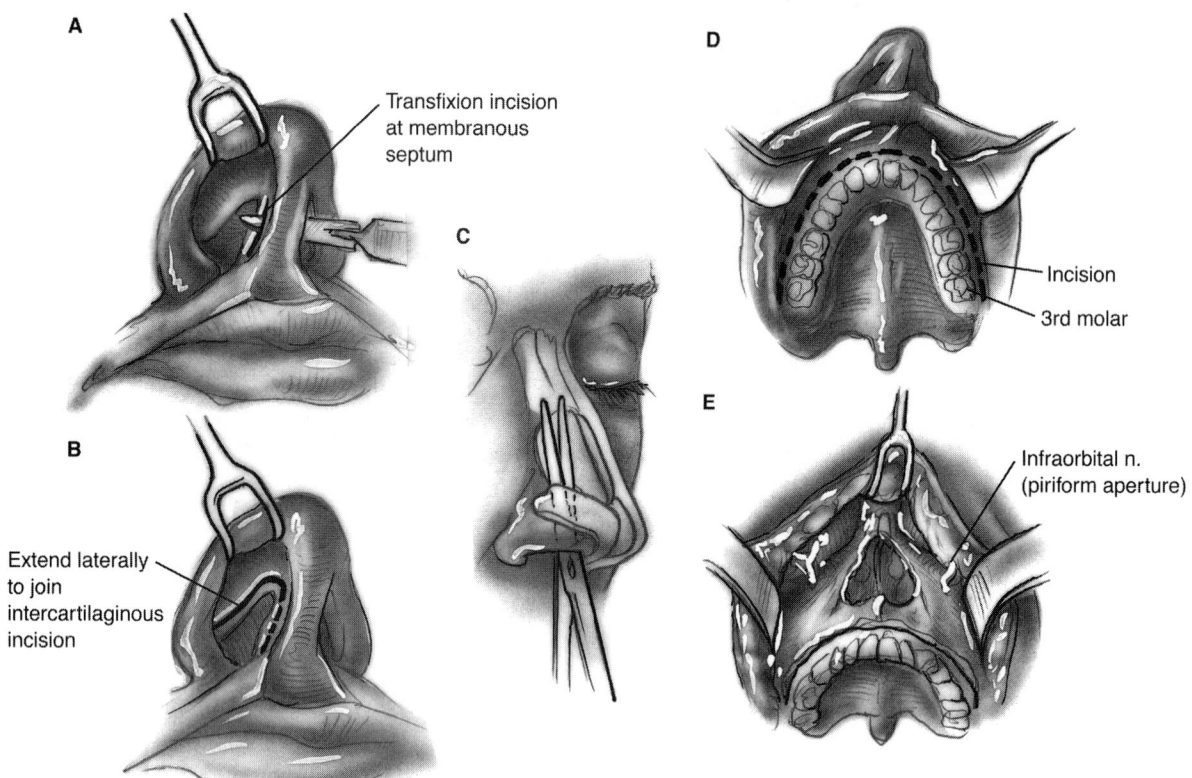

Figure 107.2   A, B: A transfixion incision is performed at the membranous septum and is extended laterally to join a transcartilaginous incision. **C:** A gingivobuccal incision is performed, extending laterally from the midline to the maxillary tuberosities. **D:** In exposing the surgical area, tenotomy scissors are introduced through the transcartilaginous incisions to dissect the skin from the nasal skeleton. The dissection over the maxilla is carried out in a subperiosteal plane. This dissection joins the nasal degloving by using sharp dissection over the piriform aperture attachments. The dissection is extended superiorly, exposing the midface skeleton. **E:** The exposure is limited by the infraorbital neurovascular bundles. The osteotomies, removal of the specimen, reconstruction, and closure are performed as described for the lateral rhinotomy.

develop, such as proptosis, diplopia, decreased visual acuity, diminished motility, chemosis, lid edema, and epiphora. CT scanning provides evidence of bony erosion, but it is not reliable in ascertaining invasion of the soft tissues. MRI better identifies soft tissue invasion, but invasion must be confirmed during surgery.

Bone erosion does not constitute an absolute indication for orbital exenteration (23). The prognosis of patients with invasion of the periorbita is dismal; therefore palliation is a more realistic goal (Table 107.9). Adjunctive radiation therapy, before or after surgery, does not seem to yield an improved prognosis.

Resection of the medial and inferior orbital walls produces severe enophthalmos and hypophthalmos, which is aggravated by resection of the periorbita. Rigid reconstruction of the bony orbit by using titanium mesh with or without calvarial bone grafts is recommended; these are then covered with local, regional, or microvascular flaps. The better to restore the orbital anatomy and to prevent lagophthalmos due to ectropion, the lateral canthus should be reattached to the corresponding anatomic site

of insertion. Ectropion may still occur because of fibrosis. The medial wall is usually resected as part of the oncologic surgery, requiring that the medial canthus be reattached to a titanium plate, as illustrated in Figure 107.3.

Cervical Metastasis

The incidence of nodal metastasis on initial presentation varies from 3% to 16%. Nodal metastases at initial presentation indicate a grim prognosis. The low incidence of nodal metastasis from sinonasal malignancies does not justify the use of elective neck dissection or radiation.

Pterygopalatine Fossa

The incidence of pterygopalatine fossa (PtPF) invasion by sinonasal tract malignancies varies from 10% to 20%. The presence of tumor in this area is considered a risk factor for local recurrence. Despite the difficulty of an en bloc resection of this area, several authors have designed approaches with sound oncologic principles, obtaining variable results.

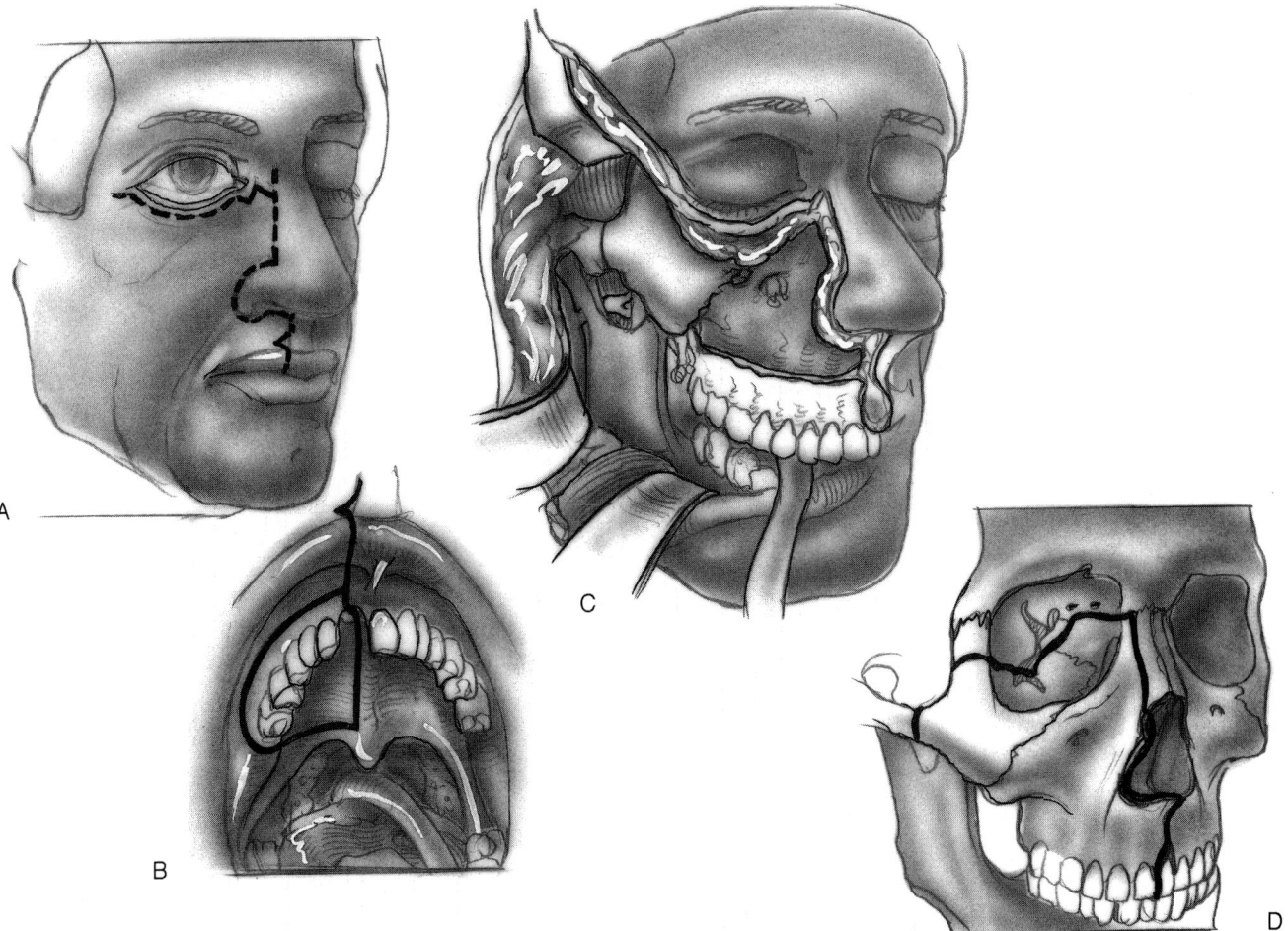

Figure 107.3 Total maxillectomy. A total maxillectomy with preservation of the orbit can be performed by using incisions identical to lateral rhinotomy incisions with a lip-splitting extension. Alternatively, a lateral rhinotomy incision may be combined with an ipsilateral degloving approach. **A:** If increased exposure is necessary, the facial incisions may be modified. The superior incision begins at the lateral canthus and extends medially, passing 3 to 4 mm below the ciliary line. The eye is protected by a temporary tarsorrhaphy stitch. This incision may be substituted by a transconjunctival incision. The subciliary limb is joined to a lateral rhinotomy incision. The orbicularis oculi muscle is incised with an inferiorly directed slant, exposing the orbital septum. The gingivobuccal incision is extended laterally to the ipsilateral maxillary tuberosity. **B:** The soft palate is incised at the junction with the hard palate, and its attachments are sharply transected. The mucoperiosteum of the hard palate is incised by following a paramedian line ipsilateral to the lesion. The paramedian strip of mucosa will be later imbricated over the bony edge of the hard palate to facilitate the fitting of a prosthesis. **C:** The orbital contents are dissected from the medial inferior and lateral walls, exposing the lacrimal sac, the anterior and posterior ethmoid arteries, and the infraorbital fissure. These are managed as described for a medial maxillectomy (Fig. 107.1). Osteotomies and removal of the specimen. **D:** The body and frontal process of the zygoma are divided with the saw. The maxilla is severed from the nasal bones with the saw, and the osteotomy is extended superiorly to the frontoethmoidal suture. A superior osteotomy is carried out posteriorly to a point 3 to 4 mm posterior to the posterior ethmoid artery. An osteotomy is performed connecting the lateral and medial wall osteotomies across the inferior orbital fissure. The hard palate is transected with a Gigli or sagittal saw. The maxilla is detached from the skull by tapping a chisel placed into the pterygomaxillary fissure in a posterosuperior direction. The superior attachments of the turbinates are sharply severed, as for a medial maxillectomy (Fig. 107.1). The specimen is removed by anteroinferior traction. Remnants of ethmoid sinus mucosa are removed in a piecemeal fashion. The coronoid process of the mandible is removed to avoid displacement of the prosthesis when opening the mandible. **E:** The exposed facial and pterygoid muscles and periorbita are lined with a split-thickness skin graft that is 0.35 to 0.45 mm thick.

(continued on next page)

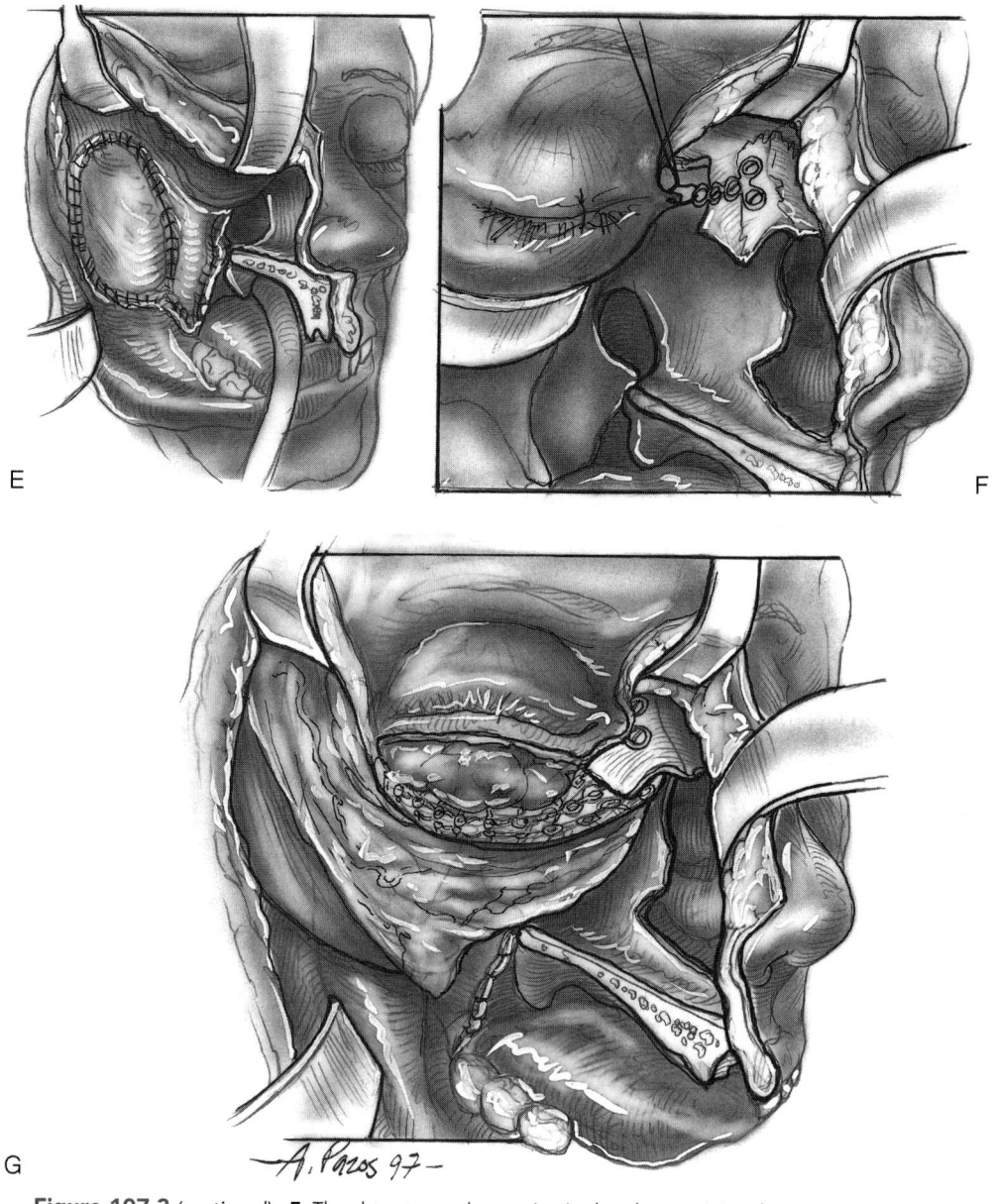

Figure 107.3 *(continued)* **E:** The obturator or denture is wired to the remaining dentition or suspended from the zygomatic arch and piriform aperture or leg screwed to the remaining hard palate. **F:** A medial canthopexy, using a Y-shape titanium plate fixed to the nasal bones. A figure-8 nonabsorbable suture is used to medialize the medial canthal tendon. **G:** The floor and medial walls of the orbit are reconstructed with titanium mesh. This is then covered by a vertically split temporalis muscle flap. The anterior half is used for the reconstruction, and the posterior half is transposed to the anterior temporal fossa to obliterate the defect.

Infratemporal Fossa and Skull Base

The skull base may be involved by tumor by direct invasion and bone erosion, by preformed pathways (e.g., cribriform plate, superior orbital fissure, foramen lacerum), or by following neural or vascular structures (e.g., V_2, V_3). The overall incidence of skull-base invasion by sinonasal malignancies appears to be about 15%. The anterior or anterolateral craniofacial resection is a well-established procedure for sinonasal tumors invading the anterior skull (Fig. 107.7). The anterior craniofacial resection may be extended laterally to join a temporal craniotomy to include the pterygoid plates, the PtPF, the infratemporal fossa, and the floor of the middle cranial fossa en bloc. Absolute contraindications for craniofacial resection are medical or nutritional problems that would eliminate the patient as a surgical candidate, presence of distant metastases, invasion of the prevertebral fascia, invasion of the cavernous sinus by a high-grade malignancy, involvement of the carotid artery in a high-risk patient (as determined by carotid-flow studies), and bilateral invasion of the optic nerves or optic chiasm.

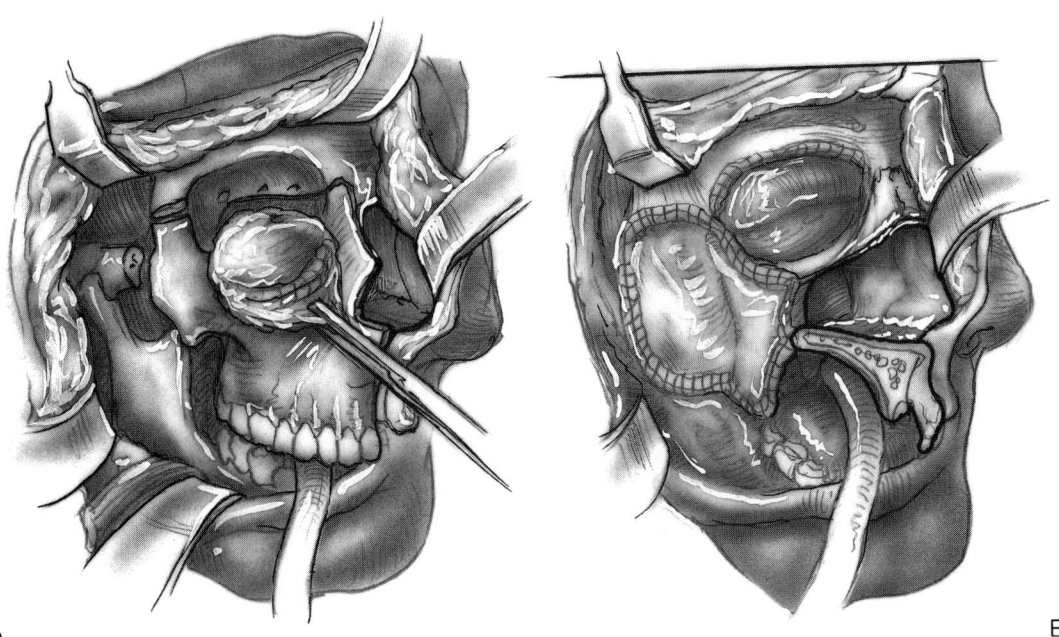

A   B

Figure 107.4 Orbital exenteration. **A:** Incisions for orbital exenteration include those described in Figure 107.3 and a supraciliary incision along the upper eyelid. These incisions allow the preservation of the lids, which can be used to line the remaining orbital cavity. If the eyelids are involved by the tumor, the incisions are modified to include their resection en bloc. The exposure proceeds as previously described (Fig. 107.3), omitting the dissection of the orbit from the inferior wall. The upper eyelid is retracted superiorly, and the periorbita is incised over the superior orbital rim. The orbit is dissected from the superior wall, identifying optic foramen and superior orbital fissure. These are infiltrated with lidocaine to block the autonomic innervation and prevent cardiac arrhythmias. The neural and vascular structures traveling through these foramina are transected after hemostasis with bipolar cautery or clamping. Inferior traction on the globe allows further visualization of the orbital floor and inferior orbital fissure. Lateral and medial wall osteotomies are connected, as in Figure 107.3D. Other osteotomies are identical to Figure 107.3D. The roof of the orbit may be lined with a skin graft or left to granulate and mucosalize. Alternatively, the cavity may be filled with a temporalis muscle flap. It should be remembered that squamous epithelium tolerates trauma (e.g., prosthesis) better than does mucosa. **B:** In exposing the surgical area, the facial flap is elevated subperiosteally. In the case of extension through the anterior wall of the antrum, the facial flap may be elevated in a subcutaneous plane, including the facial musculature in the specimen. The skin also may be resected *en bloc,* to address direct invasion by the tumor. The dissection is carried out along the lateral wall of the maxilla, and the internal maxillary artery is identified at the pterygomaxillary fissure and clipped.

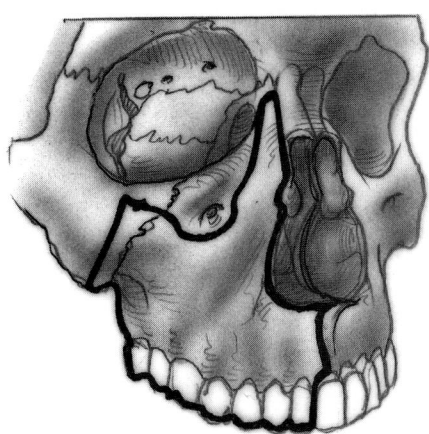

Figure 107.5 Inferior maxillectomy. Tumors confined to the floor of the antrum may be managed by partial maxillectomy. It differs from total maxillectomy in the preservation of the orbital floor and, in selected cases, of the infraorbital nerve. Bilateral maxillectomy: The procedure is performed bilaterally, as in Figure 107.3. The nasal septum may be sacrificed or preserved for suspension of the prosthesis or reconstructive flaps.

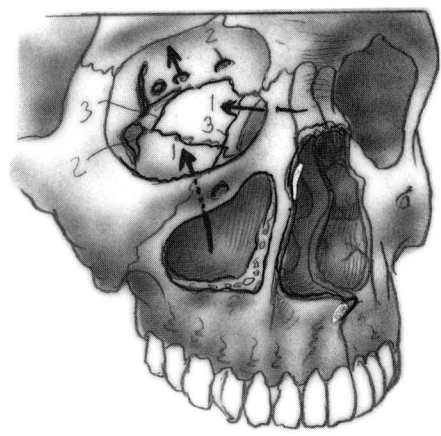

Figure 107.6 Pathways of invasion include (1) direct bony erosion (e.g., medial wall or floor), (2) perivascular or perineural invasion (e.g., infraorbital or ethmoidal neurovascular bundles), and (3) preformed pathways (e.g., infraorbital fissure, nasolacrimal duct).

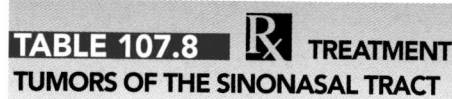

TABLE 107.8   ℞ TREATMENT
TUMORS OF THE SINONASAL TRACT

Modality	Indications
Surgery	Mainstay treatment
Radiation	Unresectable or lymphoreticular tumors, poor surgical candidates. Usually requires surgical drainage/debridement
Combination therapy	(+) margins, perineural, perivascular invasion (+) lymph nodes, recurrent tumor
Chemotherapy	Palliative role Clinical research (controlled protocols)

Resection of these areas is associated with an unacceptable morbidity and mortality rate, offers no significant palliation, and does not appear to improve survival. Relative contraindications include invasion of the dura and intracranial involvement of neural structures. These situations have a poor prognosis, but in selected cases, craniofacial resection may offer significant palliation or local control.

Improvements in the preoperative mapping of tumors with CT scan and MRI and the use of more reliable vascularized flaps for the reconstruction of the skull base have improved the surgical mortality and morbidity. However, the overall 5-year survival rate appears unchanged at 50% to 60%.

COMPLICATIONS

Surgical

The nasolacrimal duct is sacrificed during the performance of a maxillectomy, and subsequent stenosis of the lacrimal sac opening may lead to epiphora. A dacryocystorhinostomy at the time of definitive resection is an effective way to prevent this complication. Cannulation of the lacrimal canaliculi for 12 weeks is recommended.

Limitation of movement of the extraocular muscles may occur after trauma to the muscle or its motor innervation or on entrapment in the craniofacial osteotomies. The latter complication should be managed by urgent surgical release. Limitations of extraocular muscle movement due to edema or neuromuscular contusion should be managed expectantly. Diplopia may be alleviated by alternating eye patching.

The optic nerve may be compressed during the mobilization of the specimen or during craniofacial resection. High-dose steroids and emergency surgical decompression are recommended.

Enophthalmos or hypophthalmos usually develops because of the loss of the inferior orbital or medial support or both. Reconstructive techniques were previously discussed.

Radiation Therapy

The incidence of radiation complications in patients with orbit preservation is close to 100% (Table 107.10). The field included in the radiation portals for sinonasal tract tumors usually includes the anterior and posterior orbital segment. When the orbit is involved by the tumor, irradiation of the entire eye is usually necessary. Complications of the anterior globe are common with full-eye irradiation. A dry eye will decompensate rapidly, leading to severe keratitis, panophthalmitis, and blindness within 1 year. Enucleation is recommended for uncontrolled panophthalmitis or a painful eye.

If the anterior segment can be spared, patients will most likely experience delayed (3 to 5 years) loss of vision secondary to postradiation retinopathy or optic neuropathy. Although the retina and optic nerve are radioresistant, their microvasculature is not. Chemotherapy, diabetes mellitus, and atherosclerosis may have an additive effect on radiation complications. The incidence of these complications is related to total dose and fractionation. The tolerance limit seems to be around 5,000 cGy, with fractions of 200 cGy. Although they are rare at less than 3,500 cGy, their

TABLE 107.9
META-ANALYSIS OUTCOME: INVASION OF ORBIT (NED)

Study	Sparing[a]	Exenteration[b]	Significance
Som et al. 1971	—	3/27 (11%)	
Perry et al. 1988	1/2 (50%)	2/4 (50%)	
Xuexi et al. 1995	8/23 (35%)	24/88 (27%)	
Carrau et al. 1996	5/9 (56%)	6/12 (50%)	
Total	14/34 (41%)	35/131 (27%)	p > 0.05

This table demonstrates the lack of statistically significant difference in the survival rate of those patients in whom the orbit was preserved when compared with patients whose orbit was exenterated. The trend toward worst survival in those patients who required exenteration illustrates the aggressiveness of tumors that invade the periorbita.
[a]Soft-tissue invasion.
[b]No soft-tissue invasion.
Adapted from: Carrau RL, Segas J, Nuss DW, et al. Squamous cell carcinoma of the sinonasal tract invading the orbit. *Laryngoscope* 1999;109:230–235, with permission.

incidence is 50% to 65% with 6,000 to 7,000 cGy and more than 85% with 8,000 cGy.

Wound Complications

Wound complications include bleeding, infection, and loss of reconstructive flaps or skin grafts (Table 107.11). Osteoradionecrosis can occur in up to 10% of patients. The most common site of osteoradionecrosis is the maxilla. Severe osteoradionecrosis can be secondary to poor dentitia or recently extracted dentitia. We recommend the routine extraction of poor dentitia with time to recover before postoperative radiation to avoid this complication.

Postoperative infection is rare. Cellulitis should be treated with antibiotics providing broad-spectrum coverage adjusted to the culture and sensitivity results. Venous

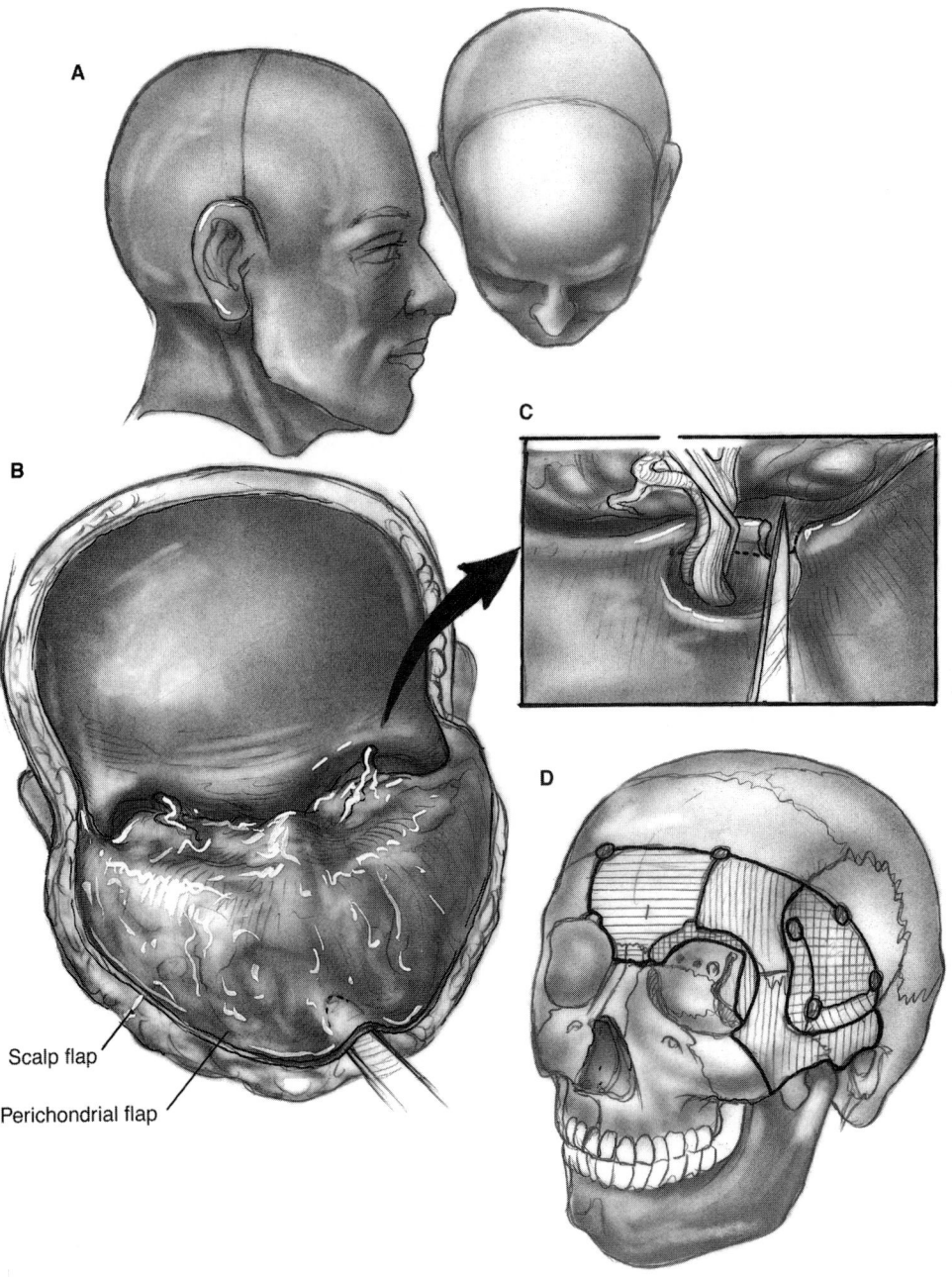

Figure 107.7 A: Bicoronal flap incision. **B:** The scalp flap is dissected anteriorly in a subperiosteal plane and laterally just above the superficial layer of the deep temporal fascia. Leaving the pericranial flap attached to the scalp flap prevents desiccation of the flap during the procedure. **C:** To expose the supraorbital rim, superior orbital cavity, and nasal bones, the supraorbital neurovascular bundle is mobilized from its notch or foramen. **D:** Orbital, cranial, and zygomatic osteotomies are performed according to the required exposure. The tumor is resected en bloc with the anterior or middle fossa skull base.

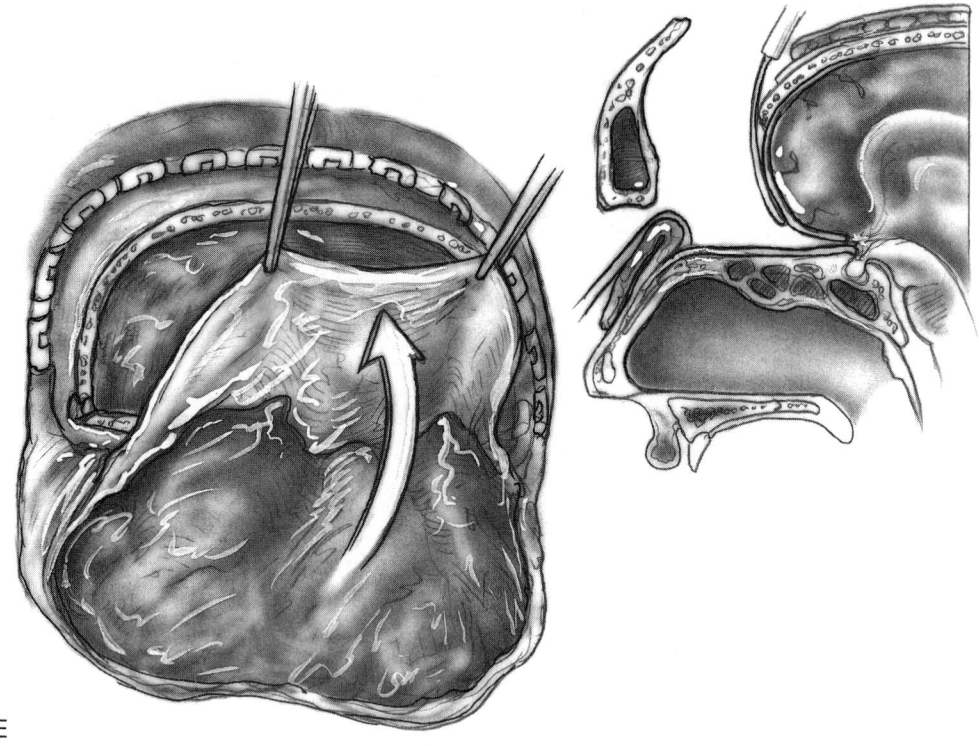

E

Figure 107.7 *(continued)* **E:** A pericranial flap is elevated and placed under the dura of anterior lobe and over the remaining bone of the anterior fossa. The craniotomy and orbital bone grafts are replaced above the pericranial flap, which separates the cranial cavity from the upper aerodigestive tract.

retrograde seeding, or even direct spread in the presence of a cerebrospinal fluid (CSF) fistula can lead to meningitis or intracranial abscess. A CT scan followed by a lumbar puncture is indicated if meningitis is suspected. Formation of crusts within the nasal cavity is a common problem and may lead to infection. Frequent irrigations with normal saline solution help with nasal hygiene.

Skull-Base Complications

Skull-base complications include CSF leak, meningitis, intracranial abscess, tension pneumocephalus, and osteomyelitis. These complications are most commonly the result of technical errors (e.g., loss of a reconstructive flap) and are surprisingly uncommon, considering that skull-base resection involves exposure of the cranial cavity to

TABLE 107.10

EFFECTS OF RADIATION ON THE EYE

Tissue	Effect	Latency	Dose
Lacrimal gland	Atrophy	>6 mo	>5,000 cGy/5–6 wk
Conjunctiva	Hyperemia	1–3 wk	≥5,000 cGy/5 wk
	May lead to secondary infection		
Cornea	Edema	1–3 wk	4,000–5,000 cGy/2–3 wk
	Chronic ulceration	Several mo	>6,000 cGy/5–6 wk
	Perforation	4–12 mo	>6,000 cGy/5–6 wk
Retina	Edema	Several wk	2,000–3,500 cGy/3–4 wk
	Retinopathy	>1 yr	5,000–6,000 cGy/5–6 wk
Lens	Cataract	1–20 yr	≥200 cGy

Adapted from Nakissa N, Rubin P, Strohl R, et al. Ocular and orbital complications following radiation therapy of paranasal sinus malignancies and review of literature. *Cancer* 1983;51:980, with permission.

TABLE 107.11 COMPLICATIONS

SINONASAL TRACT TUMORS

Problem	Treatment
Orbital	
Surgical	
Epiphora	DCR
Diplopia	Observe, release EOM if entrapped
Blindness	Perform optic nerve or orbital decompression
Enophthalmos/hypophthalmos	Support globe with bone grafts or titanium mesh or both
Radiation	
Wound	
Bleeding	Packing, arterial ligation, or embolization
Infection	Antibiotics/debridement
Loss of reconstructive flaps or skin grafts	Debridement
Skull base	
CSF leak	Observation, bed rest Reconstructive flap for persistent leak
Meningitis	Antibiotics, correct CSF leak
Pneumocephalus	Aspiration if at tension
Osteomyelitis	Antibiotics, debridement, HBO
Other	
Serous otitis media	Ventilation tube (rule out CSF leak)

CSF, cerebrospinal fluid; HBO, hyperbaric oxygen; DCR, dacryocytsorhinostomy; EOM, external oblique muscle.

aerodigestive tract flora. Treatment includes empiric intravenous antibiotics with broad-spectrum coverage, including the skin and aerodigestive flora. The antibiotics are later adjusted to the culture and sensitivity results. Further contamination or exposure of the intracranial contents to the sinonasal tract should be curtailed by the use of vascularized flaps. Free bone grafts that become infected during the early postoperative period should be removed. Late osteomyelitis or osteoradionecrosis may be managed with antibiotics and debridement limited to the affected bone. Hyperbaric oxygen treatment may be beneficial in patients with osteoradionecrosis. Intracranial abscess requires open drainage and intravenous antibiotics.

Tension pneumocephalus is treated with percutaneous aspiration and diversion of the nasal airway. The latter may be accomplished with the use of an endotracheal tube, nasal trumpets, or a tracheotomy.

EMERGENCIES ASSOCIATED WITH SINONASAL TUMORS

Bleeding

Friable or vascular tumors may lead to profuse bleeding when traumatized (e.g., biopsy), or bleeding may occur spontaneously after desiccation and breakdown of the blood vessels in the tumor (Table 107.12). Mild to moderate bleeding is managed by using the principles of treatment for anterior and posterior epistaxis. Cauterization or

packing is recommended. In the case of a massive tumor that completely occludes the nasal passages, angiography and embolization should be considered. This technique also is useful in vascular tumors, providing prompt hemostasis and facilitating surgical removal. If circumstances preclude the use of this technique, a transantral ligation of the internal maxillary artery and transorbital ligation of the ethmoidal arteries may control the bleeding. Ligation of the external carotid artery, although not as effective as internal maxillary artery ligation, may be necessary if the transantral approach is impossible. One should remember, however, that ligation of the external carotid artery will eliminate the possibility of embolization. A combination

TABLE 107.12 EMERGENCIES

SINONASAL TRACT TUMORS

Problem	Treatment
Bleeding	Cauterization/packing Arterial ligation/embolization Emergency extirpative surgery
Visual impairment	Decompression of orbit or optic nerve Radiation for lymphoreticular tumors
Infection	Antibiotics and drainage/debridement
CSF leak/ pneumocephalus	Definitive surgery, reconstructive flap

CSF, cerebrospinal fluid.

of these techniques may be required to prevent exsanguination. Uncontrollable hemostasis from a known malignancy may require emergency maxillectomy.

Vision Impairment

Sinonasal tumors may lead to blindness due to compression or stretching of the optic nerve, its arterial supply, or its venous drainage. Emergency treatment of the tumor with radiation or surgery may be necessary to prevent blindness, although it will be a moot point if the eye is going to be ultimately sacrificed.

Infection

Tumors of the sinonasal tract may obstruct sinus drainage and lead to acute bacterial sinusitis and possible orbital and intracranial complications. Secondary sinus infections must be treated with antibiotics providing broad aerobic and anaerobic coverage. Surgical drainage by endoscopic or open technique is usually required.

Cerebrospinal Fluid Leak

CSF leak may occur after destruction of the skull base and disruption of the dura mater (e.g., cribriform plate). CSF leaks are less likely to resolve spontaneously under these circumstances and therefore should be managed by prompt craniofacial resection, dural grafting, and a pericranial flap. Patients must be kept on bed rest while awaiting the operation. The use of prophylactic antibiotics is controversial. They may seem indicated in the presence of a necrotic tumor, but prolonged treatment may lead to colonization with resistant flora that will be more difficult to eradicate in case of meningitis.

HIGHLIGHTS

- Malignant tumors of the sinonasal tract constitute less than 1% of all malignancies.
- The most common clinical presentation of sinonasal tumors includes symptoms that are indistinguishable from inflammatory sinus disease: nasal airway obstruction, pain, and epistaxis. Abnormal V_1 or V_2 sensation or both strongly suggest the possibility of a tumor.
- CT or MRI is an essential component of evaluation, establishing the extent and vascularity of the tumor and its relation to neurovascular structures.
- An understanding of the variable natural history of tumors of the sinonasal tract is crucial to patient counseling and treatment planning. A wide variety of histologies may be encountered, although squamous cell carcinoma is most common.
- Rehabilitation after surgical resection may be accomplished by the use of prosthodontics or reconstructive flaps.

- Radiation is a common adjuvant to surgery for patients with squamous cell carcinoma. The response of sinonasal tract tumors to radiation therapy varies with the stage and histology of the tumor.
- Combined intraarterial cisplatin chemotherapy and radiation therapy before surgical resection offers a survival advantage in advanced squamous cell carcinoma of the paranasal sinuses.
- Bony erosion of the orbital walls does not constitute an indication for orbital exenteration.
- Patients with tumor involvement of the skull base, either in the infratemporal fossa or at the fovea ethmoidalis and cribriform plate, should be considered for craniofacial resection.
- Complications, such as CSF leak, meningitis, intracranial abscess, and tension pneumocephalus, although uncommon, are potentially devastating and must be addressed in an emergency fashion.

REFERENCES

1. Caplan LS, Hall I, Levine RS, Zhu K. Preventable risk factors for nasal cancer. *Ann Epidemiol* 2000;10:186–191.
2. Katz TS, Mendenhall WM, Morris CG, et al. Malignant tumors of the nasal cavity and paranasal sinuses. *Head Neck* 2002;24:821–829.
3. Myers EN, Fernau JL, Johnson JT, et al. Management of inverted papilloma. *Laryngoscope* 1990;100:481.
4. Kraft M, Simmen D, Kaufmann T, et al. Long-term results of endonasal sinus surgery in sinonasal papillomas. *Laryngoscope* 2003;113:1541–1547.
5. Schlosser RJ, Mason JC, Gross CW. Aggressive endoscopic resection of inverted papilloma: an update. *Otolaryngol Head Neck Surg* 2001;125:49–53.
6. Claus F, Boterberg T, Ost P, et al. Postoperative radiotherapy for adenocarcinoma of the ethmoid sinuses: treatment results for 47 patients. *Int J Radiat Oncol Biol Phys* 2002;54:1089–1094.
7. Naficy S, Disher MJ, Esclamado RM. Adenoid cystic carcinoma of the paranasal sinuses. *Am J Rhinol* 1999;13:311–314.
8. Pitman K, Prokopakis E, Aydogan B, et al. The role of skull base surgery for the treatment of adenoid cystic carcinoma of the sinonasal tract. *Head Neck* 1999;21:402–407.
9. Brandwein MS, Rothstein A, Lawson W, et al. Sinonasal melanoma: a clinicopathologic study of 25 cases and literature meta-analysis. *Arch Otolaryngol Head Neck Surg* 1997;123:290–296.
10. Thompson LDR, Wieneke JA, Miettinen M. Sinonasal tract and nasopharyngeal melanomas: a clinicopathologic study of 115 cases with a proposed staging system. *Am J Surg Pathol* 2003;27:594–611.
11. Monroe AT, Hinerman RW, Amdur RJ, et al. Radiation therapy for ethesioneuroblastoma: rationale for elective neck irradiation. *Head Neck* 2003;25:529–534.
12. Dulguerov P, Allal AS, Calcaterra TC. Ethesioneuroblastoma: a meta-analysis and review. *Lancet Oncol* 2001;2:683–690.
13. Hasegawa SL, Mentzel T, Fletcher CDM. Schwannomas of the sinonasal tract and nasopharynx. *Modern Pathol* 1997;10:777–784.
14. Hillstrom RP, Zarbo RJ, Jacobs JR. Nerve sheath tumors of the paranasal sinuses: electron microscopy and histopathologic diagnosis. *Otolaryngol Head Neck Surg* 1990;102:257.
15. Hicks J, Flaitz C. Rhabdomyosarcoma of the head and neck in children. *Oral Oncol* 2002;38:450–459.
16. Hawkins WG, Hoos A, Antonescu CR, et al. Clinicopathologic analysis of patients with adult rhabdomyosarcoma. *Cancer* 2001;91:794–803.

17. Raney RB, Meza J, Anderson JR, et al. Treatment of children and adolescents with localized parameningeal sarcoma: experience of the Intergroup Rhabdomyosarcoma Study Group protocols IRS-II through-IV, 1978-1997. *Med Pediatr Oncol* 2002;38:22–32.

18. Harvé Alsamad A, Beautru R, Gaston A, Bedbeder P, et al. Management of sinonasal hemangiopericytomas. *Rhinology* 1999;37: 153–158.

19. Kassir RR, Rassekh CH, Kinsella M, et al. Osteosarcoma of the head and neck: meta-analysis of treatment outcomes. *Laryngoscope* 1997;107:56–61.

20. Logsdon MD, Ha CS, Kavadi VS, et al. Lymphoma of the nasal cavity and paranasal sinuses: improved outcome and altered prognostic factors with combined modality therapy. *Cancer* 1997; 80: 477–488.

21. Kuhn UM, Mann WJ, Amedee RG. Endonasal approaches for nasal and paranasal sinus tumor removal. *ORL* 2001;63: 366–371.

22. Samant S, Robbins KT, Vang M, et al. Intra-arterial cisplatin and concomitant radiation therapy followed by surgery for advanced paranasal sinus cancer. *Arch Otolaryngol Head Neck Surg* 2004; 130:948–955.

23. Carrau RL, Segas J, Nuss DW, et al. Squamous cell carcinoma of the sinonasal tract invading the orbit. *Laryngoscope* 1999;109: 230–235.

Orbital Tumors

Mark A. Alford   Jeffrey A. Nerad

Wide varieties of tumors are known to occur in the orbit. Vascular, lymphoid, nervous, and mesenchymal structures are all normally found within the orbit and may give rise to primary orbital tumors. Primary lacrimal gland tumors of lymphoid and epithelial cell origin also cause orbital mass lesions. In Henderson's (1) 40-year study of orbital tumors at the Mayo Clinic, the five most common primary tumors were hemangioma, non-Hodgkin lymphoma, inflammatory tumors, meningioma, and optic nerve glioma. Wilson and Grossniklaus (2) reviewed five large series on orbital disease with a total of 4,563 orbital lesions. They found that neoplasms (primary and secondary), inflammations (Graves disease, idiopathic orbital inflammation, and infections), and other lesions composed 50%, 25%, and 25%, respectively, of the reported orbital lesions. The most common primary orbital tumors in their review were meningioma, cavernous hemangioma, and lymphoma.

The close anatomic proximity of the orbit to other important structures, including the paranasal sinuses, cranium, conjunctiva, lacrimal sac, eyelids, and globe, makes secondary invasion another common cause of orbital tumors. Secondary tumors account for approximately 12% of all orbital lesions (2) and 33% to 45% of all orbital neoplasms (1,3). The most common secondary tumors were mucoceles, squamous cell carcinoma, meningioma, vascular malformations, and basal cell carcinoma (1).

Metastatic disease, particularly adenocarcinoma of the lung and breast, may also produce orbital lesions. Between 2% and 8% of orbital tumors are due to metastatic disease (1,4). In addition to neoplasms, various inflammatory and systemic vasculitic conditions may produce orbital masses.

The incidence of orbital tumors has been studied in several long-term series. Henderson (1) found the five most common tumor groups from a series of 1,376 consecutive orbital tumors to be carcinomas (23%), cysts (12%), meningioma (10%), vascular tumors (9%), and non-Hodgkin lymphoma (8%). Shields (4), in a study of 645 orbital biopsies,

found the most common orbital tumors to be cystic lesions (30%), inflammatory masses (13%), lacrimal fossa lesions (13%), secondary tumors (11%), lymphoid tumors (10%), and vasculogenic tumors (6%).

An assortment of orbital tumors affects pediatric patients. In reported series, the exact percentages of tumors in the pediatric age group varies. However, some general patterns are clear. Most pediatric tumors are benign. Depending on the study, between 10% and 30% of childhood orbital tumors are malignant (1,5). Among the most common benign lesions are orbital dermoids, vascular tumors (capillary hemangioma and lymphangioma), optic nerve glioma, and inflammatory tumors. The most common malignant orbital tumor of children is rhabdomyosarcoma. Metastatic neuroblastoma, leukemic orbital involvement (granulocytic sarcoma), Ewing sarcoma, and extension of retinoblastoma from the globe also produce malignant orbital tumors in children.

The orbital contents are arranged in a highly organized and efficient manner with little extra room available, so almost all space-occupying lesions of the orbit produce signs and symptoms. Proptosis, the protrusion of the eye or eyes secondary to an orbital space-occupying lesion, is the most important clinical manifestation of orbital disease (Fig. 108.1; see also Color Plate 34). The characteristics of the proptosis including direction, onset, duration, and laterality are important and may aid in diagnosis. The direction of the proptosis is often described as axial versus nonaxial. Axial proptosis often occurs due to tumors inside the extraocular muscle cone (intraconal space). Nonaxial proptosis favors an extraconal position, such as the medial and inferior displacement of the globe secondary to a lacrimal gland tumor.

In general, inflammations and infections of the orbit present with acute proptosis over hours to days. Dysthyroid orbitopathy, rhabdomyosarcoma, lymphomatous lesions, and some malignant tumors have a more subacute presentation and course, worsening over a period of days. Benign

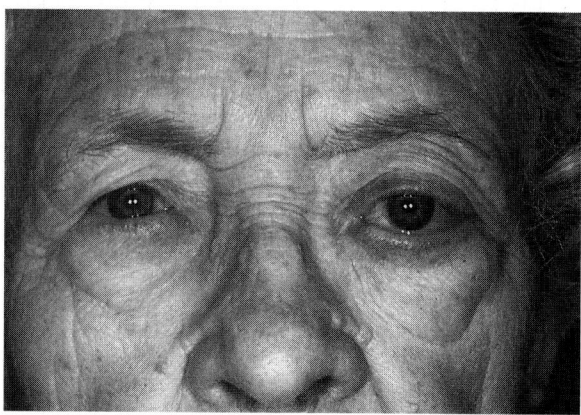

Figure 108.1 Proptosis. A patient with left-sided proptosis secondary to a metastatic orbital tumor. (See also Color Plate 34.)

tumors and cysts and some malignant tumors have a chronic course, with proptosis worsening over months to years.

Ocular motility disturbances and diplopia are common findings in orbital disease. The tumor may infiltrate the extraocular muscle or the nerve supplying the muscle, producing diplopia secondary to a motility deficit. The space-occupying tumor may also displace the globe from its normal position, causing double vision. Other signs and symptoms include vision changes, conjunctival injection and chemosis, pain, and pupillary changes.

Prompt and accurate diagnosis in addition to proper treatment can prevent loss of vision, improve motility disturbances, and in some cases increase the chances of patient survival. The goal of this chapter is to provide an overview of the most commonly encountered orbital tumors. Typical presenting characteristics and common clinical findings of each tumor are discussed to aid the otorhinolaryngologist in formulating a differential diagnosis when encountering orbital tumors.

VASCULAR TUMORS

Vascular tumors are among the most commonly encountered orbital tumors in both children and adults. Vascular tumors represent approximately 10% of all orbital tumors (2). Most vascular tumors of the orbit are benign, with cavernous hemangioma, capillary hemangioma, and lymphangioma being the most common lesions.

Cavernous Hemangioma

Cavernous hemangioma is the most common primary intraconal orbital neoplasm found in adults (6). In the Mayo Clinic study, cavernous hemangiomas were found to represent 4.3% of all orbital tumors (1). This benign tumor is more common in women and typically presents in the third to fifth decade of life. Alfred and Char (6) found that 70% of their patients with cavernous hemangiomas were

women with a mean age of 41 years at the time of diagnosis. Their patients ranged in age from 18 to 67 years.

Slowly progressive, painless, unilateral proptosis over many years is the typical presentation of patients with cavernous hemangiomas of the orbit. Significant vision loss is uncommon. Although multiple and even bilateral tumors have been reported, cavernous hemangiomas are most frequently found as isolated masses. Computed tomography (CT) and magnetic resonance imaging (MRI) findings have been shown to yield the proper diagnosis in about 95% of cases. On CT or MRI, the tumor is seen as a discrete round or oval mass without associated inflammation or infiltration of surrounding orbital structures. In 88% of cases, the tumor is located within the intraconal space (6). The tumor usually enhances with intravenous contrast. Histopathologic examination reveals an encapsulated tumor composed of multiple, large, blood-filled vascular channels lined by flattened endothelial cells.

The treatment of choice is complete surgical excision of the tumor and capsule. The prognosis for patients with cavernous hemangiomas is excellent. Recurrences are very rare even with incomplete resection. The typical intraconal location generally requires a lateral orbitotomy for complete surgical removal. In rare apical lesions, a transcranial approach may be required.

Capillary Hemangioma

Capillary hemangioma is the most common vascular tumor of the orbit and periocular tissues in infancy and childhood. This benign proliferation of endothelial cells is extremely common, and at least one lesion can be found on some part of the body in approximately 1% to 2% of all newborns. The typical superficial bright red "strawberry" mark on the eyelid or periocular skin may be an isolated finding or may be associated with orbital involvement. Deeper lesions may appear more bluish. The upper eyelid is the most common periocular location, often producing blepharoptosis. Orbital hemangiomas frequently produce proptosis and globe displacement. Approximately 5% of capillary hemangiomas are solely intraorbital, showing minimal, if any, cutaneous eyelid involvement (7).

The natural history of these lesions is well known. The capillary hemangioma is generally not present at birth, is first noted during the first month of life, and grows to its maximum size by 12 to 18 months of age. A period of stabilization occurs, followed by spontaneous involution by age 4 to 8 years. Fifty percent will involute by age 5, and approximately 90% are resolved by 7 years of age (4). There is, however, significant morbidity from these lesions because of the tumor's presence during the important period of ocular and facial development that occurs during the first decade of life. Eyelid tumors have the potential to cause deprivational and anisometropic amblyopia. Amblyopia is defined as decreased visual acuity in a structurally normal eye due to incomplete visual system development,

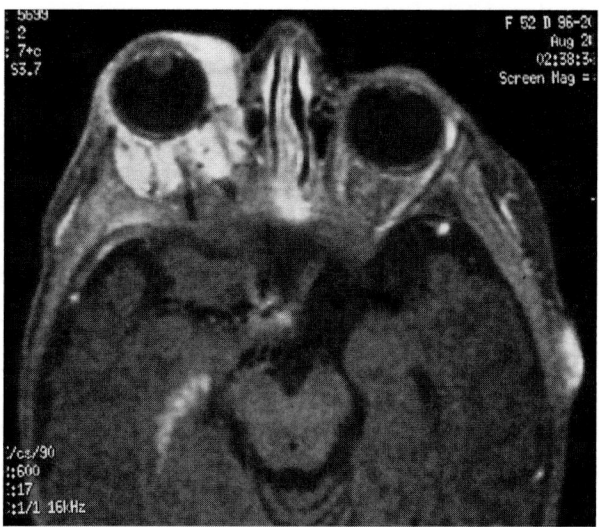

Figure 108.2 Postenhancement T1-weighted magnetic resonance image showing a capillary hemangioma of the right orbit in a neonate. Note the infiltrative nature of the tumor and the increased size of the orbit.

which can occur only during the first few years of life. Hypertrophy and stretching of the epidermal and subcutaneous tissues can lead to cosmetic cutaneous deformities. Orbital capillary hemangiomas can cause proptosis with corneal exposure, amblyopia and strabismus, optic atrophy, and bony malformations of the orbit and face.

Diagnosis is usually made on the basis of the clinical examination. Orbital involvement is best evaluated with CT or MRI. Orbital imaging shows a diffusely infiltrating nonencapsulated mass (Fig. 108.2). Capillary hemangiomas tend to conform to the surrounding orbital structures. The tumor enhances with intravenous contrast on both CT and MRI studies, confirming the lesion's vascularity. Bony erosion is not seen, but expansion of the orbital walls caused by the tumor's mass is possible. Orbital ultrasonography is also a valuable noninvasive test showing a variable pattern of high and low reflectivity.

Lesions not affecting visual or orbital development can be observed during regression as the child ages. Indications for treatment include amblyopia, proptosis with corneal exposure, optic nerve compression, and bony deformities. In many cases, the patient's parents are eager for any treatment to remove the undesirable lesion as soon as possible. The various treatment options for eyelid and orbital lesions include intralesional injections of corticosteroids, systemic corticosteroids, or careful debulking surgeries. Complete surgical removal is typically not possible.

Lymphangioma

Lymphangiomas are benign vascular malformations that may affect the ocular adnexa and orbit. They likely arise from pluripotent mesodermal tissue of the orbit and surrounding structures capable of forming vascular or lym-

phatic structures. Lymphangiomas are hemodynamically isolated from the normal orbital circulation. Histopathologically, the tumor is made up of multiple, variably sized, thin-walled, endothelial-lined vascular channels.

Rootman et al. (8) have described the location of orbital and periocular lymphangiomas as being superficial, deep, or a combination of the two. In most cases, the tumor is identified during the first decade of life. Superficial lesions are more common and involve the conjunctiva and eyelids. Tumors in this location have a better prognosis for good vision than do the deeper lesions. Orbital and eyelid lymphangiomas may also present as a soft bluish mass of the eyelid. Orbital lesions present with sudden proptosis or persistent variable proptosis. The sudden onset of proptosis is due to hemorrhage within one of the tumor's vascular channels. This spontaneous hemorrhage has been called a "chocolate cyst." If vision is not affected, these "bleeds" are observed. Lymphangiomas are also known to enlarge after an upper respiratory tract infection, resulting in increased proptosis. There is no enlargement of the lesion with a change in head position or with a Valsalva maneuver.

Diagnosis of lymphangioma is typically made with orbital imaging studies in conjunction with the clinical presentation. CT shows multiple, contiguous, dilated cystic spaces within the orbit. The radiodensity of the lobules varies with the amount of fluid and blood in each cyst (8). The cysts typically do not enhance, but rim enhancement is possible. In cases identified later in childhood, enlargement of the bony orbit is seen. MRI is likely the better study for orbital lymphangioma, allowing detailed examination of the tissue planes and cysts.

A dilated orbital vessel or varix is often confused with a lymphangioma. A varix is typically an isolated lesion that becomes symptomatic gradually. A varix is connected to the normal circulation and thus enhances with intravenous contrast and enlarges with a Valsalva maneuver.

Management of orbital and periocular lymphangioma is difficult. The infiltrative nature of these tumors makes complete resection impossible. The morbidity associated with these tumors may be quite high in some cases. Significant proptosis, corneal exposure, and optic nerve compression are all potential causes of visual loss in these patients. Surgical debulking and cyst drainage are the mainstays of treatment. Complete surgical removal is rarely possible. Other treatment options of systemic corticosteroids and radiotherapy have shown only limited results and are not recommended.

HEMATOPOIETIC TUMORS

Lymphoid Tumors

The tumors of lymphoid origin that are found in the orbit present a spectrum of disease from the benign reactive lymphoid hyperplasia to the more worrisome atypical lymphoid hyperplasia to frankly malignant orbital lymphoma.

Interestingly, the orbit does not contain lymph nodes or well-defined lymphatic vasculature, but lymphoid lesions are one of the most common orbital tumors. Lymphoid lesions of the orbit represent between 4% and 13% of all orbital tumors (2).

Orbital lymphoid lesions may be isolated to the orbital tissues or associated with systemic lymphoma. Approximately 50% of orbital lymphomas are localized to the orbit at the time of diagnosis. Approximately 15% to 25% of patients with benign reactive lymphoid hyperplasia and up to 40% of patients with atypical lymphoid hyperplasia will develop systemic lymphoma (9). Of the patients with a monoclonal malignant lymphoma of the orbit, at least one third will develop systemic disease over time. The location of the original orbital or periocular lymphoma is important in systemic prognosis. Approximately 20% of patients with lymphoid tumors of the conjunctiva developed systemic lymphoma, whereas 35% of patients with orbital tumors and 67% of patients with eyelid disease eventually developed systemic lymphoma (9). Bilateral lesions suggest systemic disease.

Orbital lymphoid lesions occur almost exclusively in adults. Most patients are between 50 and 70 years, and there is a slight female predominance. The benign and malignant lymphoid lesions present with similar findings. Most patients present with slowly progressive painless proptosis usually occurring over several weeks to a few months. These tumors are frequently located in the anterior orbit, and often a mass can be palpated along the orbital rim. The lesion may also be visible under the intact conjunctiva as a smooth, rounded, pink-orange mass ("salmon patch") (Fig. 108.3; see also Color Plate 35).

CT shows the characteristic puttylike molding of the tumor around other orbital structures. The tumor has a rather homogeneous appearance with clearly defined borders in most cases. Bony destruction is not a typical finding. Most tumors are extraconal, with the superior orbit being the most common location. The lacrimal gland is in-

volved in about 40% of cases. An affected lacrimal gland shows a smooth enlargement of its normal shape compared with the more globular or rounded enlargement seen in primary lacrimal gland neoplasms.

A generous biopsy specimen of a suspected lymphoid lesion is needed for definitive diagnosis. A portion of the biopsy specimen should be submitted to the pathologist in formalin for routine permanent section. Fresh tissue must also be submitted for sophisticated immunohistochemical studies that are required for precise cell surface marker typing for clonality. Most orbital lymphomas are of monoclonal B-cell origin. Most of the reactive orbital lymphoid lesions are composed of a majority of T cells and B cells with different cell-surface markers (polyclonal). All patients with lymphoid lesions of the orbit need a complete systemic evaluation by an oncologist, searching for systemic lymphoma. The workup should include a physical examination, complete blood count, bone marrow aspiration and biopsy, lumbar puncture, and abdominal and chest CT.

Treatment is dictated by the type of lymphoid lesion and whether there is evidence of systemic disease. Patients with isolated reactive lymphoid hyperplasia typically receive low doses of radiotherapy to the affected orbit. Isolated atypical lymphoid hyperplasia and lymphoma are treated with higher doses of radiation. Patients with systemic disease receive a combination of orbital radiotherapy and systemic chemotherapy.

Leukemia

The orbit is just one of many sites that can harbor malignant leukemic cells during the course of the disease. Approximately 10% of patients with systemic leukemia were found to have orbital involvement at the time of autopsy (1). Orbital involvement is more common in children and is often bilateral. Signs of orbital disease include a rapid onset of proptosis and inflammation that may resemble an orbital cellulitis. Spontaneous orbital hemorrhage has also been reported in association with leukemia.

A granulocytic sarcoma is a collection of immature myeloid cells, forming an obvious mass in the orbit. Historically, the tumor has been called a chloroma due to the greenish color observed when the tumor is biopsied. The pigment responsible for the distinctive color is myeloperoxidase. Granulocytic sarcomas are more common in children and may be seen in both acute and chronic myelogenous leukemias (10). In some cases, the granulocytic sarcoma precedes systemic leukemia. The most common presenting findings are painless proptosis often accompanied by a violaceous lid swelling of a few weeks' duration. As with all children with progressive proptosis, orbital imaging must be obtained urgently. In patients with an orbital granulocytic sarcoma and no sign of systemic leukemia, systemic chemotherapy is started, because all patients will eventually develop true systemic leukemia. In

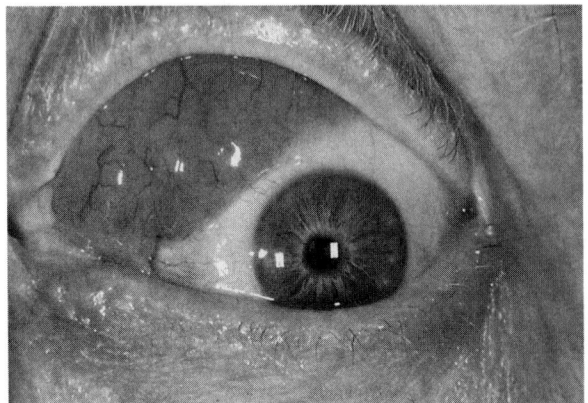

Figure 108.3 Orbital lymphoma extending under the conjunctiva of the right eye. (See also Color Plate 35.)

patients with preexisting leukemia, radiotherapy is often used to treat the orbital lesions. The prognosis for patients with granulocytic sarcoma is bleak, with most patients dying within 18 months of diagnosis.

Langerhans Cell Histiocytosis (Histiocytosis X)

Langerhans cell histiocytosis is a rare condition of proliferating Langerhans cells. The Langerhans cell is a macrophage that normally resides in the epidermis of the skin. The disease is characterized by one or more destructive bone lesions of the skull, ribs, sternum, long bones, vertebrae, or pelvis. In the disseminated form of the disease, soft tissue granulomas are also present. The orbit is rarely affected, with only 11 cases reported in the long-term Mayo Clinic study of orbital tumors (1). Most patients with Langerhans cell granulomas are children younger than 10 years. The common findings include unilateral proptosis and lateral eyelid swelling. These symptoms usually progress over a period of months. Some children present with more rapid onset of symptoms, mimicking an orbital cellulitis. The frontal and zygomatic bones are the most commonly involved orbital structures (11).

The CT appearance of this condition is quite distinctive, showing a circumscribed lytic bone lesion without sclerosis. Early in the disease, the bone appears expanded by a sharply delineated radiolucent mass. Histopathologic examination reveals the macrophage and giant cells along with a mixture of inflammatory cells.

Excision of isolated orbital bone lesions is often curative. There are also reports of spontaneous healing after biopsy. Some investigators favor postoperative radiotherapy as well. In general, the behavior of these tumors is unpredictable, and close follow-up is required. Treatment of patients with disseminated disease is more difficult. Treatment usually includes radiotherapy in combination with chemotherapy.

NEURAL TUMORS

The most common primary orbital tumors of neural origin include schwannoma, optic nerve glioma, meningioma, and neurofibroma and represent approximately 8% of all orbital tumors (1).

Schwannoma (Neurilemoma)

The schwannoma is a benign, noninvasive, peripheral nerve tumor accounting for approximately 1% of orbital tumors. Schwannomas occur primarily in adults ranging in age from 20 to 70 years (4). The patient typically presents with slowly progressive painless proptosis and diplopia. Although uncommon, progressive visual loss or a relative afferent pupillary defect may be caused by tumors located in the orbital apex.

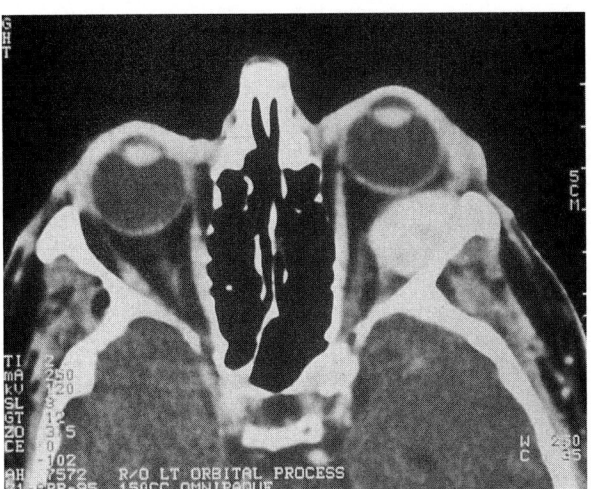

Figure 108.4 Orbital schwannoma located in the lateral portion of the left orbit in a 51-year-old man. Note the round shape and homogeneous appearance on computed tomography.

Most schwannomas are unilateral and solitary. They may arise from any nerve within the orbit. They are more commonly located in the intraconal space but may be found in any part of the orbit. CT examination shows a well-circumscribed elongated ovoid mass that displaces surrounding structures (Fig. 108.4). The lesion is commonly homogeneous. Long-standing tumors, so-called ancient schwannomas, may have areas of cystic degeneration and calcification. Schwannomas show a small degree of enhancement after intravenous contrast injection. On MRI, the tumor is hypointense on T1-weighted and hyperintense on T2-weighted images.

Histopathologic examination reveals an encapsulated tumor composed principally of Schwann cells. The Schwann cells are usually arranged as a combination of two distinctive patterns separated by variable degrees of fibrous tissue. The Antoni A pattern consists of an orderly palisading arrangement of elongated spindle-shaped cells. The Antoni B pattern is composed of a loose myxoid arrangement of ovoid or stellate cells (1).

The definitive therapy for orbital schwannomas is the complete surgical excision of the tumor and its capsule. The prognosis is excellent, with recurrences being extremely rare (12).

Optic Nerve Gliomas

The optic nerve glioma is the fifth most common primary intraorbital tumor, representing 2.4% of all orbital mass lesions in the Mayo Clinic study (1). It is also the second most common orbital tumor found in children, accounting for approximately 14% of orbital tumors in patients younger than 15 years (1). The fibrillary astrocyte is the cell responsible for optic nerve gliomas. Optic nerve gliomas are associated with neurofibromatosis in 18% to 50% of cases (13).

Most patients present in the first decade of life, with a mean age of approximately 8 years. Intraorbital optic nerve gliomas present with axial proptosis and vision loss. Frequently, young children do not report vision changes. Loss of vision in a child should be suspected if strabismus or a relative afferent pupillary defect develops. Optic nerve head edema is present early, with pallor present in long-standing disease. Gliomas located in the optic canal or chiasm may present initially with vision loss as the only finding. On CT, optic nerve gliomas appear as fusiform or lobular, isodense, homogeneous enlargements of the optic nerve (Fig. 108.5). On coronal section, the nerve cannot be separated from the tumor mass, and calcification is rare. MRI is the study of choice to evaluate extension of the tumor into the optic canal and chiasm. The glioma is hypointense relative to brain on T1-weighted images and hyperintense on T2-weighted images.

Treatment of optic nerve gliomas depends on the location of the tumor, the visual acuity, and its growth pattern. Wright et al. (13) concluded that the growth pattern of optic nerve gliomas falls into two fairly distinct groups. The first is one of indolent growth with little change in tumor size on serial examinations over many years. The other is a pattern of progressive tumor enlargement. Optic nerve meningiomas, although typically less common in children, are more aggressive than optic nerve gliomas and should be ruled out in the case of a rapidly growing optic nerve mass. Patients with tumors confined to the orbit along with good vision can be followed closely with sensitive neuroophthalmic testing and serial imaging studies. Evidence of continued growth or extension into the optic canal dictates complete resection of the optic nerve from the posterior surface of the globe to the optic chiasm. Patients with poor vision at presentation typically have the tumor and optic nerve removed via a transfrontal craniotomy for definitive diagnosis and complete resection.

Orbital Meningiomas

Primary orbital meningiomas arise from the optic nerve and represent approximately 3% of all orbital tumors (1). Of all the meningiomas found in the orbit, about 30% are primary. Most (70%) of the meningiomas of the orbit invade secondarily from the cranium and are discussed later in this chapter in the section on secondary tumors. Approximately 75% of patients with meningiomas are female (14). The disease is most common in adults in the fourth to seventh decade of life. Rarely, optic nerve meningiomas are seen in children.

Although proptosis is the most common presenting sign, seen in roughly 85% of patients with primary orbital meningiomas, visual disturbances such as decreased visual acuity and visual field defects are the more common chief complaints voiced by patients. Other findings include optic disk pallor, optic nerve head edema, diplopia, headaches, optociliary shunt vessels, and ptosis. On CT, a primary optic nerve meningioma appears as either a focal exophytic mass at any point along the optic nerve or more commonly as a fusiform enlargement of the nerve. The mass is typically homogeneous, infiltrative, and enhancing. In some cases, calcifications of the tumor in the subarachnoid space along the optic nerve tissue give the classic "railroad track" appearance. On coronal views, the normal-sized optic nerve is visible and surrounded by the tumor. As in optic nerve gliomas, MRI is the study of choice to evaluate evidence of intracranial extension.

In general, optic nerve sheath meningiomas cannot be removed from the surface of the optic nerve without causing severe vision loss. In many cases, especially in older patients, these tumors can be simply followed for evidence of intracranial extension. Radiotherapy and hormone therapy are also used in some patients. Wright et al. (14), after following 50 patients for more than 15 years, found that optic nerve meningiomas in patients younger than 40 years were more aggressive. They believed the chance of intracranial spread is considerable in these patients and recommended total excision of the tumor at an early stage.

MESENCHYMAL TUMORS

Mesodermal and Muscle Tumors

Rhabdomyosarcoma

Rhabdomyosarcoma is the most common primary malignant tumor of the orbit in children and the most common soft tissue malignancy of childhood (4). Rhabdomyosarcoma has been diagnosed in patients ranging in age from newborn to 70 years. The average age at presentation is 6 to 7 years, with 90% of patients younger than 13 years (4,15). There appears to be a slight male predominance and no racial predilection or known hereditary tendency (4).

Children typically present with progressive, painless, unilateral proptosis of a period of days to weeks. About

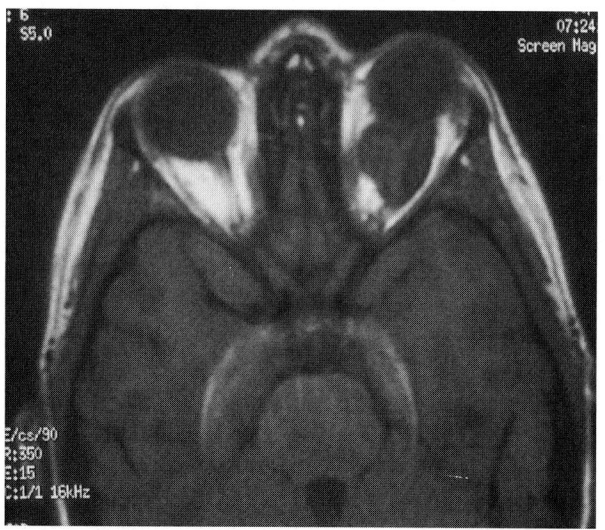

Figure 108.5 T1-weighted magnetic resonance image of an optic nerve glioma of the left orbit in a 12-year-old girl.

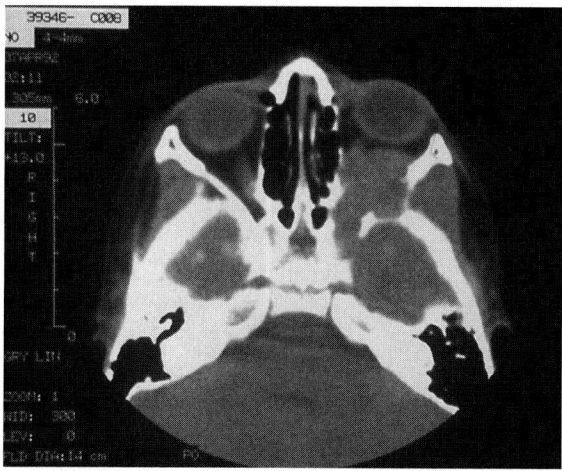

Figure 108.6 Computed tomography of rhabdomyosarcoma of the left posterior orbit in a 6-year-old girl. Note the area of bony destruction.

one third of children also present with ptosis and a palpable mass (5). The eyelid skin may be edematous and erythematous, but unlike preseptal cellulitis, the skin is not warm to the touch. Other ophthalmic findings may include conjunctival chemosis, ophthalmoplegia, choroidal folds, optic disk edema, or dilated retinal vessels. If the tumor originated in or has spread to the paranasal sinuses, symptoms of sinusitis and epistaxis may be present.

CT shows a poorly defined homogeneous orbital mass (Fig. 108.6). The tumor may arise from any location within the orbit, with about 25% being intraconal (1). Areas of bony destruction and sinus invasion may be present.

The tumor arises from primitive mesenchymal cells in the orbit. Three types of rhabdomyosarcoma have been described. Two thirds of pediatric orbital cases are of the embryonal type. The alveolar type is the most malignant form and has a predilection for the inferior orbit. The pleomorphic type is the most well-differentiated form and carries the best prognosis.

Biopsy is required for definitive diagnosis before treatment. The surgical approach should depend on the extent and accessibility of the tumor determined by the clinical examination and radiologic findings. At the time of biopsy, the largest amount of tumor that can be safely removed is taken. Fresh tissue should be sent for immunohistochemical studies. Exenteration or complete resection is not required. In biopsy-proven cases, staging and assessment of disseminated disease with bone marrow biopsy, chest radiographs, liver function tests, complete blood count, and lumbar puncture are required.

In the past, the disease was uniformly fatal. Recent advances in the treatment of rhabdomyosarcoma using a combination of chemotherapy and radiation have increased the 5-year survival rate in localized disease to approximately 90% (15). With disseminated disease, the 5-year survival decreases to 35%.

Fibro-Osseous Tumors

Fibrous Dysplasia

Fibrous dysplasia is an uncommon condition considered to be a hamartomatous malformation of unknown etiology. The condition is characterized by the replacement of normal cortical bone with a cellular fibrous stroma containing multiple nests of immature woven bone. The disease is described as monostotic when a bone or bones at a single location are involved and as polyostotic when multiple bones at different locations are affected. Orbital and facial bone involvement is more typical of the monostotic form of the disease. Orbital bone involvement may affect only one or multiple contiguous bones but typically remains unilateral. The orbital roof is the most common site of orbital involvement (16). The polyostotic form, which has been associated with Albright syndrome in a small number of cases, may affect the bones of the face but more commonly involves the ribs, sternum, and vertebrae.

The onset of the disease is typically seen in the first two decades of life. However, in some patients, the lesions are not symptomatic until much later in life. The signs and symptoms depend on which bones are involved. The most common presentation is an adolescent patient with proptosis, globe and orbit displacement, and facial asymmetry. Patients with sphenoid bone involvement may present with decreased visual acuity or visual field defects. Involvement of the maxilla may lead to upward globe displacement, nasolacrimal duct obstruction, and epiphora.

On CT, the involved bone appears thickened and deformed. Within the thickened bone are multiple areas of lucent-appearing lytic spaces and "ground glass"-appearing sclerotic zones (16). The thinner orbital bones have a cystic appearance, whereas thicker bones typically appear more sclerotic (1). Although the clinical presentation is usually adequate to make the diagnosis in a child, biopsy specimens are sometimes required for diagnosis.

It was once thought that spontaneous arrest of the disease occurred by the third decade of life. However, in some cases, progression continues into later adulthood. Although many cases can be managed with careful observation, indications for treatment include significant cosmetic deformity and vision loss secondary to compressive optic neuropathy. Treatment is surgical, with complete resection followed by immediate craniofacial reconstruction (16). In larger tumors where total resection is not possible, removal of as much of the involved bone as necessary to protect sight and correct the cosmetic deformity should be performed.

Osteoma

An osteoma is a benign tumor of bone accounting for approximately 1% of all orbital tumors (4). Osteomas are also known to arise from the bones of the paranasal sinuses. The presentation depends on the bony origin of the tumor. Most osteomas affecting the orbit originate from the frontal bone, with ethmoid and maxillary osteomas being less commonly associated with orbital findings.

Osteomas are typically unilateral solitary lesions recognized in adulthood. In patients with multiple lesions, Gardner syndrome, a familial condition associated with soft tissue tumors and colon carcinoma, must be ruled out. Patients with osteomas present with symptoms including sinusitis, dull orbital pain, facial asymmetry, globe displacement, or proptosis. Diagnosis is readily made with CT or plain films showing a smooth, rounded, or lobulated mass with a density similar to normal bone. The lesions may appear sessile or pedunculated.

Smaller asymptomatic tumors are typically followed with serial CT and clinical examinations. Larger tumors causing significant proptosis or tumors in the orbital apex compressing the optic nerve often need to be resected. The prognosis for life and vision is excellent.

Osteosarcoma

Osteosarcoma is a highly malignant tumor of bone that more commonly affects the long bones of the body but in rare cases involves the bones of the face and orbit. Recently, a gene responsible for the development of both osteosarcoma and retinoblastoma has been discovered on chromosome 13 (17). Patients present with a more rapid progression of proptosis and globe displacement when compared with benign bony tumors. Orbital pain, numbness, and vision loss have also been found to be common findings. In Henderson's (1) study of 10 patients, the median age at presentation was 41 years with a range from 16 to 64 years. CT studies show an enhancing bony mass with areas of sclerosis and lysis of bone. Areas of calcification are also seen, representing an area of new bone formation. On histopathologic examination, proliferating malignant cells are mixed with areas of immature bone.

The prognosis for patients with osteosarcoma of the orbital region is extremely poor. The treatment of choice at the present time is surgical resection along with systemic chemotherapy. However, the highly malignant nature of these tumors and the difficulty in complete resection of tumors in this area makes a cure unlikely.

LACRIMAL GLAND TUMORS

Numerous conditions are known to cause enlargement of the lacrimal gland. Mass lesions of the lacrimal gland typically produce proptosis and medial and inferior globe displacement. Most lacrimal gland masses are due to idiopathic orbital inflammatory disease and are associated with other inflammatory signs and symptoms. The findings of swelling and erythema of the lateral portion of the upper eyelid suggest inflammation of the lacrimal gland. Bacterial and viral infections of the lacrimal gland may also cause an acute dacryoadenitis. Staphylococcal and streptococcal species are the most common bacterial pathogens affecting the lacrimal gland. Viral dacryoadenitis may be seen in association with herpesvirus infections,

mumps, and mononucleosis. Chronic dacryoadenitis is caused by trachoma, syphilis, tuberculosis, and sarcoidosis.

Of the lacrimal gland masses not associated with infectious or inflammatory conditions, approximately half are caused by lymphoproliferative disorders and half by epithelial neoplasms.

The lymphoid lesions affecting the lacrimal gland include benign reactive lymphoid hyperplasia, atypical lymphoid hyperplasia, malignant lymphoma, and the leukemias. On CT examination, lymphoid lesions produce smooth enlargement and elongation of the lacrimal gland, whereas epithelial neoplasms appear more globular. Lymphoid lesions appear to mold around orbital structures and rarely show any bony changes (18).

Approximately 50% of all epithelial tumors of the lacrimal gland are benign mixed tumors (pleomorphic adenomas). The other 50% are carcinomas, including adenoid cystic carcinoma, malignant mixed carcinoma, and adenocarcinoma. Primary epithelial neoplasms of the lacrimal gland are rare, representing about 3% of all orbital tumors (2).

The benign mixed tumor of the lacrimal gland accounts for approximately 25% of all lacrimal fossa masses (4). It is composed of proliferations of both epithelial and mesenchymal elements. The tumor occurs primarily in adults ranging in age from 20 to 50 years. Patients present with slowly progressive painless proptosis, globe displacement, and upper eyelid swelling over a period of months to years. In many cases, a nontender firm mass can be palpated at the orbital rim. CT examination shows a round well-circumscribed mass in the anterior portion of the superior lateral orbit (Fig. 108.7). Pressure enlargement of the lacrimal gland fossa without bony destruction by this slow-growing tumor is almost always present.

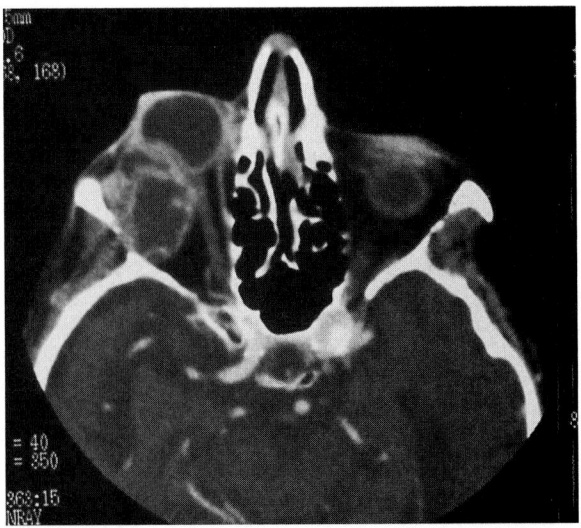

Figure 108.7 Computed tomography of a large, long-standing, benign mixed tumor of the lacrimal gland in a 90-year-old patient. Significant globe indentation is present. Corneal exposure secondary to the tumor led to a severe corneal infection and loss of the eye.

Patients presenting with findings consistent with a benign mixed tumor should undergo complete surgical excision of the tumor and its pseudocapsule through a lateral orbitotomy without a preliminary incisional biopsy. If the capsule is incised for direct biopsy or if the tumor is incompletely removed, there is a 32% rate of recurrence over the patient's lifetime, often with malignant degeneration of the tumor (18).

Adenoid cystic carcinoma is the most common malignant epithelial neoplasm of the lacrimal gland, representing about 25% of all epithelial neoplasms. Malignant mixed cell carcinomas, adenocarcinomas, and mucoepidermoid carcinomas are also found. Patients with malignant epithelial tumors of the lacrimal gland typically present with progressive proptosis of less than 12 months' duration. Pain or numbness is a very common finding and should always alert the physician to the possibility of a malignant process. Radiologic studies frequently show bony destruction associated with an enlarged lacrimal gland mass infiltrating the surrounding soft tissues. Calcification of the lesion is also more likely in malignant lesions (18).

Malignant epithelial lesions of the lacrimal gland represent a serious threat to survival, with mortality being greater than 50%. In suspected malignant lesions, incisional biopsy is indicated for definitive diagnosis. Malignant lesions require complete surgical resection. In many cases, this is achieved with exenteration, removal of adjacent bone, and postoperative radiotherapy. Distinct metastases may occur many years after excision of the primary tumor.

INFLAMMATORY TUMORS

Idiopathic orbital inflammation, also known as orbital pseudotumor, is an inflammatory condition of unknown etiology affecting various orbital tissues. In the Mayo Clinic series, idiopathic orbital inflammation constituted 4.2% of all orbital tumors and 10% of all primary orbital tumors (1). The inflammation can be diffuse or localized to specific orbital tissues, including the extraocular muscles (myositis), the lacrimal gland (sclerosing dacryoadenitis), the sclera (scleritis), or the optic nerve (perineuritis).

Idiopathic orbital inflammation has been seen in patients of all ages but is most common in adults between the ages of 30 and 70 years. The onset of symptoms typically occurs over a period of a few days, but more subacute and chronic forms have been described. Most patients present with dull and poorly localized orbital pain often exacerbated by eye movement. Proptosis is noted in 67% to 85% of patients, indicating the inflammation of retrobulbar tissues (19). Other common findings include eyelid swelling, conjunctival chemosis, and diplopia (Fig. 108.8; see also Color Plate 36). Vision loss is reported in about 20% of patients secondary to scleral, uveal, or optic nerve inflammation (20). Approximately one third of children have

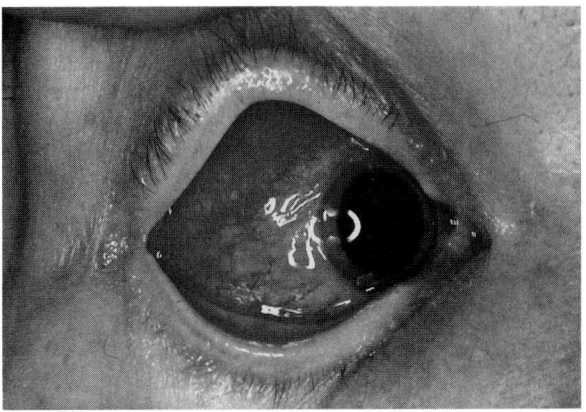

Figure 108.8 An inflamed right eye associated with idiopathic orbital inflammation. The patient complained of pain with eye movement and diplopia. (See also Color Plate 36.)

bilateral disease. Bilateral disease in an adult suggests a systemic vasculitis or lymphoproliferative disorder.

CT findings vary depending on the orbital tissues involved. Affected structures are typically enlarged, with shaggy margins surrounded by a diffuse hazy infiltrate. Enhancement is frequently noted after intravenous contrast injection. In general, multiple tissues of the orbit are affected, and this finding is highly suggestive of idiopathic orbital inflammation. Solitary mass lesions are reported but rare. In idiopathic orbital inflammation affecting the extraocular muscles, the belly of the muscle and the muscle tendon is involved. The muscle enlargement seen in thyroid-related orbital disease spares the tendon. Bony destruction is uncommon. MRI is also useful in the evaluation of idiopathic orbital inflammation. T1-weighted images show the lesions to be isointense to muscle and enhance with contrast. T2-weighted images are isointense to hyperintense to the surrounding orbital fat.

Biopsy specimens commonly show a diffuse cellular infiltrate composed of granulocytes, lymphocytes, plasma cells, and at times eosinophils. Varying degrees of fibrosis are also present. Vasculitis is not a finding consistent with idiopathic orbital inflammation.

Most patients with idiopathic orbital inflammation respond well to oral corticosteroids. A small number of cases may require more powerful immunosuppressive medications, such as cyclophosphamide or cyclosporine, or radiotherapy. In young otherwise healthy patients in whom idiopathic orbital inflammation is the most likely diagnosis from clinical and radiologic findings, an empiric trial of oral prednisone is acceptable. The response is typically dramatic, with significant improvement occurring during the first few days of therapy. Biopsy is required if the response to steroids is poor or incomplete or if the patient rebounds during the steroid taper.

Orbital vasculitis is a rare and poorly understood cause of orbital inflammation associated with many of the systemic vasculitic syndromes. The initial findings may be similar to those found in idiopathic orbital inflammation. Wegener granulomatosis, polyarteritis nodosa, giant cell arteritis, and many of the conditions causing hypersensitivity vasculitis, including systemic lupus erythematosus, are known to cause orbital inflammation. Most patients with orbital involvement present with painful proptosis and other systemic symptoms of vasculitis. In some cases, orbital findings may be the first indication of disease. The common feature found on a biopsy specimen is evidence of vasculitis. As discussed earlier, suspected idiopathic orbital inflammation that does not respond as expected to oral prednisone demands a biopsy for histologic examination. The early diagnosis of a systemic vasculitic condition may slow the progression of the disease and spare vital organs.

CYSTS

A variety of cysts is known to occur in the orbit. The most commonly encountered primary cysts are the dermoid and the simple epithelial cyst. The mucocele is the most common secondary orbital cyst and is discussed in the section on secondary orbital tumors. Dermoid and epithelial cysts accounted for approximately 2% of all orbital tumors in the Henderson (1) series and as high as 25% of all orbital tumors in the Shields (4) series. The difference is likely due to the fact that the Shields study also included dermoids of the anterior orbital rim and deep orbital lesions.

Dermoid cysts likely arise from bits of embryonic ectoderm trapped within the suture lines between the orbital bones. The superficial dermoid cysts are located most commonly at the frontozygomatic, frontoethmoid, or frontolacrimal sutures (21). The deep orbital dermoids are commonly adjacent to the sphenozygomatic or sphenoethmoid suture. Most superficial dermoid cysts are diagnosed before the age of 5 years, whereas deeper cysts can be asymptomatic until adulthood. The clinical presentation is dependent on the location of the cyst. Patients with anteriorly located dermoid cysts present with a unilateral, painless, palpable, subcutaneous mass most commonly located at the lateral portion of the eyebrow. Cysts located at the orbital rim are typically attached to the orbital bone by a small pedicle of tissue. These cysts are not attached to the overlying skin. Deeper orbital lesions present with painless progressive proptosis and globe displacement. In the cases of a spontaneous rupture, an acute inflammatory reaction develops.

CT shows a round, well-defined, thin-walled structure with a nonenhancing lumen (21). Some cysts are more irregularly shaped with less well-defined walls and cystic spaces (Fig. 108.9). Some cysts, especially those found in the deeper orbit of older patients, may show calcium deposition in the cyst wall and bony changes secondary to the pressure effect of the tumor. In rare cases, the cysts take on a dumbbell shape as they extend through the suture into the temporalis fossa, sinuses, or cranial vault. Microscopic

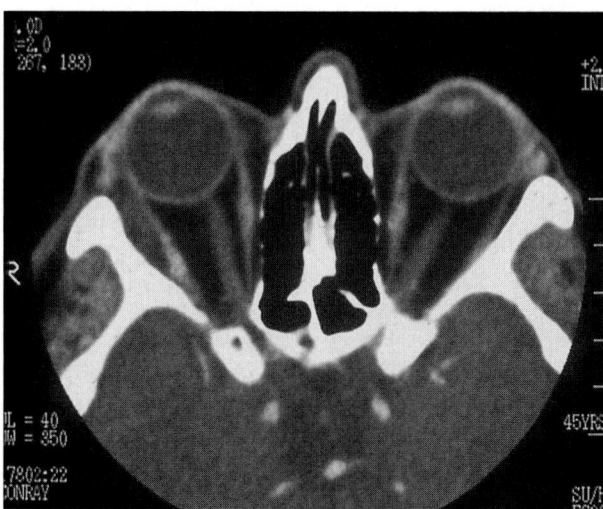

Figure 108.9 Dermoid cyst. On this computed tomography, note the mass between the lateral rectus muscle and the lateral wall on the right side.

examination reveals a cystic structure lined by stratified squamous epithelium along with the presence of dermal appendages, including hairs and sebaceous glands.

Small dermoid cysts can be followed for signs of growth, visual disturbances, or cosmetic deformity. Larger symptomatic cysts are managed with complete surgical excision without rupture of the cyst wall. The prognosis for vision is excellent for anteriorly located cysts. More posterior cysts are more difficult to remove completely and carry a slightly higher rate of recurrence.

Simple epidermal cysts are less common than dermoid cysts, representing about 1% of all orbital tumors (4). They typically appear in a slightly older age group than dermoid cysts. They likely occur because of sequestrations of conjunctival tissue in the orbit during embryologic development or are implanted after trauma. Most patients present with slowly progressive painless proptosis. Sometimes a mass can be palpated in the upper eyelid. Proptosis can be rapid and associated with eyelid swelling and erythema if the cyst ruptures. CT shows a thin-walled cystic structure without bony involvement. The preferred treatment is complete surgical excision.

SECONDARY TUMORS

Tumors arising from the structures surrounding the orbit are common causes of orbital mass lesions, accounting for 44% of all orbital tumors in the 40-year study of orbital tumors at the Mayo Clinic (1). The five most common secondary tumors affecting the orbit are mucoceles, squamous cell carcinomas, meningiomas, basal cell carcinomas, and vascular malformations (1). Secondary tumors of the orbit may spread from the paranasal sinuses, cranium, eyelids, conjunctiva, and the globe itself.

The most common mass lesion of the orbit originating in the paranasal sinuses is the mucocele. Mucoceles represent 8.3% of all orbital tumors and 18% of all secondary orbital tumors (1). Mucoceles are likely a result of sinus ostium obstruction leading to an enlarged fluid-filled sinus that first compresses and then erodes through the bony wall into the orbit. Mucoceles occur in patients of all ages, with a median age of 51 years. More than 80% of mucoceles arise from the frontal or ethmoid sinuses (22). Most patients present with a combination of unilateral proptosis, globe displacement away from the mass, lid swelling, or a palpable superonasal mass. On CT, the mucocele is seen as a well-defined homogeneous mass extending into the orbit through a bony defect associated with an opacified sinus cavity. Treatment requires drainage of the obstructed sinus, relief of the obstruction, and at times sinus obliteration.

Neoplasms of the paranasal sinuses are uncommon. However, the close proximity of the sinuses to the orbit and eye makes orbital extension common. In a study of 79 patients with sinus tumors, 45% had evidence of orbital involvement (23). It was also shown that of the patients with orbital disease, 70% had evidence of orbital extension at the time of initial presentation. Squamous cell carcinoma was by far the most common sinus tumor invading the orbit, representing 72% of all sinus tumors reported. Other tumors include inverting papilloma, adenocarcinoma, and adenoid cystic carcinoma.

The presenting ophthalmic signs and symptoms in patients with sinus tumor extension include proptosis, facial pain, globe displacement, diplopia, visual loss, epiphora, conjunctival chemosis, and a palpable orbital mass. These tumors are more common in men and are almost exclusively seen in older adults. On CT, a homogeneous mass is noted in the sinus cavity extending into the orbit. Seventy percent to 80% of patients with sinus tumors have evidence of bony destruction (23). The maxillary sinus is the site of origin in 80% of cases. Treatment involves complete surgical excision followed by radiotherapy. Early diagnosis is essential if therapy is to be effective in improving survival in patients with these tumors.

The most common tumor extending from the cranial vault into the orbit is the meningioma. In the Mayo Clinic study of orbital tumors, approximately 70% of all orbital meningiomas were of the secondary type (1). Most of these meningiomas arise from the sphenoid ridge. Most patients are women with an average age of approximately 50 years. Secondary orbital meningiomas may present as any slow-growing mass lesion of the orbit with proptosis, ocular motility disturbances, and decreased visual acuity. However, two unusual findings are also noted in some cases. One is temporalis fossa fullness seen in large tumors, and the other is boggy edema of the ipsilateral lower eyelid. Orbital and neurologic imaging with CT shows the common finding of hyperostosis of the involved bone. The soft tissue component may be present in association with the bony changes. However, MRI with gadolinium enhancement is the preferred study for evaluating the extent of the tumor. The tumor is hyperintense after contrast administration. Combined resection by an orbital surgeon and neurosurgeon is indicated for tumors compromising vision, cranial nerve function, or other vital intracranial structures.

Basal cell carcinomas, sebaceous cell carcinomas, and squamous cell carcinomas are the most common eyelid neoplasms. Basal cell carcinoma, the most common eyelid malignancy, accounts for approximately 90% of all eyelid malignancies (4). They are most commonly located on the lower eyelid and in the medial canthal area. Sebaceous cell carcinoma accounts for approximately 4% and squamous cell carcinoma for roughly 5% of all eyelid malignancies. In the Mayo Clinic study, secondary basal cell carcinomas of the orbit accounted for 2.9% of all orbital tumors (1). The usual treatment for eyelid basal cell carcinoma is surgical excision using frozen-section margins or Mohs microsurgery. As might be expected, the patients most at risk for orbital extension are those who had incomplete excision of the original lesion, received radiotherapy, or simply neglected the original lesion, allowing it to spread to the orbit. Lesions of the medial canthal area are also more commonly associated with orbital extension.

Orbital squamous cell carcinoma and sebaceous cell carcinoma arising from the eyelids are less common than basal cell carcinoma. Henderson (1) at the Mayo Clinic reported 22 (1.6%) cases of secondary orbital squamous cell carcinoma originating in the ocular adnexa of 1,376 total orbital tumors. The same study reported only four cases of orbital sebaceous cell carcinoma. The Wills Eye Hospital study of biopsied orbital masses found similar results (4).

Fixation of the skin tumor to the underlying bone of the orbital rim and ocular motility disturbances are the most important clues to orbital invasion. CT should be obtained to investigate the full extent of the orbital process. In cases of proven orbital invasion by any of these eyelid carcinomas, exenteration followed by radiotherapy is the therapy of choice.

Squamous cell carcinoma and malignant melanoma are the most common malignant lesions of the conjunctiva. Although not accounting for a significant number of orbital tumors, they are known to invade the orbit.

In adults, choroidal melanoma is the most common intraocular tumor to extend into the orbit. Approximately 8% to 10% of patients with choroidal melanoma have evidence of extrascleral extension at the time of enucleation (4). In the Mayo Clinic series, orbital extension or recurrence of uveal melanomas accounted for approximately 2% of all orbital tumors (1). Recurrence in the orbit may occur from months to many years after the initial enucleation. Treatment consists of partial or total exenteration, radiotherapy, and at times chemotherapy. The prognosis is extremely poor, with the 5-year mortality rate as high as 80%.

Retinoblastoma, a malignant neoplasm of the sensory retina, is the most common intraocular tumor in children. Orbital extension has been reported in less than

10% of cases. The most common presentation of recurrent retinoblastoma in the orbit is displacement and protrusion of the orbital implant placed after enucleation. Recurrent retinoblastoma in the orbit typically presents within 4 months of the initial enucleation (4). Treatment of orbital retinoblastoma involves a combination of surgical excision, radiotherapy, and chemotherapy.

METASTATIC TUMORS

Metastatic tumors are an important cause of orbital disease, representing approximately 8% of all orbital tumors (1). Although most patients with metastatic orbital lesions have a history of systemic cancer, orbital metastases may signal a reactivation of dormant disease or the presence of a new systemic malignancy. In 25% of cases, the orbital tumor is the presenting manifestation of an occult systemic cancer (24). Breast carcinoma is by far the most common metastatic tumor found in the orbit, accounting for almost 50% of all metastatic lesions (25). Other tumors known to metastasize to the orbit include lung carcinoma, prostate, gastrointestinal carcinoma, renal cell carcinoma, thyroid carcinoma, and malignant melanoma. The most common metastatic tumor in children is neuroblastoma.

Common presenting findings of metastatic disease of the orbit include upper eyelid ptosis, proptosis, diplopia, pain, a palpable mass, or vision loss. Interestingly, enophthalmos is seen in approximately 25% of cases, especially in scirrhous breast and prostate carcinomas (24). The average age of presentation is approximately 61 years, with most patients being female. Bilateral eyelid ecchymosis and proptosis are the most common presenting signs of orbital neuroblastoma.

Multiple patterns of metastases to the orbital structures are seen on CT examination (Fig. 108.10). The most common site of metastasis is the intraconal space, producing a well-defined infiltrative mass that enhances with intravenous contrast. The bones of the orbit are another common site of metastatic disease, producing both osteolytic and osteoblastic lesions. Prostate carcinoma is well known to produce hyperdense osteoblastic bone lesions. Carcinoma

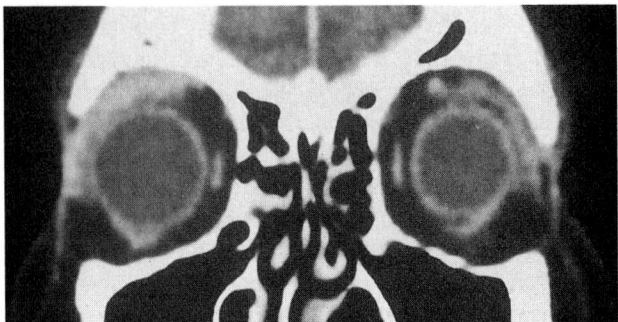

Figure 108.10 Computed tomography of metastatic breast carcinoma of the superior right orbit.

of the breast, gastrointestinal tract, and thyroid have a tendency to involve both the bone and soft tissues of the orbit. Neuroblastoma frequently causes bony destruction of the lateral orbital wall. Many of the findings present in metastatic disease mimic those of other orbital tumors. Biopsy may be required for definitive diagnosis either via orbitotomy or fine-needle aspiration.

The prognosis for patients with orbital metastases is poor, with an average survival of 10 months. Treatment modalities must be tailored to the specific tumor type and stage of the systemic disease. In general, radiotherapy is the mainstay of treatment for orbital metastatic tumors, with chemotherapy and hormonal therapy used in some cases.

CONCLUSION

The scope of disease-producing mass lesions of the orbit is broad. Both children and adults are affected by orbital tumors. The most common primary orbital tumors are meningioma, cavernous hemangioma, and lymphoma. Squamous cell carcinoma represents the most common secondary orbital neoplasm. Breast carcinoma is the most frequently encountered metastatic tumor of the orbit. Many orbital mass lesions are a result of various inflammatory conditions, including thyroid-related immune orbitopathy and idiopathic orbital inflammation. Other common orbital tumors include mucoceles and dermoid cysts. Rhabdomyosarcoma is the most common malignant tumor in children. Optic nerve glioma and capillary hemangioma are the most common benign orbital tumors in children.

The presence of proptosis, as well as its direction and duration, is the most common and important manifestation of orbital disease. In children, the most common cause of proptosis is bacterial cellulitis. In adults, the most common cause of unilateral or bilateral proptosis is thyroid-related immune orbitopathy. Benign tumors typically present with slowly progressive proptosis over many months to years. Proptosis progressing over a period of weeks to months typically is seen in malignant tumors and in thyroid disease. Infections, inflammations, and some malignant tumors present with rapidly progressive proptosis over a period of days. The history and presenting orbital findings narrow the diagnosis in most cases. The addition of orbital imaging, most commonly a CT, further refines the diagnosis. However, because of the diversity of orbital tumors, biopsy is frequently required for definitive diagnosis. In the case of a child with proptosis and an orbital mass, emergent biopsy for diagnosis is required to rule out rhabdomyosarcoma or other malignancy.

Orbital tumors are uncommon, but in some cases patients with orbital disease may present to an otorhinolaryngologist. In other cases, orbital findings may be discovered in association with sinus pathology. Early identification and appropriate treatment of these tumors can protect vision and in some cases prolong life.

HIGHLIGHTS

- A myriad of orbital tumors exist arising from every tissue type in the body.
- An orbital tumor must be ruled out in any patient presenting with proptosis.
- Thyroid orbitopathy is the most common cause of bilateral and unilateral proptosis.
- Bilateral orbital tumors are rare, with the only notable exception being lymphoid lesions.
- The most common benign orbital tumor in adults is cavernous hemangioma. The most common malignant orbital tumor in adults is lymphoma.
- The most common benign orbital tumor in children is dermoid cyst. The most common malignant orbital tumor is rhabdomyosarcoma.
- Historical clues such as pain, duration of symptoms, tempo of progression, and associated systemic illness contribute to developing a differential diagnosis.
- Signs of proptosis, nonaxial globe displacement, motility disturbance, and any associated periocular findings point to the tumor's location and refine the differential diagnosis.
- Imaging is necessary in most cases. Computed tomography is the first step in identifying physical tumor characteristics.
- Magnetic resonance imaging is useful for tumors of the optic nerve and secondary tumors such as meningioma or sinus carcinoma.
- Biopsy will be required in most cases for confirmation of the diagnosis and treatment of most orbital tumors.

REFERENCES

1. Henderson J. *Orbital tumors.* New York: Raven Press, 1994.
2. Wilson M, Grossniklaus HE. Orbital disease in North America. *Ophthalmol Clin North Am* 1996;4:539–547.
3. Rootman J. *Diseases of the orbit.* Philadelphia: JB Lippincott, 1988.
4. Shields J. *Diagnosis and management of orbital tumors.* Philadelphia: WB Saunders, 1989.
5. Volpe N, Jakobiec F. Pediatric orbital tumors. *Int Ophthalmol Clin* 1992;32:201–221.
6. Alfred P, Char D. Cavernous hemangioma of the orbit. *Orbit* 1996;15:59–66.
7. Haik B, Jacobiec F, Ellsworth R. Capillary hemangioma of the eyelid and orbit: an analysis of the clinical features and therapeutic results in 101 cases. *Ophthalmology* 1979;86:760–789.
8. Rootman J, Hay E, Graeb D. Orbital-adnexal lymphangiomas. *Ophthalmology* 1986;93:1558–1570.
9. McCormick S, Milite J. Lymphoproliferative disease of the orbit. *Ophthalmol Clin North Am* 1996;9:693–704.
10. Davis J, Parke D, Font R. Granulocytic sarcoma of the orbit. *Ophthalmology* 1985;92:1758–1762.
11. Char D, Albin A, Beckstead J. Histiocytic disorders of the orbit. *Ann Ophthalmol* 1984;16:867–873.
12. Rootman J, Goldberg C, Robertson W. Primary orbital schwannomas. *Br J Ophthalmol* 1982;66:194–204.
13. Wright J, McNabb J, McDonald W. Optic nerve glioma and the management of optic nerve tumours in the young. *Br J Ophthalmol* 1989;73:967–974.
14. Wright J, McNabb J, McDonald W. Primary optic nerve sheath meningioma. *Br J Ophthalmol* 1989;73:960–966.
15. Wharam M, Beltangady M, Hays D, et al. Localized orbital rhabdomyosarcoma. *Ophthalmology* 1987;94:251–254.
16. Moore A, Buncic J, Munro I. Fibrous dysplasia of the orbit in childhood. *Ophthalmology* 1985;92:12–20.
17. Benedict W, Fung Y, Murphree A. The gene responsible for the development of retinoblastoma and osteosarcoma. *Cancer* 1988;62:1691–1694.
18. Stewart W, Krohel G, Wright J. Lacrimal gland and fossa lesions: an approach to diagnosis and management. *Ophthalmology* 1979;86:886–895.
19. Bardenstein D. Idiopathic orbital inflammation. *Ophthalmol Clin North Am* 1996;9:659–672.
20. Kennerdell J, Dresner S. The nonspecific orbital inflammatory syndromes. *Surv Ophthalmol* 1984;29:93–103.
21. Sherman R, Rootman J, Lapointe J. Orbital dermoids: clinical presentation and management. *Br J Ophthalmol* 1984;68:642–652.
22. Lund V, Rolfe M. Ophthalmic considerations in fronto-ethmoidal mucoceles. *J Laryngol Otol* 1989;103:667–669.
23. Johnson L, Krohel G, Yeon E. Sinus tumors invading the orbit. *Ophthalmology* 1984;91:209–217.
24. Goldberg R, Rootman J. Clinical characteristics of metastatic orbital tumors. *Ophthalmology* 1990;97:620–624.
25. Freedman M, Folk J. Metastatic tumors to the eye and orbit. *Arch Ophthalmol* 1987;105:1215–1219.

Salivary Gland Neoplasms

109

Young S. Oh   David W. Eisele

Neoplasms of the salivary glands represent a diverse group of benign and malignant tumors with varying degrees of behavior. Accurate pathologic diagnosis is key to the management of these lesions because the degree of aggressiveness depends on their histologic profiles. The otolaryngologist–head and neck surgeon must understand the behavior of each tumor type to develop an appropriate treatment plan.

ANATOMY AND PHYSIOLOGY

The salivary glands are divided into the major salivary gland and the minor salivary glands. The major salivary glands consist of the paired parotid, submandibular, and sublingual glands. The minor salivary glands consist of 600 to 1,000 glands distributed throughout the upper aerodigestive tract. A commonly used classification scheme for salivary gland tumors is presented in Table 109.1.

Although the incidences vary from different series in the literature, approximately 80% of salivary gland neoplasms originate in the parotid gland, 10% to 15% develop in the submandibular gland, and the remaining tumors arise in the sublingual and minor salivary glands. The smaller the gland, the more likely the tumor will be malignant. About 80% of parotid neoplasms are benign and about 50% of submandibular tumors are benign, but fewer than 40% of sublingual and minor salivary gland neoplasms are benign (1–4). Tables 109.2, 109.3, and 109.4 list recent series in the literature detailing the incidences of neoplasms by different salivary gland type.

Ninety-five percent of salivary gland tumors occur in adults. The most common benign mesenchymal tumor in children is the hemangioma, whereas the most common benign epithelial tumor is the pleomorphic adenoma

(Table 109.5) (5). The probability of a malignancy in a child is increased if a solid nonvascular salivary mass is found. About 85% of salivary gland malignancies found in children originate in the parotid gland. Mucoepidermoid carcinoma is the most frequently encountered tumor type in this age group (Table 109.6) (5).

BENIGN NEOPLASMS

Pleomorphic Adenoma

Pleomorphic adenoma (benign mixed tumor) accounts for approximately 65% of all salivary gland tumors. These tumors are most often found in the parotid gland, followed by the submandibular gland and the minor salivary glands. They also represent the most common tumor of each type of salivary gland.

Benign mixed tumor describes the mesenchymal and epithelial components of the tumor. The gross appearance is smooth and lobular with a well-defined capsule. Microscopically, the tumor consists of epithelial and mesenchymal elements. The epithelial component forms a trabecular pattern with a mesenchymal stroma (Fig. 109.1). The mesenchymal portion may be myxoid, chondroid, fibroid, or osteoid. The stroma varies from tumor to tumor and may have a combination of any of these tissue types within it. Histologically, pleomorphic adenomas show incomplete encapsulation with pseudopod extensions. These features account for recurrence rates varying from 20% to 45% after simple enucleation (6). Appropriate surgical therapy requires resection with an adequate margin of normal tissue surrounding the tumor. Rarely, pleomorphic adenoma can metastasize and yet remain benign histologically.

TABLE 109.1

THE WORLD HEALTH ORGANIZATION'S HISTOLOGIC CLASSIFICATION OF SALIVARY GLAND TUMORS

1. Adenomas
    1.1 Pleomorphic adenoma
    1.2 Myoepithelioma (myoepithelial adenoma)
    1.3 Basal cell adenoma
    1.4 Warthin tumor
    1.5 Oncocytoma
    1.6 Canalicular adenoma
    1.7 Sebaceous adenoma
    1.8 Ductal papilloma
        1.8.1 Inverted ductal papilloma
        1.8.2 Intraductal papilloma
        1.8.3 Sialadenoma papilliferum
    1.9 Cystadenoma
        1.9.1 Papillary cystadenoma
        1.9.2 Mucinous cystadenoma
2. Carcinomas
    2.1 Acinic cell carcinoma
    2.2 Mucoepidermoid carcinoma
    2.3 Adenoid cystic carcinoma
    2.4 Polymorphous low-grade adenocarcinoma (terminal duct adenocarcinoma)
    2.5 Epithelial-myoepithelial carcinoma
    2.6 Basal cell adenocarcinoma
    2.7 Sebaceous carcinoma
    2.8 Papillary cystadenocarcinoma
    2.9 Mucinous adenocarcinoma
    2.10 Oncocytic carcinoma
    2.11 Salivary duct carcinoma
    2.12 Adenocarcinoma
    2.13 Malignant myoepithelioma (myoepithelial carcinoma)
    2.14 Carcinoma in pleomorphic adenoma (malignant mixed tumor)
    2.15 Squamous cell carcinoma
    2.16 Small cell carcinoma
    2.17 Undifferentiated carcinoma
    2.18 Other carcinomas
3. Nonepithelial tumors
4. Malignant lymphomas
5. Secondary tumors
6. Unclassified tumors
7. Tumor-like lesions
    7.1 Sialadenosis
    7.2 Oncocytosis
    7.3 Necrotizing sialometaplasia (salivary gland infarction)
    7.4 Benign lymphoepithelial lesion
    7.5 Salivary gland cysts
    7.6 Chronic sclerosing sialadenitis of submandibular gland (Kuttner tumor)
    7.7 Cystic lymphoid hyperplasia in AIDS

From Seifert G, Sobin LH. The World Health Organization's histological classification of salivary gland tumors. A commentary on the second edition. *Cancer* 1992;70:379–385, with permission.

Sites of metastasis have included the bone, lymph nodes, lung, oral cavity, pharynx, skin, liver, retroperitoneum, kidney, calvarium, the central nervous system, and paranasal sinuses (7).

TABLE 109.2

INCIDENCE OF COMMON PAROTID GLAND NEOPLASMS BY TUMOR TYPE

Tumor Type	Incidence (%)
Pleomorphic adenoma	53.3
Warthin tumor	28.3
Other benign	3.8
Total benign	**85.4**
Mucoepidermoid carcinoma	9
Adenocarcinoma	1.5
Squamous cell carcinoma	0.9
Acinic cell carcinoma	0.9
Malignant mixed tumor	0.9
Adenoid cystic carcinoma	0.5
Other malignant	0.9
Total malignant	**14.6**

From Pinkston JA, Cole P. Incidence rates of salivary gland tumors: results from a population-based study. *Otolaryngol Head Neck Surg* 1999;120:834–840, with permission.

Warthin Tumor

Warthin tumor (papillary cystadenoma lymphomatosum) is the second most common benign neoplasm of the parotid gland, accounting for 6% to 10% of all parotid tumors. The majority of Warthin tumor occurs in the parotid glands, although extraparotid sites including the cervical lymph nodes can be involved as well (8). Most cases occur in older men, but the incidence has been increasing in women, most likely related to the increased rates of smoking in women. This tumor usually presents as a slow growing mass in the tail of the parotid gland. Tumors can be multicentric in up to 21% of cases and approximately 10% are bilateral (9).

TABLE 109.3

INCIDENCE OF SUBMANDIBULAR GLAND NEOPLASMS BY TUMOR TYPE

Tumor Type	Incidence (%)
Pleomorphic adenoma	36
Other	1
Total benign	**37**
Adenoid cystic carcinoma	25
Mucoepidermoid carcinoma	12
Malignant mixed tumor	10
Adenocarcinoma	7
Squamous cell carcinoma	7
Undifferentiated carcinoma	2
Acinic cell carcinoma	<1
Total malignant	**63**

Adapted from Crabtree GM, Yarington CT. Submandibular gland excision. *Laryngoscope* 1988;98:1044 and Weber RS, Byers RM, Petit B, et al. Submandibular gland tumors: adverse histologic factors and therapeutic implications. *Arch Otolaryngol Head Neck Surg* 1990;116:1055, with permission.

TABLE 109.4
INCIDENCE OF MINOR SALIVARY GLAND NEOPLASMS BY TUMOR TYPE

Tumor Type	Incidence (%)
Pleomorphic adenoma	43
Monomorphic adenoma	4.6
Total benign	**47.6**
Adenoid cystic carcinoma	34
Mucoepidermoid carcinoma	11
Malignant mixed tumor	1.5
Adenocarcinoma	7
Squamous cell carcinoma	7
Undifferentiated carcinoma	1.5
Acinic cell carcinoma	1.5
Total malignant	**52**

From Renehan A, Gleave EN, Hancock BD, et al. Long-term follow-up of over 1000 patients with salivary gland tumors treated in a single centre. *Br J Surg* 1996;83:1751, with permission.

TABLE 109.6
MALIGNANT SALIVARY GLAND TUMORS IN CHILDREN

Tumor Type	No. of Patients
Mucoepidermoid carcinoma	108
Acinic cell carcinoma	27
Adenocarcinoma	22
Undifferentiated carcinoma	15
Sarcoma	15
Adenoid cystic carcinoma	11
Malignant mixed tumor	9
Squamous cell carcinoma	4
Other	2
Total patients	**668**
Total malignant	**32%**

From: Luna MA, Batsakis JG, El-Naggar AK. Salivary gland tumors in children. *Ann Otol Rhinol Laryngol* 1991;100:869–871, with permission.

The gross appearance of the tumor is smooth with a well-defined capsule. Cut sections reveal multiple cystic spaces of different sizes filled with thick, mucinous material. Microscopically, Warthin tumor has a characteristic appearance with a papillary epithelium with a lymphoid stroma projecting into cystic spaces (Fig. 109.2). The epithelium is a double layer of oxyphilic granular cells, with the cells of the inner layer having the nuclei oriented toward the basement membrane. The cells in the outer layer have nuclei toward the cystic space.

Treatment is complete surgical excision, with recurrence being rare.

Oncocytoma

Oncocytoma occurs almost exclusively within the parotid gland and accounts for less than 1% of all parotid neo-

plasms (10). The tumor occurs most frequently in the sixth decade of life with equal frequency between men and women.

The tumors are noncystic, firm, and rubbery. Microscopically, these neoplasms are composed of brown, plump, granular eosinophilic cells with small indented nuclei (Fig. 109.3). A mitochondria-filled cytoplasm is a characteristic finding on electron microscopy. Malignant degeneration is possible but is rare. A possible explanation for these tumors is an acquired genetic defect leading to mitochondrial dysfunction; however, an exact molecular mechanism has not been explained for this (11).

Oncocytomas usually present as a painless mass in the superficial lobe of the parotid gland and parotidectomy with facial nerve preservation is the treatment of choice.

TABLE 109.5
BENIGN SALIVARY GLAND TUMORS IN CHILDREN

Tumor Type	No. of Patients
Hemangioma	191
Pleomorphic adenoma	182
Lymphangioma	48
Neurogenic	11
Embryonal	5
Lymphoepithelial lesion	3
Cystadenoma	3
Warthin tumor	3
Other	9
Total patients	**668**
Total benign	**68%**

From Luna MA, Batsakis JG, El-Naggar AK. Salivary gland tumors in children. *Ann Otol Rhinol Laryngol* 1991;100:869–871, with permission.

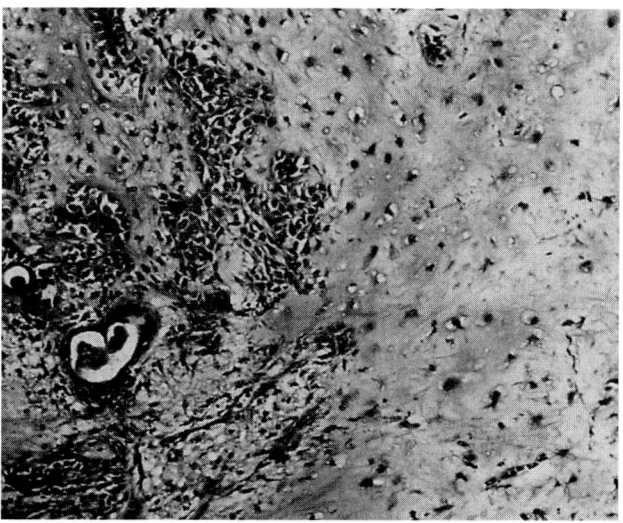

Figure 109.1 Pleomorphic adenoma. The histologic appearance shows characteristic epithelial and mesenchymal elements. (See also Color Plate 37.)

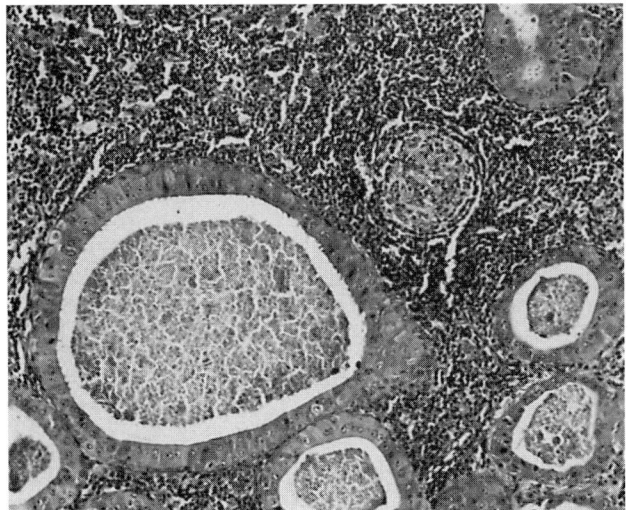

Figure 109.2 Warthin tumor. Lymphoid stroma and double-layered epithelium surround the cystic spaces.

Monomorphic Adenoma

Monomorphic adenomas include basal cell adenoma, clear cell adenoma, glycogen-rich adenoma, and other rare tumors. The most common is the basal adenoma, which is usually found in the minor salivary glands of the upper lip. The parotid gland is the most frequently involved of the major salivary glands (12).

These tumors are well circumscribed and encapsulated. Microscopically, basal cell adenomas show rows of peripheral palisading cells with a thick basement membrane. Basal cell adenomas can be confused with adenoid cystic carcinoma, and it has been suggested that adenoid cystic carcinoma may represent the malignant counterpoint of this tumor (12).

Monomorphic adenoma is considered a benign, nonaggressive tumor. Treatment consists of resection with a margin of normal tissue.

MALIGNANT NEOPLASMS

Mucoepidermoid Carcinoma

Mucoepidermoid carcinoma is the most common malignant neoplasm of the parotid gland and the second most common malignant tumor of the submandibular gland. It constitutes approximately 30% of all malignant tumors of the salivary glands (13).

Mucoepidermoid carcinomas are usually classified as low-grade or high-grade tumors. However, some authors also include an intermediate-grade as well. Low-grade tumors have a higher proportion of mucous cells to epidermoid cells. These lesions behave more like benign neoplasms but are still nevertheless capable of local invasion and metastasis. High-grade mucoepidermoid carcinomas have a higher proportion of epidermoid cells, and it may be difficult to differentiate this entity from squamous cell carcinoma. High-grade tumors are aggressive neoplasms with a high propensity for metastasis.

Low-grade tumors are usually small and partially encapsulated. High-grade neoplasms are usually larger and locally invasive. On cut sections, low-grade mucoepidermoid carcinoma may contain mucinous fluid, whereas high-grade tumors are solid. Microscopically, low-grade mucoepidermoid carcinoma demonstrates aggregates of mucoid cells separated by strands of epidermal cells (Fig. 109.4). High-grade tumors have few mucoid elements and the epidermoid cells predominate (Fig. 109.5).

The treatment of this cancer depends on the grade and stage of the tumor. For small, low-grade tumors a complete resection by parotidectomy is adequate. If all the surgical margins are clear and there are no adverse pathologic features, adjuvant radiotherapy is not needed. For high-grade mucoepidermoid carcinomas, treatment is more aggressive. For tumors of the parotid gland, complete resection by parotidectomy (sparing the facial nerve if feasible)

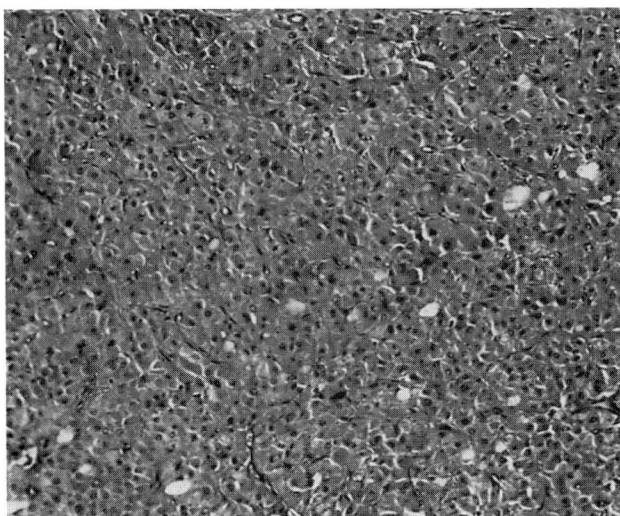

Figure 109.3 Oncocytoma. The histologic appearance is that of typical plump, granular eosinophilic cells. (See also Color Plate 38.)

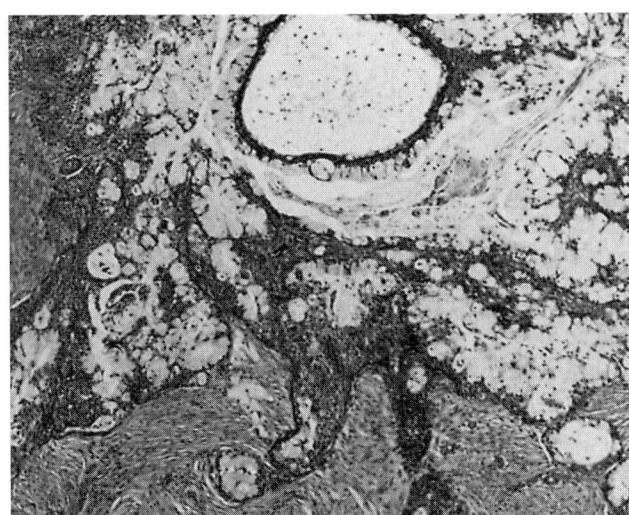

Figure 109.4 Low-grade mucoepidermoid carcinoma. Note the epithelial and glandular elements. (See also Color Plate 39.)

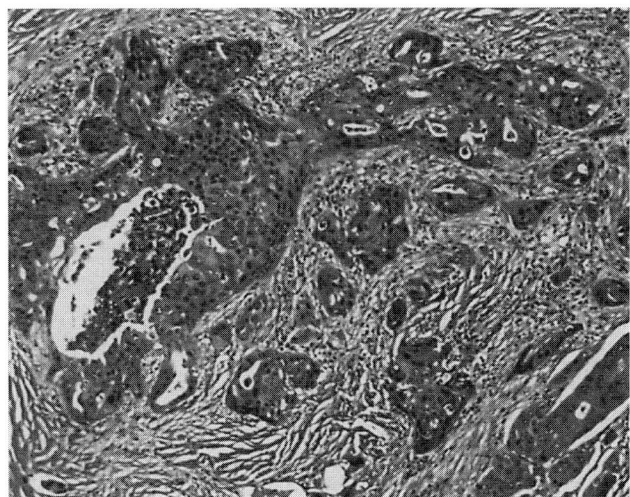

Figure 109.5 High-grade mucoepidermoid carcinoma. Note the relative lack of glandular elements. (See also Color Plate 40.)

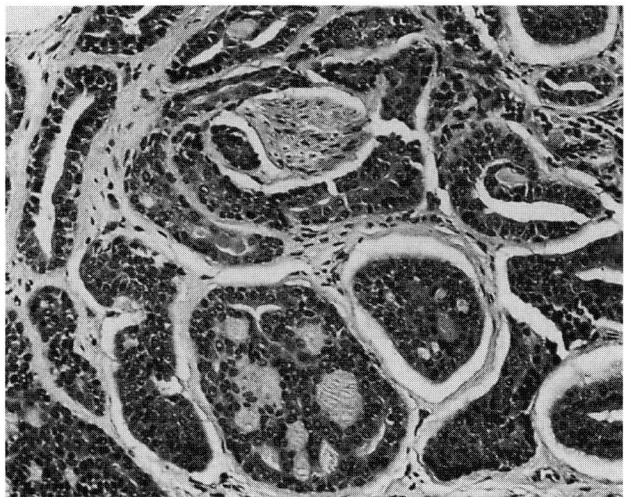

Figure 109.6 Adenoid cystic carcinoma, showing the characteristic histologic appearance with eosinophilic hyaline stroma and perineural invasion.(See also Color Plate 41.)

should be performed. Due to a high rate of occult neck metastases, an elective neck dissection should also be considered in a patient with an N0 neck (13,14). In most cases of high-grade mucoepidermoid carcinoma, radiation therapy is indicated and appears to improve local control and survival (15). Tumor grade and the status of the surgical margins seem to correlate well with prognosis.

Adenoid Cystic Carcinoma

Adenoid cystic carcinoma accounts for approximately 10% of all salivary gland neoplasms. It is the second most common malignancy of the parotid glands but is the most common malignancy of the submandibular and minor salivary glands (16). Adenoid cystic carcinoma occurs with equal frequency in men and women, usually in the fifth decade of life. Facial paralysis and pain occur as initial symptoms in a small fraction of cases.

Adenoid cystic carcinoma has a contradictory clinical course. The tumor is slow growing, but its clinical course is relentless. Multiple local recurrences can occur despite adequate surgical intervention and although regional metastatic spread is uncommon, distant spread to the lungs and bones are frequent.

Grossly, the tumor is usually monolobular and either nonencapsulated or partially encapsulated. The mass often demonstrates infiltration of surrounding normal tissue. Microscopically, adenoid cystic carcinoma has a basaloid epithelium arranged in cylindric formations in an eosinophilic hyaline stroma (Fig. 109.6). Different histologic patterns have been identified, including cribriform, solid, cylindromatous, and tubular. The solid histologic pattern appears to have a worse prognosis in terms of distant metastases and long-term survival (17).

Perineural invasion is a typical feature of adenoid cystic carcinoma. This explains the difficulty in tumor eradica-

tion despite the appearance of complete tumor removal. Complete surgical excision and postoperative radiation therapy is recommended for the management of this tumor. For select small tumors that are completely excised, however, postoperative radiation therapy may be withheld (18). There is also growing evidence that fast neutron radiotherapy may be more effective than conventional photon radiation for adenoid cystic carcinoma (19). Long-term follow-up is mandatory for these patients because of the slow, relentless disease progression.

Acinic Cell Carcinoma

Acinic cell carcinomas comprise 5% to 11% of all salivary gland cancers. The vast majority occur in the parotid gland. It affects females more often than males and occurs in the fourth to sixth decade of life. The tumor can be multicentric in 2% to 5% of cases and it ranks behind Warthin tumor for the frequency of bilateral parotid involvement (12,20).

Grossly, the well-circumscribed tumors often have a fibrous capsule. There are two populations of cells: those resembling serous acinar cells of the salivary gland and those with a clear cytoplasm. Tumors occur in several configurations, including cystic, papillary, vacuolated, or follicular. There is often a lymphoid infiltrate, and cells are characteristically positive on periodic acid–Schiff staining (Fig. 109.7).

Treatment consists of complete surgical resection. Adjuvant radiotherapy is reserved for indicators of a poor prognosis (e.g., facial nerve involvement, metastatic neck disease, and skin involvement). Elective treatment of the neck is indicated for high-grade cases of acinic cell carcinoma (20). For most cases, 5-year survival rates are excellent (20).

Adenocarcinoma

Adenocarcinoma most commonly occurs in the minor salivary glands, followed by the parotid gland. This neoplasm

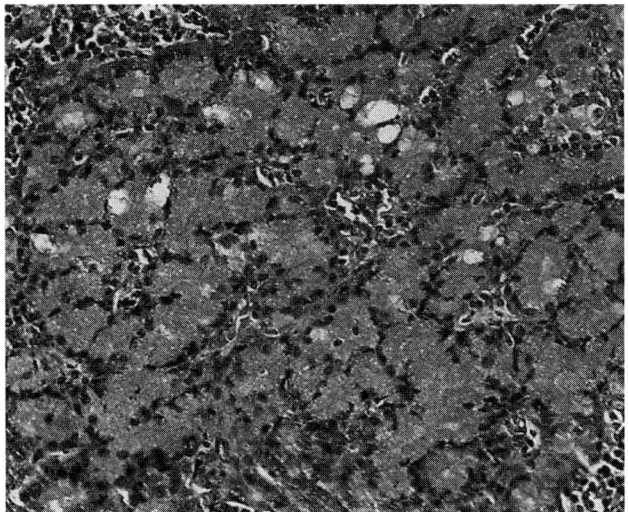

Figure 109.7 Acinic cell carcinoma. Note cells similar to serous acinar cells and cells with clear cytoplasm. (See also Color Plate 42.)

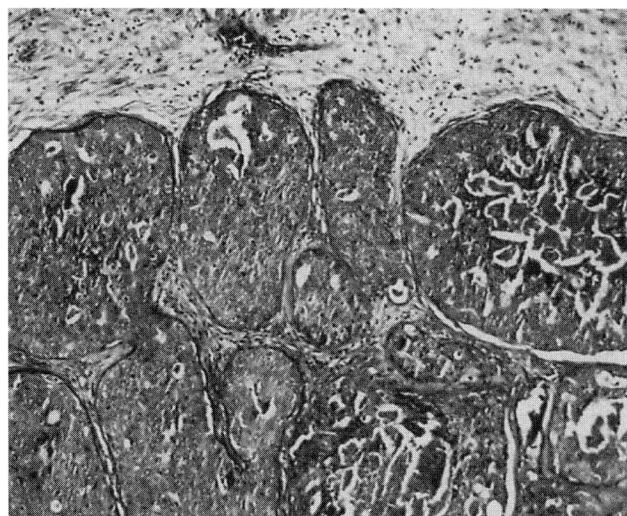

Figure 109.8 Carcinoma ex-pleomorphic adenoma is seen in a preexisting pleomorphic adenoma.

represents approximately 15% of malignant parotid neoplasms (21). Adenocarcinomas occur equally in both sexes and usually present as a palpable mass. They behave aggressively with a strong propensity to recur and metastasize.

Grossly, adenocarcinoma is firm or hard and attached to the surrounding tissue. Microscopically, the cylindric cells of variable height form papillae, acini, or solid masses. Most neoplasms produce mucus, which can be detected by mucicarmine stain. Adenocarcinoma can be differentiated from mucoepidermoid carcinoma by the lack of keratin staining. The degree of glandular formation has been used as a means of grading these tumors.

Polymorphous Low-Grade Adenocarcinoma

Polymorphous low-grade adenocarcinoma occurs almost exclusively in the minor salivary glands (22). The neoplasm most commonly occurs in the palate, buccal mucosa, and the upper lip. Women are affected more commonly than men, and most of these neoplasms occur in the sixth decade of life. The typical presentation of this tumor is of a long-standing, asymptomatic mass on the palate.

Histologically, polymorphous low-grade adenocarcinoma demonstrates a variable tumor cell differentiation and organization. Mitotic figures are unusual, as is necrosis. Tumors typically have an infiltrative growth pattern with frequent perineural invasion.

Treatment is wide local excision. Even with the presence of perineural involvement, there is no role for postoperative radiation therapy if the surgical resection is complete (22).

Carcinoma Ex-Pleomorphic Adenoma

Carcinoma ex-pleomorphic adenoma represents a malignant tumor that has arisen from a preexisting or recurrent pleomorphic adenoma. The malignant component and

metastases from this tumor are purely epithelial in origin. This malignancy represents 2% to 5% of all salivary gland tumors. Rarely, the malignancy can take the form in which the tumor contains both mesenchymal and epithelial components.

Grossly, the tumors are firm with minimal encapsulation. The lesion is widely infiltrative with regions of necrosis and hemorrhage. Microscopically, the malignant neoplasm arises in a background that is characteristic of a benign mixed tumor (Fig. 109.8). Neurovascular invasion and necrosis were frequent findings. The malignant portion of the tumor can take the form of an adenocarcinoma, salivary duct carcinoma, adenosquamous carcinoma, undifferentiated carcinoma, or other malignancy (23).

The diagnosis may be confusing because of the differing proportions of benign versus malignant elements of the tumor. Destructive, infiltrative growth is a reliable histologic finding for malignancy (12).

Local and distant metastases are common with this tumor, and, compared with other malignant salivary neoplasms, it is associated with a very poor prognosis. Prognostic factors include pathologic stage, tumor size, grade, proportion of cancer, and extent of invasion (23). Complete surgical resection with postoperative radiation therapy is the recommended treatment for this high-grade malignancy.

Squamous Cell Carcinoma

Squamous cell carcinoma of the salivary glands represents a rare neoplasm that constitutes 0.3% to 1.5% of salivary gland tumors (24). This malignancy occurs more often in the submandibular gland than the parotid gland. Proper diagnosis of squamous cell carcinoma requires exclusion of contiguous spread of a squamous cell carcinoma into the gland, metastases to the gland, and high-grade mucoepidermoid carcinoma.

These tumors usually present as firm indurated masses and occur more commonly in males, usually in the seventh decade of life. Histologically, these tumors reveal intracellular keratinization, intercellular bridges, and keratin pearl formation. However, they do not produce mucus (12).

There is a high incidence of regional and distant metastases. The prognosis for squamous cell carcinoma of the salivary gland is poor. Therapy consists of complete surgical resection and postoperative radiation therapy.

Undifferentiated Carcinoma

Undifferentiated carcinoma is a rare salivary gland malignancy. There is a high incidence of these tumors among the Inuit Eskimos of Greenland. This tumor is also closely related to infection with the Epstein-Barr virus (25). The vast majority of these tumors affect the parotid gland.

These tumors can be further subdivided into small cell undifferentiated carcinoma, large cell undifferentiated carcinoma, and lymphoepithelial carcinoma. The recommended treatment is complete surgical excision with postoperative radiation therapy. Although the lymphoepithelial variant has a good prognosis, in general, undifferentiated carcinomas are extremely aggressive with marked local invasion and early distant metastasis (26).

Sarcoma

Sarcomas arising in the parotid gland are rare (27). These aggressive malignancies occur more commonly in men than in women and usually present as an enlarging, yet painless mass. Rhabdomyosarcoma and fibrosarcoma are the most common histopathologic subtypes. Diagnosis of a primary sarcoma requires the exclusion of metastatic spread of the sarcoma to the gland or glandular invasion from local soft tissues. Primary sarcomas behave like other soft tissue sarcomas, and the prognosis correlates with tumor size, type, and degree of histopathologic differentiation (27).

Lymphoma

Primary lymphoma rarely occurs in the salivary glands. When present, it usually affects the parotid gland more commonly than the submandibular glands. The criteria necessary for the diagnosis of primary lymphoma of the salivary glands include no known extrasalivary lymphoma, histologic proof that the lymphoma involves the salivary parenchyma primarily (as opposed to secondarily from a lymph node), and architectural and cytologic confirmation of the malignant nature of the lesion (28).

ASSESSMENT AND DIAGNOSIS

Etiologic Factors

Etiologic factors for salivary gland neoplasms are not well understood. Other than Warthin tumors (29), tobacco use

has not been associated with any increased incidence of salivary gland neoplasms. In addition, alcohol consumption has not been shown to increase the risk of salivary gland neoplasms (30).

Studies have examined viruses such as the Epstein-Barr virus as etiologic factors and except for undifferentiated carcinoma, there has not been a demonstrated role for viral infection as a factor in the pathogenesis of salivary gland neoplasms (31).

Low-dose radiation has been studied as a risk factor for the development of salivary gland neoplasms. A wide range in the dosage of radiation and age of exposure has been seen. This suggests that exposure at any age and any dose may predispose one to the development of a salivary gland tumor (32). The most common benign and malignant radiation related tumors are pleomorphic adenoma and mucoepidermoid carcinoma, respectively.

Occupational exposure to wood and silica dust has been linked to an increased incidence of salivary gland malignancies (33). A diet high in dark-yellow vegetables and liver has been noted to be protective against the development of salivary gland malignancies (34).

History

Patients with salivary gland neoplasms usually present with asymptomatic masses. Benign parotid gland neoplasms typically occur in the region of the tail of the gland. Pain is unusual with benign neoplasms but can occur with associated infection, hemorrhage, or cystic enlargement. In malignant neoplasms, pain is usually indicative of neural invasion by the tumor and portends a worse prognosis than a malignant tumor that is not painful. However, pain should not be used as a reliable indicator for malignancy.

Submandibular gland neoplasms present in a similar manner as parotid tumors. Minor salivary gland tumors usually present as nonulcerated, painless masses involving the oral cavity, typically the hard or soft palate (Fig. 109.9).

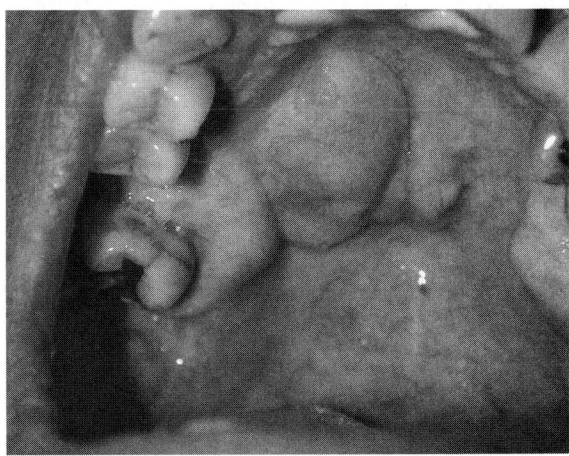

Figure 109.9 Low-grade polymorphous adenocarcinoma presenting as a smooth painless mass of the hard palate.

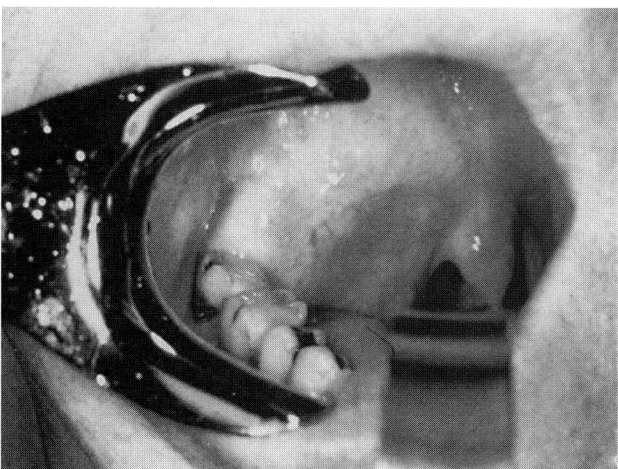

Figure 109.10 Pleomorphic adenoma of the parapharyngeal space. Note the uvular deviation to the opposite site.

Patients with nasal and paranasal sinus neoplasms usually present with advanced symptoms such as nasal obstruction or epistaxis. In the upper aerodigestive tract, minor salivary gland tumors can cause hoarseness, respiratory complaints, or dysphagia, depending on the location. Sublingual gland tumors usually present as masses in the floor of the mouth with some associated discomfort.

Tumors located in the parapharyngeal space are usually asymptomatic and first noted on routine oral examination (Figs. 109.10 and 109.11) or as a neck mass. As the tumor enlarges, alterations in speech and swallowing function may be noted.

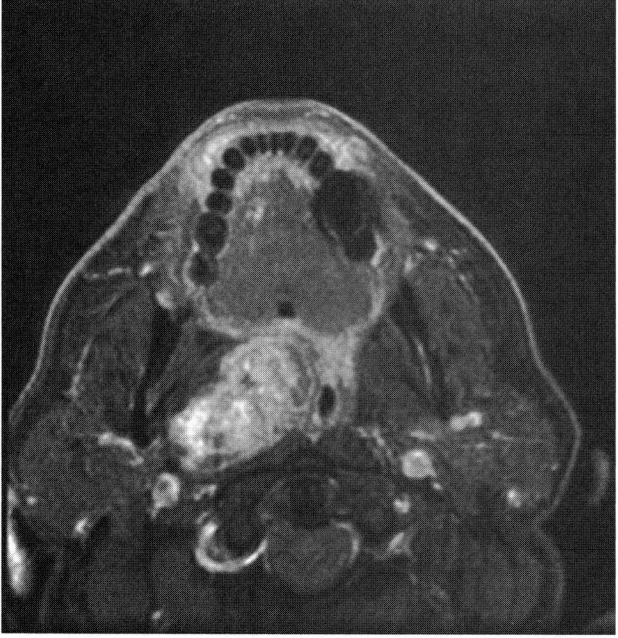

Figure 109.11 Pleomorphic adenoma of the parapharyngeal space imaged by magnetic resonance imaging.

Physical Examination

In a patient with a salivary gland neoplasm, a thorough head and neck examination is indicated. Attention should be directed to the size, location, and mobility of the tumor. The presence or absence of tenderness to the mass should be noted. Facial nerve function should also be documented. The presence of facial nerve paralysis should raise the suspicion of malignancy in the patient, although rarely, a benign tumor can cause facial nerve paralysis.

Fine-Needle Aspiration Biopsy

Fine-needle aspiration (FNA) biopsy of a salivary gland tumor is a simple and accurate aid in diagnosis. However, this technique is not uniformly accepted. Some argue that hemorrhage and in rare instances infarction at the tumor site may contribute to obscuring the final diagnosis. Also, inadequate samples and the need for multiple aspirations may delay the definitive treatment (35). Another argument made is that FNA in many instances will not change the ultimate procedure.

However, FNA does offer several advantages, including the ability to obtain a definitive diagnosis, to direct proper management, and to provide for proper preoperative patient counseling.

Radiology

Salivary gland imaging is discussed in detail in Chapter 38. In most instances, computed tomography (CT) and magnetic resonance imaging (MRI) do not differentiate benign from malignant tumors and infrequently alter the therapeutic approach to these neoplasms. Both of these imaging modalities provide similar information in aiding the diagnosis of the tumor and in terms of proper surgical planning (36). Nevertheless, useful information can be gained from imaging studies in certain instances. These include the evaluation of malignant or recurrent tumors, large neoplasms, suspected parapharyngeal space involvement, or suspected involvement of structures such as the carotid artery that would indicate unresectability.

CT and MRI are both useful for the assessment of the parapharyngeal space. The periparotid fat strip separating the deep lobe of the parotid gland from the parapharyngeal space is an important anatomic landmark and allows for the differentiation of deep lobe parotid tumors involving the parapharyngeal space from tumors that arise from ectopic salivary gland tissue in the parapharyngeal space.

Imaging studies are routinely obtained for the assessment of minor salivary gland malignancies involving the nose and paranasal sinuses. Both CT with direct coronal cuts and MRI give good information regarding the extent of the disease. CT is superior to MRI in defining bony detail, whereas MRI is useful in differentiating obstructive opacification of the paranasal sinuses from tumor involvement. Thus, the information from these studies is frequently complementary.

Other imaging modalities include ultrasound and fluorine-18 fluorodeoxyglucose positron emission tomography (PET). The roles of these studies in the evaluation of salivary gland tumors to date have not been fully defined. Both benign and malignant neoplasms can demonstrate high standardized uptake values on PET scan, thus limiting their ability to differentiate these tumors (37,38).

Diagnostic Surgery

Surgical biopsy of a parotid gland tumor should be avoided. Excisional biopsy or enucleation of parotid masses is associated with high rates of tumor recurrence, particularly for pleomorphic adenoma. The proper surgical approach for parotid neoplasms is to perform complete surgical resection by parotidectomy with identification and preservation of the facial nerve. This ensures an adequate margin of tissue surrounding the tumor. This approach is diagnostic and curative in most cases. The facial nerve is identified in all cases to allow adequate tumor excision and to avoid facial nerve injury. Open biopsy is performed rarely and usually only for an obvious malignancy in a patient who is not a surgical candidate and for whom an FNA biopsy is not diagnostic. In this situation, open incisional biopsy is useful for histopathologic diagnosis and for directing the appropriate type of palliative treatment.

Intraoral biopsy of a parapharyngeal space tumor should not be performed. This carries risks of injury to the carotid artery, risk of tumor spillage, and risk of contamination by the oral flora. A transoral or image-guided FNA biopsy usually provides the diagnosis without these risks (39).

Staging

The staging system for major salivary gland malignancies is described in Table 109.7.

Differential Diagnosis

Normal anatomic structures can be confused with salivary gland tumors. The masseter muscle, transverse process of the C1 vertebral body, and processes of the mandible can mimic parotid lesions (Fig. 109.12). Inflammatory diseases, nutritional deficiencies, and infections can cause diffuse parotid enlargement. Parotid cysts are uncommon but they may mimic tumor. Cystic lymphoepithelial lesions sometimes observed in patients who are positive for the human immunodeficiency virus may be confused with tumor.

Cutaneous malignancies can frequently metastasize to the salivary glands. Melanoma and squamous cell carcinoma account for the majority of tumors metastatic to the parotid gland or to the periparotid lymph nodes. Infraclavicular tumors can spread to the salivary glands and these include lung, kidney, breast, and colorectal cancers.

TABLE 109.7

STAGING SYSTEM FOR MAJOR SALIVARY GLAND MALIGNANCIES—AMERICAN JOINT COMMITTEE ON CANCER—2002

Primary Tumor (T)
TX: Primary tumor cannot be assessed
T0: No evidence of primary disease
T1: Tumor 2 cm or less in greatest dimension without extraparenchymal extension*
T2: Tumor more than 2 cm but not more than 4 cm in greatest dimension without extraparenchymal extension*
T3: Tumor more than 4 cm and/or tumor having extraparenchymal extension*
T4a: Tumor invades skin, mandible, ear canal, and/or facial nerve
T4b: Tumor invades skull base and/or pterygoid plates and/or encases carotid artery
*Note: Extraparenchymal extension is clinical or macroscopic evidence of invasion of soft tissues. Microscopic evidence alone does not constitute extraparenchymal extension for classification purposes.

Regional Lymph Nodes (N)
NX: Regional lymph nodes cannot be assessed
N0: No regional lymph node metastasis
N1: Metastasis in a single ipsilateral lymph node, 3 cm or less in greatest dimension
N2a: Metastasis in a single ipsilateral lymph node, more than 3 cm, but not more than 6 cm in greatest dimension
N2b: Metastasis in multiple ipsilateral lymph nodes, none more than 6 cm in greatest dimension
N2c: Metastasis in bilateral or contralateral lymph nodes, none more than 6 cm in greatest dimension
N3: Metastasis in a lymph node, more than 6 cm in greatest dimension

Distant Metastasis (M)
MX: Distant metastasis cannot be assessed
M0: No distant metastasis
M1: Distant metastasis

Stage Grouping

	T	N	M
Stage I	1	0	0
Stage II	2	0	0
Stage III	3	0	0
	1	1	0
	2	1	0
	3	1	0
Stage IVA	4a	0	0
	4a	1	0
	1	2	0
	2	2	0
	3	2	0
	4a	2	0
Stage IVB	4b	Any	0
	Any	N3	0
Stage IVC	Any	Any	1

Reproduced with permission from *AJCC Cancer Staging Manual*, 6th ed. New York: Springer-Verlag, 2002.

Necrotizing sialometaplasia is a benign lesion of salivary tissue that may be confused with a minor salivary gland tumor. Other lesions of the palate that may be mistaken for a minor salivary gland tumor include mucous retention cyst, epidermoid cyst, fibroma, and a palatine torus.

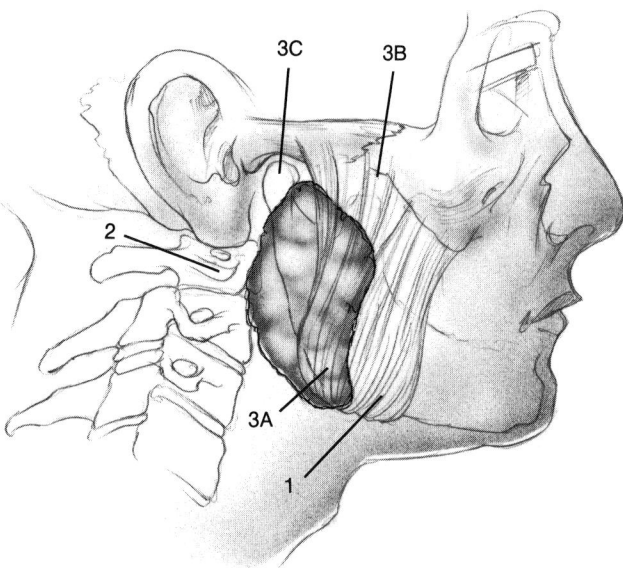

Figure 109.12 Normal anatomic structures are sometimes mistaken for parotid neoplasms. 1, masseter; 2, transverse process of C1; 3, mandibular processes: A, angle; B, coronoid; C, condyle.

MANAGEMENT

Surgery

The treatment of choice for most salivary gland neoplasms is complete surgical excision. Because most parotid tumors occur in the region of the tail of the gland and are superficial to the facial nerve, parotidectomy with identification and preservation of the facial nerve is diagnostic and curative in most cases. It is not necessary to remove the entire superficial lobe if the tumor can be removed with an adequate margin of normal tissue to ensure complete excision.

Complete excision by parotidectomy (Fig. 109.13) is usually curative for superficial low-grade malignancies (e.g., low-grade mucoepidermoid carcinoma and acinic cell carcinoma). Complete resection by parotidectomy is also recommended for high-grade malignancies. The facial nerve is to be preserved if it functions normally and is not grossly involved by tumor.

Facial nerve involvement by tumor requires facial nerve resection. Frozen sections are used to ensure negative nerve margins both proximally and distally. Immediate nerve grafting with a nerve graft is performed.

During parotidectomy for malignancy, the periparotid, upper jugular, and posterior submandibular triangle lymph nodes are inspected. Any suspicious nodes are biopsied or included in the dissection. A modified neck dissection is performed for histologically positive nodes. Also, for clinically positive cervical metastases, a neck dissection is indicated.

Parotidectomy Technique

The face and neck are prepared and draped with a transparent adhesive drape to allow for visualization of the face during the procedure. A preauricular incision is made extending inferiorly along the line of attachment of the ear lobule and curving into an upper neck crease. Alternatively, a modified facelift incision can be used for selected patients. An anterior skin flap is elevated superficial to the parotid fascia. The flap is raised to the posterior border of the masseter muscle. The tail of the parotid is then dissected from the sternocleidomastoid muscle and the posterior branch of the greater auricular nerve is preserved if possible.

The digastric muscle is then exposed as the tail of the parotid is elevated. This serves as an important landmark in identifying the facial nerve. The second plane of dissection is then developed in the pretragal region. This space is opened with blunt dissection parallel to the course of the facial nerve. This exposes the tragal pointer and opens a plane from the zygoma superiorly to just above the styloid process inferiorly. With the tail and the pretragal portions of the parotid mobilized, the remaining parotid fascial attachments to the mastoid remain and are incised. The facial nerve is then identified using the exposed anatomic landmarks (Table 109.8). If the main trunk of the facial nerve cannot be identified, then peripheral facial nerve branches can be dissected in a retrograde fashion. Alternatively, when there is significant scarring or distortion of the normal anatomy, a mastoidectomy can be performed and the facial nerve identified within the temporal bone.

After the main branch of the facial nerve is identified, individual facial nerve branches are followed peripherally and the gland is dissected off the nerve branches. After tumor removal, hemostasis is ensured and the wound closed over a closed-suction drain.

Total parotidectomy involves removal of parotid gland tissue both superficial and deep to the facial nerve. For deep lobe tumors, the facial nerve is exposed by removing the superficial lobe of the parotid gland. The deep lobe is then removed by first skeletonizing the branches of the facial nerve and removing the tissue deep to the nerve.

For parotid malignancies, the extent of the resection is determined by the extent of the disease. Frozen sections may guide the need for any additional removal of tissues.

TABLE 109.8

ANATOMIC LANDMARKS FOR FACIAL NERVE IDENTIFICATION DURING PAROTIDECTOMY

Tragal pointer
Tympanomastoid suture line
Digastric muscle attachment to digastric groove
Retrograde dissection from distal nerve branch
Nerve within temporal bone

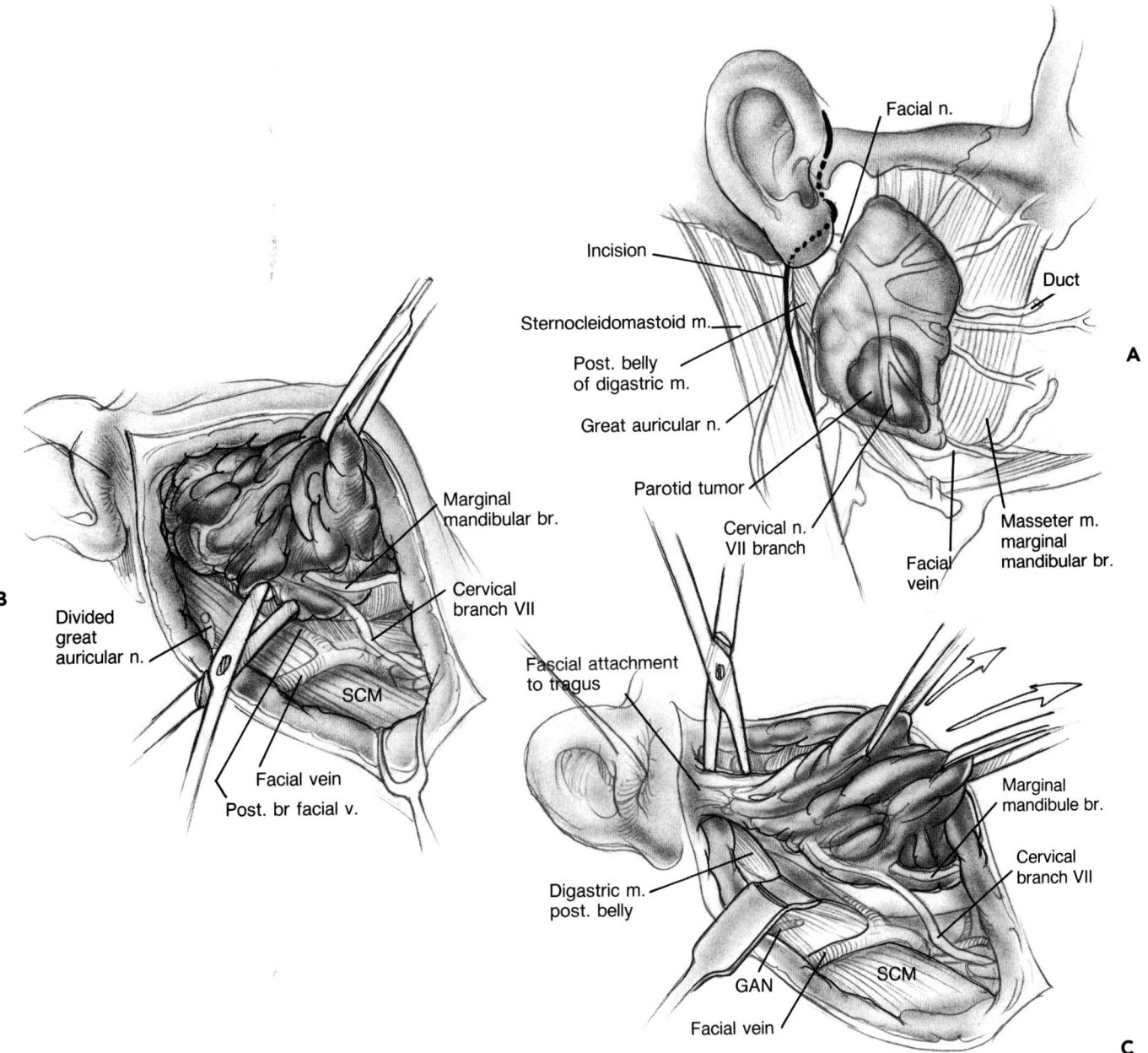

Figure 109.13   Techniques of parotidectomy. **A:** Anatomy of parotid area. **B:** Dissection of the inferior pole of the gland takes place before dissection of the facial nerve and its branches. **C:** Anterior retraction and blunt dissection above the main trunk of the facial nerve follows the mobilization of the inferior pole of the gland.

Surgical Treatment of Parapharyngeal Space Salivary Tumors

Parotid neoplasms may involve the parapharyngeal space by two routes. Round tumors extend posterior to the stylomandibular ligament. Dumbbell tumors have waistlike constrictions that form as they penetrate between the mandible and the stylomandibular ligament (Figs. 109.14 and 109.15).

Most parapharyngeal space tumors arising from ectopic salivary gland tissue can be removed by a submandibular approach. This involves mobilization of the submandibular gland to allow access to the anterior compartment of the parapharyngeal space. If further exposure is needed, stylomandibular ligament can be incised allowing for anterior retraction of the mandible. Mandibulotomy can be performed if additional exposure is necessary. Most parapharyngeal space salivary tumors can be bluntly dissected from the surrounding structures.

Text continues on page 1528.

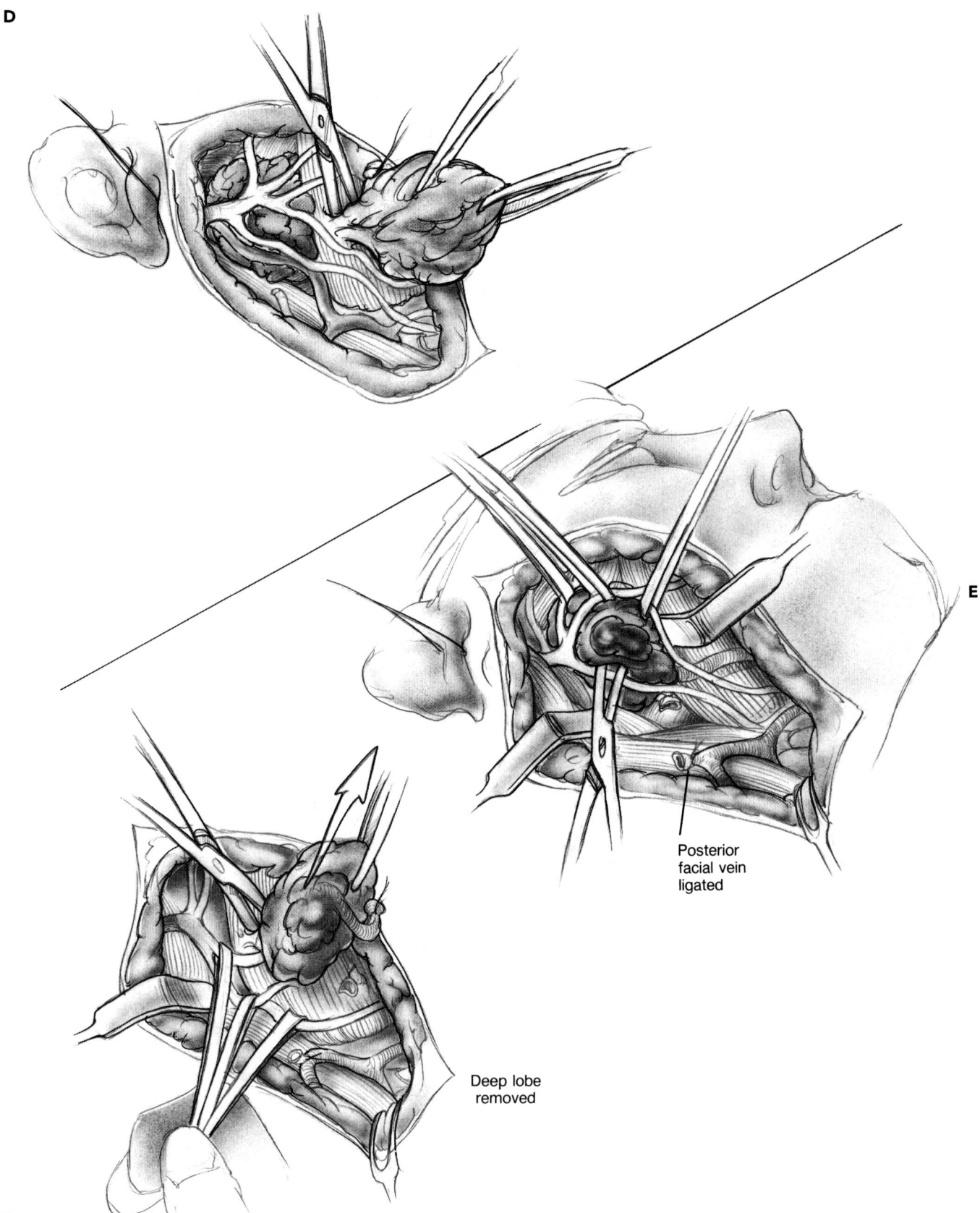

D

E

Posterior
facial vein
ligated

Deep lobe
removed

F

Figure 109.13 (*continued*)   D: All nerve branches are successively dissected and identified. Then the gland is removed in a single block. E: Deep lobe parotidectomy. Facial nerve is visualized and dissection is continued deep to it. F: The deep lobe is removed. GAN, greater auricular nerve; SCM, sternocleidomastoid muscle.

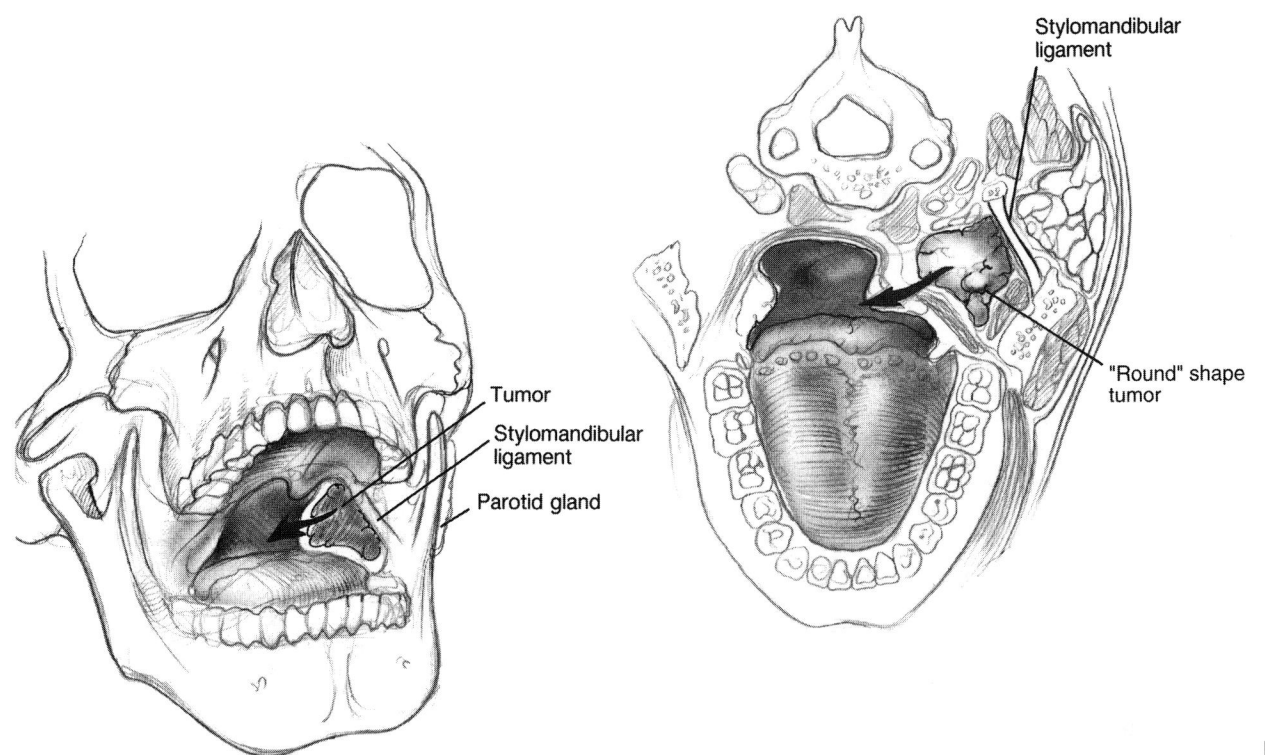

Figure 109.14 Round tumor involving the parapharyngeal space. **A:** Three-fourths view. **B:** Axial view.

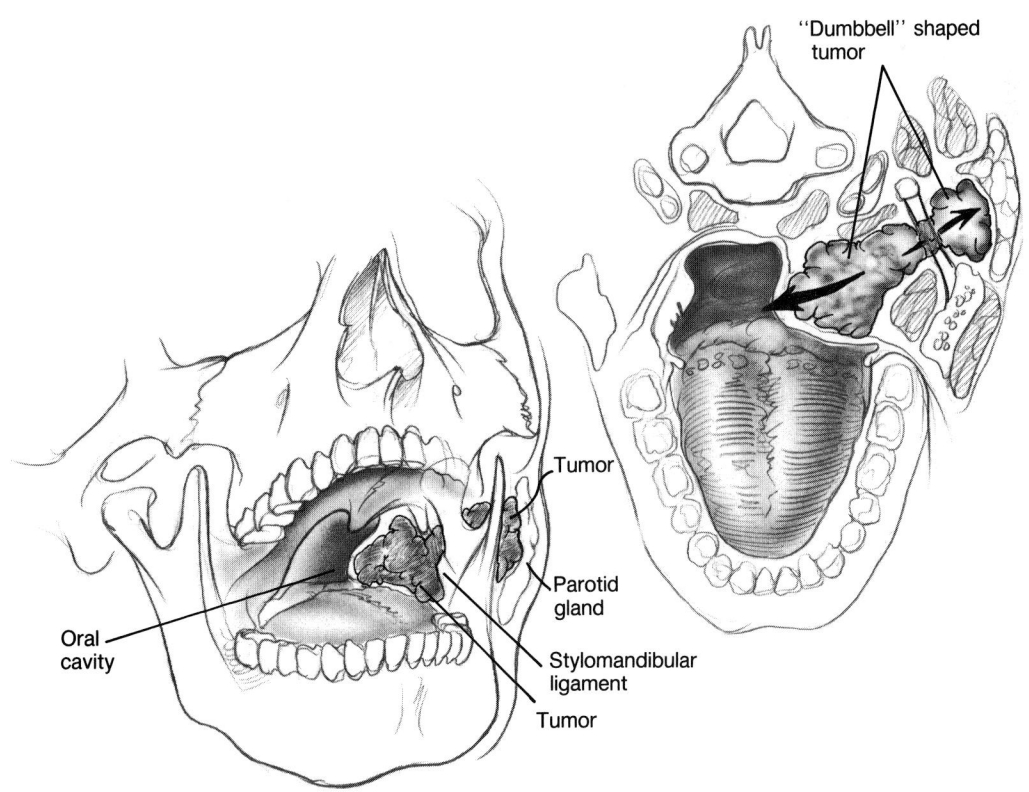

Figure 109.15 Dumbbell tumor involving the parapharyngeal space. **A:** Three-fourths view. **B:** Axial view.

Surgical Treatment of Submandibular Gland Neoplasms

Tumors involving the submandibular gland are usually limited to the gland. For benign tumors, gland excision is curative. Malignant tumors are also usually confined to the gland and surgical resection is usually confined to the contents of the submandibular triangle. All nerves are preserved unless there is evidence of tumor involvement. For malignant tumors invading the surrounding tissue, the surgical resection is extended to include the involved structures with an appropriate tumor-free margin. The involved structures may include the marginal mandibular branch of the facial nerve, the hypoglossal nerve, the lingual nerve, the mandible, the tongue, the floor of mouth, and the skin. The extent of resection depends on the extent of the disease.

Submandibular Gland Excision Technique

The neck is prepared and draped in a sterile fashion. The incision is made approximately two fingerbreadths below the inferior border of the mandible in a skin crease (Fig. 109.16). The incision is carried through the platysma muscle, and subplatysmal flaps are elevated with care to avoid injury to the marginal mandibular nerve. The superficial layer of the deep cervical fascia is divided and the anterior facial vein is divided and ligated. Elevation of this fascia exposes the submandibular gland. The dissection is then performed superiorly, and the facial artery is dived and ligated. The mylohyoid muscle is retracted anteriorly, and the gland is retracted posteroinferiorly, exposing the lingual nerve and Wharton duct. The submandibular ganglion is divided, freeing the lingual nerve. Wharton duct is then divided and ligated. The hypoglossal nerve runs superficial to the hyoglossus muscle. The hypoglossal nerve is preserved as the inferior border of the gland is dissected free. The facial artery is encountered again, and it is divided and ligated. After ensuring hemostasis, the wound is closed in layers over a drain.

Surgical Treatment of Minor Salivary Gland Neoplasms

Surgical therapy depends on the location and extent of disease. Complete surgical excision is curative for benign tumors. Adenoid cystic carcinoma most commonly involves the oral cavity, nasal cavity, and paranasal sinuses. Adenocarcinomas most commonly involve the paranasal sinuses and nasal cavities. Malignant minor salivary gland tumors involving the larynx are usually adenoid cystic carcinoma or adenocarcinoma. The surgery for malignant minor salivary gland tumors may be extensive and may require maxillectomy, craniofacial resection, mandibulectomy, laryngectomy, or tracheal resection.

Radiation Therapy

The use of radiation therapy in combination with surgery has improved the locoregional control and survival for patients with carcinoma of the major salivary glands (40,41). Because high-grade malignancies have high rates of locoregional failure, adjuvant radiotherapy is recommended for these patients. Postoperative radiation therapy also benefits patients with minor salivary gland malignancies who are at high risk for local failure (42).

Radiation therapy has been suggested for the treatment of recurrent pleomorphic adenoma. Radiation therapy has been shown to improve control of recurrent pleomorphic adenoma, but a long-term concern for this modality is the development of radiation-induced malignancies (43,44). Fast neutron radiotherapy holds promise as another modality in the treatment of recurrent pleomorphic adenoma (45).

Chemotherapy

Chemotherapy has been used in the treatment of advanced salivary gland malignancies. Presently, there is no proven benefit of adjuvant chemotherapy in improving locoregional tumor control or survival. The primary role for chemotherapy is palliation of symptomatic, unresectable disease.

Patients with unresectable malignancies who achieve a clinical response to chemotherapy often experience significant pain relief. Up to 50% of patients can see a partial or complete response.

COMPLICATIONS

Parotidectomy

There are both early and late complications of parotidectomy (Table 109.9). Partial or complete paralysis involving some or all branches of the facial nerve can occur as early complications. Facial nerve disorders are discussed in detail in Chapter 167. Temporary facial nerve paralysis involving all or just one of the branches of the nerve has occurred in 10% to 30% of all parotidectomies. Permanent facial

TABLE 109.9

COMPLICATIONS OF PAROTIDECTOMY

Early	Late
Facial nerve paralysis	Frey syndrome
Bleeding	Recurrent tumor
Infection	Poor cosmesis
Skin flap necrosis	Soft tissue deficit
Trismus	Hypertrophic scar or keloid
Sialocele	
Seroma	

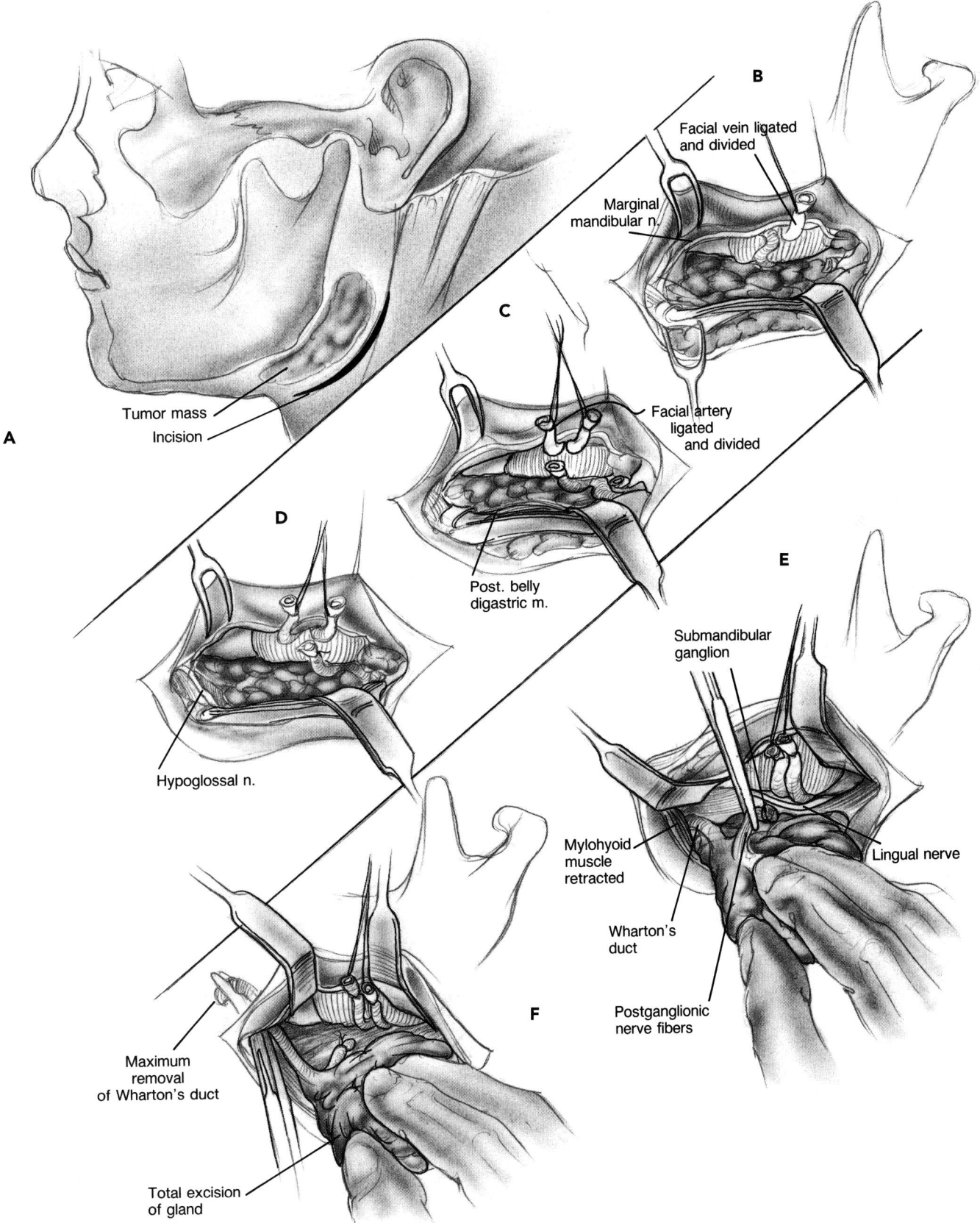

Figure 109.16 Technique for submandibular gland excision. See text for discussion.

nerve paralysis has occurred in fewer than 3% of parotidectomies. The nerve at most risk for injury during parotidectomy is the marginal mandibular branch.

The incidence of facial nerve paralysis is higher with total parotidectomy than with superficial parotidectomy. This may be related to stretch injury or interference of the vasa nervorum. Overstimulation of the nerve with a battery-powered nerve stimulator also may be responsible for a temporary paresis. Temporary paresis usually resolves from weeks to months postoperatively. Facial nerve injury is more common during reoperation for recurrent tumors. Complete nerve transection can occur during surgery and should be immediately repaired.

Continuous facial nerve monitoring during parotid surgery has been gaining popularity in recent years. Although some studies suggest a decreased incidence in temporary or permanent facial nerve paralysis (46), other studies have not demonstrated a significant difference (47,48). Despite these inconclusive results, many surgeons recommend the use of facial nerve monitoring because one can avoid the use of continuous pulse nerve stimulator and the surgeon can get continuous and instant feedback on the location and status of the nerves during dissection (46). Nerve monitoring can also be a useful adjunct in difficult cases (large tumors, reoperation, previous radiation therapy, inflammation).

Corticosteroids have been used by some surgeons in the hopes of avoiding postoperative paresis of the facial nerve by reducing edema and inflammation of the nerve. However, studies have failed to demonstrate a benefit in using perioperative corticosteroids (49).

Hemorrhage or hematoma is an uncommon complication and is usually related to incomplete hemostasis at the end of the procedure. Treatment consists of evacuation of the hematoma and surgical control of the bleeding vessels.

Infection is rare after parotidectomy and is avoided by the use of aseptic technique and careful handling of tissues. The rarity of infection is probably related to the rich vascular supply to the facial skin. Treatment of infection consists of surgical drainage, if necessary, and antibiotics.

Skin-flap necrosis is most commonly located in the distal tip of the postauricular skin flap. Care must be taken in designing this portion of the skin flap in avoiding this complication. Smoking may contribute to this complication.

Trismus may be related to inflammation and fibrosis of the masseter muscle. This complication is usually mild and self-limited with range of motion exercise of the jaw usually solving this problem.

Salivary fistula or sialocele is a relatively common complication after parotidectomy. This usually results from the cut edges of the remaining salivary gland leaking saliva and then collecting beneath the flap. This complication is usually self-limited and treated with needle aspirations. A chronic salivary fistula is rare.

Frey syndrome or gustatory sweating is a relatively common long-term complication of parotidectomy (Fig. 109.17). This complication is thought to be related to aberrant regeneration of nerve fibers from the postganglionic secretomotor parasympathetic innervation of the parotid gland to the severed postganglionic sympathetic fibers that supply the sweat glands of the skin of the face. As a result,

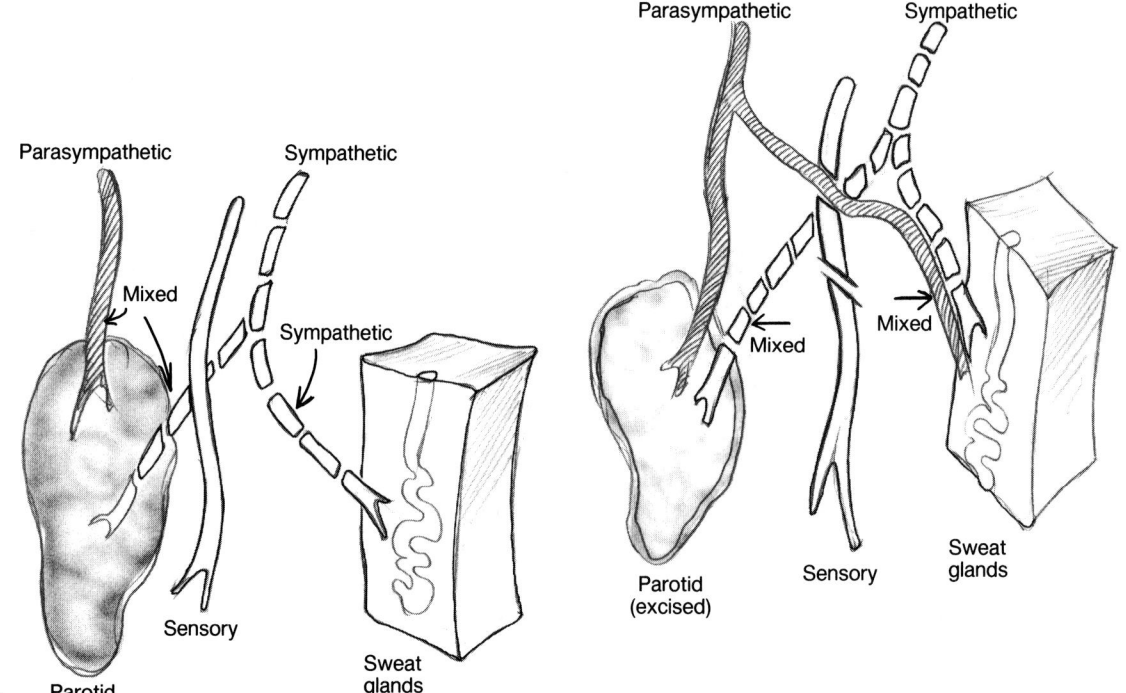

Figure 109.17   A: Normal innervation of parotid and sweat glands. **B:** Proposed mechanism of Frey syndrome.

sweating or dermal flush occurs during salivary stimulation. Frey syndrome has been reported for 30% to 60% of patients undergoing parotidectomy. Only about 10% of patients, however, have symptomatic Frey syndrome.

Most patients with Frey syndrome do not seek therapy. Medical treatment of symptomatic Frey syndrome has included topical application of antiperspirant, topical anticholinergics, and injections of botulinum toxin.

Recurrent tumor, both benign and malignant, can occur. High-grade malignancies can have a high rate of recurrence despite combined therapy. However, benign tumors such as pleomorphic adenoma recur in less than 1% of patients who are properly treated. Most recurrences occur after incomplete resection or due to tumor spillage.

There are several treatment options for recurrent pleomorphic adenoma. These include the "wait and see" approach, local tumor excision, and parotidectomy. Recurrent pleomorphic adenomas are difficult to treat because they tend to be larger than suspected, lie at a deeper level than expected, and are multicentric (50). Given this, the treatment of recurrent pleomorphic adenoma consists of total parotidectomy with facial nerve preservation and scar excision (51). A decrease in the rate of surgical control occurs with subsequent recurrences. En bloc resection with immediate nerve graft has been recommended for recurrences encasing the facial nerve. Radiation therapy, and in particular neutron radiotherapy, may be beneficial in the adjuvant setting after surgery (45).

Submandibular Gland Excision

The complications of submandibular gland excision are listed in Table 109.10. Injury to the marginal mandibular branch of the facial nerve results in loss of lip depressor function. Temporary paresis of this nerve can occur from stretch injury during retraction. Other nerves at risk include the hypoglossal nerve and lingual nerve resulting in ipsilateral tongue paralysis and anesthesia of the anterior two thirds of the tongue, respectively.

Hemorrhage, particularly from the facial artery, results in vigorous bleeding and can contribute to airway compromise. Wound reexploration and control of hemorrhage is necessary. Infection is uncommon after submandibular gland excision.

TABLE 109.10
COMPLICATIONS OF SUBMANDIBULAR GLAND EXCISION

Hemorrhage
Infection
Marginal mandibular branch of facial nerve injury
Hypoglossal nerve injury
Lingual nerve injury
Poor scar formation

TABLE 109.11
SURVIVAL RATES FOR PAROTID CARCINOMA

Type	5-yr Survival (%)	10-yr Survival (%)
Low-grade tumors		
Acinic cell carcinoma	80–90	80
Low-grade mucoepidermoid carcinoma	92–97	90–97
High-grade tumors		
Adenocarcinoma	49–75	41–60
Adenoid cystic carcinoma	45–82	28–77
Carcinoma ex-pleomorphic adenoma	50–77	30–39
Squamous cell carcinoma	42–57	57
High-grade mucoepidermoid carcinoma	35–56	28–54
Undifferentiated carcinoma	30–40	22–25

PROGNOSTIC FACTORS

The factors affecting survival for salivary carcinoma are tumor stage, location, grade, size, recurrence, and regional and distant metastasis. Facial nerve paralysis, skin involvement, pain, and gender also affect the prognosis. The staging system incorporates many of these factors and progression of disease from stage I to IV correlates with diminished survival (52).

Histopathology

Evaluation of tumor behavior based on histopathology has allowed the classification of low-grade tumors, including acinic cell carcinoma and low-grade mucoepidermoid carcinoma, and high-grade tumors, including adenocarcinoma, adenoid cystic carcinoma, carcinoma expleomorphic adenoma, squamous cell carcinoma, high-grade mucoepidermoid carcinoma, and undifferentiated carcinoma. Decreased tumor grade correlates with improved survival (Tables 109.11 and 109.12) (53,54).

TABLE 109.12
SURVIVAL RATES FOR SUBMANDIBULAR CARCINOMA

Type	5-yr Survival (%)	10-yr Survival (%)
Adenoid cystic carcinoma	77	60
Mucoepidermoid carcinoma	57	20
Adenocarcinoma	50	33
Squamous cell carcinoma	37	27

Adapted from Bhattacharyya N. Survival and prognosis for cancer of the submandibular gland. *J Oral Maxillofac Surg* 2004;62:427–430, with permission.

Tumor Size

Tumor size has been considered a major prognostic indicator for salivary gland malignancies with increased size resulting in poor prognosis and decreased survival (54,55). Increased tumor size also correlates with high rates of regional and distant metastases and increased rates of recurrence (55).

Facial Nerve Paralysis

Facial nerve paralysis associated with malignant tumor indicates a poor prognosis. Facial nerve paralysis is associated with high incidences of regional and distant metastases (55).

Skin Involvement

Invasion of surrounding tissue, including skin invasion, is associated with decreased survival (40). Skin involvement indicates advanced malignancy and requires excision of the involved structures.

Regional Lymphatic Metastases

Regional lymph node metastases are associated with poorer prognosis than for nonmetastatic disease (56,57). Elective neck dissection for the clinically negative neck is controversial, with some citing low rates of occult metastasis (56) and others advocating the elective dissection of the negative neck (58). Large tumor size and facial nerve paralysis are both associated with high incidences of regional nodal involvement (55).

Distant Metastases

Distant metastases indicate a poor prognosis. Distant metastases occur in approximately 20% of parotid malignancies and they occur most frequently in adenoid cystic carcinoma and undifferentiated carcinoma. The most common sites for distant metastases are lung, bone, and brain. The length of survival after distant failure varies according to the tumor type. The most important factors for predicting the development of distant metastases are the size of the tumor, presence or absence of regional metastases, and histologic type of tumor (55).

Pain

Pain associated with a known malignancy is an ominous symptom. This has also been found to affect survival with those with pain having a decreased survival than those without pain (59).

Recurrence

Recurrence rate for salivary gland malignancies are high for high-grade tumors. It is not clear whether or not 5-year survival rates are different between previously untreated disease and recurrent tumors (40).

Gender

Except for submandibular glands, male gender seems to be correlated with decreased survival (53,55).

Location

There appears to be no difference in survival based on the location of a malignancy within the parotid gland, but parapharyngeal space involvement by a malignancy is associated with a poor prognosis. In general, parotid malignancies have a better prognosis than salivary carcinomas arising in other locations.

For adenoid cystic carcinoma, tumors in the major salivary glands are associated with a better prognosis than those in the minor salivary glands.

HIGHLIGHTS

- Salivary gland neoplasms represent a diverse group of benign and malignant tumors.
- An accurate histopathologic diagnosis is important for guiding therapy.
- Most salivary gland tumors develop in the parotid gland.
- Low-dose radiation exposure has been implicated as an etiologic factor for salivary gland neoplasms.
- Fine-needle aspiration biopsy is an accurate method for the diagnosis of salivary gland neoplasms.
- A mass in the region of the parotid gland should be considered a salivary gland neoplasm until proven otherwise.
- Parotidectomy with identification and preservation of the facial nerve is diagnostic and curative for most parotid gland neoplasms.
- Combined surgery and radiation therapy has improved locoregional control and survival in patients with carcinoma of the major salivary glands.

REFERENCES

1. Pinkston JA, Cole P. Incidence rates of salivary gland tumors: results from a population-based study. *Otolaryngol Head Neck Surg* 1999;120:834–840.
2. Satko I, Stanko P, Longauerova I. Salivary gland tumors treated in the stomatological clinics in Bratislava. *J Craniomaxillofac Surg* 2000;28:56–61.
3. Bhattacharyya N. Survival and prognosis for cancer of the submandibular gland. *J Oral Maxillofac Surg* 2004;62:427–430.
4. Renehan A, Gleave EN, Hancock BD, et al. Long-term follow-up of over 1000 patients with salivary gland tumours treated in a single centre. *Br J Surg* 1996;83:1750–1754.
5. Luna MA, Batsakis JG, El-Naggar AK. Salivary gland tumors in children. *Ann Otol Rhinol Laryngol* 1991;100:869–871.
6. Stennert E, Guntinas-Lichius O, Klussmann JP, et al. Histopathology of pleomorphic adenoma in the parotid gland: a prospective unselected series of 100 cases. *Laryngoscope* 2001;111:2195–2200.
7. Marioni G, Marino F, Stramare R, et al. Benign metastasizing pleomorphic adenoma of the parotid gland: a clinicopathologic puzzle. *Head Neck* 2003;25:1071–1076.

8. Astor FC, Hanft KL, Rooney P, et al. Extraparotid Warthin's tumor: clinical manifestations, challenges, and controversies. *Otolaryngol Head Neck Surg* 1996;114:732–735.

9. Maiorano E, LoMuzio L, Favia G, et al. Warthin's tumor: a study of 78 cases with emphasis on bilaterality, multifocality, and association with other malignancies. *Oral Oncol* 2002;38: 35–40.

10. Stavrianos SD, McLean NR, Soames JV. Synchronous unilateral parotid neoplasms of different histologic types. *Eur J Surg Oncol* 1999;25:331–332.

11. Capone RB, Ha PK, Westra WH, et al. Oncocytic neoplasms of the parotid gland: a 16 year institutional review. *Otolaryngol Head Neck Surg* 2002;126:657–662.

12. Batsakis JG. Tumors of the major salivary glands. In: Batsakis JG, ed. *Tumors of the head and neck: clinical and pathological considerations.* Baltimore: Williams & Wilkins, 1979:1–75.

13. Boahene DK, Olsen KD, Lewis JE, et al. Mucoepidermoid carcinoma of the parotid gland: the Mayo Clinic experience. *Arch Otolaryngol Head Neck Surg* 2004;130:849–856.

14. Guzzo M, Andreola S, Sirizzotti G, et al. Mucoepidermoid carcinoma of the salivary glands: clinicopathologic review of 108 patients treated at the National Cancer Institute of Milan. *Ann Surg Oncol* 2002;9:688–695.

15. Hosokawa Y, Shinato H, Kagei K, et al. Role of radiotherapy for mucoepidermoid carcinoma of the salivary gland. *Oral Oncol* 1999;35:105–111.

16. Bradley PJ. Adenoid cystic carcinoma of the head and neck: a review. *Curr Opin Otolaryngol Head Neck Surg* 2004;12:127–132.

17. Matsuba HM, Simpson JR, Mauney M, et al. Adenoid cystic salivary gland carcinoma: a clinico-pathologic correlation. *Head Neck Surg* 1986;8:200–204.

18. Silverman DA, Carlson TP, Khuntia D, et al. Role of postoperative radiation therapy in adenoid cystic carcinoma of the head and neck. *Laryngoscope* 2004;114:1194–1199.

19. Douglas JG, Koh WJ, Austin-Seymour M, et al. Treatment of salivary gland neoplasms with fast neutron radiotherapy. *Arch Otolaryngol Head Neck Surg* 2003;129:944–948.

20. Hoffman HT, Karnel LH, Robinson R, et al. National Cancer Database report on cancer of the head and neck: acinic cell carcinoma. *Head Neck* 1999;21:297–309.

21. Spiro RH, Huvos AG, Strong EW. Adenocarcinoma of salivary origin: clinicopathologic study of 204 patients. *Am J Surg* 1982;44: 423–431.

22. Castle JT, Thompson LDR, Frommelt RA, et al. Polymorphous low grade adenocarcinoma: a clinicopathologic study of 164 cases. *Cancer* 1999;86:207–219.

23. Olsen KD, Lewis JE. Carcinoma ex-pleomorphic adenoma: a clinicopathologic review. *Head Neck* 2001;23:705–712.

24. Gaughan RK, Olsen KD, Lewis JE. Primary squamous cell carcinoma of the parotid gland. *Arch Otolaryngol Head Neck Surg* 1992; 118:798–801.

25. Sheen TS, Tsai CC, Ko JY, et al. Undifferentiated carcinoma of the major salivary glands. *Cancer* 1997;80:357–363.

26. Wang CP, Chang YL, Ko JY, et al. Lymphoepithelial carcinoma versus large cell undifferentiated carcinoma of the major salivary glands. *Cancer* 2004;101:2020–2027.

27. Luna MA, Tortoledo ME, Ordonez NG, et al. Primary sarcomas of the major salivary gland. *Arch Otolaryngol Head Neck Surg* 1991; 117:302–306.

28. Batsakis JG. Primary lymphoma of the major salivary glands. *Ann Otol Rhinol Laryngol* 1986;95:107–108.

29. Pinkston JA, Cole P. Cigarette smoking and Warthin's tumor. *Am J Epidemiol* 1996;14:183–187.

30. Muscat JE, Wynder EL. A case/control study of risk factors for major salivary gland cancer. *Otolaryngol Head Neck Surg* 1998;118: 195–198.

31. Laane CJ, Murr AH, Mhatre AN, et al. Role of Epstein-Barr virus and cytomegalovirus in the etiology of benign parotid tumors. *Head Neck* 2002;24:443–450.

32. Beal KP, Singh B, Kraus D, et al. Radiation induced salivary gland tumors: a report of 18 cases and a review of the literature. *Cancer J* 2003;9:467–471.

33. Demers PA, Kogevinas M, Bofffetta P, et al. Wood dust and sinonasal cancer: pooled reanalysis of 12 case-control studies. *Am J Ind Med* 1995;28:151–166.

34. Zheng W, Shu XO, Ji BT, et al. Diet and other risk factors for cancer of the salivary glands. A population based case control study. *Int J Cancer* 1996;67:194–198.

35. Batsakis JG, Sueige N, el-Naggar AK. Fine needle aspiration of salivary glands: its utility and tissue effects. *Ann Otol Rhinol Laryngol* 1992;101:185–188.

36. Koyuncu M, Sesen T, Akan H, et al. Comparison of computed tomography and magnetic resonance imaging in the diagnosis of parotid tumors. *Otolaryngol Head Neck Surg* 2003;129:726–732.

37. Bialek EJ, Jakubowski W, Karpinska G. Role of ultrasonography in diagnosis and differentiation of pleomorphic adenomas: work in progress. *Arch Otolaryngol Head Neck Surg* 2003;129:929–933.

38. Okamura T, Kawabe J, Koyama K, et al. Fluorine-18 fluorodeoxyglucose positron emission tomography imaging of parotid mass lesions. *Acta Otolaryngol Suppl* 1998;538:209–213.

39. Shah SB, Singer MI, Liberman E, et al. Transmucosal fine needle aspiration diagnosis of intraoral and intrapharyngeal lesions. *Laryngoscope* 1999;109:1232–1237.

40. North CA, Lee DJ, Piantadosi S, et al. Carcinoma of the major salivary glands treated by surgery or surgery plus postoperative radiotherapy. *Int J Radiat Oncol Biol Phys* 1990;18:1319–1326.

41. Harrison LH, Armstrong JG, Spiro RH, et al. Postoperative radiation therapy for major salivary gland malignancies. *J Surg Oncol* 1990;45:52–55.

42. Garden AS, Weber RS, Ang KK. Postoperative radiation therapy for malignant tumors of minor salivary glands. *Cancer* 1994;73: 2563–2569.

43. Dawson AK, Orr JA. Long-term results of local excision and radiotherapy in pleomorphic adenoma of the parotid. *Int J Radiat Oncol Biol Phys* 1985;11:451–455.

44. Dawson AK. Radiation therapy in recurrent pleomorphic adenoma of the parotid. *Int J Radiat Oncol Biol Phys* 1989;16:819–821.

45. Douglas JG, Einck J, Austin-Seymour M, et al. Neutron radiotherapy for recurrent pleomorphic adenomas of major salivary glands. *Head Neck* 2001;23:1037–1042.

46. Brennan J, Moore EJ, Shuler KJ. Prospective analysis of the efficacy of continuous intraoperative nerve monitoring during thyroidectomy, parathyroidectomy, and parotidectomy. *Otolaryngol Head Neck Surg* 2001;124:537–543.

47. Witt RL. Facial nerve monitoring in parotid surgery: the standard of care? *Otolaryngol Head Neck Surg* 1998;119:468–470.

48. Terrell JE, Kileny PR, Yian C, et al. Clinical outcome of continuous facial nerve monitoring during primary parotidectomy. *Arch Otolaryngol Head Neck Surg* 1997;123:1081–1087.

49. Lee KJ, Fee WE, Terris DJ. The efficacy of corticosteroids in postparotidectomy facial nerve paresis. *Laryngoscope* 2001;112: 1958–1963.

50. Bradley PJ. Recurrent salivary gland pleomorphic adenoma: etiology, management, and results. *Curr Opin Otol Head Neck Surg* 2001;9:100–108.

51. Stennert E, Wittekindt C, Klussmann JP, et al. Recurrent pleomorphic adenoma of the parotid gland: a prospective histopathological and immunohistochemical study. *Laryngoscope* 2004;114:158–163.

52. Spiro RH, Armstrong J, Harrison L, et al. Carcinoma of the major salivary glands: recent trends. *Arch Otolaryngol Head Neck Surg* 1989;115:316–321.

53. Bhattacharyya N. Survival and prognosis for cancer of the submandibular gland. *J Oral Maxillofac Surg* 2004;62:427–430.

54. Kokemueller H, Swennen G, Brueggemann N, et al. Epithelial malignancies of the salivary glands: clinical experience of a single institution—a review. *Int J Oral Maxillofac Surg* 2004;22:423–432.

55. Terhaard CHJ, Lubsen H, Van der Tweel I, et al. Salivary gland carcinoma: Independent prognostic factors for locoregional control, distant metastases, and overall survival: results of the Dutch Head and Neck Oncology Cooperative Group. *Head Neck* 2004; 26:681–693.

56. Korkmaz H, Yoo GH, Du W, et al. Predictors of nodal metastasis in salivary gland cancer. *J Surg Oncol* 2002;80:186–189.

57. Hocwald E, Korkmaz H, Yoo GH, et al. Prognostic factors in major salivary gland cancer. *Laryngoscope* 2001;111:1434–1439.

58. Stennert E, Kisner D, Jungehuelsing M, et al. High incidence of lymph node metastasis in major salivary gland cancer. *Arch Otolaryngol Head Neck Surg* 2003;129:720–723.

59. Spiro RH, Huvos AG, Strong EW. Cancer of the parotid gland. *Am J Surg* 1975;130:452–459.

Lip Cancer

Ramon M. Esclamado   *Michael A. Fritz*

Lip cancer is the most common malignant tumor of the oral cavity, constituting 25% to 30% of cases, and is the second most common cancer in the head and neck, following cutaneous malignancy. Its incidence in the United States is 1.8 per 100,000 population, is as high as 13.5/100,000 males in Australia, and is virtually nonexistent in parts of Asia (1,2). In a series of 350 patients, about 90% of lip carcinomas were squamous cell, and 90% occurred on the lower lip. The oral commissure is the origin of the tumor in 0.7% to 6.1% of cases (3). Lip cancer is most common in white male smokers with a fair complexion who are in their sixth decade of life. Appropriate management of this common malignancy should have as its goals maximizing survival while minimizing the functional and cosmetic morbidity associated with treatment. This requires a thorough understanding of the functional anatomy of the lips, the biologic behavior of the disease, treatment options, and reconstructive considerations.

FUNCTIONAL ANATOMY

The lips form the anterior boundary of the oral cavity and form a mobile oral sphincter that prevents dribbling of fluids and assist in mastication, deglutition, and articulation. The lips are also important aesthetically, contributing to appearance and facial expression. The anatomic extent of the lips includes only the vermilion, or that portion of the lip mucosa that contacts the opposing lip. Anteriorly, the lip ends at the vermilion border, which is the junction of the vermilion with the skin. The lower lip vermilion in repose is more everted than the upper lip. The transverse length of the upper lip is slightly longer: about 8.0 cm compared with 7.5 cm for the lower lip.

The orbicularis oris muscle is the sphincter that lies within the lip and encircles the oral aperture. Superiorly, it extends almost to the columella and attaches to the anterior nasal spine. Inferiorly, it interdigitates with the mentalis

muscles to form the mental crease. Numerous paired muscles of the facial expression insert on its lateral deep surface and contribute to oral competence and the diversity of lip movement (Fig. 110.1). The deep surface of the orbicularis oris is covered by loosely attached mucous membranes containing numerous minor salivary glands. Superficially, it is loosely attached to overlying skin.

The sensory and motor innervations of the lips are separate. The infraorbital branch of the maxillary division of the trigeminal nerve (V2) provides the major sensory supply to the skin and mucous membrane of the upper lip. The oral commissure area is supplied by the buccal branch of the mandibular division of the trigeminal nerve (V3), whereas sensation of the lower lip skin and mucosa is derived from the mental branch of the mandibular nerve. The seventh cranial nerve (facial nerve) provides the motor innervation of the lip. The upper lip musculature is supplied by the buccal branch of the facial nerve, whereas the marginal mandibular branch innervates the lower lip musculature.

The main blood supply to the lips consists of the superior and inferior labial arteries, which travel between the submucosa of the lip and the orbicularis at the level of the vermilion cutaneous junction. The vessels branch from the facial artery just lateral to the oral commissure. These paired vessels create a circumoral vascular arcade that provides the anatomic basis for the classic lip-switch procedures and other local myocutaneous flaps. Efforts should therefore be made to preserve the facial vessels when performing concomitant neck dissections (4). The arteries have accompanying veins that drain to the anterior facial vein.

The lymphatics of the lips (Fig. 110.2) begin as a fine capillary network in the vermilion border and combine to form collecting trunks. The trunks from the upper lip and commissure drain to the ipsilateral preauricular, infraparotid, submandibular, and submental lymph nodes. No contralateral drainage occurs because the embryonic fusion plane of the central frontonasal process separates the

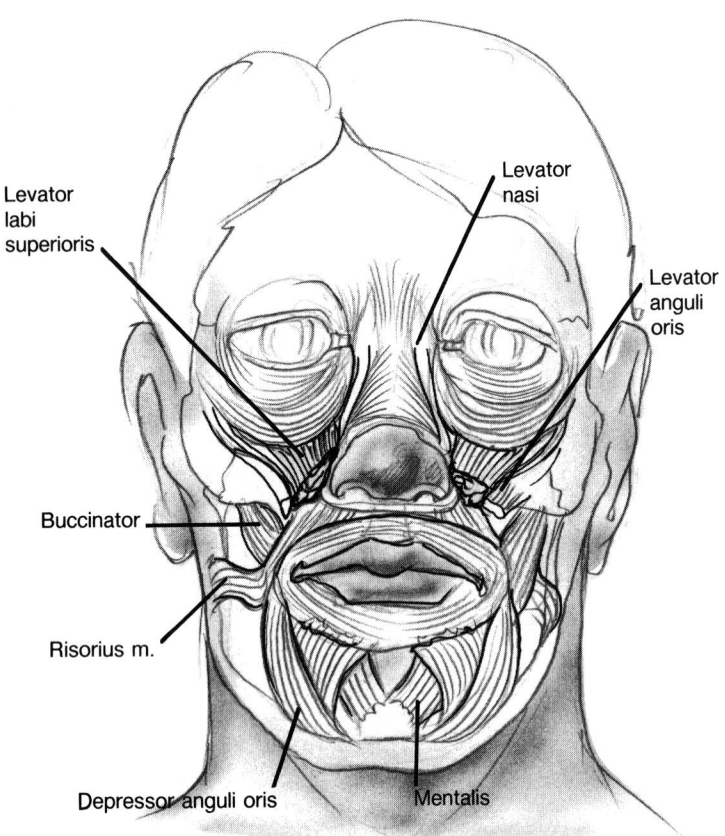

Levator
labi
superioris

Levator
nasi

Levator
anguli
oris

Buccinator

Risorius m.

Depressor anguli oris

Mentalis

Figure 110.1 Musculature of the lips. The orbicularis oris muscle is the sphincter lying within the lip and encircles the oral aperture. Numerous paired muscles of facial expression insert on its lateral deep surface to contribute to oral competence and the diversity of lip movement.

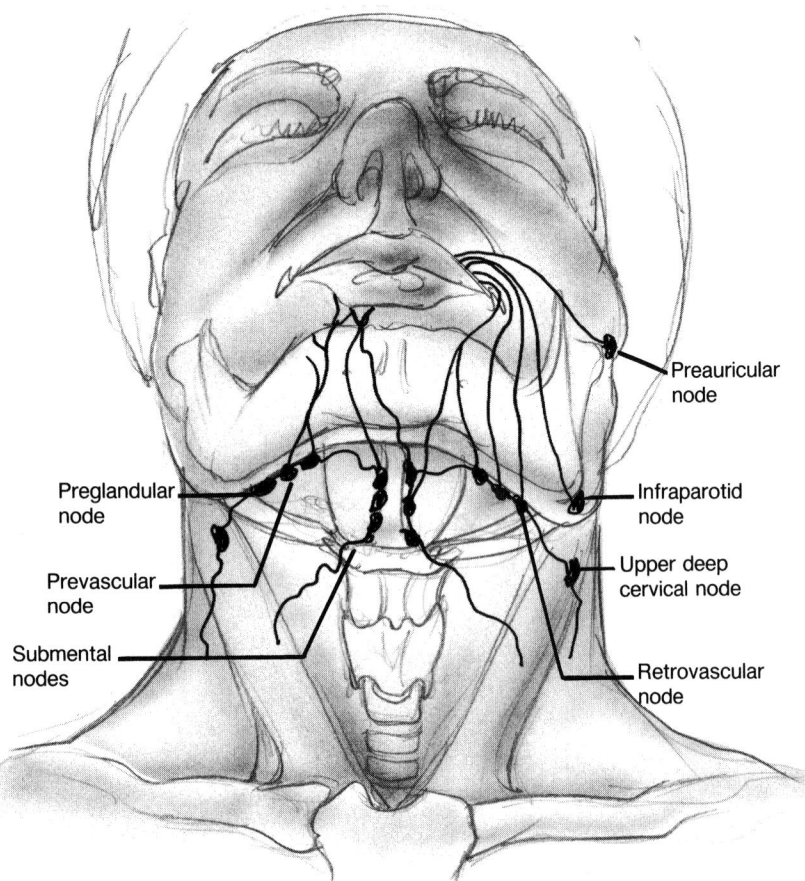

Preauricular
node

Preglandular
node

Infraparotid
node

Prevascular
node

Upper deep
cervical node

Submental
nodes

Retrovascular
node

Figure 110.2 Lymphatic drainage of the lips. Lymphatic channels of the upper lip and commissure drain to the ipsilateral preauricular, infraparotid, submandibular, and submental lymph nodes. The lower lip lymphatics drain to both ipsilateral and contralateral submental and submandibular lymph nodes. The second nodal station is the upper deep jugular nodes and occasionally the middle deep jugular nodes.

lateral maxillary processes and their associated neurovascular and lymphatic connections. The lower lip lymphatics drain to the submental and submandibular nodes. Because the mandibular processes fuse in the midline, numerous anastomoses cross the midline to drain bilaterally. Lower lip lymphatics also enter the mental foramen in 22% of patients. The second nodal station is the upper deep jugular nodes (level II) or occasionally the middle deep jugular nodes (level III).

BIOLOGIC BEHAVIOR

Lip cancer is one of the most readily curable malignancies in the head and neck. When diagnosed at an early stage, 10-year cause-specific survival is as high as 98%, with recurrence-free survival of 92.5% (5). The prominent location of the lips allows for early detection and treatment of this lesion. Characteristically, a history of crusting that bleeds on removal and a nonhealing blister for several months to years has been noted. When left untreated, the tumor progresses to involve skin of the mentum and alveolar mucosa. In advanced cases, the mandibular bone, the floor of the mouth, and the tongue can be involved, which renders the patient an oral cripple. Metastasis to cervical nodes develops with advanced lesions, and ultimately distant metastasis occurs. In a retrospective study of 1,036 patients with lip cancer (6), multivariate analysis yielded several prognostic factors predictive for significantly decreased determinate survival: patients with primary tumors larger than 3 cm, presence of cervical metastasis, poorly differentiated or undifferentiated histology, and involved surgical margins. The risk of cervical metastases is increased in large primary tumors, particularly if the oral commissure is involved, locally recurrent tumors, tumors thicker than 5 mm, poorly differentiated histology, or if perineural invasion is present (1,7,8).

The etiology is multifactorial, but prolonged exposure to sunlight is thought to play a major role. Evidence to support this view is as follows:

1. More than one third of patients have outdoor occupations.
2. Most tumors originate on the exposed vermilion of the lower lip.
3. The disease is commonly seen with second primary skin malignancies.
4. There is a higher incidence in sunny geographic locations.

Damaging effects of sun exposure are seen in adjacent tissue histologically, and leukoplakia, hyperkeratosis, and actinic cheilitis are often seen in association with the lip carcinoma (9). Pipe and cigarette smoking, poor dental hygiene, and chronic alcoholism may contribute to its development. Chronic immunosuppression also increases the risk of developing lip cancer (10).

CLINICAL EVALUATION

Lip carcinoma should be readily recognized and diagnosed. Its early stages can be indolent and protracted. As previously mentioned, the patient may present with a history of lower lip crusting that bleeds on removal or a nonhealing blister present for several months to years. Physical examination typically reveals an area of crusting with surrounding induration in an area of leukoplakia of the lower lip. In more advanced stages, a large bleeding mass may be present that can involve chin skin, the oral commissure, the upper lip, or the mandible. The integrity of the mental nerve must be evaluated even in early lesions, because tumor may track along the mental nerve and involve the mandible by direct extension, perineural invasion, or lymphatic spread into the mental foramen.

The diagnosis is established by incisional biopsy, which should include part of the deep or lateral tumor margin. This allows the pathologist to determine the pattern of invasion and the presence of perineural invasion. Ancillary radiographic studies such as a Panorex and magnetic resonance imaging (MRI) are indicated when tumor is attached to the mandible or extends over the gingiva into a tooth root, when dentition is loose, or when hypesthesia of the mental nerve is present. Ipsilateral enlargement of the mental nerve foramen is a sign of mandibular invasion via the mental nerve, and obliteration of fat in the masticator space, in the pterygopalatine fossa, or along the mandibular canal must be regarded as suspicious for tumor spread, even in the absence of gross osteolytic changes (11). An aggressive metastatic workup is not indicated in previously untreated lip carcinomas, because fewer than 2% of patients have distant metastases at the time of initial evaluation. The staging of squamous cell carcinoma of the lip, as defined by the American Joint Committee on Cancer, is outlined in Table 110.1.

Although 90% of lower lip malignancies are squamous cell carcinoma, it is important to keep in mind the

TABLE 110.1
STAGING OF SQUAMOUS CELL CARCINOMA OF THE LIP: PRIMARY TUMOR (T)

Stage	Description
TX	Primary tumor cannot be assessed
T0	No evidence of primary tumor
Tis	Carcinoma in situ
T1	Tumor 2 cm or less in greatest dimension
T2	Tumor more than 2 cm but not more than 4 cm in greatest dimension
T3	Tumor more than 4 cm in greatest dimension
T4 (lip)	Tumor invades adjacent structures (e.g., through cortical bone, inferior alveolar nerve, floor of mouth, skin of neck)

From American Joint Committee on Cancer. *Cancer Staging Manual*, 6th ed. New York: Springer, 2002, with permission.

Diagnosis	Symptoms and Signs	Tests
Squamous cell cancer	Nonhealing blister or recurrent crusting, lip induration, ulcer or mass for months to years, mental nerve numbness	Panorex CT/MRI Biopsy
Basal cell carcinoma	Pearly nodule with central dimpling, upper lip or perioral skin	Biopsy
Minor salivary gland tumor	Submucosal mass, usually upper lip	Biopsy
Keratoacanthoma	Rapid growth then spontaneous regression, may mimic squamous cell carcinoma in appearance	Incisional biopsy

TABLE 110.2 DIAGNOSIS LIP CANCER

CT, computed tomography; MRI, magnetic resonance imaging.
From Baker SR, Krause CJ. Pedicled flaps in reconstruction of the lip. *Facial Plast Surg* 1983;1:68–69, with permission.

differential diagnosis of other nonhealing ulcerative lesions of the lips, particularly when the clinical presentation is atypical for squamous cell cancer. Basal cell carcinoma is the second most common malignancy of the perioral region. Cancers of the upper lip are nearly always basal cell carcinoma (4,6). It rarely arises on lip mucosa; rather, it involves the lip by direct extension of a perioral skin lesion. This is most commonly seen with sclerosing basal cell carcinomas. These tumors usually have a distinct clinical appearance of a pearly white nodule with central dimpling, although larger tumors may appear similar to squamous cell tumors. They grow very slowly, rarely metastasize to cervical lymph nodes, and when located near embryonic fusion planes tend to track deeply into the soft tissues along these planes.

Minor salivary gland tumors of the lip are unusual; about 312 cases are reported in the literature. The age range is from 14 to 87 years. Tumors present as a smooth, firm, nonulcerated mass, and the upper lip is involved in 85% of cases. In contrast to other minor salivary gland tumors whose primary site is the lip versus other sites, only 17% of these are malignant, and the most common neoplasm, occurring 67% of the time, is a pleomorphic adenoma. Other rare malignant lesions of the lips include melanoma, microcystic adnexal carcinoma, Merkel cell carcinoma, malignant fibrous histiocytoma, and malignant granular cell tumors.

Keratoacanthoma is a benign self-limiting epithelial neoplasm that can mimic squamous cell carcinoma. It is commonly seen in patients aged 60 to 80 years. It has an initial rapid growth phase (over several weeks) to 1 to 2 cm in diameter and then stabilizes and spontaneously regresses after several weeks to months. It occurs on the lips in 8.1% of cases, appearing as an ulcerated circumscribed lesion with elevated or rolled margins, a keratinized central region, and an indurated base. It is firm in consistency, and the central keratin core can desquamate, leaving an

ulcer. Diagnosis is established by incisional biopsy, which is reported to accelerate its involution (12) (Table 110.2). Excisional biopsy, sparing as much normal tissue as possible, is indicated for persistent or enlarging lesions over several months, when squamous cell carcinoma cannot be excluded after previous incisional biopsies.

Chronic actinic changes of hyperkeratosis, leukoplakia, and angular cheilitis may be premalignant and are seen in association with squamous cell carcinoma in 46% of patients. When seen initially as an isolated lesion or if the lesion progresses in size, biopsy is indicated. Other ulcerative inflammatory lesions involving the lips, including viral stomatitis and the primary chancre of syphilis, can mimic lip carcinoma but are acute in onset, and the lip lesion heals spontaneously. A positive Wassermann reaction was associated in the past with the development of lip carcinoma, but this has been shown to be a risk factor only with multiple lip carcinomas.

MANAGEMENT

The most efficacious treatment modality for lip carcinoma is one that allows adequate treatment of the primary tumor, appropriate management of cervical lymph nodes, and successful reconstruction. The treatment plan should have the following goals:

1. Extirpate all tissue involved with cancer, both at the primary site (lips) and regional lymph nodes.
2. Maintain oral competence in terms of speech, mastication, and retention of saliva.
3. Maintain satisfactory lip cosmesis.
4. Permit early rehabilitation and return to daily activities.

Several modalities are available to treat early (stage I and II) lip cancer. Surgery and radiation therapy are equally effective in controlling early-stage lesions: 5-year determinate survival rates for lesions less than 3 cm average 90% (13). In a series of 323 patients, of which 91% were T1 or TCIS treated primarily by surgery, cause-specific survival at 10 years was 98% (5). In several large series of patients treated with primary radiation therapy, the overall locoregional control rate was 85% to 93%, and the overall 5-year actuarial survival rate was 80% to 90% (14,15). Advanced tumors (T3 and T4) and clinically palpable nodes fared poorly, with 5-year actuarial survival rates of 40% (13). A study comparing surgery versus radiotherapy concluded that cure rates are favorable with both modalities in stage 1 disease. Patients with larger tumors received radiotherapy more often and had a much poorer disease-free survival rate (14).

Radiation therapy is a low-risk noninvasive technique that avoids the potential complications associated with general anesthesia. However, the treatment time is prolonged (as much as 5 to 6 weeks), a whistle deformity may result from tissue loss and wound contracture with very large tumors, osteoradionecrosis of the mandible may develop, and future reconstructive options may be limited. Primary radiation therapy may be most useful in the treatment of early commissure lesions.

Surgical management is recommended for most patients. The oncologic, functional, and cosmetic outcome is usually excellent in early T stage disease, and the oncologic outcome is poor with primary radiation of advanced tumors, particularly when it is close to or involves the mandible. We prefer a combination of surgery and postoperative radiotherapy for stage III and IV disease and for recurrent disease after primary surgical treatment.

The standard approach to surgical resection of the primary lip lesion is full-thickness excision and careful intraoperative frozen-section evaluation of the surgical margins. The appropriate margin around a T1 primary lip tumor is controversial. A recent study reported a 2.8% local recurrence rate when a 3-mm margin normal tissue was obtained and frozen section margins were negative (16). When tumor margins are 2 mm or less, local recurrence was seen in 13% of patients, half of whom had postoperative radiation therapy (17). In T2 tumors, we advocate a 5- to 8-mm margin of normal tissue because tendency to underestimate margins is more common and reported local recurrence rates have been higher than anticipated. The primary goal of therapy is eradication of all tumor tissue, without limitation for reconstructive considerations. More advanced tumors may require resection of chin skin, mandibular bone, or oral cavity soft tissues to allow a 1- to 2-cm margin. Skin incisions should be planned so as to minimize the secondary deformity and to facilitate reconstruction but not at the expense of compromising tumor margins.

Vermilionectomy is indicated in superficial carcinoma limited to mucosa or multicentric or premalignant lesions. Recently, Mohs excision of lip carcinoma has been advocated, but this is primarily useful in stage I and II well-differentiated neoplasms that are 2.5 mm thick or less

and have no muscle involvement (18). Recently, a meta-analysis of cutaneous squamous cell cancer that included the lip showed a 5-year local recurrence rate of 10.5% in 7,022 patients with standard surgical resection versus 2.3% of 952 patients undergoing Mohs micrographic surgery (19). However, this difference may be due to selection of less advanced lesions for Mohs surgery.

The management of regional lymph nodes in patients with lip carcinoma is controversial and requires a thorough understanding of the risk of nodal metastasis, and the patterns of nodal spread. In contrast to other squamous cell carcinomas of the oral cavity, lip carcinoma uncommonly metastasizes to regional lymph nodes. However, when nodal metastasis occurs, 5-year determinate survival is decreased to 61% (6). Regional nodal metastasis is present at the time of initial diagnosis in 2% to 12% of patients, and another 3% to 13% of patients will develop delayed nodal metastasis (20). Therefore, appropriate management of the neck in lip cancer requires separate decision making for clinically palpable disease versus occult metastatic nodal disease in the newly diagnosed, untreated patient.

In patients with clinically palpable, suspicious lymph nodes, the rate of pathologically positive nodes ranges from 44% to 97% (1,8,20). If the primary tumor was on the lateral one third of the lip, the ipsilateral nodes were involved 84% of the time and were limited to level I to III (20). Bilateral or contralateral metastasis were seen 3% to 10% of patients and was usually associated with larger tumors that crossed the midline of the lower lip (1,8,20). Neck dissection of the ipsilateral side alone is recommended, if radiation therapy is planned postoperatively and includes the contralateral, undissected, clinically N0 neck. Indications for postoperative radiation therapy include a T3 or T4 primary tumor, a recurrent tumor, extracapsular spread, metastasis in multiple levels or greater than two nodes, or perineural invasion. A modified radical or radical neck dissection is performed for bulky (>3 cm) nodal disease in levels II/III, but a selective neck dissection of levels I to III is oncologically sound if the nodes are freely mobile, and postoperative radiation therapy is used for extracapsular spread, there are greater than two pathologically positive nodes, or multiple levels are involved (1,21,22).

Decision making for treating clinical N0 necks is more complex. There is limited experience with sentinel node biopsy for lip cancer, but it holds promise as in other oral cavity sites (23). T1 lesions rarely need the neck addressed, because the risk of nodal metastasis is approximately 3% (5). Our treatment philosophy is to perform ipsilateral selective neck dissection, levels I to III in N0 necks when a significant risk (20%) of occult metastasis is present. As previously mentioned, this criteria is met in large primary tumors (>3 cm), particularly if the oral commissure is involved, locally recurrent tumors, tumors thicker than 5 mm, poorly differentiated histology, or if perineural invasion is present (1,7,8). We also perform ipsilateral selective neck dissection (SND) when ipsilateral N1 disease is present, the contralateral neck is N0, and postoperative radiation therapy is not planned, or when reconstruction requires revascularized tissue transfer. Bilateral I to III SND can be performed for large primary lesions crossing the midline, but it is unnecessary if postoperative radiation will be used to treat the primary site, because the neck can be included in the treatment fields.

LIP RECONSTRUCTION

Lip reconstruction must be carefully considered when managing lip carcinomas and requires meticulous planning to achieve optimal functional and cosmetic results. The ideal reconstructive procedure should result in a lip that is sensate; has sphincter or muscle function that maintains a watertight continent seal; allows sufficient opening for food, dentures, and oral hygiene; and is aesthetically acceptable. It is not possible to satisfy all these criteria in every instance; therefore, reconstructive goals must be prioritized. The most critical component of successful reconstruction is oral continence, which is a function of sensation and two sphincteric mechanisms oriented at right angles. The deep orbicularis and buccinator muscle interplay to create an axial force that seals the lips against the teeth and the superficial orbicularis functions as a coronal sphincter, pursing and sealing the opposing lips (24). This complex relationship is best preserved when circumferential continuity of the orbicularis is maintained; however, larger defects often mandate alternative solutions to avoid compromising oral aperture size.

Appropriate evaluation and planning should include an estimate of the magnitude and location of the anticipated defect, an assessment of whether the area has been previously irradiated, the degree of laxity of the lip and adjacent check tissue, whether the patient wears dentures, and whether palpable lymph nodes may require sacrifice of the facial artery or arteries. Incisions should be placed within the circumoral relaxed skin tension lines (oriented radially), at borders of lip subunits or at boundaries such as the melolabial crease and labiomental sulcus. Tattooing the white scroll at the vermilion border with a fine needle and methylene blue dye ensures accurate postoperative realignment of this aesthetically critical boundary.

Surgical procedures to reconstitute the lip may be classified as follows (25):

1. Those that use remaining lip tissue
2. Those that borrow tissue from the opposite lip
3. Those that use adjacent tissue
4. Those that use distant flaps

Partial-Thickness Defects

Partial-thickness or mucosal loss at the vermilion only is most commonly encountered when vermilionectomy or lip shave is performed for diffuse premalignant or superficial malignant disease or preventatively in conjunction with primary tumor resection when actinic cheilitis is present in remaining lip tissue. The most commonly used method of reconstitution of lining involves submucosal dissection and advancement of labial buccal mucosa. Undermining is performed deep to minor salivary glands and superficial to the orbicularis and labial artery and it can be extended to the apex of the buccal sulcus to ensure tension-free redraping. Problems with this technique include thinning of lip, persistent deep red color of advanced mucosa (more of a problem for males), and potential inversion of hairs at the vermillion border with irritation. These drawbacks can be avoided with carbon dioxide laser lip shaves and mucosalization by secondary intention, although healing time requires 2 to 3 weeks. Other less commonly used two-stage techniques for vermillion mucosa replacement include bipedicle visor-type flaps from the undersurface of the opposing lip, ventral tongue flaps, and cross-lip mucosal flaps (26). Small vermilion deficiencies can be managed with V-Y advancement flaps.

Small partial thickness defects involving the lips are managed following basic principles of cutaneous surgery. Optimal reconstructive results are often achieved when the defect can be converted to a wedge or pentagonal defect oriented within relaxed skin tension lines. M-plasty is used when possible to avoid scars that cross the boundaries of the lip subunits. Extending resections through uninvolved vermilion and orbicularis often achieves better cosmetic results than A-to-T methods that create horizontal scars parallel to the mucocutaneous junction (26,27).

Larger partial thickness defects mandate consideration of lip subunits. Upper lip subunits include a central segment composed of the philtrum and philtral ridges and two trapezoid-shaped lateral segments (28). The lower lip consists of a single subunit. Similar to principles of nasal reconstruction, absence of the majority of a subunit is often best repaired after excision of the remaining portion. Medial advancement of lateral upper lip skin is aided greatly by the excision of perialar crescents of skin and anchoring dermis to pyriform periosteum deep to the ala. Partial thickness defects of the central segment are amenable to full-thickness skin grafting or healing by secondary intention—with the intention of narrowing the philtrum as little as possible. Patients with flat, less distinct philtral columns may be an exception to this rule (24). Large cutaneous lateral defects are optimally resurfaced with inferiorly or superiorly based melolabial transposition flaps, especially in patients with midface laxity.

Full-Thickness Defects

Isolated full-thickness defects of vermilion only (mucosa and orbicularis) are uncommon, but full-thickness deficiencies

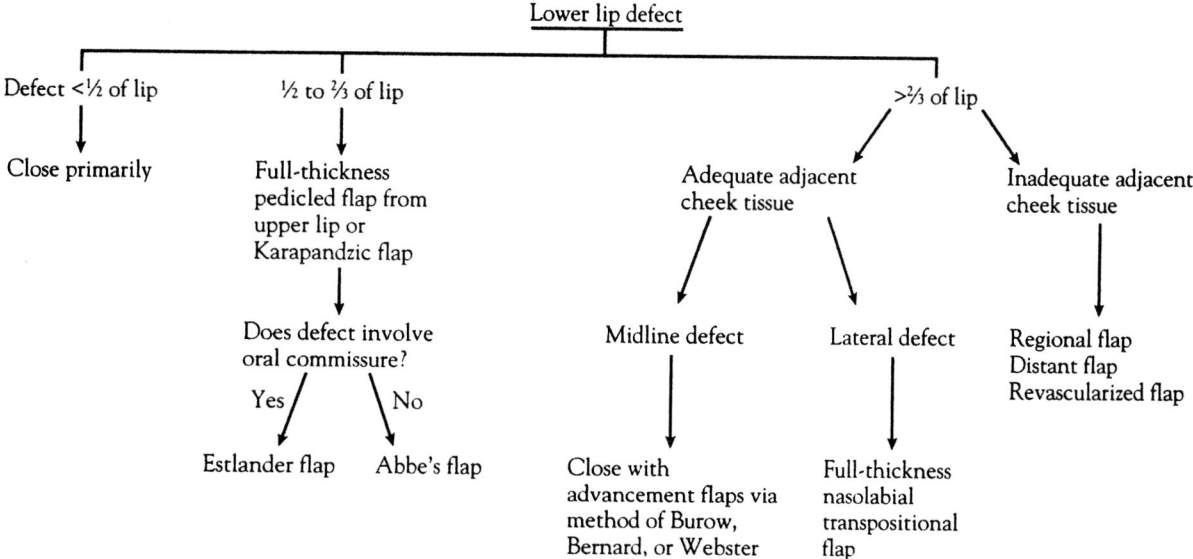

Figure 110.3 Lower lip reconstruction. (From Baker SR, Krause CJ. Pedicled flaps in reconstruction of the lip. *Facial Plast Surg* 1983;1:68–69, with permission.)

along the length of the vermilion are almost always present after extensive reconstructions with local or distant flaps. Several techniques have therefore been designed to address this issue. Small complete vermilion defects can be addressed with a full-thickness horizontal releasing incision at the vermilion-cutaneous junction of the longer portion of the remaining lip (26). Vermilion is then advanced laterally into the defect. Another option is to convert the defect to a full-thickness wedge through the cutaneous lip.

When extensive vermilion substance has been lost, a muscle-mucosal flap from the ventral surface of the tongue may be used. This flap is based posteriorly with the free edge of the flap attached to the mucocutaneous border. Two to three weeks later, the pedicle is transected at the junction of the lateral and ventral tongue, retaining muscle for bulk and mucosa for vermilion reconstruction. This technique does not limit tongue mobility; however, the newly created vermillion has a pebbled surface (25). A better alternative for more extensive defects may be the facial artery musculomucosal (FAMM) flap (29). This axial flap containing buccal mucosa, submucosa, and a small amount of buccinator muscle is based on the facial artery as it courses through the cheek lateral to the buccinator muscle and medial to other muscles of facial expression. Inferiorly based FAMM flaps incorporate the facial artery as it enters the face at the anterior edge of the masseter muscle, whereas superiorly based FAMM flaps are perfused retrograde through the angular artery. Both designs allow for a long thin flap to be harvested without compromise of viability—this both minimizes donor site morbidity and enables single-stage reconstructions of the entire vermillion. Bilateral and unilateral FAMM flaps have been used with particular success as adjuncts in total lip reconstruc-

tion for color and contour-appropriate replacement of vermilion deficiencies.

The algorithms in Figures 110.3 and 110.4 outline an excellent general approach to upper and lower lip reconstruction (25). The relative proportion of total lip length that can be excised and closed directly without distortion varies between individuals and depends on overall lip length and tissue laxity. In general, one fourth to one third of the upper lip may be closed directly with larger lateral resections sometimes amenable to direct closure. Lower lip defects of one-third to one-half lip length may be closed primarily. Shield or V excision is usually adequate with closure in three layers (mucosa, muscle, skin) and meticulous reapproximation of the orbicularis and white scroll at the vermilion border on either side of the defect.

In the lower lips, lateral advancement with incisions placed in the mental crease may be required when the defect base is broad. Every attempt should be made not to extend incisions beyond the mental crease to avoid a pointed chin deformity. Just as in partial thickness defects, full-thickness advancement in the mesial upper lip is facilitated by excising a crescent of cheek skin in the perialar region and anchoring the lateral flap to periosteum (30) (Fig. 110.5). This method is similar to that described by Diffenbach and Webster and lessens tension on remaining lip segments after primary closure (26). An Abbe flap may be used in the midline to replace the central subunit and prevent excessive tension on the wound closure.

Defects of One Third to Two Thirds of the Lip

The majority of these defects are amenable to closure using rotated or pedicled tissue from the opposing lip. Three

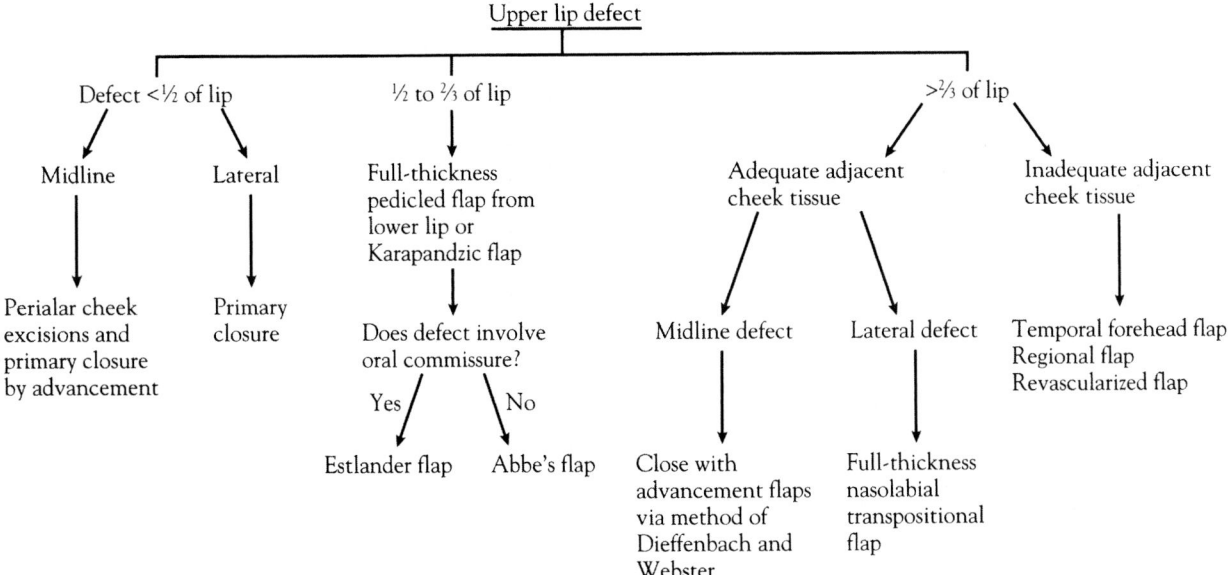

Upper lip defect

Defect <½ of lip
- Midline → Perialar cheek excisions and primary closure by advancement
- Lateral → Primary closure

½ to ⅔ of lip → Full-thickness pedicled flap from lower lip or Karapandzic flap → Does defect involve oral commissure?
- Yes → Estlander flap
- No → Abbe's flap

>⅔ of lip
- Adequate adjacent cheek tissue
  - Midline defect → Close with advancement flaps via method of Dieffenbach and Webster
  - Lateral defect → Full-thickness nasolabial transpositional flap
- Inadequate adjacent cheek tissue → Temporal forehead flap, Regional flap, Revascularized flap

Figure 110.4 Upper lip reconstruction. (From Baker SR, Krause CJ. Pedicled flaps in reconstruction of the lip. *Facial Plast Surg* 1983;1:68–69, with permission.)

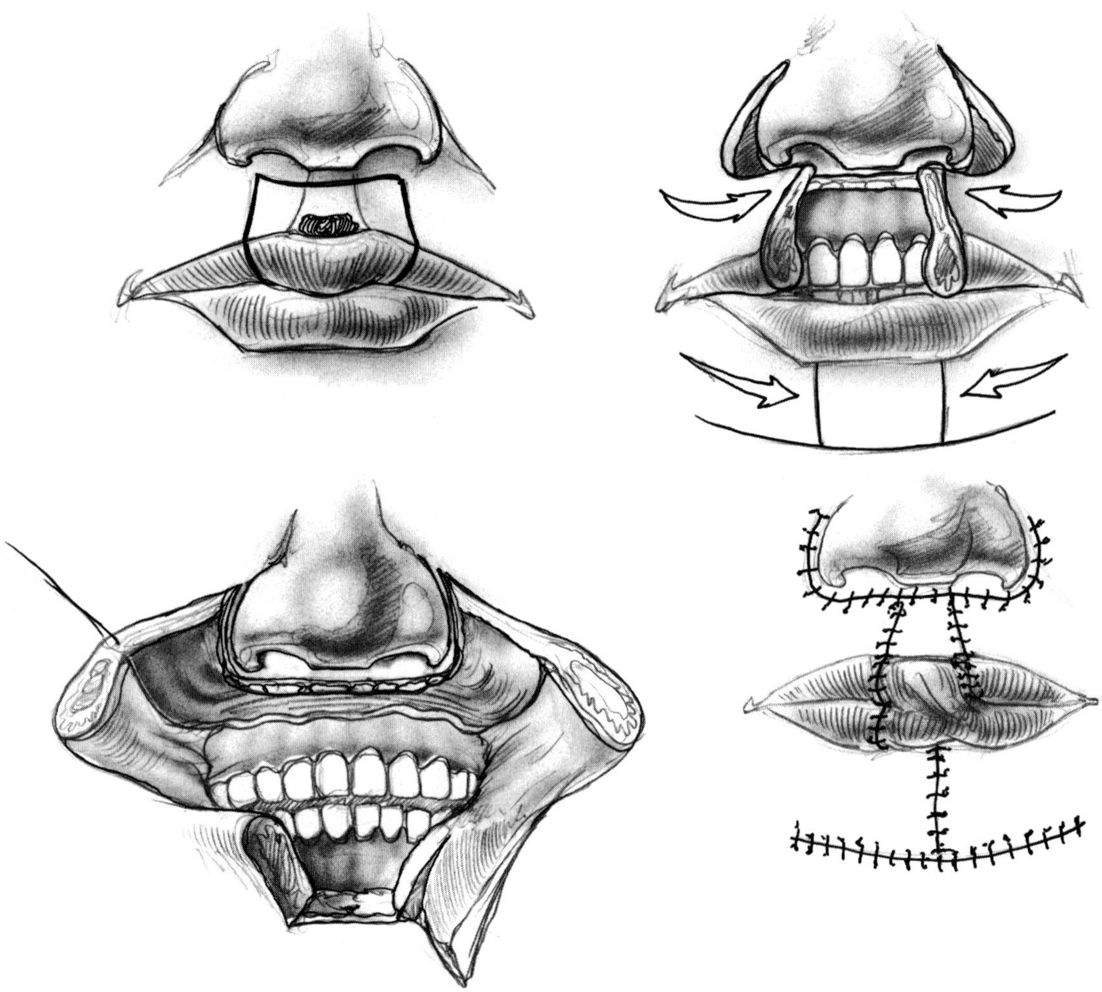

Figure 110.5 Primary closure of defects in the midline of the upper lip can be facilitated by excising crescents of cheek skin in the perialar regions. An Abbe flap can be added in the midline if the wound closure is under excessive tension.

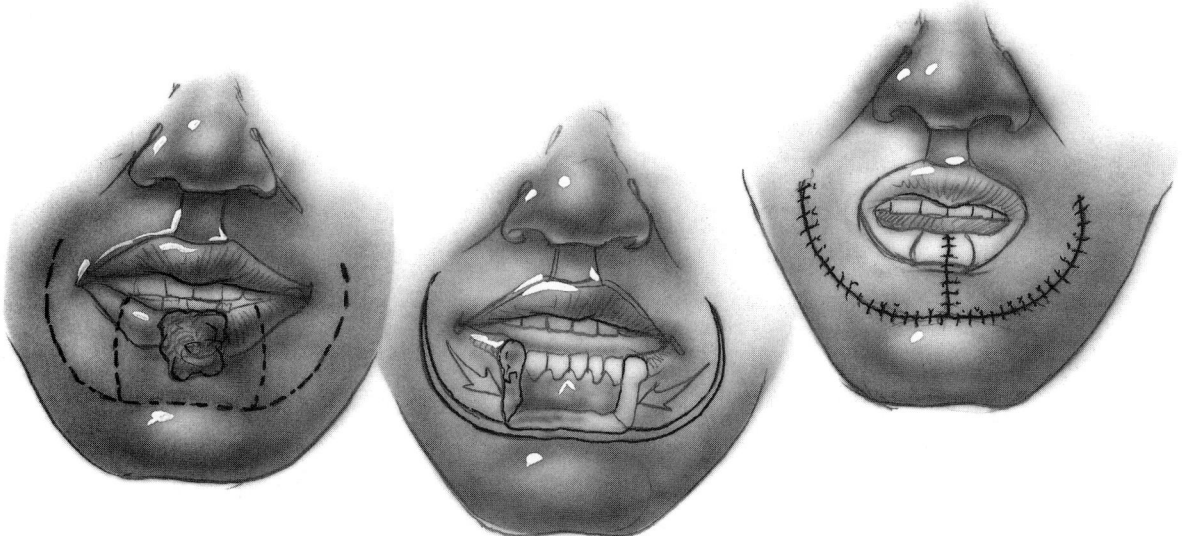

Figure 110.6 The Karapandzic labioplasty. Circumoral skin incisions are made within the nasolabial and mental creases. The orbicularis oris muscle is bluntly dissected from supporting perioral muscles, taking care to preserve the neuromuscular pedicles, which enter from the periphery. The oral mucosa usually does not require transection.

procedures constitute the majority of reconstructions in this group: the Karapandzic labioplasty, the Abbe cross-lip flap, and the Estlander cross-lip flap. Each method has advantages and disadvantages and individual surgeons favor different techniques (26,31).

The Karapandzic labioplasty, described in 1974, modified older circumoral advancement techniques to preserve vascularity, sensation, and motor innervation to the lips. This single-stage reconstructive procedure has gained popularity to become the favored reconstructive method of many surgeons for moderate-sized defects (26). This technique (Fig. 110.6) is more commonly used for lower lip defects but can be applied to upper defects as well. Circumoral incisions are begun in the mental crease and carried around the oral commissures into the melolabial sulci. An important technical point is to maintain appropriate flap width in the area of the oral commissure. Flap width is this area must approximate the height of the lip portion, which it will replace after rotation. Incisions, therefore, cannot remain within the melolabial sulcus where it runs very close to the commissures. After incisions are carried through skin and subcutaneous tissue, the lateral border of the orbicularis oris muscle is mobilized from the other supporting perioral muscles to allow rotation of segments and tension-free closure. Blunt dissection of the muscle allows identification and preservation of the superior and inferior labial arteries and the neurovascular pedicles that enter the muscle from its periphery. The underlying oral mucosa usually does not require transection for mobilization.

The advantages of the Karapandzic flap are its ease of design and the preservation of oral competence. Disadvantages include blunting of the commissures, circumoral scars,

which can be unsightly, and the potential for microstomia, which may preclude the use of dentures. One potential solution to microstomia is to initially reconstruct with this technique, accept temporary microstomia and allow tissues to stretch with time and use, then perform a cross-lip procedure to improve oral opening (31,32).

Abbe and Estlander flaps transfer full-thickness tissue between opposing lips pedicled on the labial artery. These techniques allow precise flap design, typically result in less microstomia than rotation flap reconstruction, and avoid circumoral incisions (31). Abbe flaps preserve the aesthetically important oral commissure but require a second stage for flap division. Additional disadvantages include denervation of tissue with variable reinnervation over time and the potential for pincushioning or trap door deformity in a lip segment surrounded by scars on three sides (33).

There are several important points for consideration in Abbe flap design (Fig. 110.7). Flap height should equal the height of the defect. Flap width is classically designed to be one half the width of the defect, but more modern approaches advocate reconstruction of upper lip subunit defects with like-size flaps from the lower lip when possible (28,33). Creation of the flap involves full-thickness incisions through all portions except the region of the pedicle, which consistently is found at the level of the vermilion border on the posterior surface of the orbicularis muscle just deep to the labial submucosa (34). The pedicle should be narrow to facilitate rotation and extension of anterior incisions into the vermilion allows for more accurate alignment of vermilion borders. Because the pedicle does not contain an associated major venous structure, it is important to leave a fairly wide mucosal bridge posteriorly to allow venous return. The donor site

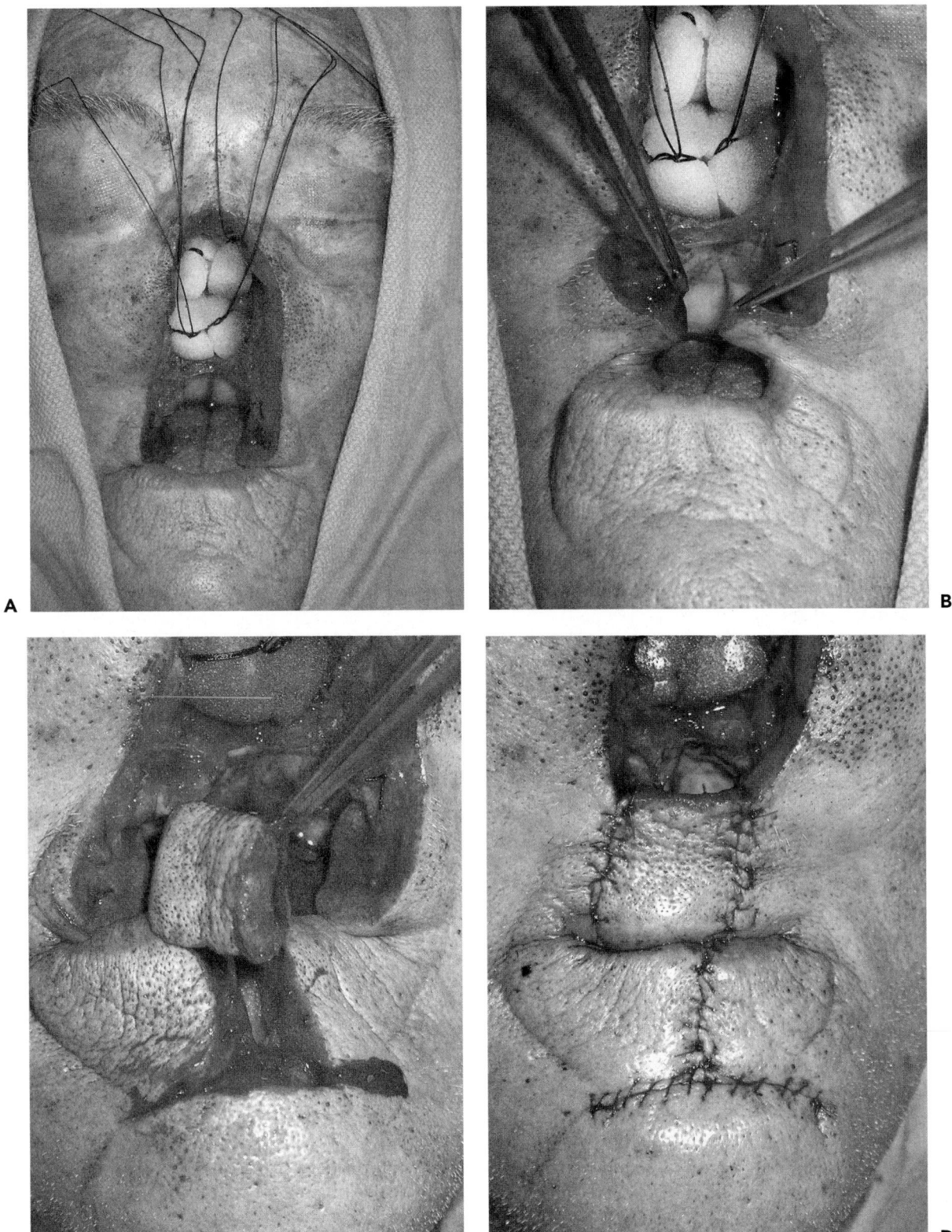

Figure 110.7 Abbe cross-lip flap for upper lip reconstruction. **A:** Patient underwent concomitant total rhinectomy (to be reconstructed with prosthesis) with central upper lip resection. **B:** Remaining lateral upper lip. **C:** Harvested flap from central lower lip. Note isolated pedicle. **D:** Flap at inset; donor site closed with lateral incisions in mental crease.

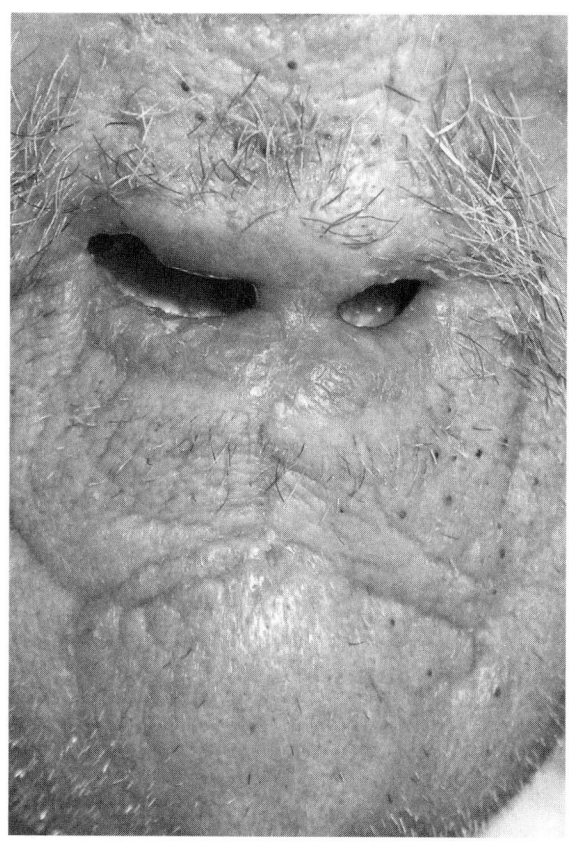

E

Figure 110.7 (*continued*) **E:** Prior to pedicle division at 3 weeks. (Photos courtesy of R. Lorenz.)

defect and flap reconstruction should be closed in three layers, with careful alignment of both orbicularis muscle and vermilion.

The Abbe flap was originally designed to close medial defects, and it can be based either medially or laterally, depending on the location of the defect and blood supply. When an Abbe flap is designed from the upper lip, lateral lip tissue should be used with medial incisions placed on the philtral ridges to camouflage donor site closure (31). This closure is facilitated by advancement of the lateral upper lip segment and excision of perialar crescents as described earlier. In general, cross-lip pedicles may be divided in 2 to 3 weeks.

The Estlander flap uses the same techniques as the Abbe flap to create a flap based a narrow labial artery pedicle approximately one half of the defect size. One exception is that the anterior incision on the pedicle side is not carried into the vermilion. Superiorly based Estlander flaps should be modified to incorporate scars within the nasolabial fold (Fig. 110.8). Donor tissue is rotated around the oral commissure to the opposing lip and therefore this single-stage procedure is only applied defects involving the commissure. This technique results in blunting of the oral commissure that, unlike the symmetric blunting of circumoral advancement, is starkly contrasted by the unviolated opposing commissure (26). As a result, secondary commissuroplasty is often performed to minimize this disparity.

Defects Greater Than Two Thirds of the Lip

Large defects of the upper lip present significant reconstructive challenges. Cross-lip flaps may be combined with lateral advancement flaps for larger central upper lip defects (Fig. 110.3), but this technique is not sufficient for total upper lip reconstruction. Modified cheek flaps that preserve neurovascular structures and the original position of the oral commissures have been used with success in reconstruction of near total and total upper lip defects (35). The main disadvantage of this technique is large transverse scars that cross the cheeks. Bilateral superiorly based composite nasolabial flaps have also provided reasonable aesthetic and functional results (36). Free temporal scalp flaps based on the superficial temporal vessels have been used with some success to import hair-bearing tissue to restore male beard patterns and provide camouflage (37). A major disadvantage of this technique is the lack of innervated tissue.

Relatively large lower lip defects can be managed with Karapandzic circumoral rotation flaps followed by cross-lip

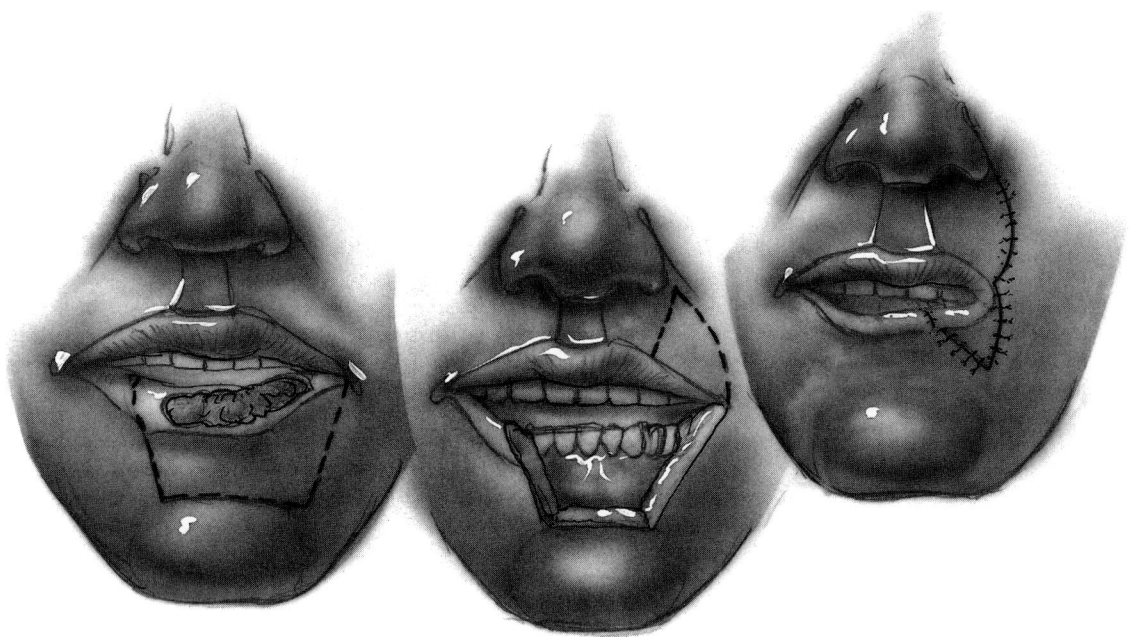

Figure 110.8 The superiorly based Estlander flap may be modified from its original description by designing the flap so that it lies within the nasolabial fold.

flaps as previously described. Midline lower lip defects may be corrected by using any of several modifications of the Bernard repair, which essentially uses full-thickness advancement flaps of adjacent cheek tissue. These techniques have the advantage of single-stage reconstruction with innervated flaps but frequently result in a tight lower lip with poor function (26,31,38).

The Webster modification of the Bernard chelioplasty employs Burow triangles whose medial vertical limbs lie within the melolabial fold (Fig. 110.9). The width of the base of the triangles is calculated so that the distance from the oral commissure to the lateral portion of the base equals one half the width of lip tissue excised. A lateral vertical limb is then drawn to complete the triangle. Skin and

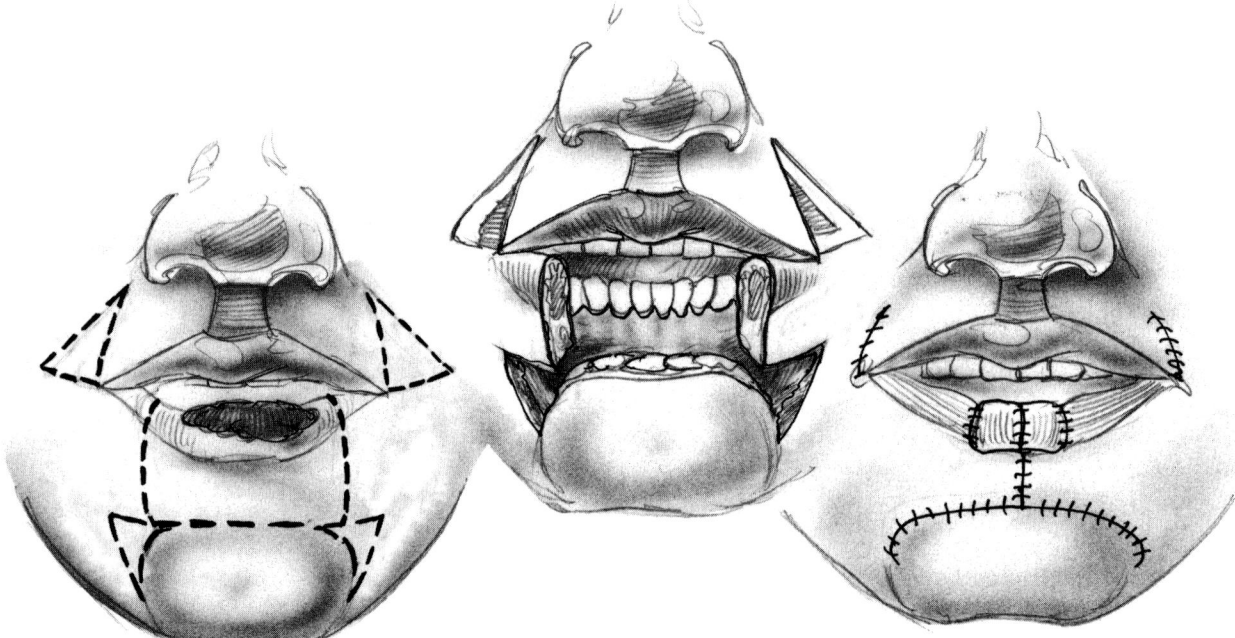

Figure 110.9 Webster modification of Bernard cheiloplasty. *Cross-hatched area* denotes mucosal flap used to create new vermilion (see text).

subcutaneous tissue only are excised from the triangles and incisions are deepened along its base, identifying and preserving the neurovascular supply to the orbicularis oris and buccinator muscles. A mucosal flap based on the superior margin of the cheek flap is elevated to create a new vermilion. Usually, incisions through skin and muscle are required around the mental crease, with Burow triangles strategically placed in the submental area to allow sufficient advancement of the cheek flaps.

Full-thickness inferiorly based nasolabial flaps have been used to reconstruct subtotal lower lip defects (31). The disadvantage of this technique is that the flaps are not innervated, and in raising the flaps, the upper lip is usually denervated. To avoid this complication, total lower lip reconstruction with skin only nasolabial flaps has been described with good aesthetic results and preservation of oral competence (39). Consistent functional reconstruction of total and subtotal defects has also been described using musculocutaneous island flaps based on the facial artery and innervated depressor anguli oris muscle (38).

Defects involving the entire lower lip and adjacent soft tissue of the cheek or chin require reconstruction with distant flaps. The composite radial forearm free flap with palmaris longus tendon has yielded reliable reconstructive results (40). The skin paddle is folded over the palmaris longus tendon to provide internal and external lip lining. The two ends of the palmaris longus tendon can be attached to medial upper lip orbicularis muscle to suspend the reconstruction and provide dynamic function (40). The lateral antebrachial cutaneous nerve can be harvested with the flap and neurotized to the stump of the mental nerve. The vermilion can be established on a deepithelialized segment of the forearm flap using a facial artery myomucosal flap as described earlier or with mucosal flaps from the tongue, upper lip, or cheek (29,40,41) (Fig. 110.10). Medical tattooing has also been used with acceptable results.

A variety of axial or myocutaneous flaps have also been described for extensive reconstructions; the pectoralis major myocutaneous flap was the most popular and dependable pedicled flap for transferring muscle and skin for a single-stage lip reconstruction before use of free vascularized flaps became routine. The pectoralis flap can be folded on itself to provide intraoral and external coverage and suspended with a fascia lata graft, but variable flap bulk, inferior tension, and the lack of sensory reinnervation result in less consistent outcomes than those provided by composite radial forearm techniques.

When the anterior mandibular arch has been resected, lower lip support requires reconstruction of the mandible. Vascularized osteomyocutaneous flaps have become the standard method of reconstructing anterior mandibular defects. The primary advantage is the ability to transfer large amounts of bone and soft tissue in an immediate single-stage reconstruction with cosmetically and functionally acceptable results. The flap selected is dependent on bone and soft tissue requirements. For anterior mandible and lip alone, a radial forearm or fibular osseocutaneous flap is an option, whereas larger defects, including the floor of the mouth, tongue, or cheek, may require use of scapular osseomyocutaneous flap or two separate free flaps (e.g., fibula and radial forearm).

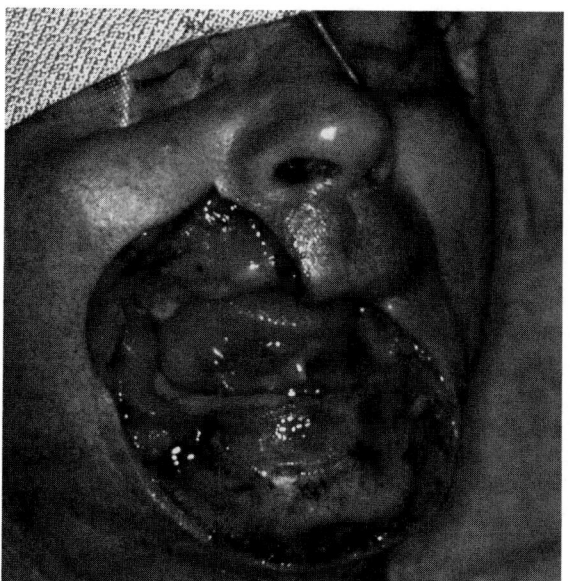
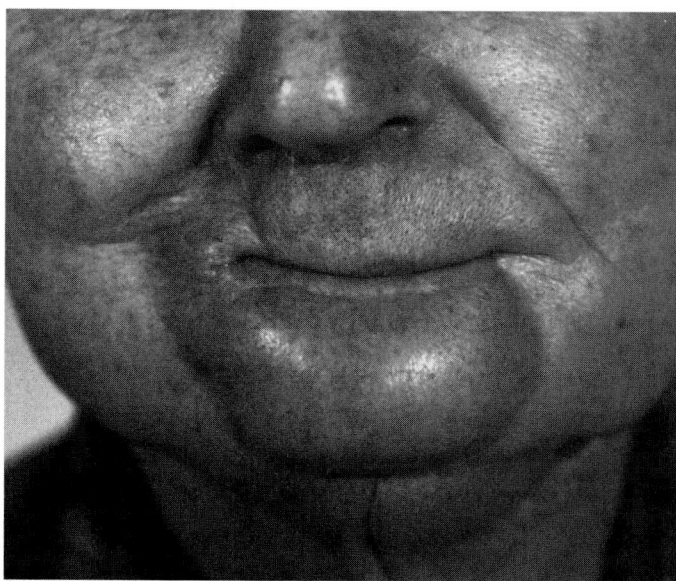

A   **B**

Figure 110.10 Radial forearm-palmaris longus reconstruction of total lower lip and one-third upper lip defect.

TABLE 110.3 **COMPLICATIONS**

LIP CANCER

Surgical
Wound infection and dehiscence
Incompetent oral sphincter
Microstomia
Poor cosmetic result

Radiation
Whistle deformity
Osteoradionecrosis

COMPLICATIONS

Complications of radiation therapy, as discussed previously, include a prolonged treatment time, with delayed rehabilitation; a whistle deformity from tissue loss and scar contracture with large tumors, which may require secondary reconstruction; osteoradionecrosis of the mandible; and limitation of future reconstructive options. Surgical complications include those associated with general anesthesia, neck dissection, and wound infection and dehiscence (Table 110.3). In regard to lip reconstruction, complications include an incompetent oral sphincter, microstomia, or poor cosmetic result. To avoid these complications, the surgeon must thoroughly understand the biologic behavior of lip carcinoma and its management principles and must carefully plan and meticulously execute the reconstructive option chosen.

EMERGENCIES

There are very few situations in which patients with lip carcinoma require emergent intervention. As previously mentioned, lip carcinoma is usually a slow-growing lesion and is usually diagnosed relatively early. Large tumors involving the tongue and the floor of the mouth may cause airway problems when general anesthesia is required; this is readily managed by initial tracheotomy under local anesthesia (Table 110.4). Patients with large tumors may be malnourished, in part due to oral incompetence, so adequate preoperative nutritional assessment is important when major resection and reconstructive procedures are contemplated.

TABLE 110.4 **EMERGENCIES**

LIP CANCER

Airway compromise with large tumors

HIGHLIGHTS

- The lips are important functionally in maintaining oral competence and aesthetically by contributing to appearance and facial expression. The lips are characterized by the vermilion, or that lip mucosa that contacts the opposite lip mucosa.
- The orbicularis oris muscle serves as the oral sphincter and is innervated by branches of the facial nerve. The blood supply is from the labial branches of the facial artery. Sensation is provided by the paired mental nerves.
- Lymphatic drainage from the lower lip is to the submental and submandibular nodes bilaterally; the upper lip drains to the ipsilateral parotid and submandibular nodes.
- Lip carcinoma is the most common malignancy of the oral cavity, composing 25% to 30% of cases. As a rule of thumb, 90% are squamous cell carcinoma, 90% occur on the lower lip, and the overall 5-year determinate survival rate is 90%. Sunlight is thought to be the principal etiologic factor in its development.
- The diagnosis is established by biopsy but is suggested by a history of recurrent crusting or a nonhealing area of lip induration noted over several months. With a high index of suspicion, lip carcinoma is easily diagnosed and successfully managed if treated in its early stages.
- Surgery and radiation therapy are equally efficacious for lesions less than 3 cm. Surgery is preferred, because it offers the advantages of tumor margin assessment, rapid rehabilitation through immediate reconstruction, and avoidance of radiation complications. For advanced lesions, surgery combined with postoperative radiation therapy is indicated.
- Indicators predictive of poor outcome are large primary tumors, mandibular involvement, mental nerve involvement, cervical node metastases, recurrent disease, and undifferentiated histology.
- The goal of lip reconstruction is to provide the patient with a sensate innervated lip that functions as a competent oral sphincter of adequate size while remaining aesthetically acceptable. Successful reconstruction requires careful preoperative planning and meticulous execution of the appropriate technique.
- Defects of less than one third of the upper lip and one half of the lower lip can be closed primarily. Defects of one third to two thirds of the lip can be closed with an Abbe-Estlander flap or Karapandzic labioplasty. Both techniques require an intact labial artery.
- When the entire lip or surrounding soft tissue or mandibular bone is resected, reconstruction requires a distant flap. The ideal technique uses revascularized fasciocutaneous or osteomyocutaneous composite flaps, which can be done in a single stage for immediate reconstruction.

REFERENCES

1. Gooris PJ, Vermey A, de Visscher JG, et al. Supraomohyoid neck dissection in the management of cervical lymph node metastases of squamous cell carcinoma of the lower lip. *Head Neck* 2002; 24:679–683.

2. Moore SR, Johnson NW, Peirce AM, Wilson DF. The epidemiology of lip cancer. *Oral Dis* 1999;5:185–195.

3. Baker SR, Krause CJ. Carcinoma of the lip. *Laryngoscope* 1980;90: 19–27.

4. Luce EA, Goldberg DP. Oncologic and reconstructive considerations in nonmelanotic skin and lip cancers. *Surg Oncol Clin North Am* 1995;5:751–784.

5. McCombe D, MacGill K, Ainslie J, et al. Squamous cell carcinoma of the lip: a retrospective review of the Peter MacCallum Cancer Institute experience 1979-88. *Aust N Z J Surg* 2000;70: 358–361.

6. Zitsch RP, Park CW, Renner GJ, Rea JL. Outcome analysis for lip carcinoma. *Otolaryngol Head Neck Surg* 1995;113:589–596.

7. Onerci M, Yilmaz T, Gedikoglu G. Tumor thickness as a predictor of cervical lymph node metastasis in squamous cell carcinoma of the lower lip. *Otolaryngol Head Neck Surg* 2000;122:139–142.

8. Vartanian JG, Carvalho AL, Filho M, et al. Predictive factors and distribution of lymph node metastasis in lip cancer patients and their implications on the treatment of the neck. *Oral Oncol* 2004; 40:223–227.

9. Bailey BJ. Management of carcinoma of the lip. *Laryngoscope* 1977;87:250–260.

10. Haagsma EB, Hagens VE, Schaaveld M, et al. Increased cancer risk after liver transplantation: a population based study. *J Hepatol* 2001;34:84–91.

11. Matzko J, Becker DG, Phillips CD. Obliteration of fat planes by perineural spread of squamous cell carcinoma along the inferior alveolar nerve. *AJNR Am J Neuroradiol* 1994;15:1843–1845.

12. de Santana EJ, Rodrigues CB, Consolaro A. Keratoacanthoma versus squamous cell carcinoma of the lower lip. *Ann Dent* 1990; 49:9–130.

13. Cerezo L, Liu FF, Tsang R, et al. Squamous cell carcinoma of the lip: analysis of the Princess Margaret Hospital experience. *Radiother Oncol* 1993;28:142–147.

14. de Visscher JGAM, Botke G, Schakenraad JACM, et al. A comparison of results after radiotherapy and surgery for stage 1 squamous cell carcinoma of the lower lip. *Head Neck* 1999;21:526–530.

15. Veness MJ, Ong C, Cakir B, Morgan G. Squamous cell carcinoma of the lip. Patterns of relapse and outcome: reporting the Westmead Hospital experience, 1980–1997. *Australas Radiol* 2001;45: 195–199.

16. de Visscher JG, Gooris PJ, Verney A, Roodenburg JL. Surgical margins for resection of squamous cell carcinoma of the lower lip. *Int J Oral Maxillofac Surg* 2002;31:154–157.

17. Babington S, Veness MJ, Cakir B, et al. Squamous cell carcinoma of the lip: is there a role for adjuvant radiotherapy in improving local control following incomplete or inadequate excision? *ANZ J Surg* 2003;73:621–625.

18. Mehregan DA, Roenigk RK. Management of superficial squamous cell carcinoma of the lip with Mohs micrographic surgery. *Cancer* 1990;66:463–468.

19. Rowe DE, Carroll RJ, Day CL. Prognostic factors for local recurrence, metastasis, and survival rates in squamous cell carcinoma of the skin, ear and lip. *J Am Acad Dermatol* 1992;26:976–990.

20. Zitsch RP III, Lee BW, Smith RB. Cervical lymph node metastases and squamous cell carcinoma of the lip. *Head Neck* 1999;21: 447–453.

21. Chepeha D, Hoff P, Taylor R, et al. Selective neck dissection for the treatment of neck metastasis from squamous cell carcinoma of the head and neck. *Laryngoscope* 2002;112:434–438.

22. Anderson PE, Warren F, Spiro J, et al. Results of selective neck dissection in management of the node-positive neck. *Arch Otolaryngol Head Neck Surg* 2002;128:1180–1184.

23. Altinyollar H, Berberoglu U, Celen O. Lymphatic mapping and sentinel lymph node biopsy in squamous cell carcinoma of the lower lip. *Eur J Surg Oncol* 2002;28:72–74.

24. Dupin C, Metzinger S, Rizzuto R. Lip reconstruction after ablation for skin malignancies. *Clin Plastic Surg* 2004;31:69–85.

25. Baker SR, Krause CJ. Pedicled flaps in reconstruction of the lip. *Facial Plast Surg* 1983;1:68–69.

26. Renner GJ. Reconstruction of the lip. In: Baker SR, ed. *Local flaps in facial reconstruction.* St. Louis: Mosby, 1995:345–396.

27. Godek CP, Weinzweig J, Bartlett SP. Lip reconstruction following Mohs' surgery, the role for composite resection and primary closure. *Plast Reconstr Surg* 2000;106:798–804.

28. Burget GC, Menick FJ. Aesthetic restoration of one-half of the upper lip. *Plast Reconstr Surg* 1986;78:583–593.

29. Pribaz JJ, Meara JG, Wright S, et al. Lip and vermillion reconstruction with the facial artery musculomucosal flap. *Plast Reconstr Surg* 2000;105:864–872.

30. Webster JP. Crescenteric peri-alar cheek excision for upper lip flap advancement with a short history of upper lip repair. *Plast Reconstr Surg* 1955;16:434–464.

31. Luce EA. Reconstruction of the lower lip. *Clin Plastic Surg* 1995; 22:109–120.

32. Kroll SS. Staged sequential flap reconstruction for large lower lip defects. *Plast Reconstr Surg* 1991;88:620–625.

33. Galyon SW, Frodel JL. Lip and perioral defects. *Otolaryngol Clin North Am* 2001;34:647–664.

34. Kroll SS. Lip reconstruction. In: Kroll SS, ed. *Reconstructive plastic surgery for cancer.* St. Louis: Mosby, 1996:201–209.

35. Chowchuen B, Surakunprapha P. Modified bilateral neurovascular cheek flaps: a new technique for reconstruction of extensive upper lip defects. *Ann Plast Surg* 2001;47:64–69.

36. Sarifakioglu N, Aslan G, Terzloglu A, Ates L. New technique of one-stage reconstruction of a large full-thickness defect in the upper lip: bilateral reverse composite nasolabial flap. *Ann Plast Surg* 2002;49:207–210.

37. Chang KP, Lai CS, Tsai CC, et al. Total upper lip reconstruction with a free temporal scalp flap: long-term follow-up. *Head Neck* 2003;25:602–605.

38. Yotsuyanagi T, Nihei Y, Yokoi K, Sawada Y. Functional reconstruction using a depressor anguli oris musculocutaneous flap for large lower lip defects, especially for elderly patients. *Plast Reconstr Surg* 1999;103:850–855.

39. Rudkin GH, Carlsen BT, Miller TA. Nasolabial flap reconstruction of large defects of the lower lip. *Plast Reconstr Surg* 2003;111: 810–817.

40. Jeng SF, Kuo YR, Wei FC, et al. Total lower lip reconstruction with a composite radial forearm-palmaris longus tendon flap: a clinical series. *Plast Reconstr Surg* 2004;113:19–23.

41. Serletti JM, Tavin ET, Moran SL, Coniglio JU. Total lower lip reconstruction with a sensate composite radial forearm-palmaris longus free flap and a tongue flap. *Plast Reconstr Surg* 1997;99:559–561.

Neoplasms of the Oral Cavity

Mark J. Jameson   *Paul A. Levine*

ANATOMY

The oral cavity is defined as the region that extends from the skin–vermilion junction of the lips to the junction of the hard and soft palate above and to the line of the circumvallate papillae below. This includes the lips, which are discussed in Chapter 110, the buccal mucosa, the upper and lower alveolar ridges, the retromolar trigone, the anterior two thirds of the tongue (oral tongue), the floor of the mouth, and the hard palate. It is divided into two sections by the alveolar ridge and teeth, the external compartment being the vestibule, and the internal compartment, the oral cavity proper.

The tissue layers of the cheek, from deep to superficial, are the mucosa, joined in continuity with the lip; the pharyngobuccal fascia, which is pierced by the parotid duct at the level of the second maxillary molar; the buccinator fat pad; the buccinator muscle; and the subcutaneous tissue and skin (1). Sensation of the cheek is provided by the second and third branches of the trigeminal nerve, and the buccinator muscle is innervated by the facial nerve (2). The lymphatics drain into the parotid compartment and level II of the neck. No finite bony or fascial planes inhibit the spread of disease.

The hard palate separates the anterior nasal vault from the oral cavity and forms the roof of the mouth. It is formed from the primary palate (the palatine process of the maxilla) and the horizontal plate of the palatine bone. The mucosa and periosteum of the hard palate are tightly adherent. The greater and lesser palatine foramina, located at the posterior and lateral junction of the hard and soft palate, convey the greater and lesser palatine vessels and nerves. The greater palatine artery anastomoses anteriorly with the nasopalatine artery (from the posterior septal branch of the sphenopalatine artery) at the incisive foramen, which lies posterior to the maxillary incisors and also conveys the nasopalatine nerve. These foramina provide potential routes for direct tumor spread from the hard palate anteriorly into the nasal cavity or posteriorly via the pterygopalatine fossa to the skull base or both. Lymphatic drainage from the posterior hard palate is to level II or retropharyngeal lymph nodes or both; the primary palate drains to level IB nodes.

V_2 provides the sensory innervation to the teeth and gingival surface of the upper alveolus via the anterior, middle, and posterior superior alveolar nerves and to the lingual surface of the upper alveolus and hard palate by the greater palatine and nasopalatine nerves. Blood is supplied to the superior alveolar ridge by the superior alveolar, nasopalatine, and greater palatine arteries, all derived from the internal maxillary system. Lymphatic drainage from the buccal superior and inferior alveolar ridges is to level IA and IB lymph nodes. Both lingual aspects drain to level II and lateral retropharyngeal nodes.

The retromolar trigone is a triangular region whose base extends across the posterior mandibular alveolus from the distal surface of the last molar and whose apex is at the maxillary tuberosity. The lateral limit of the triangle extends obliquely superiorly and laterally to the coronoid process. The medial limb blends with the anterior tonsillar pillar. Because the mucosa here is tightly adherent to the ascending ramus of the mandible, carcinoma often invades the mandibular periosteum. Referred otalgia results from innervation by V_3, the lesser palatine nerve, and the glossopharyngeal nerve. Blood is supplied by the tonsillar and ascending palatine branches of the facial artery with contributions from the dorsal lingual, ascending pharyngeal, and lesser palatine arteries (Fig. 111.1A and B). Most of the lymphatic drainage is to level II.

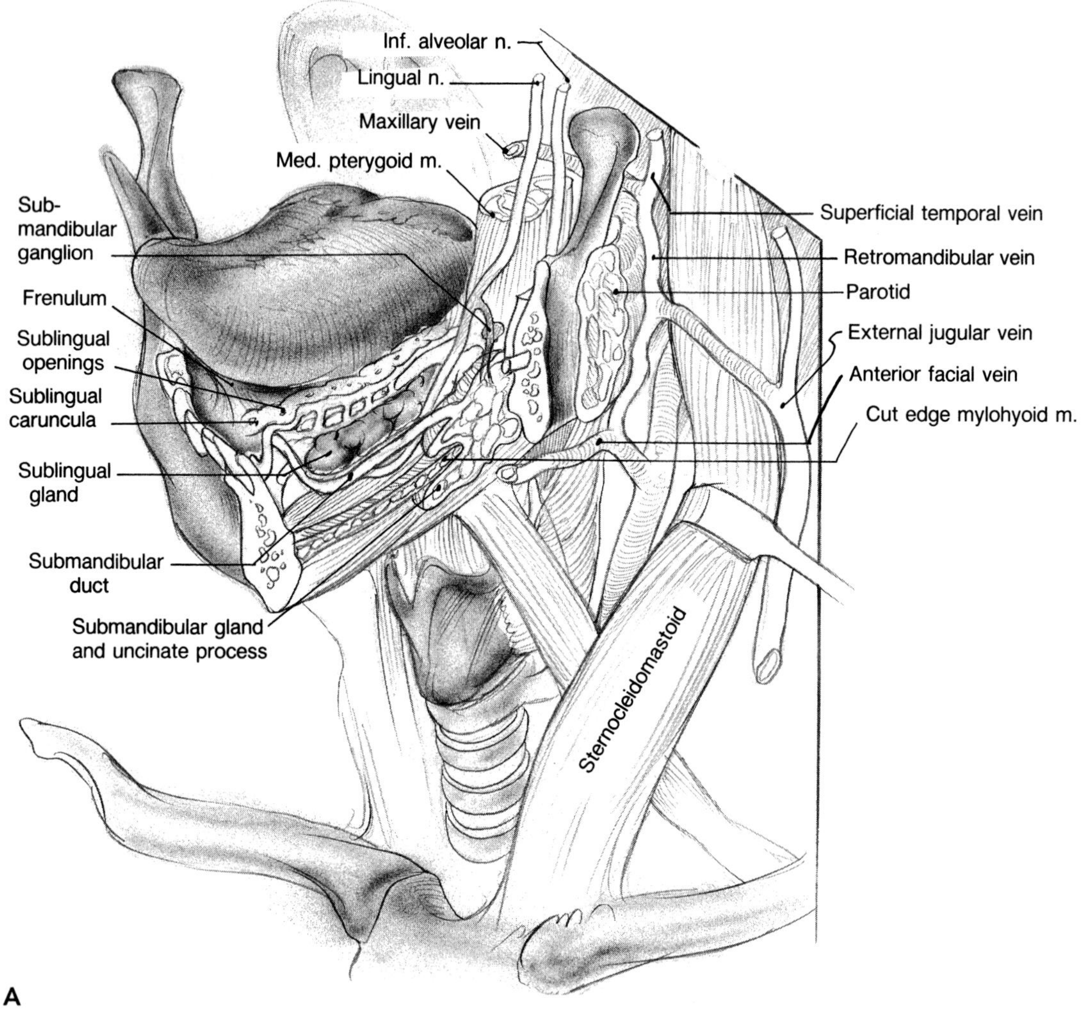

Inf. alveolar n.
Lingual n.
Maxillary vein
Med. pterygoid m.
Sub-
mandibular
ganglion
Frenulum
Sublingual
openings
Sublingual
caruncula
Sublingual
gland
Submandibular
duct
Submandibular gland
and uncinate process
Superficial temporal vein
Retromandibular vein
Parotid
External jugular vein
Anterior facial vein
Cut edge mylohyoid m.
Sternocleidomastoid

A

Figure 111.1   A: Superficial anatomic landmarks and structure of the oral cavity.
B: Deep atomic structures of the oral cavity.

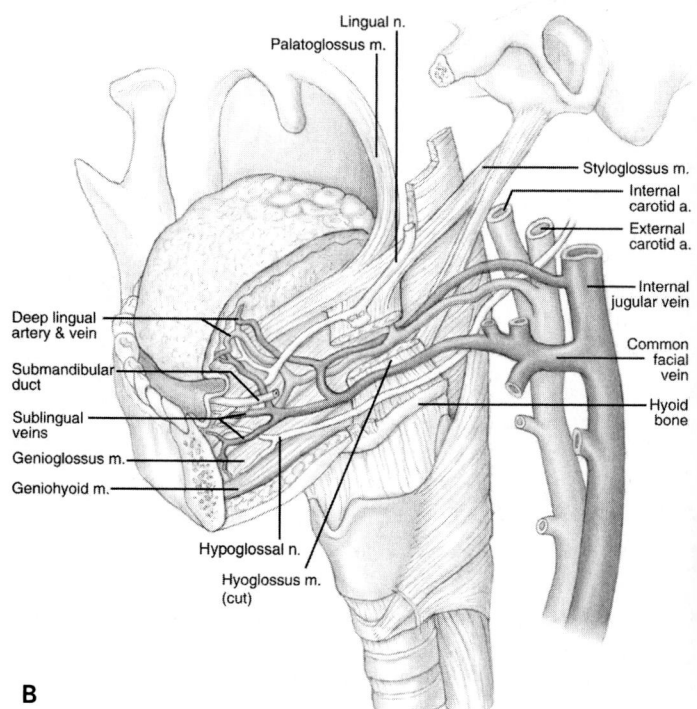

Lingual n.
Palatoglossus m.
Styloglossus m.
Internal carotid a.
External carotid a.
Internal jugular vein
Common facial vein
Hyoid bone
Deep lingual artery & vein
Submandibular duct
Sublingual veins
Genioglossus m.
Geniohyoid m.
Hypoglossal n.
Hyoglossus m. (cut)

B

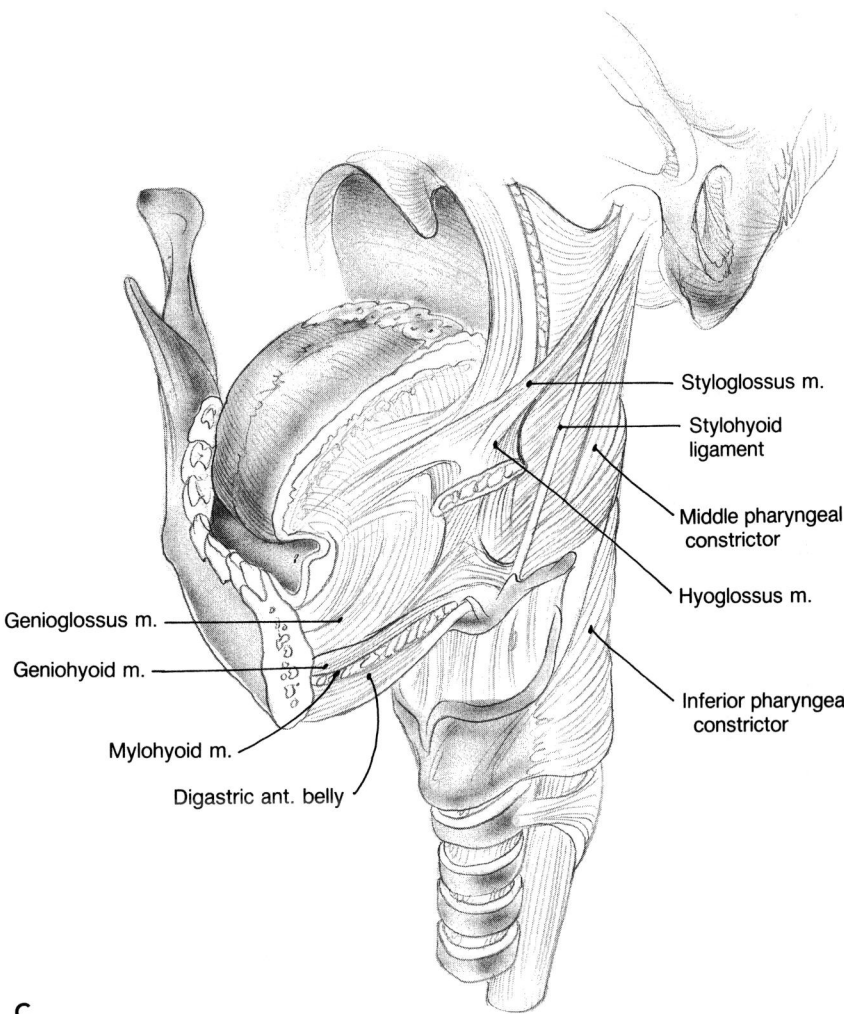

Styloglossus m.

Stylohyoid
ligament

Middle pharyngeal
constrictor

Hyoglossus m.

Inferior pharyngeal
constrictor

Genioglossus m.

Geniohyoid m.

Mylohyoid m.

Digastric ant. belly

Figure 111.1 (continued) C: Musculature
of the oral cavity.

C

The sulcus terminalis divides the tongue into an anterior
two thirds and posterior one third (3). The anterior (mobile) tongue is part of the oral cavity, and the posterior
third (base) a part of the oropharynx. The anterior ectoderm is derived from the lateral lingual swellings of the first
branchial arch, explaining the lingual nerve (V_3) sensory
innervation. The musculature of both the oral tongue and
base of the tongue is derived from the occipital myotomes
and served by the hypoglossal nerve (XII). The external
muscles of the tongue are formed by three paired groups:
the hyoglossus, styloglossus, and genioglossus. These muscles act with the intrinsic tongue musculature to assist with
articulation and deglutition. The styloglossus pulls the
tongue up and back, whereas the hyoglossus flattens it by
pulling toward the hyoid, propelling the food bolus from
the oral cavity into the oropharynx. The genioglossus pulls
the tongue forward (Figs. 111.1C and 111.2) (2,3).

Most of the tongue bulk is composed of the transverse
and vertical musculature. The motor innervation of the
tongue is the hypoglossal nerve (XII), whereas the lingual
nerve (V_3), carrying taste fibers from the chorda tympani

nerve, provides sensation for the oral tongue. Because V_3
also serves the external ear, external auditory canal, and
tympanic membrane, otalgia is often the presenting symptom for tongue cancers. The lingual artery supplies blood
to the tongue. Lymph from the tip of the tongue drains to
level IA nodes, whereas lymph from the lateral two thirds
of the tongue drains to level IB and level II nodes. The medial tongue drains directly to level III nodes (2,3). Although the tip and midline portion of the tongue, like the
tongue base, have bilateral lymphatic drainage, the lateral
aspect of the oral tongue drains to ipsilateral nodes only.

The floor of the mouth is situated between the
mandibular alveolus and the oral tongue, extending posteriorly to the anterior tonsillar pillar. It is pierced by Wharton (submandibular gland) duct orifices on either side of
the lingual frenulum. The paired sublingual glands sit on
the mylohyoid muscle between the mandible and the hyoglossus. The lingual artery supplies blood to the floor of
the mouth, and V_3 provides its innervation. A superficial
lymphatic plexus drains to both the ipsilateral and contralateral nodes, whereas the deep system drains ipsilaterally

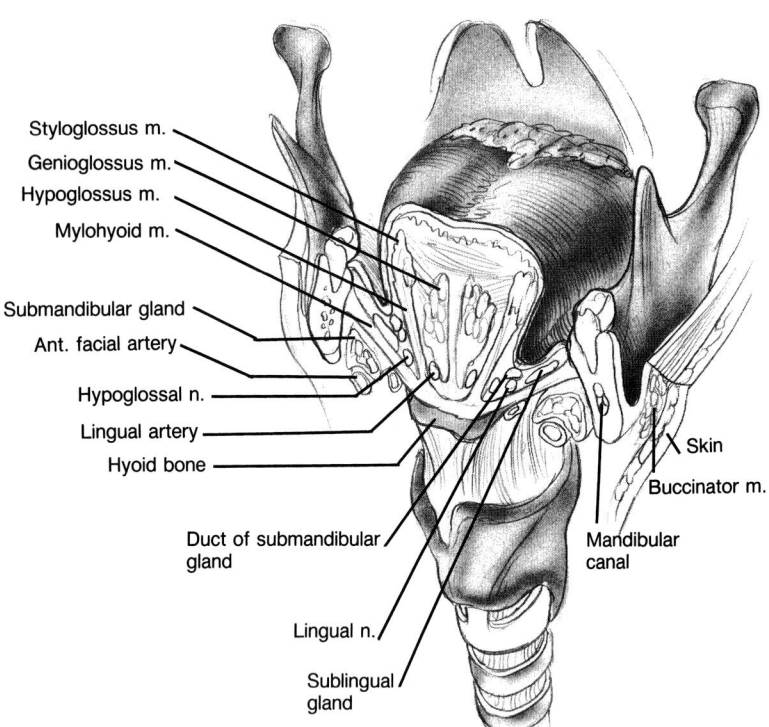

Styloglossus m.
Genioglossus m.
Hypoglossus m.
Mylohyoid m.

Submandibular gland
Ant. facial artery

Hypoglossal n.
Lingual artery
Hyoid bone

Duct of submandibular gland

Skin
Buccinator m.

Mandibular canal

Lingual n.

Sublingual gland

Figure 111.2 Intrinsic muscles of the tongue.

only. Posterior floor of mouth lymphatics drain to ipsilateral level II nodes (Fig. 111.3) (3).

EPIDEMIOLOGY AND ETIOLOGY

Although oral cavity malignancy is directly related to excessive alcohol ingestion and the use of tobacco, incidence varies significantly based on gender, geography, and ethnic differences. One constant, however, is that 95% of the malignancies of the oral cavity are squamous cell carcinoma.

According to the most recent statistics from the National Cancer Institute spanning 1997 to 2001, oral cancers had an incidence of 6.0 per 100,000 Americans, with a male-to-female ratio of 2.2:1 (4). This represents 1.6% and 0.9% of all new cancers in males and females, respectively, in this time frame. The mortality rate from oral cavity cancers was 1.6 per 100,000 or 0.6% of all cancer-related mortality. Whereas overall 5-year survival from lip cancers between 1995 and 2000 was 93%, the remainder of the oral cavity subsites had a survival of 51% to 58% (4). At the time of diagnosis, 95% of patients are older than 40 years; the average age is approximately 60 years.

Fortunately, both incidence and mortality rates are on the decline, albeit slowly. When combined with pharyngeal and salivary gland cancers, the overall incidence declined, on average, 0.5% per year from 1975 to 1993 and 2.3% per year from 1993 to 2001. Although incidence in females increased by 2.6% per year from 1975 to 1980, it has decreased 1.0% per year from 1980 to 2001. As anticipated,

based on the declining incidence, mortality rates decreased by 1.5% and 2.5% per year from 1975 to 1991 and 1991 to 2001, respectively. Unfortunately, 5-year survival rates have improved only slightly, from 53.5% in 1974 to 1994 to 58.7% in 1995 to 2000, and, whereas incidence the African-American population is similar to that of the white population, survival in the same group was only 39.0% in 1995 to 2000 (4).

Epidemiologic studies have demonstrated that the risk of developing oral cancer increases with tobacco use in a dose-dependent fashion and that alcohol use is synergistic in terms of cancer risk (5). It also was shown that, with continued smoking, patients cured of their first primary carcinoma have a 40% chance of developing either recurrence or a second head and neck cancer developing or of recurrence. It takes up to 20 years of tobacco-free existence for a reformed smoker to have the same probability of developing an oral cancer as a nonsmoker (5). It is interesting that 75% of the cases of squamous cell carcinoma of the oral cavity involve only 10% of the mucosal surfaces of the mouth. This area extends from the anterior floor of the mouth along the gingivobuccal sulcus and lateral border of the tongue to the retromolar trigone and the anterior tonsillar pillar. It has been postulated that this is due to the flow and pooling of carcinogen-contaminated saliva in these areas. This is supported by the association of snuff dipping and tobacco chewing with development of squamous cell carcinoma in areas where consistent and repeated contact with the oral mucosa has occurred (6).

Emerging evidence suggests that the human papillomavirus (HPV) may play a role in the etiology of oral cavity

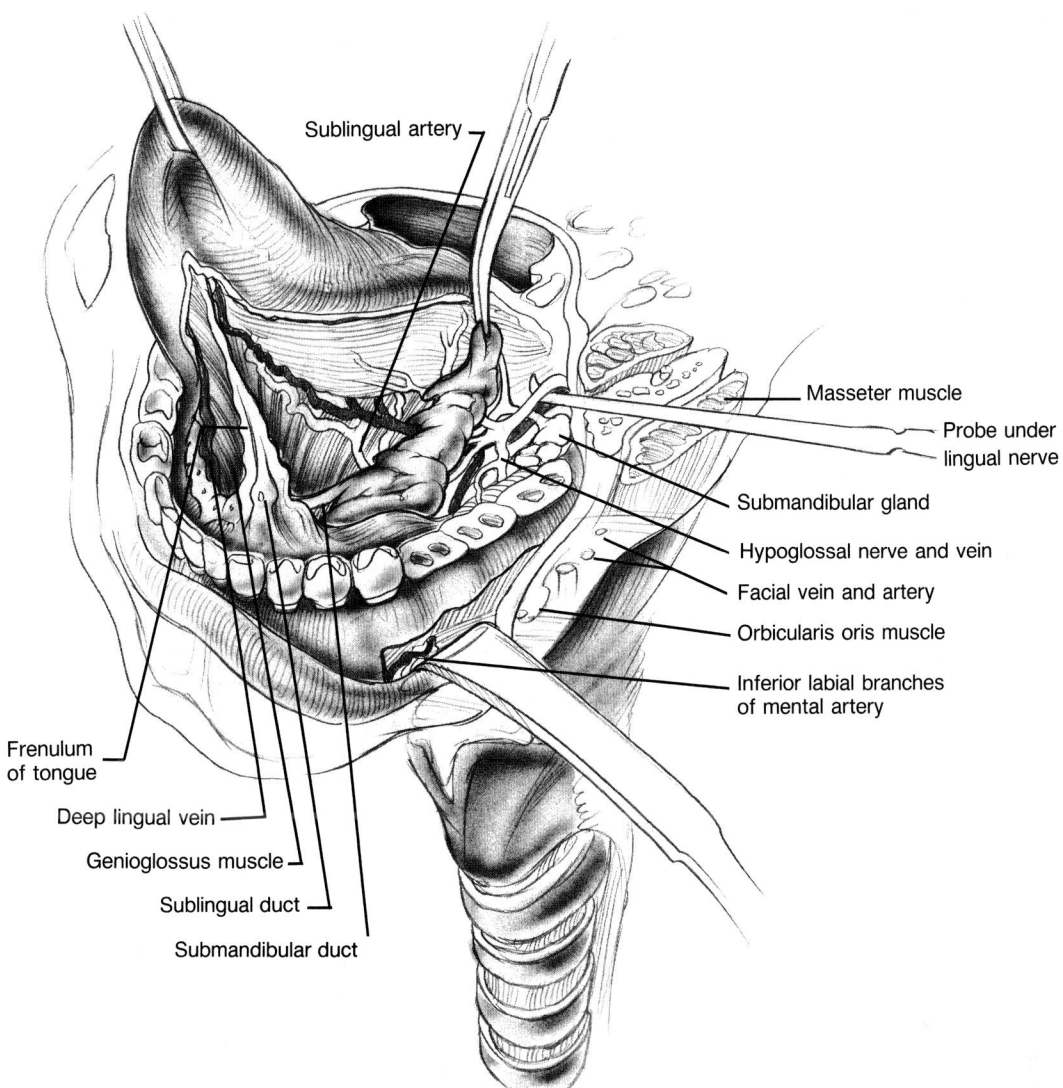

Figure 111.3 Floor of the mouth.

squamous cell carcinoma. HPV has been isolated in oral squamous cell carcinoma and, to a lesser extent, in premalignant lesions of the oral cavity (7). HPV type 16 is most common, estimated to be present in up to 15% to 25% of head and neck squamous cell carcinomas (8). HPV-positive tumors are seen in younger patients with limited or no tobacco and alcohol use, and although they tend to exhibit poor differentiation and appear at a more advanced stage, they have a better overall survival rate, likely because of their increased radiosensitivity (8). This may ultimately represent a unique subset of oral cavity cancers.

The incidence of oral cavity cancer also varies according to ethnic practices. Women in India who practice the reverse smoking of cigars, holding the burning end in the mouth and puffing continuously, have an incidence of hard palate cancer 47 times higher than that of nonsmoking women. In addition, the practice of tobacco and betelnut chewing in Asia is thought to be the reason that more than 25% of all cancers in India, Hong Kong, Taiwan, and Vietnam occur in the oral cavity. In some regions, over 50% of all cancers occur in the mouth (6).

In studies controlled for smoking, a direct relationship has been found between excessive alcohol consumption and oral cavity cancer. In American men, the synergistic effect of alcohol and nicotine increases the cancer risk 2.5-fold over the additive risk of these two habits. Because alcohol is an irritant, the theory is that repeated contact with the oral mucosa causes a chemical burn, increasing cell membrane permeability and increasing absorption of the carcinogens dissolved in alcohol. Although poor dentition and repeated mechanical irritation due to, for example, poorly fitting dentures, have been implicated as a cause of oral cancer, no conclusions concerning this relationship have been proven, nor have any correlations been conclusively found between oral cancer and nutritional deficiencies, viruses, or fungi (6).

EVALUATION AND DIAGNOSIS

Pretreatment Evaluation

Table 111.1 outlines steps in the pretreatment evaluation of neoplasms of the oral cavity, and Table 111.2 outlines steps for diagnosis. Unlike malignancies in other regions of the head and neck, such as the base of the tongue, nasopharynx, and hypopharynx, oral cavity malignancies, in general, are easily visible. Therefore it is somewhat surprising that these lesions tend to be seen initially at a greater, rather than a lesser, stage. All the standard telltale signs of head and neck malignancies apply to oral cavity cancers, including otalgia, odynophagia, bleeding, and dysphagia. These complaints may be present along with the patient's concern for inexplicable loss of teeth, oral discomfort, reduced movement of oral structures, and, if the tumor is advanced, trismus. Once a high degree of suspicion has been established and a full head and neck examination performed, a simple biopsy may be performed under local anesthesia, as long as the risk of excessive bleeding or significant tissue distortion is low. Beyond this, the physician's most important functions are to stage the full extent of the disease, rule

TABLE 111.1

PRETREATMENT EVALUATION OF NEOPLASMS OF THE ORAL CAVITY

Complete history and physical examination
  Biopsy of primary—either in office or when examined under anesthesia
  Fine-needle aspirate of possible neck metastasis—in selected cases only (open incisional/excisional biopsy not indicated)

Imaging studies
  Chest radiograph—posteroanterior and lateral
  CT/MRI of primary and neck
  Panorex or dental x-ray—to evaluate mandible invasion, if CT/MRI not performed
  Barium swallow—physician discretion

Laboratory tests
  Preanesthesia testing (per institutional guidelines)
  Baseline liver function tests

Consultations
  Radiation therapy—for adjuvant or definitive therapy considerations
  Dental—preradiation dental treatment and posttherapy cases

Optional
  Speech pathology
  Internal medicine
  Anesthesiology

Examination under anesthesia
  Direct laryngoscopy and pharyngoscopy
  Esophagoscopy
  Bronchoscopy—if indicated by chest x-ray or clinical examination
  Palpation of tongue and oro/nasopharynx

CT, computed tomography; MRI, magnetic resonance imaging.

TABLE 111.2   DIAGNOSIS

NEOPLASMS OF THE ORAL CAVITY

Complete head and neck examination
Chest x-ray and liver function tests plus additional laboratory tests dictated by patient's medical history
CT/MRI for extent of primary and possible cervical nodal evaluation
Dental evaluation
Radiotherapy evaluation
Staging endoscopy and biopsy

CT, computed tomography; MRI, magnetic resonance imaging.

out a second primary carcinoma, and evaluate the patient for any possible distant metastatic disease.

Radiologic evaluation by computed tomography (CT) or magnetic resonance imaging (MRI) is usually valuable. This must be performed before the staging endoscopy to avoid being misled by surgically induced edema of surrounding tissues. Because the mandible and its enveloping periosteum provide the only natural barrier to the spread of local disease, these studies can show the extent of disease not appreciated by physical examination. The first question, therefore, is which examination best reveals mandibular invasion?

The standard mandible series is of value only when gross transcortical tumor invasion exists, which is often appreciated on physical examination. Although Panorex images are considered superior to the standard mandible series because of excellent imaging of the mandibular body, ramus, and condyle, the symphyseal and parasymphyseal regions are poorly imaged because of spine artifact, and again, extensive bone loss is necessary to identify the lesion (9). In this setting, bone scans have been shown to be overly sensitive; periosteal inflammation due to disease proximity is represented as a suspect or positive region on the scan (9).

High-resolution CT has been the most valuable in this regard, and the recent use of CT DentaScan technology has further enhanced the anatomic detail provided by CT (9). It has been shown, however, that MRI has the same sensitivity for demonstrating cortical bone involvement, although it may not be as readily recognized by the less-skilled observer (10). In addition, MRI has been shown to be superior to contrast-enhanced high-resolution CT for evaluation of the extent of soft-tissue involvement of the tongue and the floor of the mouth, especially when using gadolinium-enhanced T_1-weighted images (11) (Fig. 111.4). Whatever technique is used, subtleties may be difficult to evaluate, especially in the face of recent previous therapy.

Imaging studies also are useful in the staging of cervical disease, especially when no palpable adenopathy is noted. Although a thorough physical examination is mandatory, combination with CT has been shown to be both more sensitive and accurate when compared with physical

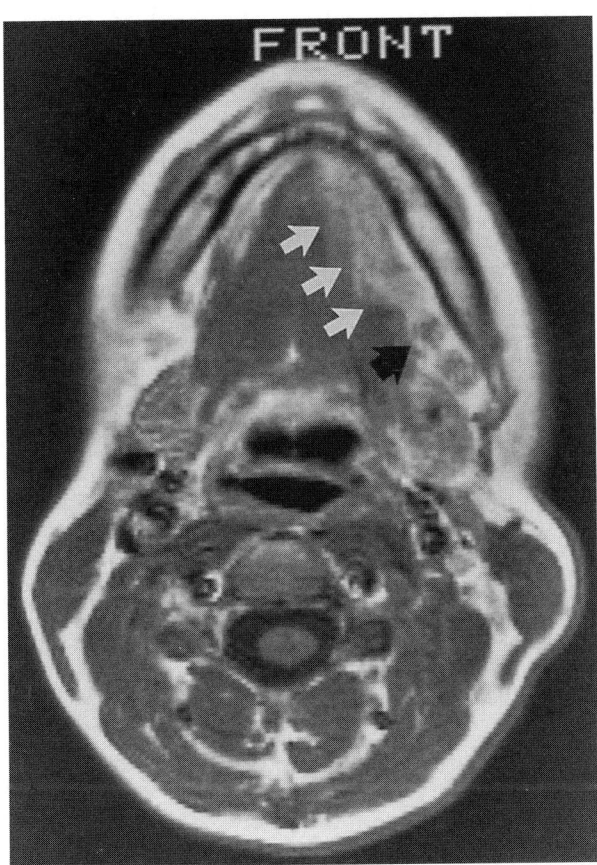

Figure 111.4 Gadolinium diethylenetriamine pentaacetic acid (Gd-DPTA)-enhanced T1 magnetic resonance image of a patient with squamous cell carcinoma of the floor of the mouth. Magnetic resonance imaging shows tumor infiltrating into the mylohyoid muscle (*white arrows*) and differentiates the infiltrated muscle from the normal muscle (*black arrow*)

than 50% (12–14). Some authors have advocated chest CT for all new head and neck cancer patients simultaneous with the CT evaluation of their primary lesion. With newer scanners, no additional contrast is required, and additional time and radiation dose are minimal (13,14). Typical chest CT protocols also adequately image the liver and will identify the vast majority of metastatic disease, potentially avoiding major surgical intervention in a subset of patients with otherwise undetected metastatic disease. However, the cost of scanning every new patient is substantial, especially when the many false positives are considered, which require further imaging, unnecessary biopsies, and potentially delayed treatment of the primary lesion. Given these concerns, an effort has been made to identify patients who are at higher risk for distant metastasis so that an aggressive imaging approach may be taken with these patients (12,13). To date, these parameters have not been fully defined.

Other imaging modalities, such as positron emission tomography (PET), may serve to evaluate, effectively and simultaneously, regional nodal disease, metastatic disease, and second primary lesions, and recent studies have shown some promise for oral cavity neoplasms (15). However, most study sizes now are small, interpretation is subjective and nonstandardized, and no clear advantage has been demonstrated over the imaging protocols described earlier.

Staging

Table 111.3 lists the criteria for clinical classification of histologically confirmed squamous cell carcinoma of the oral cavity, according to the American Joint Committee on Cancer (16).

Differential Diagnosis

As in all other regions of the head and neck, most malignancies of the oral cavity are squamous cell carcinoma. In conjunction with a strong history of tobacco and alcohol use, the presentation is either as an exophytic lesion or a nonhealing ulcer that may exhibit significant infiltrative submucosal extension by palpation. Although few other neoplasms can be mistaken for squamous carcinoma in patients with the associated history, less common neoplasms of the oral cavity also should be considered.

One benign lesion that can be mistaken by the less experienced pathologist for a well-differentiated carcinoma is the granular cell myoblastoma. This error can be made, especially in small biopsies of the lesion, because of squamous proliferation on the lesion surface and because they can show local invasion into adjacent tissue. Clinically, a neoplasm in the tongue that is not initially seen on the lateral border should be suspect for a non–squamous cell lesion.

The next group of uncommon neoplasms contains those of minor salivary gland origin; adenoid cystic carcinoma is probably the most common, but adenocarcinoma

examination alone, with a combined detection rate of greater than 90%. Criteria for determining nodal positivity, however, vary from institution to institution. At the University of Virginia, metastatic nodes must have a short-axis diameter of at least 11 mm for the jugulodigastric region and at least 10 mm for all other locations. Other evidence for positive nodal disease includes central necrosis, rim enhancement, and extracapsular spread. MRI has not been shown to be superior to CT in the evaluation of cervical disease and is significantly more expensive.

In conjunction with the endoscopic staging process, which evaluates the primary lesion and the regional nodes and rules out a regional second primary, an evaluation for distant metastatic disease and a distant second primary cancer must be performed. At present, chest radiographs and laboratory studies (including liver-function tests, alkaline phosphates, and serum calcium) are in common use to evaluate for potential lung, liver, or bone metastases or a combination of these. Patients with abnormal findings proceed to chest CT, abdominal ultrasound or CT, or bone scan as appropriate. However, recent studies have demonstrated the poor sensitivity of these screening tests, generally less

TABLE 111.3

CLINICAL CLASSIFICATION OF SQUAMOUS CELL CARCINOMA OF THE ORAL CAVITY

Primary Tumor (T)	Regional Lymph Nodes (N)	Distant Metastasis (M)

Primary Tumor (T)

Tx   Unassessable
T0   No evidence of primary tumor
Tis Carcinoma in situ
T1   Tumor 2 cm or less
T2   Tumor >2 cm but not >4 cm
T3   Tumor >4 cm
T4a Tumor invades adjacent structures (through cortical bone, into deep tongue musculature, maxillary sinus, skin)[a]
T4b Tumor invades masticator space, pterygoid plates, or skull base, and/or encases internal carotid artery

Regional Lymph Nodes (N)

NX   Unassessable
N0   No regional lymph node metastasis
N1   Single ipsilateral lymph node, 3 cm or less

N2a Single ipsilateral lymph node >3 cm but not >6 cm
N2b Multiple ipsilateral lymph nodes, none >6 cm
N2c Bilateral or contralateral lymph nodes, none >6 cm
N3   Any lymph node >6 cm

Distant Metastasis (M)

MX   Unassessable
M0   No distant metastasis
M1   Distant metastasis

Stage Grouping

M0	T1	T2	T3	T4a	T4b
N0	I	II	III	IVA	IVB
N1	III	III	III	IVA	IVB
N2	IVA	IVA	IVA	IVA	IVB
N3	IVB	IVB	IVB	IVB	IVB

All M1	IVC

[a]Superficial erosion alone of bone/tooth socket by gingival primary is not sufficient to classify a tumor as T4.

and mucoepidermoid carcinoma also can appear in this region. Because of the various mesenchymal elements in this region, sarcomas also may be present in the oral cavity. All, including rhabdomyosarcoma and liposarcoma, can be found, but because of the paucity of smooth muscle in the mouth, leiomyosarcoma is rare. Malignant fibrous histiocytoma is a rare oral cavity soft-tissue neoplasm with a poor 5-year survival rate, and the various fibromatoses can mimic low-grade sarcomas because of the associated mandibular resorption and a recurrence rate of greater than 20%. Unlike head and neck carcinomas, they occur in men younger than 30 years. In addition, both Hodgkin and non-Hodgkin lymphomas can be present in the oral cavity, as can malignant melanoma. Because of the voracity of melanoma of mucosal-lined surfaces and the lack of generalized pigmentation in the oral cavity, any pigmented lesion in a white patient, no matter how benign it appears, should be sampled for biopsy.

In this age of acquired immunodeficiency syndrome and its related diseases, it would be incomplete not to mention hairy leukoplakia of the oral cavity and Kaposi sarcoma, although neither is found in the typical head and neck patient. Kaposi sarcoma, non-Hodgkin lymphoma,

and squamous cell carcinoma, especially of the tongue, are now recognized as being prevalent in human immunodeficiency virus (HIV)-infected patients. In addition, the so-called hairy cell leukoplakia is in fact a white oral cavity lesion found to be secondary to the Epstein–Barr virus in HIV-positive patients, and it is uniquely localized to the lateral tongue border.

Precancerous Lesions and Prevention

Although leukoplakia is the most commonly noted premalignant lesion, erythroplasia carries the greater risk of malignancy. Leukoplakia is named by its "white plaque" appearance, but microscopically, it shows hyperkeratosis and dysplasia. The etiology of leukoplakia is likely related to tobacco use or repeated trauma, but the true relation between them is unclear. This is because not all leukoplakia disappears after cessation of the irritating agent; some leukoplakias that are monitored over a period of time will develop malignant changes. In addition, it has been observed that the malignant transformation rate of leukoplakia in non–tobacco users is significantly greater than that of tobacco users. Lesions with a red component are more likely to undergo malignant transformation than is uniformly white leukoplakia.

Because of the malignant potential, all white and red mucosal lesions of the oral cavity require biopsy for microscopic examination. If the lesion is benign leukoplakia and does not disappear after tobacco cessation, treatment is unclear. Surgical excision, laser excision, and similar techniques have all been used with some degree of success. Nonsurgical approaches, such as topical vitamin A therapy, also have been tried, with complete response rates in the 10% to 27% range and partial response rates in 54% to 90% of patients. The side effects were minimal, but leukoplakia recurred in 50% of patients after discontinuation of the medication (17).

MANAGEMENT

Prognostic Factors

In general, the cure rate for oral cavity lesions, except for small T1 lesions, tends not to meet the expectations of those providing the care. Although it is true that the greater the stage of the lesion, the worse the prognosis and survival, other prognostic indicators besides the size of the lesion and the extent of nodal disease may affect survival.

It is now clear that increasing tumor thickness has a significant correlation with occult nodal disease and worsening prognosis. Some debate remains about the appropriate "cutoff" thickness after which to place patients in a higher risk group and recommend elective treatment of the N0 neck. A recent report by Lim et al. (18) indicates that a tumor thickness of more than 4 mm for T1–2N0 oral tongue cancers with untreated necks is an independent predictor of late cervical metastasis, the strongest predictor of overall survival. In a large study of T1–T2 cancers in all subsites of the oral cavity, O'Brien et al. found a significant change in prognosis for tumors 4 mm thick or greater, with local control, nodal disease, and survival rates changing from 91%, 8%, and 100%, respectively, to 84%, 48%, and 74% as tumor thickness increased beyond this cutoff (19). Although several different thresholds have been proposed (19) and an absolute consensus has not been reached, the significance of tumor thickness in the oral cavity is clear, and the present data seem to support elective treatment of N0 necks for primary tumors 4 mm or more in thickness in paraffin-fixed specimens. Use of ultrasound or MRI has been proposed for preoperative assessment of tumor thickness. At present, preliminary reports support a correlation between MRI- and histology-based assessments of tumor thickness for oral tongue cancers (20).

As with other neoplasms, perineural, vascular, and lymphatic invasion bode poorly; they have been shown to predict increased risk of locoregional failure and decreased survival (21). In addition, DNA ploidy status may play a role, with aneuploid tumors conveying a worse prognosis

(22). More recently, increasing research has occurred in the field of oncogene expression in head and neck tumors. In particular, overexpression of c-erbB-2 has shown correlation with nodal disease and metastasis and worsened survival (23).

The type of squamous cell carcinoma that bears a better prognosis is verrucous carcinoma. Grossly, this is a bulky, warty lesion that occurs in older patients who chew tobacco or have poorly fitting dentures, and its diagnosis is best made by providing an accurate clinical description to the pathologist. Its behavior is relatively indolent; it tends not to metastasize, and the advancing edge appears to push the surrounding tissue rather than invade it.

Radiation Therapy

In general, radiation therapy and surgery have equal success in controlling T1 lesions of the oral cavity. Treatment options must be determined by numerous factors, including the location, the patient's physical condition and social and economic situation, and the experience of those delivering the care. Radiation therapy tends to provide a better functional result with superior speech and swallowing, but significant disadvantages of radiation therapy are diminution of taste, xerostomia, and the protracted nature of the treatment course. Unlike surgery, a curative dosage of radiation therapy requires at least 6 weeks of treatment, and this can affect the treatment choice. When considering oral cavity cancers, the highest rate of complications related to external beam radiation occurs in patients with floor-of-mouth cancer; historically, in one fourth or more of these patients, osteoradionecrosis of the mandible developed. Newer techniques such as brachytherapy and intensity-modulated radiation therapy (IMRT) allow more focused targeting and reduced complications; the possibility of treating a second primary with radiation therapy also exists with these approaches (24).

For patients requiring combined therapy, preoperative radiation therapy has not been shown to improve locoregional control compared with postoperative radiation treatment. Despite the theoretic advantages of delivering radiation preoperatively, most surgeons prefer to administer it after surgery because of the potential for improved wound healing. The first and the only large randomized study comparing these issues showed no significant difference with respect to overall survival, disease-free survival, and surgical complications (25).

Chemotherapy

Although the combination of radiation therapy and surgery provides a better chance for cure for stage III and IV disease than does either modality alone, substantial evidence suggests that the addition of concomitant chemotherapy to postoperative radiation therapy improves locoregional control and survival in these patients (26,27). Unfortunately, these studies tend to include all subsites of the head and neck, with oral cavity cancers typically representing only 15% to 25%; the results have not been stratified to demonstrate survival differences based on tumor location. Studies more focused on oral cavity primaries have, in general, been much smaller and less well controlled so that their implications for patient management are limited at best.

N0 Neck

The final general management concept is whether to irradiate an N0 neck prophylactically or, more generally, whether to be concerned with potential metastatic disease in the N0 neck. For early-stage oral cavity primary lesions, the rate of occult neck metastasis ranges from 20% to 30%. Thus these primaries require treatment of the neck, either with lymphadenectomy or radiation; this selection is often based on the choice of treatment modality for the primary lesion. With primaries that are more easily treated with radiation than with surgery, the radiation field can be expanded to treat the neck(s) simultaneously. When surgical excision of the oral-cavity primary is most appropriate, simultaneous surgical management of the neck is often most expedient. For the N0 neck, supraomohyoid neck dissection (SOHND), which removes nodes from levels I, II, and III, has been demonstrated to be appropriate (28). At many institutions, a SOHND is performed for essentially all T2 lesions and many T1 and T3 lesions, when prognostic factors warrant its use (e.g., T1 primary more than 1-cm diameter or more than 4 mm thick). If one or more positive nodes or extracapsular spread or both are detected in the lymphadenectomy specimen, patients proceed to postoperative radiation therapy. This approach reduces morbidity compared with modified radical neck dissection (MRND), but still results in a large number of unnecessary neck dissections. Byers et al. (29) raised the possibility of "skip metastases" for oral tongue cancers—occult level IV metastases that would not be addressed by a SOHND. However, this concept has been refuted by multiple studies including those of Khafif et al. (30), who demonstrated the rate of metastasis to undissected level IV was only 2% in T1–3 N0 oral tongue cancers. They also found that the rate of recurrence in the neck was not increased if level IV was only dissected when there was intraoperative suspicion of metastasis in levels II or III (30).

Thus management of the N0 neck with a T1 oral-cavity primary remains controversial. Although it has not been determined which T1 lesions are the most worrisome, it has been shown in a retrospective analysis at the University of Virginia that elective total neck irradiation provided a 95% neck control rate compared with a 38% control rate for T1 oral tongue primaries 1 cm or greater in diameter not treated with prophylactic neck irradiation (31). Given the present lack of ability to identify which primaries are most likely to metastasize, some surgeons now advocate

the use of sentinel lymph node biopsy (SLNB) to select which patients will require more extensive lymphadenectomy. The procedure involves less morbidity than neck dissection, but the question of its accuracy has not been unequivocally answered. SLNB has been validated and accepted as a useful and accurate method for lymph node staging in cutaneous melanoma and, more recently, in the management of breast cancer. A recent report by Ross et al. (32) includes a large number of SLNBs performed at multiple different centers. Their results support the viewpoint that SLNB may be useful in detecting occult neck disease; sensitivity was generally very high but was as low as 80% for floor of mouth cancers. Unfortunately, in more than half of the patients studied, SLNB was performed alone and could not be correlated with elective neck dissection. Ultimately, SLNB may prove to be an effective approach to assessment of the N0 neck, but, at present, it still requires further validation. At the time of this writing, a multiinstitutional trial is under way in the United States to address this issue.

Reconstruction

The challenge of surgery for malignancies of the oral cavity is to perform an adequate resection and then to provide the best functional reconstruction. Because of the advances in reconstruction with myocutaneous and, more recently, microvascular flaps, the choices are now more numerous, and, with appropriate selection, excellent functional results can be achieved.

Split-thickness skin grafts remain the mainstay for resurfacing small, superficial defects of the oral cavity. Full-thickness skin grafts are not widely used, and mucosal grafts of significant size would provide morbidity from the graft site, such as fibrosis with associated trismus. Tongue flaps provide readily accessible well-vascularized tissue but cause significant functional morbidity, making their use more historic than practical. The pectoralis major myocutaneous flap has been the workhorse flap for the head and neck surgeon, replacing the deltopectoral flap in this capacity because of its more durable blood supply (thoracoacromial artery vs. perforators from the internal mammary artery), more manageable residual defect (primary closure vs. split-thickness skin graft), and greater thickness. Deltopectoral flaps are now used predominantly for large skin-surface coverage, whereas pectoralis major flaps provide excellent soft tissue for large floor-of-mouth and tongue resections. If the flap is too thick, usually secondary to subcutaneous fat, the skin and fat may be discarded, and the surface can epithelialize either by secondary intention or by placement of a split-thickness skin graft.

Although the pectoralis major flap is adequate for large soft-tissue defects not involving bone, myocutaneous or osteomyocutaneous free flaps are now the reconstructive methods of choice for many oral cavity defects, particularly those that require thinner more malleable tissue or

TABLE 111.4 ℞

TREATMENT AND POSTTREATMENT FOLLOW-UP NEOPLASMS OF THE ORAL CAVITY

Surgery
  Primary—resection with adequate margins; frozen section as
    needed
    Tracheostomy as needed
    Feeding tube optional
    Surgical orientation of specimen for pathologist
  Neck—modified/radical dissection for unilateral metastatic
    disease and bilateral dissections for metastases in
    both necks
    Suction drainage
  Perioperative care
    Antibiotics
    Hospitalization for 3–10 days
    Tube feedings
    Suction drainage for necks(s)—remove when output <25–30
      mL/24-h period
    Suture removal 5–10 days postoperatively

Radiation therapy
  Indications
    Pathologically positive margins
    Perineural or intravascular spread
    Multiple histologically positive nodes in neck
    Extranodal tumor extension
    Treatment alternative for T1 and T2 lesions
    Adjuvant for T3 and T4 lesions
  Timing
    3–4 weeks after surgery completion
  Dosage
    Adjuvant: 50–60 Gy in daily 1.8- to 2.0-Gy fractions
    Curative: 60–70 Gy in daily 1.8- to 2.0-Gy fractions
    Technique: external beam, brachytherapy, or combination
  Posttreatment follow-up
  Necessity
    Risk of recurrence
    Second primary development
    Social and psychological support
  Schedule
    Year 1: every 1–3 mo
    Year 2: every 2–4 mo
    Year 3: every 3–6 mo
    Year 4: every 4–6 mo
    After 5 years: every 12 mo
  Ancillary tests
    Chest radiograph every year
    Liver function tests every year
    Thyroid function tests as indicated

bone or both. Refinements in microvascular surgery have made successful free-tissue transfer commonplace. These flaps require microvascular expertise and additional operating room time and are more difficult to perform in previously irradiated necks, but they yield superior functional and cosmetic results. Perhaps the most widely used free flap in oral cavity reconstruction is the radial forearm flap. This has the advantage of less donor-site morbidity as compared with other free flaps. In addition, decreased bulk exists compared with the pectoralis major flap,

making it suitable for oral tongue and floor-of-mouth defects. This flap may be made bilobed to increase postoperative tongue mobility. Some degree of sensation may be preserved by anastomosing the antebrachial cutaneous nerve to a recipient nerve in the wound bed (33). The goal of this maneuver is to improve swallowing function and to decrease aspiration.

If bone is required for mandibular reconstruction, fibula, iliac crest, or scapula free flaps can be used, depending on the characteristics of the defect (34); these flaps provide various combinations of bone and soft tissue/skin. Free-flap reconstruction of large palatomaxillary defects with an iliac crest–internal oblique or scapula free flap has been recently demonstrated to yield better functional and quality-of-life outcomes when compared with the standard approach of prosthetic obturator placement (35).

Fortunately, many techniques are now available to suit the needs of each patient and the skill of the head and neck surgeon. Despite the increasing popularity of free-flap techniques, the myocutaneous flaps provide the greatest reliability without the need for special surgical skills. No matter which reconstructive technique is used for large defects, the patient must be adequately counseled about alterations in speech, ability to wear dentures, swallowing, and cosmesis. Tables 111.4 and 111.5 summarize treatment and posttreatment follow-up.

Cheek

Buccal carcinoma is a relatively uncommon cancer. It is more common in India and the southeastern section of the United States, primarily because of the social habits in these regions involving oral carcinogens. Buccal carcinomas occur most commonly in 70-year-old men and are found in a region of cheek leukoplakia. The exophytic lesions may have a relatively benign appearance and may not penetrate into the soft tissues of the cheek until they are relatively large. The ulcerative lesions, however, penetrate early and make cure more difficult because of their involvement of adjacent muscle, bone, and skin. Because

TABLE 111.5 ℞

TREATMENT BY LEVEL OF STAGING NEOPLASMS OF THE ORAL CAVITY

T1 and T2 lesions: equal survival with surgical excision vs. radiation therapy
Consider patient's health, preference, mobility, and cost to patient
For larger T1 and T2 lesions with N0 neck, treat with supraomohyoid neck dissection or radiation therapy
For T3 and T4 lesions, combination therapy, either pre- or postoperative radiation therapy
Modified radical/radical neck dissection for all cases, with decision based on number of nodes, extracapsular spread, fixation to adjoining tissues/structures

no natural barriers to tumor penetration exist in the cheek, cure rates are not as good as one might expect in a region so easily inspected. In a study of 57 patients treated with surgery and radiation, Fang et al. (36) showed 3-year locoregional control and disease-specific survival to be 64% and 62%, respectively. More than half of these patients were initially seen with stage IV disease. By using multivariate analysis, only tumor invasion into the skin of the cheek had prognostic significance (36); this may simply represent a measure of tumor thickness.

As with most oral cavity neoplasms, T1 lesions can be treated either with surgery or radiation therapy, although resection and coverage of the area with a split-thickness skin graft may be more convenient and expedient. Because T1 lesions are rare, large series comparing treatment modalities cannot be found. Three-year survival rates for T1 and T2 lesions are approximately 80% and 60%, respectively, and depending on the extent of the lesions, marginal or rim mandibulectomy or partial maxillectomy or both may be necessary for adequate margins (37).

Surgery plus radiation therapy is the treatment of choice for stage III and IV disease. Three-year survival for stage III and IV disease treated with radiation therapy or surgery alone is 41% and 15%, respectively; these rates increase to 60% and 35% when surgery is combined with postoperative radiation therapy (38). The extent of resection of these larger lesions is variable, but may include resection of the maxilla or mandible, parotidectomy, neck dissection, or a combination of these. Reconstruction is with free (radial forearm) or regional myocutaneous (temporalis, pectoralis major) flaps or with an osteomyocutaneous free flap if bone is needed.

At present, we do not perform neck dissections for T1N0 lesions, but, given a greater than 40% incidence of occult neck metastases at higher T stages, it is appropriate to treat T2–4N0 necks electively (37) or when the primary exhibits poor prognostic indicators or both.

Hard Palate

Primary malignancies of the hard palate are uncommon with a relatively equal incidence of squamous cell carcinoma and salivary gland malignancies. Only in central Asian countries such as India is the incidence significant (40% of all oral cancers), due to the habit of reverse smoking. Therefore the experience at most institutions is relatively small, and certain inferences must be made concerning therapy.

It is important to recognize that tumors that appear to be of hard-palate etiology may actually be larger entities. Because the hard palate is the floor of the maxillary sinus, what appears to be a moderate-size hard-palate submucosal neoplasm could be a maxillary sinus neoplasm that has eroded through the floor. Even more extensive disease can be mistaken as a primary malignancy of the palate (Fig. 111.5). In addition, because nodal metastases are retropharyngeal, it is unnecessary to be concerned with prophylactic neck therapy. Only those patients with T4 lesions begin to approach an incidence of nodal metastases (25%) for which prophylactic neck irradiation would be considered (39). Although distant metastases are rare with squamous cell carcinoma of the hard palate, an incidence of 12% has been found in patients with salivary gland tumors (39).

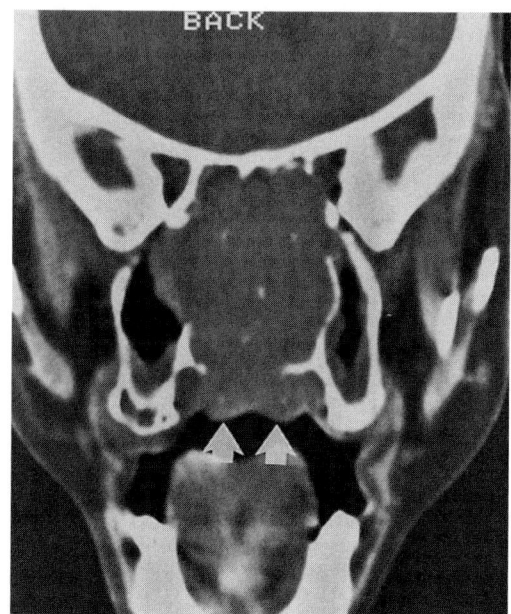
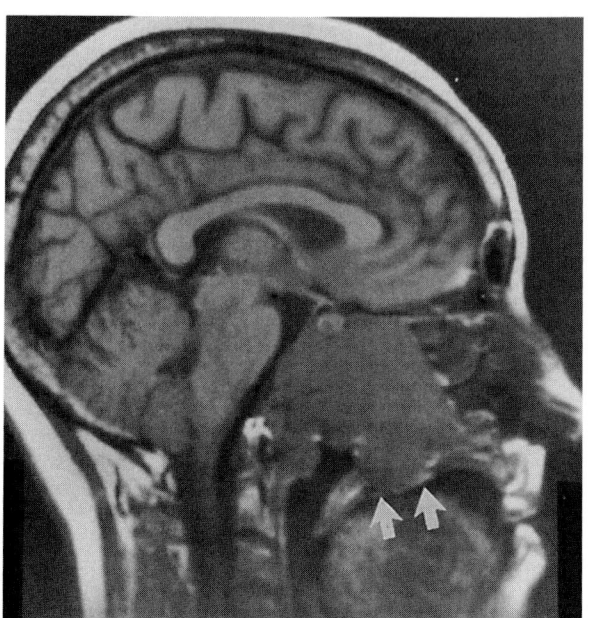

A

B

Figure 111.5 **A:** Coronal computed tomography of a patient first seen with an apparent T3 hard-palate cancer but who actually had a T4 nasopharyngeal cancer eroding through the floor of the nose. White arrows, Tumor evident in oral cavity. **B:** Sagittal magnetic resonance image showing full extent of the disease in this patient. *White arrows*, Extent of disease present in oral cavity.

Radiation therapy has been reported to be as effective as surgery in treating T1 and T2 lesions, for those of both salivary gland and squamous etiology. It is probably true, however, that T1 lesions are most easily treated by excision. For the larger T3 and T4 lesions (the 5-year survival rate decreases from 85% for a T1 lesion to 30% for a T4 lesion), the treatment of choice is a combination of surgery and radiation therapy (39). Partial or total maxillectomy is often required, and the traditional reconstruction has been with a prosthetic obturator, requiring preoperative evaluation by a prosthodontist. Newer options for reconstruction, along with a classification system for maxillary defects, have been presented by Okay et al. (40). They propose that defects involving the central hard palate or the alveolus posterior to the canine can be reconstructed with soft-tissue flaps alone; this does not interfere with standard prosthetic rehabilitation, if the ipsilateral canine and a significant number of contralateral teeth are preserved. Subtotal and total palatomaxillectomy defects yield poor results with prosthetic reconstruction, and bone-containing free flaps with osseointegrated implants for subsequent prosthetic attachment are now recommended (35,40). This approach reduces the time required to achieve dental rehabilitation, especially when postoperative radiotherapy is planned.

Retromolar Trigone

Because of the finite location of the retromolar trigone, lesions isolated to this one area are uncommon. Often they extend to the tonsil or anterior tonsillar pillar and soft palate. It is common in the analysis of these lesions to include those of the retromolar trigone with those of the palatine arch. In these circumstances, if the bulk of the disease appears to have originated in the retromolar trigone, that should be considered its site of origin.

One of the difficulties in considering therapy is the fact that this area is composed of mucosa and periosteum over the posterior and ascending ramus of the mandible. Little leeway exists to attain adequate soft-tissue margins in the mediolateral plane, and one counts on periosteal tumor resistance. In addition, the underlying mandible, because of its proximity, often must be included in the specimen. Inner-table mandibulectomies cannot be done in the same manner as in the anterior mandibular arch because of the thinness of the mandible in this region. Most patients with this tumor are initially seen with advanced disease with cervical metastases. Of 31 patients studied by Antoniades et al. (41), four were stage I or II, and 27 were initially in stage III or IV. Nodal metastases were demonstrated in 78% of ipsilateral necks, and occult metastases were found in 64% of clinically N0 necks (41).

As with most tumor sites, small T1 lesions can be treated with equal facility by either radiation therapy or surgical excision. Resection of T2 lesions usually requires resection of the soft palate, which can carry with it some deglutition morbidity. External beam irradiation is often

the treatment of choice for T1 and T2 lesions, but T3 and T4 lesions require combined therapy, with either pre- or postoperative radiation therapy. This often requires a composite resection, including a partial mandibulectomy and neck dissection. It is unnecessary to split the lower lip to accomplish this, in view of the distinct cosmetic advantage of approaching this region through a submandibular incision. Although this approach often requires sectioning of both mental nerves, sensation over the mandible is generally recovered over time. We prefer to avoid resecting the head of the condyle by making the saw cut through the condylar neck. This avoids significant bleeding, which is sometimes difficult to control, especially that from the pterygoid veins. The amount of soft tissue resected is dictated by the extent of disease but often includes the tonsillar fossa, floor of the mouth, tongue, soft palate, and buccal mucosa. Although split-thickness skin graft can be used for small defects, larger lesions generally require reconstruction with a radial forearm free flap or temporalis or pectoralis major muscle flap. When ablation results in a bony defect, a vascularized bone-containing free flap is recommended (34).

In the previously mentioned series, primary lesions were surgically excised, and ipsilateral neck dissections were performed in all patients. Masseter muscle flap or tongue flap were used for reconstruction. Postoperatively, 90% of patients received radiation therapy (51 to 58 Gy) to the primary site and neck, and adjuvant chemotherapy was offered if histologic signs of aggressive behavior were identified. The 3-year locoregional control rates were 100%, 43%, and 27% for stage I/II, III, and IV, respectively. The 3-year overall survival rate was 65.5% (41).

Alveolus

Alveolus carcinoma is a relatively rare oral cavity cancer; 80% are of the lower jaw, with most occurring in the posterior third of the dental arch. Treatment is primarily surgical, but the addition of radiation therapy is important when bony invasion, nodal metastases, or perineural invasion is present. Stage I and II disease can be treated with surgery alone, with expected 2-year disease-free survival rates of 80% and 70%, respectively. For stage III and IV disease, radiation therapy is required for the N0 neck, and a MRND with radiation therapy is indicated for positive nodal disease. When combined therapy is used, the expected 2-year survival rates are 60% and 50%, respectively, for patients with stage III and IV disease (42).

The reconstructive requirements are based on the defect size and the degree of mandibular resection required for control of the primary lesion. If adequate preoperative assessment fails to reveal mandibular invasion, then the bone must be carefully evaluated intraoperatively. If the primary tumor abuts the mandible, periosteum should be carefully removed. If the underlying bone is obviously invaded, a segmental mandibulectomy is required. If the bone appears normal and the periosteum harbors cancer cells, a minimum of marginal mandibular resection is required. After the marginal resection is performed, curetted cancellous bone may be amenable to intraoperative evaluation; a segmental resection is performed if it is positive. Multiple studies have demonstrated that frozen-section analysis of cancellous bone has acceptable sensitivity and specificity for tumor invasion (43), although the presence of excessive calcification can hinder this assay. Thus marginal mandibular resection can be used without sacrifice of oncologic principles. However, given the difficulty of confirming negative bony margins intraoperatively and given the success of reconstruction with vascularized bone-containing free flaps, some authors have recommended segmental resection and immediate free-flap reconstruction as a more reliable approach (34). Marginal resection is contraindicated when the bone has been previously irradiated, when vertical height is significantly reduced in the edentulous patient, and with gross cancellous bone involvement.

Oral Tongue

In deciding on treatment modalities for oral tongue cancer, the same factors are applicable as for most other head and neck sites. T1–2 lesions can be treated by surgery or radiation therapy, and T3–4 lesions do best with combination therapy. Radiation treatment alone achieves control rates of 86% for T1 and 75% for T2 lesions. Because of the high complication rate associated with curative doses, Wendt et al. (44) suggested a policy of initial surgery, with postoperative radiation therapy being reserved for patients with a suspected high rate of local or neck failure. Techniques for radiation therapy delivery vary. Wendt et al. (44) argued that interstitial therapy is necessary, but Wang (45) suggested that the intraoral cone electron beam boost technique provides a superior cure rate compared with interstitial implant for T1 and T2 oral lesions.

Whatever the radiotherapeutic technique used, prophylactic neck therapy is necessary for a certain subgroup of larger/more-aggressive T1 lesions, as it is for T2 lesions. Although the factors that define this group are not finalized, most surgeons now consider depth of penetration to be a key factor that dictates the necessity of neck therapy. Many also argue for prophylactic neck treatment when the primary lesions is greater than 1 cm, recognizing the poor prognostic relationship this characteristic has with neck metastases (31).

If the surgeon opts for surgical resection of an early tongue cancer, the aforementioned issues must be considered regarding prophylactic neck therapy. Although issues have been raised concerning laser versus conventional excision of these lesions, the method is purely a technical choice, because the survival rate of about 80% does not change according to technique. Laser provides no distinct oncologic advantages over a standard surgical scalpel.

The treatment of stage III and IV disease requires combination therapy to control locoregional disease better than either surgery or radiation therapy alone. Several clinical trials that have included oral tongue lesions as a small subset of the overall patient base have shown benefit from the addition of chemotherapy to standard radiation-therapy regimens (25,26). However, more-specific data are needed before the advantage of chemotherapy for these lesions is proven. Overall survival rates for patients with stage III and stage IV disease range from 30% to 35%.

As in all head and neck reconstruction, the defect-closure techniques vary from primary closure to distant flap. Greater cosmetic and functional debilitation is encountered when part of the mandible must be resected. Although the surgeon must advise the patient on the speech and swallowing deficits that accompany oral cavity resections, especially those involving the tongue and the floor of the mouth, some basic principles can be followed to minimize the level of debilitation. Tongue flaps, which provide the worst functional reconstructive results, must be avoided in view of the many choices available. Use of a split-thickness skin graft where possible provides good functional results (46). When the defects include much of the floor of the mouth and tongue, either a myocutaneous (e.g., pectoralis major) or free flap (e.g., radial forearm) must be used. For these patients, oral competence becomes a significant issue, which may be at least partially addressed by the use of a sensate radial forearm free flap (33).

Floor of Mouth

One of the problems of using radiation therapy as curative treatment for oral cavity tumors is the proximity of the mandibular arch. Although this must be considered for all oral cavity cancers, it becomes a much greater issue when treating floor-of-mouth cancers. In general, cancers of the floor of the mouth are undertreated and tend to reflect a poor stage-for-stage prognosis.

In a recent retrospective study involving 227 patients, stage I and II floor-of-mouth cancers had a 5-year disease-specific survival rate of 72% and 63%, respectively (47). As discussed earlier, elective neck dissection is typically recommended for T2 and larger or more-aggressive T1 lesions. However, in this series, Sessions et al. (47) found no survival benefit for elective neck dissection, assuming the alternative was careful follow-up with frequent assessment by physical examination and radiologic imaging. Stage III and IV lesions had disease-specific survival rates of 44% and 47%, respectively (47); these require combination therapy, which frequently involves composite resection and complex reconstruction. Treatment failures occurred at the primary site more than twice as often as did recurrence in the neck (47).

COMPLICATIONS

Table 111.6 outlines expected complications due to neoplasms of the oral cavity. From the radiotherapeutic point of view, xerostomia, mucositis, and reduced taste are the

TABLE 111.6	C	COMPLICATIONS

NEOPLASMS OF THE ORAL CAVITY

Airway obstruction: tracheotomy
Bleeding
Postoperative hemorrhage: secure airway, stabilize vital signs, return to surgery to control bleeding site
Postoperative fistula: initial local wound care and control with salivary diversion away from vascular sheath
Prevention: carotid artery coverage—dermis, muscle flap, rotation, myocutaneous, pedicle coverage
Possible secondary reconstruction of wound unhealed because of secondary infection fistula formation
Loss of reconstruction graft/flap
Split-thickness skin graft loss: local by secondary intention
Myocutaneous/muscle flap ischemia or infection: if found acutely, evaluate and correct possible tension, vascular compromise; if too late, discard and replace with secondary reconstruction
Free flap if ischemia found acutely, and Doppler evaluation shows loss of flow, return to surgery for thrombus removal from artery or vein; if too late, discard and replace with secondary reconstruction
Positive postoperative surgical margins: return to surgery for re-resection of involved margin unless technically or physically cannot be performed

expected side effects. When mucositis becomes severe enough to require a protracted treatment break, a significant risk exists that local tumor control may be compromised (48). Persistent radiation ulcers, which can appear as recurrent cancer and osteoradionecrosis of the mandible, provide significant problems for the patient. As stated earlier, complications occur most commonly with radiation therapy for cure of floor-of-mouth cancers, and the highest occurrence of osteoradionecrosis has been found when retromolar trigone tumors are treated for cure. Nonhealing ulcers can cause persistent pain unless they heal after excision of the necrotic tissue, and osteoradionecrosis of the mandible can cause persistent pain that may ultimately necessitate hyperbaric oxygen therapy or a partial mandibulectomy. Necrosis of the mandible can occur when the radiation tolerance of bone is exceeded but is more commonly related to poor dentition before radiation therapy begins. For this reason, a dentist familiar with radiation and its adverse effects must evaluate those patients before therapy. Fluoride application by the patient and dentist is necessary periodically to maintain stable dentition, and pretherapy extractions are necessary to prevent osteoradionecrosis 6 to 12 months after therapy is completed.

Surgical complications depend on the extent of surgery. The standard list for a neck dissection applies no matter what the site of the primary malignancy. Depending on the type of neck dissection performed and the skin incisions used, these might include bleeding, infection, injury to the marginal mandibular nerve leading to weakness of the corner of the mouth, injury to the hypoglossal nerve leading to a paralyzed tongue on the affected side, chylous leak (more

likely with left-neck dissection), injury to the phrenic nerve leading to a paralyzed diaphragm, brachial plexus injury (somewhat remote), numb ear, and the obvious cosmetic neck deformity. The incidence of complications is somewhat reduced with SOHND compared with MRND.

When wide local resections are performed, problems include the loss of the split-thickness skin graft or flap with delayed healing by secondary intention, fistula, exposed carotid artery, or delay in adjunctive therapy due to the need of an additional tissue flap. As the magnitude of the procedure increases, it stands to reason that the list of complications increases as well. When a flap is used, the loss of the flap and resultant fistula are the greatest concerns. For this reason, it is appropriate to protect the carotid artery if a neck dissection is to be performed. This can be done either with the spared sternocleidomastoid muscle or, if that muscle has been sacrificed, with a dermal graft or substitute (e.g., Alloderm). Exposed mandible, with the potential to lose its viability, is another concern with a lost flap, especially if an osteotomy and plate fixation have been performed for surgical access. If a rim mandibulectomy has been performed, the patient's ability to wear dentures is jeopardized. Ultimate bone necrosis or pathologic fracture is a potential complication if an inner-table mandibulectomy is necessary. If an entire segment has been resected, especially at the mentum or body, severe oral incompetence will be a problem if this segment is not replaced by a plate or bone graft. Impaired swallowing and speech ability are directly proportional to the amount of soft tissue resected. In addition to the cosmetic defects of the surgery, which can be satisfactorily masked, many functional deficits may occur.

EMERGENCIES

Emergencies specific to oral cavity malignancies are uncommon (Table 111.7). It is unusual for a patient to be first

TABLE 111.7		EMERGENCIES

NEOPLASMS OF THE ORAL CAVITY

Tongue/floor of mouth postoperative hematoma:
    if not tracheotomized, surgery for local tracheotomy, evaluation of hematoma, and control of bleeding site
Massive primary disease with airway compromise: surgery for local tracheotomy and nasogastric tube gastrostomy
Ischemia or congestion of myocutaneous flap
    If acutely found, evaluate for flap tension or mechanical impairment of vascular supply; take to surgery and correct
    If unsalvageable, remove dead flap and use alternative reconstruction technique
Ischemia or congestion of free flap
    If found acutely and loss of Doppler signal, return to surgery and remove venous/arterial thrombus and reconstitute
    If unsalvageable, remove and use alternative reconstructive technique

seen by the physician with a neoplasm so large that the airway is impaired. More frequently, endotracheal intubation can be problematic when inducing general anesthesia or after accidental decannulation postoperatively due to tumor bulk or decreased tissue mobility. The surgeon must evaluate this preoperatively and assist the anesthesiologist in achieving control of airway, whether it be via fiberoptic-guided nasal intubation or a tracheostomy under local anesthesia.

Excluding operative emergencies of neck dissection, few situations require immediate attention. One, however, is the postoperative fistula, which is characterized by erythema, edema, neck tenderness, and unexplained fever, usually 3 to 7 days postoperatively. The surgeon must recognize this early and drain and divert the saliva to prevent further tissue damage. This is especially important if the surgeon has not protected the carotid artery in a patient who has been irradiated. A chylous fistula occurring primarily in the left neck also should be recognized early to prevent excessive protein loss. Although fistulae of 500 mL or less per day can be treated with drainage, pressure, and a fat-free diet, leaks of 800 mL or more need swift surgical intervention.

THE FUTURE

One of the most disconcerting problems faced by patients who have been successfully treated for head and neck malignancy is the fact that in 10% to 40% of them, a second primary lesion will develop. These second primary tumors are the chief cause of death in patients who are successfully treated for an oral lesion (49). Although retinoids showed some initial promise for the treatment of premalignant oral lesions and prevention of second primary lesions (50), no follow-up studies have been published to demonstrate their long-term effectiveness. Other new therapies, such as growth-factor inhibitors (51), are being aggressively studied, as are new techniques for early detection with specialized optical systems (52).

The issue of how to determine whether an N0 neck is truly without disease and how to treat the N0 neck that has a significant probability of microscopic disease is still a question. As mentioned earlier, CT and MRI have helped in isolated clinical situations, but no series supports their improved efficacy over a skillful physical examination. It has been suggested that PET scanning may assist in identifying occult nodal disease not easily detectable by other imaging modalities, but at present, insufficient data warrant its routine use in assessing N0 patients.

The standard oncologic approach has been to treat all necks in which the potential incidence of metastatic disease exceeds 30%, but this means that up to seven of 10 patients with N0 necks undergo radiation therapy or neck dissection unnecessarily. Movement from MRND to selective neck dissections has reduced morbidity without sacrificing recurrence or survival rates (53). The technique of SLNB

may represent an opportunity to reduce morbidity further while still effectively identifying micrometastatic disease.

Perhaps the most interesting but difficult area of advancement is the field of biologic markers. These are molecular characteristics of oral cavity cancer cells that would allow improved prognostication, accurate staging and identification of microscopic disease, selection of appropriate therapy, and monitoring for/prevention of recurrence. A host of such markers are under investigation (54–56), and it is possible that, in the near future, rapid molecular assessment of a small biopsy specimen will help guide patients toward maximally effective therapy.

HIGHLIGHTS

- Other than the mandible periosteum, no finite bony or fascial planes inhibit tumor spread in the oral cavity.
- Lateralized lesions of the oral tongue drain to ipsilateral lymph nodes.
- In general, the cure rate for T1–2 lesions of the oral cavity is equal when treated by either radiation therapy or surgery. T3–4 lesions require combined-modality therapy.
- Because hard-palate malignancies are rare, what appears to be a hard-palate neoplasm may actually be a maxillary sinus cancer eroding through the sinus floor.
- Treatment of alveolus carcinoma is solely surgical unless bony invasion, perineural invasion, or nodal metastasis is found.
- Persistent ulcers after radiation therapy can represent either persistent tumor or radiation necrosis.
- Because large oral cavity neoplasms may complicate transoral intubation, cooperation with anesthesiologist is required to determine the best method of securing the airway.
- When treatment is warranted, selective neck dissections are appropriate for the N0 neck.

REFERENCES

1. Crafts RC. *Textbook of human anatomy*, 3rd ed. New York: John Wiley and Sons, 1985.
2. Moore KL, Dalley AF. *Clinically oriented anatomy*, 4th ed. Baltimore: Lippincott Williams & Wilkins, 1999.
3. Hollinshead WN, Rosse C. *Textbook of anatomy*, 4th ed. Philadelphia: Harper & Row; 1985.
4. Ries LAG, Eisner MP, Kosary CL, et al., eds. *SEER Cancer Stat Rev 1975–2001*. Bethesda, MD: National Cancer Institute (http://seer.cancer.gov/csr/1975–2001/), 2004.
5. Lewin F, Norell SE, Johansson H, et al. Smoking tobacco, oral snuff, and alcohol in the etiology of squamous cell carcinoma of the head and neck: a population-based case-referent study in Sweden. *Cancer* 1998;82:1367–1375.
6. Baden E. Prevention of cancer of the oral cavity and pharynx. *Ca Cancer J Clin* 1987;37:49–62.
7. Elamin F, Steingrimsdottir H, Wanakulasuriya S, et al. Prevalence of human papillomavirus infection in premalignant and malignant lesions of the oral cavity in U.K. subjects: a novel method of detection. *Oral Oncol* 1998;34:191–197.
8. Hafkamp HC, Manni JJ, Speel EJM. Role of human papillomavirus in the development of head and neck squamous cell carcinoma. *Acta Otolaryngol* 2004;124:520–526.

9. Brockenbrough JM, Petruzzelli GJ, Lomasney L. DentaScan as an accurate method of predicting mandibular invasion in patients with squamous cell carcinoma of the oral cavity. *Arch Otolaryngol Head Neck Surg* 2003;129:113–117.
10. Virapongse C, Mancuso A, Fitzsimmons J. Value of magnetic resonance imaging in assessing bone destruction in head and neck lesions. *Laryngoscope* 1986;96:284–291.
11. Phillips CD, Gay SB, Newton RL, et al. Gadolinium-enhanced MRI of tumors of the head and neck. *Head Neck* 1990;12:308–315.
12. Troell RJ, Terris DJ. Detection of metastases from head and neck cancers. *Laryngoscope* 1995;105:247–250.
13. Houghton DJ, Hughes ML, Garvey C, et al. Role of chest CT scanning in the management of patients presenting with head and neck cancer. *Head Neck* 1998;20:614–618.
14. Arunachalam PS, Putnam G, Jennings P, et al. Role of computerized tomography (CT) scan of the chest in patients with newly diagnosed head and neck cancers. *Clin Otolaryngol* 2002;27:409–411.
15. Goerres GW, Schmid DT, Gratz KW, et al. Impact of whole body positron emission tomography on initial staging and therapy in patients with squamous cell carcinoma of the oral cavity. *Oral Oncol* 2003;39:547–551.
16. Greene FL, Page DL, Fleming ID, et al., eds. *AJCC cancer staging handbook: from the AJCC cancer staging manual*, 6th ed. New York: Springer, 2002:35.
17. Gorsky M, Epstein JB. The effect of retinoids on premalignant oral lesions: focus on topical therapy. *Cancer* 2002;95:1258–1264.
18. Lim SC, Zhang S, Ishii G, et al. Predictive markers for late cervical metastasis in stage I and II invasive squamous cell carcinoma of the oral tongue. *Clin Cancer Res* 2004;10:166–172.
19. O'Brien CJ, Lauer CS, Fredrick S, et al. Tumor thickness influences prognosis of T1 and T2 oral cavity cancer: but what thickness? *Head Neck* 2003;25:937–945.
20. Lam P, Au-Yeung KM, Cheng PW, et al. Correlating MRI and histologic tumor thickness in the assessment of oral tongue cancer. *AJR Am J Roentgenol* 2004;182:803–808.
21. Kowalski LP, Medina JE. Management of the neck in head and neck cancer. nodal metastases: predictive factors. *Otolaryngol Clin North Am* 1998;31:621–637.
22. Rubio Bueno P, Naval Gias L, Garcia Delgado R, et al. Tumor DNA content as a prognostic indicator in squamous cell carcinoma of the oral cavity and tongue base. *Head Neck* 1998;20:232–239.
23. Xia W, Lau YK, Zhang HZ, et al. Strong correlation between c-erbB-2 overexpression and overall survival of patients with oral squamous cell carcinoma. *Clin Cancer Res* 1997;3:3–9.
24. Lapeyre M, Bollet MA, Racadot S, et al. Postoperative brachytherapy alone and combined postoperative radiotherapy and brachytherapy boost for squamous cell carcinoma of the oral cavity, with positive or close margins. *Head Neck* 2004;26:216–223.
25. Snow JB, Guber RD, Kramer S, et al. Randomized preoperative and postoperative radiation therapy for patients with carcinoma of the head and neck: preliminary report. *Laryngoscope* 1980;90:930–945.
26. Bernier J, Domenge C, Ozsahin M, et al. Postoperative irradiation with or without concomitant chemotherapy for locally advanced head and neck cancer. *N Engl J Med* 2004;350:1945–1952.
27. Zorat PL, Paccagnella A, Cavaniglia G, et al. Randomized phase III trial of neoadjuvant chemotherapy in head and neck cancer: 10-year follow-up. *J Natl Cancer Inst* 2004;96:1714–1717.
28. Shah JP, Candela FC, Poddar AK. The patterns of cervical lymph node metastases from squamous carcinoma of the oral cavity. *Cancer* 1990;66:109–133.
29. Byers RM, Weber RS, Andrew T, et al. Frequency and therapeutic implications of "skip metastases" in the neck from squamous cell carcinoma of the oral tongue. *Head Neck* 1997;19:14–19.
30. Khafif A, Lopez-Garza JR, Medina JE. Is dissection of level IV necessary in patients with T1-T3 N0 tongue cancer? *Laryngoscope* 2001;111:1088–1091.
31. Spaulding CA, Korb LJ, Constable WC, et al. The influence of extent of neck treatment upon control of cervical lymphadenopathy in cancers of the oral tongue. *Int J Radiat Oncol Biol Phys* 1991;21:577–581.
32. Ross GL, Soutar DS, MacDonald DG, et al. Sentinel node biopsy in head and neck cancer: preliminary results of a multicenter trial. *Ann Surg Oncol* 2004;11:690–696.
33. Urken ML, Weinberg H, Vickery C, et al. The combined sensate radical forearm and iliac crest free flaps for reconstruction of significant glossectomy-mandibulectomy defects. *Laryngoscope* 1992;102:543–558.
34. Urken ML, Buchbinder D, Costantino PD, et al. Oromandibular reconstruction using microvascular composite flaps: report of 210 cases. *Arch Otolaryngol Head Neck Surg* 1998;124:46–55.
35. Genden EM, Okay D, Stepp MT, et al. Comparison of functional and quality-of-life outcomes in patients with and without palatomaxillary reconstruction: a preliminary report. *Arch Otolaryngol Head Neck Surg* 2003;129:775–780.
36. Fang FM, Leung SW, Huang CC, et al. Combined-modality therapy for squamous carcinoma of the buccal mucosa: treatment results and prognostic factors. *Head Neck* 1997:19:506–512.
37. Bloom ND, Spiro RH. Carcinoma of the cheek mucosa: a retrospective analysis. *Am J Surg* 1980;140:556–559.
38. Nair MK, Sankaranarayanan R, Padmanabhan TK. Evaluation of the role of radiotherapy in the management of the buccal mucosa. *Cancer* 1988;61:1326–1331.
39. Chung CK, Johns ME, Cantrell RW, et al. Radiotherapy in the management of primary malignancies of the hard palate. *Laryngoscope* 1980;90:576–584.
40. Okay DJ, Gender E, Buchbinder D, et al. Prosthodontic guidelines for surgical reconstruction of the maxilla: a classification system of defects. *J Prosthet Dent* 2001;86:352–363.
41. Antoniades K, Lazaridis N, Vahtsevanos K, et al. Treatment of squamous cell carcinoma of the anterior faucial pillar-retromolar trigone. *Oral Oncol* 2003;39:680–686.
42. Wald RM, Calcaterra TC. Lower alveolar carcinoma. Arch Otolaryngol Head Neck Surg 1983;109:578–582.
43. Wax MK, Bascom DA, Myers LL. Marginal mandibulectomy vs segmental mandibulectomy: indications and controversies. *Arch Otolaryngol Head Neck Surg* 2002;128:600–603.
44. Wendt CD, Peters LF, Delcios L, et al. Primary radiotherapy in the treatment of stage I and II oral tongue cancers: importance of the proportion of therapy delivered with interstitial therapy. *Int J Radiat Oncol Biol Phys* 1990;18:1287–1292 .
45. Wang CC. Radiotherapeutic management and results of T1N0, T2N0 carcinomas of the oral tongue: evaluation of boost technique. *Int J Radiat Oncol Biol Phys* 1989;17:287–291.
46. McConnel FMS, Logemann JA, Rademaker AW, et al. Surgical variables affecting postoperative swallowing efficiency in oral cancer patients: a pilot study. *Laryngoscope* 1994;104:87–90.
47. Sessions DG, Spector GJ, Lenox J, et al. Analysis of treatment results for floor-of-mouth cancer. *Laryngoscope* 2000;110:1764–1772.
48. Maciejewski B, Withers HR, Taylor JM, et al. Dose fractionation and regeneration in radiotherapy for cancer of the oral cavity and oropharynx, Part 2: normal tissue responses: acute and late effects. *Int J Radiat Oncol Biol Phys* 1990;18:101–111.
49. Lippman SM, Hong WK. Second malignant tumors in head and neck squamous cell carcinoma: the overshadowing threat for patients with early-stage disease. *Int J Radiat Oncol Biol Phys* 1989;17:691–694.
50. Lotan R. Suppression of squamous cell carcinoma growth and differentiation by retinoids. *Cancer Res* 1994;54:1987s–1990s.
51. Myers JN, Holsinger FC, Bekele BN, et al. Targeted molecular therapy for oral cancer with epidermal growth factor receptor blockade: a preliminary report. *Arch Otolaryngol Head Neck Surg* 2002;128:875–879.
52. Sokolov K, Aaron J, Hsu B, et al. Optical systems for *in vivo* molecular imaging of cancer. *Technol Cancer Res Treat* 2003;2:491–504.
53. Ambrosch P, Kron M, Pradier O, et al. Efficacy of selective neck dissection: a review of 503 cases of elective and therapeutic treatment of the neck in squamous cell carcinoma of the upper aerodigestive tract. *Otolaryngol Head Neck Surg* 2001;124:180–187.
54. Raybaud-Diogene H, Tetu B, Morency R, et al. p53 Overexpression in head and neck squamous cell carcinoma: review of the literature. *Eur J Cancer B Oral Oncol* 1996;32B:143–149.
55. Chen IH, Chang JT, Liao CT, et al. Prognostic significance of EGFR and Her-2 in oral cavity cancer in betel quid prevalent area cancer prognosis. *Br J Cancer* 2003;89:681–686.
56. St John MA, Li Y, Zhou X, et al. Interleukin 6 and interleukin 8 as potential biomarkers for oral cavity and oropharyngeal squamous cell carcinoma. *Arch Otolaryngol Head Neck Surg* 2004;130:929–935.

Odontogenic Cysts, Tumors, and Related Jaw Lesions

Jaw Lesions

William L. Chung   *Darren P. Cox*   *Mark W. Ochs*

Odontogenic cysts and tumors comprise a unique group of lesions that have gained the interest of surgeons and pathologists because of their complex and variable history, histologic characteristics, and clinical behavior. The term *odontogenic* implies being derived from tooth-forming structures. Odontogenic cysts vary significantly in their frequency, behavior, and treatment. Odontogenic tumors are relatively uncommon lesions, representing 1% of biopsies accessioned by oral pathologists (1). Collectively, lesions of the jaws deserve considerable attention by surgeons because of their potential for tissue destruction and the related challenges they pose for reconstruction. In this chapter are reviewed the more common and clinically significant odontogenic cysts and tumors, along with several other related jaw lesions. The salient clinical, radiographic, and histologic features of each lesion are discussed, in addition to relevant treatment and prognosis.

ODONTOGENIC CYSTS

Most cysts of the oral cavity are true cysts because they contain an epithelial lining. The lining of these cysts are derived from one of three epithelial structures: (a) reduced enamel epithelium—residual epithelium that surrounds the tooth crown after enamel formation is complete; (b) rests of Malassez—remnants of the Hertwig root sheath that persist in the periodontal ligament after root formation is complete; or (c) remnants of dental lamina (rests of Serres)—islands

and strands of epithelium that originate from the oral epithelium and remain in tissues after inducing tooth development (2). Odontogenic cysts can become inflamed or infected, causing significant signs or symptoms. They can be further subclassified as either inflammatory or developmental cysts.

INFLAMMATORY CYSTS

Radicular Cyst

The radicular cyst is by far the most common type of odontogenic cyst. It develops at the apex of an erupted tooth in response to pulpal necrosis secondary to dental caries or trauma. The cyst arises from inflammatory stimulation and proliferation of the rests of Malassez. The cyst lining forms as the epithelial elements proliferate. Cellular debris within the lumen produces an osmotic gradient, and fluid is transported across the lining. This gradient slowly increases the volume of fluid inside the lumen, ultimately expanding the cyst by hydraulic pressure from within the cyst.

Clinical and Radiographic Features
Most radicular cysts, which are asymptomatic, are discovered incidentally during routine radiographic evaluation (Fig. 112.1). Radicular cysts rarely exceed 1 cm in diameter except when several adjacent teeth become devitalized as a result of trauma. Radiographically, the radicular cyst is round to ovoid, well circumscribed, and contiguous with the apex of the involved tooth.

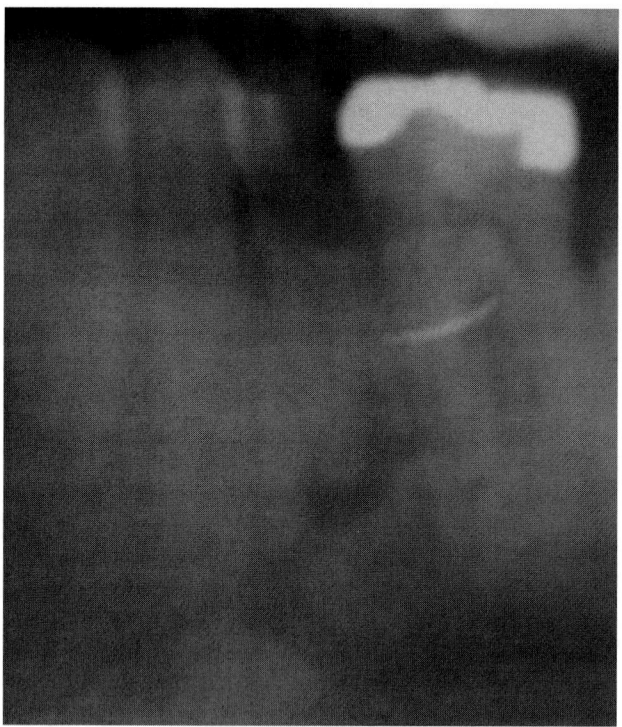

Figure 112.1 Periapical cyst. Radiograph demonstrating periapical lesion associated with grossly carious tooth # 20.

Histopathology

The cyst is lined by stratified squamous epithelium of varying thickness. The cyst wall typically supports a variable inflammatory cell infiltrate, including lymphocytes and neutrophils. The cystic lumen frequently contains necrotic cellular debris. A small percentage of radicular cysts have crescent-shaped hyaline (Rushton) bodies within the epithelial lining. Although unique to odontogenic cysts, the biologic significance of Rushton bodies is unknown. Multinucleated foreign body giant cells, cholesterol clefts, and hemosiderin may be seen throughout the connective tissue of the cyst wall.

Treatment and Prognosis

These cysts are treated by extraction of the infected tooth followed by enucleation of the cyst. Extraction of the tooth without removing the cyst may allow for persistent growth of the cyst. If the cyst is incompletely removed, a *residual* cyst can develop. Complete bony healing is typically seen within 6 months if the radicular cyst has been thoroughly removed.

DEVELOPMENTAL CYSTS

Dentigerous Cyst

The dentigerous cyst is the second most common odontogenic cyst. A dentigerous cyst must be associated with the

crown of an unerupted tooth (3). Variants exist where the cyst is seen lateral to, or completely enveloping, the associated tooth. The cyst is attached to the cervical region of the tooth, usually a mandibular third molar. Maxillary third molars, maxillary canines, and mandibular second bicuspids are also commonly involved, because these teeth are among those frequently impacted.

Clinical and Radiographic Features

Dentigerous cysts usually occur in the second and third decades with a slight male predilection. Because they are associated with an impacted tooth, the arch will appear to be missing a tooth. The cysts usually do not produce symptoms and can achieve significant size, causing bony expansion (Fig. 112.2A). The dentigerous cyst is a well-circumscribed, typically unilocular radiolucency surrounding the crown of an unerupted tooth. Mandibular cysts can displace the tooth into the ramus or the inferior border of

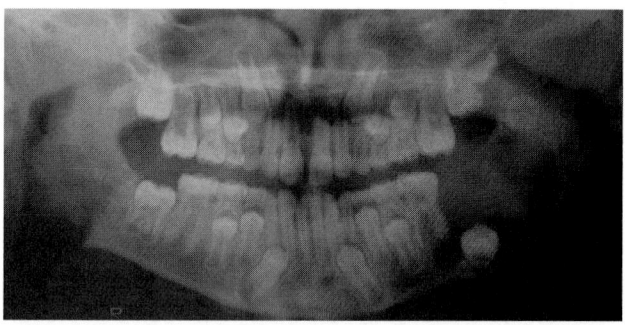

A

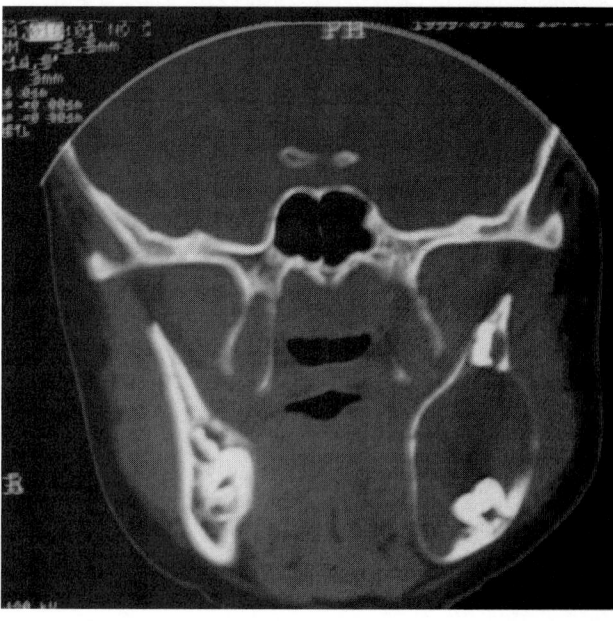

B

Figure 112.2 **A**: Dentigerous cyst. Panorex radiograph of 14-year-old who presented with facial swelling. Radiograph reveals considerable left mandibular angle and ramal involvement. Note displacement of multiple permanent teeth within lesion. **B**: Dentigerous cyst. Cyst lined by thin, stratified squamous epithelium. The cyst wall supports a moderate amount of chronic inflammation.

the mandible, whereas a maxillary cyst can displace the tooth into the maxillary sinus toward the orbital floor.

Histopathology

The cystic lumen is lined by nonkeratinized, stratified squamous epithelium that is anywhere from 2 to 10 cell layers thick (see Fig. 112.2B). It is common for the lining to be inflamed. The dentigerous cyst can share several microscopic features with the radicular cyst (e.g., Rushton bodies, cholesterol clefts, and hemosiderin deposits). Chronic dentigerous cysts may exhibit areas of keratinized epithelium, which require the lesion to be differentiated from the odontogenic keratocyst. Rarely, mucous cells can be present in the epithelial lining.

Treatment and Prognosis

Removal of the impacted tooth and thorough cyst enucleation is usually definitive therapy. When a mandibular dentigerous cyst reaches considerable size, the cyst can be marsupialized to allow for decompression and shrinkage of the cyst, with compensatory bone fill before definitive removal of the lesion. The epithelial lining can undergo transformation into an ameloblastoma, which makes timely diagnosis and treatment crucial.

Odontogenic Keratocyst

Odontogenic keratocysts (OKC), which develop from remnants of the dental lamina, can occur in any jaw location. These lesions mimic the radiographic appearance of any other odontogenic cyst and some odontogenic tumors. The mandibular ramus and posterior body are the most common locations for the OKC (Fig. 112.3A-3B). The OKC in the maxilla typically favors the posterior or canine regions. This lesion differs from other odontogenic cysts with regard to its growth potential and recurrence rate. OKC can display aggressive growth, causing bony expansion and destruction, and reports have shown recurrence rates from 5% to 60%.

Clinical and Radiographic Features

An OKC occurs over a wide age range; however, its peak incidence is within the second and third decades. When multiple OKC occur in a patient, the nevoid basal cell carcinoma syndrome (NBCCS) must be considered. This autosomal dominant syndrome will be discussed separately. Radiographically, the OKC appears as a well-circumscribed radiolucency with a distinct radiographic border. It can be either unilocular or multilocular, and many cause bony expansion or erosion of either cortex.

Histopathology

The OKC has the following distinct microscopic appearance: its lining is parakeratinized, stratified epithelium, which is six to eight cell layers thick; the luminal surface is covered by a corrugated layer of parakeratin; the basal layer is palisaded with prominent, polarized, in-

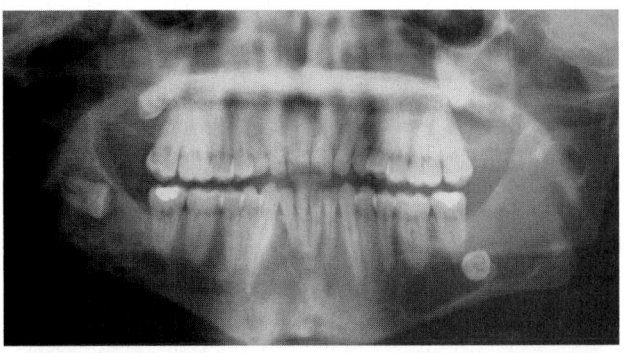

A

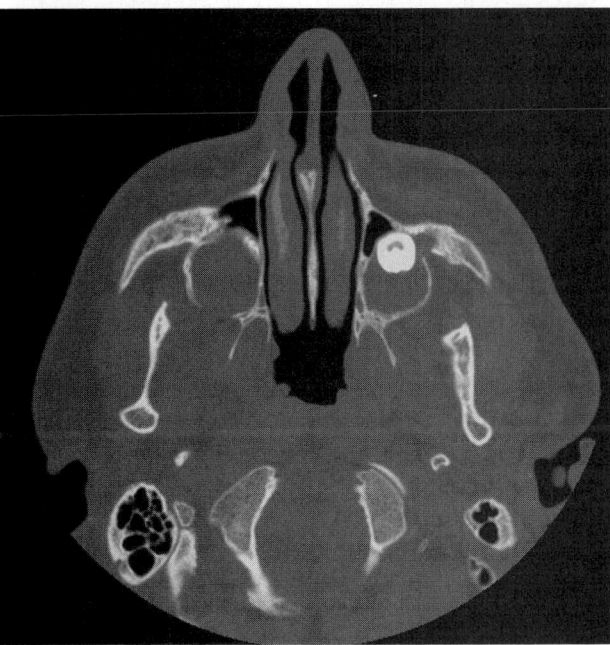

B

Figure 112.3 **A:** Odontogenic keratocyst (OKC). Panoramic radiograph of an 18-year-old man with bilateral mandibular and maxillary OKC. Patient also had nevoid basal cell carcinoma syndrome. **B:** Axial computed tomography (CT) scan of same patient, revealing bilateral maxillary lesions. Lesions were noted to extend to the orbital floors intraoperatively.

tensely stained hyperchromatic nuclei; and a lack of rete pegs. This flat epithelial-connective tissue interface results in a separation of the epithelium on processing. Desquamated parakeratin can routinely be seen in the cyst lumen. Daughter (satellite) cells may be noted in the connective tissue and may be indicative of the NBCCS.

Treatment and Prognosis

The OKC requires surgical enucleation and osseous curettage and every attempt should be made to remove it in one piece. Modified Carnoy solution is a tissue fixative that can aid in more complete lesion removal and treatment of the residual bony cavity may devitalize microscopic remnants, thus discontinuing recurrence. Some have advocated marginal resection to avoid recurrence (4). When large lesions are present, marsupialization can be performed to decompress the OKC and allow for easier removal of the cyst at a second surgery. Secondary infection, need for high patient compliance, and variable results limit the use of marsupialization techniques. Most recurrences occur within 5 years, but reports of recurrence as long as 10 years later have been documented. Thus, close follow-up is mandatory. Approximately 15% of OKC are of the orthokeratotic variety, which exhibits a far less recurrence rate (5). The orthokeratotic OKC has a prominent granular layer below a noncorrugated surface, and the basal layer is less prominent. Recurrence of OKC has been speculated based on several theories: incomplete removal of the cyst because of its thin friable membrane and adherence to adjacent tissues; residual satellite cysts following enucleation; and remnants of dental lamina not associated with the OKC in question causing de novo cyst formation.

Nevoid Basal Cell Carcinoma Syndrome (Basal Cell Nevus Syndrome, Gorlin Syndrome)

The nevoid basal cell carcinoma syndrome is an autosomal dominant inherited condition that exhibits high penetrance and variable expressivity (6,7). It is a result of a mutation of the PTCH (PATCHED) tumor suppressor gene. Patients can manifest a combination of the following clinical and radiographic features: multiple OKC of the jaws; multiple basal cell carcinomas of both exposed and non–sun-exposed areas; frontal bossing; mandibular prognathism; palmar and plantar pitting; bifid ribs; and calcification of the falx cerebri. The odontogenic keratocysts associated with NBCCS should be treated in a similar manner as an isolated OKC. Increased vigilance with 6-month or yearly clinical follow-up and imaging (panoramic radiograph or computed tomography) are warranted, however, to allow early detection of new lesions. This is particularly true of children and adolescents. Once adulthood is reached, the formation of new OKC is less problematic and the risk of basal cell carcinomas rises. Other than the skin lesions and those conditions that can be correctable, many of the other related abnormalities do not require any surgical intervention. Genetic counseling should be recommended to both the patient and family members because of the condition's autosomal dominant inheritance.

Calcifying Odontogenic Cyst (Gorlin Cyst)

Calcifying odontogenic cyst is a lesion thought to arise from remnants of the dental lamina within the gingiva or jaws. Approximately one-fourth of all calcifying odontogenic cysts (COC) occur in an extraosseous manner, within the gingiva anterior to the first molar in individuals older than 50 years (8).

Clinical and Radiographic Features
The COC behaves as most other odontogenic cysts and it has little recurrence potential. The COC has a wide age range, but the peak incidence occurs in the second decade. The lesion has a predilection for females and most are located in the anterior portion of either jaw. The extraosseous lesion can present with painless gingival expansion. These cysts are often discovered as incidental findings on routine radiographic evaluation. They initially appear lucent. As the cyst develops, calcifications can develop causing a well-circumscribed mixed radiolucent–radiopaque appearance. These opacities, however, are only seen in approximately one third to one half of all cases.

Histopathology
The COC are usually unilocular cysts lined by odontogenic epithelium. The basal layer is distinct with its columnar to cuboidal cells with hyperchromatic nuclei that are polarized away from the basement membrane. Another characteristic histologic feature of the COC is the ghost cell, an eosinophilic altered epithelial cell with loss of the nucleus that represents abnormal keratinization. With time, these ghost cells tend to become calcified, sometimes even forming calcified masses. When these cells contact the connective tissue, a foreign body reaction occurs from the release of keratin.

Treatment and Prognosis
Surgical enucleation usually results in complete resolution. The extraosseous lesions are often associated with other odontogenic tumors and, because of their low recurrence potential, are managed conservatively with lesion removal only.

Glandular Odontogenic Cyst (Sialo-Odontogenic Cyst)

The glandular odontogenic cyst was first described in 1987 (9). Although only a few cases have been reported, it is worth mentioning because of its locally aggressive behavior and its propensity to recur. This lesion is generally considered odontotogenic in origin with numerous mucus-secreting cells within its epithelial lining.

Clinical and Radiographic Features
A glandular odontogenic lesion occurs most commonly in middle-aged adults. Most glandular odontogenic cysts have been reported in the mandible, especially in the anterior region. They appear as multilocular radiolucencies and frequently cross the midline.

Histopathology
Several unique microscopic features are seen with a glandular odontogenic cyst: (a) an epithelial lining of variable thickness and a flat epithelial-connective tissue junction; (b) small microcysts and glandlike structures within the epithelial lining; and (c) a single layer of cuboidal or columnar cells lining the glandlike structures (Fig. 112.4).

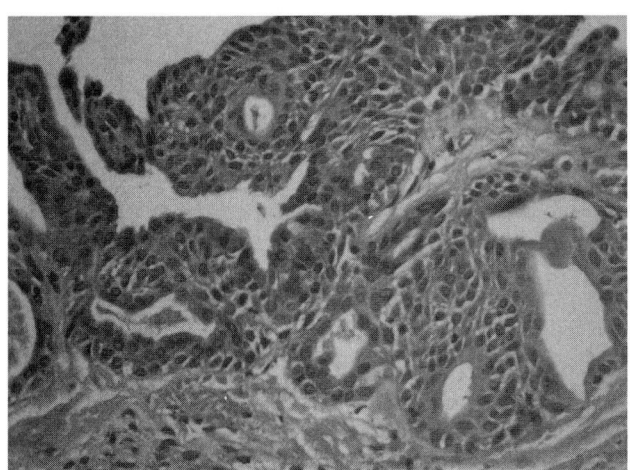

Figure 112.4 Glandular odontogenic cyst. Stratified squamous epithelium forming glandlike structures. (See also Color Plate 43.)

Treatment and Prognosis

Most glandular odontogenic cysts are amenable to enucleation and curettage. Because of its recurrence potential, however, some advocate marginal resection. Regardless, long-term follow-up is advisable.

NONODONTOGENIC CYSTS

Nasopalatine Duct Cyst (Incisive Canal Cyst)

The nasopalatine duct cyst originates from the epithelial remnants of the two embryonic nasopalatine ducts (10). Most of these cysts arise in the anterior maxilla near the incisive foramen.

Clinical and Radiographic Features

Men are affected twice as often as females, and this cyst occurs most frequently in the fourth to sixth decades. The nasopalatine duct cyst is either asymptomatic or presents as soft tissue swelling in the midline of the anterior hard palate once the lesion has perforated the bone. The lesion is typically a well-circumscribed, heart-shaped, unilocular radiolucency in the midline of the anterior palate. If the cyst reaches large proportions, it can resorb the roots of the adjacent teeth. Some normal incisive canals are radiographically wide, which can make diagnosis of this lesion less precise. It is generally accepted that any radiographic lesion greater than 6 mm should be considered a cyst and not an enlarged incisive foramen. If no soft tissue or bony swellings are present and the patient is asymptomatic, a diagnosis of nasopalatine duct cyst becomes unlikely.

Histopathology

The lining of a nasopalatine duct cyst can be either stratified squamous epithelium, ciliated columnar or cuboidal epithelium, or a combination of the two. This variable lining reflects whether the cyst has arrived from epithelium closer

to the palate (stratified squamous) or is more closely associated with the nasal cavity (ciliated columnar). The fibrous tissue contains elements of nerve and vascular tissue consistent with the surrounding incisive canal contents. Mucous glands are occasionally seen within the wall of the cyst because these glands are native to the adjacent nasal cavity.

Treatment and Prognosis

Surgical enucleation is usually curative, but can result in sacrificing the nasopalatine nerve and vessel, resulting in denervation of the mucosa of the anterior palate and maxillary incisors. Recurrence is rare.

Stafne Bone Cyst (Lingual Salivary Gland Depression, Static Bone Cyst)

The Stafne bone cyst is not a true cyst. Rather, it is a depression on the lingual aspect of the posterior body of the mandible. This condition has a pathognomonic radiographic appearance of a small ovoid, well-circumscribed radiolucency below the inferior alveolar canal in the second or third molar region. This radiographic appearance is caused by the relative thinning of the mandible. Most reported cases have occurred in males, and sialography has revealed that the depression is characteristically filled with an accessory lateral lobe of the submandibular gland, although occasionally connective tissue, adipose tissue, and lymphoid tissue have been seen (11). No treatment is required.

Idiopathic Bone Cavity (Traumatic Bone Cyst or Traumatic Bone Cavity)

The traumatic bone cavity is not a true cyst because it does not contain a true epithelial lining. It is usually found in the posterior mandible, and presents on radiograph as a less well-defined radiolucency compared with most odontogenic cysts. These lesions are typically empty on surgical exploration or contain some straw-colored fluid. No lining or tissue exists to submit for biopsy, but exploration of the lesion will be curative, because hemorrhage within the cavity will allow for granulation tissue formation and ultimate resolution of this condition.

ODONTOGENIC TUMORS

Odontogenic tumors are collectively a rare but diverse and complicated group of lesions. They arise from epithelial or mesenchymal cells, or both, associated with tooth structures. Most odontogenic tumors are true neoplasms, but some behave as hamartomatous growths. Odontogenic tumors commonly present as asymptomatic swellings, which can eventually cause bone loss, tooth displacement, and jaw expansion. They rarely cause sensory nerve dysfunction. Understanding the biologic behavior of this group of lesions will assist in choosing the appropriate treatment to best attain a cure or to optimize the outcome. The tumors discussed were selected based on their frequency, locally aggressive behavior, or likelihood of recurrence.

Odontoma

Odontomas are not true neoplasms, but rather hamartomatous growths because they form during normal tooth development, then reach a fixed size (12). The lesion contains elements of enamel, dentin, cementum, and pulp tissue. Depending on the degree of morphologic differentiation, an odontoma can be classified as either (a) compound, if the lesion resembles tooth-like structures or (b) complex, if the lesion appears as an amorphous mass.

Clinical and Radiographic Features
The odontoma is the most common odontogenic "tumor." The lesion, typically asymptomatic, is discovered on routine radiographic examination. Odontomas occur in the first two decades without any sex predilection and can block the expected eruption of a permanent tooth. Radiographically, both compound and complex odontomas are radiopaque masses and have a well-demarcated border. The compound odontoma resembles multiple tiny tooth structures, whereas the complex odontoma appears as a dense irregular mass.

Histopathology
Although reduced enamel epithelium can be present, odontomas are essentially composed of enamel, dentin, cementum, and pulp tissue. Fibrous tissue is sparse.

Treatment and Prognosis
Removal of the lesion may be necessary to rule out other lesions or if the mass is impeding the eruption of a tooth. Enucleation and curettage is considered curative and the lesion is not known to recur.

Ameloblastoma

With the exception of the odontoma, the ameloblastoma is the most common odontogenic tumor (13). It arises from any number of residual epithelial elements of tooth development: reduced enamel epithelium, rests of Serres, rests of Malassez, or the basal layer of the oral mucosa. The lesion can also develop from within a dental follicle or a dentigerous cyst. Some confusion has arisen regarding the classification schema of ameloblastomas. Most references broadly categorize ameloblastomas into one of three groups: (a) unicystic, (b) solid or multicystic, or (c) peripheral ameloblastomas. A misuse of terms or a lack of understanding of these same terms with their overlapping meanings can lead to an inadequate treatment decision, increasing the likelihood of recurrence. One example is the term *unicystic* ameloblastoma. Unicystic ameloblastoma generally implies being amenable to enucleation and curettage. An invasive ameloblastoma can be unicystic, having just one cystic space. That does not suggest, however, that this invasive lesion should be treated by enucleation and curettage merely because it was defined, properly or not, as a unicystic ameloblastoma.

Clinical and Radiographic Features
Ameloblastoma, a benign, locally aggressive neoplasm, is characterized by a slow growth pattern and can grow to profound proportions, causing gross facial deformities. It is usually asymptomatic and does not alter sensory nerve function. The posterior mandible appears to be a preferred site. The lesion has a very wide age range with a peak occurrence in the third and fourth decades, and it has no sex predilection. Radiographically, the lesion can appear as a unilocular or multilocular radiolucency, with ill-defined borders, making it difficult to determine the exact size of the lesion. Buccal and lingual cortical expansion is common, even progressing to cortical perforation (Fig. 112.5A and B). Root resorption occurs infrequently.

Histopathology
Ameloblastomas are histologically diverse. They can exhibit areas of focal variation, so adequate sampling is required. The ameloblastoma is unencapsulated, so it typically exhibits an infiltrative growth pattern into surrounding tissues. The basal cells in the epithelium are columnar and hyperchromatic and demonstrate reverse polarity, in which the nuclei move from the basement membrane pole of the cell to the opposite pole. Numerous histologic patterns have been noted in ameloblastomas; however, no current consensus exists that these different histologic patterns have different biologic behaviors (14,15). The two most frequent patterns are the follicular and plexiform (Fig. 112.5C, D).

Treatment and Prognosis
Ameloblastomas, which are limited only to the epithelial lining or proliferate only into the lumen, are treated with enucleation and curettage. No recurrence is expected in either situation. When the ameloblastoma grows into, or completely through, the connective tissue layer of the lesion or recurs, a more aggressive treatment is required. When resection is warranted, a 1.0- to 1.5-cm bony margin and one uninvolved overlying anatomic barrier margin is advocated (Fig. 112.5E) (16). When hard and soft tissue margins are negative, a cure rate of nearly 98% can be achieved. Recurrence rates as high as 90% have been reported when more aggressive ameloblastomas are inadvertently or inadequately treated with curettage. A 5-year follow-up is required; but a 10-year follow-up is prudent. When metastases have been reported, the lesions were histologically benign, as was the primary tumor. These lesions are referred to as *malignant ameloblastomas*, although they do not show cytologic features typically associated with malignancy. When the lesion is found to contain cytologic features of malignancy, it is classified as an *ameloblastic carcinoma*.

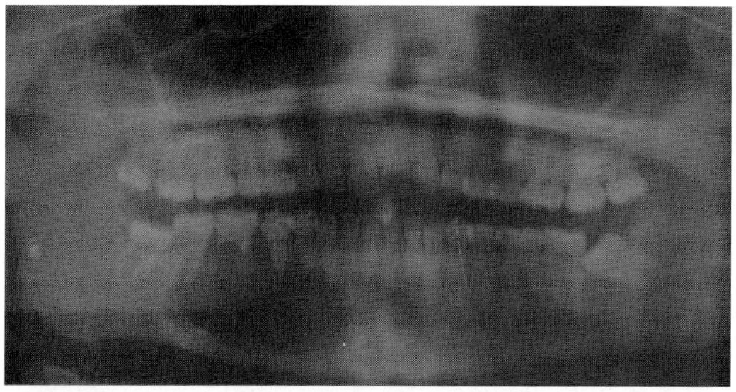

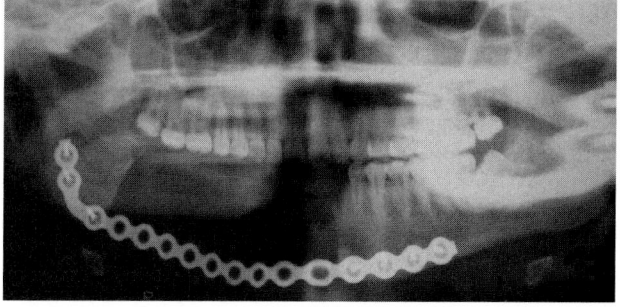

Figure 112.5 **A:** Ameloblastoma. Panoramic radiograph of 17-year-old girl with unilocular ameloblastoma of right mandible. Note resorption of multiple tooth roots in right mandible. **B:** Coronal computed tomography (CT) scan of maxillofacial bones of patient from Figure 112.4. Note extreme buccal and lingual cortical expansion of right mandible. Focal areas of perforation were noted intraoperatively. **C:** Ameloblastoma (follicular pattern). Islands of odontogenic epithelium characterized by peripheral columnar cells exhibiting reverse polarity. The central portion of these islands resemble stellate reticulum in areas. **D:** Ameloblastoma (plexiform pattern). **E:** Postoperative panoramic radiograph. Definitive reconstruction was deferred until 6 months postoperatively to avoid early recurrence. (See also Color Plate 44.)

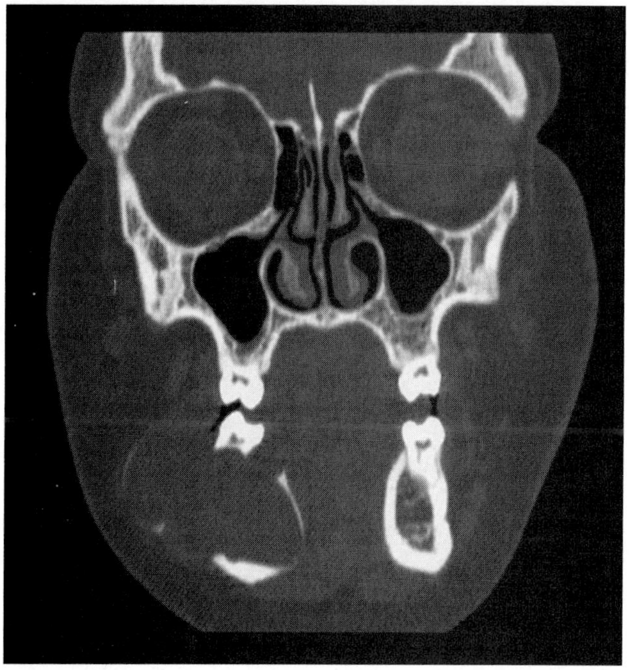

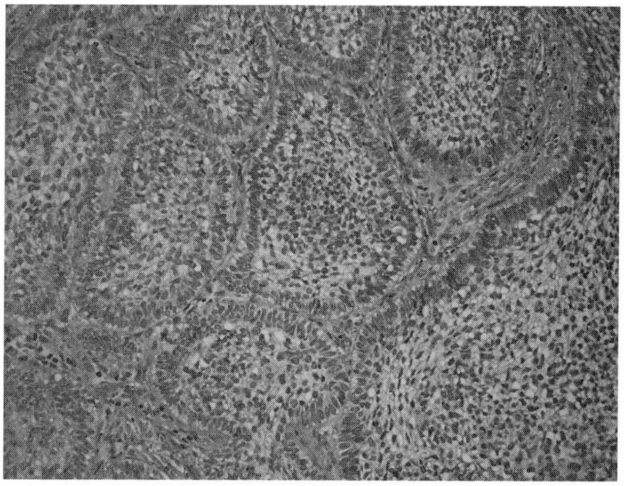

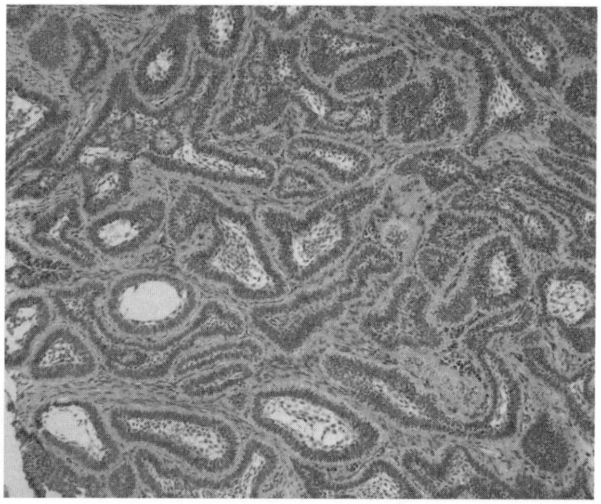

Adenomatoid Odontogenic Cyst

The adenomatoid odontogenic cyst (AOC) is a benign hamartoma of odontogenic epithelium characterized by slow, progressive growth.

Clinical and Radiographic Features
The AOC has been referred to as the "two-thirds tumor" because two-thirds are associated with an unerupted tooth, of which two-thirds are a canine; two-thirds occur in the maxilla; and two-thirds occur in young females (adolescents and teens) (17). Most AOC are less than 3 cm in diameter, but they can approach significant size and cause pain and displace tooth roots. Radiographically, the AOC usually is a well-circumscribed, unilocular radiolucency associated with an impacted tooth. Some lesions have radiographically evident small foci of calcifications.

Histopathology
The AOC is highly cellular with spindle-shaped cells in whorls or rosettes (Fig. 112.6). Enameloid material is found throughout this lesion, and the amount of calcification

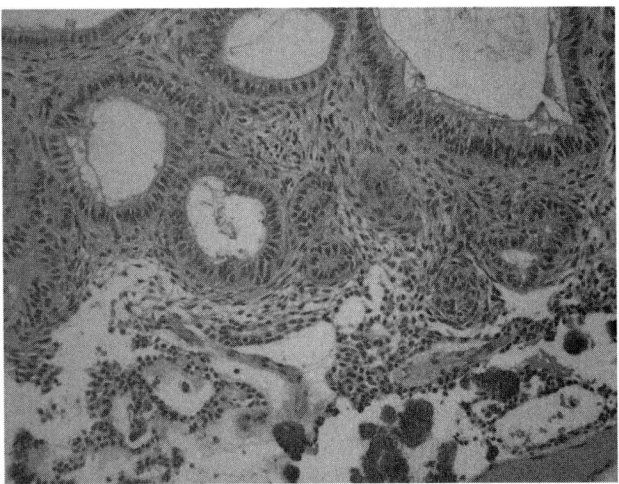

Figure 112.6 Adenomatoid odontogenic cyst. Odontogenic epithelium forming ductlike structures lined by columnar cells exhibiting reverse polarity. Calcifications, a common feature of this lesion, are seen in the lower right portion. (See also Color Plate 45.)

determines its radiographic appearance. These calcifications can resemble dentin or cementum, which validates the lesion's development from Hertwig root sheath.

Treatment and Prognosis
Recurrence is not seen in this benign encapsulated lesion, so curettage alone is curative. Bony regeneration of the defect usually occurs in about 1 year in younger patients.

Calcifying Epithelial Odontogenic Tumor (Pindborg Tumor)

The calcifying epithelial odontogenic tumor (CEOT) is a rare odontogenic tumor, representing less than 1% of all odontogenic tumors (18). It can be highly infiltrative and destructive and shares many clinical and radiographic features with the ameloblastoma. It originates from the epithelial rests of the dental lamina or reduced enamel epithelium.

Clinical and Radiographic Features
The CEOT has been reported in patients over a wide age range, but has a peak incidence in the fourth decade. It presents as a slow-growing, firm, and painless swelling, usually in the posterior mandible. The molar area is the most frequent region in either jaw. As with most other benign odontogenic tumors, the CEOT does not alter nerve function. A *peripheral* variant exists and typically presents as soft tissue swelling in the anterior aspect of the mouth. Most of these lesions appear as diffuse radiolucent lesions, unless they are large or mature; then they will exhibit areas of faint opacities consistent with the presence of calcifications in the lesion. It is typically associated with the crown of an impacted tooth. Radiographic borders are variable, ranging from distinct lines to diffuse opacified areas fusing with adjacent bone.

Histopathology
The most common pattern of the CEOT is one of sheets or strands of polyhedral epithelial cells connected by intercellular bridges. The nuclei have prominent nucleoli and can even appear pleomorphic, but this does not imply a malignant state and mitotic figures are not routinely found. Scattered calcifications are a distinct feature of the CEOT, and the calcifications form concentric rings referred to as *Liesegang rings*. Large areas of amorphous eosinophilic tissue are dispersed throughout the lesion. These areas stain positive for amyloid with Congo red, crystal violet, or thioflavin T. The prominent amyloid presence is another unique characteristic feature of the CEOT.

Treatment and Prognosis
As with the ameloblastoma, the CEOT is treated by resection, obtaining a 1-cm bony margin along with any necessary soft tissue to still achieve one layer of an uninvolved anatomic barrier. Recurrence has been reported, so long-term follow-up is recommended.

The *peripheral* variant is treated by local excision with a 5-mm margin, which should include the underlying periosteum. The remaining wound can be closed either primarily or by local advancement flaps.

Odontogenic Myxoma

The odontogenic myxoma, although a rare tumor, is worthy of mention because of its locally aggressive behavior and high recurrence rate caused by its infiltrative nature. In the jaw bones, it is derived from odontogenic ectomesenchyme and only rarely occurs in non–tooth-bearing portions of the jaws or other facial bones (19).

Clinical and Radiographic Features
The odontogenic myxoma has some clinical and radiographic features in common with the ameloblastoma. It is usually asymptomatic and slow growing, and it has the potential to displace teeth or to resorb roots, but does not alter sensory function. Although it has been reported over a wide age range, it is most commonly seen in the third decade, which is slightly younger than the peak occurrence of the ameloblastoma. The lesion has been reported in all portions of both jaws, but occurs most frequently in the posterior mandible. Radiographically, the lesion can be either a unilocular or multilocular radiolucency (Fig. 112.7). The lesion also has been described as having a "honeycomb" appearance, with its faint, wispy trabecular bone mixed within cortical plate expansion.

Histopathology
The odontogenic myxoma is an infiltrative and gelatinous tumor. It contains scant, randomly arranged, spindle-shaped mesenchymal cells within mucoid ground substance. When these lesions are noted to be more collagenous, they are referred to as myxofibromas or fibromyxomas. This

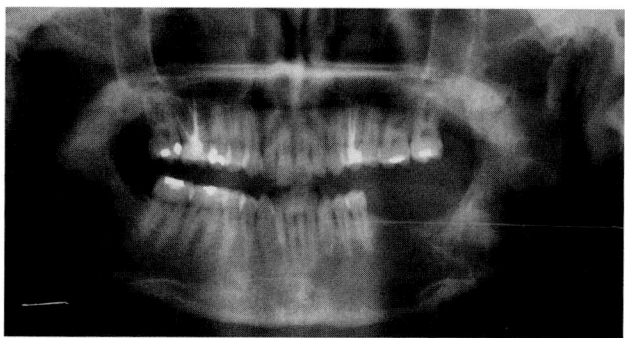

Figure 112.7 Odontogenic myxoma. Panoramic radiograph revealing diffuse, mixed radiolucent or radiopaque involvement of left hemimandible. Lesion extends from midline up to sigmoid notch.

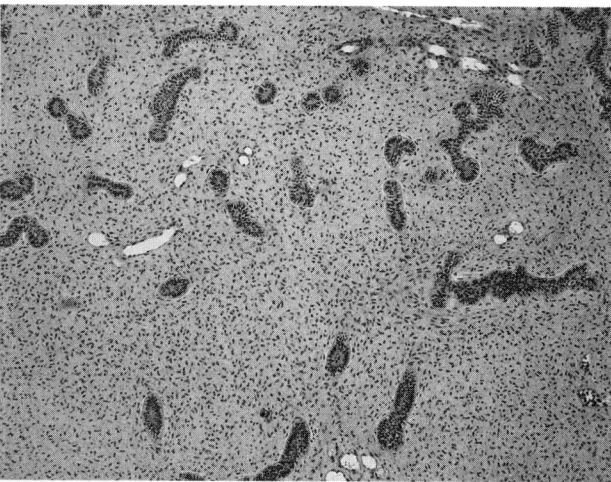

Figure 112.8 Ameloblastic fibroma. Cords of odontogenic epithelium in a background of cellular, primitive mesenchymal tissue. (See also Color Plate 46.)

classification, however, does not alter the lesion's clinical behavior.

Treatment and Prognosis

Curative treatment requires resection with a 1- to 1.5-cm bony margin and a layer of overlying soft tissue. The lesion is unencapsulated, so infiltration into adjacent bone is common, making recurrence likely if only enucleation and curettage are undertaken.

Ameloblastic Fibroma

The ameloblastic fibroma is a true neoplasm composed of both odontogenic epithelium and ectomesenchyme. The epithelium resembles dental lamina or ameloblastoma, and the mesenchyme resembles dental papilla or myxoma.

Clinical and Radiographic Features

The ameloblastic fibroma is a tumor of young patients, with rare occurrence over the age of 40. It presents as a painless swelling, usually in the posterior mandible. The lesion can be either a unilocular or multilocular radiolucency, often over an unerupted tooth and often displacing the tooth.

Histopathology

Microscopically, the tumor consists of islands of odontogenic epithelium resembling the dental lamina and cap stage of odontogenesis. This columnar epithelium is palisaded and shows striking reverse polarity identical to the ameloblastoma (Fig. 112.8). The stroma is myxoid in appearance, resembling the dental papilla, a cell-rich myxoid tissue.

Treatment and Prognosis

The ameloblastic fibroma can be cured through enucleation and curettage because it is well encapsulated. Owing to its predilection for young patients, the bony defect will repair itself within approximately 1 year. An ameloblastic

fibrosarcoma, the most common odontogenic malignancy, should be considered if this lesion recurs.

RELATED JAW LESIONS

Various nonodontogenic lesions of the jaws are worthy of mention because of their biologic behavior and indicated treatment. Some believe that these conditions are indeed odontogenic because many are only found in the jaws even though they do not reveal histologic features consistent with odontogenic-derived structures.

Torus

A torus is a developmental overgrowth rather than a tumor or hamartoma and it is thought to arise because of bone stress (20). It develops in one of two intraoral sites. When it occurs on the midline of the palate, it is termed *torus palatinus*. When tori occur on the lingual aspect of the mandible, they are typically bilateral and adjacent to the canine or bicuspid region. These are termed *torus mandibularis* or lingual tori. When a histologically similar lesion develops on the buccal aspect of either jaw, the lesion is referred to as an *exostosis*.

Clinical and Radiographic Features

The palatal torus develops after puberty. Found in approximately 20% of adults, it has a slow growth pattern. Palatal tori can either have a smooth ovoid appearance or multiple pedunculated loculations, but both presentations should have normal pink overlying mucosa. Tori can grow to large proportions, impairing speech or feeding or prohibit fabrication of a maxillary prosthesis (Fig. 112.9). Also, large lesions are often susceptible to mucosal ulceration from mastication. These larger lesions require surgical

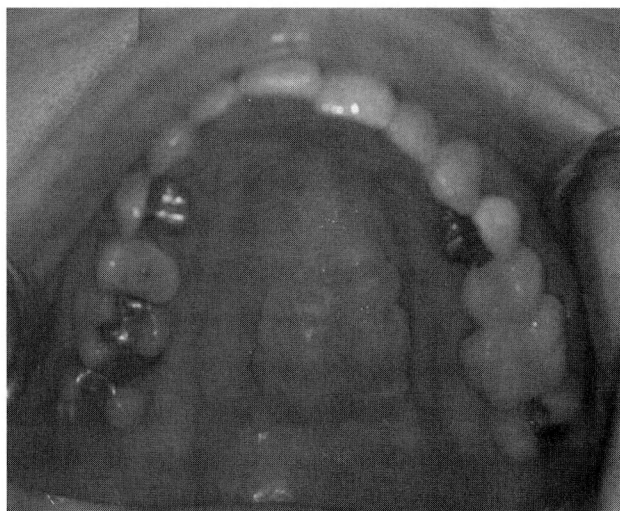

Figure 112.9   Palatal torus.

excision. A mandibular torus is commonly bilateral and also has a slow growth pattern. They too can reach sizable proportions, adversely affecting speech or feeding or the use of a lower prosthesis.

Histopathology
Tori consist of nodular masses of dense cortical, lamellar bone with central trabecular bone containing few areas of fatty marrow.

Treatment and Prognosis
Tori only require removal if they interfere with normal function or the fabrication and placement of a prosthesis such as a denture. An elliptical or double-Y–shaped mucosal incision is designed and the lesion is taken down to the level of surrounding bone with a rotary instrument. The torus can also be scored in the shape of a cross with a surgical drill then removed with an osteotome and mallet. Care must be taken not to perforate through the nasal floor, and a surgical stent can be created preoperatively so that the surgical site can be postoperatively protected from irritation from either the tongue or foods. Removal of mandibular tori requires attention to the submandibular ducts when using an osteotome and mallet to excise these lesions. A drill can be used to make vertical cuts along the inner aspect of the torus between the lesion and the alveolus. An osteotome is then used to outfracture the torus. Then, a rotary instrument is used to smooth the edges of the lingual shelf before flap closure.

Osteoma

Osteomas, hamartomas or reactive proliferations of bone, are not considered true tumors. They are composed of dense compact bone, which arises either on the surface of bone (*periosteal osteoma*) or within bone (*endosteal osteoma*). When multiple osteomas are present, consider that the patient may have *Gardner syndrome*, an autosomal dominant condition also associated with intestinal polyposis, fibromas of the skin, impacted normal and supernumerary teeth, and odontomas (21). Osteoma formation usually precedes other manifestations of the syndrome. If this syndrome is suspected, the appropriate referral should be made to rule out intestinal lesions, particularly polyps, which have a high rate of malignant transformation to colorectal cancer. The frequency of malignant transformation is essentially 100% in these patients as they reach older age.

Clinical and Radiographic Features
Slow-growing, asymptomatic exophytic bony masses, osteomas occur in either jaw in areas not typically affected by tori or exostoses. The mandibular angle is a common location. The lesion is usually an incidental finding on routine radiographic evaluation and appears as a well-circumscribed radiopaque mass.

Histopathology
Osteomas have similar microscopic features as tori or exostoses. The periosteum can be more active in the osteoma than the other two lesions.

Treatment and Prognosis
Asymptomatic single lesions can be followed clinically and radiographically. Those lesions requiring biopsy are surgically excised with little chance for recurrence.

Osteochondroma

Osteochondromas are benign hamartomas that develop most commonly in long bones, but also occur in the mandibular condyle or coronoid process (22). The lesion is believed to be associated with proliferation of epiphyseal cartilage into the surrounding tissues.

Clinical and Radiographic Features
Absence of this lesion in other portions of the mandible, skull, or facial bones serves to confirm its development in endochondral bone. Osteochondromas, which are lesions of younger patients, usually occurring in the second and third decades, are found in twice as many males as females. The lesion is slow growing and known to cause swelling and pain along with deviation of the teeth and chin pointing toward the unaffected side. Radiographically, it appears as an irregular "popcornlike" radiopaque mass on the medial side of the condyle or replacing the coronoid (Fig. 112.10A, B).

Histopathology
Osteochondromas are bony masses that have a cartilaginous cap. Endochondral ossification is noted between the cartilage and bone (see Fig. 112.10C).

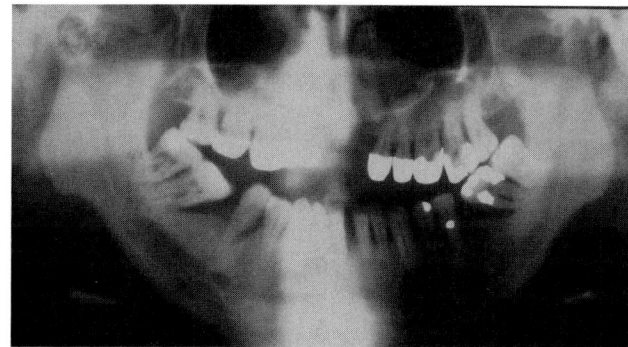

A

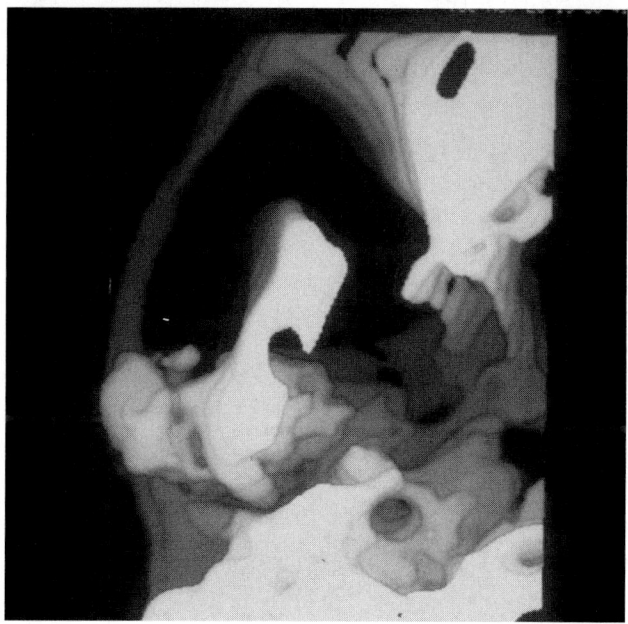

B

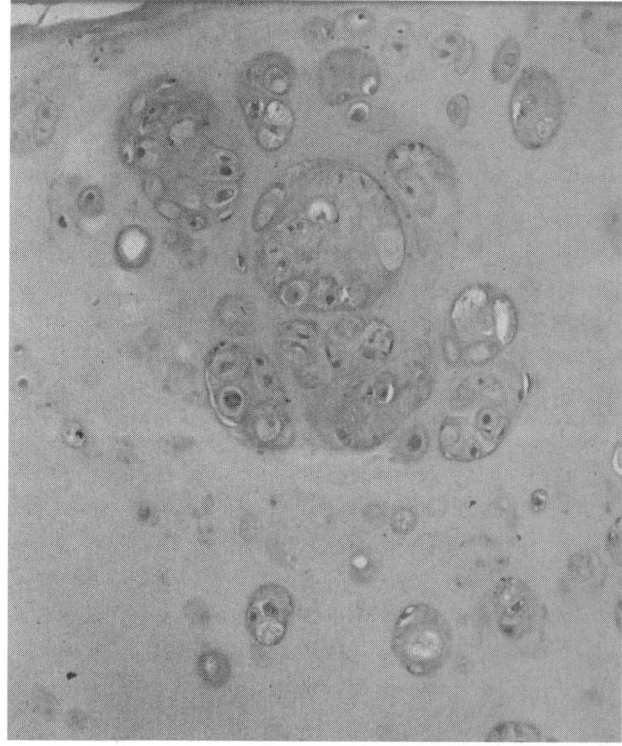

C

Figure 112.10 **A.** Osteochondroma. Panoramic radiograph of a 53-year-old man who presented with right preauricular swelling, discomfort, and left-sided shift in his occlusion. Radiograph demonstrates inhomogeneous lesion of right condyle that appears to have replaced entire normal bony architecture. **B:** Three-dimensional reformatted computed tomography (CT) scan of right side as viewed from below. Lateral and more extensive medial extension of the lesion is seen. **C:** Osteochondroma. Chondroid matrix with foci of developing osteocytes and osteoid. (See also Color Plate 47.)

Treatment and Prognosis

Lesions affecting the coronoid process are managed by a coronoidectomy with minimal removal of the attached temporalis muscle tendon. Lesions of the condyle are treated by condylectomy with a preauricular as well as a neck incision. Immediate reconstruction can be planned with either a costochondral graft or an alloplastic condyle. Recurrence is rare.

Ossifying Fibroma (Cemento-Ossifying Fibroma)

Ossifying fibromas are true benign tumors of mesenchymal origin that have a strong predilection for the tooth-bearing portion of the jaws, although they have been reported in long bones (23). This slow-growing, expansile lesion can reach enormous proportions resulting in profound facial disfigurement.

Clinical and Radiographic Features

The typical patient with an ossifying fibroma is a woman in her third to fourth decade, although the lesion has been reported over a wide age range and in both sexes. An im-

mature lesion initially presents as a radiolucency, but becomes more mixed as it matures and eventually can become completely radiopaque. More aggressive lesions expand the cortices of the jaws and frequently displace adjacent structures. In the mandible, they typically appear as a midbody growth at the inferior border of the mandible, enlarging outward and downward as if "hanging off the lower lateral border."

Histopathology

Ossifying fibromas, which are well demarcated from the surrounding bone, are composed of a dense cellular fibrous tissue layer with variable amounts of calcified trabeculae of osteoid or bone or of spherical cementumlike structures (Fig. 112.11). The ossifying fibroma is usually well circumscribed and does not exhibit diffuse infiltration of adjacent tissues.

Treatment and Prognosis

Ossifying fibromas are amenable to enucleation and curettage if detected early, or resection for larger lesions. Because these lesions do not display aggressive infiltration of

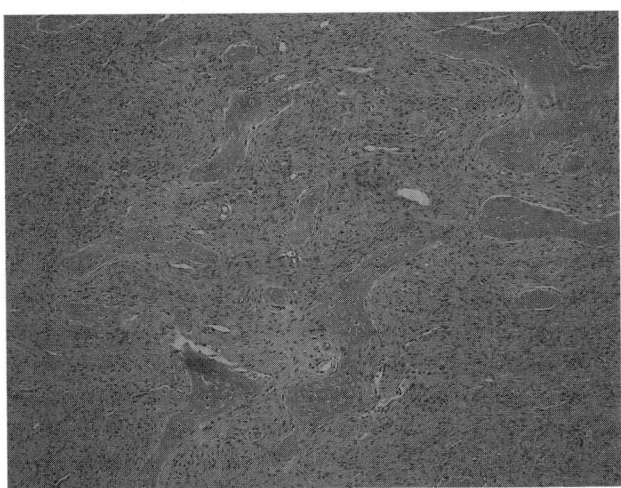

Figure 112.11 Ossifying fibroma. Irregular trabeculae of bone are seen throughout a cellular, fibrous connective tissue stroma. (See also Color Plate 48.)

surrounding tissues, for those requiring surgical resection because of large size or problematic location, a conservative 5-mm margin is appropriate and recurrence is rare. The juvenile (aggressive) ossifying fibroma, a rare variant of the above, is considered a more aggressive lesion, appearing at a younger age with a predilection for the maxilla.

Fibrous Dysplasia

Fibrous dysplasia is not a true neoplasm; rather, it is a genetically based, tumorlike condition where normal medullary bone is replaced with fibrous connective tissue mixed with irregular bony trabeculae. Fibrous dysplasia most commonly occurs in one bone (*monostotic*), or, more rarely, multiple bones (*polyostotic*). Polyostotic fibrous dysplasia can be seen as a component of *McCune-Albright syn*drome, which includes café-au-lait skin macules and multiple endocrinopathies, including hyperthyroidism or precocious puberty (24). Although genetically based, it is usually a sporadic condition involving a mutation in the α-subunit of a signal transducing G-protein.

Clinical and Radiographic Features
Fibrous dysplasia is a slow-growing, typically asymptomatic process that often produces a bony hard swelling (Fig. 112.12A–C). The condition can be self-limiting, beginning in the first decade and ceasing when the affected bone reaches maximal growth and maturation. It is capable of tooth displacement with resultant malocclusion. Early lesions are radiolucent, but become more opaque as the lesion matures. The normal medullary bone is replaced with a fine trabecular bone, giving the lesion its "ground-glass" appearance on radiographs. Fibrous dysplasia does expand the cortices but does not displace the inferior alveolar canal. The lesion margins are usually not well demarcated. Fibrous dysplasia involving the midface, calavarium,

or skullbase can cause progressive severe facial distortion and cranial nerve dysfunction via compression. In such individuals, serial visual acuity and audiology testing correlated with 1-mm cut computed tomography is warranted to monitor progression and guide timing of any necessary surgical intervention.

Histopathology
Fibrous dysplasia is seen microscopically as irregularly shaped trabeculae of woven bone in a background of a loose and cellular, fibrous connective tissue (see Fig. 112.12D). Fibrous dysplasia has a distinctive microscopic picture of abnormal bone coalescing with the normal surrounding tissue, which is in contrast with the features of the ossifying fibroma.

Treatment and Prognosis
Fibrous dysplasia does not require surgery unless the lesion is disfiguring and the patient desires a more normal and aesthetic appearance or, rarely, in cases of cranial nerve dysfunction (25). Recontouring of the affected jaw or facial bone is performed rather than resection, and surgery is usually delayed until the affected bone has reached maturity (26). Reports of sarcomatous transformation have been documented, and recurrence is more likely if the lesion is treated during an active growth period.

Central Giant Cell Lesion

The central giant cell lesion (CGCL) is a locally aggressive benign lesion that occurs in both long bones and the jaws. Jaw lesions can have similar histopathologic features as those that appear in long bones, but the biologic behavior differs. This condition has been referred to as a central giant cell reparative granuloma, but current understanding is that it does not represent a reparative process (27,28).

Clinical and Radiographic Features
The CGCL of the jaws most often are asymptomatic and are not recognized until they present as a painless swelling. A more aggressive form of the CGCL can cause pain or paresthesia. Clinically, the condition can appear as a bluish mass as a result of the thinning of the overlying bone and mucosa and its highly vascular nature. Most cases develop in the second to third decades and women outnumber men two to one. The lesion favors the anterior region of the jaws, particularly the mandible, often crossing the midline and occasionally seen bilaterally. The CGCL appears as either a well-circumscribed radiolucency or a multilocular radiolucency. Larger lesions can cause cortical expansion (Fig. 112.13A). The CGCL can also displace teeth, but root resorption is not typical.

Histopathology
The associated giant cells behave much as do osteoclasts. Multinucleated giant cells varying in size and their number

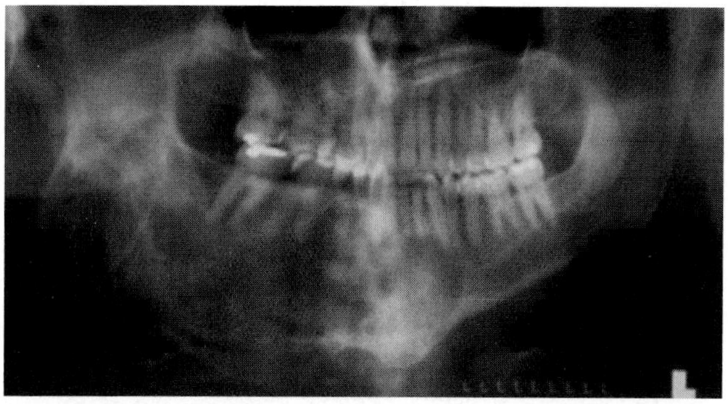

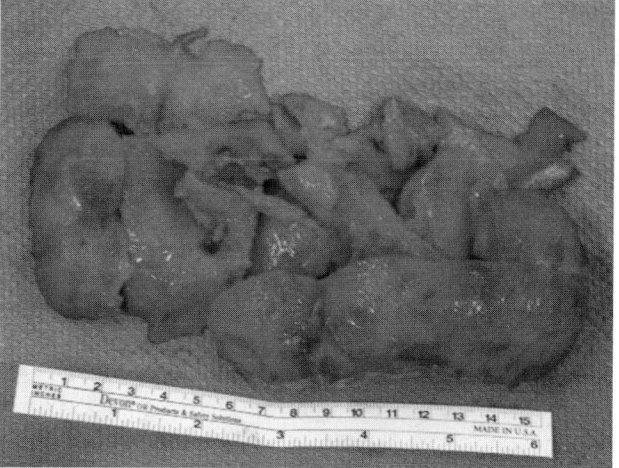

Figure 112.12 A: Fibrous dysplasia. Panoramic radiograph of 28-year-old man who presented with steadily increasing right mandibular and facial enlargement, which had been monitored over several years' time. Biopsies established diagnosis of fibrous dysplasia. **B:** Coronal computed tomography (CT) scan of maxillo-facial bones demonstrates frontal, maxillary, and mandibular bony involvement. **C:** Three-dimensional reformatted CT scan depicting the gross deformity of the right mandibular lesion. **D:** Fibrous dysplasia. Curvilinear portions of woven bone, without appositional osteoblasts, in a background of connective tissue stroma. **E:** Gross specimen of the fibrous dysplasia. (See also Color Plate 49.)

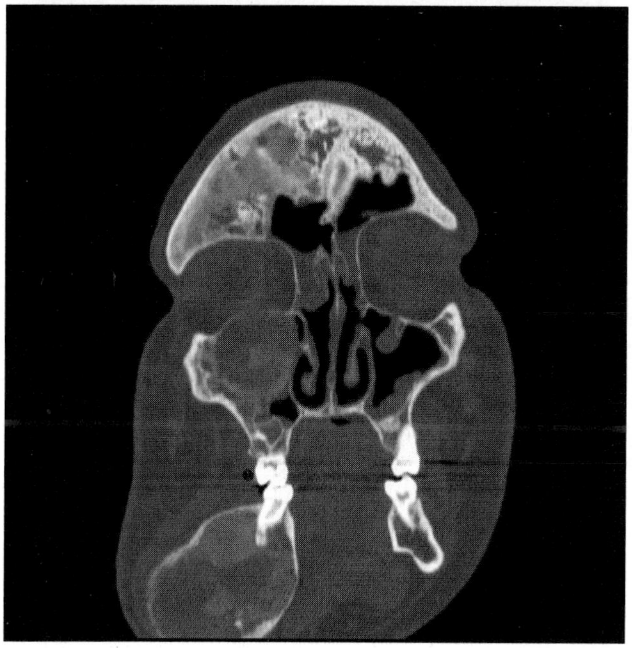

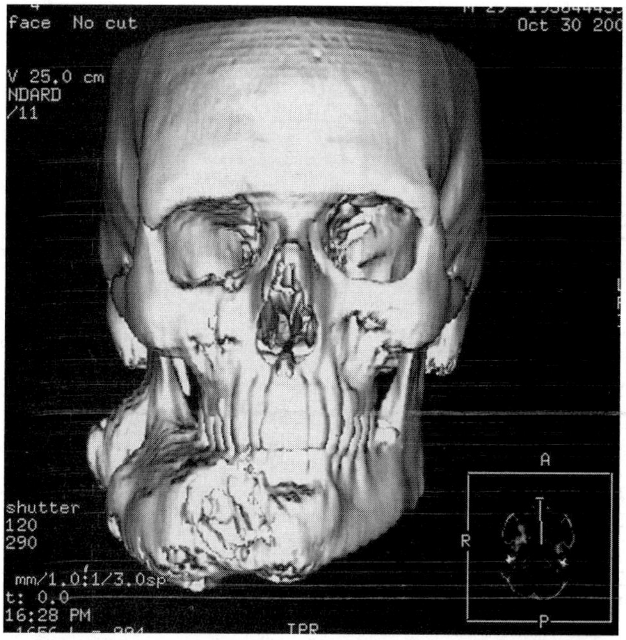

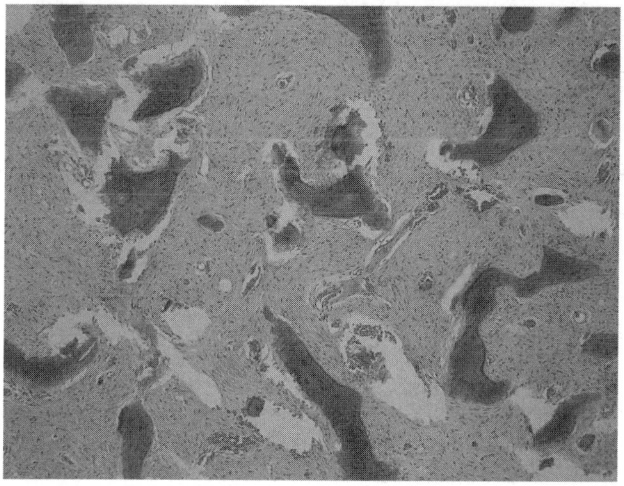

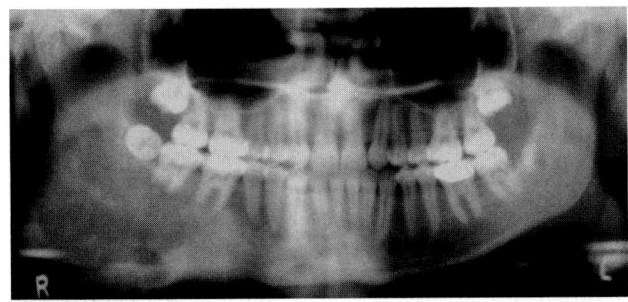

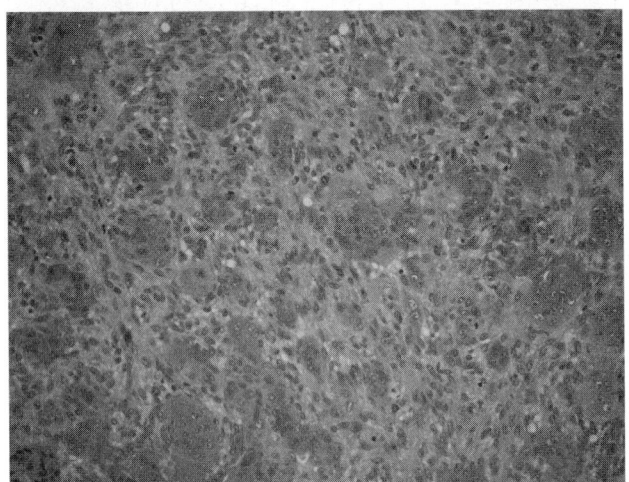

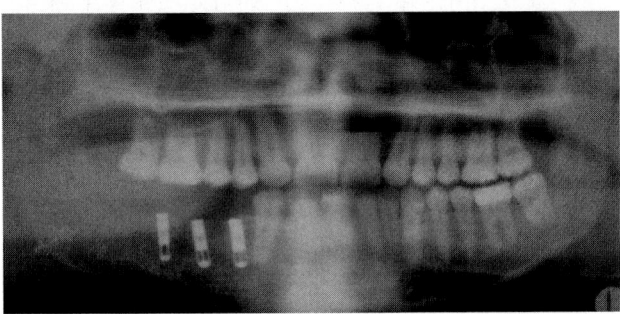

Figure 112.13 A: Central giant cell lesion. Panoramic radiograph demonstrating expansive ill-defined lesion at right angle of mandible. Patient noticed a gradually increasing swelling over the right mandible while her occlusion was shifting to the left. **B:** Central giant cell lesion. Numerous multinucleated giant cells in a background of plump, primitive mesenchymal cells. Abundant hemorrhage is seen throughout. **C:** Postoperative panoramic radiograph reveals reconstruction with an iliac crest bone graft. Endosseous implants were placed 7 months after initial graft. (See also Color Plate 50.)

of nuclei are dispersed throughout a background of spindled mesenchymal cells. The lesion is unencapsulated and fibrous tissue is also present to varying degrees (see Fig. 112.13B). Immunologic studies support the biologic behavior and notion that these giant cells represent osteoclasts. Microscopically, the CGCT is identical to several other conditions affecting the jaws, including cherubism, the Brown tumor of hyperparathyroidism, and focal areas of fibrous dysplasia. Thus, it is prudent to rule out these similar lesions if the clinical features suggest that the lesion may be something other than a CGCL.

Treatment and Prognosis

Curettage is usually curative, but recurrent or larger lesions occasionally require resection (Fig. 112.13C). Recurrence becomes an issue if the lesion is associated with difficult removal—attachment to multiple roots or neurovascular structures or larger, more vascular lesions. Several nonsurgical therapies have been reported with some degree of success. Intralesional steroid injections using triamcinolone (10 mg/mL) weekly for 6 weeks is advocated by some as a first line of therapy (29). Another reported injectable therapy is calcitonin (30). The precise mechanism of action of calcitonin on the giant cell tumor is unknown, but the giant cells have been shown to have calcitonin receptors and calcitonin somehow interferes with the progression of the tumor.

Aneurysmal Bone Cyst

The aneurysmal bone cyst (ABC) is a rare, expansile osteolytic bone lesion. It contains large blood-filled spaces that do not have an endothelial lining and, thus, is not a true cyst.

Clinical and Radiographic Features

The ABC, which commonly occurs in the first three decades of life, has a predilection for the posterior portions of the jaws. The lesions present as firm swellings that can be diffuse. Radiographically, ABC are expansile radiolucencies that can displace teeth.

Histopathology

The large blood-filled spaces are separated by connective tissue septae. Hemosiderin, bone, and osteoid can be found within the septae. Osteoclast-type, multinucleated giant cells, similar to those found in the CGCL, comprise a common feature at the periphery of the lesion.

Treatment and Prognosis

The ABC is managed by curettage, and intraoperative bleeding can become a challenge.

Vascular Malformations

Vascular malformations are developmental lesions that can affect soft tissue or bone. They do not present at birth as do hemangiomas, which are actual neoplasms. Vascular malformations can be broadly classified as either arterial (high-flow) or venous (low-flow) malformations. Arteriovenous fistulas can also be considered high-flow lesions.

Clinical and Radiographic Features

Most vascular malformations within the jaws present as slow-growing, asymptomatic, expansile lesions (31). The associated teeth become clinically mobile and can even appear elevated. Thrills or bruits can be detectable on physical examination. When the tongue is involved, lingual veins become distended. Vascular malformations take on a variable radiographic appearance. Some appear as well-circumscribed radiolucencies, whereas others appear as more mixed radiolucent–radiopaque. Tooth roots can be resorbed under high-flow lesions. A computed tomography (CT) scan or magnetic resonance imaging (MRI) should be obtained to aid in ascertaining the extent of the lesion, and angiography is performed to assist in determining the primary vascular inflow and the presence of any contralateral vascular contributions.

Histopathology
Tortuous endothelial-lined, dilated vessels comprise the microscopic appearance of this condition. Adjacent smaller feeding vessels can also be seen in some cases.

Treatment and Prognosis
Any radiolucent lesion of the jaw, which might be clinically considered a vascular malformation, requires needle aspiration before biopsy or surgery to rule out this condition. Arterial malformations are treated with preoperative selective embolization followed by resection surgery. Embolization is performed to limit the blood flow to the lesion to minimize blood loss when the lesion is excised. A variety of materials can be used to embolize these lesions: coils, polyvinyl alcohol beads, or 100% alcohol (33). Overaggressive embolization must be avoided to prevent ischemic necrosis and sloughing of tissues. Hypotensive anesthesia can also be used to further reduce intraoperative bleeding. Venous malformations can be treated with intralesional injections with coils or sclerosing agents. If adequate thrombosis is achieved, the lesion can be curettaged.

CONCLUSION

Collectively, odontogenic cysts and tumors do not occur with considerable frequency. Many of these lesions are amenable to surgical enucleation and curettage. Some of the cysts and tumors possess locally aggressive behavior and are capable of much tissue distortion and destruction. Thus, they present great challenges regarding their treatment and ultimate reconstruction, and long-term follow-up is advisable for many of these lesions because of recurrence potential.

HIGHLIGHTS

- The most common inflammatory cyst is the radicular cyst. Treatment is tooth extraction and enucleation.
- The dentigerous cyst is associated with the crown of an unerupted tooth.
- The basal cell nevus syndrome, an autosomal dominant condition, can manifest with multiple odontogenic keratocysts.

- Ameloblastoma, the most common odontogenic tumor, requires resection with a clear margin when it grows into soft tissue.
- Tori require removal only if they impair function or the use of a prosthesis.
- Asymptomatic osteoma need not be removed. Multiple osteoma may be an indication of Gardner syndrome.
- Ossifying fibroma, a benign tumor, is amenable to curettage or resection with a close margin.
- Fibrous dysplasia is not a neoplasm. Surgery is indicated in cases of disfiguration. Recontouring may be appropriate.
- Aneurysmal bone cyst is not a true cyst. Curettage is effective.

REFERENCES

1. Daley TD, Wysocki GP, Pringle GA. Relative incidence of odontogenic tumors and oral and jaw cysts in a Canadian population. *Oral Surg* 1994;77:276–280.
2. Sapp JP, Eversole LR, Wysocki GP, eds. *Contemporary oral and maxillofacial pathology.* St. Louis: Mosby-Year Book, 1997.
3. Regezi JA, Sciubba J, eds. *Oral pathology-clinical-pathological correlations,* 3rd ed. Philadelphia: WB Saunders.
4. Pogrel MA, Schmidt BL, eds. The odontogenic keratocyst. *Oral Maxillofac Surg Clin N Am* 15(3):311–461.
5. Crowley TE, Kaugars GE, Gunsolley JC. Odontogenic keratocysts: a clinical and histologic comparison of the parakeratin and orthokeratin variants. *J Oral Maxillofac Surg* 1992;50:22–26.
6. Gorlin FJ. Nevoid basal cell carcinoma syndrome. *Medicine* 1987;66:98–113.
7. Woolgar JA, Rippin JW, Browne RM. The odontogenic keratocyst and its occurrence in the nevoid basal cell carcinoma syndrome. *Oral Surg Oral Med Oral Pathol* 1987;64:727–730.
8. Buchner A. The central (intraosseous) calcifying odontogenic cyst: an analysis of 215 cases. *J Oral Maxillofac Surg* 1991;49:330–339.
9. Ramer M, Montazem A, Lane SL, et al. Glandular odontogenic cyst: report of a case and review of the literature. *Oral Surg* 1997;84:54–57.
10. Swanson KS, Kaugars GE, Gunsolley JC. Nasopalatine duct cyst: an analysis of 334 cases. *J Oral Maxillofac Surg* 1991;49:268–271.
11. Stafne EC. Bone cavities situated near the angle of the mandible. *J Am Dent Assoc* 1942;29:1969–1972.
12. Budnick SD. Compound and complex odontomas. *Oral Surg* 1976;42:501–506.
13. Ueno S, Nakamura S, Mushimoto K, et al. A clinicopathologic study of ameloblastoma. *J Oral Maxillofac Surg* 1986;44:361–365.
14. Gardner DG. A pathologist's approach to the treatment of ameloblastoma. *J Oral Maxillofac Surg* 1984;42:161–166.
15. Gardner DG, Pecak AMJ. The treatment of ameloblastoma based on pathologic and anatomic principles. *Cancer* 1980;46:2514–2519.
16. Marx RE, Stern D, eds. *Oral and maxillofacial pathology: a rationale for diagnosis and treatment.* Chicago: Quintessence Publishing, 2003.
17. Poulson RC, Greer RO. Adenomatoid odontogenic tumor: clinicopathologic and ultrastructural concepts. *J Oral Maxillofac Surg* 1983;41:818–824.
18. Franklin CD, Pindborg JJ. The calcifying epithelial odontogenic tumor: a review and analysis of 113 cases. *Oral Surg* 1976;42:753–765.
19. White DK, Chen SY, Mohnac AM, et al. Odontogenic myxoma: a clinical and ultrastructural study. *Oral Surg* 1975;39:901–917.

20. Carlson ER. Odontogenic cysts and tumors. In: Miloro M, ed. *Peterson's principles of oral and maxillofacial surgery,* 2nd ed. Hamilton, Ontario: BC Decker Inc., 2004.

21. Takeuchi T, Takenoshita Y, Kubo K, et al. Natural course of jaw lesions in patients with familial adenomatosis coli (Gardner's syndrome). *Int J Oral Maxillofac Surg* 1993;22: 226–230.

22. Vezeau PJ, Fridrich KL, Vincent SD. Osteochondroma of the mandibular condyle: literature review and report of two atypical cases. *J Oral Maxillofac Surg* 1995;53:954–963.

23. Eversole LR, Leider AS, Nelson K. Ossifying fibroma: a clinico-pathologic study of sixty-four cases. *Oral Surg Oral Med Oral Pathol* 1985;60:505–511.

24. Bolger WE, Ross AT. McCune-Albright syndrome: a case report and review of the literature. *Int J Pediatr Otorhinolaryngol* 2002;65: 69–74.

25. Chen YR, Noordhoff MS. Treatment of craniomaxillofacial fi-brous dysplasia: how early and how extensive. *Plast Reconstr Surg* 1990;86:835–844.

26. Tanner HC Jr, Dahlin DC, Childs DS Jr. Sarcoma complicating fi-brous dysplasia. Probable role of radiation therapy. *Oral Surg Oral Med Oral Pathol* 1961;14:837–846.

27. Chuong R, Kaban LB, Kozakewich H, et al. Central giant cell le-sions of the jaws: a clinicopathologic study. *J Oral Maxillofac Surg* 1986;44:708–713.

28. Ficarra G, Kaban LB, Hansen LS. Central giant cell lesions of the mandible and maxilla: a clinicopathologic and cytometric study. *Oral Surg Oral Med Oral Pathol* 1987;64:44–49.

29. Kermer C, Millesi W, Watzke IM. Local injection of cortico-steroids for central giant cell granuloma. A case report. *Int J Oral Maxillofac Surg* 1994;23:366–368.

30. deLange J, Rosenberg AJ, van den Akker HP, et al. Treatment of central giant cell granuloma of the jaws with calcitonin. *Int J Oral Maxillofac Surg* 1999;28:372–376.

31. Kaban LB, Mulliken JB. Vascular anomalies of the maxillofacial region. *J Oral Maxillofac Surg* 1986;44:203–213.

32. Perrott D, Schmidt B, Dowd C, et al. Treatment of a high-flow arteriovenous malformation by direct puncture and coil embolization. *J Oral Maxillofac Surg* 1994;52:1083–1086.

Neck Dissection

113

Jesus E. Medina

ANATOMY

Any statements about head and neck oncologic surgery must encompass a working knowledge of the anatomy of the vascular supply of the skin of the neck and the anatomic characteristics and relationships of certain structures that are commonly dealt with in the course of performing a neck dissection.

Vascular Supply to the Skin of the Neck

To avoid complications such as wound breakdown, skin flap necrosis, and exposure of the carotid artery after neck dissection, the incisions must be placed properly and the surgeon must be mindful of the vascular anatomy of the skin flaps to be created.

The skin of the anterior lateral aspect of the neck is supplied by descending branches of the facial, submental, and occipital arteries and by ascending branches of the transverse cervical and suprascapular artery (Fig. 113.1). After the platysma is pierced, these arterial branches anastomose, forming a superficial network of vessels that runs predominantly in a vertical direction. Although some or all the main arteries or their perforating branches may be ligated or divided during a neck dissection, the superficial, predominantly vertical, vascular plexus must remain intact to ensure adequate blood supply to the skin flaps.

Studies have shown that the incisions most likely to safeguard the blood supply to the skin flaps are the superiorly based apronlike incision from mastoid to mentum for combined neck dissection with intraoral procedures (Fig. 113.2A) and the apronlike incision used when a neck dissection is performed in conjunction with a laryngectomy (Fig. 113.2B).

The Y incision and the double-Y incision jeopardize the blood supply to the inferior and middle skin flaps, respectively, and suffer from placing a trifurcate incision over the carotid artery (Fig. 113.2, C and D). The modification of the Schobinger incision creates a long anterior medial flap, the tip of which may necrose as a result of the limited ascending blood supply (Fig. 113.2E). The MacFee double transverse incision transects the ascending and descending blood supply to the central part of the flap (Fig. 113.2F). This flap, however, usually fares well even in the previously irradiated patient.

Platysma Muscle

Located in the anterolateral aspect of the neck, the platysma is a wide, quadrangular, sheetlike muscle extending obliquely from the upper chest to the lower face. This muscle is located immediately deep to the subcutaneous tissue and thus provides an easily identifiable plane to raise skin flaps during neck surgery. In most neck dissections, flaps are elevated by dissecting in a plane immediately deep to the platysma; however, when the extent of the disease is such that the platysma must be left attached to the specimen, flaps can be elevated easily in a plane immediately superficial to this muscle. The beginning head and neck surgeon must remember that because of its oblique direction, the platysma does not cover a variable inferiorly based triangle in the anterior aspect and most of the posterolateral aspect of the neck. Here, flaps must be elevated in a subcutaneous plane created by the surgeon. While making the incisions for a neck dissection and elevating the skin flaps in the superolateral aspect of the neck, it is also helpful to remember the relationships of the posterior border of the platysma, which is either slightly over or anterior to the external jugular vein and the greater auricular nerve.

Marginal Mandibular Branch of the Facial Nerve

Identifying the ramus mandibularis is essential to performing an adequate excision of the lymph nodes in the

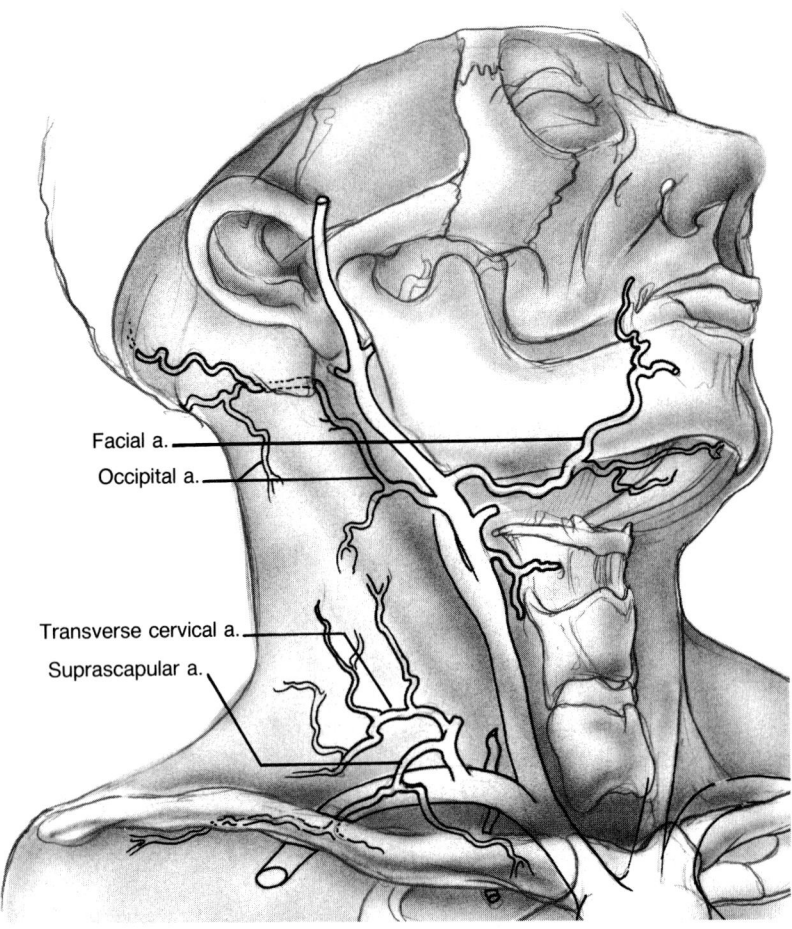

Facial a.
Occipital a.

Transverse cervical a.
Suprascapular a.

Figure 113.1 Vascular supply of the neck skin. (Adapted from Freelend AP, Rogers JH. The vascular supply of the cervical skin with reference to incision planning. *Laryngoscope* 1975;85:714, with permission.)

submandibular triangle. The practice of ligating the anterior facial vein low in the submandibular triangle and retracting it superiorly to "protect the ramus mandibularis" can also result in elevation of the prevascular and retrovascular lymph nodes, thus precluding their appropriate removal. When indicated, it is preferable to identify the nerve and thoroughly remove these lymph nodes.

The nerve can be identified about 1 cm in front of and below the angle of the mandible by incising the superficial layer of the deep cervical fascia that envelops the submandibular gland, immediately above the gland, in a direction parallel to the direction of the nerve. The incised fascia then is gently pushed superiorly, exposing the nerve that lies deep to it but superficial to the adventitia of the anterior facial vein. The submandibular retrovascular lymph nodes are usually near the nerve and must be carefully dissected away from it. As this is done, the facial vessels are exposed and can be divided.

Spinal Accessory Nerve

Below the jugular foramen, the external branch of the spinal accessory nerve is located medial to the digastric and stylohyoid muscles and lateral or immediately posterior to the internal jugular vein (IJV). Occasionally, the

uppermost portion of the nerve is posterior-medial to the vein. Then it runs obliquely downward and backward to reach the medial surface of the sternocleidomastoid muscle near the junction of its superior and middle thirds (two to three finger breadths below the tip of the mastoid). Although the nerve can continue its downward course entirely medial to the muscle (18%), more commonly it traverses it and appears in the posterior border of it (82%) (1). At this point the nerve is located above the point where the greater auricular nerve turns around the posterior border of the SCM, also known as Erbs point. The mean distance between Erb point and the spinal accessory nerve is 10.7 mm, SD ± 6.3. In all cases, the accessory nerve is above Erb point (2). From here it runs through the posterior triangle of the neck and crosses the anterior border of the trapezius muscle. The mean distance between this point and the clavicle has been measured at 51.3 mm, SD ± 17 (2). Two anatomic characteristics of this portion of the nerve are relevant in the course of a neck dissection. First, the nerve does not enter the trapezius muscle as it reaches the anterior border of it but courses along the deep surface of the muscle in close relationship with the transverse cervical vessels. Therefore, isolating the nerve to the level of the anterior border of the trapezius does not ensure its preservation during

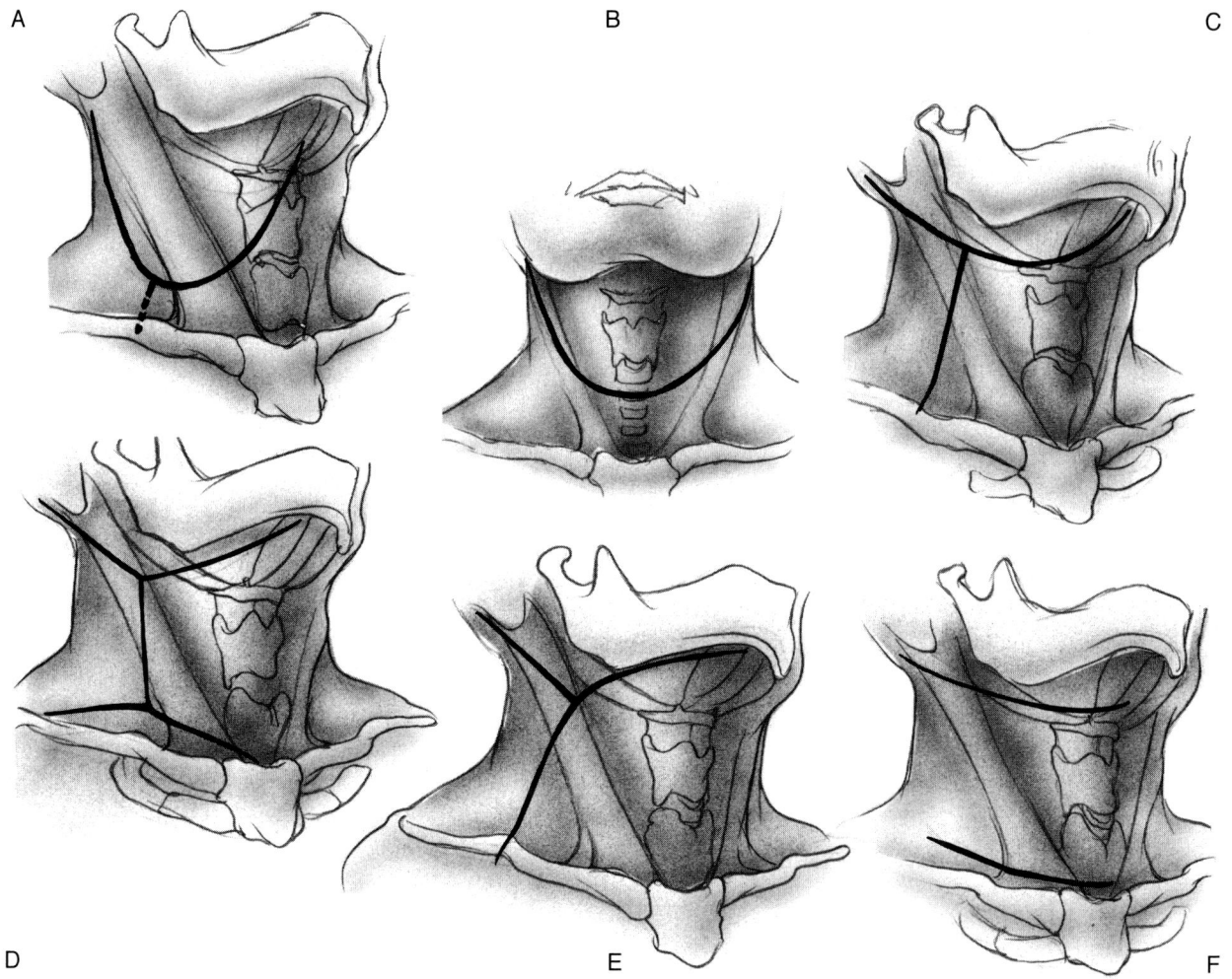

Figure 113.2 Neck dissection incisions. **A:** Latyschevsky and Freund. **B:** Freund. **C:** Crile. **D:** Martin. **E:** Babcock and Conley. **F:** MacFee.

surgical dissection below this point, particularly in a bloody operative field. Second, the spinal accessory nerve is located rather superficially as it courses through the middle and low posterior triangle of the neck, and it can be easily injured while elevating the posterior skin flaps.

Nerve to the Levator Scapulae Muscle

The levator scapulae is a triangular muscle located deep in the lateral aspect of the neck, anterior and medial to the splenius capitis muscle. It extends from the superior angle and the spine of the scapula to the transverse process of the atlas and the next three cervical vertebrae. Because one of the functions of this muscle is to draw the scapula and the shoulder upward and medially, inadvertent or unnecessary resection of the nerves to the levator during a radical neck dissection (RND) may add to the resulting deformity and functional disability of the shoulder. The levator scapulae is innervated by two or three branches of the fourth and fifth cervical nerves. From their origin in the cervical plexus,

these nerves run in an inferior and lateral direction to reach the levator in its middle third. Through most of their course, these short nerves are located deep to the fascia of the levator. Therefore, to identify and preserve them during a RND, the plane of dissection in this area of the neck must be kept superficial to the fascia of the levator.

Thoracic Duct

At the base of the neck, the thoracic duct is located to the right of and behind the left common carotid artery and the vagus nerve. From here, it arches upward, forward, and laterally, passing behind the IJV and in front of the anterior scalene muscle and the phrenic nerve. It then opens into the IJV, the subclavian vein, or the angle formed by the junction of these two vessels. The duct is anterior and medial to the thyrocervical trunk and the transverse cervical artery. Precise knowledge of these anatomic relationships is important to avoid injuring the duct during a neck dissection. It is even more important when the surgeon is called on to search for and repair a chyle leak during or after a neck dissection. To prevent a chyle leak, the surgeon also must remember that the thoracic duct may be multiple in its upper end and that at the base of the neck it usually receives a jugular, a subclavian, and usually other minor lymphatic trunks, which must be ligated or clipped individually.

Fascial Compartments of the Neck

The deep cervical fascia of the neck is divided into three layers: superficial, middle, and deep (Fig. 113.3). The superficial or investing layer surrounds the entire neck. It arises from the vertebral spinous processes and the ligamentum nuchae and encircles the entire neck to attach itself again to the spinous processes on the opposite side. This fascia divides to enclose the trapezius muscle. At the anterior border of this muscle, the two layers fuse into a single layer that crosses the posterior triangle of the neck. It divides again to surround the inferior belly of the omohyoid muscle and the sternomastoid muscle. At the lateral border of the strap muscles, it sends fibers between them before fusing in front of them as it extends onto the other side of the neck. This fascia also envelops the submandibular and parotid glands.

The middle layer of the deep cervical fascia, also called the visceral fascia, surrounds the visceral structures of the anterior portion of the neck. The deep layer of the deep cervical fascia or prevertebral fascia surrounds the deep muscles of the neck. Among them, it covers the splenius capitis, the levator scapulae, and the scalene muscles. It extends onto the other side of the neck, covering the prevertebral muscles.

The carotid sheath encircling the jugular vein, common carotid artery, and vagus nerve is formed by all layers of the deep cervical fascia. The carotid sheath originates superiorly at the jugular foramen, where it attaches to the skull base. It then follows the course of the vessels, traversing the anterior cervical triangle and extending inferiorly into the thoracic inlet.

Lymphatics of the Neck

The lymph node regions of the neck are shown in Figure 113.4. The six levels currently used encompass the complete topographic anatomy of the neck. The concept of sublevels has been introduced into the classification because certain zones have been identified within the six levels, which may have clinical significance.

Level I is divided in two sublevels. Sublevel IA (submental), which includes the lymph nodes within the triangle bound by the anterior belly of the digastric muscles and the hyoid bone. Sublevel IB (submandibular), which includes the lymph nodes within the boundaries of the anterior belly of the digastric muscle, the stylohyoid muscle, and the inferior border of the body of the mandible.

Level II (upper jugular) includes the lymph nodes located around the upper third of the IJV and adjacent spinal accessory nerve extending from the level of the skull base (above) to the level of the inferior border of the hyoid bone (below). The anterior (medial) boundary is the stylohyoid muscle (the radiologic correlate is the vertical plane defined by the posterior surface of the submandibular gland) and the posterior (lateral) boundary is the posterior border of the sternocleidomastoid muscle. Two sublevels are recognized in level II: sublevel IIA: nodes located anterior (medial) to the vertical plane defined by the spinal accessory nerve; and sublevel IIB: nodes located posterior (lateral) to the vertical plane defined by the spinal accessory nerve.

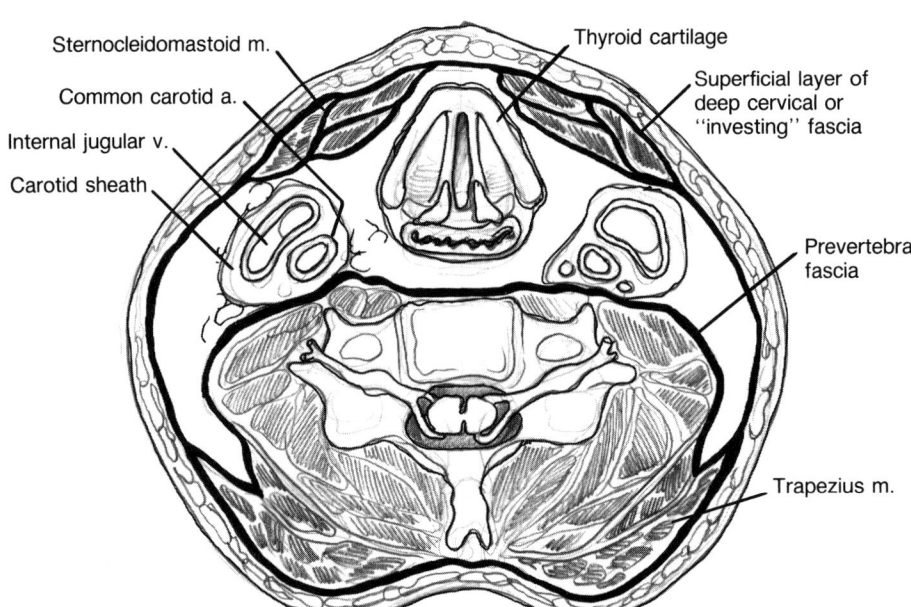

Figure 113.3 Layers of the cervical fascia.

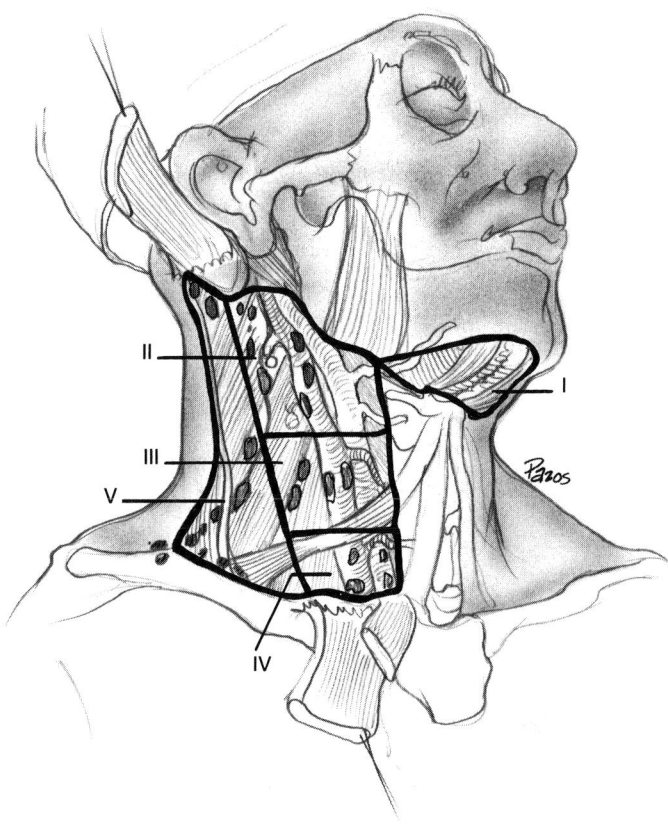

Figure 113.4 Lymph node regions of the neck.

Level III (midjugular) includes the lymph nodes located around the middle third of the IJV extending from the inferior border of the hyoid bone (above) to the inferior border of the cricoid cartilage (below). The anterior (medial) boundary is the lateral border of the sternohyoid muscle, and the posterior (lateral) boundary is the posterior border of the sternocleidomastoid muscle.

Level IV (lower jugular) encompasses the lymph nodes located around the lower third of the IJV extending from the inferior border of the cricoid cartilage (above) to the clavicle below.

Level V (posterior triangle) comprised predominantly of the lymph nodes located along the lower half of the spinal accessory nerve and the transverse cervical artery. The supraclavicular nodes are also included in posterior triangle group. The superior boundary is the apex formed by convergence of the sternocleidomastoid and trapezius muscles, the inferior boundary is the clavicle, the anterior (medial) boundary is the posterior border of the sternocleidomastoid muscle, and the posterior (lateral) boundary is the anterior border of the trapezius muscle. A horizontal plane marking the inferior border of the anterior cricoid arch separates two sublevels. Sublevel V-A, above this plane, includes the spinal accessory nodes. Sublevel V-B, below this plane, includes the nodes that follow the transverse cervical vessels and the supraclavicular nodes (with the exception of Virchow node, which is located in level IV).

Level VI (anterior compartment) Lymph nodes in this compartment include the pre- and paratracheal nodes, precricoid (Delphian) node, and the perithyroidal nodes including the lymph nodes along the recurrent laryngeal nerves. The superior boundary is the hyoid bone, the inferior boundary is the suprasternal notch, and the lateral boundaries are the common carotid arteries.

Other lymph node groups: Lymph nodes involving regions not located within these levels should be referred to by the name of their specific nodal group; examples of these are the superior mediastinum, the retropharyngeal, the periparotid, the buccinator, the postauricular, and the suboccipital lymph nodes.

PHYSIOLOGY

The trapezius is a fan-shaped muscle composed of upper, middle, and lower segments, each of which functions in a different but complementary manner. The trapezius and the other muscles that insert on the scapula stabilize and control the shoulder girdle during arm movement. The levator scapulae acts synergistically with the upper division of the trapezius to elevate the scapula; the rhomboid assists the middle part of the trapezius in retracting and stabilizing the scapula against the posterior thoracic cage. The simultaneous action of the upper and lower divisions of the trapezius muscle results in a unique rotatory action of the scapula. The upward rotation of the scapula, in combination with abduction of the arm at the glenohumeral joint, permits elevation of the arm beyond 90 degrees at the shoulder level.

Paralysis of the trapezius muscle causes a syndrome characterized by weakness and deformity of the shoulder girdle, usually accompanied by pain. The scapula is displaced inferiorly and laterally, and the entire shoulder girdle frequently drops. It also impairs the normal rotation of the scapula, restricting abduction of the affected shoulder beyond 90 degrees. The shoulder pain appears to be secondary to increased supportive demands on and strain of the levator scapulae and rhomboid muscles. Understandably, a greater degree of shoulder disability may result from a RND when the nerves to the levator scapulae muscle are severed.

DIAGNOSTIC EVALUATION

Clinical examination of the neck by palpation is not uniformly reliable in the detection of cervical lymph node metastases, particularly of lymph nodes minimally involved by tumor. The reported error rate in assessing the presence or absence of cervical lymph node metastases by palpation ranges from 20% to 51%. The factors responsible for this variation are not only the ability and experience of the examiner but also the patient's habitus and previous treatment to the neck with surgery or radiation therapy. With the advent of modern imaging techniques, it was hoped that the clinician would not have to rely solely on clinical examination to make therapeutic decisions in the treatment of the neck.

Using the histologic demonstration of metastasis in a lymph node as the gold standard, several studies have shown that computed tomography (CT), magnetic resonance imaging (MRI), and ultrasonography have a higher sensitivity and specificity than clinical examination in the detection of metastases in lymph nodes larger than 1 to 1.5 cm in diameter (3,4). Currently, these imaging techniques are not used universally in the diagnostic evaluation and staging of the neck in head and neck cancer patients; however, they do have a role in the evaluation of lymph nodes that are not easily accessible to the hands of the examiner, such as the retropharyngeal, upper mediastinal, and, in some patients, the paratracheal lymph nodes.

At the present time, a "negative" CT or MRI of the neck cannot be relied upon to withhold elective treatment of the cervical lymph nodes because they cannot detect lymph nodes smaller than 1 cm and, more importantly, because the imaging criteria to diagnose metastasis in a lymph node are not reliable. The criterion most often used to consider a cervical node positive for metastasis on CT or MRI is size of a node larger than 1 or 1.5 cm. Although a correlation exists between the size of a lymph node and the presence of histologic metastasis (Table 113.1), it is clear that not all enlarged lymph nodes contain metastatic deposit and that nodes smaller than 1 or 1.5 cm indeed can contain metastases. Thirty-three percent of all metastases from squamous cell carcinomas of the head and neck are found in lymph nodes smaller than 1 cm, 10% of tumor-positive neck dissection specimens contain only metastases less than 3 mm in diameter, and, more importantly, 25% of all clinically occult lymph node metastases are too small to be detected by any of the currently available imaging techniques (5). The presence of a central area of lucency within a node shown on CT was at one time considered equivalent to the presence of necrotic tumor within a node; however, such a finding can be caused by an artery with plaque formation or a fatty inclusion in a lymph node. Another imaging criteria used to "diagnose" metastasis in a lymph node is the shape of the node, as determined by the ratio of its short (s) and long (l) axis diameters. In a study by Steinkamp et al. (6), 730 enlarged cervical lymph nodes in 285 patients were examined using

TABLE 113.1

NODAL SIZE AND PRESENCE OF HISTOLOGIC METASTASES

Node Size (cm)	Histologic Status (%)		
	Negative	Positive	Positive with Extranodal Extension
1	67	33	14
2	38	62	26
3	19	81	49
4	12	88	71
5	0	100	76

From Hamakawa H, Fukizumi M, Bao Y. Genetic diagnosis of micrometastasis based on SCCa antigen mRNA in cervical lymph nodes of head and neck cancer. *Clin Exp Med* 1999;17:593–599, and Cachin Y. Management of cervical nodes in head and neck cancer. In: Evans P, Robin P, Fielding J, eds. *Head and neck cancer.* New York: Alan R. Liss, 1983, with permission.

ultrasound, and the l/s ratio was calculated. Histologic examination after neck dissection revealed that 95% of the enlarged cervical nodes, shown on ultrasound to have an l/s ratio of more than 2, were correctly diagnosed as benign. Nodes presenting with a more circular shape and an l/s ratio of less than 2 were diagnosed correctly as metastases with 95% accuracy. Unfortunately, multidirectional ultrasonography scanning is also hindered by the lack of specificity of morphologic criteria. Ultrasound-guided fine-needle aspiration cytology (US-FNAB) appeared more promising for the preoperative evaluation of the N0 neck because this technique enables sampling of lymph nodes as small as 3 mm in diameter and adds the advantages of cytologic evaluation (7). However, the usefulness of this technique is strongly dependent on the skill (and time) of the ultrasonographer and on the experience of the cytopathologist. Furthermore, the outcomes of a wait and see policy after negative US-FNAB have been disappointing. In a study of 92 patients with tumors of the oral cavity, staged T1 and T2, who were observed after a negative US-FNAB, metastases in neck nodes became apparent subsequently in 19 (21%) (8). This figure is troubling because the incidence of lymph node metastases in patients with such tumors, who are observed without any intervention to the neck, is about 25%.

Using 18-fluorodeoxyglucose (FDG) positron emission tomography (PET), lymph node metastases of squamous cell carcinomas of the oral cavity can be visualized with a sensitivity and specificity higher than MRI and CT. Unfortunately, current FDG-PET techniques are also limited for the detection of tumor foci smaller than 1 cm (9,10).

In an effort to overcome the limitations of current imaging techniques, particularly their inability to differentiate a tumor infiltrated lymph node from a normal or a reactive one, de Bree et al. (11) have recently experimented with radioimmunoscintigraphy (RIS), a technique in which squamous cell carcinoma specific monoclonal antibodies labeled with Technetium 99m were given intravenously to patients with squamous cell carcinoma who underwent neck dissection. Unfortunately, RIS was not superior to CT and MRI for the detection of lymph node metastases (11).

CT and MRI are valuable for the assessment of resectability of large metastatic deposits in the neck, because in most instances they can define the relationship of a metastatic tumor with critical structures, such as the common and the internal carotid artery, the cervical spine, the vertebral artery, and the brachial plexus. If tumor involvement of the common or the internal carotid artery is suspected, a systematic preoperative evaluation should include four-vessel cerebral angiography to determine the status of the contralateral carotid and to assess collateral intracerebral circulation. In addition, an attempt should be made during the angiography to measure carotid back pressure and to assess dynamically the collateral circulation by using balloon occlusion techniques while monitoring the patient for evidence of neurologic deficits under normotensive and hypotensive conditions.

Fine-Needle Aspiration

Fine-needle aspiration (FNA) has become a valuable diagnostic tool in patients with a mass in the neck in whom metastatic carcinoma is suspected. According to numerous recent reports, the specificity of FNA ranges from 94% to 100% and the sensitivity ranges from 92% to 98%. The interobserver variability between cytopathologists in one series has been reported as 8%. FNA has been found to be most accurate in the diagnosis of epithelial malignancies, achieving nearly 100% accuracy.

FNA is indicated in the patient with a solid mass in the neck when a thorough examination of the mucosal surfaces and skin of the head and neck region fails to reveal a primary tumor. FNA and a chest radiograph should constitute part of the initial evaluation of the patient with a supraclavicular mass. The cytopathology findings then can guide the clinician's search for a primary tumor below the clavicles.

Sentinel Node Biopsy

During the past decade, a number of studies from different institutions have shown that lymphoscintigraphy is feasible and reliable for the identification of the "sentinel" node or nodes in patients with squamous cell carcinoma of the upper aerodigestive tract. This technique, combined with biopsy of the sentinel nodes, may be ideal for the staging evaluation of the clinically node-negative (N0) neck. The number of sentinel nodes varies, but in a series of 48 patients studied by Ross et al. (12), the mean number of sentinel nodes harvested was 2.4. The sensitivity of the procedure is 90% when the histopathology of the sentinel node is compared with that of the neck dissection specimen. In another prospective study by Ross et al. (13), sentinel node biopsy (SNB) resulted in pathologic upstaging of the clinically N0 neck in 36% of the patients when the nodes were examined with routine hematoxylin-eosin staining; serial sectioning and immunohistochemistry upstaged an additional 8% of the cases. The detection of micrometastases can be further enhanced by using highly specific tumor markers and molecular methods (14,15). However, the applicability of these techniques in clinical practice and the prognostic and therapeutic significance of the micrometastases detected by them remains to be demonstrated in prospective clinical studies.

STAGING

At completion of the clinical evaluation of a patient with squamous cell carcinoma of the head and neck region, the disease should be classified according to stage. The staging system proposed by the American Joint Committee on Cancer in 2002 is outlined as follows:

NX: Regional lymph nodes cannot be assessed.

N0: No regional lymph node metastasis.

N1: Metastasis in a single ipsilateral lymph node, 3 cm or less in greatest dimension.

N2: Metastasis in a single ipsilateral lymph node, more than 3 cm but not more than 6 cm in greatest dimension; or in multiple ipsilateral lymph nodes, none more than 6 cm in greatest dimension; or in bilateral or contralateral lymph nodes, none more than 6 cm in greatest dimension.

N2a: Metastasis in a single ipsilateral lymph node more than 3 cm but not more than 6 cm in greatest dimension.

N2b: Metastasis in multiple ipsilateral lymph nodes, none more than 6 cm in greatest dimension.

N2c: Metastasis in bilateral or contralateral nodes no more than 6 cm in greatest dimension.

N3: Metastasis in a lymph node more than 6 cm in greatest dimension.

Staging of the neck in nasopharyngeal carcinoma patients is different because the distribution and the prognostic impact of regional lymph node spread from nasopharynx cancer, particularly of the undifferentiated type, is different from that of other head and neck mucosal cancers and justifies the use of the following scheme:

NX: Regional lymph nodes cannot be assessed.

N0: No regional lymph node metastasis.

N1: Unilateral metastasis in lymph node(s), 6 cm or less in greatest dimension, above the supraclavicular fossa.

N2: Bilateral metastasis in lymph node(s), 6 cm or less in greatest dimension, above the supraclavicular fossa.

N3: Metastasis in a lymph node(s) > 6 cm and/or to supraclavicular fossa.

N3a: Greater than 6 cm in dimension.

N3b: Extension to the supraclavicular fossa.

CLASSIFICATION OF NECK DISSECTIONS

Several cervical lymph node dissections are currently used for the surgical treatment of the neck in patients with cancer of the head and neck region. To standardize the nomenclature used to refer to these operations, it is essential to adopt a common nomenclature for the lymph node groups of the neck , such as the one outlined earlier in this chapter.

The classification of neck dissections currently recommended by the American Academy of Otolaryngology-Head and Neck Surgery takes into account primarily the lymph node groups of the neck that are removed and secondarily the anatomic structures that may be preserved, such as the spinal accessory nerve and the IJV. If the different neck dissections are analyzed from these two points of view, there are essentially three anatomic types of neck dissections: radical and modified radical, selective, and extended. This new classification is essentially the same as the 1991 version with the exception that specific names for certain types of selective neck dissection (SND) have been deleted. The rationale for this recommendation is based on the increased number of variations, which have been introduced over the past decade. A comparison of the two classifications is shown in Table 113.2.

Regardless of what name a neck dissection is given, the operative record must reflect accurately what was done in surgery in terms of the lymph node groups that were removed and the important neural and vascular structures that were removed or preserved. Furthermore, the surgeon must orient the surgical specimen for the pathologist and identify the different lymph node groups it contains. Only then can the pathologist be expected to generate a clinically and prognostically meaningful report that describes the location and number of lymph nodes examined, the number of nodes that contain tumor, and the presence or absence of extranodal extension of tumor.

Radical Neck Dissection

This operation is defined as the *en bloc* removal of the lymph node-bearing tissues of one side of the neck, from

TABLE 113.2

CLASSIFICATION OF NECK DISSECTIONS

1991 Classification	2001 Classification
1. Radical neck dissection	1. Radical neck dissection
2. Modified radical neck dissection	2. Modified radical neck dissection
3. Selective neck dissection	3. Selective neck dissection (SND):
a) Supraomohyoid	SND (I–III/IV)
b) Lateral	SND (II–IV)
c) Posterolateral	SND (II–V, postauricular, suboccipital)
d) Anterior	SND (Level VI)
4. Extended neck dissection	4. Extended neck dissection

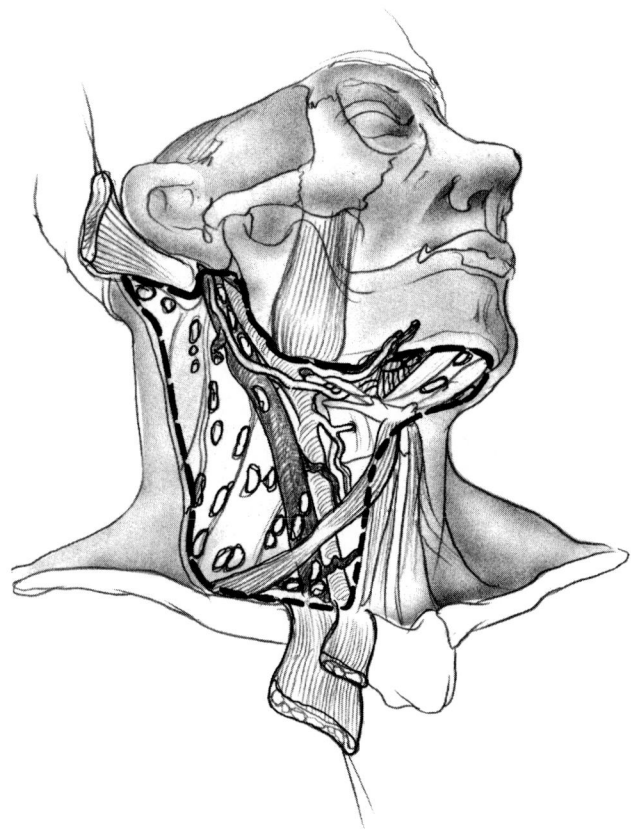

Figure 113.5 Radical neck dissection.

the inferior border of the mandible to the clavicle and from the lateral border of the strap muscles to the anterior border of the trapezius. Included in the resected specimen are the spinal accessory nerve, the IJV, and the sternocleidomastoid muscle (Fig. 113.5). A comprehensive description of the surgical technique of this operation was recently provided by McCammon and Shah (16).

Rationale

The first description of the systematic *en bloc* removal of the lymphatics of the neck was published by Crile in 1906. The operation he described came to be known as the RND. Although Crile believed that removing the IJV was essential because of the intimate relation of this structure with the lymph nodes of the neck, it is interesting to note that the drawings that illustrate his publication indicate that the spinal accessory nerve and the ansa hypoglossi were preserved. It was Martin et al. in the 1950s who championed the concept that a cervical lymphadenectomy for cancer was inadequate unless all the lymph node-bearing tissues of one side of the neck were removed and that this was impossible unless the spinal accessory nerve, the IJV, and the sternocleidomastoid muscle were included in the resection. In fact, they categorically stated "any technique that is designed to preserve the spinal accessory nerve should be condemned unequivocally."

In describing the RND, Crile contended that an *en bloc* removal of the primary tumor and the lymphatic system of the neck should be carried out in a manner similar to the Halstead operation for breast cancer. He believed that normal lymph flow is interrupted by metastasis in a lymph node, causing further tumor dissemination to occur in any direction and that a less radical "incomplete" operation would disseminate and stimulate the growth of tumor. Like Crile, Martin et al. believed that it was impossible to remove the lymphatics of the neck completely without resecting the sternocleidomastoid muscle and IJV because of the close association of the lymphatics in this area with the vein walls.

Removing the sternocleidomastoid muscle unquestionably facilitates access to the jugular vein and the removal of the lymph node-bearing tissues of the neck. In some instances, the muscle must be removed because it is involved by tumor. These considerations are as valid today as they were at the beginning of the 20th century in patients with clinically obvious lymph node metastases, particularly when the metastases are large and are located in multiple regions of the neck. However, removal of this muscle is no longer justified for ease or exposure alone.

An RND is not indicated in the absence of palpable cervical metastases (i.e., in the treatment of the N0 neck). The argument that the RND should continue to be the only dissection of the lymph nodes performed in patients with cancer of the head and neck, because it is an anatomically well-delineated operation and thus is easy to teach, is no longer valid. Currently, RNDs represent less than 20% of all neck dissections done at many institutions (17); as familiarity with the other types of neck dissection has increased so has the ability and willingness of surgeons to teach residents and fellows how to do them.

Indications

RND is indicated when there are multiple clinically obvious cervical lymph node metastases, particularly when they involve the lymph nodes of the posterior triangle of the neck and are found to involve or to be tightly related to the spinal accessory nerve. An RND is also indicated when there is a large metastatic tumor mass or when multiple matted nodes are present in the upper part of the neck. In such instances, it is unwise to preserve the sternocleidomastoid or the internal jugular or to dissect the spinal accessory nerve and risk entering the tumor. A similar situation can be created by the inflammation, hematoma, or ecchymosis that follow ill-advised excisional biopsies of neck metastases. For this reason, we often find ourselves performing a RND in such patients.

Modified Radical Neck Dissection (MRND)

This category includes modifications of the RNDs developed with the intention of reducing the morbidity of this operation by preserving one or more of these structures: the spinal accessory nerve, the IJV, or the sternocleidomastoid muscle.

The three neck dissections that can be included in this category are outlined in Table 113.2. They differ from each other only in the number of neural, vascular, and muscular structures that are preserved. Therefore, they can be subclassified as follows:

- MRND with preservation of the spinal accessory nerve
- MRND with preservation of the spinal accessory nerve and the IJV
- MRND with preservation of the spinal accessory nerve, the IJV, and the sternocleidomastoid muscle. This corresponds to the operation often called "functional neck dissection"

Modified Radical Neck Dissection with Preservation of the Spinal Accessory Nerve

This operation is defined as the *en bloc* removal of the lymph node-bearing tissues of one side of the neck, from the inferior border of the mandible to the clavicle and from the lateral border of the strap muscles to the anterior border of the trapezius, preserving the spinal accessory nerve. The IJV and the sternocleidomastoid muscle are included in the resected specimen (Fig. 113.6). The surgical technique is essentially the same as that of the RND.

Rationale. The following observations have compelled surgeons, for several decades, to explore and develop alternatives to the RND:

- The morbidity associated with the RND, especially the shoulder disability that results from the resection of the

spinal accessory nerve and, to a lesser extent, the cosmetic deformity that results from this operation, particularly when it is done on both sides of the neck
- The realization that in many instances the spinal accessory nerve is not in close proximity to the nodes grossly involved by tumor and that its preservation does not compromise the oncologic soundness of the operation.

Indications. This type of neck dissection is used in the surgical treatment of the neck of patients with clinically obvious lymph node metastases when the spinal accessory nerve is not directly involved by tumor, regardless of the number, size, and location of the involved lymph nodes. The decision to preserve the spinal accessory nerve is, therefore, a delicate intraoperative judgment call. Much like the philosophy about preservation of the facial nerve during surgery for parotid tumors, the spinal accessory nerve can be preserved whenever there is a clearly identifiable, not an artificially created, plane of dissection between the tumor and the nerve. The reported rate of recurrence in the neck when used for the treatment of the N+ neck in combination with postoperative radiation is 8.1% (18).

Modified Radical Neck Dissection with Preservation of the Spinal Accessory Nerve and the Internal Jugular Vein

In this type of dissection, the lymph node-bearing tissues of one side of the neck are removed *en bloc*, preserving the spinal accessory nerve and the IJV. This operation is seldom planned. It is done occasionally when in the course

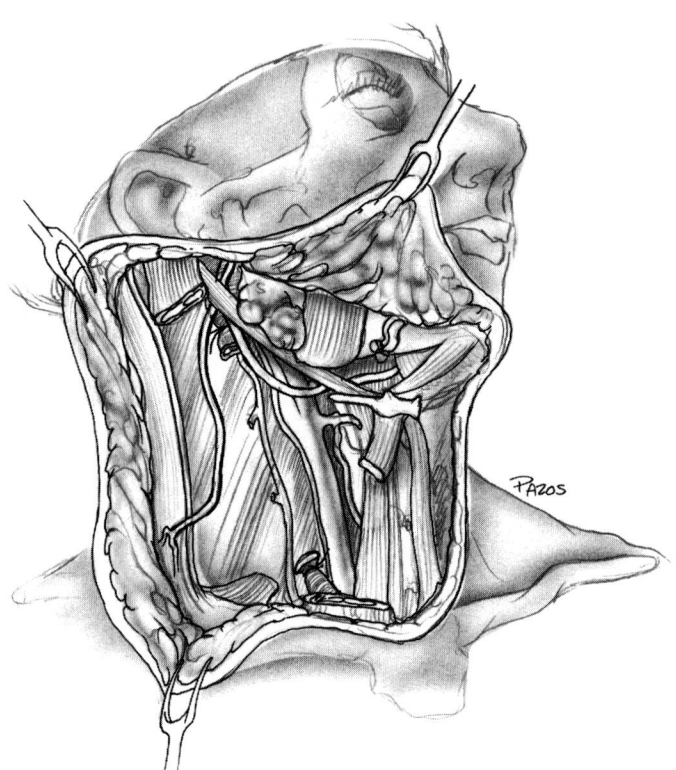

Figure 113.6 Modified radical neck dissection (type I) with preservation of the spinal accessory nerve.

of a neck dissection the metastatic tumor in the neck is noted to be adherent to the sternocleidomastoid muscle but away from the accessory nerve and the jugular vein. This situation occurs occasionally in patients with hypopharyngeal or laryngeal tumors with metastases under the middle third of the sternocleidomastoid muscle.

Modified Radical Neck Dissection with Preservation of the Spinal Accessory Nerve, the Internal Jugular Vein, and the Sternocleidomastoid Muscle

This operation consists of the *en bloc* removal of the lymph node-bearing tissues of one side of the neck, including lymph nodes levels I through V, preserving the spinal accessory nerve, the IJV, and the sternocleidomastoid muscle. The submandibular gland may or may not be removed (Fig. 113.7). A description of the operative technique of this operation, as it is currently advocated by most European surgeons, can be found in a recent publication by Gavilan (19).

Rationale. The muscular and vascular aponeurosis of the neck delimit compartments filled with fibroadipose tissue, and the lymphatic system of the neck, contained within these compartments, can be excised in an anatomic block by stripping the fascia off muscles and vessels. It should be pointed out, however, that, except for the vagus nerve contained within the carotid sheath, the nerves of the neck do not follow the aponeurotic compartment distribution. Whereas the phrenic nerve and the brachial plexus are par-

tially within a compartment, the hypoglossal and the spinal accessory nerves run across compartments. Unless these nerves are directly involved by tumor, they can be dissected free and preserved.

Indications. This operation is widely accepted, particularly in Europe, as the neck dissection of choice for the treatment of the N0 neck in patients with squamous cell carcinoma of the upper aerodigestive tract, especially when the primary tumor is in the larynx or hypopharynx. In those cases, the nodes in the submandibular triangle are at low risk of containing metastases and do not need to be removed. According to some surgeons, this operation is also indicated for the treatment of the N1 neck, when the metastatic nodes are mobile and no greater than 2.5 to 3 cm. The reported rates of recurrence in the neck with this type of neck dissection range between 0% and 16.6% for the clinically N0 neck and between 3.7% and 25% for the N+ neck (20–25).

This type of MRND is clearly the operation of choice for patients with differentiated carcinoma of the thyroid who have palpable lymph node metastases in the posterior triangle of the neck.

Selective Neck Dissections

The SND consists of the removal of only the lymph node groups at highest risk of containing metastases according to the location of the primary tumor, preserving the spinal

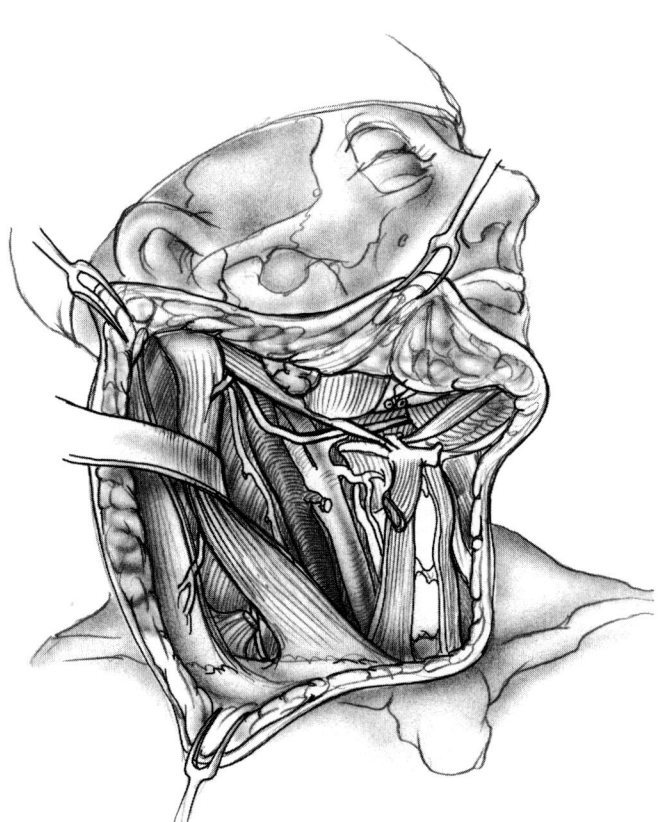

Figure 113.7 Modified radical neck dissection (type III) with preservation of the spinal accessory nerve, the internal jugular vein, and the sternocleidomastoid muscle.

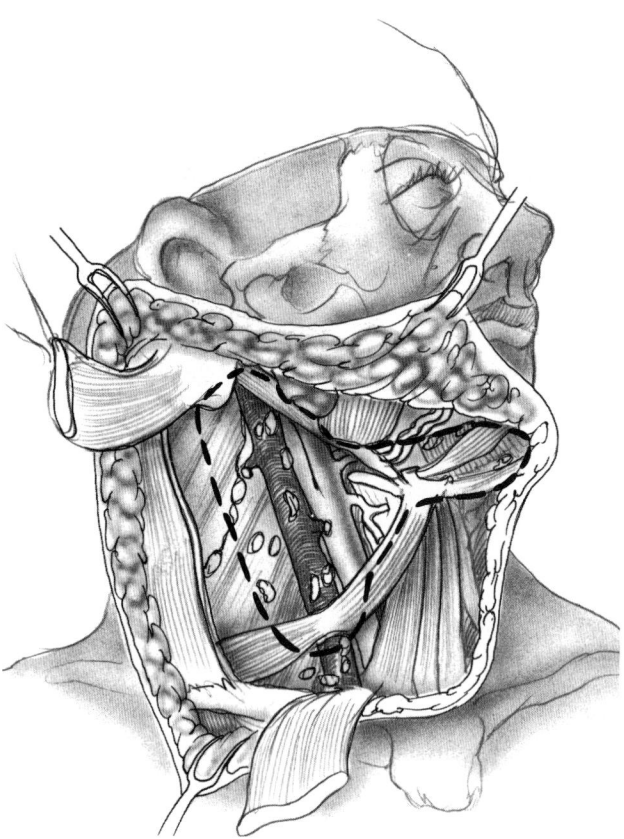

Figure 113.8 Selective neck dissection of levels I to III (supraomohyoid neck dissection).

accessory nerve, the IJV, and the sternocleidomastoid muscle. There are four main types of SNDs:

- SND of Level I to III (commonly referred to as "supraomohyoid" neck dissection) (Fig. 113.8) and SND of Levels I to IV (also referred to as "extended supraomohyoid" neck dissection). These are the neck dissections commonly used in the treatment of patients with squamous cell carcinoma of the oral cavity. The lymph nodes removed are those contained in the submental and submandibular triangles (Level I), the upper jugular region (Level II), and the midjugular region (Level III). The posterior limit of the dissection is marked by the cutaneous branches of the cervical plexus and the posterior border of the sternocleidomastoid muscle. The inferior limit is the omohyoid muscle as it crosses the IJV. Some surgeons prefer to perform a SND of Levels I to IV in cases with cancer of the oral tongue (26). For cancers of the oral cavity that are close to or involve the midline, either type of SND is done bilaterally, because the lymph nodes in both sides of the neck are at risk. These operations have been described in detail by Medina and Byers (27).
- SND of Levels II to IV (Fig. 113.9). This neck dissection, commonly referred to as the "lateral" neck dissection, is commonly used in the treatment of patients with squamous cell carcinoma of the larynx, oropharynx, and hypopharynx. It consists of the removal of the upper

(Level II), middle (Level III), and lower (Level IV) jugular lymph nodes. The superior limit of the dissection is the digastric muscle and the mastoid tip. The inferior limit is the clavicle. The anterior-medial limit is the lateral border of the sternohyoid muscle. The posterior limit of the dissection is marked by the cutaneous branches of the cervical plexus and the posterior border of the sternocleidomastoid muscle. For tumors of the supraglottic larynx and posterior pharyngeal walls, the dissection is often bilateral. A recent description of the technique for this operation has been provided by Khafif (28).

- SND of Level VI. This operation is also called "anterior" neck dissection or "central compartment" dissection. It is used in the treatment of patients with cancer of the midline structures of the anterior inferior aspect of the neck and thoracic inlet, such as the thyroid, the glottic and subglottic regions of the larynx, the pyriform sinus, and the cervical esophagus and trachea. It consists of the removal of the prelaryngeal, pretracheal lymph nodes as well as the paratracheal lymph nodes on both sides. However, using a single denomination (i.e., SND of Level VI) to refer to any dissection of the lymph nodes in this region is confusing. For instance, if the surgeon elects to remove the prelaryngeal, pretracheal and the right paratracheal lymph nodes, the operation would have the same designation as one in which only the left paratracheal nodes are removed. Therefore, until consensus is reached about grouping of the lymph nodes in this area (i.e., Level VIA and VIB), it is best to describe the operation in terms of the specific lymph nodes removed (e.g., left thyroid lobectomy with dissection of Level VI that included the pretracheal and left paratracheal nodes). These operations have been described recently by Weber et al. (29).
- SND for cutaneous malignancies of the head and neck. The extent of the regional node dissection in patients with cutaneous malignancies depends on the location of the primary lesion and the lymph node groups that are likely to harbor metastases. For skin cancers originating from the posterior scalp and the upper-lateral aspect of the neck, the operation most commonly done is a SND (Levels II to V, retroauricular, suboccipital), which is also known as the "posterolateral" neck dissection (Fig. 113.10). The superior limit of this dissection is the posterior belly of the digastric muscle and the mastoid tip anterior laterally and the nuchal line/ridge posteriorly. The inferior limit is the clavicle. The anterior-medial limit is the lateral border of the sternohyoid muscle. The posteriorlateral limit of the dissection is marked by the anterior border of the trapezius muscle inferiorly and the posterior midline of the neck superiorly (30). The regional node dissection often performed for cutaneous malignancies originating from the periauricular skin, anterior scalp, and temporal region is a SND (parotid, facial and external jugular nodes, Levels II, III, VA).

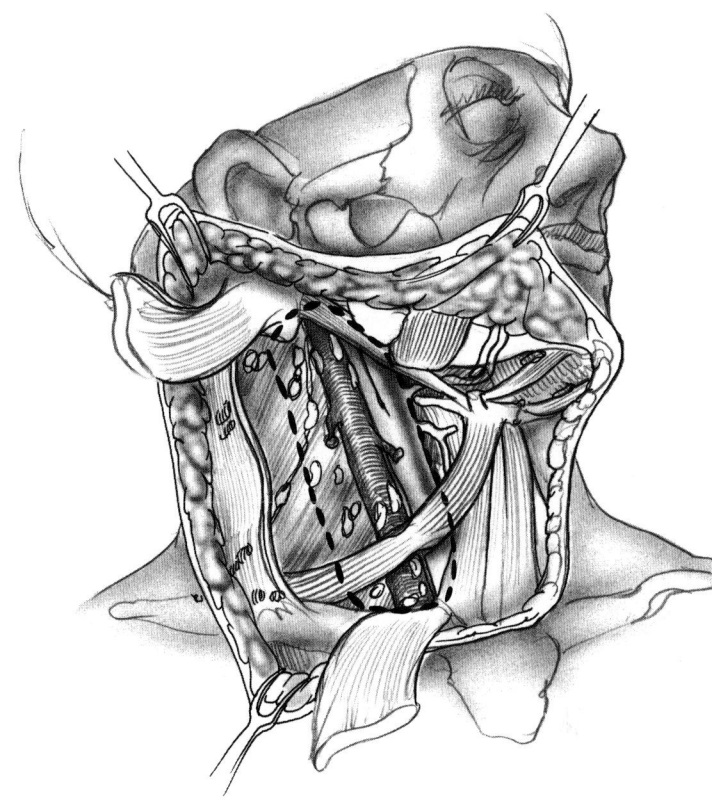

Figure 113.9   Selective Neck dissection of levels II to IV (lateral neck dissection).

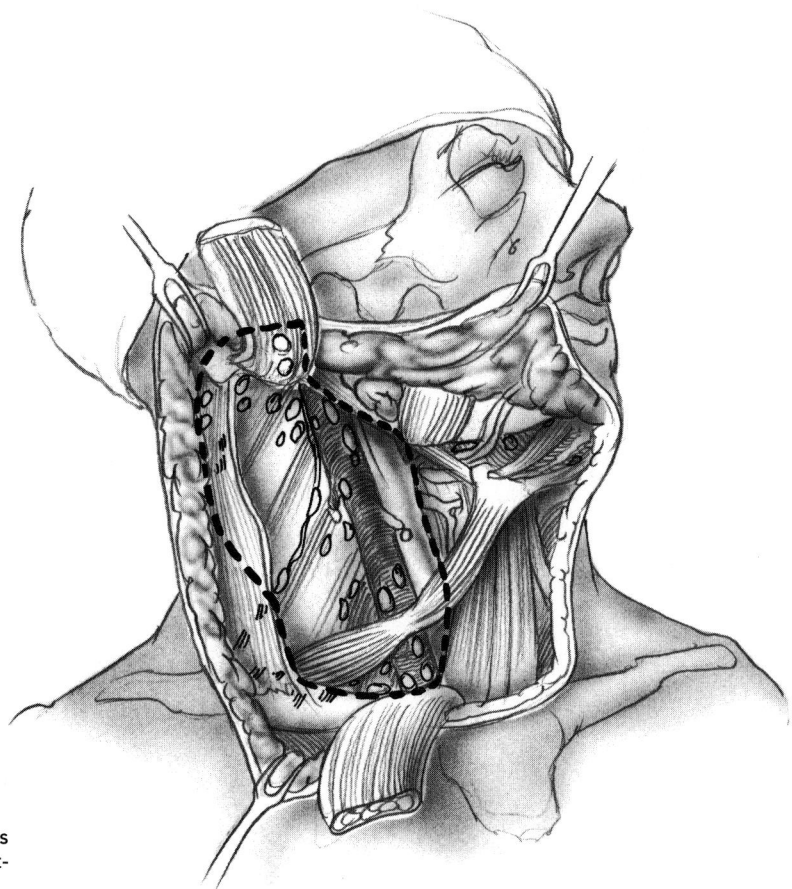

Figure 113.10   Selective neck dissection of levels II to V, retroauricular, suboccipital nodes (posterolateral neck dissection).

Rationale

In the 1960s, surgeons at The University of Texas MD Anderson Cancer Center modified the concept of the RND by selectively removing only those lymph node groups that, based on the location of the primary tumor, were at highest risk of containing metastases. Although preserving functional and cosmetically relevant structures was also a goal in the development of these operations, their current use is predicated on several concepts.

First, the concept of SND is anatomically justified. Anatomic, pathologic, and clinical investigations (26,31–41) and recent prospective studies (42,43) have demonstrated that cervical lymph node metastasis occur in predictable patterns in patients with squamous cell carcinomas of the head and neck.

The lymph node groups most frequently involved in patients with carcinomas of the oral cavity are the jugulodigastric and midjugular nodes. In addition, the nodes in the submandibular triangle are frequently involved in patients with carcinoma of the floor of the mouth, anterior oral tongue, and buccal mucosa. Furthermore, these tumors frequently metastasize to both sides of the neck, and they can skip the submandibular and jugulodigastric nodes, metastasizing first to the midjugular nodes. It has been demonstrated that in the absence of metastases to the first-echelon nodes, tumors of the oral cavity and oropharynx rarely involve the low jugular and posterior cervical nodes. Also, the nodes of the posterior triangle of the neck are not commonly involved, regardless of the site of the primary tumor and the presence or absence of metastases in the jugular nodes, conceivably because there is no retrograde flow from the jugular nodes into the spinal accessory nodes. The most compelling evidence supporting the predictability of nodal metastases from squamous cell carcinomas of the upper aerodigestive tract has been presented by Shah (38). In a retrospective study of 1,119 RNDs, he found that tumors of the oral cavity metastasized most frequently to the neck nodes in levels I, II, and III, whereas carcinomas of the oropharynx, hypopharynx, and larynx involved mainly the nodes in levels II, III, and IV.

Second, SNDs provide the surgeon with the same staging information as the more extensive radical and modified radical neck dissections. There is substantial evidence that micrometastases cannot be detected at present by noninvasive methods (44), so it is essential to dissect the neck to reduce the rate of regional recurrence and its related mortality. Thus, a SND serves as a staging procedure and can be used for decision making regarding the need for adjuvant postoperative radiation therapy. The concept of disease staging in the neck is important in patients whose primary tumors are amenable to treatment with surgery alone but who are highly likely to produce metastases to the cervical lymph nodes. Patients who have large T2N0 and T3N0 squamous cell carcinomas of the oral cavity and faucial arch region are excellent examples of this situation. Because the probability of lymph node metastasis is high in most of these patients, the neck dissection may only have the value of a staging procedure, the results of which determine whether or not postoperative radiation therapy is necessary. If the lymph nodes are histologically negative, no further therapy is indicated and the patient is treated with surgery alone. However, to make this decision with confidence, all the lymph nodes at risk of containing metastases must be evaluated. This evaluation requires dissecting both sides of the neck in patients with lesions of the anterior tongue and floor of the mouth, with the attendant morbidity of a bilateral RND. On the other hand, if the nodal metastases are multiple or the tumor extends beyond the capsule of a lymph node, the neck dissection alone is associated with a high incidence of recurrence in the neck (45,46). In these situations, the addition of postoperative radiation therapy results in better regional control of the disease (47).

Third, when SND is used for the elective treatment of the regional lymphatics, regional control and survival rates are similar to those of more extensive neck dissections (42,43,48–58).

Fourth, SNDs are associated with less postoperative morbidity. The dysfunction of the trapezius muscle produced by SNDs is minimal and, unlike that produced by the RND, is usually temporary and reversible (59–64).

Indications

SND is now the preferred type of neck dissection for the elective surgical management of the cervical lymph nodes in patients with malignant tumors of the head and neck. The effectiveness of the SND (I–III/ "supraomohyoid") and the SND (II to IV/ "lateral") in the treatment of the N0 and N1 neck in patients with squamous cell carcinoma of the upper aerodigestive tract has been evaluated in a prospective analysis of our practice in which the indications for the operations, the surgical technique, and the indications for postoperative radiation were standardized. The overall recurrence rates observed in the dissected side of the neck at 2 years, with the primary tumor under control, was 3.4% when the lymph nodes removed were histologically negative and 12.5% when multiple positive nodes or extracapsular invasion were found. These results are typical of what has been reported in the literature during the past 2 decades regarding the effectiveness of SND in the management of the N0 neck (42,43,48–58,65).

SND is being used with increasing frequency in the management of selected patients with N+ neck disease. To determine the feasibility of doing a supraomohyoid neck dissection in patients with oral cavity carcinoma who have a single clinically metastatic lymph node smaller than 6 cm (N1 and N2a), Kowalski and Carvalho (35) studied 164 oral cavity cancer patients with clinically N1 or N2a stage cancer submitted to RND. Interestingly, histopathology showed no evidence of metastatic tumor in 42.1% of the cases; metastases were found in level IV lymph nodes in only one patient (0.6%), and metastases were not found in level V nodes. Thus, these authors conclude that in patients with clinical N1 stage in whom the metastasis is at level I, a supraomohyoid neck dissection (extended or not to level IV) is feasible instead of a RND (35). Andersen et al. (66) recently reported a 10-year multiinstitutional retrospective review of pooled data from 106 previously untreated clinically and pathologically node-positive patients undergoing 129 SNDs and followed for a minimum of 2 years or until death. The neck was clinically staged as N1 in 58 patients (57.7%), N2a in 5 (4.7%), N2b in 28 (26.4%), N2c in 14 (13.2%), and N3 in 1 (0.9%). Extracapsular extension of tumor was present pathologically in 36 patients (34.0%), and postoperative radiation therapy was administered to 76 patients (71.7%). Overall, nine patients had recurrence in the neck. Six of these recurrences were in the areas of the neck that had been dissected during the SND, for a regional recurrence rate of 5.7%. The recurrence rates reported by others using SND in the N+ neck ranges from 5.5% to 11.1% (mean recurrence rate of 8.3%) (67,68). These rates are comparable to those reported after MRND or RND (18,20,21,69–72), although absolute comparison is difficult because the SND patients represented a more selected sample (47). Nonetheless, these observations support the use of SND in carefully selected patients with clinically positive nodal metastasis from squamous cell carcinoma of the upper aerodigestive tract.

Extended Neck Dissections

Any of the neck dissections described herein can be "extended" to include either lymph node groups that are not routinely removed (i.e., retropharyngeal, paratracheal, upper mediastinal) or other structures that are not routinely removed (i.e., skin of the neck, carotid artery, levator scapulae, vagus or hypoglossal nerve).

Skin, Muscles, and Nerves

In a review of 106 cases of extended neck dissections, the largest review on record in the literature, involvement of the skin occurred in 18% of cases (73). Involvement of the skin did not have a significant prognostic implication.

Tumors in the neck may involve three groups of muscles requiring extension of the neck dissection: superficial, prevertebral, and paraspinal muscles. The superficial group is composed of the strap muscles (sternohyoid, sternothyroid, and omohyoid), the mylohyoid, and the digastric/stylohyoid muscle complex. Removal of one or more of these muscles was the reason for extension of neck dissections in as many as 62% of extended neck dissections studied by Carew and Spiro (73); the digastric muscle was among the structures sacrificed in 51% of cases. The functional deficits resulting from removal of these structures are of little consequence. Their removal usually does not require reconstruction. The dissection was extended to include the prevertebral muscles in only 3% of the cases. The muscles deep to the sternocleidomastoid that may be involved by a

tumor are the splenius capitis, the levator scapulae, and the semispinalis capitis muscles. Involvement of these muscles occurs most commonly just lateral to the carotid artery. It was the reason to extend a neck dissection in 14% to 18% of cases.

Tumors may be adherent to or involve several important nerves in the neck. Because the jugulo-digastric (level II) lymph nodes are the most common site of metastases, it stands to reason that the nerve most commonly involved is the hypoglossal nerve (41%). This is followed distantly by the sympathetic chain (8%), the lingual nerve (7%), the vagus nerve (4%), the superior laryngeal nerve (3%), the phrenic nerve (3%), and the glossopharyngeal nerve (2%) (73). When a nerve is resected, it is imperative to obtain an intraoperative frozen section of the margin of resection, because perineural tumor spread is initially axial and may not result in thickening of the nerve until late (74).

Retropharyngeal Lymph Node Dissection

The retropharyngeal lymph nodes (RPLN) lie within a fat pad located behind the posterior wall of the pharynx and anterior to the prevertebral fascia and the cervical sympathetic trunk and ganglion. This fat pad extends from about the level of the carotid bifurcation to just below the skull base. The RPLN are divided into medial and lateral groups; the medial group of nodes lies behind the pharyngeal midline at a level between the first and fourth cervical vertebrae. The lateral group, better known as the nodes of Rouviere, are the nodes removed in a retropharyngeal lymph node dissection. They are contained within a sliver of fatty tissue located immediately medial to the internal carotid artery. The RPLN receive lymphatic drainage from the nasopharynx, tonsillar fossa, oropharyngeal and hypopharyngeal walls, and the posterior ethmoidal sinuses.

Clinically, involvement of the retropharyngeal nodes by tumor may be signaled by pain and stiffness in the neck. More ominous and characteristic, however, is an ipsilateral occipito-parietal headache described by the patient as pain located behind the eye. Also ominous is the presence of a Horner syndrome that results from tumor involvement of the cervical sympathetic trunk.

The highest incidence of RPLN metastases is associated with advanced cancers of the oropharynx and hypopharynx that present with neck metastases. Therefore, elective RPLN dissection is indicated when these patients are treated surgically. A RPLN dissection should also be performed in patients in whom imaging studies suggests the presence of metastases in the RPLN. A RPLN dissection should also be considered in patients with advanced cancer of the oropharynx and hypopharynx who are treated with organ preservation protocols, have an incomplete response of the tumor in the neck, and require a neck dissection. A RPLN dissection in these situations is likely to afford the patient perhaps a last opportunity to prevent recurrence in the RPLN.

Dissection of the retropharyngeal nodes can be performed separately or in continuity with the resection of the primary tumor. When it is done electively, this operation is relatively simple and it takes only a few minutes. On the other hand, when the RPLN are grossly involved by tumor, the operation may be difficult and sometimes not feasible. The proximity of the nodes to the internal carotid artery and prevertebral structures is such that these structures may be involved as soon as tumor extends beyond the capsule of the lymph nodes. The technique of retropharyngeal node dissection has been described in detail by Vasan and Medina (75).

In a retrospective study designed to assess the frequency of RPLN metastases in 774 patients with squamous cell carcinoma of the nasopharynx, oropharynx, hypopharynx, and supraglottis, using enlargement of the RPLN on CT scans as an indicator of the presence of metastases, McLaughlin et al. (76) found an overall incidence of radiologically "positive" RPLN of 9%. The highest incidence was seen in patients with cancer of the nasopharynx (74%) and the pharyngeal walls (19%). They also noted that in patients with advanced cancer of the oropharyngeal walls and hypopharynx, the incidence of radiologically positive RPLN was higher in patients with cervical metastases (N+ necks) than in those with an N0 neck (pharyngeal wall: N+ 21%, N0 16%; hypopharynx: N+ 9%, N0 0%) (76).

Amatsu et al. (77) studied 82 patients who had RPLN dissection for squamous cell carcinoma of the hypopharynx and cervical esophagus. They reported finding metastases in the RPLN in 16 patients (20%). Fourteen of these patients had hypopharyngeal cancer, and the posterior pharyngeal wall was involved in 57% of them. In keeping with the studies mentioned previously, the majority of patients with RPLN metastases had an N+ neck. However, in 15% of the patients with RPLN metastases the neck was staged N0 (77).

In these studies, the presence of RPLN metastases did not appear to influence survival (78,79). Recently, Gross et al. (80) found no statistically significant difference in the rate of local/regional recurrence, survival, or distant metastases between patients with RPLN metastases and those without them. These authors attribute this finding to more aggressive, multimodality treatment these patients frequently receive, and they advocate performing RPLN in patients with advanced tumors of the oropharynx, hypopharynx, and supraglottic larynx (80).

Paratracheal and Upper Mediastinal Lymph Node Dissection

The paratracheal lymph nodes (PTLN) are a common site of metastases for laryngeal carcinomas that involve the subglottic region and for carcinomas of the cervical esophagus. In a study that included 91 patients with carcinoma of the larynx who underwent paratracheal lymph node dissection, Weber et al. (81) found that metastases to these lymph nodes occurred more often in patients with sub-

glottic tumors (40%) and transglottic tumors (21.4%), but they also occurred in patients with glottic (13%) and supraglottic tumors (15.7%). The presence of PTLN metastases had a significant negative impact on survival. Although the survival at 48 months for the entire group of 141 patients was 60%, none of the 29 patients with PTLN metastases survived beyond 42 months ($p > 0.001$). To remove all the lymph nodes at risk of containing metastases in patients with transglottic and subglottic carcinoma, carcinoma of the cervical esophagus and trachea, and some thyroid carcinomas, a neck dissection may need to be extended to include the paratracheal and pretracheal lymph nodes. Failure to do this is probably the most common cause of stomal recurrences.

In addition, lymph node metastases from thyroid carcinoma tend to occur first in the paratracheal nodes regardless of the location of the primary within the thyroid gland (82).

Resection of the Carotid Artery

Controversy still exists about the advisability of extending a neck dissection to resect the common or the internal carotid artery. Initial reports on carotid resection showed very poor results, with approximately 50% of patients suffering either a severe stroke or death. Recent reports have shown a decrease in these events to approximately 25%, with modest improvement in survival compared with those who did not undergo resection. This is epitomized by the recent report by Freeman et al. (83) of their experience with 58 patients with neck metastasis adherent to the internal or common carotid artery. Angiography was used in patients who demonstrated fixation of the carotid artery on examination or imaging, followed by balloon test occlusion and single photon emission computer tomography (SPECT) scanning. In most patients (70%) the carotid was reconstructed with a vein graft, especially if there was insufficient collateral cerebral circulation. In addition these patients were given 15 to 20 Gy of intraoperative radiation. In their more recent cases, the carotid was permanently occluded preoperatively when possible. Unfortunately, in spite of such aggressive treatment preceded by a systematic, state-of-the-art preoperative assessment, the median disease-specific survival was 12 months and 11 patients (19%) suffered a stroke (83). The mean 1-year disease-free survival rates reported in the literature after resection and reconstruction of the carotid varies between 0% and 44% (84).

When considering resection of the carotid the surgeon must make critical preoperative, intraoperative, and postoperative decisions. Preoperative evaluation of these patients requires a clear understanding of the methods available for assessment of the cerebral circulation. Several tests are available that involve occlusion of the carotid artery with either digital pressure (Matas test) or using a balloon during arteriography. The objective of each method is to determine a "critical point" that indicates when reconstruction of the artery is necessary. With the transcranial color Doppler method the critical point is reverse flow from the external carotid artery to the internal carotid. Technetium 99m hexamethylpropyleneamine oxime brain SPECT measures cerebral perfusion. A 19% to 29% reduction in radioactivity is considered the critical point. Unlike some of the other methods, this is not a real time measurement but requires delayed imaging. Another method uses xenon in an aerosolized mixture that is inhaled by the patient, and then cerebral perfusion is measured by CT scan. Xenon is concentrated in areas of the brain that are well perfused, correlating with blood flow. Two CT scans are obtained to assess cerebral blood flow, the first one during balloon occlusion, and the second after the balloon is released. The critical point is a 25% reduction in the degree of enhancement on the first occlusion scan compared with the open study. Electroencephalography (EEG) has a distinct disadvantage compared with other methods. It does not evaluate blood flow volume to the brain directly. However, it has the advantage that it can be used intraoperatively. The critical point is a 50% attenuation of the somatosensory-evoked cortical potential in relation to the preoperative examination. Finally, stump pressure measurements can be taken during angiography to determine the pressure on the distal side of the balloon when it is occluded. The critical point is a measurement of less than 50 mm Hg. There is significant individual variability with this measurement, as it is affected by systemic blood pressure.

Intraoperatively, patients with frank involvement of the carotid wall whose preoperative evaluation indicates intolerance to carotid ligation should have the carotid reconstructed. Saphenous vein grafts are preferred over prosthetic grafts for reconstruction, and if the skin has been heavily radiated or a portion of skin over the carotid is resected, a myocutaneous flap should be used to cover the graft. There is still considerable debate regarding the routine use of intraoperative shunts, and to date there has not been a prospective study to prove their usefulness. However, shunting is clearly indicated when there is angiographic evidence of inadequate flow through the circle of Willis.

Postoperatively, delayed strokes can occur in as many as 25% of patients who have undergone carotid artery resection without reconstruction, even if they "passed" the balloon occlusion test (85). Flow from the contralateral side through the circle of Willis prevents a stroke initially. However, the resection creates an arterial stump that begins at the take-off of the middle cerebral artery and continues down to the level of the resection. This can be a site for thrombus formation, which can then propagate up into the circle of Willis. Alternatively, the thrombus may produce emboli that can travel into the distribution of the middle cerebral artery. Although these mechanisms have not been conclusively proven, many surgeons advocate the use of heparin postoperatively to prevent delayed strokes following resection of the internal carotid artery. Recommended

doses range from 5,000 units subcutaneously twice a day to full therapeutic anticoagulation (86). The benefit of anticoagulation has not been shown in a prospective controlled study.

ADJUVANT THERAPY FOLLOWING NECK DISSECTION

Numerous studies in the 1980s showed that the rate of tumor recurrence in the neck is decreased by the addition of postoperative radiation, when multiple nodes are involved at multiple levels of the neck, and when extracapsular spread (ECS) of tumor is found (87–89). Since then it has also been accepted that timing of the initiation of radiotherapy is important; delays beyond 6 weeks may compromise tumor control (88). The seminal study of Peters et al. in the early 1990s established the dose of postoperative radiation therapy that is essential to achieve optimal results. Daily fractions of 1.8 Gy, to a total dose of 57.6 Gy to the entire operative bed, is currently recommended. Sites of increased risk for recurrence, such as areas of the neck where ECS of tumor was found, should be boosted to 63 Gy (90). A prospective, randomized clinical study published in 2004 showed that the concurrent postoperative administration of chemotherapy (cisplatin 100 mg per meter squared on days 1, 22, and 43) and radiotherapy (60 to 66 Gy in 30 to 33 fractions over 6 to 6.6 weeks) significantly improved the rates of local and regional control and disease-free survival in patients with high-risk resected head and neck cancers (91). The high-risk criteria included any or all of the following: histologic evidence of metastases in two or more lymph nodes, ECS, and microscopically involved margins of resection. Although the study subjects were stratified according to the presence or absence of microscopically positive margins, the published results did not include an analysis of outcomes with and without concomitant chemotherapy in the cohort of patients with microscopically negative margins, which would have elucidated whether or not the addition of chemotherapy was beneficial to patients with high-risk neck disease. A similar study by the European Organization for Research and Treatment of Cancer, published at the same time, included patients with various clinical (primary tumor and nodal volume and nodal site) and pathologic (involved margins of resection, ECS, perineural involvement, and vascular embolism) high-risk factors related to neck metastases (92). It also showed that concomitant postoperative chemoradiation was significantly more efficacious than radiation alone in these high-risk patients. However, resection margins were positive in 30% of the patients included in the study and the design did not include an analysis focused on the neck disease factors. Nonetheless, both of these studies suggest that the addition of chemotherapy may be beneficial to patients with resectable head and neck cancers who have advanced neck metastases, N2 to N3, and to patients with N0 or N1 disease who are found to have multiple histologically positive nodes or extracapsular spread of tumor.

CURRENT CONTROVERSIES

Pertinent controversies regarding neck dissection concern the extent of SNDs, the need for postoperative radiation in patients with pathologically proven metastasis in a single cervical lymph node (pN1), and the need for and the extent of "planned" neck dissection in patients with squamous cell carcinoma of the upper aerodigestive tract who have clinically obvious neck node metastases (N+ neck) and are treated with radiation alone or in combination with chemotherapy.

Extent of Elective Selective Neck Dissection

Three issues have emerged recently regarding the extent of elective SNDs. The first two concern the need to remove routinely the nodes in level IV in patients with cancer of the oral tongue and larynx. Byers et al. (26) reported finding "skip metastases" in 15.8% of patients with oral tongue cancer. In these cases, metastases to either level IV or level III were the only manifestation of the disease in the neck. In a more recent review of 49 patients with cancer of the oral cavity staged as having N0 disease, who underwent SND of levels I to IV (extended supraomohyoid neck dissection), Crean et al. (93) found occult metastases in level IV nodes in 10% of the patients. These and other authors contend that the supraomohyoid neck dissection, therefore, is inadequate for a complete pathologic evaluation of all the nodes at risk, and they recommend dissecting the nodes in level IV when performing an elective neck dissection in patients with cancer of the oral tongue (94). The opposing point of view has been advanced by Khafif et al. (95) whose practice has been to dissect level IV only when a suspicious node is found at level III or there are multiple obviously involved lymph nodes. They reported their findings in a cohort of 58 patients with squamous cell carcinoma of the oral tongue (Stage T1 to T2 N0). The node dissections performed included levels I through III in 42 patients (69%), levels I through IV in 16 patients (26%), and levels I through V in 1 patient (5%). A positive node was found in level IV in only one instance (1/54, 1.8%), and no recurrences were observed in level IV.

The need for routine dissection of level IV nodes in patients undergoing elective SND for laryngeal cancer has recently been questioned by Khafif et al. (96). In their review of 43 patients with laryngeal squamous cell carcinoma who underwent elective SND of levels II to IV (lateral neck dissection), they found that only one patient (2.3%) had metastases in level IV nodes and that patient also had metastases in level II nodes. Others have previously reported similar observations (48). As a result, the necessity

of dissecting this nodal level in the absence of clinically detectable adenopathy has been challenged.

The third issue concerns the need to dissect the nodes in the so-called supraspinal accessory lymph node pad or submuscular recess (i.e., the fibrofatty tissue containing lymph nodes located above and behind the upper portion of the spinal accessory nerve). It has been pointed out that the prevalence of nodal metastases in the clinically N0 neck is low (1.6% to 2%) (97). Furthermore, the need to routinely dissect the "submuscular" recess has been questioned arguing that the dissection of this area of the neck is time-consuming, increases bleeding, and jeopardizes the spinal accessory nerve. Although these studies emphasize the need for care in the dissection of this region, it seems advisable to continue to dissect this area of the neck, which is so intimately related to the jugulodigastric region. Most recurrences after any type of neck dissection occur in the upper jugular region. Further studies are needed to identify better those patients in whom this area is not at risk.

Is Postoperative Radiation Beneficial in the Pathologically N$_1$ (pN$_1$) Neck?

When a single metastasis is found (pN$_1$) in a neck dissection specimen, surgery alone has been considered adequate treatment. Recently, however, regional recurrence rates from 16% to 25% have been reported with surgery alone, and it has been suggested that postoperative radiation may be beneficial (53,98). On the other hand, radiation was not found to be beneficial in a retrospective review of 58 patients with T1/T2 squamous cell carcinoma of the oral tongue treated with surgery, which included an ipsilateral SND, and were found to have metastasis in a single lymph node. These patients were treated at seven institutions and were followed for a minimum of 2 years. Twenty-two (38%) patients were treated with surgery alone, whereas 36 (62%) received postoperative radiation. In the group treated with surgery alone, two patients had recurrence at the primary site and in the neck. Of the remaining 20 patients, 6 (30%) recurred in the neck (5 contralateral and 1 simultaneous ipsilateral and contralateral). In the surgery plus radiation group, four (11%) tumors recurred in the neck, all within the operative field. The difference in the rate of recurrence in the neck for the two groups was not statistically significant. Because these results contradict the findings of two recent studies by reputable investigators, which showed benefit from radiation, a prospective, randomized study may be necessary to resolve this controversy.

"Planned" Neck Dissection After "Organ Preservation" for Squamous Cell Carcinoma of the Head and Neck

As the treatment of advanced carcinomas of the larynx and pharynx has evolved from surgery and postoperative radiation to "organ preservation" strategies with hyperfractionated radiation and more recently with various combinations of radiation and chemotherapy, a controversy has evolved regarding the management of patients with clinically obvious lymph node metastases, particularly those with advanced neck disease (N2 to N3). Some clinicians argue that a neck dissection should be carried out as part of the treatment plan, irrespective of the response of the tumor in the neck, because the clinical and pathologic responses of the tumor in the neck correlate poorly with each other (99). Other clinicians argue that this notion is obsolete and that it is not necessary to perform a "planned" neck dissection when the tumor in the neck undergoes a complete response to the treatment. The basis for this argument is that the probability of an isolated recurrence in the neck is low (5%) when these patients are observed (100,101). At the root of this controversy is our present inability to determine, preoperatively, when a complete clinical response is associated with the presence or absence of viable tumor cells. Biologic parameters, such as pretreatment tumor oxygenation status and tumor lactate concentration may be useful parameters to make such a differentiation. Likewise, PET scanning may be helpful in defining the subset of patients who are likely to benefit from a neck dissection. In a series of 12 patients studied prospectively by Rogers et al., a positive PET 1 month after radiation therapy accurately indicated the presence of residual disease in all cases; however, a negative PET indicated absence of disease in only 14% (102). More recently, the group of Lester Peters in Melbourne have suggested that FDG-PET done 12 weeks after completion of treatment with radiation or chemoradiation may be useful to determine whether posttreatment neck dissection should be omitted (103).

SEQUELAE OF NECK DISSECTION

The most notable sequelae observed in patients who have undergone a RND are related to removal of the spinal accessory nerve. The resulting denervation of the trapezius muscle, one of the most important shoulder abductors, causes destabilization of the scapula with progressive flaring at the vertebral border, drooping, and lateral and anterior rotation. The loss of trapezius function decreases the patient's ability to abduct the shoulder above 90 degrees at the shoulder. These physical changes result in the recognized shoulder syndrome of pain, weakness, and deformity of the shoulder girdle commonly associated with the RND. It should also be noted that preserving the cervical plexus contributions to the spinal accessory nerve may not decrease shoulder morbidity significantly (104). Furthermore, shoulder disability after neck dissection results not only from the spinal accessory nerve dysfunction, but also from secondary glenohumeral stiffness caused by weakness of the scapulohumeral girdle muscles and postoperative immobility.

A number of studies have demonstrated that when compared with the RND, neck dissections that preserve the spinal accessory nerve are associated with less shoulder pain (105) and better shoulder function and overall quality of life (59–63,106). However, these studies also provide evidence that even procedures that involve minimal dissection of the spinal accessory nerve can result in shoulder dysfunction. Although this dysfunction is often reversible, it behooves the surgeon to make every effort to avoid undue trauma to the nerve, particularly stretching, during any neck dissection in which the nerve is preserved. In addition, every patient who undergoes neck dissection must be questioned about the function of the shoulder and must be evaluated by a physical therapist early in the postoperative period. If any deficit is detected, the patient should be properly counseled and coached to ensure proper rehabilitation of the shoulder. Physical therapy aimed to early recovery of passive motion and to avoid the occurrence of joint fibrosis has been shown to be beneficial (107). It has also been suggested that progressive resistance exercise training may be a useful adjunct to standard physical therapy (108). It should be kept in mind, as mentioned earlier, that shoulder pain after neck dissection may not be the result of dysfunction of the spinal accessory nerve. Consequently, if a patient experiences shoulder pain after neck dissection, the trapezius muscle and active bilateral abduction of the shoulder should be examined to determine if the spinal accessory nerve is involved (109).

COMPLICATIONS OF NECK DISSECTION

In addition to the medical complications that can occur after any surgical procedure in the head and neck region, several surgical complications can be related solely or in part to neck dissection.

Infection

Following clean neck dissections, those in which the upper aerodigestive tract is not entered, wound infections are not common. Interestingly, however, a recent prospective study, designed to evaluate the effects of a prophylactic antibiotic regimen (ampicillin-sulbactam for 24 hours) on the incidence of infection after clean neck dissection, showed that the infection rate in patients that were treated with the antibiotic was 1.7% compared with a significantly higher rate (13.3%) among patients that did not receive antibiotic ($p = 0.02$) (110).

Air Leaks

Circulation of air through a wound drain is a common complication that usually is encountered during the first postoperative day. The point of entrance of air may be located somewhere along the skin incision. If the drains are connected to suction in the operating room near the completion of the wound closure, however, such an air leak usually becomes apparent then and can be corrected. Other points of entrance may not become apparent until after surgery, when the position of the neck changes or the patient begins to move. The typical example of this situation is the improperly secured suction wound drain that gets displaced, exposing one or more of the drain vents. A similar situation can occur when a skin graft to reconstruct a cutaneous defect is created in conjunction with the neck dissection. Movement of the neck can produce an air leak even after meticulous suturing of the skin graft. This can be prevented by applying an adhesive vinyl drape over the graft and surrounding skin to seal any possible air leak instead of or in addition to the bolster of gauze traditionally used to immobilize a skin graft.

Air leaks with potentially more serious consequences are those that occur through a communication of the neck wound with the tracheostomy site or through a mucosal suture line. In addition to air, contaminated secretions may be circulated through the wound. Thus, early identification of the site of leakage is desirable but may not be a simple task, and correcting it may require revision of the wound closure in the operating room.

Bleeding

Postoperative hemorrhage usually occurs immediately after surgery. External bleeding through the incision, without distortion of the skin flaps, often originates in a subcutaneous blood vessel. In most instances, this bleeding can be controlled readily by ligation or infiltration of the surrounding tissues with an anesthetic solution containing epinephrine. On the other hand, pronounced swelling or ballooning of the skin flaps in the immediate postoperative period, with or without external bleeding, must be attributed to a hematoma in the wound. If detected early, milking the drains occasionally may result in evacuation of the accumulated blood and resolve the problem. If this is not accomplished immediately or if blood reaccumulates quickly, however, it is best to return the patient to the operating room and to explore the wound under sterile conditions, evacuate the hematoma, and control the bleeding. Attempting to do this in the recovery room or at the bedside may be ill advised, because lighting may be inadequate, surgical equipment improvised, and sterile conditions precarious. Failure to recognize or to manage properly a postoperative hematoma may predispose the patient to the development of a wound infection. Although bulky pressure dressings may be useful in curtailing postoperative edema, they do not prevent hematomas and may in fact delay their recognition.

Chylous Fistula

The reported incidence of chyle fistula following neck dissection varies between 1% and 2.5%. In most patients who develop a postoperative chylous fistula, a chylous leakage is identified and apparently controlled intraoperatively (111,112). These observations behoove the surgeon to avoid injury to the thoracic duct proper and also to ligate or clip any visualized or potential lymphatic tributaries in the area of the thoracic duct, which may be accomplished with relative ease if the operative field is kept bloodless when dissecting in this area of the neck. Furthermore, as soon as the dissection of this area is completed and again before closing the wound, the area is observed for 20 or 30 seconds while the anesthesiologist increases the intrathoracic pressure.

Even the smallest leak of chylous material must be pursued seriously until it is arrested. Direct clamping and ligating may be difficult and sometimes counterproductive as a result of the fragility of the lymphatic vessels and the surrounding fatty tissue. Hemoclips are ideal to control a source of leakage that is clearly visualized. Otherwise, it is preferable to use suture ligatures with pliable material, such as 5-0 silk, that are tied over a piece of hemostatic sponge to avoid tearing. In the immediate postoperative period, serum and drainage levels of triglycerides and cholesterol obtained on the first postoperative day may be useful parameters to predict early the occurrence of a chyle fistula (112).

Management of a chyle leak noted postoperatively depends on the time of onset of the leak, the amount of chyle drainage in a 24-hour period and on the presence or absence of accumulation of chyle under the skin flaps (113). When the daily output of chyle exceeds 600 mL, especially when the chyle fistula becomes apparent immediately after surgery, and drainage is greater than 1,000 mL (111), conservative closed wound management is unlikely to succeed. In such cases, we prefer early surgical exploration before the tissues exposed to the chyle become markedly inflamed and before the fibrinous material that coats these tissues becomes adherent, obscuring and jeopardizing important structures such as the phrenic and the vagus nerves. Surgical exploration is also warranted when chyle accumulates under the skin flaps either because of inadequate drain size or because of the volume or consistency of the chyle causes partial or compete obstruction of the drains.

On the other hand, chylous fistulae that become apparent later in the postoperative period, after enteral feedings are resumed, or those that drain less than 600 mL of chyle per day, are initially managed conservatively with closed wound drainage, pressure dressings (which are cumbersome to secure in this area of the neck), repeated aspirations, and diet modifications aimed at decreasing chyle drainage while maintaining nutritional support. Usually, nutrition can be provided enterally using elemental diets supplemented with medium-chain triglycerides, which are absorbed directly into the portal circulation bypassing the lymphatic system. In some patients parenteral nutrition may be necessary (114). If these measures fail, the neck is surgically explored and the leak is identified and dealt with appropriately. Sometimes this intervention is unsuccessful and the leak persists. The use of fibrin glue and a clavicular periosteal flap may be useful to control the leak in such cases (115). Alternatively, thoracoscopic ligation of the thoracic duct in the chest may be preferable to reexploring the neck (116). In a recent report, Nyquist et al. (117) described a case in which a chylous fistula stopped draining 24 hours after the administration of octreotide (100 micrograms given subcutaneously three times a day). These authors postulate that the effect of octreotide on chylous fistulae may be due to its ability to reduce gastrointestinal and pancreatic secretions, decrease hepatic venous pressure, and reduce splanchnic blood flow, which may decrease thoracic duct flow and relative concentration of triglycerides (117).

Ipsilateral chylothorax can occur following neck dissection. Bilateral chylothorax as a complication of neck dissection is extremely rare, but it is potentially serious and sometimes fatal (118,119).

Facial or Cerebral Edema

Synchronous bilateral RNDs, in which both IJVs are ligated, can result in the development of facial edema, cerebral edema, or both. The facial edema sometimes can be dramatically severe. It appears to be a mechanical problem of venous drainage, which resolves to a variable extent with time as collateral circulation is established. It appears to be more common and more severe in patients who had previous radiation to the head and neck and in those patients in whom the resection includes large segments of the lateral and posterior pharyngeal walls. We have been able to prevent massive facial edema by preserving at least one external jugular vein whenever a bilateral RND is anticipated. The external jugular usually is separated from the tumor in the neck by the sternocleidomastoid muscle and can be dissected free between the tail of the parotid and the subclavian vein. Others have reconstructed one internal jugular using various techniques including vein with saphenous vein grafts or by using a segment of one of the resected jugular veins, distal to the site of tumor involvement (120,121). The development of cerebral edema may be at the root of the impaired neurologic function and even coma that can occur after bilateral RND. Following neck dissection, a syndrome of inappropriate secretion of antidiuretic hormone (SIADH) occurs in 8% to 30% of patients. This is a disorder in which release of antidiuretic hormone is independent of plasma osmolarity, resulting in fluid retention and development of dilutional hyponatremia. It occurs significantly more often in patients who have a history of smoking and it has been noted to resolve within 72 hours (122). It is commonly believed that synchronous, bilateral RND causes SIADH, presumably as a result of increased intracranial pressure. This belief is based mainly on the results of an experimental study published in 1978 in which occlusion of the superior vena cava in dogs resulted in increased intracranial pressure and SIADH. Using an animal model that more closely resembles the clinical condition of bilateral RND,

Khafif et al. (123) found that bilateral synchronous IJV ligation and bilateral RNDs did not result in SIADH in dogs. As these results contradict a commonly held belief in clinical practice, a prospective evaluation of the physiologic changes after bilateral RNDs is warranted. Nevertheless, it is possible that an expansion of extracellular fluids and dilutional hyponatremia that occurs in some patients after neck dissection could aggravate cerebral edema, creating a vicious cycle. In practice, this behooves the surgeon and the anesthesiologist to curtail the administration of fluids during and after bilateral RNDs. Furthermore, perioperative management of fluid and electrolytes in these cases should not be guided solely by the patient's urine output but also by monitoring central venous pressure, cardiac output, and serum and urine osmolarity.

Blindness

Blindness after bilateral RND is a rare but catastrophic complication (124). The pathogenesis of it remains unclear. In one of the few cases reported in the literature, histologic examination revealed intraorbital optic nerve infarction, suggesting intraoperative hypotension and severe venous distention as possible etiologic factors. In another case, bilateral occipital lobe infarcts were demonstrated on CT scan (125).

Apnea

Some patients may become apneic as a result of loss of their hypoxic ventilatory responses due to carotid body denervation after bilateral neck dissection.

Jugular Vein Thrombosis

Preservation of the IJV during neck dissection does not ensure its patency after surgery, particularly when radiation therapy is also used. Cotter et al. (126) used preoperative and postoperative CT or MRI on 69 patients undergoing 79 vein-sparing neck dissections. Sixty-eight veins (86%) were patent postoperatively. Interestingly, radiation therapy appears to influence patency of the IJV. Capiello et al. (127) studied the patency of the IJV following selective lateral neck dissection (LND) in a cohort of 34 patients. A preoperative baseline study of vein patency and flow by ultrasonography (US) was obtained followed by postoperative evaluations at 1 week, 1 month, and 3 months. At 1 week postoperatively, 50% of the IJVs did not present any alteration in patency, 46% had reduced flow, and 4% showed absent flow. However, at 3 months none of the patients showed evidence of IJV occlusion. Postoperative radiotherapy did not have a statistically significant impact on IJV patency ($p = 0.09$).

A recent report describes the rate of complications after planned posttreatment neck dissections in patients enrolled in organ preservation protocols. The authors conclude that the rate is similar to that previously for neck dissections

(37%) and that the rate increases when higher preoperative radiation therapy doses are used (128).

EMERGENCIES

Carotid Artery Rupture

The most feared and most commonly lethal complication after neck surgery is exposure and rupture of the carotid artery. Therefore, every effort must be made to prevent it. If the skin incisions have been designed properly, the carotid seldom becomes exposed in the absence of a salivary fistula. Fistula formation and flap breakdown are more likely to occur in the presence of malnutrition, diabetes, and prior radiation therapy, which impair healing capacity and compromise vascular supply. Faced with any of these risk factors, the surgeon must use flawless surgical technique in closing oral and pharyngeal defects. Use of perioperative antibiotics and, more importantly, free and pedicled vascularized flaps (which provide skin for closure of mucosal defects and variably bulky muscle that can protect the carotid) have rendered nearly obsolete the use of "protective" measures such as dermal grafts, levator scapulae muscle flaps, and controlled pharyngostomies.

Management of the exposed carotid depends on the likelihood of rupture, based on the length of the exposed segment, the condition of the surrounding tissues, and the size of the oropharyngocutaneous fistula. Large cutaneous defects or large high-output fistulae in previously irradiated patients are not likely to heal by secondary intention in a timely manner. The likelihood of rupture of the carotid in these conditions is extremely high. Therefore, an attempt should be made to repair the defect and to cover the carotid using well-vascularized tissue early, before the vessel has been irreversibly damaged. Whenever the carotid is exposed, it is advisable to take carotid rupture precautions:

- Warn and instruct nursing personnel and house staff about the possibility of a carotid rupture, the site of potential rupture, and the steps to be taken in the event of bleeding.
- Have compatible blood available.
- Keep appropriate surgical instruments at the bedside.

When a carotid rupture occurs, it is usually possible to stop the bleeding with manual pressure while blood and fluids are given to restore and maintain the patient's blood pressure. Only then is the patient taken to surgery. Attempts to repair the area of rupture are futile. Introducing Fogarty catheters through the area of rupture helps control the bleeding temporarily while the artery is exposed and ligated proximally and distally to the area of rupture.

Jugular Vein "Blow-Out"

This complication is seen more often because the IJV is preserved more frequently during neck dissection. Jugular vein rupture should be considered in patients undergoing primary tumor excision with MRND complicated by a pharyngocutaneous fistula. In a recent study of six patients who experienced rupture of the IJV, Cleland-Zamudio et al. (129) found that patients who have a complete circumferential dissection of the IJV low in the neck and go on to have fistulas develop may be more prone to this complication. Typically, bleeding is venous and occurs repeatedly. Treatment consists of surgical exploration and ligation of the jugular vein above and below the level of rupture.

HIGHLIGHTS

- Despite careful examination of the neck, the error rate in assessing the presence or absence of cervical lymph node metastasis ranges from 20% to 51%.
- Computed tomography and magnetic resonance imaging improve significantly the detection rate for lymph nodes larger than 1 to 1.5 cm. Ultrasonography is promising in the visualization of small nodes (3 mm) that can be sampled by fine-needle aspiration.
- Treatment of the N0 neck remains controversial, but if the primary tumor is at a high risk for metastasis, many surgeons prefer to treat the neck electively rather than to follow a course of expectant observation.
- Selective neck dissections, which remove only the lymph node groups at greatest risk of metastatic involvement, are preferable for the treatment of the N0 neck in patients whose primary tumor is treated surgically.
- Elective neck irradiation is effective in the treatment of the N0 neck in patients whose primary tumor is treated by radiation.
- Surgical treatment of the N+ neck no longer consists of a single operation.
- Comprehensive neck dissections, which remove all the lymph node regions I through V of one side of the neck, are most commonly used for the surgical treatment of the N+ neck.
- An extended neck dissection includes either lymph node groups not routinely removed or structures not routinely removed (e.g., carotid artery).
- The most notable sequela of a radical neck dissection is the "shoulder drop" that results from denervation of the trapezius muscle (supplied by the spinal accessory nerve).
- Common complications of neck dissection include air leaks, bleeding, chylous fistula, and facial/cerebral edema. Knowledge of their pathophysiology and meticulous surgical technique are essential for their prevention.
- Carotid artery rupture is the most feared complication after neck dissection. Preventive steps to protect the carotid initially include proper selection of the incision and postoperative flap coverage.
- Jugular vein rupture can occur in patients undergoing modified radical neck dissection.

REFERENCES

1. Guo C, Zhang Y, Zhang L, et al. Surgical anatomy and preservation of the accessory nerve in radical functional neck dissection. *Chin J Stomatol* 2003;38:12–15.
2. Hone S, Ridha H, Rowley H, et al. Surgical landmarks of the spinal accessory nerve in modified radical neck dissection. *Clin Otolaryngol Allied Sci* 2001;26:16–18.
3. Friedman M, Mafee M, Pacella B, et al. Rationale for elective neck dissection in 1990. *Laryngoscope* 1990;100:54–59.
4. Haberal L, Celik H, Cogmen H, et al. Which is important in the evaluation of metastatic lymph nodes in head and neck cancer: palpation, ultrasonography, or computed tomography? *Otolaryngol Head Neck Surg* 2004;130:197–201.
5. van den Brekel M, van def Waal D. The incidence of micrometastases in neck dissection specimens obtained from elective neck dissections. *Laryngoscope* 1996;106:987–991.
6. Steinkamp J, Cornehl M, Hosten N, et al. Cervical lymphadenopathy: ration of long- to short-axis diameter as a predictor of malignancy. *Br J Radiol* 1995;68:266–270.
7. van den Brekel M, Castelijns J, Stel H, et al. Modern imaging techniques and ultrasound guided aspiration cytology for the assessment of neck node metastases: a prospective comparative study. *Eur Arch Otorhinolaryngol* 1993;250:11–17.
8. Nieuwenhuis E, Castelijns J, Pijpers R, et al. Wait-and-see policy for the N0 neck in early-stage oral and oropharyngeal squamous cell carcinoma using ultrasonography-guided cytology: is there a role for identification of the sentinel node? *Head Neck* 2002;24:282–289.
9. Braams J, Pruim J, Freling N, et al. Detection of lymph node metastases of squamous-cell cancer of the head and neck with FDG-PET and MRI. *J Nucl Med* 1995;36:211–216.
10. Stokkel M, ten Broek F, Hordijk G, et al. Preoperative evaluation of patients with primary head and neck cancer using dual-head 18fluorodeoxyglucose positron emission tomography. *Ann Surg* 2000;231:229–234.
11. de Bree R, Roos J, Verel I, et al. Radioimmunodiagnosis of lymph node metastases in head and neck cancer. *Oral Dis* 2003;9:241–248.
12. Ross G, Shoaib T, Soutar D, et al. The First International Conference on Sentinel Node Biopsy in Mucosal Head and Neck Cancer and Adoption of a Multicenter Trial Protocol. *Ann Surg Oncol* 2002;9:406–410.
13. Ross G, Soutar D, MacDonald D, et al. Improved staging of cervical metastases in clinically node-negative patients with head and neck squamous cell carcinoma. *Ann Surg Oncol* 2004;11:213–218.
14. Hamakawa H, Fukizumi M, Bao Y. Genetic diagnosis of micrometastasis based on SCCa antigen mRNA in cervical lymph nodes of head and neck cancer. *Clin Exp Med* 1999;17:593–599.
15. Shores C, Xiaoying Y, Funkhouser W, et al. Clinical evaluation of a new molecular method for detection of micrometastases in head and neck squamous cell carcinoma. *Arch Otol Head Neck Surg* 2004;130:937–942.
16. McCammon S, Shah J. Radical neck dissection. *Op Tech Otolaryngol Head Neck Surg* 2004;15(3):152–159.
17. Pinsolle J, Pinsolle V, Majoufre C, et al. Prognostic value of histologic findings in neck dissections for squamous cell carcinoma. *Arch Otolaryngol Head Neck Surg* 1997;123:145–148.
18. Andersen P, Shah J, Cambronero E, et al. The role of comprehensive neck dissection with preservation of the spinal accessory nerve in the clinically positive neck. Annual Meeting of the Society of Head & Neck Surgeons, 1994(abst).
19. Gavilan J, Herranz J, Martin L. Functional neck dissection: the Latin approach. *Oper Tech Otolaryngol Head Neck Surg* 2004;15:168–175.
20. Lingeman R, Stephens R, Helmus C, et al. Neck dissection: radical or conservative. *Ann Otol Rhinol Laryngol* 1977;86:737–744.
21. Molinari R, Chiesa F, Cantu G, et al. Retrospective comparison of conservative and radical neck dissection in laryngeal cancer. *Ann Otol Rhinol Laryngol* 1980;89:578–581.
22. Joseph C, Gregor R, Davidge-Pitts K. The role of functional neck dissection in the management of advanced tumors of the upper aerodigestive tract. *S Afr J Surg* 1985;23:83–87.
23. Gavilan C, Gavilan J. Five-year results of functional neck dissection for cancer of the larynx. *Arch Otolaryngol Head Neck Surg* 1989;115:1193–1196.
24. Bocca E, Pignataro O, Oldini C. Functional neck dissection: an evaluation and review of 843 cases. *Laryngoscope* 1984;94:942–945.
25. Calearo C, Teatini G. Functional neck dissection: anatomical grounds, surgical technique, clinical observations. *Ann Otol Rhinol Laryngol* 1983;92:215–222.
26. Byers R, Weber R, Anderws T, et al. Frequency and therapeutic implications of "skip metastases" in the neck from squamous carcinoma of the oral tongue. *Head Neck* 1997;19:14–19.
27. Medina J, Byers R. Supraomohyoid neck dissection: rationale, indications and surgical technique. *Head Neck* 1989;11:111–122.
28. Khafif A. Lateral neck dissection. *Oper Tech Otolaryngol Head Neck Surg* 2004;15(3):160–167.
29. Weber R, Holsinger F. Central compartment dissection (of levels VI and VII for carcinoma of the larynx, hypopharynx, cervical esophagus, and thyroid). *Oper Tech Otolaryngol Head Neck Surg* 2004;15(3):190–195.
30. Medina J. Posterolateral neck dissection. *Oper Tech Otolaryngol Head Neck Surg* 2004;15(3):176–179.
31. Byers R, Wolf P, Ballantyne A. Rationale for elective modified neck dissection. *Head Neck* 1988;10:160–167.
32. Candela F, Kothari K, Shah J. Patterns of cervical node metastases from squamous cell carcinoma of the oropharynx and hypopharynx. *Head Neck* 1990;12:197–203.
33. Candela F, Shah J, Jaques D, et al. Patterns of cervical node metastases from squamous cell carcinoma of the larynx. *Arch Otolaryngol Head Neck Surg* 1990;116:432–435.
34. Fisch U, Sigel M. Cervical lymphatic system as visualized by lymphography. *Ann Otol Rhinol Laryngol* 1964;73:870–882.
35. Kowalski L, Carvalho A. Feasibility of supraomohyoid neck dissection in N1 and N2a oral cancer patients. *Head Neck* 2002;24:921–924.
36. Lindberg R. Distribution of cervical lymph node metastases from squamous cell carcinoma of the upper respiratory and digestive tracts. *Cancer* 1972;29:1446–1449.
37. Mukherji S, Armao D, Joshi V. Cervical nodal metastases in squamous cell carcinoma of the head and neck: what to expect. *Head Neck* 2001;23:995–1005.
38. Shah J. Patterns of cervical lymph node metastasis from squamous carcinomas of the upper aerodigestive tract. *Am J Surg* 1990;160:405–409.
39. Shah J, Candela F, Poddar A. The patterns of cervical lymph node metastases from squamous cell carcinoma of the oral cavity. *Cancer* 1990;66:109–113.
40. Skolnik E. The posterior triangle in radical neck surgery. *Arch Otolaryngol* 1976;102:1–4.
41. Wong R, Rinaldo A, Ferlito A, et al. Occult cervical metastasis in head and neck cancer and its impact on therapy. *Acta Otolaryngol* 2002;122:107–114.
42. Brazilian Head and Neck Cancer Study Group. End results of a prospective trial on elective lateral neck dissection vs type III modified radical neck dissection in the management of supraglottic and transglottic carcinomas. *Head Neck* 1999;21:694–702.
43. Buckley J, MacLennan K. Cervical node metastases in laryngeal and hyopharyngeal cancer: a prospective analysis of prevalence and distribution. *Head Neck* 2000;22:380–385.
44. Felito A, Partridge M, Brennan J, et al. Lymph node micrometastases in head and neck cancer: a review. *Acta Otolaryngol* 2001;121:660–665.
45. Ferlito A, Rinaldo A, Devaney K, et al. Prognostic significance of microscopic and macroscopic extracapsular spread from metastatic tumor in the cervical lymph nodes. *Oral Oncol* 2002;38:747–751.
46. Woolgar J, Rogers S, Lowe D, et al. Cervical lymph node metastasis in oral cancer: the importance of even microscopic extracapsular spread. *Oral Oncol* 2003;39:130–137.
47. Ferlito A, Buckley J, Shaha A, et al. Rationale for selective neck dissection in tumors of the upper aerodigestive tract. *Acta Otolaryngol* 2001;121:548–555.
48. Ambrosch P, Freudenberg L, Kron M, et al. Selective neck dissection in the management of squamous cell carcinoma of the upper digestive tract. *Eur Arch Otorhinolaryngol* 1996;253:329–335.
49. Zhang B, Xu Z, Tang P. Lateral neck dissection vs radical neck dissection in the management of supraglottic carcinoma with pathologically negative nodes. *Chin J Otorhinolaryngol* 2003;38:426–429.

50. Leon X, Quer M, Orus C et al. Selective dissection of levels II-III with intraoperative control of the upper and middle jugular nodes: a therapeutic option for the N0 neck. *Head Neck* 2001;23: 441–446.

51. Pitman K, Johnson J, Myers E. Effectiveness of selective neck dissection for management of the clinically negative neck. *Arch Otolaryngol Head Neck Surg* 1997;123:917–922.

52. Spiro R, Gallo O, Shah J. Selective jugular node dissection in patients with squamous carcinoma of the larynx or pharynx. *Am J Surg* 1993;166:399–402.

53. Byers R, Clayman G, McGill D, et al. Selective neck dissections for squamous carcinoma of the upper aerodigestive tract: patterns of regional failure. *Head Neck* 1999;21:499–505.

54. Myers E, Fagan J. Management of the neck in cancer of the larynx. *Ann Otol Rhinol Laryngol* 1999;108:828–832.

55. Davidson J, Khan Y, Gilbert R, et al. Is selective neck dissection sufficient treatment for the N0/Np+ neck? *J Otolaryngol* 1997; 26:229–231.

56. Clayman G, Frank D. Selective neck dissection of anatomically appropriate levels is as efficacious as modified radical neck dissection for elective treatment of the clinically negative neck in patients with squamous cell carcinoma of the upper respiratory and digestive tracts. *Arch Otolaryngol Head Neck Surg* 1998;124:348–352.

57. Houck J, Medina J. Management of cervical lymph nodes in squamous carcinomas of the head and neck. *Semin Surg Oncol* 1995;11:228–239.

58. Pellitteri P, Robbins K, Neuman T. Expanded application of selective neck dissection with regard to nodal status. *Head Neck* 1997;19:260–265.

59. van Wilgen C, Dijkstra P, van der Laan BF, et al. Shoulder complaints after nerve sparing neck dissections. *Int J Oral Maxillofac Surg* 2004;33:253–257.

60. Caversaccio M, Negri S, Nolte L, et al. Neck dissection shoulder syndrome: quantification and three-dimensional evaluation with an optoelectronic tracking system. *Ann Otol Rhinol Laryngol* 2003;112:939–946.

61. Zhang B, Tang P, Xu Z, et al. Functional evaluation of the selective neck dissection in patients with carcinoma of the head and neck. *Chin J Otorhinolaryngol* 2004;39:28–31.

62. Laverick S, Lowe D, Brown J, et al. The impact of neck dissection on health-related quality of life. *Arch Otolaryngol Head Neck Surg* 2004;130:149–154.

63. van Wilgen C, Dijkstra P, Nauta J, et al. Shoulder pain and disability in daily life, following supraomohyoid neck dissection: a pilot study. *J Cranio-Maxillo-Facial Surg* 2003;31:183–186.

64. Cheng P, Hao S, Lin Y, et al. Objective comparison of shoulder dysfunction after three neck dissection techniques. *Ann Otolaryngol Rhinol Laryngol* 2000;109:761–766.

65. Ambrosch P, Kron M, Pradier O, et al. A review of 503 cases of elective and therapeutic treatment of the neck in squamous cell carcinoma of the upper aerodigestive tract. *Otolaryngol Head Neck Surg* 2001;124:180–187.

66. Andersen P, Warren F, Spiro J, et al. Results of selective neck dissection in management of the node-positive neck. *Arch Otolaryngol Head Neck Surg* 2002;128:1180–1184.

67. Robbins K, Clayman G, Levine P, et al. Neck dissection classification update. Revision proposed by the American Head and Neck Society and the American Academy of Otolaryngology-Head and Neck Surgery. *Arch Otol Head Neck Surg* 2002;128:751–758.

68. Buckley J, Feber T. Surgical treatment of cervical node metastases from squamous carcinoma of the upper aerodigestive tract: evaluation of the evidence for modifications of neck dissection. *Head Neck* 2001;23:907–915.

69. Brandenburg J, Lee C. The XI nerve in radical neck surgery. *Laryngoscope* 1981;91:1851–1859.

70. Jesse RH, Ballantyne A, Larson D. Radical or modified neck dissection: a therapeutic dilemma. *Am J Surg* 1978;136:516–519.

71. Deutsch E, Skolnik E, Friedman M, et al. The conservation neck dissection. *Laryngoscope* 1985;95:561–565.

72. Mann W, Wolfensberger M, Fuller U, et al. Radical versus modified neck dissection. Cancer-related and functional viewpoints. *Laryngorhinootologie* 1991;70:32–35.

73. Carew J, Spiro R. Extended neck dissection. *Am J Surg* 1997;174: 485–489.

74. Osguthorpe J, Abel C, Lang P. Neurotropic cutaneous tumors of the head and neck. *Arch Otolaryngol* 1997;123:871–876.

75. Vasan N, Medina J. Retropharyngeal node dissection. *Oper Tech Otolaryngol Head Neck Surg* 2004;15(3):180–183.

76. McLaughlin M, Mendenhall W, Mancuso A, et al. Retropharyngeal adenopathy as a predictor of outcome in squamous cell carcinoma of the head and neck. *Head Neck* 1995;17:190–198.

77. Amatsu M, Mohri M, Kinishi M. Significance of retropharyngeal node dissection at radical surgery for carcinoma of the hypopharynx and cervical esophagus. *Laryngoscope* 2001;111:1099–1103.

78. Ballantyne A. Significance of retropharyngeal nodes in cancer of the head and neck. *Am J Surg* 1964;108:500–504.

79. Hasegawa Y, Matsuura H. Retropharyngeal node dissection in cancer of the oropharynx and hypopharynx. *Head Neck* 1994;16: 173–180.

80. Gross N, Ellington T, Wax M, et al. Impact of retropharyngeal lymph node metastases in head and neck squamous cell carcinoma. *Arch Otolaryngol Head Neck Surg* 2004;130:169–173.

81. Weber R, Marvel J, Smith P, et al. Paratracheal lymph node dissection for carcinoma of the larynx, hypopharynx and cervical esophagus. *Otolaryngol Head Neck Surg* 1993;108:11–17.

82. Khafif A, Medina J. Management of the neck in differentiated thyroid carcinoma. In: Randolph G, ed. *Surgery of the thyroid and parathyroid glands.* Philadelphia: WB Saunders, 2003:409–418.

83. Freeman S, Hamaker R, Borrowdale R, et al. Management of neck metastasis with carotid artery involvement. *Laryngoscope* 2004; 114:20–24.

84. Nemeth Z, Domotor G, Talos M, et al. Resection and replacement of the carotid artery in metastatic head and neck cancer: literature review and case report. *Int J Oral Maxillofac Surg* 2003;32: 645–650.

85. de Vries E, Sekhar L, Horton J, et al. A new method to predict safe resection of the internal carotid artery. *Laryngoscope* 1990;100: 85–88.

86. Wright J, Nicholson R, Schuller D, et al. Resection of the internal carotid artery and replacement with greater saphenous vein: a safe procedure for en bloc cancer resections with carotid involvement. *J Vasc Surg* 1996;23:775–780.

87. Johnson J, Myers E, Bedetti C, et al. Cervical lymph node metastases. *Arch Otolaryngol Head Neck Surg* 1985;111:534–537.

88. Vikram B, Strong E, Shah J, et al. Failure in the neck following multimodality treatment for advanced head and neck cancer. *Head Neck Surg* 1984;6:724–729.

89. O'Brien C, Smith J, Soong S, et al. Neck dissection with and without radiotherapy: prognostic factors, patterns of recurrence, and survival. *Am J Surg* 1986;152:456–463.

90. Peters L, Goepfert H, Kiang A, et al. Evaluation of the dose for postoperative radiation therapy of head and neck cancer: first report of a prospective randomized trial. *Int J Radiat Oncol Biol Phys* 1993;26:3–11.

91. Cooper J, Pajak T, Forastiere A, et al. Postoperative concurrent radiotherapy and chemotherapy for high-risk squamous cell carcinoma of the head and neck. *N Engl J Med* 2004;350:1937–1944.

92. Bernier J, Domenge C, Ozsahin M, et al. Postoperative irradiation with or without concomitant chemotherapy for locally advanced head and neck cancer. *N Engl J Med* 2004;350:1945–1952.

93. Crean S, Hoffman A, Potts J, et al. Reduction of occult metastatic disease by extension of the supraomohyoid neck dissection to include level IV. *Head Neck* 2003;25:758–762.

94. Ferlito A, Mannara G, Rinaldo A, et al. Is extended selective supraomohyoid neck dissection indicated for treatment of oral cancer with clinically negative neck? *Acta Otolaryngol* 2000;120:792–795.

95. Khafif A, Lopez-Garza J, Medina J. Is dissection of Level IV necessary in patients with early (T1-T3, N0) tongue cancer. *Laryngoscope* 2001;111:1088–1090.

96. Khafif A, Fliss D, Gil Z, et al. Routine inclusion of level IV in neck dissection for squamous cell carcinoma of the larynx: is it justified? *Head Neck* 2004;26:309–312.

97. Silverman D, El-Haff M, Strome S, et al. Prevalence of nodal metastases in the submuscular recess (Level IIb) during selective neck dissection. *Arch Otolaryngol Head Neck Surg* 2003;129: 724–729.

98. Yuen A, Lam K, Chan A, et al. Clinicopathological analysis of elective neck dissection for N0 neck of early oral tongue carcinoma. *Am J Surg* 1999;177:90–92.

99. Brizel D, Prosnitz R, Hunter S, et al. Necessity for adjuvant neck dissection insetting of concurrent chemoradiation for advanced head and neck cancer. *Int J Radiat Oncology Phys* 2004;58: 1418–1423.

100. Corry J, Smith J, Peters L. The concept of a planned neck dissection is obsolete. *Cancer J* 2001;7:472–474.

101. Mendenhall W, Villaret D, Amdur R, et al. Planned neck dissection after definitive radiotherapy for squamous cell carcinoma of the head and neck. *Head Neck* 2002;24:1012–1018.

102. Rogers J, Greven K, NcGuirt W, et al. Can post-RT neck dissection be omitted for patients with head and neck cancer who have a negative PET scan after definitive radiation therapy? *Int J Radiat Oncol Biol Phys* 2004;58:694–697.

103. Porcedon SV, Bartolowski E, Hicks RJ, et al. Utility of positron omission tomography for the detection of disease in residual neck nodes after (chemo) radiotherapy in head and neck cancer. *Head Neck* 2005;27:175–181.

104. El Ghani F, van den Brekel M, De Goede C, et al. Shoulder function and patient well-being after various types of neck dissections. *Clin Otolaryngol Allied Sci* 2002;27:403–408.

105. Terrell J, Welsh D, Bradford C, et al. Pain, quality of life, and spinal accessory nerve status after neck dissection. *Laryngoscope* 2000;110:620–626.

106. Kuntz A, Weymuller EJ. Impact of neck dissection on quality of life. *Laryngoscope* 1999;109:1334–1338.

107. Salerno G, Cavaliere M, Foglia A, et al. The 11th nerve syndrome in functional neck dissection. *Laryngoscope* 2002;112:1299–1307.

108. McNeely M, Parliament M, Courneya K, et al. A pilot study of a randomized controlled trial to evaluate the effects of progressive resistance exercise training on shoulder dysfunction caused by spinal accessory neurapraxia/neurectomy in head and neck cancer survivors. *Head Neck* 2004;26:518–530.

109. van Wilgen C, Dijkstra P, van der Laan BF, et al. Shoulder complaints after neck dissection: is the spinal accessory nerve involved? *Br J Oral Maxillofac Surg* 2003;41:7–11.

110. Seven H, Sayin I, Turgut S. Antibiotic prophylaxis in clean neck dissections. *J Laryngol Otol* 2004;118(3):213–216.

111. Nussenbaum B, Liu J, Sinard R. Systematic management of chyle fistula: the Southwestern experience and review of the literature. *Otolaryngol Head Neck Surg* 2000;122:31–38.

112. Erisen L, Coskun H, Basut O. Objective and early diagnosis of chylous fistula in the postoperative period. *Otolaryngol Head Neck Surg* 2002;126:172–175.

113. Kannan R, Mahajan V, Ayyappan S. Management of chyle fistulae following surgery in the neck. *Indian J Cancer* 2001;38: 117–120.

114. Morris S, Taylor S. Peripheral parenteral nutrition in a case of chyle leak following neck dissection. *J Hum Nutr Diet* 2004;17: 153–155.

115. Yoshimura Y, Kondoh T. Treatment of chylous fistula with fibrin glue and clavicular periosteal flap. *Br J Oral Maxillofac Surg* 2002;40:138–139.

116. Scott K, Simko E. Thoracoscopic management of cervical thoracic duct injuries: an alternative approach. *Otolaryngol Head Neck Surg* 2003;128:755–757.

117. Nyquist G, Hagr A, Sobol S, et al. Octreotide in the medical management of chyle fistula. *Otolaryngol Head Neck Surg* 2003; 128:910–911.

118. Jortay A, Bisschop P. Bilateral chylothorax after left radical neck dissection. *Acta Otorhinolaryngol Belg* 2001;55:285–289.

119. Kamasaki N, Ikeda H, Wang Z, et al. Bilateral chylothorax following radical neck dissection. *Int J Oral Maxillofac Surg* 2003; 32:91–93.

120. Padilla Parrado M, Galan Morales J, Abril Garcia A, et al. Bilateral neck dissection and venous reconstruction with internal saphenous vein in cancer of the larynx. *An Otorrinolaringol Ibero Am* 2002;29: 367–376.

121. Katsuno S, Ishiyama T, Nezu K, et al. Three types of internal jugular vein reconstruction in bilateral radical neck dissection. *Laryngoscope* 2000;110:1578–1580.

122. Zacay G, Bedrin L, Horowitz Z, et al. Syndrome of inappropriate antidiuretic hormone or arginine vasopressin secretion in patients following neck dissection. *Laryngoscope* 2002;112: 2020–2024.

123. Khafif A, Medina J. The syndrome of inappropriate antidiuretic hormone secretion after bilateral radical neck dissections. *Acta Otolaryngol* 2002;122:907–909.

124. Worrell L, Rowe M, Petti G. Amaurosis: a complication of bilateral radical neck dissection. *Am J Otolaryngol* 2002;23:56–59.

125. Raj P, Moore P, Henderson J, et al. Bilateral cortical blindness: an unusual complication following unilateral neck dissection. *J Laryngol Otol* 2002;116:227–229.

126. Cotter C, Stringer S, Landau S, et al. Patency of the internal jugular vein following modified radical neck dissection. *Laryngoscope* 1994;104:841–845.

127. Cappiello J, Piazza C, Berlucchi M. Internal jugular vein patency after lateral neck dissection: a prospective study. *Eur Arch Otorhinolaryngol* 2002;259:409–412.

128. Davidson B, Newkirk K, Harter W, et al. Complications from planned, posttreatment neck dissections. *Arch Otol Head Neck Surg* 1999;125:401–405.

129. Cleland-Zamudio S, Wax M, Smith J, et al. Ruptured internal jugular vein: a postoperative complication of modified/selected neck dissection. *Head Neck* 2003;25:357–360.

130. Cachin Y. Management of cervical nodes in head and neck cancer. In: Rhys Evans P, Robin P, Fielding J, eds. *Head and neck cancer.* New York: Alan R. Liss, 1983:168–177.

114

Controversies in Management of the N0 Neck in Squamous Cell Carcinoma of the Upper Aerodigestive Tract

Karen T. Pitman

The presence or absence of cervical lymph node (LN) metastasis is the most accurate predictor of cancer-related outcome for patients with head and neck squamous cell carcinoma (HNSCC) who do not have distant metastases. Cervical LN metastases diminish the disease-related survival by approximately 50%. The clinically negative neck (cN0) is defined by the absence of palpable or radiographically suspicious LNs. However, patients staged cN0 can harbor lymphatic metastases that are too small to be detected by imaging or palpation. These subclinical or occult metastases are detected on pathologic examination of cervical LNs following neck dissection. Thus, there can be discordance between the clinical and pathologic nodal stage.

Three management options are available for cN0 patients. The first is clinical observation of the neck during regularly scheduled follow-up, reserving neck dissection for patients who subsequently develop regional metastases. Staging the neck with elective neck dissection (END) or treating the neck with elective neck irradiation (ENI) are alternative options. These management options have been debated among head and neck surgeons for nearly 100 years and the controversy persists despite significant advances in imaging and surgical technique.

The magnitude of the controversy is illustrated by two studies that examined the variability in management strategies of the cN0 neck among otolaryngologists (1,2). A survey of 763 board certified otolaryngologists in the United States showed 13% of the responders would observe the neck in all cN0 patients, 66% would perform END, and 19% would recommend ENI. Of those surgeons who would operate on the cN0 neck, 21% advocate comprehensive procedures and 79% would use a selective neck dissection (SND), although there was not agreement on the extent of the selective procedure: 56% would remove levels I to III, 34% levels I to IV, and 10% other levels.

The controversy over management of the N0 neck arises for several reasons. First, radiographic imaging does not possess the accuracy required to determine if the cN0 neck contains occult metastases. END provides pathologic staging of the neck, which translates to better estimates of patient prognosis. The consequences of pathologic staging are the cost of a blanket policy of END for all cN0 patients as well as the surgical morbidity.

Second, the studies that compare END to observation of cN0 patients are retrospective and not amenable to meta-analysis. There are no prospective studies with adequate statistical power that demonstrate a statistically significant survival advantage afforded to patients managed with END. It is unlikely that prospective randomized trials will ever conclusively resolve the controversy.

This chapter explores the controversies that surround management of the cN0 neck. As a starting point, consider the following questions as related to the three management options: (a) What is the incidence of occult metastases in the cN0 neck? (b) Do occult metastases impact patient outcome? (c) How accurate are the available pre-treatment studies for detecting occult metastases?

MANAGEMENT STRATEGY FOR THE N0 NECK

Although there are advocates of a watchful waiting policy for all cN0 patients, elective treatment of the cN0 neck is advocated by most head and neck surgeons. For clinicians who opt to treat the neck electively, management decisions are based on risk-benefit analysis that weighs the incidence of occult metastases against the morbidity of treatment. The threshold most clinicians use to treat the cN0 neck is a 20% or greater risk of occult disease. The threshold of 20% is based on retrospectively performed risk-benefit analyses that were performed in the 1970's. These studies showed a survival benefit was afforded to patients with greater than 20% likelihood of metastases when END was performed. Table 114.1 shows estimates of the likelihood of occult metastases based on the site and stage of the primary tumor. Keep in mind that a threshold of 20% means a significant percent of patients will be pathologically N0 and could be said to have received unnecessary intervention.

Patient and tumor related factors also impact the decision to proceed with elective treatment of the neck. If the neck will be entered for resection of the tumor or reconstruction of the primary site, most surgeons advocate END. Accordingly, END is primarily an issue for oral cavity, oropharyngeal, and laryngopharyngeal tumors that are resected transorally or endoscopically. One could also argue that tumors that are removed with partial and total laryngectomy also present a dilemma because surgical access to remove the larynx does not overlap with the surgical field for lateral neck dissection. Many clinicians cite unreliable patient follow up as justification for elective treatment of the neck. The decision to use END versus ENI for cN0 patients is based on the modality used to treat the primary tumor. Ideally, treatment is limited to single modality therapy whenever possible.

TABLE 114.1

RISK OF OCCULT METASTASES BY SITE AND STAGE OF PRIMARY TUMOR

	Stage	Site
<15%–20%	T1	Glottis (T1/T2), retromolar trigone, gingiva, hard palate, buccal mucosa
>20%–30%	T1	Oral tongue, soft palate, pharyngeal wall, supraglottic larynx, tonsil
	T2	Floor of mouth, oral tongue, retromolar trigone, gingiva, hard palate, buccal mucosa
	T1–4	Nasopharynx, piriform sinus, base of tongue
	T2–4	Soft palate, pharyngeal wall, supraglottic larynx, tonsil
	T3–4	Floor of mouth, oral tongue, retromolar trigone, gingiva, hard palate, buccal mucosa

Modified from Mendenhall WM, Million RR. Elective irradiation for squamous cell carcinoma of the head and neck: analysis of time-dose factors and causes of failure. *Int J Radiat Oncol Biol Phys* 1986;12: 741–746, with permission.

INCIDENCE OF OCCULT METASTASES

Two methods are used to estimate the incidence of occult cervical metastases in HNSCC. The first is to review studies that have reported on the regional recurrence rate in patients who were managed with observation. Patients who develop regional metastases with control of the primary tumor can be assumed to have had occult neck disease at the time of diagnosis. Table 114.2 presents the data from several studies on regional recurrence in oral cavity lesions and suggests that the occult metastatic rate for all T stages is 40% to 50%.

The other method is to examine studies that have reported on the pathologic N stage following END. Data from several studies are shown in Table 114.3. With the exception of the hypopharynx, there is agreement among these studies for each tumor site listed. When the results of these three studies are combined the occult metastatic rate of greater than 30% for all sites listed is observed.

TABLE 114.2

REGIONAL RECURRENCE RATE: NECK OBSERVED AFTER TREATMENT OF cT1–T4, N0 ORAL CAVITY PRIMARY TUMOR

Study/Reference	Regional Metastatic Rate (%)
Yuen et al. (1997)	47
McGuirt et al. (1995)	40
Fakih et al. (1989)	66
Vandenbrouck et al. (1980)	47

TABLE 114.3

OCCULT METASTATIC RATE: PATHOLOGIC N STAGE

Primary Site	pN+ (%)		
	Pitman et al.	Byers et al.	Shah
Oral cavity	41	45	34
Oropharynx	36	39	31
Hypopharynx	36	56	17
Larynx (supraglottic/ advanced glottic)	30	26	37

When the size measurements of metastatic LNs in the END specimen are analyzed, the difficulty with clinical detection is appreciated. Many studies have shown that approximately two thirds of all metastases are less than 10 mm, 33% to 58% are less than 3 mm, and in 25% of patients, the only metastatic nodes in the neck were less than 3 mm. Additionally, extracapsular spread (ECS) occurs in 33% to 36% of occult positive nodes (3,4).

IMPACT OF OCCULT METASTASES

Many studies have sought to correlate patient outcome with the pathologic findings in the END specimen. A highly significant difference in outcome for pathologically negative (pN0) compared to pathologically positive (pN+) patients has been demonstrated in several clinical studies. Three studies (3–5) have shown a significant difference in survival when occult metastases with ECS are present. Data from another study suggests that ECS in occult nodes has the same impact as ECS in palpable nodes does. The number of pathologically positive occult LNs also correlates with survival. Patients with two or more positive nodes have significantly worse survival compared to those with less than two positive nodes (6). These studies suggest that occult metastases do have a significant impact on patient outcome and that the information obtained from pathologic staging provides accurate prognostic information.

STAGING THE CLINICALLY NEGATIVE NECK

The cN0 neck is defined as having no clinical evidence of cervical metastases. This definition has not changed since the inception of the TNM staging system for HNSCC when the neck was staged by palpation alone. What have changed are the methods that are available for evaluating the cN0 neck. The most recent version of the American Joint Committee on Cancer (AJCC) staging system states that the results of palpation *and* imaging can be used to clinically stage the neck.

Today, accurate nodal staging is a multidisciplinary diagnostic problem that starts with palpation of the neck. It is estimated that 1.0 cm is the lower size limit that LNs can be appreciated by palpation, with accuracy of between 59% and 84%. Imaging provides *anatomic* information about LNs and can detect nodes that are *suspicious* for metastases. Contemporary high-resolution imaging probably detects a certain percentage of suspicious LNs that are not appreciated on palpation and provides a slight to moderate increase in the detection rate. Histopathologic examination provides pathologic confirmation of LN metastases and detects microscopic metastases not appreciated by palpation or imaging as well as false positives identified on palpation and imaging.

If the risk of undetected occult metastases could be reduced to less than 15% with imaging, an argument could be made to observe cN0 patients. The question is whether imaging can achieve this aim.

RADIOGRAPHIC IMAGING

Imaging studies provide an assessment of LN size and shape, as well as information about the internal architecture. Suspicious LNs are spherical and greater than 1.0 to 1.5 cm. LNs that demonstrate central necrosis, surrounding soft tissue invasion, or irregular borders or groups of two or more LNs also heighten the suspicion for metastases. Imaging is also helpful in patients when palpation is less accurate. For example, patients with a thick or previously treated neck or those who are at risk for metastases to the retropharyngeal (RP) and parapharyngeal space (PPS), LN groups are best evaluated with imaging. Today computed tomography (CT), magnetic resonance imaging (MRI), ultrasound (US), and positron emission tomography (PET) scan, or any combination of these studies, are used to stage the N0 neck.

Studies that have examined the accuracy of radiographic staging must be critically assessed. Meaningful studies include only cN0 patients and corroborate radiographic findings with the results of pathologic staging.

COMPUTED TOMOGRAPHY AND MAGNETIC RESONANCE IMAGING

One of the most rigorous studies to have examined the accuracy of CT and MRI reported on 213 cN0 patients with SCC of the oral cavity, oropharynx, hypopharynx, and larynx (7). All patients had pretreatment CT and MRI of the neck and the imaging results were correlated with the results of pathologic nodal staging. The results of imaging and pathology were used to calculate the negative predictive value (NPV) and positive predictive value (PPV) for node sizes from 5.0 to 15.0 mm in 1.0-mm increments. The authors showed that a 5.0-mm node had a PPV of

44% and a NPV of 90%. This means that 56% of patients who had a positive imaging study would be pN0 and would ostensibly receive unnecessary intervention. With a NPV of 90%, 10% of patients would recur if patients with negative imaging studies were left untreated. When a 10-mm threshold for intervention was used, the PPV was 50% and the NPV was 84%. Accordingly, for every increase in LN size the false positive rate decreases, but so too does the ability to detect patients that are truly pN+. The accuracy of CT and MR were approximately equal in this study. Dr. Curtin concluded, "It is unlikely that any imaging study will distinguish normal from metastatic lymph nodes in the 5-10mm range, because nodes <5-10mm rarely show internal abnormalities that are used to distinguish suspicious lymph nodes."

A study from the Queen Mary Hospital in Hong Kong showed that metastatic nodes were present in 34% of patients who had negative imaging studies. Similarly, Habernal et al. (8) showed that there is a highly significant difference between histologic and US or CT staging of the cN0 neck ($p = .0001$). Both authors concluded that none of the currently available imaging studies were accurate enough to obviate pathologic staging of the cN0 neck.

ULTRASOUND-GUIDED FINE NEEDLE ASPIRATION

Ultrasound-guided fine needle aspiration (USGFNA) of suspicious LNs can also be used to evaluate cN0 patients. US criteria for suspicious LNs are similar to those used for CT and MRI. According to published protocols, at least one suspicious LN per patient is sampled by fine needle biopsy under US guidance. When the FNA results are positive, the neck is treated. FNA negative patients are staged N0 and followed clinically with US examination of the neck. Head and neck surgeons who use USGFNA are trained in US imaging and typically perform US examinations in the clinic. Accordingly, the low cost of the initial evaluation and follow-up and the lack of exposure to ionizing radiation make this an appealing staging modality. US also provides very accurate measurements of LN size, so it is an excellent method to detect serial changes in LNs during follow-up.

Clinicians at the Free Hospital Amsterdam studied 77 patients with T1 to T4 oral cavity lesions staged N0 by USGFNA. The lesions were excised transorally and the neck was followed at 2- to 3-month intervals. Fourteen of 77, or 18% of patients recurred regionally. Six recurrences were detected on US and eight patients presented with palpable nodes, arguing against the likelihood that US could detect LNs at an earlier stage than palpation. Ten patients (71.4%) were salvaged with neck dissection and 4 of 77 died of uncontrolled neck disease.

Other studies have compared CT to USGFNA for nodal staging and found that both studies correctly predicted 50% of the occult positive nodes with a NPV of 74% and 73%, respectively. The authors concluded that the accuracy of USGFNA and CT were equal and that they were not complimentary studies.

POSITRON EMISSION TOMOGRAPHY

PET is a functional imaging modality that has been studied for evaluation of the cN0 neck. In contrast to standard imaging techniques that provide anatomic information, PET scan with the radiolabeled glucose analog fluorodeoxyglucose (FDG) provides information about the metabolic activity of tissues. Squamous cell carcinoma cells have increased metabolic and proliferative rates. Consequently, FDG accumulates in cancer cells at increased rates relative to normal tissues.

Myers examined 14 N0 patients with PET prior to END and reported a NPV of 88% and overall accuracy of 92%. In a similar study, Kau et al. obtained preoperative PET on 70 cN0 *and* cN1 patients demonstrating a NPV of 93%. The authors suggested that the false-positive rate was influenced by conditions that increased glucose metabolism, including inflammation, sarcoidosis, and normal salivary tissue. False negatives occurred with necrotic LNs and when metastatic LNs were less than 5.0 mm. This finding suggests that a minimum amount of tumor must be present to detect a difference in glucose utilization relative to background. Because FDG uptake is proportional to the number of cells with increased glycolytic activity, it is unlikely that currently available PET imaging will detect occult metastases with the desired accuracy, for example, 3- to 5-mm nodes. Hanasono corroborated these findings and suggested that PET does not achieve the diagnostic accuracy of END.

Other studies suggest that PET and CT are complimentary studies for the cN0 patient. For example, in one study PET was not as accurate as CT for evaluating LNs near the primary tumor because of high background uptake associated with the tumor. PET was superior in cases in which there were occult metastases in the contralateral neck.

Schechter et al. (9) suggested that the modest increase in the accuracy of PET compared to CT and MRI scanning that was demonstrated in the previously discussed studies may allow it to be the most accurate imaging study currently available to detect occult neck disease.

These results suggest that no imaging study can assess the stage of the neck with 100% accuracy. This can be explained by the fact that imaging provides *anatomic* information about LNs. A positive imaging study is based on a minimum size threshold or the presence of internal abnormalities. Because a significant percentage of occult nodes are less than 5.0 mm and/or do not have aberrations of internal architecture it is unlikely that imaging is accurate enough for staging the cN0 neck. Prospective studies that correlate the pN stage with PET findings are required to determine if PET scan can reduce the risk of undetected metastases to less than 15%.

ELECTIVE NECK DISSECTION

Neck dissection is a time-honored procedure that has been used in this country for more than 100 years. Crile, who published the first description of radical neck dissection (RND) in 1906, is considered the grandfather of neck dissection. Less well known is the fact that he introduced the concept of END based on his observations that regional recurrence rates were lower in some cN0 patients whose necks were dissected electively, acknowledging the inaccuracy of clinical staging. He also advocated preservation of the spinal accessory nerve (CN XI), if it was not involved with tumor.

In 1951, Hayes Martin advocated the concept of RND. He believed that neck dissection was not an oncologic procedure unless the lymphatics of the neck were removed en bloc. He also condemned the concept of END. He described RND as en bloc removal of levels I to V that included the sternocleidomastoid muscle, CN XI, internal jugular vein, submandibular gland, omohyoid muscle, tail of parotid, and cervical plexus. In the United States, RND became the standard treatment for palpable neck dissection. Martin's precepts were not challenged until the late 1960s.

In 1963, a conservation technique was proposed by Suarez and popularized by Bocca. The rationale for preserving major structures in the neck was based on observations that the lymphatic system of the neck is contained within the adipose tissue and does not extend beyond the fascial sheaths. By removing the fascia from the sternocleidomastoid muscle, internal jugular vein, and CN XI the soft tissue containing the cervical lymphatics is completely excised. The procedure described is called a functional neck dissection and removes levels I to V while preserving major structures. Present day terminology refers to this as a comprehensive or modified radical neck dissection (MRND). Numerous studies since the introduction of MRND have shown that it is as effective as RND as a staging and therapeutic procedure if the preserved structures are not involved by tumor. Aside from the obvious functional and cosmetic advantages, MRND made simultaneous bilateral neck dissections a safe alternative to staging bilateral RNDs.

The concept of selective neck dissection (SND) emerged from the results of clinical studies suggesting that metastases proceed from the primary site to predictable first echelon nodal groups and then onto adjacent nodal basins. Retrospectively analyzing the location of occult metastases following elective MRND, Shah, Byers, and Lindberg reported on the incidence of occult metastases to specific levels from head and neck primary sites. The cervical levels that are removed for SNDs are based on this data. Thus, selective procedures remove only the cervical levels that are at risk for metastases. Although there is not unanimous agreement among clinicians about the levels to be dissected for every primary site, most clinicians remove levels I to III or I to IV for oral cavity primaries and levels II to IV for laryngeal, hypopharyngeal, and oropharyngeal primaries. The obvious advantage of SND is the reduction in surgical morbidity compared to RND and MRND. During the 1980s and 1990s most centers in the United States adopted SNDs as the preferred procedure for END.

However, even END is not a completely accurate staging procedure. Regional recurrences occur postoperatively at a rate of 3% to 6% *regardless* of the procedure used (RND, MRND, or SND). Regional recurrences can be thought of as either an error in surgical technique or in the pathologic sampling technique. If the surgeon does not completely dissect the neck or the tumor has metastasized to levels not predicted by the primary tumor, then metastatic LNs can remain in the neck. The accuracy of pathologic staging also depends on how carefully the pathologist examines the neck specimen. The detection rate is higher when cervical nodes are serially sectioned with thin cuts versus the standard procedure of bisecting LNs. Finally, some metastases are probably beyond the resolution of light microscopy. Immunohistochemical (IHC) analysis for several tumor markers in electively dissected neck specimens showed that 20% to 30% of the nodes that were pN0 on light microscopy had evidence of micrometastases on serial sectioning and IHC analysis (10,11).

CONTROVERSIES

Three controversies surround the use of END: (a) What cervical levels are removed for a specific primary tumor? (b) Is END therapeutic? (c) How does the outcome of patients managed with END compare with those whose necks are observed?

Despite studies that have showed that SNDs are as effective as comprehensive procedures for staging the cN0 neck, head and neck surgeons continue to debate the extent of the dissection required for adequate pathologic staging. The acceptance of selective procedures assumes that patterns of metastatic spread to the cervical LNs are predictable. Although this is probably true for a majority of patients, the results of preoperative lymphoscintigraphy for sentinel lymph node biopsy (SLNB) (discussed later) suggest that up to 15% to 30% of upper aerodigestive tract tumors drain to lymphatic levels that are not predicted by the tumor site and stage. These individual variations in lymphatic drainage patterns are an argument in favor of comprehensive procedures. If an END does not sample the appropriate lymphatics, the staging information will not be accurate. Procedures that remove all five levels (MRND and RND) have a higher probability of removing all of the occult metastases and have well-defined anatomic boundaries of dissection. Selective procedures are technically challenging and the anatomic limits for a specific procedure vary from surgeon to surgeon. The obvious advantage of SND is the reduction in surgical morbidity and operating time (12).

A related controversy is whether an END can be considered a therapeutic procedure. Some institutions advocate radiation therapy for all patients who are pN+. In this case, a selective procedure provides the information required to decide on the administration of adjuvant therapy. Others believe END alone is adequate treatment for patients with one or two metastatic LNs without ECS. Although most of the studies that have compared the effectiveness of MRND and SND for elective lymphadenectomy have shown no difference in outcome based on the completeness of dissection, all of the studies are retrospective and subject to the limitations of such studies. Accordingly the question has not been conclusively answered.

Elective Neck Dissection Versus Observation

Central to the debate surrounding the value of END is whether removing occult neck disease affords a survival advantage when compared to a policy of clinical observation.

Two retrospective studies published in the 1970s suggest that there is a survival benefit in patients who receive END. Ogura (13) compared the outcome of 348 patients who received therapeutic versus elective neck dissection. He showed improved 3-year survival for patients with supraglottic, piriform sinus, and base of tongue primaries who received END. In a series of more than 500 patients, Lee and Krause (14) also reported increased survival for patients who received END compared with those who required therapeutic neck dissection.

Recent studies show mixed results. Smith et al. (15) reported on the outcome of 150 patients with T1 to T4, N0 oral cavity and oropharyngeal tumors. Seventy-five patients received END based on a greater than 20% risk of occult metastases or because the neck was entered for the tumor resection or microvascular reconstruction. The other 75 patients were managed with observation based on less than 20% risk of occult disease. Despite a statistically significant difference in the regional recurrence rate, 5% for the END group and 20% for the observation group, the difference in the 5-year survival rate between the two groups was not significant. The authors did show highly significant differences in 5-year survival rates based on the number of pathologically positive nodes ($p < .001$).

Duvvuri et al. (16) compared the outcome of 359 patients with T1 to T4, N0 oral cavity and oropharyngeal tumors managed with END versus observation. The treatment groups were based on time period they were treated, for example, before or after 1990 when END was routinely used for management of the N0 neck. The 5-year overall survival between groups was not different, but the difference in the regional recurrence rate, 15% versus 27% for the END and observation groups, respectively, was highly

significant ($p < .0001$). In both studies, more patients in the END group received adjuvant radiation, a direct result of the pathologic staging information.

A similar study (17) analyzed 54 patients with T1 to T3, N0 oral cavity tumors managed with END versus observation. There was no difference in the overall survival between treatment groups. The authors recommend observation for patients with T1 tumors because there was no difference between the treatment groups for the regional recurrence rate or overall survival. However, for patients with T2 and T3 tumors, they did recommend END because the regional recurrence rate and the associated mortality were significantly higher in the group that was observed.

Other retrospective studies have shown a significant survival advantage for patients who receive END. Yuen et al. (18) reported on 63 patients with T1 and T2 oral cavity tumors. For the 33 patients managed with END, both regional recurrences and 5-year overall survival rate were significantly improved compared to the 30 patients who were observed ($p = .0008$ and $p = .01$, respectively). Despite surgical salvage of 50% of the regional recurrences in the observation group, the regional recurrence related mortality in this group was 23% compared with 3% in the SND group and this benefit translated to a significant improvement in 5-year overall survival.

In a detailed analysis of patients with T1 and T2, N0 oral tongue tumors, Haddadin et al. (19) compared the outcome of 64 patients who were observed to 37 who received END. The institutional policy was to observe the neck in all patients with T1 or T2 oral tongue tumors unless the neck was entered to resect the primary or perform reconstruction. The authors did show a trend toward improved 5-year overall survival favoring the END group. When the T2 tumors alone were analyzed a highly significant survival advantage for END ($p = .0007$) was observed. The authors also showed that the incidence of more than two LNs or ECS was significantly higher in the patients who required therapeutic neck dissection than in patients who received END, $p = .001$ and $p < .0001$, respectively. The impact of this finding is illustrated by comparing the 5-year survival of patients who were pN+ after END versus therapeutic dissections, which was 69% versus 35%, respectively ($p = .04$). Similarly, a study from Memorial Sloan Kettering Cancer Center showed that 66% of patients who developed regional recurrences during a program of observation presented with N2 or greater disease and 77% had ECS.

These studies all show significant improvements in the regional recurrence rate for patients managed with END. The benefit in terms of disease-related survival is less clear and retrospective studies will probably never conclusively answer the question. These patient cohorts are difficult to analyze because of their heterogeneity, and the number of patients who succumb to local and distant recurrences or non-cancer related causes. Hence, the number of patients who develop isolated regional recurrences in either group is small and lacks statistical power.

Although END may not show benefit when the entire cohort is analyzed, scrutinizing the outcome of pN+ patients may demonstrate a benefit. Patients with pN0 disease usually do well regardless of the treatment modality. The cohort at issue is the pN+ patients, who are the same group regardless of whether they are treated with END or observation. Anderson and Haddadin have demonstrated that high-risk pathologic findings are more common following therapeutic neck dissection. This line of indirect evidence suggests that END potentially impacts disease-related survival because LNs are removed at an earlier stage when low-risk pathologic findings are more likely.

Elective Neck Irradiation

The factors that influence the decision to irradiate the cN0 neck are similar to those for END. ENI is the treatment of choice when the primary tumor is irradiated and the risk of occult metastases is more than 20%. It is also an option for patients who are poor surgical candidates. Patients' compliance with follow-up and the morbidity of ENI are also considered. Patients who are cN0 receive substantially lower radiation doses to the neck than cN+ patients and have an associated reduction in the treatment related morbidity. The availability of conformational and intensity-modulated radiation therapy has minimized the volume of normal tissue that is included in the treatment portals, further reducing the morbidity of ENI. Mendenhall et al. (20) have reported regional recurrences in less than 5% of patients following ENI. One advantage of ENI is the ability to address groups of nodes that are not typically included in END. These include the RP and PPS LNs that are at risk of harboring occult metastases with tumors of the oropharynx, hypopharynx, nasopharynx, and nasal cavity.

A significant shortcoming of ENI is that the prognostic information from pathologic staging is not known. It is also more difficult to detect recurrences following ENI and usually the neck cannot be reirradiated.

FUTURE DIRECTIONS

More accurate, less invasive methods to evaluate the cN0 neck are active areas of investigation. SLNB and pathologic predictors of occult metastases are two techniques that demonstrate potential for clinical use in the future.

The concept of the sentinel lymph node (SLN) was introduced in 1970s by Cabanas who described it as the first-echelon LN that is most likely to contain cancer if metastases have occurred. Morton and colleagues at the John Wayne Cancer Center are credited with the development of the technique for selective identification and biopsy of the SLN in patients with intermediate thickness cutaneous melanoma (CM).

SLNB is based on the premise that metastases travel sequentially from the primary tumor to the SLN and then on to the remaining regional LNs. Therefore, the histopathologic appearance of the SLN will accurately reflect the pathologic status of the remaining regional lymphatics. This is an attractive concept because patients with pathologically negative SLNs can be spared the morbidity of regional lymphadectomy.

Since Morton's original description of the SLNB technique, numerous investigators worldwide have contributed to the evolution and refinement of the technique that is currently used. The subsequent experience with SLNB in CM has shown that the SLN can be identified in 99% of patients with sensitivity of more than 95% and false-negative rate of less than 2%. Compared with a policy of elective lymphadenectomy, SLNB has significantly decreased the morbidity of staging the regional lymphatics and has revolutionized the treatment of patients with intermediate thickness CM. Accordingly, SLNB has become the standard of care for patients with CM.

The SLNB technique begins with preoperative lymphoscintigraphy. A radiotracer is injected at four sites around the tumor and gamma camera images depict the laterality and approximate anatomic location of the SLN(s). The nuclear medicine physician marks the area(s) that corresponds to the SLN(s) on the patient's skin, which direct the surgeon to the lymphatic regions at risk. In the operating room, the surgeon uses a gamma probe transcutaneously to confirm the location of the SLN(s) and blue dye is injected intradermally. The SLN is exposed through a small skin incision and is positively identified by the presence of blue staining and/or radiotracer uptake detected by the gamma probe. Identification of the SLN with the concurrent use of blue dye and radiotracer intraoperatively increases the identification rate of SLNs and probably accounts for the accuracy observed in recent studies. The SLN(s) are removed and sent to the pathologist for histologic and IHC analysis. Therapeutic node dissection is performed only in patients whose SLN is positive.

Encouraged by the success just described many investigators have applied the technique to head and neck cancer patients who are cN0. The preliminary experience in HNSCC was summarized by Ross in 2002 and included data from 22 centers. Analysis of 316 cN0 necks showed that the SLN was identified in 95% with an overall accuracy of 90%. When the results from centers that performed less than 10 cases were excluded, the sensitivity of SLNB was 94% relative to simultaneous END. These studies demonstrated an average of two to three SLNs per neck. This and several other studies have shown that SLNB is feasible and holds promise in HNSCC. Multiinstitutional studies currently underway in the United States are the most expeditious route to accrue sufficient patients and experience to validate the technique and determine the specificity and sensitivity of SLNB compared with END.

SLNB results in a reduction in the overall morbidity and cost compared to a blanket policy of END. Advantages of SLNB specific to head and neck tumors include the ability of preoperative lymphoscintigraphy to provide accurate information on the patient's unique lymphatic drainage pattern and direct the surgeon to cervical levels that would not have been predicted by the site and stage of the primary tumor. Results of preoperative lymphoscintigraphy show that 15% of ENDs for HNSCC and 60% for head and neck CM would have been misdirected had they been based solely on classical anatomic studies (21,22). Another advantage is that SLNB is a cost-effective method for pathologic examination of select LNs. Rather than examining all of the nodes in a neck dissection specimen, SLNB identifies an average of two or three nodes per patient. This facilitates the routine use of more costly and time-consuming serial sectioning and IHC required to accurately diagnose occult metastases. Using SLNB and IHC, Ross et al. (10) showed significant improvements in the accuracy of staging the cN0 neck.

PATHOLOGIC PREDICTORS OF METASTASES

The site and stage of the primary tumor are important considerations in assessing the risk of occult metastases. Early studies suggested a direct correlation between the tumor stage and the incidence of occult metastases. Although this is true for some sites, for example, early glottic tumors, more recent studies suggest that for many sites tumor stage alone is not predictive. For example, tumor thickness has been shown to be a predictor of occult metastases for many sites and has been most intensively studied for oral cavity tumors (23,24).

Yuen et al. (25) examined several histopathologic characteristics of T1 and T2 oral tongue tumors that were correlated with occult metastases. On multivariate analysis tumor thickness was the only factor that correlated with occult metastases and 5-year survival. The pN+ rate for tumor thickness 3 mm or less was 8%. Metastases occurred in 44% of tumors between 3 and 9 mm, and in 53% of those tumors with thickness greater than 9 mm. The 5-year survival by thickness grouping was 100%, 77%, and 66%, respectively. Based on this data the authors recommend observation of the neck in patients with tumor thickness 3 mm or less, END for 3- to 9-mm tumors and radiation therapy to the primary site and neck with tumor thickness greater than 9 mm. This strategy would avoid END in 40/72 patients in this study.

These findings highlight one of the shortcomings of the current AJCC tumor staging system that is based solely on an anatomic description of the tumor. Investigators seeking to improve the prognostic capabilities of tumor staging have focused on characteristics of the primary tumor that are correlated with nodal metastases. Pathologic predictors of occult metastases that can be characterized with light microscopy, IHC, and DNA analysis are currently under active investigation.

Many studies suggest that the correlates of metastases may be different for different anatomic sites. For example, critical tumor thickness may vary depending on tumor site because the depth and caliber of the lymphatics varies throughout the mucosal sites of the head and neck. Additionally, combinations of parameters may more accurately predict the risk of metastases because it is unlikely that a single characteristic of the tumor will have a distinct cut off point in differentiating metastatic from non-metastatic disease (23,26,27).

Wolgar and Scott proposed a histologic malignancy score for oral cavity tumors based on histologic findings such as the frequency of mitotic figures, pattern of invasion, and perineural and perivascular invasion. Japanese investigators devised a scoring system based on light microscopic findings obtained from biopsy of the tumor. When this model was applied prospectively to newly diagnosed patients, metastases were accurately predicted in 87.5% of cN0 patients. Similarly, Takes et al. (28) showed that LN metastases from laryngeal tumors were accurately predicted using a combination of histologic and IHC findings ($p = .002$).

Once the characteristics of primary tumors that correlate with occult metastases have been accurately identified biologic tumor staging will be possible. The next step will be to integrate the biologic correlates of metastases into the tumor staging system. Clinicians could then make management decisions about the neck based on the results of the pretreatment biopsy and surgical intervention for staging the cN0 would have a secondary role.

CONCLUSION

Management of the cN0 neck is controversial. The pretreatment evaluation of cN0 patients aims to accurately identify patients with occult metastases who will benefit from treatment of the neck. A review of the methods that are currently in use for evaluation of the cN0 neck shows that the AJCC tumor staging system does not adequately distinguish patients with microscopic cervical metastases from N0 patients with acceptable sensitivity and specificity. Biologic tumor staging and SLNB are promising techniques that have the potential to accurately identify N0 patients before treatment is initiated. Until these investigational staging methods are refined and incorporated into a clinically useful tumor staging system, pathologic examination of the neck contents remains the most accurate method to assess the regional lymphatics.

HIGHLIGHTS

- The incidence of occult cervical metastases is greater than 20% for most head and neck mucosal sites. The exceptions are T1 tumors of the retromolar trigone, buccal mucosal, gingiva, hard palate, and T1 and T2 glottic tumors.

- The pathologic nodal status of cN0 patients is strongly correlated with the disease-related outcome.
- Radiographic imaging provides anatomic information that identifies lymph nodes that are suspicious for metastases. It does not have the accuracy to determine whether the N0 neck requires treatment.
- Elective neck dissection is currently the most accurate method to stage the cN0 neck.
- Elective neck dissection is a staging procedure that is used to guide subsequent treatment. Its therapeutic value has not been conclusively documented, although indirect evidence does appear to support a benefit compared to observation of cN0 patients.
- Elective versus therapeutic neck dissection describes the indication for neck dissection. A neck dissection is performed *electively* when there is no clinical evidence of metastases. *Therapeutic* neck dissection refers to procedures that are performed for suspicious adenopathy that is palpable or detected on radiographic imaging.
- Comprehensive versus selective neck dissection describes what cervical levels are removed. *Comprehensive* neck dissection removes levels I to V. Radical neck dissections and all three types of modified radical neck dissections are comprehensive procedures. *Selective* neck dissection removes less than five levels and are named according to the levels removed, for example, selective neck dissection I to III. Both selective and comprehensive procedures can be used for *elective* neck dissection.
- Techniques that are less invasive than elective neck dissection and more accurate than radiographic imaging for staging the cN0 neck are under active investigation and hold promise for routine clinical use in the future.

REFERENCES

1. Werning J, Heard D, Pagano C, et al. Elective management of the clinically negative neck by otolaryngologists in patients with oral tongue cancer. *Arch Otolaryngol Head Neck Surg* 2003;129:83–88.
2. Dunne AA, Folz BJ, Kuropkat C, et al. Extent of surgical intervention in case of N0 neck in head and neck cancer patients: an analysis of data collection of 39 hospitals. *Eur Arch Otorhinolaryngol* 2004;261:295–303.
3. Jose J, Coatesworth AP, MacLennan K. Cervical metastases in upper aerodigestive tract squamous cell carcinoma: histopathologic analysis and reporting. *Head Neck* 2003;25:194–197.
4. Van den Brekel M WM, van der Waal IDD, Meijer C, et al. The incidence of micrometastases in neck dissection specimens obtained from elective neck dissections. *Laryngoscope* 1996;106:987–991.
5. Pinsolle J, Pinsolle V, Majoufre C, et al. Prognostic value of histologic staging in neck dissections for squamous cell carcinoma. *Arch Otolaryngol Head Neck Surg* 1997;123:145–148.
6. Colnot DR, Nieuwenhuis EJ, Kuik DJ, et al. Clinical significance of micrometastatic cells detected by E48 (Ly-6D) reverse transcription-polymerase chain reaction in bone marrow of head and neck cancer patients. *Clin Cancer Res* 2004;10:7827–7833.
7. Curtin H, Ishwaran H, Mancuso A, et al. Comparison of CT and MR imaging in staging of neck metastases. *Radiology* 1998;207:123–130.
8. Haberal I, Celik H, Gocmen H, et al. Which is important in the evaluation of metastatic lymph nodes in head and neck cancer: palpation, ultrasonography, or computed tomography? *Otolaryngol Head Neck Surg* 2004;130:197–201.
9. Schechter NR, Gillenwater AM, Byers RM, et al. Can positron emission tomography improve the quality of care for head and neck cancer patients? *Int J Radiat Oncol Biol Phys* 2001;51:4–9.
10. Ross GL, Soutar DS, MacDonald GD, et al. Sentinel node biopsy in head and neck cancer: preliminary results of a multicenter trial. *Ann Surg Oncol* 2004;11:690–696.
11. Barrera JE, Miller ME, Said S, et al. Detection of occult cervical micrometastases in patients with head and neck squamous cell cancer. *Laryngoscope* 2003;113:892–896.
12. Sivanandan R, Kaplan M, Lee K, et al. Long-term results of 100 consecutive comprehensive neck dissections. *Arch Otolaryngol Head Neck Surg* 2004;130:1369–1374.
13. Ogura JH, Biller HF, Wette R. Elective neck dissection for pharyngeal and laryngeal cancers. *Ann Otol* 1971;80:646–651.
14. Lee JG, Krause CJ. Radical neck dissection: elective, therapeutic, and secondary. *Arch Otolaryngol* 1975;101:656–659.
15. Smith GI, O'Brien CJ, Clark J, et al. Management of the neck in patients with T1 and T2 cancer in the mouth. *Br J Oral Maxillofacial Surg* 2004;42:494–500.
16. Duvvuri U, Simental AA, D'Angelo G, et al. Elective neck dissection and survival in patients with squamous cell carcinoma of the oral cavity and oropharynx. *Laryngoscope* 2004;114:2228–2234.
17. Persky M, Lagmay V. Treatment of the clinically negative neck in oral squamous cell carcinoma. *Laryngoscope* 1999;109:1160–1164.
18. Yuen AP, Wei WI, Wong Y, et al. Elective neck dissection versus observation in the treatment of early oral tongue carcinoma. *Head Neck* 1997;19:583–588.
19. Haddadin K, Soutar D, Oliver R, et al. Improved survival for patients with clinically T1/T2, N0 tongue tumors undergoing prophylactic neck dissection. *Head Neck* 1999;21:517–525.
20. Mendenhall WM, Million RR. Elective irradiation for squamous cell carcinoma of the head and neck: analysis of time-dose factors and causes of failure. *Int J Radiat Oncol Biol Phys* 1986;12:741–746.
21. Pitman KT, Johnson JT, Brown ML, et al. Sentinel lymph node biopsy in head and neck squamous cell carcinoma. *Laryngoscope* 2002;112:2101–2113.
22. Hyde NC, Prvulovich E, Newman L, et al. A new approach to pretreatment assessment of the N0 neck in oral squamous cell carcinoma: the role of sentinel lymph node biopsy and positron emission tomography. *Oral Oncol* 2003;39:350–360.
23. Sheahan P, O'Keane C, Sheahan JN, et al. Effect of tumor thickness and other factors on the risk of regional disease and treatment of the N0 neck in early oral squamous carcinoma. *Clin Otolaryngol* 2003;28:461–471.
24. O'Brien CJ, Lauer C, Fredricks S, et al. Tumor thickness influences prognosis of T1 and T2 oral cavity cancer—but what thickness? *Head Neck* 2003;25:937–943.
25. Yuen AP, Lam KY, Lam LK, et al. Prognostic factors of clinically Stage I and II oral tongue carcinoma—a comparative study of stage, thickness, shape, growth pattern, invasive front malignancy grading, Martinez-Gimeno score, and pathologic features. *Head Neck* 2002;24:513–520.
26. Sparano A, Weinstein G, Chalian A, et al. Multivariate predictors of occult neck metastases in early tongue cancer. *Otolaryngol Head Neck Surg* 2004;131:472–476.
27. Lim SC, Zhang S, Ishii G, et al. Predictive markers for late cervical metastasis in stage I and II invasive squamous cell carcinoma of the oral tongue. *Clin Cancer Res* 2004;10:166–172.
28. Takes RP, Batenburg RJ, Schuuring E, et al. Markers for assessment of nodal metastases in laryngeal carcinoma. *Arch Otolaryngol Head Neck Surg* 1997;123:412–418.

Lymphomas of the Head and Neck

Ranjana Advani   *Charlotte D. Jacobs*

Although non-Hodgkin lymphoma (NHL) frequently involves the cervical lymph nodes, approximately 10% occur in the extranodal sites of the head and neck region. These areas include Waldeyer ring, paranasal sinuses, nasal cavity, larynx, oral cavity, salivary glands, thyroid, and orbit. The evaluation of lymphomas must be precise because therapy varies with stage, histology, and site. Lymphomas are highly curable if treated appropriately. Thus, it is imperative that the head and neck oncologist be familiar with their management.

EVALUATION AND DIAGNOSIS

The incidence of lymphoma has increased significantly over the last decade (1). Risk factors include congenital immunodeficiency disease, acquired immunodeficiency, and autoimmune disorders. The immunosuppressive regimens used for organ transplantation can cause a spectrum of lymphoproliferative disorders from oropharyngeal hyperplasia to lymphoma. Chronic infection with human immunodeficiency virus (HIV) can result in a 100-fold increased risk for lymphoma (2). Underlying Hashimoto thyroiditis is found in up to half of patients with thyroid lymphoma (3). Patients with Sjögren syndrome have an increased chance of developing lymphoma of salivary glands (4). Chinese patients in Hong Kong have a relatively high incidence of nasal lymphoma, which is closely associated with the Epstein-Barr virus (5). Recently, *Chlamydia psittaci* has been reported in association with ocular lymphomas (6).

Extranodal NHLs of the head and neck region occur predominantly in patients between 50 and 60 years of age (7). The male to female ratio is 1.6:1 with the exception of lymphomas of the salivary glands, orbit, and thyroid, which occur equally or more frequently in women.

Sites and Presenting Symptoms

More than half of extranodal head and neck lymphomas occur in Waldeyer ring; tonsils are the most common site, followed by the nasopharynx and base of tongue (7). Presenting symptoms are similar to those of squamous cancers. Tonsil lymphomas present with tonsillar swelling or throat pain. Patients with nasopharynx lymphoma often complain of cervical masses or nasal obstruction. Foreign-body sensation or sore throat are often the first symptoms of lymphomas of the base of tongue. Lymphomas are usually submucosal, differing on gross appearance from ulcerative squamous cell cancers.

About a third of head and neck lymphomas occur in extralymphatic sites, including the paranasal sinuses, nasal cavity, salivary glands, oral cavity, larynx, and orbit. Again, these mimic squamous cell cancers at presentation. Sinus lymphomas usually cause symptoms of sinusitis, whereas diplopia and exophthalmos may occur with bulky disease (8). Nasal cavity lymphomas cause obstructive symptoms and nasal bleeding; oral cavity lymphomas present with local swelling, pain, and ulcers; laryngeal lymphomas present with hoarseness, dyspnea, and dysphagia. Salivary gland lymphomas usually present with a parotid mass, although facial nerve involvement is rare. Primary lymphoma of the thyroid gland constitutes only 5% to 10% of all thyroid cancers (3). Most patients present with a rapidly enlarging thyroid mass, hoarseness, or dysphagia. Patients with orbital lymphoma usually complain of orbital swelling and may have exophthalmos on examination. Other symptoms include changes in vision, proptosis, ptosis, and pain. Visual fields are usually unaffected, and the fundi are typically benign. Patients with conjunctival disease most commonly have a palpable pink mass in the conjunctiva at presentation. Overall, approximately 15% of patients with head and neck lymphoma have neck adenopathy as a presenting complaint, whereas 12% have systemic symptoms of fever, night sweats, or weight loss. Twenty percent of patients with lymphomas have multiple sites of involvement in the head and neck region.

Diagnosis and Histologic Classification

A fine-needle aspiration (FNA) or a core biopsy is useful in the initial workup. Once a lymphoid neoplasm is suspected on the basis of a FNA or core, an open biopsy is required for definitive diagnosis of NHL. An FNA may be useful in detecting recurrent disease or histologic transformation; however, cytologic evaluation alone cannot assess whether the lymphoma is follicular or diffuse, an important factor in determining grade and prognosis. Thus, an open biopsy is preferred for the initial diagnosis. Immunohistochemical stains can help discriminate lymphoma from undifferentiated or anaplastic neoplasms: antikeratin antibodies for carcinoma, anti-S-100 protein antibodies for melanoma, and panleukocyte antibodies for lymphoma. Immunohistochemical studies can also help differentiate a benign lymphoid infiltrate from a lymphoma on light microscopy. Most NHLs express either T-cell or B-cell markers. A panel of T-cell antigens can differentiate T-cell lymphomas from hyperplasia. B-cell lymphomas express a single class of light chains (i.e., kappa or lambda), whereas hyperplasia shows an admixture of the two classes. Because immunohistochemical staining or other molecular assays, such as gene rearrangement studies to test for clonality, may perform better on fresh tissue, the pathologist should be notified if the physician entertains a diagnosis of lymphoma.

The particular histologic subtype of an NHL influences staging evaluation, therapy, and expected survival. The histologic classification of lymphomas has evolved over the years as greater understanding of molecular characteristics has allowed pathologists to identify unique entities that might have been grouped together previously. The continued changes in classification can bewilder even the most seasoned clinician. One of the most clinically useful and frequently referenced classifications was the Working Formulation, the classification scheme used in North America until the mid-1990s (9). Although it was simple, it did not take into account the relevance of the immunophenotype (i.e., B cell vs. T cell), and it did not use other correlative data (e.g., molecular genetics) to describe particular entities, demonstrate evidence of clonality, or prognosticate. In 1999, the revised European-American Lymphoma (REAL) classification distinguished lymphomas not only by histology but also by immunophenotypic, genetic, and clinical

characteristics. Subsequently a number of entities were described that were not part of the Working Formulation such as anaplastic large-cell lymphoma, marginal zone lymphomas (MALT), and mantle cell lymphoma. This system was further modified as the now universally accepted WHO classification (10).

The seemingly perpetual changes in pathologic classification can make it difficult for the practicing physician to interpret pathologic reports. Moreover, much of the literature is based on previous classification systems that might make extrapolation to current entities difficult. Nonetheless, many of the key and most common entities in the Working Formulation are still recognizable. Table 115.1 lists the Working Formulation subtypes with corresponding entities recognized in the WHO classification. The majority of this chapter references the Working Formulation primarily because of the clinical utility and because much of the literature is based on that classification system. Approximately 4% of lymphomas are composite malignancies, in which two different lymphomas occur in a single site. Approximately 10% of patients have discordant lymphomas, in which there are two distinct lymphomas at different sites. With time, lymphomas can transform, most commonly from a low- to intermediate-grade subtype.

Head and neck lymphomas are predominantly intermediate grade, whereas approximately 12% are low grade, and 16% are high grade (11). Overall, diffuse large cell is the most common subtype. Paranasal sinus and nasal cavity lymphomas are almost always intermediate- or high-grade

TABLE 115.1

HEAD AND NECK LYMPHOMAS—HISTOLOGIC CLASSIFICATION

Working Formulation (9)	WHO Equivalents (10)
Low grade	
Small lymphocytic	B-cell small lymphocytic or extranodal marginal zone
Follicular small cleaved cell	Follicular lymphoma, grade 1
Follicular mixed	Follicular lymphoma, grade 2
Intermediate grade	
Follicular large cell	Follicular lymphoma, grade 3
Diffuse small cleaved cell	Mantle cell, lymphoplasmacytic
Diffuse mixed	Diffuse large B cell, peripheral T cell
	Extranodal NK/T cell
Diffuse large cell	Diffuse large B cell, peripheral T cell
	Extranodal NK/T cell
High grade	
Immunoblastic	Diffuse large B cell, peripheral T cell
	Extranodal NK/T cell
Lymphoblastic	Lymphoblastic
Small non-cleaved cell	Burkitt lymphoma/Burkitt-like

NK, natural killer.

TABLE 115.2

HEAD AND NECK LYMPHOMAS—STAGING EVALUATION

- Pathologic review
- Complete physical examination, indirect laryngoscopy
- Complete blood count, liver function tests, LDH
- HIV test (positive risk factors)
- Chest radiograph
- CT or MRI of head and neck
- CT of chest, abdomen, and pelvis
- Upper gastrointestinal series with small bowel follow-through (Waldeyer ring)
- PET scan
- Lumbar puncture (paranasal sinus)
- Bone marrow biopsy

CT, computed tomography; LDH, lactate dehydrogenase; MRI, magnetic resonance imaging; PET, positron emission tomography.

malignancies, whereas more than half of the patients with salivary gland lymphomas have a low-grade histology (7). Most thyroid lymphomas are intermediate-grade malignancies, and a high percentage of these patients show evidence of Hashimoto thyroiditis (12). Lymphomas originating in the orbit are usually low grade and may be difficult to differentiate from nonmalignant orbital lymphoid infiltrates. Most head and neck lymphomas express B-cell markers. Lymphoblastic lymphomas and a small percentage of diffuse large cell lymphomas are of T-cell lineage. T-cell and natural killer types arise predominantly in the nasal cavity and paranasal sinuses.

Clinical Assessment

Accurate staging is imperative before initiating therapy (Table 115.2). The patient should undergo a complete history and physical examination, including indirect laryngoscopy. Computed tomography (CT) or magnetic resonance imaging (MRI) studies may more accurately assess the extent of the primary lesion in the head and neck (13). A complete blood count, liver function tests, and a lactate dehydrogenase (LDH) level are recommended. A CT scan should be obtained to evaluate mediastinal or hilar adenopathy, as well as liver, splenic, and mesenteric involvement. A positron emission tomography (PET) can be useful, particularly for imaging sites of initial bulky disease or residual masses at the completion of therapy to help confirm remission status. An association between lymphoma of Waldeyer ring and the gastrointestinal tract has been reported in 3% to 11% of patients. Hence, an upper gastrointestinal series with small bowel follow-through or upper gastrointestinal endoscopy is recommended for initial staging of these patients (14).

A posterior iliac crest bone marrow biopsy should be performed because approximately 18% of patients with extranodal head and neck lymphomas have bone marrow

involvement at presentation. This percentage is substantially higher among patients with low-grade histologies. A lumbar puncture with cerebrospinal fluid chemistry, complete cell count, and cytologic analysis is recommended at initial staging for patients with a high propensity for central nervous system involvement, which includes those with high-grade lymphoma, or those with intermediate-grade lymphoma involving paranasal sinuses, bone marrow, testes, or paraspinal areas. Because of the increased accuracy of clinical staging and the common use of chemotherapy, staging laparotomy is no longer routinely recommended.

After completion of therapy, patients should be reassessed regularly. This includes a physical examination, complete blood counts, liver function tests, LDH, and appropriate imaging studies to assess all prior sites of disease.

Staging System

After complete assessment, a stage is assigned using the Ann Arbor staging system (Table 115.3). Stage is assigned based on the sites of lymph node or organ involvement. The "E" designation indicates extralymphatic involvement of tissue adjacent to a lymph node, such as the oral cavity, salivary glands, or paranasal sinus. The stage is further denoted by "A" for patients without systemic symptoms or "B" for patients with unexplained fever, night sweats, or weight loss of more than 10% of body weight. In a series of more than 900 patients with head and neck lymphomas, 31% had stage I, 35% stage II, 14% stage III, and 19% stage IV disease (15). Only a small percentage had "B" symptoms. The majority of patients with thyroid lymphoma present with stage I or IIE disease; approximately two thirds of orbital lymphomas are stage I.

TABLE 115.3

ANN ARBOR STAGING SYSTEM

Designation	Characteristic
Stage I	Involvement of a single lymph node region (I) or of a single extralymphatic organ or site (IE)
Stage II	Involvement of two or more lymph node regions on the same side of the diaphragm (II) or localized involvement of an extralymphatic organ or site and of one or more lymph node regions on the same side of the diaphragm (IIE)
Stage III	Involvement of lymph node regions on both sides of the diaphragm (III)
Stage IV	Diffuse or disseminated involvement of one or more extralymphatic organs or tissues with or without lymph node involvement
Symptoms	
A	Absence of systemic symptoms
B	Unexplained fever, night sweats, or weight loss of more than 10% body weight

Prognostic Factors

NHL includes entities of low, intermediate, and high grades. Even within these histologic subtypes, outcomes are variable. The International Prognostic Index (IPI), published in 1993, predicts outcome for patients with aggressive diffuse large cell lymphomas based on five prognostic factors: age, performance status, LDH, number of extranodal sites, and stage (16). Recently a similar system has been developed for follicular lymphoma referred to as the Follicular Lymphoma International Prognostic Index (FLIPI) (17).

Newer technologies, such as DNA microarray analyses, have identified genes that are either over or under-expressed by lymphoma cells, and this has further differentiated patients into different risk groups even within histologies. Two distinct subtypes of diffuse large B-cell lymphoma have been identified on the basis of their pattern of gene expression by microarrays with significantly different probabilities of survival at 5 years (18).

MANAGEMENT

General Principles

The management of head and neck lymphomas should be a multidisciplinary effort by pathologists, radiologists, otolaryngologists, radiotherapists, and medical oncologists. Treatment choices depend on histologic subtype and stage. General recommendations can be made for certain subgroups (Table 115.4), but an oncologic team should individually evaluate each patient.

The primary treatment involves radiation therapy, chemotherapy, immunotherapy, or a combination of these modalities. Radiation is delivered in 200-cGy daily fractions to a total dose of 3,000 to 4,000 cGy for low-grade lymphomas and 4,900 to 5,000 cGy for intermediate-grade lymphomas. Fields are tailored for the type of tumor, location, and individual patient anatomy. The most

---

TABLE 115.4

HEAD AND NECK LYMPHOMAS—TREATMENT

Histology	Storage	Treatment Options
Low grade	I, II	Involved-field XRT
	III, IV	CVP, chlorambucil, rituximab, observation
Intermediate grade	I, II	RCHOP × 3-XRT
	III, IV	RCHOP × 6 or other combination chemotherapy
High grade	I–IV	Intensive combination chemotherapy

CVP: cyclophosphamide + vincristine +prednisone; RCHOP: rituximab + cyclophosphamide + doxorubicin + vincristine + prednisone; XRT, irradiation.

---

common field used for head and neck lymphomas is the Waldeyer field, which encompasses the lymphoid tissue of the nasopharynx, oropharynx, base of tongue, and the lymph nodes in the upper cervical, preauricular, submandibular, submaxillary, and occipital regions. The mantle field includes lymph nodes in the cervical, supraclavicular, infraclavicular, axillary, mediastinal, and hilar regions. Involved-field irradiation designates therapy that is limited to the involved lymphoid regions. Extended-field irradiation describes therapy to the involved regions and contiguous lymphoid groups.

Lymphomas are sensitive to many chemotherapeutic agents among which are cyclophosphamide, chlorambucil, vincristine, prednisone, doxorubicin (Adriamycin), bleomycin, methotrexate, and fludarabine. Chemotherapy is usually delivered in combinations in which the drugs are given in a cyclic fashion to produce the highest response rate with acceptable toxicity. In general, chemotherapy is delivered until a complete response is achieved, followed by two cycles of consolidation chemotherapy. If chemotherapy is used in combination with irradiation for early-stage disease (stage I or II), three to six cycles of chemotherapy are usually adequate. Because dose intensity is important in achieving optimal response, it is essential to deliver the highest tolerable dose of drugs on schedule. Recently, immunotherapy with an anti-CD20 antibody (rituximab) has also shown to be effective.

Many drug combinations are available for use in the treatment of lymphomas. Among commonly used regimens are the following:

CVP: cyclophosphamide, 400 mg per m^2 by mouth (PO) days 1 to 5; vincristine, 1.4 mg per m^2 intravenously (IV) day 1; prednisone, 100 mg per m^2 PO days 1 to 5; repeat every 21 days.

CHOP: cyclophosphamide, 750 mg per m^2 IV day 1; doxorubicin, 50 mg per m^2 IV day 1; vincristine, 1.4 mg per m^2 IV day 1; prednisone, 50 mg per m^2 PO days 1 to 5; repeat every 21 days.

Other regimens have added bleomycin and/or high-dose methotrexate to the previous.

Rituximab (R): 375 mg per m^2 IV per week for 4 weeks.

Specific Subtypes

Low-Grade Lymphomas, Stage I or II

Only a small percentage of lymphomas in the head and neck are low grade, early stage at presentation. Standard treatment has consisted of involved-field or extended-field radiation therapy, and most trials have not shown an advantage to adding chemotherapy. At 10 years, approximately 60% of patients are disease free, and 65% are alive. Whether or not a small proportion of these patients are cured is controversial because relapses occur even after 10 to 20 years (19). In a retrospective analysis at Stanford, a subset of patients with stage I/II follicular lymphomas were observed without any initial treatment. At a median follow-up of 7 years, more than two thirds of the patients did not require therapy. The overall survival of this group was no different from those treated initially with radiotherapy or combined modality treatment (20).

Low-Grade Lymphomas, Stage III or IV

Despite decades of research, there is no consensus as to the optimal management of follicular and low-grade lymphomas. Considerations include an alkylating agent alone, combination chemotherapy with CVP or CHOP, or a fludarabine-based regimen. With each of these regimens, approximately 60% to 80% of patients achieve a complete response. Most patients eventually relapse with only 20% to 30% of patients remaining disease-free at 10 years; however, 50% to 60% are alive with disease. Neither approach has a clear survival advantage.

Rituximab, a minimally toxic monoclonal antibody directed against the CD20 B-cell antigen, can offer a 50% response rate in low-grade lymphoma. The duration of response is about 1 year (21). This antibody is being used widely because of its activity and favorable toxicity profile. Most adverse reactions occur during the first infusion and consist primarily of fever, chills, and occasional hypotension. The possible benefit of maintenance therapy has also been evaluated in two studies using different schedules (22,23). In both, the time to progression (TTP) was longer than expected with no difference in survival rates. Forty percent of patients experienced a response of similar duration when retreated with rituximab if the initial response lasted greater than 6 months (24).

Recent randomized trials have shown superiority of rituxan-containing regimens over chemotherapy alone. In a study comparing CVP and R-CVP, the overall response rate (ORR) and time to treatment failure were in favor of the combination arm (40% vs. 80%, 7 months vs. 27 months, respectively) (25). Similar benefit has been reported using RCHOP (26). It will require a longer follow up to determine whether these observations will eventually result in a survival advantage. Given the indolent nature of the low-grade lymphomas, an acceptable approach is to observe patients until they become symptomatic with bulky adenopathy, systemic symptoms, or organ compromise. Studies comparing initial use of combination chemotherapy to no initial therapy, followed by combination chemotherapy when necessary, show no difference in survival.

Several immune-based therapies for lymphomas appear promising. The use of radioimmunotherapy has the advantage of killing not only cells to which the antibody is bound but also, as a result of the cross-fire effect, neighboring cells that may not express antigen or that are inaccessible to the monoclonal antibody. The two most commonly studied anti-CD20 monoclonal antibodies are ^{131}I-tositumomab (Bexaar) and ^{90}Y-ibritumomab

(Zevalin). Both agents are currently approved by the U.S. Food and Drug Administration for use in patients with relapsed/refractory low-grade lymphomas or those that have transformed to a higher grade lymphoma. There are notable differences between these two conjugated antibodies in their physical properties; however, both agents have similar efficacy and toxicity. The major toxicity of both is delayed myelosuppression. [131]I tositumomab was initially evaluated in patients with low-grade or transformed NHL who had at least two prior chemotherapies or refractory disease or relapse within 6 months of their most recent therapy. The ORR was 65% with 20% complete responses (CR) and a median response duration of 6.5 months (27). In a similar patient population treated with ^{90}Y-ibritumomab, the ORR was 67% with 26% CR and a median time to progression in responders of 12.9 + months (28). In a randomized trial, ^{90}Y-ibritumomab was found to have a higher CR rate compared with rituximab; however, there were no differences in response duration or TTP (29).

Intermediate-Grade Lymphomas, Stage I or II

In the past, most patients with early-stage head and neck lymphomas were treated with involved- or extended-field radiation therapy only. In a series reported from Stanford University, the disease-free survival for patients with stage I or II disease was 48% and 35%, respectively. Of those who relapsed, approximately 79% recurred distally in nodal or organ sites. Chemotherapy, predominantly CHOP, has been added to the primary treatment program, resulting in better outcome than with radiation therapy alone. Patients with only one or two sites of involvement and nonbulky disease may require fewer cycles of chemotherapy than those with advanced disease (30). For patients with stage I disease, the disease-free survival rate at five years is 80% to 100%, with an overall survival rate of 95% to 100%. For patients with stage II disease, the 5-year disease-free survival rate is 75% to 80%, and the overall survival rate 75% to 90%.

Intermediate-Grade Lymphomas, Stage III or IV

For decades CHOP has been the standard for patients with large B-cell lymphoma with stage III or IV disease. Complete response rate ranges from 50% to 85%. At 5 years, disease-free survival rates of 30% to 60% and overall survival rates of 35% to 70% have been reported. Although multiagent intensive chemotherapy appeared more effective in phase II trials, a large intergroup study failed to confirm the superiority (31). Radiation therapy is primarily used to consolidate areas of bulky disease or for urgent treatment of airway obstruction.

For intermediate-grade lymphomas, CHOP has been considered the standard against which new therapies should be compared. Although rituximab has only modest single-agent activity in intermediate-grade lymphomas, two trials have shown improvement in outcome when it is added to CHOP (32,33). In the first, patients aged 60 to

80 years of age with advanced-stage CD20 positive B-cell intermediate-grade lymphomas were randomized to CHOP or RCHOP (32). Patients randomized to RCHOP had superior CR rate (76% vs. 63%), event-free survival (57% vs. 38%), and overall survival (70% vs. 57%). Similar results have been reported recently in patients younger than 60 years (33). Cumulatively, these studies support the RCHOP as the new standard for patients with diffuse large B-cell lymphoma.

Although considerable strides have been made in treating B-cell lymphomas, the outcome of T and NK cell subtypes continues to be particularly poor (5). Long-term survival in this group is less than 20% with a high incidence of central nervous system relapse. For these patients, CHOP chemotherapy plus intrathecal methotrexate for prophylaxis should be considered. Even more intensive chemotherapy programs are being tested because of the predictably poor outcome. Because most of these patients present with extensive local disease, consolidative irradiation and prophylactic whole-brain irradiation should be considered.

Patients with advanced-stage, intermediate-grade disease who fail to respond to primary chemotherapy or relapse after treatment are unlikely to achieve a durable response to a standard second-line chemotherapy regimen. In these patients, high-dose therapy with stem cell support is the treatment of choice (34). For patients with NHLs, the source of the graft is usually autologous. Stem cells are collected from the peripheral blood or from bone marrow harvesting, cryopreserved, and reinfused following administration of high-dose therapy. This allows several-fold higher doses of chemotherapy to eradicate lymphoma that is resistant to standard doses of chemotherapy. For certain favorable subgroups of patients with recurrent disease (i.e., chemotherapy sensitive disease, age younger than 60 years, good performance status), the majority of patients enter a sustained remission.

High-Grade Lymphomas

Lymphoblastic lymphoma is most often a T-cell malignancy that presents primarily in young patients as a rapidly growing mediastinal mass, although it occasionally occurs in the head and neck region. This lymphoma spreads frequently to the central nervous system and bone marrow. Regardless of stage, combination chemotherapy, including central nervous system prophylaxis, is required. Approximately 60% of patients can be cured with an aggressive approach.

Small noncleaved cell lymphoma may appear as the Burkitt or Burkitt-like types, the latter more commonly in adults. The most effective treatment programs include combination chemotherapy with escalated doses of cyclophosphamide, doxorubicin, vincristine, prednisone, methotrexate, etoposide, cytarabine, and intrathecal methotrexate. During the first few days following initiation of therapy, these patients are at risk for tumor lysis syndrome, which is associated with hyperuricemia, hyperkalemia, hyperphosphatemia, hypocalcemia, and acute renal failure. It can occur within hours of the initiation of chemotherapy and lead to death from cardiac arrhythmias. Patients with bulky disease who may be subject to rapid lysis of large volumes of tumor should receive allopurinol, intravenous hydration, and alkalinization of the urine during the first 24 to 48 hours after therapy. With the previously described chemotherapy, approximately 65% of patients are alive at 2 years. Patients with bone marrow or central nervous system disease have considerably poorer prognoses, although the majority of patients may still be cured with intensive, leukemia-based chemotherapy protocols (35).

Thyroid Lymphomas

The majority of thyroid lymphomas are intermediate grade. Patients with stage IE or stage IIE disease should be treated with a combined-modality approach using three or six cycles of RCHOP chemotherapy in addition to radiation (30). Patients with stage III or IV disease should be treated primarily with chemotherapy. Radiation therapy has been the primary treatment for stage IE and IIE indolent thyroid lymphoma. Using extended-field irradiation that includes cervical and mediastinal nodes, the disease-free survival rate is approximately 75% at 5 years (36). Patients with poor prognostic factors—bulky tumor, extracapsular extension, fixation, and retrosternal involvement—should be treated like intermediate-grade lymphomas (37).

Orbital Lymphomas

Low-grade lymphomas confined to the orbit can be treated successfully with radiation therapy alone at 3,000 to 3,500 cGy (38). Disease-free survival is approximately 70%. In those with intermediate-grade histology or stage III or IV disease, chemotherapy should be considered. Recently, rituximab has been used as a single agent with encouraging activity (39).

Human Immunodeficiency Virus-Associated Lymphomas

The incidence of NHL is markedly increased in patients with HIV infection. Typically, these lymphomas are of intermediate- or high-grade histology with advanced stage and frequent extranodal involvement at presentation. Extranodal disease in the head and neck region may occur in up to 10% of patients with HIV-associated lymphomas. The most common sites include the gingiva, oral mucosa, parotid gland, and conjunctiva (2). Staging and treatment are similar to that of non-HIV infected patients. Overall survival is poor, however, because of the typically advanced stage of disease and inability to tolerate full doses of standard therapy.

Complications of Therapy

Radiation Therapy

The major acute toxic effect of irradiation is mucositis, which can be treated with mouthwashes and, if necessary, a break in therapy. Some patients develop dysphagia and require symptomatic treatment with antacids. Long-term toxic effects include xerostomia from salivary gland irradiation with associated chronic oral infections and dental caries. Patients should see their dentist prior to the start of radiation and use fluoride gel following irradiation. Treatment with sialogogues improves salivary flow in some patients. Hypothyroidism can occur years after irradiation, and thyroid-stimulating hormone tests should be obtained yearly.

Chemotherapy

Myelosuppression is an expected complication of chemotherapy. The most life-threatening toxic effect is neutropenia or thrombocytopenia. Neutropenia can be treated or prevented with granulocytic colony-stimulating agents (40). Nausea and vomiting occur shortly after injections of doxorubicin and cyclophosphamide and can be controlled with antiemetics. A rare, potentially serious effect of cyclophosphamide is hemorrhagic cystitis, which may present as dysuria or hematuria. Doxorubicin can cause cardiac dysfunction with eventual heart failure in patients receiving more than 550 mg per m^2. Cardiac dysfunction may occur at lower cumulative dose levels among elderly patients, those with a cardiac history, or those who have had prior mediastinal irradiation. Patients being treated with doxorubicin should have periodic evaluation of cardiac contractility.

The major toxic effects of vincristine are neurologic, resulting in peripheral neuropathy, constipation, and ileus. Patients may develop hoarseness from vocal cord dysfunction. The major complications of methotrexate—mucositis, gastrointestinal ulcerations, hematologic toxicities—can be ameliorated with leucovorin rescue. Bleomycin can cause pulmonary toxicity, predominantly an interstitial fibrosis, which occurs at doses higher than 200 mg, especially in patients with chronic pulmonary disorders. Measurement of carbon monoxide diffusion capacity can be helpful in determining early toxicity. Many agents cause alopecia, amenorrhea or azoospermia, and some, predominately the alkylators, have been associated with the development of secondary neoplasms.

THE FUTURE

The histologic evaluation and classification of lymphomas continue to evolve as pathologists develop more detailed and specific molecular markers of disease. Advances in imaging with CT, PET, or MRI have greatly enhanced the accurate assessment of head and neck lymphomas. With regard to therapy, intensity modulated radiation is being used with encouraging results. Immune-based approaches include the creation of tumor-specific vaccines administered after treatment with chemotherapy. New chemotherapeutic agents continue to be developed. The efficacy of high-dose chemotherapy and stem cell or bone marrow transplantation has been established in patients with intermediate- and high-grade lymphomas refractory to or relapsing after first-line therapy. As the treatment related morbidity and mortality have decreased substantially, efforts are underway to incorporate high-dose therapy into the primary management of patients with poor prognostic factors.

HIGHLIGHTS

- Ten percent of non-Hodgkin lymphomas of the head and neck occur in extranodal sites.
- The presenting symptoms are similar to those of squamous cell cancers.
- A biopsy is more helpful for diagnosis and histologic classification than a fine-needle aspirate.
- Special immunohistochemical stains or molecular studies can help differentiate lymphomas from other cancers or benign processes, but fresh or frozen tissue is frequently required.
- Most head and neck lymphomas are diffuse large cell, intermediate-grade lymphoma.
- Full staging should be completed before treatment planning.
- Most head and neck lymphomas are treated with combined irradiation and chemotherapy.
- Outcome is based on site, stage, histologic subtype, prognostic factors, and therapy.
- Lymphomas of the paranasal sinus have worse prognoses than those in Waldeyer ring or the thyroid, with a high incidence of relapse in the central nervous system.

REFERENCES

1. Baris D, Zahm SH. Epidemiology of lymphomas. *Curr Opin Oncol* 2000;12:383–394.
2. Singh B, Poluri A, Shaha AR, et al. Head and neck manifestations of non-Hodgkin's lymphoma in human immunodeficiency virus-infected patients. *Am J Otolaryngol* 2000;21:10–13.
3. Thieblemont C, Mayer A, Dumontet C, et al. Primary thyroid lymphoma is a heterogeneous disease. *J Clin Endocrinol Metab* 2002;87:105–111.
4. Ambrosetti A, Zanotti R, Pattaro C, et al. Most cases of primary salivary mucosa-associated lymphoid tissue lymphoma are associated either with Sjögren syndrome or hepatitis C virus infection. *Br J Haematol* 2004;126:43–49.
5. Cheung MM, Chan JK, Wong KF. Natural killer cell neoplasms: a distinctive group of highly aggressive lymphomas/leukemias. *Semin Hematol* 2003;40:221–232.
6. Ferreri AJ, Guidoboni M, Ponzoni M, et al. Evidence for an association between Chlamydia psittaci and ocular adnexal lymphomas. *J Natl Cancer Inst* 2004;96:586–594.
7. MacDermed D, Thurber L, George TI, et al. Extranodal nonorbital indolent lymphomas of the head and neck: relationship between tumor control and radiotherapy. *Int J Radiat Oncol Biol Phys* 2004;59:788–795.

8. Hon C, Kwok AK, Shek TW, et al. Vision-threatening complications of nasal T/NK lymphoma. *Am J Ophthalmol* 2002;134: 406–410.
9. The Non-Hodgkin's Lymphoma Classification Project: National Cancer Institute sponsored study of classifications of non-Hodgkin's lymphomas. Summary and description of a working formulation for classical usage. *Cancer* 1982;49:2112–2135.
10. Harris NL, Jaffe ES, Diebold J, et al. World Health Organization classification of neoplastic diseases of the hematopoietic and lymphoid tissues: report of the Clinical Advisory Committee meeting-Airlie House, Virginia, November 1997. *J Clin Oncol* 1999;17:3835–3849.
11. Hart S, Horsman JM, Radstone CR, et al. Localised extranodal lymphoma of the head and neck: the Sheffield Lymphoma Group experience (1971-2000). *Clin Oncol (R Coll Radiol)* 2004; 16:186–192.
12. Widder S, Pasieka JL. Primary thyroid lymphomas. *Curr Treat Options Oncol* 2004;5:307–313.
13. Weber AL, Rahemtullah A, Ferry JA. Hodgkin and non-Hodgkin lymphoma of the head and neck: clinical, pathologic, and imaging evaluation. *Neuroimaging Clin North Am* 2003;13:371–392.
14. Dabaja BS, Ha CS, Wilder RB, et al. Importance of esophagogastroduodenoscopy in the evaluation of non-gastrointestinal mucosa-associated lymphoid tissue lymphoma. *Cancer J* 2003;9: 321–324.
15. Jacobs C, Weiss L, Hoppe RT. The management of extranodal head and neck lymphomas. *Arch Otolaryngol Head Neck Surg* 1986;112:654–658.
16. The International Non-Hodgkin's Lymphoma Prognostic Factors Project. A predictive model for aggressive non-Hodgkin's lymphoma. *N Engl J Med* 1993;329:987–994.
17. Solal-Celigny P, Roy P, Colombat P, et al. Follicular lymphoma international prognostic index. *Blood* 2004;104:1258–1265.
18. Alizadeh AA, Ross DT, Perou CM, et al. Towards a novel classification of human malignancies based on gene expression patterns. *J Pathol* 2001;195:41–52.
19. Mac Manus MP, Hoppe RT. Is radiotherapy curative for stage I and II low-grade follicular lymphoma? Results of a long-term follow-up study of patients treated at Stanford University. *J Clin Oncol* 1996;14:1282–1290.
20. Advani R, Rosenberg SA, Horning SJ. Stage I and II follicular non-Hodgkin's lymphoma: long-term follow-up of no initial therapy. *J Clin Oncol* 2004;22:1454–1459.
21. Maloney DG. Rituximab for follicular lymphoma. *Curr Hematol Rep* 2003;2:13–22.
22. Hainsworth JD. Prolonging remission with rituximab maintenance therapy. *Semin Oncol* 2004;31:17–21.
23. Ghielmini M, Schmitz SF, Cogliatti SB, et al. Prolonged treatment with rituximab in patients with follicular lymphoma significantly increases event-free survival and response duration compared with the standard weekly x 4 schedule. *Blood* 2004;103: 4416–4423.
24. Davis TA, Grillo-Lopez AJ, White CA, et al. Rituximab anti-CD20 monoclonal antibody therapy in non-Hodgkin's lymphoma: safety and efficacy of re-treatment. *J Clin Oncol* 2000;18: 3135–3143.
25. Marcus R, Imrie K, Belch A, et al. An international multi-centre, randomized, open-label, phase III trial comparing Rituximab added to CVP chemotherapy to CVP chemotherapy alone in untreated stage III/IV follicular non-Hodgkin's lymphoma. *Blood* 2003;102:28a.
26. Hiddemann W, Dreyling MH, Forstpointner R, et al. Combined immuno-chemotherapy (R-CHOP) significantly improves time to treatment failure in first line therapy of follicular lymphoma—results of a prospective randomized trial of the German Low Grade Lymphoma Study Group (GLSG). *Blood* 2003;102:104a.
27. Kaminski MS, Zelenetz AD, Press OW, et al. Pivotal study of iodine I 131 tositumomab for chemotherapy-refractory low-grade or transformed low-grade B-cell non-Hodgkin's lymphomas. *J Clin Oncol* 2001;19:3918–3928.
28. Witzig TE. Efficacy and safety of 90Y ibritumomab tiuxetan (Zevalin) radioimmunotherapy for non-Hodgkin's lymphoma. *Semin Oncol* 2003;30:11–16.
29. Witzig TE, Gordon LI, Cabanillas F, et al. Randomized controlled trial of yttrium-90-labeled ibritumomab tiuxetan radioimmunotherapy versus rituximab immunotherapy for patients with relapsed or refractory low-grade, follicular, or transformed b-cell non-Hodgkin's lymphoma. *J Clin Oncol* 2002;20:2453–2463.
30. Miller TP, Dahlberg S, Cassady JR, et al. Chemotherapy alone compared with chemotherapy plus radiotherapy for localized intermediate- and high-grade non-Hodgkin's lymphoma. *N Engl J Med* 1998;339:21–26.
31. Fisher RI. Current therapeutic paradigm for the treatment of non-Hodgkin's lymphoma. *Semin Oncol* 2000;27:2–8.
32. Coiffier B, Lepage E, Brière J, et al. CHOP chemotherapy plus Rituximab compared with CHOP alone in elderly patients with diffuse large-B-cell lymphoma. *N Engl J Med* 2002;346:235–242.
33. Pfreundschuh MG, Trümper D, Ma A, et al. Randomized intergroup trial of first line treatment for patients <=60 years with diffuse large B-cell non-Hodgkin's lymphoma (DLBCL) with a CHOP-like regimen with or without the anti-CD20 antibody rituximab—early stopping after the first interim analysis. *Proc Am Soc Clin Oncol* 2004;22:558S.
34. Hagemeister FB. Treatment of relapsed aggressive lymphomas: regimens with and without high-dose therapy and stem cell rescue. *Cancer Chemother Pharmacol* 2002;49:S13–20.
35. Thomas DA, O'Brien S, Cortes J, et al. Outcome with the hyper-CVAD regimens in lymphoblastic lymphoma. *Blood* 2004;104: 1624–1630.
36. DiBiase SJ, Grigsby PW, Guo C, et al. Outcome analysis for stage IE and IIE thyroid lymphoma. *Am J Clin Oncol* 2004;27:178–184.
37. Ha CS, Shadle KM, Medeiros LJ, et al. Localized non-Hodgkin lymphoma involving the thyroid gland. *Cancer* 2001;91:629–635.
38. Lee JL, Kim MK, Lee KH, et al. Extranodal marginal zone B-cell lymphomas of mucosa-associated lymphoid tissue-type of the orbit and ocular adnexa. *Ann Hematol* 2005;1:13–18.
39. Sullivan TJ, Grimes D, Bunce I. Monoclonal antibody treatment of orbital lymphoma. *Ophthalmol Plast Reconstr Surg* 2004;20: 103–106.
40. Dale DC. Colony-stimulating factors for the management of neutropenia in cancer patients. *Drugs* 2002;62:1–15.

Diagnosis and Treatment of Thyroid and Parathyroid Disorders

Cristian M. Slough   *Henning Dralle*   *Andreas Machens*   *Gregory W. Randolph*

Thyroid and parathyroid surgery has evolved since the time of the Kocher, the father of modern thyroid surgery and now represents one of the most common operations in the head and neck. A thorough knowledge of neck base anatomy, attention to surgical detail, and fluency in related endocrinology are important correlates of successful thyroid and parathyroid surgery.

THYROID GLAND

Anatomy and Embryology

The thyroid gland originates from the primitive pharynx and the neural crest. An endodermal diverticulum of the floor of the primitive pharynx forms the follicular elements of thyroid tissue during the second and third weeks of fetal life. This diverticulum divides as it follows the developing heart caudally. The proximal portion withdraws and disappears leaving the foramen caecum, whereas the caudal segment develops into a bilobate structure as it descends into the neck. As a consequence of this migration into the neck the thyroglossal duct tract is formed.

Tissue from the neural crest and the fused fourth and fifth branchial pouches leads to the formation of the caudal pharyngeal complex, which includes the ultimobranchial bodies, lateral thyroid, and the upper parathyroid glands (PIV). The ultimobranchial bodies give rise to the parafollicular cells (C cells) of the thyroid that secrete calcitonin.

The main body of the thyroid gland fuses with the ultimobranchial bodies as it descends into its final position in the neck. This fusion results in parafollicular cells being restricted to a zone within the middle to upper thirds of the thyroid lobes leaving the lower poles and isthmus devoid of these cells. Therefore, medullary thyroid carcinomas (MTCs) commonly arise in the upper and middle third of the thyroid lobes.

Anomalous Development of the Thyroid

The most common anomaly of thyroid development is the persistence of the thyroglossal tract, where thyroid tissue can differentiate anywhere along its length. The pyramidal lobe, present in 30% of patients, is a caudal tract remnant. Thyroglossal cysts are formed when the epithelium of the thyroglossal duct fails to degrade.

Failure of migration can result in ectopic thyroid tissue being found anywhere along its course from the base of the tongue to the neck and beyond down to the mediastinum through excess migration associated with the heart's decent. The same pathologic processes encountered in a normal thyroid can appear in ectopic thyroid tissues, including cancer.

Lingual Thyroid

Complete arrest of the descent of the developing thyroid with resulting presence of thyroid tissue at the tongue base is termed a lingual thyroid. Histologically, the tissue resembles normal thyroid tissue but infiltration into adjacent skeletal muscle can mimic invasive carcinoma. Lingual thyroid is often the only functioning thyroid tissue in these patients. With time, most patients with lingual thyroid become hypothyroid.

Lateral Thyroid Tissue

Little controversy still exists whether lateral aberrant tissue actually represents normal thyroid tissue or metastatic thyroid carcinoma. Benign aberrant lateral thyroid tissue within the muscle and fat would not be surprising in light of the intimate relationship of the thyroid gland to mesodermal structures. However, most authors regard thyroid tissue found in the lateral neck as representing thyroid cancer and would manage it accordingly with resection of the lateral tissue and thyroidectomy. The majority of workers feel that any significant thyroid tissue within nodes lateral to the jugular vein is consistent with metastatic thyroid carcinoma. Most believe that normal thyroid follicles may occur as an embryologic rest if contained within the capsule of medially located lymph nodes, but there is controversy (1,2).

Other Ectopic Thyroid Sites

Ectopic thyroid tissue has been found in a variety of sites ranging from the heart and gallbladder to the ovaries.

Thyroglossal Duct Cysts

Persistence of the thyroglossal duct with cyst (TGDC) formation is the most common congenital cervical anomaly. Histologically, the cyst can be lined by stratified squamous or columnar epithelium and occur anywhere from the base of the tongue to the upper mediastinum. The most common clinical presentation of a TGDC is a 1- to 4-cm midline cystic mass below the hyoid bone in a child that moves on deglutination. However, a proportion arise above the hyoid in the floor of the mouth or base of the tongue; up to 20% of cysts are noted to be slightly off the midline, with a predilection for the left; and a proportion of cysts may not become clinically evident until adulthood (3). The differential diagnosis for a thyroglossal duct cyst should include submental nodes, dermoid cysts, metastatic thyroid carcinoma, pyramidal lobe nodule, branchial cleft cysts, lipomas, and sebaceous cysts, but often the definitive diagnosis is only made after surgical removal.

The goal of imaging in patients with thyroglossal duct cysts is to assess the nature of the lesion and determine if this represents the patient's only functional tissue. Although palpation of a normal gland can be used in adults, this is more difficult in children and requires preoperative imaging. Ultrasound can be used to delineate the cystic mass as well as identify a normal orthotopic thyroid gland prior to excision.

A recent study reviewed the role of computed tomography (CT) and magnetic resonance imaging (MRI) for TGDC in adults. They reported an incidence of carcinoma arising in the thyroglossal duct cyst of 1% in the adult population (4). They also found in cases of carcinoma a higher prevalence of solid soft tissue elements, and calcification were visible on CT, with calcification being the single most specific marker for carcinoma. The close association of the cyst and the hyoid bone can be helpful in confirming the diagnosis of TGDC. For these reasons we advocate the use of CT scanning in all adult patients presenting with a TGDC prior to definitive treatment.

The treatment of choice is surgical excision via a Sistrunk procedure, with specific indications including cosmesis, recurrent infection, or fistula formation. A proportion of patients may complain of dysphagia, dyspnea, or pain. Any concurrent infection of the cyst should be treated prior to surgical excision to ensure greater surgical success.

The key elements of the Sistrunk procedure, first described in 1920 (5), are removal of the central portion of the hyoid bone and excision of any proximal thyroglossal duct. A Mayo Clinic study (6) showed a recurrence rate of 4% when these techniques were adopted compared with a 50% recurrence rate when they were not. Sistrunk emphasized that due to the delicate and easily disrupted nature of the duct the proximal dissection should include a 5- to 10-mm core of tissue around the duct to avoid retraction of the structure into the soft tissue of the base of the tongue with subsequent recurrence (5). Although careful dissection is required and can include a small section of the submucosal base of tongue, entry into the oropharynx is unnecessary (7).

The procedure involves a horizontal curved linear incision made along the skin creases at the level of the cyst through the skin and platysma. A subplatysmal flap is then elevated superiorly and inferiorly to expose the strap muscles, which are subsequently separated in the midline and retracted laterally to reveal the cyst. To avoid rupturing the cyst, medial portions of the strap muscles can be incorporated into its dissection. Once the cyst is freed distally it is dissected proximally to include a 10- to 15-mm midportion of the hyoid bone together with any proximal tract above it. After the cyst is excised, the strap muscles and platysma are approximated respectively with an absorbable suture, and the wound is closed.

Higher recurrence rates have been attributed to a young age of the patient, and rupture of the cyst at the time of operation rendering dissection more difficult.

Meticulous review of the patient's previous operative record, paying particular attention to treatment of the hyoid bone and proximal tissue, and assessment of the pathology report is imperative when working on revision cases. A wide-based resection approach, with excision or further excision of the hyoid bone and a core of tissue leading to the base of the tongue should be adopted to ensure surgical success. Preoperative imaging can be particularly useful in these patients for surgical planning.

Thyroglossal Duct Cyst Carcinoma

The incidence of thyroglossal duct cyst carcinoma (TGDCC) is estimated to be approximately 1% of all TGDCs, with papillary thyroid carcinoma (PTC) comprising the majority of cases. Other variants include mixed papillary follicular, squamous cell carcinoma, and Hürthle cell carcinoma (8).

TGDCC can be difficult to distinguish from a benign TGDC preoperatively. TGDCC should be distinguished from a midline cystic metastasis from a thyroid primary process, although such a distinction is not always possible. Interestingly, MTC has not been found in any thyroglossal duct cysts, most likely due to the origin of MTC in the C cells that do not occur in the midline thyroid elements. A Mayo Clinic series has shown that 33% of patients with a TGDCC have a concurrent intrathyroidal malignant mass (9). For this reason a thyroid ultrasound can be helpful in evaluating the thyroid for occult primaries.

A Sistrunk procedure alone, when noninvasive small papillary cancer is found in a thyroglossal duct specimen with no demonstrated thyroid abnormalities on either palpation or on ultrasound evaluation, has been found to be effective in the majority of cases. We reserve thyroidectomy for patients with thyroid abnormalities either demonstrated on palpation, ultrasound evaluation, and cases of invasive or large thyroglossal duct papillary carcinomas or in cases of midline cyst nodal metastasis.

Benign Lesions

Thyroiditis

Thyroiditis comprises a diverse group of disorders that are among the most common endocrine abnormalities encountered in clinical practice. These disorders range from the extremely common chronic lymphocytic thyroiditis (Hashimoto thyroiditis) to the extremely rare invasive fibrous thyroiditis (Riedel thyroiditis). Their clinical presentations are diverse, therefore an accurate diagnosis is imperative via a rational approach including history, physical examination, laboratory evaluation, radionuclide or ultrasonographic imaging, and fine-needle aspiration (FNA) biopsy.

Chronic Lymphocytic Thyroiditis (Hashimoto Thyroiditis)

Chronic lymphocytic thyroiditis is characterized by high circulating titers of antibodies to thyroid peroxidase and thyroglobulin (Tg). Lymphocytes infiltrate the thyroid gland and ultimately result in epithelial cell damage. This immunologically mediated thyroid cell damage is responsible for thyroid gland failure and variable enlargement. High titers of antibodies directed against Tg and thyroid peroxidase (formerly called microsomal antigen) are present in patients with Hashimoto thyroiditis, and it is the thyroid peroxidase antibodies that show the highest correlation with clinical dysfunction (10). Other antibodies are often notably thyroid-stimulating hormone (TSH) receptor antibodies. These antibodies block TSH binding but do not stimulate thyroid cell function resulting in hypothyroidism in the absence of significant thyroid gland destruction (7).

Pathologically, there is lymphocytic infiltration of the thyroid tissue with formation of germinal centers. The follicular cells undergo metaplasia into larger, eosinophilic cells known as Hürthle, or Askanazy, cells, which are packed with mitochondria. These cells exhibit high metabolic activity but ineffective hormonogenesis. There is progressive fibrosis, which may be extensive. The quantity of parenchymal tissue left in the thyroid is variable, because the pathologic involvement ranges from focal regions to an entire lobe to the entire gland.

Clinical Manifestations.   Chronic lymphocytic thyroiditis most commonly presents as an incidental asymptomatic goiter in a middle-aged woman, but can occur at any age. Although chronic lymphocytic thyroiditis is the most common etiology for hypothyroidism, its systemic symptoms are only present in up to 20% of patients at the time of diagnosis (11).

Generally, a symmetrical nontender "rubbery" goiter is found on physical examination with often a palpable pyramidal lobe and occasional regional lymph node enlargement. Chronic lymphocytic thyroiditis is diagnosed by confirming the presence of either antithyroid antibodies to thyroid peroxidase (90% of cases) or to Tg (20% to 50%) (2). On imaging, patients will have patchy thyroid isotope scanning and ultrasound scanning reveals marked hypoechogenicity and heterogeneity.

Clinical Management.   All nodules larger than 1 cm within a Hashimoto gland should be evaluated with a FNA biopsy to rule out malignancy. Development of a progressive mass with a Hashimoto gland should prompt workup to rule out lymphoma. The mainstay of treatment consists of thyroid hormone replacement for hypothyroidism. Reevaluation of serum TSH concentrations should not be performed for at least 4 to 6 weeks after commencement or change in dose of thyroid hormone because of the long half-life of thyroxin; steady state concentrations of the hormone are not achieved until 4 to 6 weeks.

Suppressive thyroid hormone therapy (decreasing the serum TSH into the subnormal range) may be used in an attempt to decrease the size of a goiter. However, patients on suppression therapy should be reevaluated periodically and the dose reduced or discontinued if significant goiter reduction is not achieved because overreplacement of thyroxine may result in osteoporosis and cause cardiac dysfunction (12).

Riedel Thyroiditis

Riedel thyroiditis (Riedel struma or invasive fibrous thyroiditis) is a rare disorder of unknown etiology characterized by extensive fibrosis of the thyroid gland affecting mainly women between the ages of 30 to 60 years (female to male ratio, 3.5:1). A painless goiter in an euthyroid patient, with an extremely hard goiter on physical examination, is the most common presentation. Invasion and fixation of adjacent structures is characteristic; this fibrosis is progressive and may eventually cause compression of adjacent structures, particularly the trachea and esophagus. Riedel thyroiditis is often associated with other syndromes of focal sclerosis, such as retroperitoneal, mediastinal, and retroorbital fibrosis, and sclerosing cholangitis (13). Biopsy is necessary to exclude carcinoma. Unfortunately, fine-needle biopsy is often indeterminate. Extensive fibrosis of the gland and surrounding structures makes complete resection impossible so the mainstay of treatment is surgical resection to relieve compressive symptoms, especially over the isthmus to relieve tracheal compression. Thyroid hormone suppression therapy is ineffective so thyroid hormone replacement is indicated only if hypothyroidism is present. Medical therapies can include steroids, tamoxifen, methotrexate, and raloxifene.

Adenomas

An adenoma can be defined as a lesion that is well-circumscribed, follicle-derived, and confined to its capsule but different from the surrounding thyroid parenchyma. Also by definition adenomas will display no capsular or vascular invasion.

Follicular Adenoma

Follicular adenomas are well-circumscribed, encapsulated lesions typically considered to be of clonal growth, usually measuring 1 to 4 cm in diameter. Microscopically, several patterns can be seen including trabecular, follicular, microfollicular, and solid. These patterns may be accompanied by degenerative changes such as hemorrhage, calcification, and fibrosis.

Hürthle Cell Adenoma

Like follicular adenomas, they are circumscribed and encapsulated tumors that are homogenous and brown on cut section. Microscopically, they may show any of the patterns seen in follicular adenomas. Electron microscopy will confirm that the cells are rich in mitochondria.

Hyalinizing Trabecular Adenoma

Although similar to other types of adenomas, the cells are arranged in a trabecular pattern with little follicle formation. The nuclei of these adenomas share many features of papillary carcinomas, leading some to hypothesize that they form part of the family of papillary neoplasms.

Nodular (Adenomatous) Goiter

In nodular adenomatous goiters, the gland is diffusely enlarged and on cut surface shows extensive red-brown nodularity. Microscopically, there are coalescent nodules of different sizes, some of which are hyperplastic or dilated with dense colloid.

Goiters

The surgery of cervical and substernal goiters (SSGs) is challenging. We feel all such patients require CT (with or without contrast depending on the patient's thyroid function tests) to accurately preoperatively understand the anatomy of the goiter and its relation to the central visceral, upper chest great vessels. The presence of SSG represents in our practice a sur-gical indication. Accurate preoperative radiographic studies are essential for preoperative planning. We have proposed the following classification system for SSG (Table 116.1).

Malignant Lesions

Papillary Carcinoma

The gross appearance of PTC typically reveals a variable-sized mass, with ill-defined margins, firm consistency, whitish color, and a granular cut surface. Histologically, they form papillae and have well-known diagnostic nuclear changes. The nuclear features include subtle irregularities in the nuclear contour and size, deep nuclear grooves, and pseudoinclusions resulting from cytoplasmic invaginations. These characteristic nuclear features allow a diagnosis of PTC to be readily made on the cytologic smears obtained by FNA biopsy. Microscopically, psammoma bodies may also be seen. These are microscopic structures of concentric calcified layers of unknown origin, which are associated with up to 50% of patients with PTC.

Most papillary thyroid cancer cells retain their ability to concentrate iodine (14), produce and secrete Tg, occasionally produce thyroid hormone (15), and often express thyrotropin (TSH) receptors on their surfaces (16).

Several histologic variants of PTC exist including papillary thyroid microcarcinoma, follicular variant, encapsulated variant, diffuse sclerosing variant, oxyphilic cell variant, and two more aggressive variants—the tall-cell variant and the columnar cell variant.

A feature of PTC is its tendency for multicentric involvement of the thyroid either as a result of intrathyroidal lymph vessel spread or of true multicentric transformation of the follicular epithelium.

Extrathyroidal extension is common, with the most commonly involved sites being muscle, the recurrent laryngeal nerve (RLN), and trachea (17,18).

PTC has been shown to have lymph node involvement at presentation in 30% of cases. This number increases to in excess of 70% involvement when more extensive nodal dissection is empirically undertaken (17,18). Distant metastasis occurs less frequently in PTC than with other forms of differentiated thyroid carcinoma, occurring only in 1% to 25% of PTC patients during their illness, and in only 1% to 7% of PTC patients at the time of diagnosis (18).

Predisposing Factors

Prior exposure to ionizing radiation, particularly to the head and neck region during childhood, is the most firmly established risk factor for thyroid cancer development, particularly in children in whom the thyroid gland appears particularly vulnerable to the carcinogenic effects of ionizing radiation (22). Only 4% to 10% of patients presenting with PTC have a history of head or neck irradiation (19,20).

Several syndromes involving familial PTC have already been described. Cowden syndrome is characterized by multiple hamartomas, breast tumors, and both follicular

TABLE 116.1

SUBSTERNAL GOITER CLASSIFICATION

Type	Location	Anatomy	Prevalence
I Transcervical (sternotomy; if intrathoracic goiter, diameter > thoracic inlet diameter)	Anterior mediastinum	Anterior to great vessels, trachea, RLN	85%
II As above. Also consider sternotomy or right posterolateral thoracotomy if type IIB	Posterior mediastinum	Posterior to great vessels, trachea, RLN	15%
IIA	Ipsilateral extension		
IIB	Contralateral extension		
B1	Extension posterior to both trachea and esophagus		
B2	Extension between trachea and esophagus		
III Transcervical or sternotomy	Isolated mediastinal goiter	No connection to orthotopic gland; may have mediastinal blood supply	<1%

RLN, recurrent laryngeal nerve.
Reproduced from Randolph G. *Surgery of the thyroid and parathyroid glands*. Philadelphia: WB Saunders, 2003, with permission.

and papillary thyroid tumors. Interestingly, rates of 5% to 10% of patients with PTC have been reported to have a family history of thyroid cancer (21).

Clinical Presentation

PTC most commonly presents in young females with a palpable neck mass either in the thyroid or a palpable cervical lymph node (22). At the time of presentation, approximately one third of patients have clinically evident lymphadenopathy (22).

Follicular Carcinoma

Follicular thyroid carcinoma (FTC) represents 13% of cases of thyroid carcinoma, with approximately 700 cases annually in the United States. FTC is considered to be a more aggressive form of well-differentiated thyroid cancer compared with the more indolent PTC. The 10-year survival of patients with FTC is approximately 60% compared with the 96% 10-year survival of patients with PTC.

Grossly, FTCs are solitary tumors that vary in size and have a tan cut surface with a thick fibrous capsule. Microscopically, FTCs are more hypercellular than follicular adenomas. It is the presence of capsular and/or vascular invasion that differentiates these lesions from benign adenomas. Unfortunately, because there are no characteristic cytologic features for FTC, a definitive diagnosis on frozen section is difficult and impossible on FNA. Hematogenous spread resulting in metastases is more common in FTC than in PTC.

Two main varieties of FTC exist: minimally invasive and widely invasive. As the size of a microfollicular adenoma increases so does the risk of capsular transgression.

Predisposing Factors

Although radiation exposure has been more closely associated with the occurrence of PTC, it has also been shown in FTC. An increased incidence of FTC has been reported after the Chernobyl nuclear accident, although the majority of these radiation-induced thyroid cancers are papillary (23,24). Elevated TSH in goiter endemic areas has also been associated with FTC development.

Clinical Presentation

FTC most commonly presents as a solitary nodule or mass in the neck. In 10% to 15% of cases, distant metastasis is present at the time of diagnosis (25,26). Nodal metastases from true FTCs are much less common than for PTCs (25).

Hürthle Cell Carcinoma

Hürthle cell carcinoma (HCC) is traditionally considered a subtype of FTC characterized pathologically by the presence of oncocytes rich in mitochondria or Hürthle cells. HCC accounts for 15% of FTCs, representing just over 2% of thyroid carcinomas (27). The natural history and optimal management of HCC is difficult to elucidate due to its rarity and clinical variability.

Grossly HCCs are brown on their cut surface due to the Hürthle cells' rich mitochondrial content. Microscopically, the cells are large polygonal, follicular cells containing dense eosinophilic cytoplasm and having marked nuclear pleomorphism. Similarly to FTC, it is the presence of capsular and/or vascular invasion that separates this tumor from its benign counterpart. Consequently, as in FTC, it is impossible to exclude carcinoma in either FNA or frozen section.

Clinical Presentation

As with FTC, most patients present with a thyroid mass or nodule. Approximately 35% of patients develop distant metastasis at some time during their illness. It has also been shown to have a higher rate of lymph node metastases (6% to 9%) when compared with FTC (25). A subset of HCC may genetically overlap PTC and is associated with nodal metastasis.

Anaplastic Carcinoma

Anaplastic thyroid carcinomas (ATCs) account for less than 5% of all thyroid malignancies. These highly aggressive and almost invariably fatal carcinomas have a median survival after diagnosis of 3 to 6 months. ATC predominantly occurs in older individuals, with a peak incidence in the seventh decade (28). Distant metastasis is common and occurs most often to the lung; however, spread can occur to other organ sites, including bone, brain, and intestine.

Grossly, ATCs are often large bulky infiltrative masses that are gray-white and fibrous with areas of focal necrosis and hemorrhage. They often extend directly into the adjacent trachea and soft tissue. Microscopically, ATCs can be extensively variable with many cell types identified. The most common are spindle cell, giant cell, pleomorphic, malignant fibrous, histiocytic, and squamoid cell. The nuclei show marked pleomorphism and ample mitoses. Necrosis is frequently present and can be extensive.

Clinical Presentation

The most common presentation of ATC is a rapidly expanding neck mass or sudden change in size of preexisting goiter. However, there are many other symptoms of ATCs such as dysphagia, hoarseness, dyspnea, cough, and pain. Patients may also have a Horner syndrome secondary to sympathetic chain invasion.

Physical examination often reveals a large, firm, irregular, mass that is fixed to surrounding structures with associated cervical lymphadenopathy. Due to the high grade of the lesion, recurrent laryngeal invasion with subsequent vocal cord paralysis is common; thus, examination of the larynx is imperative. Patients may even have dyspnea or stridor secondary to bilaterally paralyzed vocal cords.

Lymphoma

Lymphoma rarely presents within the thyroid gland and only accounts for approximately 5% of thyroid malignancies (29). Lymphoma of the thyroid has a mean age at diagnosis of between 60 to 65 years, with an increased incidence in fe-

males (25). The most common thyroid lymphoma is a low- to intermediate-grade non-Hodgkin lymphoma derived from B cells. The risk of developing lymphoma in the thyroid is increased with chronic lymphocytic thyroiditis.

On cut surface, lymphomas are multinodular, with a pale tan to white surface, often with areas of focal hemorrhage and necrosis. Microscopically, there are characteristic lymphoepithelial lesions formed by the effacement of lymphoid cells against the thyroid parenchyma. Concurrent chronic lymphocytic thyroiditis is often present.

Clinical Presentation

The typical presentation of a thyroid lymphoma is a rapidly expanding thyroid mass, fixed to and compressing surrounding neck structures in the setting of a long-standing goiter or Hashimoto thyroiditis. As in ATC, the patients may also report a multitude of other symptoms including neck swelling, tenderness, hoarseness, dysphagia, neck pressure, or vocal cord paralysis (29). As the disease progresses, patients can also develop facial edema or a Horner syndrome.

Evaluation of the Thyroid Nodule

Initial Diagnostic Approach

Nodularity of the thyroid gland is common, and palpable nodules are found more often in women than in men. The main focus of the initial evaluation is to exclude malignancy (Table 116.2).

As a basic diagnostic step, all patients with thyroid nodularity should have their thyroid function assessed with a set of function tests, particularly TSH. Ultrasound has become the gold standard for evaluation of a thyroid nodule, not only for clarifying the anatomy but also for obtaining an accurate FNA result.

Preoperative Laryngoscopy

Preoperative and postoperative laryngeal examination empowers the surgeon and is essential in all cases for multiple reasons. Symptomatic assessment of vocal cord paralysis is inaccurate; up to 40% of patients with unilateral paralysis are asymptomatic (30–32). Identification of preoperative vocal cord paralysis is important in the event of contralateral nerve injury with subsequent bilateral cord paralysis.

The appropriate management of a nerve found invaded at surgery is dependent on its preoperative function. The slow progression of recurrent laryngeal nerve (RLN) infiltration with consequent vocal cord paralysis allows for accommodation by the contralateral cord. Not only does this knowledge allow accurate preoperative planning but also alerts the surgeon to obtain additional imaging to detect associated airway invasion.

Preoperative laryngeal examination is particularly vital in revision cases. One study found a preoperative vocal cord paralysis rate of 6.7% in patients who had previously undergone parathyroid surgery (33). Relying on the

TABLE 116.2 ◨ DIAGNOSIS
THYROID NODULES

History	• Commonly presents as an incidental finding on routine physical examination or cervical images
	• Usually asymptomatic but may be associated with dysphagia, voice change, dyspnea, or airway compromise
	• Patients typically euthyroid but may have hypothyroid or hyperthyroid symptoms
Physical examination	• Often a palpable nodule
	• Vocal cord mobility assessment
Laboratory evaluation	• Thyroid function tests
Radiographic evaluation	• Thyroid USS
	• Neck CT scan without contrast if necessary to delineate lymphadenopathy
	• Chest CT if substernal component
Cytologic evaluation	• Fine-needle biopsy of all nodules > 1cm

CT, computed tomography; USS, ultrasonography.

previous surgeon's operative report as an estimate of RLN injury and consequent vocal cord paralysis has also been shown to be flawed (34).

In a recent large prospective study of the United States and German Thyroid Cancer Study Group of 5,583 patients with thyroid cancer, preoperative voice abnormality was present in 8.2% but laryngoscopy was performed on only 6.1%. One of the study's main recommendations was that laryngoscopy should be performed more frequently preoperatively (35).

Imaging of the Thyroid Gland
Ultrasonography
When evaluating a thyroid mass, ultrasound is often the first imaging modality used. Although, ultrasonography (USS) is a poor predictor of malignancy and shows no functional information but is considerably more sensitive for delineation of intrathyroidal architecture than thyroid scintigraphy. The added benefit of ultrasound is that it is readily accessible, inexpensive, and noninvasive and requires no radiation exposure. It is also advantageous because it can also demonstrate any associated lymphadenopathy.

USS is able to distinguish cystic from solid lesions as well as accurately locate and measure a nodule. It determines if a nodule is solitary or part of a multinodular gland. With the use of serial ultrasound examinations, one is able to monitor disease progression, therapeutic response, and identify recurrence. Ultrasound is also capable of increasing the accuracy of FNA to more than 95% by ensuring needle position within the lesion during aspiration (36).

Despite being unable to reliably identify a thyroid malignancy, there are several ultrasonographic features that suggest a higher risk of malignancy within a nodule. These include microcalcifications and central blood flow.

Unfortunately, ultrasound is ultrasonographer dependent for both the quality of images and interpretation. Likewise, it is limited by acoustic shadowing from overlying air or bone with limited penetration in some anatomic locations. Ultrasound is poor in the evaluation of a large mass, rendering it suboptimal for large goiters.

Computed Tomography and Magnetic Resonance Imaging
In the evaluation of the thyroid gland, CT is particularly useful in identifying and delineating the full extent of any cervical lymphadenopathy and the relationship of the thyroid to surrounding cervical viscera. CT dye should be used judiciously and appropriately because administration of iodinated contrast can interfere with thyroid function testing, scanning, and radioactive iodine treatment for up to 6 to 8 weeks. It can also provoke frank hyperthyroidism in a patient with multinodular goiter and subclinical hyperthyroidism due to the large iodine load. If necessary, CT should be performed without the administration of intravenous (IV) contrast or a gadolinium-enhanced MRI can be performed. We particularly recommend the use of CT imaging of any patient who presents with associated lymphadenopathy on examination or USS, and any patient whose FNA returns positive for papillary carcinoma. We use USS to assess the central neck nodes and CT for information regarding the thyroid's relationship to central neck viscera as well as lateral neck nodal status. USS and CT are used to create a preoperative nodal map that directs nodal dissection at the time of thyroidectomy.

MRI is less commonly used for evaluation of the thyroid gland. It can be performed with a dedicated neck or surface coil, providing excellent soft tissue resolution.

Radioisotopic Scanning

The lack of reliability of thyroid scintigraphy to differentiate a benign nodule from a malignant nodule has rendered it of little use in the initial evaluation of a nodule. The two-dimensional nature of scintigraphy also allows abnormal thyroid tissue to be superimposed in front of or behind normal functioning thyroid tissue, making accurate localization difficult.

Fine-Needle Aspiration Biopsy of the Thyroid Gland
Diagnostic Categories

FNA has become the gold standard in evaluating a palpable thyroid nodule and deciding whether to proceed with surgical treatment. A survey of the members of the American Thyroid Association showed that 100% of the members would perform FNA biopsy for diagnosis of thyroid nodules (37). With the sensitivity and specificity of FNA for thyroid cancer being shown to be high, ranging from 65% to 98% and 72% to 100%, respectively, it is not surprising that it has become the test of choice for routine diagnosis and management of thyroid nodules (38–41).

FNA results can be broken down into four main groups: benign, malignant, indeterminate (suspicious), and nondiagnostic (unsatisfactory). The benign group includes colloid nodules, benign cysts, and thyroiditis. The indeterminate (suspicious) group consists of cytology that is suggestive of but not diagnostic for malignancy. The nondiagnostic (unsatisfactory) group is made up of aspirates with too few cells for diagnosis.

Benign. The benign cytologic classification represents the majority of FNA specimen results. This classification often includes a benign macrofollicular adenoma, multinodular goiter, or thyroiditis.

Malignant. The malignant group represents approximately 4% of all the thyroid FNA specimens. The most common of these is PTC. PTC lends itself well for cytologic diagnosis because its malignancy is characterized by nuclear changes including enlargement, irregular shape, grooving of the nuclear membrane, and intranuclear holes. Unfortunately, these changes occur in varying degrees, and in some cases PTC is suspected but a definitive diagnosis cannot be established so the sample will then be classified as suspicious.

Other malignancies of the thyroid that can be diagnosed on cytology include MTC and highly malignant carcinomas (ATCs and high-grade metastatic lesions). It can be difficult to distinguish between the high-grade thyroid malignancies on cytologic examination.

Suspicious. The suspicious cytologic category is used when a definite malignant diagnosis cannot be made on cytology. Malignancy is subsequently found in 10% to 50% of these patients (42). The most common cytologic diagnoses in this group include follicular neoplasm, Hürthle cell neoplasm, and suspicious for papillary carcinoma. MTC, lymphoma,

and other carcinomas can also be in this category when the cytologic findings are not conclusive for these entities.

The diagnosis of a benign or malignant follicular neoplasm or Hürthle cell neoplasm rests on the presence or absence of capsular and vascular invasion. FNA cytology can only provide an indication of a follicular neoplasm or Hürthle cell neoplasm but no information on the presence or absence of capsular and vascular invasion.

Several studies have attempted to increase the positive or negative predictive value of a suspicious aspirate by introducing other clinical information. Studies have found factors that are predictors of malignancy in this group include nodule size greater than 4 cm, solitary nodule, male sex, and fixed nodule on palpation (43,44). We recommend surgical excision of nodules in all patients with suspicious cytology. Intraoperative frozen section can be used to clarify nodules suspicious for papillary, medullary, lymphoma, and metastatic lesions. Unfortunately, frozen section cannot be used to exclude malignancy in follicular or Hürthle cell neoplasms.

Nondiagnostic. In nondiagnostic aspirates, insufficient cellular material exists to render a cytologic diagnosis. It is important to explain to patients that no information has been obtained rather than "no malignant cells were seen." Reaspiration yields diagnostic information in 50% of such patients. A nondiagnostic specimen can result for several reasons. The most common reason is inadequate sampling of the nodule. This often occurs with aspiration of a small nodule ($\leq$1.5 cm) or a cystic nodule, yielding too few follicular cells for analysis. Because malignancy has not been ruled out in these aspirates, repeat aspiration is recommended either via ultrasonographically guided FNA (USFNA) or via surgical treatment.

Procedure

An experienced clinician who is comfortable performing biopsies of the thyroid gland should always perform the FNA. Prior to the procedure the patient in placed in the supine position, the gland is palpated, and the nodule for biopsy is clearly isolated. The skin overlying the nodule is then prepped with alcohol and the patient is asked not to swallow or talk during the procedure. Local anesthesia is generally not required. A 25-gauge, $1\frac{1}{2}$-inch-long needle attached to a 10-mL disposable plastic syringe is used either attached to a mechanical syringe holder or free hand to perform the biopsy. Two techniques are recognized: the aspiration technique, in which the needle is inserted into the nodule and only after the tip is in the nodule is suction applied while the needle is moved back and forth along the long axis of the needle, or the nonaspiration technique, in which the same procedure is conducted but no suction is applied to the syringe. Both techniques dislodge cellular material into the needle hub that can then be placed on slides for cytologic diagnosis. The needle is then removed, the syringe filled with air, and the cellular material is expelled onto the slides for cytologic analysis. The slides are then air-dried, wet-fixed in 95% alcohol, or fixed with a spray fixative. To increase the diagnostic value of the procedure, normally two to four aspirations are made from different sites of the nodule, rendering two to four slides from aspiration.

Problems and Pitfalls of Fine-Needle Aspiration

Although FNA is a useful and critical adjunct in the evaluation of a thyroid nodule, there are some common limitations and pitfalls associated with this investigative modality. A common limitation is the inability to distinguish benign microfollicular adenomas from differentiated FTCs. This is also true for Hürthle cell lesions, which may represent not only an adenoma but also chronic lymphocytic (Hashimoto) thyroiditis.

A common pitfall for the cytologist is the diagnosis of papillary carcinoma. Many artifacts produced during the slide preparation may mimic the nuclear findings of papillary carcinoma. This causes the cytologist to have no choice but to call the sample suspicious for papillary carcinoma. Another pitfall is cellular atypia, which the clinician often associates with malignancy. However, nonneoplastic atypia is relatively common and most frequently seen with degenerate change, but is also seen in Hashimoto thyroiditis and postirradiation changes. It can occasionally be difficult to distinguish between MTC and lymphoma on cytology, but calcitonin staining can be helpful to identify a lesion as MTC.

Ultimately, clinical judgment overrides any cytologic diagnosis. If the history or clinical examination strongly indicates a malignancy, but the cytologic result suggests it is benign, the nodule should be surgically excised.

Ultrasonographically Guided Fine-Needle Aspiration

This procedure is particularly helpful in cases of nodules smaller than 1.5 cm in diameter, for thyroid cysts, or when a previous aspiration attempt has been unsuccessful. A large study has shown that a satisfactory diagnosis was achieved in 91.5% of cases when USFNA was used compared with in 85.9% of cases when palpation alone was used (45).

Rebiopsy

Studies have shown that routine reaspiration of cytologically benign thyroid nodules is not necessary (46,47). It is sufficient to follow a nodule with palpation alone if the FNA results are classified as benign. Reaspiration is warranted if the nodule changes in size, a cyst recurs, the palpable characteristics of the nodule change, or repeat USS shows changes since last review.

Thyroidectomy: Surgical Techniques

Initial Steps Prior to Surgery

Successful thyroid surgery implies meticulous attention to detail. This is accomplished in the setting of rigorous preoperative workup. Some key steps must be taken prior to

any thyroid surgery. Patients with hyperthyroidism should be rendered euthyroid preoperatively. Pheochromocytoma must be ruled out before surgery on patients with MTC. No paralytic agents should be used when RLN monitoring and stimulation is planned. Patients with PTC should have preoperative evaluations that not only include a thorough physical examination but also an USS and CT to create a comprehensive cervical nodal map. All patients should also have preoperative laryngoscopy. Patients with preoperative vocal cord paralysis can be evaluated with fine-cut airway CT to assess for invasion, and laryngeal, tracheal, and esophageal endoscopy can be performed at the time of thyroidectomy.

Positioning, Preparation, and Draping

The patient is placed in the supine position and after intubation the patient is positioned with the neck extended and the arms tucked and padded at the patient's side. The thyroid bag is then inflated or rolled towels are placed under the shoulders. Because optimal exposure with cosmesis is the primary goal of the incision, its position, shape, and symmetry all have important implications. The skin is marked with a sterile marking pen delineating the midline, clavicles, suprasternal notch, thyroid notch, and cricoid to guide the subsequent incision. The 4- to 5-cm incision is then marked out approximately 1 cm inferior to the cricoid cartilage, therefore placing the incision close to the isthmus of the thyroid gland. Patients with larger tumors or with short necks may require larger incisions to accommodate optimal exposure. Smaller incisions with video-assist or endoscopic approaches are being looked into presently. Small incisions may limit exposure of key anatomic locations, such as the ligament of Berry, and increase complication rates. Excessive retraction used with small incisions may lead to keloid formation.

Once fully mapped out, local anesthetic, in the form of 1% lidocaine (Xylocaine) with 1:100,000 epinephrine, is injected along the marked incision. Once injected the incision is carried down through the skin down to the platysma muscle, ensuring hemostasis at all times, then through the platysma along the whole length of the incision. After adequate hemostasis is achieved a superior subplatysma flap is raised to the level of the thyroid notch and if required an inferior flap may also be raised. The anterior jugular veins overlying the strap muscles are left down as the flap is raised and the midline is identified above the cricoid and on the upper cervical trachea below the isthmus.

Strap Muscles

The whitish midline fascial interval (linea alba) between the medial edges of the sternohyoid muscles is then dissected down to the thyroid capsule revealing the trachea above and below the thyroid isthmus. While dissecting below the isthmus, special attention must be paid to the inferior thyroid veins, which can blend to form an inferior venous plexus. If necessary these may be tied off to aid in the exposure of the trachea. During this maneuver, one must also watch for a high-riding innominate artery or a thyroid ima artery. When dissecting above the isthmus, special attention must be paid in identifying any pyramidal lobe. The pyramidal lobe normally arises from the mid portion of the isthmus and can extend cranially to varying degrees, occasionally extending up to the hyoid bone. Any prelaryngeal or Delphian nodes can be identified during this time as this region is dissected. We believe that the identification of the trachea above and below the thyroid isthmus affords a constant midline orientation throughout the rest of the case, being particularly helpful during RLN identification.

The sternothyroid is then dissected off the anterior surface of the thyroid gland, with any small bridging vessels extending from the true thyroid capsule to the undersurface of the strap muscles being identified and individually cauterized or tied. In some circumstances, a plane cannot be established easily and may represent inflammation secondary to FNA or malignant infiltration. In these circumstances, we recommend the resection of the involved segment strap muscle segment to avoid potentially leaving malignancy behind.

Lateral Thyroid Dissection

The next step is exposure of the posterolateral edge of the thyroid gland. If lateral retraction of the strap muscles does not achieve adequate exposure, they should be divided. This is best done superiorly after the lateral border of the strap muscles is identified to avoid injury to the jugular and carotid sheath contents.

A small Richardson retractor or Army-Navy retractor is then placed to retract the strap muscles laterally. At this point, a gauze sponge retracts the thyroid and laryngotracheal complex medially and anteriorly (Fig. 116.1), uncovering the middle thyroid veins and providing optimal exposure of the area posterolateral to the thyroid, where the RLN and parathyroid glands are located. The middle thyroid veins are then cleaned of adjacent tissue, ligated, and divided.

Recurrent Laryngeal Nerve

Permanent RLN paralysis rates in expert hands is in the 1% to 2% range. To successfully identify and preserve the RLN a surgeon must be familiar with its anatomy on either side of the neck. On the right side of the neck, the RLN follows an oblique course, due to its origin around the subclavian artery. However, on the left side, the RLN is in a more medial position, running along the tracheoesophageal groove after its recurrence around the ductus arteriosus. Both nerves usually pass under the inferior thyroid artery, but they may pass over it or through its branches. This relationship with the artery can be exploited in the localization of the nerve (Fig. 116.1). It is also important to note that in approximately 0.5% of patients, the right RLN can be nonrecurrent. A nonrecurrent left side is very rare because it can only occur in patients with situs inversus.

We feel that the most important rule to follow in preservation of the nerve is that no structure is cut until the RLN is identified both visually and electrically. If this single rule is adhered, RLN injury, and certainly transection, will be rare. An adjunct to this rule is a bloodless field, which allows identification of the wavelike profile and characteristic vascular strip of the RLN. Adherence to this rule can be particularly difficult in cases of goitrous enlargement; in these cases the strap muscles should be cut without hesitation if additional exposure is needed. Retraction of the thyroid and laryngotracheal complex medially can also aid exposure in these cases. However, excess retraction on the thyroid can lead to a nerve traction injury and only gentle traction should be used at all times. One must also remember that the distal course of the RLN may become

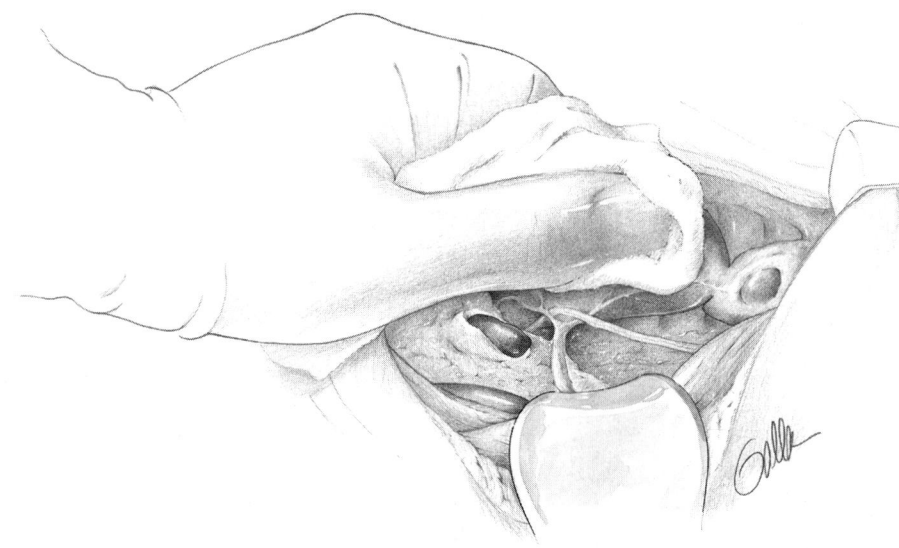

Figure 116.1 Exposure of the lateral border of the thyroid showing the relationship of the recurrent laryngeal nerve to the inferior thyroid artery and the parathyroid glands. (Reproduced from Randolph G. *Surgery of the thyroid and parathyroid glands.* Philadelphia: WB Saunders, 2003, with permission.)

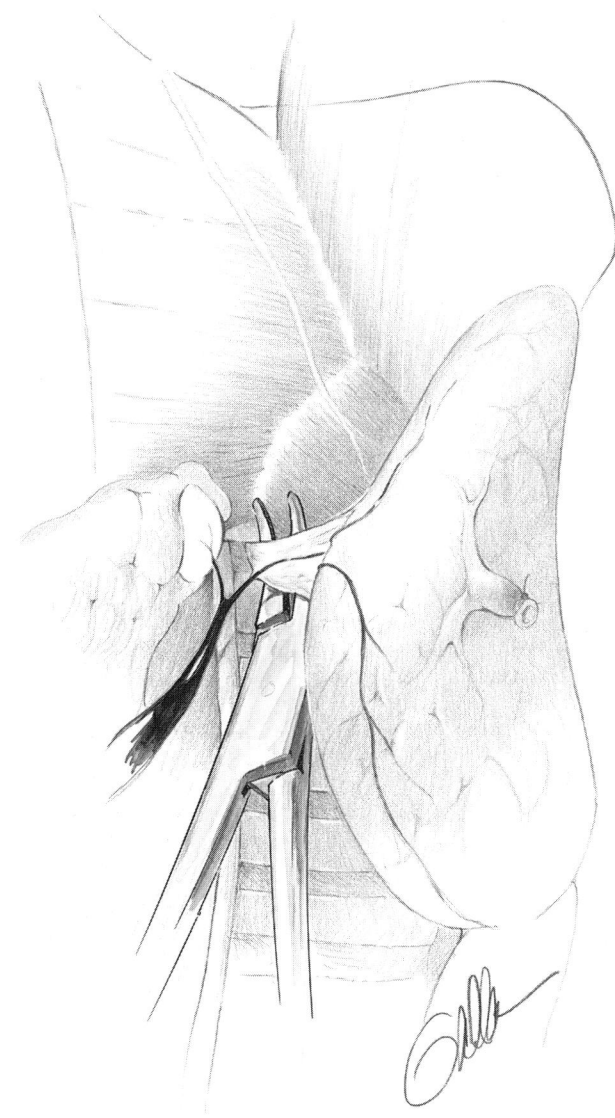

Figure 116.2 The ligament of Berry and its close association with the distal inferior thyroid artery and the recurrent laryngeal nerve. (Reproduced from Randolph G. *Surgery of the thyroid and parathyroid glands.* Philadelphia: WB Saunders, 2003, with permission.)

subject to stretch injury at the relative tethering point at the ligament of Berry because the thyroid is dissected and medially rotated from its cervical attachments (Fig. 116.2). Although hemostasis during thyroidectomy is paramount, it is important to note that after a lobe is freed from the ligament of Berry blood often oozes from this site. To control this bleeding, patience is recommended, rather than indiscriminate cautery or clamping. A neurosurgical pledget can be used to brush the area with a suction tip to allow full view of the RLN and the bleeding site. With careful discrete bipolar cautery or specific clamping of any identified bleeder, bleeding can be controlled. Any continuing minimal oozing can be controlled with Surgicel.

There are several approaches to finding and preserving the RLN. The RLN can be found in the thoracic inlet and then traced up superiorly. Typically, the nerve can be dissected in "skip" areas leaving most of its course undissected. In so doing it is important to avoid sacrifice of parathyroid blood supply. This approach is useful for revision cases in which the nerve can be found below or within prior scar. Another approach is identification of the nerve at its laryngeal entry point. Freeing up the upper pole is necessary for this approach. The superior approach is ideal for large SSG in which lateral and inferior approaches are prohibitive. The third and most common approach is the lateral approach in which the nerve is dissected at the midpole level. Identification of the nerve first just below the ligament of Berry minimizes nerve dissection and is ideal for routine first time cases (Fig. 116.3).

After the RLN is identified visually and electrically, the inferior pole is more fully dissected where it then facilitates further RLN dissection to the ligament of Berry. At that point the superior pole is dissected in its lateral aspect allowing the superior parathyroid to fall away. The superior pole is then retracted inferiorly and the external branch of the superior laryngeal nerve is visually and electrically identified on the lateral surface of the inferior constrictor muscle. The superior pole vessels are then taken. The sternothyroid muscle can be sectioned to improve access to the superior pole. Once the superior and inferior poles have been taken, the lobe is medially rotated on the trachea allowing for ligament of Berry dissection and freeing of the lobe. All thyroid tissue is then excised at the ligament of Berry in the setting of full RLN identification and visualization. Thyroid tissue is then meticulously dissected off the trachea with all vessels traversing the ligament carefully clamped, divided, and ligated.

RLN monitoring represents not only an adjunct to, and extension of, routine visual identification of the nerve but also forms an essential component in its preservation. Routine identification of the RLN is associated with lower rates of injury; we expect that monitoring, as an embellishment of visual neural identification, should help to further lower the rates of paralysis. That said, it is clear that electrical identification of the RLN should reinforce but not substitute its visual identification. Not only does RLN monitoring permit its clear identification, it also allows prognostication regarding postoperative neural function. This predictive ability is particularly helpful when a bilateral operation is being performed. RLN monitoring can be easily achieved via surface endotracheal tube electrodes. This allows passive and evoked surface electromyographic (EMG) monitoring of the left and right thyroarytenoid muscles during thyroid surgery. Recording ground and nerve stimulator surface electrodes are placed on the patient's shoulders. Endotracheal tube electrodes and grounds are interfaced with an oscilloscope through a connector box. This setup allows continuous audio and visual feedback monitoring of the thyroarytenoid laryngeal musculature.

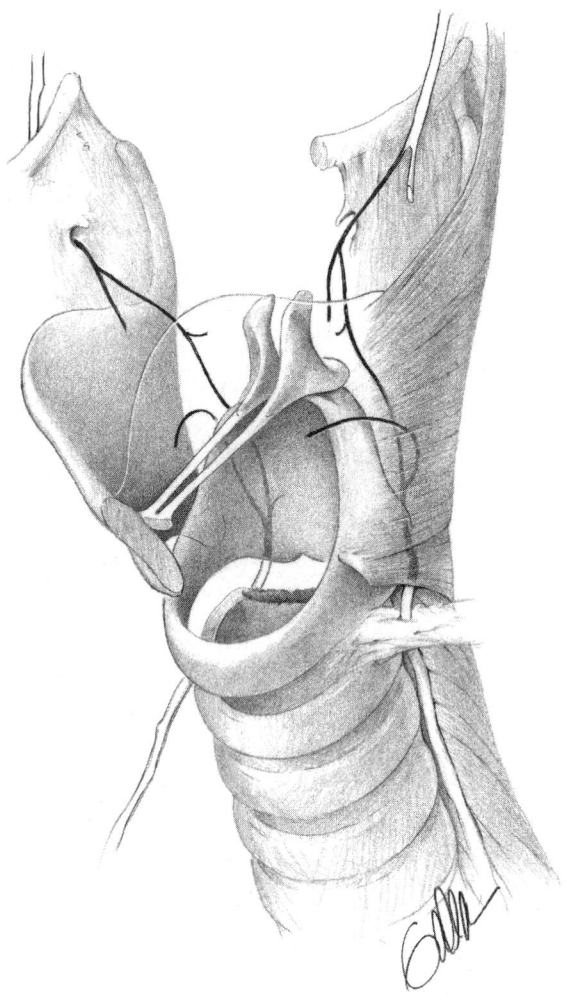

Figure 116.3 Three-dimensional view of recurrent laryngeal nerve anatomy. (Reproduced from Randolph G. *Surgery of the thyroid and parathyroid glands*. Philadelphia: WB Saunders, 2003, with permission.)

Although monitoring should be considered in all cases, it is critical in cases recognized preoperatively of having a greater risk to the RLN. These cases include cases of surgery for confirmed malignancy, requiring significant nodal resection; Graves disease and thyroiditis; SSG; operation on an only functioning nerve; and most of all revision surgery and surgery on a previously irradiated neck.

Management of Injured or Infiltrated Nerves
Infiltrated Nerves
Locally invasive PTC occurs in about 6% to 16% of cases, and the RLN represents the second most commonly affected site (48,49). In cases of RLN infiltration with carcinoma and in which the preoperative RLN function is normal, the nerve should be saved. The carcinoma should be carefully dissected off the RLN, with no gross disease left. Microscopic disease can be treated with ^{131}I and thyroxine (T_4) suppression. Careful note of this should be made in the operative note vin case reoperation is necessary. If the

RLN is found to be infiltrated with benign disease or lymphoma, it should be preserved. If preoperative RLN paralysis is present and the nerve is infiltrated with carcinoma, the nerve should be resected.

Blunt, Nontransection Injury
Work in both humans and animals suggest that should the nerve be injured bluntly or ligated it is best simply to free the nerve and not perform neurorrhaphy. Studies have shown a good recovery in cats from 3 to 8 weeks after crush injury (50).

Transected Nerve
Although management of the acutely transected nerve is controversial, most authors currently support some attempts to reinnervate the RLN with direct nerve repair or anastomosis of a branch of the ansa cervicalis. Unilateral paralysis should be deferred for 6 to 12 months to allow for optimal recovery prior to surgical rehabilitation, unless the patient is severely symptomatic. Gelfoam injection can be used as a good temporizing measure. Bilateral paralysis is a devastating complication, with most patients requiring either a tracheotomy or some procedure to widen the glottic airway.

Parathyroid Gland Preservation
A surgeon must know parathyroid embryology to successfully identify these structures, which range in their location from the mandible to the mediastinum. The parathyroids also have a clear-cut location relative to the coronal plane of the RLN in the neck (Fig. 116.4). The inferior glands lie ventral or anterior to the RLN, whereas the superior glands are dorsal or posterior. Several features of the parathyroid glands aid in their recognition; these include the glands' unique brown to reddish brown color, their softer texture compared with thyroid tissue and lymph nodes, their smooth encapsulated surface, their leaf or flattened bean shape, and their distinct hilar vessel. The best clue to the parathyroid glands, identity is their discreet gliding motion related to surrounding fat as that fat is bluntly manipulated. Another helpful feature is the discrete plane between the parathyroid and thyroid gland, unless truly intrathyroidal, allowing the parathyroid to be reflected off the thyroid surface on a laterally based vascular pedicle, with minimal bleeding.

The inferior parathyroids can normally be found within 1 to 2 cm inferior or posterolateral to the inferior pole of the thyroid, but their position is variable. The superior gland's most common location is at the level of the cricothyroid cartilage articulation often just lateral to the RLN entry point or on the lateral surface of the superior thyroid pole. The superior parathyroid glands are more constant in their position than the inferior glands.

Once the parathyroids are successfully identified, the surgeon, through the use of judicious and meticulous technique, dissects the glands off the surface of the thyroid,

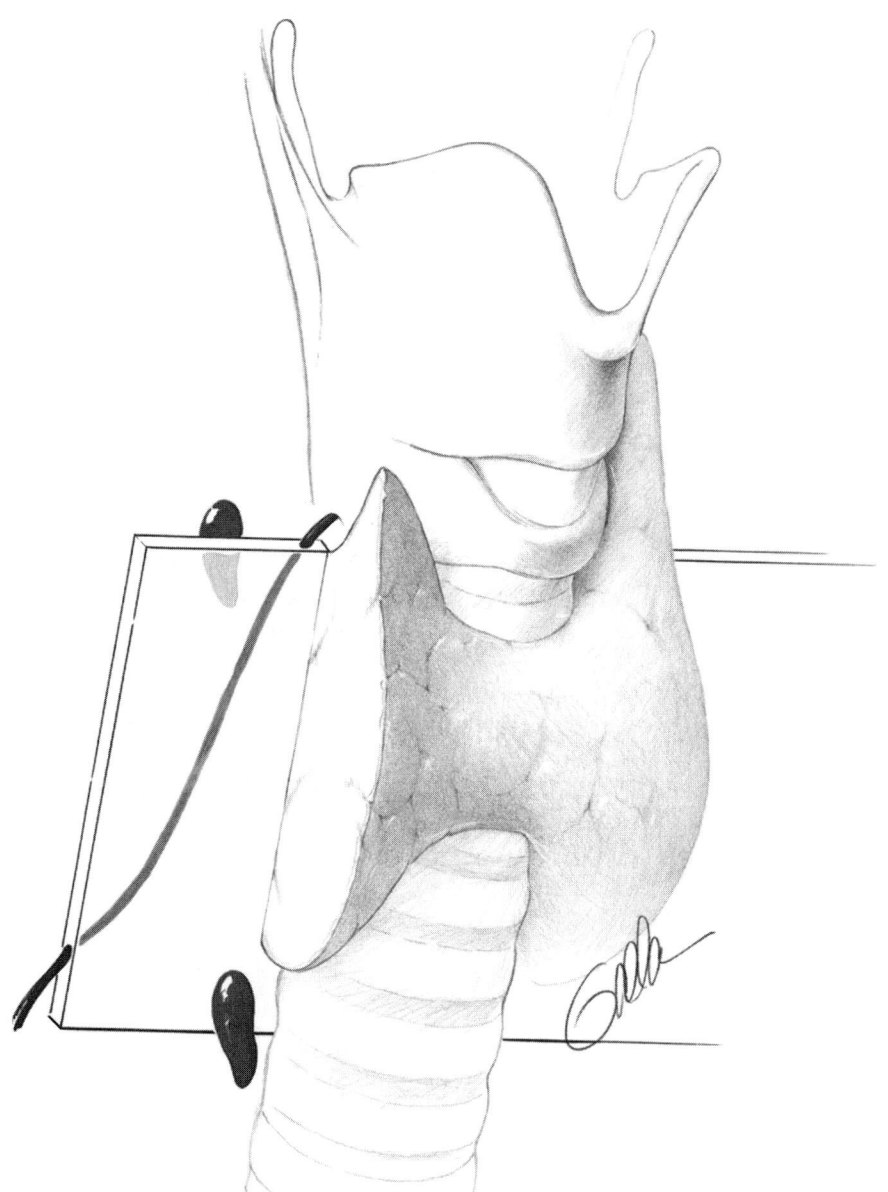

Figure 116.4 Coronal plane formed by the recurrent laryngeal nerve and its relationship to parathyroid glands. (Reproduced from Randolph G. *Surgery of the thyroid and parathyroid glands.* Philadelphia: WB Saunders, 2003, with permission.)

taking care not to ligate or injure any tissue around the parathyroid unnecessarily and by so doing ensuring the preservation of their lateral blood supply.

Parathyroid Autotransplantation

Occasionally despite attention to detail a parathyroid gland has clearly become devascularized or inadvertently removed. In these cases, autotransplantation is necessary. A small section of the suspected parathyroid gland is sent for frozen section to confirm its identity while the remaining gland is placed in sterile saline. Once frozen section confirmation is obtained, the remaining gland is divided into 1-mm^2 pieces and autotransplanted into separate muscular pockets in the sternocleidomastoid muscle of the corresponding side. Multiple pockets are used to increase the chance of successful autotransplantation, and the sites are marked with metal clips for future localization should primary hyperparathyroidism (HPT) ever develop.

Final Steps

As a final step after the specimen is removed, the neck is examined for nodal disease. The ipsilateral perithyroidal, paratracheal, and pretracheal regions are carefully examined visually and through palpation, as are the adjacent jugular nodal regions 3 and 4. Any suspicious nodal disease is excised at this point and sent for pathologic examination. Significant nodal disease in a planned hemithyroidectomy should raise the suspicion of malignancy and nodes should be sent for frozen section.

Before the thyroid specimen is sent, it is rigorously checked for any parathyroid glands on its surface. Any suspected parathyroids are carefully removed from the thyroid and a small piece sent for frozen section. Reimplantation is indicated if the frozen section confirms a parathyroid. Once this specimen is removed and checked and any nodal disease addressed, hemostasis is meticulously ensured. Particular attention is paid to the thyroid bed and platysma-skin flap with the anesthesiologist giving positive pressure ventilation (Valsalva maneuver) to elicit any venous bleeding. Scant oozing from the ligament of Berry is controlled as mentioned previously and if need be Surgicel can be placed over this region.

Extent of Thyroidectomy

A surgical plan for patients with well-differentiated thyroid cancer (WDTC) can be constructed despite the divergent information available in the literature. It is also important to not be overly dogmatic about any one approach, given the retrospective nature of the bulk of the data available.

Age and presence of metastatic disease are probably the most important prognostic determinants. Most specialists believe that the extent of treatment for WDTC should relate to the patient's risk grouping. This philosophy should be kept in mind when one is considering the extent of thyroidectomy for WDTC. The bulk of the data available suggests that the overriding principle in the surgical treatment of WDTC is that the surgeon should, at first surgery, encompass the gross disease in the thyroid and neck nodes and understand that, although present, microscopic disease in the contralateral lobe and the neck nodes has little clinical significance. Such microscopic disease is indolent and not clinically manifest in the majority of cases. Initial surgery should then encompass the palpable ipsilateral abnormality through total lobectomy and isthmusectomy, and total thyroidectomy should be considered if any gross nodules are palpated in the contralateral lobe. Intrathyroidal contralateral disease can be evaluated by preoperative sonogram and intraoperative palpation. Grossly enlarged lymph nodes should be excised. Patients with gross invasion of the trachea should be managed with segmental airway resection. Patients without contralateral nodularity or gross lymphadenopathy in the low-risk prognostic group are well treated with ipsilateral total lobectomy and isthmusectomy. Most agree that, for patients in the high-risk group, total thyroidectomy will optimize survival.

Total thyroidectomy is an excellent procedure in skilled hands. It should be offered when it does not bring with it significant morbidity. However, the feasibility of total thyroidectomy, even in experienced hands, has been questioned because residual thyroid tissue remains (typically centered at the ligament of Berry, pyramidal lobe, or superior pole) in a small but substantial fraction of patients. Thus, aggressive bilateral thyroidectomy may not obviate the need for postoperative ablation. Leaving a small contralateral lobe remnant is a reasonable option if this helps the surgeon avoid parathyroid injury. Education is required at the resident level regarding proper technique in the performance of a total thyroidectomy.

It is important to emphasize that the extent of thyroidectomy should be tailored not only to the patient's risk group and operative findings but also to the progress of the specific surgery, particularly if the contralateral lobe is not involved by cancer. If dissection of the first side has revealed two parathyroids of good color with good vascular pedicles and with an RLN that has been identified and preserved and that stimulates well electrically at the end of the dissection, contralateral thyroid surgery can be safely contemplated. If the first side has not gone well, then elective contralateral lobe resection should be deferred. We believe that parathyroid color changes associated with devascularization are not reliable for its vascularity. Characteristic blackened color change may be associated with venous disruption and implies parathyroid dysfunction. However, arterial interruption may be unassociated with this color change. RLN monitoring can help identify and dissect the RLN and can be helpful in assessing neural function at the end of surgery. An inexperienced surgeon should resist the aggressive philosophy that all patients with a diagnosis of WDTC should have total thyroidectomy. Such a philosophy will ultimately result in patient morbidity (especially in terms of permanent hypoparathyroidism) and will not likely result in survival benefit for most patients.

Postoperative Complications

Hemorrhage and Hematoma
Hemorrhage is a rare occurrence postthyroidectomy but still a very significant risk associated with the operation (Table 116.3). Hemorrhage is most likely in the presence of venous hypertension, glandular enlargement with increased vascularity, aberrant blood supply, and a substernal or intrathoracic location of the gland. Hemorrhage can be most easily avoided with the use of attention to surgical detail and careful normal inspection with a Valsalva maneuver at the time of surgery.

TABLE 116.3 COMPLICATIONS SURGERY FOR THYROID NODULES

- Hemorrhage and hematoma
- Seroma
- Infection
- Recurrent laryngeal nerve injury
- Superior laryngeal nerve injury
- Hypocalcemia
- Airway obstruction
- Others: pneumomediastinum, pneumothorax, hemothorax, and chyle leaks

Inadequate hemostasis at the time of closure or increased venous pressures at extubation due to coughing or straining are the most common causes for hematomas. Neither drains nor bulky pressure dressings will prevent the formation of a hematoma. Significant morbidity and even airway compromise may result if a definitive intervention is not instituted early to manage the hematoma. The hematoma should be explored and evacuated as soon as possible in the operating suite. Hematoma is associated with laryngeal submucosal infiltration and edema leading to glottic level obstruction. The most effective preventative measure is through meticulous attention to hemostasis throughout the case and particularly at the time of closure.

Seroma
There are several surgical situations that predispose to seroma formation including bilateral thyroid operation, particularly when a subtotal thyroid resection is performed or after removal of a large goiter. Seromas, if large enough, should be aspirated. Infected seromas require immediate and adequate drainage.

Infection
Wound infections after thyroid and parathyroid surgery is uncommon. This type of surgery is considered a "clean" procedure, and prophylactic antibiotics are not indicated.

Recurrent Laryngeal Nerve Injury
As discussed previously, injury to the RLN can occur as a result of thyroid or parathyroid surgery. Several factors have been recognized to increase the incidence of RLN injury. These include operating on a SSG, extent of thyroid resection, surgeon experience, revision thyroid or parathyroid surgery, and malignancy. Its occurrence, management, and prevention has been discussed in detail previously in the surgical technique section.

Superior Laryngeal Nerve Injury
Because of difficulties in laryngoscopic identification, the true incidence of SLN injury is difficult to quantitate. In SLN paralysis, the vocal cord may appear shorter and bowed, lying at a lower level than the contralateral normal side. The unopposed contralateral cricothyroid muscle may also cause the epiglottis and larynx to tilt to the normal side. Bilateral injury results in a more symmetrical laryngeal appearance, but the vocal cords will still appear shorter and bowed and the patient will have a breathy voice that is lowered in pitch. The only treatment for SLN injury is speech therapy.

Hypocalcaemia
One of the most common complications of thyroid and parathyroid surgery is postoperative hypocalcemia. Several factors increase its incidence and these include the extent

of resection (total > subtotal); central compartment dissection; revision cases; and surgery for SSGs, carcinoma, or Graves' disease (51,52).

All patients undergoing thyroid or parathyroid surgery should be closely monitored postoperatively for any symptoms of hypocalcemia (numbness or tingling in the lips, hands, and feet as well as a feeling of anxiety). Symptomatic hypocalcemia usually reflects a corrected calcium serum level of equal to or less than 8.0 mg/dL but may also signify a rapid decline in the serum calcium levels. For our patients who have undergone a total thyroidectomy, we recommend a serum calcium level in the recovery room and every 8 hours after that until discharge to ensure stable calcium levels. This enables us to quickly and efficaciously treat any hypocalcemia prior to any complication associated with it. Transient postoperative hypocalcemia, particularly in the first 24 hours, is common. The critical period for determining the need for supplemental calcium has been demonstrated to be in the first 24 to 72 postoperative hours (53,54). Parathyroid hormone measures within normal range at the completion of surgery predict the need for postoperative calcium.

Symptomatic hypocalcemia requires correction through oral supplementation or calcium gluconate infusion if the degree of hypocalcemia is severe. Repeated does of calcium gluconate can be given if required to maintain the corrected serum calcium levels above 8.0 mg/dL. Vitamin D is also added to the regimen if intravenous (IV) calcium gluconate is required. The patient is only discharged once an adequate dose of oral supplementation is established to maintain calcium levels above 8.0 mg/dL. A calcium level is then checked at the follow-up visit and the calcium slowly tapered off; the patient is asked to take note of any recurrence of symptoms and to contact the surgeon if symptoms recur. Some patients will require long-term calcium replacement and if so should be evaluated by an experienced endocrinologist for management.

Airway Obstruction
Whenever performing thyroid surgery on a patient who has a significant goiter, one must be aware of the special airway management problems that the goiter may present. The airway may, due to tracheal compression, already be marginal and the surgeon must be aware of the possibility of loss of the airway during induction. This situation is complicated by the fact that a tracheotomy may not be an option in many of these patients due to the goiter covering the ventral surface of the trachea. In these cases the surgeon and anesthesiologist should be prepared to use alternative methods of airway management such as the laryngeal mask airway or fiberoptic intubation. We have found that standard intubation transorally is generally straightforward despite tracheal compression. Tracheomalacia felt to result from long-standing compression by a goiter is very uncommon.

Bilateral vocal cord paralysis may result in glottic closure and airway obstruction. Their management is discussed previously.

Other Complications

Other uncommon complications include pneumomediastinum, pneumothorax, hemothorax, and chyle leaks. In most cases, the most effective method of treating complications is avoiding them. The incidence of complications can be minimized by careful preoperative evaluation, meticulous technique, and responsible postoperative care.

Postoperative Considerations

Radioiodine Therapy

Radioiodine ablation is an effective treatment used postoperatively to destroy any residual thyroid tissue. There are two main benefits for its use in thyroid carcinoma. It ablates any residual normal thyroid tissue facilitating the early detection of any recurrence by serum Tg measurement and ^{131}I whole body scanning (^{131}I WBS) and may reduce recurrence and mortality rates by eradicating any residual.

Indications

Radioiodine ablation therapy is usually given 4 to 6 weeks after surgery, but the indications for treatment are still a matter of controversy. The prognosis for patients with a WDTC of less than 1.0 to 1.5 cm is so favorable that radioiodine ablation is not clearly indicated. In these cases, the patients are clearly counseled and offered radioablation only if they request it.

In patients who have a WDTC exceeding 1.0 to 1.5 cm, the prognosis is still favorable but the perceived benefits and low-risk of side effects make radioiodine ablation an attractive option. It allows for more convenient follow up with the use of TBS and Tg measurements.

Patients with persistent or recurrent disease have a clear indication for radioiodine ablation for treating persistent neoplastic foci after any appropriate surgical intervention for gross disease.

Side Effects

The side effects of radioiodine treatment are usually minimal and transient. A dry mouth and sialadenitis are common side effects of radioiodine ablation. Nausea and gastric pain are also common side effects of radioiodine ablation. Its use is contraindicated during pregnancy and women should be advised to avoid pregnancy for 1 year after treatment with radioiodine. Despite these side effects, radioiodine has been used extensively over the years with few major complications.

Tumor Staging

Several staging and prognostic scoring systems have been developed to differentiate prognostic groups in thyroid carcinoma. The most important prognostic parameters used include age, extrathyroidal extension, sex, size of lesion, and presence of distant metastasis. We clinically use the most recent American Joint Committee on Cancer (AJCC) TNM staging classifications in our practice.

Recurrent or Persistent Disease

The benefits of treating persistent and recurrent disease are twofold. Treating metastatic disease, although not always conferring cure, has been shown to improve survival and avoid further complications associated with these metastases (i.e., pathologic fractures in bony metastasis). Early radionuclide scintigraphic diagnosis of persistent or recurrent disease, allowing prompt treatment with ^{131}I, is a critical element in improving survival and prolonging disease-free survival (55).

The preferred treatment modality for recurrent disease is often surgery if possible. For disease not amenable to surgery, ^{131}I therapy may be considered for tumors that concentrate iodine. External-beam radiotherapy can be used for disease that does not uptake iodine and cannot be treated with surgery.

Cervical Lymph Node Metastasis

Although papillary carcinoma is strongly lymphotrophic, cervical lymph node metastases at presentation seem to have no significant prognostic implication in younger patients (56,57). Microscopic disease is of limited clinical importance. This is highlighted by studies that have shown a low rate of the development of clinical disease despite a high prevalence of microscopic foci in the contralateral lobe and neck (58,59). These observations have led to the abandonment of the past recommendation of elective neck dissections in N0 patients. Although nodal metastases do not seem to worsen the overall prognosis in patients with WDTC, some studies have identified that age (>45 years) in the face of nodal metastasis does increase the risk of local recurrence and cancer-specific mortality (60–62).

The lymph nodes most commonly involved with thyroid metastasis are the paratracheal nodes. Following these, the metastasis pattern is one involving the level IV (52%), followed by the levels III, V, and II (45%, 33%, and 30%, respectively) (63). Involvement of the submandibular region without other lymph node metastasis occurs only rarely. Metastatic spread of thyroid carcinoma normally follows the previous pattern but unfortunately it does not always conform to this pattern and skip lesions can be present anywhere in the neck. Tumors exhibiting extrathyroidal extension or vascular invasion have been shown to have a higher rate of lymph node metastases (64).

We have a low threshold to perform an elective dissection of the pretracheal and the ipsilateral paratracheal nodes in all patients with papillary carcinoma. These nodes can often be removed adequately with minimal morbidity at first surgery and constitute the first echelon of lymphatic drainage for the thyroid gland. This avoids the morbidity of revision central neck dissection.

Routine elective dissection in the lateral compartment of the neck (levels II, III, IV, and V) is not indicated in N0 patients with differentiated thyroid cancer. Clear survival advantage has not been uniformly demonstrated.

In the clinically positive neck, surgical excision is the preferred treatment. Although controversy over the extent of the lymph node dissection still exists, several studies have now shown that a modified radical neck dissection (levels II to V, preserving the spinal accessory nerve, internal jugular vein, and sternocleidomastoid muscle, unless involved with cancer) is appropriate as opposed to "berry picking" (65–67). The surgical excision should be followed by ^{131}I ablation and ^{131}I therapy.

Distant Metastasis

Distant metastases occur in approximately 10% of cases of papillary and FTCs (68). They are most commonly seen with younger patients (<16 years), older patients, large tumors, extrathyroidal extension, and extensive lymph node involvement and most often involve the lung and bone (69–72).

Bone metastasis, in which the risk of orthopedic or neurologic complications is high, require surgical intervention. However, bony metastasis not amenable to surgery should be treated with external beam radiotherapy.

For multiple small lung metastasis ^{131}I therapy can be effective. At present, no chemotherapeutic agent has been shown to be effective in improving survival in patients with distant metastases.

Follow-up

Studies have shown that the average risk of tumor recurrence during long-term follow-up of patients with WDTC is approximately 15% to 35%, with 75% of recurrences and 67% of distant metastasis occurring in the first 10 years (73–75).

The exact schedule for follow-up and who should be conducting the follow-up has been controversial and very center dependent. The National Comprehensive Cancer Network (NCCN) guidelines suggest a physical examination every 3 to 6 months for 2 years and then annually if the patient is disease-free (76).

The strategy for initial follow up has traditionally relied on results of Tg and I^{123} cervical scanning obtained after withdrawal of thyroid hormone. If there is significant cervical uptake (>1% uptake), then an ablative I^{131} dose is given. One week after this ablative dose, whole body scan (WBS) is performed.

Subsequent to ablative treatment, WDTC follow-up has traditionally included TSH suppression and periodic hypothyroid Tg and WBS. Recently more emphasis has been placed on recombinant TSH-stimulated Tg and cervical USS, with a reduced weight on hypothyroid WBS. Patients after ablative treatment, with undetectable stimulated Tg

on suppressive therapy and negative cervical USS, can be safely followed. If basal Tg on suppressive therapy is elevated or becomes elevated on TSH stimulation, cervical USS and hypothyroid WBS can be considered.

Medullary Thyroid Carcinoma

MTC differs fundamentally from thyrocyte carcinomas, not only in embryology and microscopic anatomy but also in function, tumor biology, pathogenesis, and genetics. MTC can be diagnosed at a preclinical stage by a specific secretory product, calcitonin. The hereditary variant of MTC can be identified unequivocally in about 95% of patients by genetic analysis. MTC cannot be treated with radioiodine and no multimodal treatment protocol has been proven effective in advanced and/or metastatic MTC. Taken together, there is currently no available alternative to surgical treatment for curative as well as for many palliative situations.

Diagnosis

Most commonly, MTC is encountered in the lateral upper two thirds of the thyroid gland because C-cell concentrations are highest in this area. The first finding often noted clinically is a nontender mass or a circumscribed nodule arising from the thyroid gland with or without palpable lymph nodes.

In both types of MTC, sporadic and hereditary, the calcitonin concentrations reflect the secretary capacity of C cells, indicating total tumor volume (77). Patients with a nodular goiter with stimulated calcitonin levels above 100 pg/mL bear a significant risk of MTC (78). In cases of already increased basal calcitonin levels, the chance of biochemical cure has been reported to be significantly decreased, approaching 60% in node-negative patients and only 10% in node-positive MTC (79).

Imaging

Cervical high-resolution USS is the method of choice for the determination of tumor size, intrathyroidal location, and for the assessment of cervical lymph node metastases. The clinical utility of cervical USS is limited to nodes smaller than 5 mm or those that reside inside the mediastinum. Because of their superior resolution and penetration, CT and MRI better visualize widely invasive and extrathyroidal recurrences, especially after surgery in the neck or mediastinum. For the distinction between compression and invasion of the trachea, esophagus, or the carotid sheath, MRI is preferred over contrast-enhanced CT. Both imaging modalities are suitable for the detection of distant metastases. In persistent hypercalcitoninemia, [^{18}F] fluoro-2-deoxy-D-glucose positron emission tomography (^{18}FDG-PET) or recently L-Dopa-PET-CT can localize residual and recurrent tumors. Other scintigraphic methods, such as ^{131}I-MIBG-, ^{99m}Tc-DMSA-, and ^{111}In-octreotid-scintigraphy, are inferior in sensitivity to positron emission tomography.

Preoperative Evaluation

Preoperative diagnosis requires cytologic confirmation by USFNA. When postoperative calcitonin levels are less than 500 pg/mL and imaging studies have come back negative, selective venous catheterization may be able to pinpoint microscopic tumor deposits to a circumscribed area of the neck (80). Calcitonin gradients above 2.5 (central vs. peripheral) signify tumor in the drained region in 100%, whereas gradients between 1.5 and 2.5 indicate tumor in 27% of patients (81). Increased hepatic vein gradients suggest occult liver metastases (82). Selective venous catheterization is not needed when the central and lateral lymph node compartments of the neck have already been marked for systematic dissection. Superficial lung and liver metastases can be biopsied through thoracotomy and laparoscopy, respectively. Miliary hepatic metastases that had escaped various imaging modalities were confirmed in 19% (7 of 36 patients) on laparoscopy (82). In a radiologic series of 32 patients presenting with MTC, hepatic angiography was able to disclose liver metastases in 89% of patients (83).

Surgical Techniques

Total Thyroidectomy

Although some groups perform lobectomy in selected cases with genetically proven sporadic MTC, total thyroidectomy is generally accepted as the essential element of curative surgery for all forms and stages of MTC (84–88). The main reasons are that intraglandular lymphatic spread occurs even in about 10% to 20 % of sporadic MTC, and that the hereditary background is often unknown at the time of primary operation and may not even be detected during follow-up in the case of rare mutations in the RET protooncogene.

Compartment-Oriented Microdissection of Locoregional Lymph Nodes. Several recent studies revealed that locoregional lymph node colonization in MTC occurs, with only quantitative differences compared with PTC. Overall, the central neck is positive in 34% of cases with ipsilateral lateral nodes in 34% of patients (89). The contralateral cervicolateral and the infrabrachiocephalic upper mediastinal compartment are involved in 16% and 13% of primary operations and in 22% and 19% of reoperations, respectively (89). Infrabrachiocephalic upper mediastinal lymph node involvement most often is consistent with concurrent distant (micro)metastases.

The introduction of meticulous, compartment-oriented microdissection not only for primary but also for reoperative MTC represents a major step toward improved patient outcomes. This attention to nodal disease treatment has resulted in significantly improved rates of biochemical cure, defined as normalization of stimulated calcitonin levels, from 30% to 50% previously to 60% to 80% for primary operations, and from 0 to 20% to 30% to 40% for reoperations (88,90). Although it has not been proven that

the recurrence and survival in MTC can be improved by meticulous nodal surgery, several groups have demonstrated that there is a strong correlation between the number of lymph nodes involved and the postoperative basal and stimulated calcitonin levels (90). In cases of locoregional disease, removing a larger number of lymph node metastases, using the compartment-oriented microdissection technique appears to be the only effective treatment option to reduce the risk of local recurrence.

Recent data have revealed that MTC, as compared with PTC, occasionally develops systemic disease early on (91,92). In a study by Machens et al. (90), distant metastasis were found in patients with preoperative basal calcitonin levels of above 400 pg/mL at first surgery (10 pg/mL being the upper normal limit), and above 150 pg/mL in reoperative cases. Further distant metastases were present with primary tumors of 12 to 15 mm in size (primary and reoperative setting). Moreover, it was shown that the involvement of 10 or more locoregional lymph nodes or more than two compartments excluded biochemical cure. With cases of proven distant macrometastases, cervical (re)operation may be offered but would be confined to the removal of symptomatic cervical lymph nodes. Mediastinal lymph node dissection in this situation would only be included if proven radiographically.

Hereditary Medullary Carcinoma

There is no difference in survival between the familial and the sporadic form of MTC when clinicopathologic factors are adjusted for in a multivariate analysis (90,93,94). The differences in the prognosis of hereditary versus sporadic MTC are mainly caused by the high impact that early diagnosis of hereditary MTC has on survival. In 2003, the EUROMEN study convincingly showed that the progression of MTC, that is, the transition from C-cell hyperplasia (CCH) to MTC N0, and from MTC N0 to MTC N1, is directly correlated with the type of the RET mutation (95). Based on these and earlier studies, three different risk groups have been identified according to genetic risk: Level 3: (highest risk) with mutations in codon 883, 918, 922; Level 2: (high risk) with mutations in codon 634, 630, 609, 611, 618, and 620; and Level 1: (moderate risk) with mutations in codon 768, 790, 791, 804, and 891 (95–97). In cases of normal stimulated calcitonin levels, RET gene carriers should, on a prophylactic basis, be operated on at age 6 months (level 3), 5 years (level 2), and 5 to 10 years (level 1). With normal stimulated calcitonin, the risk of MTC in RET gene carriers is not more than 5% (78). Central lymph node dissection should be performed at least in all gene carriers with positive calcitonin tests. Because the risk of postoperative hypocalcemia is higher when a central node dissection is performed, the optimal time of prophylactic surgery is before the calcitonin level exceeds the normal range. In RET gene carriers with increased stimulated calcitonin, the frequency of MTC increased from 5% (with normal stimulated calcitonin) to greater than 70%.

Postoperative Considerations. Due to the often chronic course of MTC despite clinically proven metastases, the indication for chemotherapy is only given in progressive disease under the assumption that the side effects of chemotherapy do not outweigh the gain in quality of life. However, no significant benefit in terms of survival has been proven for various chemotherapeutic regimens.

As in other neuroendocrine tumors, radionuclide-based peptide receptor radiotherapy has been shown to be potentially effective in metastatic MTC. Several DOTA-labeled peptides like DOTA-TOC, DOTA-LAN, and DOTA-TATE have been developed (98–100). The effect of treatment with these substances, however, depends on the expression of the various somatostatin receptor subtypes SSTR 1 to 5.

For local control after palliative resection, external irradiation may have some benefit; however, even with this additive treatment modality, survival could not be improved (101,102).

PARATHYROID GLANDS

Anatomy and Embryology

The dorsal endoderm of third and fourth branchial pouches give rise to the inferior (PIII) and superior (PIV) parathyroid glands, respectively. With extension of the cervical spine and the descent of the heart and great vessels, the PIII migrates caudally with the thymus from the pharyngeal wall. PIII then separates from the thymus at the level of the inferior poles of the thyroid lobes. The PIV follows the migration of the ultimobranchial bodies ending at the lateral part of the main median thyroid rudiment remaining in contact with the posterior part of the middle third of the thyroid lobes. These differences in migration explain why PIV anatomic distribution is more limited than PIII.

Classically, the superior parathyroid gland is described as lying 1 cm above the intersection between the RLN and the inferior thyroid artery; however, the position of the gland does demonstrate some variability. The common ectopic locations for the superior gland include the paraesophageal or retroesophageal areas.

The inferior parathyroid gland is most often found at the lower pole of the thyroid, often within the thyrothymic ligament. Compared with the superior glands, the inferior glands enjoy a greater variability in location in the cranial-caudal axis. Knowledge of the parathyroid embryology is essential for the parathyroid surgeon.

The superior parathyroid glands obtain their blood supply from inferior or superior thyroid arteries, and their venous drainage occurs via the superior or lateral thyroid veins. The inferior glands are supplied by the inferior thy-roid artery, and its venous drainage occurs via the lateral or inferior thyroid veins.

Anomalous Development of the Parathyroid

Congenital ectopias due to variation in migration are the most common abnormality of the parathyroid gland. In addition to congenital ectopias, the surgeon must be aware of acquired ectopias that result from the migration of an enlarged gland under the influence of gravity and mechanical forces in the neck. The superior parathyroid glands have a tendency to migrate posteriorly along the posterior vertebral fascia toward the superior mediastinum. Up to 40% of adenomas may be found in such posterior positions. The inferior glands tend to migrate toward the anterior mediastinum along the pathway of the thyrothymic ligament.

Benign Lesions

Microscopically normal parathyroid glands are encapsulated structures that have a fat-rich stromal component and a parenchymal component.

Parathyroid Adenoma

Parathyroid adenomas are the most common cause of primary HPT, accounting for 80% to 90% of all cases. Parathyroid adenomas commonly occur sporadically and typically involve a single gland. They affect the superior and inferior parathyroids equally. Most adenomas are a nodule composed of chief cells arranged in cords and sheetlike arrangements, surrounded by a rim of normal, fat-cell-rich parathyroid tissue. Some of these adenomas will exhibit nodules of parenchymal cells, whereas others will consist exclusively of one homogenous cell population. Double adenomas also occur in primary HPT. Other types of adenomas include oncocytic adenomas (90% of the cells within the adenoma are oncocytes), lipoadenomas (proliferation of both parenchymal and stromal elements), microadenomas (<0.6 cm in diameter), water-clear cell adenomas (presence of cells with multiple cytoplasmic vacuoles), and atypical adenomas (features of parathyroid carcinomas but without true invasive growth).

Hyperplasia

Primary chief cell hyperplasia (PCCH) accounts for 5% to 15% of cases of primary HPT and is more common in women than in men. In PCCH, there is a proliferation of chief cells and oncocytes in multiple parathyroid glands, with an increase in parenchymal cell mass, in the absence of a known stimulus for parathyroid hormone (PTH) hypersecretion. Chief-cell hyperplasia shows variability in size of all the glands. Hyperplastic cells within the mass may be arranged in solid sheets, cords, or follicles.

Multiple gland sampling is necessary to distinguish parathyroid hyperplasia from an adenoma. Adenomas may have compressed the "rim" of normal glandular tissue. However, a "pseudorim" may be found around nodules within hyperplastic glands.

One form of hyperplasia is water-clear cell. This rare form of hyperplasia is characterized by a dark to chocolate brown color with very markedly and asymmetrically enlarged glands. Microscopically the water-clear cells are large and polygonal, with an empty appearing cytoplasm, and pseudopod-like extensions (103).

Hyperparathyroidism

Primary HPT, a primary neoplastic parathyroid glandular disorder, is characterized by elevated secretion of PTH with often but not always an increased serum calcium level. Secondary HPT is parathyroid gland hyperplasia resulting from a secondary stimulus, most commonly chronic renal failure. Tertiary HPT is a condition in which autonomous parathyroid hyperfunction develops after a metabolic defect causing secondary HPT has been corrected.

Clinical Presentation

Primary HPT is most commonly detected at routine health screening or during evaluation for an unrelated medical problem with an elevated serum calcium concentration. It occurs predominantly in women (female-to-male ratio of 3:1) between the ages of 50 and 60 years who are asymptomatic. However, complaints of weakness, easy fatigability, depression, and intellectual weariness may be reported. The physical examination is often unremarkable, with the neck showing no masses and full neuromuscular examination being normal (Table 116.4).

Preoperative Evaluation

Surgical Indications. A National Institutes of Health consensus panel and a recent workshop has recommended surgery in asymptomatic patients with HPT if there is a history of the following (104,105):

1. Serum calcium greater than 1.0 mg/dL above the upper limit of normal.
2. Marked hypercalciuria, greater than 400 mg per day.
3. Creatinine clearance less than 30% of normal.
4. Marked bone density reduction with T-score <-2.5 at any site.
5. Age less than 50 years, without symptoms.
6. Patient for whom surveillance and follow-up are difficult or impossible.

In asymptomatic young patients, surgery is justified according to the previous recommendations because multiple studies show that approximately 25% of such patients go on to develop one or more complications.

Preoperative History and Physical Examination. As with any medical condition that may require surgery, a thorough preoperative history is vital and should outline details regarding the duration and course of hypercalcemia and its symptoms. The history should include details specific to calcium-related morbidity including polydipsia, nausea and vomiting, hypertension, memory changes, depression, weight loss, renal stones, bone or joint or muscle pain, gout, pancreatitis, ulcer disease, and bone disease or fracture history.

The history of a patient with HPT must also include a detailed past medical history particularly focusing on any

---

TABLE 116.4 DIAGNOSIS
HYPERPARATHYROIDISM

History	• Symptoms of fatigue, polydipsia, nausea and vomiting, memory changes, depression, weight loss, and bone, joint, or muscle pain • History of renal stones, gout, pancreatitis, ulcer disease, and bone disease or fracture history, and hypertension • Family history of endocrine disorder
Physical examination	• Often unremarkable
Laboratory evaluation	• Thyroid function tests • Serum PTH • Serum calcium • Serum albumin • 24-hour urine creatinine and calcium • Vitamin D
Radiographic evaluation	• Thyroid USS • Bone densitometry • Technetium 99m sestamibi scan

PTH, parathyroid hormone; USS, ultrasonography.

previous history of renal disease, endocrine abnormalities, malignancies, and any previous surgery. In addition, a drug history is important as a variety of oral agents can lead to hypercalcemia such as lithium.

A careful history must also screen for multiple endocrine neoplasia (MEN) associated HPT and familial HPT. A history of pheochromocytoma and pituitary and pancreatic islet tumors as well as any family history of hypertension, endocrine tumors, calcium disorders, and any past neck, thyroid, or parathyroid surgery should be elicited. A history of radiation exposure, which increases the risk of HPT threefold, should also be revealed (106).

The physical examination is often unremarkable. However, a palpable neck nodule in this setting usually suggests an unrelated thyroid nodule or a parathyroid carcinoma. We believe not only that a physical examination is important but also that, as for thyroidectomy, a preoperative laryngeal examination with assessment of vocal cord function is imperative, particularly in the reoperative setting.

Preoperative Laboratory Workup for Primary Hyperparathyroidism. The preoperative laboratory workup for a patient with suspected HPT should always include serum calcium, intact PTH, albumin, phosphate, magnesium, and chloride. A 24-hour urine calcium and creatinine should be checked to exclude benign familial hyercalcemic hypocalciuvia (BFHH) (the diagnosis of which is made by showing a calcium/creatinine clearance ratio of less than 0.01). Renal function should be assessed with a blood urea nitrogen (BUN) and creatinine, as should an alkaline phosphatase to evaluate for active bone disease. Vitamin D levels (vit D 25 OH) can be checked because vitamin D deficiency can result in elevated PTH levels. Patients with primary HPT often will have a high chloride but a low serum phosphate, with a chloride to phosphate ratio greater than 33. Patients with a calcium level above 14 mg/dL should raise the suspicion of a parathyroid carcinoma and should be investigated accordingly.

Bone Densitometry. PTH has a catabolic effect on cortical bone and an anabolic effect on cancellous bone. The distal third of the radius provides a convenient site of cortical bone density measurement, and the lumbar spine is ideal for measurement of cancellous bone for evaluation in primary HPT (107,108). The hip region contains an equal mixture of cancellous and cortical bone, so it can also be a valuable site to evaluate during the assessment of HPT.

Preoperative Localization Tests
Ultrasonography. USS is a first-line noninvasive localization modality for the identification of parathyroid glands but is very operator dependent. Normal glands normally appear as homogenous, demarcated masses with a lower echogenicity than thyroid tissue, whereas adenomas are usually solid but occasionally have cystic elements. USS is particularly poor in detecting ectopic parathyroid glands espe-

cially in the mediastinum and tracheoesophageal region due to shadowing by larynx cartilages and sternum.

Technetium (Tc) 99m Sestamibi. Tc 99m sestamibi scanning is particularly useful in the assessment of parathyroid disease because it is quickly absorbed and retained by abnormal parathyroid tissue but is rapidly washed out from the thyroid tissue. This difference in the rate of clearance enables identification of parathyroid tissue as areas of increased uptake on delayed imaging. Sestamibi scanning enables not only detection of adenomas located in their normal anatomic position but also may detect ectopic glands. Certain conditions may reduce the accuracy of this test by retaining Tc 99m sestamibi; these include hyperplastic glands, multinodular goiter, Hashimoto thyroiditis, and thyroid adenomas, especially Hürthle cell adenomas. The accuracy of Tc 99m sestamibi scanning can be increased by combining it with single photon emission computed tomography (SPECT) (109).

Computed Tomography. The advantage of CT over USS is its ability to better visualize the anterior mediastinum (110). Unfortunately, lymph nodes, tortuous vessels, and scanning and breathing artifacts can make interpretation of CT scans for parathyroid disease difficult to interpret.

Magnetic Resonance Imaging. MRI may be more sensitive than CT in detecting parathyroid adenomas. However, it is also difficult to differentiate lymph nodes and large cervical ganglia from parathyroid adenomas.

Fine-Needle Aspiration. Although FNA is a minimally invasive test that can be used to confirm the presence of an abnormal parathyroid gland, it is limited by the skill of the cytopathologist interpreting and the small size of the adenomas. Needle rinsing for PTH helps to confirm a sampled lesion is parathyroid.

Intraoperative Parathyroid Hormone Assessment
Multiple studies have now shown that intraoperative PTH assay is a valuable tool in predicting surgical cure in patients with primary HPT (111,112). We feel its successful application relates to strict use of postexcision guidelines and avoidance of dissecting normal parathyroid glands prior to blood sampling. We recommend a 10-minute postexcision PTH sample that is both within normal limits (10 to 65 pg/mL) *and* more than 50% decreased from the initial baseline, which are the best criteria for predicting surgical cure. In cases of hyperplasia, its use can be more complex, but in general, each subsequent gland that is excised produces a progressive decrease in PTH (113).

Surgical Management of Hyperparathyroidism
A very useful landmark in the neck for parathyroid identification is their anatomic relation to the RLN. If the RLN's path in the neck is taken as a coronal plane, the upper

parathyroid glands are dorsal and the lower parathyroid glands are ventral to this plane (Fig. 116.4). In most cases, the migration paths of superior and inferior gland adenomas respect this plane. As mentioned before, the superior adenomas have a tendency to migrate into the retropharyngeal, retrolaryngeal, retroesophageal locations, and the posterior mediastinum. On the other hand, inferior adenomas tend to drift into the thymus and anterior mediastinum.

Parathyroid Vascular Anatomy

In most cases, the inferior parathyroid gland is supplied by the inferior thyroid artery and often maintains this blood supply even if the gland descends into the anterior mediastinum. However, some low-lying glands will derive their blood supply from a thymic branch of the internal mammary artery or even a direct branch off the aortic arch. The superior parathyroid gland can be supplied by the inferior thyroid artery but can be supplied by a branch from the superior thyroid artery.

Parathyroidectomy: Surgical Techniques

General Principles

There are some key principles to ensure a successful parathyroid exploration. These include the following:

1. Using a meticulous and bloodless dissection allowing safe identification of the parathyroid glands and RLN.
2. Being prepared for the need for bilateral exploration in all patients.
3. Having a low threshold to identify the RLN to protect the nerve from dissection and to help discern inferior from superior parathyroid glands.
4. Willingness to gently dissect while respecting the blood supply of a normal-appearing parathyroid to ensure that an adenoma is not attached.
5. Palpating during parathyroid exploration for a parathyroid adenoma, especially for descended superior glands that can be palpated on the prevertebral fascia.
6. Resisting the temptation to remove a normal parathyroid gland, because resection of normal parathyroid glands does not correct HPT and can result in hypoparathyroidism after subsequent successful resection of the adenoma (114).
7. Not incorporating empiric thyroidectomy during parathyroid exploration.
8. Judiciously using parathyroid biopsies to rule out multiglandular disease when intraoperative PTH is not available. If biopsy is performed, it should be taken from the distal tip of the gland, from any gland that is black or associated with questionable vascular pedicles.
9. Using intraoperative PTH assessment if available.

Surgical Technique

A parathyroid search algorithm has been devised to allow the successful identification of abnormal glands and en-sure surgical success. It relies on four steps: (1) exploration of normal parathyroid locations, (2) exploration for the missing gland, (3) fifth gland dissection, and (4) considerations for closure.

Steps 1 and 2

The location of the incision is similar to thyroidectomy but will differ if a minimally invasive technique is used. Exploration should begin on the side suggested by localization studies; however, the surgeon must always be aware that these studies may be incorrect requiring the surgeon to explore not only the other side but also common ectopic parathyroid sites.

On the side of initial exploration, the thyroid lobe is mobilized and dissection is performed close to the thyroid capsular, allowing exposure of the common locations of the parathyroid glands. The first location to explore for the superior parathyroid is the posterolateral aspect of the superior thyroid lobe, above the nerve-artery intersection, deep to the plane of the RLN. The inferior glands are commonly found adjacent to the thyroid insertion of the thyreothymic ligament within 1 cm of the lower edge of the thyroid's inferior pole.

For adequate exposure of the parathyroid glands the middle thyroid vein is divided and ligated to allow dissection of the plane lateral to the thyroid. Traction is applied for adequate rotation of the thyroid lobe and appropriate visualization of its posterior aspects (Fig. 116.1). During the initial phase of the operation, attention is paid to both exposure of normal-sized glands and identification of the adenoma. When initial dissection on one side results in a "missing" gland, one may focus further dissection toward this "missing" gland whether superior or inferior. This provides a directed organization to further dissection, outlined as follows.

Superior Gland. In many cases the superior gland occurs within 1 cm of the cricothyroid cartilage articulation. We feel it is best to orient oneself to the cricothyroid junction rather than the more variable RLN-inferior thyroid artery crossing as the first step in identifying a superior parathyroid gland. Once this junction is located it is often easiest to start by looking at the posterior edge of the upper thyroid pole. A covering fascia can frequently be found over the parathyroid glands, and transection of this outer layer makes the gland pop out or extrude from a lump of fat in this area. If despite these maneuvers the superior gland is not located, the dissection progresses around the ventral and lateroposterior thyroid surfaces, paying special attention to any clefts or prominent tubercles of the thyroid that may be concealing the parathyroid gland. The posterior aspects are brought into better view by medially rotating the upper thyroid lobe. If the gland has not been successfully identified by this point, exploration is directed to the common ectopic locations of the superior gland including the tracheoesophageal groove, lateral to or behind the esophagus, or the superior, posterior mediastinum. The superior thyroid artery can be divided for better exposure of the dorsal aspects of the upper thyroid lobe if an extended search is necessary. The superior parathyroid is rarely intrathyroidal and therefore hemithyroidectomy is seldom necessary. One must remember that the superior parathyroid can be found close to the RLN laryngeal entry point; if dissection is felt to come close to the nerve, it should be specifically identified.

Inferior Gland. When searching for the inferior parathyroid gland, the exploration should commence around the inferior and ventral aspects of the lower thyroid pole, including the thyreothymic ligament and upper parts of the thymus. If an inferior gland is not identified, the dissection proceeds cranially along the lateroposterior border of the thyroid and may even extend above the nerve-artery intersection. Inspection of the ventrolateral surface of the thyroid is imperative during the search for the inferior gland as it is frequently located adjacent to the thyroid capsule. One may consider an intrathyroidal adenoma during exploration if the remaining missing gland is inferior. If there is a suspicion the gland could be intrathyroidal an excellent option is to identify it with the use of intraoperative ultrasound. Alternatively, the suspected intrathyroidal adenoma, if palpated, will increase PTH by 150% intraoperatively (115). The intrathyroidal adenoma can be excised through a small "thyroidotomy." This avoids scarring and potential complications associated with a full lobectomy. If after all these measures, the missing inferior gland is not located, the anterior mediastinal thymus is dissected, inspected, and generally removed.

Once the abnormal gland is identified, attention should be paid to its vascular supply and identifying any lobulations of the gland, so it can be completely removed. One must also take care not to rupture the capsule of the adenoma by manipulating the gland only by its vascular stalk or connective.

Step 3: Dissection for a Fifth Gland
In the event that all four glands have been identified and appear normal and the diagnosis of HPT is correct, one must consider the possibility of a fifth gland. Identifiable supernumerary parathyroid glands occur in approximately 5% of normal individuals. In the case of a fifth gland adenoma, they are almost always in the mediastinal thymus and only rarely found in other locations (such as within the lower mediastinum, intrathyroidal, or associated with the carotid artery in the neck). Therefore, these glands are often well treated with bilateral transcervical thymic resection. One should note that in diseases such as MEN-1 and secondary HPT, a fifth gland is more common.

Step 4: Considerations for Closure
If the previous steps have been unsuccessful in locating an abnormal gland despite identification of all four glands, one should consider discontinuing the exploration. Further undirected dissection may put the blood supply of the normal parathyroids and the RLN in jeopardy. It is also important, as mentioned before, to avoid untargeted thyroidectomy. The surgeon should once again review the common locations found at reoperation to harbor pathology including thymus, para- and retroesophageal, intrathyroidal, carotid sheath, and anterior mediastinal locations. A last resort may be to individually sample the corresponding jugular veins for PTH in the hopes of identifying the side of disease. Biopsy of normal-sized glands should be performed only if absolutely necessary to confirm their identity or to rule out four-gland disease but this is discouraged because it may devascularize the gland (116). Instead, the gland should be identified as parathyroid based on morphology, consistency, and color with size used as the primary indicator of involvement in the hyperplastic process.

Reasons for Failure
Multiple series suggest that the reasons for failure at initial parathyroid exploration include incomplete exploration with missed cervical disease, missed diagnosis of multiglandular disease or double adenoma, ectopic gland, and error in initial diagnosis.

Adequate exploration and strict adherence to intraoperative PTH can keep missed cervical disease and misdiagnosed multiglandular disease to a minimum. Ectopic glands are generally rare and preoperative localization tests can help in the localization of some of these ectopic glands. Meticulous preoperative assessment should make error in diagnosis an infrequent reason for failure.

Postoperative Care
Successful surgery normally results in normalization of calcium in 48 hours postoperatively. If the patient develops symptoms of hypocalcemia or the calcium falls to 7.5 mg/dL, oral treatment should be started as for thyroidectomy. Patients with preoperative high alkaline phosphatase may demonstrate postoperative bone hunger and lower than expected calcium levels postoperatively. One must also be aware that hypomagnesemia can lead to less effective hypocalcemic treatment so this should be corrected if present during calcium replacement.

Mediastinal Adenoma

Mediastinal disease with potentially difficult access through the neck is of concern to the parathyroid surgeon. Although most mediastinal tumors are within or attached to the thymus and can be accessed from the neck, some are associated with the common carotid artery, ascending aorta, aortic arch, aortic arch branches, and pericardium. Sternotomy may be required for some of these lesions, however. Sternotomy in our practice is a planned procedure based on targeted preoperative localization studies rather than an extension of a cervical exploration.

Multiglandular Parathyroid Disease: Surgical Techniques

Patients with multiglandular parathyroid disease may have sporadic primary four-gland hyperplasia or hereditary disorders such as a MEN syndrome or a familial form of HPT. Supernumerary glands occur more commonly in hereditary causes of multigland disease. These glands are most often located in the thymic tongue.

Extent of Resection in Multigland Disease

When considering the appropriate surgery for multigland disease, the virulence of the disease process must be considered.

In these cases, the neck is explored bilaterally. All parathyroid glands are identified prior to any gland resection. Once the exploration is complete, the surgeon compares the size and gross features of all four glands. When subtotal parathyroidectomy is performed, the smallest and most normal-appearing gland can then be selected as remnant. This resection should be performed with a fresh blade and careful preservation of its vascular supply. It is important to avoid spillage of parathyroid tissue during this procedure because it may lead to seeding and recurrence elsewhere in the wound. The remnant is then assessed after 10 minutes; if there questionable viability, it should be removed and the gland next in size resected as a remnant. A nonabsorbable suture is used to mark the site of the remnant in case reexploration is necessary. Once confident of the viability of the remnant, the remaining enlarged glands are resected.

The least aggressive treatment, resection of only enlarged glands, is reserved for the least virulent multigland processes including double adenoma, sporadic four-gland hyperplasia, and MEN 2A. These processes tend to have lower recurrence rates after such conservative treatment.

More aggressive resection including subtotal parathyroid resection (i.e., $3^1/_2$ gland resection) and four-gland total parathyroidectomy (with or without autotransplantation) is recommended for patients with familial hyperplasia, neonatal HPT, MEN-1, and secondary HPT. In the most virulent forms of multigland HPT (i.e., MEN 1), to excise supernumerary glands that can cause recurrence, the bilateral cervical thymus and periglandular fat can also be excised.

Minimally Invasive Parathyroidectomy

The minimally invasive parathyroidectomy techniques range from small incision open technique to true endoscopic cervical techniques. Criteria exist (although they are constantly changing as minimal access techniques are being expanded by individual experienced workers) to identify suitable candidates for minimal access surgery parathyroidectomy; these generally include (a) accurate preoperative localization, (b) no evidence preoperatively of multigland disease, (c) first time surgery, and (d) acceptable anatomy (i.e., a short, heavy neck and an abnormally low larynx are relative contraindications). Minimal invasive techniques are now also being expanded to thyroidectomy.

Open Minimal Access Parathyroidectomy

Minimal access parathyroidectomy (MAP) involves a unilateral approach through a small incision after reliable localization studies and the use of intraoperative PTH to help ensure surgical success. The surgeon performing this procedure, as for any minimal access procedure, must be prepared to convert to a formal bilateral exploration if intraoperative PTH remains elevated or equivocal after gland resection.

Minimally Invasive Video-Assisted Parathyroidectomy

In minimally invasive video-assisted parathyroidectomy, the procedure is performed through a small incision in the neck with multiple retractors. Through the small incision (typically 2 to 3 cm), an endoscope is placed and the surgery is performed through visualization on the video monitor.

Endoscopic Parathyroidectomy

True endoscopic technique is used through multiple small stab incisions. One port is for the camera-light source and secondary port for manipulation/surgical instruments. The skin and strap muscles are elevated through gas insufflation, sometimes combined with internal retraction/elevation devices. Central and lateral cervical approaches have been described; points of access have even included the lower chest and axilla.

Parathyroid Carcinoma

Parathyroid carcinoma is an uncommon disease but every surgeon who manages primary HPT must appreciate the clinical course and treatment of this entity. Most cases occur in the fourth to sixth decades of life, and in contrast to the female predominance observed for adenomas, there are no sex differences in the incidence of carcinomas (117,118).

In parathyroid cancer, death is caused by excessive secretion of PTH, with resulting severe hypercalcemia, and not by tumor spread itself. For the best chance of cure, a wide resection of the cancer is done as the preliminary procedure. As mentioned previously, parathyroid carcinoma should be considered in any patients with HPT who have a firm perithyroid mass or extremely elevated calcium or PTH. When faced with metastatic disease, the aim of surgery is to remove as much disease as possible to lower the serum calcium as much as possible. Other treatment modalities such as bisphosphonates, chemotherapy, and radiotherapy have been unsuccessful. Although multiple operations have rarely resulted in cure, they should be attempted because they offer the best chance of palliation.

Macroscopically, parathyroid carcinomas are white, firm, ill-defined masses densely adherent to surrounding soft tissues. Microscopically, the carcinomas are composed of chief cells showing extensive pleomorphism and anaplasia arranged in solid sheet or trabecular patterns. The diagnosis of carcinoma is made with the confirmation of the presence of thick fibrous bands, mitotic activity, capsular invasion, and vascular invasion. Frozen section is unreliable in diagnosing parathyroid carcinoma so the surgeon cannot rely on it as an indicator for aggressive local resection. Parathyroid carcinoma is prone to local seeding of tumor cells if biopsied; therefore, this should be avoided if the surgeon suspects a carcinoma.

En bloc resection of the parathyroid carcinoma with a wide margin of adjacent tissue and ipsilateral tracheoesophageal groove nodal dissection is the treatment of choice for these cases. To avoid local seeding during the surgical procedure, the capsule of the tumor should remain intact. Radical neck dissections are reserved for patients with grossly enlarged cervical lymph nodes, and local invasion, or with local recurrence.

The average duration between the initial operation and death for those patients who died was 6.6 years in one study (118). The overall 5- and 10-year survival for parathyroid carcinoma is estimated at 77% and 63%, respectively (119). The reduction of mortality is greatly impacted by early diagnosis and appropriate and aggressive surgery.

HIGHLIGHTS

- Through preoperative assessment with a detailed history and physical examination, preoperative laryngoscopy, focused radiographic assessment, and cytologic evaluation are imperative.
- Radioisotopic thyroid scanning is of limited value in the assessment of a thyroid nodule in the surgical setting.
- Preoperative and postoperative laryngoscopy is essential in thyroid and parathyroid surgery.
- Recurrent laryngeal nerve monitoring is a useful adjunct in nerve identification and prognostication of postoperative function.
- The preoperative workup of hyperparathyroidism should help delineate the subtype of hyperparathyroidism, identify surgical indications, and include localization studies.
- A palpable parathyroid or greatly elevated serum calcium or parathyroid hormone should raise the suspicion of a parathyroid carcinoma.
- Superior adenomas often descend on the prevertebral fascia toward the posterior mediastinum in a paraesophageal location where palpation may help in their identification.

REFERENCES

1. Ibrahim NBM, Milewski PJ. Benign thyroid inclusions within cervical lymph nodes. *Aust N Z J Surg* 1981;51:188–189.
2. Kozol RA, Geelhoed GW, Flynn SD, et al. Management of ectopic thyroid nodules. *Surgery* 1993;114:1103–1106.
3. Walton BR, Koch KE. Presentation in management of a thyroglossal duct cyst with papillary carcinoma. *South Med J* 1997;90: 758–761.
4. Glastonbury CM, Davidson HC, Haller JR, et al. The CT and MR imaging features of carcinoma arising in thyroglossal duct remnants. *ANJR Am J Neuroradiol* 2000;21:770–774.
5. Sistrunk WE. The surgical treatment of cysts of the thyroglossal track. *Ann Surg* 1920;71:121.
6. Brown PM, Judd ES. Thyroglossal duct cysts and sinuses: results of radical Sistrunk operation. *Am J Surg* 1961;102:494–501.
7. Horisawa M, Niinomi N, Ito T. What is the optimal depth for core-out toward the foramen cecum in thyroglossal duct cyst operation? *J Pediatr Surg* 1992;27:710–713.
8. Kennedy TL, Whitaker M, Wadih G. Thyroglossal duct carcinoma: a rational approach to management. *Laryngoscope* 1998;108: 1154–1158.
9. Heshmati HM, Fatourechi V, van Heerden JA, et al. Thyroglossal duct carcinoma: a report of 12 cases. *Mayo Clinic Proc* 1997; 72:315–319.
10. Baker BA, Gharib H, Markowitz H. Correlation of thyroid antibodies and cytologic features in suspected autoimmune thyroid disease. *Am J Med* 1983;74:941–944.
11. Tunbridge WM, Brewis M, French JM, et al. Natural history of autoimmune thyroiditis. *Br Med J* 1981;282:258–262.
12. Ross DR. Subclinical thyrotoxicosis. *Adv Endocrinol Metab* 1991; 2:89.
13. Said H, Razi Hadi A, Akmal SN, et al. Tumefactive fibroinflammatory lesion of the head and neck. *J Laryngol Otol* 1988;102: 1064–1067.
14. Maxon HR. Detection of residual and recurrent thyroid cancer by radionuclide imaging. *Thyroid* 1999;9:443–446.
15. Spencer CA, LoPresti JS, Fatemi S, et al. Detection of residual and recurrent differentiated thyroid carcinoma by serum thyroglobulin measurement. *Thyroid* 1999;9:435–441.
16. Ros P, Rossi DL, Acebron A, et al. Thyroid-specific gene expression in the multi-step process of thyroid carcinogenesis. *Biochimie* 1999;81:389–396.
17. Grebe SK, Hay ID. Follicular cell-derived thyroid carcinomas. *Cancer Treat Res* 1997;89:91–140.
18. Hay ID, Klee GG. Thyroid cancer diagnosis and management. *Clin Lab Med* 1993;13:725–734.
19. McConahey WM, Hay ID, Woolner LB, et al. Papillary thyroid cancer treated at the Mayo Clinic, 1946 through 1970: initial manifestations, pathologic findings, therapy, and outcome. *Mayo Clin Proc* 1986;61:978–996.
20. Samaan NA, Maheshwari YK, Nader S, et al. Impact of therapy for differentiated carcinoma of the thyroid: an analysis of 706 cases. *J Clin Endocrinol Metab* 1983;56:1131–1138.
21. Eng C. Familial papillary thyroid cancer: many syndromes, too many genes? [Editorial] *J Clin Endocrinol Metab* 2000;85: 1755–1757.
22. Cobin RH, Gharib H, Bergman DA, et al. AACE/AAES medical/surgical guidelines for clinical practice: management of thyroid carcinoma. *Endocr Pract* 2001;7:202–220.
23. Nikiforov YE, Heffess CS, Korzenko AV, et al. Characteristics of follicular tumors and nonneoplastic thyroid lesions in children and adolescents exposed to radiation as a result of the Chernobyl disaster. *Cancer* 1995;76:900–909.
24. Pacini F, Vorontsova T, Demidchik EP, et al. Post-Chernobyl thyroid carcinoma in Belarus children and adolescents: comparison with naturally occurring thyroid carcinoma in Italy and France. *J Clin Endocrinol Metab* 1997;82:3563–3569.
25. Shaha AR, Shah JP, Loree TR. Patterns of nodal and distant metastasis based on histologic varieties in differentiated carcinoma of the thyroid. *Am J Surg* 1996;172:692–694.
26. Shaha AR, Shah JP, Loree TR. Differentiated thyroid cancer presenting initially with distant metastasis. *Am J Surg* 1997;174: 474–476.

27. Cooper DS, Schneyer CR. Follicular and Hurthle cell carcinoma of the thyroid. *Endocrinol Metab Clin North Am* 1990;19: 577–591.

28. Vassilopoulou-Sellin R, Goepfert H, Raney B, et al. Differentiated thyroid cancer in children and adolescents: clinical outcome and mortality after long-term follow-up. *Head Neck* 1998;20:549–555.

29. Mazzaferri EL, Oertel YC. Primary malignant lymphoma and related lymphoproliferative disorders. In: Mazzaferri EL, Samaan N, eds. *Endocrine tumors.* Boston: Blackwell, 1993.

30. Cunning DS. Unilateral vocal cord paralysis. *Ann Otol Rhinol Laryngol* 1955;64:487–493.

31. Huppler EG, Schmidt HW, Devine KD, et al. Ultimate outcome of patients with vocal cord paralysis of undetermined cause. *Am Rev Tuberc Pulm Dis* 1956;73:52–60.

32. Rueger BG. Benign disease of the thyroid gland in vocal cord paralysis. *Laryngosocpe* 1974;84:897.

33. Patow CA, Norton JA, Brennan MF. Vocal cord paralysis and reoperative parathyroidectomy. *Ann Surg* 1986;203:282–285.

34. Lo CY, Kwok KF, Yuen PW. A prospective evaluation of recurrent laryngeal nerve paralysis during thyroidectomy. *Arch Surg* 2000;135:204–207.

35. Hundahl SH, Cady B, Cunningham M, et al. Initial results from a prospective cohort study of 5583 cases of thyroid cancer treated in the US during 1996. United States and German Thyroid Cancer Study Group. ACS Commission on Cancer Patient Case Evaluation Study. *Cancer* 2000;89:202–217.

36. Yousem DM, Scheff AM. Thyroid and parathyroid gland pathology. *Otolaryngol Clin North Am* 1995;28:621–649.

37. Bennedbaek FN, Hegedus L. Management of the solitary thyroid nodule: results of a North American Survey. *J Clin Endocrinol Metab* 2000;85:2493–2498.

38. Gharib H, Goellner JR. Fine-needle aspiration biopsy of the thyroid: an appraisal. *Ann Intern Med* 1993;118:282–289.

39. Akerman M, Tennvall J, Biorklund A, et al. Sensitivity and specificity of fine needle aspiration cytology in the diagnosis of tumors of the thyroid gland. *Acta Cytol* 1985;29:850–855.

40. Caruso D, Mazzaferri EL. Fine needle aspiration biopsy in the management of thyroid nodules. *Endocrinologist* 1991;1:194.

41. Baloch ZW, Sack MJ, Yu GH, et al. Fine-needle aspiration of thyroid: an institutional experience. *Thyroid* 1998;8:565–569.

42. Rojeski MT, Gharib H. Nodular thyroid disease: evaluation and management. *N Engl J Med* 1985;313:428–436.

43. Schlinkert RT, van Heerden JA, Goellner JR, et al. Factors that predict malignant thyroid lesions when fine-needle aspiration is "suspicious for follicular neoplasm." *Mayo Clin Proc* 1997;72: 913–916.

44. Tuttle RM, Lemar H, Burch HB. Clinical features associated with an increased risk of thyroid malignancy in patients with follicular neoplasia by fine-needle aspiration. *Thyroid* 1998;8:377–383.

45. Danese D, Sciacchitano S, Farsetti A, et al. Diagnostic accuracy of conventional versus sonography-guided fine-needle aspiration biopsy of thyroid nodules. *Thyroid* 1998;8:15–21.

46. Lucas A, Llatjos M, Salinas I, et al. Fine-needle aspiration cytology of benign nodular thyroid disease: value of re-aspiration. *Eur J Endocrinol* 1995;132:677–680.

47. Erdogan MF, Kamel N, Aras D, et al. Value of re-aspirations in benign nodular thyroid disease. *Thyroid* 1998;8:1087–1090.

48. McCaffrey TV, Lipton RJ. Thyroid carcinoma invading the upper aerodigestive system. *Laryngoscope* 1990;100:824–830.

49. McCaffrey TV, Bergstralh EJ, Hay ID. Locally invasive papillary thyroid carcinoma 1940–1990. *Head Neck* 1994;16:165–172.

50. van Lith-Bijl JT, Mahieu HF, Stolk RJ, et al. Laryngeal abductor function after recurrent laryngeal nerve injury in cats. *Arch Otolaryngol Head Neck Surg* 1996;122:393–396.

51. Wingert DJ, Friesen SR, Iliopoulos JI, et al. Post-thyroidectomy hypocalcemia: incidence and risk factors. *Am J Surg* 1986;152: 606–610.

52. McHenry CR, Speroff, T, Wentworth D, et al. Risk factors for post thyroidectomy hypocalcemia. *Surgery* 1994;116:641–647.

53. Pattou F, Combemale F, Fabre S, et al. Hypocalcemia following thyroid surgery: incidence and prediction of outcome. *World J Surg* 1998;22:718–724.

54. Adams J, Andersen P, Everts E, et al. Early postoperative calcium levels as predictors of hypocalcemia. *Laryngoscope* 1998;108: 1829–1831.

55. Casara D, Rubello D, Saladini G, et al. Different features of pulmonary metastases in differentiated thyroid cancer: natural history and multivariate statistical analysis of prognostic variables. *J Nucl Med* 1993;34:1626–1631.

56. Noguchi S, Noguchi A, Murakami N. Papillary carcinoma of the thyroid: I. Developing pattern of metastasis. *Cancer* 1970; 26:1053–1060.

57. Cangiu M. Papillary carcinoma of the thyroid: a clinicopathologic study of 241 cases treated at the University of Florence, Italy. *Cancer* 1985;55:805.

58. Attie J. Elective neck dissection in papillary carcinoma of the thyroid. *Am J Surg* 1971;122:464–471.

59. Goepfert H, Dichtel W, Samaan N. Thyroid cancer in children and teenagers. *Arch Otolaryngol Head Neck Surg* 1984;110:72–75.

60. Schelfhout L, Creutzberg C, Hamming J. Multivariate analysis of survival in differentiated thyroid cancer: the prognostic significance of the age factor. *Eur J Cancer Clin Oncol* 1988;24:331–337.

61. Tsang T, Brierley J, Simpson W. The effects of surgery, radioiodine, and external radiation therapy on the clinical outcome of patients with differentiated thyroid cancer. *Cancer* 1998;82:375.

62. Yamashita H, et al. Extracapsular invasion of lymph node metastasis: a good indicator of disease recurrence and poor prognosis in patients with thyroid microcarcinoma. *Cancer* 1999;86: 842–849.

63. Frankenthaler RA, Sellin RV, Cangir A, et al. Lymph node metastases from papillary-follicular thyroid carcinoma in young patients. *Am J Surg* 1990;160:341–343.

64. McConahey WM, Hay ID, Woolner LB, et al. Papillary thyroid cancer treated at the Mayo clinic, 1946 through 1970: initial manifestations, pathologic findings, therapy, and outcome. *Mayo Clin Proc* 1986;61:978–996.

65. Goldman N, Coniglio J, Falk S. Thyroid cancers: I. Papillary, follicular, and Hurthle cell. *Otolaryngol Clin North Am* 1996; 29:593–609.

66. Hay ID, Bergstralh EJ, Grant CS, et al. Impact of primary surgery on outcome in 300 patients with pathologic tumor-node-metastasis stage III papillary thyroid carcinoma treated at one institution from 1940 through 1989. *Surgery* 1999;126:1173–1181.

67. Noguchi M. Impact of neck dissection on survival in well-differentiated thyroid cancer: a multivariate analysis of 218 cases. *Int Surg* 1990;75:220–224.

68. Hoie J, Stenwig AE, Kullmann G, et al. Distant metastases in papillary thyroid cancer: a review of 91 patients. *Cancer* 1988;61:1–6.

69. Dottorini ME, Vignati A, Mazzucchelli L, et al. Differentiated thyroid carcinoma in children and adolescents: a 37-year experience in 85 patients. *J Nucl Med* 1997;38:669–675.

70. Schlumberger M, De Vathaire F, Travagli JP, et al. Differentiated thyroid carcinoma in childhood: long term follow-up of 72 patients. *J Clin Endocrinol Metab* 1987;65:1088–1094.

71. Vassilopoulou-Sellin R, Klein MJ, Smith TH, et al. Pulmonary metastases in children and young adults with differentiated thyroid cancer. *Cancer* 1993;71:1348–1352.

72. Schlumberger M, Challeton C, De Vathaire F, et al. Radioactive iodine treatment and external radiotherapy for lung and bone metastases from thyroid carcinoma. *J Nucl Med* 1996;37: 598–605.

73. Mazzaferri EL, Jhiang SM. Long-term impact of initial surgical and medical therapy on papillary and follicular thyroid cancer. *Am J Med* 1994;97:418–428.

74. Pujol P, Daures JP, Nsakala N, et al. Degree of thyrotropin suppression as a prognostic determinant in differentiated thyroid cancer. *J Clin Endocrinol Metab* 1996;81:4318–4323.

75. Segal K, Raveh E, Lubin E, et al. Well-differentiated thyroid carcinoma. *Am J Otolaryngol* 1996;17:401–406.

76. Mazzaferri EL. NCCN thyroid carcinoma practice guidelines. *Oncology* 1999;13:391.

77. Cohen R, Campos JM, Salaun C, et al. Preoperative calcitonin levels are predictive of tumor size and postoperative calcitonin normalization in medullary thyroid carcinoma. Groupe d'Etude des Tumeurs à Calcitonine (GETC). *J Clin Endocrinol Metab* 2000; 85:919–922.

78. Karges W, Dralle H, Raue F, et al. Calcitonin measurement to detect medullary thyroid carcinoma in nodular goiter: German evidence-based consensus recommendation. *Exp Clin Endocrinol Diabetes* 2004;112:52–58.

79. Machens A, Ukkat J, Brauckhoff M, et al. Advances in the management of hereditary medullary thyroid carcinoma. *J Intern Med* 2005;257:50–59.

80. Lebouleux S, Baudin E, Travagli JP, et al. Medullary thyroid carcinoma. *Clin Endocrinol* 2004;61:299–310.

81. Ben Mrad MD, Gardet P, Roche A, et al. Value of venous catheterization and calcitonin studies in the treatment and management of clinically inapparent medullary thyroid carcinoma. *Cancer* 1989;63:133–138.

82. Tung WS, Vesely TM, Moley JF. Laparoscopic detection of hepatic metastases in patients with residual or recurrent medullary thyroid cancer. *Surgery* 1995;118:1024–1029; discussion 1029–1030.

83. Esik O, Szavcsur P, Szakall S Jr, et al. Angiography effectively supports the diagnosis of hepatic metastases in medullary thyroid carcinoma. *Cancer* 2001;91:2084–2095.

84. Fleming JB, Lere JE, Bouvet M, et al. Surgical strategy for the treatment of medullary thyroid carcinoma. *Ann Surg* 1999; 230:697–707.

85. Gimm O, Ukkat J, Dralle H. Determinative factors of biochemical cure after primary and reoperative surgery for sporadic medullary thyroid carcinoma. *World J Surg* 1998;22:562–568.

86. Kebebew E, Clark OH. Medullary thyroid cancer. *Curr Treat Opt Oncol* 2000;1:359–367.

87. Miyauchi A, Matsuzuka F, Hirai K, et al. Prospective trial of unilateral surgery for nonhereditary medullary thyroid carcinoma in patients without germline RET mutations. *World J Surg* 2002; 26:1023–1028.

88. Moley JF, DeBenedetti MK. Pattern of nodal metastases in palpable medullary thyroid carcinoma. *Ann Surg* 1999;229:880–888.

89. Machens A, Hinze R, Thomusch O, et al. Pattern of nodal metastasis for primary and reoperative thyroid cancer. *World J Surg* 2002;26:22–28.

90. Machens A, Schneyer U, Holzhausen HJ, et al. Prospects of remission in medullary thyroid carcinoma according to basal calcitonin level. *J Clin Endocrinol Metab* 2005;90:2029–2034.

91. Mirallie E, Vuilez JP, Bardet S, et al. High frequency of bone/bone marrow involvement in advanced medullary thyroid cancer. *J Clin Endocrinol Metab* 2005;90:779–788.

92. Szavcsur P, Gödeny M, Bajzik G, et al. Angiography-proven liver metastases explain low efficacy of lymph node dissections in medullary thyroid cancer patients. *Eur J Surg Oncol* 2005;31: 183–190.

93. Modigliani E, Cohen R, Campos JM, et al. Prognostic factors for survival and for biochemical cure in medullary thyroid carcinoma: results in 889 patients. *Clin Endocrinol* 1998;48:265–273.

94. Raue F. German medullary thyroid carcinoma/multiple endocrine neoplasia registry. German MTC/MEN Study Group. Medullary thyroid carcinoma/multiple endocrine neoplasia type 2. *Langenbecks Arch Surg* 1998;383:334–336.

95. Machens A, Niccoli-Sire P, Hoegel J, et al. European Multiple Endocrine Neoplasia (EUROMEN) Study Group. Early malignant progression of hereditary medullary thyroid cancer. *N Engl J Med* 2003;349:1517–1525.

96. Machens A, Gimm O, Hinze R, et al. Genotype-phenotype correlation in hereditary medullary thyroid carcinoma: oncological features and biochemical properties. *J Clin Endocrinol Metab* 2001;86:1104–1109.

97. Brandi ML, Gagel RF, Angeli A, et al. Consensus guidelines for diagnosis and therapy of MEN type 1 and 2. *J Clin Endocrinol Metab* 2001;86:5658–5671.

98. de Jong M, Breeman WA, Bakker WH, et al. Comparison of ^{111}In-labeled somatostatin analogues for tumor scintigraphy and radionuclide therapy. *Cancer Res* 1998;58:437–441.

99. de Jong M, Breeman WA, Bernard BF, et al. [^{177}Lu-DOTA(0), Tyr3] octreotate for somatostatin receptor-targeted radionuclide therapy. *Int J Cancer* 2001;92:628–633.

100. Virgolini I, Szilvasi I, Kurtaran A, et al. Indium-111-DOTA-Ianreotide: biodistribution, safety and radiation absorbed close in tumor patients. *J Nucl Med* 1998;39:1928–1936.

101. Brierley J, Tsang R, Simpson WJ, et al. Medullary thyroid cancer: analysis of survival and prognostic factors and the role of radiation therapy in local control. *Thyroid* 1996;6:305–310.

102. Tubiana M, Haddad E, Schlumberger M, et al. External radiotherapy in thyroid cancers. *Cancer* 1985;55:2062–2071.

103. Grimelius L, Akerström G. Parathyroid glands. In: Kovacs K, Asa SL, eds. *Functional endocrine pathology*, 2nd ed. Malden, MA: Blackwell Science, 1998.

104. National Institutes of Health. Consensus development conference statement on primary hyperparathyroidism. *J Bone Miner Res* 1991;6[suppl]:S9.

105. Bilezikian JP, Potts JT Jr, Fuleihan Gel-H, et al. Summary statement from a workshop on asymptomatic primary hyperparathyroidism: a perspective for the 21st century. *J Clin Endocrinol Metab* 2002;87:5353–5361.

106. Melton JL III. Epidemiology of primary hyperparathyroidism. *J Bone Miner Res* 1991;6:525.

107. Silverberg SJ, Shane E, de la Cruz L, et al. Skeletal disease in primary hyperparathyroidism. *J Bone Miner Res* 1989;4:283–291.

108. Bilezikian JP, Silverberg SJ, Shane E, et al. Characterization and evaluation of asymptomatic primary hyperparathyroidism. *J Bone Miner Res* 1991;6 Suppl 2:S85–S89.

109. Taillefer R, Boucher Y, Potvin C, et al. Detection and localization of parathyroid adenomas in patients with hyperparathyroidism using a single radionuclide imaging procedure with technetium-99m-sestamibi (double-phase study). *J Nucl Med* 1992;33:1801–1807.

110. Stark DD, Gooding GAW, Moss AA, et al. Parathyroid imaging: comparison of high-resolution CT and high-resolution sonography. *AJR Am J Roentgenol* 1983;141:633–638.

111. Nussbaum SR, Zahradnik RJ, Lavigne JR, et al. Highly sensitive two-site immunoradiometric assay of parathyrin, and its clinical utility in evaluating patients with hypercalcemia. *Clin Chem* 1987;33:1364–1367.

112. Kao PC, van Heerden JA, Taylor RL. Intraoperative monitoring of parathyroid procedures by a 15 minute parathormone immunochemiluminometric assay. *Mayo Clin Proc* 1994;69: 532–537.

113. Clary BM, Garner SC, Leight GS Jr. Intraoperative parathyroid hormone monitoring during parathyroidectomy for secondary hyperparathyroidism. *Surgery* 1997;122:1034–1038.

114. Akerstrom G, Rudberg C, Grimelius L, et al. Causes of failed primary exploration and technical aspects of re-operation in primary hyperthyroidism. *World J Surg* 1992;16:562–568.

115. Randolph GW, et al. Intraoperative hormonal criteria for surgical success. Syllabus for parathyroid surgery: the new millennium. Panel presentation at the 5th International Conference on Head and Neck Cancer, San Francisco, California, July 29, 2000.

116. Kaplan EL, Bartlett S, Sugimoto J, et al. Relation of postoperative hypocalcemia to operative techniques: deleterious effect of excessive use of parathyroid biopsy. *Surgery* 1982;92:827–834.

117. Wynne AG, et al. Parathyroid carcinoma: clinical and pathologic features in 43 patients. *Medicine* 1992;71:197.

118. Obara T, Fujimoto Y. Diagnosis and treatment of patients with parathyroid carcinoma: an update and review. *World J Surg* 1991;15:738–744.

119. Sandelin K, Auer G, Bondeson L, et al. Prognostic factors in parathyroid cancer: a review of 95 cases. *World J Surg* 1992;16: 724–731.

117

Nasopharyngeal Cancer

William I. Wei

Anatomically, the nasopharynx is continuous with the nasal cavities and serves as a passage for air during breathing. Because of its bony framework, it remains patent under normal circumstances. Nasopharyngeal carcinoma (NPC) is a squamous cell carcinoma (SCC) arising from the epithelial lining of the nasopharynx. This neoplasm could arise from any site in the nasopharynx and is more frequently seen at the fossa of Rosenmüller, the recess located medial to the medial crura of the eustachian tube.

A group of 14 patients with this malignancy was first reported in the English literature in 1901 (1). The first comprehensive series reporting clinicopathologic features of 114 patients with NPC in Hong Kong was published in 1941 (2).

Nasopharyngeal carcinoma is a relatively uncommon malignant disease in most countries with its age-adjusted incidence less than 1 per 100,000 (3). It occurs more frequently, however, in the Inuits of Alaska (4) and ethnic Chinese in the southern part of China, especially from the province of Guangdong. The recent reported incidence of NPC among men and women in Hong Kong in the southern part of the Guangdong province was 20 to 30 per 100,000 and 15 to 20 per 100,000, respectively (3). The incidence of NPC remains high among those Chinese who have immigrated to Southeast Asia countries or North America, but is low among those Chinese born in North America (5,6). This suggests that genetic, ethnic, and environmental factors may play a role in the etiology of the disease.

The consumption of salted fish is one of the causative factors of NPC frequently mentioned This may be related to the carcinogenic compound, nitrosamine, detected on the salted fish (7). A subsequent case-control study, however, showed that only frequent consumption of salted fish before 10 years of age is associated with increased risk of developing NPC (8).The Epstein-Barr virus (EBV) has also

been considered to play an oncogenic role in this tumor, because the EBV genome is frequently detected in the biopsy specimens of NPC (9). In view of the ubiquitous presence of this virus in the human population, it is unlikely that EBV is the only causative agent of NPC. In the first-degree relatives of patients with NPC, their incidence of developing this malignancy is six times higher than controls (10). This suggests that genetic factor might have an important role in the etiology of NPC. Comparative genomic hybridization studies have demonstrated alterations in multiple chromosomes such as the deletion of regions at 14q, 16p, 1p, and amplification of 12q and 4q (11,12). Tumor suppressive genes also have been recently located in chromosome 14q (13).

HISTOPATHOLOGY

The malignant epithelial cells of NPC are large polygonal cells with a syncytial character. Their nuclei are round or oval with scanty chromatin and distinct nucleoli. The cells are frequently intermingled with lymphoid cells in the nasopharynx, giving rise to the term lymphoepithelioma (14). Electron microscopy studies have confirmed the squamous origin of these cells, including those undifferentiated carcinomas that are a form of epidermoid SCC with minimal differentiation (15).

The histologic classification of NPC proposed by the World Health Organization (WHO) (16) in 1978 categorized tumors into three groups:

- Type I: those typical keratinizing SCC with intercellular bridges, similar to those found in the rest of the upper aerodigestive tract (Fig. 117.1).

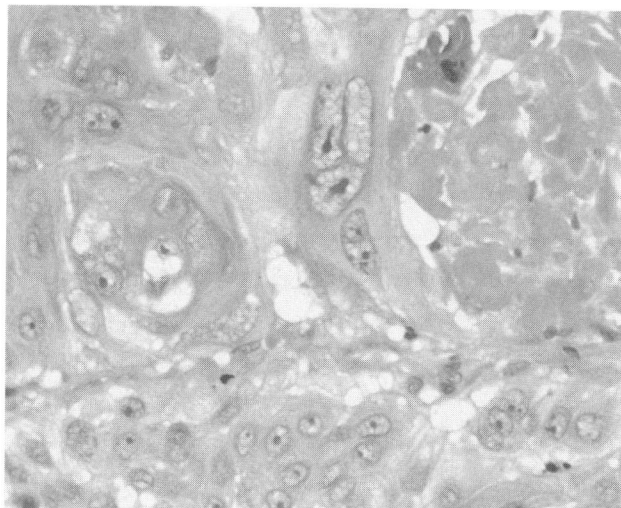

Figure 117.1 Squamous cell carcinoma of the nasopharynx. The tumor cells are large with eosinophilic cytoplasm and show features of keratinization (hematoxylin and eosin × 400). (See also Color Plate 51.)

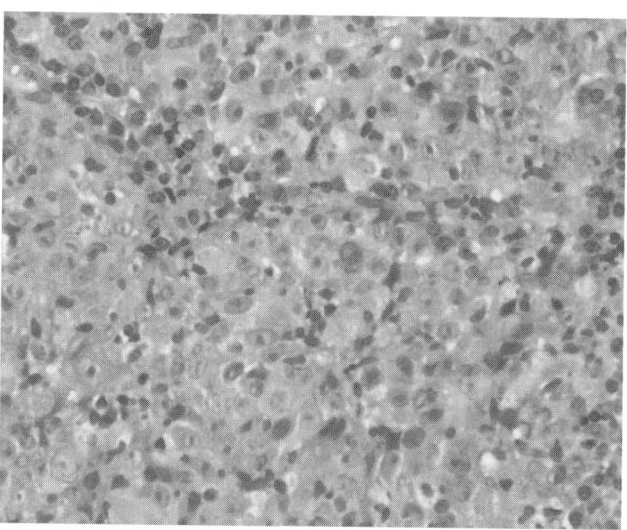

Figure 117.3 Undifferentiated carcinoma of the nasopharynx. Tumor cells are typically composed of nests or islands of pleomorphic polygonal cells with large vesicular nuclei and prominent nucleoli. The tumor nests are often surrounded by a lymphoid stroma, which is part of the nasopharyngeal stroma (hematoxylin and eosin × 400). (See also Color Plate 53.)

- Type II: nonkeratinizing epidermoid carcinomas. They show evidence of maturation but without definite squamous differentiation (Fig. 117.2).
- Type III: undifferentiated or poorly differentiated carcinomas. These cells have indistinct cell margins with hyperchromatic nuclei. (Fig. 117.3).

In North America, approximately 25% of patients with tumor have type I histology, 12% type II, and 63% type III. The corresponding histologic distribution in southern Chinese patients is 3%, 2%, and 95%, respectively (17).

An alternative classification divided tumors into two histologic types, namely squamous cell carcinomas and undifferentiated carcinomas of the nasopharyngeal type (UCNT) (18). This second classification took into consideration its

correlation with EBV serology. Patients with SCC have a lower EBV titer, whereas those with UCNT have elevated titers.

On clinical grounds, biopsies obtained from patients with NPC sometimes show a mixed histologic pattern. The recent WHO classification has taken into account this mixed pattern and also the association of the EBV with type II and III tumors. The histologic types of NPC are now classified into two groups: either as SCC or nonkeratinizing carcinomas, with the second group subdivided into differentiated and undifferentiated carcinomas (19). This new classification has also been shown to have a prognostic bearing, the undifferentiated carcinomas have a higher local tumor control rate with radiotherapy, and a higher incidence of distant metastasis (20,21).

CLINICAL PRESENTATIONS

Patients with NPC present with one or more of the four groups of symptoms. These groups of symptoms are related to the location of the primary tumor, their infiltration of structures in the vicinity of the nasopharynx, or metastasis to the cervical lymph nodes.

A tumor mass in the nasopharynx can lead to the symptoms of nasal obstruction and discharge. With a small tumor, the obstruction is unilateral and with tumor growth the symptoms can become bilateral. When the tumor ulcerates, the patient may present with epistaxis. The amount of bleeding is usually trivial and the frequent presentation is the presence of altered blood in the postnasal drip, especially in the morning.

Tumor bulk in the nasopharynx, with or without posterolateral extension into the paranasopharyngeal space, is

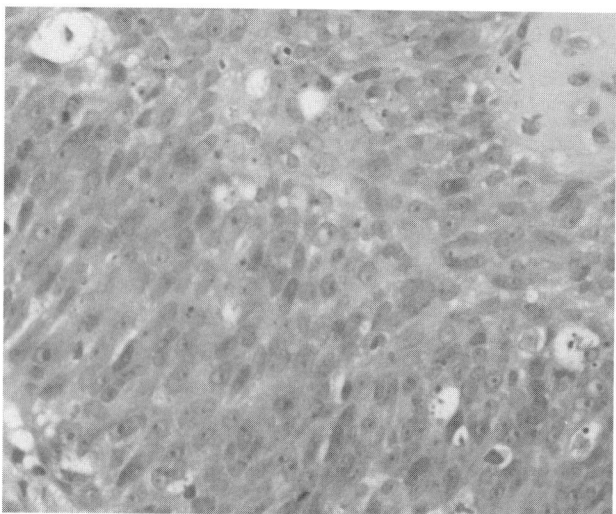

Figure 117.2 Nonkeratinizing differentiated carcinoma of the nasopharynx. The tumor cells have a papillary configuration and appear more hyperchromatic than the undifferentiated carcinoma. The nuclei at the periphery show palisading (hematoxylin and eosin × 400). (See also Color Plate 52.)

frequently associated with dysfunction of the eustachian tube. This can lead to fluid collection in the middle ear and the patients may experience unilateral conductive deafness and other otologic symptoms (e.g., otalgia and tinnitus). Serous otitis media was noted in 41% of 237 patients newly diagnosed with NPC and, thus, when a Chinese adult patient presents with this symptom, the otolaryngologist should consider the possibility of NPC (22).

When the primary tumor grows superiorly to infiltrate the skull base, the patient will experience headache. When the upward extension of tumor affects the cavernous sinus and its lateral wall, the third, fourth, and sixth cranial nerves can be affected and the patient will present with diplopia. When the tumor extends to involve the foramen ovale, the fifth cranial nerve can be affected and facial pain and numbness experienced. Cranial nerve involvement in patients with NPC is approximately 13% (23) to 30% (24), depending on disease stage.

In view of the high propensity of NPC to metastasize to cervical lymph nodes, the most frequent presenting symptom is a painless neck mass, frequently appearing in the upper neck. As the nasopharynx is a midline structure, it is not uncommon to see patients presenting with bilateral cervical lymph nodes.

Patients presenting with symptoms related to distant metastasis are relatively uncommon in NPC. Skeletal metastasis to the vertebra, liver, and lung are the sites where distant metastases are encountered.

Because of the nonspecific nature of the nasal and aural symptoms and the inconspicuous nature of the painless cervical lymph node, however, most patients with NPC have NPC diagnosed only when their tumor has reached advanced stages. A retrospective analysis of 4,768 patients showed that the symptoms at presentation were neck mass in 76%, nasal symptoms in 73%, aural symptoms in 62%, and cranial nerve palsy in 20% of patients (25). In most reports, the male-to-female ratio was 3:1 and the median age was 50 years. The presenting symptoms in young patients were similar to those of adults (26).

DIAGNOSIS

When patients present with symptoms of NPC, they should be evaluated clinically for physical signs of NPC (e.g., the presence lymph nodes in the neck, fluid in the middle ear, and cranial nerve involvement). Indirect examination of the postnasal space should be carried out with a mirror, although the anatomic variation of the nasopharynx in some patients precludes an adequate evaluation of the region. Other investigations toward the diagnosis of NPC are the estimation of antibody levels against EBV, imaging studies, and endoscopic examination of the nasopharynx and biopsy.

Serology

Epstein-Barr virus affects human in various forms. It can cause infectious mononucleosis and has also been found to be associated with Burkitt lymphoma and NPC. EBV belongs to the herpes virus family and the EBV-specific antigens can be grouped into early replicative antigens, latent phase antigens, and late antigens. In patients with NPC, their antibody, immunoglobulin A (IgA), response to the early antigen (EA) of the first group, and the viral capsid antigen (VCA) of the third group has been shown to be of diagnostic value (27).

The IgA anti-VCA is more sensitive but less specific than the IgA anti-EA. In population screening studies thousands of apparently healthy individuals, those with elevated titers of these antibodies had an incidence of harboring subclinical NPC ranging from 3% (28) to 5% (29) and their annual detection rate of NPC was 30 times higher than for the population as a whole (28). The findings were confirmed by a recent report from Taiwan in which 9,699 men were studied, who had a one-off blood sample for their EBV serology, which subsequently correlated with the cancer registry and death registry over a 15-year period. Those with elevated anti-EBV titers have a 30 times greater chance of developing NPC (30).

When a spectrum of antibodies against one of the latent phase antigens of the EBV-associated nuclear antigen (EBNA) was evaluated, both the specificity and sensitivity of the test exceeded 92% (31).

The IgA anti-VCA level has also been shown to be related to the stage of the disease, and the level may decrease following therapy (32); its value as a tumor marker in evaluating tumor eradication and detection of recurrence has not been established (33). In recent years, cell-free DNA of the EBV has been detected in patients with NPC and it has been evaluated as a tumor marker (34). It, however, has a moderate sensitivity, especially when the primary tumor is small and when radiotherapy has been given (35).

Imaging Studies

Clinical examination, together with endoscopic examination, can provide valuable information on tumor extension on the mucosal surface, but cannot determine its deep extension, including skull base erosion, and intracranial spread. This information is provided by cross-sectional imaging studies. These investigations are essential today to document the extent of the disease in the nasopharynx and in the planning delivery of radiation (36).

Computed tomography (CT) can demonstrate the soft tissue extension in the nasopharynx and laterally into the paranasopharyngeal space (37) (Fig. 117.4). It is sensitive in detecting bone erosion, especially that of the skull base. Tumor extension intracranially through the foramen ovale with perineural spread can also be detected, which provides evidence of cavernous sinus involvement without skull base erosion (38). CT can show bone regeneration after therapy, which indicates complete eradication of tumor (39).

Magnetic resonance imaging (MRI) provides multiplanar imaging abilities and is better than CT in differentiating tumor from inflammation of soft tissues. MRI is also more sensitive at evaluating retropharyngeal and deep cervical nodal metastases (40). MRI can detect bone marrow

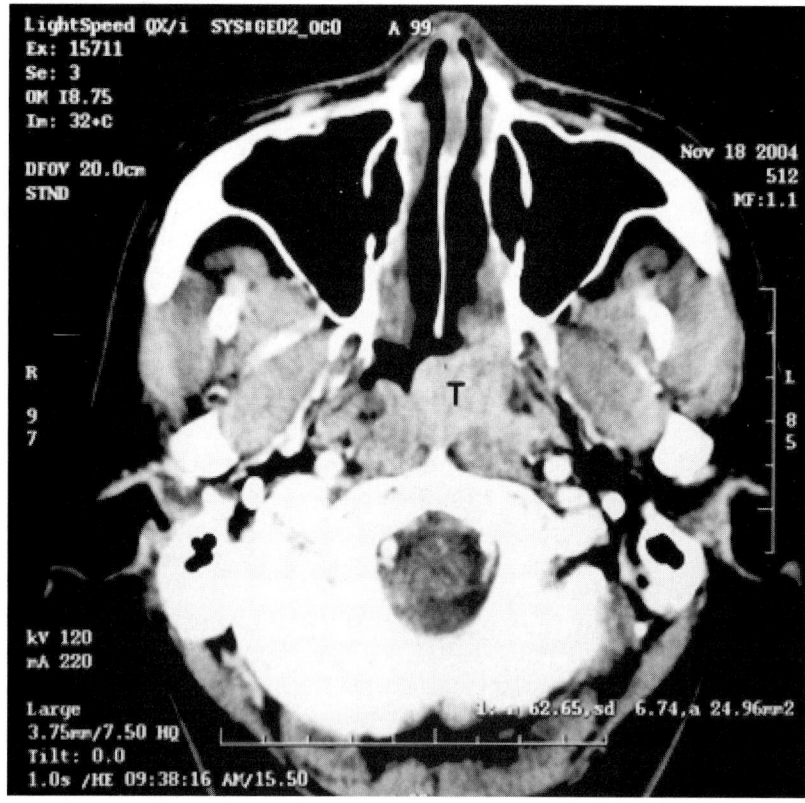

Figure 117.4 Computed tomography (axial view) showing tumor in the nasopharynx (T).

infiltration by tumors, whereas CT cannot detect this kind of infiltration unless associated bony erosion exists. It is important to detect this marrow infiltration because it is associated with an increased risk of distant metastases (41). MRI, however, cannot evaluate details of bone erosion, and CT should be performed when the status of the skull base needs to be evaluated.

Another contribution of cross-sectional imaging studies in NPC is toward the therapeutic aspects. Because CT or MRI determines the primary tumor extent with unprecedented precision, it enables radiotherapy treatment to be designed and administered more accurately and effectively, resulting in an improved outcome (42). This is particularly applicable recently with the intensity modulated radiotherapy (IMRT),

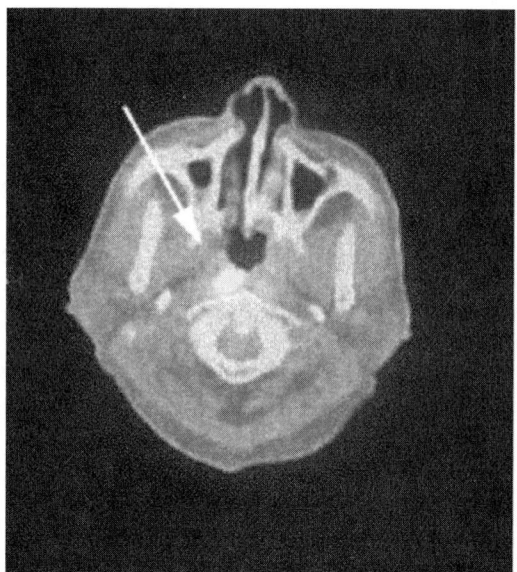
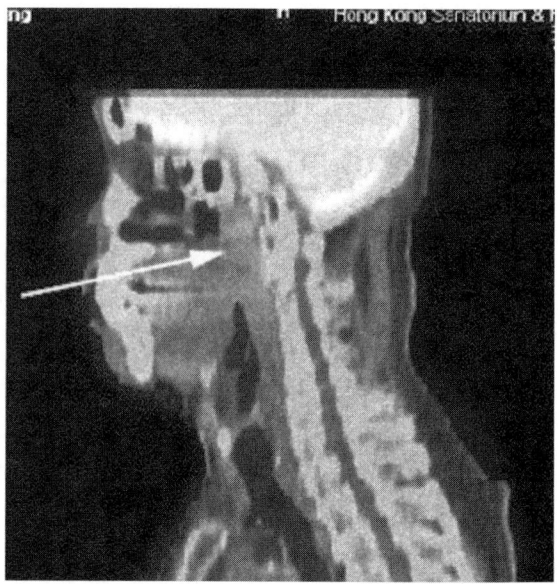

A

B

Figure 117.5 **A:** Axial view of positron emission tomography superimposed with computed tomography image, showing increased activity at the primary site in the nasopharynx signifying presence of tumor (*arrow*). **B:** Sagittal view of the same patient. (See also Color Plate 54.)

which makes use of composite CT–MRI targets (43), and this enables radiotherapy to be targeted even more accurately onto tumor while sparing adjacent normal tissues.

Both CT and MRI, however, have relatively low sensitivity in detection of tumor recurrence (44) because recurrent NPC after radiotherapy can exhibit a range of signal intensities and contours, and these can be difficult to interpret (45). Positron emission tomography (PET) is reported to be more sensitive than cross-sectional imaging studies in detecting persistent and recurrent NPC (46), both at the primary site and in the neck (Fig. 117.5)

The precise detection of distant metastases at diagnosis is difficult. Studies have concluded that bone scans, liver scintigraphy (47), and marrow biopsy (48) are of little value. They should only be used for those patients with high risk of distant spread (e.g., those with N3 disease) (49).

Endoscopic Examination

A confirmed diagnosis of NPC requires a positive biopsy taken from the tumor in the nasopharynx. The nasopharynx can be adequately examined under topical anesthesia with endoscopes. The rigid Hopkin telescopes, both 0° and 30°, give an excellent view of the nasopharynx on the insertion side (Figs. 117.6 and 117.7). In cases of a deviated septum, a 70° endoscope inserted through the opposite nasal cavity can also provide adequate visualization of the tumor. This 70° endoscope inserted behind the soft palate allows visualization of the roof of nasopharynx and both eustachian tube openings (Fig. 117.8). These rigid endoscopes do not have a suction or biopsy channel. Blood and mucus covering the tumor should be removed by a separate suction device for a clear view of the pathology. Biopsy forceps should also be inserted along side the endoscope to take a biopsy of the tumor under direct vision.

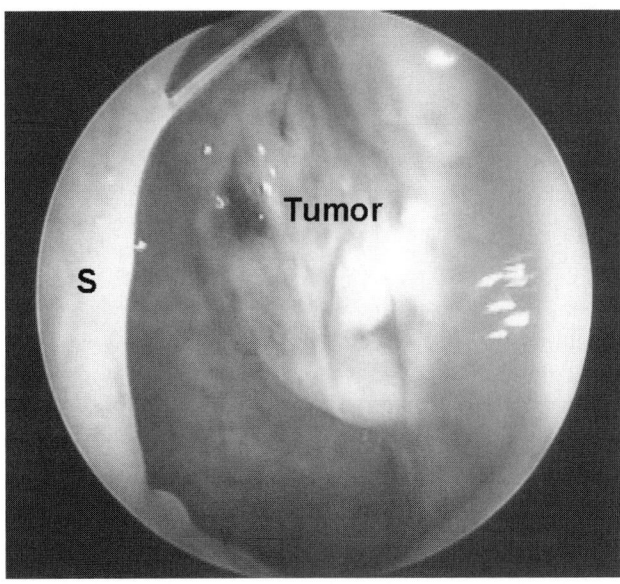

Figure 117.7 Rigid endoscope (30°) inserted through the left nasal cavity of the same patient and tumor in the nasopharynx identified (*Tumor*). The posterior edge of the septum is visible (*S*).

The flexible endoscope allows thorough examination of the entire nasopharynx, even when it is inserted through one nasal cavity. Its tip can be maneuvered behind the nasal septum to the opposite side. It has a suction channel and a biopsy forceps can be inserted through it to take a biopsy of the tumor under direct vision. Despite all these advantages, the visual image gathered with the flexible endoscope is inferior to that of the rigid endoscope and the size of the biopsy

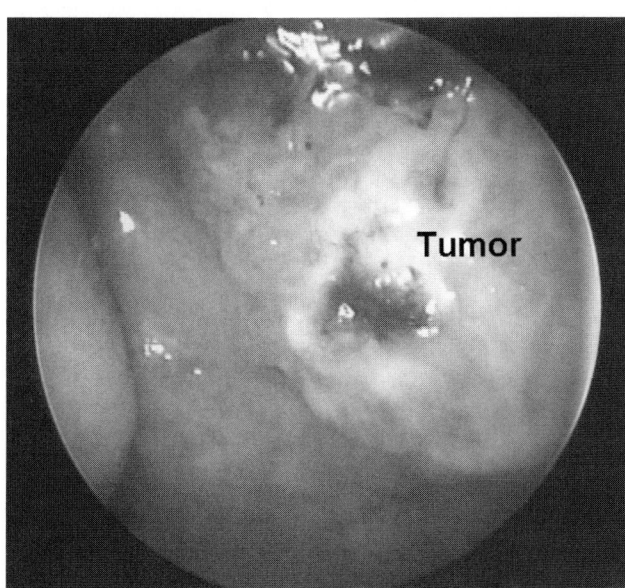

Figure 117.6 Rigid endoscope (0°) inserted through the left nasal cavity and tumor in the nasopharynx is identified (*Tumor*).

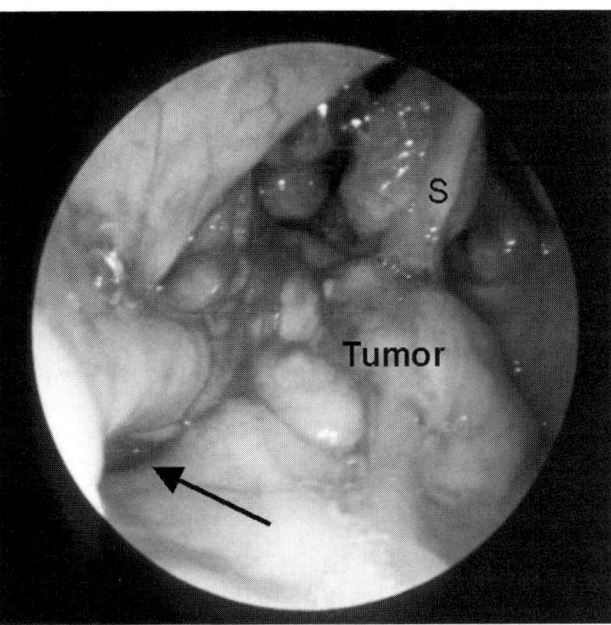

Figure 117.8 Rigid endoscope (70°) inserted through the oral cavity, inspecting the nasopharynx from below. Posterior edge of the nasal septum (*S*) right eustachian tube orifice (*arrow*) and nasopharyngeal tumor can be seen extending from the right lateral wall onto the roof of the nasopharynx (*Tumor*).

forceps is also small; thus only suboptimal tissue may be obtained. Sometimes, a larger biopsy forceps can be inserted by the side of the flexible endoscope to obtain more substantial amount of tissue for histologic examination.

STAGING

The different clinical staging systems for NPC each have their merits. The American Joint Committee on Cancer/Union Internationale Contre le Cancer (AJCC/UICC) system, preferred in America and Europe, follows the usual patterns of staging for head and neck malignancies (Table 117.1), whereas Ho's system (50), which is frequently used in Asia, has its nodal classification, reflecting better prognostic significance (Table 117.2).

Incorporating experiences gained from various centers around the world and taking into account a number of prognostic factors, including skull base erosion, involvement of cranial nerves, tumor extension to paranasopharyngeal space, and the location and size of the cervical nodes, a revised AJCC/UICC staging system was published in 1997. Stage T1 tumor in the new staging system includes both T1 and T2 classified under the old system. The new stage T2 tumors cover those that had extended to the nasal fossa, oropharynx, or paranasopharyngeal space. The new stage T3 tumor includes those that had extended to the skull base or other paranasal sinuses. The new stage T4 tumors cover those that had extended into the infratemporal fossa, orbit, hypopharynx, and cranium, or to the cranial nerves. For cervical lymph node, stage N1 under the new system refers to unilateral nodal involvement; stage N2 bilateral nodal disease that had not reached N3 designation, irrespective of the size, number, and anatomic location of the nodes. N3 refers to lymph nodes larger than 6 cm (N3a) or nodes that had extended to the supraclavicular fossa (N3b) (51). This new staging system has enabled disease to be staged more precisely according to the extensiveness of NPC and has been shown to predict survival (52,53).

TREATMENT

Radiotherapy

In view of the nasopharynx location, lying in close proximity to important structures, and the infiltrative nature of NPC, surgical resection of the primary tumor is challenging. NPC, however, is radiosensitive and, thus, radiotherapy has been the primary treatment modality for decades. Radiotherapy, although effective, can also produce undesirable complications because NPC at the base of skull is surrounded by the brain stem, spinal cord, pituitary-hypothalamic axis, temporal lobes, eyes, middle and inner ears, and parotid glands. All these organs limit the amount of radiation that can be delivered to the tumor. Because NPC tends to infiltrate and spread toward these

TABLE 117.1

AMERICAN JOINT COMMITTEE ON CANCER STAGING FOR NASOPHARYNGEAL CANCER

Tumor in nasopharynx (T)

T1	Tumor confined to the nasopharynx
T2	Tumor extends to soft tissues of oro-pharynx and/or nasal fossa
T2	a without parapharyngeal extension
T2	b with parapharyngeal extension
T3	Tumor invades bony structures and/or paranasal sinuses
T4	Tumor with intracranial extension and/or involvement of cranial nerves, infratemporal fossa, hypopharynx, or orbit

Regional Lymph Nodes (N)
The distribution and the prognostic impact of regional lymph node spread from nasopharynx cancer, particularly of the undifferentiated type, is different than that of other head and neck mucosal cancers and justifies use of a different N classification scheme.

NX	Regional lymph nodes cannot be assessed
N0	No regional lymph node metastasis
N1	Unilateral metastasis in lymph node(s), 6 cm or less in greatest dimension, above the supraclavicular fossa
N2	Bilateral metastasis in lymph node(s), 6 cm or less in greatest dimension, above the supraclavicular fossa
N3	Metastasis in a lymph node(s)
	N3a greater than 6 cm in dimension
	N3b extension to the supraclavicular fossa

Distant Metastasis (M)

MX	Distant metastasis cannot be assessed
M0	No distant metastasis
M1	Distant metastasis

Stage grouping

Stage 0	T1s	N0	M0
Stage I	T1	N0	M0
Stage IIA	T2a	N0	M0
Stage IIB	T1	N1	M0
	T2	N1	M0
	T2a	N1	M0
	T2b	N0	M0
	T2b	N1	M0
Stage III	T1	N2	M0
	T2a	N2	M0
	T2b	N2	M0
	T3	N0	M0
	T3	N1	M0
	T3	N2	M0
Stage IVA	T4	N0	M0
	T4	N1	M0
	T4	N2	M0
Stage IVB	Any T	N3	M0
Stage IVC	Any T	Any N	M1

From Fleming ID, Cooper JS, Henson DE, et al., eds. *AJCC cancer staging manual*, 5th ed. Philadelphia: Lippincott-Raven, 1997:33–35, with permission.

dose-limiting organs, it is difficult to shield these structures without compromising the dose delivered to the primary tumor. Because of the high incidence of occult neck node involvement, the neck is usually included in the radiation field electively (54). Good locoregional

TABLE 117.2

HO STAGING FOR NASOPHARYNGEAL CANCER

T: Primary tumor
T1:   Tumor confined to nasopharynx (space behind choanal
        orifices and nasal septum and above posterior margin
        of soft palate in resting position)
T2:   Tumor extended to nasal fossa, oropharynx, or adjacent
        muscles or nerves below base of skull
T3:   Tumor extended beyond T2 limits and subclassfied as
        follows:
T3a: Bone involvement below base of skull (floor of
        sphenoid sinus is included in this category)
T3b: Involvement of base of skull
T3c: Involvement of cranial nerve(s)
T3d: Involvement of orbits, laryngopharynx (hypopharynx),
        or infratemporal fossa

N: Regional lymph nodes
        N0: No node palpable or nodes thought to be benign
        N1: Node(s) wholly in upper cervical level, bounded
        below by the skin crease extending laterally and
        backward from or just below thyroid notch (laryngeal
        eminence)
N2:   Node(s) palpable between crease and supraclavicular
        fossa, the upper limit being a line joining the upper
        margin of the sternal end of the clavicle and the angle
        formed by the lateral surface of the neck and the supe-
        rior margin of the trapezius
N3:   Node(s) palpable in the supraclavicular fossa and/or
        skin involvement in the form of carcinoma en cuirasse
        or satellite nodules above the clavicles

M: Metastases
        M0: No hematogenous metastases
        M1: Hematogenous metastases present, and/or lymph
        nodal metastases below the clavicle

Stage grouping
  I   T1, N0
  II   T2 and/or N1
  III   T3 and/or N2
  IV   N3 (any T)
  V   M1

From Ho JH. *Stage classification of nasopharyngeal carcinoma: a re-view.* International Agency for Research on Cancer, Publication No. 20, 1978;99–113, with permission.

control can be achieved and once locoregional relapse occurs, an increased risk exists of developing distant metastases (55).

Radiotherapy for NPC usually starts with large lateral opposing faciocervical fields that cover the primary tumor and the upper neck lymphatics in one volume, with matching lower anterior cervical field for lower neck lymphatics. When the spinal cord dose reaches 40 to 45 Gy, two options exist for the second phase of treatment. The delivery of radiation can either be changed from the original fields to lateral opposing facial fields with another anterior facial field for the primary tumor, with matching anterior cervical field for the neck lymphatics (50). Alternatively, radiation treatment can be continued using the lateral opposing faciocervical fields, but these fields are reduced in size to avoid the spinal cord, while the superior-posterior lymphatic are treated with electron fields (56,57).

In general, the radiation dose given to the primary tumor is in the range of 65 to 75 Gy and that to the involved neck nodes is 65 to 70 Gy. For elective radiation of node-negative neck, the dose given is 50 to 60 Gy. This treatment has successfully controlled T1 and T2 tumors in 75% to 90% of cases, and T3 and T4 tumors in 50% to 75% of cases (58,59). Nodal control is achieved in 90% of patients with N0 and N1 diseases, but the regional control rate drops to 70% for N2 and N3 cases (58).

For T1 and T2 tumors, employing a booster dose using intracavitary brachytherapy has improved tumor control by 16% (60). Although stereotactic radiosurgery has also been used to deliver the booster dose (61), the hypofractionated treatment is associated with undesirable side effects and is probably better reserved for the treatment of persistent and recurrent disease (62).

The major limitations of two-dimensional planning for NPC can now be eliminated with three-dimensional conformal radiotherapy and IMRT (63,64). When the tumor extension is close to the dose-limiting organs, IMRT is distinctly useful because it further improves the dose differential between the tumor and the dose-limiting organs (65,66). IMRT also eliminates the dose uncertainty problem at the junction between the primary tumor and neck lymphatic target volumes, because it enables the primary tumor and the upper neck nodes to be treated in one volume.

Excellent locoregional control has been achieved with IMRT in the management of NPC (67). Following IMRT, prospective study has confirmed the recovery of salivary functions within 2 years (68). Satisfactory results were also achieved with IMRT for recurrent NPC, and the degree of short-term control was encouraging (69). The limitation of IMRT remains its precision in determining the junction of tumor and the adjacent normal structures. Until the optimal safety margin that needs to be covered between gross tumor and adjacent tissues is established, the planning of clinical target volume for IMRT should be performed cautiously.

Other attempts to enhance the results of radiotherapy include accelerated fractionation (70), accelerated hyperfractionation (71), and a combination of one or other of these treatments with chemotherapy (72,73).

Chemotherapy

For the management of NPC cases, especially those with advanced locoregional disease, chemotherapy has been applied in combination with radiotherapy. Chemotherapy, consisting of cisplatin, can be given before, during, or after radiation; thus there were studies that reported results on neoadjuvant, concurrent, and adjuvant chemotherapy with radiotherapy, respectively.

The Intergroup 1997 study first showed that using chemotherapy with radiotherapy improved overall survival when compared with using radiotherapy alone (74). This study included many patients with well-differentiated carcinoma and initially doubts were raised whether it was applicable to NPC in the endemic areas. A subsequent study from Taiwan confirmed the benefit of this approach (75).

Two neoadjuvant studies (76,77) reported improvement in relapse-free survival, but not improvement in overall survival, whereas two others reported no improvement in survival (78,79). The two prospective, randomized studies on adjuvant chemotherapy reported no improvement, either in relapse-free survival and overall survival (80,81).

General agreement now is that, for advanced diseases, concurrent chemoradiotherapy is useful, whereas other forms of combination therapy require further evaluation. To improve the results of concurrent chemoradiotherapy, a study on neoadjuvant chemotherapy followed by concomitant chemoradiotherapy has reported excellent overall survival and acceptable toxicity (82). In view of the ototoxicity of cisplatin, other chemotherapeutic agents have been used. A study reports on the concurrent use of cisplatin and radiotherapy, followed by adjuvant ifosfamide, 5-fluorouracil (5FU), and leucovorin in patients with stage IVb NPC. Although these patients had more advanced disease, treatment outcome was comparable to other platinum-based adjuvant chemotherapy studies and the compliance rate was acceptable (83).

Follow-Up

The health-related quality of life for those patients with NPC who survived, in general, is impaired (84,85). Late complications appear in the long-term survivors and these are the results of radiation on the dose-limiting organs adjacent to the nasopharynx and neck nodes. These sequelae include neuroendocrine (86) and auditory (87) complications, xerostomia leading to poor oral and dental hygiene (88,89), radiation-induced soft tissue fibrosis (90), and carotid artery stenosis (91). Debilitating neurologic complications include temporal lobe necrosis (92), cranial nerve palsies (93), and other less obvious side effects such as memory (94), and cognitive (95) and neuropsychological dysfunctions (96). Cisplatin-based chemotherapy adds other otologic side effects (97).

Complete remission of NPC following treatment can be monitored with clinical examination, endoscopic examination with or without biopsy, and imaging studies. Studies comparing PET with MRI or CT to detect persistent and recurrent tumor have reported PET to be superior (98,99). Early detection of locoregional relapses is important because these tumors are still amenable to salvage when detected early (100). In cases of persistent disease, in either the nasopharynx or neck 10 weeks after completion of the initial therapy, then salvage treatment should be considered (101).

Management of Persistent or Recurrent Disease

Although concomitant chemoradiation is effective in the management of NPC, local or regional failure presenting as persistent or recurrent tumor still occurs. To attain a high salvage rate, early detection and therapy are essential. PET is superior to CT (99) and MRI (98) in detecting persistent or recurrent disease in the nasopharynx, and any malignancy can usually be confirmed with biopsy through endoscopic examination. Persistent or recurrent tumor in the neck node after chemoradiotherapy, however, is notoriously difficult to confirm, because only clusters of tumor cells are present in some lymph nodes (102).

Aggressive treatment for locally recurrent NPC is warranted because, although survival after retreatment for extensive disease remains poor, it is still longer than for those managed with supportive treatment only. For patients with NPC, even in cases of synchronous locoregional failures, aggressive treatment should be considered for selected patients (103).

Persistent or Recurrent Tumor in Neck Lymph Nodes

Following combined chemoradiation for NPC, isolated failure in the neck was reported to be less than 5% (104). If cancer persists or recurs in the cervical lymph nodes, as evidenced by fine-needle aspiration cytology, imaging studies, or progressive enlargement of the lymph nodes, salvage therapy is indicated. When managed with another course of external radiotherapy, the reported overall 5-year survival rate was only 19.7% (105). Radical neck dissection as a form of surgical salvage has been reported to achieve a 5-year tumor control rate of 66% in the neck and a 5-year actuarial survival of 38% (106). For those persistent or recurrent tumors in the neck nodes, pathologic studies have shown extensive disease involvement of the local tissue. Malignant cells could be seen to extend outside the capsule of the lymph nodes and lying close to the accessory nerve and the internal jugular vein. Many lymph nodes that appeared free of tumor were found to harbor malignant cells. Tumor clusters were seen in the sternomastoid muscle and other tissue in the neck. A radical neck dissection was considered essential for salvage when malignant tumor were found in the neck nodes.

When tumor in the neck node extends beyond the confines of the lymph node, brachytherapy should be applied to the tumor bed in addition to radical neck dissection. With this adjuvant therapy, a similar tumor control rate has been reported when compared with radical neck dissection done for less extensive neck disease (107).

Persistent or Recurrent Tumor in the Nasopharynx

Persistent or recurrent disease in the nasopharynx after the initial radical dose of radiation can still be managed with a second course of external radiotherapy with a larger radiation dose. A salvage rate of 32% has been reported, although the cumulative incidence of late sequelae after repeated irradiation was 24%, with a treatment mortality of 1.8% (108). The complications arising from the second dose of external radiotherapy affects significantly the quality of life of these patients. To alleviate this high incidence of complications resulting from repeated irradiation, alternative salvage measures have been introduced. These include stereotactic radiotherapy, brachytherapy, and surgical resection. These treatment options are useful only when the persistent or recurrent tumor is small and localized in the nasopharynx.

Stereotactic Radiotherapy

The local tumor control rate achieved with stereotactic radiotherapy for management of persistent or recurrent tumor was 72% at 2 years (62) and 86% at 3 years (109). In general, fewer patients have been treated with this modality (110) and long-term follow-up information on local control rate, survival rate, and incidence of complication has to be documented before this method can be applied widely for the management of these cases.

Brachytherapy

With the application of brachytherapy in the management of persistent or recurrent nasopharyngeal carcinoma, the radiation source is inserted directly into the tumor. The radiation dose is highest at the source and declines gradually with increasing distance from the tumor. Thus this allows the delivery of a high therapeutic radiation dose to the persistent or recurrent tumor in the nasopharynx while the surrounding tissue was irradiated with a much smaller dose.

The brachytherapy radiation source also delivers radiation at a continuous rate and this gives radiobiological advantage over fractionated external radiation. Intracavitary brachytherapy has been used for NPC, both as a boost of the primary treatment and for persistent or recurrent disease (111). The radiation source was placed either in a tube or a mould and then inserted into the nasopharynx. Good results achieved with the intracavitary brachytherapy have been reported (112). In view of the irregular contour of the primary tumor within the nasopharynx, however, it is difficult to apply the radiation source accurately to provide a tumoricidal dose to the whole tumor. To circumvent this problem, radioactive interstitial implants have been used to treat small localized persistent or recurrent tumor in the nasopharynx (113).

Radioactive gold grains (^{198}Au) are frequently used as a brachytherapy source. Gold grains can be implanted either transnasally or using the split-palate approach (114). The split-palate approach gives the surgeon a direct view of the tumor and enables the precise implantation of the desired number of gold grains permanently into the tumor (Fig. 117.9). Thus, the exact dosimetry of radiation can be achieved for salvage. For tumors localized in the nasopharynx, without bone invasion, this method has provided effective salvage with minimal morbidity. The surgical procedure is simple and less than 10% of patients may develop a small palatal fistula, which can be managed conservatively or repaired later with a palatal flap (115). Lead shields, however, have to be used in the operating room to reduce the radiation hazards of health care workers. When gold grain implants were used to treat persistent and recurrent tumors after radiotherapy, the reported 5-year local tumor

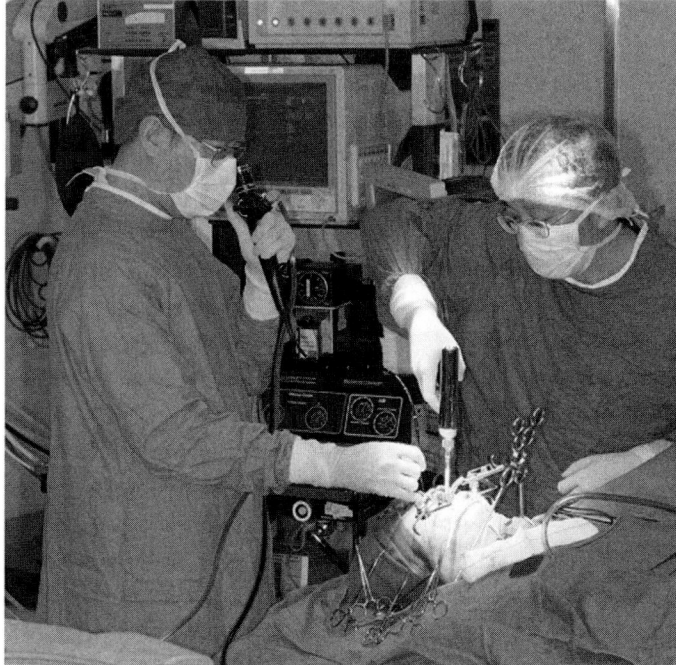
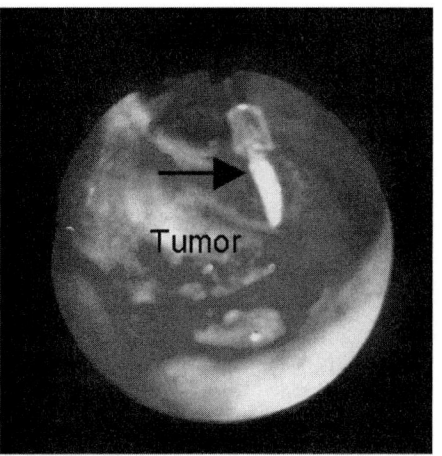

Figure 117.9 A: The surgeon (left), after splitting the palate, holds a flexible endoscope placed in the nasopharynx to provide illumination and guidance. The oncologist (right) uses the gold grain applicator to insert the radioactive grains directly into the tumor. **B:** Endoscopic view showing the tip of the gold grain applicator (*arrow*) before inserting into the tumor (*Tumor*).

control rates were 87% and 63%, respectively, and the corresponding 5-year, disease-free survival rates were 68% and 60%, respectively (116).

Nasopharyngectomy

When the persistent or recurrent tumor in the nasopharynx has extended to the paranasopharyngeal space or is too bulky for brachytherapy to be successful, the next salvage option is surgery. Nasopharyngectomy is effective in the eradication of localized disease in selected patients.

The nasopharynx is located in the central part of the head. It is difficult to expose the region adequately to carry out an oncologic resection of a tumor situated in the nasopharynx that has extended to its vicinity. Various approaches have been used to expose the nasopharynx for salvage nasopharyngectomy. The brain and the spinal cord render superior and posterior approaches not practical. The transantral and midfacial deglove procedures to reach the nasopharynx from the front do not provide adequate exposure of the whole nasopharynx. These anterior approaches, even with the downfracture of the hard palate, expose only the posterior wall of the nasopharynx and not the lateral walls. Fisch described an approach to the nasopharynx from the lateral aspect, through the infratemporal fossa (117). This route of entry started with a radical mastoidectomy and various important structures have to be mobilized, including the internal carotid artery, the fifth cranial nerve, and the floor of the middle cranial fossa. The resultant morbidities are not negligible and it mainly exposes the lateral wall of the nasopharynx on the side of the surgery and not the entire nasopharynx.

The nasopharynx can be approached from the inferior aspect using the transpalatal, transmaxillary, and transcervical approach (118,119). This approach is useful for tumors located in the central and posterior wall of the nasopharynx (Fig. 117.10). For more extensive tumors, especially those situated on the lateral wall (Fig. 117.11), the dissection of the paranasopharyngeal space is difficult from the inferior aspect and the internal carotid artery has to be protected. The anterolateral approach to the nasopharynx or the maxillary swing procedure has also been used for salvage nasopharyngectomy. Following osteotomies, the maxilla bone attached to the anterior cheek flap can be swung laterally as one osteocutaneous complex (120) (Fig. 117.12). This exposes the entire nasopharynx and the paranasopharyngeal space so that an oncologic surgical procedure can be carried out. The operative procedure, which is similar to a maxillectomy (Fig. 117.13), provides good control of the internal carotid artery. The mortalities associated with these salvage surgical procedures have been generally low and acceptable. As all these patients had previously had radical radiotherapy; complete wound healing might take some time and many patients developed trismus. In general, as long as the persistent or recurrent tumor can be resected with a clear margin, the long-term results have been satisfactory. The 5-year actuarial control of tumors in the nasopharynx following salvage nasopharyngectomy has been reported to be

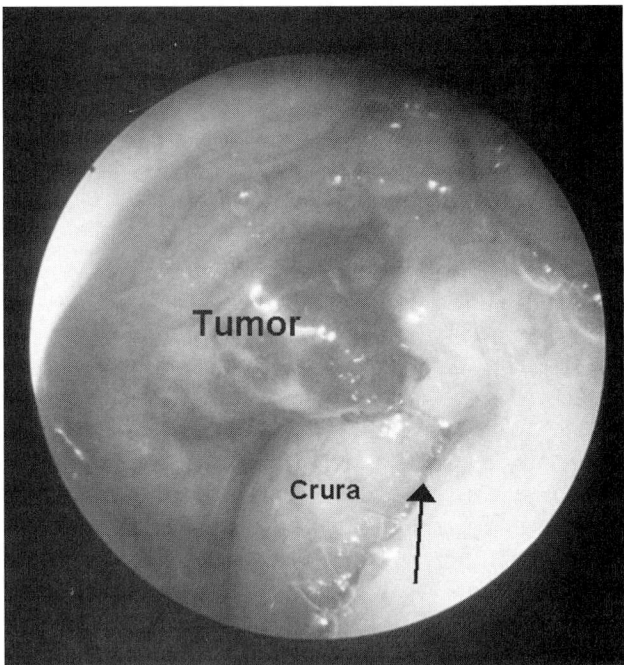

Figure 117.10 Endoscopic view showing recurrent tumor in the central posterior wall (*Tumor*). Opening of the eustachian tube (*arrow*) and medial crura (*Crura*) can be seen.

approximately 65%, and the 5-year, disease-free survival rate is approximately 54% (121,122).

External Radiotherapy and Concurrent Chemotherapy

For more advanced or extensive tumors localized in the nasopharynx, a second course of external radiotherapy might be required for salvage (123). Based on the experience

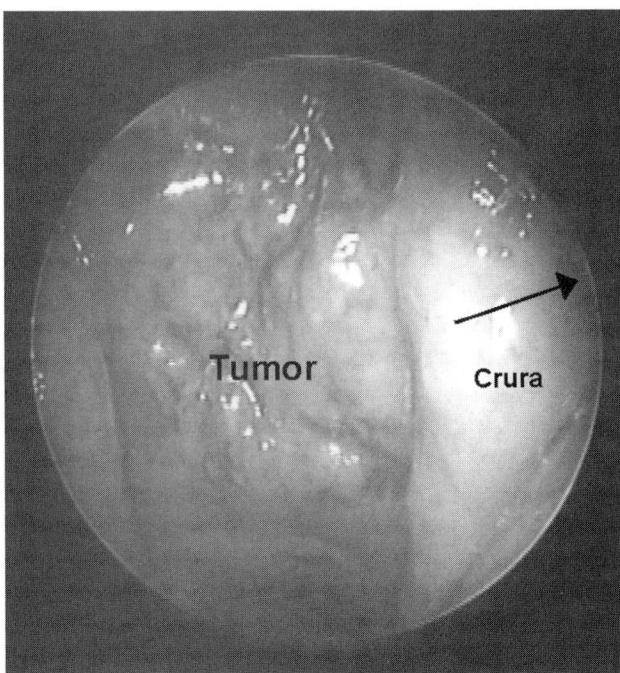

Figure 117.11 Endoscopic view showing recurrent tumor (*Tumor*) in the posterior wall and fossa of Rosenmüller encroaching onto the medial crura of the eustachian tube (*Crura*). The opening of the eustachian tube (*arrow*) is shown.

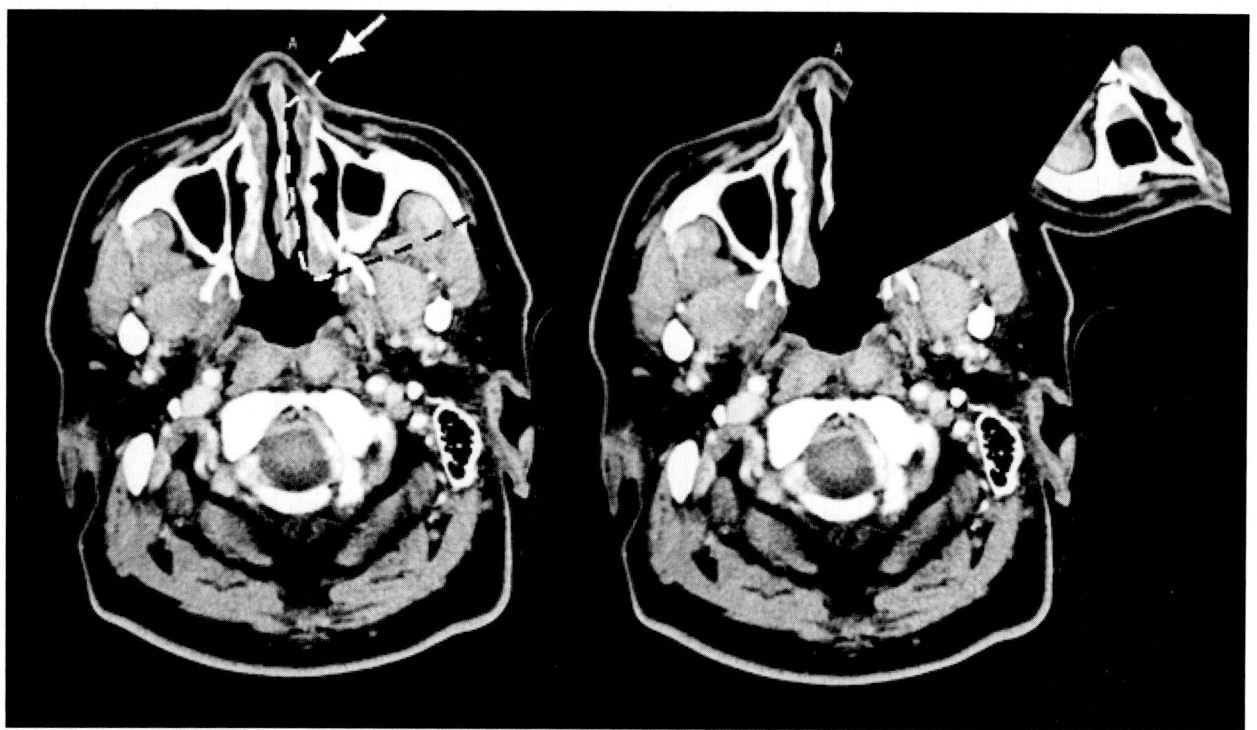

Figure 117.12 Schematic computed tomography. **A:** Planned osteotomies of the maxilla and the posterior part of the nasal septum (*arrow* and *broken line*). **B:** The maxilla is swung laterally while still attached to the cheek flap.

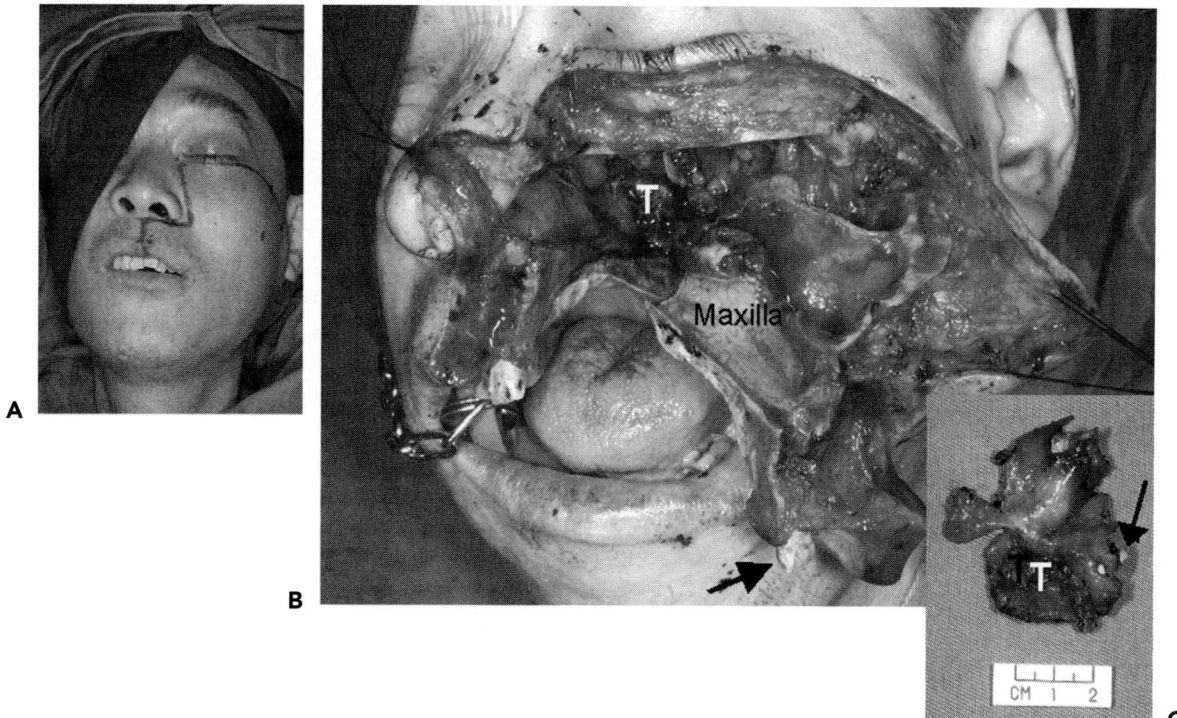

Figure 117.13 **A:** Facial incision for maxillary swing approach to the nasopharynx. **B:** The left maxilla is swung laterally to expose the nasopharynx with recurrent tumor (*T*). The maxilla and the left central incisor tooth (*arrow*) are shown. **C:** Nasopharyngectomy specimen showing tumor (*T*). The eustachian tube opening is marked with a yellow tube (*arrow*).

gained with the use of concurrent chemotherapy and radiotherapy as the primary treatment modality for NPC, a second course of external radiotherapy administered concurrently with chemotherapy has been tried. This treatment reportedly has a 5-year actuarial overall survival rate of 26%, although the risk of major late toxicities was significant (124). The use of precision radiotherapy (e.g., IMRT) might improve the therapeutic outcome without damaging the surrounding normal tissue; the overall survival rate, however, depends on the incidence of distant metastasis, which is an issue in patients with recurrent disease after the initial therapy.

Distant Metastasis

The most effective treatment for patients with NPC with distant metastasis is to use cisplatin-based combination chemotherapy. Cisplatin and infusional 5FU is currently the standard treatment, achieving a 66% to 76% response rate (125). The aim of this form of therapy is essentially palliative, although long-term, disease-free survivors have been reported (126). A number of phase II studies on the newer agents have been reported (127,128). More intensive combinations give a higher response rate but are also usually associated with increased toxicities (129).

For the few selected patients with localized metastases to the lungs, resection of the pulmonary metastases can result in prolonged tumor control (130). For patients with localized metastasis to the mediastinal nodes, the application of radiotherapy and chemotherapy can also result in more prolonged tumor control (131).

FUTURE THERAPEUTIC POSSIBILITIES

As nasopharyngeal carcinoma is closely associated with Epstein-Barr virus, this gives additional opportunities for other therapeutic possibilities. Gene therapy, using a novel replication-deficient adenovirus vector, has been reported to increase cytotoxicity through apoptosis (132). Immunotherapy approaches include the therapeutic augmentation of cytotoxic T lymphocytes responses (133), and adoptive transfer of autologous EBV-specific cytotoxic T cells has also been reported (134). Further clinical trials with longer follow-up periods are required to document their efficacy.

HIGHLIGHTS

- Nasopharyngeal carcinoma is most commonly encountered in ethnic Chinese and Inuits of Alaska.
- Undifferentiated carcinoma of the nasopharynx is associated with elevated antibodies against Epstein-Barr virus.
- The most frequent presenting symptom is a painless neck mass.
- For advanced tumor, concurrent chemoradiotherapy is often prescribed.
- Nasopharyngectomy is effective in treatment of some patients with localized persistent or recurrent disease after initial therapy.

REFERENCES

1. Jackson C. Primary carcinoma of the nasopharynx. A table of cases. *JAMA* 1901;37:371–377.
2. Digby KH, Fook WL, Che YT. Nasopharyngeal carcinoma. *Br J Surg* 1941;28:517–537.
3. Parkin DM, Whelan SL, Ferlay J, et al., eds. *Cancer incidence in five continents*, Vol. VII. International Agency for Research on Cancer, Publication No. 143, 1997;814–815.
4. Nielsen NH, Mikkelsen F, Hansen JP. Nasopharyngeal cancer in Greenland. The incidence in an Arctic Eskimo population. *Acta Pathol Microbiol Scand* [A] 1977;85:850–858.
5. Dickson RI, Flores AD. Nasopharyngeal carcinoma: an evaluation of 134 patients treated between 1971–1980. *Laryngoscope* 1985;95:276–283.
6. Buell P. The effect of migration on the risk of nasopharyngeal cancer among Chinese. *Cancer Res* 1974;34:1189–1191.
7. Fong YY, Chan WC. Bacterial production of di-methyl nitrosamine in salted fish. *Nature* 1973;243:421–422.
8. Yu MC, Ho JH, Lai SH, et al. Cantonese-style salted fish as a cause of nasopharyngeal carcinoma: report of a case-control study in Hong Kong. *Cancer Res* 1986;46:956–961.
9. zur Hausen H, Schulte-Holthausen H, Klein G, et al. EBV DNA in biopsies of Burkitt tumors and anaplastic carcinomas of the nasopharynx. *Nature* 1970;228:1056–1058.
10. Yu MC, Garabrant DH, Huang TB, et al. Occupational and other non-dietary risk factors for nasopharyngeal carcinoma in Guangzhou, China. *Int J Cancer* 1990;45:1033–1039.
11. Fang Y, Guan X, Guo Y, et al. Analysis of genetic alterations in primary nasopharyngeal carcinoma by comparative genomic hybridization. *Genes Chromosomes Cancer* 2001;30:254–260.
12. Chen YJ, Ko JY, Chen PJ, et al. Chromosomal aberrations in nasopharyngeal carcinoma analyzed by comparative genomic hybridization. *Genes Chromosomes Cancer* 1999;25:169–175.
13. Cheng Y, Ko JM, Lung HL, et al. Monochromosome transfer provides functional evidence for growth-suppressive genes on chromosome 14 in nasopharyngeal carcinoma. *Genes Chromosomes Cancer* 2003;37:359–368.
14. Godtfredsen E. On the histopathology of malignant nasopharyngeal tumors. *Acta Pathol Microbiol Scand* 1944;55 (Suppl): 38–319.
15. Prasad U. Cells of origin of nasopharyngeal carcinoma: an electron microscopical study. *J Laryngol Otol* 1974;88:1087.
16. Shanmugaratnam K, Sobin LH. Histological typing of upper respiratory tract tumors. In: Shanmugaratnam K, Sobin LH, eds. *International histological classification of tumours*, No 19. Geneva: World Health Organization, 1978:32–33.
17. Nicholls JM. Nasopharyngeal carcinoma: classification and histological appearances. *Adv Anat Pathol* 1997;4:71–84.
18. Michaeu C, Rilke F, Pilotti S. Proposal for a new histopathological classification of the carcinomas of the nasopharynx. *Tumori* 1978;64:513–518.
19. Shanmugaratnam K, Sobin LH. Histological typing of tumors of upper respiratory tract and ear. In: Shanmugaratnam K, Sobin LH, eds. *International histological classification of tumours*, 2nd ed. Geneva: World Health Organization, 1991:32–33.
20. Reddy SP, Raslan WF, Gooneratne S, et al. Prognostic significance of keratinization in nasopharyngeal carcinoma. *Am J Otolaryngol* 1995;16:103–108
21. Marks JE, Philips JL, Menck HR. The National Cancer Data Base report on the relationship of race and national origin to the histology of nasopharyngeal carcinoma. *Cancer* 1998;83:582–588.
22. Sham JS, Wei WI, Lau SK, et al. Serous otitis media. An opportunity for early recognition of nasopharyngeal carcinoma. *Arch Otolaryngol Head Neck Surg* 1992;118:794–797.
23. Sham JS, Cheung YK, Choy D, et al. Cranial nerve involvement and base of the skull erosion in nasopharyngeal carcinoma. *Cancer* 1991;68(2):422–426.
24. Turgut M, Erturk O, Saygi S, et al. Importance of cranial nerve involvement in nasopharyngeal carcinoma. A clinical study comprising 124 cases with special reference to clinical presentation and prognosis. *Neurosurg Rev* 1998;21:243–248.
25. AW Lee, W Foo, SC Law, et al. Nasopharyngeal carcinoma: presenting symptoms and duration before diagnosis. *Hong Kong Med J* 1997;3:355–361.

26. Sham JS, Poon YF, Wei WI, et al. Nasopharyngeal carcinoma in young patients. *Cancer* 1990;65:2606–2610.

27. Ho HC, Ng MH, Kwan HC, et al. Epstein-Barr-virus-specific IgA and IgG serum antibodies in nasopharyngeal carcinoma. *Br J Cancer* 1976;34:655–660.

28. Zeng Y, Zhang LG, Wu YC, et al. Prospective studies on nasopharyngeal carcinoma in Epstein-Barr virus IgA/VCA antibody-positive persons in Wuzhou City, China. *Int J Cancer* 1985;36:545–547.

29. Sham JS, Wei WI, Zong YS, et al. Detection of subclinical nasopharyngeal carcinoma by fibreoptic endoscopy and multiple biopsy. *Lancet* 1990;335:371–374.

30. Chien YC, Chen JY, Liu MY, et al. Serologic markers of Epstein-Barr virus infection and nasopharyngeal carcinoma in Taiwanese men. *N Engl J Med* 2001;345:1877–1882.

31. Cheng WM, Chan KH, Chen HL, et al. Assessing the risk of nasopharyngeal carcinoma on the basis of EBV antibody spectrum. *Int J Cancer* 2002;97:489–492.

32. Henle W, Ho JH, Henle G, et al. Nasopharyngeal carcinoma: significance of changes in Epstein-Barr virus-related antibody patterns following therapy. *Int J Cancer* 1977;20:663–672.

33. Lynn TC, Tu SM, Kawamura A Jr. Long-term follow-up of IgG and IgA antibodies against viral capsid antigens of Epstein-Barr virus in nasopharyngeal carcinoma. *J Laryngol Otol* 1985;99:567–572.

34. Lo YM, Chan LY, Lo KW, et al. Quantitative analysis of cell-free Epstein-Barr virus DNA in plasma of patients with nasopharyngeal carcinoma. *Cancer Res* 1999;59:1188–1191.

35. Wei WI, Yuen AP, Ng RW, et al. Quantitative analysis of plasma cell-free Epstein-Barr virus DNA in nasopharyngeal carcinoma after salvage nasopharyngectomy: a prospective study. *Head Neck* 2004;26:878–883.

36. Chong VF, Mukherji SK, Ng SH, et al. Nasopharyngeal carcinoma: review of how imaging affects staging. *J Comput Assist Tomogr* 1999;23:984–993.

37. Sham JS, Cheung YK, Choy D, et al. Nasopharyngeal carcinoma: CT evaluation of patterns of tumor spread. *AJNR Am J Neuroradiol* 1991;12:265–270.

38. Chong VF, Fan YF, Khoo JB. Nasopharyngeal carcinoma with intracranial spread: CT and MR characteristics. *J Comput Assist Tomogr* 1996;20:563–569.

39. Fang FM, Leung SW, Wang CJ, et al. Computed tomography findings of bony regeneration after radiotherapy for nasopharyngeal carcinoma with skull base destruction: implications for local control. *Int J Radiat Oncol Biol Phys* 1999;44:305–309.

40. Dillon WP, Mills CM, Kjos B, et al. Magnetic resonance imaging of the nasopharynx. *Radiology* 1984;152:731–738.

41. Cheng SH, Jian JJ, Tsai SY, et al. Prognostic features and treatment outcome in locoregionally advanced nasopharyngeal carcinoma following concurrent chemotherapy and radiotherapy. *Int J Radiat Oncol Biol Phys* 1998;41:755–762.

42. Cellai E, Olmi P, Chiavacci A, et al. Computed tomography in nasopharyngeal carcinoma. Part II: Impact on survival. *Int J Radiat Oncol Biol Phys* 1990;19:1177–1182.

43. Emami B, Sethi A, Petruzzelli GJ. Influence of MRI on target volume delineation and IMRT planning in nasopharyngeal carcinoma. *Int J Radiat Oncol Biol Phys* 2003;57:481–488.

44. Chong VF, Fan YF. Detection of recurrent nasopharyngeal carcinoma: MR imaging versus CT. *Radiology* 1997;202:463–470.

45. Ng SH, Chang JT, Ko SF, et al. MRI in recurrent nasopharyngeal carcinoma. *Neuroradiology* 1999;41:855–862.

46. Yen RF, Hung RL, Pan MH, et al. 18-fluoro-2-deoxyglucose positron emission tomography in detecting residual/recurrent nasopharyngeal carcinomas and comparison with magnetic resonance imaging. *Cancer* 2003;98:283–287.

47. Kraiphibul P, Atichartakarn V, Clongsusuek P, et al. Nasopharyngeal carcinoma: value of bone and liver scintigraphy in the pretreatment and follow-up period. *J Med Assoc Thai* 1991;74:276–279.

48. Sham JS, Chan LC, Loke SL, et al. Nasopharyngeal carcinoma: role of marrow biopsy at diagnosis. *Oncology* 1991;48:480–482.

49. Kumar MB, Lu JJ, Loh KS, et al. Tailoring distant metastatic imaging for patients with clinically localized undifferentiated nasopharyngeal carcinoma. *Int J Radiat Oncol Biol Phys* 2004;58:688–693.

50. Ho JHC. An epidemiologic and clinical study of nasopharyngeal carcinoma. *Int J Radiat Oncol Biol Phys* 1978;4:182–198.

51. Lee AW, Foo W, Law SC, et al. Staging of nasopharyngeal carcinoma: from Ho's to the new UICC system. *Int J Cancer* 1999;84:179–187.

52. Cooper JS, Cohen R, Stevens RE. A comparison of staging systems for nasopharyngeal cancer. *Cancer* 1998;83, 213–219.

53. Özyar E, Yildiz F, Akyol FH, et al. Comparison of AJCC 1988 and 1997 classifications for nasopharyngeal carcinoma. *Int J Radiat Oncol Biol Phys* 1999;44:1079–1087.

54. Lee AW, Sham JS, Poon YF, et al. Treatment of stage I nasopharyngeal carcinoma: analysis of the patterns of relapse and the results of withholding elective neck irradiation. *Int J Radiat Oncol Biol Phys* 1989;17:1183–1190.

55. Kwong D, Sham J, Choy D. The effect of loco-regional control on distant metastatic dissemination in carcinoma of the nasopharynx: an analysis of 1301 patients. *Int J Radiat Oncol Biol Phys* 1994;30:1029–1036.

56. Mesic JB, Fletcher GH, Goepfert H. Megavoltage irradiation of epithelial tumors of the nasopharynx. *Int J Radiat Oncol Biol Phys* 1981;7:447–453.

57. Hoppe RT, Goffinet DR, Bagshaw MA. Carcinoma of the nasopharynx. Eighteen years' experience with megavoltage radiation therapy. *Cancer* 1976;37:2605–2612.

58. Chua DT, Sham JS, Wei WI, et al. The predictive value of the 1997 American Joint Committee on Cancer stage classification in determining failure patterns in nasopharyngeal carcinoma. *Cancer* 2001;92:2845–2855.

59. Lee AW, Poon YF, Foo W, et al. Retrospective analysis of 5037 patients with nasopharyngeal carcinoma treated during 1976–1985: overall survival and patterns of failure. *Int J Radiat Oncol Biol Phys* 1992;23:261–270.

60. Levendag PC, Lagerwaard FJ, de Pan C, et al. High-dose, high-precision treatment options for boosting cancer of the nasopharynx. *Radiother Oncol* 2002;63:67–74.

61. Le QT, Tate D, Koong A, et al. Improved local control with stereotactic radiosurgical boost in patients with nasopharyngeal carcinoma. *Int J Radiat Oncol Biol Phys* 2003;56:1046–1054.

62. Chua DT, Sham JS, Kwong PW, et al. Linear accelerator-based stereotactic radiosurgery for limited, locally persistent, and recurrent nasopharyngeal carcinoma: efficacy and complications. *Int J Radiat Oncol Biol Phys* 2003;56:177–183.

63. Waldron J, Tin MM, Keller A, et al. Limitation of conventional two dimensional radiation therapy planning in nasopharyngeal carcinoma. *Radiother Oncol* 2003;68:153–161.

64. Cheng JC, Chao KS, Low D. Comparison of intensity modulated radiation therapy (IMRT) treatment techniques for nasopharyngeal carcinoma. *Int J Cancer* 2001;96:126–131.

65. Wu VW, Kwong DL, Sham JS. Target dose conformity in 3-dimensional conformal radiotherapy and intensity modulated radiotherapy. *Radiother Oncol* 2004;71:201–206.

66. Hsiung CY, Yorke ED, Chui CS, et al. Intensity-modulated radiotherapy versus conventional three-dimensional conformal radiotherapy for boost or salvage treatment of nasopharyngeal carcinoma. *Int J Radiat Oncol Biol Phys* 2002;53:638–647.

67. Lee N, Xia P, Quivey JM, Sultanem K, et al. Intensity-modulated radiotherapy in the treatment of nasopharyngeal carcinoma: an update of the UCSF experience. *Int J Radiat Oncol Biol Phys* 2002;53:12–22.

68. Kwong DL, Pow EH, Sham JS, et al. Intensity-modulated radiotherapy for early-stage nasopharyngeal carcinoma: a prospective study on disease control and preservation of salivary function. *Cancer* 2004;101:1584–1593.

69. Lu TX, Mai WY, Teh BS, et al. Initial experience using intensity-modulated radiotherapy for recurrent nasopharyngeal carcinoma. *Int J Radiat Oncol Biol Phys* 2004;58:682–687.

70. Lee AW, Sze WM, Yau TK, et al. Retrospective analysis on treating nasopharyngeal carcinoma with accelerated fractionation (6 fractions per week) in comparison with conventional fractionation (5 fractions per week): report on 3-year tumor control and normal tissue toxicity. *Radiother Oncol* 2001;58:121–130.

71. Franchin G, Vaccher E, Talamini R, et al. Nasopharyngeal cancer WHO type II-III: monoinstitutional retrospective analysis with

standard and accelerated hyperfractionated radiation therapy. *Oral Oncol* 2002;38:137–144.

72. Wolden SL, Zelefsky MJ, Kraus DH, et al. Accelerated concomitant boost radiotherapy and chemotherapy for advanced nasopharyngeal carcinoma. *J Clin Oncol* 2001;19:1105–1110.

73. Jian JJ, Cheng SH, Tsai SY, et al. Improvement of local control of T3 and T4 nasopharyngeal carcinoma by hyperfractionated radiotherapy and concomitant chemotherapy. *Int J Radiat Oncol Biol Phys* 2002;53:344–352.

74. Al-Sarraf M, Leblanc M, Giri PG, et al. Chemoradiotherapy versus radiotherapy in patients with advanced nasopharyngeal cancer: phase III randomized intergroup study 0099. *J Clin Oncol* 1998; 16:1310–1317.

75. Lin JC, Jan JS, Hsu CY, et al. Phase III study of concurrent chemodiotherapy versus radiotherapy alone for advanced nasopharyngeal carcinoma: positive effect on overall and progression-free survival. *J Clin Oncol* 2003;21:631–637.

76. International Nasopharynx Cancer Study Group VUMCA I trial. Preliminary results of a randomized trial comparing neoadjuvant chemotherapy (cisplatin, epirubicin, bleomycin) plus radiotherapy vs. radiotherapy alone in stage IV(> or = N2, M0) undifferentiated nasopharyngeal carcinoma: a positive effect on progression-free survival. *Int J Radiat Oncol Biol Phys* 1996;35: 463–469.

77. Ma J, Mai HQ, Hong MH, et al. Results of a prospective randomized trial comparing neoadjuvant chemotherapy plus radiotherapy with radiotherapy alone in patients with locoregionally advanced nasopharyngeal carcinoma. *J Clin Oncol* 2001;19: 1350–1357.

78. Chua DT, Sham JST, Choy D, et al. Preliminary report of the Asian-Oceanian Clinical Oncology Association randomized trial comparing cisplatin and epirubicin followed by radiotherapy versus radiotherapy alone in the treatment of patients with locoregionally advanced nasopharyngeal carcinoma. *Cancer* 1998;83: 2270–2283.

79. Hareyama M, Sakata K, Shirato H, et al. A prospective, randomized trial comparing neoadjuvant chemotherapy with radiotherapy alone in patients with advanced nasopharyngeal carcinoma. *Cancer* 2002;94:2217–2223.

80. Rossi A, Molinari R, Boracchi P, et al. Adjuvant chemotherapy with vincristine, cyclophosphamide, and doxorubicin after radiotherapy in local-regional nasopharyngeal cancer: results of a 4-year multicenter randomized study. *J Clin Oncol* 1988;6: 1401–1410.

81. Chi KH, Chang YC, Guo WY, et al. A phase III study of adjuvant chemotherapy in advanced nasopharyngeal carcinoma patients. *Int J Radiat Oncol Biol Phys* 2002;52:1238–1244.

82. Oh JL, Vokes EE, Kies MS, et al. Induction chemotherapy followed by concomitant chemoradiotherapy in the treatment of locoregionally advanced nasopharyngeal cancer. *Ann Oncol* 2003; 14:564–569.

83. Chua DT, Sham JS, Au GK. A concurrent chemoirradiation with cisplatin followed by adjuvant chemotherapy with ifosfamide, 5-fluorouracil, and leucovorin for stage IV nasopharyngeal carcinoma. *Head Neck* 2004;26:118–126.

84. Fang FM, Chiu HC, Kuo WR, et al. Health-related quality of life for nasopharyngeal carcinoma patients with cancer-free survival after treatment. *Int J Radiat Oncol Biol Phys* 2002;53:959–968.

85. McMillan AS, Pow EH, Leung WK, et al. Oral health-related quality of life in southern Chinese following radiotherapy for nasopharyngeal carcinoma. *J Oral Rehabil* 2004;31:600–608

86. Lam KS, Tse VK, Wang C, et al. Effects of cranial irradiation on hypothalamic-pituitary function—a 5-year longitudinal study in patients with nasopharyngeal carcinoma. *Q J Med* 1991;78:165–176.

87. Ho WK, Wei WI, Kwong DL, et al. Long-term sensorineural hearing deficit following radiotherapy in patients suffering from nasopharyngeal carcinoma: a prospective study. *Head Neck* 1999;21: 547–553.

88. Pow EH, McMillan AS, Leung WK, et al. Salivary gland function and xerostomia in southern Chinese following radiotherapy for nasopharyngeal carcinoma. *Clin Oral Invest* 2003;7: 230–234.

89. Pow EH, McMillan AS, Leung WK, et al. Oral health condition in southern Chinese after radiotherapy for nasopharyngeal carcinoma: extent and nature of the problem. *Oral Dis* 2003;9:196–202.

90. Leung SF, Zheng Y, Choi CY, et al. Quantitative measurement of post-irradiation neck fibrosis based on the young modulus: description of a new method and clinical results. *Cancer* 2002;95: 656–662.

91. Cheng SW, Ting AC, Lam LK, et al. Carotid stenosis after radiotherapy for nasopharyngeal carcinoma. *Arch Otolaryngol Head Neck Surg* 2000;126:517–521.

92. Lee AW, Kwong DL, Leung SF, et al. Factors affecting risk of symptomatic temporal lobe necrosis: significance of fractional dose and treatment time. *Int J Radiat Oncol Biol Phys* 2002;53:75–85.

93. Lin YS, Jen YM, Lin JC. Radiation-related cranial nerve palsy in patients with nasopharyngeal carcinoma. *Cancer* 2002;95:404–409.

94. Lam LC, Leung SF, Chan YL. Progress of memory function after radiation therapy in patients with nasopharyngeal carcinoma. *J Neuropsychiatry Clin Neurosci* 2003;15:90–97.

95. Cheung M, Chan AS, Law SC, et al. Cognitive function of patients with nasopharyngeal carcinoma with and without temporal lobe radionecrosis. *Arch Neurol* 2000;57:1347–1352.

96. Lee PW, Hung BK, Woo EK, et al. Effects of radiation therapy on neuropsychological functioning in patients with nasopharyngeal carcinoma. *J Neurol Neurosurg Psychiatry* 1989;52:488–492.

97. Kwong DL, Sham JS, Au GK, et al. Concurrent and adjuvant chemotherapy for nasopharyngeal carcinoma: a factorial study. *J Clin Oncol* 2004;22:2643–2653.

98. Yen RF, Hung RL, Pan MH, et al. 18-fluoro-2-deoxyglucose positron emission tomography in detecting residual/recurrent nasopharyngeal carcinomas and comparison with magnetic resonance imaging. *Cancer* 2003;98:283–287.

99. Kao CH, Tsai SC, Wang JJ, et al. Comparing 18-fluoro-2-deoxyglucose positron emission tomography with a combination of technetium 99m tetrofosmin single photon emission computed tomography and computed tomography to detect recurrent or persistent nasopharyngeal carcinomas after radiotherapy. *Cancer* 2001;92:434–439.

100. Chua DT, Sham JS, Kwong DL, et al. Locally recurrent nasopharyngeal carcinoma: treatment results for patients with computed tomography assessment. *Int J Radiat Oncol Biol Phys* 1998;41: 379–386.

101. Kwong DL, Nicholls J, Wei WI, et al. The time course of histologic remission after treatment of patients with nasopharyngeal carcinoma. *Cancer* 1999;85:1446–1453.

102. Wei WI, Ho CM, Wong MP, et al. Pathological basis of surgery in the management of postradiotherapy cervical metastasis in nasopharyngeal carcinoma. *Arch Otolaryngol Head Neck Surg* 1992; 118:923–929.

103. Chua DT, Wei WI, Sham JS, et al. Treatment outcome for synchronous locoregional failures of nasopharyngeal carcinoma. *Head Neck* 2003;25:585–594.

104. Huang SC, Lui LT, Lynn TC. Nasopharyngeal cancer: study III. A review of 1206 patients treated with combined modalities. *Int J Radiat Oncol Biol Phys* 1985;11:1789–1793.

105. Sham JS, Choy D. Nasopharyngeal carcinoma: treatment of neck node recurrence by radiotherapy. *Australas Radiol* 1991;35: 370–373

106. Wei WI, Lam KH, Ho CM, et al. Efficacy of radical neck dissection for the control of cervical metastasis after radiotherapy for nasopharyngeal carcinoma. *Am J Surg* 1990;160:439–442.

107. Wei WI, Ho WK, Cheng AC, et al. Management of extensive cervical nodal metastasis in nasopharyngeal carcinoma after radiotherapy: a clinicopathological study. *Arch Otolaryngol Head Neck Surg* 2001;127:1457–1462.

108. Lee AW, Law SC, Foo W, et al. Retrospective analysis of patients with nasopharyngeal carcinoma treated during 1976–1985: survival after local recurrence. *Int J Radiat Oncol Biol Phys* 1993;26: 773–782.

109. Yau TK, Sze WM, Lee WM, et al. Effectiveness of brachytherapy and fractionated stereotactic radiotherapy boost for persistent nasopharyngeal carcinoma. *Head Neck* 2004;26:1024–1030.

110. Xiao J, Xu G, Miao Y. Fractionated stereotactic radiosurgery for 50 patients with recurrent or residual nasopharyngeal carcinoma. *Int J Radiat Oncol Biol Phys* 2001;51:164–170.

111. Wang CC, Busse J, Gitterman M. A simple afterloading applicator for intracavitary irradiation of carcinoma of the nasopharynx. *Radiology* 1975;115:737–738.

112. Law SC, Lam WK, Ng MF, et al. Reirradiation of nasopharyngeal carcinoma with intracavitary mold brachytherapy: an effective means of local salvage. *Int J Radiat Oncol Biol Phys* 2002;54: 1095–1113.

113. Harrison LB, Weissberg JB. A technique for interstitial nasopharyngeal brachytherapy. *Int J Radiat Oncol Biol Phys* 1987;13: 451–453.

114. Wei WI, Sham JS, Choy D, et al. Split-palate approach for gold grain implantation in nasopharyngeal carcinoma. *Arch Otolaryngol Head Neck Surg* 1990;116:578–582.

115. Choy D, Sham JS, Wei WI, et al. Transpalatal insertion of radioactive gold grain for the treatment of persistent and recurrent nasopharyngeal carcinoma. *Int J Radiat Oncol Biol Phys* 1993;25: 505–512.

116. Kwong DL, Wei WI, Cheng AC, et al. Long term results of radioactive gold grain implantation for the treatment of persistent and recurrent nasopharyngeal carcinoma. *Cancer* 2001;91: 1105–1113.

117. Fisch U. The infratemporal fossa approach for nasopharyngeal tumors. *Laryngoscope* 1983;93:36–44.

118. Fee Jr WE, Roberson Jr JB, Goffinet DR. Long-term survival after surgical resection for recurrent nasopharyngeal cancer after radiotherapy failure. *Arch Otolaryngol Head Neck Surg* 1991;117: 1233–1236.

119. Morton RP, Liavaag PG, McLean M, et al. Transcervico-mandibulo-palatal approach for surgical salvage of recurrent nasopharyngeal cancer. *Head Neck* 1996;18:352–358.

120. Wei WI, Lam KH, Sham JS. New approach to the nasopharynx: the maxillary swing approach. *Head Neck* 1991;13:200–207

121. Fee Jr WE, Moir MS, Choi EC, et al. Nasopharyngectomy for recurrent nasopharyngeal cancer: a 2- to 17-year follow-up. *Arch Otolaryngol Head Neck Surg* 2002;128:280–284.

122. Wei WI. Nasopharyngeal cancer: current status of management. *Arch Otolaryngol Head Neck Surg* 2001;127:766–769.

123. Leung TW, Tung SY, Sze WK, et al. Salvage radiation therapy for locally recurrent nasopharyngeal carcinoma. *Int J Radiat Oncol Biol Phys* 2000;48:1331–1338.

124. Poon D, Yap SP, Wong ZW, et al. Concurrent chemoradiotherapy in locoregionally recurrent nasopharyngeal carcinoma. *Int J Radiat Oncol Biol Phys* 2004;59:1312–1318.

125. Wang TL, Tan YO. Cisplatin and 5-fluorouracil continuous infusion for metastatic nasopharyngeal carcinoma. *Ann Acad Med Singapore* 1991;20:601–603.

126. Fandi A, Bachouchi M, Azli N, et al. Long-term disease-free survivors in metastatic undifferentiated carcinoma of nasopharyngeal type. *J Clin Oncol* 2000;18:1324–1330.

127. Chua DT, Sham JS, Au GK. A phase II study of capecitabine in patients with recurrent and metastatic nasopharyngeal carcinoma pretreated with platinum-based chemotherapy. *Oral Oncol* 2003; 39:361–366.

128. Ngan RK, Yiu HH, Lau WH, et al. Combination gemcitabine and cisplatin chemotherapy for metastatic or recurrent nasopharyngeal carcinoma: report of a phase II study. *Ann Oncol* 2002;13: 1252–1258.

129. Taamma A, Fandi A, Azli N, et al. Phase II trial of chemotherapy with 5-fluorouracil, bleomycin, epirubicin, and cisplatin for patients with locally advanced, metastatic, or recurrent undifferentiated carcinoma of the nasopharyngeal type. *Cancer* 1999;86: 1101–1108.

130. Cheng LC, Sham JS, Chiu CS, et al. Surgical resection of pulmonary metastases from nasopharyngeal carcinoma. *Aust N Z J Surg* 1996;66:71–73.

131. Kwan WH, Teo PM, Chow LT, et al. Nasopharyngeal carcinoma with metastatic disease to mediastinal and hilar lymph nodes: an indication for more aggressive treatment. *Clin Oncol (R Coll Radiol)* 1996;8:55–58.

132. Li JH, Chia M, Shi W, et al. Tumor-targeted gene therapy for nasopharyngeal carcinoma. *Cancer Res* 2002;62:171–178.

133. Duraiswamy J, Sherritt M, Thomson S, et al. Therapeutic LMP1 polyepitope vaccine for EBV-associated Hodgkin disease and nasopharyngeal carcinoma. *Blood* 2003;101(8):3150–3156.

134. Chua D, Huang J, Zheng B, et al. Adoptive transfer of autologous Epstein-Barr virus-specific cytotoxic T cells for nasopharyngeal carcinoma. *Int J Cancer* 2001;94:73–80.

135. Ho JH. *Stage classification of nasopharyngeal carcinoma: a review.* International Agency for Research on Cancer, Publication No. 20, 1978;99–113.

136. Fleming ID, Cooper JS, Henson DE, et al., eds. *AJCC Cancer staging manual*, 5th ed. Philadelphia: Lippincott-Raven, 1997: 33–35.

Oropharyngeal Cancer

118

Christopher H. Rassekh   Hadi Seikaly

Cancer of the oropharynx is relatively uncommon, accounting for fewer than 1% of all new cancers. National cancer data is reported in a way that combines oral cavity sites with oropharyngeal sites, making the exact incidence of specific oropharyngeal primary site cancers somewhat difficult to determine. It has been estimated that just over 28,000 cases of oral cavity and pharyngeal cancer will be diagnosed in the United States in 2004 (1). Approximately one third of these will be expected to arise in the oropharynx. Its peak incidence is between the sixth and seventh decades of life; however, cases in the fifth and fourth decades of life are not uncommon. The disease has a distinct male predominance, but recent data show an increased incidence among women. Squamous cell carcinoma (SCC) and its variants account for more than 90% of malignant oropharyngeal lesions. The most important etiologic factor continues to be the prolonged exposure to tobacco and alcohol. Treatment of this disease is complex, and a team including a head and neck surgeon, reconstructive surgeon, radiation oncologist, medical oncologist, prosthodontist, and speech and language pathologist offers the patient the best opportunity for comprehensive treatment.

ANATOMY

The oropharynx is the midportion of the pharynx that connects the nasopharynx and oral cavity to the hypopharynx. It extends from an imaginary horizontal plane through the hard palate to another through the hyoid bone (Fig 118.1). Anteriorly, it opens to the oral cavity through the oral isthmus and is bound by the circumvallate papillae, anterior tonsillar pillars, and the junction of the hard and soft palates. Clinically, the oropharynx is divided into lateral walls or tonsillar regions, posterior wall, base of tongue, and soft palate. The pharyngeal walls are made of multiple layers: the mucosa, submucosa, pharyngobasilar fascia, constrictor muscles (superior and upper fibers of middle), and buccopharyngeal fascia. The superficial anatomy of the lateral walls includes the anterior tonsillar pillars with palatoglossus muscles, tonsillar fossae, posterior tonsillar pillars with palatopharyngeal muscles, and a small portion of lateral pharyngeal walls. The palatine tonsils lie in the tonsillar fossae, when present, and has an irregular surface filled with crypts, which are blind tubules of epithelium that invaginate deep within the tonsil.

The soft palate is a fibromuscular structure that projects posteriorly and downward into the oropharynx. It is composed of the palatine aponeurosis, which forms the skeleton; the tensor veli palatini, levator veli palatini, and uvular; palatoglossus; and palatopharyngeal muscles. The base of the tongue lies anteriorly in the oropharynx and extends from the circumvallate papillae to the pharyngoepiglottic and glossoepiglottic folds. The lingual tonsils lie superficial and lateral on either side and cause its mucosal surfaces to be irregular.

Most of the oropharynx is supplied with sensory and motor innervation through the glossopharyngeal (cranial nerve IX) and vagus (cranial nerve X) nerves. The hypoglossal nerve (cranial nerve XII) supplies motor innervation to the base of the tongue, and the trigeminal nerve (V2, V3) provides the motor and most of the sensory innervation to the soft palate.

The oropharynx is abundantly supplied with blood from most branches of the external carotid artery. The lymphatic drainage is primarily through levels II and III, with central structures such as the tongue base, soft palate, and posterior pharyngeal wall draining to both sides of the neck. The posterior pharyngeal wall and tonsillar region also drain to the retropharyngeal nodes, which in turn drain to the upper level II nodes.

The oropharynx is surrounded on three sides by potential fascial spaces. The retropharyngeal space is an area of loose connective tissue lying between the buccopharyngeal fascia of the pharynx and the alar layer of the prevertebral

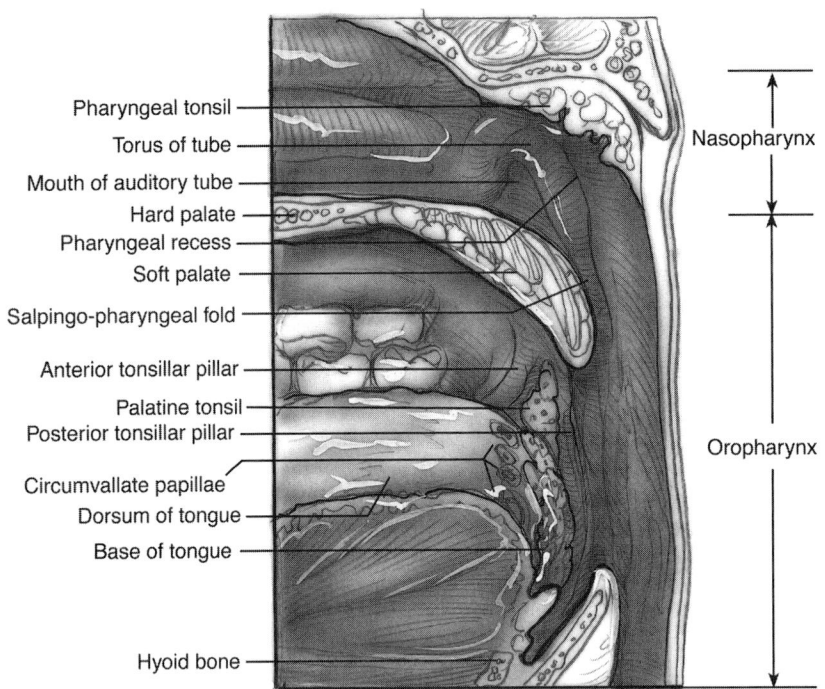

Pharyngeal tonsil

Torus of tube

Mouth of auditory tube

Hard palate

Pharyngeal recess

Soft palate

Salpingo-pharyngeal fold

Anterior tonsillar pillar

Palatine tonsil

Posterior tonsillar pillar

Circumvallate papillae

Dorsum of tongue

Base of tongue

Hyoid bone

Nasopharynx

Oropharynx

Figure 118.1 Surface anatomy of the oropharynx.

fascia. It extends from the skull base to the superior mediastinum and communicates with the parapharyngeal space laterally. The parapharyngeal space is defined by fascial planes extending from the skull base to the greater cornu of the hyoid bone and lying lateral to the pharyngeal walls. It has the shape of an inverted pyramid, and its boundaries include the skull superiorly, pterygomandibular raphe anteriorly, prevertebral fascia posteriorly, and the pharynx medially. The lateral boundary is the most complex and is formed by the fascia overlying the medial pterygoid muscle, a portion of the mandible, deep lobe of the parotid, and the posterior belly of the digastric muscle. This fascia extends superiorly, incorporating the stylomandibular ligament and fuses with the strong interpterygoid fascia to attach to the skull base in a line passing medial to the foramen ovale and spinosum. It also separates the parapharyngeal space from the infratemporal fossa and masticator space and places the trigeminal nerve within the latter (2). The parapharyngeal space can be further divided by a layer of fascia running from the tensor veli palatini muscle to the styloid and its related structures into two compartments. The prestyloid compartment contains fat, variable portions of the deep lobe of the parotid, and a small branch of the trigeminal nerve to the tensor veli palatini. The poststyloid compartment contains the carotid artery, jugular vein, cranial nerves IX to XII, sympathetic chain, and lymph nodes.

There are multiple aspects of oropharyngeal anatomy that are clinically important. The irregular surfaces of the tongue base and the tonsils make it difficult to identify small tumors. The vagus and glossopharyngeal nerves have tympanic and auricular branches (Jacobson and Arnold nerves), which cause the referred otalgia associated with tumors of this area.

The retropharyngeal and parapharyngeal spaces also serve as potential routes for cancer spread. Surgical margins may be difficult to achieve in some patients because of superior extension from the soft palate or oropharyngeal walls to the nasopharynx. Tumors that involve the palate or tonsillar pillar may invade or encase bone of the mandible or maxilla and the muscles of mastication when disease extends to the retromolar trigone, hard palate, or floor of mouth or becomes advanced in the parapharyngeal space.

PHYSIOLOGY

The oropharynx is essential for normal speech production, respiration, and deglutition. These functions require rapid, coordinated neuromuscular events of structures in the pharynx. Understanding these events is crucial for appropriate reconstruction and minimization of the sequelae associated with surgery.

Deglutition is the most complex of these functions and can be arbitrarily subdivided into four phases: (a) oral preparatory, (b) oral, (c) pharyngeal, and (d) esophageal. The oropharynx plays an important role in the first three phases. The soft palate is pulled forward while the tongue base is slightly elevated during both oral phases to prevent food from spilling prematurely into the pharynx. The food bolus at the end of the oral phase is propelled between the tongue and palate, past the tongue base and faucial arches, triggering the pharyngeal phase. This phase culminates with the propulsion of the food bolus into the esophagus through the following events: (a) velopharyngeal closure, (b) elevation and closure of the larynx, (c) contraction of the pharyngeal muscles and retraction of the tongue base, and (d) opening of the cricopharyngeal region. The major driving force of the bolus through the pharyngeal phase is the pressure developed by the tongue base; pharyngeal contraction and peristalsis serve mostly to clear the residual material present at the end (3).

Cancer surgery of the oropharynx may result in poor speech production, dysphagia, or aspiration. This is usually a result of velopharyngeal incompetence, pharyngeal stenosis, inappropriate functioning of the tongue base because of tethering or volume reduction, decreased pharyngeal contraction, or delayed triggering of the pharyngeal swallow because of decreased sensation. Most of these undesirable sequelae can be avoided with proper patient selection for surgery, appropriate reconstruction, and vigorous postoperative therapy.

ETIOLOGY

SCC of the head and neck is known to arise from the accumulation of multiple genetic alterations to genes important to the regulation of cellular growth and death. These alterations, which may be inherited but are more often acquired from exposure to environmental agents, provide the cell with a selective growth advantage. The cells then undergo further selection, which eventually results in a clone that overcomes the normal growth controls and host defenses to establish the tumor (4).

Multiple environmental factors are associated with SCC of the oropharynx, the most important of which are prolonged exposure to tobacco and alcohol. The effect of these agents is dose related, and concurrent exposure is synergistic, resulting in a risk that is greater than the sums of the risks of either one alone (5). Viruses have been shown to be a probable etiologic agent in development of SCC. The most extensively studied virus is human papillomavirus (HPV). HPV has been shown to be present in a subset of tonsillar cancers, many of which lacked the usual risk factors of tobacco and alcohol (6–9). Dietary factors such as vitamin deficiency, poor nutrition, poor oral hygiene, syphilis, occupational exposure, and previous irradiation also have been implicated as etiologic agents, but their effects are overshadowed by those of tobacco and alcohol.

Immunosuppression due to heredity, transplantation, or human immunodeficiency virus (10,11) may accelerate the development of SCC, lymphoma, and other tumors of the oropharynx by impairing normal immune surveillance mechanisms.

HISTOPATHOLOGY

Premalignant lesions occur in the oropharynx but to a lesser extent than in the oral cavity. These lesions are seen most commonly on the soft palate and anterior tonsillar pillars and include leukoplakia, erythroplakia, and lichen planus.

SCC and its variants account for more than 90% of malignant oropharyngeal lesions. The spindle cell variant is clinically and biologically similar to SCC, whereas others behave differently. Verrucous carcinoma is a fungating, slow-growing tumor with well-differentiated keratinizing epithelium and rare cellular atypia or mitosis on histology. These lesions erode into deep structures and rarely metastasize. Lymphoepithelioma grows rapidly and readily metastasizes. These lesions usually occur in the tonsillar region of young adults that do not have the typical risk factors. Adenoid squamous, adenosquamous, and basaloid SCCs are rare and highly aggressive variants, with the latter two having a propensity for early regional and distant metastasis. Lymphomas from the Waldeyer throat ring (usually the non-Hodgkin type), minor salivary gland tumors, mucosal melanomas, and sarcomas are other malignant lesions found in the oropharynx.

Some benign lesions, such as minor salivary gland tumors, pseudoepitheliomatous hyperplasia, necrotizing sialometaplasias, Crohn disease, papillomas, pyogenic granulomas, and median rhomboid glossitis may clinically mimic malignant lesions. They can often be diagnosed by history and physical examination but ultimately may require a biopsy.

NATURAL HISTORY

Prolonged exposure of the upper aerodigestive surfaces to carcinogens results in molecular changes throughout the mucosa. With time, certain areas may undergo further change, giving rise to premalignant and malignant lesions. This concept of "field cancerization" or "condemned mucosa" applies to all mucosal head and neck cancers and results in the high rates of second primaries in patients with oropharyngeal cancer (12) (Table 118.1).

SCC usually starts on the surface and spreads superficially, deeply, and submucosally. Invasion of vessels and thick fascia such as the prevertebral fascia or periosteum is uncommon until late stages, but perineural invasion may occur at any time. Bone involvement is also rare, occurring in only 17% of the lesions (13). Invasion into the parapharyngeal and retropharyngeal spaces allows easy spread to the skull base and neck with possible involvement of the internal carotid artery, cranial nerves IX through XII, and the sympathetic chain. Invasion of the masticator and infratemporal spaces results in trismus and possible involvement of the trigeminal nerve or any of its branches.

Lymphatic metastases at presentation are common because the oropharynx is richly supplied with lymphatics and the tumors are generally advanced (14) (Table 118.1).

Oropharyngeal cancers tend to metastasize in an orderly fashion from superiorly located first echelon nodes (level II, III, and retropharyngeal) inferiorly. This orderly

TABLE 118.1

THE INCIDENCE OF NODAL DISEASE AT PRESENTATION, SECOND PRIMARIES, AND DISTANT METASTASIS

Site	Palpable Nodes at Presentation	Second Primary[a]	Distant Metastasis[b]
Base of tongue	72%	19%	18%
Tonsillar region	58%	25%	15%
Soft palate	45%	26%	7.5%
Posterior wall	52%	29%	11%

[a]Incidence of synchronous and metachronous second primaries.
[b]Incidence of distant metastasis with control above the clavicles.

metastasis may be altered by obstruction of the lymphatic channels caused by inflammation, previous surgery, radiation, or large metastatic deposits. Oropharyngeal cancers have a tendency to metastasize to both necks, especially if the lesion is central. The rate of occult neck metastases in the clinically negative neck is estimated at greater than 20% for all lesions larger than T1.

Distant metastases are rare at presentation, occurring in 2% to 5% of patients, but with control of the disease above the clavicles, the incidence of overt distant metastasis increases (12,15) (Table 118.1). The most common sites affected by distant metastases are lung, liver, and bones.

DIAGNOSIS

History

A complete history, including a review of systems, past medical history, and social and family history, is essential in planning the proper therapy. Oropharyngeal cancer patients tend to have a prolonged history of tobacco and alcohol abuse and consequently suffer from cardiac, pulmonary, and liver disease.

Patients with oropharyngeal cancer tend to present with advanced disease because early lesions are usually asymptomatic. Pain and dysphagia are the most common presenting symptoms. Neck node enlargements are usually present at presentation but are the primary symptom in only 30% of the patients. Other symptoms include otalgia, foreign-body sensation, dysarthria, hemoptysis, and weight loss. Trismus and numbness in the distribution of V3 should alert the clinician of the possible involvement of the masticator space and mandible.

Physical Examination

A complete physical and a thorough head and neck examination should be routinely performed on all patients. Systematic visualization of all the mucosal surfaces of the upper aerodigestive tract is essential due to the field cancerization phenomenon. This examination is greatly facilitated by the use of a fiberoptic nasopharyngoscope,

especially in patients with trismus. The mandibular range of motion and cranial nerve function are also examined, with deficiencies indicating extension into the mandible, parapharyngeal, or masticator spaces. Palpation of the primary tumor to judge the extent of the lesion and submucosal spread is always performed. All the neck levels are systematically evaluated, and size, location, and fixation of nodes are noted. The patient's dentition is also assessed because restoration or extraction may be required before initiation of treatment.

Investigations

The extent of the tumor, neck metastasis, distant metastasis, and the medical condition of the patient should be assessed completely before a treatment plan is devised or implemented. The following radiologic studies are recommended:

1. Chest radiograph: to evaluate the lungs for metastasis, second primary tumors, and chronic changes associated with tobacco use.
2. Computed tomography (CT) and magnetic resonance imaging (MRI): These modalities are extremely useful but should not be used indiscriminately. They are indicated in the assessment of advanced-stage tumors or when involvement of the mandible, parapharyngeal space, prevertebral fascia, neck nodes, or retropharyngeal nodes is suspected. CT scanning is better suited for evaluating bony structures. MRI is best at evaluating soft tissue involvement, such as the tongue base, parapharyngeal space, or prevertebral fascia.
3. Panorex: This helps in detecting mandibular involvement and assessing the dentition of the patient.
4. Special tests: Barium swallow is performed on patients with dysphagia if esophagoscopy is not planned. Angiography with the balloon test occlusion and cerebral blood flow evaluation should be considered if the tumor involves the carotid and resection is contemplated. Positron emission tomography (PET) scan is now used extensively in cancer of the aerodigestive tract. However, its exact role in cancer at various oropharyngeal subsites is still not yet clear.

Laboratory evaluation of oropharyngeal cancer patients includes a complete blood count, blood chemistry, liver function tests, and an electrocardiogram. Nutritional evaluation may be included in this regimen if indicated by the patient's physical status.

Tissue diagnosis is obtained with fine-needle aspiration of enlarged nodes and/or biopsy of the oropharyngeal lesion. This can usually be performed in the office or clinic, but biopsy should be reserved for endoscopy in patients with trismus, tenuous airway, or lesions that are not easily accessible transorally.

Staging Endoscopy

Patients with epithelial primary tumors should undergo examination under anesthesia irrespective of the size of the tumor or the adequacy of the initial assessment. Complete visualization and palpation of the tumor greatly facilitates the assessment of submucosal spread and invasion of surrounding structures such as the prevertebral fascia and mandible, especially in patients with trismus. A thorough search for a synchronous second primary tumor, which occurs in approximately 8% of patients (15), is conducted via systematic examination of the upper aerodigestive tract and esophagus. Bronchoscopy is optional in patients with normal chest radiographs (16), but we usually perform a tracheobronchoscopy, because small lesions in the trachea or hilum are not readily seen on routine radiographs. Biopsies are performed at the end of the endoscopy to allow the examination to proceed unhindered by bleeding from the biopsy site. If lymphoma is suspected, the pathologist should be notified in advance and an adequate sample of tissue is submitted fresh to allow for receptor typing. The teeth are evaluated and restored or extracted as needed at the end of the procedure. The findings of endoscopy and tumor mapping then are recorded on preprinted forms with diagrams, and the patient is staged. Table 118.2 shows the tumor staging for the oropharynx. Many patients with oropharyngeal cancer present initially with an unknown primary with a cervical metastasis. Panendoscopy is crucial in these patients and tonsillectomy is recommended if the primary tumor is not

---

TABLE 118.2

TUMOR (T) STAGING FOR THE OROPHARYNX

Stage	Description
Tx:	Carcinoma in situ
T1:	Tumor 2 cm or less in greatest dimension
T2:	2–4 cm in greatest dimension
T3:	Greater than 4 cm in greatest dimension
T4a:	Tumor invades the larynx, deep/extrinsic muscles of the tongue, medial pterygoid, hard palate, or mandible
T4b:	Tumor invades lateral pterygoid muscle, pterygoid plates, lateral nasopharynx, skull base, or carotid artery

Greene FL, Page DL, Fleming ID, et al. AJCC Cancer Staging manual, 6th ed. New York: Springer, 2002.

TABLE 118.3   🄳 DIAGNOSIS
OROPHARYNGEAL CANCER

1. History
   Alcohol and tobacco abuse
   Pain and dysphagia
2. Physical
   Nodal enlargement
   Trismus
   Cranial nerve deficits
3. Biopsy of the primary lesion and fine needle aspiration of enlarged nodes
4. Imaging studies
   Chest radiograph
   CT scan/MRI
   Panorex
   PET scan
5. Laboratory studies
   Complete blood count and chemistry
   Liver function tests
   ECG
6. Examination under anesthesia
   Examination of all the aerodigestive mucosa for second primaries
   Assessment of submucosal spread, mandibular invasion, and tumor fixation

---

CT, computed tomography; MRI, magnetic resonance imaging; ECG, electrocardiography; PET, positron emission tomography.

---

found (Table 118.3). The neck staging and stage groupings are the same as other sites of the head and neck.

TREATMENT

The treatment of oropharyngeal cancer patients is complex, and a team including a head and neck surgeon, reconstructive surgeon, radiation oncologist, medical oncologist, prosthodontist, and speech and language pathologist offers the patient the best opportunity for a comprehensive treatment plan. The surgeon must consider an array of factors when deciding on the optimal regimen for the individual patient. These include the type of treatment needed for the primary tumor and the neck, the modality best suited for functional preservation or restoration, the general medical condition of the patient, and, most important, the patient's preferences. The availability of facilities, expertise, and social support also play a role (Table 118.4). All patients should be counseled and aided in cessation of smoking and alcohol consumption at the time of diagnosis.

Squamous Cell Carcinoma

Surgery and radiation therapy, alone or combined, have been the mainstays of treatment for squamous cell oropharyngeal cancer. Newer approaches using concurrent chemotherapy with radiotherapy for advanced cancers of the oropharynx are gaining popularity. Currently, multicenter

TABLE 118.4 ℞ **TREATMENT OROPHARYNGEAL CANCER**

1. Team approach
2. Primary tumor treatment
   a. T1 and T2: surgery or radiation
   b. T3 and T4: combined modality (chemoradiation or surgery and postoperative radiation)
3. Neck treatment
   a. N0 and N1: surgery or radiation
   b. N2 and N3: combined modality (surgery and postoperative chemoradiation or chemoradiation and planned neck dissection)
   c. Both sides of neck are treated with central lesions
   d. Retropharyngeal nodes are always treated

TABLE 118.5

INDICATIONS FOR POSTOPERATIVE RADIATION (+/− CHEMO)

Tumor factors
1. Close or involved resection margins
2. Perineural or vascular invasion
3. T3
4. T4
Neck factors
1. Clinically N0 or N1 neck
   a. Two or more histologically positive nodes
   b. Histologically positive nodes at multiple sites
   c. Perineural or vascular invasion
   d. Extracapsular nodal spread
2. N2
3. N3

prospective trials data using organ preservation strategies for oropharyngeal carcinoma have not been as extensively validated as those for laryngeal cancer. One meta-analysis of more than 70 randomized trials demonstrated a small significant benefit on survival when chemotherapy is added to locoregional treatment (17). This favorable effect, however, was mainly due to concomitant or alternating chemoradiation use, with adjuvant and neoadjuvant chemotherapy providing no added benefit. A nonsignificant negative effect of chemotherapy on survival also was found in the organ preservation trials (17). Subsequent studies have demonstrated that concurrent chemoradiation offers good local and regional control, with similar survival rates compared with surgery and postoperative radiotherapy for advanced oropharyngeal carcinoma (18–22). One randomized trial did show a significant survival increase for patients by adding concurrent carboplatin and 5-fluorouracil to radiotherapy (22). Thus, routine use of concurrent chemotherapy and radiotherapy is now advocated as the preferred approach for organ preservation protocols. There are some data to suggest that chemotherapy and radiotherapy actually is more effective than surgery and postoperative radiotherapy (21). Although a recent cooperative group trial showed a benefit from adding chemotherapy to postoperative radiotherapy for high-risk patients, some patients cannot tolerate such intense treatment (23).

Primary Tumor

Surgery or radiation alone is equally effective for T1 and T2 oropharyngeal cancers. Regardless of which modality is used initially, the other may be used for salvage, resulting in high local control rates. Deeply infiltrative lesions and those that extend beyond the anterior tonsillar pillars or that have significant involvement of the base of the tongue are not controlled well with external beam radiation alone; therefore, primary surgery or the addition of brachytherapy or chemotherapy is preferred (24–26). Postoperative radiation is indicated if after resection the margins are involved or close or if the tumor exhibits aggressive behavior (27,28) (Table 118.5). The decision to treat even the smallest oropharyngeal primary with surgery alone is difficult because of the high risk of occult lymph

node metastasis in even very early stage lesions. Stage T3 and T4 tumors are best controlled with surgery and postoperative radiation, but concurrent chemoradiation or hyperfractionated radiotherapy are now reasonable alternatives for patients, especially those whose morbidity from surgery is deemed too high to tolerate the procedures and regain function.

Neck

All patients with oropharyngeal SCC more extensive than T1 require some treatment of the neck because of the high rate of clinically positive nodes and occult nodal metastasis at presentation. The choice of initial treatment modality (surgery or radiation) for the neck and retropharyngeal nodes is usually dictated by that used for the primary tumor. Stage N0 and N1 neck disease are effectively controlled with a single modality, but neck dissection has the added benefit of providing pathologic staging. The use of selective neck dissection in ruling out regional spread following transoral excision of the primary is not as reliable in oropharyngeal cancer as in oral cancer. This is due to the less predictable lymphatic pathways and the increased difficulty accessing the retropharyngeal nodes. For this reason, radiotherapy is often used even when the primary is treated surgically. Combined modality results in better regional control in stage N2 and N3 neck disease (23). Both necks should be treated when there is clinical disease in one side of the neck, the lesion is central, or crosses the midline. The retropharyngeal nodes must always be considered in the neck treatment plan.

Squamous Cell Variants and Other Oropharyngeal Cancers

The spindle cell variant is clinically and biologically similar to SCC, whereas the others behave differently and deserve further discussion. Verrucous carcinoma requires a wide local excision. Lymphoepitheliomas are treated primarily with radiation therapy regardless of stage because they are exquisitely sensitive to this modality. Surgery is reserved for salvage or persistent neck disease. Adenoid squamous, adenosquamous, and basaloid SCCs are best controlled with combined surgery and radiation. Primary tumors arise in the tonsillar fossae, tonsillar pillars, soft palate, posterior pharyngeal wall, and the base of tongue and vallecula. The tonsil fossa is the most common site with all other sites together accounting for less than half of the cases. Although there are some specific features that distinguish these primary sites, this chapter addresses the entire group of oropharyngeal cancers together, highlighting the specific surgical points for each subsite. There is significant overlap between subsites in terms of behavior and management. In fact, many tumors involve more than one subsite in the pharynx.. The reader is directed to other more specific cancer textbooks and journal articles cited in this chapter for more details about the specific management of each subsite.

Lymphomas are treated with chemotherapy and radiation (29). Malignant minor salivary gland tumors usually behave as their counterparts in the major salivary glands and are treated with wide local excisions with or without postoperative radiation. Melanomas and sarcomas are treated with wide local excision, and neck dissection is used for nodal involvement or surgical access.

Nonsurgical Management

Nonsurgical management consists of radiotherapy with or without concurrent chemotherapy. Most chemotherapy regimens are based on platinum agents. The radiation course usually consists of delivering a dose of 60 to 70 Gy through an external-beam shrinking field to the primary lesion and necks over a 6- to 7-week period. Other strategies, such as brachytherapy, hyperfractionation, and electron boost to the neck, are used in some centers to enhance the effectiveness of radiation therapy in more advanced lesions. Alternative methods of delivering radiation therapy, such as conformal and intensity-modulated radiation therapy (IMRT), have been described recently. These techniques require further development and study but have the potential to improve targeting of radiation to the tumor and high-risk areas with relative sparing of normal tissues such as salivary glands (30,31). Following nonsurgical organ preservation, patients who presented with N2 and N3 disease should probably undergo a neck dissection (32), but if a complete clinical response is obtained, there are data to support a watchful waiting approach as this usually predicts a complete histologic response (33).

Surgery

Primary Tumor

Most oropharyngeal tumors are amenable to surgical excision but become relatively unresectable after extension into the poststyloid parapharyngeal compartment, prevertebral fascia, or involvement of the carotid artery. Successful extirpation of oropharyngeal cancers hinges on good exposure and wide resection margins (1 to 2 cm),

because these tumors have the propensity for submucosal spread. Frozen-section clearance obtained of all the margins, including the depth of the resection. Patients with microscopically positive margins that are found intraoperatively or postoperatively after the permanent sections are examined should undergo 1-cm reresection of the involved margin if possible and adjuvant radiation therapy. Extensive tumors also may require management of the larynx for oncologic or aspiration purposes.

Oropharyngeal cancers can be resected through three surgical approaches: transoral, transpharyngeal, and transmandibular. The optimal approach depends on the size and site of the tumor.

Transoral Approaches

Oral. The oral approach to the oropharynx involves resection of the tumor through the open mouth with no external incisions. Caution should be exercised before recommending this approach because it provides limited exposure. It may be indicated for small (T1), superficial, or exophytic cancers of the upper or anterior sites of the oropharynx, such as lesions of the soft palate, anterior tonsillar pillar, and posterior wall. The surgeon must ensure that there is good visualization of not only the entire tumor but a 1- to 2-cm resection perimeter surrounding it on all sides, including the deep margin. Trismus, height of the mandible, and presence of teeth may further hinder visualization, making adequate resection almost impossible. Resections through this approach are quick and have minimal morbidity, but visualization of the posterior and deep resection margins tends to be very poor. For tumors that are difficult to access, the CO_2 laser is sometimes a valuable tool. Although tumors of the soft palate and tonsil may be removed with cautery, the laser is more precise. For tumors of the posterior pharyngeal wall and posterior tongue base and vallecula, otherwise inaccessible lesions may be resected transorally by using the laser and microscope. Recently, a large group of patients treated with laser resection for carcinoma of the base of tongue was reported (34). In this series, the local control was 100% for T1 and T2 lesions. Local failure occurred in 20% of patients with advanced primaries, but 5-year disease-free survival was 73% and function was preserved in the majority. This represents an interesting alternative to major open surgery and chemoradiation for advanced cancer and an adjunct to the armamentarium for early tumors.

Mandibular Lingual Release. The mandibular lingual release approach to the oropharynx is indicated for lesions confined mostly to the base of the tongue. The technique involves a standard apron flap elevated in the subplatysmal plane to the lower border of the mandible. Neck dissections are performed as needed. An incision is made through the lingual mucoperiosteum and the periosteum at the lower edge of the mandible (Fig. 118.2A). The anterior mandibular muscles are released with the periosteum from the inner

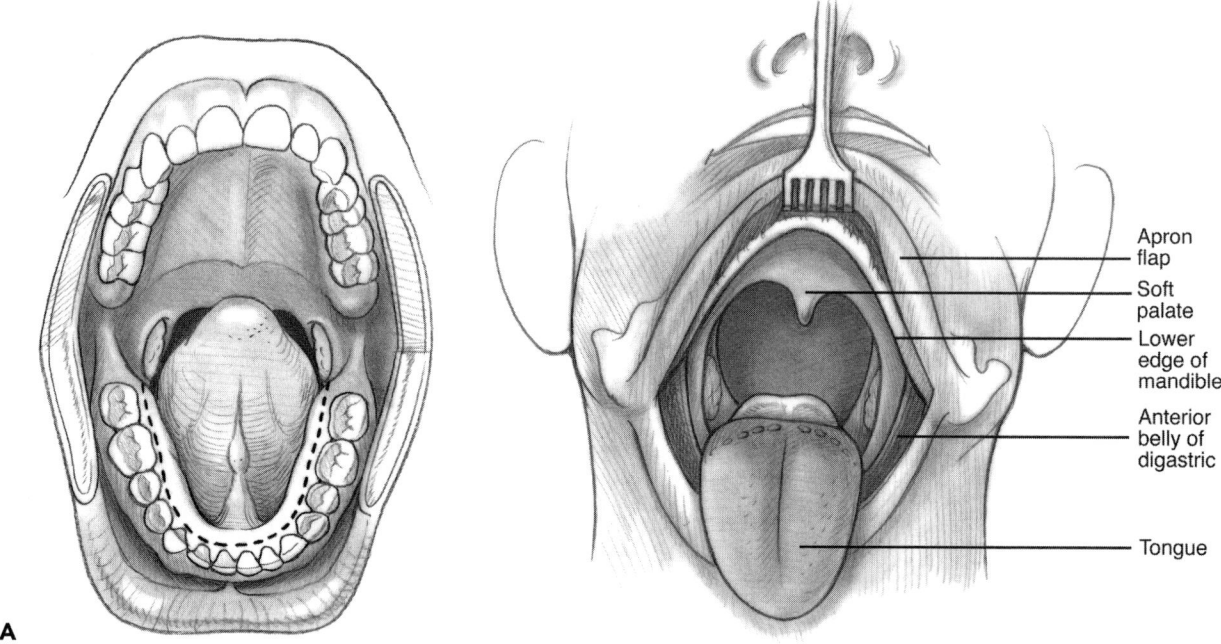

Apron
flap
Soft
palate
Lower
edge of
mandible
Anterior
belly of
digastric

Tongue

A   B

Figure 118.2 Mandibular lingual release. **A:** An incision is made through the lingual mucoperiosteum and the periosteum at the lower edge of the mandible. **B:** The anterior mandibular muscles are released with the periosteum from the inner mandibular table, delivering the tongue and floor of mouth into the neck.

mandibular table, delivering the tongue and floor of mouth into the neck. The lesion can then be resected with excellent direct visualization (Fig. 118.2B). This approach does not require mandibulotomy or a lower lip split, but it offers less access to the lateral pharynx and parapharyngeal spaces than the transmandibular approaches. The lingual arteries, lingual nerves, and hypoglossal nerves are also at risk for damage.

Transpharyngeal Approaches

Suprahyoid Pharyngotomy. The suprahyoid approach is useful for small tumors of the base of the tongue and pharyngeal walls. The pharynx is entered through the vallecula, and the resection is performed from the neck with preservation of the lingual arteries and the hypoglossal nerves (Fig. 118.3). The pharyngotomy also can be extended laterally and inferiorly along the thyroid ala to widen the exposure. This approach results in an excellent functional and cosmetic outcome, but the visualization of the superior margin in larger tumors is inadequate and there is a risk of cutting into cancer if there is extensive involvement of the tongue base or vallecula.

Lateral Pharyngotomy. The lateral pharyngotomy may be used for small lesions of the base of the tongue and pharyngeal walls. The pharynx is entered posterior to the thyroid ala on the least affected side. The hypoglossal and superior laryngeal nerves are dissected and retracted superiorly and inferiorly. Once the pharynx has been entered, the larynx is retracted to the opposite side, providing a good

view of the entire posterior pharyngeal wall, opposite lateral wall, and base of the tongue (Fig. 118.4A). Further superior exposure can be achieved by extending the pharyngotomy across the vallecula or by combining this approach with a lateral mandibulotomy (Fig. 118.4B). The disadvantages of this approach are the limited superior visualization and the risk of damage to the hypoglossal and superior laryngeal nerves. The lateral mandibulotomy also results in transection of the inferior alveolar nerve.

Transmandibular

Midline Labiomandibular Glossotomy. The midline labiomandibular glossotomy is rarely used and is useful only for small midline posterior pharyngeal wall cancers that are too low to reach through a transoral approach or small midline tongue base lesions. The approach involves splitting of the lip (35), gingiva, mandible, and anterior tongue in the midline. The incision can be carried through the base of tongue down to the hyoid bone if wide exposure of the posterior wall is required (Fig. 118.5). Bleeding and neurologic deficits are minimal because the hypoglossal nerves and lingual arteries are usually not disrupted. However, the approach does not provide access to the parapharyngeal space or lateral oropharyngeal sites.

Mandibular Swing Approach. The mandibular swing approach provides wide exposure to the entire oropharynx and allows an en bloc resection of the cancer and the draining nodes. It can be used for resecting a variety of

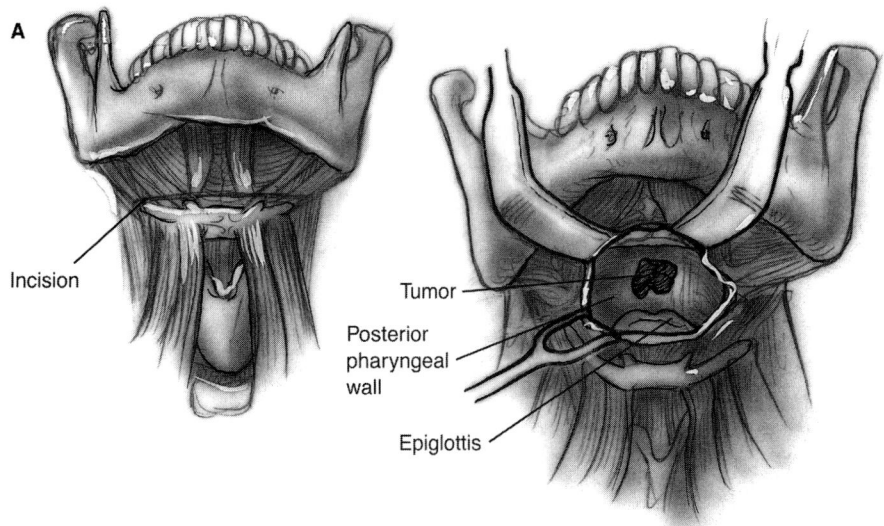

A

Incision

Tumor

Posterior
pharyngeal
wall

Epiglottis

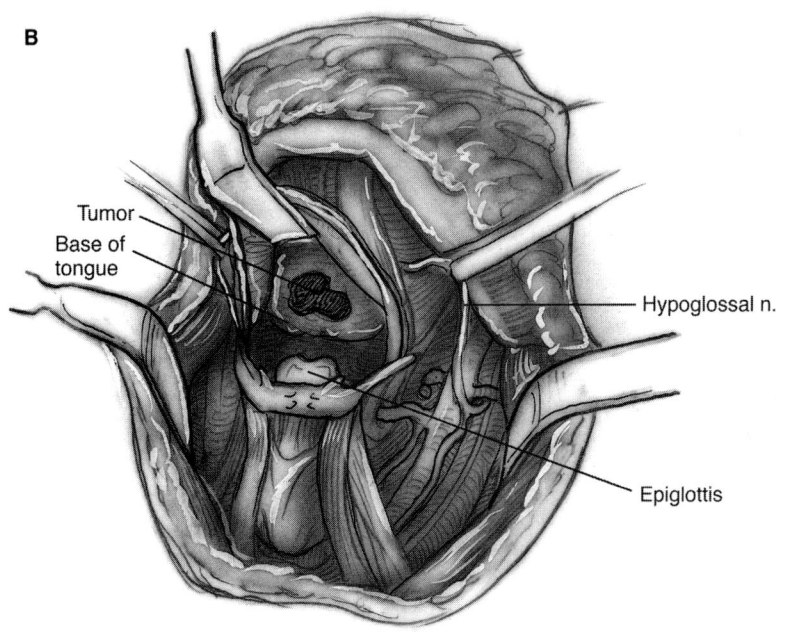

B

Tumor

Base of
tongue

Hypoglossal n.

Epiglottis

Figure 118.3 Suprahyoid pharyngotomy. **A:** Incision above the hyoid through the vallecula with exposure of the posterior pharyngeal wall. **B:** Exposure of the tongue base.

oropharyngeal cancers that do not involve the mandible, especially those that include multiple sites and the parapharyngeal space. The technique involves a standard apron flap elevated in the subplatysmal plane to the lower border of the mandible. Neck dissections are performed as needed, identifying the carotid sheath structures and lingual and hypoglossal nerves in the process. The lip then is split. Visor flaps to preserve the continuity of the lip should not be used because they require division of both mental nerves and result in suboptimal posterior exposure. The osteotomy is performed anterior to the mental nerve on the ipsilateral side through the site of a missing or extracted tooth. Lateral osteotomies that are posterior to the mental foramen are not recommended because they result in the division of the

inferior alveolar nerve and have more limited exposure. A full-thickness soft tissue cut then is made through the floor of the mouth and continued posteriorly to the anterior margin of resection, transecting the lingual nerve if needed. The mandibular segments and tongue are distracted, exposing the tumor and parapharyngeal space (Fig. 118.6). Closure of the soft tissue defect usually requires a flap, and the mandible is reapproximated using compression plates. The main disadvantage of using this approach is the potential sacrifice of the whole hemimandible if unsuspected mandibular involvement that is not amenable to a marginal resection is found after the mandibulotomy. This problem can be avoided in most cases by careful evaluation at endoscopy and review of the imaging modalities.

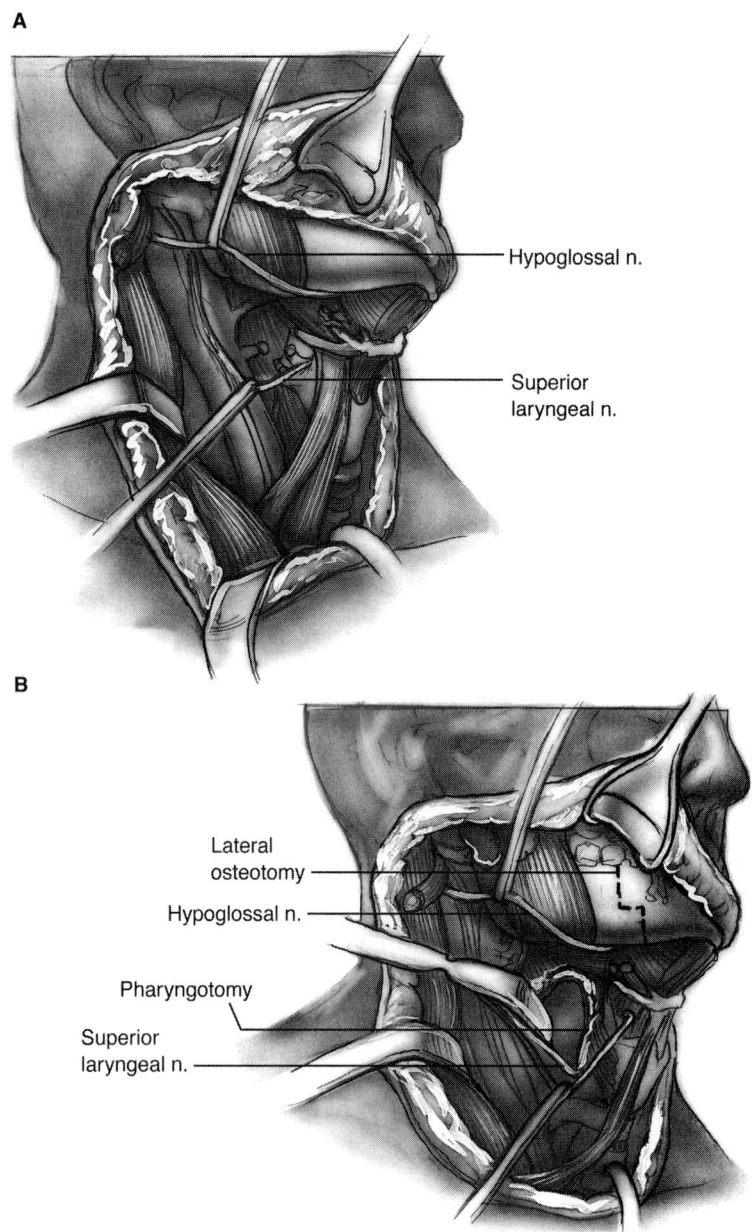

A

Hypoglossal n.

Superior
laryngeal n.

B

Lateral
osteotomy

Hypoglossal n.

Pharyngotomy

Superior
laryngeal n.

Figure 118.4 Lateral pharyngotomy. **A:** Retraction of the hypoglossal and superior laryngeal nerves. **B:** Exposure of the lower oropharynx and the hypopharynx. Further superior exposure is obtained with lateral mandibulotomy.

Mandibulectomy. Oropharyngeal composite resection with mandibulectomy is used in advanced cancers in which there is overt bony invasion or in situations in which mandibular invasion cannot be ruled out. Usually, the resection is preceded by a neck dissection, leaving the specimen attached to the inferior border of the angle of the mandible. The lip is divided and a cheek flap is developed by performing a full-thickness incision through the buccogingival sulcus. The uninvolved outer periosteum of the mandible may be left on the cheek flap. The anterior mandibular cut is performed well clear of the tumor (1 to 2 cm), preserving as much of the mandibular body as possible, and frozen sections of the inferior alveolar nerve are obtained. However, the entire mental canal must be re-sected, placing the mandibular body osteotomy anterior to the mental foramen, if there is overt mandibular canal invasion or hypesthesia in the inferior alveolar distribution, or if the nerve is positive on frozen section, because there is no reliable method of assessing bony tumor extension intraoperatively. The cranial mandibular cuts are placed along the ramus, but resection of the coronoid process and the condyle may be required with extensive tumors. The mandible then is retracted laterally, and the remaining tumor cuts are performed (Fig. 118.7). The main disadvantage of this approach is the resultant functional and cosmetic deficits, especially if the defect is closed primarily. Mandibulectomy and mandibulotomy approaches compare favorably (36).

A

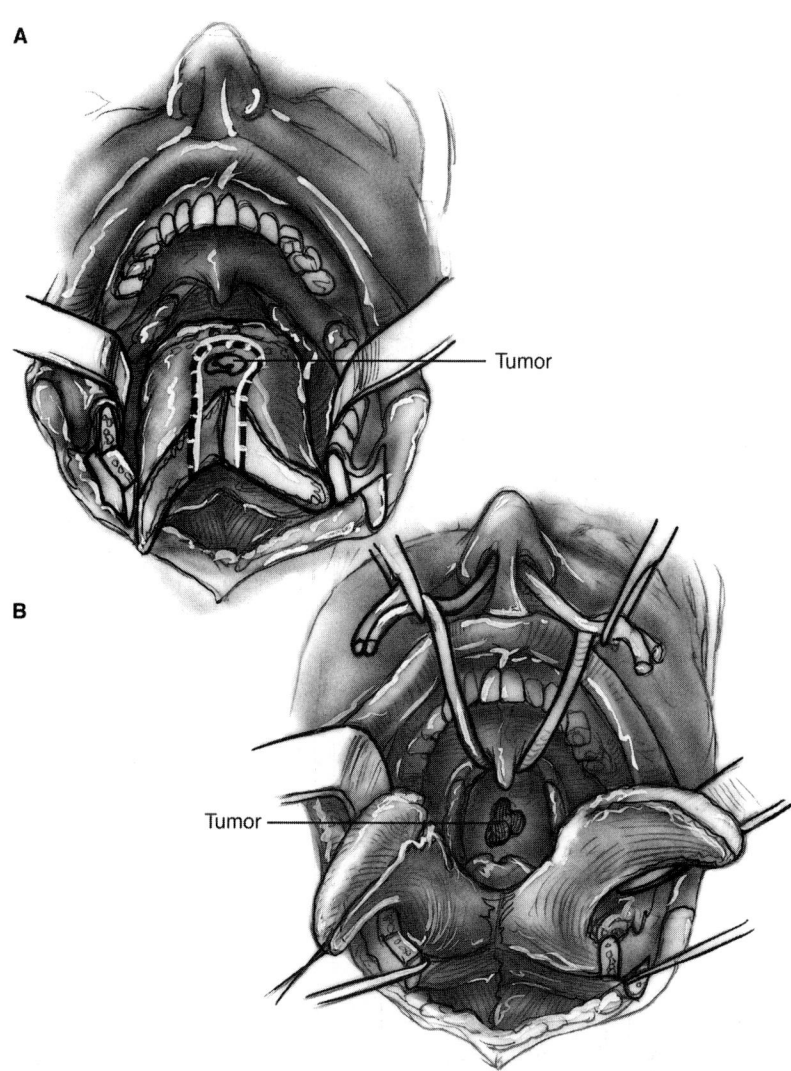

Tumor

B

Tumor

Figure 118.5 Midline labiomandibular glosso-tomy. **A:** The lip, mandible, and tongue are split in midline for a base of tongue lesion. **B:** Exposure of the posterior pharyngeal wall after division of the tongue base.

RECONSTRUCTION

The reconstruction of oropharyngeal cancer defects has been revolutionized in the past two decades by the development of pedicled regional myocutaneous flaps and free tissue transfer. The objective of modern reconstruction is to restore the integrity of the oropharynx and its essential functions of deglutition, respiration, and speech production.

Successful reconstruction requires the surgeon to have a detailed knowledge of the various reconstructive techniques and an understanding of their limitations. A variety of techniques have been described over the years (Table 118.6), but none has achieved the ideal reconstruction of replacing the resected structure with tissue that matches its form and function. The reconstructive capabilities at present are limited to restoration of integrity, bulk, and sensation, but the complex motor functions of the oropharynx cannot be duplicated.

The use of local flaps has decreased significantly in the past two decades as a result of the limited amount of tissue they provide and their inferior functional results

when compared with regional flaps and free tissue transfer. The regional flaps reliably provide abundant well-vascularized tissue that can be used for single-stage reconstruction, they are easy to harvest, and they do not require microvascular expertise. Their disadvantages include the limited superior reach, bulk, and the significant rate of marginal necrosis of the distal skin, especially with pectoralis major flaps. They also can rarely be tailored to reconstruct a defect that involves multiple sites. The free microvascular flaps overcome most deficiencies of the regional flaps and have the added advantage of sensory or motor reinnervation. The use of free tissue transfer along with conservative approaches to the mandible significantly decrease morbidity and length of hospitalization and result in improved function at a cost comparable with regional myocutaneous flaps (37–39). The main disadvantages of free microvascular flaps that have prevented them from wide acceptance by head and neck surgeons are the prolongation of operative time and the need for special expertise. A free skin graft is also often a very viable method (39).

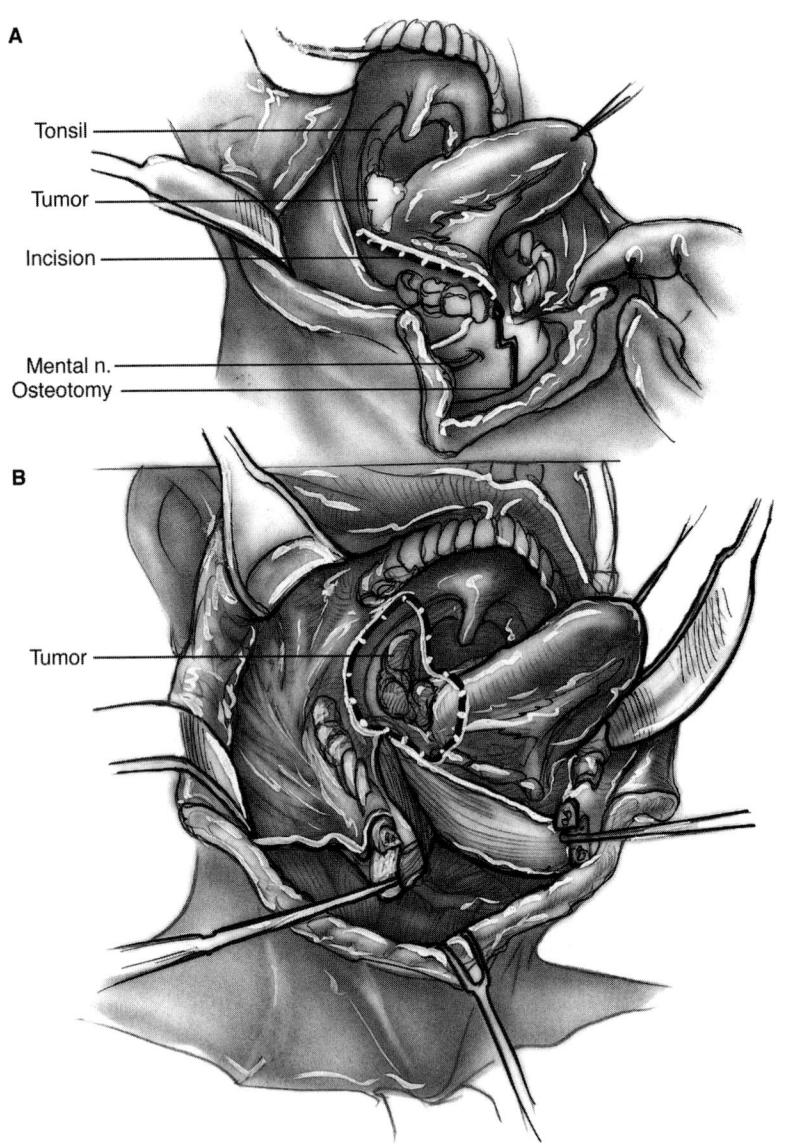

A

Tonsil

Tumor

Incision

Mental n.
Osteotomy

B

Tumor

Figure 118.6   Mandibular swing approach. **A:** Osteotomy is placed anterior to the mental foramen. **B:** The full thickness of the floor of the mouth is incised. The mandibular segments are then retracted laterally, allowing good access to the oropharyngeal structures and parapharyngeal space.

The other component essential for successful reconstruction is an intimate understanding of the ablated tissue's functional and cosmetic capacities. The tongue base is the structure most important to the function of the oropharynx, because it is responsible for pharyngeal closure during the oral phase and is the main driving force of the bolus through the pharyngeal phase (3). Optimal functional restoration requires the presence of at least one intact hypoglossal nerve and lingual artery to allow for mobility and survival of the remaining tongue. The reconstruction must restore some of the bulk, the glossopharyngeal fold, and ensure continued mobility of this organ (40,41). The pharyngeal walls help generate the pressure needed for appropriate movement of the food bolus and clear material remaining in the pharynx after a swallow. The remaining pharynx and the tongue can easily compensate for these functions after partial resection (42); therefore, a reconstruction that maintains the integrity of the pharynx and function of the base of the tongue is required. The soft palate is the most important component of the velopharyngeal mechanism, which also includes the lateral and posterior pharyngeal walls. Restoration of the soft palate's complex dynamic fibromuscular structure is not possible, but good velopharyngeal function is obtained if the reconstruction allows for the closure of the nasopharynx with swallowing and an opening of no more than 20 mm^2 during speech (43). Defects that involve multiple sites provide a considerable challenge, and elaborate techniques often are required to achieve the reconstructive objectives because of the different requirements of each site. Patients with extensive defects involving most of the oropharyngeal walls or tongue base may require laryngeal manipulation to prevent chronic aspiration, and their function is usually suboptimal, even after adequate reconstruction.

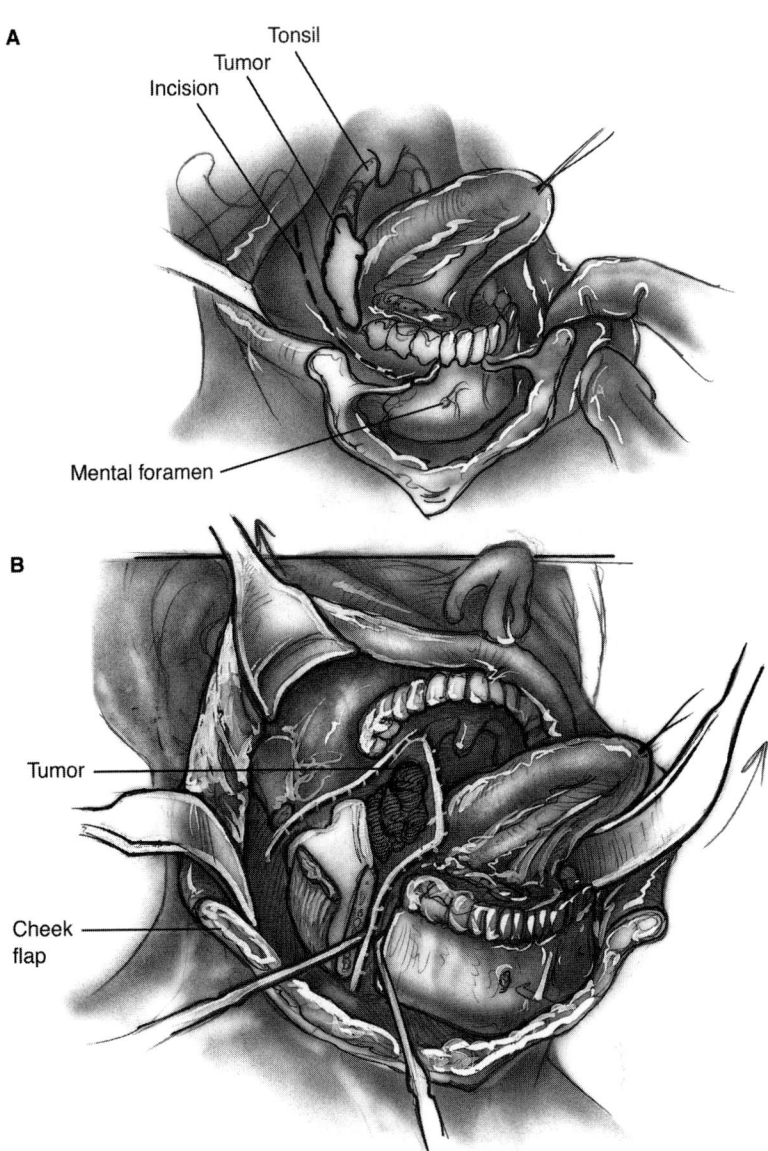

Figure 118.7 Mandibulectomy. **A:** A cheek flap is developed through a full-thickness incision of the gingivobuccal sulcus, exposing the mandible. **B:** The mandibular cuts are made well clear of the tumor and anterior to the mental foramen if the mandibular canal or inferior alveolar nerve are involved with tumor. The mandible is then retracted laterally and the soft-tissue cuts are performed.

Soft Tissue Reconstruction

Choosing the appropriate reconstruction requires an individualized treatment plan based on careful consideration of all pertinent tumor-, defect-, and patient-related factors. Generally, the least complex method that restores function and form is selected. Sensory reinnervation of the flaps is preferred whenever feasible, because pharyngeal function may benefit from such a reconstruction. Small defects of the pharyngeal walls up to 3 cm in largest dimension and those less than one third the volume of the tongue base can be closed, primarily by a split-thickness skin graft, or left to granulate if not open into the neck with minimal functional deficits. Larger lesions require some form of reconstruction, because primary closure results in poor function due to tongue tethering or pharyngeal stenosis. Free fasciocutaneous flaps are well suited for these reconstructions, especially when the defect involves multiple sites, such as the pharyngeal wall, soft palate, and tongue base. The thin and pliable nature of these flaps is ideal for pharyngeal wall reconstruction, and bulk for the tongue base may be obtained by deepithelializing and burying part of the flap (41) (Fig. 118.8). Adequate reconstruction with myocutaneous regional flaps is achieved when the defect is mostly base of tongue, but these flaps tend to be too bulky for pharyngeal wall or soft palate reconstruction, especially when mandibular continuity is maintained. In these situations, regional myofascial flaps are better suited because of the decreased bulk.

Small defects of the soft palate that can be removed with partial-thickness resection and preservation of the posterior mucosa may be left to granulate with excellent functional results. Full-thickness defects are best reconstructed with fasciocutaneous flaps that are folded onto themselves and sutured to the remaining nasal and oral

TABLE 118.6

OPTIONS FOR SOFT TISSUE AND MANDIBULAR RECONSTRUCTION OF OROPHARYNGEAL DEFECTS

A. Soft tissue
 1. Primary closure/secondary intention
 2. Split-thickness skin grafts
 3. Local flaps
  Tongue flaps
  Pharyngeal flaps
  Palatal and cheek flaps
 4. Regional flaps
  Pectoralis major
  Latissimus dorsi
  Trapezius
  Platysma and sternocleidomastoid myocutaneous flaps
  Others (temporal, temporalis, masseter, pericranial, deltopectoral flaps)
 5. Free microvascular flaps
  Fasciocutaneous (forearm, lateral thigh, lateral arm, and scapular)
  Latissimus dorsi
  Rectus abdominis
 6. Prosthetics
B. Mandible
 1. None
 2. Plate
 3. Pedicled osseous flaps (rib, scapula, clavicle, and calvarium)
 4. Free osteocutaneous flaps (fibula, iliac crest, scapula, radial forearm, and clavicle)

aspects of the soft palate (Fig. 118.8). Surgical adhesions are fashioned between the neopalate and the posterior pharyngeal wall to narrow the adynamic reconstructed segment of the velopharyngeal complex when the defect involves more than half the soft palate. Alternatively, a combination of fasciocutaneous flaps and pharyngeal

flaps also can be used (44,45). These reconstructions result in immediate and excellent function in most cases and may be further augmented with a prosthesis if needed after the radiation mucositis resolves. The use of prosthetics only is also an option, with good results obtained when the defect involves the total palate, movement of the residual velopharyngeal complex exists, and the patient has good supporting tissue to anchor the palatal device properly (40). The main disadvantage of prosthetics is the potential delay in function because definitive obturation cannot be performed until postoperative healing is complete and the acute radiation changes resolve.

Mandibular Reconstruction

Oropharyngeal cancers rarely invade the mandible, and with the use of mandibular preservation techniques, segmental resections are infrequent. The options for primary mandibular reconstruction are listed in Table 118.6 and are discussed in detail in Chapter 162. Lateral mandibular defects can be reconstructed with bone containing free flaps, but newer generation reconstruction plates with soft tissue reconstruction have been shown to be an alternative for some patients (46).

COMPLICATIONS

Complications related to the management of oropharyngeal cancer patients are the same as those of any head and neck cancer patient and are listed in Table 118.7. Surgical complications are more likely in patients previously treated with radiotherapy. Radiotherapy complications can be reduced by using IMRT, but caution is advised as altered patterns of local recurrence have been reported in patients treated with IMRT (47).

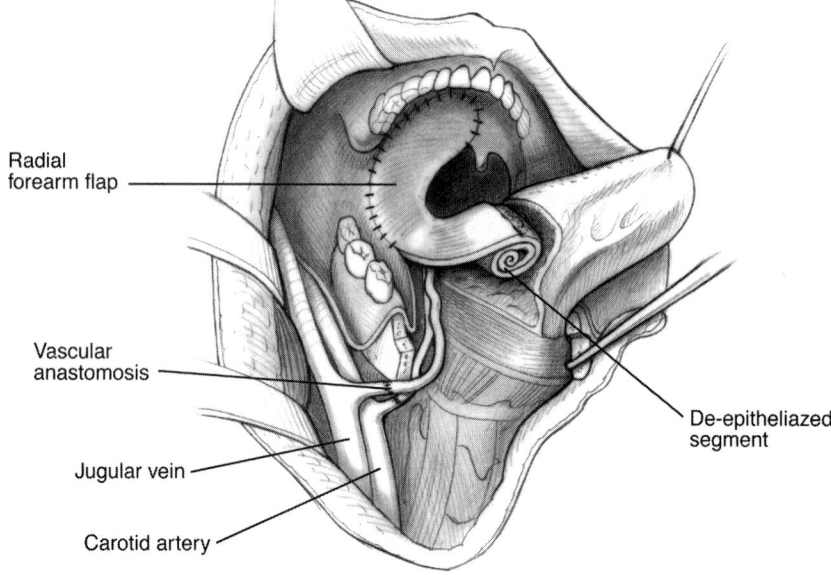

Figure 118.8 Reconstruction of the pharyngeal wall and tongue base with radial forearm fasciocutaneous flap. The distal flap is deepithelialized and rolled on itself to replace tongue base volume. The proximal flap is folded onto itself and sutured to the remaining nasal and oral aspects of the soft palate.

Radial forearm flap — Vascular anastomosis — Jugular vein — Carotid artery — De-epitheliazed segment

TABLE 118.7 COMPLICATIONS OROPHARYNGEAL CANCER TREATMENT

1. Radiation
    - Mucositis
    - Xerostomia
    - Taste dysfunction
    - Dysphagia
    - Fibrosis
    - Ulceration and tissue necrosis
    - Osteoradionecrosis of the mandible
    - Hypoglossal palsy
2. Surgical
    - A. Approach related
        - Damage to teeth
        - Damage to nerves
        - Cerebral embolism and carotid artery thrombosis
    - B. Resection and reconstruction related
        - Hemorrhage
        - Wound infection and dehiscence
        - Positive resection margin
        - Pharyngocutaneous fistula
        - Aspiration
        - Dysphagia
        - Poor speech
        - Velopharyngeal incompetence
        - Eustachian tube dysfunction
        - Nonunion and osteomyelitis of the mandible
        - Malocclusion and TMJ dysfunction

TMJ, temporomandibular junction.

EMERGENCIES

The most urgent problems that arise in oropharyngeal cancer patients are airway obstruction, bleeding, and free flap vascular compromise after reconstruction (Table 118.8). Airway obstruction is usually due to large exophytic tumors or edema from treatment. Imminent obstruction should be managed with a tracheotomy in the operating room with an anesthesiologist experienced in fiberoptic intubation. Bleeding from the tumor is usually controlled with selective cautery or embolization, but surgery with ligation of the carotid artery or its branches may be required in extreme situations. When free tissue transfer is used to reconstruct the surgical defect, any signs of arterial or venous compromise require immediate exploration of the vessels in an attempt to salvage the failing flap.

TABLE 118.8 EMERGENCY CARE

1. Airway obstruction
2. Bleeding
3. Free tissue transfer vascular compromise

TABLE 118.9 FOLLOW-UP SCHEDULE AFTER COMPLETION OF TREATMENT

Years Posttreatment	Follow-up
1st	1–3 mo
2nd	2–4 mo
3rd	3–6 mo
4th and 5th	4–6 mo
After 5th	Every 12 mo

FOLLOW-UP

Oropharyngeal cancer patients require close observation initially to detect recurrences, and lifelong follow-up after to identify second primaries. A general follow-up schedule after completion of treatment is provided in Table 118.9 (19). Chest radiographs, liver enzymes, and thyroid-stimulating hormone levels are obtained as indicated. Chemoprevention with retinoids is beneficial in this patient population, but their use is not widespread because of the high rate of toxicity (48).

PROGNOSIS

Table 118.10 shows the expected actuarial 5-year survival of patients with oropharyngeal cancers (49). As previously mentioned, for selected groups, better results have been reported. Patients with early stage cancer die of unrelated diseases or second primary tumors, because they are usually cured of their index tumor, whereas patients who have advanced disease often die of locoregional recurrence or distant metastasis. Patients with advanced disease treated with surgery and postoperative radiotherapy can be expected to have approximately a 50% 3-year survival and greater than 70% local control rate (50). The results are very similar with concurrent chemoradiation (21).

TABLE 118.10 THE 5-YEAR SURVIVAL OF OROPHARYNGEAL CANCER PATIENTS BY STAGE

Stage	5-Year Survival
1	67%
2	46%
3	31%
4	32%

NEW AND DEVELOPING TREATMENTS

The continued discovery of more active chemotherapeutic agents and refinement of diagnostic and reconstructive techniques offer hope of improving cure rates and postoperative function of oropharyngeal cancer patients. The exciting development of salivary preservation radiation protocols (IMRT) (30,31) and the recent use of surgical submandibular gland transfer have the potential of eliminating xerostomia and greatly enhancing the patient's quality of life after treatment (51). PET scan has allowed detection of occult metastatic disease and persistent disease following nonsurgical therapy and may help in the future to guide the extent of surgery and the role of adjuvant therapy (52). Lymphoscintigraphy and sentinel node mapping and biopsy for oral cancer is now being studied in a multicenter cooperative group trial in the United States. Preliminary experience also suggests that it may be feasible in oropharyngeal carcinomas (53). Properly conducted quality of life studies with larger patient numbers will help predict functional outcomes for different treatments and help determine which patients would be better served with a nonsurgical approach (40,45,54). Finally, targeted therapies, some of which are currently under investigation, will hopefully also improve patient selection for different therapeutic modalities. For example, for advanced disease, there may be molecular markers available soon that will indicate which patients would be better served with surgery and which patients will have a good response to nonsurgical therapy (55–58).

HIGHLIGHTS

- Cancer of the oropharynx is relatively uncommon, affecting mostly heavy smokers and drinkers; oncogenic HPV subtypes play a role, especially in nonsmokers.
- Squamous cell carcinoma and its variants account for 90% of primary malignant oropharyngeal lesions, whereas lymphomas, minor salivary gland tumors, melanomas, and sarcomas make up the rest.
- The concept of "field cancerization" or "condemned mucosa" applies to all mucosal head and neck cancers and is the reason for the high rate of second primaries in oropharyngeal cancer patients.
- The complete visualization and palpation of the tumor under general anesthesia greatly facilitates the assessment of submucosal spread, invasion of surrounding structures such as the prevertebral fascia and mandible, and identification of second primary tumors.
- Surgery or radiation alone are equally effective for T1 and T2 oropharyngeal cancers, but primary surgery or the addition of brachytherapy or chemotherapy are preferred for deeply infiltrative lesions and those that extend beyond the anterior faucial arch or have significant involvement of the base of tongue. T3 and T4 lesions are best controlled with a combined modality.

- Almost all patients with oropharyngeal squamous cell cancers require some treatment of the neck because of the high rate of clinically positive nodes and occult nodal metastasis at presentation.
- N0 and N1 are usually adequately treated with a single modality, whereas a combined modality results in better regional control in N2 and N3 neck disease. Treatment often includes both necks and retropharyngeal nodes. Sentinel node mapping remains investigational.
- Successful extirpation of oropharyngeal cancers hinges on good exposure and wide resection margins because these tumors have the propensity for submucosal spread. Mandibular sparing procedures are used whenever possible.
- The appropriate reconstruction requires an individualized treatment plan based on careful consideration of all pertinent tumor-, defect-, and patient-related factors. Generally, the least complex method that restores function and form is selected. If good function cannot be maintained with surgery, a nonsurgical approach should be considered.
- Oropharyngeal cancer patients require close observation initially to detect recurrences, and life-long follow-up afterward to identify second primary tumors. Patients with early-stage cancer die of unrelated diseases or second primary tumors, whereas those with advanced disease die of locoregional recurrence or distal metastasis

REFERENCES

1. Jemal A, Tiwari RC, Murray T, et al.; American Cancer Society. Cancer statistics, 2004. *CA Cancer J Clin* 2004;54:829.
2. Curtin HD. Separation of the masticator space from the parapharyngeal space. *Radiology* 1987;163:195–204.
3. McConnel FMS, Cerenko D, Jackson RT, et al. Timing of major events of pharyngeal swallowing. *Arch Otolaryngol Head Neck Surg* 1998;114:1413–1418.
4. Myers JN. Molecular pathogenesis of squamous cell carcinoma of the head and neck. In: Myers EN, Suen JY, eds. *Cancer of the head and neck.* Philadelphia: WB Saunders, 1996:5–16.
5. Mashberg A, Boffetta P, Winkelman R, et al. Tobacco smoking, alcohol drinking and cancer of the oral cavity and oropharynx among US veterans. *Cancer* 1993;72:1369–1375.
6. Brandsma JL, Abramson AL. Association of papillomavirus with cancers of the head and neck. *Arch Otolaryngol Head Neck Surg* 1989;115: 621–625.
7. Klussman JP, Weissenborn SJ, Wieland U, et al. Prevalence, distribution and viral load of human papillomavirus 16 DNA in tonsillar carcinomas. *Cancer* 2001;92:2875–2884.
8. Gillison ML, Koch WM, Capone RB, et al. Evidence for a causal association between human papillomavirus and a subset of head and neck cancers. *J Natl Cancer Inst* 2000;92:709–720.
9. Strome SE, Savva A, Brisset AE, et al. Squamous cell carcinoma of the tonsils: a molecular analysis of HPV associations. *Clin Cancer Res* 2002;8:1093–1100.
10. Singh B, Balwally AN, Shaha AR, et al. Upper aerodigestive tract squamous cell carcinoma. The human immunodeficiency virus connection. *Arch Otolaryngol Head Neck* 1996;122:639–643.
11. Chandler SW, Rassekh CH, Rodman SM, et al. Immunohistochemical localization of interleukin-10 in human oral and pharyngeal carcinomas. *Laryngoscope* 2002;112:808–815.
12. Zelefsky MJ, Harrison LB, Armstrong JG. Long-term treatment results of postoperative radiation therapy for advanced stage oropharyngeal carcinoma. *Cancer* 1992;70:2388–2395.
13. Tsue TT, McCulloch TM, Girod DA, et al. Predictors of carcinomatous invasion of the mandible. *Head Neck* 1994;16:116–126.

14. Jesse RH, Fletcher GH. Metastasis in cervical lymph node from oropharyngeal carcinoma treatment and results. *AJR Am J Roentgenol* 1963;90:990–996.

15. Chung TS, Stefani S. Distant metastases of carcinoma of tonsillar region: a study of 475 patients. *J Surg Oncol* 1980;14:5–9.

16. Maisel RH, Vermeersch H. Panendoscopy for second primaries in the head and neck cancer. *Ann Otol* 1981;90:460–464.

17. Pignon JP, Bourhis J, Domenge C, et al. Chemotherapy added to locoregional treatment for head and neck squamous-cell carcinoma: three meta-analyses of updated individual data. *Lancet* 2000;355:949–955.

18. Brizel DM, Albers ME, Fisher SR, et al. Hyperfractionated irradiation with or without concurrent chemotherapy for locally advanced head and neck cancer. *N Engl J Med* 1998;338:1798–1804.

19. Machtay M, Rosenthal DI, Hershock D, et al. Organ preservation therapy using induction plus concurrent chemoradiation for advanced resectable oropharyngeal carcinoma: University of Pennsylvania Phase II trial. *J Clin Oncol* 2002;20:3964–3971.

20. Olmi P, Crispino S, Fallai C, et al. Locoregionally advanced carcinoma of the oropharynx: conventional radiotherapy vs. accelerated hyperfractionated radiotherapy vs. concomitant radiotherapy and chemotherapy—a multicenter randomized trial. *Int J Radiat Oncol Biol Phys* 2003;55:78–92.

21. Mantz CA, Vokes EE, Stenson K, et al. Induction chemotherapy followed by concomitant chemoradiotherapy in the treatment of locoregionally advanced oropharyngeal carcinoma. *Cancer J* 2001;7:140–148.

22. Calais G, Alfonsi M, Bardet E, et al. Randomized trial of radiation therapy versus concomitant chemotherapy and radiation therapy for advanced-stage oropharynx carcinoma. *J Natl Cancer Inst* 1999;91:2081–2086.

23. Cooper JS, Pajak TF, Forastiere AA, et al. Radiation Therapy Oncology Group 9501/Intergroup. Postoperative concurrent radiotherapy and chemotherapy for high-risk squamous-cell carcinoma of the head and neck. *N Engl J Med* 2004;350:1937–1944.

24. Leborgne JH, Leborgne F, Barlocci LA, et al. The place of brachytherapy in the treatment of carcinoma of the tonsil with lingual extension. *Int J Radiat Oncol Biol Phys* 1986;12:1787–1792.

25. Lee RW, Mendenhall WM, Parsons JT, et al. Carcinoma of the tonsillar region: a multivariate analysis of 243 patients treated with radical radiotherapy. *Head Neck* 1993;15:283–288.

26. Mendenhall WM, Amdur RJ, Stringer SP, et al. Radiation therapy for squamous cell carcinoma of the tonsillar region: a preferred alternative to surgery? *J Clin Oncol* 2000;18:2219–2225.

27. Houck JR, Shaha A. Oropharynx. In: Medina JE, Chairman. *Clinical practice guidelines for the diagnosis and management of cancer of the head and neck.* Presented at the meeting of the American Society for Head and Neck Surgery and the Society of Head and Neck Surgeons. Los Angeles: The American Society for Head and Neck Surgery, 1996:25–29.

28. Galati LT, Myers EN, Johnson JT. Primary surgery as a treatment for early squamous cell carcinoma of the tonsil. *Head Neck* 2000;22:294–296.

29. Nathu RM, Mendenhall NP, Almasri NM, Lynch JW. Non-Hodgkin's lymphoma of the head and neck: a 30-year experience at the University of Florida. *Head Neck* 1999;21:247–254.

30. Chen KS, Majhail N, Huang CJ, et al. Intensity-modulated radiation therapy reduces late salivary toxicity without compromising tumor control in patients with oropharyngeal carcinoma: a comparison with conventional techniques. *Radiother Oncol* 2001;61:275–280.

31. Smith RV, Goldman SY, Beitler JJ, et al. Decreased short-and-long-term swallowing problems with altered radiotherapy dosing used in an organ-sparing protocol for advanced pharyngeal carcinoma. *Arch Otolaryngol Head Neck Surg* 2004;130:831–836.

32. Brizel DM, Prosnitz RG, Hunter S, et al. Necessity for adjuvant neck dissection in setting of concurrent chemoradiation for advanced head-and-neck cancer. *Int J Radiat Oncol Biol Phys* 2004;58:1418–1423.

33. Clayman GL, Johnson CJ 2nd, Morrison W, et al. The role of neck dissection after chemoradiotherapy for oropharyngeal cancer with advanced nodal disease. *Arch Otolaryngol Head Neck Surg* 2001;127:135–139.

34. Steiner W, Fierek O, Ambrosch P, et al. Transoral laser microsurgery for squamous cell carcinoma of the base of the tongue. *Arch Otolaryngol Head Neck Surg* 2003;129:36–43.

35. Rassekh CH, Janecka IP, Calhoun KH. Lower lip splitting incisions: anatomic considerations. *Laryngoscope* 1995;105[8 Pt 1]:880–883.

36. Christopoulos E, Canan R, Segas T, et al. Transmandibular approaches to the oral cavity and oropharynx—a functional assessment. *Arch Otolaryngol Head Neck Surg* 1992;118:1164–1167.

37. O'Brien CJ, Nettle W, Lee KK. Changing trends in the management of carcinoma of the oral cavity and oropharynx. *Aust N Z J Surg* 1993;63:270–274.

38. Tsue TT, Desyatnikova SS, Deleyiannis FW, et al. Comparison of cost and function in reconstruction of posterior oral cavity and oropharynx. Free vs pedicled soft tissue transfer. *Arch Otolaryngol Head Neck Surg* 1997;123:731–737.

39. Sabri A. Oropharyngeal reconstruction: current state of the art. *Curr Opin Otolaryngol Head Neck Surg* 2003;11:251–254.

40. Friedlander P, Caruana S, Singh B, et al. Functional Status after primary surgical therapy for squamous cell carcinoma of the base of the tongue. *Head Neck* 2002;24:111–114.

41. Salibian AH, Allison GR, Krugman ME, et al. Reconstruction of the base of tongue with the microvascular ulnar forearm flap: a functional assessment. *Plast Reconstruct Surg* 1995;96:1081–1089.

42. Walther EK. Dysphagia after pharyngolaryngeal cancer surgery. Part 1: pathophysiology of postsurgical deglutition. *Dysphagia* 1995;10:275–278.

43. Curtis TA, Beumer J III. Speech, velopharyngeal function, and restoration of soft palate defects. In: Curtis TA, Beumer J III, Marunick MT, eds. *Maxillofacial rehabilitation prosthodontic and surgical consideration.* St. Louis: Ishiyaku EuroAmerica, 1996: 285–329.

44. Brown JS, Zuydam AC, Jones DC, et al. Functional outcome in soft palate reconstruction using a radial forearm free flap in conjunction with a superiorly based pharyngeal flap. *Head Neck* 1997;19:524–534.

45. Seikaly H, Rieger J, Wolfaardt J, et al. Functional outcomes after primary oropharyngeal cancer resection and reconstruction with the radial forearm free flap. *Laryngoscope* 2003;113:897–904.

46. Blackwell KE, Lacombe V. The bridging lateral mandibular reconstruction plate revisited. *Arch Otolaryngol Head Neck Surg* 1999;125:988–993.

47. Eisbruch A, Marsh LH, Dawson LA, et al. Recurrence near base of skull after IMRT for head-and-neck cancer: implications for target delineation in high neck and for parotid gland sparing. *Int J Radiat Oncol Biol Phys* 2004;59:28–42.

48. Hong WK, Lippman SM, Itri LM, et al. Prevention of second primary tumors with isotretinoin in squamous cell carcinoma of the head and neck. *N Engl J Med* 1990;323:795–801.

49. Pugliano FA, Piccirillo JF, Zequeira MR, et al. Clinical severity staging system for oropharyngeal cancer: five-year survival rates. *Arch Otolaryngol Head Neck Surg* 1997;123:1118–1124.

50. Denittis AS, Machtay M, Rosenthal DJ, et al. Advanced oropharyngeal carcinoma treated with surgery and radiotherapy: oncologic outcome and functional assessment. *Am J Otolaryngol* 2001;22:329–335.

51. Seikaly H, Jha N, Harris JR, et al. Long-term outcomes of submandibular gland transfer for prevention of postradiation xerostomia. *Arch Otolaryngol Head Neck Surg* 2004;130:956–961.

52. Greven KM, Williams DW 3rd, McGuirt WF Sr, et al. Serial positron emission tomography scans following radiation therapy of patients with head and neck cancer. *Curr Opin Otolaryngol Head Neck Surg* 2003;11:251–254.

53. Ross G, Shoaib T, Soutar DS, et al. The use of sentinel node biopsy to upstage the clinically N0 neck in head and cancer. *Arch Otolaryngol Head Neck Surg* 2002;128:1287–1291.

54. Gillespie MB, Brodsky MB, Day TA, et al. Swallowing-related quality of life after head and neck cancer treatment. *Laryngoscope* 2004;114:1362–1367.

55. Ritchie JM, Smith EM, Summersgill KF, et al. Human papillomavirus infection as a prognostic factor in carcinomas of the oral cavity and oropharynx. *Int J Cancer* 2003;104:336–344.

56. Hannisdal K, Boysen M, Evensen JF. Different prognostic indices in 310 patients with tonsillar carcinomas. *Head Neck* 2003;25: 123–131.

57. Friesland S, Mellin J, Munck-Wikland E, et al. Human papilloma virus (HPV) and p53 immunostaining in advanced tonsillar carcinoma-relation to radiotherapy response and survival. *Anticancer Res* 2001;21(IB):529–534.

58. Dahlstrand H, Dahlgren L, Lindquist D, et al. Presence of human papillomavirus in tonsillar cancer is a favourable prognostic factor for clinical outcome. *Anticancer Res* 2004;24:1829–1835.

Hypopharyngeal Cancer

119

Seungwon Kim   Randal S. Weber

Cancer of the hypopharynx constitutes only 5% to 10% of malignancies of the upper aerodigestive tract and yet cancer of this region presents the head and neck surgeon with a difficult challenge. The complex anatomy and the functional importance of this region require a multidisciplinary approach that incorporates the care of head and neck surgeons, medical oncologists, radiation oncologists, and speech pathologists. The pathologic features of hypopharyngeal cancer are often unfavorable and are marked by multicentricity, submucosal spread, and early unilateral or bilateral lymph node metastasis. Furthermore, patients with hypopharyngeal cancer often present with advanced disease and severe malnutrition that complicate their care. For these reasons, the overall prognosis of patients with hypopharyngeal cancer remains poor.

Recent advances in surgical reconstruction and refinements of chemotherapeutic and radiotherapy regimens, however, have resulted in better palliation and improved disease-free interval. The advances in microvascular reconstruction have expanded the role of curative surgical resections and these advances have been accompanied by the development of organ preservation protocols with chemotherapy and radiotherapy. Faced with this continuing evolution in the care of patients with hypopharyngeal cancer, the clinician must be familiar with the various anatomic, pathologic, and clinical aspects of hypopharyngeal cancer when formulating the most appropriate treatment.

ANATOMY

The hypopharynx extends from the level of the hyoid bone to the lower border of the cricoid cartilage. It is funnel-shaped and is in continuity with the oropharynx superiorly

and the cervical esophagus inferiorly (Fig. 119.1). The hypopharynx is divided into three subsites: pyriform sinuses laterally, the posterior pharyngeal wall posteriorly, and the postcricoid area anteriorly (Fig. 119.2). The pyriform sinuses

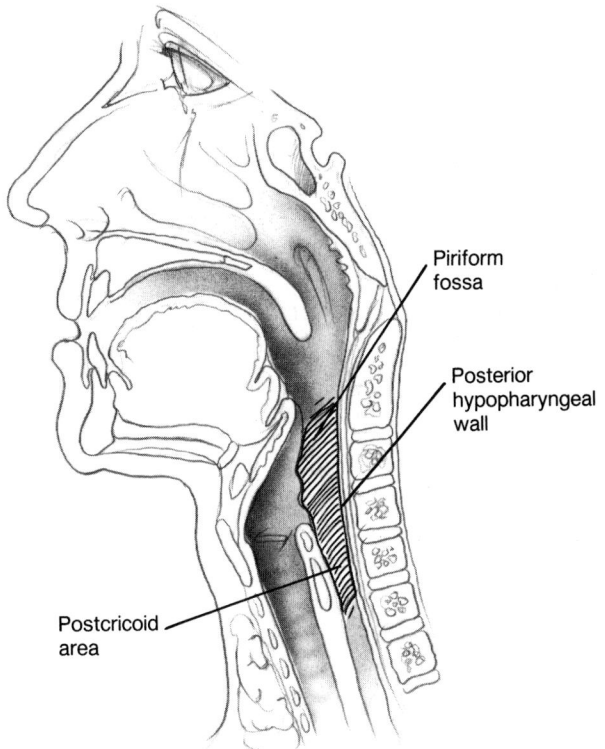

Piriform fossa

Posterior hypopharyngeal wall

Postcricoid area

Figure 119.1 The hypopharyngeal region extends from a point at the superior edge of the body of the hyoid bone down to the inferior aspect of the cricoid cartilage; it is composed of the piriform fossa, the posterior hypopharyngeal wall, and the postcricoid area.

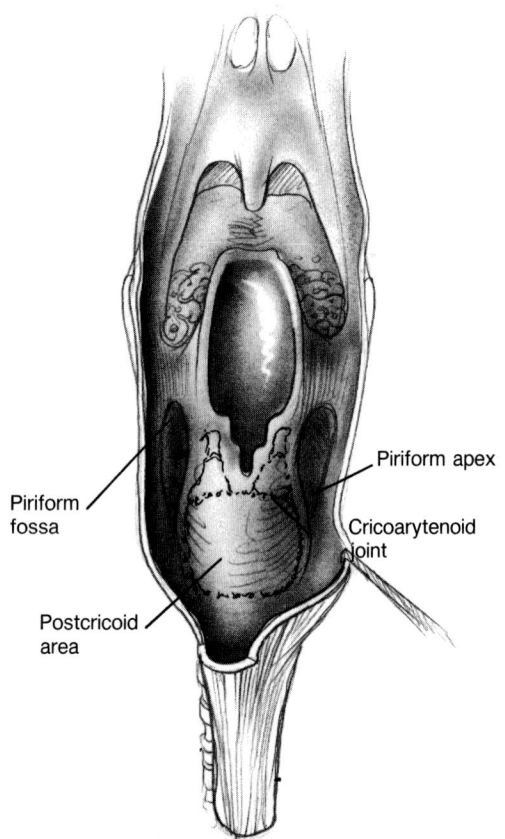

Figure 119.2 The piriform apex is at the junction between the inferior aspect of the piriform fossa and the postcricoid region. It marks the location of the cricoarytenoid joint.

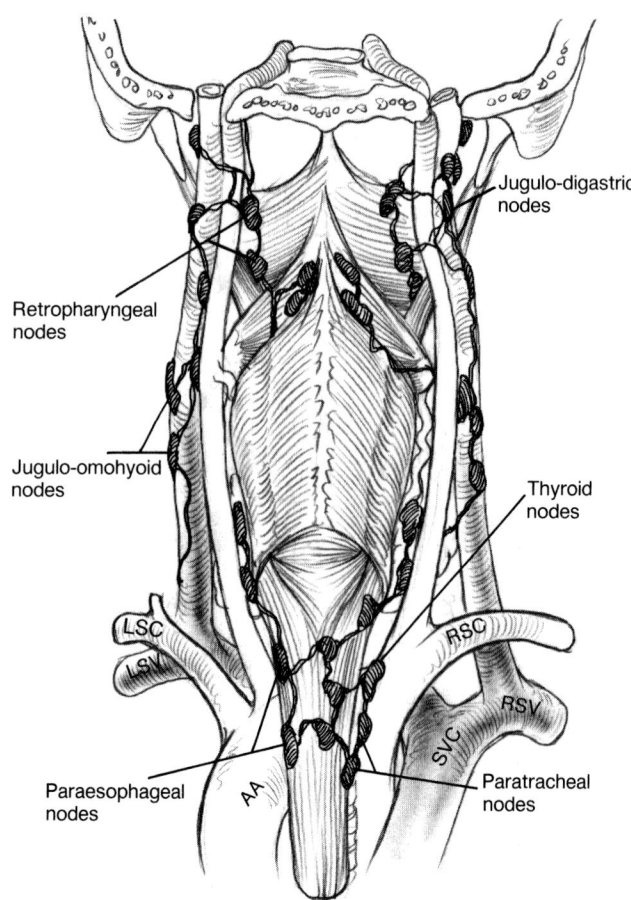

Figure 119.3 The primary lymph node drainage of the hypopharynx. Cancers of the superior hypopharynx metastasize to the jugulodigastric and retropharyngeal nodes, whereas those of the inferior hypopharynx, including the piriform apex, metastasize to the jugulo-omohyoid, paraesophageal, paratracheal, and thyroid lymph nodes. AA, aortic arch; LSC, left subclavian artery; LSV, left subclavian vein; RSC, right subclavian artery; RSV, right subclavian vein; SVC, superior vena cava.

extend from the pharyngoepiglottic folds superiorly to an apex inferiorly at the level of the true vocal cords. The lateral boundaries of the pyriform sinuses are formed by the thyroid cartilages and the thyrohyoid membrane. The medial boundaries are formed by the larynx. The posterior pharyngeal wall forms the second subunit of the hypopharynx. The third subunit of the hypopharynx, the postcricoid area, extends from the posterior surface of the arytenoids mounds to the inferior border of the cricoid cartilage and forms the anterior boundary of the hypopharynx.

The vascular supply of the hypopharynx is derived from the great vessels of the neck and includes branches of the superior thyroid, lingual, and ascending pharyngeal arteries. Sensory innervation of the hypopharynx is supplied by the glossopharyngeal and the vagus nerves via the pharyngeal plexus and the internal branches of the superior laryngeal nerve. The vagus nerve also gives rise to the Arnold nerve, which provides sensory innervation to the external auditory canal and accounts for referred otalgia caused by hypopharyngeal lesions. Motor innervation to the inferior constrictor muscle is via the pharyngeal plexus, whereas the terminal branches of the recurrent laryngeal nerve innervate the cricopharyngeus muscle.

It is important to note that the hypopharynx has an extensive lymphatic drainage system (Fig. 119.3). The lymphatic drainage can be divided into anterior and posterior drainage pathways. The anterior pathway drains the larynx and the pyriform sinuses through the thyrohyoid membrane along with the superior laryngeal artery. This pathway then drains into the subdigastric, upper, middle, and inferior jugular nodes. The second lymphatic group of channels drains the posterior pharyngeal wall to the retropharyngeal and upper and middle jugular nodes through the inferior constrictor muscle. Retropharyngeal metastasis can occur as high as the level of the skull base. Furthermore, inferior pyriform sinuses also drain through the cricothyroid membrane along the recurrent laryngeal nerve into paratracheal nodes (1). Bilateral lymphatic metastases are common, especially for lesions on the medial wall of the pyriform sinuses and the posterior pharyngeal wall (2).

DIAGNOSIS

History

Common presenting symptoms for hypopharyngeal cancer patients are odynophagia, dysphagia, and otalgia. Dysphagia is usually progressive and difficulty with liquids as well as solids suggests an advanced lesion. The patient may also complain of repeated throat clearing or globus sensation. Persistent unilateral otalgia in the presence of normal otoscopic examination mandates an endoscopic evaluation of the hypopharynx. Dyspnea and hoarseness, findings of late-stage disease, may be caused by direct laryngeal invasion or involvement of the recurrent laryngeal nerve.

Detailed medical history, a thorough review of systems, and a review of the tobacco and alcohol history are essential in formulating an appropriate treatment plan. Many patients with hypopharyngeal cancer will have pulmonary or cardiac comorbidities, which can influence their therapy. Significant malnutrition may also be present because of inadequate diet or excessive alcohol consumption (Table 119.1).

Physical Examination

Before performing a detailed head and neck examination, much information can be gained from assessing the general status of the patient. The presence of hoarseness, mild dyspnea, or stridor suggests laryngeal involvement and gives information regarding the state of the airway. Poor nutritional status may be evident by loose clothing, skin pallor, loss of turgor, and the general condition of the skin and nails.

A thorough head and neck examination is mandatory for all patients. Examination of the oral cavity includes the evaluation of the dentition, because many patients require definitive dental care before radiation therapy. The oral cavity should also be examined for the presence of leukoplakia or a second primary lesion. Evaluation of the hypopharynx and the larynx can then be performed with an indirect mirror examination. The upper pyriform sinuses, the aryepiglottic fold, and the arytenoids can be visualized as well. The apex of the pyriform sinus, however, may be obscured by pooled secretion. The presence of edema and erythema on these structures suggest tumor involvement.

Examination of the neck should be undertaken in a systematic fashion to adequately assess all cervical lymph node levels. Hypopharyngeal cancers have a high rate of cervical lymph node metastasis and accurate assessment of the cervical lymph node status is critical in treatment planning.

Despite advances in imaging techniques, palpation of the neck remains an important diagnostic tool in the detection of cervical metastasis. Palpation of the larynx may reveal extralaryngeal spread of the tumor, whereas loss of laryngeal crepitus suggests postcricoid involvement. Cranial nerve examination is also an integral part of the head and neck examination. Neurologic deficits can be the re-

TABLE 119.1	**DIAGNOSIS**

HYPOPHARYNGEAL CANCER

History
- Treated for pharyngitis
- Tobacco and ethanol abuse
- Weight loss
- Dehydration
- Odynophagia
- Dysphagia
- Hoarseness
- Dyspnea
- Otalgia
- Neck mass
- Airway obstruction
- Support group status

Physical
- Weight loss or cachexia
- Decreased skin turgor
- Hyporesonant voice
- Hoarseness
- Stridor
- Status of dentition
- Indirect examination with mirror
- Flexible fiberotic laryngoscopy
- Full neck examination

Radiology
- Chest radiograph
- Barium swallow
- CT or MRI of the neck

Laboratory
- Complete chemistries
- Staging endoscopy and biopsy
- Control of airway
- Complete paralysis
- Gross characteristics of tumor
- Three-dimensional relationships of tumor
- Biopsy
- Determination of inferior border
- Esophagoscopy
- Bronchoscopy, if warranted

CT, computed tomography; MRI, magnetic resonance imaging.

sult of direct tumor involvement or be caused by other concurrent disease. Vocal cord paralysis can be caused by the tumor invasion of the paraglottic space, cricoarytenoid joint, or the recurrent laryngeal nerve. Hypoglossal nerve deficit can also occur from nerve invasion by tumor from adjacent metastatic lymph node with extracapsular extension. Fiberoptic laryngoscopy is invaluable in evaluating a patient with suspected tumor of the upper aerodigestive tract because it allows direct visualization of the tumor and assessment of the motor and sensory function of the larynx and hypopharynx. The use of Valsalva maneuver frequently facilitates the visualization of the pyriform sinuses and the evaluation of superficial lesions. Vocal fold mobility should be carefully assessed because any impairment suggests laryngeal involvement. The status of the laryngeal airway can also be evaluated with this technique, allowing for planning of airway management in the operating room at the time of biopsy or treatment.

Radiology

In general, computed tomography (CT) will offer adequate evaluation of the primary tumor as well as the status of the cervical lymph nodes. If further soft tissue delineation is required, magnetic resonance imaging (MRI) can be used. The lengthy image acquisition time required by MRI, however, can lead to motion-induced artifacts and image degradation. This is especially true in patients with moderate compromise of the upper airway or patients with difficulty handling secretions who cannot tolerate the supine position for prolonged periods. Assessment of the laryngeal cartilage for tumor invasion can be performed with both CT and MRI. The accuracy of CT for detection of laryngeal cartilage invasion varies from reported sensitivity of 46% to 91% and specificity of 80% to 91% (3–5). MRI offers comparable rates of detection of laryngeal cartilage invasion with the sensitivity ranging from 89% to 94% and the specificity ranging from 74% to 88% (3–6). In a prospective study of 44 patients with hypopharyngeal carcinoma, Zbaren et al. (6) studied the ability of CT and MRI to detect laryngeal cartilage invasion. MRI was more sensitive in detecting neoplastic invasion of the laryngeal cartilage than CT (97% vs. 68%), although MRI was less specific than CT (62% vs. 84%). No difference was seen between the overall accuracy of CT and MRI in detecting neoplastic invasion of the laryngeal cartilages (78% vs. 75%). Because of practical reasons, however, CT remains the more frequently used method of imaging in most centers.

Imaging studies to assess for a second primary tumor of the lungs or distant metastatic disease should be considered in patients with head and neck cancer. For patients with early-stage disease, a chest radiograph may suffice. The risk of distant metastases, however, increases with higher nodal stage (7,8). Patients with three or more lymph node metastases have almost a 50% risk of developing distant metastases (8). For these patients, CT of the chest is preferable to chest radiographs because CT offers superior sensitivity and specificity in detecting pulmonary metastasis (9,10). In patients with advanced nodal disease who are at risk for distant metastases, 18-fluorodeoxyglucose positron-emission tomography (FDG-PET) is another mode of imaging that can be used. One advantage that FDG-PET may have over other modes of imaging is the ability to perform whole-body imaging for detection of distant metastases at the time of initial diagnosis. The accuracy of FDG-PET in detecting distant metastases in the lungs appears to be comparable to that of chest CT (approximately 80% for FDG-PET vs. 90% for chest CT) (11). Teknos et al. (12) studied the usefulness of CT of the chest compared with FDG-PET in 12 consecutive patients with stage III and IV head and neck cancer. Of these 12 patients, 4 had hypopharyngeal

squamous cell carcinoma (SCC). Of the 3 of the 12 patients who had biopsy-proved pulmonary metastases, FDG-PET could detect the metastatic disease in all 3 of these patients. In contrast, chest CT detected only one of the three patients with pulmonary metastases. Further investigation, however, is needed to determine the cost-effectiveness of FDG-PET versus chest CT as a routine imaging procedure in newly diagnosed patients with advanced head and neck cancer.

Barium swallow can be useful for identifying a second primary tumor of the esophagus. Special studies (e.g., bone scan) are not routinely indicated unless the patient complains of bone pain or if hematological or chemical analysis indicates bone metastasis.

PATHOLOGY

As with cancers of other sites in the head and neck, squamous cell carcinomas comprise more than 95% of hypopharyngeal cancers (13). Most hypopharyngeal cancers arise from the pyriform sinuses (66% to 75%) followed by the posterior pharyngeal wall (20% to 30%) (14). Cancer arising from the postcricoid area is least common (1% to 5%) (Table 119.2). A strong association is found with excessive alcohol and tobacco consumption. Gastroesophageal reflux (GERD) has also received much attention as a possible cause of hypopharyngeal cancer (15). The peak incidence is in the sixth to seventh decade of life, with a higher incidence in men. An exception is patients with Vinson-Plummer disease, who are mostly women and the development of postcricoid carcinomas in these patients is independent of tobacco or alcohol history (16).

Patterns of Spread

A distinguishing feature of hypopharyngeal cancer is the common finding of submucosal spread (17). In fact, this mode of extension should be anticipated in every hypopharyngeal cancer and it is not uncommon to have submucosal

TABLE 119.2

HYPOPHARYNGEAL CANCER: STAGING (EASTERN VIRGINIA MEDICAL SCHOOL EXPERIENCE)

Location	No. (%)	Stage			
		I	II	III	IV
Piriform fossa	63 (64)	11	10	24	18
Posterior wall	30 (30)	5	15	8	2
Postcricoid	4 (4)	—	—	3	1

Eastern Virginia Medical School experience of 97 previously untreated patients, 1972–1985.

extension of 5 to 10 mm. Submucosal spread is more common in tumors located in the inferior hypopharynx adjacent to the cervical esophagus than in lesions of the superior hypopharynx. This is thought to be caused by the rich density of lymphatic channels near the pharyngoesophageal junction. The frequent finding of submucosal spread requires a wide surgical margin, especially inferiorly, when resecting a hypopharyngeal tumor. Skip lesions are also a common finding in hypopharyngeal cancer. It is difficult, however, to determine pathologically whether these lesions share the same origin as the primary tumor or if these lesions represent a second primary lesion.

Postcricoid tumors are often advanced at the time of diagnosis and tend to grow circumferentially. Involvement of the cervical esophagus by inferior extension is a frequent finding. Because of the proximity of the cricoid cartilage, the cricoarytenoid joints, and the cricoarytenoid muscles, invasion into these structures is also common. Postcricoid tumors also often involve the thyroid gland, and paratracheal and paraesophageal nodes (Fig. 119.4) (18,19). Overall, up to 40% of patients with postcricoid tumors will have regional metastatic disease (20).

Tumors of the pyriform sinuses often present at an advanced stage. Lateral spread of the tumor involves the thyroid cartilage and soft tissues of the neck. Medial extension of the tumor will involve the larynx and the paraglottic space (Fig. 119.5). Involvement of the cricoarytenoid joint or the recurrent laryngeal nerve results in hypomobile or immobile true vocal cord. Posteriorly, the tumor can spread to and along the posterior pharyngeal wall into the contralateral pyriform sinus. Pyriform sinus cancers are accompanied by high (50% to 80%) rates of regional lymph node metastases, most commonly to the jugulodigastric nodes (21,22). In a review of 79 patients with pyriform sinus cancer who had radical neck dissection for clinically N+ neck cancer, Candela et al. (22) found a 72% incidence of lymph node metastasis in level II and III, and a 47% incidence of lymph node metastasis in level IV. The percentage of neck dissection specimen with pathologically positive nodes in level I and V were only 6.3% and 7.6%, respectively (22). Furthermore, bilateral metastasis is more common with lesions of the medial wall of the pyriform sinus than the lateral wall. Johnson et al. (2) noted that regional recurrences in the contralateral neck were more frequent with lesions of the medial wall compared with lesions of the lateral wall of the pyriform sinus.

Tumors of the posterior pharyngeal wall tend to be exophytic without invasion of the prevertebral fascia. Therefore,

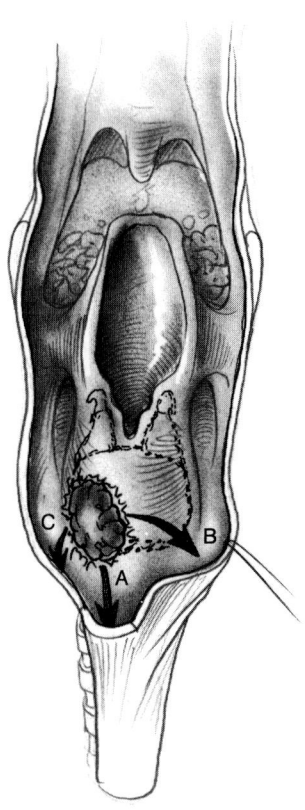

Figure 119.4 Lymph node and submucosal spread of postcricoid cancer. Submucosal spread inferiorly **(A)** can be extensive, and these lesions frequently metastasize to the paratracheal, thyroid, and paraesophageal nodes **(B and C)**.

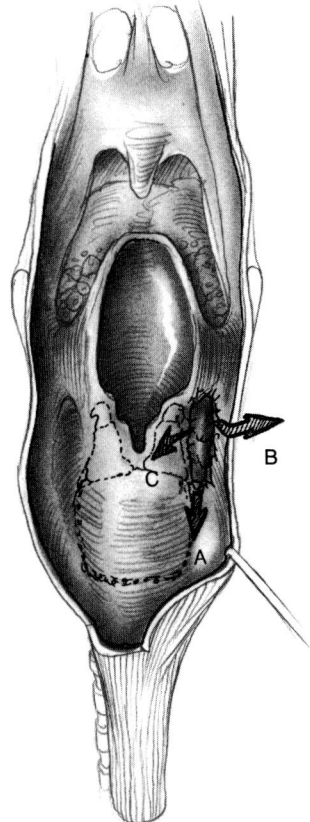

Figure 119.5 Lymph node and submucosal spread of piriform fossa cancer. Submucosal spread inferiorly **(A)** can involve the piriform apex and then metastases to the paratracheal, paraesophageal, thyroid, and jugulo-omohyoid nodes **(B)**. Medial extension **(C)** involves the arytenoid and perilaryngeal compartments.

early lesions of the posterior pharyngeal wall are amenable to surgical resection. Tumors that have invaded the prevertebral fascia are generally not considered to be curative with surgical resection. Because of the midline location of these tumors, when regional metastasis does develop, bilateral metastasis is common. The first echelons of nodes draining the posterior hypopharyngeal wall are levels II and III, and the retropharynx (23). Metastases to retropharyngeal nodes have been reported in 42% to 67% of patients with tumors of the posterior pharyngeal wall (24,25). Overall, the incidence of cervical nodal disease is between 35% and 45% (23,26).

Molecular Pathology

Although hypopharyngeal SCC often display clinically distinct behavior when compared with other sites of head and neck, molecular features that are specific for hypopharyngeal cancers have not yet been identified. The most common genetic abnormality found in head and neck cancer, including the hypopharynx, is mutation in the *p53* tumor suppressor gene (27). Cyclin D1, a protooncogene, has been reported to be overexpressed in hypopharyngeal cancer, but this finding is not specific to cancers of the hypopharynx (28). Although the overexpression of several genes (e.g., MMP2) and glucose transporter 1 has been suggested to correlate with poor prognosis in patients with hypopharyngeal cancer, the evidence is not conclusive (29,30). Attempts to correlate oncogenes such as *ras*, *myc*, and *C-erb/neu* with tumor phenotype, behavior, and response to therapy have not been successful. Chromosomal aberrations known as losses of heterozygosity are frequently found in chromosomes 3p, 17p, 13q, 11q, 6p, 8p, and 14q (31).

Staging

In the sixth edition of the American Joint Committee on Cancer (AJCC) Cancer Staging Manual, T4 lesions of the hypopharynx have been divided into T4a (resectable) and T4b (unresectable), leading to the division of the stage IV into stage IVA and stage IVB. Patients with distant metastatic disease are classified as stage IVC, regardless of the tumor (T) or node (N) stage. The staging system proposed by the American Joint Committee on Cancer for hypopharyngeal cancer is as follows:

T1: Tumor limited to one subsite of hypopharynx and is 2 cm or less in greatest dimension

T2: Tumor invades more than one subsite of hypopharynx or an adjacent site, or is more than 2 cm but not more than 4 cm

T3: Tumor is more than 4 cm in greatest dimension or with fixation of hemilarynx

T4: Tumor invades thyroid or cricoid cartilage, hyoid bone, thyroid gland, esophagus, or central compartment soft tissue

NX: Regional lymph nodes cannot be assessed

N0: No regional lymph node metastasis

N1: Metastasis in a single ipsilateral lymph node is 3 cm or less in greatest dimension

N2a: Metastasis in a single ipsilateral lymph node is more than 3 cm but not more than 6 cm in greatest dimension

N2b: Metastasis in multiple ipsilateral lymph nodes, none is more than 6 cm in greatest dimension

N2c: Metastasis in bilateral or contralateral lymph nodes, none is more than 6 cm in greatest dimension

N3: Metastasis in a lymph node is more than 6 cm in greatest dimension

MX: Distant metastasis cannot be assessed

M0: No distant metastasis

M1: Distant metastasis

MANAGEMENT

Treatment of patients with hypopharyngeal cancer is complex and requires the consideration of several factors. Disease factors, including the extent of the primary disease and the status of the cervical lymph nodes as well as the patient's performance status, pulmonary reserve, and comorbidity, must be considered. For early-stage diseases (T1–T2) of all the subsites of the hypopharynx, definitive radiation therapy is a reasonable therapeutic option (Table 119.3). Larynx-conserving surgeries can also be considered for highly selected patients. Adequate tumor resection, however, should never be compromised by procedures that attempt to preserve the larynx. For advanced cancers of the hypopharynx (T3–T4), surgical resection followed by postoperative radiation therapy remains the standard therapeutic

TABLE 119.3

HYPOPHARYNGEAL CANCER: 5-YEAR SURVIVAL BY LYMPH NODE STATUS (EASTERN VIRGINIA MEDICAL SCHOOL EXPERIENCE)[a]

Node Location (n)	Negative (n)	Positive (n)	5-Year Survival (%)
Piriform fossa (63)	14	49	8/14 (57)
			11/49 (22)
Posterior wall (30)	7	23	5/7 (71)
			12/23 (52)
Postcricoid (4)	1	3	1/1 (100)
			0/3 (0)
Totals	22	75[b]	14/22 (63)
			23/75 (30)

[a]Eastern Virginia Medical School 1972–1985; 97 patients.
[b]Bilateral nodes in 10 of 97 (10%) of entire group or 10 of 75 (13%) of those with positive nodes. Only 1 of 10 (10%) survived 5 years.

choice. Organ preservation protocols, which can achieve laryngeal preservation in 30% to 40% of the patients without compromising survival, have become valid therapeutic options for patients with advanced lesions.

Posterior Hypopharyngeal Wall Cancer

Lesions of the posterior hypopharyngeal wall are often exophytic and do not invade the prevertebral fascia until advanced. These pathologic features allow resection of early lesions of posterior hypopharyngeal wall. At M.D. Anderson Cancer Center, however, the early lesions of the posterior hypopharyngeal wall are most often treated with radio-

therapy. Radiotherapy may offer superior functional outcome compared with surgery because the pharyngeal plexus is invariably removed during the surgical resection, which can lead to aspiration because of the loss of propulsion and coordination of swallowing. Furthermore, even the early lesions of posterior hypopharyngeal wall will require postoperative radiotherapy to cover the retropharyngeal lymph nodes because of the high risk of metastases in these nodes (24).

When surgical resection is used for these early lesions, approaches can be via lateral or suprahyoid pharyngotomy (Fig. 119.6). Median labiomandibular glossotomy can be used for small lesions of the upper posterior pharyngeal

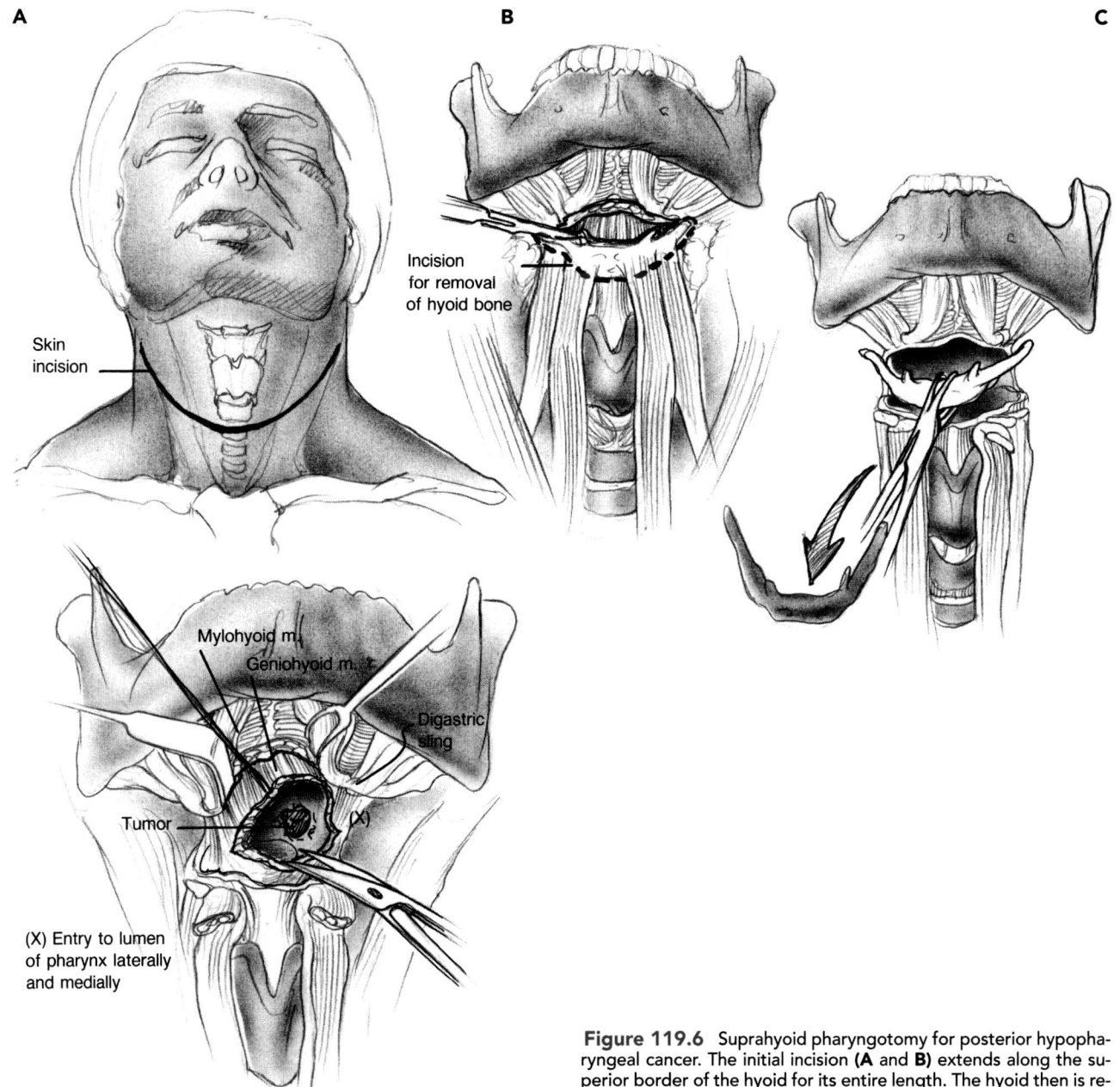

A

Skin incision

B

Incision for removal of hyoid bone

C

D

Mylohyoid m.
Geniohyoid m.
Digastric sling
Tumor
(X)
(X) Entry to lumen of pharynx laterally and medially

Figure 119.6 Suprahyoid pharyngotomy for posterior hypopharyngeal cancer. The initial incision (**A** and **B**) extends along the superior border of the hyoid for its entire length. The hyoid then is removed (**C**) to facilitate completion of the pharyngotomy (**D**).

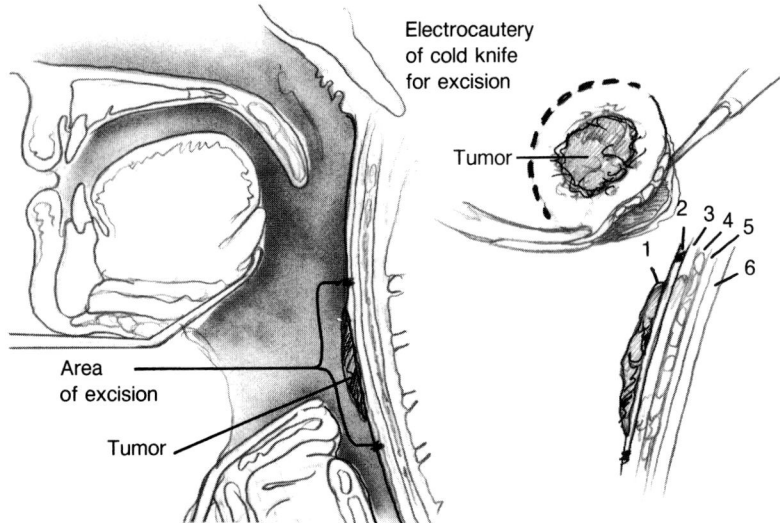

Figure 119.7 Suprahyoid pharyngotomy for posterior hypopharyngeal cancer. After the hyoid is removed and the pharyngotomy completed, superior and inferior retraction provides excellent exposure for wide excision of the cancer. *1*, tumor; *2*, mucosa; *3*, constrictor; *4*, longus colli; *5*, retropharyngeal space; *6*, prevertebral fascia.

wall but can result in significant morbidity. To approach these lesions via suprahyoid pharyngotomy, first the larynx is exposed and then the vallecula is entered at the midline. The incision is then extended laterally along the greater cornua of the hyoid bone. Because the dissection is extended laterally, care must be taken to avoid injury to the hypoglossal nerve and the superior laryngeal neurovascular bundle. This incision provides good exposure of the posterior hypopharyngeal wall. The tumor of the posterior pharyngeal wall can be excised at this time (Fig. 119.7). When excising a tumor on the posterior pharyngeal wall, the incision should be taken down to the level of the prevertebral fascia. The prevertebral muscles, if involved, can also be resected, but this finding portends low probability of local control with surgical resection. If a retropharyn-

geal node is noticed intraoperatively to have metastatic disease, retropharyngeal node dissection should be performed. If the retropharyngeal nodes are clinically negative and surgical resection is performed for the primary lesion, adjuvant radiotherapy must be delivered to the retropharyngeal lesion following the resection.

Reconstruction of the surgical defect can be undertaken with spit-thickness skin graft (Fig. 119.8). The skin graft can be held in place by a bolster dressing, which can then be removed transorally in 7 to 10 days. If the resection site is on the posterolateral wall of the hypopharynx, lateral pharyngotomy alone or in combination with suprahyoid pharyngotomy may be used (Figs. 119.9 and 119.10). In these cases, reconstruction can be accomplished with a pectoralis myofascial flap, rectus myocutaneous flap, or bipedicled

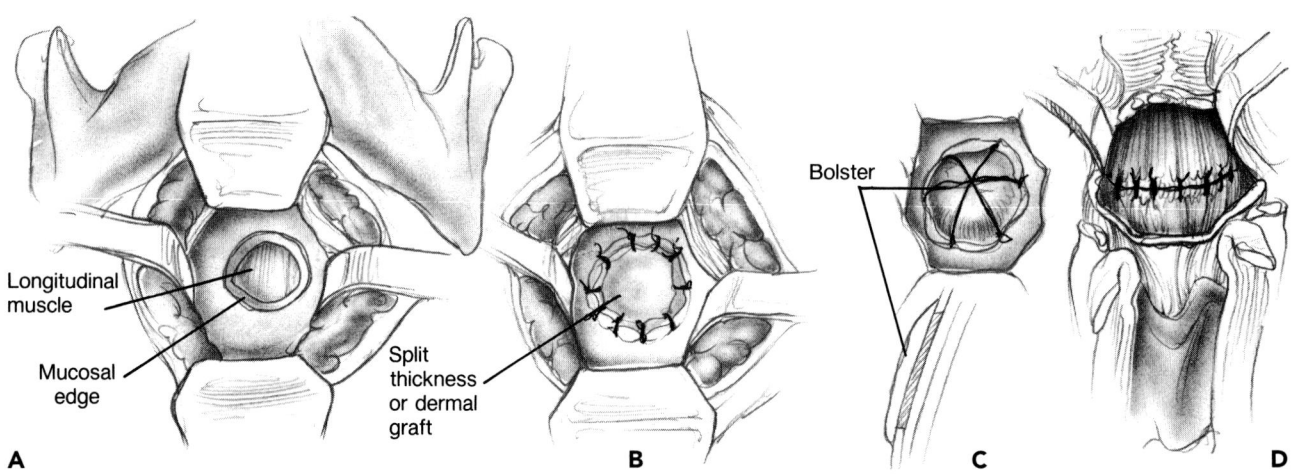

Figure 119.8 Suprahyoid pharyngotomy for posterior hypopharyngeal cancer. The incision is usually carried down to the prevertebral fascia **(A)**, which acts as the surgical plane for excision. The defect is then covered with a split-thickness or dermal skin graft **(B)**. This is held in place with a bolster **(C)** of nylon sheeting stuffed with cotton balls. The pharyngotomy is closed in layers, avoiding suture ligation of the hypoglossal and superior laryngeal nerves **(D)**.

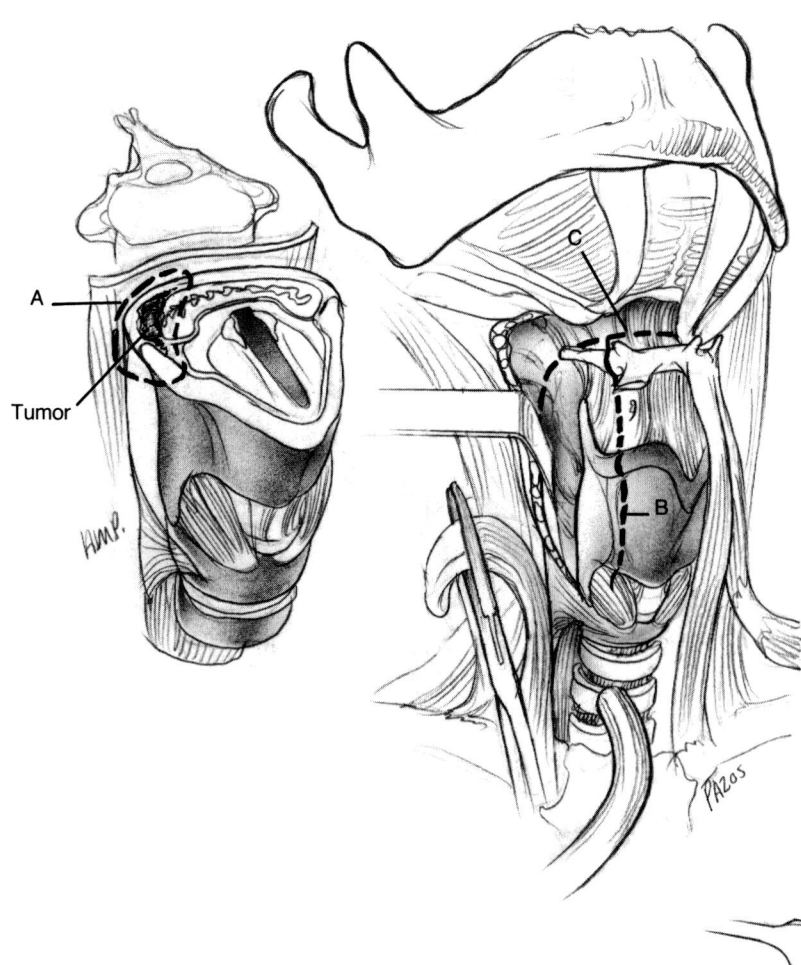

Figure 119.9 Combined suprahyoid and lateral pharyngotomy for posterolateral hypopharyngeal cancer. These cancers (**A**) are approached by excising the posterior third of the thyroid cartilage and combining the anterolateral pharyngotomy incision (**B**) with the suprahyoid incision (**C**).

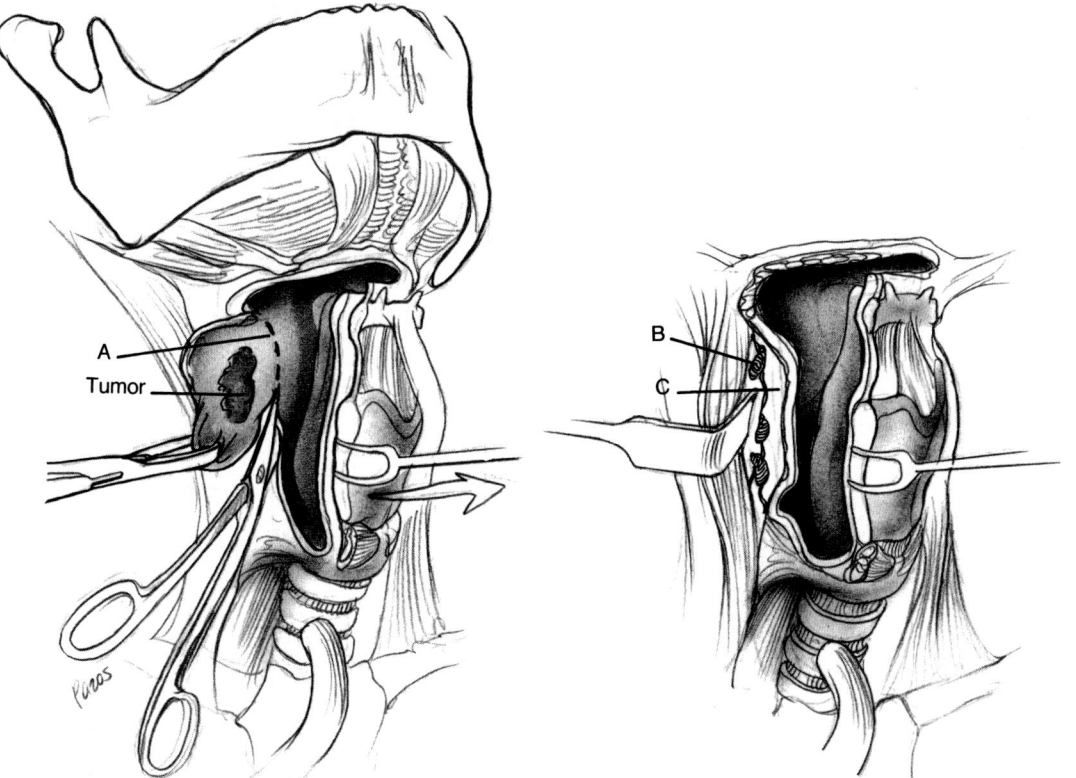

Figure 119.10 Combined suprahyoid and lateral pharyngotomy for posterolateral hypopharyngeal cancer. The final incision (**A**) is made under direct vision. The cervical sympathetic ganglion (**B**) should be preserved if it is not involved with the cancer. Reconstruction can be accomplished by using a portion of the prevertebral muscle (**C**) as a backing for a skin graft.

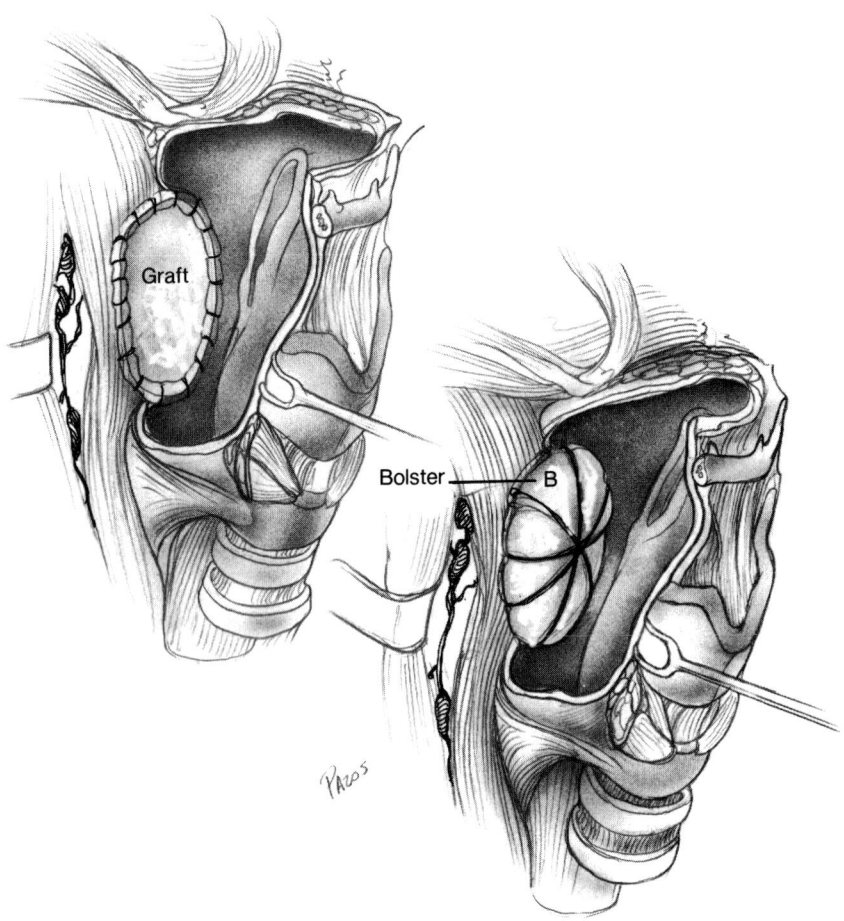

Figure 119.11 Combined suprahyoid and lateral pharyngotomy for posterolateral hypopharyngeal cancer. The split-thickness or dermal skin graft is sutured to the prevertebral muscle **(A)** and held in place with a nylon mesh and cotton-ball bolster **(B)**.

prevertebral muscle flap with split-thickness skin graft (Figs. 119.11 and 119.12). Care should be taken, however, to ensure that the bulkiness of the muscle flap does not interfere with swallowing. For larger defects, reconstruction via jejunal free flap or radial forearm free flap can be considered.

T1 and T2 Pyriform Sinus Cancer

Radiotherapy is preferred for the early hypopharyngeal cancers: T1 and T2 pyriform sinus cancer (32,33). These lesions are amenable to radiotherapy with high cure rates,

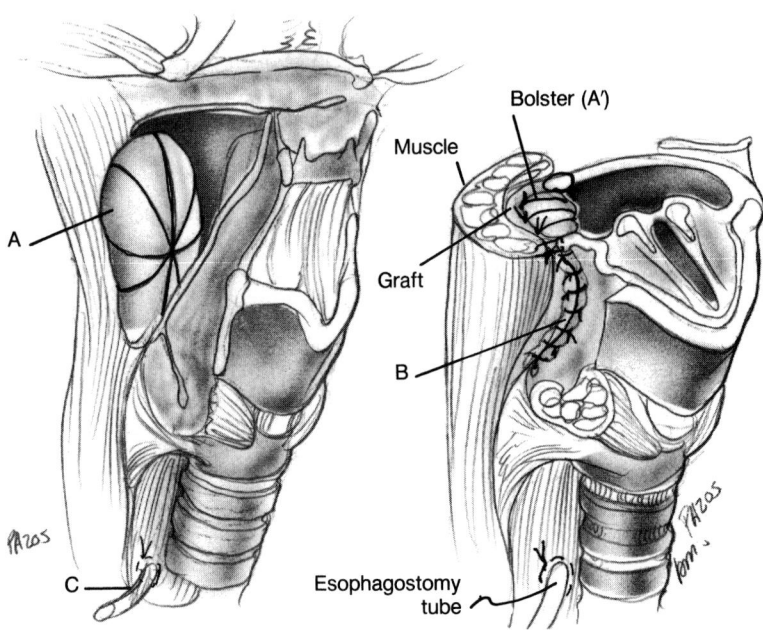

Figure 119.12 Combined suprahyoid and lateral pharyngotomy for posterolateral hypopharyngeal cancer. After the steps illustrated in Figures 119.9 through 119.11, the prevertebral muscle is mobilized as a bipedicled flap for medial rotation of the skin graft–bolster combination **(A)**. The bolster is sutured in place with long sutures from the graft. A watertight closure of the pharyngotomy **(B)** is then accomplished, and a feeding esophagostomy is placed **(C)**.

especially for the exophytic tumors. Because postoperative adjuvant radiotherapy is often indicated for early hypopharyngeal cancers, single modality therapy in the form of definitive radiotherapy is preferred over surgical resection with postoperative adjuvant irradiation. Surgical salvage can be used for those patients who fail radiation therapy, although higher complication rates are expected. When radiotherapy is the primary therapeutic modality, the radiation field should also include the regional lymphatic basins at risk, including bilateral cervical and retropharyngeal lymph nodes.

Surgical procedures that preserve the larynx may also be appropriate for early lesions of the medial wall of the pyriform sinuses or the pharyngoepiglottic fold (34). The lesion, however, must not involve the apex of the pyriform sinus or the postcricoid area, and the movement of the ipsilateral vocal cord must not be impaired. Patients also must have (a) good pulmonary reserve, (b) no cartilage involvement, and (c) no extension to the apex of the pyriform sinus. Keep in mind that only 2% of patients with hypopharyngeal cancer will be candidates for conservation surgery.

Resection of these tumors can be achieved with partial pharyngolaryngectomy (Figs. 119.13 to 119.15). This procedure combines supraglottic laryngectomy with the resection of the involved pyriform sinus. The exposure of the larynx is similar to that for supraglottic laryngectomy. The vallecula is then entered on the contralateral side. With the tumor in view, the incision is then extended to the ipsilateral vallecula and inferiorly along the posterior aspect of the ipsilateral pyriform sinus. The contralateral aryepiglottic fold is divided and this incision is extended inferiorly into the laryngeal ventricle and forward to the anterior commissure (Fig. 119.16).

An incision is then made vertically down the interarytenoid space to the superior border of the cricoid cartilage. This incision is extended superiorly and anteriorly across the vocal process and anteriorly through the ventricles. Finally, this incision is joined to the incision from the contralateral side above the anterior commissure (Fig. 119.16).

The last cuts to be made are at the apex of the pyriform sinus at the posterior border with the tumor in direct visualization. The vocal cord remnant needs to be brought back into a midline position and this can be accomplished by suturing the vocal process remnant to the upper edge of the cricoid cartilage. The resulting hypopharyngeal defect can be closed by suturing the tongue base to the thyroid perichondrium on the ipsilateral side. A second layer of closure can be accomplished using the strap muscles (Figs. 119.17 and 119.18).

Another conservation laryngeal surgery that can be used for early lesions of the hypopharynx is the supracricoid hemilaryngectomy (35). This procedure can be used for lesions of the anterior part, the lateral wall, the medial wall, and the aryepiglottic fold. Laccourreye et al. (35) reviewed

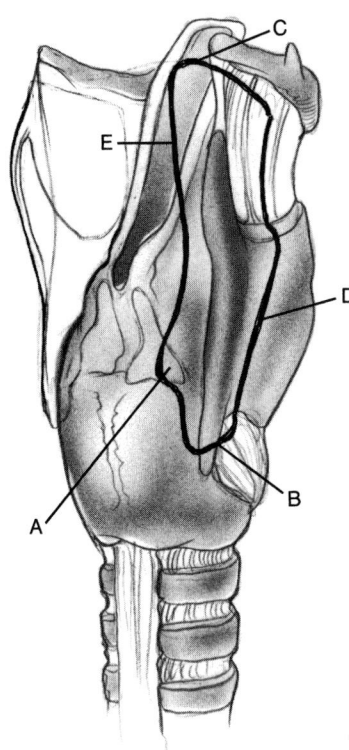

Figure 119.13 External surgical anatomic projections of the piriform fossa. The piriform apex **(A)** is just above the cricothyroid articulation at the inferior cornu **(B)**. The superior border is at the inferior margin of the hyoid bone **(C)**. The anterior border is at the junction of the anterior and posterior halves of the thyroid cartilage **(D)**. The posterior edge of the thyroid cartilage marks the posterior border of the piriform fossa **(E)**.

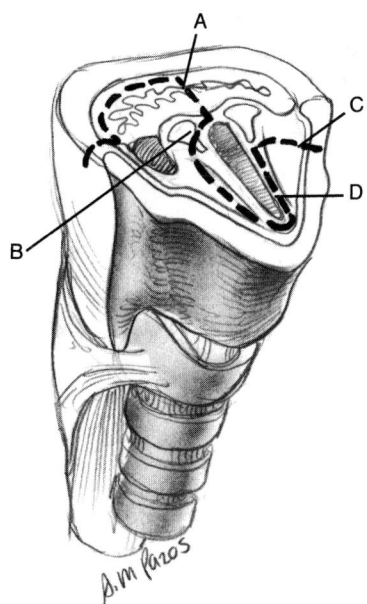

Figure 119.14 Partial laryngopharyngectomy (PLP) for cancer of the superior piriform fossa. The key elements of the PLP involve an interarytenoid incision **(A)** that extends across the vocal process **(B)** on the ipsilateral side and an incision in the aryepiglottic fold **(C)** and ventricle **(D)**, similar to that used for supraglottic laryngectomy on the contralateral side.

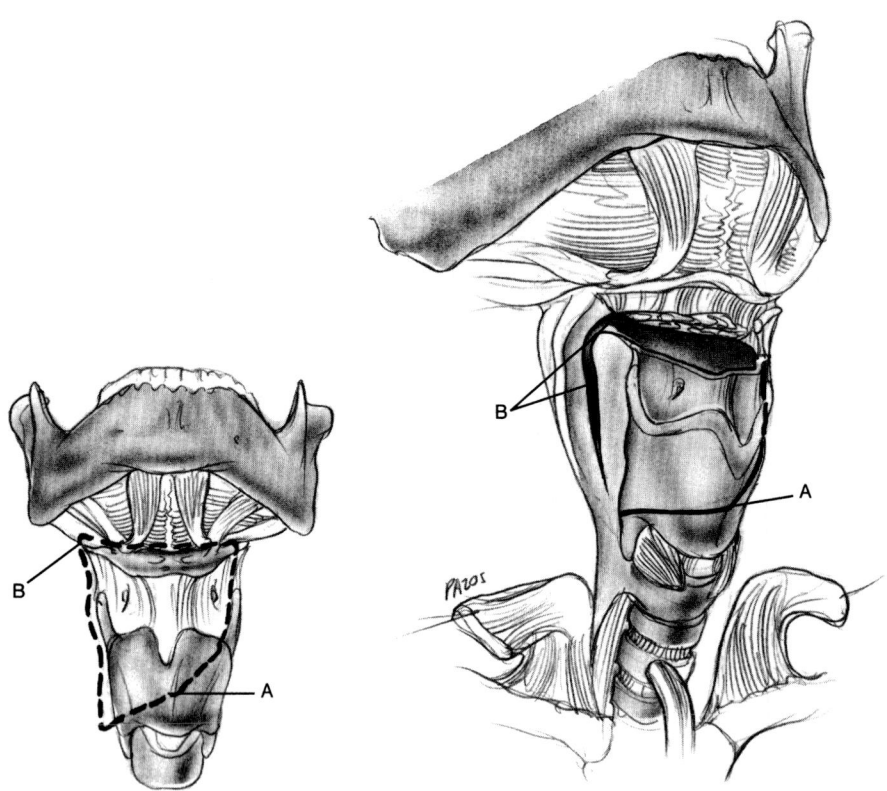

Figure 119.15 Partial laryngopharyngectomy for cancer of the superior piriform fossa. The cartilage cuts begin at a point above the anterior commissure (**A**) and extend laterally and inferiorly on the ipsilateral side and laterally and superiorly on the contralateral side. The pharynx is entered through a combination of suprahyoid and lateral pharyngotomy incisions (**B**).

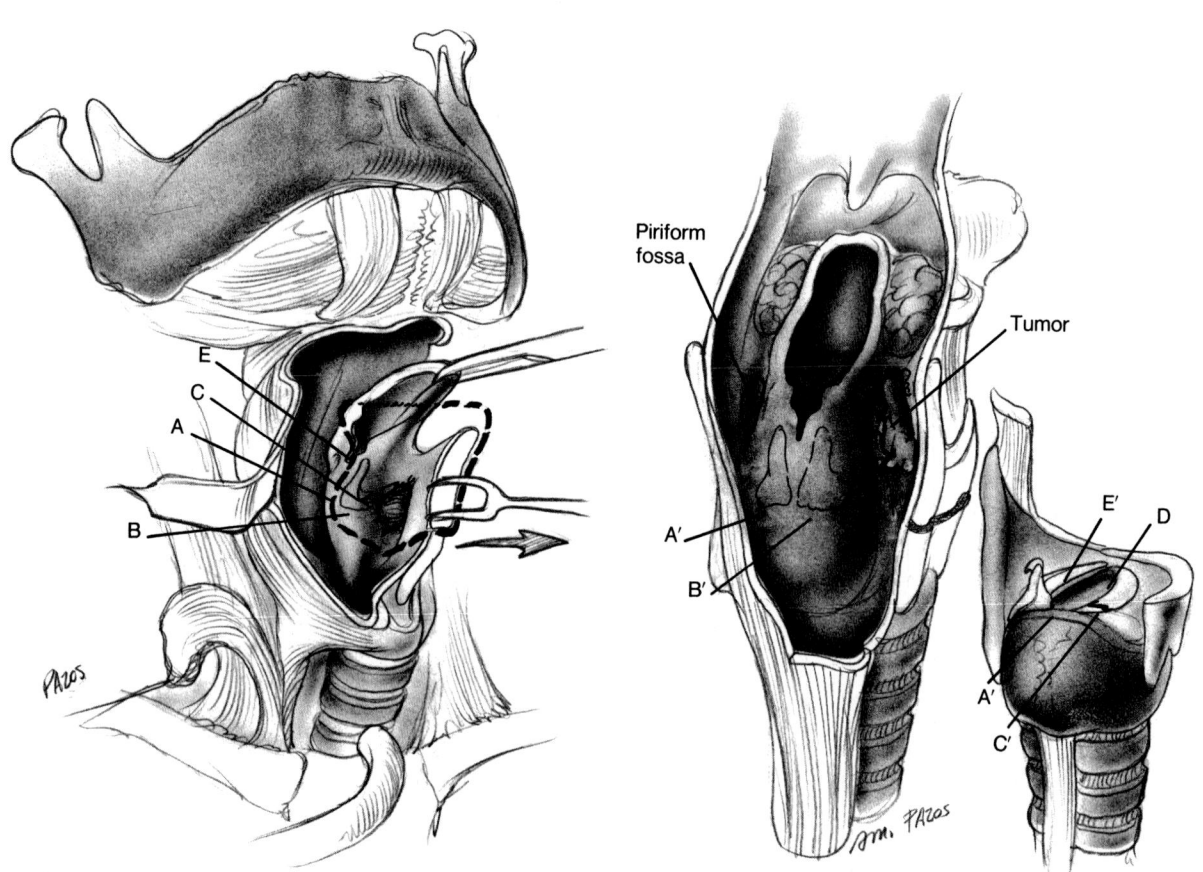

Figure 119.16 Partial laryngopharyngectomy for cancer of the superior piriform fossa. The interarytenoid incision (**A**) is carried down to the cricoid cartilage through the cricoarytenoid joint (**B**), across the vocal process (**C**), and anteriorly through the ventricle (**D**). The contralateral aryepiglottic fold and ventricular incisions (**E**) also extend forward to the anterior commissure.

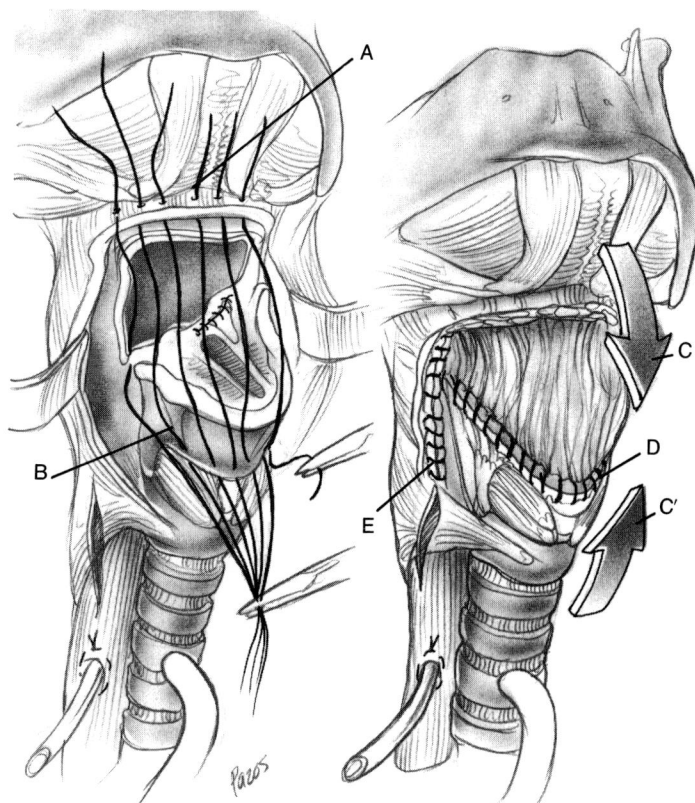

Figure 119.17 Partial laryngopharyngectomy for cancer of the superior piriform fossa. A watertight closure of the pharyngotomy is accomplished with a combination of sutures from the tongue base **(A)** to the thyroid perichondrium **(B)**. Head flexion allows tongue base and laryngeal relaxation **(C)** with closure of the horizontal segment of the pharyngotomy **(D)**. The lateral pharyngotomy is sutured vertically **(E)**.

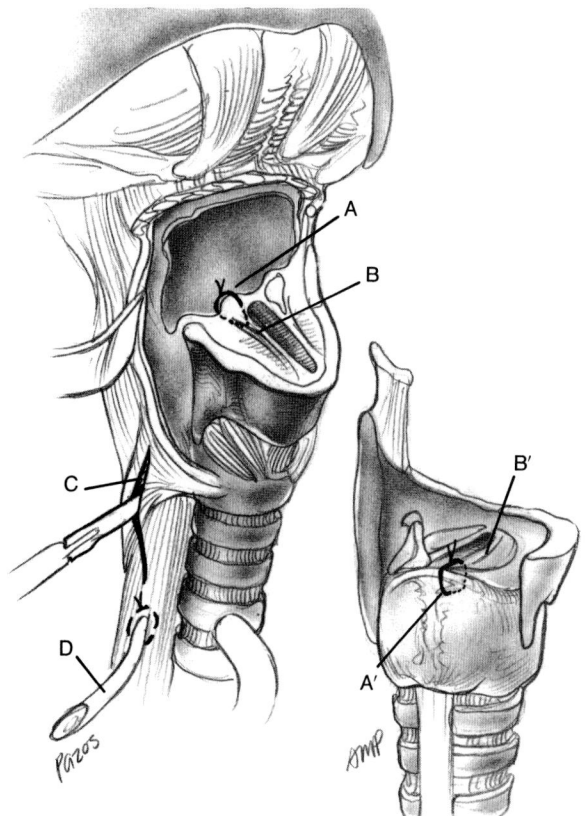

Figure 119.18 Partial laryngopharyngectomy for cancer of the superior piriform fossa. The vocal cord retention suture **(A)** is placed through the lateral aspect of the vocal process remnant, through the cricoid cartilage, then tied down to bring the cord **(B)** to the midline. A cricopharyngeal myotomy **(C)** is performed, and a feeding esophagostomy tube **(D)** placed.

the outcome of 34 patients with T2 lesions of the pyriform sinus who were treated with induction chemotherapy, followed by supracricoid hemilaryngectomy and postoperative radiotherapy. The 5-year actuarial local control rate was reported to be 97%. All but one of the patients were decannulated with average decannulation time of 7 days. Deglutition was achieved in 31 of 34 patients by the end of the first postoperative month. Aspiration pneumonia occurred in seven patients, however, and three of the seven patients required a temporary gastrostomy because of persistent aspiration-related problems.

T3 and T4 Pyriform Sinus Cancers

Surgery with postoperative radiation therapy remains the gold standard for patients with T3 and T4 cancers of the pyriform sinus. Conservation surgery is not possible for T3 and T4 tumors of the pyriform sinus and these tumors require total laryngectomy with partial pharyngectomy. When the lesions approach the apex of the pyriform sinus, it is important to remember the propensity of hypopharyngeal tumors for submucosal extension. Lesions with extension into the cervical esophagus will also require cervical esophagectomy. If the tumor extends into the thoracic esophagus, total esophagectomy followed by gastric pull-up reconstruction is indicated. Direct extension of tumors into the thyroid gland is also common and, therefore, surgical resections of T3 and T3 hypopharyngeal tumors should also include ipsilateral thyroidectomy. Because of the high incidence of paratracheal lymph node metastasis, unilateral paratracheal lymph node dissection should be performed (1). For advanced lesions that cross the midline or extend into the cervical esophagus, total thyroidectomy and bilateral paratracheal node dissections are indicated. Postoperative radiation therapy for advanced lesions of the pyriform sinus results in significantly improved local control compared with surgery alone (36,37). An organ preservation approach with chemoradiation is also a valid alternative option to total laryngopharyngectomy.

Cancer of the Postcricoid Region

Patients with cancers of the postcricoid area often do not present until the lesion is advanced. These lesions are often associated with invasion of the cricoid cartilage and cricoarytenoid muscle, and inferior extension into the cervical esophagus. Cancer of the postcricoid area, therefore, requires total laryngectomy, partial pharyngectomy, and often cervical esophagectomy followed by postoperative radiation therapy (38). Organ preservation approaches using chemotherapy with radiation therapy can be considered for patients who do not desire a total laryngectomy.

Cancer of the Neck

Cancer of the neck can be addressed with radiation therapy or neck dissection, depending on the therapeutic modality selected for the primary lesion. Regardless of the treatment modality, the high rate of cervical metastasis in hypopharyngeal cancer mandates the treatment of the neck. Lymph node metastases are associated with hypopharyngeal cancer in about 75% of the cases, with bilateral disease present in 10% of patients (Table 119.4). Treatment of the ipsilateral neck may be adequate for early lesions (T1 and T2) and le-

sions of the lateral pharyngeal wall. Advanced lesions or lesions that approach or involve the midline, however, require treatment of both sides of the neck.

Hypopharyngeal cancer most frequently metastasizes to cervical lymph nodes in level II, III, and IV. In a retrospective review of 126 patients with hypopharyngeal carcinoma who had radical neck dissections, Shah (39) examined the incidence of metastatic disease in each cervical lymph node level within the neck dissection specimens. In patients with clinically N0 neck cancer, 75% had pathologic positive nodes in levels II and III. When the neck cancer was clinically N+, 78%, 75%, and 47% of the neck dissection specimens had pathologically positive nodes at levels II, III, and IV, respectively. Therefore, elective neck dissection in patients with hypopharyngeal cancer should cover cervical lymph node levels II, III, and IV.

Paratracheal lymph nodes, or level VI, must also be addressed in advanced lesions of the hypopharynx. Weber et al. (1) retrospectively analyzed the incidence of paratracheal lymph node metastases in 141 patients with advanced lesions of the larynx and the hypopharynx. Metastatic disease in the paratracheal lymph nodes was present in 8.3% of the patients with cancer of the hypopharynx. Furthermore, survival analysis showed that the presence of paratracheal lymph node metastasis had a statistically significant negative impact on the survival of these patients. Based on these findings, Weber et al. recommended elective dissection of the paratracheal nodes for patients with advanced lesions of the hypopharynx. For unilateral hypopharyngeal cancers that do not approach the midline, unilateral paratracheal node dissection and ipsilateral thyroidectomy will suffice. When the advanced lesions cross the midline or extend into the cervical esophagus, however, total thyroidectomy and bilateral paratracheal node dissections are indicated (1). If bilateral dissections are performed, one or two parathyroid glands are identified and reimplanted in the sternocleidomastoid muscle or the forearm after histologic confirmation.

TABLE 119.4

HYPOPHARYNGEAL CANCER: 5-YEAR SURVIVAL BY STAGE[a]

Location No.	Stage				
	I	II	III	IV	Overall
Piriform fossa (63)	6/11	5/10	7/24	1/18	19/63
	54%	50%	29%	5%	30%
Posterior wall (30)	5/5	11/15	1/8	0/2	17/30
	100%	75%	12%	0%	56%
Postcricoid (4)			1/3	0/1	1/4
			33%	0%	25%
Totals	11/16	16/25	9/35	1/21	37/97
	68%	64%	25%	4%	38%

[a]Eastern Virginia Medical School, 1972–1985; 97 patients.

Involvement of retropharyngeal nodes is a concern in patients with cancer of the posterior pharyngeal wall. Ballantyne (24) was first to note the high risk of retropharyngeal metastatic disease in patients with posterior pharyngeal wall lesions. In his review of 48 patients with pharyngeal wall lesions, the retropharyngeal nodes were positive of metastatic disease in 20 of 48 (42%) patients. In addition, only the retropharyngeal nodes were positive in 5 of 20 patients. Hasegawa et al. (40) and Amatsu et al. (25) found incidences of retropharyngeal node metastasis of 67% and 57%, respectively, in patients with carcinomas of the posterior pharyngeal wall. All of these patients had retropharyngeal node dissection as part of their surgical management, regardless of the status of these nodes. These data suggest that the retropharyngeal nodes need to be treated in patients with lesions of the pharyngeal wall even when the nodes are clinically negative. For patients treated with primary radiotherapy, the radiation field should cover the retropharyngeal nodes. When the management consists of surgery and planned postoperative radiation, the retropharyngeal nodes do not require dissection unless radiographic evidence of disease in this area exists or if an involved node is encountered intraoperatively.

Role of Chemotherapy and Radiation Therapy in Hypopharyngeal Cancer

As mentioned, definitive radiation therapy is the treatment of choice for patients with T1 and T2 hypopharyngeal cancers, although it is arguable that radiation therapy results in better function than larynx-conserving procedures. With radiation therapy, the 5-year local control rate for patients with T1 and T2 hypopharyngeal cancers ranges from 70% to 100% (32,33). In cases of T3 and T4 hypopharyngeal cancer, however, radiation therapy is used most commonly as postoperative adjuvant therapy. The use of postoperative radiation therapy results in improvement in locoregional control from approximately 28% to 43% when compared with surgery alone. Furthermore, postoperative radiation therapy produces improved locoregional control when compared with preoperative radiation therapy (21,36). In a study by the Radiation Therapy Oncology Group (RTOG), patients with locally advanced SCC of the oral cavity, oropharynx, supraglottic larynx, and the hypopharynx were randomized to receive preoperative radiation therapy followed by surgery, postoperative radiation therapy 4 weeks following surgery, or definitive radiation therapy with salvage surgery, if necessary. Patients with hypopharyngeal cancers constituted 26% of the study group. Although subset analysis for hypopharyngeal cancer was not available, the locoregional control for all sites combined was superior for postoperative radiation therapy than for preoperative radiation therapy (37).

Chemotherapy as sole therapy is not indicated in the treatment in hypopharyngeal cancer. Although no studies have yet examined the role of chemotherapy as a definitive therapy specifically in hypopharyngeal cancer, several studies have examined the role of induction chemotherapy for SCC for all sites of head and neck cancer combined (41,42). The percentage of patients with hypopharyngeal cancer in these studies ranged from 17% to 27%. These studies, however, demonstrated no improvement in survival or locoregional control with the use of induction chemotherapy.

Concurrent chemoradiotherapy, on the other hand, has shown survival benefit in patients with advanced head and neck cancer. The Meta-Analysis of Chemotherapy in Head and Neck Cancer collaborative group performed meta-analysis of 63 trials between 1965 and 1993 involving 10,741 patients comparing the effects of neoadjuvant, concurrent, or adjuvant chemotherapy on overall survival (43). This study found a survival benefit of 8% at 2 and 5 years with concurrent chemoradiotherapy, whereas induction and adjuvant chemotherapy had no impact on survival.

Supported by data such as these, the European Organization for Research and Treatment of Cancer (EORTC) performed a study of the effectiveness of chemotherapy and radiotherapy when used sequentially as an organ-preserving alternative to total laryngectomy for patients with advanced (T3 and T4) hypopharyngeal cancer (44). In this study, patients were randomized to induction chemotherapy followed by definitive radiation therapy or total laryngectomy followed by postoperative radiation therapy. No statistical differences were seen in local control rates between the two arms, although larynx conservation was possible in up to 42% of the patients. Furthermore, the median (25 vs. 44 months) and 3-year survival rates (43 vs. 57 months) were higher in the larynx preservation group. Although quality of life data from this study are lacking, the study showed that larynx conservation protocols using induction chemotherapy followed by definitive radiation therapy is a legitimate option in patients with advanced hypopharyngeal cancer who desire to avoid a total laryngectomy.

Another relevant issue regarding an organ preservation approach is whether concurrent chemoradiation therapy is better than induction chemotherapy followed by radiotherapy. This issue was examined for laryngeal cancer in the intergroup R91-11 study in which patients with advanced laryngeal cancer were randomized to receive concurrent chemoradiation therapy, induction chemotherapy followed by radiation therapy, or radiation therapy alone (45). This study showed that concurrent chemoradiation therapy yielded superior locoregional control than did induction chemotherapy followed by radiotherapy. It remains to be studied whether concurrent chemotherapy is the next step in the evolution of organ preservation protocol for patients with hypopharyngeal cancer. A follow-up to the EORTC trial is currently in progress to answer this question.

An issue relevant to the use of concurrent chemoradiotherapy is its role in the postoperative adjuvant setting. For patients at high risk of local recurrence, the treatment of choice has been surgery combined with postoperative radiotherapy. The RTOG 9501 study and the EORTC trial 22931, however, examined the role of postoperative concurrent chemoradiotherapy in patients with head and neck cancer (46,47). In both of these studies, patients who had had surgical resection of the primary tumor and were noted to be high risk for treatment failure were randomized to receive postoperative radiotherapy or postoperative concurrent chemoradiotherapy. High risk of treatment failure was defined in the RTOG study as histologic evidence of involvement of two or more lymph nodes, extracapsular invasion, or positive margins. In addition to these features, the EORTC study extended the high-risk criteria to include vascular invasion, perineural invasion, any pT3 or pT4 disease, or tumor stage of 1 or 2 with a nodal stage of 2 or 3 and no distant metastasis. Patients with hypopharyngeal cancers constituted 20% of both the radiotherapy group and the concurrent chemoradiotherapy group in the EORTC study, whereas the hypopharynx was the primary site in 12% of the radiotherapy group and 7% of the concurrent chemoradiotherapy group in the RTOG study. Both studies showed that postoperative concurrent chemoradiotherapy increased the 2-year local and regional control compared with the postoperative radiotherapy group (increase by 10% and 11% in RTOG and EORTC studies, respectively). Only the EORTC study was able to demonstrate an increase in the survival (53% in the postoperative concurrent chemoradiotherapy group vs. 40% in the postoperative radiotherapy group). It should be noted that the incidence of severe, early side effects was higher in the combination therapy group compared with the radiotherapy alone group. Therefore, patients at high risk for treatment failure after surgical resection should benefit from adjuvant concurrent chemotherapy, provided the patient is able to tolerate the intensity of the combined treatment.

PROGNOSIS

As a group, the overall survival rate of patients with hypopharyngeal cancer ranges from 35% to 40% (Table 119.5). Kraus et al. (48) retrospectively reviewed 132 patients who had surgery and postoperative therapy for hypopharyngeal cancer and reported 5-year overall and disease-free survival of 30% and 41%, respectively. Kim et al. (49) found comparable 5-year and disease-free survival of 46.8% and 47.4%, respectively, in their retrospective review of 73 patients with hypopharyngeal cancer. The presence of regional lymph node metastasis, however, will have significant negative influences on these figures (see Table 119.4) (50). Kraus et al. (48) reported that the 5-year disease-free survival was 54% in patients with N0 or N1

TABLE 119.5 ℞ TREATMENT HYPOPHARYNGEAL CANCER

Surgery
  Suprahyoid pharyngotomy
  Partial laryngopharyngectomy
  Laryngectomy
  Pharyngectomy
  Partial cervical esophagectomy
  Skin graft
  Free flap
  Gastric interposition
  Feeding tube
  Neck dissection
  Superior mediastinal dissection
Radiotherapy
  T1, some T2
  Postsurgical
Chemotherapy
Chemoradiation
High-dose intraarterial chemotherapy and radiotherapy
Must treat the necks even in patients without palpable metastases

disease, but was decreased to 20% in patients with N2 or N3 disease.

Posterior Hypopharyngeal Wall

For all stages of posterior pharyngeal wall cancer, the 5-year survival rate ranges from 35% to 44% when treated with surgery and postoperative radiotherapy (48,51). Although radiation therapy is effective for the early lesions of the pharyngeal wall, surgery combined with adjuvant radiotherapy is superior for advanced lesions. Meoz-Mendez et al. (52) reported a 49% failure rate for T3 and T4 tumors of the pharyngeal walls 1 year after treatment with radiotherapy alone but a 25% failure rate for similar lesions treated with surgery and postoperative radiotherapy (52). Similarly, Kim et al. (49) reported 5-year survival rates of 15.7% in patients treated with radiotherapy only and 46.8% for those treated with surgery and postoperative radiotherapy.

Pyriform Sinus

The reported 5-year disease-free survival for cancer of the pyriform sinus ranges from 40% to 60%. Consensus in the literature is that patients with early lesions of the pyriform sinus can be treated with either radiotherapy or conservation laryngeal surgery. For advanced lesions of the pyriform sinus, however, radiotherapy alone offers poor rates of local control compared with surgery followed by adjuvant radiotherapy. Spector et al. (53) retrospectively reviewed the treatment result of 408 patients with cancer of the pyriform sinus and reported that radiation therapy combined with conservation surgery was more curative than with radiation alone (71% vs. 27%, respectively). Similarly, Vandenbrouck et al. (54) reviewed the outcome results of 199 patients treated with surgery and postoperative radiotherapy and 153 patients treated with radiotherapy alone. The 5-year survival was reported as 33% and 14% for the combined treatment group and the radiotherapy group, respectively. The locoregional recurrence rate was also lower for the combined treatment group at 44% vs. 17.5% for the radiotherapy group. El Badawi et al. (21) compared the recurrence rate above the clavical in patients treated with surgery alone versus those treated with surgery and postoperative radiotherapy. The recurrence rate above the clavicle was 39% following surgery alone, as opposed to recurrence rate of 11% following surgery and postoperative radiotherapy.

Postcricoid Area

Prognostic data in the literature specifically for the postcricoid area are limited. As with other subsites of hypopharynx, radiotherapy alone may be adequate for early lesions but surgical resection with postoperative radiotherapy offers superior outcomes. Farrington et al. (55) reported cause-specific 5-year survival of only 22% in patients with cancer of the postcricoid area treated with primary radiotherapy. This study also found that survival decreased significantly with lesions more than 2 cm in length. For tumors greater than 4 cm in length, the survival at 5 years was less than 5%. Vocal cord paralysis was also found to be a poor prognostic factor.

Stell et al. (56) reported a 38% 5-year survival in patients with cancer of the cricoid area treated with either primary radiotherapy or surgery. The patients treated with primary radiotherapy had mostly T1 and T2 lesions and those treated with surgery had tumors greater than 5 cm, positive regional disease, or recurrent lesions after primary radiotherapy. From these data, the authors suggest that for advanced lesions of the postcricoid area, surgical resection offers a superior outcome compared with radiotherapy.

Harrison and Thompson (13) reviewed a series of 101 patients with hypopharyngeal cancer treated with surgical resection, gastric pull-up reconstruction, and postoperative radiotherapy. Of lesions, 66% were located in the postcricoid area. The 5-year survival was reported to be 58% in this study. Although the result of this series is more favorable than the survival rates reported in other studies, it emphasizes the need for combined therapy in advanced lesions of the postcricoid area.

RECONSTRUCTION

For small defects resulting from the resection of small lesions, primary closure or skin grafts can be sufficient. Tubing the remaining pharyngeal mucosa to achieve primary closure should be discouraged when less than 2 cm of the mucosa remains, however, because of concerns of stricture. In this situation, the subtotal defect can be repaired in a patch-fashion using the pectoralis major myocutaneous flap or fasciocutaneous flaps such as the radial forearm free flap or the anterolateral thigh flap (57,58). Another option is to excise the remaining mucosa and perform a circumferential reconstruction. In general, the pectoralis major flap should not be used for hypopharyngeal reconstruction when the larynx is spared. The bulk and the immobile nature of the pectoralis major flap may predispose these patients to intractable aspiration.

Reconstruction following total pharyngectomy is best accomplished with the use of microvascular, free tissue transfer. The reconstructive option of choice is the free jejunal graft or tubed fasciocutaneous free flap such as radial forearm free flap or anterolateral thigh flap (59,60). Defects from the nasopharynx to the thoracic inlet can be reconstructed with this method. The free jejunal graft, which allows early deglutition, is associated with a low incidence of stenosis and fistula (59,60). When total pharyngoesophagectomy is required, the reconstructive method of choice is the gastric pull-up procedure (61). The need for major abdominal surgery and posterior mediastinal dissection, however, results in operative morbidity of 50% and mortality rates of 10% (13). Another option in this situation is the use of pedicled jejunum or colonic interposition. Because these pedicled enteric reconstructions often display arterial insufficiency at the distal end of the enteric conduit (oral end), graft necrosis and anastomotic leakage can occur. To circumvent this problem, "supercharging" of the arterial supply to the distal end of the enteric conduit can be performed where additional vascular supply to this area is established via microvascular anastomosis. In this fashion, the pedicled jejunum will have vascular supply from the original vascular pedicle as well as the augmented vascular supply to the distal end of the conduit (62,63). When the "supercharge" technique was used to augment the vascular supply to enteric conduits in 82 cases of pharyngeal and esophageal reconstructions, Sekido et al. (63) reported a graft failure rate of only 2%. Regardless of which method of reconstruction is used, oncologic safety should not be compromised in favor of a particular reconstructive option.

Comparison of functional outcomes after hypopharyngeal reconstruction is difficult because of the lack of uniformity in assessment of these parameters in various studies. In general, restoration of G-tube independent swallowing following reconstructions with either fasciocutaneous flaps or enteric flap (e.g., jejunal free flap) can be achieved in greater than 85% of the patients (64–67). Some studies suggest, however, that jejunal free flap can result in better swallowing ability compared with radial forearm free flap. In a study by Disa et al. (67), the ability to tolerate unrestricted diet following hypopharyngeal reconstruction with either radial forearm free flap or jejunal free flap was examined. Although the jejunal free flap was reserved for reconstructing circumferential defects only, this method resulted in a higher percentage of patients tolerating an unrestricted diet than those having radial forearm free flap reconstruction (66% vs. 51%) (67).

Restoration of speech following hypopharyngeal reconstruction can be achieved with the use of tracheoesophageal puncture (TEP). The quality of TEP speech following hypopharyngeal reconstruction, however, is usually inferior to TEP speech in patients after laryngectomy who did not require hypopharyngeal reconstruction. The vocal quality of patients who have had hypopharyngeal reconstruction is often described as low pitch and "wet" (68). Multiple studies also show that, although the fundamental frequency and the intensity level of TEP speech were not statistically different between those who required hypopharyngeal reconstruction and those who did not, the group having reconstruction consistently scored lower on various qualitative parameters (69,70). Nevertheless, it should be emphasized that adequate and dependable voice restoration can be achieved in most patients following hypopharyngeal reconstructions.

COMPLICATIONS

In general, complications associated with major surgeries in other sites of head and neck cancer also apply to the postoperative period following laryngopharyngectomy (Tables 119.6 and 119.7). Most early complications following resection of hypopharyngeal tumors are the result of leakage at the site of pharyngeal closure. The preoperative nutritional status of the patient, history of prior radiation therapy, as well as the type of reconstructive option used may all influence the development of pharyngeal fistula. Intraoperative factors such as tight closure caused by inadequate available mucosa or the presence of tumor at the resection margin will also lead to the development of pharyngeal fistula. Infection, hemorrhage, and breakdown of skin wounds are also common in these high-risk patients.

Airway obstruction is usually a concern in the early postoperative period of patients who are tracheostomy-dependent. Good nursing care and diligent suctioning of the tracheostomy tube can circumvent these problems. A late complication following surgery for hypopharyngeal cancer is aspiration, which if severe, can lead to pneumonia. Swallowing rehabilitation under the supervision of a

TABLE 119.6   **COMPLICATIONS**
WOUND INFECTION

Hemorrhage
Fistula
Aspiration
Stricture

TABLE 119.7   **EMERGENCY CARE**

Obstruction
Airway
Tracheotomy
Laser debulking
Esophagus
Feeding tube
Fluid resuscitation
Disimpaction
Hemorrhage
Isolate source
Angiography
Embolization
Surgical ligation

speech or swallowing therapist is mandatory for these patients. Swallowing difficulties can also be the result of stenosis after circumferential reconstructions and may require repeated dilation in an outpatient setting.

HIGHLIGHTS

- Patients with hypopharyngeal cancer often have medical problems associated with tobacco use, alcohol abuse, and malnutrition.
- Pathologic characteristics of hypopharyngeal cancer include propensity for submucosal spread and satellite lesions.
- Lymphatic drainage of the inferior hypopharynx includes the paratracheal lymph nodes. The retropharyngeal lymph nodes are also often involved in hypopharyngeal lesions, especially for lesions of the posterior hypopharyngeal wall.
- High incidence of cervical metastasis mandates the treatment of cervical lymphatic basins, including the retropharynx, by radiotherapy or neck dissection in virtually all stages of hypopharyngeal cancer.
- Although early lesions of the posterior hypopharyngeal wall can be surgically resected, this invariably leads to functional compromise because of the removal of the pharyngeal plexus. Therefore, definitive radiation therapy may be more appropriate for these lesions.
- Surgical resection (total laryngectomy with partial or total pharyngectomy) with adjuvant radiotherapy remains the gold standard for treatment of advanced hypopharyngeal lesions. Organ-preservation approaches using chemotherapy and radiotherapy, however, have become established as valid therapeutic alternatives for patients with advanced hypopharyngeal lesions.
- Many types of reconstructive methods are available for hypopharyngeal reconstruction. The optimal choice of reconstruction depends on the surgeon's experience and the technique that will result in the most functional result.
- Successful restoration of function including swallowing and tracheoesophageal speech is often possible following hypopharyngeal reconstruction.

REFERENCES

1. Weber RS, Marvel J, Smith P, et al. Paratracheal lymph node dissection for carcinoma of the larynx, hypopharynx, and cervical esophagus. *Otolaryngol Head Neck Surg* 1993;108:11–17.
2. Johnson JT, Bacon GW, Myers EN, et al. Medial vs lateral wall pyriform sinus carcinoma: implications for management of regional lymphatics. *Head Neck* 1994;16:401–405.
3. Castelijns JA, Gerritsen GJ, Kaiser MC, et al. Invasion of laryngeal cartilage by cancer: comparison of CT and MR imaging. *Radiology* 1988;167:199–206.
4. Becker M, Zbaren P, Laeng H, et al. Neoplastic invasion of the laryngeal cartilage: comparison of MR imaging and CT with histopathologic correlation. *Radiology* 1995;194:661–669.
5. Becker M, Zbaren P, Delavelle J, et al. Neoplastic invasion of the laryngeal cartilage: reassessment of criteria for diagnosis at CT. *Radiology* 1997;203:521–532.
6. Zbaren P, Becker M, Laeng H. Pretherapeutic staging of laryngeal carcinoma: clinical finding, computed tomography and magnetic resonance imaging compared with histopathology. *Cancer* 1996;77: 1263–1273.
7. Merino OR, Lindberg RD, Fletcher GH. An analysis of distant metastases from squamous cell carcinoma of the upper respiratory and digestive tracts. *Cancer* 1977;40:145–151.
8. Leemans CR, Tiwari R, Nauta JJ, et al. Regional lymph node involvement and its significance in the development of distant metastasis in head and neck carcinoma. *Cancer* 1993;71:452–456.
9. de Bree R, Deurloo EE, Snow GB, et al. Screening for distant metastases in patients with head and neck cancer. *Laryngoscope* 2000;110:397–401.
10. Houghton DJ, Hughes ML, Garvey C, et al. Role of chest CT scanning in the management of patients presenting with head and neck cancer. *Head Neck* 1998;20:614–618.
11. Wax MK, Myers LL, Gabalski EC, et al. Positron emission tomography in the evaluation of synchronous lung lesions in patients with untreated head and neck cancer. *Arch Otolarygol Head Neck Surg* 2002;128:703–707.
12. Teknos TN, Rosenthal EL, Lee D, et al. Positron emission tomography in the evaluation of stage III and IV head and neck cancer. *Head Neck* 2001;23:1056–1060.
13. Harrison DF, Thompson AE. Pharyngolaryngoesophagectomy with pharyngogastric anastomosis for cancer of the hypopharynx: review of 101 operations. *Head Neck Surg* 1986;8:418–428.
14. Marks JE, Smith PG, Sessions DG. Pharyngeal wall cancer: a reappraisal after comparison of treatment methods. *Arch Otolaryngol* 1985;111:79–85.
15. Ward PH, Hanson DG. Reflux as an etiological factor of carcinoma of the laryngopharynx. *Laryngoscope* 1988;98:1195–1199.
16. Carpenter RJ 3rd, DeSanto LW, Devine KD, et al. Cancer of the hypopharynx. Analysis of treatment and results in 162 patients. *Arch Otolaryngol* 1976;102:716–721.
17. Ho CM, Ng WF, Lam KH, et al. Submucosal tumor extension in hypopharyngeal cancer. *Arch Otolaryngol Head Neck Surg* 1997;123: 959–965.
18. Hirano M, Kurita S, Tanaka H. Histopathologic study of carcinoma of the hypopharynx: implications for conservation surgery. *Ann Otol Rhinol Laryngol* 1987;96:625–629.
19. Kirchner JA, Owen JR. Five hundred cancers of the larynx and pyriform sinus. Results of treatment by radiation and surgery. *Laryngoscope* 1977;87:1288–1303.
20. Hahn SS, Spaulding CA, Kim JA, et al. The prognostic significance of lymph node involvement in pyriform sinus and supraglottic cancers. *Int J Radiat Oncol Biol Phys* 1987;13:1143–1147.
21. El Badawi SA, Goepfert H, Fletcher GH, et al. Squamous cell carcinoma of the pyriform sinus. *Laryngoscope* 1982;92:357–365.
22. Candela FC, Kothari K, Shah JP. Patterns of cervical node metastases from squamous carcinoma of the oropharynx and hypopharynx. *Head Neck* 1990;12:197–203.
23. Jones AS, Stell PM. Squamous carcinoma of the posterior pharyngeal wall. *Clin Otolaryngol* 1991;16:462–465.
24. Ballantyne AJ. Principles of surgical management of cancer of the pharyngeal walls. *Cancer* 1967;20:663–667.
25. Amatsu M, Mohri M, Kinishi M. Significance of retropharyngeal node dissection at radical surgery for carcinoma of the hypopharynx and cervical esophagus. *Laryngoscope* 2001;111:1099–1103.
26. Teichgraber JF, McConnel FM. Treatment of posterior pharyngeal wall carcinoma. *Otolaryngol Head Neck Surg* 1986;94:287–290.
27. Somers KD, Merrick MA, Lopez ME, et al. Frequent *p53* mutations in head and neck cancer. *Cancer Res* 1992;52:5997–6000.
28. Masuda M, Hirakawa N, Nakashima T, et al. Cyclin D1 overexpression in primary hypopharyngeal carcinoma. *Cancer* 1996;78: 390–395.
29. Repassy G, Forster-Horvath C, Juhasz A, et al. Expression of invasion markers CD44v6/v3, NM23 and MMP2 in laryngeal and hypopharyngeal carcinoma. *Pathol Oncol Res* 1998;4:14–21.
30. Mineta H, Miura K, Takebayashi S, et al. Prognostic value of glucose transporter 1 expression in patients with hypopharyngeal carcinoma. *Anticancer Res* 2002;22:3489–3494.
31. van der Riet P, Nawroz H, Hruban RH, et al. Frequent loss of chromosome 9p21-22 early in head and neck cancer progression. *Cancer Res* 1994;54:1156–1158.
32. Mendenhall WM, Parsons JT, Cassisi NJ, et al. Squamous cell carcinoma of the pyriform sinus treated with radical radiation therapy. *Radiother Oncol* 1987;9:201–208.
33. Fein DA, Mendenhall WM, Parson JT, et al. Pharyngeal wall carcinoma treated with radiotherapy: impact of treatment technique and fractionation. *Int J Radiat Oncol Biol Phys* 1993;26: 751–757.
34. Hamoir M, Ledeghen S, Rombaux P, et al. Conservation surgery for laryngeal and hypopharyngeal cancer. *Acta Otorhinolaryngol Belg* 1999;53:207–213.
35. Laccourreye O, Merite-Drancy A, Brasnu D, et al. Supracricoid hemilaryngopharyngectomy in selected pyriform sinus carcinoma stage as T2. *Laryngoscope* 1993;103:1373–1379.
36. Frank JL, Garb JL, Kay S, et al. Postoperative radiotherapy improves survival in squamous cell carcinoma of the hypopharynx. *Am J Surg* 1994;168:476–480.
37. Tupchong L, Scott CB, Blitzer PH, et al. Randomized study of preoperative versus postoperative radiation therapy in advanced head and neck carcinoma: long-term follow-up of RTOG study 73-03. *Int J Radiat Oncol Biol Phys* 1991;20:21–28.
38. Harrison DF. Pathology of hypopharyngeal cancer in relation to surgical management. *J Laryngol Otol* 1970;84:349–367.
39. Shah JP. Patterns of cervical lymph node metastasis from squamous carcinomas of the upper aerodigestive tract. *Am J Surg* 1990;160:405–409.
40. Hasegawa Y, Matsuura H. Retropharyngeal node dissection in cancer of the oropharynx and hypopharynx. *Head Neck* 1994;16: 173–180.
41. Head and Neck Contract Program. Adjuvant chemotherapy for advanced head and neck squamous cell carcinomas. *Cancer* 1987;60:301.
42. Laramore GE, Scott CD, al-Sarraf M, et al. Adjuvant chemotherapy for resectable squamous cell carcinomas of the head and neck: report on intergroup study 0034. *Int J Radiat Oncol Biol Phys* 1992;23:705–713.
43. Pignon JP, Bourhis J, Domenge C, et al. Chemotherapy added to locoregional treatment for head and neck squamous-cell carcinoma: three meta-analysis of updated individual data. *Lancet* 2000;355:949–955.
44. Lefebvre JL, Chevalier D, Luboinski B, et al. Larynx preservation in pyriform sinus cancer: preliminary results of a European Organization for Research and Treatment of Cancer phase III trial. *J Natl Cancer Inst* 1996;88:890–899.
45. Forastiere AA, Berkely B, Moshe M, et al. Phase III trial to preserve the larynx: induction chemotherapy versus concomitant chemoradiotherapy versus radiotherapy alone, Intergroup Trial R91-11 (abst). *Proc Am Soc Clin Oncol* 2001;20:20a.
46. Cooper JS, Pajak TF, Forastiere AA, et al. Postoperative concurrent radiotherapy and chemotherapy for high-risk squamous-cell carcinoma of the head and neck. *N Engl J Med* 2004;350:1937–1944.
47. Bernier J, Domenge C, Ozsahin M, et al. Postoperative irradiation with or without concomitant chemoradiotherapy for locally advanced head and neck cancer. *N Engl J Med* 2004;350:1945–1952.
48. Kraus DH, Zelefsky MJ, Brock HA, et al. Combined surgery and radiation therapy for squamous cell carcinoma of the hypopharynx. *Otolaryngol Head Neck Surg* 1997;116:637–641.
49. Kim S, Wu HG, Heo DS, et al. Advanced hypopharyngeal carcinoma treatment results according to treatment modalities. *Head Neck* 2001;23:713–717.

50. Lefebvre JL, Castelain B, De la Torre JC, et al. Lymph node invasion in hypopharynx and lateral epilarynx carcinoma: a prognostic factor. *Head Neck Surg* 1987;10:14–18.
51. Julieron M, Kolb F, Schwaab G, et al. Surgical management of posterior pharyngeal wall carcinomas: function and oncologic results. *Head Neck* 2001;23:80–86.
52. Meoz-Mendez RT, Fletcher GH, Guillamondegui OM, et al. Analysis of the results of irradiation in the treatment of squamous cell carcinomas of the pharyngeal walls. *Int J Radiat Oncol Biol Phys* 1978;4:579–585.
53. Spector JG, Session DG, Emami B, et al. Squamous cell carcinoma of the pyriform sinus: a nonrandomized comparison of therapeutic modalities and long-term results. *Laryngoscope* 1995;105:397–406.
54. Vandenbrouck C, Eschwege F, De la Rochefordiere A, et al. Squamous cell carcinoma of the pyriform sinus: retrospective study of 351 cases treated at the Institut Gustave-Roussy. *Head Neck Surg* 1987;10:4–13.
55. Farrington WT, Weighill JS, Jones PH. Post-cricoid carcinoma (ten-year retrospective study). *J Laryngol Otol* 1986;100:79–84.
56. Stell PM, Carden EA, Hibbert J, et al. Post-cricoid carcinoma. *Clin Oncol* 1978;4:215–226.
57. Rees RS, Ivey GL 3rd, Shack RB, et al. Pectoralis major musculocutaneous flaps: long-term follow-up of hypopharyngeal reconstruction. *Plast Resconst Surg* 1986;77:586–591.
58. Anthony JP, Singer MI, Mathes SJ. Pharyngoesophageal reconstruction using the tubed free radial forearm flap. *Clin Plast Surg* 1994;21:137–147.
59. Theile DE, Robinson DW, McCafferty GJ. Pharyngolaryngectomy reconstruction by revascularized free jejunal graft. *Aust N Z J Surg* 1986;56:849–852.
60. Reece GP, Schusterman MA, Miller MJ, et al. Morbidity and functional outcome of free jejunal transfer reconstruction for circumferential defects of the pharynx and cervical esophagus. *Plast Reconstr Surg* 1995;96:1307–1316.
61. Hartley BE, Bottrill ID, Howard DJ. A third decade's experience with the gastric pull-up operation for hypopharyngeal carcinoma: changing patterns of use. *J Laryngol Otol* 1999;113:241–243.
62. Nagawa H, Seto Y, Nakatsuka T, et al. Microvascular anastomosis for additional blood flow in reconstruction after intrathoracic esophageal carcinoma surgery. *Am J Surg* 1997;173:131–133.
63. Sekido M, Yamamoto Y, Minakawa H, et al. Use of the "supercharge" technique in esophageal and pharyngeal reconstruction to augment microvascular blood flow. *Surgery* 2003;134:420–424.
64. Coleman JJ 3rd, Tan KC, Searles JM, et al. Jejunal free autograft; analysis of complications and their resolution. *Plast Recontr Surg* 1989;84:589–595.
65. Oniscu GC, Walker WS, Sanderson R. Functional results following pharyngolaryngoesophagectomy with free jejunal graft reconstruction. *Eur J Cardiothorac Surg* 2001;19:406–410.
66. Scharpf J, Escalmado RM. Reconstruction with radial forearm flaps after ablative surgery for hypopharyngeal cancer. *Head Neck* 2003;25:261–266.
67. Disa JJ, Pusic AL, Hidalgo DA, et al. Microvascular reconstruction of the hypopharynx: defect classification, treatment algorithm, and functional outcome based on 165 consecutive cases. *Plast Reconstr Surg* 2003;111:652–660.
68. Surkin MI, Lawson W, Biller HF. Analysis of the methods of pharyngoesophageal reconstruction. *Head Neck* 1984;6:953–970.
69. Mendelsohn M, Morris M, Gallagher R. A comparative study of speech after total laryngectomy and total laryngopharyngectomy. *Arch Otolaryngol Head Neck Surg* 1993;119:508–510.
70. Deschler DG, Doherty ET, Reed CG, et al. Tracheoesophageal voice following tubed free radial forearm flap reconstruction of the neopharynx. *Ann Otol Rhinol Laryngol* 1994;103:929–936.

Cervical Esophageal Cancer

120

Jonas T. Johnson

ANATOMY

The cervical esophagus is that area of the esophagus situated superior to the manubrium. The superior margin is the cricopharyngeus muscle, and its inferior limit is the suprasternal notch. The precise length of the cervical esophagus varies; some patients with severe kyphosis have little or no esophagus superior to the sternum.

The esophagus is covered throughout by a layer of stratified squamous epithelium. Beneath the mucosa is a submucosal or areolar layer, then a muscular layer composed of an external longitudinal and an internal circular layer. In the cervical esophagus, this muscular layer is striated muscle (in contrast to the lower esophagus, which is largely smooth muscle). The arterial supply of the cervical esophagus is derived from the thyroid branch of the thyrocervical trunk; the venous drainage is to the inferior thyroid vein. The nervous supply is derived from the vagus nerve via the recurrent laryngeal nerve and from the sympathetic trunks. The parasympathetic and sympathetic fibers form plexuses between the layers of the muscular coat, which serve to mediate peristalsis.

The lymphatic drainage of the cervical esophagus goes to the paratracheal nodes, from where they can pass either superiorly to join the lymphatics of the pharynx and terminate in the internal jugular chain of nodes or inferiorly to drain into the superior mediastinum.

PHYSIOLOGY

Active participation in swallowing is the function of the cervical esophagus. The cricopharyngeus muscle, located at the superior aspect of the cervical esophagus, serves as the upper esophageal sphincter. Coordinated reflex relaxation of the cricopharyngeal muscle is critical to the normal physiology of swallowing. Dilatation of the cricopharyngeus results in initiation of the esophageal peristaltic wave. Normal resting tone of the cricopharyngeus serves to prevent or reduce reflux of esophageal contents into the hypopharynx.

EPIDEMIOLOGY

Carcinoma of the esophagus accounts for less than 1% of newly diagnosed malignancies in the United States each year, but the incidence varies greatly around the world (1). Approximately 14,000 new cases are diagnosed annually; cancer of the cervical esophagus is only a fraction of this total. Approximately13,000 deaths per year are attributed to esophageal cancer (1). Cancer of the esophagus is 80 times more common in the Middle East, southern and eastern Africa, and northern China (2). Alcohol and tobacco use has a clear-cut causative relationship to the risk of esophageal carcinoma. In one study, the risk for a heavy smoker was 4.5 times that of a nonsmoker, nondrinker, whereas that of the heavy drinker was 11 times the risk. The apparent synergy between tobacco and alcohol use is demonstrated by the fact that the risk in people who both smoke and drink heavily is over 100 times (3).

Some studies have suggested that nitrosamines may be associated with increased risk of carcinoma of the esophagus (4). Tylosis, an autosomal-dominant trait in which marked thickening of the palms and soles occurs, has been associated with a high risk of developing esophageal carcinoma by age 65 (8). Similarly, patients with a history of head and neck cancer or achalasia have an increased incidence of carcinoma of the esophagus. Development of an esophageal carcinoma has been widely reported in a significant percentage of patients with a primary tumor on another mucosal site in the head and neck. In addition, a patient with cervical esophageal cancer has an increased risk of developing a second primary carcinoma in either the lung or upper aerodigestive tract.

Most tumors involving the cervical esophagus either extend distally into the thoracic esophagus or originate in the hypopharynx with extension into the cervical esophagus. Carcinoma limited to the cervical esophagus is rare. Diagnostic maneuvers must be aimed at identifying the full extent of tumor involvement so that therapeutic planning and reconstruction, when excision is appropriate, can be appropriately coordinated.

The tumor most commonly encountered in the cervical esophagus is squamous cell carcinoma (5). Adenocarcinoma occasionally is encountered in the esophagus, but it arises either from gastric mucosa found near the gastroesophageal junction or in mucous glands embedded in the epithelium of the esophagus. Barrett esophagus (the columnar epithelium associated with long-standing reflux esophagitis) has been associated with adenocarcinoma. An estimated 5% of people with gastroesophageal reflux may develop Barrett esophagus, and 5% of that group may develop a malignancy (6). These lesions are almost always in the distal esophagus. Adenocarcinoma of the cervical esophagus has been reported arising in heterotopic gastric mucosa (7).

EVALUATION

Clinical Presentation

Dysphagia is the primary symptom of cervical esophageal carcinoma (9). This rather common complaint, however, mimics several more common and innocuous problems and is often overlooked until the patient develops dysphagia to solid food or complete obstruction of the alimentary tract, with resultant weight loss leading to cachexia and, occasionally, aspiration pneumonia.

The diagnosis of esophageal carcinoma should be considered in a patient with a history of persistant dysphagia. Failure of antireflux medications may prompt early evaluation. The most common abnormal finding is a neck mass (21%) (9). Laryngoscopy may show pooling of secretions in the hypopharynx. Vocal cord paralysis is an indication of involvement of the recurrent laryngeal nerve by direct transmural penetration of the nerve by tumor. Bilateral vocal cord paralysis can precipitate sudden airway hunger or dyspnea on exertion; transmural penetration of the trachea by tumor should be considered an extremely late sign.

As mentioned, esophageal squamous cell carcinoma presence is frequently associated with head and neck cancer. It is felt that this is attributable to exposure to common carcinogens, the most important of which are alcohol and tobacco. In one report of 25 patients with synchronous head and neck malignancy and esophageal squamous cell carcinoma, gender distribution, tumor location, and histologic findings were similar in the two groups. The patients with synchronous cancer were younger than those who had a solitary tumor. Five-year survival rates for patients treated for synchronous tumors (17%) did not differ from those for patients treated for a solitary tumor (14%) (10). Efforts have been made to determine if paired tumors share common origin. Another study of 16 patients with head and neck cancer and esophageal cancer patterns of allelic loss on chromosomal arms 3p, 9p, and 17p was undertaken. In 14 of these cases (87%), the paired tumors had discordant patterns of allelic loss, suggesting that these tumors are not clonally related (11).

Laboratory Tests

Diagnostic efforts include cine-esophagography, computed tomography (CT), or magnetic resonance imaging (MRI), and endoscopic evaluation with biopsy.

Barium cine-esophagography should be used routinely to evaluate patients with cervical dysphagia. Tumor presence can be suggested by the characteristic irregularity of the mucosa. The fluoroscopist may often suspect transmural penetration of tumor with involvement of adjacent structures. He or she should note mobility with peristalsis of the esophagus as it relates to fixed structures such as the vertebral column. Contrast cine-esophagography offers the radiologist the opportunity to determine if the esophagus is fixed to the prevertebral fascia, a sign of relative inoperability. Contrast esophagoscopy is probably superior to CT or MRI in delineating the cephalocaudal extent of mucosal involvement. Patients presenting with complete or near-complete obstruction of the esophagus should not undergo contrast swallowing studies because of the potential for aspiration.

Both contrast-enhanced CT and MRI are potentially useful to define the depth of tumor invasion and the presence of adenopathy (12,13).

Diagnostic Surgery

Endoscopic evaluation under general anesthesia affords the surgeon the opportunity to assess the superior margin of the tumor and its relationship to the posterior aspect of the cricoid cartilage and arytenoid cartilages. Esophagoscopy may also give the surgeon the opportunity to evaluate the distal extent of mucosal disease. Patients with obstruction or near-total obstruction of the esophageal lumen often cannot be safely instrumented, however, and the distal limits of the lesion must be estimated using imaging techniques. Biopsy should be obtained for histologic confirmation.

Patients with severe weight loss and near-total esophageal obstruction should be offered early gastrostomy or jejunostomy. Care should be taken, however, to assure that this maneuver will not compromise subsequent reconstructive alternatives. For instance, insertion of gastrostomy can interfere with gastric pull-up. When circumstances permit, a small-diameter feeding tube can occasionally be inserted via the

<table>
<tr><td>

TABLE 120.1   **D** DIAGNOSIS
ESOPHAGEAL CARCINOMA

History
  Tobacco abuse
  Alcohol abuse
  Achalasia
  Plummer-Vinson syndrome
  Prior head and neck cancer

Physical examination
  Vocal cord paralysis
  Endoscopy
  Obstruction of lumen
  Irregular mucosa

Radiography
  Video esophagography
  Magnetic resonance imaging
  Computed tomography
  Ultrasound-guided fine-needle aspiration

</td></tr>
</table>

nasogastric route at the time of endoscopic evaluation. Under some circumstances, complete contrast esophagography can be undertaken in patients with near-total obstruction and aspiration by pulling the nasogastric tube into the proximal esophagus and instilling barium.

Metastasis to lymph nodes is an important aspect of staging in patients presenting with cancer of the cervical esophagus. Potentially, nodes in the cervical chains, superior mediastinum, or celiac drainage basin may be involved. Reports suggest that ultrasound-guided fine-needle aspiration biopsy is effective in making this assessment of cervical nodes (14). Endoscopic ultrasound-guided biopsy may be appropriate in patients with mediastinal or celiac nodes (15). Ultrasonography may play a useful role in the decision to perform cervical lymph node dissection in patients with esophageal cancer. Table 120.1 provides a summary of diagnostic considerations.

Staging

Staging of carcinoma of the cervical esophagus is identical to that for the intrathoracic esophagus. Tis indicates carcinoma in situ. Tumor that involves 5 cm or less of esophageal length without obstruction and that demonstrates neither circumferential nor transmural involvement is T1. A T2 tumor involves more than 5 cm of esophageal length without extraesophageal spread, or any tumor that produces obstruction or involves the entire circumference of the esophagus without extraesophageal spread. T3 is any tumor with extraesophageal spread.

The nodal classification system differs from the system used for head and neck sites. N0 indicates no clinically palpable nodes. N1 indicates mobile unilateral nodes, and N2 indicates bilateral mobile nodes. Fixed nodes are designated N3.

MANAGEMENT

Treatment planning must include consideration of the cephalocaudal extent of the tumor, transmural penetration to involve adjacent structures, laryngeal involvement, presence or absence of metastatic disease, and the reconstructive alternatives available should surgery be undertaken. Table 120.2 summarizes the treatment options.

Efforts directed at patients with incurable cancer of the cervical esophagus are frustrated by esophageal obstruction, with resultant aspiration and, eventually, life-threatening pneumonia. Nutrition can be maintained through tube feedings, most often established through gastrostomy. Aspiration of upper aerodigestive tract secretions, however, can create symptoms that require intervention. The final common denominator is death by aspiration and pneumonia. The misery accompanying this slowly progressive disease caused by aspiration of saliva often requires surgical intervention. With alimentary tract obstruction, all secretions must be expectorated and patients find they can neither assume the supine position nor sleep comfortably. Tracheotomy affords improved nursing care; however, laryngotracheal separation may be required to allow the patient to recline and sleep comfortably. In this regard, we have found the technique described by Lindeman to be effective (Fig. 120.1) (16). It can be done under local anesthesia with limited morbidity. It results in a permanent tracheostome and subsequent absence of laryngeal speech, but most patients find it far superior to chronic terminal aspiration.

Esophagectomy or laryngopharyngoesophagectomy for patients with incurable carcinoma of the cervical esophagus is rarely indicated. It offers little improvement in quality of life or duration of life over performance of the Lindeman procedure alone. In some patients, dysphagia can be palliated with endoscopic dilatation and insertion of an esophagus bypass tube (17,18).

Nonoperative Management of Cervical Esophageal Cancer

Advanced Esophageal Carcinoma
Patients with evidence of metastatic disease should be considered incurable and treated with palliative intent, as should patients with transmural involvement of the prevertebral fascia, trachea, or carotid arteries.

<table>
<tr><td>

TABLE 120.2   **R** TREATMENT
ESOPHAGEAL CARCINOMA

Extension to postcricoid area mandates laryngectomy
Involvement of thoracic esophagus mandates total
  esophagectomy
Gastric pull-up is the preferred reconstruction
Chemotherapy and radiation are used for palliation of patients
  with advanced carcinoma

</td></tr>
</table>

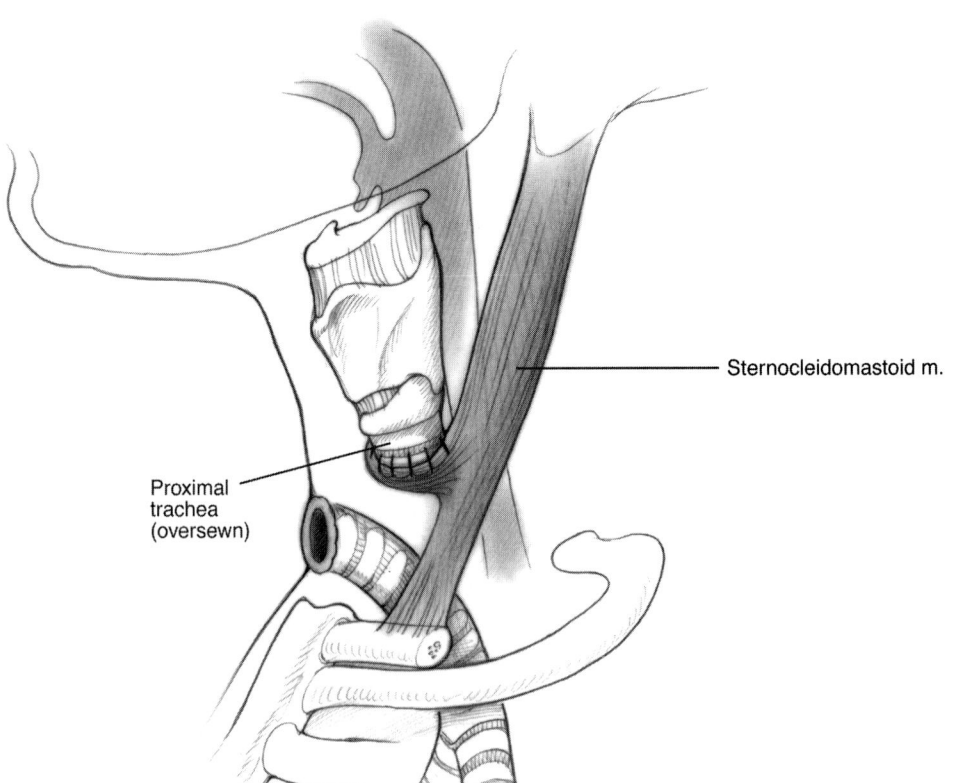

Sternocleidomastoid m.

Proximal
trachea
(oversewn)

Figure 120.1 The Lindeman procedure effectively achieves total aerodigestive separation by creating an endotracheal stoma. The proximal trachea is oversewn. This suture line should be reinforced with a muscle flap developed from the adjacent sternocleidomastoid muscle.

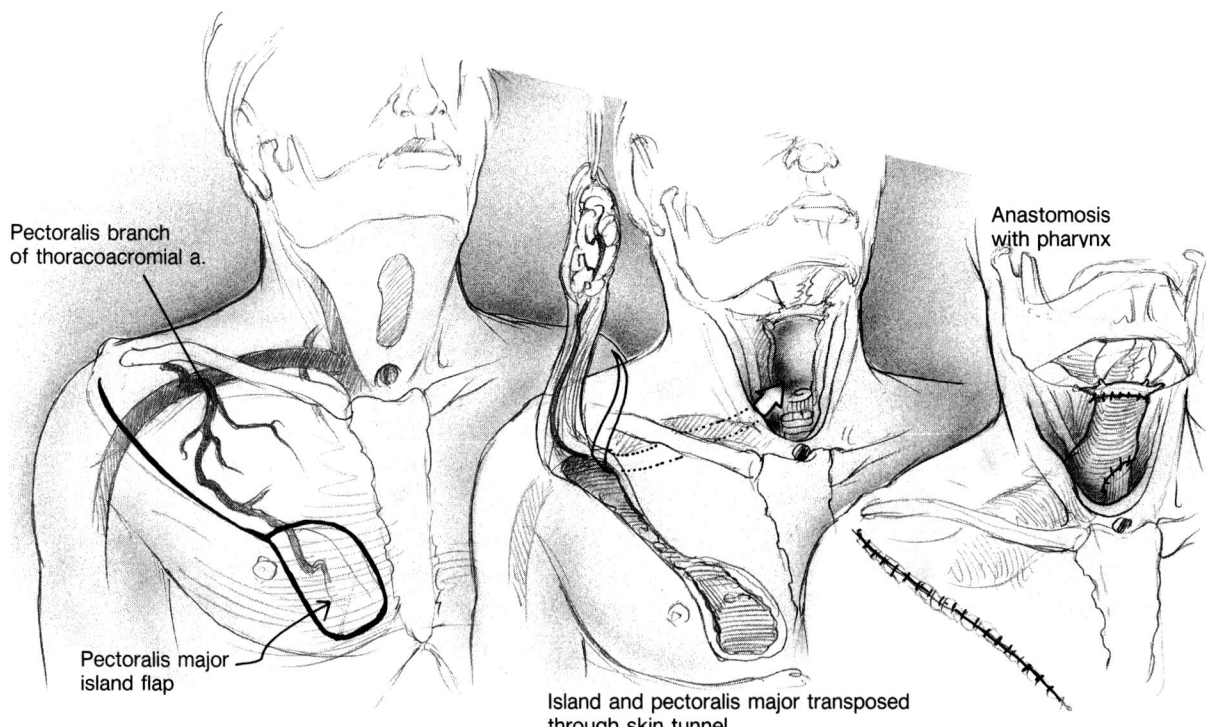

Pectoralis branch
of thoracoacromial a.

Pectoralis major
island flap

Island and pectoralis major transposed
through skin tunnel

Anastomosis
with pharynx

Figure 120.2 The pectoralis major myocutaneous flap has had widespread success in single-stage primary reconstruction of major head and neck wounds. The bulk of this flap is a relative disadvantage in reconstructing the cervical esophagus.

Advances in the management of solid tumors with combination chemotherapy and radiation therapy have resulted in several encouraging reports. Protocols using 5-fluorouracil and cisplatin with concurrent radiation therapy have resulted in complete local response in 91% of patients. Projected 5-year survival was 55% (19–23).

Operative Cervical Esophageal Carcinoma

Unfortunately, it is rare to encounter small, discrete, well-circumscribed, squamous cell carcinoma of the cervical esophagus. Photodynamic therapy (PDT), however, may be especially effective in patients with superficial lesions (24). Lesions involving the postcricoid mucosa or with transmural involvement of the recurrent laryngeal nerve or proximal trachea and cricoid are best treated with resection requiring total laryngopharyngectomy with resection of the cervical esophagus.

From a historical perspective, reconstruction of defects involving the total cervical esophagus or, more commonly, defects that involve the larynx, pharynx, and esophagus have presented surgeons with a formidable challenge. Staged reconstruction of pharyngoesophageal defects has become largely relegated to historical perspective.

The survival rate of patients requiring total cervical esophageal reconstruction for advanced carcinoma of the hypopharynx and cervical esophagus is poor. Two-year disease-free survival rates are poor (9% to 39%) (25,26). The surgeon cannot predict with accuracy which patients will have disease control, but from a statistical point of view it is clear that most patients are being treated with palliation. The introduction of safe, reliable one-stage reconstructive techniques represents a major advance because it allows meaningful palliation. Painful, obstructing tumors causing aspiration can be resected, aerodigestive separation accomplished, and reconstruction performed in a single stage. When this can be accomplished without significant complications, truly meaningful palliation has been achieved. It remains for future researchers to develop effective adjuvant therapies to improve the survival rate for those patients afflicted with this disease. Modern reconstructive alternatives allow circumferential replacement of the pharynx in a single stage.

Tubed pedicle flaps offer the potential of reconstruction with tissue that can be acquired from the adjacent region (e.g., pectoralis major or latissimus dorsi myocutaneous flaps) (Fig. 120.2).

The major advantages of pectoralis major flap reconstruction are that it avoids an intraabdominal procedure, reduces operating time, and does not require repositioning of the patient for flap harvest. Disadvantages include difficulty tubing the flap into a 360-degree conduit because of excessive bulk, which can lead to fistula formation, delayed wound healing, and the postoperative sequela of stenosis. These complications can be greatly reduced or avoided, however, by using a bypass salivary stent; the flap is tubed around the stent, which is left in place for approximately 2 weeks postoperatively (27,28).

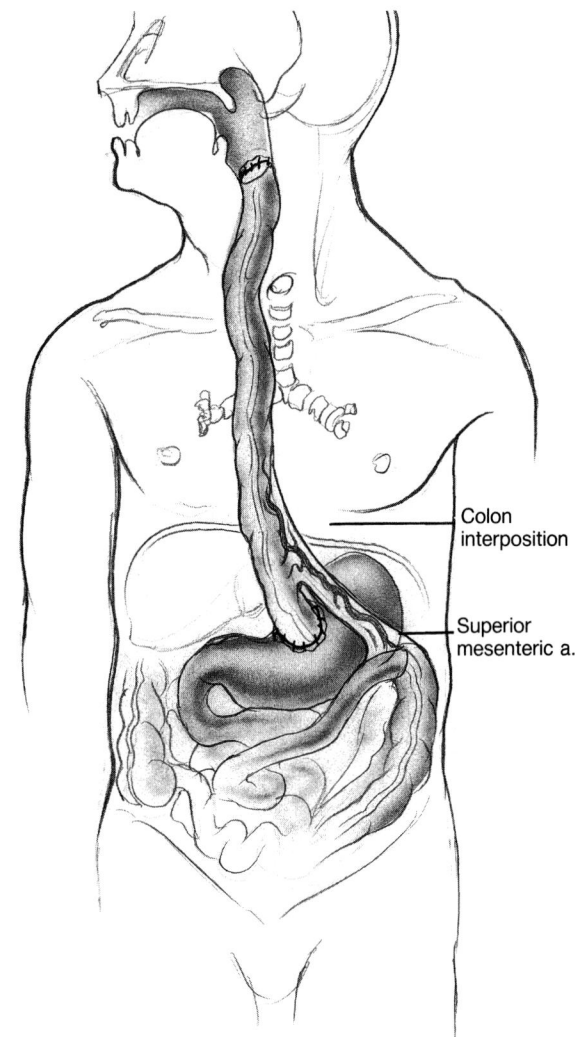

Figure 120.3 Colon interposition allows one-stage reconstruction or bypass of the entire esophagus. A high incidence of septic complications is associated with this procedure.

The esophagus can be replaced or bypassed with colon. The right colon is mobilized on the superior mesenteric artery. Under most circumstances, this allows an anastomosis to be made in the pharynx. The distal colon is then brought to the stomach. This technique (Fig. 120.3) has been used for over 50 years. Potential advantages are the one-stage reconstruction with no need for microvascular technology. Colon interposition, however, has been associated with a significant incidence of postoperative infection, sometimes resulting in operative mortality. Accordingly, the colon is usually placed in a subcutaneous pocket anterior to the sternum, so that if necrosis occurs, it would be less likely to result in a life-threatening complication. Colon interposition is not ideally suited for reconstruction of the cervical esophagus and is not currently considered a first-choice reconstructive alternative.

Gastric pull-up and pharyngogastric anastomosis (Fig. 120.4) offers several distinct advantages, chief of which is the creation of a single anastomosis. The stomach is brought

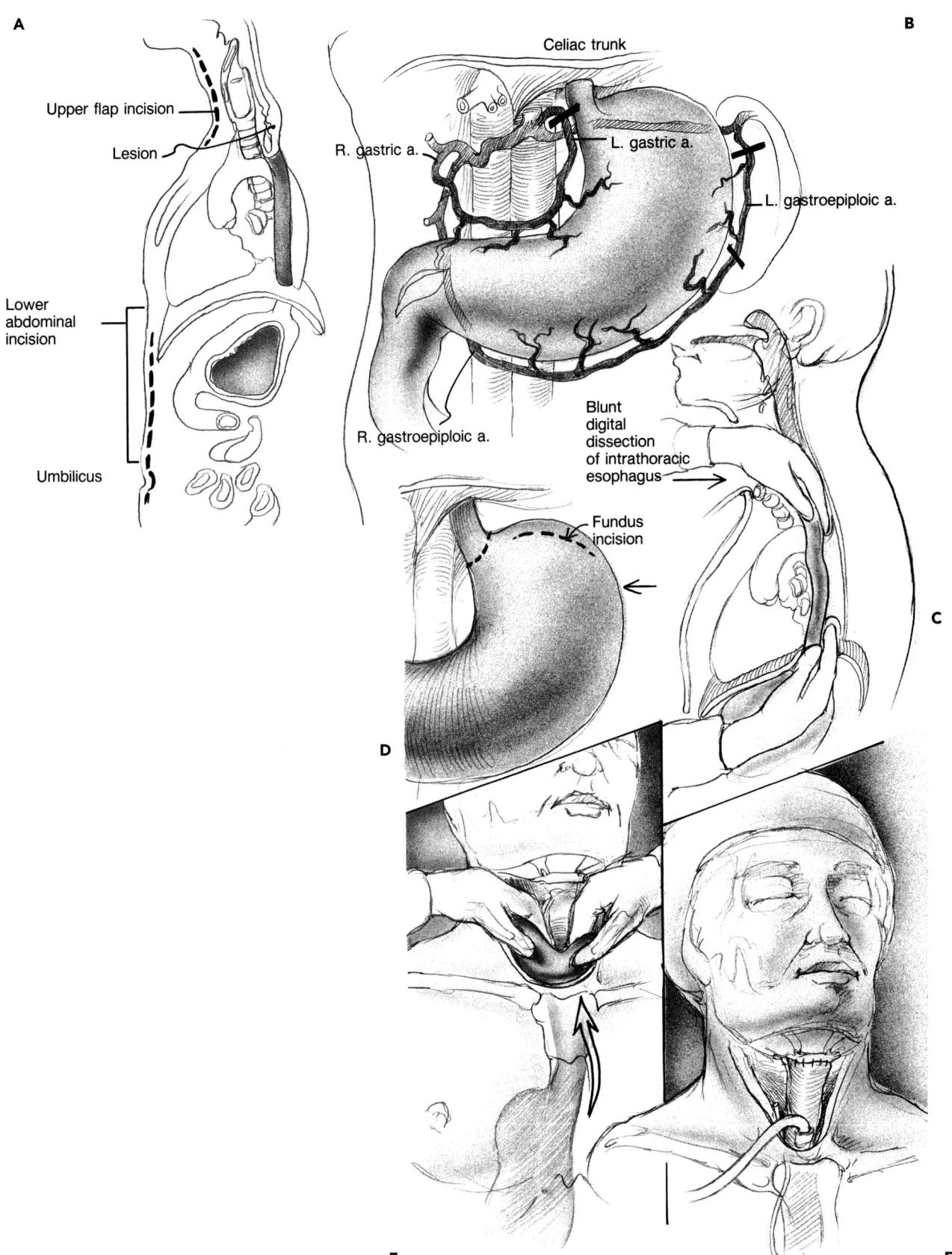

A

Upper flap incision

Lesion

Lower abdominal incision

Umbilicus

B

Celiac trunk

R. gastric a.

L. gastric a.

L. gastroepiploic a.

R. gastroepiploic a.

Blunt digital dissection of intrathoracic esophagus

Fundus incision

C

D

E

F

Figure 120.4 **A:** Gastric pull-up with pharyngogastric anastomosis is commonly used to reconstruct total esophageal defects. **B:** The intraabdominal procedure includes vagotomy with pyloroplasty. The duodenum is mobilized with the Kocher maneuver. **C:** The esophagus is removed without thoracotomy, using bimanual transabdominal and transcervical dissection. The stomach is brought up through the chest into the neck in the posterior mediastinum. **D:** The fundus is opened to provide the greatest length for anastomosis. **E:** Fundus in neck. **F:** Fundus surgery.

through the posterior mediastinum using blunt dissection without thoracotomy. The duodenum is mobilized using a Kocher maneuver. This allows the fundus of the stomach to be anastomosed in the nasopharynx, if necessary. Vagotomy and pyloroplasty are required. A jejunostomy tube is inserted at the time of the abdominal procedure and used during convalescence. The principal disadvantage of this procedure is the morbidity incurred during the mediastinal part of the procedure, which often results in pneumothorax or hemothorax. These problems can be managed with thorocostomy tubes. Pulmonary contusion is managed expectantly, and the cardiorespiratory system is supported in the intensive care unit. The operative mortality rate is an estimated 5% to 15% (26,29).

Long-term gastrointestinal complaints following gastric pull-up include early satiety, emesis, and dumping. Stricture of the pharyngogastric anastomosis can occur. Stricture is most commonly associated with anastomotic leakage. A prospective randomized clinical study evaluated one- versus two-layer anastomoses. The anastomotic leakage rate was similar (19% in the two groups); however, the incidence of fibrotic stricture following the one-layer anastomosis was significantly reduced when compared with the stricture in the group having a two-layer procedure (30). Other investigators have indicated that postoperative leakage at the anastomosis and a stapled, rather than a hand-sewn, anastomosis are independent risk factors for the development of a stricture (31). Factors such as preoperative irradiation therapy and diabetes mellitus are reported to be not significant (32).

A potential advantage is that gastric pull-up with pharyngogastric anastomosis gives the surgeon the opportunity to undertake total esophagectomy, which encompasses lesions that extend below the sternum, and may allow the surgeon to obtain the widest possible margin on the mucosal lesion.

Free transfer of jejunum to reconstruct the cervical esophagus remains a technique of choice in patients who do not require resection of esophagus caudal to the thoracic inlet (33). Laparoscopic harvest of the jejunal free flap has been described (34). Jejunal autograft can be used to reconstruct the cervical esophagus without laryngectomy in well-selected cases. This technique is inappropriate with a tumor that involves the postcricoid larynx; laryngectomy is then necessary. Similarly, this technique is inappropriate for patients with extension into the thoracic esophagus. This highly selected group of patients is characterized by a diagnosis of non–squamous cell carcinoma. The propensity for submucosal spread in patients with squamous carcinoma almost always requires a more extended and radical resection to achieve free surgical margins. Fasciocutaneous free flaps (e.g., the radial forearm and lateral thigh) are also reconstructive options in this select group of patients. The main advantage of these flaps over free jejunal transfer is that laparotomy is avoided with its associated potential for intraabdominal complications (35).

TABLE 120.3 COMPLICATIONS ESOPHAGEAL CARCINOMA

Complication	Management
Wound infection	Drain to prevent
Fistula	Prompt repair with free flap is recommended

Successful first-stage operations are achieved in 95% to 97% of patients (36,37). Postoperative fistulae occur in 8% to 19%, of which most healed spontaneously without further surgical intervention.

COMPLICATIONS

Wound separation and associated fistula formation is the complication seen most often in patients having cervical esophagectomy (Table 120.3). Adequate drainage must be established as soon as a subcutaneous collection is identified. Ideally, the drains should be placed intraoperatively so that the purulent material does not compromise good tracheal toilet. Most fistulae that develop in patients who have not received prior radiation therapy will close spontaneously. Healing by secondary intention may take 4 to 6 weeks, however, and it is often associated with the development of stenosis of the pharyngeal lumen. Fistulae that develop in patients who have received prior high-dose radiation therapy may require secondary reconstructive efforts. No single technique is uniformly appropriate or successful. In general, the newer techniques of free tissue transfer are associated with the highest success rates, but these techniques are the most technically demanding; they require the longest operative time and have the greatest potential for postoperative morbidity. Mobilizing local tissue in patients who have had prior radiation therapy is almost always frustrated by recurrent fistulization. Accordingly, the use of healthy vascularized tissue is always suggested. Persistent stenosis of the distal suture line occurs approximately 15% of the time and will usually respond to dilatation.

EMERGENCIES

Sudden development of a postoperative hematoma is most often evidenced by rapid wound swelling and bright red blood flowing from the wound drains (Table 120.4). This most often indicates a displaced vascular ligature; however, in the setting of a microvascular reconstruction, hematoma can indicate anastomotic disruption. Immediate return to the operating room for wound exploration is indicated.

Vascular thrombosis following free tissue transfer for repair of the cervical esophagus must be managed as an

TABLE 120.4 ✚ EMERGENCY CARE ESOPHAGEAL CARCINOMA	
Problem	**Management**
Hematoma	Explore and evacuate promptly
Vascular thrombosis of microvascular percutaneous anastomosis	Monitor with Doppler

emergency. Microvascular anastomoses must be carefully monitored to determine the adequacy of the vascular reconstruction. In the case of vascular compromise, the patient must be moved expeditiously to the operating room and the microvascular anastomosis reexplored. Our experience has been that more than 90% of jejunal autografts can be salvaged using this technique.

IMPORTANT RECENT INFORMATION

Fractionated high dose rate (HDR) brachytherapy alone has been reported as an effective method of palliation in advanced esophageal tumors (38). An alternative palliative approach may be photodynamic therapy (PDT) (24).

Postoperative anastomotic leakage is the single most important source of morbidity following either pharyngogastric anastomosis or jejunal interposition. Hand-sewn anastomoses seem to be more reliable (31) when a pharyngogastric anastomosis is used; a single-layer closure is as reliable as a two-layer closure and is less frequently associated with anastomotic stenosis (30).

Recent advances in minimally invasive surgical procedures have prompted investigators to consider laparoscopic and thoracoscopic surgery for esophagectomy. These ideas serve as a challenge to developments in the future management of cancer of the cervical esophagus (39).

HIGHLIGHTS

- The incidence of carcinoma of the esophagus is markedly increased in patients who use tobacco and alcohol or have achalasia, Plummer-Vinson syndrome, or a history of prior head and neck carcinoma.
- Assessment with endoscopy and contrast radiography offers the best estimate of the cephalocaudal extent of the tumor.
- Magnetic resonance imaging gives the most accurate assessment of transmural penetration of the tumor and evidence of metastatic adenopathy.
- Superior extension to the postcricoid area dictates the need for concurrent laryngectomy.
- Extension through the cervical esophagus to involve the thoracic esophagus indicates the need for total esophagectomy.

- Defects requiring total pharyngoesophageal reconstruction are best managed with gastric mobilization and pharyngogastric anastomosis.
- A single-layer anastomosis is as reliable as a two-layer closure and is associated with fewer strictures.
- Defects requiring repair of the pharynx and cervical esophagus can be managed with free tissue transfer, including jejunal interposition, facsiocutaneous flaps, and omentum.
- Concurrent chemoradiation may result in disease control and preserve esophageal function in more than half of patients.
- Either HDR brachytherapy or PDT may offer palliation for patients with near total obstruction.

REFERENCES

1. Jemal A, Tiwari RC, Murray T, et al. Cancer statistics, 2004. *CA Cancer J Clin* 2004;54:8–29.
2. Dunham LJ, Bailar JC. World maps of cancer mortality rates and frequency ratios. *J Natl Cancer Inst* 1968;41:155–203.
3. Wynder EL, Bross IJ. A study of etiological factors in cancers of the esophagus. *Cancer* 1961;14:389–413.
4. Yang CS. Research on esophageal cancer in China: a review. *Cancer Res* 1980;40:2633–2644.
5. Jones AS, Roland NJ, Hamilton J, et al. Malignant tumors of the cervical esophagus. *Clin Otolaryngol* 1996;21:49–53.
6. Sjogren RW Jr, Johnson LF. Barrett's esophagus. *Am J Med* 1983; 74:313–321.
7. Triboulet JP, Mariette C, Chevalier D, et al. Surgical management of carcinoma of the hypopharynx and cervical esophagus: analysis of 209 cases. *Arch Surg* 2001;136(10):1164–1170.
8. Harper PS, Harper RMJ, Howel-Evans AW. Carcinoma of the esophagus with tylosis. *Q J Med* 1970;39:317–333.
9. Kelley DJ, Wolf R, Shaha AR, et al. Impact of clinicopathologic parameters on patient survival in carcinoma of the cervical esophagus. *Am J Surg* 1995;170:427–431.
10. Wind P, Roullet MH, Quinaux D, et al. Long-term results after esophagectomy for squamous cell carcinoma of the esophagus associated with head and neck cancer. *Am J Surg* 1999;178: 251–255.
11. Califano J, Leong PL, Koch WM, et al. Second esophageal tumors in patients with head and neck squamous cell carcinoma: an assessment of clonal relationships. *Clin Cancer Res* 1999;5:1862–1867.
12. Schmafuss IM. Imaging of the hypopharynx and cervical esophagus. *Magn Reson Imaging Clin N Am* 2002;10(3):495–509.
13. Roychowdhury S, Loevner LA, Yousen DM, et al. MR imaging for predicting neoplastic invasion of the cervical esophagus. *Am J Neuroradiol* 2000;21(9):1681–1687.
14. Natsugoe S, Yoshinaka H, Shimada M, et al. Assessment of cervical lymph node metastasis in esophageal carcinoma using ultrasonography. *Ann Surg* 1999;229:62–66.
15. Giovannini M, Monges G, Seitz JF, et al. Distant lymph node metastases in esophageal cancer: impact of endoscopic ultrasound-guided biopsy. *Endoscopy* 1999;31:536–540.
16. Snyderman CH, Johnson JT. Laryngotracheal separation for intractable aspiration. *Ann Otol Rhinol Laryngol* 1988;97:466–470.
17. Segalin A, Granelli P, Bonaviana L, et al. Self-expanding esophageal prosthesis. Effective palliation for inoperable carcinoma of the cervical esophagus. *Surg Endosc* 1994;8:1343–1345.
18. Loizou LA, Rampton D, Brown SG. Treatment of malignant strictures of the cervical esophagus by endoscopic intubation using modified endoprostheses. *Gastrointest Endosc* 1992;38:153–164.
19. Carey RW, Hilgenberg AD, Wilkins EW, et al. Preoperative chemotherapy followed by surgery with possible postoperative radiotherapy in squamous cell carcinoma of the esophagus:

evaluation of the chemotherapy component. *J Clin Oncol* 1986;4: 697–701.

20. Seitz JF, Giovannini M, Padaut-Cesana J, et al. Inoperable non-metastatic squamous cell carcinoma of the esophagus managed by concomitant chemotherapy (5-fluorouracil and cisplatin) and radiation therapy. *Cancer* 1990;66:214–219.

21. Coia LR, Engstrom PF, Paul A. Nonsurgical management of esophageal cancer: report of a study of combined radiotherapy and chemotherapy. *J Clin Oncol* 1987;5:1783–1790.

22. Stuschke M, Stahl M, Wilke H, et al. Induction chemotherapy followed by concurrent chemotherapy and high-dose radiotherapy for locally advanced squamous cell carcinoma of the cervical oesophagus. *Oncology* 1999;57:99–105.

23. Burmeister B, Dickie G, Smithers BM, et al. Thirty-four patients with carcinoma of the cervical esophagus treated with chemoradiation therapy. *Arch Otolaryngol Head Neck Surg* 2000;126:205–208.

24. Moghissi K, Dixon K. Photodynamic therapy (PDT) in esophageal cancer: a surgical view of its indications based on 14 years of experience. *Technology in Cancer Research & Treatment* 2003;2(4):319–326.

25. Marmuse JP, Guedon C, Koka VN. Gastric tube transposition for cancer of the hypopharynx and cervical oesophagus. *J Laryngol Otol* 1994;108:33–37.

26. Cahow CE, Sasaki CT. Gastric pull-up reconstruction for pharyngo-laryngo-esophagectomy. *Arch Surg* 1994;129:425–429.

27. Spriano G, Pellini R, Roselli R. Pectoralis major myocutaneous flap for hypopharyngeal reconstruction. *Plast Reconstr Surg* 2002;110:1408–1416.

28. Shektman A, Silver C, Strauch B. A re-evaluation of hypopharyngeal reconstruction: pedicled flaps versus microvascular free flaps. *Plast Reconstr Surg* 1997;100:1691–1696.

29. Schusterman MA, Shestak K, DeVries EJ, et al. Reconstruction of the cervical esophagus: free jejunal transfer versus gastric pull-up. *Plast Reconstr Surg* 1990;85:16–21.

30. Zieren HU, Muller JM, Pichlmaier H. Prospective randomized study of one- or two-layer anastomosis following esophageal resection and cervical oesophagogastrostomy. *Br J Surg* 1993;80: 608–611.

31. Honkoop P, Sierseman PD, Tilanus HW, et al. Benign anastomotic strictures after transhiatal esophagectomy and cervical esophagogastrostomy: risk factors and management. *J Thorac Cardiovasc Surg* 1996;111:1141–1146; discussion 1147–1148.

32. Dewar L, Gelfand G, Finley RJ, et al. Factors affecting cervical anastomotic leak and stricture formation following esophagogastrectomy and gastric tube interposition. *Am J Surg* 1992;163: 484–489.

33. Bhathena HM. Free jejunal transfer for pharyngo-esophageal reconstruction. *Acta Chirurgiae Plasticae* 2002;44(4):120–123.

34. Wadsworth JT, Futra N, Eubanks TR. Laparoscopic harvest of the jejunal free flap for reconstruction of hypopharyngeal and cervical esophageal defects. *Arch Otolaryngol Head Neck Surg* 2002;128(12):1384–1387.

35. Robb GL, Lewin JS. Speech and swallowing outcomes in reconstructions of the pharynx and cervical esophagus. *Head Neck* 2003;25:232–244.

36. Omura K, Misaki T, Watanabe Y, et al. Reconstruction with free jejunal autograft after pharyngolaryngoesophagectomy. *Ann Thorac Surg* 1994;57:112–117; discussion 117–118.

37. Reece GP, Schusterman MA, Miller MJ, et al. Morbidity and functional outcome of free jejunal transfer reconstruction for circumferential defects of the pharynx and cervical esophagus. *Plast Reconstr Surg* 1995;96:1307–1316.

38. Sur RK, Levin CV, Donde B, et al. Prospective randomized trial of HDR brachytherapy as a sole modality in palliation of advanced esophageal carcinoma—an International Atomic Energy Agency study. *Int J Radiat Oncol Biol Phys* 2002;53(1):127–133.

39. Luketich JD, Nguyen NT, Weigel T, et al. Minimally invasive approach to esophagectomy. *J Soc Laparoendosc Surg* 1998;2:243–247.

Early Glottic and Supraglottic Carcinoma: Endoscopic Techniques

121A

Steven M. Zeitels

Although hoarseness is the most frequent symptom associated with glottic cancer, most patients have had this symptom for many years, while dysplastic mucosa undergoes malignant degeneration (1). Tobacco smoking is accepted as the primary risk factor associated with laryngeal cancer. This deduction was made, in part, because larynx cancer was a rare disease until the 20th century. Shortly after the introduction of mass-produced cigarettes in the early 1900s, premalignant glottal epithelium was described along with escalating frequency of laryngeal cancer (2).

Solis-Cohen (3) was probably the first individual to cure cancer of the larynx by performing a transcervical vertical partial laryngectomy in 1869 for what was probably early glottic cancer. Fraenkel (4) reported the first successful transoral (mirror guided) resection of laryngeal cancer in 1886. Radiotherapy, introduced in the late 19th century, gained progressive popularity through the 20th century. Despite the fact that endolaryngeal surgery (5–11) and radiotherapy (XRT) (12) are equally successful in curing the early disease, radiotherapy became the dominant treatment modality because of the concern of many surgeons that their individual skills were not comparable to those reporting the endoscopic techniques, especially with regard to voice preservation. Tables 121A.1 through 121A.4 review diagnosis and staging, treatment, complications, and emergencies associated with early glottic cancer.

RADIOTHERAPY FOR EARLY GLOTTIC CANCER

Radiotherapy is a mainstay of treatment for early glottic cancer, especially among those who do not feel comfortable with microlaryngoscopic resection methods and associated reconstructive techniques. Patients who cannot be adequately exposed during staging endoscopy are ideal candidates for radiotherapy. The optimal clinical scenario for using XRT in early glottic cancer is diffuse superficial disease (T1b, T2b) in which surgical intervention would disrupt the basic architecture of both vocal folds, the anterior commissure tendon, or the laminae propria.

The disadvantages of XRT include treatment of noncancerous vocal-fold tissue (T1a, T2a), which frequently results in scarring of the mucosa of the normal vocal fold with associated dysphonia (13). Typically, the saccular glands are included in the treatment field so that associated mucosal dryness can lead to further disruption in glottal vibratory function and severe hoarseness. Administering radiotherapy to younger patients is a relative contraindication because it is a single-use treatment and a significant risk for metacronous lesions exists. In addition, a theoretic risk exists for radiation-induced cancer (14). Finally, radiation is more expensive than endoscopic resection (15).

TABLE 121A.1 DIAGNOSIS
STAGING

Laryngeal examination and videostroboscopy
Panendoscopy with biopsy and mapping of the tumor
Computed tomography scan of the neck with contrast
Chest x-ray study
Comprehensive chemistry panel, including liver function tests
Complete blood count

PHONOMICROSURGICAL TREATMENT OF EARLY GLOTTIC CANCER

The goal of endoscopic treatment of an isolated T1 lesion of the musculo-membranous vocal fold is eradication of the disease with maximal preservation of the normal layered microstructure (epithelium and laminae propria). This management minimizes oncologically sound margins (10,11,16–18) and institutes creative reconstruction (11,19) to optimize the postoperative airway, voice, and deglutition. This approach results in optimal postoperative voice without compromising oncologic cure. The universal modular glottiscope was designed specifically to perform endolaryngeal resection of glottic cancer (20). It has a number of advantages for exposing the tumor as well as for tangential tissue dissection.

Four basic procedures are based on the depth of excision (Fig. 121A.1a,b) (10,11,18): (a) dissection just deep to the epithelial basement membrane and superficial to the superficial lamina propria for epithelial atypia and microinvasive cancer; (b) dissection within the superficial lamina propria (SLP) microinvasive cancer that is not attached to the vocal ligament; (c) dissection between the deep lamina propria (vocal ligament) and the vocalis muscle for lesions that are attached to the ligament but not through it; and (d) dissection within the thyroarytenoid muscle for lesions penetrating the vocal ligament and invading the vocalis. This approach can be fine-tuned further by performing partial resections of any of the layered microstructure. The specimen is always oriented for whole-mount histologic

TABLE 121A.2 TREATMENT

Endoscopic phonosurgery
Suspend the larynx
Ensure adequate exposure of the lesion
Employ microscope
Vasoconstriction and hydrodissection of lesion using
    adrenaline injection
Partial cordectomy
Partial laryngectomy
Reconstruction of the larynx using medialization techniques
    (fat, Gore-Tex)

TABLE 121A.3 COMPLICATIONS

Hemoptysis subsequent to reconstruction
Hematoma
Airway edema
Airway obstruction
Dysphonia
Aspiration
Positive surgical margins
Laryngeal stenosis
Scarring
Extrusion of Gore-Tex implant

analysis and frozen-section margin assessment is used selectively to verify a complete excision.

If dissection is performed in the SLP, cold instruments facilitate precise tangential dissection around the curving vocal fold (10,11,16,17). This allows for maximal preservation of the SLP and for pliability of the regenerating epithelium. Dissection between the vocal ligament and the vocalis muscle can be performed equally well with cold instruments alone or with assistance by the laser. Dissection within the muscle is performed most precisely with the CO_2 laser, which allows for improved visualization because of its hemostatic cutting properties.

Subepithelial saline-epinephrine infusion into Reinke space (18) (Fig. 121A.2) improves preexcisional assessment of lesion depth. If the tumor has invaded the vocal ligament, the SLP at the perimeter of the lesion will distend, creating a contour depression in the region of the cancer. Assessment of invasion depth is also enhanced by palpation of the cancer. The subepithelial infusion assists with the surgeon's technical execution of the surgery in a number of other ways:

1. The infusion facilitates mucosal incisions by improving visualization of the lateral border of the lesion and by distending the SLP so that the overlying epithelium is under tension.
2. The infusion also increases the depth of the superficial lamina propria, which facilitates less traumatic dissection in this layer and leads to regenerated epithelium that is more flexible.
3. The epinephrine and hydrostatic pressure of the infusion vasoconstrict the microvasculature in the SLP and this improves visualization and a precise dissection.
4. If the laser is used, the saline acts as a heat sink, which decreases thermal trauma to the normal vocal-fold tissue.

TABLE 121A.4 EMERGENCIES

Bleeding
Airway obstruction

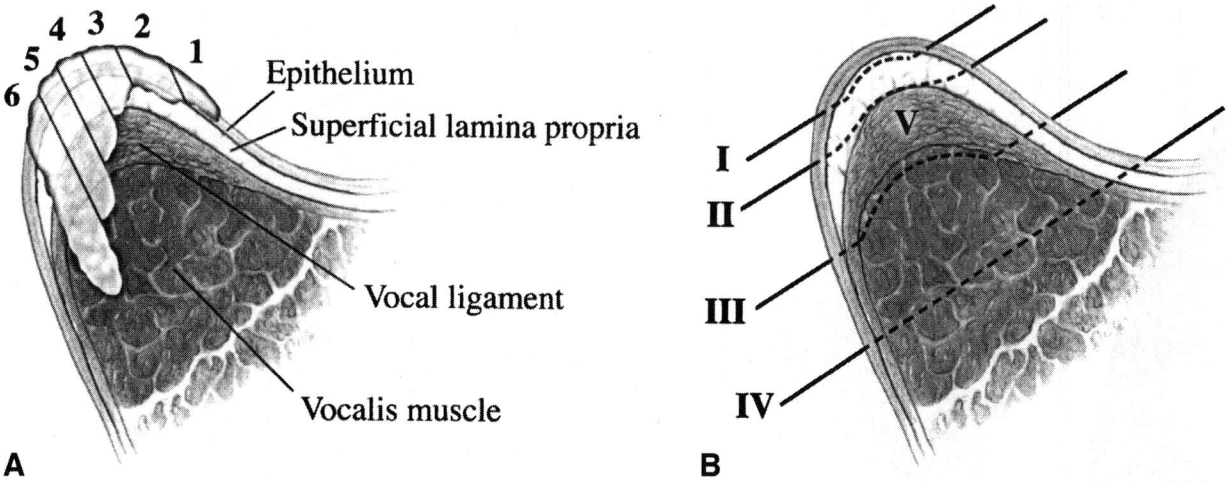

Figure 121A.1   A: Various depths of neoplastic invasion despite, which is indeterminable based on surface appearance. **B:** Various options for ultra-narrow margin resection based on depth of tumor invasion. (Reprinted from Hartig G, Zeitels SM. Optimizing voice in conservation surgery for glottic cancer. *Oper Tech Otolaryngol Head Neck Surg* 1998;9:214–223.)

ENDOSCOPIC VERTICAL PARTIAL LARYNGECTOMY

If adequate endoscopic exposure can be achieved, transoral partial laryngectomy is usually feasible for confined glottic disease with limited subglottic or supraglottic extension (21). Extensive subglottic and supraglottic extension can dramatically compound the difficulty in performing an on-cologically sound resection. Because impaired mobility implies deep invasion in the musculature of the paraglottic space or the cricoarytenoid joint, detailed radiographic imaging (computed tomography [CT], magnetic resonance imaging [MRI]) is often helpful toward procedure planning.

As with all endoscopic procedures, exposure is of paramount importance for the successful completion of the surgery. The largest laryngoscope that can be inserted into the patient with a suitable suspension device is used. The universal modular glottiscope (20) is designed to facilitate the resection of the anterior and lateral glottis because its shape simulates the contours of the inner thyroid laminae. After obtaining adequate endoscopic exposure, the tumor is inspected under high magnification to determine the limits of the resection before distortion of the specimen. This three-dimensional perspective is often enhanced by the use of telescopes.

Subsequent to histologic confirmation of cancer, the CO_2 laser is used with a microspot (0.2 to 3 mm) to outline the area of excision. Typically, the vestibular folds and infrapetiole region of the supraglottis must be resected before cancer removal to facilitate adequate exposure of the anterolateral limits of the lesion (22,23). Laryngeal forceps are used to retract the true vocal fold medially, while the CO_2 laser is used in a repeated pulsed mode (~0.1 second interval and duration) at approximately 2.5 to 4 watts. The

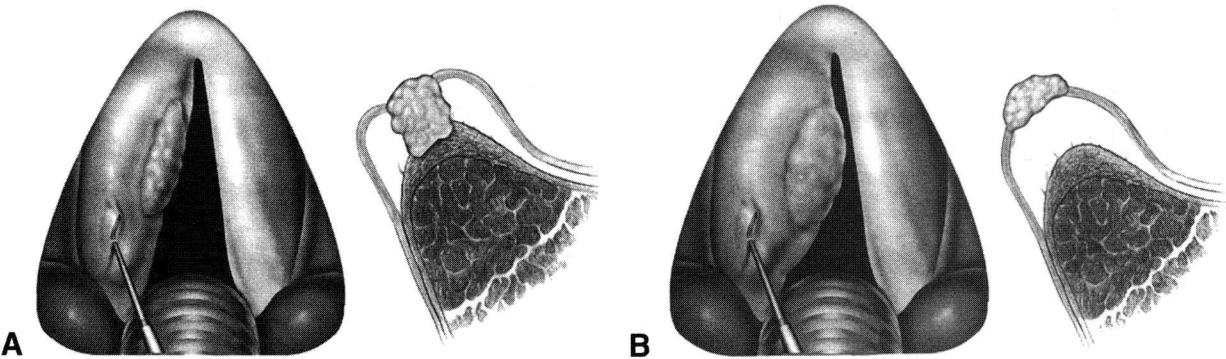

Figure 121A.2   A: The subepithelial infusion reveals tumor invasion into the vocal ligament. **B:** The subepithelial infusion lifts the lesion, which has microinvasion through the epithelial basement membrane. This enhances the precision of the procedure and facilitates maximal preservation of the vocal folds layered microstructure. (Reprinted from Hartig G, Zeitels SM. Optimizing voice in conservation surgery for glottic cancer. *Oper Tech Otolaryngol Head Neck Surg* 1998;9:214–223.)

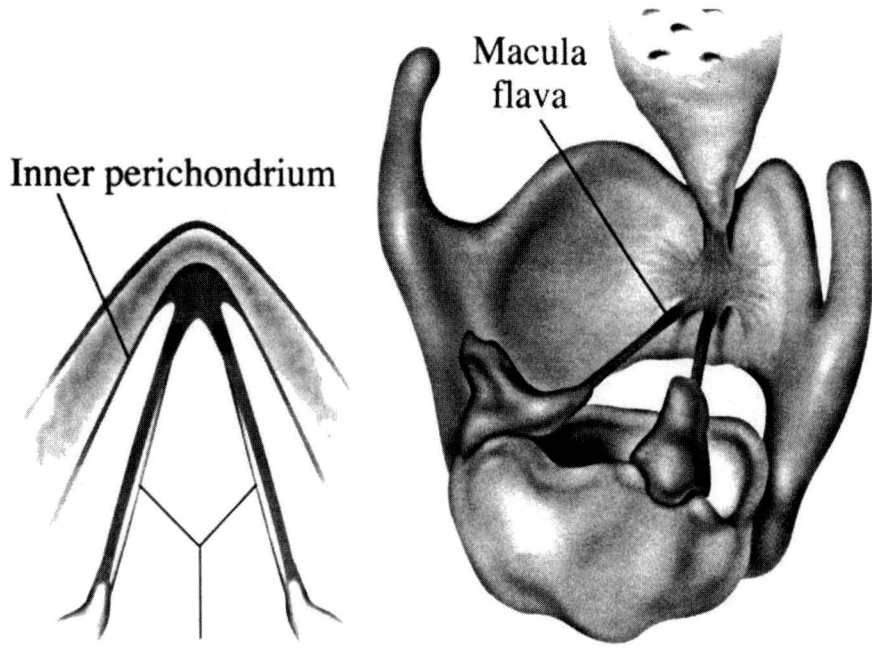

Inner perichondrium

Macula flava

Superficial lamina propria

Figure 121A.3 Ligamentous composition of the anterior commissure tendon. (Reprinted from Hartig G, Zeitels SM. Optimizing voice in conservation surgery for glottic cancer. *Oper Tech Otolaryngol Head Neck Surg* 1998;9: 214–223.)

counter-traction provided by the forceps is invaluable in completing the dissection accurately and expeditiously. Removal of the entire vocal fold including, the anterior commissure and arytenoids, can be done as is necessary.

ENDOSCOPIC TREATMENT OF GLOTTIC CARCINOMA IN THE ANTERIOR COMMISSURE

The anterior commissure tendon, or Broyle ligament, is a confluence of the vocal ligament, the thyroepiglottic ligament, the conus elasticus, and the internal perichondrium of the thyroid ala (Fig. 121A.3). A misconception is that T1 cancers at the anterior commissure have a great predilection for understaging and many of these lesions have occult invasion of the thyroid cartilage (T4 stage). This is based on the misunderstanding that the anatomy of the dense anterior-commissure ligament is a less-resilient tumor barrier than the adjacent thin thyroid perichondrium (Fig. 121A.4). Kirchner and Carter (25) and Kirchner himself (26) have made clear that T1a and T1b carcinomas rarely erode through Broyle ligament to invade thyroid cartilage. Anterior commissure tumors that have thyroid cartilage invasion typically display cephalad surface invasion of the infrapetiole region of the supraglottis or caudal surface invasion of the subglottis (both T2 by surface staging criteria).

Divergent opinion is found regarding whether cancer can be endoscopically eradicated from the anterior commissure. The proscriptions imposed by some are based primarily on the difficulty in obtaining adequate surgical exposure in this

area (27). The rate-limiting factors for resection of early cancer in the anterior commissure are the true extent of the disease (Is it invading cartilage?) and the endoscopic exposure required to encompass the lesion (11,22,24). Davis et al. (28) demonstrated that cancer could be removed from the anterior commissure; however, it required great skill to excise the lesion without vaporizing the specimen. Vaporizing cancer without clear resection margins is an inadequate surgical oncologic technique. This factor, as well as

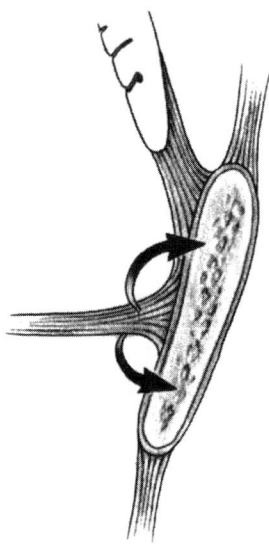

Figure 121A.4 Pattern of caudal and cephalad spread of cancer into thyroid cartilage at the anterior commissure. (Reprinted from Hartig G, Zeitels SM. Optimizing voice in conservation surgery for glottic cancer. *Oper Tech Otolaryngol Head Neck Surg* 1998;9:214–223.)

underestimating the extent of disease, probably led to the reported failures by a number of investigators (27,29).

If one accepts Kirchner's histopathologic data regarding the invasion pattern of T1 glottic cancer, no reason exists to believe that an adequate soft-tissue resection of small-volume soft-tissue disease is not adequate treatment. This premise is further substantiated by a number of reports that did not find a correlation between anterior commissure involvement with T1 glottic cancer and failure of radiotherapy as a curative modality (30).

A number of investigators have established that glottic cancer in the anterior commissure can be removed effectively by endoscopic techniques (24,31,32). The problem with any surgical approach that requires the resection of the entire anterior commissure (for true T1a, T1b, and T2 lesions) is that the structural integrity of both vocal folds is disrupted, which often results in a poor voice. Lesions that are invading cartilage, which are T4 by stage, require open partial laryngectomy and are not suitable for endoscopic excision alone. An endoscopic exploration of the infrapetiole region of the supraglottis allows for definitive determination about whether a presumed T1 lesion has cartilage invasion (T4) (22,23). This procedure facilitates precise staging (without disarticulating Broyle ligament), commensurate management, and optimal post-treatment voice quality.

GLOTTIC RECONSTRUCTION SUBSEQUENT TO ENDOLARYNGEAL CANCER RESECTION

Preoperative laryngeal stroboscopy is valuable in determining the location of pliable glottal mucosa, which is the primary determinant of post-treatment voice quality (33). If normal superficial lamina propria exists in one vocal fold, a normal conversational-level voice (11) can typically be achieved with phonomicrosurgical resection (10,17,23) and, as necessary, reconstruction of the excavated neocord (34,35). Voice restoration is achieved by reconstituting the lost paraglottic soft tissue resulting from the resection to restore aerodynamic valvular competency. The preserved thyroid lamina serves as a buttress from an augmentation and can be done by means of lipoinjection (35,36) or Gore-Tex medialization (35,37). Gore-Tex is an ideal laryngoplasty implant for cancer defects because it can be varied continuously during phonotary gestures, which enhance optimal precise reconstruction. As necessary, a laryngofissure (35) can be performed to sublux one thyroid lamina within the other to close anterior defects that result from resection of the anterior commissure tendon. This approach differs from classic prior models of open partial laryngectomy reconstruction in which the cartilage was removed so that the soft tissue would collapse into the glottal aperture to restore aerodynamic competency during phonation.

The primary advantages of the secondary framework reconstruction after an initial endoscopic resection are that

the procedure is done under local anesthesia to effect phonatory feedback and *tuning* of the voice. In addition, a tracheotomy is not needed for the resection or reconstruction and hospitalization is shorter because both the transoral resection and the transcervical reconstruction typically require hospitalization for only one night.

The goal of a glottal reconstruction is to create midline straight neocord to provide a surface for the normal vocal fold to vibrate against during phonation. Normal conversational-level voicing is usually achieved if aerodynamic competence is reestablished and viable superficial lamina propria exist to oscillate in the noncancerous vocal fold. In the future, postresection phonation will be further improved by the placement of subepithelial biomaterials and tissue grafts that simulate the rheology of normal glottal mucosa (38,39).

HIGHLIGHTS

- Most early glottic cancer can be resected endoscopically with minimal difficulty.
- Phonomicrosurgical resection, which can be repeated, preserves all future treatment options.
- A normal conversation-level voice can be achieved by performing a narrow margin resection and, as necessary, phonosurgical reconstruction.
- The primary value of laryngeal stroboscopy in glottic cancer is to determine where there is residual pliable normal glottal mucosa (epithelium and underlying superficial lamina propria) because this soft tissue is the primary determinant of the potential vocal outcome.
- The goal of phonosurgical reconstruction is medialization of the postresection neocord to reestablish aerodynamic glottal competency.

REFERENCES

1. Zeitels SM, Healy GB. Laryngology and phonosurgery: past present and future. *N Engl J Med* 2003;349: 882–892.
2. Jackson C. Cancer of the larynx: is it preceded by a recognizable precancerous condition? *Trans Am Laryngol Assoc* 1922;44:182–201.
3. Solis-Cohen J. Clinical history of surgical affections of the larynx. *The Medical Record* 1869;4:244–247.
4. Fraenkel B. First healing of a laryngeal cancer taken out through the natural passages. *Archiv fur Klinische Chirurgie* 1886;12:283–286.
5. Lynch RC. Intrinsic carcinoma of the larynx, with a second report of the cases operated on by suspension and dissection. *Trans Am Laryngol Assoc* 1920;40:119–126.
6. LeJeune FE. Intralaryngeal operation for cancer of the vocal cord. *Ann Otol Rhinol Laryngol* 1946;55:531–536.
7. Lillie JC, DeSanto LW. Transoral surgery of early cordal carcinoma. *Trans Am Acad Ophthalmol Otolaryngol* 1973;77:92–96.
8. Strong MS. Laser excision of carcinoma of the larynx. *Laryngoscope* 1975;85:1286–1289.
9. Vaughan CW, Strong MS, Jako GJ. Laryngeal carcinoma: transoral treatment using the CO_2 laser. *Am J Surg* 1978;136:490–493.
10. Zeitels SM. Phonomicrosurgical treatment of early glottic cancer and carcinoma in situ. *Am J Surg* 1996;172:704–709.
11. Zeitels SM, Hillman RE, Franco RA, et al. Voice and treatment outcome from phonosurgical management of early glottic cancer. *Ann Otol Rhinol Laryngol* 2002;111(Suppl 190):1–20.

12. Cragle SP, Brandenburg JH. Laser cordectomy or radiotherapy: cure rates, communication, and cost. *Otolaryngol Head Neck Surg* 1993;108:648–653.
13. Lehman JJ, Bless DM, Brandenburg JH. An objective assessment of voice production after radiation therapy for stage I squamous cell carcinoma of the glottis. *Otolaryngol Head Neck Surg* 1988;98: 121–129.
14. DeSanto LW. Selection of treatment for in situ and early invasive carcinoma of the glottis. In: Albert PW, Bryce DB, eds. *Workshops from the Centennial Conference on Laryngeal Cancer.* New York: Appleton-Century-Crofts, 1976:146–150.
15. Myers EN, Wagner RL, Johnson JT. Microlaryngoscopic surgery for T1 glottic lesion: a cost-effective option. *Ann Otol Rhinol Laryngol* 1994;103:28–30.
16. Zeitels SM. Microflap excisional biopsy for atypia and microinvasive glottic cancer. *Oper Tech Otolaryngol Head Neck Surg* 1993;4: 218–222.
17. Zeitels SM. Premalignant epithelium and microinvasive cancer of the vocal fold: the evolution of phonomicrosurgical management. *Laryngoscope* 1995;105(Suppl 67):1–51.
18. Zeitels SM. Vocal fold atypia/dysplasia and carcinoma. In: *Atlas of phonomicrosurgery and other endolaryngeal procedures for benign and malignant disease.* San Diego: Singular, 2001:177–218.
19. Zeitels SM, Jarboe J, Franco RA. Phonosurgical reconstruction of early glottic cancer. *Laryngoscope* 2001;111:1862–1865.
20. Zeitels SM. A universal modular glottiscope system: the evolution of a century of design and technique for direct laryngoscopy. *Ann Otol Rhinol Laryngol* 1999;108(Suppl 179):1–24.
21. Zeitels SM, Dailey SH, Burns JA. Technique of en bloc endoscopic fronto-lateral laryngectomy for glottic cancer. *Laryngoscope* 2004; 114:175–180.
22. Zeitels SM. Infrapetiole exploration of the supraglottis for exposure of the anterior glottal commissure. *J Voice* 1998;12:117–122.
23. Hartig G, Zeitels SM. Optimizing voice in conservation surgery for glottic cancer. *Oper Tech Otolaryngol Head Neck Surg* 1998; 9:214–223.
24. Desloge RB, Zeitels SM. Endolaryngeal microsurgery at the anterior glottal commissure: controversies and observations. *Ann Otol Rhinol Laryngol* 2000;109:385–392.
25. Kirchner JA, Carter D. Intralaryngeal barriers to the spread of cancer. *Acta Otolaryngology* (Stockh) 1987;103:503–513.
26. Kirchner JA. What have whole organ sections contributed to the treatment of laryngeal cancer? *Ann Otol Rhinol Laryngol* 1989;98: 661–667.
27. Wolfensberger M, Dort JC. Endoscopic laser surgery for early glottic carcinoma: a clinical and experimental study. *Laryngoscope* 1990;100:1100–1105.
28. Davis RK, Jako GJ, Hyams VJ, et al. The anatomic limitations of CO2 laser cordectomy. *Laryngoscope* 1982;92:980–984.
29. Krespi Y, Meltzer CJ. Laser surgery for vocal cord carcinoma involving the anterior commissure. *Ann Otol Rhinol Laryngol* 1989; 98:105–109.
30. Mendenhall W, Parsons JT, Stringer SP, et al. Management of Tis, T1, T2 squamous cell carcinoma of the glottic larynx. *Am J Otolaryngol* 1994;15:250–257.
31. Steiner W. Results of curative laser microsurgery of laryngeal carcinomas. *Am J Otolaryngol* 1993;14:116–121.
32. Eckel H, Thumfart WF. Laser surgery for the treatment of larynx carcinomas: indications, techniques, and preliminary results. *Ann Otol Rhinol Laryngol* 1992;101:113–118.
33. Colden D, Zeitels SM, Hillman RE, et al. Stroboscopic assessment of vocal-fold atypia and early cancer. *Ann Otol Rhinol Laryngol* 2001;110:293–298.
34. Zeitels SM. Optimizing voice after endoscopic partial laryngectomy. *Otolaryngol Clin N Am* 2004;37:627–636.
35. Zeitels SM, Jarboe J, Franco RA. Phonosurgical reconstruction of early glottic cancer. *Laryngoscope* 2001;111:1862–1865.
36. Burns JA, Kobler JB, Zeitels SM. Micro-stereo-laryngoscopic lipoinjection: practical considerations. *Laryngoscope* 2004;114:1864–1867.
37. Zeitels SM, Mauri M, Dailey SH. Medialization laryngoplasty with Gore-Tex for voice restoration secondary to glottal incompetence: indications and observations. *Ann Otol Rhinol Laryngol* 2003; 112:180–184.
38. Jia X, Burdick JA, Kobler J, et al. Synthesis and characterization of in situ crosslinkable hyaluronic acid-based hydrogels with potential application for vocal fold regeneration. *Macromolecules* 2004; 37:3239–3248.
39. Klemuk S, Titze IR. Viscoelastic properties of three vocal-fold injectable biomaterials at low audio frequencies. *Laryngoscope* 2004; 114:1597–1603.

Early Glottic and Supraglottic Carcinoma:

Vertical Partial Laryngectomy and Laryngoplasty

Byron J. Bailey

Laryngeal cancer originates on the true vocal cord about 75% of the time. If properly managed, it should be among the most curable malignancies of the aerodigestive tract. Hoarseness that persists for more than 2 weeks is a strong early warning to the patient and the physician that appropriate diagnostic steps must be taken. When laryngeal cancer is suspected, diagnosed, and managed at this early stage, treatment by endoscopic surgery, partial laryngectomy, or radiation therapy should achieve cure rates of 90% or more. The management issues in glottic carcinoma are local control, effective management of suspected or known metastatic cervical lymph nodes, patient education concerning carcinogenic substances (usually smoking cessation therapy), and patient follow-up for the possibility of residual laryngeal cancer or second primary lesions. Tumors arising on the arytenoid cartilage, in the subglottic region, or in the supraglottic portion of the larynx do not cause hoarseness until they are quite large and often are diagnosed at a later stage. They have a lower cure rate because delayed diagnosis is associated with diminished therapeutic effectiveness of surgery or radiation therapy. Patient survival is the key issue in management, and preservation of life is given a higher priority than preservation of laryngeal function.

Recent advances in laryngeal reconstruction after vertical partial laryngectomy (VPL) have enhanced the quality of life for patients cured of their cancer. This chapter discusses the principles used in managing early glottic cancer using VPL and laryngoplasty (laryngeal reconstruction) and analyzes the results obtained from several reports. Indications and contraindications for various forms of VPL are summarized. In general, early glottic carcinoma can be managed without total laryngectomy and without the procedures that reduce vocal quality or rely on radiation therapy with its inherent problems. A broad surgical armamentarium now includes endoscopic excision, laser resection, and open surgical excision, with a number of reconstructive or rehabilitative techniques to enhance postoperative function. The rationale for early VPL and laryngoplasty is explained, and the advantages associated with this group of procedures are clarified.

BIOLOGY OF LARYNGEAL CANCER

Recent advances in molecular biology and genetics have increased our understanding of the basic biological mechanisms that influence the development of laryngeal malignancy and its clinical course. Recent reports that show promise of practical clinical utility include the following:

- The immortalizing enzyme, telomerase, has been linked to carcinogenesis and its confirmed presence in laryngeal cancer specimens may provide a novel molecular marker, especially for diagnosing persistent malignancy after radiation failure (1).

- A form of hyaluronidase, PH-20, which is expressed in primary laryngeal cancer tissue, is elevated even more in metastatic lesions, such that it can serve as a useful tumor marker and have prognostic value (2).
- Using polymerase chain reaction techniques, herpes simplex virus DNA was found in 75% of laryngeal cancers, but only in 25% of oral cancers and in no control biopsy tissue, suggesting that it may be a cocarcinogen in some patients (3).
- Mutations of the p53 gene have been found to correlate with the clinical outcome of patients with laryngeal cancer. The predictive power of p53 gene mutations is an area of high research interest at this time (4).
- Retinoblastoma protein expression negativity is associated with a higher likelihood of lymph node metastasis and a significantly lower 5-year survival rate (5).
- Low levels of cyclin D1 can be detected by immunohistochemical staining of paraffin-embedded specimens.
- Low levels of cyclin D1 correlate with radio-resistant early-stage larynx carcinoma (6).

DIAGNOSTIC ASSESSMENT

Patients with early glottic carcinoma are assessed preoperatively to confirm the diagnosis of cancer, to rule out the presence of synchronous second primary tumors, to determine whether regional lymph nodes may be involved, and to evaluate the patient's suitability for various forms of treatment with particular attention to pulmonary function.

History establishes the duration and progression of symptoms. Most patients with early glottic carcinoma have a history of cigarette smoking, and it is important to document the duration and dosage of this exposure. Some cofactors, such as ethanol intake, laryngopharyngeal reflux disease, and occupational exposure to fumes or other carcinogens, are significant. A history of any pulmonary or cardiovascular disease requires clarification. Chronic medical problems, medications being taken, and allergies are noted.

Physical examination is the key to accurate diagnosis and proper patient selection for specific types of treatment:

- Listen carefully to the acoustical features of the patient's voice.
- Assess swallowing and respiration grossly during your examination.
- Assess thoroughly the head and neck region, giving particular emphasis to the appearance of the nasal and oral mucous membranes.
- Palpate the tongue and examine indirectly the hypopharynx, tongue base, and larynx.

- Examine carefully the nasopharynx for signs of infection, chronic inflammation, and neoplasm.
- Inspect and palpate the neck with particular attention to the laryngeal cartilages, thyroid gland, and deep jugular lymph node chain.

Physical examination reveals that most early glottic tumors arise on the membranous portion of the true vocal cord, with about 20% of tumors extending to the supraglottis, about 20% extending 5 mm or more below the glottic margin, and about 25% extending to the anterior commissure.

The introduction of various fiberoptic and lens instruments for endoscopy in office practice has been extremely advantageous. These instruments allow photographic or videotape documentation of pathology; they allow observations to be made by several people at about the same time; and they are tolerated better by patients. Video imaging can be used for patient education as well as providing permanent documentation of the lesion and preoperative vocal function. Acoustic analysis of vocal function is receiving widespread attention, and most likely advances in this area will enhance diagnostic capability in the near future. Interpretation of the visual image continues to be challenging, particularly in distinguishing the degree of vocal cord mobility when impairment exists and the depth of tumor invasion is based on the mucosal wave.

Differentiating a bulky glottic tumor without fixation from a true cord fixation secondary to vocalis muscle invasion can be difficult. The key to visualization is persistence until an adequate impression of the surface extent of the lesion and a conceptualized impression of the three-dimensional extent of the tumor have been achieved.

Radiographic studies are often helpful in preoperative evaluation of patients with glottic carcinoma. Computed tomography (CT) can be extremely valuable in demonstrating invasion and destruction of thyroid cartilage. Deep laryngeal soft-tissue infiltration by tumor can be difficult to detect on physical examination but it is demonstrable on CT scans. High-resolution CT improves the accuracy of preoperative staging for laryngeal carcinoma and should be a part of the preoperative assessment of patients with advanced cancer, but its role in early glottic lesions is less clear. Combining radiographic assessment with physical examination should result in diagnostic staging accuracy between 90% and 95%.

The entire hypopharynx, base of the tongue, cervical esophagus, and piriform sinus regions are assessed carefully at direct laryngoscopy. The interior of the larynx is searched carefully for any second areas of involvement or occult tumor spread. A biopsy of the tumor should be taken for diagnosis, and the surrounding tissue should be evaluated as well for possible areas of dysplasia or carcinoma *in situ*. This "mapping" of epithelial changes is a key element in therapeutic planning (Table 121B.1).

TABLE 121B.1	DIAGNOSIS
EARLY GLOTTIC CARCINOMA	

History
  Tobacco
  Ethanol

Symptoms
  Hoarseness
  Dysphagia
  "Lump in throat"

Examination
  Listen to voice
  Palpate neck and larynx
  Use indirect laryngoscopy

Computed tomography scan

Direct laryngoscopy
  Biopsy the lesion
  Map the larynx

TREATMENT

The treatment options for early glottic carcinoma include endoscopic surgical excision (using traditional microsurgical instrumentation or laser), thyrotomy with cordectomy, hemilaryngectomy, VPL with laryngoplasty, and radiation therapy. Adjuvant chemotherapy has been shown to have a beneficial impact on survival even with early glottic cancer (7). The spectrum of diseases encountered includes dysplasia, carcinoma in situ, microinvasive carcinoma, and invasive epidermoid carcinoma. Verrucous carcinoma is the most common variant, and other types of malignancy are rare. The key to effective treatment is to match the therapy with the nature and extent of the malignancy in a manner that does not compromise cure rate but preserves maximal laryngeal function.

We emphasize the importance of approaching conservation laryngeal surgery as we would approach otologic surgery. Preoperative plans should be made carefully, and all laryngeal pathology along with the specific health and needs of the patient should be evaluated thoroughly. Surgical intervention must emphasize meticulous adherence to Halsted's surgical principles. Postoperatively, there should be minimal raw surface area, and the use of keels is recommended to prevent postoperative stenosis.

After mapping the lesion histologically to acquire a thorough understanding of the tumor and surrounding tissue, the surgeon should have a relatively clear idea of the tumor in a three-dimensional sense. Whatever technique is used, the larynx should be entered as far away from the tumor as possible to use frozen-section margins to determine the adequacy of resection and to approach any laryngeal surgery performed as if it were the only chance for cure.

Severe Dysplasia and Carcinoma *In Situ* (Squamous Intraepithelial Neoplasia)

The diagnosis of noninvasive glottic carcinoma cannot always be made easily. Pathologic changes range from early atypia to carcinoma *in situ* (Fig. 121B.1), and the description and categorization of these lesions can vary among observers. At some point, the cellular components lose their orderly progression of maturation, and mitosis becomes so frequent that the pathologist is comfortable with the diagnosis of malignancy. This point varies among pathologists, and the confidence level in making the diagnosis of carcinoma *in situ* is a function of the pathologist's experience and the level of communication between surgeon and pathologist. Careful histologic evaluation and clinical follow-up have led many pathologists and surgeons to conclude that severe dysplasia and carcinoma *in situ* have the same prognosis, with about one of three of these lesions progressing eventually to invasive carcinoma when the management is limited to a single excisional biopsy. Severe dysplasia and carcinoma *in situ* are defined recently in more accurate terminology as "squamous intraepithelial neoplasia, grade 3 (SIN III)" to reflect both the histologic features and the biologic behavior of these lesions (8). Therefore, when a diagnosis of severe dysplasia or carcinoma *in situ* is made and when the site of the lesion involves the true vocal cord, microscopic suspension laryngoscopy with precise excision of the lesion and a closely monitored program of follow-up are indicated. Vocal cord stripping has been replaced by microlaryngeal laser surgery or microflap dissection techniques in an effort to reduce the amount of scarring. The patient must be convinced of the necessity to discontinue smoking and ethanol intake and to maintain a schedule of regular visits for indirect laryngoscopy following a pattern of careful assessment every 2 or 3 months for at least 5 years.

When any postoperative voice change or visible pathology is noted by the patient or surgeon, repeat vocal cord biopsy is indicated. Such cases should not be managed in this manner if the patient refuses to cooperate with the follow-up program. Patients should be advised that some reports recommend radiation therapy initially and others advise radiation therapy if there is a recurrence after the initial excision. We propose that radiation therapy is indicated when lesions are bilateral or extend to involve the supraglottic or subglottic region. Other reports conclude that more failures are associated with radiation therapy than with surgical management of severe dysplasia or carcinoma *in situ*.

Microinvasive Carcinoma

Recently, considerable attention has been given to the relatively small number of patients with glottic carcinoma who show evidence of only superficially invasive cancer. This diagnosis is made when the pathologist notes that

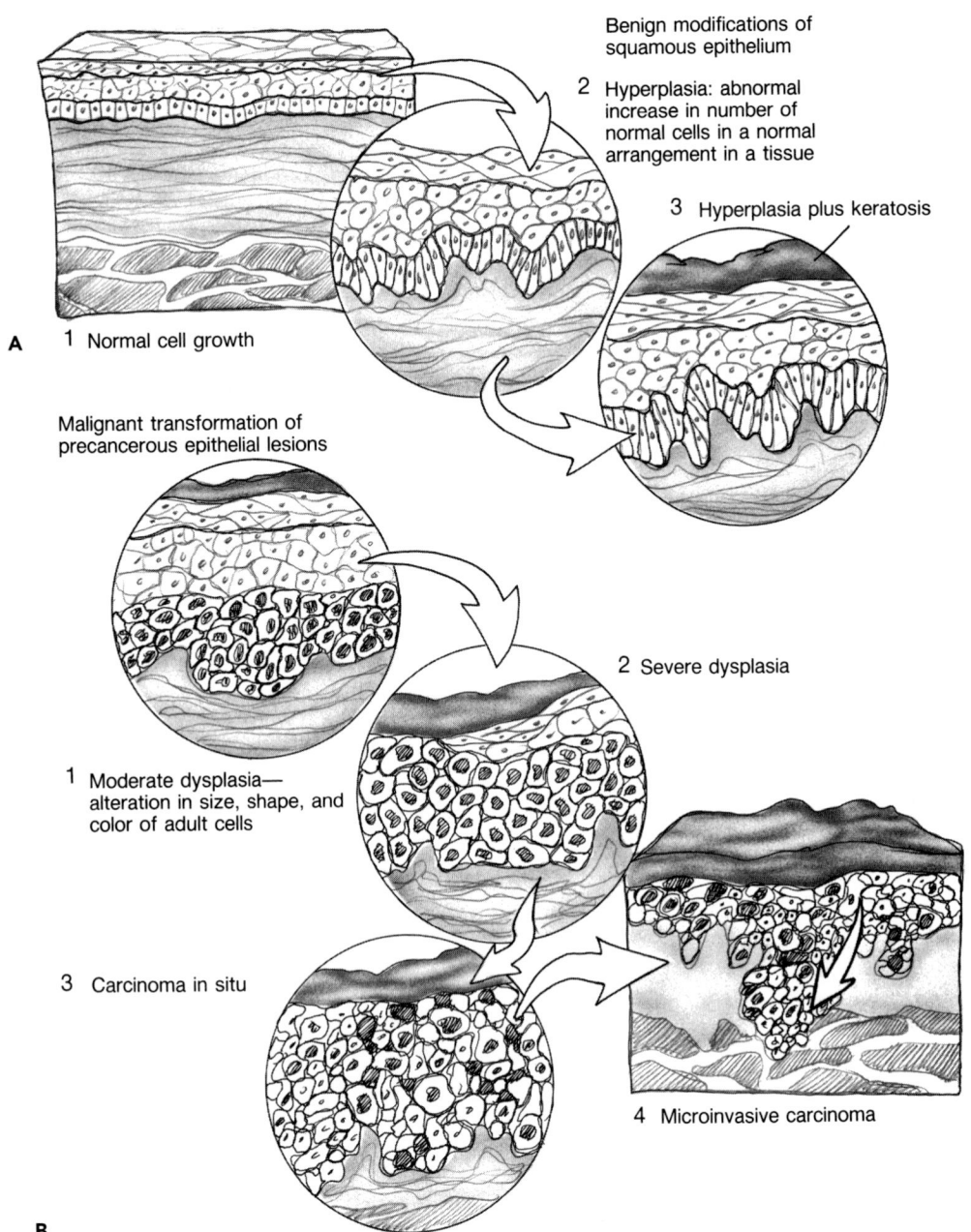

Figure 121B.1 **A:** Benign modifications of squamous epithelium. **B:** Malignant transformations of precancerous epithelial lesions.

malignant cells extend through the basement membrane of the vocal cord epithelium but do not invade the vocalis muscle. In this relatively small patient population (usually no more than 5% of the total laryngeal cancer group), a more conservative form of management is indicated.

Microinvasive carcinoma can be managed by endoscopic excisional biopsy using a microflap technique, by laser excision endoscopically, or by radiation therapy. We prefer a protocol consisting of microscopic suspension laryngoscopy and sequential vocal cord excision every 3 months until two consecutive epithelial specimens can be confirmed to be free of malignant cells. We then monitor

these patients with indirect laryngoscopy every 2 to 3 months. If any suspicious epithelial changes or significant voice changes are noted, we repeat the suspension microlaryngoscopy and biopsy.

Invasive Epidermoid Carcinoma

Early invasive glottic carcinoma can be treated by endoscopic excision, laser excision, thyrotomy with cordectomy, hemilaryngectomy, VPL with laryngoplasty, or radiation therapy. Traditionally, radiation therapy has been offered as the preferred treatment for invasive epidermoid carcinoma involving the membranous portion of the mobile true vocal cord. Recently, some studies have challenged that approach, and endoscopic excision with or without the laser has been found to be equally safe and effective. Late recurrence of carcinoma and the development of second primary tumors are issues of great importance and mandate a pattern of close follow-up, regardless of the treatment chosen.

Radiation therapy is the primary treatment for glottic carcinoma in Scandinavia, with total or partial laryngectomy used for salvage of those patients who have recurrence of cancer. In other parts of the world, surgeons report wider use of VPL for early glottic carcinoma and for advanced T2 glottic lesions. Endoscopic laser excision is used frequently in Germany and Italy.

Verrucous Carcinoma (Ackerman Tumor)

Verrucous carcinoma can be distinguished histologically from other well-differentiated squamous cell carcinomas. This tumor is characterized by its rough, shaggy surface, a rounded, pushing margin, and no metastasis. Smaller lesions can be excised endoscopically; larger tumors are managed by partial laryngectomy. This tumor is less radiosensitive than ordinary squamous cell carcinoma, but radiation therapy is a reasonable alternative for treating larger tumors; total laryngectomy is reserved for large lesions that do not respond to radiation therapy.

Treatment Options for Early Glottic Cancer

The goals of any treatment chosen for early glottic carcinoma include (a) complete removal of all malignant disease; (b) preservation of function (respiration, deglutition, phonation, sphincteric function, airway protection); and (c) predictable and reliable rehabilitation of the patient. These goals can be achieved most consistently when patients and their lesions are matched with the most appropriate treatment.

Recent reports have described large series of early glottic carcinomas that were managed effectively by endoscopic surgical excision (9–11). Success with these lesions requires understanding of the limitations of endoscopic resection combined with diagnostic accuracy that permits proper patient selection.

Microlaryngoscopic surgery has been confirmed by others to be safe and effective management for T1 glottic lesions, and it also has been noted to be a cost-effective option (8).

Open Partial Laryngectomy

The term *open partial laryngectomy* refers to a group of procedures that include midline thyrotomy and cordectomy, standard hemilaryngectomy, and VPL with laryngoplasty. In these procedures, the larynx is approached through the neck and exposed for surgical entry. The larynx is entered by one of several optional techniques. With the tumor under direct vision, either a limited excision of the true vocal cord (cordectomy), traditional hemilaryngectomy (excision of about 50% of the endolarynx with the overlying thyroid cartilage), or some other form of VPL is performed (Fig. 121B.2). Our preference is a type of VPL that preserves the overlying thyroid cartilage and reconstructs the surgical defect by means of a bipedicle muscle flap or an imbrication type of procedure.

Cordectomy is used primarily for early lesions that do not extend to the anterior commissure or involve the region of the arytenoid cartilage. Hemilaryngectomy is used for larger lesions (T1 and T2); VPL and laryngoplasty can be used for transglottic or very extensive bilateral glottic carcinoma.

Indications for VPL and laryngoplasty are tumor involvement of the anterior commissure, extension to involve the vocal process of the arytenoid cartilage, selected superficial transglottic lesions, and carcinoma recurring after radiation therapy. The contraindications for any of these procedures include a fixed vocal cord, involvement of the posterior commissure, invasion of both arytenoid cartilages, bulky transglottic lesions, and lesions invading the thyroid cartilage. Hemilaryngectomy is not as safe or as effective as frontolateral partial laryngectomy when the anterior commissure is involved.

Several published series have shown that VPL and hemilaryngectomy offer patients better cure rates than radiation alone. In addition, growing documentation of results refute the belief that surgery accomplishes its success at the expense of voice preservation, whereas radiation therapy does not.

When used properly, VPL is as effective as total laryngectomy in controlling cancer because of the predictable spread of tumor along known lymphatic pathways. Postoperative laryngeal function is enhanced by the use of various forms of reconstruction of the surgical defect so that the soft tissue removed has been replaced and the lumen of the airway has been relined by epithelium without granulation tissue. Calcaterra (12) prefers to reconstruct the glottis with bilateral omohyoid muscle flaps (Fig. 121B.3). He has observed that this tissue can be tailored along with investing fascia so that the repair is ideal for small anterior commissure defects.

Hemilaryngectomy

In standard hemilaryngectomy, the larynx is exposed by a vertical or horizontal skin incision in the skin over the thyroid cartilage (Fig. 121B.4). The strap muscles are retracted, and the thyroid cartilage perichondrium is divided vertically in the midline. The thyroid cartilage is cut in the exact center, allowing entry into the laryngeal lumen at the anterior commissure. The tumor can be visualized and excised with an adequate cuff of normal tissue. The specimen usually includes most of the true

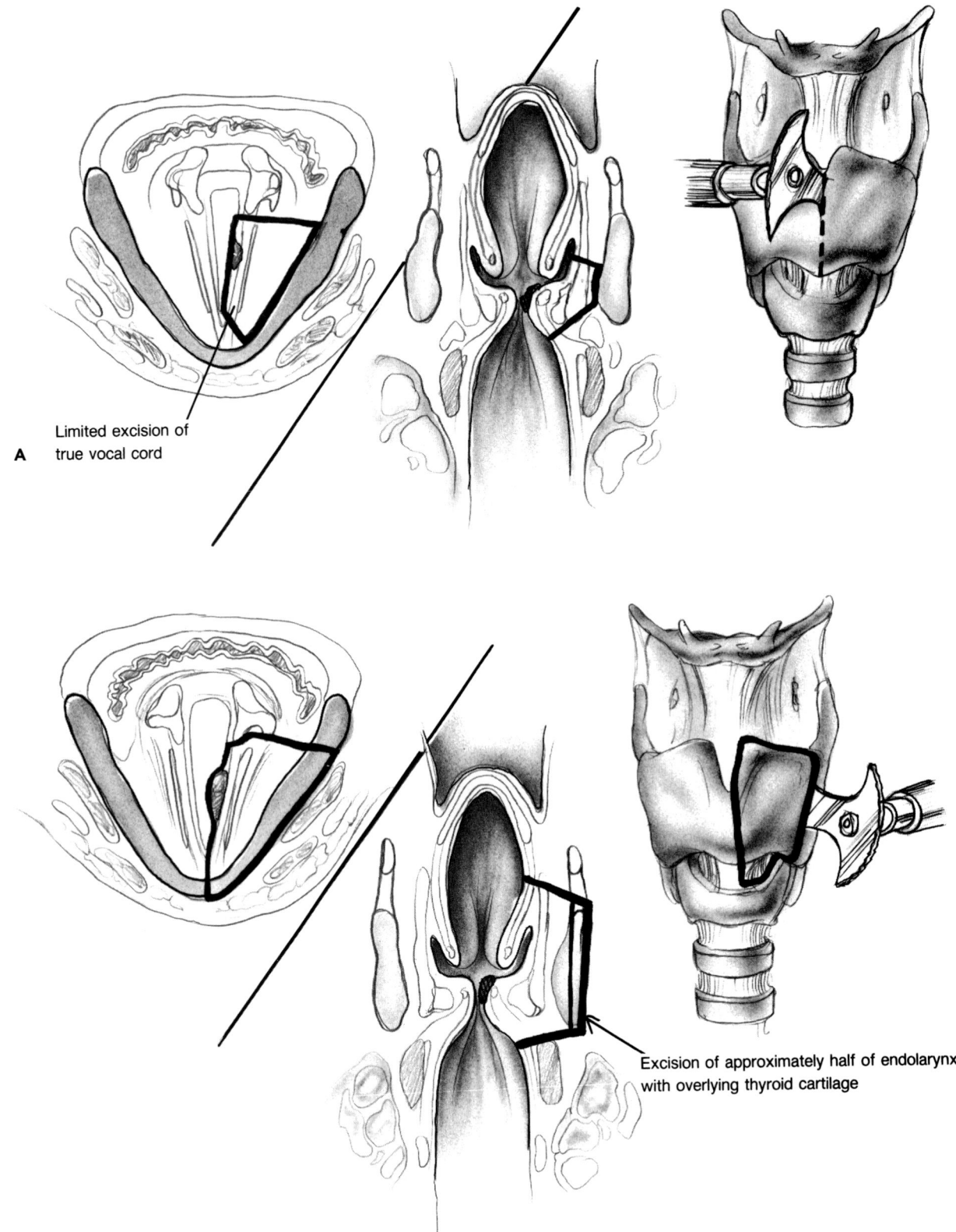

A   Limited excision of true vocal cord

B   Excision of approximately half of endolarynx with overlying thyroid cartilage

Figure 121B.2 Types of partial laryngectomy procedures. **A:** Open partial laryngectomy (cordectomy). **B:** Vertical partial laryngectomy (hemilaryngectomy, including thyroid cartilage).

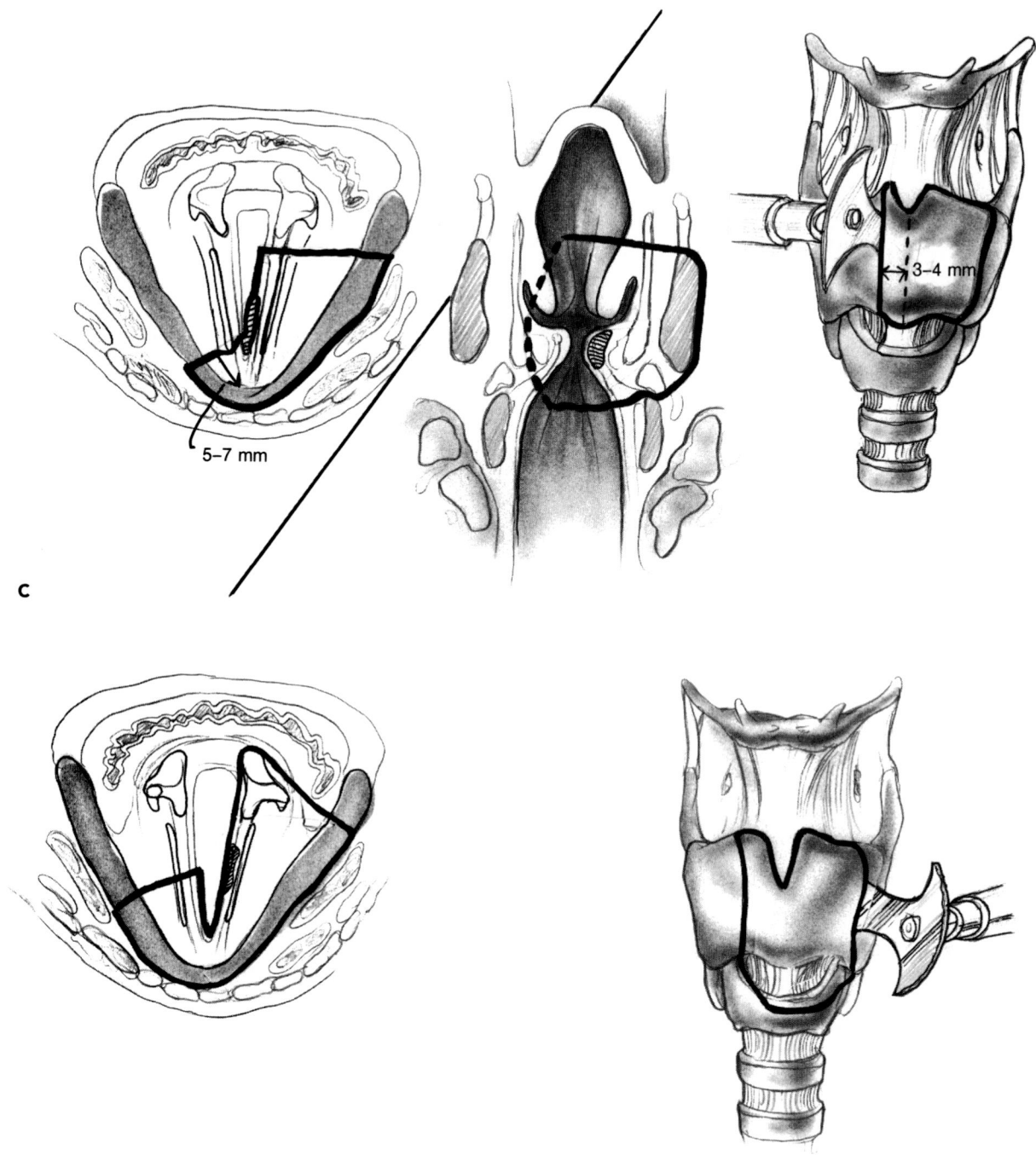

Figure 121B.2 (*continued*)   **C:** Frontal vertical partial laryngectomy. **D:** Extended frontolateral vertical partial laryngectomy, including arytenoid cartilage and portion of cricoid cartilage cephalic margin.

vocal cord (often including the arytenoid cartilage region). The overlying thyroid ala is included with the tumor, with the external thyroid perichondrium serving as the deep margin of the resection. The adjacent mucosa of the piriform sinus region can be elevated and rotated into the surgical defect to cover some of the raw surgical surface. Hemilaryngectomy is less safe and less effective than frontolateral laryngectomy if the glottic cancer approaches or involves the anterior commissure.

Vertical Partial Laryngectomy and Laryngoplasty

Vertical partial laryngectomy with laryngoplasty usually begins with the patient under local anesthesia. A transverse incision is made one fingerbreadth below the cricoid cartilage in a direction parallel with the natural skin creases of the neck skin (Fig. 121B.5). A tracheotomy is performed, an endotracheal tube is inserted, and general endotracheal anesthesia is induced. The initial incision is extended laterally and then curved superiorly to the extent necessary to

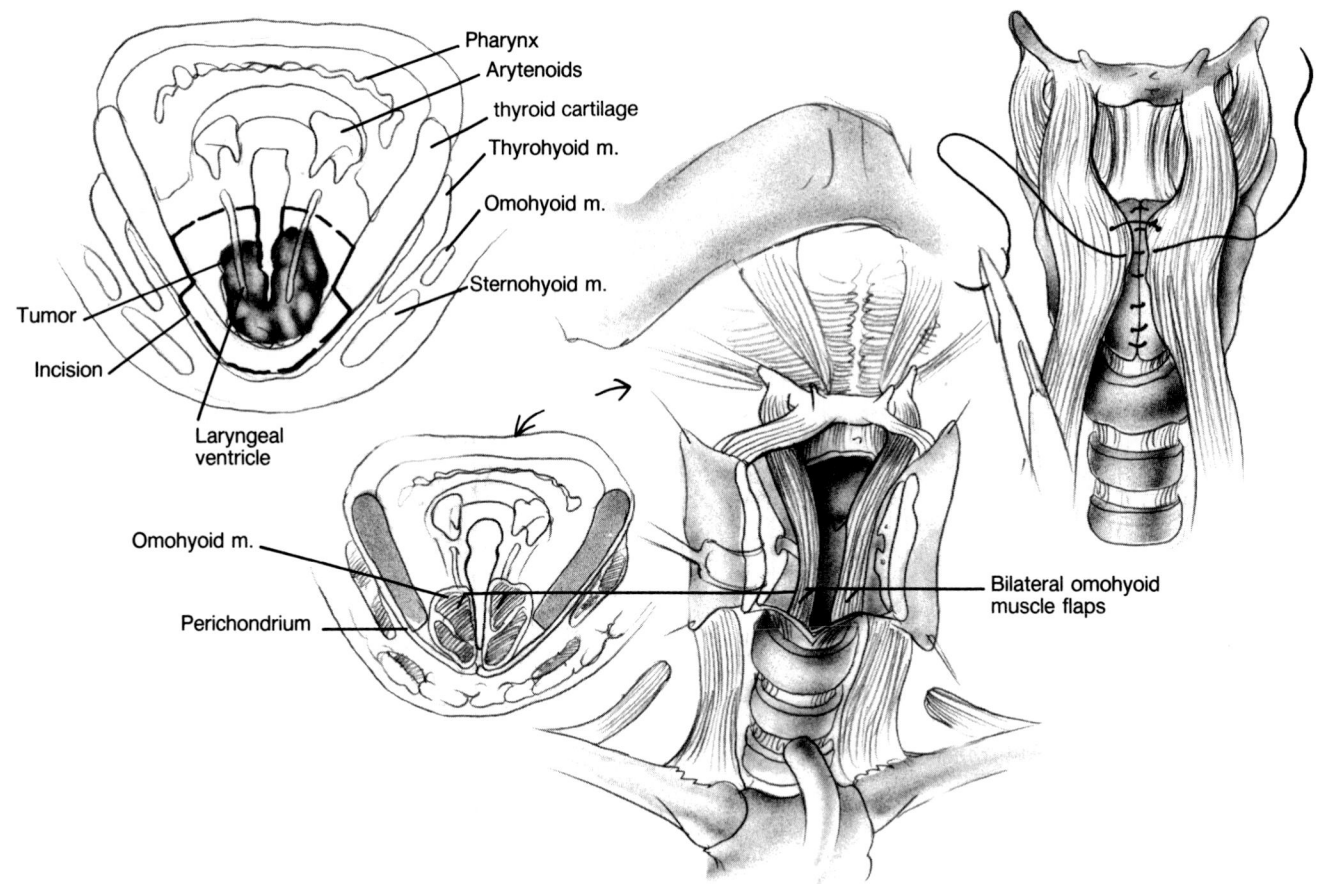

Figure 121B.3 Partial laryngectomy with bilateral omohyoid muscle flap reconstruction. (Redrawn from Biacabe B, Crevier-Buchman L, Hans S, et al. Vocal function after vertical partial laryngectomy with glottic reconstruction by false vocal fold flap: durational and frequency measures. *Laryngoscope* 1999;109:698–704; with permission.)

create a superiorly based flap that permits exposure up to the level of the hyoid bone. The flap is developed deep to the platysma, and the cervical lymph node chains are explored in search of nodal metastases. Any suspicious nodes are sent for frozen-section analysis.

An incision is made in the midline between the two sternohyoid muscles, and the external thyroid perichondrium is divided in the midline. Curved incisions through the perichondrium pass along the superior margins of the thyroid alae and laterally along the inferior margins of the thyroid alae. The external perichondrium is elevated carefully to a point parallel with the superior and inferior thyroid cornua.

For unilateral lesions that do not involve the anterior commissure, the thyroid cartilage is divided in the midline and the tumor is visualized (Fig. 121B.6). The internal thyroid perichondrium then is elevated from the deep surface of the thyroid alae, and the tumor is excised with a cuff of normal tissue. The lower half of the false vocal fold and all of the true cord (including the arytenoid region, when necessary) are excised.

To reconstruct the surgical defect, a bipedicle muscle flap (sternohyoid, sternothyroid, and thyrohyoid muscles) is created. This flap then is transposed to lie deep to the remaining thyroid ala with the carefully preserved external thyroid perichondrium serving as the lining of the laryngeal lumen. Frozen-section analysis of the margins of the surgical defect confirms the adequacy of the resection.

For bilateral lesions, including tumors that involve the anterior commissure, the advantage of VPL is the increased extent of surgical resection that can be accomplished. It is possible to remove the entire endolaryngeal circumference except for one arytenoid region and the posterior commissure. Reconstruction is achieved by use of bilateral bipedicle muscle flaps.

When the anterior commissure is involved, a central segment of thyroid cartilage is isolated and removed en bloc with the tumor specimen (Fig. 121B.7). The procedure begins in the same manner as for unilateral lesions, but two paramedian incisions are used rather than a single midline cartilage incision. The internal thyroid perichondrium is elevated laterally, and the laryngeal lumen is

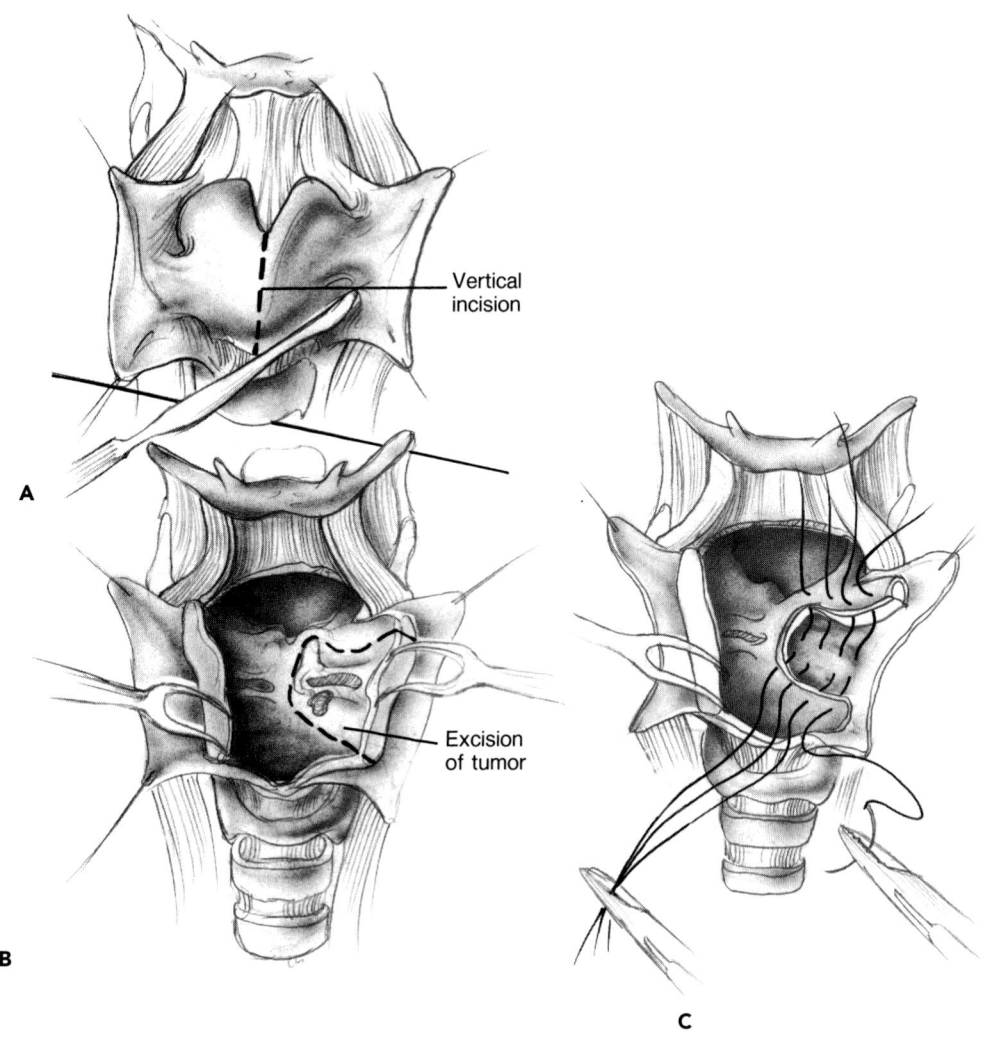

Figure 121B.4 Hemilaryngectomy (specimen includes overlying thyroid cartilage). **A:** Vertical incision for hemilaryngectomy. **B:** Excision of tumor with adequate cuff of normal tissue, arytenoid cartilage, and thyroid ala. **C:** Sutures in place for closure.

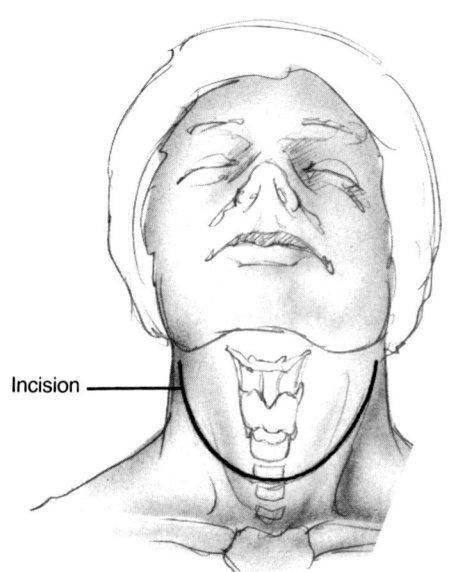

Figure 121B.5 Vertical partial laryngectomy. The preferred incision is made in the skin crease.

entered away from the tumor on the side of lesser tumor involvement. The incisions are extended carefully, allowing the surgeon to open the laryngeal lumen much like opening a book. This permits tumor visualization and allows the surgeon to cut around the margin of the tumor and excise it with an adequate margin of normal tissue.

Bilateral bipedicle muscle flaps are developed and transposed so that they lie deep to the two thyroid cartilage alae. This reconstructive technique results in two raw surfaces adjacent to each other, and the two flaps must be separated by an anterior commissure keel during the healing phase (about 3 weeks). We use a keel of Silastic (polymeric silicone) sheeting that is about the size of a large postage stamp. The keel is fashioned so that three anterior limbs are created; these are tacked down with 3-0 absorbable sutures to the soft tissue outside the larynx. The keel is removed about 3 weeks after surgery by direct laryngoscopy, limiting adhesions of the anterior commissure.

Small anterior commissure lesions can be resected with preservation of the posterior true vocal cords and arytenoid cartilages. The overlying thyroid cartilage must be included

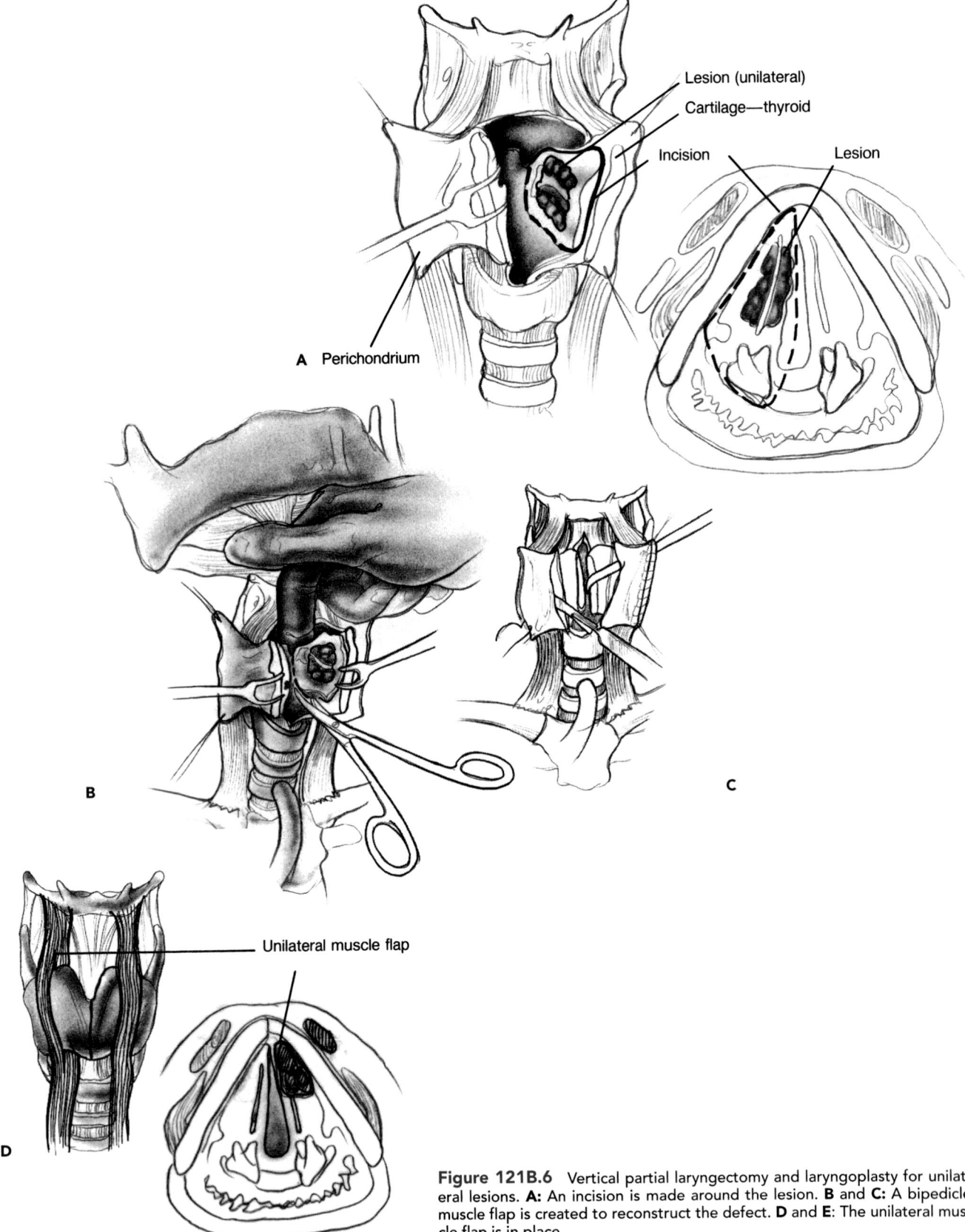

Figure 121B.6 Vertical partial laryngectomy and laryngoplasty for unilateral lesions. **A:** An incision is made around the lesion. **B** and **C:** A bipedicle muscle flap is created to reconstruct the defect. **D** and **E:** The unilateral muscle flap is in place.

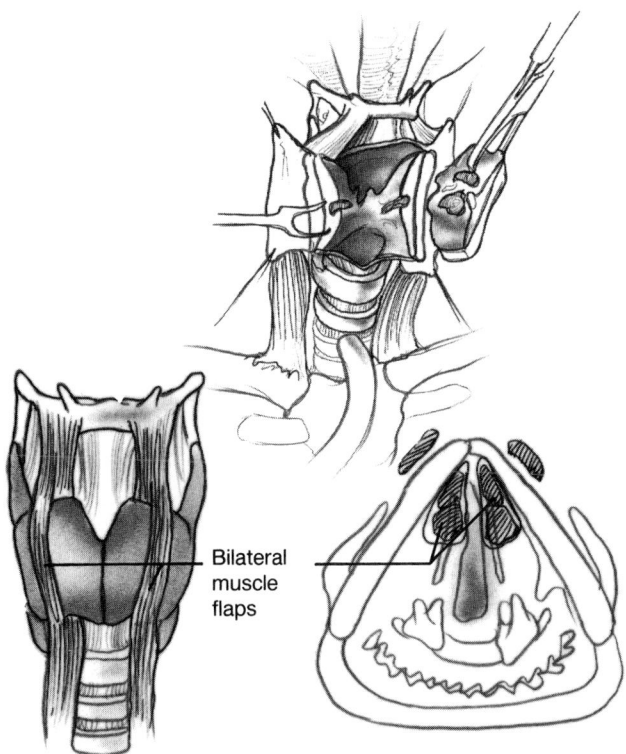

Figure 121B.7 Vertical partial laryngectomy and laryngoplasty for anterior commissure and bilateral lesions. When the anterior commissure is involved, a central segment of thyroid cartilage is removed *en bloc* with the tumor.

en bloc with the tumor because of the direct insertion of the vocalis tendons into the adjacent cartilage. This area of ligamentous insertion is called the Broyles tendon and is a pathway for direct tumor extension into the cartilage. The curability of radiation therapy is hampered in this situation, and a surgical approach is preferred (Fig. 121B.8).

Reconstruction can be achieved by dissecting the adjacent triangular epiglottic petiole free and pulling it inferiorly into the triangular surgical defect. This tissue is sutured in place, and the lateral margins are approximated as the wound is closed. The presence of the remaining true cords and both functioning arytenoid cartilages provides the basis for excellent functional rehabilitation.

Managing postradiation tumor recurrence is an appropriate indication for partial laryngectomy in certain circumstances (13,14). The oncologic safety and effectiveness of this approach have been confirmed when strict patient selection criteria are observed. Biller and Lawson (15) recommend this approach when the following criteria are met:

- The lesion is limited to one true vocal cord (anterior commissure *may* be involved).
- The body of the arytenoid is free of tumor.
- Subglottic tumor extension is no more than 5 mm.
- A mobile cord is present.
- Cartilage is not invaded.
- The recurrent cancer correlates closely with the original primary lesion.

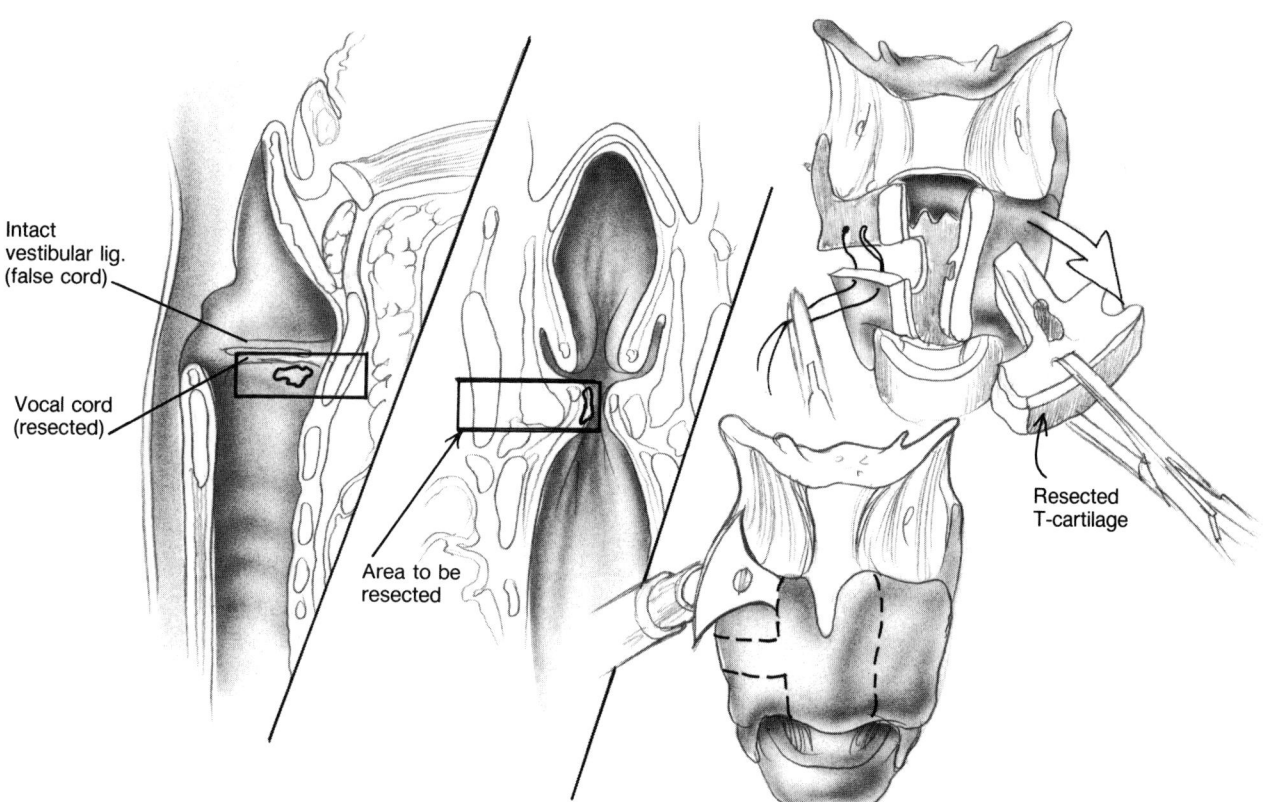

Figure 121B.8 Surgical resection of anterior commissure for small localized tumors in this region.

Most recurrent carcinomas do not meet these criteria, and total laryngectomy is usually necessary to manage this situation adequately. This is the strongest argument against a general strategy of managing all early glottic carcinoma cases with radiation therapy and reserving surgical procedures for radiation therapy failures.

The management of recurrent cancer after previous partial laryngectomy can be individualized according to the specific analysis of each case. Superficial recurrent cancer (often a second primary lesion arising in adjacent mucosa), if extensive, can be managed by radiation therapy. A second partial laryngectomy has been possible in almost 50% of the patients we have seen. Local recurrences (or second primary lesions) arise in about 10% of the patients treated. Deep or extensive instances of recurrent glottic cancer require total laryngectomy.

Persistent edema following radiation therapy for laryngeal carcinoma strongly suggests the possibility of residual cancer. If edema persists beyond 6 months, the surgeon must confirm by a definitive biopsy the presence or absence of malignancy.

Vertical Partial Laryngectomy Procedures

Vertical partial laryngectomy for large T1 glottic cancers is used by Olsen and his colleagues at the Mayo Clinic (16). Anterior commissure involvement is the primary indication in their institution, and they use VPL for tumors as large as those extending from the arytenoid cartilage on one side to the anterior third of the opposite cord. They note better patient survival and fewer total laryngectomies for salvage when VPL is selected rather than radiation therapy in these patients.

Biller and Lawson (15) reported the surgical management of 15 patients who presented with epidermoid carcinoma with vocal cord fixation (and another 11 patients with marked limitation of cord motion). Tumor-free control was achieved in 19 of these 26 patients (73%) at 2 years. Extended hemilaryngectomy was performed, including resection of the cephalic portion of the cricoid cartilage. Subglottic extension is the limiting factor, and the surgeon should expect a complication rate higher than that observed with standard hemilaryngectomy.

Imbrication laryngectomy refers to a procedure in which the surgeon accomplishes a through-and-through excision of a horizontal segment of the larynx. The caudal and cephalic laryngeal margins then are rejoined, preserving the cartilaginous support and soft-tissue planes of the larynx (Fig. 121B.9). The investigators claim high cancer control rates and good postoperative vocal function with this technique (17).

Another approach involves the use of a thyroid cartilage flap in conjunction with a bipedicle sternohyoid muscle flap to reconstruct the defect after VPL. Good functional results are reported in their patients, even when the arytenoid cartilage had to be resected or when radiation therapy had been used initially (18).

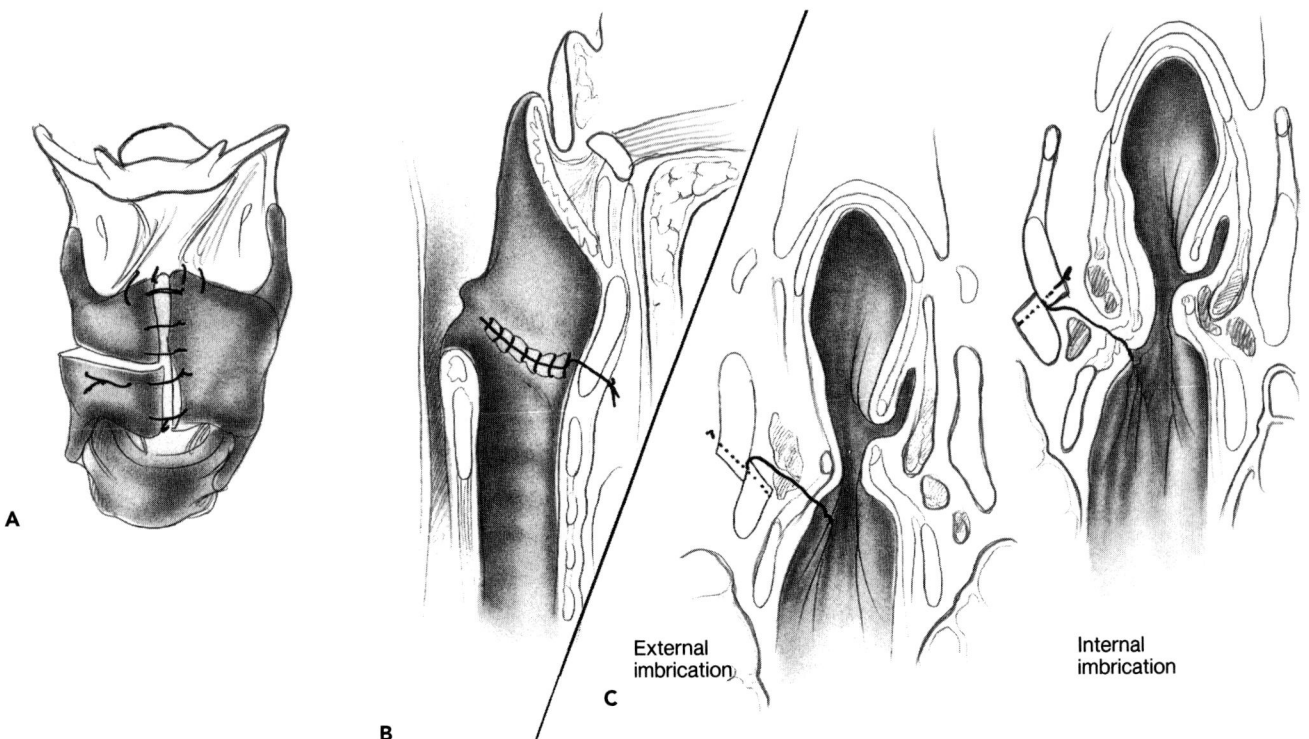

Figure 121B.9 Imbrication laryngectomy. **A** and **B:** Caudal and cephalic margins rejoined. **C:** External imbrication. **D:** Internal imbrication.

COMPLICATIONS

The complications following surgical management of early glottic carcinoma are those conditions and known risks that follow surgical procedures involving the upper airway. Early recognition and effective management are essential.

Early

Early complications include problems associated with the temporary tracheotomy that is usually required. These are subcutaneous emphysema, hemorrhage, tracheotomy tube obstruction (lumen occlusion or tube angulation or mal-positioning), and accidental decannulation. The laryngeal or tracheotomy wound can become infected or colonization can occur around the tracheotomy tube or laryngeal stent or keel if such a device is used. During the early postoperative phase, aspiration and dysphonia are observed routinely. Persistence of these problems beyond 3 weeks should be considered evidence of complicating factors.

Positive resection margins on frozen-section analysis should be managed by wider local excision in most instances. In an alternative strategy, partial laryngectomy is followed by radiation therapy when the margin is questionable or shows severe dysplasia, but the problem of questionable tumor margins continues to be investigated; evidence is inconclusive at this point. Positive margins on permanent section during the postoperative period after the patient has been returned to the ward raises additional questions concerning further management. By sending strips of tissue adjacent to the margins of the original resection, we have decreased this complication. Some proponents argue for postoperative radiation when this condition is encountered, whereas others argue that close observation is sufficient and will result in early detection of any residual disease. These decisions require individual thought, planning, and patient concurrence.

Late

Late complications include persistent aspiration, lingering infection (chondritis), laryngeal stenosis, severe hoarseness, granulation tissue formation, and tumor recurrence. After hemilaryngectomy, some patients have persistent aspiration, with a reported incidence of 6% to 10% failure to recover normal deglutition in several series of patients. Surgeons have tried to correct this problem by injecting various materials in the region of the surgical defect, but this has been generally unsuccessful because of extensive fibroses. Gax collagen has been reported to be useful because it can be injected slowly, under high pressure through a 27-gauge needle into the scar tissue bed of the defect. Persistent aspiration has not been observed with VPL and laryngoplasty. Extensive resection for bilateral glottic carcinoma can be expected to produce significant dysphonia but results in a postoperative voice that may be superior to tracheal esophageal, esophageal, or prosthetic speech.

Information is accumulating regarding voice quality after VPL:

- More involvement of supraglottic structures in the production of voice is seen than was previously appreciated.
- The vocal range is restricted.
- The importance of arytenoid function preservation is better understood.

These findings correlate closely with our personal observations and underscore the fundamental importance of sparing at least one functional arytenoid cartilage and reconstituting the glottic sphincter in the region of the vocal fold resection.

Recent studies compared voice quality after laser excision of glottic cancer with that following radiation therapy. Rydell et al. (19) found voice quality to be better after radiotherapy, whereas McGuirt et al. (20) found that vocal quality was about the same in patients with similar staging. A recent report by Biacabe et al. (21) described in detail the improved vocal results that can be achieved using a false vocal fold mucosal flap to reconstruct the glottis after VPL.

Delayed decannulation or ability to decannulate patients after partial laryngectomy is unusual. In most series, it is noted in only 3% to 5% of patients. This complication can be avoided in some patients by careful attention to the principles of conservation surgery and preservation of all uninvolved tissue. We strongly advise preserving one functional arytenoid cartilage and avoiding the extension of the surgical resection into the region of the epiglottis. Careful selection of patients who fail radiation therapy for salvage with hemilaryngectomy yields high rates of tumor control with retention of vocal function. These patients tend to have higher complication rates and slower recovery, but the final results are encouraging.

Tumor recurrence is generally related to inappropriate patient selection for surgery. The two common causes for failure with hemilaryngectomy are the inability to recognize the inferior margin of the tumor and the spread of cancer outward through the cricothyroid membrane. For cases of T1 glottic cancer that were managed endoscopically, the recurrence rate is reported to be about 12%.

Recurrence rates and complication rates are higher in obese patients after radiation therapy for early vocal cord carcinoma when radiation treatment is given with anterior oblique ports. Some strongly advise that primary conservation laryngeal surgery yields much better results.

EMERGENCIES

Emergent situations associated with early glottic carcinoma are extremely rare. The major concern is that patients with laryngeal carcinoma usually have a history of heavy smoking and ethanol ingestion, which introduces significant risk factors for general anesthesia during the diagnostic endoscopy and biopsy session. Thorough assessment of general health, medications, and chronic cardiovascular and pulmonary pathology is key to a favorable outcome at this stage.

Following surgical management of early glottic carcinoma, the major emergencies are those of airway obstruction and aspiration. During the immediate postoperative period, observation and protection of the airway are crucial nursing responsibilities. After the first 72 hours, airway obstruction associated with the surgical procedure rarely poses problems. The persistent aspiration of saliva and pharyngeal contents predisposes to pneumonia and is a likely precursor to fatality if this condition is overlooked. During the immediate postoperative period, aspiration can be managed by collagen injection, but this approach is not technically feasible after 6 to 8 weeks. Additional rare emergency situations are cardiovascular problems and pulmonary insufficiency.

FRONTIERS OF KNOWLEDGE

Our ability to assess and treat early glottic carcinoma would be enhanced by additional scientific information from clinical trials addressing several topics. The following are needed:

- A prospective, randomized, multicenter clinical trial comparing the various forms of surgical management and, in particular, laser management with radiation therapy for early glottic carcinoma
- Clarification of the therapeutic effectiveness and safety of photodynamic therapy
- Clarification of the precise indications and limitations for each of the forms of surgical intervention that have been proposed for early glottic carcinoma

---

HIGHLIGHTS

- Laryngeal cancer arises on the vocal cords in 75% of cases, and hoarseness is an early warning symptom, suggesting cancer when it persists for more than 2 weeks.
- Laryngeal lymphatic anatomy underlies the effective surgical treatment of early glottic carcinoma.
- Laryngeal function includes airway protection, respiration, phonation, and sphincteric activity, and surgical procedures to treat laryngeal cancer must consider all four functions.
- Serial section of cancerous larynges has provided understanding of the pathophysiology of early vocal cord cancer.
- Most membranous vocal cord (glottic) carcinomas extend to the supraglottic region (20%), to the subglottic region (20%), or to the anterior commissure (25%).

- Early glottic carcinoma limited to the membranous portion of the vocal fold can be cured using endoscopic surgical excision, thyrotomy with cordectomy, hemilaryngectomy, VPL with laryngoplasty, and radiation therapy.
- About one of six patients with severe dysplasia or carcinoma *in situ* will develop invasive carcinoma if the only therapy used is a single vocal cord excision or biopsy.
- Microinvasive carcinoma of the true vocal fold can be managed by sequential endoscopic excisional biopsy, endoscopic laser excision, or radiation therapy.
- The goals of treatment for early glottic carcinoma are (a) complete removal of all malignant disease, (b) preservation of function, and (c) predictable and reliable rehabilitation of the patient.
- Indications for VPL and laryngoplasty are anterior commissure involvement, extension to the vocal process of the arytenoid cartilage, selected superficial transglottic lesions, and recurrent cancer after radiation therapy.
- Partial laryngectomy for recurrent cancer after radiation therapy must meet the following criteria: (a) lesion limited to one cord (may involve the anterior commissure); (b) body of arytenoid cartilage free of tumor; (c) subglottic extension no more than 5 mm; (d) mobile cord; (e) no cartilage invasion; and (f) recurrence correlating with initial tumor.
- Early complications after partial laryngectomy include subcutaneous emphysema, bleeding, and tracheotomy tube occlusion.

REFERENCES

1. Curran AJ, Gullane PJ, Irish J, et al. Telomerase activity is upregulated in laryngeal squamous cell carcinoma. *Laryngoscope* 2000; 110(part 1):391–396.
2. Godin DA, Fitzpatrick PC, Scandurro AB, et al. PH2O: a novel tumor marker for laryngeal cancer. *Arch Otolaryngol Head Neck Surg* 2000;126:402–404.
3. Pou AM, Vrabec JT, Jordan J, et al. Prevalence of herpes simplex virus in malignant laryngeal lesions. *Laryngoscope* 2000;110 (part 1):194–197.
4. Chomchai JS, Du W, Sarkar FH, et al. Prognostic significance of p53 gene mutations in laryngeal cancer. *Laryngoscope* 1999;109: 455–459.
5. Dokiya F, Ueno K, Ma S, et al. Retinoblastoma protein expression and prognosis in laryngeal cancer. *Acta Otolaryngol* 1998;118: 759–762.
6. Yoo SS, Carter D, Turner BC, et al. Prognostic significance of cyclin D1 protein levels in early-stage larynx cancer treated with primary radiation. *Int J Cancer* 2000;90(1):22–28.
7. Laccourreye O, Bassot V, Brasnu D, et al. Chemotherapy combined with conservation surgery in the treatment of early larynx cancer. *Curr Opin Oncol* 1999;11(3):200–203.
8. Flint PW. Minimally invasive techniques for management of early glottic cancer. *Otolaryngol Clin N Am* 2002;35(5):1055–1066.
9. Kim DR, Kevin H, Smith ME. Endoscopic vertical partial laryngectomy. *Laryngoscope* 2004;114(2):236–240.
10. Zeitels SM, Dailey SH, Burns JA. Technique of en bloc laser endoscopic frontolateral laryngectomy for glottic cancer. *Laryngoscope* 2004;114(1):175–180.
11. Gallo A, deVincentiis M, Manciocco V, et al. CO2 laser cordectomy for early-stage glottic carcinoma: a long-term follow-up of 156 cases. *Laryngoscope* 2002;112(2):370–374.

12. Calcaterra TC. Bilateral omohyoid muscle flap reconstruction for anterior commissure cancer. *Laryngoscope* 1987;97:810.
13. Makiko T, Nibu K, Nakao K, et al. Partial laryngectomy to treat early glottic cancer after failure of radiation therapy. *Arch Otolaryngol Head Neck Surg* 2002;182(8):909–912.
14. Mooney WW, Cole IF, Albsoul N, et al. Salvage vertical partial laryngectomy for radiation failure in early glottic carcinoma. *Australian and New Zealand Journal of Surgery* 2002;72(10): 746–749.
15. Biller HF, Lawson W. Partial laryngectomy for vocal cord cancer with marked limitation or fixation of the vocal cord. *Laryngoscope* 1986;96:61.
16. Olsen KD, DeSanto LW. Partial laryngectomy—indications and surgical technique. *Am J Otolaryngol* 1990;11:153.
17. Lui C, Ward PH, Pleet L. Imbrication reconstruction following partial laryngectomy. *Ann Otol Rhinol Laryngol* 1986;95:567.
18. Burgess LPA, Yim DWS, Thyroid cartilage flap reconstruction of the larynx following vertical partial laryngectomy: an interim report. *Laryngoscope* 1988;98:605.
19. Rydell R, Schalen L, Fex S, et al. Voice evaluation before and after laser excision vs. radiotherapy of T1A glottic carcinoma. *Acta Otolaryngol (Stockh)* 1995;115:560.
20. McGuirt WF, Blalock D, Koufman JA, et al. Comparative voice results after laser resection or irradiation of T1 vocal cord carcinoma. *Arch Otolaryngol Head Neck Surg* 1994;120:951.
21. Biacabe B, Crevier-Buchman L, Hans S, et al. Vocal function after vertical partial laryngectomy with glottic reconstruction by false vocal fold flap: durational and frequency measures. *Laryngoscope* 1999;1.09: 698–704.

Early Glottic and Supraglottic Carcinoma: Open Supraglottic and Supracricoid Partial Laryngectomy

Gregory S. Weinstein   *Ollivier Laccourreye*   *Christopher H. Rassekh*

Two basic types of supracricoid partial laryngectomy (SCPL) exist: one in which the epiglottic and preepiglottic space are resected, and one in which they are spared. In both cases, both true and false cords and the entire thyroid cartilage are resected, and at least one arytenoid cartilage must be spared. For glottic carcinoma a procedure is used in which the epiglottis and preepiglottic space are spared and the space is reconstructed by suturing the cricoid cartilage to the epiglottis and hyoid bone and tongue base; this procedure is known as a cricohyoidoeopiglottopexy (CHEP). A procedure in which the epiglottis and preepiglottic space are resected is used for supraglottic and transglottic carcinomas in which this space is reconstructed by suturing the cricoid cartilage to the hyoid and tongue base: this procedure is known as a cricohyoidopexy (CHP) (1,2).

The open supraglottic partial laryngectomy (SGPL) is performed by resecting the upper portion of the thyroid cartilage, the epiglottis and preepiglottic space, and the false cords. The hyoid bone is resected only if it is involved by carcinoma. The reconstruction, known as a thyrohyoidopexy (THP), is performed by suturing the thyroid cartilage to the hyoid and tongue base. The difference between the SCPL with CHP and the SGPL alone is that in the SCPL with CHP the entire thyroid cartilage and the true cords are resected. The SGPL is used for selected supraglottic carcinomas (3).

This chapter focuses on early glottic and supraglottic carcinomas (T1N0 and T2N0), which can be treated either with SCPL with CHEP or CHP and those that can be treated with SGPL alone. Tables 121C.1 through 121C.4

TABLE 121C.1 ▧ DIAGNOSIS

History
Physical examination
　Careful examination of mobilities (vocal cord and arytenoid separately)
　Neck examination

Computed tomography
　Cartilage involvement, preepiglottic space, subglottis, neck nodes.
　　Panendoscopy, with careful telescopic and microscopic tumor mapping and careful attention to arytenoid and subglottis
Chest radiography assessment of pulmonary reserve

TABLE 121C.2 ℞ TREATMENT

T1 and T2 glottic cancer
Endoscopic with or without laser
Vertical partial laryngectomy
Supracricoid partial laryngectomy with CHEP
Radiotherapy

T1 and T2 supraglottic cancer
Endoscopic with laser, including formal laser SGPL
Open SGPL
SCPL-CHP
Radiation alone for stage I and II

CHEP, cricohyoidoepiglottopexy; SGPL, supraglottic partial laryngectomy; SCPL-CHP, supracricoid partial laryngectomy–cricohyoidopexy.

TABLE 121C.3 C COMPLICATIONS

Bleeding
Infection
Rupture of closure stitches
Pneumonia
Positive surgical margin

TABLE 121C.4 EMERGENCIES

Airway distress secondary to tracheostomy displacement
Bleeding

---

review diagnosis, treatment, complications, and emergencies associated with these conditions.

FUNDAMENTAL CONCEPTS

It is important to note that, although the T-staging system is useful for predicting the outcome following nonsurgical organ preservation approaches (e.g., radiation or chemotherapy and radiation), the four T categories are too broad to have value in planning for surgical organ preservation with either open or endoscopic approaches. The organ preservation surgeon must have the skill to accurately assess both the surface and deep extent of the cancer so that the cancer can be placed on a spectrum of lesions, from small to large, and to correlate this with a spectrum of surgical procedures that can be used to preserve the larynx (4). Figures 121C.1 and 121C.2 show the *organ preservation surgery spectra* for

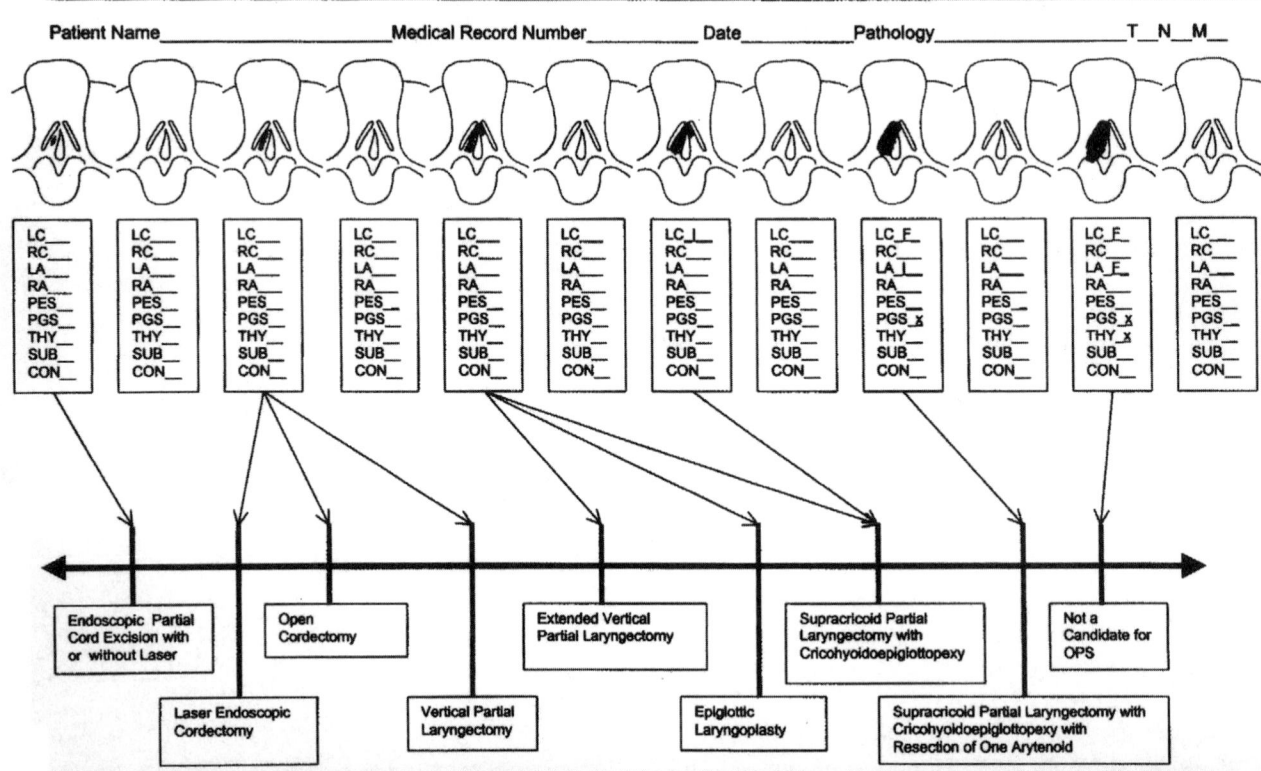

Figure 121C.1 Organ preservation surgery spectrum for glottic carcinoma.

Patient Name_____Medical Record Number_____ Date_____ Pathology_____ T__N__M__

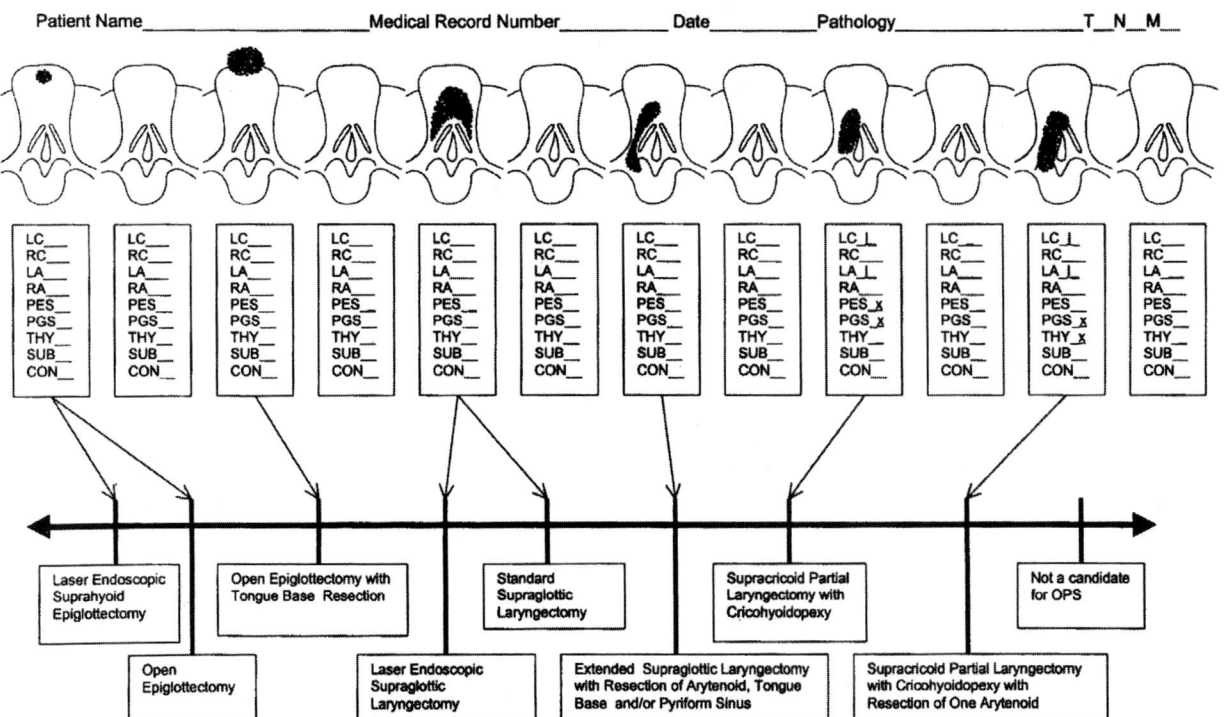

LC: left vocal cord mobility; RC: right vocal cord mobility; LA: left arytenoid mobility; RA: right arytenoid mobility; PES: preepiglottic space involvement; PGS: paraglottic space invasion; THY; early radiologic evidence of thyroid cartilage invasion; SUB: subglottic extension > 1m at midcord, or > 0.5 cm posterior cord level; CON: tumor and non-tumor contraindications. At the top of the form is a series of schematic diagrams of the larynx with additional descriptors in the text box below. At the bottom of the form is the spectrum of organ preservation surgeries that are applicable. Representative cancers are shown in a spectrum from least extensive on the left through most extensive on the right. The mucosal extent is documented on the schematic. Mobility is documented with either a "blank" for normal mobility, "I" for impaired mobility, and "F" for fixation. An "x" documents involvement of the preepiglottic space, paraglottic space, thyroid cartilage, and a tumor- or non-tumor-related contraindication. This form may be used in surgical planning by drawing the lesion into a blank laryngeal schematic, in the appropriate place on the spectrum.

Figure 121C.2 Organ preservation surgery spectrum for supraglottic carcinoma.

glottic carcinoma and supraglottic carcinoma, respectively. The clinician can utilize these spectra by placing the cancer being assessed along the laryngeal schematics at the top and see which surgical technique may be useful. These spectra are useful teaching aids for residents and fellows, as well.

Another important concept is the idea of the cricoarytenoid unit (Fig. 121C.3). In the conservation surgery paradigm, in which the accepted open partial laryngectomies were the vertical partial laryngectomy and the open SGPL, the main focus was on the vocal cord itself. With the transition to the organ preservation surgery paradigm, which includes SCPL as well as the tranoral laser techniques, the focus shifts to the cricoarytenoid unit. The cricoarytenoid unit is considered the fundamental functional unit of the larynx. It includes one arytenoid cartilage with its associated cricoarytenoid musculature and recurrent and superior laryngeal nerves. Preservation of one cricoarytenoid unit with the associated cricoid ring allows for speech and swallowing without a permanent tracheostomy.

The SCPL and SGPL are fundamentally similar procedures (Fig. 121C.4 through 121C.15). They are all horizontal partial laryngectomies, which means that entry into the

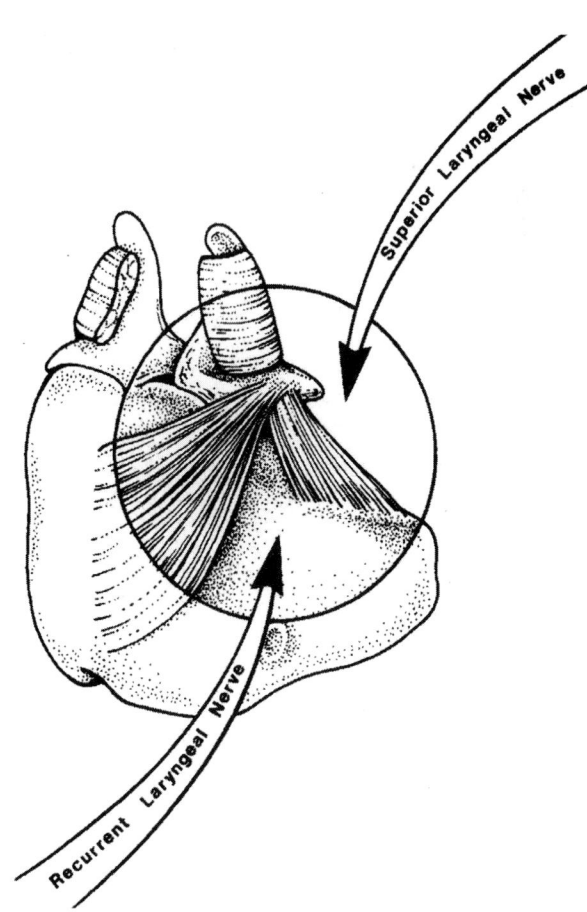

Figure 121C.3 The cricoarytenoid unit.

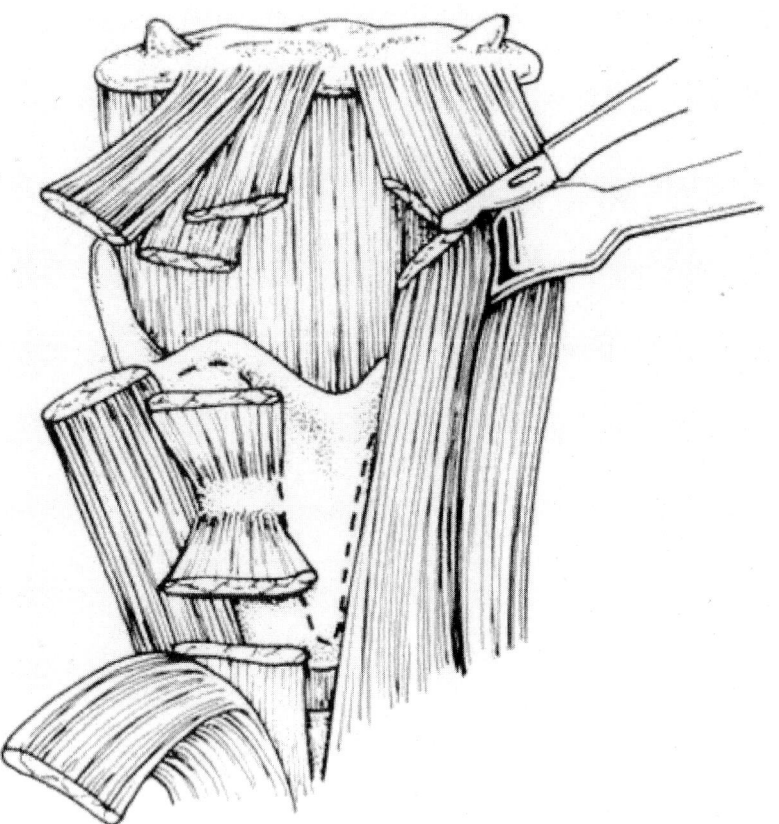

Figure 121C.4 Transection of the strap muscles, which is the same for supraglottic partial laryngectomy (SCPL) with cricohyoidoeopiglottopexy (CHEP) and cricohyoidopexy (CHP).

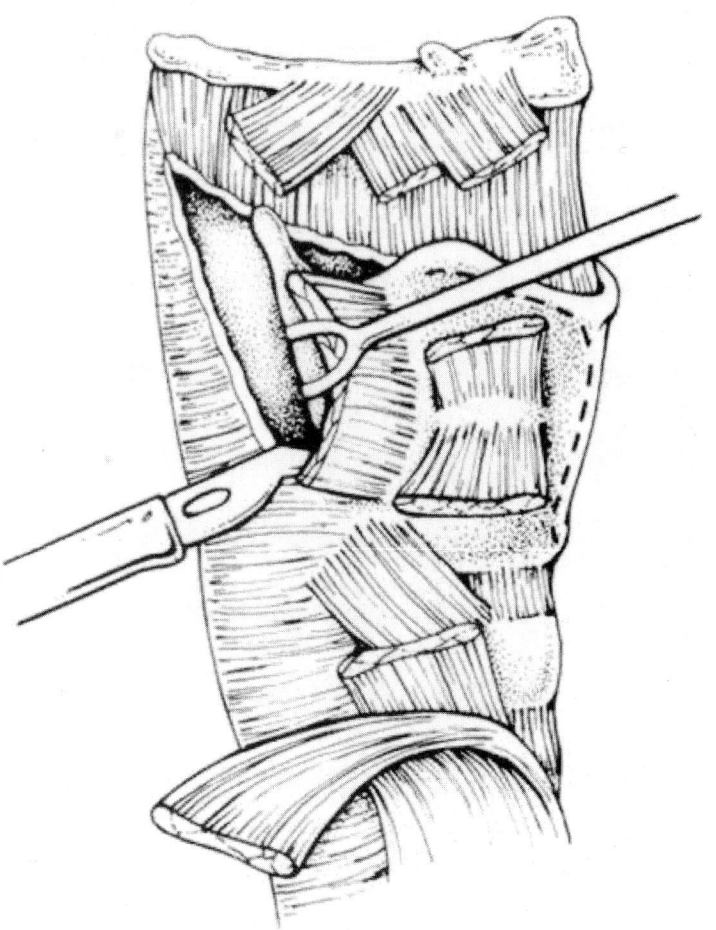

Figure 121C.5 Transection of the constrictor muscles, which is the same in the supraglottic partial laryngectomy (SCPL) with cricohyoidoeopiglottopexy (CHEP) and cricohyoidopexy (CHP).

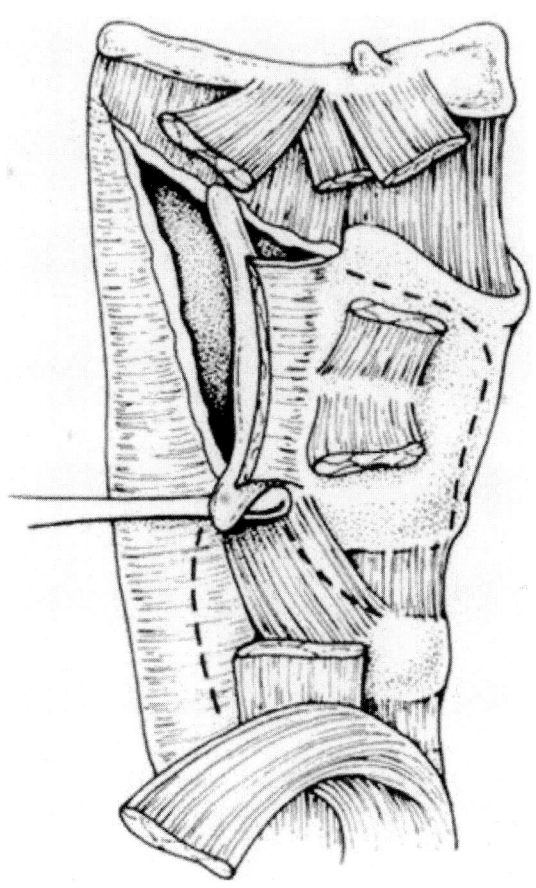

Figure 121C.6 Disarticulation of the cricothyroid joint, which is the same for supraglottic partial laryngectomy (SCPL) with cricohy-oidoeopiglottopexy (CHEP) and cricohyoidopexy (CHP).

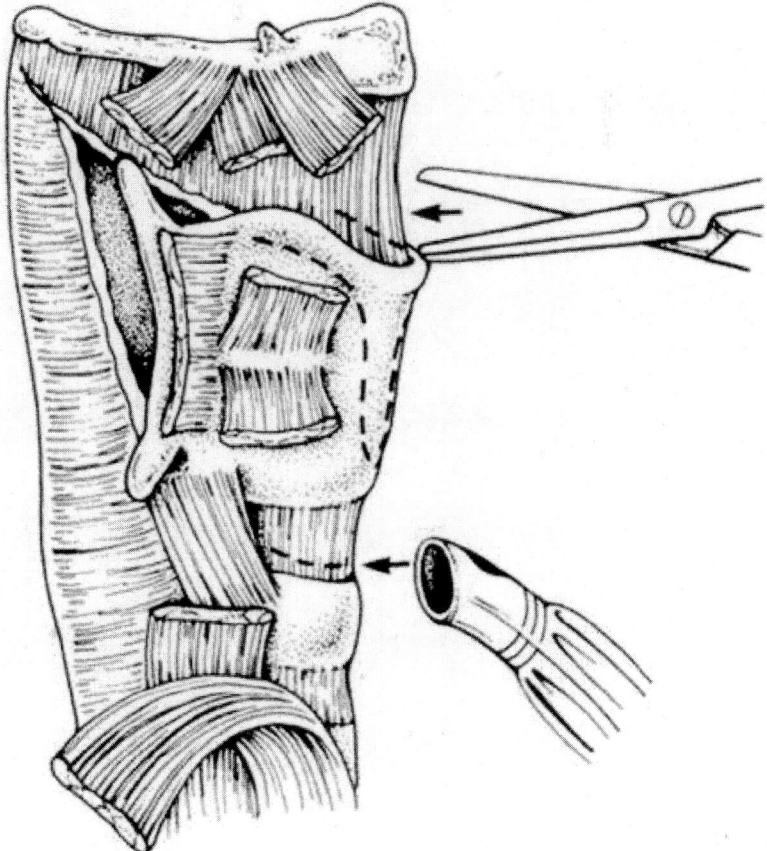

Figure 121C.7 Horizontal cricothyroidectomy and entry into the larynx just above the thyroid notch, which is done in supraglottic partial laryngectomy (SCPL) with cricohyoidoeopiglottopexy (CHEP).

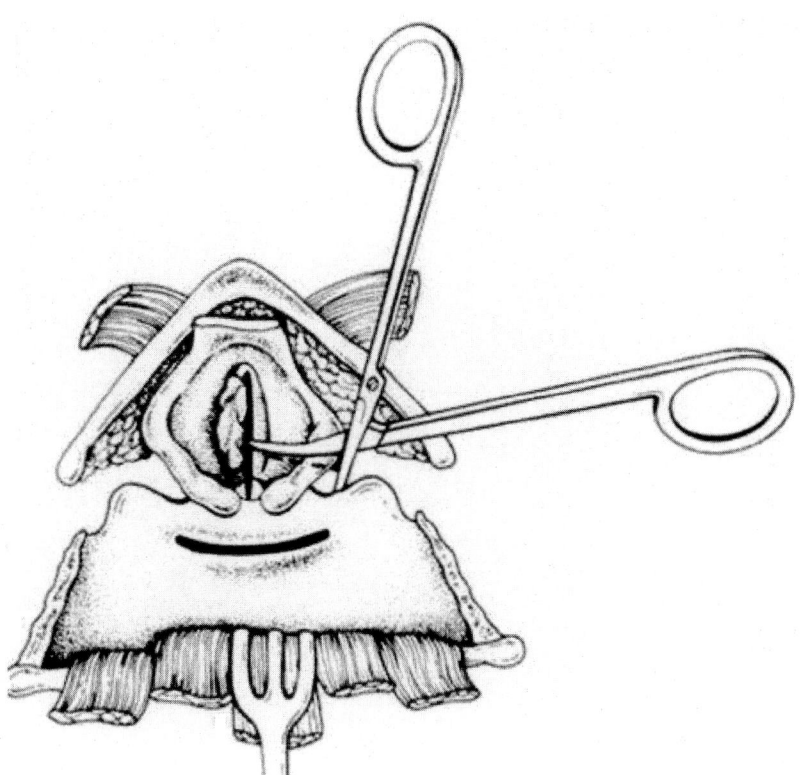

Figure 121C.8 The view during the supraglottic partial laryngectomy (SCPL) with cricohyoidoeopiglottopexy (CHEP) is now looking into the larynx from the top of the bed and one scissor blade is in the space between the inner thyroid cartilage and previously elevated inner thyroid perichondrium starting on the side with least tumor.

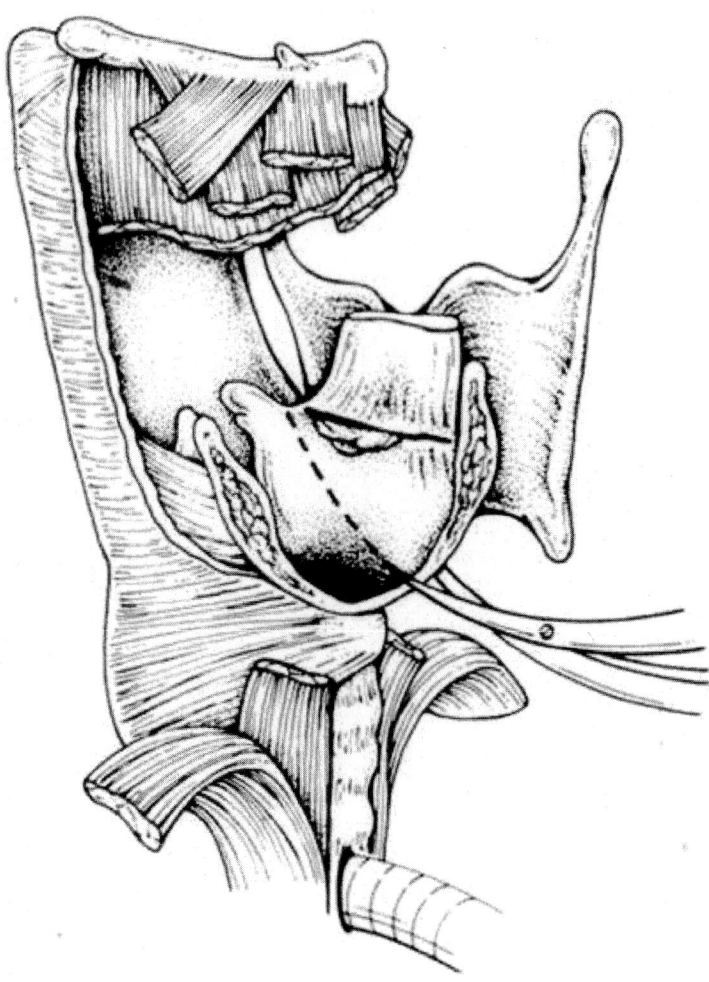

Figure 121C.9 The larynx is opened during the supraglottic partial laryngectomy (SCPL) with cricohyoidoeopiglottopexy (CHEP) on the anterior spine of the thyroid cartilage, like opening a book, and the resection is completed.

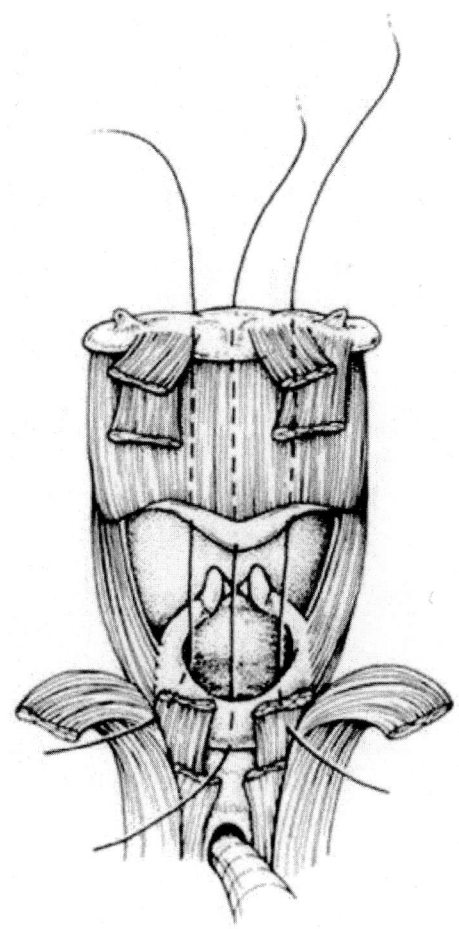

Figure 121C.10 The closure is begun during the supraglottic partial laryngectomy (SCPL) with cricohyoidoeopiglottopexy (CHEP) with three stitches placed, one in the midline and the remaining two placed 1 cm from the midline on either side.

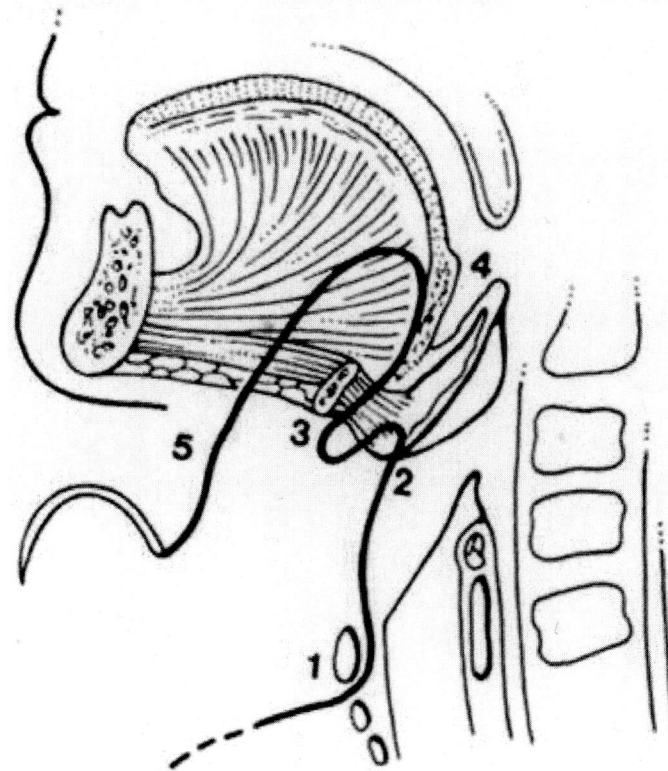

Figure 121C.11 The suture placement during supraglottic partial laryngectomy (SCPL) with cricohyoidoeopiglottopexy (CHEP): (*1*) submucosally around the cricoid cartilage, then (*2*) through the petiole of the epiglottis, then (*3*) back into the preepiglottic space and around the hyoid bone, (*4*) deep into the tongue base, and then (*5*) out through the suprahyoid musculature.

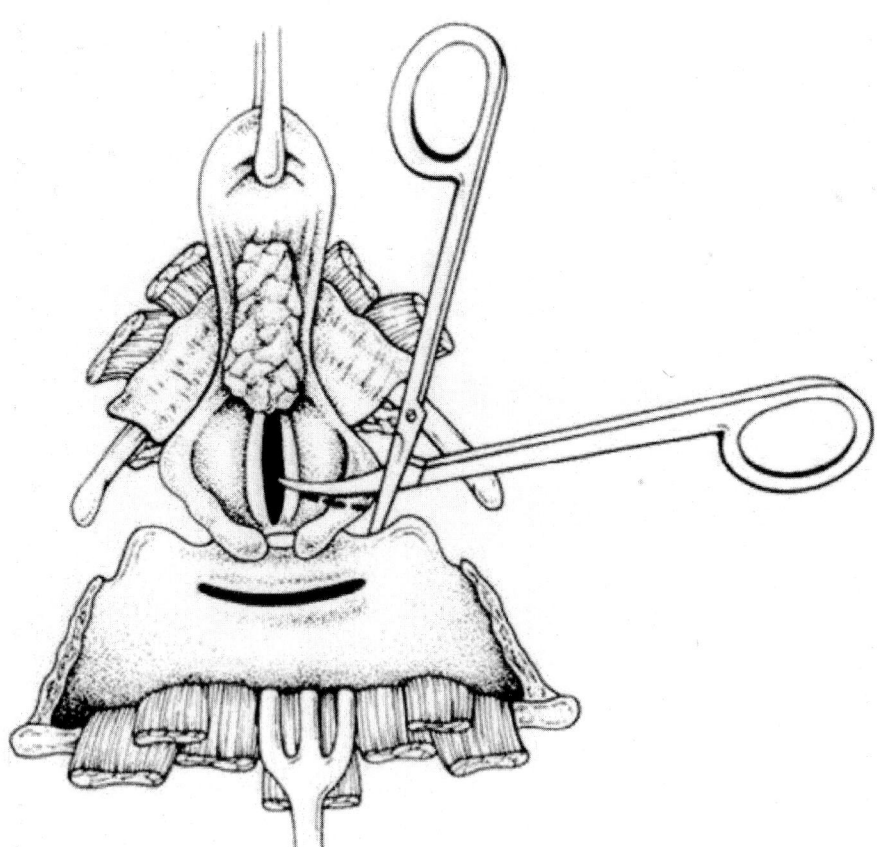

Figure 121C.12 The view during the supraglottic partial laryngectomy (SCPL) with cricohyoidoeopiglottopexy (CHEP) is now looking into the larynx from the top of the bed and one scissor blade is in the space between the inner thyroid cartilage and previously elevated inner thyroid perichondrium starting on the side with least tumor.

larynx and exposure of the cancer before resection is via a horizontal laryngotomy, either just below the hyoid bone as in the case of SGPL and SCPL with CHP, or just above the false cords as in the case of the SCPL with CHEP. Conceptually, the three operations can be thought of as variations in which the resection cuts are shifted either superiorly to encompass the epiglottis or inferiorly to encompass the remainder of the thyroid cartilage and glottic level. In both SCPL with SGPL or CHP and SGPL alone, it is important and feasible to save both superior laryngeal nerves to allow for functional rehabilitation (5). Finally, another similarity is in the closure used. Each is closed with three (number one) Vicryl sutures passed first submucosally around the cricoid cartilage (SCPL), then either around the hyoid and tongue base (SCPL with CHP or SGPL) or through the petiole of the epiglottis and then around the hyoid and tongue base (SCPL with CHEP) (Figs. 121C.11, 121C.15, and 121C.16). The height of the thyroid cartilage that remains after SGPL is about the same as the cricoid cartilage, making the three stitch closure for the SGPL and the SCPL similar from a technical standpoint. In both SCPL and SGPL, this effectively resuspends the cricoid cartilage and cricoarytenoid unit so that it is in the proper position. Following placement of these three large sutures, mucosa-to-mucosa approximation exists between the epiglottis and cricoid cartilage (SCPL with CHEP), the tongue base

and cricoid cartilage (SCPL with CHP), or the tongue base and true cords (SGPL). In all cases, this closure allows for position of the central aspect of the tongue base over the airway to help prevent aspiration and direct the food bolus laterally in the intact pyriform sinuses.

Although our discussion is limited to N0 disease to focus on "early" glottic and supraglottic carcinoma, neck disease deserves some mention. The glottis and supraglottis are very distinct in terms of the risk of lymph node metastasis. There is a paucity of lymphatics at the level of the glottis, which makes the chance of a T1 carcinoma having lymph node metastasis almost nonexistent, and the chances of a T2 glottic carcinoma having lymph node metastasis rare (6,7). When metastases do occur at the glottic level, they occur ipsilaterally. No indication exists to treat the neck for T1N0 glottic carcinoma, and the role of ipsilateral neck dissection is controversial for T2N0 glottic carcinoma. Alternatively, the rich lymphatics at the level of the supraglottis make bilaterally metastasis more common, and it is not uncommon, even in the N0 carcinoma of the neck, to discover occult metastatic nodes at the time of bilateral neck dissection. The standard is to offer bilateral selective neck dissection for T1N0 and T2N0 supraglottic carcinoma (8). This discussion also has significant bearing on treatment planning. Because glottic carcinoma has such a low propensity for lymph node metastasis, the

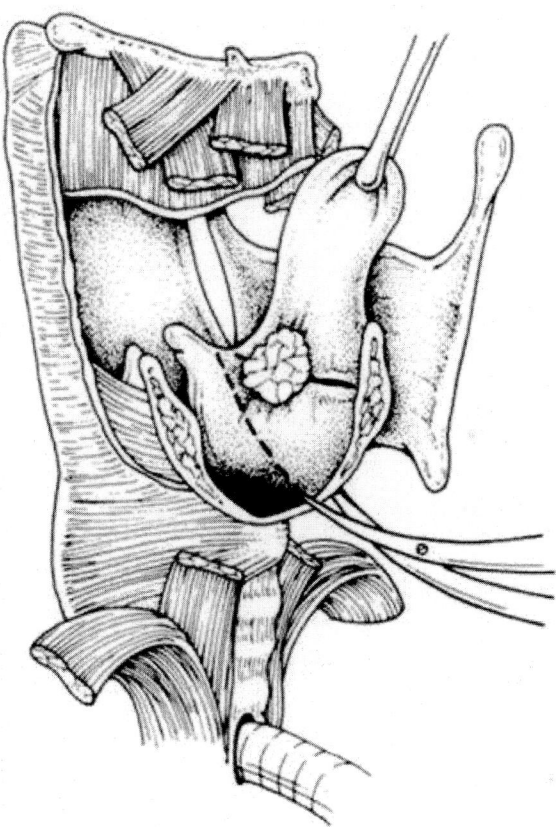

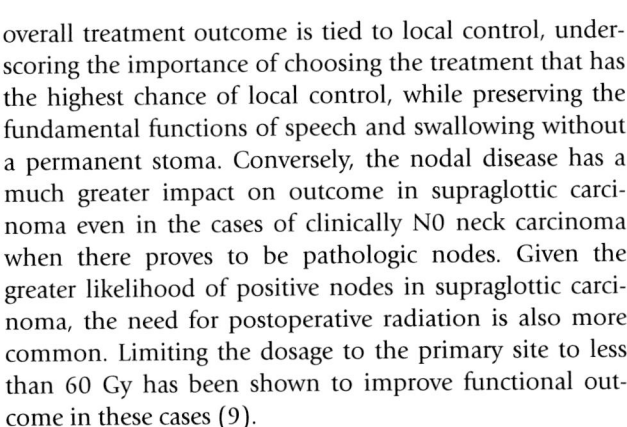

Figure 121C.13 The larynx is opened during the supraglottic partial laryngectomy (SCPL) with cricohyoidoeopiglottopexy (CHEP) on the anterior spine of the thyroid cartilage, like opening a book, and the resection is completed.

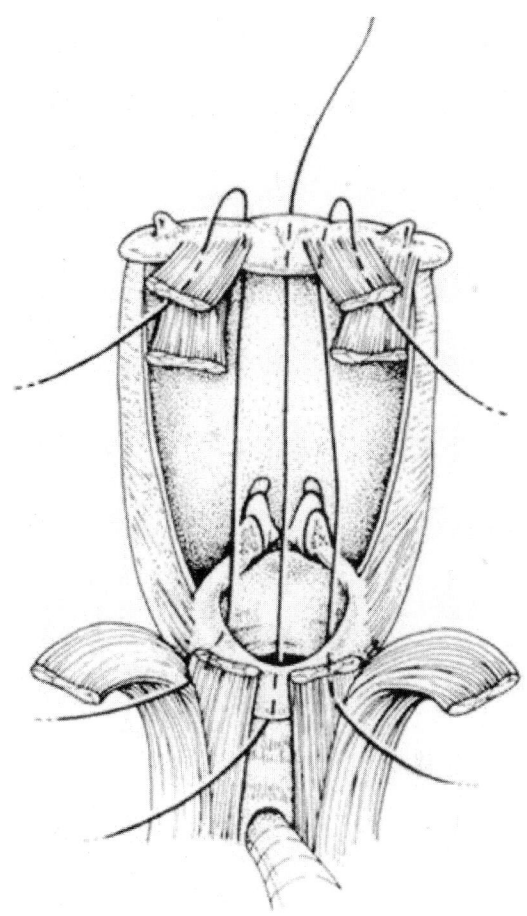

Figure 121C.14 The closure is begun during the supraglottic partial laryngectomy (SCPL) with cricohyoidoeopiglottopexy (CHEP) with three stitches placed, one in the midline and the remaining two placed 1 cm from the midline on either side.

overall treatment outcome is tied to local control, underscoring the importance of choosing the treatment that has the highest chance of local control, while preserving the fundamental functions of speech and swallowing without a permanent stoma. Conversely, the nodal disease has a much greater impact on outcome in supraglottic carcinoma even in the cases of clinically N0 neck carcinoma when there proves to be pathologic nodes. Given the greater likelihood of positive nodes in supraglottic carcinoma, the need for postoperative radiation is also more common. Limiting the dosage to the primary site to less than 60 Gy has been shown to improve functional outcome in these cases (9).

Previously. the indications for SCPL were limited to those lesions that had less than 1 cm of subglottic extension at the midcord level (10,11). Recent data indicate that cancers with less than 1.5 cm of extension into the subglottis at the midcord level do not have diffuse invasion of the cricoid cartilage, allowing for oncologically sound resection of these cancer, with the adjacent portion of the thyroid cartilage (12). This effectively broadens the indications for the SCPL by including cancers with 1.5 cm

of subglottic extension. Fixation of the arytenoid cartilage, however, remains a contraindication because of the significant risk of involvement of the cricoid cartilage at the level of the joint (13).

EARLY GLOTTIC CARCINOMA

If we define early glottic carcinoma as limited to T1N0 and T2N0 carcinoma, then the role for SCPL with CHEP for early glottic carcinoma is in the management of T2 glottic carcinomas. No role exists for SCPL with CHEP for T1a glottic carcinoma. Although a role is seen for SCPL with CHEP in radiation failures that fit the criteria for T1b glottic carcinoma, untreated T1b carcinomas can be successfully treated nonsurgically, with radiation or with surgery with less radical organ preservation surgical (OPS) approaches (e.g., endoscopic laser resection), with less morbidity, and, therefore, OPS approaches are favored in these early lesions. Nonetheless, given the inherent limitations of the staging system, at times a surgeon may be dealing

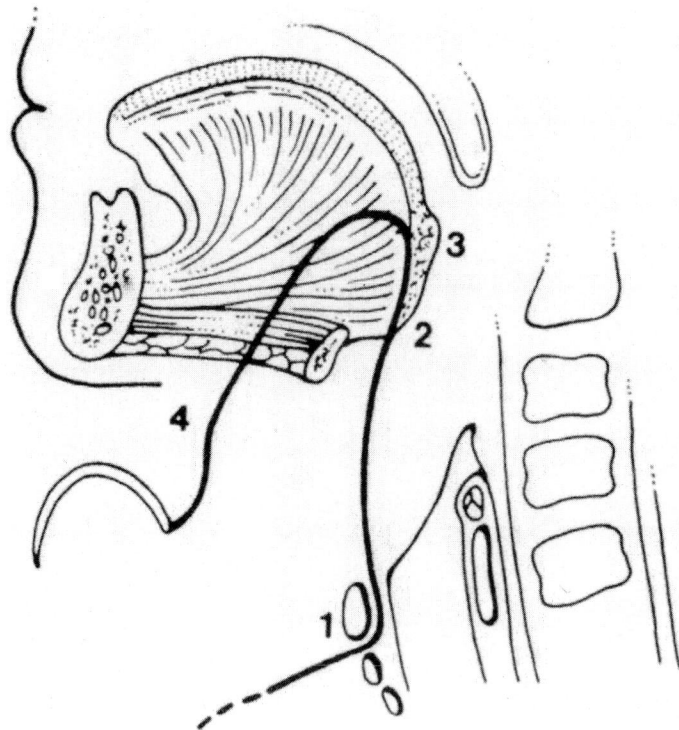

Figure 121C.15 The suture placement during supraglottic partial laryngectomy (SCPL) with cricohyoidoeopiglottopexy (CHEP) is placed (*1*) submucosally around the cricoid cartilage, then (*2*) submucosally into the tongue base, then (*3*) deep into the tongue base, and then (*4*) out through the suprahyoid musculature.

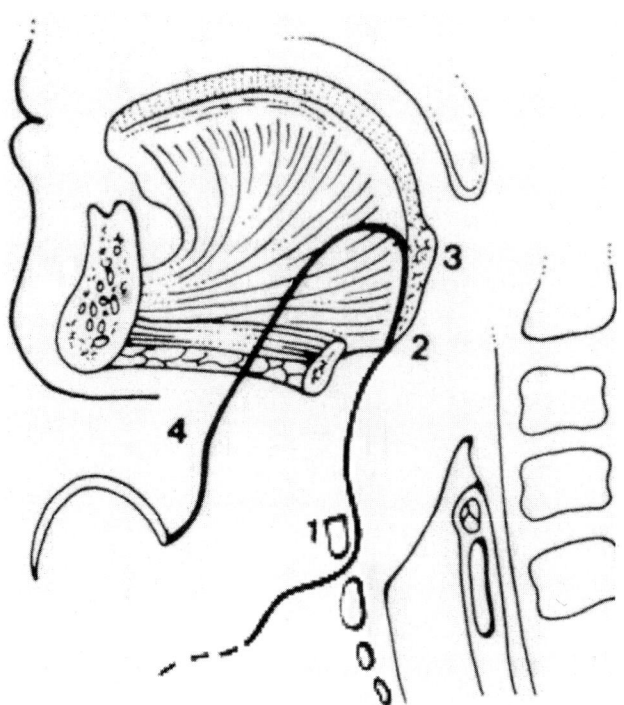

Figure 121C.16 The suture placement during supraglottic partial laryngectomy (SGPL) is placed (*1*) submucosally around the remaining inferior portion of the thyroid cartilage, then (*2*) submucosally into the tongue base, then (*3*) deep into the tongue base, and then (*4*) out through the suprahyoid musculature.

with a lesion that is borderline between T1b and T2, and, in these cases, it may be reasonable to consider a SCPL with CHEP. Nonetheless, the following discussion is limited to T2 glottic carcinomas.

A number of options exist for the management of T2 glottic carcinoma. Overall, radiation therapy alone yields a local control of approximately 70%, with retrospective studies indicating that the local control following radiation is worse in the T2 category (13a). Although endoscopic transoral laser resection in expert hands yields local control in the 90% range for T1a glottic carcinomas, the local control for T2b carcinomas is in the 60% to 70% range. This is a lower local control rate compared with SCPL with CHEP (14–16). In addition, to achieve these types of local control with endoscopic transoral laser resection for T2 glottic carcinoma, the surgeon must be willing to resect widely, down to the thyroid and cricoid cartilages (14). The SCPL with CHEP yields consistent local control rates of greater than 90% in a large number of studies (10,17,18). Although the advantage the SCPL with CHEP has over radiation therapy alone is superior local control (and possible advantages in terms of survival), the long-term voice quality following SCPL with CHEP is permanent hoarseness. Nonetheless, survival is compromised among the approximately 30% of patients who have local failure following radiation therapy for T2 glottic carcinoma (19). It is also inappropriate to irradiate a T2 glottic carcinoma and suggest to patients that if local failure occurs they will be salvaged with a laryngeal-sparing surgery because total laryngectomy is required for most patients who fail radiation therapy (19). Radiation therapy, transoral laser resection, or SCPL with CHEP is a reasonable option for T2a glottic carcinoma. When counseling the patient, however, it should be stressed that SCPL with CHEP offers a better chance for long-term laryngeal preservation than radiation and, possibly, improved survival, but that the voice quality will be worse with the surgical approach. For T2b glottic carcinomas, the lower local control rates for radiation therapy and transoral laser resection make SCPL with CHEP the better option.

The oncologic contraindications for SCPL with CHEP are (a) cancers arising in the anterior commissure or ventricle, which have a propensity for early invasion of the preepiglottic space (these may be resected with SCPL-CHP); (b) cancers of the glottis with fixation of the ipsilateral arytenoid cartilage; (c) cancers of the glottis with 1.5 cm of subglottic extension reaching the upper border of the cricoid cartilage or invading the cricoid cartilage; (d) glottic cancers involving the posterior commissure; and (e) glottic cancers involving the outer perichondrium of the thyroid cartilage or having extralaryngeal spread (10).

EARLY SUPRAGLOTTIC CARCINOMA

If we limit our discussion to T1N0 and T2N0 supraglottic carcinomas, then OPS, including endoscopic laser supraglottic partial laryngectomy, open supraglottic laryngectomy, and supracricoid partial laryngectomy can be expected to have local control in the 90% range, whereas with radiation therapy alone the local control is approximately 20% less (3,8,11,20–24). In addition, as with glottic carcinoma, Parsons et al. (25) noted a 5-year survival of 30% in patients who failed locally after radiation therapy for all T stages of supraglottic carcinoma.

Currently, SGPL as a surgical option is limited because of the advent of transoral laser SGPL. This is because comparable local control rates are seen for open versus transoral laser SGPL. In addition, a decrease was seen in acute morbidity following transoral laser SGPL by avoiding a tracheostomy in almost all cases in which the transoral approach was used, as well as faster swallowing rehabilitation following the transoral approach. The only indication for currently using open SGPL for T1 or T2 supraglottic carcinoma are cases in which the head and neck anatomy precludes endoscopic exposure of the larynx adequate for transoral laser SGPL. The oncologic contraindications include (a) cricoid or thyroid cartilage invasion; (b) cancer invasion of the mucosa of the arytenoid cartilage; (c) cancer invasion of the posterior or anterior commissure; (d) impaired mobility or fixation of the vocal cord; (e) malignant invasion of the base of the tongue closer than 1 cm to the circumvallate papillae; (f) impaired motion of the tongue base, indicating deep cancer invasion; and (g) invasion of the floor of the mouth in carcinomas with vallecular involvement.

Although a variety of technical maneuvers have been forwarded to quantify "exposure" during laryngoscopy, the practical approach is to perform a separate endoscopy at which time a percutaneous gastrostomy, if indicated, can also performed. At that time, the surgeon can also assess whether the larynx can be adequately exposed for the transoral laser SGPL, which is scheduled for a subsequent surgical date. If the patient's larynx cannot be exposed adequately for transoral laser SGPL, then an open SGPL can be performed at the later date. Closed laryngoscopes do not allow for adequate exposure of the supraglottis for laser resection, with the exception of the occasional use of the Lindholm scope (Storz, Tuttlingen, Germany). Rudert (26) modified the bivalving laryngoscope originally described by Weerda et al. (27) into a Storz supraglottiscope in which the lateral plates of its spatulas can be positioned to keep the border of the tongue obscuring the operative field.

The SCPL with CHP is used for selected T2 supraglottic carcinomas that have extension from the supraglottis to the glottic level (1).

The oncologic contraindications for SCPL with CHP include (a) arytenoid cartilage fixation; (b) infraglottic extension of tumor more than 15 mm anteriorly (cricothyroid membrane), more than 5 mm posterolaterally, or reaching the superior border of the cricoid cartilage; (c) extensive preepiglottic space invasion with clinical evidence of bulging beneath the vallecula mucosa or extension through the thyrohyoid membranes; (d) tumor abutting the hyoid bone that would require resection of this bone; (e) cricoid cartilage invasion; (f) involvement of the pharynx or interarytenoid fixation; and (g) external thyroid cartilage perichondrial invasion and extralaryngeal spread of tumor. Expected local control rates for SCPL with CHP are in the 90% range (28).

Given the higher reported local control rates with primary surgery for T1N0 and T2N0 supraglottic carcinoma than for nonsurgical organ preservation regimens such as radiation therapy, OPS should be the primary treatment modality when no contraindication exists.

ORGAN PRESERVATION SURGERY FOR RADIATION FAILURES

Special considerations are necessary when using SGPL or SCPL with either CHEP or CHP in patients who have a recurrence following radiation therapy. First, the surgeon must try to discern what the original size and extent of the cancer was before radiation. Unless the surgeon actually saw the lesion before radiation, this will always only be a "best guess." The assessment and description of laryngeal cancers are so subjective that relying on the prior description is fraught with difficulty. Prior radiographs of early lesions are only useful to confirm that indeed the initial lesion was small, but they are inadequate reflection of what the true extent of the mucosal disease before radiation. A "rule of thumb" is that if the original lesion was described as too large for the operation now being contemplated, in almost all cases, the procedure should not done. The problem with this approach is when the prior physician has described the lesion as extensive and now a minute lesion is present. In these cases, use judgment and discuss the issues with the patient and, in rare instances, go ahead with the organ-sparing surgery if instincts lead to the conclusion that such is appropriate. If the cancer was originally described as small and it is still small enough for organ preservation surgery, proceed with the organ-sparing approach. Nonetheless, the literature and experience teach that cancers are almost never smaller following radiation failure and this should be factored into the decision-making process (19). The second consideration is the appearance of the laryngeal and pharyngeal mucosa. If massive edema and swelling exist and restrict arytenoid cartilage or cord mobility, then the surgeon should do a total laryngectomy. Again, this is not a "black and white" situation, and borderline cases require that judgment must be used. The less experience the surgeon has, the less risk should be taken in this regard. Although prior chemoradiation is not in and of itself a contraindication, the reality is that following chemoradiation most patients will have so much edema and laryngeal dysfunction that it is simply uncommon that the patient will be eligible for the organ-preserving surgery. In addition, most patients who have chemoradiation had larger cancers before radiation so they hardly ever have recurrences that are amenable to organ preservation surgery.

During the operation, the surgeon must be liberal with frozen sections because a positive margin on permanent section will require return to the operating room for total laryngectomy. In these types of cases, in particular, the surgeon should take the specimen to the pathology bench, ink the specimen, and get frozen sections from the suspicious locations of the main specimen. Once the specimen is removed, small frozen sections from the patient will not allow sampling from the highest risk areas. In all cases, explain to the patient during the consent process that intraoperative conversion to total laryngectomy may be needed.

Postoperatively, the expectation should be a delay in functional rehabilitation, with resumption of swallowing occurring in the 6-week range rather than the 3-week range, as in SCPL. In addition, tracheal decannulation will be delayed to approximately 4 to 6 weeks, because of the expected increased laryngeal edema. Local failure in the radiation setting for SCPL has been higher than that reported for patients without prior treatment, but is comparable to total laryngectomy (25,29–31). In conclusion, although few patients are candidates for organ preservation surgery in the postradiation setting, it is reasonable to proceed to such when surgery can spare the larynx.

Some points concerning SGPL in the setting of postradiation failure deserve special attention. First, the literature and clinical experience show us that patients who were candidates for SGPL before radiation are almost never

candidates for SGPL following failure (32). This is because of the reasons outlined above concerning the increased size of the cancer at the time of the recurrence as well as issues related to laryngeal edema. Although almost all supraglottic radiation failures require total laryngectomy, SCPL with CHP offers wider oncologic margins than SGPL, but it also removes more mucosa and thyroid cartilage that has been damaged by the radiation.

FUTURE DIRECTIONS

New textbooks are published because of our constantly changing knowledge of how diseases are best treated. Kuhn (33) has noted that major changes in science do not occur by evolution, but by revolution. Ideas that are so radical and different than what was thought to be "truth" shatter the former theories and shift us to a new paradigm or worldview. The two most recent clinical developments that have shifted the paradigm for surgical organ preservation are SCPL and transoral laser resections. What will be the next revolution to change the management of early glottic and supraglottic carcinoma? Three areas of clinical research may give us a glimpse into the future. First is the use of exclusive chemotherapy. Chemotherapy alone has been shown to control early laryngeal carcinoma, avoiding the morbidity of either surgical organ preservation and radiation therapy (34,35). Second, interstitial photodynamic therapy, which presently is used for solid tumors outside the head and neck area and for palliation in the head and neck, may prove of value in avoiding the morbidity of traditional resections (36). Third, new work being pioneered in the area of transoral robotic surgery (TORS) may allow us to overcome the limitations of laser surgery. TORS involves transoral robotic resections that use a minimum of three robotic arms to complete the procedure (37) (Fig. 121C.17).

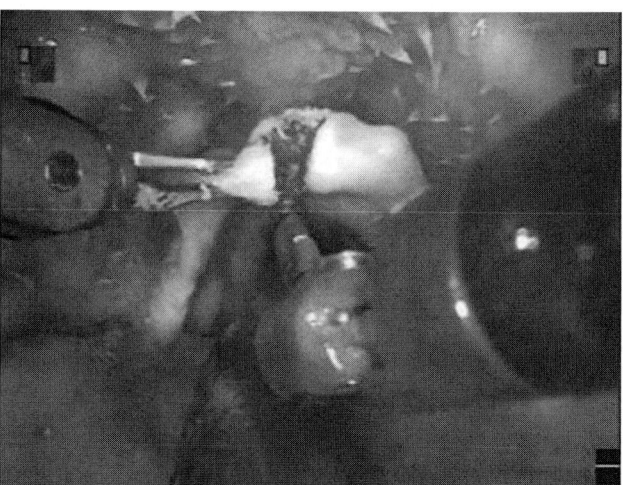

Figure 121C.17 Using electrocautery to transect the epiglottis in the midline during transoral robotic surgery (TORS) supraglottic laryngectomy in the canine model.

Laser surgery is inherently limited by the need for keeping the area being resected within the line of sight of the laser, the source of which is far from the tissues being resected (i.e., the laser is outside the patient). TORS offers the potential advantages over the transoral laser techniques including increased precision at the time of resection, increased freedom of movement because the technology allows the use of two hands for surgical resection, which overcomes the line of site limitations of the laser and filtration of tremor (37–39). Which, if any, of these will be the basis for the next paradigm shift in the management of early laryngeal carcinoma, of course, is unknown. We will await the next version of this chapter to answer those questions.

HIGHLIGHTS

- Two basic types of SCPL exist: the CHEP for selected glottic carcinomas and the CHP for selected supraglottic carcinomas.
- The basic functional unit of the larynx that allows for speech and swallowing without a tracheostomy is the cricoarytenoid unit.
- Glottic and supraglottic treatment spectra are more specific than T staging for choosing the appropriate organ preservation surgical procedure.
- For T2b glottic carcinomas, the lower local control rates for radiation therapy and transoral laser resection make SCPL with CHEP the better option.
- The only indication for currently using open SGPL for T1 or T2 supraglottic carcinoma is cases in which the head and neck anatomy precludes adequate endoscopic exposure of the larynx for transoral laser SGPL.
- Expected local control rates for SCPL with CHP for T2 supraglottic carcinoma with extension to the glottic level are in the 90% range.

REFERENCES

1. Laccourreye O, Weinstein G. Supracricoid partial laryngectomy with cricohyoidoepiglottopexy. In: Weinstein GS, Laccourreye O, Brasnu D, Laccourreye H, eds. *Organ preservation surgery for laryngeal cancer.* San Diego: Singular Publishing Group, 1999:73–94.
2. Brasnu D, Hartl DM, Laccourreye, H. Supracricoid partial laryngectomy with cricohyoidopexy. In: Weinstein GS, et al., eds. *Organ preservation surgery for laryngeal cancer.* San Diego: Singular Publishing Group, 1999:127–143.
3. DeSanto LW. Cancer of the supraglottic larynx: a review of 260 patients. *Otolaryngol Head Neck Surg* 1985;93(6):705–711.
4. Weinstein GS, Laccourreye O. Organ preservation surgery of the larynx: a new paradigm. In: Weinstein GS, et al., eds. *Organ preservation surgery for laryngeal cancer.* San Diego: Singular Publishing Group, 1999:5.
5. Rassekh CH, Driscoll BP, Seikaly H, et al. Preservation of the superior laryngeal nerve in supraglottic and supracricoid partial laryngectomy. *Laryngoscope* 1998;108(3):445–447.
6. Johnson JT, Myers EN, Hao SP, et al. Outcome of open surgical therapy for glottic carcinoma. *Ann Otol Rhinol Laryngol* 1993;102(10):752–755.
7. McGavran, MH, Bauer WC, Ogura JH. The incidence of cervical lymph node metastases from epidermoid carcinoma of the larynx and their relationship to certain characteristics of the primary tumor. *Cancer* 1961;4:55–66.
8. Lutz CK, Johnson JT, Wagner RL, et al. Supraglottic carcinoma: patterns of recurrence. *Ann Otol Rhinol Laryngol* 1990;99(1):12–17.
9. Laccourreye O, Hans S, Borzog-Grayeli A, et al. Complications of postoperative radiation therapy after partial laryngectomy in supraglottic carcinoma: a long-term evaluation. *Otolaryngol Head Neck Surg* 2000;122(5):752–757.
10. Laccourreye H, Laccourreye O, Weinstein G, et al. Supracricoid laryngectomy with cricohyoidoepiglottopexy: a partial laryngeal procedure for glottic carcinoma. *Ann Otol Rhinol Laryngol* 1990;99:421–426.
11. Laccourreye H, Laccourreye O, Weinstein G, et al. Supracricoid laryngectomy with cricohyoidopexy: a partial laryngeal procedure for selected supraglottic and transglottic carcinomas. *Laryngoscope* 1990;100:735–741.
12. Sparano A, Chernock R, Feldman M, et al. Extending the inferior limits of supracricoid partial laryngectomy: a clinicopathological correlation. *Laryngoscope* 2005;115(2):297–300.
13. Brasnu D, Laccourreye H, Dulmet E, et al. Mobility of the vocal cord and arytenoid in squamous cell carcinoma of the larynx and hypopharynx: an anatomical and clinical comparative study. *Ear Nose Throat J* 1990;69(5):324–330.
13a. Motta G, Esposito E, Motta S, et al. CO(2) laser surgery in the treatment of glottic cancer. *Head Neck* 2005;27(7):566–573; discussion 573–574.
14. Eckel HE. Local recurrences following transoral laser surgery for early glottic carcinoma: frequency, management, and outcome. *Ann Otol Rhinol Laryngol* 2001;110(1):7–15.
15. Peretti G, Piazza C, Bolzini A, et al. Endoscopic CO_2 laser excision for tis, T1, and T2 glottic carcinomas: cure rate and prognostic factors. *Otolaryngol Head Neck Surg* 2000;123(1):853–858.
16. Steiner W. Results of curative laser microsurgery of laryngeal carcinomas. *Am J Otolaryngol* 1993;14(2):116–121.
17. Chevalier D, Laccourreye O, Brasnu D, et al. Cricohyoidoepiglottopexy for glottic carcinoma with fixation or impaired motion of the true vocal cord: 5-year oncologic results in 112 patients. *Ann Otol Rhinol Laryngol* 1997;106:365–369.
18. Piquet JJ, Chevalier D. Subtotal laryngectomy with cricohyoido-epiglotto-pexy for the treatment of extended glottic carcinomas. *Am J Surg* 1991;162(October):357–361.
19. Viani L, Stell PM, Dalby JE. Recurrence after radiotherapy for glottic carcinoma. *Cancer* 1991;67(3):577–584.
20. Spriano G, Antognoni P, Piantanida R, et al. Conservative management of T1-T2N0 supraglottic cancer: a retrospective study. *Am J Otolaryngol* 1997;18(5):299–305.
21. Coates HL, DeSanto LW, Devine KD, et al. Carcinoma of the supraglottic larynx. A review of 221 cases. *Arch Otolaryngol* 1976;102(11):686–689.
22. Lee NK, Goepfert H, Wendt CD. Supraglottic laryngectomy for intermediate-stage cancer: U.T. M.D. Anderson Cancer Center experience with combined therapy. *Laryngoscope* 1990;100(8):831–836.
23. Chevalier D, Piquet JJ. Subtotal laryngectomy with cricohyoidopexy for supraglottic carcinoma: review of 61 cases. *Am J Surg* 1994;168:472–473.
24. de Vincentiis M, Minni A, Gallo A, et al. Supracricoid partial laryngectomies: oncologic and functional results. *Head Neck* 1998;20(6):504–509.
25. Parsons JT, Mendenhall WM, Stringer SP, et al. Salvage surgery following radiation failure in squamous cell carcinoma of the supraglottic larynx. *Int J Radiat Oncol Biol Phys* 1995;32(3):605–609.
26. Rudert H. Equipment for CO_2 laser surgery. *HNO* 1989;37(2):76–77.
27. Weerda H, Pedersen P, Meuret G. A new distending laryngoscope for diagnosis and microsurgery of the larynx. *Laryngoscope* 1983;93(5):639–641.
28. Bron L, Brossard E, Monnier P, et al. Supracricoid partial laryngectomy with cricohyoidoepiglottopexy and cricohyoidopexy for glottic and supraglottic carcinomas. *Laryngoscope* 2000;110(4):627–634.
29. Spriano G, Pellini R, Romano G, et al. Supracricoid partial laryngectomy as salvage surgery after radiation failure. *Head Neck* 2002;24(8):759–765.
30. Makeieff M, Venegoni D, Mercante G, et al. Supracricoid partial laryngectomies after failure of radiation therapy. *Laryngoscope* 2005;115(2):353–357.

31. Laccourreye O, Weinstein G, Naudo P, et al. Supracricoid partial laryngectomy after failed laryngeal radiation therapy. *Laryngoscope* 1996;106(4):495–498.

32. Rodriguez-Cuevas S, Labastida S, Gonzalez D, et al. Partial laryngectomy as salvage surgery for radiation failures in T1-T2 laryngeal cancer. *Head Neck* 1998; 20(7):630–633.

33. Kuhn TS. *The structure of scientific revolutions*, 2d ed. Chicago: University of Chicago Press, 1970:xii, 210.

34. Laccourreye O, Veivers D, Bassot V, et al. Analysis of local recurrence in patients with selected T1-3N0M0 squamous cell carcinoma of the true vocal cord managed with a platinum-based chemotherapy-alone regimen for cure. *Ann Otol Rhinol Laryngol* 2002;111(4):315–321.

35. Laccourreye O, Veivers D, Hans S, et al. Chemotherapy alone with curative intent in patients with invasive squamous cell carcinoma of the pharyngolarynx classified as T1-T4N0M0 complete clinical responders. *Cancer* 2001;92(6):1504–1511.

36. Lou PJ, Jager HR, Jones L, et al. Interstitial photodynamic therapy as salvage treatment for recurrent head and neck cancer. *Br J Cancer* 2004;91(3):441–446.

37. Weinstein GS, O'Malley BW Jr, Hockstein NG, et al. Transoral robotic surgery (TORS): supraglottic laryngectomy in the canine model. *Laryngoscope* 2005;115(7):1315–1319.

38. Hockstein NG, Nolan JP, O'Malley BW Jr, et al. Robot-assisted pharyngeal and laryngeal microsurgery: results of robotic cadaver dissections. *Laryngoscope* 2005;115(6):1003–1008.

39. Hockstein NG, Nolan JP, O'Malley BW Jr, et al. Robotic microlaryngeal surgery: a technical feasibility study using the daVinci surgical robot and an airway mannequin. *Laryngoscope* 2005;115(5): 780–785.

Advanced Cancer of the Larynx

122

Richard V. Smith   *Marvin P. Fried*

The treatment of advanced laryngeal cancer requires recognition of the fundamental role the larynx plays in helping to define that which makes us human. If the clinician were to assume that the larynx is simply the sum of all its parts, the treatment of advanced laryngeal cancer would be quite simple. One would remove the larynx and create a tracheopharyngeal junction that would not allow aspiration and would recreate speech with some prosthetic technique. However, such an oncologically sound approach is often an unacceptable alternative for most patients and can be quite socially isolating.

Historically, before the turn of the eighteenth century, surgery was the only modality available for the treatment of these neoplasms. First developed in the late 1700s for the removal of papillomas, the laryngofissure offered surgeons the first open approach to debulk laryngeal tumors. Other approaches followed with the introduction of the suprahyoid and thyrohyoid laryngotomies. Until Billroth performed the first total laryngectomy on a school teacher in 1873, no method existed by which the surgeon could remove a tumor as a compartmental dissection. Interestingly, it took until well into the twentieth century for this procedure to be accepted as safe and therapeutic. Before such surgeons as Gluck, Sorenson, Solis-Cohen, Krause, and Martin, total laryngectomy was thought to be an interesting exercise with a very high perioperative mortality rate and low probability of curing the cancer. With better protection of the airway, antibiotics, fluid replacement, and other advances in surgical science, the operation became quite safe. Martin was responsible for much of the work that ultimately led to the acceptance of total laryngectomy as a safe and effective tool for the treatment of advanced laryngeal cancer. For the next 20 to 30 years, this procedure became the gold standard against which all other surgical

procedures and other modalities were measured. Removal of the larynx has been looked on with some degree of skepticism by patients and some physicians, and some have questioned whether the treatment is worse than the disease. McNeil et al. (1), in the much quoted fireman's study, made the issue of laryngeal preservation even more clear by finding that some patients would accept a 20% decline in survival rather than lose their voice box.

The larynx, as much as any structure in the body, is a critical component of what defines us as a human. Much of our socialization, expression of feelings, and interaction with our environment comes from this portion of the airway. The larynx may have as its fundamental purpose the separation of the airway from the alimentary tract, but it also allows the movement of air over the special sense organs that permit us to taste and smell. Not only are these senses critical for us to enjoy and immerse ourselves in our world, but they also help to protect us from danger in our environment, such as the bitter taste of poisonous foods and scent of smoke warning of a fire. The voice also is critical for daily function, communicating our feelings, and who we are. It therefore comes as no surprise that the loss of the larynx is thought to be one of the greatest fears of any patient with head and neck cancer. It is for these reasons that most of the research on the treatment of these tumors during the latter half of this century has centered on laryngeal preservation. Current reconstructive techniques, in association with appropriate preoperative counseling, allow reintegration into society in a meaningful way after total laryngectomy, and some of the initial stigmata of laryngectomees have been eliminated. Advances in partial laryngeal surgery also have allowed subtotal removal of the larynx with disease cure and preservation of function as well. The ultimate goal of every clinician treating advanced laryngeal tumors should be to preserve the speech and swallowing functions of all patients with larynx cancer while offering the highest chance for cure.

EPIDEMIOLOGY

Cancer of the larynx remains the second most common head and neck malignancy, constituting 25% of all tumors. In 2002, 8,900 new cases of larynx cancer were predicted, with a 3.5:1 male-to-female ratio and a total of 3,700 cancer deaths associated with these malignancies. A steady decrease in the total number of new cases has been noted and a gradual leveling of the gender ratio from 6:1 in 1973 to the current figure, as gender patterns in tobacco and alcohol consumption equalize. Interestingly, however, no overall change in survival has occurred since the 1970s, leveling at approximately a 65% 5-year survival for all stages. Eighty-five percent of laryngeal cancers can be attributed to smoking and alcohol, with alcohol playing a greater role in supraglottic cancers when compared with glottic or subglottic cancers. A strong dose–response relation exists between these substances, which are synergistic when they are used together, and the ultimate development of cancer. This disease is primarily one of advancing age, with the highest incidence occurring in the sixth and seventh decades of life. One might have expected the numbers of late-stage laryngeal cancers to have declined over the years, given the greater awareness of high-risk patients. However, a review of more than 350 laryngeal cancers treated in Mexico City revealed that more than two thirds of patients were initially seen with T3 or T4 disease.

ANATOMY

The understanding and treatment of laryngeal cancer is predicated on a detailed knowledge of the complex anatomy of this region. The larynx is divided into supraglottic, glottic, and subglottic regions (Fig. 122.1). The supraglottic region extends from the tip of the epiglottis to the apices of both ventricles and includes both false vocal cords, the lingual and laryngeal surfaces of the epiglottis, the laryngeal surfaces of the arytenoids, and both aryepiglottic folds but not the mucosa overlying the hyoepiglottic ligament in the vallecula. Inferiorly, the saccule and the lateral and superior surfaces of the ventricle are included in the supraglottic larynx. The glottic region contains both true vocal cords, the floor of the ventricle, the anterior commissure, and the interarytenoid area. The subglottic region extends from 10 mm inferior to the apex of the laryngeal ventricle to the lower border of the cricoid cartilage, and is remarkable for the ease of extralaryngeal extension in this laryngeal compartment.

Advanced laryngeal cancers may blur the distinctions between these regions, but even advanced tumors may remain confined to one anatomic site, more commonly seen in the supraglottic region. Dye studies have shown this compartmentalization in lymphatics, vasculature, and anatomic barriers, and histologic studies have confirmed the existence of connective tissue barriers to cancer spread. Barriers include the thyroid and cricoid cartilages with their overlying perichondrium, the conus elasticus, the quadrangular membrane, the ventricle, the thyrohyoid membrane, and the hyoepiglottic ligament, and a ventricular membrane has been described (2). The thyroepiglottic ligament and

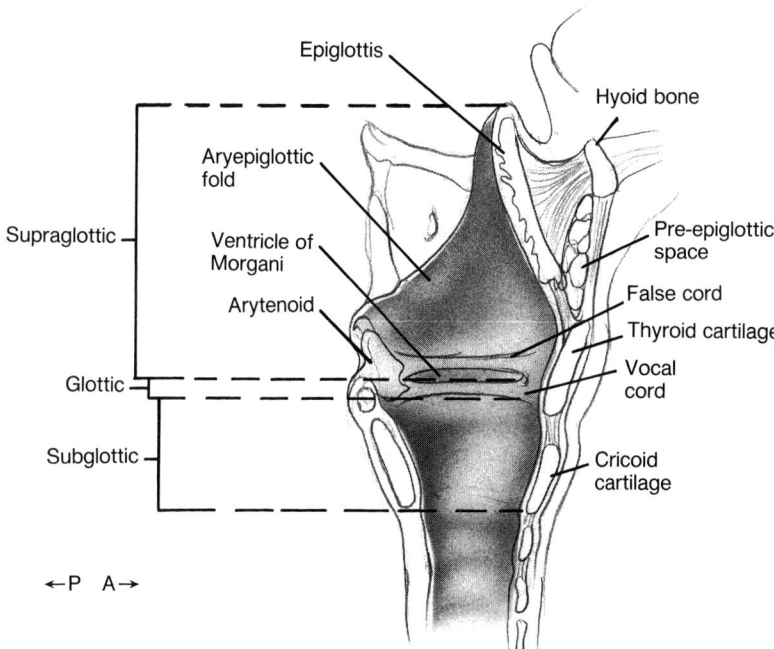

Figure 122.1 Midline sagittal section of the larynx demonstrating the supraglottic and glottic regions, as well as the preepiglottic space.

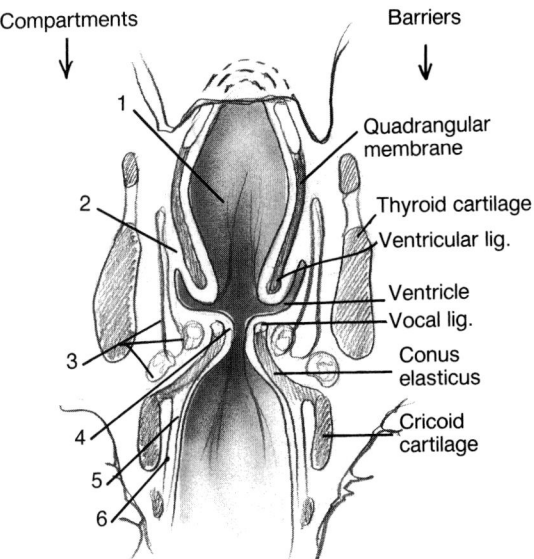

Figure 122.2 Coronal view of the larynx at the mid-cord level demonstrating barriers to tumor spread as well as spaces through which tumor may spread more easily. Compartments: *1*, supraglottic area; *2*, portion of paraglottic space continuous with preepiglottic space; *3*, paraglottic space; *4*, Reinke space; *5*, subglottic space; *6*, cricoid area.

the anterior commissure tendon offer little resistance to tumor spread (Fig. 122.2), and anterior commissure lesions are notorious for thyroid cartilage involvement and upstaged tumors due to their deep extension. The larynx drains into levels 2, 3, and 4 within the neck, and laryngeal lesions are known for their propensity to spread bilaterally or contralaterally. In addition, the pretracheal and paratracheal lymph nodes are important in the management of glottic and subglottic tumors, as they may be the primary-echelon lymph nodes for these primary sites.

PATTERNS OF SPREAD

Anatomic studies confirm the existence of laryngeal spaces or compartments within which cancer can spread more freely and through which cancer may spread out of the larynx. Tumors initially tend to spread by the path of least resistance into these preexisting compartments, such as the preepiglottic space or the paraglottic space. The preepiglottic space is bound by the hyoepiglottic ligament superiorly, the thyroid cartilage and the thyrohyoid membrane anteriorly, and the epiglottis and thyroepiglottic ligament posteriorly. Cancer involving the preepiglottic space may have access to the soft tissues of the neck by means of the dehiscences in the thyrohyoid membrane created by the superior laryngeal vessels and nerves, or they may involve the glottis or subglottis through involvement of the paraglottic space.

The paraglottic space is lateral to the ventricles, between the laryngeal introitus and the medial wall of the pyriform sinus, and is the posterolateral extension of the preepiglottic space. Thus the preepiglottic and paraglottic spaces

form a horseshoe-shaped fatty space surrounding the internal laryngeal structures. Infiltration of the paraglottic space will allow tumors to involve the supraglottic, glottic, and subglottic regions. Tumors that involve this space and are superior and inferior to the ventricle are referred to as *transglottic tumors*. Invasion of this space also is associated with a high rate of subglottic or extralaryngeal spread of tumor. In a study by Kirchner (3), 31 of 52 transglottic cancers invaded the laryngeal framework. The proximity of the thyroid cartilage and cricothyroid membrane to this space explains this finding (Figs. 122.3 through 122.5). In addition, tumors of this space will often follow the lateral aspect of the conus elasticus to the superior border of the cricoid, subsequently breaking through the cricothyroid membrane to access the extralaryngeal soft tissues and thyroid gland.

Other areas have a propensity to spread locally as well. Tumors at the anterior commissure tend to spread to the anterior subglottis and invade the thyroid cartilage because of the lack of thyroid perichondrium in the region of the anterior commissure tendon. This anatomic defect allows easy access to the cartilage, as the perichondrium is the primary barrier to its involvement. Subglottic tumors will frequently invade the laryngeal cartilages (e.g., four of eight in Kirchner's study), often are first seen late in the

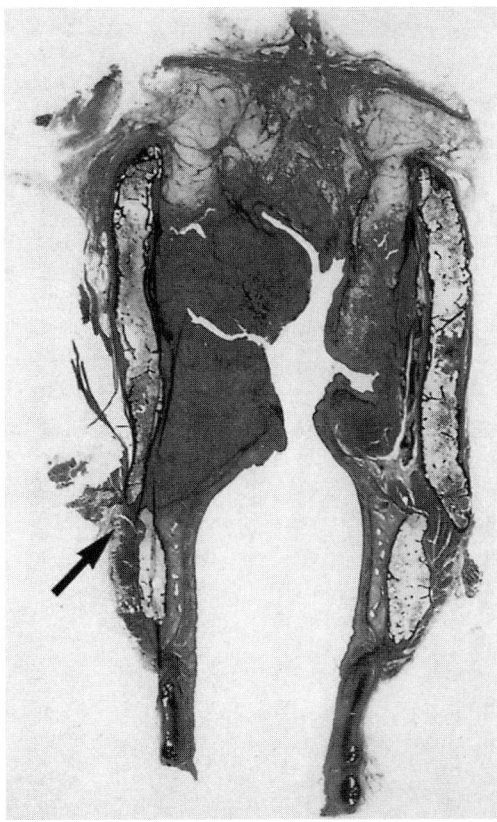

Figure 122.3 Transglottic cancer growing toward the cricothyroid space (*arrow*). This pattern was observed in 16 of 19 transglottic growths in Kirchner's study. (Reprinted from Kirchner JA. One hundred laryngeal cancers studied by serial section. *Ann Otol* 1969;78:689–709, with permission.)

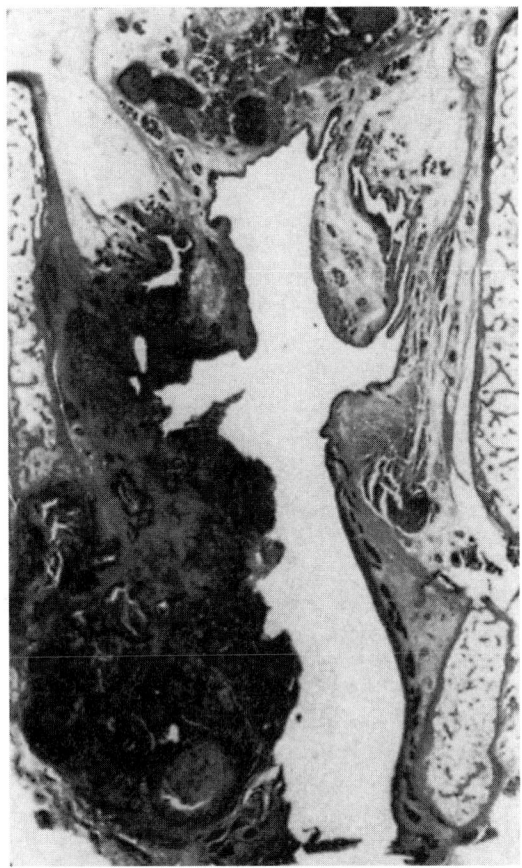

Figure 122.4 Transglottic cancer destroying the cricoid ring and the lower edge of the thyroid ala. (Reprinted from Kirchner JA. One hundred laryngeal cancers studied by serial section. *Ann Otol* 1969;78:689–709, with permission.)

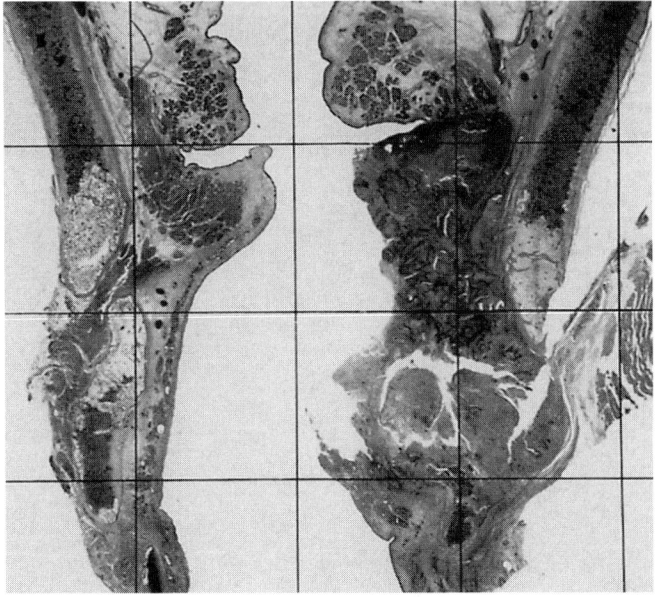

Figure 122.5 Glottic cancer invading and destroying cricoid ring.

course of the disease, and are associated with a poor prognosis. Primary subglottic tumors are relatively rare, with most subglottic disease representing extensions of glottic or supraglottic primaries.

The patterns of lymphatic spread have been described well by many authors, for both clinically negative and clinically positive necks. Nodal metastases are more common in supraglottic cancers than in glottic cancers, although a high rate of nodal metastases exists for subglottic primaries as well. Larger tumor surface area and advanced stage also are associated with increased regional metastases. Tumors of the supraglottic larynx spread primarily to levels 2 and 3 before involving level 4. Glottic tumors metastasize to the delphian, or pretracheal, lymph node as well as to levels 2, 3, and 4. Subglottic tumors commonly spread to the pretracheal, paratracheal, and level 3 and 4 lymph nodes. It is unusual for laryngeal cancers of any site to metastasize to the submandibular and submental regions in the absence of significant tongue invasion, and level 5 is infrequently involved as well. This has led to the recent trend to address levels 2, 3, and 4 primarily, with surgical management of the pre- and paratracheal lymph nodes for advanced glottic and subglottic carcinoma (4). The anterior lateral neck dissection therefore remains the standard for these lesions. With advanced neck disease of N2 or N3, however, a more traditional complete lymphadenectomy, such as a modified radical or radical neck dissection, is more appropriate.

STAGING

Advanced carcinomas of the larynx are defined not only by the extent of invasion of the primary tumor but also by the nodal status and the presence or absence of distant metastases. These factors are the basis for our current American Joint Committee on Cancer (AJCC) staging of the larynx. For purposes of this chapter, we define a laryngeal cancer as advanced if the AJCC stage is III or IV, as these tumors will generally require multimodality therapy.

Crucial to the determination of whether a laryngeal tumor is T3 is the assessment of vocal cord motion. A fixed vocal cord most frequently indicates deep invasion into the laryngeal musculature, although direct invasion into the cricoarytenoid joint is possible from a subglottic or postcricoid tumor. In addition, radiographic invasion of the preepiglottic space denotes a T3 tumor in the supraglottic larynx. The T4a tumors of the supraglottis and glottis invade through the cartilaginous framework of the larynx, most often in ossified portions of the cartilage, or have spread outside the confines of the larynx. The ossification of the cartilaginous portions of the adult larynx is critical to the understanding of laryngeal cancer spread, as invasion of the thyroid lamina can allow remote intralaryngeal tumor spread through the trabecular bone portions of the thyroid cartilage. The subglottis is slightly different, as a T4a tumor needs only to invade into the thyroid or cricoid cartilages or involves the structures beyond the larynx or both. In all cases of larynx cancer, a T4b tumor invades the prevertebral space, encases the carotid artery, or invades mediastinal structures.

The current system of laryngeal staging, which considers the size and location of the primary and regional disease, the presence of vocal cord fixation, extralaryngeal spread, or distant metastases, is, at best, a simplified assessment of outcome based on only a few clinical indicators. Pathologic examinations have shown that the clinical staging of a laryngeal cancer is underestimated at 25% to 40%. Advanced cancers of the larynx are most often understaged because early cartilage invasion cannot be assessed clinically.

Many other important prognostic factors related to the primary tumor are not currently considered in the tumor-node-metastasis (TNM) staging system. These include the presence of perineural or intralymphatic invasion, spindle cell or basal cell variants, poor differentiation, elevated DNA content, a high Ki67 or PCNA (proliferating cell nuclear antigen) score, expression of the c-*myc* oncogene or int-2 gene (5,6), the presence of circulating immune complexes, and overexpression of mutant p53 protein. The presence of high levels of mutant p53 has clearly been associated with diminished survival (7). Other genetic markers are becoming more commonly measurable as technology improves. However, the common flaw of individual genetic abnormalities is their lack of consistency, limiting their ability to act as reliable prognostic factors across a population. Therefore assessments of global gene-expression patterns may prove more useful and reliable, as they assess the entire specimen and a multitude of genes from many functional families. Studies of cDNA microarray expression patterns have been shown to distinguish clinical outcome in patients who are equivalent with respect to TNM staging (8).

With respect to regional staging, size and number of nodes are important factors in estimating prognosis and serve as the basis for the current N-stage criteria. Critical regional prognostic factors, however, such as the lowest level of involvement, number of levels with metastases, and the presence of extracapsular nodal spread are all ignored by the current staging system. Several of these primary and regional factors, considered both individually and together, have been shown to be more predictive than the criteria currently in use, and these factors have led to current alterations in postoperative recommendations for adjuvant therapy. Studies from the United States and Europe have demonstrated a benefit to adding chemotherapy to postoperative adjuvant radiotherapy for neck disease, although the toxicity of such therapy is certainly increased (9,10). The inclusion criteria for these studies were factors considered high risk, including the involvement of two or more regional lymph nodes, extracapsular nodal disease, or involved margins (9) or these factors plus perineural or vascular tumor involvement (10). The locoregional control was improved in the chemotherapy group, 82% versus 72% (*p* =0.01) and 82% versus 69%

for the respective studies. The trade-off for this improvement is an increase in serious toxicity; Cooper et al. (9) showed 77% grade 3 or higher toxicity in the chemoradiotherapy group (including four deaths) and 34% in the radiotherapy-alone group, and Bernier et al. (10) reported severe side effects in 41% of the chemoradiotherapy patients compared with 21% of the radiation-only patients.

Other staging systems have been proposed. Kleinsasser suggested that all tumors with any change in mobility of the vocal cord should be staged as either T3 or T4. Some staging systems have been proposed that use a high-resolution computed tomographic (CT) scan to determine the total volume of a tumor. This information can then be used to assist in the choice of therapy. In treating advanced head and neck cancer by using accelerated superfractionated radiation, Johnson et al. found local control rates to be 92% at 36 months if tumor volumes were less than or equal to 35 cc, and 34% at 36 months if tumor volumes were greater than 35 cc. CT and magnetic resonance imaging (MRI) also allow us to assess more accurately the involvement of laryngeal subsites. This is critical because sites may differ in their propensity for local or regional spread, recurrence, and, ultimately, prognosis. In the future, newer staging systems that incorporate subsites as well as other prognostic variables will help us to stage laryngeal tumors more accurately. Ferlito et al. (4) proposed a five-part system composed of separate criteria for clinical-diagnostic (cTNM), surgical evaluation (sTNM), pathologic (pTNM), retreatment (rTNM), and autopsy (aTNM). Perhaps one further classification could be added: for cellular/molecular studies (cmTNM). Other aspects of a patient are included in the clinical staging system proposed by Picarillo et al. (11). This was the first to include comorbidity into a comprehensive staging system, which they found to be a more accurate assessment for predicting a particular individual's treatment outcome with a certain tumor burden.

Clearly, not all advanced-stage lesions of equal AJCC staging are alike. This leaves the clinician with many factors to consider that are not typically addressed in the standard AJCC staging. All these factors eventually must be coalesced into a new staging system so that a treatment plan can fit more accurately a particular patient's health and volume of disease. For the time being, we are left with the need to decide whether a particular tumor is favorable or unfavorable, based on proven prognostic indicators, and if the patient's comorbidity makes the disease state more advanced than the same tumor in a patient who is otherwise healthy (Table 122.1) (12).

EVALUATION AND DIAGNOSIS

History

All patients need to have a comprehensive medical history. This should include a careful assessment of the current problem, medical history, social history with a quantification of

TABLE 122.1

STAGING OF ADVANCED LARYNGEAL CANCER

The primary

Supraglottic

T3	Tumor limited to the larynx with fixation of the larynx and/or invasion of any of the following:
	Postcricoid area
	Preepiglottic space
	Paraglottic space
	Minor thyroid cartilage invasion (inner cortex)
T4a	Tumor invades through thyroid cartilage and/or invades tissue beyond the larynx (trachea, strap muscles, extrinsic tongue muscles, thyroid, or esophagus)
T4b	Tumor invades prevertebral space, encases the carotid artery, or invades the mediastinal structures

Glottic

T3	Tumor confined to the larynx with vocal cord fixation and/or paraglottic space involvement or minor thyroid cartilage invasion (inner cortex)
T4a	Same as for supraglottis
T4b	Same as for supraglottis

Subglottic

T3	Tumor confined to larynx with vocal cord fixation
T4a	Tumor invading cricoid or thyroid cartilages, and/or into tissues beyond the larynx
T4b	Same as for supraglottis

Regional disease

N2a	Metastasis in a single ipsilateral lymph node, >3 cm but ≤ 6 cm in greatest dimension
N2b	Metastasis in multiple ipsilateral lymph nodes, none >6 cm
N2c	Metastasis in bilateral or contralateral lymph nodes, none >6 cm
N3	Metastasis in a lymph node >6 cm in greatest dimension

Distant disease

Mx	Presence of distant metastases cannot be assessed
M0	No distant metastasis
M1	Distant metastasis

Staging of advanced cancers

III	T3, N0 or N1, M0
IVA	T4a, N0 or N1, M0
	T1-4a, N2, M0
IVB	T4b, any N, M0
	Any T, N3, M0
IVC	Any T, Any N, M1

From AJCC. *AJCC Cancer Staging Manual*, 6th ed. New York: Springer, 2002.

prior smoking and drinking habits, family history to include epithelial tumors, and a review of systems. In addition, patients first seen with advanced cancer of the larynx have significant derangements of the normal function of the larynx. Patients may have a hoarse voice (e.g., glottic cancer), a muffled/hot potato voice (e.g., supraglottic cancer), aspiration pneumonia, dysphagia, odynophagia, hemoptysis, shortness of breath, stridor, sore throat, or otalgia. Patients often have lost a significant amount of weight because of impaired deglutition or because of the advanced stage of their cancer. Unfortunately, many early symptoms are closely associated with more common benign conditions. Therefore, an inherent tendency exists for the late recognition of a more serious problem in this region.

Smoking and alcohol are strongly associated with laryngeal cancer, with an almost linear correlation between the number of cigarettes smoked per day and the age-standardized mortality rate. Alcoholics also are at an increased risk of developing laryngeal cancer, with a synergistic effect of the interaction between tobacco and alcohol that results in a geometric progression of risk with increased dose and exposure. A few groups, including metal workers, asbestos workers, textile processors, and certain construction workers, may be at increased risk of laryngeal cancer from occupational exposures. Antioxidants such as vitamin A and its derivatives (i.e., β-carotene and retinoids) appear to have a protective effect, and there is an increased risk of laryngeal cancer in patients deficient in these substances. However, long-term trials with chemoprevention, using retinoids and other compounds, have not proven effective or have had significant toxicities. Therefore, no accepted chemopreventive regimen exists, and this area remains a fertile ground for continued research.

Physical Examination

An adequate office or bedside physical examination, with a comprehensive head and neck examination, is essential. One must assess the extent of tumor, vocal cord mobility, patency of the airway, extralaryngeal involvement, and extent of regional spread before more definitive examination with the patient under general anesthesia in the operating room. A mirror examination gives the best global view of the larynx and tongue base, but proper evaluation of the anterior commissure may be difficult, depending on the shape and position of the epiglottis. Fiberoptic flexible laryngoscopy offers a closer look at individual areas and an opportunity for video and photographic recording of the visible pathology.

Today, physicians of all disciplines involved in the treatment of these tumors must have a fiberoptic endoscope available to examine patients. The clinician should perform both a mirror and a fiberoptic examination to obtain as much visual information as possible while the patient is awake. One should be careful to assess fully the mucosa of the entire upper respiratory tract for second primary tumors, leukoplakia, erythroplasia, and signs of gastroesophageal reflux. Palpation of the laryngeal cartilages may reveal extension of tumor outside the larynx. Loss of laryngeal crepitus (i.e., the "click" when moving the larynx from side to side) indicates possible postcricoid invasion. Palpation of the floor of the mouth, oral tongue, base of the tongue, vallecula, and tonsillar region allows assessment of the total depth of the tumor.

The neck also must be carefully examined for adenopathy, documenting the location, mobility, size, and proximity or attachment of the nodes to adjacent structures. Nodal disease can appear in the prelaryngeal (delphian) node (level 6), levels 2, 3, 4, or the thyroid gland. In the presence of massive neck disease or base-of-tongue involvement, the submental, submandibular, and spinal accessory nodes also may become involved as a result of blockage of the normal lymphatic pathways by advanced disease. The neck should be examined bimanually from behind the patient, allowing the examiner's fingers to compress the lymphatic regions against the deep musculature as well as between the fingers for a more thorough examination. The submandibular region should be examined bimanually from the front of the patient, with one hand palpating the floor of the mouth.

The integrity of the airway must always be assessed. This should take place through visualization, auscultation of stridor, and assessment of the use of accessory muscles of respiration. This allows the clinician to determine the need for a tracheotomy as well as the obstacles the airway presents for treatment.

Preoperative Evaluation

Nutritional assessment, dental evaluation, pulmonary evaluation, and a metastatic workup should be performed preoperatively on these patients (Table 122.2). Many patients who have advanced laryngeal cancer are malnourished, but

TABLE 122.2   DIAGNOSIS

LARYNGEAL CANCER

History	Risk factors, duration of symptoms, associated medical conditions, symptoms of metastatic disease
Physical examination	Status of airway, extent of primary tumor, appearance of tumor (e.g., fungating, ulcerating, nodular), vocal cord fixation, neck disease
Diagnostic endoscopy and biopsy	Map primary and assess for skip areas, thoroughly palpate neck under general anesthesia, perform biopsy within and beyond the borders of the tumor
Laboratory tests	
Albumin, transferrin	Assess nutritional status
Calcium	Hypercalcemia may signify metastatic disease
Alkaline phosphatase	Elevated with bony metastasis, liver disease, and other conditions
Electrolytes, creatinine, blood count	Routine preoperative screening
Imaging studies	
CT scan of neck with contrast	Useful in delineating subglottic extension, cartilaginous involvement, extralaryngeal spread, and nodal disease
CT scan of chest/chest radiograph	Helps detect metastatic disease as a separate primary in the chest
MRI	Most useful in detecting occult nodal disease—not if already have obtained a neck CT
PET	Evaluate occult neck disease or distant metastases
Other studies	
Pulmonary function tests	Preoperative evaluation of pulmonary reserve, especially important if conservation surgery is planned

CT, computed tomography; MRI, magnetic resonance imaging; PET, positron emission tomography.

the practice of preoperative nutritional optimization should not interfere with the timely initiation of definitive therapy. Consideration of a gastrostomy (percutaneous or open) is included in the preoperative plan to ensure that the patient is moving toward and will achieve a noncatabolic state. Pulmonary function tests and an arterial blood gas measurement on room air are important because these patients, as a result of their tobacco history, often have obstructive pulmonary disease. If conservation surgery is planned, pulmonary function is important to assess. Although many advocate pulmonary function tests, no standards have been developed to provide a cut-off on which patients can, or cannot, tolerate the physiologic changes accompanying conservation laryngeal surgery. Most clinicians are satisfied if the patient is capable of walking up a flight of stairs without stopping. All patients must have an anteroposterior and lateral chest radiograph to assess their lung parenchyma for chronic obstructive pulmonary disease changes and to look for second primary tumors. Many have advocated routine chest CT in these patients, rather than a screening chest radiograph, although either is appropriate at this time. All tumors with pharyngeal involvement require an evaluation of the patient's entire esophagus, either endoscopically or with a barium swallow, although the frequency of second esophageal primaries makes routine assessment of the esophagus prudent.

Appropriate imaging of the laynx and neck is critical to assess the disease state as well. Obtaining a CT or an MRI scan from the skull base to clavicles with and without intravenous contrast agents is important to detect both intralaryngeal and extralaryngeal spread of tumor and cartilage invasion and to evaluate the extent of regional metastases. Imaging, therefore, is important in the accurate staging of larynx cancer, as this is the only way to assess the preepiglottic and paraglottic spaces other than at the time of surgery. The current staging system does permit the inclusion of radiographic criteria to develop the ultimate clinical stage. With advanced nodal disease, the scan may help to determine the relation of large metastases to the paraspinal muscles, cervical spine, or carotid artery. A scan is particularly important in the detection and evaluation of local and regional recurrences after primary radiation therapy. Physical examination alone may not be able to differentiate neoplastic changes from acute inflammation or radiation fibrosis. MRI is more sensitive for subtle changes in soft tissues, and therefore may be more useful in the detection of recurrent disease or in the evaluation of the tongue base. Positron emission tomography (PET) scanning, as a whole, has similar positive predictive value to that of CT or MRI when used in the initial workup of a patient, with the exception of identfying occult metastases outside the head and neck. PET is useful for differentiating recurrent laryngeal cancer from laryngeal radionecrosis (13), and its most promising use is in the ability to identify recurrent tumor in the absence of clinically obvious disease. One must view with caution, however, the positive results of PET scan taken within 3 to 4 months

of radiotherapy completion, as the inflammation from the treatment may give a false-positive PET result. In the future, PET also may be useful to quantify responses to chemotherapy in advanced lesions, because it assesses tumor metabolism. For a patient with advanced laryngeal cancer, particularly patients who have large or low neck metastases, a CT scan of the chest should be considered to evaluate the mediastinum as well as for a more comprehensive examination of the lung parenchyma, searching for additional primary tumors or distant metastases.

Further evaluation and planning should be based on the treatment plan and physical findings. If a neck mass is present, a fine-needle aspiration should be planned to assess involvement of the cervical nodes and may obviate the need for an endoscopic biopsy to make the diagnosis. Ultimately, however, surgical endoscopy is required to assess definitively the extent of the tumor for proper treatment planning. An open biopsy into a regional mass, which will cause contamination of the skin, subcutaneous tissues, and other adjacent structures, should be avoided, as the risk of regional failure may be increased in these cases. If a laryngectomy is planned, preoperative consultation with a speech therapist must not be overlooked so that the patient will be better prepared for the loss or impairment of speech and change in deglutition. It is an opportunity for the patients to learn more about the new airway and swallowing passage, and they also will be shown the many possible ways of restoring their function. Plans for immediate, primary, or delayed, secondary, surgical voice-restoration procedures also should be discussed at that time. All outside studies and pathology slides must be reviewed before any further diagnostic steps or examination under anesthesia.

Diagnostic Surgery

Clearly, no definitive treatment can be started without a biopsy-proved pathologic diagnosis of the primary site. Once all the clinical information has been obtained, each patient will need to have a full head and neck examination under anesthesia for biopsy and definitive tumor staging. Intraoperative laryngoscopy and esophagoscopy are the basic tools used for staging, with bronchoscopy being held for appropriate cases. Passive mobility of both vocal cords should be assessed, and appropriate biopsies taken. If any concern is present about the adequacy of the specimen, frozen-section analysis should be performed to ensure that representative tissue has been obtained. The tumor must be mapped out carefully, and a tumor diagram should be filled out, clearly indicating the sites of involvement. All additional lesions must be examined via biopsy as well, which is critical if partial laryngectomy is being considered. Flexible or rigid esophagoscopy should be performed to assess the patient thoroughly for skip lesions, second primary tumors, and the extent of cervical esophageal involvement. As technology improves, image-guided techniques, such as intraoperative MRI or ultrasonography, may allow localization and biopsy of tumors deep to the visible surface, and virtual endoscopy may be more useful in assessing areas of secondary involvement.

With the patient fully relaxed under general anesthesia, palpation of the neck can reveal subtle findings not apparent during the office examination, allowing more accurate regional staging. Often lymph nodes deep to the sternocleidomastoid muscle cannot be palpated while the patient is awake and guarding against pain. After the endoscopy has been completed, an open or percutaneous endoscopic gastrostomy and dental extractions can be performed to expedite the start of treatment. No type of laryngectomy should be planned without a biopsy-proven pathologic diagnosis.

Differential Diagnosis and Pathology

Squamous cell carcinoma remains the most common malignancy of the larynx, accounting for more than 90% of cancers occurring in this region. Nevertheless, many inflammatory and neoplastic lesions can mimic their appearance, and unless a definitive biopsy is obtained, an inappropriate therapeutic plan can be initiated. Certain granulomatous diseases, including tuberculosis, sarcoidosis, Wegener granulomatosis, blastomycosis, and histoplasmosis, can have the gross appearance of cancer, often appearing as a fungating or ulcerative mass. Verrucous carcinoma and respiratory papilloma are difficult to differentiate at times, both having a wartlike, papillary appearance. Granular cell tumors can appear in the larynx, and they usually affect a younger group of patients. The overlying epithelium of these tumors shows pseudoepitheliomatous hyperplasia, which can be difficult to distinguish from truly invasive neoplasms. Paragangliomas, plasmacytomas, and carcinoid tumors also occur in the larynx. Tumors of minor salivary gland origin are most often malignant, and these are most commonly found in the supraglottic larynx; however, they occasionally may involve the glottic or subglottic regions. Other carcinomas that must be excluded include small cell (oat cell) neuroendocrine carcinoma and adenocarcinoma, not otherwise specified. More rarely, benign and malignant soft-tissue neoplasms, such as chondromas, chondrosarcomas, spindle cell sarcomas, and rhabdomyosarcomas, may occur in the larynx. Various forms of lymphoma also may involve the larynx at any site. Sarcomas, minor salivary gland cancers, and lymphoma most often are first seen as submucosal masses rather than as ulcerative, mucosa-based lesions. It also is important to remember that the larynx can be a site of secondary spread from an extrinsic structure such as the thyroid gland. Aggressive cancers of the thyroid can easily invade the larynx and appear to be advanced laryngeal primary tumors. Rarely, the larynx can be a site of a distant metastasis.

Multidisciplinary Care

Every patient with a new head and neck primary tumor should be seen and evaluated in a multidisciplinary tumor

clinic. This should include representatives from speech therapy, dentistry, social service, radiation, medical, and surgical oncology departments, with other services involved as needed, including plastic/reconstructive surgery, palliative care, radiology, pathology, or others. Each specialist must perform a complete examination and have the opportunity to become familiar with the patient's problem. When all pertinent information concerning history, physical examination, review of pathology slides, and radiologic examinations is available, every patient should be presented to a multidisciplinary head and neck tumor planning group. It is helpful for several members of each specialty to be present for this meeting so that the patient can benefit from the input of many cancer specialists. This is particularly important for the patient with advanced tumors, because often several different competing treatment options have similar outcomes. No patient should be treated on the basis of any single individual's personal experience, because this might lead to care on the basis of a clinician's bias to one modality or anecdotal knowledge base.

MANAGEMENT

Natural History Without Treatment

As with all head and neck malignancies, any stage of laryngeal cancer may be seen at presentation. Minimal involvement of the vocal fold causes hoarseness that may persist unchanged, or with little progression, even in the presence of vocal cord fixation. The degree of dysphonia has no correlation to the extent of tumor within the larynx. Hemoptysis is more common with supraglottic than with glottic tumors, in which extension to the tongue base is associated with increased vascularity. Furthermore, lateral or preepiglottic space extension can cause infiltration into branches of the external carotid artery with subsequent massive bleeding.

Airway obstruction usually signifies advanced disease because of tumor bulk, diminished vocal cord motion, active inflammation, or infection. Tumors involving the subglottis may be small and may obstruct the airway because of the confined circumferential space. In any case, the airway must be established and secured. This has direct bearing on the subsequent treatment because of concerns of tumor seeding and stomal recurrence. Ideally, if practical and appropriate, endoscopic debulking of a laryngeal primary is preferable to a tracheotomy, which should be reserved for the most severe cases of laryngeal obstruction.

Medical complications may arise secondary to a primary laryngeal cancer. Aspiration producing pneumonia can occur as a result of an incompetent glottis from vocal cord fixation or tumor bulk, particularly when swallowing liquids. The patient tries to avoid aspiration by limiting the quantity of food and liquid ingested, leading to inanition, which further compounds the problem. Fixation of tumor to surrounding structures limits vertical laryngeal mobility, making it difficult to complete the pharyngeal component of swallowing and initiate the esophageal phase. This is especially true in malignancies involving the epiglottis and aryepiglottic folds. Infiltration of the pharyngeal musculature or disruption of sensory and motor innervation also can lead to dysphagia and to local and referred pain to the ear. Ultimately, if left untreated, advanced laryngeal cancer can cause the patient's death by bleeding, malnutrition, aspiration, or airway obstruction. Occasionally, the primary lesion may remain relatively quiescent, whereas regional and distant disease proliferates. This can lead to the overall decline of the patient and death from infection in the context of multisystem failure. In addition, paraneoplastic syndromes may develop, resulting in hypercalcemia, diarrhea, or other systemic symptoms.

Treatment

The primary goal of treatment of advanced cancers of the larynx is to cure the patient, with preservation of speech and swallowing being significant secondary goals. The sacrifice of the larynx should be avoided if possible, although patient preference and appropriate selection based on tumor characteristics are important. It is, therefore, imperative that treatment decisions center on both of these objectives. The currently available treatment modalities include external beam radiation, chemotherapy, surgery, or a combination of any of these. The treatment of advanced laryngeal lesions most often requires the use of at least two of these modalities. Occasionally, a T3 laryngeal lesion with early N1 or N0 regional disease may be treated with one modality: surgery or radiation. It is of paramount importance that the patient be brought into the decision-making process from the very beginning so that he or she can make an informed decision between several options for treatment. Advanced laryngeal

cancer forces modifications of normal voice, respiration, and deglutition regardless of therapy. In contrast to treating smaller laryngeal lesions, normalcy is not restored and survival rates are not as good, with 5-year survival ranging from 30% to 60% in these advanced cases (12). It should not be surprising to the clinician that most patients who are given the opportunity to preserve the larynx will choose either a nonsurgical alternative or a more functional subtotal resection. It is therefore critical that the physician not allow personal anecdotal preferences to enter into the decision-making process. Currently, every patient who is eligible should be offered the opportunity to select a course of treatment that preserves the larynx. Evidence is clear that attempts to preserve the larynx do not compromise the prognosis of the patient if treatment is administered in the proper multidisciplinary setting with proper monitoring.

The variables of location of the primary tumor (e.g., supraglottic, glottic, or subglottic) and the presence of nodal metastases preclude recommending any one therapeutic regimen for all patients. Apart from well-described surgical procedures, many different chemoradiation protocols are currently being offered throughout the world. Furthermore, many studies are ongoing, and many questions about the best combination of therapy remain to be answered. It appears, from the publication of the RTOG 91-11 trial comparing radiotherapy, neoadjuvant chemoradiotherapy, and concomitant radiotherapy, that concomitant chemoradiotherapy offers the best local control among these modalities used in an organ-sparing fashion, with larynx preservation in 70%, 75%, and 88%, respectively (14). Unfortunately, little uniformity is found from institution to institution in the use of surgery or radiation therapy for any specific site or stage of disease (Table 122.3). Radiotherapy

TABLE 122.3 Rx TREATMENT
LARYNGEAL CANCER

Condition	High Points
Advanced supraglottic cancers	Because of high rate of lymphatic spread, inclusion of the cervical lymphatics in the treatment regimen is necessary Partial laryngectomy may be performed in certain cases Consent for total laryngectomy must be obtained If partial laryngectomy is planned, adequate pulmonary and cardiac function is necessary Radiation therapy may be used as a primary modality, but it is less effective than surgery for large lesions or for tumors with palpable neck disease Combined therapy (surgery and postoperative irradiation) gives higher cure rates than either modality alone Combined chemotherapy and radiotherapy is more effective than radiation alone
Advanced glottic cancers	Airway control by intubation or debulking preferred for obstructing lesions For most T3 and T4 glottic lesions, total laryngectomy is the treatment of choice Partial laryngectomy may be possible in selected T3 tumors Planned postoperative radiotherapy improves survival in advanced lesions
Advanced subglottic cancers	Airway control by intubation or laser debulking is preferred for obstructing lesions Total laryngectomy with paratracheal node dissection is the rule Planned postoperative radiotherapy should be used for advanced lesions

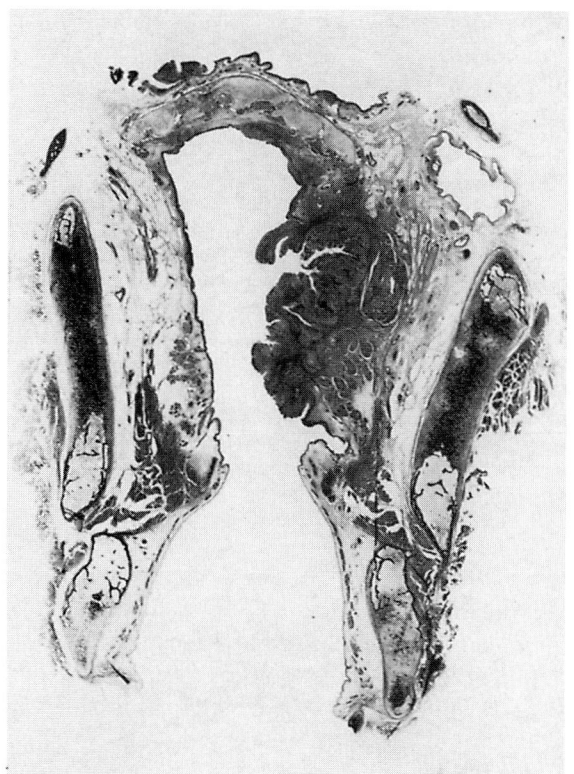

Figure 122.6 Supraglottic cancer showing no tendency to cross the ventricle in either this or other sections. (Reprinted from Kirchner JA. One hundred laryngeal cancers studied by serial section. *Ann Otol* 1969;78:689–709, with permission.)

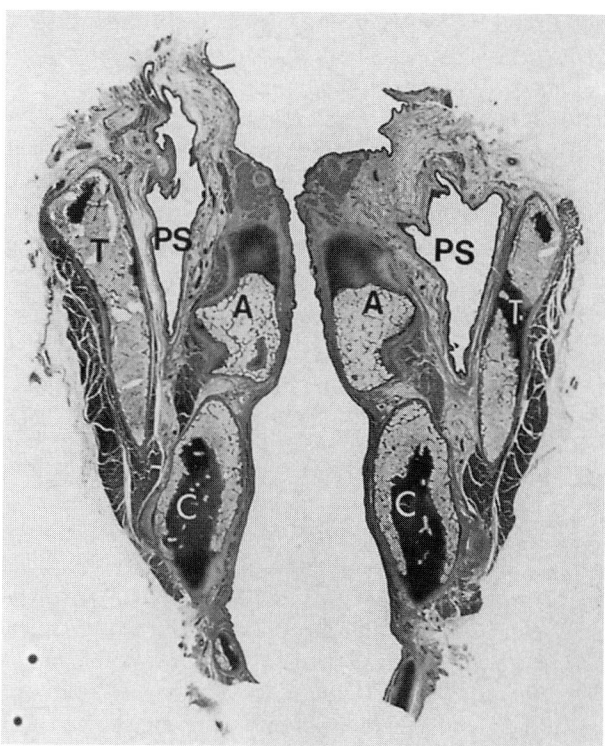

Figure 122.7 Coronal section of posterior larynx, showing proximity of arytenoid cartilage (*A*) to upper edge of cricoid (*C*). Subglottic extension of cordal cancer in this area, even for only a few millimeters, can invade the cricoid cartilage, changing an early lesion to an advanced one. *T*, thyroid cartilage; *PS*, piriform sinus. (Reprinted from Kirchner JA, Som ML. Clinical significance of the fixed vocal cord. *Laryngoscope* 1971;81:1029, with permission.)

alone, even for early and late supraglottic cancers, was curative in 43% of patients (15). Although 60% of the 410 patients in this series with supraglottic carcinoma obtained tumor control, only 44% retained their larynges.

The most important determinant of survival is the extent of regional involvement. Several studies have shown an inverse relation between the extent of neck disease and ultimate local control. Involvement of the preepiglottic space, the cartilages, or the soft tissues of the neck is associated with an even higher rate of lymphatic spread to the prelaryngeal and deep cervical nodes (Figs. 122.6 and 122.7). Cervical node metastases are uncommon in purely

glottic tumors, but in transglottic, supraglottic, and subglottic tumors, the incidence is higher (Table 122.4). Given the abundant bilateral lymphatic drainage, treatment of both sides of the neck should coincide with treatment of the primary cancer.

Today appropriate questions are being asked by many individuals and organizations about the cost and quality of the treatment of head and neck patients. Given the wide variation of the treatment of advanced laryngeal lesions, it has become difficult to promote and defend any one treatment method as the most efficacious and cost-effective

TABLE 122.4
RISK OF LARYNGEAL CANCER METASTASIS TO THE NECK

| Primary Site | Investigation | Incidence (%) of Metastasis by Stage | | | | |
		T1	T2	T3	T4	All T
Supraglottis	Shah and Tollefsen	40	42	55	65	51
	Bocca et al.	25	31		42	32
Glottis	Jesse				39	
	Daly and Strong	5	8	15		
Subglottis	Harrison					50[a]

[a]Involvement of paratracheal nodes.

choice. Because follow-up evaluation of nonsurgical treatments has shown long-term functional consequences, recent efforts have focused on quality-of-life issues in differing treatments with similar cure rates. Traditionally, nonsurgical trials have evaluated their adverse events in the early periods after therapy. However, late toxicities, predominantly swallowing and related functions, have persisted in these patients (16). What follows is a distillation of the current management options based on reported experiences and our preferences.

Advanced Supraglottic Lesions

Stage III and IV carcinoma of the supraglottic larynx may represent advanced primary or regional disease. As defined earlier, this implies fixation of the vocal cord, extension to the postcricoid area, preepiglottic space, extralaryngeal spread, or it may represent the presence of lymph node metastases. The supraglottis is rich in lymphatic channels, and the incidence of clinically palpable and occult, unilateral or bilateral regional metastases varies from 25% to 75%. Treatment of these lesions must incorporate the elective or therapeutic treatment of the neck, either surgical or nonsurgical.

Although surgery and radiation therapy are effective as single modalities for treating early primary tumors and regional metastases, individually they are far less effective for more-advanced lesions. This creates concerns about partial laryngeal surgery, which includes the supraglottic laryngectomy, the supracricoid partial laryngectomy, or a near-total laryngectomy. A partial laryngectomy without radiation can yield excellent functional results; however, when such partial laryngeal surgery is combined with postoperative radiation, the functional results and the likelihood of decannulation are poor. So when postoperative radiation is considered from the outset, we must proceed with caution with these conservation procedures. The critical factor in assessing the impact of postoperative radiotherapy is the need to irradiate the remnant larynx. If the primary site can be adequately addressed with partial laryngeal surgery, and the neck addressed with neck dissection and postoperative radiotherapy, surgery remains a viable, appropriate, and excellent option. The best lesions for this form of surgery are those for which a high probability exists that a partial laryngectomy and bilateral neck dissection will be all that is necessary.

Current practices have been extending the use of supraglottic laryngectomy for the management of these tumors. A growing body of knowledge advances the use of endoscopic resections in these patients. In general, endoscopic supraglottic laryngectomy has been reserved for T1 and T2 lesions of the supraglottic larynx. However, as experience has broadened, patients with T3 and T4 disease also have been managed endoscopically. The key to the success of such an approach is to achieve pathologically negative margins. When negative margins are achieved, this can lead to local control in 83% of cases

TABLE 122.5

CLINICAL INDICATIONS FOR PARTIAL OR TOTAL LARYNGECTOMY

Documented laryngeal malignancy
Airway obstruction related to massive cancer
Severe aspiration after partial laryngectomy
Radiation necrosis
Persistent tumor after chemotherapy or radiation therapy in a patient with histologically documented persistence or recurrence
Adjunct to removal of tumor of tongue base, cervical esophagus, or thyroid carcinomas
Clinical, radiographic, or endoscopic evidence of absence of multiple aerodigestive tract malignancies
Absence of distant metastatic disease (conditional, as a palliative laryngectomy is occasionally indicated)

(17). However, one must always address the necks in these patients, and these findings may necessitate chemotherapy and radiotherapy for high-risk disease (9,10). In spite of this, the standard from which all other procedures must be measured remains the total laryngectomy (Table 122.5).

The following are partial surgical procedures and their indications.

1. *Supraglottic laryngectomy.* This procedure removes the glottis to the level of the midportion of the laryngeal ventricle (the entire supraglottic larynx) and the preepiglottic space and leaves a portion of the thyroid cartilage and both arytenoids intact. Endoscopic supraglottic laryngectomy may not result in the complete removal of all the structures highlighted. The indications for supraglottic laryngectomy include the following: supraglottic cancers classified as T3 because of preepiglottic space invasion, minimal medial piriform sinus involvement above the level of the true cords, no extension to the vocal cord; and patients must be in good general health with reasonable pulmonary reserve. Patients with a single arytenoid involved also may be appropriate for this procedure. The patient also must understand that findings at surgery may necessitate a total laryngectomy, and all patients undergoing any type of conservation laryngeal surgery should be consented for total laryngectomy as well. The expected functional outcome includes normal speech and eating with a supraglottic swallowing pattern.

2. *Supracricoid partial laryngectomy with cricohyoidopexy.* This method adds to the standard supraglottic procedure by extending the resection to include the entire thyroid cartilage. One or more of the following structures can be resected: an arytenoid and a portion of the upper cricoid. One functional arytenoid must be preserved. The indications for this procedure include supraglottic tumors classified as T3 because of vocal cord fixation, preepiglottic space invasion, paraglottic involvement, or limited invasion of the thyroid alae. The patient

should be in good general health with good pulmonary reserve, and the expected functional outcomes include decannulation and the recovery of speech and deglutition. However, these outcomes may require an extended period of rehabilitation.

3. *Near-total laryngectomy.* A single arytenoid cartilage is preserved to produce a lung-powered voice through a tracheoesophageal conduit (Fig. 122.8). Almost the entire larynx is resected, leaving the patient with a permanent tracheostomy. Subglottic extension below the cricoid ring or failure of radiation therapy is a contraindication to this procedure. The indications for this procedure are large T3 or T4 lesions not amenable to a supraglottic or supracricoid resection with one uninvolved arytenoid and ventricle, patients with lesions amenable to a standard supraglottic procedure but with poor cardiopulmonary function, or patients with unilateral transglottic tumors with cord fixation. The functional outcomes include a permanent tracheostomy, usable speech fistula, and normal swallowing. It is important to note that this procedure is very technically challenging, and few have been able to incorporate this successfully into their practice.

Despite the currently available preoperative diagnostic testing, no consistently reliable method exists to assess the degree of tumor extension completely in many patients. Therefore when a partial procedure is planned, the surgeon must describe the planned procedure to the patient with the option that a total laryngectomy may be required. The

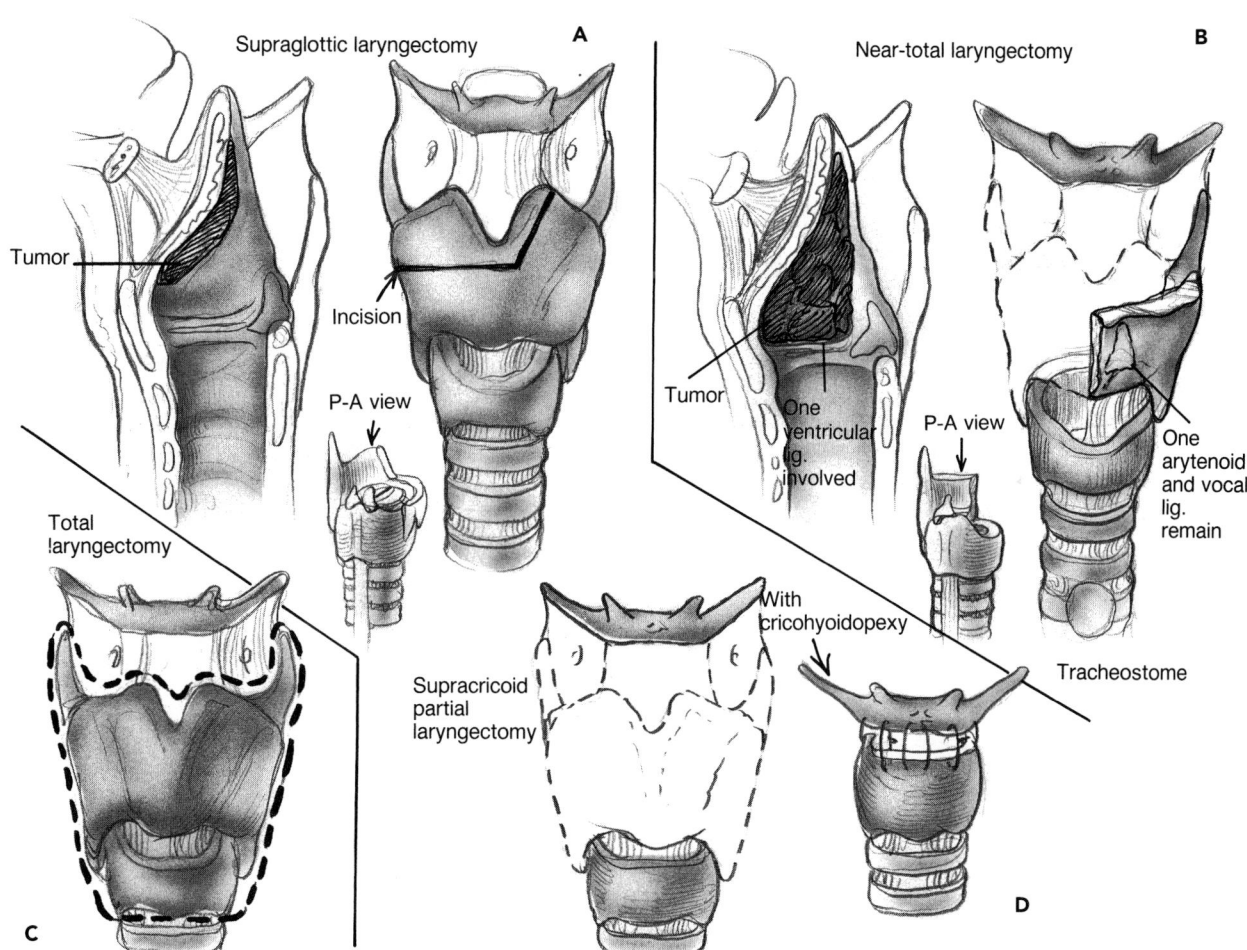

Figure 122.8 Supraglottic laryngectomy. Excision involves supraglottic portion of ipsilateral thyroid cartilage, supraglottic larynx, including aryepiglottic folds, false vocal cords, and epiglottis. **A:** For complete excision of the preepiglottic space, the hyoid bone must be removed. Excision may be extended to include one but not both arytenoids. Adequate pulmonary reserve is essential. **B:** Near-total laryngectomy is performed for advanced cancers of the larynx. It requires a permanent tracheostomy but preserves a voluntary voice. One arytenoid should be free of cancer, and the patient's pulmonary reserve should be adequate. **C:** Total laryngectomy is performed for advanced cancers of the larynx and for patients with inadequate pulmonary reserve. Excision involves the entire thyroid and cricoid cartilages as well as the hyoid bone. **D:** Supracricoid partial laryngectomy with cricohyoidopexy. This procedure resects the entire thyroid lamina and is indicated for most extensive glottic lesions that preserve some degree of vocal fold mobility with a single mobile arytenoid preserved. This operation allows vocalization without a permanent tracheostomy.

final decision for functional surgery can be made only at the time of surgery with the benefit of direct visualization and frozen-section pathologic confirmation. If the patient is not willing to give consent for these procedures, a limited resection should be avoided. Poor pulmonary function and cardiac reserve negate conservation surgery. Failure of prior full-course radiation therapy is not an absolute contraindication to the partial laryngeal procedures, as supracricoid laryngectomies and endoscopic supraglottic laryngectomies have been successfully used in these patients with excellent long-term functional results. If the surgical criteria are met, control of disease at the primary site is comparable with other modalities of treatment, and survival is improved. These criteria define more-favorable lesions, so the improvement in survival reflects the more limited nature of the primary tumor.

Total laryngectomy must be considered in any patient who does not fulfill the criteria for partial laryngectomy or for whom irradiation, with or without chemotherapy, is not a reasonable option. Indications for this procedure include the following:

All T3 cancers not amenable to supraglottic or supracricoid laryngectomy
All T4 cancers not amenable to supracricoid or near-total laryngectomy
Tumors with extensive involvement of the thyroid or cricoid cartilage
Invasion of the surrounding soft tissue of the neck
Extension beyond the posterior third of the base of tongue

Functional outcome includes the ability to swallow. Speech is created via esophageal speech, a tracheal–esophageal prosthesis, or a handheld mechanical aid such as an electrolarynx.

The Neck

Regular patterns of lymphatic involvement have been observed in laryngeal carcinoma. For the supraglottic larynx, the lymph node levels most often involved are levels 2, 3, and 4. If surgery is to be the modality of choice for the primary tumor, a bilateral lateral selective neck dissection would be the treatment of choice for the N0 patient (4,18). Lutz et al. (19) found the most common site of recurrence in their 11-year review of patients treated for supraglottic carcinoma at the Pittsburgh Eye and Ear Infirmary to be the contralateral undissected neck (83%). Only 2% recurred at the primary site. Therefore the data from this article and others led to the common practice of bilateral neck treatment, either surgical or nonsurgical. The node-positive neck will often necessitate a more definitive neck dissection (modified radical or radical neck dissection), although an accumulating body of literature validates selective neck dissection for the management of select N1 nodal disease. For N0 or N1 regional disease, radiation

has been shown to be equivalent to surgery in its ability to sterilize the neck.

Adjuvant Radiation

Postoperative radiation can be needed when factors that place the patient at a higher risk of recurrence are found either at the primary site or at regional sites. Factors that would necessitate postoperative treatment include positive margins; T4 lesions; N2 or N3 neck disease or evidence of extracapsular lymph node spread; perineural or vascular invasion; metastases to inferior tracheoesophageal, lower jugular, or mediastinal nodes; multiple levels of nodal involvement; and subglottic extension. Recent data have supported the use of postoperative chemotherapy and radiotherapy in patients who are at high risk of recurrence in the neck, usually defined as those with extracapsular extension or multiple positive lymph nodes (9,10). In both these studies, an improvement in overall survival was seen when chemotherapy was added to the postoperative radiotherapy. However, significantly more toxicity was found when chemotherapy was added. Ultimately, the clinician and the patient will have to weigh the risks and benefits of this added toxicity.

Radiation as the Definitive Modality

Radiation as the first modality of therapy has been advocated to preserve an intact larynx. The results of the RTOG 91-11 trial, however, suggest that this is a relatively less effective alternative when compared with chemotherapy and radiotherapy in combination (14). Another way to look at the data, however, is to conclude that radiotherapy alone, in advanced larynx cancer, did result in locoregional control in 61% of the patients, and laryngeal preservation, in 70%. These data certainly support the use of this modality in patients who cannot tolerate the more aggressive concomitant chemoradiotherapy. Radiation alone has been generally relegated to those who cannot, or will not, undergo surgical removal of their advanced larynx cancer. In T4 larynx cancer, radiotherapy alone is generally thought to be inferior to surgery with adjuvant radiotherapy. This was demonstrated by Weems et al. (20), who found that 60% of T3 and 31% of T4 cancers were controlled with radiation alone compared with 94% of T3 and 83% of T4 cancers treated with surgery and postoperative radiation. Some surgeons advocate radiation for the definitive treatment of these advanced lesions. Studies during the 1970s and 1980s revealed a control that ranged from 18% to 74%. Some authors advocated initial radiation treatment with salvage surgery for all stage III and IV disease, describing a 67% locoregional control rate with irradiation at 3 years, increasing to 85% with surgical salvage of recurrences. Selected T3, small-volume cancers can be treated effectively with radiation alone.

The ideal patients for this treatment are the same as those who would be considered for conservation surgery. Massive tumors (i.e., >4 cm in greatest diameter), large nodal metastases, T4 lesions, and a tracheotomy for airway obstruction before any treatment are some indications of the need for combined modality treatment. Patients with significant extralaryngeal spread and marked tongue involvement (>1 cm) are excluded from most nonsurgical trials. Findings on pretreatment CT can be helpful in predicting local control for T3 cancers treated with radiation, and some studies have been undertaken on the relation between tumor volume and radiotherapy response. In general, tumors greater than 3.5 cc on CT have a lower probability of local control with radiotherapy alone. Perhaps the emerging three-dimensional imaging techniques will be of even greater predictive value.

If irradiation is chosen as the sole treatment, close follow-up with reevaluation of the larynx must be continued for the first 3 years. It can be extremely difficult to pick out an early recurrence in the face of a great deal of postirradiation swelling. For this reason, if any suggestive change is noted in the examination, or if new pain develops, it is mandatory that the patient undergo an evaluation under general anesthesia with biopsy to rule out a recurrence. In addition, PET scanning has shown particular promise in this area, recurrent larynx cancer after nonsurgical therapy, and should be included as part of the workup if possible. Failure to ascertain recurrence can be a major problem, and at times it can substantially diminish a patient's chance of survival.

Hypothyroidism may occur as a consequence of thyroidectomy at the time of laryngectomy, from radiation therapy alone, or both. The combination of the two will cause hypothyroidism in as many as 70% of these patients (21). Decreased thyroid function delays wound healing and causes mental depression; it must be considered in cases of postoperative pharyngocutaneous fistulae. Delayed hypothyroidism may occur 6 months to 1 year after completion of treatment of the laryngeal cancer and must be kept in mind when new symptoms become evident.

The issue as to whether a particular fractionation scheme improves survival from laryngeal cancers is currently under study. Over the years, twice-daily therapy has yielded gradual improvement in outcome, especially for T3 lesions. The most recent assessment of radiation therapy alone is the RTOG 91-11 trial comparing radiotherapy alone, with neoadjuvant chemotherapy, or with concomitant chemoradiotherapy, and has shown improved local control in the chemotherapy arms, most significantly in the concomitant group (14).

Survival

Despite this aggressive approach, the survival rate for stage IV supraglottic cancer is rarely better than 50%, even with combined treatment. Clearly, we need to continue the effort to find more effective treatments to improve survival without destroying a patient's ability to lead a reasonably normal life. It should also be remembered that the initial VA study (22) and the follow-up RTOG 91-11 (14) study demonstrated that chemotherapy and radiotherapy have survival rates similar to those with total laryngectomy in these patients.

ADVANCED GLOTTIC LESIONS

Some aspects of glottic cancers distinguish them from their supraglottic and subglottic counterparts. Glottic tumors benefit from a limited lymphatic flow, which leads to fewer regional metastases. The choice of treatment for T3 glottic cancers entails an understanding of the many causes of vocal cord fixation. Loss of mobility of the glottis can be caused by tumor invasion into the thyroarytenoid muscle or cricoarytenoid joint, by fixation of the vocal cord to the thyroid cartilage perichondrium, and more rarely by invasion of the recurrent laryngeal nerve. T3 glottic lesions are therefore a mixed group of tumors of very different pathologic potential. Mendenhall et al. divide T3 and T4 glottic cancers into relatively favorable and unfavorable lesions. Lesions confined mostly to one side of the larynx with minimal airway obstruction are favorable. To this we would add the truly exophytic tumor lacking deeply invasive spread. They define unfavorable lesions as those with extensive bilateral disease, to which we would add any tumor with extensive submucosal spread, extralaryngeal involvement, extensive cartilage invasion, and subglottic extension below the level of the upper edge of the cricoid.

Patients with favorable lesions may be candidates for several treatment options. These include either primary radiation, chemoradiotherapy, partial laryngectomy, or total laryngectomy. Results for these highly selected patients can be comparable with those with smaller lesions, with cure rates higher than 80%. Patients with unfavorable lesions should be offered either a total laryngectomy with postoperative radiation or concurrent chemoradiotherapy with possible surgical salvage. When counseled about treatment options other than a total laryngectomy, the patient with a favorable lesion must understand that a total laryngectomy still may be necessary at some point during, or after, treatment. When using this approach, salvage laryngectomy is an effective way to address residual disease, with similar control rates if the patient initially had radiotherapy, neoadjuvant chemoradiotherapy, or concomitant chemoradiotherapy (23).

A review of the Gainesville experience with T3 glottic cancers revealed the choice of initial therapy to have no effect on survival. Patients treated with initial surgery followed by postoperative radiation had survival rates similar to those of patients receiving definitive radiation, with surgery held for salvage. The radiation group had an 84%

survival compared with 82% for the surgery group. Many reviews have reported on patients with T3 tumors undergoing primary radiation. Local control rates have varied from 50% to 77%. Interestingly, T4 cancers treated initially with either surgery or radiation also were found to have similar chances of survival. Primary radiation with surgical salvage leads to a 5-year survival of between 38% and 49%; total laryngectomy and postoperative radiation provide a similar survival range of 30% to 54%. These data are in concordance with chemoradiotherapy data, which show similar disease-free and survival rates when comparing this with total laryngectomy (22). When considering surgery, the decision for less-than-total laryngectomy must be based on the findings at direct laryngoscopy, the results of radiographic studies, and findings at the time of surgical exploration. The following factors, when present, preclude a partial vertical laryngectomy: (a) subglottic extension to the level of the cricoid, although partial cricoid resection is feasible; (b) bilateral arytenoid involvement; and (c) obvious cartilage invasion or spread to the extralaryngeal soft tissues.

Extensive partial resections, including near-total laryngectomy and supracricoid partial laryngectomy with closure by cricohyoidopexy, are further modifications that allow wide or total thyroid cartilage removal with voice preservation when appropriately chosen. Great care must be taken not to jeopardize the potential for cure in a vain attempt at vocal salvage.

To improve the criteria for treatment, Yuen et al. attempted to identify factors that influence local and regional control of these tumors. Their results indicated that a high histologic grade (i.e., undifferentiated tumors), subglottic extension of more than 1 cm, histologically confirmed positive lymph nodes, and the performance of a tracheotomy before definitive treatment were features associated with higher failure rates above the clavicles. Postoperative planned radiation therapy is advised for these patients as a minimum, and with the current information, some of these patients may need chemotherapy as well.

Radiation or Surgery?

Debate continues about the role of primary surgery or primary radiotherapy in cases of glottic cancer. Primary radiation therapy has been advocated for patients who are relatively easy to examine for possible tumor recurrence, who agree to close follow-up after completion of treatment, and who recognize the potential need for a laryngectomy after the treatment has been completed. It is our recommendation that primary radiation as a single therapy be limited to the patient with a favorable T3 lesion (i.e., low tumor volume) or patients who cannot tolerate chemotherapy and are unwilling to consider total laryngectomy. Clearly, these patients are also candidates for a partial laryngectomy, and it is our belief that patients who are candidates for partial laryngeal surgery that will preserve a good-quality voice should undergo such a procedure. Certainly, however, if the patient

has a favorable primary tumor with bulky nodal disease, then up-front nonsurgical treatment with surgical salvage may be more appropriate. It is likely that such a case will require surgery to the neck as well as the chemoradiotherapy. The ultimate decision of whether to proceed with a given treatment will rest with the patient and the surgeon, the surgeon's familiarity with these procedures, and his or her comfort performing the procedure. Whether twice-daily radiation improves tumor control or influences survival continues to be under study. Some believe that twice-daily treatment has not significantly improved these results. It also is clear that total dose delivered is important. Wang et al. (24), in a review of 162 patients with T3 laryngeal and hypopharyngeal carcinomas, all treated with twice-daily therapy, showed 5-year actuarial local control rates of 83% with a total dose of more than 70 Gy and of 65% with a total dose of less than 67 Gy. Prognostically, women fare better than men after radiation therapy, and the recurrence rate among men older than 60 years is significantly lower than that among men younger than 60 years.

Tumors that extend out of the confines of the larynx (T4) carry a high probability of cervical metastases and require aggressive therapy to the primary site and neck. Emergency tracheotomy is required in almost one third of these patients; if performed before definitive treatment, it is associated with diminished survival. It is frequently not possible to evaluate the degree of infiltration to surrounding structures, making the consideration of partial laryngectomy unlikely. For this reason, standard treatment is total laryngectomy with resection of any contiguous region and the ipsilateral neck lymphatics, if appropriate. Bilateral neck therapy, either neck dissections or neck irradiation, must be considered in all cases of advanced glottic cancer. If surgery is to be performed, the dissected levels must include the paratracheal lymphatics as well as levels 2, 3, and 4. Postoperative radiation therapy should be planned based on the adequacy of the resection and tumor characteristics.

In explaining total laryngectomy to the patient, it must be emphasized that removal of the larynx is not equivalent to aphonia. The reconstructive options, such as voice prostheses, mucosal shunts, and electronic devices, will permit the patient to communicate and function in society. Laryngectomy support groups also help in this often difficult transition, and often local chapters of laryngectomy associations or support groups for people with cancer are available, all of whom provide an important social network for these patients.

Total laryngectomy is the procedure of choice for tumor recurrence if radiation therapy was delivered in curative doses for a larger tumor or if a partial laryngectomy was the first operation. Occasionally, partial laryngectomy procedures are possible for T3 recurrent glottic cancers. However, the recurrence rates are high, and close follow-up is required to maximize survival if additional surgical salvage is required. Total laryngectomy remains the standard against which all other treatments are measured.

Adjuvant Radiation

The indications for postoperative radiation are similar to those for supraglottic cancers.

The Neck

Palpable cervical nodes can be found in about 30% of patients; an additional 10% have occult metastatic disease. The most likely regions to be involved include the jugular chain and paratracheal and pretracheal groups. Once large metastases appear, the ability to predict the pattern of flow no longer exists, and lymph nodes in unusual locations will begin to become involved. Typically, as for supraglottic cancer, the posterior and submandibular triangles are spared before the occurrence of paradoxical lymphatic flow. When cervical nodes are apparent, treatment should include the appropriate therapeutic neck dissection. Disease advanced beyond the N1 stage will likely require either a modified radical or a radical neck dissection, although neck dissections for glottic cancer must address only levels 2, 3, and 4 in the vast majority of cases (4). For occult or early N1 disease, a selective anterolateral dissection that includes levels 2, 3, 4, and 6 will address the lymph nodes at greatest risk for tumor spread. Radiation remains equally effective for the sterilization of the N0 and N1 neck.

ADVANCED SUBGLOTTIC CANCER

No feasible partial resections exist for this region. Regional metastases are frequent and bilateral. Often the paratracheal and pretracheal lymph nodes are the first to become involved, with frequent involvement of the thyroid gland. The middle and lower jugular regions also are at risk. Total laryngectomy with postoperative radiation remains the current standard for the treatment of these lesions. For patients who refuse surgery, primary radiation or concomitant chemoradiotherapy can be offered. Reports by Guedea and Ward (25) reveal that this course of treatment for T3/T4 cancers sometimes can be successful. However, the protocols for organ preservation in laryngeal cancer often do not apply to primary subglottic carcinomas, as they commonly have significant extralaryngeal extension (a contraindication to most organ-sparing protocols) (14). Subglottic cancers have a higher incidence of stomal recurrence after total laryngectomy. This may be related to tumor seeding during surgery, submucosal tracheal involvement, or undissected paratracheal lymphatics. Such a recurrence is very difficult to cure, although mediastinal dissection is approriate in selected individuals with limited stomal disease and an excellent performance status. The resection may have a very high perioperative morbidity and mortality rate, precluding its routine use. Therefore postoperative irradiation is advocated in subglottic cancers, and the fields must extend into the mediastinum and to the stomal skin to miminimize the risk of recurrence.

CHEMOTHERAPY AND ORGAN PRESERVATION

Over the past 15-year period, treatment options available to patients with advanced laryngeal cancer have changed significantly. Based on the early phase II and III trials in the 1980s by Al-Sarraf and colleagues at Wayne State University, cisplatin and 5-fluorouracil have become the backbone of all current organ-preservation protocols. In an attempt to improve survival and increase the likelihood of organ preservation, various regimens of adjuvant, neoadjuvant, and concomitant chemoradiation were developed and clinically tested. Neoadjuvant or induction protocols begin with chemotherapy and then are followed by either radiation or surgery, depending on tumor response. The landmark induction study for laryngeal cancer was the multiinstitutional, randomized clinical trial reported by the Cooperative Studies Program of the Department of Veterans Affairs (22). Patients in this study were assigned to receive either three cycles of chemotherapy (i.e., with cisplatin and 5-fluorouracil) and radiation therapy or surgery and radiation therapy. The clinical tumor response was assessed after two cycles of chemotherapy, and patients with a response received a third cycle followed by definitive irradiation (i.e., 66 to 76 Gy). Patients in whom no tumor response was found or who had locally recurrent cancers after chemotherapy and radiation therapy underwent salvage laryngectomy. After a median follow-up of 33 months, the estimated 2-year survival rate for both groups was 68%. More local recurrences and fewer distant metastases were found in the chemotherapy group than in the surgery group. Overall, the disease-free interval and survival remained unchanged. Disease-free interval was actually lower for patients treated with chemotherapy because of the local recurrences. Nevertheless, the larynx was preserved in 66% of surviving patients, although this represented only 31% of the entire group. At 3 years, 40% of the patients randomized to the chemotherapy arm were alive, disease free, and with an intact larynx (22). In addition, several randomized trials have shown that induction chemotherapy can improve survival for patients with unresectable disease. Taxanes also have been added to the treatment of advanced head and neck cancers in general, some of which are laryngeal primaries. These protocols have shown similar results, and the routine addition of taxanes is not standard at this time. Additional trials will be conducted to assess the ultimate indications for its addition.

One added feature of neoadjuvant therapy is that it allows monitoring of the initial response to treatment, leaving all conventional options open. In a retrospective review, Lecanu et al. (26) found that they were able to perform conservation surgery on some partial responders to chemotherapy who were initially deemed candidates for total laryngectomy. They found survival rates to be no less in this group than in the complete responder/radiation or total laryngectomy groups. Similarly, Laccourreye et al. (27), in a retrospective review of 60 patients, found that neoadjuvant chemotherapy allowed the mobilization of a fixed arytenoid in 10 patients. These patients then became amenable to supracricoid partial laryngectomy with cricohyoidopexy. Others have cautioned against the routine use of neoadjuvant chemotherapy because of the delay in definitive locoregional treatment.

Concomitant chemoradiation therapy has added an entirely new dimension to organ preservation. The chemotherapeutic agent acts as a radiation sensitizer while providing a systemic antineoplastic effect. The addition of chemotherapy to the radiation therapy markedly increases the toxicity in these patients, with high-grade toxicity noted in 82% of the patients receiving concurrent chemoradiotherapy compared with 61% in the radiation-only patients described by Forastiere et al. (14). The incidence of surgical complications in the patients in this trial did not, however, increase significantly in the chemotherapy groups (23). Adjuvant chemotherapy has not been shown to improve survival and is, therefore, rarely added to the treatment regimen. Nevertheless, it does not delay definitive therapy to the primary site and regional nodes because it is given after the "definitive" therapy.

Intraarterial chemotherapy, as described by Robbins et al. (28), allows delivery of very high doses of cisplatin, through angiographically placed microcatheters, to the tumor bed. Systemic effects are minimized by a concurrent intravenous administration of sodium thiosulfate, a chemotherapeutic rescue agent. Subsequently, they treated 29 patients with previously untreated stage IV head and neck cancer, five of whom had laryngeal cancer, with a regimen combining intraarterial cisplatin, intravenous sodium thiosulfate, and once-daily radiotherapy (total dose, 62 to 70 Gy). A pathologic complete response was seen in 23 of 24 evaluable patients. The local effects from this regimen can be severe, and a 41% rate of severe mucositis was seen in this patient group. Follow-up studies on larger cohorts of patients have confirmed both the efficacy and the toxicity of this treatment for head and neck cancer patients. The late toxicities of xerostomia and potentially severe dysphagia also must be addressed during the pretreatment counseling of these patients. All of these studies showed significant toxicities, and the ultimate ability of the physician and patient to tolerate and manage these complications will dictate the treatment course in any particular patient.

IMPROVING PROGNOSIS

Over the past quarter century, the survival rate for advanced laryngeal cancer has not significantly improved, despite advances in surgery and radiation therapy. The only method shown to increase cure is the earlier detection of tumors, with resulting lower staging, which can be achieved by defining the groups at risk (i.e., heavy smokers, tobacco chewers, and alcohol drinkers) and by performing screening laryngoscopy or evaluation at the initial appearance of symptoms. Heightened public awareness is mandatory for this to be accomplished and must include educating primary care physicians to avoid unnecessary delay—no symptoms of hoarseness should be present for more than 3 weeks before referral to a specialist.

Another area with potential for improved prognosis is the prevention or reversal of cellular alterations induced by carcinogens. This approach has been partially effective in various head and neck malignancies, including laryngeal cancer, with the use of vitamin A and β-carotene, which appear to stabilize squamous epithelium. The identification of persons at risk also may be possible by analysis of genetically controlled sensitivity to environmental carcinogens. For example, young adults with head and neck cancer have been shown to express increased susceptibility to mutagen-induced chromosome damage. Gene therapy, although in its infancy, holds some promise. Most studies show responses in only a small percentage of patients treated, but promise is seen in using gene therapy as an adjunctive modality. The combination of defining persons who are genetically susceptible, diminishing carcinogenic exposure, and promoting cancer inhibitors, in addition to offering effective treatment options, holds the best hope for improved survival and quality of life. The future also may allow therapies that alter the patient's genetic profile, rendering the patient less susceptible to cancer and more susceptible to other anticancer therapies. The study of a tumors' global gene expression, methylation status, or proteomic expression may ultimately prove the best way to stratify treatment regimens in the future, rather than relying on the rather crude staging parameters we are currently using.

COMPLICATIONS

Complications of Surgery

Surgical complications include hematoma, hypothyroidism, aspiration pneumonia, wound infection, hypocalcemia, and fistula (Table 122.6). Small pharyngocutaneous fistulae often close with local wound care and nasogastric or gastrostomy tube feeding, with the patient allowed nothing to eat by mouth until no further drainage is apparent. However, these fistulae will occasionally require adjuvant surgical procedures, which may include debridement and local closure, regional tissue transfer, or free tissue transfer to address chronic, nonhealing fistulae. We do not advocate the routine use of radiographic swallowing studies to determine when a patient can be fed orally. In general, patients who have not been previously irradiated can be safely fed on postoperative day 5 to 7, and those with prior irradiation, by postoperative day 7 to 10. Debate continues regarding the timing of oral feeding, with some authors advocating feeding as early as postoperative day 3 in uncomplicated cases, and others advocating delaying feeding for 10 to 14 days. This is largely an issue of personal preference and experience. Large fistulae or wound disruptions with or without

TABLE 122.6

SURGICAL COMPLICATIONS

Early
- Hematoma
- Aspiration pneumonia
- Wound infection
- Hypocalcemia
- Pharyngocutaneous fistula
- Chyle fistula
- Wound dehiscence
- Carotid artery exposure with blow-out
- Medical: pulmonary, cardiac, nutritional, electrolyte

Late
- Pharyngeal stricture
- Stomal stenosis
- Stomal recurrence
- Carotid blow-out
- Hypothyroidism

impending vascular rupture necessitate flap closure. One should assure no metabolic derangements, such as nutritional depletion or hypothyroidism, before additional surgical procedures. If such derangements are found, then they should be appropriately corrected.

Additional complications may be prophylactically addressed with appropriate medical intervention or surgical technique. Wound infections are best prevented with prophylactic antibiotics, which include coverage of anaerobic and aerobic bacteria found in the upper digestive tract. The carotid artery may be protected either by the sternocleidomastoid muscle or, in the case of radical dissections, a dermal graft or muscle flap, although these adjuncts are increasingly less common. Debate still exists regarding trifurcate incisions, with some advocating against them, and others in favor of their use when required. Those who argue against them contend that the vascularity of the trifurcation tips is compromised and therefore will lead to an increased incidence of wound breakdown/dehiscence at the trifurcation site. If a trifurcate incision is chosen, care must be taken to place the trifurcation away from the carotid artery, thus minimizing the chances of carotid exposure.

Late complications include pharyngeal stricture, stomal stenosis, and hypothyroidism. Tracheal stoma stenosis can be minimized by avoiding tension on the trachea, cutting the medial heads of the sternocleidomastoid muscle, beveling the transected trachea, and avoiding trauma to the stomal area with suctions and laryngectomy tubes. Infections and irradiation also predispose to stenosis. Strictures are best avoided by ensuring that enough tissue is available to prevent a tight pharyngeal closure. A regional or free flap should be considered whenever minimal mucosa remains after the resection, although as little as 3 cm of residual pharyngeal mucosa may provide an adequate closure.

Complications occur with increased frequency when surgery is performed for salvage after radiation treatment,

with the rate of postoperative complications as high as 60%. In a separate study of salvage laryngectomy, McCombe (29) found a 39% incidence of fistula, compared with 4% when surgery was done primarily. Poor surgical technique, a lack of meticulous tissue handling, prolonged surgery, poor nutritional status of the patient, advanced stage of the lesion, and extensive resection have all been shown to increase the likelihood of complications.

Complications of Radiation

The acute effects of radiation are numerous. They include hoarseness, edema, dysphagia, odynophagia, mucositis, thick secretions, and skin breakdown, all of which typically subside within 6 to 8 weeks after treatment ends. At times, these side effects can be so severe that they necessitate the interruption of treatment, which has a negative impact on overall prognosis. Recent trials with radioprotectants have demonstrated a decline in the frequency and severity of acute toxicities, such as mucositis, and late toxicities, such as xerostomia. In the future, such a focus on concurrent radioprotection of normal tissues, through pharmacologic agents or altered treatment schemes (intensity-modulated radiation therapy), may significantly reduce treatment-related complications. Late effects include chondronecrosis; fibrosis of skin, soft tissue, and mucous membranes; severe dryness; stricture; hypothyroidism; trismus; and rarely a secondary neoplasm such as a sarcoma. Persistent laryngeal edema, the most frequent late complication of radiation therapy, is related to the dose given, the volume treated, the size of the original tumor, the performance of a neck dissection, and the patient's continued use of cigarettes and alcohol. About 50% of patients complain of a lump in the throat from arytenoid edema. Chondronecrosis is a rare complication but should heighten the concern for persistent or recurrent cancer and may require a total laryngectomy, even if no tumor can be demonstrated in a biopsy specimen. Irradiated laryngeal tissue is susceptible to infection immediately after treatment and for the subsequent years. This is due to the poor blood supply to the cartilage, arteriosclerosis associated with aging, destruction caused by the prior tumor, and irradiation. The need for repeated biopsies to assess any recurrent tumor also may lead to perichondritis, which only compounds the problem and may result in the need for a total laryngectomy for functional reasons.

Emergency Surgery

If the patient is first seen with impending airway obstruction, a secure airway must be obtained immediately (Table 122.7). If possible, the patient should be orotracheally intubated awake, laser debulked, or tracheotomized under local anesthesia. Tracheotomy should be avoided if at all possible, because many studies from the 1960s and 1970s showed an increased incidence of stomal and peristomal recurrence after laryngectomy when a preoperative

TABLE 122.7 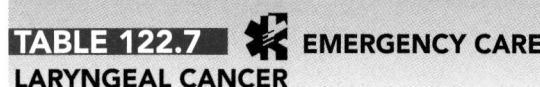 **EMERGENCY CARE LARYNGEAL CANCER**

Goal	Action
Airway control	Intubation with or without laser resection of endolaryngeal tumor is preferred
	Tracheotomy is performed if intubation is not possible
	"Emergency laryngectomy" is rarely done

or emergency tracheotomy had been performed. An opposing view was put forward by Rubin et al. (30), who demonstrated that preoperative and emergency tracheotomies were not related to stomal recurrence. Despite these findings, and because an increased incidence of stomal recurrence after endotracheal intubation has never been documented, we recommend avoiding emergency tracheotomy if endotracheal intubation is possible. An effective alternative is laser debulking, which will successfully restore the airway, provide tissue for diagnosis, and allow nonoperative definitive therapy without a tracheotomy. This may be performed with jet ventilation or after intubation with a small laser-safe endotracheal tube. Some surgeons have performed emergency laryngectomy in the setting of impending airway obstruction, although this is not recommended. No evidence of a decreased incidence of stomal recurrence has been presented with the use of this procedure; however, an emergency laryngectomy does not allow preoperative laboratory and imaging studies to be performed and does not properly prepare the patient for the loss of the larynx. Moreover, the surgeon must rely on a frozen-section pathologic diagnosis that can be inaccurate. A decision for total laryngectomy is made more safely on a diagnosis confirmed by permanent section.

HIGHLIGHTS

- Patients may accept a 20% decrease in overall survival to save their larynx.
- Vocal cord fixation implies invasion of the thyroarytenoid muscle and possibly the lateral and posterior cricoarytenoid and interarytenoid muscles, the cricoarytenoid joint, or perineural space.
- Careful preoperative evaluation requires complete endoscopy, histologic assessment of the extent of the tumor, and CT scans to assist in the evaluation of degree of invasion.
- Tracheotomy and emergency laryngectomy based solely on frozen-section diagnosis should be avoided.
- Partial laryngectomy based on oncologically sound principles can be performed for carefully selected patients with T3 (stage III) laryngeal carcinomas.

- Endoscopic laser partial laryngectomy is an alternative to manage T3 and selected T4a tumors, and may be selectively, and successfully, applied to cases of radiation failure.
- Organ preservation with a chemoradiation protocol or definitive radiation is an appropriate option for initial therapy, the choice of which is stage dependent.
- Total laryngectomy remains the accepted standard of treatment for advanced laryngeal cancer and should not be considered a defeatist option.
- Postoperative radiation therapy improves survival for advanced laryngeal cancer.
- Treatment of the neck for palpable or occult metastatic disease must be considered for all advanced laryngeal cancer.
- Postoperative complications increase with prior high-dose preoperative radiation therapy.
- Hypothyroidism can occur after surgery, radiation therapy, or both.
- Improved prognosis necessitates earlier diagnosis.

REFERENCES

1. McNeil BJ, Weichselbaum R, Pauker SG. Speech and survival: tradeoffs between quality and quantity of life in laryngeal cancer. *N Engl J Med* 1981;305:982–987.
2. Beitler JJ, Mahadevia PS, Silver CE, et al. New barriers to ventricular invasion in paraglottic laryngeal cancer. *Cancer* 1994;73:2648–2652.
3. Kirchner JA. *Atlas on the surgical anatomy of laryngeal cancer.* San Diego: Singular Publishing Group, 1998.
4. Ferlito A, Silver CE, Rinaldo A, et al. Surgical treatment of the neck in cancer of the larynx. *ORL* 2000;62:217–225.
5. Welkoborsky HJ, Hinni M, Dienes HP, et al. Predicting recurrence and survival patients with laryngeal cancer by means of DNA cytometry, tumor front grading, and proliferating markers. *Ann Otol Rhinol Laryngol* 1995;104:503–510.
6. Truelson JM, Fisher S, Beals TE, et al. DNA content and histologic growth pattern correlate with prognosis in patients with advanced squamous cell carcinoma of the larynx. *Cancer* 1992;70:56–62.
7. Bradford CR, Zhu S, Poore J, et al. p53 mutation as a prognostic marker in advanced laryngeal carcinoma. *Arch Otolaryngol Head Neck Surg* 1997;123:605–609.
8. Belbin TJ, Singh B, Barber I, et al. Molecular classification of head and neck squamous cell carcinoma using cDNA microarrays. *Cancer Res* 2002;62:1184–1190.
9. Cooper JS, Pajak TF, Forastiere AA, et al. Postoperative concurrent radiotherapy and chemotherapy for high-risk squamous-cell carcinoma of the head and neck. *N Engl J Med* 2004;350:1937–1944.
10. Bernier J, Domenge C, Ozsahin M, et al. Postoperative irradiation with or without concomitant chemotherapy for locally advanced head and neck cancer. *N Engl J Med* 2004;350:1945–1952.
11. Picarillo JF, Wells CK, Sasaki CT, et al. New clinical severity staging system for cancer of the larynx: five year survival rates. *Ann Otol Rhinol Laryngol* 1994;103:83–92.
12. AJCC. *AJCC Cancer staging manual,* 6th ed. New York: Springer, 2002.
13. McGuirt WF, Greven KM, Keyes JW, et al. Laryngeal radionecrosis versus recurrent cancer: a clinical approach. *Ann Otol Rhinol Laryngol* 1998;107:293–296.
14. Forastiere AA, Goepfert H, Maor M, et al. Concurrent chemotherapy and radiotherapy for organ preservation in advanced laryngeal cancer. *N Engl J Med* 2003;349:2091–2098.
15. Johansen LV, Grau C, Overgaard J. Supraglottic carcinoma: patterns of failure and salvage treatment after curatively intended

radiotherapy in 410 consecutive patients. *Int J Radiat Oncol Biol Phys* 2002;53:948–958.

16. Smith RV, Kotz T, Beitler JJ, et al. Long term swallowing problems following organ preservation therapy with concomitant radiation therapy and intravenous hydroxyurea: initial results. *Arch Otolaryngol Head Neck Surg* 2000;126:384–389.

17. Iro H, Waldfahrer F, Altendorf-Hofman A, et al.Transoral laser surgery of supraglottic cancer: follow-up of 141 patients. *Arch Otolaryngol Head Neck Surg* 1998;124:1245–1250.

18. Brazilian Head and Neck Cancer Study Group. End results of a prospective trial on elective lateral neck dissections vs. type III modified radical neck dissection in the management of supraglottic and transglottic carcinomas. *Head Neck* 1999;21:694–702.

19. Lutz CK, Johnson JT, Wagner RL, et al. Supraglottic carcinoma: patterns of recurrence. *Ann Otol Rhinol Laryngol* 1990;99:12–16.

20. Weems DH, Mendenhall WM, Parsons JT, et al. Squamous cell carcinoma of the supraglottic larynx treated with surgery and/or radiation therapy. *Int J Radiat Oncol Biol Phys* 1987;13:1483–1487.

21. Mercado G, Adelstein DJ, Saxton JP, et al. Hypothyroidism: a frequent event after radiotherapy and after radiotherapy with chemotherapy for patients with head and neck carcinoma. *Cancer* 2001;92:2892–2897.

22. Department of Veterans Affairs Laryngeal Cancer Study Group. Induction chemotherapy plus radiation compared with surgery plus radiation in patients with advanced laryngeal cancers. *N Engl J Med* 1991;324:1685–1690.

23. Weber RS, Berkey BA, Forastiere A, et al. Outcome of salvage total laryngectomy following organ preservation therapy: the radiation therapy oncology group trial 91-11. *Arch Otolaryngol Head Neck Surg* 2003;129:44–49.

24. Wang CC, Nakfoor BM, Spiro IJ, et al. Role of accelerated fractionated irradiation for supraglottic carcinoma: assessment of results. *Cancer J Sci Am* 1997;3:88–91.

25. Guedea F, Parsons JT, Mendenhall WM, et al. Primary subglottic cancer: results of radical radiation therapy. *Int J Radiat Oncol Biol Phys* 1991;21:1607–1611.

26. Lecanu JB, Monceaux G, Perie S, et al. Conservative surgery in T3-T4 pharyngolaryngeal squamous cell carcinoma: an alternative to radiation therapy and to total laryngectomy for good responders to induction chemotherapy. *Laryngoscope* 2000;110:412–416.

27. Laccourreye O, Brasnu D, Biacabe B, et al. Neo-adjuvant chemotherapy and supracricoid partial laryngectomy with cricohyoidopexy for advanced endolaryngeal carcinoma classified as T3-T4: 5-year oncologic results. *Head Neck* 1997;20:595–599.

28. Robbins KT, Storniolo AM, Hryniuk WM, et al. "Decadose" effects of cisplatin on squamous cell carcinoma of the upper aerodigestive tract, II: clinical studies. *Laryngoscope* 1996;106:37–42.

29. McCombe AW, Jones AS. Radiotherapy and complications of laryngectomy. *J Laryngol Otol* 1993;107:130–132.

30. Rubin J, Johnson JJ, Myers EM. Stomal recurrence after laryngectomy: interrelated risk factor study. *Otolaryngol Head Neck Surg* 1990;103:805.

Voice Rehabilitation after Laryngectomy

123

Mark I. Singer   Carla D. Gress

The operative procedure of total laryngectomy separates the airway from the digestive tract and establishes a permanent tracheostoma at the base of the neck. The pharynx is reconstituted by simply closing the mucosa or, in more complex cases, by interposing skin flaps to preserve an adequate lumen for swallowing. Although the process of swallowing is simplified without the larynx, sound production is lost. The threat of voicelessness has a profound and devastating effect on laryngeal cancer patients. Several voice-restoring methods have been proposed and are reviewed.

ANATOMY OF THE OPERATIVE DEFECT

Total laryngectomy or wide-field laryngectomy includes removal of the supraglottic larynx and hyoid bone, intrinsic larynx, portions of the pharynx, the strap muscles, one or more rings of the trachea, and part or all of the thyroid gland. The resection may include neck dissection, upper mediastinal lymph node dissection, and portions of the tongue base. The actual resection of the larynx requires entrance into the pharynx, determined by the location of the primary disease. It is desirable to make an entry away from the tumor and yet have complete visualization of the disease. The resulting defect, a pharyngotomy, consists of varying amounts of pharyngeal and esophageal mucosa, constrictor muscle remnants, and tongue base. The usual closure of this defect is primary. The geometry of closure ("T," "Y," "I," or horizontal suture line) is determined by the amount of residual tissue, resultant tension, and the surgeon's experience.

The usual approach to laryngectomy separates the pharyngeal constrictor muscles at the oblique line of the thyroid cartilage (Fig. 123.1). Specifically this includes the inferior pharyngeal constrictor and cricopharyngeus muscles. The separated constrictors are used as the third or external layer in the conventional three-layer closure of the pharynx. The junction of the pharynx and esophagus has been studied by speech pathologists as the sound source for alaryngeal speech and is called the "PE" segment, the pseudoglottis, or the CP (cricopharyngeus). It is difficult to predict resultant voice or quality because of variations in anatomy, tumor extent, muscle bulk, and operative technique. Pharyngeal closure after laryngectomy is generally concerned with controlling secretions, swallowing, and prevention of fistula formation. Recently, attention has been directed to alaryngeal voice acquisition and the possibilities for maximizing the results by changing the reconstructive technique (1,2).

MECHANICS OF VOICE RESTORATION

When the patient is healed and able to swallow after the laryngectomy, three possibilities for speech rehabilitation exist: the artificial larynx (electrolarynx), esophageal speech, and tracheoesophageal speech.

Artificial Larynx

The artificial larynx is an instrument that serves as a voicing source. The most common types are placed against a supple point on the neck and introduce a mechanical sound into the tissues and air spaces of the vocal tract. This sound, emanating from the mouth, is articulated by the structures of the remaining vocal tract (the tongue, lips, and teeth) as understandable speech. The artificial larynx is rapidly learned and does not delay or interfere with the acquisition of other forms of alaryngeal speech.

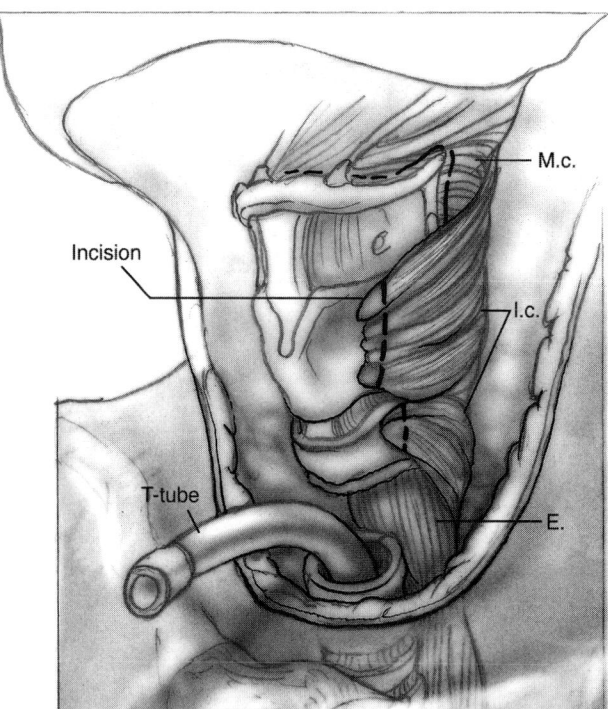

Figure 123.1 Separation of the pharyngeal constrictors from the larynx. *E*, esophagus; *Ic*, inferior constrictor; *Mc*, middle pharyngeal constrictor.

A second type of artificial larynx uses a tube adapter to direct the sound to the oral cavity, where it can be articulated with some reduction in intelligibility. This is useful for patients whose necks do not transmit the electrical sound or in the immediate postoperative period when the neck is healing. Most of the intraoral tube devices are electrically powered, although a few air-powered (pneumatic) instruments use the patient's exhaled air to activate a sound source of vibrating elastic bands. A newer device consists of an electric sound source that is housed in a denture and is activated by a hand control or by the tongue (3).

The artificial larynx or electrolarynx has the advantages of low cost, availability, short learning time, and loudness. Its disadvantages are the dependence on batteries, mechanical sound, conspicuous appearance, loss of hands-free speech, and hygiene of the intraoral tubes or dental appliance. It also relies on the use of batteries and is often not covered by insurance policies. Nevertheless, many laryngectomized patients use the artificial devices as the primary method for speech communication.

Esophageal Speech

Esophageal speech is another recommended method for alaryngeal speech rehabilitation, and variations of the technique have been known for more than 100 years. The most successful users (5% to 30% of laryngectomy patients) have natural voice quality with fluency and intelligibility, free of extraneous noise from the stoma or facial–oral gestures. The characteristic esophageal voice

is low in fundamental frequency (~65 Hz), is of short duration, and requires some effort to produce. The patient learns to insufflate the esophagus, usually under the direction of a speech pathologist or another patient with a laryngectomy. The most common method involves trapping air in the mouth or pharynx and then injecting it into the esophagus by the propulsive action of the tongue. The air may be stored in the esophagus and the stomach. With diaphragmatic effort, the air refluxes through the esophagus and crosses the upper esophageal sphincter. The mucosa of this region is vibrated by the released air and produces a characteristic belch-like sound. This sound issues from the mouth, in similar fashion to that from the artificial larynx, and is articulated by the tongue, lips, and teeth. Rapid repetitive movements of injection and release produce fluent and understandable speech.

In the second method for esophageal speech insufflation, the patient relaxes the upper esophageal sphincter and introduces air into the esophagus by inhaling during the increased negative intrathoracic pressure of inspiration. This is less common than the injection method and is characterized by breathy voice quality and less intensity. Successful esophageal speech is preferred to the artificial larynx because it is less conspicuous and does not require the use of hands, is more natural sounding, and the patient is independent of devices. The critical problem with esophageal speech is its low acquisition rate and the extended learning period.

Shunts and Valves

From the time of the first laryngectomies, it was known that tracheal air during exhalation can be shunted to the pharynx or esophagus through a planned fistula or tract, and this pulmonary-driven insufflation can produce effective speech (Figs. 123.2 and 123.3) (4–6). The same principles of speech production apply with articulation at the oral cavity and sound produced in the upper esophageal sphincter. The shunts, however, introduced a new series of problems that limited their wide application. Particularly after radiation, mucosal-lined tracts are difficult to maintain, and patency is compromised by stenosis at the level of the tracheal or pharyngeal meatus. Continued salivary flow through them often causes inflammation, breakdown, and sometimes necrosis. Patency of the shunt to tolerate airflow at resistances of 35 to 45 cm H_2O/LPS for natural speech production also allows salivary reflux into the trachea. Chronic salivary soiling of the upper airway with tracheoesophageal shunts makes their use hazardous in patients with compromised pulmonary reserve.

For this reason, some investigators developed mechanical valves to divert the secretions from the trachea or attempted to devise biologic valves (sphincters) for airway protection (Fig. 123.4) (3). Most of these efforts failed because of valve incontinence or stenosis. Radiation therapy is a relative contraindication to techniques that rely on tissue valving.

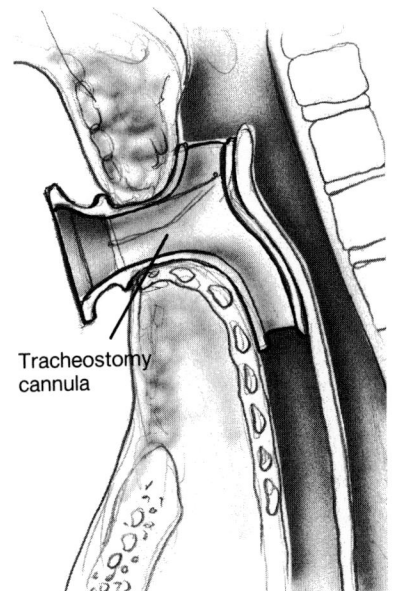

Figure 123.2 Modified tracheostomy cannula for air diversion to the pharynx.

Prosthetic replacements for the larynx had a brief lifespan in the early 1960s. Synthetic valves of Teflon or Dacron were sewn into canine tracheas, but these procedures failed because of the inability to place prosthetic material in a contaminated airway for long-term incorporation and the failure to clear the secretions effectively from the valves and trachea.

Duckbill Voice Prosthesis

The creation of a successful, surgical voice-restoration technique did not occur until the introduction of the tracheoesophageal puncture (TEP) by Singer and Blom in 1979.

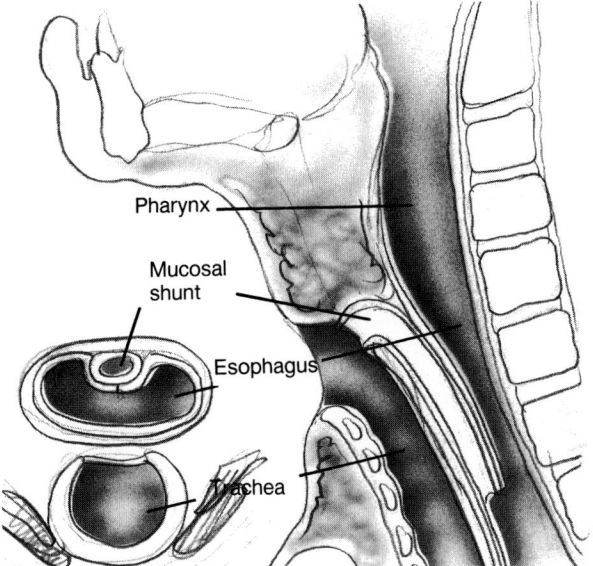

Figure 123.3 Mucosal shunt for voice restoration proposed by Conley.

It was proposed as a secondary salvage technique for those who failed to produce esophageal speech or those who were displeased with the electrolarynx voice. A removable silicone tube was developed in 1978 that would maintain an endoscopically placed tracheoesophageal puncture and would serve as a one-way valve (Figs. 123.5 and 123.6) (7). The design called for a simple valve that was biologically compatible, removable, and inexpensive. The initial caliber was 3.3 mm (14 French), and the simplest valve concept was a slit through the long axis of the tube. The end opposite the stent/valve was open with a second window on the inferior (ventral) surface.

This early voice prosthesis was called a "duckbill" valve to describe the action of the slit valve, and it became known as the "duckbill voice prosthesis." The silicone tube was well tolerated by the trachea and esophagus, with a low incidence of foreign-body reaction. A retention collar was added to the valve end to maintain its position in the puncture tract.

The puncture can be placed primarily (at the time of laryngectomy) or secondarily (after laryngectomy) without contraindication of radiation therapy. The puncture permits a direct midline communication from the posterior trachea to the anterior esophagus at a location inferior to the cricopharyngeus muscle and pharyngeal constrictor muscles. The location at the tracheostoma permits direct visibility for the patient and clinician.

The prosthesis functions by allowing exhaled air to enter the esophagus. After the esophageal reservoir is filled, a continuous air stream flows superiorly toward the pharynx and vibrates the mucosa of the upper esophageal segment, producing sound. This is an intense sound and is continuous because of the efficiency of the respiratory system to maintain volume and pressure for voice. When phonation is finished and airflow stops, the valve slit closes and prevents pharyngeal secretions from entering the airway. Taking advantage of the mechanics of normal breathing, the patient can vary voicing efforts, and more natural phrasing is possible. Measurements of intensity, fundamental frequency, and speaking rate confirm that tracheoesophageal speech is more acoustically similar to normal laryngeal speech and is more intelligible and acceptable than standard esophageal speech (8–10). Initially, patients learn to cover the tracheostoma manually, and with varying pressure, they achieve a fluent voice with little air escape or masking noise.

A second valve was later developed for closing the tracheostoma for phonation (11). The higher airflows for tracheoesophageal voice production close a curled valve diaphragm against a plastic housing. With normal respiration, two-way flow through the valve is possible. This allows natural speech that is inconspicuous without the hands and is quieter. The tracheostoma valve can be attached by using an adhesive to the peritracheal skin or to a silicone tube (laryngectomy tube) that is inserted into the tracheostoma (12). Use of a tracheostoma valve

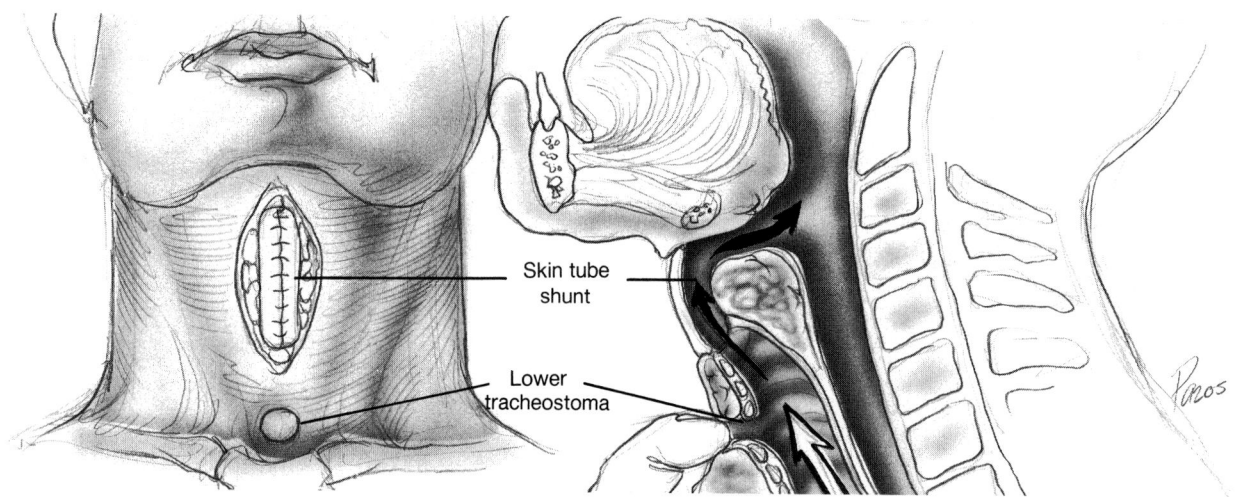

Figure 123.4   Skin tube shunt from the trachea to the hypopharynx (Asai procedure).

requires varying intratracheal pressures. It cannot be used in patients who have impaired respiratory function, such as chronic obstructive pulmonary disease. The adhesive attachment of the tracheostoma housing requires a meticulous technique to ensure a long-lasting seal. Although desirable, the tracheostoma valve is effective for only 25% to 30% of the laryngectomized population (13).

The early experience and a growing population of tracheoesophageal speakers rapidly accrued a group of voice failures estimated at 25% to 40% (the numbers varied depending on the criteria for successful voice acquisition)

(14). A proposed solution was the development of a low-pressure voice prosthesis (8) (Fig. 123.7). The design consideration was to reduce airflow resistance to that of the larynx itself (30 cm H_2O/LPS), which requires less effort for voicing. A further refinement has been to increase the diameter of the prosthesis from the standard 16F to 20F, permitting increased airflow with a resultant increase in loudness. Numerous prosthetic devices are currently on the market, including in-dwelling prostheses, designed to meet individualized patient requirements for aerodynamic characteristics, length of wear, ease of insertion, and prevention of aspiration.

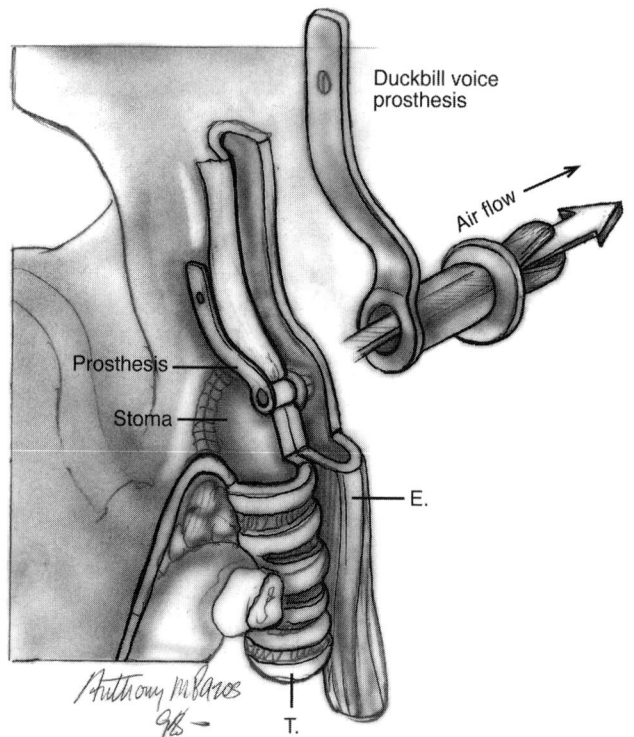

Figure 123.5   Duckbill (slit-valve) voice prosthesis.

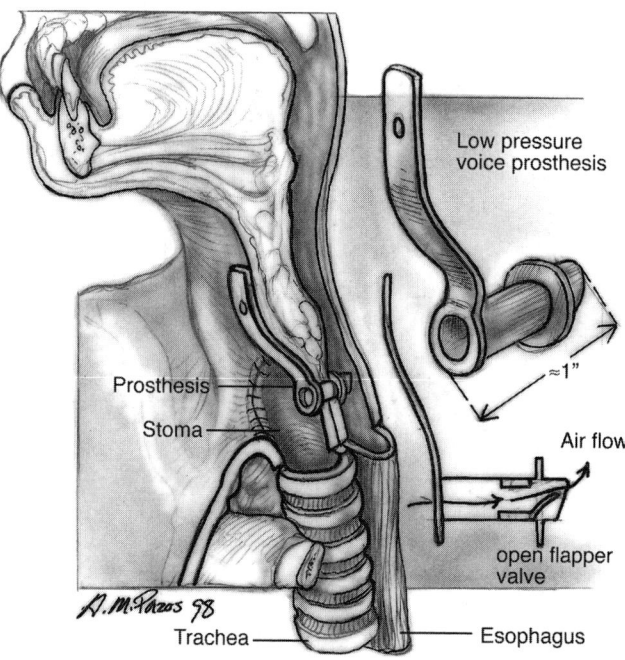

Figure 123.6   Voice prosthesis in place in the tracheoesophageal puncture.

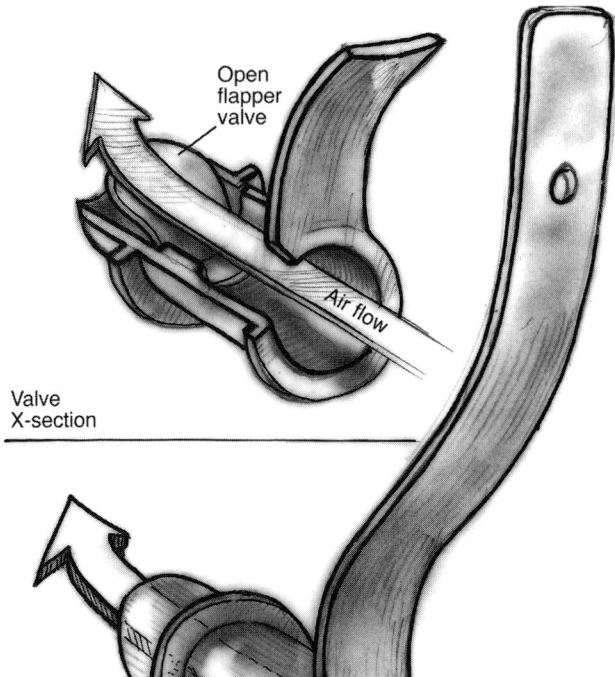

Figure 123.7 Low-pressure (trap-valve) voice prosthesis.

PATIENT EVALUATION FOR SECONDARY TRACHEOESOPHAGEAL PUNCTURE CANDIDACY

In the general survey of the laryngectomized patient, the initial stage of disease, operative technique, use of radiation therapy, and reconstruction methods should be noted. The patient's health, age, and physical status are assessed. Relative concerns that may reduce the success of voice restoration are pharyngeal stricture with symptomatic dysphagia, radiation therapy exceeding 6,500 cGy, malnutrition, diabetes, dementia, and severe chronic obstructive pulmonary disease.

The physical examination includes a careful head and neck examination with attention to stomal hygiene, patient's dexterity, as well as overall motivation and interest in voice restoration. The patient's inability to use and care for the prosthesis due to impaired mental status or decrease in manual dexterity due to age, arthritis, or neurologic insult/disease has been overcome with the introduction of the indwelling prosthesis. Bilateral severe sensorineural hearing loss and limited pulmonary function are also relative contraindications to TEP because the patient cannot hear the TE voice, and limited pulmonary air restricts the fluency and volume of speech, respectively (6).

The stoma should be free of a cannula if possible and at least 1.0 cm in one dimension. Microstomia makes it difficult to place the prosthesis and may compromise the airway because of the prosthesis size. If microstoma exists, the stoma should be dilated and stented with a laryngectomy tube or revised by Z-plasty. Patients who have undergone

radiation therapy whose tissues appear to be at risk are better managed by the former method. However, the posterior wall of a laryngectomy tube can be fenestrated to allow the use of voice prosthesis and laryngectomy tube together.

A preoperative esophageal insufflation test is important in predicting the likelihood of successful secondary tracheoesophageal speech. It estimates the possibility of dysfluency from pharyngeal constrictor spasm (15,16). The TEP crosses the upper tracheostoma and enters the esophagus inferior to the reconstituted cricopharyngeus muscle and upper esophageal sphincter. The distention of the esophagus that occurs with air ingestion results in a reflexive increase in tone in the pharyngeal constrictor muscles. This finding was described in early manometric studies of the region in normal, nonlaryngectomized patients (17). Insufflation of the esophagus in the clinical setting requires placement of a catheter through the nose into the upper esophagus. Air is introduced into the esophagus either by an external source or by adapting the tube to a special connector fixed to the tracheostoma. After air enters the esophagus and is released, voice production and connected speech are attempted, which may result in sound (i.e., ah, a low-pitched rumble, or eructation) or in a series of connected words, as in counting. The fluency of speech should be assessed carefully, observing any air trapping, which, if complete, will cause gastric filling, distention, discomfort, and even vagal syncope. One of four responses is obtained after the insufflation test: fluent, sustained voice production with minimal effort indicating relaxed pharyngoesophageal muscles; a breathy, hypotonic voice indicating the absence of pharyngeal constrictor muscle tone; hypertonic voice characterized by intermittent production of effortful speech with gastric distention and posttrial burping; and spasm characterized by no production of voice even with substantial pulmonary air flow. Despite these possible responses to esophageal insufflation, no definitive guidelines exist for successful duration of speech, airflow, or desirable pressures (pharyngeal or intratracheal). Some patients may have increased pharyngeal constrictor tonicity during tracheoesophageal voicing, but no reliable data show the incidence of patients who will succeed despite equivocal catheter insufflation testing. Furthermore, dysfluency on insufflation testing may be due to causes unrelated to pharyngoesophageal spasm, including postradiation tissue edema or the presence of recurrent disease. Therefore esophageal insufflation testing may be considered a subjective evaluation of esophageal distention and should not be used as the sole method for determining the need for open-neck exploration and pharyngeal constrictor relaxation.

Pharyngoesophageal spasm, suspected with a dysfluent speech pattern on insufflation testing, may be confirmed by anesthetic block of the pharyngeal plexus. The most effective method for analysis combines radiographic assessment with a plexus block. The patient is evaluated by videofluoroscopy with a barium-coated pharynx and

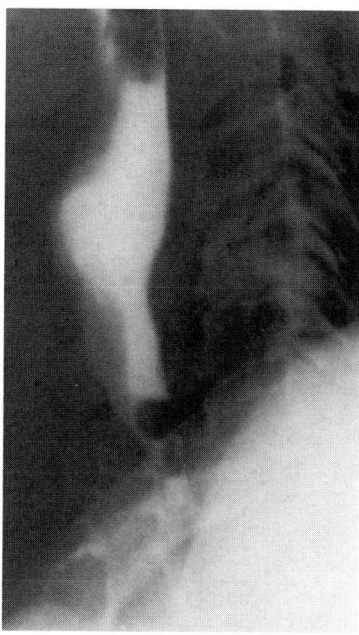

Figure 123.8 Lateral radiograph demonstrating the constrictor mass during esophageal distention. (Reprinted from Singer MI, Blom ED. A selective myotomy for voice restoration after total laryngectomy. *Arch Otolaryngol* 1981;107:670–673; with permission.)

esophagus; the lateral view is preferred. An at-rest view is first obtained to review the morphology of the neo-pharynx and to rule out stricture, fistula tract, or persistent neoplasm. Several views during voicing are taken. The pharynx is examined for the mass of constrictors, seen in the retropharyngeal radiographic plane as a bar (Fig. 123.8) (18). Note the axial length with reference to the proximity to the tongue base and its overall breadth.

The study is followed by the pharyngeal plexus block with local anesthesia (150 to 200 mg of 2% lidocaine without epinephrine). The anesthetic is injected with a 23-gauge, 1.5-inch needle placed at the level of the pre-vertebral fascia and then extracted 1 to 2 mm before injection. The neck skin is entered at the level of C2–C3 immediately parapharyngeal and medial to the carotid sheath. After 3 to 5 minutes, the patient is instructed to attempt voicing, which is nearly always effective, effort-less, and fluent. The voicing dynamics are now analyzed by fluoroscopy. The typical appearance shows a reduc-tion in the mass of the constrictor muscles, including the axial length. In effect, the pinchcock effect of the con-strictors during esophageal distention is temporarily blocked by the anesthetic and is readily documented by the radiographic examination. This indicates that the use of botulinum toxin A, pharyngeal constrictor myotomy, or pharyngeal plexus neurectomy will most likely be suc-cessful in treating pharyngoesophageal spasm.

Secondary voice restoration should be delayed until 6 weeks after laryngectomy, 6 to 8 weeks after postope-rative radiation therapy, or until the peristomal skin has

recovered from radiation toxicity, and at least 1 month after recovery from reconstruction of a total laryngophary-ngectomy or total laryngopharyngoesophagectomy defect and adjunctive therapies. Patients after reconstruction sho-uld also undergo barium swallow to evaluate the reconstr-uctive changes and the presence of a stricture.

DIFFERENTIAL DIAGNOSIS

The diagnostic problem is to evaluate voice failures after TEP (Table 123.1). The largest percentage of patients is the group who reflexively elevate the upper esophageal sphincter pressure during esophageal distention above the threshold for voice fluency. The patients may be capable of only a few syllables, a fluent "ah" or counting up to only 5 or 6, but also may exhibit considerable effort to voice, with the characteristic appearance and results of the Valsalva maneuver. Some patients initially demonstrate the Valsalva pattern. By using breath control and internal feed-back, they can reduce esophageal distention and the resultant upper esophageal sphincter tonicity.

This dysfluent speech pattern may change over a 4- to 6-week period, but if it has not improved (and ≥15% to 25% will not change), further investigation and possible intervention are required. Voice is reassessed by the open-tract test, in which the voice prosthesis is removed and the patient tries to speak. This is successful in only a few patients, which demonstrates that the failure is the result of the unfavorable mechanics of the voice prosthesis. The device may be too long or too short. Confirmation of cor-rect fitting length can be assessed by flexible endoscopic evaluation of the esophagus while the patient is asked to prolong phonation. If the voice retains a strained quality after assuring a proper fit, switching to a prosthesis with low-resistance characteristics and larger diameter (20F) helps reduce the resistance to airflow and results in less effort for most patients.

The patient with persistent voice failure with the open-tract test should be evaluated systematically by using video fluoroscopic examination and pharyngeal constrictor local anesthetic block. It is unusual for voice failure to occur from a morphologic abnormality of the pharynx or stricture or

---

TABLE 123.1
EVALUATION OF TRACHEOESOPHAGEAL SPEECH FAILURE

Prosthesis failure: position, size, type, patency
Reflex pharyngeal constricture spasm
Nonvibrating pharyngoesophageal segment: radiation-induced, edema, reconstructed segment
Puncture closure
Inadequate air supply: decreased respiratory support, improper stoma occlusion

the angle of the prosthesis. If the air is directed to the distal esophagus, it will regurgitate superiorly to the pharynx as the esophagus distends. If the pharynx is tubular and rigid (common with skin-flap pharyngeal reconstruction), the voice may be breathy or whisper-like. Myocutaneous flap reconstructions are characterized by decreased pitch, judged as "wet," and can be slow to initiate because of the inertia introduced by the bulk of the flap (19,20).

The free microvascular transfer of a segment of jejunum represents another problem. The segment of intestine is often redundant and traps air and secretions. This also is complicated by the intrinsic tonicity of the intestine, which impedes free egress of air across the grafted segment. Although a myotomy of the jejunal wall has been suggested, evidence of its efficacy remains to be documented. Although gastric transposition introduces mechanical complexity at the level of the tracheostoma, no increased risks have been described by puncture at this level into the stomach. The resultant airflow is unimpeded, and the pitch is low, with a characteristic hollow voice (21).

SURGICAL TECHNIQUE

The TEP is readily established secondarily by using an endoscopic technique (4). A rigid esophagoscope is introduced with the patient under general anesthesia through the laryngectomized pharynx and into the upper thoracic esophagus (Fig. 123.9). Mucosal irregularity, stricture, or ulceration at the level of the cervical esophagus should be noted. At the tracheostoma, the esophagoscope is rotated 180 degrees from introduction, with the longer side of the bevel now opposed to the posterior trachea. A window on this surface facilitates the puncture.

The membranous trachea is palpated through the stoma, ensuring that the esophagoscope is against the posterior trachea. Transillumination of the trachea is not usually helpful for the precise placement of the puncture. A puncture location is identified 5 mm from the superior trachea, and the window on the esophagoscope is aligned with this point. A 14-gauge needle is curved and introduced through the wall of the trachea, corresponding with the endoscope window. Direct vision through the esophagoscope allows direction of the needle into the lumen of the endoscope. Puncture of the posterior esophageal wall and its possible sequelae are prevented by the posterior wall of the esophagoscope.

With the needle in place, a 16-gauge intravenous catheter is threaded through the needle until the catheter is retrieved at the mouth. The needle is withdrawn, and with the catheter in place as a guide, the puncture is dilated carefully with a small hemostat. The catheter is attached to a urethral catheter (14F), filiform, or other gradually tapered device. With continuous traction at the mouth, the intravenous catheter/dilating catheter is pulled retrograde through the esophagus and hypopharynx, "trailing" the esophagoscope into the oral cavity. At this point, the intravenous catheter is released, and it must be ensured that no significant bleeding is present; then the esophagoscope is reinserted. The integrity of the anterior esophageal wall at the site of the puncture is examined, and, with the tip of the endoscope, the dilating catheter is directed into the distal esophagus. A suture is placed at the lateral tracheostoma to tie the dilating catheter in place.

The patient may be released on an ambulatory basis and permitted to resume a normal diet. Neither analgesics nor antibiotics are used. The patient can use an electrolarynx or limited esophageal voice. The stoma requires increased hygiene, and increased tracheal secretions are expected. In some cases, a temporary laryngectomy may be inserted for better stoma maintenance. The prosthesis is usually fitted in 2 days.

Fitting and placement of the voice prosthesis is simple. The first step in fitting is to remove the dilating catheter from the puncture that was placed in the operating room, and serially dilate the puncture by using catheters to 18F to ease placement of the measuring device, and measure the distance across the puncture (Fig. 123.10). The vocal tract

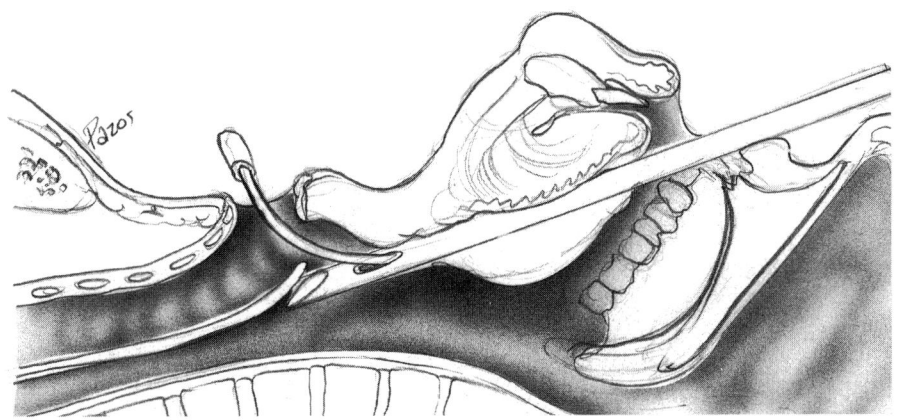

Figure 123.9 Endoscopic voice restoration (tracheoesophageal puncture).

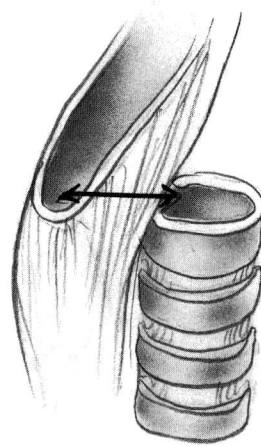

Figure 123.10 Fitting distance from the posterior trachea to the anterior esophagus.

is tested before placing the prosthesis by covering the tracheostoma and introducing air with exhalation. Patients will voice easily, and most will be capable of connected speech. The second step is the actual insertion of the voice prosthesis. The prosthesis is fixed to an inserter and introduced into the puncture at an angle corresponding to the presentation of the retention collar, end on. The collar will pass with slight resistance into the esophageal lumen; when fully entered, it will unfold, and a locking sensation is detectable.

The voice prosthesis is oriented by vertical placement of the silicone strap above the tracheostoma. It is fixed to the skin with paper adhesive tape. Efforts to produce and sustain voice may now begin with the prosthesis in position. The next steps vary from patient to patient and include instruction in careful stoma occlusion for efficient airflow, proper hygiene practices and management of secretions, varying breath control and diaphragmatic pressure, diminishing injection behavior from esophageal voice, experience with prosthesis cleaning and replacement, and guidelines for emergency situations. Long-term success in voice restoration requires that the patient fully comprehend the importance of maintaining the puncture at all times and diligently observing the prosthesis for signs of failure.

The initial prosthesis design required that it be removed and cleaned daily. However, this placed a great responsibility on the patient, possibly contributing to failure and complications, particularly in those with limited dexterity. Several indwelling devices with improved retention capabilities have been introduced more recently. The physician or speech pathologist must perform placement, because the insertion and removal techniques can be traumatizing to the tissues, and special instruments are sometimes required. The prosthesis remains in place and is cleaned externally until a new prosthesis is needed. Candidiasis results in premature failure of the prosthesis (usually valve degradation with aspiration of liquids through the prosthesis) but can be managed effectively with nystatin oral suspension (22).

TABLE 123.2

MANAGEMENT OF DYSFLUENT SPEECH

Use correct-size prosthesis with optimal airflow characteristics
Perform pharyngeal constrictor myotomy, neurectomy, or Botox injection
Allow edema to subside, provide external pressure
Dilate the puncture or repuncture
Speech therapy

Patients with persistent pharyngoesophageal spasm after a successful primary or secondary TEP can be secondarily treated with a pharyngeal constrictor myotomy (Table 123.2) (14), a pharyngeal constrictor neurectomy, or botulinum toxin A injection to reduce the tonicity of the upper esophageal sphincter. The myotomy is undertaken with a dilator (36F) in place in a manner analogous to a cricopharyngeal myotomy for dysphagia in patients with an intact larynx. Complications of this procedure are few but include salivary leakage and fistula formation, hypotonic voice, and esophageal reflux.

A secondary pharyngeal constrictor neurectomy (23) is approached in a fashion similar to the pharyngeal constrictor myotomy. The pharynx is distended with a mercury-filled dilator. Surgery is performed on the opposite side of the neck if a previous radical neck dissection has occurred. The parapharyngeal tissues are dissected to the level of the prevertebral fascia. The pharynx is rotated away from the carotid sheath, exposing the posterolateral wall of the pharyngoesophagus.

A careful dissection of the fascia overlying the constrictor muscles is done, directing the dissection superiorly to the base of the tongue, where a key landmark is encountered, the middle pharyngeal constrictor muscle. The main branches of the pharyngeal plexus are found at the junction of the middle and inferior pharyngeal constrictor muscles, where they course before dividing and innervating the underlying constrictor muscle fibers. When the branches of the pharyngeal plexus are stimulated, a fine contraction in the constrictor muscles is produced that moves from superior to inferior. After the pharyngeal plexus is identified, which represents one to three nerve branches at this level, the fibers are electrocoagulated and divided. The procedure is performed unilaterally. The wound is then drained away from the stoma and closed. The patient may resume a normal postoperative diet, and speech rehabilitation may begin the following day.

Botulinum toxin A may be injected under electromyographic guidance or fluoroscopy into the pharyngeal constrictor muscles to correct spasm (24). Its effect usually occurs within 72 hours after injection and may require repeated injections approximately every 6 months. This method is the preferred method of choice for most patients, particularly for poor surgical candidates and for those who do not wish additional surgery.

VOICE RESTORATION DURING LARYNGECTOMY

Maves and Lingeman (25) and Hamaker et al. (26) were the first to introduce TEP as a primary technique at the time of laryngectomy. Patient-selection criteria are essentially the same as those for secondary TEP. If a patient is indecisive regarding primary TEP, a puncture can be performed and then allowed to close if the patient does not wish TE speech. Placing a TEP primarily requires the careful construction of the tracheostoma and a pharyngeal constrictor relaxation procedure. The surgical steps include incision (laryngectomy), followed by tracheostoma construction, TEP, unilateral pharyngeal constrictor myotomy or pharyngeal plexus neurectomy, and buttressing the tracheoesophageal party wall (26).

After laryngectomy, the stoma is constructed. The optimal tracheal diameter is ≥3 cm to prevent stenosis. The midline inferior skin flap is sewn to the midline anterior tracheal ring by using half vertical mattress sutures, which allow coverage of the cartilage. Interrupted sutures are placed at 5-mm intervals on either side of the midline, pulling the trachea laterally. This creates a straight, horizontal membranous trachea, which is sewn to the superior skin flap. If the trachea is smaller than 3.0 cm, a stomaplasty is performed (27).

The TEP is placed after the stoma is constructed and before the pharynx is closed (26). The upper tracheal rings are fixed anteriorly and inferiorly to the skin flap rather than through a concentric skin defect. After stabilizing the tracheostoma, a right-angled hemostat is placed against the membranous trachea 1 cm from the tracheal edge by way of the open pharynx (Fig. 123.11). The membranous trachea is incised transversely for 3 to 4 mm to permit the tips of the hemostat to protrude into the tracheostoma. The tracheoesophageal common wall should not be separated; if this occurs, it should be closed to prevent saliva from dissecting into this space. The tip of the hemostat is used to direct a 16F silicone Foley catheter into the esophagus to serve as a stent for the TEP and as a convenient feeding tube.

Management of the pharyngeal constrictor muscles to prevent pharyngeal spasm is the key to successful TE speech. A very reliable method for preventing spasm, if done properly, is a pharyngeal constrictor myotomy. The pharynx is rolled over a tubular structure, most often a finger or dilator, and the muscles are incised vertically in the posterior midline of the pharynx from the level of the puncture to the tongue base. The muscles are cut to the level of the submucosa. If bleeding occurs, careful use of bipolar cautery is recommended. If an inadvertent pharyngotomy is made, the mucosa is repaired at this time. If flap reconstruction of the pharynx is performed, the segment of muscle from the puncture site to the inferior flap is myotomized (26,27).

An alternative method that can be performed to prevent pharyngeal spasm is a unilateral pharyngeal plexus

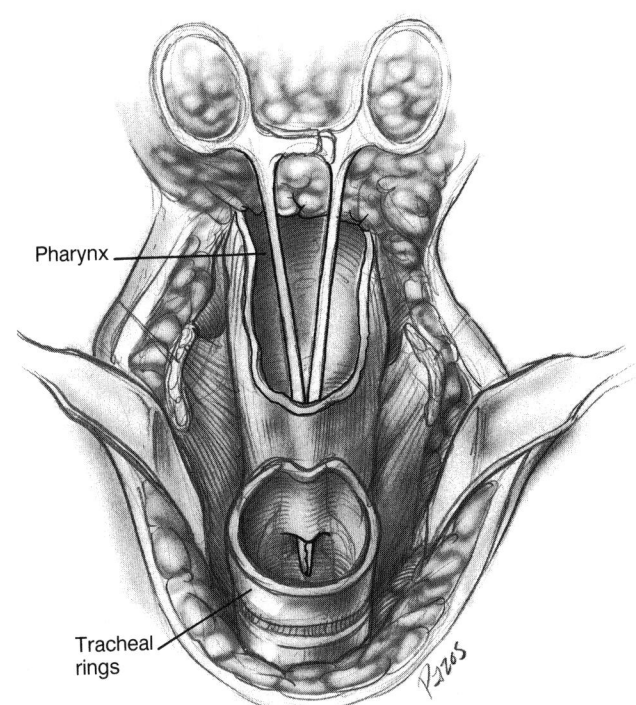

Figure 123.11 Primary placement of the tracheoesophageal puncture via the pharyngotomy.

neurectomy (10). The neurectomy is less traumatic to the pharyngeal wall, effectively reduces the increase in wall tension (sphincter spasm) during esophageal distention, and preserves the elasticity and vascularity of the constrictor muscles. This is performed after neck dissection while the larynx is in place (Fig. 123.12). The cornu of the thyroid cartilage and the greater cornu of the hyoid bone form a space that includes the middle pharyngeal constrictor muscle and the muscular hiatus through which the plexus fibers travel. The nerves are electrically stimulated for identification, coagulated, and divided as previously mentioned. This method also is useful when the pharynx is already closed and a myotomy was inadvertently not performed.

The party wall usually separates ~3 to 5 mm above the site of the puncture. The party wall is buttressed by using interrupted sutures of 3-0 chromic or 4-0 vicryl, which obliterates this space. This prevents the collection of saliva in this area if a fistula develops and helps to maintain the integrity of the posterior stoma. If separation of the party wall extends below the area of the planned puncture, then the puncture is delayed, as this can lead to pocket formation with abscess and loss of the posterior tracheal wall (26,27).

RESULTS

Many variables have been studied by various clinicians to predict those patients who will achieve successful TE speech with primary or secondary puncture. However, no consensus has been reached among these studies. We reviewed 128 patients over a 9-year period who had under-gone primary

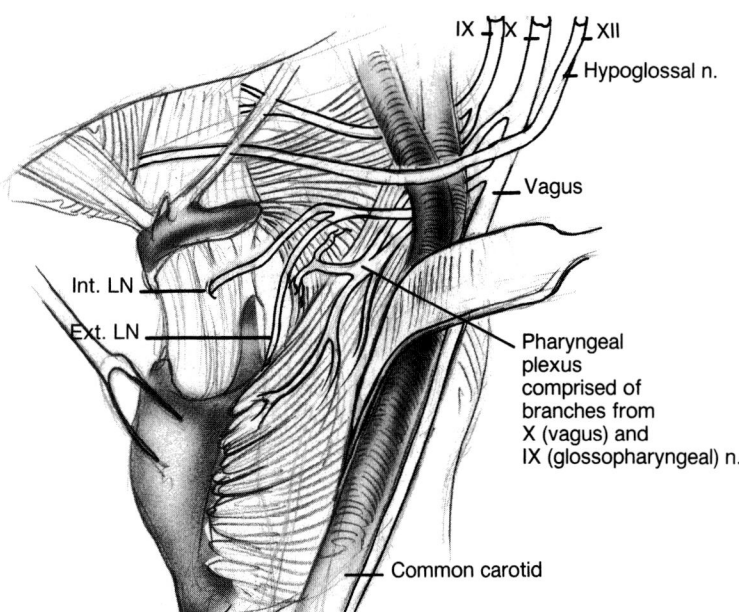

Figure 123.12 Surgical anatomy of the pharyngeal plexus during laryngectomy.

voice restoration during laryngectomy (20). Two 4-year periods were analyzed. In the earlier group of 48 patients, 29% experienced voice failure, which was reduced to 13% by revision procedures. The more current group failed 15% of the time, with revision reducing it to 9%. This finding represents an improving trend for voice rehabilitation, with the development of improved voice prostheses, more effective patient training, and refinement of the operative techniques. Speech after laryngectomy was successful 10 to 35 days postoperatively (average, 22 days). Tracheostoma stenosis occurred in 4%, and closure of the TEP occurred in 10% of cases because of extrusion of the prosthesis, radiation therapy, or inadequate stoma hygiene (Table 123.3).

The shape of the low-pressure voice prosthesis (trapdoor valve) has introduced a problem that has affected the acceptability of this device. The tapered or obturator tip of the duckbill prosthesis gave way in the

new design to a short bevel and retention collar, which complicated insertion of the prosthesis into the lumen of the esophagus. In many cases, the retention collar resides within the lumen of the puncture tract itself, producing a scarred ridge anterior to the meatus of the esophageal puncture. Stenosis of the esophageal meatus, difficult voicing, and eventual extrusion of the prosthesis may occur with closure of the fistula. Insertion can be eased by placing the prosthesis tip and the folded retention collar into half of a gelatin capsule, thus creating a rounded tip for introduction into the puncture tract. Some prostheses bypass these insertion problems by using retrograde introduction of the prosthesis via a special guidewire or catheter.

Other puncture problems include tracheal granulation tissue (treated with cautery or laser), prolapse of esophageal mucosa through the TEP, or leakage at the TEP and aspiration. Aspiration of the prosthesis itself has occurred in 3% to 5% of users and is prevented by careful instruction and modification of the method for patient insertion or by using the indwelling devices. The significant problem and hazard of aspiration through the TEP is usually managed by reconstructing the tracheoesophageal common wall by interposing a sternocleidomastoid muscle flap (Fig. 123.13) or, in heavily irradiated patients, placing a pectoralis major myofascial flap (20).

Voice Quality

It is important for potential TE speech users to have realistic expectations. The goal of voice restoration is to provide fluent, effortless, and intelligible speech. The quality of voice cannot be controlled. Patients should realize that a learning curve is associated with TE speech, and it generally improves over time (28).

TABLE 123.3 **C COMPLICATIONS**

Epidural abscess or vertebral osteomyelitis secondary to violation of posterior esophageal wall during secondary tracheoesophageal puncture (TEP)
Mediastinitis secondary to dissection of party wall
Loss of the puncture site by dislodgment of the catheter placed at the time of puncture
Partial or complete extrusion of the prosthesis
Migration of the puncture site
Formation of granulation tissue
Stomal or pharyngoesophageal stenosis
TEP dilation
Aspiration of saliva and foods through puncture site
Esophageal prolapse
Tracheostoma prolapse

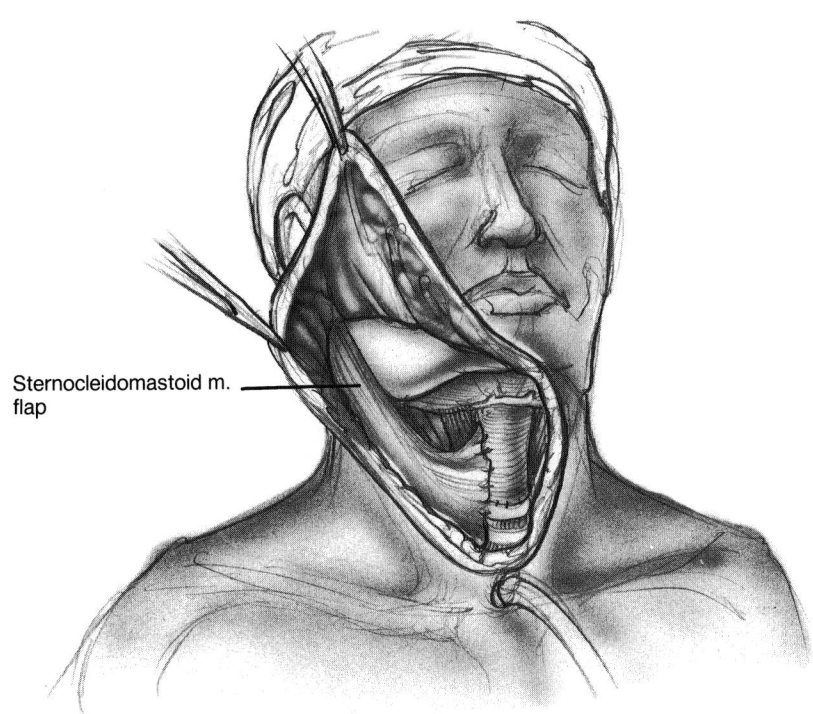

Sternocleidomastoid m.
flap

Figure 123.13 Sternocleidomastoid muscle flap augmentation of the tracheoesophageal common wall.

Acoustic analysis of TE speech has been compared with laryngeal, esophageal, and electrolarynx speech by many. The fundamental frequency, intensity, and rate of TE speech approximate those of normal speech. In a study by Robbins et al. (29), esophageal and TE speakers were analyzed for intensity, frequency, and rate of speech production. TE speech was found to be more similar to laryngeal speech than to esophageal speech. When compared with esophageal speech, it gives superior voice quality in reference to volume and phrase length and is much easier to learn. The rate of speech is faster, and the intelligibility is superior to that acquired by using the artificial larynx or esophageal speech (30). However, in the presence of noise, a lower rate of listener intelligibility of TE speech is found compared with laryngeal speech.

The prevention of pharyngeal spasm is paramount to the production of successful TE speech. Acoustic analysis of TE speech was studied after three different surgical methods used to address the pharynx: pharyngeal plexus neurectomy, pharyngeal constrictor myotomy, and unilateral pharyngeal plexus neurectomy with a drainage myotomy limited to the cricopharyngeus. Patients undergoing pharyngeal plexus neurectomy had the highest fundamental frequency, which may be the result of the residual resting tone in the pharyngoesophageal segment. Management of the pharynx with neurectomy may be desirable in women undergoing laryngectomy with voice restoration.

Tracheoesophageal speech has been rated the most desirable form of alaryngeal speech by both speech pathologists and patients (31) and is the preferred method of alaryngeal speech by naïve listeners.

EMERGENCIES

Two urgent conditions may result for prosthesis users and should be attended to without delay (Table 123.4). For patients who routinely change their prostheses, the inability to insert the tip of the prosthesis and collar into the lumen of the esophagus may occur, which results initially in increased voice resistance and, in some cases, complete loss of voice. The TEP tract will close from the esophagus externally, and it will be impossible after 24 to 48 hours to reenter the lumen. If this occurs, the TEP can be serially dilated with plastic catheters ranging from 10F to 18F and then stented with a flexible catheter for several hours before the voice prosthesis is replaced. If available, urethral dilators are an effective instrument for TEP dilatation. Dilatation must be performed with as little resistance as possible because it is possible to dissect into the tracheoesophageal common wall and enter the anterior mediastinum.

The second urgent condition is aspiration of the voice prosthesis. This condition usually occurs when patients attempt to replace the device in the TEP, and a cough is stimulated. The most common location for device

TABLE 123.4 ℞ EMERGENCIES

Aspiration of prosthesis
Airway obstruction
Tracheoesophageal necrosis
Voice prosthesis incompetence

impaction is at the level of the upper right mainstem bronchus and carina. This usually is well tolerated, but an uncomfortable dyspnea is present. Furthermore, in the resultant anxiety, the TEP is not stented, and tracheal aspiration of saliva may occur. This complication can be prevented in most cases by providing detailed instruction in emergency techniques at the time of initial prosthesis fitting. Should aspiration of the prosthesis occur, the patient should first securely stent the puncture and then attempt to bend over as far as possible and cough out the prosthesis. Deep inhalations should be avoided because the result may be deeper penetration of the prosthesis into the airway. In the event of failure, the patient should go to an emergency medical facility as soon as possible. The size of the prosthesis prevents it from occluding the airway; patients will experience only moderate dyspnea with aspiration of the prosthesis.

The most efficient method for prosthesis retrieval is to use topical anesthesia and a rigid open or flexible bronchoscope with grasping forceps. After removing the foreign body, the TEP is stented with an 18F catheter for 24 hours before reinserting the prosthesis. The patient should avoid the changing process and should be introduced to the appropriate clinician follow-up team.

THE FUTURE

Laryngeal transplantation is currently under investigation. Animal studies have shown that canine laryngeal allografts can be physiologically reinnervated, which suggests that human larynges can be successfully innervated. However, additional research regarding the immunogenicity and function of transplanted larynges must be performed (32).

HIGHLIGHTS

■ Tracheoesophageal puncture avoids mucosalizing the passageway between the trachea and the esophagus. Its primary advantage over previous shunt and reconstructive procedures after total laryngectomy is to avoid aspiration or stenosis of the shunt.
■ The silicone voice prosthesis does not produce voice. Sound is produced by vibration of the pharyngoesophageal mucosa under air pressure.
■ Tracheoesophageal speech is more acoustically similar to normal laryngeal speech and more intelligible than standard esophageal speech.
■ Restoration of the voice after total laryngectomy must not compromise the established principles of surgical oncology.
■ Airway contamination is avoided by placing an effectively functioning voice prosthesis, which is a one-way valve.
■ Upper esophageal sphincter spasm occurs during esophageal distention secondary to air charging of this structure.

■ Esophageal insufflation testing via a catheter may simulate the patient's response to esophageal distention. Nevertheless, in the absence of effective data, esophageal insufflation should not be used exclusively for planning eventual neck exploration for treatment of spasm.
■ The initial application of the voice prosthesis requires varying breath control, which may be difficult for the esophageal speech user.
■ Tracheoesophageal speech dysfluency may be the result of pharyngeal constrictor tonicity, excessive resistance to airflow by a prosthesis with high-resistance characteristics, or tissue changes related to edema, fibrosis, or recurrent disease.
■ The primary placement of the TEP during total laryngectomy requires the addition of pharyngeal constrictor relaxation to ensure the development of fluent speech.

REFERENCES

1. Anthony JP, Deschler DG, Dougherty ET, et al. Long-term functional results after pharyngoesophageal reconstruction with the radial forearm free flap. *Am J Surg* 1994;168:441–445.
2. Kelly KE, Anthony JP, Singer MI. Pharyngoesophageal reconstruction using the radial forearm fasciocutaneous flap: preliminary results. *Otolaryngol Head Neck Surg* 1994;111:16–24.
3. Ultra Voice. Malvern, PA: Health Concepts.
4. Conley JJ, DeAmesti F, Pierce MK. A new surgical technique for vocal rehabilitation of the laryngectomized patient. *Ann Otol Rhinol Laryngol* 1958;67:655–664.
5. Asai R. Laryngoplasty after total laryngectomy. *Arch Otolaryngol* 1972;95:114–119.
6. Staffieri M, Serafini I. La riabilitazione chirurgica della voce er della respirazione dopo laringectomia totale. Presented at the 29th National Congress of the Associazione Otologi Ospedaliere Italiana. Bologna: Associazione Otologi Ospedaliere Italiana, 1976:1–222.
7. Singer MI, Blom ED. An endoscopic technique for voice restoration after total laryngectomy. *Ann Otol Rhinol Laryngol* 1980;89:529–533.
8. Robbins J, Fisher HB, Blom ED, et al. Selected acoustic features of tracheoesophageal, esophageal, and laryngeal speech. *Arch Otolaryngol* 1984;110:670–672.
9. Callanan VP, Toma A, Baldwin DL, et al. A comparison of patient preferences and voice production between esophageal voice, Provox valve and the indwelling Blom-Singer valve for post laryngectomy voice rehabilitation. In: Algaba J, ed. *Surgery and prosthetic voice restoration after total and subtotal laryngectomy.* Amsterdam: Elsevier Science, 1996:327–331.
10. Bertino G, Bellomo A, Miani C, et al. Spectrographic analysis of tracheoesophageal vs. esophageal speech. In: Algaba J, ed. *Surgery and prosthetic voice restoration after total and subtotal laryngectomy.* Amsterdam: Elsevier Science, 1996:333–338.
11. Blom ED, Singer MI, Hamaker RC. Tracheostoma valve for postlaryngectomy voice rehabilitation. *Ann Otol Rhinol Laryngol* 1982;91:576–578.
12. Barton D, DeSanto LW, Pearson BW, et al. An endostomal tracheostomy tube for leakproof retention of the Blom-Singer stomal valve. *Otolaryngol Head Neck Surg* 1988;99:38–41.
13. Grolman W, Schouwenburg PF, de Boer MF, et al. First results with the Blom-Singer adjustable tracheostoma valve. *ORL J Otorhinolaryngol Relat Spec* 1995;57:165–170.
14. Singer MI, Blom ED, Hamaker RC. Further experience with voice restoration after total laryngectomy. *Ann Otol Rhinol Laryngol* 1981;90:498–502.
15. Blom ED, Singer MI, Hamaker RC. An improved esophageal insufflation test. *Arch Otolaryngol Head Neck Surg* 1985;111:211–212.
16. Lewin JS, Baugh RF, Baker SR. An objective method for prediction of tracheoesophageal speech production. *J Speech Hear Disord* 1987;52:212–217.

17. Creamer B, Schlagel JF. Motor responses of the esophagus to distention. *J Appl Physiol* 1957;10:498–504.
18. Singer MI, Blom ED. A selective myotomy for voice restoration after total laryngectomy. *Arch Otolaryngol* 1981;107:670–673.
19. Deschler DG, Doherty ET, Reed CG, et al. Tracheoesophageal voice following tubed free flap reconstruction of the neopharynx. *Ann Otol Rhinol Laryngol* 1994;103:929–936.
20. Hilgers FJM, Hoorweg JJ, Kroon BBR, et al. Prosthetic voice rehabilitation with the Provox system after extensive pharyngeal resection and reconstruction. In: Algaba J, ed. *Surgery and prosthetic voice restoration after total and subtotal laryngectomy.* Amsterdam: Elsevier Science, 1996:111–119.
21. Maniglia AJ, Leder SB, Goodwin WJ Jr, et al. Tracheogastric puncture for vocal rehabilitation following total pharyngolaryngoesophagectomy. *Head Neck Surg* 1989;11:524–527.
22. Blom ED. *Correct use of nystatin.* Carpenteria, CA: Health Technologies, 1995.
23. Singer MI, Blom ED, Hamaker RC. Pharyngeal plexus neurectomy for alaryngeal speech rehabilitation. *Laryngoscope* 1986;96:50–53.
24. Zormier MM, Meleca RJ, Simpson ML, et al. Botulinum toxin injection to improve tracheoesophageal speech after total laryngectomy. *Otolaryngol Head Neck Surg* 1999;120:314–319.
25. Maves MD, Lingeman RE. Primary vocal rehabilitation using the Blom-Singer and Panje voice prosthesis. *Ann Otol Rhinol Laryngol* 1982;1:458-460.
26. Hamaker RC, Singer MI, Blom ED, et al. Primary voice restoration at laryngectomy. *Arch Otolaryngol* 1985;111:182–186.
27. Blom ED, Hamaker RC. Tracheoesophageal voice restoration following total laryngectomy. In: Myers EN, Suen JY, eds. *Cancer of the head and neck,* 3rd ed. Philadelphia: WB Saunders; 1996:839–852.
28. Hotz MA, Baumann A, Schaller I, et al. Success and predictability of Provox voice rehabilitation. *Arch Otolaryngol Head Neck Surg* 2002;128:687–691.
29. Robins J, Fisher HA, Blom ED, et al. Selected acoustic features of tracheoesophageal, esophageal and laryngeal speech. *Arch Otolaryngol* 1984;110:670–672.
30. Williams S, Watson B. Speaking proficiency variation according to method of alaryngeal voicing. *Laryngoscope* 1987;97:737–739.
31. Culton GL, Gerwin JM. Current trends in laryngectomy rehabilitation: a survey of speech-language pathologists. *Otolaryngol Head Neck Surg* 1998;118:458–463.
32. Berke GS, Ye M, Block RM, et al. Orthotopic laryngeal transplantation: is it time? *Laryngoscope* 1993;103:857–864.

Tracheal Tumors

124

K. Robert Shen   Douglas J. Mathisen

Primary tracheal tumors are rare. Approximately 2.7 new cases of tracheal tumors per million persons are estimated to occur annually. Few institutions have been able to accumulate enough experience to allow definitive conclusions, and the rarity of these tumors often leads to a delay in diagnosis and inappropriate initial treatment. A high degree of suspicion still is needed to make the diagnosis early, especially because many patients appear to have normal chest radiographs.

Modern surgical techniques allow reconstruction at any level of the airway (1–10). Operations for proximal tumors can spare the larynx, and operations for distal tumors allow reconstruction of the carina. Surgeons dealing with tracheal tumors must be familiar with these techniques, release maneuvers to reduce anastomotic tension, the biologic characteristics of the tumors, and alternatives to resection. Meaningful long-term follow-up data are lacking. Because numbers of patients are small and the biologic behavior of the tumors is variable, definitive data are few. Even one of the more common tumors, adenoid cystic carcinoma (ACC), is notorious for its prolonged clinical course and insidious tendency to recur after many years (8,11). Our experience involves treatment of 318 patients with primary tracheal tumors over 40 years (8,12). This experience is the largest in the world and allows certain inferences, but even these data are inconclusive for the reasons mentioned.

RADIOLOGIC EVALUATION

The primary diagnostic modalities for tracheal abnormalities are radiologic studies and bronchoscopy. All too often, a plain chest radiograph is considered normal, but closer inspection shows tracheal column abnormality. Relatively simple radiologic techniques without contrast media can delineate tracheal abnormalities (13). The location and linear extent of the lesion, extratracheal involvement, and amount of airway not involved in the process can be determined. In addition to standard views of the chest in various projections and centered high enough to show tracheal detail, anteroposterior filtered tracheal views of the entire airway from the larynx to the carina are obtained. A lateral neck view obtained with a soft-tissue technique with the patient swallowing and the neck hyperextended to bring the trachea above the clavicles is useful for defining abnormalities in the upper trachea.

Fluoroscopy shows functional asymmetry of the vocal cords and provides information about the extent of the lesion. Only spot radiographs usually are needed. Polytomography (anteroposterior and lateral views) can give additional detail, particularly of mediastinal involvement. Barium esophagography can help define esophageal involvement by extrinsic compression or invasion. Computed tomography (CT) offers little over conventional radiography, except to define an extratracheal component. Magnetic resonance imaging (MRI) offers the advantage of sagittal and coronal views of the trachea. Resolution is less than that of CT, however, and the cost is much greater. For these reasons, we rarely use MRI. Spiral or helical CT has been advocated (14,15). It offers the advantage of multiplanar and three-dimensional reconstruction with the resolution of conventional CT.

AIRWAY MANAGEMENT

Crucial to the management of all problems of the trachea is the ability to control the airway. Tracheal tumors can manifest as airway obstruction. Endotracheal intubation can be impossible and even dangerous because it can cause complete airway obstruction, especially among patients with high tracheal lesions. Simple maneuvers to elevate the head of the patient, cool mist and oxygen administration, and careful sedation can gain control of the airway. Control is best accomplished in the operating room, where an assortment of rigid bronchoscopes, dilators, biopsy forceps, and instruments for emergency tracheostomy are readily available (16,17).

Every effort is made to design an anesthetic plan that permits extubation at the end of the procedure (18). This technique should include placement of an epidural catheter preoperatively as well as the use of total intravenous anesthesia (TIVA). This strategy relies on short-acting hypnotics, narcotics [e.g., Remifentanil (*Ultiva*), GlaxoSmithKline] and paralytic agents [e.g., Cisatracurium (*Nimbex*), GlaxoSmithKline] to permit adequate respiratory drive on completion of the surgery.

Initial evaluation is performed with a rigid bronchoscope carefully inserted through the vocal cords and stopping just proximal to the level of obstruction. Rigid telescopes are inserted through the bronchoscope to assess the obstruction. Most tumors, even those causing near-total obstruction, allow a rigid bronchoscope to be passed beyond them. After the status of the distal airway has been assessed, the tumor can be partially removed with biopsy forceps to determine consistency and vascularity. For most tumors, the tip of the rigid bronchoscope can be used to "core out" most of the tumor. The tumor then can be grasped with biopsy forceps and removed. If bleeding occurs, the bronchoscope can be passed into the distal airway for ventilation and to tamponade the bleeding. Direct application of epinephrine-soaked pledgets helps to control persistent oozing. Rarely have we had to resort to cautery with insulated electrodes in these situations. Some surgeons advocate routine use of a laser to relieve obstruction and coagulate bleeding sites, but we have found use of a laser time consuming, expensive, and rarely advantageous compared with the mechanical technique.

Endotracheal removal of malignant tumors, mechanically or with a laser, is only a temporary measure. Using these techniques for emergencies (Table 124.1) allows thorough evaluation and elective surgical treatment. Many patients with low-grade tumors are taking high doses of steroids, having been treated for refractory "asthma." When an airway is established, glucocorticoids can be tapered and discontinued, and a surgical procedure can be performed without the threat of impaired healing. Repeated coring of the tumor may be needed during steroid tapering.

Similar airway control maneuvers can be used at the time of elective surgery, even if the patient has a stable airway. This allows assessment of the distal airway, placement of an endotracheal tube, and provision of an adequate lumen to prevent accumulation of carbon dioxide early in the procedure. During tracheal resection, the tube can be

pulled back or removed and a sterile, cuffed endotracheal tube (e.g., a flexible, armored Tovell tube) can be inserted into the distal airway. Sterile connecting tubing is passed to the anesthesiologist to allow ventilation of the patient. The Tovell tube can be removed whenever necessary for suctioning or placement of sutures. The patient should be breathing spontaneously at the end of the procedure so that extubation can be performed in the operating room. Intraoperative, high-frequency ventilation has been used with equal success, but we are satisfied with the technique described. In certain complex carinal resections however, high-frequency ventilation is especially useful.

TUMOR CLASSIFICATION

Approximately two thirds of primary tracheal tumors are of two histologic types: squamous cell carcinoma (SCC) and ACC, formally called cylindroma (Table 124.2). The

TABLE 124.2

CHARACTERISTICS OF 270 PATIENTS WITH PRIMARY TRACHEAL CARCINOMA

	ACC	SCC	χ^2 p Value
Sex			
Female	53%	32%	0.004
Male	46%	68%	
Mean age (median), years	49(47)	61(62)	
Comorbidities (%)			
Smoker	45	89	<0.001
Hypertension	17	29	0.02
EtOH use	5	18	<0.001
Past MI	2	13	0.001
Diabetes mellitus	2	12	0.002
Steroid use	7	7	0.812
Angina	3	6	0.238
Arrhythmia	3	5	0.356
Prior stroke	2	3	0.702
Prior cancers (%)			
Lung	1	15	<.0001
Larynx	0	7	0.001
Head and neck	0	4	0.024
Colon	1	1	0.562
Prostate	1	1	0.562
Oropharynx	0	1	0.156
Other	0	7	0.001
Symptoms (%)			
Dyspnea	65	50	0.014
Cough	55	52	0.626
Hemoptysis	29	60	<0.001
Wheeze	44	27	0.003
Stridor	21	27	0.200
Hoarseness	10	13	0.495
Dysphagia	7	7	0.812
Fever	7	4	0.184
Other	12	14	0.495

ACC = adenoid cystic carcinoma; EtOH = alcohol; MI = myocardial infarction; SCC = squamous cell carcinoma.

TABLE 124.1   EMERGENCIES

- Tracheoarterial fistula
- Pneumothorax
- Acute pulmonary edema

most common type of surgically treated malignant tracheal tumor is ACC (8,11,19–25). If surgically and nonsurgically managed tumors are included, SCC has the highest incidence (26). The remaining one third is a heterogeneous group of malignant and benign tumors. A variety of cervical and mediastinal forms of carcinoma can involve the trachea, including tumors of the larynx, thyroid, lung, and esophagus. In rare instances, neoplasms can metastasize to the submucosa of the trachea or to the mediastinum with secondary invasion of the trachea. Carcinoma of the breast or mediastinal lymphoma sometimes invades the trachea.

In our original series (8), 70 (35%) of the 198 patients had primary SCC of the trachea or carina, 80 (40%) had ACC, and the other 48 (24%) had a variety of benign and malignant lesions. SCC can be exophytic or ulcerative, multiple, and scattered over a considerable length of trachea. The tumor metastasizes to the regional lymph nodes and, in its more aggressive and late forms, invades mediastinal structures. Its progress appears to be more rapid than that of ACC. Many patients have returned with a second primary squamous cell carcinoma, usually of the lung or oropharynx.

Adenoid cystic carcinoma typically has a prolonged course of clinical symptoms. After treatment, many years can pass before recurrence. ACC can extend over long distances submucosally in the airways and perineurally. It spreads to regional lymph nodes but less frequently than does SCC. Although it can invade the thyroid or the muscular layers of the esophagus by contiguity, ACC that has not been disturbed surgically frequently displaces mediastinal structures before actually invading them. Metastasis to the lungs is not uncommon. Metastatic lesions can grow slowly over many years and remain asymptomatic until they are huge. Metastasis to bone and other organs also occurs.

Tumors other than SCC and ACC, although representing only about one third of this population, are a multitude of tumor types with various degrees of malignancy; they include epithelial and mesenchymal neoplasms (Table 124.3). In patients presenting with multiple squamous papilloma, the lesions were not resected but were removed by means of cryotherapy, electrocoagulation, or laser treatment, depending on current technology. One patient with pleomorphic adenoma years earlier had had excision of a similar tumor from a salivary gland. No evidence of metastasis was seen, and the lesion, therefore, was classified as a primary tracheal lesion. A patient who had rhabdomyosarcoma had an isolated pedunculated lesion without extratracheal penetration, but he had cervical rhabdomyosarcoma managed by means of radical operation and intensive irradiation 6 years earlier without evidence of local recurrence. No other foci developed, but this may have been a secondary lesion. The plexiform neurofibroma and the two paragangliomas were involved inextricably with the airway wall and appeared to have originated there. The vascular malformations involved arterial

TABLE 124.3

PRIMARY TRACHEAL TUMORS OTHER THAN SQUAMOUS CELL AND ADENOID CYSTIC CARCINOMA

Type	Patients (N)
Benign	
Squamous papilloma	4
Multiple	1
Solitary	3
Pleomorphic adenoma	2
Granular cell tumor	2
Fibrous histiocytoma	1
Leiomyoma	2
Chondroma	2
Chondroblastoma	1
Schwannoma	1
Paraganglioma	2
Hemangioendothelioma	1
Vascular malformation	2
Intermediate	
Carcinoid	10
Mucoepidermoid	4
Plexiform neurofibroma	1
Pseudosarcoma	1
Malignant	
Adenocarcinoma	1
Adenosquamous carcinoma	1
Small-cell carcinoma	1
Atypical carcinoid	1
Melanoma	1
Chondrosarcoma	1
Spindle cell sarcoma	2
Rhabdomyosarcoma	1

and venous components throughout the neck and mediastinum, but had localized intraluminal obstructing protrusions. The small-cell carcinoma was confined to the trachea without any involvement or adherence of lung. The melanoma appeared to be solitary without any previous known skin lesions, and without evidence of retinal or other primary tumor. Additional patients with tumors of apparently mediastinal origin were excluded from review.

We recently conducted a retrospective study of 270 patients diagnosed with primary ACC or SCC of the trachea seen at Massachusetts General Hospital between 1962 and 2002 (12). As shown in Table 124.2, patients with SCC were more likely to be male, smokers, and have prior cancers of the respiratory tract. In contrast, patients with ACC had a slight female predominance (72 women, 63 men). In our series, SCC predominated among patients in the sixth or seventh decade of life, similar to the incidence of SCC of the lung. The mean age of patients with SCC was 61 years. ACC, on the other hand, was distributed among patients 20 to 69 years of age, with a slight peak in the fifth decade. The mean age of patients with ACC was 49 years, with a median of 47 years. Other primary tracheal tumors have an almost even male-to-female distribution and a scattered age distribution because of the variety of types.

Tumors can secondarily involve the trachea. Papillary and follicular carcinomas of the thyroid and mixed varieties of the two can invade the trachea, usually at the level of the isthmus (7). A patient with hemoptysis can have carcinoma of the thyroid. Invasion of the trachea by thyroid carcinoma is best managed by means of resection with airway reconstruction. Localized extension of tumor also may necessitate partial esophageal resection or radical resection, including laryngectomy with mediastinal tracheostomy. More commonly, invasion is found after thyroidectomy for carcinoma during which the surgeon became aware of shaving of the tumor from the trachea. In such cases, concurrent or early resection of the involved trachea is considered.

SIGNS AND SYMPTOMS

Tracheal tumors can manifest insidiously. The most common symptoms and signs are cough, hemoptysis, and signs of progressive airway obstruction, including shortness of breath on exertion, wheezing and stridor, and dysphagia or hoarseness. Wheezing can cause errors in diagnosis. It is not commonly appreciated that wheezing can be a predominant symptom of a tracheal tumor for a prolonged period. A conventional chest radiograph usually shows clear lung fields, and on this basis, the physician assumes that no organic mass lesion is present. Patients often are treated for adult-onset asthma. Hemoptysis may not be pursued aggressively if the chest radiographic findings appear normal. A tracheal tumor also can manifest as unilateral or bilateral recurrent episodes of pneumonitis, which respond to antibiotic treatment but then recur.

Signs and symptoms vary with tumor type. Hemoptysis is prominent among patients who have SCC, and it usually leads to earlier diagnosis. Among our 270 patients with adenoid cystic or SCC, hemoptysis was a presenting symptom in 60% of patients with SCC, and 29% of patients with ACC. Hoarseness as an early symptom can signify advanced disease. ACC more often has dyspnea and wheezing or stridor as a predominant symptom, and diagnosis is often delayed. In our most recent series (12), the mean duration of symptoms was 12.2 months, with longer durations in ACC and in tumors later found to be unresectable (resected ACC 18.3 months, resected SCC 4.54 months; unresectable ACC 23.7 months, unresectable SCC 7.58 months; $P < 0.001$). For some benign tumors or low-grade malignant tumors of the trachea, the mean duration for presumption of an incorrect diagnosis was 4 years.

DIAGNOSIS

Diagnosis long after symptoms begin is the rule rather than the exception. Many patients first come to medical attention with a troublesome cough, dyspnea on exertion,

---

TABLE 124.4   📖 **DIAGNOSIS**

Symptoms
  Cough
  Dyspnea on exertion
  Stridor
Most common histology
  Squamous cell carcinoma
  Adenoid cystic carcinoma

---

and eventually wheezing and stridor (Table 124.4). Normal lung fields on chest radiographs usually lull the physician into a sense of security. The patient frequently receives a misdiagnosis of asthma. Only after hemoptysis or recurrent focal pneumonia occurs is bronchoscopy performed. For a few patients, flow-volume curves show loss of peaks, a finding that suggests upper airway obstruction (19). If tumor is suspected, simple radiologic studies without contrast medium usually show the location and extent of the tumor (14). It is as important to outline the extent of the grossly uninvolved airway remaining for reconstruction as it is to define precisely the extent of the tumor. The function of the larynx also is studied fluoroscopically. Bronchoscopy can be performed cautiously as a separate procedure if it is especially indicated. If the tumor appears to be highly obstructing, or if it appears to be an exceedingly vascular lesion, biopsy is not performed until arrangements have been made for a definitive surgical approach with the same anesthesia.

Definitive bronchoscopy is performed at projected resection if an accurate frozen-section pathologic diagnosis can be obtained. A flexible bronchoscope is useful for looking beyond an extensive tumor, especially at the carinal level, to check the possibility of distal infiltration, as occurs with ACC. Caution must be exercised during flexible bronchoscopic examinations of outpatients with a tumor producing high-grade obstruction. Secretions, bleeding, or swelling can precipitate sudden airway obstruction. The patient can die if adequate facilities are not available to secure the airway.

ANESTHETIC TECHNIQUE

Slow induction may be needed if a high degree of airway obstruction exists. Slow induction is preferable to paralysis of respiration with a consequent urgent need to establish an airway. The surgeon is available with an array of rigid bronchoscopes, including pediatric and adult sizes, as induction is begun. The residual airway through which the patient is breathing can be as little as 2 or 3 mm in diameter. In most cases, tumors are not circumferential, unlike the circumferential stenosis that occurs with some inflammatory lesions. After bronchoscopy, a small endotracheal tube often can be insinuated past a highly obstructive tumor. In other cases, the tube is left above the tumor. In rare instances, it is necessary to "nibble away" bits of tumor with a biopsy forceps to enlarge the channel for tube passage. Because of their size and inflexibility, double lumen endotracheal tubes often present difficulties in these procedures. As such, an extra-long, flexible, armored, single lumen endotracheal tube is used, which can be advanced into a mainstem bronchus to provide one-lung ventilation as indicated. As surgical resection proceeds, the remaining mainstem bronchus is intubated across the operative field with a sterile endotracheal tube connected to sterile tubing passed off to the anesthesiologist. A plan of intermittent ventilation then proceeds to allow precise placement of anastomotic sutures. This is done by close cooperation of surgeon and anesthesiologist. As the end-to-end tracheobronchial anastomosis is reapproximated and the sutures are tied, the original endotracheal tube is advanced into the bronchus allowing uninterrupted ventilation. Secondary anastomosis (end of bronchus to side of trachea) can then be completed. The endotracheal tube is removed, and the patient should be breathing spontaneously at the end of the procedure. Particularly if the trachea has been greatly shortened, it is undesirable to have even a low-pressure cuff lying in contact with the anastomosis. Alternative ventilatory techniques such as high frequency (jet) ventilation (27) and independent lung ventilation are options with which both surgeon and anesthesiologist should be knowledgeable. Cardiopulmonary bypass, although feasible, should be discouraged during carinal resection and reconstruction in adults and older children as a consequence of the incremental morbidity associated with the procedure. Cardiopulmonary bypass is of no use whatsoever in upper tracheal resection.

SURGICAL TECHNIQUE

Treatment options are summarized in Table 124.5.

The patient must be positioned to allow full access to the operative field needed. A cervical collar incision is used for relatively limited tumors in the upper half of the trachea.

TABLE 124.5 ℞ TREATMENT

Rigid bronchoscopy
Endotracheal débridement
Formal resection
  End-to-end anastomosis
    Coated polyglactin suture
    Tension free
  Traction sutures
    Hilar release
    Suprahyoid release
  Innominate protection
    Strap muscle flap

Partial sternal division through a vertical midline extension provides greater access to the upper mediastinum (Fig. 124.1). If the larynx must be exposed, this can be done from beneath the upper flap of the collar incision or through a second, short horizontal incision above the hyoid bone. If the tumor appears to be somewhat longer, or of a type that can prove more extensive (e.g., ACC), the patient must be positioned for further extension of the incision into the right fourth interspace to the posterior axillary line. For this reason, the right arm is best draped and kept within the field so that it can be moved back and forth. The preferred approach to tumors of the lower trachea and carina is through a high right posterolateral thoracotomy. The right arm is draped and kept in the operative field. The field includes the entire neck for access to the hyoid region, larynx, and trachea for possible cervical mobilization and laryngeal release. In rare cases, individualized incisions are designed. If subtotal removal of the trachea or a laryngotrachiectomy is necessary, a long, somewhat lower, horizontal incision is used. A vertical incision is avoided to preserve the possibility of mediastinal tracheostomy (28). This step rarely is needed but must be planned.

In dissection of the tumor, an effort is made to take as much tissue from around the level of tumor as possible, limited as it may be. The trachea is approached above and below the lesion, and these areas are cleared first. If the primary lesion is a malignant tumor of the thyroid gland, strap muscles may have to be included *en bloc*, and partial neck dissection may be needed. With other primary tumors of the upper trachea, resection of one or both lobes of the thyroid on the side on which the tumor is based is performed to avoid the possibility of exposing tumor that may have invaded the tracheal wall at that point. Each operation must be individualized and approached with caution.

The surgical approach to malignant tumors contrasts to the approach to benign disease of the trachea, in which dissection remains close to the trachea and scar-encased recurrent laryngeal nerves may not be visualized. In surgery for tumors, the nerves are identified far from the location of the tumor and followed toward the area of tumor. Sometimes it is necessary to sacrifice a recurrent laryngeal nerve because of its involvement with tumor, even if no functional paralysis is evident. Special care must be exerted in the right transthoracic approach not to injure the left recurrent laryngeal nerve as the aortic surface is approached from the right side. Adjacent lymph nodes are included with the dissection, but only limited node dissection can be done without endangering the blood supply of the trachea (29). This blood supply enters segmentally, principally from the branches of the inferior thyroid artery above, and from the bronchial arteries below. Vascular contributions also arise from the internal mammary artery, the highest intercostal artery, and esophageal branches. It is critical not to dissect around the trachea for any great distance if that portion of trachea is to be left in the patient.

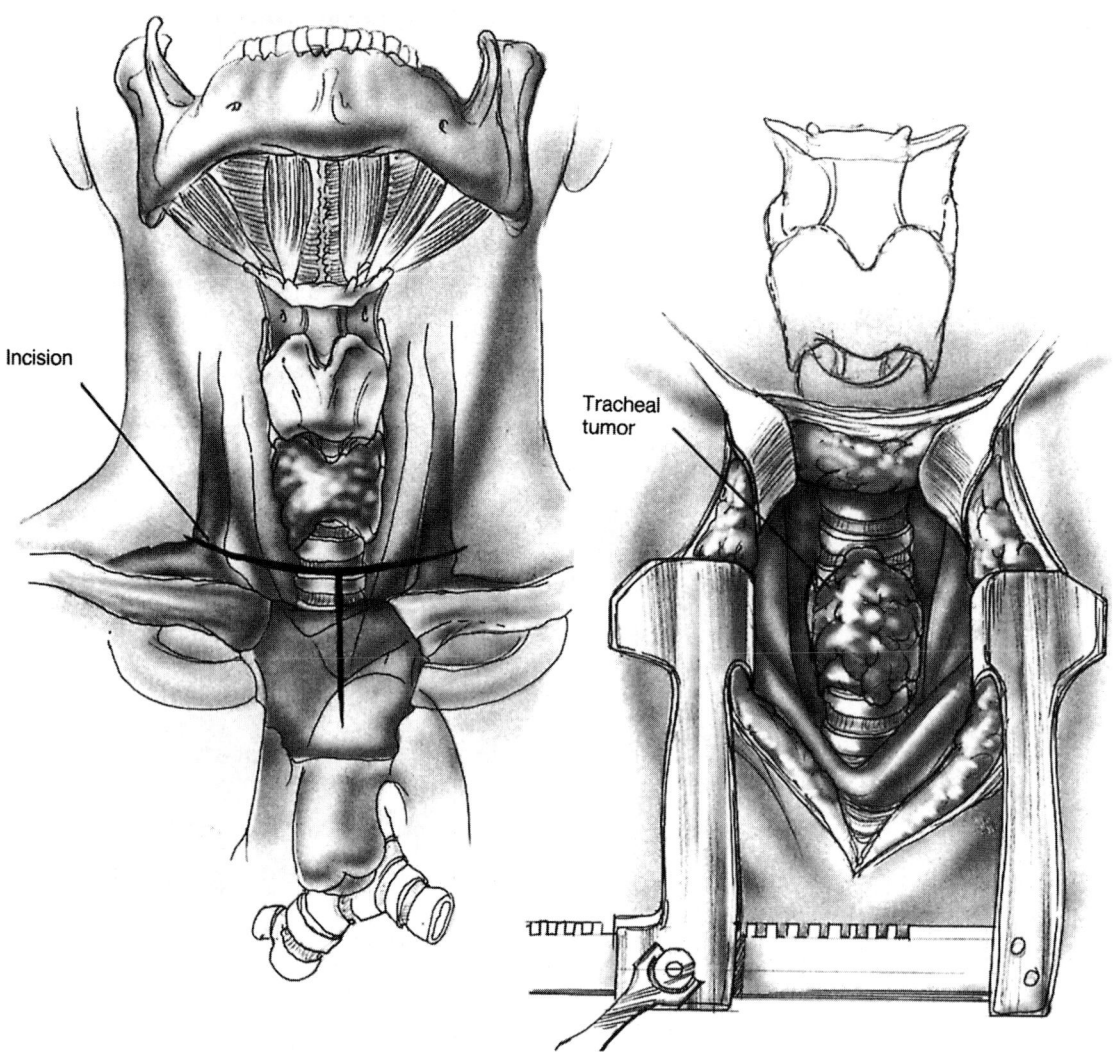

Incision

Tracheal
tumor

Figure 124.1   A cervical incision is used for most tracheal resections. A T incision with upper ster-notomy can be used to expose the distal trachea.

As a matter of safety, it is best not to circumferentially free more than 1 or 2 cm of tracheal length if the tissue is to remain in the patient. Devascularization can cause necrosis and stenosis.

The entire pretracheal plane is freed bluntly to the carina and often down the anterior surface of the proximal right and left main bronchi. Care is taken to spare the lateral pedicles, which contain the blood supply. After the apparent lower extent of tumor has been identified, lateral traction sutures of 2-0 polyglactin 910 are placed through the full thickness of the tracheal wall in the anteroposterior midline on either side (3 o'clock and 9 o'clock positions), at the distance estimated to be 1 cm or more distal to the eventual line of transection. A previously prepared, flexible, sterile endotracheal tube is available in the field along with sterile connecting anesthesia tubing.

The trachea is opened transversely, distal to the lower margin of the tumor, and the lumen is cautiously inspected (Fig. 124.2). If the incision is not sufficiently distal

to the tumor, a lower level is selected. The trachea is transected cleanly and transversely. Intubation is performed across the operative field. A sliver of tissue can be taken from the distal resection margin at the point closest to the tumor and sent for immediate frozen-section analysis to determine whether the distal margin is adequate. The anesthesia tube from above is withdrawn at this point. If the line of resection in the trachea is close to the cricoid cartilage, it is advisable to suture a catheter to the tip of the endotracheal tube so that if the tube is withdrawn above the vocal cords, it can be easily pulled down again later. An assistant is assigned the job of stabilizing the endotracheal tube in the distal trachea. That person keeps the tip from passing into the right main bronchus and frequently suctions blood that puddles above the cuff. Blood that seeps past the cuff into the distal tracheobronchial tree can produce shunting after the operation.

The specimen end of the divided trachea can be grasped with a forceps and placed on tension to facilitate upward

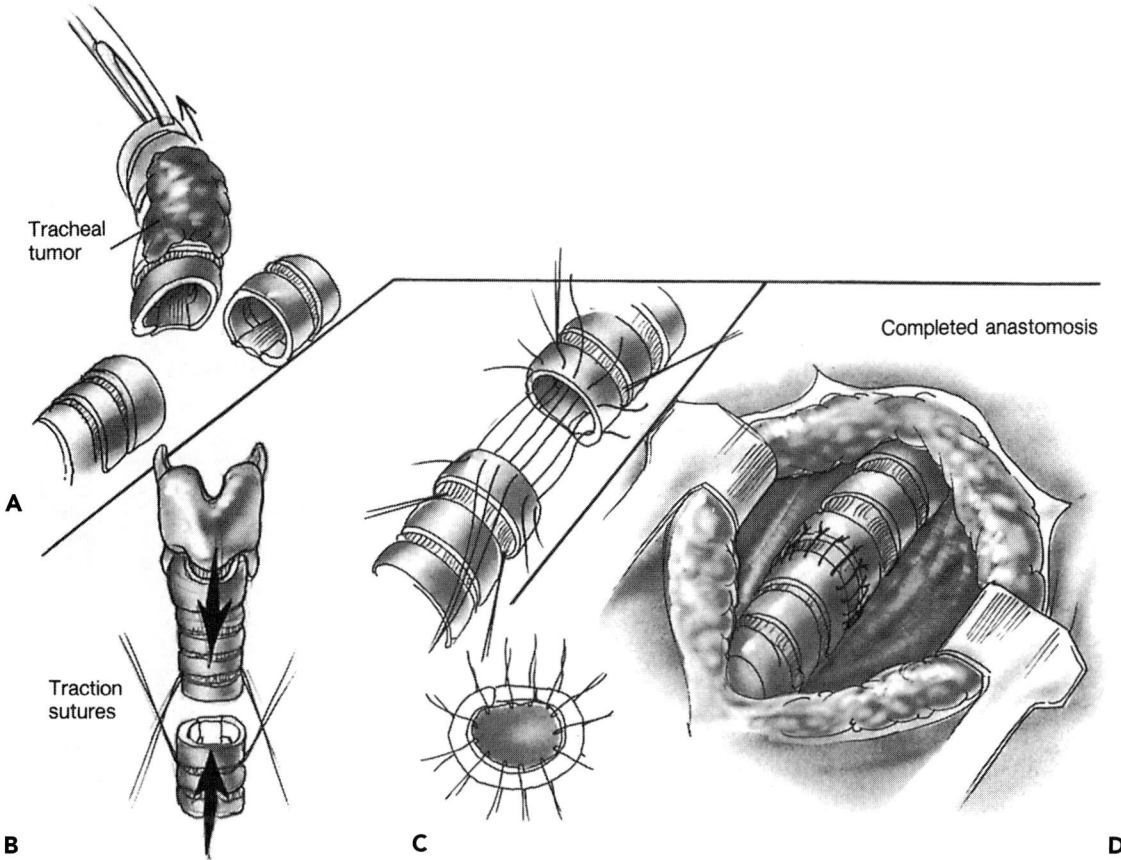

Figure 124.2 **A:** The trachea is divided just above and below the tumor. **B:** Traction sutures are pulled to approximate the two ends. **C:** Interrupted 4-0 polyglactin 910 sutures are placed circumferentially. **D:** All sutures are tied to complete the anastomosis.

dissection. If the tumor is somewhat lower, it is better to perform the transection above the tumor and leave the tumor in place with an endotracheal tube passed beyond it to provide a reasonable handle until a clean line for transection can be established below the tumor. Lateral traction sutures are placed in the airway above the level of transection, as they were below. If the transection is high, the sutures can be placed in the larynx rather than in the trachea. It sometimes is necessary to bevel obliquely a portion of the lower larynx, such as half or more of the cricoid cartilage. If the esophageal wall is involved, as shown in preoperative barium swallow examination, esophagoscopy or inspection of the operative field, partial- or full-thickness resection of the anterior or anterolateral esophageal wall may be necessary. The esophagus is reconstructed with two layers of interrupted 4-0 silk sutures over a nasogastric tube. A pedicled strap muscle is useful for reinforcement.

After removal of the specimen and establishment of negative transection margins at either end, reconstruction can begin. The surgeon and assistant both draw together the tracheal traction sutures on their respective sides while the anesthetist tentatively flexes the neck (Fig. 124.2). The chin is brought down in an arc toward the sternum. Gentle

traction on the lateral sutures approximates the two ends. No absolute rule exists about how much trachea can be resected and how much approximation can be achieved in this manner. In operations on young, relatively thin patients, 60% of the trachea can be resected, and simple end-to-end anastomosis can be done without excessive tension. In operations on older, heavy patients, in whom the angle of the trachea is different, it may be impossible to bring the ends together in this way, even after only 3 cm has been resected. When excessive tension is applied, the likelihood of separation or stenosis increases markedly in operations on adults. Probably less tension is safe for juvenile patients. Intraoperative clinical appraisal of tension is essential in determining the extent of resection. If further relaxation is needed, a variety of maneuvers can be used. Suprahyoid laryngeal release or Montgomery release is particularly effective, especially after resection of the proximal trachea (30). A length of 1 to 2.5 cm can be obtained, primarily anteriorly where the length is needed most.

Anastomosis is performed with fine, strong, absorbable suture material of 4-0 polyglactin, preferably coated (Fig. 124.2). Use of this suture material has reduced to zero the incidence of suture-line granuloma, a sharp contrast with early experience (31). All sutures are placed individually in a circumferential manner beginning in the posterior aspect and proceeding toward the anterior, first on one side and then on the other (Fig. 124.2). These sutures are placed at approximately 4-mm intervals, 3 mm back from the cut edge of the trachea. Anterolaterally, they pass through cartilage. No effort is made to pass sutures submucosally. The sutures are sequentially clipped carefully to the drapes so that they do not become confused. Once all sutures are placed, the endotracheal tube is removed from across the operative field, and the proximal endotracheal tube is readvanced distally. The patient's head and neck are supported securely in the flexed position. The lateral traction sutures are tied to approximate the tracheal ends without telescoping them. The anastomotic sutures are tied from front to back on both sides, and the ends of each are cut as they are tied. Saline solution is placed in the wound, the endotracheal tube cuff is deflated, and the anastomosis is tested for air tightness. In some operations, the thyroid isthmus is sutured over a high anastomosis, or other tissue is placed over it. If the innominate artery has not been deliberately skeletonized, no particular need exists for interposition of muscle between it and the operative field. If any question arises, it may be better to interpose a pedicled strap muscle or other tissue. Closure is in the usual manner. The sternum is wired if it has been partially divided, and the other tissues are closed in layers after insertion of soft suction drains. If possible, extubation is done while the patient is on the operating table.

If the tumor involves the carina, various reconstructive techniques are used (Fig. 124.3). Unless the tumor is small, it is rarely feasible to reconstruct it by means of approximation of the right or left main bronchus to form a new carina and then attaching it to the trachea. This suturing method anchors the carina low in the mediastinum, and if more trachea has been excised, approximation is not possible. More commonly, the right or left main bronchus is sutured to the trachea in an end-to-end manner, and anastomosis of the other bronchus to the lower portion of the tracheal wall laterally above the initial anastomosis is performed.

The principles and technique of anastomosis are as described previously for tracheal resection. Intraoperative management of the airway is more difficult and requires close cooperation with the anesthesiologist. Jet ventilation has been useful in some complicated reconstructions. All intrathoracic anastomoses are covered with a second layer of pedicled pleura or pericardial fat pad, as in sleeve lobectomy. It is important to interpose tissue between the airway suture line and adjacent pulmonary vessels. Omentum is used only if irradiation has been used.

A recurrent laryngeal nerve involved by tumor is sacrificed. The nerves usually are identified and carefully saved, if possible. Local paratracheal lymph nodes are excised with the specimen, if possible. Extensive lymph node dissection is not performed because it can destroy the blood supply to the residual trachea. The extent of resection usually is determined by frozen section examinations to ensure that

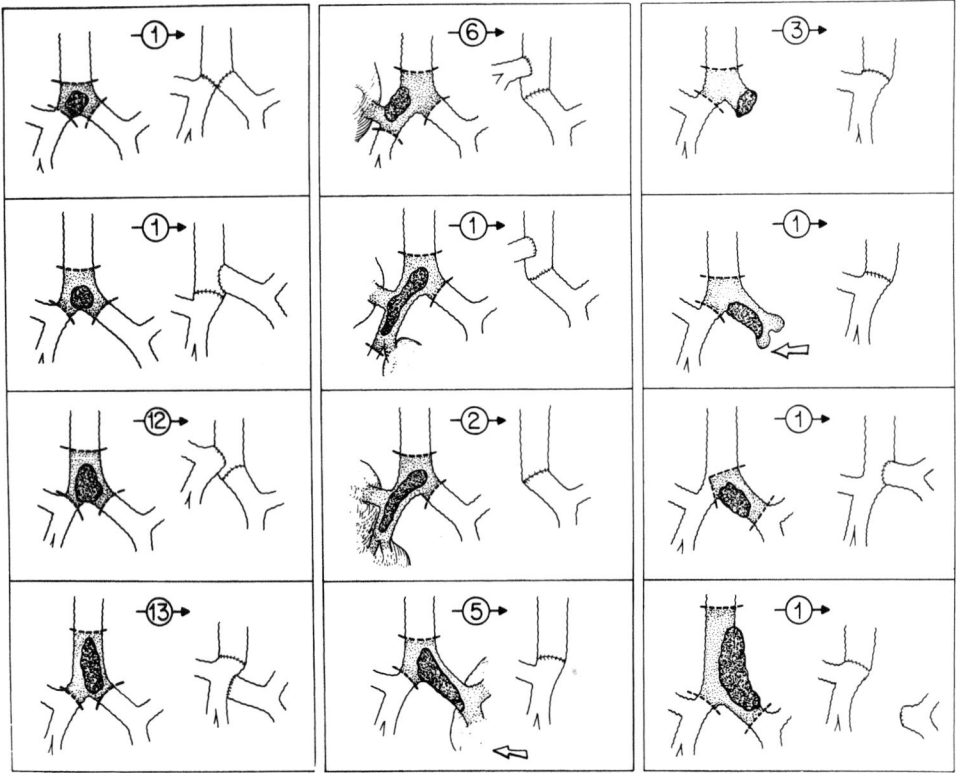

Figure 124.3 Twelve possible carinal resections.

TABLE 124.6
PRIMARY TRACHEAL TUMORS

Variable	Squamous	Adenoid Cystic	Other	Total
Number of lesions	135	135	48	318
Percentage of total	42.5	42.5	15	100
Resected	90 (67%)	101(75%)	43 (90%)	234 (74%)
Unresectable	45 (33%)	34 (25%)	5 (5%)	84 (26%)
Trachea	59	44	28	131
Laryngotracheal	6	9	2	17
Tracheal with permanent tracheostomy	5	7	0	12
Carinal without pulmonary resection	18	23	13	54
Carinal with pulmonary resection	2	18	0	20
Staged procedure	2	6	0	8

the margins are clear. ACC, in particular, can extend so far that total resection of microscopic tumor may be impossible. Irradiation for microscopically positive margins is effective in preventing local recurrence.

RESULTS

Of the 318 lesions in the Massachusetts General Hospital series, 234 were removed by means of resection and reconstruction of trachea or carina, laryngotracheal resection with or without cervicomediastinal exenteration, or staged reconstruction with excision of the tumor in the hope of restoring airway continuity with cervical cutaneous tubes (Table 124.6). Contraindications precluded resection in 34 (25%) patients with ACC and 45 (33%) patients with SCC. Unresectable tumors were found during thoracotomy in 11 patients and cervical or cervicomediastinal exploration in 6. The primary contraindication to resection was locoregional disease in more than 90% of patients with unresectable lesions, whereas distant metastases were present in less than 7% (Table 124.7). This report focuses on

TABLE 124.7
CONTRAINDICATIONS TO RESECTION IN UNRESECTED PATIENTS

Reason for Contraindication (%)	ACC (n = 34)	SCC (n = 45)
Extent of airway involvement	68	67
Extent of regional disease	23	24
Distant disease	6	7
Medical contraindication	0	2
Patient choice	3	0

ACC = adenoid cystic carcinoma; SCC = squamous cell carcinoma.

the 234 patients who had resection and primary reconstruction. Eight patients had staged reconstruction. These procedures were performed when the extent of possible surgical resection was being explored. Because of complications, high mortality, and the small number of patients who could participate to completion, the procedure was abandoned. Most patients who did not have resection had radiation therapy.

Surgical Approach

Operations were planned flexibly so that the approach would be adequate if more trachea than anticipated were involved by tumor. Upper tracheal tumors were explored through a cervical collar incision, with the option to extend exposure through the upper sternum. For midtracheal tumors, the option was kept open to extend the incision through full median sternotomy with the possibility of a transpericardial approach or by means of a trapdoor incision through the right fourth interspace. Most often, lower tracheal tumors were approached through right thoracotomy. The earliest operations were performed electively through a trapdoor incision, which allows access to the entire trachea. Median sternotomy with a transpericardial approach was used, but it offered less adequate exposure for extensive tumors. Carinal resection was approached principally through a right posterolateral thoracotomy, in a few selected patients through a left thoracotomy, and for three patients through a bilateral thoracotomy if carinal reconstruction with combined left pneumonectomy was anticipated. The modes of reconstruction are diagrammed in Figure 124.3.

Technical Features

In operations on 10 patients (1 with squamous tumor, 3 with ACC, and 6 with other tumors), laryngoplasty (partial resection of the larynx) was necessary to establish adequate margins around a tumor. The operations were individualized. The trachea was tailored appropriately to mortise into the irregular defect made in the larynx. The recurrent laryngeal nerve was protected. This type of resection has been described in detail for management of secondary invasion of the airway by carcinoma of the thyroid (7).

Adjunctive procedures were used to decrease tension on the anastomosis, in addition to pretracheal dissection and cervical flexion. Laryngeal release was performed on seven patients having tracheal resection and on five having carinal resection. We have since concluded that laryngeal release does not generally translate into relaxation after carinal resection. It can be useful, however, in the treatment of patients having extensive resection of the midtrachea and carina. Hilar release, which involves a U-shaped incision in the pericardium beneath the inferior pulmonary vein, or complete circumcision of the pericardium around the hilum, was performed on 12 patients having transthoracic tracheal resection and 23 patients having carinal resection. Four patients with ACC having carinal resection had both laryngeal and hilar releases.

Ten patients had various degrees of thyroidectomy to encompass tumors. Seven patients with tracheal tumors and two with carinal tumors had lateral removal of the esophageal wall, either muscularis alone or full thickness of the wall. The recurrent laryngeal nerve was deliberately sacrificed in four tracheal resections and in one carinal resection because of tumor involvement. Three patients who had squamous carcinoma and one patient who had sarcoma had omental pedicles brought up substernally for reinforcement of the suture line. All of these patients had previously had high-dose irradiation. Two patients who had tracheoesophageal fistula caused by ACC and were expected to have long survival periods had colonic esophageal bypass with exclusion of the fistula.

Operative Complications

Anastomotic complications, fatal and nonfatal, occurred in 28 patients (14.6%; separation 7.3%, stenosis 3.1%, granulations 2.1%, tracheoarterial fistula 1.0%, necrosis 0.5%, and other 0.5%). Postoperative tracheostomy was required in 17 patients. Four patients had suture-line granuloma in the era before absorbable sutures were used. These patients were treated by bronchoscopic means. One patient, who had had laryngoplasty, had elevation of the posterior mucosal flap, which healed in place after brief intubation.

One esophageal fistula occurred after transthoracic tracheal resection with extensive full-thickness resection of the esophageal wall. A small fistula healed spontaneously. Vocal cord paralysis, reversible with time in some cases, occurred among eight patients having tracheal or carinal resection for squamous carcinoma and among three patients having tracheal or carinal resection for ACC. Six patients experienced aspiration on deglutition, principally after laryngeal

TABLE 124.8	🄲 COMPLICATIONS	
Anastomotic complications	14.6%
Separation	7%
Stenosis	3%
Granuloma	2%
Vocal cord paralysis	
Aspiration	

release necessitated by extended resection. Most cases of aspiration resolved with time, although temporary gastrostomy was needed in rare instances. One patient, who had had transthoracic tracheal resection, had a small empyema that was managed with drainage. One patient had postsurgical Guillain-Barré syndrome.

Two patients had acute pulmonary edema after carinal resection with right pneumonectomy. Three others had pneumonia. One patient who had carinal resection with anastomosis of the right main bronchus and exclusion of the left lung had hypoxemia. The pulmonary artery had not been ligated. Left pneumonectomy later was needed to remove the nonfunctioning but shunting lung.

Other complications are listed in Table 124.8.

Operative Deaths

The hospital mortality was 10% (10/101) in ACC, and 4.9% (4/90) in SCC. The highest mortality occurred among patients having carinal resection for ACC, probably because of excessive tension after extended resection for this infiltrating disease (5). Overall hospital mortality after carinal resection was 16% compared with 3.9% after tracheal resection and 0% after laryngotracheal resection. As can be seen in Table 124.7, 69% of carinal resections were performed for ACC compared with only 27% performed for SCC.

Mortality (five of eight patients) was unacceptably high among the patients having staged reconstruction, and the procedure has been abandoned. Of nine patients who had exploration alone, three died. One death after exploration was caused by hemorrhage from the innominate artery after establishment of a mediastinal tracheostomy in continuity. Two deaths were caused by respiratory failure. Two deaths after staged reconstruction were caused by anastomotic separation, one was caused by respiratory failure, one by hemorrhage from the innominate artery, and one by hypoxemia related to the use of cardiopulmonary bypass with extensive manipulation of the right middle and lower lobes to accomplish reconstruction in a patient with only a left upper lobe on the opposite side.

Long-Term Survival

Overall survival for all patients with primary tracheal carcinoma was 84% at 1 year, 45% at 5 years, and 25% at 10 years. Mean survival time was 38 months with resected

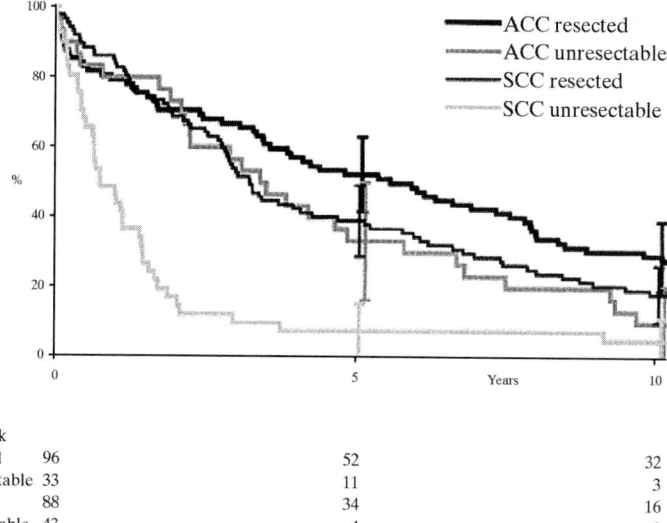

Figure 124.4 Actuarial overall survival by resection status and tumor type. ACC, adenoid cystic carcinoma; SCC, squamous cell carcinoma. (From Gaissert HA, Grillo H, Shadmehr B, et al. Long-term survival after resection of primary adenoid cystic and squamous cell carcinoma of the trachea and carina. *Ann Thorac Surg* 2004;78:1889–1897, with permission.)

Patients at risk

ACC resected	96	52	32
ACC unresectable	33	11	3
SCC resected	88	34	16
SCC unresectable	43	4	2

SCC, 8.8 months with unresectable SCC, 69 months with resected ACC, and 41 months with unresectable ACC. Figure 124.4 depicts the survival by tumor type and resection status. At 5 years, 39.1% of patients with resected and 7.3% of patients with unresectable SCC survived. Five-year survival was 52.4% for resected and 33.3% for unresectable ACC. A comparison of survival after laryngotracheal, tracheal, and carinal resections is shown in Figure 124.5. Despite higher hospital mortality after carinal resection, differences in long-term survival between these types of resection were not significant.

Survival according to airway margin status is depicted in Figures 124.6 and 124.7. Complete resection with negative airway margins resulted in higher survival compared with incomplete resection or unresectable tumors for both

ACC and SCC, although in SCC there were few patients with tumor-bearing airway margins and the difference from tumor-free margins was not significant. In ACC, the survival after incomplete resection separates from unresectable tumors after 10 years; we know of no survivor beyond 13 years in the unresectable group, whereas survival after incomplete resection at 15 years was 14.5%.

The logistic multivariate analysis of resected patients (Table 124.9) identified ACC, complete resection, and negative resection margins to be associated with 5-year survival and ACC, complete resection, and age to be associated with 10-year survival. Sensitivity analyses showed that either negative pathologic airway margins or complete resection, as determined by the surgeon, were associated with improved survival when run in separate models.

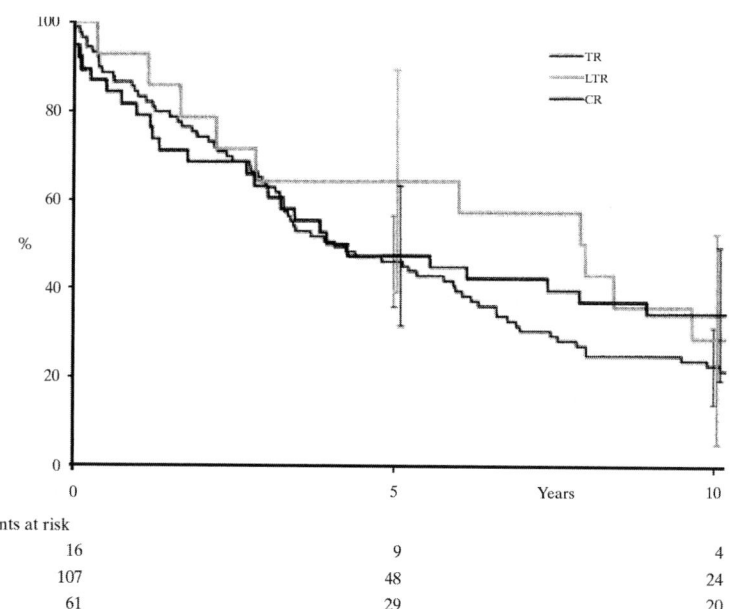

Figure 124.5 Actuarial survival by type of resection. (CR, carinal resection; LTR, laryngotracheal resection; TR, tracheal resection. (From Gaissert HA, Grillo H, Shadmehr B, et al. Long-term survival after resection of primary adenoid cystic and squamous cell carcinoma of the trachea and carina. *Ann Thorac Surg* 2004;78:1889–1897, with permission.)

Patients at risk

LTR	16	9	4
TR	107	48	24
CR	61	29	20

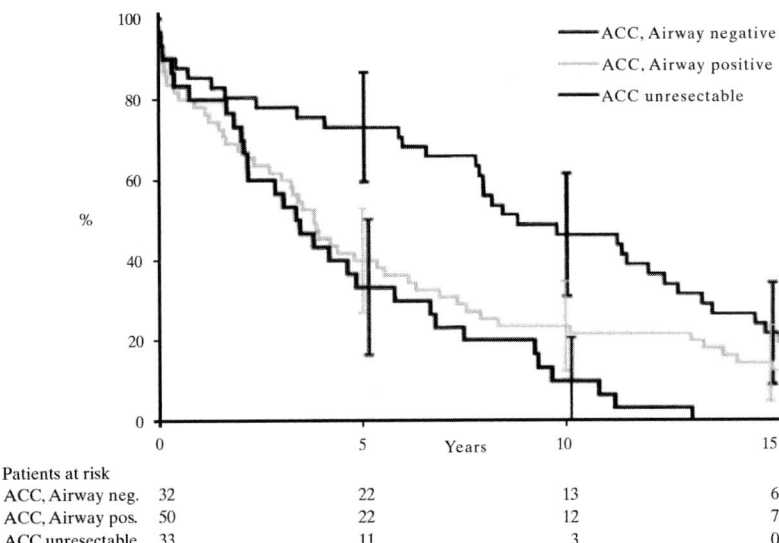

Figure 124.6 Actuarial survival in adenoid cystic carcinoma by airway margin. Note 15-year observation interval. ACC, adenoid cystic carcinoma. (From Gaissert HA, Grillo H, Shadmehr B, et al. Long-term survival after resection of primary adenoid cystic and squamous cell carcinoma of the trachea and carina. *Ann Thorac Surg* 2004;78: 1889–1897, with permission.)

As expected in the heterogeneous group of other tumors, statistical results for outcome are good because many of these tumors were benign or low-grade malignant lesions. One of the 11 carcinoids was highly atypical and had metastasized to regional lymph nodes in a malignant manner. All mucoepidermoid tumors behaved benignly. Adenocarcinoma occurred in the membranous wall of the carina of a child in the base of a cyst but had not recurred in more than 3.5 years. The one patient with adenosquamous carcinoma had a tumor that involved the larynx to such an extent that it could not be saved. The patient died of metastasis 4.7 years later. One patient with small-cell carcinoma confined to the trachea had subsequent chemotherapy and irradiation because of the histologic appearance of

the tumor. He was without recurrence 3.7 years after resection. The one patient with melanoma had no history of cutaneous lesions and no current cutaneous or retinal lesions, but the follow-up period was brief. No other metastatic disease had been detected. It is believed that this was indeed a primary lesion of the airway. The patient who had pseudosarcoma was free of disease 19 years later. Several patients who had this disease in the era before extended tracheal resection was performed died of strangulation because of local growth without metastasis. The chondrosarcoma was a low-grade lesion, but the patient died of pulmonary metastasis slightly more than 5 years after resection. The patient with rhabdomyosarcoma died of osteogenic sarcoma, probably because of radiation treatment

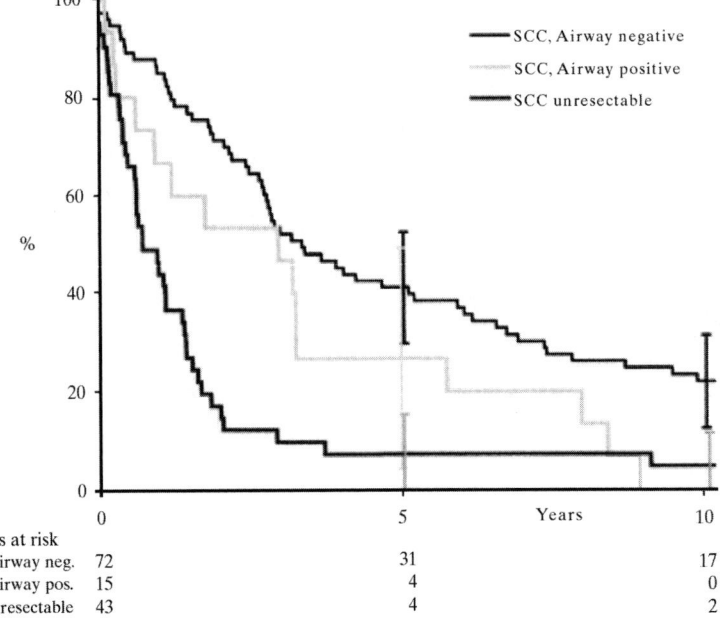

Figure 124.7 Actuarial survival in squamous cell carcinoma by airway margin. SCC, squamous cell carcinoma. (From Gaissert HA, Grillo H, Shadmehr B, et al. Long-term survival after resection of primary adenoid cystic and squamous cell carcinoma of the trachea and carina. *Ann Thorac Surg* 2004;78:1889–1897, with permission.)

TABLE 124.9

INFLUENCE OF PERIOPERATIVE VARIABLES ON SURVIVAL AT 5 AND 10 YEARS

		Overall	Survival at 5 years		Survival at 10 years	
	No.	Average/ Percent	Bivariate OR (CI)	Multivariate OR (CI)	Bivariate OR (CI)	Multivariate OR (CI)
Histology						
ACC	101	53%	2.59 (1.34–5.01)	8.76 (2.44–31.41)	3.19 (1.53–6.67)	7.58 (2.13–26.95)
SCC (REF)	90	47%	1.00	1.00	1.00	1.00
p			0.005	0.009	0.002	0.0017
Tumor length	177	2.8 (±1.4)	0.84 (0.67–1.06)	0.76 (0.54–1.06)	0.85 (0.66–1.09)	0.75 (0.54–1.06)
p			0.147	0.1016	0.208	0.1005
Type of resection						
CR	175	92%	3.59 (0.75–17.21)	8.10 (0.95–69.46)	2.29 (0.49–10.68)	2.523 (0.34–18.62)
LTR/TR (REF)	16	8%	1.00	1.00	1.00	1.00
p			0.11	0.0563	0.292	0.364
Age	189	54.8 (±15.4)	0.98 (0.96–1.00)	0.98 (0.95–1.01)	0.96 (0.93–0.98)	0.96 (0.92–0.99)
p			0.063	0.1898	<0.001	0.0109
Resection						
Complete	76	41%	2.69 (1.36–5.33)	31.93 (3.92–260.33)	3.04 (1.33–6.92)	1.55 (0.24–10.06)
Other (REF)	110	59%	1.00	1.00	1.00	1.00
p			0.005	0.0012	0.008	0.6469
Lymph node status						
Not positive	149	78%	0.27 (0.12–0.59)	0.60 (0.21–1.73)	0.26 (0.10–0.69)	0.55 (0.14–2.15)
Positive (REF)	42	22%	1.00	1.00	1.00	1.00
p			0.001	0.3469	0.007	0.3923
Smoker						
No	67	35%	1.00	1.00	1.00	1.00
Yes	124	65%	1.06 (0.54–2.08)	1.35 (0.52–3.52)	1.04 (0.49–2.21)	1.56 (0.51–4.70)
p			0.868	0.5394	0.912	0.4345
Airway margin						
Negative	115	60%	0.71 (0.36–1.39)	7.13 (1.04–48.73)	0.64 (0.30–1.40)	9.55 (1.48–61.72)
Other (REF)	76	40%	1.00	1.00	1.00	1.00
p			0.316	0.0452	0.264	0.0178

ACC = adenoid cystic carcinoma; CI = confidence interval; CR = carinal resection; LTR = laryngotracheal resection; OR = odds ratio; REF = reference; SCC = squamous cell carcinoma; TR = tracheal resection.

for cervical rhabdomyosarcoma in early childhood. The other death from tumor was that of a patient who had spindle cell sarcoma of the carina.

Five patients with other tumors had operations for the same tumors before referral. Three had carcinoids that had been removed incompletely and had recurrences 10 to 14 years later. An 8-year-old patient who had malignant fibrous histiocytoma had had incomplete resection in a local plastic procedure at the carina. She remained free of disease for 3 years after carinal resection but was not available for follow-up evaluation. A 19-year-old patient who had a fibrous tumor of the carina had had pneumonectomy with residual tumor left at the carina. He was free of disease almost 2 years after carinal resection. Two patients were not available for follow-up evaluation: One had low-grade spindle cell sarcoma and had participated in follow-up evaluation for 10 years without recurrence. The other had solitary squamous papilloma and had had follow-up evaluation for 7 years without recurrence. One patient who had granular cell tumor high in the trachea involving the

lower posterior larynx was later found to have a concurrent granular cell tumor of the bronchus intermedius, which was removed by means of sleeve resection.

Recurrence

The first patient who had resection of the carina for ACC in this series was free of disease until recurrence at the suture line 17 years later. Because resection margins and lymph nodes had been negative, no irradiation had been performed. Bronchoscopic follow-up examinations had been terminated after 10 years. Because this type of tracheal carcinoma has a proclivity for a long clinical course and late recurrence, it is more difficult to interpret results of resection. Table 124.10 lists vital status and recurrence in 177 operative survivors. Of 55 patients with recurrence, the site was locoregional only in 26, distant in 16, combined in 7, and unstated in 7 patients. New primary malignancy was observed in 14 patients. In SCC, lung cancer occurred in 6, head and neck carcinoma in 2, and leukemia,

TABLE 124.10

VITAL STATUS AND RECURRENT DISEASE IN 177 PATIENTS SURVIVING TRACHEAL RESECTION FOR PRIMARY CARCINOMA

	ACC (n)	SCC (n)	Total (%)
Died of disease	17	23	23
Died without evidence of disease	8	19	15
Died, unknown status	5	14	11
Alive with disease	11	4	8.5
Alive without evidence of disease	34	24	33
Incomplete follow-up	16	2	10
Total	91	86	100

ACC = adenoid cystic carcinoma; SCC = squamous cell carcinoma.

TABLE 124.11

LENGTH AND DEPTH OF RESECTED TUMORS, AND STATUS OF RESECTION MARGINS

Descriptor	ACC	SCC
Tumor length (cm), mean (95% confidence interval)	3.2(2.9–3.5)	(2.1–2.7)
Tumor depth (%)		
Mucosa and submucosa	4.9	27
Limited to airway wall	17	24
Peritracheal soft tissue	60	31
Adjacent organ	15	13
Depth not known	3.0	4.4
Margin status (%)		
Only tracheal margin positive	8	10
Only radial margin positive	29	22
Tracheal and radial margin positive	51	8
Any tracheal margin positive	59	18
Total positive margins	93	40

Any tracheal margin was positive if either cephalad or caudad tracheal margins, or mainstem bronchial margin contained tumor. Total positive margins denote tumor involving or approaching within 1 mm either the radial or tracheal surgical margin.
ACC = adenoid cystic carcinoma; SCC = squamous cell carcinoma.

colon, prostate, and other tumor in 1 patient each; in ACC, lung and breast cancer developed in 1 patient each.

Effect of Tumor at Resection Margins and in Lymph Nodes

The finding of tumor at the resection margins, even through frozen section during the operation, has particular importance in airway reconstruction. Because of the requisite for reconstruction, it is sometimes impossible to resect more airway without endangering the safety of the anastomosis by causing excessive tension. Extensive regional lymph node dissection can destroy the blood supply to the trachea. Loss of blood supply can cause necrosis at the anastomosis followed by irreparable stenosis. Therefore, only immediately adjacent regional lymph nodes are blocked out with the specimen. Others can be sampled for prognostic information.

Length and depth of resected tumors and status of resection margins are listed in Table 124.11. ACC were longer and extended more often into peritracheal soft tissues or to adjacent organs, most commonly the esophageal muscle coat. Tumor, therefore, was more often present at or close to the radial resection margin, and tracheal margins frequently contained microscopic tumor. Of patients with ACC, 59% had positive airway margins, in contrast to only 18% with SCC.

Table 124.12 shows the lymph node status in the 191 patients having tracheal resection for primary carcinoma. Selective sampling established lymph node metastasis in 19.4% (37/191) of patients, most commonly from peritracheal and subcarinal stations; nodal biopsies were not obtained in 35%. Figure 124.8 shows the survival according to lymph node status. Lymph node-positive SCC had a markedly lower survival than tumors without nodal metastasis. No correlation was noted between lymph node status and survival in ACC. A retrospective French multicenter study of 208 patients did not find a decrease in survival

for patients with positive lymph nodes(24), which we observed in SCC. Our logistic multivariate analysis of patients having lesions resected (Table 124.9) did not find lymph node involvement predictive of survival. These seemingly conflicting data were based on small numbers of lymph node-positive patients, and the multivariate analysis may have attributed any effect on outcome to squamous histology. The multivariate analysis did not establish other variables of disease extent as predictors of survival in either tumor, such as tumor depth or tumor length. These findings indicate the problems in characterizing basic oncologic relationships in primary tracheal carcinoma because of its low incidence and suggest a current lack of data to formulate a precise staging system.

TABLE 124.12

LYMPH NODE STATUS IN 191 PATIENTS UNDERGOING TRACHEAL RESECTION FOR PRIMARY CARCINOMA

	ACC (n)	SCC (n)	Total (%)
No lymph node biopsy	45	22	35
Tumor-free lymph nodes	43	44	45
One lymph node positive	8	16	13
More than one lymph node positive	5	8	7
Total	101	90	100

ACC = adenoid cystic carcinoma; SCC = squamous cell carcinoma.

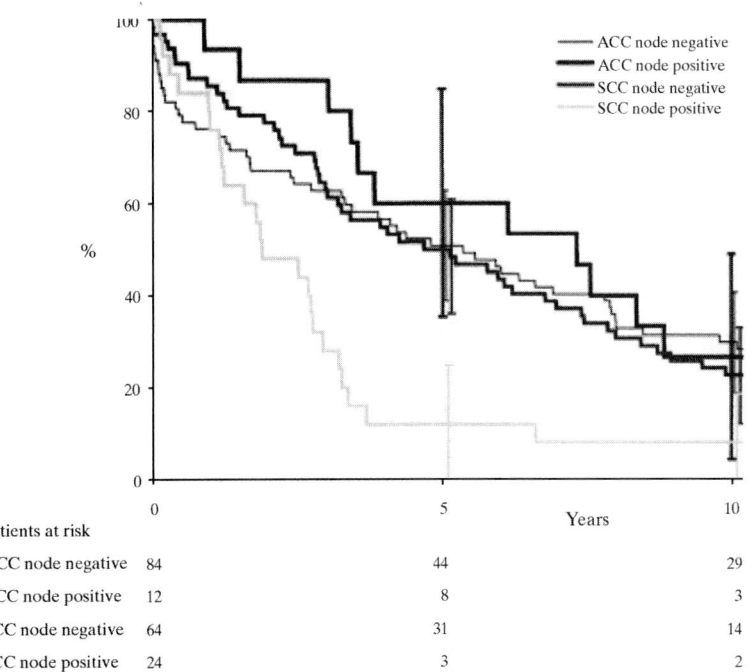

Figure 124.8 Actuarial survival of primary tracheal carcinoma by lymph node status. ACC, adenoid cystic carcinoma; SCC, squamous cell carcinoma. (From Gaissert HA, Grillo H, Shadmehr B, et al. Long-term survival after resection of primary adenoid cystic and squamous cell carcinoma of the trachea and carina. *Ann Thorac Surg* 2004;78: 1889–1897, with permission.)

Patients at risk			
ACC node negative	84	44	29
ACC node positive	12	8	3
SCC node negative	64	31	14
SCC node positive	24	3	2

Positive lymph nodes in SCC were found more commonly among patients who later died with cancer than among those who survived without cancer. Invasive carcinoma at the resection margin is of graver consequence than is in situ carcinoma: four of five patients with invasive carcinoma died. All six patients with in situ disease were free of disease. Almost all patients had radiation therapy in doses from 4,500 to 6,500 cGy. Because irradiation was administered in many centers, it was impossible to control for dosage or portal differences. With ACC and positive margins, lymph nodes, or both, little difference was seen compared with results among patients who had negative margins and nodes. Because of the proclivity of this tumor to extend for long distances submucosally and perineurally, the finding of malignant cells far from the gross tumor is all too common. The surgeon often must compromise total resection for safety. All of these patients now have postoperative irradiation. Suture-line recurrences thus far have been rare. Late recurrences have developed in lung, bone, liver, or brain. Irradiation of unresected tumor, however, is all but uniformly characterized by local recurrence within 3 to 5 years, despite early good response.

Other Squamous Cell Carcinomas

A total of 16 patients who had resection of squamous carcinoma of the trachea had a history, concurrent finding, or later occurrence of SCC in the respiratory tract. One had concurrent SCC of the tongue. One patient had carcinoma of the larynx and was treated before tracheal resection, and a second later had carcinoma of the larynx. In one patient, a second primary carcinoma of the trachea developed at a different level. Seven patients had had lobectomy or pneumonectomy for squamous carcinoma of the lung; five of these patients later had SCC of the lung. Of these 12 patients, 2 of whom had two primary squamous carcinomas of opposite lungs at extended intervals, 3 died of recurrent tracheal carcinoma, 1 died of recurrence of previous carcinoma of the lung, 1 died of a later carcinoma of the lung, and 1 died of a second primary carcinoma of the lung and had had tracheal resection between the two pulmonary episodes. Four patients who had pulmonary resection before or after tracheal resection were living without disease 2.5 to 15 years after the tracheal episode.

Role of Irradiation

In view of the narrow margins that often can be obtained in tracheal resection, even when the margins and lymph nodes are histologically negative, it is prudent to use postoperative irradiation to managing SCC and ACC of the trachea. Both tumors are radiosensitive, particularly ACC. After recurrence of ACC 17 years after resection in a patient who did not have irradiation, it appeared wiser to use irradiation after surgery. Irradiation alone has been argued to be appropriate primary therapy for carcinoma of the trachea. We compared results among patients who had resection with or without subsequent radiation therapy with those among patients who received radiation therapy alone as primary treatment. A few also had exploration. The principal reason for assigning patients to the radiation therapy category was extent of tumor. This, however, frequently was longitudinal extension and did not necessarily indicate a large mass. The number of patients dead of disease

TABLE 124.13

SURVIVAL AFTER THERAPY FOR TRACHEAL TUMORS

Tumor Type	Patients Dead from Carcinoma (N)	Patients Alive > 1 yr Without Disease (N)
Squamous		
Resection (± irradiation)	11	18
Irradiation (± exploration)	16	1
Adenoid cystic		
Resection (± irradiation)	7	38
Irradiation (± exploration)	9	3

TABLE 124.14

PALLIATIVE VALUE OF OPERATION AND IRRADIATION FOR SQUAMOUS CELL TRACHEAL CARCINOMA

Time to Death After Treatment (mo)	Irradiation Only	Resection with Irradiation
<12	5	1
12–24	3	2
24–36	1	4
36–48	0	4
>48	1	0

and those alive without disease for more than 1 year for each type of tracheal carcinoma and for each treatment method (operation and irradiation versus irradiation alone) are listed in Table 124.13. These patients were seen over many years, which diminished the precision of the comparison.

Of the patients with SCC of the trachea who had surgical resection followed by radiation therapy, 11 patients died of carcinoma of the trachea. Eighteen were alive longer than 1 year without evidence of disease. In marked contrast, 16 patients for whom radiation therapy was essentially the only treatment method were dead of carcinoma. One was alive approximately 7 years after treatment.

Patients who had ACC had been divided into those who died of carcinoma and those who were alive without known disease. Analysis was more difficult for these patients because the disease can have long periods of apparent control after operation or irradiation. Among patients treated with operation and usually postoperative radiation therapy, 7 were dead of carcinoma and 38 were alive without known disease. With irradiation alone, 9 were dead of carcinoma, and only 3 were alive without evidence of disease.

In an effort to determine whether a palliative benefit to patients who undergo operation exists, given its risks, in combination with radiation therapy compared with radiation therapy alone, survival of patients with squamous carcinoma having one or the other treatment method but who died of carcinoma was examined. Table 124.14 shows the number of surviving patients in 12-month periods. The results of radiation therapy alone are much like those obtained for SCC of the lung, most patients having a recurrence in 2 years. In contrast, resection with radiation therapy provides 2 to 4 years of survival. Because the course of ACC is so prolonged, we examined similar treatment groups with the same endpoint of death from SCC or ACC but compared median and average survival periods in months (Table 124.15). Resection combined with irradiation, given the limits of this nonrandomized comparison,

tripled survival time for SCC and at least a tripled survival time for ACC.

Results of analysis of this 40-year experience with surgical management of primary tumors of the trachea appear to confirm and extend conclusions based on previously reported experiences. Eschapasse (19) collected information on 152 primary tracheal tumors from multiple teams in France and the Soviet Union. In 1974, he described 121 patients surgically treated; 75 of these patients had reconstruction after cylindrical resection and anastomosis (47 cases) or carinal resection (28 cases). In 121 operations, 13 deaths occurred. Of 19 patients who had adenoid cystic tumors, five were alive and free of disease for 3 to 9 years, and 11 of 27 patients who had SCC were alive and free of disease for 7 months to 16 years.

Pearson et al. (21) reported on surgical treatment of 44 patients between 1963 and 1983. Of the patients who had reconstruction, 29 including 16 sleeve resections and 13 carinal resections, 2 deaths occurred. Nine patients with adenoid cystic carcinoma were alive without disease 1 to 20 years after the operation, 3 had died of other disease in 6 to 18 years, and 2 were alive with disease. Of 6 patients with SCC who had resection, 4 were alive 6 to 56 months after treatment.

TABLE 124.15

DURATION OF SURVIVAL AFTER IRRADIATION OR RESECTION

Treatment	Survival Time (mo)	
	Median	Average
Squamous cell carcinoma		
Irradiation only	10	11
Resection (± irradiation)	34	31
Adenoid cystic carcinoma		
Irradiation only	28	39
Resection (± irradiation)	118	107

In 1987, Perelman and Koroleva (23) reported on a 20-year experience (1963–1983) with 116 open operations on 135 patients; 75 were treated by sleeve resection (41 cases) or carinal resection (34 cases); 11 deaths occurred. The overall survival rate for SCC was 27% at 3 years and 13% at 5 and 10 years. For ACC, the overall survival rate was 71% at 3 years, 66% at 5 years, and 56% at 10 and 15 years.

In 1996, Maziak et al. (11) updated their 32-year experience (1963-1995), specifically with ACC. Among the 38 patients, 32 were treated with resection and reconstruction. Three patients died within 30 days of the operation (9%). Among the 14 patients who had complete resection, the mean survival period was 9.8 years. For the 15 with incomplete resection, the mean survival period was 7.5 years. For the 6 treated with irradiation only, the mean survival time was 6.2 years.

Regnard et al. (24) reported the results of treatment of 208 patients with tracheal tumors collected from 26 centers in France. Their series included 94 patients with SCC, 4 with adenocarcinoma, 65 with ACC, and 45 patients with miscellaneous tumors. The overall operative mortality rate was 10.5%. For ACC, 5- and 10-year survival rates were 73% and 57%. For tracheal cancer, the corresponding survival rates were 47% and 36%. Among the patients with tracheal cancer, the 5-year survival rates for complete and incomplete resections were 55% and 25%. Postoperative radiation therapy was used to treat 59% of patients who had tracheal cancer and 43% of patients who had ACC. The authors believed that the benefit of postoperative radiation therapy was inconclusive, except among patients with incomplete resection of tracheal cancers.

Rafaely and Weissberg (25) reported on 22 tracheal resections for tumor. One operative death occurred. Of the 12 survivors with ACC, 2 patients, both of whom did not have radiation therapy, died of metastatic spread. Nine patients who had irradiation were living free of tumor. Among the five patients with squamous cell tumor, one died of another cause, one has local recurrence and was alive and receiving radiation therapy 3.3 years after the operation, and three were without disease 5 to 11 years postoperatively.

Several therapeutic recommendations appear to be justified by our experience and the data from other studies. First, benign primary tumors of the trachea and tumors of intermediate aggressiveness are best managed by means of surgical resection with reconstruction of the airway. Second, primary SCC and ACC of the trachea are best managed by resection if primary reconstruction can be accomplished safely. Most patients with tracheal cancer, in contrast to peripheral lung cancer, have limited disease when symptoms occur and, therefore, are good candidates for surgical therapy. Resection probably should be followed by full-dose mediastinal irradiation in most cases. Third, malignant primary tracheal tumors of other types should be resected if resection allows safe primary reconstruction. Irradiation probably should be administered postoperatively to most patients. Surgical mortality and morbidity undoubtedly can be improved in the years ahead. It appears judicious that extensive tracheal reconstruction, in particular that of the carina, be accomplished in centers that specialize in this type of surgery.

HIGHLIGHTS

- Use of gentle, controlled inhalational induction with a volatile anesthetic to allow spontaneous ventilation is the best technique for operations on patients with tracheal stenosis.
- Use of a rigid bronchoscope and biopsy forceps to core out a tracheal neoplasm is a rapid, safe technique to open an airway obstructed with tumor.
- Diagnosis of tracheal tumors requires a high degree of suspicion because many patients have normal chest radiographs.
- Current staging methods have limited accuracy in defining the locoregional extent of disease.
- Adenoid cystic carcinoma and squamous cell carcinoma are the two most common tracheal tumors.
- Adenoid cystic carcinoma is best managed by tracheal resection and postoperative radiation therapy, even if the margins are negative.
- Incomplete resection because of positive tracheal margins continues to be justified in selected patients with adenoid cystic carcinoma in the hands of experienced surgeons
- Squamous cell carcinoma is best managed with tracheal resection and postoperative irradiation, even if the margins are negative.
- Tracheal reconstruction is performed by direct end-to-end anastomosis with fine absorbable sutures; this avoids suture line granuloma.
- Anastomotic tension is avoided by use of traction sutures, dissection of the pretracheal plane, flexion of the neck, hilar release, and suprahyoid release, when necessary
- Bronchoplastic techniques allow proximal and distal resection with preservation of the larynx and reconstruction of the carina.
- Long-term survival after resection and irradiation is possible, but careful long-term follow-up evaluation is mandatory, especially for adenoid cystic carcinoma, which can recur many years later.

REFERENCES

1. Grillo HC. Surgery of the trachea. In: Keen G, ed. *Operative surgery and management,* 2nd ed. Bristol, UK: Wright, 1987:776–784.
2. Grillo HC. The trachea. In: Ravitch MM, Steichen FM, eds. *Atlas of general thoracic surgery.* Philadelphia: WB Saunders, 1988: 293–331.
3. Pearson FG. Resection of the trachea for stricture. In: Jackson JW, ed. *Rob and Smith's operative surgery,* 3rd ed. London: Butterworths, 1978:373–380.
4. Grillo HC. Primary reconstruction of airway after resection of subglottic and upper tracheal stenosis. *Ann Thorac Surg* 1982;33:39–58.
5. Grillo HC. Carinal reconstruction. *Ann Thorac Surg* 1982;34: 356–373.
6. Pearson FG, Brito-Filomeno L, Cooper JD. Experience with partial cricoid resection and thyrotracheal anastomosis. *Ann Otol Rhinol Laryngol* 1986;95:582–585.

7. Grillo HC, Zannini P. Resectional management of airway invasion by thyroid carcinoma. *Ann Thorac Surg* 1986;42:287–298.
8. Grillo HC, Mathisen DJ. Primary tracheal tumors: treatment and results. *Ann Thorac Surg* 1990;49:69–77.
9. Mitchell JD, Mathisen DJ, Wright CD, et al. Clinical experience with carinal resection. *J Thorac Cardiovasc Surg* 1999;117:39–53.
10. Kutlu CA, Goldstraw P. Tracheobronchial sleeve resection with the use of a continuous anastomosis: results of one hundred consecutive cases. *J Thorac Cardiovasc Surg* 1999;117:1112–1117.
11. Maziak DE, Todd TRJ, Keshavjee SH, et al. Adenoid cystic carcinoma of the airway: thirty-two-year experience. *J Thorac Cardiovasc Surg* 1996;112:1522–1532.
12. Gaissert HA, Grillo H, Mathisen D, et al. Long-term survival after resection of primary adenoid cystic and squamous cell carcinoma of the trachea and carina. *Ann Thorac Surg* 2004;78:1889–1897.
13. Weber AL, ed. Symposium on the larynx and trachea. *Radiol Clin North Am* 1978;16:179–341.
14. Whyte RI, Quint LE, Kazerooni EA, et al. Helical computed tomography for the evaluation of tracheal stenosis. *Ann Thorac Surg* 1995;60:27–30.
15. LoCicero J III, Costello P, Campos CT, et al. Spiral CT with multiplanar and three-dimensional reconstructions accurately predicts tracheobronchial pathology. *Ann Thorac Surg* 1996;62:811–817.
16. Mathisen DJ, Grillo HC. Endoscopic relief of malignant airway obstruction. *Ann Thorac Surg* 1989;48:469–475.
17. Daddi G, Puma F, Avenia N, et al. Resection with curative intent after endoscopic treatment of airway obstruction. *Ann Thorac Surg* 1998;65:203–207.
18. Behringer EC, Wilson RS. Tracheal resection and reconstruction. In: Cohen E, ed. *The practice of thoracic anesthesia.* Philadelphia: JB Lippincott, 1995:531–561.
19. Eschapasse H. Les tumeurs tracheales primitives: traiement chirurgical. *Rev Fr Mal Respir* 1974;2:425–430.
20. Perelman M, Koroleva N. Surgery of the trachea. *World J Surg* 1980;4:583–593.
21. Pearson FG, Todd TRJ, Cooper JD. Experience with primary neoplasms of the trachea and carina. *J Thorac Cardiovasc Surg* 1984;88:511–518.
22. Xu LT, Sun ZF, Li ZJ, et al. Clinical and pathologic characteristics in patients with tracheobronchial tumor: report of 50 patients. *Ann Thorac Surg* 1987;43:276–278.
23. Perelman MI, Koroleva NS. Primary tumors of the trachea. In: Grillo HC, Eschapasse H, eds. *International trends in general thoracic surgery.* Vol. 2. Philadelphia: WB Saunders, 1987:91–106.
24. Regnard JF, Fourquier P, Levasseur P. Results and prognostic factors in resections of primary tracheal tumors: a multicenter retrospective study. The French Society of Cardiovascular Surgery. *J Thorac Cardiovasc Surg* 1996;111:808–824.
25. Rafaely Y, Weissberg D. Surgical management of tracheal tumors. *Ann Thorac Surg* 1997;64:1429–1433.
26. Allen MS. Symposium on intrathoracic neoplasms. VI: malignant tracheal tumors. *Mayo Clin Proc* 1993;68:680–684.
27. El-Baz N, El-Ganzouri A, Gottschalk W et al. One-lung high-frequency pressure ventilation for sleeve pneumonectomy: an alternative technique. *Anesth Analg* 1981;60:683–686.
28. Grillo HC, Mathisen DJ. Cervical exenteration. *Ann Thorac Surg* 1990;49:401–408.
29. Salassa JR, Pearson BW, Payne WS. Gross and microscopical blood supply of the trachea. *Ann Thorac Surg* 1977;24:100–107.
30. Montgomery WW. Suprahyoid release for tracheal anastomosis. *Arch Otolaryngol* 1974;99:255–260.
31. Grillo HC, Zannini P, Michelassi F. Complications of tracheal reconstruction: incidence, treatment, and prevention. *J Thorac Cardiovasc Surg* 1986;91:322–328.

Vascular Tumors of the Head and Neck

125

Umamaheswar Duvvuri   **Ricardo L. Carrau**   **Amin B. Kassam**

Vascular tumors of the head and neck constitute a heterogeneous group of neoplasms that have in common their origin from the vascular system and a marked propensity for bleeding after trauma or during excision. Their clinical presentation, however, varies widely. Although some vascular tumors cause little apparent problem or disfigurement, others are locally aggressive or even malignant.

For this chapter, we will follow Batsakis' classification (Table 125.1). It is a broad classification that divides vascular tumors of the head and neck into benign and malignant and includes syndromes that have vascular lesions as important components.

BENIGN TUMORS

Benign tumors can be localized or generalized. Mulliken and Glowacki (1) classify benign tumors as hemangiomas or vascular malformations.

Localized Tumors

Hemangioma

The most common localized benign vascular tumor of the head and neck is the hemangioma, which can present in a number of forms. Although clinicians continue to refer to these lesions as "strawberry or cavernous hemangiomas," Mulliken and Young's classification (1) was adopted at the 1996 meeting of the International Society for the Study of Vascular Anomalies. In this classification, the lesions are classified according to histologic characteristics and biological behavior. Hemangiomas can be present at birth (30%) or appear a few weeks after birth. Hemangiomas have a female predilection with a male-to-female ratio of 1:6. It typically affects the skin of the head and neck and can remain quiescent or undergo a period of rapid growth. Some hemangiomas involve deeper structures and have a more

---

TABLE 125.1

VASCULAR TUMORS OF THE HEAD AND NECK (BATSAKIS)

Benign tumors
  Localized
    Hemangioma
    Lymphangioma
    Angiofibroma
  Generalized
    Angiomatosis
    Cystic hygroma
  Inflammatory
  Arteriovenous fistula, aneurysm
  Telangiectasia, phlebectasia

Syndromes
  Osler-Weber-Rendu
  Sturge-Weber
  Maffucci
  Von Hippel-Lindau

Malignant neoplasms
  Angiosarcoma
  Hemangiopericytoma
  Paraganglioma
    Carotid
    Vagus
    Larynx
    Jugular
    Tympanic

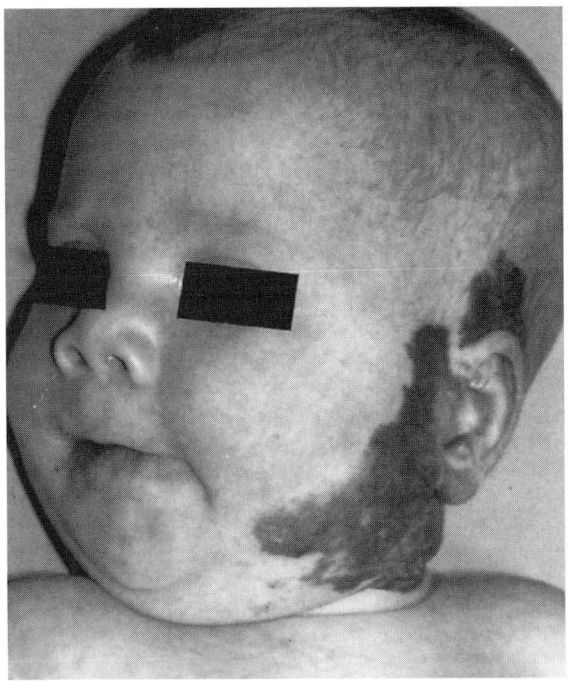

Figure 125.1 Cavernous hemangioma of the cheek of an infant. The lesion grew and stridor occurred, owing to subglottic hemangioma. Both lesions regressed spontaneously without formal treatment.

aggressive course (Fig. 125.1). Clinically, hemangiomas have a rapid proliferation in the first year of life characterized by endothelial cell hyperplasia and generally involute spontaneously. The rate of involution can vary, ranging from 6 to 12 years. Histologically, hemangiomas demonstrate rapidly proliferating endothelial cells with frequent mitoses and the presence of mast cells.

Hemangiomas can affect both the cutaneous surfaces of the head and neck and also the mucosal surfaces (Fig. 125.2). Neonates with cutaneous hemangiomas who present with respiratory distress or stridor may have

a laryngeal or subglottic lesion (Fig. 125.3). These lesions are submucosal, soft, and compressible and are usually are located in the left posterolateral subglottis. Because the overlying mucosa is normal, the hemangioma may not be the usual red or pink color so characteristic of the cutaneous lesions. Approximately half of the children with laryngeal hemangiomas have an associated cutaneous hemangioma. In adults, when a laryngeal hemangioma is diagnosed, the lesion usually is located in the supraglottis. Hoarseness is the most common symptom; bleeding and respiratory compromise are less common (2). Subglottic hemangiomas can be managed with systemic corticosteroid therapy, intralesional corticosteroid therapy, CO_2 laser resection, tracheotomy, interferon, laryngotracheoplasty, or they may simply be observed (3).

Many hemangiomas that initially appear stable can become proliferative with age. In general, however, a rapid growth phase of these tumors is almost always followed by gradual involution. An initial period of observation is recommended for most localized hemangiomas. Family members may press the surgeon when the tumor is growing aggressively only to find that, given time, the tumor gradually shrinks. Indications for early intervention include massive, ulcerative, or grossly disfiguring lesions; blockage of the visual field by a large hemangioma around the eyelids; bilateral auditory compression with resulting hearing loss; or evidence of airway compromise. Tumors with high vascular flow can lead to high-output cardiac failure and may require immediate treatment.

Therapeutic options include surgical excision, but this is infrequently used because of large tumor size and the resulting disfigurement. Surgical extirpation of lesions with high flow can be complicated by life-threatening hemorrhage. Various forms of lasers have been successfully used to extirpate or debulk hemangiomas. Hemangiomas with both superficial and deep components, or large lesions often require combined therapy with laser and surgical re-

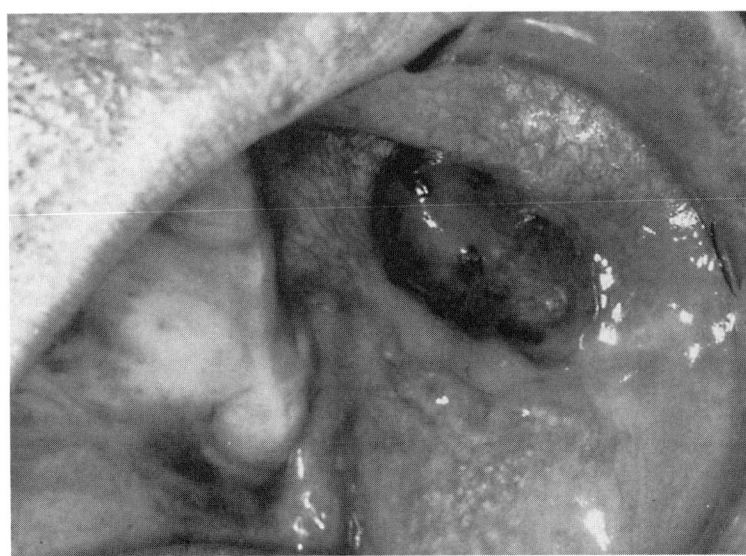

Figure 125.2 Cavernous hemangioma of the buccal mucosa. The patient was concerned about malignancy. The lesion was excised.

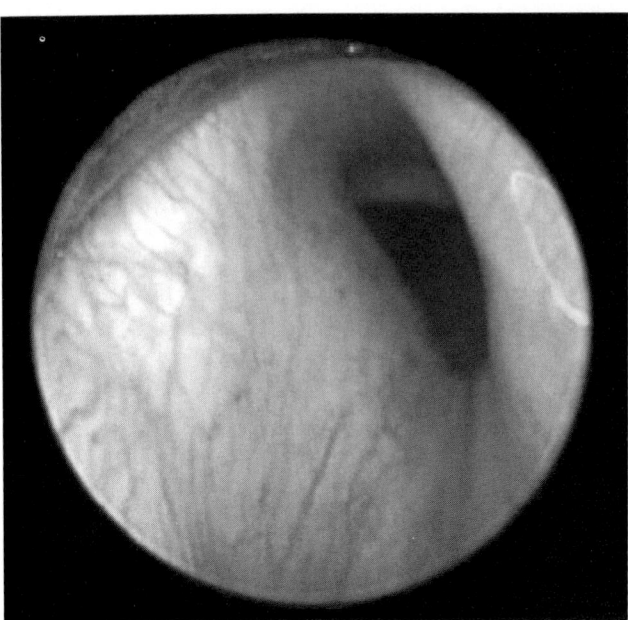
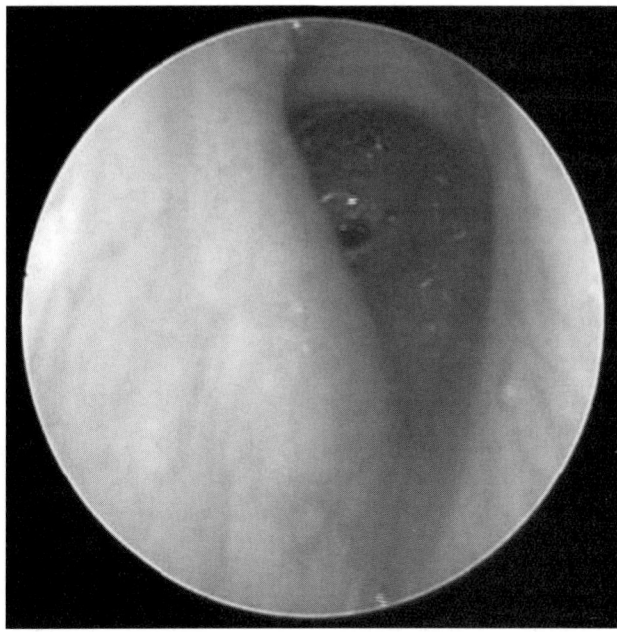

A   B

Figure 125.3   A: Child with a subglottic hemangioma resulting in airway compromise. **B:** Change a few weeks after intralesional steroid therapy. Open excision/tracheotomy was averted because the lesion shrunk substantially after treatment. (Images courtesy of David L. Mandell, MD, Children's Hospital of Pittsburgh, Pittsburgh, PA).

section. The timing of intervention depends on the clinical history and status of the hemangioma. Residual lesions after involution can be excised and any residual scar can be revised to improve cosmesis.

Intralesional or systemic corticosteroids may reduce rapid growth, but a rebound effect can occur when the medication is stopped. Systemic complications limit the use of high doses or long-term use of corticosteroids. Corticosteroid therapy typically extends for a 3- to 4-week course, with a gradual taper within 8 weeks. Patients who do not respond to initial treatment with corticosteroids rarely benefit from further steroid therapy. These patients can be treated with interferon, either interferon alpha-2a or alpha-2b (4,5). Most patients receiving daily subcutaneous doses of interferon alpha-2a are associated with a high rate of success and low recurrence rate after discontinuation of therapy. Interferon alpha-2a, however, is associated with systemic side effects that include liver enzyme elevation, renal failure, bone marrow suppression, and gait, posture, and fine-motor deficits. Intralesional sclerotherapy has been largely abandoned because of concerns regarding the scarring of the local site and adjacent tissue and inconsistent effects on proliferating hemangiomas.

Port-Wine Stains (Nevus Flammeus)

Although often classified as an intradermal hemangioma, the histology and clinical presentation of nevus flammeus more appropriately places it in the vascular malformation group. Microscopic examination shows that nevus flammeus contains vessels with mature endothelial lining and no hypercellularity (6). Nevus flammeus is present at

birth, grows proportionately with other structures, and rarely proliferates (1). Its association with sensory nerves, particularly the trigeminal nerve, is a well-recognized phenomenon. Port-wine stains initially present as pink, flat, and sharply demarcated lesions, but later become nodular and develop a darker scarlet or purple color (6,7). Treatment aims to improve the cosmesis for which tattooing, surgical excision, camouflage with cosmetics, and multiple other techniques have been reported (6,8). Laser therapy (used mainly in Europe) seems to be effective in selected cases (9). As with hemangioma, the association of nevus flammeus with various syndromes must be considered.

Vascular Malformations

Mulliken and Glowacki classified the different types of vascular malformations according to the types of vessels involved by the lesion, namely, arterial, arteriovenous, venous, capillary, and lymphatic. By definition, all vascular malformations are present at birth. They can manifest themselves at different stages of life, however, as the result of vascular ectasia caused by trauma, sepsis, or endocrinologic changes. Vascular malformations do not exhibit a gender bias. Vascular malformations do not have a proliferative phase, but they do grow with age and can undergo spontaneous involution. Histoanalysis reveals flat, normal-appearing endothelial cells with ectatic vessels.

Vascular malformations can be divided in low-flow and high-flow varieties. Venous and lymphatic malformations, which are low-flow lesions, are soft to palpation. High-flow lesions, which are firm to palpation and often show palpable pulsation, are warm to the touch. Surgery may be

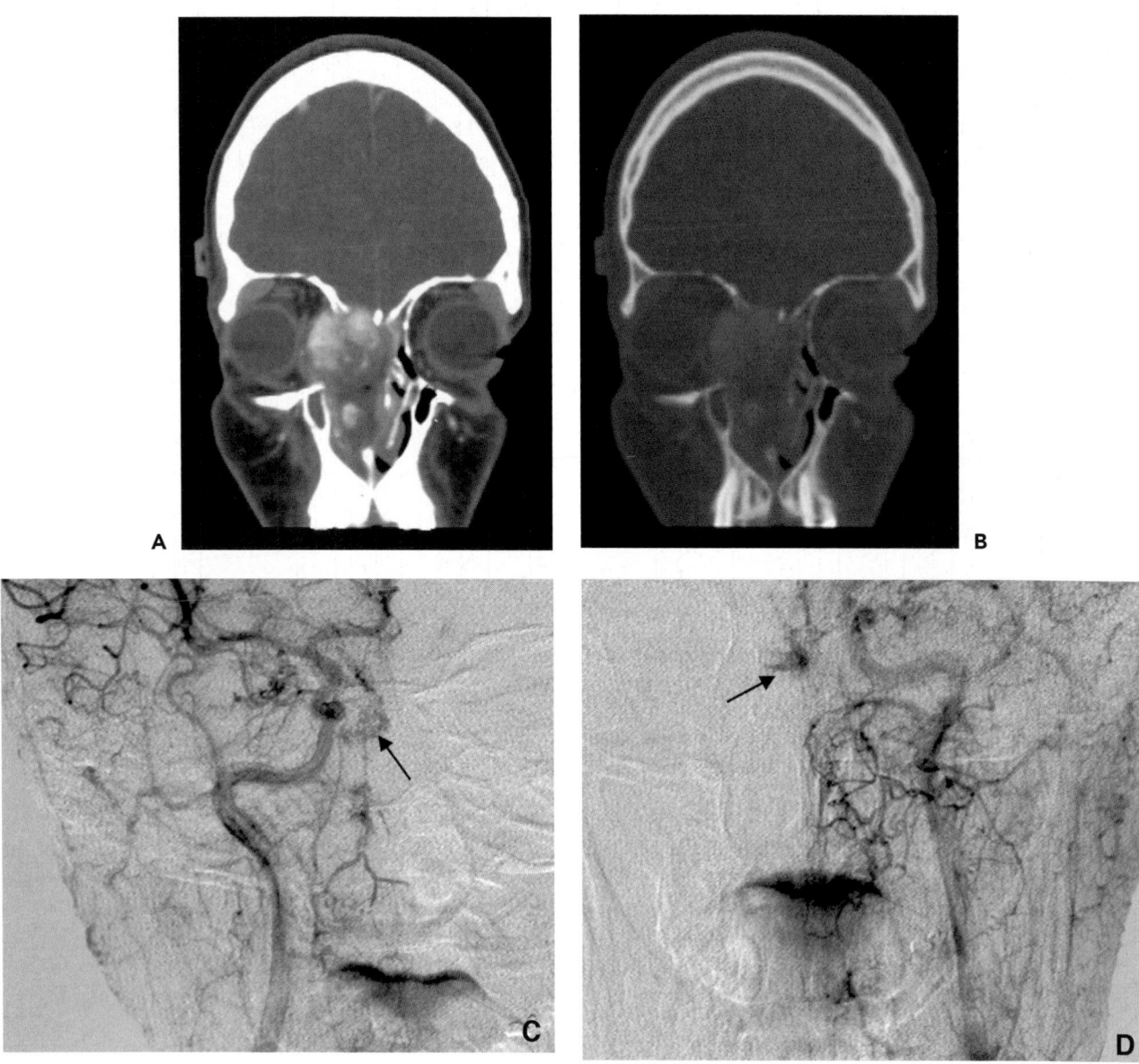

Figure 125.4 Vascular malformation of the skull base in a 24-year-old patient who presented with massive epistaxis. **A** and **B** show computed tomography (CT) images with soft tissue and bone algorithms, respectively. Destruction of the skull base and medial orbital wall is apparent. **C** and **D** show angiographic images; the *arrow* points to the vascular blush of the lesion. No dominant feeding vessels were identified for embolization. This lesion was resected through an endoscopic approach.

necessary to improve cosmesis and avoid pyschosocial trauma to a child. Low-flow venous and capillary lesions can be treated with laser therapy (superficial or interstitial) and some can be treated with surgery as the only modality. High-flow lesions can be managed with embolization followed by surgical resection (5) (Fig 125.4). Intralesional angiography and embolization using permanent or sclerosing agents have shown promising results (5).

Lymphangioma

Lymphangioma is a vascular malformation involving the lymphatic vessels. Its clinical presentation varies, but typi-

cally it consists of multiple papules on the skin or mucous membranes or a painless swelling that can resemble a lipoma in consistency (6,10). Lymphangiomas of the head and neck are most commonly found in the neck and the mucosal surfaces of the oral cavity, particularly the tongue. They can cause passive deformation of the facial skeleton because of their growth pattern. A lymphangioma always extend beyond its clinical extent. Magnetic resonance imaging (MRI) and, to a lesser degree, ultrasound help to better define the true extent and involvement of adjacent structures (11).

Multiple treatments have been advocated for lymphangiomas, including surgical resection, sclerosing agents,

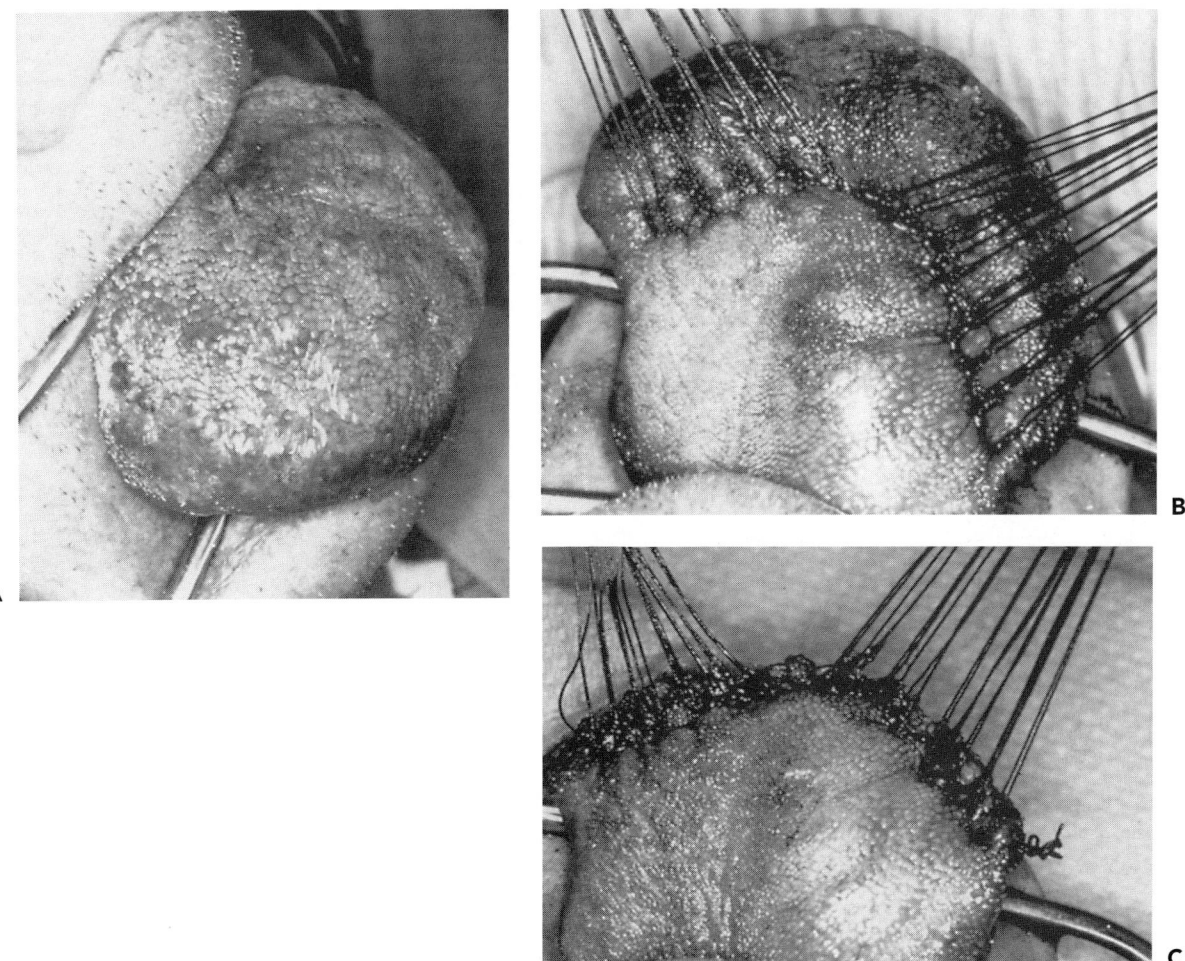

Figure 125.5 A: Hemangioma-lymphangioma of the tongue. **B:** Isolation of anterior tongue with hemostatic sutures. **C:** Hemangioma-lymphangioma has been resected with minimal blood loss, owing to the hemostatic effect of the sutures.

intralesional and systemic corticosteroids, and laser ablation therapy. Bardach (10) designed a technique for resection of large tumors of the anterior tongue using circumferential sutures (Fig. 125.5). The lymphangioma is isolated with absorbable sutures to then isolate the protruding portion of the tongue or other structures. Blood loss is minimal and healing is not a problem because of the rich blood supply.

Juvenile Angiofibroma

Juvenile angiofibroma (JA) develops exclusively in male adolescents, who usually present with epistaxis, nasal obstruction, or both. Unilateral middle ear effusion, proptosis, diplopia, cheek swelling with or without pain, or sinusitis should alert the physician to the possibility of this diagnosis and the need for a nasal endoscopic examination. Histologically, JA consists of multiple vascular channels surrounded by fibrous connective tissue. It originates in the basisphenoidal suture just superior to the sphenopalatine foramen and can extend to the posterior choana, the pterygopalatine fossa, the infratemporal fossa,

and, following preformed pathways, the orbit, and occasionally the cranial cavity.

Physical examination of patients suspected to have a JA should include a complete cranial nerve examination and an endoscopic evaluation of the nasal cavity and nasopharynx. Typically, the angiofibroma appears as a reddish, smooth polypoid mass. Otoscopic examination may demonstrate a middle ear effusion or a retracted tympanic membrane secondary to eustachian tube dysfunction. A computed tomography (CT) scan defines the bony architecture of the sinonasal tract and the skull base and is the preferred imaging evaluation. The use of contrast media during the imaging provides an accurate depiction of the vascularity and stage of the tumor. Its appearance is so characteristic that a biopsy is rarely needed to corroborate the diagnosis. MRI complements CT in cases of intracranial, intraorbital, or infratemporal extension. MRI better defines the interfaces of tumor with the surrounding soft tissue and helps to differentiate tumor from edematous mucosa and retained sinonasal secretions (Fig. 125.6). Biopsy is only necessary in cases presenting with rapid growth or with an atypical pattern of extension.

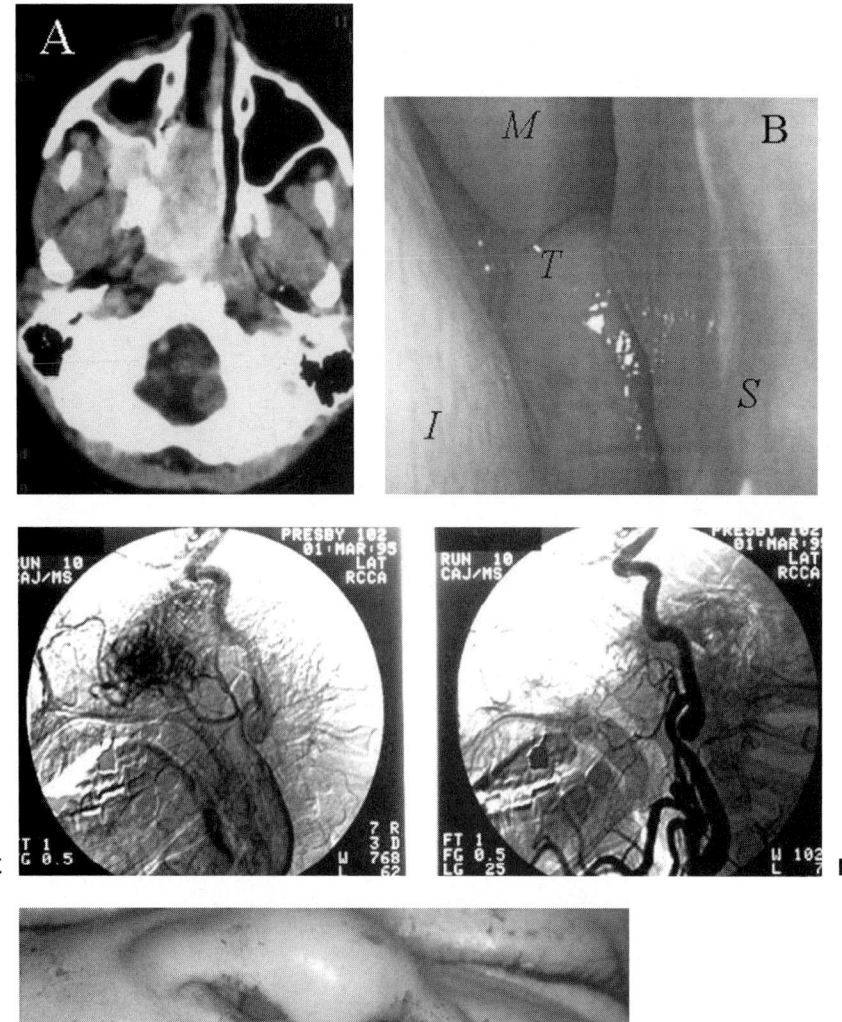

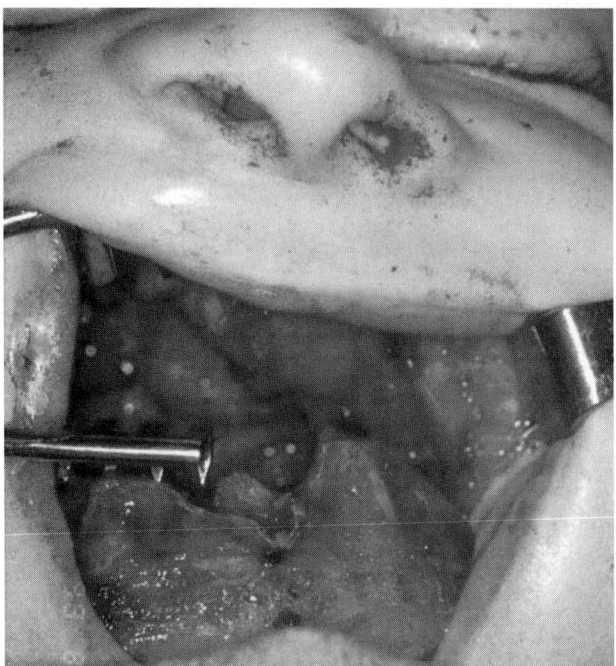

Figure 125.6 **A:** Axial computed tomographic scan at the level of the maxillary sinus shows nasopharyngeal angiofibroma occupying the right nasal cavity. The point of origin from the right medial pterygoid plate is visible. **B:** Endoscopic view of the lesion in the right nasal cavity. *S,* nasal septum: *I,* inferior turbinate: *M,* middle turbinate: *T,* tumor. **C:** Lateral subtraction angiogram shows vascular blush of the nasopharyngeal angiofibroma originating from the terminal branches of the internal maxillary artery. **D:** Lateral subtraction angiogram after embolization of the angiofibroma to reduce its blood supply. Both diagnostic angiography and embolization were accomplished at the same sitting. **E:** Resection of the angiofibroma through a facial degloving incision, with a LeFort I osteotomy.

Biopsy may be necessary to differentiate JA from lesions such as rhabdomyosarcoma or olfactory neuroblastoma that may have a similar clinical presentation. It is generally not necessary to biopsy these tumors. In the event that preoperative imaging in combination with an accurate history and physical examination are inconclusive, however, an incisional biopsy may be necessary. The surgeon should anticipate significant bleeding; thus, it is safer to perform the biopsy in the operating room with the patient under general endotracheal anesthesia. If bleeding is encountered, electrocautery may be helpful in obtaining hemostasis. Alternatively, anterior or posterior packing of the nose may be necessary to control tumor bleeding.

Arteriography delineates the vascular supply; however, it is not necessary to confirm the diagnosis; thus, its main indication is to provide a means for preoperative embolization. Most commonly, the feeding vessels arise from the external carotid artery system (internal maxillary and ascending pharyngeal arteries), but the internal carotid artery can contribute to the blood supply of large tumors or to those that have intraorbital or intracranial extension. Large lesions, or those that approach the midline, can receive blood supply from the contralateral vessels. Therefore, angiography should include the internal and external carotid systems bilaterally. Embolization of the pertinent vessels is completed in a single stage.

Embolization does carry the risk of cerebral embolization because of the presence of anastamoses that connect the internal and external carotid systems. Visual loss can result from accidental embolization of the ophthalmic artery. Surgery ideally follows embolization within 24 hours to take advantage of the maximal hemostatic effect and avoid the inflammatory reaction produced by the embolization.

Surgery is the mainstay of therapy for JA. Irradiation and chemotherapy should be considered, however, for patients who are poor surgical candidates or who have JA with massive intracranial extension. The surgical approach depends on the staging of the tumor. Commonly used options include an endoscopic transnasal approach, the transpalatal approach, and transmaxillary approach, with or without facial degloving. More recently, endoscopic techniques have been developed to approach tumors (12,13; see Chapter 32) that are well defined and of moderate size. This provides the patient with a superior cosmetic result and minimizes the morbidity that can accompany an external approach.

Generalized Tumors

The generalized tumor category of benign vascular tumors of the head and neck includes diseases such as angiomatosis and cystic hygroma, both of which are closely related to lymphangioma (Fig. 125.7). Cystic hygroma consists of painless masses covered by normal skin that is present at birth or that appears in early infancy. Cystic hygroma of the posterior triangle of the neck has been associated with hydrops fetalis, Turner syndrome, chromosomal aneuploidy, other congenital malformations, and fetal death. In view of this association, genetic analysis is indicated when a baby is born with a cystic hygroma (14). Cystic hygromas enlarge gradually and never involute. They have extensive infiltration that extends beyond the apparent clinical boundaries; therefore, CT or MRI usually is advocated to delineate lesion extent. Mainstay therapy for cystic hygroma is complete surgical excision. If the

tumor is intimately associated with vital structures, maximal excision sparing these structures is recommended. Recurrences are not uncommon and repeat surgical intervention may be required. A detailed preoperative discussion of this possibility, as part of the informed consent, is prudent. Careful follow-up evaluation and periodic MRI can identify an early recurrence, facilitating the surgical re-excision and minimizing cosmetic and functional deficits.

Inflammatory Tumors

Inflammatory tumors include granuloma pyogenicum and granuloma gravidarum. These lesions seem to develop as an exaggerated response to relatively minor trauma. Simple excision is usually curative, although a shave-excision followed by laser photocoagulation of the base seems to be an effective alternative (15). For septal hemangiomas, which are often broadly based, the resection may need to include the perichondrium of the septal cartilage.

Arteriovenous Fistula or Aneurysm

Arteriovenous (AV) fistula or aneurysm (vascular malformation) typically manifests as a pulsatile, painless mass and can appear with or without a history of trauma. Disfigurement can be produced by the gradual facial enlargement caused by large arteriovenous malformations (Fig. 125.8). The extent of an AV malformation determines its clinical presentation. Some patients have a palpable thrill or audible bruit only but, in large AV fistulas, a high output cardiac failure may be produced. Surgical excision is curative, but many lesions are inaccessible or associated with unacceptable morbidity. Likewise, embolization of these lesions may not be advisable because of the high vascular flow. Interventional angiography and balloon occlusion may be necessary.

Telangiectasias

In the head and neck region, telangiectasias of clinical significance are most commonly associated with hereditary hemorrhagic telangiectasia (HHT) or Osler-Weber-Rendu disease. This disorder is transmitted in an autosomal dominant manner, thus, it affects both genders equally. Diagnosis of HHT requires the presence of a triad of characteristics: telangiectatic lesions, inheritance of the disease, and hemorrhage from the lesions. Epistaxis is the hallmark of this disease, but oral bleeding is a common and important component of it. Cutaneous and mucosal lesions often develop in early youth, manifesting problems during the second and third decades of life. Telangiectasias are common over the facial skin, particularly the cheeks and, less commonly, the scalp, fingers, ears, toes, and nail beds. Management of intranasal lesions is based on reducing the number of telangiectasias or occluding the nasal cavity to eliminate the desiccating effects of airflow. The most successful

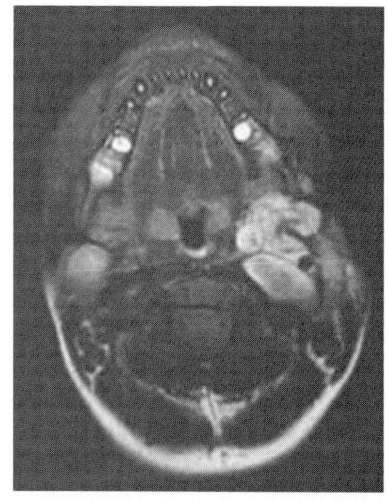

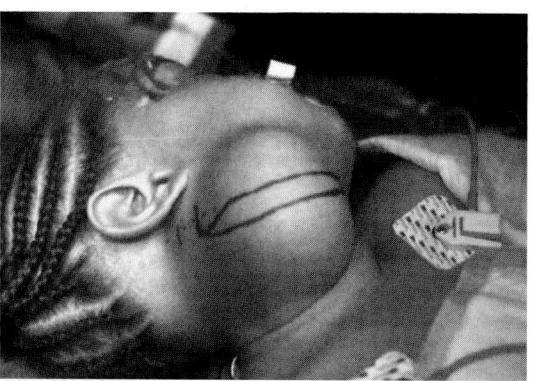

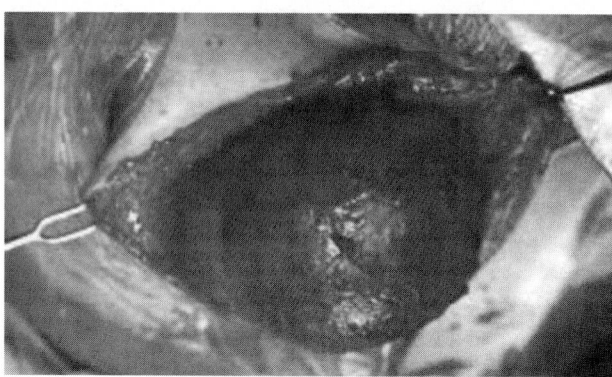

Figure 125.7 **A:** Magnetic resonance imaging scan shows cystic hygroma of the left submandibular space. **B:** Preoperative photograph of another patient with a submandibular cystic hygroma. **C:** Intraoperative photograph showing dissection of the mass from the submandibular gland. (Images courtesy of David L. Mandell, MD, Children's Hospital of Pittsburgh, and Barton F. Branstetter IV, MD, University of Pittsburgh Medical Center, Pittsburgh, PA.)

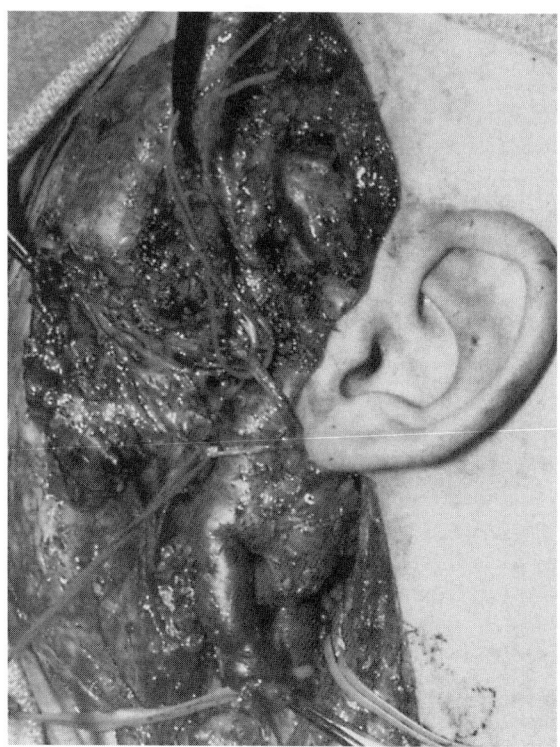

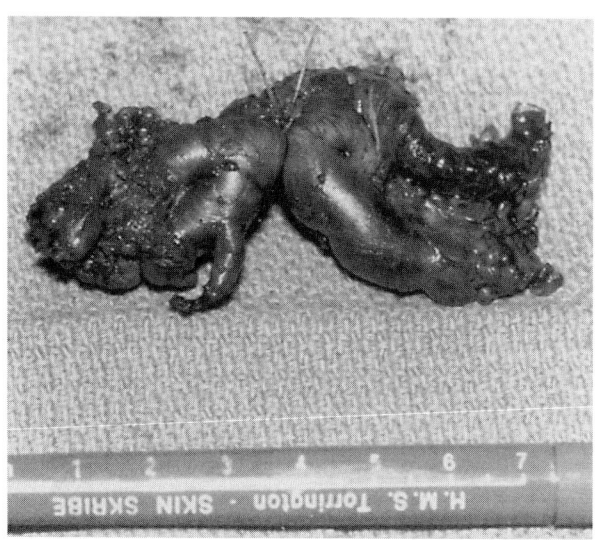

Figure 125.8 **A:** Arteriovenous malformation of the cheek. This patient had symptoms of high-output cardiac failure caused by the amount of blood flow through the lesion. Marked dilatation of the distal external carotid artery branches is evident. The facial nerve has been dissected. **B:** Resected specimen.

procedures for septal telangiectasias are nasal occlusion and septal dermoplasty. Septal dermoplasty is technically difficult, and revisions may be necessary. Occlusion of the nose by a local lap is effective but poorly accepted by the patients. Temporary occlusion with a sponge or cotton ball packing is a simple and useful technique. Repeated laser treatment is of variable effectiveness but often is the preferred initial treatment. Other treatments (e.g., use of creams containing estrogen or other hormones) can have some effectiveness.

MALIGNANT TUMORS

Malignant vascular tumors are extremely rare. Angiosarcoma, Kaposi sarcoma, malignant paraganglioma, and malignant hemangiopericytoma are recognized malignant vascular tumors. The latter two categories, however, are usually benign tumors that can be potentially malignant, although their course is highly variable.

Angiosarcoma

Angiosarcoma is an extremely rare malignant tumor of the vascular endothelial cells (16). It arises predominantly in the scalp, although the neck, mouth, and antrum can be affected in that order of frequency. Angiosarcomas most commonly occur during middle part of life but can arise at the extremes of age (Fig. 125.9). In general, these are rapidly growing neoplasms, although they can present with an insidious onset associated with minimal symptoms. The clinical course after diagnosis is relatively rapid. Less than 50% of patients are cured by surgical excision and those who die usually do so within 3 years after diagnosis. Radiation therapy offers some palliation. Accurate identification of neoplasm margins is particularly difficult for the clinician. Because the tumor consists of blood vessels, it is also difficult for the pathologist. This often results in an incomplete resection.

Hemangiopericytoma

Hemangiopericytomas arise from hemangiopericytes, which are myoepithelial cells of the capillary system. The musculoskeletal system and skin are the most frequent sites of origin. Hemangiopericytoma must be regarded as an unpredictable neoplasm with malignant potential (16). Tumors can be partially or completely encapsulated, but aggressive tumors can manifest gross infiltration and can have a friable, hemorrhagic character. Treatment is wide surgical excision with careful mandatory surveillance. Radiation therapy offers a palliative effect but is not recommended as part of the initial treatment unless positive margins or unresectable lesions are apparent.

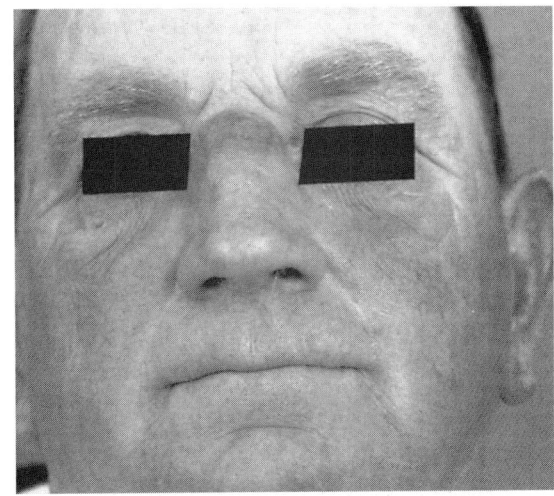

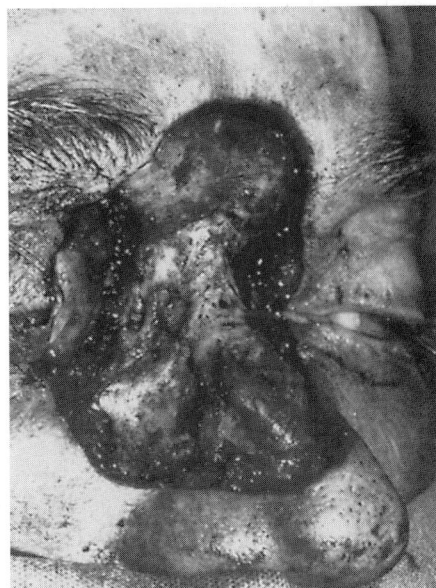

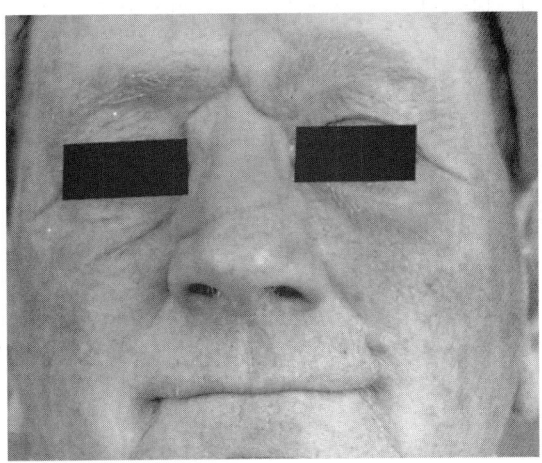

Figure 125.9 A: Angiosarcoma of the nasal dorsum. **B:** Extent of resection by means of micrographic controlled excision. Tumor extended onto each medial canthus in addition to the glabella. **C:** Result after reconstruction with a median forehead flap.

Kaposi Sarcoma

Kaposi sarcoma is more common among patients with acquired immunodeficiency syndrome. Clinically, Kaposi sarcoma presents as a nonpruritic, painless, flat or nodular, pigmented lesion on any skin or mucosa of the head and neck region. The lesions are often purple among white persons and nearly black among persons with darker pigmentation. Cutaneous lesions present mainly a cosmetic concern, but mucosal lesions of the upper aerodigestive tract often cause functional problems related to pain, bleeding, and obstruction. Treatment is geared toward treatment of the underlying immunosuppressive disorder, which is the most important prognostic factor. Local treatment is done to improve local control, reduce symptoms, and improve cosmesis. Radiation therapy and chemotherapy, which are effective local treatments, are associated with significant morbidity. Intralesional injection of vinblastine, interferon, cryotherapy, and laser excision can be helpful in the management of small tumors (17). Systemic therapy is indicated for patients with systemic visceral or pulmonary disease, or those with extensive mucocutaneous involvement (> 10 new lesions in 1 month). The current mainstay of systemic treatment is liposomal anthracyclines (doxorubicin or daunorubicin) with or without combination therapy (vinblastine, bleomycin). Systemic etoposide and paclitaxel have also been used (17).

Paraganglioma

Paragangliomas are neuroendocrine tumors derived from the extra-adrenal paraganglia of the autonomic nervous system. Paraganglia tend to be distributed symmetrically and segmentally. Each paraganglion in the head and neck is composed of two cell types: granule-storing chief cells and Schwannlike satellite cells. Paraganglia of the head and neck and the superior mediastinum closely resemble the carotid bodies and, typically, are related to arterial vasculature and cranial nerves. Some branchiomeric paraganglia, including the carotid and aortic bodies, mediate chemosensory reflexes and are sensitive to changes in pH and arterial oxygen tension.

In the head and neck region, paraganglionic tissue is distributed in the aortic arch, the superior and inferior laryngeal paraganglia, the carotid body, the vagal body, and the jugulotympanic region (Fig. 125.10). Paraganglia also occur in the posterior nasal region and in the orbit. In general, carotid body tumors are the most common paragangliomas in the head and neck, followed in order by tumors of the jugulotympanic, intravagal, laryngeal, nasal, nasopharyngeal, and orbital areas. A definite incidence of multicentricity and a familial distribution are found. The incidence of bilaterality and multicentricity of these tumors increases from about 3% normally to 26% among persons with a familial distribution (18).

Familial paragangliomas account for 10% to 15% of cases. They are frequently multiple and bilateral and are detected at an early age. The gene for familial paraganglioma has been identified as the *PGL1* gene and is on the 11q23 locus. This gene is transmitted in an autosomal dominant pattern with genomic imprinting. Affected males have a 50% chance of having an affected child, but females will only pass the inactivated gene to the next generation.

Grossly, paragangliomas appear as sharply demarcated polypoid masses with a "rubbery" consistency. Under light microscopy, paraganglioma cells form distinctive cell balls, Zellballen, that are separated from each other by fibrovascular stroma. The tumor cells are generally homogeneous in their appearance and nuclear polymorphism, mitotic activity, and necrosis are rare.

Paragangliomas are commonly found incidentally during a routine physical examination. A careful family history for tumors of the head and neck should be part of the initial evaluation. Critical to the physical examination, are a detailed cranial nerve and otologic examination. Paragangliomas can be biochemically active and 1% to 3% of them can secrete catecholamine. Biochemical testing is advocated for those patients who present with symptoms. Evaluation and diagnosis include CT, MRI, and, for some patients, CT or MR arteriography and venography. MRI with contrast, the initial imaging modality of choice to evaluate paragangliomas, defines the soft tissue boundaries and the vascular characteristics of the tumor itself. High-resolution CT scanning with contrast is a reasonable alternative for the initial imaging of the tumors or can be used to better define the bony anatomy of the skull base, middle ear, and lateral temporal bone. Magnetic resonance angiography is noninvasive and provides detailed mapping of the involved vessels and identification of additional neoplasms. Interventional arteriography allows the assessment of the collateral circulation, but it is mainly indicated as a means for preoperative embolization.

If embolization is to be performed, superselective angiography is most helpful (19). Angiography of both the internal and external carotid systems is important to rule out bilateral tumors. [111]Indium pentetreotide scanning has been used to detect familial paragangliomas. This method uses a radionuclide that labels the abundant somatostatin receptors found in paraganglionic tumors. This method also allows for the detection of multifocal tumors in other parts of the body. Telischi et al. (20) have used octreotide scintigraphy to detect primary and concurrent paragangliomas and suggest that this method may be useful in preoperative planning. Imaging findings are diagnostic and biopsy usually is unnecessary.

Carotid Body Tumors

A normal carotid body measures 5 mm by 2.5 mm and is located at the bifurcation of the common carotid artery.

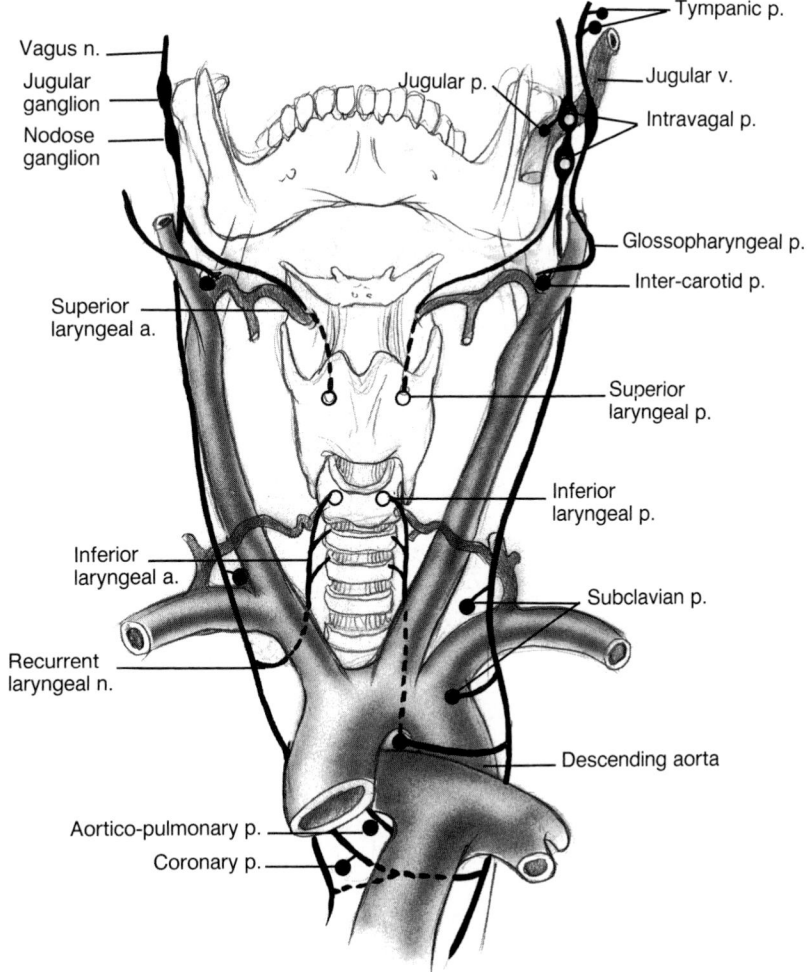

Figure 125.10 Distribution and location of paraganglia in the head and neck.

Most carotid body paragangliomas manifest as asymptomatic, slowly enlarging, nontender neck masses of the anterolateral neck at the level of the hyoid bone. A cranial neuropathy may be the presenting finding.

Clinically, a carotid body tumor can produce a bruit on auscultation and is freely mobile in a lateral direction but fixed in a cephalic-caudal direction. About 10% of carotid body tumors extend into the peripharyngeal region to produce a mass in the oropharyngeal wall. The differential diagnosis includes aneurysms of the carotid system and vagal or sympathetic chain neurilemmoma. A pathognomonic imaging finding is widening of the carotid bifurcation by a well-defined vascular tumor (Lyre sign). Most carotid body tumors are clinically benign, but a small percentage can manifest regional or distant metastasis and, thereby, are classified as malignant. As with other paragangliomas, no clear histologic characteristics determine malignancy (18).

The risks of arterial injury during resection increase with increasing tumor size. Observation is a reasonable alternative for patients with seemingly stable tumors, for the elderly, and for those in whom surgery may be associated with a high incidence of postoperative cranial neuropathies. Ra-

diation therapy should be considered for those patients with progressive tumors with high surgical risks. More recently, gamma knife radiosurgery has been used to treat paragangliomas, but its long-term results are not yet available (21).

The operative procedure allows early identification and isolation of the proximal and distal carotid vascular tree (Fig. 125.11). The potential for vascular replacement surgery is considered in every case. A saphenous venous graft or synthetic material can be used for reconstruction. The lower extremity is prepared if vascular reconstruction of the internal carotid artery is a possibility. Alternatively, a superficial temporal artery to middle cerebral artery bypass may be performed. A subadventitial plane can be developed in which the carotid body tumor is removed from the bifurcation and internal carotid artery. The external carotid artery is sacrificed to mobilize the inferior margin of the tumor, in most cases. If the tumor is considered malignant, regional lymphadenectomy in conjunction with excision can be performed (Fig. 125.12). If possible, the cranial nerves are preserved, and every attempt is made to leave the vascular tree intact. Unintentional entrance into the artery is repaired, only if it is a simple injury.

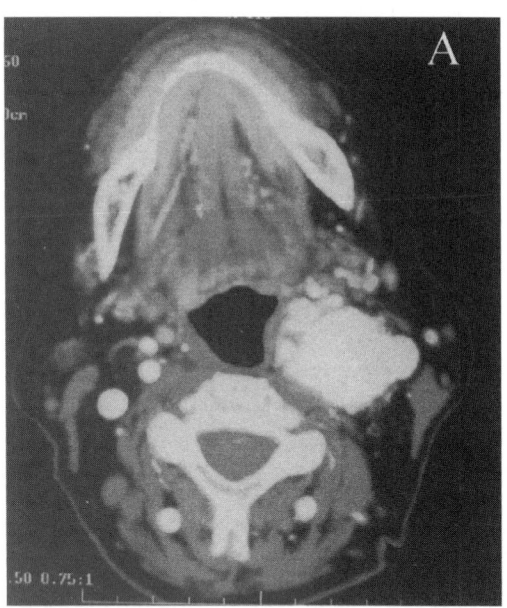

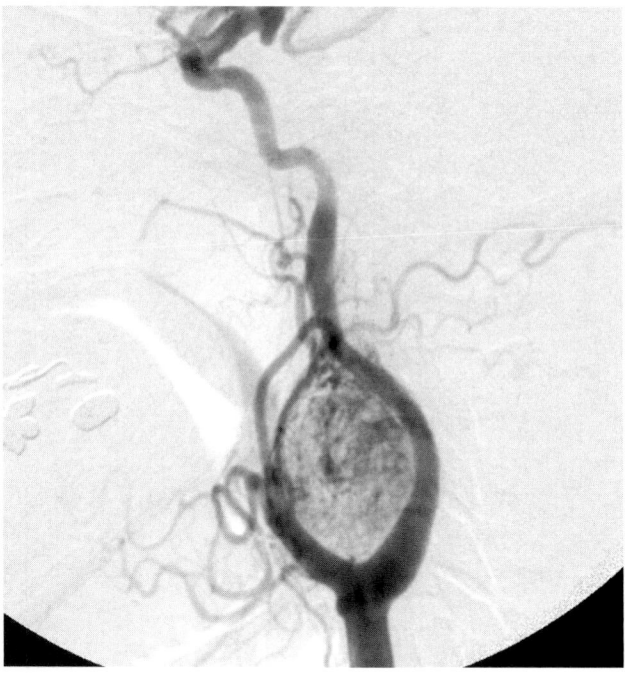

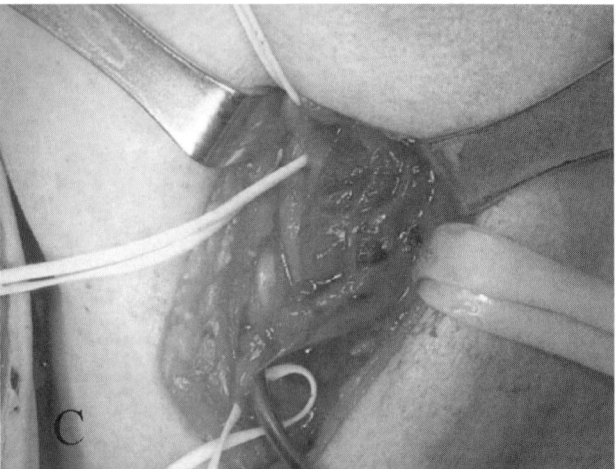

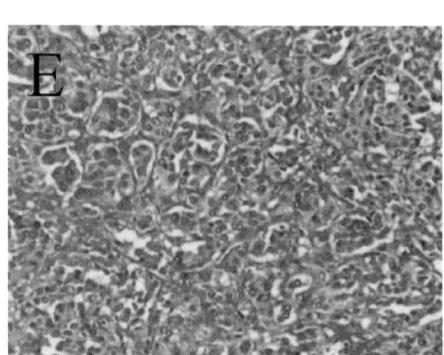

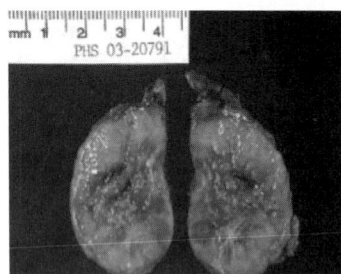

Figure 125.11   A: Contrast enhanced computed tomography (CT) scan showing a carotid body tumor. **B:** Anterior carotid arteriogram showing a carotid body tumor at the carotid bifurcation and displacement of the carotid vessels (Lyre sign). **C:** Intraoperative photograph shows carotid body tumor. **D:** Gross photograph demonstrating the tumor. **E:** Histology section stained with hematoxylin and eosin showing the characteristic Zellballen. (See also Color Plate 55.)

Formal grafting is required if a larger defect has to be bridged. Some patients tolerate carotid resection without reconstruction. Preoperative balloon occlusion testing during angiography can provide important information. Some authors have advocated preoperative embolization in an effort to minimize blood loss. Embolization, however, can lead to scarring and hamper the dissection in the subadventitial plane. It is not routinely used at our institution.

The mortality rate for carotid body tumors is approximately 8%. Posttreatment recurrence is unusual but has been reported to occur at a rate of approximately 10% among those observed for as long as 26 years. Early

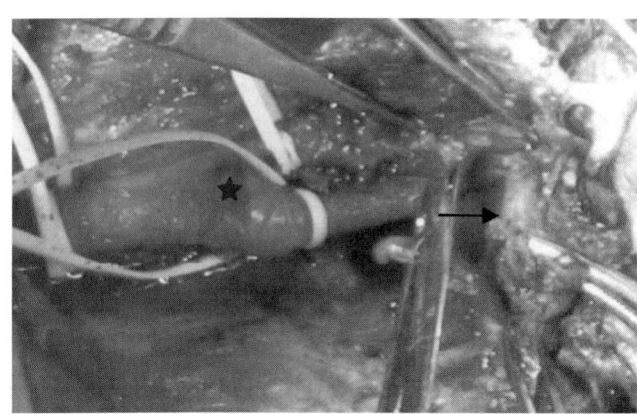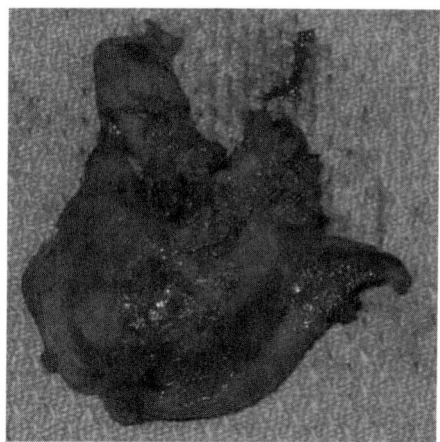

Figure 125.12 A: Malignant glomus vagale tumor as evidenced by metastasis to cervical lymph nodes. Tumor removal included both neck carotid system dissection. The carotid bifuration is marked with an *asterisk*, and the tumor is marked with an *arrow*. **B:** The resected tumor, which measures 4.5 cm in size.

operation is desirable because the procedure can be less extensive and is generally better tolerated. Close observation with repeated imaging can be an option for an elderly person with a small, asymptomatic paraganglioma.

Glomus Jugulare

Juguloparaganglioma is also known as glomus tympanicum tumor, tympanic body tumor, glomus jugulare, or tumor of the ear of the carotid body type. Paraganglioma is the most common neoplasm of the middle ear and is second to neurilemmoma in frequency of tumors involving the temporal bone. Often, the patient seeks medical attention because of pulsatile tinnitus or hearing loss. A typical finding in the middle ear cavity is a reddish mass behind the tympanic membrane, although it is not always present. A high-riding jugular bulb or carotid artery that is exposed to the middle ear can mimic a glomus jugulare tumor. In general, the anatomic location of the glomus jugulare contributes to symptoms related to the middle ear or erosion of the lesion into the cranial vault.

As with carotid body tumor, its blood supply and multicentricity is ascertained by CT and CT arteriography or MR angiography. Interventional angiography is reserved for those patients who require preoperative embolization. Operative procedures are designed to remove the tumor, preserving hearing and facial nerve function. The surgical approach addresses the potential routes of tumor spread from the area of the jugular bulb. Surgical steps include the control of the internal carotid artery (ICA) and wide exposure of the tumor margins including removal of tumor from the ICA and posterior cranial fossa. Although surgery is the mainstay of treatment, radiation therapy can have a palliative role in the management of recurrent disease or persistent disease and in the treatment of patients at high risk.

Vagal Paraganglioma

Vagal paraganglioma, or vagal body tumor, typically arises from nests of paraganglionic tissue within the perineurium of the vagus nerve immediately below or at the level of the ganglion nodosum. Vagal paragangliomas can be distinguished from carotid body tumors (CBT) as they displace the ICA anteriorly and medially, whereas CBT usually splay the bifurcation of the common carotid artery. These tumors can extend into the jugular foramen in a "dumbbell" fashion or extend caudally (18).

Surgical resection is the mainstay treatment, although asymptomatic or bilateral tumors may be observed. Sacrifice of the vagus nerve is usually needed and even in the rare case in which the vagus can be spared, function is never preserved (Fig. 125.13). The consequent laryngeal or pharyngeal paralysis requires surgical rehabilitation in the form of a medialization laryngoplasty with or without an arytenoid adduction procedure or pexy. Swallowing therapy is also needed to optimize the compensatory function of the remaining laryngopharynx. The risk for vascular injury increases with tumor size, because large tumors can impinge or surround the ICA at the skull base.

Angiolymphoid Hyperplasia

Angiolymphoid hyperplasia merits brief mention because it can cause diagnostic confusion. It is an angiomatous neoplasm similar to a hemangioma with a reactive histologic pattern. It can mimic other vascular tumors (22).

SYNDROMES

Many of the vascular lesions described herein are associated with clinical syndromes. Early detection and diagnosis

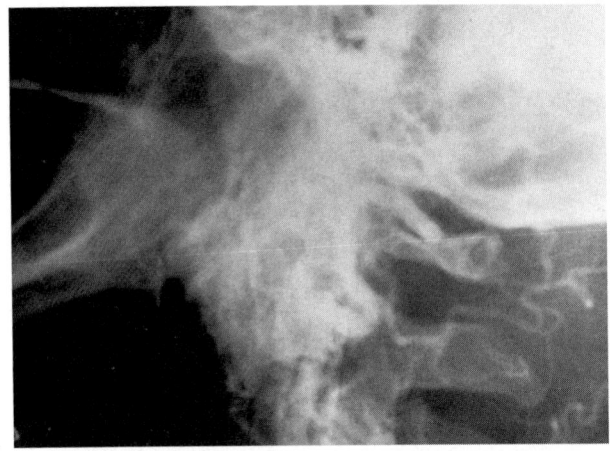

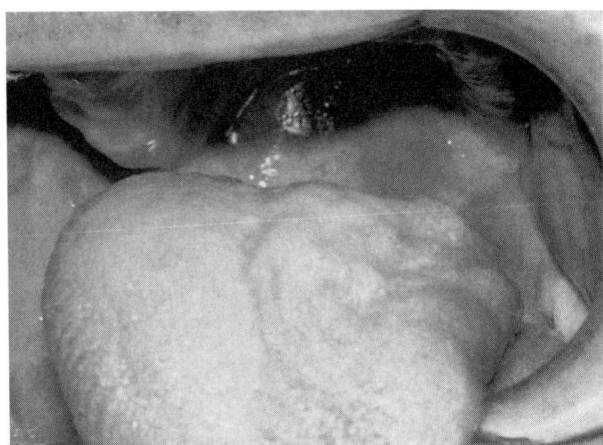

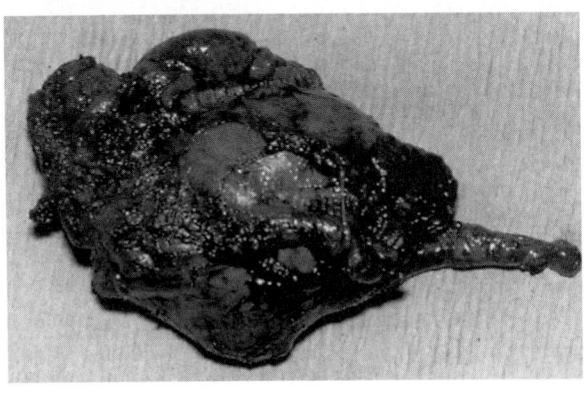

Figure 125.13 A: Lateral carotid arteriogram shows vagal paraganglioma. **B:** Inspection of oral cavity shows paresis of hypoglossal nerve. **C:** Resected specimen has tumor enveloping the vagus nerve.

facilitates their treatment and optimizes the outcome. Several important syndromes with vascular components are listed in summary below.

Osler-Weber-Rendu Syndrome (Hereditary Hemorrhagic Telangiectasia)

Multiple telangiectasis of the skin and mucous membranes

Occasional gastrointestinal and central nervous system involvement

Autosomal dominant inheritance

Sturge-Weber Syndrome

Port-wine stain usually over trigeminal nerve distribution

Ipsilateral meningeal vascular malformations that may or may not have calcifications

Possible association with seizure disorder and mental retardation

Maffucci Syndrome

Multiple cavernous hemangiomas

Dyschondroplasia with shortening and deformity of the involved bones

Occasional visceral vascular lesions

Twenty-five percent incidence of chondrosarcoma

Von Hippel-Lindau Disease

Hemangiomas of the cerebellum and retina
Cysts of the kidney and pancreas

HIGHLIGHTS

- Hemangioma is the most common localized benign vascular tumor
- Hemangiomas demonstrate a marked proliferative phase that is usually followed by a period of involution over the course of years.
- Vascular malformations, which are congenital, are usually present at birth. They do not proliferate rapidly and do not involute.
- Lymphangioma often involves the oral cavity mucosa or tongue. The lesions usually are more extensive than what they appear to clinical examination.
- Angiofibroma consists of a rich network of vascular channels surrounded by connective tissue. Surgical excision is the preferred treatment.
- Cystic hygroma is characterized by multiple cystic, clear compartments resembling a cluster of grapes. The lesion arises between the axilla and the midface and tends to enlarge with time. Complete removal is often not achievable.
- Arteriovenous fistulae or aneurysms present as pulsatile, painless masses with or without an audible or palpable

thrill or cardiac failure. Balloon occlusion or surgical excision is often necessary.

- Angiosarcoma and hemangiopericytoma are malignant vascular tumors that most commonly arise in the scalp, mouth, and antrum.
- Paragangliomas are derived from neural crest cells. The most common paragangliomas in the head and neck are the carotid body tumor, glomus jugulare, and glomus tympanicum.
- Carotid body tumors arise at the bifurcation of the carotid artery. Surgical excision may require replacement or repair of the internal carotid artery with a venous or synthetic graft.
- Glomus jugulare tumors commonly involve the middle ear or the lateral skull base. Computed tomography and arteriography are critical to plan the details of surgical excision.

REFERENCES

1. Mulliken JB, Young AE. *Vascular birthmarks: hemangiomas and malformations.* Philadelphia: WB Saunders, 1988.
2. Bridger GP, Nassar VH, Skinner HG. Hemangioma in the adult larynx. *Arch Otolaryngol Head Neck Surg* 1970;92:493–501.
3. Rahbar R, Nicollas R, Roger G, et al. The biology and management of subglottic hemangioma: past, present, future. *Laryngoscope* 2004;11:1880–1891.
4. Greene AK, Rogers GF, Mulliken JB. Management of parotid hemangioma in 100 children. *Plast Reconstr Surg* 2004;113:53–60.
5. Buckmiller LM. Update on hemangiomas and vascular malformations. *Curr Opin Otolaryngol Head Neck Surg* 2004;12:476–487.
6. Werner JA, Dunne A-A, Lippert BM, et al. Optimal treatment of vascular birthmarks. *Am J Clin Dermatol* 2003;4(11):745–756.
7. Warner M, Suen JY, ed. *Hemangiomas and vascular malformations of the head and neck.* New York; Wiley-Liss, 1999.
8. Demiri EC, Pelissier P, Genin-Etcheberry T, et al. Treatment of facial hemangiomas: the present status of surgery. *Br J Plast Surg* 2001;54:665–674.
9. Gupta G, Bilsland D. A prospective study of the impact of laser treatment on vascular lesions. *Br J Dermatol* 2000;143(2):356–359.
10. Bardach J. Pediatric plastic and reconstructive surgery of the head and neck. In: Bluestone CD, Stool SE, eds. *Pediatric otolaryngology.* Philadelphia: WB Saunders, 1990:694–717.
11. Donnelly LF, Adams DM, Bisset III GS. Vascular malformations and hemangiomas: a practical approach in a multidisciplinary clinic. *AJR Am J Roentgenol* 2000;174:597–608.
12. Mann WJ, Jecker JP, Amedee RG. Juvenile angiofibromas: change in surgical concepts over the last 20 years. *Laryngoscope* 2004;14:291–293.
13. Carrau RL, Snyderman CH, Kassam AB, et al. Endoscopic and endoscopic-assisted surgery for juvenile angiofibroma. *Laryngoscope* 2001;111:483–487.
14. Baena N, De Vigan C, Cariati E et al. Prenatal detection of rare chromosomal autosomal abnormalities in Europe. *Am J Med Genet* 2003;118A(4):319–327.
15. Kirschner RE, Low DW. Treatment of pyogenic granuloma by shave excision and laser photocoagulation. *Plast Reconstr Surg* 1999;104:1346–1349.
16. Sturgis EM, Potter BO. Sarcomas of the head and neck region. *Curr Opin Oncol* 2003;15:239–252.
17. Wheeland RG, Bailin PL, Norris MJ. Argon laser photocoagulative therapy of Kaposi's sarcoma: a clinical and histopathologic evaluation. *J Dermatol Surg Oncol* 1985;11:1180–1185.
18. Pellitteri PK, Rinaldo A, Myssiorek D, et al. Paragangliomas of the head and neck. *Oral Oncol* 2004;40:563–575.
19. Hunsicker RC, Koch TJ, Folander H. Superselective embolization in two cases of laryngeal paraganglioma. *Otolaryngol Head Neck Surg* 1995; 113: 126–130.
20. Telischi FF, Bustillo A, Whiteman ML, et al. Octreotide scintigraphy for the detection of paragangliomas. *Otolaryngol Head Neck Surg* 2000;122:358–362.
21. Huo JS, Chen JCT, Yu C, et al. Gamma knife radiosurgery for benign cavernous sinus tumors: quantitative analysis of tumor outcomes. *Neurosurgery* 2004;54:1385–1394.
22. Don DM, Ishimaya A, Johnstone AK, et al. Angiolymphoid hyperplasia with eosinophilia and vascular tumors of the head and neck. *Am J Otolaryngol* 1996;17:240–245.

Cranial-Base Surgery

126

Peter D. Costantino   Ahmed S. Ismail   Ivo P. Janecka

Over the past 15-year period, cranial-base surgery has evolved from a group of dissimilar surgical procedures into a well-established surgical subspecialty with its own journal and representative societies. This evolution began in the early 1960s with an original report by Ketcham et al. (1) on the use of a combined intracranial and transfacial approach to the anterior cranial base to manage cancer of the paranasal sinuses. Lewis and Page (2) followed with a description of the modern technique of temporal bone resection. The high mortality associated with these procedures limited the original applications and slowed evolution of cranial-base surgery during the 1960s and 1970s. This situation changed during the 1980s, when cranial-base surgery and the technology supporting it expanded greatly. Factors responsible for this progression included new methods of accurate computer-aided imaging of the cranial base, reliable anesthetic techniques that allowed safe and long operations, new dynamic studies for the evaluation of cerebral blood flow (CBF) and prediction of the safety of carotid artery resection, and development of reliable vascularized flaps for reconstruction of large defects at the base of the skull. These developments, more than any single method of surgical resection, made contemporary cranial-base surgery possible. Cranial-base surgery is now an interdisciplinary field that has elements of neurosurgery, head and neck surgery, neurootology, and plastic reconstructive surgery. The hallmark of contemporary cranial-base surgery is a team approach whereby experts of various backgrounds interact for the comprehensive care of the patient.

The purpose of this chapter is to provide a general review of the techniques most commonly used in cranial-base surgery. To understand these techniques and the applications, knowledge of the anatomic features of the cranial base, the function of the related neurovascular structures, and the lesions that arise therein is needed. This information is reviewed, as is management of the most common complications of resection at the base of the skull. It should be emphasized that this chapter is far from a comprehensive treatise on cranial-base surgery. It should instead be regarded as an educational starting point for motivated surgical residents and clinicians.

NEUROANATOMIC CONSIDERATIONS

In no other area of the body are so many important neurologic and vascular structures in such proximity as in the cranial base. Three-dimensional mastery of the relations between the structures is critical to the performance of safe, successful cranial-base surgery. Because of the density of neurologic structures in this region, tumors frequently cause site-specific neurologic deficits. For example, one of the earliest signs of tumor extension into the cavernous sinus is sixth cranial nerve palsy that causes an inability to abduct the affected eye. In this situation, infiltration of the cranial nerve by tumor is ipsilateral to the functional deficit. Most sensory and motor lesions of the cranial nerves manifest themselves ipsilaterally. Only motor lesions within the spinal cord (pyramidal tract) produce ipsilateral deficits. Sensory deficits originating within the spinal cord (spinothalamic tract) are contralateral to the causative lesion.

Arterial Supply

The arterial supply of the central nervous system depends on the paired internal carotid and vertebral arteries (Fig. 126.1). After the internal carotid arteries pass through the petrous portion of the temporal bone and cavernous sinus, they ramify into the anterior and middle cerebral arteries, which supply most of the cerebrum. The vertebral arteries join in the midline to form the unpaired basilar artery, which is immediately ventral to the pons in the region of the clivus. The basilar artery forms the paired posterior cerebral, anterior inferior cerebellar, and posterior cerebellar

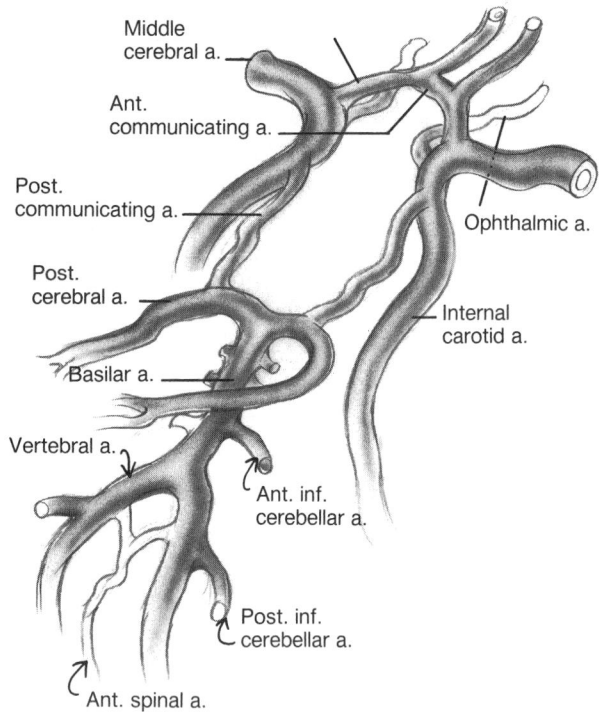

Figure 126.1 The basilar artery and the arteries of the circle of Willis.

Occlusion of the posterior inferior cerebellar artery causes lateral medullary syndrome, characterized by a loss of pain and temperature sensation ipsilaterally on the face and contralaterally on the body. Ipsilateral Horner syndrome (ptosis, small pupil, and facial anhidrosis), nystagmus, cerebellar dysfunction, vertigo, hoarseness, difficulty swallowing, and loss of ipsilateral taste also occur with this syndrome.

Venous Drainage System

The venous drainage of the intracranial space is through the dural sinuses. The largest is the midline superior sagittal sinus, which usually is confluent at the torcular herophili with both of the paired transverse sinuses (Fig. 126.2). Drainage of the superior sagittal sinus can be to only one of the transverse sinuses if those sinuses are not confluent at the torcular. The transverse sinuses are continuous with the paired sigmoid sinuses. The superior petrosal sinus joins the sigmoid sinus at its junction with the transverse sinus; the smaller inferior petrosal sinus empties into the jugular bulb. The petrosal sinuses drain the cavernous sinuses. The vein of Labbe, which drains the temporal lobe, enters the transverse sinus at a point medial to the superior petrosal sinus. If the vein of Labbe is occluded, substantial temporal lobe edema can occur.

Within the temporal bones, the sigmoid sinuses become continuous with the internal jugular veins at the jugular bulb. Sacrifice of only one sigmoid sinus without a preoperative venous study usually is possible without risk of cerebral edema. If both the sigmoid sinus and jugular vein must be sacrificed on one side, potentially preventing

arteries. The cerebellar arteries also supply portions of the brainstem. The anterior (carotid) circulation is joined to the posterior (vertebral) circulation by the posterior communicating arteries. These arteries and the anterior communicating arteries form the circle of Willis.

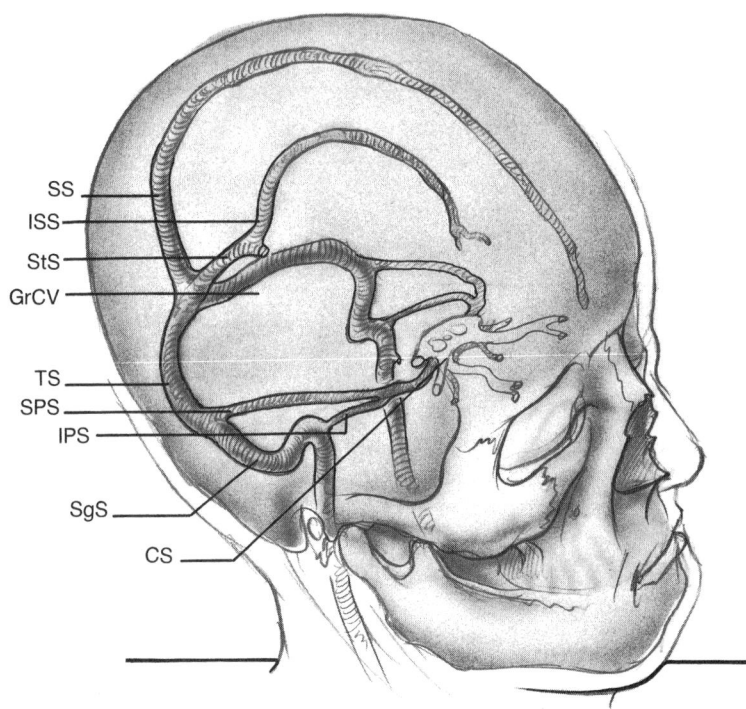

Figure 126.2 The venous drainage system of the brain. The confluence of the paired transverse sinuses and sagittal sinus is at the torcular herophili. The sagittal sinus can be patent with both or only one transverse sinus at the torcular. *CS,* cavernous sinus; *GrCV,* great cerebral vein; *IPS,* inferior petrosal sinus; *ISS,* inferior sagittal sinus; *SgS,* sigmoid sinus; *SPS,* superior petrosal sinus; *SS,* sagittal sinus; *TS,* transverse sinus.

drainage through the superior and inferior petrosal sinuses, a preoperative venous study must be done to confirm cross-flow at the torcular herophili to avoid cerebral edema. It is critical that the interrelations of the superior and inferior petrosal sinuses, the sigmoid sinus, and the torcular be understood to avoid potentially serious and entirely preventable complications due to venous outflow obstruction after tumor resection.

Ventricular Cerebrospinal Fluid Drainage System

The ventricular system (Fig. 126.3) of the neuraxis serves to carry cerebrospinal fluid (CSF) from its site of production at the choroid plexus, located within the large paired lateral ventricles, to the single midline third ventricle. The third ventricle empties into the single midline fourth ventricle through the foramen of Sylvius. The fourth ventricle is located at the level of the pons and cerebellum. This location is important because two common tumors of the base of the skull, acoustic neuroma and clival chordoma, can compress the drainage ports from the fourth ventricle and cause hydrocephalus.

After it leaves the fourth ventricle, CSF enters the subarachnoid space and eventually is resorbed by the arachnoid villi along the walls of the superior sagittal sinus. If these arachnoid villi become clogged with blood or fibrous exudate, as can occur in the postoperative or posttraumatic

period, hydrocephalus can develop. This situation is most frequently identified after development of a postoperative CSF leak that is refractory to standard methods of repair. Although this resorptive disjunction of the arachnoid villi usually is transient, it can become long lasting or permanent and can necessitate use of an external CSF drain (external ventricular drain) or an internal shunt, usually tunneled subcutaneously through the scalp to the intraperitoneal space.

NEUROPHYSIOLOGY

Intracranial Pressure Relations

The intracranial space is considered a closed compartment in which a change in one physiologic value, such as intracranial pressure (ICP), changes other values such as CBF, intracranial venous blood volume, or the amount of intracranial CSF. Normal ICP is less than 200 mm water in a recumbent person. ICP is not affected by changes in mean arterial blood pressure (MAP) as long as these changes remain within the range of 60 to 150 mm Hg MAP. CBF is autoregulated to remain in the range of 45 mL per 100 g brain tissue per minute, or ~750 mL/min in a healthy adult, when MAP remains within this range. If MAP exceeds or falls below this range of 60 to 150 mm Hg, autoregulation is overwhelmed, and CBF increases or decreases commensurately (3). Increases in ICP, if not controlled or compensated through CSF leak, can decrease CBF and cause cortical ischemia.

Unlike blunt head injuries, in which the intracranial compartment remains closed, cranial-base surgery frequently produces defects within the cranium. An increase in ICP is rare; however, disturbances in the ability of the arachnoid villi to absorb CSF can cause hydrocephalus, manifested primarily as CSF leak rather than symptoms of increased ICP. Unlike an increase in ICP, cortical edema is common after cranial-base surgery. This edema usually is caused by prolonged or excessive retraction of the brain during tumor resection. The presence of large amounts of edema fluid correlates highly with a postoperative course complicated by a short-term decrease in mental function and long-term neurologic deficit. The most effective way to manage postoperative cortical edema is prevention by means of removal of large segments of the calvarium and base of the skull to obviate brain retraction during tumor resection (4). The importance of this concept in the performance of competent and safe cranial-base surgery cannot be overstated.

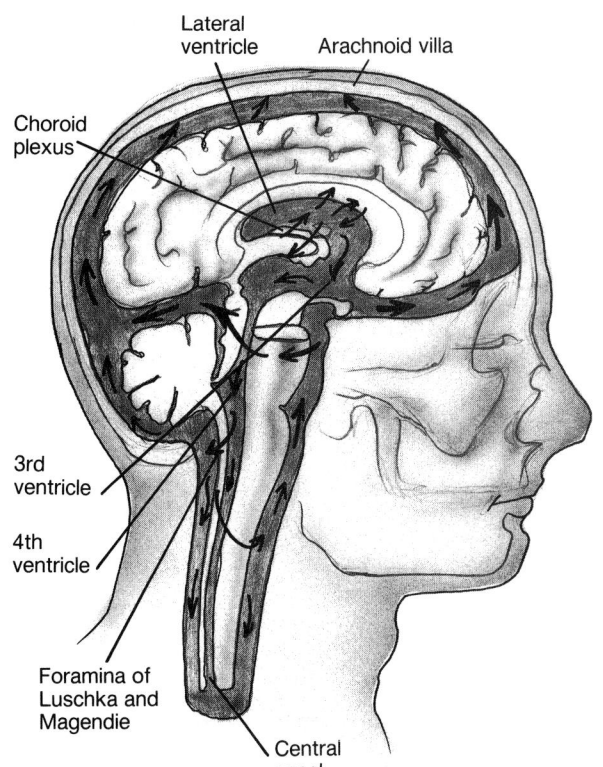

Figure 126.3 Pathways of cerebrospinal fluid circulation.

Labels on figure:
Lateral ventricle
Arachnoid villa
Choroid plexus
3rd ventricle
4th ventricle
Foramina of Luschka and Magendie
Central canal

Cerebral Blood Flow

Cerebral blood flow is extremely sensitive to changes in $Paco_2$. Hypercapnia causes a linear increase in CBF, and

TABLE 126.1

NEUROPHYSIOLOGIC EFFECTS OF ANESTHETIC AGENTS

Anesthetic	Mean Arterial Pressure	Cerebral Blood Flow	Cerebrovascular Autoregulation	Intracranial Pressure
Inhalation				
Halothane	∅∅∅	≠≠≠	Abolished	≠≠
Enflurane	∅∅∅	≠≠	Abolished	≠≠
Isoflurane	∅∅∅	≠≠	Maintained	≠≠
Nitrous oxide	∅	∅∅	Maintained	NC
Intravenous				
Barbiturates	∅∅∅	∅∅	Maintained	∅∅
Etomidate	∅∅	∅∅	Maintained	∅∅
Narcotics	∅∅	∅	Maintained	NC

NC, no change; ∅∅∅, marked decrease; ∅∅, moderate decrease; ∅, slight decrease; ≠≠≠, marked increase; ≠≠, moderate increase; ≠, slight increase.

hypocapnia causes the reverse effect. Maintaining an intraoperative $PaCO_2$ between 20 and 30 mm Hg is the primary method of minimizing cerebral edema caused by vascular engorgement. CBF is directly affected by all inhalational anesthetics. These agents alter autoregulation by increasing CBF with increased concentration of anesthetic. Narcotics, barbiturates, etomidate, and benzodiazepines, however, cause varying decreases in CBF with increased dosage (Table 126.1). Anesthetic technique is therefore critical in preventing increased ICP, minimizing cerebral edema, and maintaining adequate CBF (5).

Cerebrospinal Fluid Production

Production and resorption of CSF are under tight autoregulation; the result is a fairly stable volume of intracranial CSF under normal conditions. The normal amount of CSF in an adult is ~150 to 200 mL. CSF is produced at a rate of ~20 mL/hr (500 mL/day); the total volume of CSF is replaced every 8 hours. The amount of CSF resorbed cannot be controlled pharmacologically, but the amount produced can be altered with carbonic anhydrase inhibitors such as acetazolamide. Acetazolamide decreases production of CSF, thereby decreasing ICP and assisting in maintaining CBF.

INTRAOPERATIVE MONITORING

Intraoperative monitoring has proved indispensable in both routine and complex operations on the cranial base (6). This field involves numerous monitoring techniques with varying degrees of usefulness, depending on the surgical procedure and the type and location of the tumor. From a practical standpoint, two types of intraoperative monitoring frequently are used—monitoring of somatosensory evoked potentials (SSEPs) and tracking of electromyographic

potentials of the cranial motor nerves considered at risk during surgery. Monitoring of SSEPs is useful in tracking the general status of the neuraxis by means of electric stimulation of the peripheral nerves, such as the median or peroneal, and recording the cortical responses. Changes in the SSEP waveform, especially in operation in the region of the brainstem, can reflect unfavorable manipulation or ischemia. Changes in SSEP waveforms can precede development of a permanent neurologic deficit; therefore, monitoring can warn the surgeon of impending permanent damage.

Electromyographic monitoring is specific to the motor nerve at risk and can be used to monitor the status of cranial nerves III, IV, VI, VII, X, XI, and XII. It is most useful in monitoring the intraoperative status and location of the facial nerve. The use of needle electrodes for this purpose allows reliable identification and preservation of even small branches of cranial nerve VII. Other important neurophysiologic monitoring techniques are listed in Table 126.2.

EVALUATION

Imaging Studies

Computed tomography (CT) and magnetic resonance imaging (MRI) are essential in the preoperative planning of cranial-base procedures. These two modalities often are complementary in the information that they provide. MRI shows greater soft-tissue detail, but CT is superior for visualizing the craniofacial skeleton and calcified tissues at the base of the skull. Complete CT evaluation of the cranial base consists of axial and coronal images with soft-tissue and bone algorithms. MRI is particularly useful because tissue types and tumors can be differentiated on the basis of signal response (Table 126.3). MRI can generate sagittal images, which is not possible with most CT techniques. Magnetic resonance angiography can provide useful vascular

TABLE 126.2
INTRAOPERATIVE NEUROPHYSIOLOGIC MONITORING TECHNIQUES

Structure Monitored	Monitoring Modality	Usefulness
Cranial nerve II	Visual evoked response	Investigational
	Direct optic nerve potential	Investigational
Cranial nerve III, IV, VI	Ocular muscle EMG nerve stimulation	Useful
Cranial nerve VII	Facial muscle EMG with direct nerve stimulation	Very useful
Cranial nerve VIII	Cochlear action potential	Investigational
	BSER	Useful
	Direct nerve action potential	Useful
Cranial nerve X	Sound-activated monitoring of vocal cord	Investigational
Cranial nerve XI	Trapezius muscle EMG	Useful
Cranial nerve XII	Tongue EMG	Useful
Temporal lobe (during retraction)	BSER from opposite side	Very useful
Brainstem	BSER from contralateral side	Very useful
Cervicomedullary junction	SSEP	Useful

EMG, electromyography; BSER, brainstem-evoked response; SSEP, somatosensory-evoked potential.

information in a noninvasive manner without use of intravenous or intraarterial contrast material.

Because biopsy often cannot be performed on tumors of the cranial base, preoperative diagnosis often is based on other methods. Current imaging techniques clearly define tumor location. Because many types of tumors of the cranial base are site specific, this information can narrow the range of histologic types of the tumor (Table 126.4). The particular radiographic appearance of a tumor in light of its location usually allows accurate tumor-type identification before histologic examination is possible (7).

Positron emission tomography can be performed at a few medical centers. This technique depicts actual cellular activity in the brain, primarily through detection of labeled glucose taken up by the tissues under examination. Although this technique eventually may be useful for identification of primary tumors within the neuraxis, it is most appropriate for evaluation of response to adjuvant therapy after histologic identification and resection of a tumor. It also can be useful in detecting tumor recurrence at an early stage, thereby prompting stereotactic biopsy and early use of adjuvant measures such as stereotactic radiation. In the primary setting, positron emission tomography is less useful than CT or MRI.

Cerebrovascular Evaluation

The purpose of cerebrovascular evaluation is to determine the functional adequacy of CBF. It includes temporary balloon occlusion (TBO) test, which is used to simulate carotid clamping or permanent ligation with respect to development of neurologic deficits. For this purpose, the TBO test usually is combined with a neurologic examination or more objective or quantitative examination, such as xenon CT. Temporary occlusion of the carotid artery is achieved with an intraarterial balloon catheter inserted during cerebral angiography. If neurologic signs develop during the 10 to 20 minutes of occlusion, the result is considered a failure, and the patient cannot undergo carotid resection. Because 10% to 15% of patients who pass the TBO test have cerebral ischemia after carotid resection, a second test, xenon-enhanced CT, is performed.

Xenon CT involves inflation of the intraarterial balloon within the internal carotid artery and allows the patient to

TABLE 126.3
APPEARANCE OF NORMAL TISSUES WITH MAGNETIC RESONANCE IMAGING

Sequence	Bone	Fat	Water[a](CSF)	Muscle	Brain (white)	Brain (gray)
T_1-weighted	Very dark	Very bright	Dark	Intermediate	Bright	Dark
T_2-weighted	Very dark	Dark	Very bright	Intermediate	Dark	Bright

[a]CSF, cerebrospinal fluid.
Increased water content increases the brightness of T_2-weighted images. Therefore, inflammation tends to be brighter than tumor tissue on T_2-weighted images, depending on the amount of edema.

TABLE 126.4

TUMORS INVOLVING THE CRANIAL BASE[a]

Anterior cranial base
  Benign
    Meningioma
    Juvenile angiofibroma
    Fibroosseous lesions
  Malignant
    Squamous cell carcinoma
    Esthesioneuroblastoma

Middle cranial base
  Benign
    Meningioma
    Pituitary adenoma
    Chordoma
    Craniopharyngioma
  Malignant
    Nasopharyngeal carcinoma
    Squamous cell carcinoma (paranasal sinus extension)
    Adenoid cystic carcinoma

Posterior cranial base
  Benign
    Glomus tumors (paraganglioma)
    Meningioma
    Chordoma
    Schwannoma, neuroma
  Malignant
    Squamous cell carcinoma (otogenic)

[a]The tumors listed represent those most likely to occur in the indicated location.

breathe a xenon–oxygen mixture. Xenon is radiodense and diffuses into the bloodstream, serving as a marker for cerebral perfusion. The digital data generated during CT can be used to determine the amount of blood flow to regions of the brain before and after TBO. With this method, a decrease in blood flow after TBO of the carotid artery can be quantified. These data have led to the development of criteria to quantify the carotid resection and the need for reconstruction of the internal carotid artery, usually with a saphenous vein interposition graft. The criteria and a decision-making algorithm are shown in Table 126.5. Although xenon CT coupled with the TBO test has increased the safety of carotid resection, it does not entirely eliminate the risk of postoperative ischemia. About 2% of patients who pass the xenon CT–TBO test have a neurologic deficit after carotid resection. The most important disadvantages of xenon CT are limited availability and expense. Less-sophisticated testing has been combined with the TBO test to enhance ascertaining which patients can pass the TBO test, only to have a postoperative ischemic deficit after resection of the carotid artery. One such method is use of electrocardiography during TBO. This technique has proved useful in several studies in decreasing the risk of delayed cerebral ischemia to less than 7% (8).

Radionuclide injection and brain scanning in conjunction with TBO testing to visualize underperfused portions of the cortex also have proved useful. In some studies, this combination has yielded results comparable with those of xenon CT evaluation of cerebrovascular sufficiency. It must be noted that even if a patient passes a TBO test, real risk of delayed cerebrovascular ischemia persists unless the carotid system is bypassed before tumor removal or is reconstructed after resection.

SURGICAL ANATOMY

The base of the skull can be divided into three regions—the anterior, middle, and posterior segments. These three regions are distinct in anatomic features, spectrum of pathologic lesions, and surgical approaches used to treat them.

TABLE 126.5

CEREBROVASCULAR EVALUATION AND TREATMENT OPTIONS: BALLOON OCCLUSION TEST OF INTERNAL CAROTID ARTERY

Nature of Occlusion	Neurologic Deficit	No Neurologic Deficit (Xenon CT-CBF Study)	
		Reduction of CBF 15–35 mL/100 g/min	No reduction of CBF >35 mL/100 g/min
Hemodynamic stroke risk			
• Brief temporary occlusion	Mild–moderate	None	None
	High	Mild	Mild
• Prolonged temporary occlusion	High	Moderate to high	None
	ST–MCA bypass	ST–MCA bypass	ICA–ICA short vein graft (benign tumors)
Permanent	ST–MCA and direct vein graft	ICA–ICA vein graft	No reconstruction (malignant tumors)
Management options if artery must be occluded	ECA–MCA long vein graft		

CT, computed tomograpy; CBF, cerebral blood flow; ST–MCA, superficial temporal artery–middle cerebral artery; ICA–ICA, internal carotid artery–internal carotid artery; ECA–MCA, external carotid artery–middle cerebral artery.

TABLE 126.6

FORAMINA OF THE BASE OF THE SKULL

Foramen	Structures Transmitted
Cribriform plate	Olfactory nerve (CN I)
Foramen cecum	Occasional small vein; origin of sagittal sinus
Optic canal	Optic nerve (CN II); ophthalmic artery
Superior orbital fissure	Cranial nerves III, IV; ophthalmic division of trigeminal nerve (CN, V_1); VI, superior ophthalmic vein
Inferior orbital fissure	Maxillary division of trigeminal nerve (CN V_2); zygomatic branch of trigeminal nerve; filaments from pterygopalatine branch of the maxillary nerve; infraorbital vessels; anastomosis between inferior ophthalmic vein and pterygoid venous plexus
Foramen rotundum	Maxillary division of trigeminal nerve (CN V_2)
Foramen ovale	Mandibular division of trigeminal nerve (CN V_3)
Foramen spinosum	Middle meningeal artery
Sulcus tubae auditivae	Lodges cartilaginous part of auditory (eustachian) tube
Foramen lacerum	Closed inferiorly by a fibrocartilaginous plate that contains the auditory tube; upper part traversed by the internal carotid artery
Carotid canal	Internal carotid artery
Stylomastoid foramen	Facial nerve (CN VII); stylomastoid artery
Jugular foramen	Beginning of the internal jugular vein; cranial nerves IX, X, XI
Internal acoustic meatus	Facial nerve (CN VII); vestibuloacoustic nerve (CN VIII)
Hypoglossal canal	Hypoglossal nerve (CN XII)
Foramen magnum	Spinal cord (medulla oblongata); spinal accessory nerves (CN XI); vertebral arteries; anterior and posterior spinal arteries; occipitoaxial ligament

CN, cranial nerve.

The foramina of the base of the skull and the structures that pass through each region are listed in Table 126.6.

The Scalp

Knowledge of the layers of the scalp and its vascular supply is essential in planning surgical incisions that preserve potential reconstructive flaps and maximize primary wound healing. The three most important layers are the pericranium, the galea, and the temporoparietal fascia (9). The blood supply to the pericranium and galea is primarily from the supraorbital and supratrochlear arteries. The galea also receives its blood supply from the supraorbital and supratrochlear arteries as well as the superficial temporal artery. It can be used alone or in combination with pericranium as a reconstructive flap for the anterior fossa. When a galeal flap is elevated, the risk of causing ischemic necrosis of the forehead skin is present, particularly if the forehead has been exposed to therapeutic radiation. In this setting, cranial-base reconstruction is performed with flaps other than galeal–pericranial tissue. If a pericranial flap has been used, a galeal flap cannot be used. The quality, vascularity, and quantity of tissue available from the galea alone for revision reconstruction would be inadequate. It is in this setting that microvascular transfer, usually consisting of a radial forearm or rectus abdominis flap, would be most appropriate. For most patients who have not undergone surgery or radiation therapy, a pericranial flap alone is adequate, and the galea need not be elevated from the overlying cutaneous tissue of the forehead. A bicoronal incision is placed substantially posterior to the hairline so that a sufficient length of pericranium can be preserved anterior to the incision to serve as a useful reconstructive flap.

The final scalp-derived flap for reconstruction of cranial-base defects is the temporoparietal fascial flap. Unlike the temporalis muscle flap, which is a separate entity and is based on the deep temporal vascular system, the temporoparietal fascial flap receives its blood supply from the superficial temporal vessels. Both a temporalis muscle flap and a temporoparietal fascial flap can be raised simultaneously from the same side of the head for reconstruction. The temporoparietal flap is elevated off the subcutaneous tissue of the lateral scalp over the temporal and parietal regions. This flap cannot be used if that area of the scalp has been exposed to therapeutic radiation because of the high probability of scalp loss after removal of the underlying temporoparietal fascial blood supply from the overlying cutaneous tissues. This flap is about 10 cm wide and as long as 16 cm long. It can be tunneled into the nasopharynx, the orbit, the posterior anterior fossa, the middle fossa, and mastoid or temporal defects. The thin, supple nature of the flap coupled with its robust blood supply and minimal donor-site morbidity make it valuable for reconstruction of lateral defects of the cranial base (9). Unlike transposition of a temporalis muscle flap, use of a temporoparietal fascial flap does not produce contour deformity in the temporal region. Flap survival depends on preservation of the integrity of the superficial temporal vessels during placement of bicoronal incisions and scalp flap elevation.

Anterior Cranial Base

The intracranial surface of the anterior cranial base extends from the frontal bone, over the orbital roofs, to the anterior (superior) edge of the greater wing of the sphenoid bone. The frontal poles of the brain rest on the anterior cranial base. The frontal sinus is in the frontal bone, and its posterior wall forms the anterior limit of the anterior cranial base. The foramina of the anterior cranial are the cribriform plate, through which pass the filamentous olfactory nerves (cranial nerve I) into the nasal cavity. The olfactory bulbs rest on the cribriform plate and connect these cranial nerves to the brain. The keel-like crista galli divides the cribriform plate in the midline. It is immediately just posterior to the foramen cecum, which marks the origin of the sagittal sinus. The roof of the ethmoidal and sphenoidal sinuses form the floor of the anterior cranial base between the orbits. The portion of the ethmoidal sinuses that contributes to the anterior floor of the base of the skull is called the *fovea ethmoidalis*. The fovea ethmoidalis, not the cribriform plate, is the most common location of iatrogenic defects and CSF leaks through the floor of the anterior cranial base after ethmoidal sinus surgery.

Extracranial landmarks that help to identify the floor of the anterior cranial base are the anterior and posterior ethmoidal arteries. A line joining the anterior to the posterior ethmoidal arteries usually identifies the level of the floor of the anterior cranial base. If ethmoidal sinus surgery is limited to a level below this line, unintentional entrance into the intracranial space usually can be avoided. The optic nerve (just before it enters the optic canal) is located ~5 mm posterior to the posterior ethmoidal artery. The relation of these ethmoidal vessels to each other and the optic nerve is shown in Fig. 126.4. The planum sphenoidale is the roof of the sphenoidal sinus. It contributes to the most posterior limit of the anterior cranial base. Immediately lateral to the planum sphenoidale are the optic canals, the intracranial openings of which also demarcate the posterior limit of the anterior cranial base.

Middle Cranial Base

The intracranial surface of the middle cranial base is composed of the greater wing and body of sphenoid bone, the petrous bone anterior to the petrous ridge, and the squamous portion of the temporal bone. The temporal lobes of the brain occupy most of the middle cranial base. A separate location exists for the pituitary gland, which is lodged in the sella turcica. The sella turcica is below the optic chiasm and behind the posterior wall of the sphenoidal sinus. The sphenoidal sinus usually is well pneumatized in adults,

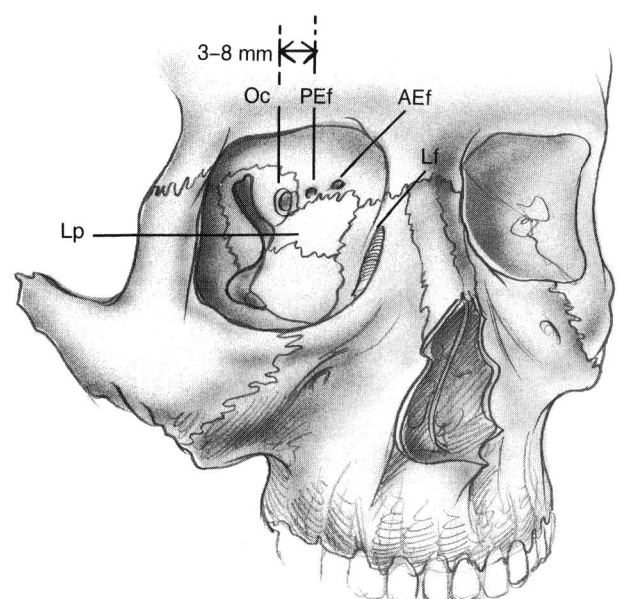

Figure 126.4   The ethmoidal foramina that transmit the anterior and posterior ethmoidal arteries mark the roof of the ethmoidal sinuses, above which lie the anterior cranial base and brain. *AEf*, anterior ethmoidal foramen; *Lf*, lacrimal fossa; *Lp*, lacrimal papyracea of ethmoid bone; *Oc*, optic canal; *PEf*, posterior ethmoidal foramen.

and access to the sella can be gained through this sinus with a transsphenoidal approach. If the sinus is not well pneumatized, ease of access to the sella can be affected.

The three types of sphenoidal sinus are shown in Fig. 126.5. The sellar type of sinus is the most common, with the presellar and conchal (nonpneumatized) sinuses occurring in decreasing frequency (10). The transsphenoidal approach provides access to the middle, not the anterior, cranial base. On either side of the sella turcica is the cavernous venous sinus, a common site for tumor involvement in lesions of the base of the skull. The cavernous sinus is composed of a rich network of venous channels that drain the tissues of the midface. It contains the internal carotid artery and cranial nerves III, IV, V_1, V_2, and VI (Fig. 126.6). The cavernous sinus itself is drained by the paired superior and inferior petrosal sinuses.

The internal carotid artery is the most important arterial structure within the cranial base, and its three-dimensional course must be appreciated. The internal carotid artery becomes encased in the petrous portion of the temporal bone after it enters the carotid canal at the base of the skull. It first proceeds in a vertical direction until it passes medially to the osseous eustachian tube, where the artery bends in an anteromedial direction to form the horizontal segment. It is not uncommon for the osseous eustachian tube to be dehiscent where it is in contact with the internal carotid artery. The horizontal segment ends as the carotid artery turns vertically to pass alongside the lateral wall of the sphenoidal sinus. The impression of the internal carotid

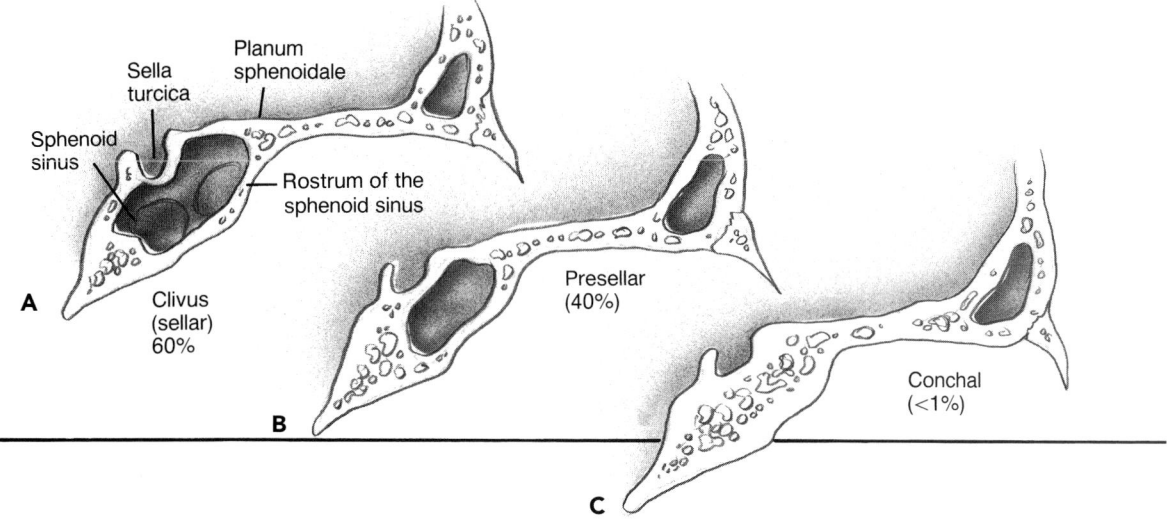

Figure 126.5 Sagittal view of the sphenoidal sinus and sella turcica shows the anatomic variants—sellar type (**A**), presellar (**B**), and nonpneumatized (**C**). Lack of nonpneumatization of a sphenoidal sinus can be a contraindication to transsphenoidal access to the sella turcica.

artery within the lateral wall of the sinus usually can be seen with endoscopy. The internal carotid artery traverses the cavernous venous sinus just before entering the intracranial space.

In approaches to the horizontal segment of the internal carotid artery through the middle fossa, the artery can be located first by means of identification of the greater superficial petrosal nerve (GSPN). The GSPN supplies parasympathetic innervation to the parotid gland after its fibers synapse in the otic ganglion. The course of the GSPN is directly above and in the same direction as the horizontal portion of the petrous portion of the internal carotid artery. The GSPN is the most reliable intracranial landmark for the petrous portion of the internal carotid artery (11). The superior orbital fissure is a point of egress for several important intracranial structures (Fig. 126.7). The inferior orbital fissure does not open into the cranial cavity but opens into the pterygopalatine fossa. The inferior orbital fissure is formed by close approximation of the posterior wall of the maxillary sinus to the base of the skull; no direct intracranial connection exists. Numerous neural and vascular foramina are found in the middle cranial base.

The extracranial surface of the middle cranial base comes into contact with several regions—the temporal fossa, the infratemporal fossa, the pterygopalatine fossa, and the poststyloid (paranasopharyngeal) space. The temporal fossa is filled with the temporal muscle, which extends from its fanlike origin on the squamous portion of the temporal bone to its insertion on the coronoid process of the mandible. This muscle, based on the deep temporal arteries, is the reconstructive flap most commonly used in cranial-base surgery. The deep temporal arteries are branches of the internal maxillary artery, which is just medial to the condylar neck of the mandible. The deep temporal artery provides the primary blood supply for the temporalis muscle (Fig. 126.8). The temporalis muscle reaches its insertion site on the coronoid process of the mandible by passing under the zygomatic arch. It is below this arch that the temporal fossa becomes the infratemporal fossa.

The infratemporal fossa is bounded anteriorly by the posterior buttress of the malar eminence and maxillary sinus, posteriorly by the glenoid fossa, mandibular neck, and condyle, and medially by a plane extending from the

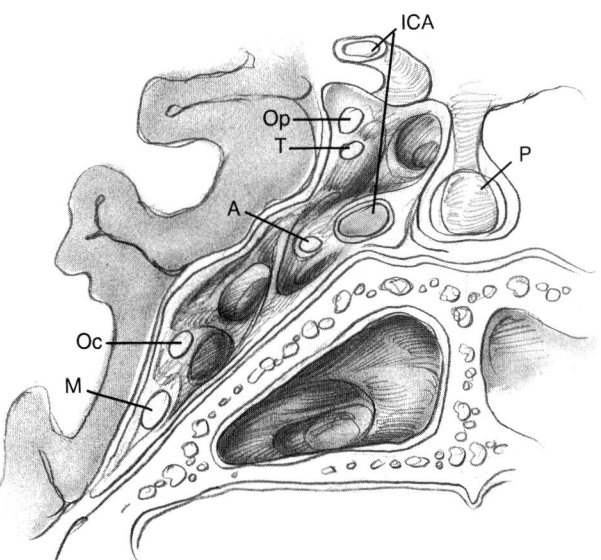

Figure 126.6 The cavernous venous sinus and the structures that pass through it. *Oc*, oculomotor nerve III; *Op*, ophthalmic nerve; *P*, pituitary gland; *T*, trochlear nerve; *A*, abducent nerve VI; *ICA*, internal carotid artery; *M*, maxillary nerve V₂.

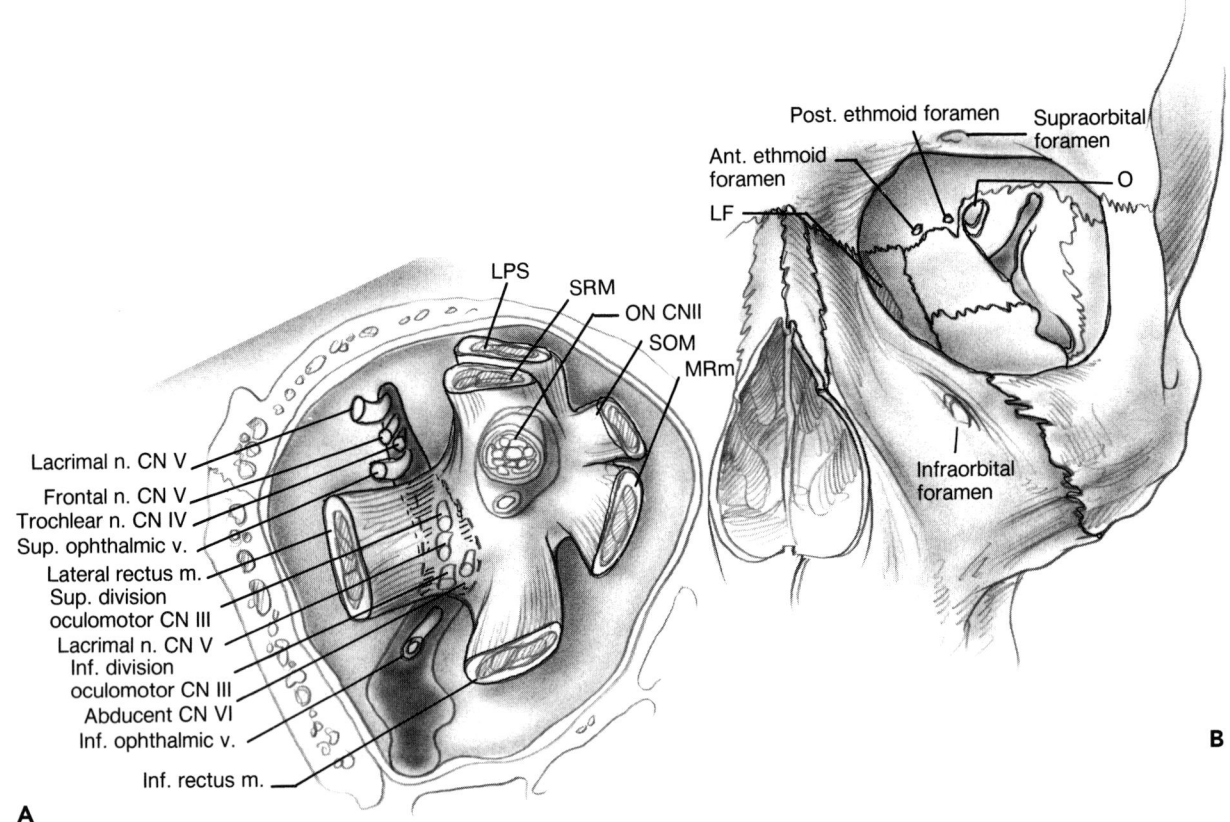

Figure 126.7 The orbital fissures and foramina **(A)** and the structures that pass through them **(B)**. *LF,* lacrimal fossa; *LPS,* levator palpebrae superioris muscle; *MRm,* medial rectus muscle; *O,* optic foramen; *ON CNII,* optic nerve; *SOM,* superior oblique muscle; *SRM,* superior rectus muscle.

lateral pterygoid plate to the spine of the sphenoid bone. In addition to the insertion of the temporalis muscle, the pterygoid muscles are contained in this fossa. Only two surgically important foramina are found in the infratemporal fossa—the foramen ovale, through which passes the third division of the trigeminal nerve, and the foramen spinosum, which transmits the middle meningeal artery. The eustachian tube exits the base of the skull just medial to the spine of the sphenoid bone at the junction of the infratemporal fossa and poststyloid space.

The pterygopalatine fossa is the space between the posterior wall of the maxillary sinus and pterygoid plates. This narrow fossa contains the foramen rotundum, through which the second division of the trigeminal nerve exits the cranial vault. This fossa contains the vidian nerve (also called the nerve of the pterygoid canal), which is formed by contributions of the lesser petrosal (parasympathetic) and deep petrosal (sympathetic) nerves. The vidian nerve passes through the pterygoid canal to synapse in the pterygopalatine ganglion, where it provides autonomic innervation to the nasal cavity, nasopharynx, and lacrimal glands.

The poststyloid space, located behind a plane that connects the medial pterygoid plate to the styloid process,

contains the entrance to the carotid canal and jugular foramen. An important group of structures is centered at the spine of the sphenoid bone. The spine is medial to the glenoid fossa, just anterior to the carotid canal, immediately behind and slightly lateral to the foramen spinosum and foramen ovale, and lateral to the cartilaginous insertion of the eustachian tube into the base of the skull (Fig. 126.9). The spine of the sphenoid bone is the most consistent and reliable extracranial landmark for locating the internal carotid artery where it enters the petrous portion of the temporal bone (12).

Posterior Cranial Base

The posterior cranial base extends from the petrous ridge posteriorly to the occipital bones. This region includes the clivus, which is centrally located between the foramen magnum and the petrous tips. Meningioma and chordoma can originate here. Normal anatomic openings in the posterior cranial base include the internal auditory canal, foramen magnum, hypoglossal canal, and jugular foramen. Venous sinuses (petrous, sigmoid, and transverse) run along the periphery of the posterior fossa.

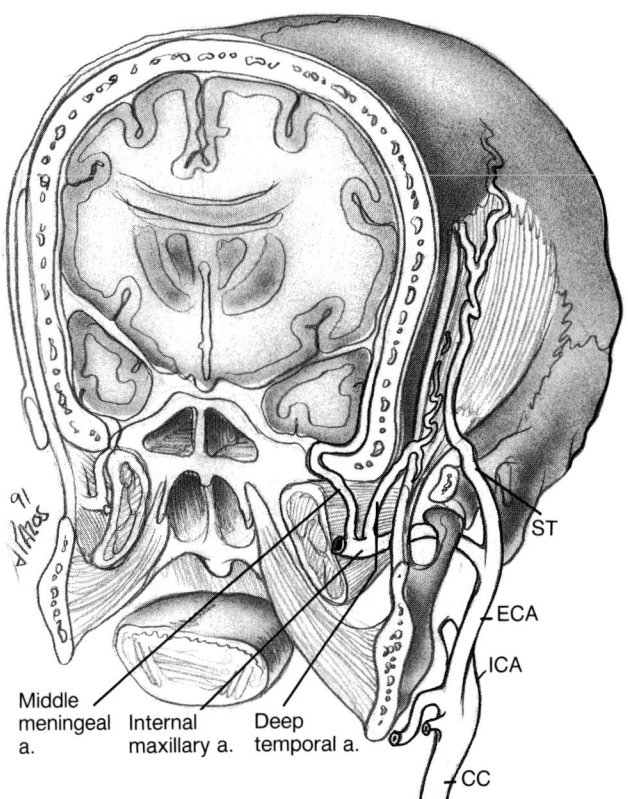

Figure 126.8 Coronal section of the temporal fossa, anterior view, shows the deep temporal artery that provides the blood supply to the temporalis muscle. The superficial temporal vessels have only a minimal contribution to the blood supply of the temporalis muscle. The middle meningeal artery passing through the foramen spinosum is evident. *ST*, superficial temporal artery; *CC*, common carotid artery; *ECA*, external carotid artery; *ICA*, internal carotid artery.

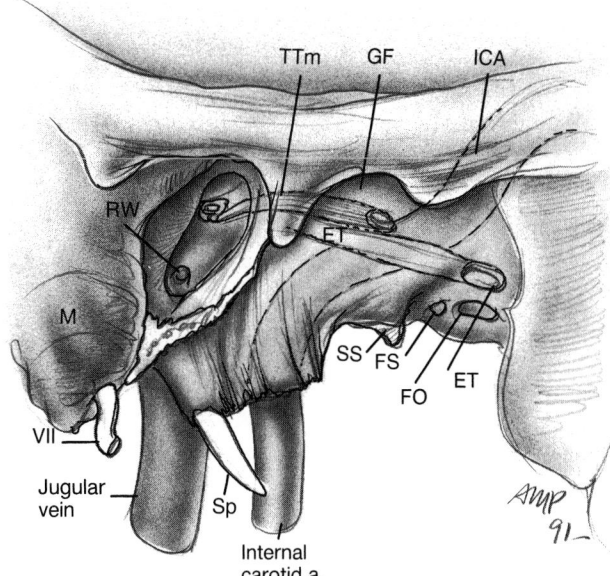

Figure 126.9 View of the internal carotid artery through the glenoid fossa shows how the artery is close to the medial surface of the eustachian tube, where it begins to turn in an anteromedial direction to form the horizontal segment of the artery. *ET*, eustachian tube; *FO*, foramen ovale; *FS*, foramen spinosum; *GF*, glenoid fossa; *M*, mastoid bone; *RW*, round window; *Sp*, styloid process; *SS*, sphenoid spine; *TTm*, tensor tympani muscle.

MANAGEMENT OF CRANIAL-BASE TUMORS

Surgical Approaches

Approaches to the cranial base are tailored to a region and type of lesion (Table 126.7).

Anterior Cranial Base

Tumor involvement of the anterior cranial base usually is caused by contiguous spread from the paranasal sinuses, nasal cavity, or nasopharynx. Approaches to this region traditionally involve exposing these tumors both intracranially (bicoronal incision and bifrontal craniotomy) and through the midface (Weber–Fergusson incision). Experience with the subcranial approach (supraorbital rim and glabellar osteotomies) can allow removal of even large paranasal sinus tumors without facial incisions. Avoidance of facial incisions gives the patient a substantial aesthetic advantage.

Access to the intracranial anterior base of the skull usually is gained through a bicoronal incision positioned sufficiently behind the hairline to preserve an expanse of

pericranium and galea adequate for use as a reconstructive flap. Scalp incisions that track the anterior hairline are avoided because they do not contribute to exposure, tend to be aesthetically unacceptable, particularly for men, and can shorten the length of vascularized pericranium available for

TABLE 126.7
APPROACHES TO THE CRANIAL BASE

Anterior cranial base
    Basilar subfrontal with or without facial incisions (craniofacial approach)
    Transfrontal sinus

Middle cranial base
    Transoral, transseptal, transsphenoidal approach to the sella
    Subtemporal–infratemporal fossa (preauricular)
    Subtemporal–infratemporal fossa (postauricular)
    Facial translocation
    Midfacial split
    Facial degloving
    Mandibular split procedure
    Palatal split procedure
    Le Fort I osteotomy with or without transseptal exposure

Posterior cranial base
    Extreme lateral approach
    Transoral approach to craniovertebral junction
    Palatal split procedure
    Translabyrinthine approach
    Retrosigmoid approach
    Suboccipital approach

reconstructive application. The superficial temporal artery is preserved as the bicoronal incision is brought down over the temples in front of the ears. Preservation of these vessels allows use of a temporoparietal fascial flap for cranial-base reconstruction. This flap is elevated from the undersurface of the posterior temporal and anterior parietal scalp. The temporoparietal fascial flap is most useful in reconstruction of middle fossa (infratemporal fossa) and sphenoidal sinus defects. It is entirely separate from the temporalis muscle flap and the pericranial flap. The usefulness of the temporoparietal fascial flap is discussed later.

After incision and preservation of the superficial temporal artery, the deep tissues of the forehead can be elevated anteriorly to the level of the superior orbital rims in a plane deep to the pericranium. Care is taken to preserve the supraorbital and supratrochlear vessels, because they provide blood to the pericranium, which is an important reconstructive flap. This flap is useful in anterior cranial-base surgery and can be used to resurface the floor of the anterior cranial fossa completely. The usefulness of this flap in sealing complex defects of the sphenoidal sinus and sphenoidal rostrum is limited. Use of the flap in conjunction with a separately elevated temporoparietal fascial flap is advised. The combination of these two flaps to manage complex sphenoidal sinus defects can decrease the risk of postoperative CSF fistula. If thought and attention are not given to preservation of the vessels that supply these flaps before incision and scalp elevation, the potential for use of the flaps is jeopardized. The importance of these vascularized flaps in preventing potentially devastating postoperative complications cannot be overemphasized.

Bifrontal craniotomy can be performed to expose the dura over the frontal poles; the removed section of calvarium usually corresponds to area 1 in Fig. 126.10. A separate segment of bone containing the glabella and supraorbital rims can be removed between the supraorbital foramen (Fig. 126.10, area 2) to provide direct anterior exposure of the ethmoidal sinuses and to maximize exposure of the subfrontal base of the skull and minimize brain retraction during tumor removal. With experience, use of the subfrontal extension can allow removal of selected tumors of the paranasal sinus without use of facial incisions. Facial incisions such as lateral rhinotomy and the Weber–Fergusson incision can be avoided in most instances when endoscopic sinus or midfacial degloving approaches are used. After bifrontal craniotomy with or without subfrontal extension, the frontal poles and overlying dura can be separated from the bony cranial base to allow transection of the olfactory nerve connections through the cribriform plate. Olfactory-sparing operations are possible, but we believe that they contribute to acute or delayed postoperative formation of CSF fistulae. In most instances, the patient is told to expect permanent anosmia as a result of surgery. With elevation of the frontal dura and transection of the olfactory poles, exposure can be gained as far posteriorly as the planum sphenoidale and optic chiasm. The sphenoidal

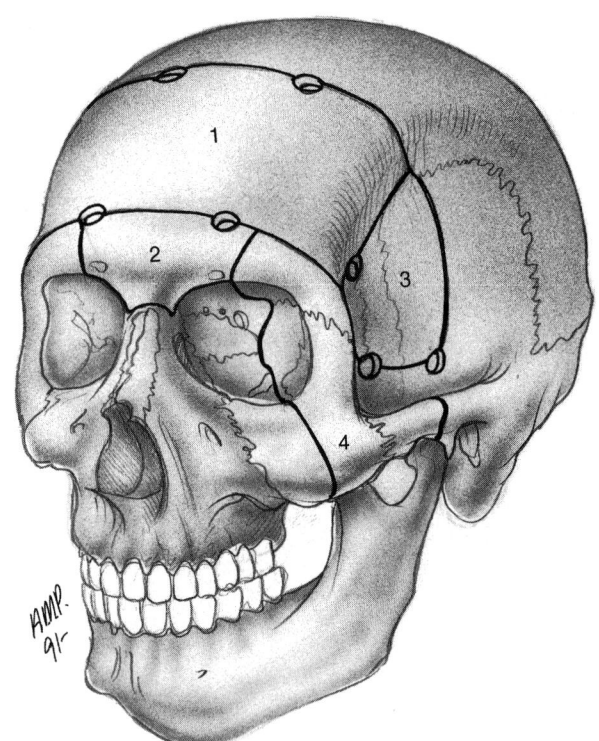

Figure 126.10 The potential areas of temporary bone removal for the basal subfrontal or subtemporal–infratemporal fossa approaches to the cranial base.

sinus can be entered through the planum sphenoidale (its roof), and the optic nerves can be exposed by means of opening the optic canals medially and superiorly (Fig. 126.11). The intracranial portion of the tumor can be circumscribed with additional osteotomies through the ethmoidal air cells.

Facial incisions often are used as part of a combined craniofacial resection if both intracranial and transfacial exposure of the tumor is needed. Lateral rhinotomy is useful in exposing the superior limit of the nasal cavity and paranasal sinuses for complete tumor removal. This is particularly true if the tumor is malignant or the surgeon has not performed many operations on the base of the skull. Lateral rhinotomy can be easily combined with periorbital incisions, either subciliary or transconjunctival, to allow orbital exenteration if the periorbital septum has been breached by the malignant tumor.

Alternative methods of exposing the nasal cavity and nasopharynx that do not entail facial incisions include facial degloving and the transpalatal approach. These approaches are useful when tumor spread does not involve the paranasal sinuses. These techniques have the advantage of avoiding facial scars, but they provide much more limited exposure of the upper vault and ethmoidal sinuses than do approaches that entail lateral rhinotomy (13).

The central anterior cranial base usually is reconstructed with a pericranial flap. Pericranium alone usually is adequate. The use of galea is avoided, because elevation of the

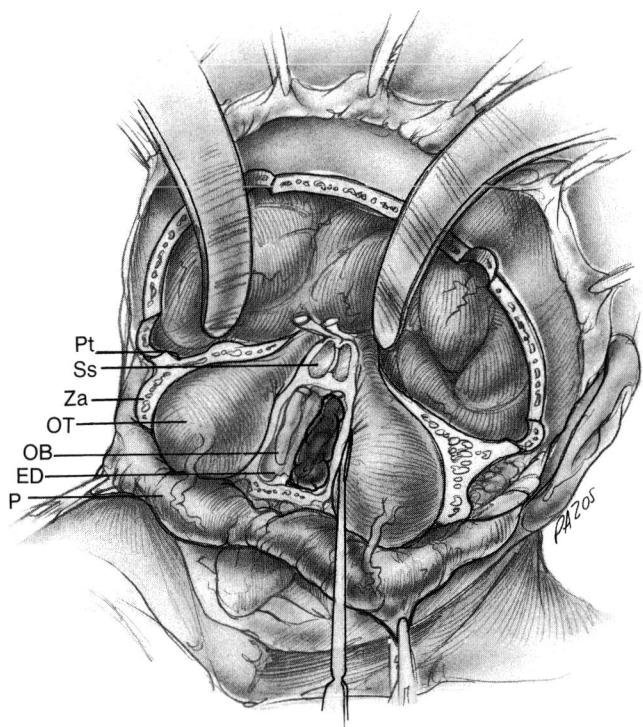

Pt
Ss
Za
OT
OB
ED
P

Figure 126.11. Basal subfrontal approach to the anterior cranial base. The brain has been retracted posteriorly after bifrontal craniotomy, the orbital roofs have been removed, the sphenoidal sinus has been entered, and the course of the optic nerves defined. The ethmoidal region is ready for resection with or without the aid of a facial incision, depending on the extent of tumor within the nasal vault. *ED,* ethmoid bone and dura; *OB,* transected olfactory bulbs; *OT,* orbital tissues; *P,* pericranium; *Pt,* pterion; *Ss,* sphenoidal sinus; *Za,* zygomatic arch.

galea can cause devascularization of the forehead, especially if the superficial temporal arteries have been transected bilaterally. Dural defects are closed separately before reconstruction of the cranial base with the pericranial flap. Dural defects are best repaired with autogenous materials, such as fascia lata or pericranium, or with semisynthetic preparations such as acellular dermis. Care is taken during dural repair to achieve a watertight closure. The pericranium can be turned intracranially and tacked to the periphery of the resection defect with sutures. Skin grafts have proved successful in bridging defects of the anterior cranial base, but vascularized tissue usually is preferable.

Bone grafts rarely are necessary to prevent herniation of brain into the nasal cavity. Adequate support of the frontal poles usually is provided by the dura and pericranium alone. Bone grafts can be considered when a substantial portion of the bone covering the orbits has been removed. Soft-tissue reconstruction of the orbital roof can allow the transmission of vascular pulsation from the brain to the eyes. These orbital pulsations can be extremely disturbing to patients in the extended postoperative period. If bony orbital volume and structural integrity are not reestablished, high risk of enophthalmos exists because of posterior–superior retraction of

the intraorbital soft tissues within the expanded orbital space. This cosmetic deformity is particularly unacceptable and difficult to correct secondarily. A temporalis muscle flap or temporoparietal fascial flap can be used together with the pericranial flap to reconstruct lateral extensions of defects of the anterior cranial base. Exposed pericranium within the nasal cavity usually becomes covered with mucosa within several weeks, so skin-graft coverage is unnecessary.

Middle Cranial Base

A multitude of transoral, transfacial, and transtemporal approaches to the middle cranial base have been described, but the concepts embodied by most of these approaches can be illustrated with three basic procedures—the transsphenoidal approach, the infratemporal fossa approach, and the facial translocation or maxillotomy procedure (14). Selection of a particular approach depends on the exact location of the tumor and its histologic type. The transsphenoidal approach (Fig. 126.12) is limited to midline tumors affecting the posterior nasal cavity, nasopharynx, sphenoidal sinus, and sella turcica. These lesions usually are histologically benign. Tumors that arise in the petroclival portions of the middle cranial base and involve the petrous carotid artery, such as meningioma and chordoma, usually can be resected through a variant of the infratemporal fossa approach (Fig. 126.13). In contrast, non-midline tumors arising in the paranasal sinuses and nasopharynx often are malignant. They necessitate greater exposure to achieve clear surgical margins than can be reliably provided with either the transsphenoidal or the infratemporal fossa approach. In this setting, facial translocation provides superior exposure of the infratemporal fossa, nasopharynx, and external part of the middle cranial base (Fig. 126.14).

Transsphenoidal Approach to the Sella Turcica

Transsphenoidal exposure of the sella usually is achieved through a transoral gingivobuccal incision that provides wide exposure of the piriform aperture (Fig. 126.12A). A mucoperichondrial flap can be elevated on one side of the cartilaginous septum. The opposite layer of mucoperichondrium and the anterior cartilaginous septum can be reflected laterally to expose the osseous septum. This osseous septum can be resected to expose the sphenoidal rostrum. At this point, the sphenoidal sinus can be entered through its anterior face. An opening large enough to visualize the entire sinus can be safely made (Fig. 126.12B). The bulge of the sella turcica in the posterior superior limit of the sinus can be identified, and the bone over the sella carefully removed with an osteotome to expose the dura over the pituitary gland in preparation for tumor resection by the neurosurgeon. After resection, the sella and possibly the sphenoidal sinus can be filled with a free fat or fascial graft to minimize the risk of CSF leak. Closure is achieved by allowing the mucoperichondrium and cartilaginous

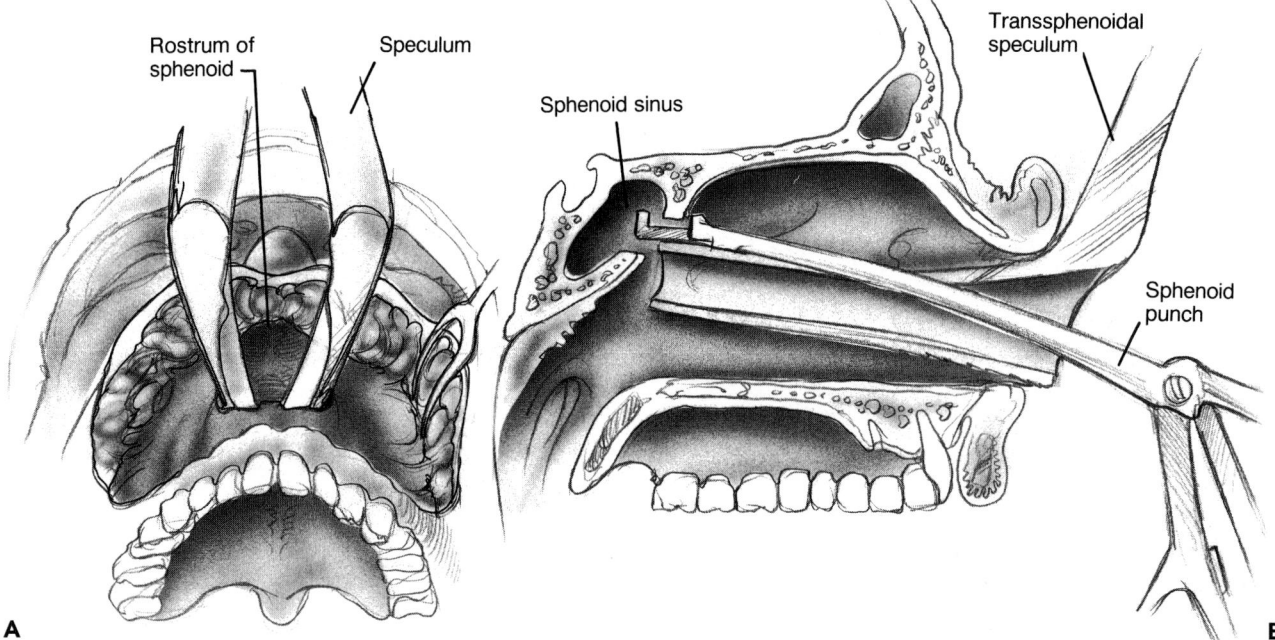

Figure 126.12 Anterior **(A)** and lateral **(B)** views show a transsphenoidal speculum in place for a transoral transsphenoidal approach to the sella turcica. The sphenoidotomy in **B** is being widened with a punch in preparation for entrance into the sella proper.

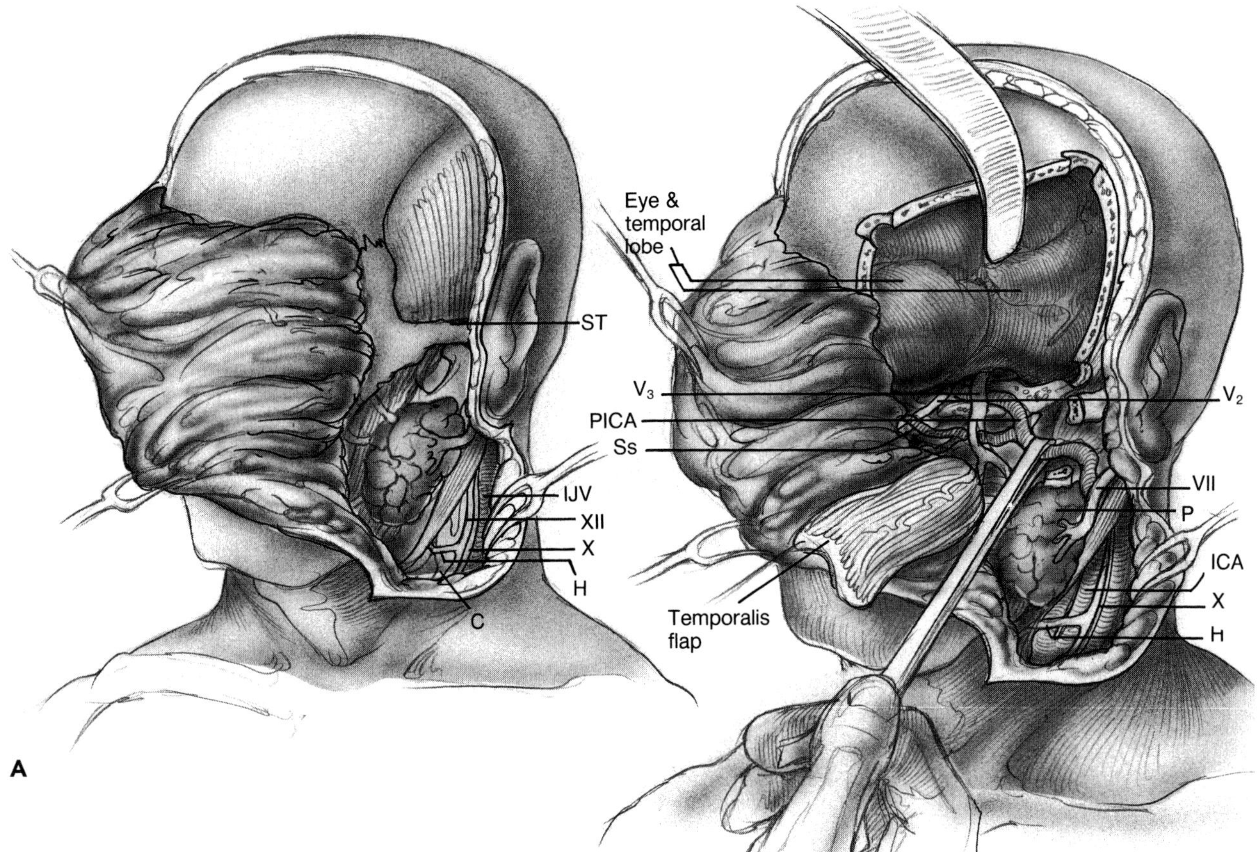

Figure 126.13 Preauricular infratemporal fossa approach to the cranial base. **A:** Before osteotomy and craniotomy. **B:** After craniotomy, zygomaticoorbital osteotomy, and exposure of the petrous portion of the internal carotid artery. *C,* carotid artery; *H,* hypoglossal nerve; *ICA,* internal carotid artery; *P,* parotid gland; *PICA,* petrous internal carotid artery; *ST,* superficial temporal artery.

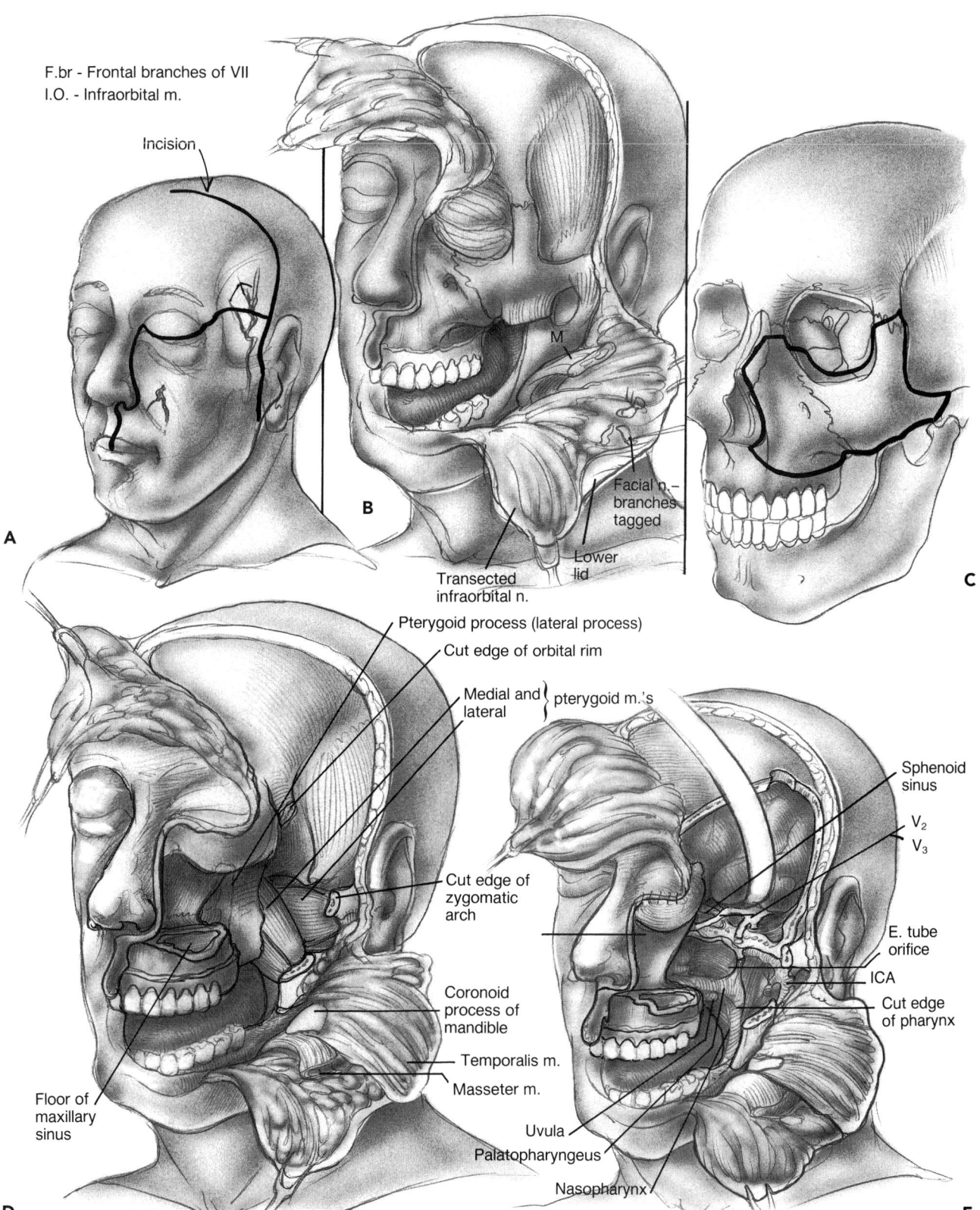

Figure 126.14 Facial translocation approach to the cranial base. **A:** The necessary facial incision lines and the course of the frontal branches of the facial nerve are evident. **B:** The facial flaps have been elevated to expose the facial skeleton and transected nerves tagged for later reanastomosis. **C:** *Shaded area* shows the region of bone removed as a single unit for access to the nasopharynx and cranial base. **D:** The bone has been removed, and the nasopharynx and pterygoid plates have been exposed. **E:** Craniotomy has been performed to provide additional access to the intracranial space, petrous internal carotid artery, and cavernous sinus.

septum to reappose each other. The nasal cavity can be filled bilaterally with light packing, and the gingivobuccal incision can be closed with absorbable suture material.

Although the transsphenoidal approach is used primarily to manage pituitary tumors, variants of this technique can be used to resect a limited number of other lesions, primarily benign, that occur in the midline of the posterior nasal cavity and sphenoidal sinus, such as chordoma or craniopharyngioma. The extent of the central cranial-base exposure can be increased greatly if the previously described technique is combined with Le Fort I osteotomy of the maxilla (15). This osteotomy separates the superior dental arch from the midface at a level just superior to the roots of the teeth. A wide gingivobuccal incision provides access for osteotomy. The result is downward pivoting of the entire palate and superior dental arch based on the maxillary tuberosities. Care must be taken to preserve the palatine nerve and artery in the posterior aspect of each side of the disarticulated palate. "Down-fracturing" of the palate provides wide exposure of the clivus, craniocervical junction, and nasopharynx. After tumor resection, the palate can be returned to anatomic position and held in place with titanium miniplates. Exact occlusion can be restored by means of drilling the holes for these plates before performing Le Fort I osteotomy.

Infratemporal Fossa

Most tumors of the middle cranial base are not midline, and approaches other than those previously described are necessary for removal. One procedure designed for tumors invading the petroclival portions of the middle cranial base is the infratemporal fossa approach (16). Several variations of this approach share several features. The temporal and infratemporal regions are reached through a preauricular or postauricular incision that extends onto the cervical region and the scalp in a hemicoronal or bicoronal manner, which allows exposure of the temporalis muscle, the orbitozygomatic complex of the facial skeleton, the parotid gland, and the facial nerve (Fig. 126.13A). Exposure of the parotid gland and facial nerve often is unnecessary, and the inferior extent of the preauricular incision can be limited to the level of the tragus.

Removal of the orbitozygomatic segment of bone (Fig. 126.10, area 4) allows elevation of the temporalis muscle from the temporal fossa to gain access to the infratemporal fossa. Further exposure can be gained with retraction of the condylar head and synovial capsule of the temporomandibular joint in an inferior direction. If extensive distraction of the temporomandibular joint is necessary, it usually is preferable to remove the mandibular neck and condylar head. Postoperative mandibular dysfunction, such as trismus and limited mandibular excursion, is less common when the neck and head of the mandible are removed without replacement than when the temporomandibular joint is widely distracted or the mandibular neck and head are replaced. Care is taken during transection

of the mandibular neck not to injure the blood supply to the temporalis muscle (the internal maxillary and deep temporal vessels), which is just medial to the mandibular neck. After this maneuver, the glenoid fossa and spine of the sphenoid bone can be visualized with the foramina ovale and spinosum.

Frontotemporal craniotomy can be performed (Fig. 126.10, area 3) to elevate the brain. The petrous portion of the internal carotid artery is immediately medial to the osseous eustachian tube as it enters the carotid canal. Here the petrous carotid artery can be uncovered by means of careful removal of bone. During bone removal, the facial nerve and otic capsule must be protected, because they are immediately superior and posterior to the genu of the internal carotid artery. When fully uncovered, the internal carotid artery can be mobilized to allow access to the medial petroclival structures. The sphenoidal sinus can be entered between the second and third divisions of the trigeminal nerve, or the third division can be transected to provide wider access to the cavernous sinus for tumor removal (Fig. 126.13B). Access to the nasopharynx by this approach usually is limited, especially in attempts to resect a malignant tumor.

Reconstruction of the defect usually is achieved with either an ipsilateral temporalis muscle or a temporoparietal fascial flap, which is turned into the resultant defect. If these flaps are no longer available, as in postresection tumor recurrence, free microvascular tissue transfer is performed. Reconstruction of the bony base of the skull in this region usually is not necessary. Large defects can be structurally enhanced with titanium mesh, but this step is reserved for massive defects, which are rare. Adequate temporalis and temporoparietal fascial flaps usually are available for these defects. These two flaps are entirely separate and derive a blood supply from separate sources. They therefore can be raised simultaneously from the same side of the head. The temporalis flap is fed by the deep temporal vessels that emanate from the internal maxillary artery. The temporoparietal fascial flap is supplied entirely by the superficial temporal artery and vein.

Advantages of use of a temporalis muscle flap include ease of elevation (minimal technical skill is needed), bulk, and durable blood supply. Disadvantages include risk of compromise of the deep temporal vessels during infratemporal fossa dissection and inability to reach consistently beyond the midline in the region of the sphenoidal sinus and nasopharynx. The temporoparietal fascial flap is much less bulky and more supple than the temporalis muscle flap, so insetting into the subcranial base of the skull is easier. The blood supply of the temporoparietal fascial flap is not jeopardized by infratemporal fossa dissection, because the flap emanates from the external carotid system. Most important, the temporoparietal fascial flap can be tunneled beyond the midline to manage defects of the sphenoidal sinus and nasopharynx. This substantially improves the ability of the flap to seal possible sites of CSF leakage. The main disadvantages of the temporoparietal fascial flap are the technical skill needed for elevation and the time needed for complete development of the flap on its preauricular pedicle. However, the security that this flap provides in the repair of defects of the sphenoidal sinus and nasopharynx is well worth the time and effort needed to elevate the flap. We believe that use of the temporoparietal fascial flap is the single greatest factor in decreasing our overall CSF leakage rate to less than 4%.

Facial Translocation and Maxillotomy Approaches

If wide exposure of the middle cranial base, infratemporal fossa, pterygopalatine fossa, and nasopharynx is necessary, the facial translocation procedure or the maxillotomy approach can be considered (17). The main disadvantage of these approaches is the need for facial incisions (Fig. 126.14A). This disadvantage is more than balanced by the wide exposure of the middle cranial base and nasopharynx. Although the facial-translocation procedure originally was described to include transection of the frontal branches of the facial nerve, this incision and the resultant frontal motor deficit can be avoided in most tumor resections.

Facial translocation, in the classic description, is begun with the facial incisions shown in Fig. 126.14A. After this step, the three or four frontal branches of the facial nerve are tagged and transected to allow elevation of the facial flaps (Fig. 126.14B). The facial nerve branches are reanastomosed at the end the procedure. Return to function is expected within 6 months (17). To achieve complete cheek-flap reflection, the infraorbital nerve must be transected. If reanastomosis of the cut infraorbital nerve stumps is possible, the stumps are tagged before transection. The lacrimal system is transected in preparation for osteotomy. Osteotomy to remove the anterior face of the maxillary sinus in continuity with the zygoma is performed with a reciprocating saw (Fig. 126.14C). After this segment of bone is removed, direct access to the infratemporal fossa can be obtained. With this approach, tumor resection can proceed in an extracranial manner (Fig. 126.14D), or subtemporal craniotomy–craniectomy can be performed to gain access to intracranial tumor extension (Fig. 126.14E). Complete en bloc resection of the pterygoid plates and nasopharyngeal mucosa can be achieved with this approach. The sphenoidal sinus, cavernous sinus, petrous carotid artery, and petroclival portions of the base of the skull can be reached through this surgical field. When necessary, the nasal septum can be removed to obtain wide exposure of the contralateral nasal cavity. The translocation procedure can be performed bilaterally through a midfacial incision (midfacial split approach) to provide unparalleled bilateral access to the middle cranial base.

Reconstruction after facial translocation usually is done with a temporalis muscle flap, whether or not a craniotomy has been performed. This flap is positioned within the infratemporal fossa and below the central cranial base and tacked into place with sutures. If the temporalis flap is inadequate for the defect or if its blood supply has been compromised, a free microvascular muscle transfer is done. Once adequate vascularized soft tissue has been placed into the resection defect, the zygomatic–maxillary bone segment can be replaced. This bone usually is secured with titanium microplates to achieve immediate rigid fixation. The lacrimal system is reconstructed with silicone stents, which are left in place for 4 to 6 weeks postoperatively. The wound is closed in standard manner after the infraorbital nerve has been reimplanted into the soft tissue of the cheek, if possible, and the frontal branches of the facial nerve have been reanastomosed. The functional and cosmetic results after this extensive exposure usually are excellent.

Posterior Cranial Base

Approaches to the posterior cranial base are mentioned only briefly, because most of these procedures fall under the domain of neurosurgeons or neurotologists. Neurotologic procedures, such as the transmastoid–translabyrinthine and retromastoid–retrosigmoid approaches, provide access to the jugular-bulb and cerebellopontine-angle regions of the posterior cranial base. The traditional neurosurgical approach to this region has been through suboccipital craniotomy with the patient sitting. The extreme lateral approach allows wide access to the jugular foramen, lateral foramen magnum, and inferolateral clivus (18). In this approach, retrolabyrinthine, transsigmoid, and low suboccipital craniectomies are used for exposure. The otolaryngologist often is involved in the temporal bone portion of the dissection, but most of the procedure is performed by a neurosurgeon.

MINIMALLY INVASIVE TECHNIQUES OF SKULL-BASE SURGERY

Use of Navigation Systems

The use of navigation systems has proven to be an invaluable addition to surgery of the cranial base, whether performed via open technique or endoscopically. This imaging guidance is "real time" in providing anatomic and position data during surgical approaches to many anterior, middle, and posterior cranial fossa lesions. As a consequence, complications during surgery should, theoretically, decrease, and safety should increase. In situations in which endoscopic surgery is used, navigation is required for the successful performance of the procedures. Several different systems are now available, all of which are frameless, allowing the surgeon to visualize on a monitor four different views simultaneously: the coronal, sagittal and axial CT scan images at the same time as the real-time surgical endoscopic or microscopic view. It is then possible to compare the surgically visualized anatomy with the same anatomy of the CT scans. The unique aspect of the *frameless system* is that the surgeon knows by looking at the monitor exactly where his instruments are during surgery on the CT visualization. Initially, axial CT images are obtained of the craniofacial structures with the patient wearing a special headset. The CT images are then processed and downloaded onto the computer, where the coronal and sagittal views are reconstructed and displayed simultaneously on a monitor in the operating room (OR) along with the endoscopic view. At the time of surgery, the system is taken to the OR, and the CT scan is visualized on the monitor while the surgeon inserts a special probe into the nose. The position of the probe can thus be visualized on the monitor by using standard surgical endoscopic instruments. Thus the position of the probe inside the nose can be pinpointed exactly and visualized precisely on the navigation system as cross-hairs. As a result, the surgeon can precisely orient himself or herself to the anatomy, both on the CT scan and with the endoscopic view, and can dramatically reduce potential complications during the surgery. In addition, the navigation system is very helpful in teaching cases with residents who may need additional navigational tools. With the navigation system, the x-ray exposure to medical personnel is not an issue, and the information gained is three-dimensional, so the localization of important structures is more precise (19). With this new frameless version of the navigational system, the surgical field became wider and nonobstructed with the system frame. Body positioning became much easier as the patient's head need not be immobilized on the operating table.

Endoscopic Endonasal Cranial-Base Skull-Base Surgery

Pure endoscopic endonasal cranial-base surgery has been recommended for limited, resectable lesions of the anterior, middle, and posterior skull base that are confined to the 2-cm-wide area of the midline of the skull base, as

- It takes advantage of the otorhinolaryngologic experience in the functional endoscopic surgery of the nasal and paranasal sinus and the base of the skull with a better view of all median and paramedical anatomic structures.
- It is less traumatic than the traditional open approaches or the microscopic transsphenoidal approach using the endonasal retractor and postoperative packing.
- The hospital stay and hence the surgery cost are reduced significantly (20,21).

Although the sinonasal endoscopy was introduced by Hirshmann (22) as early as 1901 by using a modified cystoscope, the first to use the microscope assisted by the endoscope in a transsphenoidal operation was Guiot in 1963 (23). Functional endoscopic sinus surgery was introduced in the 1980s (24), and endoscopic sinus surgery has been popularized as the surgical treatment of choice for sinonasal problems (25,26). The use of sinonasal endoscopy has been expanded to include repair of CSF leakage from the anterior cranial fossa and removal of benign anterior skull base mass that has an intracranial extension from sinus pathology.

Most recently, endoscopic sinus surgery has been reported for the management of primary intracranial lesions of the anterior, middle, and posterior skull base.

Three endonasal approaches were described and have become routinely used: (a) paraseptal approach, (b) middle meatal approach, and (c) middle turbrinectomy approach. The choice of the approach depends mainly on the site and size of the lesion and the surgeon preference in the reconstruction process (20,22).

- The paraseptal approach is made between the middle turbinate and nasal septum; the middle turbinate is displaced laterally, and the nasal septum is detached contralaterally. Bilateral ethmoidectomy is performed to reach the skull base.
- The middle meatal approach is made through the middle meatus between the middle turbinate and the orbit. When medial displacement of the middle turbinate, uncinectomy, bilateral ethmoidectomy, and anterior sphenoidectomy are performed, the skull base is exposed. It has a narrower surgical corridor than the paraseptal approach.
- The middle turbinectomy approach provides a wider operating corridor leading to the anterior fossa skull base by bilateral ethmoidectomy. Anterior sphenoidectomy will provide access to the middle and posterior skull base as well. The loss of supportive structures in the nasal cavity to hold fat grafts and titanium mesh in place can be a drawback of this approach when anterior skull base is reconstructed. The paraseptal and middle meatal approaches are used mainly for lesions on the contralateral side and they are preferred more than the middle turbinectomy approach when reconstruction with a fat graft is expected. Endoscopic endonasal transsphenoidal surgery had been proved safe and effective, in experienced hands, not only for adults but even in children. The minimal invasiveness of this procedure, compared with the transcranial or transsphenoidal microsurgical approaches, makes it ideal for the treatment of several pediatric pathologic conditions as pituitary adenoma, in which it is essential to preserve the anatomic and functional integrity of hypothalamic–pituitary axis, both to assure a normal growth and to maintain a good sinonasal viability (27). This endonasal endoscopy provided excellent surgical exposure from the cribriform plate at the anterior fossa to the foramen magnum, the lower clivus, and upper cervical vertebrae (24). When an endoscopic endonasal transsphenoidal approach has been used in various pituitary lesions, the endoscopic technique has proved to be advantageous in providing wider exposure at the perisellar region and upper clivus (28).

Surgery of the Cavernous Sinus and Clival Tumors

These approaches also are being used for management of cavernous sinus tumors, where such procedures are considered minimally invasive. Most often, tumors involving the cavernous sinus have been surgically treated through radical surgical approaches as face-splitting maxillectomy, transcranial lateral skull-base approaches, petrosal approaches, or transoral approaches. Although having been used for removal of clival tumors, the conventional microscopic transsphenoidal approach provides a narrow surgical corridor limiting surgical exposure at the clivus. With the use of the endoscopic endonasal transsphenoidal approach, we can manage tumors of anterior skull base and cavernous sinus (chordoma, meningioma, chondrosarcoma, and chondromas) that are not adherent to the carotid artery or dura. The ideal head positioning for the endoscopic endonasal transsphenoidal approach to the clivus and posterior fossa is 15 degrees flexion of the forehead–chin line (21). Endoscopic exposure ranges from the floor of the cribriform plate to the foramen magnum in the vertical dimension and about 15 mm on both sides of the midline between the carotid arteries in the transverse dimension. When an endoscope is adopted during microscopic transsphenoidal surgery, similar visualization may be attainable as well (28). However, the use of retractors restricts the maneuverability of surgical instruments and restricts the horizontal field dimensions. At the level of the cavernous sinus, the lateral horizontal plane of the field is limited by the carotid artery, but further exposure could be attained up to the foramen ovale and foramen rotundum. At the level of the sellar floor, the abducent nerve lies lateral to the carotid artery, and at the lower clivus, the hypoglossal nerve is the lateral limit. The petrous apex and jugular bulb also are accessible through this endonasal approach. Access to the dorsum sella is somewhat hindered by the pituitary gland. Bone removal was made mainly by the use of high-speed drill. The clival venous plexus can be problematic. However, it is often obliterated by the tumor expansion. Dural bleeding is usually controlled by bipolar, monopolar suction–coagulation or absorbable gelatin (Gelfoam), whereas bone bleeding is managed with bone wax. This minimally invasive endoscopic endonasal technique has proved excellent surgical exposure to the midline clivus and posterior fossa with minimal morbidity intrinsic to the nature of transsphenoidal surgery. The potential problems with endoscopic endonasal anterior skull-base surgery are postoperative CSF leaks, neurovascular compression by the intracranial fat graft, infection related to the semicontaminated field of the nasal cavity, difficulty in controlling massive intraoperative bleeding when it happens, technical difficulties related to the intrinsic learning curve, and sinonasal complications. The possibility of postoperative CSF leaks and difficulty with reconstruction of the cranial base remain the major potential problems.

Endoscopic Transoral Surgery of the Skull Base
Endoscopically assisted transoral surgery has been described as alternative microsurgical techniques for transoral approaches to the anterior cervicomedullary junction.

When used with intraoperative fluoroscopy or the navigation system, it provides a safe method for anterior decompression of the cervicomedullary junction area without the need of hard palate resection, or extended maxillectomy. It also enables the surgeon to observe residual tumor cells in areas that could not be viewed by using the operative microscope. A Dingman retractor with a rubber guard is placed over the teeth and used to keep the mouth open, while self-retaining retractors are attached to the Dingman retractor to depress the tongue. When needed, soft palate split could be performed. The distance of incision is from the clivus superiorly to the level of C3 inferiorly, and the lateral exposure should be limited to 15 mm from the midline so as not to injure the hypoglossal nerves, vertebral arteries, or eustachian tubes. With the endoscope, the optics and illumination are in the field of the resection at the level of the abnormality. By the use of a 30-degree endoscope, the clivus is clearly visualized, and by rotating the endoscope, a wider field is obtained. The extended viewing angle of the endoscope lens (fish-eye effect) can be used to inspect hidden but important anatomic structures without applying additional retraction.

ADJUVANT THERAPIES

Benign neoplasms of the cranial base are not routinely managed with radiation therapy after resection, with the exception of unresectable or recurrent meningioma. Tumor growth of these lesions can be decreased greatly with external-beam or stereotactically targeted radiation therapy. Radiation therapy is most frequently considered an adjunctive modality after resection of malignant tumors of the cranial base. Most patients undergoing cranial-base surgery for recurrent malignant disease have received a full course of external-beam radiation therapy. In this situation, brachytherapy often is used as an effective method of delivering an additional therapeutic dose to the site of recurrent disease after salvage surgery. Brachytherapy relies on implanted percutaneous catheters temporarily loaded with a radioactive source, such as iridium, several days after surgery (29). This technique allows accurate delivery of radiation with respect to dose and anatomic location. Usually, 3,000 to 5,000 cGy can be delivered by this technique over a period of several days while the overlying skin and surrounding normal structures are spared. After the therapeutic dose has been delivered, the radioactive source and percutaneous catheters are removed.

A gamma knife, also known as *stereotactic radiation* or *radiosurgery,* can be used after cranial-base tumor resection. Although called *surgery,* the procedure does not involve any incisions and is actually a form of radiation therapy that entails computer-controlled focusing of many small beams of radiation on the region of the base of the skull that contains the tumor. This spares the overlying skin and nearby neurologic structures from the collateral damage usually inflicted by external-beam radiation therapy. Because the stereotactic beam is guided with CT or MRI data, it is extremely accurate with respect to the shape and volume of the treated tissue (37). Lesions of the sella are particularly amenable to treatment with a gamma knife when complete resection is impossible. Whereas many tumors of the cranial base extend too far interiorly to be attacked with a gamma knife, newer forms of stereotactically focused body irradiation now allow management of tumors that extend inferior to the base of the skull.

Chemotherapy has not proved useful in the management of solid tumors of the base of the skull in adults. Pediatric rhabdomyosarcoma, however, has proved chemosensitive. Chemotherapy along with radiation therapy often is used when this tumor occurs at the base of the skull. Biologic modifiers and immunotherapy are under investigation.

COMPLICATIONS

Complications that occur during and after cranial-base surgery are summarized in Table 126.8.

Cerebrospinal Fluid Fistula

Postoperative leakage of CSF, and the risk of meningitis, is the most common complication after cranial-base surgery.

As many as 20% of extensive resections of the cranial base entail a CSF leak (29). To determine the treatment course, two primary questions must be answered: Is it a high-flow or a low-flow leak? Where is it coming from? If active flow of CSF can be seen coming from the wound, ear canal, or nasal cavity, it is a high-flow leak. If CSF is found on dressings in the form of a halo sign, but flow cannot be actively seen, it is a low-flow leak. The halo sign occurs when a mixture of CSF and blood is absorbed onto dressings or bed linens. As the CSF and blood mixture spreads out onto the absorbent surface, a dark ring of blood chromatographically forms around a more lightly stained center, forming a halo.

High-flow CSF leaks usually are managed by means of direct closure in the OR as soon as is feasible. If the location of the leak is not evident, CT cisternography is performed to localize the source of the spinal fluid. A CT cisternogram involves injection of a radiopaque intrathecal contrast agent before CT to locate the source of the leak. If the leak is low flow, nonoperative measures can be used. A lumbar spinal drain is placed, and approximately 150 mL of spinal fluid per day is removed (50 mL every 8 hours) to eliminate flow through the defect and allow it to seal. The egress of CSF through the lumbar drain must be strictly controlled so that it does not become excessive. Draining too much CSF can cause air entrainment into the cranial vault through cranial-base defects. The result is pneumocephalus. The development of tension pneumocephalus can cause life-threatening

TABLE 126.8   **POTENTIAL COMPLICATIONS**
CRANIAL-BASE SURGERY

Category	Complication	Treatment Options
Mass lesions	Brain edema	Mannitol, diuretics, barbiturate coma, occasionally lobectomy
Vascular	Carotid or vertebral artery rupture	Reexploration and repair or occlusion
	Arterial thrombosis	Microvascular bypass
		Anticoagulation
	Arterial dissection	Anticoagulation
	Cerebral infarction	Induced hypertension
	Venous thrombosis	Volume expansion
		Diuretics, heparinization
	Air embolism	Left lateral decubitus position, occlusion of venous defect
Other cerebral	Seizures	Anticonvulsants
Cerebrospinal fluid	Cerebrospinal fluid leakage—wound, ear, nose nasopharynx	Reexploration and repair; spinal fluid drainage; vascularized flap
Infections	Meningitis	Antibiotics
	Wound abscess	Drainage
	Epidural, subdural, or brain abscess	Antibiotics
Wound	Flap necrosis	Local or distant flap repair
Cranial nerve palsy	Cranial nerves I through XII	Nerve reconstruction
		Compensatory procedures (e.g., vocal cord injection)
		Rehabilitation
Metabolic	Diabetes insipidus	Fluid replacement, vasopressin
	Syndrome of inappropriate antidiuretic hormone secretion	Fluid restriction, hypertonic saline solution

brain compression. If a low-flow leak has not stopped within 5 days, reoperation usually is necessary.

Sometimes it is difficult to determine whether the fluid collected is CSF. This can occur when CSF is leaking into the nasal cavity through the eustachian tubes or through a defect in the floor of the anterior fossa. Fluid that contains glucose probably is CSF, because nasal secretions do not contain glucose as does CSF. This test is not specific, however, because serous exudate from the surgical wound often is mixed with nasal mucus in the same area as the suspected leak. Because serum contains glucose, a risk of misidentifying nasal secretions as spinal fluid exists owing to glucose contamination from the serum. The presence of a CSF leak can be most specifically confirmed by means of testing for the protein β_2-transferrin. Only three body fluids contain this protein: CSF, perilymph, and the vitreous fluid of the eye. All these areas are essentially extensions of the neuraxis. Because the amount of perilymph is small and vitreous contamination is highly unlikely (and would be recognized clinically), the presence of β_2-transferrin almost confirms the presence of CSF.

Meningitis

Meningitis is a nonspecific term denoting inflammation of the meninges of the brain. This inflammation can be localized or diffuse and can have various causes (viral, bacterial, or aseptic chemical). Regardless of the etiologic agent, the symptoms of diffuse meningeal irritation are similar. The patient becomes ill, a headache develops, sometimes with nausea and vomiting, and mental status decreases. A stiff neck and positive Kernig sign (pain in the hamstring muscles on attempted extension of the leg after flexion of the thigh) are common. A differentiating feature is marked pyrexia, which occurs in bacterial or viral meningitis but usually is absent if the origin is aseptic. In this setting, CT is performed to rule out increased ICP and is followed by lumbar puncture with CSF sampling. Analysis and culture

of CSF are the best method of ascertaining the cause of meningeal irritation (Table 126.9).

After cranial-base surgery, meningitis usually is aseptic or bacterial. Viral meningitis is not a factor in the postoperative period. Postsurgical aseptic meningitis is caused by meningeal irritation from surgical manipulation, blood, and blood breakdown products. This form of meningitis usually is self-limited and necessitates no specific treatment after the diagnosis is confirmed through CSF analysis and culture.

No single group of patients is more at risk of bacterial meningitis than are those undergoing cranial-base surgery. Defects of the cranial base often are large and in gravity-dependent locations, which is a predisposing factor for CSF leak. The presence of a CSF fistula close to the paranasal sinuses is an added source of bacterial contamination for the development of meningitis. The etiologic organisms associated with various types of meningitis are listed in Table 126.10. Bacterial meningitis is managed

TABLE 126.10
TYPES OF MENINGITIS AND CAUSATIVE ORGANISMS

Type	Organism	Appearance[a]
Spontaneous	*Escherichia coli*	Gram-negative rods
Neonatal	*Haemophilus*	Gram-negative rods
Pediatric	*Meningococcus*	Gram-negative cocci
Adult	Pneumococcus	Gram-positive cocci
	Meningococcus	Gram-negative cocci
Posttraumatic[b]	*Staphylococcus aureus*	Gram-positive cocci
	Pneumococcus	Gram-positive cocci
	S. aureus	Gram-positive cocci
Postoperative[b]	Enterococcus	Gram-positive cocci

[a]Gram positive, blue; gram negative, red.
[b]With or without a cerebrospinal fluid leak.

TABLE 126.9
CEREBROSPINAL FLUID EVALUATION FOR MENINGITIS

Characteristics	Normal	Aseptic (chemical)	Bacterial
Color	Clear	Clear	Cloudy
Gram stain	Negative	Negative	Bacteria present
Protein	<40 mg/100 mL[a]	Normal to slightly elevated	Elevated
Glucose	45–80 mg/100 mL	Normal	Decreased
RBC	None	None	None
WBC	0–5 cells/mL		Elevated
Pressure (recumbent)	<200mm H_2O	Normal to slightly elevated	Elevated

[a]A traumatic lumbar puncture can introduce red blood cells (RBCs) into the cerebrospinal fluid (CSF). In this setting, for every 700 RBCs, usually one white blood cell (WBC) is present, and the protein is elevated by 1 mg/100 mL. This should be taken into account when interpreting CSF-analysis results. The presence of polymorphonuclear leukocytes should be considered abnormal until proven otherwise, because normal CSF contains only lymphocytes and monocytes.

with intravenous antibiotics selected to cover the specific antibiotic sensitivities of the organism, as determined by means of culture.

Surgical Management of Postoperative Cerebrospinal Fluid Fistula

Unlike spontaneous or posttraumatic CSF fistula, postoperative leaks almost always necessitate surgical closure. Spontaneous leaks frequently necessitate closure, but some can be managed by conservative means. Posttraumatic leaks frequently close with conservative therapy alone. Postsurgical leaks, unless they are low flow without use of a lumbar drain or ventriculostomy, are not managed conservatively. The patient is returned to the OR without delay for reexploration of the wound. At reexploration, the technical options for closure depend on factors such as the exact site of the leak, a history of radiation therapy, the size of the defect, the continuity of the defect with mucosa-lined cavities, the available reconstructive flaps, and the technical ability of the surgeon.

Although a movement toward endoscopic management of CSF fistula has occurred, this technique is rarely appropriate for acute leaks caused by resection at the base of the skull. Fistulae after cranial-base surgery usually necessitate reexploration of the resection site and closure or reclosure of areas that had appeared to be sealed during the ablative procedure. These leaks usually necessitate application of vascularized tissue. The exception is isolated sphenoidal sinus defects usually caused by transsphenoidal hypophysectomy. Never is a patient with CSF leakage treated by means of long-term lumbar drainage or administration of antibiotics. Lumbar drainage for longer than 5 days generally is contraindicated. If any leak, regardless of causation, persists longer than 5 days, operative closure is pursued. Long-term use of antibiotics does not prevent meningitis and specifically increases the risk of meningitis or wound infection with resistant microorganisms.

The method and materials used for closure depend on the site of the leak. One of the most common sites of CSF leakage is the sphenoidal sinus after transsphenoidal hypophysectomy. In this situation, endoscopically directed closure with sealing agents such as fibrin glue or hydroxyapatite cement or autografts such as fat and fascia become useful. Fibrin glue is particularly effective in sealing low-flow CSF leaks. High-flow leaks are managed with lumbar drainage before placement of fibrin glue. When the leak involves the sphenoidal sinus, a useful technique entails use of free autogenous fat to fill the sphenoidal sinus in combination with the fibrin glue. The fibrin glue immediately seals the leak, and the fat ensures long-term obliteration of the sinus to prevent delayed leakage after resorption of the fibrin glue. Fibrin glue was first used as a hemostatic agent in the early 1900s. It was applied as an adhesive in the 1940s. Since the 1980s, highly concentrated forms have been used as a tissue sealant and adhesive. Use of nonautogenous fibrin glue carries the risk of disease transmission comparable with that of use of fresh frozen plasma. Use of autogenous fibrin glue does not pose this risk, but it is time-consuming to formulate the glue, and the seal frequently is not as durable as that obtained with prefabricated, nonautogenous fibrin glue. The actual fibrin sealant is formed when fibrinogen and thrombin are combined in the presence of factor XIII with calcium as a required catalyst. The fibrin plugs the CSF fistula and serves as a matrix for proliferation of fibroblasts into the wound, enhancing healing. Fibrinolysis can occur when fibrin glue is exposed to excess amounts of plasma. Because the thin layer of scar tissue generated by fibrin glue alone can be eroded by the constant pressure of the CSF pulsations, it is best to combine the glue with an autogenous fat or fascial graft to enhance long-term stability.

Instead of fibrin glue, hydroxyapatite cement can be applied to the sphenoidal sinus. This material has the advantage that once set, it forms a hard barrier to future CSF leakage. Several types of hydroxyapatite cement have individual strengths and weaknesses. These materials are mixed with a dilute acid aqueous solution that causes setting of the calcium phosphate reactants. Setting usually occurs in 8 to 15 minutes, depending on the preparation. Once set, these materials stay water sensitive for 4 to 6 hours and can be dissolved during this period by excess blood or CSF. Hemostasis and temporary (12 hours) use of a lumbar drain is recommended when these materials are applied, regardless of the specific type of hydroxyapatite cement. In all cases, the resultant hydroxyapatite is water insoluble and, when in contact with viable bone, acts as a scaffold onto and into which bone can grow slowly. This ingrowth takes months to years, particularly among older adults with lower metabolic bone turnover. The material must be applied directly to the surface of viable bone, hence the requirement that all mucous membrane within the sphenoidal sinus be removed. If the membrane is not removed and the cement is applied to it, the cement does not adhere immediately and can serve as a source of chronic mucosal inflammation. These cement preparations are not applied to leaks within the ethmoidal sinuses, because entrapment of mucosa is unavoidable, and success is doubtful. An important feature of all of these hydroxyapatite-based biomaterials is the absolute requirement that the surgeon be familiar with their use before applying them in the demanding setting of a CSF leak. Experience is needed in other types of reconstruction of open cranial defects before a surgeon attempts use of these cements to repair CSF leaks.

In addition to the previously mentioned sealants, an essential component of prevention and management of CSF fistulae is reestablishment of the continuity of the dura. If the dura is sealed, no fistula can occur, regardless of the bony defect of the cranial base. A number of new materials are available for this purpose, such as preserved bovine pericardium and acellular dermis. Both of these materials can be used to patch dural defects, but acellular dermis has the advantage of undergoing conversion to dura-like tissue.

Both materials carry risk of viral disease transmission, but this risk is much less than that of CSF leak. Unlike use of preserved homograft dura, use of acellular dermis poses no risk of transmission of a slow brain virus. Virus particles have not been found, even in the dermis of infected persons. Acellular dermis is our choice for essentially all duraplasties. It is best if all of these dural replacement materials are covered with vascularized tissue because they can be contaminated before developing their own vascular supply and lose integrity.

Cranial Nerve Deficits

The most debilitating cranial nerve deficits are those of nerves VII, IX, and X (29). Combined paralysis of cranial nerves III, IV, and VI results in total ophthalmoplegia of the affected globe. This combination, called *cavernous sinus syndrome,* is not uncommon after aggressive dissection of cavernous sinus tumor. Cavernous sinus syndrome also can be accompanied by unilateral conjunctival injection and edema due to obliteration of cavernous sinus blood flow. The result is decreased venous drainage from the globe. An uncommon variant of this syndrome also can be caused by midfacial cutaneous infection, usually of the nose, that has spread to the cavernous sinus through the connecting veins. Cavernous sinus syndrome caused by infection has a high mortality. Early diagnosis, aggressive antibiotic therapy, and anticoagulation are the primary means of successful treatment.

Nerves paralyzed from surgical manipulation have substantial regenerative capacity. This is particularly true of the facial nerve when paralysis is caused by surgical displacement but not transection. After infratemporal fossa approaches that necessitate extensive transposition of the extratemporal facial nerve, temporary (4 to 6 weeks) facial paralysis is common. This may be the result of temporary nerve ischemia or temporary mechanical nerve compression. Prolonged recovery may be accompanied by some asymmetry and synkinesis, which can be decreased by means of facial nerve–movement retraining in the postoperative period.

When the lower cranial nerves (primarily IX and X) are compromised, the combination of vocal cord and swallowing dysfunction can occur (30). If the tumor had slowly compromised the function of these nerves before resection, many patients show little or no functional deficit after unilateral resection. If loss of function has been abrupt, the patient has difficulty after surgery. This is particularly true of elderly patients, who often need a tracheostomy and a feeding tube. Early placement of a gastrostomy, even at the original resection, is both prudent and comfortable. Early use of thyroplasty can greatly limit risk of aspiration in the postoperative period.

Fluid and Metabolic Disturbances

Two clinically important electrolyte disturbances can occur in the postoperative period. Both are caused by abnormal secretion of antidiuretic hormone (vasopressin) from the neurohypophysis. These two disturbances are diabetes insipidus and the syndrome of inappropriate secretion of antidiuretic hormone (SIADH) (Table 126.11).

Diabetes insipidus usually occurs after severe head trauma or after the removal of pituitary or hypothalamic tumors. This disorder is caused by a secretion of antidiuretic hormone in inadequate amounts. This limits the ability to retain free water, which is manifested by polyuria, dehydration, hypovolemia, and polydipsia. Urine output greater than 250 mL for 2 consecutive hours suggests diabetes insipidus in the postoperative period. If diabetes insipidus is suspected, urine and serum laboratory studies are performed. The diagnosis of diabetes insipidus is confirmed if

TABLE 126.11

POSSIBLE ELECTROLYTE DISTURBANCES AFTER CRANIAL-BASE SURGERY

Laboratory Value	Diabetes Insipidus	SIADH
Serum osmolality	Increase	<280 mOsm/kg
Urine osmolality	<150 mOsm/kg	Increased
Serum sodium	>150 mEq/L	<135 mEq/L
Urine sodium	Decreased	>25 mEq/L
Urine specific gravity	<1.005	>1.015
Circulating free water	Decreased	Increased
Volume of urine output	>250 mL/h for more than 2 h[a]	<30 mL/h[b]

SIADH, syndrome of inappropriate antidiuretic hormone secretion.
[a]The onset of diabetes insipidus usually is heralded by urine output >250 mL/h for 4 consecutive hours; the first sign of SIADH usually is serum sodium concentration <135 mEq/L.
[b]In a euvolemic patient.

serum level of sodium exceeds 150 mEq/L, the urine is dilute with a specific gravity less than 1.005, and urine osmolality is between 50 and 150 mOsm/kg.

Therapy for mild diabetes insipidus is fluid and electrolyte replacement. If dehydration, electrolyte disturbances, or discomfort becomes a problem because of the quantity of urine output, pharmacologic control can be instituted. Vasopressin or one of its analogues can be given to control urine output. Because diabetes insipidus usually is self-limited in duration, pharmacologic support usually is temporary.

The opposite situation exists with SIADH, which also is caused by head trauma or intraoperative manipulation. This syndrome is caused by numerous conditions that affect the brain, such as stroke, systemic metabolic disturbances, or intracranial bleeding. High levels of antidiuretic hormone cause an inability to eliminate free water; the result is hyponatremia and hypoosmolality. The laboratory criteria for diagnosis of SIADH are a serum level of sodium less than 135 mEq/L, elevated urine level of sodium (>25 mEq/L), serum osmolality less than 280 mOsm/kg, and a urine osmolality elevated in relation to serum osmolality.

Management of SIADH consists of fluid restriction to a maximum of 1,000 mL/day. Severe cases of hyponatremia can be corrected with 3% (hypertonic) saline solution. Care is taken to limit the increase in serum level of sodium to 12 mEq/L/day to prevent central nervous system damage. Diuretics such as furosemide can be used as an adjunct for eliminating free water. The effect of antidiuretic hormone on the renal tubules can be blocked with demeclocycline. Like diabetes insipidus, postoperative SIADH usually is self-limited in duration.

EMERGENCIES

The four most common postoperative emergencies are listed in Table 126.12.

Postoperative Cerebral Edema

Postoperative cerebral edema is inevitable after brain manipulation. The degree of edema depends on the amount and duration of surgical retraction. Surgical approaches that minimize brain retraction have an intrinsic advantage over those that entail cortical elevation or retraction. Because

TABLE 126.12

POSTOPERATIVE EMERGENCIES

Postoperative cerebral edema
Hematoma and vascular emergencies
Air embolism
Postoperative seizures

of the rigid confinement of the cranial cavity, cerebral edema can compromise cerebral blood supply, and symptomatic cerebral edema always must be controlled. Treatment options include hyperventilation, intravenous mannitol, and corticosteroids. Barbiturate coma can be induced if cerebral edema becomes severe. The hallmark of cerebral edema is development of focal or lateralizing neurologic signs or a decrease in mental status. These changes usually become evident several hours after surgery but can begin as late as several days postoperatively. Infusion CT is useful for diagnosis.

Hematoma and Vascular Emergencies

Postoperative hematoma can cause a mass effect, a rapid decrease in level of consciousness, focal or lateralizing neurologic signs, brain compression, infarction, and herniation. Any epidural, subdural, or intraparenchymal collection of blood must be identified as soon as possible. All patients undergoing cranial-base surgery need CT within 24 hours of the operation, preferably the morning after. If a collection of blood is found, treatment usually involves reoperation and evacuation.

Vascular complications always are a possibility when the petrous carotid artery is exposed or replaced. These complications can take the form of arterial wall dissection, pseudo-aneurysm formation, or thrombosis due to surgical manipulation. When the artery is replaced, usually with a saphenous vein interposition graft, the vessel is particularly at risk of thrombotic occlusion. The risk of intracranial bleeding usually precludes use of postoperative anticoagulants to treat patients undergoing cranial-base surgery. Because patients who need interposition grafts usually are those least able to tolerate prolonged arterial occlusion due to cerebrovascular insufficiency, early diagnosis of inadequate blood flow is critical. Patients undergoing segmental replacement of the internal carotid artery need cerebral angiography and CT the morning after surgery to confirm adequate flow through the graft. Prophylactic bypass of the carotid system sometimes is performed at a separate operation before tumor resection so that anticoagulants can be used until the graft matures without the risk of intracranial bleeding.

Air Embolus

When craniotomy is performed, venous sinuses within the diploë of the skull are opened to the air. These bony venous channels can be the source of entrance of air into the systemic venous circulation. Although this can occur with any type of craniotomy, it is most likely to occur when the patient is in the sitting position used for a posterior fossa approach. During operations at the cranial base, entrance into the sigmoid sinus, jugular bulb, or jugular vein also can allow air to enter the venous circulation. A fairly large amount of air is necessary to interfere with cardiac function,

TABLE 126.13 ℞ TREATMENT
POSTOPERATIVE SEIZURE

Drug	Indication	Dose
Diazepam	Ongoing seizure activity or status epilepticus May cause respiratory depression; stops seizures, but does not prevent them; follow with loading dose of phenytoin or phenobarbital	10 mg, IV, every 20 min
Phenytoin	Ongoing seizure activity, status epilepticus, or oral seizure prophylaxis Does not depress respiration; can cause hypotension; do not give faster than 50 mg/min; therapeutic blood levels 10–20 µg/mL; causes nystagmus on lateral gaze at therapeutic levels	Treatment: 15 mg/kg, IV, over 30–45 min Prophylaxis: 300 mg/d, IV or by mouth
Phenobarbital	Seizure prophylaxis Marked sedative effect in adults; therapeutic blood level (adult): 20–40 µg/mL	60 mg twice a day, IV or by mouth
Carbamazepam	Seizure prophylaxis Can cause blood dyscrasia, leukopenia, and liver dysfunction; also can be used to manage trigeminal neuralgia; therapeutic blood levels	100–200 mg IV or by mouth, 2 to 3 times a day

but circulatory compromise can occur with volumes as low as 30 mL. This situation can occur during radical neck dissection when the internal jugular vein is entered anywhere along its length.

Sometimes the first sign of air embolism is difficulty maintaining blood pressure or a churning sound heard by the anesthesiologist over the precordium. In this ominous situation, the wound is filled with wet packing, the surgical field is covered completely, and the patient is turned to the head-down, left lateral decubitus position. This position prevents further entrance of air by means of increasing venous pressure in the head and neck and trapping air in the right side of the heart to minimize embolization to the lungs. This position is maintained until circulatory stability returns or aspiration of the air can be achieved with a transvenous catheter. The source of the air leak is sealed as quickly as possible after circulatory stabilization.

Postoperative Seizures

Many cranial-base procedures involve manipulation or resection of the temporal lobe, a region of the brain that is particularly epileptogenic. Postoperative antiseizure prophylaxis is routine. If seizures do arise, they are controlled quickly, because prolonged seizure activity can increase ICP, exacerbate cerebral edema, and cause cortical damage due to metabolic disturbances. Initial control of seizure activity is attempted with intravenous agents such as phenytoin, phenobarbital, or diazepam. If seizures are refractory to intravenous drugs and status epilepticus persists, general anesthetic agents are considered. Once seizures have been controlled, oral prophylactic antiseizure therapy can be begun. The loading doses and maintenance schedules

for commonly used antiseizure medications are listed in Table 126.13. While maintenance antiseizure medications are being given, the epileptogenic source is investigated. CT is mandatory to evaluate for possible postoperative hematoma or infarction. Levels of electrolytes in the serum, arterial blood gases, and level of glucose in the serum are measured to evaluate for a metabolic cause.

HIGHLIGHTS

- Lesions of the anterior region are mainly squamous cell carcinoma originating in the paranasal sinus.
- Most middle region lesions are nasopharyngeal carcinoma (extracranial) or meningioma (intracranial).
- The most common lesions of the posterior region are acoustic schwannoma and meningioma of the cerebellopontine angle. Osseous lesions of the second cervical vertebra can cause symptoms of compression of the lower brainstem.
- Measurement of CBF with a TBO test in conjunction with xenon-enhanced CT increases the safety of carotid resection or replacement in selected cases.
- The sphenoid spine is the most consistent landmark for locating the internal carotid artery before entrance into the cranial base. Knowing the location of the sphenoid spine also helps identify the location of the foramen spinosum, foramen ovale, and eustachian tube.
- The most important short-term complications of cranial-base surgery are CSF leak, meningitis, and cortical edema.
- The most important and most debilitating long-term complications of cranial-base surgery are caused by cranial nerve dysfunction, especially lower cranial nerve palsy (swallowing and vocal cord function).

- Although meningioma does not metastasize and is histologically benign, its behavior can be aggressive. Numerous recurrences can cause profound neurologic deficits and even death.
- Wide access can be gained to the middle region of the cranial base through the facial translocation procedure while the appearance and function of the face are preserved.
- Cranial-base surgery offers the greatest benefit when performed as a primary therapeutic modality. Early diagnosis is essential.

REFERENCES

1. Ketcham AS, Wilkins RH, VanBuren JM, et al. A combined intracranial facial approach to the paranasal sinuses. *Am J Surg* 1963;106:698.
2. Lewis JS, Page R. Radical surgery for malignant tumors of the ear. *Arch Otolaryngol* 1966;83:114.
3. Jackson CG, ed. *Surgery of skull base tumors.* New York: Churchill-Livingstone, 1991.
4. Sekhar LN, Schramm VL, Jones NF, et al. Operative exposure and management of the petrous and upper cervical internal carotid artery. *Neurosurgery* 1986;19:967.
5. Sekhar LN, Sen CN, Jho HD, et al. Surgical treatment of intracavernous neoplasms: a 4-year experience. *Neurosurgery* 1989;24:18.
6. Sclabassi RJ, Krieger DN, Weisz DJ, et al. Methods of neurophysiological monitoring during cranial base tumor resection. In: Sekhar LN, Janecka IP, eds. *Surgery of cranial base tumors.* New York: Raven Press, 1993:83–98.
7. Hirsch W, Curtin UD. MRI and CT in the evaluation of skull base masses. In: Sekhar LN, Janecka IP, eds. *Surgery of cranial base tumors.* New York: Raven Press, 1993:15–32.
8. Costantino PD, Russell EJ, Reisch D, et al. Ruptured petrous carotid aneurysm presenting with otorrhagia and epistaxis. *Am J Otol* 1991;12:378–383.
9. Cheney ML, Varvares MA, Nadol JB Jr. The temporoparietal fascial flap in head and neck reconstruction. *Arch Otolaryngol Head Neck Surg* 1993;119:618–625.
10. Fahlbusch R, Buchfelder M. The transsphenoidal approach to invasive cellar and clival lesions. In: Sekhar LN, Janecka IP, eds. *Surgery of cranial base tumors.* New York: Raven Press, 1993:337–358.
11. Glasscock ME. Management of aneurysms of the petrous portion of the internal carotid artery by resection and primary anastomosis. *Laryngoscope* 1983;93:1445.
12. Sen CN, Sekhar LN. An extreme lateral approach to intradural lesions of the cervical spine and foramen magnum. *Neurosurgery* 1990;27:197.
13. Krause CJ, Baker SR. Extended transantral approach to pterygomaxillary tumors. *Ann Otol* 1982;91:391–398.
14. Janecka IP. Classification of facial translocation approach to the skull base. *Otolaryngol Head Neck Surg* 1995;112:579–585.
15. Crockard HA. Anterior approaches to lesions of the upper cervical spine. In: *Clinical neurosurgery: the Congress of Neurological Surgeons.* 1988:34:389.
16. Fisch U, Pillsbury HS. Infratemporal fossa approach to lesions in the temporal bone and base of the skull. *Arch Otolaryngol* 1979;105:99.
17. Janecka IP, Sen CN, Sekhar LN, et al. Facial translocation: a new approach to the cranial base. *Otolaryngol Head Neck Surg* 1990;103:413.
18. Vikram B, Strong EW, Shah J, et al. A non-looping afterloading technique for interstitial implants of the base of tongue. *Int J Radiat Oncol Biol Phys* 1981;7:419–426.
19. Ohhashi G, Kamio M, Abe T, et al. Endoscopic transnasal approach to the pituitary lesions using a navigation system (Insta-Track System): technical note. *Minim Invas Neurosurg* 2002;45:120–123.
20. Jho HD, Ha HG. Endoscopic endonasal skull base surgery: part 1: the midline anterior fossa skull base. *Minim Invas Neurosurg* 2004;47:1–8.
21. Jho HD, Ha HG. Endoscopic endonasal skull base surgery: part 3: the clivus and posterior fossa. *Minim Invas Neurosurg* 2004;47:16–23.
22. Messerklinger W. Background and evolution of endoscopic sinus surgery. *Ear Nose Throat J* 1994;73:449–450.
23. Guiot G, et al. Explorations endoscopiques intracranniennes. *Presse Med* 1963;71:1225–1228.
24. Kennedy DW. Functional endoscopic sinus surgery technique. *Arch Otolaryngol* 1985;111:643–649.
25. Senior BA, Kennedy DW, Tanabodee J, et al. Long-term results of functional endoscopic sinus surgery. *Laryngoscope* 1998;108:151–157.
26. Stammberger H. Endoscopic endonasal surgery: concepts in treatment of recurring rhinosinusitis, Part 1: anatomic and pathologic considerations. *Otolaryngol Head Neck Surg* 1986;94:143–146.
27. Carrau RL, Snyderman CH, Kassam AB, et al. Endoscopic and endoscopic-assisted surgery for juvenile sangiofibroma. *Laryngoscope* 2001;111:483–487.
28. Batay F, Vural E, Karasu A, et al. Comparison of exposure obtained by endoscope and microscope in the extended trans-sphenoidal approach. *Skull Base* 2002;12:119–124.
29. Sen C, Snyderman CH, Sekhar LN. Complications of skull base operations. In: Sekhar LN, Janecka IP, eds. *Surgery of cranial base tumors.* New York: Raven Press, 1993:831–840.
30. Snyderman CH, Johnson JT. Rehabilitation of swallowing. In: Sekhar LN, Janecka IP, eds. *Surgery of cranial base tumors.* New York: Raven Press, 1993:819–824.

Surgical Techniques to Enhance Prosthetic Rehabilitation

127

Mark S. Chambers   *James C. Lemon*   *Jack W. Martin*

This chapter presents current concepts regarding oral and facial prosthetic rehabilitation and oncologic principles associated with the care of patients with head and neck cancer. Multidisciplinary therapeutic techniques are commonly used in the care of patients with advanced disease of the head and neck. The surgical technique is used to eliminate local disease and aid in preserving function and mobility and physical appearance. Hence, collaboration and team efforts among the head and neck surgeon, maxillofacial prosthodontist, and reconstructive surgeon are vital to patient's quality of life.

Before the surgical procedure, the team specialists formulate plans and preparations for prosthetic rehabilitation. Clear and open communication between the head and neck surgeon and the maxillofacial prosthodontist is of utmost importance for successful prosthetic rehabilitation (1–5). Early dental intervention can help reduce future inpatient care by treatment of oral infection sites and by decreasing risk factors for oral complications, such as osteoradionecrosis. For this reason, patients are referred to the maxillofacial prosthodontist as early as possible for evaluation of their oral and dental condition and for discussion of treatment options in prosthetic rehabilitation. In some cases, for instance, ablated structures can be replaced immediately with prostheses that restore function and improve appearance. The primary head and neck surgeon integrates this information into the treatment plan. Essentially, rehabilitation of function and improved physical appearance, as well as reduction of posttreatment sequelae, are the primary aims after elimination of disease (6,7).

ORAL AND DENTAL ANATOMY

Head and neck surgeons have a thorough knowledge of oral and dental anatomy that makes communication with the maxillofacial prosthodontist ideal in assisting with rehabilitation. For example, it is crucial that the surgeon know which teeth are to be extracted for the surgical procedure so that the maxillofacial prosthodontist can plan and fabricate an immediate or postoperative prosthesis. The universal numbering system of teeth is used for this purpose. In this system, the teeth of adults are numbered sequentially from 1 to 32, starting with the right maxillary third molar, going to the left maxillary third molar, continuing with the opposing left mandibular third molar, and finishing with the right mandibular third molar (Fig. 127.1) (8).

Anatomic landmarks important in prosthetic rehabilitation in edentulous maxillary and mandibular arches are shown in Figure 127.2. In the maxilla, the tuberosity, alveolar ridge, and hard palate are the important supporting tissues for prostheses. The important mandibular landmarks are the alveolar ridge, retromolar pad, and buccal shelf. Preserving, enhancing, or reconstructing these tissues is important for prosthesis support and retention, and periodontally

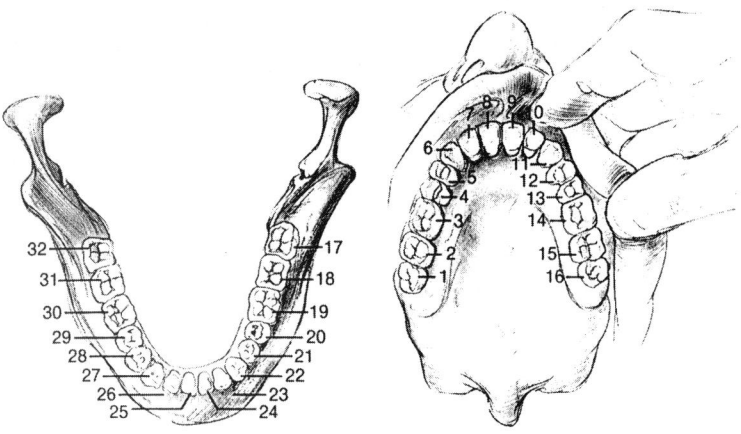

Figure 127.1 Universal numbering system for identification of teeth.

healthy teeth are essential for prosthesis retention and support. Conservation of the supporting tissues, if possible, after eliminating disease, is a priority (9,10).

ORAL AND DENTAL EVALUATION

A preoperative evaluation should include the patient's medical history, intercurrent illnesses, preoperative oral and dental status, previous chemotherapy or radiation treatment, and other factors (e.g., age, nutritional status, and history of tobacco and alcohol use) (5,11,12). The oral and dental evaluation is part of the routine head and neck examination. The head and neck surgeon will identify acute or chronic pathologic conditions related to the dentition or supporting structures, such as advanced periodontal disease, gross dental caries, tissue irritation from poorly fitting prostheses, and poor oral hygiene (5). Gross caries, plaque, and calculus formation on teeth indicate poor oral hygiene, possibly periodontal disease, and a precipitating factor for sepsis. Oral and dental abnormalities are documented during the initial medical examination (7). The patient is then referred to a maxillofacial prosthodontist for further evaluation and treatment.

The initial oral and dental examination by the prosthodontist confirms the existence of acute and chronic oral

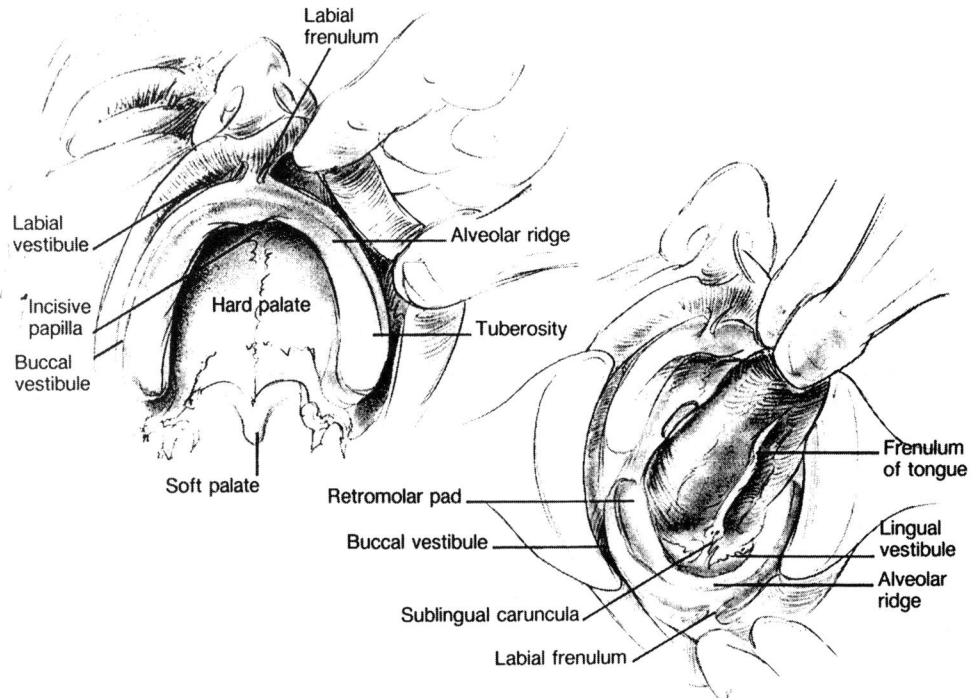

Figure 127.2 Areas that can support prostheses are preserved, if disease removal allows. In the maxilla, these areas include the tuberosity, alveolar ridge, and hard palate. In the mandible, they are the retromolar pad, alveolar ridge, and buccal shelf.

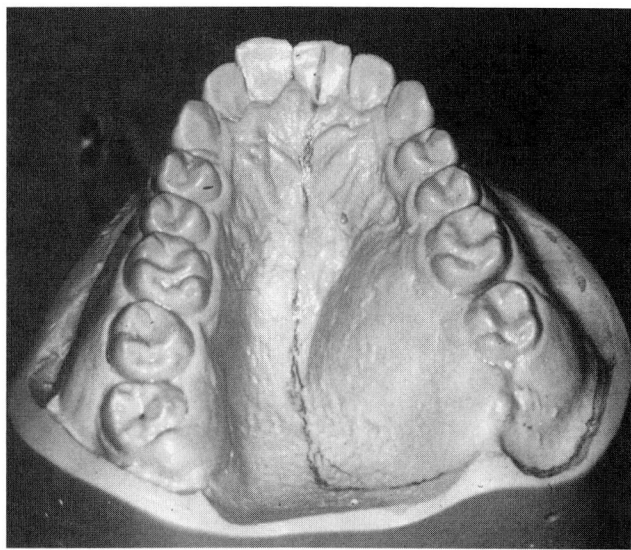

Figure 127.3 A cast obtained at the initial dental examination can be used to fabricate a surgical prosthesis. The surgeon has outlined the planned resection across the hard palate. Anterior hard palate is retained to support the prosthesis.

pathologic conditions, such as dental abscess, teeth with advanced periodontal disease, or dental calculus causing gingivitis (5,7). Diagnostic radiographs are taken, as indicated or requested. The more common diagnostic imagings used in an oral and dental examination are the panoramic, periapical, bitewing, and occlusal radiography. A panoramic radiograph shows the overall topographic features of the dentition, maxilla, mandible, sinuses, nasal cavity, and temporomandibular joints (5,13,14). These radiographs can be of great value to the head and neck surgeon in diagnosis of bony invasion by tumor of the maxilla or mandible and are easily obtained from most dental offices. Stone casts obtained from impressions of the maxilla and mandible during the initial dental visit can be useful if surgical prosthesis (intraoral or extraoral or both) is needed, such as a surgical obturator for a patient who has maxillectomy (Fig. 127.3) (15,16). Teeth having a poor or uncertain prognosis are identified and extracted before or during the primary ablative surgical procedure.

PRINCIPLES AND INFORMATION FOR THE SURGEON

Patients who have radiation therapy to the head and neck that includes the major salivary glands, have reduced salivary flow (xerostomia) in varying degrees and increased susceptibility to dental caries and oral infection (5). The severity of the morbidity is related to radiation dose, volume of tissue treated, and age of the patient when treated (5,7). These patients need to be placed on an anticaries preventive regimen (i.e., fluoride). Numerous studies have shown that fluoride reduces radiation decay of teeth if

used in a systematic, predictable manner (5,6,17). Caries is an important consideration for patients with autoimmune- or radiation-induced xerostomia (Fig. 127.4) (5,17). Reducing the risk of dental infection while maintaining optimal oral health can decrease the risk of osteoradionecrosis or a septic condition in the care of a patient who has radiation therapy or chemotherapy (3,6,18–23).

Some patients with head and neck cancer need removable prostheses to replace surgically removed anatomic structures (2,5,16). Usually, three phases of prosthetic rehabilitation occur: surgical, interim, and definitive. Each phase includes fabrication or modification of a prosthesis. These phases span several months to a year. Surgical and interim prostheses may have to be adjusted frequently while tissues are healing (1,15). Such prostheses are used to restore oral contour and function immediately after maxillectomy. A common problem associated with maxillary obturator prostheses is leakage of fluid around the prosthesis and through the nose. Speech and swallowing can be compromised but, in most cases, can be corrected immediately during the postoperative period.

Most patients are hesitant about starting oral and dental hygiene postoperatively because they fear disturbing the surgical site. Meticulous oral, dental, and prosthetic hygiene is highly encouraged for immediate practice after head and neck surgery (1,24). Routine oral and dental hygiene can be initiated 2 weeks after surgery; oral care can be limited to oral lavage and rinses (1,5,6,24).

Postoperative physiotherapy is a consideration in rehabilitation, and suitable techniques can be discussed with, and explained to, the patient before surgery and reinforced postoperatively. Such therapy can maintain the oral opening and allow the patient better access to the surgical defect and to the rest of the oral cavity (1,24,25). Opening exercises with wooden tongue blades or sophisticated oral opening devices (e.g., TheraBite oral opening device; Atos Medical Co., Milwaukee, WI) can be effective in maintaining

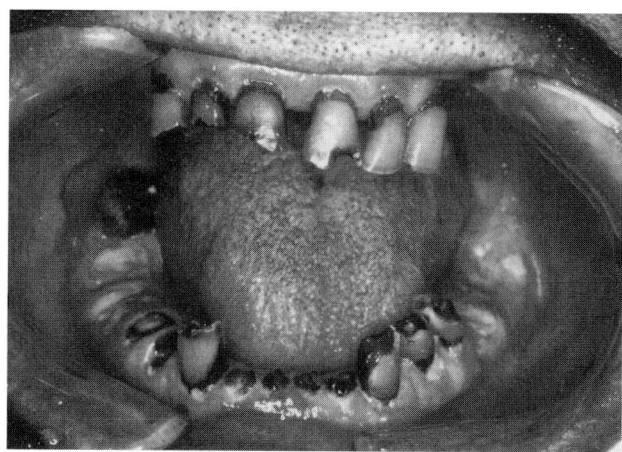

Figure 127.4 Radiation-induced xerostomia can cause a rapid onset and progression of rampant dental caries and osteoradionecrosis.

or restoring oral opening following surgery (1). Reduced mobility of the jaw is a serious and sometimes painful condition that prohibits patients from doing simple tasks such as chewing, swallowing, speaking, or maintaining oral hygiene. Pain can be persistent and coupled with limited functioning; furthermore, patients' quality of life is significantly affected. The TheraBite is a jaw mobilization device designed to help restore proper jaw opening. This comfortable, patient-controlled device utilizes repetitive passive motion and stretching and does so in an anatomically correct pattern (1,5). The above features achieve two positive outcomes: (a) increased jaw opening by stretching connective tissues, mobilizing joints, strengthening muscles, and (b) reduction of pain and inflammation by activating anti-inflammatory properties. A physiotherapist may be helpful in more complex cases to implement electrotherapy, ultrasound, and other advanced techniques, as needed (1,6,25).

Complications vary and depend on the patient's oral and dental status, type of malignancy, and type of therapy. Thorough oral and dental assessment and treatment by a maxillofacial prosthodontist can greatly minimize oral complications and promote healthy oral and dental outcome.

SURGICAL TECHNIQUES TO ENHANCE PROSTHETIC REHABILITATION

Maxilla

Lesions of the maxillary sinus, hard palate, and oral alveoli can cause postoperative speech and swallowing problems that can be reduced or eliminated with careful surgical planning (1). The dental cast obtained at the initial dental visit is used in discussion with the surgeon for the surgical procedure and fabrication of the prosthesis. Several surgical techniques can be incorporated into maxillectomy to improve prosthetic rehabilitation. The most common surgical techniques include the following:

1. Alveolar cuts are made through the socket of an extracted tooth or an edentulous space to prevent iatrogenic bone loss and to ensure the longevity of the tooth next to this cut (1,6,16).
2. When making the palatal cut, as much of the premaxilla as possible is spared. The premaxilla is important for the support and retention of a prosthesis (Fig. 127.5). If the tumor is in the anterior region of the sinus, it may be possible to spare the maxillary tuberosity on the side of the defect, which would also increase prosthetic support.
3. A split-thickness skin graft or allogenic material is placed in the maxillary defect (1,26). A skin graft provides an excellent scar tissue band for retention of the prosthesis and decreases mucous secretion and crust formation in the ablated sinus; the result is improved hygiene (Fig. 127.6).

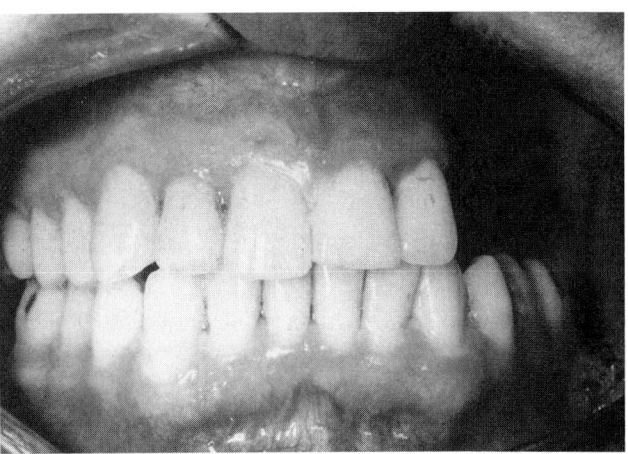

Figure 127.5 The maxillectomy incision is made through the socket of tooth 11 to retain the premaxilla. Some surgeons routinely make a midline incision between teeth 8 and 9; this reduces the amount of supporting tissue.

4. The palatal mucosa, if not affected by disease, can be retained and wrapped around the midline portion of the palatal cut.
5. Removal of the inferior and middle turbinates allows extension of the prosthesis into the defect area (Fig. 127.7). If not removed, the turbinates can be irritated by the prosthesis (1,6).
6. Consideration is given to removing the mandibular molars on the side of the maxillectomy. These teeth can cause a hygiene problem and are essentially nonfunctional after maxillectomy (24).
7. The Weber-Fergusson incision is used for access in a maxillectomy; however, an intraoral approach is increasingly being used to eliminate the facial incision. This makes manipulation of the lip and cheek easier for the dentist and patient during postoperative prosthetic procedures (1,5,9,15,26).

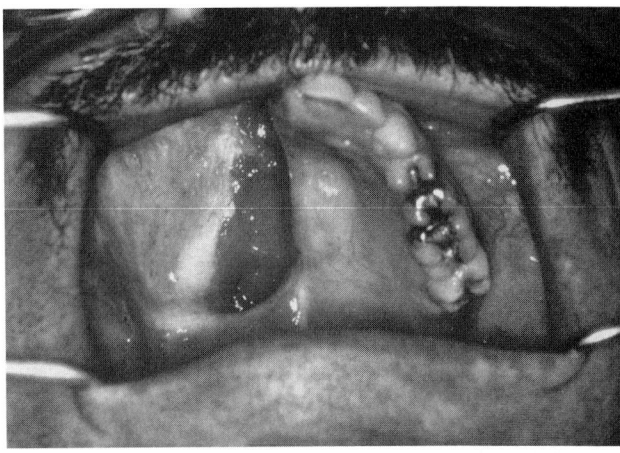

Figure 127.6 Lining the maxillary defect with split-thickness skin grafts makes hygiene of the defect easier. The palatal mucosa has been retained and used to line the cut edge of the palatal defect. This provides excellent support for a maxillary prosthesis.

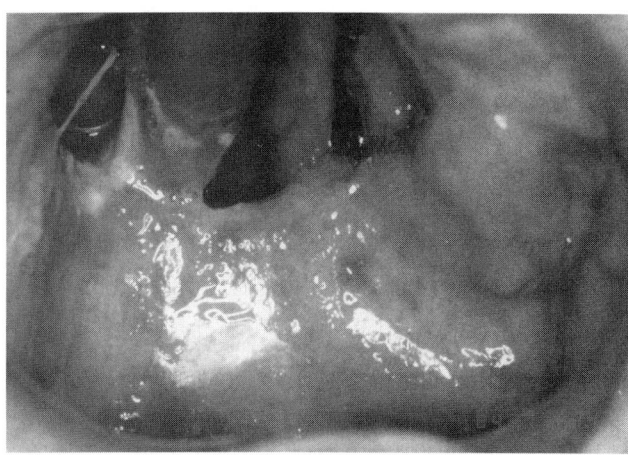

Figure 127.7 Proper extension of the prosthesis into the defect is impeded by the turbinate and nasal septum; the result is reduced retention of the prosthesis. Compromise of the border seal of the defect causes leakage of food and liquid into the nasal cavity.

8. A surgical obturator prosthesis is placed to restore the oral contour for immediate function and good postoperative appearance. This prosthesis supports the surgical packing and can be either fixed to the remaining teeth with surgical wire or retained with a bone screw in an edentulous patient (Fig. 127.8). Use of an obturator can eliminate the need for a nasogastric tube and decreases the duration of postoperative rehabilitation. The obturator maintains proper lip and cheek support during healing and helps to reduce contracture of scar tissue. When the surgical packing is removed, usually within 3 to 5 days of the procedure, the surgical obturator can be converted into an interim prosthesis. Use of a surgical prosthesis can improve the patient's mental outlook (1,9,15,26).

The three distinct phases of maxillary obturator rehabilitation are surgical, interim, and definitive (1). The size and location of the surgical defect, dentition status, and supporting surface area of remaining palate and overlying structures determine the stability and retention of an obturator (1,2,5,6,10,27). As the size of the defect increases and the residual palatal tissues decrease, stability and functionality of the prosthesis reduce significantly because of fewer teeth for direct clasp retention or surface area to engage undercuts (1,2,5,6,10,27).

Some clinicians suggest that maxillary defects should be closed completely using free-tissue grafts (1,6,28,29). Function and cosmesis can be effectively restored with surgical reconstruction. This method does occlude the surgical defect but can preclude prosthetic rehabilitation and can become a challenge if fistulation develops or flap bulkiness occurs, thus, disallowing oral function and prosthetic placement. This is an excellent alternative for patients who do not desire a prosthesis after a maxillectomy (1,6,28,29).

Soft Palate

When some soft palate is removed in the surgical procedure, the surgeon must consider whether the remaining soft palate will be functional. It is easier to rehabilitate a patient's speech and swallowing if the soft palate is removed totally (Fig. 127.9) (1,6). If the remaining soft palate is nonfunctional, rehabilitation can be difficult or even impossible. Sometimes a thin strip of soft palate can be useful for prosthesis retention in a patient with limited supporting tissue (1,2,9). Primary irradiation of the soft palate can cause palatal incompetency because of fibrosis and tumor necrosis. Patients with this problem can regurgitate liquid and food through the nose, and speech can

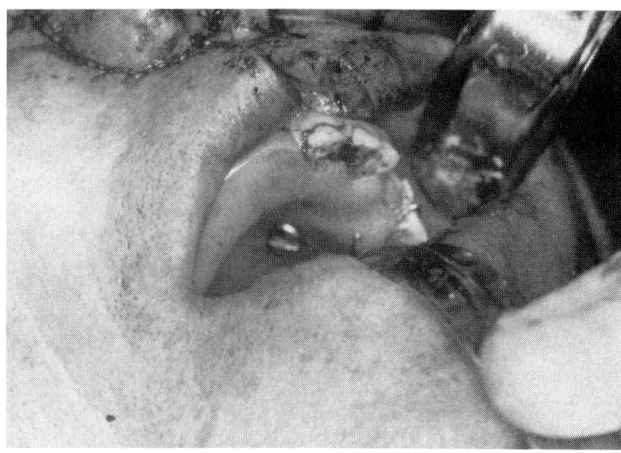

Figure 127.8 Surgical obturator is retained with a bone screw. The surgical obturator maintains stent and graft placement. It is removed 5 to 7 days after surgery, and an interim obturator prosthesis is placed.

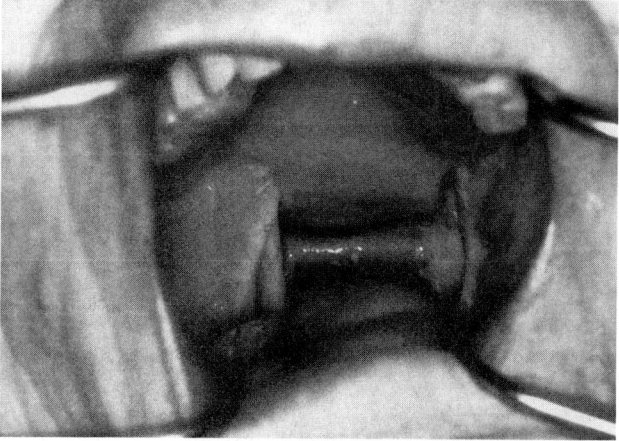

Figure 127.9 Definitive obturator prosthesis in a patient with total soft palate resection. The posterior roll of tissue near the palatal extension of the prosthesis is the posterior pharyngeal wall, which moves in speech and swallowing and compensates for the missing soft palate by closing the nasal cavity during function.

be affected (6,9). In this situation, prosthetic rehabilitation can be impossible because of poor access to the oral pharynx.

Mandible

Over the last 20 years, many advances in head and neck surgical techniques, plate technology, and microvascular surgery have improved the functional and esthetic restoration in patients with head and neck cancer (1,11,30). The significant challenge to the surgeon during mandibular surgery is to re-establish an anatomic structure that is essential in verbalization, oral competence, mastication, deglutination, airway support, and facial appearance (1,30,31). Mandibular reconstruction can be accomplished with alloplastic materials, soft tissue coverage of mandibular reconstruction plates, nonvascularized bone grafts, free flaps and vascularized bone flaps, and osteocutaneous free flaps with the fibula, scapula, iliac crest, and radial forearm (11,30–32). Each type includes the overlying muscle, soft tissue, and skin. Microvascular free tissue transfer has revolutionized mandibular reconstruction because it has predictable results, even when a patient has a mandibulectomy with postoperative radiation.

A fibular graft appears to be the most adaptable for prosthetic rehabilitation. It supplies the length and quality of bone to reconstruct defects of the mandible (30–39) and is an excellent recipient for dental implants and prostheses. Most patients who have had mandibular reconstruction have inadequate vestibular depth, a bulky load-bearing tissue base over the reconstructed alveolar ridge, and physiologic characteristics insufficient for adequate retention and support of a prosthesis. Two procedures routinely used to correct these problems are (a) vestibuloplasty with placement of a split-thickness skin graft and (b) placement of dental implants (1,2,6,40,41).

Patients treated for mandibular neoplasia may need surgical stents, arch bars, or both to reposition the mandibular segments before surgical reconstruction. If the normal association of the mandibular segments with the glenoid fossa and maxilla is not maintained, prosthetic rehabilitation can be limited or even impossible (1). The maxillary teeth opposing the mandibular reconstruction may have to be removed to prevent trauma to bone and soft-tissue flaps. When reconstruction is not indicated in the care of a patient who has had mandibulectomy, removal of the condyle and ramus on the affected side prevents migration of these structures toward the maxilla. Such movement can adversely affect prosthetic rehabilitation.

Primary reconstruction after marginal mandibulectomy (alveolectomy) can be done with a split-thickness skin graft. Skin grafts are important because they provide a sound tissue base for a prosthesis and separate the floor of the mouth from the buccal mucosa (Fig. 127.10) (26). When the tongue, floor of the mouth, or both are sutured

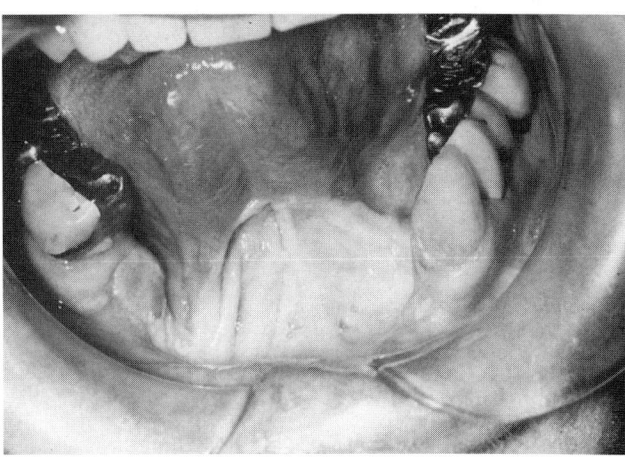

Figure 127.10 Split-thickness skin grafts placed during a primary surgical procedure separate the floor of the mouth from the labial mucosa. The remaining alveolus is used to support a prosthesis.

to the buccal or labial mucosa, prosthetic rehabilitation is limited, if not impossible (2). As with the maxilla, conservation of the supporting tissue in the mandible, as removal of disease allows, is important.

Tongue

Tumors involving the tongue often require extensive resection of bone and soft tissue, resulting in functional and cosmetic morbidity (1,2,5,6,16,42). The degree of speech impediment depends on the extent to which the tongue function is affected. Resection of large portions of the tongue prevents its interaction with other oral structures. This loss compromises the articulation and deglutition as a result of damaged motor or sensory innervation with impaired mobility (16). If the mandible has been involved in the resection, during mastication, the entire envelope of motion occurs on the surgical defect side, resulting in challenged efficiency of chewing and swallowing. Speech and swallowing dysfunction are common problems in patients after glossectomy. Palatal augmentation prostheses that are approximated to the maxilla conform to residual or reconstructed tongue movements and help normalize speech (improving specific sounds) and swallowing (Fig. 127.11) (1,6). At times, however, when the palatal vault is lowered sufficiently for swallowing, speech is adversely affected. This can be addressed with two alternating prostheses: one that is optimal for swallowing and one that is optimal for speech (43). The assistance of a speech pathologist in fabricating the augmentation prosthesis optimizes results. Tongue prostheses can be fabricated but, in general, they have poor function for the patient. Several types of flaps can be used to restore the tongue; although nonfunctional, they reduce space in the oral cavity and make prosthetic fabrication easier and more effective (1,16,42,44).

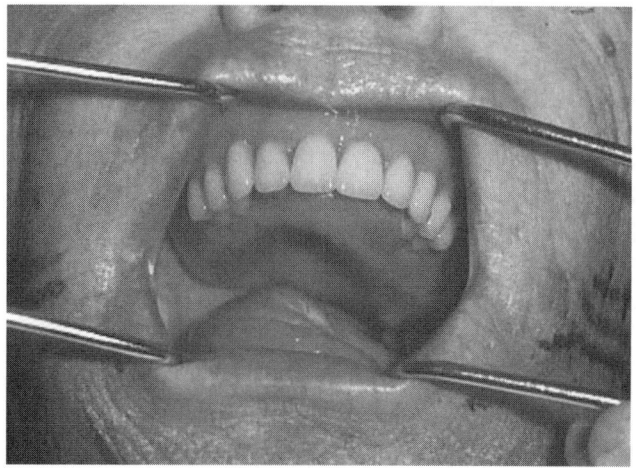

Figure 127.11   Palatal augmentation prosthesis is designed to bring the palate down to the residual or reconstructed tongue for function in speech and swallowing.

EXTRAORAL LESIONS

Lesions involving facial structures can necessitate prosthetic rehabilitation. The reconstructive surgeon must understand both the limitations of facial prostheses and the surgical techniques that enhance success (45). Prostheses can be made from a variety of materials, such as polymethyl methacrylate or urethane-backed, medical-grade silicone. These prostheses are retained with adhesives and tissue undercuts or, in some cases, extraoral osseointegrated implants (1,45). Facial and intraoral prostheses can be connected with magnets. The aesthetic result depends on the amount of tissue removed, type of reconstruction, morbidity of adjunctive treatment (radiation and chemotherapy), and the physical characteristics of the tissue base available to support and retain the prostheses (6,46).

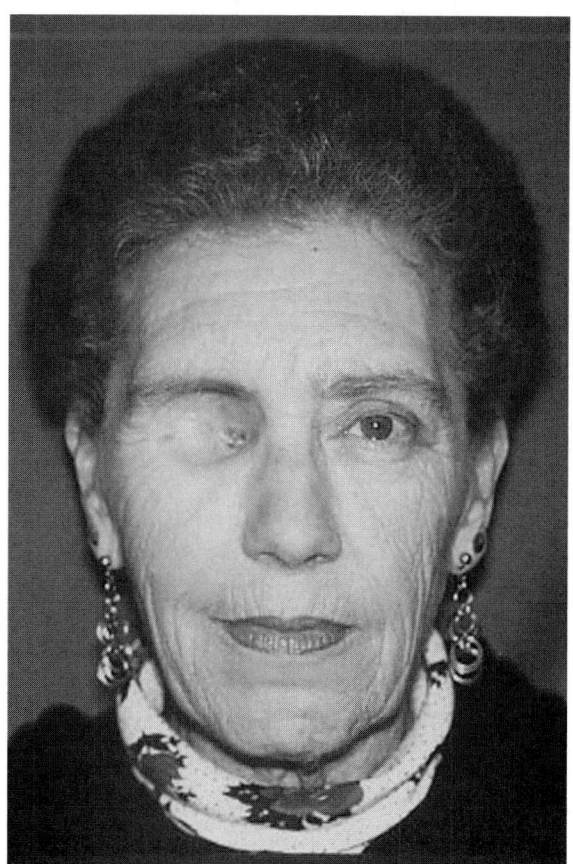

A

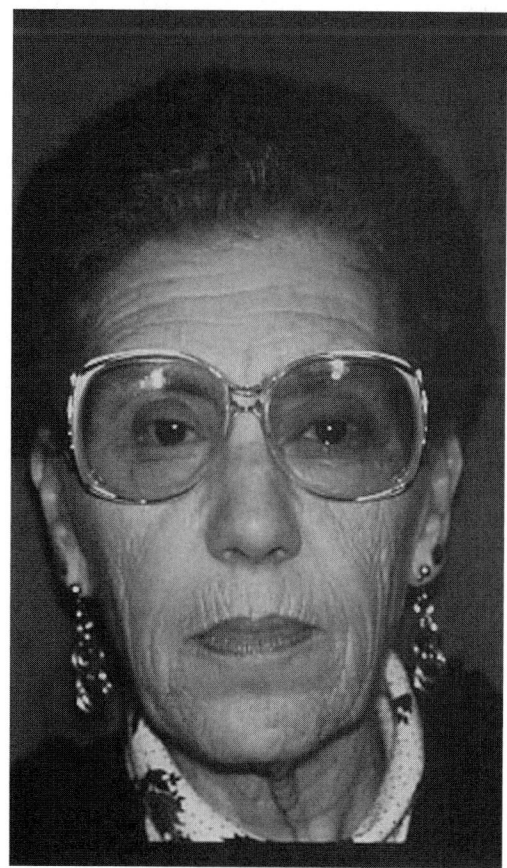

B

Figure 127.12   A: Orbital exenteration is reconstructed with split-thickness skin graft. This technique allows extension of the prosthesis into the defect to improve retention and support. **B:** The customized definitive orbital prosthesis is made of silicone material.

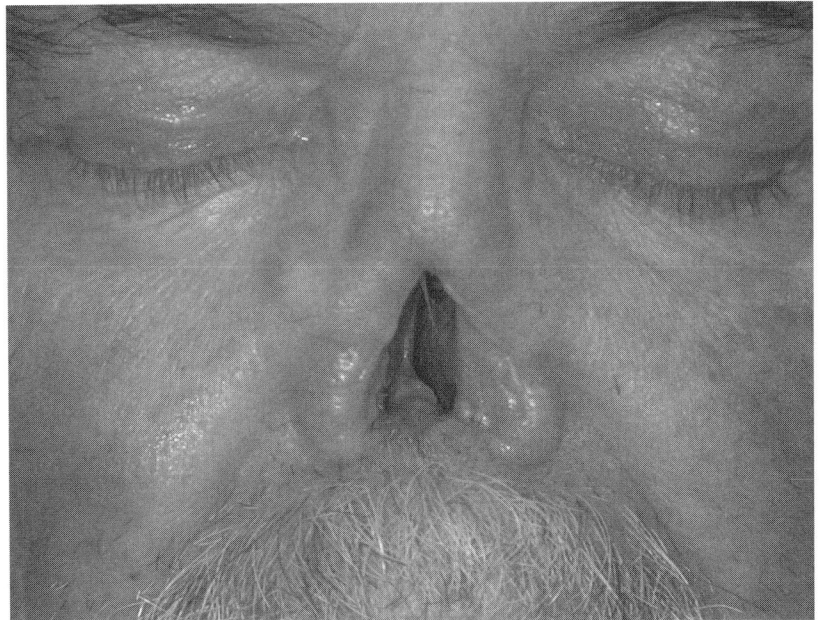

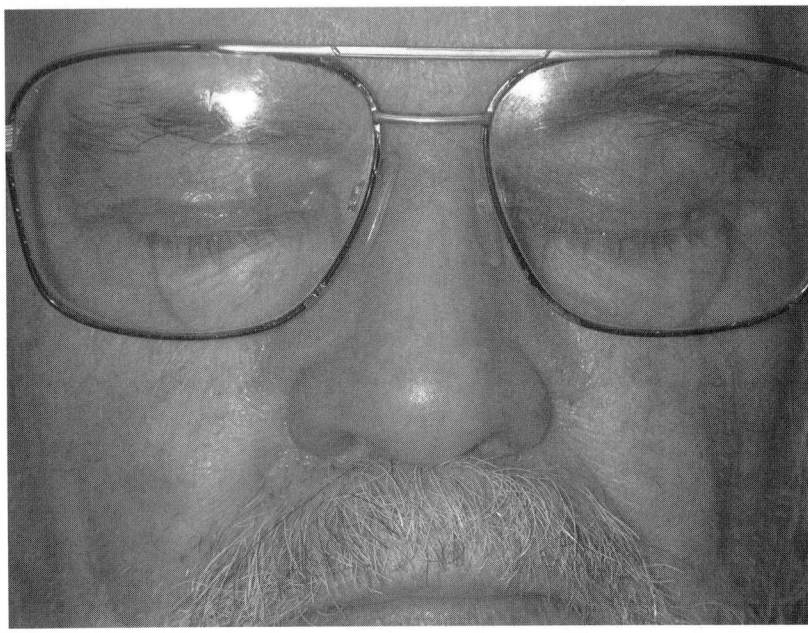

Figure 127.13 **A:** Skin graft at the base of the nose immobilizes the borders of the defect and provides a good base for prosthesis placement. **B:** The nasal prosthesis is positioned onto the underlying skin and retained by a biocompatible adhesive. The patient's glasses help conceal the superior prosthetic margins.

Orbit

In total orbital exenteration, several surgical considerations can improve prosthetic rehabilitation. The eyelid is resected while the position of the eyebrow is maintained. Sharp or rough bony margins are smoothed and rounded. If possible, the infraorbital bony margin is reconstructed. A split-thickness skin graft is placed into the area of the defect to cover exposed bone. Hygiene becomes easier for the patient, and the prosthesis can be extended into the defect for greater orientation and stability (Fig. 127.12) (1,45).

Nose

Resection of lesions involving the nose can necessitate partial or total nasal restoration. The nasal spine is left intact, if possible, for stability of the nasal prosthesis. Unsupported tissue tags are removed, because they can make impression techniques difficult and can compromise the final prosthesis. A split-thickness skin graft is placed over the resected bone margins to increase the stability of the nasal prosthesis (2,45). Grafts or flaps are used to maintain the position of the upper lip (Fig. 127.13).

Ear

Operations on the ear vary from subtotal resection to total auriculectomy. It is easier to replace a complete ear than a partial ear. With a total replacement, the maxillofacial prosthodontist has more freedom in shape, size, and location of the prosthesis. First, the recipient area must be flat or concave. Convexities from excessive tissue bulk can hamper esthetic results. Second, skin devoid of hair provides a good adhesive base, although a split-thickness skin graft is better. Tissue pockets assist in orientation and stabilization of the prosthesis and allow the margins to extend in a zero-degree emergence profile (1,45). If tissue can be spared, the tragus is the first choice. It is a good separate landmark that is not easily displaced (1,45). The tragus allows the anterior margin of the prosthesis to be hidden behind the posterior flexure.

Hair, angle of the helical rim, or both provide posterior margin concealment. The inferior half of the soft-tissue pinna is of little or no use. Because it lacks cartilaginous support, the lobe of the auricle is normally drawn down and away from the head. It is difficult to capture this effect in an impression, and bilateral symmetry usually cannot be achieved. The lobe margin is difficult to maintain and can be troublesome when the patient attempts to insert or place the prosthesis.

The superior half of the auricle has better cartilaginous support yet tends to become distorted after the operation. This distortion is accentuated when the residual auricle is rotated and used to close the defect. A preserved portion of the root of the helix is a good landmark and support for eyeglasses. This area can help later in vertical support of the prosthesis. The anterior superior helical rim is left in place, if possible. Posterior regions can be grafted (Fig. 127.14).

Although surgical techniques can enhance the recipient tissue bed for the prostheses, the main concern of the treating surgeon is elimination of disease.

OSSEOINTEGRATED DENTAL IMPLANTS

Osseointegrated dental implants have become an excellent alternative to conventional prosthetic rehabilitation (1,6,40,41,47). The principle of osseointegration of commercially pure titanium through the intermediary of the layer of titanium oxide and integration with surrounding bone opened a completely new field of clinical application for biotechnology in prosthetic dentistry (48,49). Implant designs fall into three main categories: endosseous, subperiosteal, and transosteal. More than 50 implant subtypes are available from which the prosthodontist can choose for patient rehabilitation (40,48). Additionally, numerous abutments are available that range from fixed (cemented) and fixed-removable (screw or clip retained) designs to removable affixed by O-rings, clips, or snap designs (40). The most common implants used today are endosseous

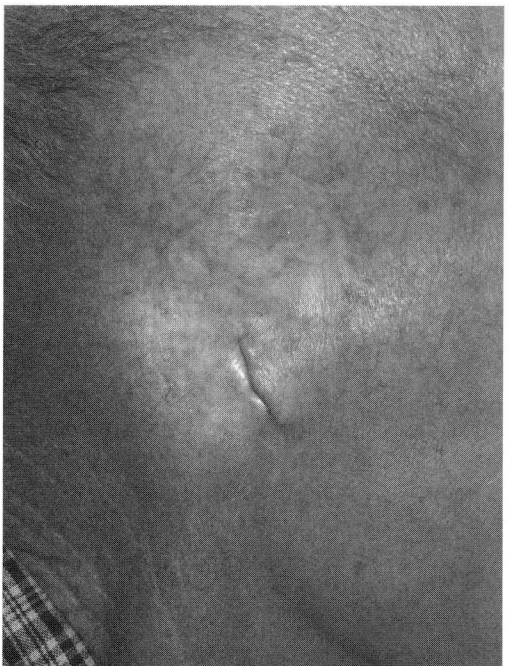
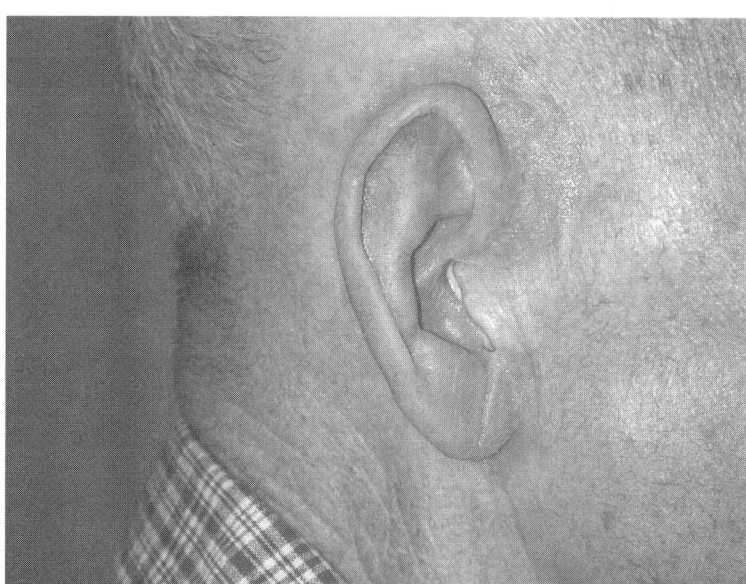

A   B

Figure 127.14 A: The tragus has been preserved following an auriculectomy and will hide the anterior margins of an auricular prosthesis. **B:** Complete ear prosthesis is retained by adhesive. The prosthesis can be worn for 3 or 4 days at a time before removal for cleaning.

implants that are surgically inserted into the maxillae or mandible and integrate with the surrounding bone (41). Endosseous implants have provided the support, retention, and stability that are greatly needed in compromised oral cavities following tumor ablative procedures (41).

Several common terms are used today in oral implantology: dental implant, endosteal dental implant, abutment, and osseointegration (48). A dental implant is a device specially designed to be placed surgically within or on the mandibular or maxillary bone in providing resistance to displacement of a overlying prosthesis. It can be placed transgingivally or fully embedded subgingivally (48). The endosteal dental implant is an implant of which part is anchored within the maxillary or mandibular bone (48). An abutment is a component connected to the endosteal part of the dental implant that allows retention or support of a dental implant (48). The abutment connects the fixture (implant) to a superstructure and overlying prosthesis (40,41,48). Osseointegration is a direct structural and functional connection between vital bone and the surface of a load-carrying implant (48,49). Finally, the endosseous dental implants can be divided into different categories according to their shape, surface characteristics, chemical composition, or the way the implant is inserted into the bone (48).

Meticulous surgical and prosthetic planning is required before implant placement (1,41). If adequate supporting tissues exist or can be established, patients can function satisfactorily with routine prostheses, or they may be considered for implants if the recipient sites are appropriate. Several types of implants are currently available for intraoral and extraoral maxillofacial uses (1,6,46). Most implants used in maxillofacial prosthetics are made of titanium, cylindrically designed, and use threads that anchor them in the bone. Such implants are produced in a variety of lengths and widths. In most of these implant systems, placement involves a two-stage procedure. The first stage, performed under local or general anesthesia, is the placement of the

implant into the bony recipient site (1,40,41). Placement is performed in a very precise fashion to ensure the least amount of damage to the adjacent bone and soft tissue, particularly in irradiated tissues. Following placement, the implant is covered primarily by the initial tissue flap and allowed to integrate with the bone for 12 or more weeks. The purpose is to promote perimplant integration with the implant interface, as described previously. Confirmed osseointegration, by radiographic and clinical interpretation, implies a direct and lasting connection between vital bone and the titanium implant of defined surface topography and geometry (1,6). In the second stage, only the superior portion of the implant is uncovered and an abutment, usually made of titanium alloy, is placed onto the implant (1). This connection will join the implant to the prosthesis. The number of implants, type of retention, and prosthetic design are at the discretion of the restoring prosthodontist. In general, the prosthesis is fabricated so that it can be easily removed by the patient and allows maintenance and proper oral hygiene (Fig. 127.15). Most patients who have had intraoral irradiated treatment have the maxillofacial area restored by removable prostheses (1,46). For those patients, rehabilitation with implants can be successfully restored with an overlying removable prosthesis using ball abutments and O-ring attachments embedded in the prosthesis.

Implants can be placed during or after the primary reconstructive procedure if the host bone has acceptable cortical plates suitable for implant fixation (50,51). The fibula tissue graft is an excellent recipient site for such implants (30). The fibula free flap provides a long segment of bone and can include a large fasciocutaneous component (30,31,36–39). As such, this versatile flap can be harvested as an osteomyocutaneous flap or a purely osseous flap. The pedicle runs the length of the fibula, with perforators extending to the skin paddle (30,31,36–39). It provides the longest segment of bone currently available for harvest; up to 26 cm can be taken without affecting leg function. Many bony defects of

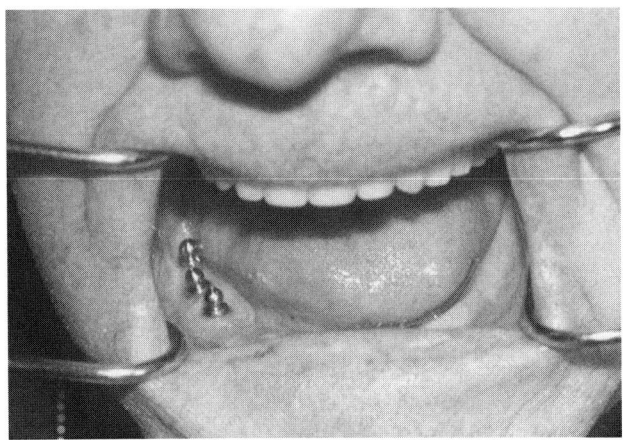

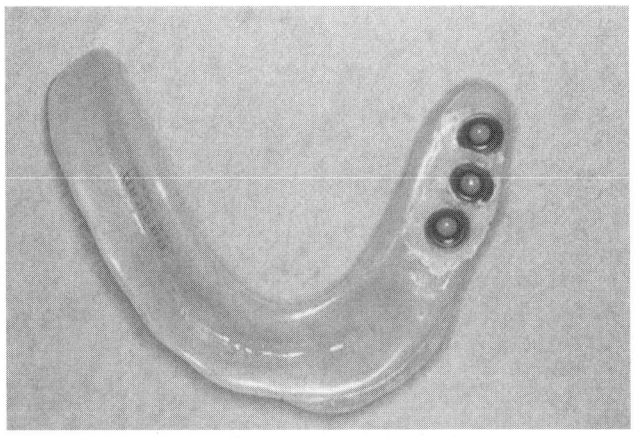

A

B

Figure 127.15   A: Endossesous implants placed in a mandible reconstructed with a fibula osteocutaneous flap. **B:** Implant-retained mandibular prosthesis revealing O-ring retainers on the tissue surface of the prosthesis that will engage ball attachments intraorally.

the head and neck region are well suited for reconstruction with a fibula free flap. Functional rehabilitation can be optimal. Patients who have osseointegrated implants placed in the fibula graft can have near-normal mastication and speech re-established (30,31). In most cases, implant placement is best accomplished during a secondary procedure when a premade surgical stent can guide the prosthodontist in aligning and positioning the implants (1). Patients who have received postoperative radiation in proximity to the proposed implant site may be poor candidates for it, because of hypovascularity in the volume of tissue radiated and may benefit from hyperbaric oxygen therapy before implant placement (19,52–57).

The goals of prosthetic rehabilitation with implants include predictability and simplicity. Fabrication of a fixed implant prosthesis often involves methods and materials that are complicated and increase costs to the restoring dentist and patient. Additional prosthetic components and additional appointments to complete the prosthesis can create unnecessary inconveniences; therefore, a removable prosthesis should be considered initially in treatment planning for a patient with maxillofacial deficits (1,41). Aside from patient factors, decision-making on the type of implant to use, restoring materials, and prosthetic rehabilitation should be based on evidence from clinical protocols and facts of corporate products.

COMPLICATIONS

Oral and dental complications are usually associated with preexisting conditions that cause their initiation and persistence (5). The three sites in the oral cavity that are a focus of these complications are the mucosa, periodontium, and teeth. If oral and dental complications develop during chemotherapy (e.g., periodontal abscesses), they can potentially lead to systemic involvement (Table 127.1) (1,5,6). Complications from radiation therapy to the head and neck usually are either acute (e.g., treatment-related mucositis or dermatitis) or chronic (e.g., hypovascularity, xerostomia, dental decay) (1,58–62). Irradiation can adversely affect cellular elements of bone, which can limit the potential for wound maintenance and the ability to heal after a traumatic event (1,5,19). Infections in the oral cavity can complicate postoperative recovery time, significantly compromise any reconstructive graft to a point of failure, and delay effective adjunctive therapy (e.g., radiation therapy or chemotherapy).

Other complications can be related to poor communication between members of the health care team (1). Some patients are not referred to a dentist because they are edentulous. These patients, however, may have poorly fitting prostheses, impacted or abscessed teeth (diagnosed by radiographs), or bone disease that can affect postoperative rehabilitation. In all cases, patients who have head and neck surgery should be monitored closely by the health care team.

TABLE 127.1 **COMPLICATIONS**

ORAL COMPLICATIONS RELATED TO CANCER THERAPY

Chemotherapy
Acute: Primary (direct) effects
  Mucosal barrier injury
    Mucosal thinning and ulceration (mucositis)
  Swallowing difficulty
  Nausea
Chronic: Secondary effects (i.e., bone marrow suppression)
  Oral infection: soft and hard tissue
  Oral bleeding
  Pancytopenia

Radiation therapy
Acute: Primary (direct) effects
  Mucosal barrier injury: site specific
    Mucosal thinning and ulceration (mucositis)
  Alteration of taste and smell
  Infection
  Dermatitis
Chronic: Secondary effects (i.e., salivary gland dysfunction)
  Xerostomia
  Dental caries
  Abnormal bony development
  Fibrosis
  Trismus
  Osteoradionecrosis

Head and neck surgery
Acute: Primary (direct) effects
  Infection
  Discomfort
  Bleeding
  Edema
Chronic: Secondary effects
  Trismus
  Iatrogenic salivary gland dysfunction
  Postmaxillectomy sinus drainage
  Skin contracture
  Oral discontinuity

Regularly scheduled appointments with the dental practitioner are essential for monitoring oral and dental hygiene, proper fit of prostheses, and, most importantly, disease recurrence. If a patient complains of a sudden loss of oral opening ability, the clinician should consider recurrence of disease in their differential diagnoses (1,6,7).

Patients with head and neck cancer can experience significant changes of the oral anatomy and physiology as a sequela of disease or treatment; specifically, masticatory performance and swallowing efficiency of patients treated for head and neck cancer can be altered (1,5,63). One study by Marunick and Mathog (63) objectively analyzed the masticatory and swallowing threshold performance of head and neck patients following prosthodontic rehabilitation of intraoral defects, revealing a significant improvement. This study proposed techniques in evaluating success of masticatory factors of prosthetic rehabilitation, such as dentition and occlusion, denture stability, biting forces, temporomandibular joint status, range of motion, and salivary function (63).

EVIDENCE-BASED PROSTHETIC REHABILITATION

Improvements in dental implants, biomaterials, bioengineering, and surgical preservation techniques increase the retention, stability, and longevity of prosthetic rehabilitation and, ultimately, a patient's quality of life (1,6,64). The use of osseointegrated implants and guided tissue regeneration (i.e., synthetic membranes) procedures in patients who have had irradiation therapy have great promise (47,65). The cellular and metabolic changes in the irradiated bone can affect both the qualitative and quantitative aspects of osseointegration (1,46). Important factors in successful dental restoration are the influence of radiation dose, delivery system (e.g., intensity modulated radiation therapy, IMRT), implant biomaterials, time from radiation therapy to implant surgery, the experience of the prosthodontist, fixture and abutment lengths, appropriate implantation sites, and type of prosthetic retention on implant survival. In addition, the benefit of osteogenesis and angiogenesis of hyperbaric oxygen therapy, in conjunction with reconstructive techniques, in the patient having had irradiation therapy is also being studied (52–57). New physiotherapy methods are being developed to improve the postoperative function of patients with head and neck cancer (1,5). Tissue engineering, sterolithography, and rapid prototyping technology has recently resulted in the successful formation of new tissue equivalents of bone and cartilage that will enhance prosthetic rehabilitation in the future (65–68).

HIGHLIGHTS

- Maxillofacial prosthodontics is the branch of dentistry responsible for rehabilitation of intraoral and extraoral surgical defects.
- Preservation techniques during surgery can improve the effectiveness of prosthetic rehabilitation.
- The oral and dental status of patients scheduled for radiation therapy or chemotherapy is assessed before treatment and is followed closely thereafter.
- Dental radiographs (e.g., periapical, occlusal, and panoramic views) are useful in evaluating malignant disease and infection of the oral cavity.
- If the soft palate is involved in surgical resection, the entire soft palate may have to be removed to improve prosthetic rehabilitation.
- Skin grafting of maxillectomy defects improves hygiene and prosthetic rehabilitation.
- The inferior and middle turbinates are removed during maxillectomy.

- A fibular graft is an excellent choice for surgical reconstruction and prosthetic rehabilitation (i.e., placement of osseointegrated implants after mandibulectomy).
- Split-thickness skin grafts are used in reconstruction of facial defects to immobilize tissue and provide a stable tissue base for the prosthesis.
- The eyelid is removed and eyebrow position maintained in orbital exenteration.
- Unsupported tissue tags are removed in auriculectomy and rhinectomy.
- Optimal prosthetic rehabilitation requires close communication between all members of the treatment team.
- Oral and dental complications are usually associated with preexisting conditions.

REFERENCES

1. Chambers MS, Lemon JC, Martin JW, et al. Oral rehabilitation of patients with head and neck cancer. In: Myers EN, Suen JY, Myers JN, et al., eds. Cancer of the head and neck, 4th ed. Philadelphia: WB Saunders, 2003:Chapter 29.
2. Lemon JC, Martin JW, Jacob RF. Prosthetic rehabilitation. In: Weber RS, Miller MJ, Goepfert H, eds. Basal and squamous cell skin cancers of the head and neck. Baltimore: Williams & Wilkins, 1996:305–312.
3. King GE, Jacob RFK, Martin JW. Oral and dental rehabilitation. In: Johns ME, ed. Complications in otolaryngology head and neck surgery. Philadelphia: BC Decker, 1986:131.
4. Van Blarcom CW. The glossary of prosthodontic terms. J Prosthet Dent 2005;94:51.
5. Chambers MS, Toth BB, Martin JW, et al. Oral and dental management of the cancer patient: prevention and treatment of complications. Support Care Cancer 1995;3:168–175.
6. Martin JW, Lemon JC, King GE. Maxillofacial restoration after tumor ablation. In: Schusterman MA, ed. Clinics in plastic surgery. Philadelphia: WB Saunders, 1994:87–96.
7. Lingeman RE, Singer MJ. Evaluation of the patient with head and neck cancer. In: Sven JY, Myers EN, eds. Cancer of the head and neck. New York: Churchill Livingstone, 1981:15.
8. Fuller JL, Deneky GE. Concise dental anatomy and morphology, 2nd ed. Chicago: Mosby Year Book, 1984:9.
9. Beumer JP, Curtis TA. Restoration of acquired hard palate defects. In: Maxillofacial rehabilitation: prosthodontic and surgical considerations. St. Louis: Mosby, 1979:188.
10. Okay DJ, Genden E, Buchbinder D, et al. Prosthodontic guidelines for surgical reconstruction of the maxilla: a classification system of defects. J Prosthet Dent 2001;86:352–363.
11. Smith JE, Ducic J. Mandibular reconstruction, plating. Available at: http:// www.emedicine.com (ent topic743); June 11, 2003.
12. Silverman S. Oral cancer: complications of therapy. Oral Surg Oral Med Oral Pathol Oral Radiol Endod 1999;88:122–126.
13. Langland OE, Langlois RP, Morris CR. Principles and practice of panoramic radiology. Philadelphia: WB Saunders, 1982:131–156.
14. Blaschbe DP, Osborn AG. The mandible and teeth. In: Bergeron RT, Osborn AG, San PM, eds. Head and neck imaging. St. Louis: Mosby, 1984: 279.
15. Martin JW, Jacob RF, Larson DL, et al. Surgical stents for the head and neck cancer patient. Head Neck Surg 1984;7:44.
16. Curtis TA, Beumer J. Restoration of acquired hard palate defects: etiology, disability, and rehabilitation. In: Beumer J, Curtis TA, Firtell DN, eds. Maxillofacial rehabilitation: prosthodontic and surgical considerations. St. Louis, CV Mosby, 1979:188–243.
17. Fleming TJ. Oral tissue changes of radiation oncology and their management. Dent Clin North Am 1990;34:233–237.
18. Marx RE, Johnson RP. Studies in the radiobiology of osteoradionecrosis and their clinical significance. Oral Surg Oral Med Oral Pathol Oral Radiol Endod 1987;64:379–390.

19. Marx RE. Radiation injury to tissue. In: Kindwall EP, ed. *Hyperbaric medicine Practice.* Flagstaff, AR: Best Publishing, 1994:447–503.

20. Marx RE, Ehler WJ, Tayapongsak P, et al. Relationship of oxygen dose to angiogenesis induction in irradiated tissue. *Am J Surg* 1990;160:519–524.

21. Marx RE, Johnson RP, Kline SN. Prevention of osteoradionecrosis: a randomized prospective clinical trial of hyperbaric oxygen versus penicillin. *J Am Dent Assoc* 1985;11:49–54.

22. Ang E, Black C, Irish J, et al. Reconstructive options in the treatment of osteoradionecrosis of the craniomaxillofacial skeleton. *Br J Plast Surg* 2003;56:92–99.

23. Marx RE, Johnson RP. Problem wounds in oral and maxillofacial surgery: the role of hyperbaric oxygen. In: Davis JC, Hunt TK, eds. *Problem wounds: the role of oxygen.* New York: Elsevier, 1988: 65–123.

24. Martin JW, Austin JR, Chambers MS, et al. Postoperative care of the maxillectomy patient. *ORL Head Neck Nurs* 1994;12:15–20.

25. Barrett NV, Martin JW, Jacob RF, et al. Physical therapy techniques in the treatment of the head and neck patient. *J Prosthet Dent* 1988;59:343.

26. Teichgraeber J, Larson DL, Castaneda O, et al. Skin grafts in intraoral reconstruction: a new stenting method. *Arch Otolaryngol Head Neck Surg* 1984;101:463.

27. Aramany MA. Basic principles of obturator design for partially edentulous patients. Part II: design principles. *J Prosthet Dent* 1978;40:656–662.

28. Olsen KD, Meland N, Ebersold MJ, et al. Extensive defects of the sino-orbital region: results with microvascular reconstruction. *Arch Otolaryngol Head Neck Surg* 1992;118:828–833.

29. Kuriloff DB, Sullivan MJ. Revascularized tissue transfers in head and neck surgery. In Bailey BJ, ed. *Head and veck surgery—otolaryngology.* Philadelphia: Lippincott-Raven; 1998: 2345–2387.

30. Schusterman MA, Reece GP, Miller MJ, et al. The osteocutaneous free fibula flap. Is the skin paddle reliable? *Plast Reconstr Surg* 1992;90:787.

31. Winslow CD, Wax MK. Tissue transfer: Fibula. Available at: http://www.Emedicine.com. Accessed August 28, 2003.

32. Cordeiro PG, Wolfe SA. The temporalis muscle flap revisited on its centennial: advantages, newer uses, and disadvantages. *Plast Reconstr Surg* 1996;98:980–987.

33. Ioannides C, Fossion E, Boeckx W. Surgical management of the osteoradionecrotic mandible with free vascularized composite flaps. *J Craniomaxillofac Surg* 1994;22(6):330–334.

34. Lydiatt DD, Lydiatt WM, Hollins RR, et al. Use of free fibula flap in patients with prior failed mandibular reconstruction. *J Oral Maxillofac Surg* 1998;56(4):444–446.

35. Shaha AR, Cordeiro PG, Hidalgo DA, et al: Resection and immediate microvascular reconstruction in the management of osteoradionecrosis of the mandible. *Head Neck* 1997;19(5):406–411.

36. Anthony JP, Rawnsley JD, Benhaim P. Donor leg morbidity and function after fibula free flap mandible reconstruction. *Plast Reconstr Surg* 1995;96(1):146–152.

37. Disa JJ, Cordeiro PG. The current role of preoperative arteriography in free fibula flaps. *Plast Reconstr Surg* 1998;102(4): 1083–1088.

38. Hidalgo DA. Fibula free flap mandibular reconstruction. *Clin Plast Surg* 1994;21(1):25–35.

39. Urken ML, Cheney ML, Sullivan MJ. Fibula free flaps. In: Urken ML, Cheney ML, Sullivan MJ, et al. *Atlas of regional and free flaps for head and neck reconstruction.* New York, NY: Raven Press, 1995.

40. Lee MB. Implants. Available at: Webmaster@cincinnati-oralsurgery.com. Support Central. Accessed April 2003.

41. Eckert SE, Desjardins RP. The impact of endosseous implants on maxillofacial prosthetics. In: Taylor TD, ed. *Clinical maxillofacial prosthetics.* Chicago: Quintessence 2000:145–153.

42. Godoy AJ, Perez DG, Lemon JC, et al. Rehabilitation of a patient with limited oral opening following glossectomy. *Int J Prosthodont* 1991;4:70–74.

43. Shimodaira K, Yoshida H, Yusa H, et al. Palatal augmentation prosthesis with alternative palatal vaults for speech and swallowing: a clinical report. *J Prosthet Dent* 1998;80:1–3.

44. Cantor R, Curtis T. Prosthetic management of edentulous mandibulectomy patients. Part II: Clinical procedures. *J Prosthet Dent* 1971;25:546.

45. Howard G, Osguthorpe JD. Concepts in orbital reconstruction. *Otolaryngol Clin North Am* 1997;30:541–562.

46. Granstöm G, Tjellström A, Branemark PI, et al. Bone anchored-reconstruction of the irradiated head and neck cancer patient. *Otolaryngol Head Neck Surg* 1993;108:334–343.

47. Hong WL, Chu SA, Dam JG, et al. Oral rehabilitation using dental implants and guided bone regeneration. *Ann Acad Med Singapore* 1999;28:697–703.

48. Scortecci GM. Introduction to oral implantology in restorative dentistry. In: Scortecci GM, Misch CE, Benner KU, eds. *Implants and restorative dentistry.* New York: Martin Dunitz Ltd, 2001:1–25.

49. Branemark PI, Zarb G, Albrektsson T. Tissue-integrated prostheses. In: Branemark PI, ed. *Osseointegration in clinical dentistry.* Chicago: Quintessence 1985:1–50.

50. Lemon JC, Chambers MS, Wesley PJ, et al. Rehabilitation of a midface defect with reconstructive surgery and facial prosthetics: a case report. *Int J Oral Maxillofac Implants* 1996;11:101–105.

51. Benner KU. Morphological aspects of oral implantology. In: Scortecci GM, Misch CE, Benner KU, eds. *Implants and restorative dentistry.* New York: Martin Dunitz Ltd, 2001:26–46.

52. Ferguson BJ, Hudson WR, Farmer JC. Hyperbaric oxygen for laryngeal radiation necrosis. *Ann Otol Rhinol Laryngol* 1987;96:1–6.

53. Tibbles PM, Edelsberg JS. Hyperbaric-oxygen therapy. *N Engl J Med* 1996;334(25):1642–1648.

54. Feldmeier JJ, Jelen I, Davolt DA, et al. Hyperbaric oxygen as a prophylaxis for radiation induced delayed enteropathy. *Radiother Oncol* 1995;35:138–144.

55. Feldmeier JJ, Davolt DA, Court WS, et al. Histologic morphometry confirms a prophylactic effect for hyperbaric oxygen in the prevention of delayed radiation enteropathy. *Undersea Hyperb Med* 1998;25(2):93–97.

56. Feldmeier JJ, Newman R, Davolt DA, et al. Prophylactic hyperbaric oxygen for patients undergoing salvage for recurrent head and neck cancers following full course irradiation. *Undersea Hyperb Med* 1998;25(Suppl):10 (abst).

57. Ueda M, Kaneda T, Takahashi H. Effect of hyperbaric oxygen therapy on osseointegration of titanium implants in irradiated bone: a preliminary report. *Int J Oral Maxillofac Implants* 1993;8:41–44.

58. Chambers MS, Garden AS, Kies MS, et al. Radiation-induced xerostomia in patients with head and neck cancer: pathogenesis, impact on quality of life, and management. *Head Neck* 2004;26: 796–807.

59. Eisbruch A, Ten Haken RK, Kim HM, et al. Dose, volume, and function relationships in parotid salivary glands following conformal and intensity-modulated irradiation of head and neck cancer. *Int J Radiat Oncol Biol Phys* 1999;45:577–587.

60. Chao KS, Deasy JO, Markman J, et al. A prospective study of salivary function sparing in patients with head-and-neck cancers receiving intensity-modulated or three-dimensional radiation therapy: initial results. *Int J Radiat Oncol Biol Phys* 2001;49:907–916.

61. Rubenstein EB, Peterson DE, Schubert M, et al. Clinical practice guidelines for the prevention and treatment of cancer therapy-induced oral and gastrointestinal mucositis. *Cancer* 2004;100 (9 Suppl):2026–2046

62. Sonis ST, Elting LS, Keefe D, et al. Perspectives on cancer therapy-induced mucosal injury: pathogenesis, measurement, epidemiology, and consequences for patients. *Cancer* 2004;100(9 Suppl): 1995–2025.

63. Marunick MT, Mathog RH. Mastication in patients treated for head and neck cancer: a pilot study. *J Prosthet Dent* 1990;63: 566–573.

64. Kornblith AB, Zlotolow IM, Gooen J, et al. Quality of life of maxillectomy patients using an obturator prosthesis. *Head Neck* 1996; 18:323–334.

65. Thompson RC, Mikos AG, Beahm EB, et al. Guided tissue fabrication from periosteum using preformed biodegradable polymer scaffolds. *Biomaterials* 1999;20:2007–2018.

66. Miller MJ, Goldberg DP, Yasko AW, et al. Guided bone growth in sheep: a model for tissue-engineered bone flaps. *Tissue Eng* 1996; 2:51–59.

67. Reitemeier B, Notni G, Heinze M, et al. Optical modeling of extraoral defects. *J Prosthet Dent* 2004;91(1):80–84.

68. Eppley BL. The accuracy of stereolithography in planning craniofacial bone replacement. *J Craniofac Surg* 2003;14(6):934–935.

Otology

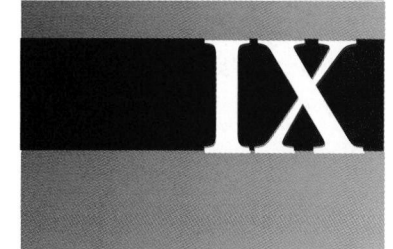

IX

Barry E. Hirsch   *Arun K. Gadre*

Development of the Ear

128

Michael J. Wareing   *Anil K. Lalwani*   *Robert K. Jackler*

The development of the structures necessary for transmission of sound information from the environment to the auditory cortex is a complex and interwoven process. An understanding of the major developmental steps and their interrelations is desirable because therein lies the key to understanding many conditions encountered by otolaryngologists. Awareness of the developmental process alerts the surgeon to anatomic associations and explains important departures from normal.

Abnormal development is important for its clinical effects, but it also has a role in unraveling the complexities of normal development. The critical period of ear development begins in the third week after fertilization, the inner ear appearing first. The inner, middle, and outer portions of the ear have different embryologic origins, and development can be arrested at any stage. The result is a range of abnormalities from mild to severe. In view of the different origins, a disorder in one part does not necessarily signify a disorder in another, but proximity in terms of time of development, originating tissue, anatomic characteristics, and function does mean that multiple malformations are possible. The disorders can be caused by an inborn genetic error, either inherited or spontaneous, or by a teratogenic influence during organogenesis. The tissues of the head and neck are derived from all three layers of the embryo—ectoderm, mesoderm, and endoderm. The neural crest cells play a special role in the head and neck, where they constitute most of the skeletal and connective tissue. These cells arise from the ectodermal layer at the junction where the neural tube begins to fold. All divisions of the ear contain some neural crest tissue. The mesodermal proportion in the head and neck is less than that in the rest of the body.

The story of ear development goes back to the time life itself was in its infancy. Fish seem to be the first hearing organisms, with development of a hearing organ from an internal balance organ. Even at this early evolutionary stage, the hair-cell design now so widespread was in use. Both amphibians and reptiles inherited the balance labyrinth of fish but went on to develop auditory labyrinths of their own, having branched from the line of fish before acquisition of a hearing organ. The need to hear in air resulted in development of a conductive apparatus to correct the impedance mismatch of sound arriving in air but having to be transmitted into the liquid of the labyrinth. Mammalian design continued from the basic reptilian design with, in particular, the addition of rows of hair cells, an independent cochlear nerve, changes in the middle-ear conduction system, and protective external auditory canals (1). Throughout this work, we separate development of the ear into its component parts as an aid to understanding. It is important, however, to remember that these changes occur in a simultaneous manner. An overview of ear development is presented in Table 128.1.

AURICULAR DEVELOPMENT

In keeping with its recent evolutionary appearance, the auricle of the external ear begins its development later than do other components of the ear. From the fifth week of gestation, three hillocks arise on the first branchial (mandibular) arch (hillocks 1, 2, and 3), and three arise on the second branchial (hyoid) arch (hillocks 4, 5, and 6) on either side of the first branchial cleft (Fig. 128.1).

TABLE 128.1

OVERVIEW OF EAR DEVELOPMENT

Fetal Age (wk)	Outer Ear	Middle Ear	Inner Ear
3			Otic placode develops. VC ganglia appear.
4	EAC begins.	Tubotympanic recess is apparent	Otocyst present.
5	Hillocks become evident.	Ossicles begin to condense in mesenchyme.	Otocyst begins to divide into vestibular and cochlear areas. Semicircular canals begin to outpouch; VC ganglion divides.
6	All hillocks are distinct.	Malleus and incus are identifiable as cartilaginous models.	Superior SCC completed. Utricle and saccule are present; cochlear duct begins.
7			Maculae present; sensory ridges in the cochlea appear.
8	Auricle has identifiable structure; deep meatus is apparent as epithelial strand.	Incudomalleolar and incudostapedial joints form.	Ductus reuniens is identifiable; $1^1/_2$ cochlear turns; cristae present. Vacuoles develop in vascular precartilage surrounding membranous labyrinth; cartilaginous model of otic capsule forms.
9		Tympanic membrane has trilaminar structure.	Nerve fibers enter sensory epithelium; oval window develops.
10		Stapes loses annular form; facial nerve runs through middle ear.	$2^1/_2$ cochlear turns.
11			Hair cells present in cochlea; synaptic connections are present.
12		Tympanic ring begins to ossify.	Otoconial membrane is present; cochlear duct changes to triangular shape.
16		Malleus, incus, and stapes begin to ossify.	Ossification of the otic capsule begins.
18	Auricle has adult form.		
20	Meatal plug begins to disintegrate.	Tympanic cavity begins to open.	Cochlear duct reaches full length; membranous labyrinth is full size.
22		Antrum begins to develop.	Tunnel of Corti present at all levels; basal turn of cochlea is functional.
23			Otic capsule ossification is complete.
24			Perilymphatic space is completed.
26		Facial nerve makes second genu in adult position.	
28	EAC is fully open.		
30		Malleus and incus are ossified.	
34		Ossicles lie within open middle ear space. Mastoid air cells begin to develop.	

VC, vestibulocochlear; SCC, semicircular canal; EAC, external auditory canal.

Hillocks 1 and 6 are the first to be identifiable separately, but by the sixth week, all are distinct. The lobule also can be identified on the second arch. By the eighth week, the auricle has an identifiable structure, and the contributions of the hillocks to the adult form can be recognized: hillock 1, tragus; hillock 2, crus helicis; hillock 3, ascending helix; hillock 4, horizontal helix, upper portion of scapha, and antihelix; hillock 5, descending helix, middle portion of the scapha, and antihelix; and hillock 6, antitragus and inferior aspect of the helix (2). Although this is the majority view, uncertainty exists about the origin of the crus helicis and ascending helix; some believe these structures can arise from the second arch (3). By approximately 18 weeks gestation, the auricle has achieved essentially adult form, although it continues to grow in childhood with changes continuing into late adult life.

Developmental Anomalies

A wide spectrum of pinna deformity exists, from anotia, in which no development occurs, to a small but normally formed pinna. Microtia encapsulates the wide spectrum

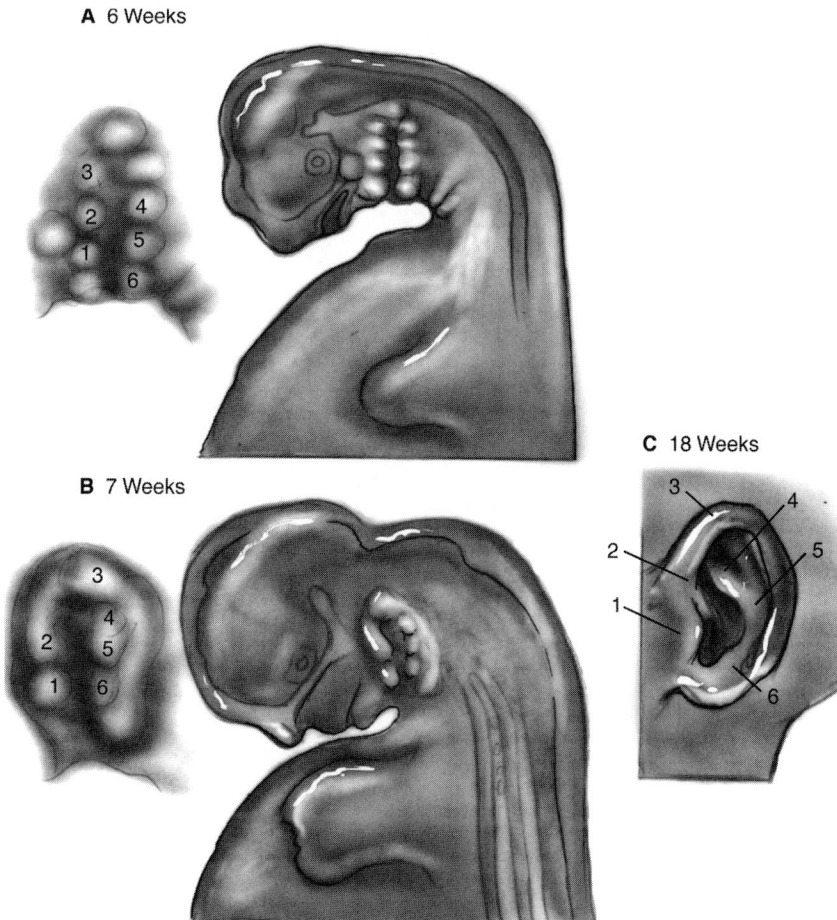

Figure 128.1 Development of the auricle. **A:** Six hillocks form on the first and second branchial arches. All can be identified at 6 weeks' gestation. **B:** Seven-week stage. **C:** By 18 weeks, the adult form is recognizable.

between anotia and normality. The superior portion of the auricle usually is severely malformed or absent. The presence of a deformity of the pinna can indicate further defects of the auditory system. Although this is less common with some minor deformities, severe cases of microtia and anotia are almost always associated with atresia of the external auditory canal and defects of the middle ear (see later). Auricular abnormalities also are present in all the common chromosomal abnormalities and thus are useful markers of these conditions (4). Classification of deformities of the pinna and treatment are discussed in Chapter 180.

DEVELOPMENT OF THE EXTERNAL AND MIDDLE EAR

External Auditory Canal

The external auditory canal begins to form in the fourth week of gestation (Fig. 128.2). The first branchial cleft, between the first and second branchial arches, widens, and the ectoderm proliferates to form a pit, which comes into apposition with the endoderm of the first pharyngeal pouch. This pit is the forerunner of the cartilaginous external auditory canal. This arrangement is temporary, because mesenchymal growth separates the cleft and the pouch.

The deep portion of the external auditory canal is apparent from the eighth week of gestation as a strand of epithelial cells running down to the disk-shaped precursor of the tympanic membrane (3). At approximately 28 weeks' gestation, this epithelial core has canalized from the medial to the lateral aspect to allow communication with the tympanic membrane. The epithelial core is the precursor of the bony external auditory canal.

Tympanic Membrane

The tympanic membrane has a trilaminar origin of ectoderm from the floor of the first branchial cleft laterally as the epidermal layer, endoderm of the first pharyngeal pouch medially as the mucosal layer, and neural crest mesenchyme with cephalic mesoderm interposed as the fibrous layer (5). It is almost horizontal initially but gradually tilts to lie in the adult position at approximately 3 years of age. The bone of the tympanic ring, derived from neural crest mesenchyme, begins to ossify at approximately 3 months.

Middle Ear Cavity

The cavity and lining of the middle ear and eustachian tube develop from the expanding terminal end of the first

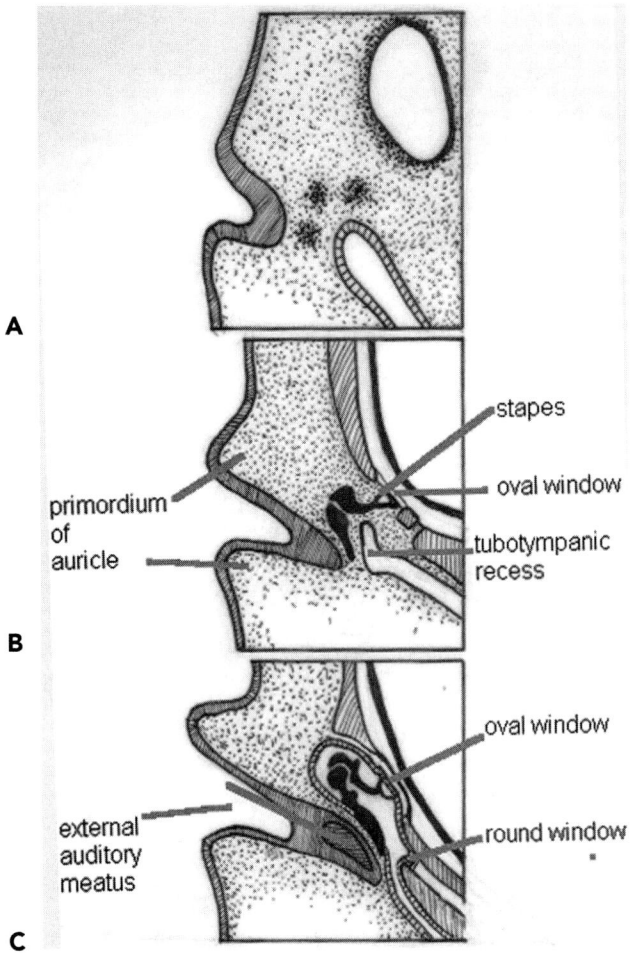

Figure 128.2 Development of the middle ear and ear canal.
A: Week 5. **B:** Week 10. **C:** Week 27.

Ossicles

The exact origin of the ossicles has long been debated. It is certain that the main source is the neural crest mesenchyme of the first and second branchial arches—the Meckel cartilage (first arch) and Reichert cartilage (second arch). The otic capsule has a role in formation of the stapes footplate (8). It is generally agreed that the head of the malleus and the body and short process of the incus are formed from the Meckel cartilage and are initially continuous with the cartilaginous mandible. The mandibular branch of the trigeminal nerve is the nerve of the first arch; thus it supplies the tensor tympani muscle, also a derivative of the first branchial arch. The long process of the incus, handle of the malleus, stapes superstructure, and tympanic surface of the stapes footplate are derived from the Reichert cartilage. The facial nerve is the nerve of the second arch; this supplies the stapedius muscle. The vestibular surface of the footplate is a derivative of the mesoderm of the otic capsule, as is the anular ligament (3) (Fig. 128.3).

The malleus and incus are first formed as cartilaginous models from the sixth week of gestation. They begin to ossify in week 16, and ossification is almost complete by week 30. The stapes appears slightly before the malleus and incus. It is initially ring shaped and penetrated by the stapedial artery, the artery of the second arch, which regresses. By 10 weeks, the stapes has already started to assume the familiar stirrup shape. By the time ossification begins from a solitary center at 16 weeks, the structure is a model of the future stapes. It is reduced in bulk throughout fetal life to develop its slender architectural form.

Maldevelopment

The spectrum of abnormal development in congenital atresia of the external auditory canal parallels the fact that the canal is present, albeit short, and then is absent before achieving the adult form. In the most severe cases of atresia, a bony mass replaces the tympanic ring and forms the lateral wall of the middle ear cavity, the condyle of the mandible lying more posteriorly. In membranous atresia, which is less common, a fibrous mass replaces the external auditory canal. The mildest form of abnormality is stenosis of the external auditory canal, common in Down syndrome, which can be difficult to diagnose unless complications such as proximal cholesteatoma, caused by trapped debris, supervene. Congenital atresia is unilateral in 70% of cases (9).

A further consideration with atresia is the presence of coexisting abnormalities of either the pinna or the middle ear. Associated auricular abnormality exists in 94% of cases of atresia, and the middle ear is frequently deranged (10), in part because all these structures are derived from the first two branchial arches and the intervening branchial cleft. Consequent are further abnormalities of branchial arch derivatives, such as the mandible. Among

pharyngeal pouch with a small contribution from the second pharyngeal pouch. This is apparent in the fourth week of gestation as the tubotympanic recess, which is positioned against the ectoderm of the infolding branchial groove. In the fifth and sixth weeks, the mesenchyme between the branchial cleft and the developing inner ear has condensations destined to become the ossicles. The tympanic cavity continues to develop as the continuing expansion of the endodermal pouch surrounds the ossicles and their supporting structures. It remains a slitlike structure until the fifth month but begins to expand such that the ossicles lie within an open tympanic space by the eighth month (6). Continuation of the tympanic cavity from the epitympanum into the antrum begins at 22 weeks and is complete at birth. Formation of the mastoid air cell system begins late in fetal life; the antrum is present at birth, and continues throughout childhood. The pattern and extent of pneumatization are highly variable. Pneumatization of the petrous pyramid, present in 30% of temporal bones, does not begin until the third year of life (7). At birth, the mastoid tip is not developed but expands through the tractional effect of the sternocleidomastoid attachment.

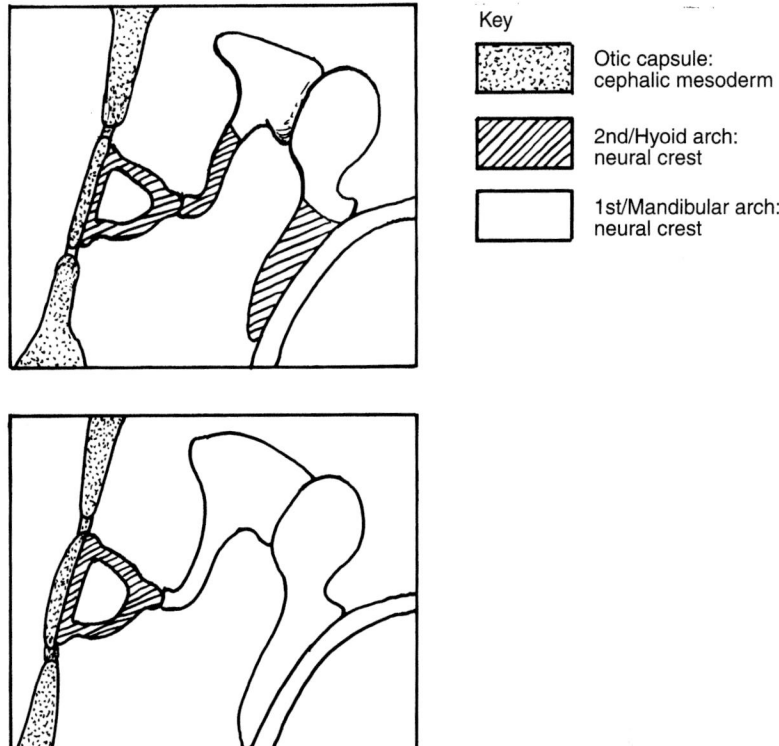

Key

░░░░░ Otic capsule:
       cephalic mesoderm

///// 2nd/Hyoid arch:
       neural crest

□□□□□ 1st/Mandibular arch:
       neural crest

Figure 128.3 Origin of the ossicles—two interpretations.

children with microtia or anotia, 20% to 40% have an identifiable syndromal malformation, such as hemifacial microsomia, Treacher Collins syndrome (mandibulofacial dysostosis), or Goldenhar (oculoauriculovertebral) syndrome (4,11). These syndromal malformations are discussed in Chapter 99.

Ossicular abnormalities also encompass a wide spectrum, from a rudimentary ossicular mass to minor morphologic defects. Middle ear deformities without coexisting outer ear defects are unusual, occurring among fewer than 10% of children with congenital conductive defects (12). This may, however, be an underrepresentation, with cases undiagnosed or ascribed to acquired causes. The malleus is always fixed to a bony atretic plate if present, and incudomalleolar fusion or fixation is a common defect. Stapedial abnormalities are less common. In particular, the footplate can have normal mobility, even with a severe coexisting abnormality, because of its separate development from the otic capsule (13).

Persistent stapedial artery is a condition with an interesting embryologic background, although only approximately 50 cases have been reported worldwide. The stapedial artery is the remnant of the second arch artery, which courses from the aortic sac to the dorsal aorta. This artery regresses at approximately 10 weeks' gestation, and its role is assumed by the precursors of the internal and external carotid arteries. When the artery persists, a vessel arises from the internal carotid artery in the hypotympanum, which courses through the crura of the stapes to the

fallopian canal. It enters the fallopian canal and courses forward to the geniculate ganglion and to the dura. The clinical interest is in cases in which middle ear surgery has been undertaken to manage presumptive otosclerosis or for cochlear implantation (14). Another condition with an embryologic basis is congenital cholesteatoma. This condition is caused by failure of atrophy of epidermoid formation in the anterior mesotympanum.

Although the inner ear develops separately, still an approximately 10% incidence of coexisting inner and middle-outer ear abnormalities is found (13). Careful assessment of the auditory system is mandatory if one is alerted to problems by maldevelopment of the auricle or ear canal. Classification and management of congenital atresia are discussed in Chapter 137.

DEVELOPMENT OF THE FACIAL NERVE

The facial nerve is extremely important in surgical anatomy of the ear. The complex course of the nerve is a result of development of the structures that surround it. The facioacoustic primordium appears in the third week of gestation and has split into distinct seventh and eighth cranial nerves by the fifth week. The facial nerve supplies second arch structures, in particular the muscles of facial expression. Secretomotor and special sensation fibers also are derived from the nervus intermedius, which is distinct by the seventh week. The chorda tympani has appeared in the fourth week, running to the first arch, before supplying sensation to the anterior two thirds of the tongue. The greater superficial petrosal nerve appears in the sixth week. The nerve to the stapedius is identifiable by the seventh week (15). The first genu can be considered the result of the nerve's being pushed forward by the developing otic capsule. The fallopian canal is derived from the mesoderm of the otic capsule. More distally, the fallopian canal is formed partly by the Reichert cartilage (8). In the tenth week, the facial nerve makes its second genu in the middle ear, and its relation to the structures of the external and middle ear is far more anterior than in adults. By week 26, partial closure of the fallopian canal by bone is found, and the nerve has moved posteriorly, coming to lie in a position comparable with that in adults. In a manner similar to its being pushed forward by the otic capsule proximally, the nerve is pulled posteriorly by the growing tympanic ring and structures of the posterior tympanum and pulled inferiorly by the developing meatus and mastoid system. The facial nerve comes to lie between the tympanic and mastoid portions of the temporal bone. Even at birth, the facial nerve, which exits through the superficially positioned stylomastoid foramen, is more superficial than it is in the final adult position, which is attained by means of growth of the mastoid tip.

Maldevelopment

In ears with congenital defects of the outer or middle ear, the implication of this pattern of development is that the facial nerve lies more anteriorly and superficially in the lateral temporal bone. Often this means that the expected position of a new external meatus is crossed by the facial nerve (Fig. 128.4). In atretic ears, the facial nerve is abnormal in as many as 50% of cases (13).

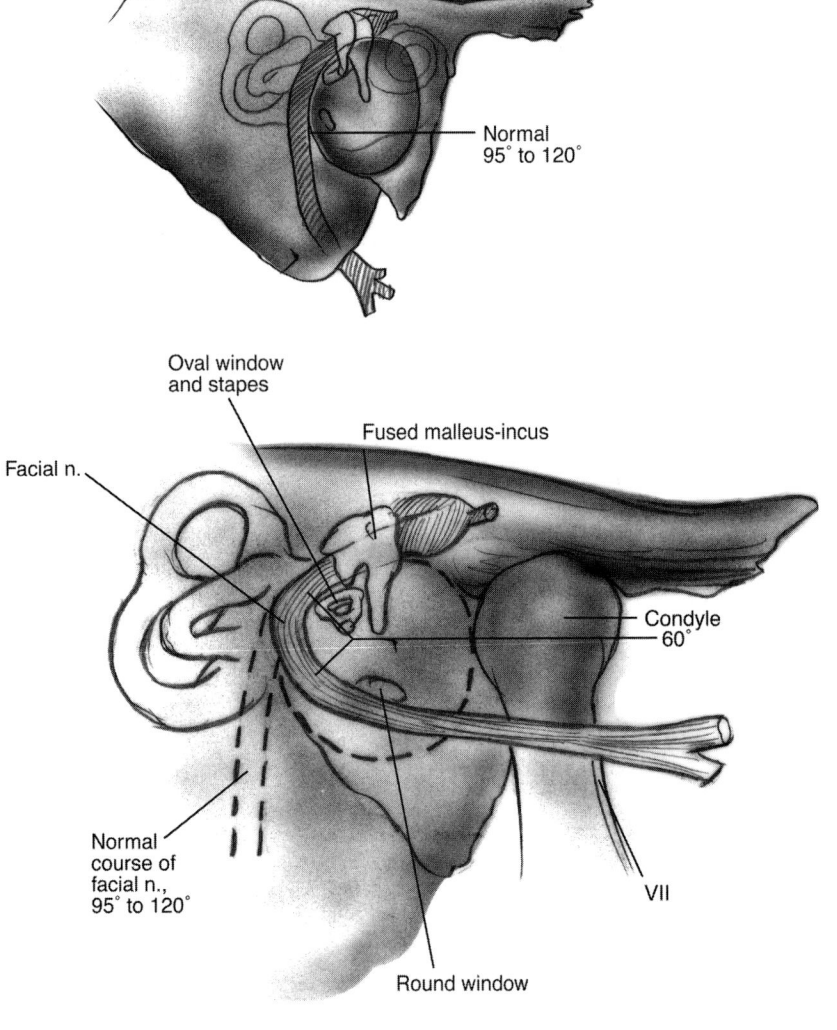

Figure 128.4 The facial nerve is anterior and superficial in atretic ears.

Some congenital disorders of the stapes are related to abnormal development of the facial nerve. Anterior displacement of the nerve at the 6-week stage can prevent the developing stapes from coming into contact with the otic capsule; the result is rudimentary formation (16). The facial nerve also can divide around the stapes. Dehiscence of the fallopian canal is common enough for it to be considered a normal variant, present in approximately 25% of temporal bones. The most common site is above the oval window, although sufficient dehiscence to allow prolapse over the oval window is much less common.

DEVELOPMENT OF THE INNER EAR

Membranous Labyrinth

The internal ear phylogenetically predates the other components of the ear and is accordingly the first part to develop. At the end of the third week of gestation, the otic placode can be differentiated on the lateral surface of the cephalic end of the embryo as a thickening of ectoderm in contact with hindbrain portion of the closing neural tube. The neural tube, also derived from ectoderm, is destined to become the central nervous system. This contact is short-lived. By the time the neural tube closes, a layer of thin ectoderm separates it from the neural epithelium. The placode invaginates itself to become a pit and a closed sac, the otocyst or otic vesicle, the precursor of the membranous labyrinth (Fig. 128.5). Positioned between the second and

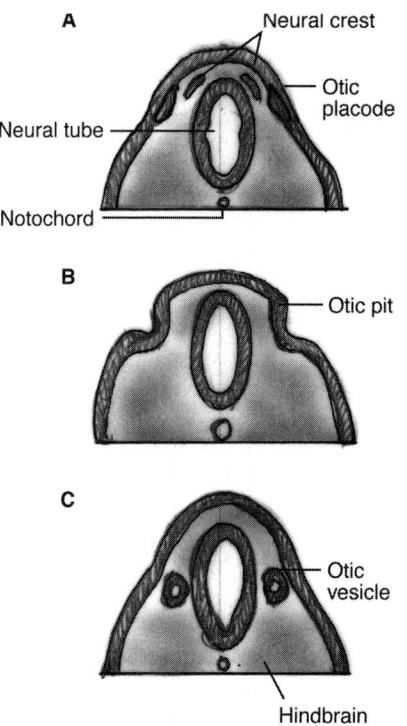

Figure 128.5   A–C: Early development of the inner ear in the third and fourth weeks of gestation—formation of the otocyst from the otic placode.

third branchial arches, it is predictable that the otocyst is supplied by the eighth cranial nerve. It migrates inward, changing shape and growing dramatically so that it achieves adult form by the tenth week and adult size by 20 weeks (17) (Fig. 128.6).

The otocyst lengthens more than it widens. The cranial portion becomes marked off as the developing endolymphatic duct. The caudal portion is destined to become the cochlear duct, and the intermediate portion, the utriculosaccular area, is the vestibular precursor. These distinctions are discernible in the fifth week of gestation. The vestibular portion begins to take shape slightly before the cochlear portion, in keeping with its older phylogenetic status. From the utricular part of the vestibular pouch, three outpocketings appear, which are converted, through fusion of the central epithelium, into semicircular canals. The superior canal is completed first, in the sixth week. The posterior canal is next to be completed, and the lateral canal is last. The utricle and saccule start to develop in the sixth week and form the utriculosaccular duct. The cochlear duct also begins to grow from the saccule in the sixth week with recognizable narrowing of the communication; the ductus reuniens is visible by the eighth week. The cochlear duct grows rapidly, having 1.5 turns at 8 weeks and the full 2.5 turns at 10 weeks, although it does not reach full length until 20 weeks (2).

The sensory epithelia of the vestibular system, the three cristae and two maculae and the organ of Corti in the cochlea, are derived from the ectodermal epithelium of the otocyst. These six areas, which initially are close together, develop in the wall of the membranous labyrinth (3). The maculae develop in the seventh week of gestation by means of intense proliferation of the epithelium accompanied by cell differentiation. The distinctive cells and otoconial membrane are apparent by week 12. Development of the cristae parallels this event; they are distinguishable at 8 weeks and have reached adult form at 23 weeks.

The sensory epithelium of the cochlea begins to develop in the seventh week as the duct itself grows and begins to coil. Lying on the medial wall, the layers of the epithelium organize into two ridges and spiral along the length of the cochlea. The larger inner ridge differentiates into the inner hair cells and tectorial membrane. The smaller outer ridge differentiates into the outer hair cells (18). The supporting cells arise from both ridges. The hair cells are identifiable from week 11, the inner hair cells appearing marginally before the outer hair cells at the same position along the basilar membrane (6). Hair-cell development is initially apparent in the midbasal region of the cochlea and moves toward the apex, maturation of the base preceding that of the apex by 1 to 2 weeks, although the most basal portion of the cochlear lags slightly behind the midbasal portion. The supporting cells develop in the same direction, and at the 21-week stage, the tunnel of Corti is present at all levels. At approximately this time, the organ of Corti becomes functional, at least in its basal

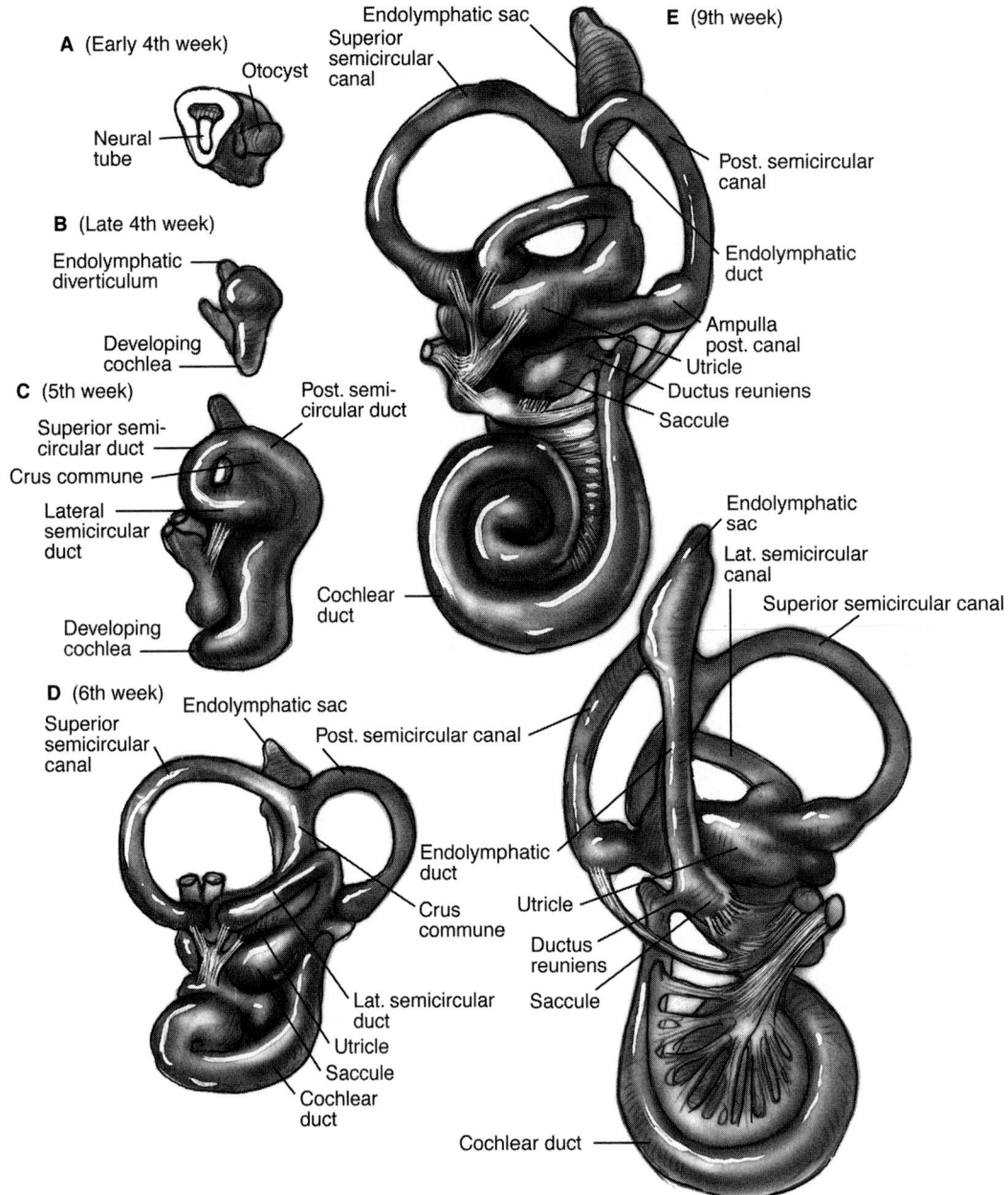

A (Early 4th week)

Otocyst

Neural tube

B (Late 4th week)

Endolymphatic diverticulum

Developing cochlea

C (5th week)

Superior semi-circular duct

Crus commune

Lateral semicircular duct

Developing cochlea

Post. semi-circular duct

Cochlear duct

D (6th week)

Superior semicircular canal

Endolymphatic sac

Post. semicircular canal

Endolymphatic duct

Crus commune

Lat. semicircular duct

Utricle

Saccule

Cochlear duct

Endolymphatic sac

Superior semicircular canal

E (9th week)

Post. semicircular canal

Endolymphatic duct

Ampulla post. canal

Utricle

Ductus reuniens

Saccule

Endolymphatic sac

Lat. semicircular canal

Superior semicircular canal

Utricle

Ductus reuniens

Saccule

Cochlear duct

Figure 128.6   A–E: Development of the membranous labyrinth from gestational weeks 4 through 9.

turn (2). The shape of the cochlear duct changes starting at approximately week 12 from oval to triangular, the changes first happening in the basal turn. The surrounding mesoderm of the osseous labyrinth participates in this process. The endolymphatic duct and sac are the only parts of the inner ear that continue to grow into the third trimester. Full size is not attained until adulthood (19).

Development of Innervation of the Membranous Labyrinth

The facioacoustic primordium appears in the third week of gestation. It does not, however, have a uniform origin. The

vestibulocochlear ganglia arise from ectoderm of the primitive otocyst, having split away from the epithelium in the third week. Although destined to innervate different portions of the inner ear, the vestibulocochlear ganglia appear to arise from a common site on the otic epithelium. The neural crest is a small additional source of supporting cells of the ganglion (5).

From the vestibulocochlear ganglia, fibers grow toward their destined target organs, the inductive process driven by the target organs. While the otocyst is dividing into its vestibular and cochlear portions, the vestibulocochlear ganglion divides into a superior and an inferior division. The fibers of the superior division pass to innervate the superior and lateral ampullae of the semicircular canal and the utricle. The inferior division sends fibers to the posterior ampulla and the saccule. The remaining portion becomes the spiral ganglion of the cochlea (2). As the cochlear duct grows and coils, the ganglion follows it to give its characteristic configuration. At approximately the ninth week, nerve fibers grow to enter the sensory epithelium, and synaptic connections are identifiable as the hair cells begin to differentiate in week 11. The inner hair cells are innervated before the outer hair cells; afferent innervation precedes efferent innervation, and the basal turn precedes the apex in development (18).

Development of the Osseous Labyrinth

The most important aspect of development of the perilymph-filled osseous labyrinth is a resorptive process in the mesoderm that separates the membranous labyrinth from the developing bony otic capsule. In the eighth week of gestation, the vascular precartilage that surrounds the membranous labyrinth develops vacuoles in its structure that coalesce to leave the perilymphatic space. This process begins around the utricle and saccule and progresses outward from there. The part around the cochlear duct destined to be the scala tympani precedes the scala vestibuli, and development is further advanced in the basal turn than in the apical turn. The perilymphatic space is completed by week 24 (8). The origin of the precartilage is cephalic mesoderm with a small contribution from neural crest cells. The cephalic mesoderm contributes to the basilar membrane, Reissner membrane, and the stria vascularis, which also has cells derived from the neural crest (20,21).

Development of the Otic Capsule

It is remarkable that the bony otic capsule achieves its adult size by week 22 of gestation. Arising from cephalic mesoderm, a precartilaginous precursor appears in the seventh week. From week 8 to week 16, the developing labyrinth is surrounded by an enlarging cartilaginous model, which ossifies in three layers over a 7-week period from a total of 14 centers (7,8). Solidification is completed in the early postnatal stage; the petrous (stony) nature of the otic capsule results from the compactness of the bone of the original ossification centers. The oval (vestibular) window is formed where the developing stapes abuts the cartilaginous model of the otic capsule in the ninth week. This section becomes the vestibular surface of the footplate. The rim of the footplate and the facing rim of the window, derivatives of the otic capsule precursor, do not turn into bone but remain cartilage; the intervening tissue becomes the anular ligament. The round (tympanic) window forms adjacent to the basal turn of the cochlea, where cartilage is not turned into bone but is converted into the fibrous tissue of the secondary tympanic membrane.

The vestibular aqueduct forms around the endolymphatic duct and sac but is late in achieving full ossification (8). The cochlear aqueduct forms in the mesoderm, which ossifies to become the otic capsule, and is first apparent as an outpouching of the subarachnoid space. Progressive ossification causes curving and lengthening of the cochlear aqueduct, which has two sections. The otic capsule section, which has a narrow cochlear opening just inside the round window membrane, becomes progressively narrower from its appearance in the fourth month to the ossification of the otic capsule at week 23. The medial petrous apex portion enlarges throughout the third trimester, and it is in this section that postnatal elongation of the cochlear aqueduct takes place. The length in a newborn infant is 3.5 mm; the average length in an adult is 10 mm (22). The internal acoustic meatus forms around the vestibulocochlear nerve and internal auditory blood vessels as well as the facial nerve. The facial nerve, however, is cranial to the eighth nerve, and its path is deflected by the growing otic capsule, although the bony fallopian canal proximal to the second genu is of otic capsule derivation. The adult position of the facial nerve in the internal acoustic meatus is in the anterosuperior quadrant.

Maldevelopment

A practical categorization divides inner ear anomalies into those affecting the osseous and membranous labyrinth and those affecting the membranous labyrinth alone (23). As many as 20% of patients with congenital sensorineural hearing loss (SNHL) fall into the first category, which can be identified with radiologic techniques (24,25). In the absence of histologic confirmation, however, accurate categorization ultimately reflects the sensitivity of the contemporary imaging modality (26). Inner ear abnormalities can be caused by arrested or aberrant development (Table 128.2). The variable but frequent coexistence of deformities involving the component parts of the labyrinth suggests a number of different factors can be involved: The anomaly can be genetically predetermined, an insult can occur before the fifth week, or the separate portions of the developing system can be variably susceptible to teratogenic insult.

The most common histopathologic finding in congenital deafness is cochleosaccular dysplasia due to incomplete development of the caudal portion of the otocyst, the pars inferior, first described by Scheibe in 1892 (24). The organ of Corti typically is partially or completely missing, the cochlear duct and saccule are collapsed, and the stria vascularis is degenerated. The utricle and semicircular canals are normal. The normality can be explained in part by the earlier development of the vestibular system. Basal-turn dysplasia is the mild end of this spectrum. Complete membranous labyrinthine dysplasia (Bing–Siebenmann) is rare and is the most severe membranous abnormality.

Most combined membranous–osseous labyrinth abnormalities appear to be caused by arrested development

TABLE 128.2

CLASSIFICATION OF CONGENITAL INNER EAR MALFORMATIONS

Malformations limited to the membranous labyrinth
 Complete membranous labyrinthine dysplasia
  (Bing-Siebenmann)
 Limited membranous labyrinthine dysplasia
  Cochleosaccular dysplasia (Scheibe)
  Cochlear basal turn dysplasia
Malformations of the osseous and membranous labyrinth
 Complete labyrinthine aplasia (Michel)
 Cochlear anomalies
  Cochlear aplasia
  Cochlear hypoplasia
  Common cavity
  Incomplete partition (Mondini)
 Labyrinthine anomalies
  Semicircular canal dysplasia
  Semicircular canal aplasia
 Aqueductal anomalies
  Enlargement of the vestibular aqueduct
  Enlargement of the cochlear aqueduct
 Internal auditory canal abnormalities
  Narrow internal auditory canal
  Wide internal auditory canal

From Jackler RK. Congenital malformations of the inner ear. In: Cummings CW, Fredrickson JM, Harker LA, et al. *Otolaryngology: head and neck surgery.* St. Louis: Mosby–Year Book, 1993:2576–2771, with permission.

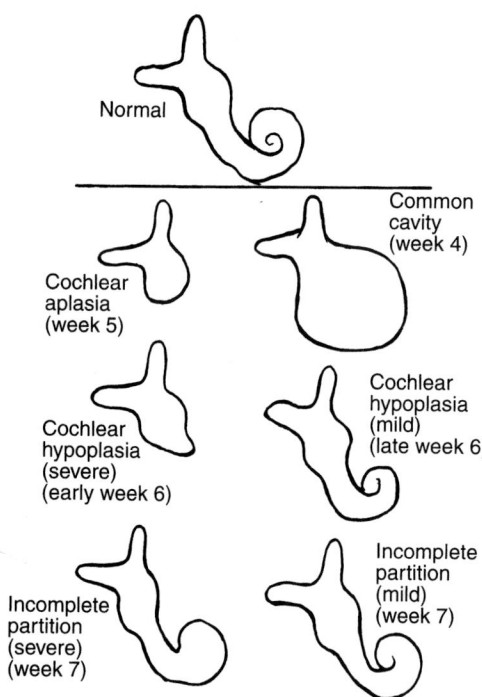

Figure 128.7 Stages of cochlear maldevelopment.

between the fourth and eighth weeks of gestation. The appearance of most malformed ears is in accord with the stages of labyrinthine development (Fig. 128.7). The most severe abnormality, complete aplasia (Michel malformation), is extremely rare and presumably is caused by failure of the otic vesicle to develop. Cochlear aplasia, hypoplasia, and incomplete partition are a spectrum occurring from arrest at gestational weeks 5, 6, and 7. The common cavity can arise from arrest at 4 weeks or can be caused by later aberrant development. Dysplasia of the semicircular canals is caused by failure of central epithelial fusion and is 4 times as common as aplasia of the semicircular canals. The lateral semicircular canal (LSCC) is most commonly affected because it develops later, and lateral dysplasia of the semicircular canals can occur as the sole abnormality. Approximately 40% of ears with osseous cochlear abnormalities have concomitant abnormalities of the semicircular canals (23). Bilateral involvement with osseous inner ear deformities is the rule, the same morphologic abnormality occurring in both ears (23).

An enlarged vestibular aqueduct is the most common radiologically detectable abnormality of the inner ear and may be due to acquired or genetic influences (27). The vestibular duct may be abnormally broad and short because of premature arrest of development or as a consequence of increased cerebrospinal fluid pressure. As part of the genetic Pendred syndrome, large vestibular aqueduct can be associated with disturbance of thyroid organification resulting

from mutations in *SLC26A4*, a chloride-iodide transporter gene (28).

Whereas the vestibular aqueduct forms around an ectodermal structure, the cochlear aqueduct is a secondary structure around a mesodermal derivative. Developmental aberrations of the otic capsule are expected to cause absence of rather than enlargement of the cochlear aqueduct. It is likely that radiographic enlargement of the cochlear aqueduct is an exceedingly rare or even nonexistent malformation (22). Absence of the cochlear aqueduct is as yet unreported.

Of all the inner ear structures, the internal auditory canal is most variable in size, length, and configuration. Absence of a bony partition between a large bulbous lateral end of the canal and the inner ear is associated with stapes gusher (DFN3). Because of a mutation in a developmental transcription factor gene *POU3F4*, this finding contraindicates stapedectomy for congenital stapes fixation. A narrow internal auditory canal can indicate failure of development of the eighth cranial nerve. If the internal auditory canal has a diameter less than 3 mm and normal facial function is present, it is likely that only the facial nerve is present. This condition is a contraindication to cochlear implantation (29).

The ability to identify maldevelopment of the inner ear is dependent on the sensitivity of radiologic imaging and experience of the clinician reviewing the images (30). Morphologic abnormalities of the bony labyrinth are identified in approximately 20% to 40% of patients with childhood SNHL undergoing temporal bone computerized tomography (CT) scan. Although the identification of severe morphogenetic

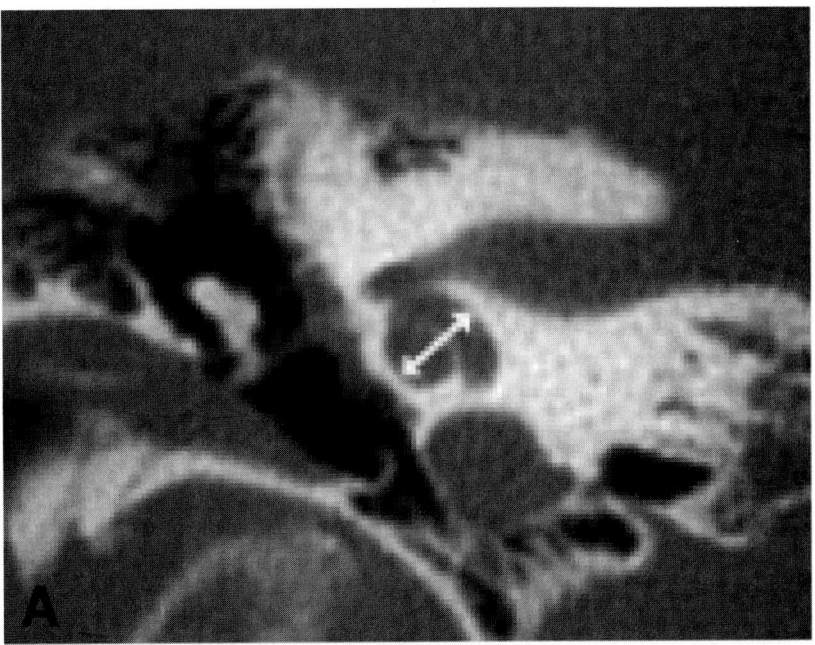

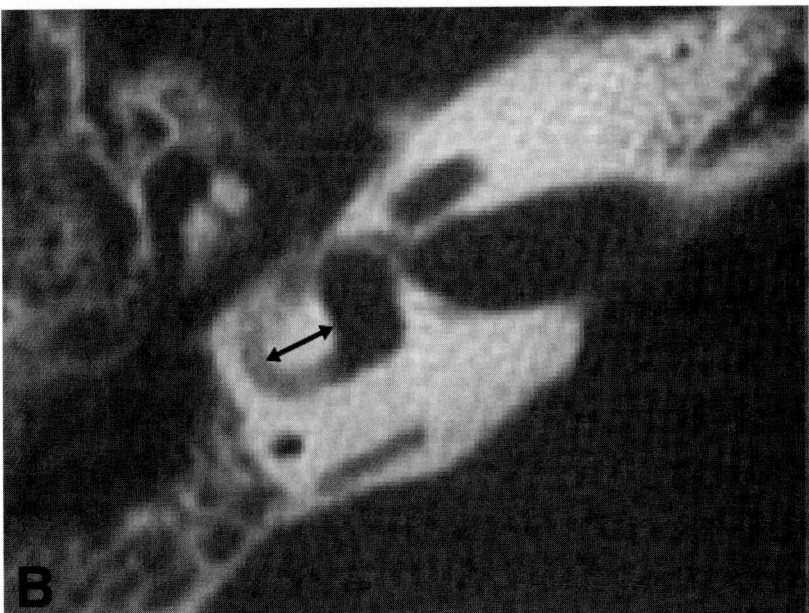

Figure 128.8 A, B: Routine measurements on computerized tomography of the temporal bone of the cochlear height on coronal images **(A)** and the bony island of the lateral semicircular canal on axial images **(B)** will complement visual analysis and greatly aid in the identification of inner ear malformations.

malformations such as complete labyrinthine aplasia or Michel deformity and common cavity deformity is not difficult (accounting for only 1% of abnormalities), the detection of milder radiologic abnormalities is dependent on the experience of the clinician. Nearly one third of these less-severe dysplasias are missed by simple visual inspection of the radiologic images. Introduction of standardized measurements of inner ear structures, such as the dimension of the vestibular aqueduct and the internal auditory canal, and more recently, the vertical height of the cochlea on coronal scan and of the central bony island within the LSCC on axial scan or temporal bone CT can complement visual analysis and greatly aid in the identification of inner ear malformations (Fig. 128.8) (30).

CONTROL OF EAR DEVELOPMENT

Molecular–genetic techniques with knockout and mutant animals have helped to elucidate the development of the ear. Development of both the outer and the middle ear is controlled by genes that affect first and second branchial arch identity as well as hindbrain segmentation and identity. Genetic defects range from the complete absence of structural elements to hypomorphism or duplication. New cartilage elements can arise. The phenotypes are not neatly arranged by branchial arch, reflecting functional redundancy in the system.

Invagination and inward movement of the otocyst are under control of external tissue interactions, particularly the hindbrain. Information from knockouts and mutants shows that the genes that control hindbrain segmentation, especially rhombomeres 5 and 6, and genes expressed in neural crest cells influence inner ear development. The inner ear consequently has an indirect requirement for neural genes also expressed in ear tissue. Absence of these genes can cause dramatic changes in inner ear development. For example, inactivation of the transcription factor gene *Hoxa1* produces a primitive cystic inner ear. The vestibular and cochlear apparatus are under separate genetic control; the *Pax2* knockout mouse has a normal vestibular apparatus but has no cochlea or spiral ganglion. The LSCC seems particularly sensitive to genetic perturbations, which is in accord with its being the most commonly abnormal semicircular canal. The various structural elements of the otic vesicle are under independent genetic control for specification, morphogenesis, or both (31).

- of the bony otic capsule ossifies from 14 centers between week 16 and week 23. It is adult size at 22 weeks.
- Congenital inner ear abnormalities are divided into those affecting the membranous labyrinth alone and those affecting both the bony and membranous labyrinths. The latter appear to be caused by arrested development between weeks 4 and 8 of gestation. They account for only 20% of cases of abnormality but can be diagnosed with imaging techniques.

HIGHLIGHTS

- The auricle develops from six ectodermal hillocks arising from the first and second branchial arches. Most of the adult pinna is of second arch origin.
- The ectoderm of the first branchial cleft forms the external auditory canal. The cartilaginous canal forms first and the bony canal later, from medial to lateral, at 28 weeks. The outer layer of the tympanic membrane is derived from this source.
- The tympanic cavity is derived from the first pharyngeal pouch and develops from the fourth week of gestation. It remains a slitlike structure as the endodermal pouch surrounds the ossicles and their supports to the fifth month and expands so the ossicles lie in a cavity in the eighth month.
- The ossicles develop from the neural crest mesenchyme of the first and second branchial arches, except for the vestibular surface of the footplate and the anular ligament, which arise from the mesoderm of the otic capsule.
- The facial nerve comes to lie in its adult position only late in fetal life. It consequently is anterior and superficial in ears with congenital malformations of the middle or outer ear.
- The membranous labyrinth develops from the otic placode. It invaginates to become the otocyst, subdivides into vestibular and cochlear compartments, and grows and dramatically changes shape to achieve adult form at 10 weeks and adult size at 20 weeks of gestation.
- The organ of Corti becomes functional in its basal turn at approximately 20 to 24 weeks.
- The vestibulocochlear ganglia are derived from the otic placode. They innervate six areas of neuroepithelial ectoderm on the wall of the membranous labyrinth that become the three cristae, two maculae, and the spiral organ of Corti.
- The perilymphatic space forms by means of resorption of precartilage from week 8 to week 24. The cartilage model

REFERENCES

1. Peck JE. Development of hearing, I: phylogeny. *J Am Acad Audiol* 1994;5:291–299.
2. Sulik KK. Embryology of the ear. In: Gorlin RJ, Toriello HV, Cohen MM, eds. *Hereditary hearing loss and its syndromes.* New York: Oxford University Press, 1995:22–42.
3. Van De Water TR, Noden DM, Maderson PFA. Embryology of the ear: outer, middle and inner. In: Alberti PW, Ruben RJ, eds. *Otologic medicine and surgery.* New York: Churchill Livingstone, 1988:3–28.
4. Carey JC. External ear. In: Stevenson RE, Hall JG, Goodman RM, eds. *Human malformations and related anomalies.* New York: Oxford University Press, 1993:193–220.
5. Noden DM. Cell movements and control of patterned tissue assembly during craniofacial development. *Development* 1988;103(suppl):121–140.
6. Peck JE. Development of hearing, II: embryology. *J Am Acad Audiol* 1994;5:359–364.
7. Nager GT. *Pathology of the ear and temporal bone.* Baltimore: Williams & Wilkins, 1993.
8. Donaldson JA, Duckert LG, Lambert PM, et al. *Anson-Donaldson surgical anatomy of the temporal bone.* New York: Raven Press, 1992.
9. De La Cruz A, Linthicum FHJ, Luxford WM. Congenital atresia of the external auditory canal. *Laryngoscope* 1985;95:421–427.
10. Jafek BW, Nager GT, Strife J, et al. Congenital aural atresia: an analysis of 311 cases. *Trans Am Acad Ophthalmol Otol* 1975;80:588–595.
11. Kaye C, Rollnick BR, Hauck WW, et al. Microtia and associated anomalies: statistical analysis. *Am J Med Genet* 1989;34:574–578.
12. Bergstrom L. Assessment and consequence of malformation of the middle ear. In: Gorlin RJ, ed. *Morphogenesis and malformation of the ear: birth defects.* Original article series XVI(4). New York: Alan R. Liss, 1980:217–241.
13. Cressman WR, Pensak MI. Surgical aspects of congenital aural atresia. *Otolaryngol Clin North Am* 1994;27:621–632.
14. Wardrop P, Kerr AIG, Moussa SA. Persistent stapedial artery preventing successful cochlear implantation. *Ann Otol Rhinol Laryngol* 1987;128(suppl 12):443–445.
15. Sataloff RT. Embryology of the facial nerve and its clinical applications. *Laryngoscope* 1990;100:969–984.
16. Lambert PR. Congenital absence of the oval window. *Laryngoscope* 1990;100:37–40.
17. Streeter GL. The histogenesis and growth of the otic capsule and its contained periotic tissue spaces in the human embryo. *Carnegie Contrib Embryol* 1910;7:5–54.
18. Pujol R. Morphology, synaptology and electrophysiology of the developing cochlea. *Acta Otolaryngol (Stockh)* 1985;421(suppl):5–9.
19. Fisher NA, Curtin HD. Radiology of congenital hearing loss. *Otolaryngol Clin North Am* 1994;27:511–531.
20. Hilding WJ, Ginzberg RD. Pigmentation of the stria vascularis. *Acta Otolaryngol (Stockh)* 1977;84:24–37.
21. Van De Water TR. Tissue interactions and cell differentiation: neurone-sensory cell interaction during otic development. *Development* 1988;103(suppl):185–193.
22. Jackler RK, Hwang PH. Enlargement of the cochlear aqueduct: fact or fiction? *Otolaryngol Head Neck Surg* 1993;109:14–25.
23. Jackler RK, Luxford WM, House WF. Congenital malformations of the inner ear: a classification based on embryogenesis. *Laryngoscope* 1987;97(suppl 40):2–14.

24. Jackler RK. Congenital malformations of the inner ear. In: Cummings CW, Flint PW, Harker LA, et al., eds. *Otolaryngology–head and neck surgery.* St. Louis: Elsevier Mosby, 2005:4398–4421.
25. Carey JC. Inner ear. In: Stevenson RE, Hall JG, Goodman RM, eds. *Human malformations and related anomalies.* New York: Oxford University Press, 1993:231–236.
26. Purcell DD, Fischbein N, Lalwani AK. Identification of previously "undetectable" abnormalities of the bony labyrinth with computed tomography measurement. *Laryngoscope* 2003;113:1908–1911.
27. Jackler RJ, De La Cruz A. The large vestibular aqueduct syndrome. *Laryngoscope* 1989;99:1238–1243.
28. Li XC, Everett LA, Lalwani AK, et al. A mutation in PDS causes non-syndromic recessive deafness. *Nat Genet* 1998;18:215–217.
29. Papsin BC. Cochlear implantation in children with anomalous cochleovestibular anatomy. *Laryngoscope* 2005;115(suppl 106):1–26.
30. Purcell D, Johnson J, Fischbein N, et al. Establishment of normative cochlear and vestibular measurements to aid in the diagnosis of inner ear malformations. *Otolaryngol Head Neck Surg* 2003;128:78–87.
31. Fekete DM. Development of the vertebrate ear: insights from knockouts and mutants. *Trends Neurosci* 1999;22:262–269.

129

Anatomy and Physiology of Hearing

John H. Mills   *Samir S. Khariwala*   *Peter C. Weber*

This chapter provides a brief summary of the most basic features of the anatomy and physiology of the ear. It is divided into sections on the external and middle ear, cochlea, and central nervous system (CNS). The focus is on the anatomic and physiologic bases of audition with an effort directed at functional features. Surgical anatomy, vasculature, and eustachian tube function are not discussed.

EXTERNAL EAR

The external ear consists of the pinna (auricle) and the external auditory canal from the meatus to the tympanic membrane (Fig. 129.1). The pinna of humans is composed mostly of cartilage and has no useful muscles. The center of the pinna, the concha, leads to the external auditory meatus, which is about 2.5 cm long. The lateral third of the canal is the cartilaginous portion. It contains cerumen-producing glands and hair follicles. The remaining medial two thirds is the bony portion, including an epithelial lining over the tympanic membrane (1).

The external ear and the head have a passive but important role in hearing because of their acoustic properties. The concha, or bowl of the auricle, has a resonance of about 5 kHz, and the irregular surface of the pinna introduces other resonances and antiresonances. These acoustic features are useful to help differentiate whether sound sources are in front of the listener or behind.

The external auditory canal (EAC) is essentially a tube that is open at one end and closed at the other; thus the EAC behaves like a quarter-wave resonator. The resonant frequency (f_0) is determined by the length of the tube; the curvature of the tube is irrelevant. For a tube of 2.5 cm, the resonant frequency is approximately 3.5 kHz:

$$f_0 = \text{Velocity of sound @ } 350\text{m/s}/(4 \times 2.5 \text{ cm})$$

A flat, wide-band sound measured in a sound field is changed considerably by the acoustic properties of the head and external ear. As Figure 129.2 demonstrates, a gain of about 15 dB occurs in the 3-kHz range of the human, cat, and chinchilla, and 10 dB between 2 and 5 kHz. The acoustic properties of the external ear are one of the reasons noise-induced hearing losses occur first and most prominently at the 4-kHz frequency region (boilermaker notch).

In addition to the prominence of noise-induced hearing loss in the 4-kHz region, the acoustic properties of the head and external ear have an important role in several hearing functions. In localization of sound sources, the head acts as an attenuator at frequencies at which the width of the head is greater than the wavelength of the sound. Thus at frequencies greater than 2 kHz, a *head shadow effect* occurs, in which interaural intensity differences of 5 to 15 dB are used to localize sound sources. At lower frequencies, at which the wavelength of the sound is larger than the width of the head, little attenuation is provided by the head. Interaural time differences (~0.6 ms for sound to travel across the head) are the salient cues for localization. The head-shadow effect is the reason right-handed hunters using rifles and shotguns have larger hearing losses in their left ears than in their right ears and vice versa. The muzzle of the gun, where the acoustic energy is greatest, is closer to the left ear, and the right ear is protected by the head-shadow effect.

The 10- to 15-dB gain provided by the external ear in the 3- to 5-kHz region is useful for improving the detection

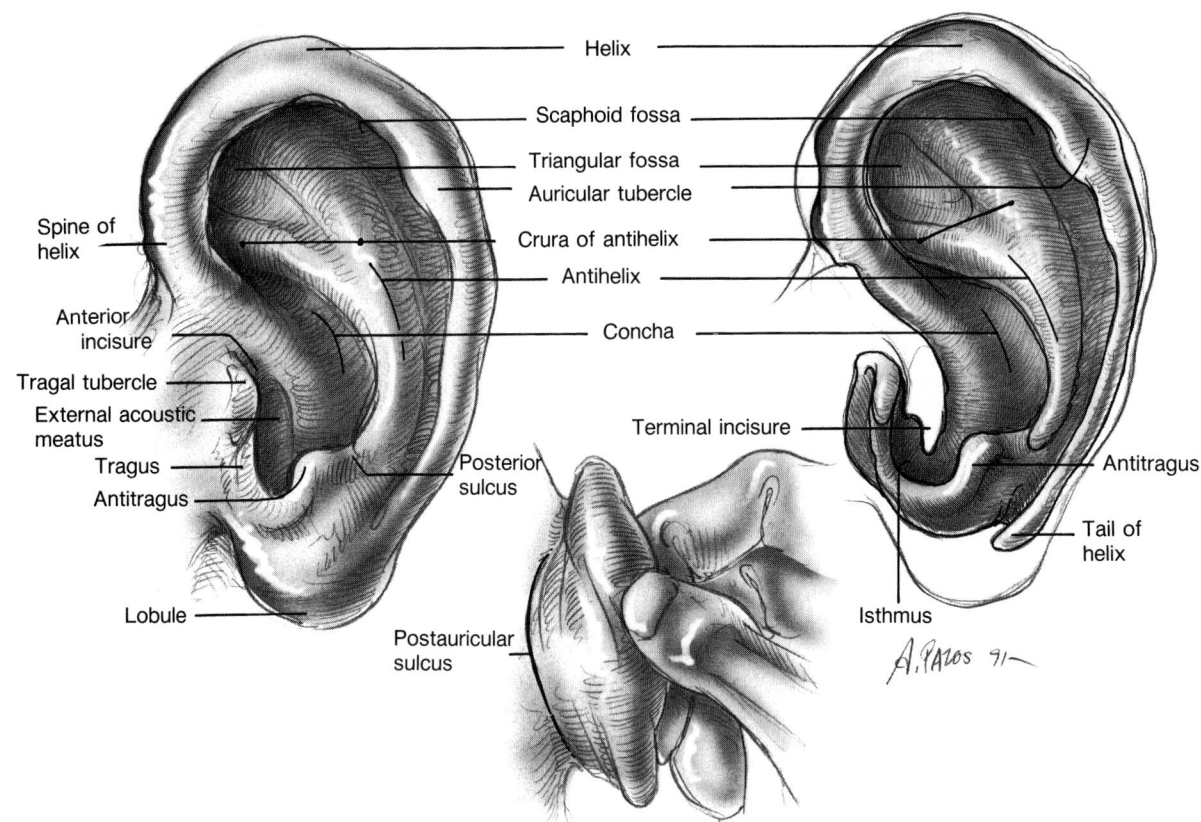

Figure 129.1 External ear.

and recognition of low-energy, high-frequency sounds such as voiceless fricatives. The importance of the acoustic properties of the external ear and head is reflected in hearing-aid design and evaluations. Finally, the resonance of the external canal is approximately 8 kHz in infants and decreases to adult values after approximately 2.5 years of age. This developmental feature has several

clinical implications, especially for sound-field testing and for hearing-aid design and evaluation of infants.

MIDDLE EAR

The middle ear transmits acoustic energy from the air-filled EAC to the fluid-filled cochlea. It functions as an impedance-matching device inasmuch as it couples the low impedance of air to the high impedance of the fluid-filled cochlea. The impedance match is achieved in three ways. The first and most important factor is that the effective vibratory area of the tympanic membrane is approximately 17 to 20 times greater than the effective vibratory area of the stapes footplate (Fig. 129.3). A second factor involves the lever action of the ossicular chain. The arm of the long process of the incus is shorter, by a factor of 1.3, than the length of the manubrium and neck of the malleus. A third and minor factor is the shape of the tympanic membrane. The combined result of these three factors is a pressure gain of approximately 25 to 30 dB. The variance in published measurements of the transformer ratio is noteworthy. With the exception of studies of acoustic impedance of the ear, most data are from studies of human cadavers, with all of their shortcomings, or of animals, usually cats. In addition to its role in the transfer of power to the inner ear, the tympanic

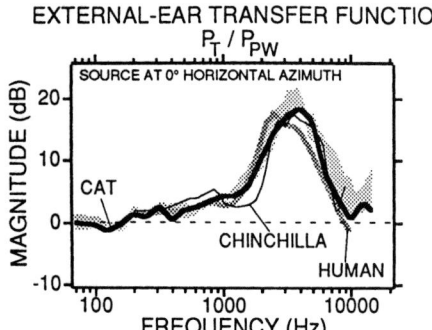

Figure 129.2 Ratio of sound pressure measured at the tympanic membrane to sound pressure measured in a sound field. Acoustic properties of the head, pinna, and external auditory meatus in three species (cat, chinchilla, and human). (From Rosowski JH. The effects of external and middle ear filters on noise-induced hearing loss. *J Acoust Soc Am* 1991;90:124, with permission.)

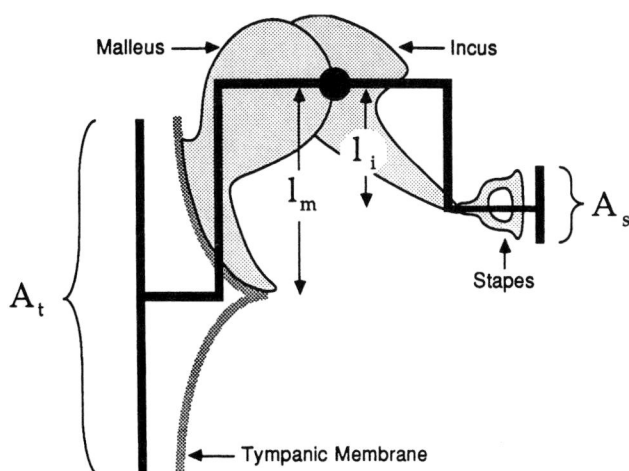

Figure 129.3 Schematic of ossicular chain and tympanic membrane shows the differences in area and vibratory pattern of the ossicles. (From Relkin EM. Introduction to the analysis of middle ear function. In: Jahn HF, Santos-Sacchi J, eds. *Physiology of the ear.* New York: Raven Press, 1988:103, with permission.)

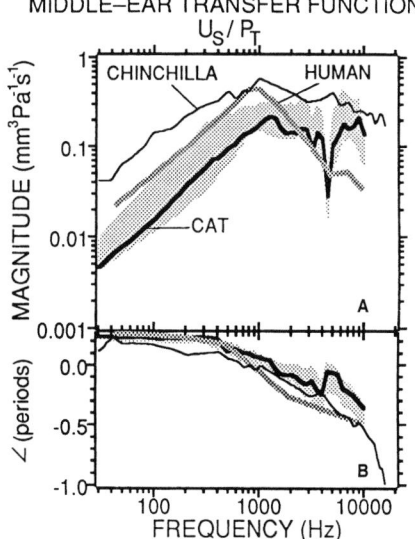

Figure 129.4 A: Transfer function of the middle ear in chinchilla, cat, and human. *Ordinate* is the ratio of the volume velocity of the stapes to sound pressure at the tympanic membrane. **B:** Phase shift of stapes footplate in relation to tympanic membrane. (From Rosowski JH. The effects of external and middle ear filters on noise-induced hearing loss. *J Acoust Soc Am* 1991;90:124, with permission.)

membrane protects the middle ear space from foreign material of the ear canal and maintains the air cushion that prevents insufflation of foreign material from the nasopharynx through the eustachian tube.

The vibratory behavior of the ossicular chain is described in Figure 129.3. The transformer action of the tympanic membrane and ossicular chain provides for relatively efficient transfer of power to the inner ear, and the fidelity of sound transmission across the middle ear is outstanding. Distortion of sound signals does not occur in the middle ear, even for input signals with sound levels greater than 130 dB sound pressure level (SPL).

The middle ear, including the tympanic membrane, ossicular chain with supporting ligaments, and middle ear space, can be viewed as a passive mechanical system with both mass and compliant elements and therefore resonant properties. This linear system is coupled to the cochlea, which contributes a large resistance. The result is a middle ear system that is highly damped and linear and has a wide frequency response. The input–output function or transfer function of the middle ear is shown in Figure 129.4A. The ratio of the volume velocity of the stapes to sound pressure at the tympanic membrane increases in humans to approximately 800 to 900 Hz, which is the resonant frequency of the middle ear, and decreases at higher frequencies. Phase shift or time lag between movement of the tympanic membrane and the stapes generally increases with frequency (Fig. 129.4B). Although the middle ear is an impressive system in terms of frequency response, linearity, and transformer properties, considerably less than half of the power entering the middle ear actually reaches the cochlea because of the absorption of energy by the ligaments and middle ear. As shown in Figure 129.5, the human middle ear is particularly inefficient at frequencies greater than 2 kHz, especially in comparison with the ears

of cats and chinchillas. It also is important to recall that a 50% loss of power is a loss of only 3 dB.

Auditory function is profoundly affected by cochlear impedance as well as the combined acoustic effects of the head, external ear, and middle ear. The combined effects of the acoustic properties of the head, external ear, and middle ear, as well the input impedance of the cochlea, have a profound effect on auditory function. For example, these factors determine the shape of the audibility curve and therefore the frequency range of human hearing (Fig. 129.6). For example, humans do not

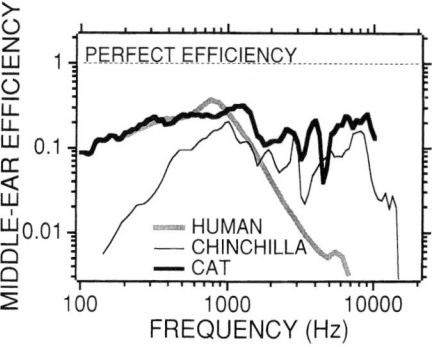

Figure 129.5 Efficiency of the transfer of power through the middle ear. For all species shown, less than half the power that enters the middle ear actually reaches the cochlea. Energy loss is caused by absorption by the tympanic membrane, ossicular ligaments, and middle ear. (From Rosowski JH. The effects of external and middle ear filters on noise-induced hearing loss. *J Acoust Soc Am* 1991;90:124, with permission.)

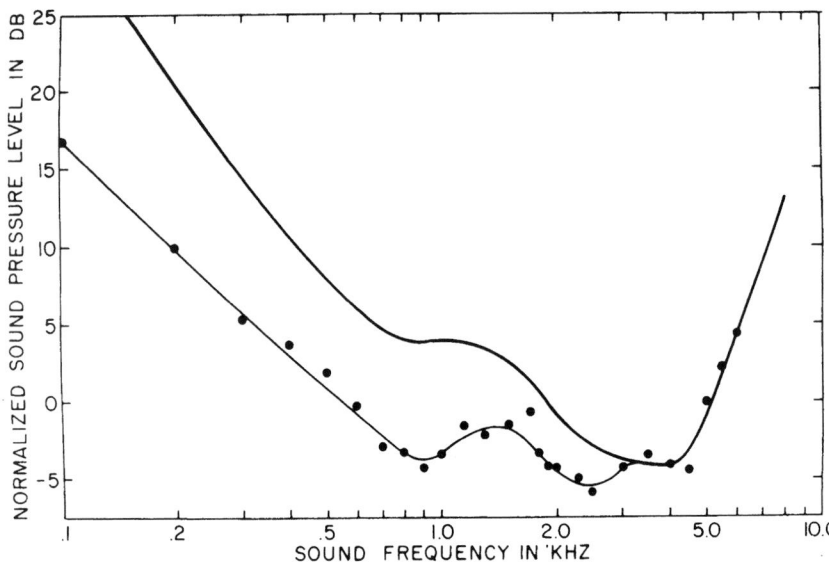

Figure 129.6 Comparison between overall outer and middle ear transfer function (*circles, lower curve*) and median threshold of audibility. (From Zwislocki JJ. The role of the external and middle ear in sound transmission. In: Turner D, ed. *The nervous system, human communication and its disorders.* Vol 3. New York: Raven Press, 1975:45, with permission.)

detect and recognize sounds greater than approximately 20 kHz because such high-frequency sounds are not transmitted efficiently through the middle ear to the cochlea. A second example of this sound transformation is shown in Figure 129.7, in which the spectrum of a cannon measured in a sound field is compared with the spectrum of the cannon by the time it is transformed and shaped by the acoustic properties of the external ear, head, middle ear, and input impedance of the cochlea. Low-frequency energy is not transmitted to the cochlea, and the frequency region of greatest energy concentration is 3 to 4 kHz. Thus, these acoustic properties are primarily responsible for the ability of intense low-frequency sounds (measured in a

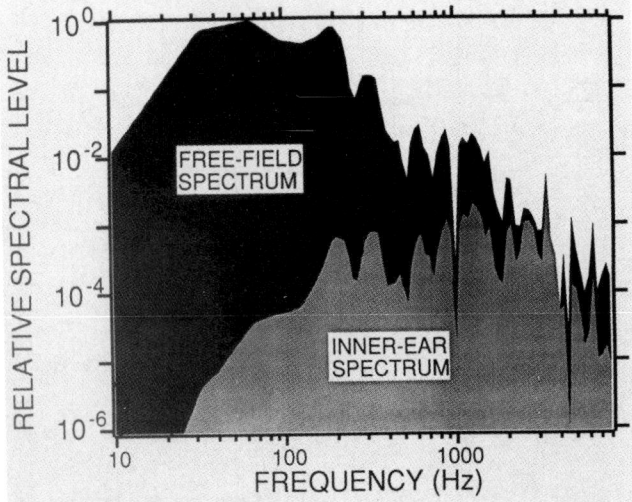

Figure 129.7 A comparison of the relative power spectra of impulses produced by a cannon and measured in a free field with the power that actually reaches the cochlea of a cat. (From Rosowski JH. The effects of external and middle ear filters on noise-induced hearing loss. *J Acoust Soc Am* 1991;90:124, with permission.)

sound field) to produce high-frequency hearing losses and injuries in the basal region of the cochlea.

Two striated muscles, the tensor tympani and the stapedius, are located in the middle ear. The former attaches to the malleus and is innervated by the trigeminal nerve. The stapedius muscle attaches to the stapes and is innervated by the stapedial branch of the facial nerve. Noticeably the stapedius and tensor tympani muscles are the smallest striated muscles in the body and also have a high innervation ratio, that is, nerve fibers per muscle fiber. Although no question remains that contraction of these muscles affects sound transmission through the middle ear, the details of the effect and the extent of the influence of the middle ear muscles are still not fully understood. A number of disparate functions have been attributed to the middle ear muscles.

One function of the middle ear muscles is to protect the cochlea from loud sounds (2). When sounds louder than approximately 80 dB SPL are presented monaurally or binaurally, consensual (bilateral) reflex contraction of the stapedius muscle occurs. This contraction increases the stiffness of the ossicular chain and tympanic membrane, attenuating sounds less than approximately 2 kHz. Although the tensor tympani contracts as part of a startle response, acoustic reflex data from human subjects with neurologic involvement of cranial nerves V and VII suggest that the tensor tympani does not normally respond to intense acoustic stimulation. Laboratory and field studies of noise-induced hearing loss have shown convincingly that the stapedial reflex protects the cochlea, particularly from low-frequency (<2 kHz) sounds in excess of 90 dB. Inasmuch as the latency of the acoustic reflex is greater than 10 ms, the cochlea may be unprotected from short-duration, unanticipated impulsive sounds.

The following functions have been attributed to the middle-ear muscles. Some of these functions include providing strength and rigidity to the ossicular chain; contributing to the blood supply of the ossicular chain; reducing physiologic noise caused by chewing and vocalization; improving the signal-to-noise ratio for high-frequency signals, especially high-frequency speech sounds such as voiceless fricatives, by means of attenuating high-level, low-frequency background noise; functioning as an automatic gain control and increasing the dynamic range of the ear; and smoothing out irregularities in the middle-ear transfer function.

COCHLEA

The human cochlea is a coiled, bony tube approximately 35 mm long, divided into the scala vestibuli, scala media, and scala tympani (Fig. 129.8). The scalae vestibuli and tympani contain perilymph, an extracellular fluid-like material with a potassium concentration of 4 mEq/L and a sodium concentration of 139 mEq/L. The scala media is bounded by the Reissner membrane, the basilar membrane and osseous spiral lamina, and the lateral wall. It contains endolymph, an intracellular-like fluid with a

potassium concentration of 144 mEq/L and a sodium concentration of 13 mEq/L. The scala media has a positive direct current (DC) resting potential of approximately 80 mV that decreases slightly from base to apex. This endocochlear potential is produced by the heavily vascularized stria vascularis of the lateral wall of the cochlea. The sodium–potassium–adenosine triphosphatase (Na^+-K^+-ATPase) pumps in a number of specialized cells of the stria vascularis contribute to this potential (3).

Acoustic energy enters the cochlea through the piston-like action of the stapes footplate on the oval window and is coupled directly to the perilymph of the scala vestibuli. The perilymph of the scala vestibuli communicates with the perilymph of the scala tympani through a small opening at the apex of the cochlea known as the *helicotrema*. The organ of Corti rests on the basilar membrane and osseous spiral lamina (Fig. 129.9). The basilar membrane is approximately 0.12 mm wide at the base and increases to approximately 0.5 mm at the apex. The major components of the organ of Corti are the outer and inner hair cells, supporting cells (Deiters, Hensen, Claudius), tectorial membrane, and the reticular lamina–cuticular plate complex (Fig. 129.10). Supporting cells provide structural and

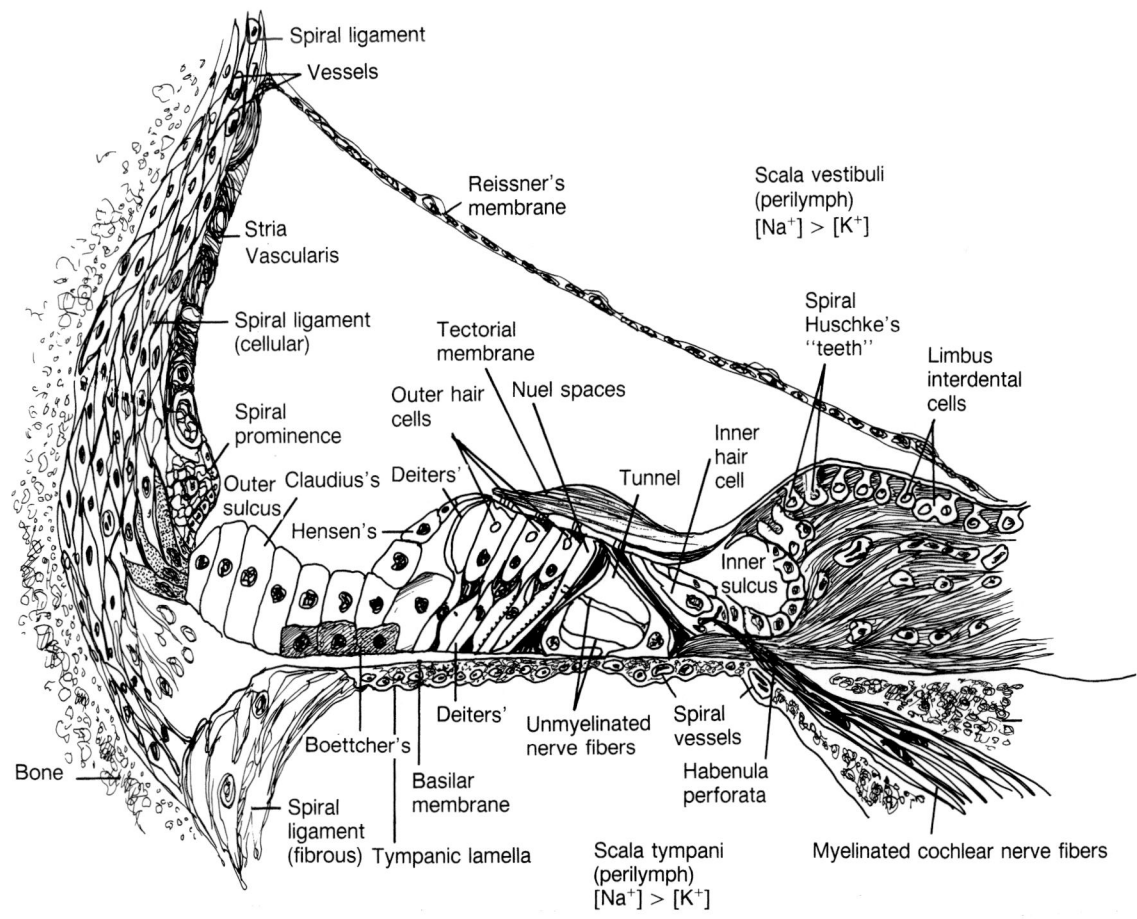

Figure 129.8 Midmodiolar view of cochlear duct. (Redrawn from Hawkins JE Jr. Hearing: anatomy and acoustics. In: Best C, Taylor NB, eds. *The physiological basis of medical practice*, 8th ed. Baltimore: Williams & Wilkins, 1966:347, with permission.)

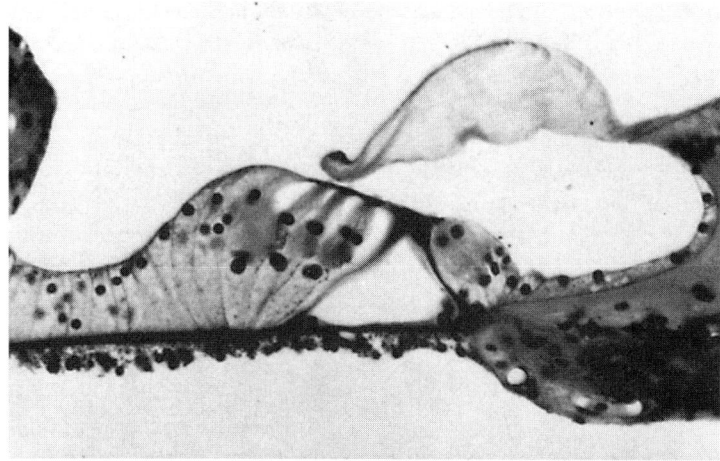

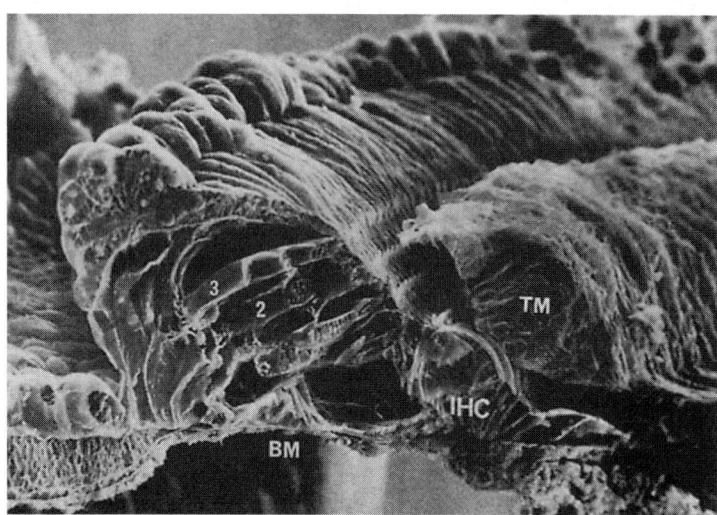

Figure 129.9 **A:** The organ of Corti of a cat in conventional midmodiolar section. Both sensory cells and supporting elements are evident. **B:** Photograph obtained through scanning electron microscope shows a corresponding specimen from a guinea pig. The inner hair cell (IHC) and three rows of outer hair cells (*1, 2, 3*) are visible. *BM*, basilar membrane; *TM*, tectorial membrane. (From Bredberg G, Ades W, Engstrom H. Scanning EM of the normal and pathologically altered organ of Corti: inner ear studies. *Acta Otolaryngol (Stockh)* 1972;301(suppl): 48, with permission.)

metabolic support for the organ of Corti. The phalangeal processes of the Deiters cells form tight cell junctions of the reticular lamina.

Outer and inner hair cells of the organ of Corti are important in transduction of mechanical (acoustic) energy into electrical (neural) energy. Outer hair cells are radically different from inner hair cells. Figure 129.11 and Table 129.1 detail these differences (4). In addition to the morphologic differences between outer and inner hair cells, neural innervation is different (Fig. 129.12). The spiral ganglion, the cell body of the auditory nerve, sends axons to the cochlear nucleus of the brainstem, whereas the dendrite projects through the osseous spiral lamina. Of the 50,000 neurons that innervate the cochlea, 90% to 95% synapse directly on inner hair cells. These are called *type I neurons*. Each inner hair cell is innervated by approximately 15 to 20 type I neurons. In contrast, 5% to 10% of the 50,000 neurons innervate the outer hair cells (*type II neurons*). Each type II neuron branches to innervate approximately 10 outer hair cells. In addition to the afferent innervation pattern of the cochlea, approximately 1,800 efferent fibers, originating from the ipsilateral and contralateral superior olivary complex, project to the cochlea (Fig. 129.13).

Transduction is initiated by displacement of the basilar membrane in response to displacement of the stapes due to acoustic energy. The displacement pattern of the basilar membrane is a traveling wave (Fig. 129.14). The basilar membrane is stiffer at the base than in the apex. The stiffness component is distributed continuously. Therefore, the traveling wave always progresses from base to apex. The maximal amplitude of basilar membrane displacement varies as a function of stimulus frequency. Traveling waves produced by high-frequency sounds (10 kHz) have maximal displacement near the base of the cochlea, whereas the waves to low-frequency sounds (125 Hz) have the maximum toward the apical region. Traveling waves generated by high-frequency sounds do not reach the apical region of the cochlea, whereas waves to low-frequency sounds can travel the entire length of the basilar membrane.

In the past, the mechanical traveling wave was considered a broadly tuned response, with finer tuning introduced subsequently by transduction, the auditory nerve, and the CNS. Data obtained with sensitive recording and detection methods, however, have shown that the traveling wave has an extremely sharply tuned response (Fig. 129.15) and that many of the remarkable frequency-selective abilities of the

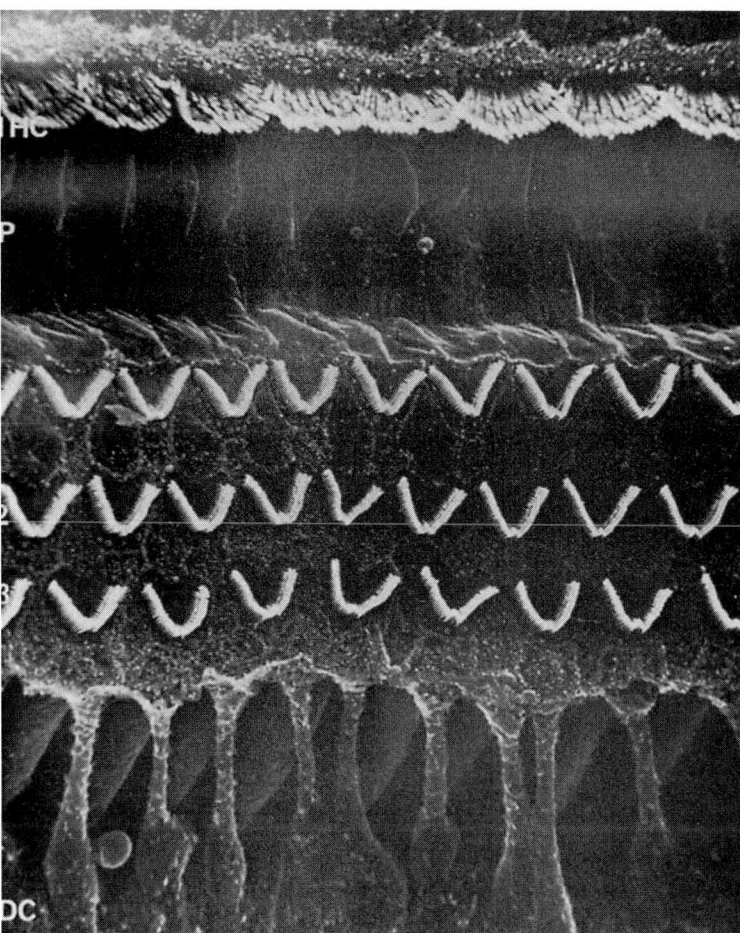

Figure 129.10 Scanning electron micrograph shows upper surface of organ of Corti with tectorial membrane removed. Modiolus is toward the *top.* Three rows of outer hair cells (*1, 2, 3*) with their characteristic V- or W-arranged stereocilia and a single row of inner hair cells (*IHC*) with slightly curved rows of stereocilia are visible. Inner and outer hair cells are separated by heads of pillar cells (*P*). Phalangeal processes of third row of Deiters cells (*DC*) are visible because Hensen cells have been removed. (From Bredberg G, Ades W, Engstrom H. Scanning EM of the normal and pathologically altered organ of Corti: inner ear studies. *Acta Otolaryngol (Stockh)* 1972;301(suppl):52, with permission.)

ear can be explained by the mechanical properties of the cochlea.

The mechanism by which the sharply tuned peak is generated within the mechanical traveling wave involves an enhancement known as the *cochlear modifier.* This is an activity of the outer hair cells that enhances the motion of the basilar membrane at frequencies near the best frequency of the particular cochlear location. This enhancement contributes to the fine frequency-selective abilities of the ear and to the sensitivity of the ear and ability to detect extremely faint sounds. The notion of an active process in the cochlea, the cochlear amplifier, is supported by the phenomenon of *otoacoustic emissions.* That is, when a short-duration signal is presented to the ear, an echo emanating from the cochlea can be recorded in the external auditory meatus. Because the energy of the echo can be greater than the energy of the short-duration signal, an active process, the cochlear amplifier, is assumed. Factors that may contribute to the cochlear amplifier include motility of outer hair cells and the mechanical properties of the stereocilia and tectorial membrane.

The stereocilia–hair cell complex is critical to transduction. Stereocilia are bundles of actin filaments that form

tubes and are inserted into the cuticular plate. They also are cross-linked between themselves. Stereocilia of inner hair cells probably do not contact the tectorial membrane, but those of outer hair cells are in direct contact. Deflection of the stereocilia by the traveling wave opens and closes nonspecific ion channels at the tips of the stereocilia, resulting in current flow (potassium) into the sensory cell. The flow of potassium ions into the sensory cell is modulated by the opening and closing of ion channels of the stereocilia. The potassium flux is caused by the endocochlear potential of +80 mV added to the negative intracellular potentials of hair cells. The resulting intracellular depolarization causes an enzyme cascade involving calcium. This ultimately leads to the release of chemical transmitters, and the subsequent activation of the afferent nerve fibers.

Although the notion of the cochlea as an active rather than a passive organ is no longer debated, specific details of the cochlear amplifier and the biologic basis of its operation are under active investigation. One point of view attributes the cochlear amplifier to the ability of hair cells to contract and lengthen in response to electrical signals, a property called *somatic electromotility.* A protein named *prestin* has been identified in outer hair cells and is considered to be

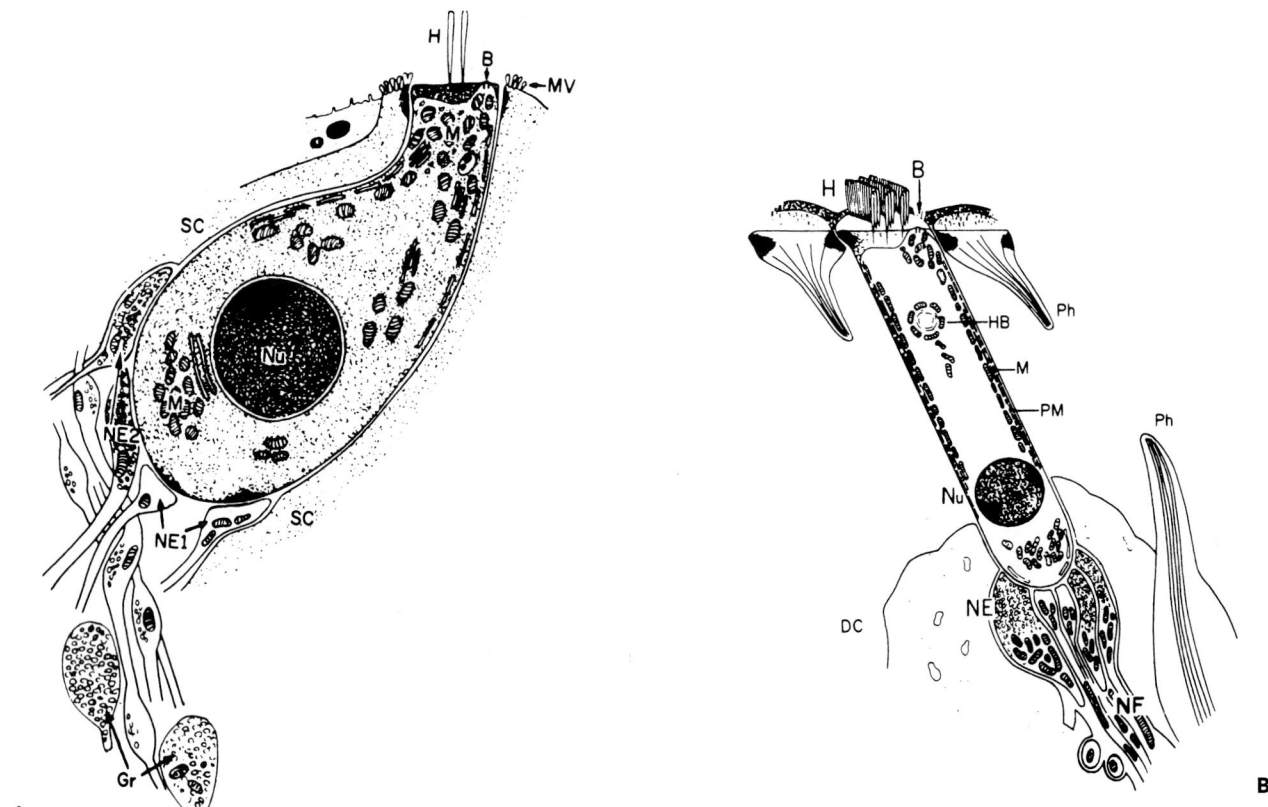

Figure 129.11 Differences in structure, ultrastructure, and innervation between inner **(A)** and outer **(B)** hair cells. *B*, Basal body; *D*, Deiters cells; *H*, stereocilia; *M*, mitochondria; *MV*, microvilli; *NE1*, afferent endings (cochlear nerve); *NE2*, efferent endings (olivocochlear bundle); *Nu*, nucleus; *SC*, supporting cells. (From Engstrom H, Ades HW, Hawkins JE Jr. In: Neff WD, ed. *Contribution to sensory physiology.* Vol 1. New York: Academic Press, 1965:67, with permission.)

the motor protein of outer hair cells and the driving force of electromotility of hair cells (5). Another point of view focuses on rapidly acting potassium and calcium ion channels presumed to be the basis of the cochlear amplifier and its regulation (6). A third approach suggests that a collection of motor proteins within a hair cell can generate oscillations that depend on the elastic properties of the cell (7). The foregoing approaches are nonlinear models that involve rapidly acting calcium channels. Specification of the biologic basis of the cochlear amplifier (nonlinearity) is important inasmuch as many forms of hearing loss involve loss of the cochlear amplifier.

The neurotransmitters of the afferent and efferent systems are the subject of intense study. In regard to the afferent system, analysis of excitatory amino acid receptor expression by the techniques of reverse transcriptase–polymerase chain reaction, in situ hybridization, and immunochemical analysis indicates that glutamate is the afferent neurotransmitter. Glutamate has been detected in both spiral ganglion cells and sensory cells (8). The principal transmitter substance of cochlear efferent fibers is acetylcholine. It is possible that the organ of Corti is mechanically modified by means of motility changes of outer hair cells under the influence of the efferent system. Acetylcholine acts on receptors to

produce hyperpolarization of the cell membrane and doubling of the input conductance of the cell. The acetylcholine receptor has both muscarinic and nicotinic features. In addition to acetylcholine, γ-aminobutyric acid and several neuroactive peptides are neurotransmitters for the efferent system (9,10).

Gross Cochlear Potentials

Four gross (extracellular) potentials can be recorded in the cochlea (11)—endolymphatic (endocochlear) potential, cochlear microphonic, summating potential, and whole-nerve action potential (Fig. 129.16). Unlike the other cochlear potentials, the endolymphatic potential is not generated in response to acoustic stimulation; rather, it is a DC potential of 80 to 100 mV recorded in the scala media. It arises from the stria vascularis of the lateral wall of the cochlea. The stria vascularis is considered to be the energy source, or "battery," of the cochlea, crucial for transduction. The nature of the energy source is related to the heavy vasculature of the stria vascularis and to the Na^+-K^+-adenosine triphosphatase (ATPase). This pump has been localized to several types of cochlear cells, including marginal cells of the stria vascularis, outer sulcus cells, and fibrocytes near

TABLE 129.1
STRUCTURE AND INNERVATION OF INNER AND OUTER HAIR CELLS

Characteristic	Inner Hair Cells	Outer Hair Cells
Number	3,500	12,000
Shape	Flask	Cylindrical
Stereocilia		
No. of hair cells	Few	Many
Arrangement	Three or four rows; rows slightly curved	Six or seven rows; rows arranged in V or W shape
Attachment to tectorial membrane	None or loosely connected	Longest stereocilia firmly embedded
Ultrastructure		
Position of nucleus cell body	Center	Base
Cytoplasmic organelles	Scattered	Adjacent to cell membrane
Presynaptic specializations	Large	Small or absent (synaptic bars and vesicles)
Glycogen content	Low	High
Relation to supporting cells	Completely surrounded	Supported only at surface and base
Afferent innervation		
Ganglion cells	Type I	Type II
Number of ganglion cells	27,000	2,100
Hair cell-to-ganglion cell ratio	1.8:1	5.7:1
Efferent innervation		
Source	Lateral superior olivary complex	Medial superior olivary complex
Postsynaptic target	Afferent dendrites	Base of hair cell

From Neely JG, Dennis JM, Lippe WR. Anatomy of the auditory end organ and neural pathways. In: Cummings CW, ed. *Otolaryngology–head and neck surgery*. St. Louis: Mosby, 1986:2571, with permission.

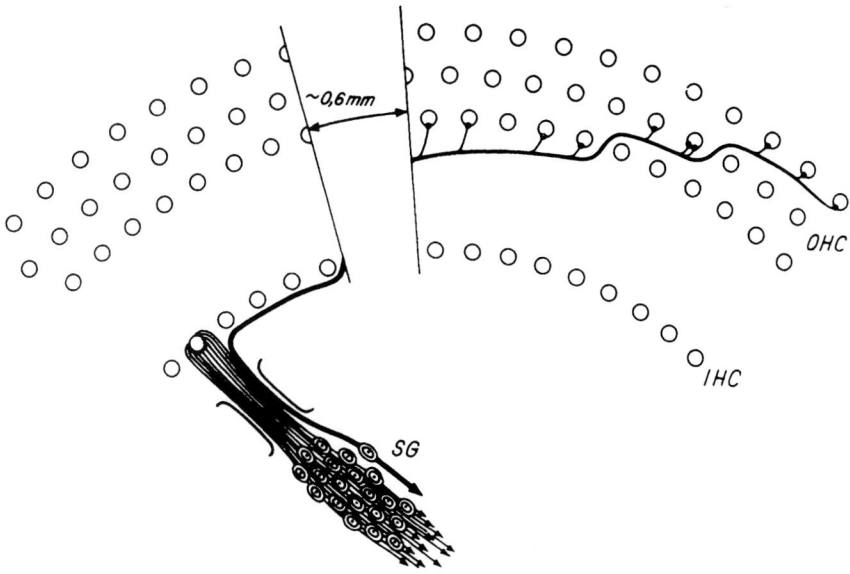

Figure 129.12 Schematic view from above shows the surface of the organ of Corti. The distribution of cochlear nerve fibers to inner (*IHC*) and outer (*OHC*) hair cells is evident. Basal end of cochlea is toward the *right*. Most spiral ganglion cells (*SG*) synapse with inner hair cells. Each ganglion cell innervates only one hair cell; many ganglion cells contact each hair cell. Only approximately 5% of spiral ganglion cells innervate outer hair cells. Each fiber travels basally for some distance before sending branches to several outer hair cells. (From Spoendlin H. The afferent innervation of the cochlea. In: Naunton RF, Fernandez C, eds. *Evoked electrical activity in the auditory nervous system*. New York: Academic Press, 1978:29, with permission.)

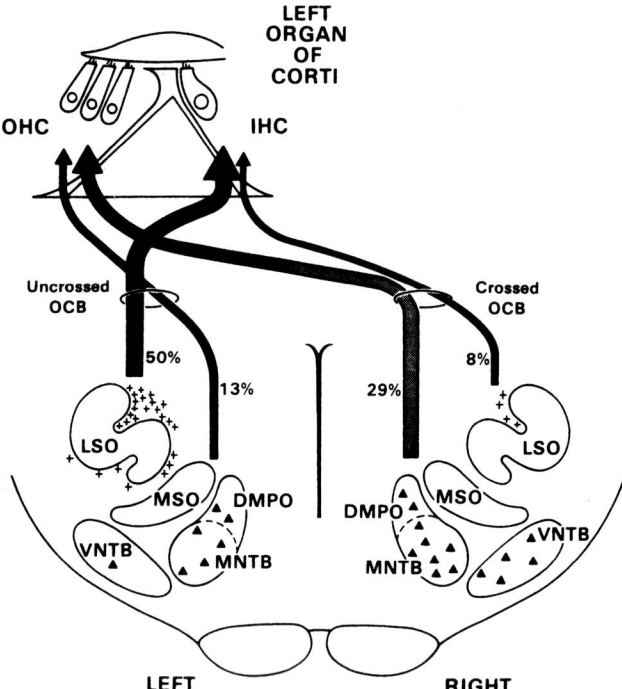

Figure 129.13 Schematic shows origin and distribution of efferent fibers of the olivocochlear bundle. *Crosses*, Small olivocochlear bundle neurons; *triangles*, large olivocochlear bundle neurons. The *number* of each kind of symbol, relative widths of *lines*, and *percentages* indicate the proportion of total olivocochlear projection to one cochlea that arises from each cell group. Efferent fibers to outer hair cells originate from large cells in the medial portion of the superior olivary complex. Approximately 70% of the projection to outer hair cells comes from the contralateral side of the brain. Projection to inner hair cells arises from small cells in the lateral region of the superior olive. Most of these fibers (85%) originate on the ipsilateral portion of the brain. Data are from studies with cats. *DMPO*, dorsomedial preolivary nucleus; *IHC*, inner hair cells; *LSO*, later superior olivary nucleus; *MNTB*, medial nucleus of the trapezoid body; *MSO*, medial superior olivary nucleus; *OCB*, olivocochlear bundle; *OHC*, outer hair cells; *VNTB*, ventral nucleus of the trapezoid body. (From Warr B. The olivocochlear bundle: its origins and terminations in the cat. In: Naunton RF, Fernandez C, eds. *Evoked electrical activity in the auditory nervous system.* New York: Academic Press, 1978:60, with permission.)

the attachment of the Reissner membrane and in the spiral ligament. Whereas Na^+-K^+-ATPase must play a significant role in ion transport in the cochlea, the nature of the energy source and the details of the ion exchange remain active research issues (3).

Malfunctioning of the mechanisms involved in production of endolymph and the endolymphatic potential can produce hearing loss, sometimes called *metabolic presbycusis.* When the flow of endolymph through the ductus reuniens is blocked, endolymphatic pressure increases, and hydrops occurs.

The cochlear microphonic is an alternating current (AC) voltage usually recorded within the cochlea or near the round window. It represents the potassium ion current flow through mainly the outer hair cells; that is, the electrical resistance of outer hair cells is altered by the motion of the basilar membrane. When stereocilia are bent away from the modiolus, the resistance of the hair cells decreases. The result is an increase in current flow and a small decrease in endolymphatic potential. When stereocilia are bent toward the modiolus, resistance increases and current flow decreases with an accompanying increase in the endolymphatic potential. The corresponding voltage fluctuations, the cochlear microphonic, depend on the presence of outer hair cells. Unlike neural potentials, the waveform of the cochlear microphonic mirrors the motion of the basilar membrane. The summating potential is a DC potential recorded in the cochlea in response to sound. It follows the envelope of the stimulating sound. Recordings of this DC potential can be made in the scala tympani, media, or vestibuli and in some circumstances from a gross electrode in the human ear canal. The potential can be positive or negative, and it can reverse polarity, depending on electrode location or stimulus frequency and level. The summating potential probably has several origins, but it largely reflects the DC shifts caused by stimulus-driven intracellular potentials of outer hair cells. Inner hair cells contribute to these to a lesser extent.

The whole-nerve or compound action potential arises from the all-or-none discharge of auditory nerve fibers. The

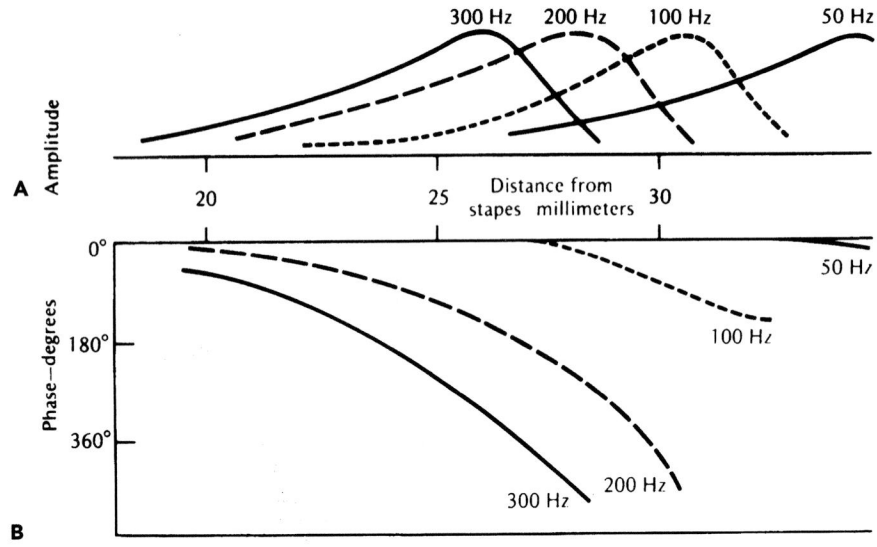

Figure 129.14 **A:** Amplitude of basilar membrane motion as a function of distance from the base of the cochlea to a 200-Hz tone. *Top:* instantaneous displacement of basilar membrane at successive time intervals (*solid lines*); displacement envelope (*dashed line*). *Bottom:* instantaneous velocity of basilar membrane at successive time intervals (*solid lines*); velocity envelope (*dashed line*). **B:** Relative amplitude of vibration at different points along the basilar membrane for four different frequencies. *Bottom,* phase lag at different points along the basilar membrane for four different frequencies. (From Von Bekesy G. *Experiments in hearing.* New York: John Wiley & Sons, 1960, with permission.)

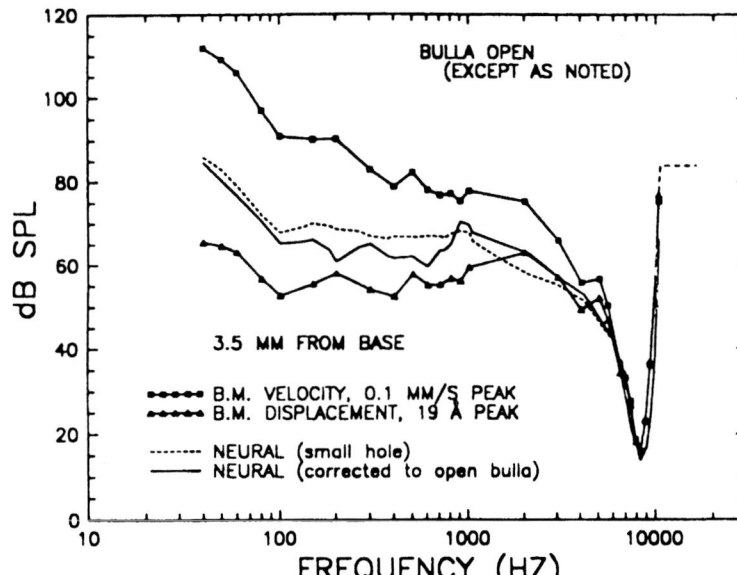

figure 129.15 Comparison of mechanical tuning of the basilar membrane and neural tuning of an afferent fiber of the auditory nerve. (From Ruggero MA, Rich NC, Robles L, et al. Middle ear response in the chinchilla and its relationship to mechanics at the base of the cochlea. *J Acoust Soc Am* 1990;87:1612, with permission.)

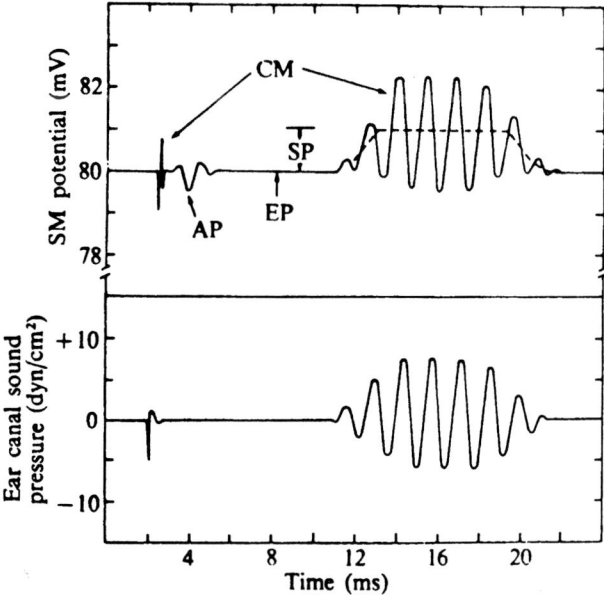

Figure 129.16 Schematic shows cochlear potentials recorded in the scala media in response to typical acoustic stimuli. All waveforms are approximately to scale. **Bottom:** Time waveforms of sound pressure in the ear canal for a click and a 750-Hz tone burst obtained with a probe-tube microphone. *Positive* and *negative* pressures refer to condensation and rarefaction, respectively, with the static value of atmospheric pressure subtracted out. An acoustic pressure of 5 dyne/cm² is equivalent to 88 dB SPL, referred to as 0.0002 dyne/cm² (20 Pa). **Top:** Resulting time waveform of the potential recorded in scala media by a single micropipette in the basal turn. The voltage is referenced to the neck of the animal. Ordinate is discontinuous to allow closer inspection of stimulus-related waveforms on the 80-mV endocochlear potential (*EP*), that is, the whole-nerve action potential (*AP*), the cochlear microphonic (*CM*), and the summating potential (*SP*). At low frequencies, the phase of the cochlear microphonic waveform leads that of the sound pressure at the eardrum. (From Schmiedt RA. Basic techniques for the measurement of cochlear potentials. In: Beagley HA, ed. *Auditory investigation: the scientific and technological basis.* Oxford: Clarendon Press, 1979:211, with permission.)

compound action potential is recorded most effectively with a gross electrode placed near the round window or auditory nerve and with high-frequency signals with rapid onsets. Such signals produce synchronous neural activity, which is summed to become the compound action potential waveform. The amplitude of the compound action potential increases with stimulus intensity over a 40- to 50-dB range, whereas latency decreases as stimulus intensity is increased. At high levels, a second peak sometimes is observed that probably reflects activity of the cochlear nucleus. The compound action potential can be clinically recorded with scalp electrodes or electrodes in the external meatus or by means of a transtympanic approach in which an electrode is placed near the round window niche. The ratio of the amplitude of the summating potential to the amplitude of the compound action potential has been used as an indicator of perilymphatic fistula, but the validity of this indicator is doubtful.

EIGHTH NERVE PHYSIOLOGY

The auditory nerve has approximately 30,000 fibers in humans and approximately 50,000 in cats. Perhaps one of the most important research findings in recent years was the observation that 90% to 95% of neurons (type I, radial fibers) innervate inner hair cells, whereas 5% to 10% (type II, outer spiral fibers) innervate to the outer hair cells (Fig. 129.12). Most, if not all, recordings from auditory nerve fibers are from the larger type I fibers in contact with inner hair cells. These radial fibers have bipolar cell bodies in the spiral ganglion. Outer spiral fibers are monopolar and unmyelinated. Most recordings of single units of the auditory nerve are obtained by means of inserting a microelectrode into the auditory nerve where it exits the internal auditory meatus. The most basic measures of auditory nerve function are spontaneous rates, tuning curves, and intensity (rate-level) functions.

Most auditory nerve fibers in mammals discharge in the absence of acoustic stimulation. The nerve fibers have been classified into three categories on the basis of rate of spontaneous discharge—high (18 to 120 spikes per second), medium (0.5 to 18 spikes per second), and low (0 to 0.5 spikes per second). Fibers with high rates of spontaneous activity respond to auditory signals at lower levels than do fibers with medium or low rates of spontaneous activity. In other words, the most-sensitive fibers have the most-spontaneous activity. Fibers with high spontaneous rates have thick dendrites that tend to terminate on the side of inner hair cells facing outer hair cells. Fibers with low and medium spontaneous rates have thin dendrites that terminate on the side of the inner hair cell facing the modiolus. Ongoing studies indicate that fibers with high rates of spontaneous activity have different terminations in the auditory CNS (cochlear nucleus) than do fibers with low rates of spontaneous activity. In other words, spontaneous activity of nerve fibers is not random but is proving to be anatomically and functionally significant (12–15). The tuning curve of a single auditory nerve fiber is perhaps the most basic measure of auditory nerve function. A tone burst controlled in frequency and level is presented. The level is adjusted until a criterion change (one or two spikes per second) in firing rate is detected. Tone bursts covering a wide range of frequencies are used, and the lowest level of signal is recorded for a given frequency that produces a specific rate of discharge. The resulting isoresponse curve is called a *tuning curve.*

Figure 129.17 shows tuning curves for six different fibers. The sharp tip of the tuning curve identifies the best,

or characteristic, frequency of the fiber. Units with low characteristic frequency are fibers that innervate inner hair cells in the apical region of the cochlea, fibers with high characteristic frequency innervate inner hair cells from the basal region, and so on. Tuning curves are described according to the frequency of the tip or characteristic frequency, the high- and low-frequency side, and the tail. Fibers with a characteristic frequency less than 1 kHz are roughly V shaped. Fibers with a higher characteristic frequency have an obvious tip at the characteristic frequency and a tail that extends to the low frequencies. The high side of a tuning curve is the frequency region greater than characteristic frequency. As characteristic frequency increases, the high side of the tuning curve becomes steeper with a slope or rejection rate that can exceed 500 dB per octave. The characteristics of tuning curves of auditory nerve fibers are strikingly similar to isoamplitude curves of a mechanical traveling wave (Fig. 129.15).

Injury or damage to sensory cells, including stereocilia, can alter the shape of tuning curves dramatically (Fig. 129.18). The lower right portion of the figure shows that when outer hair cells are destroyed, the tuning curve of auditory nerve fibers from normal inner hair cells is changed in several ways. The sensitive tip region is missing; that is, the threshold of the fiber is elevated by approximately 40 to 45 dB. The high-frequency side no longer has a steep slope, and the low-frequency side becomes slightly more sensitive, or hypersensitive. The characteristic frequency of the fiber appears to be much lower in frequency, and the band width of the fiber appears broader. The upper left portion of Figure 129.18 shows the consequences of partial injury to the stereocilia of outer hair cells. A threshold shift of approximately 30 dB occurs, but a short, sharply tuned tip remains, and the low-frequency tail is again hypersensitive. Irregularities in this tuning curve may explain monaural diplacusis; that is, a tone in one ear (800 Hz) has two pitches, for example, one at 800 Hz and a second at approximately 2.8 kHz.

The upper left portion of Figure 129.18 shows a tuning curve in which stereocilia of inner hair cells are damaged or in disarray, whereas most of the stereocilia of outer hair cells appear normal or nearly so. The threshold of the unit is elevated approximately 30 dB, but the tuning curve is approximately normal. The lower left portion of the figure shows responses to signals in a narrow range of frequencies only at sound levels greater than 90 dB SPL. In this case, sensory cells are present, but stereocilia of inner hair cells are destroyed, and those of outer hair cells are destroyed or in disarray. Thus normal neural activity, including sensitivity (detection of faint sounds) and frequency-resolving power, depends on intact outer hair cells and normal stereocilia.

Although thresholds of auditory nerve fibers are related to the rate of spontaneous discharge, most afferent nerve fibers (60%) have high spontaneous rates and thresholds within 20 dB greater than the thresholds for the animal. The remaining low-spontaneous fibers have thresholds that cover

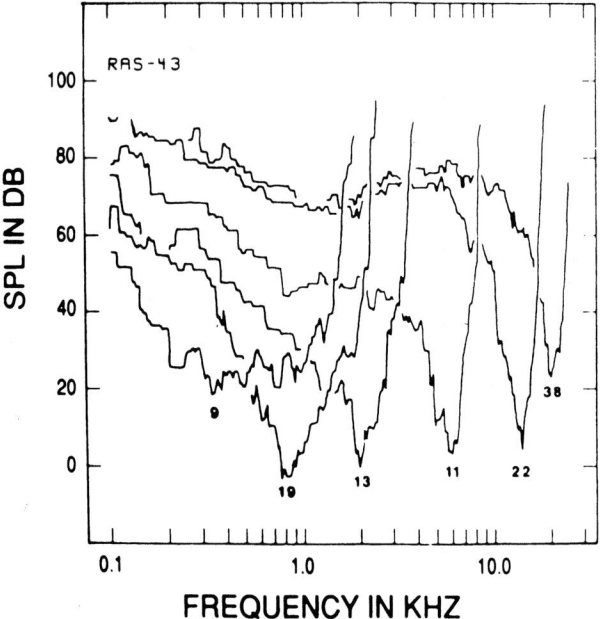

Figure 129.17 Tuning curves obtained from single fibers in the auditory nerve of a 6-month-old gerbil (CG-9) raised in quiet. Fiber numbers given in sequence during the experiment are at the *tips* of the curves. (From Schmiedt RA, Mills JH, Adams K. Tuning and suppression in auditory nerve fibers of aged gerbils raised in quiet or noise. *Hear Res* 1990;45:221, with permission.)

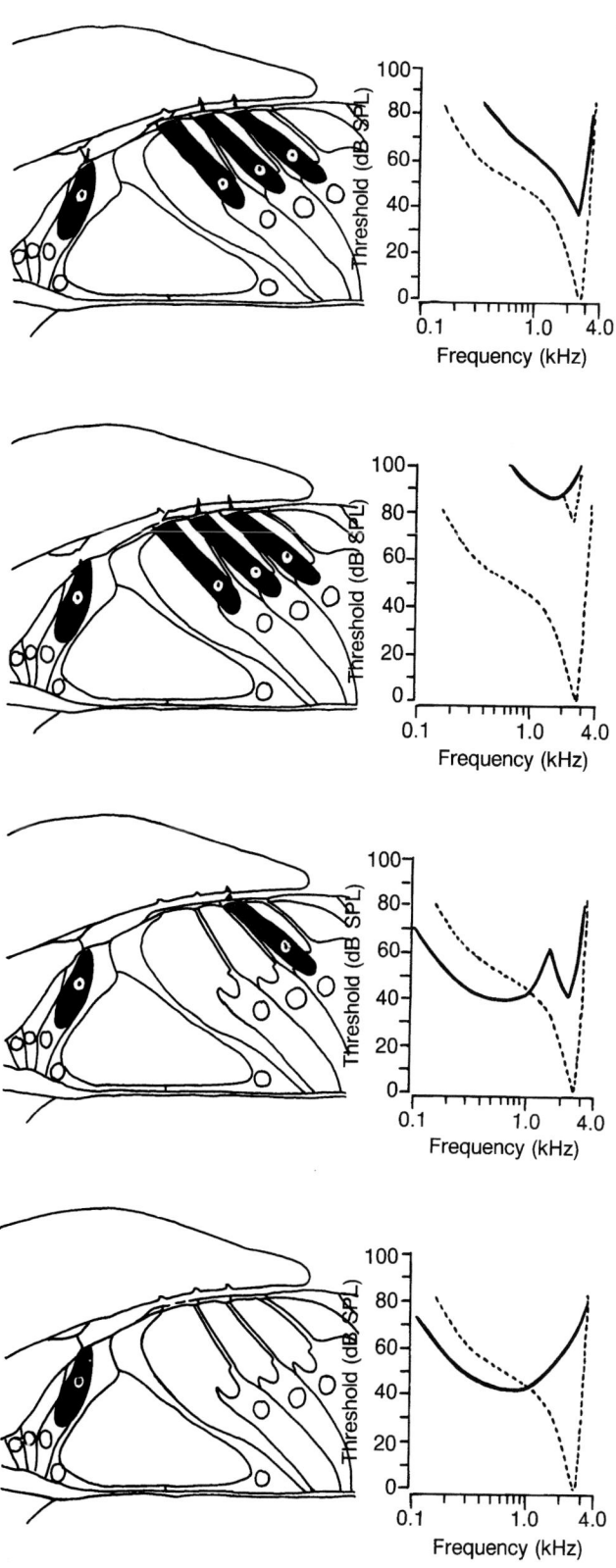

Figure 129.18 Tuning curves of single units of the auditory nerve with different degrees and types of acoustic injury to the sensory cells, including stereocilia. *Dotted line,* normal; *solid line,* after injury. (Redrawn from Liberman MC, Dodds LW. Single neuron labeling and chronic cochlear pathology III: stereocilia damage and alterations of threshold tuning curves. *Hear Res* 1984;16:55, with permission.)

approximately 60 dB. The dynamic range of most auditory nerve fibers is approximately 30 dB from threshold to saturation (Fig. 129.19), although some low-spontaneous fibers have a much wider dynamic range. Given the dynamic range of human hearing (0 dB SPL to ≥100 dB SPL), the auditory system must have neurons the thresholds of which cover a wide range and have firing rates that also cover a wide range of intensities. The ability of the human ear to respond appropriately to sounds over a 120-dB range (10,12) is remarkable. One way is with low-spontaneous fibers; another is recruitment of fibers of characteristic frequency.

One of the most common features of sensorineural hearing loss is recruitment of loudness. Figure 129.20 gives an explanation. It is assumed that loudness depends on the total activity of the auditory nerve. As Figure 129.20A shows, the number of fibers activated increases slowly as intensity is increased, and only the tips of tuning curves are activated. As the intensity increases further, the tails of the tuning curves are encountered, and the number of fibers activated increases rapidly. In the case of sensorineural hearing loss, the tips of the tuning curves are missing, and the fibers are not activated until the level of the signal is sufficient to reach the tails of the tuning curves. Abruptly, many fibers then are abruptly activated simultaneously.

NONLINEAR PROPERTIES OF THE EAR

Some of the outstanding features of the middle ear transformer are its linear properties, but the outstanding features of the cochlea and auditory nerve are the nonlinear characteristics. Perhaps the most studied nonlinearities are combination tones, described herein in relation to cochlear emissions, and two-tone rate suppression, as recorded in auditory nerve fibers.

Two-tone rate suppression is the reduction in firing rate produced by one tone when a second tone is introduced. Figure 129.21 shows a tuning curve with a suppression area outlined above the characteristic frequency of the nerve fiber and an area below the characteristic frequency of the fiber. Tones presented in the dotted or suppression areas in the figure reduce the firing rate caused by the probe tone. Both the excitor and suppressor tones are presented simultaneously, and because little or no time lag is associated with this phenomenon nor is any evidence available that it is neurally produced, the effect is called *suppression* rather than inhibition. Two-tone suppression in single units is reflected in the compound action potential. Figure 129.21 (right) shows tuning curves of the compound action potential with suppression areas shown in the dotted areas. In this case, the amplitude of the compound action potential is altered by the suppressing signal, whereas in the single-unit case (left), the firing rate of a neuron is reduced by an arbitrary amount (20%). The single-unit and compound action potential suppression areas are similar. Inasmuch as two-tone suppression can be

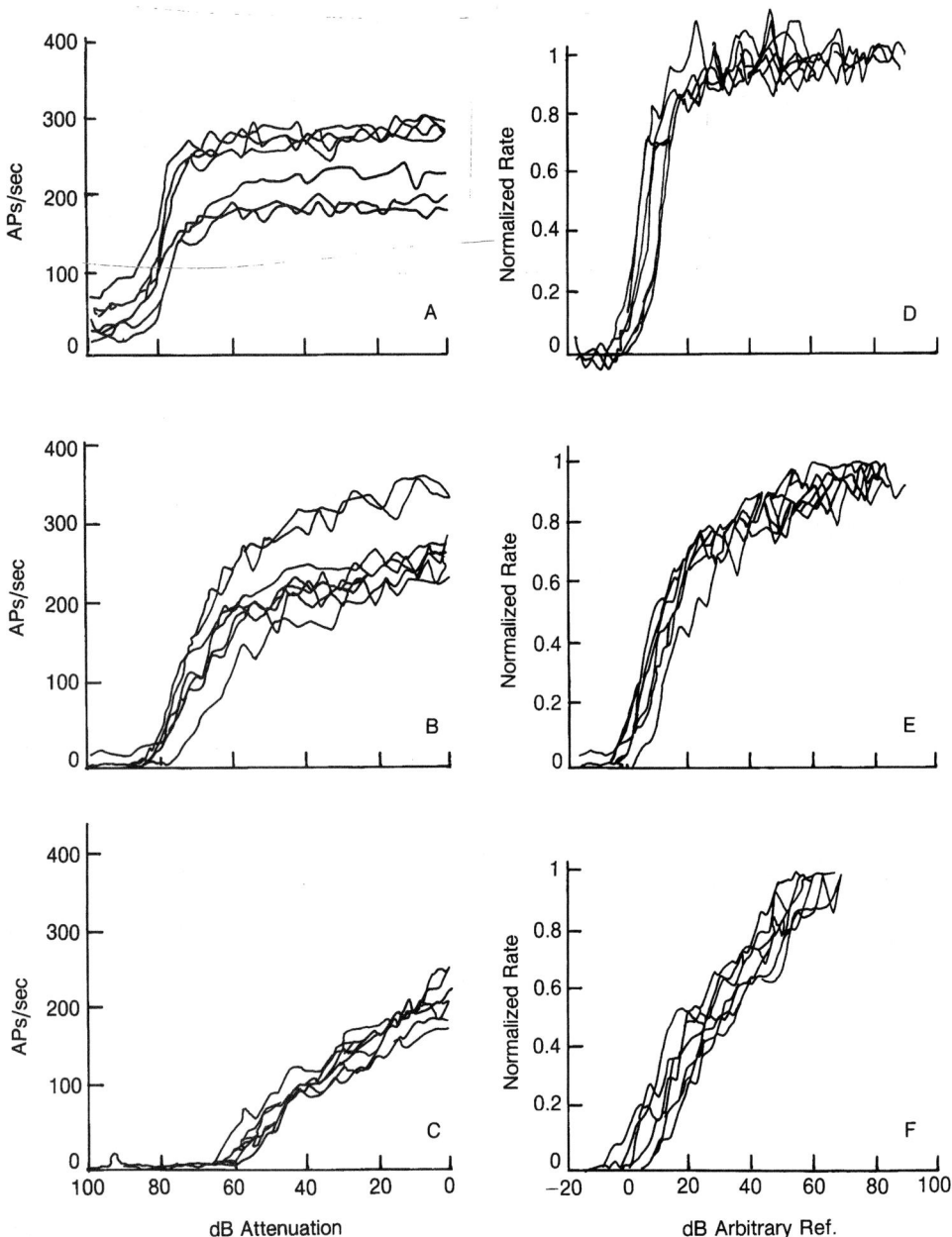

Figure 129.19 Examples of the three types of rate-intensity function. **A:** Saturating. **B:** Sloping saturation. **C:** Straight. For all units, characteristic frequency (*CF*) varies between 16 and 24 kHz, and maximum sound level varies between 104 and 115 dB SPL. **D–F:** Normalized rate–intensity functions for the fibers in **A, B,** and **C.** (Redrawn from Winter IM, Robertson D, Yabs GK. Diversity of characteristic frequency rate-intensity functions in guinea pig auditory nerve fibers. *Hear Res* 1990;45:191, with permission.)

observed in the DC intracellular response of inner hair cells, it is probable that two-tone suppression originates in the active nature of cochlear mechanics and before the inner hair cells.

In the presence of sensorineural hearing loss caused by exposure to noise or to ototoxic drugs, two-tone rate suppression is severely affected, if at all measurable. Two-tone rate suppression appears normal or nearly so in cases of cochlear hearing loss in which the sensory cells, including

stereocilia, are normal or nearly so, but the stria vascularis is affected. The latter scenario leads to presbycusis (16).

Otoacoustic emissions (OAEs) are sounds that are detected in the ear canal when the tympanum receives vibrations transmitted through the middle ear from the cochlea. OAEs provide support for the notion that the cochlea is not just a passive receiver of acoustic energy but can also generate or amplify sounds. Several different types of OAEs are found (17). *Spontaneous* OAEs occur in

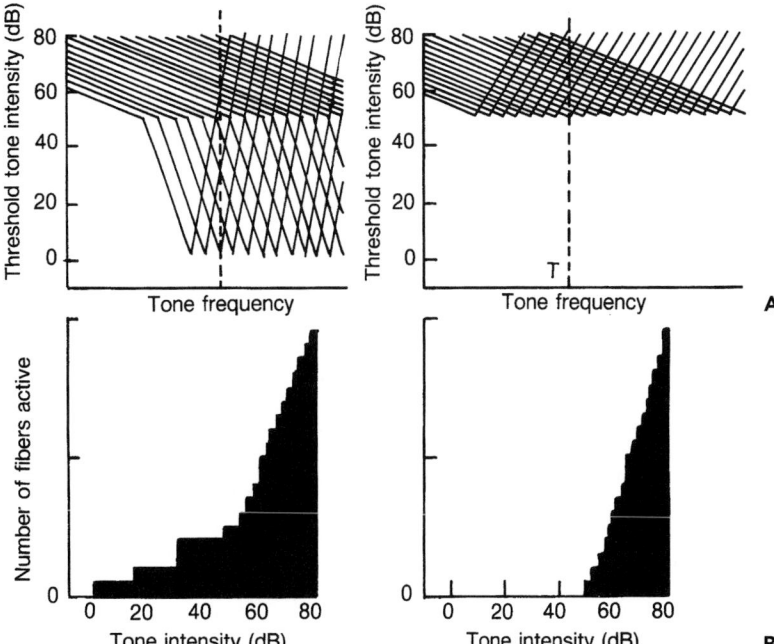

Figure 129.20 Neural explanation of one mechanism of loudness recruitment. **A:** Normal ear. **B:** Loudness in an abnormal ear grows abnormally quickly with intensity once the threshold is reached because the tips of the tuning curves are missing. (From Evans EF. The sharpening of cochlear frequency selectivity in the normal and abnormal cochlea. *Audiology* 1975;14:419, with permission.)

the absence of acoustic stimulation and are typically highly stable pure tones of –10 to 30 dB SPL, which are found in 30% to 40% of healthy young ears (18,19). The precise frequency of a spontaneous OAE does not imply an origin at a precise place in the cochlea, but only a particular coincidence of travel time and reflection from an ill-defined region of high outer cell activity. Spontaneous OAEs can be recorded over long periods with only minor but seemingly systematic variations in frequency and amplitude.

A second class of OAEs are produced after exposure to an acoustic signal. *Transient-evoked* OAEs (TEOAE) are made via a probe placed in the ear canal. The oscillatory sound pressure waveform seen in TEOAE responses actually corresponds to the motion of the eardrum resulting from pressure fluctuations generated within the cochlea (Fig. 129.22). Although stimulatory clicks excite the entire cochlea, TEOAE responses can be used to give frequency-specific information about the cochlea through splitting of the responses into different frequency bands. TEOAEs are highly sensitive to cochlear pathology in frequency-specific manner. Frequencies at which hearing thresholds exceed 20 to 30 dB hearing loss (HL) are typically absent in the TEOAE response (20,21). Because of their sensitivity to cochlear dysfunction, TEOAEs have found widespread application in newborn hearing screening programs (22).

Distortion-product OAEs also are used widely in clinical situations. The TEOAE and DPOAE techniques complement each other. DPOAEs offer a wider frequency range of observation with less sensitivity to minor and subclinical conditions in adults. When two primary tones, F1 and F2,

are presented to the cochlea, several distortion products are produced. The most prominent of all these intermodulation distortion products is the cubic distortion tone, 2F1-F2. Measurement of DPOAEs at multiple stimulus levels can establish the OAE "growth rate." Healthy ears tend to exhibit a DPOAE growth rate of 1 dB of OAE per 1 dB of stimulus or less. Ears with some impairment show steeper growth. Single DPOAE results can be misleading, and results must be averaged across a range of frequencies. The DPOAE is easily recordable in patients with a normal middle ear system (23).

AUDITORY CENTRAL NERVOUS SYSTEM

The ascending and descending auditory pathways are described briefly herein in relation to auditory evoked potentials. Schematics of the afferent and efferent pathways are shown in Figs. 129.23 and 129.13, respectively. These diagrams oversimplify the system but provide a rough introduction to the auditory CNS and its complexity. All eighth-nerve afferent fibers stop at the level of the cochlear nucleus. Five major cell types are found within the cochlear nucleus, each with distinct cell morphologic and physiologic features, such as response to stimulus onset, stimulus offset, and frequency modulation. From the cochlear nucleus, most fibers cross the brainstem to the contralateral superior olivary complex; a much smaller number of fibers run to the ipsilateral superior olivary complex.

The superior olivary complex is considered the first center in the ascending auditory system, where inputs from both

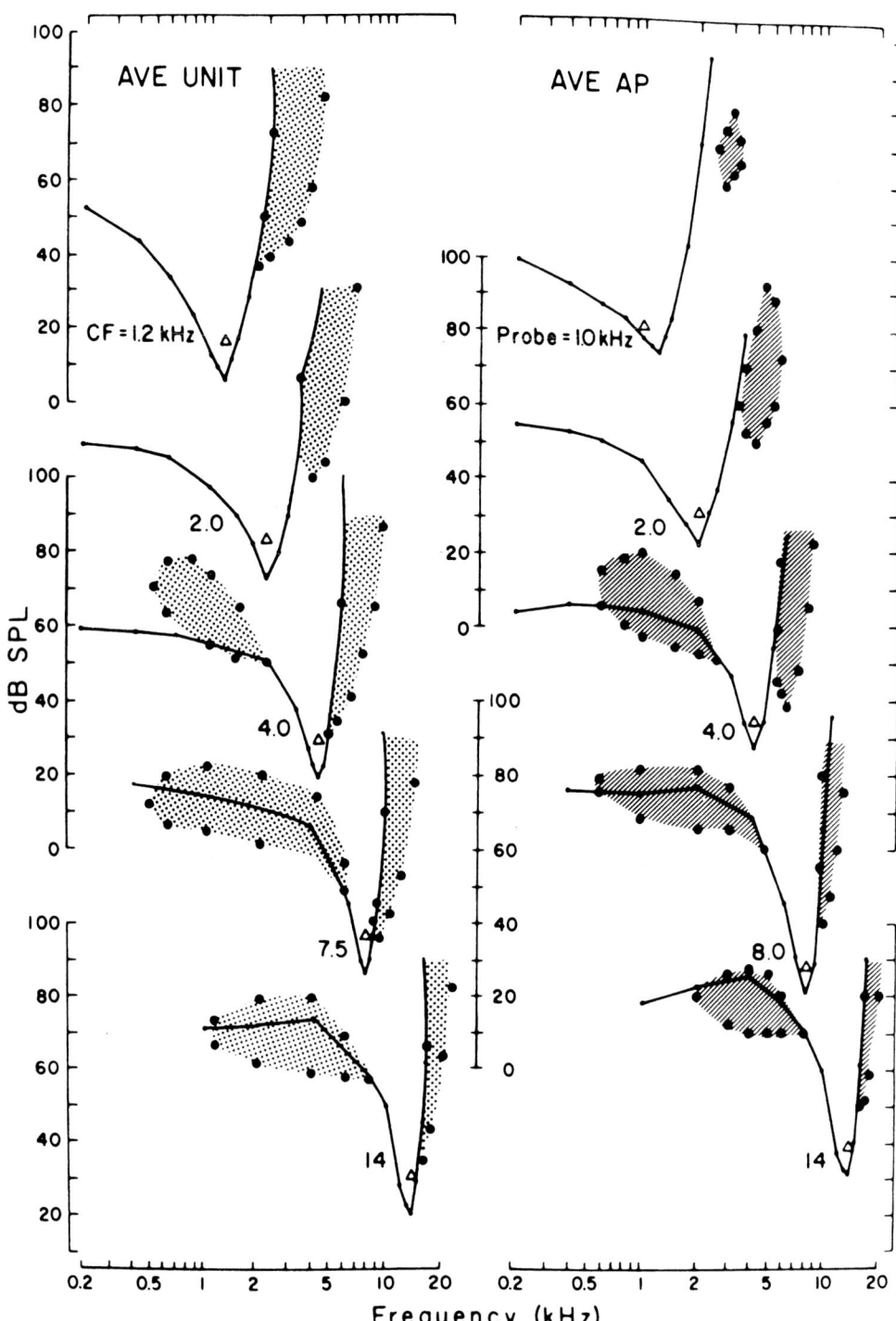

Figure 129.21 Left: Excitatory tuning curve (*circles*) and two-tone suppression areas (*shaded*) for a single auditory nerve fiber. Tones presented in the suppression areas decrease the firing rate to the excitatory tone. **Right:** Tuning and suppression of the compound action potential (CAP). (From Harris DM. Action potential suppression, tuning curves and thresholds: comparison with single fiber data. *Hear Res* 1979;1:133, with permission.)

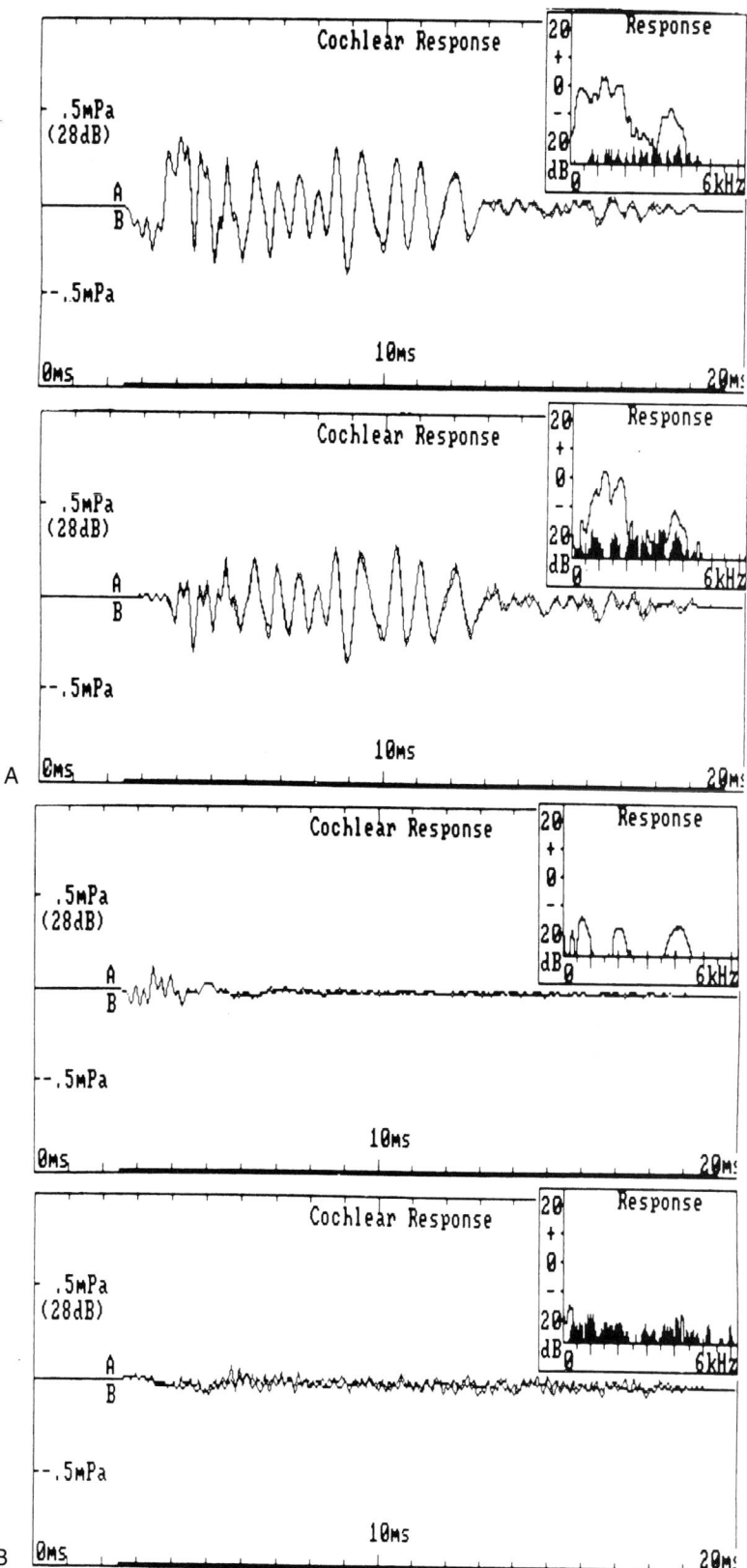

Figure 129.22   Cochlear echoes, also called *stimulated cochlear emissions*, from a normal ear **(A)** and a deaf ear **(B).** (From Kemp DT, Ryan S, Bray P. Otoacoustic emission analysis and interpretation for clinical purpose. *Adv Audio* 1990;12:77–92, with permission.)

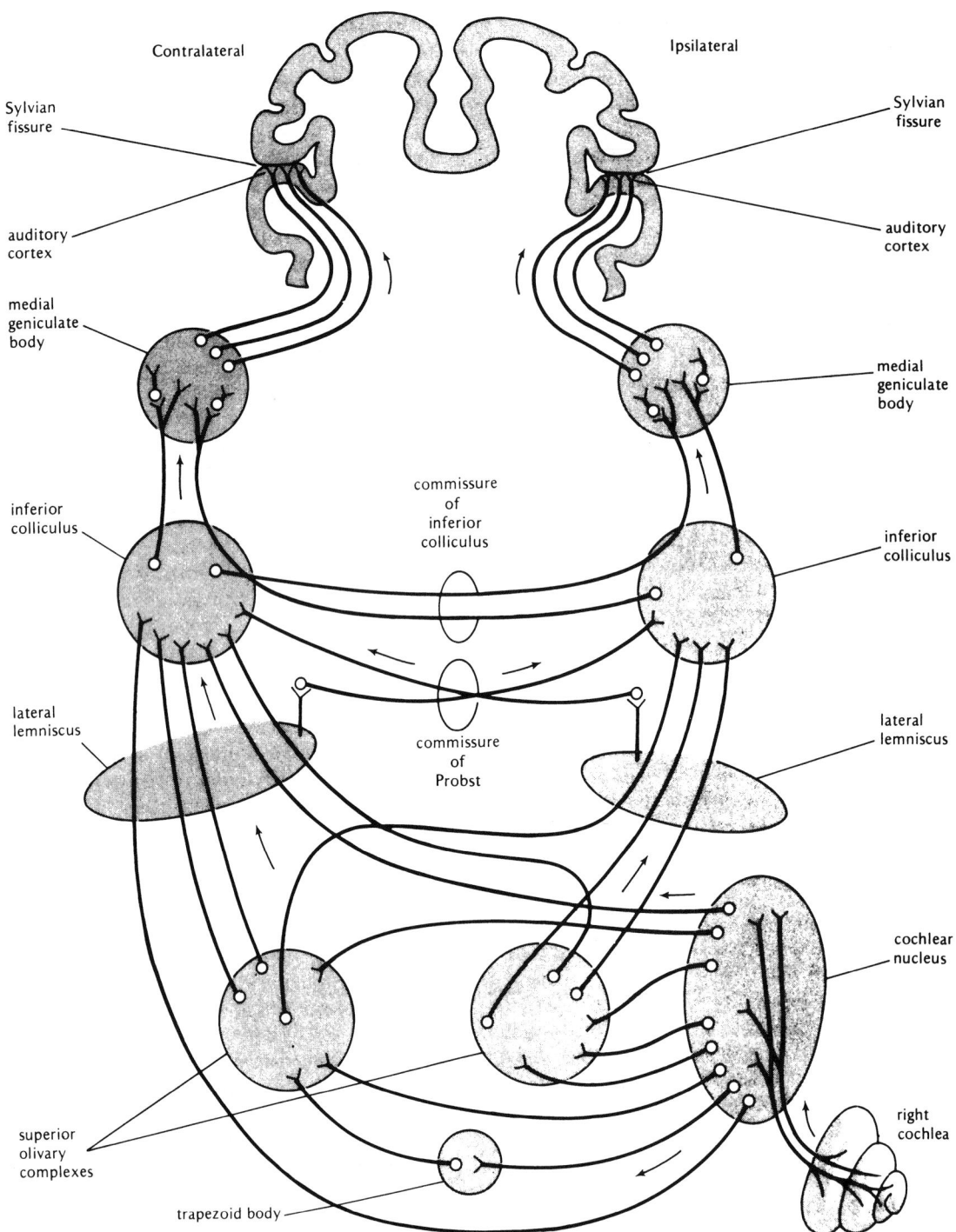

Figure 129.23   Highly schematic diagram of the ascending (afferent) pathways of the central auditory system from the right cochlea to the auditory cortex. No attempt is made to show the subdivisions and connections within the various regions, cerebellar connections, or connections with the reticular formation. (From Yost WA, Neilsen *DW. Fundamentals of hearing*, 2nd ed. New York: Holt, Rinehart & Winston, 1985:121.)

ears converge. Auditory nuclei above the superior olivary complex can be excitatory or inhibitory with inputs from each ear. Stimulation of the contralateral ear typically is excitatory to cell bodies of the auditory CNS, whereas stimulation of the ipsilateral ear is inhibitory. As shown in Figure 129.13, the medial superior olivary complex is the

origin of the crossed efferent fibers that terminate on outer hair cells, whereas the lateral superior olivary complex is the origin for the uncrossed efferent fibers that terminate on inner hair cells. Although many functions have been attributed to the efferent auditory system, especially protecting the cochlea from loud sounds, the functions of the system are unknown; those that have been proposed are easily debated (24).

The inferior colliculus is a complex nucleus with at least 18 major cell types and at least five areas of specialization. It is involved in probably all forms of auditory behavior, including differential sensitivity for frequency and intensity, loudness, and binaural hearing. The inferior colliculus is clearly more than a relay center. The medial geniculate body of the thalamus sends projections to the auditory cortex, but its specific functions are unknown.

The auditory cortex is located in the sylvian fissure of the temporal lobe; many secondary auditory areas are clustered around the primary area. In each area, the cells are tonotopically organized in a columnar manner, each column having a special attribute. The cells in one column can have different tuning at a similar characteristic frequency, whereas another column can be associated with intensity encoding, another with providing inhibitory responses to stimulation of one ear and excitatory responses of the other ear, and so on. As is common for thalamic connections with the cortex, nuclei within the medial geniculate body that send fibers to the auditory cortex also receive fibers from the same area of the cortex. Bilateral le-

sions of the temporal lobe have been shown to produce wide-ranging effects (cortical deafness, in which several auditory behaviors are severely affected, including speech discrimination, localization of sound, temporal processing of information, and the detection of faint, short-duration signals) (25). Another important feature of the auditory system is its tonotopic nature. From the basilar membrane to the auditory cortex, the system is organized spatially with respect to frequency. Each place on the basilar membrane responds best to a specific frequency—high-frequency sounds are localized to the base, and low-frequency sounds, to the apex. The tonotopic organization of the cochlea is preserved at the cochlear nucleus. Figure 129.24 shows that as an electrode penetrates the cochlear nucleus, fibers with different characteristic frequencies are contacted, and the characteristic frequencies form an orderly progression. Similar data exist at all nuclei of the auditory CNS, including the auditory cortex.

The most obvious clinical application of basic information on the auditory CNS involves interpretation of evoked potentials. The auditory brainstem response (ABR) is one component of auditory evoked potentials. The existence of the ABR was first reported by Sohmer and Feinmesser in

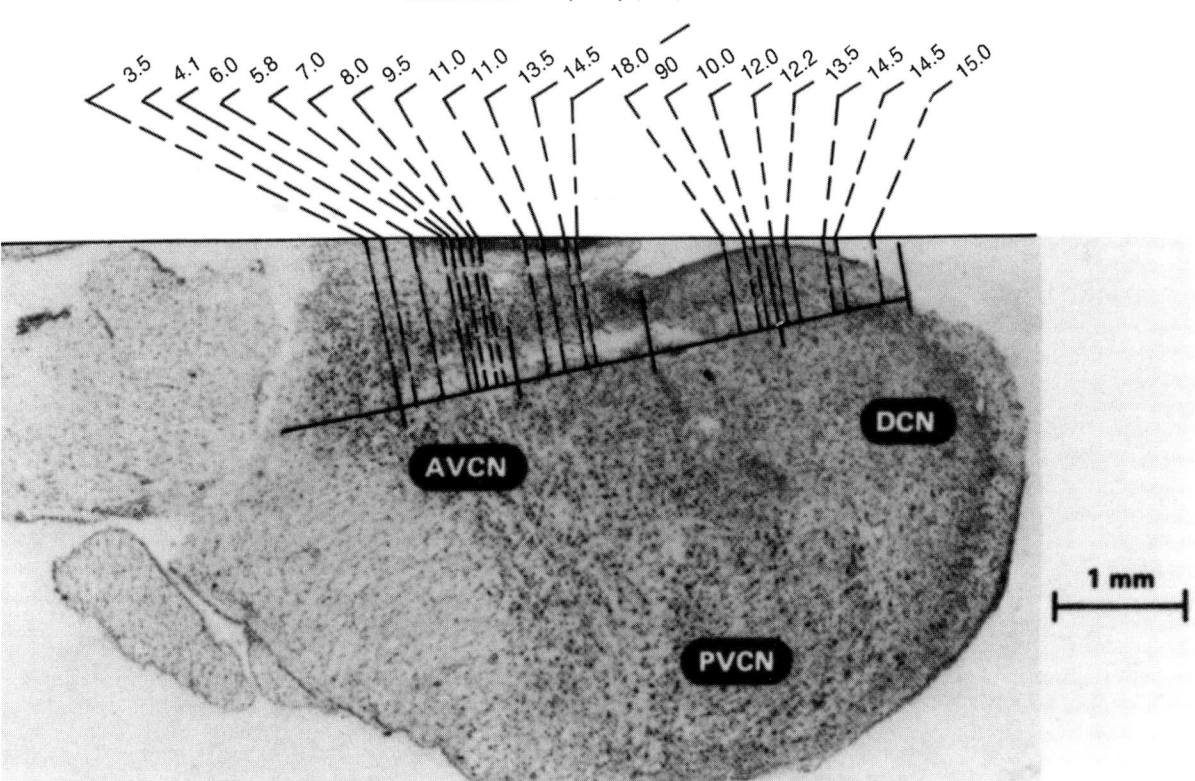

Figure 129.24 Cross section of cochlear nucleus shows the track made by electrode penetration. The characteristic frequencies of neurons recorded from various points within the anteroventral cochlear nucleus (*AVCN*) and dural cochlear nucleus (*DCN*) show that the spatial separation of frequency is maintained within those two divisions of the cochlear nucleus. *PVCN*, posteroventral cochlear nucleus. This tonotopic organization is maintained throughout the central auditory system. (Redrawn from Rose JE, Galambos R, Hughes JR. Microelectrode studies of the cochlear nuclei of the cat. *Bull Johns Hopkins Hosp* 1959;104:211, with permission.)

1967 (26). The ABR is recorded from electrodes attached to various positions on the head. The ABR consists of a series of seven waves occurring within about 10 milliseconds after stimulus onset. The convention in the United States is to label wave peaks with Roman numerals. It is generally accepted that the ABR is generated by the auditory nerve and subsequent fiber tracts and nuclei within the auditory brainstem pathways. It is widely believed that each wave is generated as follows: wave I and II are the eighth nerve, III is cochlear nucleus, IV is superior olive/lateral lemniscus, and V is lateral leminiscus/inferior colliculus.

The ABR is generated by a click stimulus because it yields the clearest response. The ABR is used clinically both in the estimation of auditory sensitivity and in otoneurologic assessment. In this way, it can be used to detect lesions along the auditory nerve and brainstem pathways. The study can be performed regardless of state of wakefulness, and the result is unaffected by most medications. As a result, children are often tested while under sedation or during sleep.

The field of clinical objective audiometry has recently gained an additional technique in the auditory evoked response battery. The *auditory steady-state response* (ASSR) promises to be a valuable study in the workup of auditory dysfunction. Unlike ABRs, which are obtained through the use of transient stimuli, ASSRs are evoked by using sustained continuous tones. The tones are frequency specific because the continuous tones do not have spectral distortion problems as do brief tone bursts or click (27). Of note, ASSR also can be performed regardless of the state of wakefulness.

There are several advantages of ASSR over ABR. First, ASSR is a better technique for evaluating hearing aid performance because hearing aids and cochlear implants process continuous stimuli with less signal distortion than transient stimuli. Furthermore, ASSR can provide threshold information in a frequency-specific manner at intensity levels of 120 dB or greater (28,29). This allows differentiation of severe and profound hearing loss, which cannot be accomplished with ABR. This characteristic of ASSR may allow it to be used in assessing pediatric patients for cochlear implant candidacy (30). Last, ASSR has been shown to be more time efficient by determining more thresholds in a shorter time compared with ABR (31). Future research and clinical use are likely to solidify the status of ASSR in the audiologic armamentarium.

The neuroanatomic features of the system are complicated. Processing of neural information probably involves both parallel and serial processing. The former is anatomically described by a single fiber with ramifications to many target areas. Serial processing involves a fiber going to one target, which in turn goes to another target, and so forth. In the auditory CNS, both serial and parallel processing are involved. Because the auditory CNS is a highly redundant, complicated, and extremely powerful system, interpretation of evoked-potential data, and of other CNS neural data, is not straightforward.

HIGHLIGHTS

- The acoustic properties of the head and external ear are important, particularly because they provide cues for localizing sources of sound.
- The middle ear acts as a transformer between air and the fluid-filled cochlea and provides a sound pressure gain of 25 to 30 dB. The combined effect of the acoustic properties of the head, external ear, and middle ear, and the input impedance of the cochlea determine the frequency range of human hearing.
- The cochlea is a coiled bony tube approximately 35 mm long and divided into three compartments—the scala tympani, scala vestibuli, and scala media. The scalae tympani and vestibuli contain perilymph and are connected through the helicotrema at the apex of the cochlea. The scala media contains endolymph and has a positive DC resting potential of approximately 80 mV, which arises from Na^+-K^+-ATPase pumps in the stria vascularis.
- The auditory transducer is the organ of Corti, which contains sensory cells (three rows of outer hair cells and one row of inner hair cells). Deflection of stereocilia (hairs) of the sensory cells by a mechanical traveling wave starts transduction.
- A traveling wave, from the base toward the apex of the cochlea, arises in response to piston-like movement of the stapes. The traveling wave has a sharply tuned peak at the base for high-frequency sound that progresses toward the apex as frequency decreases.
- Deflection of stereocilia by the traveling wave opens and closes ion channels; the result is current flow (potassium ion) into the sensory cell. The potassium flux arises from the +80 mV endocochlear potential added to the negative intracellular potential of inner and outer hair cells. The resulting depolarization causes an enzyme cascade that releases chemical transmitters and activates afferent nerve fibers.
- Approximately 90% to 95% of the radial nerve fibers (type I) innervate inner hair cells. Approximately 5% to 10% (type II, outer spiral fibers) are connected to outer hair cells. Each inner hair cell is innervated by 15 to 20 type I neurons. Each type II neuron branches to innervate approximately 10 outer hair cells. Approximately 1,800 efferent fibers project to the sensory cells from the ipsilateral and contralateral superior olivary complexes.
- The most basic measure of auditory nerve function is the tuning curve of a single auditory nerve fiber. Tuning curves of single fibers of the nerve are strikingly similar to tuning curves of the mechanical traveling wave. Injury to sensory cells and stereocilia alters the features of tuning curves, including sensitivity and sharp tuning.
- The middle ear system is passive and linear in response to signals as great as 130 dB SPL, but the inner ear is an active system with its own amplifier and is nonlinear. These properties allow the inner ear to respond to a wide range of intensities and provide the basis for suppression phenomena.
- Although the efferent auditory system is well developed, the functional significance is not well understood. It may have a role in the cochlear transduction and in protecting the cochlea from overexposure to intense sound.

REFERENCES

1. Tonndorf J. The external ear. In: Jahn HF, Santos-Sacchi J, eds. *Physiology of the ear.* New York: Raven Press, 1988:4–20.
2. Moller A. The acoustic middle ear muscle reflex. In: Keidel WD, Neff WD, eds. *Handbook of sensory physiology.* New York: Springer-Verlag, 1974:5:312–329.
3. Schulte BA, Adams JC. Distribution of immunoreactive Na$^+$, K$^+$-ATPase in gerbil cochleas. *J Histochem Cytochem* 1989;37:127–135.
4. Neely JG, Dennis JM, Lippe WR. Anatomy of the auditory end organ and neural pathways. In: Cummings CW, ed. *Otolaryngology–head and neck surgery.* St. Louis: Mosby, 1986.
5. Zheng J, Shen W, He DZ, et al. Prestin is the motor protein of cochlear outer hair cells. *Nature* 2000;405:149–155.
6. Eguiluz VM, Ospeck M, Choe Y, et al. Essential nonlinearities in hearing. *Physiol Rev Lett* 2000;84:5232–5235.
7. Camalet S, Duke T, Julicher F, et al. Auditory sensitivity provided by self-tuned critical oscillations of hair cells. *Proc Natl Acad Sci U S A* 2000;97:3183–3188.
8. Niedzielski AS, Safieddin S, Wenthold RJ. Molecular analysis of excitatory amino acid receptor expression in the cochlea. *Audiol Neurootol* 1997;2:79–91.
9. Sewell W. Neurotransmitters and synaptic transmission, In: Dallas P, Popper A, Fay R, eds. *The cochlea.* Berlin: Springer-Verlag, 1996:503–523.
10. Housley GD, Ryan AE Cholinergic and purinergic neurohumoral signalling in the inner ear: a molecular physiological analysis. *Audiol Neurootol* 1997;2:92–110.
11. Schmiedt RA. Basic techniques for the measurement of cochlear potentials. In: Beagley HA, ed. *Auditory investigation: the scientific and technological basis.* Oxford: Clarendon Press, 1979:211–232.
12. Liberman MC, Dodds LW, Pierce S. Afferent and efferent innervation of the cat cochlea: quantitative analysis with light and electron microscopy. *J Comp Neurol* 1990;301:443–451.
13. Fekete DM, Rouiller EM, Liberman MC, et al. The central projections of intracellularly labeled auditory nerve fibers in cats. *J Comp Neurol* 1984;229:432–440.
14. Leake PA, Synder RL. Topographic organization of the central projections of the spiral ganglion in cats. *J Comp Neurol* 1989;281:612–629.
15. Liberman MC. Effects of chronic de-efferentation on auditory nerve response. *Hear Res* 1990;49:209–221.
16. Schmiedt RA, Mills JH, Adams JC. Tuning and suppression in auditory nerve fibers of aged gerbils raised in quiet or noise. *Hear Res* 1990;45:221–229.
17. Probst R. Otoacoustic emissions: new aspects of cochlear mechanics and inner ear pathophysiology. In: Pfaltz CR, ed. *Advances in otorhinolaryngology.* Basel: Karger, 1990.
18. Penner MJ, Zhang T. Prevalence of spontaneous otoacoustic emissions in adults revisited. *Hear Res* 1997;103:28–34.
19. Burns EM, Arehart KH, Campbell SL. Prevalence of spontaneous otoacoustic emissions in neonates. *J Acoust Soc Am* 1992;91:1571–1575.
20. Glattke TJ, Robinette MS. Transient evoked otoacoustic emissions. In: Robinette RM, Glattke T, eds. *Otoacoustic emissions: clinical applications,* 2nd ed. New York: Thieme, 2002:95–115.
21. Harris FP, Probst R. Otoacoustic emissions and audiometric outcomes. In: Robinette RM, Glattke T, eds. *Otoacoustic emissions: clinical applications,* 2nd ed. New York: Thieme, 2002:213–242.
22. Prieve BA. Otoacoustic emissions in neonatal screening. In: Robinette RM, Glattke T, eds. *Otoacoustic emissions: clinical applications,* 2nd ed. New York: Thieme, 2002:348–374.
23. Kemp DT. Otoacoustic emissions, their origin in cochlear function, and use. *Br Med Bull* 2002;63:223–241.
24. Liberman MC. The olivocochlear efferent bundle and susceptibility of the inner ear to acoustic injury. *J Neurophysiol* 1991;65:123–132.
25. Jerger J, Weikers NJ, Sharbrough FW, et al. Bilateral lesions of the temporal lobe. *Acta Otolaryngol (Stockh)* 1969;258(suppl):1.
26. Sohmer H, Feinmesser M. Cochlear action potentials recorded from the external ear in man. *Ann Otol Rhinol Laryngol* 1967;76:427–436.
27. Lins OG, Picton TW. Auditory steady state responses to multiple simultaneous stimuli. *Electroencephalogr Clin Neurophysiol* 1995;95:420–432.
28. Rans G, Dowell RC, Richards FW, et al. Steady state evoked potential and behavioral hearing thresholds in a group of children with absent click evoked auditory brainstem response. *Ear Hear* 1998;19:48–61.
29. Swanepoel D, Hugo R, Roode R. Auditory steady state responses for children with severe to profound hearing loss. *Arch Otolaryngol Head Neck Surg* 2004;130:531–535.
30. Zwolan TA. Cochlear implants. In: Katz J, ed. *Handbook of clinical audiology,* 5th ed. Baltimore: Lippincott Williams & Wilkins, 2002:740–757.
31. Swanepoel D, Schmulian D, Hugo R. Establishing normal hearing with the dichotic multiple-frequency auditory steady state response compared with auditory brainstem response protocol. *Acta Otolaryngol* 2004;124:62–68.

Vestibular Function and Anatomy

130

Shawn D. Newlands   *Conrad Wall III*

The vestibular system, defined as the peripheral vestibular motion detectors and related central nervous system structures, senses motion in space and converts that motion into information that the remainder of the central nervous system can use to generate appropriate motor reflexes or facilitate complex processes such as the coordination of head, eye, and trunk movements or updating one's perception of his or her orientation in the world. The vestibular system, like the auditory system, converts physical stimuli into neural signals, but the vestibular system detects angular and linear acceleration, rather than sound. The vestibular system is present in all vertebrates and many invertebrates. Yet, despite the importance of spatial orientation in all mobile animals, the vestibular system is largely underappreciated until a malfunction occurs, at which point patients present to a physician, often an otolaryngologist, for treatment and education. This chapter discusses the anatomy of the peripheral vestibular system, the biophysics of sensory transduction, vestibular hair cell types and physiology, vestibular afferent types and physiology, and the organization of sensory inputs to the central nervous system, but it is only an introduction to this important, complex system.

The complexity of challenges presented to the vestibular system on a daily basis is elucidated with a simple example. Figure 130.1 follows an office worker through the simple processes of looking for a book on a shelf. She pushes her chair back, stands, and turns left to face the shelf. She then tilts her head (right ear down) to scan the book titles. One way to describe the motion the worker's head makes between the two positions is to decompose the movement into linear (straight-line) motion and angular (rotational) motion, by considering a path made by the center of her head. In this example, the linear motion can be described as backing away from the desk 2 m, with a leftward motion of 3 m and an upward motion of 1 m (Fig. 130.1B). In terms of rotary motion, the woman pitches her head upward 40 degrees from looking down at the paper to looking horizontal. She turns 90 degrees to the left around a vertical axis to face the bookshelf. She then tilts her head 75 degrees toward the right-ear-down position to read the book titles (Fig. 130.1A). Thus, the motion the worker uses to complete the movement between the starting and ending positions can be characterized by three linear movements and three angular movements.

The vestibular system must be able to detect both linear and angular motion in order for the brain to estimate the orientation of the body in space. An important additional piece of information needed for orientation is the direction of gravitational pull or the gravity vector. Among other things, the knowledge of the orientation of gravity allows humans to maintain a vertical stance. Even in the previous simple example, there is not only a complex interaction between the motions of the head, eyes, and body relative to one another, all of which use information generated by the vestibular system, but there is a visual, somatosensory, and vestibular system interaction that allows the worker to know her orientation relative to her surroundings.

GROSS ANATOMY OF THE VESTIBULAR SYSTEM

Vertebrates have what amounts to an inertial guidance system made up of multiple sensors of linear acceleration and multiple sensors of angular acceleration in each inner ear.

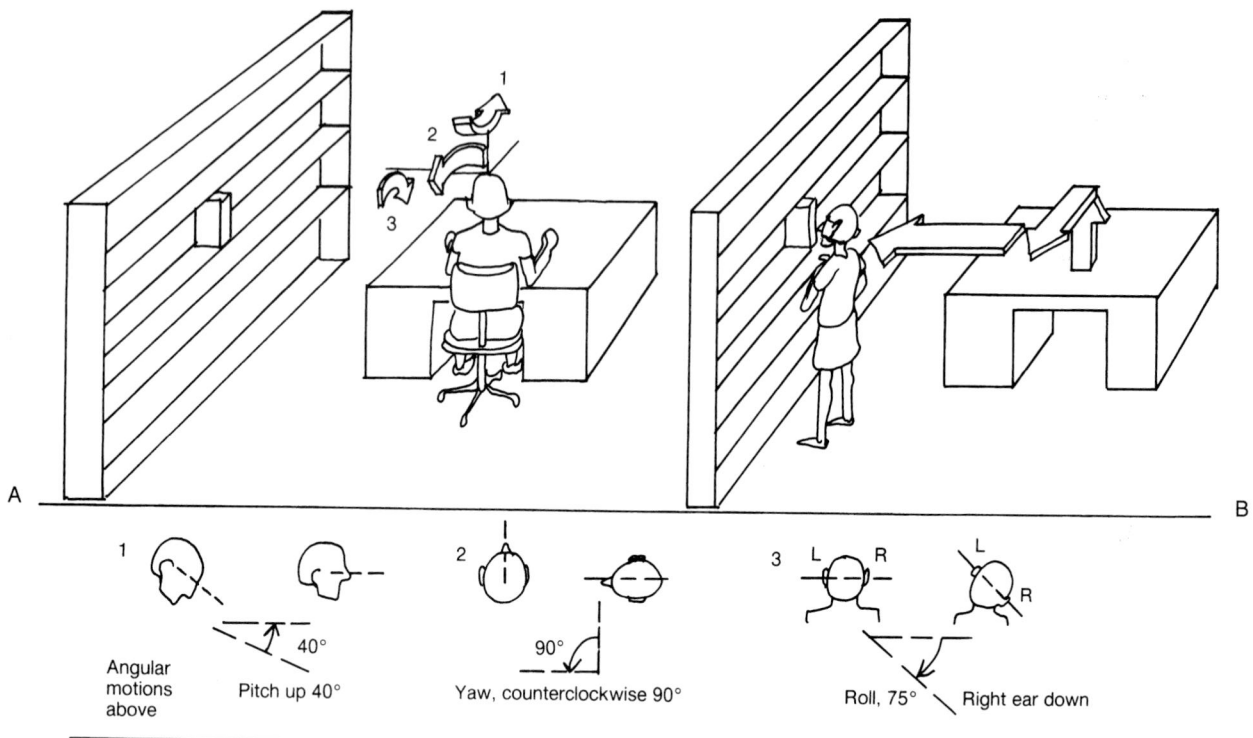

Figure 130.1 Angular and linear motion associated with moving the head from one point in space to another. **A:** Worker seated at desk. **B:** Worker moves from desk to bookcase and tilts head to read book title. The angular motion needed is shown in **A**, the linear motion in **B**.

This guidance system, the vestibular labyrinth, is housed in a portion of the otic capsule in the petrous portion of the temporal bone. The bony labyrinth is the thick bone of the otic capsule that houses the membranous labyrinth suspended in perilymph. The membranous labyrinth holds endolymphatic fluid and the neuroepithelial structures of sensory transduction. The perilymphatic and endolymphatic spaces of the labyrinth are continuous with those of the cochlea; therefore, the composition and homeostatic mechanisms of the perilymph and endolymph discussed in the cochlea chapter (Chapter 129) apply to the vestibular system as well. As in the cochlea, proper function of the vestibular system depends on the unique composition of these fluids.

The vestibular labyrinth is a paired structure, with the right and left labyrinth mirroring one another. Subdivisions of the vestibular labyrinth include the three semicircular canals: the lateral or horizontal canal, the posterior canal, and the anterior or superior canal, all of which detect angular accelerations. The geometric layout of the canals is shown in Figure 130.2. The horizontal canals lie parallel to the line between the external auditory canal and the outer canthus of the eye, which is inclined 30 degrees above the horizontal axial plane. The vertical canals are roughly at right angles to the horizontal canals and to each other. When looking down at the top of the head, the anterior canal is oriented at approximately 45 degrees off mid-

sagittal and 45 degrees anterior to the intraaural line. The posterior canal is aligned roughly 45 degrees behind the intraaural line; thus, the anterior canal on the left is roughly parallel to the posterior canal on the right, and the left posterior canal and the right anterior canal are similarly aligned.

At one end of the bony canal, there is a swelling known as the ampulla; this swelling houses both the crista ampullaris and the cupula. The ampullated end of the lateral semicircular canal is at the anterior end of the canal; the ampulla of the superior semicircular canal is also anterior, and the ampulla of the posterior semicircular canal is lateral. The nonampullated end of the lateral semicircular canal enters the vestibule posterolaterally. The nonampullated ends of the posterior and superior semicircular canals join to form the common crus and enter the vestibule posteromedially.

Housed in the vestibule are the otolith organs—the utricle and the saccule—which detect linear acceleration. Neither organ is perfectly planar, but the utricle is primarily aligned parallel to the earth and is roughly aligned with the ipsilateral horizontal canal (Fig. 130.3). At rest, the saccule is perpendicular and at right angles to the utricle. The sensitivity of detection of translational acceleration is greatest in the plane of the macula. Thus, the utricular macula is sensitive in the horizontal plane, and the saccular macula is sensitive in the sagittal plane.

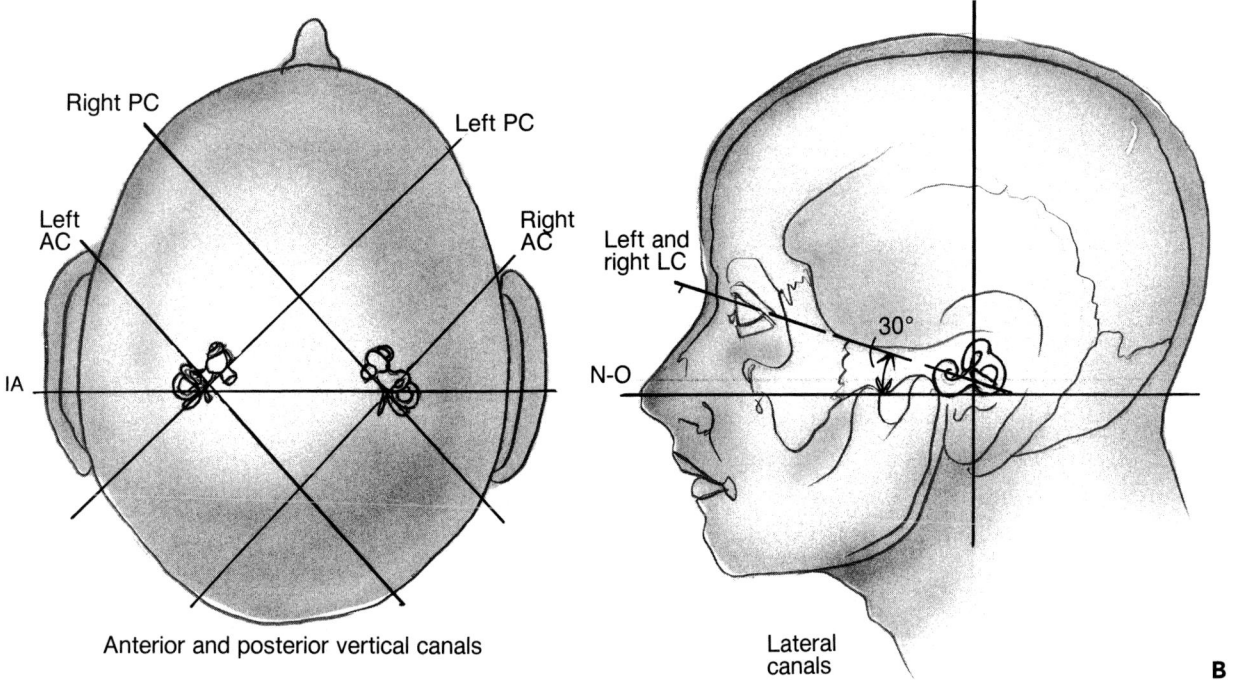

Figure 130.2 **A:** Orientation of the vertical canals in the human head. **B:** Plane of the lateral semicircular canals. AC, anterior vertical semicircular canal; IA, interaural; LC, lateral semicircular canal; N-O, nasal-occipital axis; PC, posterior vertical semicircular canal.

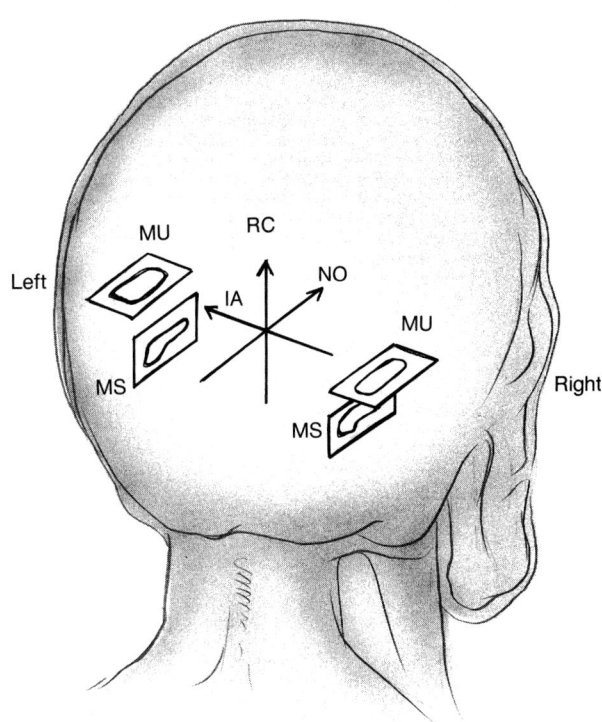

Figure 130.3 Approximate planar layout of the otolith organs. MS, Macular saccule; MU, macular utriculi; IA, interaural axis; NO, nasal-occipital axis; RC, rostral-caudal axis.

BASIC PHYSICS OF MECHANOTRANSDUCTION

Both the linear (utricle and saccule) and the angular (semicircular canal) acceleration sensors for the inner ear use a three-step process to convert accelerations of the head into useful information for the nervous system (Fig. 130.4). The elements used in these three steps are inertial mass, one or more sensory hair cells, and the nerve fibers connected to the hair cells through synaptic junctions. Figure 130.4A shows the system at rest (no acceleration). Figure 130.4B shows the response when the system is accelerated to the left. The resulting rightward movement of the mass (M) relative to the sensory hair cell deflects the sensory hairs, depolarizes the cell body, and increases the discharge rate of the attached nerve fiber.

The term inertial mass invokes Newton's second law, which relates the acceleration ($\vec{a}$) of an object possessing mass to the force ($\vec{F}$) needed to accelerate said object. For linear acceleration, Newton's second law can be written $\vec{F} = M\vec{a}$. The arrows above F and a indicate vector quantities having both magnitude and direction. In accelerometers, acceleration is measured by measuring the force created on a mass during the movement. Mass also is subject to the force of gravitational attraction ($\vec{g}$). Thus, the total force generated on an object possessing mass is $\vec{F} = M(\vec{a} - \vec{g})$. The quantity ($\vec{a} - \vec{g}$) is called specific force, and this equation shows that mass does not differentiate linear acceleration from gravitational attraction.

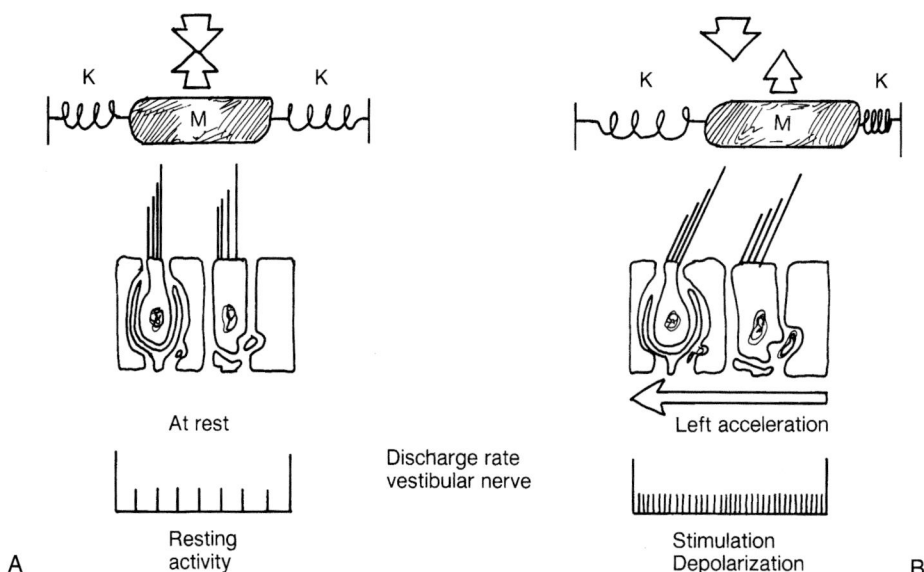

Figure 130.4 Elementary model of vestibular motion sensor. **A:** Head at rest. **B:** Head accelerating to the left. The seismic mass (*M*) is suspended by two restoring spring forces (*K*). Acceleration to the left displaces the mass to the right relative to the hair cells. This displacement increases the discharge rate of the afferent fibers attached to them.

For the saccule and utricle, the inertial mass is accounted for by the calcium carbonate crystals, or otoconia, minus the buoyancy of the fluid surrounding them. For the semicircular canal, the angular equivalent of seismic mass, the moment of inertia (J), is provided by the liquid that fills the inside of the torus-shaped tube of the membranous labyrinth. In the case of angular acceleration, Newton's second law ($\vec{T} = J\vec{a}$, where $\vec{a}$ is angular acceleration) relates the angular acceleration to the amount of torque ($\vec{T}$) produced by acceleration. This torque is not affected by linear acceleration.

Acceleration, linear or angular, produces a force, or torque, on a mass that is in opposition to a springlike restoring force. Hook's law states that the force generated by a spring ($\vec{F}$) is proportional to the amount it is deflected ($\vec{x}$): $\vec{F} = K\vec{x}$, where K is the so-called spring constant. Therefore, there is specific displacement ($\vec{x}$) of a mass, the deflection of which is resisted by a springlike force: $\vec{x} = M\vec{a}/K$. It is this deflection that is sensed by hair cells.

NEUROEPITHELIUM

The sensory hair cells in the membranous labyrinth are similar to those in the cochlea in that both detect small deflections and transmit the information provided by the displacement to the central nervous system (Fig. 130.5). However, significant differences are found between the cochlea and the vestibular neuroepithelia. The vestibular hair cell body is surrounded by supporting and other hair

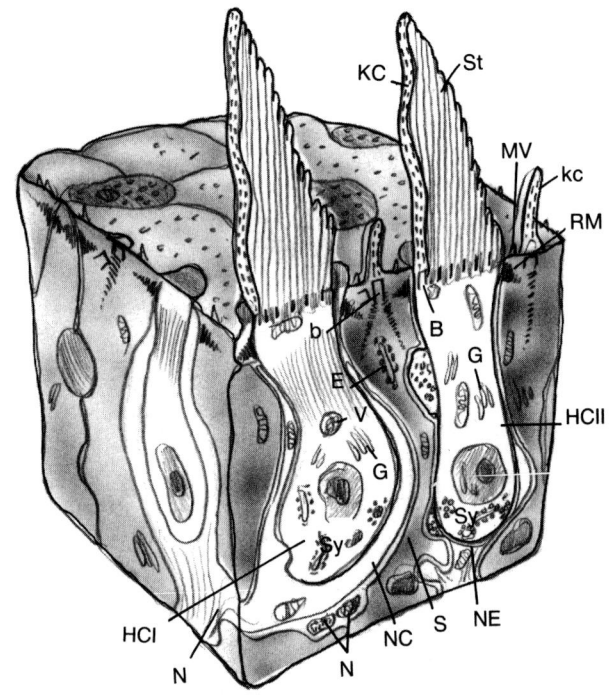

Figure 130.5 Vestibular sensory epithelium and its innervation. HCI, type I hair cell; HCII, type II hair cell; St, stereocilia; KC, kinocilia [kc, modified kinocilia and roots (b) of supporting cells, (S)]; N, nerve fiber; NC, nerve chalice; NE, nerve endings; Sy, synaptic structures; G, Golgi membranes; RM, multivesicular reticular membrane; E, endoplasmic reticulum; MV, microvilli; V, vesicle; B, basal body. (Modified from Spoendlin HH. The ultrastructure of the vestibular sense organ. In: Wolfson RJ, ed. *The vestibular system and its diseases.* Philadelphia: University of Pennsylvania Press, 1966:39, with permission.)

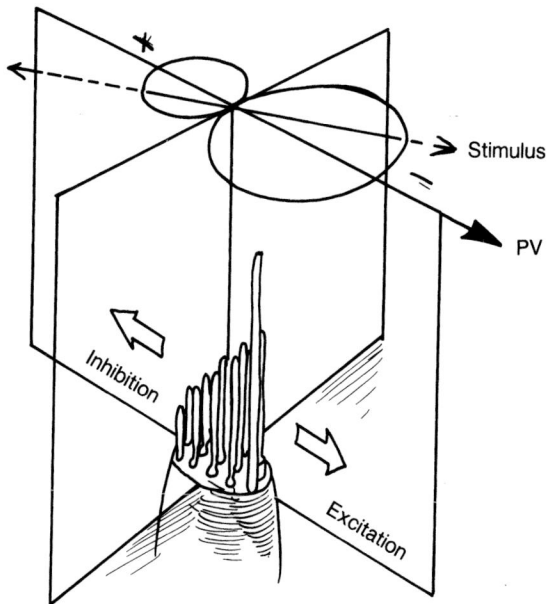

Figure 130.6 Directional sensitivity of the hair cell approximating a cosine function of stimulus direction. The output varies as the cosine of the angle between the direction of maximum sensitivity and the applied displacement. PV, polarization vector. (Modified from Loewenstein WR. *Handbook of sensory physiology.* Vol. 1. *Principles of receptor physiology.* New York: Springer-Verlag, 1971:415, with permission.)

cells. Sensory bundles extend from the apical surface of the vestibular hair cell body and are usually in contact with a gelatinous membrane, the motion of which is affected by displacement of the mass element: either the cupula of the semicircular canal or the otolithic membrane for the utricle and saccule. These sensory hair bundles have two distinct ciliary types. The kinocilium is the tallest cilia and is near the edge of the top of the hair cell. Kinocilia are not found on cochlear hair cells. The position of the kinocilium determines the orientation of the hair cell. There are many stereocilia, arranged in columns and rows, and the closer they are to the kinocilium, the taller they are. This arrangement produces an orderly array of stereocilia and a means by which alignment of an individual hair cell can be determined by its so-called morphologic polarization vector, which is shown as an arrow in Figure 130.6. Experimental data show that a functional axis of alignment corresponds with the morphologic one. It is in this axis that a cell responds most vigorously to the displacement of the stereocilia. Displacement of the stereocilia perpendicular to the polarization axis causes no change in the resting potential of the hair cells. On any one sensory organ, neighboring hair cells tend to have polarization vectors that are aligned.

The electrical potential inside the body of hair cells differs from that of the fluids surrounding them because of active transport at the cell membrane. Bending the stereocilia on top of the cell toward the kinocilium opens potassium channels and temporarily increases the resting

potential, depolarizing the cell. Deflection away from the kinocilium hyperpolarizes the cell. The channels responsible for transduction are located at the top of stereocilia in the utricle and are opened by relative motion of the stereocilia (1). The hair cells release a neurotransmitter (believed to be glutamate) that is excitatory to the hair cell afferents with which they connect. At rest, there is a baseline release of the neurotransmitter. This release is important because not only does deflection of the hair cell bundle toward the kinocilium (depolarizing the hair cell) increase transmitter release, but deflection of the hair cell bundle away from the kinocilium (hyperpolarizing the hair cell) reduces transmitter release. Thus, one hair cell detects both acceleration and deceleration along the axis of the morphologic polarization vector.

There are two morphologically and physiologically distinct types of hair cell bodies: type I or chalice hair cells and type II or cylindrical hair cells. The body of a type I hair cell is entirely engulfed by one afferent terminal. Efferent innervation is indirect, as the efferent nerve has its synapse on the afferent nerve ending. Type II hair cells can have one or more afferent nerve endings on the body of the cell. Type II hair cells can also be directly or indirectly innervated by vestibular efferent terminals. Type I and type II hair cells are not evenly distributed throughout the neuroepithelium of either the semicircular canal ampullae or the utricular maculae. As discussed later, they are innervated by different classes of vestibular afferents.

The neuroepithelium contains other cell types as well. Supporting cells have the nuclei located at the basal end of the sensory epithelial, above the basement membrane. These cells are believed to make and secrete the extracellular macromolecules of the cupula and otolith membrane. Dark cells can be found at the margins of the transitional epithelium surrounding the neuroepithelium. These dark cells are located directly above pigmented cells and are thought to produce the ionic composition of the endolymph.

MICROANATOMY AND BIOPHYSICS OF THE SEMICIRCULAR CANALS

The semicircular canal is a membranous structure shaped like a torus or hollow doughnut (Fig. 130.7). Maximum sensitivity is to rotation in the plane of the torus. At one end of the torus, there is an enlargement, the ampulla. A gelatinous flap, the cupula, completely seals one side of the ampulla from the other. Because the cupula is elastic, any pressure difference causes it to deflect. The interior of the torus is filled with endolymph, a liquid with the density and viscosity of water. The membranous portion of the canal is attached to the temporal bone. When the head is turned, the membranous labyrinth moves with it, but the endolymph inside has an inertial mass that tends to oppose the turning motion. This oppositional force causes pressure buildup across the cupula, deflecting the cupula

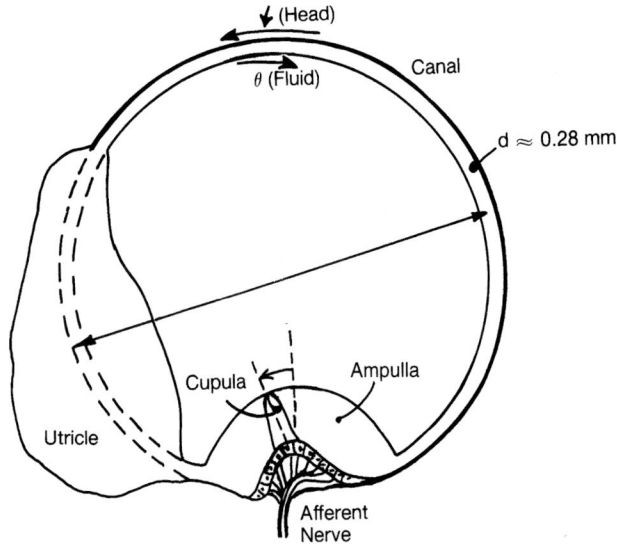

Figure 130.7 Semicircular canal. (Modified from Milsum J. *Biological control systems analysis*. New York: McGraw-Hill, 1966, with permission.)

from its equilibrium position. Within the physiologic range of motion, this deflection most nearly resembles the motion of the head of a drum or clamped diaphragm when pressure is uniformly applied to one side.

Cilia are embedded in the gelatinous cupula. As the cupula is deflected, the stereocilia bend either toward or away from the kinocilium, producing an increase or decrease, respectively, in the firing rate of the vestibular nerve. The kinocilia are parallel to the long axis of the canal. In the lateral semicircular canal, hair cells are arranged such that the kinocilia are closest to the vestibule; maximal excitation occurs with ampullopetal flow of endolymph. In the posterior and superior semicircular canals, this arrangement is reversed—the kinocilium are farthest from the vestibule. Thus, ampullofugal flow is excitatory.

The crista ampullaris has been divided into central, intermediate, and peripheral zones. In humans and other mammals, type I hair cells are relatively more common in the central zone than in the intermediate and peripheral zones (2). In contrast, type II cells are relatively less common in the central zone than in other zones.

More than half a century ago, Steinhausen constructed a biophysical model of the semicircular canal known as the *torsion pendulum model*. The behavior of this model is determined by the mass of the endolymph, the viscous damping properties of the endolymph, and the springlike restoring force of the cupula. Estimates of these physical properties and knowledge of the geometric properties of the semicircular canal allow observers to relate deflection of the cupula to angular acceleration of the head. With this model, it can be predicted that cupular deflection is proportional to head velocity over a frequency bandwidth of approximately 0.1 to 10 Hz. Above and below this fre-

quency bandwidth, the cupular deflection is not as great, and the sensitivity of the semicircular canal to velocity decreases. At 0 Hz, which corresponds to constant-velocity rotation, the torsion-pendulum model predicts there will be no response at all. The prediction made with this model agrees with the perception of a person who is turned at a constant velocity around a vertical axis. Subjects sense initial acceleration, but in the absence of other cues such as vision, subjects feel they are no longer rotating after 30 to 60 seconds. Rotating subjects who are suddenly brought to a full stop feel a sensation of turning in the opposite direction. This sensation is due to the inertia of the endolymph, which continues to rotate, deflecting the cupula in the direction opposite to that experienced with the initial rotation. Reflexive eye movements measured during these steps of velocity mirror the sensation felt by the subjects and are the basis of cupulometry used in the Bárány test and other tests of the vestibuloocular reflex.

MICROANATOMY AND BIOPHYSICS OF THE OTOLITH ORGANS

All the sensors in the vestibular system combine a mass element connected to sensory hair cells (Fig. 130.4). In the case of the otolith organs (utricle and saccule), the mass is composed of calcium carbonate crystals known as otoconia that are embedded in a gelatinous supporting substrate. Displacement of this structure due to linear acceleration or change in orientation with respect to gravity affects a number of sensory hair cells. Each cell has a polarization vector oriented in a slightly different direction, making each one maximally sensitive to acceleration in that particular direction (Fig. 130.8).

The calcium carbonate crystals are suspended in the otolith membrane. Under this membrane are a number of sensory hair cells, each of which can have one or more afferent connections to the vestibular nerve. The drawing in Figure 130.8 is an exploded view. In reality, the stereocilia from the hair cells are in direct contact with the otolith membrane. In Figure 130.8, each of the sensory hair cells has a polarization vector with a small arrow indicating its direction of maximal excitation in the plane. The large arrow at the top of the otolithic mass represents linear acceleration that deflects the otolith mass in the direction of the arrow. Hair cells that have polarization vectors aligned with the arrow and in the same direction are excited maximally, whereas hair cells that have polarization vectors perpendicular to the acceleration are not stimulated.

In the maculae of the utricle and saccule, type I hair cells are relatively more prevalent close to the striola than in the peripheral zone areas. The striola is a zone that runs the length of the macula, is about 100 microns wide, and divides the macula into the medial and lateral extra striola zones. The orientation of the hair cells on either side of the striola is roughly 180 degrees out of phase. Because the

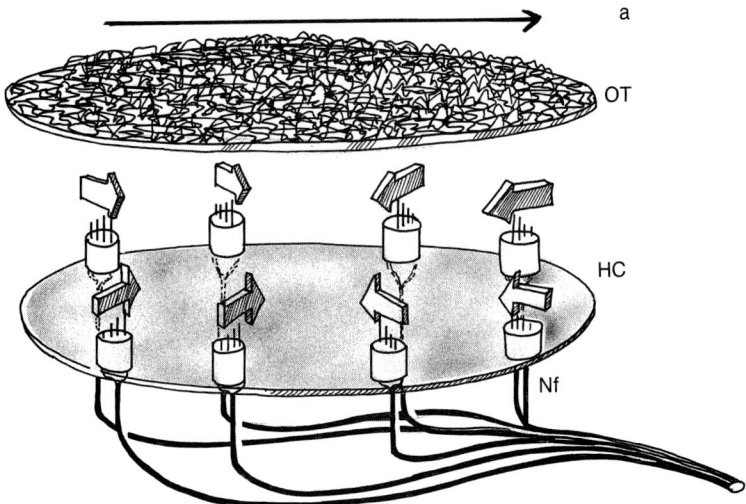

Figure 130.8 Simplified otolith organ. The otoconial mass (OT) is suspended above the sensory hair cells (HC) in an exploded view. Each hair cell is innervated by one afferent nerve fiber (Nf). These nerve fibers join together to form a branch of the vestibular nerve. Each hair cell has a *small arrow* above it that corresponds to the direction of its functional polarization vector. This *arrow* is always pointing in the direction of the kinocilium. The *long arrow* above the otolithic mass is a linear acceleration vector. The response of hair cell depends on the cosine of the direction between its polarization vector and linear acceleration (a).

striola is C-shaped in the utricle, orientation vectors of hair cells in the utricle are aligned in all directions of the plane of the utricular macula (Fig. 130.9).

It is from an array of these hair cells that the brain can estimate the magnitude and direction of linear acceleration. If all polarization vectors were identically aligned, it would be impossible to determine the magnitude and direction of an acceleration vector in the plane of the otolithic macula. At least two different orientations are needed to resolve the vector in two dimensions. At least three separate orientations are needed to resolve the magnitude and direction of an acceleration vector in three dimensions.

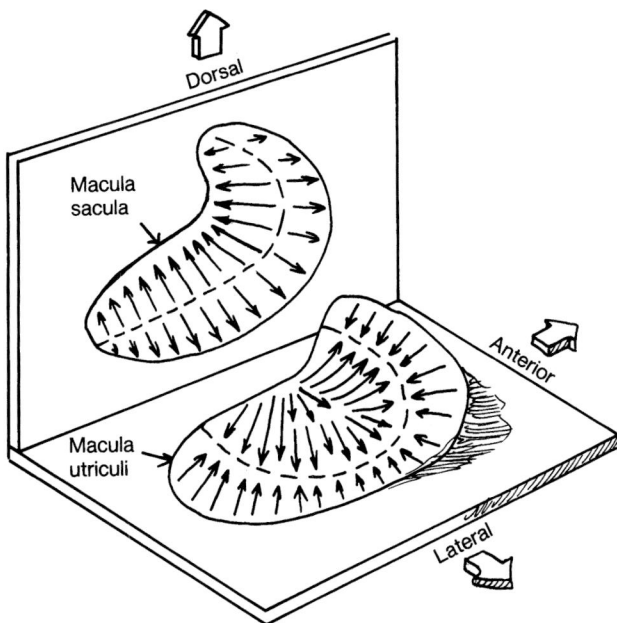

Figure 130.9 Polarization of hair cells on the otolith organs. Direction of *arrows* indicates direction of hair deflection that excites hair cells in that region of the receptor surface. (Modified from Barber HO, Stockwell CW, *Manual of electronystmography*, 2nd ed. St. Louis: Mosby, 1980:31 Fig. 2-21.)

As in the simple example described earlier, each otolith organ has sensory hair cells arranged in a wide variety of orientations of its polarization vectors (Fig. 130.9). Because of this architecture, the asymmetries inherent in the sensitivity of a single hair cell can be canceled out within one otolith organ itself. The orientation of the polarization vectors is toward the striola in the utricular macula and away from the striola in the saccular macula. The right and left otolith organs, like semicircular canals, have mirror symmetry around the sagittal plane. The exact neural connections of the otolith organs have not been as extensively studied as those of the pairs of semicircular canals. Thus, the exact circuitry for resolving linear acceleration in three-dimensional space has not been determined.

A simplified model of the response of the otolith organ to linear acceleration and changes in orientation with respect to gravity can be made with a mass, a spring, and a damper (Fig. 130.4). In this case, the mass is the otoconia macula minus the buoyant force placed on it by the surrounding endolymph. The spring and the damping factors come from the viscoelastic properties of the gelatinous structure in which the otoconia are embedded.

The response characteristics of the otolith organs can be predicted with the above model. Although the specific gravity of the otoconia has been found to be 2.7 times that of the endolymph, the damping forces of the otolithic membrane are more difficult to measure. These damping forces prevent oscillation of the otolith membrane in response to a given linear acceleration. However, when direct recordings are taken from otolith afferents, physiologic performance deviates from that predicted in the model. There are two types of neuronal otolith afferent populations that can be defined that are similar to those in the semicircular canals. The first population appears to respond to head position, and its responses closely follow those predicted with the model for sinusoidal stimulation at frequencies up to 0.1 Hz. A second population of neurons encodes information on linear acceleration. These

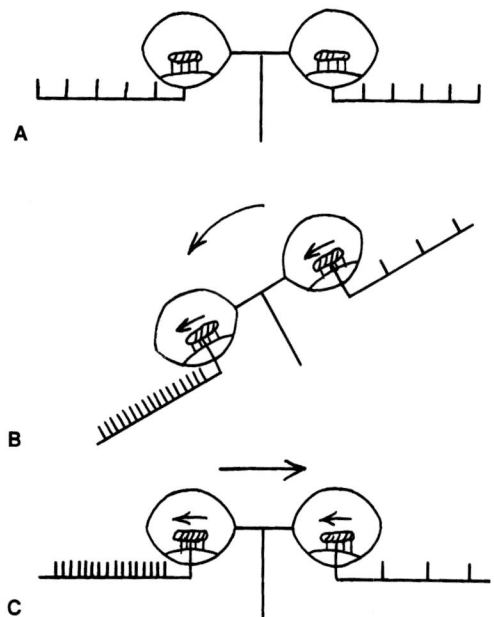

A

B

C

Figure 130.10 Modulation of the pulse interval by shearing of the utricular otolith membrane of the vertebrate vestibular organ. **A:** Horizontal position at rest. **B:** Tilted to the left. **C:** During linear acceleration to the right. (Modified from Barlow JS. Inertia navigation as a basis for animal navigation. *J Theor Biol* 1990;6:76, with permission.)

neurons display increasing gain in proportion to higher-frequency stimuli.

Figure 130.10 shows, theoretically, how two otolith organs operating in the same plane react to head tilt or to acceleration of the head in the plane of the otolithic macula. If there is no acceleration in that plane, the nerve firing rate of each otolith organ is constant and equal. When the head is tilted to the left, the firing rate of the nerve innervating the left otolith organ increases, while the firing rate of the nerve innervating the right otolith organ decreases. Maximum sensitivity is obtained by means of subtracting the firing rate of the right nerve from that of the left. Acceleration of the head to the right causes deflection of both otoconia to the left in a manner similar to a head tilt to the left. This acceleration produces an increase of the firing rate of the left nerve and decrease in the firing rate of the right nerve. This model (Fig. 130.10) shows that the asymmetry present in one hair cell innervating an otolith organ can be canceled by combining it with a signal from a hair cell that has the same polarization factor in the other side. It also shows that the otolith organs are influenced by both tilt orientation with respect to gravity and linear acceleration.

Einstein recognized that an ambiguity presented between linear acceleration and gravity, and in aviation, is a problem during the acceleration of takeoff, when pilots have trouble differentiating the acceleration of the airplane from the gravity vector. Because translational motion in one direction creates the same inertial force as gravity to

tilt in the opposite direction (Fig. 130.10), this problem is known as a tilt-translational ambiguity. Recent research has demonstrated that the central nervous system uses semicircular canal information (activated during tilt but not during translation) in combination with the otolith input to distinguish, for example, tilting the head upward versus accelerating forward as in a car, sled, or airplane (3). This mechanism works poorly at low frequency rotations. In the circumstance where the rotational component of the motion is at low frequency (<0.1 Hz), the brain uses visual or tactile information to help interpret the otolith's signal. In the absence of non-otolith input, such as vision or rotation at frequencies above 0.1 Hz, the system defaults to interpreting linear acceleration as tilt (or gravity). Returning to the aviation example, fighter pilots taking off from an aircraft carrier deck at night will feel as if they are tilted backwards during forward acceleration. The natural correction for this feeling is to steer the plane downward, which could result in disaster.

VESTIBULAR AFFERENTS

Based on the anatomy of peripheral termination, there are three distinct vestibular afferent types: calyx, dimorphic, and bouton. Calyx afferents terminate exclusively on type I hair cells at the calyx endings. Calyx endings may terminate on one or several hair cells. Dimorphic afferents have both calyx endings on type I hair cells and bouton endings on type II hair cells. Dimorphic afferents are likely the most prevalent. Bouton afferents have only bouton endings and thus only terminate on type II hair cells. These three afferent types differ immunohistochemically. Calrentinin, a calcium binding protein, is seen only in calyx afferents; peripherin, which is an intermediate filament protein, is seen in bouton afferents; and neither of these markers is seen in dimorphic afferents.

There are other anatomic distinctions between these afferent types. Calyx afferents have characteristically thick axons, whereas bouton afferents are thinner. Dimorphic afferents, however, can be thick or thin. The processes to the calyx endings are thicker than the processes to the bouton endings. The distribution of the three fiber types is also characteristic. Calyx afferent endings are found in the central zone of the crista ampullaris, whereas dimorphic afferents terminate in the central, intermediate, and peripheral zones, and bouton fibers terminate in the peripheral zone. Similarly, utricular calyx afferents terminate in the striola region, whereas dimorphic afferent terminals are seen throughout the macula and bouton afferents and generally terminate peripherally.

Afferents also differ in their discharge regularity, conduction velocity, and sensitivity to vestibular and galvanic stimulation. Although response gains, conduction velocity, and discharge regularity over a population of neurons all fall along a continuum, based on these characteristics, vestibular afferents fall into three general groups that correspond well with the three groups (calyx, dimorphic, and bouton) determined by peripheral morphology. Calyx afferents innervating the central ampulla or striola are large fibers that are irregularly firing, sensitive to galvanic stimulation, and have a low sensitivity to angular motion. Dimorphic afferents may have thick or thin axons. Those terminating more centrally tend to have thicker axons and are irregularly firing, galvanically sensitive, and sensitive to (rotational or linear) stimulation. Dimorphic afferents terminating peripherally (either in the macula or crista) and bouton afferents tend to be thinner fibers with lower galvanic and natural stimulation thresholds and are regularly firing with slower conduction velocities (4). These different afferent types may be of more interest than just physiologic curiosity. The high sensitivity irregular afferents are sensitive to small perturbations but have nonlinear dynamics because they readily silence when the head moves in the inhibitory direction. These afferents may be best suited for quick, nonlinear reflexes such as vestibulospinal responses to inhibit a fall. In contrast, the linear characteristics of the thinner, more regular afferents are appropriate for linear vestibular reflexes, like the vestibuloocular reflex, that must work over a wide range of frequencies and peak velocities (5).

Both semicircular canal afferents and otolith afferents are cosine tuned, which means they have one best characteristic response vector. For utricular afferents, these vectors can lie anywhere in the horizontal plane and are dependent on the orientation vector of the hair cells that they innervate. The response of the afferent is proportional to the cosine angle between the direction of stimulation and the orientation vector of the afferent. Similarly, the rotational vector of maximum stimulation for semicircular canal afferents is in the plane of rotation of the canal. The response of the fiber decreases as cosine of the angle between the plane of rotation and the canal plane. The cosine tuning of the afferent is consistent with the fact that transmitter release by hair cells is proportional to the cosine of the angle between the displacement of the hair cell bundle and the direction of stimulation (Fig. 130.6). Thus, both the hair cells and the afferents are cosine tuned. The coding of the vestibular system is such that the direction of stimulation is encoded by the afferent population stimulated, and the intensity of the movement is encoded by the intensity of the response of the stimulated afferent.

All of the vestibular epithelium are also innervated by vestibular efferent neurons. These neurons have cell bodies in the brainstem in areas around the genu of the facial nerve. Their fibers in humans run mixed with the vestibular afferent fibers and can terminate either presynaptically (on type II hair cells) or postsynaptically on calyx or bouton endings. The function of the vestibular efferent system in mammals is unknown.

VESTIBULAR BRAINSTEM

Vestibular afferents are bipolar neurons that have cell bodies in the inferior and superior Scarpa (vestibular) ganglion. The peripheral (dendritic) processes of these neurons exit the neuroepithelium and collect in the inferior and superior vestibular nerves. The inferior division includes neurons from the posterior canal and saccule, and the anterior division includes utricular, horizontal canal, and anterior canal afferents (Fig. 130.11). Axonal branches of primary afferent ramify in the vestibular nuclei. Afferent terminals from the different end organs primarily innervate the various divisions of the vestibular nuclei, although terminations are seen in the cerebellum and other brainstem nuclei as well. The precise terminations by end organ (semicircular canal or otolith) in the central nervous system are similar in many species (6). Not only does the brainstem region receive convergent output from different branches of the vestibular nerve, but individual neurons receive afferent input from one, two, or more end organs (canal ampullae or otolith maculae). Thus, the vestibular nuclei integrate information from multiple ipsilateral receptors.

There are four major vestibular nuclei in the brainstem: the lateral (Deiters), superior, medial, and inferior (spinal, descending) nuclei. In addition, there are several minor

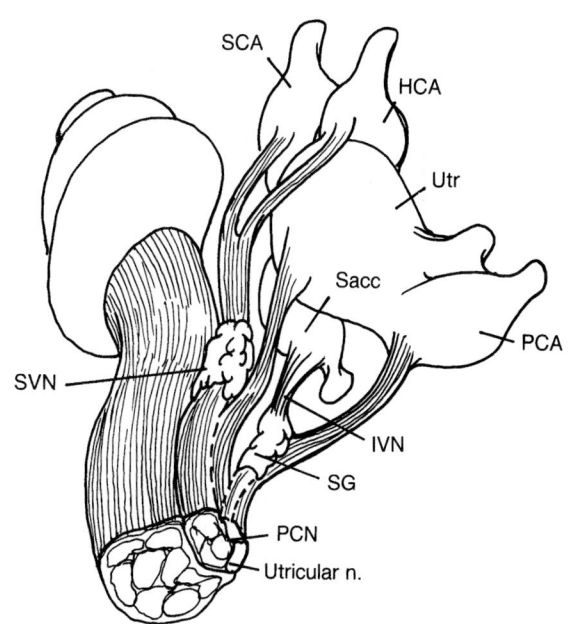

Figure 130.11 Peripheral vestibular innervation. *Dark fibers* represent bundles of large-diameter neurons. HCA, Horizontal canal ampulla; SCA, superior (anterior) vertical canal ampulla; PCA, posterior vertical canal ampulla; PCN, posterior canal innervation; Sacc, saccule; SG, Scarpa ganglion cells; SVN, IVN, superior and inferior vestibular nerve trunks; utr, utricle. (Modified from Gacek RR. The course in central termination of first order neurons supplying vestibular end organs in the cat. *Acta Otolaryngol (Stock)* 1969;[Suppl 254]:1, with permission.)

vestibular nuclei, including nucleus y, that are identified in various species by various investigators. The vestibular nuclei not only receive vestibular information but other information pertaining to spatial orientation as well. These inputs include optokinetic signals through the accessory optic system, neck proprioceptive signals, and Purkinje cell projections from the cerebellar cortex. From the vestibular nuclei, vestibular signals are passed throughout the central nervous system. The dominant output of the vestibular nuclei are to the ocular motor nuclei, via the medial longitudinal fasciculus and the ascending tract of Deiters; to the spinal cord, via the medial and lateral vestibulospinal tracts; to the cerebellum, via the cerebellar peduncles; and to the contralateral vestibular nuclei, via the vestibular commissural system. Other pathways connect the vestibular nuclei with the autonomic system, which has implications in motion sickness and blood pressure control, and with the thalamus.

One important function of the vestibular commissural system is inhibition. Experimental data show that the discharge frequencies of neurons excited during ipsilateral angular acceleration are also excited due to a decrease of crossed inhibition, which is caused by a decrease in discharge rate from the contralateral paired semicircular canal. This reciprocal mechanism is the basis of the so-called push-pull connection that increases the sensitivity of the system through use of the difference in signals between the functionally paired semicircular canals (left horizontal–right horizontal, left anterior–right posterior, left posterior–right anterior) in either ear. In this way, the paired canals complement one another and tend to cancel out the asymmetries inherent in the hair cell transduction mechanisms and afferent firing patterns mentioned earlier. The neural signals from these pairs of canals converge in a synergistic way in the nervous system, allowing the system to function even in the presence of a complete unilateral lesion. However, responses in patients with unilateral lesions are more asymmetric than those among healthy persons given high enough angular acceleration to reveal these inherent asymmetries, which are apparent when the push-pull redundancy is not available.

The best studied vestibular reflex is the vestibuloocular reflex. Vestibuloocular reflexes are of two types: compensatory reflexes that stabilize gaze during motion and orienting reflexes that align the eye with the gravitational vector. One of the challenges for the nervous system is to translate signals from the semicircular canal planes into coordinates appropriate for effector action. Those who study the vestibular system use an external frame of reference, as shown in Figure 130.3. Linear acceleration or rotational acceleration occurs around three axes that are perpendicular to each other: the interaural or pitch axis, the nasal-occipital or roll axis, and the rostral-caudal or yaw axis. The vestibule-oculo-motor system, however, is thought to use a coordinate system based on the orientation of the three pairs of semicircular canals. Experiments

have shown that stimulation of afferent branches of the eighth cranial nerve that come exclusively from one semicircular canal produces reflexive eye movements that tend to rotate around the axis of greatest sensitivity for that canal. The three agonist-antagonist pairs of eye muscles themselves do not produce eye movements that completely correspond to these axes of orientation of the semicircular canals. Thus, there is a distribution of signals from the semicircular canals to produce compensatory eye movement of the desired magnitude and direction.

According to a simplified analysis, the connection between the three pairs of semicircular canals and the three pairs of eye muscles can be described with a set of nine constant coefficients. First-order analysis indicates that the translation of incoming vestibular systems needed to produce compensatory eye movement is a relatively simple operation for the brain to perform. This operation is contrasted to the more complicated series of commands that must be given when signals from the vestibular system are used to stabilize the head on the neck or the body with leg muscles.

The nervous system can adapt its response by comparing vestibular input to other sensory input. When the head moves, the vestibuloocular reflex tends to stabilize the image of an object in space on the retina by producing an eye movement compensatory to the head movement. At any time, the functional anatomic connections needed to stabilize an object can be thought of as a set of nine constant coefficients that distribute the incoming vestibular systems to the ocular motor neurons to form the reflexive eye movement response. For example, the motion of the head 10 degrees to the right produces eye movement 10 degrees to the left.

Provisions have been made in the nervous system for this response to adapt when necessary, owing to factors such as disease or aging. One such example is people with myopia who wear eyeglasses. If the magnification of the lens is 1.2 times, rotation of the head 10 degrees to the right produces rotation of the world as viewed by the eye 12 degrees to the left and therefore demands a corresponding reflexive eye movement 12 degrees to the left. The nervous system makes this form of adaptive change to resolve a conflict between afferent inputs, in this case vestibular and visual inputs. In this example, the nervous system can correspondingly increase the amount of eye movement produced for a given head movement so that the error between the head motion input and eye motion response is reduced to nearly zero. This gain plasticity requires participation of the flocular lobe of the cerebellum.

CURRENT VESTIBULAR ISSUES

Like most fields in basic sciences, the vestibular system is actively studied in a number of excellent laboratories. Among the many actively investigated areas are the pharmacology of the vestibular periphery, interactions between active head movements and the passive vestibular reflexes, the role of vestibular signals in spatial orientation, the function of vestibular efferent system, physiologic and cellular mechanisms of adaptation and compensation after vestibular injury, and the adaptation of the vestibular system to microgravity. In addition, efforts are ongoing to develop prosthetic devices to aid patients with vestibular deficits. This research holds the promise of improving our understanding of this vital, well conserved, and underappreciated "sixth" sensory system.

HIGHLIGHTS

- The vestibular system is an inertial guidance system in vertebrates. It is composed of two or more sensors of linear acceleration and three or more sensors of angular acceleration in each inner ear. The right and left inner ear structures are mirror images of each other.
- Vestibular motion sensors use inertial elements connected to sensory hair cells. Both linear and angular acceleration sensors in the inner ear use a three-step process to convert accelerations of the head into useful information for the nervous system. The elements in these three steps are inertia, sensory hair cells, and nerve fibers connected to the hair cells.
- Vestibular organs are arranged by pairs in functional planes. The right and left lateral semicircular canals lie in the same plane. The other four vertical canals lie in planes nearly perpendicular to the plane of the horizontal canal pair. The anterior vertical canal on one side is in nearly the same plane as the posterior vertical canal on the other, forming a functional pairing of the semicircular canals. The otolith organs are similarly paired.

- Head movement produces compensatory reflexive eye movement. When the head moves, the vestibuloocular reflex tends to stabilize the image of an object in space on the retina by producing eye movement compensatory to the head movement.
- Vestibular sensory hair cells are arranged in orderly arrays. The orientation of a hair cell is defined by the orientation of its kinocilia. This orientation is known as *morphologic polarization*. A corresponding physiologic attribute is called *functional polarization*, which means the hair cell is the most sensitive to displacement along its anatomically defined polarization vector.
- As the cochlea is sensitive to a frequency range of sounds, the semicircular canal is sensitive to a frequency range of angular accelerations. The canal itself has a bandwidth of approximately 0.10 to 10.0 Hz. The normal function of the brain is to extend low-frequency performance to about 0.01 Hz. This range still does not include 0 Hz, which corresponds to constant-velocity rotation.

REFERENCES

1. Hudspeth AJ, Logothetis NK. Sensory systems. *Curr Opin Neurobiol* 2000;10:631–641.
2. Merchant SN, Velazquez-Villasenor L, Tsuji K, et al. Temporal bone studies of the human peripheral vestibular system. Normative vestibular hair cell data. *Ann Otol Rhinol Laryngol Suppl* 2000;181:3–13.
3. Angelaki DE, Dickman JD. Gravity or translation: central processing of vestibular signals to detect motion or tilt. *J Vestibular Res* 2003;13:245–253.
4. Goldberg JM. Afferent diversity and the organization of central vestibular pathways. *Exp Brain Res* 2000;130:277–297.
5. Minor LB, Lasker DM, Backous DD, et al. Horizontal vestibuloocular reflex evoked by high-acceleration rotations in the squirrel monkey. I. Normal responses. *J Neurophysiol* 1999;82:1254–1270.
6. Newlands SD, Perachio AA. Central projections of the vestibular nerve: a review and single fiber study in the Mongolian gerbil. *Brain Res Bull* 2003;60:475–495.

Balance Function Tests 131

Colin L. W. Driscoll   J. Douglas Green, Jr.

Balance is maintained through complex interaction of the vestibular, visual, and somatosensory information that is combined within the brainstem to generate a motor response correcting the perturbation. Abnormalities within any portion of the system can cause a sensation of imbalance or dizziness. Dizziness is one of the most common reasons for seeking medical evaluation, and the otorhinolaryngologist is often the primary contact. Evaluating patients for dizziness can be frustrating for both patient and physician. The symptoms are difficult for patients to describe, the differential diagnosis is broad, and many tests have to be considered. An understanding of the balance tests currently available and the pathophysiologic principles on which they are based improves treatment of these challenging patients. The particular approach to dizziness is affected by type of practice, available resources, and patient population.

The main goals of the diagnostic evaluation are to determine the location and severity of lesions within the balance system and to help formulate and guide a treatment plan. The etiologic evaluation of the balance system dysfunction necessitates compilation of other data, including those from a comprehensive history and physical examination and other directed laboratory and radiologic examinations. In most cases, clues revealed during the history and physical examination lead to a diagnosis, and treatment can begin without additional testing. Balance function testing should be interpreted in light of the history and physical exam findings and often provides confirmatory information as to pathophysiologic processes involved. Formal balance function testing provides information as to the site and side of the lesion, to ascertain who is likely to benefit from vestibular rehabilitation, to assess recovery of vestibular function, and to document contralateral function when a destructive procedure is contemplated. Clinical decision support systems have been described to help office personnel determine which patients may need balance function testing (1).

This chapter reviews tests for assessing the balance system (Table 131.1). These balance system tests, usually administered by an audiologist or trained technician, require specialized equipment and dedicated space. The basic physiologic principles of the tests are reviewed.

ELECTRONYSTAGMOGRAPHY

The electronystagmography (ENG) test battery is the workhorse of balance function testing. It is a combination of tests that together provide complementary information about the vestibular and oculomotor systems. Rather than a diagnosis, the tests provide data that must be used in conjunction with the findings of the history, physical examination, and other studies to determine a diagnosis. The ENG battery typically consists of the vestibular and oculomotor tests listed in Table 131.2.

The ENG tests are based on the well-studied neurophysiologic characteristics of the vestibulo-ocular reflex. Motion of the head, or simulated motion through labyrinthine stimulation, produces compensatory eye movement. These eye movements are observable and recordable responses that provide the basis for interpretation of the various tests. Changes in eye position are recorded by means of taking advantage of the natural difference in electrical charge between the cornea (+) and the retina (−), the corneal-retinal potential. Electrodes record the changes in potential when the eye moves [electrooculography (EOG)]. The advantages of this recording technique are low cost, ease of administration, noninvasiveness, avoidance of head restraint, and extensive experience in interpreting the data. The technique does have technologic limitations. The signal is susceptible to changes in skin resistance due to perspiration, interference from eye-blink artifacts, and a poor signal-to-noise ratio. Although abnormal eye movements can be revealed by means of direct visualization during testing, it is preferable in most cases to

TABLE 131.1 ⬛ 𝕀ℝ **DIAGNOSIS**
BALANCE TESTS

Electronystagmography
Rotary chair, sinusoidal harmonic acceleration
Vestibular autorotation test
Computerized dynamic posturography
Vestibular evoked myogenic potentials
Dynamic visual acuity

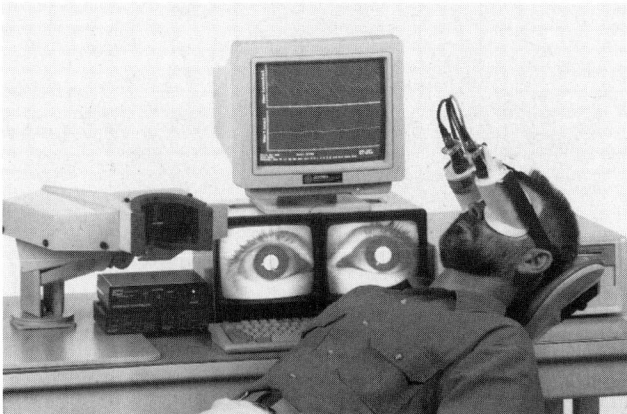

Figure 131.1 System in which small video cameras are used to observe and record eye movement. (From Jedmed Instrument Company, St. Louis, with permission.)

have quantifiable data to characterize the abnormalities. Furthermore, some parts of the test require that the eyes be closed to prevent fixation suppression. Nystagmus is the primary ocular movement measured and is defined by its direction (horizontal, vertical, or torsional) and velocity (degrees per second). Direction is determined by the fast component, and velocity is calculated from the slow-phase component.

New technologies for observing and recording eye movement continue to be developed (2,3). Video ENG systems, vidoenystagmography, are now available that use small video cameras to observe and monitor horizontal, vertical, and torsional eye movement during vestibular evaluations (Fig. 131.1). With this system, tests that require the patient to move are performed with a lightweight goggle assembly. Pursuit, gaze, and saccade testing can be performed with an oculomotor module with tracking targets for each eye. The eyes are illuminated with near-infrared light that is not visible to the patient but allows the cameras to pick up and project images of the eyes on video monitors. This system has several advantages over traditional ENG testing techniques. Nonelectrode eye movement recording eliminates artifacts, the need for frequent recalibration, and impedance testing. Vertical eye movements can be accurately recorded. Torsional eye movements can be visualized and recorded without fixation suppression. Disconjugate eye movements are more easily identified. A portable unit allows testing at home, in an intensive care unit, or at any other remote location. The disadvantages are high cost, need to wear goggles, and unfamiliarity with the equipment. Most companies that

manufacture ENG equipment now offer a videonystagmography system to make use of these advantages.

Virtual reality testing systems are being developed and promise to provide a means to produce visual stimuli that were previously impossible (4). Images can be produced on a visual display, and because the system is software driven, the images can be manipulated quickly and with tremendous flexibility. For example, cross-axis stimulation (head motion in one plane and eye motion in another) becomes easy to perform.

The sequence of ENG tests is important to prevent obtaining misleading results. For example, testing for benign paroxysmal positional vertigo is performed at the beginning of the test series to avoid fatiguing of the response. The tests must be performed with proper attention to detail and accurate calibration. Patient anxiety, fatigue, lack of cooperation, and medications can adversely affect test results.

Interpretation of ENG results is critical to proper diagnosis and treatment and should be performed by qualified audiologists and physicians who are trained and familiar with the equipment being used for testing. Increasingly, specialists in other fields, chiropractors, and poorly trained medical doctors are investing in ENG equipment in hopes of financial gain, often without knowledge of how to interpret the ENG test results and how to apply them in clinical practice. It is essential that otorhinolaryngologists offering ENG testing be familiar with interpretation of the results. Several excellent courses are available to otorhinolaryngologists offering ENG testing within their offices.

Spontaneous and Gaze Nystagmus

Spontaneous nystagmus refers to nystagmus that is present without visual or vestibular stimulation. Spontaneous nystagmus can sometimes be seen only with loss of visual fixation (e.g., milder forms of spontaneous vestibular nystagmus) or may be seen with both eyes open and with loss of

TABLE 131.2 ⬛ 𝕀ℝ **DIAGNOSIS**
ELECTRONYSTAGMOGRAPHY TEST BATTERY

Vestibular Subtests	Oculomotor Subtests
Spontaneous nystagmus	Pursuit system evaluation
Gaze nystagmus	Saccadic system
Positional nystagmus evaluation	Optokinetic system evaluation
Positioning nystagmus	Fixation system evaluation
Fistula test	
Bithermal caloric tests	

visual fixation (e.g., congenital nystagmus and severe vestibular nystagmus). Spontaneous nystagmus can be observed both at the bedside and in the vestibular laboratory. However, although reduction of visual fixation can be achieved easily in the laboratory using infrared video goggles or EOG with eye closure, at the bedside, achieving a reduction in visual fixation while still maintaining an ability to observe eye movements can be challenging. Observing a patient's eye with an ophthalmoscope while the other eye is occluded allows the examiner to assess spontaneous nystagmus with reduced visual fixation. The most common type of spontaneous nystagmus, that is, spontaneous vestibular nystagmus, occurs with unilateral peripheral vestibular lesions. Spontaneous vestibular nystagmus is always unidirectional and increases when the patient gazes in the direction of the quick component of the nystagmus. This gaze dependent change in nystagmus intensity is called "Alexander's Law." As noted previously, loss of visual fixation also increases the magnitude of spontaneous vestibular nystagmus. Thus, judicious use of gaze direction and presence or absence of visual fixation can aid the examiner both at the bedside and in the laboratory in judging whether or not a spontaneous nystagmus is a result of a vestibular abnormality. Failure of fixation suppression is highly suggestive of a central pathologic condition.

Gaze nystagmus, also known as gaze-evoked nystagmus, is a bidirectional nystagmus with right beating nystagmus on right gaze and left beating nystagmus on left gaze. Many patients with gaze-evoked nystagmus also will manifest an up-beating nystagmus on upward gaze. Note that down-beating nystagmus in any gaze position, even in downward gaze, is not considered a component of gaze-evoked nystagmus and should be regarded as a manifestation of a central nervous system abnormality at the level of the craniocervical junction unless proven otherwise. Gaze-evoked nystagmus can be seen in normal individuals when horizontal gaze exceeds 30 degrees from the straight-ahead position. Thus, it is best to limit the amount of gaze deviation when assessing a patient for gaze-evoked nystagmus to less than 30 degrees. Gaze-evoked nystagmus occurs as a result of inadequate gaze-holding, thereby leading to a slow drift of the eyes back toward the straight ahead gaze position with the drift interrupted intermittently by rapid, nystagmus fast phases in the direction of gaze. Bidirectional gaze-evoked nystagmus is always a result of a central nervous system abnormality and never is the result of a peripheral vestibular abnormality. There are many etiologies for gaze-evoked nystagmus. The most common cause of gaze-evoked nystagmus is a medication effect (e.g., from anticonvulsants).

Positional and Positioning Tests

Positional tests are designed to detect the response to changes in direction of gravitational force. The patient is moved slowly into a series of stationary positions with the eyes closed, and presence or absence of nystagmus is assessed. The nystagmus can be either fixed or direction changing. If nystagmus is elicited in the positional tests, the entire body is turned to determine whether neck torsion is responsible. Interpretation of results is controversial and necessitates consideration of the number of positions that elicit nystagmus and the velocity of the nystagmus. Positional nystagmus of peripheral origin can fatigue with repeated testing, is usually direction fixed, and often is associated with caloric weakness. The direction of nystagmus caused by a peripheral lesion typically does not change independently of head movement (5). Direction-changing nystagmus without an accompanying change in head position indicates the presence of a central disorder.

The positioning test used most often is the Dix-Hallpike maneuver. The patient is rapidly moved from sitting to supine with the head turned and hanging below the level of the table. If nystagmus is elicited, the maneuver is repeated to determine the existence of fatigability. A response that fatigues suggests a peripheral problem. The patient's eyes are kept open to allow the examiner to evaluate for torsional nystagmus, which can indicate benign positional vertigo due to loose otoconia within the labyrinth. Torsional nystagmus cannot be recorded with conventional ENG. Head hanging to the right produces counterclockwise torsional nystagmus, and head hanging to the left produces clockwise torsional nystagmus. A variant of benign positional vertigo affecting the horizontal semicircular canal produces pure horizontal nystagmus.

Bithermal Caloric Tests

Bithermal caloric tests are used to evaluate the function of the horizontal semicircular canals. Changes in temperature stimulate fluid flow (equivalent to a very slow frequency of only 0.002 to 0.004 Hz) within the horizontal semicircular canal; if the system is functioning, nystagmus is elicited. The very slow frequency of stimulation is not a condition normally experienced during daily life. Each ear is tested independently, and the responses are compared.

Caloric testing is performed with the patient supine and head elevated 30 degrees. The external auditory canal is irrigated directly with 250 mL of water at 7 degrees above and below body temperature for 30 seconds. An alternative is to place a small, distensible balloon in the ear canal and fill it with water (closed-loop system). Ocular movements are recorded for approximately 2 minutes, beginning with stimulation. Fixation suppression is evaluated during this time. The slow-phase velocity of elicited nystagmus is calculated and recorded as an objective measure of the response. Warm and cool air irrigation or a closed-loop system can be substituted for direct irrigation if the tympanic membrane is perforated. The responses of the right and the left ears are compared. A difference greater than 20% usually is considered abnormal and is reported as left- or right-sided weakness. The total right-beating responses is

---

TABLE 131.3 ℞ DIAGNOSIS
ELECTRONYSTAGMOGRAPHY INTERPRETATION

Findings suggestive of a central disorder
Spontaneous or positional nystagmus with normal caloric results
Direction-changing nystagmus independent of stimulus changes
Failure of fixation suppression
Bilateral reduced or absent caloric responses without a history of labyrinthine or middle ear disease
Abnormal saccade or pursuit results, especially with normal caloric results
Hyperactive caloric responses (loss of cerebellum-generated inhibition)

Findings suggestive of a peripheral disorder
Unilateral caloric weakness
Bilateral caloric weakness with a history of labyrinthine disease or administration of ototoxic drugs
Fatiguing positional nystagmus
Intact fixation suppression response
Direction-fixed nystagmus

Modified from Kramer PD, Roberts DC, Shelhamer M, et al. A versatile stereoscopic visual display system for vestibular and oculomotor research. *J Vestib Res* 1998;8:363–379, with permission.

compared with the total left-beating responses, and the result is reported as a right or left directional preponderance. A difference greater than 30% is considered significant. Abnormal directional preponderance without unilateral weakness suggests a central pathologic condition. The results indicating central or peripheral disorders are summarized in Table 131.3.

A monothermal caloric screening test has been suggested to minimize procedure time and patient discomfort. This test has been criticized for a high false-negative rate. However, the results of a study by Jacobson et al. (6) suggest that if appropriate failure criteria are used, the sensitivity reaches 93% and the specificity 98%. Patients who fail the screening test need conventional bithermal testing.

Patients with a complete unilateral or bilateral caloric loss should be tested with ice caloric irrigation of the affected ear(s). Frequently, nystagmus can be elicited with this stronger stimulus. Ice caloric stimulation is uncomfortable for the patient and should be limited in use. It should be noted that the absence of caloric response to warm, cool, or ice water irrigations cannot be taken as an indication of complete lack of function. This should be confirmed by rotational chair testing.

Electronystagmography Fistula Test

If a fistula exists between the middle ear space and the inner ear fluid, application of positive or negative pressure in the external ear canal may produce a fluid shift resulting in nystagmus. Objective nystagmus or a clear subjective response suggests a perilymph fistula or dehiscence of the horizontal or superior semicircular canal.

Saccadic System

The saccadic system is used to move a target from the periphery of the retina to the fovea. Targets more than 20 degrees from the line of sight are normally located by means of a combination of eye and head movement, called *gaze saccade* (7). This test is performed while the patient sits facing a light bar and keeps his or her head stationary. Lights on the bar are activated to the left and right of center by 10 to 20 degrees, and the patient is asked to shift gaze to each new target. Electrooculographic recording techniques are used. Latency, maximum velocity, duration, gain (overshoot or undershoot), refixation saccade, glissade (postsaccadic drift, or slip of the eye), and other variables are measured and observed.

Abnormal saccades can be caused by lesions in a wide variety of locations. However, they are most commonly caused by a central pathologic disorder rather than a peripheral vestibular one. An abnormal saccadic response can be caused by lesions in the cerebellum (dorsal cerebellar vermis), brainstem (particularly the paramedian pontine reticular formation and medial longitudinal fasciculus), or ocular muscles and nerves. Cerebellar lesions typically manifest as saccadic overshoot or undershoot dysmetria. Dysmetria is an error in range, rate, or direction in performance of precision voluntary movement. It usually is found through past pointing in a finger-to-nose test (8). Different patterns of abnormalities and testing paradigms can help to localize a lesion (9). Age, fatigue, lack of attention, sedatives, drug intoxication (phenytoin), and other factors can cause slow saccades or increase latency.

Pursuit System

The smooth pursuit system stabilizes images of moving objects on the fovea (7). Healthy persons can pursue an object moving at a velocity of about 30 degrees per second. At faster rates, the image can slip, and a corrective saccade is used to catch up. Smooth pursuit usually is tested with sinusoidal stimuli, such as a pendulum, light-emitting diodes, or a laser, with a frequency range of 0.2 to 0.7 Hz and a horizontal range less than 20 degrees to the left and right. Electrooculographic techniques are used to record gain, phase lead or lag, symmetry, and other variables. Because the smooth pursuit system is distributed throughout the brainstem and cerebellum, anatomic localization is not possible (9). If age, alertness, medications, and congenital nystagmus are eliminated as causes of abnormal test results, a central cause is suggested. Saccadic pursuit suggests cerebellar disease. Reduced bilateral gain can be caused by a brainstem lesion. Patients with Alzheimer disease and schizophrenia can perform worse with sinusoidal stimuli than with fixed velocity stimuli (9).

Optokinetic System

The optokinetic system differs slightly from the pursuit system in that it allows persons to keep the visual field in focus while they or most of the environment are moving. The vestibulo-ocular reflex alone is not adequate to generate compensatory eye movements at low frequency. In clinical testing, this effect is achieved by keeping the patient stationary and moving the environment. About 90% of the visual field must be filled with the target to avoid simply testing the pursuit system. A rotating drum with thin vertical stripes or stripes projected on the wall are common stimuli. The patient is instructed to look straight ahead. As the targets pass by, there should be small amplitude excursions of the eye (stare nystagmus). If the patient fixes on the target, longer excursions occur, and the pursuit system is being tested (look nystagmus) (9). Separating the smooth pursuit system and the optokinetic system can be even more difficult. Experiments indicate that both systems are responsible for eye movement during stimulation. If, however, the lights are extinguished, the smooth pursuit system response drops to zero almost instantly. With the lights out, patients continue to have nystagmus for approximately 25 seconds. It is believed that this nystagmus [optokinetic afternystagmus (OKAN)] is caused by the optokinetic system alone (7). Because of the contribution of the pursuit system, it is not possible to conclude that the optokinetic system is normal without having nystagmus for approximately 25 seconds following optokinetic stimulation.

The optokinetic system is widely distributed throughout the brainstem and cerebellum; therefore, abnormalities are not site specific. Absence or asymmetry of the OKAN occurs with peripheral vestibular lesions. Bilateral labyrinthectomy profoundly reduces or eliminates OKAN (10). These findings suggest an interaction between the vestibuloocular reflex and the optokinetic system (7). The OKAN becomes asymmetric after unilateral vestibular ablation; the result is stronger and more prolonged nystagmus directed at the side of the lesion (10). A problem is that the sensitivity in identifying unilateral vestibular disease is not high (10). In a study involving 12 patients who had undergone removal of acoustic neuroma, OKAN helped identify the side of the lesion for only 7 of the

patients (10). Baloh et al. (11) found abnormal test results among patients with cerebellar atrophy.

Optokinetic testing is not routinely used but can be indicated as a confirmatory examination when abnormal pursuit is identified. Combining the results of OKAN with those of rotary testing can be helpful in determining the side of the lesion. Another potential use might be to exclude vestibular disease, especially for patients who cannot undergo caloric testing (10). As more is learned about the production of optokinetic nystagmus, clinical usefulness can expand.

ROTARY CHAIR, SINUSOIDAL HARMONIC ACCELERATION

Rotational testing paradigms offer the theoretic ability to test the semicircular canals under more physiologic, that is, higher frequency, conditions than can be achieved with caloric testing. The stimulus can be precisely controlled and is repeatable. Because both ears are tested simultaneously, the results reflect the integrated function of both ears (12). In this test, the rotary chair is oscillated from side to side at a series of preprogrammed rates (Fig. 131.2). The acceleration frequencies tested range from 0.01 to 1.28 Hz with a maximum velocity of 50 degrees per second.

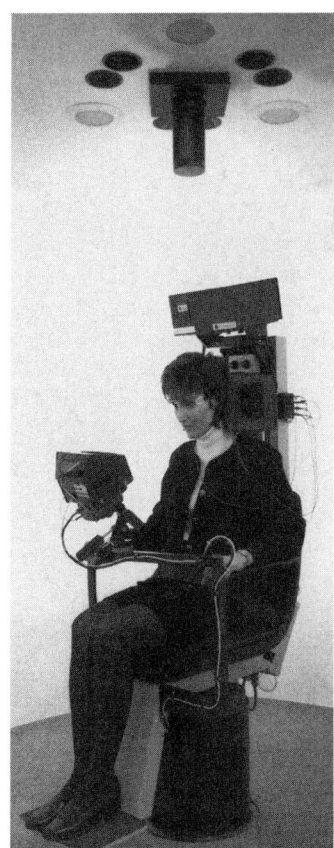

Figure 131.2 Rotary chair apparatus with patient in position for testing.

More rapid rotational velocities may result in head slippage adversely affecting test results. An infrared camera is mounted to the chair to monitor the patient and eye movement. Mental alerting tests are used, as in ENG. As the chair begins to rotate to the right, standard EOG techniques are used to record slow compensatory eye movement to the left. Saccadic eye movement returns the eye to a central position. This movement is eliminated mathematically, and slow-phase movement is compared with chair movement. Three basic characteristics are measured—phase, gain, and symmetry of eye movement. Testing is comfortable for the patient and takes approximately 15 minutes.

Interpretation of the results requires integration with complementary data and the clinical history. Symmetry represents a comparison between the peak slow-wave velocity when the patient is rotated to the left and the peak slow-wave velocity with rotation to the right. For a patient with acute, uncomplicated unilateral peripheral weakness, the symmetry measure shows weakness on the affected side. A problem is that symmetry can be misleading in many cases. Spontaneous nystagmus, irritation of the labyrinth, vestibular compensation, and cerebellar lesions can produce erroneous data. The value of symmetry alone as an indicator of the side of a lesion is controversial. Caution is needed in interpretation of the results. Symmetry often improves with compensation after a vestibular insult and can be useful for monitoring recovery (11). Asymmetry or directional predominance can also be seen with migraine-associated dizziness, a common form of dizziness.

The phase variable is the relation between maximum chair velocity and maximum slow-phase velocity. Eye velocity typically leads chair velocity, the so-called phase lead. The phase lead often is exaggerated among patients with central or peripheral vestibular disease. If abnormal, this value is nonlocalizing. Some laboratories also include a step test in addition to sinusoidal acceleration testing described previously. In the step test, the system time constant is measured by varying the speed at which the chair rotates. This test can be performed simultaneously with the sinusoidal acceleration testing, providing additional vestibulo-ocular reflex information.

Gain is the ratio of maximum eye velocity to maximum chair velocity. A gain of one indicates that slow-phase eye velocity equals chair velocity and is opposite in direction. If there is no eye movement, the gain is zero. A problem is that gain can fluctuate markedly with changes in alertness. Consistent testing is critical to obtain valid results. The gain values used in calculating phase and symmetry must be accurate. Low gain values alert the physician that the results may be inaccurate. Depressed gain values under good testing conditions suggest bilateral peripheral lesions. Abnormally high gain can indicate the presence of a cerebellar lesion that is decreasing vestibular inhibition. Another caution is that there can be considerable differences in results between laboratories, depending on the specific data analysis algorithms used and operator intervention (13).

Rotary testing is useful to (a) monitor changes in vestibular function over time, especially bilateral lesions or lesions due to vestibular toxicity, (b) monitor compensation after acute injury, and (c) identify residual labyrinthine function for patients with no response during caloric testing or low-frequency rotary chair testing (12,14).

Off-vertical-axis rotation is a variation of rotary chair evaluation (15). The testing procedure is similar, except that the chair can be tilted 30 degrees. Earth horizontal axis (barbecue spit) rotation is another variation. The proposed advantage is that otolith function is incorporated into the response. The role of this type of testing is being investigated. Data suggest that a single labyrinth is sufficient to produce normal semicircular canal–otolith interaction; therefore, the value of the test may be limited (15). Another modification is to test unilateral otolith-ocular response. During constant angular rate rotation, the patient is displaced laterally on the rotating turntable, so that one labyrinth becomes aligned with the rotary axis and the second (eccentric) labyrinth is solely exposed to inertial acceleration (16).

VESTIBULAR AUTOROTATION TEST

The vestibular autorotation test is a method of evaluating the vestibuloocular reflex (head-shaking nystagmus) that has distinct clinical and practical advantages over rotary chair testing and ENG (2,17–21). Patients are wired with conventional EOG electrodes to record horizontal and vertical eye movement and are fitted with a lightweight headband containing an EOG amplifier and rotational velocity sensor. The patient is instructed to fix on a target and to rotate the head in synchrony with an auditory cue. The auditory cue accelerates to a maximum of 6 Hz and maintains this velocity for 13 seconds for a total test time of 18 seconds. The test is repeated three times in the horizontal and vertical dimensions. Phase, gain, and symmetry data are collected over the frequency range of 2 to 6 Hz (17).

The vestibular autorotation test has several attractive characteristics. The vestibular system is evaluated at frequencies more physiologic than the ultralow frequencies used in conventional ENG or rotary chair testing (20,22–24). The vestibular autorotation test can be performed efficiently, does not require dedicated space, is portable, allows testing in the vertical plane, and is well tolerated by patients. A potential disadvantage is that it includes the cervical-ocular reflex, but this is thought to be an unimportant contribution at the frequencies used. Vestibular autorotation testing also requires patients to rotate their heads appropriately, which may be problematic for elderly patients or patients with cervical pathology. Interpretation of the results is the same as with ENG and rotary chair testing. The clinical value of headshake nystagmus in evaluating dizziness has been challenged. Jacobson et al. (21) reported a sensitivity of only 27% and a specificity of 85%.

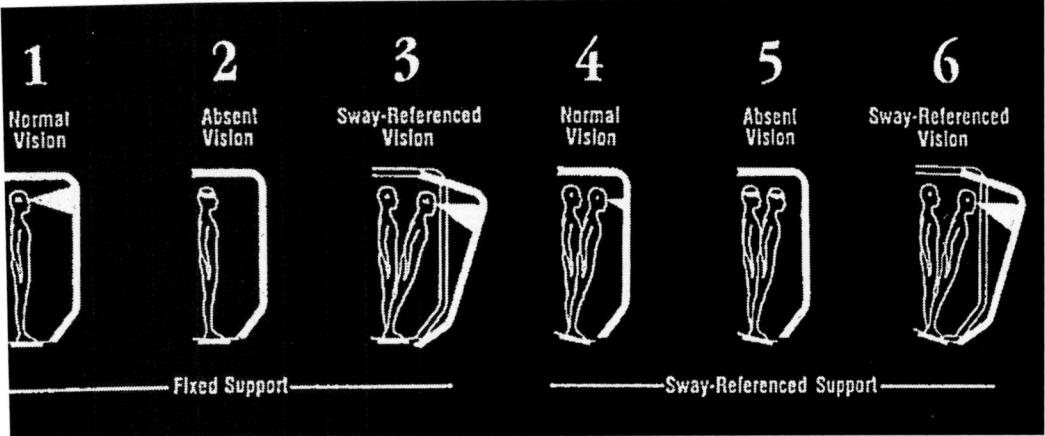

Figure 131.3 Sensory organization testing conditions for posturography. (From NeuroCom International, Clackamas, OR, with permission.)

DYNAMIC POSTUROGRAPHY

Computerized dynamic posturography came into the clinical realm in 1985 with the introduction of the Equitest system developed by NeuroCom. Posturography consists of two tests—the sensory organization test and the movement coordination test. The sensory organization test protocol calls for evaluation under six conditions in which sensory and proprioceptive inputs are varied (Fig. 131.3). During the sensory organization test portion, the patient's

anterior and posterior body sway is recorded, and a performance index is calculated on a scale of 0% to 100% (fall, 0; no sway, 100). During the movement coordination test, the patient stands quietly on a platform, with the visual surround fixed (Fig. 131.4). The platform then undergoes a series of translational and rotational movements. The principal measurement recorded is the latency to onset of active recovery from destabilizing perturbation. Amplitude and symmetry of the neuromuscular responses also are recorded.

Several classification systems to assist with interpretation of results have been proposed (25). Table 131.4 summarizes one system (9). Although these patterns seem to suggest the site of the lesion, the test is not designed or suited for this purpose. A patient with abnormal scores on tests 5 and 6 can have a central or peripheral vestibular disorder. Patients with a compensated unilateral peripheral vestibular dysfunction

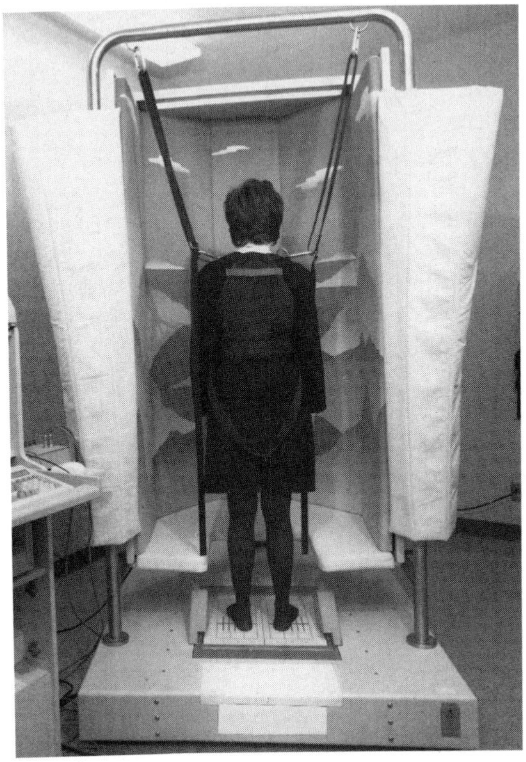

Figure 131.4 Posturography platform with patient in position. Harness is used to prevent injury due to falls.

TABLE 131.4 **D** DIAGNOSIS
CLASSIFICATION OF ABNORMAL SENSORY PATTERNS

Pattern	Abnormal Condition (Test No.)
Vestibular dysfunction	5 and 6
Visual vestibular dysfunction	4, 5, and 6
Visual preference	3 and 6 or 6 alone
Visual preference and vestibular dysfunction	3, 5, and 6
Somatosensory and vestibular dysfunction	2, 3, 5, and 6
Severe dysfunction	Abnormal scores on four or more conditions not covered above
Aphysiologic or functional dysfunction	1, 2, 3, and 4 or any combination with normal 5 and 6

have normal performance on tests 5 and 6. A patient with abnormal scores on conditions 1, 2, 3, and 4 is more likely to have a nonvestibular lesion or functional disorder (aphysiologic sway). A diagnosis of functional disorder is suggested when test results on the more difficult conditions (tests 4, 5, and 6) are equal to or better than those recorded during testing of the easier conditions (tests 1, 2, and 3).

The postural evoked responses in the movement coordination test portion of the evaluation are useful in validating the sensory responses and in identifying a central pathologic disorder. The tests are based on the automatic muscle responses thought to be triggered by proprioceptive changes. The response requires normal muscle, nerve, spinal cord, cerebellar, brainstem, and cortical function and is thus a diffusely distributed response. It is likely that the response is modulated by vestibular and other sensory input.

The most common test for perilymphatic fistula is ENG of the vestibuloocular reflex. Dynamic posturography offers an alternative testing strategy that eliminates potentially confounding effects from the visual and proprioceptive systems. Dynamic posturography can eliminate visual and somatosensory input and therefore better isolate the vestibular apparatus. Positive and negative pressures can be applied to the external auditory canal by means of standard tympanometry techniques, and postural adjustments can be analyzed (23). This test can be more sensitive than the traditional ENG fistula test (26,27). However, lack of a definitive test for the existence of a perilymph fistula impedes development of a clear relation.

Posturography can be combined with standard electromyographic techniques. Electromyography is beneficial in identifying particular muscle response patterns triggered by changes in visual or somatosensory input controlled by the computerized dynamic posturography apparatus. These testing strategies are most useful in research aimed at understanding the complex interactions that allow maintenance of postural control.

Posturography is especially beneficial in documenting overall postural stability and in identifying particular balancing strategies. It is useful for vestibular rehabilitation and for monitoring improvement or decompensation. The computerized dynamic posturography evaluation is comfortable for patients, and they feel that their balance is being thoroughly tested. The test results correlate more closely than those of other balance function test results with the Dizziness Handicap Inventory, which is a subjective measure of overall balance limitations (28).

PEDIATRIC TESTING

Vestibular testing of children presents several challenges. Mental alerting, lack of tolerance of uncomfortable stimuli, inability to follow verbal commands, and inability to remain still all make testing difficult. Modifications of the standard adult ENG battery allow oculomotor, positional, and caloric testing (29). Simultaneous minimal caloric irrigations improve tolerability by reducing the degree of induced nystagmus and time of the procedure. Of course, the data obtained are not as informative as those provided by alternate binaural testing. Closed-loop irrigation systems can improve tolerance. Vestibular autorotation testing can prove useful in children, but more experience is needed. Rotational chair testing can be performed on most children, and very young children can sit on a parent's lap. Computerized dynamic posturography can be performed on older children, but normative data are not available. Most testing protocols can be shortened to minimize testing time and improve compliance.

VESTIBULAR EVOKED MYOGENIC POTENTIALS

Standard caloric testing performed as part of an ENG battery evaluates the superior vestibular nerve because the lateral semicircular canal is being stimulated. A relatively new test can be performed using equipment traditionally used for auditory brainstem response testing to evaluate the function of the inferior vestibular nerve. Colebatch and Halmagyi (30) described the electromyographic response of the neck musculature to a loud, ipsilateral, broad band click. The afferent limb of the response is thought to be due to stimulation of the saccule with transmission via the inferior vestibular nerve to the brainstem and vestibular nuclei. The efferent limb of the response is via the spinocerebellar tract with the response typically recorded on the ipsilateral sternocleidomastoid muscle. The desire for inferior vestibular nerve evaluation has greatly increased the use of this test, which is termed the vestibular evoked myogenic potential (VEMP).

As experience with VEMP accumulates, the limitations and benefits of testing are becoming more apparent. Patients older than 60 years may have a reduced response in VEMP amplitude, which is thought to potentially be due to deterioration of saccular function (31). Pathologic changes in the brainstem, such as multiple sclerosis, may result in delayed potentials with variability noted in the response of the test to common conditions such as acoustic neuromas, Ménière disease, and vestibular neuritis (32). Surprisingly, early Ménière disease frequently demonstrates normal VEMP responses with progressive loss of the potentials with disease progression.

DYNAMIC VISUAL ACUITY

Movement of the head causes significant retinal slip and loss of visual acuity unless the vestibulo-ocular reflex produces an appropriate compensatory response. Patients with dizziness frequently complain of visual blurring and unsteady visual sensations, particularly with head movement. The lack of visual stability on the retina can be quite disconcerting to patients and may prove dangerous for patients during driving. Several commercial devices are available that can assess dynamic visual acuity. These tests use a rotational velocity sensor in combination with a computer screen to evaluate vision during head movement, giving a functional assessment of the vestibulo-ocular reflex in both horizontal and vertical planes (33).

Age does seem to affect dynamic visual acuity results with older patients demonstrating reduction in visual stability. Although some variability has been noted, the test does show good sensitivity and specificity in distinguishing normal patients from those with abnormalities. Patients with bilateral vestibular deficits were shown to have a greater degree of reduction in comparison with unilateral vestibular deficits and patients with nonvestibular dizziness. Surprisingly, oscillopsia did not correlate with abnormalities on vertical dynamic visual acuity in patients with bilateral vestibular loss. This seems to be due to the central preprogramming and the predictability of the head movements. Recent studies demonstrate recovery of the dynamic visual acuity following deterioration after traumatic brain injury associated with dizziness (34).

SUMMARY

Table 131.5 summarizes the typical findings for several common disorders and conditions.

TABLE 131.5 **DIAGNOSIS**
BALANCE FUNCTION FINDINGS IN COMMON DISORDERS

Disorder	Electronystagmography	Rotational Tests	Posturography	VEMP	DVA
Ménière disease	Early: Normal or reduced caloric responses Nystagmus may be in either direction Late: Reduced or absent caloric responses	Normal or decreased gain or phase or both	Typically normal, may be profoundly abnormal in bilateral disease Movement coordination tests are usually normal	Early: Frequently normal amplitude potentials Late: Variable but reduced peak amplitude with normal latency	Early: Frequently normal between episodes Late: Reduced acuity
Benign paroxysmal positional vertigo	Positive Dix–Hallpike sign (torsional nystagmus)	Normal	Normal		
Cerebellar disease	Normal caloric responses Abnormal fixation suppression, increased gain and abnormal saccades, or pursuit	Symmetric responses with phase lead		Prolonged latency	
Bilateral ototoxicity	Absent caloric responses No spontaneous or positional nystagmus Normal results of oculomotor testing	Markedly reduced gain	Vestibular deficit pattern (falls on conditions 5, 6) May be unable to stand for test because of poor balance Normal latency on movement coordination tests		Severely reduced acuity

REFERENCES

1. Kinney WC. Web-based clinical decision support system for triage of vestibular patients. *Otolaryngol Head Neck Surg* 2003;128: 48–53.
2. Ng M, Davis LL, O'Leary DP. Autorotation test of the horizontal vestibulo-ocular reflex in Ménière's disease. *Otolaryngol Head Neck Surg* 1993;109:339–412.
3. Waldorf RA. ENG testing method emerges from video-based technology. *Hear Instrum* 1994;45:16–17.
4. Kramer PD, Roberts DC, Shelhamer M, et al. A versatile stereoscopic visual display system for vestibular and oculomotor research. *J Vestib Res* 1998;8:363–379.
5. Teter DL. The electronystagmography test battery and interpretation. *Semin Hear* 1983;4:11–21.
6. Jacobson GP, Calder JA, Rupp KA, et al. Reappraisal of the monothermal warm caloric screening test. *Ann Otol Rhinol Laryngol* 1995;104:942–945.
7. Schwarz DWF, Tomlinson RD. Physiology of the vestibular system. In: Jackler RK, Brackmann DE, eds. *Neurotology*. St. Louis: Mosby–Year Book, 1994:59–98.
8. Haring RD, Simmons FB. Cerebellar defects detectable by electronystagmography calibration. *Arch Otolaryngol* 1973;98: 14–17.
9. Shepard NT, Telian SA. *Practical management of the balance disorder patient*. San Diego: Singular Publishing Group, 1991.
10. Hain TC, Herdman SJ, Holliday M, et al. Localizing value of optokinetic afternystagmus. *Ann Otol Rhinol Laryngol* 1994;103:806–811.
11. Baloh RW, Jenkins HA, Honrubia V, et al. Visual-vestibular interaction and cerebellar atrophy. *Neurology* 1979;29:116–119.
12. Mathog RH. Testing of the vestibular system by sinusoidal angular acceleration. *Acta Otolaryngol (Stockh)* 1972;74:96–103.
13. Goebel JA, Hanson JM, Fishel DG, et al. Interlaboratory variability of rotational chair test results. *Otolaryngol Head Neck Surg* 1994;110:400–405.
14. Cyr DG, Möller CG, Moore GF. Clinical experience with the low-frequency rotary chair test. *Semin Hear* 1989;10:172–190.
15. Furman JMR, Schor RH, Kamerer DB. Off-vertical axis rotational responses in patients with unilateral peripheral vestibular lesions. *Ann Otol Rhinol Laryngol* 1993;102:137–143.
16. Clarke AH, Engelhorn A. Unilateral testing of utricular function. *Exp Brain Red* 1998;121:457–464.
17. O'Leary DP, Davis LL. High-frequency autorotational testing of the vestibulo-ocular reflex. *Neurol Clin* 1990;8:297–312.
18. Hain TC, Fetter M, Zee DS. Head-shaking nystagmus in patients with unilateral peripheral vestibular lesions. *Am J Otolaryngol* 1987;8:36–47.
19. Goebel JA, Hanson JM, Langhofer LR, et al. Head-shake vestibulo-ocular reflex testing: comparison of results with rotational chair testing. *Otolaryngol Head Neck Surg* 1995;112:203–209.
20. Panosian MS, Paige GD. Nystagmus and postural instability after headshake in patients with vestibular dysfunction. *Otolaryngol Head Neck Surg* 1995;112:399–404.
21. Jacobson GP, Newman CW, Safadi I. Sensitivity and specificity of the head-shaking test for detecting vestibular system abnormalities. *Ann Otol Rhinol Laryngol* 1990;99:539–542.
22. Grossman GE, Leigh RJ, Abel LA, et al. Frequency and velocity of rotational head perturbations during locomotion. *Exp Brain Red* 1988;70:470–476.
23. Grossman GE, Leigh RJ. Instability of gaze during locomotion in patients with deficient vestibular function. *Ann Neurol* 1990;27: 528–532.
24. O'Leary DP, Davis LL, Maceri DR. Vestibular autorotation test asymmetry analysis of acoustic neuromas. *Otolaryngol Head Neck Surg* 1991;104:103–109.
25. Hamid MA, Hughes GB, Kinney SE. Specificity and sensitivity of dynamic posturography: a retrospective analysis. *Acta Otolaryngol Suppl (Stockh)* 1991;481:596–600.
26. Black FO, Lilly DJ, Peterka RJ, et al. The dynamic posturographic pressure test for the presumptive diagnosis of perilymph fistulas. *Neurol Clin* 1990;8:361–374.
27. Shepard NT, Telian SA, Niparko JK, et al. Platform pressure test in identification of perilymphatic fistula. *Am J Otol* 1992;13:49–54.
28. Jacobson GP, Newman CW, Hunter L, et al. Balance function test correlates of the Dizziness Handicap Inventory. *J Am Acad Audiol* 1991;2:253–260.
29. Cyr DG, Brookhouser PE, Valente M, et al. Vestibular evaluation of infants and preschool children. *Otolaryngol Head Neck Surg* 1985;93:463–468.
30. Colebatch JG, Halmagyi GM. Vestibular evoked potentials in human neck muscles before and after unilateral vestibular deafferentation. *Neurology* 1994;42:1635–1636.
31. Su HC, Huang TW, Young YH, et al. Aging effect on vestibular evoked myogenic potential. *Otol Neurotol* 2004;25:977–980.
32. Murofushi T, Matsuzake M, Mizuno M. Vestibular evoked myogenic potentials in patients with acoustic neuromas. *Arch Otolaryngol Head Neck Surg* 1998;124:509–512.
33. Herdman SJ, Tusa RJ, Blatt P, et al. Computerized dynamic visual acuity test in the assessment of vestibular deficits. *Am J Otol* 1998;19:790–796.
34. Gottshall K, Drake A, Gray N, et al. Objective vestibular tests as outcome measure in head injury patients. *Laryngoscope* 2003; 113:1746–1750.

Assessment of Peripheral and Central Auditory Function

132

James W. Hall III   Patrick J. Antonelli

In recent years, researchers have introduced new techniques and strategies for assessment of the auditory function in adults. Pure-tone audiometry, immittance measurement (tympanometry and acoustic reflexes), and calculation of word recognition scores continue to be important in hearing assessment, and the traditional audiogram is useful in summarizing the results of basic audiologic assessment. Clinical audiology, however, now also includes other behavioral and electrophysiologic test procedures. For example, electrocochleography (ECochG) can contribute to the diagnosis of Ménière disease. Auditory brainstem response (ABR) offers a readily accessible and relatively inexpensive means of estimating hearing sensitvity in infants and young children, and of identifying retrocochlear auditory dysfunction. Otoacoustic emissions (OAE), because of unique sensitivity and specificity to cochlear dysfunction, have become an integral component of the clinical audiologic test protocol. And, within recent years, the auditory steady-state response (ASSR) has emerged as a valuable addition to the pediatric audiologic test battery. A variety of speech and nonspeech behavioral measures and several cortical auditory evoked responses are available for clinical assessment of central auditory nervous system dysfunction and associated auditory processing disorders.

Working closely with audiologists, the otolaryngologist has a critical role in ascertaining if a patient is at risk of hearing loss, in initiating diagnostic auditory assessment, and in implementation of timely and appropriate medical or surgical intervention. This chapter summarizes current techniques and strategies for hearing assessment among adults.

The authors emphasize the use of a test battery that maximizes diagnostic accuracy and efficiency and minimizes test time and cost. A glossary of common audiologic terms and abbreviations is provided at the end of the chapter.

BASIC AUDIOLOGIC TEST BATTERY

Pure-Tone Audiometry

Pure-tone audiometry is the most common measurement of hearing sensitivity. Stimuli are pure tones (sinusoids) at octave frequencies typically from 250 Hz to 8,000 Hz and, often, two interoctave frequencies (3,000 Hz and 6,000 Hz). Interoctave hearing loss is a characteristic of commonly encountered problems, such as noise-induced cochlear dysfunction. High-frequency audiometry for stimulus frequencies greater than 8,000 Hz (up to 20,000 Hz) is technically feasible and clinically useful to certain populations, such as patients at risk for ototoxicity. Test results in many clinics are graphed on an audiogram. Two versions of audiograms are illustrated in Fig. 132.1. All audiograms include at the minimum a graph for plotting hearing threshold levels as a function of the frequency of pure-tone signals, although the exact format and symbols vary.

The unit of stimulus intensity is the decibel (dB), a logarithmic unit. The intensity of any sound is defined by the ratio of its sound pressure, or sound intensity, to a reference sound pressure, or sound intensity. The reference sound pressure is the amount of pressure against the eardrum,

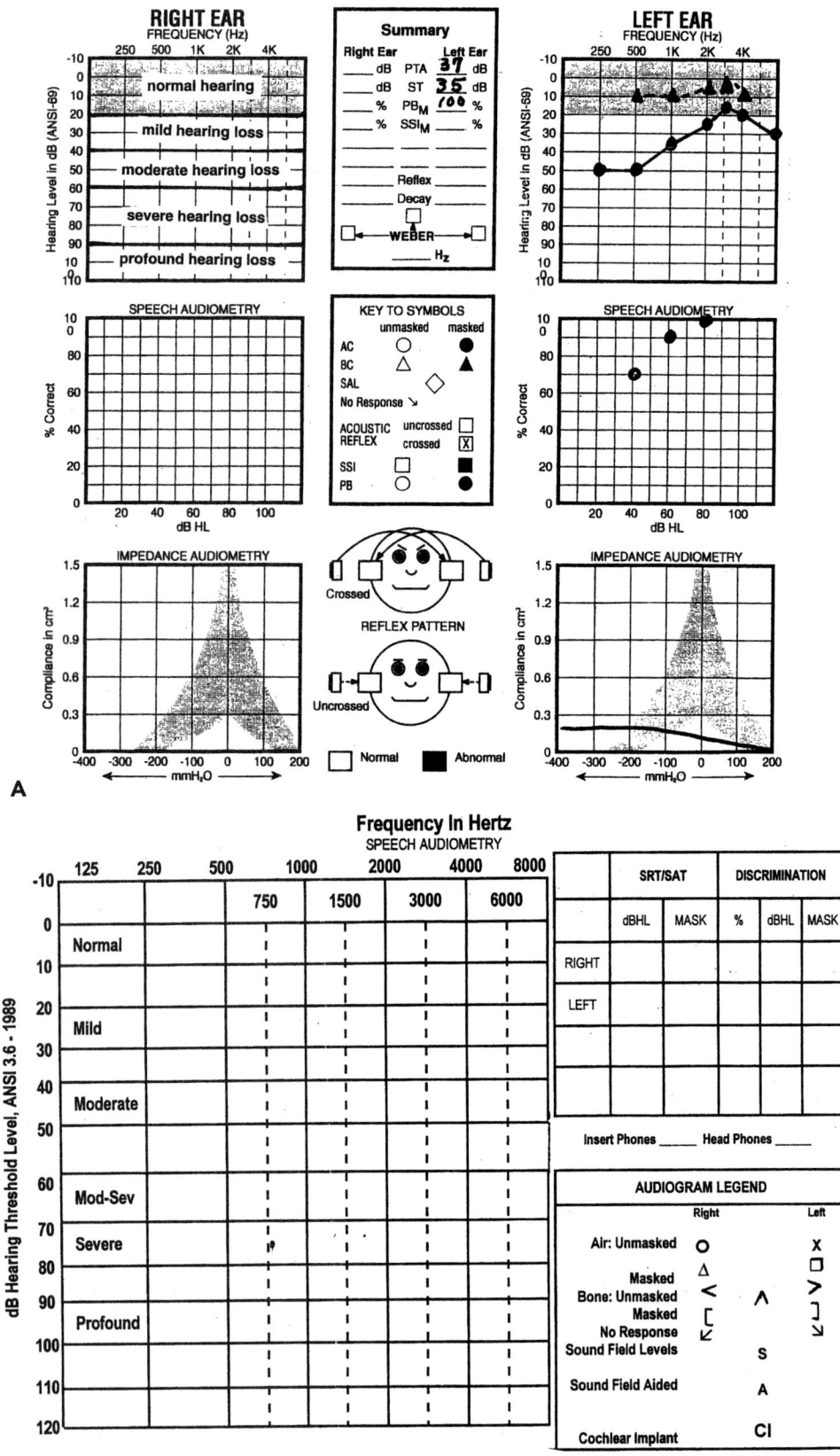

Figure 132.1 Two examples of audiogram forms. **A:** The separate ear form has sections for reporting results for pure-tone audiometry (*top*), speech audiometry (*center*), and aural immittance measurement (*bottom*). Masking is indicated by *filled symbols*. Left-ear findings typify conductive hearing loss. **B:** The traditional audiogram form utilizes symbols (see audiogram legend) for each of 13 signal presentation types. It does not permit graphic display of immittance or speech measurement findings.

caused by air molecules when a sound is present, that vibrates the eardrum and can just be detected by a normal human ear. Briefly, the relation for sound intensity is described as dB = 10 $\log_{10}$ (sound intensity/reference intensity), or for sound pressure as dB = 20 $\log_{10}$ (sound pressure/reference pressure). The reference sound pressure is defined as decibels sound pressure level (dBSPL) and is derived from one of two physical quantities: (a) 0.0002 dyne/cm^2, 20 micropascals root mean square or (b) 2×10^{-5} Newtons/m^2 root mean square.

Clinically, the intensity of sound is described in decibels hearing level (dB HL), a biologic reference level, rather than in sound pressure level. On an audiogram (see Fig. 132.1), the decibel scale has as its reference 0 dB, which is described as *audiometric 0*. This is the standard for the intensity level that corresponds to the mean normal hearing threshold level, the minimal detectable intensity for each test frequency for persons with normal hearing. Another common unit for expressing sound intensity is decibels sensation level (dB SL), which is intensity of the stimulus in decibels above an individual's hearing threshold. For example, a word recognition test can be administered at an intensity level of 40 dB SL (40 dB above the person's pure-tone average).

In audiologic assessment of adults, hearing thresholds for tonal or speech signals are measured separately for each ear with earphones (air-conduction stimulation). Insert earphones (ER3A) are now the transducer of choice for routine audiologic assessment. They offer distinct advantages over traditional supraaural earphones, including increased comfort, reduced likelihood of ear canal collapse, greater interaural attenuation, and greater acceptance by young children. In addition, insert earphones contribute in a significant way to the control of infection in a clinical setting, as the insert portion is disposable. Pure-tone audiometry can be performed with stimuli presented with a bone-conduction oscillator or vibrator placed on the mastoid bone. During pure-tone audiometry, all equipment must meet the specifications of the American National Standards Institute (ANSI). Periodic equipment calibration and validation is necessary. Testing is conducted according to clinical adaptations of psychoacoustic methods (1). Patients are instructed to listen carefully for the tones and to respond, usually by pushing a button that activates a response light on the audiometer or by raising a hand, every time they believe they hear a tone. To minimize interference by ambient background acoustic noise, pure-tone audiometry always is performed with the patient in a double-walled, sound-treated room that meets ANSI specifications.

The clinically normal region on an audiogram is 0 to 20 dB HL, although for children, hearing threshold levels exceeding 15 dB should be considered abnormal. Thresholds in the 20 to 40 dB HL region constitute mild hearing loss, 40 to 60 dB HL thresholds define moderate loss, and threshold levels greater than 60 dB HL are considered

severe hearing loss (2). As a reference, the intensity level of whispered speech close to the ear is less than 25 dB HL. Conversational speech is in the 40 to 50 dB HL region, and a shouted voice within 1 foot (30 cm) of the ear is at a level of about 80 dB HL. The most important frequencies for understanding speech are 500 through 4,000 Hz, although higher frequencies can contribute to discrimination between certain speech sounds. Hearing sensitivity within the speech frequency region often is summarized by means of calculation of the pure-tone average (PTA; hearing thresholds for 500, 1,000, and 2,000 Hz divided by 3 and reported in decibels). A four-frequency PTA including 3,000 Hz is required by the American Academy of Otolaryngology—Head and Neck Surgery.

Audiometric results are valid only when the patient's responses are caused by stimulation of the test ear. If a sound greater than 40 dB HL is presented to one ear through air conduction (AC) with supraaural earphones and cushions (resting on the outer ear), the acoustic energy can cross over from one side of the head to the other and stimulate the ear not being tested. The main mechanism of crossover is presumed to be bone-conduction stimulation caused by vibration of the earphone cushion against the skull at high-stimulus intensity levels. The amount of sound intensity needed before crossover occurs is a reflection of interaural attenuation, that is, the sound insulation between the two ears provided by the head. Interaural attenuation is usually about 50 dB for lower test frequencies and 60 dB for higher test frequencies, such as those contributing to the ABR. Interaural attenuation is considerably higher for insert earphones (2). With bone-conduction stimulation, interaural attenuation is less than 10 dB. In clinical circumstances, the examiner needs to assume conservatively that interaural attenuation for bone-conducted signals is 0 dB. In other words, even a very faint sound presented to the mastoid bone of one ear by a bone-conduction vibrator can be transmitted through the skull to either or both inner ears. Perception of this bone-conducted signal depends on the patient's sensorineural hearing sensitivity in each ear.

Masking is the audiometric technique used to eliminate participation of the ear not being tested whenever air- and bone-conduction stimulation exceeds interaural attenuation. An appropriate noise (narrow band noise for pure-tone signals and speech noise for speech signals) is presented to the ear not being tested when the stimulus is presented to the test ear. With adequate masking, any signal crossing over to the ear not being tested is masked by the noise. The level of masking noise presented to the ear not being tested must exceed the threshold of hearing for that ear. Excess levels of masking noise must be avoided because the noise can cross back over to the ear being tested. Selection of appropriate masking can be difficult, especially when there is bilateral hearing loss (2). Indeed, patients with severe bilateral conductive hearing loss may present the "masking dilemma," that is, when enough masking to the nontest ear actually crosses over to the test ear and interferes with accurate estimation of hearing threshold. An otolaryngologist interpreting audiologic results must verify that appropriate masking was used if testing was not performed by an audiologist.

Knowledge of the type of hearing loss, determined by means of comparison of the hearing thresholds for air- and bone-conduction signals, is useful in classifying a hearing loss as sensorineural (no air-bone gap), conductive [normal bone conduction (BC) and a loss by air conduction], or mixed (loss by BC with a superimposed air-bone conduction gap).

Configuration refers to hearing loss as a function of the test frequency. With a sloping configuration, hearing is better for low frequencies and then becomes poorer for higher frequencies. The most common pattern associated with sensorineural hearing loss is a deficit in thresholds for higher test frequencies. The configuration can be gently sloping from low to high frequencies, be precipitously decreasing above a high-frequency cutoff, such as 2,000 Hz, or be characterized by a notching deficit within a certain frequency region, such as 4,000 Hz. A rising configuration is typified by relatively poor hearing for low-frequency stimuli and better hearing for the high frequencies. A rising configuration can be caused by varied types of middle-ear abnormalities. An exception to the typical association of conductive hearing loss with rising configuration is Ménière disease (see Chapter 156). Ménière disease is one cochlear abnormality that may produce a rising configuration. A flat audiometric configuration often is recorded from patients with mixed hearing loss; that is, both sensorineural and conductive components are present. Other configurations, such as the midfrequency "cookie bite" pattern, are encountered in clinical practice. Test–retest variability in clinical pure-tone threshold estimation is typically ±5 dB.

Guidelines for Evaluation of Hearing Handicap

The results of pure-tone audiometry are adequately summarized in an audiogram and with the terms just defined, such as PTA and the degree, configuration, and type of hearing loss. It also is possible to quantify hearing loss in percentage units according to published and accepted guidelines (3). This approach sometimes is necessary in medicolegal cases or when a patient seeks compensation for hearing loss. According to the guidelines of the American Academy of Otolaryngology Committee on Hearing and Equilibrium and the American Council of Otolaryngology Committee on the Medical Aspects of Noise, *permanent hearing impairment* is defined as follows: "A change for the worse in either structure or function, outside the range of normal, is permanent impairment. . . . Permanent impairment is due to any anatomic or functional abnormality that produces hearing loss" (3). This is differentiated from

TABLE 132.1

GUIDELINES FOR CALCULATING PERCENTAGE OF MONAURAL HEARING IMPAIRMENT[a]

DSHL[b]	Percentage	DSHL	Percentage
100	0.0	240	52.5
105	1.9	245	54.4
110	3.8	250	56.2
115	5.6	255	58.1
120	7.5	260	60.0
125	9.4	265	61.9
130	11.2	270	63.8
135	13.1	275	65.6
140	15.0	280	67.5
145	16.9	285	69.3
150	18.8	290	71.2
155	20.6	295	73.1
160	22.5	300	75.0
165	24.4	305	76.9
170	26.2	310	78.8
175	28.1	315	80.6
180	30.0	320	82.5
185	31.9	325	84.4
190	33.8	330	86.2
195	35.6	335	88.1
200	37.5	340	90.0
205	39.4	345	93.8
210	41.2	350	93.8
215	43.1	355	95.6
220	45.0	360	97.5
225	46.9	365	99.4
230	48.9	370	100.0
235	50.6		(or greater)

[a]American Academy of Otolaryngology Committee on Hearing and Equilibrium and the American Council of Otolaryngology Committee on the Medical Aspects of Noise.
[b]From the audiogram, find the decibel sum of the hearing threshold levels (DSHL) of 500, 1,000, 2,000, and 3,000 Hz.

permanent hearing handicap, which is defined as follows: "The disadvantage imposed by an impairment sufficient to affect a person's efficiency in the activities of daily living is a permanent handicap" (3). The guidelines also detail the approach for converting hearing handicap for one or both ears into a percentage. The first step is to determine the degree of sensorineural hearing loss for four test frequencies (500, 1,000, 2,000, and 3,000 Hz) from the audiogram (Table 132.1). The next step is to follow the guidelines for computation of percentage hearing loss:

If the monaural percent figure is the same for both ears, that figure expresses the percent hearing handicap. If the percent monaural hearing impairments are not the same, apply the formula:

$$(5 \times \% [\text{better ear}]) + (1 \times \% [\text{poorer ear}]) / 6 = \% \text{ hearing impairment}$$

The interoctave test frequency—3,000 Hz—in the calculation of percentage of hearing handicap is very important.

It is good clinical practice to routinely obtain hearing thresholds from each ear for the 3,000 Hz frequency. This frequency is included in the formula for hearing loss (3) because much of the spectral information vital for speech understanding is within the 2,000 to 3,000 Hz region. Percentage of binaural hearing handicap is easily calculated with a detailed tabular matrix that relates the four-frequency degree of sensorineural hearing loss for the better versus poorer ear (4).

Speech Audiometry

The purpose of speech audiometry is to determine how well a person hears and understands speech signals. Speech audiometry procedures usually are performed to measure hearing sensitivity (thresholds in decibels) for words or to estimate the ability to recognize words (speech discrimination). Spondee reception threshold, also called *speech threshold*, is the softest intensity level at which a patient can correctly repeat words approximately 50% of the time. Spondee words, two-syllable words with equal stress on each syllable, such as *hot dog, baseball*, and *eardrum*, are presented to the patient monaurally through earphones. The technique is comparable with the method for determining pure-tone thresholds described earlier.

Because PTA reflects hearing threshold levels in the speech frequency region and speech threshold is measured with a speech signal, one can expect close agreement between the PTA and the speech threshold. If the difference between PTA and speech threshold exceeds ±7 dB, there is reason to suspect that one or both of the measures are invalid. An unusually good speech threshold relative to PTA, such as speech threshold of 5 dB and PTA of 45 dB, immediately alerts the examiner to the possibility of nonorganic hearing loss, such as malingering. With cooperative adult patients, particularly if pure-tone hearing thresholds are within the normal region (500 to 4,000 Hz), there is probably little or no clinical benefit in measuring speech thresholds. Test time can be saved with no loss of diagnostic information by excluding speech threshold measurement from the test battery for such patients.

Speech recognition for phonetically balanced (PB) words is a common clinical approach for estimating a person's ability to hear and understand speech (2). A list of 25 or 50 single-syllable words typically are presented to the patient through earphones at one or more fixed intensity levels. The percentage of words correctly repeated by the patient is calculated by the examiner. One ear is tested at a time. Within the list of words, specific speech sounds (*phonemes*) occur approximately as often as they would in everyday conversation, that is, they are PB. Traditionally, these words were spoken into a microphone by the examiner while the level was monitored with a volume unit meter. The words were routed to the patient through an audiometer after selection of the test ear and desired intensity level. This is an outdated and poor clinical practice

because it lacks standardization and consistency and increases the variability of test outcome. For adult patients, it almost always is possible and always is preferable to use professionally produced, commercially available speech materials, presented with a tape recorder or compact disk player and an audiometer (2). Diagnostic speech audiometry is described later.

Audiometry is typically performed by a clinically licensed audiologist with a graduate degree (Masters, or Doctor of Audiology) from an accredited academic institution. Audiometric technicians, commonly nurses or other members of an otolaryngologist's clinic staff, have been employed to maximize availability of testing coverage and to minimize cost. Although testing by such individuals may be excellent, handling difficult situations, such as masking and interaural attenuation, may prove problematic. Similarly, self-administered, computer-automated audiometers (e.g., Otogram,™ by Tympany, Stafford, TX) have seen tremendous growth in popularity in recent years. Early studies have shown good reliability between conventional, audiologist-administered and self-administered, computer-automated audiometry, but clinical experience with these newer modalities is limited (5,6).

Aural Immittance (Impedance) Measurement

Aural immittance (impedance) measurement is an important part of the basic audiometric test battery. *Immittance* is a term derived from the words for two related techniques for assessing middle-ear function—*im*pedance and ad*mittance*. These techniques have been used clinically since 1970 (7). The external ear canal is sealed with a soft rubber probe tip. The probe tip is connected to a device that produces a tone delivered toward the eardrum. Middle-ear impedance or admittance is calculated from the intensity and other physical properties, such as phase, of the tone in the ear canal. A middle ear (tympanic membrane and ossicular system) with low impedance (higher admittance) more readily accepts the acoustic energy of the probe tone. A middle ear with abnormally high impedance (lower admittance) caused by, for example, fluid in the middle-ear space tends to reject energy flow. Thus, impedance (admittance) characteristics of the middle ear system can be inferred objectively with this technique and related to well-known patterns of findings for various pathologic conditions of the middle ear.

Tympanometry

Tympanometry is the dynamic recording of middle-ear impedance, as air pressure in the ear canal is systematically increased or decreased. The technique is a sensitive measure of the integrity of the tympanic membrane and of middle-ear function (Fig. 132.2). Compliance (the reciprocal of stiffness) of the middle ear, the dominant component of immittance, is the vertical dimension of a tympanogram.

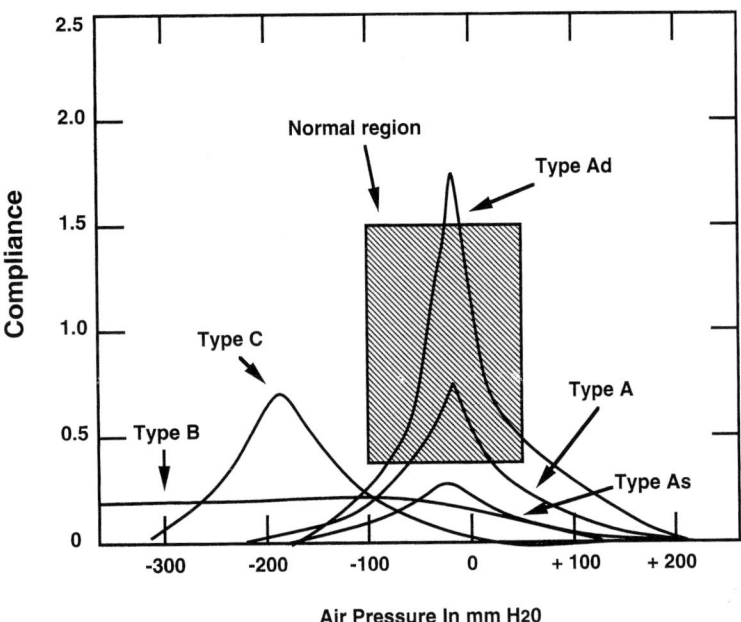

Figure 132.2 Classification system for tympanograms. (Modified from Jerger JF. Clinical experience with impedance audiometry. *Arch Otolaryngol* 1970;92:11–24, with permission.)

Tympanometry is popular clinically because it requires little technical skill and only several seconds to perform. It is an electrophysiologic, as opposed to behavioral, method that does not depend on cooperation of the patient, and it is a highly sensitive index of middle-ear function. Tympanometric patterns, in combination with audiographic patterns, allow differentiation and classification of middle-ear disorders.

The most clinically widespread approach to describing tympanograms was described first by Jerger in 1970 (7). There are three general types of tympanogram—A, B, and C. A normal, or type A, tympanogram has a distinct peak in compliance within 0 to −100 mm water (dPa) in the ear canal (see Fig. 132.2). To be classified as normal, the location of the compliance peak on the pressure dimension and the height of the peak must be within normal range, as indicated in Fig. 132.2 by the stippled area. On a type B tympanogram, there is no peak in compliance, but there is a flat pattern, with little or even no apparent change in compliance as a function of pressure in the ear canal. This pattern is most often associated with the presence of fluid within the middle-ear space (otitis media), although other middle-ear disorders also can produce a type B tympanogram. Although a type B tympanogram can appear to be recorded from ears with perforated tympanic membranes, technically this finding is invalid because the perforation prevents the change in ear canal pressure needed for tympanometry. Like type A recordings, type C tympanograms have a distinct peak in compliance, but the peak is within the negative pressure region beyond −100 mm water (dPa). This pattern usually occurs among patients with eustachian-tube dysfunction and inadequate ventilation of the middle-ear space. It often precedes acquisition of a type B tympanogram in the development of otitis media.

A variation of a type A tympanogram is type A_s (see Fig. 132.2). The *s* stands for shallow. Peak compliance is less than the lower normal limit of compliance. That is, middle-ear impedance is abnormally high. The type A_s pattern is common among patients with fixation of the ossicular chain, including some patients with the diagnosis of otosclerosis. In contrast, with an unusually steep and high-compliance tympanogram (type A_d for *deep*), the peak can exceed the upper compliance limits of the equipment. A type A_d tympanogram occurs among patients with disruption of the ossicular chain, which leaves the middle ear extremely mobile and overly compliant; that is, there is little impedance. In the absence of serious hearing loss, this tympanographic pattern usually is associated with minor tympanic membrane abnormality, such as atrophy. At the beginning of a tympanometric examination, high positive or negative pressure is introduced into the ear canal. This essentially decouples the middle ear system from the measurement. If the impedance device records an abnormally large equivalent volume of air (2 cm or more in an adult, or twice the volume recorded for the other ear) between the probe tip and presumably the eardrum at this stage in the procedure, the integrity of the eardrum is questioned. That is, the immittance device is recording not only ear canal volume but also volume of the middle-ear space. This test finding is consistent with perforation of the tympanic membrane or the presence of an open (patent) middle-ear ventilation tube.

Acoustic Stapedial Reflex Measurement

The stapedius muscle within the middle ear is the smallest muscle in the body. Measurement of contractions of the stapedius muscle in response to high sound-intensity levels (usually 80 dB or greater) is the basis of the acoustic reflex. Acoustic reflex measurement is clinically useful for estimating hearing sensitivity and for differentiating sites of auditory disorders, including the middle ear, inner ear, eighth cranial nerve, and auditory brainstem (2,8). The afferent portion of the acoustic reflex arc is the eighth cranial nerve. Complex brainstem pathways lead from the cochlear nucleus on the stimulated side to the region of the motor nucleus of the seventh cranial (facial) nerve on both sides (ipsilateral and contralateral to the stimulus) of the brainstem. The efferent portion of the arc is the seventh cranial nerve, which innervates the stapedius muscle. The muscle contracts, causing increased stiffness (decreased compliance) of the middle ear system. The small change in compliance that follows stapedius muscle contraction within 10 ms is detected with the probe and immittance device, much as compliance changes are detected during tympanometry.

Acoustic reflex measurement is useful clinically because it quickly provides objective information on the status of the auditory system from middle ear to brainstem. Distinctive acoustic reflex patterns for ipsilateral and contralateral stimulation and measurement conditions characterize middle-ear, cochlear, eighth-nerve, brainstem, and even facial-nerve dysfunction (see lower portion of Fig. 132.1A). Acoustic reflexes are typically abnormal or absent if they are recorded when there is a conductive hearing loss in the probe ear. Analysis of the pattern for acoustic reflex findings is also useful in assessing the site of lesion for patients with facial nerve paralysis. Comparison of acoustic reflex threshold levels—the lowest stimulus-intensity level that activates the reflex—for tonal versus noise signals allows estimation of the degree of cochlear hearing loss (2). This technique is especially valuable in the care of children and difficult-to-test patients.

AUDITORY EVOKED RESPONSES

Auditory Brainstem Response

Auditory evoked responses are electrophysiologic recordings of responses to sounds. With proper test protocols, the responses can be recorded clinically from activation of all levels of the auditory system, from cochlea to cortex (8). Among these responses, the ABR, which neurologists often call the brainstem auditory evoked response (BAER), is used most often clinically. An ABR recording is shown schematically in Figure 132.3. The ABR is generated with transient acoustic stimuli (clicks or tone bursts) and detected with surface electrodes (disks) placed on the forehead and near the ears (earlobe or within the external ear canal). The ABR represents minimal electrophysiologic activity (less than 1 µV) within electroencephalographic activity that is 100 times larger in amplitude. With a commercially available, computer-based device, it is possible

to present rapidly (20 to 30 per second) thousands of sound stimuli and, by means of signal averaging, to detect reliable ABR waveforms in a matter of minutes.

Extensive research has shown that the ABR wave components arise from the eighth cranial nerve and auditory regions in the caudal and rostral brainstem (Fig. 132.3). Wave I unquestionably represents the synchronously stimulated compound action potentials from the peripheral portion (cochlear end) of the eighth cranial nerve. Wave II may arise from the eighth nerve but near the brainstem (the central end). Waves I and II are generated by structures ipsilateral to the ear stimulated. All later ABR waves have multiple generators within the auditory brainstem. Wave III, which usually is prominent, is generated within the caudal pons with likely contributions from the cochlear nuclei, trapezoid body, and superior olivary complex (8). The most prominent and rostral component of the ABR—wave V—is thought to arise in the region of the lateral lemniscus as it approaches the inferior colliculus, probably contralateral to the ear stimulated.

The ABR is not a test of hearing. It reflects synchronous firing of a subset of onset neurons within the auditory system. In ABR waveform analysis, the first objective is to assure that the response is reliably recorded. At the minimum, two replicated waveforms are averaged. If the response cannot be replicated, the test protocol is modified, and technical problems are considered and systematically ruled out. When the existence of a response that can be replicated is confirmed, reproducible absolute latencies for each wave component and relative (interwave) latencies between components are calculated in milliseconds. These latency data for each ear are assessed for symmetry (wave V within 0.4 ms between ears) and compared to appropriate normative data (8).

Common ABR waveform patterns are illustrated in Figure 132.4. A well-formed and clear wave I at a delayed latency value for the maximum stimulus intensity level is characteristic of conductive or mixed hearing loss. When wave I is small and poorly formed but interwave latency values are within normal limits (the wave I–V latency value less than 4.60 ms), high-frequency sensory (cochlear) hearing loss is suspected. Delayed interwave latency values are the signature of retrocochlear auditory dysfunction. Abnormal delays (e.g., >2.40 ms) between the early wave components (I–III) are consistent with posterior fossa lesions that involve the eighth cranial nerve or lower brainstem, whereas prolonged latency of waves III through V (e.g., >2.45 ms) suggests intraaxial auditory brainstem dysfunction.

A primary goal in any neurodiagnostic evaluation of ABR is to record a clear and reliable wave I component. Wave I is the benchmark for peripheral auditory function. Subsequent interwave latencies offer indices of retrocochlear (eighth-cranial-nerve and brainstem) function that are relatively unaffected by conductive or sensory hearing loss. The likelihood that wave I is recorded is enhanced through

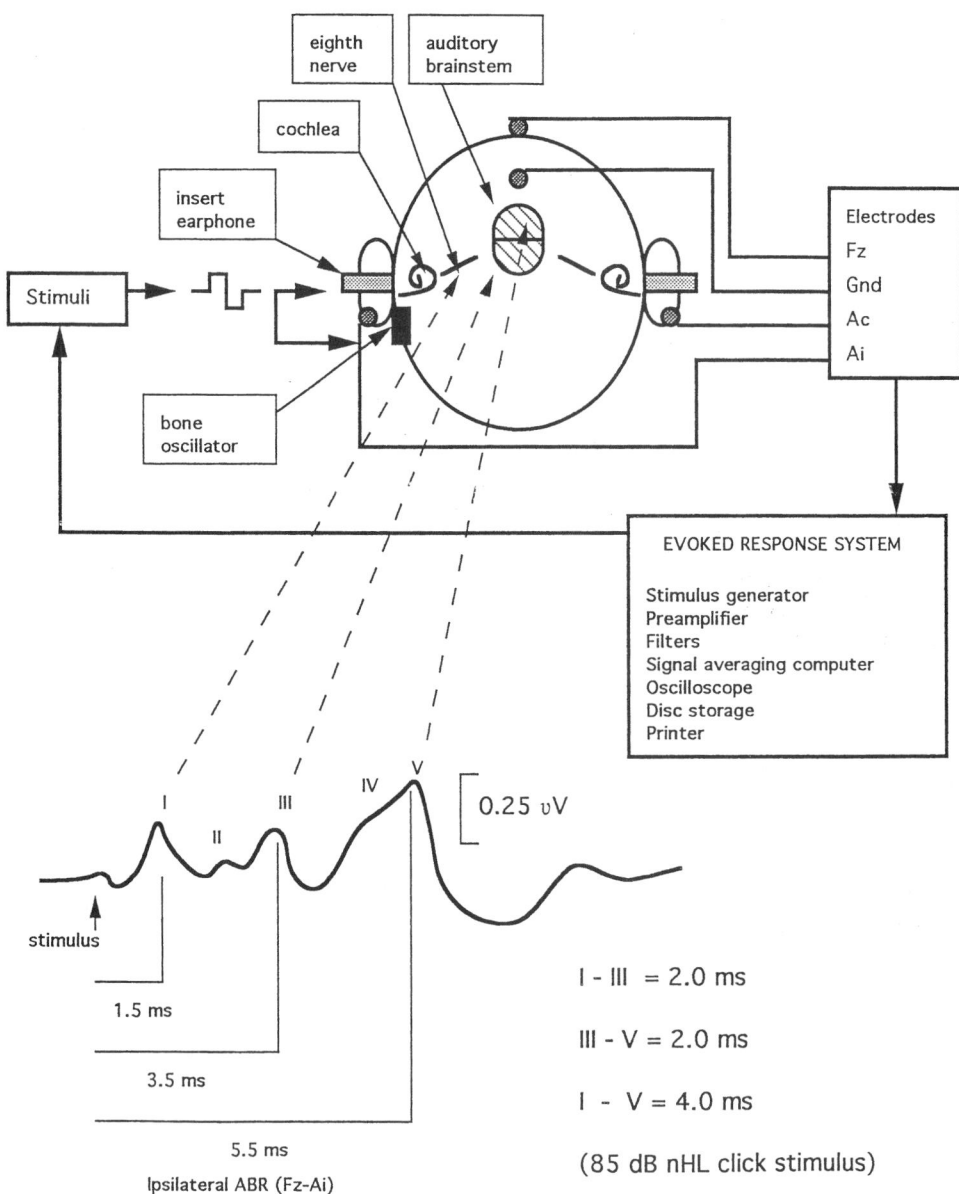

Figure 132.3 Schematic shows the instrumentation for recording the auditory brainstem response (ABR) and important relations between auditory anatomic features and waveform components. A simple strategy for analysis of ABR waveform in neurodiagnosis also is shown.

use of ear canal or tympanic membrane electrode designs and through alterations in the test protocol, such as a slower stimulus rate, rarefaction stimulus polarity, and maximum stimulus intensity level (8).

Reports on ABR dating to the late 1970s have confirmed that waveforms evoked by high-intensity signals yield neurodiagnostic information about cochlear and retrocochlear auditory function. The data can be used in the identification of retrocochlear disorders, such as acoustic neuroma, with an accuracy that exceeds 95%, at least for medium to large tumors. With the development of sophisticated neuroradiologic techniques, such as magnetic resonance imaging (MRI) with enhancement, and earlier diagnosis of smaller tumors, the sensitivity of ABR has dropped (9). In

addition, an inexpensive fast-spin echo MRI is technically feasible and available clinically as a neuroradiologic screening procedure for detection of retrocochlear pathology.

False-negative ABR outcomes can occur in a small percentage of individuals with normal hearing and among patients at risk of retrocochlear auditory dysfunction, usually attributable to the presence of small intracanicular vestibular schwannomas. The poor results are evidence of the relatively poorer sensitivity of ABR than that of MRI to mass lesions. False-positive outcomes of MRI also have been reported among patients with normal ABR results and no surgical evidence of tumor, however (10). It must be kept in mind that ABR is a measure of function, whereas computed tomography and conventional MRI are measures of

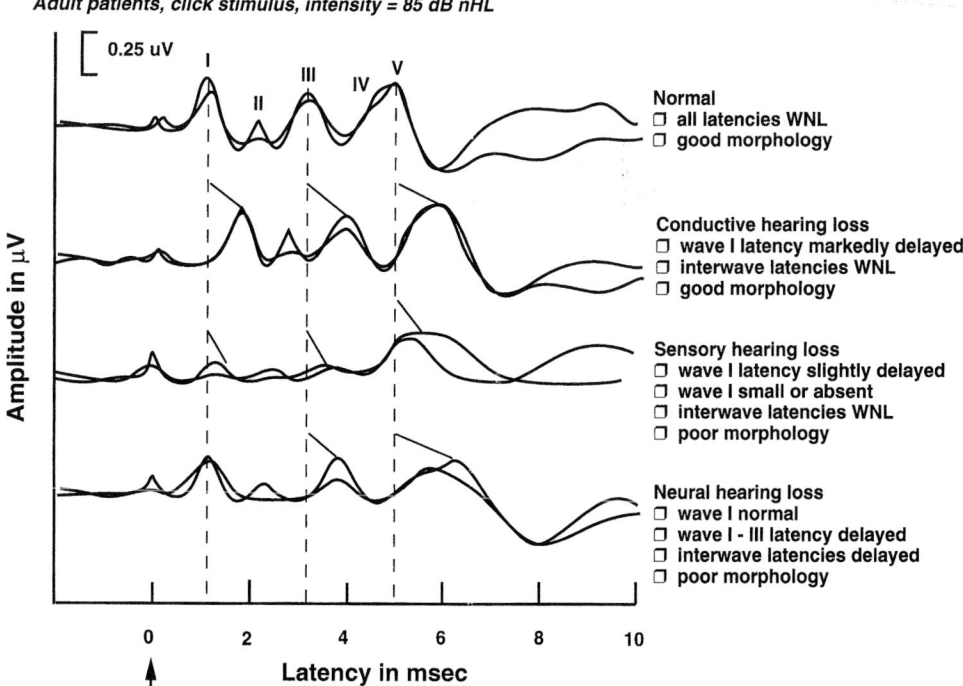

Adult patients, click stimulus, intensity = 85 dB nHL

Figure 132.4 Auditory brainstem response patterns associated with various types of auditory dysfunction. Information about dysfunction can be inferred from the latency of specific waves and overall structure of the waveforms.

structure (see Chapter 147). Assessment of ABR continues to be a readily available, relatively inexpensive, and reasonably sensitive procedure for initial diagnostic evaluation of eighth-nerve and auditory brainstem status in the care of patients with retrocochlear signs and symptoms. ABR is particularly useful in patients for whom concerns are limited to larger tumors, such as the elderly and the medically infirm. As described in Chapter 131, assessment of ABR can also be valuable in electrophysiologic monitoring of the eighth-cranial-nerve and auditory-brainstem function during neurotologic operations such as vestibular nerve section and posterior tumor removal.

The application of ABR in the estimation of hearing sensitivity in infants and young children is now essential (8). With the emergence of universal newborn hearing screening, children at risk for hearing loss are identified at birth. Research on the benefits of early intervention for hearing loss in infants (11) argues strongly for the diagnosis of hearing loss and the beginning of hearing aid use before a child is 6 months old. Appropriate hearing aid fitting, however, requires information on hearing sensitivity at specific frequencies within the range of hearing critical for understanding speech. Unfortunately, it is not possible to obtain behavioral estimates of hearing sensitivity (an audiogram) at such a young age. By performing ABR recordings with frequency-specific signals (tone bursts), hearing thresholds can be estimated electrophysiologically, and infant hearing aid fitting can be accomplished within months after birth. Electrophysiologic estimation of hearing sensitivity with

ABR does have one serious clinical constraint, however. The maximum intensity level is only about 80 dB for very brief (transient) click-and-tone-burst signals used to elicit the ABR. Therefore, the ABR cannot be used to estimate hearing sensitivity in the severe-to-profound range of impairment. Accurate and early hearing aid fitting is, of course, critical for infants with serious hearing loss.

A relatively recent clinical electrophysiologic measure, the auditory steady-state response (ASSR), has proven useful for these infants (8). The ASSR is an auditory response similar to the ABR. It is, however, elicited with pure-tone signals (steady-state signals), rather than transient signals (clicks or tone bursts). The pure-tone signals are altered with rapid modulation of the amplitude and, sometimes, frequency. The pure-tone signal activates the cochlea at the specific frequencies (e.g., 1,000 Hz or 500 Hz) and provides the type of information on hearing available with the audiogram. In addition, energy at the modulation rate (e.g., 80/s) is generated in the auditory system and can be detected automatically with sophisticated algorithms for signal detection. The major clinical advantage of ASSR is the ability to estimate hearing sensitivity at discrete frequencies for children with hearing loss exceeding 80 dB HL. Thus, the ABR and ASSR can be used in combination to define any degree of hearing loss in children at any age, including infants soon after birth. Analysis of ASSR findings can also contribute to the early and confident identification of infants who are likely candidates for cochlear implantation.

Electrocochleography

For more than 30 years, electrocochleography (ECochG) has been used to assess peripheral auditory function. The examination is performed most often for intraoperative monitoring of cochlear and eighth-nerve status and in the diagnosis of Ménière disease (8). Optimal ECochG waveforms are recorded with a small needle electrode placed through the tympanic membrane and on the promontory, although electrode placement on the tympanic membrane or, to a lesser extent, in the ear canal, can be clinically useful. Stimulus and acquisition criteria for ECochG have been well defined for decades. The three major components of the ECochG are the cochlear microphonic, summating potential, and action potential. The cochlear microphonic and summating potential reflect cochlear bioelectric activity. The action potential is generated by synchronous firing of distal afferent eighth-nerve fibers and is equivalent to ABR wave I (Fig. 132.5). The typical ECochG analysis technique in neurotology requires determination of the amplitude of the summating potential (SP) and the action potential (AP) from a common baseline. The ratio of the summating potential to the action potential (SP/AP) is calculated and reported as a percentage. Normal ranges and cutoffs for SP/AP ratio have been reported for each electrode type. Abnormal SP/AP ratio values are defined as more than 50% for the ear canal electrode type, more than 40% for a tympanic membrane

electrode, and more than 30% for a transtympanic needle electrode (8).

Among patients with Ménière disease, the characteristic ECochG finding is abnormal enlargement of the relation between the component amplitudes of the summating potential and the action potential. With the tympanic membrane electrode technique, the sensitivity of ECochG in the diagnosis of endolymphatic hydrops is 57%; the specificity was 94% in a series of 100 patients (12). Only 3 of 30 patients had false-positive results. Thus, according to this data, an abnormally enlarged SP/AP ratio is highly suggestive of endolymphatic hydrops. In the study (10), the likelihood of an abnormal ECochG SP/AP ratio was statistically higher as hearing loss increased and when hearing loss fluctuated. Similar elevations in the SP/AP ratio have, however, been reported in both perilymph fistula (13–15) and autoimmune inner ear disease (16,17).

Cortical Auditory Evoked Responses

More than a dozen subtypes of auditory evoked responses can be recorded beyond the brainstem, from auditory regions of the thalamus, hippocampus, internal capsule, and cortex. Prominent among them in clinical audiology are the auditory middle latency response (AMLR), the auditory late response (ALR), and the P300 response (8). Cortical auditory evoked responses were reported as early as the 1930s. In fact, all of the above-noted responses were well described before the ABR was discovered.

Cortical auditory evoked responses are characterized by longer latencies (100 to 300 ms) than ECochG waveforms and ABR because they arise from more rostral regions of the auditory central nervous system (CNS) and depend on multisynaptic pathways. Amplitudes of the cortical responses are considerably larger (2 to 20 times) than those of the earlier responses because they reflect activity evoked from a greater number of neurons. Measurements are distinctly different for the cortical versus cochlear or brainstem responses. For example, stimulus rate must be slower and physiologic filter settings lower. As a rule, stimulus intensities are moderate, rather than high. Cortical-evoked responses are best elicited with longer duration, and therefore frequency-specific, tonal stimuli, rather than the click stimuli optimal for ECochG and ABR. The analysis time must extend beyond the expected latency of the response (more than 300 ms) for cortical responses. Recording electrode sites also are different for cortical responses. More emphasis is given to scalp sites over the hemispheres and less to electrode sites near the ears.

The AMLR consists of a prominent positive voltage (labeled *Pa*) component in the 25- to 30-ms region. When recorded with electrodes located over the temporal-parietal region, the AMLR is generated by pathways leading to the primary cortex and from this region of the temporal lobe. The ALR occurs later in time, with major peaks (N1 and P2) appearing within the time frame of 100 to 200 ms.

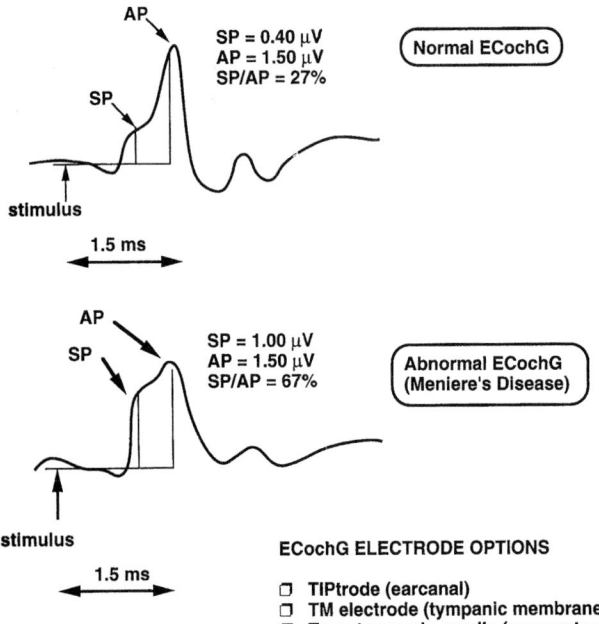

Figure 132.5 Electrocochleography waveforms show normal relation of summating potential (*SP*) and action potential (*AP*) and abnormally enlarged SP/AP relation for a patient with Ménière disease. Absolute and relative amplitude values for the SP and AP components and the criteria for definition of a normal response vary greatly for different electrode sites (ear canal versus tympanic membrane versus promontory).

A variety of types of signals can be used to elicit the ALR, including speech (e.g., phonemes \da\ and \ga\). The AMLR and ALR are now undergoing considerable investigation for the electrophysiologic assessment of children and adults and the documentation of effectiveness of intervention (e.g., auditory training, hearing aids, and cochlear implants) for communication impairment (18).

The P300 response is recorded with what is typically called the *oddball paradigm*. Two types of stimuli are used. One—the frequent stimulus—is presented often, in a predictable manner. The other—the rare or deviant stimulus—is presented infrequently and pseudorandomly. The rare stimuli account for less than 20% of the total stimuli presented. The patient is instructed to ignore the frequent stimuli and to attend to the rare stimuli. The waveform for the frequent stimulus is essentially an auditory late response consisting of a positive peak of 5 to 10 μV within the 150 to 200 ms region. In contrast, the waveform averaged from the attended rare stimuli is characterized normally by a large positive peak in the 300 ms region, hence the term *P300 response*. Presumed generators of the P300 response include regions of the medial temporal lobe (hippocampus) that are important in auditory attention.

OTOACOUSTIC EMISSIONS

Otoacoustic emissions (OAE) are low-intensity sounds produced by the cochlea either spontaneously, or more commonly, in response to an acoustic stimulus. A moderate-intensity click or an appropriate combination of two tones can evoke outer hair cell movement, or motility (2,19). Outer hair cell motility affects basilar membrane biomechanics; the result is a form of intracochlear energy amplification and cochlear tuning for precise frequency resolution. Outer hair cell motility generates mechanical energy within the cochlea that is propagated outward through the middle ear system and the tympanic membrane to the ear canal. Vibration of the tympanic membrane produces an acoustic signal (the OAE), which can be measured with a sensitive microphone.

There are two broad classes of OAE—spontaneous and evoked. Spontaneous otoacoustic emissions (SOAE) occur among only approximately 60% of persons with normal hearing. They are measured in the external ear canal when there is no external sound stimulation. A marked sex effect has been confirmed for SOAE—women have SOAE at twice the rate of men. Evoked otoacoustic emissions, elicited by moderate levels (50 to 80 dB SPL) of acoustic stimulation in the external ear canal, are generally classified according to characteristics of the stimuli used to elicit them or characteristics of the cochlear events that generate them. Stimulus-frequency otoacoustic emissions (SFOAE), which are technically difficult to record, are the least studied of the evoked OAE.

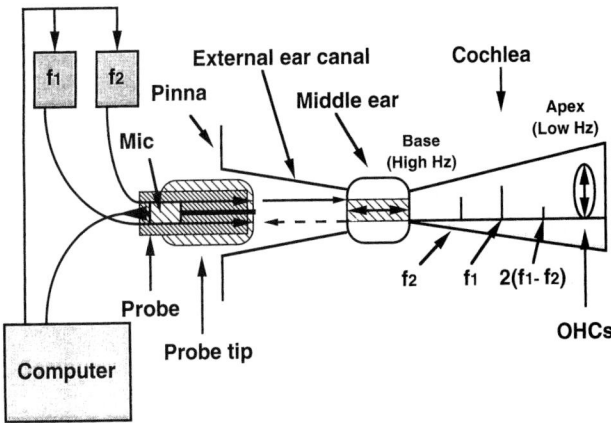

Figure 132.6 Equipment and procedure for measurement of distortion product otoacoustic emissions (DPOAEs). The two stimulus frequencies (f_1, f_2) are presented to the ear with a soft probe (*inward-pointing arrows*). The DPOAEs (at the frequency $2f_1$–f_2) produced by the outer hair cells are propagated outward through the middle ear to the external ear canal. Amplitude of DPOAE in dBSPL is plotted as a function of the frequency of the stimuli (the f_2 stimulus).

Distortion-product otoacoustic emissions (DPOAE) are produced when two pure-tone stimuli at frequencies f_1 and f_2 are presented to the ear simultaneously (Fig. 132.6). The most robust DPOAE occurs at the frequency determined by the equation $2f_1 - f_2$, whereas the actual cochlear frequency region assessed with DPOAE is between these two frequencies and probably close to the f_2 stimulus for recommended test protocols (2,12). With all instruments commercially available for recording DPOAE, amplitude detected in the ear canal and described in dBSPL is plotted as a function of the frequencies of the stimuli in a DPOAE-gram. Transiently evoked otoacoustic emissions (TEOAE) are elicited with brief acoustic stimuli such as clicks or tonebursts. Although there are distinct differences in the methods for recording DPOAE and TEOAE, and the exact cochlear mechanisms responsible for generation are different, each type of evoked OAE is being incorporated into routine auditory assessment of children and adults (2,19).

When outer hair cells are structurally damaged or at least nonfunctional, OAEs cannot be evoked with acoustic stimuli. Among patients with mild cochlear dysfunction, OAEs can be recorded, but amplitudes are below normal limits for some or all stimulus frequencies. Some patients with abnormal OAEs that indicate cochlear dysfunction have normal pure-tone audiograms, and OAEs provide information about auditory function at far more frequencies (up to 20 per octave) than does an audiogram. An example of these advantages is a patient with tinnitus but normal audiologic findings (12). Abnormal OAEs are expected in the frequency region represented by the tinnitus. Up to 30% of a population of outer hair cells can be damaged without substantially affecting a simple audiogram (20). In such cases, abnormal OAE findings are invariably recorded. Conversely, OAEs may be recorded in individuals with

TABLE 132.2

CLINICAL APPLICATIONS OF OTOACOUSTIC EMISSIONS

Children

Newborn hearing screening
- Diagnostic pediatric audiology
- Monitoring ototoxicity
- Assessment of auditory processing disorders
- Assessment of suspected functional (nonorganic) hearing loss

Adults

Early detection of noise-induced cochlear dysfunction
- Monitoring of cochlear status in potential ototoxicity
- Differentiation of cochlear versus retrocochlear auditory dysfunction
- Assessment in suspected functional (nonorganic) hearing loss
- Confirmation of cochlear dysfunction in patients with tinnitus

From Hall JW III. *Handbook of Otoacoustic Emissions.* San Diego: Singular Publishing Group, 2000, with permission.

severely impaired auditory function, either as a result of mass lesion on the auditory nerve (21) or auditory neuropathy (22). The noninvasive nature of OAE recording, coupled with accuracy and objectivity in assessing cochlear, especially outer hair cell, function suggests diverse potential clinical applications that range from auditory screening to sensorineural diagnosis (2,19). A listing of clinical applications and their rationale is provided in Table 132.2.

ASSESSMENT OF AUDITORY PROCESSING DISORDERS

Myklebust in 1954 wrote, "Hearing is a receptive sense . . . and essential for normal language behavior" (23). He also wrote, "The diagnostician of auditory problems in children has traditionally emphasized peripheral damage. It is desirable that he also include considerations of central damage" (23). He explained that "central deafness [central auditory processing disorder] is a deficiency in transmitting auditory impulses to the higher brain centers while receptive aphasia [language disorder] is a deficiency in the interpretation of these impulses after they have been delivered" (23). During this era, Bocca et al. (24) reported that surgically confirmed central auditory system abnormalities can be detected with sufficiently sensitive audiologic procedures. These pioneering observations and studies have been validated by many clinical investigations. There are now a variety of behavioral and electrophysiologic techniques for the assessment of peripheral and central auditory system function, including auditory processing disorders (APDs) involving the peripheral or central auditory system. The term *auditory processing disorder* is used to describe a deficit in the perception or complete analysis of auditory information attributable to central auditory nervous system dysfunction, usually at the level of the cerebral cortex (2,25). Central auditory processing takes place before language processing or comprehension.

Risk Factors for Central Auditory Nervous System Dysfunction

The Joint Committee on Infant Hearing (26) has delineated a number of indicators associated with sensorineural and conductive hearing loss among neonates and infants. Some of these indicators, such as in utero infection, bacterial infection, asphyxia, hyperbilirubinemia, and head trauma, as well as other neurologic insults in infancy (intraventricular hemorrhage and hydrocephalus) can be associated with central as well as peripheral auditory nervous system dysfunction. The joint committee identified an important indicator, one of interest to primary care professionals: "parent/caregiver concern regarding hearing, speech, language, and/or developmental delay" (26). Additional indications for evaluation of children for APD are teachers' concerns about hearing, recurrent middle-ear disease, language impairment, attention deficit disorder with or without hyperactivity, reading delay, and learning disabilities. Central auditory nervous system dysfunction can coexist with any of these disorders. Among adults, risk factors for central auditory nervous system dysfunction include but are not limited to advanced age and history or clinical evidence of stroke, head injury, brain neoplasms, Alzheimer disease, and other disorders affecting the central nervous system. A good clinician always considers the possibility of central auditory dysfunction when a patient describes hearing problems that do not conform with audiographic findings.

Auditory Processing Disorders Test Battery

The central auditory system consists of auditory regions within brainstem and midbrain, the thalamus, and the cerebral cortex, specifically the Heschl gyrus on the superior gyrus of the temporal lobe. The auditory evoked responses described earlier are useful in the assessment of the central auditory nervous system (2,8). Assessment for APD typically is conducted with a battery of behavioral tests that have proven sensitivity to central auditory dysfunction. In most cases, peripheral auditory function is normal. The overall goal is to measure reliable performance for each ear on a series of speech audiometric procedures (including a dichotic word test), such as dichotic digits, a dichotic sentence test, and a speech-in-competition test, and reliable performance with binaural stimulation on one or more nonspeech measures, such as pitch pattern sequence and duration pattern tests. Auditory evoked responses are recorded if specifically requested by the referring practitioner or if there are any concerns about the reliability or interpretation of behavioral test performance. Findings of evaluations for APD are compared with age-corrected normative data. Minimal criteria for confirmation of APD are scores less than the age-corrected normal region (more than 2.5 standard deviations below the mean) for one or both ears for at least two different procedures performed on a child with normal results of peripheral auditory tests.

In constructing an APD test battery, it is wise to rely on procedures not apt to be influenced by linguistic, cognitive, or attention disorders. Interpretation of APD test results is most straightforward when deficits are unilateral. The findings confirm that the patient has understood the task and that the outcome is not caused by a linguistic, cognitive, or attention disorder. A pronounced unilateral abnormality, specifically a marked left-ear deficit, is one of the most common patterns of APD test battery findings. Another rather definite APD test-battery pattern is reduced performance apparent only on difficult portions of a test. This finding implies an auditory as opposed to linguistic, cognitive, or strictly attentional explanation for the child's poor performance. Other important features of a clinically feasible APD test battery are (a) resistance to the influence of even slight peripheral auditory dysfunction, (b) availability of adequate age-matched normative data, and (c) use of professionally produced test materials recorded on tape or a compact disk. Earlier concerns about the usefulness of APD assessment with rudimentary procedures lacking these criteria were justifiable. Now, however, there are clinically feasible and commercially available procedures for testing children and adults (2). In addition, children with auditory processing disorders of auditory nervous system development and functional improvement following the completion of computer-based and conventional auditory training programs provide recent evidence (18).

INDICATIONS FOR DIAGNOSTIC AUDIOLOGIC ASSESSMENT

Children

Hearing loss, regardless of causation, affects the speech and language development of infants and young children. Communication deficits can occur within the first 6 months of life. Hearing loss among preschool and school-age children interferes with educational development. Identification of hearing loss at birth and prompt and appropriate intervention before the age of 6 months are essential if a child is to reach his or her communicative and educational potential (9). Pediatricians and primary care physicians have the responsibility of testing a child's hearing at regular intervals during the first 5 years of life (27). Otolaryngologists and audiologists must coordinate efforts in properly and promptly assessing and managing hearing loss among children.

Adults

The first suspicion of hearing loss among adults occurs while a medical history is being obtained. The patient cites hearing loss as the chief symptom, or close questioning reveals that the patient has difficulty hearing, especially difficulty understanding speech. Sometimes this problem is apparent or is most noticeable only under specific conditions, such as when the patient is speaking on the telephone or conversing in noisy environments or conversing with certain persons, such as children or women, whose voices tend to be fainter and higher pitched than those of men. The medical history can provide other information that suggests risk of hearing loss, such as exposure to damaging levels of recreational or work-related noise or administration of ototoxic medications. Specific symptoms, such as tinnitus or vertigo, or physical findings of otologic abnormalities or of other pathologic conditions associated with auditory system involvement, also indicate the need for audiologic assessment.

GLOSSARY

ABLB Alternate binaural loudness balance. A traditional diagnostic auditory procedure for detecting loudness recruitment used in differentiating cochlear from retrocochlear auditory dysfunction in unilateral hearing loss. The task is to balance the sensation of loudness for the better versus poorer hearing ear. Loudness recruitment is a cochlear auditory sign.

ABR (BAER) Auditory brainstem response (brainstem auditory evoked response). Electrical activity, evoked (stimulated) by sounds of very brief duration, that arises from the eighth cranial nerve and auditory portions of the brainstem. Usually recorded from the surface of the scalp and external ear with disk-type electrodes and processed with a fast-signal-averaging computer. Wave components are labeled with Roman numerals and described according to latency in milliseconds after the stimulus and amplitude in microvolts from one peak to the following trough.

AC Air conduction. Audiometric signals presented through earphones to the ear canal. The difference in pure-tone thresholds for air-conducted versus bone-conducted signals. With calibrated audiometers, the normal ear and the sensorineurally impaired ear show no air-bone gap; conductive hearing losses are characterized by an air-bone gap.

ASSR Auditory steady-state response. An electrophysiologic measure similar to the ABR, but elicited with pure-tone signals (versus transient signals for ABR) that are modulated rapidly in amplitude and frequency. Electrophysiologic activity in the brain is generated by the signal modulation and detected automatically with a sophisticated processing algorithm.

audiologist A hearing care professional educated and trained clinically to measure the function of the auditory system and to provide nonmedical care of persons with auditory and communicative losses. Minimal educational requirements and professional credentials for audiologists are a Master's degree, or Doctor of Audiology (Au.D.), and state licensure.

BC   Bone conduction. Audiometric signals presented to the skull, such as mastoid bone or forehead, by means of an oscillator.

BCL   Békésy comfortable loudness. A Békésy audiometry procedure conducted at a comfortable loudness level as opposed to threshold level. Békésy audiometry An audiometric procedure performed with a Békésy audiometer for differentiating cochlear and retrocochlear auditory dysfunction. Békésy audiometry is based on comparison of responses to pulsed and continuous tones varied across a wide frequency range. Jerger classified four patterns of Békésy responses.

BOA   Behavioral observation audiometry. A pediatric behavioral audiometry procedure in which motor responses to sounds such as eye opening and head turning are detected by a trained observer.

configuration   The shape or pattern of an audiogram. Shows how hearing loss varies as a function of the audiometric test frequency. The three main configurations are rising (a low-frequency loss), sloping (a high-frequency loss), and flat (hearing thresholds are similar for all audiometric frequencies).

crossover   Property by which sound stimulus presented to one ear (test ear) travels around the head (by means of air conduction) or across the head (by means of bone conduction) to stimulate the other ear (nontest ear). See *interaural attenuation* and *masking dilemma*.

dB HL   Decibels hearing level. A decibel scale referenced to accepted standards for normal hearing (0 dB is average normal hearing for each audiometric test frequency).

dB nHL   Decibels normal hearing level. A decibel scale used in ABR measurement referenced to average behavioral threshold for the click stimulus of a small group of normal-hearing subjects.

dB SL   Decibels sensation level. Sound intensity described in reference to an individual patient's behavioral threshold for an audiometric frequency or another measure of hearing threshold, such as the speech reception threshold.

dB SPL   Decibels sound pressure level. A decibel scale referenced to a physical standard for intensity, such as 0.0002 dyne/cm^2.

dichotic   Simultaneous presentation of a different sound to each ear.

DPgram, DPOAEgram   A graph of distortion product otoacoustic emission amplitude in the ear canal (dBSPL) as a function of the frequencies of the stimulus tones (Hz).

DPOAE   Distortion product otoacoustic emission.

ECochG   Electrocochleography. Recording of evoked responses originating from the cochlea (the summating potential, the cochlear microphonic, and the eighth cranial nerve [the action potential]).

ENG   Electronystagmography. A test of vestibular function in which nystagmus is recorded with electrodes placed near the eyes during stimulation of the vestibular system.

ENoG   Electroneurography. Recording of myogenic activity of the facial muscles, usually in the nasolabial fold, in response to electrical stimulation of the facial nerve as it exits the stylomastoid foramen.

interaural attenuation   Insulation to the crossover of sound (acoustic or mechanical energy) from one ear to the other provided by the head. Varies depending on whether the signal is presented by air conduction (interaural attenuation more than 40 dB) or bone conduction (interaural attenuation less than 10 dB). Insert earphones offer maximum interaural attenuation.

malingering   Feigning or exaggerating a hearing loss. Also called *functional or nonorganic hearing loss*.

masking (masker)   A controlled background noise presented usually to the ear not being tested in an audiometric procedure to prevent a response from that ear caused by crossover when interaural attenuation is exceeded.

masking dilemma   A problem encountered in audiometric assessment of patients with severe conductive hearing loss. The level of masking noise necessary to overcome the conductive component and adequately mask the ear not being tested exceeds interaural attenuation levels. The masking noise can cross over to the ear being tested and mask the signal, such as a pure tone or speech. In the masking dilemma, enough masking is too much masking. The masking dilemma can be reduced by the use of insert earphones. The sensory acuity level test also is helpful for measuring ear-specific bone conduction hearing thresholds for patients who present the masking dilemma.

MCL   Most comfortable level. The intensity level of a sound perceived as comfortable.

MLD   Masking level difference. An audiometric procedure used to compare a threshold response with masking noise presented in phase as opposed to out of phase with a pure tone or speech signal. Release from masking is a normal phenomenon reflecting auditory brainstem integrity.

OAE   Otoacoustic emissions. Sounds generated by energy produced by the outer hair cells in the cochlea and detected with a microphone placed in the external ear canal.

PB   Phonetically balanced. Word lists developed in the late 1940s that contain all the phonetic elements of general American English speech that occur with the approximate frequency of occurrence in conversational speech.

PI   Performance intensity. A measure of speech recognition or understanding as a function of the intensity level of the speech signal. See *rollover*.

PTA   Pure-tone average. The arithmetic average of hearing threshold levels for 500, 1,000, and 2,000 Hz, or the speech frequency region of the audiogram. The PTA should agree within ±7 dB with the speech reception threshold.

rollover   A decrease in speech recognition performance, in percentage correct, at high signal-intensity levels as opposed to lower levels. Rollover is an audiometric sign of retrocochlear auditory dysfunction.

SAL   Sensory acuity level. An audiometric procedure developed by Jerger for assessing bone-conduction hearing among patients with serious conductive hearing loss. Air-conduction thresholds are determined without masking and with masking presented by bone conduction to the forehead. The size of the masked shift in hearing thresholds corresponds to the degree of the conductive hearing loss component.

SAT   Speech awareness threshold (speech detection threshold, **SDT**). The lowest intensity level at which a person can detect the presence of a speech signal. The SAT approximates the best hearing level in the 250- to 8,000-Hz audiometric frequency region.

SISI   Short increment intensity index. A clinical procedure developed by Jerger for assessing the ability to detect a 1-dB increase in intensity. A high SISI score is consistent with cochlear auditory dysfunction.

S/N   Signal-to-noise. The signal-to-noise ratio is the difference between the intensity level of a sound or electrical event and background acoustic or electrophysiologic energy.

SRT   Speech reception level. The lowest intensity level at which a person can accurately identify a speech signal, such as two-syllable spondee words. See *PTA*.

SSI   Synthetic sentence identification. A measure of central auditory function that involves identification of syntactically incomplete sentences (a closed set of 10 sentences) presented simultaneously with a competing message (an ongoing story about Davy Crockett).

SSW   Staggered spondaic word test. A measure of central auditory function developed by Katz in which spondee words are presented dichotically.

tone decay test   A clinical measure of auditory adaptation in which a tone is presented continuously to an ear with a hearing loss until it becomes inaudible. There are numerous versions of tone decay tests. Excessive tone decay is a sign of retrocochlear auditory dysfunction.

TROCA   Tangible reinforcement operant conditioning audiometry. A pediatric behavioral audiometry technique used to reinforce a response to auditory signals with food. TROCA is used mainly in the care of children with mental retardation or developmental delay.

UCL (LDL)   Uncomfortable level (loudness discomfort level). The intensity level of a sound perceived as too loud.

VRA   Visual reinforcement audiometry. A pediatric behavioral audiometry procedure used to reinforce localization responses to acoustic signals with a visual event, such as an animal playing.

HIGHLIGHTS

- Pure-tone audiometry is the most common measure of hearing sensitivity.
- Masking is the audiometric technique used to eliminate participation of the ear not being tested whenever air- and bone-conduction stimulation exceeds interaural attenuation.
- Speech audiometry procedures usually are performed to measure hearing sensitivity (thresholds in decibels) for words or to estimate word recognition, such as speech discrimination, ability.
- *Immittance* is a term derived from the words for two related techniques of assessing middle-ear function (impedance and admittance), techniques that have been used clinically since 1970.
- Tympanometry is the dynamic recording of middle-ear impedance as air pressure in the ear canal is systematically increased or decreased.
- Acoustic reflex measurement is useful clinically because it can quickly provide objective information about the status of the auditory system from middle ear to brainstem.
- Extensive research has shown that the ABR wave components arise from the eighth cranial nerve and auditory regions in the caudal and rostral brainstem.
- Optimal ECochG waveforms are recorded with a small needle electrode placed through the tympanic membrane onto the promontory, although placement on the tympanic membrane and to a lesser extent the ear canal also is clinically useful.
- Otoacoustic emissions are low-intensity sounds produced by the cochlea in response to an acoustic stimulus.
- Indicators of sensorineural or conductive hearing loss among neonates and infants include intrauterine infection, bacterial infection, asphyxia, hyperbilirubinemia, and head trauma, as well as neurologic insults during infancy.
- No single measure of auditory function is adequate for comprehensive hearing assessment.
- Hearing loss, regardless of causation, affects the speech and language development of infants and young children.

REFERENCES

1. Carhart R, Jerger JF. Preferred method for clinical determination of pure-tone thresholds. *J Speech Hear Disord* 1959;24:330–345.
2. Hall JW III, Mueller HG III. *Audiologists' desk reference.* Vol. I. San Diego: Singular Publishing Group, 1997.
3. American Academy of Otolaryngology Committee on Hearing and Equilibrium and the American Council of Otolaryngology Committee on the Medical Aspects of Noise. Guide for the evaluation of hearing handicap. *JAMA* 1979;11:2055–2059.
4. Mueller HG III, Hall JW III. *Audiologists' desk feference.* Vol. II. San Diego: Singular Publishing Group, 1998:700–714.
5. Henry JA, Flick CL, Gilbert A, et al. Reliability of computer-automated hearing thresholds in cochlear-impaired listeners using ER-4B Canal Phone earphones. *J Rehabil Res Dev* 2003;40:253–264.
6. Henry JA, Flick CL, Gilbert A, et al. Reliability of hearing thresholds: computer-automated testing with ER-4B Canal Phone earphones. *J Rehabil Res Dev* 2001;38:567–581.
7. Jerger JF. Clinical experience with impedance audiometry. *Arch Otolaryngol* 1970;92:11–24.
8. Hall JW III. *The new handbook of auditory evoked responses.* Boston: Allyn & Bacon, 2005.
9. Ruckenstein MJ, Cueva RA, Morrison DH, et al. A prospective study of ABR and MRI in the screening for vestibular schwannomas. *Am J Otol* 1996;17:317–320.
10. Loftus B, Wazen JJ. A false-positive gadolinium-enhanced MRI: acoustic neuroma versus cochleovestibular neuritis. *Otolaryngol Head Neck Surg* 1990;103:299.
11. Yoshinaga-Itano C, Sedley AL, Coulter DK, et al. Language of early- and later-identified children with hearing loss. *Pediatrics* 1998;102:1161–1171.
12. Pou AM, Hirsch BE, Durrant JD, et al. The efficacy of tympanic electrocochleography in the diagnosis of endolymphatic hydrops. *Am J Otol* 1996;17:607–611.
13. Sass K, Densert B, Magnusson M. Transtympanic electrocochleography in the assessment of perilymphatic fistulas. *Audiol Neurootol* 1997;2:391–402.
14. Badr-el-Dine M, Gerken GM, Meyerhoff WL. Loss of perilymph affects electrocochleographic potentials in the guinea pig. *Am J Otol* 1994;15:717–722.
15. Campbell KC, Abbas PJ. Electrocochleography with postural changes in perilymphatic fistula. Animal studies. *Ann Otol Rhinol Laryngol* 1994;103:474–482.
16. Kakigi A, Sawada S, Takeda T, et al. Electrocochleographic findings in cases of autoimmune disease with sensorineural deafness. *Auris Nasus Larynx* 2003;30:349–354.
17. Bouman H, Klis SF, Meeuwsen F, et al. Experimental autoimmune inner ear disease: an electrocochleographic and histophysiologic study. *Ann Otol Rhinol Laryngol* 2000;109:457–466.
18. Hayes EA, Warrier CM, Nicol TG, et al. Neural plasticity following auditory training in children with learning problems. *Clin Neurophysiol* 2003;114:673–684.
19. Hall JW III. *Handbook of Otoacoustic Emissions.* San Diego: Singular Publishing Group, 2000.
20. Bohne BA, Clark WW. Growth of hearing loss and cochlear lesion with increasing duration of noise exposure. In: Hamernik RP, Henderson D, Salvi R, eds. *New perspectives on noise-induced hearing loss.* New York: Raven Press, 1982:283–301.
21. Norman M, Thornton AR, Phillips AJ, et al. Otoacoustic emissions recorded at high rates in patients with confirmed acoustic neuromas. *Am J Otol* 1996;17:763–772.
22. Rapin I, Gravel J. "Auditory neuropathy": physiologic and pathologic evidence calls for more diagnostic specificity. *Int J Pediatr Otorhinolaryngol* 2003;67:707–728.
23. Myklebust HR. *Auditory disorders in children: a manual for differential diagnosis.* New York: Grune & Stratton, 1954.
24. Bocca E, Calearo C, Cassinari V. A new method for testing hearing in temporal lobe tumors. *Acta Otolaryngol* 1954;44:219–221.
25. Jerger J, Musiek F. Report of the Consensus Conference on the diagnosis of auditory processing disorders in school-aged children. *J Am Acad Audiol* 2000;11:467–474.
26. Joint Committee on Infant Hearing. Year 2000 position statement: principles and guidelines for early hearing detection and intervention. *Am J Audiol* 2000;9:9–29.
27. American Academy of Pediatrics Task Force on Newborn and Infant Hearing. Newborn infant hearing: diagnosis and intervention. *Pediatrics* 1999;103:527–529.

Neurophysiologic Intraoperative Monitoring

133

Matthew R. O'Malley   *Brian A. Moore*   *David S. Haynes*

The primary goal of intraoperative neurophysiologic monitoring is the preservation of nerve integrity and function. In selected applications, neurophysiologic monitoring may allow for the prediction of postoperative functional impairment. Table 133.1 depicts the ideal requirements for an intraoperative neurophysiologic monitor. These criteria are imperative to the utility of any intraoperative monitoring system. Intraoperative neurophysiologic monitoring has been employed in numerous surgical scenarios throughout the body. The purpose of this chapter is to acquaint the reader with currently available techniques of neurophysiologic monitoring, primarily as they relate to the surgical management of temporal bone and posterior fossa pathology.

The growth of otology, neurotology, and skull base surgery has allowed the surgical extirpation of intratemporal and retrocochlear pathology while attempting seventh and eight cranial nerve preservation. Intraoperative monitoring, along with advanced microsurgical techniques, has led to the expectation of cranial nerve preservation in many instances. This chapter will discuss the indications, techniques, and potential controversies of intraoperative auditory and facial nerve monitoring.

AUDITORY SYSTEM MONITORING

The primary goal of most otologic and neurotologic procedures is the eradication of disease while minimizing atten-

dant morbidity. When considering acoustic neuromas and skull base tumors, many surgeons regard the preservation of hearing a secondary, yet significant, goal, even in patients with functional hearing in the contralateral ear. Advances in diagnostic capabilities, specifically the routine use of contrast-enhanced MRI, have likely resulted in the more frequent detection of small tumors. Enhanced detection, coupled with advances in the surgical armamentarium, including intraoperative neurophysiologic monitoring, has increasingly made preservation of hearing a reasonable goal. Further, the likelihood of certain disease processes, such as neurofibromatosis type II, to produce bilateral lesions highlights the benefits of attempted hearing preservation.

Until the characterization of the human auditory evoked potentials (AEP) in 1971 by Jewett and Williston, no techniques existed for intraoperative monitoring of the auditory nerve, and this technology was not applied to surgical cases until 1978 (1,2). Intraoperative eighth nerve monitoring has since been used during vestibular schwannoma resection, vestibular nerve section, facial nerve exploration, skull base procedures including excision of temporal bone paraganglioma, endolymphatic sac operations, cochlear implantation, and microvascular decompression of the fifth, seventh, and eighth cranial nerves.

Although each of the aforementioned procedures places the auditory system at risk, acoustic neuroma resection carries the highest risk of postoperative hearing impairment (3). Many patients with vestibular schwannoma initially present

TABLE 133.1

CHARACTERISTICS OF THE IDEAL NEUROPHYSIOLOGIC MONITOR

Function in the operating room in the presence of other electrical devices, such as air drills and anesthesia machines, with minimal dysfunction or artifact.

Function safely so that even if dysfunction does occur, no harm to the patient can occur.

Incorporate straightforward and reproducible setup and monitoring procedures to avoid delay in preparation for the procedure and to minimize errors in data analysis, operative time, and cost.

Accurately and continuously monitor the cranial nerve (end organ, peripheral system) at risk for intraoperative injury.

Exhibit sufficient sensitivity and specificity to detect intraoperative changes in the system being monitored for surgical alterations, without unnecessary false alarms.

Rapidly alert the surgeon in sufficient time to alter surgical technique to minimize trauma to the system at risk.

In the case of intraoperative facial nerve monitoring, allow the surgeon to receive feedback through auditory, visual (electromyographic tracing, oscilloscope), or a combination of stimuli, so that the surgeon can monitor the facial nerve without the mandatory assistance of trained personnel, if desired.

with sensorineural hearing loss, which is believed secondary to cochlear dysfunction induced by internal auditory artery insufficiency, or by cochlear nerve dysfunction caused by pressure, atrophy, or tumor invasion. Surgical techniques, such as the middle fossa approach and the suboccipital (retrosigmoid) approach, have been designed to minimize the hearing loss associated with the translabyrinthine approach, but even these measures preserve some degree of hearing in only 28% to 87% of patients (4). Comparatively, approximately 10% to15% of patients undergoing microvascular decompression of the fifth, seventh, and eighth cranial nerves will experience hearing loss (5).

During surgery, the auditory system may be injured via direct injury to the cochlea, through labyrinthine artery injury with resultant cochlear ischemia, or via cochlear nerve stretching, compression, transection, or thermal injury as a result of drilling, cautery, or surgical dissection. As such, the auditory system may be injured at the cochlea, anywhere along the course of the eighth nerve, and at the brainstem. Because of the variable coverage of the central glial segment of the nerve that often extends to the internal auditory canal (IAC), the auditory nerve may be even more fragile than other cranial nerves, rendering it particularly susceptible to stretch or thermal injuries (6). Operative manipulation causing varying degrees of neural conduction block accounts for approximately 30% to 44% of the hearing impairment in posterior fossa surgery (7,8). In acoustic neuroma resection, hearing may also be jeopardized by the size of the tumor, its degree of involvement with the nerve fibers or blood supply, the location of the lesion, and its extent into the posterior fossa (9,10). When applied to acoustic neuroma resection, the goals of intraoperative auditory monitoring are twofold: to warn the surgeon when his or her surgical manipulation may be causing auditory system injury and to predict postoperative hearing function.

Auditory System Monitoring Techniques

There are three primary types of intraoperative auditory monitoring—brainstem auditory evoked potentials (BAEP),

also known as auditory brainstem response (ABR); electrocochleography (ECochG); and auditory nerve compound action potential (ANCAP), which is also known as direct eighth nerve monitoring (DENM) or cochlear nerve action potential (CNAP) monitoring. Although these techniques are described separately for purposes of discussion, when clinically applied to intraoperative monitoring of the auditory system, each may be used alone, or in combination with each other.

Following an auditory stimulus, the components and neural connections in the auditory system respond with electrical potentials that may be measured; these evoked potentials provide the foundation for neurophysiologic eighth nerve monitoring. Each of the techniques provides useful information about auditory system integrity and function, and each provides level-specific responses, as seen in Figure 133.1.

Auditory Brainstem Response (ABR)

The least invasive method of eighth nerve monitoring, ABR, is a commonly utilized modality. Because of the relatively large distance between the recording electrodes and the actual generators of the response, ABR is known as a far-field technique. Stimuli, often in the form of "clicks" or tone bursts, are presented to the ear through transducers or special earphones, and responses from components of the auditory system are recorded from the scalp or external auditory canal with high-gain, low-noise electroencephalogram amplifiers. When compared to near-field monitoring techniques (e.g., ECochG, DENM), ABR provides a low-amplitude signal that requires extensive, time-consuming averaging for useful interpretation.

Measuring the ABR provides five peaks, moving from distal (cochlea) to proximal (brainstem) along the auditory pathway. The first two peaks (I and II) are believed to arise from activity along the distal and proximal cochlear nerve, whereas peak III corresponds to the cochlear nucleus; peak IV corresponds to the superior olive, and peak V corresponds to the lateral lemniscus and inferior colliculus (11). Examining the intraoperative waveforms and the

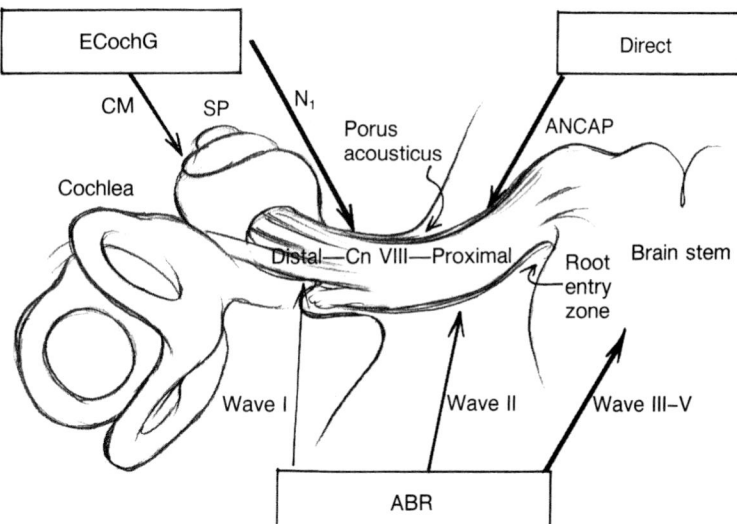

Figure 133.1 Schematic shows level-specific responses obtained with electrocochleographic, auditory brainstem response, and direct auditory nerve compound action potential recordings.

latency intervals reveals potential damage to the hearing apparatus and signal conduction. Deviations from the baseline recording are analyzed relative to surgical manipulations, indicating potential damage to the cochlea or the nerve. Because of the extensive signal averaging involved in ABR monitoring, minutes may lapse between an offensive manipulation and the presence of changes in the baseline recording. The surgeon must then retrospectively evaluate the recent operative actions and provide a corrective action, if possible. The time lag between surgical manipulation and subsequent detection of ABR abnormalities is likely the most significant limitation to this technique. Though digital filtering allows more rapid averaging and notification (3), the implementation of recent advancements in ABR has yet to yield improved functional outcomes (12).

Intraoperative changes in the ABR may include any of the following: desynchronization of wave V; diminished amplitude or elimination of waves I, III, or V; and lengthening of the I to V latency (3,8,13). Any of these responses may arise during retraction, exposure, and dissection, indicating potential trauma to the auditory system. Nontraumatic maneuvers like opening the dura will alter the conduction patterns of the ABR and appear as changes on the monitor; in these situations, an intraoperative baseline may need to be reestablished prior to manipulation of the auditory system. Stretching the nerve, as may occur with cerebellar retraction, elicits an increase in the wave V latency, as well as in the I to V latency interval (14). A more severe injury, such as a contusion or complete transection, will eliminate wave V (5).

In addition to the time lag between offensive manipulation and signal deviation mentioned earlier, an additional drawback of the ABR is that, in order to successfully utilize this technique, the patient should have a useful preoperative ABR. Some patients with absent preoperative ABR waveforms can be monitored with other techniques (e.g., DENM), and a significant percentage of these patients can

ultimately achieve hearing preservation (15). One report has described a series of nine patients with absent preoperative ABR waveforms who were successfully monitored with DENM. Seven of the nine patients ultimately achieved hearing preservation (15). Last, ABR can be affected by hypothermia, certain volatile anesthetics, blood in the middle ear, the tumor or disease process itself, as well as surgical manipulations away from the cochlear nerve such as retraction, irrigation, drilling, and opening of the dura (16–18).

Electrocochleography

When auditory monitoring is performed near the source of the signal (near-field technique) the signal is more robust and can be obtained quicker with fewer sweeps and less required averaging. Electrocochleography (ECochG) is a near-field technique that monitors the most peripheral components of the auditory system. Auditory stimuli are delivered to the cochlea commonly in the form of a wideband click, composed of many frequencies that stimulate the entire cochlea. Figure 133.2 shows a typical ECochG setup, with an insulated transtympanic recording needle electrode placed on the promontory of the middle ear. To improve intraoperative stability, the electrode may first be placed through the tragus (19). External auditory canal electrodes are also available, but their distance from the recording targets minimizes the amplification advantage of this near-field technique. Figure 133.3 shows an ECochG tracing from a patient undergoing removal of a vestibular schwannoma. If the recording electrode is placed closer to the origins of the response, less noise is encountered, allowing more rapid signal generation (within 10 s) with less required averaging (9,14). ECochG can be used to monitor the cochlear microphonic, as well as the summating potential and eighth nerve action potentials arising from a stimulus.

The cochlear microphonic (CM) is an alternating current response generated by the hair cells of the organ of Corti; it mirrors the waveform of the sound stimulus. Also

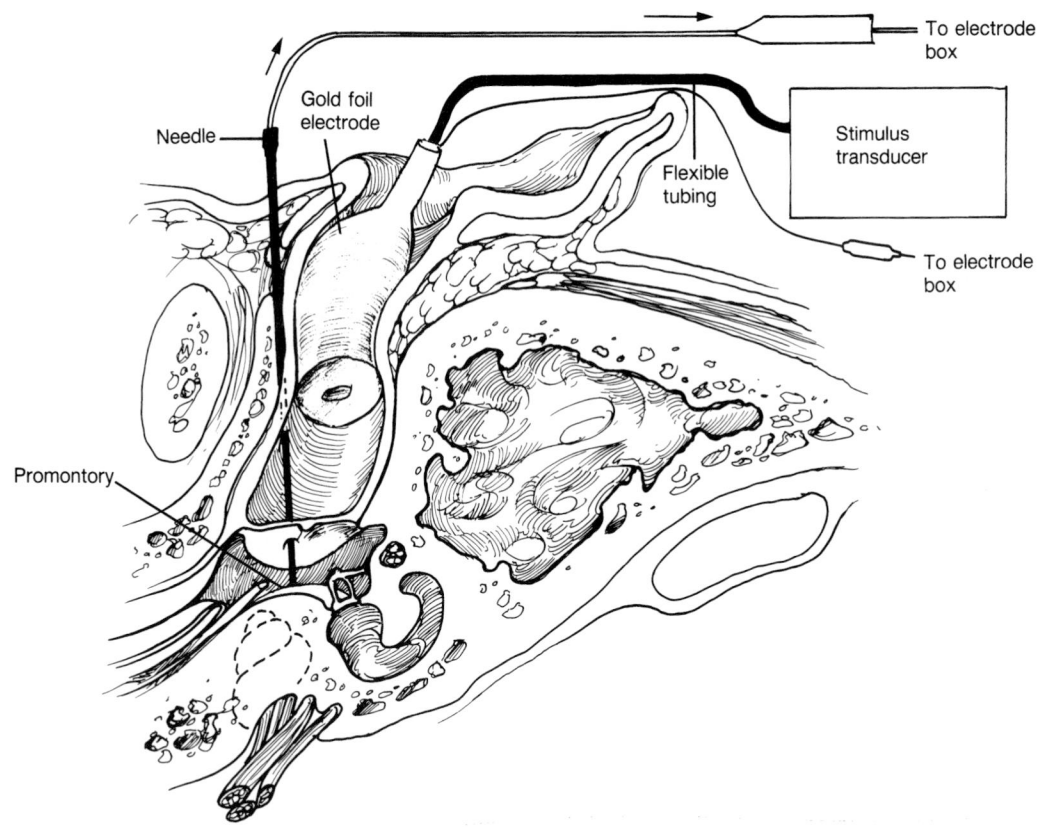

Figure 133.2 Schematic shows placement of intraoperative transtympanic needle electrode through tragus. A gold foil electrode sound delivery system is in the distal portion of the ear canal.

generated by the hair cells, the summating potential (SP) typically occurs throughout the duration of the stimulating acoustic event and typically is negative for all stimulus frequencies and intensities. It may represent asymmetry in the basilar membrane caused by pressure differences between the scala media and scala vestibuli, indicating changes in endolymphatic fluid. The compound action potential (CAP) of the auditory nerve represents the summed response of synchronous discharges from several thousand individual nerve fibers and is most representative of responses from the basal turn of the cochlea.

The first component of the action potential is known as N1 and is analogous to wave I of the ABR. Differentiation of the summating potential from the compound action potential, which are normally superimposed on one another, may be accomplished by increasing the click rate. With higher click rates, the eighth nerve compound action potential will decrease because the stimulus frequency is shorter than the refractory period for each neuron contributing to the CAP. The N1 latency is inversely related to the stimulus rate, whereas its amplitude is directly related to the stimulus rate (20).

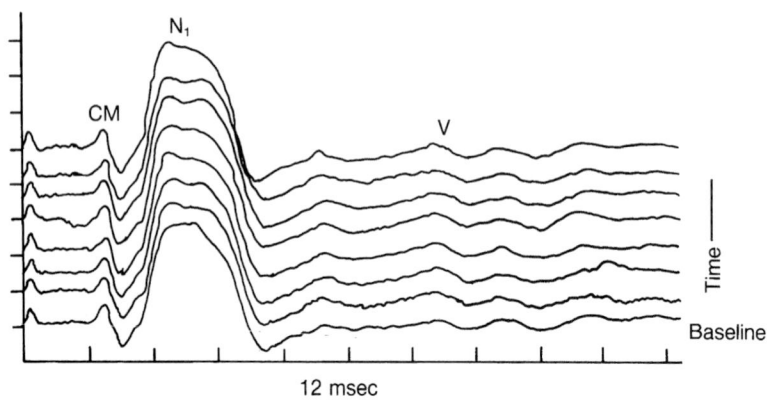

Figure 133.3 Intraoperative transtympanic electrocochleographic recordings of a patient undergoing removal of acoustic tumor. *CM*, cochlear microphonic; N_1, action potential of eighth cranial nerve.

Clinically, ECochG may best sense changes in cochlear blood supply. Reduced amplitude or loss of the ECochG action potential is believed to indicate injury to the labyrinthine (internal auditory) artery (21). Decreased amplitude, or prolonged latency, of N1 or the CM has also been associated with postoperative hearing loss. In fact, any change in the cochlear microphonic may indicate cochlear pathophysiology, potentially indicating postoperative hearing loss. An abrupt change in ECochG tracings may indicate vascular compromise, either by direct injury or vasospasm. Because less signal averaging is required, surgeons are alerted to damaging maneuvers or situations more quickly than with ABR (10).

Potential drawbacks of ECochG monitoring arise from its invasiveness, difficulty of appropriate needle placement, and potential for intraoperative dislodgement of the electrode (5). Transtympanic needle placement may increase the risk of postoperative cerebrospinal fluid otorrhea (9). More significantly, ECochG may not be sensitive to intraoperative changes that occur medially within the cerebellopontine angle (5). Also, the persistence of intraoperative and postoperative ECochG signals despite cochlear nerve section has been well documented. Utilizing intraoperative ECochG, Silverstein et al. demonstrated signal persistence for 25 minutes after cochlear nerve section (22,23). In a patient evaluated both preoperatively and postoperatively, Ohashi et al. (24) documented compound action potentials three years after cochlear nerve resection. Because of limitations encountered with ECochG use, and the suspicion that use of ECochG alone may not be as effective as other means of monitoring (14), the use of ECochG as the sole means of intraoperative monitoring has been reported with less frequency in recent years.

Direct Eighth Nerve Monitoring

Direct monitoring of the cochlear nerve action potential seeks to circumvent some of the potential problems with ABR and ECochG recording. Since its introduction by Moller and Jannetta in the 1980s, DENM has gained increasing acceptance (25). In this technique, a monopolar or bipolar electrode is placed directly on or near the cochlear nerve, ideally medial to the lesion and even in the lateral recess of the fourth ventricle adjacent to the cochlear nucleus (26). Various electrodes, ranging from cotton wicks on malleable wires to self-retaining devices, have been devised (27). A reference electrode is then placed in the musculature of the surgical wound. Click stimuli are administered to the ear as in the previously described systems, eliciting a characteristic waveform with an initial positive peak (N1), as in Figure 133.4. Because the compound action potential is very large in this near-field technique, there is little to no need for signal averaging, and the feedback to the surgeon can be nearly instantaneous, usually within seconds (14).

Regarded as the most sensitive available eighth nerve monitoring modality, this technique can be employed

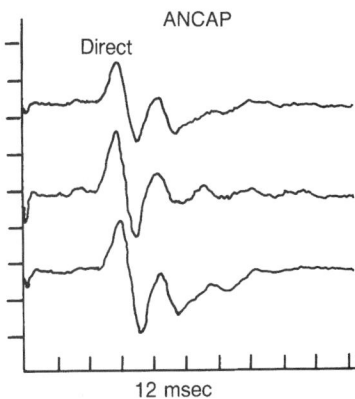

Figure 133.4 Intraoperative recording shows direct auditory nerve compound action potential of a patient undergoing retrolabyrinthine vestibular nerve section.

even in cases in which patients have poor or absent ABR tracings. The preservation of hearing in patients with absent ABR, monitored by DENM alone, has been well documented (15).

The response to certain injuries corresponds to ABR changes in that moderate injury will decrease the CNAP amplitude, with complete loss occurring with severe contusion or transection. Stretching the nerve will increase the N1 latency, and diminished N1 amplitude may be the first sign of mechanical or thermal injury to the nerve (14). Analyzing the morphology and latency of CNAP components provides information regarding the mechanism of injury and gives the surgeon insight into which maneuvers are beneficial and which are harmful to hearing. Monitoring with bipolar recording electrodes promotes identification and mapping of the nerve and its subdivisions, as well as recognition of cleavage plains between an acoustic tumor and surrounding tissue (28,29). However, DENM requires adequate exposure of the nerve, which may be limited by the lesion, or by the approach used. Because of the variations in exposure provided by the different approaches, techniques have been devised to allow direct eighth nerve monitoring for most approaches, including the middle cranial fossa approach (30).

Despite the advantage of more rapid feedback, and the suggestion of improved rates of hearing preservation (31), some surgeons have been reluctant to embrace this technique. The placement of the electrode can be challenging under certain conditions. Once placed, the electrode can become a cumbersome impediment as it lies in the surgical field.

Armed with an understanding of the fundamental techniques of intraoperative auditory system monitoring, the surgeon may then decide which modalities, if any, will be applicable to the planned surgical procedure.

Applications and Benefits

Auditory system monitoring, regardless of the technique employed, has been associated with improved outcomes following certain otologic and neurotologic procedures. Successful use of auditory monitoring has been reported during resection of acoustic neuromas, vestibular nerve section, endolymphatic sac surgery, cochlear implantation, and microvascular decompression of cranial nerves (32–34). In general, nearly all studies investigating the utility of a particular intraoperative monitoring technique have suggested that the technique under investigation can be associated with improved outcomes. Although such claims have been supported by retrospective analyses (35), the validation of intraoperative auditory monitoring with a prospective trial comparing monitored patients with unmonitored patients will likely never be achieved. The overwhelming majority of data supporting the use of intraoperative monitoring of the auditory system comes from retrospective analyses, and some are quite convincing (31).

Comparing the results of hearing preservation surgeries across studies or institutions is inherently difficult for a number of reasons. First, the selection criteria for patients undergoing hearing preservation surgery can differ dramatically between institutions. Tumor size, preoperative hearing ability, and the surgeon's experience in removing such tumors are only some of the frequently encountered variables. Additionally, the intraoperative monitoring technique used is not constant and neither is the interpretation or surgical response. Last, the most significant limitation may be the variability as to what is ultimately considered preservation of hearing. Some studies regard any detectable hearing as preservation, whereas others use more selective criteria to indicate those with truly functional hearing. A recent review demonstrated that substantial variations in published rates of hearing preservation can be achieved simply by manipulating the definition of success (36). Standardized schemes for reporting results have been developed, but even these are disputed and are not uniformly applied (36,37).

Beyond these difficulties, advancements in diagnostic and operative technologies have reduced the utility of comparing current results with results from the premonitoring era. Probably because of the prevalence of contrast-enhanced MRI scanning, today's surgeon encounters a greater number of small tumors and is afforded a greater opportunity to preserve hearing (38).

Though comparing studies evaluating the success of hearing preservation surgery remains difficult, the use of intraoperative auditory monitoring has been associated with improved results. Many surgeons have reported monitoring to be useful, and a substantial body of literature supports the use of intraoperative auditory monitoring in the appropriate setting. Consequently, the use of intraoperative auditory monitoring has become common in hearing preservation surgery in many major centers.

Despite the previously described weaknesses of ABR, intraoperative monitoring with this technique has been associated with an increased likelihood of hearing preservation during resection of acoustic neuromas (8,39,40). A retro-

spective analysis by Slavit and colleagues (41) demonstrated improved preservation of hearing in patients monitored by ABR while undergoing acoustic neuroma resection, particularly when their tumors were less than 1–2 cm. Other authors have shown in a prospective, randomized fashion, that the implementation of corrective actions based on ABR changes can significantly improve the rate of functional hearing preservation (42).

Several studies have attempted to evaluate the prognostic value of intraoperative ABR (43). Although few findings have gained universal agreement as to their significance, certain intraoperative ABR patterns have been correlated with postoperative hearing. Persistence of waves I and V at the conclusion of the procedure has been associated with hearing preservation, whereas the presence of wave V has been associated with serviceable hearing (10,14). Similarly, complete elimination or irreversible and progressive loss of waves I and V indicates a high likelihood of postoperative hearing loss (3,43).

Unfortunately, preservation of wave I or V does not guarantee preserved postoperative hearing, as auditory function may disappear postoperatively, despite its presence in the immediate postoperative period, possibly reflecting postoperative cochlear artery spasm (44). Loss of intraoperative ABR recordings does not always mean that hearing is completely lost or unserviceable postoperatively. Variable reversible loss of ABR tracings has been associated with varied hearing outcomes (43). Figure 133.5 shows a series of intraoperative ABR recordings on a 52-year-old male who had undergone resection of an intracanalicular acoustic neuroma via a middle fossa approach. Tracing A1 shows a baseline intraoperative recording. During dissection of a tumor within the fundus of the internal auditory canal, there is a prolongation of wave I to III latency, seen in tracing A2. Further tracings, A3 through A5, show progressive deterioration of the ABR recording. Yet, this patient's preoperative (Fig. 133.6) and postoperative audiogram (Fig. 133.7) showed preservation of serviceable hearing.

Auditory brainstem responses have also been monitored in patients undergoing cochlear implantation, with intraoperative ABR recordings used to assist in the programming of the device, a process termed neural response telemetry (NRT) (34). A decrease in auditory morbidity has also been noted following posterior fossa microvascular decompression of cranial nerves in which intraoperative ABR has been used (45).

ECochG and direct eighth nerve monitoring have also proven useful in the operating room. ECochG, particularly the summating potential, has also been useful in surgery for Ménière disease, as sac decompression has precipitated a decrease in previously elevated SPs in several patients (33). Loss of the action potential recorded during ECochG has strongly correlated with postoperative hearing impairment. A comparison of monitored and nonmonitored patients undergoing acoustic neuroma resection demonstrated

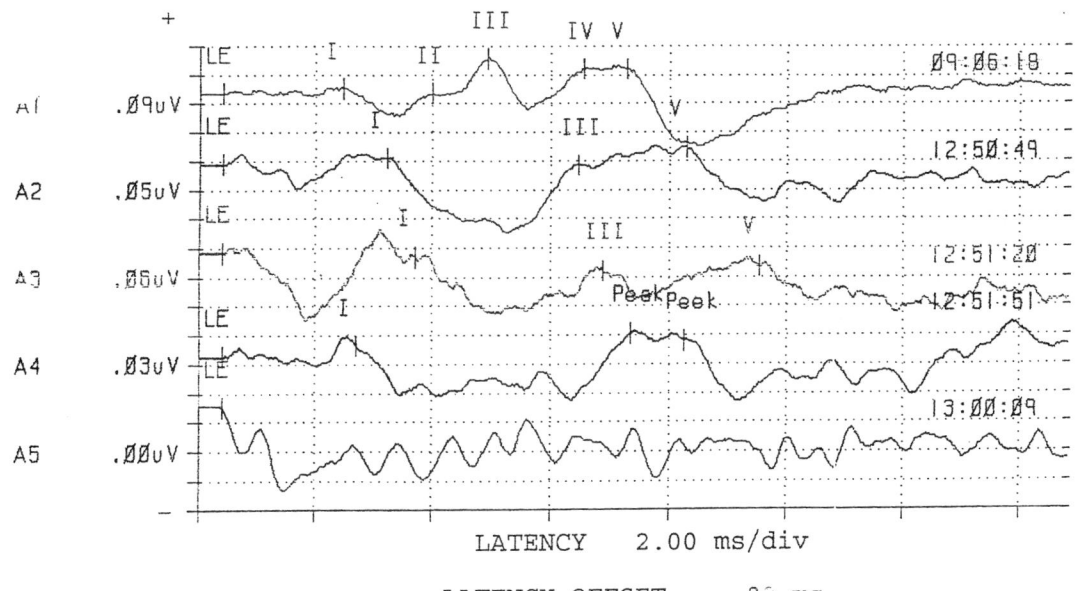

| LATENCIES (ms) | | | | | | | | |
	I	II	III	IV	V	RarV	ConV	Peak	Peek
A1	1.64	3.17	4.10	5.72	6.45				
A2	2.39		5.64		7.46				
A3	2.88		6.04		8.71				
A4	1.87							6.51	7.44
A5									

Figure 133.5 Intraoperative ABR tracings of a patient with preserved hearing after excision of intracanalicular acoustic neuroma. *A1*, baseline; *A2*, prolongation of I through III latency; *A3–A5*, additional intraoperative deterioration.

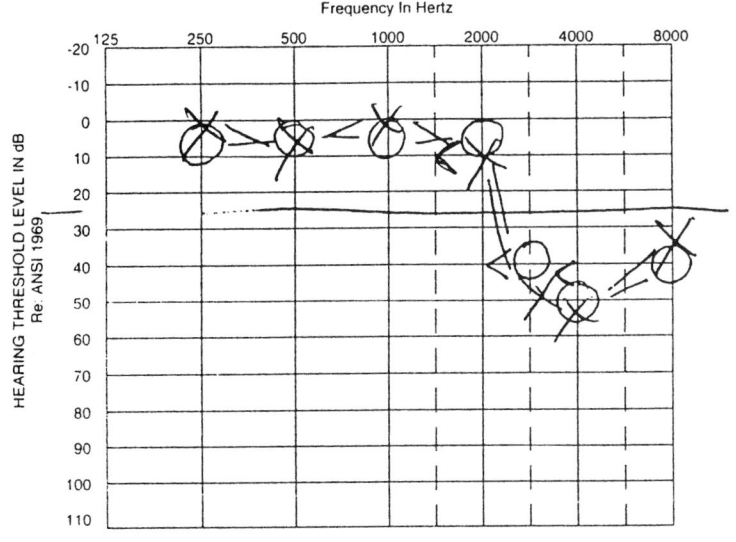

SPEECH AUDIOMETRY						
	PTA	SRT	SDT	HL/PB	HL/PB	LIST
Right		5		65dB 96%		
Left		10		65dB 96%		
SF						

Figure 133.6 Preoperative audiometric findings for patient in Figure 133.5.

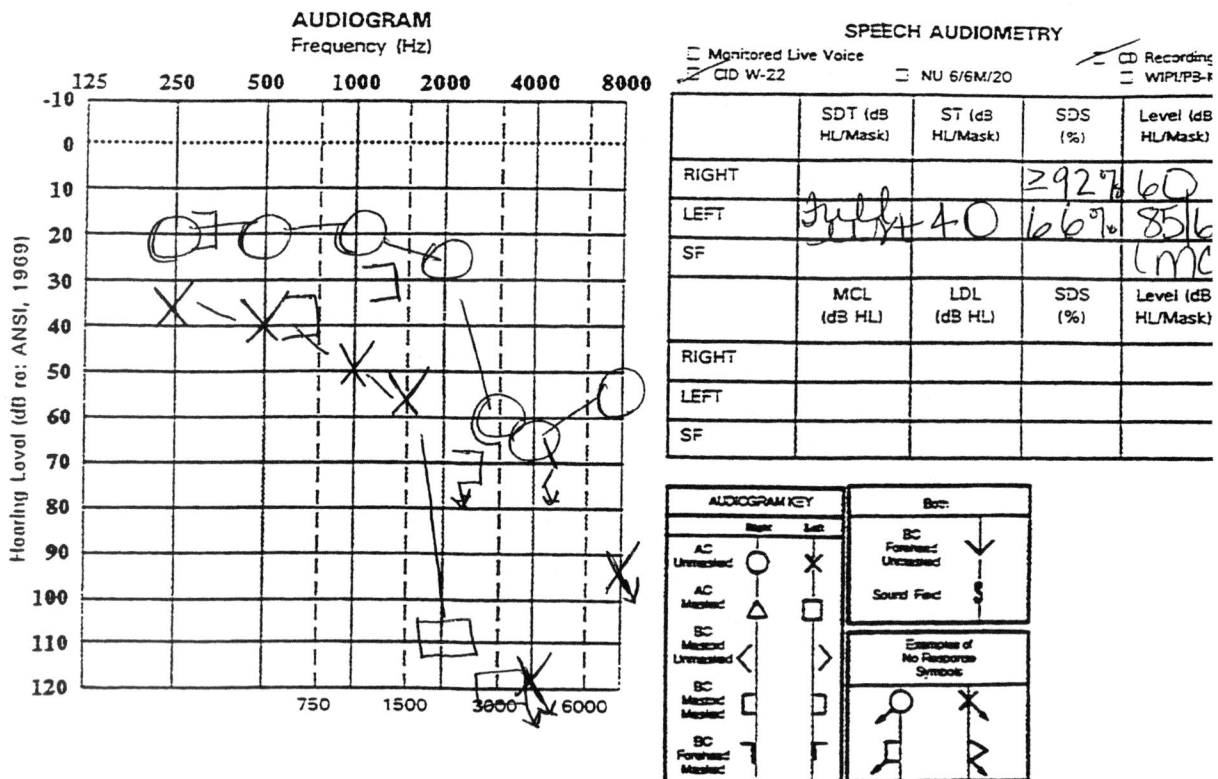

Figure 133.7 Postoperative audiometric findings for patient in Figure 133.5. *SF*, sound field; *MCL*, most comfortable loudness; *LDL*, loudness discomfort level; *SDS*, speech discrimination score; *SDT*, speech-detection threshold; *AC*, air conduction; *BC*, bone conduction; *ST*, spondee threshold.

a significantly improved outcome for those in the monitored group (35). The use of ECochG as the sole monitoring means in vestibular schwannoma resection has been reported (14), but because of advancements in other techniques, such reports have become less common in recent years. Because of the limitations of ECochG in detecting certain types of lesions, ECochG may be a useful adjunct to other monitoring techniques that provide a broader picture of hearing pathways (9,40,46).

Direct eighth nerve monitoring has recently emerged as perhaps the most useful technique, assisting in the surgical dissection and providing a reasonably accurate gauge of postoperative hearing (47). The information provided by DENM is presented in real time, allowing the surgeon to correct for the offending maneuver. Potential difficulties with securing the electrode have largely been overcome utilizing a variety of techniques (27,48). The placement of an electrode can be challenging, if not infeasible, however, when applied to tumors with cerebellopontine angle involvement (31).

Most recent studies that have evaluated DENM compared to other monitoring techniques have concluded that DENM offered superior monitoring and improved outcomes (14,29,31). Perhaps the most convincing of these studies compared 22 ABR-monitored patients with 44 DENM-monitored patients and demonstrated a statistically significant improvement in hearing preservation

rates (defined as preservation of any retained hearing) in those monitored with DENM. When comparing the preservation of serviceable hearing, the results did not achieve statistical significance, but the trend pointed toward DENM (27% for ABR, 43% for DENM). DENM has also been shown to be a sensitive prognostic tool. Preservation of the CNAP has been associated with hearing preservation in 78% of patients (48); conversely, lack of an action potential response at the completion of the procedure carries a very poor prognosis for postoperative hearing preservation (9,14,48).

Intraoperative direct eighth nerve action potential monitoring has been shown to provide better postoperative auditory function compared to patients monitored with ABR (29,31,49) or ECochG (10,48). The technical difficulty of placing and operating around electrodes, as well as the limited space available in the setting of large tumors, continue to limit the acceptance of direct auditory AP monitoring (5).

Combined Approaches and Horizons

Because individual cochlear nerve–monitoring modalities have limitations and weaknesses in their clinical applications, some surgeons have combined various modalities. Combinations of near- and far-field techniques help create a complete picture of the auditory system, beginning with the cochlea and the distal eighth nerve and including the brainstem and higher centers. Some investigators have described the simultaneous use of ABR and ECochG in determining the site and origin of detected changes in the auditory system, whereas others advocate ABR and CNAP monitoring (9,19).

When monitoring patients undergoing acoustic neuroma removal with both ABR and ECochG monitoring, Schalke and colleagues reported an overall hearing preservation rate of 51% (50). The loss of ECochG signal in this study indicated postoperative deafness (26/26 patients). However, 25% of patients with an absent postoperative ABR, but preserved ECochG, demonstrated serviceable postoperative hearing. The use of ABR combined with CNAP has been evaluated by many groups, and very good rates of hearing preservation have been documented (29,48,51). The utility of ABR in cases monitored with CNAP has been called into question, however, as one study demonstrated no advantage for patients monitored with ABR and CNAP compared to CNAP alone (48).

Rapid feedback and improved sensitivity of the more recently developed techniques have improved the clinical applications of this technology, but all responses must be critically viewed in relation to the surgical procedure. Table 133.2 depicts pertinent data on each method of eighth nerve monitoring. Eighth nerve monitoring cannot serve as a replacement for preoperative planning, meticulous surgical technique, and a detailed knowledge of regional anatomy.

Despite the difficulties and weaknesses of intraoperative auditory monitoring in otologic and neurotologic procedures, expanding technological frontiers, including distortion product otoacoustic emissions, have continued to increase the use of eighth nerve monitoring. Otoacoustic emissions have been investigated as potential intraoperative monitors of the auditory system, with promising results, primarily because of their exquisite sensitivity to changes in cochlear blood flow (52,53). Recent studies have confirmed the potential utility of this technique (54), but further evaluation is required to assess its impact on outcomes. Although the future appears bright for eighth nerve monitoring, it still trails facial nerve monitoring in applications and acceptance.

INTRAOPERATIVE FACIAL NERVE MONITORING

Facial nerve injury with resultant paresis or paralysis is a devastating complication of otologic surgery. Morbidity from this injury depends on the site of the injury as well as the degree of injury to the facial nerve. The degree of injury may range from a mild, partial paresis of brief duration, to permanent injuries with significant sequela. Temporary or partial paralysis may result in long-term cosmetic deformities, including synkinesis, atrophy, or bothersome facial twitching. Permanent facial paralysis may result in extensive cosmetic deformity or severe functional deficits, leading to oral incompetence and, in extreme cases, corneal injuries and blindness. Facial nerve injury is the most feared complication of otologic surgery and the second most common reason for malpractice litigation in otolaryngology (55).

Facial nerve injury can occur during any otologic or neurotologic procedure, but certain procedures such as acoustic neuroma excision, revision mastoid surgery, and repair of congenital malformations carry a relatively greater risk. Although most otolaryngologists are familiar with normal facial nerve anatomy, the nerve may be altered in its course or obscured by tumor, fibrosis, cholesteatoma, granulation tissue, bleeding, and even spinal fluid. The incidence of facial nerve paralysis resulting from otologic and neurotologic procedures has declined over the past few decades, likely because of the advent of the operative microscope, high-speed surgical drill, advanced microsurgical techniques, and intraoperative facial nerve monitoring (IOFNM). Prior to these advances, the incidence of facial nerve paralysis following mastoid surgery was as high as 15% (56). An estimate reported by Wiet suggests that the incidence of facial nerve injury

TABLE 133.2

INTRAOPERATIVE AUDITORY EVOKED POTENTIAL RECORDING OPTIONS

Options	Amplitude (μV)	No. of Sweeps	Time (s) @20/s
Surface-recorded ABR	0.1–0.5	500–1,500	25–75
ET-ECochG	0.3–1.0	250–1,200	12–60
TT-ECochG	5–15	40–100	2–5
Direct extradural	10–20	5–15	<1
Direct ANCAP	15–30	1–5	<1

ABR, auditory brainstem response; ET, extratympanic; ECochG, electrocochleography; TT, transtympanic; ANCAP, auditory nerve compound action potential.

ranges from 0.6% to 3.6% of all otologic cases, and 4% to 10% of revision cases (55). Another, more recent, review found an incidence of 1.7% in 1,024 consecutive mastoidectomies (57).

The importance of facial nerve monitoring during otologic and neurotologic surgery extends beyond merely avoiding untoward outcomes. Because of its intricate involvement with the structures of the temporal bone, the facial nerve often serves as an invaluable landmark in performing certain operations. Identification of the facial nerve promotes orientation in the complex three-dimensional anatomy of the temporal bone and comprises an essential step in procedures such as vestibular nerve section.

Facial Nerve Injury

There are many mechanisms by which the facial nerve can be injured during otologic and neurotologic surgery. Possible sources of trauma are listed in Table 133.3.

The facial nerve is potentially at risk for injury during any otologic and neurotologic procedure. Resection of acoustic neuromas places the facial nerve at the greatest risk, primarily because of the limited access to the intracranial facial nerve, the narrow confines of the internal auditory canal, the absence of a fibrous protective layer of epineurium, and the tendency for the tumor to splay the nerve fibers. Most facial nerve injuries during resection of acoustic neuromas occur medial to the porus acousticus at the mid-cerebellopontine angle, where it may be injured from surgical dissection or compression by the mass (58).

Excluding acoustic neuroma surgery, the most common site of iatrogenic injury occurs in the lower tympanic segment, followed by the mastoid segment. During otologic surgery, the tympanic segment, mastoid segment, and second genu are most easily injured (59). In a review of the experience at the House Ear Clinic, 57% of the iatrogenic facial nerve injuries occurred during mastoidectomy, with or without tympanoplasty. Of note, 14% of the patients studied sustained an injury to the facial nerve during tympanoplasty, and an additional 14% were injured during the

removal of bony exostoses from the ear canal (60). Therefore, caution must be exercised in all otologic and neurotologic procedures to minimize the chance of inadvertent injury to the facial nerve. Intraoperative facial nerve monitoring serves as a useful adjunct to a detailed knowledge of normal and variant temporal bone anatomy, careful preoperative planning, and meticulous surgical technique.

History

The first reported case of facial nerve monitoring during a neurotologic procedure was by Krause in 1898, who noted that electrical stimulation, or "unipolar faradic irritation," of the nerve resulted in facial movement (61). Throughout the first half of the twentieth century, other surgeons used similar techniques, employing either direct observation of the facial muscles or having an assistant manually palpate the face during dissection or electrical stimulation. In 1965, Jako developed a photoelectric sensing device that detected light transmission through the cheek when placed inside the mouth, activating an audible signal and further refining intraoperative facial nerve monitoring (62). Some surgeons went as far as securing bells to the faces of their patients in the hopes that facial movement would produce an audible alert (63). Hampered by poor sensitivity and reliability, few of the early devices gained widespread acceptance.

Electromyography (EMG) was first employed as a method of facial nerve monitoring by Delgado et al. in 1979. Intraoperative stimulation of the nerve triggered responses that were detected by surface electrodes and displayed on an oscilloscope (64). In an attempt to improve recognition of facial nerve stimulation, Sugita and Kobayashi (65) devised a method to transduce facial movement to an auditory signal that could be heard by the surgeon and operating room personnel. In 1984, Moller and Jannetta (66) combined EMG, a constant voltage stimulator, and auditory signal in IOFNM. Other innovative pioneers such as Silverstein, Nadol, Prass, Wiet, Kartush, and Brackmann contributed to the expansion of facial nerve monitoring technology by incorporating useful modifications to existing systems (67–71). The addition of combined visual and auditory signals to represent facial nerve stimulation, insulated stimulator probes, and insulated burrs and microinstruments has not only increased the utility of facial nerve monitoring, but also simplified the practical application of such technologies.

Facial Nerve Monitoring Systems

Several types of facial nerve monitors are currently available. Most of these systems monitor facial nerve integrity by detecting facial muscle contractions. Some systems utilize mechanical pressure sensors to detect facial muscle activity resulting from manipulation, trauma, or directed stimulation of the nerve with a specially designed probe;

TABLE 133.3

TYPES OF FACIAL NERVE INJURY

Transection
Direct trauma from surgical dissection
Direct trauma from surgical drill
Stretch
Compression
Thermal damage from drilling, cautery, laser, irrigation
Vascular compromise
Direct or indirect injury from the ultrasonic aspirator
Edema of the nerve in the fallopian canal from surgical dissection

TABLE 133.4
OBJECTIVES OF INTRAOPERATIVE FACIAL NERVE MONITORING

Early identification of the facial nerve in the temporal bone, internal auditory canal, cerebellopontine angle, or extratemporal portion during surgical dissection

Differentiation of the facial nerve from other structures in the surgical field, such as tumor, granulation tissue, or fibrosis

Differentiation of the facial nerve from other nerves in the cerebellopontine angle (trigeminal, cochlear, superior, and inferior vestibular nerves)

Rapid notification of the surgeon about trauma or pending trauma to the nerve

Reduction of trauma to the nerve during dissection of acoustic neuroma or cholesteatoma, as well as during procedures that require transposition or rerouting of the nerve

Early warning to the surgeon of an aberrant course of the nerve, or of unsuspected dehiscence of the nerve

Evaluation of nerve integrity at the completion of the procedure and prediction of postoperative function

Efficient identification of the site and degree of neural degeneration in patients undergoing facial nerve exploration for mass or paralysis[a]

[a]Silverstein H, Smouha EE, Jones R. Routine intraoperative facial nerve monitoring during otologic surgery. *Am J Otol* 1988;9:269–275.

others rely on videoanalysis of facial movements (71,72). Still others examine facial nerve action potentials, recorded either in an orthodromic (proximal to distal) or antidromic (distal to proximal) manner. Currently, the most common method of IOFNM measures EMG potentials. By monitoring the electrical activity of the target muscle, EMG systems reflect the activity and integrity of the innervating nerve (56). Although EMG systems have been shown to be more sensitive to facial nerve stimulation than movement sensors, a role still exists for mechanical–pressure sensing monitors in routine otologic cases (73). Videoanalysis, though not as sensitive as EMG, also remains an area of active research (72,74). Regardless of the system used, intraoperative monitoring systems should meet certain criteria (Table 133.1) and assist in performing certain tasks (Table 133.4) (29).

Electromyography and Evoked Electromyography

An EMG is performed by placing a pair of needle electrodes into a target muscle of the monitored nerve. In the case of IOFNM, the facial musculature is monitored, typically both the orbicularis oculi and the orbicularis oris muscles in the two-channel setup; a third channel placed in the contralateral face or the trapezius muscle may be used as a reference electrode. The potential difference between each electrode pair is subsequently amplified and displayed on an oscilloscope. Electrical activity of the muscle will appear as biphasic waveforms on the oscilloscope tracing. The motor unit potential reflects the electrical response of a single muscle fiber to a single efferent nerve fiber. When the response of an entire muscle group to an efferent motor nerve is considered, it is termed the collective action potential (CAP) or the compound muscle action potential (CMAP). Changes in neural activity may occur during operative dissection near the facial nerve and

during manipulation of the nerve, altering the baseline neural activity and propagating compound action potentials that appear as deflections on the oscilloscope (58).

Electromyographic activity appears in four primary forms: random muscle activity, a pulsed response coinciding with electrical stimulation, repetitive (train) activity, and nonrepetitive (burst, neurotonic discharge) activity (73). Repetitive EMG activity manifests as multiple responses from multiple motor units following a single stimulus. Such repetitive activity occurs following stretch injury or transmitted thermal injury to the nerve, actions that precipitate prolonged depolarization of the facial nerve beyond its threshold for generating an action potential. In this setting, the nerve will continue to fire until repolarization occurs or nerve activation can no longer be sustained. Repetitive activity, or train activity, typically does not occur until several seconds or minutes have passed following the initial event, although it may indicate complete or ongoing damage to the nerve. Conversely, nonrepetitive EMG activity closely follows direct mechanical or electrical stimulation, making it more helpful to otologic and neurotologic surgeons in locating and identifying the facial nerve (5). Although quite effective in identifying the facial nerve and alerting operating room personnel to the potential of nerve injury, no reliable correlation has been established between the magnitude or duration of the EMG response and the presence, if any, of facial nerve injury. Similarly, a normal baseline EMG tracing may signify the absence of trauma to the nerve or an injured nerve unable to respond to noxious stimuli (75). With this in mind, EMG tracings should continuously be viewed in the context of the surgical procedure.

Facial nerve monitoring systems may be enhanced by the addition of stimulation probes that can assist in nerve identification and, ideally, preservation. Stimulation of the facial nerve can occur directly with the use of the stimulus

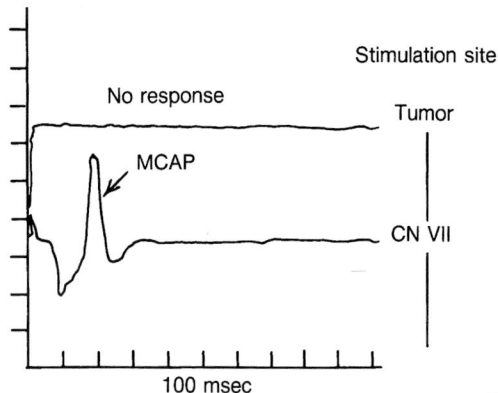

Figure 133.8 Intraoperative recordings of evoked electromyography of the facial nerve in response to stimulation of the seventh cranial nerve and tumor.

probe or indirectly as a result of surgical manipulation. Stimulation probes deliver a stimulus of preset intensity and pulse duration to the facial nerve and are designed to function in a constantly changing surgical environment. The effects of bleeding or accumulation of other fluids such as irrigation, perilymph, endolymph, and cerebrospinal fluid may be minimized by insulating the probe flush to the tip (75). The stimulus intensity level is chosen to give the maximum neuromuscular response with the least amount of delivered current. When the nerve is directly stimulated by the probe via a depolarizing current, the resulting compound action potential of the facial muscle is recorded by EMG, identifying the location of the facial nerve (Fig. 133.8). To achieve this aim, either monopolar or bipolar stimulating probes may be used.

Bipolar probes offer the advantage of being more selective by stimulating a smaller region of the nerve, allowing more precise localization. Unfortunately, bipolar stimulation depends on appropriate alignment of the bipolar tip in contact with the nerve. Such precise orientation is difficult, if not impossible, to achieve in the tight confines of the posterior fossa or on a small exposed area of the intratemporal segment of the facial nerve. Despite the theoretical advantages, practical application of bipolar stimulators in otologic and neurotologic surgery has been limited (3,58).

Because the selectivity offered by the bipolar stimulator is less an issue in surgical fields containing one, or few, nerves of interest, monopolar stimulators are more widely used in facial nerve monitoring. When stimulus intensity approximates the nerve threshold level, a monopolar electrode can achieve spatial orientation of less than 1 mm. Several methods of monopolar stimulation have been developed. A thin, malleable probe that has been insulated to the tip and looks much like an unsharpened pencil has been fashioned by Prass and Luders. This design allows the probe to deliver a stimulus to the tissue in question with minimal risk of collateral spread (76,77). Yingling and Gardi (3) developed a probe with a ball electrode capping an insulated, flexible platinum-iridium tip, allowing for

stimulation of the nerve in obscured areas where the flush tip may not be able to gain sufficient contact with the nerve. Kartush (78) devised a set of dissecting instruments that allow for simultaneous operating in the surgical field and stimulation of the facial nerve. By applying continuous electrical current to the bur and insulated microsurgical instruments, Silverstein (71) has further advanced the armamentarium of intraoperative facial nerve monitoring.

Stimulating probes may be either constant current or constant voltage systems. Bleeding, soft tissue, tumor, cholesteatoma, and spinal fluid may shunt current from the stimulus probe away from the nerve, creating variations in electrode impedance. To continue to depolarize the nerve, the constant current stimulator must be increased to higher levels in the face of increased resistance. Potential damage to the nerve may occur by stimulating the nerve with a constant current device in a changing operative environment when suctioning or control of bleeding eliminates the resistance of the fluid because a greater current than intended may be delivered to the nerve. On the other hand, constant voltage systems deliver current based on the intrinsic resistance of the nerve according to Ohm's law, adjusting current accordingly and limiting the effect of shunting on these systems. Although the total current changes as the operative milieu changes, the current delivered to the nerve remains more stable in constant voltage systems (3). Despite the theoretical differences in the two systems, no specific clinical advantage of either system has been found (76).

Direct Facial Nerve Monitoring

In addition to EMG monitoring of compound action potentials resulting from facial nerve stimulation, techniques for direct monitoring of neural transmission exist. Unlike EMG, direct monitoring systems follow compound nerve action potentials (CNAPs) as they progress down the nerve itself. Antidromic, or distal-to-proximal, potentials may also be monitored, allowing real-time detection of facial nerve injury or conduction blockade (79,80). Direct monitoring does, however, require the attachment of electrodes to the nerve directly, a technically challenging and potentially deleterious activity. Further, direct monitoring of CNAPs is limited by the smaller field potentials created by depolarization of nerve fibers, resulting in diminished sensitivity.

Anesthesia and Facial Nerve Monitoring

In the course of routine anesthesia, anesthesiologists commonly use muscle end plate blocking agents. To block postsynaptic nicotinic receptors, these agents act as antagonists (nondepolarizing) or agonists (depolarizing) at the end plate receptor. Nondepolarizing agents may be short acting or long acting. Atracurium, vecuronium, and mivacurium typically induce paralysis for up to 30 minutes, whereas pancuronium and tubocurarine may last up to one hour. Meanwhile, succinylcholine, the most common depolarizing agent, is extremely short acting, exerting its effects for 5 to 10 minutes. Paralysis that results from the use of these agents interferes with the recording of EMG potentials during IOFNM. Therefore, nondepolarizing agents are typically contraindicated in cases in which intraoperative facial nerve monitoring is planned, with the exception of succinylcholine for induction, because of its short duration of effect. If facial nerve action potentials, either orthodromic or antidromic, will be monitored, however, such neuromuscular blocking agents may be used.

At our institution, patients who are to undergo intraoperative facial nerve monitoring are intubated with a short-acting muscle relaxant, typically succinylcholine. This short-acting agent has a plasma half-life of 3.5 minutes and allows complete recovery from neuromuscular blockade within 15 minutes. The time period in which the facial muscles are paralyzed is generally insignificant in otologic cases, as it occurs during positioning, prepping, and routine exposure, when the facial nerve generally is not at risk. After the effects of the muscle paralysis have dissipated, anesthesia is maintained with a combination of inhalational or intravenous agents.

Local anesthesia can also impair the use of facial nerve monitoring. At The Otology Group of Vanderbilt, we routinely use 2% lidocaine with epinephrine at the beginning of the procedure, both at the site of the incision and in the ear canal when indicated. The advantages of this injection are improved hemostasis and analgesia, possibly limiting the amount of narcotic analgesia required for patient comfort. Care is taken during the injection of the local anesthetic to avoid potential paralysis of the facial nerve that would interfere with the facial nerve monitoring. The surgeon's index finger is placed on the mastoid tip during injection to avoid deep injection of lidocaine near the stylomastoid foramen. Care is also taken to not overaggressively inject the ear canal, especially in the posterior–inferior aspect. No anterior injections are made or required. Many surgeons have encountered the unnerving transient postoperative facial paralysis that resolves within several hours and can be attributed to the activity of local anesthetic (81).

We have utilized this method of anesthesia with great success in operations in which IOFNM is used. We do not use partial muscle paralysis during monitored cases at our institution. Because a partially paralyzed muscle fatigues rapidly, multiple successive stimuli may lead to progressively smaller evoked EMG amplitudes, causing potential problems when using the stimulus probe, as well as diminished sensitivity of the continuous EMG monitor. Partial paralysis monitored by nerve "twitches" is unnecessary during otologic and neurotologic surgery.

Indications for Intraoperative Facial Nerve Monitoring

A list of surgical procedures that should be considered for intraoperative facial nerve monitoring can be found in

TABLE 133.5

POTENTIAL INDICATIONS FOR INTRAOPERATIVE FACIAL NERVE MONITORING

Acoustic neuroma and tumors of the cerebellopontine angle
Vestibular nerve section
Repair of congenital aural atresia
Skull base surgery
Microvascular decompression of the fifth, seventh, and eighth cranial nerves
Cochlear implantation
Labyrinthectomy
Endolymphatic sac surgery
Facial nerve decompression
Mastoidectomy
Tympanoplasty
Canalplasty
Stapedectomy
Parotidectomy
Excision of glomus tumors

Table 133.5. We have applied the routine use of the facial nerve monitor in all otologic and neurotologic cases, as the facial nerve is potentially at risk in all such situations. In addition, some authors have advocated the use of IOFNM when residents are involved in otologic surgery (82). A recent survey of 223 American otolaryngologists showed that 66% use IOFNM at least some of the time for otologic procedures (chronic ear surgery, or stapedectomy) (83).

The use of IOFNM in acoustic neuroma removal is routine at many institutions and should be employed when possible (84). In an impressive study, Hammerschlag and Cohen (85) reported a significant and substantial reduction (14.5% to 3.6%) in the frequency of facial nerve paralysis following the implementation of monitoring in cerebellopontine angle surgery. Though the benefits of IOFNM for acoustic neuroma surgery and posterior fossa surgery have been established, the role of monitoring in routine otologic procedures is less well defined. As recent surveys have demonstrated, the use of monitoring in such cases is not universal. In his survey, Greenberg et al. (83) found that 46% of surgeons never use facial nerve monitoring for mastoidectomy or stapedectomy. A study of surgeons in the United Kingdom similarly found that a substantial percentage of surgeons never use monitoring for mastoidectomy (38%) or stapedectomy (85%) (86). The question as to whether IOFNM should be employed in "routine" otologic cases has been raised. The fear that surgeons may gain a false confidence in their skills and knowledge based on their use of intraoperative facial nerve monitors reflects a broader concern from many in the otolaryngology community that over-reliance on this technology could, in fact, lead to iatrogenic facial nerve injuries, particularly in situations when the monitor fails to recognize the nerve. In addition, there has been some reluctance in the otolaryngology community to declare IOFNM as the standard of care in otologic surgery. At the time of this writing, the decision to utilize IOFNM for otologic surgery remains at the discretion of the surgeon (87,88).

The use of the facial nerve monitor can never take the place of planning, experience, and a thorough knowledge of the anatomy of the temporal bone and posterior fossa. Several general principles regarding the facial nerve during otologic and neurotologic surgery should be employed:

1. Obtain and maintain thorough knowledge of the ear, temporal bone, and posterior fossa. Temporal bone lab dissection is essential in gaining this knowledge and expertise. Understand the three-dimensional anatomy of the facial nerve in the temporal bone. Appropriate courses are available throughout the United States for practicing physicians if they have no routine access to a formal temporal bone lab.
2. Treat the facial nerve as if it is dehiscent until proven otherwise, especially in the tympanic segment, superior to the oval window.
3. Expect any type of anatomic variation of the facial nerve, especially in revision cases.
4. Use meticulous surgical technique at all times.
5. Always be well prepared—identify preoperatively cases in which the facial nerve may be at greater risk (i.e., congenital atresia).
6. Routinely examine the monitoring system to ensure that all parts are in working order, and understand the physiologic basis of your particular system.

Benefits and Applications

Numerous studies support the use of intraoperative facial nerve monitoring in performing acoustic neuroma and skull base surgery, but as has been suggested, the utility of this technology extends beyond the internal auditory canal and cerebellopontine angle. Facial nerve monitoring has been reported as beneficial in nearly all surgical procedures that place the facial nerve at risk. The benefits of such adaptations have been well documented.

Removal of Acoustic Neuromas and Tumors of the Cerebellopontine Angle
The benefits of IOFNM in acoustic neuroma surgery have been clearly established. Intraoperative facial nerve monitoring allows identification of the nerve in the internal auditory canal or cerebellopontine angle before the nerve is clearly visualized through the use of stimulating probes or stimulating microsurgical instruments; similar techniques allow mapping of the course of the facial nerve during dissection. Based on feedback provided by the monitoring system, the surgeon is able to adjust the microsurgical technique to minimize injury or trauma to the nerve. Since the advent of IOFNM, several reports have extolled the advantages of facial nerve monitoring in acoustic tumor and CPA surgery, each citing improved facial nerve outcome, espe-

cially in removing large tumors (85,89–96). By indicating trauma to the contents of the internal auditory canal, IOFNM may even improve hearing preservation (97).

Additionally, IOFNM may be used to predict postoperative facial nerve function (98–100). Low-level stimulation of the facial nerve with either constant current or constant voltage probes should produce contraction of the facial musculature, if the nerve is intact. Measuring the sustained ongoing EMG activity as well as the magnitude of muscle contraction following stimulation has been shown to predict facial nerve function following tumor removal in certain patients (101). Similarly, intraoperative facial nerve stimulation–current threshold determination can be useful in predicting the ultimate facial nerve outcome, with lower stimulating thresholds reflecting a better facial nerve result (102,103). Proximal absolute EMG amplitudes, as well as the proximal-to-distal compound muscle action potential ratios, may also be predictive of facial nerve function in the immediate postoperative period (104,105). Caution must be exercised, however, in relying solely on the prognostic value of IOFNM in cases of postoperative weakness or paralysis, for patients with poor initial results and less-than-ideal stimulation parameters may eventually manifest excellent recovery of facial nerve function (106). In addition to surgical manipulation, facial nerve outcomes depend on the preoperative function, the size of the tumor, its location, the adherence of the nerve to the tumor, the extent of facial nerve compression, and the degree of vascular compromise present.

Posterior Fossa, Middle Fossa, and Skull Base Procedures
Vestibular nerve section, microvascular decompression of the fifth, seventh, and eighth cranial nerves, and lateral skull base surgery comprise additional areas in which IOFNM is beneficial. Extrapolating from the benefits of identification and limited damage offered by IOFNM, Moller and Jannetta described a method of microvascular decompression of the facial nerve for hemifacial spasm that utilizes the monitoring system. The details of this procedure may be found elsewhere, but simply stated, the ongoing presence of abnormal responses to facial nerve stimulation indicates continued compromise of the nerve. Decompression, therefore, is continued until the abnormal responses abate, indicating removal of the offending vessel from the nerve (107,108). Facial nerve monitoring promotes improved identification of the offending vessel, decreasing the need for re-exploration. In addition, IOFNM has been shown to improve facial nerve function following the infratemporal fossa approach for extirpation of lesions of the lateral skull base (109). New horizons in IOFNM for posterior and middle cranial procedures include resection of arteriovenous malformations using EMG techniques for mapping cranial nerve nuclei on the brainstem surface (110).

Chronic Ear Surgery and Revision Mastoid Surgery

Previous operations and alterations in normal landmarks increase the level of difficulty in removing extensive cholesteatoma and in revision mastoidectomy. Cholesteatoma, otorrhea, granulation tissue, fibrosis, and other disease processes that necessitate the procedure also can obscure the facial nerve and its landmarks. The facial nerve can be dehiscent in up to 57% of patients without cholesteatoma or previous operations (111). Exposure of the nerve during prior operations or from erosion of the fallopian canal by cholesteatoma further heightens the chances of encountering an exposed facial nerve. Intraoperative facial nerve monitoring will alert the surgeon to the presence of dehiscent nerve segments and aid in mapping the nerve to allow focused surgical dissection (112). Some studies suggest that monitoring in this setting will often detect a dehiscence before it is visualized (82). The success of monitoring in this setting has been documented, and one group has reported 1,200 consecutive cases without facial nerve injury (112). Additionally, a recent cost-effectiveness study concluded that using facial nerve monitoring in both primary and revision surgery was the most cost-effective approach (113). Our current practice is to utilize IOFNM monitoring on all cases for CSOM, including tympanoplasty and mastoidectomy, both initial and revision.

Stapedectomy

The most common site for a dehiscence in the fallopian canal occurs in the tympanic segment. The intimate relationship between the oval window and the tympanic segment of the facial nerve demands that extreme caution be exercised in performing a stapedectomy, as a dehiscent facial nerve may be present. Although this is not a contraindication to performing the operation, IOFNM may alert the surgeon to a dehiscent nerve during surgical dissection or laser stapedectomy. Injuries to the nerve during this procedure are rare, but they have been reported (111). Any steps taken to minimize this occurrence, including IOFNM, may be beneficial to the patient. Though the use of IOFNM for otologic surgery remains the choice of the individual surgeon, our current practice is to use facial nerve monitoring in all middle ear cases, routine or complicated, including stapedectomy.

Pediatric Otology

Iatrogenic facial nerve injury is equally, if not more, devastating in the pediatric population. Although the physical consequences of such an injury are the same, the emotional damage may be magnified in children. The facial nerve occupies a similar position in children as in adults, but some subtle differences related to development exist. Because the development of the facial nerve is intimately related to the development of the temporal bone, the facial nerve will not typically reach its adult course until mastoid development is complete (age 2). Facial nerve development is complete by approximately age 4 (114). Any abnormality of the inner, middle, or external ear, or of the mastoid, may presage an abnormal course for the facial nerve (115). Given the potential for an aberrant nerve course, combined with the long-term consequences of an iatrogenic injury, intraoperative facial nerve monitoring may be beneficial in any pediatric otologic procedure, excepting tympanostomy and tube placement.

Congenital Aural Atresia

Iatrogenic facial nerve injury comprises the greatest concern held by parents, patients, and surgeons regarding repair of congenital aural atresia. This risk, particularly in unilateral cases, dissuades many otologic surgeons from attempting these complicated operations. In these patients, the facial nerve is typically located more anterior and superior than in normal subjects. A wide range of other anomalies have also been reported (116). The incidence of iatrogenic facial paralysis during repair of congenital aural atresia ranges from 0% to 8% (117). Published reports primarily reflect the experience of the authors in their own series, though, most with extensive experience in this type of surgery. Jahrsdoerfer describes five instances where the facial nerve is vulnerable to injury during atresia surgery (Table 133.6). From his experience, the nerve is most likely to be injured during canalplasty when drilling through the inferoposterior aspect of the dense atretic bone (117). McKinnon and Jahrsdoerfer (118) report routinely employing IOFNM during these operations.

CONCLUSIONS

Intraoperative neurophysiologic monitoring has undergone significant improvements since its nascence in the twentieth century, but it remains a relatively new technology, with its applications still in the early stages of development. Preservation of hearing and facial nerve function is paramount in many otologic and neurotologic procedures. Though the preservation of hearing has yet to reach the same level of success achieved in preservation of the facial nerve function, the technology is ad-

---

TABLE 133.6

LIKELY TIMES FOR IATROGENIC INJURY DURING REPAIR OF ATRESIA

Skin incision
Dissection in the glenoid fossa
Canalplasty with drilling of atretic bone, especially posteroinferiorly
- Transposition of the nerve to improve access to the stapes footplate and oval window
Preauricular soft-tissue dissection for auricular repositioning during mastoidectomy

vancing, and further improvement seems likely. We have elucidated numerous procedures in which IOFNM, as well as eighth nerve monitoring, are advantageous. Despite the lack of a consensus opinion on the applications for intraoperative monitoring of the facial and auditory nerves, the procedures discussed here may be rendered more safe and efficient through the use of neurophysiologic monitoring, with improved chances of normal facial function and hearing. Nevertheless, intraoperative neurophysiologic monitoring should serve only as an adjunct to, not a replacement for, extensive preoperative planning, a thorough knowledge of temporal bone anatomy and its common variants, and meticulous surgical technique.

HIGHLIGHTS

- Auditory compromise during surgery can occur via direct injury to the cochlea, internal auditory artery, or the labyrinthine artery, or as a result of cochlear nerve stretching, compression, transection, or thermal injury.
- Electrocochleography (ECochG), auditory brainstem response testing (ABR), and direct eighth nerve monitoring (DENM) are all techniques used in intraoperative auditory system monitoring.
- ECochG best measures the integrity of cochlear blood supply.
- Direct eighth nerve action potential monitoring can be used in patients who have an absent preoperative ABR.
- ABR is a far-field technique, whereas ECochG and DENM are near-field techniques.
- Facial nerve injury may occur as a result of transection; direct trauma from drilling, using the ultrasonic aspirator, or dissection; stretch; compression; thermal injury from drilling, cautery, or the laser; vascular compromise; or edema of the nerve from regional dissection.
- The facial nerve may be monitored by mechanical-pressure sensing devices, electromyography (EMG), and direct monitoring of action potentials.
- Monitoring systems may be augmented by the addition of stimulating probes and dissecting instruments that help identify and map the facial nerve.
- IOFNM should assist the surgeon in identifying the facial nerve, rapidly notify the surgeon when trauma occurs, warn the surgeon as to an aberrant nerve course, evaluate neural integrity at the conclusion of the procedure, and help predict postoperative facial nerve function.
- Unless facial nerve action potentials comprise the sole source of IOFNM, avoid the use of nondepolarizing muscle relaxants during anesthesia.
- IOFNM has proven useful in improving facial nerve outcomes during removal of acoustic neuromas and tumors of the cerebellopontine angle, particularly in larger tumors.
- Additional applications of IOFNM include vestibular nerve section, skull base surgery, microvascular decompression, cochlear implantation, repair of congenital aural atresia, stapedectomy, and chronic ear surgery.

REFERENCES

1. Jewett DL, Williston JS. Auditory evoked far fields averaged from the scalp of humans. *Brain* 1971;94:681–696.
2. Levine RA, Montgomery WW, Ojemann RJ. Evoked potential detection of hearing loss during acoustic neuroma surgery. Abstract. *Neurology* 1978;28:339.
3. Yingling CD, Gardi JN. Intraoperative monitoring of facial and cochlear nerves during acoustic neuroma surgery. *Otolaryngol Clin North Am* 1992;25:413–448.
4. Kaylie DM, Gilbert E, Horgan MA, et al. Acoustic neuroma surgery outcomes. *Otol Neurotol* 2001;22:686–689.
5. Harper CM, Daube JR. Facial nerve electromyography and cranial nerve monitoring. *J Clin Neurophys* 1999;15:206–216.
6. Lang J. Anatomy of the brainstem and lower cranial nerves, vessels, and surrounding structures. *Am J Otol* 1985;6(suppl):1–19.
7. Colletti V, Fiorino FG, Mocella S, et al. ECoG, CNAP, and ABR monitoring during acoustic neuroma surgery. *Audiology* 1997;37:27–37.
8. Matthies C, Samii M. Management of vestibular schwannomas (acoustic neuromas): the value of neurophysiology for evaluation and prediction of auditory function in 420 cases. *Neurosurgery* 1997;40:919–929.
9. Zappia JJ, Wiet RJ, O'Connor CA, et al. Intraoperative monitoring in acoustic neuroma surgery. *Otolaryngol Head Neck Surg* 1996; 115:98–106.
10. Nadol JB Jr., Levine R, Ojemann RG, et al. Preservation of hearing in surgical removal of acoustic neuromas of the internal auditory canal and cerebellopontine angle. *Laryngoscope* 1987;97:1287–1294.
11. Moller AR. *Evoked potential intraoperative monitoring.* Baltimore: Williams and Wilkins, 1988.
12. Schmerber S, Lavielle JP, Dumas G, et al. Intraoperative auditory monitoring in vestibular schwannoma surgery: new trends. *Acta Otolaryngol* 2004;124:53–61.
13. Schramm J, Mokrusch T, Fahlbusch R, et al. Detailed analysis of intraoperative changes monitoring brainstem acoustic evoked potentials. *Neurosurgery* 1988;22:694–702.
14. Battista RA, Wiet RJ, Paauwe L. Evaluation of three intraoperative auditory monitoring techniques in acoustic neuroma surgery. *Am J Otol* 2000;21:244–248.
15. Roberson JB, Jackson LJ, McCauley JR. Acoustic neuroma surgery: absent ABR does not contraindicate attempted hearing preservation. *Laryngoscope* 1999;109:904–910.
16. Kileny PR, Niparko JK. Intraoperative monitoring of auditory and facial functions in neurotologic surgery. *Adv Otolaryngol Head Neck Surg* 1988;2:55–60.
17. Kaga K, Takiguchi T, Mayokai K, et al. Effects of deep hypothermia and circulatory arrest on the auditory brainstem responses. *Arch Otorhinolaryngol* 1979;225:199–205.
18. Manninen P, Lam A, Nicholas J. The effects of isoflurane and isoflurane-nitrous oxide anesthesia on brainstem auditory evoked potentials in humans. *Anesth Analg* 1985;64:43–47.
19. Prass RL, Kinney SE, Lüders H. Transtragal, transtympanic electrode placement for intraoperative electrocochleographic monitoring. *Otolaryngol Head Neck Surg* 1987;97:343–350.
20. Eggermont JJ. Electrocochleography. In: Keidel WD, Neff WD, eds. *Handbook of sensory physiology—Vol. V: Auditory system, Part 3: clinical and special topics.* Berlin: Springer-Verlag, 1976.
21. Wazen JJ. Intraoperative monitoring of auditory function: experimental observations and new applications. *Laryngoscope* 1994;104:446–455.
22. Silverstein H, McDaniel AB, Norrell H. Hearing preservation after acoustic neuroma surgery using intraoperative direct eighth cranial nerve monitoring. *Am J Otol* 1985;6(suppl):99–106.
23. Levine RA, Ojemann RG, Montgomery WW, et al. Monitoring auditory evoked potentials during acoustic neuroma surgery: insights into the mechanism of hearing loss. *Ann Otol Rhinol Laryngol* 1984;93:116–123.
24. Ohashi T, Ochi K, Kinoshita H, et al. Electrocochleogram after transaction of vestibulo-cochlear nerve in a patient with a large acoustic neurinoma. *Hearing Res* 2001;154:26–31.
25. Moller AR, Jannetta PJ. Compound action potentials recorded intracranially from the auditory nerve in man. *J Exp Neurol* 1981;74:862–874.

26. Moller AR. Monitoring auditory function during operations to remove acoustic tumors. *Am J Otol* 1996;17:452–460.

27. Cueva RA, Morris GF, Prioleau GR. Direct cochlear nerve monitoring: first report on a new atraumatic, self-retaining electrode. *Am J Otol* 1998; 19:202–207.

28. Nguyen BH, Javel E, Levine SC. Physiologic identification of eighth nerve subdivisions: direct recordings with bipolar and monopolar electrodes. *Am J Otol* 1999;20:522–534.

29. Colletti V, Fiorino FG. Advances in monitoring of seventh and eighth cranial nerve function during posterior fossa surgery. *Am J Otol* 1998;19:503–512.

30. Roberson J, Senne A, Brackmann D, et al. Direct cochlear nerve action potentials as an aid to hearing preservation in middle fossa acoustic neuroma resection. *Am J Otol* 1996;17:653–657.

31. Danner C, Mastrodimos B, Cueva RA. A comparison of direct eighth nerve monitoring and auditory brainstem response in hearing preservation surgery for vestibular schwannoma. *Otol Neurotol* 2004;28:826–832.

32. McDaniel AB, Silverstein H, Norrell H. Retrolabyrinthine vestibular neurectomy with and without monitoring of eighth nerve potentials. *Am J Otol* 1985;4(suppl):23–26.

33. Arenberg IK, Kabayashi H, Obert AD, et al. Intraoperative electrocochleography of endolymphatic hydrops surgery using clicks and tone bursts. *Acta Otolaryngol Suppl* 1993; 504: 58–67.

34. Brown CJ, Abbas PJ, Fryauf-Bertschy H, et al. Intraoperative and postoperative electrically evoked auditory brainstem responses in nucleus cochlear implant users: implications for the fitting process. *Ear Hearing* 1994;15:168–176.

35. Nedzelski JM, Chiang CM, Cashman MZ, et al. Hearing preservation in acoustic neuroma surgery: value of monitoring cochlear nerve action potentials. *Otolaryngol Head Neck Surg* 1994;111:703–709.

36. Sanna M, Kharis T, Russo A, et al. Hearing preservation surgery in vestibular schwannoma: The hidden truth. *Ann Otol Rhinol Laryngol* 2004;113:156–163.

37. Committee on Hearing and Equilibrium guidelines for the evaluation of hearing preservation in acoustic neuroma (vestibular schwannoma). American Academy of Otolaryngology—Head and Neck Surgery Foundation, Inc. *Otolaryngol Head Neck Surg* 1995;113:179–180.

38. Kanzaki J, Inoue Y, Ogawa K. The learning curve in post-operative hearing results in vestibular schwannoma surgery. *Auris Nasus Larynx* 2001;28:209–213.

39. Harper CM, Harner SG, Slavit DH, et al. Effect of BAER monitoring on hearing preservation during acoustic neuroma resection. *Neurology* 1992;42:1551–1553.

40. Ojemann RG, Levine RA, Montgomery WM, et al. Use of intraoperative auditory evoked potentials to preserve hearing in unilateral acoustic neuroma removal. *J Neurosurg* 1984;61:938–948.

41. Slavit DH, Harner SG, Harper M, et al. Auditory monitoring during acoustic neuroma removal. *Arch Otolaryngol Head Neck Surg* 1991;117:1153–1156.

42. Strauss C, Bischoff B, Neu M, et al. Vasoactive treatment for hearing preservation in acoustic neuroma surgery. *J Neurosurg* 2001;95:771–777.

43. Neu M, Strauss C, Romstock J, et al. The prognostic value of intraoperative BAEP patterns in acoustic neurinoma surgery. *Clin Neurophysiol* 1999;110:1935–1944.

44. Schwartz DM, Gennarelli TA. Delayed sensorineural hearing loss following uncomplicated neurovascular decompression of the trigeminal root entry zone. *Am J Otol* 1990;11:95–98.

45. Radtke RA, Erwin CW, Wilkins RH. Intraoperative brainstem auditory evoked potentials: significant decrease in postoperative morbidity. *Neurology* 1989;39:187–191.

46. Levine RA, Ojemann RG, Montgomery WW, et al. Monitoring auditory evoked potentials during acoustic neuroma surgery: insights into the mechanism of the hearing loss. *Ann Otol Rhinol Laryngol* 1984;93:116–120.

47. Stanton SG, Cashman MZ, Harrison RV, et al. Cochlear nerve action potentials during cerebellopontine angle surgery: relationship of latency, amplitude, and threshold measurements to hearing. *Ear Hearing* 1989;10:23–30.

48. Jackson LE, Roberson JB Jr. Acoustic neuroma surgery: use of cochlear nerve action potential monitoring for hearing preservation. *Am J Otol* 2000;21:249–259.

49. Kveton JF. The efficacy of brainstem auditory evoked potentials in acoustic tumor surgery. *Laryngoscope* 1990;100:1171–1173.

50. Schlake HP, Milewski C, Goldbrunner RH, et al. Combined intra-operative monitoring of hearing by means of auditory brainstem responses (ABR) and transtympanic electrocochleography (ECochG) during surgery of intra- and extrameatal acoustic neurinomas. *Acta Neurochir (Wien)* 2001;143:985–996.

51. Yamakami I, Oka N, Yamaura A. Intraoperative monitoring of cochlear nerve compound action potential in cerebellopontine angle tumour removal. *J Clin Neurosci* 2003;10(5):567–570.

52. Telischi FF, Widick MP, Lonsbury-Martin BL, et al. Monitoring cochlear function intraoperatively using distortion product otoacoustic emissions. *Am J Otol* 1995;16:597–608.

53. Telischi FF, Mom T, Agrama M, et al. Comparison of auditory-evoked brainstem response wave I to distortion-product otoacoustic emissions resulting from changes to inner ear blood flow. *Laryngoscope* 1999;109:186–191.

54. Morawski K, Namyslowski G, Lisowska G, et al. Intraoperative monitoring of cochlear function using distortion product otoacoustic emissions (DPOAEs) in patients with cerebellopontine angle tumors. *Otol Neurotol* 2004;25:818–825.

55. Wiet RJ. Iatrogenic facial paralysis. *Otolaryngol Clin North Am* 1982;15:773–781.

56. May M, Wiet RJ. Iatrogenic injury: Prevention and management. In: May M, ed. *The facial nerve.* New York: Thieme, 1986.

57. Nilssen E, Wormald P. Facial nerve palsy in mastoid surgery. *J Laryngol Otol* 1997;111:113–116.

58. Selesnick SH. Optimal stimulus duration for intraoperative facial nerve monitoring. *Laryngoscope* 1999;109:1376–1385.

59. Mancini F, Taibah AK, Falcioni M. Otitis media: surgical principles based on pathogenesis. *Otolaryngol Clin North Am* 1999;32(3):567–583.

60. Green JD Jr., Shelton C, Brackmann DE. Iatrogenic facial nerve injury during otologic surgery. *Laryngoscope* 1994;104:922–925.

61. Krause F. *Surgery of the brain and spinal cord,* Vol. II. New York: Rebman, 1912.

62. Jako GJ. Facial nerve monitor. *Trans Am Acad Ophthalmol Otolaryngol* 1965;69:340–343.

63. Williams JD, Lehman R. Bells against palsy. *Am J Otol* 1988;9:81–82.

64. Delgado TE, Buchheit SG, Rosenholtz HR. Intraoperative monitoring of facial muscle evoked responses obtained by intracranial stimulation of the facial nerve: A more accurate technique for facial nerve dissection. *Neurosurgery* 1979;4:418–421.

65. Sugita K, Kobayashi S. Technical and instrumental improvements in the surgical treatment of acoustic neuromas. *J Neurosurg* 1982;57:747–752.

66. Moller AR, Jannetta PJ. Preservation of facial function during removal of acoustic neuromas: use of monopolar constant-voltage stimulation and EMG. *J Neurosurgery* 1984;61:757–760.

67. Silverstein H, Rosenberg S. Intraoperative facial nerve monitoring. *Otolaryngol Clin North Am* 1991;24:709–725.

68. Metson R, Thornton A, Nadol JB, et al. A new design for intraoperative facial nerve monitoring. *Otolaryngol Head Neck Surg* 1988;98:258–261.

69. Prass R, Kinney SE, Hardy RW, et al. Acoustic (loudspeaker) facial electromyographic monitoring: part II—use of evoked EMG activity during acoustic neuroma resection. *Otolaryngol Head Neck Surg* 1987;97:541–551.

70. Kartush JM, Niparko J, Bledsoe S, et al. Intraoperative facial nerve monitoring: A comparison of stimulating electrodes. *Laryngoscope* 1985;95:1536–1540.

71. Silverstein H. Microsurgical instruments and nerve stimulator-monitor for retrolabyrinthine vestibular neurectomy. *Otolaryngol Head Neck Surg* 1986;94:409–411.

72. Filipo R, De Sata E, Bertoli GA. Intraoperative videomonitoring of the facial nerve. *Am J Otol* 2000;21:119–122.

73. Bendet E, Rosenberg SI, Willcox TO, et al. Intraoperative facial nerve monitoring: A comparison between electromyography and mechanical-pressure monitoring techniques. *Am J Otol* 1999;20:793–799.

74. Filipo R, Pichi B, Bertoli A, et al. Video-based system for intraoperative facial nerve monitoring: comparison with electromyography. *Otol Neurotol* 2002;23:594–597.

75. Prass RL. Iatrogenic facial nerve injury—the role of facial nerve monitoring. *Otolaryngol Clin North Am* 1996;29:265–275.

76. Prass R, Luders H. Constant current versus constant-voltage stimulation. *J Neurosurg* 1985;62:622–623.

77. Kartush JM, Niparko JK, Bledsoe SC, et al. Intraoperative facial nerve monitoring: a comparison of stimulating electrodes. *Laryngoscope* 1985;95:1536–1540.

78. Kartush JM. Electroneurography and intraoperative facial monitoring in contemporary neurotology. *Otolaryngol Head Neck Surg* 1989;101:496–503.

79. Richmond IL, Mahla M. Use of antidromic recording to monitor facial nerve function intraoperatively. *Neurosurgery* 1979;4:418–421.

80. Colletti V, Fiorino FS, Policante Z, et al. New perspectives in intraoperative facial nerve monitoring with antidromic potentials. *Am J Otol* 1997;18:249–251.

81. Silverstein H, Smouha EE, Jones R. Routine intraoperative facial nerve monitoring during otologic surgery. *Am J Otol* 1988;9:269–275.

82. Pensak ML, Willging JP, Keith RW. Intraoperative facial nerve monitoring in chronic ear surgery: a resident training experience. *Am J Otol* 1994;15:108–110.

83. Greenberg JS, Manolidis S, Stewart MG, et al. Facial nerve monitoring in chronic ear surgery: US practice patterns. *Otolaryngol Head Neck Surg* 2002;126:108–114.

84. National Institutes of Health. *Consensus statement: acoustic neuroma.* NIH Consensus Development Conference, Bethesda, MD, December 11–13, 1991.

85. Hammerschlag PE, Cohen NL. Intraoperative monitoring of facial nerve function in cerebellopontine angle surgery. *Otolaryngol Head Neck Surg* 1990;103:681–684.

86. Saravanappa N, Balfour A, Bowlder A. Use of laser, otoendoscopy and facial nerve monitoring in otological surgery: United Kingdom survey. *J Laryngol Otol* 2003;117:751–755.

87. Roland PS, Meyerhoff WL. Intraoperative electrophysiological monitoring of the facial nerve: is it standard of practice? *Am J Otol* 1994;15:267–270.

88. Silverstein H, Rosenberg SI, Wilcox TO Jr., et al. Letter to the editor. *Am J Otol* 1994;15:121–122.

89. Harner SG, Daube JR, Ebersold MJ, et al. Improved preservation of facial nerve function with the use of electrical monitoring during removal of acoustic neuromas. *Mayo Clin Proc* 1987;62:92–102.

90. Benecke J, Calder H-B, Chadwick G. Facial nerve monitoring during acoustic neuroma removal. *Laryngoscope* 1987;97:697–700.

91. Kwartler JA, Luxford WM, Atkins J, et al. Facial nerve monitoring in acoustic tumor surgery. *Otolaryngol Head Neck Surg* 1991;104:814–817.

92. Nissen AJ, Sikand A, Welsh JE, et al. A multifactorial analysis of facial nerve results in surgery for cerebellopontine angle tumors. *ENT—Ear Nose Throat J* 1997;76:37–40.

93. Harner SG, Daube JR, Beatty CW, et al. Intraoperative monitoring of the facial nerve. *Laryngoscope* 1988;98:209–212.

94. Uziel A, Benezech J, Frerebeau P. Intraoperative facial nerve monitoring in posterior fossa acoustic neuroma surgery. *Otolaryngol Head Neck Surg* 1993;108:126–134.

95. Silverstein H, Rosenberg S, Flanzer J, et al. Intraoperative facial nerve monitoring in acoustic neuroma surgery. *Am J Otol* 1993;14:524–532.

96. Kartush JM, Lundy LB. Facial nerve outcome in acoustic neuroma surgery. *Otolaryngol Clin North Am* 1992;25:623–647.

97. Kartush JM, LaRouere MJ, Graham MD. Intraoperative facial nerve monitoring during posterior skull base surgery. *Skull Base Surgery* 1991;1:85–92.

98. Magliulo G, Zardo F. Facial nerve function after cerebellopontine angle surgery and prognostic value of intraoperative facial nerve monitoring: a critical evaluation. *Am J Otolaryngol* 1998;19:102–106.

99. Berges C, Fraysse B, Yardeni E, et al. Intraoperative facial nerve monitoring in posterior fossa surgery: prognostic value. *Skull Base Surgery* 1993;3:214–216.

100. Zeitouni AG, Hammerschlag PE, Cohen NL. Prognostic significance of intraoperative facial nerve stimulus thresholds. *Am J Otol* 1997;18:494–497.

101. Beck DL, Atkins JS Jr., Benecke JE Jr., et al. Intraoperative facial nerve monitoring: Prognostic aspects during acoustic tumor removal. *Otolaryngol Head Neck Surg* 1991;104:780–782.

102. Silverstein H, Willcox TO Jr., Rosenberg SI, et al. Prediction of facial nerve function following acoustic neuroma resection using intraoperative facial nerve stimulation. *Laryngoscope* 1994;104:539–544.

103. Zeitouni AG, Hammerschlag PE, Cohen NL. Prognostic significance of intraoperative facial nerve stimulus thresholds. *Am J Otol* 1997;18:494–497.

104. Sobottka SB, Schackert G, May SA, et al. Intraoperative facial nerve monitoring predicts facial nerve outcome after resection of vestibular schwannoma. *Acta Neurochir (Wien)* 1998;140:235–243.

105. Goldbrunner RH, Schlake HP, Milewski C, et al. Quantitative parameters of intraoperative electromyography predict facial nerve outcomes for vestibular schwannoma surgery. *Neurosurgery* 2000;46:1140–1146.

106. Axon PR, Ramsden RT. Intraoperative electromyography for predicting facial function in vestibular schwannoma surgery. *Laryngoscope* 1999;109:922–926.

107. Moller AR, Jannetta P. Monitoring facial EMG during microvascular decompression operations for hemifacial spasm. *J Neurosurg* 1987;66:681.

108. Halnes S, Torres F. Intraoperative facial nerve monitoring during decompressive surgery for hemifacial spasm. *J Neurosurg* 1991;74:254.

109. Leonetti JP, Brackmann DE, Prass RL. Improved preservation of facial nerve function in the infratemporal fossa approach to the skull base. *Otolaryngol Head Neck Surg* 1989;101:74–78.

110. Chang SD, Lopez JR, Steinberg GK. Intraoperative electrical stimulation for identification of cranial nerve nuclei. *Muscle Nerve* 1999;22:1538–1543.

111. Welling DB, Glasscock ME, Gantz BJ. Avulsion of the anomalous facial nerve at stapedectomy. *Laryngoscope* 1992;102:729–733.

112. Olds MJ, Rowan PT, Isaacson JE, et al. Facial nerve monitoring among graduates of the Ear Research Foundation. *Am J Otol* 1997;18:507–511.

113. Wilson L, Lin E, Lalwani A. Cost-effectiveness of intraoperative facial nerve monitoring in middle ear or mastoid surgery. *Laryngoscope* 2003;113:1736–1745.

114. Schaitkin BM, Shapiro A, May M. Disorders of the facial nerve. In: Lalwani AK, Grundfast KM, eds. *Pediatric otology and neurotology.* Philadelphia: Lippincott-Raven, 1998: 457–475.

115. Jahrsdoerfer RA. The facial nerve in congenital middle ear malformations. *Laryngoscope* 1981;91:1217–1224.

116. Schuknecht HF. Congenital aural atresia. *Laryngoscope* 1989;99:908–917.

117. Jahrsdoerfer RA, Lambert PR. Facial nerve injury in congenital aural atresia surgery. *Am J Otol* 1998;19:283–287.

118. McKinnon BJ, Jahrsdoerfer RA. Congenital auricular atresia: update on options for intervention and timing of repair. *Otolaryngol Clin North Am* 2002;35:877–890.

Imaging Studies of the Temporal Bone

134

John A. Butman   *Nicholas J. Patronas*   *Hung Jeffrey Kim*

High-resolution computed tomography (CT) and magnetic resonance imaging (MRI) allow otolaryngologists and radiologists to examine the complex anatomy of the temporal bone in exquisite detail, and thereby reveal a broad spectrum of pathology. CT and MRI are complementary, as CT affords sharp submillimeter resolution of osseous structures, and MRI shows fluid and soft tissue components with comparable resolution. When imaging is performed for evaluation of hearing loss, choice of CT or MRI is primarily dependent on whether the hearing loss is conductive (CHL) or sensorineural (SNHL). CT is best suited for CHL, whereas MRI is best suited for the evaluation of retrocochlear SNHL. When the question is bone destruction from inflammation or metastasis, CT is the modality of choice. When the question is perineural invasion or intracranial extension of disease, MRI is the modality of choice. In complex cases, both CT and MRI may be necessary, and, in some instances, additional information may be gleaned by nuclear medicine studies [e.g. bone scintigraphy or positron emission tomography (PET)] or interventional cerebral angiography.

COMPUTED TOMOGRAPHY TECHNIQUE

CT is performed by rotating an X-ray source around the body and acquiring projections from multiple different angles (1). To generate a two-dimensional cross-sectional image, different reconstruction algorithms are used to estimate the density of the tissue that has been traversed by the X-ray beam, measured in Hounsfield Units (HU). On this scale, air is −1,000 HU, water is 0 HU, soft tissues are 10 to 100 HU, and cortical bone is typically greater than 1,000 HU. The high-resolution algorithm used for temporal bone imaging results in extremely sharp bone margins, allowing fractures, ossicular joints, and other fine details to be shown (Fig. 134.1), but it does make images much noisier, so that soft tissue contrast and enhancement may not be discernible (Fig. 134.2). The slice thickness of routine clinical temporal bone CT should range from 0.5 mm to 1.5 mm, and the field of view (FOV) should be 9 cm to 12 cm. CT window width must be large (~ 4,000 HU), so that texture of bone may be revealed.

The orbitomeatal line, extending from the inferior orbital rim to the external auditory canal, is used as a horizontal reference. Axial and coronal sections are acquired 30 degrees and 120 degrees above this line, respectively. Helical (or spiral) techniques performed with single or multislice scanners allow for overlapping slices to be reconstructed. Such scans allow for coronal reformations that may sometimes substitute for direct coronal acquisitions.

MAGNETIC RESONANCE IMAGING TECHNIQUE

MRI scanners detect signal emitted by the protons (hydrogen nuclei) of fat and water in the body following excitation with a radiofrequency pulse (2). The intensity of this signal is influenced by the local tissue environment, which determines the spin-lattice (T1) and spin-spin (T2) relaxation times. Adjusting the parameters of MRI pulse sequences allows either T1 or T2 relaxation to have a dominant effect on the MR signal, resulting in T1- or T2-weighted (T1W or T2W) images. On T2W images, fat and water are bright or

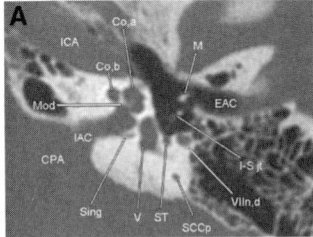 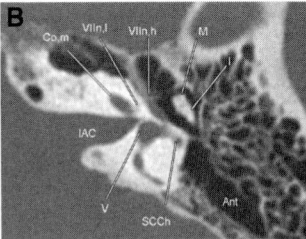 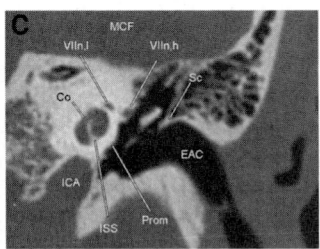 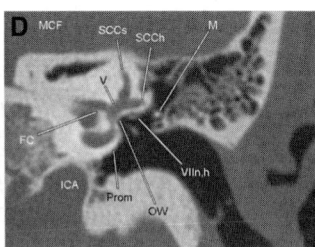

Figure 134.1   Normal computed tomographic (CT) temporal bone anatomy. Axial CT at the mid-cochlear level **(A)** and more superiorly at the horizontal semicircular canal (SCC) level **(B).** Coronal CT at the level of the cochlea **(C)** and more posteriorly at the vestibule **(D).** Ossicular chain: On axial CT **(A),** the manubrium of the malleus and long process of the incus appear as two dots. Both stapes crura can be seen. On more superior axial CT **(B),** the head of the malleus and the body of the incus appear as an "ice-cream cone," representing the "scoop" and the "cone," respectively. Facial nerve: On anterior coronal section **(C),** the labyrinthine and horizontal segments appear as a paired "snake eyes" structure. Note the thin plate of bone covering the horizontal segment **(D),** which may normally be dehiscent. It is identified just inferior to the horizontal SCC on coronal sections. The descending canal widens at the level of the sinus tympani as the canal is shared with the stapedius muscle **(A).** AICA, anterior inferior cerebellar artery; Ant, mastoid antrum; Co, Cochlea (a, apical, b, basal, m, middle turns); CoP, cochlear partition; CPA, cerebellopontine angle cistern; EAC, external auditory canal; FC, falciform crest; IAC, internal auditory canal; ICA, internal carotid artery; I, incus; I-S jt, incudostapedial joint; M, malleus; MCF, middle cranial fossa; Mod, modiolus; OW, oval window; Prom, promontory; Sc, scutum; ScV, scala vestibuli; ScT, scala tympani; SCC, semicircular canal (h, horizontal, p, posterior, s, superior); Sing, canal for singular nerve; ST, sinus tympani; V, vestibule; VA, vestibular aqueduct; VIIn, facial nerve VII (i, intracanalicular or meatal, d, descending or vertical, g, geniculate, h, horizontal or tympanic, l, labyrinthine).

"hyperintense." On T1W images, fat is bright, tissues are intermediate in signal, and water is dark or "hypointense."

Because the inner ear and internal auditory canal (IAC) are fluid-filled, high-resolution T2W images based on spin and gradient, echo techniques define these structures to best advantage (Fig. 134.3) (3). High-resolution spin-echo–based techniques include 2D and 3D fast spin echo (FSE) and fast recovery FSE. Gradient-echo–based techniques include 3D balanced fast-field echo (FFE), fast-imaging employing steady-state acquisition (FIESTA), true fast induction of steady-state precession (FISP), and constructive interference in the steady state (CISS). Although some of these techniques may be specific to certain scanner makes and models, all can produce high-resolution T2-weight-

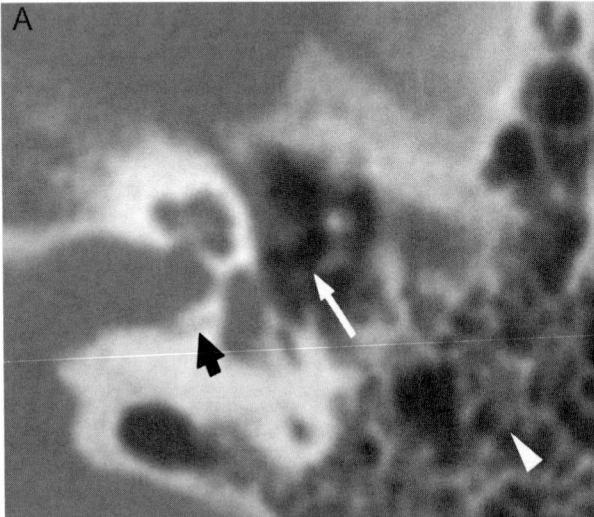 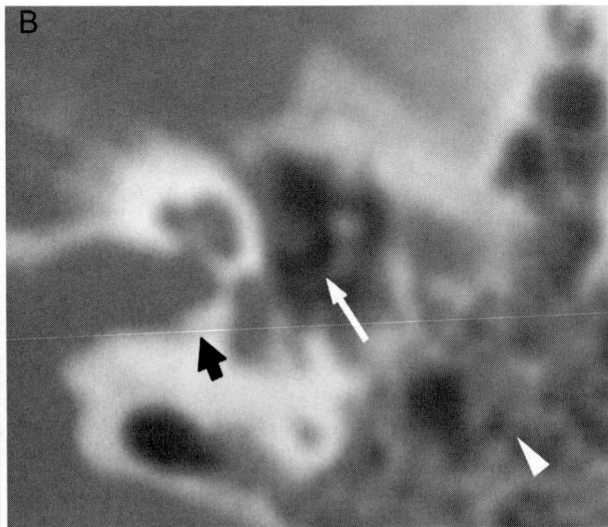

Figure 134.2   Temporal bone computed tomography (CT) scan requires high-resolution reconstruction kernels "bone algorithms" as well as "bone window" settings. Temporal bone CT was obtained with 1 mm collimation (slice thickness) and 12 cm FOV (field of view). The same CT raw data was processed with a "bone algorithm" to generate the image in **(A)** and a "soft tissue algorithm" to generate the image in **(B).** Both are displayed with "bone windows" (WL = 250, WW = 3,500). Note the marked difference in fine detail. Compare the appearance of the canal for the singular nerve (*black arrow*), the incudostapedial joint (*thin white arrow*), and mastoid septations (*white arrowhead*).

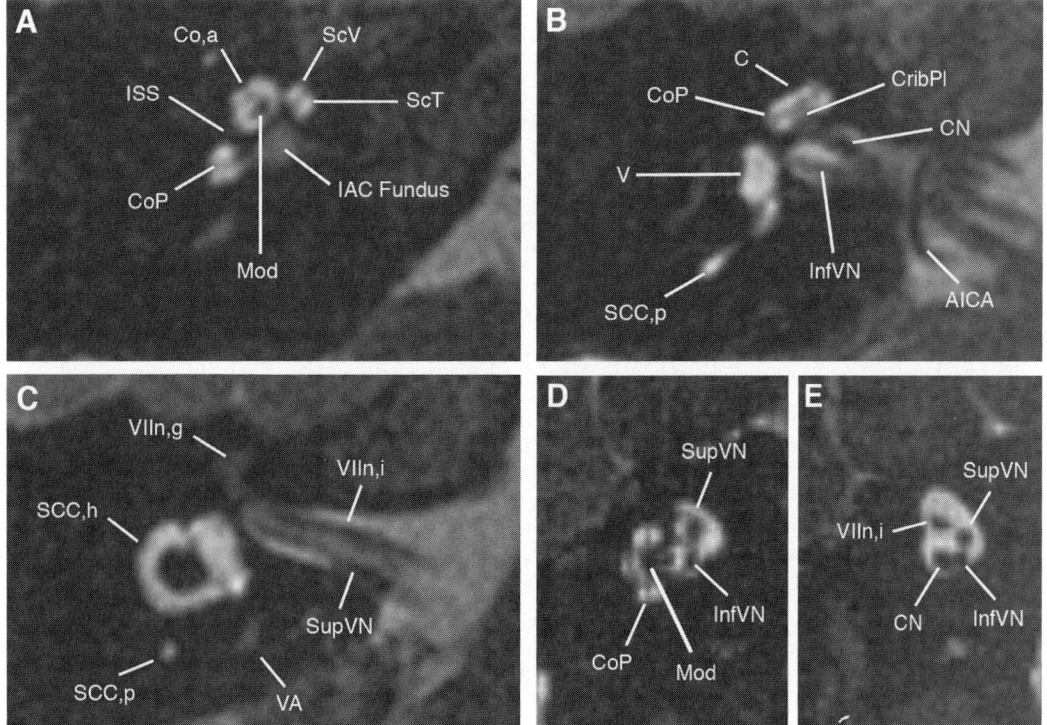

Figure 134.3 Fast imaging employing steady-state acquisition (FIESTA) magnetic resonance image (MRI) of the internal auditory canal (IAC) and labyrinth, axial **(A–C)** and sagittal sections **(D,E)**. CSF, perilymph, and endolymph are hyperintense (*bright*); all other tissues are hypointense (*dark*). Internal architecture of the cochlea is better seen on FIESTA MRI than on computed tomography (CT) (i.e., cochlear partition, modiolus). The normal vestibular aqueduct is usually faintly seen on FIESTA, in contrast to FSE T2W, where it is hyperintense. All four components of the eighth nerve are readily identified on sagittal FIESTA. Refer to Figure 134.1 legend for abbreviation key.

ing (bright fluid) to view the fine structure of the labyrinth.

Gadolinium-based contrast agents shorten T1 relaxation times, so that leak of intravenously injected contrast into tissue causes increase in signal or "enhancement" on T1W images. Because of the blood-brain barrier, these contrast agents do not rapidly leak into brain parenchyma, cochlea, and cranial nerves; hence, there is no enhancement on T1W. One can reliably confirm that contrast has been administered when hyperintense signal is present in the nasal mucosa on T1W images.

Because of the strong magnetic fields used in MR, any metal has the potential to produce image artifacts, physically heat up, or abruptly displace, posing a hazard to the patient. For this reason, certain otologic implants have been considered to be contraindications to MRI. The MRI compatibility of stapes implants must be assessed on a case-by-case basis, according to manufacturer recommendations (4). Although cochlear implants have been considered absolute contraindications to MRI, newer devices address this limitation. Low-field (0.2 Tesla) MRI has been performed in patients with the Med-El Combi® 40+ cochlear implant without adverse effect on the patient or the device (5). The cochlear Nucleus®

24 Contour allows for temporary surgical explantation of the magnet, so that MRI may be performed at field strengths of up to 1.5 Tesla (6).

EXTERNAL AUDITORY CANAL

The bony external auditory canal (EAC) consists of the tympanic bone forming the anterior, inferior, and part of the posterior wall of the external canal and the squamous temporal bone forming the roof. The soft tissue that covers the bone is extremely thin. Thickening of the EAC lining on CT usually simply represents cerumen, but this should be evaluated by direct visualization.

Congenital Anomalies of the External Ear Canal

Congenital aural anomalies result from a developmental defect of the first and second branchial arches and usually involve malformations of both the auricle and external canal (7). Failure of the epithelial cells of the first branchial groove to canalize leads to EAC atresia or

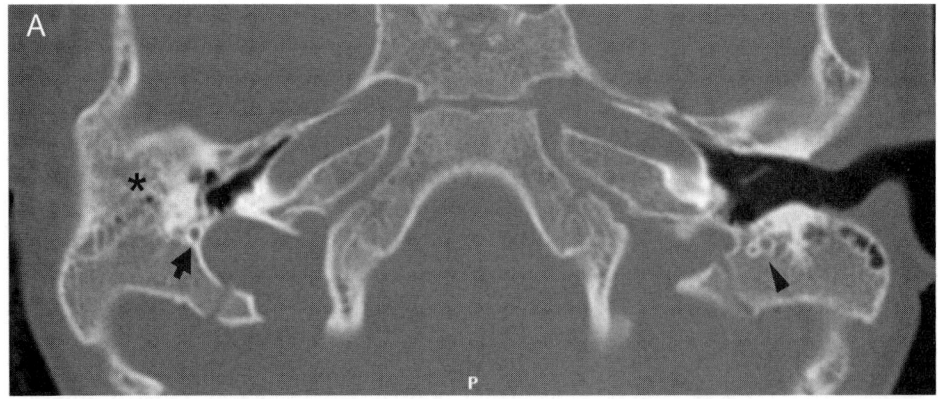

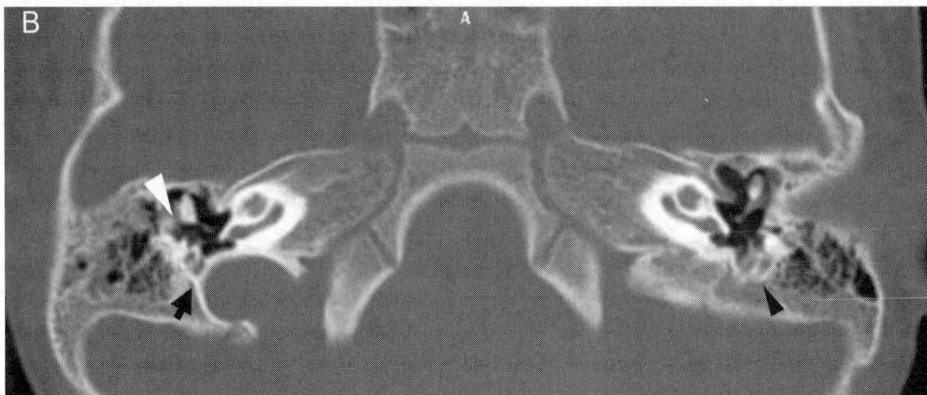

Figure 134.4   External auditory canal (EAC) atresia. Axial computed tomography (CT) scan shows **(A,B)** absence of the right EAC (*asterisk*—**B**). There is fusion of a deformed malleus to an atretic plate (*white arrowhead*). The cochlea is normal. The vertical segment of the facial nerve courses more anteriorly on the right (*black arrow*) than on the left (*black arrowhead*).

stenosis. As the first pharyngeal pouch develops at the same time, anomalies of the middle ear and mastoid are almost always associated with congenital aural atresia or stenosis.

High-resolution CT is the single most important imaging study to plan surgical repair of aural atresia (7). If possible, CT is deferred until 5 years of age, to allow for adequate development of temporal bone structures. A surgical rating scale based on CT determines whether a patient is a good candidate for an aural atresia repair (8). The following structures are assessed on CT: (a) the stapes, (b) oval window, (c) round window, (d) mastoid pneumatization, (e) middle ear pneumatization, (f) course of the facial nerve, (g) incudomalleal complex (h) bony vs. membranous atresia, and (i) normal inner ear morphology (Fig. 134.4) (7). Inner ear malformation is unusual and may exclude a patient from aural atresia repair if SNHL is present. Identification of the stapes is the most important CT finding associated with successful surgical outcome (8).

Syndromic aural atresias (e.g., Treacher Collins syndrome, Goldenhar syndrome) are more commonly asso-

ciated with severe middle ear and inner ear malformations (8).

Benign Neoplasms

Cholesteatoma and Keratosis Obturans
Cholesteatomas rarely occur within the EAC and should be differentiated from keratosis obturans, both of which present with chronic otalgia and otorrhea (9). EAC cholesteatomas are typically unilateral and present in older patients. Squamous debris and granulation tissue accumulate in the ear canal, accompanied by focal bone erosion demonstrated on CT. In contrast, keratosis obturans usually occurs in younger patients with a history of sinusitis and bronchiectasis. Unlike the focal bony erosion associated with an EAC cholesteatoma, the CT finding of keratosis obturans is diffuse widening of the EAC (Fig. 134.5).

Exostoses and Osteomas
Exostoses and osteomas are common benign bony tumors of the external canal (10). Exostoses are typically multiple

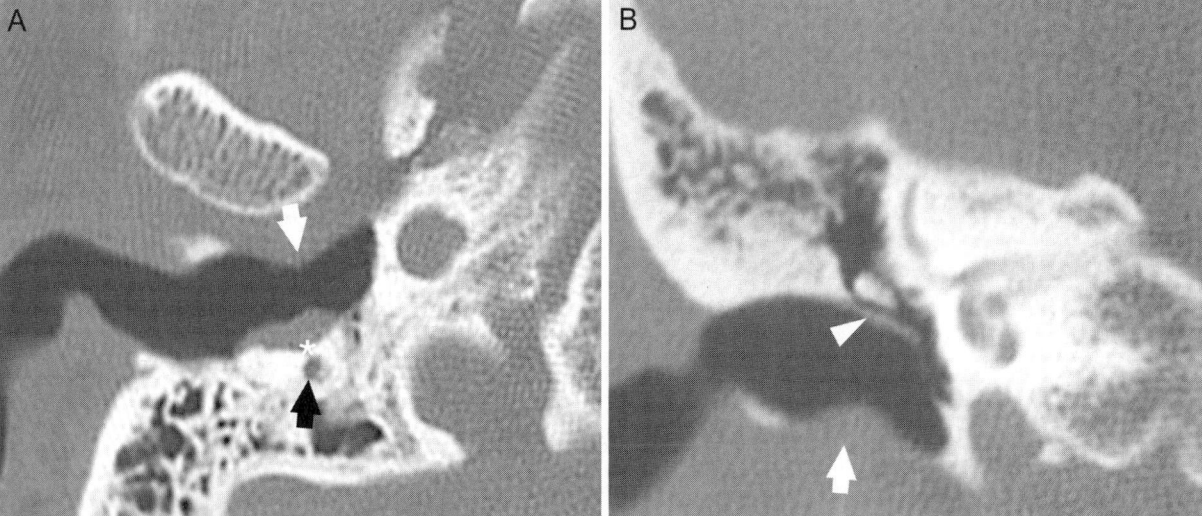

Figure 134.5 Keratitis obturans, following debridement. Smooth erosion of the bony external auditory canal (EAC) (*white arrows*) on axial **(A)** and coronal computed tomography **(B).** Note the thickened tympanic membrane (*white arrowhead—***B**). Note the incidental cerumen (*white asterisk—***A**) in the EAC anterior to the fallopian canal (*black arrow—***A**) that contains the vertical segment of the facial nerve.

and bilateral and are often found in patients with a chronic history of prolonged exposure to cold water, as is seen in swimming or diving. Exostoses are classically broad-based lesions that arise from the medial aspect of the bony EAC, near the tympanic annulus and along the tympanomastoid and tympanosquamous suture lines. In contrast, osteomas are typically solitary and unilateral. Osteomas are pedunculated and are found in the lateral bony EAC (Fig. 134.6) (10). These can sometimes be distin-

guished on imaging as marrow extends into an osteoma, whereas exostoses have the appearance of uniform cortical bone.

Malignant Neoplasms

Malignant tumors that primarily arise within the EAC are rare and include squamous cell carcinoma, basal cell carcinoma, and ceruminous gland tumors (11). Secondary

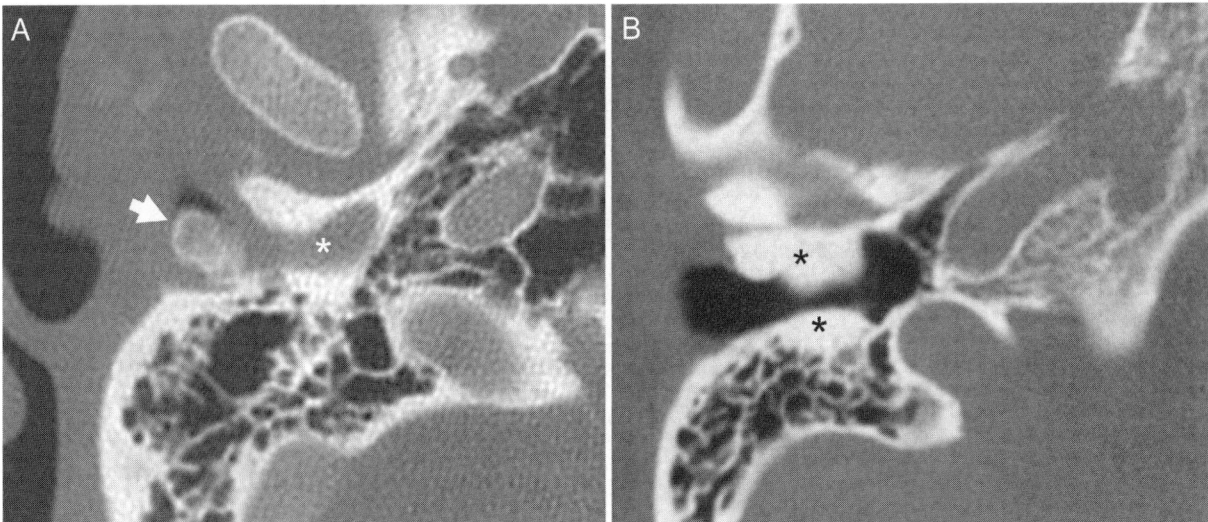

Figure 134.6 Osteoma **(A)** vs. exostosis **(B).** Dense cortical bone and low density of central marrow is apparent in the laterally based osteoma (*white arrow—***A**). Contrast this with the medial location and the high density of the exostoses (*black asterisks—***B**). The osteoma arises from the tympanomastoid suture and partially occludes the EAC, which is filled with cerumen (*white asterisk—***A**).

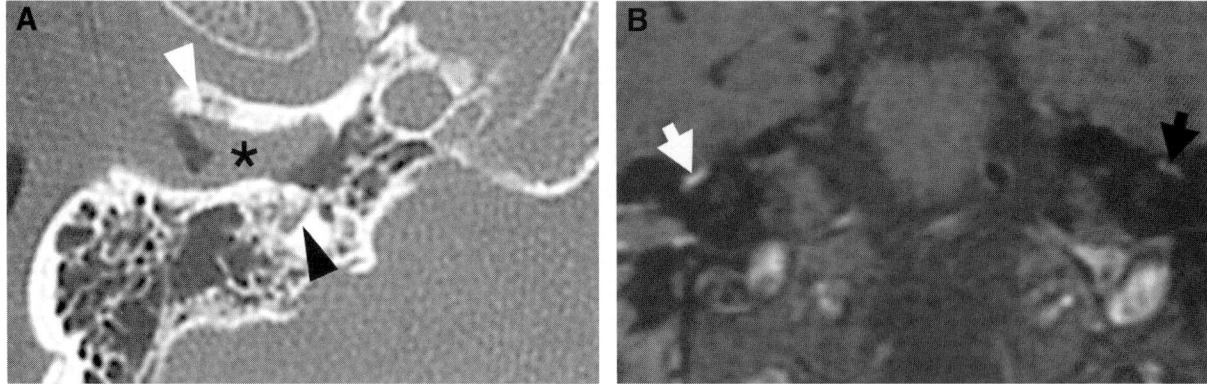

Figure 134.7 Squamous cell carcinoma. Axial CT **(A)** and coronal T1-weighted magnetic resonance imaging (T1W MRI) with contrast **(B).** Soft tissue mass in the right auditory canal (*black asterisk—A*). Note the focal bony erosion involving the anterior aspect of the bony external ear canal (*white arrowhead—A*). Extension into the vertical segment of the fallopian canal (*black arrowhead*) results in facial nerve paresis. On T1W postcontrast MRI, the perigeniculate facial nerve on the right enhances because of perineural invasion (*white arrow—B*). Contrast this with the normal appearance of the perigeniculate facial nerve on the left (*black arrow—B*).

malignant tumors of the EAC are more common, involving the EAC by direct extension from adjacent tissues (e.g., skin or parotid). Although the hallmark of malignant tumors on imaging is irregular bone destruction associated with a soft tissue mass, this is nonspecific.

EAC malignancies can easily extend anteriorly through the fissure of Santorini to the parotid gland, into the middle ear though the tympanic membrane, and into the mastoid cavity through the tympanomastoid suture line. Both CT and MRI may be used to define the full extent of disease (Fig. 134.7). MRI is essential for defining perineural invasion.

One diagnostic dilemma is that of a destructive bone lesion in the cancer patient who has received radiation. It is quite difficult for CT or MRI to distinguish between recurrent metastatic disease and osteoradionecrosis.

Infectious and Inflammatory Diseases

Uncomplicated external otitis is usually self-limiting, and CT or MRI are rarely required for this condition. In the elderly diabetic or immunocompromised individual particularly, however, the potentially life-threatening necrotizing or malignant otitis externa can develop, and this may extend to involve adjacent soft tissues and the skull base (12).

CT can demonstrate the subtle bony erosion and involvement of the mastoid and middle ear cavity (Fig. 134.8). MRI is better for demonstrating the development of skull

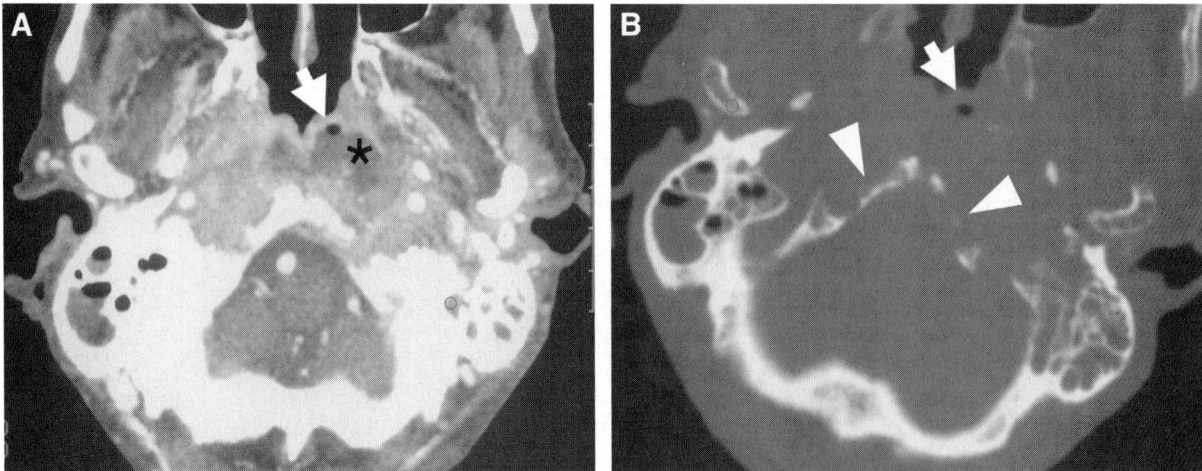

Figure 134.8 Malignant otitis externa. Axial computed tomography scan with contrast shows heterogeneously enhancing tissue throughout the prevertebral soft tissues anterior to the skull base. Fluid density (**A**—*asterisk*) and gas (*white arrows*) indicate abscess formation. Note the extensive osseus destruction of the clivus and jugular foramina (**B**—*arrowheads*).

base osteomyelitis, as well as potential intracranial involvement.

Both MRI and CT have difficulties monitoring the response of osteomyelitis to therapy. Single photon emission computed tomography (SPECT) using Technetium-99m methylene diphosphonate (MDP), Gallium-67 scintigraphy, or Indium-111 tagged white blood cells may be used for post-treatment assessment (13).

MIDDLE EAR, MASTOID, AND PETROUS APEX

Infectious and Inflammatory Diseases

Otitis Media and Mastoiditis

Mastoid and middle ear effusions are often incidental findings on MRIs of the brain performed for a number of reasons, including those performed in healthy volunteers. In particular, they are commonly present in chronically intubated patients. The presence of a unilateral mastoid effusion in an adult should, however, prompt a careful assessment of the nasopharynx for an occult mass. Often, a unilateral mastoid effusion is identified in the setting of radiation-induced eustachian tube dysfunction as an incidental finding in patients with brain tumor or head and neck cancer. These effusions are hyperintense on T2W and

hypointense on T1W images and do not enhance with contrast. Mastoid septations and the ossicular chain are intact. Enhancement with contrast suggests the presence of active inflammation (e.g., mastoiditis). Chronic infections can lead to bone thickening and sclerosis, resulting in calcification of the tympanic cavity and membrane (tympanosclerosis). Erosion of mastoid septations is best demonstrated on CT and indicates the transition to coalescent mastoiditis resulting from enzymatic resorption of bone (Fig. 134.9) (14).

Extracranial extension of mastoiditis can occur (15): A subperiosteal abscess can develop as a result of direct extension through the thin trabecular bone in the lateral mastoid cortex. Spread along the zygomatic root forms a preauricular abscess. Erosion through the mastoid tip forms a Bezold abscess medial to the sternocleidomastoid muscle.

Intracranial complications of mastoiditis, such as dural venous sinus thrombosis, abscesses (epidural, subdural, and intracerebral), and meningitis are best evaluated by MRI (15).

Dural Sinus Thrombosis

Mastoiditis can be complicated by sigmoid sinus thrombosis caused by a retrograde thrombophlebitis (16). The thrombus may then propagate in an antegrade fashion into the internal jugular vein or retrograde into the

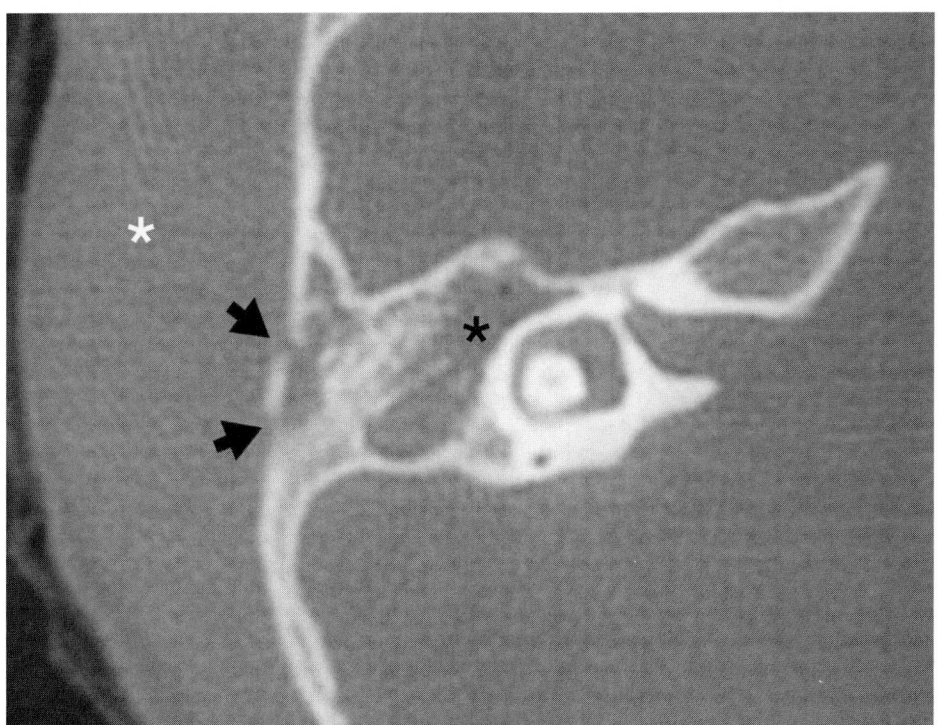

Figure 134.9 Coalescent mastoiditis with subperiosteal abscess. Axial computed tomography scan in a child shows the completely opacified mastoid (*black asterisk*) and the poorly defined irregular osseous mastoid septations. Frank disruption of the cortical bone of the mastoid is present (*black arrows*), and there is marked soft tissue swelling of the overlying subcutaneous tissues (*white asterisk*). (Courtesy of Dr. Alex Grevendulis.)

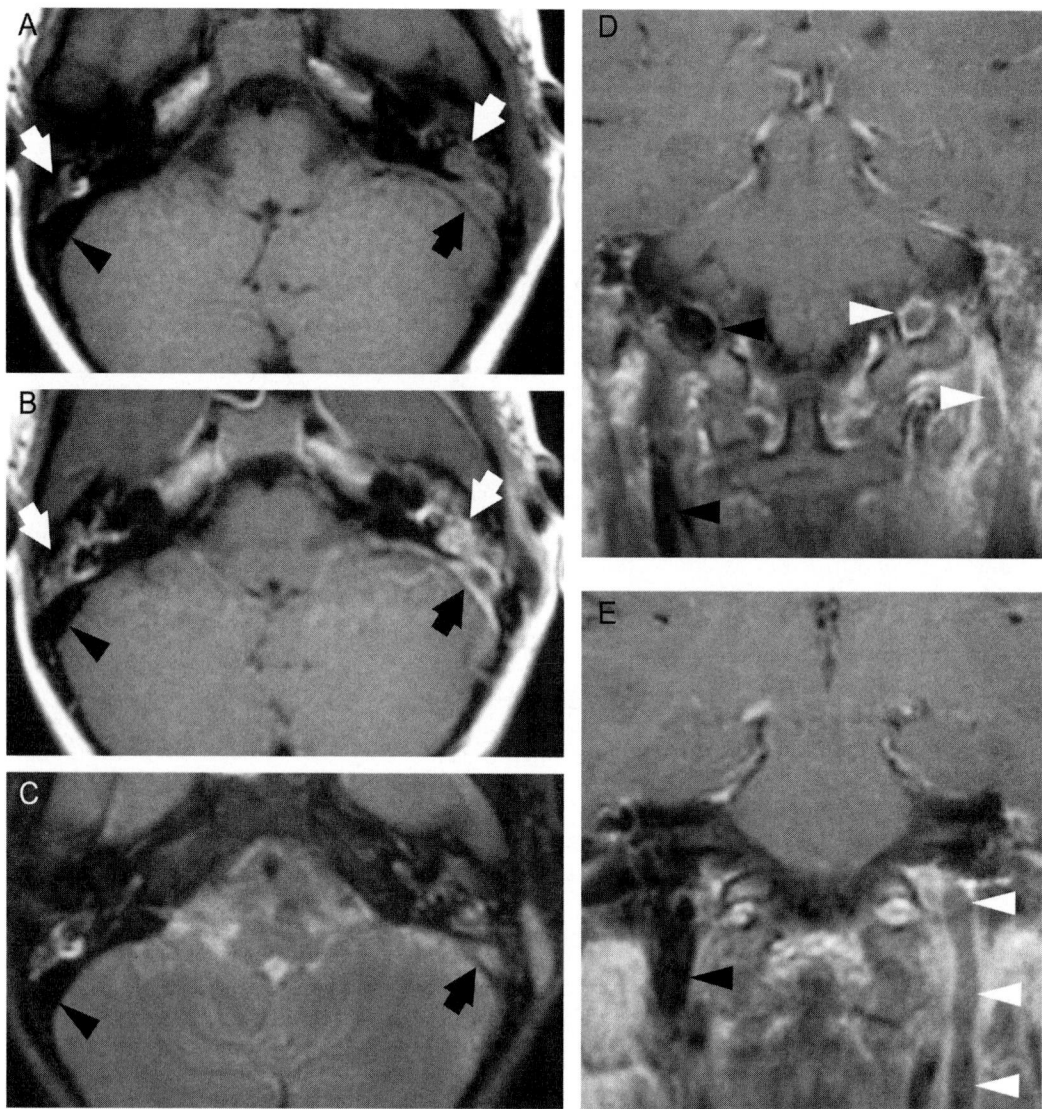

Figure 134.10 Mastoiditis complicated by sigmoid sinus thrombosis. Mastoiditis is evident as enhancing tissue in both middle ears (*white arrows*) on axial T1-weighted (T1W) pre- **(A)** and postcontrast **(B)** magnetic resonance imaging (MRI). Thrombus in the sigmoid sinus (*black arrows*) is isointense on T1W **(A)** and T2-weighted (T2W) **(C)** with enhancement of the surrounding dura **(B)**. Flow void results in absence of signal from the normal sigmoid sinus on the right (*black arrowheads*). On coronal T1W postcontrast MRI, flow void is seen in the normal right jugular bulb and internal jugular vein (*black arrowheads—***D,E**). Isointense thrombus with marked enhancement of the walls of the jugular bulb and internal jugular vein are seen on the left (*white arrowheads—***D,E**).

transverse or superior sagittal and straight sinuses. Sigmoid dural venous sinus thrombosis can be detected with contrast-enhanced CT or with MRI (Fig. 134.10). On CT, acute thrombus may be hyperdense. On standard spin-echo T1W and T2W images, flow voids are present in the sinuses, making them hypointense. When flow is extremely slow or there is frank thrombus, signal becomes isointense. Contrast enhances the dura surrounding the thrombus on both CT and MR, but not the thrombus itself. Chronic thrombus will vascularize and therefore enhance.

Petrositis

Apical petrositis can occur not only in the pneumatized petrous apex (30% to 35%), but also in the nonpneuma-tized petrous apex as an osteomyelitis (15). The classic triad of Gradenigo syndrome (retro-orbital pain, sixth-nerve palsy, and chronic otorrhea) is now quite rare. CT reveals the opacified petrous apex cells with lysis of bony septations. MRI usually shows peripheral meningeal enhancement at the petrous apex as the adjacent dura becomes thickened and covered with granulation tissue.

Cholesterol Granuloma (Cholesterol Cyst)

Chronic inflammatory mucosal secretions can become trapped within the pneumatized petrous apex to form a cholesterol granuloma (17). Similar to a paranasal muco-cele, the cholesterol granuloma is expansile, so that CT demonstrates opacification and smooth expansion of the

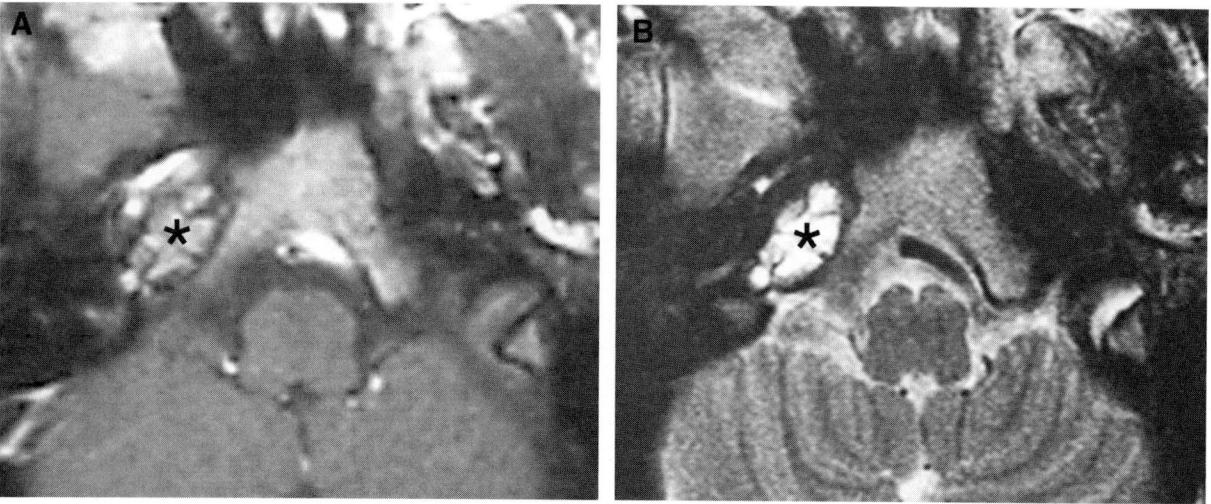

Figure 134.11 Cholesterol granuloma. Magnetic resonance imaging (MRI) shows an expansile lesion (*asterisks*) in the right petrous apex, with increased MR signal on noncontrast T1-weighted (T1W) **(A)** and T2-weighted (T2W) **(B)** images due to presence of methemoglobin in the cyst.

cortical margins of the petrous apex. High signal on both T1W and T2W MRI images are characteristic of a cholesterol granuloma (Fig. 134.11). The hyperintensity on T1W images is likely attributable to methemoglobin from microhemorrhage and distinguishes the cholesterol granuloma from simple fluid, apicitis, or cholesteatoma that are hypointense on T1W MRI. Deposition of ferritin and hemosiderin may result in T1 and T2 hypointensity within the cholesterol granuloma.

Acquired Cholesteatoma

Acquired cholesteatomas are (usually small) inclusions of squamous epithelium that are highly erosive and found in the middle ear and mastoid cavity (18). Attic cholesteatomas arise from retraction of the pars flaccida and grow into the Prussak space and between the lateral attic wall and the head of the malleus. They may displace the malleus medially and extend posteriorly to involve the posterolateral attic and antrum. Since CT cannot distinguish soft tissue or fluid from a cholesteatoma, the diagnosis is only definitive on CT when characteristic bone erosion is seen. Erosion of the scutum is the earliest sign, best detected on coronal CT (Fig. 134.12). Eventually, ossicular chain destruction may be seen. The long process of the incus is most commonly involved, followed by the body of the incus and the head of the malleus (18).

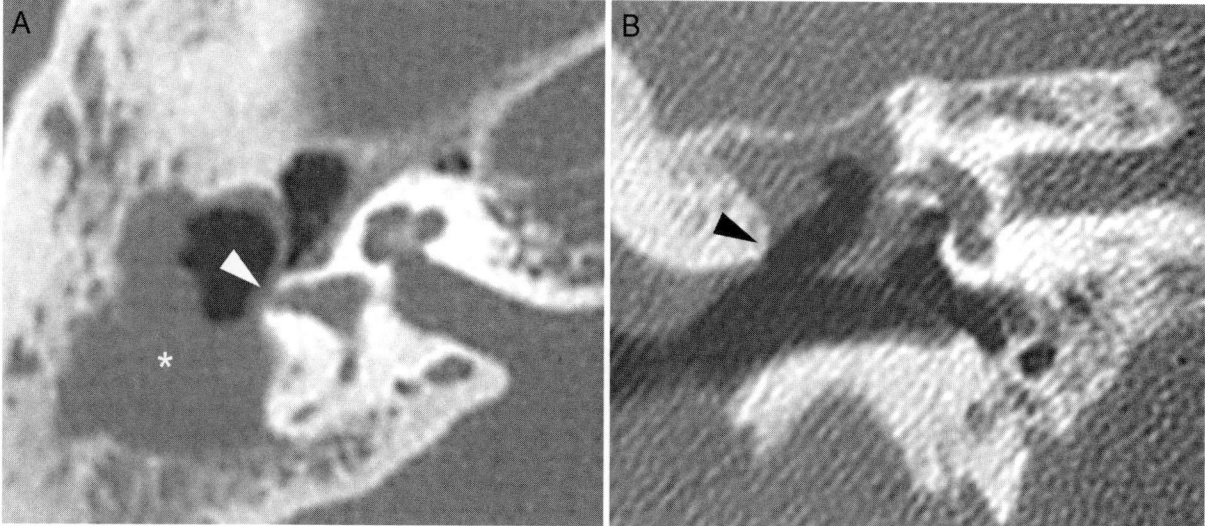

Figure 134.12 Cholesteatoma. Large soft-tissue density mass expands the mastoid antrum and erodes adjacent bony septations (*asterisk—***A**) and scutum (*black arrowhead—***B**). Note the fistula into the lateral SCC (*white arrowhead—***A**).

Cholesteatomas arising from the pars tensa usually originate from posterosuperior tympanic retraction and progress posteriorly to involve the facial recess and sinus tympani. These lesions can extend medial to the ossicular chain. These cholesteatomas commonly erode the long process of the incus and superstructure of the stapes.

A labyrinthine fistula may develop from chronic cholesteatomas. The most common site for a fistula to occur is the lateral semicircular canal (Fig. 134.12). Less often, pars tensa cholesteatomas can cause a cochlear fistula at the promontory area located between the round and oval windows. Facial nerve paresis is rarely associated with cholesteatomas. This is caused by either bony erosion of the fallopian canal or inflammation on the facial nerve, most commonly at the tympanic segment.

Most cholesteatomas of the middle ear and mastoid are poorly characterized by MRI. On T1W MRI, rim enhancement may be seen with contrast administration. They are moderately hyperintense on T2W images. Granulation tissue associated with cholesteatomas cannot be differentiated from a recurrent cholesteatoma on a noncontrast CT. This differentiation can be made with a contrast MRI exam, though, because granulation tissue will enhance, whereas a cholesteatoma will not. When a cholesteatoma is suspected of extending outside the temporal bone, MRI is indicated. In such cases of extensive disease, diffusion-weighted imaging may distinguish cholesteatoma from other destructive lesions (19). Diffusion-weighted imaging is a low-resolution technique and prone to artifact in regions of air tissue interfaces, particularly the temporal bone, however, and should be interpreted with caution in this region. It is of more value in evaluating intracranial epidermoid tumors. (See the section Internal Auditory Canal and Cerebellopontine Angle Lesions, on page 1981).

Tumors of the Middle Ear

The differential diagnosis of a mass in the middle ear includes glomus tumor, cholesteatoma, schwannoma, adenoma, and numerous other rare entities (Fig. 134.13). Variants of normal anatomy, such as an aberrant internal carotid artery and a dehiscent high-riding jugular bulb, can also present as a mass-like lesion in the hypotympanum.

Paraganglioma/Glomus Tympanicum

Paragangliomas in the tympanic cavity are termed *glomus tympanicum* and arise from the glomus bodies along Jacobson nerve (a branch of the glossopharyngeal nerve) or more rarely from Arnold nerve (a branch of the vagus nerve) (20). The glomus tympanicum tumor is the most common primary tumor of the middle ear. Small glomus tympanicum appear as small soft tissue masses on the cochlear promontory and must be distinguished from the aberrant stapedial artery, which also courses over the promontory. Since they present as small lesions, they are usually best demonstrated

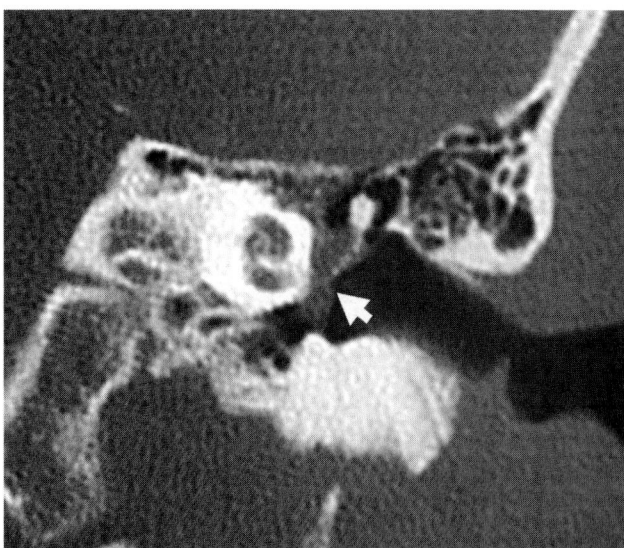

Figure 134.13 Middle ear adenoma. On coronal computed tomography, a soft tissue mass (*white arrow*) is shown in the anterior aspect of the left mesotympanum between the cochlea and malleus.

on CT (Fig. 134.14), although dramatic contrast enhancement can be seen on MRI.

Congenital Cholesteatoma or Epidermoid

A congenital cholesteatoma or epidermoid is a rare tumor of the middle ear and is believed to arise from aberrant epithelial embryonic rests left behind in the middle ear (21). Like the acquired cholesteatoma, it is lined by keratinizing stratified squamous epithelium that gradually enlarges in

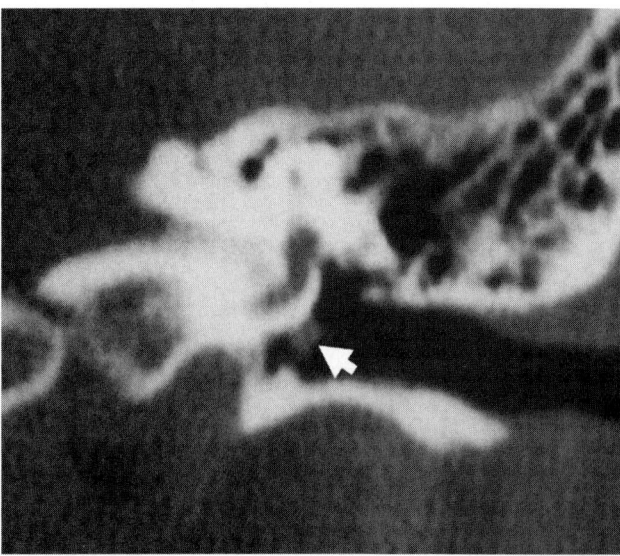

Figure 134.14 Glomus tympanicum. Coronal computed tomography demonstrates a soft tissue mass (*white arrow*) on the promontory of the left cochlea. This presented as a red mass in the hypotympanum on otoscopy.

the air spaces inside the middle ear and mastoid cavity. There is a distinct propensity for its occurrence in the anterosuperior mesotympanum, near the eustachian tube opening.

INNER EAR

Congenital Anomalies

About 20% of patients with congenital sensorineural hearing loss have morphologic anomalies detectable by CT or MRI (22). Developmental insults in weeks four through eight of gestation, when the labyrinth forms, result in various degrees of deformity.

Michel aplasia, the complete absence of the inner ear, results from developmental arrest at the third week (Fig. 134.15). The "common cavity" deformity, a confluence of an ill-developed cochlea and vestibular organ, results from a disruption during the fourth and fifth weeks (Fig. 134.16). An arrest during the fifth or sixth week of gestation results in cochlear aplasia or cochlear hypoplasia, respectively.

The Mondini cochlear deformity consists of a failure to properly partition the cochlea so that the interscalar septum is absent and the modiolus is poorly formed or "deficient." On CT and MRI, the cochlear apex appears "bulbous." High-resolution T2W MRI depicts the modiolar deficiency well. The Mondini cochlear deformity is almost

always associated with an enlarged vestibular aqueduct, as in Mondini's original description (Fig. 134.17).

The semicircular canals develop between the sixth and eighth week of gestation. Because the superior and posterior semicircular canals develop before the horizontal semicircular canal, horizontal semicircular deformities are the most common vestibular organ deformity discovered. (Fig. 134.18).

The most common inner ear abnormality detected by CT in individuals with congenital SNHL is the enlarged vestibular aqueduct (EVA) (23). MRI clearly demonstrates the enlargement of the endolymphatic duct and sac that underlies the expansion of the bony vestibular aqueduct (Fig. 134.19). The vestibular aqueduct is considered to be enlarged when it is greater than 1.5 mm wide (approximately the width of the posterior semicircular canal), measured at the midpoint between the common crus and the external aperture.

Some inner ear anomalies are associated with absence of the bony partition between the IAC and vestibule. Stapes surgery is contraindicated in this situation, as a cerebrospinal fluid (CSF) "gusher" may develop upon a manipulation of the stapes (24). Rarely, the IAC can be narrow (1 to 2 mm), implying the absence of the cochlear nerve (Fig. 134.15). Absence of the cochlear nerve, which may be confirmed by high-resolution MRI, represents one of the few absolute contraindications for cochlear implantation.

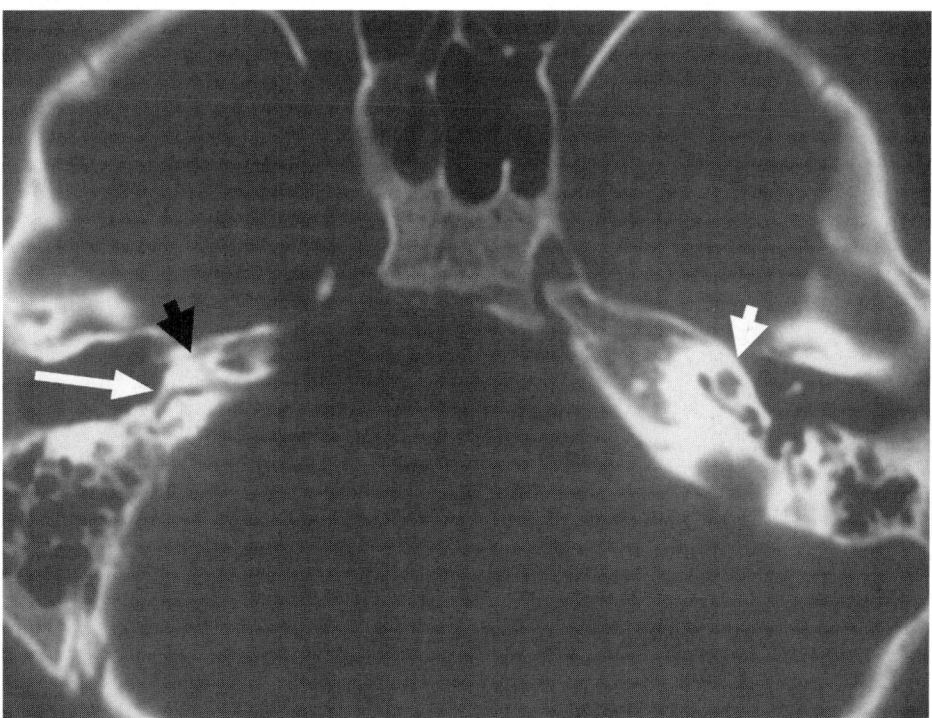

Figure 134.15   Michel aplasia. The labyrinth is absent on the right (*black arrow*), whereas the left cochlea is normal on computed tomography (*white arrow*). The right internal auditory canal is narrow and contains only the facial nerve (*thin white arrow*). The volume of the right petrous temporal bone is smaller than that of the left.

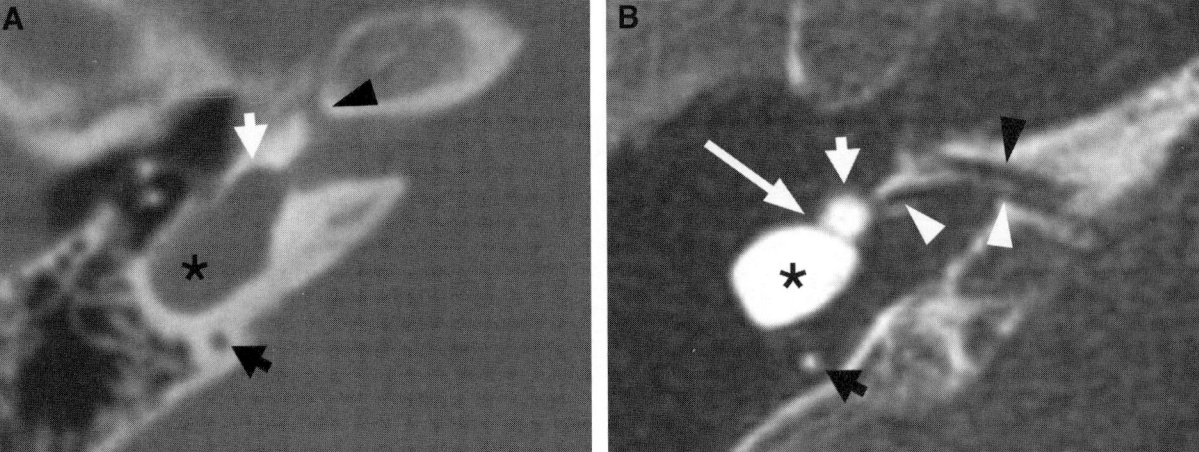

Figure 134.16 Common cavity deformity on computed tomography (CT) **(A)** and fast imaging employing steady-state acquisition (FIESTA) magnetic resonance imaging (MRI) **(B)**. A septation (*thin white arrow—B*) seen on FIESTA divides the primitive cochlea anteriorly (*white arrow—A,B*) from the fused vestibule and semicircular canals posteriorly (*black asterisk*). Note that a portion of the posterior semicircular canal has formed (*black arrows*). Note the anomalous course of the common cochleovestibular nerve (*white arrowheads*) in the internal auditory canal. Note the labyrinthine segment of the fallopian canal on CT (*black arrowhead—A*) and the facial nerve in the internal auditory canal (*black arrowhead—B*).

An absence of a small portion of bone in the otic capsule over the superior semicircular canal is referred to as superior semicircular canal dehiscence (25). This dehiscence may give rise to a distinct syndrome of sound- or pressure-induced vertigo (Tullio phenomenon) and air to bone gap on audiometric threshold testing. High-resolution (0.5 mm) collimation dramatically improves the sensitivity for detecting such dehiscences relative to 1 mm collimation

(Fig. 134.20). Oblique reformats in the plane of the semicircular canal are also beneficial in identifying the dehiscence.

Inflammation and Hemorrhage

Labyrinthitis presents as SNHL, vertigo, or tinnitus usually because of viral or autoimmune disease, although neoplasm,

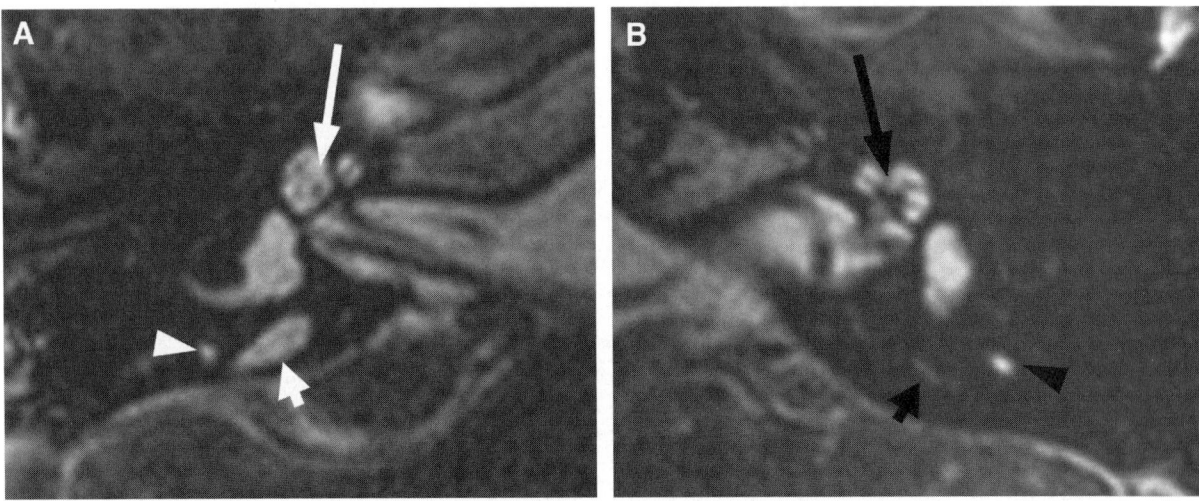

Figure 134.17 Enlarged vestibular aqueduct with modiolar dysplasia (Mondini malformation). Fast imaging employing steady-state acquisition (FIESTA) magnetic resonance image (MRI) of right inner ear **(A)** shows enlarged endolymphatic sac expanding the vestibular aqueduct (*thick white arrow*) as compared with the normal posterior SCC (*arrowheads*). The osseous spiral lamina and modiolus (*thin white arrow*) are hypoplastic. Compare with the normal FIESTA MRI of the left inner ear **(B)**. Note that the vestibular aqueduct is typically only faintly visualized on FIESTA (*thick black arrow*) and normal cochlea and modiolus (*thin black arrow*).

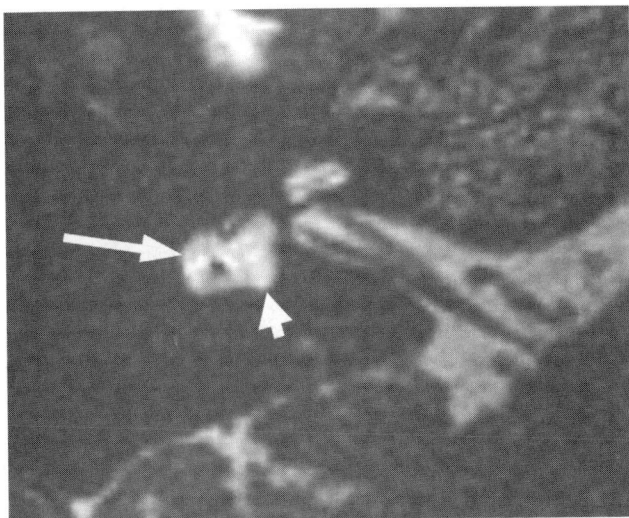

Figure 134.18 Lateral semicircular canal anomaly. fast imaging employing steady-state acquisition (FIESTA) magnetic resonance imaging (MRI) shows partial fusion of the horizontal SCC (*thin white arrow*) with the vestibule (*white arrow*). Both appear bulbous.

trauma, or bacterial infection may be causative (26). The primary role of MRI is to rule out other pathologies, as MRI is usually normal in patients with labyrinthitis. Labyrinthitis, however, can be identified on MRI as diffuse enhancement of the normally nonenhancing labyrinth (Fig. 134.21). Hemorrhagic labyrinthitis or intralabyrinthine hemorrhage is readily identified as hyperintense signal on pre-contrast T1W images but is not identifiable on CT (Fig. 134.22) (27). Hemorrhage may be accompanied by a variable degree of T2W hypointensity that is often best appreciated on high-resolution gradient-echo–based MR sequences (e.g., CISS, FIESTA). Fibrosis of the membranous labyrinth develops

with chronic labyrinthitis, also resulting in T2 hypointensity in the normally bright fluid of the labyrinth. This may be detected on MRI prior to the detection of frank labyrinthitis ossificans on CT (28) and is most useful when assessing the patency of the cochlea in planning cochlear implantation in patients with profound hearing loss following meningitis.

Neoplasms

Intralabyrinthine Schwannoma
The vestibular schwannoma, typically found in the IAC can extend into the labyrinth (29). Rarely, a schwannoma can be entirely confined within the cochlea or vestibule. Because it is characterized by intense enhancement within the labyrinth on MR, it may be indistinguishable from labyrinthitis (Fig. 134.23).

Endolymphatic Sac Tumor
The endolymphatic sac tumor (ELST) is benign, but locally aggressive. The ELST characteristically arises from the vestibular aqueduct and is detectable at early stages on CT by erosion of the walls of the aqueduct (30). As the tumor enlarges, it may extend into the otic capsule, cerebellopontine angle (CPA), and jugular foramen. Spicules of bone may be seen on CT, similar to a glomus jugulare tumor. On MR, T1 and T2 hyperintense foci are present within or adjacent to the ELST, reminiscent of a cholesterol granuloma and suggesting hemorrhage (Fig. 134.24). A solid T1 isointense–enhancing component may also be present. Notably, high signal in the labyrinth indicates intralabyrinthine hemorrhage, which may be the earliest manifestation of the ELST, causing symptoms even when the tumor itself is radiographically occult (Fig. 134.22) (31).

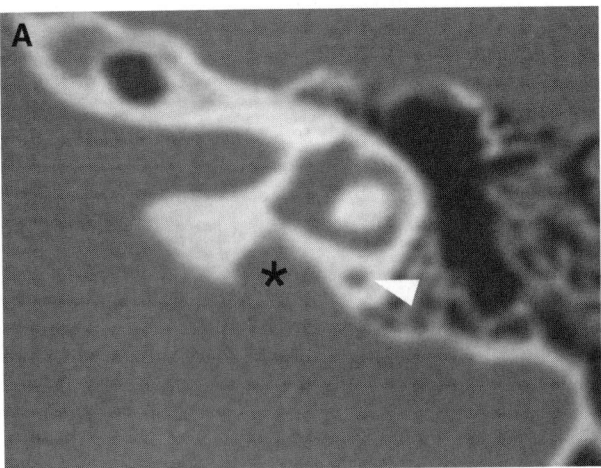
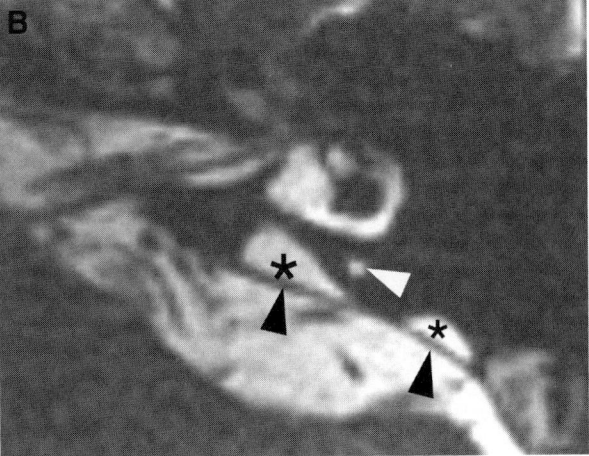

Figure 134.19 Enlarged vestibular aqueduct. Axial computed tomography (CT) **(A)** and fast imaging employing steady-state acquisition (FIESTA) **(B)** demonstrate an abnormally enlarged left vestibular aqueduct (*asterisks*) medial and posterior to the normal posterior SCC (*white arrowheads*). The dura overlying the dilated endolymphatic sac is seen on FIESTA magnetic resonance imaging (MRI) (*black arrowheads*), but the contents of the aqueduct are indistinguishable from the posterior fossa on CT.

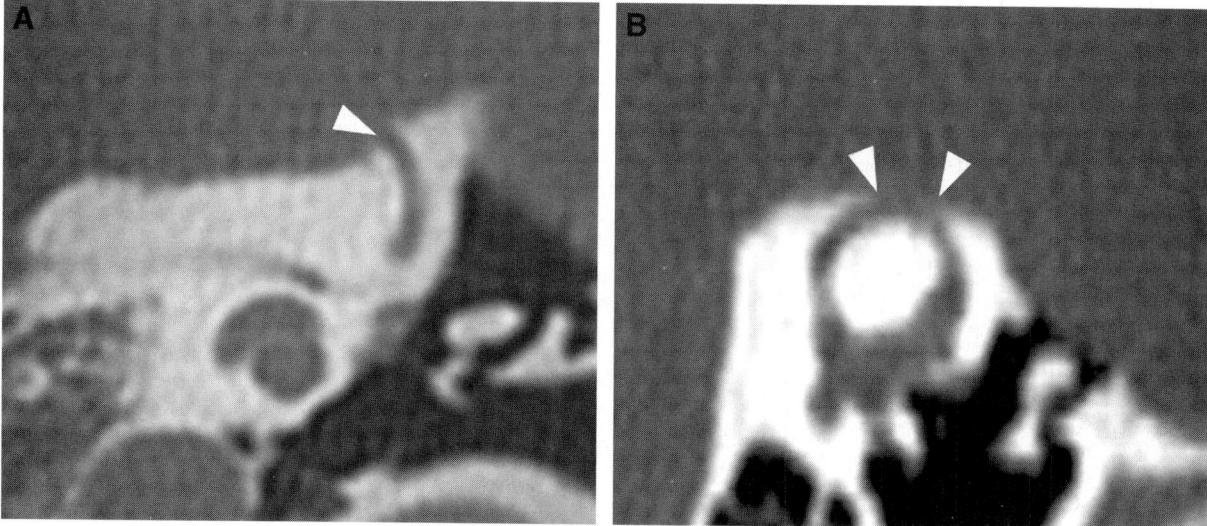

Figure 134.20 Superior semicircular canal (SCC) dehiscence. Direct coronal 0.625 mm computed tomography (**A, B**) shows dehiscence of the left superior SCC (*white arrowheads*). Double oblique reformat along the plane of the superior SCC shows that the bony dehiscence extends slightly more than 2 mm.

Otodystrophies

Bony disorders involving the otic capsule and temporal bone are best evaluated by CT. Otosclerosis (otospongiosis) is a condition in which the enchondral bone around the otic capsule is replaced by multiple foci of spongy vascular irregular bone, resulting in hearing loss (32) . The spongy bone later becomes calcified and sclerotic. The most commonly involved site is anterior to the oval window (fistula ante fenestrum), where a small radiolucent plaque may develop. Otosclerosis involving the otic capsule results in demineralization along the basal turn of the

cochlea, identifiable by the "double ring sign" on CT (Fig. 134.25A). Even more extensive demineralization of the otic capsule can be seen in osteogenesis imperfecta, with a similar appearance (33) (Fig. 134.25B). "Obliterative otosclerosis" is rare and is usually limited to the round window and basal turn of the cochlea. The diagnosis of otosclerosis is usually based on clinical and audiologic findings, and thus a CT is not routinely indicated.

Other primary bone diseases such as Paget disease, fibrous dysplasia (Fig. 134.26), and osteoporosis can affect the temporal bone but rarely involve the otic capsule and are less likely to cause SNHL.

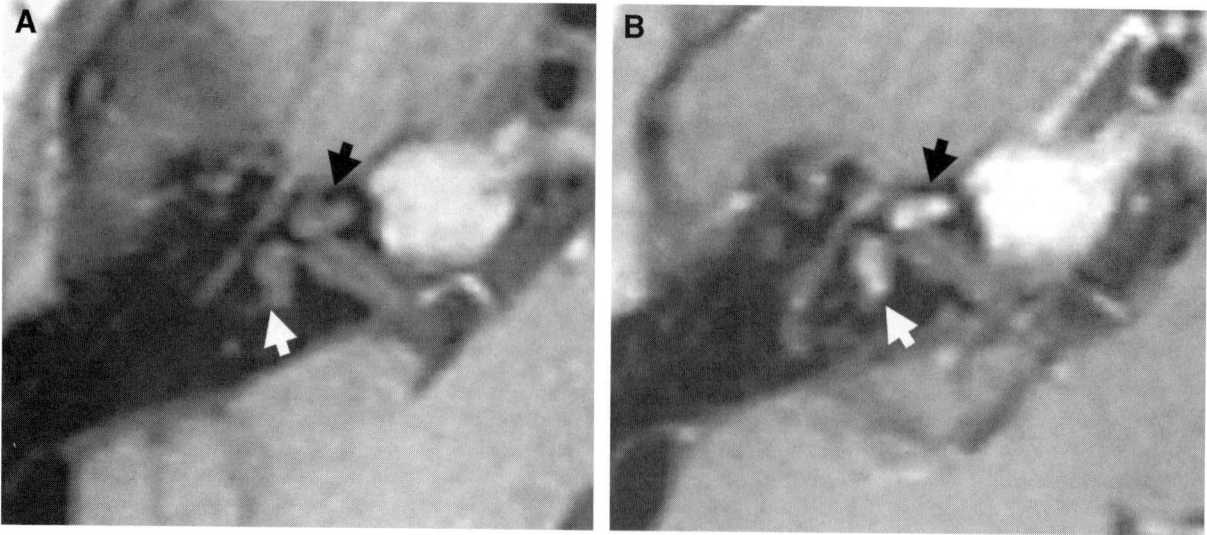

Figure 134.21 Labyrinthitis. T1-weighted magnetic resonance image (T1W MRI) with (**B**) and without (**A**) contrast shows dramatic enhancement of the cochlea (*black arrows*) and vestibule (*white arrows*), indicating labyrinthitis.

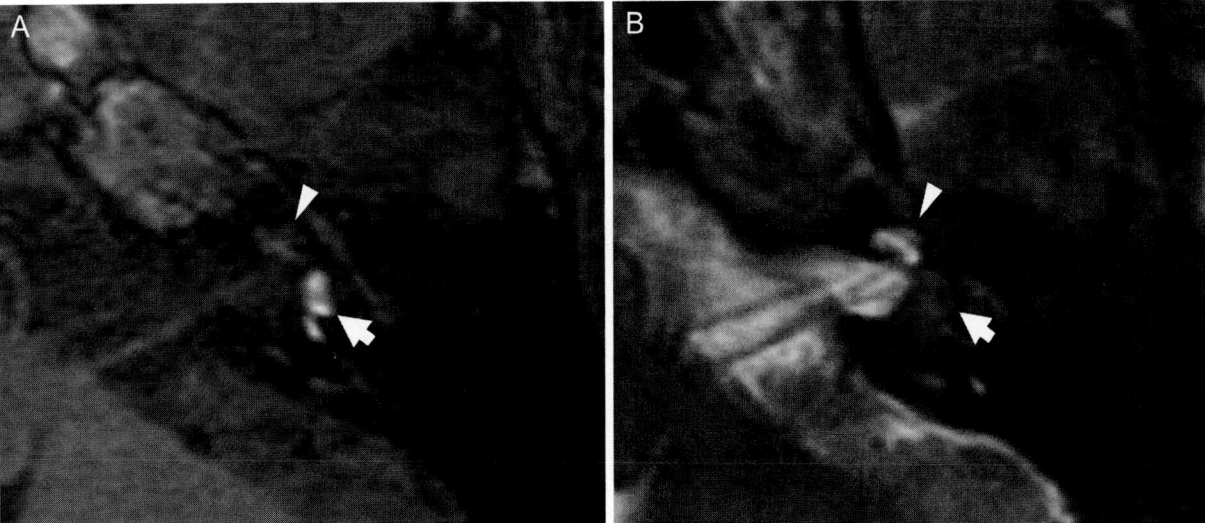

Figure 134.22 Intralabyrinthine hemorrhage in a patient with endolymphatic sac tumor (*not shown*). Hyperintense signal on noncontrast T1-weighted magnetic resonance image (T1W MRI) fills the vestibule and a portion of the posterior SCC (*white arrow*—**A**). On fast-spin echo T2-weighted magnetic resonance image (T2W MRI) (*white arrow*—**B**) the vestibule is poorly visualized because of signal loss from blood. Note the normal appearance of the cochlea on both the noncontrast T1W and T2W MRI (*white arrowheads*—**A,B**).

Otologic Implants

Stapes Prosthesis

CT is used to evaluate new vertigo or SNHL in patients with stapes prostheses. The etiology of delayed or recurrent hearing loss, including reparative granuloma formation, prosthesis subluxation, and regrowth of otosclerosis, can often be detected (Fig. 134.27) (34).

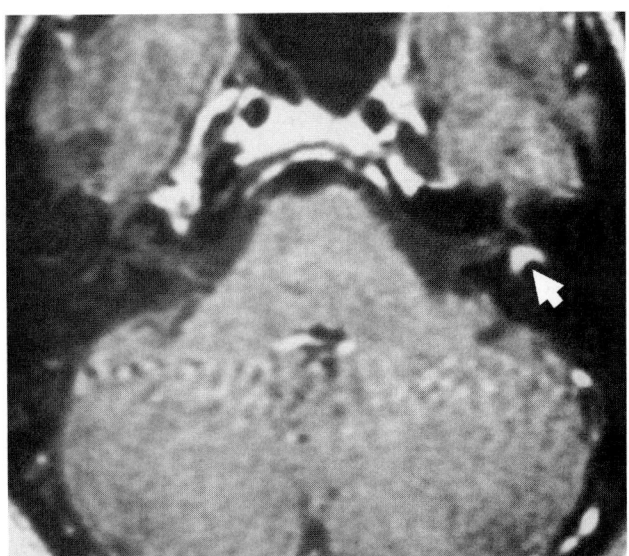

Figure 134.23 Intralabyrinthine schwannoma. T1-weighted postcontrast magnetic resonance image depicts an abnormally enhancing lesion within the left vestibule (*white arrow*). Note that the imaging findings may be indistinguishable from labyrinthitis.

Cochlear Implantation

Prior to cochlear implantation, it is important to identify labyrinthitis ossificans, which may alter the surgical approach and impact prognosis. MRI and CT are very specific (~90%) in identifying a patent membranous cochlea, but are relatively insensitive (30 to 40%). Therefore, usage of both CT and MRI have been advocated (28). With cochlear malformations or a narrow IAC, MRI can identify the presence of the cochlear division of the eighth cranial nerve in the internal auditory canal, a prerequisite for a successful implantation (Fig. 134.3D,E).

Plain film radiography or helical CT may be used to assess the placement of a cochlear implant. The "cochlear view" radiograph is obtained with the X-ray tube angled 50° from the midsagittal plane, such that the beam is in the same plane as the orbitomeatal line (35).

TEMPORAL BONE TRAUMA

CT is essential to characterize temporal bone fractures, which are classified as longitudinal, transverse, or mixed according to their orientation relative to the long axis of the petrous bone (36). Fluid in the middle ear may represent hemotympanum or cerebrospinal fluid (CSF) leak. Integrity of the ossicular chain should be carefully assessed. Entry of fracture lines into the otic capsule, fallopian canal, and tegmen should be noted.

Longitudinal fractures are more common (~75%). They originate in the mastoid process or posterior portion of the squamous temporal bone and follow the path of least

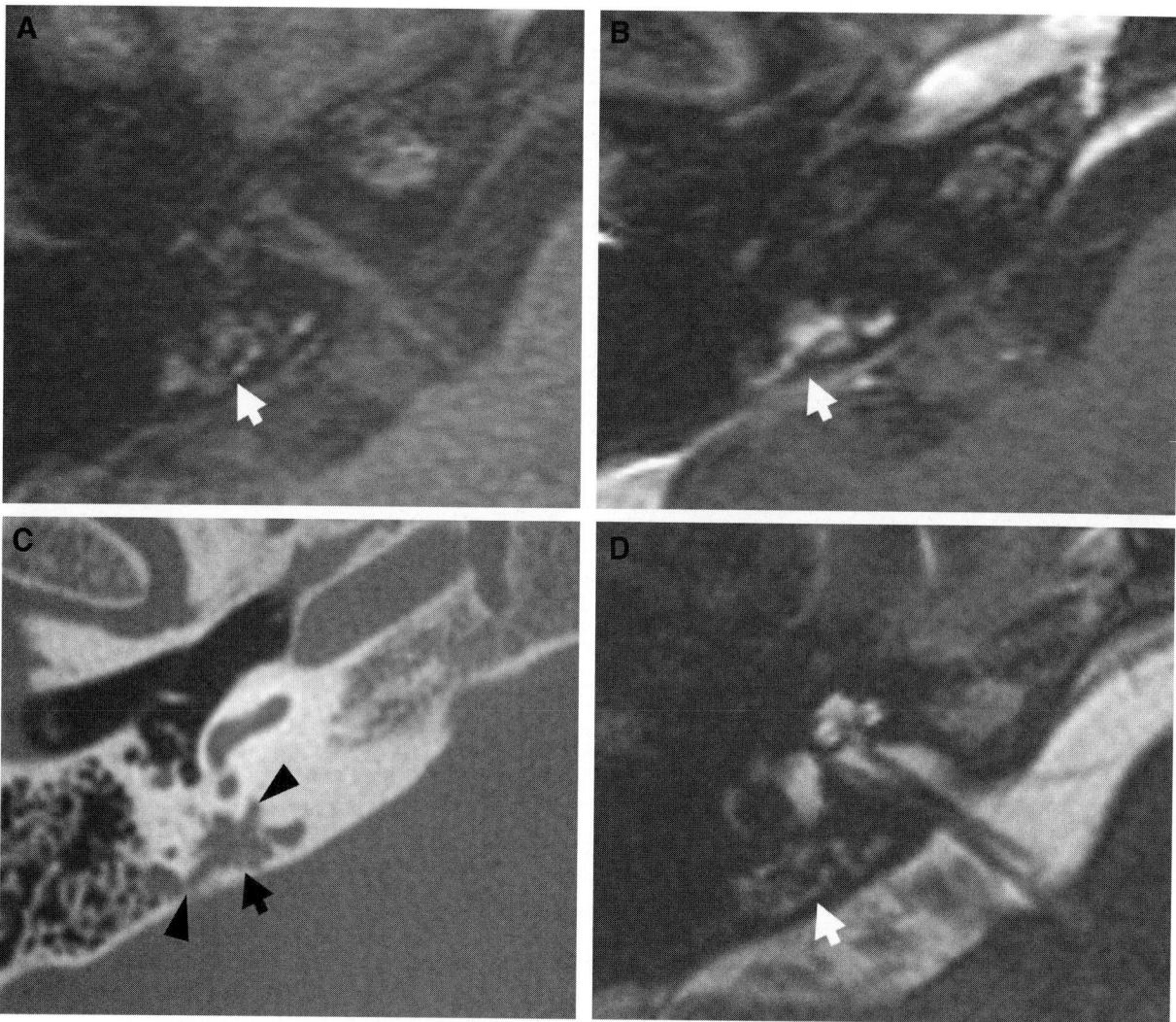

Figure 134.24 Endolymphatic sac tumor. T1-weighted (T1W) precontrast **(A)** and postcontrast **(B)** magnetic resonance image (MRI) show a hyperintense enhancing lesion (*white arrow,* **B**) in the right petrous bone at the expected position of the endolymphatic sac. Note hyperintensity (*white arrows,* **A, D**) on precontrast T1W **(A)** and T2-weighted (T2W)**(D)** MRI caused by hemorrhagic and proteinaceous elements of the tumor. Computed tomography demonstrates erosion of temporal bone (*black arrow—***C**) adjacent to the vestibular aqueduct (*black arrowheads—***C**), which is characteristic of this tumor.

resistance to the petrous apex, disrupting the ossicular chain and exiting through the perigeniculate ganglion region of the facial nerve (Fig. 134.28A). Otic capsule injury is rare. These fractures commonly accompany a ruptured tympanic membrane and hemotympanum. The persistent conductive hearing loss after a closure of tympanic membrane perforation and resolution of hemotympanum implies ossicular injury.

Transverse temporal bone fractures course perpendicular to the long axis of the petrous bone (Fig. 134.28B). They commonly begin near the jugular foramen or foramen magnum and extend to the middle cranial fossa. The fracture line usually involves the bony labyrinth and results in profound sensorineural hearing loss and vertigo.

Facial nerve injury typically occurs at the labyrinthine segment or the perigeniculate ganglion region.

FACIAL NERVE

CT is excellent for demonstrating the facial nerve bony canal within the temporal bone, and it is the modality of choice for evaluating bony erosion around the facial canal by a tumor or inflammation, such as a cholesteatoma (37). MRI depicts the seven segments of the facial nerve itself as it courses from the CPA to the stylomastoid foramen and is excellent for evaluating inflammatory and neoplastic processes of the facial nerve.

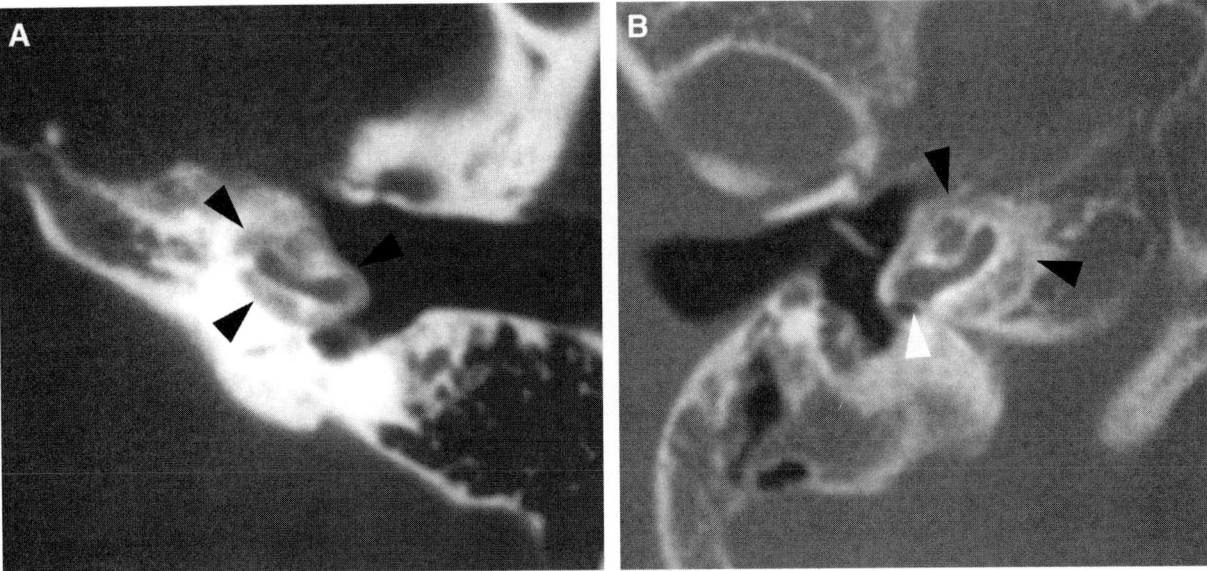

Figure 134.25   Otosclerosis **(A)** vs. osteogenesis imperfecta **(B)**. Marked demineralization (*black arrowheads*—**A,B**) of the otic capsule around the cochlea is seen as radiolucency (decreased attenuation) on axial computed tomography. Note the obliterated round window (*white arrowhead*—**B**). (Figure A modified from Swartz JD, Harnsberger HR. *Imaging of the temporal bone*, 3rd ed. New York: Thieme, 1998, with permission.)

Neoplasms

Facial nerve schwannomas are rare, accounting for less than 1% of all temporal bone tumors (38). Although this neoplasm can arise anywhere along the facial nerve, it is most often identified near the geniculate ganglion. As with other schwannomas, the facial nerve schwannoma en-

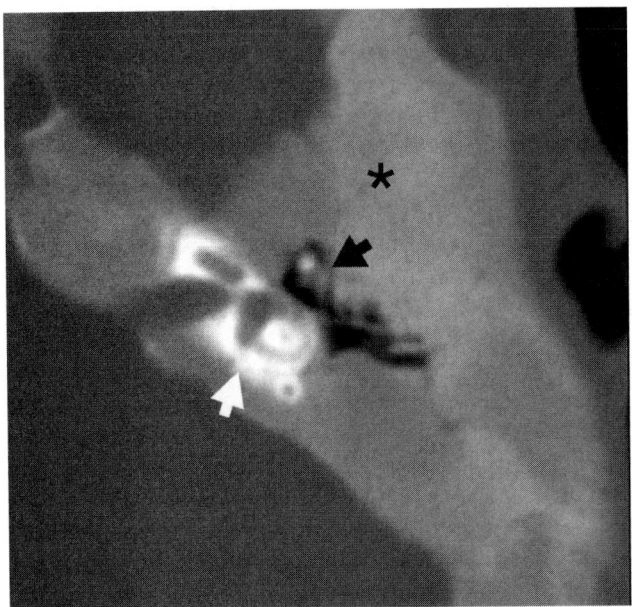

Figure 134.26   Fibrous dysplasia. Characteristic "ground glass" appearance of fibrous dysplasia on axial computed tomography (*asterisk*). Note that the otic capsule is spared (*white arrow*) and that the dysplastic bone encroaches upon the ossicles in the epitympanum (*black arrrow*).

hances homogenously on postcontrast T1W MRI. Because the tumor is slow growing, it may be identified by a well-corticated expansion of the geniculate fossa on CT, without frank erosion.

A hemangioma of the facial nerve is a nonencapsulated vascular lesion that most commonly originates at the level of the geniculate ganglion (38). Unlike the facial nerve schwannoma, the hemangioma presents with facial paresis when the lesion is small. CT findings of a facial nerve hemangioma are a soft tissue mass in the perigeniculate area with irregular, poorly defined, bony margins or spicules of bone within the lesion (39). The MRI shows enhancing lesions that are usually hypo- to isointense on T1W images, and hyperintense on T2W images.

Many malignancies such as squamous cell carcinoma or adenoid cystic carcinoma can extend into the temporal bone along the facial nerve. Although CT may demonstrate an enlarged canal, contrast-enhanced MRI is considered more sensitive in defining this perineural extension (Fig. 134.7B).

Inflammation

An acute onset of facial nerve palsy of unknown etiology is usually considered to be Bell palsy, and imaging evaluation is typically deferred unless the palsy does not resolve in two months, is recurrent, or is slowly progressive. When Bell palsy is imaged during the acute phase, pathologic enhancement of the facial nerve may be seen (Fig. 134.29). Because the normal geniculate ganglion and the anterior tympanic segments often enhance on MRI, this normal enhancement should not be mistaken for pathology (37).

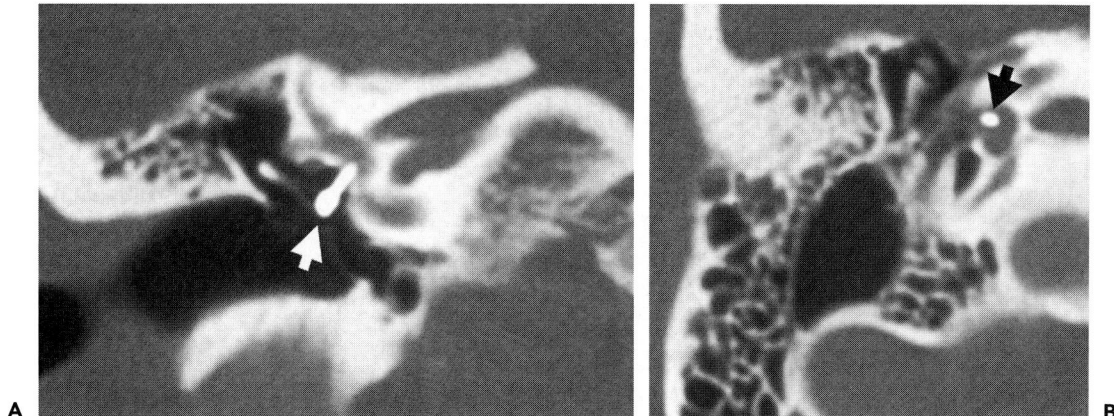

Figure 134.27   Improperly sized stapes prosthesis. Coronal computed tomography (CT)**(A)** shows stainless steel bucket stapes prosthesis (*white arrow—***A**) excessively protruding into the vestibule. Axial CT **(B)** shows the tip of the prosthesis deeply embedded in the vestibule (*black arrow—***B**).

Focal enhancement of the facial nerve in the distal portion of the IAC is, therefore, a distinctive finding in Bell palsy.

VASCULAR ANOMALIES AND DISEASES

Pulsatile tinnitus often prompts imaging to identify vascular anomalies or temporal bone pathology that may be responsible (40). In addition to MRI, MR angiography may help define anomalous vasculature, and MR venography may identify venous thrombosis. Objective tinnitus should prompt evaluation with catheter angiography when clinical suspicion is high for a vascular lesion such as dural arteriovenous fistulas.

Normal Vascular Variants

When the cervical portion of the internal carotid artery fails to develop, an enlarged inferior tympanic artery enters the middle ear through the tympanic canaliculus to join the caroticotympanic artery to form the horizontal petrous portion of the internal carotid artery (41). This aberrant internal carotid artery crosses the mesotympanum, and can be easily mistaken as a glomus tumor by otoscopic exam. This anomaly is commonly associated with persistent stapedial artery. On CT, portions of the bony carotid canal are absent, namely the vertical segment and the posterolateral wall of the horizontal segment (Fig. 134.30). The anterior tympanic segment of the facial nerve canal can be also enlarged because of an associated persistent stapedial artery.

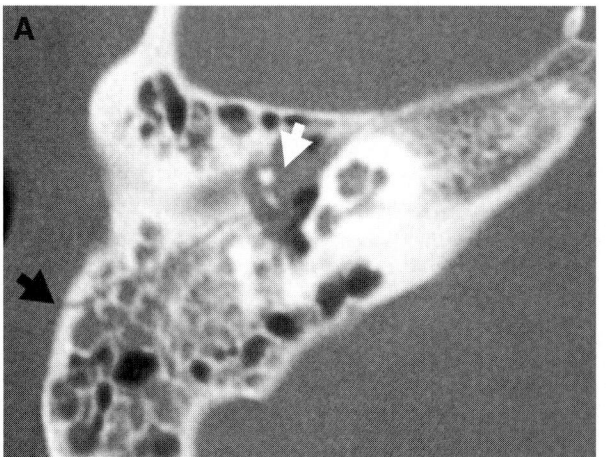
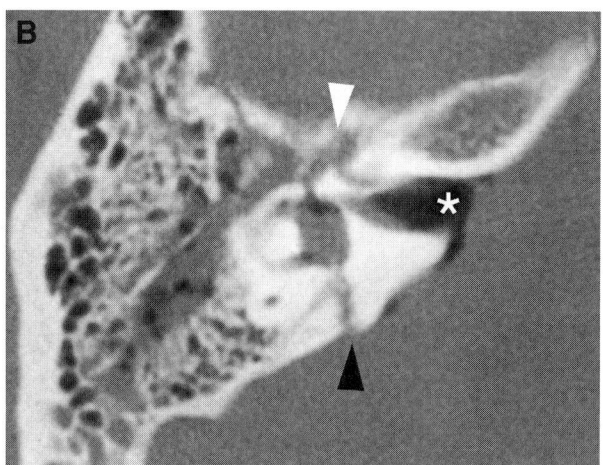

Figure 134.28   Longitudinal **(A)** vs. transverse **(B)** fractures of the temporal bone. In the longitudinal fracture **(A)**, a fracture line begins in the lateral mastoid (*black arrow*) and parallels the long axis of the temporal bone. The ossicular chain is disrupted and laterally displaced (*white arrow*). The otic capsule is spared. In contrast, the transverse fracture (*black arrowhead*, **B**) is perpendicular to the long axis of the temporal bone. The fracture line extends through the otic capsule (*white arrowhead*). Note the low attenuation of air in the labyrinth and internal auditory canal (*asterisk*), and bony fragments (*black arrowhead*) in the facial canal.

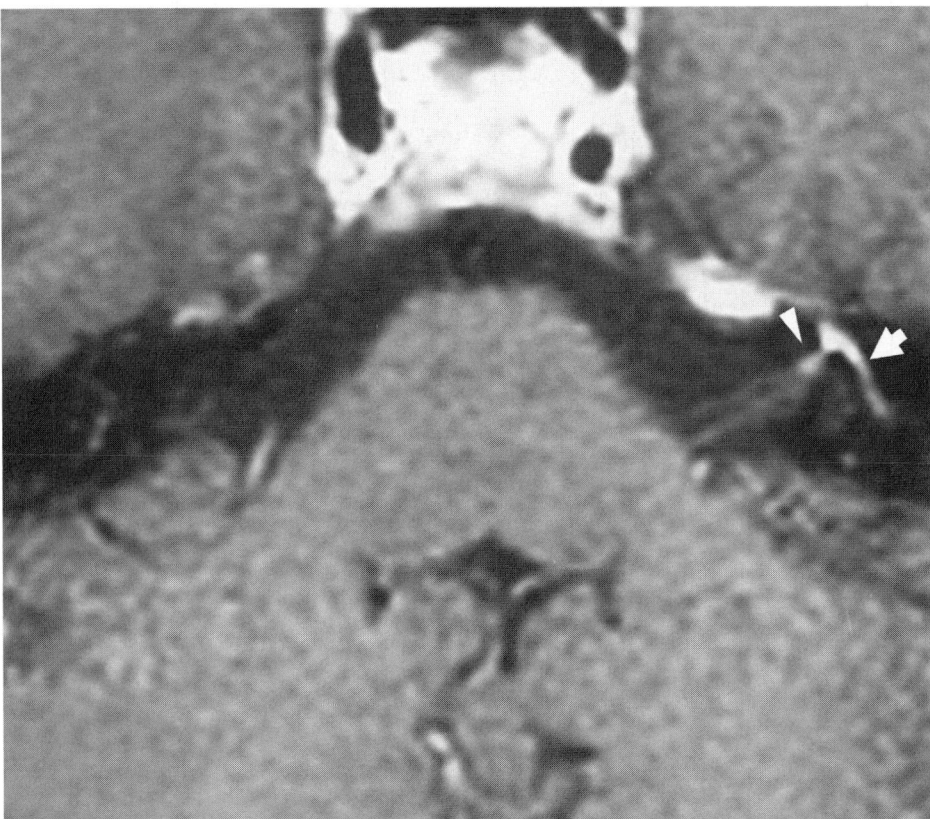

Figure 134.29 Idiopathic facial nerve paralysis (Bell palsy). T1-weighted (T1W) postcontrast magnetic resonance image (MRI) reveals abnormal enhancement of the labyrinthine segment of the left facial nerve (*white arrowhead*). The geniculate ganglion and the tympanic segment (*white arrow*) of the left facial nerve also demonstrate an abnormal enhancement pattern.

On MRA and conventional angiography, the aberrant internal carotid artery appears to be more posteriorly and laterally displaced than the normal internal carotid artery.

The persistent stapedial artery is rare and occurs when the second branchial artery fails to regress by the third month of gestation (41). In the middle ear, it courses between the stapes crura and along the anterior tympanic segment of the facial nerve canal to exit the facial hiatus and forms the middle meningeal artery. On CT, the foramen spinosum is absent, and the anterior tympanic segment of facial canal is enlarged (Fig. 134.30).

An asymmetrically enlarged jugular bulb occurs most commonly on the right; the cortical margin around the jugular foramen is preserved. A jugular bulb is considered to be high riding if its superior limit is above the floor of the IAC. When the bone covering a high-riding jugular bulb is dehiscent, it can present as a vascular mass behind the tympanic membrane. A jugular diverticulum is suspected when a superior part of the jugular bulb bulges outward from the lumen. Schwannoma of lower cranial nerves can produce smooth enlargement of the jugular foramen margins on CT scans, and its uniformly enhancement on contrast T1W MRI easily distinguish it from the normal variant enlarged jugular bulb.

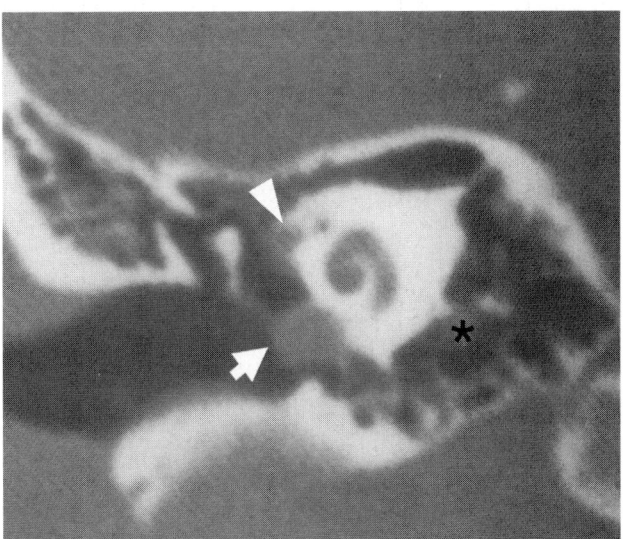

Figure 134.30 Aberrant internal carotid artery and persistent stapedial artery. Coronal computed tomography shows a hypotympanic mass (*white arrow*) consistent with an aberrant internal carotid artery. Note the tympanic segment of the facial nerve canal is enlarged (*white arrowhead*) because of the presence of a persistent stapedial artery. Note the absence of the vertical portion of the internal carotid artery in its expected location under the cochlea (*asterisk*). (Modified from Swartz JD, Harnsberger HR. *Imaging of the temporal bone*, 3rd ed. New York: Thieme, 1998, with permission.)

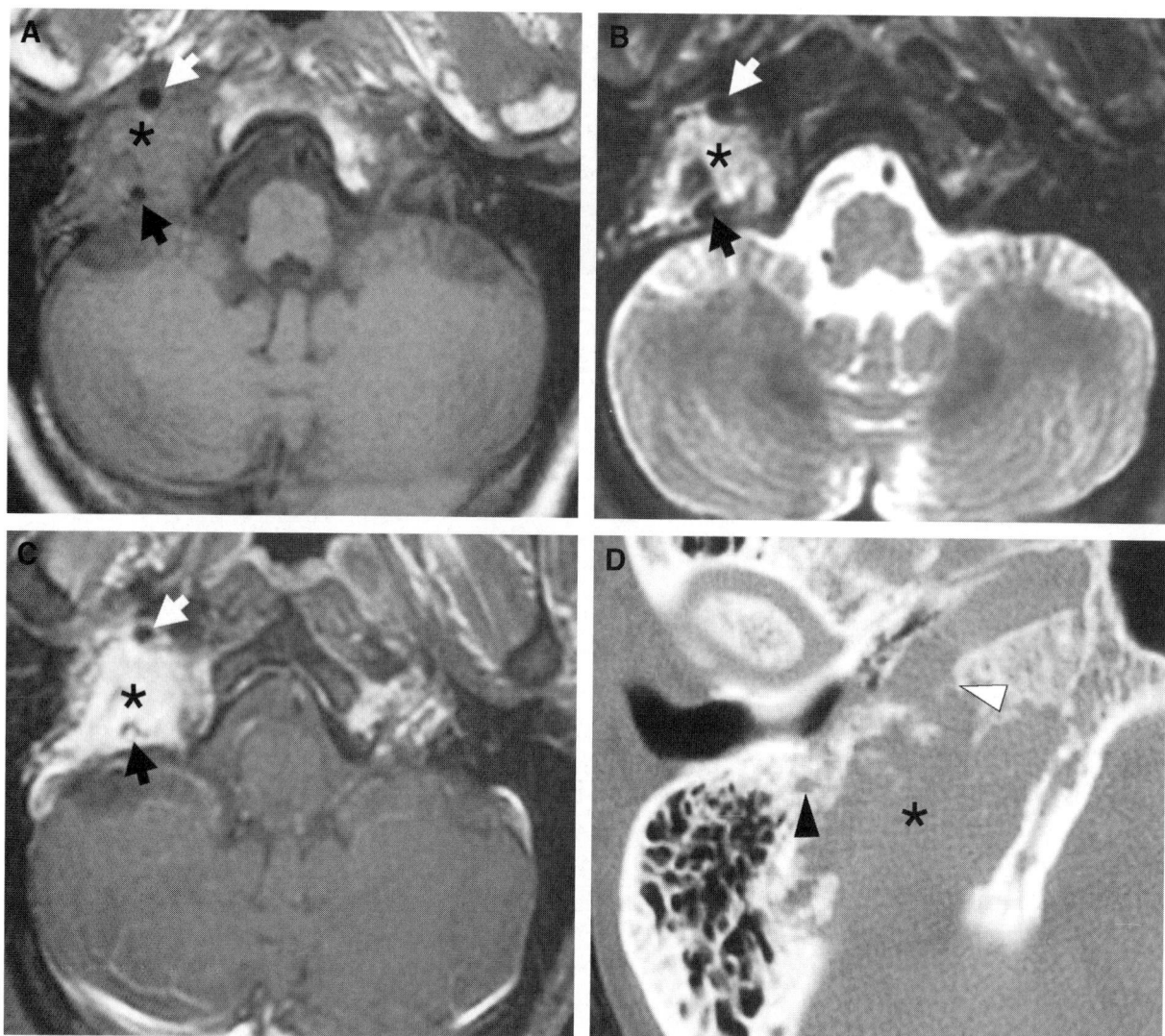

Figure 134.31 Glomus jugulare. A mass is present in the jugular foramen (*black asterisks*). It is hypointense on T1-weighted magnetic resonance image (T1W MRI) **(A)**, and hyperintense on T2-weighted magnetic resonance image (T2W MRI) **(B)**, and enhances dramatically on postcontrast T1W MRI **(C)**. Note the anterior displacement of the carotid flow void (*white arrows*) and a large flow void posteriorly (*black arrows*) within the tumor. Axial computed tomography **(D)** shows irregular bony erosion extending into the petrous portion of carotid artery canal (*white arrowhead*). Note the vertical segment of the facial nerve just lateral to the tumor (*black arrowhead*).

Vascular Neoplasms

A paraganglioma of the temporal bone is the most common tumor associated with pulsatile tinnitus (20,42). This tumor arises from the glomus bodies of the glossopharyngeal and vagus nerves, and so is also referred to as a "glomus tumor." These lesions usually grow by local invasion along paths of least resistance, such as air cells, vascular channels, and foramina. Multiple glomus tumors can be found, especially in familial cases. MRI can best demonstrate the soft tissue extent of the tumor, especially when intracranial extension is suspected (Fig. 134.31). Because these tumors are extremely vascu-

lar, they vigorously enhance with contrast. On T2W MRI, rapid flow in intratumoral vessels appear as black "flow voids," resulting in a characteristic "salt and pepper" appearance in larger tumors. CT is extremely helpful for obtaining information on bony surgical landmarks and extent of bony erosion (Fig. 134.31). CT can detect subtle bony changes in hypotympanum and distinguish between the glomus jugulare from glomus tympanicum confined to the middle ear. For large glomus jugulare tumors, angiography is performed before a surgery to delineate the vascular supply of the tumor, search for multicentric tumors, and preoperatively embolize the tumor, if feasible.

Other Vascular-Related Conditions

A dural arteriovenous fistula is an acquired artery-to-vein shunt in the dura matter and can lead to intracranial hypertension, cerebral hemorrhage, and focal neurologic deficits. When the thrombosed dural sinus recanalizes, a direct arteriovenous connection can be formed between the meningeal branches of the external carotid artery and the recanalized dural venous sinus. MRI or MRA may not be sensitive enough to detect a small dural arteriovenous fistula. In patients with objective pulsatile tinnitus, selective angiography of the external carotid artery may need to be performed to detect a vascular fistula (43). Intra-arterial embolization may be required for treatment. Petrous internal carotid artery aneurysm is a rare cause of pulsatile tinnitus. The aneurysm can produce smooth expansion of the horizontal carotid canal on CT scan and complex MR signals on T1W MRI from rapidly flowing blood in the lumen and the presence of thrombus.

INTERNAL AUDITORY CANAL AND CEREBELLOPONTINE ANGLE LESIONS

The IAC contains the vestibulocochlear nerve, facial nerve, nervus intermedius, labyrinthine artery, and sometimes a loop of the anterior inferior cerebellar artery (AICA). The IAC is a lateral extension of the CPA cistern, and so is lined by dura and filled with CSF. MRI is the gold standard for evaluating the IAC and CPA and has also replaced the auditory brainstem evoked response (ABER) as the method of choice in screening patients with unilateral SNHL for vestibular schwannoma (44). In this context, various forms of a limited MRI have been proposed as sufficient for screening purposes (45). However, limited studies have the potential drawback of failing to detect intralabyrinthine and inflammatory lesions as well as central nervous system (CNS) pathology (46). Therefore, a complete contrast-enhanced MRI study of IAC and brain is recommended for patients with sensorineural hearing loss or vertigo, with or without associated neurologic findings (47).

Neoplasms

Formerly known as "acoustic neuroma," the most common tumor (85%) of the CPA is the vestibular schwannoma (VS), a benign tumor that arises from the vestibular portion of the eighth cranial nerve (47). Bilateral VS is the hallmark of neurofibromatosis type 2. Typically, the VS presents as progressive SNHL and tinnitus, but 10% of patients may present with sudden SNHL.

Schwannomas are usually isointense to hypointense to brain on T1W and isointense to slightly hyperintense on T2W. Enhanced T1W images show a homogeneously enhancing mass centered near the porous acusticus with an IAC extension (Fig. 134.32). The classic configuration is a conical projection from the IAC, with exophytic growth into the CPA. Both high-resolution T2W and contrast-enhanced T1W techniques can detect extremely small lesions, as small as 2 mm in size (Fig. 134.33). Note that a segmental enhancement of the vestibular nerve may occur with a neuritis, mimicking a small VS. Both cystic and hemorrhagic areas may be seen associated with larger tumors, but calcification is rare (47).

The main differential consideration in this region is the meningioma, which accounts for less than 10% of CPA tumors (47). Signal characteristics of meningiomas and schwannomas are quite similar, isointense to brain on

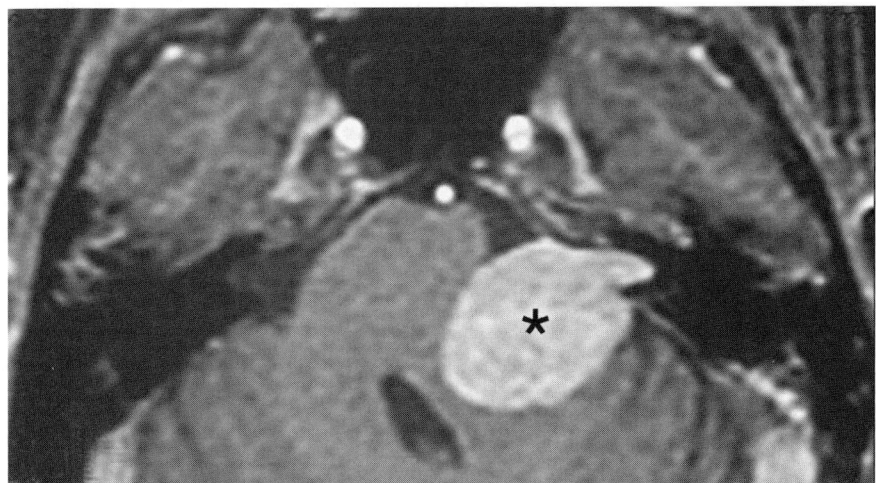

Figure 134.32 Vestibular schwannoma (VS). T1-weighted postcontrast magnetic resonance image (MRI) shows a large enhancing mass (asterisk) in the left cerebellopontine angle (CPA), extending out from the internal auditory canal (IAC). Note the compression of the cerebellum and brainstem, and distortion of the seventh ventricle.

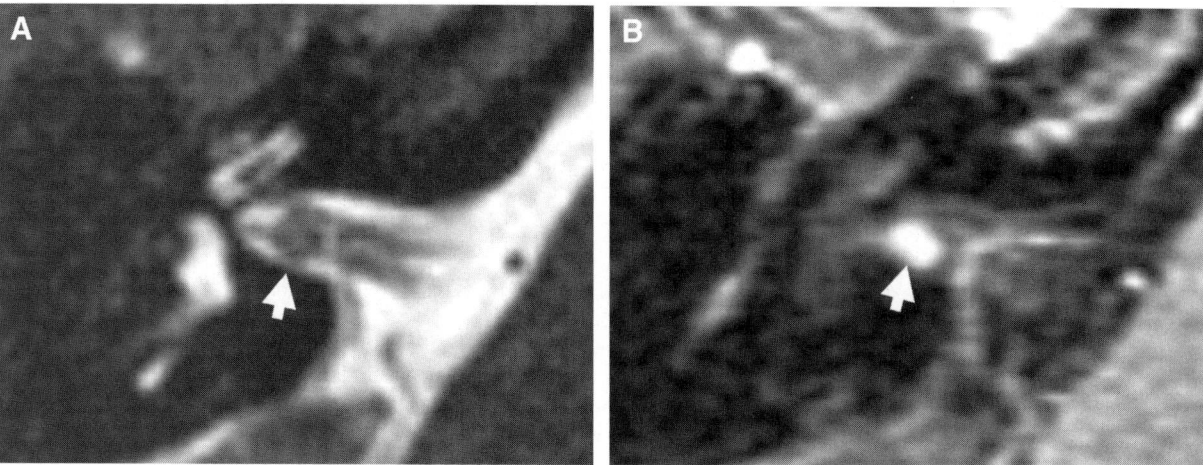

Figure 134.33 Vestibular schwannoma (VS). Asymptomatic 2.5 mm VS in a patient with neurofibromatosis type 2. It is seen as a "filling defect" on fast imaging employing steady-state acquisition (FIESTA) (*white arrow*—**A**) and more conspicuously as an enhancing lesion on postcontrast T1-weighted magnetic resonance image (T1W MRI) (*white arrow*—**B**).

T1W and T2W MRI and both homogeneously enhanced. Meningioma tends to have T1WMR signals more similar to brain parenchyma than schwannoma. Other distinguishing characteristics include the presence of internal cysts in large VS, the broad-based dural attachment and "dural tail" of the meningioma, and site of origin (IAC versus posterior petrous bone) (Fig. 134.34). Dense calcification (hypointense on T2W images) may be seen in the meningioma. Note that CT is much more sensitive than MRI for the detection of calcification.

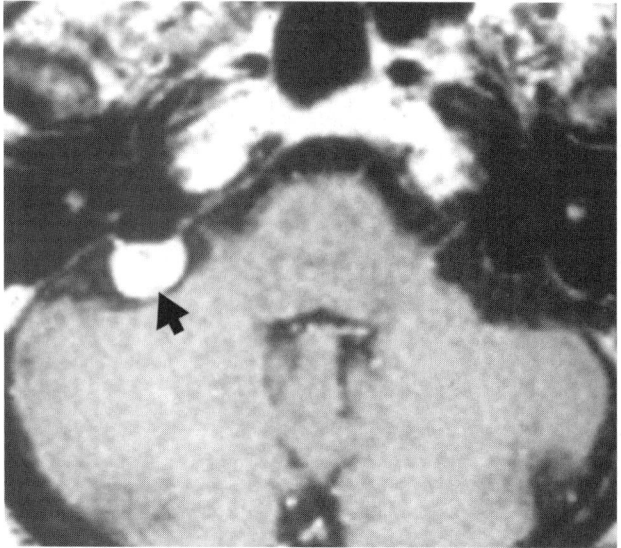

Figure 134.34 Meningioma. T1-weighted postcontrast magnetic resonance image demonstrates a uniformly enhancing mass (*black arrow*) in the right cerebellopontine angle. Note the broad-based dural attachment on the petrous bone and small dural tails.

Congenital Lesions

Cystic lesions of the CPA include the epidermoid tumor or cyst (also known as congenital cholesteatoma) and the arachnoid cyst. (48). Both are recognized by mass effect and distortion of neural structures, as their signal appears identical to that of CSF on standard T1W and T2W images. Neither lesion enhances. Arachnoid cysts arise from duplication or entrapment of arachnoid membranes, and their content truly matches that of CSF. Epidermoids, in contrast, contain stratified squamous epithelium, and certain sequences MRI techniques such as diffusion-weighted imaging, FIESTA and FLAIR (fluid-attenuated inversion recovery) may reveal signal that does not follow that of CSF, hence distinguishing these lesions from arachnoid cysts (Fig. 134.35). Epidermoids tend to insinuate into clefts and dissect into natural tissue planes.

Another congenital lesion of the CPA and IAC is the lipoma, identified by the hyperintense fat signal on T1W images (49). Because of this, it can easily be misinterpreted as an enhancing lesion (e.g., VS) if the precontrast T1W image is not inspected. Suppression of MR by applying a fat saturation pulse will confirm its diagnosis (Fig. 134.36).

Leptomeningeal Disease

Leptomeningeal disease involving the IAC may represent infection, inflammation, or neoplasm, and the MRI findings of leptomeningeal enhancement as seen on postcontrast MRI is nonspecific (50). Although FLAIR may be more sensitive than T1W imaging in the detection of meningeal disease, high FLAIR signal is often seen in the CPA because of normal CSF pulsations. Therefore, high signal on FLAIR in the CPA should be interpreted with

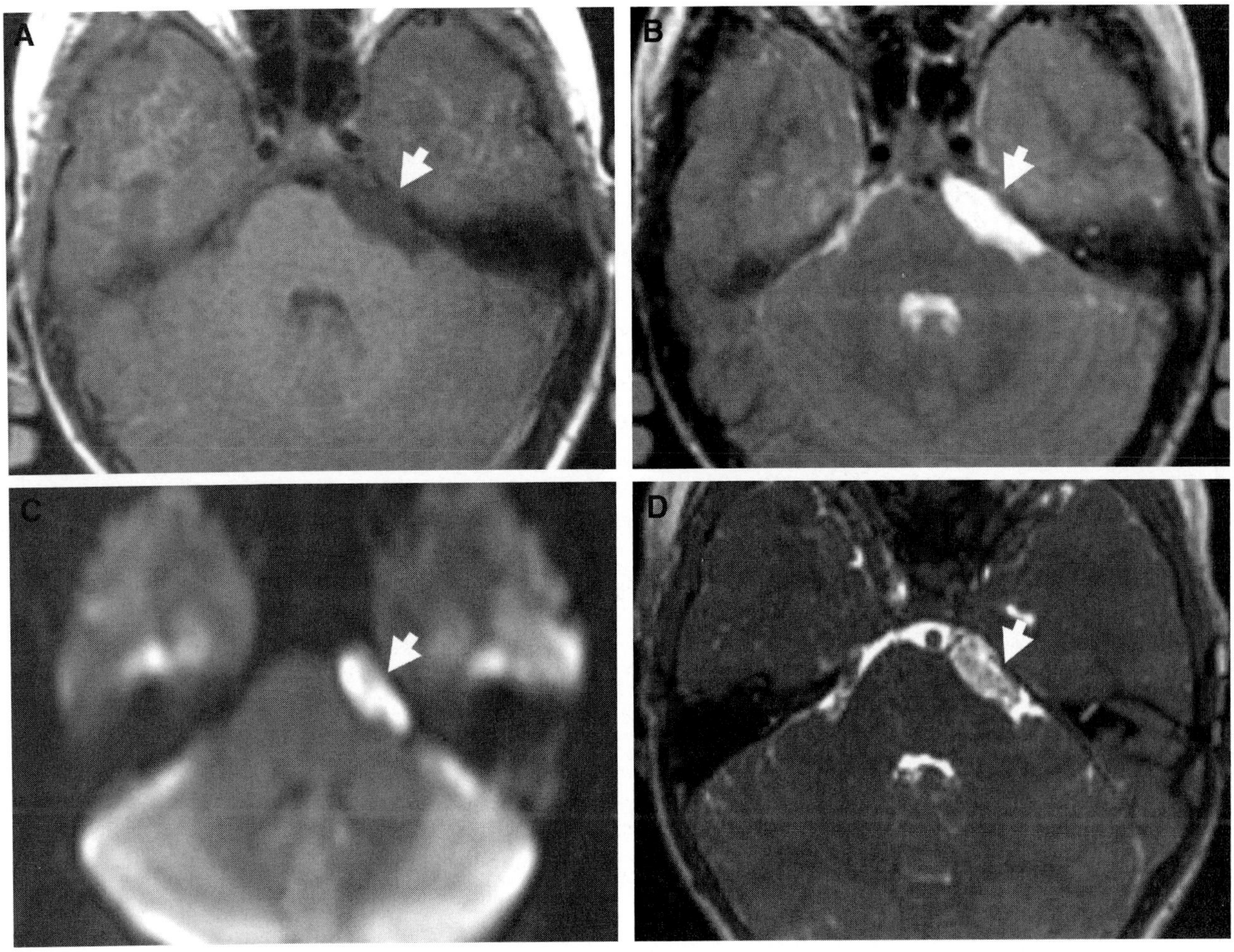

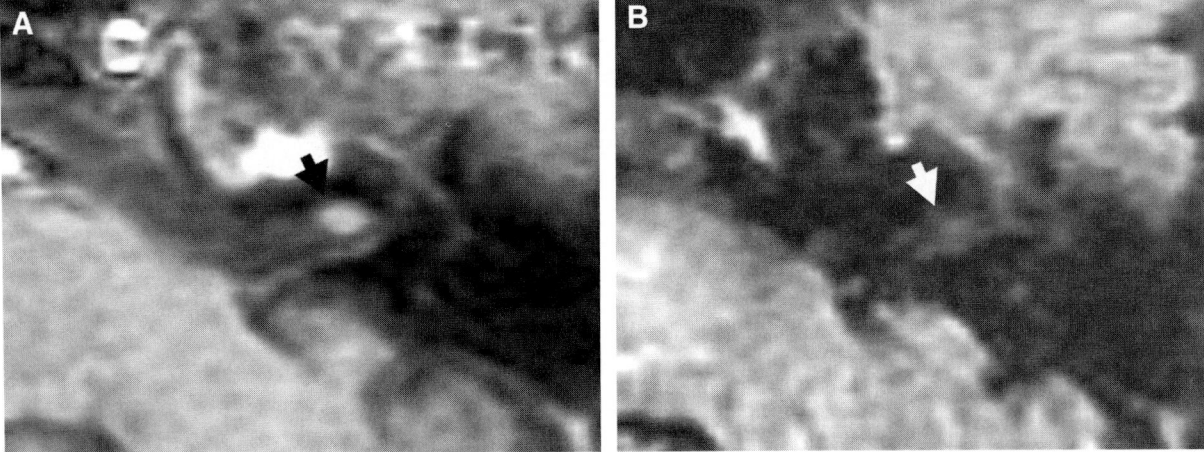

Figure 134.35 Epidermoid. Magnetic resonance image shows enlargement of the left cerebello-pontine angle (CPA) (*white arrows*), with mass effect on the brainstem. Signal matches that of cerebrospinal fluid (CSF) on T1-weighted **(A)** and T2-weighted **(B)** images. Hyperintensity on diffusion-weighted imaging **(C)** and hypointensity on fast imaging employing steady-state acquisition (FIESTA) **(D)** differentiates the epidermoid from an arachnoid cyst.

Figure 134.36 Internal auditory canal (IAC) lipoma. A hyperintense lesion (*black arrow*—**A**) in the anterior aspect of the right IAC is seen on noncontrast T1-weighted magnetic resonance image. FLAIR with fat saturation completely suppresses signal from the lesion, confirming lipoma (*white arrow*—**B**).

caution. Enhancement of the meninges entering the CPA is also commonly seen with intracranial hypotension following intracranial surgeries or lumbar punctures.

HIGHLIGHTS

- In the evaluation of hearing loss, CT is best suited for evaluating atypical CHL, particularly in congenital cases, osteodystrophies, or for the purposes of surgical planning.
- In the evaluation of hearing loss, MRI is best suited for evaluating retrocochlear SNHL. MRI is used for routine screening for VS in cases of asymmetric SNHL.
- CT is used to evaluate bone integrity as an indicator of various pathologies such as cholesteatoma, coalescent mastoiditis, malignancies, and trauma.
- Both CT and high-resolution T2W MRI demonstrate the morphology of congenital labyrinth malformations. When considering cochlear implantation, MRI additionally provides information on the presence of eighth cranial nerve and patency of the cochlear duct.
- Intralabyrinthine pathologies are sometimes demonstrable using high-resolution T2W or contrast-enhanced T1W MRI.
- MRI is essential for evaluating intracranial lesions as well as temporal bone and skull base lesions that may have intracranial extension. MRI characterizes the extent of disease and provides differential diagnoses based on MR signal characteristics.

REFERENCES

1. Alexander AE Jr, Caldemeyer KS, Rigby P. Clinical and surgical application of reformatted high-resolution CT of the temporal bone. *Neuroimag Clin North Am* 1998;8:631–650.
2. Sabnis EV, Mafee MF, Chen R, et al. Magnetic resonance imaging of the normal temporal bone. *Top Magn Reson Imaging* 2000;11:2–9.
3. Casselman JW, Kuhweide R, Ampe W, et al. Pathology of the membranous labyrinth: comparison of T1- and T2-weighted and gadolinium-enhanced spin-echo and 3DFT-CISS imaging. *AJNR Am J Neuroradiol* 1993;14:59–69.
4. Syms AJ, Petermann GW. Magnetic resonance imaging of stapes prostheses. *Am J Otol* 2000;21:494–498.
5. Wackym PA, Michel MA, Prost RW, et al. Effect of magnetic resonance imaging on internal magnet strength in Med-El Combi 40+ cochlear implants. *Laryngoscope* 2004;114:1355–1361.
6. Heller JW, Brackmann DE, Tucci DL, et al. Evaluation of MRI compatibility of the modified nucleus multichannel auditory brainstem and cochlear implants. *Am J Otol* 1996;17:724–729.
7. Yeakley JW, Jahrsdoerfer RA. CT evaluation of congenital aural atresia: what the radiologist and surgeon need to know. *J Comput Assist Tomogr* 1996;20:724–731.
8. Jahrsdoerfer RA, Yeakley JW, Aguilar EA, et al. Grading system for the selection of patients with congenital aural atresia. *Am J Otol* 1992;13:6–12.
9. Persaud RA, Hajioff D, Thevasagayam MS, et al. Keratosis obturans and external ear canal cholesteatoma: how and why we should distinguish between these conditions. *Clin Otolaryngol* 2004;29:577–581.
10. Agarwal A, Deschler DG, Baker KB. Exostoses of the external auditory canal. *Am J Otol* 1999;20:807–808.
11. Moody SA, Hirsch BE, Myers EN. Squamous cell carcinoma of the external auditory canal: an evaluation of a staging system. *Am J Otol* 2000;21:582–588.
12. Sreepada GS, Kwartler JA. Skull base osteomyelitis secondary to malignant otitis externa. *Curr Opin Otolaryngol Head Neck Surg* 2003;11:316–323.
13. Seabold JE, Simonson TM, Weber PC, et al. Cranial osteomyelitis: diagnosis and follow-up with In-111 white blood cell and Tc-99m methylene diphosphonate bone SPECT, CT, and MR imaging. *Radiology* 1995;196:779–788.
14. Antonelli PJ, Garside JA, Mancuso AA, et al. Computed tomography and the diagnosis of coalescent mastoiditis. *Otolaryngol Head Neck Surg* 1999;120:350–354.
15. Wetmore RF. Complications of otitis media. *Pediatr Ann* 2000;29:637–646.
16. Van den Bosch MA, Vos JA, de Letter MA, et al. MRI findings in a child with sigmoid sinus thrombosis following mastoiditis. *Pediatr Radiol* 2003;33:877–879.
17. Pisaneschi MJ, Langer B. Congenital cholesteatoma and cholesterol granuloma of the temporal bone: role of magnetic resonance imaging. *Top Magn Reson Imaging* 2000;11:87–97.
18. Yates PD, Flood LM, Banerjee A, et al. CT scanning of middle ear cholesteatoma: what does the surgeon want to know? *Br J Radiol* 2002;75:847–852.
19. Aikele P, Kittner T, Offergeld C, et al. Diffusion-weighted MR imaging of cholesteatoma in pediatric and adult patients who have undergone middle ear surgery. *AJR Am J Roentgenol* 2003;181:261–265.
20. Mafee MF, Raofi B, Kumar A, et al. Glomus faciale, glomus jugulare, glomus tympanicum, glomus vagale, carotid body tumors, and simulating lesions. Role of MR imaging. *Radiol Clin North Am* 2000;38:1059–1076.
21. Potsic WP, Korman SB, Samadi DS, et al. Congenital cholesteatoma: 20 years' experience at The Children's Hospital of Philadelphia. *Otolaryngol Head Neck Surg* 2002;126:409–414.
22. Casselman JW, Offeciers EF, De Foer B, et al. CT and MR imaging of congenital abnormalities of the inner ear and internal auditory canal. *Eur J Radiol* 2001;40:94–104.
23. Davidson HC, Harnsberger HR, Lemmerling MM, et al. MR evaluation of vestibulocochlear anomalies associated with large endolymphatic duct and sac. *AJNR Am J Neuroradiol* 1999;20:1435–1441.
24. Kumar G, Castillo M, Buchman CA. X-linked stapes gusher: CT findings in one patient. *AJNR Am J Neuroradiol* 2003;24:1130–1132.
25. Belden CJ, Weg N, Minor LB, et al. CT evaluation of bone dehiscence of the superior semicircular canal as a cause of sound-and/or pressure-induced vertigo. *Radiology* 2003;226:337–343.
26. Hegarty JL, Patel S, Fischbein N, et al. The value of enhanced magnetic resonance imaging in the evaluation of endocochlear disease. *Laryngoscope* 2002;112:8–17.
27. Weissman JL, Curtin HD, Hirsch BE, et al. High signal from the otic labyrinth on unenhanced magnetic resonance imaging. *AJNR Am J Neuroradiol* 1992;13:1183–1187.
28. Gleeson TG, Lacy PD, Bresnihan M, et al. High resolution computed tomography and magnetic resonance imaging in the preoperative assessment of cochlear implant patients. *J Laryngol Otol* 2003;117:692–695.
29. Kennedy RJ, Shelton C, Salzman KL, et al. Intralabyrinthine schwannomas: diagnosis, management, and a new classification system. *Otol Neurotol* 2004; 25:160–167.
30. Mukherji SK, Albernaz VS, Lo WW, et al. Papillary endolymphatic sac tumors: CT, MR imaging, and angiographic findings in 20 patients. *Radiology* 1997;202:801–808.
31. Lonser RR, Kim HJ, Butman JA, et al. Tumors of the endolymphatic sac in von Hippel-Lindau disease. *N Engl J Med* 2004;350:2481–2486.
32. Valvassori GE. Imaging of otosclerosis. *Otolaryngol Clin North Am* 1993;26:359–371.
33. Alkadhi H, Rissmann D, Kollias SS. Osteogenesis imperfecta of the temporal bone: CT and MR imaging in Van der Hoeve-de Kleyn syndrome. *AJNR Am J Neuroradiol* 2004;25:1106–1109.
34. Kosling S, Bootz F. CT and MR imaging after middle ear surgery. *Eur J Radiol* 2001;40:113–118.

35. Xu J, Xu SA, Cohen LT, et al. Cochlear view: postoperative radiography for cochlear implantation. *Am J Otol* 2000;21:49–56.
36. Swartz JD. Temporal bone trauma. *Semin Ultrasound CT MR* 2001;22:219–228.
37. Jager L, Reiser M. CT and MR imaging of the normal and pathologic conditions of the facial nerve. *Eur J Radiol* 2001;40:133–146.
38. Falcioni M, Russo A, Taibah A, et al. Facial nerve tumors. *Otol Neurotol* 2003;24:942–947.
39. Salib RJ, Tziambazis E, McDermott AL, et al. The crucial role of imaging in detection of facial nerve haemangiomas. *J Laryngol Otol* 2001;115:510–513.
40. Sismanis A. Pulsatile tinnitus. *Otolaryngol Clin North Am* 2003;36:389–402, viii.
41. Lau CC, Oghalai JS, Jackler RK. Combination of aberrant internal carotid artery and persistent stapedial artery. *Otol Neurotol* 2004;25:850–851.
42. Noujaim SE, Pattekar MA, Cacciarelli A, et al. Paraganglioma of the temporal bone: role of magnetic resonance imaging versus computed tomography. *Top Magn Reson Imaging* 2000;11: 108–122.
43. Shin EJ, Lalwani AK, Dowd CF. Role of angiography in the evaluation of patients with pulsatile tinnitus. *Laryngoscope* 2000; 110:1916–1920.
44. Schmidt RJ, Sataloff RT, Newman J, et al. The sensitivity of auditory brainstem response testing for the diagnosis of acoustic neuromas. *Arch Otolaryngol Head Neck Surg* 2001;127:19–22.
45. Daniels RL, Swallow C, Shelton C, et al. Causes of unilateral sensorineural hearing loss screened by high-resolution fast spin echo magnetic resonance imaging: review of 1,070 consecutive cases. *Am J Otol* 2000;21:173–180.
46. Annesley-Williams DJ, Laitt RD, Jenkins JP, et al. Magnetic resonance imaging in the investigation of sensorineural hearing loss: is contrast enhancement still necessary? *J Laryngol Otol* 2001;115: 14–21.
47. Swartz JD. Lesions of the cerebellopontine angle and internal auditory canal: diagnosis and differential diagnosis. *Semin Ultrasound CT MR* 2004;25:332–352.
48. Bonneville F, Sarrazin JL, Marsot-Dupuch K, et al. Unusual lesions of the cerebellopontine angle: a segmental approach. *Radiographics* 2001;21:419–438.
49. Bigelow DC, Eisen MD, Smith PG, et al. Lipomas of the internal auditory canal and cerebellopontine angle. *Laryngoscope* 1998;108:1459–1469.
50. Tsuchiya K, Katase S, Yoshino A, et al. FLAIR MR imaging for diagnosing intracranial meningeal carcinomatosis. *AJR Am J Roentgenol* 2001;176:1585–1588.

Infections of the External Ear

135

Christopher J. Linstrom   *Frank E. Lucente*

Otolaryngologists see many patients with infections of the external ear. The infections may be categorized by location and cause, and classified by time course as acute, subacute, and chronic. Before discussing the individual disease processes, we review the normal anatomy and physiology of the external ear.

ANATOMY AND PHYSIOLOGY

The external ear is composed of the auricle and external auditory canal. Both contain elastic cartilage derived from mesoderm and a small amount of subcutaneous tissue, covered by skin with its adnexal appendages (1,2). There is fat but no cartilage in the lobule. The auricle is derived from six hillocks, three each from branchial arches I and II (Fig. 135.1). During normal gestation, the cartilaginous hillocks merge to form the auricle, and with selective growth of the mandible, the auricle rises from its original position near the lateral commissure of the mouth to the temporal area

The external auditory canal is derived from the first ectodermal branchial groove between the mandibular (I) and hyoid (II) arches (2,3). The epithelium lining this groove contacts the endoderm of the first pharyngeal pouch, thus forming the tympanic membrane, the most medial extent of external auditory canal. Connective tissue of mesodermal origin is found between ectoderm and endoderm and becomes the fibrous layer of the tympanic membrane (2). Because of its origin, the external auditory canal, including the lateral surface of the tympanic membrane, is derived from ectoderm and is lined by squamous epithelium.

The process of canalization is complete by about week 12 of gestation, at which time the canal fills with epithelial tissue. The canal ordinarily recanalizes by about week 28 of fetal life (3).

The external auditory canal may be thought of in two sections. The outer 40% is cartilaginous and contains a thin layer of subcutaneous tissue between the skin and cartilage. The inner 60% is osseous, is formed primarily by the tympanic ring, and contains very scant soft tissue between the skin, periosteum, and bone. The average length of the adult external auditory canal is 2.5 cm. Because of the oblique position of the tympanic membrane, the posterosuperior part of the canal is about 6 mm shorter than the anteroinferior portion (1). The junction of the cartilaginous and bony portions of the canal is a narrowed section termed the *isthmus*.

The tragus and antitragus form a partial barrier to the entrance of macroscopic foreign bodies. Laterally to medially, the canal curves slightly superiorly and posteriorly in a gentle S shape. The canal can be thought of as pointing toward the nose; thus, the auricle needs to be pulled gently upward, outward, and backward to straighten the canal for examination. Three macroscopic defense mechanisms protect the external auditory canal and lateral surface of the tympanic membrane: the tragus and antitragus, the skin with its cerumen coat, and the isthmus of the canal.

The skin of the cartilaginous canal contains many hair cells and sebaceous and apocrine glands such as cerumen glands (Fig. 135.2). Together, these three adnexal structures provide a protective function and are termed the *apopilosebaceous unit*. Glandular secretions combine with sloughed squamous epithelium to form an acidic coat of cerumen, one of the primary barriers to infection of the canal. An invagination of the epidermis forms the outer wall of the hair follicle, and the hair shaft forms the inner wall. The follicular canal is the space between these two structures. The alveoli of the sebaceous and apocrine

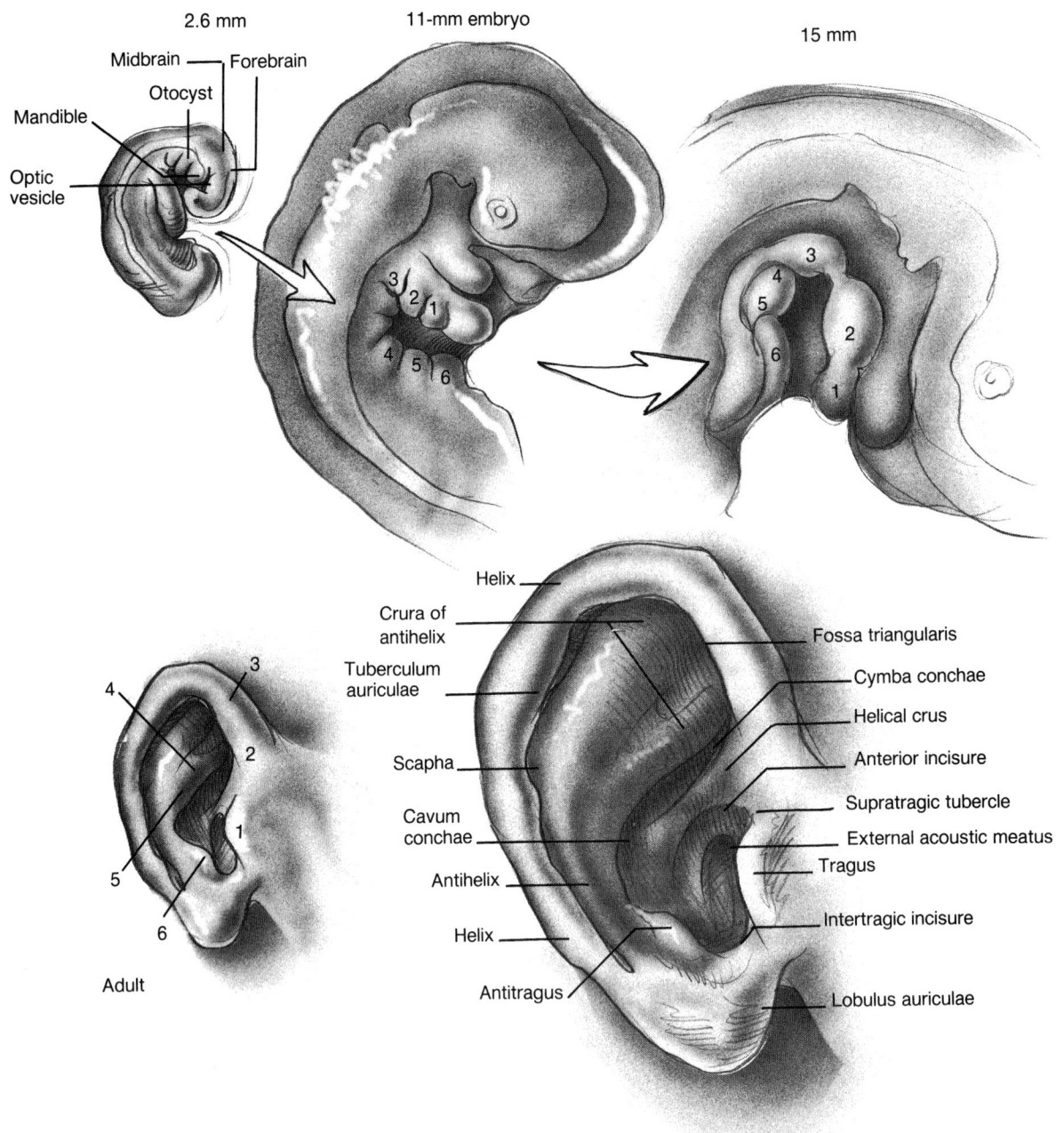

Figure 135.1 The auricle is formed from six auricular hillocks, three each from branchial arches I and II.

glands empty into short, straight excretory ducts, which drain into follicular canals. Obstruction of any part of the ductal system predisposes to infection.

The canal is normally a self-protecting and self-cleansing structure. The cerumen coat gradually works its way past the isthmus to the lateral part of the canal and sloughs externally. Instrumentation and excessive cleansing of the canal disturb this primary protective barrier and may lead to infection. Individual variations in the anatomy of the canal or the consistency of the cerumen produced may predispose some people to wax accumulation.

The canal interfaces on all but its lateral surface. Medially, it is bound by the tympanic membrane and squamosa of the temporal bone, which when intact is a good barrier to the spread of infection. In the presence of a tympanic membrane perforation, infection may spread back and forth from the middle ear cleft to the external auditory canal. The horseshoe-shaped tympanic ring and squamosa separate the canal from the middle cranial fossa. Rarely is this the direct mechanism of intracranial extension of infection. The posterior bony canal serves as the anterior boundary of the mastoid cavity. Several vessels penetrate

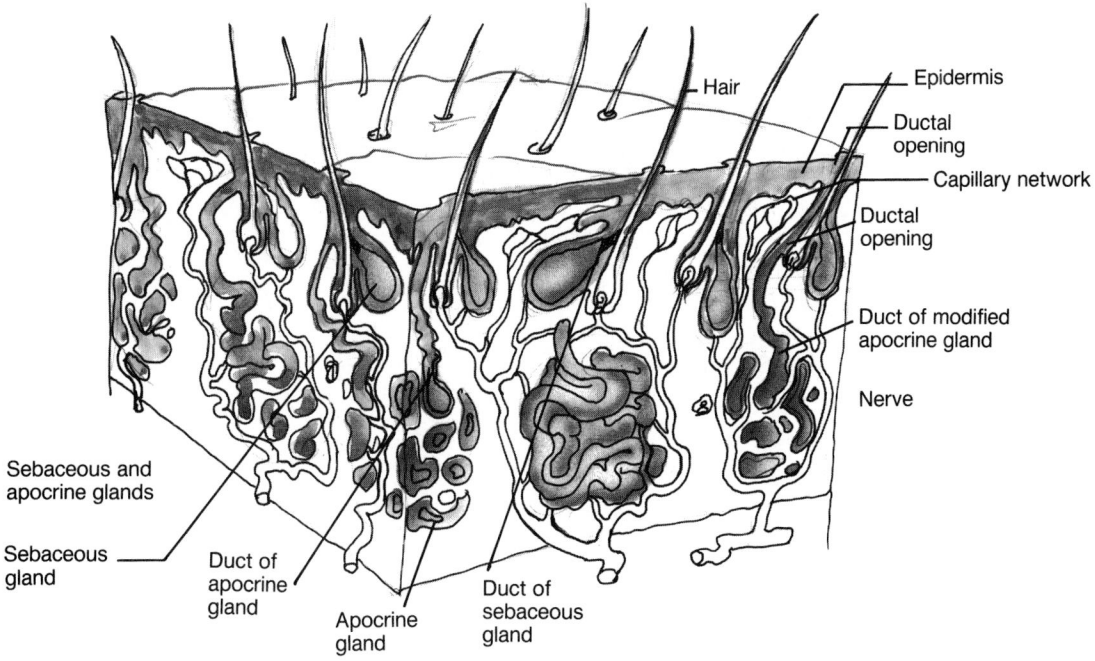

Figure 135.2 Microscopic view of the normal apopilosebaceous unit, demonstrating drainage of the secretions of the sebaceous and modified apocrine glands into the follicular canal of the hair follicle.

the canal, especially along the tympanomastoid suture. These may be involved in the hematogenous extension of infection from the canal to the mastoid segment. Posterior to the cartilaginous canal lies dense connective tissue overlying the mastoid, which may become secondarily infected.

Superiorly, the canal is bound by the infratemporal fossa and base of the skull. Infections extending through the roof of the canal may extend into these structures. Anteriorly, the canal is bordered by the temporomandibular joint and the parotid gland.

The lymphatic drainage of the canal is an important channel for the spread of infection. Anteriorly and superiorly, the canal drains to the preauricular lymphatics in the parotid gland and the superior deep cervical nodes. The inferior portion of the canal drains into the infra-auricular nodes near the angle of the mandible. Posteriorly, the lymphatics drain into the postauricular nodes and the superior deep cervical nodes. The auricle and external auditory canal receive their arterial supply from the superficial temporal and posterior auricular branches of the external carotid artery (1). Venous drainage from the auricle and meatus is via the superficial temporal and posterior auricular veins. The former joins the retromandibular vein, which usually divides and joins both jugular veins; the latter joins the external jugular but may also drain to the sigmoid sinus through the mastoid emissary vein (1).

Sensation to the auricle and external auditory canal is supplied from cutaneous and cranial nerves, with contributions from the auriculotemporal branches of the trigeminal (V), facial (VII), glossopharyngeal (IX), and vagus (X) nerves and the greater auricular nerve from the cervical

plexus (C2–3). The vestigial extrinsic muscles of the ear, anterior, superior, and posterior auricular, are supplied by the facial nerve (VII) (1).

OTITIS EXTERNA

Otitis externa is a spectrum of infection of the external auditory canal. The appearance of the canal varies according to the time course of infection: acute, subacute, or chronic.

Acute otitis externa is an infection of the canal caused by a break in the normal skin or cerumen protective barrier, often occurring in the milieu of elevated humidity and temperature. Although commonly called swimmer's ear, acute otitis externa may be caused by anything that results in the removal of the protective lipid film from the canal, allowing bacteria or fungal organisms to enter the apopilosebaceous unit. It usually begins with itching in the canal and is commonly caused by instrumenting the canal with a cotton swab or fingernail. This temporarily relieves itching but allows proliferation of bacteria in locally macerated skin and sets up an itch-scratch cycle. The warm, dark, moist setting of the canal is now a perfect medium for rapid bacterial growth. Later, pain ensues as the swollen soft tissues of the canal distract the periosteal lining of the bony canal. As the disease progresses, purulent discharge begins, and the auricle and periauricular soft tissues may become involved.

In patients in whom the disease does not resolve after treatment, a subacute or chronic form may occur. This condition may be likened to eczema and is a spectrum of disease ranging from mild drying and scaling of the canal skin to complete obliteration of the canal by chronically infected hypertrophic skin.

History

The history and functional inquiry should include information regarding the length of time, the number of occurrences, the nature and severity of pain, antecedent otologic disease, previous auricular instrumentation or trauma (especially the use of cotton-tipped applicators or forceful aural irrigation), and any predisposing factors such as diabetes or radiotherapy or any condition causing immunosuppression. Any previous otologic or head and neck surgery is noted.

Pain, fullness, itching, and hearing loss are the four major symptoms of external otitis, although not every patient has each symptom (4). Throughout the examination, the examiner should remember the innervation of the external auditory canal and recall that pain from other areas of the upper aerodigestive tract may be referred to the ear.

Physical Examination

On initial inspection, look at the ear itself and then at its relation to the head. Is it red, swollen, protruding? Is there obvious discharge? Are the auricle and periauricular tissues normal in appearance or lichenified, with a heaping up of the normal epidermal architecture? Is there erythema or cellulitis spreading to the periauricular tissues, face, and neck? A gentle tug upward and backward will usually confirm the clinical suspicion. Although not an infallible rule, the patient with acute otitis externa usually will not tolerate this maneuver; patients with acute otitis media often will.

To make the correct diagnosis of infections of the external canal and to follow the clinical response to treatment, clean the canal thoroughly and examine it under good illumination. A hand-held otoscope will often suffice for a quick examination, but all instrumentation of the ear is best done under the microscope with the patient lying supine in the chair, in anticipation of a possible vasovagal response mediated by Arnold nerve, a branch of cranial nerve X.

Although topical and local anesthesia may be tried before cleansing, they are usually of little effect in hyperemic macerated tissue and no substitute for reassurance and patience. Using graduated specula will often ease the patient into a complete examination. The canal may be cleaned with suction, a cerumen loop, or alligator forceps. The choice of instruments is unimportant. Gentleness and thoroughness are very important.

Bacteriology

The usual pathogens responsible for acute otitis externa are *Pseudomonas aeruginosa*, *Proteus mirabilis*, staphylococci, streptococci, and various gram-negative bacilli. For the mild or uncomplicated infection, culture of the canal is ordinarily not taken, because it will usually demonstrate a mixed pattern of growth. For recalcitrant infections, culture may identify a predominant organism and assist in the choice of antibiotic therapy.

Staging

Senturia et al. (4) divided the clinical course of external otitis into the following stages: preinflammatory; acute inflammatory, which can be mild, moderate, or severe; and chronic inflammatory. Typically, the preinflammatory stage begins when the stratum corneum becomes edematous because of the removal of the protective lipid layer and acid mantle from the canal, resulting in plugging of the apopilosebaceous unit. As obstruction continues, a sense of fullness and itching begins. The disruption of the epithelial layer allows invasion of bacteria that either reside in the canal or are introduced on foreign objects inserted into the canal, such as a cotton swab or a dirty fingernail. This produces the acute inflammatory stage, which is accompanied by pain and tenderness of the auricle. In the earliest stage, the skin of the external auditory canal shows mild erythema and minimal edema (Fig. 135.3). A small amount of clear or slightly cloudy secretion may be seen in the canal. As pain and itching increase, the patient progresses

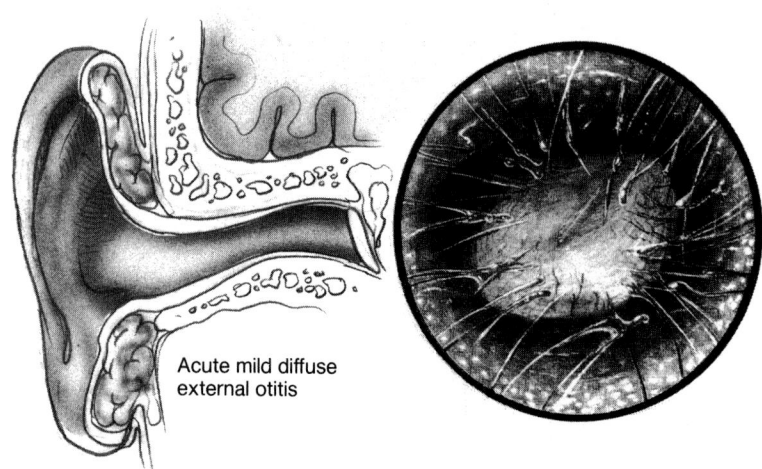

Acute mild diffuse external otitis

Figure 135.3 Otitis externa, acute inflammatory stage. Mild erythema and edema of the canal skin are seen. Clear secretions may be viewed in the canal. (From Senturia BA, Marcus MD, Lucente FE. *Diseases of the external ear*, 2nd ed. New York: Grune & Stratton, 1980, with permission.)

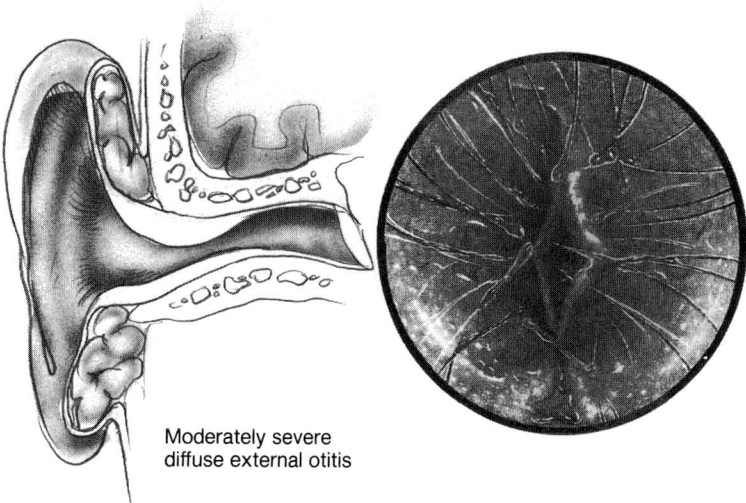

Figure 135.4 Otitis externa, moderate acute inflammatory stage. The external auditory canal is more edematous than in the acute stage, approaching obliteration of the lumen, with a more profuse exudate. (From Senturia BA, Marcus MD, Lucente FE. *Diseases of the external ear*, 2nd ed. New York: Grune & Stratton, 1980, with permission.)

Moderately severe diffuse external otitis

to the moderate stage, in which the canal shows more edema and a thicker more profuse exudate (Fig. 135.4).

Further progression of the inflammation in the absence of treatment produces the severe inflammatory stage, characterized by increased pain and obliteration of the lumen of the canal. A profuse, purulent exudate and edema of the canal skin may obscure the tympanic membrane. In addition, small white papules are often visible on the surface of the canal skin. *P. aeruginosa* or another gram-negative bacillus can almost always be cultured at this stage. In the severe stage, the physician often sees evidence of extension of infection beyond the canal to involve the adjacent soft tissues and cervical lymph nodes (Fig. 135.5).

In the chronic inflammatory stage, the patient experiences less pain but more profound itching. The skin of the external canal is thickened, and superficial flaking may be seen (Fig. 135.6). The auricle and concha often show secondary changes, such as eczematization, lichenification, and superficial ulceration. This condition is likened to eczema and may range from mild drying and thickening of the canal to complete obliteration of the external canal by chronically infected hypertrophic skin (Table 135.1).

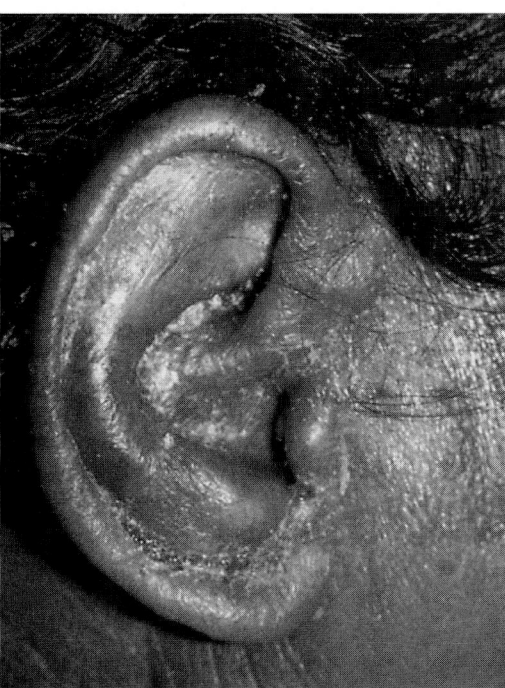

Figure 135.5 Otitis externa, severe stage. Infection extends beyond the limits of the canal to involve adjacent soft tissues and cervical lymph nodes. Erythema of the conchal skin and scaliness are secondary to profuse drainage.

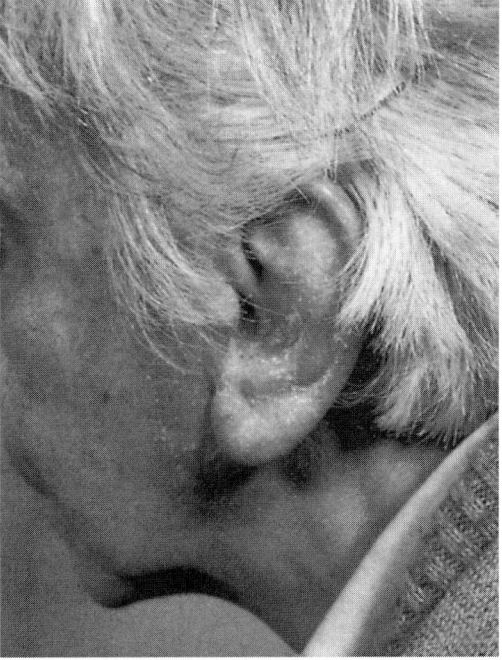

Figure 135.6 Otitis externa, chronic inflammatory stage. The skin of the external canal is thickened, and superficial flaking may be seen. The surrounding skin of the auricle may show secondary changes such as eczematization, lichenification, and superficial ulceration.

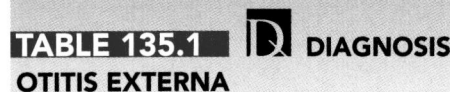

TABLE 135.1   DIAGNOSIS

OTITIS EXTERNA

History
Pain Fullness Itching
Discharge

Physical examination
Preinflammatory
Mild erythema, edema
Acute inflammatory
Auricular tenderness
Erythema
Edema
Discharge
Chronic inflammatory
Thickening, flaking of canal skin
Eczematization
Ulceration

Laboratory
Culture
P. aeruginosa
P. mirabilis
Staphylococcus sp.
Streptococcus sp.

Radiology
Rarely indicated

Differential Diagnosis

The differential diagnosis of conditions that are similar to external otitis is large and includes necrotizing otitis externa, bullous external otitis, granular external otitis, perichondritis, chondritis, relapsing polychondritis, furunculosis, and carbunculosis, as well as many dermatoses, such as psoriasis and seborrheic dermatitis. All have features in common with acute and chronic external otitis yet have enough dissimilarities to be considered distinct clinical entities.

Carcinoma involving the external auditory canal may present as infection, and in its earliest stages is often mistaken for infection and treated inappropriately. The most common malignant neoplasm of the external ear is squamous cell carcinoma, although other primary carcinomas, such as basal cell carcinoma, malignant melanoma, ceruminous adenoma or adenocarcinoma, adenoid cystic and metastatic carcinomas to the temporal bone with extension to the external auditory canal such as breast, prostatic, small (oat) cell, and renal cell carcinomas, have been described. The occurrence of pain in an old previously stable mastoid cavity is the hallmark of carcinoma and must be excluded by biopsy and other investigations.

Natural History

The natural history of untreated acute otitis externa is one of increasing pain, swelling, and discharge from the canal. The infection may spread to the adjacent periauricular soft tissues, face, and neck. In an immunocompromised patient, what began as an isolated superficial infection of the apopilosebaceous unit of the external auditory canal may progress to perichondritis, chondritis, cellulitis, and erysipelas. Rich lymphatic and hematogenous drainage pathways favor the spread of infection to local and regional sites in the head and neck. Few patients progress to such an advanced stage before seeking medical attention.

The natural history of chronic otitis externa is far less dramatic than its acute counterpart. The chronic scaling and itching in the canal predispose to manipulation of the canal, excoriation, and repeated episodes of acute otitis externa. With time, the canal skin may become lichenified, and ultimately the canal may become completely obliterated.

Medical Treatment

The four fundamental principles in the treatment of external otitis in all stages (5) are frequent and thorough cleaning, judicious use of appropriate antibiotics, treatment of associated inflammation and pain, and recommendations regarding the prevention of future infections. In any stage of infection, thorough cleaning is a priority. Meticulous debridement of exfoliated debris, purulence, and cerumen will do as much if not more than simply placing the patient on ear drops. In the preinflammatory stage, a complete cleaning may be all that is required. In the absence of purulence, a brief course of an acidifying drop such as aluminum sulfate–calcium sulfate (Domeboro) is efficacious in discouraging bacterial or fungal growth.

Treatment of the acute inflammatory stage varies with the extent of disease. In the mildest form, cleaning as described previously is indicated. An antibiotic otic drop is recommended to cover what is probably a *Pseudomonas* infection. There is an emerging body of evidence that the fluoroquinolone preparations with or without steroids (ciprofloxacin, ofloxacin, dexamethasone, hydrocortisone (Cipro HC, Ciprodex, Floxin)] may have advantages over the neomycin/polymyxin/hydrocortisone preparations (Cortisporin or Coly-Mycin S Otic) (6,7).

At this time, no significant antibiotic resistance has been shown to emerge due to the use of the fluoroquinolone ototopic medications (8).

At this stage, edema of the external auditory canal should not be severe, and the patient should be able to instill drops into the ear by tilting the head to the side or by lying down with the involved ear upright.

Moderate Stage

In the moderate stage of inflammation, edema of the canal may interfere with the instillation of drops. The physician should then insert a wick into the canal and instill drops on it. Often the canal may accommodate two or even three wicks. As the wick expands, it presses the soft tissues and periosteum toward the nondistended position; this alone may relieve pain. All instrumentation of the ear is best done under the microscope. The wick is removed by the physician at the time of reexamination. If the edema has not been significantly reduced, repacking is indicated. Antibiotic drops should be continued for at least 2 to 3 days after the cessation of pain, itching, and drainage, so that complete eradication of infection may be ensured.

In the moderate stage, an oral analgesic is often prescribed because pain can be pronounced. Caution the patient to avoid manipulation of the canal. Teach swimmers to towel dry the concha and lateral canal, to shake water out of the canal, or to instill an acidifying drop after swimming. If the infection has not spread beyond the boundaries of the external canal, the use of oral antibiotics will be of little if any value. A final office visit is important to ensure that the infection has completely resolved and the canal is back to its normal state.

Severe Stage

In the severe stage, infection usually extends beyond the limit of the canal. In addition to the cleaning, packing, and use of antibiotic drops as discussed previously, attend to any soft-tissue involvement by using an oral antibiotic with broad-spectrum coverage. Successive generations of the cephalosporins widen gram-negative coverage at the expense of gram-positive coverage.

In addition to anti-*Pseudomonas* eardrops, common choices of oral antibiotics are antistaphylococcal penicillins, first-generation cephalosporins, or one of the antipseudomonal fluoroquinolones such as ciprofloxacin or levofloxacin. The fluoroquinolone antibiotics are effective against *Pseudomonas* species but at present are not approved for use in patients under age 18 because of the risk of arthropathy formation (6). Multiple reports over the last 10 years have indicated the safe use of ciprofloxacin in the pediatric patient with little if any increased development of arthopathy over adults. The fluoroquinolones remain contra-indicated, however, except in extraordinary circumstances, such as in the treatment of respiratory disease in children with cystic fibrosis. (9)

Warm soaks (normal saline or diluted aluminum sulfate–calcium acetate solution) are also useful in the treatment of the crusting and edema involving the auricle and surrounding skin. Culture of the canal is indicated only for the severe stage or for patients who have previously been treated without resolution. Treatment is generally continued for 10 to 14 days if there is a good response. In rare patients who do not respond to this regimen, hospitalization, vigorous daily local care, repeat culturing, and intravenous antibiotics are indicated.

Chronic Stage

The chronic stage of external otitis is manifested by marked thickening of the skin of the external auditory canal caused by long-standing infection. Examination reveals flakes of dry scaly skin in the canal. Although removal of debris is recommended, this may be difficult due to the narrowing of the lumen of the canal. Repeated

cleaning and instillation of antibiotics and steroids are indicated. Triamcinalone acetonide 0.25% cream or ointment (Kenalog) or dexamethasone sodium phosphate 0.1% (Decadron, Pred Forte 1%) ophthalmic drops may be used.

In all cases of acute or chronic external otitis, instruct the patient to avoid future infections by not placing any object or instrument into the canal. These often excoriate the canal skin and push debris further into the canal rather than remove it. Patients who have repeated infections despite adhering to these measures are best advised to use an acidifying drop composed of equal measures of vinegar and water, or ethyl alcohol and water, when exposed to high humidity. Alternatively, an acidifying power such as boric acid may be used. Custom-made ear molds are useful for these patients.

Recalcitrant Otitis Externa

The physician will be able to judge very quickly which patients are responding. If no progress is made in the office, the rare patient may have to be admitted as an inpatient. Toilet of the ear should be performed under the microscope, frequently (at least daily) and carefully. Look for subtle signs of chronic middle ear disease—granulation tissue or the opening of a tiny perforation. The latter may be obscured by a swollen tympanic membrane, giving a "fish-mouth" appearance to the perforation. A "sewer cap" of crust on the drum may reveal a cholesteatoma underneath. Examine every part of the auricle. Look for signs of underlying chondritis or perichondritis, especially diffuse crusting or exudative weeping. Culture the ear. Examine the periauricular tissues carefully to look for signs of spreading infection. Computed tomography of the temporal bones may give additional information. Look for opacification of the mastoid and signs of bony erosion.

Place the patient on daily aural drops, preferably one covering *P. aeruginosa*, and intravenous antibiotics with gram-positive and gram-negative coverage. A cephalosporin together with an aminoglycoside is a logical combination. Therapy should be tapered according to culture and sensitivities. Severely swollen ears may calm down with steroids.

Many recalcitrant infections occur because of noncompliance or chronic instrumentation of the canal skin. The patient should be counseled to amend bad habits. Treat these patients exactly as those with severe otitis externa, but as inpatients. This will allow intravenous antibiotics to be given and will ensure local care (Tables 135.2 and 135.3).

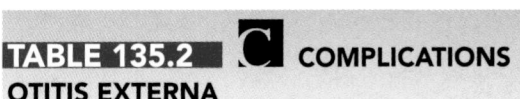

TABLE 135.2 COMPLICATIONS

OTITIS EXTERNA

Cellulitis
Erysipelas
Perichondritis
Chondritis
Chronic nonresolving infection

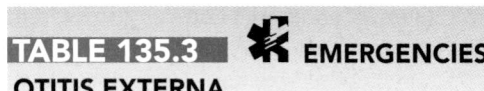

TABLE 135.3   **EMERGENCIES**
OTITIS EXTERNA

Unresolving pain, despite local care
    Admit to hospital
    Analgesia
    Control inflammation

Cranial neuropathy with external otitis
    Consider necrotizing external otitis

Surgical Management of Hypertrophic Chronic Otitis Externa

When such local measures are insufficient to eradicate infection and reestablish the lumen of the canal, it is necessary to remove the involved canal skin and any adjacent involved cutaneous or cartilaginous tissue. This is very rarely required and may be performed through the canal but is better done through a postauricular incision, which allows visualization of the involved tissues. A generous amount of conchal cartilage is removed to effect a wide meatoplasty. The bony canal is enlarged with a drill. Take care to protect the facial nerve in its vertical segment; the use of an intraoperative facial nerve monitor facilitates this. The canal is resurfaced with a split-thickness (8:1,000 inch) skin graft that is temporarily held in place with stents or packing.

It is the experience of many otolaryngologists that even the most recalcitrant infection can be managed if the four basic principles—thorough cleaning, antibiotic treatment, pain control, and instruction of the patient—are meticulously followed. There is no substitute for thorough and repeated local care (Table 135.4).

NECROTIZING (MALIGNANT) EXTERNAL OTITIS

This potentially life-threatening disease should be viewed within the larger context of osteomyelitis of the temporal bone and skull base. Thanks in large part to newer anti-*Pseudomonas* antibiotics, chief among them the fluoro-

TABLE 135.4   **TREATMENT**
OTITIS EXTERNA

Medical
    Frequent thorough cleaning
    Antibiotic coverage
        Drops
        Oral
        Intravenous as needed
    Treat inflammation, pain
    Recommendations for prevention

Surgical
    Excise involved canal skin
    Perform wide meatoplasty
    Resurface canal with split-thickness skin graft

quinolones, necrotizing external otitis (NEO) is not as prevalent as it was even a decade ago. By no means is it a disease of the past, especially among diabetics; the immunocompromised, especially HIV+ patients; and the elderly. The otolaryngologist must still keep NEO within the differential diagnosis of a refractory external ear infection in the patient at risk.

Toulmouche (10) described a case of progressive osteomyelitis of the temporal bone in 1838 that was probably the first reported case of NEO. In 1959 Melzer and Kelleman (11) described a case of progressive *Pseudomonas osteomyelitis* of the temporal bone and skull base. Chandler (12–16) is credited with the clinical description of what he termed malignant otitis externa in 1968 and thereafter. He believed that radical surgical debridement of the ear and adnexal structures offered the only hope of a cure. Although many early cases ended in the death of the patient, the entity does not involve carcinoma and thus the more appropriate term used today is NEO. Advances in both early radiological imaging and, more importantly, anti*Pseudomonas* medications have significantly altered the natural history of this disease.

Diagnosis

The diagnosis of NEO is made in a patient with the appropriate history, physical examination, and supporting laboratory findings. Four salient features are found (17): persistent otalgia for longer than 1 month; persistent purulent otorrhea with granulation tissue for several weeks; diabetes mellitus, another immunocompromised state, or advanced age; and cranial nerve involvement. The disease that begins in the external auditory canal may pass through preformed channels: anteriorly through the fissures of Santorini and posteroinferiorly through the stylomastoid foramen to the jugular bulb and skull base. The disease may pass through thrombosed veins and along the route of the facial nerve anteriorly and inferiorly toward both the petrous apex and the skull base.

Other diseases to be included in the differential diagnosis include severe acute otitis externa, squamous cell carcinoma, glomus jugulare tumor, cholesteatoma, nasopharyngeal carcinoma, Hans-Schüller-Christian disease, eosinophilic granuloma, Wegener granulomatosis, clival chordoma, and meningeal carcinoma (18). The physician's index of suspicion should be high so that no patient is denied aggressive treatment when appropriate (Table 135.5).

Clinical and Radiographic Findings

NEO usually begins as an acute external otitis that does not resolve despite medical therapy, as described previously. The history is significant for a long-standing infection of the external canal accompanied by aural discharge and severe deep-seated pain. The disease is usually found in elderly diabetic patients in poor metabolic control, although it may be found in any chronically ill, debilitated,

TABLE 135.5 ▯ DIAGNOSIS
NECROTIZING EXTERNAL OTITIS

History
    Persistent otalgia
    Persistent purulent otorrhea, granulations
    Diabetes mellitus, advanced age, immunocompromised state
    Cranial neuropathy(ies)

Physical examination
    Granulations in external canal
    Purulent discharge seen
    +/− cranial neuropathy, especially cranial nerve VII

Culture
    Pseudomonas sp.[a]
    Pseudomonas aeruginosa[a]

Radiology
    Nuclear (gallium, technetium)
    CT with contrast
    MRI with contrast

CT, computed tomography; MRI, magnetic resonance imaging.
[a]Almost always.

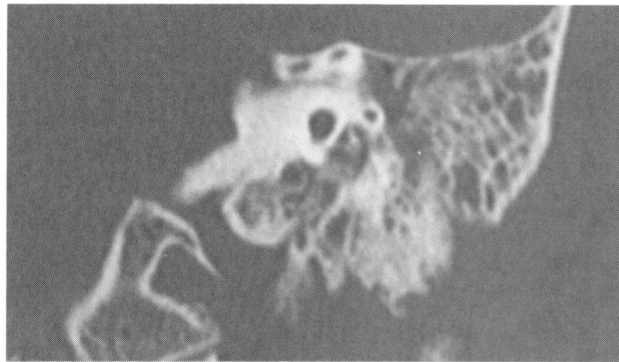

Figure 135.7 Coronal computed tomography scan of a patient with left necrotizing otitis externa.

or immunocompromised patient (19). The HIV status of the patient should be known.

On physical examination, most patients with NEO usually but not invariably have granulation tissue visible in the inferior aspect of the canal or even extruding from it. This may obscure the tympanic membrane. It is rare to see granulation tissue in patients with routine otitis externa; however, granulations are common in an acute exacerbation of chronic otitis media with perforation of the tympanic membrane. The skin of the canal is often erythematous, indurated, and sometimes macerated. Purulent secretions are common.

The causative organism is almost always *P. aeruginosa*, although other organisms such as *P. mirabilis*, *Aspergillus fumigatus*, *Proteus* sp., *Klebsiella* sp., and *Staphylococcus* sp. have been isolated (13,20–23). Fungal infections causing NEO are less commonly associated with diabetes but are found more commonly in patients who are immunocompromised in other ways, especially by HIV disease (24).

The natural history of NEO is one of relentless progression to involve the cranial nerves, especially the facial nerve. Pain is inexorable and is deep seated. Damiani et al. (25) reported that the most commonly involved cranial nerves were VII (75%), X (70%), and XI (56%). More recent reports have estimated the facial nerve to be involved in at least one fourth of patients, with less frequent involvement of cranial nerves IX, X and XI (24).

CT of the temporal bone with contrast is the initial radiograph to be done, yielding excellent bony detail with less precise information about soft tissue. It may define subtle bony changes such as erosion of the anterior canal wall with involvement of the temporomandibular joint and erosion of the tympanic ring and base of the skull. It may demonstrate soft tissue thickening and mastoid clouding. An important radiological feature on coronal CT of the

temporal bone is effacement of the tympanic ring (Fig. 135.7). The fat plane in the subtemporal triangle near the stylomastoid foramen may be effaced (26).

Magnetic resonance imaging (MRI) yields very little information about bone, which appears as a silhouette. MRI without and with gadolinium enhancement may be advantageous in defining the medial extent of soft tissue disease at the skull base. Dural enhancement and involvement of the medullary bone spaces are seen with central-skull-base invasion (24). Underlying cerebral involvement is easily visualized with gadolinium-enhanced MRI. The patency of the dural sinuses and great vessels of the neck may be assessed in a noninvasive fashion with magnetic resonance angiography or venography. Changes seen on MRI do not resolve with clinical improvement. Thus, MRI is a useful diagnostic tool to assess the extent of disease but is not a useful tool in following the clinical course of NEO (27).

Technetium-99m bone scanning and gallium-67 scanning have been advocated in the evaluation of NEO (21,24). Their sensitivity for the presence of infection is far greater than their specificity for the cause (Fig. 135.8).

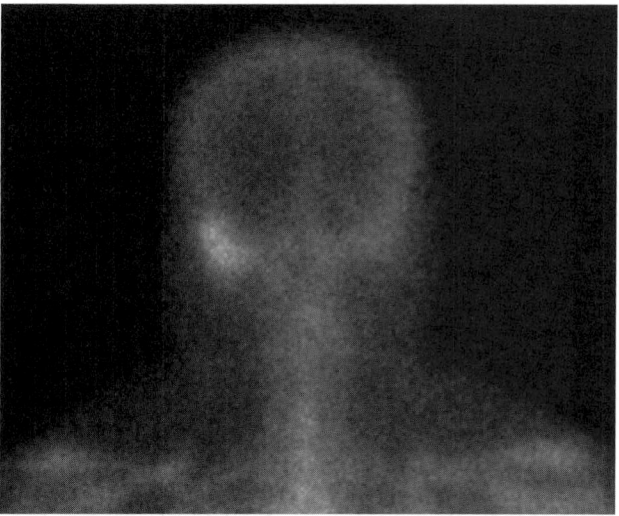

Figure 135.8 Bone scan of a patient with necrotizing otitis externa.

Tc-99m scanning gives excellent information about bone function but poor information about bone structure. A positive scan is thought to represent osteoblastic activity as little as 10% above normal (21). The scan is positive in acute and chronic osteomyelitis and in areas of active bone repair without infection, as in trauma. Increases in Tc-99m uptake between 4 and 24 hours postinjection is the most sensitive indicator of temporal bone osteomyelitis (28). Its use in the evaluation of NEO is complementary to that of Ga-67 scanning. Ga-67 is thought to be incorporated into proteins and polymorphonucleocytes at sites of active infection as a Ga-67–lactoferrin complex (21). It will highlight an acute infective focus but not the full extent of an osteomyelitic process. As treatment progresses, the Ga-67 scan will revert to normal (negative). The Tc-99m scan will lag behind for many months. Baseline studies of both are thus recommended, and sequential imaging is used to monitor the response to therapy. Indium-111–labeled leukocyte (In-WBC) planar scintigraphy has been demonstrated to yield better results for the detection of osteomyelitis than either planar or tomographic Ga-67 and/or Tc-99m–methyline diphosphonate and may replace the former two radionuclide modalities in the evaluation of NEO-suspected patients (22). It is best to consult with whomever will be performing the radionuclide study, though, to determine which of these choices will be best.

Medical Treatment

Swab and/or tissue cultures of the external auditory canal should be obtained. If present, granulations should be biopsied and sent to rule out carcinoma or another pathological entity. *P. aeruginosa* is almost always cultured. *Pseudomas* is frequently the predominant organism, so the patient is treated with anti-*Pseudomonas* antibiotics for an extended period, often for 6 weeks or more. Because of the synergy achieved with the use of 2 antibiotics, one an antipseudomonal antibiotic and the other an aminoglycoside, monotherapy is discouraged in the treatment of NEO. Usually two anti-*Pseudomonas* antibiotics are chosen from several alternatives, including gentamicin or tobramycin with or without ticarcillin or piperacillin. Alternative antibiotics include mezlocillin or azlocillin, ceftazidime, imipenem, aztreonam, amikacin, norfloxacin, and ciprofloxacin or any of the other appropriate anti-*Pseudomonas* fluoroquinolones. If an aminoglycoside is chosen, peak and trough levels and hearing must be carefully monitored. It is wise to treat in concert with an infectious disease colleague to help select those medications that will be of greatest benefit with the least toxicity.

Because of the high tissue levels seen with oral fluoroquinolones, the apparent incidence of NEO has fallen. The physician should not be lulled into a false sense of security, however. Many patients with poor microvasculature, especially diabetics, may achieve cidal concentrations of an antibiotic solely with intravenous administration. Patients refractory to intravenous administration of antibiotic may require surgical control of the infected site. Emergence of resistance to ciprofloxacin has been reported in 20% of long-term (6 weeks or more) therapy for osteomyelitis (29). Outside of cystic fibrosis and severe infections in which no other treatment is possible, the only pediatric situations where fluoroquinolones are superior to standard treatments for children are typhoid fever, severe shigella dysenteries and enterobacteria meningitis. Thus, fluoroquinolones should still be reserved for second-line use in pediatrics because of the potential emergence of resistant strains and because they have been shown to cause arthropathy in the weight-bearing joints of immature animals (9).

An early clinical feature of success in treatment is the cessation of pain, and patients may be tempted to discontinue therapy once this occurs. Regardless of the choice of medication or mode of delivery, patients must understand that they will require meticulous aural toilet and antibiotic treatment for at least 6 weeks and vigorous management of diabetes.

Either in the hospital or in the office, the ear is debrided carefully under the microscope on a regular basis until granulations have subsided. The patient is placed on anti-*Pseudomonas* otic drops and appropriate systemic antibiotics. Diabetes is aggressively managed, usually with the aid of an internist or endocrinologist. The diet is carefully monitored with the aid of the nutritionist.

Hyperbaric oxygen has been advocated by Shupak et al. (30), but Chandler et al. (15) were unsure of its value. Hyperbaric oxygen is thought to facilitate osteoneogenesis and to promote repair of diseased bone. The cost and inconvenience of hyperbaric oxygen therapy have limited its availability. Its use is recommended for advanced disease with significant skull base or intracranial involvement, recurrent disease, and infections refractory to antibiotic treatment (24).

Surgical Treatment

Most patients can be managed medically, and the role of surgery in NEO remains controversial. Surgical debridement of tissue and osteomyelitic bone is usually reserved for patients who do not respond to conventional therapy. Progression of pain despite aggressive medical therapy, persistence of granulations, and the development of cranial nerve involvement are all ominous signs that call for more aggressive medical therapy and possibly surgical intervention.

With the onset of clinical facial weakness, early surgical removal of granulations and, when necessary, decompression of the descending facial nerve have given excellent return of function. The primary surgical goal is to excise the underlying necrosis and to replace it with vascularized tissue. Serial electroneuronography (ENOG) has been used to determine the electrical degeneration of the VII nerve in patients with clinical facial paralysis. An ENOG showing

TABLE 135.6 ℞ TREATMENT
NECROTIZING EXTERNAL OTITIS

Medical
Hospital admission
Intravenous antibiotics
Daily cleaning, debridement

Surgical
Excise granulations +/− middle ear exploration
+/− mastoidectomy
+/− facial nerve decompression
+/− temporal bone resection if no response

more than 90% electrical degeneration of the clinically involved facial nerve may support surgical decompression of the involved segment of the nerve.

John and Cheesman (31) have advocated wide local excision of infected cartilage and soft tissues if pain persists after medical treatment or if facial palsy occurs. Reines and Schindler (32) have reported three cases in which subtotal temporal bone resection was performed to gain access to the primary focus of infection and provide adequate drainage. Surgical treatment including abscess drainage, debridement of sequestra, and more extensive resection should be individualized depending upon the patient's overall health status and response to more conservative measures (33).

Mortality remains significant, especially in the immunocompromised patient. Progression of disease results in severe unremitting pain within the ear and at the base of the skull and extension of infection to the mastoid, parotid, lower cranial nerves, and transverse and sigmoid sinuses. Osteomyelitis of the skull base may lead to meningitis, brain abscess, and death. Meyerhoff et al. (34) reported an overall mortality of 37% before the introduction of combined carbenicillin and gentamicin and 23% afterward. With multiple cranial neuropathies, Babiatzki and Sadé (18) and Damiani et al. (25) have reported mortality rates of 60% and 61%, respectively. Poor prognostic factors include facial paralysis, polyneuropathy, and intracranial extension (35).

The diagnosis and management of patients with NEO remains an otoloryngologic challenge. Perhaps the greatest

TABLE 135.7 COMPLICATIONS
NECROTIZING EXTERNAL OTITIS

Cranial neuropathy (VII and lower)
Progression despite aggressive local care, including hyperbaric oxygen therapy (to mastoid, parotid, lower cranial nerves, base of skull, dural venous sinuses, brain)
Meningitis
Brain abscess
Death

TABLE 135.8 EMERGENCIES
NECROTIZING EXTERNAL OTITIS

Any complications in Table 135.7 (in living patient)
Change antibiotic
Increase level of daily care
Consider surgery

advance in its treatment has been the recognition of NEO as a distinct entity and a clear understanding of its pathophysiology. A team approach involving the cooperation of otolaryngology, endocrinology, and infectious disease may enhance the overall outcome (Tables 135.6 to 135.8). The devastating disease reported by Chandler (12) in his classic 1968 article has significantly changed. The advent of the fluoroquinolones and other anti-*Pseudomonas* antibiotics has significantly lowered the morbidity and mortality associated with NEO.

CONDITIONS RELATED TO EXTERNAL OTITIS

Several other infectious and inflammatory diseases are included in the differential diagnosis of otitis externa.

Radiation-Induced Otitis Externa

Another form of otitis externa occasionally occurs after radiotherapy of the region of the external ear. The predominant symptoms result from the inflammation and infection that occur when radiotherapy weakens local defense mechanisms and resident bacteria flourish. When limited to the skin of the external auditory canal, treatment measures with particular attention to water avoidance are appropriate. In its worst form of osteoradionecrosis, sequestra of devitalized tissue must be removed and replaced with vascularized tissue.

Bullous External Otitis

Bullous external otitis is a very painful condition in which vesicles or bullae are noted in the bony portion of the external canal. The vesicles are commonly hemorrhagic and should not be ruptured, because secondary infection may ensue. Because *Pseudomonas* may be one of the causative organisms, appropriate otic drops are recommended. Packing and irrigation of the canal should be avoided, because they tend to prolong the course of this disease.

Granular External Otitis

Granular external otitis often resembles the earliest stage of NEO in that there may be small granular plaques or pedunculated granulations in the external canal. This condition may occur in patients who have not been fully treated for a previous episode of external otitis. After topical or local anesthesia, removal of granulation tissue, placement of a wick in the canal, and the instillation of antibiotic drops will usually resolve the problem. Oral antibiotics should be given if the infection extends beyond the canal. If the patient is diabetic or debilitated, the diagnosis of NEO is entertained and treated appropriately.

Perichondritis and Chondritis

Perichondritis, inflammation of the perichondrium, and chondritis, inflammation of cartilage, may follow or complicate infections of the external auditory canal or result from accidental or surgical trauma to the auricle. The condition is painful, and the patient often complains of severe itching deep within the canal. With time, the skin over the affected area becomes crusted with squamous debris, and the involved cartilage begins to weep. The ear is indurated and erythematous; often the canal swells shut. The surrounding soft tissues of the face and neck may become involved.

In the mildest stages, thorough debridement and treatment with topical and oral antibiotics are generally sufficient. If these measures do not succeed, the ear is debrided again, and cultures are taken. Appropriate treatment for common pathogens, especially *Pseudomonas*, is begun and tapered according to culture results. Ciprofloxacin is a logical choice for moderate stages, combined with an anti-*Pseudomonas* drop such as gentamicin or a fluoroquinolone drop.

If the infection spreads to involve regional soft tissues and lymphatics, the patient should be hospitalized and parenteral treatment with adequate coverage for *Pseudomonas* begun. In difficult cases, the ear should be cultured before starting treatment. With recalcitrant infections, ask the help of an infectious disease consultant. At every stage of the disease, frequent and thorough debridement of the canal is essential. The metabolic requirements of cartilage are low, and its blood supply is appropriately diminished. Once infection has become established in the perichondrium or cartilage, it is extremely difficult to treat. If subacute or chronic infection evidenced by inexorable weeping continues, surgical intervention is indicated. This is best done in the operating room under controlled conditions.

The affected area is cleansed and injected with local anesthetic containing epinephrine. Skin flaps are appropriately planned and the dissection taken down to the affected cartilage. If it has lost its normal "pearly white" appearance, it is most likely necrotic and should be excised. Often necrosis extends farther than can be grossly visualized. Small irrigation drains are placed beneath the flaps and sutured to the skin. The skin flaps are closed. The drainage ports are irrigated with antibiotic irrigation such as bacitracin (50,000 U of bacitracin dissolved in 250 mL

of normal saline). The drains are advanced as the condition resolves. Parenteral antibiotics, otic drops, and aggressive local care continue until the infection has resolved.

Relapsing Polychondritis

Relapsing polychondritis is an intermittently progressive disease marked by inflammatory destruction of cartilage. Although thought to be an autoimmune disorder, the exact cause is unknown. Cartilage of the external ear, larynx, trachea, bronchi, and nose may be involved. Symptoms are episodic, with fever, anemia, erythema, swelling, pain, and an elevated sedimentation rate during acute episodes. As the disease progresses, symptoms of increasing respiratory obstruction become apparent. Labyrinthine disturbances are rarely present. The diagnosis is made on the basis of the history and physical examination, supported by an elevated sedimentation rate. Biopsy of involved cartilage may show necrosis, inflammation, and fibrosis. Treatment is with oral corticosteroids.

Furunculosis and Carbunculosis

Furunculosis and carbunculosis are conditions resulting from gram-positive infections, usually staphylococcal, of the hair follicles. The primary lesion is usually a small well-circumscribed pustule that may enlarge to become a furuncle or merge with several similar lesions to form a carbuncle. The infection occurs most commonly at the junction of the concha and canal skin.

For treatment to be successful, any accumulated infectious material must be removed. Spontaneous drainage can often be encouraged by the use of warm soaks, supplemented by topical and oral antibiotics. If this fails to relieve obstruction of the canal, incision and drainage under local anesthesia are indicated.

Infectious Eczematoid Dermatitis

Infectious eczematoid dermatitis results from the drainage of contaminated or purulent material from the middle ear into the floor of the external ear and adjacent infra-auricular skin (Fig. 135.9). This drainage causes a secondary infection or an autosensitization phenomenon manifested by crusted plaques in the canal. Treatment is directed at control of the underlying middle ear infection. Supportive treatment of the external canal reaction consists of removal of accumulated debris, application of sterile saline soaks to the crusted areas, and application of an antibiotic cream or ointment.

Otomycosis

Otomycosis is a fungal infection of the skin of the external canal. Although fungi may be the primary pathogens, they are usually superimposed on chronic bacterial infection of

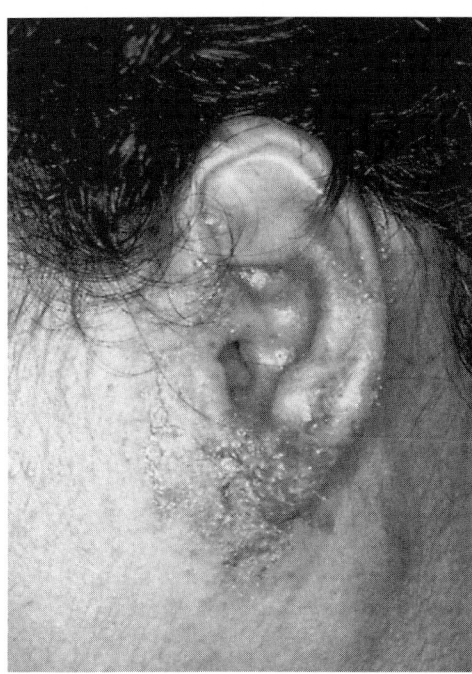

Figure 135.9 Infectious eczematoid dermatitis with inflammation and crusting of the skin of the canal and auricle secondary to drainage of purulent material through a tympanic membrane perforation in a patient with chronic otitis media.

the external canal or middle ear. Secondary otomycosis tends to recur if the underlying primary infection is not controlled. All fungi have three basic growth requirements: moisture, warmth, and darkness. Altering moisture will discourage fungal growth. *Aspergillus* species are the most common, and pruritus is the primary clinical manifestation. Physical examination commonly shows a white, black, or dotted gray membrane. Thorough cleaning with removal of the matted fungal debris is supplemented by the topical application of an acidifying solution such as aluminum sulfate–calcium acetate (Domeboro) or by a drying powder such as boric acid. Clotrimazole cream or solution (Lotrimin) may also be used. In the presence of a tympanic membrane perforation or pressure-equalizing tube, clotrimazole drops or lotion may be very painful. Thorough cleaning and drying therapies such as powders are best. Metacresyl acetate (Cresylate) may be painted on the margin of a perforation or an infected ventilation tube. This is best done under the microscope. Be careful not to allow this medication to enter the middle ear cleft, because it is quite irritating. In recalcitrant infections, a foreign body such as a ventilation tube acts as the nidus for infection and should be removed. Tympanoplasty is best performed to close a perforation that intermittently drains with a superimposed fungal infection.

Gentian violet is usually well tolerated in patients with mastoid cavities, although it is best left out of the middle ear cleft in the presence of a perforation. Because it will permanently stain skin and clothing, small amounts are used with adequate protection of the surrounding area.

Many patients with refractory otomycotic infections may have had previous mastoid surgery. Often the canal wall is down. Because of moderate to severe hearing loss, the patient must wear a hearing aid with a closed mold. This is a significant problem, because the patient relies on the aid virtually all day and is reluctant to leave the instrument out. Carefully explain the problem to the patient, meticulously debride the ear, and use a drying agent such as boric acid powder, chloromycetin-sulfanilamide-fungizone (amphotericin B) powder or chloromycetin-sulfanilamide-tinactin (tolnaftate) powder; this will often help clean up the cavity. Ointments in cavities with closed hearing aids may promote fungal growth because of the accumulation of moisture. In refractory cases, gentian violet or metacresyl acetate (Cresylate) is used topically.

Herpes Zoster and Herpes Simplex

Herpes zoster and herpes simplex are viruses known to affect the external auditory canal. The patient initially experiences a period of burning, pain, or localized headache, and vesicles usually appear within several days. When vesicles coalesce and rupture, crusts are formed. Herpes zoster tends to appear unilaterally in a dermatomic distribution. Involvement of the facial nerve may produce paresis or paralysis (herpes zoster oticus or Ramsay Hunt syndrome). Treatment is supportive, with topical application of a drying agent, such as hydrogen peroxide for crusts. The status of the facial nerve is carefully followed; surgical decompression of the facial nerve may be a consideration. Many patients excoriate the blisters, and bacitracin ointment or a suitable substitute should be applied to prevent superinfection. Acyclovir, famcyclovir and valacyclovir have been shown to ameliorate herpetic infections, especially herpes zoster oticus. The latter two have easier dosing schedules and are better absorbed orally than acyclovir. Also, famcyclovir reduces the duration of postherpetic neuralgia. However, it will cause a transitory rise in hepatic enzyme production and must be used with caution.

Dermatoses

Allergic and irritant contact dermatoses may mimic diffuse external otitis. These result when the susceptible patient comes in contact with any type of agent that can produce a cutaneous response. Irritants may be absolute, so noxious that a reaction occurs in everyone exposed (e.g., strong acids or alkalis), or relative, noxious to susceptible individuals, usually after repeated exposures (e.g., soaps and the plastic mold of a hearing aid). Allergic contact dermatitis refers to delayed hypersensitivity reactions resulting from substances such as poison ivy, nickel compounds (earrings), and rubber compounds (headphones). The typical reaction presents as erythema, weeping, and vesiculation accompanied by itching. The patient may produce a secondary infection by scratching. Treatment consists of removal of the causative agent and the use of topical steroids and astringents. Topical or systemic antibiotics are indicated for the treatment of infection. Systemic steroids may be indicated for severe cases. In rare cases, for example, the patient with a cochlear implant and hypersensitivity to plastic, the external, ear-level receiver/stimulator may be painted with a different material or covered with a cloth casing to separate it from the skin.

EXTERNAL EAR DISEASE IN THE HUMAN IMMUNODEFICIENCY VIRUS–INFECTED PATIENT

Among the external ear manifestations in HIV disease is Kaposi sarcoma, which presents with reddish-blue lesions typically described as hemorrhagic nodules (36). The lesions may be discrete or confluent. Although chemotherapy, radiotherapy, and interferon-α have been used for therapy, treatment of auricular and canal lesions is rarely necessary.

Infections of the external ear in HIV-infected patients include both typical and atypical pathogens. Recurrent herpetic infections and *Pneumocystis carinii*–infected aural polyps have been reported in the external auditory canal as a result of chronic otitis media (37).

Another external ear manifestation of HIV disease is seborrheic dermatitis, which tends to be more widespread and refractory to treatment than the same condition in noninfected patients. Necrotizing external otitis in the HIV+ patient adds another level of concern regarding its treatment. An infectious disease consultant should be involved in the overall care of the HIV+ patient.

CONCLUSION

With a thorough knowledge of the normal embryology, anatomy, and physiology of the external ear, together with an understanding of the natural history of the various common disease processes that occur in this location, treatment of the patient with external ear disease becomes logical. However, it is not always easy. Most conditions can be managed with the recommendations outlined in this chapter. There is no substitute for patience and thoroughness.

HIGHLIGHTS

■ An understanding of the various disease entities occurring in the external ear is predicated on a knowledge of the embryology, anatomy, and physiology of the canal.
■ Infection and blockage of the apopilosebaceous unit are the precursors of infectious otitis externa.
■ Otitis externa presents as a spectrum of disease and may be classified into preinflammatory, acute inflammatory, and chronic inflammatory stages.

■ Four principles form the basis of treatment for all stages of infection of the external ear: thorough cleaning, antibiotic therapy, control of inflammation and pain, and recommendations to prevent infection. Of these, thorough cleaning is the cornerstone of therapy.
■ Recalcitrant and recurrent otitis externa must be treated aggressively with daily local care and antibiotics, often in the hospital. Patience and thoroughness are needed for successful treatment.
■ Surgery is rarely indicated for infections of the external canal but may be required to reverse the natural course of chronic disease.
■ NEO is a disease occurring in immunosuppressed patients. It must enter the differential diagnosis of any patient with nonresolving acute external otitis.
■ There are four hallmarks of NEO: persistent otalgia; persistent otorrhea and granulation tissue; diabetes mellitus, advanced age, or immunocompromised state; and cranial nerve involvement.
■ NEO must be treated aggressively with proper radiographic imaging to map the extent of disease, meticulous local care control of diabetes or immunodeficiencies (when possible), and antibiotics. Surgery is rarely required. Mortality remains significant with cranial nerve involvement.
■ Many infectious and inflammatory conditions related to external otitis occur in the ear. Therapy is based on treatment of the underlying condition.

REFERENCES

1. Hollinshead WH. *Anatomy for surgeons: the head and neck,* 3rd ed. Vol. 1. Philadelphia: Harper& Row, 1982:159–163.
2. Anson BJ, Donaldson JA. *Surgical anatomy of the temporal bone,* 3rd ed. Philadelphia: W.B. Saunders, 1981:28.
3. Hughes GB, Pensak ML. *Textbook of clinical otology.* New York: Thieme-Stratton, 1997.
4. Senturia BA, Marcus MD, Lucent FE. *Diseases of the external ear,* 2nd ed. New York: Grune & Stratton, 1980.
5. Lucente FE. External otitis. In: Gates GA, ed. *Current therapy in otolaryngology—head and neck surgery, 6th ed.* New York: Elsevier Science, 1997.
6. Roland PS, Pien FD, Henry DC, et al. Efficacy and safety of topical ciprofloxacin/dexamethasone versus neomycin/polymyxin B/hydrocortisone for otitis externa. *Curr Med Res Opin* 2004;8:1175–1183.
7. Myer CM III. *Ear Nose Throat J.* 2004;83(Suppl):9–11.
8. Weber PC, Roland PS, Hannley M, et al. The development of antibiotic resistant organisms with the use of ototopical medications. *Otolaryngol Head Neck Surg.* 2004;130(3 Suppl)S89–S94.
9. Gendrel D, Chalumeau M, Moulin F, et al. Fluoroquinolones in paediatrics: a risk for the patient or for the community? *Lancet Infect Dis* 2003;9:537–546.
10. Toulmouche MA. Observations d'otorrhee cérébrate suivis des reflexions. *Gazette Med Paris* 1838;6:422–426.
11. Meltzer PE, Kellemen G. Pyocyaneus osteomyelitis of the temporal bone, mandible and zygoma. *Laryngoscope* 1959;60:1300–1316.
12. Chandler JR. Malignant external otitis. *Laryngoscope* 1968;78:1257–1294.
13. Chandler JR. Malignant external otitis: further considerations. *Ann Otol Rhinol Laryngol* 1977;86:417–428.
14. Chandler JR. Pathogenesis and treatment of facial paralysis due to malignant otitis externa. *Ann Otol Rhinol Laryngol* 1972;81:648–656.

15. Chandler JR, Grobman L, Quencer R, et al. Osteomyelitis of the base of the skull. *Laryngoscope* 1986;96:245–251.
16. Chandler JR. Malignant external otitis and osteomyelitis of the base of the skull. *Am J Otol* 1989;10:108.
17. Kimmelman CP, Lucente FE. Use of ceftazidime for malignant external otitis. *Ann Otol Rhinol Laryngol* 1989;98:721.
18. Babiatzki A, Sadé J. Malignant external otitis. *J Laryngol Otol* 1987;101:205–210.
19. Geerlings SE, Hoepelman AM. Immune dysfunction in patients with diabetes mellitus (DM). *FEMS Immunol Med Microbiol* 1999;28:259–265.
20. Strauss M, Aber RC, Conner GH, et al. Malignant external otitis: long-term (months) antimicrobial therapy. *Laryngoscope* 1982;92:397–406.
21. Weber PC, Seabold JE, Graham SM, et al. Evaluation of temporal and facial osteomyelitis by simultaneous In-WBC/Tc-99m-MDP bone SPECT scintigraphy and computed tomography scan. *Otolaryngol Head Neck Surg* 1995;113:36–41.
22. Cunningham M, Yu LY, Turner J, et al. Necrotizing otitis externa due to *aspergillus* in an immunocompromised patient. *Arch Otolaryngol Head Neck Surg* 1988;114:554–556.
23. Cohen D, Friedman P. The diagnostic criteria of malignant external otitis. *J Laryngol Otol* 1987;101:216–221.
24. Gangadar SS, Kwartler JA. Skull base osteomyelitis secondary to maliganant otitis externa. *Current Opin Otol HN Surg* 2003;1:316–323.
25. Damiani JM, Damiani KK, Kinney FE. Malignant external otitis with multiple cranial nerve involvement. *Am J Otol* 1979;2:115.
26. Murray ME, Britton L: Osteomyelitis of the skull base: the role of high resolution CT in diagnosis. *Clin Radiol* 1994;49:408–411.
27. Grandis JR, Curton HD, Yu VL. Necrotizing (malignant) external otitis: prosective comparison of CT and MR imaging and follow-up. *Radiology* 1995;196:499–504.
28. Hardoff R, Gipa S, Uri N, et al. Semiquantitative skull planar and SPECT bone scintigraphy in diabetic patients: differentiation of necrotizing (malignant) external otitis from severe external otitis. *J Nucl Med* 1994;35:411–415.
29. Gilbert D, Tice AD, Marsh PK, et al. Oral ciprofloxacin therapy for chronic contiguous osteomyelitis caused by aerobic gram-negative bacilli. *Am J Med* 1987;82:254.
30. Shupak A, Greenberg E, Hardoff R, et al. Hyperbaric oxygenation for necrotizing (malignant) otitis externa. *Arch Otolaryngol Head Neck Surg* 1989;115:1470.
31. John AC, Cheesman AD. Malignant otitis externa. *Hosp Update* 1979;5:589.
32. Reines JM, Schindler RA. The surgical management of recalcitrant malignant external otitis. *Laryngoscope* 1980;90:369.
33. Pedersen HB, Rosborg J: Necrotizing external otitis: aminoglycoside and β-lactam antibiotic treatment combined with surgical treatment. *Clin Otolaryngol* 1997,22:271–274.
34. Meyerhoff WL, Gates GA, Montalbot PJ. *Pseudomonas* mastoiditis. *Laryngoscope* 1977;87:483.
35. Amorosa L, Modugno GC, Pirodda A. Malignant external otitis: review and personal experience. *Acta Otolaryngol Suppl* 1996;521:3–16.
36. Gherman CR, Ward RR, Bassis ML. Pneumocystis carinii otitis media and mastoiditis as the initial manifestation of the acquired immuno-deficiency syndrome. *Am J Med* 1988;85:250.
37. Lucente FE. Acquired immunodeficiency syndrome (AIDS) In: Lucente FE, Lawson W, Novick N, eds. *The external ear*. Philadelphia: W.B. Saunders, 1995:95.

Neoplasms of the Ear and Lateral Skull Base

136

Bradley P. Pickett   *James P. Kelly*

This chapter provides an overview of neoplasms that affect the temporal bone and the external ear. These neoplasms are usually identified on the basis of their location, and this convention is adopted in this chapter. Classification based on location offers a relatively straightforward outline of tumor types that is useful in the differential diagnosis (Table 136.1, Fig. 136.1). Neoplasms of the pinna and the external auditory canal and the middle ear, mastoid, and temporal bone are discussed in this context. When extensive neoplasms occupy more than one anatomic location, however, or when the same pathology arises in more than one location, classification based solely on the site of origin of the neoplasm becomes confusing. In these instances, it is preferable to consider the cell type that gives rise to the neoplasm and the sites that contain this particular cell type or the sites into which the neoplasm migrates or grows. Paragangliomas and hemangiomas are examples of this type of neoplasm. Because a detailed discussion of each neoplasm is beyond the scope of this chapter, the reader is encouraged to examine the recommended readings and references. It should be borne in mind that the causes of neoplasms of the temporal bone and the external ear are in most instances unknown. Therefore, the growth patterns of neoplasms, presenting symptoms and signs, the prognosis for individuals affected by them, and current modes of surgical and medical therapy are the principal areas of concern in this chapter.

NEOPLASMS OF CELL-SPECIFIC ORIGIN

Paraganglioma

Paragangliomas of the temporal bone arise from glomus bodies that occur in the adventitia of the jugular bulb, along the course of the tympanic branch of the glossopharyngeal nerve (Jacobson nerve) and along the course of the auricular branch of the vagus nerve (Arnold nerve). Glomus bodies are part of the diffuse neuroendocrine system. Histologically, they are identical to the carotid body and are similar to the autonomic ganglia of the adrenal medulla. Glomus bodies consist of clusters of chief cells supplied by a network of arterioles, venules, and both afferent and efferent nerve terminals. They are more accurately referred to as paraganglia, because they appear to play a role as neuromodulators or monitors of vascular activity. Chief cells have neurosecretory granules that contain norepinephrine and dopamine, suggesting that the release of granule contents into the vascular system helps to regulate cardiorespiratory function, modify local blood distribution, and maintain thermoregulation. Unlike the carotid body and the adrenal medulla, however, paraganglia of the temporal bone play an uncertain role in these neuroendocrine functions. Paraganglia of the temporal bone are distinguished from other components of the diffuse neuroendocrine system, such as the adrenal medulla, by their lack of affinity for chromium salts used in certain histologic stains. They are therefore categorized as nonchromaffin paraganglia. Chief cells of paraganglia arise from neural crest cells that migrate with sympathetic ganglia during embryonic development (1). Adult temporal bones usually have only two or three paraganglia, but on occasion there may be more, particularly during the fifth decade of life. Most paraganglia of the temporal bone are found in the anterolateral region of the jugular fossa and within the middle ear. Neoplastic transformation of paraganglia can occur in either location. Paragangliomas that originate in the middle ear are termed glomus tympanicum tumors. Paragangliomas that originate in association in the jugular fossa are termed glomus jugulare tumors.

TABLE 136.1

NEOPLASMS OF THE EAR AND LATERAL SKULL BASE

Neoplasms of cell-specific origin
Paraganglioma
  Glomus tympanicum
  Glomus jugulare
Epidermoid
  External auditory canal and middle ear (cholesteatoma)
  Internal auditory canal, petrous apex, and cerebellopontine angle
Vascular neoplasm
  Hemangioma
  Hemangiopericytoma
Hematologic malignancy
  Lymphoma
  Plasmacytoma
  Leukemia

Neoplasms of the pinna and external auditory canal
Cutaneous carcinoma
  Squamous cell carcinoma
  Basal cell carcinoma
Malignant melanoma
Glandular neoplasm
  Ceruminous adenoma
  Ceruminous adenocarcinoma
  Pleomorphic adenoma
  Adenoid cystic carcinoma
Osteoma and exostosis
Miscellaneous neoplasm
  Merkel cell carcinoma
  Squamous papilloma
  Pilomatrixoma
  Myxoma
  Auricular endochondrial pseudocyst
  Chondrodermatitis nodularis chronica helicis (Winkler disease)

Neoplasms of the middle ear, mastoid, and temporal bone
Adenomatous neoplasm
  Benign middle ear adenoma
  Endolymphatic sac tumor
Langerhans cell histiocytosis
  Eosinophilic granuloma
  Hand-Schüller-Christian disease
  Letterer-Siwe disease
  Sarcoma
  Rhabdomyosarcoma
  Chondrosarcoma
  Ewing sarcoma
  Osteogenic sarcoma
  Fibrosarcoma
Chordoma
Congenital neoplasm
  Dermoid
  Teratoma
  Choristoma
Cholesterol granuloma

Neoplasms of the internal auditory canal and cerebellopontine angle
Schwannoma
  Vestibular schwannoma
  Facial nerve schwannoma
  Trigeminal schwannoma
  Jugular foramen schwannoma
Meningioma
Lipoma
Metastases

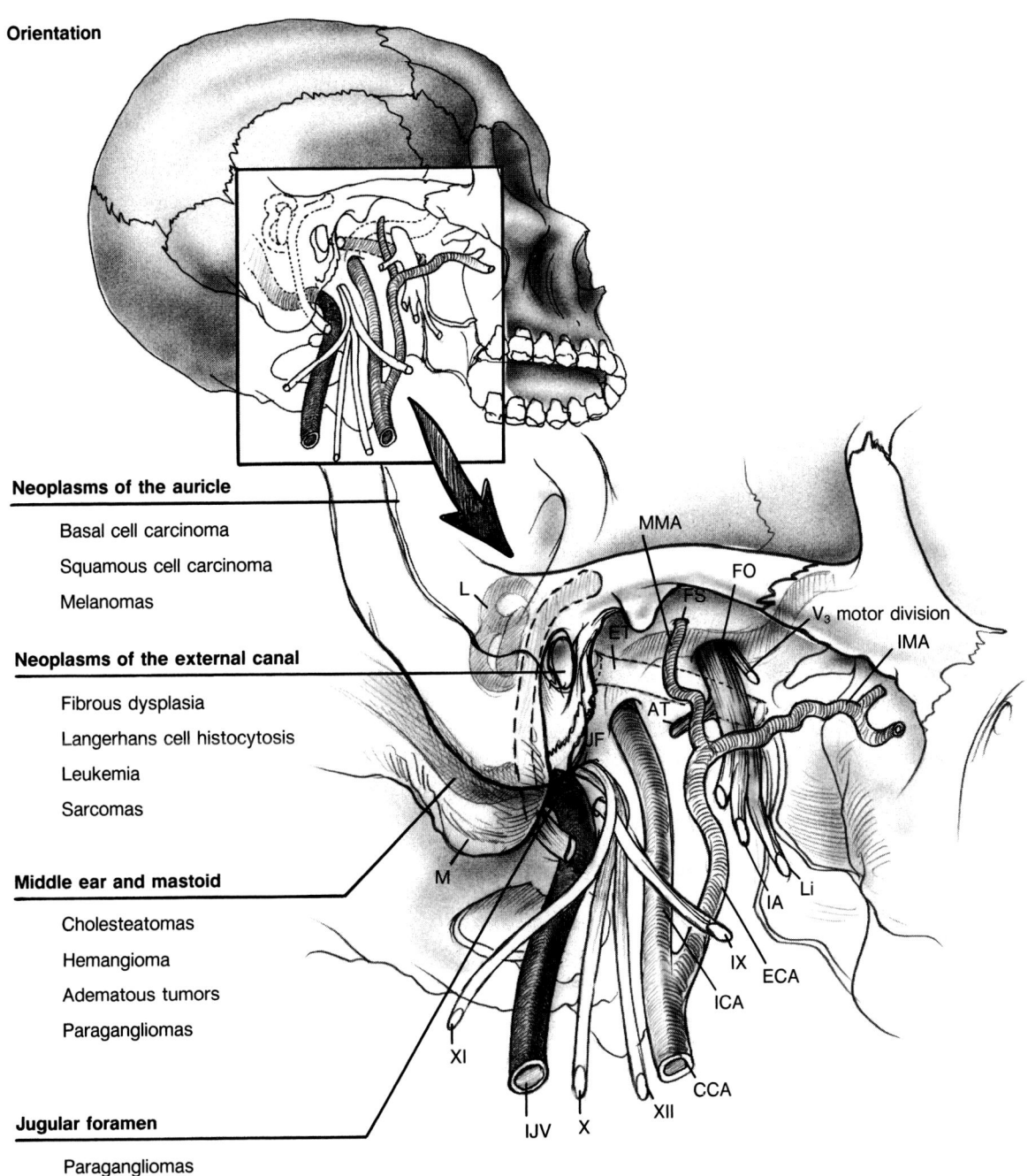

Orientation

Neoplasms of the auricle

Basal cell carcinoma

Squamous cell carcinoma

Melanomas

Neoplasms of the external canal

Fibrous dysplasia

Langerhans cell histocytosis

Leukemia

Sarcomas

Middle ear and mastoid

Cholesteatomas

Hemangioma

Adematous tumors

Paragangliomas

Jugular foramen

Paragangliomas

Nerve sheath tumors

Sarcomas

Figure 136.1 Anatomy of the lateral skull base and common locations of neoplasms found in this region. AT, auriculotemporal nerve; CCA, common carotid artery; ECA, external carotid artery; ET, eustachian tube; FO, foramen ovale; FS, foramen spinosum; IA, inferior alveolar nerve; ICA, internal carotid artery; IJV, internal jugular vein; IMA, internal maxillary artery; JF, jugular foramen; L, labyrinth; Li, lingual nerve; M, mastoid process; MMA, middle meningeal artery; V_3 motor division, mandibular division of the trigeminal nerve IX, glossopharyngeal nerve; X, vagus nerve; XI, accessory nerve; XII, hypoglossal nerve.

Although they are often described as rare, paragangliomas are the most common true neoplasm of the middle ear and are considered the most common pathologic condition involving the jugular foramen. Paragangliomas occur most frequently in whites and predominate on the left side.

Females are affected by paragangliomas more frequently than males (6:1). Although the peak incidence occurs during the fifth decade of life, paragangliomas may present from infancy to old age. Tumors that arise in very young patients should generate additional concern, because they tend to be more aggressive, are more commonly multifocal, and are more likely to secrete vasoactive substances (1). Approximately 5% to 10% of patients with paraganglioma eventually present with multiple tumors, but when paragangliomas occur as a familial form of an autosomal dominant disorder, multicentricity may occur in as many as 50% of patients. Genetic analysis of patients with familial paragangliomas shows defects on chromosome loci 11q13.1 and 11q22-23, and some evidence suggests that sporadic head and neck paragangliomata have a similar molecular pathogenesis (2,3). Although the chief cells of paragangliomas have neurosecretory granules that store catecholamines, only 1% to 3% of these tumors actively secrete norepinephrine. Catecholamines are much more likely to be secreted by glomus jugulare tumors than by glomus tympanicum tumors. Opinions vary regarding the need to screen for functionally active temporal bone paraganglioma, but all tumor patients who present with a history of flushing, frequent diarrhea, palpitations, headaches, poorly controlled hypertension, orthostasis, or excessive perspiration should have serum catecholamine levels measured and 24-hour collection of urine for analysis of vanillylmandelic acid and metanephrine.

The growth patterns of paragangliomas of the temporal bone are determined by the sites of tumor origin and by regional anatomy. Clinical manifestations are related to tumor extent and vascularity. Paragangliomas are generally slow-growing neoplasms. The time interval between initial symptoms and diagnosis may approach a decade. *Glomus tympanicum* tumors usually originate on the promontory of the cochlea. As they grow, they follow the path of least resistance. First, the tumor enlarges to fill the middle ear and to envelope the ossicles. Patients present at this stage with conductive hearing loss and pulsatile tinnitus caused by direct transmission of vascular pulsations from the highly vascularized tumor to the ossicles. Pulsatile tinnitus is the most common presenting symptom for patients with temporal bone paragangliomas. Because glomus tympanicum tumors enlarge within the middle ear cavity, patients with these tumors generally present with pulsatile tinnitus at an earlier stage than patients with glomus jugulare tumors. The tympanic membrane often remains intact as a glomus tympanicum tumor grows, but the tumor may displace the membrane laterally. If tumor extends through the tympanic membrane into the external auditory canal, patients may present with otalgia or bloody otorrhea. As glomus tympanicum tumors enlarge further, they may extend into the mastoid antrum via the aditus ad antrum, into the facial recess, or into the retrofacial air cell tract. At this stage, the tympanic and mastoid portions of the facial nerve may become involved with tumor. The tumor may grow anteriorly into the eustachian tube and inferiorly into the infralabyrinthine air cell tract. When the tumor causes bone erosion in the hypotympanum, the jugular fossa or the vertical portion of the petrous carotid artery may be exposed. It is difficult to distinguish an extensive

glomus tympanicum tumor of this kind from a glomus jugulare tumor. Patients with extensive tumors may present with multiple cranial nerve neuropathies.

Glomus jugulare tumors arise in the jugular fossa and are usually large before patients become symptomatic. Compression of neurovascular structures in the jugular fossa and extension medially along the skull base to the hypoglossal canal can lead to cranial nerve neuropathies manifesting as dysphagia, dysphonia, aspiration, and dysarthria. Erosion of the jugular fossa anteriorly and superiorly exposes the petrous carotid artery and allows tumor to invade the middle ear, causing conductive hearing loss and pulsatile tinnitus. Intracranial extension occurs when glomus tumors grow into the eustachian tube and extend into the peritubal air cell tract or follow the petrous carotid artery into the petrous apex, the cavernous sinus, and the middle cranial fossa, resulting in facial hypesthesia. Glomus jugulare tumors may involve the posterior cranial fossa when they extend medially along the skull base or through the infralabyrinthine air cell tract. A patient with extensive tumor that compresses the cerebellum and the brainstem in the posterior fossa may present with ataxia and imbalance.

On gross examination, paragangliomas are deep red, firm, rubbery masses that bleed profusely during manipulation. The microscopic appearance of paraganglioma is distinctive. Clusters of chief cells, termed *zellballen*, are enclosed by fibrous septa and supporting cells within a vascular network. Unmyelinated nerve fibers may be identified, but they are scarce when compared with normal paraganglia (1). Nuclear pleomorphism and hyperchromatism are prominent in chief cells but do not appear to indicate malignant growth. Variable cranial nerve invasion may occur, a feature that has significance during surgical removal of the tumor mass. Metastases of paragangliomas are uncommon. They occur in association with only 3% to 4% of paragangliomas and are most often found in the regional lymph nodes, lungs, liver, spleen, and bone.

Paragangliomas of the temporal bone can usually be diagnosed on the basis of findings on physical exam and characteristic features found on imaging studies. Otoscopic examination of a middle ear paraganglioma frequently demonstrates a reddish-blue pulsatile mass medial to the inferior tympanic membrane. Positive pressure during pneumatic otoscopy causes blanching of the mass, a phenomenon known as the Brown sign. The pulsatile nature of the tumor can be diminished with ipsilateral carotid artery compression, a phenomenon known as the Aquino sign. Objective tinnitus may be apparent if auscultation over the mastoid or infra-auricular area reveals an audible bruit. When tumor extends through the tympanic membrane, otoscopic examination shows a hemorrhagic aural polyp. Tumors involving the jugular foramen can be identified when lower cranial nerve palsies develop. Jugular foramen syndrome, also termed Vernet syndrome, arises when tumor growth affects cranial nerves IX, X, and XI and causes paresis or paralysis of the muscles innervated by these nerves. Villaret syndrome is a combination of jugular foramen syndrome with Horner syndrome in patients with more extensive disease. Patients with paragangliomas that erode the carotid canal and compromise the sympathetic plexus present with Horner syndrome (miosis, ptosis, anhydrosis, and enophthalmos). If facial nerve weakness or paralysis exists, it denotes extensive involvement of the middle ear and mastoid. Tuning fork tests or complete audiometric evaluation in these patients shows conductive hearing loss and on rare occasions sensorineural hearing loss. Ataxia or rostral cranial nerve palsies are disquieting signs that indicate involvement of the posterior cranial fossa or cavernous sinus.

Diagnostic imaging studies offer essential information for the evaluation of patients with temporal bone paragangliomas. These studies provide diagnostic facts and details about tumor extent and regional anatomy that are essential in planning surgery. High-resolution computed tomography (HRCT) of the temporal bone uses a thin-section bone algorithm and is usually the first imaging study ordered to evaluate a patient suspected of having a temporal bone paraganglioma. HRCT can identify the tumor origin accurately when the bony partition between the jugular fossa and the hypotympanum is intact. In this instance, a glomus jugulare tumor that erodes the jugular fossa and involves lower cranial nerves can be distinguished from a glomus tympanicum tumor that occupies the middle ear. Without this bony partition, it may be difficult to identify the origin of a temporal bone paraganglioma. Erosion of the caroticojugular spine that separates the jugular bulb and the petrous carotid artery usually indicates a glomus jugulare tumor. If the spine is eroded and the carotid canal is exposed, involvement of the petrous carotid artery is likely. HRCT also helps to identify other lesions that should be excluded, such as a dehiscent jugular bulb or an aberrant internal carotid artery. Obliteration of the fallopian canal indicates adherence of tumor to the facial nerve or invasion of the nerve by tumor. Intracranial extension can also be identified, but magnetic resonance imaging (MRI) is better than HRCT to evaluate the relationship between paraganglioma and adjacent soft tissue structures. MRI will not only identify intracranial extension but may help differentiate between intradural and extradural extension. MRI signal characteristics can be diagnostic for paragangliomas showing vascular flow voids within the tumor, the so-called salt and pepper pattern. Magnetic resonance angiography and magnetic resonance venography can show intraluminal involvement of the petrous carotid artery or occlusion of the jugular vein and sigmoid sinus. However, these studies are usually not useful for most large tumors because formal angiography will be necessary. MRI of the neck offers enough detail to screen for multicentric disease such as carotid body tumors or glomus vagale tumors, but positron emission tomography and octreotide scintigraphy have been advocated to increase the sensitivity of screening for multicentric lesions and recurrent disease (4,5).

The principal therapeutic modality is complete surgical excision of the tumor. Secreting tumors must be treated with adjunctive α and β blockade. If surgical therapy is deemed appropriate, small tumors isolated to the promontory can be removed via the transcanal or hypotympanotomy approach. More advanced lesions of the middle ear and mastoid can be exposed with an extended facial recess approach through the mastoid. Large paragangliomas should be evaluated preoperatively with four-vessel angiography. Angiography is combined with embolization using polyvinyl alcohol or intravascular coils 1 or 2 days before surgery to decrease intraoperative blood loss, shorten duration of the procedure, and reduce postoperative morbidity. If sacrifice of the internal carotid artery is anticipated, balloon occlusion studies and single photon emission computed tomography (CT) or xenon CT studies can be combined with angiography to assess cerebral cross-circulation. Glomus jugulare tumors are approached via transmastoid-transcervical exposure of the jugular bulb and jugular foramen. Large tumors require limited facial nerve rerouting or formal infratemporal fossa dissection through this approach. In some cases, more extensive temporal bone dissection is necessary to eradicate tumor that has spread to the petrous apex. This may necessitate removal of part or all of the labyrinth. Intracranial extension requires a combined neurosurgical-neurotologic procedure. Postoperative cranial nerve palsies are not uncommon, and some patients require follow-up care to assist with facial reanimation, deglutition, and phonation. Alternatives to surgical therapy for primary, recurrent, or persistent disease includes external beam radiation therapy and stereotactic radiosurgery. Radiation has little effect on the primary tumor cells, the chief cells, but it causes obliterative endarteritis in tumor vessels, which can stop tumor growth. Control of tumor growth and stabilization of neurologic symptoms with stereotactic radiosurgery occurs in greater than 90% of patients who have been monitored for less than 10 years, but longer follow-up is needed to establish the efficacy of this therapy (6).

Epidermoid (Cholesteatoma)

Epidermoids are soft tissue masses caused by aberrant accumulation of keratin debris within a sac of squamous epithelium. They are termed masses rather than neoplasms because they are not strictly cellular growths. Depending on where they arise in the ear or in the lateral skull base, epidermoids may be the result of squamous epithelial migration or implantation, congenital entrapment during embryogenesis, or metaplasia of a mucosal lining. The nomenclature used to describe these masses is determined in part by both the site of origin and by pathogenesis. For example, masses that arise from congenital epithelial rests and occur in the petrous apex, in the internal auditory canal, or in the cerebellopontine angle are generally referred to as epidermoids. Masses that are the result of epithelial migration from the tympanic membrane into the middle ear or from traumatic implantation deep to the skin of the external auditory canal are called cholesteatoma. One exception to this terminology is congenital cholesteatoma, which usually refers to an epithelial sac that arises within the middle ear when congenital epithelial rests become trapped during development. No matter where they originate or how they arise, all have similar histology and growth potential.

Middle ear cholesteatomas are generally distinguished as two types, congenital and acquired. *Congenital* middle ear cholesteatoma occurs in the presence of an intact tympanic membrane, whereas acquired masses are associated with perforation or retraction of the tympanic membrane. Congenital masses are thought to originate from embryonic rests of what is termed the epidermoid formation in the anterosuperior quadrant of the middle ear cleft (7). *Acquired* cholesteatomas consist of transposed keratinizing squamous epithelium in the middle ear, epitympanum, or mastoid. They are by far the more common of the two types and probably result from eustachian tube dysfunction and/or deficient tympanic membrane structure that leads to the formation of a retraction pocket in the tympanic membrane, which traps epithelium and leads to the accumulation of keratin debris in the middle ear. Acquired aural cholesteatoma may extend to the petrous bone or to the cranial cavity, but most lesions of the petrous apex and the cerebellopontine angle are thought to be of congenital origin. Cholesteatoma of the external auditory canal could conceivably result from congenital rests of tissue trapped deep to the skin of the canal, but most canal wall cholesteatomas occur after traumatic implantation of epithelium subsequent to external trauma or otologic surgery. Patients with cholesteatoma of the middle ear and the external auditory canal most often present with purulent otorrhea and conductive hearing loss. Patients with congenital cholesteatoma, however, may not present with otorrhea because the tympanic membrane is usually intact.

Epidermoids represent approximately 1% of all intracranial tumors and most occur in the cerebellopontine angle. Approximately 3% to 4% of all cerebellopontine angle tumors are epidermoids. Squamous metaplasia within the temporal bone or intradural space has been proposed in the histogenesis of these lesions, but developmental entrapment of ectodermal rests is more likely to be the cause. Because squamous epithelium at the periphery of the epidermoid is the only viable proliferating tissue, they grow very slowly when compared with solid benign neoplasms of similar dimensions. Epidermoids enlarge by expanding to fill empty spaces such as the cerebellopontine angle, the internal auditory canal, or air cells that occupy the petrous apex. These masses are infiltrative, and they grow to a relatively large size before they begin to compress or displace adjacent structures. Additionally,

epidermoids tend to incite a localized inflammatory reaction that causes the lining to become densely adherent to juxtaposed brainstem or cerebellum. Local neurovascular structures become enveloped by epidermoids instead of being displaced or compressed, and neurologic function may be altered when the vascular supply of a nerve is compromised by the infiltrative process. Most patients become symptomatic in a very gradual manner, and their symptoms are related to the location of the mass. Patients with internal auditory canal or cerebellopontine angle epidermoids often present with imbalance and hearing loss like patients with vestibular schwannoma. However, epidermoids are more likely than vestibular schwannoma to cause facial weakness or hemifacial spasm. Epidermoids are also more likely to compromise the trigeminal nerve, causing diminished facial sensation or facial pain. Intracranial extension of these lesions may also manifest as diplopia or headache.

All epidermoids and cholesteatomas exhibit a similar morphologic appearance. The friable lesions are either smooth and cystic with a round or oval appearance or nodular and irregular. The lining of the sac is usually whitish in color and spongy in consistency. Histologically, the cyst is lined with a benign keratinizing squamous epithelium consisting of three components: the sac or epithelial matrix, the perimatrix, and the contents of the cyst. All normal layers of typical squamous epithelium may be identified within the epithelial matrix. The contents of the cyst include fully differentiated laminated keratin. Acquired and congenital lesions can often be distinguished because acquired cholesteatomas have a thicker matrix layer and have proliferation of inflammatory cells within the sac and at its periphery.

Diagnosis of cholesteatoma is usually made during otologic examination, whereas epidermoids are usually diagnosed from radiographic imaging studies. Congenital epidermoids are frequently identified as an asymptomatic mass in the anterosuperior quadrant of the middle ear. Patients with acquired disease have keratin debris, granulation polyps, or purulent material emanating from the mouth or opening of the sac. Clinical findings in patients with epidermoids include facial weakness or paralysis and sensorineural hearing loss when the lesion involves the internal auditory canal and/or the cerebellopontine angle. Facial hypesthesia and abducens nerve palsy occur when epidermoids invade the anterior petrous apex. HRCT of the temporal bone in patients with epidermoids shows a well-defined homogeneous mass that sometimes contains areas of calcification. MRI is diagnostic, showing a well-circumscribed nonenhancing mass that has low signal intensity on T1-weighted images and high signal intensity on T2-weighted images. Diffusion weighted images may be used to differentiate epidermoids from other lesions such as arachnoid cysts.

Management of cholesteatomas of the external auditory canal and middle ear is addressed in other chapters in this text. Optimal treatment of epidermoids of the skull base includes complete surgical excision. This often requires a posterior fossa or middle fossa craniotomy, but transtemporal approaches may be indicated, especially in patients with nonserviceable hearing in the ipsilateral ear. Because the capsule of the mass may be densely adherent to the brainstem or intracranial vascular structures, complete removal of epidermoids of the skull base is extremely difficult or even impossible. Complete excision is possible in only half of all patients with epidermoids, and additional postoperative cranial nerve deficits are found in most of these patients (8). Recurrence can be expected in at least 30% of patients when subtotal removal is carried out.

Hemangioma and Hemangiopericytoma

Hemangiomas are benign vascular proliferations that arise from capillaries, arterioles, or venules. They are classified according to the type of vessel from which they originate: capillary hemangioma, cavernous hemangioma, and venous hemangioma. It is unclear whether they represent true neoplasms or hyperplastic growth of normal tissue occurring in an appropriate anatomic location. Hemangiomas are reported to occur in a variety of locations involving the external ear and lateral skull base, namely the external auditory canal and tympanic membrane, the middle ear, the internal auditory canal, and the geniculate segment of the facial nerve. Tumors are spongy red or purple nodular masses. On microscopic examination they show thin-walled vascular channels that contain blood and are small or intermediate in size. These channels are not surrounded by an elastic or muscular layer. Clinical presentation varies depending on tumor location. Hemangiomas of the external auditory canal and tympanic membrane have been reported when patients present with mild conductive hearing loss and aural fullness. Patients with middle ear tumors are often asymptomatic, but they can also present with conductive hearing loss, aural fullness, and pulsatile tinnitus. Otologic examination reveals a vascular intratympanic mass that can be confused with a paraganglioma, an adenomatous tumor, or an aberrant vascular anatomy. Preoperatively, hemangiomas of the internal auditory canal may be difficult to distinguish from vestibular schwannomas when patients present with unilateral sensorineural hearing loss. However, accompanying facial nerve dysfunction is more characteristic of hemangioma, even when tumors are small. Imaging studies help to differentiate intracanalicular lesions when hemangiomas show calcium stippling, which is characteristic of an osseous hemangioma. Geniculate hemangiomas are the most common temporal bone hemangioma and perhaps the most intriguing. They consistently arise from the superior aspect of the geniculate ganglion, probably from vascular plexuses on the surface of the nerve, and extend into the floor of the middle cranial fossa. Even though the tumor is generally extraneural, they sometimes infiltrate the nerve or are associated with a localized inflammatory response that causes the tumor to adhere tightly to the nerve sheath. This intimate relationship with the facial nerve accounts for the frequently associated facial nerve dysfunction, indicated by paralysis, twitching, or spasm of the facial musculature, even when tumors are very small. Treatment of hemangioma is complete surgical excision. Resection of lesions from the external canal and the middle ear is usually straightforward, but it may be unnecessary in pediatric patients who are asymptomatic because these lesions often involute spontaneously. When hemangioma is associated with the facial nerve, however, proper management is controversial. If facial paralysis exists, tumor resection with nerve grafting may be appropriate. If facial nerve function is normal or only mildly compromised, early excision when the tumor can be peeled off the nerve while preserving function may be preferable. However, most reported cases show that this is usually not possible. Because most geniculate hemangiomas grow very slowly, observation may be the most appropriate management until severe dysfunction or facial paralysis occurs.

Hemangiopericytoma is a rare vascular tumor derived from pericytes that line the outside surface of capillary basal lamina. They can occur wherever capillaries are found. Less than 20% of hemangiopericytomas occur in the head and neck, and fewer than 10 cases have been reported in which the tumor originated in the temporal bone. The middle ear, jugular fossa, and petrous bone were the apparent sites of origin of the tumors that occurred in the temporal bone. Symptoms include hearing loss, otorrhea, and cranial nerve deficits. Hemangiopericytoma can occur in patients of any age, but it is most frequent in patients in their fifth decade, affecting males and females equally. Tumors are soft or rubbery and pale gray or white in color. The metastatic rate for primary temporal bone tumors is lower and is estimated to be 15% to 20%. On microscopic examination, hemangiopericytomas are circumscribed pseudoencapsulated cellular tumors containing thin-walled vascular spaces separated by sheets of polyhedral and spindle-shaped cells. Tumors with malignant behavior may display nuclear pleomorphism, lymphocytic infiltration, and lack of vascular spaces. Wide excision is the treatment of choice, but external beam radiation therapy, stereotactic radiosurgery, or chemotherapy may be used to treat extensive, recurrent, or inoperable tumors.

Lymphoma, Plasmacytoma, and Leukemia

Lymphoma is a neoplasm of the lymphoreticular system that may involve the temporal bone either as a secondary lesion after metastatic spread or as a primary lesion causing focal disease. Neoplastic infiltration of the middle ear, the facial nerve, the eighth cranial nerve, and the bone marrow of the petrous apex is not an uncommon finding during postmortem examination of temporal bones from patients with systemic lymphoma. However, most patients are asymptomatic unless lymphomatous infiltration results in middle ear effusion or hemorrhage and conductive hearing loss. Tucci et al. (9) were the first to report two cases of primary temporal bone B-cell lymphoma that involved the middle ear. Staging evaluation in both patients revealed no evidence of distant or disseminated disease. Since this initial report, a number of instances of primary B-cell and T-cell non-Hodgkin lymphoma and Hodgkin lymphoma of the middle ear, mastoid, and internal auditory canal have been identified (10,11). In these case reports, the most common symptoms were conductive hearing loss, otalgia, otorrhea, fevers, sensorineural hearing loss, and facial nerve weakness from perineural invasion. Physical examination showed middle ear effusion or middle ear masses and facial paresis. Once diffuse lymphoma has been ruled out, most patients with primary lymphoma of the temporal bone do well after chemotherapy and/or radiation therapy. The role of surgery in these patients is to obtain tissue for diagnosis.

Extramedullary plasmacytoma of the temporal bone is a rare neoplasm that is thought to arise from plasma cells in the submucosal stroma of the middle ear. These are solitary lesions that occur outside the bony medullary spaces, and they are less likely to develop into disseminated disease or into multiple myeloma when compared with solitary osseous plasmacytomas. Extramedullary plasmacytomas occur in all age groups but are most frequent in the sixth and seventh decades. Patients present with aural fullness or otalgia, hearing loss, and tinnitus, and physical examination reveals a thickened tympanic membrane with an intratympanic mass or an aural polyp. Microscopic examination of these fleshy masses shows sheets of monotonous round cells that are typical of plasma cells. Nuclear and cellular atypia is variable and defines tumor differentiation and grade. Tumor grade, however, is not necessarily predictive of tumor behavior. When biopsy specimens confirm the diagnosis of extramedullary plasmacytoma, patients should be evaluated for disseminated disease or multiple myeloma. This evaluation includes serum and urine analysis for monoclonal antibodies, peripheral smear examination, bone marrow biopsy, and skeletal radiographic survey. Chemotherapy is indicated for disseminated disease, but extramedullary plasmacytoma isolated to the temporal bone is usually successfully treated with external beam radiation therapy.

Leukemia may involve the temporal bone by infiltrating marrow spaces and the tympanomastoid cavity or by causing hemorrhage within the middle or inner ear. In leukemia patients, marrow spaces in the temporal bone are frequently infiltrated by leukemic cells, but this rarely results in clinical manifestations. Infiltration of the middle ear and mastoid air cells is less common but results in symptomatic effusions. Patients with acute or chronic myelogenous leukemia may develop larger consolidated infiltrates that form solid tumors known as granulocytic sarcomas or chloromas. They consist of immature granulo-

cytes and contain myeloperoxidase that gives the lesion a green hue, hence the name chloroma. Most chloromas occur in children with leukemia. Leukemic infiltrates can involve the cochlea causing sensorineural hearing loss, but inner ear injury more likely results from local hemorrhage. Treatment of systemic leukemia that infiltrates the temporal bone requires appropriate chemotherapy and management by a hematologist/oncologist. Chloroma responds best to external beam radiation therapy.

NEOPLASMS OF THE PINNA AND EXTERNAL AUDITORY CANAL

Cutaneous Carcinoma

Basal cell carcinoma is a cutaneous malignancy that comprises approximately one fifth of neoplasms that involve the ear and temporal bone. This common lesion is generally found in adult patients and is usually diagnosed for the first time during the sixth decade of life. Most basal cell carcinomas occur on the pinna or in the periauricular area, where they are more common than squamous cell carcinoma, whereas only about 15% arise in the external auditory canal where squamous cell carcinoma is far more common. Actinic exposure is thought to be the most important factor that initiates this neoplastic transformation because the periauricular areas and the auricular helix, which receive the most sun exposure, are especially susceptible. Males are affected approximately twice as often as females. The noduloulcerative lesion that appears on the pinna is similar to basal cell carcinomas found in other areas of the body. It is characterized by locally infiltrating nodular growth with a rolled border and a central crusting ulcer. This neoplasm appears to be well circumscribed, but there may be subcutaneous extension with indistinct clinical margins. Distant or regional metastases are extremely rare. Histologic examination shows a rim of palisading basaloid cells at the tumor margin with central necrosis and ulceration. Most of the tumor is quite cellular, making it simple to make a diagnosis and to identify the tumor margin. However, 25% of basal cell carcinomas that involve the skin of the external ear are morpheaform or sclerosing subtypes. They are distinguished from the more common noduloulcerative lesions by linear strands of basaloid cells that infiltrate the subcutaneous layers of the skin and are accompanied by a fibrous matrix. The linear strands are diffuse within the fibrous matrix, and consequently the margin of the morpheaform type of basal cell carcinoma is indistinct.

Basal cell carcinoma of the ear is a slow-growing neoplasm, and the diagnosis is readily obtained by inspection and biopsy. If untreated, these low-grade malignancies progressively enlarge and infiltrate peripherally into the periauricular tissues or medially into the external auditory canal, the middle ear, and the mastoid. Morpheaform lesions are especially troublesome because they infiltrate along deep tissue planes. Extension into the temporal bone may remain undetected until the malignancy is far advanced. Basal cell carcinoma is best treated with complete surgical excision. However, the risk of recurrence for auricular basal cell carcinoma is high compared with other sites in the head and neck because deep invasion often occurs. Mohs micrographic surgery appears to be the most successful technique to minimize recurrence and to conserve nonneoplastic tissue. Radiation therapy is used as palliative therapy or as adjunct therapy for extensive or recurrent tumors.

Squamous cell carcinoma that involves the ear and lateral skull base is most often a cutaneous neoplasm that originates from the skin of the pinna or external auditory canal. A much smaller portion of these malignancies originates from the middle ear, presumably from metaplastic middle ear mucosa. The average age at diagnosis of squamous cell carcinoma of the pinna is the late sixties, whereas primary external auditory canal lesions generally present 10 to 15 years earlier. Tumors that originate in the middle ear affect adults in an intermediate age group at an average age of 60 years. Patients with squamous cell carcinoma of the ear and temporal bone comprise 24% of patients with squamous cell carcinoma of the head and neck. Most of these tumors originate on the pinna. Like basal cell carcinoma, more than half of these occur on the helix, which receives the greatest actinic exposure. Sun exposure and cold injury certainly predispose patients to this malignancy, but other factors such as radiation exposure and chronic infection are thought to play an etiologic role. For squamous cell carcinoma that originates in the middle ear, chronic otitis media and human papillomavirus are proposed to be important elements in the pathogenesis of malignancy (12).

Squamous cell carcinoma of the pinna is a scaly, irregular, indurated maculopapular lesion. Very often the surface of the erythematous lesion is ulcerated with either a crust or serosanguinous exudate. Patients with squamous cell carcinoma of the external auditory canal often present with hemorrhagic otorrhea that has been treated for years as otitis externa. In older patients, chronic bloody drainage and sudden onset of deep ear pain suggest an invasive malignancy. Ipsilateral facial nerve deficit is another indication of invasive malignancy. Extensive involvement of the external auditory canal or the middle ear results in conductive hearing loss, but deep invasion that extends into the internal auditory canal, the cerebellopontine angle, or the labyrinthine capsule may cause sensorineural hearing loss. Metastasis to cervical or parotid lymph nodes occurs more frequently when the primary neoplasm is located in the bony portion of the external auditory canal. Histologic examination shows proliferative pleomorphic spindle-shaped epidermal cells with keratin pearls and intercellular bridges that are typical features of squamous cell carcinoma. A less aggressive form of squamous cell carcinoma

of the pinna, called adenoid squamous cell carcinoma, shows similar histologic features, but there is nodular proliferation of epidermoid cells that show prominent glandular patterns. These lesions are invasive but slow growing, and they rarely metastasize.

The diagnosis of squamous cell carcinoma of the pinna is easily made with a biopsy, but many middle ear and external auditory canal malignancies are far advanced by the time of diagnosis. Biopsy is advisable whenever middle ear or external canal infections fail to respond to appropriate medical therapy. Untreated carcinoma of the pinna will likely spread laterally to periauricular areas or medially into the external auditory canal. The prognosis declines when external canal lesions extend medially into the tympanic bone or through the tympanic membrane and into the middle ear. Tumor in the middle ear extends anteriorly into the eustachian tube and carotid canal and posteriorly into the mastoid air cell system. From the carotid canal, squamous cell carcinoma can invade the petrous apex, the anterior skull base, and the cavernous sinus. The inner ear is generally resistant to invasion, but tumor in the mastoid may penetrate the dural plate and extend into the posterior cranial fossa.

The treatment of squamous cell carcinoma of the ear and lateral skull base, even for less advanced tumors, should be aggressive because recurrence rates are high (13). Complete surgical resection is favored whenever possible. Complete resection of lesions of the pinna is most easily achieved with Mohs micrographic surgical techniques. Carcinoma that invades the temporal bone requires radiation therapy in addition to temporal bone resection. In most cases, regional lymph nodes need to be addressed (14). Chemotherapy is sometimes offered as adjuvant or palliative therapy but has not yet been shown to increase survival.

Melanoma

Malignant melanoma of the external ear is a cutaneous neoplasm that originates from melanocytes in the epidermis or dermis of the pinna. Melanomas account for only 4% to 5% of malignant cutaneous neoplasms, yet more than 50% of deaths from cutaneous malignancies are caused by melanoma. The external ear is the site of origin for approximately 10% of all primary melanomas of the head and neck and 1% of all melanomas, with the helix and antihelix being the most common location of the original lesion. Primary melanoma of the external auditory canal is extremely rare, and melanoma of the middle ear is most likely to be metastatic disease or the result of regional extension. The average age at diagnosis of melanoma of the pinna is 50 years, but this disease affects all age groups except for young children. Men are affected by melanoma at least three times more often than women, and fair-skinned individuals with blonde or red hair, blue eyes, and freckled skin are predisposed to the disease. Sun exposure, specifically repeated intense exposure causing severe solar injury, has a role in the pathogenesis of this neoplasm. Melanoma is five times more common in the Southwestern United States when compared with the Northeast. The incidence of melanoma in all areas of the world appears to be increasing annually. Atmospheric ozone depletion may be responsible for some of this increase, but heightened awareness of skin malignancy by patients and by medical professionals enhances the likelihood of detection. Patients may also be genetically predisposed to melanoma. First-degree relatives of patients with melanoma have twice the risk of developing this malignancy, and inherited disorders, such as familial dysplastic nevus syndrome, also increase the risk of developing melanoma.

Melanomas have a radial growth phase during which they grow in diameter and a vertical growth phase during which dermal invasion occurs. Melanomas are divided into three types based on appearance and potential for dermal invasion. *Superficial spreading melanoma* is the most common type. It starts as a regular dark pigmented macule that becomes nodular and ulcerated once the vertical growth phase begins. The radial growth phase is intermediate in length and is estimated to last anywhere from 1 to 6 years. Pigmented round epithelioid melanocytes grow in nests invading the epidermis during the radial growth phase and the dermis during the vertical growth phase. Many of these lesions will incite an inflammatory response. *Nodular melanoma* is the most aggressive of the three types. These darkly pigmented nodules grow rapidly and invade the dermis early on. On histologic examination, atypical melanocytes are both spindle shaped and epithelioid in nature and the surrounding inflammatory response is minimal. *Lentigo maligna*, the third type of melanoma, is a macular lesion with variable pigmentation that tends to have a prolonged radial growth phase before dermal invasion occurs. A lentigo consists of pigmented spindle cells that are usually confined to the epidermis, and there may be a surrounding inflammatory response.

The diagnosis of melanoma is suspected when pigmented lesions change color or texture, increase rapidly in size, or ulcerate. Prompt excisional biopsy is recommended for all suspicious pigmented lesions because early melanoma is curable. Tumor thickness is critical to establish the prognosis, but nodular configuration, ulceration, and regional or distant metastases all indicate a poor prognosis. Once the dermis is invaded, the probability of regional or distant metastases increases. Unfortunately, one third of patients have cervical node involvement at presentation. In the past, tragus and anterior pinna lesions were thought to metastasize to the parotid gland and to high anterior cervical lymph nodes, whereas posterior pinna lesions were thought to spread to the mastoid bone and occipital and posterior cervical nodes. However, this correlation between melanoma location and nodal drainage is inconsistent, and sentinel node mapping using lym-

phoscintigraphy is becoming the primary method of identifying nodal drainage patterns (15).

The treatment of choice for malignant melanoma of the external ear is complete surgical excision with at least a 1- to 2-cm margin because satellite lesions can occur. The treatment of metastatic disease to the neck is somewhat controversial (16). Elective neck dissection is generally not recommended for early lesions measuring less than 0.76 mm in thickness, whereas lymphadenectomy may offer survival advantage and better local control for intermediate lesions measuring approximately 0.8 to 4.0 mm. The risk of regional or distant metastases for lesions more than 4.0 mm in thickness is greater than 70%. Thus, elective neck dissection is of uncertain benefit. Lymphoscintigraphy with sentinel node biopsy may help to make the decision regarding neck dissection for patients with clinically negative necks. Functional neck dissection is usually recommended for the control of regional disease in all patients with lymph node metastases. High-dose interferon-alpha-2b is recommended for patients with lymph node positive disease. Other adjuvant therapy including immunomodulation therapy, vaccination, high-dose fractionated radiation therapy and chemotherapy have not been shown to improve survival but continue to be investigated (17).

Glandular Tumors

Glandular tumors of the external auditory canal are rare benign neoplasms that are thought to arise exclusively from the ceruminous glands of the canal. It is true that nearly all glandular tumors of the external auditory canal arise in the lateral membranous portion of the canal where ceruminous and sebaceous glands predominate, but both ceruminous and sebaceous glands are categorized as apocrine glands, meaning that glandular cells release secretions by pinching off and liberating the secretion-rich portion of the cell. Some glandular tumors of the external ear canal, however, seem to arise from eccrine glands. These are glands that secrete by releasing secretory granules. Ceruminous glands might give rise to eccrine gland tumors if they also had some eccrine function. Electron microscopy suggests that ceruminous glands do indeed release secretory granules and may have eccrine function. They might then be better classified as apocrine glands and thus might be the origin of all glandular tumors of the external auditory canal.

It is possible to distinguish at least four different histologic types of glandular tumors of the external auditory canal. *Ceruminous adenoma* clearly arises from ceruminous glands. Histologically, it consists of well-differentiated proliferating ceruminous glands that form solid, cystic, and papillary patterns. The glands have a cuboidal or columnar cell layer of apocrine origin and an outer spindle-cell layer of myoepithelial origin. These tumors may be more common in males, and the average age of patients at presentation is 61 years. These nonencapsulated benign neoplasms do not invade surrounding structures. *Ceruminous adenocarcinoma,* on the other hand, is an invasive neoplasm that can metastasize to regional lymph nodes. Histologically, this tumor is nearly identical to a benign adenoma, and it may be difficult to distinguish benign and malignant forms based on microscopic anatomy. However, in some cases, microscopic examination of malignant lesions shows anaplasia, nuclear pleomorphism, mitotic figures, and perivascular or perineural invasion. The primary distinguishing features are regional metastases and invasion into surrounding tissues. Like adenomas, adenocarcinomas are more common in males, but they are diagnosed at an earlier age, averaging 48 years. *Pleomorphic adenoma* of the external auditory canal is similar to neoplasms of the salivary glands, which are eccrine glands, and consists of both epithelial and mesenchymal elements. These benign tumors affect males and females equally, and the average age at diagnosis is 51 years. *Adenoid cystic carcinoma* is the most common glandular neoplasm of the external auditory canal. The cell type that gives rise to these tumors when they occur in the external auditory canal is uncertain. Histologically, these tumors are similar to malignant salivary gland tumors. They lack a capsule and consist of small hyperchromatic cells arranged in cribriform, tubular, or solid patterns. Perineural invasion and invasion along deep tissue planes are prominent features. Regional lymph node metastases are not uncommon, and distant metastases can occur in any vascularized organ, but the lung is the most common site of distant disease. Adenoid cystic carcinoma is more common in females and is diagnosed on average at 43 years of age.

Glandular tumors usually present as asymptomatic soft tissue masses in the membranous external auditory canal. Once the canal is occluded, conductive hearing loss or secondary otitis externa may result. Malignant lesions are more likely to ulcerate or to cause otalgia. Both benign and malignant tumors grow along the path of least resistance, extending laterally out the meatus or medially through the tympanic membrane and into the middle ear. Invasive malignant tumors also extend radially through auricular cartilage and the fissures of Santorini into the parotid gland or into surrounding periauricular tissue. Medial extension with erosion of tympanic membrane or temporal bone is also indicative of malignancy. Diagnosis is made on the basis of microscopic examination of biopsy specimens. To distinguish between benign and malignant ceruminous tumors, biopsy specimens should be large enough to identify deep tissue invasion. HRCT of the temporal bone and MRI of soft tissue around the lateral skull base can be helpful in this respect also. Benign tumors are treated with wide local excision and reconstruction of the external auditory canal. Because of high recurrence rates, especially in cases of adenoid cystic carcinoma, treatment of malignant lesions should be aggressive. Lateral temporal bone resection with parotidectomy and postoperative radiation therapy is appropriate for early lesions. Larger malignant tumors require a more extensive temporal bone resection and cervical lymph node dissection in addition to parotidectomy and postoperative radiation therapy.

Osteomata and Exostoses

Osteomata and exostoses are benign bony growths that involve the external auditory canal. Some controversy exists about whether these are separate entities or actually variations of the same pathologic process, but most sources suggest that osteoma and exostosis are clinically and histologically distinct. Osteomata are solitary pedunculated osseous lesions that are smooth and round and originate on the tympanosquamous and tympanomastoid suture lines inside the bony external auditory canal. Patients in almost any age group may present with these neoplasms, but most are middle-aged adults at presentation, and women appear to be affected more often than men. The etiology of osteomata is unknown. Clinically, most patients are unaware of the neoplasm until it is incidentally discovered during otologic examination. When the tumor is sufficiently large, patients may experience conductive hearing loss or recurrent bouts of otitis externa. Histologically, osteomata consist of lamellar bone around trabeculated cancellous bone that contains marrow spaces or fibrovascular tissue. The bone is lined with periosteum and keratinizing stratified squamous cell epithelium. The diagnosis is made during otologic examination when palpation reveals a pearly white or erythematous tender bony growth fixed within the bony canal. Surgical removal of symptomatic tumors requires either a transcanal or a postauricular approach for exposure. Osteomata are removed with a drill while preserving as much skin as possible. Split-thickness skin grafts are used to cover exposed tympanic bone when necessary.

Exostoses are broad-based osseous lesions that occur around the circumference of the medial aspect of the bony external auditory canal. They occur as multiple lesions and are often bilateral. Most patients are diagnosed in their teens or as young adults, and exostoses are far more common in males. The occurrence of exostoses is strongly correlated with exposure to cold water and is therefore thought to result from cold-induced periostitis. Like patients with osteomata, most are asymptomatic until the external auditory canal is occluded or nearly occluded and the diagnosis is made during otologic examination. Histologically, exostoses differ from osteomas. Exostoses consist of parallel layers of subperiosteal bone containing no or only poorly developed trabeculated fibrovascular channels. Surgical removal of exostoses is usually more challenging than the removal of osteomata. Generally, a postauricular approach is required, and facial nerve monitoring is recommended because the distal mastoid portion of the facial nerve is at risk during drilling of the posteroinferior aspect of the bony canal. Skin flaps are developed to expose the bony lesions, and they are removed with a drill while preserving the skin. Split-thickness skin grafts may be necessary to prevent postoperative cicatrix formation.

Miscellaneous Neoplasms of the Pinna and External Auditory Canal

Merkel cell carcinoma is a rare but highly malignant cutaneous neuroendocrine tumor that has many characteristics in common with small cell carcinoma of the lung. Fifty percent of these tumors are found in the head and neck, and most that involve the external ear are found in the external auditory canal instead of the pinna. Lesions seem to occur on sun-exposed areas of skin or in patients who are immunosuppressed. The average patient is 65 years old and presents with a rapidly growing, firm, painless nodule that is red, pink, or blue in color. Metastases to regional lymph nodes are present in more than half of patients, and distant pulmonary, hepatic, skeletal, and neurologic metastases occur in approximately 30%. Biopsy specimens show cords, strands, and clusters of round cells in the dermis. Like small cell carcinoma of the lung, these cells have uniform basophilic oval nuclei and stain positively with labeled antibodies to vasoactive intestinal peptide and neuron-specific enolase. Merkel cell carcinoma may be distinguished from amelanotic malignant melanoma, lymphoma, or metastatic carcinoma on the basis of these immunohistochemical staining characteristics. Aggressive therapy is indicated because local recurrence rates approach 50%, metastatic potential is high, and nearly half of patients fail to survive more than 5 years (18). Wide local excision with a 2- to 3-cm margin or Mohs micrographic surgery is recommended, along with prophylactic or therapeutic lymph node dissection to address drainage basins in the parotid gland and in the neck. Radiation therapy is advisable in all cases. Chemotherapy, like that used for small cell carcinoma of the lung, may offer additional therapeutic benefit for patients with extensive or widely metastatic disease.

Squamous cell papilloma is a benign epithelial neoplasm that occurs in the external auditory canal and is thought to result from infection by human papillomavirus type 6. Most squamous cell papillomas are fungiform lesions with narrow stalks. Microscopic examination shows well-differentiated squamous cells proliferating on the periphery of a fibrous tissue core. Papillomas are treated by complete excision or laser ablation. *Pilomatrixoma*, also termed calcifying epithelioma of Malherbe, is another benign tumor that may be found in the membranous portion of the external auditory canal or on any hair-bearing skin of the ear such as the lobule. These are solitary cystic lesions that originate from primitive hair matrix cells and are most commonly found in children. Histologically, the wall of the tumor consists of basaloid cells interposed with connective tissue septa surrounding a central region of degenerative debris containing ghost or shadow cells, keratin, and calcified material. These lesions are easily removed and usually do

not recur. *Myxomas* of the external canal and pinna are rare neoplasms of unknown etiology. Generally, they are well-circumscribed tumors attached to the skin by a pedicle, but they can erode the bony canal wall. Histology shows stellate or spindle-shaped cells in a mucoid matrix of hyaluronic acid. If not completely excised, these tumors tend to recur. Myxoma of the external ear may also be a manifestation of systemic complex myxomatous disease. *Auricular endochondrial pseudocysts* are cystlike degenerations of auricular cartilage that are thought to result from recurrent minor trauma. These are tumorlike lesions that occur in young adults and are often confused with auricular hematomas. Pathogenesis is thought to be related to minor trauma when small amounts of serous fluid collect between auricular cartilage and the perichondrium. In time, the internal surface of the perichondrium generates a layer of cartilage that encloses the serous fluid. There is no epithelial or endothelial lining and no associated inflammation. Auricular endochondrial pseudocysts can be difficult to eliminate. They may require aspiration and injection of a sclerosing agent or incision and drainage with curettage and obliteration with a sclerosing agent. *Chondrodermatitis nodularis chronica helicis (Winkler disease)* is an inflammatory condition of unknown etiology. Caucasian adult males are most commonly afflicted and the problem manifests as painful papules or nodules on the free border of the helix or on the antihelix. Within the lesions there is a chronic inflammatory infiltration of the perichondrium, often with focal degeneration or deformity of the underlying cartilage. The lesions can be successfully treated with wide excision, deep shave of the underlying cartilage, or intralesional injections with steroid.

NEOPLASMS OF THE MIDDLE EAR, MASTOID, AND TEMPORAL BONE

Adenomatous Tumors

Since they were first described over a century ago, classification of adenomatous tumors of the middle ear and mastoid has been the subject of controversy. The clinical course of these rare tumors is highly variable, and attempts have been made to identify tumor subtypes so that neoplastic behavior can be predicted and appropriate treatment implemented. Much of the debate about tumor classification focuses on whether the varied microscopic anatomy can be correlated with the tissue of origin and tumor growth potential. It has been suggested, based on immunohistochemical analysis, that all adenomatous tumors of the temporal bone arise from pluripotential undifferentiated neural crest cells that have migrated to the middle ear (19). This would not explain why some adenomatous lesions develop into malignant tumors, whereas others remain benign. Currently, most evidence suggests two distinct types of primary adenomatous neoplasms of the temporal bone, *benign adenoma,* which arises from the mucosa of the middle ear, and *aggressive papillary tumor,* which arises from the endolymphatic sac.

Benign adenomas of the middle ear are rare nonaggressive neoplasms that are most commonly found in adolescents and young adults, affecting males and females equally. As discussed previously, middle ear adenomas seem to arise from the glandular elements of the middle ear mucosa, but what initiates their histogenesis is unknown. Histology of these tumors often reveals benign glandular proliferation, and it has been suggested that benign adenomas represent reactive hyperplasia and not true neoplasm. However, in most reports there is no history of otitis media or any other source of inflammation. Adenomas are rubbery fibrous tumors that are white, gray, or reddish-brown in color. Microscopic examination shows cuboidal or columnar endothelial cells arranged in single-layered glandular structures. Some tumors have trabecular or ribbonlike architecture with sheets of endothelial cells lying adjacent to one another. Nuclei are round or oval and lack mitotic figures or other features of dysplasia. Immunohistochemical staining shows positive staining for synaptophysin, chromogranin, and serotonin, suggesting a neuroectodermal origin for the tumor. Patients most often present with a middle ear mass and an intact tympanic membrane, but tumors can extend through the tympanic membrane or into the mastoid. Generally, there is no bony erosion and no other sign of malignant aggressive growth. Excisional biopsy is recommended, and recurrence is unlikely.

Endolymphatic sac tumors are rare aggressive papillary tumors of the middle ear. Fewer than 100 cases have been reported since they were first described by Heffner in 1989 (20). The age of the patient at the time of diagnosis ranges from 15 to 71 years, with a mean of 41 years. There appears to be no predilection for right- versus left-sided tumors, and a review of the literature suggests that they occur more frequently in females. The time between the onset of symptoms and diagnosis of the tumor is variable and ranges from 1 month to 23 years, with an average of approximately 9 years.

The association between aggressive papillary tumor of the middle ear and von Hippel-Lindau disease was first suggested by Eby et al. in 1988 (21). von Hippel-Lindau disease is an autosomal dominant disorder associated with a defect on chromosome 3p25-26 (22). The disease manifests itself as multiple hemangioblastomas of the retina and central nervous system accompanied by renal cysts, renal carcinoma, pheochromocytoma, pancreatic cysts, papillary cystadenomas of the epididymis, and endolymphatic sac tumor. The prevalence of this disease is estimated to be 1 in 35,000 to 1 in 40,000. Endolymphatic sac tumors associated with von Hippel-Lindau disease are clinically and histologically identical to endolymphatic sac tumors in patients without this disease. However, the incidence of endolymphatic sac tumor is higher in patients with von

Hippel-Lindau disease, and there are more bilateral tumors. Approximately 11% of patients with von Hippel-Lindau disease have endolymphatic sac tumor (23). However, as many as 60% of patients with von Hippel-Lindau disease who also have hearing loss may eventually develop an endolymphatic sac tumor. Therefore, it is prudent to screen for endolymphatic sac tumor in patients with von Hippel-Lindau disease because early diagnosis allows prompt therapy.

Endolymphatic sac tumors are highly vascular friable polypoid masses. Bony invasion is characteristic of these tumors, and infiltrated bone appears to be completely replaced by fibrotic portions of the invasive tumor. On microscopic examination, endolymphatic sac tumors contain both papillary and cystic components. The cellular structure of the papillary component resembles the rugose portion of normal endolymphatic sac epithelium. The epithelial lining of an endolymphatic sac tumor consists of a single cell layer of either low cuboidal or low columnar cells. The nuclei of endolymphatic sac tumor cells are typically aligned in a uniform fashion. Nuclear pleomorphism and mitotic activity are uncommon histologic findings in these tumors. The lumen of the cystic component of the tumor contains a proteinaceous material. This material may be indistinguishable from thyroid colloid. Consequently, it is important to use thyroglobulin staining to distinguish metastatic papillary thyroid carcinoma from endolymphatic sac tumor. The underlying stroma in endolymphatic sac tumors contains an abundant capillary vascular supply that may have the appearance of a second epithelial layer. Immunohistochemical analysis of normal endolymphatic sac tissue provides additional support for the theory that adenomatous tumors of the temporal bone arise from the endolymphatic sac. Normal endolymphatic sac tissue and tissue from endolymphatic sac tumors both stain positively for S-100, a neuron-specific protein; for vimentin, an intermediate filament protein; and for neuron-specific enolase.

The clinical manifestations of endolymphatic sac tumors are best understood on the basis of tumor origin and potential routes of spread. The endolymphatic sac is located in the posterior-medial plate of the petrous bone approximately midway between the sigmoid sinus and the internal auditory canal. The sac consists of both a proximal and distal segment. The proximal or rugose portion of the sac is contiguous with the endolymphatic duct and lies within the posterior portion of the petrous bone. This portion of the sac is covered in part by the bony operculum. The distal portion of the sac is located between the dura mater proper and the periosteal portion of the dura mater within the posterior cranial fossa. Both histologic and radiologic studies suggest that the proximal portion of the sac gives rise to tumors.

Endolymphatic sac tumors extend along the endolymphatic duct in the direction of the bony labyrinth. Destruction of the labyrinth results in unilateral sensorineural hearing loss, tinnitus, and vertigo. From the endolymphatic duct, an endolymphatic sac tumor may erode into the vestibule, the posterior semicircular canal, and the mastoid cavity. Once in the mastoid cavity, these tumors follow the retrofacial air cell tract to encompass the facial nerve or to involve the jugular bulb. The middle ear may become involved when tumor enveloping the facial nerve extends anteriorly. From the middle ear cavity, tumor may erode superiorly through the tegmen tympani into the middle fossa, medially to involve the otic capsule, or laterally through the tympanic membrane to involve the external auditory canal. Because of these routes of spread, involvement of the facial nerve and the middle ear space are common clinical findings. On rare occasion, anterior extension of an endolymphatic sac tumor along the petrous ridge into the petrous apex and cavernous sinus has been reported. Anterior extension into Meckel cave and the internal auditory canal may lead to involvement of cranial nerves V, VII, and VIII. Extension into the cerebellum and into the posterior cranial fossa accounts for the high incidence of ataxia and headaches in patients with advanced lesions. Finally, inferior extension to the region of the jugular foramen accounts for the clinical findings of hoarseness, weakness of the sternocleidomastoid muscle, and palatal dysfunction.

The diagnosis of an endolymphatic sac tumor is usually made by screening audiometry in conjunction with temporal bone imaging studies. Audiograms from patients with endolymphatic sac tumors usually reveal a sensorineural hearing loss. On occasion a conductive hearing loss may be caused by extension of the tumor into the middle ear cavity. CT shows a soft tissue mass on the posterior petrous face with erosion of adjacent regions of the temporal bone. On bone windows, these tumors commonly contain stippled, reticular, or spiculated areas of calcification. Endolymphatic sac tumors have an "expansile" appearance that helps to differentiate them from other aggressive neoplasms of the temporal bone such as metastatic tumors and high-grade chondrosarcomas that have a less regular pattern of bony destruction. Unenhanced T1-weighted images on MRI studies reveal a pattern of signal intensity that varies with tumor size. In general, endolymphatic sac tumors show increased signal intensity on T1-weighted images, but tumors greater than 3 cm in diameter display multiple intratumoral foci of increased intensity and have a "speckled" appearance. In contrast, tumors less than 3 cm in diameter often have a circumferential rim of increased signal intensity. This rim of high signal intensity is probably generated by breakdown products of subacute hemorrhage found at the periphery of tumors. This characteristic finding on unenhanced T1-weighted imaging is dissimilar to other more common tumors of the petrous apex. Endolymphatic sac tumors enhance with intravenous contrast, but the degree and type of enhancement obtained with this technique varies from tumor to tumor. On T2-weighted imaging, endolymphatic sac tumors contain scattered areas of increased signal intensity. Flow voids are found in 80% of endolymphatic sac tumors and appear to be related to tumor size.

Limited therapeutic experience with endolymphatic sac tumor suggests that optimal control and cure may be achieved by complete resection. Most endolymphatic sac tumors, however, are quite large at the time of diagnosis and may involve the entire lateral skull base. Subtotal resection combined with regularly scheduled radiologic follow-up examinations with revision surgery for significant tumor progression is an alternate treatment option. However, because most patients with endolymphatic sac tumors are young adults, unacceptably high morbidity is likely to develop with incomplete resection. To minimize morbidity and mortality, complete tumor resection using modern techniques in skull base surgery should be attempted in most patients with endolymphatic sac tumors. Because these tumors are quite vascular, preoperative embolization plays a role in all but the smallest tumors. Radiation therapy and chemotherapy are used almost exclusively as palliative treatments for endolymphatic sac tumors that cannot be resected completely.

Langerhans Cell Histiocytoses

Langerhans cell histiocytoses, also called Langerhans cell tumors, are a group of neoplasms characterized by idiopathic histiocytic and eosinophilic proliferation. Until recently, these tumors were discussed as three separate disease entities: Letterer-Siwe disease, Hand-Schüller-Christian disease, and eosinophilic granuloma. These disorders are now considered to represent three different manifestations of the same disease. However, the use of these names persists mainly as an aid in categorizing the location and extent of disease. In the case of eosinophilic granuloma, the mass is usually localized, whereas in Hand-Schüller-Christian disease and Letterer-Siwe disease, the disease tends to be disseminated. All forms of this disorder are characterized by proliferation of Langerhans histiocytes. These are cells that are derived from monocytes in the bone marrow but are normally found in the epidermis. Langerhans cell histiocytes proliferation is an aggressive and sometimes malignant disease process that seems to occupy a continuum between the two extremes: histiocytic malignant lymphoma and benign reactive lymph node hyperplasia. Thus, these lesions are more accurately described as tumorlike proliferations, and the lesions may merely be the result of imbalanced immunoregulation. Eosinophils associated with histiocytosis, in cases of eosinophilic granuloma are believed to be incidental and may be a secondary reaction that accompanies abnormal proliferation of Langerhans cells. All forms of this disease may involve the temporal bone and lateral skull base.

Eosinophilic granuloma presents as a unifocal bony lesion, usually involving the flat bones of the skull, specifically the frontal and temporal bones, and the mandible. Patients are generally children and young adults with complaints of chronic or recurrent middle and external ear infection. White males are affected more frequently than other groups. The tumor is characterized by a localized collection of histiocytes, in polygonal and sheet formation, and eosinophils that cause resorption of bone, producing a radiolucent lesion. Diagnosis is confirmed by bone scan and open biopsy. This disease process is considered to be the localized form of Langerhans cell histiocytosis. Treatment of eosinophilic granuloma is surgical excision, with radiation therapy for recurrent lesions.

Otologic manifestations of *Hand-Schüller-Christian disease* include chronic purulent middle and external ear disease and hearing impairment. This is also a disease of children and young adults. Typically, there are numerous bony lesions of the skull and axial skeleton. Multifocal involvement of the abdominal viscera and cutaneous lesions indicate a particularly poor prognosis. In CT images, the osteolytic lesions are described as punched-out defects or moth-eaten holes. In addition, there is a triad that exists in approximately 10% of the patients, consisting of bone lesions, diabetes insipidus, and exophthalmos. Invasion of the temporal bone occurs frequently and is often bilateral. Biopsy helps establish the diagnosis, showing sheets of polygonal histiocytes admixed with eosinophils, plasma cells, and lymphocytes, which is the characteristic microscopic finding in these lesions. This is considered to be a chronic disseminated form of Langerhans cell histiocytosis. Treatment includes medical therapy with vinblastine and corticosteroids or radiation therapy. Despite treatment, the mortality rate approximates 30%.

Letterer-Siwe disease affects infants and manifests as hepatosplenomegaly, lymphadenopathy, bleeding diathesis, anemia, cutaneous lesions, and multiorgan dysfunction secondary to histiocyte proliferation and infiltration. This is the acute disseminated form of Langerhans cell histiocytosis. The temporal bone may be involved and patients may present with ear pain and/or otorrhea (18% to 61%). Treatment consists of chemotherapeutic agents, but the disease is almost uniformly fatal in 1 to 2 years.

Sarcoma and Chordoma

Sarcomas of the lateral skull base are exceptionally rare neoplasms; however, in children they are the most common primary malignancy of the temporal bone. Rhabdomyosarcoma is the most common of these neoplasms, accounting for 30% of sarcomatous temporal bone tumors and 4% to 7% of all temporal bone malignancies. Ninety percent of patients with rhabdomyosarcoma are younger than 10 years, with the average age at presentation of 4.5 years. Pluripotential mesenchymal cells in the middle ear and eustachian tube give rise to this neoplasm. Most patients present with chronic otorrhea and otalgia that fails to respond to appropriate medical therapy. Otologic

examination reveals a friable aural polyp, hemorrhagic aural discharge, and/or mastoid swelling. Facial weakness or paralysis is not uncommon early in the disease process and may indicate a malignant process. Regional lymph node metastases are unusual, but distant metastases to lungs, liver, brain, and bone are present in 14% of patients at the time of presentation. Rhabdomyosarcoma is divided into several histologic types: embryonal, botryoid, alveolar, and pleomorphic. The *embryonal type* is the most common. Microscopic features of embryonal rhabdomyosarcoma are small round and spindle-shaped primitive mesenchymal cells in a loose myxoid or compact pattern. Longitudinal or cross-striations characteristic of rhabdomyosarcoma may or may not be evident in the embryonal subtype. *Alveolar rhabdomyosarcoma*, which has a poorer prognosis, consists of sheets of round, oval, or straplike cells arranged in a trabecular pattern surrounding empty alveolar compartments. *Pleomorphic rhabdomyosarcoma* is composed of anaplastic multinucleated spindle cells that form whorls and fascicles with longitudinal striations. Most *botryoid tumors* are histologically classified as embryonal, and the term botryoid refers to their gross appearance resembling a grape cluster. Radiologic imaging of the temporal bone shows a soft tissue in the middle ear and mastoid with surrounding bony destruction. With this type of clinical presentation, the diagnosis is confirmed with biopsy specimens. Attempts at radical surgical excision offer no survival advantage for this highly malignant neoplasm, and therefore current treatment includes limited surgical intervention, external beam radiation therapy, and chemotherapy. Survival has improved with the use of contemporary adjuvant therapy, and 5-year failure-free survival exceeds 60% (24).

Chondrosarcoma of the skull base is thought to arise from persistent islands of embryonal cartilage rests that occur near cranial base synchondroses. Patients in nearly all age groups can be afflicted by this relatively low-grade sarcoma, but it is most common in young adults in their fourth and fifth decades of life. Males and females are affected equally. The petroclival region near foramen lacerum and the petrous apex is perhaps the most common location of origin. Patients present with headache and symptoms suggesting cranial nerve compromise such as diplopia, hoarseness, dysphagia, facial dysesthesia, and hearing loss. Cranial nerve examination often confirms the neurologic deficits in symptomatic patients. Histologic diagnosis of sarcoma can be difficult without clinical features or radiologic findings that suggest malignancy because benign cartilage shows varying patterns of cellularity and heterogeneity that may be interpreted as anaplastic. Like rhabdomyosarcoma, there are a number of histologic subtypes of chondrosarcoma, and prognosis varies depending on histologic subtype and grade of differentiation. Imaging studies show bony destruction of the skull base lateral to the midline and enhancement of the tumor mass when contrast is injected. Surgical excision is the primary therapeutic modality for chondrosarcoma, but complete excision is often not possible and recurrences are common. Both radiation therapy and chemotherapy are of unproved benefit.

Ewing sarcoma, osteogenic sarcoma, and fibrosarcoma are rarely reported to occur in the temporal bone. *Ewing sarcoma* of the temporal bone is an aggressive but rare malignancy that occurs in patients younger than 20 years. Patients present with signs and symptoms much like those of other temporal bone sarcomas, and imaging studies show a well-circumscribed soft tissue lesion eroding into the surrounding bone. Ewing sarcoma is a cellular tumor that is readily diagnosed during microscopic examination of biopsy specimens. Because no more than 20 cases of Ewing sarcoma of the temporal bone have been recorded in the world literature, the prognosis is uncertain. Limited experience, however, shows that metastatic disease does not occur, and favorable outcomes can be obtained with combined temporal bone resection, radiation therapy, and chemotherapy. *Osteogenic sarcoma* of the temporal bone is highly malignant but fortunately exceedingly rare. Most patients are between the ages of 10 and 30 years, and males are affected more often than females by a ratio of 3:2. Few cases of radiation-induced osteogenic sarcoma have been reported, but in most instances there is no clear etiology. Patients present with rapidly progressive painful swelling in the periauricular area. Temporal bone resection along with radiation therapy and chemotherapy are advocated, but this disease appears to be uniformly fatal. *Fibrosarcoma* of the temporal bone can occur in infants, and nearly one third of infants with this neoplasm present at birth. Lymph node metastases may occur in 10% of pediatric patients, but 5-year survival rates are greater than 80% after surgical treatment. The prognosis for adults is not as favorable. Regional lymph node metastases occur in 50%, and radiation-induced fibrosarcoma in adults is a lethal neoplasm (25).

Skull base chordomas are low- to intermediate-grade malignancies that result from defective embryonic remnants of the notochord. During embryonic development, the cranial aspect of the notochord begins in the sphenoid bone just posterior to the sella turcica. As the notochord is followed inferiorly, it exits the bone traveling along the clivus in the soft tissue adjacent to the nasopharyngeal mucosa and reenters the basiocciput skull base before coursing inferiorly into the odontoid process and vertebral bodies. The cranial aspect of the notochord gives rise to stalks that project into the subendothelial tissue of the nasopharynx and intracranially along the ventral aspect of the brainstem. Therefore, chordoma not only occurs in the clivus but also as a primary intracranial or nasopharyngeal soft tissue tumor. Patients of all age categories may have chordomas, but they are most likely to occur in males between the ages of 35 and 45 years. On gross examination, tumors are covered with a pseudocapsule and have a characteristic lobular configuration. They are gray and semitranslucent and contain gelatinous material. Chordomas are divided into histologic subtypes, but the main microscopic features are stellate, intermediate, and vacuolated physaliphorous or soap-bubble cells in a mucoid matrix growing in nests, cords, or trabeculae. Immunohistochemical staining is positive for cytokeratin and epithelial membrane antigen, which helps to distinguish chordoma from chondrosarcoma. Metastases are unusual, and most chordomas grow slowly and insidiously, eroding the skull base and compromising regional neurovascular structures. Headache, diplopia, and visual deficits are the most common presenting complaints, and physical examination usually reveals oculomotor function abnormalities, especially abducens nerve palsy. When chordoma originates or extends into the nasopharynx, patients can present with upper airway obstruction and a nasopharyngeal mass. In many cases, the diagnosis can be obtained from imaging studies and cytologic evaluation of a transnasal fine-needle aspirate. CT images show bony erosion of the clivus or basiocciput in the midline instead of lateral erosion that is more characteristic of chondrosarcoma. The soft tissue component of the tumor is heterogeneous on MRI, usually demonstrating low signal intensity on T1-weighted images and high signal intensity on T2-weighted images. CT and MR images both show signal enhancement after injection of contrast material. The primary mode of therapy is surgical excision via transoral-transpalatal or infratemporal fossa approach, but complete resection is often not feasible and recurrence is common. Postoperative proton beam radiation therapy may improve survival and prolong disease-free intervals.

Dermoid, Teratoma, and Choristoma

Dermoids, teratomas, and choristomas are mass lesions that result from errors in fetal development. These tumors are distinguished on the basis of the embryologic germ layer from which they are derived. *Dermoids* of the temporal bone are cystic lesions derived from the ectoderm that are more correctly classified as congenital inclusions and not true neoplasms. When they occur in the middle ear, the mastoid, or the eustachian tube, they are thought to originate at a point where the first branchial cleft, the anlage of the external auditory canal, lies adjacent to the first branchial pouch, the anlage of the middle ear and the eustachian tube. This location may be significant because it suggests that the histogenesis of dermoids is related to incomplete closure at the lines of fusion between branchial elements or to traumatic introduction of inappropriate germinal layers into the middle ear. However, dermoids may also occur in the petrous apex.

Dermoid cysts are pink or white pedunculated tumors. They have both ectodermal and mesodermal components. They are lined by keratinizing stratified squamous epithelium that contains hair follicles, sebaceous glands, smooth muscle, and adipose tissue. Most patients present as infants or children with hearing loss, otorrhea, dizziness, or upper airway obstruction, and examination reveals a middle ear mass that may extend through the eustachian tube and into the nasopharynx. The growth rate of these cysts is variable, but they eventually become symptomatic and require removal.

Teratomas of the temporal bone are extremely rare and differ significantly from dermoid cysts. They are considered to be true neoplasms that arise from pluripotential stem cells that originate near the notochord. These pluripotential cells may differentiate into types of tissue derived from any of the three embryonic germinal layers. The type of tissue into which they differentiate is generally not native to the site where they occur. Tumors are firm polypoid or cystic lesions that may contain stratified squamous epithelium, respiratory and gastrointestinal endothelium, cartilage, skeletal muscle, glandular tissue, neural tissue, and, surprisingly, even mature teeth. Tumors are graded in relation to tissue differentiation. Malignant undifferentiated forms exist, but they have never been reported in the temporal bone. Patients present at birth or in early childhood, often with large rapidly growing tumors, and their symptoms include facial paralysis, hearing loss, and airway obstruction. Imaging studies show a heterogenous tumor that may contain calcifications. Teratomas can be cured with complete resection but this may require radical transtemporal or infratemporal fossa approaches to achieve adequate surgical exposure for curative resection.

Choristoma is a term that is used to describe normal tissue that occurs in a nonnative location. When choristoma occurs in the middle ear, this generally refers to salivary tissue, although sebaceous glands and neural tissue have been reported (26,27). Choristomas are probably derived from rests of salivary tissue trapped in the middle ear during development. These rests mature into small masses but have no neoplastic potential. Choristomas are pink or tan lobular masses located lateral to the long process of the incus and medial to the manubrium, and some have been associated with anomalies of the ossicles or the intratemporal portion of the facial nerve. Histologic examination reveals mature ectopic salivary gland tissue. Patients may have conductive hearing loss, but most are asymptomatic. They usually present with a middle ear mass that was incidentally discovered during routine otoscopic examination. Choristomas have little if any growth potential and only require incisional or excisional biopsy to confirm diagnosis.

Cholesterol Granuloma

Cholesterol granuloma of the petrous apex is not a true neoplasm but rather a mass lesion that results from a reactive process within the temporal bone. It can be diagnosed from imaging studies and should be included in the differential diagnosis when evaluating temporal bone masses. Cholesterol granuloma was first described more than 100 years ago as dark blue discoloration of the tympanic membrane and was called an "idiopathic hematotympanum." This condition occurred in patients with eustachian tube dysfunction and was often accompanied by chronic otitis media or cholesteatoma. It was hypothesized that cholesterol granuloma occurs as a consequence of four factors: interference with drainage of the middle ear, hemorrhage, obstruction of ventilation, and foreign body reaction to cholesterol crystals derived from hemoglobin catabolism. Evidence in support of this hypothesis has been provided by animal experiments. Cholesterol granuloma can be produced by injecting cholesterol into the middle ear or by occluding the eustachian tube (28). Cholesterol granuloma of the petrous apex, whereas not necessarily associated with otitis media or cholesteatoma, probably results from a similar pathophysiologic process. It is found in pneumatized petrous bones that occur in 30% of patients. The process starts when ventilation of petrous air cells is disrupted secondary to temporal bone trauma, eustachian tube dysfunction, or mucosal edema. Inflammation or trauma of the petrous bone may cause hemorrhage into the air cells of the petrous apex, and because there is no effective drainage pathway, detritus from the hemorrhage accumulates in the air cells. The membranes of degenerating red blood cells appear to be the primary source of cholesterol crystals, which subsequently initiate a foreign body reaction. Inflammation from the foreign body reaction increases hemorrhage and mucosal edema, promoting the inflammatory cycle and allowing the granuloma to enlarge. An alternative theory for cholesterol granuloma pathogenesis proposes that these lesions result when expanding aircell tracts lined with mucosa interface with marrow spaces in the petrous apex. Coaptation between the mucosal lining and the exposed marrow results in a progressive sustained hemorrhage from the marrow spaces and this leads to cyst formation and expansion (29). It is not surprising that histologic examination of cholesterol granuloma shows cholesterol crystals surrounded by multinucleated giant cells, round cell infiltration, and hemosiderin-laden macrophages. Cholesterol granuloma may be confined to the petrous bone and may be asymptomatic. Alternatively, it may extend into the posterior cranial fossa and cause an abducens nerve palsy, diplopia, facial pain, facial weakness or twitching, headache, dizziness, tinnitus, and hearing loss. The diagnosis of cholesterol granuloma may be made by MRI, which shows a smooth-walled, nonenhancing, expansive lesion that has high signal intensity on both T1-weighted and T2-weighted images. The mainstay of surgical therapy is simple drainage, allowing permanent aeration of the cavity. However, some controversy exists about whether the fibrous wall of the cyst requires removal to achieve long-term cure.

NEOPLASMS OF THE INTERNAL AUDITORY CANAL AND CEREBELLOPONTINE ANGLE

Schwannoma

Schwannomas of the temporal bone and the skull base are benign neoplasms that arise from the sheaths of cranial nerves. Available evidence suggests that these tumors arise from Schwann cells alone and not other nerve components. Therefore, terms such as acoustic neuroma are not appropriate. The etiology of schwannoma is unclear, but it has been suggested that neoplastic growth occurs preferentially at the junction between the central and peripheral components of the cranial nerves. Myelin is formed by oligodendrocytes in the intracranial portion of a cranial nerve, and as the nerve enters the skull base, there is a transition to a Schwann cell sheath. This transition occurs in a region called the Obersteiner-Redlich zone, which is variable in location in different cranial nerves. It has also been proposed that schwannomas may arise in locations with the greatest concentration of Schwann cells. For vestibular schwannomas this would be Scarpa ganglion, whereas for jugular foramen schwannomas this would be the superior and inferior ganglia of the glossopharyngeal nerve, the jugular and nodose ganglia of the vagus nerve, or the junction of cranial and spinal components of the spinal accessory nerve. What causes the proliferation of Schwann cells is not known, but genetic aberrations, such as those associated with neurofibromatosis type 2 (NF2), may be associated with neoplastic transformation. NF2 appears to be the result of a defect on the long arm of chromosome 22, which is responsible for the production of a tumor suppressor protein called merlin (30). Exactly what this protein does to inhibit Schwann cell proliferation is uncertain (31). NF2 is an autosomal dominant disorder, and patients may have a functioning copy of the tumor suppressor gene on their intact chromosome. However, production of merlin is terminated when a mutation occurs on the intact chromosome 22, and this is when NF2 patients develop schwannomas. For the same sequence of events to occur in a patient without NF2, mutations must occur on the long arm of both chromosomes. Thus, neoplastic transformation in cases of sporadic schwannoma is a much less likely event.

Schwannomas of the temporal bone can be categorized as vestibular, facial, trigeminal, and jugular foramen tumors. Vestibular schwannomas are by far the most common, comprising approximately 7% of all intracranial tumors and 80% of cerebellopontine angle tumors. They occur in about 1 of 100,000 patients per year. Because they usually arise in the vicinity of the vestibular ganglion, most vestibular schwannomas begin inside the internal auditory canal. Isolated intralabyrinthine schwannomas do occur, as do cochlear schwannomas, but they are extremely rare. Vestibular schwannomas expand centrally from the internal auditory canal into the cerebellopontine angle and may compress the pontine brainstem and the cerebellum. Therefore, the most common symptoms with which patients present are unilateral hearing loss, tinnitus, and dysequilibrium. Vestibular schwannomas may also extend anteriorly within the cerebellopontine angle, compressing the trigeminal nerve and causing facial hypesthesia or paresthesia, but neuralgia is infrequent. Large tumors will eventually result in hydrocephalus with headache, visual impairment, and alterations of mental status if the tumor is left untreated.

Facial nerve schwannomas differ from vestibular schwannomas in that they can arise anywhere along the nerve from the oligodendrocyte-Schwann cell junction to the most distal aspect of the extratemporal facial nerve. Most commonly, however, they arise from the perigeniculate, tympanic, or mastoid segments of the nerve. Multiple nerve segments are usually involved by the time these lesions are diagnosed. Facial weakness or paralysis that progresses gradually over weeks or months is the most common presentation. Patients may also present with facial twitching and synkinesis. Twenty percent of patients with facial nerve schwannoma may present with acute facial paralysis, suggesting Bell palsy. Conductive hearing loss, tinnitus, or otalgia occur when neoplasms extend into the middle ear.

Trigeminal schwannomas are rare lesions that usually originate from the gasserian ganglion and may expand into posterior and/or middle cranial fossae. Patients present with facial neuralgia, paresthesia, or hypesthesia in one or more divisions of the trigeminal nerve. Retroorbital pain may be another complaint. When motor function is affected, patients describe difficulty when chewing.

Jugular foramen schwannomas arise within the jugular fossa from the sheaths of cranial nerves IX, X, and XI. Because they grow vertically along the path of least resistance, intracranial and extracranial extension of the tumor is variable. Vagus nerve origin seems most frequent, followed by glossopharyngeal origin, but it is often difficult to identify the nerve from which the tumor is derived. Patients present with dysphagia, aspiration, hoarseness, or shoulder weakness. If there is significant intracranial extension, patients may note hearing loss, tinnitus, imbalance, or headache.

On gross and microscopic examination, all temporal bone schwannomas are generally the same. They are tan, yellow, or pale gray rubbery masses with varying amounts of surface vascularity. As they enlarge, schwannomas displace adjacent soft tissue structures and may become tightly adherent to these structures. They appear to have a fibrous capsule, but histologic examination shows that the capsule may be so thin that tumor cells oppose surrounding tissue directly. Tumor cells are spindle-shaped and are arranged in both Antoni type A and type B patterns. The type A pattern consists of densely packed spindle cells with aligned or palisading nuclei, termed Verocay bodies. The type B pattern, on the other hand, is characterized by spindle cells that are loosely arranged in a myxoid stroma. Cystic degeneration, necrosis, and hemorrhage are often noted, especially in larger tumors. Nuclear pleomorphism and hypercellularity might appear consistent with malignancy, but malignant degeneration of schwannomas is highly unusual.

Radiographic imaging studies may provide the diagnosis, but physical examination reveals functional deficits caused by the tumor. Otologic exam is generally normal unless a facial nerve schwannoma presents as a retrotympanic mass. In patients with cervical extension of jugular fossa schwannomas, head and neck examination may show an anterosuperior neck mass, sternocleidomastoid muscle weakness, or bulge of the lateral pharyngeal wall, suggesting a mass in the parapharyngeal space. Cranial nerve examination showing palatal weakness and vocal cord paralysis is also indicative of a jugular fossa lesion. When decreased corneal reflexes, facial hypesthesia, and masseter muscle weakness are apparent, trigeminal schwannoma or other cerebellopontine schwannomas that compress the trigeminal nerve may be the cause. Facial nerve dysfunction suggests facial nerve schwannoma rather than vestibular schwannoma, but audiometric evaluation helps to differentiate the two lesions. Sensorineural hearing loss is more common in patients with vestibular schwannoma, whereas conductive hearing loss is more common in patients with facial nerve schwannoma. The preliminary diagnosis of schwannoma is made when the deficits discovered on physical examination correlate with findings from imaging studies. MRI shows a lesion with low signal intensity on T1-weighted images that enhances following injection with intravenous contrast. HRCT of the temporal bone shows expansion or erosion of the fallopian canal and extension into the middle ear in patients with facial nerve schwannomas. HRCT also helps to define skull base anatomy preoperatively in patients with jugular foramen schwannomas.

Management of temporal bone schwannomas is beyond the scope of this chapter. Suffice it to say that patients generally have three therapeutic options: surgical excision, stereotactic radiation therapy, or observation. Complete surgical excision is the only curative therapy available at this time. The major disadvantage is morbidity associated with cranial nerve injury, cerebrospinal fluid leak, and central nervous system damage. Advanced technology for treating patients with schwannomas using stereotactic radiosurgery has now been available for 15 years. Long-term follow-up in patients treated with lower radiation dosages (10 to 14 Gy) using more accurate tumor targeting technology shows that complications can be minimized while tumor growth is controlled in approximately 95% (32). It is generally not recommended for patients with tumors greater than 3 cm in diameter and who are symptomatic with significant brainstem compression. Observation as a management option is based on data

suggesting that more than 60% of vestibular schwannomas, especially intracanalicular tumors, grow very slowly, remain stable in size, or involute during long-term follow-up (33). All three therapeutic options play a role in the management of patients with temporal bone schwannomas.

Meningioma

Meningiomas are neoplasms that arise from the arachnoid layer of the meninges. More specifically, temporal bone meningiomas arise from arachnoid cell granulations that cluster at the tips of arachnoid villi inside dural venous sinuses and at foramina, such as the internal auditory canal, the jugular fossa, the geniculate ganglion, and the bony sulci near the greater and lesser superficial petrosal nerves. Meningiomas are common neoplasms and constitute between 13% and 20% of all intracranial tumors and approximately 10% of all cerebellopontine angle tumors. The incidence of meningioma increases with age, with the highest incidence rate (40 per 100,000) in individuals older than 65 years. Children and even infants can have meningiomas, but fortunately this is rare. In children, boys are affected as often as girls, and their tumors are generally more aggressive, growing rapidly and becoming relatively large before they are diagnosed. In adults, women with meningioma outnumber men by at least 2 to 1, especially in the older age groups. The most frequent location for meningioma of the lateral skull base is on the posterior aspect of the petrous bone between the superior and inferior petrosal sinuses. Less commonly, meningioma presents as a tumor that is confined to the internal auditory canal, and in rare cases meningioma presents as an extracranial neoplasm in the middle ear, the external auditory canal, or the infratemporal fossa.

The etiology of meningioma is the subject of controversy. The relationship between severe head injuries and subsequent development of meningioma a number of years later was first suggested by Cushing in the 1920s when he observed that meningiomas occur directly beneath a previous skull fracture. In most patients, however, there was no history of trauma or the injury may have occurred at a site distant from the tumor. Subsequent epidemiologic studies have failed to show a causal relationship between trauma and the occurrence of meningioma. Genetic factors have some role in the pathogenesis of meningioma because inherited tumors occur in patients with NF2. In fact, aberrations involving chromosome 22 occur in almost 50% of patients with sporadic meningiomas, and abnormalities have also been identified on chromosomes 1 and 14 (34). Radiation exposure seems to be clearly linked to the occurrence of meningioma. The most convincing evidence of this is the discovery that children who were treated with low-dose radiation for tinea capitis in the 1950s were almost 10 times more likely to develop meningioma. As the radiation dose increases, the risk of developing a tumor seems to rise. Hormonal stimulation, specifically from progesterone and possibly from estrogen, is thought to have a role in the genesis and progression of meningioma. This has been suggested because meningioma is more common in women, there are estrogen and progesterone receptors in meningioma, meningiomas seem to change size during pregnancy and during the menstrual cycle, and there may to be a link between meningioma and breast cancer, which also has estrogen and progesterone receptors. The details relating estrogen or progesterone release and meningioma growth are unclear, but such an association could have consequences related to prevention, detection, and treatment of this tumor.

Meningiomas are well-circumscribed, firm, rubbery, nodular masses that invade dural lining, dural sinuses, and neurovascular channels. One fourth of these tumors are flat, so-called en-plaque tumors that invade adjacent bone and incite an osteoblastic reaction referred to as hyperostosis. Most meningiomas are benign, but approximately 5% have malignant characteristics. These tumors show anaplastic histologic features and may invade the adjacent brain. Metastatic disease is highly unusual. The clinical presentation of meningioma is variable and depends on where the tumor is located within the temporal bone or skull base. Meningioma of the internal auditory canal is difficult to distinguish from vestibular schwannoma, which is more common. Both neoplasms present with unilateral sensorineural hearing loss and tinnitus, but auditory complaints occur more frequently in patients with vestibular schwannoma. Conversely, meningioma is more likely to cause facial twitching, weakness, or paralysis. Meningioma that originates on the posterior petrous face expands into the posterior cranial fossa, compressing the cerebellum and brainstem. These patients present with imbalance or vertigo and difficulty with fine motor movements. When these tumors become very large, they may cause hydrocephalus and elevated intracranial pressure resulting in headaches, nausea, vomiting, lethargy, and somnolence. Petrous apex lesions may extend onto the clivus, into the cavernous sinus, or through Meckel cave and into the middle cranial fossa. Extensive tumors in these locations can cause trigeminal neuralgia, facial hypesthesia, visual disturbance, and headache. Jugular fossa meningiomas may cause dysphonia, aspiration, and dysphagia, whereas physical examination shows palatal weakness, pooling of hypopharyngeal secretions, and vocal cord paresis. Geniculate ganglion and petrosal nerve tumors result in facial weakness or paralysis, and conductive hearing loss may occur when tumor extends to fill the middle ear.

The diagnosis is based on histopathologic findings and imaging characteristics that are consistent with meningioma. Histologic features that mark meningioma include polygonal and spindle-shaped cells arranged in nests, vascular spaces, and psammoma bodies, which are spherical concretions consisting of calcium salts. However, the microscopic appearance of meningioma is highly variable. Consequently, meningiomas are classified as endotheliomatous, fibrous, transitional, angiomatous, and sarcomatous depending on predominant cell shape, stromal content, tumor vascularity, and nuclear anaplasia. Further, the World Health Organization classifies meningiomas based on histologic characteristics, cellular atypia, and evidence of brain invasion. Both methods to classify meningiomas may provide prognostic information. In many cases, imaging characteristics on CT and MRI are diagnostic. Meningiomas are hyperdense or isodense compared with surrounding brain on CT images, and they exhibit homogeneous enhancement after contrast injection. Calcification within the tumor or associated hyperostosis support the diagnosis of meningioma. Vestibular schwannomas are, on the other hand, isodense or hypodense to brain, and they exhibit inhomogeneous enhancement and lack of calcification or hyperostosis. MR images reveal the broad-based eccentric nature of meningioma and may sometimes show obvious dural or dural sinus origin. The margin of the tumor may elongate and flatten out along the bone, termed the dural tail. MRI of vestibular schwannoma is more likely to show erosion of the internal auditory canal where the tumor originates and pronounced enhancement with injection of intravenous contrast. Intracanalicular lesions are difficult to distinguish on any imaging study.

The mainstay of treatment for meningiomas is surgical removal, and complete surgical removal is the only curative treatment available at this time. Resection is recommended for most patients with accessible tumors, especially if the patient has symptoms and there are no medical contraindications to surgery. The tumor should be removed with a wide margin of meninges and adjacent bone. Preoperative angiography helps to identify the major feeding vessels of the tumor and may be combined with embolization to reduce operative blood loss. Despite efforts at total resection, recurrence rates for meningioma are relatively high. Even when the entire tumor with a margin of dura and bone are removed, meningiomas recur in almost 10% of patients. The most important features to consider when estimating the probability of surgical cure are tumor location, which may allow complete resection, and lack of malignant characteristics. For patients who are not candidates for surgery, who have residual disease after surgery, who have recurrent or unresectable disease, or who have meningiomas that show malignant characteristics, radiation therapy should be considered. Recent clinical studies examining the efficacy of radiosurgical treatment of skull base meningiomas are encouraging. Ten- and fifteen-year follow-up data show local tumor control in more than 90% of patients (35). Local control in radiosurgery patients may be better when meningiomas are treated with radiosurgery alone compared with patients treated with radiosurgery postoperatively. Current research focuses on hormonal treatment, targeted chemotherapy, gene therapy using adenovirus vectors, and other forms of medical therapy that might help to arrest tumor growth and prevent recurrences.

Lipoma

Lipomas of the internal auditory canal and the cerebellopontine angle are rare but potentially problematic tumors that may originate from the aberrant differentiation of neural crest cells into adipocytes. Bigelow et al. (36) provide the most comprehensive review of this subject in their multiinstitutional study and review of the world literature. They recorded 84 documented cases of lipoma of the internal auditory canal and cerebellopontine angle and studied the clinical findings in each case. Patients ranged in age from 7 months to 82 years, with an average age of 40 years. Tumors predominated in males by a ratio of 2:1. Lipomas measured from 1 to 26 mm in diameter with a mean of 11 mm. Three patients presented with bilateral tumors. Ninety-two percent of patients were symptomatic. They most often presented with hearing loss, dizziness, tinnitus, and headache. Lipomas are fatty masses that may envelop the neurovascular structures of the internal auditory canal and cerebellopontine angle. Large lipomas may be adherent to the lateral aspect of the brainstem. Some lipomas have highly vascularized outer surfaces and are more accurately classified as angiolipomas. Biopsy specimens show benign mature adipocytes and varying amounts of fibrous tissue. Lipomas may infiltrate cranial nerves and surround component fascicles of nerve fibers.

Lipomas have unique imaging characteristics. Therefore, a definitive diagnosis can be obtained from an MRI. On MRI, lipomas are similar to subcutaneous fat with high signal intensity on T1-weighted images and diminished signal intensity on T2-weighted images. T1-weighted images do not enhance with injection of intravenous contrast because the tumor signal is near saturation. MRI with fat suppression further confirms the diagnosis. Follow-up for most patients with unresected tumors has been short, and thus the rate of growth of lipoma, thought to be very slow, is unknown. The only documented instance of the growth of a lipoma involves a patient with a 2-cm tumor that was biopsied but not removed. The tumor enlarged 15% over an 8-year period. Review of surgical outcomes shows that complete tumor resection is possible in only one third of patients and 68% suffer postoperative neurologic deficits. Forty-three percent of postoperative patients have improvements in symptoms, but only 19% have improvement with no new neurologic deficits. From this experience, it is clear that expectant management is advisable in most cases. Surgical therapy should be reserved for patients with progressive or disabling symptoms.

METASTATIC DISEASE OF THE TEMPORAL BONE AND LATERAL SKULL BASE

Temporal bone metastases resulting from distant malignancies are an infrequent but not insignificant occurrence. In the largest series of patients with temporal bone metastases studied to date, 47 metastases to the temporal bone were documented at autopsy in a population of 212 individuals with primary nondisseminated malignant neoplasms (37). The most common sites of origin of temporal bone metastases in order of decreasing frequency are breast, lung, kidney, gastrointestinal tract, larynx, prostate gland, and thyroid gland. The incidence of bilateral involvement may exceed 50%. Metastatic involvement of the temporal bone may occur as the first evidence of distant malignant disease, first presenting as hearing loss and later as facial paralysis or dysequilibrium. There is usually a conductive hearing loss that may be accompanied by pain. More frequently, temporal bone involvement is occult and occurs late in the course of disease. Tumor cells may accumulate preferentially in area of bone with sluggish blood flow, including the marrow and aerated regions. Areas of the temporal bone that show a predilection for metastatic disease include the petrous apex, the mastoid, and the internal auditory canal. The bony labyrinth appears to resist neoplastic invasion because inner ear involvement is uncommon.

Metastatic disease should be considered as a possible cause of hearing loss in a patient with a clinical history of malignant neoplasm. This is especially true in patients with rapidly growing temporal bone lesions associated with progressive neurologic symptoms.

HIGHLIGHTS

- Paragangliomas of the temporal bone arise from nonchromaffin paraganglia, or glomus bodies, which are part of a diffuse neuroendocrine system. Glomus jugulare tumors arise within the jugular fossa, and glomus tympanicum tumors arise along the course of the tympanic branch of cranial nerve IX (Jacobson nerve) and along the course of the auricular branch of cranial nerve X (Arnold nerve).

- Temporal bone and cerebellopontine angle epidermoids are aberrant collections of keratin debris within a sac of squamous epithelium. They result from entrapment of ectodermal rests during embryogenesis and therefore are categorized as congenital lesions. Epidermoids expand to fill empty spaces and incite a localized inflammatory reaction. Thus, they are usually large and very adherent to surrounding structures by the time they are treated with surgery.

- Patients with cutaneous carcinomas of the external auditory canal may present with symptoms similar to those of patients with chronic otitis externa. However, chronic bloody drainage and sudden onset of deep ear pain indicate the possibility of malignancy and suggest the need for biopsy.

- Melanoma accounts for more that 50% of deaths from cutaneous malignancies. Excisional biopsy for early diagnosis is the key first step to optimize therapeutic outcomes. Sentinel node mapping using lymphoscintigraphy is becoming the primary method of identifying nodal drainage patterns for these neoplasms and high-dose interferon-alpha-2b may benefit patients with lymph node metastases.

- Aggressive papillary tumors of the middle ear appear to be derived from the pars rugosa portion of the endolymphatic sac. They are slow growing but aggressive tumors that erode and spread extensively throughout the temporal bone and often recur after surgical treatment. Endolymphatic sac tumors occur in more than 10% of patients with von Hippel-Lindau disease, and therefore these patients require screening.

- Embryonal rhabdomyosarcoma accounts for 30% of sarcomatous temporal bone neoplasms and is the most common sarcoma of this region. It is derived from pluripotential mesenchymal cells that differentiate into primitive skeletal muscle cells. Most patients are younger than 12 years and present with hemorrhagic aural drainage, a friable aural polyp, mastoid swelling, and facial nerve dysfunction. Current therapy includes limited surgical intervention, external beam radiation therapy, and chemotherapy.

- Chordomas result from defective embryonic remnants of the notochord. They are semitranslucent neoplasms that contain gelatinous material and are histologically characterized by clusters of physaliphorous (soap-bubble) cells in a mucoid matrix. Most chordomas occur in the clivus, but some originate or extend laterally into the petrous apex.

- Schwannomas of the lateral skull base are neoplasms that arise from Schwann cells at the transition zone between central myelin-producing oligodendrocytes and peripheral myelin-producing Schwann cells. What initiates the growth of these neoplasms is unknown, but aberrations or mutations on the long arm of chromosome 22, such as those that occur in NF2, are linked to these neoplasms.

- Microscopic examination of schwannomas is characterized by spindle-shaped cells arranged in Antoni type A and type B patterns. The type A pattern consists of densely packed cells with palisading nuclei, termed Verocay bodies. The type B pattern consists of loosely arranged spindle cells in a myxoid stroma.

- Meningiomas are neoplasms that arise from the arachnoid layer of the meninges. Imaging studies of cerebellopontine angle meningiomas show homogeneous enhancement of a broad-based eccentric neoplasm that may contain speckled calcifications and may initiate a local hyperostotic reaction. Vestibular schwannomas, conversely, often exhibit heterogeneous enhancement and are "mushroom shaped," showing internal auditory canal origin and erosion.

REFERENCES

1. Gulya AJ. The glomus tumor and its biology. *Laryngoscope* 1993;103:7–15.
2. Petropoulos AE, Luetje CM, Camarata PJ, et al. Genetic analysis in the diagnosis of familial paragangliomas. *Laryngoscope* 2000;110:1225–1229.
3. Bikhazi PH, Messina L, Mhatre AN, et al. Molecular pathogenesis in sporadic head and neck paraganglioma. *Laryngoscope* 2000;110:1346–1348.
4. Hoegerle S, Ghanem N, Altehoefer C, et al. 18F-DOPA positron emission tomography for the detection of glomus tumours. *Eur J Nucl Med Mol Imaging* 2003;30:689–694.
5. Bustillo A, Telischi FF. Octreotide scintigraphy in the detection of recurrent paragangliomas. *Otolaryngol Head Neck Surg* 2004;130:479–482.
6. Maarouf M, Voges J, Landwehr P, et al. Stereotactic linear accelerator-based radiosurgery for the treatment of patients with glomus jugulare tumors. *Cancer* 2003;97:1093–1098.
7. Levine J, Wright C, Pawlowski K, et al. Postnatal persistence of epidermoid rests in the human middle ear. *Laryngoscope* 1998;108:70–73.
8. Talacchi A, Sala F, Alessandrini F, et al. Assessment and surgical management of posterior fossa epidermoid tumors: report of 28 cases. *Neurosurgery* 1998;42:242–251.
9. Tucci D, Lambert P, Innes D. Primary lymphoma of the temporal bone. *Arch Otolaryngol Head Neck Surg* 1992;118:83–85.
10. Hill N, Little B, Vasan N, et al. Cerebellopontine angle lymphoma presenting as chronic mastoiditis. *J Laryngol Otol* 2000;114:618–620.
11. Merkus P, Copper MP, Van Oers MH, et al. Lymphoma in the ear. *ORL J Otorhinolaryngol Relat Spec* 2000;62:274–277.
12. Marioni G, Altavilla G, Busatto G, et al. Detection of human papillomavirus in temporal bone inverted papilloma by polymerase chain reaction. *Acta Otolaryngol* 2003;123:367–371.
13. Moody SA, Hirsch BE, Myers EN. Squamous cell carcinoma of the external auditory canal: an evaluation of a staging system. *Am J Otol* 2000;21:582–588.
14. Chu A, Osguthorpe JD. Nonmelanoma cutaneous malignancy with regional metastasis. *Otolaryngol Head Surg* 2003;128:663–673.
15. Cole MD, Jakowatz J, Evans GR. Evaluation of nodal patterns for melanoma of the ear. *Plast Reconstr Surg* 2003;112:50–56.
16. Pockaj BA, Jaroszewski DE, DiCaudo DJ, et al. Changing surgical therapy for melanoma of the external ear. *Ann Surg Oncol* 2003;10:689–696.
17. Terando A, Sabel MS, Sondak VK. Melanoma: adjuvant therapy and other treatment options. *Curr Treat Options Oncol* 2003;4:187–199.
18. Poulsen M. Merkel-cell carcinoma of the skin. *Lancet Oncol* 2004;5:593–599.
19. Torske KR, Thompson LD. Adenoma versus carcinoid tumor of the middle ear: a study of 48 cases and review of the literature. *Mod Pathol* 2002;15:543–555.
20. Heffner D. Low-grade adenocarcinoma of probable endolymphatic sac origin: a clinicopathologic study of 20 cases. *Cancer* 1989;64:2292–2302.
21. Eby T, Makek M, Fisch U. Adenomas of the temporal bone. *Ann Otol Rhinol Laryngol* 1988;97:605–612.
22. Choo D, Shotland L, Mastroianni M, et al. Endolymphatic sac tumors in von Hippel-Lindau disease. *J Neurosurg* 2004;100:480–487.
23. Lonser RR, Kim HJ, Butman JA, et al. Tumors of the endolymphatic sac in von Hippel-Lindau disease. *N Engl J Med* 2004;350:2481–2486.
24. Hawkins DS, Anderson JR, Paidas CN, et al. Improved outcome for patients with middle ear rhabdomyosarcoma: a children's oncology group study. *J Clin Oncol* 2001;19:3073–3079.
25. Daw NC, Mahmonud HH, Meyer WH, et al. Bone sarcomas of the head and neck in children: the St. Jude Children's Research Hospital experience. *Cancer* 2000;88:2172–2180.
26. Gyure DA, Thompson LD, Morrison AL. A clinicopathological study of 15 patients with neuroglial heterotopias and encephaloceles of the middle ear and mastoid region. *Laryngoscope* 2000;110:1731–1735.

27. Nelson E, Kratz R. Sebaceous choristoma of the middle ear. *Otolaryngol Head Neck Surg* 1993;108:372–373.
28. Main T, Shimada T, Lim D. Experimental cholesterol granuloma. *Arch Otolaryngol* 1970;91:356–359.
29. Jackler RK, Cho M. A new theory to explain the genesis of petrous apex cholesterol granuloma. *Otol Neurotol* 2003;24:96–106.
30. Xiao GH, Chernoff J, Testa JR. NF2: the wizardry of merlin. *Genes Chromosomes Cancer* 2003;38:389–399.
31. Halum SL, Erbe CB, Friedland DR, et al. Gene discovery using a human vestibular schwannoma cDNA library constructed from a patient with neurofibromatosis type 2. *Otolaryngol Head Neck Surg* 2003;128:364–371.
32. Landy HJ, Markoe AM, Wu X, et al. Safety and efficacy of tiered limited-dose gamma knife stereotactic radiosurgery for unilateral acoustic neuroma. *Stereotact Funct Neurosurg* 2004;82:147–152.
33. Raut VV, Walsh RM, Bath AP, et al. Conservative management of vestibular schwannomas- second review of a prospective longitudinal study. *Clin Otolaryngol* 2004;29:505–514.
34. Lopez-Gines C, Cerda-Nicolas M, Gil-Benso R, et al. Association of loss of 1p and alterations of chromosome 14 in meningioma progression. *Cancer Genet Cytogenet* 2004;148:123–128.
35. Mendenhall WM, Morris CG, Amdur RJ, et al. Radiotherapy alone or after subtotal resection for benign skull base meningiomas. *Cancer* 2003;98:1473–1482.
36. Bigelow D, Eisen M, Smith P, et al. Lipomas of the internal auditory canal and cerebellopontine angle. *Laryngoscope* 1998;108:1459–1469.
37. Gloria-Cruz T, Schachern P, Paparella M, et al. Metastases to temporal bones from primary nonsystemic malignant neoplasms. *Arch Otolaryngol Head Neck Surg* 2000;126:209–214.

Congenital Aural Atresia

137

Paul R. Lambert

Atresia of the ear canal with middle ear anomalies can occur in isolation or in association with microtia or craniofacial dysplasia. The reported incidence is 1 in 10,000 to 20,000 births. Genetic transmission occurs in many of the syndromes that include aural atresia (e.g., Treacher Collins syndrome), but it is rarely found in cases of isolated atresia. Aural atresia is bilateral in approximately one third of the cases, and each side can vary in complexity (1).

The evaluation and treatment of aural atresia present a number of challenges to the otologic surgeon. First, overall hearing must be assessed and the need for immediate amplification determined. The second challenge is to formulate a long-term rehabilitation strategy. The key component of this challenge is to determine if surgical correction of the atresia is appropriate. This decision process requires the integration of results from audiometric and radiographic studies with a qualitative assessment of the patient's functional hearing status and the probability of restoring serviceable hearing. If surgery is recommended, the last challenge becomes the operative procedure itself, which is made complex by abnormal development of the temporal bone. This fact places the facial nerve and labyrinth at a greater risk than encountered in routine temporal bone surgery and complicates the healing process, particularly for canal patency. This chapter reviews the concepts and protocols necessary to meet these challenges successfully.

EMBRYOLOGY

Placed in the context of congenital aural atresia, a general knowledge of the embryologic development of the ear is fascinating and essential for understanding the altered surgical anatomy. Development of the first pharyngeal pouch, the first and second branchial arches, the first branchial cleft, and the otic capsule must all be considered in this discussion.

External Auditory Canal

The external ear canal is derived from the first branchial groove and initially is represented by a solid core of epithelial cells that extends down to the area of the tympanic ring and first pharyngeal pouch. This core of cells remains in place until the middle trimester of fetal life, a time when most structures of the inner, middle, and outer ear are well differentiated. At this point, absorption of the epithelial cells begins, progressing in a medial to lateral direction. If this canalization process is arrested prematurely, it is possible to have a more normally developed tympanic membrane and bony external ear canal associated with an atretic or very stenotic membranous canal, a situation that predisposes to canal cholesteatoma formation as the trapped squamous epithelium continues to desquamate.

The medial portion of the external ear canal is formed by the tympanic bone. This structure begins to ossify in the third embryonic month, eventually forming the tympanic ring and osseous ear canal; the latter structure continues its lateral growth during the first and second postnatal years. Malformation of the tympanic bone produces atretic bone at the level of the tympanic membrane and results in atresia of the ear canal (2). The mandibular condyle articulates with this rudimentary tympanic bone.

Mastoid and Middle Ear

The eustachian tube, middle ear, and mastoid air cells are derived from the first pharyngeal pouch. Although the middle ear cavity and mastoid air cells are smaller than normal in patients with aural atresia, no anatomic or clinical studies show impaired eustachian tube function in these ears. Pneumatization of the mastoid is a late embryologic event, starting at the seventh or eighth month and continuing into postnatal life. A well-pneumatized mastoid usually indicates good middle ear development, including size of the tympanum and formation of the ossicles. The relationship between middle ear development and degree of differentiation of the pinna is disputed (3).

The ossicles, except for the vestibular portion of the stapes footplate, are formed from the first and second branchial arches. The external ear canal and tympanic membrane are derived from the first branchial cleft. Isolated branchial arch (ossicular) or branchial cleft (external ear canal) deformities are possible, but usually these malformations occur in combination (2). Other branchial arch defects may occur, especially mandibular hypoplasia. Because the membranous labyrinth is derived from the ectodermal otocyst, sensorineural and vestibular function should be normal. The stapes footplate is formed in part from the otic capsule, and in most cases it is normally developed in ears with congenital atresia. It is uncommon to encounter a fixed stapes footplate in the usual major congenital ear malformation, although the superstructure is frequently deformed. This information is important, because the stapes is often partially obscured by the lateral ossicular mass or the facial nerve in atretic ears, and its normal mobility may be difficult to determine with certainty.

Absence of the stapes footplate and oval window can occur, but this is usually encountered in a patient with a patent external ear canal and normal-appearing tympanic membrane rather than in a patient with aural atresia (4). It has been suggested that this condition is caused by abnormal development of the facial nerve (5,6). By the fifth to sixth week of gestation, the horizontal and vertical segments of the facial nerve are evident (6). If anterior displacement of the facial nerve occurred at this time, the nerve could become interposed between the otic capsule and the stapes blastema, which is beginning to grow toward the otic capsule. This would interfere with further stapes development, resulting in a rudimentary ossicle attached to the incus. Continued growth of the stapes toward the otic capsule could result in the rudimentary crura becoming embedded in the displaced facial nerve (4). Because the stapes never contacts the otic capsule, an oval window does not form. With further anterior displacement of the facial nerve, it is possible for that structure to course across the promontory, inferior to the region of the oval window (4). It has been hypothesized that displacement of the facial nerve occurs because of underdevelopment of the first branchial arch (5). This results in a compensatory overshifting of the second branchial arch, and its nerve follows this shift, assuming a more anterior position.

Facial Nerve

Facial nerve abnormalities are common in cases of aural atresia (7,8). Bony dehiscence of the fallopian canal frequently occurs, and the facial nerve may also take an anomalous course. Typically, the facial nerve makes an acute angle at the second genu, crossing the middle ear in a more anterior and lateral direction to exit into the glenoid fossa. This abnormal position of the mastoid segment of the facial nerve places it at jeopardy when drilling the posterior inferior portion of the new external ear canal. As the facial nerve exits the skull, it may lie just deep to the area of the tragus. Inadvertent injury to the nerve can occur if undermining of the auricle is necessary to better align the meatus and newly created external ear canal. A correlation between the degree of microtia and the extent of facial nerve abnormality has been observed (3,9).

CLASSIFICATION

Patients with congenital aural atresia are classified on the basis of auricular development and external canal/middle ear development. Deformity of the auricle is straightforward and is divided into three grades (10). Grade I microtia represents a minor malformation, with the auricle being smaller than normal but with all parts discernible. In grade II microtia, the auricle is represented by a curving or vertical ridge of tissue. In grade III microtia, any resemblance to an auricle is lost, and only a small rudimentary soft tissue structure is present.

Classification of the external canal/middle ear deformity has been more problematic because of the various parameters that have been used, including clinical examination, radiographic findings, surgical observations, or histopathologic studies. Ombredanne (11) proposed dividing congenital aural atresia into two groups only, major and minor malformations. This classification scheme is attractive because of its simplicity and clinical utility. With minor modifications, the following descriptions reflect Ombredanne's criteria.

Major Malformation

In the major malformation group, the external ear canal and tympanic membrane are usually absent, although cases of severe canal stenosis are also included. A small rudimentary tympanic membrane attached to a bony septum is occasionally seen in the canal stenosis patients, but typically the stenosis prevents visualization of the medial aspect of the ear canal. The size of the middle ear space is reduced, and the malleus and incus are deformed, fused, and fixed to the atretic bone. In severe cases, the middle ear space is very hypoplastic, and ossicles are rudimentary or absent. Dehiscence or displacement of the facial nerve can be expected in most major malformations.

Grade II or III microtia is common, and inner ear function is usually normal.

Minor Malformation

The significant defect in the minor malformation group involves the middle ear. A conductive hearing loss exists because of absence or deformity of one or more ossicles or fixation of the ossicular chain. Abnormalities of the stapes may be more severe in the minor malformation group than in the major group. The middle ear space and tympanic membrane are normal or only slightly smaller. The external ear canal is patent but may be mildly stenotic. Dehiscence or displacement of the facial nerve can occur, and the pinna is normally developed or only slightly deformed.

PATIENT EVALUATION

Most cases of major congenital ear malformations are evident at birth because of microtia or other craniofacial anomalies. Patients with a normal or only slightly deformed pinna and a stenotic or blindly ending external auditory canal, however, may escape diagnosis for years. Unilateral minor congenital ear malformations with a patent ear canal and normal tympanic membrane can be more difficult to diagnose and may be discovered only with routine hearing screening in school.

When initially evaluating an infant or young child with congenital aural atresia, there are two principal objectives. First, one must assess the overall hearing status and need for immediate amplification. Second, one must formulate a treatment plan that provides for consultation with members of other specialties (e.g., plastic surgery, genetics, developmental pediatrics) and for acquisition of data necessary to make further recommendations for rehabilitation and possible surgery.

PHYSICAL EXAMINATION

The initial focus of the physical examination is on overall craniofacial development, because abnormalities or syndromes involving the first or second branchial arch may be associated with the aural atresia. Careful palpation of the mandible may reveal a mild hemifacial microsomia not immediately obvious on inspection. Development of the palate and other intraoral structures should be assessed. The degree of microtia is observed, as is mastoid development. The caliber of the external auditory canal should be graded as normal, stenotic (i.e., mild or severe), blindly ending, or completely atretic. If possible, the tympanic membrane is examined otoscopically. Displacement of the malleus handle (usually anteriorly) or a bony shelf extending from the posterior canal wall may exist. Mobility of the tympanic membrane and malleus handle is determined.

In the case of a child, achievement of neurologic milestones, such as speech and ambulation, is assessed by history and direct observation. This information can provide insight into auditory and vestibular development. Each major division of the facial nerve is carefully examined and any weakness observed. It is rare to encounter a paresis or paralysis involving the entire hemiface, although there is occasionally involvement of the lower face or lip area. The most common anomaly of facial function is a congenital absence of the depressor anguli oris muscle.

Audiometric Evaluation

Auditory assessment in patients with unilateral atresia is usually straightforward. Behavioral audiometry can be used in most cases, although auditory brainstem response testing may be necessary in young infants or children who are difficult to test. Patients with bilateral atresia present more of a challenge because of the masking dilemma. In such cases, it is essential to determine the level of cochlear function in each ear to prevent operating on an only-hearing ear or on an ear with little or no potential for hearing improvement. It is unsafe to assume that cochlear function is normal bilaterally, even if inner ear development appears normal by computed tomography (CT). Objective data are needed, and bone conduction auditory brainstem response testing can provide this (12).

Wave I of the auditory brainstem response is generated by the distal portion of the auditory nerve. There is minimal crossover of this small potential to the contralateral ear, and it is thus best measured by a recording electrode ipsilateral to the stimulated side. When recording simultaneously from both ears with surface electrodes, the presence of a wave I should represent the response from the ear being stimulated only. Although stimulation of each ear independently is not possible with a bone-conducted signal, the wave I response is ear specific, thereby allowing differential assessment of cochlear function.

If the ear canals are patent, electrocochleography can be used in a similar way to obtain ear-specific information. Instead of surface electrodes, a transtympanic, tympanic membrane, or canal electrode are possible, providing a more robust wave I response.

Computed Tomography

CT of the temporal bone is necessary in all patients being considered for surgery. It is also recommended in patients with stenosis of the external auditory canal to examine for possible cholesteatoma formation. To completely assess middle ear development, projections in the axial (i.e., parallel to the line from the infraorbital rim to the external meatus) and coronal (i.e., parallel to the ramus of the mandible) planes are necessary. For example, the body of the malleus and incus, the incudostapedial joint, and the round window are best seen by axial scans, but the stapes, the oval window, and the vestibule are best delineated by coronal scans; both projections are necessary to follow the course of the facial nerve.

Assuming normal sensorineural function has been confirmed audiometrically, the decision to operate depends primarily on the degree of middle ear development, as reflected by the size of the tympanum and status of the ossicles. CT is also important for assessing the development of the cochlear and vestibular labyrinths because their appearance can influence middle ear surgery. For example, an enlarged vestibule and horizontal semicircular canal suggest the possibility of an abnormal communication between the perilymph and cerebrospinal fluid. In such cases, manipulation of the stapes should be avoided.

The course of the facial nerve usually can be delineated by CT. The inability to define this structure precisely, however, is not a contraindication to surgery, assuming the other criteria for middle ear development are met.

Cholesteatoma can occur in association with congenital aural atresia. Occasionally, sufficient canalization of the external canal occurs such that a space develops in the medial end of the bony canal. Because the lateral end of the canal remains atretic or stenotic, the potential for cholesteatoma formation exists. Early in the development of this problem, symptoms such as pain or drainage from the ear canal or a fistulous track may be absent, and the diagnosis can only be made by CT.

Temporal bone CT is performed near the time of operation. Radiographic studies on infants are usually not recommended because the information is rarely applicable to immediate rehabilitative plans. In very young children, poor patient cooperation often necessitates anesthesia or results in a suboptimal study that must be repeated later. Almost all patients with cholesteatoma formation are older than 3 years, which is another reason to delay the CT evaluation until the patient is beyond that age (13).

MEDICAL MANAGEMENT

Unilateral Atresia

No immediate medical intervention is necessary in the young child discovered to have unilateral atresia, assuming there is normal hearing in the contralateral ear. The parents can be reassured that speech, language, and intellectual development will proceed normally. Preferential seating in school is advised, but a hearing aid is not recommended because of poor acceptance by most children and because of the small benefit to overall audition. Many adults, however, find the consequences of unilateral hearing loss from atresia to be a significant aggravation at work and in social settings, and they more readily accept hearing aids. In patients with atresia of the ear canal, a bone-conduction hearing aid must be used. If the canal is only stenotic, an air-conduction aid is preferred because of cosmesis, improved sound localiza-

tion (i.e., stimulation of one cochlea only), broader frequency response, less sound distortion, and comfort.

Bilateral Atresia

Early amplification is essential in infants with bilateral atresia. Initial medical and audiologic evaluations can be completed within the first few months of life and a bone-conduction hearing aid fitted soon thereafter.

SURGICAL MANAGEMENT

Unilateral and Bilateral Atresia Repair

Although most otologic surgeons would consider atresia repair in bilateral cases, many are reluctant to operate on unilateral atresias. The issue is not the unilateral aspect of the hearing loss because most otologic surgeons will explore the middle ear of a child with a large unilateral conductive hearing loss due to other causes (e.g., trauma, infection). The concern is the degree and predictability of hearing improvement that can be achieved, potential lifetime care of a mastoid cavity, and the risk to the facial nerve in atresia surgery. These concerns have prompted many surgeons to recommend delaying surgery in unilateral cases until adulthood, when patients can make their own decision based on the risks and benefits.

An improvement in the hearing threshold to 25 dB or better eliminates the handicap of unilateral hearing loss. This degree of hearing improvement is not possible in all atresia patients, but it can be achieved in at least 50% of carefully selected patients. A mastoid cavity is not created if the "anterior" surgical approach is used, and risk to the facial nerve is minimized by understanding the abnormal development of this structure and by using intraoperative facial nerve monitoring. I and others contend that the benefits of binaural hearing and the possibility of achieving that goal are sufficiently great to offer corrective surgery to carefully selected children with unilateral atresia (9,14).

Patients with bilateral atresia present less of a surgical dilemma. The goal in these cases is to restore sufficient hearing so that amplification is no longer needed. In contradistinction to ear selection for other otologic disorders, the "best" (as determined by CT evaluation) ear is selected for the initial surgical procedure. Most surgeons recommend operating as the child approaches school age and, depending on the hearing result, on the second ear within the next several years. Although the selection criteria are not as stringent as in unilateral cases, careful patient screening is essential for routinely satisfactory results.

Selection Criteria

Most patients undergoing atresia repair have a residual conductive deficit of at least 10 dB. Sensorineural function should be normal to achieve binaural hearing in unilateral cases or to obviate the need for a hearing aid in bilateral cases. Normal or near-normal sensorineural function in the contralateral ears is also important to avoid operating on the better hearing ear.

Although audiometric criteria can be defined quantitatively, the real art of patient selection is centered on the CT evaluation of the middle ear. Hypoplasia of the middle ear space, ranging from mild to severe, occurs in most cases of congenital atresia, and ossicular development can be expected to correlate directly with middle ear size. The risk of surgical complications will be minimized and the chances for a successful hearing result are increased if the middle ear and mastoid size are at least two thirds of the normal size and if all three ossicles, although deformed, can be identified (Figs. 137.1 and 137.2). CT demonstration of the oval and round windows and a near-normal course of the facial nerve further define the ideal surgical candidate. The relationship of the facial nerve to the oval window (i.e., normally positioned or overhanging) and the position of the vertical segment are noted. Anterior displacement of the vertical segment of the nerve restricts access to the middle ear space, reducing the chance for a successful

hearing result and increasing the chance of facial nerve injury. A grading system that quantifies the developmental status of the ear has been shown to predict postoperative hearing results (Table 137.1) (15). In unilateral atresia cases, only the ideal candidates are selected; in bilateral cases, the minimal criteria are a middle ear of at least one half normal size and the presence of an ossicular mass. Overall, only about 60% of patients with aural atresia are surgical candidates.

Often the CT findings can be anticipated by the physical examination. For example, poor middle ear development is more frequently seen in patients with craniofacial deformities than in patients with isolated aural atresia. Patients with Treacher Collins syndrome often have truly bizarre middle ear findings. In general, the better developed the auricle, the larger and better developed the middle ear.

Timing of Surgery

If elected, surgery can be performed as early as 6 to 7 years of age. By this time, accurate audiometric tests have been obtained, pneumatization of the temporal bone is well advanced, and most children are able to cooperate with

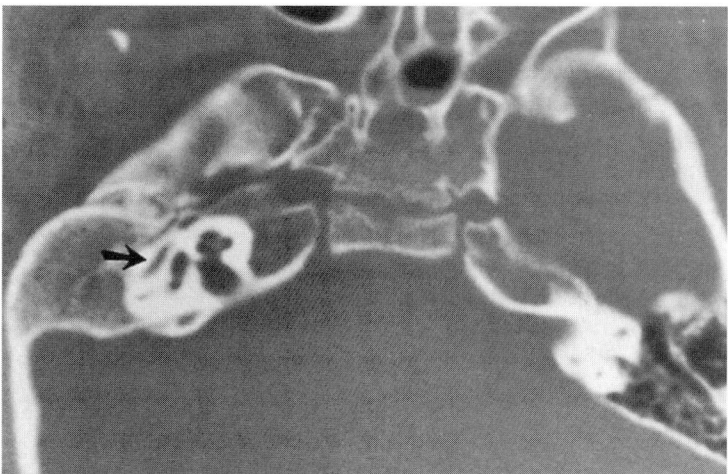

A

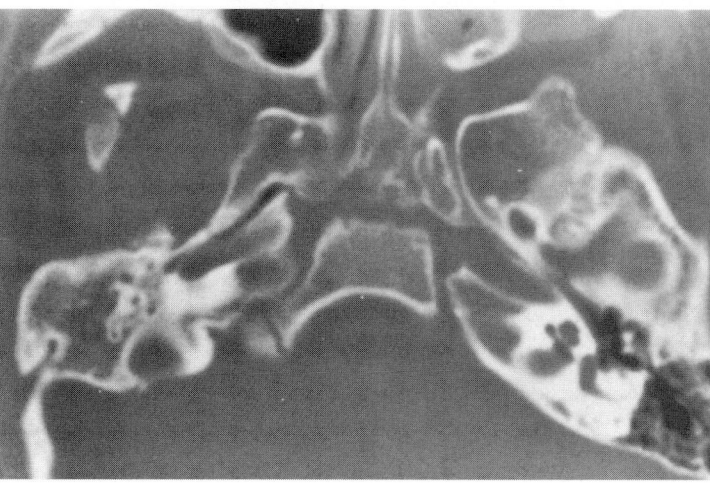

B

Figure 137.1 **A:** Computed tomography from a patient with right congenital aural atresia. There is normal inner ear development, but the middle ear is almost non-existent (*arrow*). **B:** Notice a comparable section through the normal left ear. This patient is not a candidate for surgery.

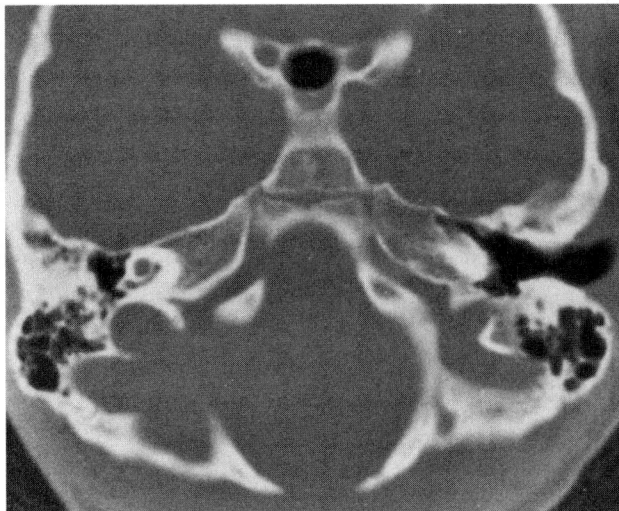
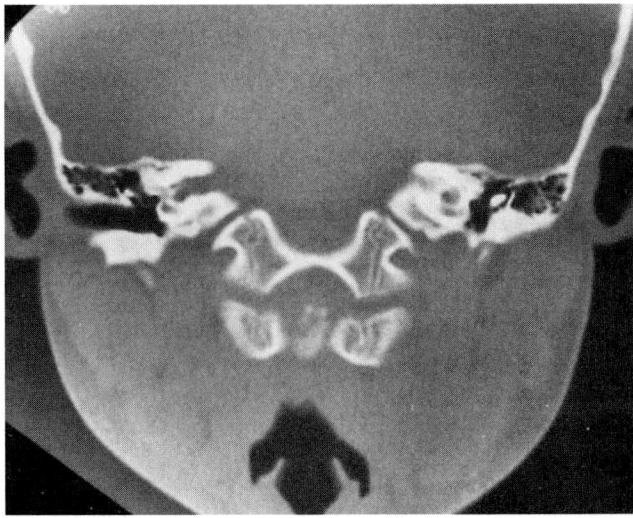

A   B

Figure 137.2   A: Axial computed tomography from a patient with right congenital aural atresia. The middle ear space is more than 50% of normal size. The ossicular mass is not seen on this section, but it was identifiable on other scans. Notice the solid atretic bone anterior to the mastoid air cells. **B:** Coronal computed tomography from a patient with left congenital aural atresia. There is good development of the middle ear space. The fused heads of the malleus and incus are seen, and on other sections, an oval window with stapes was imaged. Based on radiographic findings, both patients are candidates for surgery.

postoperative care. This timing also permits microtia repair to be well under way.

In microtia patients requiring major external ear reconstruction, it is reasonable for the reconstructive surgeon to operate first. This ensures a virgin field without scars or compromised blood supply, optimizing survival of the implanted auricular framework. The overall cosmetic result should also be better without the restriction of having to reconstruct the auricle around a bony canal drilled in the temporal bone. Typically, the otologic surgery is performed midway through the multistaged microtia repair, after the auricular framework has been implanted and the

lobule transposed but before the tragus is reconstructed and the auricle is elevated from the side of the head. Although the reconstructed auricle may not be centered exactly over the created bony canal, it can be repositioned with appropriate undermining so that the meatus and external canal are aligned.

Cholesteatoma

Patients with cholesteatoma, regardless of CT or audiometric findings, should undergo surgery to eradicate the disease process and, if possible, improve hearing. Patients with stenosis of the external canal who are at risk for cholesteatoma formation should also be considered for surgery. Cole and Jahrsdoerfer (13) reviewed a series of 50 patients (54 ears) with an average canal diameter of 4 mm or less and found that 50% of them developed a cholesteatoma. Patient age and exact canal size were important variables in predicting disease. For example, no cholesteatomas were found in patients younger than 3 years, and bone erosion and middle ear involvement from a canal cholesteatoma were not encountered in patients younger than age 12. The preponderance of cholesteatomas developed in canals 2 mm or less in diameter. Beginning in young adolescence, individuals with severe canal stenosis are at a particular risk for cholesteatoma formation [i.e., 10 of 11 ears in the series reported by Cole and Jahrsdoerfer (13)]. The usual presenting symptom in these patients is drainage from the ear canal or from a fistula track postauricularly.

Given these data on the risk of canal cholesteatomas, management protocols can be set forth. Patients with stenosis extensive enough to prevent adequate cleaning of the

---

TABLE 137.1

JAHRSDOEFER GRADING SYSTEM FOR CONGENITAL AURAL ATRESIA

Parameter	Points[a]
Stapes present	2
Oval window patent	1
Middle ear space	1
Facial nerve	1
Malleus/incus complex	1
Mastoid pneumatization	1
Incus-stapes connection	1
Round window	1
External ear appearance	1

[a]Total points: 8, good prognosis; 7, fair prognosis; 6, marginal candidate; 5, poor prognosis.
From Jahrsdoerfer RA, Yeakley JW, Aguilar EA, et al. Grading system for the selection of patients with congenital aural atresia. *Am J Otolaryngol* 1992;13:6–12, with permission.

canal and examination of the tympanic membrane should have CTs by age 4 or 5, even if there is no aural drainage. Assuming a cholesteatoma is not found, several options are available, depending on middle ear development. If the CT findings are favorable with regard to hearing improvement, canal and middle ear surgery is advised at this time. Canaloplasty alone is offered to patients with unfavorable middle ear findings. If the parents are uncomfortable with surgery, a CT should be obtained every few years to rule out cholesteatoma development. Periodic CTs are not necessary in patients with a completely atretic ear canal, given the rarity of cholesteatoma formation in that setting.

SURGICAL TECHNIQUE

There are two basic surgical approaches for repair of aural atresia: the mastoid approach and the anterior approach. In the mastoid approach the sinodural angle is first identified and followed to the antrum (16–18). The facial recess is opened and the incudostapedial joint separated. The atretic bone is then removed. In the anterior approach, as popularized in this country by Jahrsdoerfer (3), exposure of the mastoid air cells is limited. Drilling is confined to an area defined by the temporomandibular joint anteriorly, the middle cranial fossa dura superiorly, and the mastoid air cells posteriorly. An advantage of the anterior approach is that a large mastoid cavity with its attendant problems of debris accumulation and infection is avoided. There is also less surgical manipulation in the area of the mastoid

segment of the facial nerve, and the more cylindrical contours of the new canal with limited mastoid exposure facilitate placement of the split-thickness skin graft. For these reasons, the anterior approach is preferred and is the technique described here. Facial nerve monitoring is used.

Incision

A postauricular incision is used to expose the mastoid bone. The soft tissues are elevated anteriorly until a depression is encountered. In most major malformations, this depression is the temporomandibular joint, although occasionally a stenotic bony ear canal may be encountered. Dissection within this area may be necessary to differentiate between the two, but the manipulation should be limited because the facial nerve frequently exits the skull into the glenoid fossa.

Drilling a Canal

In most atretic ears, a tympanic bone remnant is not identified, but occasionally it is present and clearly demarcated from the surrounding cortex (Fig. 137.3). In such instances, the atretic bone serves to direct the drilling for the external canal. Even when not identified, there is sufficient space between the glenoid fossa anteriorly and the mastoid air cells posteriorly for a canal. Ideally, drilling is confined to the area just lateral to the middle ear space, and the initial entrance to the middle ear is in the epitympanum. This is accomplished by using the middle cranial

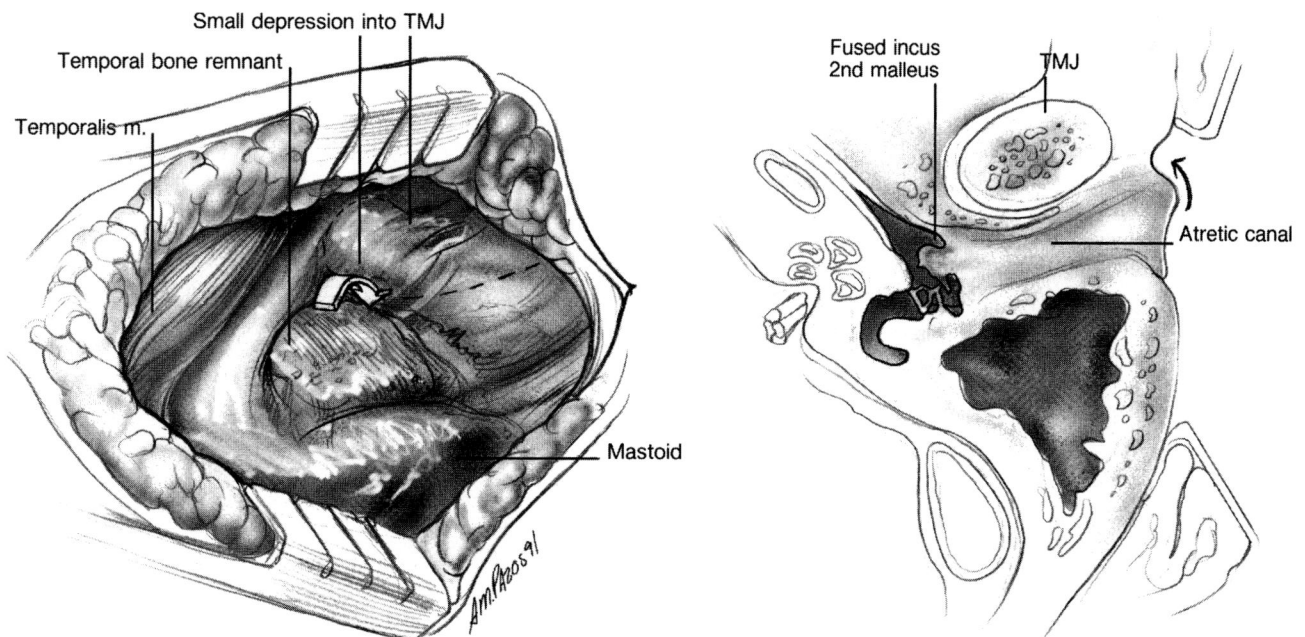

Figure 137.3 **A:** Through a postauricular incision, the soft tissues have been elevated to reveal the mastoid cortex and the atretic bone (tympanic bone remnant). Notice the depression anterior to the atretic bone, which represents the temporomandibular joint (TMJ). **B:** Axial section.

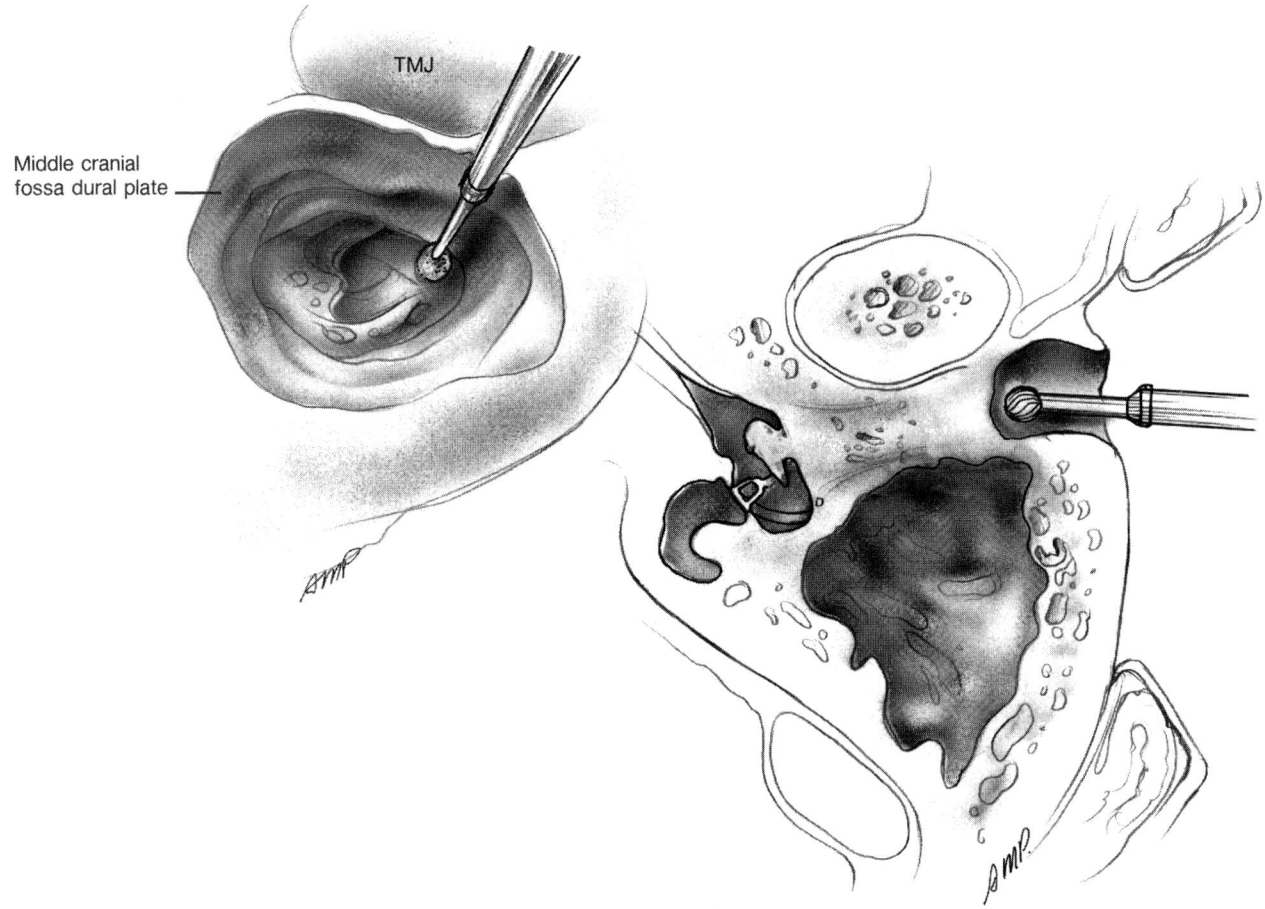

Figure 137.4   The initial stage of drilling an external auditory canal is shown. Landmarks for the canal include the middle cranial fossa dura superiorly, the temporomandibular joint (TMJ) anteriorly, and the mastoid air cells posteriorly.

fossa dura as the superior landmark and the temporomandibular joint as the anterior landmark. The bone removed is usually solid but may be cellular in areas (Fig. 137.4). The posterior wall of the glenoid fossa should be very thin to maximize anterior exposure and to limit opening into the mastoid air cells. As the middle cranial fossa dura plate is followed medially, the epitympanum will be entered and the fused heads of the malleus and incus identified (Fig. 137.5). Concentrating the drilling superiorly along the middle cranial fossa has the advantage of protecting the facial nerve because that structure always lies medial to the ossicular mass in the epitympanum. Because of the more acute angle the facial nerve may take at the second genu, it is vulnerable to injury as the external canal is enlarged in the posteroinferior direction. In this area, the nerve may lie lateral to the middle ear cavity in addition to being anteriorly displaced.

Exposure of the Ossicular Chain

The malleus neck or deformed manubrium is typically fused to the atretic bone. To free the ossicular chain, this overlying bone is thinned carefully with a diamond burr and then completely removed with an incudostapedial joint knife or small hook. Periosteum underlying the atretic bone is still attached to the malleus and should be sharply excised with a microknife or microscissors, or vaporized with the laser. Care is taken to limit trauma to the inner ear by drilling or excessive manipulation of the ossicular chain. The incudostapedial joint is not routinely separated.

Except for the fossa incudis, which may be left intact, bone should be completely removed around the ossicles, leaving at least a 2- to 3-mm space between these structures and the adjacent canal wall. The atretic bone should be removed so that the ossicular mass is centered in the new canal (Fig. 137.6). To ensure proper draping of the fascia and split-thickness skin graft, the canal walls should be smooth and without ledges lateral to the ossicular mass.

Middle Ear Surgery

The stapes may be partially obscured because of the contracted middle ear cavity, the malformed lateral ossicular mass, or the overlying facial nerve. Usually, enough of that

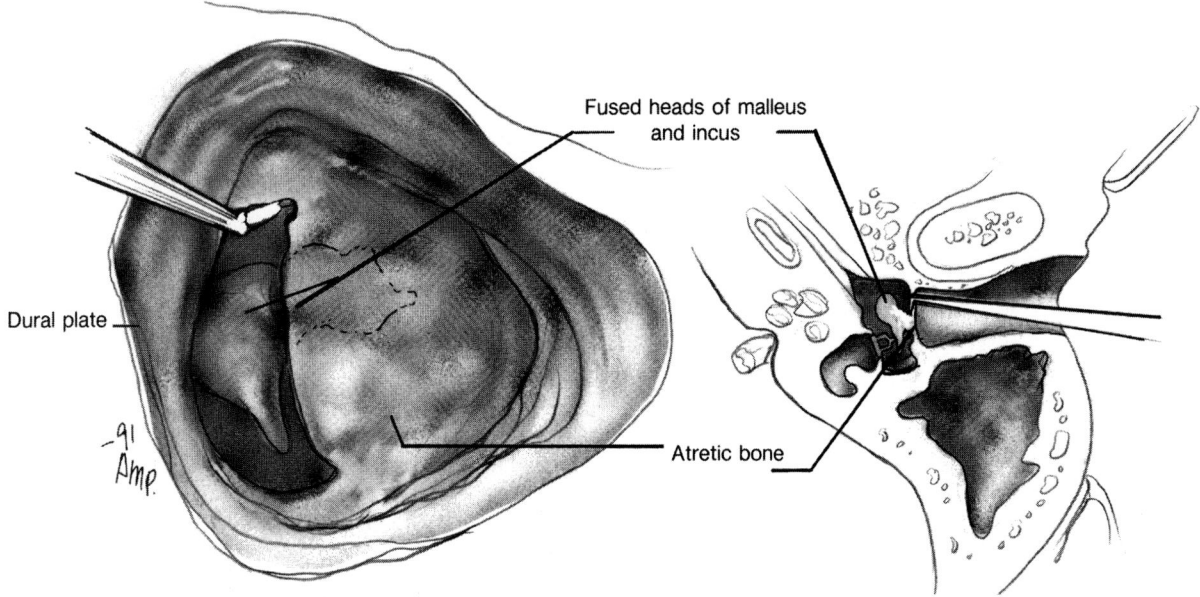

Figure 137.5   The epitympanum is entered by following the middle cranial fossa dura medially. The atretic bone over the fused malleus-incus complex is thinned with a diamond burr and removed with a right-angle hook.

ossicle can be seen to assess its mobility and the integrity of the incudostapedial joint. Although the stapes is often small, with delicate misshapen crura, a normal oval window and stapes footplate are anticipated. The lateral ossicular mass is maintained in position and not removed to obtain a better view of the stapes. In most cases, the ossicular chain, although deformed, is mobile, and hearing results may be better when the chain is left intact instead of interpositioning a prosthesis or autograft material (9).

Tympanic Membrane Grafting

A thin fascia graft is placed over the mobilized ossicular chain. Because the manubrium of the malleus is either absent or very deformed, it is difficult to anchor the graft beneath the ossicular chain. Absence of a tympanic membrane remnant or annulus further predisposes to lateralization. Several techniques can be used to prevent this potential complication. First, the graft can be tucked

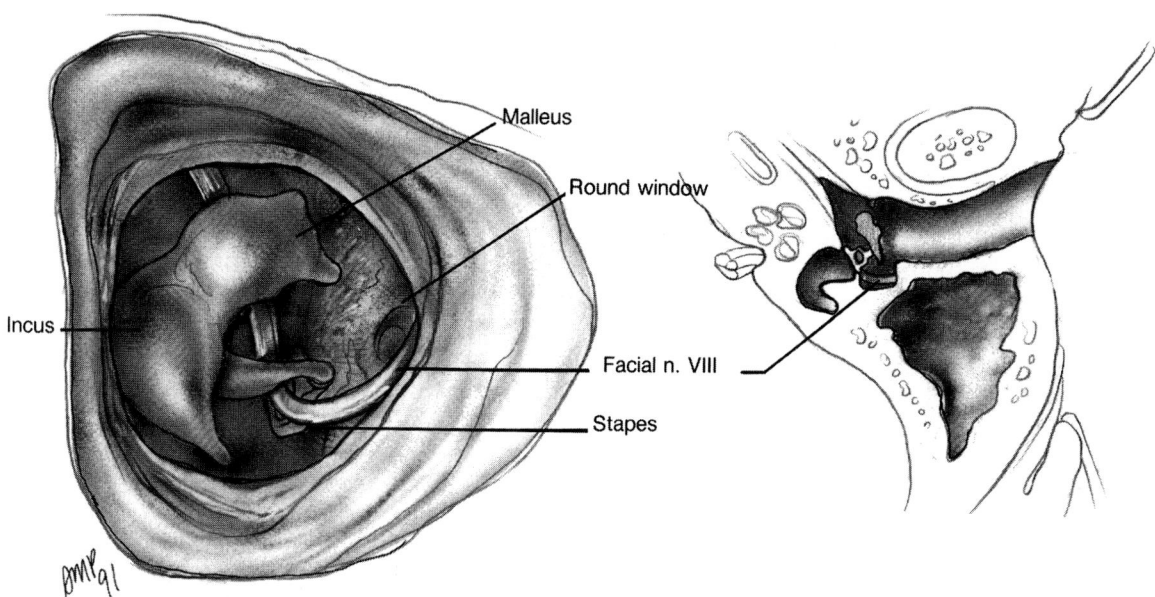

Figure 137.6   The ossicular mass is fully exposed. Notice the more acute angle of the facial nerve at its genu.

beneath the anterior and superior bony ledges of the canal wall. If the ledges are too shallow to stabilize the graft, a sulcus several millimeters deep can be drilled in the anterior canal wall medial to the level of the ossicles. A second technique to avoid lateralization involves covering the fascia graft with the split-thickness skin graft of the canal and then placing a Silastic button that has been contoured to the circumference of the canal on top of the covered ossicles (19).

Meatoplasty

The auricle is undermined and the deep soft tissue debulked from the approximate area of the meatus. Leaving only a small amount of subcutaneous tissue around the meatus limits the length of the membranous canal and helps prevent stenosis. When possible, an anteriorly based thin skin flap is raised over the planned meatal opening. This skin flap is subsequently used to cover a portion of the anterior membranous canal. The auricle is returned to its normal anatomic position to check for alignment of the meatus and the bony canal. Frequently, the meatus appears to be offset anteriorly or inferiorly. In such cases, further undermining of the auricle is necessary so that it can be positioned without tension more posteriorly and superiorly. A strip of skin can be excised from the postauricular incision to help maintain the auricle in its new location. The facial nerve is vulnerable to injury if extensive soft tissue undermining is necessary because prior auricular reconstruction may have caused scarring and tethering of the extratemporal facial nerve in a more superficial position.

Skin Grafting

A skin graft 0.010-inch thick is taken from the upper thigh or upper arm and used to line the canal. To determine the proper configuration of the split-thickness skin graft, several measurements of the canal are made with a 2-0 silk suture. Typically, the resulting skin graft is shaped like a hexagon and is approximately 4 by 6 cm. To facilitate graft placement at the level of tympanic membrane and to ensure eversion of the skin edges, multiple small wedges are excised from the medial portion of the graft; the graft is also pie crusted.

With the ear retracted forward, the split-thickness skin graft is positioned in the bony canal so that it overlaps the fascia graft (Fig. 137.7). Completely covering the fascia graft with the skin graft is acceptable and may facilitate epithelialization of the new tympanic membrane. A silastic disc (0.04 inches thick), approximating the diameter of the bony canal, is placed on the fascia graft to help prevent lateralization. Stabilization of the split-thickness skin graft within the canal is achieved by placing Merocel wicks which are then hydrated with an otic drop (Fig. 137.8). After the bony canal

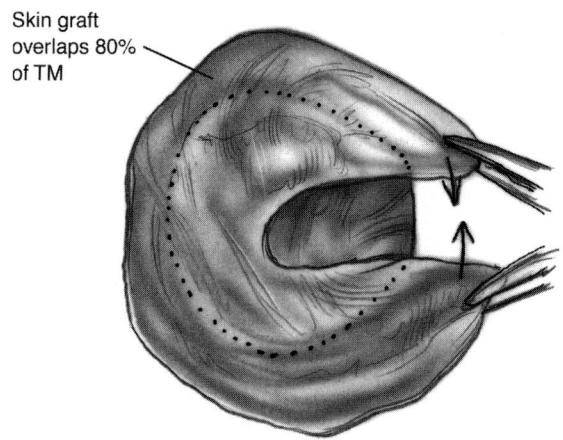

Figure 137.7   Placement of the split-thickness skin graft.

has been fully packed, the ear is returned to its normal anatomic position, and the postauricular incision is closed with subcuticular sutures. Working through the meatus, the lateral end of the split-thickness skin graft is grasped and pulled through the meatal opening. It is trimmed as necessary and sutured in place. Additional packing with Merocel is used to fill the lateral soft tissue portion of the canal. Oral antibiotics are not required.

The initial packing of the split-thickness skin graft in the bony canal prevents it from being dislodged during the final step of suturing the graft to the meatal skin. The placement of the graft in the bony canal while the ear is reflected forward provides maximal exposure, ensuring that

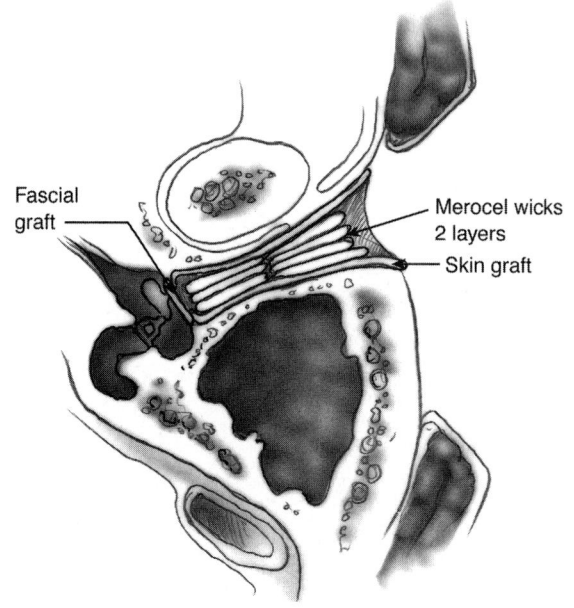

Figure 137.8   The fascia graft for the tympanic membrane has been placed and the split-thickness skin graft is being positioned within the ear canal. These grafts are stabilized by layered packing (axial view).

all the canal is covered and that the split-thickness skin graft has been positioned accurately relative to the fascia graft. The previously elevated skin flap from the area of the meatus is sutured to a cuff of periosteal tissue near the temporomandibular joint (TMJ) to cover a portion of the anterior membranous canal.

Postoperative Care

Approximately 10 days postoperatively, the ear canal packing and silastic disc are removed. Complete take of the split-thickness skin graft is anticipated at this time. If any granulation tissue is seen, antibiotic-soaked pieces of Gelfoam are placed within the canal and the patient is instructed to keep these moist for the next 7 to 10 days.

SURGICAL FINDINGS

Ossicles

In major atresia cases, the expected finding is a fused and deformed malleus-incus complex. The malleus is typically more deformed than the incus and has a short manubrium (Fig. 137.9). The site of ossicular fixation is most commonly between the malleus neck or shortened manubrium and the atretic bone. In minor malformations, the incus and malleus are less deformed and may be completely normal. If abnormal, ossicular fixation in the epitympanum and/or a deformed manubrium or incus long process is common.

In atretic ears, the stapes is usually small and delicate with misshapen crura. Stapes fixation is uncommon. The incudo-stapedial joint may also appear fragile and occasionally may exist as only a fibrous connection. The facial nerve may encroach on the stapes, partially obscuring the footplate. Complete visualization of the stapes may also be impaired by the overlying ossicular mass.

Fixation of the stapes, severe deformity of the stapes, or even absence of the stapes and oval window may be encountered in minor malformation cases. These abnormalities, although rare, are more common in patients with a patent external auditory canal and normal tympanic membrane than in patients with major atresia of the ear.

Facial Nerve

Facial nerve abnormalities are common in major atresia patients. The anticipated abnormalities include complete dehiscence of the tympanic segment, inferior displacement of the tympanic segment, and anterior and lateral displacement of the mastoid segment. The last abnormality frequently obscures the round window. Although the course of the facial nerve is often aberrant, predictable abnormalities are the rule and help guide the surgeon. The degree of external ear deformity provides some indication of facial nerve development, with a higher incidence of facial nerve anomalies occurring in patients with more severe microtia (3,4).

Aberrant facial nerves are frequently encountered in ears with minor malformations, and the abnormalities may even be more severe than those seen in atresia cases. The most common findings include dehiscence or inferior displacement of the tympanic segment. In several cases, a facial nerve coursing across the middle portion of the promontory, well inferior to the oval window, has been observed. In all patients with a congenital conductive hearing loss, even if the pinna, external auditory canal, and tympanic membrane are normal, an abnormal facial nerve should be anticipated and appropriate facial nerve monitoring and surgical care exercised.

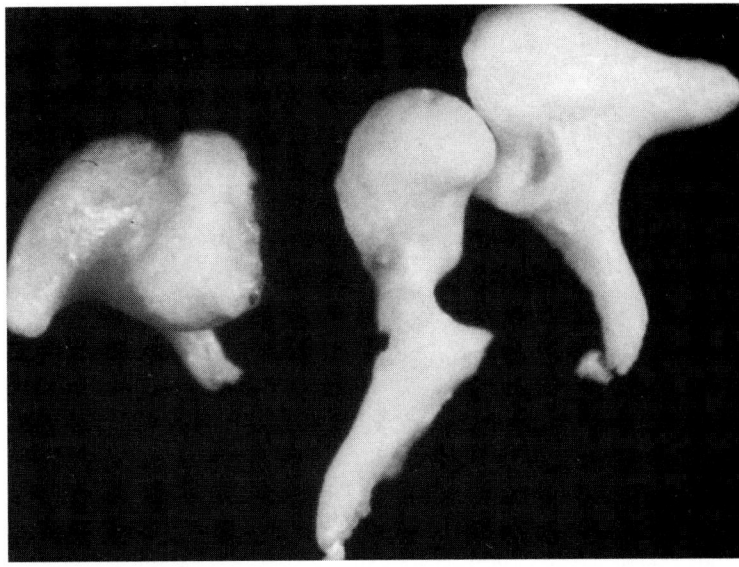

Figure 137.9 The typical appearance of a fused malleus-incus complex is shown (*left*). Notice that this complex is smaller than the normal malleus and incus (*right*) and that the malleus is more deformed than the incus.

HEARING RESULTS

It is difficult to compare hearing results from various series because of differences in classifying congenital ears, in selection criteria, in reporting hearing results, and in the length of follow-up. In general, an initial postoperative hearing level of 30 dB or better can be achieved in approximately 50% to 75% of major congenital atresia patients; a hearing level of 20 dB or better is possible in 15% to 50% of these patients. Bellucci (2) reported a hearing level of at least 30 dB in 55% of 71 patients followed for at least 2 years. Schuknecht (20) reported similar success in 30 patients with mean follow-up of 1.3 years. Thirty percent of Schuknecht's patients had a hearing level of 20 dB or better. Nager and Levin (16) reported that 70% of 23 patients treated over a 17-year period had a hearing level of at least 30 dB. Mattox and Fisch (21) found at least a 30-dB improvement in air-conduction thresholds in 45% of 11 patients followed a minimum of 2 years. De la Cruz and colleagues (18,22) reported 56 patients with a 6-month follow-up and observed that 53% had a conductive deficit of 20 dB or less and 73% had a deficit of 30 dB or less. In a follow-up series involving 77 ears, air-bone gap closure to less than 30 dB was achieved in 60% of cases (23). In 2003, De la Cruz and Teufert (24) reported a 30-dB or less conductive hearing loss in 58.5% of 116 ears with short-term follow-up, which decreased to 50.8% with longer-term (= 6 months) observation. Lambert (9) reported that 67% of 15 patients followed for at least 1 year had a speech reception threshold of 30 dB or better; the mean improvement in the hearing level was 30 dB. Jahrsdoerfer (3) found that 65% of 17 patients followed for 2 months to 8 years had a pure-tone average of 30 dB or less. In a more recent series of 86 patients, Jahrsdoerfer (15) reported a postoperative hearing level at 1 month of 25 dB or better in 71%. Lambert (25) reported data comparing early (less than 1 year) and longer term (1.0 to 7.5 years, mean follow-up 2.8 years) hearing results after surgery for congenital aural atresia. This study involved 59 consecutively operated ears. In the early postoperative period, a speech reception threshold (SRT) of less than 25 dB was achieved in 60% and an SRT of less than 30 dB in 70%. With longer-term follow-up, 46% of patients maintained an SRT of less than 25 dB.

COMPLICATIONS

Given the fact that near-normal hearing is not universally achieved even in carefully selected atresia patients, the surgical complications must be carefully compared with the merits of atresia surgery. The two potential serious complications are sensorineural hearing loss and facial nerve paralysis. Other complications that can occur include canal stenosis, chronic infection, and recurrent conductive hearing loss.

It should be recognized that revision surgery is often required after congenital aural atresia repair. In the series by Lambert (25) in which patients were followed for an average of 2.8 years, one third of the patients did require revision surgery. Stenosis of the ear canal and lateralization of the tympanic membrane were the most common problems encountered. After revision surgery, approximately half of these patients did achieve a speech reception threshold of 25 dB or better with at least 1 year of follow-up.

Labyrinthine Injury

The anterior surgical approach limits exposure of mastoid air cells, thus minimizing potential injury to the horizontal semicircular canal. High-frequency sensorineural hearing loss has been noted in some patients postoperatively, although a loss in the speech frequencies is rare (9,17, 20,22,26). Because the ossicular mass is connected to the atretic bone, energy from drilling will be transmitted to the inner ear in all atresia cases regardless of the approach. This may be of less consequence, however, than direct manipulation of the ossicular chain by instruments or the drill. Care in removing the final portion of atretic bone from the ossicular chain is particularly important in the anterior approach, because the incudostapedial joint is not disarticulated.

Facial Nerve Injury

The abnormal development of the temporal bone in cases of aural atresia places the facial nerve at increased vulnerability. Understanding the anomalies of the facial nerve likely to be encountered and the use of facial nerve monitoring, however, enable the surgeon to proceed with confidence. Temporary facial paralysis has occurred rarely. This complication has usually resulted from transposition of the facial nerve to gain access to the oval window (20,27). Facial paresis or paralysis has not been observed in recent series in which facial nerve monitoring has been used (9,22).

Jahrsdoerfer and Lambert (28) have reported a 1% incidence of facial paresis in more than 1,000 patients who had undergone congenital aural atresia surgery.

Potential damage to the facial nerve can be minimized by adhering to several surgical guidelines. First, as the atretic bone is removed, the drilling should be concentrated superiorly along the middle cranial fossa dural plate, entering the middle ear first in the epitympanum. The facial nerve is protected in this approach, because it will always lie medial to the ossicular heads. Second, care should be exercised as the canal is enlarged in the posterior-inferior direction because of the more anterior and lateral course of the mastoid segment. Injury to the facial nerve can also occur in its extratemporal segment, as the postauricular incision is made, or as the auricle is undermined to align the soft tissue meatus and the created bony canal.

Canal Stenosis

Some narrowing of the new external auditory canal, particularly in its lateral or soft tissue segment, develops in as many as 25% of patients. If a large meatus (i.e., approximately twice normal size) has been made, this narrowing is of little consequence. Occasionally, a significant stenosis occurs, trapping squamous epithelium and causing infection. In such cases, attempts to dilate the canal with soft or hard stents are usually ineffective, and a secondary meatoplasty with skin grafting is necessary. This potential problem can be minimized by generously debulking soft tissue from the auricle before the meatoplasty, thus decreasing the length of the membranous canal. Coverage of all exposed bone and soft tissue by the split-thickness skin graft is also essential to prevent granulation tissue formation and subsequent stricture. The use of the meatal skin flap to cover a portion of the anterior membranous canal obviates a circumferential split-thickness skin graft (STSG) at the meatal opening and may also help prevent stenosis.

In some patients, the lateral canal may be narrowed by displacement of the pinna rather than by fibrous proliferation. Because the reconstructed auricle has more mass and less muscular and soft tissue support than the normal pinna, it can shift, usually anteriorly or inferiorly, after surgery. This shift causes a malalignment of the meatus and bony canal. If there is concern about proper alignment of the membranous and bony canals during the atresia surgery, a permanent suspension suture from the framework of the auricle to the mastoid periosteum or to a hole drilled in the mastoid cortex is placed.

Chronic Infection

Normal migration of keratin debris is lacking in the skin-grafted ear canal. Protective secretions from sebaceous and apocrine glands are also absent. As a consequence, the incidence of canal infections is higher than in the normal ear. The cylindrical contour of the canal and absence of a mastoid defect achieved with the anterior surgical approach minimize debris accumulation. A widely patent meatus and membranous canal are important for aeration and cleaning, which may be required once or twice annually. Most patients are not restricted with regard to water activities.

Conductive Hearing Loss

Persistent or recurrent conductive hearing loss is the most common negative outcome in aural atresia surgery. The causes of the former are varied and include inadequate mobilization of the ossicular mass from the atretic bone, an unrecognized incudo-stapedial joint discontinuity, or a fixed stapes footplate. Wide exposure of the ossicular mass at surgery is necessary to ensure chain mobility and to facilitate assessment of chain integrity. Recurrence of a conductive hearing loss after an initial satisfactory improvement in air-conduction thresholds is usually secondary to refixation of the ossicular chain or to tympanic membrane lateralization. At least a 2- to 3-mm wide area of bone removal around the ossicular mass (except at the fossa incudis) is desirable, because bony regrowth can occur, especially in children. Anchoring the fascia graft beneath a bony ledge and/or the use of a Silastic disc helps minimize graft lateralization. The incidence of tympanic membrane perforation or middle ear adhesions approximates that encountered in routine tympanoplastic procedures.

Bone-Anchored Hearing Implant

A bone-anchored hearing aid is an alternative rehabilitative strategy for patients with unilateral or bilateral aural atresia, and especially for those patients who are marginal or poor surgical candidates. This approach uses an osseointegrated titanium fixture, placed in the mastoid area, to which a sound processor is attached percutaneously. The osteointegration allows more efficient transfer of sound than can be achieved with a traditional bone conduction hearing aid (29). As in patients with otosclerosis, a hearing aid option should be discussed in tandem with surgical intervention

CONCLUSIONS

The objective in congenital ear surgery is to create a functional pathway by which sound can reach the cochlear fluids. Although simple in concept, this type of surgery presents a true challenge to the otologic surgeon. A thorough knowledge of the anatomic variations that can occur with abnormal development of the temporal bone is essential, and the nuances of audiometric and radiographic interpretation must be mastered.

HIGHLIGHTS

- During the fifth to seventh month of embryogenesis, the solid core of epithelial cells representing the external auditory canal canalizes, beginning medially and progressing laterally. If incomplete, this process can result in a stenotic membranous canal laterally, with a more normal caliber bony canal and tympanic membrane medially. This condition predisposes to cholesteatoma formation within the ear canal.

- Congenital ear malformations can be classified as major or minor. The significant defect in the minor malformation group involves the middle ear, especially the ossicular chain. In most cases of microtia and atresia of the ear canal, the cochlear and vestibular labyrinths are normally formed.

- In major atresia cases, the stapes is usually small with misshapen crura. The footplate is usually intact and mobile.

Hearing results that are consistently excellent cannot yet be achieved in atresia surgery, but with adherence to strict selection criteria and with further refinements in surgical technique, this goal is realistic.

- The facial nerve is often aberrant in major congenital ear malformations. Dehiscence of the tympanic segment with or without inferior displacement is often seen. The mastoid segment of the facial nerve often makes a more acute angle at the second genu, resulting in anterior and lateral displacement; it may obscure the round window.
- Bilateral congenital atresias can present a masking dilemma during audiometric testing. Bone-conduction auditory brainstem response can provide objective data on ear-specific cochlear function in these cases and help with operative selection.
- In cases of major atresia, the middle ear space should be greater than 50% of normal size, and all three ossicles, although deformed, should be visible.
- The principal landmarks in the anterior approach for aural atresia are the middle fossa dura superiorly, the temporomandibular joint anteriorly, and the mastoid air cells posteriorly.
- With proper patient selection in cases of major atresia, it is possible to achieve a hearing level of 25 dB or better in approximately 50% to 70% of patients.
- The most frequent complications in congenital atresia surgery are canal stenosis and failure to achieve an adequate hearing level. The latter can occur because of inadequate mobilization of the ossicular mass from the atretic bone, lateralization of the tympanic membrane graft, or refixation of the ossicular chain by bony regrowth or fibrous tissue.

REFERENCES

1. Jafek BW, Nager GT, Strife J, et al. Congenital aural atresia: an analysis of 311 cases. *Trans Am Acad Ophthalmol Otolaryngol* 1975;80: 588–592.
2. Bellucci RJ. Congenital aural malformations: diagnosis and treatment. *Otolaryngol Clin North Am* 1981;14:95–124.
3. Jahrsdoerfer RA. Congenital atresia of the ear. *Laryngoscope* 1978;88[Suppl 13]:1–46.
4. Lambert PR. Congenital absence of the oval window. *Laryngoscope* 1990;100:37–40.
5. Gerhardt HJ, Otto HD. The intratemporal course of the facial nerve and its influence on the development of the ossicular chain. *Acta Otolaryngol* 1981;91:567–573.
6. Jahrsdoerfer RA. Embryology of the facial nerve. *Am J Otol* 1988; 9:423–426.
7. Crabtree JA. The facial nerve in congenital ear surgery. *Otolaryngol Clin North Am* 1974;7:505–510.
8. Jahrsdoerfer RA. The facial nerve in congenital middle ear malformations. *Laryngoscope* 1981;91:1217–1224.
9. Lambert PR. Major congenital ear malformations. *Ann Otol Rhinol Laryngol* 1988;97:641–649.
10. Marx H. Die Missbildungen des Ohres. *Handb Spez Path Anat Hist* 1926;12:620–625.
11. Ombredanne M. Chirugie des surdites congenitales par malformation ossiculaires. *Acta Otorhinolaryngol Belg* 1971;25:837–840.
12. Tucci DL, Ruth RA, Lambert PR. Use of the bone conduction ABR wave I response in determination of cochlear reserve. *Am J Otolaryngol* 1990;11:119–124.
13. Cole RR, Jahrsdoerfer RA. The risk of cholesteatoma in congenital aural stenosis. *Laryngoscope* 1990;100:576–582.
14. Jahrsdoerfer RA. Reconstruction of the ear canal. In: English GM, ed. *Otolaryngology*, Vol. 4. Philadelphia: JB Lippincott, 1990:1–7.
15. Jahrsdoerfer RA, Yeakley JW, Aguilar EA, et al. Grading system for the selection of patients with congenital aural atresia. *Am J Otolaryngol* 1992;13:6–12.
16. Nager GT, Levin LS. Congenital aural atresia: embryology, pathology, classification, genetics, and surgical management. In: Paparella MM, Shumrick D, eds. *Otolaryngology*. Philadelphia: WB Saunders, 1980;1303–1344.
17. Glasscock ME III, Schwaber MK, Nissen AJ, et al. Management of congenital ear malformations. *Ann Otol Rhinol Laryngol* 1983;92: 504–509.
18. De la Cruz A, Linthicum FH Jr, Luxford WM. Congenital atresia of the external auditory canal. *Laryngoscope* 1985;95:421–427.
19. Jahrsdoerfer RA, Cole RR, Gray LC. Advances in congenital aural atresia. In: *Advances in otolaryngology—head and neck surgery*, Vol. 5. St. Louis: Mosby-Year Book, 1991:1–5.
20. Schuknecht HG. Congenital aural atresia. *Laryngoscope* 1989;99: 908–917.
21. Mattox DE, Fisch U. Surgical correction of congenital atresia of the ear. *Otolaryngol Head Neck Surg* 1986;94:574–577.
22. Malony TB, De la Cruz A. Surgical approaches to congenital atresia of the external auditory canal. *Otolaryngol Head Neck Surg* 1990;103:991–1001.
23. Chandrasekhr SS, De la Cruz A. Surgery of congenital aural atresia. *Am J Otol* 1995;16:713–717.
24. De la Cruz A, Teufert KB. Congenital atresia surgery: long term results. *Otolaryngol Head Neck Surg* 2003;129:121–127.
25. Lambert PR. Congenital aural atresia: stability of surgical results. *Laryngoscope* 1998;108:1801–1805.
26. Jahrsdoerfer RA. Congenital malformation of the ear. *Ann Otol Rhinol Laryngol* 1980;89:348–352.
27. Jahrsdoerfer RA, Hall JW. Congenital malformations of the ear. *Am J Otol* 1986;7:267–269.
28. Jahrsdoerfer RA, Lambert PR. Facial nerve injury and congenital aural atresia surgery. *Am J Otol* 1998; 19:283–287.
29. Lustig L, Arts HA, Brackmann D, et al. Hearing rehabilitation using the BAHA bone-anchored hearing aid: results in 40 patients. *Otol Neurotol* 2001;22:328–334.

Intratemporal and Intracranial Complications of Otitis Media

138

J. Gail Neely   H. Alexander Arts

EVALUATION AND DIAGNOSIS

Definition and Classification

A complication of otitis media is defined as spread of infection beyond the confines of the pneumatized spaces of the temporal bone and their attendant mucosa (1). The four intratemporal and six intracranial complications characteristically considered during discussion of this topic are addressed in this chapter. Table 138.1 lists these complications.

Pathophysiology

Details of the pathophysiology in each of these complications of otitis media are unknown, and because of their rarity, no systematic studies have been undertaken in most of these complications. However, these complications still do arise even today in the United States and other developed countries at rates similar to underdeveloped countries (2).

It is important to understand the anatomy in which these infections exist, their routes of spread, and the characteristic patterns of disease. However, the primary pathogenesis seems to be a complex interaction among the specific organisms involved and the host (3). An important host response leading to complication is the production of granulation tissue that becomes obstructive to drainage and aeration and destructive of bone and the consequent development of an anaerobic environment. Important mi-

crobiologic factors seem to pivot about the synergistic pathogenicity of anaerobic organisms (4). Occasionally, the excessively invasive characteristics of *Haemophilus influenzae* type B become important.

Precursors to Complications

Early clinical signs of an impending complication provide some information about the pathogenesis (Table 138.2). With the exception of meningitis, most complications originate from subacute or chronic infection (Table 138.3). Therefore, it is important to be alert to the persistence of an acute infection beyond 2 weeks or the recurrence of symptoms within a 2- to 3-week period, which suggests that the infection is not controlled and is becoming subacute. Additionally, an acute exacerbation of a chronic infection may allow an invasive acute infection to penetrate previous bony barriers that have been eroded by chronic infection and granulations. Fetid discharge concomitant with an acute exacerbation suggests an uncontrolled deep-seated bone erosive infection and increased numbers of anaerobic and microaerophilic organisms.

The epidemiology and microbiologic behavior of the organisms found in complications offer perhaps some insight into the pathogenesis and pathophysiology of these complications (Table 138.4). For example, infections with *Streptococcus pneumoniae* and nontypable *H. influenzae* are the most common causes of acute suppurative otitis media (5). Only about 4% of otitis media is caused by infection

TABLE 138.1 COMPLICATIONS

OTITIS MEDIA

I. Intratemporal
   A. Mastoiditis (most common intratemporal complication from acute otitis media)
      1. Associated with subperiosteal abscess
      2. Associated with inferior deep neck abscess (Bezold)
      3. "Masked" mastoiditis
   B. Petrositis
   C. Labyrinthitis[a]
      1. Serous or toxic
      2. Suppurative
         a. Otogenic
            Acute
            Chronic
         b. Meningogenic
   D. Facial paralysis (second most common intratemporal complication from acute otitis media)
      1. Associated with acute infection
      2. Associated with subacute or chronic infection

II. Intracranial
   A. Extradural granulation tissue and/or abscess (most common intracranial complication from chronic infection)
   B. Sigmoid sinus thrombophlebitis
      1. Nonoccluding
      2. Occluding
   C. Brain abscess
      1. Cerebritis
      2. Latent period
      3. Abscess
      4. Termination
   D. Otitis hydrocephalus (associated with occluding sigmoid sinus thrombophlebitis)
   E. Meningitis (most common intracranial complication from acute otitis media)
      1. Associated with acute infection
         a. Hematogenous
         b. Associated with congenital CSF leaks through otitic capsule (e.g., severe Mondini), adjacent to otic capsule (e.g., geniculate ganglion, Hyrtle "fissure"), or distant to otitic capsule (e.g., meningoencephaloceles) (16)
         c. Poststapedectomy or postcraniectomy or posttraumatic CSF leaks
      2. Associated with subacute or chronic infection
         a. Dural erosion
         b. Cholesteatoma labyrinthine fistula
   F. Subdural abscess

CSF, cerebrospinal fluid.
[a] Schuknecht HF. Pathology of the ear, 2nd ed. Philadelphia: Lea & Febiger, 1993.

with *H. influenzae* type B; however, pediatric patients with otitis media occurring simultaneously with meningitis or other central nervous system infections were found to have an unusually high incidence of *H. influenzae* type B (6).

Uncomplicated chronic otorrhea characteristically cultures *Pseudomonas aeruginosa, Staphylococcus aureus,* and a variety of other gram-negative organisms, such as *Proteus* sp., *Klebsiella* sp., and *Escherichia coli.* In contrast, mastoiditis associated with chronic suppurative otitis media frequently is foul smelling and in addition contains *Bacteroides fragilis* (5). Multiple organisms are found in 57% of chronically draining ears with cholesteatoma, with an average of three different organisms. However, if these ears are foul smelling, characteristically 5 to 11 organisms are found, always including both anaerobes and aerobes. Mal-

odorous discharge is a significant early sign of complication. Anaerobic organisms are a major cause of foul-smelling discharge. *Moraxella catarrhalis,* previously a reasonably uncommon organism in the middle ear, is emerging as a common pathogen for acute suppurative otitis media (5).

β-Lactamase-producing organisms, such as *S. aureus, H. influenzae, B. catarrhalis,* and *Bacteroides* sp., not only survive β-lactam antibiotics but may also protect other potentially penicillin-susceptible pathogens from penicillin and other β-lactam antibiotics. Anaerobic organisms have recently been shown to play major roles in pathogenic synergism by protecting against host defenses, creating suitable environments for other organisms, and inactivating antibiotics (3,4).

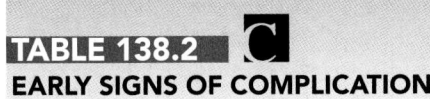

TABLE 138.2

EARLY SIGNS OF COMPLICATION

Impending complication
    Persistence of acute infection for 2 weeks
    Recurrence of symptoms within 2 weeks
    Acute exacerbation of chronic infection, especially if fetid
    Fetid discharge during treatment
    Haemophilus influenzae type B or anaerobes

Early or obvious signs/symptoms of complication (associated complication)
    Fever associated with a chronic perforation (intracranial complication or extracranial cellulitis)
    Pinna displaced inferolaterally and/or edema of the posterosuperior canal wall skin (mastoiditis associated with subperiosteal abscess)
    Retroorbital pain on side of infected ear (petrositis)
    Vertigo and nystagmus in a patient with an infected ear (labyrinthitis)
    Facial paralysis on the side of an infected ear (facial paralysis)
    Headache and/or lethargy (intracranial)
    Papilledema (otitic hydrocephalus; brain abscess; meningitis)
    Meningismus (meningitis)
    Focal neurologic signs and/or seizure (brain abscess)
    Catastrophic neurologic signs (subdural abscess; meningitis)

PATTERNS OF DISEASE

Complications tend to follow fairly predictable patterns; for example, with the exception of meningitis in infants and young children and some cases of facial paralysis, which may be associated with acute suppurative otitis

TABLE 138.3

PATTERNS OF DISEASE

Origin of complication
Acute infection
    Meningitis—infants and young children
    Meningitis—adults or children with occult CSF leaks
    Facial paralysis—children more commonly
    Labyrinthitis
    Subdural abscess—infants more commonly
Subacute or chronic infection
    Mastoiditis
    Petrositis
    Facial paralysis
    Labyrinthitis
    Extradural abscess and granulations
    Sigmoid sinus thrombophlebitis
    Brain abscess
    Otitic hydrocephalic
    Meningitis
    Subdural abscess

Patterns of associated diseases in usual sequence
Mastoiditis or petrositis
    Extradural granulation tissue and/or abscess
    Sigmoid sinus thrombophlebitis
    Brain abscess or otitic hydrocephalus
Meningitis
    Subdural abscess—infants more commonly

CSF, cerebrospinal fluid.

media, most complications tend to be associated with sub-acute or chronic middle ear infection (Table 138.3). In subacute or chronic infections, mastoiditis characteristically is the initial complication. Petrositis is almost never seen without mastoiditis. Facial paralysis and labyrinthine fistulization most often result from chronically infected ears with cholesteatoma. The close proximity of the sigmoid sinus to the large air cells adjacent to its lateral surface, which are most distant from the eustachian tube, makes it particularly susceptible to bone-eroding granulations in a subacutely or chronically infected ear. Infection adjacent to the dura of the sigmoid sinus may incite an intraluminal mural thrombus (7). If in the presence of infection, the sigmoid sinus becomes obstructed, intracranial hypertension, known as otitic hydrocephalus, may result. Retrograde thrombophlebitis may extend intracerebrally, resulting in a brain abscess. Subdural abscesses from suppurative ear disease are extremely rare; these abscesses are most often found in infants with meningitis. The meningitis, of course, can result from suppurative ear disease.

Diagnosis

High Index of Suspicion

The diagnosis of an impending or manifest intratemporal or intracranial complication of otitis media is contingent on a high index of suspicion. Because antibiotic therapy may have a masking effect on the significant signs and symptoms of complications, a high level of clinical awareness is important for early diagnosis. If the patient is not improving sufficiently with medical management, radioimaging followed by any necessary surgical procedure is the required course of action (8). Key to the differential is the discovery of a host response or microorganism deviation from the usual

TABLE 138.4
BACTERIOLOGY[a, b]

Acute suppurative otitis media (in order of prevalence)
1. *Streptococcus pneumoniae*—most common
2. *Haemophilus influenzae* (nontypable)
3. *Moraxella catarrhalis* (emerging common pathogen)
4. Others, far less common
   a. Group A streptococci
   b. *Staphylococcus aureus* (infrequent)
   c. Gram-negative bacilli (infrequent)

Acute mastoiditis (in order of prevalence)
1. *Streptococcus pneumoniae*
2. *Pseudomonas aeruginosa* (6)
3. Group A beta-hemolytic *Streptococci* (e.g., *Streptococcus pyogenes*)
4. Coagulase-negative *Staphylococcus* species
5. Others, less common
   a. *S. aureus*
   b. *Proteus* species
   c. *Bacteroides* species

Chronic otorrhea with or without cholesteatoma (in order of prevalence)
1. Mixed aerobic (also occasionally including *S. pneumoniae*) and anaerobic organisms
   a. Foul-smelling ears (especially cholesteatomas) may grow 5–11 organisms; always anaerobes *and* aerobes
2. *Pseudomonas aeruginosa* (most common aerobe)
3. *S. aureus* and *Staphylococcus epidermidis*
4. Other aerobic organisms, including *Proteus* species, *Klebsiella* species, and *Escherichia coli*
5. Various anaerobic organisms, including *Bacteroides fragilis*

Intracranial abscesses (brain and subdural) of otogenic origin (mixed cultures)
Streptococcus sp.
Staphylococcus sp.
Proteus sp.
Anaerobic organisms (*Peptococcus, Peptostreptococcus, B. fragilis*)

Bacterial meningitis in children
S. pneumoniae
H. influenzae type B
Neisseria meningitidis

---

[a] Fairbanks DN. *Antimicrobial therapy in otolaryngology—head and neck surgery,* 11th ed. Alexandria, VA: American Academy of Otolaryngology—Head and Neck Surgery Foundation, 2003.
[b] Phillips EJ, Simor AE. Bacterial meningitis in children and adults. Changes in community-acquired disease may affect patient care. *Postgrad Med* 1998;103(3):102–122.

onset, progression, and recovery of a noncomplicated infection (Tables 138.2 and 138.5). The presence of any one of the five conditions listed in Table 138.2 suggests the possibility of an impending complication and requires diligence in attempting rapid resolution of the infection and follow-up of the patient to normalcy.

Obvious or Generalized Suggestive Signs

When faced with a list of 10 possible complications, of which several may coexist, it is helpful to approach the menu of possibilities using several initial filters of thought and observation (Table 138.2).

1. The first filter is "obvious complications" consisting of mastoiditis with concomitant subperiosteal abscess, labyrinthitis, facial paralysis, and meningitis. That narrows the list from 10 to 7. Pinna displacement inferolaterally and edema of the posterior superior canal wall skin are highly suggestive of mastoiditis; their absence, however, does not rule out "masked" mastoiditis. Vertigo and nystagmus in a patient with an infected ear suggest serous or suppurative labyrinthitis with or without a labyrinthine fistula from cholesteatoma (chronic labyrinthitis). Facial paralysis on the side of an infected ear strongly suggests that infection is the cause of the paralysis. Meningismus is an obvious sign of meningeal irritation and is easily detected, except in infants and in the elderly or debilitated patient.

2. The second filter is retroorbital pain. This filter narrows the list of 7 down to 6. A patient with petrositis has retroorbital pain but usually does not have abducens paralysis, which is the third of the triad of Gradenigo syndrome. The absence of retroorbital pain reasonably tends to obviate the diagnosis of petrositis. However, retroorbital pain is not a symptom that most patients spontaneously report; it must be specifically elicited.

TABLE 138.5 ▯ DIAGNOSIS

SUBTLE DISEASE

"Masked" mastoiditis
- Persistent or recurrent pain 2 weeks after specific antibiotic treatment in ear with non–air-containing mastoid
- Radiographic evidence of coalescence

Extradural granulation tissue and/or abscess
- Exposure during surgery

Sigmoid sinus thrombophlebitis
- MRI intensity signal changes with time and technique in sinus
- Exposure during surgery

Brain abscess
During initial cerebritis
- Headache and lethargy for 3–5 days, spontaneous recovery
- MRI evidence of localized cerebral edema

During latent period
- Almost impossible to diagnose, even with MRI

During manifest abscess
- Focal neurologic deficit and/or seizure
- MRI evidence of enhancing hyperintense area surrounding a hypointense center

Otitic hydrocephalus
- Headache and lethargy
- Severe papilledema
- No evidence of meningitis
- No evidence of brain abscess on MRI
- Documentation of increased intracranial pressure

MRI, magnetic resonance imaging.

Additionally, petrositis can result in other regions of referred unexplained head pain.

3. The third filter is symptoms and signs of subdural abscess. Characteristically, subdural infection creates both a mass effect and an irritative focus and results in catastrophic rapidly progressive neurologic signs and symptoms. The fact that subdural abscesses are so rarely associated with ear infections and, when present, are so catastrophic tends to reduce the list down to 5.

4. The fourth filter is generalized evidence of increased intracranial pressure, or focal neurologic lesions. Headache and lethargy are early signs of intracranial complications. Papilledema is an obvious sign of an intracranial complication with increased intracranial pressure; however, it may easily go undetected unless the examiner does a funduscopic examination. Focal neurologic signs, seizures, or catastrophic neurologic signs such as coma are obvious signs of intracranial complications. Fever in association with a chronically draining ear is an early sign of intracranial complication or extracranial cellulitis.

Systematic Approach (Tables 138.2, 138.3, and 138.5)

Mastoiditis

Mastoiditis may present in association with a subperiosteal abscess, commonly lateral to the mastoid cortex,

medial to the concha of the pinna, and rarely into the neck through the medial tip cells as in Bezold abscess. It may also present as "masked mastoiditis." The advent of antibiotics has made the diagnosis and definition of mastoiditis more difficult. Classically, the term mastoiditis referred to acute coalescent mastoiditis with subperiosteal abscess lateral to the mastoid cortex occurring 2 weeks after onset of acute suppurative otitis media. The patient would be febrile and, in some cases, toxic; radiographs would demonstrate extensive bone destruction in the mastoid region of pneumatization, characteristically lateral to the sigmoid sinus. Just before extensive subperiosteal abscess formation, marked edema, erythema, and tenderness over the mastoid postauricularly and sagging of the posterosuperior canal wall skin from edema were found. Classically, patients with chronic mastoiditis presented with fetid purulent chronic discharge, boring pain, and occasional radiographic evidence of irregular lytic lesions in the temporal bone lateral to the sigmoid sinus surrounded by hyperostotic areas. Today, the signs and symptoms may be much less obvious; antibiotics may obscure the presentations but may not prevent the complication (9). Persistent or recurrent pain may be the only symptom or sign of "masked" mastoiditis. Computed tomography (CT) has expanded our ability to identify early bone-destructive lesions in the mastoid. However, meningitis, facial paralysis, brain abscess, otitic hydrocephalus, sigmoid sinus thrombophlebitis, and extradural abscess all may occur with little or no CT evidence of bone destruction.

The best diagnostic algorithm is based on the comparison of the expected clinical course and an appreciation that complications progress medially much more often than laterally. A person with acute suppurative otitis media should be expected to respond within 3 to 5 days to appropriate antibiotic therapy; within 2 weeks, the purulent-appearing effusion in the middle ear should convert to a more seromucinous appearance. The ear should clear and aerate within 1 to 3 months without recurrence of symptoms. There should be no posterosuperior canal wall skin edema nor postauricular edema or tenderness and certainly no subperiosteal abscess displacing the pinna inferolaterally.

If there is no response to antibiotics within the first week, mastoiditis should be considered possible. If there is postauricular edema, subperiosteal abscess, or recurrence of pain—even mild—within 2 to 3 weeks after onset of acute suppurative otitis media, mastoiditis should be considered imminent. Risk factors for complications also include a more rapidly aggressive course than expected, younger age, and radiographic evidence of previous significant infections with resultant hyperostosis ("sclerosis").

If these ominous signs appear, myringotomy for culture and sensitivity for aerobes and anaerobes and high-resolution CT of the temporal bone should be done. Appropriate antibiotic therapy for 2 to 3 weeks and close periodic examination, usually on a weekly basis, are necessary until the patient and the mastoid x-ray films have completely reverted to normal. It is not an unusual event for the middle ear to clear with myringotomy and antibiotics and for the mastoid to remain opacified and non–air containing. This condition continues to raise the specter of "masked" mastoiditis behind an obstructed aditus ad antrum or tympanic isthmus. If symptom free, the patient may be followed longer; however, if symptoms, such as deep boring but subtle pain are present, mastoidectomy may be considered. Magnetic resonance imaging (MRI) with gadolinium may be useful to detect early extradural abscess formation and sigmoid sinus thrombophlebitis.

Chronic mastoiditis with osteitis should be suspected when persistent fetid discharge is found despite local and systemic treatment. If the discharge persists despite treatment after 2 weeks, a diagnosis of chronic mastoiditis with osteitis should be presumed. High-resolution CT may be helpful to identify subtleties of osteitic bone destruction, but it is usually disappointing. MRI with gadolinium may identify early deeper complications; however, in most cases, the diagnosis is made clinically, and surgical intervention is appropriate at this point.

Petrositis

Petrositis has become exceptionally rare, but still occurs, even in the classic triad of Gradenigo, that is, retroorbital pain, abducens paralysis, and ipsilateral acute or chronic otitis media. Petrositis may occur even in a nonpneumatized, sclerotic, or diploic petrous apex. Diagnosis of petrositis is made in a similar fashion to that of mastoiditis, with the additional symptom of retroorbital pain and evidence of petrous apex bone distructions. Abducens paralysis is extremely rare and is not necessary to make the diagnosis.

Labyrinthitis

Labyrinthitis characteristically is viral-induced endolabyrinthitis and is not potentially fatal. However, labyrinthitis secondary to middle ear infection can be fatal if suppurative labyrinthitis and, subsequently, meningitis occur. Therefore, each call from the emergency department to see a patient in whom severe vertigo and hearing loss occur simultaneously requires the clinician to determine whether the middle ear is normal. Experimental and human experience with acute and chronic otitis media reveals serous labyrinthitis and endolymphatic hydrops are fairly frequent complications of suppurative middle ear disease. However, suppurative labyrinthitis is extremely rare and potentially fatal. These conditions may occur together or separately. Cholesteatomas may erode the otic capsule, creating perilymph fistulae that may cause mechanical cochlear effects, serous labyrinthitis, and a preformed pathway for acute infection to enter the labyrinth; therefore, vertigo in the presence of a cholesteatoma must be evaluated immediately and very carefully.

Until recently, diagnosis of labyrinthitis was made on clinical grounds. Serous labyrinthitis, in which toxic or metabolic products of bacteria or the host inflammatory response enter the inner ear through the round window membrane or cholesteatoma-induced fistula, results in sensorineural loss and vertigo with nystagmus. However, the degree of loss is not total, and some recovery is possible. Conversely, suppurative labyrinthitis from the entrance of bacteria into the labyrinth through the same route creates similar symptoms but profound losses that never resolve and result in extensive inner ear and spiral ganglia cell loss. Hegarty et al. (10) have found evidence of labyrinthine disease by contrast-enhanced MRI; this technique may prove to be helpful in the future to confirm the presumptive diagnosis of labyrinthitis.

Facial Paralysis

The major diagnostic challenge in facial paralysis from the suppurative ear disease is to identify the possibility of a nerve-destructive lesion versus neuropraxia from toxicity or slight compression and edema. Facial paralysis from acute suppurative otitis media may not be destructive. However, facial paralysis in the presence of a subacute infection, acute coalescent mastoiditis, masked mastoiditis, petrositis, or chronic suppurative otitis media, with or without cholesteatoma, may well be destructive, particularly in the tympanic segment.

The typical topognostic techniques for site-of-lesion identification are useful to confirm the intratemporal site of lesion. Degree-of-lesion techniques, such as the nerve excitability test, the maximum nerve excitability test, electroneurography, and electromyography, are extremely important, although imperfect, tools to identify a nerve-destructive lesion. MRI with gadolinium is useful in identifying neoplastic and inflammatory lesions of the facial nerve but as yet cannot determine the degree of lesion. The most useful tool of all is a detailed careful history of the patient's current illness and past medical history of ear disease with a specific attempt to define the exact pathophysiology that may be involved with each case. It is probably prudent to err on the side of assuming a nerve-destructive lesion when in doubt and plan to explore the nerve.

Cholesteatoma is by far the most common cause of facial paralysis. The lesion characteristically is most common in the tympanic and upper mastoid segments; however, the labyrinthine segment also may be involved in deep petrous cholesteatomas. Degeneration and inflammation are variably present in the localized area of the facial nerve and may be partially or more rarely completely destructive of the facial nerve. Granulation tissue that invades the epineurium is more dangerous than cholesteatoma matrix; granulation tissue may infiltrate between nerve fibers and, if surgically pursued, may result in transection of the nerve.

Extradural Granulation Tissue or Abscess

In our experience and that of others, extradural granulation tissue or abscess can be, and usually is, completely occult preoperatively (2). Even intraoperatively, huge extradural abscesses may be missed unless painstaking care is taken to observe the dura of the middle fossa and posterior fossa, particularly over the sigmoid sinus, through thin bone. It is not necessary to remove the bone completely to see whether the dura is normal or abnormal. If there is any question or if the dura appears abnormal, it is necessary to remove the bone and inspect the dura directly. In every case of operable disease, extradural granulation tissue should be expected.

MRI is proving to be superior to CT in demonstrating intracranial suppurative lesions and may ultimately prove to be able to identify small collections of extradural granulation tissue and abscess. Larger extradural empyemas demonstrate a hypointense rim representing displaced dura adjacent to a hyperintense collection.

Sigmoid Sinus Thrombophlebitis

Lateral or sigmoid sinus thrombophlebitis may be totally asymptomatic or may be associated with the classic intermittently spiking ("picket fence") fever, gross signs of toxemia, torticollis, and septic embolization. The thrombus can rarely propagate into the internal jugular vein and jugular bulb, creating a jugular foramen syndrome or be associated with retrograde thrombosis of cerebral veins, leading to brain abscess and/or infarction (11). Should the vein of Labbé be thrombosed, speech and language deficits might occur; severe neurologic consequences, such as coma or death might follow. Prothrombotic factors, such as elevated levels of lipoprotein apolipoprotein [Lp(a)], antibodies to beta 2-glycoprotein and to cardiolipin, and heterozygosity for factor V Leiden mutation, may predispose patients to sigmoid sinus thrombosis during acute otitis media (12). If the sinus is obstructed, it can create serious degrees of intracranial hypertension. It is associated with overlying granulation tissue or cholesteatoma.

MRI with and without gadolinium has proved to be an exceptionally good diagnostic tool to identify at least major degrees of sigmoid sinus thrombophlebitis by the presence of increased intraluminal signal on all planes with all pulse sequences.

Brain Abscess

Diagnosing a brain abscess may be difficult or impossible, depending on the stage of abscess formation and its clinical presentation. It may present with fever, headache, and seizures but is usually not so obvious. A manifest abscess may present as a seizure, loss of consciousness, or a focal neurologic deficit. The abscess may be associated with increased intracranial pressure.

A brain abscess has four clinical stages. A wide range of excellent CT, MRI, gross, and histologic images may be found through Google, image tab, brain abscess (www.google.com). The first stage is invasion (initial encephalitis), manifested by low-grade fever, drowsiness, or loss of ability to concentrate, and headache associated with a general feeling of malaise. These symptoms are subtle and frequently overlooked and spontaneously resolve after several

days. The second stage, localization (latent or quiescent abscess), is clinically silent, with no symptoms and possibly lasting for weeks. During the third stage, enlargement (manifest abscess), an actual abscess forms in the region of the previous cerebritis and produces focal symptoms of a mass lesion, seizures, or loss of consciousness. In the fourth stage, termination (rupture of the abscess), the abscess ruptures into the ventricle or into the subarachnoid space. This results in a rapidly progressive, frequently fatal, outcome.

CT and MRI with gadolinium easily identify a hypointense center with a hyperintense capsule about a formed abscess. MRI offers additional precision in identifying extraparenchymal (intraventricular or subarachnoid) spread of the abscess. Newer sequences such as diffusion-weighted magnetic resonance imaging (DW-MRI) have proven to be useful in detection and surveillance of an abscess (13,14).

The real dilemma is in having a high enough index of suspicion to obtain an MRI to detect the developing abscess in stages I or II or to detect an asymptomatic manifest abscess in stage III. Again, the most useful tool is a careful, thoughtful history and physical examination with attention to clinical indicators that suggest an impending complication, which can easily include a brain abscess (Table 138.2). If there is any suspicion that a complication may be occurring, an MRI is advised. Because brain abscesses take several weeks to manifest, the examiner should remember that if an MRI was ordered initially, a repeat MRI should be done 2 to 3 weeks later and, occasionally, again 2 to 3 weeks after the second time if the index of suspicion remains high.

Otitic Hydrocephalus

Otitic hydrocephalus is defined as increased intracranial pressure secondary to acute or chronic middle ear infection without evidence of meningitis or subdural or brain abscess. It characteristically presents as headache and lethargy in a patient with an ear infection. MRI easily identifies sigmoid sinus thrombosis with total occlusion. Papilledema is most often present; however, papilledema is not always an adequate predictor of increased intracranial pressure.

Meningitis

Bacterial meningitis with its three clinical and associated cerebrospinal fluid (CSF) stages is fairly easy to diagnose because of its presentation of headache, fever, neck rigidity, and abnormal reflexes such as Kernig (inability to completely extend the leg) or Brudzinski (active flexion of the hip and knee when the neck is passively forward flexed) sign.

The major diagnostic dilemma is to identify the route of spread to the meninges and the organism involved with otologic-associated meningitis. Most cases are in children and occur by hematogenous dissemination of invasive organisms such as *H. influenzae* type B. Pneumococcal meningitis and otitis media are usually considered concomitant manifestations of a systemic infection (15). However, in a child with rapid onset of meningitis within hours of an acute suppurative otitis media in which the offending organism is *S. pneumoniae* or nontypable *H. influenzae* and in which the child has a unilateral or bilateral congenital sensorineural hearing loss and possible vestibular deficit, a Mondini malformation should be suspected. These malformations allow abnormal communication from the middle ear to the CSF through the stapes footplate or round window to the vestibule or cochlea, respectively, and ultimately the internal auditory meatus. They are easily identified on high-resolution CT. Adults similarly presenting with rapid onset of meningitis and acute suppurative otitis media in ears with normal hearing or conductive hearing loss must be suspected of having a communicating meningoencephalocele through the middle fossa or, occasionally, the posterior fossa dura or an occult CSF leak about the geniculate ganglion or through a patent Hyrtl (tympanomeningeal) fissure (16,17).

Adults or children with meningitis associated with chronic suppurative otitis media should be suspected of having extension of infecting organisms directly through the dura. Meningitis has been reported following acute otitis media following stapedectomy and following cochlear implantation (18,19). Additionally, it is possible for bacteria to enter the meninges through the labyrinth by a cholesteatoma-induced fistula.

Subdural Abscess

Subdural abscesses are rare but are much more common with sinusitis than with otitis media. Because of the mass effect and the close proximity to cerebral cortex, marked focal irritative neurologic deficits, seizures, and rapid loss of consciousness may be the presenting symptoms; more subtle presentations can occur.

CT with intravenous contrast can detect these lesions as hypodense (but more dense than CSF) extracerebral collections with an enhancing medial border; however, these may be missed with CT. MRI without contrast may show these as low intensity on T1-weighted images and high intensity on T2-weighted images. However, MRI with intravenous gadolinium (GD-DTPA) is more sensitive to detect these lesions and tends to demarcate the abscess as a rim of enhancement (20).

Bacteriology

The final step in diagnosis in all complications is the identification of the specific organisms involved in both the ear and in the complication (Table 138.4). It is important to remember that cultures from the discharge from the external auditory canal, middle ear, and mastoid and the intracranial complication may differ; therefore, independent and systematic cultures from these various sites, as they become available, are important in guiding antibiotic therapy.

MANAGEMENT

Management of complications of otitis media is the identification of each organism involved in both the ear and other sites with the complication, followed by culture-specific antibiotics and surgery for the ear and the complication (Table 138.6). The primary objectives of treatment are to eradicate the infecting organism, to remove destructive and obstructing granulation tissue, and to promote drainage in both the ear and the site of complication. Initial antibiotics suggested for site of complications are listed in Table 138.6. The patient is promptly admitted to the hospital, and antibiotics are administered parenterally. Mastoidectomy "appropriate for the ear disease," as seen in Table 138.6, refers to the three major categories of surgical approaches to and through the mastoid: intact canal wall technique with facial recess approach to the middle ear; modified radical mastoidectomy in which at least the eustachian tube and usually the complete middle ear are separated from the external environment by a fascia graft; and radical mastoidectomy in which the tympanic membrane, malleus, incus, and posterior and superior osseous canal wall have been removed and not reconstructed. The technique used in a specific case is best left to the experience and judgment of the surgeon involved and the particular nuances of the case.

It is important to remember that unusual diseases, such as Wegener granulomatosis, blastomycosis, tuberculosis, neoplasia, fungi, and histiocytosis X, especially in the immunocompromised patient, can present as bacterial complications. Therefore, laboratory studies and tissue biopsy are more than just routine in the management of these patients.

Mastoiditis

Controversy exists as to whether all cases of acute mastoiditis require surgical intervention. There is evidence that medical treatment alone can result in an appropriate outcome. However, there is compelling evidence derived from the study of complications of suppurative ear disease that more serious or fatal complications can arise from inadequately treated or diagnosed infections, especially if follow-up is inadequately astute. Therefore, it is advised that surgically skilled and experienced otologic surgeons be consulted in these cases. Certainly surgical intervention in cases of chronic mastoiditis is necessary.

Petrositis

Lateral transmastoid, perilabyrinthine approaches to exenterate disease and drain the petrous apex are usually sufficient to resolve the infection. However, if clinical signs and symptoms of persistent infection continue, a middle fossa approach to the petrous apex may be necessary.

TABLE 138.6 ℞ TREATMENT COMPLICATIONS OF OTITIS MEDIA

Initial antibiotics (5,34)

Appropriate initial antibiotics, followed by culture-specific antibiotics for the ear and the complication

Acute (subacute) mastoiditis from acute otitis media
• Vancomycin IV plus ceftriaxone (Rocephin) IV

Mastoiditis from chronic otitis media
• Ciprofloxacin PO with or without clindamycin
• Piperacillin/tazobactam IV (Zosyn)

Meningitis or intracranial complication from acute otitis media (34)
• Ceftriaxone

Meningitis or intracranial complication from chronic mastoiditis (34)
• Cefotaxime

Surgery and other treatment

Acute or subacute mastoiditis
• Large myringotomy
• Mastoidectomy, intact canal wall technique with large facial recess approach to middle ear and removal of middle ear granulations

Chronic mastoiditis
• Tympanoplasty and mastoidectomy, intact canal wall technique, with large facial recess approach to middle ear and removal of middle ear granulations and cholesteatoma, if present
• Tympanoplasty and modified radial mastoidectomy and removal of middle ear granulations and cholesteatoma, if present

Petrositis
• Lateral, transmastoid, perilabyrinthine approaches to the deep petrous infected site
• Middle fossa, extradural approaches, with or without lateral approaches, to otherwise unreachable or recalcitrant deep petrous infected site

Labyrinthitis from acute otitis media
• Myringotomy

Labyrinthitis from subacute or chronic infection
• Mastoidectomy (appropriate for the ear disease and experience of the surgeon)
• Petrosectomy, if necessary
• Repair of labyrinthine fistula, if present

Facial paralysis from acute otitis media
• Myringotomy

Facial paralysis from subacute or chronic infection
• Mastoidectomy (appropriate for the ear disease)
• Exploration of facial nerve to thinned fallopian canal bone and/or to nerve epineurial sheath. DO NOT OPEN NERVE SHEATH, ESPECIALLY PERINEURIUM.
• Petrosectomy, if necessary

Extradural abscess/granulations
• Mastoidectomy (appropriate for the ear disease)
• Exposure of all diseased dura to normal dura
• Removal of pus and excess dural granulations. DO NOT PERFORATE DURA.

Sigmoid sinus thrombophlebitis
• Mastoidectomy (appropriate for disease)
• Exposure of all diseased dura to normal dura
• Removal of excess extradural granulations
• Palpate sinus, extraluminally. Small needle aspiration may be appropriate for further diagnosis. DO NOT PERFORATE MEDIAL DURAL WALL.
• It is not ordinarily necessary to open sinus to remove clot; however, if pus in sinus, it may be necessary to evacuate pus, trying not to establish blood flow
• If demonstrated emboli from sinus (rare), it may be necessary to evacuate septic thrombus and anticoagulate (23)

Otitic hydrocephalus
• Treatment of sigmoid sinus thrombophlebitis
• Lower intracranial hypertension
• Monitor vision carefully

Brain abscess
• Mastoidectomy (appropriate for disease)
• Exposure of all diseased dura to normal dura
• Removal of excess dural granulations
• Evaluation of dural integrity
• Concomitant neurosurgical consultation for management of brain abscess; often antibiotics only

Meningitis from acute otitis media
• Myringotomy
• Repair of Mondini malformation (with intralabyrinthine fascia and cartilage oval window occlusion to hold fascia) or meningoencephalocele (with intracranial fascia and cartilage tegmen defect occlusion to hold fascia), if present (rare)

Meningitis from subacute or chronic infection
• Mastoidectomy (appropriate for disease)
• Exposure of all diseased dura to normal dura
• Removal of excess dural granulations
• Evaluation of dural integrity; repair of dural defect if present (rare)

Subdural abscess from acute otitis media
• Myringotomy
• Neurosurgical consultation for management of subdural abscess

Subdural abscess from subacute or chronic infection
• Mastoidectomy (appropriate for disease)
• Exposure of all diseased dura to normal dura
• Removal of excess dural granulations
• Neurosurgical consultation for management of subdural abscess

IV, intravenous; PO, by mouth.

Labyrinthitis

The treatment of labyrinthitis from acute otitis media is focused on clearing the middle ear infection as rapidly as possible with antibiotics and with myringotomy. Labyrinthitis from subacute or chronic infection requires exenteration of middle ear and mastoid disease. Cholesteatoma matrix over fistulae of the semicircular canals may be removed if extreme care is taken not to tear the membranous labyrinth. It should be noted that deep fistulae or those into the cochlea may not result in a good outcome and may destroy the ear if the cholesteatoma matrix is removed. Leaving a small piece of matrix on the fistula and returning at a later date in a sterile ear, or marsupializing the area, may be a more appropriate way of managing these difficult cases. However, hearing deterioration still may occur. It is prudent to cover these patients prophylactically with antibiotics in an attempt to avoid suppurative labyrinthitis and meningitis.

Facial Paralysis

Treatment of facial paralysis from acute otitis media is directed at clearing the middle ear infection as rapidly as possible with antibiotics and myringotomy. Usually more extensive treatment is not necessary, unless the infection persists or there is evidence of neural degeneration.

In most cases of subacute or chronic infection, particularly with evidence of neural degeneration, surgical intervention is necessary. Early intervention is important for a good outcome (21). The purpose of the surgery is to clear the middle ear and mastoid infection as rapidly as possible and to remove granulations near the facial nerve. To do this, thinning the fallopian canal bone to a point where the sheath may be inspected through thin bone is important. If the sheath is involved with cholesteatoma or granulation tissue, careful removal of this cholesteatoma matrix or granulation tissue is worthwhile. It should be emphasized that removing granulation tissue, which can be interspersed among nerve fibers, can easily cause surgical destruction of the complete cross-section of the nerve. To avoid this, resection deeper than the plane of the most lateral surface of the nerve is not recommended. Because the nerve sheath, particularly the perineurium, is a barrier to infection and because neural tissue, per se, lacks resistance to infection, it is very important not to incise the sheath of the nerve.

Extradural Abscess or Granulation Tissue

Management of extradural granulation tissue and abscess begins with discovery. It depends on a careful inspection of the dura of the tegmen tympani, tegmen mastoideum, sigmoid sinus, and posterior fossa bone medial to Trautmann triangle (22). The dura may be properly inspected by thinning the bone carefully; the bone does not need to be removed to identify normal or abnormal dura. However, it is imperative to extend the mastoidectomy to these limits; simply sculpturing the bone along the plane of the tegmen and sigmoid sinus is not satisfactory. If the dura appears normal in these areas, no additional work is necessary. If the dura is abnormal, the bone should be removed over the abnormal dura until normal dura is encountered. If an abscess is encountered, exposure satisfactorily drains the abscess. Excess granulation tissue should be removed with a blunt instrument, scraping parallel with the plane of the dura. Care must be taken not to perforate the dura; some granulation tissue will necessarily be left. No further surgical treatment is necessary.

Sigmoid Sinus Thrombophlebitis

The treatment of sigmoid sinus thrombophlebitis, partially obstructive or totally obstructive, is predominantly to expose diseased dura and remove excess granulation tissue. If otitic hydrocephalus is present from a totally obstructed, inflamed sigmoid sinus, the treatment additionally involves lowering intracranial hypertension and monitoring vision carefully (discussed later in the section on otitic hydrocephalus). The presence of a septic thrombus, or one that releases septic or aseptic emboli, is unusual. In these situations, carefully aspirating or opening the sigmoid sinus and evacuating the septic and friable thrombus may be appropriate; care must be taken not to violate the medial dural sinus wall. If bleeding from the proximal sigmoid sinus occurs, it can usually be controlled by extradural compression of the sinus with Surgicel placed between the bone of the sigmoid sulcus and the most lateral aspect of the dural sinus. Ligation of the internal jugular vein to avoid further embolization of tissue or material used to control surgical bleeding might be required. Intraluminal Surgicel can be sparingly used if necessary, but only after ligation of the internal jugular vein has been performed; however, it may increase sepsis in severely infected cases. Ligation or hemostatic stapling of the sinus may be done but usually results in CSF egress from the puncture holes, which is usually inadvisable in infected cases. The use of heparin may be helpful (23).

Brain Abscess

Management of brain abscess requires surgical intervention in the ear and treatment of the brain abscess, with neurosurgical consultation. Surgical treatment of the brain abscess, such as aspiration, may occur simultaneously with the surgical approach to the ear, or it may precede the ear surgery if the intracranial problem is of such severity that it would best be done first. Increased intracranial pressure may occur. In these cases, it is probably prudent to lower the intracranial pressure and aspirate the abscess before surgical approach to the ear. Intravenous antibiotics are the predominant treatment of brain abscess and are occasionally recommended as the exclusive treatment. However, shorter hospital stays, better isolation of the offending organisms, and better early and long-term results may be obtained by antibiotics and a surgical approach to the abscess.

Surgical approaches to the abscess include aspiration, open drainage, and excision. It is generally thought that aspiration is satisfactory, except in cases in which air is found within the intracranial abscess; air within the abscess is indicative of a direct extension from a pneumatized space to the abscess. In cases of direct extension, CT-guided, percutaneous, transmastoid drainage of the abscess has been effective. Epilepsy and epileptic foci may occur and seem to be more frequent after excision of the abscess; thus, anticonvulsant prophylaxis may be appropriately considered.

Otitic Hydrocephalus

Treatment of otitic hydrocephalus requires mastoidectomy appropriate for the disease, exposure of all diseased dura to normal dura, and removal of excess extradural granulation tissue. A gentle insertion of a hypodermic syringe or a small opening of the sinus may be advisable to identify an intraluminal septic thrombus or abscess. This thrombus, however, is often identifiable from the clinical picture of a high, spiking, intermittent fever, although a masked abscess is possible. Usually, the thrombus is highly organized and fibrotic. It is not advisable to attempt to do a thrombectomy, except enough to evaluate an abscess, because of the potential of releasing emboli and rupturing the sinus intracranially. If intraluminal partial thrombectomy is necessary, the internal jugular vein must be ligated. Generally, managing the mastoid is all that is required surgically. Management of otitic hydrocephalus extends for months beyond the initial surgical approach to the sinus. It is designed to medically lower intracranial hypertension and monitor the patient's condition carefully for progressive blindness and brain herniation; a ventricular shunt may be required.

Initial treatment with acetazolamide, prednisone, and repeated lumbar punctures may not satisfactorily lower the intracranial hypertension. Furosemide and mannitol tend to act synergistically, result in more rapid lowering of intracranial pressure, and remain in effect for a longer period of time than either agent used alone. The combined use of mannitol and intermittent withdrawal of CSF fluid also creates some synergism. However, the effect of mannitol may last for only about 4 hours, and the effect of CSF withdrawal may lower the pressure for only about 1 hour. High-dose barbiturates have been found to effectively lower resistant intracranial hypertension (24). Percutaneous lumboperitoneal shunts are effective on a long-term basis for reducing intracranial hypertension. Occasionally, all these measures, including lumboperitoneal shunting, fail to reverse progressive visual deterioration; in these cases, fenestration of the optic nerve sheath has proved to be effective (25). In rare situations, a venous bypass from one lateral sinus to the jugular vein might prove to be effective (26).

Monitoring visual change in these patients includes monitoring not only visual acuity but visual fields. Occasionally, visual field reduction precedes visual acuity change.

Meningitis from Acute Otitis Media

Intravenous antibiotics and myringotomy are the mainstays of treatment for acute bacterial meningitis associated with acute otitis media. However, in instances in which a Mondini malformation or a spontaneous meningoencephalocele is diagnosed, repair of the Mondini malformation or meningoencephalocele is necessary toward the end of the meningitis treatment. It is probably prudent to extend the treatment a little longer to cover the perioperative period.

Despite effective antibiotic treatment, about one third of meningitis survivors suffer neurologic sequelae such as behavioral disorders, mental retardation, and deafness,

which are thought to be caused by inflammatory mediators such as the cytokines. Dexamethasone has recently been shown to reduce these inflammatory sequelae and not to interfere with antibiotic treatment (27).

Meningitis from Subacute or Chronic Mastoiditis

In meningitis from subacute or chronic mastoiditis, a direct extension into the meninges is more often the case; thus, resistant gram-negative and anaerobic organisms are encountered. Third-generation cephalosporins, especially intravenous ceftriaxone (Rocephin) and cefotaxime (Claforan), penetrate the blood–brain barrier well and are good initial choices (5,28).

Surgically, it is important to exenterate the ear disease carefully, expose all diseased dura, and remove excess dural granulation tissue. It is also imperative to carefully inspect the dura that is diseased for perforation and to evacuate any immediately associated abscesses on either side of the dura. The timing and planning of these operations, concomitantly or sequentially, immediately or delayed, necessarily must be done by the otologic surgeon and neurosurgeon. Small dural repairs, even in the face of infection, can easily be done through the middle ear and mastoid during initial surgery.

Subdural Abscess

The management of subdural abscess from acute otitis media consists in clearing the ear infection as rapidly as possible with intravenous antibiotics and myringotomy and treating the subdural abscess. Subdural empyemas from subacute or chronic ear infections require mastoidectomy, appropriate for the disease, and careful exploration on the dura with removal of excess granulation tissue. Treatment of subdural abscess usually requires drainage from separate burr holes or craniotomy and definitely the institution of long-term parenteral antibiotics.

COMPLICATIONS OF TREATMENT

Table 138.7 summarizes possible complications of treatment.

Complications of Inadequate Antibiotics or Drainage

Complications arising from treatment are predominantly those of omission, inadequate treatment, or missed diagnoses. The resulting complications can be one or more of the 10 complications of suppurative ear disease. It is important to remember that undertreated complications are more likely to extend medially into the intracranial cavity than externally.

| TABLE 138.7 | | COMPLICATIONS TREATMENT |

Inadequate treatment or failure to treat aggressively

Mastoiditis
- Subperiosteal abscess
- Osteitis/osteomyelitis of skull
- Petrositis
- Facial paralysis
- All intracranial complications

Petrositis
- Osteitis/osteomyelitis of skull
- Carotid rupture
- Facial paralysis
- All intracranial complications

Labyrinthitis
- Progressive sensorineural hearing loss
- Delayed endolymphatic hydrops
- Benign paroxysmal positional vertigo
- Suppurative labyrinthitis
- Meningitis
- Facial paralysis

Facial paralysis
- Permanent destruction of facial nerve
- Labyrinthine fistula

Extradural granulation and/or abscess
- All intracranial complications

Sigmoid sinus thrombophlebitis
- Propagation of thrombus to sagittal sinus and/or internal jugular vein
- Pulmonary emboli
- Brain abscess
- Otitic hydrocephalus

Brain abscess
- Meningitis
- Ventriculitis
- Brain herniation
- Diffuse cerebritis/multiple abscesses
- Seizure disorder
- Focal neurologic deficits
- Death

Otic hydrocephalus
- Blindness
- Brain herniation
- Death

Meningitis
- Brain abscess
- Subdural abscess
- Retardation
- Deafness
- Multiple neurologic deficits
- Death

Subdural abscess
- Seizures
- Coma
- Local neurologic deficits
- Meningitis
- Death

Complications of surgical exenteration and drainage

During myringotomy
- Canal skin laceration
- Excessive laceration of tympanic membranes
- Fracture of ossicles
- Laceration of jugular bulb
- Laceration of internal carotid artery
- Oval or round window traumatic fistula
- Facial nerve laceration
- Meningitis

During mastoidectomy
- Wound infection
- Dural perforation
- Cerebrospinal otorrhea or rhinorrhea
- Brain herniation
- Laceration of sigmoid sinus
- Facial nerve contusion or laceration
- Ossicular disruption
- Sensorineural hearing loss
- Labyrinthine fistula
- Excessive blood loss

During petrosectomy
- Same as mastoidectomy, with increased risk
- Laceration of internal carotid artery
- Temporal lobe infarction

During facial nerve exploration
- Same as mastoidectomy, with increased risk
- Total destruction of facial nerve

During management of labyrinthine fistula by cholesteatoma
- Deterioration of inner ear if matrix remains
- Sudden loss of inner ear function during matrix removal
- Meningitis

During labyrinthectomy
- Certain loss of hearing and unilateral balance function
- Same as mastoidectomy, with increased risk, especially facial nerve injury

During lumbar puncture
- Brain herniation
- Spinal headache
- Lower extremity neural deficit
- Meningitis

During removal of dural granulation tissue
- Cerebrospinal otorrhea
- Meningitis

During sigmoid sinus exploration
- Hemorrhage externally
- Hemorrhage into posterior fossa
- Cardiac or pulmonary emboli
- Air emboli

During aspiration of brain abscess
- Meningitis
- Ventriculitis
- Cerebritis
- Intracerebral hemorrhage

During subdural drainage
- Meningitis
- Cerebral contusion or infarction

Complications of Surgery

The second group of complications of treatment are those secondary to surgical exenteration and drainage procedures (Table 138.7). All the complications that may arise from middle ear and mastoid surgery may certainly occur in addition when treating these complications. However, because of the extensive nature of the disease, which includes excessive granulation tissue and unusual patterns of bone erosion, the surgical risks are increased both to the structures within the temporal bone and to those within the cranium. A few of these complications deserve special mention.

Excessive Blood Loss

Excessive blood loss, particularly in children, can be an unexpected complication from mastoidectomy. The granulation tissue can be extremely vascular in acute or subacute mastoiditis, and 250 to 300 mL of blood can be lost rapidly during the course of mastoidectomy. This blood loss continues until all the granulation tissue is removed. If the anatomy, or the skill of the operator, hinders rapid mastoidectomy and if excessive blood loss is still occurring, it is probably most prudent to stop the operation at that point and return at a later date after the antibiotics have had a longer period during which to work.

Brain Herniation

Brain herniation deserves special mention, both as a potential complication of disease or as a complication of diagnostic or therapeutic intervention. It is well known that lumbar puncture in the presence of elevated intracranial pressure, particularly with evidence of a mass lesion, can result in respiratory arrest, cervical cord compression, transtentorial herniation with cerebral and brainstem compression, and infarction. Papilledema is not always an adequate predictor of dangerous intracranial hypertension or a possible complication from lumbar puncture. Several important landmarks seen on CT or MRI that help identify patients at risk for brain herniation are lateral shift of midline structures, loss of suprachiasmatic and basilar cisterns, obliteration of the fourth ventricle, and obliteration of the superior cerebellar and quadrigeminal plate cisterns with sparing of the ambient cistern. Immediate neurosurgical attendance during any necessary lumbar puncture in these cases is prudent.

Brain herniation is diagnosed by MRI or CT, demonstrating such things as herniation of the cerebellar tonsils into the foramen magnum, herniation of the temporal lobe, uncus herniation filling the homolateral perimesencephalic cistern, and the disappearance of the perimesencephalic cistern. Auditory brainstem responses and particularly somatosensory evoked potentials have also been found to be sensitive to increased intracranial pressure; severe brain injury may occur if intracranial pressure exceeds 30 mm Hg, which requires decompression within 1.5 hours (29). Some of the effective measures to reduce in-

tracranial hypertension are discussed under the section on management of otitic hydrocephalus earlier in this chapter.

Pulmonary Emboli

Pulmonary emboli, a very rare potential complication of sigmoid sinus thrombophlebitis, may manifest suddenly and catastrophically with cardiovascular and respiratory collapse; on the other hand, onset may be subtle. Ventilation-perfusion scanning using radioisotope-labeled gases has become the standard of early diagnosis. Pulmonary angiography is reserved for confirmation. Anticoagulation is appropriate. Thrombolysis is not usually recommended (30).

Air Embolism

Air embolism is possible during manipulation of the sigmoid sinus. Air embolism during surgery can result in coma and seizures, a variety of decerebrate conditions, cortical blindness, and cardiovascular and pulmonary collapse with significant lung injury. Air embolism creates sudden right heart failure, which may intraoperatively respond to occluding the venous bleeding, turning the patient onto the left side, placing the table in Trendelenburg, aspirating air from the central venous catheter, flooding the wound with saline, giving 100% oxygen and stopping nitrous oxide administration, possibly administering dobutamine or ephedrine, and providing supportive measures for hypotension and arrhythmias (31). The mainstay of longer treatment is hyperbaric oxygen administered as rapidly as possible.

EMERGENCIES

Table 138.8 summarizes emergencies that can arise in suppurative ear disease.

Definition

All the complications of suppurative ear disease represent emergencies. However, a few emergencies require special mention. In these conditions, immediate assessment or treatment is required to avoid or minimize significant morbidity or mortality. These may be considered true emergencies.

Emergent Presentation of Disease

Vertigo and Nystagmus with Ear Infection

The patient presenting with acute vertigo, nystagmus, and associated decrease in hearing must be evaluated immediately for the presence or absence of middle ear or mastoid infection. If such infection is present or if a cholesteatoma is present, there is an immediate potential for suppurative labyrinthitis followed by meningitis within minutes to hours. It is not possible to initially separate serous

2054 Section IX: Otology

TABLE 138.8	✚ EMERGENCIES
SUPPURATIVE EAR DISEASE	

Vertigo and nystagmus with ear infection
- Labyrinthitis

Facial paralysis with ear infection
Headache and lethargy/coma
- Brain abscess
- Otitic hydrocephalus
- Meningitis
- Subdural abscess
- Brain herniation with increased intracranial pressure

Seizure
- Brain abscess
- Meningitis
- Subdural abscess

Focal neurologic deficits
- Brain abscess
- Subdural abscess

Meningismus
- Meningitis
- Ventriculitis
- Subdural abscess

Sudden cardiovascular collapse
- Pulmonary embolus
- Air embolus

Sudden catastrophic bleeding
- Carotid rupture (red, pulsatile)
- Sigmoid or jugular (darker, nonpulsatile)

Reduction of visual fields or acuity
- Otic hydrocephalus

labyrinthitis from suppurative labyrinthitis, and it is not possible to presuppose with confidence that suppurative labyrinthitis will not occur. Affected patients should be immediately admitted to the hospital and placed on appropriate antibiotic therapy and local care to the ear as previously mentioned. As the condition resolves, the patient may be allowed to leave the hospital on continued therapy, if necessary.

Facial Paralysis with Ear Infection
Patients presenting with lower motoneuron facial paralysis associated with an acutely or chronically infected ear must be assessed immediately for a neural destructive lesion. These patients are best treated initially in the hospital with intravenous antibiotics and surgery, if appropriate. Except for myringotomy, which should be done immediately in the presence of an acute suppuration, mastoidectomy and additional surgical interventions are best delayed until appropriate levels of antibiotics are reached.

Headache and Lethargy/Coma
Patients in coma are immediately recognized as being in an emergent condition, regardless of the cause. However, patients with ear infections complaining of headache or lethargy at presentation or in the recent past must be evaluated immediately for brain abscess, otitic hydrocephalus, meningitis, and subdural abscess.

Seizure
A patient presenting with seizure after a recent, past, or current acute or chronic ear infection is suspected of having a brain abscess. In many cases, the ear infection will have resolved, but a careful history may reveal a protracted unusual course during the resolution. Occult or quiescent cholesteatomas are not infrequent in this group of patients.

Focal Neurologic Deficits
All patients presenting with focal neurologic deficits require immediate and careful evaluation. Expert evaluation of the ears and paranasal sinuses is imperative to avoid delayed diagnosis of subtle or occult infections capable of producing brain abscesses and subdural abscesses that may lead to these deficits.

Meningismus
Meningismus is an obvious sign of meningeal irritation and an obvious emergency. Meningitis is the most common cause of meningismus; however, ventriculitis from a ruptured brain abscess or the presence of a subdural abscess may present in this fashion. Again, a careful and expert history and physical examination of the ears and paranasal sinuses are necessary. Patients with meningismus should be immediately admitted to the hospital for further evaluation and treatment.

Emergencies During Treatment
Brain herniation, air embolus, and thromboembolus are conditions of greatest urgency and have already been discussed in detail in the section on complications.

Carotid Rupture
Rupture of the internal carotid artery into a radical mastoid cavity or into the middle ear behind an intact drum is a rare and extremely urgent condition, which is obvious to all present. However, identification of a patient inclined to carotid rupture through the ear is much more subtle. Candidates for carotid rupture are those in whom the internal carotid artery, just anterior to the cochlea, is exposed to the atmosphere or persistent infection as a result of destruction, removal of the osseous carotid canal by surgical intervention, or disease, particularly osteoradionecrosis with infection, malignancy, or necrotizing "malignant" external otitis. Occasionally, it is necessary to remove a portion of the carotid canal to completely remove disease. Next, it is imperative to cover the carotid with tissue such as fat, fascia, or a myocutaneous flap.

Rupture of the carotid can be controlled with finger pressure until the definitive control of the area by balloon embolization or ligation above and below the perforation. After this, healthy viable tissue should be placed over the rupture site and carotid.

Reduction of Visual Fields or Acuity

Patients with intracranial complications, particularly obstructive thrombophlebitis of the sigmoid sinus, may present with increased intracranial pressure or may develop increased pressure during evaluation and treatment. Reduction of visual fields or visual acuity is truly an emergency. The treatment has been discussed in the section on management of otitic hydrocephalus. The point of emphasis here, however, is that increased intracranial pressure may occur during treatment or, if present initially, may persist for months with fluctuations despite treatment. Therefore, careful monitoring of the visual fields and visual acuity is necessary throughout the evaluation and management course until the complication has completely resolved.

FUTURE OPPORTUNITIES

The area of intracranial and intratemporal complications is wide open for systematic investigation. Very little is known about the pathophysiology of these complications. The answer may lie with the nature of invasive organisms and the pathogenic synergism of anaerobic and microaerophilic microbes and biofilm formation. The host response surely plays a role; this is most obvious with immunocompromised persons. However, less obvious is the differential ability of some persons to generate excessive amounts of obstructive and destructive granulation tissue.

The rarity of many of these conditions makes investigation of the complication in the total organism extremely difficult; however, important questions that relate to these complications and are germane to common problems, such as otitis media with effusion or chronic otitis media with perforation, can be asked. What are the conditions under which the surface epithelium is ulcerated? What mediators differentially incite granulation tissue? What is synergistic with these mediators? What turns them off after they have begun? How do organisms move from one tissue plane to another? An excellent example of basic science investigation leading to a progressive understanding of the pathophysiology of cholesteatoma is the life work of Chole (32).

HIGHLIGHTS

- There are 10 basic complications of suppurative ear disease, 4 intratemporal and 6 intracranial.
- Clinical signs of impending complications are the persistence or recurrence of acute infection within 2 weeks of treatment or the persistence of fetid discharge despite treatment.

- Persistent low-intensity pain of 1 week's duration during specific antibiotic treatment for suppurative otitis media strongly suggests the diagnosis of "masked mastoiditis."
- Retroorbital pain during ear infection, a key sign of petrositis, often is not voluntarily shared; it must be specifically elicited from the history.
- Extradural granulation tissue over the sigmoid sinus is predictable in mastoiditis and is the key to three additional intracranial complications (sigmoid sinus thrombophlebitis, brain abscess, otitic hydrocephalus).
- Anaerobes are frequently found in masked mastoiditis or mastoiditis with subperiosteal abscess and are not found in acute otitis media.
- The organism most frequently causing meningitis, associated with acute suppurative otitis media, is *Streptococcus pneumoniae*.
- *Streptococcus faecalis*, *Proteus* sp., and *Bacteroides fragilis* are most frequently found in brain abscesses.
- *Pseudomonas aeruginosa*, *Bacteroides* sp., and anaerobic streptococci are most commonly found in association with cholesteatoma.
- The absence of, or resolution of, a subperiosteal abscess may allow a serious intracranial complication to develop because of an unrecognized and undertreated mastoiditis.
- Proper surgical care of most intracranial and intratemporal complications requires visualization through thin bone or actual exposure of the dura of the middle fossa and sigmoid sinus. Failure to do this can result in misdiagnosis and undertreatment of serious intracranial complications.
- A call to see a patient with peripheral vertigo, nystagmus, and hearing loss is a true emergency until it is established that the middle ear is normal.

REFERENCES

1. Neely JG. Facial nerve and intracranial complications of otitis media. In: Jackler RK, Brackmann DE, eds. *Neurotology*, 2nd ed. Philadelphia: Elsevier, Mosby, 2005:912–925.
2. Greenberg J, Manolidis S. High incidence of complications encountered in chronic otitis media surgery in a U.S. metropolitan public hospital. *Otolaryngol Head Neck Surg* 2001;125:623–627.
3. Relman D, Falkow S. A molecular perspective of microbial pathogenicity. In: Mandell G, Bennett J, Dolin R, eds. *Mandell, Douglas, and Bennett's principles and practice of infectious disease*, Vol. 1, 5th ed. Philadelphia: Churchill Livingstone, 2000:2–12.
4. Finegold S. Anaerobic bacteria: general concepts. In: Mandell G, Bennett J, Dolin R, eds. *Mandell, Douglas, and Bennett's principles and practice of infectious disease*, Vol. 2. Philadelphia: Churchill Livingstone, 2000:2518–2575.
5. Fairbanks DN. *Antimicrobial therapy in otolaryngology-head and neck surgery*, 11th ed. Alexandria, VA: American Academy of Otolaryngology-Head and Neck Surgery Foundation, 2003.
6. Bluestone CD. Clinical course, complications and sequelae of acute otitis media. *Pediatr Infect Dis J* 2000;19(5):S37–S46.
7. Agarwal A, Lowry P, Isaacson G. Natural history of sigmoid sinus thrombosis. *Ann Otol Rhinol Laryngol* 2003;112:191–194.
8. Shiao A-S, Guo Y-C, Hsieh S-T, Tsai T-L. Bacteriology of medically refractory acute otitis media in children: a 9-year retrospective study. *Int J Pediatr Otorhinolaryngol* 2004;68:759–765.
9. Luntz M, Brodsky A, Nusem S, et al. Acute mastoiditis—the antibiotic era: a multicenter study. *Int J Pediatr Otorhinolaryngol* 2001;57:1–9.

10. Hegarty J, Patel S, Fischbein N, et al. The value of enhanced magnetic resonance imaging in the evaluation of endocochlear disease. *Laryngoscope* 2002;112:8–17.

11. Ozer E, Sivasli E, Bayazit YA, et al. Otogenic cerebral venous infarction: a rare complication of acute otitis media. *Int J Pediatr Otorhinolaryngol* 2003;67:1019–1021.

12. Kornreich L, Yaniv I, Tamary H. Prothrombotic factors in children with otitis media and sinus thrombosis. *Laryngoscope* 2004;114:90–95.

13. Mikami T, Saito K, Kato T, et al. Detection and characterization of the evolution of cerebral abscesses with diffusion-weighted magnetic resonance imaging—two case reports. *Neurol Med Chir (Tokyo)* 2002;42(2):86–90.

14. Leuthardt E, Wippold FN, Oswood M, Rich K. Diffusion-weighted MR imaging in the preoperative assessment of brain abscesses. *Surg Neurol* 2002;58:395–402.

15. Rasmussen N, Johnsen N, Bohr V. Otologic sequelae after pneumococcal meningitis: a survey of 164 consecutive cases with a follow-up of 94 survivors. *Laryngoscope* 1991;101:876–882.

16. Neely JG. Classification of spontaneous cerebrospinal fluid middle ear effusion: review of 49 cases. *Otolaryngol Head Neck Surg* 1985;93:625–634.

17. Gulya AJ, Schuknecht HF. *Anatomy of the temporal bone with surgical implications,* 2nd ed. New York: Parthenon Publishing Group, 1995.

18. Arnold W, Bredberg G, Gstottner W, et al. Meningitis following cochlear implantation: pathomechanisms, clinical symptoms, conservative and surgical treatments. *ORL J Otorhinolaryngol Relat Spec* 2002;64:382–389.

19. Nielsen T, Thomsen J. Meningitis following stapedotomy: a rare and early complication. *J Laryngol Otol* 2000;114:781–783.

20. Komori H, Takagishi T, Otaki E, et al. The efficacy of MR imaging in subdural empyema. *Brain Dev* 1992;14:123–125.

21. Harker L, Pignatari S. Facial nerve paralysis secondary to chronic otitis media without cholesteatoma. *Am J Otol* 1992;13:372–374.

22. Glasscock ME, Shambaugh GE, Johnson GD. *Surgery of the ear,* 4th ed. Philadelphia: WB Saunders, 1990.

23. Lin D, Reeck J, Murr A. Internal jugular vein thrombosis and deep neck infection from intravenous drug use: management strategy. *Laryngoscope* 2004;114:56–60.

24. Wilberger J, Cantella D. High-dose barbiturates for intracranial pressure control. *New Horiz* 1995;3:469–473.

25. Friedman D, Jacobson D. Idiopathic intracranial hypertension. *J Neuroophthalmol* 2004;24(2):138–145.

26. Sekhar L, Tzortzidis F, Bejjani G, et al. Saphenous vein graft bypass of the sigmoid sinus and jugular bulb during the removal of glomus jugulare tumors. Report of two cases. *J Neurosurg* 1997;86:1036–1041.

27. Lutsar I, Friedland I, Jafri H, et al. Factors influencing the anti-inflammatory effect of dexamethasone therapy in experimental pneumococcal meningitis. *J Antimicrob Chemother* 2003;52:651–655.

28. Singh J, Burr B, Stringham D, et al. Commonly used antibacterial and antifungal agents for hospitalised paediatric patients: implications for therapy with an emphasis on clinical pharmacokinetics. *Paediatr Drugs* 2001;3:733–761.

29. Kawahara N, Sasaki M, Mii K, et al. Reversibility of cerebral function assessed by somatosensory evoked potentials and its relation to intracranial pressure—report of six cases with severe head injury. *Neurol Med Chir (Tokyo)* 1991;31:264–271.

30. Buller H, Agnelli G, Hull R, et al. Antithrombotic therapy for venous thromboembolic disease: the Seventh ACCP Conference on Antithrombotic and Thrombolytic Therapy. *Chest* 2004;126[3 Suppl]:401S–428S.

31. Archer D, Pash M, MacRae M. Successful management of venous air embolism with inotropic support. *Can J Anaesth* 2001;48:204–208.

32. Chole R, Faddis B. Evidence for microbial biofilms in cholesteatomas. *Arch Otolaryngol Head Neck Surg* 2002;128:1129–1133.

Middle Ear and Temporal Bone Trauma

139

Rodney Diaz   Hilary A. Brodie

Temporal bone trauma can result in significant morbidity and, rarely, mortality. The temporal bone houses or encapsulates many important structures, all of which are at risk of injury with trauma to the temporal bone: These include the facial nerve, vestibulocochlear nerve, cochlea and labyrinth, ossicular chain, tympanic membrane, external auditory canal, temporomandibular joint, lower cranial nerves, jugular vein, and carotid artery. Damage to each anatomic structure can lead to distinctive long- and short-term sequelae.

Adjacent intracranial structures such as the temporal lobe and meninges, abducens nerve, and brainstem may also be injured with temporal bone fracture. Fracture of the temporal bone can expose intracranial contents to the external world, resulting in cerebrospinal fluid (CSF) fistula, meningitis, and brain herniation.

In addition to inducing neurotologic manifestations by direct injury to these structures, temporal bone fractures can have associated intracranial complications such as epidural or subdural hematomas, intraparenchymal contusion or hemorrhage, cerebral edema, posttraumatic encephalopathy, and elevated intracranial pressure. Neurotologic symptoms can also result from shearing strain within the brain tissue with disruption of vessels, axons, dendrites, and synapses (1).

EPIDEMIOLOGY

Injury to the lateral skull has increased with the advent of modern technology: The leading cause of temporal bone fracture is involvement in motor vehicle accidents (2). In the past, 75% of motor vehicle accidents resulted in a head injury. The increased use of seatbelts and the advent of frontal and side curtain airbags may, however, alter these statistics in the future. When the head trauma is of sufficient magnitude to fracture the skull, 14% to 22% of those injured sustain a temporal bone fracture (3,4). In the largest series of temporal bone fractures reported to date, 31% of the temporal bone fractures in the general population resulted from motor vehicle accidents (2). Assault was the second most common cause, followed by falls and motorcycle accidents. Pedestrian injuries, bicycle accidents, gunshot wounds, all terrain vehicle accidents, sports injuries, and miscellaneous injuries accounted for a quarter of all cases (2) (Fig. 139.1). The most common injury etiology in temporal bone fractures specific to the pediatric population is equally divided between motor vehicle accidents and falls (between 30% to 60% each) (5–9).

Temporal bone fractures are reported to occur across all age groups with more than 70% of fractures occurring in second, third, and fourth decades of life (2). These fractures occur predominantly in males, with a 3:1 to 4:1 ratio of males to females affected (2,10). The predisposition to temporal bone fractures in males is attributed not to an inherent structural weakness of the male skull versus the female skull but rather to biased involvement of males in many of the above at-risk activities. This is evidenced by the fact that head injuries in general also follow a 4:1 male to female ratio (10).

In a prospective study of 350 consecutive patients treated for head trauma, 10% were found to have temporal

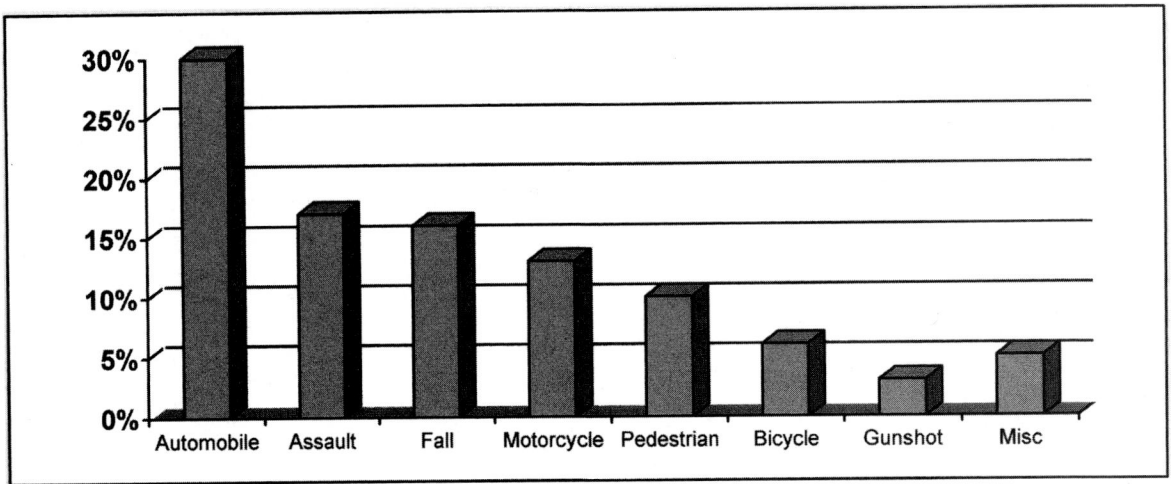

Figure 139.1   Cause of injury.

bone fractures on radiographic evaluation using helical computed tomography (CT), whereas only 6% manifested clinical signs of temporal bone fracture on primary evaluation (10). Large retrospective reviews at Level I trauma centers have found an incidence of temporal bone fracture in 2% to 4% of consecutive head injury patients (11,12).

Eight percent to 29% of patients with temporal bone fractures sustain them bilaterally (2,10,13,14).

PATHOPHYSIOLOGY

The temporal bones are pyramidal structures in the thick bone of the skull base and consequently require a great force to fracture. Early studies of static loading of the lateral skull estimated fracture thresholds of 300 to 800 kg (15). More recent dynamic loading studies have estimated the force of lateral impact required to fracture the temporal bones of fresh cadavers at 6,000 to 8,000 N, or approximately 1,300 to 1,800 lb (16,17). Comparison of data from static versus dynamic loading experiments indicates an increase in force tolerance by a factor of two under dynamic loading (18). Such fractures typically take the path of least resistance, which is along structurally weakened points such as the various foramina perforating the skull base.

Sixty percent of temporal bone fractures are categorized as open fractures presenting with bloody otorrhea, brain herniation, or CSF draining from the ear canal, eustachian tube, or penetrating wound site (2). These patients are at greater risk for meningitis than those without evidence of an intracranial connection. In addition, those patients with fractures traversing the otic capsule are at even still greater risk of meningitis, sometimes delayed for years or decades, due to an inability of the otic capsule enchondral bone to remodel and heal (19–21). Pollak et al. (20) reported a 51-year-old man who died of meningitis who had suffered an otic capsule disrupting fracture in childhood.

The histopathology of his temporal bone revealed pus in the middle ear extending through an unhealed fracture line across the otic capsule. The fracture line contained a loose fibrous tissue. Membranous bone, such as that along the tegmen, has the capability to form callous and heal, whereas the enchondral bone of the otic capsule does not. Fractures through the otic capsule will generally only partially fill with fibrous tissue, although the surface may potentially seal with periosteal bone reaction (20) (Fig. 139.2).

Trauma to the temporal bone often results in one or more neurotologic complications, depending on the severity of injury and type of fracture, and can vary between adult and pediatric populations. Table 139.1 summarizes incidence of common complications of temporal bone fractures in the general and pediatric populations (2,6).

CLASSIFICATION

Temporal bone fractures have traditionally been divided into transverse and longitudinal fractures, based on the relationship of the fracture line to the axis of the petrous ridge (11,22,23). Some authors argue that the majority of fractures are actually oblique as opposed to longitudinal and/or are quite frequently mixed (24,25). This anatomic classification scheme is being replaced with a new structural scheme classifying fractures by whether they disrupt or spare the otic capsule, the bone housing the cochlea and semicircular canals (2,26,27) (Figs. 139.3, 139.4, and 139.5).

Fractures that spare the otic capsule typically involve the squamosal portion of the temporal bone and the posterosuperior wall of the external auditory canal. The fracture passes through the mastoid air cells and middle ear and fractures the tegmen mastoideum and tegmen tympani. The fracture proceeds anterolateral to the otic capsule, typically fracturing the tegmen in the region of the

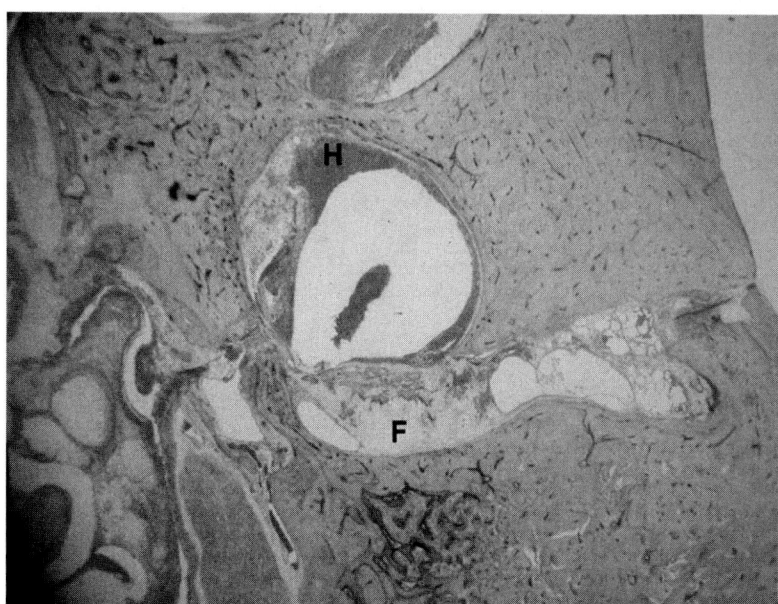

Figure 139.2 Histopathology of a patient who died of meningitis several decades following an otic capsule disrupting temporal bone fracture. F, fibrosis with a small amount of ossification within the fracture line in the otic capsule; H, hemorrhage and purulence. (See also Color Plate 56.)

facial hiatus. Otic capsule sparing fractures typically result from a blow to the temporoparietal region.

Otic capsule disrupting fractures pass through the otic capsule generally proceeding from the foramen magnum across the petrous pyramid and otic capsule. The fracture will often pass through the jugular foramen, internal auditory canal, and the foramen lacerum. These fractures do not typically affect the ossicular chain or the external auditory canal (28). Otic capsule disrupting fractures generally result from blows to the occipital region.

Longitudinal fractures are reported to comprise 70% to 90% of temporal bone fractures with the remaining 10% to 30% categorized as transverse (11,24,26,28–31). In two large series using the newer classification scheme, only 2.5% to 5.8% of fractures disrupted the otic capsule (2,25). This would suggest that many fractures that are oriented perpendicular to the petrous ridge do not actually cross the otic capsule. Many of the otic capsule disrupting fractures are actually oriented in the longitudinal plane (25).

TABLE 139.1

INCIDENCE OF COMMON COMPLICATIONS OF TEMPORAL BONE FRACTURES IN THE GENERAL AND PEDIATRIC POPULATIONS

Complication	General	Pediatric
Facial nerve injury	7%	6%
CSF fistula	17%	28%
Meningitis	2%	0.7%
Hearing loss	24%	33%
Conductive HL	21%	43%
Sensorineural HL	57%	52%
Mixed HL	22%	5%

CSF, cerebrospinal fluid; HL, hearing loss.

The traditional schema of anatomic designation of fracture type was first extensively used in biomechanical studies of cadaveric skull deformation, without correlation to functional outcome (23). In contrast, the newer structural schema underscores the importance of otic capsule involvement in heralding neurotologic sequelae. Otic capsule disrupting fractures have a much higher incidence of facial nerve paralysis than otic capsule sparing fractures (30% to 50% vs. 6% to 13%) (2,25). In addition, Fisch reported a much higher incidence of nerve disruption in fractures involving the otic capsule (32). There is a two- to 10-fold increase in CSF fistula in otic capsule disrupting fractures as well as a much greater risk of intracranial injuries, compared with otic capsule sparing fractures (2,25,27). Fractures that disrupt the otic capsule will almost always result in a sensorineural hearing loss, although there are reported exceptions to the rule (33). Hearing loss in otic capsule sparing fractures tends to be conductive or mixed (2,27). Historically, sensorineural hearing loss has been associated with transverse rather than longitudinal fracture type, but in a recent study this correlation was not borne out but rather inverted: longitudinal fractures were three times as likely to be associated with sensorineural hearing loss as were transverse fractures (27). This study demonstrated a statistically significant difference in complication rates involving facial nerve injury, CSF fistula, and conductive hearing loss when 155 temporal bone fractures were categorized with the structural schema of otic capsule sparing versus disrupting fracture types, while demonstrating no statistical significance when using the traditional classification schema of longitudinal versus transverse fracture types.

The newer classification scheme emphasizes functional outcome and better prognosticates those temporal bone fractures that will exhibit neurotologic manifestations. In

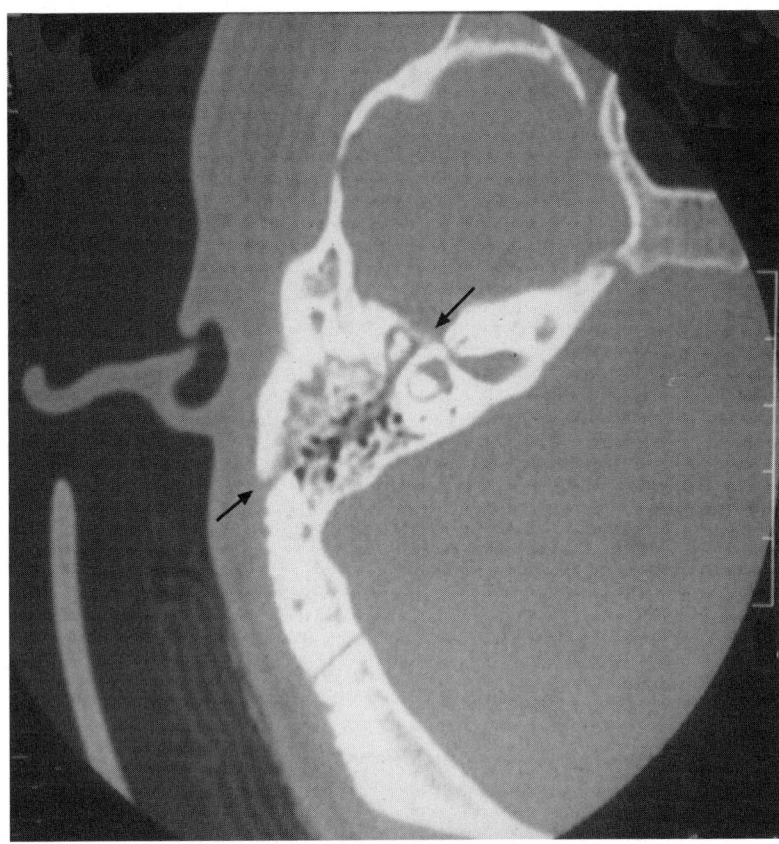

Figure 139.3 Axial cut high-resolution computed tomography demonstrating a longitudinally oriented fracture that is sparing the otic capsule. Black arrows point along the fracture line.

addition to the predictive value for various complications and comorbidities, categorization of fractures into otic capsule sparing and disrupting injuries guides the indications for surgical intervention for CSF fistula and facial paralysis as well as the surgical approach to be used in their repair.

EVALUATION

It is uncommon for temporal bone fractures to occur in isolation of other bodily injury, and consequently the initial evaluation and management is focused on the urgent

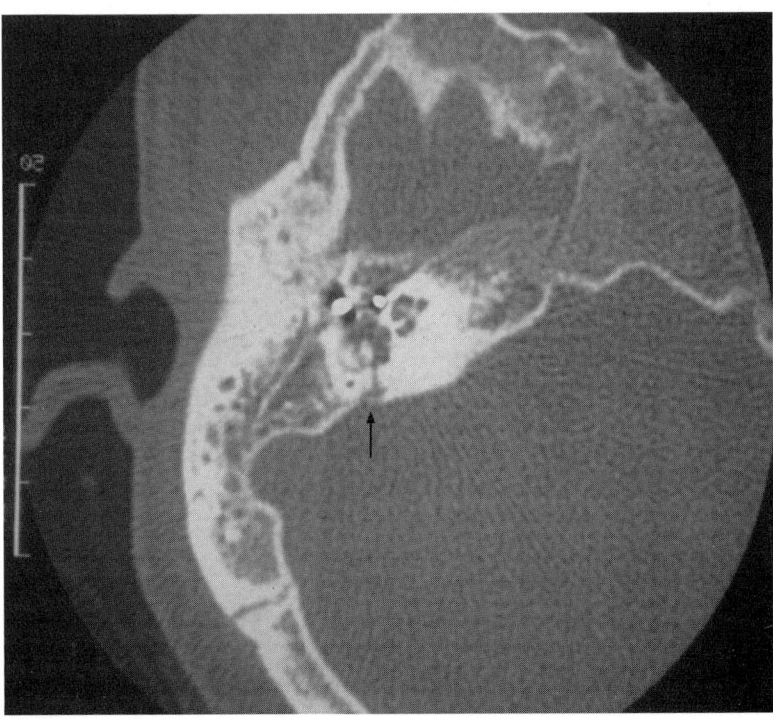

Figure 139.4 Axial cut high-resolution computed tomography demonstrating a transverse oriented fracture, secondary to a gunshot injury, disrupting the otic capsule. The black arrow points to the fracture line.

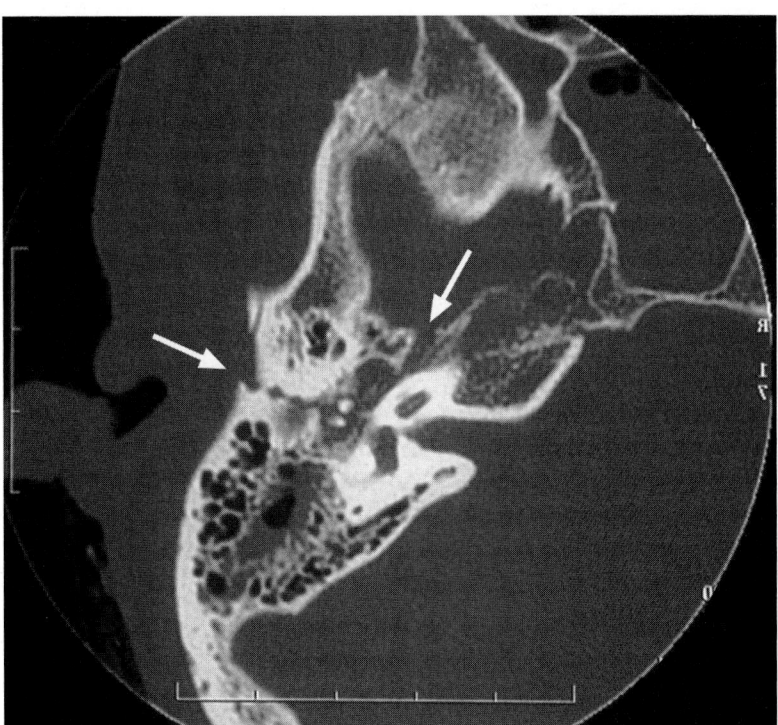

Figure 139.5 Axial cut high-resolution computed tomography demonstrating a mixed oriented fracture that spares the otic capsule. The white arrows point to the fracture lines.

life-threatening issues of securing an airway, controlling hemorrhage, evaluating the neurologic status, and stabilizing and evaluating the cervical spine. Following or concurrent with this evaluation, the neurotologic examination is performed. It is extremely important to assess facial nerve function in the emergency room as early as possible, prior to the administration of muscle relaxants, as discussed later. The ear examination focuses on the condition of the auricle, ear canal, tympanic membrane, and middle ear.

Clinical Evaluation

The auricles are inspected for lacerations and hematomas. Lacerations are closed after thorough cleaning and debridement of exposed cartilage. Hematomas are drained and pressure bolsters are sutured in place to close the dead space and prevent a recollection of blood. Untreated, the auricular hematomas will result in an auricular chondropathy or "cauliflower ear."

Battle sign is seen in the presence of basilar skull fractures, including temporal bone fractures. Extravasation of blood from the emissary vein leads to ecchymosis over the mastoid bone and mastoid tip. This sign may be present in the initial clinical assessment but more often appears in a delayed fashion days after the injury.

The ear canal is inspected for fractures along the roof, CSF otorrhea, degree of hemorrhage, and the presence of brain herniation. The ear is examined as aseptically as possible. Blood and cerumen in the ear canal should never be debrided with irrigation. Following stabilization in the emergency room and transfer to the ward or intensive care unit, the ear can be more carefully examined with the aid

of an operating microscope. Typical findings include fractures along the scutum and roof of the external auditory canal and/or tympanic membrane perforations. Hemotympanum or bloody otorrhea are almost invariably present and are two of the most common signs of temporal bone fracture (Figs. 139.6, 139.7, and 139.8).

The integrity of the tympanic membrane is assessed, as is the presence of hemotympanum. Hemotympanum and any associated serous effusion generally resolve spontaneously, with resolution of concomitant conductive hearing loss, within 4 to 6 weeks and simply require observation. Traumatic tympanic membrane perforations generally heal spontaneously as well, and consequently no acute intervention is necessary.

Hearing is initially assessed clinically at the bedside with a progressively louder whispered voice. Tuning fork examination is useful in delineating conductive from sensorineural hearing loss. Pure tone and speech audiometry are not typically necessary in the acute setting and are obtained after the patient is stabilized. However, in the presence of complications of facial paralysis or CSF fistula in which surgical intervention may be necessary, preoperative audiometry is necessary as results will dictate the options available for management within the treatment algorithm, as discussed later.

The neurotologic examination should note the presence or absence of nystagmus as well as the type of nystagmus. Peripheral vertigo generally manifests with horizontal or rotatory nystagmus and is suppressible with visual fixation. Central vertigo may present with vertical or direction-changing nystagmus that fails to suppress and may even enhance with fixation. The most common type of vertigo

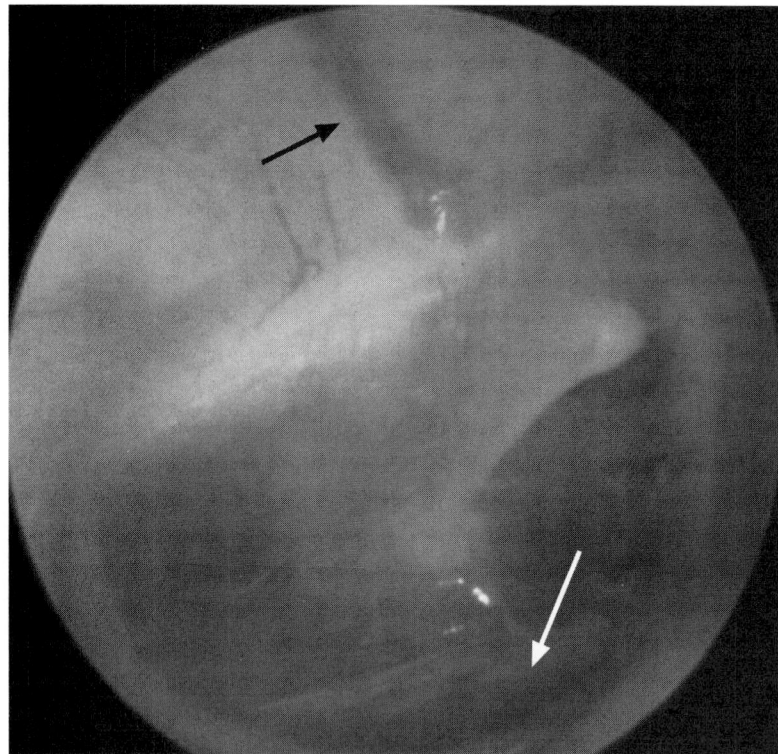

Figure 139.6 Otoscopic image demonstrating a nondisplaced fracture along the scutum *(black arrow)*. Blood is layering out inferiorly *(white arrow)*.

following head trauma is benign paroxysmal positional vertigo (BPPV) (34). BPPV classically manifests with latent-onset, transient rotatory nystagmus and concomitant vertigo with the Dix-Hallpike maneuver (34,35). The nystagmus occurs with the affected ear down. There is a 2- to 10-second latency followed by 10 to 30 seconds of rotatory nystagmus in the geotropic direction—that is, with the

upper half of the globe rotating in fast phase direction toward the ground. On returning to an upright sitting position, a second bout of vertigo with nystagmus in the counter-rotatory direction is often seen. The nystagmus is fixed in direction and is fatigable with repeated maneuvers. In contrast, central positional vertigo induces direction changing nystagmus, which has no latency and is

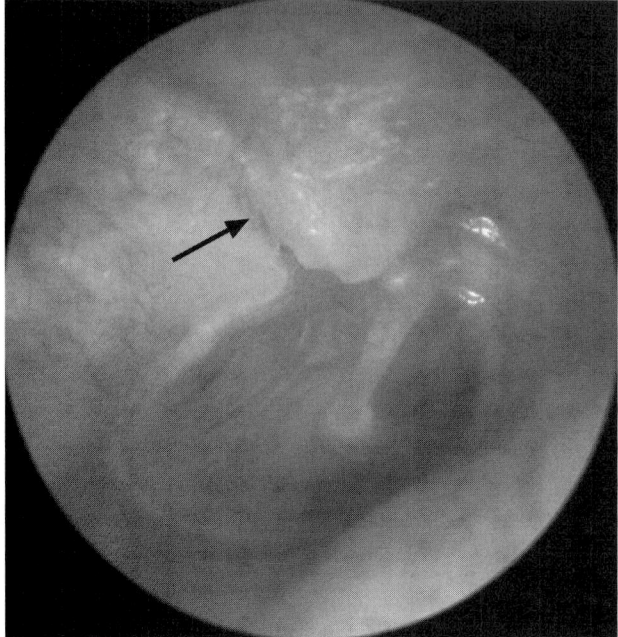

Figure 139.7 Otoscopic image demonstrating a displaced fracture along the scutum *(black arrow)*. (See also Color Plate 57.)

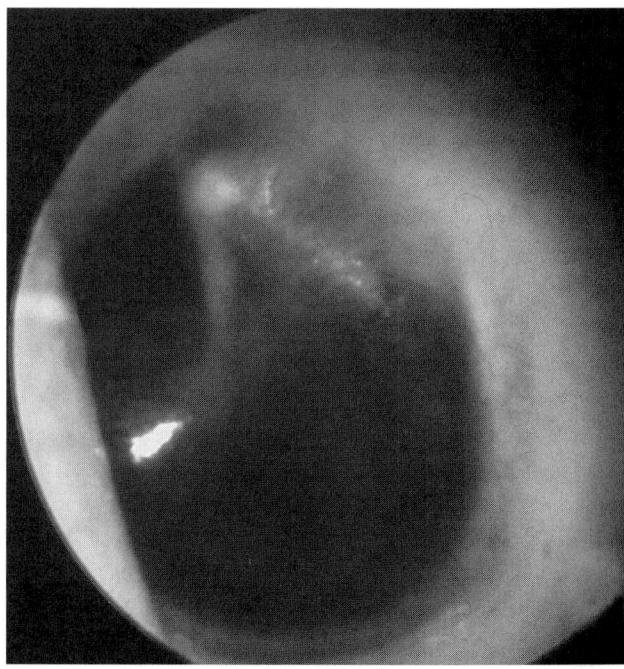

Figure 139.8 Otoscopic image demonstrating a hemotympanum. (See also Color Plate 58.)

nonfatigable. Interestingly, the incidence of vertigo does not closely correlate with the severity of the trauma (36).

Electronystagmography (ENG) is helpful in categorizing and localizing the vestibular injury; however, as with audiometry, it is typically not obtained in the acute setting. The vast majority of posttraumatic vertigo resolves spontaneously. If the symptoms persist following discharge from the hospital, an ENG can be obtained to help clarify diagnosis on an outpatient basis.

The fistula test, which consists of applying positive and negative pressure in the ear canal with a pneumatic otoscope, is also not performed in the acute setting. Application of positive and negative pressure in the potential setting of CSF fistula, and/or communication with the labyrinth if the fracture is otic capsule disrupting, increases the risk of iatrogenic injury from introduction of infection or air into the intracranial space or inner ear. This risk outweighs any potential diagnostic benefit in the acute setting. If the patient continues to experience vertigo or is experiencing fluctuating or progressive hearing loss longer than 1 week after the injury, a perilymph fistula is suspected and a fistula test is then performed. The continued presence of spontaneous nystagmus following traumatic injury to the temporal bone is also suggestive of a perilymph fistula. The fistula test should not be performed if there is evidence of a persistent CSF fistula or infection in the middle ear.

Radiographic Evaluation

Patients with severe head trauma of the magnitude required for a temporal bone fracture will generally already have had a CT scan of the head to assess for intracranial hemorrhage and other intracranial injuries. Temporal bone fractures can typically be discovered on standard head CT alone and can be traditionally classified as either longitudinal, transverse, or mixed or categorized with the more clinically significant otic capsule sparing versus disrupting classification, as discussed previously.

Additional imaging of the temporal bone with axial and coronal high-resolution CT scanning (HRCT) is indicated in the presence of facial paralysis, signs of CSF otorrhea or rhinorrhea, disruption of the superior wall of the external auditory canal or scutum with potential trapping of epithelium (Fig. 139.9), or suspected vascular injury. HRCT of the temporal bones is also indicated if surgical intervention is required in the management of a neurotologic complication.

HRCT proves an invaluable tool for management decision making in the setting of immediate onset, complete facial paralysis: A finding of bony impingement of the facial nerve and fallopian canal, either by bony spicules or by translocation of fracture components, is an indication for facial nerve exploration and decompression. In contrast, delayed-onset or incomplete facial paralysis alone does not require further radiologic evaluation with HRCT.

Hearing loss alone, whether conductive or sensorineural, in the absence of other complications also does not warrant

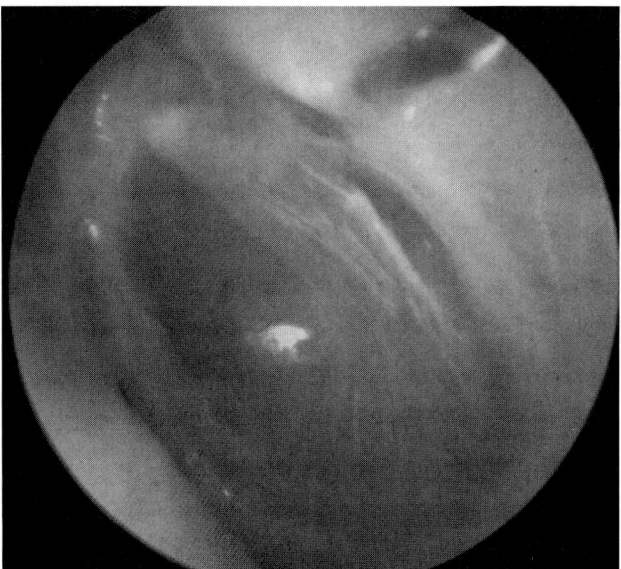

Figure 139.9 Otoscopic photograph demonstrating a distracted fracture along the roof of the external auditory canal and scutum allowing for potential in growth of canal skin.

additional temporal bone imaging in the acute setting. Demonstration of a transverse fracture or otic capsule disrupting fracture in the setting of anacusis or profound sensorineural hearing loss will not alter the treatment plan. However, preoperative assessment with CT scanning in patients with a conductive hearing loss of sufficient magnitude to warrant exploration and ossicular reconstruction may provide useful information that may influence the surgical approach.

Ossicular discontinuity following temporal bone trauma can often be imaged on HRCT; types of discontinuities most easily identifiable on HRCT are incus dislocation and malleoincudal subluxation (37). In complete incus dislocation, the position of the incus can be quite variable: residing in the epitympanum lateral to the malleus head (causing a "Y" configuration when viewed on coronal cuts), within the external auditory canal, or even not visible at all (presumably extruded from the body or "lost" within the mastoid air cells). Partial dislocation of the incus and subluxation of the malleoincudal joint creates a diastasis of the malleus head "ice cream scoop" from the incus body "cone," with or without rotation of the incus body, on axial imaging. Incudostapedial subluxation and stapes fracture are difficult to ascertain on CT.

Posttraumatic sensorineural hearing loss is highly correlated with otic capsule disrupting fractures, but many cases present with no radiologic findings. In these cases, an impulsive disruption of the membranous labyrinth, termed cochlear concussion, is theorized (38). Intralabyrinthine hemorrhage is an etiology that can be imaged and is seen as a region of signal hyperintensity within the vestibule and cochlea on noncontrast T1-weighted magnetic resonance (MR) imaging if performed acutely (39,40).

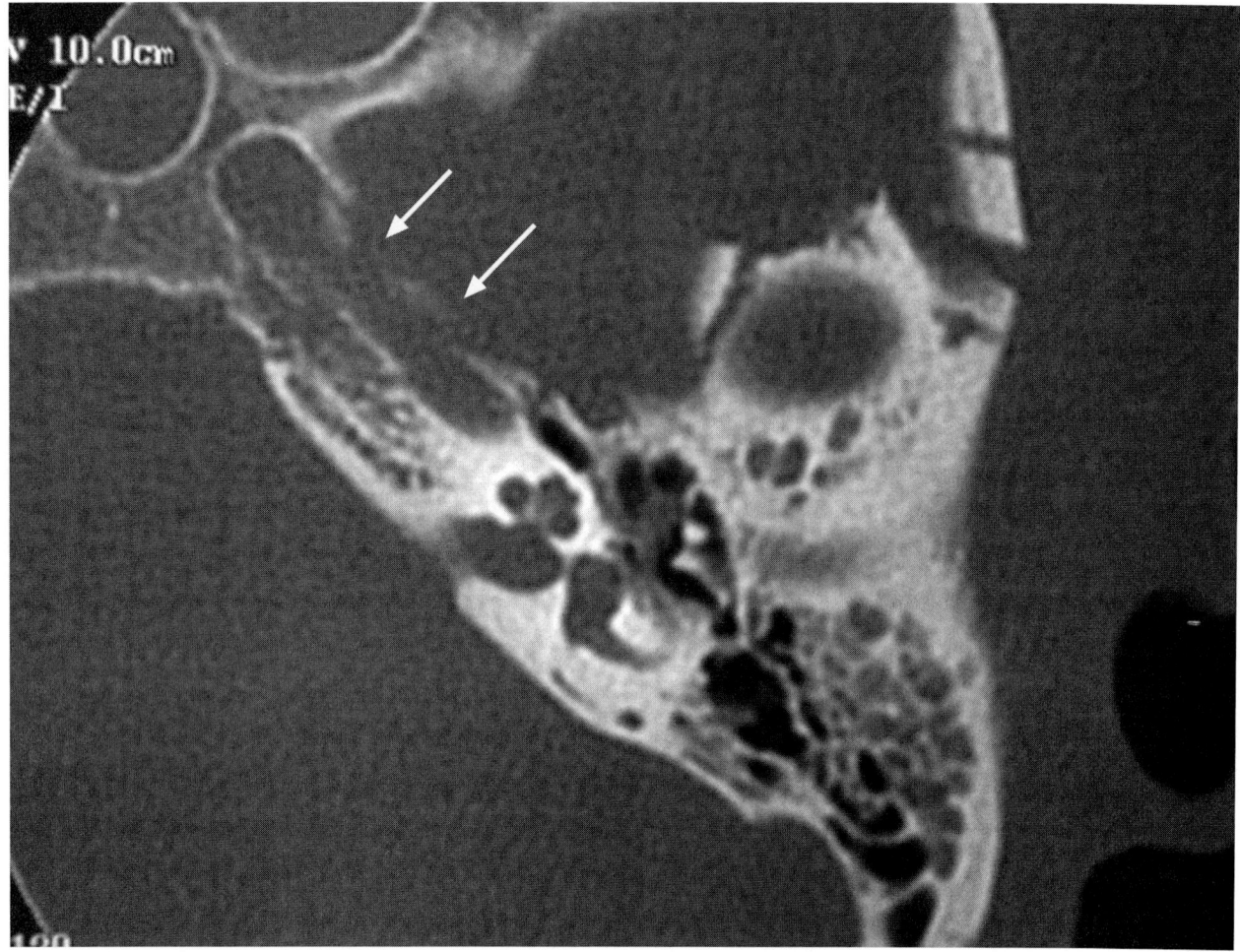

Figure 139.10   Axial cut high-resolution computed tomography demonstrating a fracture along the carotid canal. White arrows point to the fractured carotid canal.

Similarly, identification of perilymph fistula is usually not directly possible on radiographic imaging, but this diagnosis can be suggested when recognition is made of otic capsule disrupting fracture, stapes fracture, loss of stapes bone, or pneumolabyrinth in the setting of persistent fluctuating hearing loss and vertigo (37,41).

The role of HRCT in the evaluation of potential carotid artery injuries is unclear. Resnick et al. (42) reported a 5% incidence of carotid injury in basilar skull fractures if the fracture spares the carotid canal and an 18% incidence of carotid injury in patients with fractures through the carotid canal seen on HRCT. However, Kahn et al. (43) argue that, in an asymptomatic patient, HRCT demonstration of a fracture through the carotid canal yields no valuable additional information. Subsequent angiography performed in cases of asymptomatic carotid canal fractures yielded no evidence of carotid artery injury and provided no clinical utility (43). Consequently, in patients sustaining a temporal bone fracture, who are neurologically intact, HRCT and angiography are not required. On the other hand, if there are any transient or persistent neurologic deficits in patients

with basilar skull fractures, HRCT of the temporal bone together with CT angiography is indicated (Fig. 139.10). MR angiography can also be considered for screening evaluation of the petrous carotid artery.

Conventional skull radiography, including Schuller, Towne, Chamberlain, Stenvers, and basal views as well as tomograms, have been supplanted by HRCT scanning and no longer play a role in the evaluation of patients suspected of having a temporal bone fracture.

In evaluating temporal bones for fracture on CT, care must be taken to avoid mistaking normal anatomic structures for fracture lines. Extrinsic suture lines (petro-occipital, temporo-occipital, occipito-mastoid sutures), intrinsic suture lines (tympanomastoid, tympanosquamous, petrotympanic fissures), and intrinsic channels (cochlear aqueduct, vestibular aqueduct, glossopharyngeal nerve/glossopharyngeal sulcus, subarcuate artery/petromastoid canal, singular nerve/singular canal, Arnold nerve/mastoid canaliculus, Jacobsen nerve/inferior tympanic canaliculus, and greater superficial petrosal nerve/facial hiatus) may all mimic fracture lines within the temporal bone (37). Knowledge of their anatomic relationships and distinction with true fracture lines is necessary to prevent incorrect interpretation of CT imaging.

MANAGEMENT

The morbidity and mortality associated with temporal bone fractures results from injuries to the structures passing through the temporal bone or abutting the temporal bone as described previously. The most common complications include facial nerve injury, CSF fistula, sensorineural hearing loss, conductive hearing loss, vertigo, cholesteatoma formation, and stenosis of the ear canal. In addition, rare complications may occur, including abducens nerve injury, trigeminal nerve injury, Horner syndrome, carotid injury, sigmoid sinus thrombosis, traumatic porencephalic cyst formation, and intracranial dislocation of the mandibular condyle (12,44–49).

Facial Nerve Injury

Facial paralysis is a severely disfiguring complication of temporal bone fractures. Six percent to 7% of temporal bone fractures result in facial paralysis. This figure represents data based on large prospective and retrospective series of all consecutive patients treated for head injury or temporal bone fracture, thereby avoiding previous systematic bias toward overreporting of clinical complications (2,10). Of these facial nerve injuries, one fourth are complete. The incidence of facial nerve injury in temporal bone fractures of the pediatric population is 3% to 9%, comparable to that of the adult population (5,8,9).

The incidence of facial paralysis in the literature has previously been reported as high as 30%. However, this estimation is exaggerated due to sampling error: Simple, uncomplicated temporal bone fractures without facial nerve injury are often not referred for otolaryngologic consultation. The incidence of facial paralysis in the literature has also been overestimated by including patients in retrospective reviews who have been referred to a tertiary care center for management of complications of temporal bone fractures such as facial paresis. Because the entire pool of temporal bone fracture patients had not been included in prior statistics, the reported incidence of complications has previously been quite biased.

If head trauma patients are carefully evaluated in the emergency room on admission, prior to the administration of muscle relaxants, 27% of facial nerve injuries will present with immediate-onset facial paralysis; 73% will have facial motion in the initial examination and subsequently deteriorate (2). The latency in onset of facial palsy ranges from 1 to 16 days. It is crucial to differentiate "delayed onset" from "delayed diagnosis." Delayed onset of facial paralysis is defined as documented facial function in the emergency room that subsequently deteriorates. A delayed diagnosis of facial paralysis occurs when the patient is given a paralytic agent and intubated prior to examination of facial function. In this situation, an assessment of facial function is delayed until extubation. These patients should be categorized as unestablished onset and treated similar to the immediate-onset patients. In one large series, 10% of patients fell into this unestablished onset category (50).

Many aspects in the management of facial nerve injury remain controversial. One of the main issues to be resolved is the indication for surgical exploration. Because the vast majority of traumatic facial palsies resolve spontaneously, the decision of which injuries to explore is based on prognostic factors for poor outcome. The factors that are assessed in predicting recovery of facial function include timing of onset (delayed vs. immediate onset), severity of the injury (penetrating vs. nonpenetrating), and the presence of associated infection.

The delay of onset of paralysis following temporal bone fracture is the most important of the predictive factors. In one series of 37 delayed-onset facial palsies, five were lost to follow-up and the remainder recovered to a House-Brackmann grade I or II (2). McKennan and Chole described their experience with 17 patients with immediate-onset facial paralysis and 19 patients with delayed-onset paralysis (51). Complete spontaneous recovery of facial function occurred in 94% of the patients with delayed-onset paralysis. The one remaining patient had a House-Brackmann grade II recovery. In contrast, 8 out of the 17 immediate-onset paralysis patients had facial nerve transections.

Turner (52) reviewed a large series of traumatic facial paralysis treated conservatively. His article included 36 immediate-onset and 34 delayed-onset facial palsies. Complete recovery occurred in 94% of the delayed-onset cases and 75% of immediate-onset palsies. The one patient with delayed-onset paralysis who had no recovery of function developed the facial palsy coincident with acute otitis media. Maiman et al. (53), in contrast, found no correlation between immediate- or delayed-onset facial paralysis, treated nonsurgically, and outcome. However, 44 out of 45 of their patients (including both immediate and delayed onset) had satisfactory recovery. Review of the previously mentioned literature argues strongly against surgical exploration and decompression of delayed posttraumatic and facial paralysis. The natural course of delayed facial paralysis is almost always recovery of facial function to a House-Brackmann grade I or II. There are no convincing data in the literature that demonstrate that surgical intervention in delayed-onset paralysis will increase the probability of complete recovery of function.

May (54) describes the difficulty in differentiating immediate from delayed-onset facial paralysis. He explored reportedly delayed-onset palsies and found on occasion a severed nerve. This observation highlights the necessity of careful examination in the emergency room prior to chemical paralysis. Even in comatose patients, painful stimuli will generally induce a symmetric grimace when both facial nerves are intact; unilateral weakness of all facial branches implies a peripheral (i.e., facial nerve) lesion, whereas selective weakness of the lower branches with bilateral temporal branch sparing implies a central lesion, proximal to the facial nucleus. Admittedly, information regarding facial nerve function immediately following an injury is not always available. Sometimes the examination is omitted due to attention to other life-threatening complications or because the patient has already received muscle relaxants with intubation. Some patients are not responsive to pain and a grimace cannot be induced. The critical issue is whether or not any facial function has been identified. If facial function is present in the emergency room and subsequently deteriorates, our experience is that the patient will recover without surgical treatment. When reliable information from the emergency room is unavailable, the patient is never documented to have facial function, and the diagnosis of facial palsy is delayed by a few days, these cases must be categorized as "unknown onset" and considered with the immediate-onset group when considering management options.

The degree of facial nerve injury is also a critical factor in guiding the management algorithm. Incomplete paresis rarely fails to completely resolve spontaneously unless an additional insult to the nerve, such as infection, occurs (2). Consequently, only patients with complete paralysis of immediate or unknown onset are considered for surgical exploration.

The degree of injury can be assessed not only clinically with facial motion but also with electrodiagnostic testing using the Hilger facial nerve stimulator, evoked electromyography (EEMG), also known as electroneuronography (ENoG), and standard electromyography (EMG). The role of electrodiagnostic testing is to assist the clinician in differentiating a neuropraxic injury from a neural degenerative injury and to assess the proportion of degenerated axons. Nerves sustaining a neuropraxic injury proximal to the stimulated portion of the nerve maintain electrical stimulability at all times following the injury. Partial or complete disruption of the nerve results in Wallerian degeneration and consequent decrease or loss of stimulability. However, Wallerian degeneration occurs in a delayed fashion, and the distal segment of the nerves maintains electrical stimulability for 3 to 5 days postinjury (55). Consequently, electrodiagnostic testing cannot reliably differentiate a neuropraxic injury from a laceration of the nerve for up to 3 to 5 days.

Sunderland classified nerve fiber injuries in five categories (56). The first-degree injury is an anatomically intact nerve fiber with a conduction blockade (neuropraxia). These lesions tend to recover completely. The second-degree injury transects the axons but maintains an intact endoneurium (axonotmesis). Again, these lesions also tend to resolve without subsequent deficits. The third-degree injury transects the axon and endoneurium but maintains an intact perineurium (neurotmesis). Aberrant regeneration can occur with third-degree injuries, leaving patients with some weakness and synkinesis. Fourth-degree injuries transect the entire nerve trunk but maintain an intact epineural sheath (neurotmesis). Loss of the conduit of the epineural sheath allows regenerating axons to cross into adjacent fascicles, resulting in a loss of topographic organization. A proportion of the regenerating fibers are also lost due to the healing process and scarring. These lesions result in a high incidence of residual weakness, synkinesis, and hyperkinesis. Complete transection of the entire nerve trunk and epineurium is classified as a fifth-degree injury (neurotmesis) and is associated with poor spontaneous recovery, if any, depending on the degree of diastasis of the nerve stumps

The Hilger facial nerve stimulator is used to perform both the minimal nerve excitability test (NET) as well as the maximal stimulation test (MST). The facial nerve is stimulated percutaneously adjacent to the stylomastoid foramen and the various distal branches. In NET, the branches of the facial nerve are stimulated on both the injured side and on the contralateral side, which serves as a control. The current used is incrementally increased just until threshold is reached, manifested by facial twitching, and this threshold level is recorded for each side individually. A threshold difference of 3.5 mA or greater between the affected and nonaffected sides of the face suggests significant neural degeneration. The test is most useful between three and 14 days postinjury in patients with dense facial paralysis to differentiate between neuropraxic and neurodegenerative injuries. The testing is unnecessary in incomplete paralysis in which there is almost always 100% recovery.

May et al. (57) argues that the MST provides a more reliable estimation of the degree of degeneration. In the MST, stimulation of the nonaffected, control side is performed similar to in the NET, but the intensity of the stimulus is further increased until the amount of facial contraction plateaus or is limited by patient intolerance. The affected, injured side is then stimulated with the same current amplitude, and the degree of contraction is subjectively assessed by the physician and compared with that of the unaffected side of the face. The difference in contraction is expressed as equal, mildly decreased, markedly decreased, or no response. The latter two categories are associated with poorer prognosis. Similar to NET, MST is most useful between 3 and 14 days postinjury in patients with dense facial paralysis. Again, any volitional movement of the face would indicate an intact nerve trunk and supersede any electrical testing.

EEMG has been popularized by Fisch and termed ENoG. ENoG differs from EEMG only in the use of bipolar stimulating and recording electrodes (58). Both techniques measure the evoked compound muscle action potential (CAP) and provide similar information to the MST but in an objective fashion. The stimulating bipolar electrodes are placed adjacent to the stylomastoid foramen, and the recording bipolar electrodes in the nasolabial crease. The peak-to-trough amplitude of the CAP is measured on both sides, and the diminution in amplitude of the CAP on the paretic side as compared with the control side is indicative of the percentage of degenerated nerve fibers. EEMG has been demonstrated to be the most accurate electrodiagnostic test for prognostic information (59). Fisch (60) reported that patients in whom the degeneration on EEMG reaches 90% within 6 days of onset of a traumatic facial paralysis have a poorer outcome and consequently should be decompressed. Sillman et al. (61) demonstrated a significant association between a CAP decline of greater than 90% and poor recovery of function for idiopathic paralysis but demonstrated no significant association between CAP decline of greater than 90% and clinical outcome in traumatic paralysis.

The value of EMG in the acute management of traumatic facial paralysis remains controversial. Standard monopolar EMG is performed by insertion of an EMG electrode into the muscle and the spontaneous electrical activity recorded. Two types of information are obtainable: voluntary activity and fibrillation potentials. If voluntary activity is present in the acute postinjury period, the patient has a very high probability of good recovery (61). However, May et al. (62) reported only 75% accuracy in predicting a poor recovery and 62% accuracy in predicting a favorable result. Fibrillation potentials result from denervation of the muscle but are delayed 2 to 3 weeks following the injury and consequently offer little additional information to guide therapy in the acute setting (63).

After defining the at-risk population for poor recovery of function, the next question to answer is: does surgical intervention alter the outcome? In 1944, Turner (52) reported on 69 patients with varying degrees of facial paralysis following temporal bone trauma. Thirty of these patients had complete facial paralysis, all of which were treated nonoperatively. This group of patients was unbiased in that none of his series underwent surgical decompression. Good recovery occurred in 63% of the patients, incomplete recovery with synkinesis in 23%, and poor recovery in 13%. Maiman et al. (53) reported on the outcome of 21 patients with post-traumatic complete facial paralysis. Full recovery occurred in 52% of the patients and incomplete recovery in 43%. One patient had a poor outcome. Brodie and Thompson (2) had eight patients with complete paralysis who met criteria for facial nerve decompression who, for a variety of reasons, did not undergo surgical exploration. Seven of the eight patients had good recovery of function and one patient had a poor outcome. The combined rate of good recovery of function with conservative, nonsurgical management, in the previous three studies is 63%.

In contrast, analysis of six case series studies of patients undergoing surgical decompression for complete facial nerve paralysis revealed a combined rate of good recovery of facial function of 51%. This figure excludes severed facial nerves. The criteria to be included in the surgical groups were that the nerves were no longer stimulable with the Hilger facial nerve stimulator or demonstrated greater than 90% degeneration within 6 days or 95% degeneration within 14 days on EEMG/ENoG.

The outcomes in facial nerve function for patients who underwent conservative, nonsurgical management versus those undergoing facial nerve decompression in various series are summarized in Table 139.2 (2,50,52,53,64–67).

It is difficult to compare the recovery rates of facial nerve function in patients undergoing surgical and nonsurgical management. The patients included in the observation studies did not necessarily meet the same criteria as

TABLE 139.2

FACIAL NERVE OUTCOMES FOLLOWING COMPLETE FACIAL PARALYSIS

Treatment	n	Good (HB I or II)	Incomplete (HB III or IV)	Poor (HB V or VI)	Transected nerve
Nonoperative					
Turner	30	19	7	4	
Maiman	21	11	9	1	
Brodie	8	7	0	1	
RATE:		63%	27%	10%	
Operative					
Kamerer	62	18	15	9	20
Lambert	17	11	0	0	6
Coker	12	5	4	1	2
Brodie	6	4	0	2	0
Darrouzet	65	25	26	5	9
Yeoh	6	4	1	1	0
RATE:		51%	35%	14%	(22%)

those included in the surgical decompression studies, thereby potentially artificially inflating the positive outcomes in patients treated nonsurgically. In an extensive review and analysis of the literature, Chang and Cass (68) concluded that there are no studies that prove or disprove the efficacy of facial nerve decompression.

Because Wallerian degeneration is not documented on electrodiagnostic testing for 3 to 5 days following the axonotmesis or neurotmesis, surgical intervention is delayed until several days after the nerve has degenerated. Although decompression of the facial nerve prophylactically in acoustic neuroma surgery has been proven efficacious, the decompression is performed prior to Wallerian degeneration having occurred (69). Demonstrating that decompression of a posttraumatic nonsevered nerve is efficacious remains to be proven in a randomized prospective study.

The key factor in the decision to surgically explore a facial nerve is whether the nerve is suspected of being severed, crushed, or impaled with bone fragments. The incidence of transected nerves in the largest series ranges from 6% to 45% (50,64–66,70). The high frequency of severed nerves in some of these reports is biased by patient selection, as discussed previously. Patients are referred to the tertiary centers performing nerve explorations when they fail to spontaneously recover. However, the vast majority of patients do not have a transected nerve and therefore recover spontaneously and are not referred to tertiary centers.

The probability of severing the facial nerve is actually quite low, but the outcome of a transected nerve following observation alone is poor. Therefore, an attempt should be made to identify patients with crushed, impaled, or otherwise transected nerves, because these are the patients who would most benefit from surgical intervention. Electrodiagnostic testing of nerves with complete paralysis can only differentiate injuries that have undergone Wallerian degeneration from those which have not (i.e., Sunderland II to V vs. Sunderland I degree injuries). Because one cannot differentiate a Sunderland fifth-degree injury (severed nerve) from a second-, third- or fourth-degree injury on the basis of electrodiagnostic testing, exploration is warranted only in patients with complete, immediate-onset paralysis in whom electrical stimulability is lost: It is these patients who are at greatest risk for crushed, partially severed, or transected nerves.

The site of injury to the facial nerve in temporal bone fractures is in the perigeniculate region in 80% to 93% of patients (32,64,65). Lambert and Brackmann (64) found a second lesion in 4 out of 21 patients in the mastoid segment. Accordingly, the approach used for the nerve exploration must expose these two regions. Fisch (60) advocates a translabyrinthine approach for transverse fractures and a combined transmastoid/middle cranial fossa approach for longitudinal fractures. May (71) described a transmastoid/supralabyrinthine approach to the region of the geniculate ganglion for facial nerve decompression. Goin (72) studied this approach in cadaveric temporal bones and found that he could consistently expose the distal labyrinthine segment and geniculate ganglion. However, the fundus of the internal auditory canal (IAC) could be exposed in only 60% of the temporal bones. Yanagihara (73) applied the transmastoid/ supralabyrinthine approach in 36 patients. Only five temporal bone fractures in his series of 41 patients required a middle cranial fossa approach to expose the geniculate region.

The translabyrinthine approach is advocated for facial nerve exploration in patients with profound hearing loss. The approach provides excellent exposure for decompression, nerve rerouting with direct reanastomosis, and cable grafting. In otic capsule sparing fractures with ossicular discontinuity, the nerve is explored via a transmastoid/ supralabyrinthine approach. This approach generally requires dislocation of the incus and ossicular reconstruction at the completion of the operation. If the patient has any contralateral hearing loss or the anatomy is not conducive for supralabyrinthine exposure, a middle cranial fossa approach is used.

Timing of facial nerve repair has in the past been controversial. McCabe (74) advocated repairing the nerve within the first 3 days or delaying facial nerve reanastomosis for 20 days postinjury. This recommendation was based on the observation that regeneration and axoplasmic flow were greatest at 3 weeks postinjury. Barrs (75) studied the timing of facial nerve repair in micropigs and found no advantage of waiting the 3 weeks until the neuronal cell body metabolic activity was maximal. This animal model did not show a statistically significant difference in electrophysiologic testing between nerves grafted throughout various times within three months of transection.

Fisch (76) advocates exploration when the ENoG indicates 90% degeneration occurring within 6 days. He argues that decompression should be performed early to minimize further degeneration. May (54) also advocates early exploration. His series demonstrated a correlation between better results and shorter interval between injury and repair.

Late exploration for potentially severed nerves is still indicated, but the role of late decompression remains controversial. Quaranta et al. (77) reported on nine patients decompressed 2 to 3 months after sustaining their temporal bone fractures. Seventy-eight percent recovered to a House Brackmann grade I or II at 1 year post-decompression. The question as to whether these patients would have recovered spontaneously to the same degree remains unanswered. Clearly, if the nerve was severed and not approximated, spontaneous recovery to a House Brackmann grade I or II would not occur. In that scenario, a House-Brackmann grade VI would be anticipated.

The range in latency to recovery of facial function varies from 1 day to 1 year. Fifty-nine percent of facial palsies that recover spontaneously do so within 1 month and 88% recover by 3 months postinjury (2).

Summary of Facial Nerve Treatment Algorithm

Patients with delayed-onset facial paralysis are placed on a 2-week course of systemic corticosteroids (unless medically contraindicated) and observed. Although there is no data in the literature supporting or contradicting this recommendation, the rational for corticosteroid use is based on antiinflammatory activity and the assumption that neural edema is the primary factor in the progression of injury in the traumatized, nontransected nerve (58) (Fig. 139.11).

Patients with complete paralysis of immediate onset are tested with the Hilger nerve stimulator between days 3 and 7 postinjury. If stimulability is present to any degree (implying a physically intact nerve), the patients are observed. If the nerve loses all stimulability within 1 week of the injury, facial nerve exploration is recommended.

Facial nerve injuries occurring in an otic capsule disrupting fracture are typically explored via a translabyrinthine approach: The translabyrinthine approach affords the most direct, complete access to the entire length of the intratemporal facial nerve, and in fractures that cause a profound sensorineural hearing loss, the approach does not engender any significant morbidity than that already sustained.

In otic capsule sparing fractures, two surgical approaches are used. In patients in whom excellent intrinsic exposure of the intratemporal facial nerve can be achieved, that is, with well-aerated mastoid air cell systems or with ossicular discontinuity, a transmastoid/supralabyrinthine approach is chosen. If the patient has a poorly aerated mastoid air cell system or total facial nerve decompression cannot be achieved by the transmastoid/supralabyrinthine approach, a combined transmastoid/middle cranial fossa approach is used. If a severed facial nerve is encountered using the transmastoid/supralabyrinthine approach and inadequate exposure for cable grafting occurs, a middle cranial fossa approach is performed.

The transmastoid facial nerve decompression begins with a complete mastoidectomy skeletonizing the tegmen mastoideum superiorly, the sigmoid sinus posteriorly, and the posterior external auditory canal (EAC) wall anteriorly. The antrum is opened, exposing the short process of the incus and the lateral semicircular canal. The semicircular canals are then skeletonized. The facial recess is opened and the facial nerve is skeletonized from the second genu to the stylomastoid foramen. If there is any evidence of bony trauma in this region, a complete decompression is performed; however, the nerve sheath is not incised. The buttress to the incus is subsequently removed, followed by removal of the incus, and the tympanic portion of the nerve is decompressed. If there is adequate room to proceed, a supralabyrinthine decompression of the intralabyrinthine portion of the facial nerve is performed. A laceration of the facial nerve in this region is cable grafted with a section of the greater auricular nerve. The cable graft is placed in the bony channel of the fallopian canal abutting the sharply incised edges of the facial nerve. To improve exposure, the tegmen can be drilled to eggshell thickness and retracted superiorly. If the exposure remains inadequate, a middle fossa craniotomy is performed. If the fracture involves the proximal portion of the intralabyrinthine segment of the facial nerve, a middle fossa craniotomy is performed.

To begin the middle fossa craniotomy, the squamosal portion of the temporal bone is exposed by extending the postauricular skin incision in a "lazy S" shape up toward the vertex, first extending anteriorly, then posteriorly. The temporalis fascia is reflected inferiorly and the temporalis muscle is split vertically and elevated off of the squamosal portion of the temporal bone. The soft tissue dissection and exposure should extend underneath the zygomatic arch to allow adequate exposure for the craniotomy. Self-retaining retractors are adjusted to hold both muscle and skin. A bone window is created with large cutting and then diamond burrs, taking care to avoid lacerating the underlying dura. This bone window is 4 by 4 cm in size and placement is set with the inferior border at the level of the zygomatic root, with two thirds of the window anterior and one third posterior to the vertical plane of the EAC. A rongeur or drill is used to remove any remaining bone at the inferior edge of the craniotomy down to the level of the floor of the middle cranial fossa. This allows the optimal surgical line of site with minimal temporal lobe retraction. The House-Urban middle fossa retractor is engaged with the prongs in the edge of the craniotomy. The blade is gradually advanced, as the dura is elevated off the floor of the middle fossa. It is common to encounter dural venous bleeding at the anterior extent of the dissection. This can usually be controlled with a hemostatic agent such as Surgicel or Oxycel. The fracture line and hematoma are generally encountered in the region of the facial hiatus, consistent with the notion of fracture lines following natural foramina within the temporal bone.

The landmarks in the middle fossa are the middle meningeal artery at the foramen spinosum, the greater superficial petrosal nerve at the facial hiatus, and the arcuate eminence. The geniculate ganglion may be exposed without a bony covering on the floor of the middle cranial fossa, so care should be exercised during dural elevation. The landmark for the superior semicircular canal is the arcuate eminence, but the precise location of the canal does not uniformly correspond with the arcuate eminence. The canal may have very little bone coverage and be seen as a blue line after simple dural elevation, or there may be a large number of air cells between the canal and the surface of the tegmen. A coronal CT scan may be helpful in ascertaining this relationship: The association of the contours of the middle fossa floor to the superior semicircular canal as well as the distance between the two can be assessed.

Identification of the internal auditory canal and intralabyrinthine portion of the facial nerve can be accomplished in any of numerous ways. House (78) and Glasscock (79) advocated identifying the greater superficial petrosal nerve and following this to the geniculate ganglion. Fisch (80)

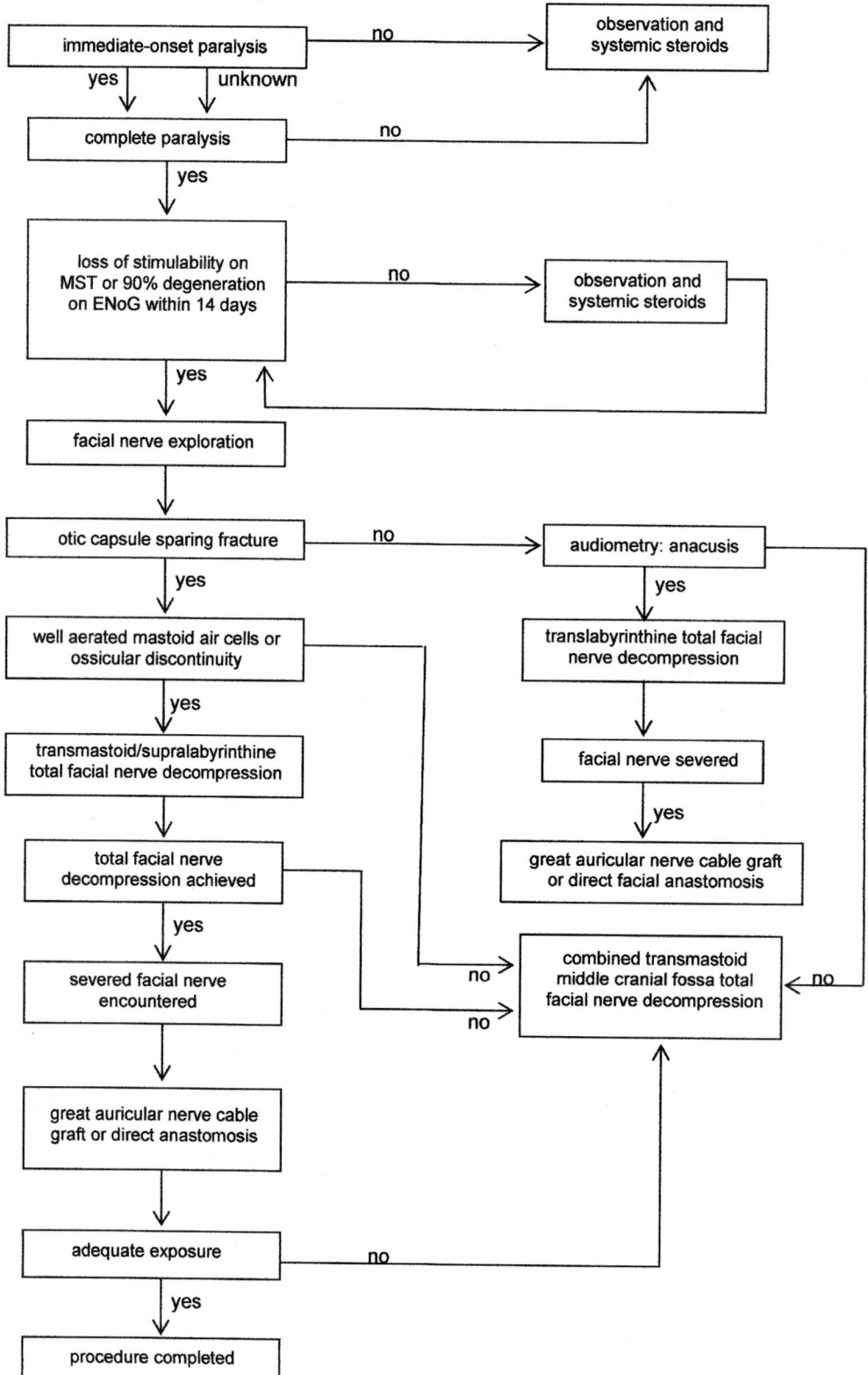

Figure 139.11   Management of traumatic facial paralysis.

suggested using the relationship of the superior semicircular canal to find the internal auditory canal. The internal auditory canal is located within the meatal plane that lies within a 60-degree angle from the plane of the superior semicircular canal. Portmann et al. (81) report finding the internal auditory canal (IAC) 8- to 12-mm anteromedial to the location of the superior semicircular canal in the direction parallel to the petrous ridge. The tegmen tympani may be opened with ensuing identification of the ossicles and tympanic portion of the facial nerve, which can then be followed retrograde toward the geniculate ganglion. The method of Garcia-Ibanez is a reliable technique that can provide extended exposure if required (82).

Once oriented with one or more of the previously stated approaches, the bone over the superior semicircular canal is removed using suction irrigation and diamond burrs. A light medial to lateral stroke is used until the blue line of the superior canal is identified. After the superior canal has been identified, dissection proceeds along the meatal plane, which is the bone within a 60-degree angle from the blue line of the superior canal. Drilling within the confines of this plane will reduce the risk of inadvertent injury to the cochlea. Much wider drilling may be performed medially, whereas at the lateral extent of the IAC there is very little space between the cochlea and ampulla of the superior semicircular canal. The burr should hug the line of the superior canal as bone removal progresses. The dissection will appear quite deep before the IAC is encountered. Bone can be removed 180 degrees around the IAC close to the porus acusticus, but the exposure becomes more limited as the dissection proceeds to the lateral aspect of the IAC. An eggshell thickness of bone should be left over the IAC. The last step in exposure of the canal is careful removal of this bone, and copious irrigation to remove bone dust.

At the most lateral extent of the IAC, the vertical crest or "Bill bar" is identified, with the facial nerve anteriorly and the superior vestibular nerve posteriorly. The dura of the IAC is incised in a longitudinal fashion, along the posterior edge, away from the facial nerve. If the facial nerve is lacerated, the proximal edge is freshened with micro scissors. The nerve graft is secured proximally with a single 9-0 nylon suture and distally placed into the bony channel of the tympanic portion of the fallopian canal. A piece of temporalis fascia is placed over the graft. Bone wax is used to fill exposed air cells. A piece of temporalis muscle is placed in the bony defect, and the pedicled temporalis fascia flap is reflected over the floor of the middle cranial fossa. The temporal lobe is released, compressing the fascia over the bony defect. The bone flap is replaced within the craniotomy window, and the temporalis muscle is reapproximated, leaving a gap inferiorly where the temporalis fascia passes. Skin is closed in two layers.

Cerebrospinal Fluid Fistulae

CSF fistulae and the potential for meningitis are among the most serious of complications from temporal bone fractures. CSF fistulae occur in 17% of temporal bone fractures (2). CSF fistulae in otic capsule sparing fractures typically occur through the floor of the middle cranial fossa (tegmen tympani and tegmen mastoideum) into the epitympanum, antrum, and mastoid air cell tract. The CSF will flow out the ear canal if the tympanic membrane is disrupted or into the eustachian tube, resulting in CSF rhinorrhea. In otic capsule disrupting fractures, CSF flows from the posterior cranial fossa through the disrupted otic capsule into the middle ear.

A unique characteristic of a fracture through the otic capsule is the absence of healing. The otic capsule is adult size at birth and undergoes minimal remodeling throughout life (83). Following a fracture, fibrous tissue will partially fill the crevice, and the adjacent periosteal bone may seal off the fracture but the enchondral bone itself will not heal (19,21). This fibrous scar affords a potential tract for an infection of the middle ear cleft to spread to the intracranial space, leaving the patient at continued risk for meningitis even years after the initial injury.

The onset of CSF leakage following trauma was delayed for greater than 1 week in 28% of the 192 cases surveyed by Lewin (84). Immediate CSF leak results from separation of dural fibers in a traumatized region of dura adjacent to a fracture site. In contrast, delayed CSF leak has been theorized to occur from (a) herniation of meningocele or meningoencephalocele (often termed brain fungus or fungus cerebri) into the fracture site, followed by delayed atrophy of the brain fungus or delayed resolution of elevated intracranial pressure and retraction of brain fungus out of the fracture site or (b) resolution of hematoma previously obstructing the outflow of CSF through the fracture site.

The CSF fistula will continue to leak until fibroblastic proliferation creates a fibrous barrier that closes the subarachnoid space or the sinus or air cell mucosa covers the bony defect (85). However, in the early stages of repair, the fibrous barrier is weak and the mucosal barrier remains fragile. If the CSF pressure gradient is greater than the healing tensile strength of these vulnerable barriers the leak will continue. The tenuous, newly formed barrier may be easily ruptured by increased nasopharyngeal pressure or Valsalva (86). Therefore, the importance of enforcing relatively mundane precautions such as avoiding nose blowing, avoiding strenuous physical activity or physical therapy, keeping the head of the bed elevated, and avoiding constipation cannot be overemphasized.

A CSF fistula is suspected when clear watery drainage is noted in the ear canal or from the nose. Otorhinorrhea will often drain down the back of the throat. The rate of flow of the discharge will usually increase with exertion or leaning forward. Consequently, when evaluating a patient for a suspected CSF fistula, the patient is asked to lean forward with the neck flexed, collecting nasal discharge into a sterile container. Patients often complain of headaches that are dull, continuous, and bilateral. The origin of aural and nasal drainage is often obscured by concurrent bleeding or lysis of old blood clot. Once a nasal discharge is suspected of being CSF, it can be differentiated from watery rhinitis, lacrimal secretions or serosanguinous discharge on the basis of its composition. CSF has elevated glucose, decreased protein, and decreased potassium concentration levels than nasal secretions. Qualitative tests such as those using glucose oxidase test strips (Clinitest) have been shown to lack specificity and result in a substantial proportion of false positives (87). Quantitative glucose, protein, and potassium determinations are more accurate in diagnosing a CSF fistula.

A noninvasive technique for identifying and localizing a CSF fistula using protein electrophoresis for beta-2 transferrin was first described by Meurman (88). The beta-2 isoform of transferrin, a protein involved in iron transport, is confined to CSF, perilymph, and aqueous humor, whereas the beta-1 isoform is found globally in serum, nasal secretions, saliva, and tears. Nasal and otic secretions with CSF contamination exhibit an additional band on immunofixation electrophoresis than noncontaminated counterparts. In addition to being noninvasive, a major advantage of this technique is the small amount of fluid specimen required for the test: Recommended specimen volume is typically 0.5 mL, and beta-2 transferrin can be detected in sample specimens as small as 50 μL. False-positive results are rare and occur in patients with alcoholic cirrhosis, inborn errors of glycoprotein metabolism, or genetic transferrin variants, in which transferrin allelic variants with similar electrophoretic mobility to the beta-2 isoform are present in sera (89). In these cases, collection and electrophoresis of a concurrent serum sample, which would contain beta-1 as well as beta-2-like bands, can help avoid a falsely positive result interpretation.

Other minimally invasive techniques for detection of CSF otorrhea or rhinorrhea are currently being developed, including detection of beta-trace protein, or prostaglandin D synthase (90,91). Beta-trace protein is synthesized in the meninges and has a 20- to 40-fold increase in concentration in CSF compared with serum. New nephelometric assays of beta-trace protein are being developed and have shown a specificity and sensitivity of CSF detection comparable to that of current beta-2 transferrin assays (92,93). In addition, the nephelometric technique is comparatively inexpensive and rapid, increasing its potential for further development and use in the clinical setting.

HRCT will generally demonstrate the potential sites of a CSF fistula. When a fracture is seen but the exact site of the fistula has not been identified, CT cisternography with intrathecal contrast (Omnipaque) can be quite useful. HRCT will show a bony defect in 70% of patients with a CSF fistula (94). When a defect cannot be demonstrated by HRCT, rarely will CT cisternography or radionuclide cisternography detect a site of leakage (94). Radionuclide scans tend to lack sensitivity and specificity.

Intrathecal fluorescein is a sensitive and specific test for investigating the presence of a CSF fistula. Following a lumbar puncture, 0.5 mL of a 5% solution of fluorescein is mixed with 10 mL of the patient's CSF and reinjected. Any subsequent otorrhea or rhinorrhea can be collected on micropledgets and examined under a Wood lamp for green fluorescence. Although occasional reports of neurotoxicity (e.g., paraparesis and grand mal seizures) following intrathecal injection of fluorescein appear in the literature, these complications are very infrequent, occurred at higher doses of fluorescein than is currently recommended, and have never resulted in permanent damage (86,95,96). No persistent side effects or complications have been reported with the current recommended dosing. Fluorescein is frequently successful in localizing fistulas when all other methods have failed and can be used intraoperatively to aid in the actual repair of the fistula (96–98). Therefore, the continued usage of fluorescein may be justified and the risks of increased morbidity following failure to locate a CSF fistula preoperatively may outweigh the risks involved in its use.

None of the localizing techniques described previously are useful if the CSF leak is quiescent at the time of investigation.

The incidence of meningitis in patients with CSF leaks ranges from 2% to 88% (2,86,99–102). The wide range in incidence is a result of multiple factors, the most significant of which is the duration of leakage (86,100,102,103). Mincy (102) and Leech and Patterson (100) compared the incidence of meningitis in patients with CSF leaks continuing 7 days or less to those persisting for more than 7 days. Leech and Patterson found only a 5% incidence of meningitis in patients with CSF fistulae of less than 7 days duration, and Mincy reported a similarly low incidence of meningitis in his group of 11%. The incidence of meningitis in patients with leakage for more than 7 days in Leech and Patterson's series was 55%, and in Mincy's series was 88%. Spetzler and Wilson (103) demonstrated a 33% incidence of meningitis in persistent fistulae, and Grahne (86) found 54% of his patients with chronic CSF leakage developed meningitis.

Many studies over the past 25 years have demonstrated no benefit of prophylactic antibiotics in temporal bone fractures in the absence of CSF fistulas (100,101,104–110). The incidence of meningitis in this group is quite low. Rathore (111) pooled the data from many of these studies and found a 4% incidence of meningitis in patients with basilar skull fractures receiving prophylactic antibiotics and a 3% incidence in patients not receiving prophylactic antibiotics. Brodie and Thompson (2) demonstrated a 1% incidence of meningitis in 578 patients with temporal bone fractures and no CSF fistulae. Hoff et al. (104) conducted a prospective randomized trial assigning patients with temporal bone fractures into a prophylactic antibiotic treatment group or to a no antibiotic group. None of the patients in either group developed meningitis. All of these studies conclude that prophylactic antibiotics are not indicated, given the low incidence of meningitis in temporal bone fractures without a CSF fistula and the lack of evidence demonstrating any benefit to prophylactic antibiotics in this situation.

However, the risk of meningitis is significantly higher in patients with temporal bone fractures when CSF fistulae are present. Consequently, the role of prophylactic antibiotics must be examined in relation to this subset of trauma patients. Multiple studies over the past three decades have concluded that prophylactic antibiotics did not have a statistically significant effect on the incidence of meningitis in patients with CSF fistulae (101,103,105,106,110,112).

However, the number of patients included in the various studies was inadequate for valid statistical analysis. Reevaluation of the literature over the past 25 years using a meta-analysis revealed a statistically significant reduction in meningitis using prophylactic antibiotics in patients with CSF fistula; 320 patients were included in the analysis (113). The incidence of meningitis in patients with posttraumatic CSF fistulae treated with prophylactic antibiotics was 2.1%. In patients who did not receive prophylactic antibiotics, the incidence of meningitis was significantly higher at 8.7% ($p < .02$). Individually, none of the studies included in the meta-analysis demonstrated a statistically significant effect of prophylactic antibiotics, which points out the pitfall of statistical analysis with inadequate numbers of patients.

In addition to the inadequate numbers of patients in these prior studies, there are significant problems inherent in this type of retrospective study. How do we define adequate prophylaxis? Do 3 days of perioperative antibiotics for repair of a concomitant open femur fracture constitute adequate prophylaxis of a CSF fistula that persists for 5 days? Do therapeutic antibiotics for a concurrent infection constitute adequate prophylaxis of a CSF fistula? One very important risk factor increasing the risk of meningitis in patients with CSF fistulae is the presence of a concurrent infection. Brodie and Thompson (2) found a 20% incidence of meningitis in patients with concurrent infection and a 3% incidence of meningitis in the absence of concurrent infection. In that study, in the absence of concurrent infection, no patients receiving prophylactic antibiotics developed meningitis within the first month postinjury. Clearly, these confounding variables must be controlled in a prospective multiinstitutional study to adequately address the question of the efficacy of prophylactic antibiotics.

The most common infecting organisms in meningitis occurring in the presence of a CSF fistula reported in the literature are *Streptococcus pneumoniae* followed by *Streptococcus* and *Haemophilus influenzae* (101,114,115). Fifty-seven percent to 85% of posttraumatic fistulas that are treated conservatively cease leaking within 1 week (84,102). Because acute posttraumatic CSF fistulae are associated with a high probability of early spontaneous closure and a low incidence of meningitis, they can be treated conservatively for 7 to 10 days. This treatment includes total bed rest with elevation of the head of the bed; stool softeners; instructions to avoid nose blowing, sneezing, and straining; and repeat lumbar punctures or lumbar drain if the leak persists. All of these measures are directed at maintaining the CSF pressure gradient below the healing tensile strength of the healing barrier. Due to the increased risk of meningitis following persistent CSF fistulae, surgical closure of fistulae persisting greater than 7 to 10 days is recommended.

Closure of Cerebrospinal Fluid Fistulae

The approach chosen to close a CSF fistula is influenced by many factors, including the status of hearing in the affected

and contralateral ears, the presence of brain herniation through the tegmen, and the location of the fistula. The treatment algorithm is presented in Fig. 139.12. In a patient with a fracture of the otic capsule resulting in profound sensorineural hearing loss, obliteration of the mastoid and middle ear and canal overclosure is recommended (116,117). The ear canal, tympanic membrane, incus and malleus, and middle ear mucosa are all excised. The external auditory meatus is closed in two layers, and a complete mastoidectomy is performed. The mucosa of the eustachian tube is inverted and a muscle plug is inserted. The incus is then inserted as well, wedging the muscle into place. The eustachian tube and fracture line are covered by temporalis fascia, and the mastoid cavity and middle ear are obliterated with an abdominal fat graft.

The approach for closure of a fistula resulting from an otic capsule sparing fracture is dictated by the location of the fracture along the floor of the middle cranial fossa, the presence of brain herniation, and the status of the ossicular chain. Fistulae which occur posterolaterally in the middle cranial fossa are accessible through a complete mastoidectomy and can be repaired by sealing the mastoid cavity off from the epitympanum and middle ear by placing a temporalis fascia graft over the antrum, facial recess, and retrofacial air cell tracts. A second fascia graft is placed over the fistula and the mastoid cavity is obliterated with a fat graft.

Fistulae that occur more medially or anteriorly along the tegmen tympani or are associated with brain herniation are addressed with a combined approach. When the temporal lobe herniates through the tegmen, the damaged brain is debrided via the transmastoid approach and the remaining brain and dura are elevated back up into the middle fossa by way of the middle fossa craniotomy. Temporalis fascia is placed over the floor of the middle cranial fossa. If a bony defect is present in the tegmen, the craniotomy bone window is split or thinned with a burr and placed along the floor of the middle cranial fossa superior to the fascia to prevent subsequent prolapse. A piece of Gelfilm is inserted through the mastoid cavity and antrum and placed over the top of the ossicles in the epitympanum to avoid adhesions and postoperative conductive hearing loss.

In the case of a fistula through the tegmen tympani in a patient with an ossicular discontinuity and the absence of brain herniation, the fistula can often be closed via a transmastoid approach alone. A tragal cartilage graft is inserted superior to the superior EAC wall extending to the tympanic portion of the facial nerve. The cartilage graft seals off the epitympanum and prevents herniation of tissue into the middle ear. The epitympanum is filled with a temporalis fascia graft.

Additional techniques have been advocated by other authors. Glasscock et al. (118) have advocated an intradural as opposed to an extradural approach for large defects, arguing that a better closure can be achieved intradurally. Kveton et al. reported on the successful closure of

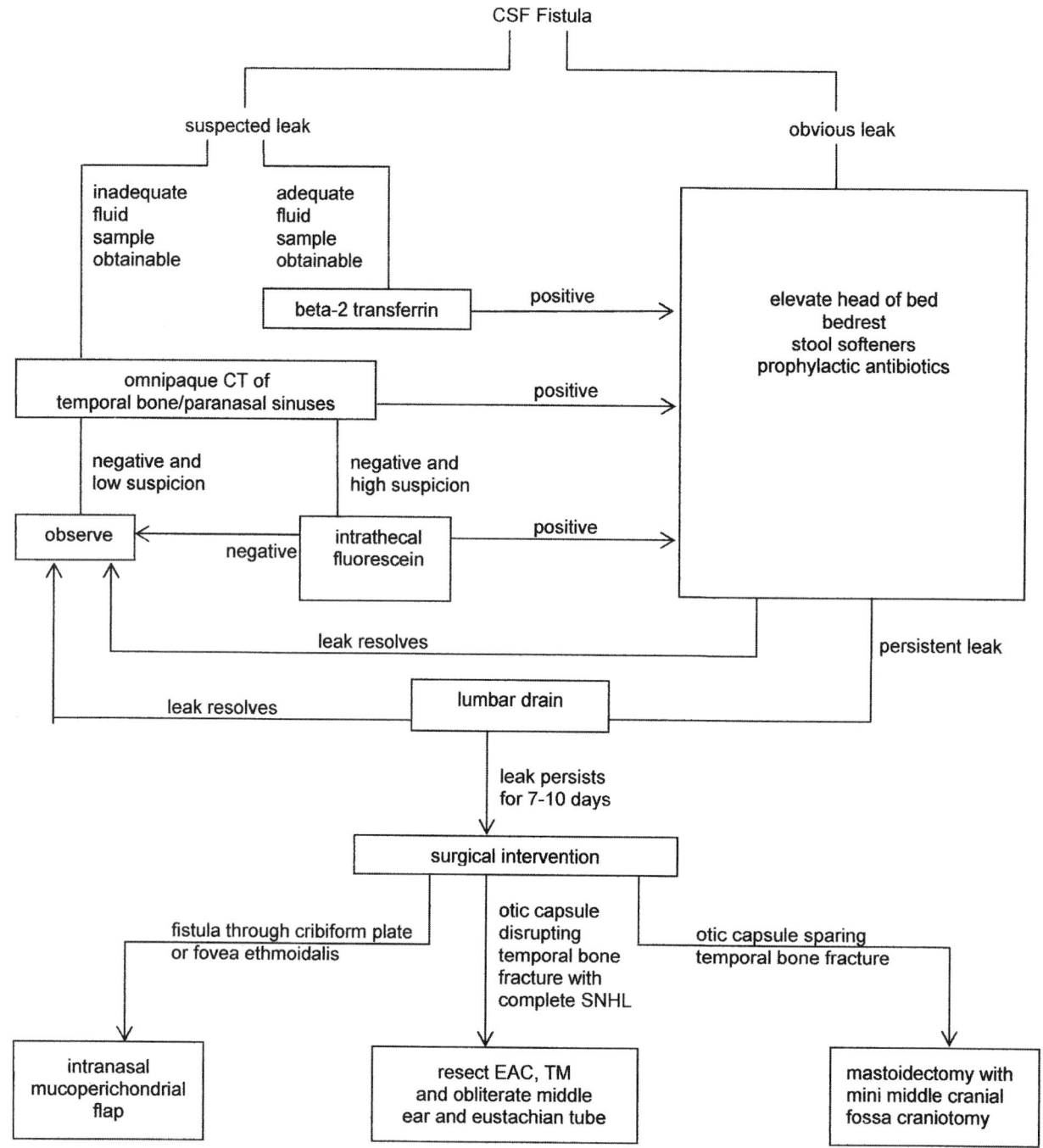

Figure 139.12 Treatment algorithm for closure of a cerebrospinal fluid fistula.

13 cases of CSF leak using hydroxyapatite cement through a transmastoid approach, in addition to reporting successful closure of 106 out of 109 temporal bone defects of all types (119,120). This approach is highly successful in closing CSF leaks following translabyrinthine removal of acoustic neuromas but care must be taken in traumatic CSF leaks where the field is much more contaminated. Placement of a foreign body in a potentially contaminated wound increases the chance of infection. One of the other potential complications of closure of tegmen CSF fistulae

with hydroxyapatite cement is conductive hearing loss, which may occur if any of the cement migrates to the ossicular chain.

There is a high risk of EAC stenosis and cholesteatoma formation when the ear canal is severely traumatized, as seen with gunshot wounds to the temporal bone (121,122). In this situation, the CSF fistulae are generally closed with resection of the EAC and tympanic membrane and obliteration of the mastoid and middle ear as described above. Extreme care is taken to avoid leaving any fragments of epithelium that may subsequently lead to cholesteatoma formation. All mucosa is removed and the eustachian tube and external meatus are closed as described previously.

Hearing Loss

Temporal bone trauma can cause a conductive hearing loss, sensorineural hearing loss, or mixed loss. Otic capsule sparing fractures extend along the roof of the EAC, often tearing the tympanic membrane in the region of the notch of Rivinus. The fracture proceeds along the tegmen tympani and in 20% of patients disrupts the ossicular chain (11). The most common injuries to the ossicular chain are subluxation of the incudostapedial joint (82%) and dislocation of the incus (57%) followed by fracture of the stapes crura (30%) (123). The majority of stapedial fractures do not occur in isolation but are associated with incus dislocations (11). Fixation of the ossicles in the epitympanum (25%) and fracture of the malleus (11%) occurs less frequently (123). One third of the patients will have multiple concomitant middle ear pathologies.

The pattern of ossicular injuries can be explained by the structural features specific to each ossicle. The malleus is well supported by the tensor tympani tendon, the epitympanic ligaments, and the tympanic membrane. The stapes, being the smallest and lightest bone in the body, is comparatively well supported by the stapedius muscle tendon and annular ligament. In contrast, the incus is relatively heavy, situated with articulating joints on both ends, and is supported by only minor posterior and superior ligaments, thereby making it the ossicle most commonly involved in posttraumatic discontinuity.

Almost universally, patients with temporal bone fractures will experience a hemotympanum with associated conductive hearing loss. Over a few days to few weeks postinjury, the middle ear will reaerate with resolution of the hearing loss that was attributable to the middle ear fluid. Factors that increase the duration of the middle ear fluid include endotracheal intubation, associated craniofacial fractures, nasogastric tube placement, and the presence of a CSF leak. Eighty percent of cases of conductive hearing loss will resolve spontaneously without the need for surgical intervention (124).

Residual conductive hearing loss following resolution of the hemotympanum and healing of the tympanic membrane suggests the possibilities of ossicular fracture or discontinuity. The indications for exploratory tympanotomy and ossicular reconstruction are conductive hearing loss greater than 30 dB that persists for more than 2 months postinjury. However, if the conductive hearing loss is in an only-hearing ear, surgery is contraindicated. The audiogram in a mixed hearing loss must be critically assessed to establish the true potential benefit of ossicular reconstruction. If the bone conduction thresholds are more than 30 dB worse than in the contralateral ear, reconstruction, even with an excellent closure of the conductive component

of the hearing loss, will provide minimal subjective improvement. In this scenario, the patient would still require a hearing aid to attain usable hearing in the surgical ear. Consequently, unless the mixed loss is profound and the patient cannot benefit preoperatively from a hearing aid, ossicular reconstruction is not recommended.

The most conducive injury for ossicular reconstruction is a dislocation of the incudostapedial joint. In this situation, an Applebaum hydroxyapatite prosthesis is inserted between the long process of the incus and capitulum of the stapes, generally resulting in near closure of the air-bone gap. Dislocation of the entire incus requires bridging the gap between the stapes superstructure and the manubrium of the malleus. A sculpted incus interposition graft is preferred in this situation, although a variety of incus strut replacement and partial ossicular replacement prostheses are available and suitable for this type of reconstruction. The incus interposition is accomplished by drilling a cup in the end of the short process of the incus that will fit over the capitulum of the stapes. The long process of the incus is removed and the body sculptured. The articular surface is fashioned to fit under the manubrium. If, in addition to the incus dislocation, the stapes superstructure is fractured, the long process of the incus is left intact and the body and short process sculptured. The superior surface of the body of the incus is fashioned to rest under the manubrium and the long process sits on the footplate. A variety of total ossicular replacement prostheses are also available for this purpose as well.

A unique problem occurs when the stapes superstructure is fractured but the incus remains connected to the malleus. These patients are good candidates for a laser stapedotomy. The hearing results following ossicular reconstruction for traumatic ossicular disruption are superior to those performed for chronic otitis media. Hough and Stuart report closure of the air-bone gap to within 10dB in 78% of patients and complete closure in 45% (123).

Otic capsule disrupting fractures typically result in severe to profound sensorineural hearing loss. In addition, bilateral temporal bone fractures can also result in bilateral profound sensorineural hearing loss (125). In addition to the risk of sensorineural hearing loss from temporal bone trauma, patients who sustain closed head injuries in general, with or without temporal bone fracture, are at risk of acute sensorineural hearing loss that can further progress with time (126). Multiple pathogenic mechanisms can contribute to posttraumatic deafness: disruption of the membranous labyrinth, avulsion or trauma to the cochlear nerve, interruption of the cochlear blood supply, hemorrhage into cochlea, and perilymphatic fistula. Another proposed mechanism is endolymphatic hydrops resulting from obstruction of the endolymphatic duct by the temporal bone fracture (127). Acoustic trauma associated with temporal bone fractures and incus dislocations frequently contributes to a sensorineural component to a mixed hearing loss; 50% of patients with traumatic incus dislocations will have at least 10 dB of sensorineural hearing loss as well, and 18% will have more than 30 dB of loss (128). The loss occurs primarily in the 2,000 to 4,000 Hz range. The prognosis for recovery of function in patients with anacusis or profound deafness is extremely poor; however, patients with moderate to severe loss may have some recovery (124,129). Patients who are experiencing progressive or fluctuating sensorineural hearing loss, suggestive of a possible underlying perilymphatic fistula, may benefit from exploration and patching of the fistula (130).

Cholesteatoma and External Auditory Canal Stenosis

Cholesteatoma formation may occur many years after a temporal bone fracture (121,131). There are four pathogenic mechanisms responsible for posttraumatic cholesteatoma formation: (a) epithelial entrapment in the fracture line, (b) in-growth of epithelium through the unhealed fracture line or rent in the tympanic membrane, (c) traumatic implantation of tympanic membrane skin into the middle ear, and (d) trapping of epithelium medial to a stenosis of the EAC. The typical location for cholesteatoma resulting from epithelium trapped within the fracture line is in the epitympanum and antrum. The fracture line along the posterior superior canal wall and scutum expands and then closes trapping the canal skin. As the trapped skin grows, it expands into the epitympanum and antrum forming a cholesteatoma. The in-growth of epithelium through a displaced fracture line may also extend into the same region. Traumatic implantation of tympanic membrane skin will result in cholesteatoma formation within the mesotympanum. Blast injuries can result in displacement of keratinizing stratified squamous epithelium into the mastoid air cells, mesotympanum, epitympanum, and even intracranially (132). The fourth mechanism of cholesteatoma formation, trapping of epithelium medial to an EAC stenosis, results in a canal cholesteatoma. Posttraumatic canal cholesteatomas are the most preventable by careful follow-up, debridement, and stenting when narrowing progresses. Early intervention with stenting at the onset of the stenosis can effectively prevent a problem that is much more difficult to address once the stenosis is mature. The ear canal can be dilated with the insertion of increasing numbers of Merocel sponge packs (i.e., Oto-wick, Schindler pack) saturated with antibiotic solution, replaced every few days. Once the canal is adequately dilated, a larger Merocel sponge is inserted to maintain the lumen. A large vented custom ear mold is occasionally required to maintain the lumen in the long term following severe canal injuries. The mold is used throughout the day for 3 to 6 months. When the stenosis is complete and dilation is not possible, a canalplasty and possible tympanoplasty are required. A lateral stenosis of the EAC should not be allowed to persist, even if completely benign in appearance,

because of the very high probability of cholesteatoma formation.

Posttraumatic cholesteatoma involving the attic, antrum, or mastoid air cells will often grow for many years prior to detection. Until the cholesteatoma involves the ossicular chain with resultant conductive hearing loss, grows laterally causing effacement of the posterior external auditory canal or postauricular sulcus eroding into the labyrinth causing vertigo or sensorineural hearing loss, compresses the facial nerve resulting in facial paresis, or grows into the middle ear cleft and can be visualized on physical examination, the growth will go undetected.

Vascular Injuries

Injuries to the intratemporal carotid artery are rare but potentially life-threatening complications. Bloody otorrhea is a common presentation in temporal bone fractures, and the ear canal is not usually packed initially unless significant hemorrhage is present and must be controlled. In such cases, injury to the petrous portion of the carotid artery should be suspected and the patient taken immediately to either the operating room for carotid ligation or the angiography suite for balloon occlusion.

CT angiography or MR angiography is indicated in patients with focal transient or persistent neurologic deficits. In patients with significant hemorrhage from the ear or nose or with rapid neurologic deterioration, traditional interventional angiography is indicated for confirmation of carotid injury as well as immediate therapeutic intervention if necessary.

HIGHLIGHTS

- A newer classification system of temporal bone fracture emphasizes functional outcome: otic capsule sparing versus disrupting injuries.
- Assessment of facial nerve function as soon as possible facilitates clinical decision making.
- The majority of temporal bone fractures are incurred in auto accidents; multiple concurrent injuries are the rule and must be evaluated.
- The most common complications of temporal bone fractures are facial nerve injury, cerebrospinal fluid leak, hearing loss, vertigo, cholesteatoma formation, and ear canal stenosis.
- Delayed-onset facial paralysis merits steroid administration and observation.
- Immediate-onset facial paralysis requires nerve stimulation. If the nerve will stimulate, observation is recommended. If the nerve will not stimulate, the nerve should be explored.
- The use of prophylactic antibiotics in this setting is controversial.
- Most posttraumatic cerebrospinal fluid leaks close spontaneously. Surgical closure is required for persistent fistula.

REFERENCES

1. Makashima K, Sobel SF, Snow JB Jr. Histopathologic correlates of otoneurologic manifestations following head trauma. *Laryngoscope* 1976;86:1303–1314.
2. Brodie HA, Thompson TC. Management of complications from 820 temporal bone fractures. *Am J Otol* 1997;18:188–197.
3. Nageris B, Hansen MC, Lavelle WG, et al. Temporal bone fractures. *Am J Emerg Med* 1995;12:211–214.
4. Virapongse C, Bhimani S, Sarwar M. Radiography of the abnormal ear. In: Taveras JM, Ferrucci JT, eds. *Radiology: diagnosis-imaging-intervention*, Vol. III. Philadelphia: JB Lippincott, 1987;9:1–19.
5. Lee D, Honrado C, Har-El G. Pediatric temporal bone fractures. *Laryngoscope* 1998;108:816–821.
6. McGuirt WF Jr. Stool SE. Temporal bone fractures in children: a review with emphasis on long-term sequelae. *Clin Pediatr (Phila)* 1992;31:12–18.
7. Williams WT, Ghorayeb BY, Yeakley JW. Pediatric temporal bone fractures. *Laryngoscope* 1992;102:600–603.
8. Glarner H, Meuli M, Hof E, et al. Management of petrous bone fractures in children: analysis of 127 cases. *J Trauma* 1994;36:198–201.
9. Ort S, Beus K, Isaacson J. Pediatric temporal bone fractures in a rural population. *Otolaryngol Head Neck Surg* 2004;131:433–437.
10. Exadaktylos AK, Sclabas GM, Nuyens M, et al. The clinical correlation of temporal bone fractures and spiral computed tomographic scan: a prospective and consecutive study at a level I trauma center. *J Trauma* 2003;55:704–706.
11. Cannon CR, Jahrsdoerfer RA. Temporal bone fractures: review of 90 cases. *Arch Otolaryngol* 1983;109:285–288.
12. Ghorayeb BY, Rafie JJ. Fractures of the temporal bone. An evaluation of 123 cases. *J Radiol* 1989;70:703–710.
13. Tos M. Course of and sequelae to 248 petrosal fractures. *Acta Otolaryngol* 1973;75:353–354.
14. Griffin JE, Altenau MM, Schaefer SO. Bilateral longitudinal temporal bone fractures: a retrospective review of seventeen cases. *Laryngoscope* 1979;89:1432–1435.
15. Messerer O. *Uber Elasticitat und Festigkeit der Menschlichen Knochen*. Stuttgart, Germany: Verlag der JG Cotta Oschen Buchhandlung,, 1880.
16. Travis LW, Stalnaker RL, Melvin JW. Impact trauma of human temporal bone. *J Trauma* 1977;17:761–766.
17. Yoganandan N, Pintar FA, Sances AJ, et al. Biomechanics of skull fracture. *J Neurotrauma* 1995;12:659–668.
18. Yoganandan N, Pintar FA. Biomechanics of temporo-parietal skull fracture. *Clin Biomech (Bristol, Avon)* 2004;19:225–239.
19. Perlman HB. Process of healing in injuries to the capsule of labyrinth. *Arch Otolaryngol* 1939;29:287–305.
20. Pollak AM, Pauw BKH, Marion MS. Temporal bone histopathology: resident's quiz. *Am J Otol* 1991;12:56–58.
21. Sudhoff H, Linthicum Jr FH. Temporal bone fracture and latent meningitis: temporal bone histopathology study of the month. *Otol Neurotol* 2003;24:521–522.
22. Ulrich K. Verletzungen des Gehororgans bei Schadel-Basisfrakturen. *Acta Otolaryngol (Stockh)* 1926;S4:1–50.
23. Gurdjian ES, Webster JE, Lissner HR. Deformation of the skull in head injury studied by stresscoat technique. *Surg Gynecol Obstet* 1946;83:219–233.
24. Ghorayeb BY, Yeakley JW. Temporal bone fractures: longitudinal or oblique? The cases for oblique temporal bone fractures. *Laryngoscope* 1992;102:129–134.
25. Dahiya R, Keller JD, Litofsky NS, et al. Temporal bone fractures: otic capsule sparing versus otic capsule violating clinical and radiographic considerations. *J Trauma* 1999;47:1079–1083.
26. Kelly KE, Tami TA. Temporal bone and skull trauma. In: Jackler RK, Brackmann DE, eds. *Neurotology*. St. Louis: Mosby, 1994:1127–1147.
27. Ishman SL, Friedland DR. Temporal bone fractures: traditional classification and clinical relevance. *Laryngoscope* 2004;114:1734–1741.
28. Wiet RJ, Valvassori GE, Kotsanis CA, et al. Temporal bone fractures. *Am J Otol* 1985;6:207–215.
29. Tos M. Course of and sequelae to 248 petrosal fractures. *Acta Otolaryngol (Stockh)* 1973;75:253–254.
30. Healy GB. Hearing loss and vertigo secondary to head injury. *N Engl J Med* 1982;306:1029–1031.
31. Fredrickson JM, Griffith AW, Lindsay JR. Transverse fractures of the temporal bone. *Arch Otolaryngol* 1963;78:770–784.
32. Fisch U. Facial paralysis in fractures of the petrous bone. *Laryngoscope* 1974;84:2141–2154.
33. Vrabec JT. Otic capsule fracture with preservation of hearing and delayed-onset facial paralysis. *Int J Pediatr Otorhinolaryngol* 2001;58(2):173–177.
34. Schuknecht HF. Mechanism of inner ear injury from blows to the head. *Ann Otol Rhinol Laryngol* 1969;78:253–262.
35. Dix MR, Hallpike CS. The pathology symptomatology and diagnosis of certain common disorders of the vestibular system. *Proc R Soc Med* 1952;45:341–354.
36. Ylikoski J, Palva T, Sanna M. Dizziness after head trauma: clinical and morphologic findings. *Am J Otol* 1982;3:343–352.
37. Swartz JD. Temporal bone trauma. *Semin Ultrasound CT MR* 2001;22:219–228.
38. Morgan WE, Coker NJ, Jenkins HA. Histopathology of temporal bone fractures: implications for cochlear implantation. *Laryngoscope* 1994;104:426–432.
39. Casselman JW. Temporal bone imaging. *Neuroimaging Clin North Am* 1996;6:265–289.
40. Jang CH, Kim YH. Sudden hearing loss in intralabyrinthine haemorrhage in a child. *J Laryngol Otol* 2004;118:450–452.
41. Gross M, Ben-Yaakov A, Goldfarb A, et al. Pneumolabyrinth: an unusual finding in a temporal bone fracture. *Int J Pediatr Otorhinolaryngol* 2003;67:553–555.
42. Resnick DK, Subach BR, Marion, DW. The significance of carotid canal involvement in basilar cranial fractures. *Neurosurgery* 1997;40:1177–1181.
43. Kahn JB, Stewart MG, Diaz-Marchan PJ. Acute temporal bone trauma: utility of high-resolution computed tomography. *Am J Otol* 2000;21:743–752.
44. Abrunhosa J, Goncalves P, dos Santos JG, et al. Traumatic porencephalic cyst and cholesteatoma of the ear. *J Laryngol Otol* 2000;114:864–866.
45. Ozveren MF, Uchida K, Erol FS, et al. Isolated abducens nerve paresis associated with incomplete Horner's syndrome caused by petrous apex fracture—case report and anatomical study. *Neurol Med Chir (Tokyo)* 2001;41:494–498.
46. Barron RP, Kainulainen VT, Gusenbauer AW, et al. Fracture of glenoid fossa and traumatic dislocation of mandibular condyle into middle cranial fossa. *Oral Surg Oral Med Oral Pathol Oral Radiol Endod* 2002;93:640–642.
47. Lee GY, Halcrow S. Petrous to petrous fracture associated with bilateral abducens and facial nerve palsies: a case report. *J Trauma* 2002;53:583–585.
48. Spanio S, Baciliero U, Fornezza U, et al. Intracranial dislocation of the mandibular condyle: report of two cases and review of the literature. *Br J Oral Maxillofac Surg* 2002;40:253–255.
49. van der Linden WJ. Dislocation of the mandibular condyle into the middle cranial fossa: report of a case with 5 year CT follow-up. *Int J Oral Maxillofac Surg* 2003;32:215–218.
50. Darrouzet V, Duclos JY, Liguoro D, et al. Management of facial paralysis resulting from temporal bone fractures: our experience in 115 cases. *Otolaryngol Head Neck Surg* 2001;125:77–84.
51. McKennan KX, Chole RA. Facial paralysis in temporal bone trauma. *Am J Otol* 1992;13:167–172.
52. Turner JWA. Facial palsy in closed head injuries. *Lancet* 1944;246:756–757.
53. Maiman OJ, Cusick JF, Anderson AJ, et al. Nonoperative management of traumatic facial nerve palsy. *J Trauma* 1985;25:644–648.
54. May M. Trauma to the facial nerve. *Otolaryngol Clin North Am* 1983;16:661–670.
55. Fisch U. Prognostic value of electrical tests in acute facial paralysis. *Am J Otol* 1984;5:494–498.
56. Sunderland S. Some anatomical and pathophysiological data relevant to facial nerve injury and repair. In: Fisch U, eds. *Facial nerve surgery*. New York: Aesculapius, 1977:47–61.
57. May M, Harvey JE, Marovitz WF, et al. The prognostic accuracy of the maximal stimulation test compared with that of the nerve excitability test in Bell's palsy. *Laryngoscope* 1971;81:931–938.
58. Fisch U. Surgery for Bell's palsy. *Arch Otolaryngol* 1981;107:1–11.
59. May M, Klein SR, Taylor FH. Idiopathic (Bell's) facial palsy: natural history defies steroid or surgical treatment. *Laryngoscope* 1985;95:406–409.

60. Fisch U. Management of intratemporal facial nerve injuries. *J Laryngol Otol* 1980;94:129–134.
61. Sillman JS, Niparko JK, Lee SS, et al. Prognostic value of evoked and standard electromyography in acute facial paralysis. *Otolaryngol Head Neck Surg* 1992;107:377–381.
62. May M, Blumenthal F, Klein SR. Acute Bell's palsy: prognostic value of evoked electromyography, maximal stimulation, and other electrical tests. *Am J Otol* 1983;5:1–7.
63. Sittel C, Stennert E. Prognostic value of electromyography in acute peripheral facial nerve palsy. *Otol Neurotol* 2001;22:100–104.
64. Lambert PR, Brackmann DE. Facial paralysis in longitudinal temporal bone fractures: a review of 26 cases. *Laryngoscope* 1984;94:1022–1026.
65. Coker NJ, Kendall KA, Jenkins HA, et al. Traumatic intratemporal facial nerve injury: management rationale for preservation of function. *Otolaryngol Head Neck Surg* 1987;97:262–269.
66. Kamerer DO. Intratemporal facial nerve injuries. *Otolaryngol Head Neck Surg* 1982;90:612–615.
67. Yeoh TL, Mahmud R, Saim L. Surgical intervention in traumatic facial nerve paralysis. *Med J Malaysia* 2003;58:432–436.
68. Chang JCY, Cass S. Management of facial nerve injury due to temporal bone trauma. *Am J Otol* 1999;20:96–114.
69. Sargent EW, Kartush JM, Graham MD. Meatal facial nerve decompression in acoustic neuroma resection. *Am J Otol* 1995;16:457–464.
70. Fisch U. Facial paralysis in fractures of the petrous bone. *Laryngoscope* 1974;84:2141–2154.
71. May M. Total facial nerve exploration: transmastoid, extralabyrinthine, and subtemporal indications and results. *Laryngoscope* 1979;89:906–917.
72. Goin OW. Proximal intratemporal facial nerve in Bell's palsy surgery: a study correlating anatomical and surgical findings. *Laryngoscope* 1982;92:263–271.
73. Yanagihara N. Transmastoid decompression of the facial nerve in temporal bone fracture. *Otolaryngol Head Neck Surg* 1982;90:616–621
74. McCabe BF. Facial nerve grafting. *Plast Reconstr Surg* 1970;45:70–75.
75. Barrs DM. Facial nerve trauma: optimal timing for repair. *Laryngoscope* 1991;101:835–848.
76. Fisch U. Current surgical treatment of intratemporal facial palsy. *Clin Plast Surg* 1979;178:347–361.
77. Quaranta A, Campobasso G, Piazza F, et al. Facial nerve paralysis in temporal bone fractures: outcomes after late decompression surgery. *Acta Otolaryngol* 2001;121:652–655.
78. House WF. Surgical exposure tot he internal auditory canal and its contents through the middle cranial fossa. *Laryngoscope* 1961;71:1363–1385.
79. Glasscock M. Middle fossa approach to the temporal bone. *Arch Otolaryngol* 1969;90:41–57.
80. Fisch U. Transtemporal surgery of the internal auditory canal. *Adv Otorhinolaryngol* 1970;17:202–239.
81. Portmann M, Cohandon F, Castel JP, et al. [Neurotomy of the 8th cranial pair via the temporal fossa]. *Rev Laryngol Otol Rhinol (Bord)* 1969;90:700–715.
82. Garcia-Ibanez E, Garcia-Ibanez JL. Middle fossa vestibular neurectomy: a report of 373 cases. *Otolaryngol Head Neck Surg* 1980;88:486–490.
83. Schuknecht HF, Gulya AJ. *Anatomy of the temporal bone with surgical implications.* Philadelphia: Lea & Febiger, 1986.
84. Lewin W. Cerebrospinal fluid rhinorrhea in nonmissile head injuries. *Clin Neurosurg* 1964;12:237–252.
85. Hirsch D. Successful closure of cerebrospinal fluid rhinorrhea by endonasal surgery. *Arch Otolaryngol* 1952;56:1–12.
86. Grahne B. Traumatic cranionasal fistulas persistent cerebrospinal fluid rhinorrhea and their repair with frontal sinus osteoplasty. *Acta Otolaryngol* 1970;70:392–400.
87. Kogoy J, Trieff NM, Winkelmann P, et al. Glucose in nasal secretion: diagnostic significance. *Arch Otolaryngol* 1972;95:225–229.
88. Meurman OH, Irjala K, Suonpaa J, et al. A new method for the identification of cerebrospinal fluid leakage. *Acta Otolaryngol* 1979;87:366–369.
89. Sloman, AJ, Kelly RH. Transferrin allelic variants may cause false positives in the detection of cerebrospinal fluid fistulae. *Clin Chem* 1993;39:1444–1445.
90. Felgenhauer K, Schadlich HJ, Nekic M. Beta-trace protein as marker for cerebrospinal fluid fistula. *Klin Wochenschr* 1987;65:764–768.
91. Bachmann G, Nekic M, Michel O. Clinical experience with beta-trace protein as a marker for cerebrospinal fluid. *Ann Otol Rhinol Laryngol* 2000;109:1099–1102.
92. Petereit HF, Bachmann G, Nekic M, et al. A new nephelometric assay for beta-trace protein (prostaglandin D synthase) as an indicator of liquorrhea. *J Neurol Neurosurg Psychiatry* 2001;71:347–351.
93. Arrer E, Meco C, Oberascher G, et al. Beta-trace protein as a marker for cerebrospinal fluid rhinorrhea. *Clin Chem* 2002;48:939–941.
94. Stone JA, Castillo M, Neelon B, et al. Evaluation of CSF leaks: high-resolution CT compared with contrast-enhanced CT and radionuclide cisternography. *Am J Neuroradiol* 1999;20:706–712.
95. Briant TDR, Snell D. Diagnosis of cerebrospinal rhinorrhea and the rhinologic approach to its repair. *Laryngoscope* 1967;77:1390–1409.
96. Charles DA, Snell D. Cerebrospinal fluid rhinorrhea. *Laryngoscope* 1979;89:822–826.
97. Calcaterra TC. Extracranial surgical repair of cerebrospinal rhinorrhea. *Ann Otol* 1980;89:108–116
98. Morley TP, Wortzman G. The importance of the lateral extensions of the sphenoidal sinus in post-traumatic cerebrospinal rhinorrhea and meningitis. *J Neurosurg* 1965;22:326–332.
99. Hughes GB, Glasscock ME III, Hays JW, et al. Cerebrospinal fluid leaks and meningitis following acoustic tumor surgery. *Otolaryngol Head Neck Surg* 1982;90:117–125.
100. Leech PI, Paterson A. Conservative and operative management of cerebrospinal fluid leakage after closed head injury. *Lancet* 1973;1(7811):1013–1015.
101. MacGee EE, Cauthen JC, Brackett CE. Meningitis following acute traumatic cerebrospinal fluid fistula. *J Neurosurg* 1970;33:312–316.
102. Mincy JE. Post-traumatic cerebrospinal fluid fistula of the frontal fossa. *J Trauma* 1966;6:618–622.
103. Spetzler RF, Wilson CB. Management of recurrent CSF rhinorrhea of the middle and posterior fossa. *J Neurosurg* 1978;49:393–397.
104. Hoff JT, Brewin A, Sang H. Antibiotics for basilar skull fractures. *J Neurosurg* 1976;44:649.
105. Zrebeet HA, Huang PS. Prophylactic antibiotics in the treatment of fractures at the base of the skull. *Del Med J* 1986;58:741–748.
106. Frazee RC, Mucha P, Farnell MB, et al. Meningitis after basilar skull fracture. *Postgrad Med* 1988;83:267–274.
107. Einhorn A, Mizrahi EM. Basilar skull fractures in children. *Am J Dis Child* 1978;132:1121–1124.
108. Hellings TS, Evans LL, Fowler DL, et al. Infectious complications in patients with severe head injury. *J Trauma* 1988;28:1575–1577.
109. Ignelzi RJ, VanderArk GD. Analysis of the treatment of basilar skull fractures with and without antibiotics. *J Neurosurg* 1975;43:75–85.
110. Dagi TF, Meyer FB, Poletti CA. The incidence and prevention of meningitis after basilar skull fracture. *Am J Emerg Med* 1983;3:295–298.
111. Rathore MH. Do prophylactic antibiotics prevent meningitis after basilar skull fracture. *Pediatr Infect Dis J* 1991;10:87–88.
112. Klastersky J, Sadeghi M, Brihaye J. Antimicrobial prophylaxis in patients with rhinorrhea or otorrhea: a double blind study. *Surg Neurol* 1976;6:111–114.
113. Brodie HA. Prophylactic antibiotics for post-traumatic cerebrospinal fluid fistulae. A meta-analysis. *Arch Otolaryngol Head Neck Surg* 1997;123:749–752.
114. Applebaum E. Meningitis following trauma to the head and face. *JAMA* 1960;173:1818–1822.
115. Kaufman BA, Tunkel AR, Pryor JC, et al. Meningitis in the neurosurgical patient. *Infect Dis Clin North Am* 1990;4:677–701.
116. Kveton JF. Obliteration of the mastoid and middle ear for severe trauma to the temporal bone. *Laryngoscope* 1987;97:1385–1387.
117. Coker NJ, Jenkins HA, Fisch U. Obliteration of the middle ear and mastoid cleft in subtotal petrosectomy. Indications, technique and results. *Ann Otol Rhinol Laryngol* 1986;95:5–11.
118. Glasscock ME III, Dickins JRE, Jackson CG, et al. Surgical management of brain tissue herniation into the middle ear and mastoid. *Laryngoscope* 1979;89:1743–1754.

119. Kveton JF, Goravalingappa R. Elimination of temporal bone cerebrospinal fluid otorrhea using hydroxyapatite cement. *Laryngoscope* 2000;110:988–990.

120. Kveton JF, Coelho DH. Hydroxyapatite cement in temporal bone surgery: a 10 year experience. *Laryngoscope* 2004;114:33–37.

121. McKennan KX, Chole RA. Post-traumatic cholesteatoma. *Laryngoscope* 1989;99:779–782.

122. Kronenberg J, Ben-Shoshan J, Modan M, et al. Blast injury and cholesteatoma. *Am J Otol* 1988;9:127–130.

123. Hough JVD, Stuart WD. Middle ear injuries in skull trauma. *Laryngoscope* 1968;78:899–937.

124. Tos M. Prognosis of hearing loss in temporal bone fractures. *Laryngol Otol* 1971;85:1147–1159.

125. Atkin G, Watkins L, Rich P. Bilateral sensorineural hearing loss complicating basal skull fracture. *Br J Neurosurg* 2002;16:597–600.

126. Bergemalm PO. Progressive hearing loss after closed head injury: a predictable outcome? *Acta Otolaryngol* 2003;123:836–845.

127. Rizvi SS, Gibbin KP. Effect of transverse temporal bone fracture on the fluid compartment of the inner ear. *Ann Otol Rhinol Laryngol* 1979;88:741–748.

128. Dommerby H, Tos M. Sensorineural hearing loss in post-traumatic incus dislocation. *Arch Otolaryngol* 1983;109:257–261.

129. Podoshin L, Fradis M. Hearing loss after head injury. *Arch Otolaryngol* 1975;101:15–18.

130. Lyos AT, Marsh MA, Jenkins HA, Coker NJ. Progressive hearing loss after transverse temporal bone fracture. *Arch Otolaryngol Head Neck Surg* 1995;121:795–799.

131. Freeman J. Temporal bone fractures and cholesteatoma. *Ann Otol Rhinol Laryngol* 1983;92:558–560.

132. Goldfarb A, Eliashar R, Gross M, Elidan J. Middle cranial fossa cholesteatoma following blast trauma. *Ann Otol Rhino Laryngol* 2001;110:1084–1086.

Cholesteatoma

140

Ted A. Meyer   *Chester L. Strunk, Jr.*   *Paul R. Lambert*

Cholesteatomas are cystlike, expansile lesions of the temporal bone lined by stratified squamous epithelium that contain desquamated keratin. They most frequently involve the middle ear and mastoid, but they may develop anywhere within the pneumatized portions of the temporal bone. They may be congenital (infrequently) or acquired.

The accumulation of keratin may cause infection, otorrhea, bone destruction, hearing loss, facial nerve paralysis, a labyrinthine fistula, and intracranial complications such as epidural and subdural abscesses, parenchymal brain abscesses, meningitis, and thrombophlebitis of the dural venous sinuses.

Cholesteatoma is a misnomer originally coined by Johannes Mueller in 1838 when he described "layered pearly tumor of fat, which was distinguished from other fat tumors by the biliary fat or cholesterin that is interspersed among the sheets of polyhedral cells" (1). Cholesteatomas do not contain fat, and they do not usually contain cholesterin. Nevertheless, the term remains, despite a more appropriate term suggested by Schuknecht: keratoma.

The matrix of a cholesteatoma is composed of fully differentiated squamous epithelium resting on connective tissue. The deeper layers of the epithelium of a cholesteatoma matrix show activity in the form of downgrowths into the underlying connective tissue. There is always a layer of granulation tissue in contact with bone. This layer of granulation tissue elaborates various enzymes such as collagenase resulting in bone destruction.

CONGENITAL CHOLESTEATOMA

Congenital cholesteatoma is defined by Derlacki and Clemis (2) as an embryonic rest of epithelial tissue in the ear without tympanic membrane perforation and without a history of ear infection. Levenson et al. (3,4) have modified the definition of a congenital cholesteatoma to include a normal pars flaccida and pars tensa, no history of prior otorrhea, and no history of prior otologic procedures. Prior episodes of otitis media without otorrhea are not criteria for excluding congenital origin. Two thirds of the middle ear congenital cholesteatomas are seen as a white mass in the anterior-superior quadrant (Fig. 140.1). They may also be found within the tympanic membrane and in the petrous apex. The mean age at presentation for a congenital middle ear cholesteatoma is 4.5 years, with a male to female preponderance of 3:1 (4).

The pathogenesis of congenital cholesteatomas is incompletely understood. In a review of the development of the epibranchial organs, Teed (5) noted an ectodermal epithelial thickening that developed in proximity of the geniculate ganglion, medial to the neck of the malleus. This mass of epithelial cells soon undergoes involution to become mature middle ear lining. Teed believed that if involution failed to take place, this formation could be the source of a congenital cholesteatoma. In pursuit of this theory, Michaels (6,7) undertook a review of fetal human temporal bones and identified a squamous cell tuft present from 10 to 33 weeks of gestation in 37 of 68 specimens studied. He termed this structure the *epidermoid formation* and noted it to be located in the anterosuperior wall of the developing middle ear cleft. Failure of the epidermoid formation to involute could be the basis for the development of cholesteatomas in the anterior mesotympanum (8–10). Other investigators implicate ectodermal migration or even metaplasia of the middle ear mucosa in the pathogenesis of congenital cholesteatomas (11,12).

ACQUIRED CHOLESTEATOMA

Acquired middle ear cholesteatomas come in two varieties: primary or retraction pocket cholesteatoma and secondary cholesteatoma. Cholesteatomas that arise from retraction

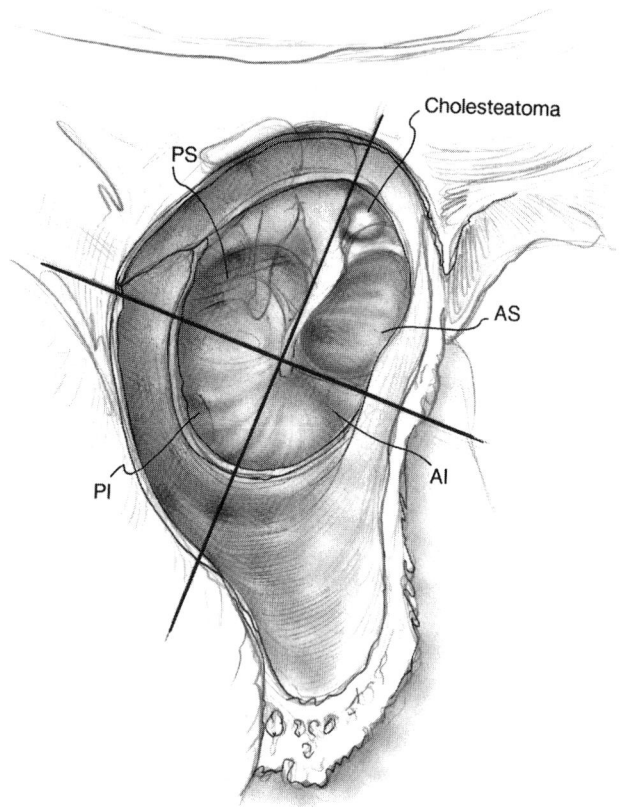

Figure 140.1 Congenital cholesteatoma of the anterior-superior quadrant. AI, anterior inferior; AS, anterior superior; PI, posterior inferior; PS, posterior superior.

pockets are known as primary acquired cholesteatomas on the basis that infection has not given rise to the cholesteatoma. Several theories have been advanced to explain the formation of primary acquired or attic retraction cholesteatomas, including invagination of the pars flaccida, basal cell hyperplasia, otitis media with effusion, and perforation of the pars flaccida membrane with epithelial ingrowth (Table 140.1). Patients with cleft palates are particularly prone to the development of primary acquired attic cholesteatomas (13–17).

The invagination theory is supported by the observations of Aschoff in 1897 and Wittmaack in 1933 (18).

TABLE 140.1

PATHOGENESIS OF CHOLESTEATOMAS

Primary acquired cholesteatomas
  Invagination theory
  Basal cell hyperplasia theory
  Otitis media with effusion theory
  Epithelial invasion theory

Secondary acquired cholesteatomas
  Implantation theory
  Metaplasia theory
  Epithelial invasion theory

They proposed that an infantile sterile otitis media neonatorum or nonbacterial otitis media develops soon after birth. Before it has had time to resorb, a permanent fibrosis and thickening of the embryonic subepithelial tympanic connective tissue occurs resulting in blockage of the attic causing a localized negative pressure with retraction of the pars flaccida. The fibrosis and thickening in the attic blocks the normal process of pneumatization of the epitympanum and antrum and decreases the pneumatization of the mastoid process and petrous portions of the temporal bone throughout the patient's life. This small dimplelike retraction of the pars flaccida that cannot be reduced by inflation of the eustachian tube is the first stage in the development of an attic cholesteatoma.

A second method by which a small retraction pocket may develop is from longstanding otitis media with effusion (Fig. 140.2). Bluestone and Klein (13) demonstrated that in children with attic retractions, the eustachian tube constricts rather than dilates with swallowing. This results in impaired ventilation of the middle ear and mastoid air cell system and fluctuating or sustained high negative middle ear pressures. Negative middle ear pressure caused by eustachian tube dysfunction can result in retraction of the pars flaccida and collection of desquamated debris.

Like primary acquired cholesteatomas, several pathogenic mechanisms may contribute to the formation of secondary acquired cholesteatomas (Table 140.1). The implantation theory, the metaplasia theory, and the epithelial invasion theory have all been advanced as possible mechanisms involved in cholesteatoma formation. The implantation theory describes the formation of a cholesteatoma by the iatrogenic implantation of skin into the middle ear or eardrum as a result of surgery, a foreign body, or a blast injury. Cholesteatomas may develop secondary to a myringotomy for ventilating tube placement or a tympanoplasty procedure. They occur as a result of epithelial migration or displacement through the myringotomy or from the displacement of a flap of the tympanic membrane into the middle ear at the time of a tympanoplasty. Secondary acquired cholesteatomas are also thought to arise from a perforation as a result of acute necrotic otitis media in childhood (19).

The metaplasia theory describes the transformation of columnar epithelium to keratinized stratified squamous epithelium secondary to chronic or recurrent otitis media. Support for this theory comes from changes that occur in the bronchi in the face of chronic irritation and infection. However, metaplasia is not thought to be a significant cause of cholesteatoma in humans (20). The epithelial invasion theory involves the invasion of the middle ear by skin from the meatal wall of the outer drum surface through a marginal perforation or an attic perforation (21). This is supported by experimental evidence demonstrating that epithelial cells migrate along a surface until they encounter another epithelial surface, at which point they stop migrating; this is known as contact inhibition.

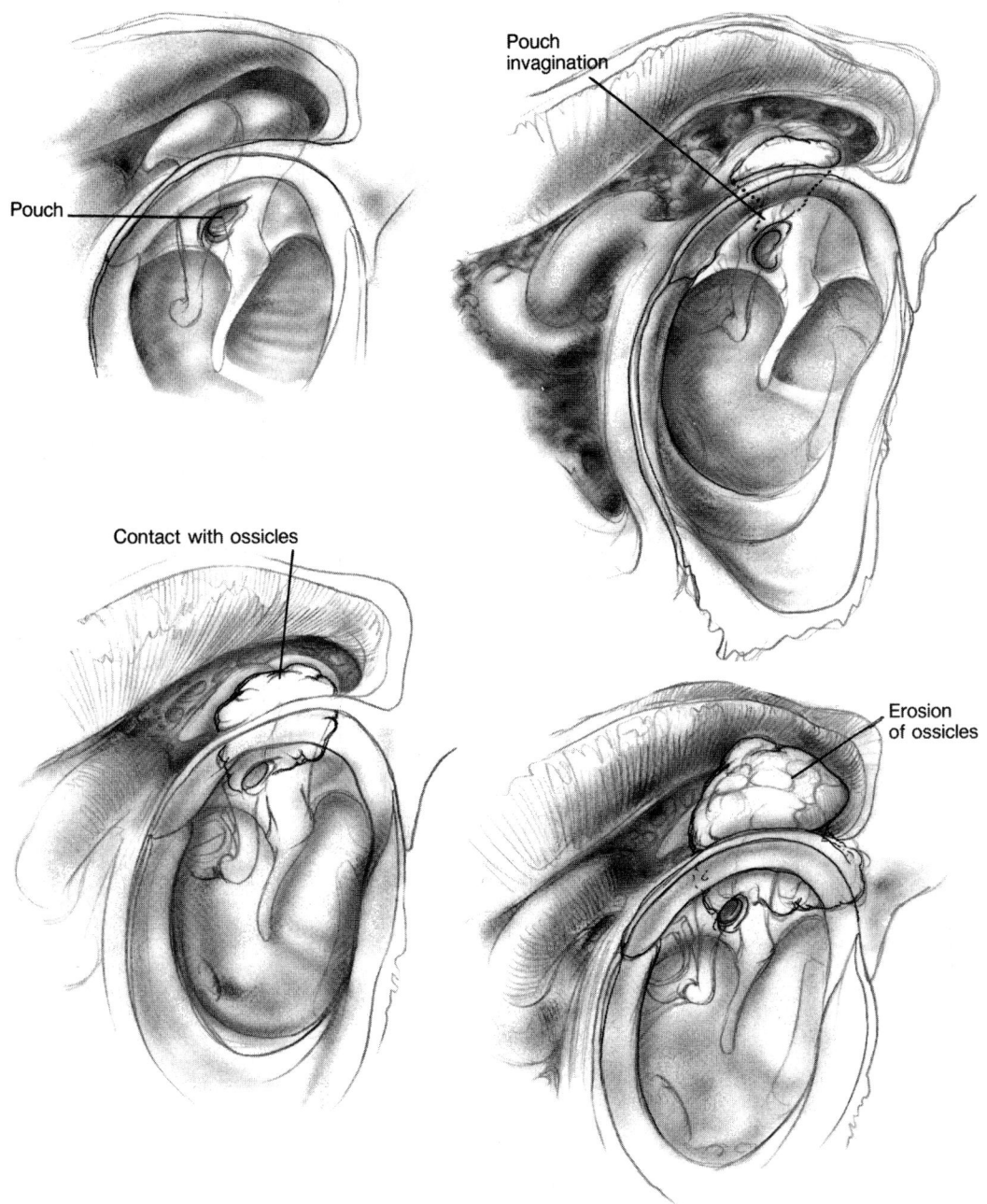

Figure 140.2 Evolution of an attic cholesteatoma.

If the middle ear mucosa were destroyed by infection, then this would allow for epithelial migration from a marginal perforation. This is the generally accepted theory for the formation of secondary acquired cholesteatomas of the posterior-superior tympanic membrane.

A unique feature that cholesteatoma and tympanic membrane epithelium have in common is migration. No other epithelium tested, including skin, vocal cord, and oral epithelium, has shown the locomotion present with tympanic membrane epithelium and cholesteatoma (22). Once a retraction pocket develops, the epithelial migratory pattern is altered and keratin accumulates. This is the second stage in

the development of a cholesteatoma. The sac slowly enlarges by accumulation of keratin and other debris until the walls of the attic are reached. Once this point is reached, bone resorption occurs. Three factors appear to be involved in the process of bony resorption: (a) *mechanical,* related to pressure generated by the expansion of cholesteatoma as it accumulates increasing amounts of keratin and purulent debris (23–25); (b) *biochemical,* due to bacterial elements (endotoxins), products of the host's granulation tissue (collagenase, acid hydrolases), and substances related to the cholesteatoma itself (growth factors, cytokines) (26–34); and (c) *cellular,* predominantly induced by osteoclastic

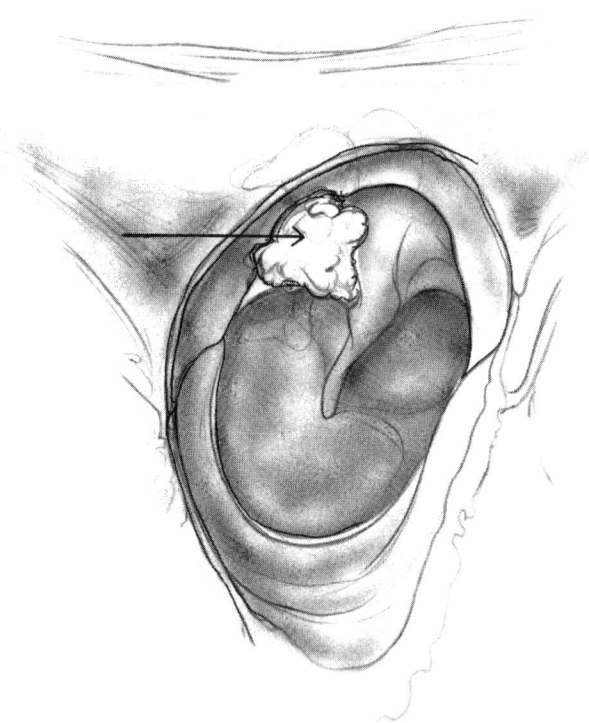

Figure 140.3 Infected cholesteatoma of the attic eroding the scutum (*arrow*).

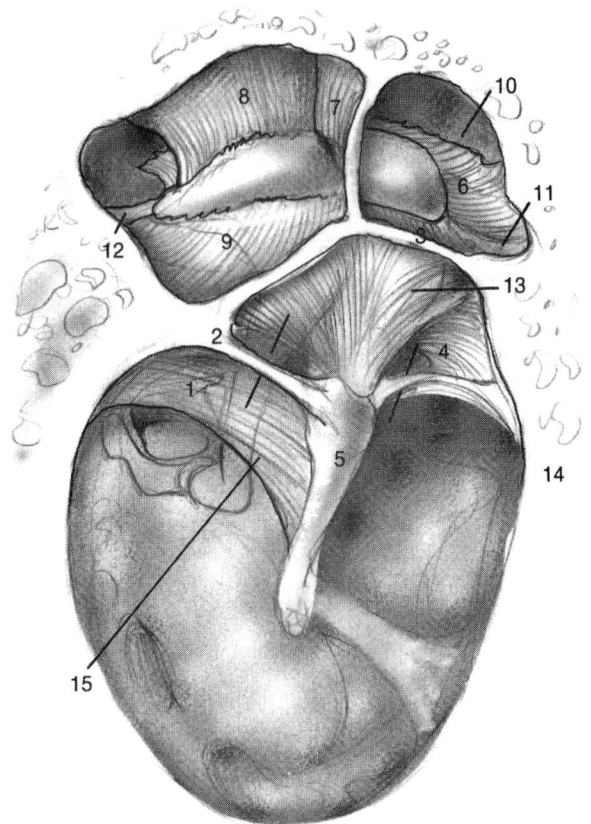

Figure 140.4 Spaces and pouches on the middle ear defined by various ligaments and folds. 1, posterior mallear fold; 2, posterior tympanic stria; 3, lateral mallear fold; 4, anterior tympanic membrane stria; 5, malleus (short process); 6, tensor fold; 7, superior mallear fold; 8, superior incudal fold; 9, lateral incudal fold; 10, anterior epitympanic space; 11, anterior mallear ligament; 12, postincudal ligament; 13, Prussak's space; 14, anterior pouch (VT); 15, posterior pouch of von Troeltsch.

activity (35–37). It is likely that bone destruction in cholesteatoma results from a combination of these factors, but clarification is needed regarding their specific roles.

Multinucleated osteoclasts within the subepithelial matrix of a cholesteatoma release acid phosphatase, collagenase, and other proteolytic enzymes that resorb the bone products. The osteoclasts may be further activated by infection, pressure, and Langerhans cells through an immune mechanism. Cholesteatoma debris is a favorite culture medium for bacteria from the external meatus, including staphylococci, *Pseudomonas aeruginosa*, *Proteus*, *Enterobacter*, aerobic and anaerobic nonhemolytic streptococci, diphtheroid bacilli, and *Aspergillus* molds. When the cholesteatoma becomes infected from water contamination, a foul-smelling discharge ensues. An active infected cholesteatoma will resorb bone at a faster rate.

The ability of cholesteatomas to erode bone is what makes them particularly dangerous (Fig. 140.3). Their expansion is dictated by space available, their migratory tendency, and their internal desquamation. Pressure alone may cause bone resorption to take place.

SURGICAL ANATOMY

Cholesteatomas are channeled along characteristic pathways by ligaments and folds. During the third to fifth fetal months, endothelial-lined sacs develop from evaginations of the first brachial pouch to form the tympanic cavity mucosal folds and ossicular suspensory ligaments. These sacs

contact each other, defining the various pouches, spaces, and compartments that divide the middle ear (Fig. 140.4).

The most common locations of origin of cholesteatomas in decreasing frequency are the posterior epitympanum, the posterior mesotympanum, and the anterior epitympanum (38). Epitympanum cholesteatomas originate in a shallow pocket that lies between the pars flaccida of the tympanic membrane and the neck of the malleus. This pouch, known as Prussak's space, has as its floor the lateral process of the malleus and its associated mucosal folds lying in the horizontal plane. Cholesteatomas most commonly exit Prussak's space by the posterior route: the cholesteatoma penetrates the superior incudal space lateral to the body of the incus. From there, it traverses the aditus ad antrum to enter the mastoid (Fig. 140.5). The cholesteatoma may reach the middle ear by descending through the floor of Prussak's space into the posterior space of von Troeltsch, a pouch lying between the tympanic membrane and the posterior mallear fold, the inferior edge of which contains the chorda tympani nerve (Fig. 140.4). This pouch contains a medial, superior, and lateral wall but is open to the mesotympanum

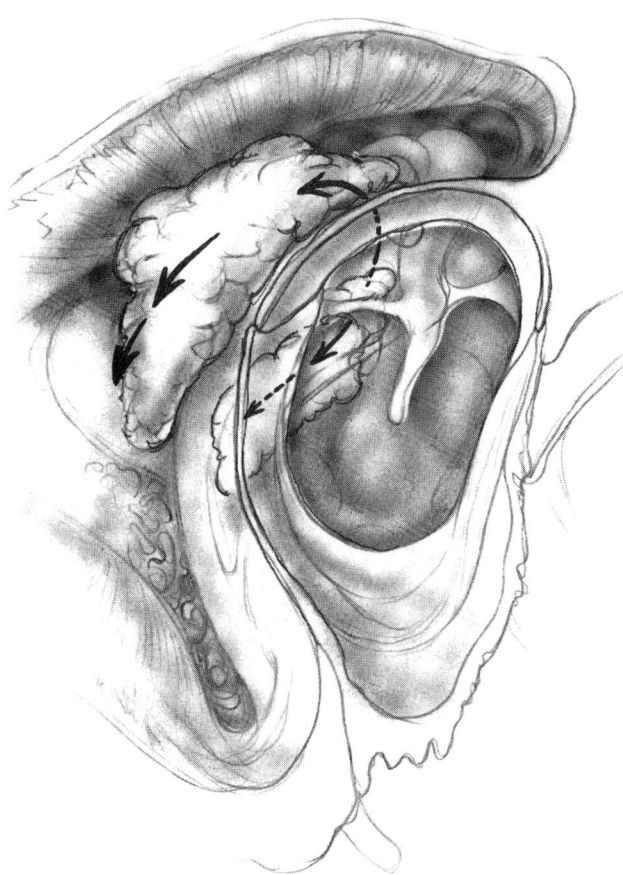

Figure 140.5 Posterior epitympanic cholesteatoma passing through the superior incudal space and the aditus ad antrum.

inferiorly toward the posterior mesotympanum. Cholesteatomas in this region may involve the stapes, round window, sinus tympani, and facial recess.

The second most common site of origin of cholesteatomas is the posterior mesotympanum (Fig. 140.6). The pars tensa retracts into the mesotympanum to form a cholesteatoma sac that passes medial to the malleus and the incus. Cholesteatomas in this region invade the sinus tympani and facial recess. The sinus tympani lies between the facial nerve and the medial wall of the mesotympanum. The facial recess is bounded by the fossa incudis and the facial nerve medially and the chorda tympani nerve laterally. Both areas are difficult to access surgically (Fig. 140.7) and are common sites of residual cholesteatoma.

Anterior epitympanic cholesteatomas develop as a retraction pocket anterior to the malleus head. The anterior epitympanic space or supratubal recess is limited anteriorly by the middle cranial fossa, the petrous tip, and the root of the zygoma; posteriorly by a bony ridge, termed the *cog*, extending to the cochleariform process; superiorly by the middle cranial fossa; and laterally by the tympanic bone and chorda tympani nerve. The floor of the anterior epitympanum is intimately associated with the horizontal portion of the facial nerve. Cholesteatomas in this region

can therefore cause a facial paresis or paralysis (39). Anterior epitympanic cholesteatomas extend to the supratubal recess of the middle ear via the anterior pouch of von Troeltsch, a shallow pouch lying between the tympanic membrane and the anterior mallear fold (Fig. 140.8). If the area anterior to the malleus head is not explored thoroughly during tympanomastoidectomy, cholesteatomas in this region can be overlooked.

PREVENTION

A retraction pocket secondary to eustachian tube dysfunction precedes the development of acquired cholesteatoma. It is good practice to aggressively manage such retraction pockets. A tympanostomy tube should be inserted early in an effort to resolve the negative middle ear pressure and to return the tympanic membrane to a neutral position (Fig. 140.9). However, many retraction pockets persist after tube placement. If the retraction pocket adheres to the ossicles or surrounding structures, it will not reverse. Similarly, if the tympanic membrane has been retracted for a long time and loses all its elasticity, it will not revert to a normal appearance. Tube placement is best done under general anesthesia, where the retraction pocket may be seen to distend as the patient is masked with positive-pressure ventilation. A T-tube or some other long-term ventilation tube is often necessary. If the retraction pocket does not distend with positive pressure ventilation, then it should be examined carefully to determine the extent and depth of the pocket. Mirror examination or the use of a 90-degree telescope may be used to see hidden borders of the pocket. Most retraction pockets extend into the epitympanum or sinus tympani. If the pocket persists despite tympanostomy tube placement, then surgical exploration may be indicated.

PREOPERATIVE EVALUATION

The presence of a cholesteatoma requires surgical management unless advanced age or poor health prohibits an operation. Both congenital and acquired cholesteatomas are asymptomatic during early development. Careful questioning of a patient with a middle ear cholesteatoma often reveals many years of subtle ear symptoms, beginning with a progressive hearing loss (usually unilateral). Unilateral hearing loss may be ignored until the cholesteatoma becomes infected secondary to water contamination or an upper respiratory infection, producing a foul-smelling otorrhea. When an infected cholesteatoma is present or there is bone destruction, the purulent discharge tends to be thick, scanty, and fetid. An occasional patient will ignore the disease until impending complications develop, heralded by the onset of pain, bloody otorrhea, vertigo, headache, facial paresis, or the appearance of a polyp at the meatus.

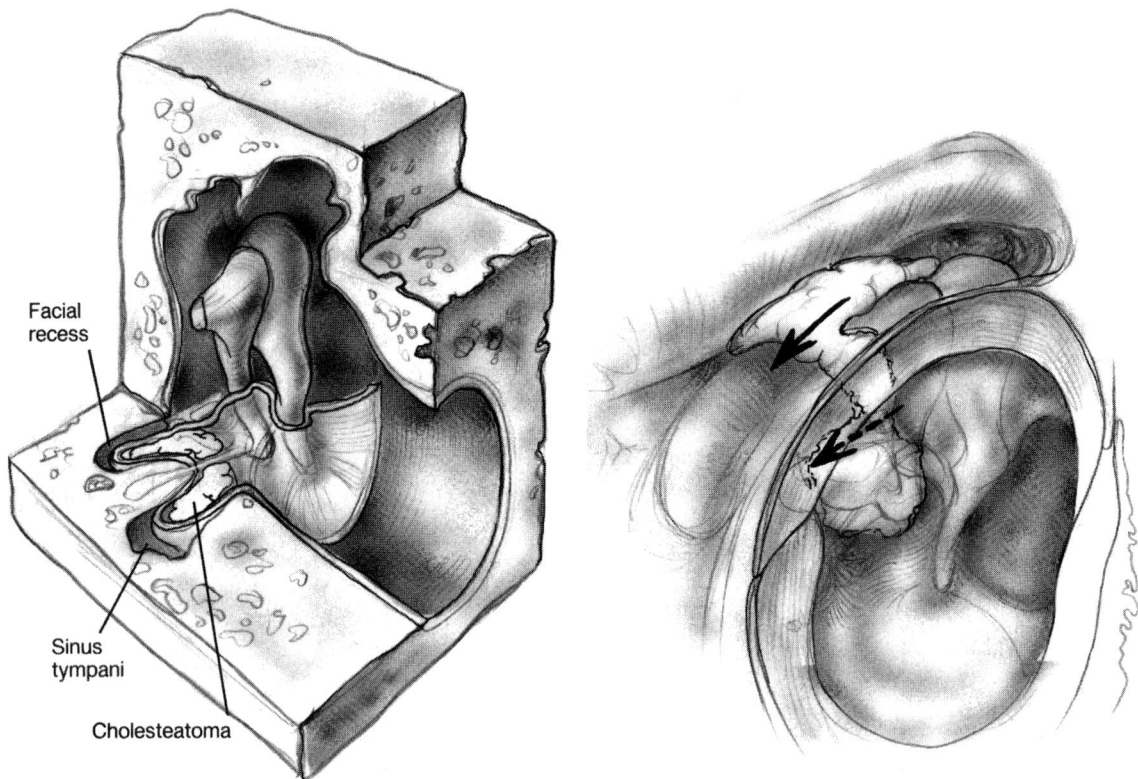

Facial
recess

Sinus
tympani

Cholesteatoma

Figure 140.6   Posterior mesotympanic cholesteatoma invading the sinus tympani and facial recess.

The microscopic examination of the ear is the most important diagnostic maneuver in evaluating the presence of a cholesteatoma. The ear must first be meticulously cleaned with cotton-tipped applicators or suction. Acquired cholesteatomas will be noted in the attic or Shrapnell area and in the posterior-superior region, where they are usually associated with erosion of the bony canal. Granulation tissue may arise from the diseased bone of the outer attic wall or scutum or from the posterior bony wall of the external auditory meatus, where it overhangs the facial recess. A polyp consisting of a mass of edematous granulation tissue may protrude through an attic defect. The polyp may continue to enlarge and in fact may extrude through the meatus. If the disease is very extensive, the entire attic and mastoid antrum will be filled with granulation tissue, and the underlying bone will become necrotic and friable over a wide area. General anesthesia may be required in children to perform an adequate examination. Pneumatic otoscopy

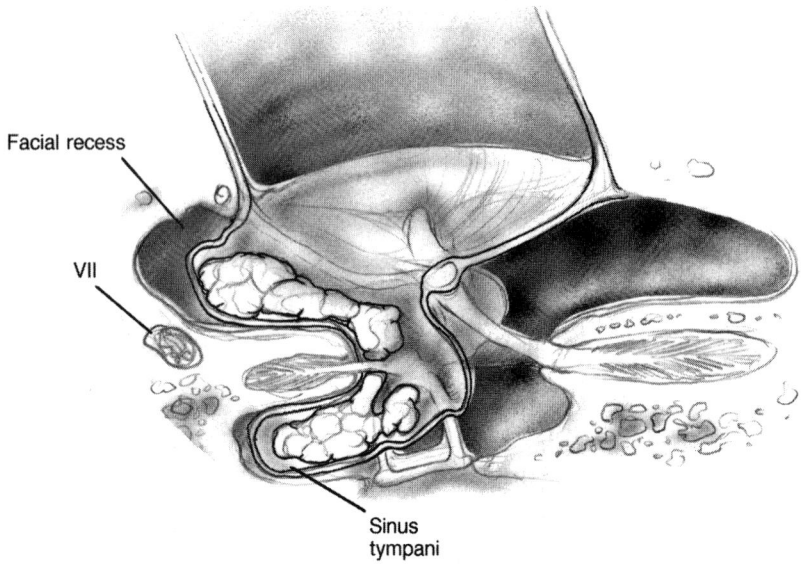

Facial recess

VII

Sinus
tympani

Figure 140.7   Posterior mesotympanic cholesteatoma involving the facial recess and sinus tympani. VII, facial nerve.

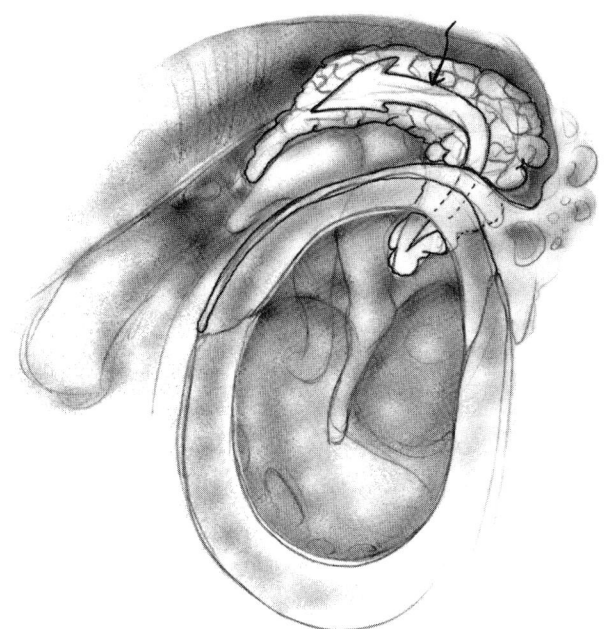

Figure 140.8 Anterior epitympanic cholesteatoma (*arrow*) with extension to the geniculate ganglion.

should be performed in every patient with a cholesteatoma. A positive fistula response characterized by vertigo and nystagmus is very suggestive of erosion into the inner ear, especially the horizontal semicircular canal or less commonly the cochlea. Infected cholesteatomas characterized by fetid, foul-smelling otorrhea and cholesteatomas associated with polyps should be initially managed medically. Dry ears are much easier to operate on than wet, infected ears. Polyps can be removed with great care in the clinic with

microscopic visualization by using a snare, suction, or small cup forceps, or they may be cauterized. They should never be aggressively pulled out by grasping them because they may be connected to an important underlying structure such as an ossicle or the facial nerve. A vasoconstricting agent applied to a wick will control bleeding. An attic cholesteatoma may be obscured by a crust that looks like cerumen. Removing the crust reveals a whitish keratin mass typical of a cholesteatoma.

Weber and Rinne tests using a 512-Hz tuning fork should be performed and correlated with the audiogram. Preoperative and postoperative audiometric evaluations are essential and should include air and bone thresholds, speech reception threshold, and word recognition. A conductive deficit in excess of 35 dB indicates ossicular discontinuity, usually secondary to destruction of the long process of the incus or the capitulum of the stapes. Alternatively, only a mild conductive hearing loss may be present despite incus erosion if sound is passing through the cholesteatoma directly to the stapes.

The surgical preparation of the patient with an infected cholesteatoma begins with a topical antibiotic drop. Oral quinolones such as ciprofloxacin and levofloxacin are effective with *P. aeruginosa* but are often unnecessary. For medical therapy to be effective, aural toilet is essential. Irrigating the ear with half-strength white vinegar can be effective in controlling infection.

Successful surgical management of cholesteatoma includes exteriorization and removal of all trapped keratinizing epithelium. The goals of surgery should be carefully reviewed with the patient preoperatively. The primary objectives of surgery are a safe, dry ear, with hearing

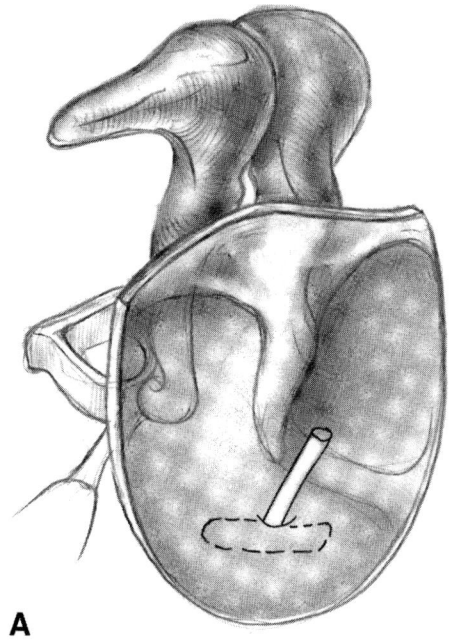

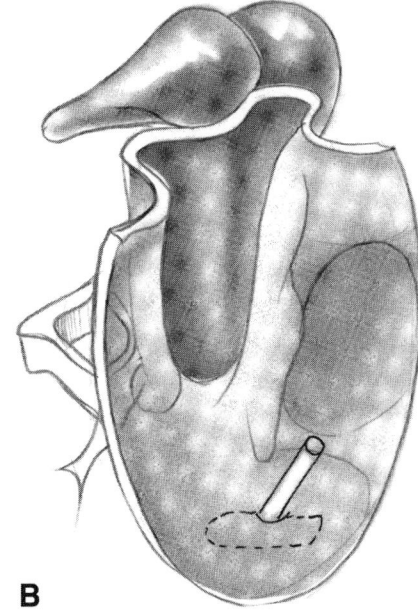

A   **B**

Figure 140.9 **A**: Reversal of a posterosuperior retraction pocket with a tympanostomy tube. **B**: Persistence of a retraction pocket despite tympanostomy tube placement.

TABLE 140.2

SURGICAL GOALS FOR CHOLESTEATOMA

Treat complications
Remove diseased tissue
Obtain a dry "safe" ear
Preserve normal anatomy
Improve hearing

improvement a secondary goal. Specific goals include the following (Table 140.2):

1. Treating complications that have already supervened (extradural abscess, brain abscess, facial nerve palsy, and labyrinthitis)
2. Removing diseased bone, mucosa, granulation polyps, and cholesteatoma to allow drainage and prevent extension of disease to vital structures
3. Stopping the discharge permanently
4. Preserving as much normal anatomy as possible (e.g., posterior canal wall)
5. Preserving or improving hearing

Patients should be carefully counseled about the possible adverse outcomes of surgery: facial paralysis, dysgeusia, vertigo, further hearing loss, tinnitus, recurrent and residual cholesteatoma, cerebrospinal fluid (CSF) leak, and meningitis. The chronic nature of the disease and the need for prolonged follow-up should be stressed. If a mastoid cavity is created, water precautions and the possible need for cavity debridement every 6 to 12 months must be mentioned. The need for second-stage procedures for residual cholesteatoma or ossicular chain reconstruction should be discussed with the patient and performed when appropriate.

Thin-section (1-mm) computed tomography (CT) scans without contrast, taken in the coronal and axial projections, are often of value in the preoperative assessment of cholesteatomas. It must be emphasized that routine CT scanning is not advocated for cholesteatoma diagnosis, although several alterations of temporal bone anatomy frequently are associated with it. Among these, erosion of the scutum and expansion of the antrum within areas of air cell breakdown and soft tissue density are characteristic. Other features may include ossicular destruction, erosion of the facial canal, mastoid tegmen dehiscence, and erosion into the otic capsule, especially over the horizontal semicircular canal. CT scanning is important in complicated disease and in the evaluation of cholesteatomas and other masses behind an intact tympanic membrane or when the clinical history correlates poorly with physical findings.

SURGICAL MANAGEMENT

Surgical treatment of the mastoid in patients with cholesteatoma has gradually evolved. Before the develop-

ment of the surgical microscope and the electric drill, significant morbidity, including facial paralysis, profound sensorineural hearing loss, and dural tears, attended surgery of the temporal bone. Understandably, otologic surgeons of that day were reluctant to pursue complete removal of cholesteatomas, so a philosophy of exteriorization of cholesteatomas without complete removal emerged. This led to progressive hearing loss and chronically draining ears, requiring constant supervision.

To avoid cavity problems altogether, the canal-wall-up (CWU) facial recess approach was developed. The posterior canal wall was preserved at all costs. A second stage was planned in 6 to 18 months for removal of residual disease and reconstruction of the ossicular chain. Experience with this philosophy over the past 20 years has resulted in a rethinking of this position by many prominent otologists. A high rate of recidivism approaching 36% in some series (40–46) has resulted in a more individualized approach. Instead of using the same procedure on every ear with cholesteatoma, the procedure is adapted to the extent of disease. The specific operation is determined by local ear factors, general medical factors, and the skill of the surgeon. The local ear factors include the extent of the cholesteatoma, presence of a fistula, clinical assessment of eustachian tube function, degree of mastoid pneumatization, and the degree of neurosensory hearing loss in both ears. General factors include the patient's general medical condition, occupation, and reliability (Table 140.3). The CWU procedure involves preserving the posterior canal wall with or without a posterior tympanotomy (facial recess approach). The posterior tympanotomy is performed through a triangle bounded by the fossa incudis, facial nerve, and chorda tympani nerve. The CWU procedure is indicated in patients with a well-pneumatized mastoid and middle ear space. Relative contraindications to the CWU procedure include a sclerotic mastoid, a labyrinthine fistula, an only hearing ear, and poor eustachian tube function (47–49).

The canal-wall-down (CWD) procedure involves taking down the posterior canal wall to the vertical facial nerve and

TABLE 140.3

DETERMINANTS OF OPERATIVE TECHNIQUE FOR CHOLESTEATOMA

Local factors
   Presence of a fistula
   Extent of disease
   Eustachian tube function
   Mastoid pneumatization
   Hearing status of both ears

General factors
   General medical condition
   Occupation
   Reliability

Skill and experience of the surgeon

TABLE 140.4

SURGICAL APPROACHES TO CHOLESTEATOMA

Canal-wall-up
  Complete mastoidectomy
  Facial recess approach

Canal-wall-down
  Modified radical mastoidectomy
  Radical mastoidectomy

Other
  Atticotomy
  Bondy procedure
  Canal-wall-reconstruction

TABLE 140.5

COMPLICATIONS AND EMERGENCIES CHOLESTEATOMA

Conductive and sensorineural hearing loss
Labyrinthine fistula
Vertigo
Facial paralysis
Intratemporal infection
Intracranial infection
Brain herniation

marsupializing the mastoid into the external ear canal. In a CWD procedure, all accessible air cells are meticulously exenterated. CWD procedures can be divided into those in which the middle ear space is preserved (modified radical mastoidectomy) and those in which the middle ear space is eliminated and the eustachian tube plugged (radical mastoidectomy). A more limited procedure is the atticotomy, which involves the removal of the lateral wall of the epitympanum (scutum) to the limits of the cholesteatoma. To prevent recurrent cholesteatoma, the atticotomy defect is blocked with cartilage. A more extensive attic cholesteatoma that is lateral to the ossicles and accompanied by a sclerotic mastoid may be managed with a Bondy procedure. This involves the removal of the scutum and portion of the posterior canal wall with preservation of the ossicles and middle ear space. The bony defect is not reconstructed; rather, the cholesteatoma matrix is exteriorized. A patient with a cholesteatoma and poor eustachian tube function as evidenced by absence of middle ear aeration and a sclerotic mastoid should have a CWD procedure (Table 140.4).

Several variations of a canal-wall-reconstruction (CWR) procedure have recently been developed to improve exposure and removal of cholesteatoma as in a CWD approach while retaining the benefits of an intact canal wall (improved hearing and avoidance of the bowl cavity) (50–64). In these procedures, a complete mastoidectomy including a facial recess is performed and the posterior canal is removed. The cholesteatoma, the ossicles, and the tympanic membrane are addressed, and the posterior canal wall is replaced. Some surgeons opt to fill the mastoid cavity with bone pate or hydroxyapatite, whereas others leave it open as in a CWU procedure. These techniques have even been used to "repair" radical mastoid cavities. See Chapter 141 for a more complete description of surgical approaches to the mastoid.

COMPLICATIONS AND EMERGENCIES

As cholesteatomas expand and become infected, they cause ossicular chain destruction, exposure of the membranous labyrinth, tegmen dehiscence, exposure of the facial nerve,

and infection of the mastoid and intracranial spaces (Table 140.5).

Hearing Loss

Some degree of ossicular chain erosion occurs in most cases of cholesteatoma. Attic cholesteatomas involve the head of the malleus and body of the incus early. As the cholesteatoma expands inferiorly, the lenticular process of the incus and the stapes superstructure are eroded. Pars tensa cholesteatomas that develop from a posterior-superior retraction pocket also involve the lenticular process of the incus and the stapes superstructure. When both of these bones are involved, the hearing loss can be as great as 50 dB. However, if a natural myringostapediopexy develops, then loss may be as little as 20 dB. One should always assume that the ossicular chain is intact in a patient with a cholesteatoma. Cholesteatoma on the lateral surface of the incus can be removed using microsurgical ear instruments without disturbing the ossicular chain. Involvement of the medial surface of the incus often requires removal of the incus by first separating the incudostapedial joint, then the incudomallear joint. Cholesteatoma extending medial to the head of the malleus into the anterior epitympanic space (or supratubal recess) usually requires removal of the incus and the head of the malleus. Removal of cholesteatoma from the stapes should be done last by dissecting parallel with the stapedius tendon in a posterior to anterior direction to avoid dislocating the footplate and causing sensorineural hearing loss. One should avoid superior or inferior movement as well as depression of the stapes. The tympanic membrane is grafted to seal the middle ear, and Silastic sheeting is placed over the promontory to prevent adhesions. A second-stage procedure is performed in 6 to 18 months to remove residual cholesteatoma and reconstruct the ossicular chain. If cholesteatoma removal is certain and the mucosal involvement is minimal, the ossicular chain can be reconstructed at the primary procedure.

Labyrinthine Fistula

A labyrinthine fistula may be found in up to 10% of patients with long-standing cholesteatomas or in revision cases. One should suspect a fistula in patients with chronic ear disease who have sensorineural hearing loss and/or vertigo induced by noise or pressure changes in the middle ear. A positive fistula test with manipulation of the external canal may be present, although its absence does not exclude a fistula. Suppurative labyrinthitis with complete loss of hearing and vestibular function may occur secondary to a fistula from a cholesteatoma. High-resolution, thin-section CT of the temporal bone may reveal a fistula of the semicircular canals or the basal turn of the cochlea. Fistulae of the horizontal semicircular canal are most common (65). The procedure of choice in labyrinthine fistulae is a modified radical (CWD) mastoidectomy. This avoids leaving residual disease concealed in the mastoid cavity and necessitating the patient to undergo multiple procedures. Management of the matrix covering the fistula depends on several factors, including the infection status of the ear, the degree of sensorineural hearing loss in the involved ear as well as the opposite ear, the size and location of the fistula, and the surgeon's skill. In the patient with a fistula of the only hearing ear, a CWD procedure is performed and the matrix is left intact over the fistula. Attempting to remove it places the patient at significant risk for a permanent total sensorineural hearing loss. If the opposite ear has normal hearing and eustachian tube function, then the surgeon can be more selective in management. If the fistula involves one of the semicircular canals and the mastoid is small, then a CWD mastoidectomy, leaving the matrix on the fistula, is appropriate. If there is a small semicircular canal fistula and the mastoid cavity is large, then the skillful surgeon may elect to perform an intact canal wall procedure, remove the matrix, cover the fistula with fascia, and plan a second procedure. If the hearing is normal, then the matrix covering extensive fistulae of the vestibule or cochlea should be left alone. If cochlear function is profoundly depressed, the matrix should be removed and the fistula covered with fascia. The removal of matrix over the fistula and then immediately covering it with fascia should be the last part of the procedure. Suction should not be used around the fistula site; only blunt dissection is appropriate. If the semicircular canal is inadvertently opened by a drill, then the iatrogenic fistula should be immediately covered with fascia. Parenteral antibiotics and steroids may be helpful. Postoperative vertigo is a sign of labyrinthine and cochlear trauma. A bone-conduction audiogram may be depressed immediately but may recover in 4 to 6 weeks in some cases.

Facial Paralysis

Facial paralysis in patients with cholesteatoma may develop acutely due to infection or slowly due to chronic expansion. In either case, surgery should be performed as soon as the paralysis is recognized. High-resolution, thin-section CT with both axial and coronal scanning will localize the involvement. A common site of nerve involvement is the geniculate ganglion (66). A mastoidectomy with facial recess approach will expose the horizontal and vertical

portions of the facial nerve. Removing the cholesteatoma and decompressing the facial nerve are sufficient if the nerve is anatomically intact; opening the sheath of the facial nerve is unnecessary. A middle fossa approach is required for cholesteatomas involving the petrous apex. Intravenous antibiotics and high-dose steroids are helpful. The House-Brackmann facial nerve grading system should be used to assess the degree of facial paralysis, and the intraoperative use of a facial nerve stimulator/monitor is helpful. Iatrogenic injury of the facial nerve at the pyramidal turn may occur with drilling of the mastoid. The horizontal segment of the facial nerve may be injured during blunt removal of the cholesteatoma in the middle ear. Immediate repair is performed when the injury is recognized, and decompression of the facial nerve for several millimeters on either side of the injured segment is recommended. A delayed facial paralysis within a few days of surgery indicates minor trauma, with recovery expected within 6 weeks. These patients are treated like those with idiopathic facial paralysis and given high-dose steroids. Antiviral therapy may also be beneficial.

Infections

Serious infections associated with cholesteatoma include periosteal abscess, lateral sinus thrombosis, meningitis, and intracranial abscess. A high-resolution, thin-section, contrast-enhanced CT scan is performed. Infections of this nature occur in less than 1% of all cholesteatomas because of the widespread use of antibiotics and the tendency to operate earlier. The most dangerous type of infected cholesteatomas are those where drainage through the external auditory canal is obstructed by an inflamed and narrow canal. The egress may be further blocked by mucosal edema, squamous debris, or a polyp. Early intervention to remove cholesteatoma and provide adequate drainage is required.

Periosteal abscess may develop behind a cholesteatoma and inflammation that is blocking the aditus ad antrum or from an extensive cholesteatoma that erodes through the mastoid cortex. It presents as an inflamed, fluctuant postauricular mass. High-dose antibiotics are begun and adjusted according to needle aspiration culture results. Surgery is performed after 24 to 48 hours of antibiotics. It is important to be aware that the dura or lateral sinus may be exposed by disease.

Lateral sinus thrombosis may occur from an infected cholesteatoma. It presents with a characteristic high, spiking fever in a picket-fence pattern. Treatment requires high-dose antibiotics and surgery similar to management of lateral sinus thrombosis in association with acute coalescent mastoiditis. If the cholesteatoma is extensive, a CWD mastoidectomy should be performed (66).

Patients who develop headaches on the side of a cholesteatoma should have a CT scan to rule out an impending intracranial complication. Pain and headache may arise from involvement of dura by the cholesteatoma, by a developing epidural abscess, or because of loculated abscess. Cerebellar or temporal lobe abscesses may exhibit only mild symptoms such as low-grade fever, mild ataxia, or mental changes. Intracranial abscesses should be managed by the neurosurgeon after beginning intravenous antibiotics. After control of the intracranial problem, the otologist can then manage the ear disease. See Chapter 138 for more information on intracranial complications.

Brain Herniation

Brain herniation may develop following previous mastoid procedures presenting as an encephalocele or meningoencephalocele through a defect in the tegmen tympani or tegmen mastoideum. The etiology is thought secondary to aggressive drilling that exposes and traumatizes the dura during previous mastoid surgery. Subsequent brain herniation can be prevented by carefully inspecting any exposed dura for injury. If a tegmen defect is small and the dura is intact, no further treatment is necessary. If there is a disruption in the integrity of the dura with or without a CSF leak, repair is necessary. Many of these defects can be successfully treated from the mastoid. One should circumferentially elevate the dura from the tegmen with a blunt instrument and remove 1 mm of bone from around the site of injury to expose normal-appearing dura. Bleeding is controlled with low-energy bipolar cautery rather than monopolar cautery to avoid injury and thrombosis of cerebral vessels. The surgeon should circumferentially insert temporalis fascia, cut larger than the defect, between the dura superiorly and the tegmen inferiorly. Defects larger than a few millimeters require conchal cartilage or a bone chip for support to prevent herniation. If an established encephalocele or meningoencephalocele is encountered, it should be removed. A biopsy is needed to confirm brain tissue and rule out a malignancy. One should carefully dissect the circumference of the mass to identify its site of origin. In most cases, the encephalocele in the epitympanum or mastoid is necrotic and functionless. The herniated brain tissue is removed to the level of the tegmen and dural defect and repaired as described previously. For larger defects, a mini-craniotomy is performed by making an opening in the squamosa laterally, just above the plane of the tegmen. The dura can then be elevated off the floor of the middle fossa and the defect repaired with fascia and cartilage or bone.

HIGHLIGHTS

- The only epithelium that migrates is that of the tympanic membrane and cholesteatoma.
- The posterior epitympanum is the most common location for acquired cholesteatomas.
- Posterior mesotympanic cholesteatomas are common sites of residual cholesteatoma; epitympanic cholesteatomas are common sites of recurrent cholesteatoma.

- Posterior mesotympanic and epitympanic retraction pockets should be managed with either a ventilating tube or a cartilage-supported tympanoplasty if the pocket is adherent.
- Aural polyps can be snared but should not be pulled aggressively because they may be attached to an ossicle or the facial nerve.
- An ideal candidate for a canal-wall-up mastoidectomy is a patient with a well-pneumatized mastoid and a cholesteatoma limited to the posterior mesotympanum and antrum.
- The operative approach chosen is dictated by the disease and the hearing status of the contralateral ear.
- Removal of cholesteatoma from the stapes should be done last by dissecting parallel with the tendon.
- One should assume that the incudostapedial joint is intact unless proved otherwise by direct inspection.
- Patients with cholesteatomas who develop new headaches on the same side should have a CT scan to evaluate a potential intracranial problem.

REFERENCES

1. Kuhn A. Das Cholesteatom des Ohres. *Zeitschr Ohrenheilk* 1891; 21:231.
2. Derlacki EL, Clemis JD. Congenital cholesteatoma of the middle ear and mastoid. *Ann Otol Rhinol Laryngol* 1965;74:706–727.
3. Levenson MJ, Michaels L, Parisier SC, et al. Congenital cholesteatomas in children: an embryologic correlation. *Laryngoscope* 1988;98:949–955.
4. Levenson MJ, Michaels L, Parisier SC. Congenital cholesteatomas of the middle ear in children: origin and management. *Otolaryngol Clin North Am* 1989;22:941–954.
5. Teed FW. Cholesteatoma verum tympani (its relationship to the first epibranchial placode). *Arch Otolaryngol* 1936;24:455–474.
6. Michaels L. An epidermoid formation in the developing middle ear: possible source of cholesteatoma. *J Otolaryngol* 1986;15:169–174.
7. Michaels L. Origin of congenital cholesteatoma from a normally occurring epidermoid rest in the developing middle ear. *Int J Pediatr Otorhinolaryngol* 1988;15:51–65.
8. Karmody CS, Byahatti SV, Blevins N, et al. The origin of congenital cholesteatoma. *Am J Otol* 1998;19:292–297.
9. Lee TS, Liang JN, Michaels L, et al. The epidermoid formation and its affinity to congenital cholesteatoma. *Clin Otolaryngol Allied Sci* 1998;23:449–454.
10. Wang RG, Hawke M, Kwok P. The epidermoid formation (Michaels' structure) in the developing middle ear. *J Otolaryngol* 1987;16:327–330.
11. Aimi K. Role of the tympanic ring in the pathogenesis of congenital cholesteatoma. *Laryngoscope* 1983;93:1140–1146.
12. Fisch U. 'Congenital' cholesteatomas of the supralabyrinthine region. *Clin Otolaryngol Allied Sci* 1978;3:369–376.
13. Bluestone CD, Klein JO. Intratemporal complications and sequelae of otitis media. In: Bluestone CD, Stool SE, eds. *Pediatric otolaryngology*. Philadelphia: WB Saunders, 1990:521–526.
14. Sheahan P, Blayney AW, Sheahan JN, et al. Sequelae of otitis media with effusion among children with cleft lip and/or cleft palate. *Clin Otolaryngol Allied Sci* 2002;27:494–500.
15. Goldman JL, Martinez SA, Ganzel TM. Eustachian tube dysfunction and its sequelae in patients with cleft palate. *South Med J* 1993;86:1236–1237.
16. Dominguez S, Harker LA. Incidence of cholesteatoma with cleft palate. *Ann Otol Rhinol Laryngol* 1988;97[6 Pt 1]:659–660.
17. Vartiainen E, Karja J. Bilateral chronic otitis media. *Arch Oto Rhino Laryngol* 1986;243:190–193.

18. Wittmaack K. Wie entsteht ein genuines Cholesteatoma? *Arch Ohren Nasen Dehlkopfh* 1933;137:306.
19. Glasscock ME. Pathology and clinical course of inflammatory disease of the middle ear. In: Shambaugh G, Glasscock ME, eds. *Surgery of the ear*. Philadelphia: WB Saunders, 1990:178.
20. Vennix PP, Kuijpers W, Tonnaer EL, et al. Cytokeratins in induced epidermoid formations and cholesteatoma lesions. *Arch Otolaryngol Head Neck Surg* 1990;116:560–565.
21. Palva T, Karma P, Makinen J. The invasion theory in cholesteatoma and mastoid surgery. In: Sade J, ed. *Cholesteatoma and mastoid surgery. Proceedings of the Second International Conference on Cholesteatoma and Mastoid Surgery*. Amsterdam: Kugler Publications, 1982:249–264.
22. Michaels L. Biology of cholesteatoma. *Otolaryngol Clin North Am* 1989;22:869–881.
23. Orisek BS, Chole RA. Pressures exerted by experimental cholesteatomas. *Arch Otolaryngol Head Neck Surg* 1987;113:386–391.
24. Wolfman DE, Chole RA. Osteoclast stimulation by positive middle-ear air pressure. *Arch Otolaryngol Head Neck Surg* 1986;112:1037–1042.
25. Chole RA, McGinn MD, Tinling SP. Pressure-induced bone resorption in the middle ear. *Ann Otol Rhinol Laryngol* 1985;94[2 Pt 1]:165–170.
26. Tanaka Y, Kojima H, Miyazaki H, et al. Roles of cytokines and cell cycle regulating substances in proliferation of cholesteatoma epithelium. *Laryngoscope* 1999;109[7 Pt 1]:1102–1107.
27. Yetiser S, Satar B, Aydin N. Expression of epidermal growth factor, tumor necrosis factor-alpha, and interleukin-1alpha in chronic otitis media with or without cholesteatoma. *Otol Neurotol* 2002;23:647–652.
28. Akimoto R, Pawankar R, Yagi T, et al. Acquired and congenital cholesteatoma: determination of tumor necrosis factor-alpha, intercellular adhesion molecule-1, interleukin-1-alpha and lymphocyte functional antigen-1 in the inflammatory process. *J Oto-Rhino-Laryngol Related Specialties* 2000;62:257–265.
29. Albino AP, Reed JA, Bogdany JK, et al. Increased numbers of mast cells in human middle ear cholesteatomas: implications for treatment. *Am J Otol* 1998;19:266–272.
30. Albino AP, Kimmelman CP, Parisier SC. Cholesteatoma: a molecular and cellular puzzle. *Am J Otol* 1998;19:7–19.
31. Amar MS, Wishahi HF, Zakhary MM. Clinical and biochemical studies of bone destruction in cholesteatoma. *J Laryngol Otol* 1996;110:534–539.
32. Bujia J, Kim C, Ostos P, et al. Role of interleukin 6 in epithelial hyperproliferation and bone resorption in middle ear cholesteatomas. *Eur Arch Oto-Rhino-Laryngol* 1996;253(3):152–157.
33. Yan SD, Huang CC. The role of tumor necrosis factor-alpha in bone resorption of cholesteatoma. *Am J Otolaryngol* 1991;12:83–89.
34. Iino Y, Toriyama M, Ogawa H, et al. Cholesteatoma debris as an activator of human monocytes. Potentiation of the production of tumor necrosis factor. *Acta Oto-Laryngol* 1990;110:410–415.
35. Hamzei M, Ventriglia G, Hagnia M, et al. Osteoclast stimulating and differentiating factors in human cholesteatoma. *Laryngoscope* 2003;113:436–442.
36. Jung JY, Chole RA. Bone resorption in chronic otitis media: the role of the osteoclast. *J Oto-Rhino-Laryngol Related Specialties* 2002;64:95–107.
37. Chole RA. Cellular and subcellular events of bone resorption in human and experimental cholesteatoma: the role of osteoclasts. *Laryngoscope* 1984;94:76–95.
38. Jackler RK. The surgical anatomy of cholesteatoma. *Otolaryngol Clin North Am* 1989;22:883–896.
39. Chu FW, Jackler RK. Anterior epitympanic cholesteatoma with facial paralysis: a characteristic growth pattern. *Laryngoscope* 1988;98:274–279.
40. Cruz OL, Kasse CA, Leonhart FD. Efficacy of surgical treatment of chronic otitis media. *Otolaryngol Head Neck Surg* 2003;128:263–266.
41. Silvola J, Palva T. One-stage revision surgery for pediatric cholesteatoma: long-term results and comparison with primary surgery. *Int J Pediatr Otorhinolaryngol* 2000;56:135–139.
42. Stangerup SE, Drozdziewicz D, Tos M, et al. Recurrence of attic cholesteatoma: different methods of estimating recurrence rates. *Otolaryngol Head Neck Surg* 2000;123:283–287.
43. Darrouzet V, Duclos JY, Portmann D, et al. Preference for the closed technique in the management of cholesteatoma of the middle ear in children: a retrospective study of 215 consecutive patients treated over 10 years. *Am J Otol* 2000;21:474–481.
44. Vartiainen E. Factors associated with recurrence of cholesteatoma. *J Laryngol Otol* 1995;109:590–592.
45. Rosenfeld RM, Moura RL, Bluestone CD. Predictors of residual-recurrent cholesteatoma in children. *Arch Otolaryngol Head Neck Surg* 1992;118:384–391.
46. Brown JS. A ten year statistical follow-up of 1142 consecutive cases of cholesteatoma: the closed vs. the open technique. *Laryngoscope* 1982;92:390–396.
47. Brackmann DE. Tympanoplasty with mastoidectomy: canal wall up procedures. *Am J Otol* 1993;14:380–382.
48. Dawes PJ, Leaper M. Paediatric small cavity mastoid surgery: second look tympanotomy. *Int J Pediatr Otorhinolaryngol* 2004;68:143–148.
49. McDonald TJ, Cody DTR. Surgery of the temporal bone air cell system: mastoid and petrosa. *Otolaryngol Head Neck Surg* 1986;4:3081.
50. Gantz BJ, Wilkinson EP, Hansen MR. Canal wall reconstruction typanomastoidectomy with mastoid obiteration. *Laryngoscope* 2005;115:1734–1740.
51. Babighian G. Posterior and attic wall osteoplasty: hearing results and recurrence rates in cholesteatoma. *Otol Neurotol* 2002;23(1):14–17.
52. Black B. Mastoidectomy elimination. *Laryngoscope* 1995;105[12 Pt 2 Suppl 76]:1–30.
53. Dornhoffer JL. Retrograde mastoidectomy with canal wall reconstruction: a single-stage technique for cholesteatoma removal. *Ann Otol Rhinol Laryngol* 2000;109:1033–1039.
54. Grote JJ, van Blitterswijk CA. Reconstruction of the posterior auditory canal wall with a hydroxyapatite prosthesis. *Ann Otol Rhinol Laryngol Suppl* 1986;123:6–9.
55. Hartwein J, Hormann K. A technique for the reconstruction of the posterior canal wall and mastoid obliteration in radical cavity surgery. *Am J Otol* 1990;11:169–173.
56. Hosoi H, Murata K, Kimura H, et al. Long-term observation after soft posterior meatal wall reconstruction in ears with cholesteatoma. *J Laryngol Otol* 1998;112:31–35.
57. Ikeda M, Yoshida S, Ikui A, et al. Canal wall down tympanoplasty with canal reconstruction for middle-ear cholesteatoma: post-operative hearing, cholesteatoma recurrence, and status of re-aeration of reconstructed middle-ear cavity. *J Laryngol Otol* 2003;117:249–255.
58. Leatherman BD, Dornhoffer JL, Fan CY, et al. Demineralized bone matrix as an alternative for mastoid obliteration and posterior canal wall reconstruction: results in an animal model. *Otol Neurotol* 2001;22:731–736.
59. Magliulo G, Ronzoni R, Vingolo GM, et al. Reconstruction of old radical cavities. *Am J Otol* 1992;13:288–291.
60. Magliulo G, D'Amico R, Forino M. Reconstruction of the posterior auditory canal with hydroxyapatite-coated titanium. *J Otolaryngol* 2001;30:330–333.
61. Mercke U. The cholesteatomatous ear one year after surgery with obliteration technique. *Am J Otol* 1987;8:534–536.
62. Roberson JB Jr, Mason TP, Stidham KR. Mastoid obliteration: autogenous cranial bone pate reconstruction. *Otol Neurotol* 2003;24:132–140.
63. Takahashi H, Hasebe S, Sudo M, et al. Soft-wall reconstruction for cholesteatoma surgery: reappraisal. *Am J Otol* 2000;21:28–31.
64. Wiet RJ, Harvey SA, Pyle MG. Canal wall reconstruction: a newer implantation technique. *Laryngoscope* 1993;103:594–599.
65. Farrior JB. *Surgery for cholesteatoma: complications in otolaryngology-head and neck surgery*. Toronto: BC Decker, 1986.
66. Harker LA, Koontz FP. Bacteriology of cholesteatoma: clinical significance. *Trans Sect Otolaryngol* 1977;84[4 Pt 1]:ORL-683–686.

Surgery of the Mastoid and Petrosa

141

Richard A. Chole   *Hilary A. Brodie*   *Abraham Jacob*

HISTORY

Surgery of the mastoid and petrosa developed as a treatment for suppurative ear disease (1). Infections of the ear were recorded as early as 380 BC in the Hippocratic Canon. Near the turn of the 16th century, Fabricius Hildanus reported a case of spontaneous drainage from a postauricular abscess for which he advocated early incision and drainage. Riolan the Younger described a procedure akin to mastoidectomy in 1649, and John Luis Petit performed the first surgical trephination of the mastoid in 1774. Petit described exposing the mastoid cortex, performing a trephination, and then enlarging the surgically created fistula. J.G.H. Fielitz reported five such cases in 1785. The procedure fell into disrepute, however, after the sensational death of the Danish physician Johanne Gust Von Berger in 1792. He died of meningitis 12 days after a mastoidectomy performed by Koelpin and Callisen. Fortunately, however, Schwartze repopularized the operation in 1873. Since then, technologic advancements such as the operating microscope, the high-speed drill, and specialized microsurgical instruments have led to significant advances in the treatment of mastoid disease. Regions of the skull base previously thought to be inaccessible such as the petrous apex, the course of the facial nerve, the endolymphatic sac, and the cerebellopontine angle were now within reach. Indications for these procedures (Table 141.1) include acute otologic infections (Chapter 138), chronic infections with or without cholesteatoma (Chapters 138 and 140), trauma (Chapter 139), facial nerve disorders (Chapter 144), vestibulopathy (Chapter 156), and tumors of the skull base (Chapter 136).

SURGICAL TECHNIQUE: MASTOIDECTOMY

Incisions

The two principal incisions used for access to the mastoid cortex are the postauricular incision of Wilde and the endaural incision of Lempert. The postauricular incision provides better overall exposure and allows complete access to the mastoid tip. In adults, the incision is placed 8 to 10 mm posterior to the postauricular sulcus where it is hidden by the pinna. This incision can be placed more posteriorly for wider exposure as might be necessary during translabyrinthine access to the cerebellopontine angle. It should not be placed directly in the postauricular crease, however, because this creates a deep, difficult to clean postauricular furrow. In children younger than 2 years, the inferior portion of this incision must be placed more posteriorly than in adults (Fig. 141.1). This is because the tympanic ring in children is underdeveloped, mastoid pneumatization is incomplete, and the stylomastoid foramen is quite shallow. Therefore, the facial nerve is vulnerable to injury. The surgeon should also keep in mind that congenital anomalies of the temporal bone can result in highly variable facial nerve position.

The postauricular incision is first outlined with a marking pen and infiltrated with a mixture of local anesthetic and epinephrine. The skin and subcutaneous tissues are incised sharply down to the temporalis fascia (superior to the inferior temporal line) and down to the periosteum overlying the mastoid cortex (inferior to the inferior temporal line). The ear flap is elevated anteriorly to identify the posterior edge of the external ear canal. Additional elevation

TABLE 141.1
CLINICAL INDICATORS FOR MASTOIDECTOMY

Strategy
Indicators (one of the following)
   Persistent or recurrent otorrhea
   Persistent or recurrent ear pain
   Conductive hearing loss
   Tympanic membrane perforation and/or cholesteatoma
   Acute mastoiditis with osteitis
   Neoplasm of temporal bone
   Fracture of temporal bone with CSF leak
   Facial nerve paralysis requiring decompression of the facial nerve
Laboratory tests (as indicated)
Audiogram
Other tests (as indicated)
Type of anesthesia (as indicated)
Location of service (as indicated)

Process
Criteria for discharge
   Recovery from anesthesia
   Absence of significant vertigo
   Absence of signs of meningitis or toxic shock syndrome

Outcome
Results
Follow-up
   Healing of mastoid cavity if present
   Healing of surgical wound
   Resolution of presenting symptoms
   Evaluation of hearing

CSF, cerebrospinal fluid.
The American Academy of Otolaryngology–Head and Neck Surgery and the American Society for Head and Neck Surgery have published Clinical Indicators for surgical procedures. These Clinical Indicators are educational statements that have been drafted to assist surgeons in their practice and to promote discussion. These Indicators are not practice guidelines nor do they represent standards of practice with which individuals must conform.

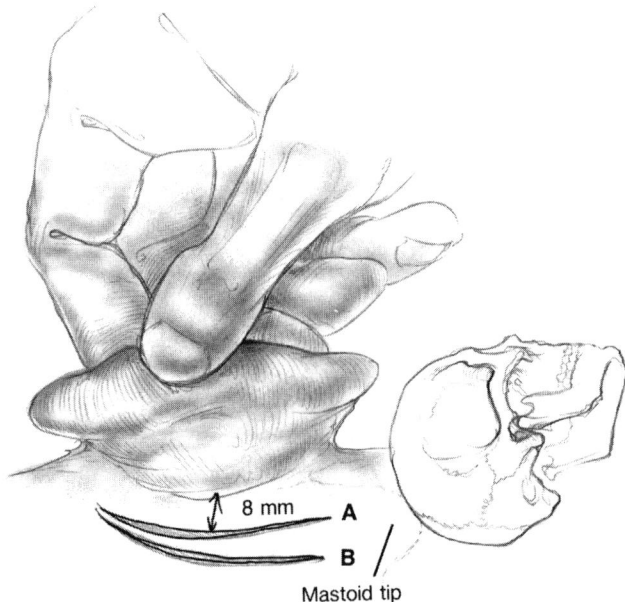

Figure 141.1   Placement of postauricular incisions in adults **(A)** and infants **(B)**.

superior to the ear canal exposes the root of the zygoma. Posterior to the ear canal, the postauricular muscle and pericranial soft tissues are incised and elevated in the same plane as described above. This dissection is carried to the mastoid tip. Care must be taken not to dissect anterior to the tip because this endangers the facial nerve in the stylomastoid foramen. Unless the mastoid tip is to be removed, the sternocleidomastoid muscle's insertion onto the tip should not be severed. This minimizes postoperative discomfort. Thus far, the skin and soft tissues of the pinna have been laid anteriorly, but the periosteum still remains attached to the mastoid cortex.

The mastoid cortex is now exposed to start the drilling process. A T-shaped incision is made through the soft tissues and periosteum overlying bone. The superior limb of the "T" is placed along the inferior temporal line (inferior margin of the temporalis muscle) starting at a point just superior to the anterior-superior ear canal. This incision extends posteriorly as far as is needed for adequate exposure. An

inferior limb to the "T" is fashioned from the mastoid tip to the superior limb just described. Periosteal elevators are then used to elevate the periosteum of the mastoid cortex toward the posterior margin of the ear canal (Fig. 141.2). Superior to the ear canal, the periosteum should be elevated anteriorly along the zygomatic root. Inferior to the ear canal, the surgeon should elevate periosteum to the anterior margin of the superior aspect of the mastoid tip. If the tip is to be removed, the surgeon must remove all the periosteum from its surface. Taking a few moments to get this anterior extension superiorly and inferiorly will allow the ear to be held forward easily when using self-retaining retractors. The periosteum can also be elevated somewhat down the ear canal to release tension and prevent a canal laceration.

The suprameatal spine of Henle marks the lateral extent of the posterior-superior bony ear canal. Self-retaining retractors should be placed to hold the auricle forward. The surgeon has raised two anteriorly based flaps: (a) the pinna and subcutaneous tissues and (b) the deeper musculoperiosteal tissues. This deeper flap can be used to partially obliterate the mastoidectomy cavity at the end of a canal-wall-down mastoidectomy (2). After an intact canal wall mastoidectomy, however, both layers should be closed to maintain a patent meatus and a properly positioned auricle.

Endaural incisions were first described by Kessel in 1885 and later popularized by Lempert (3) in 1938. These incisions expose a limited portion of the mastoid cortex. First, a posterior canal wall incision is made from the 12-o'clock to the 6-o'clock position just medial to the bony cartilaginous junction (Lempert I incision). From the 12-o'clock position of the Lempert I incision, a medial to lateral incision is

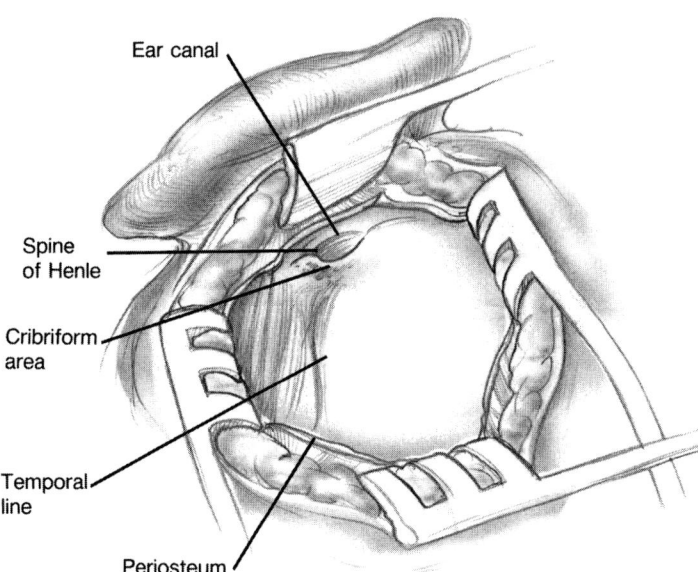

Figure 141.2 The periosteum is elevated off the mastoid cortex, exposing the posterior wall of the external auditory canal.

made into the incisura between the tragus and root of the helix (Lempert II incision). A relaxing incision is then made at the inferior margin of the Lempert I incision (in a medial to lateral direction). This allows the posterior ear canal and conchal skin to be mobilized (Fig. 141.3). The skin, soft tissues, muscle, and periosteum over the mastoid cortex are elevated using Lempert elevators and a self-retaining retractor placed. Indications for this incision include simple mastoidectomy in very poorly pneumatized temporal bones, atticotomies, canalplasties, and in some tympanoplasties. The endaural incision is closed in a layered fashion approximating deep tissues and then skin.

Surface Landmarks

The inferior temporal line (linea temporalis) defines the inferior limit of the temporalis muscle and provides a topographic landmark for the floor of the middle cranial fossa. Inferior to the temporal line is a protuberance at the posterosuperior margin of the ear canal called the suprameatal spine of Henle. Macewen triangle (cribrose area) is a depressed pit just posterior to the spine of Henle and serves as a topographic landmark for the underlying mastoid antrum. The antrum is typically located 15 mm medial to the cribrose area. The zygomatic root is palpable superior to the ear canal. The bony ear canal is made up of both tympanic and squamous bone. The anterior, inferior, and posterior-inferior walls of the external auditory canal are formed by the tympanic bone. The region between the tympanosquamous and tympanomastoid suture lines (i.e., the posterior-superior bony ear canal) is made of squamous bone. The canal skin in this region is thicker and more vascular than the inferior canal skin. When creating a laterally based conchal flap, this thickened "vascular strip"

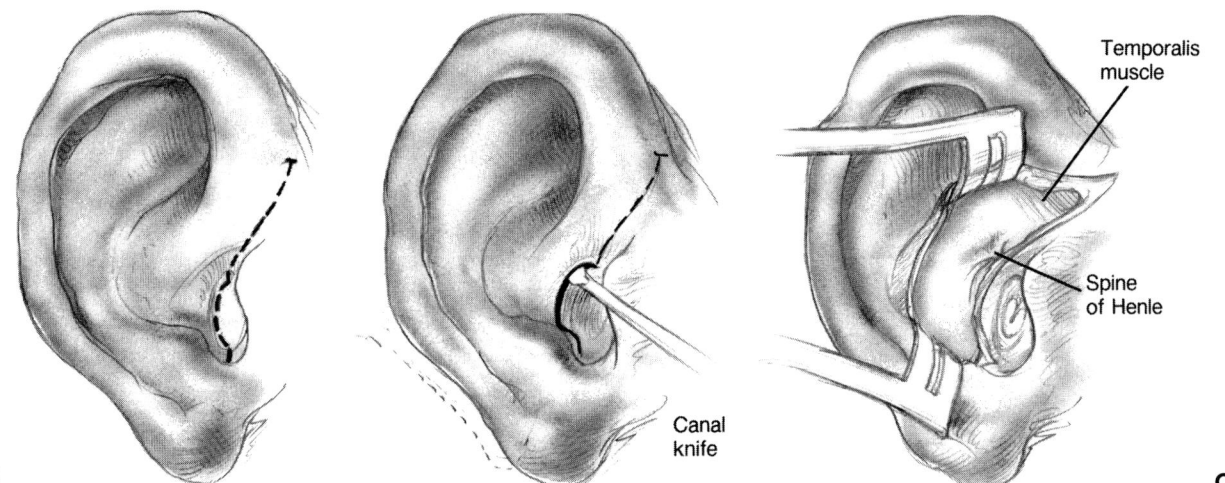

A,B
C

Figure 141.3 **A:** Endaural incision. **B:** Separation of bony cartilaginous junction. **C:** Mastoid exposure via an endaural incision.

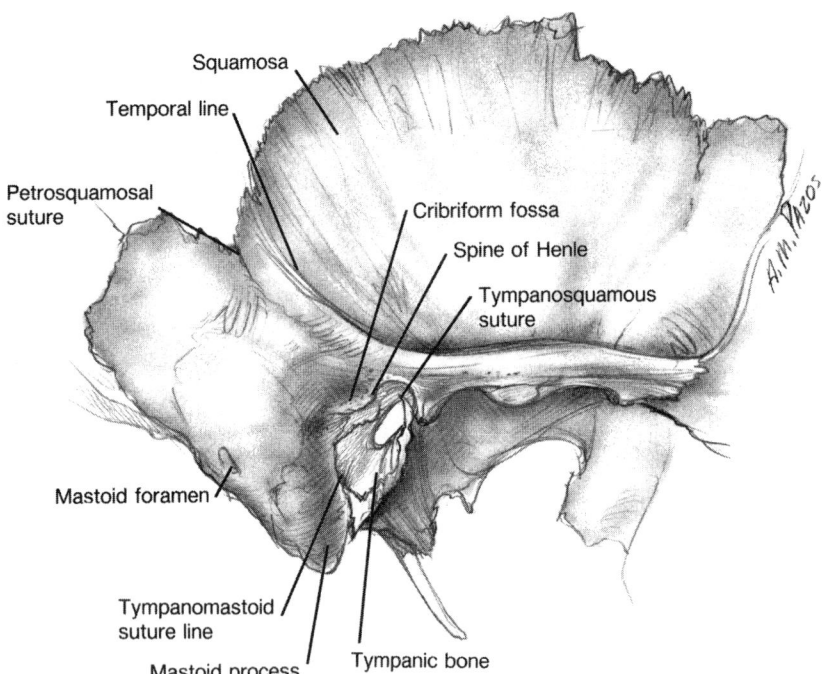

Figure 141.4 Surface anatomy of the adult temporal bone.

is elevated and preserved. The surface anatomy of the adult and young child's temporal bone differs. Children younger than 2 years have immature tympanic rings and poorly developed mastoids (Figs. 141.4 and 141.5). In children or adults with canal atresia, maldevelopment of the tympanic bone may result in a facial nerve that exits directly from what appears to be the mastoid cortex (4).

Types of Mastoidectomy

The ear canal is made up of a cylinder of skin contained within a bony cylinder. In the normal ear, the tympanic membrane is the medial boundary for those cylinders. During routine office examination, it is not possible to see

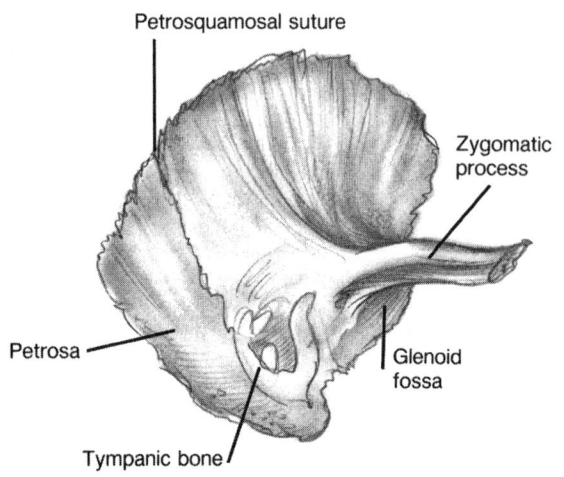

Figure 141.5 Surface anatomy of the infant temporal bone.

the epitympanum or mastoid region when the canal wall is intact. This is because the scutum blocks visualization of the epitympanum, and the posterior canal wall blocks access to the mastoid cavity. Therefore, removing the superior and posterior aspects of the bony canal allows direct access to the epitympanum and mastoid. This has the advantage of more thorough postoperative examination of the ear in the office. However, it leaves patients with cavities that require lifelong maintenance.

Mastoidectomy procedures can be categorized as canal-wall-up and canal-wall-down operations. Canal-wall-up procedures include the so-called simple mastoidectomy and the complete mastoidectomy with and without a facial recess approach. Canal-wall-down operations include the radical mastoidectomy, the modified radical mastoidectomy (MRM), and the Bondy MRM. The radical mastoidectomy removes the posterior and superior bony ear canal as well as the tympanic membrane, malleus, and incus. The stapes is usually preserved. The eustachian tube is packed, and no middle ear space remains. The entire cavity becomes lined with squamous epithelium. The radical mastoidectomy is "modified" when a tympanic membrane and mucosa-lined middle ear space are reconstructed. This is accomplished by placing a graft from the anterior annulus to the facial ridge. Ossicular reconstruction can also be performed during a MRM. The Bondy MRM is performed when disease spares the middle ear and only involves the epitympanum and mastoid. The scutum and posterior bony ear canal are removed to exteriorize the antrum and epitympanum, but the middle ear is not entered. Tympanoplasty and ossicular reconstruction can be performed whether the canal wall is taken down or left intact.

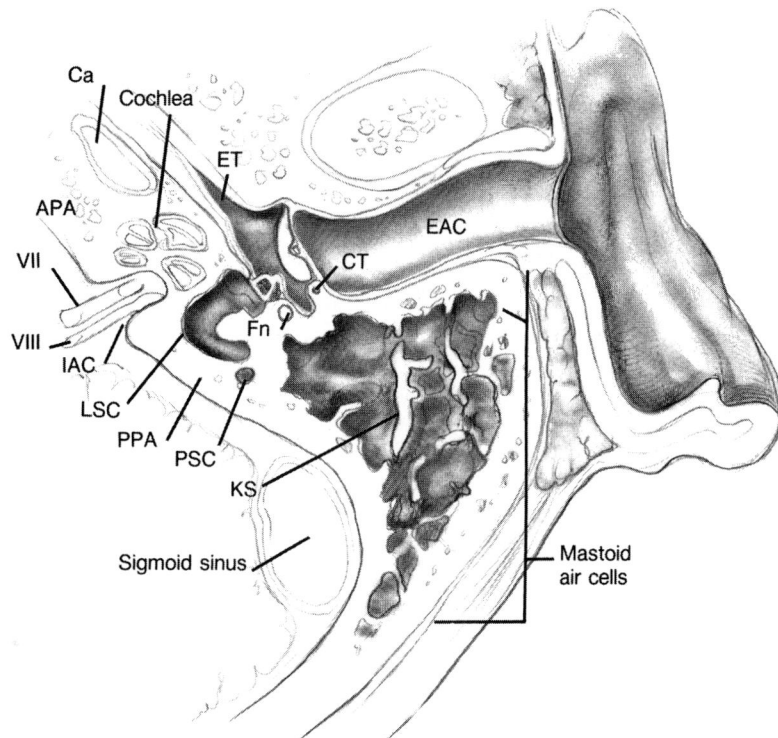

Figure 141.6 Axial section of a right adult temporal bone. VII, seventh cranial nerve; VIII, eighth cranial nerve; APA, anterior petrous apex; Ca, carotid artery; CT, chorda tympani; EAC, external auditory canal; ET, eustachian tube; Fn, facial nerve; IAC, internal auditory canal; KS, Körner septum; LSC, lateral semicircular canal; PPA, posterior petrous apex; PSC, posterior semicircular canal.

Simple Mastoidectomy

A simple mastoidectomy has limited usefulness; it is most commonly used to drain acute mastoid infections that do not respond to antibiotics. The procedure involves removing the mastoid cortex, drilling through the lateral air cells, and entering the antrum. The remainder of the air cell system is not drilled.

Complete Mastoidectomy

The complete mastoidectomy affords access to the antrum, attic, labyrinth, endolymphatic sac, and vertical segment of the facial nerve (Fig. 141.6). All the air cells along the tegmen, sigmoid sinus, facial nerve, and semicircular canals are removed. The epitympanum is made accessible though the aditus ad antrum, and the incus and head of the malleus can be inspected directly. The incus and the head of the malleus may be removed for greater access to the supratubal recess.

Using the postauricular incision, the ear is laid forward and the mastoid cortex exposed as described above. The temporal line, spine of Henle, cribrose area, and posterior ear canal are used as the initial landmarks for drilling. The location of the mastoid antrum can be approximated by the intersection of a horizontal and vertical line drawn tangential to the superior and posterior margins of the external auditory canal. A large cutting burr and suction/irrigation are used to begin the mastoidectomy. Cortical bone is removed inferior to the middle fossa dura (tegmen mastoideum); the posterior edge of the bony ear canal is delineated; and the

sigmoid sinus is identified. It is important to widely saucerize the mastoidectomy bowl by removing any overhanging edges. This permits more light to enter the cavity and allows the surgeon to bring in his instruments at an angle rather than directly along his line of sight. After determining the level of the tegmen, all air cells lateral to the sigmoid sinus should be removed to see the blue hue of the sinus through thin bone. The sinodural angle, marking the posterior-superior limit of the mastoid cavity, is then opened. Drilling proceeds medially along the tegmen toward the epitympanum. Keeping this anterior-superior portion of the dissection as the deepest portion of the cavity avoids inadvertent injury to the facial nerve. Korner septum is a plate of bone lateral to the antrum, and it represents the posterior extension of the petrosquamous suture line within the mastoid (5) (Fig. 141.7). The superior aspect of Korner septum must be removed to enter the mastoid antrum. The floor of the antrum, the horizontal semicircular canal, is a vital landmark that must be clearly visualized (Fig. 141.8). The labyrinth, made of otic capsule bone, usually appears slightly yellow when compared with the surrounding (white) membranous bone.

Once the antrum is entered, the dissection moves anteriorly into the epitympanum to find the incus. The posterior ear canal must be thinned although excessive thinning may lead to delayed dissolution of this structure. Identifying the posterior incudal ligament (often seen as a white streak through thin bone just inferior to the fossa incudus) is a useful landmark. In addition, by flooding the antrum with clear irrigant, the surface of the fluid forms a lens that

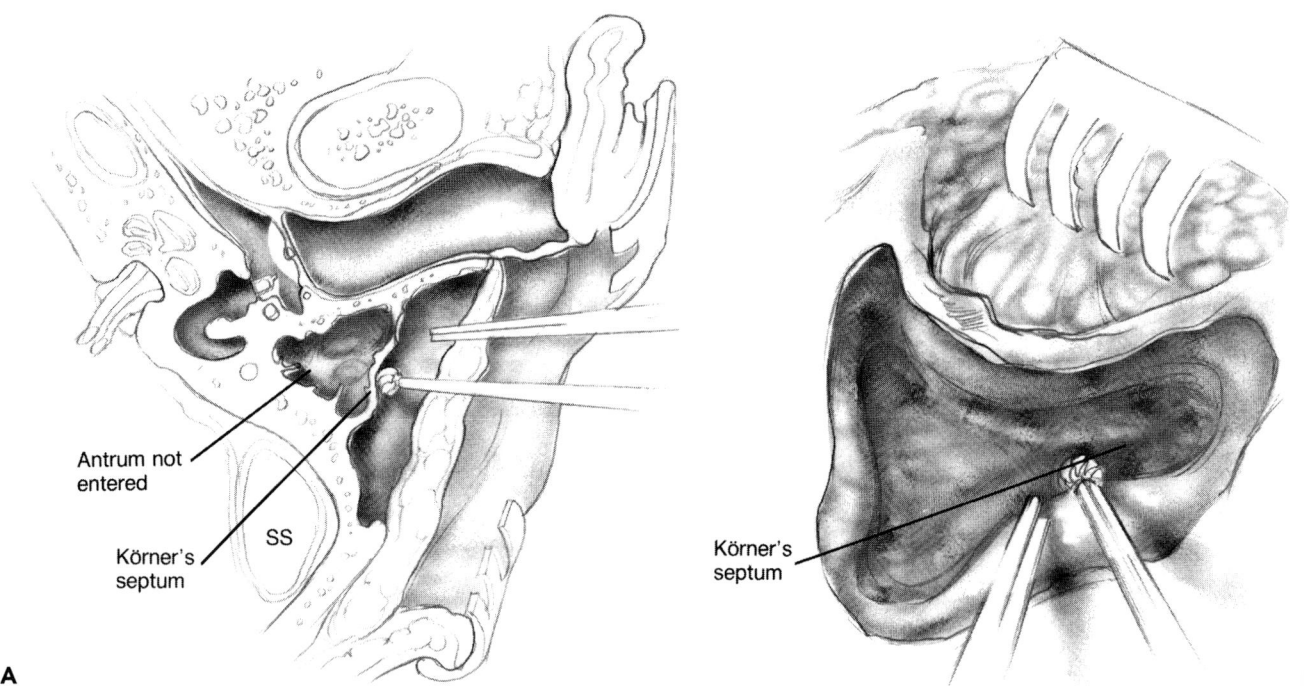

Figure 141.7 Körner septum. **A:** Axial section view of Körner septum. **B:** Lateral surgical view of Körner septum. SS, sigmoid sinus.

will bend light from the microscope and allow the surgeon to see the incus before actually coming upon it (Fig. 141.8). Touching the incus with a rotating burr must be avoided because transmission of high-frequency mechanical energy to the inner ear can cause sensorineural hearing loss. Once the body of incus is identified, removing the bone lateral to the ossicles (between the tegmen tympani and superior ear canal) opens the epitympanum. Carrying this dissection anteriorly will expose the head of the malleus.

Having found the antrum, the horizontal semicircular canal, and the incus, attention can now be directed to finding the facial nerve. The bony external auditory canal is

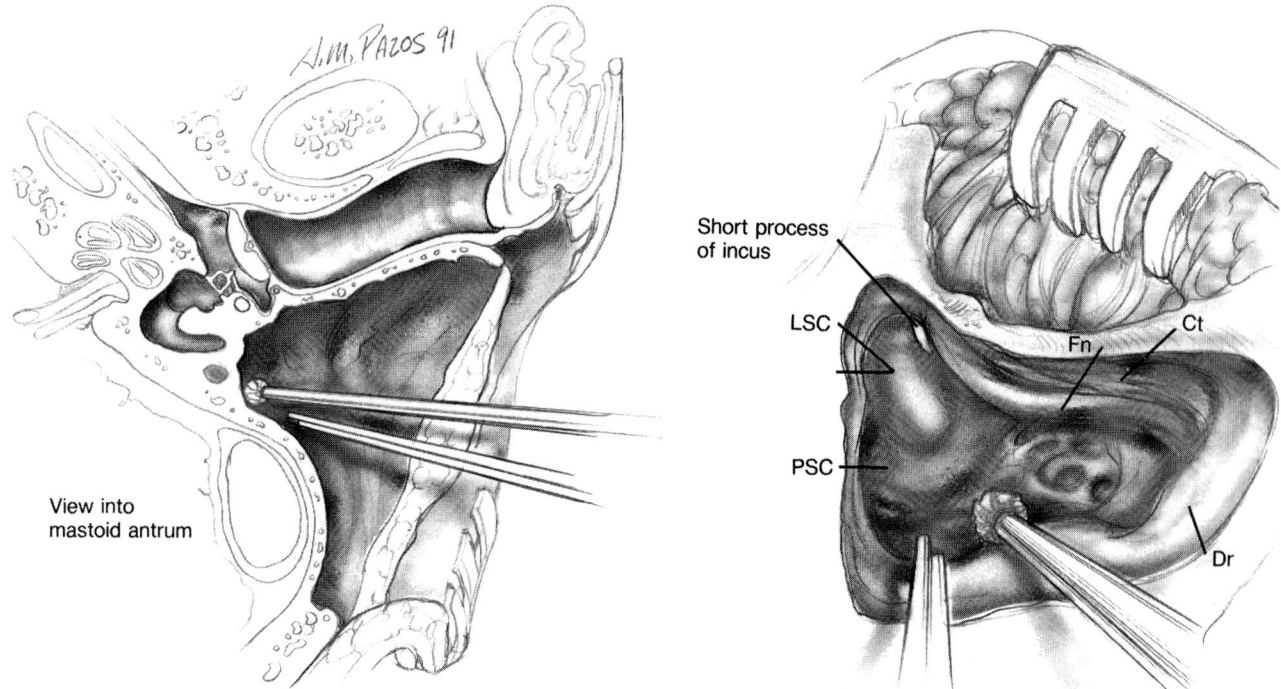

Figure 141.8 Simple mastoidectomy. **A:** Axial section view of mastoid cavity. **B:** Lateral surgical view of mastoid cavity. Ct, chorda tympani; Dr, digastric ridge; Fn, facial nerve; LSC, lateral semicircular canal; PSC, posterior semicircular canal.

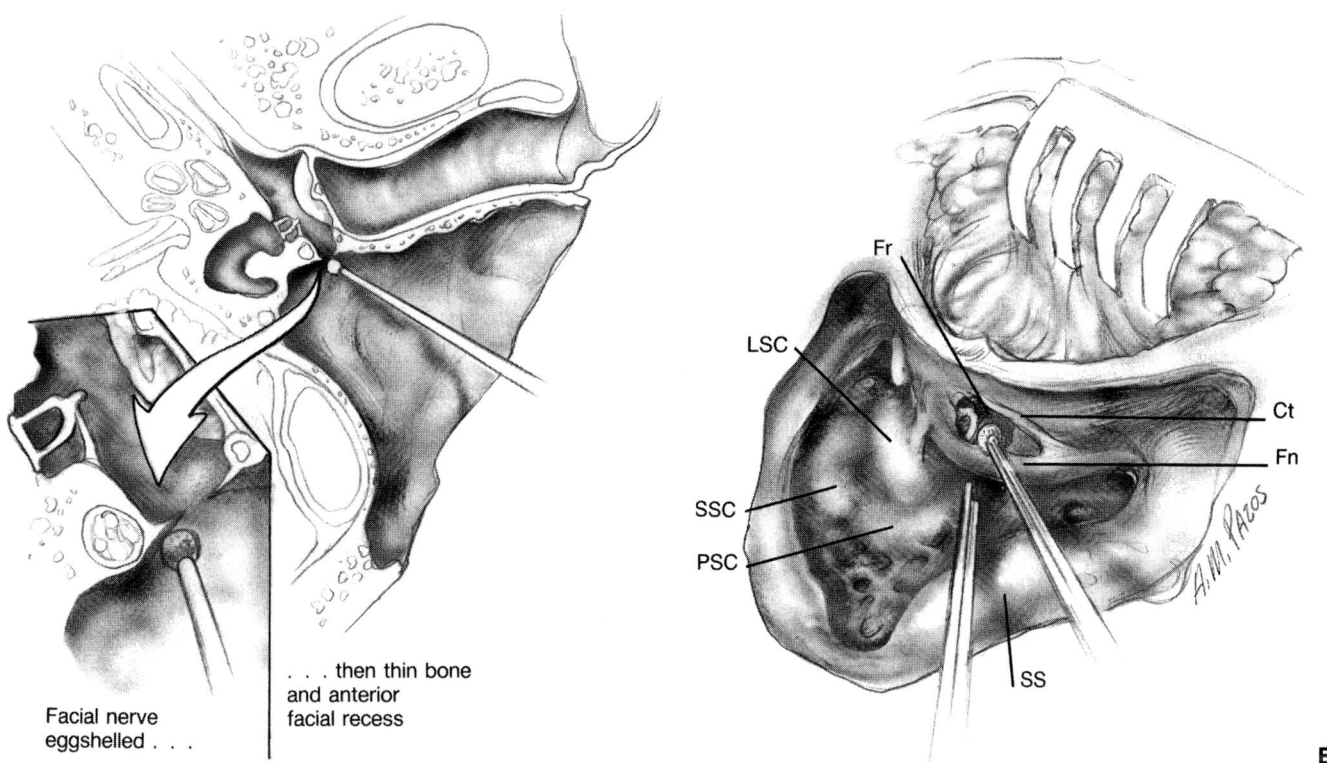

A
Facial nerve
eggshelled . . .

. . . then thin bone
and anterior
facial recess

B

Figure 141.9 Facial recess approach. **A:** Axial view. **B:** Surgical view. Ct, chorda tympani; Fn, facial nerve; Fr, facial recess; LSC, lateral semicircular canal; PSC, posterior semicircular canal; SS, sigmoid sinus; SSC, superior semicircular canal.

progressively thinned from a lateral to medial direction. As this dissection proceeds medially, facial recess air cells anterior to the facial nerve will be encountered. The second genu of the facial nerve is immediately anterior and inferior to the midpoint of the horizontal canal, just medial to the short process of the incus. A 4-mm diamond burr and copious irrigation are used to make wide strokes from the incus superiorly toward the stylomastoid foramen along the presumed course of the facial nerve. Adequate irrigation prevents thermal injury to the nerve. The nerve should be visualized through thin bone but not completely exposed. As the facial nerve is traced inferiorly, the branch-point of the chorda tympani nerve will be found (Figs. 141.8 and 141.9). The chorda can then be traced anteriorly and superiorly.

All of the cells within the mastoid tip should be exenterated. The posterior belly of the digastric muscle inserts medially on the mastoid tip. Identifying the muscle through egg-shelled bone is referred to as the "digastric ridge," which is actually a surgically created landmark (Fig. 141.8). The fascia enveloping the digastric muscle is continuous anteriorly with the fibrous tissue surrounding the facial nerve at the stylomastoid foramen. Therefore, following the digastric ridge anteriorly in the mastoid tip is one way to find the facial nerve. Infralabyrinthine (retrofacial) air cells are those cells medial to the facial nerve, superior to the jugular bulb, and inferior to the posterior semicircular canal. They should be exenterated if disease is found within them or if either the jugular bulb or endolymphatic sac needs to be exposed.

Following a complete mastoidectomy the surgeon should thoroughly irrigate the cavity to remove bone dust, which may otherwise result in ossicular fixation. The complete mastoidectomy cavity should consist of a well-defined tegmen tympani and tegmen mastoideum superiorly, a clearly delineated sigmoid sinus posteriorly, an open sinodural angle, well-visualized semicircular canals, an intact posterior ear canal wall, and the facial nerve seen through thin bone.

Complete Mastoidectomy with a Facial Recess Approach

The facial recess is an aerated extension of the posterior-superior middle ear space. Medial to the tympanic annulus and lateral to the fallopian canal, it allows access to the middle ear from the mastoid cavity. Some surgeons use the term "posterior tympanotomy" to describe a facial recess approach. The facial recess is a triangular opening bordered posteromedially by the facial nerve, anterolaterally by the chorda tympani nerve, and superiorly by the fossa incudis (Fig. 141.9). An open facial recess provides access to the ossicles, stapedial tendon, round window, tympanic segment of the facial canal, and cochleariform process (6).

There are numerous indications for performing a posterior tympanotomy. These include transmastoid cochlear implantation, presence of cholesteatoma within both the middle ear and mastoid, chronic otomastoiditis with granulation tissue or cholesterol granuloma, and tumors within the middle ear and mastoid.

In the anterior epitympanum, a projection of bone extending inferiorly from the tegmen tympani (the cog) can obscure disease in the supratubal recess (7). The presence of granulation tissue, cholesteatoma, or tumor in the anterior epitympanum and supratubal recess requires removal of the incus, head of the malleus, and the cog for exposure. The incudostapedial joint must first be disarticulated through the facial recess before removing the incus and malleus head. Opening the facial recess can also improve aeration of the mastoid by providing an alternate route for air from the eustachian tube to enter the mastoid (other than the aditus ad antrum). Inadequate aeration or loculation of the mastoid cavity may result in recurrent retraction pocket formation, mucocele formation, or chronic otomastoiditis. One way to test for adequate aeration of the mastoid cavity is to fill the middle ear with saline and watch for flow into the mastoid. When the incus has been removed, rarely is a facial recess approach required for aeration.

When thinning the posterior canal wall, the facial recess is encountered medially. It is first noted as a color change (darker appearing bone) anterior to the facial nerve just inferior to its second genu. The facial nerve lies medial and inferior to the tip of the short process of the incus. The second genu of the facial nerve usually forms an angle of 95 to 125 degrees; it usually makes a gentle curve rather than an abrupt turn. The nerve may descend directly through the mastoid in a caudal direction, or it may deviate from the vertical by 5 to 35 degrees. The temporal bone is a three-dimensional structure. The facial nerve travels laterally as it moves inferiorly through its vertical segment. The nerve is lateral to the posteroinferior tympanic annulus in 65% of cases (8).

The surgeon should be aware of potential facial nerve anomalies. Dehiscence of the facial nerve is reported to occur in 55% to 57% of temporal bones (9). The facial nerve is dehiscent approximately 50% of the time in its tympanic segment just superior to the oval window. Other areas of possible dehiscence include the geniculate ganglion, facial recess, tympanic sinus, and the retrofacial region inferior to the labyrinth. Bone erosion secondary to

cholesteatoma may also create dehiscence in the fallopian canal. Before encountering the nerve, the vasa nervorum can be appreciated through the egg-shelled bone overlying the nerve. The most common site of injury to the facial nerve in mastoid surgery is inferior to the lateral semicircular canal just beyond the second genu (9).

At a variable point along its descent toward the stylomastoid foramen, the facial nerve gives off the chorda tympani nerve. This nerve travels in an anterior, superior, and lateral direction. Facial nerve anomalies can include a chorda that branches from the facial nerve after it exits from the stylomastoid foramen, a bifid facial nerve, or a nerve coursing through the middle ear space just inferior to the oval window (10). Once the chorda tympani nerve is identified, the bone between the chorda and the facial nerve may be removed with a small diamond burr and copious irrigation. This opens the facial recess (Fig. 141.9). If additional exposure is required, the chorda may be sacrificed and the facial recess extended inferiorly—an extended facial recess approach. Care must be taken to identify the fibrous annulus of the tympanic membrane and to avoid inadvertent injury to the eardrum or medial ear canal.

Intact Canal Versus Canal-Wall-Down Mastoidectomy

Both the open (canal-wall-down) and the closed (intact canal with facial recess) procedures have advantages and disadvantages. Judgment as to which procedure to perform depends on the nature of the disease, the reliability of the patient, and the experience of the surgeon (Table 141.2).

The intact canal wall approach offers several advantages over open (canal-wall-down) techniques. First, there is no mastoid cavity to care for. Patients with cavities often require regular office debridement, may have a difficult time fitting hearing aids, need to adhere to water precautions, and have meatoplasties that may be cosmetically unappealing. An intact canal procedure also allows for a more physiologic ossicular reconstruction with a deeper, better-aerated middle ear. Some authors, however, have found no significant benefit in

TABLE 141.2

OPEN VERSUS CLOSED TECHNIQUES FOR MASTOIDECTOMY

	Advantages	Disadvantages
Intact wall	Physiologic tympanic membrane position Deep middle ear No mastoid bowl	Residual cholesteatoma may be occult Recurrent cholesteatoma may occur in attic Delayed canal breakdown Incomplete exteriorization of facial recess Second stage often required
Canal-wall-down	Residual cholesteatoma visible on follow-up Recurrent cholesteatoma is rare Total exteriorization of facial recess	Mastoid bowl maintenance can be a lifelong problem Middle ear is shallow and difficult to reconstruct Position of pinna may be altered Second stage sometimes required

hearing results for intact canal wall mastoidectomy compared with canal-wall-down procedures (11,12).

There are several potential disadvantages to the intact-canal-wall approach. First, there is an increased risk of residual or recurrent disease. Widely varying results using a canal-wall-up mastoidectomy have been reported in the literature. However, most of the larger series reveal residual cholesteatoma in 20% to 35% of cases and recurrent disease in 5% to 20% (12–20). This is in contrast to results for open procedures in which there is a 2% to 17% rate of residual disease and a 0% to 10% chance for recurrence (12–14,19–22). The most common site for residual disease is the sinus tympani (18). A second potential although uncommon problem with the intact canal wall procedures is delayed breakdown of the posterior canal wall. This is due to compromised blood supply from overthinning the bone. A third disadvantage is an inability to see the mastoid cavity in the office for surveillance. Some surgeons routinely perform a "second look" operation 6 to 12 months after the initial procedure. A staged ossicular reconstruction can also be done at that time. Careful patient selection is vital. Intact-canal procedures should be performed in reliable patients who will follow-up regularly in the office.

Radical Mastoidectomy

The radical mastoidectomy is the most aggressive of the open cavity mastoid procedures. The classical radical mastoidectomy involves a canal-wall-down mastoidectomy combined with complete removal of the tympanic membrane, annulus, malleus, incus, and all middle ear mucosa. The eustachian tube is stripped of mucosa and obliterated with packing (fascia, muscle or bone). The goal of radical mastoidectomy is to establish a dry, open cavity devoid of

secretory epithelium. Before the advent of tympanoplasty, this radical procedure was by far the most common open procedure. However, it is rarely performed today. Most surgeons prefer to do a MRM with reconstruction of a middle ear space and sound conduction apparatus. If disease permits, a graft can be placed isolating the eustachian tube and round window from the middle ear, creating a cava minor reconstruction. However, there are still some indications for a radical mastoidectomy. These include unresectable cholesteatoma with extension down the eustachian tube, cholesteatoma with erosion into the cochlea or labyrinth, or patients who have had multiple failed MRMs.

The procedure involves performing a complete (intact canal) mastoidectomy with identification of all the landmarks discussed previously. The superior and posterior canal walls are then removed with a cutting burr and suction-irrigation. Prior to encountering the ossicles, the incudostapedial joint is separated and the head of the malleus and incus are removed. The canal wall can then be lowered to the level of the facial nerve. The stapes is preserved. A diamond burr with copious irrigation is used as the facial nerve is approached. All the mastoid and middle ear mucosa is stripped, and the eustachian tube is packed with muscle, fascia, or synthetic materials. The mastoid tip is removed below to the level of the digastric ridge. Care should be taken to lower the facial ridge, remove overhanging edges, and lower the inferior canal wall so as to prevent a dependent mastoid tip. To reduce the depth of the cavity, the perimeter is well saucerized.

Modified Radical Mastoidectomy

The radical mastoidectomy operation has been "modified" when a middle ear space is reconstructed (Fig. 141.10). The

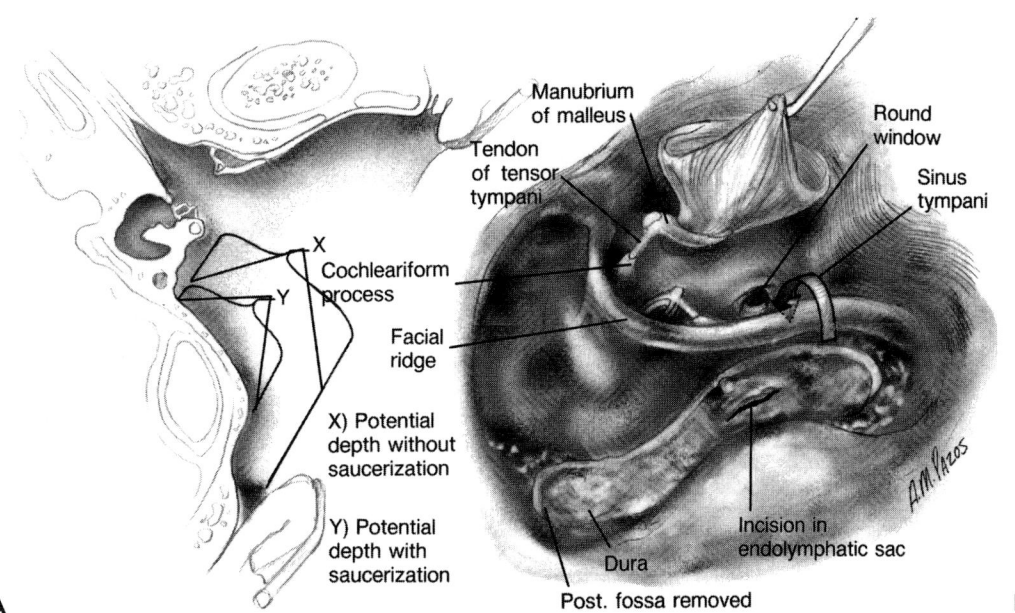

A **B**

Figure 141.10 Completed canal-wall-down modified radical mastoidectomy. **A:** Axial view. **B:** Surgical view with location of endolymphatic sac.

MRM begins with a complete mastoidectomy. The decision to take the canal wall down is then based on the extent of disease (Table 141.2). Most of the bone lateral to incus can be removed quickly with a large cutting burr and the scutum made flush with the anterior canal wall. Because the facial nerve is medial to the incus, it is protected. The bone immediately lateral to the ossicles must be removed carefully with microinstruments rather than the drill. This avoids direct contact between the rotating burr and ossicular chain. Alternately, the incudostapedial joint may be separated and the incus and head of the malleus removed. The posterior and inferior portions of the remaining ear canal are then removed. The bone, lateral to the facial nerve, called the "facial ridge," is drilled down to the level of the nerve.

A few technical points deserve mention. Once the bulk of the posterior ear canal has been removed with cutting burrs, the vertical segment of the facial nerve is found by lowering the facial ridge with a diamond burr. The nerve should be seen through thin bone. Actual exposure of the facial nerve should be avoided, however, because this puts it at risk. With radical mastoidectomies and MRMs, the mastoid cortex must be well saucerized and the mastoid tip removed. This precludes a deep cavity with overhanging edges that can be difficult to cleanse. Saucerization makes the cavity shallow by allowing surrounding soft tissues to prolapse inward. The inferior portion of the tympanic ring should be lowered so it is flush with the hypotympanum. This prevents the formation of a dependent mastoid tip that collects debris. An anterior canal wall canalplasty should be performed to better expose the anterior tympanic sulcus. An incision is made in the anterior canal wall just lateral to the tympanic annulus, the skin is raised in a retrograde manner back to the bony cartilaginous junction, and the bone sculpted as necessary. One should use a large diamond burr with constant suction-irrigation to avoid entering the glenoid fossa.

After mastoid surgery has been completed, the middle ear space is reconstructed. A fascia graft is laid from the anterior annulus to and over the facial ridge. The graft must be well supported by absorbable Gelfoam. Surgeons may elect to place Silastic or Gelfilm over the promontory to prevent adhesions between the drum and middle ear mucosa. Although the middle ear is shallow in open techniques, there is usually sufficient space to perform an ossiculoplasty.

The Bondy Modified Radical Mastoidectomy

The Bondy procedure (23), first suggested by Körner (5) in 1899, is a variation of the MRM. Therefore, by definition, this is a canal-wall-down procedure. It can be performed through either an endaural or postauricular incision. This operation is used in cases of large attic cholesteatomas in which the middle ear has been spared of disease. An atticotomy is performed first. The entire scutum is removed to expose the epitympanum, marsupialize the cholesteatoma,

and debride its keratin content. The medial wall of the cholesteatoma matrix is left in place over the body of the incus and head of the malleus in the epitympanum. This seals the middle ear space. If the cholesteatoma is seen extending around the ossicles, the surgeon must be prepared to perform a more traditional MRM.

If involvement of the middle ear is in question preoperatively, a high-resolution computed tomography (CT) scan of the temporal bone with axial and coronal views may help determine whether a Bondy procedure is indicated. This operation is reserved for those ears with large primary acquired cholesteatomas in which hearing is preserved and the ossicular chain is free of disease. A Bondy mastoidectomy is a particularly useful technique in cases with cholesteatoma and a labyrinthine fistula, especially in an only hearing ear. After the procedure, keratin can be debrided in the office while leaving the medial matrix of the cholesteatoma intact over the fistula. The surgeon must be vigilant, however, during each office examination. If cholesteatoma appears to extend into the middle ear, this finding should be verified with CT imaging. A traditional MRM would then become necessary.

MEATOPLASTY AND MASTOID OBLITERATION

The most important factors in avoiding a chronically draining cavity are adequate removal of disease during surgery, designing a properly shaped mastoid cavity, and creating a wide external auditory meatus.

Mastoid Obliteration

Following canal-wall-down mastoidectomy, the patient is left with a cavity. The keratinizing squamous epithelium that lines the mastoid bowl is prone to collecting debris and should be cleaned on a regular basis. Many patients must adhere to lifelong water precautions to minimize risk of infection. Some technical considerations help to limit postoperative complications in a canal-wall-down mastoidectomy (2,24–30). Wide saucerization of the mastoid bowl allows the surrounding soft tissues to prolapse into and partially obliterate the cavity. Lowering the facial ridge and performing a generous meatoplasty also helps. Avoiding a dependent mastoid tip prevents accumulation of debris in this difficult to clean area. Lowering the bony canal wall and inferior annulus flush with the hypotympanum facilitates in-office access to the dependent areas of the mastoid.

Some surgeons obliterate the mastoidectomy cavity in more formal ways. Originally described by Mosher (27), the Palva flap has been used successfully in obliterating mastoid cavities (2). This flap is a long, laterally based postauricular musculoperiosteal flap that is rotated into cavity at the end of the procedure. Postmortem histologic examination of temporal bones from patients who underwent mastoid obliteration with the Palva flap has demonstrated viable muscle, fat, collagen, and richly vascularized tissue years after the procedure. There can be some atrophy, however, over the 5-year period after mastoidectomy. This may result in progressive widening of some cavities (29,31). Other potential flaps that could be used to obliterate the mastoid bowl include an anteriorly based temporalis muscle flap or a temporalis fascia flap based on superficial temporal artery pedicle (the Hong Kong flap) (25,32). Such flaps provide bulk, cover exposed bone, recruit a blood supply, and provide a surface for epithelial migration. Palva (30) has advocated the use of bone pâté and bone chips for obliterating the mastoid defect. It is important to collect the bone pâté from cortical bone, before entering the diseased portions of the mastoid. This pâté is laid into the cavity at the end of the case and flaps rotated over it. All bone pâté must be completely covered by fascia or the Palva flap. Osteoneogenesis then results in further reduction of the size of the mastoid cavity (31) over time.

Grote and Blitterswijk (32) have described reconstructing the posterior canal wall with porous hydroxyapatite. It is packaged as a preformed prosthesis, which can then be covered with a vascularized flap (33,34). Others have used cartilage for canal wall reconstruction. Montandon et al. (24) recommended combining the canal-wall-up procedure with mastoid obliteration using a fat graft as a means of avoiding recurrent disease. They also exteriorize the attic into the ear canal.

Meatoplasty

Enlarging the external auditory meatus is a necessary part of canal-wall-down procedures. It promotes aeration and epithelialization, facilitates effective postoperative care, and makes office debridement of the cavity much easier. An adequate meatoplasty also reduces the depth of the bowl. Several techniques to enlarge the external auditory meatus have been devised. Each involves removing some conchal cartilage and drapes the posterior meatal skin into the mastoid bowl (Fig. 141.11).

An excellent meatoplasty can be performed by connecting superior and inferior Lempert endaural incisions with the postauricular incision. The superior cut is brought out laterally into the tragal incisura while the inferior cut is curved just medial to the antitragus. This creates a laterally based composite flap made of conchal cartilage and meatal skin. Varying amounts of this cartilage can be removed (through the postauricular incision), leaving behind thin conchal skin that drapes into the mastoid bowl. Adequate resection of cartilage and appropriate positioning of the posterior canal skin are vital. The meatus can be maintained open by placing absorbable sutures from the remaining conchal cartilage and perichondrium to the postauricular periosteum. Three sutures are usually placed: one posterosuperiorly, one directly posterior, and the third posteroinferiorly. The sutures are not tied until all three have been properly placed. These tacking sutures prevent postoperative protrusion of the auricle and collapse of the meatus.

This meatoplasty technique can be adapted to individual reconstructive needs. Portmann (35) describes a three-flap technique that maximizes canal epithelium in appropriate cases. The meatus can be enlarged superiorly by only removing cartilage at the base of the helix as it joins the concha. The surgeon should tailor the extent of cartilage removal to the size and shape of the postmastoidectomy cavity.

ENDOSCOPY

Endoscopes often see where the microscope cannot. The surgeon's view through the operating microscope depends on a clear line of sight. A 1.7- to 2.8-mm, 30-degree rigid telescope, however, can look around a corner to visualize the facial recess, sinus tympani, or epitympanum. It can also be used to assess the depth of retraction pockets and determine the extent of cholesteatomas. Some authors have advocated the use of endoscopes for second-look procedures following intact canal wall tympanomastoidectomies (36–38). Rosenberg et al. (37) reported that endoscopic findings correlated well with open surgical exploration in ten out of ten patients. The role of endoscopy will continue to expand in the otologic and neurotologic applications as surgeons become more comfortable with their use and larger studies confirm their efficacy.

ENDOLYMPHATIC SHUNT

In 1927, Guild (39) proposed that endolymph in the inner ear may flow from the cochlea to the endolymphatic sac. It was near this time that Portmann (40) first incised the endolymphatic sac in the treatment of Ménière disease. Interestingly, however, not until a decade later did Hallpike and Cairns (41) demonstrate the histopathology of endolymphatic hydrops in patients with Ménière disease. Since then multiple procedures have been designed to "shunt" endolymph from the endolymphatic sac for the treatment of intractable Ménière disease. House (42) advocated shunting endolymph from the sac to the subarachnoid space by placing a specially designed shunt tube through the medial wall of the endolymphatic sac. Shea (43) described drainage of endolymph from the sac into the mastoid cavity using a Teflon film. Shambaugh (44) believed decompression of the sac without incision yielded the same results. Shunts from the endolymphatic sac into the mastoid have been established using Silastic strips or specially manufactured valves (45,46). Successful control of vertigo is reported in a majority of patients regardless of the technique used, but some have questioned the efficacy of these procedures (47) (see Chapter 156).

Exposure of the endolymphatic sac requires a complete mastoidectomy. The facial nerve is clearly identified and

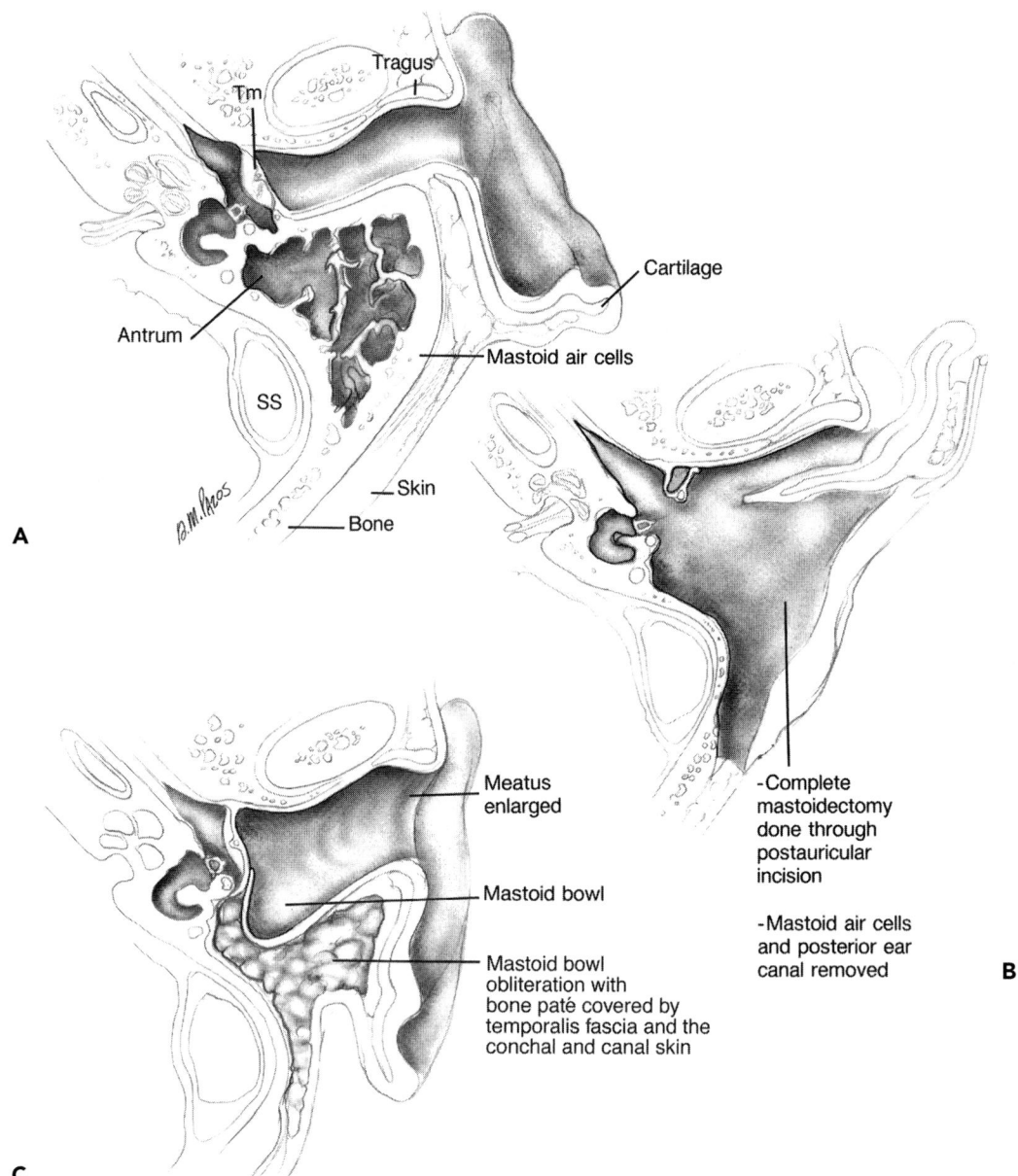

Figure 141.11 Meatoplasty following canal-wall-down mastoidectomy. **A:** Axial view of unoperated temporal bone. SS, sigmoid sinus; Tm, tympanic membrane. **B:** Axial view of temporal bone after canal-wall-down mastoidectomy. **C:** Axial view after meatoplasty and partial obliteration of mastoid bowl with muscle-periosteal flap.

traced from the second genu through its vertical segment. The posterior semicircular canal is identified, and the posterior fossa plate between the sigmoid sinus and the posterior semicircular canal is thinned. The inferior crus of the posterior semicircular canal does not extend more than 12 mm inferior to the tip of the incus (48). The sigmoid sinus is followed inferiorly toward the jugular bulb. As the posterior fossa plate is thinned, the endolymphatic sac comes into view just posteroinferior to the posterior semicircular canal. This structure appears as a thickened, white area of dura. The bone overlying the sac must be removed, and its lateral wall is incised (Fig. 141.12). Because the "lumen" of the endolymphatic sac is a labyrinth of small, interconnected lu-

mina, space for the shunt is created by blunt dissection. The surgeon should place a sickle knife or similar instrument into the sac and palpate the operculum. An anterior sigmoid sinus may completely overlie the endolymphatic sac. In such cases, the sinus can be decompressed and retracted posteriorly for visualization of the sac. One should be vigilant for the presence of a high jugular bulb. This does not usually impair access to the sac but its presence limits the amount of space available to the surgeon inferior to the posterior semicircular canal. The patient should be well secured to the bed; decompressing the posterior fossa plate and endolymphatic sac often requires that the patient be rotated maximally toward the surgeon.

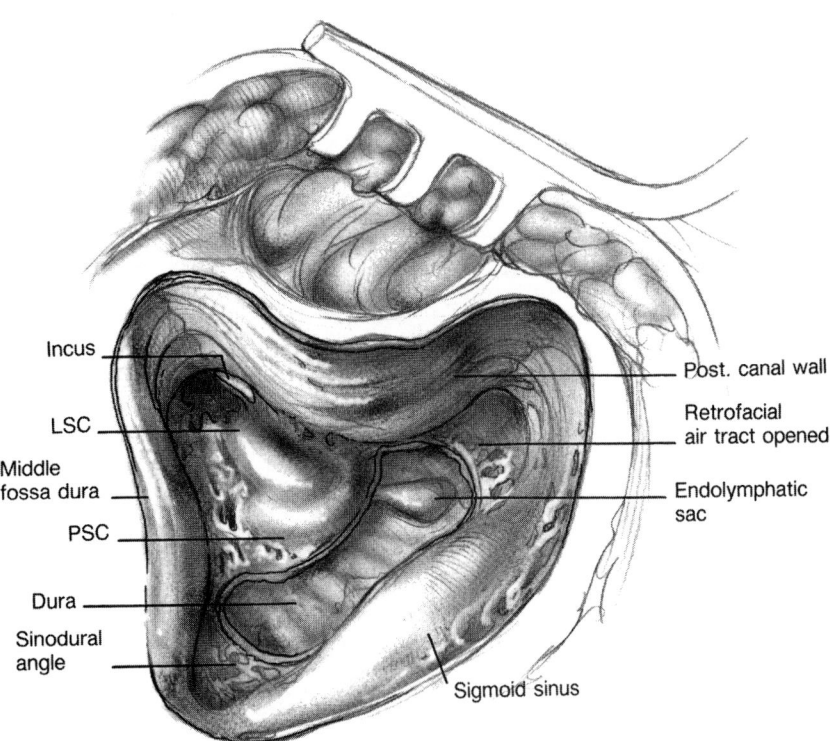

Incus

LSC

Middle
fossa dura

PSC

Dura

Sinodural
angle

Post. canal wall

Retrofacial
air tract opened

Endolymphatic
sac

Sigmoid sinus

Figure 141.12 Transmastoid exposure of endolymphatic sac. LSC, lateral semicircular canal; PSC, posterior semicircular canal.

PETROUS APICECTOMY

Infections of the mastoid and middle ear can spread to the anterior and medial segment of the temporal bone known as the petrous apex. Petrous apicitis is classically characterized by deep retroorbital pain, abducens nerve palsy, and otorrhea (Gradenigo syndrome). Cranial nerves V, VI, and VII may become involved (49,50). Surgical access to the petrous apex becomes necessary for drainage of expanding cholesterol granulomas and mucosal cysts, exenteration of infected air cells, removal of cholesteatomas, and biopsy of various mass lesions.

The petrous apex takes the form of a truncated pyramid (Fig. 141.13) divided into an anterior and posterior portion by a coronal plane through the internal auditory canal. Thirty percent of posterior petrous apices and 9% of anterior apices are pneumatized (50). The petrous tip is in close relation to Dorello canal and Meckel cave. Dorello canal, formed by the petrous apex, clivus, and petrosphenoidal (Gruber) ligament, contains the abducens nerve. The trigeminal fossa (Meckel cave), in the floor of the middle cranial fossa, houses the trigeminal (Gasserian) ganglion. Given this anatomy, it is easy to see why diseases here can compromise cranial nerves V and VI.

The classic procedures designed to access the posterior petrous apex include the transmastoid infralabyrinthine approach and the translabyrinthine approach. Procedures used to access the anterior petrous apex include the infracochlear approach, the transotic approach, the middle fossa approach, and an anterior approach through the glenoid fossa (Fig. 141.14). Other procedures including the transcanal anterior approach (51), endoscope-assisted

approach (52), and an image-guided approach through the sphenoid sinus (53) have also been described. Sparing the otic capsule surgically is preferred in patients with serviceable hearing.

Fortunately, most lesions in the petrous apex require drainage rather than en bloc resection. An isolated middle cranial fossa approach can be used when the disease involves the anterior petrous apex but spares the middle ear and mastoid. Unfortunately this approach does not allow for dependent drainage. Details regarding the middle fossa approach are beyond the scope of this chapter. In brief, however, the pathology is approached from an extradural, superior direction after creating a temporal craniotomy. The temporal lobe is retracted superiorly. The internal auditory canal is delineated with small diamond burrs as the key surgical landmark. Bone anterior to the internal auditory canal and medial to the carotid artery is removed to access the lesion.

The classic infracochlear approach provides direct surgical access to the petrous apex. A postauricular incision is made and the ear raised forward in the usual manner. A wide superiorly based tympanomeatal flap is elevated using canal incisions in the 10-o'clock and 2-o'clock positions. The flap should be relatively long so as to cover the enlarged tympanic ring created by the procedure. This flap is folded into the anterior-superior quadrant and a canaloplasty is performed lowering both the inferior tympanic ring and the floor of the external auditory canal. The infracochlear air cell tract must then be identified. It is initially bordered by the basal turn of the cochlea superiorly, the vertical segment of the internal carotid artery anteriorly, and the jugular bulb inferiorly. A 1- or 2-mm diamond burr and

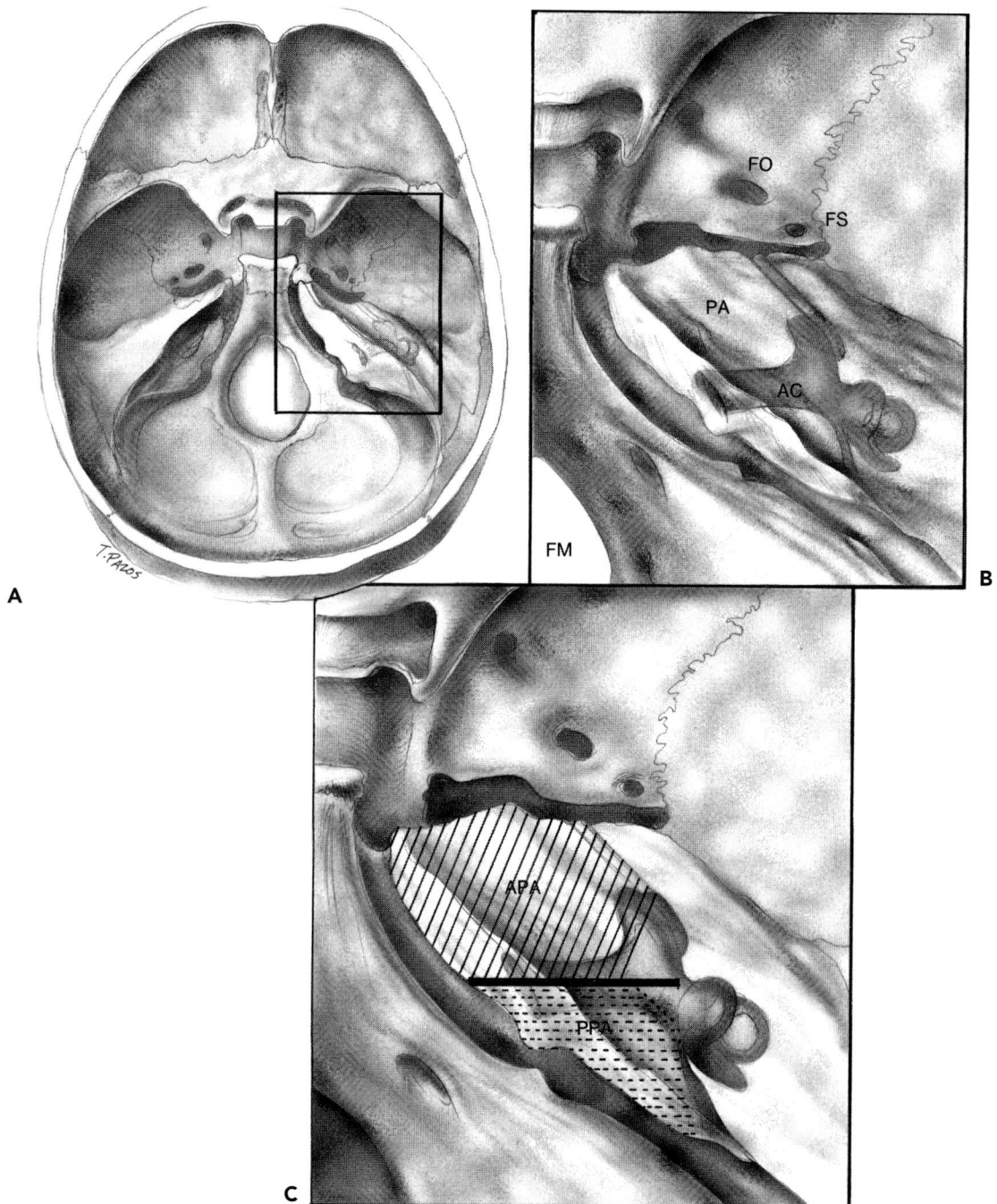

Figure 141.13 A: Superior view of base of skull. **B:** The petrous apex with the relative location of the internal auditory canal and labyrinth. **C:** Petrous apex divided into the anterior and posterior portions. APA, anterior petrous apex; PPA, posterior petrous apex.

suction irrigation are used to open the air cells of this tract. Once the biopsy or drainage procedure is complete, a silastic stent can be placed into the pathway to facilitate aeration. The tympanomeatal flap is returned to its anatomic position, and the ear is closed in the usual manner. A high-riding jugular may prohibit use of this approach.

The transmastoid, infralabyrinthine approach to the petrous apex necessitates a complete mastoidectomy and precise delineation of the facial nerve. The canal wall may

be maintained in patients with adequate mastoid development and pneumatization. The infralabyrinthine air cell tract is located inferior to the posterior semicircular canal, superior to the jugular bulb, and medial to the facial nerve. This tract is opened in an anterior and medial direction. The route passes inferior to the internal auditory canal and through the cochlear aqueduct, which must be plugged to prevent a postoperative cerebrospinal fluid (CSF) leak. The lesion in question should be exteriorized or biopsied, and

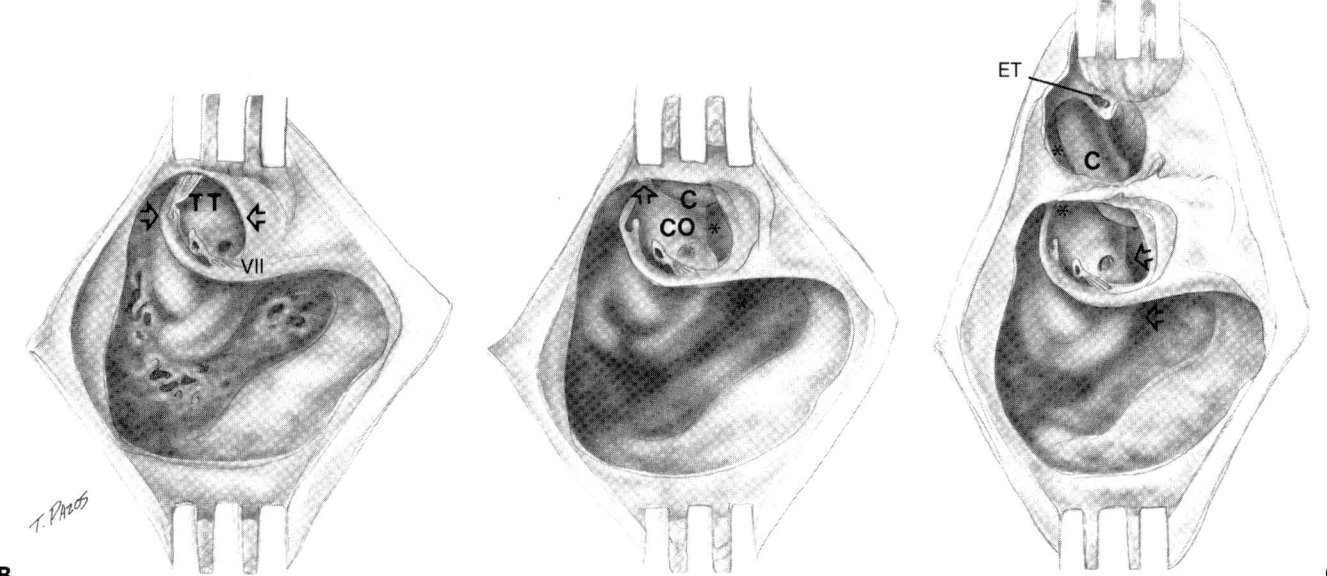

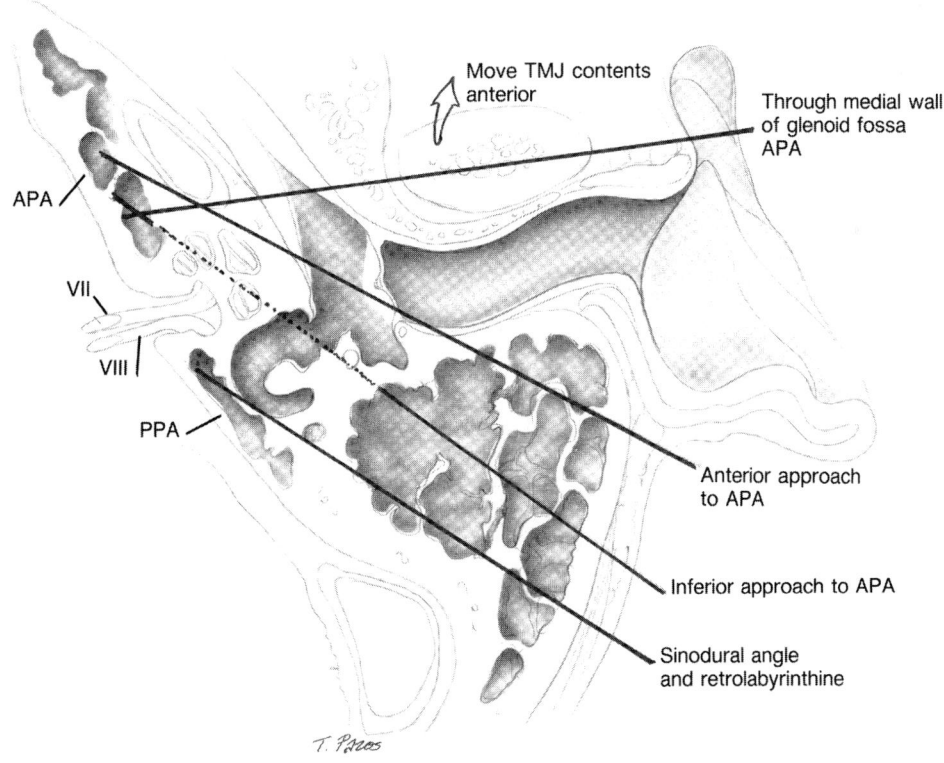

Figure 141.14   A: Access to the posterior apex air cells. **B:** Access to the petrous apex via the infra-labyrinthine air cell tract. **C:** Anterior approach to the anterior petrous apex through the glenoid fossa. **D:** Axial view of the temporal bone demonstrating the approaches to the petrous apex. VII, seventh cranial nerve; VIII, eighth cranial nerve; APA, anterior petrous apex; C, carotid artery; CO, cochlea; ET, eustachian tube; PPA, posterior petrous apex. (From Chole RA. Petrous apicitis: surgical anatomy. *Ann Otol Rhinol Laryngol* 1985;94:251, with permission.)

a silastic stent placed. Adequate review of preoperative high-resolution CT scans will determine whether this tract is present and of reasonable caliber for access.

Patients with large lesions and no serviceable preoperative hearing are candidates for the transotic approach. This route provides superior access for complete removal of mass lesions such as cholesteatomas. The procedure begins with a radical mastoidectomy and removal of the stapes suprastructure. The semicircular canals are drilled away as is the cochlea. Great care is taken to delineate and protect the facial nerve (superior and posterior), petrous carotid (anterior), jugular bulb (inferior), and internal auditory canal. The surgeon dissects in an anterior and medial direction. Should a patent cochlear aqueduct be encountered, it must be plugged with bone wax at the end of the case. After removing the mass in question, most surgeons choose to obliterate the cavity with fat, plug the eustachian tube, and close off the external auditory canal.

Gerek and colleagues (51) describe a transcanal approach for drainage of limited lesions in the anterior petrous apex. Using cadaver dissections, they suggest elevation of a wide, superiorly based tympanomeatal flap followed by a generous anterior and inferior canalplasty. The vertical segment of the petrous carotid is exposed and traced for 5 to 10 mm. The cortical bone anterior to the cochlea, between it and the internal carotid artery, is then drilled. These authors report that an air cell tract to the anterior petrous apex is present in this location with mean anterior-posterior diameter, height, and length of 4.7, 3.2, and 14.7 mm, respectively.

If greater exposure of the anterior apex is required, the complete apicectomy of Ramadier and Lempert may be performed (54–56). The glenoid fossa must be exposed and the mandibular condyle can either be removed or displaced anteriorly. This provides access to the medial wall of the glenoid fossa. In the classically described procedure, the anterior external auditory canal wall is removed. However, it can be preserved in most cases. The position of the petrous carotid must be kept in mind as the medial wall of the glenoid fossa is removed using diamond burrs and suction-irrigation. All bone between the carotid artery and the dura of the middle cranial fossa is removed (Fig. 141.14C). Complete exenteration of the anterior petrous apex is impossible without performing a labyrinthectomy, but, in most cases, drainage of infected cells is sufficient to reverse the suppurative process (Fig. 141.14D).

COMPLICATIONS AND EMERGENCIES (TABLE 141.3)

Facial Nerve Injury

The facial nerve is at risk in its labyrinthine, tympanic, and mastoid segments during otologic surgery. The nerve not only takes a tortuous, sometimes-anomalous course through the temporal bone, but its canal may also be dehiscent. Heat

TABLE 141.3   COMPLICATIONS: MASTOID SURGERY

Perioperative complications
  Facial nerve injury
  Sensorineural hearing loss
  Postoperative infection
  Dysgeusia
  Brain herniation
  Cerebrospinal fluid leakage
  Bleeding

Delayed complications
  Posterior canal breakdown
  Perichondritis
  Blue-domed cyst
  Mucosalization of mastoid bowl
  Stenosis of external canal

generated by a diamond burr can injure the nerve without direct mechanical trauma. Constant suction-irrigation helps dissipate thermal energy and prevent this complication. Landmarks such as the antrum, horizontal semicircular canal, short process of the incus, fossa incudus, cochleariform process, oval window, pyramidal process, chorda tympani, and digastric ridge help to locate the nerve. However, such landmarks may be absent or altered during procedures for congenital atresia or cases requiring revision surgery. Intraoperative facial nerve monitoring may be helpful in reducing the risk of iatrogenic trauma.

If the facial nerve is traumatized during surgery, the extent of injury should be assessed both by direct observation and electrical testing. The region of the suspected injury should be examined by decompressing the nerve 5 to 10 mm proximal and distal to the site of injury. It should be exposed in a 180-degree fashion. If facial muscle contraction can be elicited by stimulation with 0.5 mA or less proximal to the injured area, further treatment is unnecessary. Systemic corticosteroids may be helpful in the postoperative period to minimize swelling. If facial movement can be elicited by stimulation of the nerve distally but not proximal to the injury, the extent of nerve disruption determines the next course of action. If only a few fibers are damaged, they may simply be returned to their anatomic position. Significant disruption of the nerve, however, requires either direct reanastomosis or cable grafting. When greater than 50% of the facial nerve was disrupted, Green and colleagues obtained a House-Brackmann Grade III recovery using direct reanastomosis and Grade IV with cable grafting (57). Direct repair may require facial nerve rerouting, which itself may compromise nerve function.

Unexpected facial paralysis noted postoperatively requires prompt attention. Weakness without frank paralysis has a good prognosis and can be treated with a tapering course of steroids. However, complete facial paralysis in patients where the nerve was never formally identified presents a diagnostic dilemma. Local anesthetics administered preoperatively may be responsible for immediate postoperative facial palsy. Therefore, surgical exploration should be deferred for a few hours and the patient reassessed. If complete paralysis persists, early exploration is indicated. The nerve must be clearly identified, and, if traumatized, the surgeon should decompress it or perform the necessary repair.

Hearing Loss

Iatrogenic hearing loss may be conductive or sensorineural. Undetected disruptions of the tympanic membrane or ossicular chain may cause a conductive hearing loss. Sensorineural hearing loss can result from a variety of causes. Acoustic trauma from a loud drill or suction squeal near the footplate may cause hearing loss. Transmission of high frequency mechanical energy from contact between the drill and the ossicular chain also causes sensorineural hearing loss. If such contact is unavoidable, the surgeon should first disarticulate the incudostapedial joint. Inadvertent entry into the inner ear (semicircular canal, oval or round window, cochlea, etc.) and loss of perilymph/endolymph may result in hearing loss. The surgeon must be especially cautious when operating on an only hearing ear (58). If faced with cholesteatoma matrix overlying the stapes footplate or a horizontal semicircular canal fistula, removing this matrix may result in a sensorineural hearing loss. The options here include completely removing the cholesteatoma, exteriorizing the matrix, or simply leaving a small part of cholesteatoma behind. The surgeon may elect the latter option and perform a second operation in 6 to 12 months. At that time, the residual cholesteatoma matrix (now a small pearl) can be removed. This second procedure is usually safer because the field is no longer infected and visualization much improved.

Vestibular Injury

Injury to the labyrinth during tympanomastoid surgery can result from direct trauma or from postoperative infection. Ears affected by serous labyrinthitis often recover function over time and may benefit initially from steroid therapy. Suppurative labyrinthitis, however, usually destroys vestibular function. Complete unilateral vestibulopathy usually results in acute vertigo. This resolves over the next few days to weeks as central compensation occurs. Some patients are left with mild disequilibrium that improves slowly with vestibular rehabilitation. Chronic disequilibrium may occur in those patients who do not undergo successful central compensation. Some patients may also experience delayed benign positional vertigo. These patients may be treated with repositioning maneuvers and vestibular rehabilitation.

Infection

Postoperative infection continues to pose a threat to successful outcomes in otologic surgery. Immediate concerns include dehiscence of the postauricular incision, failure of the tympanoplasty grafts, and necrosis of the external auditory canal skin flaps. Perichondritis requires debridement of necrotic cartilage and administration of parenteral antibiotics. Other potential complications include suppurative labyrinthitis, facial nerve palsy, epidural or subdural abscess, meningitis, sigmoid sinus thrombosis, otitic hydrocephalus, and brain abscess. If an ear is grossly infected preoperatively, antibiotics may be administered based on cultures and sensitivity data. Intraoperative irrigation with antibiotic solutions may also be of benefit. For most otologic procedures, however, preoperative prophylactic antibiotic therapy is not indicated. In a recent review by Verschuur and colleagues, they concluded that there was no role for the use of prophylactic antibiotics in clean and clean-contaminated otologic procedures (59).

Dysgeusia

Dysgeusia resulting from injury to the chorda tympani nerve may be quite distressing to some patients. Symptoms such as a metallic taste in the mouth usually improve with time, but patients must be warned that these taste alterations may persist. This may be of particular concern for those needing a keen sense of taste or flavor in their professions. Traumatized chorda tympani nerves tend to result in more prolonged dysgeusia than cutting the nerve.

Cerebrospinal Fluid Leakage and Encephalocele

The terms meningocele, encephalocele, and meningoencephalocele refer to herniation of meninges, brain matter, or both outside their normal confines. In the course of thinning the tegmen tympani and tegmen mastoideum, small areas of dura may become exposed. This is generally of little consequence. However, if larger areas of dura are exposed or lacerated, CSF, meninges, and brain tissue may enter into the mastoid cavity. Elderly patients are at particular risk because the dura tends to thin with advancing age.

Encephaloceles usually present with CSF otorrhea, CSF rhinorrhea, a persistent clear effusion behind an intact tympanic membrane, hearing loss due to mass effect (fluid and brain matter), or infections such as meningitis and encephalitis. A CSF leak can occur, however, without herniation of meninges or brain matter. High-resolution CT scans with axial and coronal views help define bony defects in the tegmen or posterior fossa plate, and magnetic resonance imaging (MRI), with its excellent soft tissue resolution, distinguishes brain from fluid, cholesteatoma, or cholesterol granuloma. MRI is also useful in evaluating the integrity of the dura. β_2-transferrin assays, capable of detecting minute quantities of CSF, help with the diagnosis.

Conservative options for managing CSF leaks include bed rest, stool softeners, and placement of a lumbar drain for controlled CSF removal. When such measures fail or if the patient becomes infected, surgical options are necessary. Repairing an encephalocele requires resection of devitalized tissue followed by reconstruction of the defect. If the damage is recognized during the initial procedure, the defect can be repaired at that time. Dura is elevated in a circumferential manner around the defect and a fascia graft placed intracranially between the dura and bone. Other materials available to the surgeon in place of fascia include pericranium, Alloderm, homograft pericardium, or DuraGen. More fascia, cartilage, bone, or commercially available alloplastic materials can then be placed against the defect from within the mastoid. If the CSF leak or encephalocele is recognized postoperatively, the precise location of the defect and the patient's hearing status dictate the surgical approach. An audiogram and imaging should be obtained. Options include transmastoid, middle fossa, or combination techniques. For small defects, a mini middle fossa craniotomy can be used. The temporal lobe is elevated and a sheet of temporalis fascia is placed below the dural defect. The window of bone harvested in the craniotomy is thinned and inserted between the fascia and the floor of the middle cranial fossa. Approaching the dura carefully using diamond burrs rather than cutting burrs helps to prevent these injuries.

Bleeding/Air Embolism

Most bleeding from the sigmoid sinus or jugular bulb can be controlled easily using Gelfoam or Surgicel pledgets covered by a small cottonoid. However, a significant laceration places the patient at risk for secondary complications such as air embolism or thrombosis of the sigmoid sinus. Once the bleeding is controlled, the potential for air embolism must be entertained. An air bubble in the venous system that becomes trapped within the right ventricle can result in cardiopulmonary arrest. The early signs of air embolism include increased end-expiratory carbon dioxide, hypotension, and abnormal cardiac sounds. The surgical field should be flooded with saline immediately and the patient should be placed in the Trendelenburg (head-down) position to minimize further ingress of air into the vascular system. Placement in the left lateral position can help to reposition the air bubble into the right atrium or vena cava. If cardiovascular compromise is still present after these maneuvers, the air must be aspirated from the vena cava using a central venous catheter.

Injury to the carotid artery during tympanomastoid surgery requires immediate hemostasis by direct occlusion. Once the bleeding is temporarily controlled, options include direct repair of the vessel, ligation proximally in the neck with occlusion distally, angiography with embolization or placement of coils, and angiography with stenting. Even with these interventions, the patient remains at risk for stroke.

Delayed Complications

Other complications of mastoid surgery include delayed posterior external ear canal wall breakdown, perichondritis, cholesterol granulomas, mucosalization of the mastoid bowl, and external auditory canal stenosis.

HIGHLIGHTS

- Postauricular incisions allow excellent exposure of the mastoid cortex. The inferior portion of the incision must be placed more posteriorly in young children to avoid facial nerve injury.
- The mastoid antrum is located directly medial to Macewen triangle.
- The temporal line provides a topographic landmark for the tegmen and floor of the middle fossa.
- The surgeon must thoroughly saucerize the mastoid cavity during a canal-wall-down mastoidectomy.
- Facial nerve variations and anomalies are common within the temporal bone, especially in patients with congenital ear malformations.
- The posterior musculoperiosteal flap, known as the Palva flap, has been successful in obliterating mastoid cavities especially in conjunction with bone pate.
- Saucerization, removal of the mastoid tip, obliteration techniques, and a large meatoplasty are vital to obtaining a clean, dry ear in canal-wall-down mastoidectomies.
- Disadvantages of intact canal wall procedures include an increased risk of occult residual and recurrent disease.
- The endolymphatic sac can be located inferiorly between the posterior semicircular canal and the sigmoid sinus.
- The anterior petrous apex can be opened through the anterior epitympanum, the hypotympanum, and the middle cranial fossa.

REFERENCES

1. Politzer A. *History of otology*, Vol 1. Phoenix, AZ: Callumella Press, 1981 (translated from the original German edition of 1907).
2. Palva T. Surgery of chronic ear without cavity. *Arch Otolaryngol* 1963;77:570–580.
3. Lempert J. Improvement of hearing in cases of otosclerosis: new one-stage surgical technique. *Arch Otolaryngol* 1938;28:42–97.
4. Nager GT, Proctor B. The facial canal: normal anatomy, variations and anomalies. II. Anatomical variations and anomalies involving the facial canal. *Ann Otol Rhinol Laryngol Suppl* 1982;97 [Suppl]:45–61.
5. Körner O. *Die eitrigen erkrankungen des Schlafenbeins*. Wiesbaden: Bergmann, 1899.
6. Jackler RK. The surgical anatomy of cholesteatoma. *Otolaryngol Clin North Am* 1989;22:883–896.
7. Horn KL, Brackmann DE., Luxford WM, et al. The supratubal recess in cholesteatoma surgery. *Ann Otol Rhinol Laryngol* 1986;95:12–15.
8. Litton WB, Krause CJ, Anson BA, et al. The relationship of the facial canal to the annular sulcus. *Laryngoscope* 1969;79:1584–1604.
9. Green JD Jr, Shelton C, Brackmann DE. Iatrogenic facial nerve injury during otologic surgery. *Laryngoscope* 1994;104:922–926.
10. Baxter A. Dehiscence of the fallopian canal: an anatomic study. *J Laryngol Otol* 1971;85:587–594.

11. Cook JA, Krishnan S, Fagan PA. Hearing results following modified radical versus canal-up mastoidectomy. *Ann Otol Rhinol Laryngol* 1996;105:379–383.

12. Hirsch BE, Kamerer DB, Doshi S. Single-stage management of cholesteatoma. *Otolaryngol Head Neck Surg* 1992;106:351–354.

13. Roden D, Honrubia VT, Wiet R. Outcome of residual cholesteatoma and hearing in mastoid surgery. *J Otolaryngol* 1996;25:178–181.

14. Sadé J, Berco E, Brown M. Results of mastoid operations in various chronic ear diseases. *Am J Otol* 1981;3:11–20.

15. Wright WK. A concept for management of otitis cholesteatoma. In: McCabe B, Sadé J, Abramson M, eds. *Cholesteatoma, First International Conference*. Birmingham, AL: Aesculapius, 1981:374–379.

16. Smyth GDL. Postoperative cholesteatoma in combined approach tympanoplasty: Fifteen year report on tympanoplasty. Part I. *J Laryngol Otol* 1967;90:597–621.

17. Glasscock ME, Miller GM. Intact canal wall tympanoplasty in the management of cholesteatoma. *Laryngoscope* 1976;86:1639–1657.

18. Palva T, Karma P, Palva A. Cholesteatoma surgery: canal down and mastoid obliteration. In: McCabe B, Sadé J, Abramson M, eds. *Cholesteatoma, First International Conference*. Birmingham, AL: Aesculapius, 1977:363–367.

19. Ojala K. Late results of obliteration operation in chronic otitis media. *Acta Ophthalmol Otorhinolaryngol* 1979;47:4.

20. Charachon R, Gratacap B, Tixier C. Closed versus obliteration technique in cholesteatoma surgery. *Am J Otol* 1988;9:286–292.

21. Cody DT, McDonald TJ. Mastoidectomy for acquired cholesteatoma: follow-up to 20 years. *Laryngoscope* 1984;94:1027–1030.

22. Gristwood RE. Chronic otitis media with epidermoid cholesteatoma: a discussion of some points of controversy concerning surgical management. *Clin Otolaryngol Allied Sci* 1976;1:337–342.

23. Bondy G. Totallaufmeisselung mit Erhaltung bon Trommelfull und Gehorknochelchen. *Monatsschr Ohrenheilk* 1910;44:15.

24. Montandon P, Benchaou M, Guyot JP. Modified canal wall-up mastoidectomy with mastoid obliteration for severe chronic otitis media. *ORL J Otorhinolaryngol Relat Spec* 1995;57:198–201.

25. Van Hasselt CA, Lui KC, Tong MC. The Hong Kong vascularized temporalis fascia flaps for optimal, mastoid cavity reconstruction. *Rev Laryngol Otol Rhinol (Bord)* 1995;116:57–60.

26. Irving RM, Gray RF, Moffat DA. Bone pate obliteration or revision mastoidectomy: a five-symptom comparative study. *Clin Otolaryngol* 1994;19:158–160.

27. Mosher HP. A method of filling the excavated mastoid with a flap from the back of the auricle. *Laryngoscope* 1911;21:1158–1163.

28. Palva T, Palva A, Karja J. Cavity obliteration and ear canal size. *Arch Otolaryngol* 1970;92:366–371.

29. Palva T, Makinen J. The meatally based musculoperiosteal flap in cavity obliteration. *Arch Otolaryngol* 1979;105:377–380.

30. Palva T. Mastoid obliteration. *Acta Otolaryngol (Stockh)* 1979;360 [Suppl]:152–154.

31. Ojala K, Sorri M, Sipila P, Vainio-Mattila J. Correlation of postoperative ear canal volumes with obliteration material and with volume of operation cavity. *Arch Otorhinolaryngol* 1982;234:37–43.

32. Grote JJ, van Blitterswijk CA. Reconstruction of the posterior auditory canal wall with hydroxyapatite. *Ann Otol Rhinol Laryngol* 1986;123[Suppl]:6–9.

33. Black B. Mastoidectomy elimination. *Laryngoscope* 1995;105 [Suppl 76]:1–30.

34. Black B, Kelly S. Mastoidectomy reconstruction: revascularizing the canal wall repair. *Am J Otol* 1994;15:91–95.

35. Portmann M. Meatoplasty and chonchoplasty in cases of open techniques. *Laryngoscope* 1983;93:520–522.

36. McKennan KX. Endoscopic transcutaneous mastoidectomy for evaluation of residual epitympanic/mastoid cholesteatoma. *Am J Otol* 1993;14:362–368.

37. Rosenberg SI, Silverstein H, Hoffer M, et al. Use of endoscopes for chronic ear surgery in children. *Arch Otolaryngol Head Neck Surg* 1995;121:870–872.

38. Bottrill ID, Poe DS. Endoscope-assisted ear surgery. *Am J Otol* 1995;16:158–163.

39. Guild SR. The circulation of endolymph. *Am J Anat* 1927;39:57–81.

40. Portmann M. Vertigo: surgical treatment by opening the saccus endolymphaticus. *Arch Otolaryngol* 1927;6:309–319.

41. Hallpike CS, Cairns H. Observations of the pathology of Ménière's syndrome. *J Laryngol Otol* 1938;53:625–655.

42. House WF. Subarachnoid shunts for drainage of endolymphatic hydrops: a preliminary report. *Laryngoscope* 1962;72:713–729.

43. Shea JJ. Teflon film drainage of the endolymphatic sac. *Arch Otolaryngol* 1966;83:316–319.

44. Shambaugh GE Jr. Surgery of the endolymphatic sac. *Arch Otolaryngol* 1966;83:305–315.

45. Paparella MM, Hanson DG. Endolymphatic sac drainage for intractable vertigo (method and experiences). *Laryngoscope* 1976;86:697–703.

46. Arenberg IK, Stahle J, Glasscock ME, et al. Endolymphatic sac valve surgery: I. The technique. *Laryngoscope* 1979;89[Suppl 17]:1–20.

47. Thomsen J, Bretlau P, Tos M, et al. Placebo effect in surgery for Ménière's disease: a double-blind, placebo-controlled study on endolymphatic sac shunt surgery. *Arch Otolaryngol* 1981;107:271–277.

48. Shea DA, Chole RA, Paparella MM. The endolymphatic sac: anatomical considerations. *Laryngoscope* 1979;89:88–94.

49. Gradenigo G. Ueber die Paralyse de Nercus Abducens bei Otitis. *Arch Ohrenheilkunde Rhinolaryngol* 1907;74:149–158.

50. Chole RA, Donald PJ. Petrous apicitis: clinical considerations. *Ann Otol Rhinol Laryngol* 1983;93:544–551.

51. Gerek M, Satar, B, Yazar F, et al. Transcanal anterior approach for cystic lesions of the petrous apex. *Otol Neurotol* 2004;25:973–976.

52. Mattox DE. Endoscopy-assisted surgery of the petrous apex. *Otolaryngol Head Neck Surg* 2004;130:229–241.

53. Dinardo LJ, Pippin GW, Sismanis A. Image-guided endoscopic transsphenoidal drainage of select petrous apex cholesterol granulomas. *Otol Neurotol* 2003;24:939–941.

54. Chole RA. Petrous apicitis: surgical anatomy. *Ann Otol Rhinol Laryngol* 1985;94:251–257.

55. Ramadier J. Exploration de la pointe du rocher par la coie du canal carotidien. *Ann Otolaryngol* 1933;4:422–444.

56. Lempert J. Complete apicectomy: a preliminary report of a new technic. *N Y State J Med* 1936;36:1210–1218.

57. Green JD, Shelton C, Brackmann DE. Surgical management of iatrogenic facial nerve injuries. *Otolaryngol Head Neck Surg* 1994;111:606–610.

58. Schuknecht HF, Gacek RR. Surgery on only-hearing ears. *Trans Am Acad Ophthalmol Otolaryngol* 1973;77:257–266.

59. Verschuur HP, de Wever WW, van Benthem PP. Antibiotic prophylaxis in clean and clean-contaminated ear surgery. *Cochrane Database Syst Rev* 2004;3:CD003996.

142

Reconstruction of the Tympanic Membrane and Ossicular Chain

Charles M. Luetje II

The critical issue in tympanic membrane and ossicular chain reconstruction is the ability to manage any situation with a surgical technique applicable to the specific problem. The surgeon must not rely on one methodology for all abnormalities. An inventory of skills and surgical techniques that can successfully correct any otologic abnormality is essential. Previously learned stereotypical surgical techniques must be blended to solve any unusual conditions encountered.

Rather than concentrating on a "stereotypical technique" for tympanic membrane reconstruction, this chapter concentrates on surgical treatment of three specific pathologic tympanic membrane abnormalities: central perforations, posterior sinus tympani retraction difficulties, and erosion of the lateral attic wall by cholesteatoma. Ossicular chain reconstruction is discussed, emphasizing techniques successfully used by the author.

A short discussion of preoperative assessment, intraoperative related issues, and postoperative management precedes the technical aspects of the chapter. However, it merely highlights some philosophies of patient management and is not meant to be definitive. The strength of this chapter is intended to be technical. The purpose is to explain points designed to enhance successful tympanoplasty surgery and augment existing surgical skills.

PREOPERATIVE ASSESSMENT

The importance of historical information cannot be minimized. This includes the status of the contralateral ear. Age at onset, drainage, eustachian tube function, and previous surgery are the key historical factors. Surgeons must rely on their own interpretation of what information the patient provides. Information gathered by the nurse assistant, medical student, resident, fellow, or even a questionnaire is useful but does not replace a thorough understanding of the historical pathology obtained by the operating surgeon.

Microscopic examination is the most important aspect of the initial evaluation. It should be accomplished with the patient in the supine position. This allows an assessment of ear canal size in the surgical position, bend of the neck, shoulder elevation, anticipated comfort of the surgeon in a seated surgical position, and patient tolerance for examination. The contralateral ear is carefully examined first and serves as a point of reference. The status of the middle ear mucosa in the surgical ear will dictate topical preoperative treatment. The extent of perforation, type of cholesteatoma if present, continuity of the lateral attic wall, presence of tympanosclerosis, status of the annulus and ossicles, segmental middle ear aeration, and physiology of the ear canal skin are evaluated. Preoperative cultures and x-ray films are of questionable value. If feasible, the accompanying spouse or relatives are asked if they want to observe the pathology through the microscope.

Based on the pathology, surgical discussion ensues and includes the possibility for staging the operation for ossicular chain reconstruction. In general, staging the operation is based on the extent of mucosal disease and destruction by cholesteatoma. It is better to clean up the diseased ear and then reconstruct the ossicular chain at a second stage when the first operation is accompanied by extensive disease. There are no hard and fast rules as to which situations dictate the decision for staging. It is a judgment call that relies on experience and training of the surgeon. However, if in doubt, one should stage.

One caveat: In general, with experience, careful microscopic examination will give its own history so that errors in the patient's story and even outside operative reports can be clarified. It is not uncommon to read an operative report that says one thing and to have your examination reveal something different than expected. This is why careful supine microscopic examination is the most important part of the preoperative assessment.

Surgical candidacy is based on the presence of drainage, recurrent infection, and/or hearing loss, not just because an asymptomatic perforation exists. The goals of surgery should be a safe dry ear, an intact tympanic membrane, improved hearing, and if possible a single operation.

Audiometric evaluation includes tuning fork testing by the surgeon, air-bone-speech audiometry, and an index of suspicion for Tullio phenomenon. The last may be a subtle sign for a labyrinthine fistula. There is little indication for tympanometry.

Preoperative management includes elimination of active infection, if possible. This is best accomplished by careful microscopic debridement of desquamated epithelium, cerumen, crusting of dried exudate, and any other debris. This is followed by initiation of topical antibiotic/steroid drops two to three times daily followed by blow drying the ear with a hair drier on the low heat setting. Return appointments may be necessary for further microscopic treatments. In some cases that are resistant to topical antibiotics, elimination of the antibiotics and the use of equal parts of white vinegar and rubbing alcohol may be used followed by blow-drying. Occasionally, all efforts are unsuccessful and proceeding to surgery is appropriate.

At the time of discussing the proposed surgical procedure, the anticipated benefits and potential risks are provided to the patient and significant family members, if present. Informed consent is obtained in writing after answering all questions and providing additional information by way of office booklets or other printed materials specific to the proposed surgery.

INTRAOPERATIVE APPROACH

The author's preferences for configuring the operating room setup are described.

The scrub nurse is across from the surgeon, and the microscope is at the top of the patient's head. If the patient is under general anesthesia, the anesthesiologist sits on the same side as the surgeon toward the foot of the bed. Lidocaine with epinephrine is injected, and the ear is prepared for 2 to 3 minutes allowing the preparation solution to enter into the ear. Ondansetron (Zofran) 16 mg and dexamethasone (Decadron) 8 mg are given intravenously, usually at the

start of surgery, to prevent postoperative nausea and vomiting. After removal of disease, chronically infected and draining ears are usually irrigated with antibiotic solution. Piperacillin-tazobactam sodium (Zosyn) 3.375 g in 20 mL of saline or a similar antibiotic solution is irrigated through the mastoid and middle ear. A few milliliters of the same solution are injected into the surrounding subcutaneous soft tissue. Methylprednisolone sodium succinate (Solu-Medrol) irrigation follows. Occasionally, ceftriaxone sodium (Rocephin) 1 g is given intravenously. I prefer not to use silastic in the middle ear even if the surgery is to be staged for reconstruction because of fibrous reaction. Gelfilm is used instead and normal aeration of the middle ear ensues. Drains are not used and the only "packing" is a half cylinder of Gelfoam posteriorly and Cortisporin ointment. A running absorbable subcuticular suture is used for skin closure, Steri-Strips are placed over the incision and a mastoid dressing applied.

POSTOPERATIVE CARE

Postoperative care begins when the patient leaves the operating room, accompanied to the recovery room by the surgeon, followed by visiting the family, distribution of surgical photographs, and dictation of the operative note. Discharge occurs the day of surgery, and the mastoid dressing is removed the next day by the patient or family. Similarly, the Steri-Strips are removed in 1 week. A small piece of cotton in the ear canal is changed as needed until bleeding stops and then the ear is left open to the air. Patients are allowed to wash their hair after the dressing comes off but must keep the ear dry. There are no limitations of activity. Oral antibiotics, such as quinolones or cephalosporins, are given for 5 days, and extra-strength acetaminophen or ibuprofen is usually sufficient for pain.

The first postoperative check is at 6 weeks, at which time the dried Gelfoam and antibiotic ointment placed at surgery are removed. No antibiotic drops are used before this visit. The tympanic membrane should be healed if a medial graft has been placed or nearly healed if a lateral graft has been placed. Steroid antibiotic drops may be necessary at this point in the presence of delayed healing due to granulation tissue. An audiogram is obtained. Patients may begin to perform Valsalva maneuvers and to blow their nose; some may swim. They are instructed to return in 3 months for another audiogram and recheck. Usually, annual visits are scheduled thereafter.

TECHNICAL CONSIDERATIONS

Tympanic Membrane Reconstruction

The following discussion addresses three pathologic conditions and their correction rather than routine grafting techniques. Whatever technique is used by the surgeon, it can be modified based on the presenting pathology.

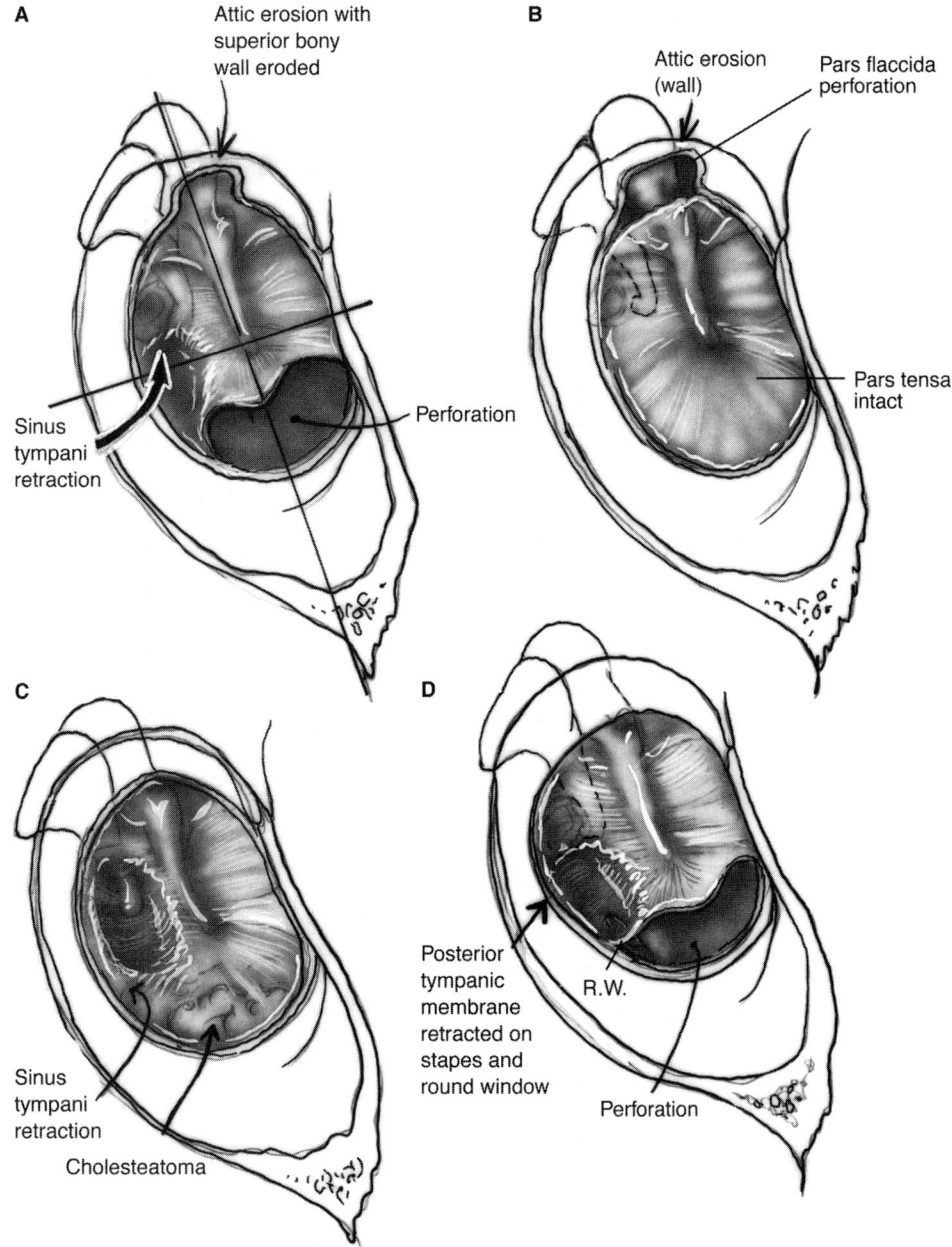

A Attic erosion with superior bony wall eroded

Sinus tympani retraction

Perforation

B Attic erosion (wall)   Pars flaccida perforation

Pars tensa intact

C Sinus tympani retraction

Cholesteatoma

D Posterior tympanic membrane retracted on stapes and round window

R.W.

Perforation

Figure 142.1 **A:** Composite of tympanic membrane perforation pathology. **B:** Eroded lateral attic wall with pars flaccida perforation. **C:** Posterior sinus tympani retraction disease. **D:** Inferior central perforation with posterior retraction. RW, round window.

Figure 142.1 shows three different pathologic abnormalities of the tympanic membrane: attic retraction cholesteatoma under an eroded lateral attic wall, sinus tympani retraction cholesteatoma, and central perforation. Each of these requires different and specific surgical consideration.

Central Perforation

Central perforation in the absence of cholesteatoma is technically the easiest tympanic membrane defect to repair, but should the graft fail, having to explain the outcome to the patient creates a difficult situation. It can be managed by lateral or medial grafting techniques predi-

cated on surgical methods familiar to the surgeon using modifications dictated by the given pathology. I prefer a medial graft, or underlay, technique (1,2). Regardless of the approach, an important objective to achieving successful repair of this perforation is elimination of a prominent anterior canal wall bony overhang, if present, to secure the graft anteriorly.

Medial Graft Technique

A vascular strip posteriorly is elevated in retrograde fashion and connected with the postauricular incision. The anterior canal wall skin is elevated in a retrograde fashion from just lateral to the fibrous annulus out to the meatus. The skin is left intact and protected by folding it laterally, keeping it out of the way. The anterior canal wall bony overhang is then removed with a cutting burr under constant suction and irrigation. The entire fibrous annulus should be easily visible at completion of this step.

A Rosen needle or sickle knife is used to elevate the fibrous annulus away from the bony annulus anteriorly from the 1-o'clock to the 5-o'clock position (right ear, and the reciprocal imaginary clock face positions for the left). The mucoperiosteum of the eustachian tube is incised and separated from the fibrous annulus, leaving it like a bowstring, attached above and below to the bony annulus. Epithelium is left on its surface, because the graft will be positioned medial to the fibrous annulus.

Surgery then proceeds in routine fashion, preparing the ear for grafting according to the procedural steps necessary for medial grafting. It is the author's preference to perform a mastoidectomy on almost every patient to inspect the heads of the ossicles, the epitympanum, and aditus ad antrum. This adds little time and no morbidity to the patient. The results of tympanoplasty are more favorable when a mastoidectomy is accomplished because this additional exposure ensures there is no disease beyond the middle ear space (3).

In general, unless the ear is dry and the middle ear mucosa normal, the middle ear and mastoid are irrigated, after removal of disease, first with 3.375 g of piperacillin-tazobactam in 20 mL of saline and then with 40 mg of methylprednisolone sodium succinate, before graft placement. It is noteworthy that, with antibiotic irrigation and postoperative oral antibiotics for 5 days, the incidence of postoperative infection in chronic ear surgery has been zero in the author's experience. A previous report indicated antibiotics were of insignificant value (4).

Figure 142.2 depicts the technique of securing the medial graft anteriorly (5). It is my preference to use Gelfilm over the promontory and not Silastic. The fascia is then brought medial to the umbo and medial to the anterior fibrous annulus. The anterior fibrous annulus is displaced posteriorly with a Rosen needle and a no. 3 Baron suction used between the fibrous annulus and the bony annulus to pick up the graft and pull it up and onto the anterior bony canal wall. The fibrous annulus is released from the Rosen needle and the fascia straightened out over the bony canal wall. The fibrous annulus is then replaced into its original position but with the fascia between it and its bony annular seat. The anterior canal wall skin flap is then returned to overlap the fascia.

Lateral Graft Technique

A vascular strip posteriorly is elevated in retrograde fashion and connected with the postauricular incision. The anterior canal wall skin is removed for later placement followed by removal of the anterior overhanging bony canal wall (6). With this technique, total removal of

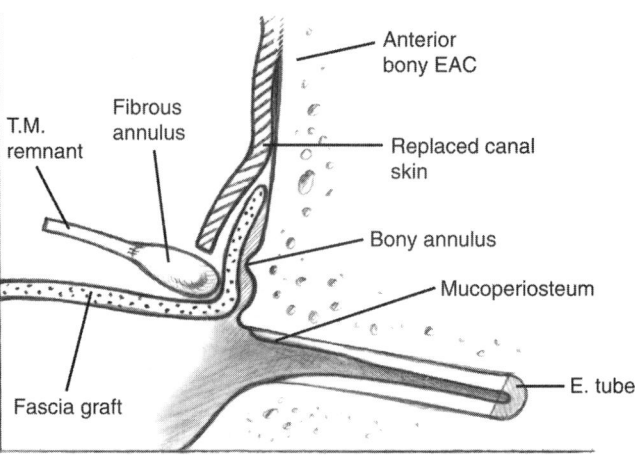

Figure 142.2 Cross-section of surgical technique for placement of fascia graft medial to the fibrous annulus anteriorly, lateral to the bony annulus and up onto the bony anterior canal wall, covered by canal epithelium.

squamous epithelium from the tympanic membrane remnant surface is mandatory. The most crucial area is in the anterior sulcus at the annulus. Thus, anterior canal wall bone removal is a necessity in almost all cases. The fibrous annulus should be easily visible throughout its entirety.

A Rosen needle or sickle knife is used to elevate the fibrous annulus away from the bony annulus anteriorly from the 1-o'clock to the 5-o'clock position (for the right ear and the reciprocal imaginary clock face positions for the left). The mucoperiosteum of the eustachian tube is kept intact with the fibrous annulus and elevated away from the bone of the eustachian tube for a few millimeters. A shelflike pocket over the fibrous annulus, medial to the bony annulus and between the bone of the eustachian tube and mucoperiosteum, is created for later graft placement anteriorly.

Surgery then proceeds in routine fashion, preparing the ear for grafting according to the technical choices for lateral grafting. A mastoidectomy is performed on almost every patient to inspect the aditus ad antrum, heads of the ossicles, and the epitympanum. Piperacillin-tazobactam and methylprednisolone sodium succinate irrigations are used as described previously.

Figure 142.3 illustrates the technique of graft placement with the lateral graft technique. Gelfilm is placed over the promontory. After the graft has been brought up medial to the malleus, the anterior aspect of the graft is teased into the fibrous annulus-mucoperiosteal shelf pocket with a Rosen needle. Placement of the graft in this fashion helps prevent lateralization of the graft in the anterior sulcus, a complication that may accompany the lateral graft technique. One can see the importance of not leaving any squamous epithelium on the fibrous annulus. After the graft is in its ideal position, the canal wall skin is replaced so that it

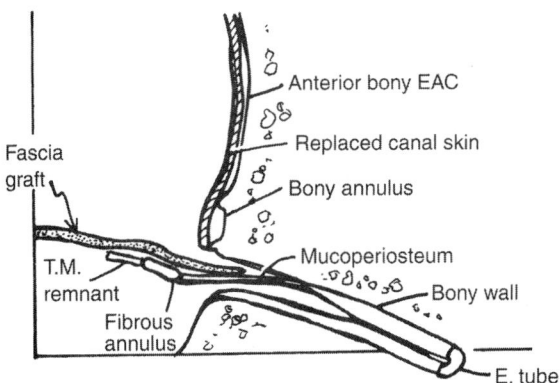

Figure 142.3 Cross-section of surgical technique for placement of fascia graft lateral to the fibrous annulus anteriorly and onto the shelf of intact mucoperiosteum of the eustachian tube.

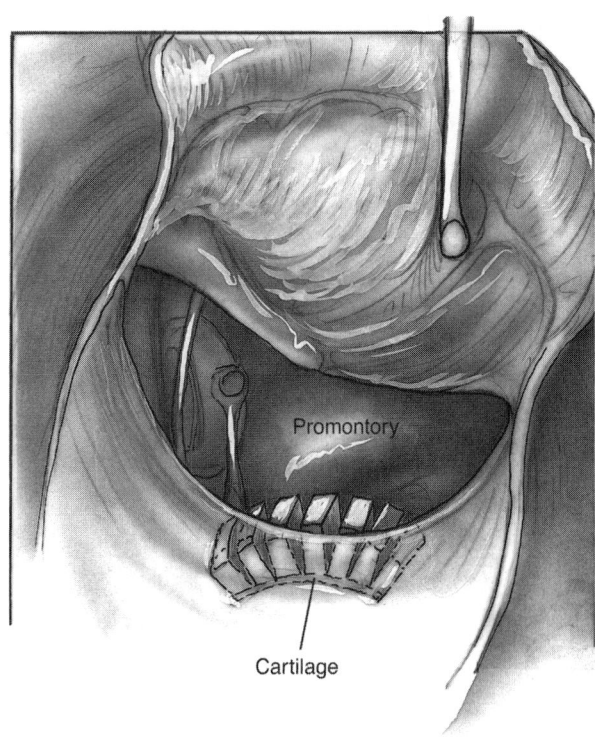

Figure 142.4 Surgeon's view, scored cartilage, incised convex surface toward the middle ear, in place and blocking the sinus tympani to prevent future retraction.

abuts but does not overlap the fascia graft at the bony annulus.

Sinus Tympani Retraction Cholesteatoma

Sinus tympani retraction cholesteatoma is perhaps technically the most difficult case for surgery because it involves working in an area that is usually not well visualized. It is not mandated that these cases must undergo a radical mastoidectomy for removal of disease. With diligent dissection and use of Crabtree elevators (Bausch & Lomb Surgical, San Dimas, CA) and the facial recess approach, disease can be removed.

Working through the ear canal via a postauricular approach and after the ear canal skin and bone have been managed, the posterior fibrous annulus is elevated from superiorly to inferiorly. Middle ear dissection begins inferiorly. Usually the area of adhesive retraction begins at the anterior aspect of the round window niche. The area of retraction is freed and separated from the tympanic membrane anteriorly. The monomeric adhesion is elevated toward the sinus tympani. Gentle tedious elevation of the retraction pocket epithelium is continued superiorly out of the sinus tympani up to the stapes and cranial nerve VII. Once free from the sinus tympani, an intact canal wall mastoidectomy and facial recess approach to the middle ear are completed. Confirmation of total cholesteatoma removal is obtained by visual inspection through a widely opened facial recess and repeated sweeping passes of the Crabtree elevator through the sinus tympani. Although I do not think it necessary, endoscopy has been used to provide additional inspection of the area.

The key is to prevent recurrence of the same problem. Although poorly understood and despite anterior middle ear aeration, both preoperatively and postoperatively, retraction can still recur into the sinus tympani over time. Efforts should be directed toward prevention of recurrence in all cases, because no one can predict in which cases this process will recur.

A piece of tragal cartilage is then removed, leaving the perichondrium intact on one surface. The cartilage is contoured into an ovoid rectangle. The surface without the perichondrium is scored down to but not through the perichondrium (7). The tension of the attached perichondrium on the other side produces a convexity on the scored side. With the convexity toward the promontory the cartilage is then placed into the middle ear and positioned from the posterior aspect of the oval window niche to the posterior aspect of the round window niche, thereby blocking the entrance into the sinus tympani (Figs. 142.4 and 142.5). The cartilage should fit snugly against the medial side of the posterior bony external canal wall and bone of the middle ear between the oval and round window niches. Grafting is then accomplished without regard to the scored cartilage.

The scored cartilage does not interfere with any reconstruction of the ossicular chain or with any aspect of surgical decision making. Residual cholesteatoma, if total removal is not accomplished, will eventually make its way around the cartilage.

Lateral Attic Wall Erosion Cholesteatoma

Lateral attic wall erosion cholesteatoma is the most common type of cholesteatoma causing a tympanic membrane defect. Other than perhaps a small congenital cholesteatoma, all cholesteatomas will usually require

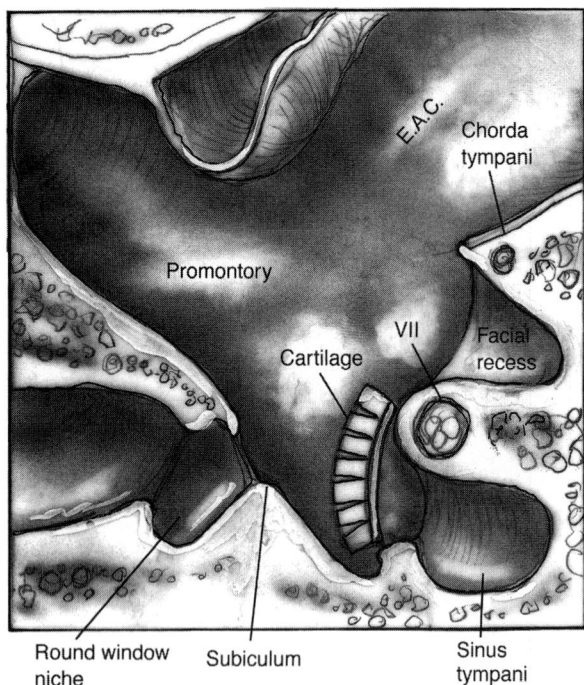

Figure 142.5 Cross-section depicting placement of the scored cartilage blocking entrance into the sinus tympani.

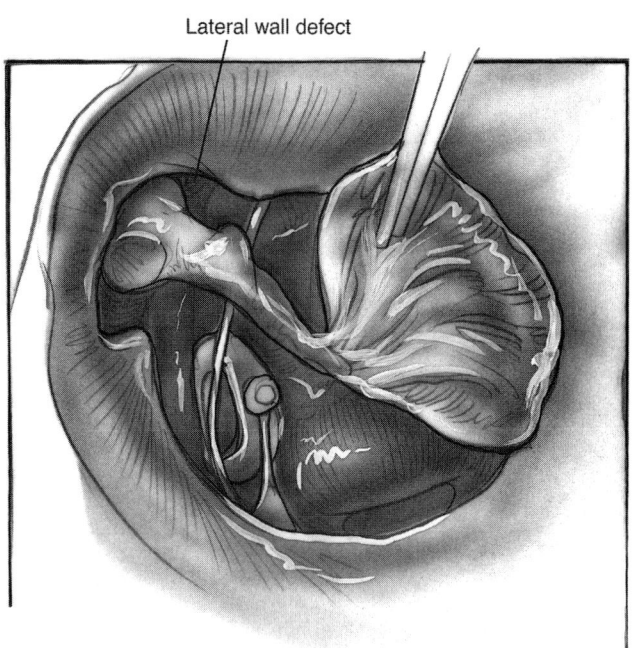

Figure 142.6 Anterior and posterior elevation of pars tensa with attached fibrous annulus, maintaining the attachment to the umbo of the malleus.

tympanic membrane repair. The key to success in these cases is to reconstruct the lateral attic wall with cartilage. Usually the inferior aspect of the tympanic membrane is intact, and frequently the anterior middle ear is aerated. Thus, the target of surgery is the epitympanum and mastoid, which calls for a different and tailored approach.

Through a postauricular approach, via the ear canal, attention is directed toward superior elevation of the fibrous annulus anteriorly and posteriorly. The posterior fibrous annulus is elevated first out of the bony annulus followed by the anterior annulus. Elevation inferiorly pulls the tympanic membrane off the short process of the malleus and onto the long process. At this point, a tympanic membrane flap is developed down to but not off the umbo. This provides excellent exposure of the upper two thirds of the mesotympanum, anteriorly and posteriorly to the level of the umbo (Fig. 142.6).

The pars flaccida area and cholesteatoma under the eroded lateral attic wall are then approached. As much cholesteatoma as possible is removed via the middle ear without enlarging the eroded lateral attic wall defect. An intact canal wall mastoidectomy and facial recess approach are then performed and total removal of cholesteatoma accomplished. At the completion of cholesteatoma removal, the Crabtree elevator is swept across the medial aspect of the lateral attic wall to remove any remaining fragments of squamous epithelium.

The lateral attic wall is then reconstructed with tragal cartilage (Fig. 142.7) (8). The perichondrium is left in contact on one surface. The perichondrium is elevated to the superior edge allowing it to lie on the bony lateral

wall, holding from above the cartilage in the defect in the scutum. The key point, however, is to have the cartilage fixed snugly against the malleus neck so that it will not retract. If the malleus has been removed, the cartilage may extend to the fallopian canal. If the inferior edge of the

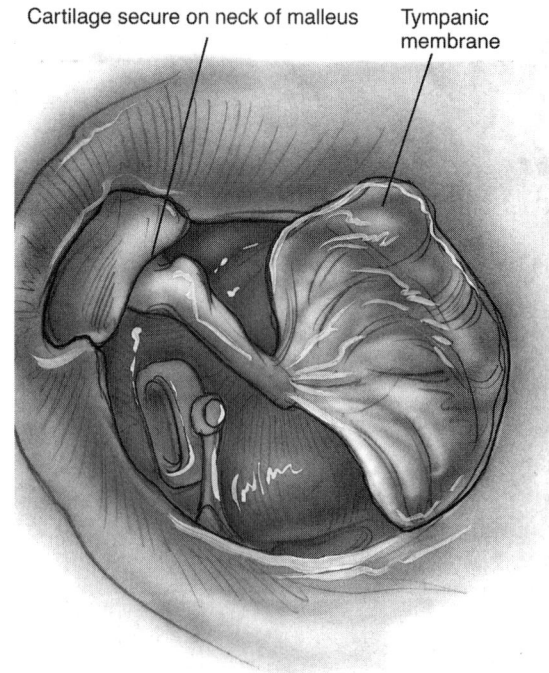

Figure 142.7 Tragal cartilage reconstruction of the lateral attic wall, noting the cartilage resting on the neck of the malleus at the short process.

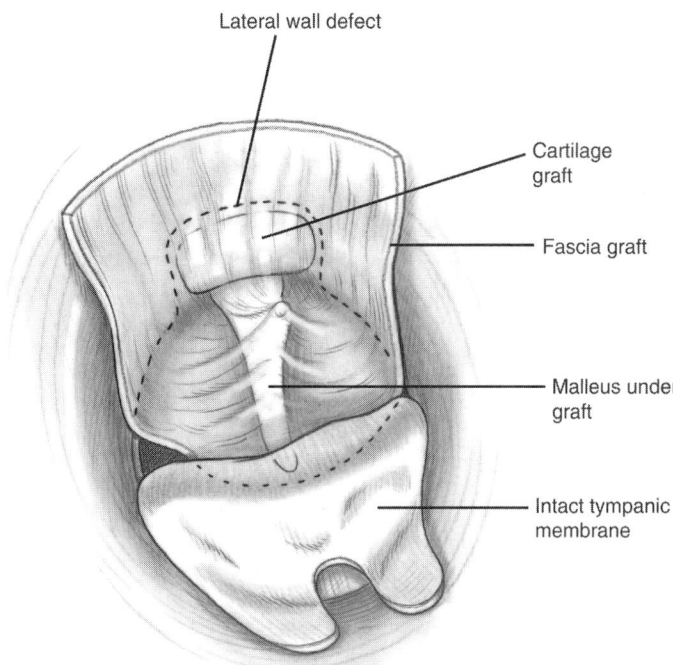

Figure 142.8 Fascia graft placement extending down from the external canal wall, over the reconstructed lateral attic wall, saddled over the neck of the malleus and medial to the tympanic membrane.

cartilage is free to retract back into the defect, the original type of retraction may recur. Cartilage against the malleus neck will not affect hearing.

As seen in Fig. 142.8, a "saddle blanket" graft is placed over the superior bony external canal and lateral attic walls. The graft then saddles itself over the malleus long process to the umbo and extends inferiorly and medially to the tympanic membrane remnant. When the tympanic membrane remnant flap is replaced, the graft becomes secured by adherence to the pars tensa after it is reflected back into its anatomic position.

As can be seen from the foregoing description, specific surgical techniques can be incorporated into routine operative procedures to achieve successful repair of the tympanic membrane. An important goal is to prevent slowly developing long-term recurrences and failures. The issue is not whether a medial or lateral graft technique is used but what can be done with each technique to increase the likelihood of success.

Ossicular Chain Reconstruction

Early versions of Plasti-Pore partial ossicular replacement prostheses (PORPs) and total ossicular replacement prostheses (TORPs) resulted in unacceptable extrusion rates. The use of cartilage interposed over the prosthesis platform helped reduce the extrusion rate. The tissue integration properties of the more recent hydroxyapatite prostheses seem to have eliminated the necessity for cartilage protection, but extrusion problems have not been eliminated (9). Smith & Nephew ENT (now Gyrus ENT, Bartlett, TN) introduced HAPEX, a homogeneous com-

posite of particulate hydroxyapatite and high-density polyethylene blended in a 40:60 ratio, by volume (10). Subsequently, they incorporated porous coralline (from sea coral) hydroxyapatite (Interpore International, Irvine, CA) as a head on a HAPEX shaft for PORPs and TORPs (11,12). Titanium prostheses are under investigation (13,14).

Because of unacceptable extrusion rates, in 1987 I introduced a method of reconstruction from stapes to graft or drum using autogenous cartilage remaining attached by its perichondrium (15). This was called the perichondrial double cartilage block (DCB) and replaced the PORP. No extrusions have been demonstrated using this technique in more than 20 years despite occasional cases of severe atelectasis. Although new materials continue to be introduced to "improve" PORP reconstruction, I have not abandoned the DCB technique because of excellent hearing results and long-term stability. It is simple, safe, and autogenous.

Double Cartilage Block

The advantage of the DCB is that it can be used for reconstruction during primary surgery for a draining ear (16) or with a tympanotomy for a conductive hearing loss. It is especially suited for atelectatic retraction problems. There is no fear of extrusion. This autogenous reconstruction will tolerate a total atelectatic situation with surprisingly little associated hearing loss. It is simple to perform, the tissue is always available, the technique is dependable, and it usually results in air-bone closure to within 5 to 15 dB.

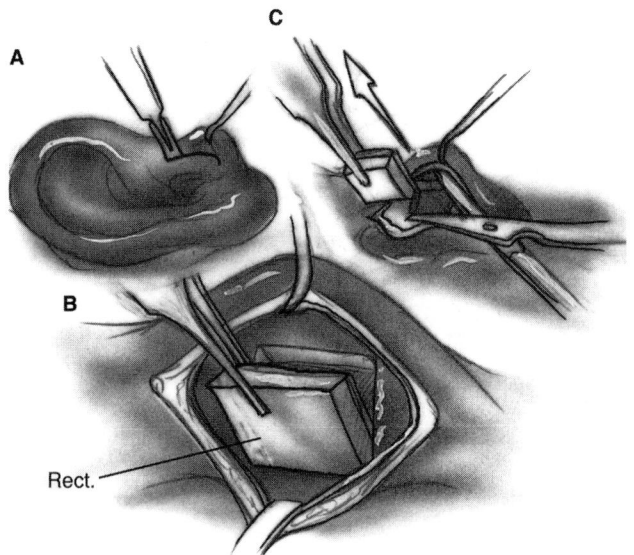

Figure 142.9 A–C: Obtaining tragal cartilage for double cartilage block ossicular reconstruction.

A piece of tragal cartilage is obtained from an incision on the posterior aspect of the tragus (Fig. 142.9), leaving the perichondrium intact on the posterior side. The cartilage is fashioned into a rectangle (Fig. 142.10) and incised to but not through the perichondrium so that the cartilage with attached perichondrium will fold on itself. An acetabulum for the capitulum stapes is made in one of the blocks. The perichondrium prevents the blocks of cartilage from slipping. More spring in the DCB may be gained by not cutting quite all the way through the

cartilage. The autograft DCB is then placed between the undersurface of the graft or tympanic membrane and the acetabulum of the stapes. Additional height can be obtained with a triple cartilage block, (Fig. 142.11) but this is rarely necessary.

Total Ossicular Replacement Prosthesis

The Plasti-Pore TORP is an ideal prosthesis because it can be cut, it is stiff but not brittle, and a suture can be passed through it. However, it is highly erosive and will extrude through the tympanic membrane, a graft, or even the stapes footplate unless protected. Care must be taken so there is no contact between the articular surfaces and the prosthesis. If contact surfaces are protected, it will provide excellent results without extrusion, nearly closing the air-bone gap in some cases. Careful measurements are obtained from the stapes footplate to the undersurface of the graft or tympanic membrane using a stapes measuring rod or other similar instrument from which distance measurements can be inferred. The prosthesis and oversewn platform cartilage should tent the tympanic membrane or graft to provide good tension.

The TORP platform is trimmed so that there is only enough platform to support a 7-0 silk suture. The small platform and slightly broader coverage of cartilage are crucial. Tragal cartilage is obtained through a small incision on the posterior surface of the tragus. The cartilage is placed on a cutting block and the perichondrium stripped from its surface and saved in the Gelfoam press. The TORP with its trimmed platform is grasped with a fine thumb forceps and a 7-0 silk placed through the platform undersurface and out the top. The suture is placed through the

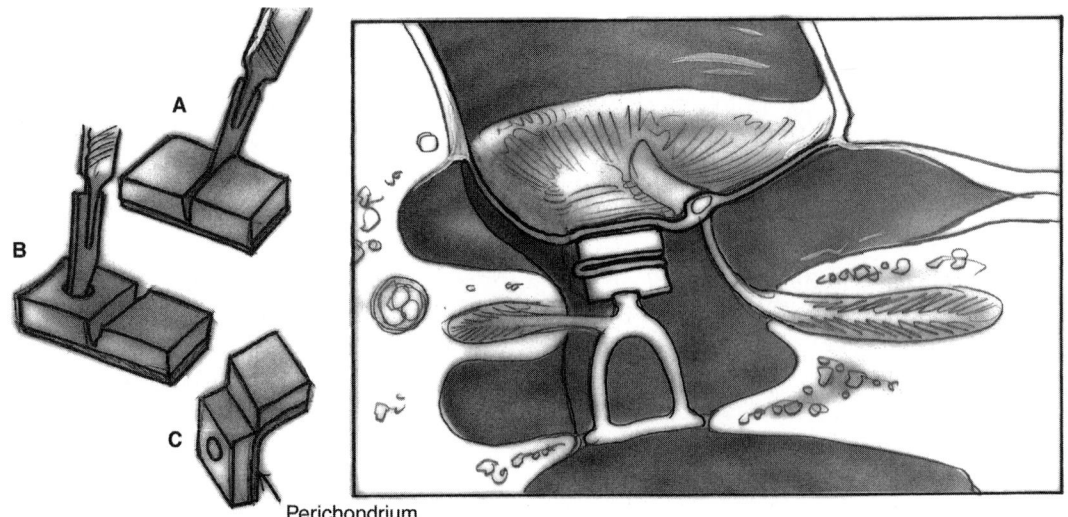

Figure 142.10 Composite of cartilage preparation **(A–C)**, incising cartilage to, but not through, the attached perichondrium and final placement of the double cartilage block with attached perichondrium onto stapes, slightly elevating the tympanic membrane (grafted or not).

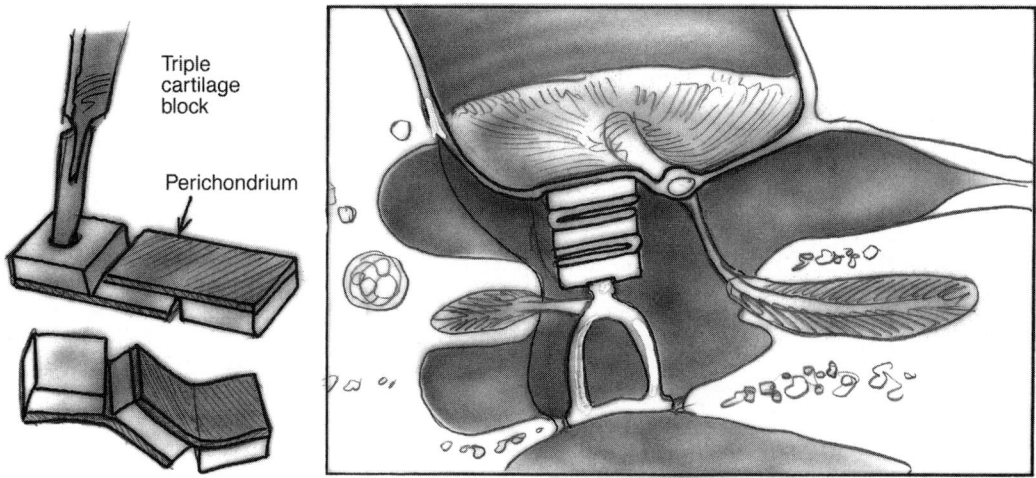

Figure 142.11 Composite of preparation to obtain additional height and placement using a triple cartilage block.

cartilage and back through to the original side. The loop should be only 1 to 2 mm. The suture goes back through the top of the platform to its underside and cinches down the cartilage when tied around the TORP shaft. Cartilage is then trimmed to within 1 mm of the platform, keeping the platform edge protected from contacting the graft or tympanic membrane. The shaft is then cut according to the measurement obtained for total prosthesis length.

The perichondrium is placed over the footplate, and the TORP is inserted. The shaft is seated into the center of the perichondrium, covering the footplate and the prosthesis is rotated up under the tympanic membrane or graft (Fig. 142.12). A notch is cut into the oversewn cartilage to fit under the malleus. This keeps the prosthesis from migrating posteriorly to the scutum (Fig. 142.13). The tensor tympani is cut to increase the lateral mobility of the malleus long process. In addition, the prosthetic assembly should be under slight tension between the graft and/or tympanic membrane and perichondrial tissue over the footplate.

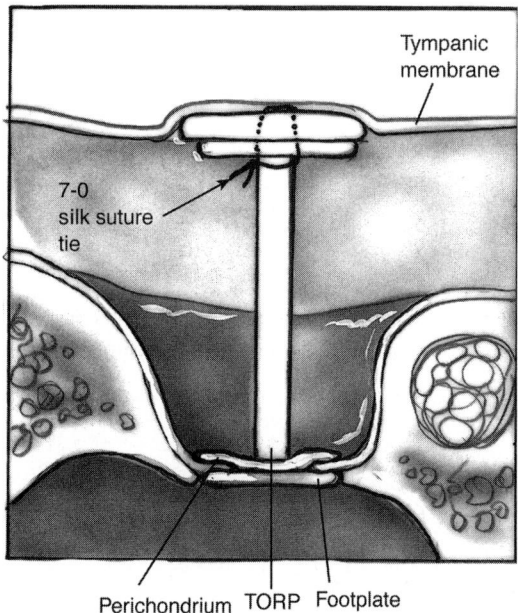

Figure 142.12 Total ossicular replacement prosthesis, positioned on the stapes footplate covered with pressed tragal perichondrium, when the malleus is not present.

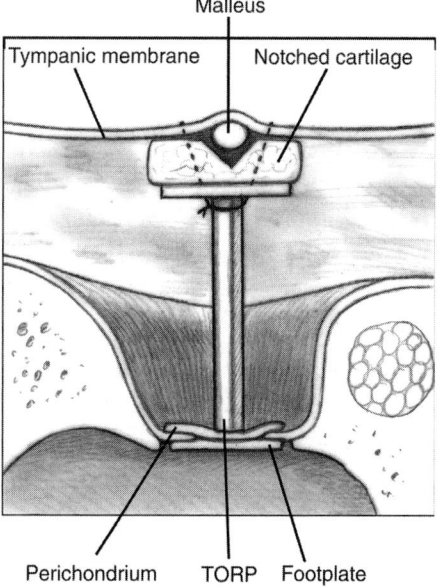

Figure 142.13 Total ossicular replacement prosthesis with incised oversewn cartilage, notched to fit under the malleus handle to prevent migration.

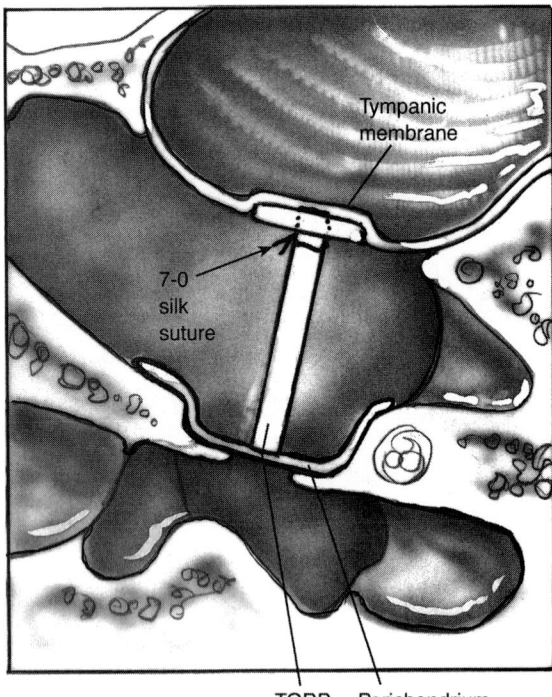

Figure 142.14 Total ossicular replacement prosthesis positioned over an open vestibule covered by pressed perichondrium.

If a stapedectomy has been necessary and the TORP extends to an opened vestibule, a separate piece of larger pressed perichondrium must be used to cover the vestibule (Fig. 142.14). Accurate measurements in this case are extremely important. The prosthesis should be prepared before the vestibule is opened to minimize exposure time. Air-bone gap closure to within 5 to 10 dB can usually be accomplished in these cases.

SUMMARY

Careful attention to detail can produce excellent results from reconstruction of the tympanic membrane and ossicular chain. It is more important to possess knowledge of variations in surgical techniques than to be constrained by a stereotypical operation for every case. Anterior fixation of tympanic membrane grafts is important for healing in perforations that extend to the annulus. Recurrence of sinus tympani retraction cholesteatoma can be prevented by the use of contoured, strategically positioned cartilage. Lateral attic wall defects should be reconstructed with a cartilage graft. DCB reconstruction from the stapes to the undersurface of the tympanic membrane or graft gives a high percentage of improved hearing while avoiding the possibility of prosthesis extrusion. TORP reconstruction is effective and extrusion less likely if the surface of any prosthesis that articulates with the tympanic membrane or graft is protected by cartilage and is not adherent to the posterior ear canal wall.

REFERENCES

1. Hough JVD. Tympanoplasty with the interior fascial graft technique and ossicular reconstruction. *Laryngoscope* 1970;80:1385–1413.
2. Glasscock ME. Tympanic membrane grafting with fascia: overlay vs undersurface technique. *Laryngoscope* 1973;83:754–770.
3. McGrew BM, Jackson CG, Glasscock ME. Impact of mastoidectomy on simple tympanic membrane perforation repair. *Laryngoscope* 2004;114:506–511.
4. Jackson CG. Antimicrobial prophylaxis in ear surgery. *Laryngoscope* 1988;98:1116–1123.
5. Bailey HAT. Maintenance of the anterior sulcus-tympanic membrane relationships in tympanoplastic surgery. *Laryngoscope* 1976;86:179–184.
6. Sheey JL, Glasscock ME. Tympanic membrane grafting with temporalis fascia. *Arch Otolaryngol* 1967;86:391–402.
7. Luetje CM. Prevention of sinus tympani retraction following tympanoplasty. *Arch Otolaryngol Head Neck Surg* 1994;120:1395–1396.
8. Luetje CM. Utility of autograft tragal cartilage in tympanoplasty and ossicular reconstruction. In: Friedman M, Pulec J, eds. *Operative techniques in otolaryngology—head and neck surgery.* Philadelphia: WB Saunders, 1995:1819–1827.
9. Macias JD, Glasscock ME, Widick MH, et al. Ossiculoplasty using the black hydroxylapatite hybrid ossicular replacement prostheses. *Am J Otol* 1995;16:718–721.
10. Swain RE, Beale B. *HAPEX: a bioactive hydroxylapatite/polyethylene composite suitable for otologic applications.* Bartlett, TN: Smith & Nephew ENT, 1995.

11. Swain RE, Beale B. *HyCor 200: a coralline hydroxylapatite biomaterial used in ossicular replacement surgery.* Bartlett, TN: Smith & Nephew ENT, 1996.
12. Jahn AF. Experimental applications of porous (coralline) hydroxylapatite in middle ear and mastoid reconstruction. *Laryngoscope* 1992;102:289–299.
13. Martin AD, Harner SG. Ossicular reconstruction with Titanium prostheses. *Laryngoscope* 2004;114:61–64.

14. Gardner EK, Jackson CG, Kaylie DM. Results with Titanium ossicular reconstruction prostheses. *Laryngoscope* 2004;114: 65–70.
15. Luetje CM. Perichondrial attached double cartilage block: a better alternative to the PORP. *Laryngoscope* 1987;97:1106–1108.
16. Harvey SA, Lin SY. Double cartilage block (DCB) ossiculoplasty in chronic ear surgery. *Laryngoscope* 1999;109:911–914.

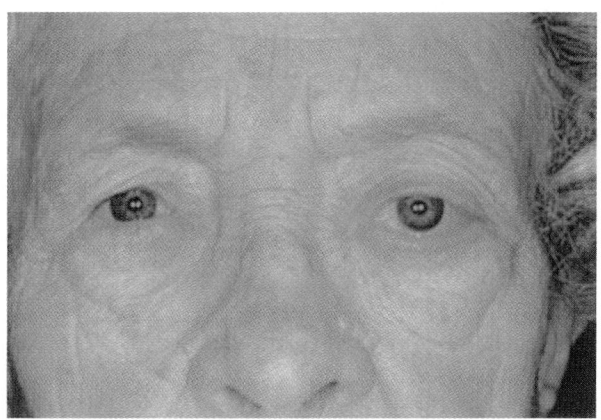

COLOR PLATE 34 Proptosis. A patient with left-sided proptosis secondary to a metastatic orbital tumor. (See Fig. 108.1.)

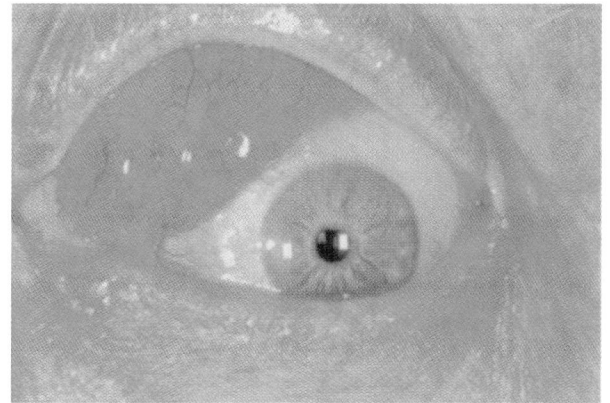

COLOR PLATE 35 Orbital lymphoma extending under the conjunctiva of the right eye. (See Fig. 108.3.)

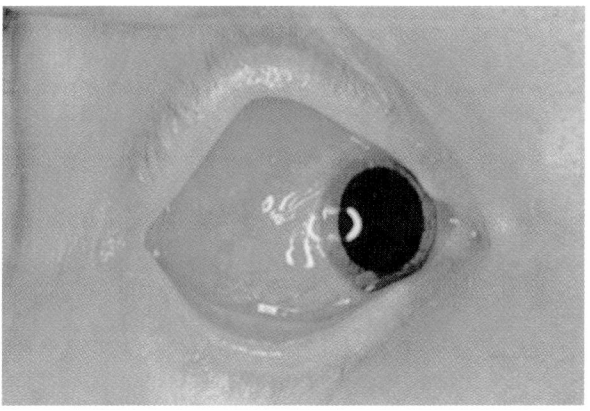

COLOR PLATE 36 An inflamed right eye associated with idiopathic orbital inflammation. The patient complained of pain with eye movement and diplopia. (See Fig. 108.8.)

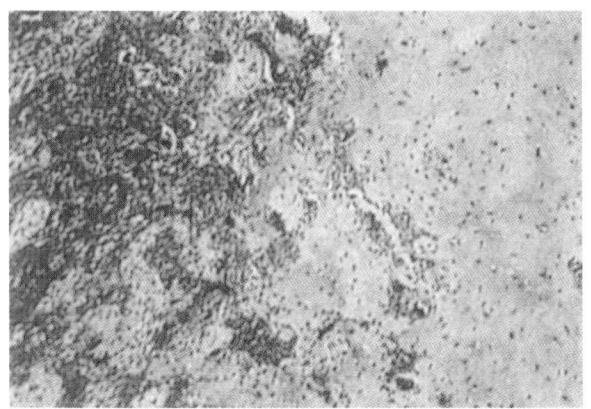

COLOR PLATE 37 Pleomorphic adenoma. The histologic appearance shows characteristic epithelial and mesenchymal elements. (See Fig. 109.1.)

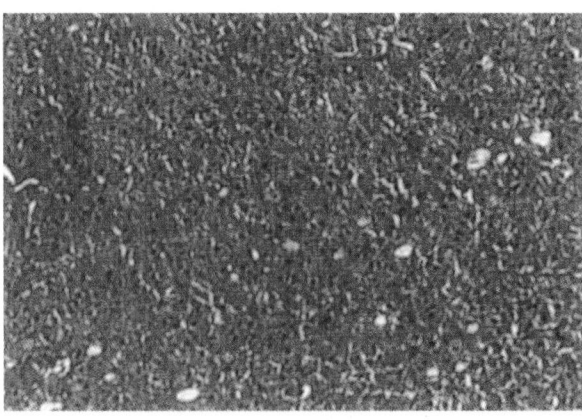

COLOR PLATE 38 Oncocytoma. The histologic appearance is that of typical plump, granular eosinophilic cells. (See Fig. 109.3.)

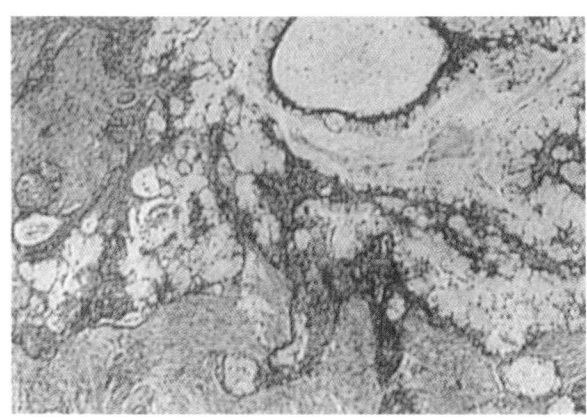

COLOR PLATE 39 Low-grade mucoepidermoid carcinoma. Note the epithelial and glandular elements. (See Fig. 109.4.)

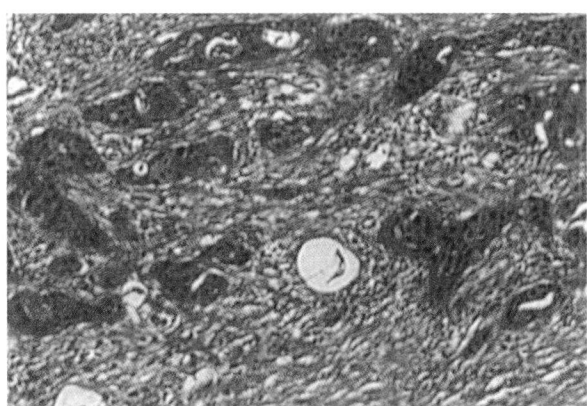

COLOR PLATE 40 High-grade mucoepidermoid carcinoma. Note the relative lack of glandular elements. (See Fig. 109.5.)

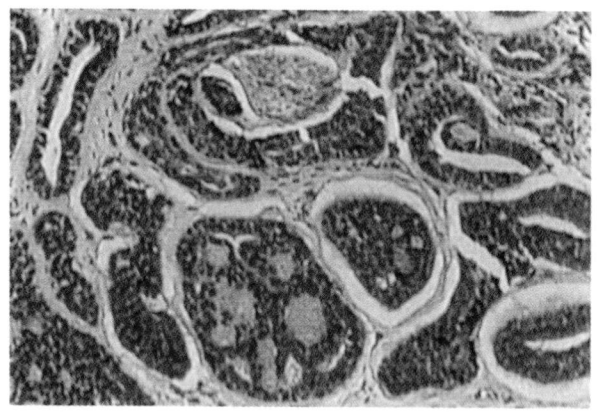

COLOR PLATE 41 Adenoid cystic carcinoma, showing the characteristic histologic appearance with eosinophilic hyaline stroma and perineural invasion. (See Fig. 109.6.)

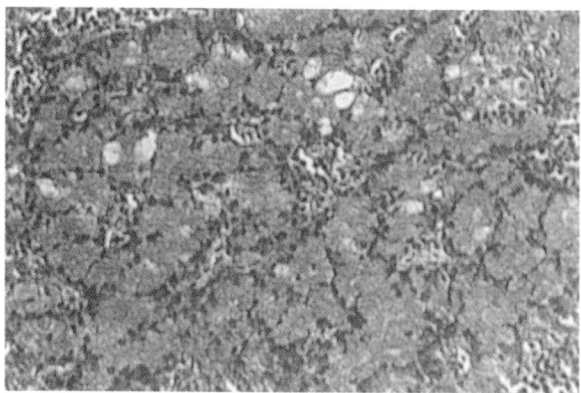

COLOR PLATE 42 Acinic cell carcinoma. Note cells similar to serous acinar cells and cells with clear cytoplasm. (See Fig. 109.7.)

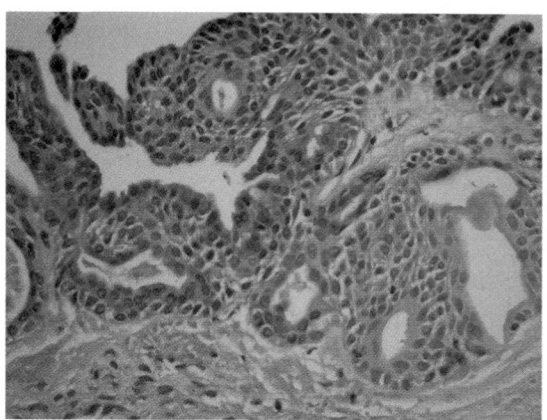

COLOR PLATE 43 Glandular odontogenic cyst. Stratified squamous epithelium forming glandlike structures. (See Fig. 112.4.)

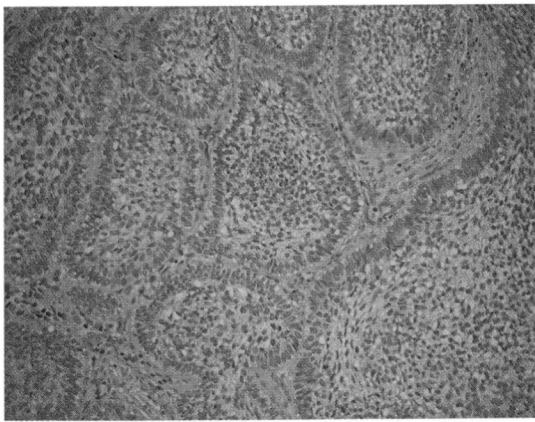

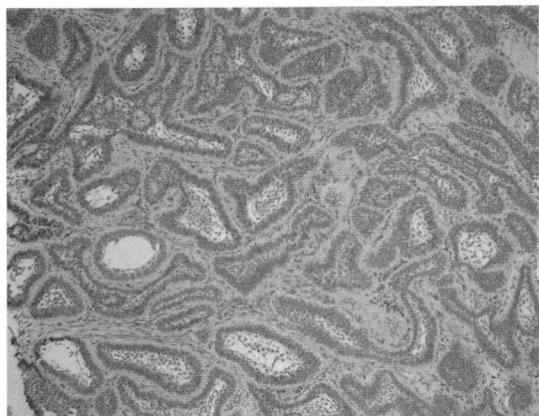

COLOR PLATE 44 C: Ameloblastoma (follicular pattern). Islands of odontogenic epithelium characterized by peripheral columnar cells exhibiting reverse polarity. The central portion of these islands resemble stellate reticulum in areas. **D:** Ameloblastoma (plexiform pattern). (See Fig. 112.5.)

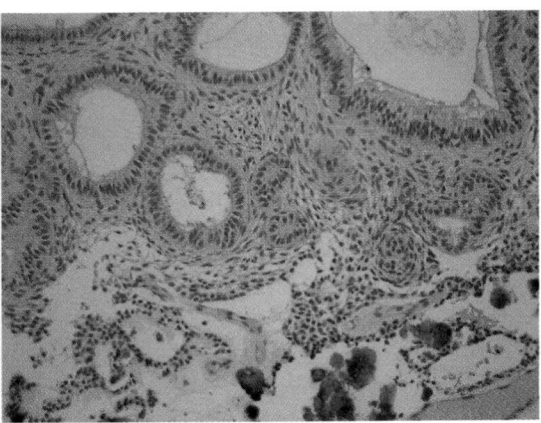

COLOR PLATE 45 Adenomatoid odontogenic cyst. Odontogenic epithelium forming ductlike structures lined by columnar cells exhibiting reverse polarity. Calcifications, a common feature of this lesion, are seen in the lower right portion. (See Fig. 112.6.)

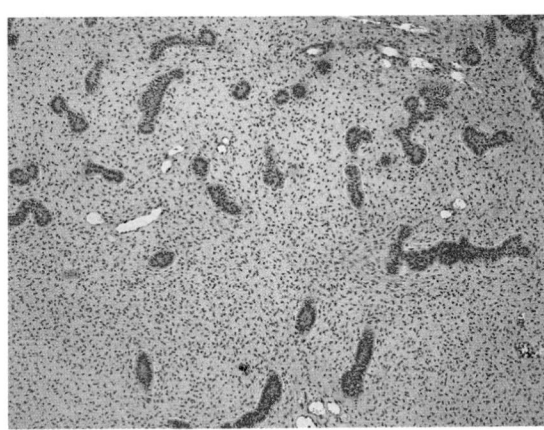

COLOR PLATE 46 Ameloblastic fibroma. Cords of odontogenic epithelium in a background of cellular, primitive mesenchymal tissue. (See Fig. 112.8.)

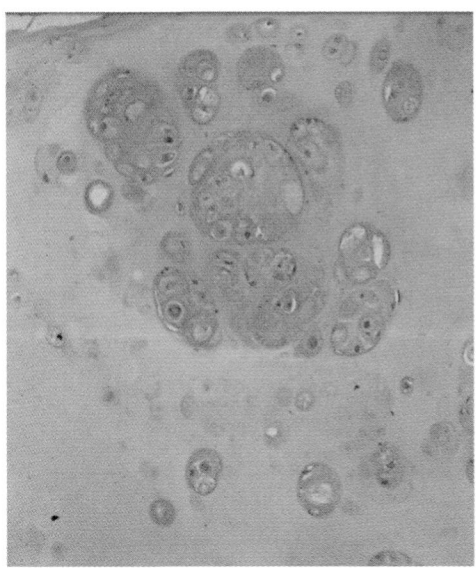

COLOR PLATE 47 Osteochondroma. Chondroid matrix with foci of developing osteocytes and osteoid. (See Fig. 112.10.)

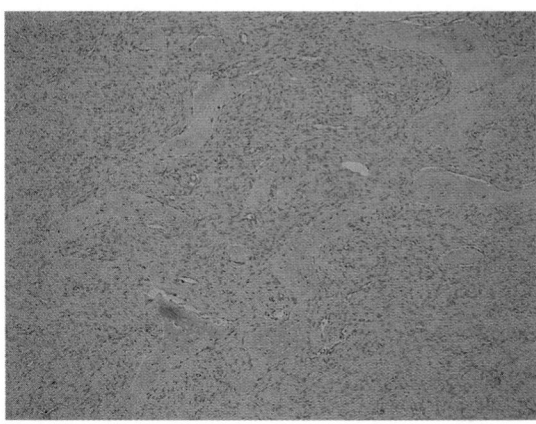

COLOR PLATE 48 Ossifying fibroma. Irregular trabeculae of bone are seen throughout a cellular, fibrous connective tissue stroma. (See Fig. 112.11.)

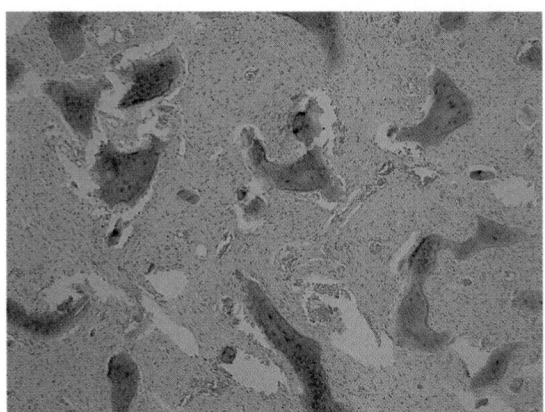

COLOR PLATE 49 Fibrous dysplasia. Curvilinear portions of woven bone, without appositional osteoblasts, in a background of connective tissue stroma. (See Fig. 112.12.)

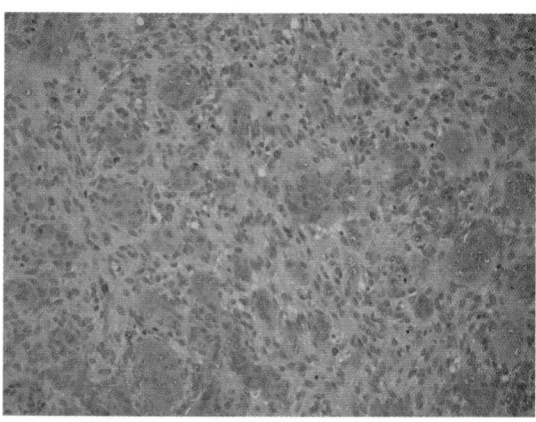

COLOR PLATE 50 Central giant cell lesion. Numerous multinucleated giant cells in a background of plump, primitive mesenchymal cells. Abundant hemorrhage is seen throughout. (See Fig. 112.13.)

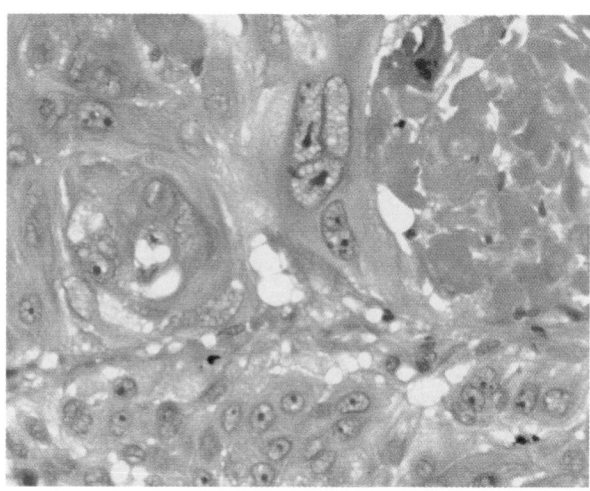

COLOR PLATE 51 Squamous cell carcinoma of the nasopharynx. The tumor cells are large with eosinophilic cytoplasm and show features of keratinization (hematoxylin and eosin × 400). (See Fig. 117.1.)

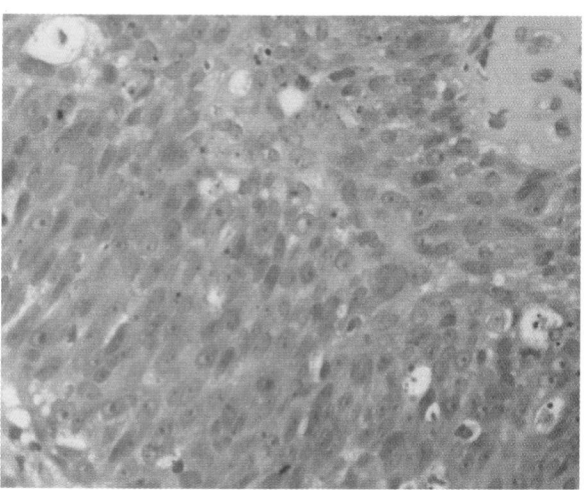

COLOR PLATE 52 Nonkeratinizing differentiated carcinoma of the nasopharynx. The tumor cells have a papillary configuration and appear more hyperchromatic than the undifferentiated carcinoma. The nuclei at the periphery show palisading (hematoxylin and eosin × 400). (See Fig. 117.2.)

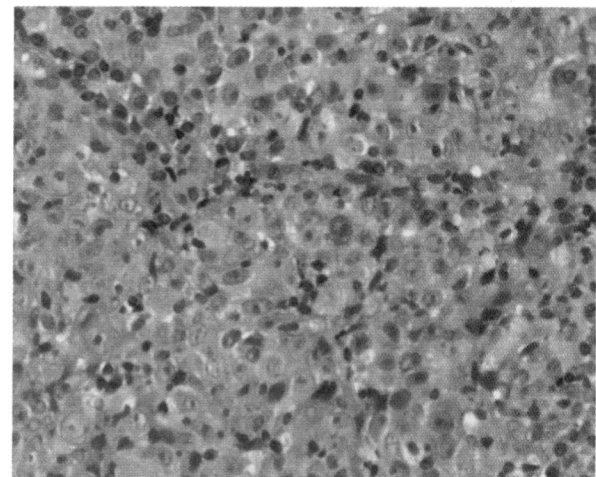

COLOR PLATE 53 Undifferentiated carcinoma of the nasopharynx. Tumor cells are typically composed of nests or islands of pleomorphic polygonal cells with large vesicular nuclei and prominent nucleoli. The tumor nests are often surrounded by a lymphoid stroma, which is part of the nasopharyngeal stroma (hematoxylin and eosin × 400). (See Fig. 117.3.)

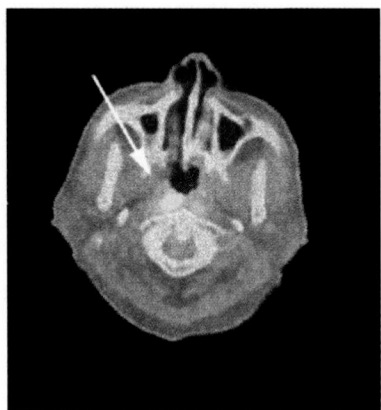
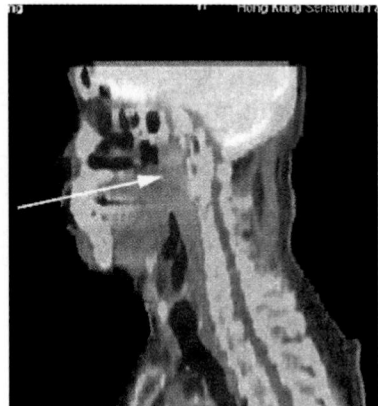

COLOR PLATE 54 A: Axial view of positron emission tomography superimposed with computed tomography image, showing increased activity at the primary site in the nasopharynx signifying presence of tumor (*arrow*). **B:** Sagittal view of the same patient. (See Fig. 117.5.)

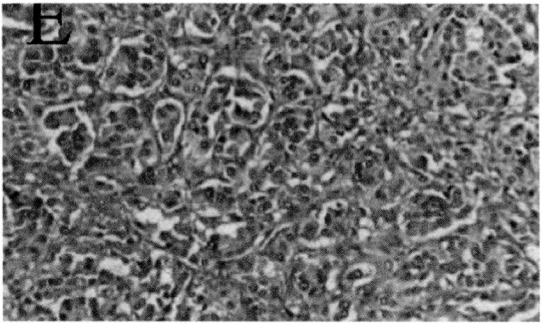

COLOR PLATE 55 Histology section stained with hematoxylin and eosin showing the characteristic Zellballen. (See Fig. 125.11.)

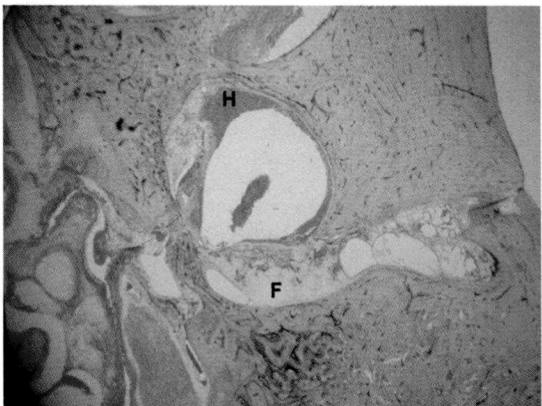

COLOR PLATE 56 Histopathology of a patient who died of meningitis several decades following an otic capsule disrupting temporal bone fracture. F, fibrosis with a small amount of ossification within the fracture line in the otic capsule; H, hemorrhage and purulence. (See Fig. 139.2.)

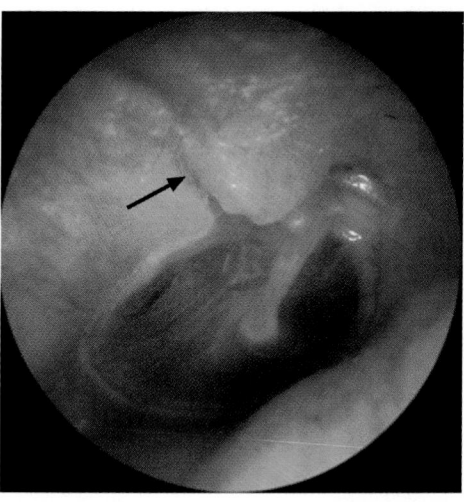

COLOR PLATE 57 Otoscopic image demonstrating a displaced fracture along the scutum (*black arrow*). (See Fig. 139.7.)

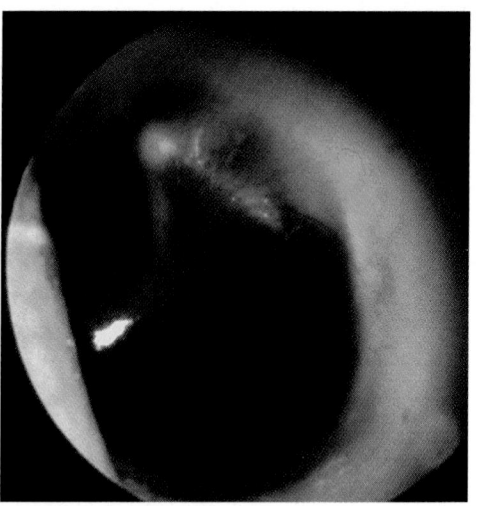

COLOR PLATE 58 Otoscopic image demonstrating a hemotympanum. (See Fig. 139.8.)

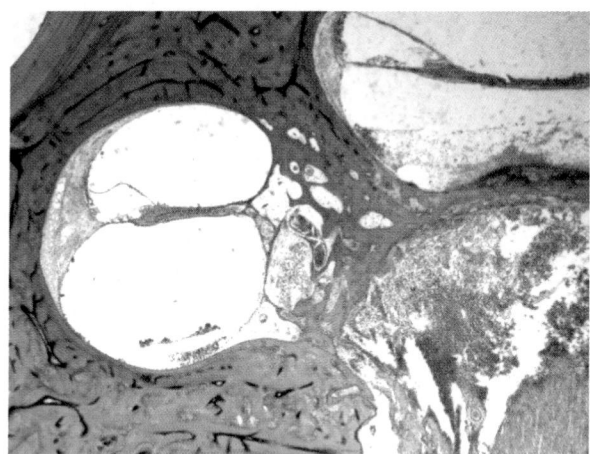

COLOR PLATE 59 A 26-year-old man sustained a gunshot wound to the ear. At 66 years, he developed an otitis media in the injured ear and meningitis that caused his demise. Histopathology of his opposite temporal bone shows the presence of labyrinthitis resulting from pyogenic meningitis. (See Fig. 146.2.) (Photograph courtesy of Fred H. Linthicum Jr., MD and Jose N. Fayad, MD of the Eccles Temporal Bone Laboratory at the House Ear Institute, Los Angeles.)

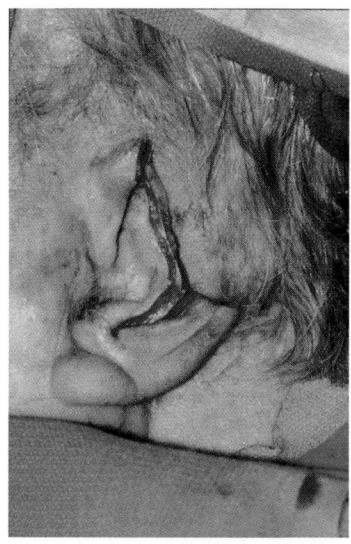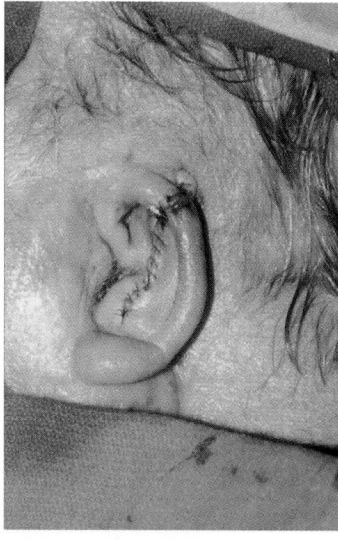

COLOR PLATE 60 B: Planned chondrocutaneous advancement flap. **C:** Flap sutured into position. (See Fig. 163.13.)

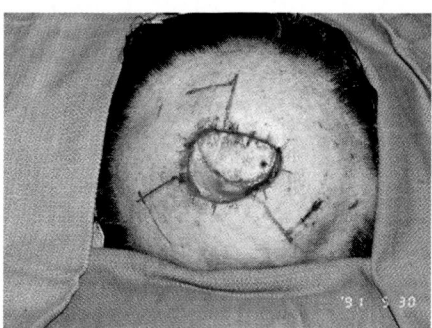

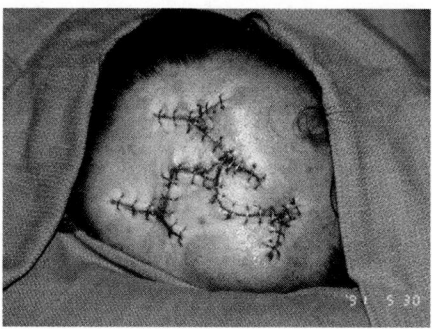

COLOR PLATE 61 B: Triple rhomboid flap designed. **D:** Immediately after surgery. **E:** Six months after surgery. (See Fig. 163.14.)

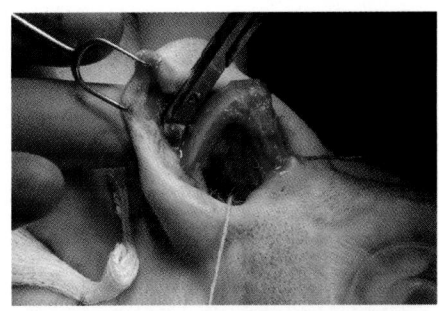

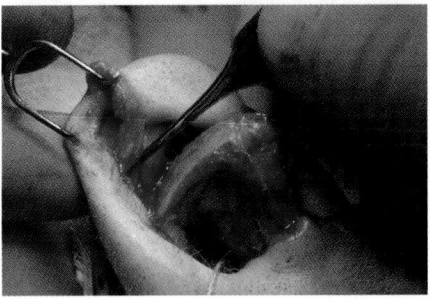

COLOR PLATE 62 Proper insertion of alar rim grafts. (See Fig. 173.22.)

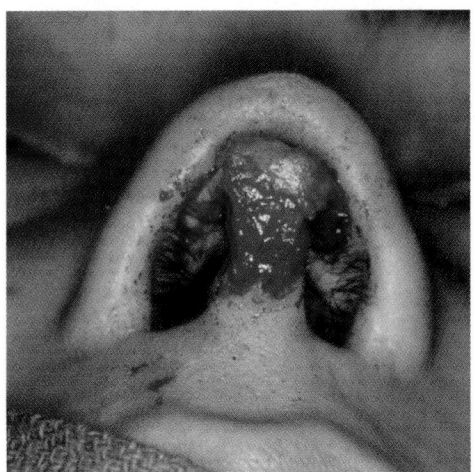

COLOR PLATE 63 Perichondrium covering nasal tip grafts to prevent postoperative graft visibility. (See Fig. 173.23.)

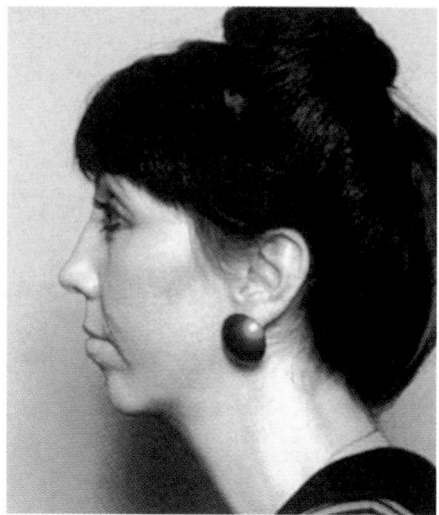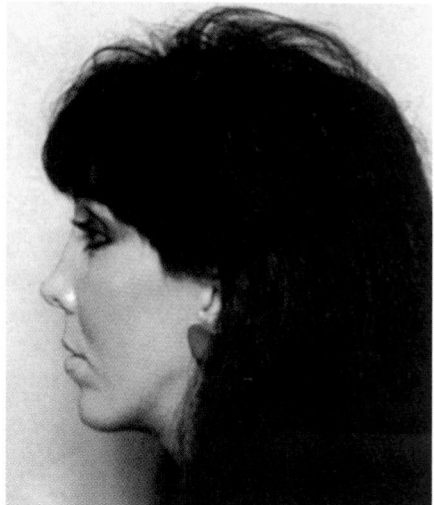

COLOR PLATE 64 This patient had a facelift, rhinoplasty, chin augmentation, and malar implants. **A:** Preoperative view: patient with flattened malar prominence and receding chin. **B:** Postoperative view: facelift with chin implant and cheek implant. Notice the malar prominence and strong chin with shallow melolabial fold. (See Fig. 181.12.)

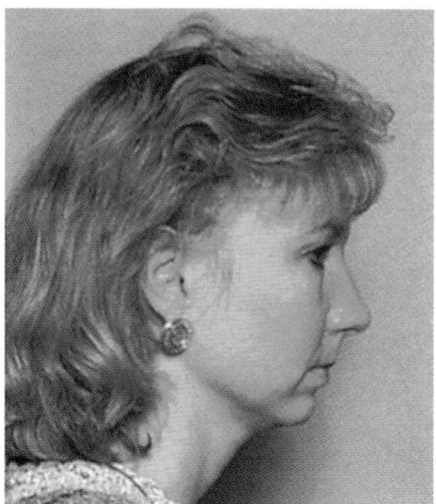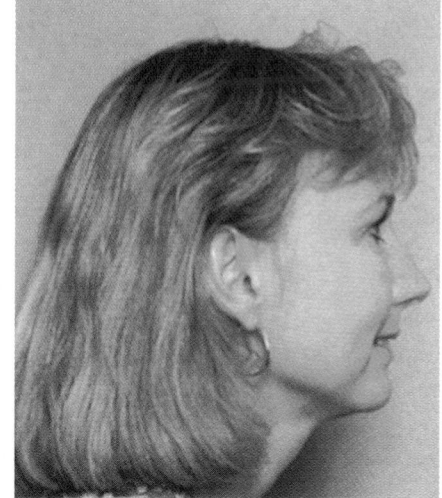

COLOR PLATE 65 Chin augmentation alone. **A:** Preoperative view: hypoplastic mandible makes the nose appear prominent. **B:** Postoperative view: chin implant. The nose appears to be in better proportion to the rest of the face. (See Fig. 181.16.)

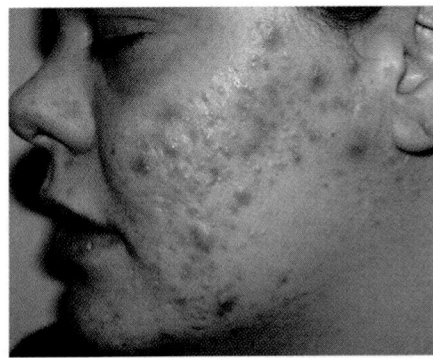

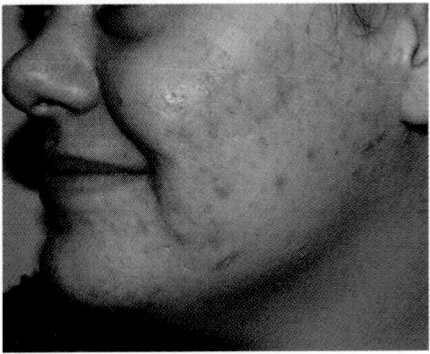

COLOR PLATE 66 A: This patient had significant acne and acne scarring. **B:** After four treatments with the 1450-nm laser (Smooth-beam, Candela Laser, Wayland, MA) she had a significant improvement in her facial acne and a reduction in her acne scarring. (See Fig. 182B.2.)

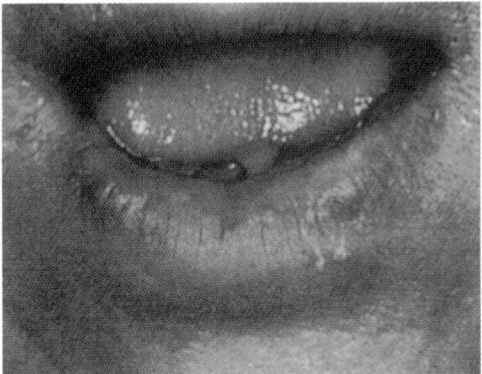

COLOR PLATE 67 Actinic cheilitis. (See Fig. 183.1.) (Reprinted from McKee P, duVivier A. *Atlas of clinical dermatology.* London: Gower, 1986, with permission.)

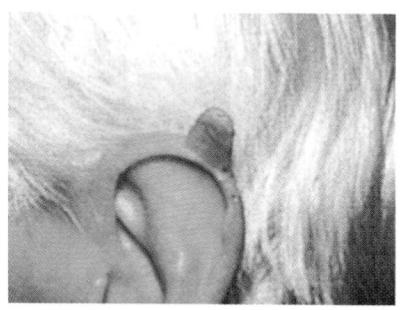

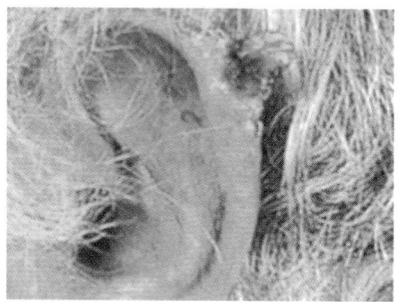

COLOR PLATE 68 Cutaneous horn. (See Fig. 183.2.) (Reprinted from McKee P, duVivier A. *Atlas of clinical dermatology*. London: Gower, 1986, with permission.)

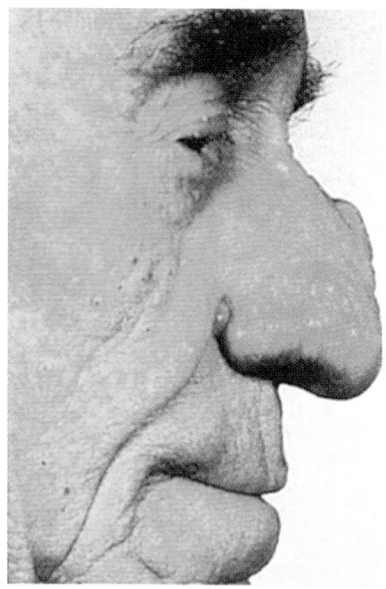

COLOR PLATE 69 Rhinophyma. (See Fig. 183.3.) (Reprinted from McKee P, duVivier A. *Atlas of clinical dermatology*. London: Gower, 1986, with permission.)

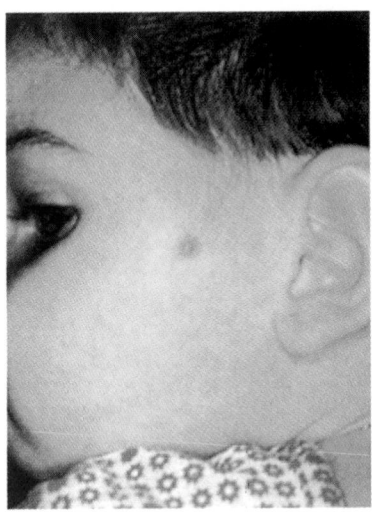

COLOR PLATE 70 Pilomatricoma. (See Fig. 183.4.) (Reprinted from McKee P, duVivier A. *Atlas of clinical dermatology*. London: Gower, 1986, with permission.)

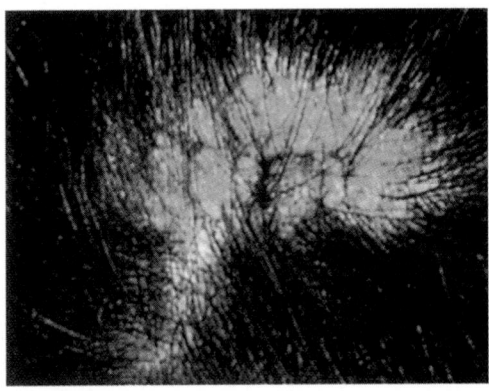

COLOR PLATE 71 Nevus sebaceus. (See Fig. 183.5.) (Reprinted from McKee P, duVivier A. *Atlas of clinical dermatology*. London: Gower, 1986, with permission.)

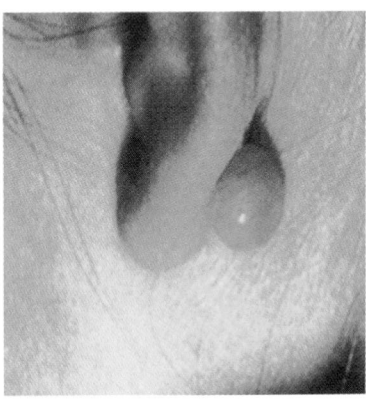

COLOR PLATE 72 Keloid. (See Fig. 183.7.) (Reprinted from McKee P, duVivier A. *Atlas of clinical dermatology*. London: Gower, 1986, with permission.)

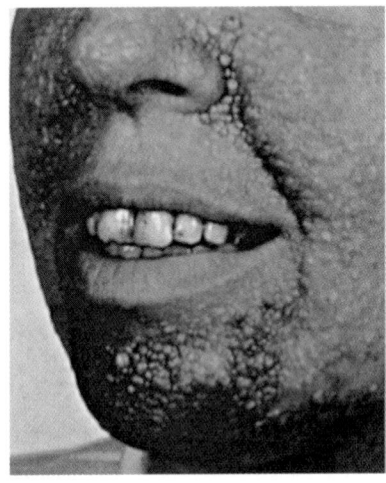

COLOR PLATE 73 Adenoma sebaceum. (See Fig. 183.8.) (Reprinted from McKee P, duVivier A. *Atlas of clinical dermatology*. London: Gower, 1986, with permission.)

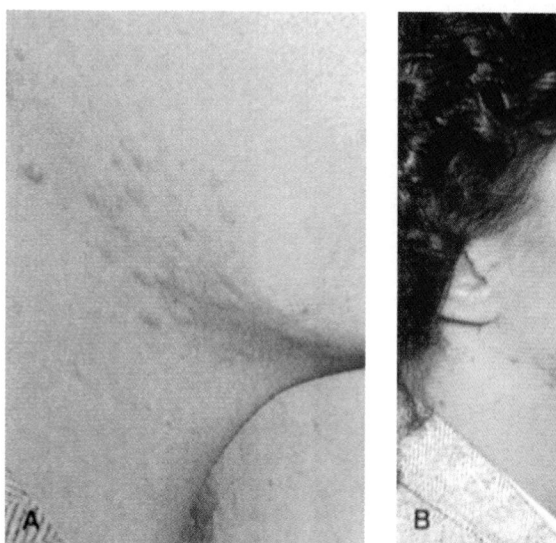

COLOR PLATE 74 Multiple leiomyomas. (See Fig. 183.9.) (Reprinted from McKee P, duVivier A. *Atlas of clinical dermatology.* London: Gower, 1986, with permission.)

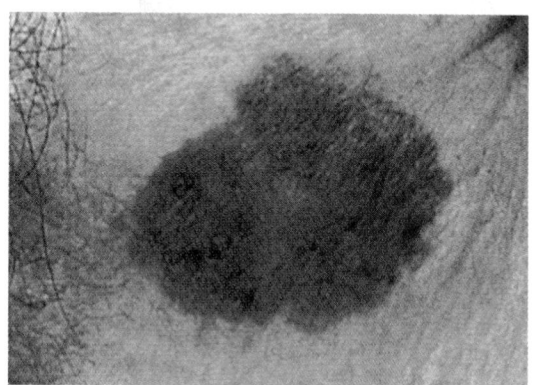

COLOR PLATE 75 Lentigo senilis. (See Fig. 183.14.) (Reprinted from McKee P, duVivier A. *Atlas of clinical dermatology.* London: Gower, 1986, with permission.)

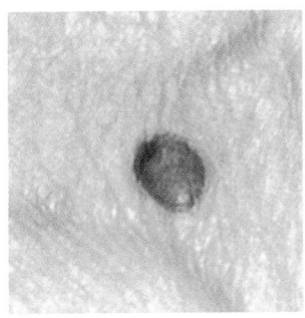

COLOR PLATE 76 Blue nevus. (See Fig. 183.16) (Reprinted from McKee P, duVivier A. *Atlas of clinical dermatology*. London: Gower, 1986, with permission.)

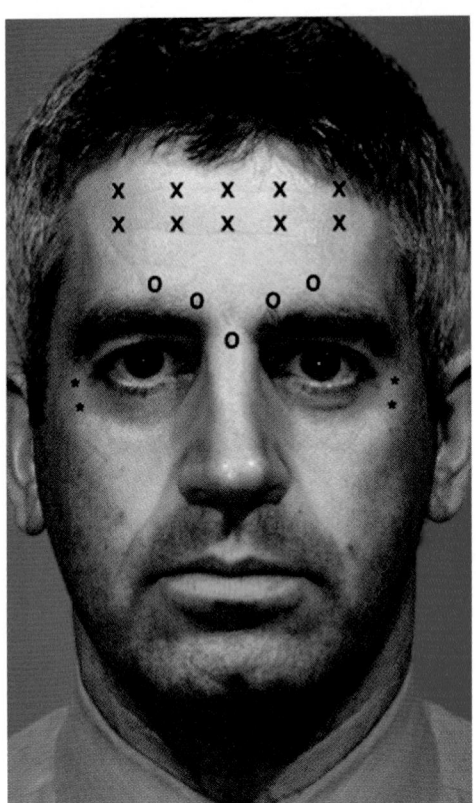

COLOR PLATE 77 Typical injection points for transverse forehead rhytids (*X*), glabellar rhytids (*O*), and lateral periorbital rhytids (asterisk). (See Fig. 185.2.)

Otosclerosis

143

Peter S. Roland   Ravi N. Samy

Otosclerosis (OS) is a fibrous osteodystrophy of the human otic capsule; no animal models exist. Its clinical manifestations are primarily conductive hearing loss (CHL), although sensorineural hearing loss (SNHL) and mixed hearing loss (MHL) can also occur. The disease process causes abnormal resorption and deposition of bone. OS is noted clinically in 1% of the Caucasian population; it is transmitted in an autosomal dominant fashion but with incomplete penetrance. Females appear to be affected more often than males (2:1 ratio) (1).

In 1873, Schwartze described a reddish hue behind an intact tympanic membrane (TM), which is due to the increased vascularity of the cochlear promontory in active OS lesions (the phase known as otospongiosis). This finding is named after him and is known as Schwartze sign. It is seen in 10% of patients with OS. In 1881, von Troltsch noted abnormalities of the middle ear mucosa in this disease and was the first to use the term OS. In 1893, Politzer described OS as a primary disease of the otic capsule, rather than a condition related to previous episodes of inflammatory ear disease, as originally thought (1).

The clinical entity of OS was further described by Bezold (1908), when he discussed its historical, physical, and audiometric findings. In 1912, Siebenmann discussed the possibility of OS causing SNHL. Since that time, numerous etiologies of OS have been suggested, including hereditary, endocrine, biochemical, metabolic, infectious (e.g., measles), traumatic, vascular, and even autoimmune factors. In fact, Lopez-Gonzalez and Delgado (2) suggested that oral vaccination with type II collagen may mitigate the autoimmune reaction in those susceptible to OS through hyposensitization. It is also possible that interplay of these different factors exist and vary from individual to individual, while causing the same pathologic and clinical findings. In other words, OS may be the common, final pathway of a clinically and genetically heterogeneous group of disorders (1).

EMBRYOLOGY

The maturation of the bony labyrinth plays a role in the pathogenesis of OS. The otic capsule arises from mesenchyme surrounding the otic vesicle at 4 weeks of embryologic development. At 8 weeks, the cartilaginous framework is begun. At 16 weeks, endochondral bony replacement of this framework begins in 14 identifiable centers. In some people, complete bony replacement does not occur and leaves cartilage in certain locations. One of these regions, the fissula ante fenestram, is anterior to the oval window (OW) and is usually the last area of endochondral bone formation in the labyrinth. According to temporal bone studies, this region is affected in 80% to 90% of patients with OS. In 1985, Schuknecht and Barber reported other areas of predilection for otosclerotic lesions, such as the border of the round window (RW), the apical medial wall of the cochlea, the area posterior to the cochlear aqueduct, the region adjacent to the semicircular canals, and the stapes footplate itself (which is derived from otic capsule, as opposed to the superstructure, which is a branchial arch derivative) (1).

HISTOLOGY

There are three forms of otosclerotic lesions: otospongiosis (early phase), transitional phase, and OS (late phase). The early, active phase lesions consist of histiocytes, osteoblasts, and the most active cell group, the osteocytes. The osteocytes resorb bone around preexisting blood vessels, which causes widening of the vascular channels and dilation of the microcirculation. Otoscopic or microscopic exam can reveal the reddish hue caused by these lesions (Schwartze sign if seen on clinical examination). As osteocytes become more involved, these areas grow rich in amorphous ground substance and deficient in mature collagen, resulting in formation of new spongy bone. With hematoxylin-eosin (H&E) staining, this new spongy bone appears densely blue. This was described in 1914 by Manasse and is known as the blue mantles of Manasse. Interestingly, mantles are found in up to 20% of normal temporal bones. On electron microscopy, the foci of perivascular bony invasion coalesce as the lesions enlarge within the otic capsule (1).

The predominant finding in the late phase of OS is the formation of sclerotic, dense bone in areas of previous bony resorption. The vascular spaces that were once dilated are narrowed due to bony deposition. Within each temporal bone containing OS, lesions can be found in early, transitional, and late phases, although the overall histologic status of the developing lesions is fairly uniform. Although OS begins in endochondral bone, as the spongiosis and sclerosis continue, the endosteal and periosteal layers also become involved (1).

PATHOPHYSIOLOGY

The areas of OS involvement dictate the clinical presentation. The most common type involves the stapes and accounts for those cases in which CHL is the presenting symptom. The CHL is due to fixation of the stapes footplate, usually beginning at the fissula ante fenestram (Fig. 143.1). Progressive involvement of the footplate can create a thick focus of OS that fills the OW niche (obliterative OS) (1).

If OS involves only the footplate and spares the annular ligament, minimal fixation may occur. Such a thickened footplate is called a biscuit footplate. Because of minimal fixation, biscuit footplates can become mobilized inadvertently during a stapes procedure, placing the patient at a higher risk of postoperative SNHL. The RW is involved in 30% of all clinical cases of OS; complete closure of this niche is uncommon (1).

Whether OS can cause SNHL has been an area of dispute. Some patients with OS have a greater amount of SNHL than expected considering their age and history of noise exposure. The mechanism for the SNHL is possibly the liberation of toxic metabolites into the inner ear with resultant injury to neuroepithelium, vascular compromise, or direct extension of lesions into the cochlea, causing disruption of electrolytes and changes in basilar membrane mechanics. SNHL is usually associated with significant stapedial OS, although some otologists contend that isolated pure SNHL can be seen without associated CHL. The latter presentation is also known as cochlear OS (3).

Shambaugh (3) has suggested seven criteria to identify patients suffering from SNHL due to OS:

1. Schwartze sign in either ear
2. Family history of OS
3. Unilateral CHL consistent with OS and bilateral, symmetric SNHL
4. Audiogram with a flat or "cookie-bite" curve with excellent discrimination
5. Progressive pure cochlear loss beginning at the usual age of onset for OS
6. Computed tomography (CT) scan showing demineralization of the cochlea typical for OS
7. Stapedial reflex demonstrating the biphasic "on-off effect" seen before stapedial fixation

Dizziness occurs in up to 30% of patients with OS. Otologists have seen OS lesions in the lateral semicircular canal during fenestration procedures (which have been replaced by the stapedectomy/stapedotomy). The vestibular symptoms are usually not severe, but objective evidence can be obtained with electronystagmographic (ENG) testing. Dizziness associated with OS has been termed OS inner ear syndrome. It is important to differentiate this disorder from Ménière disease or superior semicircular canal dehiscence (SSCD). An absolute contraindication for stapedectomy/

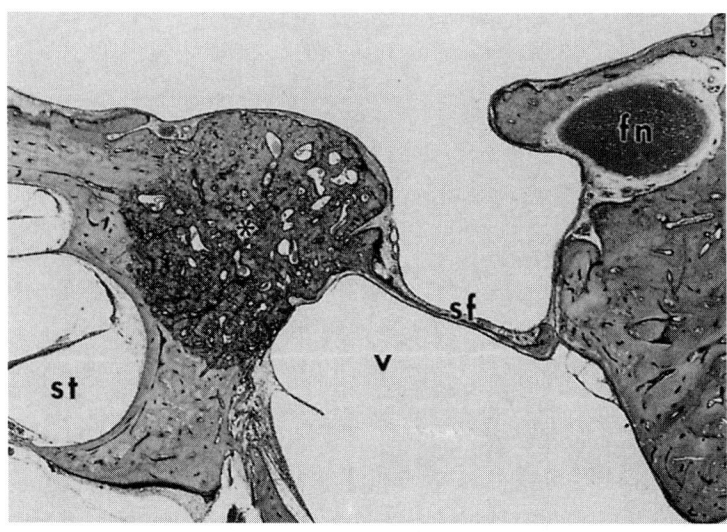

Figure 143.1 Photomicrograph of temporal bone section in a 79-year-old white man demonstrating a mature otosclerotic focus (∗) involving the promontory and anterior stapes footplate (*sf*). *st*, scala tympani; *v*, vestibule; *fn*, facial nerve. (×20.) (Courtesy of M.M. Paparella, director, and S. Lamey, coordinator, Otopathology Laboratory, University of Minnesota.)

stapedotomy is Ménière disease. When the endolymphatic space is dilated (endolymphatic hydrops), the saccule may be enlarged to the point that it adheres to the undersurface of the stapes footplate. A stapes procedure can injure the saccule and produce profound SNHL. The distinction between OS inner ear syndrome and other causes of dizziness is based on differences in clinical presentation. Rarely does the inner ear syndrome of OS cause well-defined episodes of severe rotational vertigo, nausea, vomiting, and fluctuating SNHL. Dizziness in OS inner ear syndrome is milder but more persistent; low-frequency SNHL is generally not present (1).

In 2004, Mikulec et al. (4) reported on eight patients with presumed OS/unilateral CHL that did not improve after a stapes procedure. These patients were ultimately found to have SSCD. In contrast to typical SSCD patients, these patients had only CHL and no vestibular symptoms. One should keep this entity in mind, especially in a patient with CHL and pressure or sound-induced vertiginous symptoms.

EPIDEMIOLOGY

OS is transmitted in an autosomal dominant fashion with incomplete penetrance (25% to 40%). The degree of penetrance is related to the distribution of lesions in the otic capsule. Some lesions are not located where they can cause clinical symptoms. About 10% of Caucasians have histologic findings of OS. However, of those with histologic changes, only 12% have clinical symptoms; thus, overall, this represents about 1% of the Caucasian population. In the Japanese and South American populations, the incidence is 50% of that in Caucasians. The African-American population has fewer cases of OS; only 1% demonstrate histologic findings of the disease. In all races, when one ear is affected, the contralateral ear shows histologic involvement 80% of the time. Generally, the lesions occur in similar anatomic locations and at similar histologic phases. The age at which symptoms become apparent is variable due to the insidious progression of hearing loss, but hearing loss often begins between the ages of 15 and 45 years. The average age at presentation is 33 years (1).

About 60% of patients with clinical OS report a family history of this condition. The remaining 40%, as suggested by Morrison and Bundey (5), make up a collection of cases that fall into one of the following categories:

1. Autosomal dominant inherited cases with failure of penetrance in other family members
2. Phenocopies
3. New mutations
4. Those rare cases transmitted by alternate modes of inheritance (i.e., autosomal recessive)

OS has been reported to advance more rapidly in females than males, although no difference has been noted in age at onset. A recent study by Clayton et al. (6) examined the relationship in elderly women between osteoporosis and OS; both diseases show some similarities, including an association with the COL1A1 gene. The study showed that a much higher percentage of women with OS also had osteoporosis as compared with a similar aged group with only presbycusis ($p < .0007$). Juvenile OS may progress more rapidly than the adult form. Hormonal factors may play a role; some females with OS appear to have their condition worsen during pregnancy. Estrogen receptors have been noted in the OS plaques. However, more recent data by Dr. William Lippy (unpublished data) minimizes the association between pregnancy and worsening of OS.

HISTORY AND PHYSICAL EXAMINATION

Patients with OS usually present with a slowly progressive hearing loss over a period of years. Patients may describe hearing speech more easily in noisy situations. The CHL improves the signal to noise ratio by subduing background noise (paracusis of Willis). Tinnitus is present in 75% of patients. A complete head and neck examination is performed to rule out concurrent otolaryngologic abnormalities. Otomicroscopic examination with pneumatic insufflation is done of the external auditory canal (EAC) and TM to assess for the presence of a middle ear effusion or mass, cholesteatoma, or TM retraction. The physical appearance of the TM is normal in most patients with OS. A Schwartze sign may be present. The tuning fork examination should confirm a CHL. The Rinne test should demonstrate bone conduction to be better than air conduction (Rinne -) in patients contemplating a stapes procedure. In the initial phases of the disease, CHL may be limited to the 256 Hz tuning fork. As footplate fixation progresses, the 512 Hz and 1024 Hz tuning forks will "convert" or "flip" as well. The amount of air-bone gap required to flip the forks are about 10 to 15 dB for the 256 Hz tuning fork and 20 to 25 dB for the 512 Hz tuning fork. The Weber test should lateralize to the ear with the greater degree of CHL, although this test is also affected by concurrent SNHL (1).

AUDIOLOGIC TESTING

The main objective measurement in OS is the hearing test (Fig. 143.2). On the audiogram, OS is seen as a widening air-bone gap that usually begins in the low frequencies. Variable degrees of SNHL may also be present. Bone conduction may show a 20 dB loss at 2000 Hz and a 5 dB loss at 500 Hz and 4000 Hz. Such an apparent depression of bone conduction at 2000 Hz is known as Carhart notch, which is most commonly seen in OS but can be seen in other types of CHL. This notch is an artifact of the audiogram and disappears after a stapedectomy. It is secondary

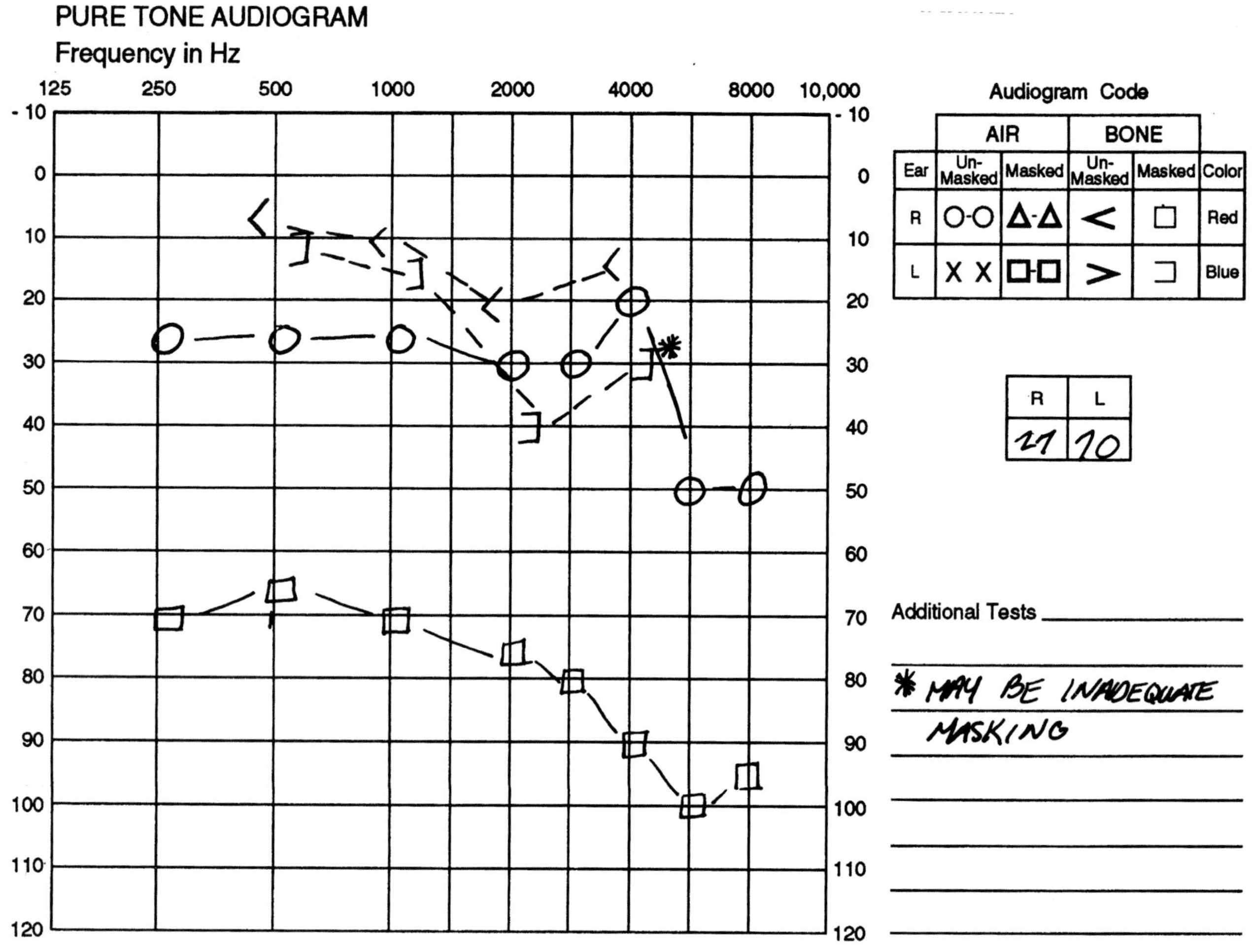

PURE TONE AUDIOGRAM
Frequency in Hz

Audiogram Code					
	AIR		BONE		
Ear	Un-Masked	Masked	Un-Masked	Masked	Color
R	O-O	Δ-Δ	<	☐	Red
L	X X	☐-☐	>	☐	Blue

R	L
27	70

Additional Tests _____

* MAY BE INADEQUATE MASKING

SPEECH HEARING TESTS

TEST		R	L	BIN	SF
Sp. Reception Threshold (SRT)		20 db	65 db	db	db
Sp. Discrim. Scores	80 db HL	100 %	/ %	%	%
(PB)	90 db HL	/ %	100 %	%	%
	_____ db HL	%	%	%	%
Most Comfortable Loudness (MCL)		db	db	db	db
Loudness Discomfort Level (LDL)		db	db	db	db

SSI TEST	R	L
at _____ db HL	%	%
at _____ db HL	%	%
at _____ db HL	%	%

Figure 143.2 Audiogram of a 27-year-old white woman with otosclerosis demonstrating near-maximum conductive hearing loss in the left ear and Carhart notch at 2000 Hz in both ears. Notice that discrimination remains at 100% in both ears.

to stapes fixation and a resultant change in the resonance of the bony capsule (1).

Speech discrimination is usually excellent. Impedance can show reduced TM compliance (type A or As). Stapedial reflexes can also be normal or abnormal, depending on the degree of fixation. With early stapes fixation, a characteristic abnormal decrease in impedance may be noted at the onset and offset of the eliciting signal. This is the on-off

effect of OS. Vestibular testing should be included when dizziness is present. Although there are not characteristic findings for OS inner ear syndrome, findings or a clinical history suggestive of SSCD or Ménière disease will alter treatment planning (1).

High-resolution CT scans can help identify or confirm patients with OS. These scans can also assess the ossicular chain in addition to the bony labyrinth (cochlea, semicircular canals). Radiolucent areas in and around the cochlea are noted early in the course of the disease, creating the "halo sign." Diffuse sclerosis is found in mature cases. Negative results on the CT scan are not diagnostic because some patients have disease below the capabilities of scanning protocols. The CT can also be helpful to rule out middle ear masses, vascular anomalies, or facial nerve abnormalities but is not an essential part of the workup (1).

DIFFERENTIAL DIAGNOSIS

The differential diagnosis should include other causes of CHL or MHL. A history of progressive CHL or MHL in the absence of history of trauma or infection but with the presence of a normal TM limits the possibilities. However, a definitive diagnosis can only be made during exploratory tympanotomy. The most common conditions that mimic OS are those that result in ossicular discontinuity or exert a mass effect on the TM or ossicles. A history of recurrent chronic otitis media suggests an ossicular discontinuity due to incus necrosis. The TM may be normal or thickened or atrophic in cases of chronic infection. The TM in these ears is sometimes abnormally compliant, which can be manifested as a type Ad tympanogram. Fibrous union of the incudostapedial (IS) joint can produce an air-bone gap wider in the high frequencies than in the lower frequencies (1).

Congenital stapedial footplate fixation presents at an earlier age than does juvenile OS. De la Cruz noted in his series that congenital footplate fixation was detectable at age 3, whereas juvenile OS was not detectable until about age 10 (7). In lateral ossicular chain fixation, the malleus and/or incus become fixed in the epitympanum (usually at the superior malleolar ligament), resulting in immobility of all the ossicles; this can occur congenitally or may be acquired through tympanosclerosis. The entire ossicular chain must be examined with every exploratory tympanotomy to avoid overlooking this lesion. Tympanosclerosis can mimic OS, but a history of recurrent otitis media or placement of tympanostomy tubes is usually present. In addition, the TM is often thickened with associated myringosclerosis. Persistent middle ear effusion, neoplasms of the middle ear and EAC (such as glomus tumors or facial nerve tumors), and chronic suppurative otitis media with and without cholesteatoma can also cause CHL. Audiometry and physical examination should help make the diagnosis apparent (1).

Paget disease (osteitis deformans) is a disease with diffuse bony involvement that is histologically similar to OS. In contrast to OS, Paget disease begins in the periosteal layer and involves the endochondral bone last. Temporal bone involvement can produce SNHL, but stapes involvement or fixation rarely occurs (1).

Osteogenesis imperfecta (van der Hoeve-de-Kleyn syndrome) is an autosomal dominant defect of osteoblast activity resulting in multiple fractures. Stapes fixation and

TABLE 143.1   DIAGNOSIS OTOSCLEROSIS

History
 Progressive hearing loss
 Family history of otosclerosis
 Tinnitus
 Possible vestibular symptoms (rule out Ménière or SSCD)
 Otitis media/otorrhea (absent)
 Head trauma (absent)

Physical examination
 Tympanic membrane (normal)
 Schwartze sign
 Rinne test (negative at 256 and 512 Hz)
 Weber test (lateralizes to side with greater CHL)

Ancillary studies
 Audiogram (assess for CHL, mixed HL, SNHL, Carhart notch)
 Tympanometry (type A or As; absent or on-off stapedial reflex)
 Imaging (CT scan showing radiolucent areas around bony labyrinth)

CHL, conductive hearing loss; CT, computed tomography; HL, hearing loss; SNHL, sensorineural hearing loss; SSCD, superior semicircular canal dehiscence.

unique blue sclera are also found in 40% to 60% of affected patients. Stapes surgery can be performed in these patients, usually with results similar to those in patients with OS (Table 143.1) (1).

MANAGEMENT

Ninety percent of patients with histologic evidence of OS are asymptomatic; active lesions usually mature without stapedial fixation or cochlear loss. In the symptomatic patient, slowly progressive CHL and SNHL usually begin by age 20. The disease may advance more rapidly at times, possibly depending on environmental factors. Periods of progress may be followed by periods of quiescence. The CHL stabilizes at a maximum of 50 to 60 dB (1).

AMPLIFICATION

Patients with hearing loss secondary to OS should be offered the option of amplification with typical hearing aids as an alternative to observation or surgery. Unilateral or bilateral hearing aids may provide effective treatment. Some patients may not be suitable candidates for surgery, making amplification the only reasonable option. Another option is to use a bone conduction hearing aid. The one that is currently used in the United States is the bone-anchored hearing aid (BAHA, Entific). It bypasses the ossicular chain and amplifies sound that stimulates the cochlea directly through bone conduction. McClarnon et al. (8) reported that of subgroups examined for satisfaction, patients receiving the BAHA for congenital aural atresia tended to have the highest satisfaction rate; those receiving the BAHA for single-sided deafness (e.g., acoustic neuroma patients) had the lowest satisfaction rate. Patients with OS tended to fall in the middle.

Although amplification avoids potential risk of profound hearing loss that could occur from surgery, it is not capable of providing many of the benefits or patient satisfaction of successful operation. Hearing aids are usually not used at night. The canal occlusion effect, difficulties with feedback, and the physical sensation of the device within the EAC are disagreeable and have a negative impact on patient satisfaction. In addition, most insurance companies cover the costs of surgery but few cover the costs of hearing aids, which include batteries and a finite lifespan of 3 to 5 years.

For those with severe to profound SNHL bilaterally due to OS, cochlear implantation is an option. However, Rotteveel et al. (9) reported that partial electrode insertions, misplacement of the electrode, and inadvertent facial nerve stimulation are more likely than in patients without OS and normal cochlear anatomy.

MEDICAL MANAGEMENT

Medical therapy can be considered for all patients with OS, whether they are managed by observation, amplification, or surgery. In 1923, Escot was the first to suggest the use of calcium fluoride for the treatment of OS. Shambaugh (3) predicted stabilization of OS lesions with the use of sodium fluoride. Fluoride ions replace the usual hydroxyl radical, forming a more stable fluorapatite complex instead of a hydroxyapatite crystal. The fluorapatite complex resists osteoclastic action and is confirmed by histologic evidence. Thus, fluoride consumption may help retard the progression of OS related CHL, SNHL, and dizziness.

The recommended dosage of sodium fluoride is 20 to 120 mg per day. Evaluation of efficacy may be based on the disappearance of Schwartze sign (if it was present), stabilization of hearing, and improvement in the CT appearance of the otic capsule. Side effects of this therapy are usually minor and gastrointestinal related (nausea) but may affect patient compliance; these effects can be minimized by lowering the dose or using enteric-coated tablets. Occasionally, a patient complains of joint, muscle, or bone pain, which usually resolves with temporary discontinuation of therapy. Rarely, fluid retention, cutaneous eruptions, and eye problems occur. Using this treatment regimen, 80% of patients improve or show no worsening of their symptoms (Table 143.2) (1).

SURGICAL MANAGEMENT

Although Rosen introduced the stapes mobilization procedure in 1953, most otologists replace the stapes superstructure with a prosthesis (due to less chance of recur-

TABLE 143.2	C COMPLICATIONS
OS SURGERY	

Intraoperative
  Bleeding (high jugular bulb, tympanomeatal flap, persistent
    stapedial artery, mucoperiosteum)
  Facial nerve injury ($<1\%$)
  Perilymph gusher
  Fracture/dislocation of incus
  Floating footplate

Postoperative
  Acute otitis media
  TM perforation
  CHL (middle ear effusion, displaced prosthesis, incus erosion)
  SNHL, vertigo, tinnitus (due to intraoperative trauma,
    labyrinthitis, reparative granuloma, perilymph fistula)
  Facial nerve palsy (local anesthetic, intraoperative trauma,
    delayed Bell palsy)

CHL, conductive hearing loss; OS, otosclerosis; SNHL, sensorineural hearing loss; TM, tympanic membrane.

rence of fixation) (10). The stapedectomy was popularized by John Shea in the late 1950s (11). He removed the entire footplate and placed a vein graft to close off the vestibule. The stapes superstructure was reconstructed with a polyethylene prosthesis. Others modified this procedure by using a combined fat or connective tissue and wire prosthesis or by using gelatin sponge to seal the vestibule; a wire prosthesis was then placed on top of the gelatin material. The use of this material in replacement of the footplate is no longer used due to high risk of reparative granuloma formation postoperatively, which frequently results in a significant amount of SNHL. Partial stapedectomies have also been performed (instead of a total stapedectomy). Further modifications of these procedures have been described, but the essential principles have remained the same for almost 50 years (1).

PATIENT SELECTION AND CONTRAINDICATIONS

The clinical circumstances favoring successful stapes procedures include unacceptable conductive hearing loss (CHL), a negative Rinne test (BC > AC) at 512 Hz, and good speech discrimination. When maximal CHL due to OS coexists with significant SNHL, detection of the bone line and conductive component can be difficult due to the limits of the audiometer. The situation is worse with bilateral MHL. Air-conduction thresholds may be present at very reduced levels (90 to 100 dB) or entirely absent. A history of progressive hearing loss should raise suspicion that OS may be involved. Suspicion should be heightened if discrimination scores or the ability to function appears much better than one would expect with such a high degree of hearing loss. The presence of As tympanograms, abnormalities of stapedial reflex, or a family history of OS should raise suspicion even further. Use of the tuning forks may also separate advanced OS from SNHL of other causes (1).

A CT scan will sometimes permit a diagnosis of advanced OS when an audiometric test is inconclusive. If advanced OS is suspected, exploratory tympanotomy should be considered. Stapedectomy in such a setting can produce meaningful results. Air-conduction thresholds and discrimination scores can be improved enough to allow amplification to work (1).

Age is a consideration in contemplating surgery. In addition, the pediatric patient is not allowed to provide consent, although he or she may provide assent to the procedure; this can potentially be a medicolegal issue in a patient who suffers postoperative profound SNHL. The very young patient has a higher incidence of OW reclosure after a successful initial procedure. Although revision can be performed, a secondary procedure in any patient has a decreased success rate and a greater risk for postoperative SNHL. De la Cruz noted that in addition to being manifest at an earlier age, congenital footplate fixation is less likely to have a positive family history (7). Half of the children with juvenile OS had a positive family history, but only 10% of those children with congenital footplate fixation had other family members with CHL. Patients with X-linked conductive hearing loss have a high incidence of poststapedectomy profound SNHL due to a perilymph [cerebrospinal fluid (CSF) leak] gusher. The incidence of congenital anomalies of the malleus and incus was substantially higher in children with congenital footplate fixation (25%) than in children with juvenile OS (3%). This difference in abnormalities of the remainder of the ossicular chain probably accounts for the poorer results. Eighty-two percent of the children with juvenile OS had closure of the air-bone gap to within 10 dB. This is in contrast to children who had congenital footplate fixation; only 44% had closure within 10 dB. Very young children with OS are also at greater risk postoperatively due to their increased incidence of otitis media and eustachian tube dysfunction.

Age is an important variable for surgical outcome; poorer results in the high-frequency range have been seen in older patients who have undergone stapes surgery. However, Meyer and Lambert (12) reviewed the recent literature and reported that primary and revision stapedectomy are still felt to be good options in the elderly. Lifestyle and occupation are important factors in selecting patients for stapedectomy. Persons whose activities include repeated exposure to barometric pressure changes (e.g., scuba diver) may be at greater risk for postoperative fistulae and prosthesis dislocation. Patients whose work or hobbies dictate excellent balance should be considered questionable candidates for surgery. Those in whom taste is of the utmost importance (e.g., chefs, vintners) should also be recommended to have amplification instead of surgery, due to the risk of stretching or cutting the chorda tympani nerve.

Patients with otologic complaints not attributed to their OS must be carefully evaluated. For example, patients with Ménière disease and OS have a greater risk of cochlear hearing loss after stapedectomy. Patients with TM perforations and OS should have their perforations successfully repaired before attempted stapedectomy (i.e., staging of the ear). The incidence of severe to profound SNHL is much greater if stapedectomy is performed in an ear with a perforation. Patients with a history of severe eustachian tube dysfunction or a history of cholesteatoma are not good candidates for stapedectomy. Those with canal exostoses that are obstructing surgical access should have them removed before the stapedectomy. Surgical intervention on the better-hearing ear or only-hearing ear is a relative contraindication. The presence of a middle ear infection or effusion is an absolute contraindication to removal of the footplate (1).

The worse hearing ear should be approached first. The likelihood of achieving serviceable hearing in a unilateral MHL is an important consideration. Improved communication in such a patient may not be achieved after elimination of the CHL due to the continued SNHL. Some surgeons believe that significant high-frequency SNHL after stapedectomy in the first ear contraindicates attempting the second. A minimum of approximately 6 months should elapse before attempting surgery on the second ear due to the small but present risk of sudden postoperative hearing loss (1).

PATIENT COUNSELING

Observation, fluoride use, and a trial of hearing aid use is discussed with every patient, whether he or she has CHL or MHL. The patient must understand the elective nature of the procedure. The patient must be candidly informed of the risk of stapedectomy (postoperative deafness of less than 2%).

Stretching or contusion of the chorda tympani nerve can produce alteration of taste (or rarely, dryness of the mouth). When these symptoms occur, they are usually self-limited and disappear in a few weeks or months. A severely stretched or contused chorda tympani nerve may produce more symptoms than one that is divided. Dehiscence of the fallopian canal over the OW can permit exposure or prolapse of the facial nerve. If the nerve is traumatized or injured during the stapes procedure, facial nerve palsy can result. However, facial nerve paralysis occurs less than 1% of the time. There are reported cases of delayed facial palsy occurring after stapes procedures; this may be due to reactivation of the herpes simplex virus and a Bell palsy occurring (1).

A postoperative TM perforation may occur 2% of the time as a consequence of trauma or vascular injury to the TM flap. Acute balance disturbance is common after stapedectomy. It usually resolves in 3 to 7 days. Long-term balance disturbances or vertigo rarely occur. Sparano et al. (13) reported that 85% of patients with tinnitus improved after stapedectomy (with 52.5% reporting complete resolution, 12.5% reporting no change, and 2.5% reporting worsening of their tinnitus).

SURGICAL TECHNIQUE

A well-performed stapes procedure is gratifying for both surgeon and patient. However, stapedectomies are one of the most technically challenging procedures performed by an otologist. One concern about current resident training is the lack of stapedectomies performed. Prior to graduation, the average number of cases a resident performs as the operating surgeon is three. Vrabec and Coker (14) proposed that the number of surgical OS cases per surgeon could be decreasing due to the use of measles vaccination and because the number of surgeons able to perform the surgery has increased significantly over the past 30 years. The pros and cons of local versus general anesthesia must be presented to the patient. Although general anesthesia is often easier for the patient and surgeon, local anesthesia may be safer to the patient (systemically) and to hearing preservation. Local anesthesia allows the patient to provide feedback about whether any dizziness is occurring during the procedure, allowing the surgeon to terminate the procedure momentarily or permanently. The patient can also let the surgeon know about the status of hearing improvement or loss intraoperatively.

Two keys to stapes surgery are adequate exposure and adequate hemostasis. Preoperatively, the ear canal and TM are carefully inspected for evidence of inflammation or infection that would dictate postponement of the procedure. The patient can also be consented for use of endaural or postauricular approaches if the ear canal is too small for a transcanal approach. Intraoperatively, the ear is prepped and draped in the usual sterile fashion. Canal vibrissae may be trimmed to improved operative exposure. Trauma to the drum or the canal from the preparation can occur, making the procedure more difficult. The canal is injected with local (1% lidocaine with 1:100,000 epinephrine) for both anesthetic and vasoconstrictive effect. The largest speculum that can be placed is used; in adults, a 7-mm speculum can usually be placed. Some surgeons prefer to use a black speculum as opposed to a silver speculum; the black color absorbs light and is less likely to reflect light from the microscope back to the surgeon. It is often possible to dilate the ear canal during the case with progressively larger speculums as well. Due to the finesse required during this surgery, some advocate the use of a speculum holder, freeing up both hands to concentrate on the procedure. The flap is elevated from the 6 o'clock to 12 o'clock position. The superior exposure is important to allow inspection of the epitympanum and lateral ossicular chain

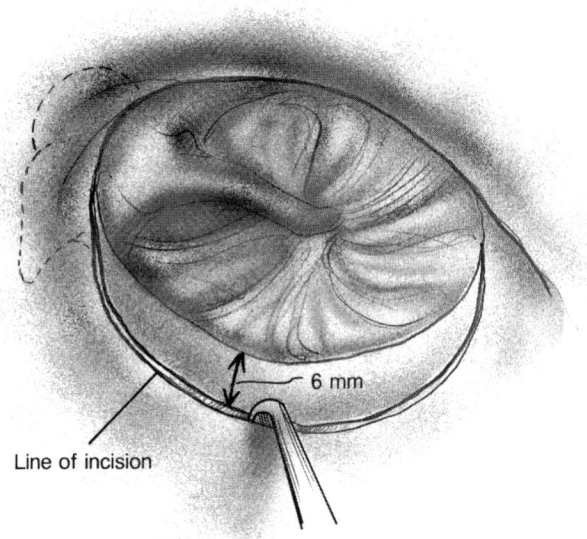

Figure 143.3 Typical design for a tympanomeatal flap.

if needed. The flap is approximately 6-mm wide, as measured from the fibrous annulus. This flap must be sufficient to cover any bony defect created by curetting the scutum (Fig. 143.3) (1).

The TM is elevated with the fibrous annulus (Fig. 143.4). The chorda tympani nerve is identified and preserved if possible. Enough scutum (the medial most posterior-superior EAC wall) is removed to visualize the OW, pyramidal process, and facial nerve (tympanic segment) (Fig. 143.5). The scutum may be removed either with a sharp curette or drill. Care is taken to assess whether the facial nerve has an aberrant course or if the nerve is dehiscent or overhanging too much to allow the procedure to continue. Prior to assessing stapes movement, the lateral ossicular chain is assessed for

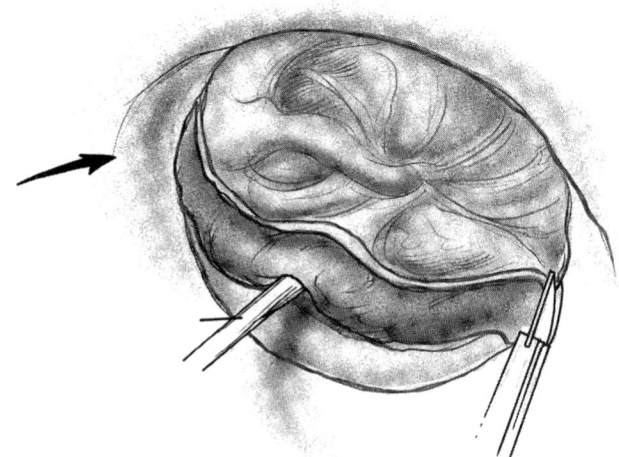

Figure 143.4 Technique for tympanomeatal flap elevation. The skin is elevated to the tympanic sulcus and then the annulus is elevated from the sulcus.

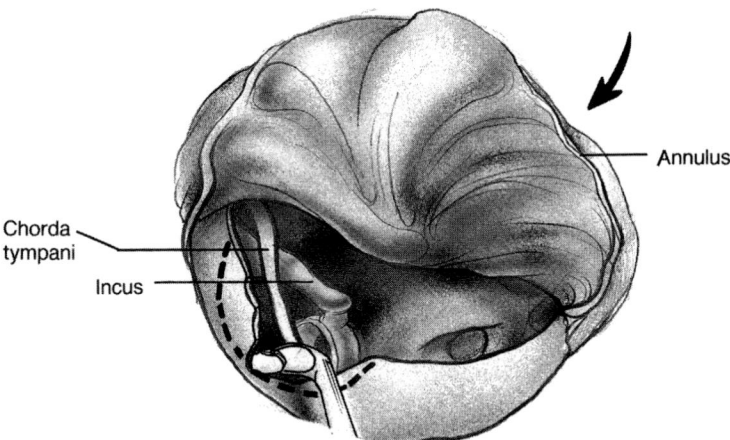

Figure 143.5 The tympanomeatal flap is now elevated. The dotted line indicates the area of bone removal for exposure to the oval window.

normal motion; one needs to rule out other causes of preoperative CHL. The stapes superstructure and footplate are palpated. A RW reflex can also be assessed. The stapedial tendon is cut. The IS joint is then divided (1).

Instead of a stapedectomy, a stapes mobilization can be performed by palpation of the footplate. This is performed typically in a selected group of patients, those in whom a small focus of OS can be seen and in whom improved stapes mobility can be clearly demonstrated. This technique can also be used in cases of tympanosclerosis. Poe (20) described a minimally invasive mobilization using an endoscope and the argon laser to potentially avoid the placement of a prosthesis; he called the procedure a stapedioplasty. However, refixation is common (1).

Typically, however, a stapedectomy is done. The stapes superstructure can be down-fractured toward the promontory. Some surgeons prefer to create a control hole in the footplate prior to manipulating the stapes itself. Whether one should perform a total stapedectomy, partial stapedectomy, or stapedotomy depends on the surgeon. Anterior

crurotomy with partial stapedectomy, as described by Hough in 1960, requires removal of only the anterior footplate and crus (15). This procedure is helpful in the patient with isolated anterior fixation at the fissula ante fenestram. The footplate is fractured in its midportion, and only the anterior half is removed. A connective tissue graft is then placed over the exposed area. The IS joint is not disturbed. The stapedial tendon is not divided, which makes this technique of potential benefit to patients working in a noisy environment.

Because in most patients more extensive stapedial fixation is found, a stapedectomy/stapedotomy is needed. Both require dividing the stapedial tendon with a laser or sharp instrument (e.g., sickle knife or otologic scissors) and placing a control hole in the footplate before separation of the IS joint (Fig. 143.6). The superstructure of the stapes is fractured and extracted (Fig. 143.7). The entire footplate is then removed in a piecemeal fashion using small right-angle hooks of varying sizes (Fig. 143.8). Care is taken to avoid injuring the inner ear now that the vestibule has

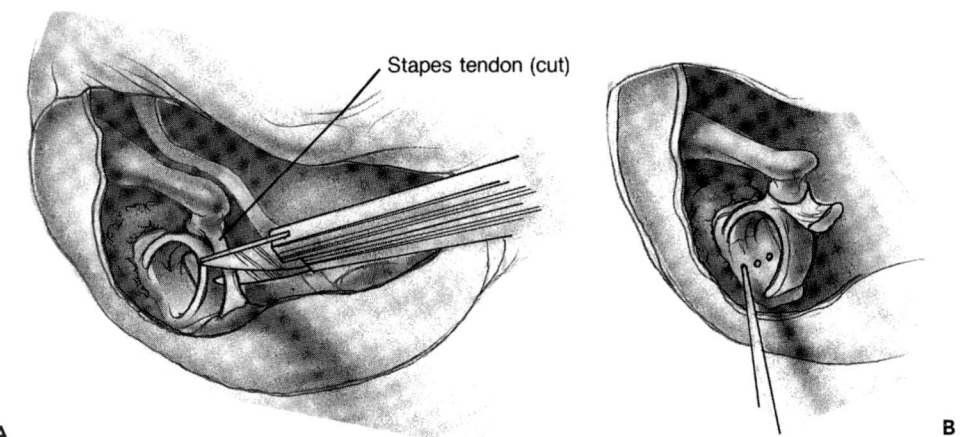

Figure 143.6 **A:** The tympanomeatal flap is now elevated, and bone has been removed. The stapedial tendon is lysed by a pair of microscissors. **B:** Control holes are placed in the stapedial footplate.

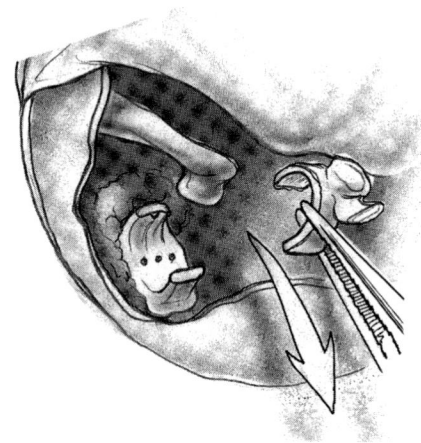

Figure 143.7 The stapedial superstructure is removed after fracturing of the anterior and posterior crus.

been exposed. Perilymph may be suctioned in an area away from the vestibule. However, one must avoid direct suctioning in the vestibule and a resultant dry vestibule, which has a risk of postoperative deafness. The OW is

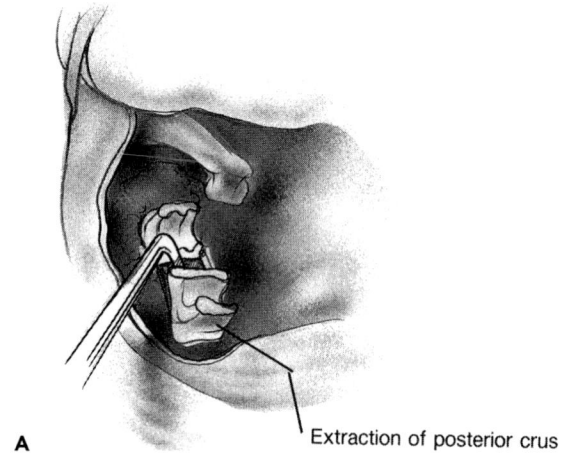

A

Extraction of posterior crus

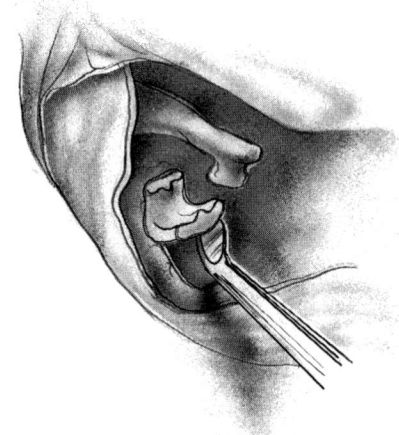

B

Figure 143.8 **A:** The posterior half of the stapedial footplate is removed with a sharp pick. **B:** The anterior half of the stapedial footplate is removed by a joint knife or Hough hoe.

sealed with a graft, and the prosthesis is placed (Fig. 143.9). The most common tissue types used are dorsal hand vein graft, tragal perichondrium, and fascia. Schmerber et al. (16) recently reported that use of the vein graft (as opposed to perichondrium) showed better postoperative air-bone gap closure and a lower incidence of postoperative SNHL.

Some cases of OS have formation of exuberant sclerotic bone that fills and obliterates the OW. Obliterative OS is encountered less commonly now than previously. When present in one ear, obliterative OS is present in the contralateral ear in 50% of cases. Obliterative OS requires thinning of the thickened footplate before creation of a fenestration and prosthesis placement. Thinning is usually accomplished with a small electrical or hand drill, which can also be used to perform the fenestration. The fenestra is usually 0.8 to 1.0 mm in diameter. A prosthesis is then placed through the fenestra into the vestibule. The vestibule is sealed by placing soft tissue around the prosthesis. However, some surgeons use just a blood seal with the stapedotomy approach. Ayache et al. (17) demonstrated a 62% success rate (with closure of the air-bone gap to 10 dB or less) in the drill-out procedure.

As experience grew with the drill-out procedure for obliterative OS, some otologists began using the stapedotomy technique in all their patients with OS. The surgical technique involves creating a fenestra in the midportion of the stapes using a drill, picks, or laser. Perkins was the first to use the laser in the treatment of OS (1980) (18). Since his original description, several types of lasers have been used: argon, potassium-titanyl-phosphate (KTP), erbium-YAG, and carbon dioxide. Each laser has its advantages and disadvantages. Those who use a laser believe it is less traumatic to the footplate and vestibule, perhaps decreasing the risk of postoperative SNHL. Typically, however, no difference has been shown between different types of lasers in terms of safety and efficacy or between lasers and the use of a drill or microinstruments. Buchman et al. (19) confirmed this in a relatively recent study; they performed a retrospective review of patients undergoing argon laser or carbon dioxide laser stapedotomy (approximately 60 patients in each group). No difference was seen in the incidence

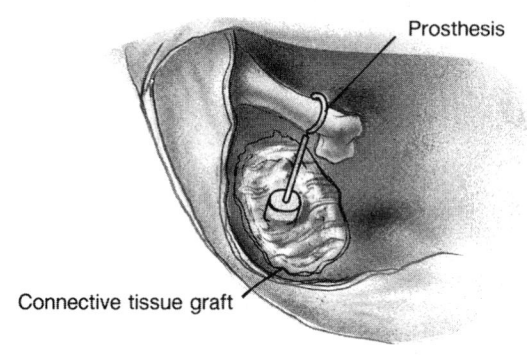

Prosthesis

Connective tissue graft

Figure 143.9 Prosthesis in place.

of postoperative complications, hearing improvement, or speech discrimination. The surgeon's operative experience and skill are considered the most important factors in determining the success and incidence of complications.

After a stapedotomy or stapedectomy is performed, a piston prosthesis is then positioned. Longstanding results of the stapedotomy procedure have been comparable to a total stapedectomy. Some reports suggest a decrease in postoperative cochlear deafness and improvement in the air-bone gap closure above 2000 Hz with stapedotomy. Stapedotomy and partial stapedectomy may show better postoperative hearing at higher frequencies (4000 Hz) than total stapedectomy; however, total stapedectomy may show better gains at lower frequencies (250 Hz and 500 Hz) (1).

Numerous stapes prostheses have been developed since John Shea popularized the stapedectomy procedure. Early prostheses with a sharp or beveled end were found to cause a prohibitive number of postoperative fistulae. The designs that have proved most effective include a connective tissue OW graft and piston prosthesis. Tissue can be obtained from tragal perichondrium, dorsal hand vein graft, or temporalis fascia. The graft is combined with a variety of prosthetic designs, such as a wire Teflon piston or a Robinson-type bucket-handle prosthesis, which has a wire loop that is placed over the lenticular process of the incus. If the stapedotomy procedure is performed, the prosthesis is positioned, and connective tissue is placed around the prosthesis base to seal the vestibule (Fig. 143.9). A recent addition to the variety of available stapes prosthesis is a heat-activated self-crimping prosthesis (the SMart prosthesis: Gyrus, London, UK).

After completion of the desired procedure, the TM flap is returned to its normal anatomic position. The EAC may be dressed in a variety of ways (e.g., packed with gelatin sponge, antibiotic ointment), depending on the surgeon's preference. The use of perioperative antibiotics is common, despite the lack of statistical evidence of their benefits. Perioperative steroids may be used to reduce the incidence of anesthesia induced nausea and vomiting.

In the immediate postoperative period, the patient is asked to avoid lifting and straining for about 1 month. Nose blowing should be discouraged. The patient should also cough or sneeze with the mouth open, to reduce the risk of increased middle ear pressure and displacement of the TM. The patient is kept on dry ear precautions until the healing of the TM is completed. In some patients, immediate hearing improvement is noted. Other patients report a slower hearing improvement with associated vestibular symptoms, probably due to serous labyrinthitis. Balance disturbances usually resolve within 1 to 2 days but occasionally linger for a few weeks. A postoperative audiogram is obtained 3 months after surgery, allowing enough time for middle ear fluid and blood to resorb. Postoperative hearing results reveal closure of the air-bone gap to within 10 dB of the preoperative bone-conduction level in 90% of patients.

About 10% of patients experience either worsening hearing or no improvement. About 2% of patients suffer persistent and profound SNHL. Recent evidence has suggested a progressive high-frequency SNHL in some post-stapedectomy patients. It is unclear whether this is due to cochlear OS or long-term postsurgical effects.

The otolaryngologist should be aware of certain complicating factors associated with stapes surgery. Anatomic variations of the middle ear sometimes alter the surgical procedure. Occasionally, a high or dehiscent jugular bulb is encountered. If it is injured, the middle ear must be packed to tamponade the bleeding before continuing with surgery. Continued or persistent bleeding may require termination of the procedure. One must be sure that the bleeding is due to a jugular bulb and not an aberrant internal carotid artery. A persistent stapedial artery that courses in the obturator foramen of the stapes can be a complicating factor due to its bleeding potential. This artery is the embryologic remnant of the second branchial arch. To gain access to the footplate, the vessel must be divided or the procedure will need to be aborted. Blood that enters the vestibule increases the risk of postoperative SNHL (1).

Careful and complete inspection of the middle ear should be performed at each exploratory tympanotomy. Other causes of CHL, such as malleus head fixation, can be associated with OS. Malleus head fixation can be congenital or caused by immobility of the ossicular chain, allowing for ankylosis to the attic wall. Mobilization of the malleus can be achieved by applying a malleus nipper to the neck of the malleus but only after the IS joint has been severed. Unfortunately, mobilization is often followed by refixation. In addition, this will not address lateral chain fixation; the malleus and incus may still need to be freed.

A dehiscent and abnormally low facial nerve can at times obscure the OW. If footplate removal and prosthesis placement can be achieved safely, surgery should continue. If the surgeon believes the nerve is in jeopardy, the procedure should be aborted.

A profuse perilymph gusher (i.e., CSF leak) can be encountered. This finding is believed to be due to a patent cochlear aqueduct and is seen more frequently on the left than the right side. It is more common in congenital footplate fixation. Complete stapes footplate removal in the presence of a gusher increases the risk of postoperative cochlear deafness. The fenestration (control hole) placed before footplate removal should allow for early identification of this problem. Stapedotomy, or careful and controlled footplate removal with a connective tissue seal, can then be performed. At times, a lumbar drain may be needed to decompress the subarachnoid space to allow for adherence of the graft to the OW (1).

Fracture of the incus long process can occur during stapedectomy. It may follow separation of the IS joint, placement of the prosthesis, or curettage of the scutum. Usually, the prosthesis can be placed on the remaining incus, but a malleus to OW prosthesis may be needed.

Some recommend staging the procedure and coming back at a later time to allow the incus to heal and be used in the future, because a malleus to OW prosthesis is more difficult to place and typically has poorer postoperative results (1).

It is difficult to remove a nonfixed (floating) stapedial footplate after the crural arches have been fractured. Attempts to manipulate the footplate may push it downward into the vestibule. This is a case in which the laser may be used to atraumatically remove or ablate the footplate. In addition, one of the purposes of the control hole made before fracturing the crura is to provide access to the footplate, if it accidentally becomes mobilized. Small right angle hooks or needles can be placed through the hole to lift the footplate out of the vestibule. An alternative strategy for managing a floating footplate is to drill a shallow groove in the inferior part of the OW niche. A small hook can then be passed beside the footplate to remove it. If all or part of the footplate is significantly depressed into the vestibule, it is best left there. Attempts to remove it can result in significant SNHL. A connective tissue graft and prosthesis can be placed lateral to the depressed footplate. In this setting, postoperative disequilibrium can be expected but is usually self-limiting (1).

The use of a local anesthetic such as lidocaine can cause intraoperative or postoperative vertigo. Lateral canal stimulation from irrigation fluids can cause vertigo, as can chemical irritation of the labyrinth from the local anesthetic. Palpation of the footplate can directly cause vertigo from mechanical stimulation of the underlying vestibule. An overly long prosthesis can stimulate the saccule (1).

TM tears should be avoided. If a small tear occurs, it can be repaired with a leftover piece of the OW grafting material. Persistent postoperative perforations should be repaired within 4 to 6 weeks after surgery to prevent any problems with transcanal contamination of the middle ear and a subsequent otitis media and SNHL (1).

The most common cause for failure of stapedectomy has been prosthesis displacement, with or without incus erosion. Other causes of failure are footplate refixation, perilymph fistula, otosclerotic regrowth, and lateralization of the OW membrane. Patients need to be informed that revision surgery is usually not as successful as primary surgery. The possibility of postoperative cochlear deafness is also more common with revision surgery. Patients who seem to achieve better results in revision procedures are those who experienced an initial improvement in hearing followed by a gradual worsening of the air-bone gap over a period of several months or a year (1) (Table 143.3).

COMPLICATIONS/PITFALLS

Complications after stapes surgery can occur immediately or months to years later. Vertigo or dizziness immediately after surgery is usually due to loss of perilymph, surgical trauma, or serous labyrinthitis. This symptom generally subsides within a few days. If dizziness does not improve within the first postoperative week, the use of corticos-

TABLE 143.3

CLINICAL INDICATORS FOR STAPEDECTOMY

Strategy
Indicators (one of the following)
    Conductive hearing loss without other source of conductive abnormality (e.g., perforated TM, serous otitis media)
Laboratory tests (required)
    Audiogram with air-bone gap, speech reception threshold, and discrimination scores
Other tests (as indicated)
    Impedance audiometry
Type of anesthesia (as indicated)
Location of service (as indicated)

Process
Criteria for discharge
    Recovery from anesthesia
    Absence of significant vertigo
    Ability to ambulate without assistance
    Absence of signs of infection
    Absence of significant ear drainage

Outcome
Results
Follow-up
    Improvement in hearing
    Healing of tympanic membrane

TM, tympanic membrane.
The American Academy of Otolaryngology-Head and Neck Surgery and the American Society for Head and Neck Surgery have published clinical indicators for surgical procedures. These clinical indicators are educational statements that have been drafted to assist surgeons in their practice and to promote discussion. These indicators are not practice guidelines nor do they represent standards of practice with which individuals must conform.

teroids may be of some benefit. Persistent vertigo may be due to a depressed footplate fragment, long prosthesis, OW fistula, or a reparative granuloma. Benign paroxysmal positional vertigo can also be seen during the postoperative course due to surgical injury to the utricle. This is usually self-limiting and resolves within several months (1).

Acute otitis media is a rare postoperative complication; if it does occur, it poses a serious threat to hearing in the operated ear. The newly created OW partition allows a middle ear infection to quickly involve the labyrinth (suppurative labyrinthitis) and potentially meningitis. Historically, a beveled prosthesis on a gelatin sponge appeared to increase the risk of suppurative labyrinthitis. Intensive systemic antibiotic therapy for otitis media is begun immediately; if diagnosed early, the condition may improve without significant sequelae (1).

A reparative granuloma occurs after approximately 1% of stapedectomies. It usually becomes manifest within 7 to 15 days after surgery, but it can occur as late as 6 weeks postoperatively. The hallmark of reparative granuloma is progressive SNHL after earlier postoperative hearing improvement. The granuloma can also be associated with vertigo, aural fullness, or tinnitus. The TM appears thickened, and the posterior aspect is erythematous. The audiogram reveals a MHL that often is most severe in the high frequencies. The discrimination score is usually significantly lower than expected from the degree of hearing loss. If this complication is suspected, antibiotics and corticosteroids can be given. If the symptoms or hearing loss continue, surgical exploration is indicated. A CT scan can be helpful in the diagnosis of this process and to assess the status of the prosthesis/vestibule. Findings at surgery include a significant amount of granulation tissue around the OW. Histologically, evidence of acute and chronic inflammation is found. Treatment involves removal of the OW seal and prosthesis with replacement using a different material. In the past, this reaction was felt to be due to the use of gelatin sponge as the OW sealant or the presence of powder on operating gloves. The overall outcome of this potentially devastating process is related to early diagnosis and treatment (1).

Perilymph fistulae may occur in the early postoperative period or may be seen many years later. The initial complaints usually include fluctuating or progressive hearing loss associated with tinnitus or vertigo. A history of sudden barometric pressure change or trauma may also be reported but is not necessarily diagnostic. Fistula testing by pneumatic otoscopy may be helpful. Audiometric testing usually reveals the expected SNHL, although fistulae rarely occur without hearing loss. The most important factor in diagnosis is a high clinical index of suspicion. If a fistula is thought to be present, conservative measures may be appropriate (particularly in the immediate postoperative period, because surgical exploration is difficult except for the most experienced otologic surgeon). These conservative measures can include the use of acetazolamide and bed rest for 5 days. If symptoms continue, exploratory surgery with grafting of the OW is indicated. Findings at surgery may include a displaced prosthesis with or without an obvious fistula. Postoperative expectations include stabilization of the SNHL and resolution of the dizziness (1).

Persistent or progressive CHL can follow stapedectomy. Loosening or displacement of the prosthesis, resorption of the incus long process, adhesions around the prosthesis, and further OS lesions can produce postoperative CHL. Significant hearing loss may warrant surgical exploration. It must be remembered that removal of the prosthesis is associated with a higher incidence of SNHL and a poorer rate of closure of the air-bone gap (1).

HIGHLIGHTS

- Otosclerosis is a primary disease of the otic capsule that causes progressive conductive hearing loss, sensorineural hearing loss, or mixed hearing loss.
- The disease is present histologically in 8% to 10% of the Caucasian population, but only 12% of patients with histologic changes actually present with clinical symptoms.
- Histologically, the disease begins by bone resorption around vascular channels and later matures as dense, sclerotic bone.

- Patients suffering from otosclerosis typically present with a slowly progressive hearing loss over a period of years.
- The physical appearance of the tympanic membrane is typically normal.
- The audiogram remains the key to diagnosis, revealing a conductive hearing loss or mixed hearing loss in most cases.
- Surgical therapy remains the mainstay of treatment for conductive hearing loss from otosclerosis; however, this is an elective procedure. Patients must be given the alternative of amplification. Medical treatment can be given to all patients.
- Postoperative hearing results reveal closure of the air-bone group to within 10 dB of the preoperative bone-conduction level in 90% of patients.
- The possibility of postoperative cochlear deafness is much higher with revision surgery when compared with primary stapedectomies.

REFERENCES

1. Roland PS, Meyerhoff WL. Otosclerosis. In: Bailey BJ, ed. Otolaryngology—head and neck surgery, 3rd ed. Philadelphia: Lippincott Williams & Wilkins, 2001:1829–1841.
2. Lopez-Gonzalez MA, Delgado F. Oral vaccine in otosclerosis. *Med Hypotheses* 2000;54:216–220.
3. Shambaugh G. Clinical diagnosis of cochlear (labyrinthine) otosclerosis. *Laryngoscope* 1965;75:1558–1562.
4. Mikulec AA, McKenna MJ, Ramsey MJ, et al. Superior semicircular canal dehiscence presenting as conductive hearing loss without vertigo. *Otol Neurotol* 2004;25:121–129.
5. Morrison A, Bundey S. The inheritance of otosclerosis. *J Laryngol Otol* 1970;84:921–932.
6. Clayton AE, Mikulec AA, Mikulec KH, et al. Association between osteoporosis and otosclerosis in women. *J Laryngol Otol* 2004;118:617–621.
7. De la Cruz A, Angeli S, Slattery W. Stapedectomy in children. *Otolaryngol Head Neck Surg* 1999;120:487–492.
8. McLarnon CM, Davison T, Johnson IJ. Bone-anchored hearing aid: comparison of benefit by patient subgroups. *Laryngoscope* 2004;114:942–944.
9. Rotteveel LJ, Proops DW, Ramsden RT, et al. Cochlear implantation in 53 patients with otosclerosis. *Otol Neurotol* 2004;25:943–952.
10. Rosen S. Mobilization of the stapes to restore hearing in otosclerosis. *N Y J Med* 1953;53:2650–2653.
11. Shea JJ. Fenestration of the oval window. *Ann Otol Rhinol Laryngol* 1958;67:932–951.
12. Meyer TA, Lambert PR. Primary and revision stapedectomy in elderly patients. *Curr Opin Otolaryngol Head Neck Surg* 2004;12:387–392.
13. Sparano A, Leonetti JP, Marzo S, et al. Effects of stapedectomy on tinnitus in patients with otosclerosis. *Int Tinnitus J* 2004;10(1):73–77.
14. Vrabec JT, Coker NJ. Stapes surgery in the United States. *Otol Neurotol* 2004;25:465–469.
15. Hough JV. Partial stapedectomy. *Ann Otol Rhinol Laryngol* 1960;69:571–596.
16. Schmerber S, Cuisnier O, Charachan R, et al. Vein versus tragal perichondrium in stapedotomy. *Otol Neurotol* 2004;25:694–698.
17. Ayache D, Sleiman J, Plovin-Gaudon I, et. al. Obliterative otosclerosis. *J Laryngol Otol* 1999; 113:512–514.
18. Perkins RC. Laser stapedotomy for otosclerosis. *Laryngoscope* 1980;90:228–240.
19. Buchman CA, Fucci MJ, Robertson JB Jr, et al. Comparison of argon and CO_2 laser stapedotomy in primary otosclerosis surgery. *Am J Otolaryngol* 2000;21: 227–230.
20. Poe DS. Laser-assisted endoscopic stapedectomy: a prospective study. *Laryngoscope* 2000;110[5 Pt 2 Suppl 95]:1–37.

Acute Paralysis of the Facial Nerve

144

Jeffrey T. Vrabec   Newton J. Coker

Acute facial palsy is a common diagnostic problem encountered by the otolaryngologist, but its presentation often provokes consternation on the physician's part. This reaction stems from our limited knowledge of facial nerve pathology, from the shortcomings of currently popular electrophysiologic tests in defining nerve injury, and from the controversy surrounding the management of facial palsy. This chapter presents contemporary opinions on management of acute facial palsy.

ANATOMY AND PHYSIOLOGY OF THE FACIAL NERVE

The seventh cranial nerve is a complex motor/sensory nerve consisting of special visceral afferent, general visceral efferent, and special visceral efferent fibers (Fig. 144.1) (1). The special visceral afferent fibers convey the sense of taste from the sensory receptors on the anterior two thirds of the tongue and project via the lingual and chorda tympani nerves to the geniculate ganglion and, hence, via the nervus intermedius to the tractus solitarius.

The general visceral afferent fibers constitute a parasympathetic system with three subsets of postsynaptic fibers. The preganglionic fibers arise in the superior salivatory nucleus. One subset of fibers exits the facial hiatus within the greater superficial petrosal nerve to synapse at the sphenopalatine ganglion. Postsynaptic fibers then innervate the lacrimal and palatine glands. Another subset of preganglionic fibers within the lesser petrosal nerve synapses at the otic ganglion; the postsynaptic fibers provide secretory supply, in part, to the parotid gland. The third subset of this parasympathetic system exits the temporal bone along the chorda tympani nerve and passes along the lingual nerve to synapse at the submandibular ganglion. The postsynaptic fibers then provide the secretory supply to the submandibular and sublingual glands.

The special visceral efferent fibers arise within the facial motor nucleus and pass through the temporal bone, except for the fibers to the stapedius muscle, to exit the stylomastoid foramen and innervate the auricular, posterior belly of the digastric, stylohyoid, and platysma muscles and the superficial facial musculature.

Evidence that the sensory afferent fibers provide sensation from the external auditory canal and proprioception from the face is contradictory. These fibers are thought to account for the otalgia experienced in Bell palsy and the vesicular eruption in herpes zoster infection.

The intracranial segment of the facial nerve and the nervus intermedius exit the brainstem in a recess adjacent to the pons, cross the cerebellopontine angle medial to the vestibuloacoustic nerve, and enter the internal auditory canal. The meatal segment of the facial nerve and the intermedius nerve occupy the anterior-superior quadrant within the canal and enter the fallopian canal at the meatal foramen superior to the crista transversa and anterior to the crista verticalis (Bill's bar). The labyrinthine segment of the nerve courses 2 to 4 mm within the narrowest part of the fallopian canal to the geniculate ganglion, where the nerve makes an acute turn of 40 to 80 degrees (external or first genu) to enter the middle ear. Coursing posteriorly and slightly inferiorly above the cochleariform process and the oval window, the tympanic segment (11 mm) curves into the second (pyramidal) turn inferior to the horizontal semicircular canal. This turn has a more obtuse angle of 110 to 120 degrees. The mastoid segment then descends 13 mm vertically to the stylomastoid foramen. There are several branches of the nerve in its intratemporal course. At the

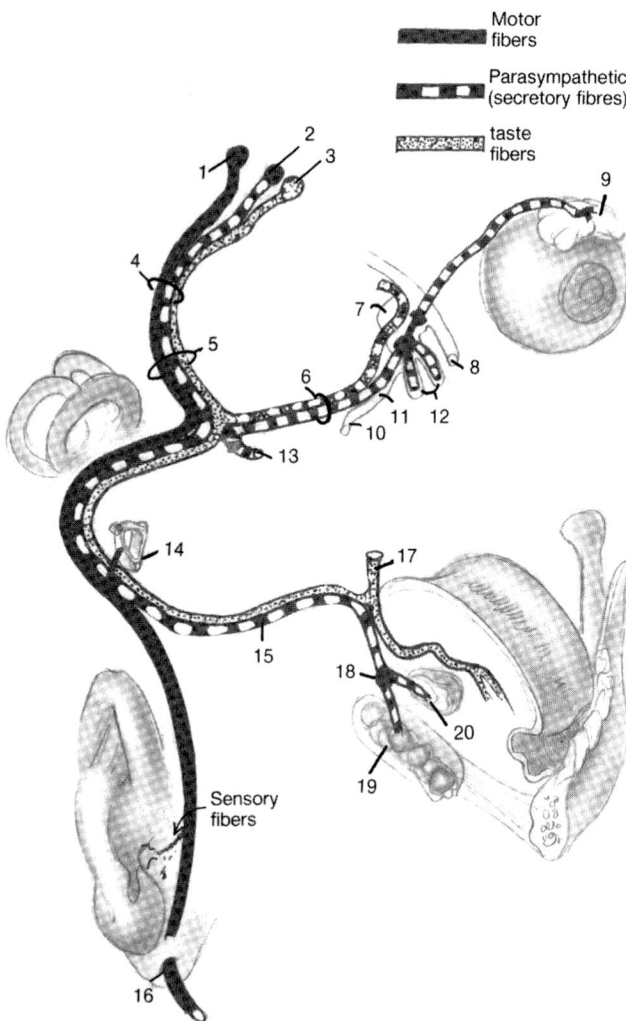

Motor fibers

Parasympathetic (secretory fibres)

taste fibers

Sensory fibers

Figure 144.1 Efferent and afferent tracts of cranial nerve VII. The projection of the sensory fibers from the external auditory canal is undetermined. *1*, Nucleus of facial nerve; *2*, superior salivary nucleus; *3*, solitary tract; *4*, porus acusticus internus; *5*, meatal foramen; *6*, greater petrosal nerve; *7*, sphenopalatine ganglion; *8*, maxillary nerve; *9*, lacrimal gland; *10*, deep petrosal nerve; *11*, vidian nerve; *12*, innervation of glands of nose and palate; *13*, anastomosis with minor petrosal nerve; *14*, stapedial nerve; *15*, chorda tympani; *16*, stylomastoid foramen; *17*, lingual nerve; *18*, submandibular ganglion; *19*, submandibular gland; *20*, sublingual gland. (Modified from Miehlke A. *Surgery of the facial nerve*, 2nd ed. Baltimore: Urban & Schwarzenburg, 1973;19, with permission.)

geniculate ganglion, the greater superficial petrosal nerve courses anterior and medially. The branch to the stapedius muscle arises from the proximal mastoid segment, whereas the chorda tympani exits the distal mastoid segment. The nerve to the digastric is the first branch distal to the stylomastoid foramen. The special visceral efferent fibers constituting the extracranial segment enter the posterior parotid gland and undergo secondary and tertiary branching. These fibers ultimately innervate the five regions of mimetic musculature: temporal, zygomatic, buccal, mandibular, and cervical. The peripheral branches of the nerve are the most variable in location.

SURGICAL ANATOMY

Knowledge of the intratemporal anatomy of the facial nerve and the associated landmarks is critical to safe otologic surgery. The surgical approach to different segments of the nerve varies if middle and inner ear structures are to be preserved. When hearing is good, the meatal and labyrinthine segments of the nerve are approached via the middle cranial fossa (Fig. 144.2). This allows access to the internal auditory canal and/or geniculate ganglion. Important landmarks include the arcuate eminence, meatal plane, facial hiatus, and greater superficial petrosal nerve. The location of the internal canal and meatal segment is approximated by bisection of the angle formed between the plane of the superior semicircular canal (arcuate eminence) and the greater superficial petrosal nerve. The nerve occupies the anterior quadrant of the internal auditory canal.

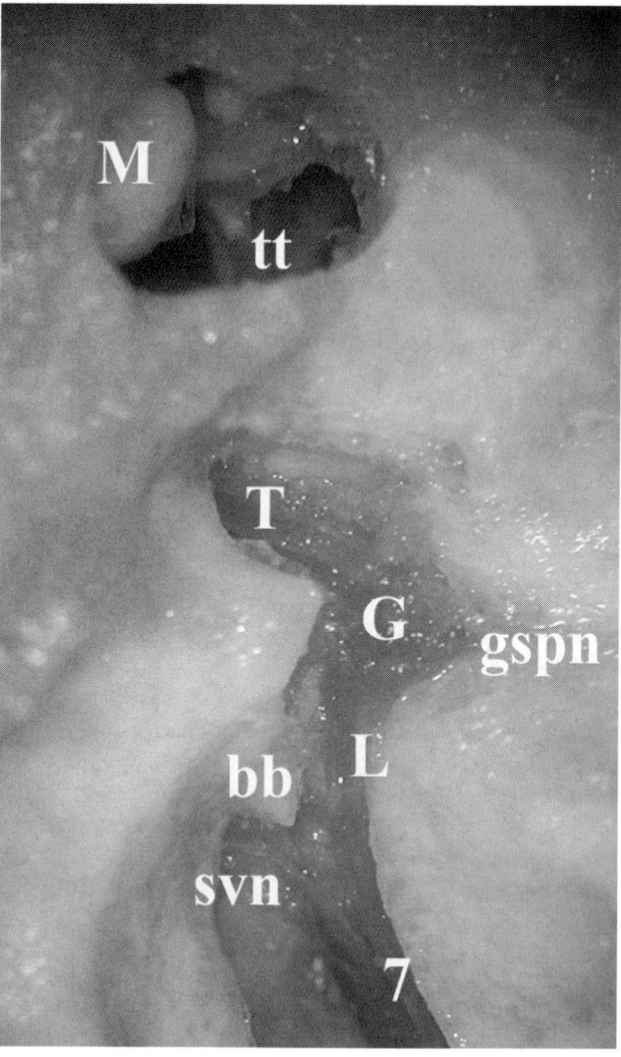

Figure 144.2 Surgical anatomy of the facial nerve in the middle cranial fossa. *7*, Facial nerve in the internal auditory canal; *L*, labyrinthine segment; *G*, geniculate ganglion; *T*, tympanic segment; *M*, malleus; *tt*, tensor tympani; *bb*, Bill's bar; *svn*, superior vestibular nerve.

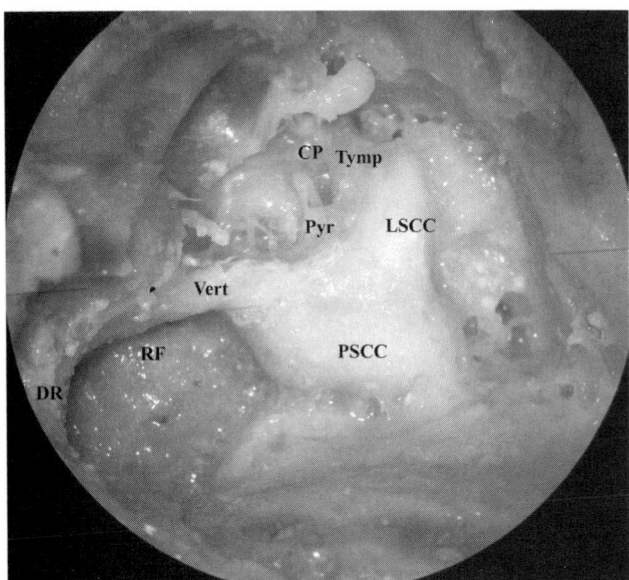

Figure 144.3 Surgical landmarks to the facial nerve in the middle ear and mastoid. *LSCC*, lateral semicircular canal; *PSCC*, posterior semicircular canal; *DR*, digastric ridge; *RF*, retrofacial air cells; *Vert*, vertical segment proximal to stylomastoid foramen; *Tymp*, tympanic segment; *CP*, cochleariform process; *Pyr*, pyramidal eminence.

Important landmarks for identification of the tympanic segment in the middle ear are the cochleariform process and the oval window. The nerve is located superior to these structures and inferior to the horizontal semicircular canal. The upper mastoid segment lies posterior and medial to the chorda tympani and medial to the facial recess air cell tract. The stapedius muscle and posterior semicircular canal are medial to the facial nerve. The lower mastoid segment is at the same level as the digastric ridge (Fig. 144.3), lateral to the retrofacial air cell tract. The mastoid segment of the nerve can be identified by removing the bone from the posterior aspect of the external auditory canal, thereby exposing the nerve on its lateral aspect. The surgeon should expect the nerve along a line drawn between the horizontal semicircular canal and digastric ridge.

When hearing preservation is not an issue, the entire intratemporal course of the nerve can be exposed via the translabyrinthine approach. The mastoid segment is defined as discussed previously. Removal of the labyrinth allows skeletonization of the tympanic segment along its superior aspect. The labyrinthine segment is located just anterior and superior to the ampulla of the superior canal. The internal auditory canal is identified medial to the vestibule. In the lateral end of canal, the facial nerve is separated from the superior vestibular nerve by the vertical crest (Bill's bar).

Anomalies of the Facial Nerve

Anomalies of the facial nerve are rare, but their existence makes even the most experienced otologic surgeon wary. The most common "anomaly" is a dehiscence in the facial canal, which exposes the nerve to injury during temporal bone surgery. The most common location is the tympanic segment over the oval window, followed by the geniculate ganglion and the mastoid segment adjacent to the retrofacial air cells (2). The intratemporal course of the nerve is usually constant, but variations do occur. Deviations in the labyrinthine segment are exceedingly uncommon; usually the finding in this area is a difference in the angulation of the nerve between the meatal foramen and the geniculate ganglion, which relates to the depth of the internal auditory canal below the floor of the middle fossa. In the tympanic segment, the nerve may prolapse against the arch of the stapes, bifurcate around the stapes, or course below the oval window. Below the horizontal semicircular canal, the nerve may curve more acutely, making the prominent turn more susceptible to injury during an antrotomy. In the mastoid segment, bifurcations and trifurcations are exceedingly rare, but when duplication exists, the nerves occupy separate bony canals and exit individual foramina. Anomalies of the fallopian canal are suspect in congenital atresia of the middle ear and anomalies of the otic capsule. Thin-section high-resolution computed tomography (CT) of the facial canal is recommended to provide as much preoperative information as possible about the course of the facial nerve.

Topographic Organization of the Facial Nerve

Spatial orientation of the intracranial or intratemporal efferent and afferent fibers is unlikely, based on animal studies by Thomander et al. (3) and Gacek and Radpour (4). For years, clinical investigators proposed sites of lesion identification within the temporal bone according to the degree of muscle weakness in different regions of the face or the dysfunction of the nonmotor fibers. The nerve was presumed to have spatial orientation of the motor axons equivalent to the organization in the facial motor nucleus and cortex. This lack of intratemporal organization makes interfascicular repair of the nerve proximal to the stylomastoid foramen impractical. Synkinesis is inevitable with any reanastomosis or nerve grafting procedure.

Arterial Supply to the Facial Nerve

Both the carotid and vertebrobasilar arterial systems vascularize the intratemporal facial nerve (5). The labyrinthine artery, a branch of the anterior inferior cerebellar artery, provides the blood supply to the nerve within the internal auditory canal. The petrosal artery, a branch of the middle meningeal, supplies the nerve in the perigeniculate region and anastomoses with the stylomastoid artery, which feeds the mastoid and tympanic segments. The intratemporal facial nerve has a rich extrinsic anastomotic network to prevent ischemia, except in the labyrinthine segment at the junction between the carotid and vertebrobasilar systems.

EVALUATION

History

A careful history narrows the scope of the differential diagnosis and reduces the number of laboratory studies necessary to establish the cause. First, the onset of the paralysis is defined as sudden, delayed or gradual. Sudden refers to acute deterioration of facial function over a few days, either with or without an antecedent event. Delayed refers to acute deterioration in close temporal relationship with an antecedent event, though facial function is normal immediately following the event. Gradual refers to progressive loss over a period of weeks or longer. These definitions assume normal function prior to onset. When rapid deterioration occurs in a nerve exhibiting abnormal function, the onset is considered gradual or progressive unless there has been a lengthy period of stable facial function. A recovery of function followed by a long period of stable function is required to designate the palsy as recurrent.

Next, the degree of paralysis is designated as complete or incomplete. This is often of great prognostic importance. Incomplete paralysis or paresis is usually associated with good prognosis for recovery, unless a neoplasm is diagnosed. Complete paralysis typically caries a guarded prognosis for return of normal facial movement, especially when accompanied by electrical evidence of complete degeneration.

Associated symptoms provide additional diagnostic clues. Numbness in the middle and lower face, otalgia, hyperacusis, diminished tearing, and an alteration in taste are common in Bell's palsy and Ramsay Hunt syndrome. Intense ear pain and a vesicular eruption are the hallmarks of herpes zoster oticus. Sensorineural hearing loss and vertigo are symptoms of advanced disease involving the labyrinth, the internal auditory canal, or brainstem.

Recurrent facial palsy also may indicate a tumor, although some persistent dysfunction is likely in between episodes of worsening function. More common causes of recurrent palsy include Bell's palsy and Melkersson-Rosenthal syndrome. About 7% of patients with Bell's palsy develop recurrent palsy, with half of recurrences on the ipsilateral side (6). Melkersson-Rosenthal syndrome is often familial, and the first episode of facial palsy usually occurs before 20 years (7). Associated findings include facial edema, particularly of the upper lip; fissured tongue; and migraine headaches.

Any thorough history encompasses other medical conditions that may be incriminated in the differential diagnosis of the palsy: cancer; sarcoidosis; autoimmune disorders; and previous surgeries in the posterior fossa, temporal bone, or parotid.

Physical Examination

The physical examination includes a complete head and neck evaluation with microscopic examination of the ear, a thorough assessment of the upper aerodigestive tract, and

TABLE 144.1
ASSESSMENT OF FACIAL PALSY

History
  Onset
  Duration
  Rate of progression
  Recurrent or familial
  Associated symptoms
  Major medical illness or previous surgery
Physical examination
  Complete head and neck evaluation
  Microscopic otoscopy
  Upper aerodigestive tract examination
  Cranial nerve assessment (III–XII)
  Palpation of parotid gland and neck
  Neurologic evaluation
  Cerebellar signs
  Motor
  Facial palsy
  Complete vs. incomplete (paresis)
  Segmental vs. uniform involvement
  Unilateral vs. bilateral
  Schirmer test
Laboratory studies
  Pure-tone and speech audiometry
  Electrophysiologic tests
  Nerve excitability test (NET)
  Maximal stimulation test (MST)
  Electroneurography (ENoG)
  Electromyography (EMG)
  Radiographic studies
  Computed tomography
  Magnetic resonance imaging
Other considerations
  Complete blood cell count and differential with sedimentation rate
  Serum antibody tests
  Serum antinuclear antibody (ANA) and rheumatoid factor (RF)
  Chest x-ray radiograph
  Lumbar puncture with cerebrospinal fluid assay

a cranial nerve assessment (III through XII) (Table 144.1). Obvious physical findings confirm many infectious, neoplastic, and traumatic diagnoses. Otorrhea, purulent middle ear effusion or obvious cholesteatoma indicate an infectious etiology. Slowly progressive weakness, temporal bone or parotid mass lesion, or segmental weakness (some branches paralyzed while others are spared) suggest a neoplasm. Contusion or laceration over the distribution of the extracranial nerve, Battle's sign (mastoid ecchymosis), or hemotympanum are evidence of trauma. Multiple cranial nerve deficits typically indicate an advanced intracranial or skull base infection, extensive neoplasm involving the temporal bone, or a neurologic disorder, such as Guillain-Barré syndrome.

The examination focuses on the motor function of the facial nerve. One should compare the range of facial movement between the affected and unaffected sides. The subject should attempt a broad range of facial expressions while the examiner watches for movement in each of the

TABLE 144.2
DIFFERENTIAL DIAGNOSIS OF THE COMMON ACUTE FACIAL PALSIES

Infection
  Bell palsy (herpes simplex mononeuritis)
  Herpes zoster oticus (Ramsay Hunt syndrome)
  Otitis media with effusion
  Acute suppurative otitis media
  Coalescent mastoiditis
  Chronic otitis media
  Malignant otitis externa (skull base osteomyelitis)
  Tuberculosis
  Lyme disease[a]
  Acquired immunodeficiency syndrome
  Infectious mononucleosis
Trauma
  Temporal bone fractures[a]
  Birth trauma
  Facial contusions/lacerations
  Penetrating wounds, face and temporal bone
  Iatrogenic injury
Neoplasia
  Cholesteatoma
  Glomus jugulare or tympanicum
  Carcinoma (primary or metastatic)
  Facial neuroma
  Schwannoma of lower cranial nerves
  Meningioma
  Leukemia
  Histiocytosis
  Rhabdomyosarcoma
Congenital
  Compression injury
  Möbius syndrome
  Lower lip paralysis
Idiopathic
  Recurrent facial palsy
  Melkersson-Rosenthal syndrome
Metabolic and systemic
  Sarcoidosis[a]
  Guillain-Barré syndrome[a]
  Autoimmune disorders

[a]May present with bilateral palsy.

major branches of the nerve. The subject is asked to raise the eyebrows, close the eyes as tightly as possible, wrinkle the nose, smile broadly, pucker, or grimace. A common error is to attribute the movement in the upper eyelid due to the levator palpebrae superioris muscle (cranial nerve III) to facial nerve function and to misrepresent the finding as a facial paresis.

The more common causes of acute facial paralysis are outlined in Table 144.2. Over half of the presentations are due to Bell's palsy. Trauma is the second most common etiology, producing about 20% of cases. The palsy is not Bell in the presence of any of the following: signs of tumor, vesicles, multiple cranial nerve involvement, temporal bone infection, trauma, palsy at birth, signs of a central nervous system lesion, and acute infectious mononucle-

osis. Bilateral facial nerve involvement occurs in less than 1% of patients who have facial palsy. Common etiologies include brainstem tumors, intracranial infection, Guillain-Barré syndrome, or Lyme disease (8).

Laboratory Studies

Based on the mixed afferent-efferent function of cranial nerve VII, the once-popular topographic testing (Schirmer test, stapedial reflex assessment, electrogustometry, and salivary flow) for determining the site of the lesion and for prognostication is obsolete. CT and magnetic resonance imaging (MRI) better demonstrate the site of the lesion. Prognosis for return of motor function is best established by serial electrophysiologic testing. The Schirmer test remains useful to quantitate the amount of tearing in the involved eye. Reduced tear secretion suggests the need for aggressive treatment to protect the cornea.

Several studies may be indicated in the evaluation of acute facial paralysis (Table 144.1), depending on the findings in the history and physical examination. Because of numerous problems arising within the temporal bone and the proximity of the seventh and eighth cranial nerves in the posterior fossa, pure tone and speech audiometry is recommended in all cases of facial palsy.

When examination shows the paralysis to be complete, electrophysiologic studies are done to establish the end point of degeneration and prognosis for recovery. Imaging is essential in any case when the etiology is uncertain or the paralysis is recurrent or atypical. High-resolution CT of the temporal bone is the study of choice for assessment of the fallopian canal. Any potential cause of facial paralysis associated with bone destruction (mastoiditis, cholesteatoma, tumors, temporal bone trauma) is seen best on CT. MRI is most useful when infectious or neoplastic involvement of the nerve (idiopathic facial palsy, herpes zoster oticus, facial schwannoma) is suspected. When the diagnosis is uncertain, other laboratory studies can be considered to exclude blood dyscrasias, autoimmune disorders, Lyme disease, sarcoidosis, and central nervous system diseases.

PATHOPHYSIOLOGY OF NERVE INJURY

One of the greatest shortcomings in our understanding of neural degeneration and regeneration is the lack of knowledge of events occurring at the molecular level after insult. Current electrophysiologic tests cannot differentiate the levels of injury; hence, prognostication is limited, which explains why a completely degenerated nerve can have either totally normal recovery or none at all.

Classically, nerve injury is described in terms of neurapraxia, axonotmesis, or neurotmesis. Neurapraxia results when a lesion compresses the flow of axoplasm from the somata to the distal axons. The nerve is viable and recovers normal function when the blockade is removed. On testing a neurapraxic nerve, the nerve excitability test (NET), the maximal stimulation test (MST), and electroneurography (ENoG) or evoked electromyography demonstrate normal findings, and electromyography (EMG) fails to show voluntary motor action potentials, because these cannot be conducted across the blockade.

Axonotmesis describes a state of Wallerian degeneration distal to the lesion characterized by the preservation of endoneural sheaths of the motor axons. Electrically, if the axonotmesis is complete and pure, the NET, MST, and ENoG will indicate rapid and complete degeneration. The EMG will not demonstrate voluntary motor units, and after 10 to 14 days, myogenic fibrillation potentials become evident. As long as the endoneural tubules are preserved, regeneration to the original motor end plates will proceed until recovery is total.

In neurotmesis, the lesion leads to Wallerian degeneration and the loss of endoneural tubules. Consequently, the electrophysiologic tests yield results similar to those found in axonotmesis; however, the outcome is less predictable. The regeneration process depends on the completeness of injury to all connective tissue components of the nerve, including the endoneurium, the perineurium binding the axons into fascicles, and the epineurium enclosing the fascicles into a common nerve. Loss of endoneural tubules ensures a synkinetic result if regeneration occurs. Furthermore, the growth of neurofilaments is governed by conditions at the injury site and can be hindered by ischemia and scar.

Sunderland (9) outlines five levels of neural injury based on the integrity of the connective tissue components. According to this scheme, first-degree injury is equivalent to neurapraxia; second-degree injury, to axonotmesis; and third through fifth degrees, to neurotmesis. The third, fourth, and fifth degrees of injury correspond to loss of endoneurium; loss of endoneurium and perineurium; and loss of endoneurium, perineurium, and epineurium, respectively. This classification helps to explain the discrepancies in recovery and the oddities of electrophysiologic testing, but the levels must be differentiated after the nerve has undergone regeneration. The resulting grades of facial weakness and synkinesis reflect the underlying neural insult (Table 144.3).

TABLE 144.3
CLASSIFICATION OF RECOVERY FROM FACIAL PARALYSIS

Grade	Characteristics
I. Normal	Normal facial function in all areas
II. Mild dysfunction	Gross
	Slight weakness noticeable on close inspection
	May have very slight synkinesis. At rest, normal symmetry and tone
	Motion
	Forehead: moderate-to-good function
	Eye: complete closure with minimal effort
	Mouth: slight asymmetry
III. Moderate dysfunction	Gross
	Obvious, but not disfiguring difference between the two sides
	Noticeable but not severe synkinesis, contracture, or hemifacial spasm
	At rest, normal symmetry and tone
	Motion
	Forehead: slight-to-moderate movement
	Eye: complete closure with effort
	Mouth: slightly weak with maximum effort
IV. Moderately severe dysfunction	Gross
	Obvious weakness and/or disfiguring asymmetry. At rest, normal symmetry and tone
	Motion
	Forehead: none
	Eye: incomplete closure
	Mouth: asymmetric with maximum effort
V. Severe dysfunction	Gross
	Only barely perceptible motion. At rest, asymmetry
	Motion
	Forehead: none
	Eye: incomplete closure
	Mouth: slight movement
VI. Total paralysis	No movement

From House JW, Brackmann DE. Facial nerve grading system. *Otolaryngol Head Neck Surg* 1985;93:146–147, with permission.

TABLE 144.4
ELECTROPHYSIOLOGIC TESTS

Test	Indication	Interpretation	Limitation
Nerve excitability test	Complete paralysis <3 wk duration	≤3.5 mA threshold difference: prognosis good	Not useful in first 3 days after onset or during recovery
Maximal stimulation test	Same as NET	Marked weakness or no muscle contraction: advanced degeneration with guarded prognosis	Not objective
Electroneurography	Same as NET and MST	<90% degeneration: prognosis good;≥90%: prognosis in question	False-positive results in deblocking phase
Electromyography	Acute paralysis less than 1 wk duration	Active mu: intact motor axons	Cannot assess degree of degeneration or prognosis for recovery
	Chronic paralysis greater than 2 wk duration	mu + fibrillation potentials: partial degeneration	
		Polyphasic mu: regenerating nerve	

MST, maximal stimulation test; mu, motor units; NET, nerve excitability test.

Electrophysiologic Tests

The currently popular tests used to establish prognosis for return of function are the NET, MST, ENoG, and EMG. Serial testing can establish the end point of degeneration, but any one test given at one point in time during the paralysis provides only limited information. The tests are complementary and when used appropriately can accurately describe the completeness of degeneration. The indications, interpretations, and limitations of these tests are outlined in Table 144.4.

General rules apply to the use of these tests. The NET, MST, and ENoG are most applicable in the evaluation of acute paralysis (i.e., while the nerve is in the degenerative phase). During degeneration, the NET will demonstrate increasing side-to-side threshold differences, the MST greater degrees of facial weakness, and the ENoG lower percentages of intact motor axons. The results will reach a nadir or end point, and the nerve will enter the recovery phase. This may be evident immediately on clinical examination or may be delayed, depending on the cause and extent of nerve injury. The tests provide no pertinent information during a paresis, as the existence of facial movement on examination indicates that the nerve is intact and primarily neurapraxic, and the prognosis for recovery at that particular point in time is good. The most common causes of acute facial paralysis (Bell's palsy, trauma, infection) produce nerve degeneration within the first 3 weeks after onset of palsy, and the NET, MST, and ENoG provide the most accurate information within this time frame. Nevertheless, when the neurapraxic axons begin recovery, asynchronous depolarization, differing conduction velocities in the motor axons, poor summation of the myogenic action potentials, and poor muscular contraction can give a false-positive report of nerve status and even may suggest that the nerve has completely degenerated.

EMG in combination with NET, MST, and ENoG greatly aids in eliminating these false-positive results, as the demonstration of voluntary active motor units confirms the integrity of intact axons in the recovery phase. This test is useful in the earliest phase of degeneration, as the presence of motor units indicates an intact nerve with incomplete injury. Within the first 3 days after onset of complete paralysis, the results of NET, MST, and ENoG yield little useful information, because Wallerian degeneration distal to the stimulation areas has not occurred; the results always indicate incomplete degeneration and good prognosis (10). Because of this limitation, the prognosis cannot be established by using NET, MST, or ENoG until the sixth or seventh day after onset of paralysis. The primary limitation of EMG is the inability to differentiate a totally neurapraxic nerve from a completely degenerated one in the acute phase of degeneration. Nevertheless, the EMG is complementary in the evaluation of acute paralysis and essential in the evaluation of longstanding paralysis. The presence of myogenic fibrillation potentials and the absence of voluntary motor units denote complete nerve degeneration, the coexistence of both fibrillation potentials and motor units indicates an incomplete lesion, and the appearance of polyphasic motor units signifies a regenerating nerve.

In the NET, the current thresholds required to elicit just-visible muscle contraction on the normal side of the face are compared with those values required over corresponding sites on the side of the paralysis. The current, measured in milliamperes, is delivered percutaneously in a square-wave pulse of 0.3-ms duration at a rate of one per second over the main trunk and branches of the facial nerve. A side-to-side threshold difference is calculated for the respective sites of stimulation. A side-to-side difference of 3.0 to 3.5 mA is compatible with advanced degeneration. Lauman and Jongkees (10) found reversible nerve dysfunction for values below 3.5 mA and an unfavorable prognosis for differences exceeding 3.5 mA.

The MST is a modification of the NET that uses a level of current sufficient to depolarize all motor axons underlying the stimulating probe (11). The facial muscular responses are graded subjectively according to the degree of contraction (equal, slightly decreased, markedly decreased, or absent). Markedly decreased or absent facial movement signifies advanced degeneration. When the response to MST remains normal for 10 days, 88% of patients have complete return and 12% fair return of facial function. If the response is decreased, 73% have complete return of function. If the response is lost, return does not begin until the fourth month.

Introduced by Esslen and popularized by Fisch (12), ENoG allows quantitative analysis of nerve degeneration. A supramaximal level of current applied with bipolar electrodes percutaneously over the main trunk of the facial nerve creates synchronous depolarization of the motor axons, thereby evoking a compound myogenic action potential in the facial musculature that is recorded with bipolar surface electrodes (Fig. 144.4). The peak-to-peak amplitude of this potential is directly proportional to the number of intact motor axons. Compared with the amplitude of potential evoked on the normal side, it can be used to calculate the percentage of intact axons. Greater than 90% degeneration indicates a poor prognosis for immediate or complete restoration of facial function. Traumatic injuries undergoing more than 90% degeneration within 6 days of the injury represent complete lesions. In Bell's palsy, patients exceeding 95% degeneration within the first 2 weeks of onset fall into the guarded prognostic category (13).

It is important for the clinician to understand potential sources of testing error. Naturally, the level of experience of the physician or technician performing the test is a significant variable. Two testing paradigms are used for ENoG: standard lead placement and optimal lead placement (OLP). The former test places recording electrodes at the same anatomic location on both sides of the face, usually at the lateral edge of the nasolabial crease and lateral and inferior to the oral commissure. The OLP technique uses repeated repositioning of recording electrodes until the maximal response is detected. The use of electrode paste and the amount of pressure applied to the stimulating and recording electrodes can influence results of any method of electrical testing. Patient factors such as age, obesity, and sex may also influence NET test results.

Coker et al. (14) compared the results of NET and ENoG testing in patients with acute facial paralysis. The study intended to assess correlation of results of the two tests. They found that the tests display an exponential relationship, not a linear one. The highest levels of correlation were seen when OLP technique was used in ENoG testing.

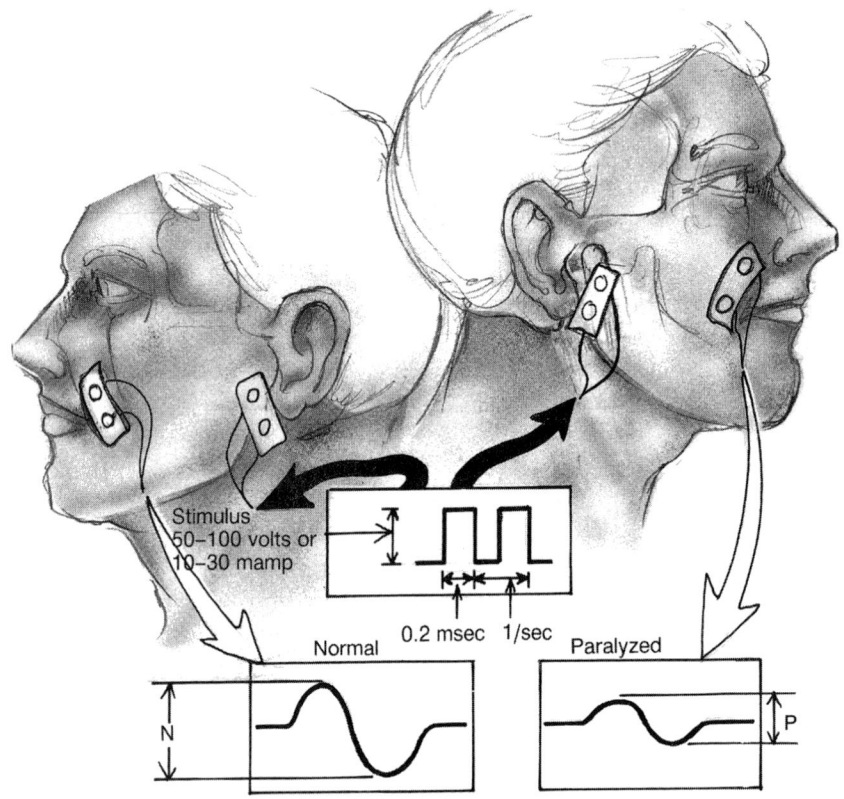

Figure 144.4 Clinical electroneurography in the assessment of acute facial paralysis. Percentage of viable motoneurons = P/N ×100. (Modified from Coker NJ, Fordice JO, Moore S. Correlation of the nerve excitability test and electroneurography in acute facial paralysis. *Am J Otol* 1992;13:127–133, with permission.)

There were no instances of measurable compound action potential on OLP ENoG and no response on NET. The lack of exact correlation between the two tests illustrates the inability to achieve consistent synchronous depolarization of viable axons, which the authors suggest may be explained by a deblocking phenomenon or partial demyelination; however, greater NET differences are predictive of a diminished response on ENoG. The authors concluded that the two tests are complementary in assessment of acute facial paralysis.

BELL'S PALSY

The term *Bell's palsy* has been used to describe a facial paralysis of acute onset and limited duration, the etiology of which was deemed idiopathic. This diagnosis could be made only after exclusion of all other possible etiologies. Despite these constraints on establishing the diagnosis, Bell's palsy is the most common diagnosis given to patients with acute facial paralysis.

The incidence of Bell's palsy is between 30 and 45 cases per 100,000 per year (15,16). The incidence varies with age, being rare in children and greatest between the ages of 15 and 45. Some find incidence increasing with age, whereas others find a decreasing incidence after age 60. The incidence appears greater in arid climates and during winter months.

The clinical picture is defined by rapid onset of the facial palsy, minimal associated symptoms, and spontaneous recovery. Facial nerve dysfunction developing over several weeks or months is not Bell's palsy. Peitersen (16) characterized the natural history of untreated Bell palsy. Thirty percent of patients develop only a paresis, and 94% of these patients recover without sequelae. The other 70% developed a complete paralysis, with only 61% of this group achieving full recovery. Time to return of movement is associated with ultimate recovery. Some return of facial tone or movement is seen in 85% of all patients within 3 weeks. Full recovery is typically achieved by 2 months. Patients who develop complete paralysis may not have return of function for 3 to 5 months. The longer the delay until some recovery is evident, the greater the likelihood of adverse sequelae, including synkinesis, residual weakness, and muscle spasms. Other factors that are associated with poor recovery include advanced age and pain at presentation. Peitersen (16) expressed final outcome using a modification of the Jongkees grading system. Extrapolation of his findings to the more familiar (in the United States) House-Brackmann scale reveals an estimated 71% of all patients achieving grade I and 12% grade II outcome.

Histopathologic studies of patients with Bell's palsy were reviewed by Liston and Kleid (17). The reported findings are not uniform, reflecting the different periods from onset of paralysis to nerve examination, methods of preparation, portion of the nerve studied, and possibly etiology of the facial paralysis. Most recent reports, however, demonstrate inflammatory infiltrates throughout the course of the facial nerve. Vascular thrombosis is generally not observed, although intraneural hemorrhage is seen occasionally.

It has long been postulated that the herpes simplex virus (HSV) is the infecting agent in Bell's palsy. Recent investigations provide convincing evidence to support this theory. The development of polymerase chain reaction techniques has allowed identification of HSV in the geniculate ganglion. Murakami et al. (18) sampled endoneurial fluid and muscle from patients undergoing decompression surgery for Bell's palsy and Ramsay Hunt syndrome. Control specimens were obtained during repair of the facial nerve after trauma, excision of parotid malignancies, and facial neuromas. Samples from 10 of 13 patients who had Bell's palsy were positive for HSV, whereas none of the controls showed evidence of the virus. Eight of nine patients with Ramsay Hunt syndrome had evidence of varicella-zoster virus, but none had HSV.

Additional support is given by replication of the clinical syndrome in an animal model. Sugita et al. (19) produced transient facial palsy in an animal model by inoculation with HSV. In this experiment, HSV was inoculated into the auricle or lateral tongue. Paralysis developed in 56% of animals inoculated in the auricle and 20% inoculated in the tongue. The paralysis developed 6 to 9 days later and persisted for 3 to 7 days. Spontaneous resolution occurred in all cases. Histopathology revealed significant edema and inflammation about the geniculate ganglion. HSV antigens could be isolated from the nerve, geniculate ganglion, and facial motor nucleus in some of the animals that developed paralysis. Antigen could not be detected on the contralateral side in any animal.

Because of the high rate of spontaneous recovery, it is difficult to prove that medical or surgical intervention improves recovery in patients with Bell's palsy. The most widely used intervention is corticosteroid treatment. Stankiewicz (20) reviewed the literature on steroid treatment in 1987. No irrefutable study showing efficacy of steroid treatment existed at that time; however, he concluded steroids may prevent denervation, speed recovery, lessen synkinesis, and prevent progression of paralysis. A subsequent meta-analysis of prospective, randomized studies comparing corticosteroids with placebo found a significant increase in probability of full recovery in those individuals with complete facial paralysis who received steroids (21). The addition of antiviral medications may provide additional benefit, although conclusive evidence is lacking. Adour et al. (22) investigated the addition of acyclovir to a regimen of steroid treatment in a double-blind study. Patients were randomized to receive either acyclovir 2,000 mg per day in five doses and prednisone or placebo and prednisone. All patients initiated this trial within 3 days of onset of the paralysis. Only 20% of patients progressed to complete paralysis (House-Brackmann grade VI) within 2 weeks of onset, and these were evenly distributed between the two treatment groups. Acyclovir-treated patients demonstrated less evidence of degeneration as measured by MST and a lower incidence of unsatisfactory recovery (House-Brackmann grades III and IV). Hato et al. (23) found improved outcomes using a combination of prednisolone and acyclovir compared with historical controls treated with prednisolone alone.

Selection of a medical regimen for any patient with Bell's palsy must consider potential side effects of medications, concurrent illness, and the patient's wishes. Treatment must be initiated promptly for maximal efficacy. The treatment effect is greatest for those patients with complete paralysis, but waiting for a mild weakness to progress undermines the efficacy of the treatment regimen. Prednisone is most commonly started at 1 mg/kg/day in divided doses for 7 days. A gradual taper over the next week is optional. Antivirals can be added if treatment is initiated within the first 72 hours, beyond this time additional efficacy is not likely. Valacyclovir is given at a dose of 1,000 mg three times daily for 7 days or famciclovir may be given at 750 mg three times daily.

Debate continues as to how to manage best those patients who progress to severe electrical degeneration despite medical intervention. Those patients who display greater than 90% degeneration on ENoG in the first 2 weeks of the paralysis recover to House-Brackmann grade I or II function only 50% of the time (24). Although histopathologic studies demonstrate inflammatory involvement of the entire nerve, it is postulated the maximal nerve injury occurs at the meatal foramen. In this location, the nerve occupies a greater proportion of the lumen of the fallopian canal than elsewhere. Further support for this theory was given by Fisch and Esslen (12), who confirmed the presence of a conduction block proximal to the meatal foramen in 11 of 12 patients undergoing total facial-nerve decompression. Surgical intervention thus is directed at unroofing the labyrinthine segment of the nerve via a middle fossa approach. Incision of the epineurium is advocated by some for additional neural decompression. Decompression of the mastoid and tympanic segments of the nerve has no effect on recovery of facial function.

Gantz et al. (24) presented the results of a prospective multiinstitutional trial of middle fossa decompression. Criteria for entry into the study were development of more than 90% degeneration on ENoG (OLP technique) within 14 days of onset of the paralysis and no voluntary motor unit potentials on EMG. Patients meeting these criteria were offered middle fossa decompression. Patients self-selected treatment, choosing either surgical decompression or continued medical treatment. Good outcome (House-Brackmann grade I/II) was achieved in 91% of the surgical patients versus only 42% in the medical treatment only group. Patients who progressed to a complete paralysis but did not develop more than 90% degeneration achieved a final House-Brackmann grade I in 89% of

cases. They concluded that the 90% degeneration threshold on ENoG accurately separates patients into a good or poor prognostic category. In addition, middle fossa decompression of the labyrinthine segment (including the geniculate ganglion and internal auditory canal) performed within 14 days of onset of paralysis significantly improves outcome in those patients with a poor prognosis. Decompression performed after 14 days provides no additional benefit. None of the patients in the medical treatment group received antiviral therapy; however, the potential benefit of antivirals is in preventing progression to severe degeneration. Antivirals are not expected to provide additional benefit once severe degeneration has occurred.

HERPES ZOSTER OTICUS

Varicella-zoster virus establishes a latent infection in many cranial nerve ganglia at the time of the initial infection. Years later, the latent virus is reactivated by an unknown mechanism. Reactivation of latent virus within the geniculate ganglion produces herpes zoster oticus or Ramsay Hunt syndrome. The patient presents with acute facial paralysis and severe ear pain and a vesicular eruption of the external auditory canal and concha. The pain often precedes the facial paralysis by a few days. Associated symptoms of sensorineural hearing loss and vestibular dysfunction are present in more than 30% of patients.

Ramsay Hunt syndrome is the second most common cause of acute facial paralysis with an annual incidence about one tenth that of Bell palsy. The incidence increases with age. The prognosis for spontaneous recovery of normal facial function is poorer than in Bell palsy (25). Satisfactory return of facial movement occurs in about 50% of patients; others will suffer varying grades of weakness, synkinesis, contractures, and spasm. Unlike Bell palsy, in which degeneration proceeds rapidly within the first 2 weeks after onset, degeneration of the facial nerve in herpes zoster oticus may evolve more slowly over the course of 3 weeks. When the degeneration is total, regeneration requires 3 to 6 months before facial movement becomes evident on clinical examination.

Jackson et al. (26) reported intraoperative findings in a patient with Ramsay Hunt syndrome demonstrating no return of function after 1 year. An excisional biopsy demonstrated a sharp demarcation between normal and devitalized nerve in the labyrinthine segment. Proximal and distal portions of the nerve appeared grossly normal. This observation suggests an increased susceptibility of the labyrinthine segment to inflammation-induced degeneration.

Management of herpes zoster oticus includes intervention directed at the underlying viral infection and associated complications. As stated earlier, antiviral therapy must be initiated promptly for maximal effectiveness. Acyclovir has proven to be of benefit in treatment of herpes zoster infections, demonstrating reduction in pain and shortening time to resolution of skin lesions. Varicella-zoster virus is less sensitive to acyclovir than HSV; thus, higher doses are required. Poor absorption of acyclovir by the oral route can be circumvented by intravenous administration or by substituting oral valacyclovir. The latter drug is metabolized to acyclovir, improving bioavailability by threefold to fivefold. Valacyclovir is given at a dose of 1,000 mg three times a day for 7 days. Steroids are usually given at the same doses as in Bell palsy. Few studies have examined the benefits of both steroids and antiviral therapy in herpes zoster oticus, but preliminary reports are encouraging (27,28). The role of surgical decompression remains investigational. It is difficult to identify those with a poor prognosis because electrical test data are less well established than in Bell palsy.

OTITIS MEDIA AND FACIAL PALSY

Facial palsy can present as a complication of acute suppurative otitis media, otitis media with effusion, chronic otitis media, and mastoiditis. Infection involving the fallopian canal leads to inflammation and neural edema. Immediate treatment should be directed toward eradicating the infection. When a middle ear effusion is present, myringotomy is performed promptly to drain the middle ear space. Cultures of the middle-ear aspirate direct antibiotic therapy against the offending organism.

The incidence of facial palsy in acute otitis media is approximately 1:20,000 cases (29). Most cases are seen in children due to the greater incidence of otitis media in the pediatric population. The prognosis of facial palsy in acute otitis media is excellent. Recovery of facial function begins rapidly in conjunction with resolution of infection. Operative management is usually limited to myringotomy and tube.

Facial paralysis in association with chronic otitis media or cholesteatoma carries a more ominous prognosis. The development of the paralysis is often more insidious. Aural toilet and antibiotics are initiated promptly. If the tympanic membrane is intact, myringotomy is performed. CT is recommended to evaluate the fallopian canal before surgery. Suspicion of intracranial complications is appropriate in this setting. Tympanomastoid surgery is necessary to remove infected tissues from the middle ear mastoid, provide drainage of the mastoid, establish better long-term ventilation of the middle ear and mastoid, restore the ossicular chain, and repair the tympanic membrane. The facial nerve is inspected carefully. Granulation tissue, cholesteatoma matrix, and infected bone are removed. This effectively decompresses the nerve. Incision of the epineurium is not advised. Facial nerve function is most likely to improve in those cases in which onset of paralysis

is acute and treatment is prompt. Facial paralysis that has been present for several weeks or more rarely improves despite aggressive management.

TRAUMA

Facial nerve injuries occur in a variety of ways, including blunt or penetrating trauma and iatrogenic harm. Management differs according to extent of injury, though the severity of the injury is not always easy to establish. History, physical examination, imaging, and electrophysiologic testing are all important in determining the probability of spontaneous recovery.

Immediate evaluation of the motor function of the facial nerve after trauma to the head and neck provides key information. All facial nerve branches should be inspected carefully to document movement. If a paresis is present, spontaneous return of satisfactory facial function will occur without intervention. Soft tissue swelling and ecchymosis impair the assessment of facial movement; thus, repeated examination is often necessary. Immediate complete paralysis indicates a severe nerve injury and warrants surgical exploration in cases of penetrating trauma.

Electrophysiologic testing in employed when the severity of injury is uncertain. The presence of voluntary motor units on EMG establishes continuity of the nerve, and this test may be performed at any time. Evoked EMG or ENoG testing is usually deferred for several days after the injury to avoid a false positive evoked response. Severe nerve injuries lead to rapid and complete degeneration, characterized by the absence of both voluntary and evoked responses. Predicting spontaneous recovery in traumatic lesions remains imprecise; additional data correlating the rate of neural degeneration on ENoG and spontaneous recovery is needed.

Pure-tone and speech audiometry is necessary for intratemporal lesions to document the type and degree of hearing loss. Imaging is usually limited to high-resolution CT scan, with the intent of defining any fractures traversing the fallopian canal. MRI or angiography is indicated if a major vascular injury is suspected, as with penetrating injuries at the skull base. Cervical spine films are requested if neck injury is suspected.

The recommended management of injuries with complete facial paralysis is outlined in Table 144.5 (30). For extracranial lacerations, the transected trunk or major branches should be repaired as soon as practical. This usually requires either direct end-to-end anastomosis or interpositional grafting, preferably at the time of soft tissue closure. Branches medial to the lateral canthus of the eye rarely need repair because of the rich cross-anastomotic connections of the nerve in the midface. Observe patients who have closed soft tissue injuries for resolution of the paralysis.

TABLE 144.5

MANAGEMENT OF TRAUMATIC INJURIES WITH COMPLETE FACIAL NERVE PARALYSIS

Mechanism of Injury	Tests	Critical Result	Management
Intratemporal Injury			
Blunt trauma	CT	Fracture involving fallopian canal	
(temporal bone fracture)	NET	>3.5 mA difference	
ENoG		>90% degeneration	
	EMG	Absent volitional activity	Surgical exploration if all of above present
	Audiometry	Conductive loss	Transmastoid–middle fossa approach
		Sensorineural loss—severe	Translabyrinthine approach
	History	Delayed onset	Observation
Penetrating trauma	Follow algorithm above, add:		
	Angiography	Suspicion of major vascular injury	Endovascular or open repair
Iatrogenic	History	Immediate onset	Surgical exploration
		Delayed onset (>3 days)	Observation
Extratemporal Injury			
Penetrating trauma	Physical examination		Exploration and repair
Blunt trauma	Physical examination		Observation
Iatrogenic	History	Suspected transection by report	Exploration and repair
		Nerve intact	Observation

CT; computed tomography; EMG, electromyography; ENoG, electroneurography; NET, nerve excitability test.

Temporal bone fractures are the most common cause of traumatic injury to the facial nerve. The fractures are categorized according to involvement of the otic capsule (31). Fewer than 5% of all temporal bone fractures involve the otic capsule. However, facial nerve injury occurs in half of all otic capsule fractures. Otic capsule sparing fractures are associated with facial paralysis in less than 10% of cases. Most injuries occur in the perigeniculate region. Less commonly, the nerve is injured in the upper mastoid segment by the fracture in the posterior osseous external auditory canal.

Once the injured segment of the nerve is identified, an operative approach is selected according to residual hearing. The middle fossa approach provides complete access to the perigeniculate region in those patients with good hearing. A transmastoid approach with a posterior tympanotomy allows examination of the tympanic and mastoid segments of the nerve. If profound sensorineural hearing loss is present, a translabyrinthine approach allows access to all segments of the nerve.

Blunt injuries rarely result in nerve transection. The most common findings are edema and contusion (intraneural hemorrhage) (Fig. 144.5) (30). The injured segment is inspected and any bone impaling or compressing the nerve is removed. Additional decompression of the fallopian canal may be performed proximal and distal to the injury. Intraneural hematomas are evacuated after incision of the epineural sheath. Complete transection of the nerve requires rerouting of the nerve with direct end-to-end anastomosis or an interpositional graft if direct anastomosis is not feasible.

Gunshot injuries of the temporal bone produce facial nerve paralysis in more than half of all cases (32). This unique form of penetrating injury often produces severe neural damage. The nerve can be directly involved (i.e., transected) or secondarily injured by the kinetic energy imparted by the projectile or by the bony fragmentation of the temporal bone. The most common sites of injury are the mastoid and tympanic segments of the nerve. When the nerve is transected, interpositional grafting is advised. Determining extent of injury may be difficult, because the damage is often more extensive along the proximal and distal segments than anticipated. As a result, outcome of facial function is poorer than in blunt temporal bone fractures.

The incidence of facial nerve injury during middle ear and mastoid surgery is much less than 1%. Delayed onset paresis (more than 3 days postsurgery) is more common but usually due to viral reactivation (33). The most common site of iatrogenic injury is the tympanic segment adjacent to the oval window (34). The nerve is more susceptible in this region because it is the most common site of fallopian canal dehiscence. The next most common site of injury is the mastoid segment. At times, cholesteatoma and granulation tissue obscure landmarks, increasing the risk of nerve injury. When in doubt, remove diseased tissue to confirm the location of the horizontal semicircular canal, digastric ridge, and incus to aid facial nerve dissection. Iatrogenic injury frequently results in complete transection of the nerve. Once again, end-to-end anastomosis or interpositional graft is required to restore continuity. Partial injuries, involving 50% of the diameter of the nerve

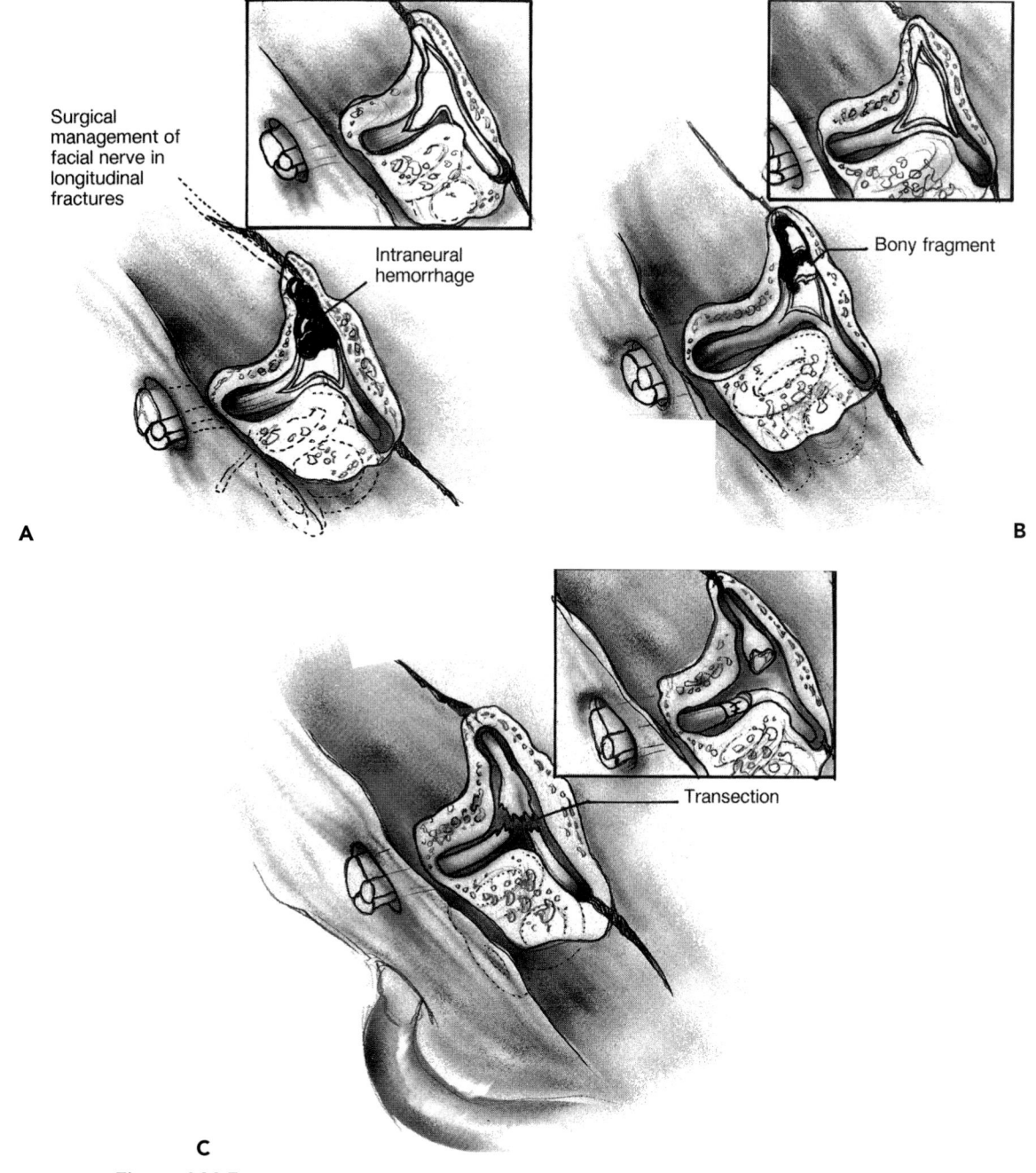

Figure 144.5 Pathogenesis of facial nerve injuries in longitudinal fractures of the temporal bone. Management includes **(A)** evacuation of intraneural hematomas, **(B)** removal of bony spicules, and **(C)** reanastomosis of transsectional injuries. (Modified from an illustration by Jim Schmidt.)

or less, are best treated by decompression proximal and distal to the injury.

Nerve anastomosis is accomplished using interrupted epineural sutures of a 9-0 monofilament, such as nylon. General principles of neurorrhaphy attempt to maximize the number of regenerating axons sprouting across the anastomotic site and include the following. All neural tissue is handled atraumatically by using microinstruments designed for neural repair. Approximation of nerve endings is done best under the illumination and magnifica-

tion of the operating microscope. Exact end-to-end approximation is performed without tension on the anastomosis.

Interpositional grafts are used when a direct end-to-end anastomosis creates tension or when segments of the nerve are missing or severely damaged. Donor nerves for use in grafting include the greater auricular, median antebrachial cutaneous, and sural nerves (Fig. 144.6). Resulting sensory deficits are modest and show some improvement with time.

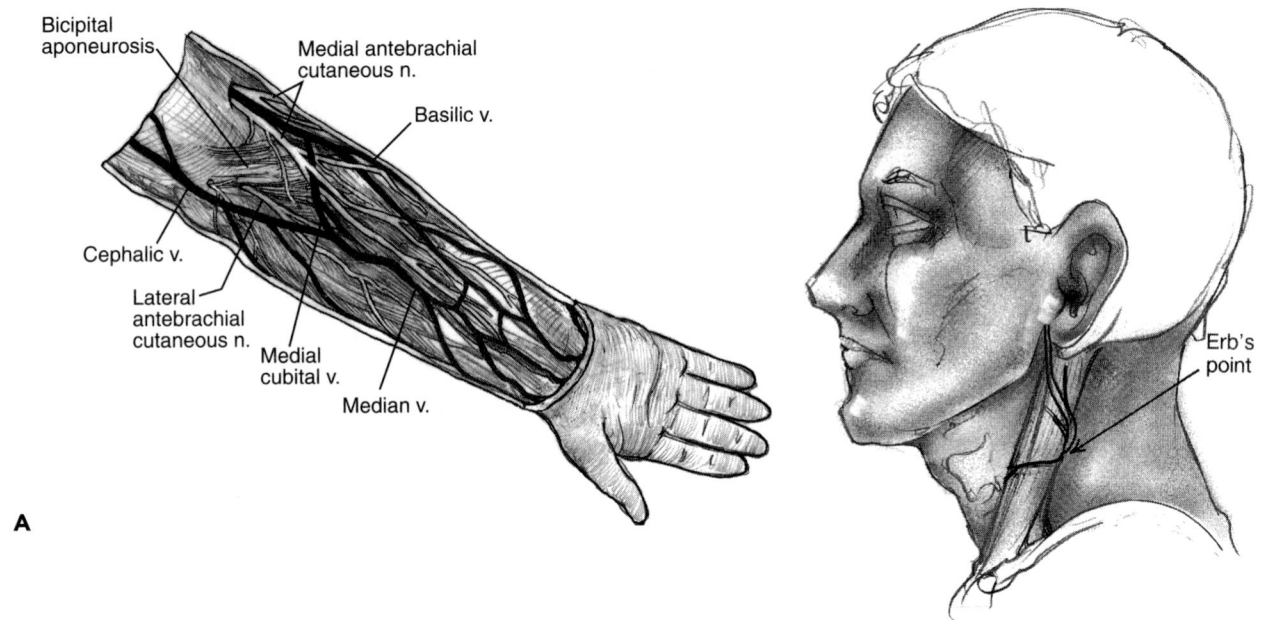

Figure 144.6   Popular interpositional grafts for repair of the facial nerve include the medial antebrachial cutaneous and greater auricular nerves.

TUMORS OF THE SKULL BASE AND FACIAL NERVE

Tumors rarely present with acute facial paralysis. It is estimated that only 5% of tumors involving the facial nerve present in this manner. Opinions differ on the guidelines for obtaining radiographic evaluation in patients with acute facial paralysis, but certain circumstances do increase the probability of neoplastic discovery, including the following:

- A paresis evolving slowly over a period exceeding 3 weeks
- Coexistence of facial twitching with an evolving paresis
- Development of chronic, unilateral eustachian tube dysfunction in a patient with no prior history of chronic middle ear disease
- Presence of multiple cranial-nerve deficits
- No return of facial function when the process has had an opportunity for regeneration
- Recurrent palsy on the same side
- Presence of a neck or parotid mass
- History of cutaneous malignancy

Several benign and malignant tumors can involve the facial nerve along its intracranial, intratemporal, or extracranial course. The most common tumor of the nerve is the facial schwannoma. Initial symptoms vary, depending on the involved segment of the nerve. Tumors involving only the cerebellopontine angle or internal auditory canal portions of the nerve will present with hearing loss or tinnitus. Intratemporal tumors often present with a slowly evolving facial paralysis, middle-ear mass, or conductive hearing loss. Extratemporal tumors present as a parotid mass and rarely exhibit any facial nerve dysfunction. All segments of the nerve may be involved, although the geniculate and labyrinthine segments are most common (35). Excision usually requires the use of interpositional grafting for restoration of continuity (36). One of the most difficult decisions on discovery of the tumor is the timing of management. In the geriatric population, a small tumor with minimal facial or middle-ear involvement is best observed. In the young patient, the tumor is best resected and the nerve grafted. If the tumor is allowed to grow, more motor axons will undergo degeneration with irreversible changes in both the axons and muscle end plates, such that any neural reinnervation technique will be compromised. A grade III return of facial function is the best result anticipated from grafting, so the patient needs preparation for a less than perfect outcome.

Skull-base tumors present an array of management problems regarding the facial nerve, and the otologic surgeon must be capable of any number of procedures to preserve the integrity of the nerve: transposition, rerouting, division and reanastomosis, interpositional grafting, and cranial nerve crossover. Anterior transposition of the facial nerve spares the greater superficial petrosal nerve and preserves normal tearing and is preferred for benign tumors of the infralabyrinthine compartment. Posterior transposition provides access to the petrous apex. Division and reanastomosis may aid exposure to the parapharyngeal space, but it should be avoided, as any transection of the nerve followed by neural anastomosis will result in synkinesis or mass movement. When the tumor is benign, the continuity of the nerve should be preserved by mobilization techniques. Exceptions to this rule include facial nerve schwannomas, which usually require resection of nerve with interpositional grafting; a benign tumor invading the nerve (e.g., cranial-nerve schwannomas, paragangliomas, cholesteatoma); and a recurrent tumor adherent to the nerve, which necessitates excision of the nerve to ensure complete tumor removal.

Malignant tumors involving nerve require excision with a tumor-free margin. Exceptions include patients with normal or slightly impaired facial function and the following tumors: lymphomatous and leukemic invasion of the nerve and low-grade malignancies of the parotid. These tumors are removed while sparing the nerve.

FACIAL PALSY IN THE NEWBORN

The differential categories for facial palsy in the newborn include traumatic and congenital etiologies. Trauma may be evident by facial contusion, ecchymosis over the mastoid or course of the extracranial nerve, or a hemotympanum. The mechanism of injury is proposed to be compressional due to molding of the head in passage through the birth canal or to the use of forceps. Within the first 3 days of life, a complete paralysis should undergo electrical stimulation to demonstrate muscle contraction or evoked myogenic potentials. If trauma is not so evident, the information gained from the electrical tests provides conclusive evidence of neuromuscular integrity. For later presentations, NET, MST, and ENoG should be used initially, followed by EMG if myogenic responses are absent. The EMG may demonstrate insertional muscle activity, intact motor units, fibrillation potentials, or polyphasic motor units indicative of incomplete injury. The prognosis for spontaneous regeneration is excellent and surgical exploration is not recommended unless the nerve has had an opportunity for recovery (37).

Congenital palsy most commonly presents as a unilateral weakness of the lower lip and can be associated with other anomalies. Kobayashi (38) found no relationship of this limited form of palsy to the use of teratogenic drugs, rubella, birth trauma, or hereditary factors. Complete congenital paralysis is rare and has been described as a result of congenital absence of the motor portion of the facial nerve and facial musculature or agenesis of the facial motor nucleus (39). Associated findings in Möbius syndrome include unilateral or bilateral and complete or incomplete facial weakness, unilateral or bilateral abducens nerve palsy, and deformities of the extremities; those of thalidomide embryopathy include limb and ear anomalies and abducens nerve palsy. Congenital paralysis is best left untreated until late childhood, because muscle transfers and fascial slings are often necessary for improved cosmesis. Because of the good skin turgor, the eye uncommonly

requires protective measures to prevent exposure keratitis in the child.

EYE CARE

The most common complication after the onset of facial paralysis is corneal desiccation. Complete paralysis, diminished tearing, loss of corneal sensitivity due to trigeminal nerve involvement, and absent Bell phenomenon are poor prognostic signs. At the onset, the patient should be warned of the evidence for corneal irritation: itching, redness, foreign-body sensation, and visual blurring. Rubbing the eye is a sure sign of corneal irritation. Measures recommended for protection include the liberal use of ophthalmic lubricants, closure of the eye with tape at night, use of moisture chambers or shielded glasses, and avoidance of wind, vents, and fans. Patient education and aggressive treatment usually prevent the development of ulcers or scarring. If symptoms persist, ophthalmologic consultation is advised. Surgical treatment of the eye is rarely necessary in acute and temporary palsies. Longstanding paralysis, corneal hypesthesia, and nerve repair with grafts are examples of situations likely to require adjunctive management of the eye. Gold weight implants, canthoplasty, tarsorrhaphy, and upper eyelid springs are among the available surgical options.

HIGHLIGHTS

- Cranial nerve VII is composed of special visceral afferent, general visceral efferent, and special visceral efferent fibers, which provide taste, lacrimation, and mimetic functions respectively.
- The middle-ear and mastoid landmarks to the location of the facial nerve include the cochleariform process, the oval window, the horizontal semicircular canal, the chorda tympani nerve, and the digastric ridge.
- A paresis does not warrant electrophysiologic tests (nerve excitability test, maximal stimulation test, electroneurography), because the prognosis for recovery is good until the palsy is complete. Serial testing of a complete paralysis in the acute phase of degeneration provides the most accurate information on nerve injury and prognosis for recovery. Electromyography is the most reliable test for the evaluation of longstanding paralysis.
- Bell's palsy accounts for more than half of acute facial palsy presentations. Any of the following make the diagnosis of Bell's palsy less probable: a paresis evolving over a period exceeding 3 weeks, signs of neoplasia, trauma along the course of the nerve, vesicles on the head or neck, multiple cranial nerve involvement, temporal bone infection, palsy at birth, signs of central nervous system lesion, and failure to have any evidence of recovery 6 months after onset.

- Bell's palsy patients demonstrate return to normal or near normal function in 83% of cases without treatment. Experimental and clinical data implicate herpes simplex virus as the likely causative agent. Medical therapy commonly includes steroids and antivirals, although the ability of these agents to alter prognosis remains controversial.

- The varicella-zoster virus can produce facial paralysis. The hallmark of this infection is a vesicular eruption over the distribution of sensory afferent neurons of the cervical plexus or cranial nerves V, VII, IX, or X. The prognosis for functional recovery is poorer than in patients with Bell's palsy. Antiviral therapy is recommended.

- For facial palsy presenting as a complication of infection, the immediate treatment should be directed toward eradicating the infection.

- Temporal bone fractures are the most common cause of traumatic injury to the facial nerve. Most injuries involve the nerve in the perigeniculate region or in the tympanic segment above the oval window. The most common finding at surgical exploration is contusion.

- The preferred order of procedures used to preserve the integrity of motor function of the facial nerve is transposition or rerouting, division and reanastomosis, interpositional grafting, and cranial nerve crossover (XII to VII or XI to VII). Any anastomosis or grafting of the intracranial or intratemporal facial nerve will have synkinesis as a result.

REFERENCES

1. Anson BJ, Harper DG, Warpeha RL. Surgical anatomy of the facial canal and facial nerve. *Ann Otol* 1963;72:713–734.
2. Nager GT, Proctor B. Anatomical variations and anomalies involving the facial canal. *Ann Otol Rhinol Laryngol* 1982;91[Suppl]:45–57.
3. Thomander L, Aldskogius H, Grant G. Motor fibre organization in the intratemporal portion of a cat and rat facial nerve studied with the horseradish peroxidase technique. *Acta Otolaryngol (Stockh)* 1982;93:397–405.
4. Gacek RR, Radpour S. Fiber orientation of the facial nerve: an experimental study in the cat. *Laryngoscope* 1982;92:547–556.
5. Blunt MJ. The blood supply of the facial nerve. *J Anat* 1954;88:520–526.
6. Pitts DB, Adour KK, Hilsinger RL. Recurrent Bell's palsy: analysis of 140 patients. *Laryngoscope* 1988;98:535–540.
7. Levenson MJ, Ingerman M, Grimes C, et al. Melkersson-Rosenthal syndrome. *Arch Otolaryngol* 1984;110:540–542.
8. Keane JR. Bilateral seventh nerve palsy: analysis of 43 cases and review of the literature. *Neurology* 1994;44:1198–2002.
9. Sunderland S. *Nerve and nerve injuries,* 2nd ed. New York: Churchill Livingstone, 1978.
10. Lauman EPJ, Jongkees LBW. On the prognosis of peripheral facial paralysis of endotemporal origin. *Ann Otol Rhinol Laryngol* 1963;72:621–636.
11. May M, Harvey JE, Marovitz WF, et al. The prognostic accuracy of the maximal stimulation compared with that of the nerve excitability test in Bell's palsy. *Laryngoscope* 1971;81:931–938.
12. Fisch U, Esslen E. Total intratemporal exposure of the facial nerve. *Arch Otolaryngol* 1972;95:335–341.
13. Fisch U. Prognostic value of electrical tests in acute facial paralysis. *Am J Otol* 1984;5:494–498.
14. Coker NJ, Fordice JO, Moore S. Correlation of the nerve excitability test and electroneurography in acute facial paralysis. *Am J Otol* 1992;13:127–133.
15. Campbell KE, Brundage JF. Effects of climate, latitude, and season on the incidence of Bell's palsy in the US Armed Forces, October 1997 to September 1999. *Am J Epidemiol* 2002;156:32–39.
16. Peitersen E. Bell's palsy: the spontaneous course of 2,500 peripheral facial nerve palsies of different etiologies. *Acta Otolaryngol Suppl* 2002;549:4–30.
17. Liston SL, Kleid MS. Histopathology of Bell's palsy. *Laryngoscope* 1989;99:23–26.
18. Murakami S, Mizobuchi M, Nakashiro Y, et al. Bell palsy and herpes simplex virus: identification of viral DNA in endoneurial fluid and muscle. *Ann Intern Med* 1996;124:27–30.
19. Sugita T, Murakami S, Yanagihara N, et al. Facial nerve paralysis induced by herpes simplex virus in mice: an animal model of acute and transient facial paralysis. *Ann Otol Rhinol Laryngol* 1995;104:574–581.
20. Stankiewicz JA. A review of the published data on steroids and idiopathic facial paralysis. *Otolaryngol Head Neck Surg* 1987;97:481–486.
21. Ramsey MJ, DerSimonian R, Holtel MR, Burgess LP. Corticosteroid treatment for idiopathic facial nerve paralysis: a meta-analysis. *Laryngoscope* 2000;110:335–341.
22. Adour KK, Ruboyianes JM, Von Doersten PG, et al. Bell's palsy treatment with acyclovir and prednisone compared with prednisone alone: a double-blind, randomized, controlled trial. *Ann Otol Rhinol Laryngol* 1996;105:371–378.
23. Hato N, Matsumoto S, Kisaki H, et al. Efficacy of early treatment of Bell's palsy with oral acyclovir and prednisolone. *Otol Neurotol* 2003;24:948–951.
24. Gantz BJ, Rubinstein JT, Gidley P, et al. Surgical management of Bell's palsy. *Laryngoscope* 1999;109:1177–1188.
25. Sweeney CJ, Gilden DH. Ramsay Hunt syndrome. *J Neurol Neurosurg Psychiatry* 2001;71:149–154.
26. Jackson CG, Johnson GD, Hyams VJ, et al. Pathologic findings in the labyrinthine segment of the facial nerve in a case of facial paralysis. *Ann Otol Rhinol Laryngol* 1990;99:327–329.
27. Murakami S, Hato N, Horiuch J, et al. Treatment of Ramsay Hunt syndrome with acyclovir-prednisone: significance of early diagnosis and treatment. *Ann Neurol* 1997;41:353–357.
28. Kinishi M, Amatsu M, Mohri M, et al. Acyclovir improves recovery rate of facial nerve palsy in Ramsay Hunt syndrome. *Auris Nasis Larynx* 2001;28:223–226.
29. Ellefsen B, Bonding P. Facial palsy in acute otitis media. *Clin Otolaryngol* 1996;21:393–395.
30. Coker NJ, Kendall KA, Jenkins HA, et al. Traumatic intratemporal facial nerve injury: management rationale for preservation of function. *Otolaryngol Head Neck Surg* 1987;97:262–269.
31. Brodie HA, Thompson TC. Management of complication from 820 temporal bone fractures. *Am J Otol* 1997;18:188–197.
32. Duncan NO, Coker NJ, Jenkins HA, et al. Gunshot injuries of the temporal bone. *Otolaryngol Head Neck Surg* 1986;94:47–56.
33. Vrabec JT. Delayed facial palsy following tympanomastoid surgery. *Am J Otol* 1999;20:26–30.
34. Green JD, Shelton C, Brackmann DE. Iatrogenic facial nerve injury during otologic surgery. *Laryngoscope* 1994;104:922–926.
35. Vrabec JT, Guinto FC, Nauta HJ. Recurrent facial neuromas. *Am J Otol* 1998;19:99–103.
36. Lipkin AF, Coker NJ, Jenkins HA, et al. Intracranial and intratemporal facial neuroma. *Otolaryngol Head Neck Surg* 1987;96:71–79.
37. Bergman I, May M, Wessle HB, et al. Management of facial palsy caused by birth trauma. *Laryngoscope* 1986;96:381–384.
38. Portmann M, Miehlke A, Kobayashi T. Congenital facial palsy. In: Fisch U, ed. *Facial nerve surgery.* Birmingham: Aesculapius, 1977:578–584.
39. Nisenson A, Isaacson A, Grant S. Masklike facies with associated congenital anomalies (Möbius syndrome). *J Pediatr* 1955;46:255–261.

145

Otologic Manifestations of Systemic Disease

Alexander J. Schleuning Jr.[†]   *Peter E. Andersen*
Karen J. Fong   *Samuel P. Gubbels*

A variety of systemic disorders can manifest as otologic complaints. The symptoms may be part of the progression of an already detected systemic disorder, or they may present as the initial complaint of a patient who has a previously unrecognized systemic disease. Because the list of diseases that may affect the temporal bone is large, the otolaryngologist–head and neck surgeon must maintain a high index of suspicion when evaluating patients with otologic complaints.

The disorders discussed here focus on diseases that are primarily systemic but may have manifestations within the middle ear and temporal bone. These include, but are not limited to, infectious processes, autoimmune diseases, disorders of bone, metabolic, and granulomatous diseases (Table 145.1).

INFECTIOUS DISEASES

Herpes Simplex

Primary herpes simplex virus occurs in patients without prior immunity to the virus, primarily infants and children. It may manifest as gingivostomatitis, keratoconjunctivitis, or meningoencephalitis. The causative agent is a DNA virus. The vesicular eruption can involve the skin of the auricle and external ear. Herpetic external otitis is self-limiting, and treatment is primarily symptomatic, consisting of analgesics and topical or systemic antibiotics for secondary infection.

Medical therapy is most effective when started during the prodrome phase of the infection. The effectiveness of oral acyclovir in speeding healing of the lesions has been well documented and may be considered in some cases (1). Current recommendations for a primary infection are 400 mg of acyclovir three times a day for 7 to 10 days. Prophylactic dosage for those patients with frequent recurrence is 400 mg twice a day. Alternative agents include valacyclovir 2 g twice daily for one day, or famciclovir 500 mg three times daily for 7 days.

Varicella-Zoster

Varicella-zoster is a DNA virus of the herpes family that causes two distinct clinical diseases: varicella (chickenpox), and herpes zoster (shingles). Chickenpox is an extremely contagious disease that most often affects children. Transmission is believed to be respiratory, and the attack rate is greater than 90%. Primary infection in adults is associated with a 20% rate of varicella pneumonia. The maculopapular exanthem often involves the skin of the auricle. Because this infection is self-limited, no specific therapy is indicated unless there are complications, and treatment should be directed at supportive measures only. Hearing loss after chickenpox is not uncommon but is usually due to a secondary bacterial infection causing a conductive hearing loss (CHL). Herpes zoster oticus, or Ramsay Hunt syndrome, is believed to result from reactivation of latent

TABLE 145.1
SYSTEMIC DISEASES

Infectious
  Herpes simplex
  Varicella-zoster
  Mumps
  Measles
  Syphilis
  Lyme disease
  Leprosy
  Tuberculosis
  Human immunodeficiency virus

Immunologic
  Wegener granulomatosis
  Relapsing polychondritis
  Discoid lupus erythematosus
  Systemic lupus erythematosus
  Polyarteritis nodosa
  Rheumatoid arthritis
  Autoimmune inner ear disease

Metabolic
  Gout
  Ochronosis
  Mucopolysaccharidoses

Diseases of bone
  Osteogenesis imperfecta
  Osteopetrosis
  Paget disease
  Fibrous dysplasia

Idiopathic
  Histiocytosis X

herpes zoster virus within the geniculate ganglion. It presents with hearing loss and facial nerve paresis due to nerve inflammation. A vesicular eruption may be seen on the auricle and external auditory canal in the areas of sensory innervation by the facial nerve. The eruption may be accompanied by intense pain. If facial nerve paralysis develops, in most cases it manifests 1 to 2 days after the vesicular eruption, and histologic examination of the facial nerve will reveal active neuronitis. In some cases, patients may experience auditory or vestibular symptoms due to spread of the inflammatory reaction to the eighth nerve complex (2). Treatment of immunocompetent hosts is generally recommended (3) because some studies have shown improved facial nerve outcomes and rates of recovery when acyclovir was used in addition to steroid treatment for Ramsay Hunt syndrome (4). Immunocompromised patients are at highest risk for complications, including secondary bacterial infection, pneumonia, corneal lesions, myocarditis, and nephritis. Use of glucocorticoids to prevent postherpetic neuralgia is controversial. Treatment for varicella in patients who require it is 20 mg per kg body weight up to 800 mg orally four times per day for 5 days. Zoster also can be treated with acyclovir 800 mg orally five

times a day for 7 to 10 days. An equally effective alternative, valacyclovir, the active metabolite of acyclovir, may be used. The adult dose of valacyclovir is 1,000 mg three times a day for 7 days (5). A vaccine for varicella was introduced in 1995 in the United States and has resulted in a significant decrease in varicella-related hospitalizations and hospital charges for adults and children. (6) The effect of the vaccine on the incidence of Ramsay Hunt syndrome is unknown.

Mumps

Mumps is caused by an RNA paramyxovirus and is transmitted by salivary secretions, usually via the respiratory tract. Manifestations include salivary adenitis, epididymoorchitis, pancreatitis, thyroiditis, polyarthritis, and myocarditis. Mumps infection causes hearing loss in 5 of 10,000 patients and affects both sexes with equal frequency (7). The hearing loss is unilateral 80% of the time and tends to develop suddenly toward the end of the parotitis. Tinnitus and aural fullness are commonly seen, and the hearing loss tends to be more pronounced in high frequencies. Vestibular symptoms may be seen and usually resolve over several weeks. The hearing loss is usually permanent but has been reported to resolve in some cases (8). Limited forms of the disease are possible, with some patients demonstrating only some of the many possible manifestations of the infection. There is no specific treatment for infections with the mumps virus, although corticosteroids have been reported to help diminish fever and pain resulting from parotid and testicular swelling. Vaccination provides protection to 75% to 95% of persons, and central nervous system complications are not a proven complication of the vaccine.

Measles

Measles (rubeola) is caused by an RNA virus and is highly contagious, the attack rate being greater than 90%. It was a common cause of acquired sensorineural hearing loss (SNHL) before the advent of the measles vaccine, accounting for 3% to 10% of acquired deafness in children. Hearing loss occurs in fewer than 0.1% of all measles infections. Since the introduction of current vaccination strategies, hearing loss secondary to measles has been drastically reduced. Measles-associated SNHL is usually bilateral and begins abruptly at the same time as the macular rash. Forty-five percent of patients develop profound hearing loss, whereas the remainder have mild to moderate hearing loss. The hearing loss may be asymmetric and tends to be maximal at higher frequencies. Tinnitus and vertigo may be present. Measles-associated hearing loss is permanent, and about 70% of affected patients have absent or diminished vestibular responses (9). Other complications of measles include pneumonia (seen most often in children), myocarditis, mesenteric adenitis, and encephalomyelitis.

Gamma globulin can alter the course of the disease and mitigate the symptoms to some degree.

The measles virus has also been implicated by some to play a causative role in the development of otosclerosis (10–15). Since the late 1980s, multiple groups have reported both electron microscopic and immunohistochemical evidence of the presence of measles virus proteins in the osteocytes of otosclerotic foci (10–12). More recent evidence has used reverse transcriptase polymerase chain reaction and polymerase chain reaction to isolate measles virus genomic RNA and DNA fragments from temporal bone specimen with histologic evidence of otosclerosis (13–15). Other investigators have failed to corroborate these findings using similar techniques (16). Ongoing research may further elucidate the role of the measles virus in otosclerosis.

Syphilis

The middle ear and mastoid may be affected by both congenital and acquired syphilis. The causative organism is the spirochete *Treponema pallidum*. During latent syphilitic infection, middle ear and mastoid osteitis is seen with a leukocytic infiltration of the ossicles and temporal bone. Tertiary syphilis is characterized by the gumma, a granulomatous lesion with central necrosis and obliterative arteritis. The gumma may affect the middle ear with tympanic membrane perforation and a granular appearance of the middle ear mucosa.

Labyrinthine involvement in acquired syphilis can occur in either the secondary or tertiary stages. Hearing loss during the secondary stage is usually abrupt, bilateral, and rapidly progressive, whereas vestibular symptoms are unusual. Patients also may complain of rash characteristic of secondary syphilis and headache. Lymphadenopathy and cranial nerve palsies may be detected on examination. Examination of the cerebrospinal fluid (CSF) shows a lymphocytosis with elevated total protein and normal glucose levels (17). Hearing loss occurring during tertiary syphilis is asymmetric and fluctuating. Progressive tinnitus and vertigo also may occur. A positive fistula test (the Hennebert sign) may be seen. Loss of speech discrimination may be out of proportion to the pure-tone thresholds. During tertiary syphilis, the CSF usually shows minimal lymphocytosis and the total protein level may be normal or elevated (18). Diagnosis of both secondary and tertiary syphilitic hearing loss requires the presence of a positive serum fluorescent treponemal antibody absorption test (FTA-ABS) or microhemagglutination assay–*Treponema pallidum* (MHA-TP). Treatment for acquired syphilitic hearing loss consists of penicillin given either as benzathine penicillin (2.4 million units intramuscularly weekly for 6 to 12 weeks) or as aqueous penicillin (600,000 U intramuscularly daily for 6 to 12 weeks). Azithromycin treatment has been used with some success though recent development of macrolide resistance has been reported and it is no longer recommended

as therapy (19). Prednisone (30 to 60 mg per day on alternate days) should be given for 3 to 6 months and tapered slowly. Prednisone should be increased or restarted if hearing deteriorates during or after tapering. Long-term maintenance therapy with prednisone may be necessary in some patients. Fifty percent of patients with acquired syphilitic hearing loss show some improvement of their hearing with this therapy (20).

Lyme Disease

Lyme disease is caused by infection with the spirochete *Borrelia burgdorferi* and is transmitted by certain species of ticks. In the United States, Lyme disease is commonly transmitted by the *Ixodes pacificus* tick on the west coast and the *Ixodes dammini* tick on the east coast. The disease has a worldwide distribution and is endemic in many parts of the United States. It is especially prevalent in the northeastern and midwestern United States, where it is usually spread by the nymphal *Ixodes scapularis* tick. The initial sign of Lyme disease is often a rash (erythema migrans) at the site of the tick bite, commonly the thigh, groin, or axilla. The rash develops from days to a month following the bite in 20% of patients. It generally begins as red macules or papules, which enlarge to form patches with or without areas of normal-appearing skin. Other early symptoms include severe headache, neck stiffness, fever, chills, myalgias, and profound fatigue. Late symptoms may include multiple neuropathies, arthritis, meningitis, and myocarditis. Patients may present to the otolaryngologist with facial paralysis, temporal mandibular joint pain, tinnitus, SNHL, sudden hearing loss, otalgia, facial pain, cervical adenopathy, vertigo, Ménière-like symptoms, and headache. It has become evident that Lyme disease is a common cause of facial paralysis; in one series, more than 50% of cases of acute facial paralysis among children were found to be caused by Lyme disease. The facial paralysis usually resolves slowly over 6 to 12 months. Until a highly sensitive and specific test has been developed, diagnosis of Lyme disease will be based primarily on clinical and epidemiologic evidence. Isolation of the causative agent in culture is considered the gold standard for diagnosis. However, this has not been met in most case series of Lyme borreliosis. The reliability of other methods of diagnosis is open to question. A two-step serologic approach has been proposed. A positive or equivocal enzyme-linked immunosorbent assay or indirect immunofluorescence assay is followed on the same serum sample by an immunoblot test that can detect immunoglobulin M (IgM) and IgG antibodies. Less commonly used tests are Western blot analysis testing for the presence of *B. burgdorferi* surface proteins, polymerase chain reaction to amplify DNA specific to the spirochete, and cultures of biopsy or aspirate material (21,22).

Although most manifestations of Lyme disease will resolve spontaneously without treatment, antibiotics are often used to hasten the resolution of symptoms and prevent disease progression. Early Lyme disease responds well to a number of single-agent oral therapies, including doxycycline, amoxicillin, penicillin, tetracycline, or cefuroxime axetil. Treatment is usually continued for 14 days. Use of tetracycline to treat disease suggestive of early Lyme disease also is effective against Rocky Mountain spotted fever and ehrlichiosis. Children younger than the age of 9 and pregnant or lactating women should not receive tetracyclines (22).

Leprosy

Leprosy, or Hansen disease, is endemic in tropical countries, such as India, Brazil, Burma, Madagascar, Nepal, and Mozambique which account for 83% of the registered cases (23). Patients may present with the disease long after leaving an endemic country, highlighting the importance of recognition even in the United States. Within the United States, more than 90% of diagnosed patients have lived in foreign countries where the disease is endemic, but endemic cases have been reported in Texas, Louisiana, Hawaii, and California. Between 1984 and 1993, 2,217 cases were reported in the United States.

The disease is caused by *Mycobacterium leprae* (Hansen bacillus). Cases are divided into groups based on clinical, histologic, and immunologic findings. The attack rate can be as high as 10% among spouse-spouse and parent-child contacts over a prolonged period. The nasal mucosa is thought to be the primary site of transmission from infected persons. The bacteria can infect the nasal mucosa, leading to mucosal swelling and rhinorrhea. Exposure to armadillos is another possible mode of transmission. Presentation typically is with skin lesions, weakness, numbness, or ulceration in an area of anesthesia on an extremity. Patients with borderline cases present with eye pain, skin lesions, acute palsy, leprosy reaction with neuropathic pain, or a systemic febrile illness. The nervous, cutaneous, and ocular involvement can lead to extremity mutilation, leonine features, and keratoconjunctivitis. The face is frequently involved, and the lesions are typically hyposthenic, hairless, and dry. The bacillus has a propensity to infect nerves, and the immune response to infection causes the nerves to thicken considerably. The greater auricular nerve, ulnar nerve, peroneal nerve, and radial nerve are commonly affected. The greater auricular, peroneal, and ulnar nerves should be palpated for evidence of enlargement (24). Lesions of the external ear occur in 70% of patients and consist of infiltrating nodules, loss of cartilage, and ulceration. Diagnosis is made on the basis of the presence of one or more of the following: hypopigmented or reddish patches with definite loss of sensation, thickened peripheral nerves and skin, or nerve biopsies showing acid-fast bacilli in modified mononuclear or epithelioid cells called lepra cells (25). When present in large numbers, the bacilli have a "cigar bundle" appearance on staining. Leprosy is classified as tuberculoid, borderline tuberculoid, borderline, borderline lepromatous, or lepromatous depending on the extent and nature of the clinical findings (26). Spontaneous fluctuations in the clinical state are termed leprosy reactions and are of two types: Type 1 reaction or reversal reaction is caused by a spontaneous increase in T-cell reactivity in peripheral nerves and skin lesions producing edema and painful inflammation of involved sites (27). The type 2 reaction or erythema nodosa leprosum (ENL) reaction is characterized by a toxic systemic inflammatory reaction secondary to immune complex deposition and occurs only in borderline lepromatous or lepromatous leprosy (28). Hansen disease is treated with combinations of dapsone, clofazimine and rifampin with the duration of treatment being determined by the degree of involvement (25). Management of type 1 leprosy reactions are with high doses of prednisolone (27), whereas type 2 reactions are managed preferably with thalidomide unless contraindicated (29). Thalidomide use continues to be highly regulated in the United States.

Tuberculosis

Tuberculosis is a communicable disease caused by *Mycobacterium tuberculosis*. Since the introduction of isoniazid in 1952, the incidence of tuberculosis in the United States has decreased from 84,304 in 1953 to 22,201 in 1985. Since then, the incidence increased until 1995, when 22,860 cases were reported, and has subsequently steadily decreased to 14,874 in 2003.

In the United States, tuberculosis is largely a disease of the human immunodeficiency virus (HIV)-infected, immigrant, and disadvantaged populations. The increase has been greatest in those infected with HIV, which also has been implicated as a factor in the rapid increase in multidrug-resistant strains of *M. Tuberculosis*. Transmission most commonly is due to aerosolized respiratory secretions expelled by the cough of an infected person. Most infected people become asymptomatic carriers. Immunocompetent people have a 5% to 10% lifetime risk of developing clinical disease (30). Those with both *M. tuberculosis* and HIV infection have a 5% to 10% annual risk of developing clinical disease and most often present with pulmonary disease. *M. tuberculosis* can affect multiple sites in the head and neck, including the larynx, pharynx, oral cavity, nasal cavity, salivary glands, cervical spine, middle ear, and mastoid. Cervical lymphadenopathy is seen in 5% to 10% of all patients with tuberculosis. Aural tuberculosis may present as facial paralysis, persistent aural discharge, refractory chronic otitis media, profuse granulation tissue, bone sequestra or necrosis, perichondritis, or failed otologic surgery (31). Otitis media caused by infection with *M. tuberculosis* may result from hematogenous and lymphatic routes of spread from pulmonary infection or from an ascending infection through the eustachian tube from the nasopharynx. *Mycobacterium bovis, Mycobacterium avium,* and *Mycobacterium fortuitum* also have been reported to cause otitis media. The infection is generally painless, most commonly with otorrhea from a tympanic membrane perforation. Occasionally, multiple small tympanic membrane perforations may be present. Facial paralysis occurs in 10% of adults and 35% of children with tuberculous otitis media and generally responds to medical treatment. (32,33). CHL due to ossicular destruction occurs early along with jugular lymphadenopathy. SNHL and labyrinthitis may occur as later manifestations. Patients may have draining sinus tracts in 20% of cases (34). The middle-ear mucosa appears granular or polypoid, and bony sequestra may form. Computed tomography generally shows complete soft tissue opacification of the middle ear and mastoid cavity, with bony erosion and possible fistula formation as findings only in advanced stages (33). A presumptive diagnosis of tuberculosis is histologic demonstration of acid-fast organisms in exudate or tissue preparations. A definite diagnosis is made by isolation and identification of *M. tuberculosis* in culture from a diagnostic specimen. Staining and culture of aural discharge in tuberculous otitis media or mastoiditis is infrequently positive and it may be necessary to obtain tissue for culture (35). It is critical that tissue specimens intended for culture not be placed in formalin. Newer techniques based on the polymerase chain reaction amplification of specific DNA sequences may allow for diagnosis of mycobacterial species and identification of mutations associated with drug resistance in a matter of hours (36). Treatment of aural tuberculosis consists primarily of administration of standard multidrug antituberculous chemotherapy, but surgery may sometimes be needed to remove intractably pathologic tissue and sequestrated bone (37), especially when an otologic complication such as facial paralysis or extradural abscess has occurred. Some have suggested that failure to respond, as measured by continued otorrhea, to appropriate medical therapy is also an indication for surgical management. (38). Initial multidrug treatment with isoniazid (5 to 10 mg/kg/day up to 300 mg), rifampin (10 mg/kg/day up to 600 mg), and pyrazinamide (15 to 25 mg/kg/day up to 2.5 g/day) for 6 months is recommended for uncomplicated, susceptible extrapulmonary disease. Pyridoxine (25 to 50 mg daily) is often added to regimens that include isoniazid. Alternative regimens should be used with any drug-resistant strains or complicated cases (39). Inadequate therapy due to poor patient compliance and improper dosing by physicians are the most common causes for development of drug resistance (40). An emergence in multiple drug resistant strains of *M. tuberculosis* underscores the importance of testing sensitivities and ensuring compliance with medical treatment.

Human Immunodeficiency Virus

Otologic complaints in patients infected with HIV, a single-stranded RNA retrovirus, are common. In one study, 34% of patients infected with HIV complained of aural fullness, 32% of dizziness, 29% of hearing loss, 26% of tinnitus and 23% of otalgia (41). HIV does not seem to involve the ear directly, but it deserves mention because immunocompromised patients are more susceptible to opportunistic infections. Otitis externa is a common otologic problem associated with HIV infection. *Pseudomonas aeruginosa* is the most common causative agent, with *Proteus* and *Aspergillus* species being less common (42). Treatment is the same as in the immunocompetent patient, with removal of debris and topical antibiotic drops with coverage for *Pseudomonas*. Polyps of the external auditory canal can be manifestations of both *Pneumocystis* and tuberculous infections. Diagnosis is made by tissue biopsy and treatment is appropriate therapy directed at the infecting agent resulting in rapid resolution of the polyp (43). Recurrent acute otitis media and serous otitis media are common otologic problems in the HIV-infected population. Acute otitis media is more common in the pediatric HIV-infected population when compared with the noninfected population. The pathogens are similar to that seen in the immunocompetent population, with the addition of opportunistic organisms. Serous otitis media occurs in up to 80% of the pediatric HIV-infected population and may be more common in the adult population (42). Nasopharyngeal masses secondary to adenoid hypertrophy, lymphoma, and nasopharyngeal carcinoma can cause eustachian tube dysfunction, otitis media with effusion, and CHL (44). SNHL in HIV-infected patients has a prevalence of 21% to 41% and can be attributed to a variety of causes, including otosyphilis, cryptococcal infection, ototoxic medications, cytomegalovirus infection, herpes simplex virus infection, primary or metastatic central nervous system neoplasms, and direct infection by HIV (43). Kaposi sarcoma (KS), a spindle cell neoplasm, can involve the internal ear canal (IAC), middle ear, and external ear. Differentiation of KS from bacillary angiomatosis, a newly described lesion associated with the *Bartonella* organism, is important because the latter can be treated with antibiotics whereas the former requires surgical extirpation or intralesional chemotherapy as treatment (42).

IMMUNOLOGIC DISEASES

Wegener Granulomatosis

Wegener granulomatosis (WG) is an immunologically mediated systemic disease of unknown etiology. The presence of circulating and deposited immune complexes, granulomas, and vasculitis support an autoimmune phenomenon. It is associated with the triad of necrotizing granulomas of the upper and lower respiratory tract, focal necrotizing glomerulonephritis, and systemic vasculitis of small arteries and veins. Prior to the use of effective medical therapy, the prognosis was poor, with a 90% 2-year mortality rate.

Because it is such a rare disease, the true incidence is difficult to determine. The male-to-female ratio is approximately 1:1 and is seen almost exclusively in whites. It can present at any age, with 15% of patients younger than 19 years. The mean age of onset is approximately 40 years (45). The most common symptoms involve the upper and lower respiratory tract and include sinus pain, bloody rhinorrhea, septal ulceration, cough, dyspnea, pleuritic chest pain, and nodular infiltrates on chest radiographs. The nasal cavity and paranasal sinuses are involved in 85% to 100% of cases. Renal disease is present in 85% of cases and is the greatest cause or morbidity and mortality. Other generalized symptoms include fever, malaise, weight loss, and arthralgias.

Otologic involvement is seen in approximately 35% of cases and can occasionally be the first and only sign of the disease. The most common otologic manifestations are facial or postauricular pain, otitis media with effusion, acute otitis media, hearing loss (both conductive and sensorineural), and vertigo. Facial nerve palsy has been reported as an initial clinical symptom (46,47). Serous otitis media with conductive hearing occurs most frequently and may result from eustachian tube obstruction from luminal granulomata or from nasopharyngeal inflammation or ulceration. Some patients may present with chronic serous otitis media, which will resolve with successful treatment and may be used as an indicator of remission or recurrence. Chronic suppurative otitis media occurs in 24% of patients with WG and can be associated with notable postauricular pain and otorrhea. (48). Perforations of the tympanic membrane, sometimes multiple, may be seen and can be confused with otitis media caused by *M. tuberculosis* (49).The etiology of the SNHL is still unknown but may be related to immune complex deposits in the cochlea, vasculitis of the vasa vasorum of the cochlea, or pressure on the acoustic nerve by a granulomatous lesion. The sensorineural loss may be accompanied by tinnitus possibly occurring in the setting of a coexistent CHL. Vertigo may be due to central nervous system involvement or immune complex deposits within the inner ear (46), although the low incidence of vertigo compared with the high incidence of SNHL in patients with WG suggests vestibular compensation (50).

Involvement of the external ear occurred in 3 of 112 patients in one series (49). External ear involvement consists of diffuse, erythematous swelling of the pinna during active phases of the disease. Positive laboratory findings are an elevated erythrocyte sedimentation rate, anemia, hematuria, elevated serum creatinine, and presence of serum antineutrophil cytoplasmic antibody (ANCA). Using immunofluorescent technique, it is possible to distinguish a c-ANCA (cytoplasmic pattern) from a p-ANCA (perinuclear pattern). Cytoplasmic ANCA is found in 90% of patients with active WG and in 60% of cases with limited disease, whereas p-ANCA can be found in other vasculitis and idiopathic glomerulitis (48). When cANCA

immunofluorescence is combined with anti-PR3 (cytoplasmic antibody) enzyme-linked immunosorbent assay (ELISA) the sensitivity and specificity rise to 90% and 98%, respectively (51).

The chest radiograph may reveal pulmonary lesions. Biopsy of the lesions reveals necrotizing granulomatous vasculitis. However, obtaining a good biopsy specimen is often difficult and is often nondiagnostic, especially with nasal lesions. Left untreated, WG is a fatal disease. Treatment of choice is corticosteroids and immunosuppressives such as cyclophosphamide, azathioprine, or methotrexate. Long-term remission is achieved in more than 90% of patients, especially in patients who have not yet developed major renal damage. The use of trimethoprim-sulfamethoxazole has been reported to induce remission in refractory cases and to help maintain remission (52,53), but its use remains controversial.

Relapsing Polychondritis

Relapsing polychondritis is a rare disorder characterized by episodic inflammation of cartilaginous structures. Autoimmune mechanisms appear to be responsible for relapsing polychondritis. The disease can involve any cartilaginous structure, especially those of the ear, nose, trachea, larynx, ribs, and eustachian tubes. Episcleritis, arthropathies, anemia, weight loss, myalgias, and fever also are associated with the disease. Over time the recurrent inflammation can lead to atrophy, scarring, and distortion of the involved cartilage. The disease is slightly more common in women than in men, with the average age of onset in the forties. Otologic manifestations of relapsing polychondritis consist of a red, tender, edematous pinna with sparing of the external ear canal, thus differentiating the condition from external otitis. Diagnosis is primarily clinical, and biopsy of the acutely inflamed pinna should be avoided because of the risk of infection. When necessary, biopsy of affected cartilage shows chondrolysis, chondritis, and perichondritis. During the active phase, there is infiltration of the cartilaginous matrix with inflammatory cells. Later, the cartilage is replaced by granulation tissue and eventually fibrous tissue (54). Laboratory findings may include an elevated erythrocyte sedimentation rate, anemia, and a positive rheumatoid factor. Corticosteroids have been effective in the treatment of relapsing polychondritis. The use of dapsone, indomethacin, and salicylates has been successful (55). Treatment with methotrexate also has been described (56).

Chronic Discoid Lupus Erythematosus

Chronic discoid lupus erythematosus (DLE) is a condition that causes raised erythematous lesions on the skin of the head, neck, and chest. It is a common form of lupus erythematosus that is limited to the skin in 90% of cases. The cause is unknown, but demonstration of immune complexes in the dermal–epidermal junction suggests an autoimmune phenomenon. The typical lesion is a well-circumscribed, raised lesion on the ear, face, neck, or chest that slowly enlarges and is pruritic. Scarring and hypopigmentation may develop over time. Patients with DLE have a 80% to 90% 15-year survival rate. Most patients with poor outcomes have kidney involvement. No specific treatment exists, but topical corticosteroids may be helpful. Above all, the patient should be protected against sun exposure. About 5% of patients progress to systemic lupus erythematosus (57).

Polyarteritis Nodosa

Polyarteritis nodosa is a necrotizing vasculitis of small- and medium-diameter arteries. Diagnosis is based on biopsy showing polymorphonuclear neutrophils infiltrating all layers of the vessel wall and perivascular areas, which leads to intimal proliferation and degradation of the vessel wall. Chronic lesions usually reveal a mononuclear cell infiltrate. Immunofluorescence studies reveal a deposition of immune complexes within vessel walls. The lesions are segmental and tend to affect the areas of arterial bifurcation. Angiography of affected organs reveals small aneurysms, particularly at branch points of vessels. As the lesions heal, there may be collagen deposition with narrowing or occlusion of the vessel. Hepatitis B surface antigen can be demonstrated in the serum of 30% to 40% of patients. Average age of onset is 45 years, with a male-to-female ratio of 2.5:1. Signs and symptoms are typically nonspecific: fever, weight loss, and malaise. Specific complaints may be related to the organ involved. Serologic testing may show an elevated leukocyte count, anemia of chronic disease, an elevated sedimentation rate, and the presence of ANCA. Common systemic complaints are ecchymosis of the skin, myocardial ischemia, bowel infarction, renal failure, and hypertension. The middle ear may be affected by polyarteritis nodosa. The predominant otologic symptom is usually hearing loss, which can be either conductive or sensorineural. Facial nerve paralysis may be associated with hearing loss. Treatment consisting of systemic corticosteroids combined with cyclophosphamide has been reported to result in long-term remission rates of up to 90%, but the prognosis for patients with multiorgan system involvement is poor (58,59).

Rheumatoid Arthritis

Rheumatoid arthritis (RA) is a chronic multisystem disease of unknown etiology. The characteristic feature is persistent inflammatory synovitis causing progressive cartilage and bone destruction within joints. It affects about 1% of the population and is three times more common in women than in men. Presentation is usually in the fourth or fifth decade of life. There is an association with expression of human leukocyte antigen DR4 locus (HLA-DR4) and increased risk for RA. Most patients have symptoms of fatigue, anorexia, muscular weakness, and myalgias prior

to arthritic complaints. Laboratory studies often reveal an elevated sedimentation rate, normochromic normocytic anemia, and the presence of rheumatoid factor. Rheumatoid factors typically tested are immunoglobulin M (IgM) autoantibodies to the Fc portion of IgG. This test is not specific for RA and is seen in a number of other diseases as well as in 5% of healthy persons. However, the titer can be of prognostic importance. Patients with high titers tend to have more severe disease. Treatment involves aspirin, nonsteroidal antiinflammatory drugs, glucocorticoids, immunosuppressive therapy, and surgery. RA can involve the external or middle ear. Rheumatoid nodules are both cutaneous and subcutaneous and may involve the external ear. These nodules are painful, raised lesions with necrotic centers. Treatment is the same as for other systemic manifestations of the disease. In patients who have RA, both conductive and SNHL can occur, and they have a significantly higher incidence of SNHL than normal persons, possibly due to autoimmune inner-ear disease. Abnormal middle ear mechanics has been proposed as a possible cause of the CHL seen in these patients. Laxity of the middle ear transducer mechanism, due to involvement of the ossicular suspensory ligaments and the incudomalleolar and incudostapedial joints, has been proposed as the cause of the CHL seen in patients with RA (60,61).

VOGT-KOYANAGI-HARADA SYNDROME

Voyt-Koyanagi-Harada (VKH) syndrome or uveomeningoencephalitic syndrome is a rare systemic disorder involving many organ systems, including the eye, ear, and integumentary and nervous systems. VKH syndrome has a predilection for darkly pigmented races such as American Indians, Asians, and Hispanics and typically presents in the second to fifth decades of life (62). The cause of VKH syndrome is unknown though autoimmune etiology has been implicated. Cell culture (63) and immunohistologic studies (64) suggest a delayed type hypersensitivity against melanocytes that express class II major histocompatibility complex (MHC) might be responsible for the inflammatory process in VKH.

VKH syndrome occurs in three phases, the first being the meningoencephalitis phase characterized by generalized weakness, hemiparesis, hemiplegia, dysarthria, and aphasia after a viral-like illness. The second phase occurs 3 to 5 days later and is characterized by loss of visual acuity, eye pain, tinnitus, and hearing loss. As the uveitis subsides, the disease enters a convalescent phase characterized by cutaneous findings such as poliosis involving the eyebrow and eyelashes, vitiligo, and alopecia, which tend to be permanent (65). Diagnosis of VKH is based on the presence of bilateral iridocyclitis, posterior uveitis, CSF pleocytosis, or tinnitus and cutaneous findings.

Treatment of VKH syndrome includes systemic corticosteroids with the addition of immunosuppressives for cases failing to respond. Surgical therapy for glaucoma may be necessary for some patients (66). Prompt referral to an ophthalmologist for evaluation and management of patients with idiopathic hearing loss, tinnitus, and signs of active uveitis is essential.

Autoimmune Inner Ear Disease

Autoimmune inner ear disease, first described by McCabe in 1979 (67), is a disease characterized by fluctuating progressive SNHL that is responsive to immunosuppressive drugs and is associated with positive findings of immune system activation on nonspecific tests. Patients tend to be in young adulthood to early middle age and have otologic symptoms that persist for months to years. Hearing loss is bilateral and often asymmetric, and approximately half of the patients experience vestibular symptoms. The ear appears normal on examination. Patients may have other systemic autoimmune diseases, such as systemic lupus erythematosus, RA, or polymyositis.

Diagnosis of autoimmune inner ear disease is based on rapidly progressive bilateral, often fluctuating hearing loss, which is unresponsive to conventional therapy but improves with immunosuppressive drugs. There are frequently associated systemic autoimmune disorders, positive "screening" test results such as serum cryoglobulins, elevated erythrocyte sedimentation rate, or positive antinuclear antibodies. Western blot analysis of the sera from patients with progressive SNHL has revealed the presence of an antibody against an inner-ear antigenic epitope with a molecular weight of 68 kd (68). In a recent study, antibody to the 68-kd protein was detected in serum from 89% of patients with actively progressing SNHL and none of the 25 patients with inactive disease. Furthermore, patients who were antibody positive responded to steroid treatment more often than those who were antibody negative (69). Further studies have reported that this 68-kd antigen is associated with heat shock protein (HSP)-70 (70,71). Western blot analysis for the 68-kd inner-ear antigen is a useful adjunct in the diagnosis and management of progressive SNHL. Treatment is with high-dose immunosuppressive drugs, usually corticosteroids. Cyclophosphamide and methotrexate have been used as alternatives to systemic corticosteroids. After hearing is stabilized, immunosuppressive therapy is gradually tapered, and the dose is increased only if hearing worsens. Some patients may require long-term maintenance therapy.

METABOLIC DISORDERS

Gout

Gout is a disorder of purine metabolism that causes abnormally high levels of uric acid. Urates are deposited in the tissues, causing arthritis and tophaceous nodules. Patients may be categorized as either overproducers (with abnormally high production of uric acid) or underexcreters (with abnormally low renal excretion of uric acid). The disease is most common among men in the fourth or fifth decade of life. The tophus found on the auricle may be confused with a rheumatoid nodule; however, when squeezed, it exudes a chalky white material. Therapy is directed toward the specific disorder. Overproducers are treated with allopurinol, which inhibits urate production. Underexcreters are treated with uricosuric drugs such as probenecid (72). Small helical nodules do not require treatment.

Ochronosis

Ochronosis, a form of alkaptonuria, is an autosomal-recessive disorder of homogentisic acid metabolism. Affected persons accumulate homogentisic acid, which is oxidized to a black compound that adheres to cartilage and thus discolors the ear, fingers, buccal mucosa, and nose. The urine of affected persons turns black on exposure to sunlight. Presentation is typically in the third decade of life. Osler sign, pigmentation of the sclera, is a common cause for presentation. The pigment also can accumulate in the mucosa of the upper aerodigestive tract. Treatment consists of a low-protein diet to prevent accumulation of homogentisic acid (73).

Mucopolysaccharidoses

The mucopolysaccharidoses are a group of storage diseases characterized by inherited deficiencies of enzymes needed for degradation of mucopolysaccharidoses. Hunter syndrome is caused by a lack of gamma-iduronidase and is inherited in an X-linked fashion. Hurler syndrome is caused by a deficiency of the same enzyme but is inherited as an autosomal-recessive disease. Morquio syndrome is caused by a deficiency of N-acetylgalactosamine-6-sulfatase or of beta-galactosidase. Hearing loss in the mucopolysaccharidoses is usually mixed with the conductive component due to eustachian tube dysfunction and resulting serous otitis media. Some studies recommend the placement of long-term ventilation tubes if tympanostomy is indicated given a higher anesthetic risk seen in this patient population (74). The cause of the sensorineural loss is uncertain but may be due to abnormal lipid metabolism within nerve cells (75).

DISEASES OF BONE

Osteogenesis Imperfecta

Osteogenesis imperfecta (OI), or van der Hoeve-deKleyn syndrome, is an autosomal-dominant disorder of connective tissue that can result in a high susceptibility to fractures, even with slight trauma. The disease is caused by mutations in either of the two chains that form type I procollagen, the major structural protein of bone, skin, and tendons. The severity of OI ranges from a lethal form in the perinatal period to a form mild enough to elude clinical detection. Frequent fractures, bowed limbs, vertebral body compression, and scoliosis are common problems for these patients. Type I OI, the mildest form, is inherited as an autosomal-dominant trait and is associated with hearing loss, multiple fractures, and blue sclera. The incidence of type I OI is about 1 in 30,000. Type II OI is lethal *in utero* or shortly after birth and has a reported incidence at birth of 1 in 60,000. Types III and IV are intermediate in severity between types I and II. They are less severe than type II, and the sclerae are only slightly bluish in infancy and white in adulthood. Type III tends to become more severe with age and can be inherited as either an autosomal-recessive or autosomal-dominant trait. Type IV is inherited as an autosomal-dominant trait and is similar to type I except that the sclerae are normal. Both CHL and SNHL can occur in OI and are found in 90% of subjects older than 30 years (76). The CHL is associated with blue sclera, whereas severe SNHL usually is associated with gray or white sclera. CHL is caused by involvement of the ossicles with pathologic fractures of the long process of the incus or stapes crura. The stapes footplate may be involved but is not always fixed (Fig. 145.1). Hearing restoration can be accomplished with either amplification or surgery (77). Stapedectomy can give results similar to that seen in otosclerosis but is a very delicate procedure due to the fragility of the ossicles, hypervascularity of the promontory mucosa, and an obliterated or mobile stapes footplate.(78) Some studies have suggested better results after

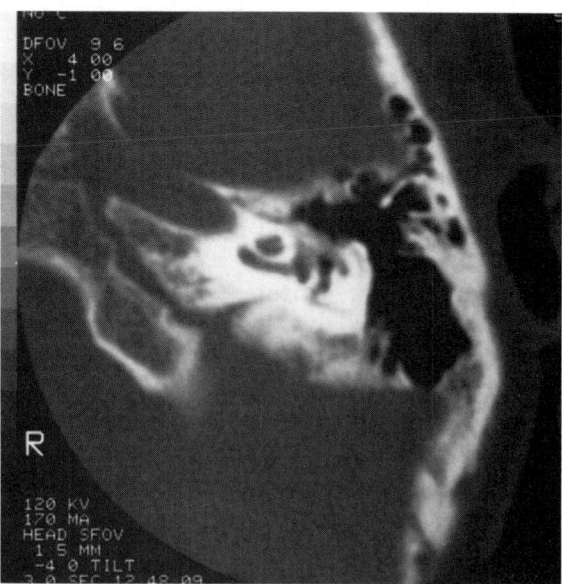

Figure 145.1 Osteogenesis imperfecta of the temporal bone in a 9-year-old boy with conductive hearing loss. This is an axial computed tomogram of the left temporal bone. There is exuberant otospongiosis of the middle-ear cleft and surrounding temporal bone with involvement of the cortical bone. (Photo courtesy of J. Michael Talbot, M.D.)

stapedotomy in patients with type I osteogenesis imperfecta than in the other types (79).

Osteopetrosis

Osteopetrosis is an inherited disorder causing faulty remodeling of bone. It can have either a dominant or a recessive pattern; the recessive type is more severe. The dominant form is characterized by progressive enlargement of the head and mandible and long-bone clubbing. Progressive cranial neuropathies are caused by nerve compression at the foramina, resulting in optic atrophy, trigeminal hypoesthesia, recurrent facial paralysis, and SNHL. The recessive form is characterized by the aforementioned features, with the addition of hepatosplenomegaly and mental retardation; death usually occurs by the second decade.

CHL may be secondary to thickening of the bone of the ossicles, meso- and epitympanum, and fixation of the stapes footplate (80,81). Recurrent facial nerve paralysis is caused by compression of the nerve along its intratemporal course. Facial paralysis may be relieved by total facial nerve decompression (82).

Paget Disease

Paget disease, or osteitis deformans, is a chronic, often progressive disorder of bone metabolism. It is characterized by bony hypertrophy and remodeling due to increased activity of both osteoclasts and osteoblasts. The etiology is unknown. It affects 3% of the population older than 40 years and up to 11% of those older than 80 years (83). Men are affected four times more frequently than women, and onset is usually in the sixth decade of life. Paget disease of the temporal bone can cause a combination of SNHL and CHL. No consistently identified pathologic changes have been found to account for the hearing loss. It is believed that both types of losses are caused by changes in bone density, mass, and geometry that dampen the normal hearing mechanisms of both the middle and inner ear. The losses are not believed to be due to ossicular fixation or compression of the cochlear nerve (84).

Otologic symptoms include hearing loss, tinnitus, and mild vestibular complaints. The facial nerve is not affected. Audiograms show mixed hearing loss with downsloping bone conduction. The conductive loss ranges from 20 to 30 dB. The SNHL in Paget disease appears to be related to generalized loss of bone mineral density of the otic capsule (85). Other signs include calvarial enlargement, enlargement of the superficial temporal artery, elevated serum alkaline phosphatase, and typical findings on radiographic studies.

Radiographic findings include thickening of the calvarium with a mixture of dense and radiolucent areas of fibrosis, areas of cortical erosion, and characteristic coarse bony trabeculae (Fig. 145.2). Treatment includes the use of calcitonin and etidronate disodium to decrease osteoclast

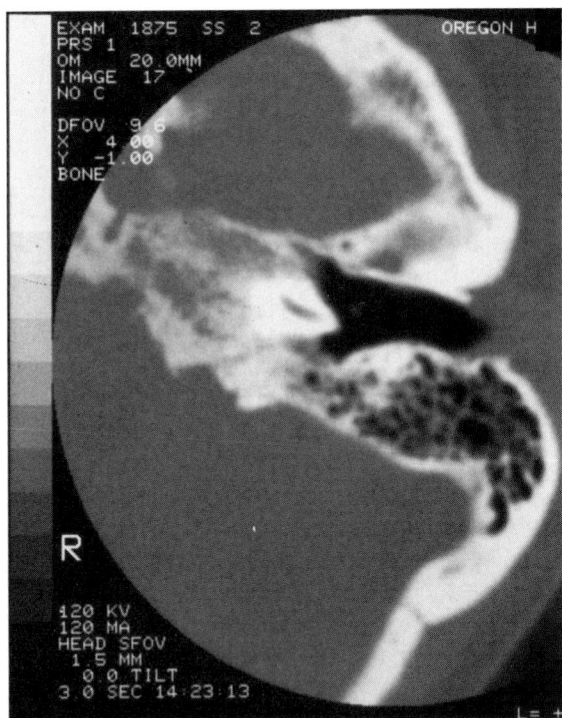

Figure 145.2 Paget disease of the temporal bone in a 68-year-old woman. This axial computed tomogram shows the multiple patchy densities visible in the petrous apex, which are typical of this disease. The thickening of the bone and involvement of the cortex are other classic features of Paget disease. (Photo courtesy of J. Michael Talbot, M.D.)

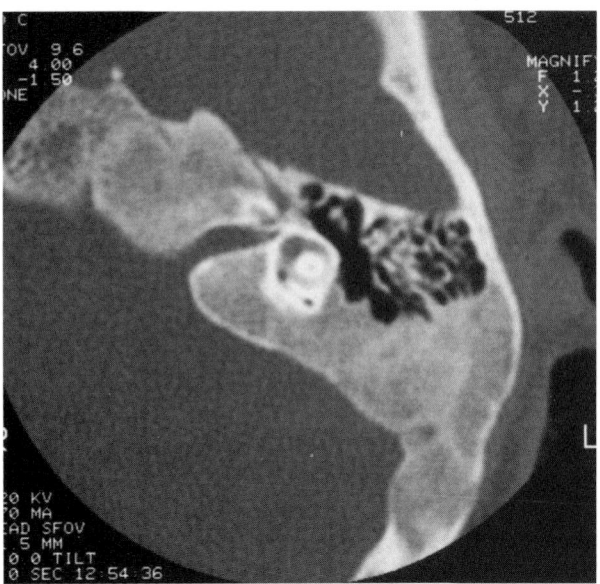

Figure 145.3 Fibrous dysplasia of the temporal bone in a 27-year-old woman with bilateral temporal bone involvement. This axial computed tomogram demonstrates the expansion of the medullary cavity with fibrous tissue and bony spicules, whereas the overlying cortical bone remains intact. (Photo courtesy of J. Michael Talbot, M.D.)

activity. The CHL caused by Paget disease is not considered amenable to surgical intervention (70).

Fibrous Dysplasia

Fibrous dysplasia is an idiopathic disorder that is characterized by replacement of normal cancellous bone by spicules of woven bone in a fibrous stroma. Involvement of the temporal bone results in painless progressive enlargement of the squamosa, mastoid, and external canal. The disease may be monostotic, polyostotic, or part of the McCune-Albright syndrome of polyostotic fibrous dysplasia, precocious puberty, and abnormal skin pigmentation. Monostotic fibrous dysplasia accounts for 70% of cases and tends to present in late childhood; lesions often become quiescent after puberty. The monostotic form is most common and usually involves the ribs, skull, proximal femur, and tibia (86). Polyostotic disease tends to present earlier, and the lesions may progress into the third and fourth decades of life. Although McCune-Albright syndrome is seen almost exclusively in females, a few cases have been reported in males (87). It presents earliest due to the endocrine abnormalities. The skeletal lesions are polyostotic, typically with a unilateral distribution. The areas of atypical skin pigmentation tend to be large, flat areas of hyperpigmentation, usually on the neck and torso. Hyperthyroidism

is the most common associated endocrinopathy, seen in 5% of patients with McCune-Albright syndrome.

Craniofacial involvement is seen in 10% to 30% of monostotic disease and 50% to 100% of polyostotic disease. The temporal bone is affected in 18% of cases with craniofacial involvement (Fig. 145.3). The most common presenting symptoms of temporal bone fibrous dysplasia are CHL (80%), progressive occlusion of the external auditory canal (85%), and canal cholesteatoma (40%) (88). Facial nerve paralysis or paresis and SNHL are other possible complications. Most CHL is due to stenosis of the external auditory canal, but involvement of the ossicular chain also may be a cause. SNHL may be attributable to involvement of the otic capsule or the internal auditory canal. Indications for surgical treatment of patients with fibrous dysplasia of the temporal bone include CHL and cholesteatoma secondary to external auditory canal stenosis. Recovery of SNHL by surgical decompression in a patient with narrowing of the internal auditory canal by fibrous dysplasia has been reported (89). Radiation therapy is contraindicated because of an increased rate of spontaneous neoplastic transformation to sarcomatous lesions.

IDIOPATHIC DISEASES

Langerhans Cell Histiocytosis

Langerhans cell histiocytosis refers to a group of idiopathic diseases, including eosinophilic granuloma, Hand-Schüller-Christian disease, and Letterer-Siwe disease. Lichtenstein, in 1953, recognized all three of these conditions as being of histiocyte origin and coined the name histiocytosis X, which is now more accurately known as Langerhans cell histiocytosis. The disease is characterized by an accumulation of histiocytes, lymphocytes, and eosinophils in the skin, bone marrow, lymph nodes, lung, liver, thymus, spleen, and central nervous system. The presence of the Langerhans cell, which is normally found in the dermis, is characteristic of the disease. These cells usually contain cytoplasmic inclusion bodies known as Birbeck granules. Most patients with Langerhans cell histiocytosis have a deficiency of suppressor lymphocytes and an elevated amount of helper lymphocytes. Definitive diagnosis is made by showing the presence of Birbeck granules on electron microscopy or immunohistochemical testing showing the presence of CD1 antigen (90). Patients are usually children, and mortality is about 10%, usually in those with multisystem disease. Adverse prognostic factors include onset before the age of 2 years, the degree of soft tissue involvement, and involvement of vital organs.

Head and neck involvement is seen in 73% of cases. The sites of involvement include the cranial vault, external auditory canal, temporal bone, cervical lymph nodes, maxilla, and mandible. Presenting symptoms can include otorrhea, aural granulation tissue, mastoid swelling, deafness, collapse of the external auditory canal, and swelling of the mandible or maxilla. Complications include SNHL, facial nerve paresis, and secondary infection.

Treatment is based on extent of disease. Systemic disease is often treated initially with steroids. Those who do not respond may be treated with etoposide, vincristine, or vinblastine. Topical or intralesional steroids may be used for localized lesions. Surgical debulking may be of use in cases of auditory canal stenosis or nerve impingement but often is done for biopsy purposes only. Patients who have involvement of the external auditory canal skin who do not respond to topical steroids may benefit from mustine otic drops, which have been shown to be efficacious (90). Radiation for lesions of the temporal bone has been used, but it carries the risk of radiation-induced malignancy.

Eosinophilic granuloma is a unifocal process that occurs in children and young adults. It consists of an osteolytic lesion in the femur, pelvis, vertebrae, ribs, skull, or temporal bone. Temporal bone symptoms include pain, swelling, purulent otorrhea, and CHL. Radiographs show a destructive lesion within the temporal bone. Radiation therapy is curative, and prognosis is excellent.

Hand-Schüller-Christian disease is similar to eosinophilic granuloma but is a multifocal process. It occurs in children younger than 5 years, who may experience systemic symptoms such as fever, anorexia, and weight loss. Splenomegaly, exophthalmos, or diabetes insipidus is seen in 50% of patients. The prognosis is less favorable than that of patients with eosinophilic granuloma, and low-dose chemotherapy may be needed in some cases to control systemic symptoms.

Letterer-Siwe disease is a rapidly progressive fulminant form of Langerhans cell histiocytosis that occurs in children younger than 3 years and demonstrates a rapidly fatal course. Systemic manifestations are prominent, for example, hepatosplenomegaly, adenopathy, coagulopathy, and skin lesions. Death occurs from bleeding or infection caused by bone marrow failure from replacement by immature histiocytes (91).

Treatment depends on the severity of disease. Surgery, radiation therapy, and chemotherapy all have been used.

HIGHLIGHTS

- Acquired sensorineural hearing loss from measles occurs in fewer than 0.1% of cases and begins at the time of the macular rash. In 45% of cases, this loss is bilateral and profound.
- Treatment of acquired syphilitic hearing loss consists of benzathine penicillin (2.4 million units) intramuscularly weekly for 6 to 12 weeks. Prednisone 30 to 60 mg every other day for 3 to 6 months is given as well.
- Fifty percent of cases of acute facial paralysis among children are caused by Lyme disease.
- Diagnosis of Lyme disease is based on a history of a tick bite and the finding of elevated antibodies for the organism *Borrelia burgdorferi*.
- Tubercular otitis is painless and is associated with single to multiple large (tympanic membrane) perforations with a pale granular or polypoid middle-ear mucosa.
- Otologic involvement can occasionally be the first and only presenting sign of Wegener granulomatosis. Facial or postauricular pain, otitis media with effusion, hearing loss, and vertigo are the most common manifestations.
- Relapsing polychondritis to the external ear is diagnosed by a painful red ear without involvement of the external canal.
- The nodules of rheumatoid arthritis that appear on the pinnae are painful and raised and have a necrotic center.
- The nodules of gout, although painful when squeezed, exude a white, chalky material.
- Paget disease is four times more common in men than in women, and hearing loss is generally nonoperable, even when a conductive loss is noted. Onset is usually in the sixth decade of life.
- Patients who have osteogenesis imperfecta generally have either conductive or sensorineural hearing loss.
- Conductive hearing loss is associated with blue sclera, whereas severe neurosensory hearing loss usually is associated with gray or white sclera.

REFERENCES

1. Arbesfeld DM. Cutaneous herpes simplex virus infections. *Am Fam Phys* 1991;43:1655–1664.
2. Aleksic SN, Budzilovich GN, Lieberman AN. Herpes zoster oticus and facial paralysis (Ramsay-Hunt syndrome): clinico-pathologic study and review of literature. *J Neurosci* 1973;20:149–159.
3. Morrow MJ. Bell's palsy and herpes zoster oticus. *Curr Treat Options Neurol* 2000;2:407–416.

4. Kanishi M, Amatasu M, Mohri M, et al. Acyclovir improves recovery rate of facial nerve palsy in Ramsay Hunt syndrome. *Auris Nasus Larynx* 2001;28:223–226.

5. Beutner KR, Friedman DJ, Forszpaniak C, et al. Valciclovir compared with acyclovir for improved therapy for herpes zoster in immunocompetent adults. *Antimicrob Agents Chemother* 1995;39:1546–1553.

6. Davis MM, Patel MS, Gebremariam A. Decline in varicella-related hospitalizations and expenditures for children and adults after introduction of varicella vaccine in the United States. *Pediatrics* 2004;114:786–792.

7. Everberg G. Deafness following mumps. *Acta Otolaryngol* 1957;48:397–403.

8. Vuori M, Lahikainen EA, Peltonen T, et al. Perceptive deafness in connection with mumps: a study of 298 servicemen suffering from mumps. *Acta Otolaryngol* 1962;55:231–236.

9. Shambaugh GE, Hagens EW, Holderman JW, et al. Statistical studies of the children in the public schools for the deaf. *Arch Otolaryngol* 1928;7:424–513.

10. McKenna MJ, Mills BG, Galey FR, Et al. Filamentous structures morphologically similar to viral nucleocapsids in otosclerotic lesions in two patients. *Am J Otol* 1986;7:25–28.

11. McKenna MJ, Mills BG. Immunohistochemical evidence of measles virus antigens in active otosclerosis. *Otolaryngol Head Neck Surg* 1989;101:415–421.

12. McKenna MJ, Adams K. Immunohistochemical demonstration of measles fusion and phosphor protein antigens in active otosclerosis. In: McCabe BF, Veldman JE, Mogi G, eds. *Proceedings of the Third International Academic Conference on Immunobiology in Otology, Rhinology and Laryngology.* New York: Kugler, 1992:101–107.

13. Niedermeyer H, Arnold W, Neubert WJ, et al. Evidence of measles virus RNA in otosclerotic tissue. *ORL J Otorhinolaryngol Relat Spec* 1994;56:130–132.

14. McKenna MJ, Kristiansen AG, Haines J. Polymerase chain reaction amplification of a measles virus sequence from human temporal bone sections with active otosclerosis. *Am J Otol* 1996;7:827–830.

15. Niedermeyer HP, Arnold W, Neubert WJ, et al. Persistent measles virus infection as a possible cause of otosclerosis: state of the art. *Ear Nose Throat J* 2000;79:552–558.

16. Bozorg Grayeli A, Palmer P, Tran Ba Huy P, et al. No evidence of measles virus in stapes samples from patients with otosclerosis. *J Clin Microbiol* 2000;38:2655–2660.

17. Saltiel P, Melmed CA, Portnoy D. Sensorineural deafness in early acquired syphilis. *Can J Neurol Sci* 1983;10:114–116.

18. Nadol JB. Hearing loss of acquired syphilis: diagnosis confirmed by incudectomy. *Laryngoscope* 1975;85:1888–1897.

19. Lukehart SA, Godomes C, Molini BJ, et al. Macrolide resistance in Treponema pallidum in the United Stated and Ireland. *N Engl J Med* 2004;351:154–158.

20. Rothenberg R. Syphilitic hearing loss. *South Med J* 1979;72:118–120.

21. Magnarelli LA. Current status of laboratory diagnosis for Lyme disease. *Am J Med* 1995;98:105–145.

22. Nadelman RB, Wormser GP. Lyme borreliosis. *Lancet* 1998;352:557–565.

23. World Health Organization (WHO). *Report on third meeting of the WHO technical advisory group on the elimination of leprosy.* Geneva: WHO, 2002, WHO/CDS/CPE/CEE/2002.29.

24. Wathen PI. Hansen's disease. *South Med J* 1996;89:647–652.

25. WHO Expert Committee on Leprosy, *World Health Organ Tech Rep Ser* 1998;874:1–43.

26. Ridley DS, Jopling WH. Classification of leprosy according to immunity: a five group system. *Int J Lepr* 1997;68:255–273.

27. Britton WJ. The management of leprosy reversal reactions. *Lepr Rev* 1998;69:225–234.

28. Lockwood DNJ. The management of erythema nodosum leprosum: current and future options. *Lepr Rev* 1996;67:253–259.

29. Jakeman P, Smith WCS. Thalidomide in leprosy reaction. *Lancet* 1994;343:432–433.

30. Bayer R, Dupuis L. Tuberculosis, public health, and civil liberties. *Annu Rev Public Health* 1995;16:307–326.

31. Robertson K, Kumar A. Atypical presentations of aural tuberculosis. *Am J Otolaryngol* 1995;16:294–302.

32. Singh B. Role of surgery in tuberculous mastoiditis. *J Laryngol Otol* 1991;105:907–915.

33. Vaamonde P, Castro C, Garcia-Soto M. Tuberculous otitis media: a significant diagnostic challenge. *Otolaryngol Head Neck Surg* 2004;130:759–766.

34. Cleary KR, Batsakis JG. Mycobacterial disease of the head and neck: current perspective. *Ann Otol Rhinol Laryngol* 1995;104:830–833.

35. Kulkami NS, Goapl GS, Ghaisas SG, Gupte NA. Epidemiological considerations and clinical features of ENT tuberculosis. *J Laryngol Otol* 2001;115:555–558.

36. Kapur V, Li L, Hamrick MR, et al. Rapid mycobacterium assignment and unambiguous identification of mutations associated with antimicrobial resistance in *Mycobacterium tuberculosis* by DNA sequencing. *Arch Pathol Lab Med* 1995;119:131–138.

37. Weiner GM, O'Connell JE, Pahor AL. The role of surgery in tuberculous mastoiditis: appropriate chemotherapy is not always enough. *J Laryngol Otol* 1997;111:752–753.

38. Saunders NC. Tuberculous mastoiditis: when is surgery indicated. *Int J Pediatr Otorhinol* 2002;65:59–63.

39. Gilbert DN. *The Sanford guide to antimicrobial therapy,* 34th ed. Hyde Park, VT: Antimicrobial Therapy, Inc. 2004:85–92.

40. Iseman MD. Treatment of multidrug-resistant tuberculosis. *N Engl J Med* 1993;329:784–791.

41. Chandresekhar SS. Otologic and audiologic evaluation of HIV infected patients. *Am J Otolaryngol* 2000;21:1–9.

42. Lalwani AK, Sooy CD. Otologic and neurotologic manifestations of acquired immunodeficiency syndrome. *Otolaryngol Clin North Am* 1992;25:1183–1197.

43. Truitt TO, Tami TA. Otolaryngologic manifestations of human immunodeficiency virus infection. *Med Clin North Am* 1999;83:303–315.

44. Stern JC, Lin P-T, Lucente FE. Benign nasopharyngeal masses and human immunodeficiency virus infection. *Arch Otol* 1990;116:206–208.

45. Fauci AS. The vasculitis syndromes. In: Braunwald E, Fauci AS, Isselbacher KJ, et al., eds. *Harrison's online.* New York: McGraw-Hill, 1999.

46. Rinaldo A, Sacilotto C, Mannara GM, et al. Wegener's granulomatosis presenting with otologic manifestations. *J Otolaryngol* 1999;28:347–350.

47. Fenton JE, O'Sullivan TJ. The otological manifestations of Wegener's granulomatosis. *J Laryngol Otol* 1994;108:144–146.

48. Bradley PJ. Wegener's granulomatosis of the ear. *J Laryngol Otol* 1983;97:623–626.

49. McCaffrey TV, McDonald TJ, Facer GW, et al. Otologic manifestations of Wegener's granulomatosis. *Otolaryngol Head Neck Surg* 1988;88:586–593.

50. Fenton JE, O'Sullivan TJ. The otological manifestation of WG. *J Laryngol Otol* 1994;108:144–146.

51. Goeken JA. Antineutrophil cytoplasmic antibody—a useful serological marker for vasculitis. *J Clin Immunology* 1991;11:605–612.

52. Isreal HL. Sulfamethoxazole-trimethoprim therapy for Wegener's granulomatosis. *Arch Intern Med* 1988;148:2293–2295.

53. Fukuda K, Yuasa K, Uchizono A, et al. Three cases of Wegener's granulomatosis treated with an antimicrobial agent. *Arch Otolaryngol Head Neck Surg* 1989;115:515–518.

54. McCaffrey TV, McDonald TJ, McCaffrey LA. Head and neck manifestations of relapsing polychondritis: review of 29 cases. *Otolaryngology* 1978;1:473–478.

55. Martin J, Roenigk HH, Lynch W, et al. Relapsing polychondritis treated with dapsone. *Arch Dermatol* 1976;112:1272–1274.

56. Park J, Gowin KM, Schumacher HR Jr. Steroid sparing effect of methotrexate in relapsing polychondritis. *J Rheumatol* 1996;23:937–938.

57. Prystowsky SD, Gilliam JN. Discoid lupus erythematosus as part of a larger disease spectrum: correlation of clinical features with laboratory findings in lupus erythematosus. *Arch Dermatol* 1975;111:1448–1452.

58. Peitersen E, Carlsen B. Hearing impairment of the initial symptom of polyarteritis nodosa. *Acta Otolaryngol* 1966;61:189–195.

59. Dudley JP, Goodman M. Periarteritis nodosa and bilateral facial paralysis. *Arch Otolaryngol* 1969;90:139–146.

60. Ozcan M, Larakus MF, Gunduz OH, et al. Hearing loss and middle ear involvement in rheumatoid arthritis *Rheum Int* 2002;22(1):16–19.

61. Raut VV, Cullen J, Cathers G. Hearing loss in RA. *J Otolaryngol* 2001;30:289–294.

62. Ohno S, Char DH, Kimura SJ, et al. Vogt-Koyanagi-Harada syndrome. *Am J Ophthalmol* 1977;83:735–740.
63. Minoda H, Sakai J, Suguira M, et al. High inducibility of Epstein-Barr virus replication in B lymphocytes in Vogt-Koyanagi-Harada disease. *Nippon Ganka Gakkai Zasshi* 1999;103:289–296.
64. Norose K, Yano A, Aosai F, et al. Immunologic analysis of cerebrospinal fluid lymphocytes in Vogt-Koyanagi-Harada disease. *Invest Ophthalmol Vis Sci* 1990;31:1210–1216.
65. Mondkar SV, Biswas J, Ganesh SK. Analysis of 87 cases with Vogt-Koyanagi-Harada disease. *Jpn J Ophthalmol* 2000;44:296–301.
66. Forster DJ, Rao NA, Hill RA, et al. Incidence and management of glaucoma in Vogt-Koyanagi-Harada syndrome. *Ophthalmology* 1993;100:613–628.
67. McCabe BF. Autoimmune sensorineural hearing loss. *Ann Otol Rhinol Laryngol* 1979;88:585–589.
68. Harris JP, Sharp P. Inner ear autoantibodies in patients with rapidly progressive sensorineural hearing loss. *Laryngoscope* 1990;100:516–524.
69. Moscicki RA, San Margin JE, Quintero CH, et al. Serum antibody to inner ear proteins in patients with progressive hearing loss: correlation with disease activity and response to corticosteroid treatment. *JAMA* 1994;272:611–616.
70. Billings PB, Keithley EM, Harris JP. Evidence linking the 68 kilodalton antigen identified in progressive sensorineural hearing loss patient sera with heat shock protein 70. *Ann Otol Rhinol Laryngol* 1995;104:181–188.
71. Bloch DB, San Martin JE, Rauch SD, et al. Serum antibodies to heat shock protein 70 in sensorineural hearing loss. *Arch Otol Head Neck Surg* 1995;121:1167–1171.
72. Wyngaarden JB, Kelley WN. *Gout and hyperuricemia.* New York: Grune & Stratton, 1979.
73. LaDu BN. Alcaptonuria. In: Stanbury JB, Wyngaarden JB, Fredrickson DS, eds. *The metabolic basis of inherited disease,* 2nd ed. New York: McGraw-Hill, 1966:303–317.
74. Motamed M, Thorne S, Narula A. Treatment of OME in children with mucopolysaccharidoses. *Int J Ped Otorhinolaryngol* 2000;53:121–124.
75. Zechner G, Altman F. The temporal bone in Hunter's syndrome (gargoylism). *Arch Klin Exp Ohren-Nasen Kehlkopfheilkd* 1968;192:137–144.
76. Prockop DJ, Kuivaniemi H, Tromp G. Inherited disorders of connective tissue. In: Braunwald E, Fauci AS, Isselbacher KJ, et al., eds. *Harrison's online.* New York: McGraw-Hill, 1999.
77. Armstrong BW. Stapes surgery in patients with osteogenesis imperfecta. *Ann Otol Rhinol Laryngol* 1984;93:634–635.
78. Albahnasawy L, Kishore A, O'Reilly BF. Results of stapes surgery on patients with osteogenesis imperfecta. *Clin Otol* 2001;26:473–476.
79. Van der Rijt AJ, Cremers CW. Stapes surgery in osteogenesis imperfecta: results of a new series. *Otol Neurotol* 2003;24:717–722.
80. Milroy CM, Micheals L. Temporal bone pathology of adult-type osteopetrosis. *Arch Otolaryngol* 1990;116:79–84.
81. Wahab Hamed AA, Linthicum FH Jr. Temporal bone osteopetrosis. *Otol Neurotol* 2004;25:635.
82. Hammersma H. Osteopetrosis (marble bone disease) of the temporal bone. *Laryngoscope* 1970;80:1518–1539.
83. Davies D. The temporal bone in Paget's disease. *J Laryngol Otol* 1970;84;553–560.
84. Khetarpal U, Schuknecht HF. In search of pathologic correlates of hearing loss and vertigo in Paget's disease: a clinical and histopathologic study of 26 temporal bones. *Ann Otol Rhinol Laryngol* 1990;99[Suppl]:1–16.
85. Monsell EM. The mechanism of hearing loss in Paget's disease of bone. *Laryngoscope* 2004;114:598–608.
86. Cohen A, Rosenwasser H. Fibrous dysplasia of the temporal bone. *Arch Otolaryngol* 1969;89:447–459.
87. Nager GT, Kennedy DW, Kopstein E. Fibrous dysplasia: a review of the disease and its manifestations in the temporal bone. *Ann Otol Rhinol Laryngol* 1982;[Suppl 92]:1–52.
88. Megerian CA, Sofferman RA, McKenna MJ, et al. Fibrous dysplasia of the temporal bone: ten new cases demonstrating the spectrum of otologic sequelae. *Am J Otol* 1995;16:408–419.
89. Morrissey DD, Talbot JM, Schleuning AJ. Fibrous dysplasia of the temporal bone: reversal of sensorineural hearing loss after decompression of the internal auditory canal. *Laryngoscope* 1997;107:1336–1340.
90. Christen HJ, Bartlau N, Hanefeld F, et al. Peripheral facial palsy in childhood—Lyme borreliosis to be suspected unless proven otherwise. *Acta Paediatr Scand* 1990;79:1219–1224.
91. Irving RM, Broadbent V, Jones NS. Langerhans' cell histiocytosis in childhood: management of head and neck manifestations. *Laryngoscope* 1994;104:64–70.

Infections of the Labyrinth

146

Arun K. Gadre   C. Y. Joseph Chang   Kamalakar C. Gadre

A detailed discussion of the anatomy of the inner ear is covered elsewhere. However, a few salient features that are relevant to the topic are discussed here. The inner ear comprises the membranous labyrinth with its contained potassium-rich endolymph. The membranous labyrinth is suspended within the bony labyrinth and floats in the sodium rich perilymph. The bony labyrinth and its contained perilymph protect the contained delicate membranous labyrinth, in much the same manner as the skull and cerebrospinal fluid (CSF) protect the brain. When compared with the eye, the inner ear is protected from the environment and physically unconnected to it. Consequently, infections of the inner ear are relatively uncommon. A variety of organisms (mainly viral and bacterial, and sometimes fungal) can invade the labyrinth, resulting in labyrinthitis. The term labyrinthitis therefore includes both cochleitis and vestibulitis. Certain organisms may have the propensity to cause damage in one or another division of the labyrinth, and symptoms and signs so produced may reflect this differential propensity. Once acute inflammation sets in the four cardinal signs of acute inflammation occur. These were listed by the first century AD by the Roman writer Celsus and include *calor* (heat), *rubor* (redness), *dolor* (pain), and *tumor* (swelling), and to these Virchow added a fifth clinical sign namely *functio laesa* or loss of function. In the inner ear, although one cannot directly perceive warmth, erythema, or edema, certain imaging modalities [e.g., magnetic resonance imaging (MRI) with gadolinium] make these effects apparent. The inner ear is devoid of pain fibers, hence patients do not complain of pain when they have an isolated labyrinthitis. On the other hand, loss of function, which is often severe and punctuated by deafness, tinnitus, and vertigo, is most pronounced.

This chapter is designed to deal chiefly with infections that are specific to the labyrinth. Although there may be some overlap, labyrinthitis that results from otitis media or systemic disease are discussed in other chapters. Since the publication of the previous edition of this book, there has been a considerable increase in our understanding of the pathologic processes involved in labyrinthitis. These have been included in this chapter.

LABYRINTHINE FORM AND FUNCTION

Anatomy

Infections can enter the sterile environment of the labyrinth through five potential avenues. These include the two windows between the middle and inner ear, namely the oval and round windows, the cochlear aqueduct, the internal auditory canal, and hematogenous spread via the circulatory system. The first and perhaps the most common route for the spread of infection is from the middle ear. Here the labyrinth abuts on the middle ear space at the oval and round windows. Of these, the round window is thought to be the predominant route for the spread of infections from the middle ear into the inner ear. Although infections of the middle ear are extremely common, those of the inner ear are relatively infrequent. The three-layered round window membrane may also serve as a barrier to the spread of infection from the middle ear.

The perilymph communicates with the CSF through the cochlear aqueduct and the internal auditory canal. Consequently, vectors of meningitis can extend into the inner ear by direct continuity between the CSF and the perilymph. The cochlear aqueduct is trumpet shaped. It begins at a tiny orifice situated on the medial wall of the basal turn of the scala tympani and runs in a plane, parallel and inferior to the internal auditory canal. It ends at a more flared out end situated at the medial aspect of the jugular foramen. Its patency decreases with age due to progressive obliteration with time. Eighty-two percent of subjects younger than 16 years have patent cochlear aqueducts, whereas only 30% of those older than 60 years have aqueducts that are patent (1). The anterior inferior quadrant of the internal auditory canal ends laterally at the cribrose area through which the cochlear nerve enters the cochlea. These foramina may form a potential route for the passage of particulate matter and bacteria from the CSF into the inner ear. The neural elements within the internal auditory canal may also form a route for the spread of neurotropic viruses. Blood-borne pathogens can gain access into the inner ear by way of labyrinthine blood vessels, which are branches of the anterior inferior cerebellar artery. A rich plexus of capillaries is observed in the stria vascularis, which can harbor these blood-borne pathogens. Thrombosis of the end arteries from infection is also detrimental to the integrity of the end organ. Organisms can infect the spiral ganglion after gaining access to the inner ear vasculature (1).

Physiology

The reader is referred to the chapters on cochlear and vestibular physiology for details. Infectious processes that disrupt the endocochlear potential, tectorial membrane, hair cells, neurons, or neural structures cause auditory dysfunction. In general, auditory nerve dysfunction is manifested by a loss of speech discrimination out of proportion to the degree of pure-tone hearing loss and by auditory brainstem response (ABR) abnormalities, such as wave delay, poor wave morphology, or poor repeatability of waveforms. Interaural asymmetry of tonic discharge of vestibular fibers is perceived as rotatory motion, and hyperactivity or hypoactivity in one labyrinth produces an imbalance that is perceived as vertigo. When sudden unilateral loss of vestibular function occurs, as in labyrinthitis, there is an initial decrease in the spontaneous activity of the vestibular nuclei of the ipsilateral side. This is mediated by cerebellar inhibition or by contralateral vestibular inhibition. With compensation spontaneous activity recovers, and this in turn is associated with functional recovery. In the acute phase of vestibular injury the vegetative symptoms such as nausea and vomiting persist for about 3 days. By the end of the first week most patients are able to ambulate and are essentially recovered by 1 month. Recovery takes longer in older individuals compared with young adults (1).

MENINGITIS AND LABYRINTHITIS

There is a close relationship between meningitis and labyrinthitis. Middle ear infections can also result in the passage of organisms into the inner ear. It must be remembered that not every case of meningitis results in labyrinthitis. However, a high index of suspicion is important to make the diagnosis. The etiology is often bacterial, but viral and fungal etiologies are also known to occur. A fundamental difference between the outcome of viral and bacterial infections is the propensity of bacterial infections to result in labyrinthitis ossificans. Viral infections cause damage to the hair cells but tend to spare the endosteum. In the case of bacterial infections on the other hand, the damaged endosteum reacts with deposition of osteoid, which can then ossify and produce changes of labyrinthitis ossificans. Labyrinthitis ossificans is not known to occur with any degree of regularity in the face of viral labyrinthitis (2). As will be seen later, this has important clinical implications in the management and timing of rehabilitation in patients with labyrinthitis (*vide infra*).

Bacterial Meningitis

Most victims are in the pediatric age group, although persons of any age may be affected. As mentioned previously, organisms can gain access through the cribrose area or the cochlear aqueduct.

Etiology

In 1978, Nadol reported that *Haemophilus influenzae*, *Neisseria meningitidis*, and *Streptococcus pneumoniae* accounted for 71% of the cases of nonfatal, bacterial meningitis among patients older than 2.5 years (3). The introduction of the *H. influenzae* type B (Hib) vaccine in 1990 has resulted in a drastic reduction of cases of *H. influenzae* meningitis and epiglottitis. Between the years 1985 to 1995, the average annual number of cases of *H. influenzae* meningitis in a pediatric population decreased by 90.5% (4). This decrease has permitted the emergence of *S. pneumoniae* as the predominant etiologic organism. Other causative organisms included β-streptococcus, *Escherichia coli*, *Citrobacter* species, *Enterococcus* species, *Mycobacterium tuberculosis*, *Salmonella* species, *Klebsiella pneumoniae*, *Pasteurella* species, *Staphylococcus aureus*, and *Listeria monocytogenes* (4).

Bacterial meningitis is the most common cause of labyrinthitis ossificans and profound acquired bilateral sensorineural hearing loss (SNHL) in childhood (3,5,6). The incidence of hearing loss following meningitis ranges from 6% to 37% and 5% have profound deafness (3,7–12). Although most victims have stable thresholds over time, about 3% show improved, worsened, or fluctuating hearing losses over time (13). Site-of-lesion testing supports a cochlear disorder rather than retrocochlear abnormality (3,13).

Although *Streptococcus*, *H. influenzae*, and *N. meningitidis* accounted for approximately 67% of all cases of nonfatal meningitis in the pediatric population (4), these same three organisms were related to 83% of the cases of hearing loss. Of the three organisms, the greatest incidence of hearing loss is due to *S. pneumoniae* (31%) and the lowest is with *H. influenzae* (6%). The mortality rate of *S. pneumoniae* meningitis (19% in children and 20% to 30% in adults) is also the highest of the three organisms (14,15).

Woolley and colleagues (4) assessed the risk factors for hearing loss in childhood meningitis using multiple logistic regression. They found low CSF glucose levels, computerized tomographic (CT) evidence of increased intracranial pressure, *S. pneumoniae* as the causative organism, male sex, and (perhaps) nuchal rigidity to be the only factors significantly predictive of subsequent hearing loss. Prompt initiation of appropriate therapy is also thought to be important to the risk of hearing loss, because auditory/vestibular damage occurs early in the course of the infection (4). It also has been suggested that the initial bacteremia precipitates the eventual hearing loss before any symptoms or signs develop (13).

Pathology

Four primary pathologic correlates of labyrinthitis are associated with meningitis: acute toxic labyrinthitis, acute suppurative labyrinthitis, chronic labyrinthitis, and labyrinthine sclerosis. The incidence of partial labyrinthine ossification has been reported to be as high as 80% in patients with profound postmeningitic deafness (12). A cellular infiltrate is seen to occur within hours to 3 days following infection in experimental animals (16,17). Changes of inflammation can be seen in the perilymphatic space even in the absence of bacteria (18). Considerable advances have been made in understanding the molecular pathophysiology of bacterial meningitis, particularly its role in the induction of meningeal inflammation and inner ear complications of meningitis (19,20). Cytokines (e.g., interleukin 1b and tumor necrosis factor-α) are believed to be important in meningeal inflammation. Another recent study in the rat model has demonstrated that reactive nitrogen species (RNS) mediated cochlear damage and a breakdown of the blood–labyrinth barrier (BLB) during meningogenic pneumococcal labyrinthitis. However adjunctive treatment with the peroxynitrite scavenger uric acid and manganese(III) mesotetrakis(4-benzoic acid)-porphyrin (MnTBAP) significantly reduced breakdown of the BLB when compared with the use of ceftriaxone alone (21). This same group also demonstrated the otoprotective nature of *N*-acetyl-*L*-cystine and Mn(III)tetrakis(4-benzoic acid)-porphyrin (MnTBAP) in meningitis-associated hearing loss in the rat model (22).

Three characteristic stages have been observed once labyrinthitis supervenes: acute inflammation, fibrosis, and ossification (23). Endolymphatic hydrops is associated with all but the end-stage labyrinthine sclerosis. With progression and mineralization of osteoid, and remodeling, the perilymphatic and then endolymphatic spaces get obliterated. Although hearing loss may occur soon after the onset of meningitis, complete ossification occurs a year after the infection (24). In a recent study, Tinling et al. (25) have demonstrated that osteoid deposition occurred as early as

3 days after infection in the gerbil model. This observation has important implications for the performing of cochlear implantation early if a patient should develop profound bilateral hearing loss on the heels of an episode of bacterial meningitis. This observation also has implications for future research with regard to the timing of medical intervention if prevention of neo-ossification is desired.

Evaluation and Management

The history and clinical findings are often dependent on the interval between the occurrence of meningitis and the request for consultation by the primary care physician or neurologist. If meningitis occurs in the presence of middle ear infection, the findings of an inflamed ear drum, fluid in the middle ear, or the presence of mucopurulent drainage or a cholesteatoma are often evident. (However, when the patient is examined months or years following the meningitis, tympanic membrane findings may be remarkably bland.) Medical intervention with antibiotics should then be commenced without delay, and surgical treatment appropriate for the otologic condition should be performed as soon as the patient is stable to undergo the procedure. Even when the patient is very ill, a myringotomy and cultures can be obtained at the bedside. Prior to any kind of surgical intervention including the performance of a myringotomy, it is important (where possible) to obtain a pure-tone audiogram and if possible vestibular testing. These together with CSF cultures helps with the use of targeted antibiotic therapy. Although other causes such as history of hyperbilirubinemia and kernicterus, ototoxic antibiotics, hypoxia, hyperpyrexia, and infectious and hereditary causes are considered, it is important to educate the patient or the caregiver that hearing loss is likely to be the result of the disease process. Although ototoxic antibiotics may be implicated in the causation of hearing loss, it is incumbent upon the otolaryngologist to educate the patient that these must sometimes be used to save the patient's life. Also patients who are bedridden may not complain of vertigo or imbalance problems caused by ototoxic medications until they are well enough to walk. Monitoring of antibiotic levels on a routine basis can help reduce this complication.

The use of methods to test hearing that do not require patient participation, in particular otoacoustic emissions (OAEs) and ABRs, have found increasing application in monitoring hearing loss. They have the advantages that the test can be performed early and may have predictive implications as well. Audiometric evaluation should be performed as soon as feasible in the acute stage and may have some predictive value. OAEs with tympanometry are recommended for young children (4); ABR testing is performed if OAEs are suspicious for hearing loss. Patients with normal ABRs in the first few days of hospitalization are unlikely to develop a SNHL (13); however, it should be remembered that a normal ABR can be misleading, because it reflects hearing only in the 2,000- to 4,000-Hz range (4). It is important to obtain behavioral audiometry as soon as possible (4).

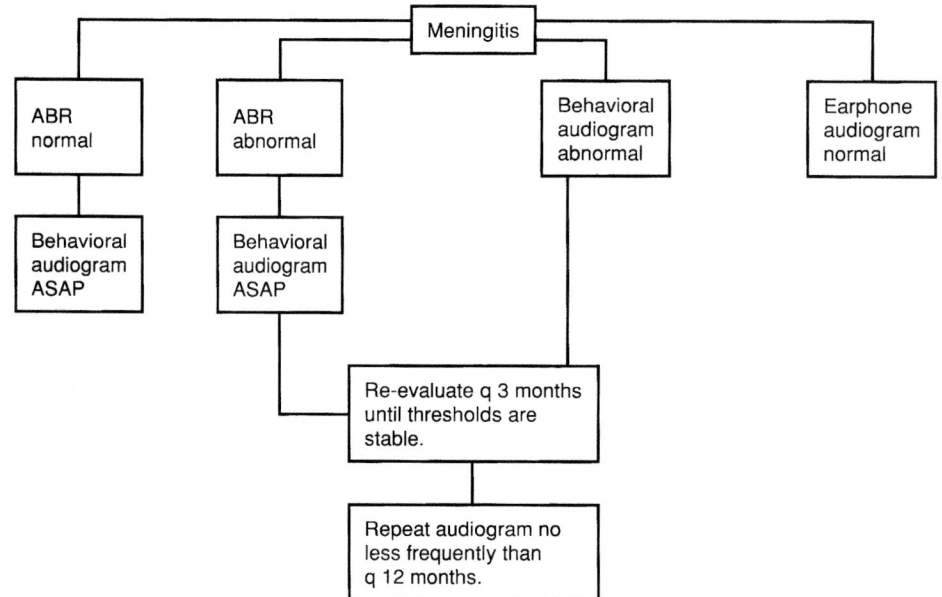

Figure 146.1 Follow-up protocol for the postmeningitic child. Otoacoustic emissions may be used as a screening test prior to auditory brainstem response testing.

Vestibular testing often is omitted, but it must be considered, even if imbalance is not the presenting complaint. In some cases, despite improvement in auditory acuity, a complete absence of vestibular response may persist (13).

Corticosteroids, specifically dexamethasone, have been evaluated for their ability to modulate the development of meningeal inflammation. Dexamethasone is effective in diminishing neurologic deficits (including SNHL) in pediatric *H. influenzae* meningitis (26,27); similar efficacy for adult meningitis remains to be demonstrated (27). With respect to pediatric *S. pneumoniae* meningitis, its neurologic complications may not be so tractable. In one meta-analysis, dexamethasone therapy was protective only if administered prior to, or concurrent with, parenteral antibiotics (26). Also, in one retrospective, nonrandomized study of 180 children with pneumococcal meningitis, dexamethasone "was not associated with a beneficial effect" (28). Hartnick et al. (29) reviewed the relationship between administration of steroids at the time of diagnosis of bacterial meningitis and the development of labyrinthitis ossificans. Of the 32 patients studied, they analyzed the data on 10 children requiring cochlear implantation who developed profound deafness from bacterial meningitis. All four patients who failed to receive steroids at the time of the initial illness developed labyrinthitis ossificans, but only one in six patients who received steroids during their initial illness developed the condition. This patient received steroids 3 days after admission. Hence, timing of administration of steroids may be just as important as the dose administered. Although steroid administration may not prevent deafness, it appears likely that its prompt use may prevent labyrinthitis ossificans, making the cochlea more amenable to the insertion of a cochlear implant. Such findings, combined

with the predominance of *S. pneumoniae* in pediatric meningitis, emphasize the importance of continuing research into other therapeutic avenues for averting hearing loss. A number of animal models of experimental pneumococcal meningitis have been developed and have shown the importance of pneumolysin as a cause of cochlear damage (30); prevention/amelioration of SNHL by combined administration of dexamethasone, ketorolac, and ampicillin (31); and diminished neuronal cell death with treatment with a broad-spectrum caspase inhibitor (N-benzyloxycarbonyl-Val-Ala-Asp-fluoromethyl-ketone, or, Z-VAD-Fmk) (32).

Brookhouser and colleagues (13) suggested a protocol for the follow-up of the postmeningitic child (Fig. 146.1). OAE screening may have a complementary role to ABR testing. Richardson et al. (33) evaluated OAE screening as compared with the gold standard of ABR testing, in a population of 124 children recovering from meningitis. They found OAE screening to have a sensitivity of 1.00 (95% confidence interval, 0.59 to 1.00), a specificity of 0.91 (0.85 to 0.97), a positive predictive value of 0.44 (0.2 to 0.7), and a negative predictive value of 1.00 (0.96 to 1.00).

The issue of the appropriateness of cochlear implantation remains a subject of debate; a 1-year trial of amplification is suggested because aidable hearing may exist, even though there is an initially profound SNHL without improvement in the unaided thresholds over time (13). Spontaneous recovery of profound postmeningitic hearing loss has been reported in the literature although this is an exceedingly rare event (34). Aso and Gibson (35) argue that recovery of profound hearing loss is extremely unlikely, and these patients should receive a cochlear implant as soon as possible. They recommend waiting 9 months in patients with residual hearing. More recently, there has been a tendency among otologists to favor early cochlear implantation in these patients because the surgery is rendered more difficult and the hearing results are poorer once ossification of the cochlea supervenes (36). In cases in which hearing loss is the result of pyogenic meningitis, it is important to perform both high-resolution computed tomography of the temporal bone and T2-weighted, gradient-echo sequences in magnetic resonance tomography to allow early detection of loss of fluid in the fibrotic stages of cochlear ossification (37). Additionally, imaging studies also helps rule in or out the presence of a congenital inner ear abnormality that is often associated with a higher incidence of meningitis. In the case of the post-meningitic adult, particularly if seen several years after the insult, the selection of the appropriate auditory rehabilitation modality is made more readily (Fig 146.2).

Viral Meningitis

Although viral infections of the labyrinth are recognized as potential causes of hearing loss or imbalance, it has been difficult to link viral meningitis to these complaints. Nadol (3) found that none of 304 cases of aseptic meningitis developed a hearing loss. Hearing loss in this subset of patients with meningitis is not as prevalent as in those with bacterial meningitis. The treatment of the hearing loss involves treatment of the condition. Hearing loss caused by varicella-zoster meningitis, which responded to treatment with acyclovir, has been reported (38).

Fungal Meningitis

Fungal organisms, such as *Cryptococcus neoformans, Aspergillus* species, *Candida albicans,* and *Coccidioides immitis,* were causative agents in only 1.3% of the cases of meningitis reported in the Massachusetts General Hospital between 1962 and 1975 (3). One can anticipate an increasing number of patients with fungal meningitis with the current human immunodeficiency virus (HIV) epidemic. Immunocompromised cancer and transplant patients are also at risk for the development of fungal meningitis.

Histopathologic studies support a neural involvement in fungal meningitis, demonstrating granulomas in the internal auditory canal and Rosenthal canal (3). Although limited audiologic data exist, fungal meningitis appears to be associated with retrocochlear lesions rather than the cochlear hearing losses seen with bacterial meningitis (3). The hearing loss following cryptococcal meningitis might be largely reversible (39). Because there are so few data on hearing loss related to fungal meningitis, it seems reasonable to recommend evaluation and management similar to that for bacterial meningitis until further information is available (Table 146.1).

Viral Labyrinthitis

Many viruses produce systemic or localized illness. It would therefore be safe to assume that they are involved in

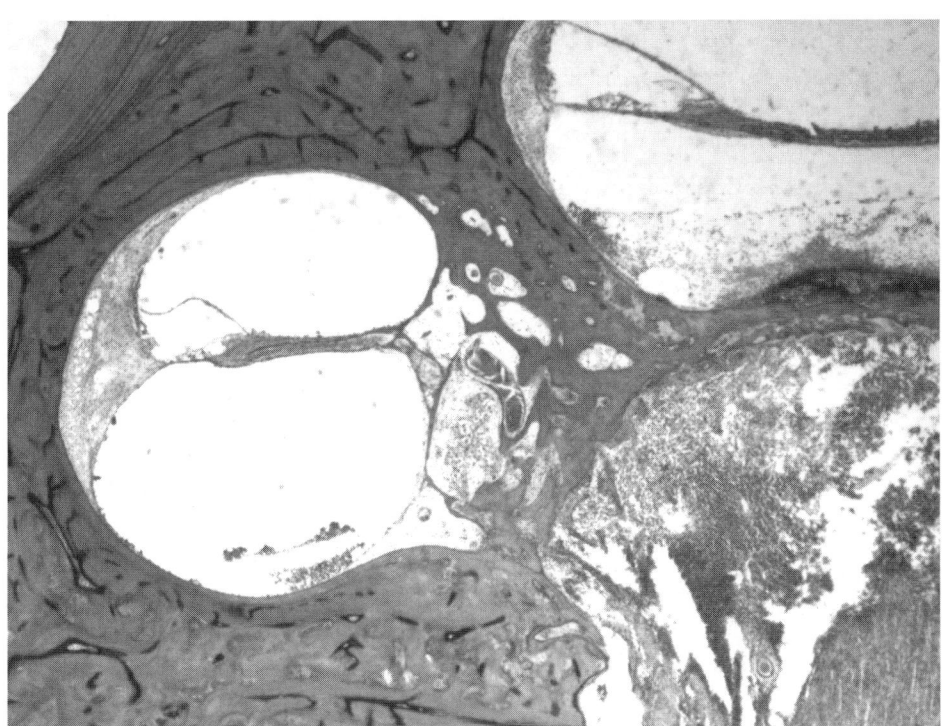

Figure 146.2 A 26-year-old man sustained a gunshot wound to the ear. At 66 years, he developed an otitis media in the injured ear and meningitis that caused his demise. Histopathology of his opposite temporal bone shows the presence of labyrinthitis resulting from pyogenic meningitis. (Photograph courtesy of Fred H. Linthicum Jr., MD and Jose N. Fayad, MD of the Eccles Temporal Bone Laboratory at the House Ear Institute, Los Angeles.) (See also Color Plate 59.)

TABLE 146.1

HEARING LOSS RELATED TO BACTERIAL OR FUNGAL MENINGITIS

Circumstance	Strategy
Diagnosis	History, especially noting ototoxic medications, perinatal risk factors, hereditary factors, or otologic infections; examination should exclude serous otitis media, acute otitis media, chronic otitis media; audiogram, ABR, and vestibular testing, as appropriate
Treatment	Antimicrobials as appropriate for the etiologic agent; steroids to combat meningeal inflammation; cochlear implantation (?); auditory rehabilitation
Complications	Sensorineural hearing loss and imbalance
Emergency	Diagnosis and immediate institution of therapy to avert sensorineural hearing loss

ABR, auditory brainstem response.
Adapted from Dodge PR, Davis, H, Feigin RD, et al. Prospective evaluation of hearing impairment as a sequela of acute bacterial meningitis. *N Engl J Med* 1984;311:869, with permission.

the causation of labyrinthitis. However evidence for their occurrence by way of satisfying of Koch's postulates remains elusive. Only two viruses—cytomegalovirus (CMV) and the mumps virus—have actually been isolated and cultured from the inner ear of affected humans (40,41).

Circumstantial evidence incriminates viruses as the likely culprits in cochleovestibular dysfunction. This includes the association of acute cochleovestibular dysfunction with a viral illness (e.g., influenza, upper respiratory infection), viral seroconversion with acute-stage titers higher than convalescent antibody titers, and histopathologic studies of acute cochleovestibular dysfunction that show changes reminiscent of known viral disease. These have failed to show evidence suggesting bacterial infection, vascular abnormalities, or labyrinthine membrane rupture (42–45), which are also speculative causes of inner ear dysfunction.

Perinatal Viral Labyrinthitis

Maternal rubella during the first trimester of pregnancy and congenital CMV infection are the most widely recognized antenatal viral infections, associated with perinatal signs and symptoms including hearing loss. The patient's history is generally of little help in making a diagnosis of viral labyrinthitis, and the manifestations of German measles is often forgotten or passed-off for another condition and hence not documented. The examination should probe for the stigmata of viral infection. Assays should be performed for urinary sediment and virus isolation, antiviral immunoglobulin M (IgM) from the infant's serum or umbilical cord, and viral isolation from throat culture or amniotic fluid. Hearing assessment should include a pure-tone audiogram (in patients who are old enough to undergo behavioral testing), OAEs and ABR as appropriate, and possibly vestibular testing. With the universal adoption of a hearing screening program, the presence of these hearing losses is more often picked up, and early intervention is instituted. Consequently, cochlear implantation, sometimes as early as at 6 months of age, is being actively investigated.

Cytomegalovirus

Congenital CMV is the most common intrauterine infection and affects between 0.4% and 2.3% of live-born infants in the United States (46–48). Only 10% to 15% of those infected exhibit clinical evidence of congenital infection at birth, but this group is more likely to experience sequelae, including SNHL, cognitive motor and visual deficits, and seizures. Approximately half the children with symptomatic CMV infection develop hearing loss, and the majority develop continued postnatal deterioration of the deficit (48,49). Symptomatic CMV infection, also called cytomegalic inclusion disease, accounts for only 1% to 2% of all congenital CMV infections and is manifested by hemolytic anemia, hepatosplenomegaly, jaundice, and purpura (40,41). Between 30% and 65% of the infants who survive the neonatal period develop a severe, relatively symmetric SNHL that is most pronounced in the high frequencies (40,50). In some instances, an initially moderate SNHL may progress over the first decade of life (40). Onset of hearing loss is often delayed (up to 6 years of age) and the course is frequently progressive and fluctuating (51). Disseminated disease at birth—as evidenced by petechiae, hepatosplenomegaly, intrauterine growth retardation, thrombocytopenia, or hepatitis—is predictive of hearing loss. In contrast, clinical evidence of central nervous system (CNS) involvement at birth is not associated with increased likelihood of developing hearing loss (49). A surprising finding in this study was that though children with microcephaly develop hearing loss, microcephaly was not a predictor of hearing loss. There is also an association between the amount of urinary excretion of CMV at birth and the percentage of patients developing hearing loss, which supports the position that disseminated disease at birth is more important in the development of hearing loss than is isolated neurologic involvement. This finding helps in the counseling of parents of children born with congenital CMV. The viral load in urine and blood early infancy was predictive of hearing loss with a substantial number of children demonstrating progression of hearing loss during childhood (52).

CMV, a member of the herpesvirus group, is a large, DNA-containing virus. Its name derives from the characteristic light microscopic changes it induces in infected cells, including cytomegaly (up to 25 mm in diameter) and intranuclear (acidophilic) and cytoplasmic (basophilic) inclusion bodies (53). When latent within cells, it can escape microscopic visualization and remaining detectable only by special histochemical techniques (53). Inclusion-laden cells are seen at pathology within the membranous labyrinth.

Cochlear alterations, most severe in the basal turn, include hydrops or collapse of the Reissner membrane and inclusion bodies in the cells of the stria vascularis and the endolymphatic surface of the Reissner membrane (40). The route of labyrinthine invasion remains controversial, although there is some evidence supporting the idea of a viremic spread to the modiolar vessels with subsequent involvement of the spiral ganglion cells (53,54). Although CMV has been demonstrated in the endothelial structures of the endolymphatic space, CMV has been detected in the perilymph by quantitative real-time polymerase chain reaction (55). Children of immune mothers are just as likely to develop congenital CMV infection as children of non-immune mothers. This suggests that the latent virus in the mother can be reactivated and cross the placenta to infect the fetus (40). There is a high risk of postnatal transmission of human CMV to the infant via breast milk because many seropositive mothers have virus reactivation during lactation and shedding of the virus in breast milk. Previous studies have demonstrated that the rate of transmission by consuming CMV-positive breast milk is as high as 38% in the preterm infant (56,57). However, early results indicate that CMV-positive breast milk does not have a negative effect on neural development and hearing in this group of patients (58).

Asymptomatic CMV infection constitutes the bulk of neonatal disease, and 8% to 15% of affected infants can be expected to have a mild to moderate SNHL, although unilateral and bilateral profound losses have been reported (40,50). The diagnosis of congenital CMV infection is suggested by the radiographic demonstration of intracerebral calcium deposits in a microcephalic child (41). The history obtained from the mother, although it may help exclude the possibility of a rubella infection, generally is not helpful in the case of congenital CMV infection because most maternal infections are asymptomatic (40). Because 97% of the infantile cases are asymptomatic, there are none of the physical stigmata of cytomegalic inclusion disease. Laboratory testing is helpful in establishing the diagnosis. "Owl-eye" bodies, representing infected renal tubular cells that have the virally induced intranuclear inclusions, can be identified on microscopic examination of fresh urinary sediment only during the first week of life. Isolation of CMV from fresh urine during the first 3 weeks of life can clinch the diagnosis in symptomatic and asymptomatic cases;

saliva, blood, or other tissue can be used, but they have lower viral concentrations. *The diagnosis of congenital CMV infection is difficult to establish after the first year of life because normal infants can become infected asymptomatically, shed virus in their urine, and develop antibody titers.* Fortunately, it is unusual for a CMV infection acquired after birth to cause SNHL (40). Early diagnosis is important because there may be effective therapy. In a phase II trial, Whitley et al. (59) reported hearing improvement or stabilization in 16% of 30 babies with symptomatic congenital CMV infection with ganciclovir therapy. In a follow-up landmark study, Kimberlin et al. (60), concluded that ganciclovir therapy begun in the neonatal period in symptomatically infected infants with CMV infection prevented hearing deterioration at 6 months and may prevent hearing deterioration beyond 1 year. Almost two thirds of the patients on ganciclovir develop neutropenia, and white cell counts must be monitored while on this medication (60).

Monitoring of auditory function is probably best done according to the timetable for postmeningitic SNHL (Fig. 146.1), with similar recommendations for amplification. The recommendations may need to be modified according to concomitant mental or physical handicaps. As reported by Fowler et al. (50), only 5.2% of all infants with congenital CMV infection had hearing loss at birth. They found late-onset hearing loss in an additional 3.2% of children at 1 year of age and in an additional 7% by 6 years of age.

Rubella

Rubella as a cause of hearing loss continues to remain a problem in developing countries, but in an era when international travel is increasingly frequent, it must be considered in the United States as well. In fact, most recent literature on the subject is from developing countries. In the not too distant past, large epidemics have occurred in the United States at 6- to 8-year intervals. This cycle was interrupted in 1969 with the introduction of the rubella vaccination program. In addition, there have been no epidemics reported in the United States since the 1964 to 1965 pandemic (61). Rubella is caused by an RNA-containing virus, which produces a disease similar to measles (rubeola). It is less severe than measles and is sometimes referred to as German measles. It consists of rash, adenopathy, fever, and malaise. The presence of postauricular and occipital lymphadenopathy with a maculopapular rash that tends to remain discrete and rarely coalesces should raise suspicion of the disease. If rubella infection is acquired *in utero*, it produces multiple malformations, including those of the temporal bone. The usual findings on histopathologic examination of involved temporal bones, although not specific for rubella, include cochleosaccular degeneration and strial atrophy (41). There are no experimental studies that shed light on the route of viral entry to the labyrinth.

The most recent epidemic of congenital rubella occurred in 1965 and resulted in deafness in more than

12,000 infants (40). Vaccination has decreased the incidence of congenital rubella dramatically, and most papers on the subject are now from populations who do not have access to or are not vaccinated. Like congenital CMV infections, congenital rubella infections occur in symptomatic and asymptomatic forms. The symptomatic form (i.e., the rubella syndrome) implies infection in the first trimester of pregnancy and produces hearing loss in about 50% of the patients. It also results in congenital cardiac malformations, visual loss (e.g., cataracts, glaucoma, retinitis, microphthalmia), osteitis, motor deficits, thrombocytopenic purpura, hepatosplenomegaly, icterus, anemia, low birth weight, and cerebral damage and mental retardation. It is rare to see birth defects in the child if the mother is infected after the fourth month of pregnancy. The asymptomatic form arises from infection during the second or third trimesters of pregnancy, is silent at birth, and is associated with hearing loss in 10% to 20% of those affected (40). Unlike CMV, the rubella virus does not appear to have the ability to reactivate from a latent phase and cross the placenta to infect the fetus of an immune mother. Although the rubella vaccine, if given to a nonimmune pregnant woman, can cross the placental barrier to infect the fetus, the risk of subsequent hearing loss is small (40). Symptomatic rubella should be considered in evaluating an infant who has hearing loss associated with cardiac abnormalities or cataracts. The mother may recall a rubella-like infection, although the history of a rash-associated illness during pregnancy is not considered reliable for the diagnosis (40). Often this is not the case and the mother may have no recollection of the illness during pregnancy.

Physical examination of the child is usually unrevealing, except for symptomatic cases in which the physician may observe associated malformations. Laboratory testing is useful in the diagnosis of congenital rubella infections and includes the isolation of the rubella virus from the urine of the infant during the first few weeks of life. Isolation of rubella virus from throat cultures, detection of anti-rubella IgM antibodies in the neonatal serum, or documentation of an increasing titer of antirubella antibody during the first few months after birth can independently substantiate the diagnosis of congenital rubella. The diagnosis of congenital rubella has been established *in utero* by the isolation of the rubella virus from amniotic fluid, which also has been performed for congenital CMV infection (40).

Children afflicted with hearing loss from intrauterine infection generally have bilateral, although possibly asymmetric, SNHL. It is most often profound (55% of patients), with severe (30%) or mild to moderate (15%) deficits occurring less frequently (40). In some patients, the hearing loss may progress (40). Generally, all frequencies are affected equally, with a middle frequency (500 to 2000 Hz) accentuation existing in some cases (40). Speech discrimination may be poor. A central site of lesion has been hypothesized as operative in children with normal pure-tone thresholds but poor speech development (40).

As with CMV infections, vestibular testing may document a hypoactive vestibular response or frank unilateral or bilateral canal paresis (40). Management is similar to that outlined (Fig. 146.1) for postmeningitic SNHL.

Postnatal Viral Labyrinthitis

Based on clinicopathologic studies, Schuknecht (42) developed a classification of neurolabyrinthitis describing the labyrinthine disorders thought to be related to viruses for the reasons cited earlier. This classification delineates acute viral labyrinthitis (acute cochlear labyrinthitis, acute vestibular labyrinthitis, and acute cochleovestibular labyrinthitis), acute viral neuritis (acute cochlear neuritis, acute vestibular neuritis, and acute cochleo-vestibular neuritis), and delayed endolymphatic hydrops (ipsilateral, contralateral, and bilateral) (42). As observed earlier, viral labyrinthitis is not generally associated with labyrinthitis ossificans.

Neurolabyrinthitis

Acute viral labyrinthitis describes involvement of the auditory or vestibular end organs, and acute neuritis refers to a disruption of cochlear or vestibular peripheral nerve function. With current diagnostic methods, it is not always possible to differentiate labyrinthitis from neuritis, although for the cochlea, site-of-lesion testing, including speech discrimination testing, recruitment testing, OAEs, and ABR testing, may suggest an answer. Because therapy is not altered by the distinction, this pathologic detail has limited practical relevance.

Acute Cochlear Labyrinthitis and Neuritis

Acute cochlear labyrinthitis of viral etiology afflicts about 10 of 100,000 persons annually in the United States (43). This rate probably varies from year to year according to the virulence of the viruses affecting the population. Acute cochlear labyrinthitis, also referred to as idiopathic sudden sensorineural hearing loss (ISSNHL), has been defined as the loss of at least 30 dB of hearing in at least three contiguous frequencies in fewer than 3 days in an otherwise healthy person (43).

Many viruses have been implicated in ISSNHL, particularly the influenza B, mumps, rubeola, CMV, and varicella-zoster viruses (43). Primary infection and host-virus interaction have been hypothesized as mechanisms leading to the hearing loss (43). The SNHL sustained initially may vary from mild to profound. Although it is usually unilateral, it may be bilateral or sequential. Histopathologic examination most commonly shows a loss of cochlear hair cells, most severe at the basal turn, with relative preservation of other elements of the cochlear duct and the spiral ganglion neurons. Documentation of changes consistent with acute cochlear neuritis is rare, with only one patient showing solely total atrophy of the cochlear neurons in the affected ear (42). In a recent study from the same laboratory, loss of hair cells and supporting cells within the organ of Corti, with or without atrophy of the tectorial membrane, stria vascularis, spiral limbus, and cochlear neurons was the commonest finding (62). Vascular etiology was thought to be the cause in only one ear. The authors summarized that membrane breaks, perilymph fistulae, or vascular occlusion were generally not the cause of ISSNHL. They have put forth an intriguing hypothesis that cellular stress pathways involving nuclear factor-[kappa] B within the cochlea may be involved (62). MRI may be useful in the identification of neuritis, similar to Bell palsy or herpes zoster oticus.

ISSNHL is one of the few true emergencies in otology because prompt initiation of appropriate therapy may improve or totally reverse the hearing loss. The patient usually complains of the sudden onset of hearing loss, noticed during the day or on first arising in the morning, and experiences concomitant aural fullness or tinnitus. Pain is not associated with ISSNHL. The otolaryngologist must ensure that there is no prior history of surgical, head, or pressure-induced trauma. About 50% of these patients recall a recent viral infection (e.g., upper respiratory infection, herpes-type cold sore). The patient also may complain of disequilibrium or true vertigo. A complete examination should include neurologic evaluation to establish that there are no other cranial neuropathies and to detect any nystagmus. Otologic examination is mandatory and reveals normal external auditory canals and tympanic membranes bilaterally.

Laboratory testing is performed to exclude other possible causes for ISSNHL, but a full audiometric evaluation is the key initial step (43). The audiometric configuration has prognostic value (63). Vestibular testing by electronystagmography (ENG) also has prognostic value; patients with normal ENGs have a statistically greater likelihood of hearing recovery than do those with abnormal ENGs (e.g., directional preponderance, canal paresis, or absent vestibular response) (63). A labyrinthitis that is severe enough to involve the vestibular system in addition to the cochlea (i.e., acute cochleovestibular labyrinthitis) is expected to cause a more severe cochlear deficit. The possibility of a vestibular schwannoma should be excluded by gadolinium-enhanced magnetic resonance (MR) scanning. In a retrospective study of 182 patients with sudden or progressive SNHL of unknown etiology, serologic tests for herpes simplex and varicella-zoster viruses (IgM and IgG titers), Lyme disease, syphilis, and HIV were performed. The infection screening was positive in only 1 of 182 patients (0.6%) and this patient was diagnosed with latent syphilis (64). Based on this study, the authors recommended that infection screening be limited to patients with suspect histories or symptomatologies, except for patients with a diagnosis of syphilis.

If the patient is seen within the first 10 days after onset of the SNHL, high-dose corticosteroid therapy is begun, barring any medical contraindications, and is tapered over the next 12 days (63). Aspirin is forbidden, and antacids or proton pump inhibitors are administered concomitantly. In a double-blind, randomized, prospective, placebo-controlled study, corticosteroid therapy enhanced the likelihood of hearing recovery in the intermediate hearing loss range of ISSNHL (63). The efficacy of valacyclovir (1 g three times a day) in conjunction with corticosteroid therapy with prednisone has demonstrated that valacyclovir has no beneficial effect in the treatment of sudden SNHL (65). Similar findings have been reported by others using acyclovir (66,67). The role of steroids administered intratympanically is also being explored. In a small number of patients, Chandrasekhar (68) demonstrated both safety and efficacy of intratympanic dexamethasone in the management of ISSHL.

Carbogen (i.e., 95% oxygen and 5% carbon dioxide) inhalational therapy is an unproved modality of treatment, as is the administration of dextran or other vasodilating agents. Dextran administration has resulted in the death of at least one patient treated for ISSNHL, which is not a life-threatening disorder. The prognosis for hearing recovery can be quantified using information such as patient age, audiometric configuration, and electronystagmographic findings (69). Prompt treatment with steroids (i.e., within 14 days of onset) was felt to be most important for the recovery of hearing (70). Patients who are seen long after the onset of ISSNHL or in whom the hearing does not recover should receive appropriate hearing aid evaluation and fitting. Patients must also be provided with information about hearing protection in the better hearing ear. They must be urged to report to their otologist immediately, if any deterioration of hearing in this ear is perceived. Yearly audiograms are advised.

Acute Vestibular Labyrinthitis or Neuritis

The syndrome of acute, prolonged vertigo of peripheral origin is commonly called vestibular neuritis, although terms such as vestibular neuronitis, labyrinthitis, neurolabyrinthitis, and unilateral vertigo of unknown etiology have also been used (71). It is also sometimes referred to as epidemic vertigo and is a relatively common disorder. The fact that the condition often has a viral prodrome, that it occurs in epidemics, that it may affect several members of a family, and that it occurs most often in spring and early summer all support a viral etiology (71). The patient may recall a recent influenza-like illness, an upper respiratory infection, or contact with others suffering from vertigo (72).

It is defined as the sudden, unilateral loss of vestibular function without associated auditory or CNS symptoms in an otherwise healthy adult (72). There are single-attack and multiple-attack forms of the disease (72). In contrast to ISSNHL, in which the cochlear end organ is more commonly involved than the cochlear nerve, isolated atrophy of the vestibular nerves is the rule on histopathologic examination of cases of vestibular neuritis and atrophy of the vestibular end organs is rare (e.g., a single case in the Massachusetts Eye and Ear Infirmary temporal bone collection) (42,72). The histopathologic changes seen in cases of vestibular neuritis are thought to be most compatible with a viral cause because they closely mimic the alterations seen with herpes zoster infection of the vestibular system (72).

Coates suggested diagnostic criteria for vestibular neuritis: an acute, unilateral peripheral vestibular disorder without an associated hearing loss, occurrence predominately in middle age, a single episode of severe and prolonged vertigo, decreased caloric response in the involved ear, and complete subsidence of the symptoms within 6 months (72). These criteria were deemed too restrictive, and a chronic form of the disease is recognized as consisting of recurrent episodes of disequilibrium frequently associated with persistent or intermittent unsteadiness (72).

Entities to be considered in the differential diagnosis include Ménière disease, vestibular schwannoma, and cerebellar infarction in particular. The attacks of Ménière disease are usually shorter than those of vestibular neuritis and usually are associated with auditory symptoms. A cerebellar infarction may present with acute vertigo and increased intracranial pressure. MR scanning may be the only way to differentiate acute vestibular neuritis from a vestibular schwannoma, although retrocochlear signs on audiometric testing are expected with schwannoma.

The typical history consists of the sudden onset of acute vertigo, which is severe with acute vestibular labyrinthitis and of variable severity with acute vestibular neuritis. There are no associated CNS or auditory symptoms. The vertigo may be severe enough to precipitate nausea and vomiting. The acute phase of the disease generally lasts several days to a few weeks as the mechanisms of vestibular compensation adjust, and complete recovery is expected within 6 months. The multiple-attack variant manifests with recurring episodes of vertigo, although the attacks are milder and briefer than those of the single-attack form (72). A common feature of vestibular neuritis is selective damage to the superior part of the vestibular labyrinth (horizontal and superior semicircular canals and utricle) with a sparing of the inferior part supplied by the inferior vestibular nerve (73). Positional vertigo, like that of benign paroxysmal positional vertigo, may therefore appear in the recovery phase even though the superior and horizontal canals have no function (71). In the acute phase, physical examination reveals a visibly ill, usually middle-aged patient with pallor, diaphoresis, and cold, clammy skin. Movement tends to aggravate the dizziness and may precipitate emesis. Complete examination generally reveals only spontaneous nystagmus. The patient may or may not be able to stand. When they can stand they can do so without support. Cranial nerve examination should be unremarkable and, except for the unsteadiness expected for an acute labyrinthine disorder, there should be no cerebellar abnormalities.

Audiometric evaluation is obtained to document the absence of any auditory deficit or an asymmetric auditory deficit. Electronystagmographic testing in the acute phase may show only intense spontaneous nystagmus, but it also may document a unilateral decreased vestibular response or absent vestibular response. Appropriate imaging is performed to exclude the diagnosis of cerebellar infarction if there are cerebellar signs or a vestibular schwannoma. The diagnosis of vestibular neuritis is usually made clinically, and on the basis of the appearance of the nystagmus, a positive head thrust test, and a negative neurologic examination, one can be confident of the diagnosis of unilateral peripheral vestibulopathy (74). It must be remembered that the positive head-thrust test (as evidenced by a catch up saccade) may occur with brainstem infarction involving the root entry zone of the eighth cranial nerve and is not pathognomonic for peripheral lesions alone; however, this pathology of the brainstem is more often associated with other neurologic findings such as facial and contralateral body hypesthesia, facial weakness, Horner syndrome, and occasional speech and swallowing dysfunction.

Treatment consisting of vestibular suppressants (Table 146.2), hydration, and antiemetics is supportive only, anticipating the patient's gradual recovery through compensation. After the first few days of the acute episode, the vestibular suppressant therapy can be tapered to minimize its potential effect on the compensatory mechanisms (75). A few patients with the multiple-attack form of the disease may have sufficient symptoms to warrant vestibular nerve section (Table 146.3). Because the pathophysiology is uncertain there is no established treatment and symptomatic therapy is often used. The main classes of drugs used are antihistamines, anticholinergic agents, antidopaminergic agents, and gamma aminobutyric acid-enhancing (GABAergic) agents (74, 75). Two recent randomized clinical trials found that dimenhydrinate (50 mg) was more efficacious than lorazepam (2 mg) and that dimenhydrinate was as efficacious as droperidol in an emergency room setting (76,77). During the acute phase it is useful to administer this drugs intramuscularly or intravenously. All medications are sedating, and must not be administered when

TABLE 146.2
THERAPY FOR VERTIGO

Treatment	Dosage
Severe	
Dramamine (dimenhydrinate)	50 mg i.m. every 6 h
Innovar (droperidol/fentanyl citrate)	0.5–2.0 mL, one dose, i.v. or i.m.
Mild to moderate	
Valium (diazepam) and	2 mg orally t.i.d.
Robinul (glycopyrrolate)	2 mg orally b.i.d.
Antivert (meclizine)	25–50 mg orally every 6 h
Dramamine (dimenhydrinate)	50 mg orally every 4 h

i.m., intramuscularly; i.v., intravenously; t.i.d., three times daily; b.i.d., twice daily.

TABLE 146.3

POSTNATAL VIRAL LABYRINTHITIS

Circumstance	Strategy
Diagnosis	History should especially survey for viral illness; examination is generally but not specifically helpful; tests include those considered for ISSNHL
Treatment	Corticosteroids, vestibular suppressants; carbogen and early treatment with acyclovir are experimental; vestibular nerve section
Emergency	Sudden hearing loss is a true otologic emergency

ISSNHL, idiopathic sudden sensorineural hearing loss.

a high level of alertness is required. These medications should be stopped once the acute phase has passed and vestibular rehabilitation program must be started as quickly as possible. In one small controlled study, corticosteroids were more effective than placebo in treating the acute symptoms of vestibular neuritis (78).

MUMPS, MEASLES, AND VARICELLA-ZOSTER INFECTIONS

Discussion of the third category of neurolabyrinthitis, delayed endolymphatic hydrops, is best preceded by a review of the temporal bone manifestations of mumps, rubeola (measles), and varicella-zoster infections.

Mumps

The mumps virus is a paramyxovirus that causes a symptom complex of parotitis, orchitis, meningoencephalitis and, in 0.05% of cases, hearing loss (40). The hearing loss usually occurs at the end of the first week of the parotitis; it is unilateral in 80% of the patients; and it can range from a mild, high-frequency SNHL (i.e., more severe impact on the basal turn of the cochlea) to a profound SNHL (40,41). Vestibular involvement is uncommon. The mumps virus has been isolated from the perilymph of a patient with parotitis-associated sudden SNHL (40). Evidence supports the hypothesis that a subclinical mumps infection can cause ISSNHL in an otherwise healthy person (41,43,44).

Histopathologic examination of available temporal bones has shown alterations, most severe basally, of the cochlear duct structures, including atrophy of the organ of Corti and stria vascularis with collapse of the Reissner membrane (41). Associated findings include deformation and detachment of the tectorial membrane and moderate loss of spiral ganglion cells in the basal turn; the vestibular structures appear unscathed (41). Experimental mumps

labyrinthitis suggests that perilymph contamination from CSF leads to labyrinthine involvement. In humans, the late development of deafness is thought to be consistent with labyrinthine involvement from CSF, but mumps meningitis has not been correlated with the development of SNHL (3,40).

Countries in which the mumps vaccine is routinely administered (such as the United States) have achieved nearly complete elimination of mumps deafness (79). Such coverage is not global, so mumps remains a diagnostic consideration for the United States–based otolaryngologist, as is the case for many other diseases that have been essentially eliminated in the United States by immunization.

A unilateral hearing loss may go undetected in childhood until school screening is performed, and the diagnosis is not made as easily as when the patient is seen in the acute phase of the disease. The examiner may need to perform a complete investigation for other potential causes of unilateral SNHL (e.g., trauma, tumor). The physical examination generally is unrevealing, except for the stigmata of parotitis in the acute phase of the illness.

In the acute phase, the mumps virus may be isolated from the throat or from the CSF; the diagnosis also may be confirmed by documenting a fourfold change in mumps antibody titers between acute (i.e., onset and 1 month after illness) and convalescent (i.e., 3 months after onset) levels (40,43). Audiometric testing should be performed to document the degree of hearing loss sustained; the hearing loss is cochlear rather than retrocochlear. Electronystagmographic testing can reveal vestibular hyporeactivity or an absent vestibular response, even in patients without a history of dizziness (40).

Although ISSNHL has been related to the mumps virus and steroid therapy has proved beneficial in a subset of ISSNHL patients, no data exist to support such therapy for acute parotitis and SNHL. Studies are needed to evaluate steroid and antiviral therapies (Table 146.4).

Measles

The rubeola virus is an RNA myxovirus, similar in structure to the mumps virus, which gives rise to the clinical syndrome of measles (i.e., morbilli) consisting of rash, conjunctivitis,

TABLE 146.4

MUMPS LABYRINTHITIS

Circumstance	Strategy
Diagnosis	History of viral illness is important, as is parotid swelling found during examination; testing should include audiogram
Treatment	Indeterminate for acute stage; appropriate amplification for late stage

TABLE 146.5
MEASLES LABYRINTHITIS

Circumstance	Strategy
Diagnosis	History of viral illness important; examination should look for xanthematous rash, Koplik spots, conjunctivitis, and acute otitis media; testing should include throat culture, comparing acute and convalescent rubeola titers, immunofluorescence of epithelium, audiogram, electronystagmographic results
Treatment	Indeterminate for acute stage; appropriate amplification for late stage

and buccal mucosal lesions known as Koplik spots. Permanent SNHL, occurring in fewer than 0.1% of these patients, is usually bilateral, although it may be asymmetric, worst in the high frequencies, and mild to moderate (55% of patients) or profound (45%) (40,41). Loss of vestibular function, manifested by reduced or absent caloric responses, occurs in as many as 72% of patients (40). The development of the measles vaccine has markedly decreased the incidence of measles-related acquired hearing loss, which in the 1930 to 1950 literature was estimated to account for 4% to 10% of the cases of childhood-acquired SNHL (40,41).

The characteristic alterations induced by the measles virus consist of multinucleated giant cells known as Warthin-Finkeldey cells. Temporal bone findings associated with measles labyrinthitis include atrophy of the organ of Corti, which is worst at the basal aspect of the cochlea or culminates in its complete absence. There are associated degenerative changes in the spiral ganglion, stria vascularis, and tectorial membrane and collapse of the Reissner membrane (41). In the pars superior, the cristae and maculae exhibit atrophy of their neurosensory elements (41).

Animal models of measles labyrinthitis demonstrate viral infection of the spiral ganglion, organ of Corti, and vestibular ganglion cells, with the characteristic multinucleated giant cells (40). Much of the same anamnestic data are acquired as in the evaluation for mumps-associated SNHL. In the acute phase, physical examination demonstrates the exanthematous rash of measles, Koplik spots (i.e., small white foci representing necrotic lesions of the buccal mucosa in the region of Stensen ducts), and mild conjunctivitis. Rarely, there may be an associated acute otitis media, but it is not a cause of bilaterally profound SNHL (41).

The diagnosis of measles in the acute stage can be determined by isolating the rubeola virus from throat cultures, documenting a fourfold increase in the titers of antibody to the rubeola virus between the acute and convalescent sera, or immunofluorescent staining of the exfoliated epithelium from the oropharynx or conjunctiva, which can demonstrate rubeola antigen (40). Audiometric evaluation usually reveals an asymmetric SNHL that is more severe for the high

frequencies (40). ENG, including caloric testing, can document the presence and severity of vestibular dysfunction.

There is no clear documentation that steroid or antiviral therapy can benefit acute disease by preventing or ameliorating the SNHL. Long-term management consists of hearing aid evaluation and fitting or possibly cochlear implantation in the most severely affected cases (Table 146.5).

Varicella-Zoster

The varicella-zoster virus is a member of the herpesvirus group, a DNA viral family that also includes herpes simplex types I and II, CMV, and Epstein-Barr virus. Characteristic of its group, it can reactivate from a latent state to cause symptoms (80). Primary infection with the virus is manifested clinically as chickenpox, with a characteristic pustular rash, and although hearing loss may develop, it generally is due to an associated otitis media (40).

Herpes zoster oticus (i.e., Ramsay Hunt syndrome) was described by James Ramsay Hunt in 1907 and develops when the latent virus is reactivated and consists of variable severity of facial nerve paralysis, SNHL, and vertigo in association with a painful vesicular rash of the external auditory canal and concha (41). It is not established that the activated virus arises from the geniculate ganglion as is commonly hypothesized; alternative theories hypothesize an initial encephalomeningomyelitis that secondarily spreads from the CSF to the labyrinth (41).

Inflammatory neuritis of the facial, cochlear, and vestibular nerves is the predominant finding in herpes zoster oticus (40,41). Associated findings include atrophy of cochlear neurons and of the sensorineural elements of the vestibular labyrinth, collapse of the Reissner membrane, and fibrous tissue and neo-ossification in the perilymphatic compartment of the lateral semicircular canal (40,42). The herpesvirus family, including the varicella-zoster virus, has been implicated in the development of ISSNHL without associated vesicular eruption or facial nerve paralysis (80).

The patient must have a history of previous chickenpox, and there should be a vesicular rash of the external ear to diagnose herpes zoster oticus, although herpes zoster can

TABLE 146.6
VARICELLA-ZOSTER INFECTION

Circumstance	Strategy
Diagnosis	History of chickenpox in the past and immunocompromise; testing should include isolation of virus from vesicles, varicella-zoster antibody titers (acute and convalescent), audiogram; auditory brainstem response, and electronystagmographic and facial nerve testing
Treatment	Corticosteroids, acyclovir, amplification

be reactivated without a rash (40). Patients may be iatrogenically immunocompromised or may have an HIV infection disrupting immune function. The examination should document the degree of facial nerve dysfunction and any vesicular eruption. Occasionally, the external auricular rash may present as a severe external otitis, obscuring more medial structures. Varicella-zoster virus can be isolated from vesicular fluid to establish the diagnosis; acute and convalescent antibody titers, if documenting a fourfold change, also can establish the diagnosis.

Various degrees of SNHL develop in about 6.5% of the patients with Ramsay Hunt syndrome. The hearing loss is worst in the high frequencies and can have characteristics of a sensory or neural lesion (40,41). ABR testing usually documents cochlear neuritis. Electronystagmographic testing may reveal a reduced or absent vestibular response in the involved ear. Recently, two cases were reported wherein cochleovestibular symptoms outweighed the facial nerve symptoms and presumably represent reactivation of the virus in the spiral and/or vestibular ganglion (81). In the only prospective study of patients with Ramsay Hunt syndrome, 14% developed vesicles after the onset of facial palsy, and some never develop vesicles at all but had a fourfold increase in antibodies to varicella-zoster virus. Therefore, some patients who have "Bell palsy" may have the so-called *zoster sine herpete* (82).

Corticosteroids and a 7- to 10-day course of famciclovir or acyclovir have been used in the treatment of varicella-zoster infections. The natural history of the disease is consistent with some recovery of auditory and vestibular function over several weeks, but severe SNHL rarely recovers completely (40,41). To what extent medical therapy alters this prognosis is undetermined (Table 146.6).

DELAYED ENDOLYMPHATIC HYDROPS

Schuknecht (42), in his classification of neurolabyrinthitis, proposed that ipsilateral, contralateral, or bilateral endolymphatic hydrops may be a delayed manifestation of some viral labyrinthine infections. Due to the subclinical nature of the viral injury to the resorptive mechanism of the endolymphatic sac, eventually a fluctuating SNHL or episodic vertigo becomes evident.

The history typically comprises an early childhood loss of cochlear or vestibular function in one or both ears, temporally related in many cases to mumps, an upper respiratory illness, or influenza (42). Many years later, symptoms of progressive endolymphatic hydrops appear. For example, a child sustaining a unilateral, profound SNHL in association with mumps may many years later develop a fluctuating hearing loss in the contralateral, apparently normal ear and would be diagnosed as having contralateral delayed hydrops.

Audiometric testing documents the degree of and fluctuation in the SNHL. ABR testing is consistent with a cochlear lesion. Electrocochleographic findings have not been reported. Electronystagmographic testing demonstrates a variable degree of loss of unilateral or bilateral vestibular function. Therapy is the same as for Ménière disease and is dictated according to the predominant symptoms (Table 146.7).

TABLE 146.7
DELAYED ENDOLYMPHATIC HYDROPS

Circumstance	Strategy
Diagnosis	History of cochleovestibular insult, fluctuating hearing loss or episodic vertigo; examination results are generally nonspecific; testing should include an audiogram, auditory brainstem response, and electronystagmogram, perhaps electrocochleography
Treatment	Same as for Ménière disease

HUMAN IMMUNODEFICIENCY VIRUS LABYRINTHITIS

A variety of auditory and vestibular complaints have been reported in patients with acquired immunodeficiency syndrome (AIDS). In one prospective study of 50 HIV-infected patients [Centers for Disease Control and Prevention (CDC) categories A through C], Chandrasekhar and colleagues (83) reported that 32% complained of dizziness, 29% of hearing loss, and 26% of tinnitus, among a variety of otologic symptoms. The pathogenetic mechanisms underlying these complaints require further study for elucidation (84,85). The relative importance of the HIV infection itself as opposed to its associated opportunistic infections and the therapeutic measures used to combat these infections, as well as the HIV infection, require further study for resolution (39,84). McNaghten et al. (86) reviewed the data in the Adult Spectrum of HIV Disease (ASD) project, which is a multicenter medical record review surveillance initiative conducted in 11 U.S. cities. They reported that the prevalence of hearing loss in this population was 0.8%. This study most likely underestimates the true prevalence because audiometry was not performed on these patients. This number therefore represents the minimum prevalence in this cohort of patients.

Etiology

Light microscopic evaluation of temporal bones from patients whose deaths stemmed from AIDS and its complications have variably shown cryptococcosis of the inner ear and internal auditory canal (in patients who have concomitant cryptococcal meningitis), CMV-associated inclusion bodies in the internal auditory canal and inner ear, and, in one patient, a deposit of Kaposi sarcoma. In many cases, there are no histopathologic alterations (87,88). Electron microscopic studies by Pappas and colleagues (89,90) documented HIV-like particles, with apparent budding, in a variety of cochlear and vestibular epithelial and connective tissue cells. Clinical correlates to these histopathologic findings do not exist currently, however.

Although CMV, adenovirus type 6, and herpes simplex type I virus have variably been recovered from the inner-ear fluids of AIDS patients, no associated inflammatory changes have been seen on histopathologic examination (88). The dearth of inflammatory changes led Davis and colleagues (88) to hypothesize that either the viral infections were nonpathogenic or that they were terminal events and that the immunosuppression of the AIDS prevented the mounting of any immune response.

Evaluation and Management

Clinical audiometric studies of patients with AIDS, including routine audiometry, OAEs, and ABR testing (91), have shown that mild SNHLs are common, but severe hearing

losses may also occur, especially in the low and high frequencies. One case-control study of 99 HIV-infected patients (92) found that 29% of patients demonstrated a measurable hearing loss (by portable audiometric evaluation); individuals 35 years of age or older also appeared to demonstrate an association between hearing loss and anti-retroviral therapy. ABR patterns occasionally suggested a retrocochlear site of lesion, and OAEs revealed diminished responses in most AIDS patients (91). As pointed out by Soucek and Michaels (91), AIDS; ototoxicity of the medications used in the treatment of AIDS and its complications; or concomitant infection, especially by CMV, *Cryptococcus*, and *Treponema pallidum*, were all potential factors in precipitating the auditory dysfunction. Accordingly, it appears that until more is known about AIDS and the labyrinth, the evaluation of such patients for auditory or vestibular dysfunction should consider the full differential diagnostic spectrum. A recent paper demonstrated that HIV-positive individuals can benefit from cochlear implantation without increased surgical risk and, although their performance was varied, as a group the hearing results were good (93).

SYPHILITIC LABYRINTHITIS

Incidence and Etiology

Syphilis was a common disease before the development of penicillin. The incidence in the developed world ranges from 0.4 per 100,000 in Canada to 1.35 per 100,000 in Germany (94). According to the CDC, in 1995 more than 68,000 cases of syphilis were detected in adults in the United States; the highest syphilis rates were reported in the eight southern states (95). Higher incidences are reported in East European countries. The etiologic agent of syphilis is *T. pallidum*, and the disease has a wide variety of clinical manifestations, earning it the name of the great mimicker. Syphilis can be classified into congenital and acquired forms. Acquired syphilis is further divided into primary, secondary, and tertiary forms. SNHL develops in the congenital and acquired forms with variable frequency and with or without vestibular symptoms (41). Congenital syphilis manifests as late (tardive) or early (infantile) forms.

Early congenital syphilis is generally fatal, and the cochleovestibular involvement pales in comparison with the systemic manifestations. Late congenital syphilis can present with a sudden SNHL in childhood that is generally symmetric and profound, and although there usually are associated vestibular symptoms, parental documentation is often inaccurate (96). In 51% of these patients, SNHL appears suddenly and asymmetrically between the ages of 25 and 35 years, shows a variable rate of progression and fluctuation, and may be associated with episodic vertigo and tinnitus (96).

SNHL can develop in the primary (rarely), secondary, latent (early and late), and tertiary forms of acquired syphilis (41,96). The cochleovestibular symptoms arising in early acquired syphilis have been related to a basilar meningitis that involves the eighth cranial nerve and that manifests as a suddenly appearing, rapidly progressive bilateral hearing loss with vestibular symptoms of lesser degree.

Patients who develop cochleovestibular symptoms with late acquired syphilis present in a fashion essentially identical to that of late congenital syphilis. Here, however, vertigo is often the presenting complaint, and the initial hearing loss may be so asymmetric as to appear unilateral (96). There is no pathognomonic pattern of symptoms for luetic otitis, and a wide variety of manifestations are the rule (96). Luetic otitis should be considered in the differential diagnosis of vestibular labyrinthitis, vestibular neuritis, ISSNHL, Ménière disease, and autoimmune SNHL.

Temporal bone histopathologic alterations are similar for the congenital and acquired forms of syphilis, particularly if comparing early and late stages of each form, and are characterized by mononuclear leukocytic infiltrates and obliterative endarteritis (41). Inflammatory fibrosis with round cell infiltration can obliterate the endolymphatic sac and duct and cause the development of hydrops (41,96). Gummas, central necrosis, and lymphocytic infiltrates are most frequent in the vestibular otic capsule and can result in degeneration of the sensory and neural structures of the labyrinth and the eighth cranial nerve (41,96). Gummatous involvement of the ossicles can precipitate conductive hearing loss.

Temporal bone osteitis with round cell infiltration is typical of late latent, tertiary, and late congenital syphilis, and the acute lymphocytic meningitis of secondary syphilis may be accompanied by an acute syphilitic labyrinthitis (41).

Evaluation and Management

Any unexplained SNHL or vertigo should be evaluated for the possibility of a syphilitic infection. In a population of adult patients with unexplained SNHL, 6.5% had associated positive fluorescent treponemal antibody absorption (FTA-ABS) tests compared with a 2% prevalence among the control population; 7% of patients with symptoms of Ménière disease had positive FTA-ABS results (97). Denial by the patient of a prior history or treatment of a syphilitic infection is not sufficient to rule out the diagnosis (97). The physical examination generally is unremarkable except for signs of hearing loss and imbalance. It is unusual to see the hallmark manifestations of severe and untreated congenital syphilis: bossing of the skull, saber shins, Hutchinson teeth, moon molars, interstitial keratitis, and snuffles (41).

The Hennebert sign (i.e., positive fistula test with an intact tympanic membrane) and Tullio sign (i.e., vertigo and nystagmus precipitated by loud noise exposure like a Barany box) are associated with congenital syphilis. These phenomena probably reflect inner ear fluid movement in response to pressure or sound, permitted by the presence of a bony semicircular canal fistula (41). The Hennebert sign has been related to endolymphatic hydrops in general and may be related to fibrous attachment of the vestibular membranes to the stapes footplate; the typical Hennebert response consists of a few beats of nystagmus over the course of one second or longer (41). Syphilitic otitis generally results in a bilateral hearing loss, which is not necessarily symmetric, may fluctuate, and may progress to a profound hearing loss. Most patients with syphilitic otitis demonstrate an abnormal elevated summating potential:action potential (SP:AP) ratio on electrocochleographic testing (98). ABR testing can demonstrate pathologic interpeak latencies and reduction of the amplitude of wave V (97). Electronystagmographic testing can be expected to demonstrate a vestibular disturbance in 80% of patients that is consistent with peripheral rather than central vestibular injury (98). The most common abnormality demonstrated on electronystagmographic testing is a decreased vestibular response (99). Congenital syphilitics demonstrate the greatest severity of electronystagmographic alterations and the highest incidence of bilateral abnormalities (99).

Serologic testing is used to determine the presence of nontreponemal [i.e., phospholipid, Venereal Disease Research Laboratory (VDRL), cardiolipin, or "nonspecific"] and treponemal antibodies (100). The CDC has approved four tests for phospholipid antibodies: the rapid plasma reagin (RPR) test, the VDRL slide test, the untreated serum reagin test, and the toluidin red unheated serum test (100). The RPR and VDRL tests are flocculation tests; their greatest sensitivity is for the secondary stage of syphilis, and they often are falsely negative in the early and late stages of syphilis (85).

Treponemal antibody tests are more useful in the diagnosis of syphilitic otitis (e.g., the FTA-ABS). False-positive results can occur in connective tissue diseases, leprosy, infectious mononucleosis, and pregnancy. Autoimmune screening tests, such as the erythrocyte sedimentation rate, lupus erythematosus prep, antinuclear antibody, and serum electrophoresis, are helpful in differentiating the false positives resulting from connective tissue disease and in evaluating the possibility of autoimmune SNHL. More recently, Murphy and colleagues (101) have demonstrated the utility of the treponemal Western blot as a confirmatory test for syphilis in patients with rheumatic disease. According to the World Health Organization (102), all patients who have syphilis should be tested for HIV.

No treatment regimen has been assessed for efficacy in the recovery of hearing or balance function in a blinded, prospective, randomized study. Previous studies have indicated that 35% to 50% of treated patients improve, particularly in their speech discrimination scores (85).

The doubling time of the treponeme in late syphilis is prolonged to 90 days, a fact that suggests that the treponemicidal levels of antibiotic should be maintained for at least 3 months (85). Penicillin G has the greatest antitreponemal activity and a single intramuscular injection of 2.4 million units of its benzathine preparation is sufficient for the therapy of cochleovestibular dysfunction in association with early luetic otitis (85).

Unfortunately, the penetration of uninflamed meninges by penicillin is poor, and the obliterative endarteritis of luetic otitis may impede antibiotic access to the temporal bone. For the late forms of luetic otitis, initial outpatient therapy consists of a 3-week course of 1.8 million units of procaine penicillin G on a daily basis, with 500 mg of probenecid orally every 6 hours, as recommended for the treatment of neurosyphilis (85). Therapy can be extended for a full 3 months with 2.4 million units of benzathine penicillin G given intramuscularly on a weekly basis.

Doxycycline, tetracycline, erythromycin, or ceftriaxone may be substituted for penicillin, but they do not have the same antitreponemal activity (Table 146.8) (85,102). Corticosteroid therapy, specifically prednisone, constitutes the second arm of therapy for luetic otitis, because of its salutary effect on the febrile component of the Jarisch-Herxheimer reaction and the desired antiinflammatory effects on the endolymphatic sac and the vessels of the temporal bone (Table 146.9). Prednisone therapy consists of 1 mg/kg each day in divided doses, with a maximal recommended dose of 80 mg each day for 1 month. Then the patient is assessed, and if improvement has occurred, it is tapered to a maintenance level; if no benefit has been derived, it is tapered and discontinued. Long-term maintenance therapy comprises twice the daily dose given on an alternate-morning basis, preferably before 8 AM. Aspirin is forbidden for fear of the development of gastric bleeding, and antacid use is encouraged.

In a recent report of a series of six cases with otosyphilis, improvement of symptoms was achieved in all but one case of congenital syphilis. A close working relationship between the otolaryngologist and dermatologist was stressed to ensure prompt identification and treatment of these patients (103). The expert opinion of a specialist in infectious diseases should also be sought.

TABLE 146.8
ALTERNATE SYPHILIS THERAPY

Treatment	Dosage
Primary/secondary syphilis	
Doxycycline	100 mg orally b.i.d. for 14 days
Erythromycin	500 mg orally q.i.d. for 14 days
Ceftriaxone	250 mg i.m. for 14 days
Late syphilis	
Tetracycline	500 mg orally q.i.d. for 30 days
Erythromycin	500 mg orally q.i.d. for 30 days
Doxycycline	200 mg orally q.i.d. for 20 days

b.i.d., twice daily; q.i.d., four times daily.
Reprinted from 1998 Guidelines for treatment of sexually transmitted diseases. *MMWR* 1997;47:1, with permission.

TABLE 146.9
LUETIC LABYRINTHITIS

Circumstance	Strategy
Diagnosis	History of unexplained vertigo or sensorineural hearing loss; examination is usually nonspecific, but the Hennebert sign or Tullio sign is occasionally observed; testing includes audiogram, auditory brainstem response, serology, and electronystagmography, perhaps electrocochleography
Treatment	2.4 million U of benzanthine penicillin G i.m. for early stage; 1.8 million U of procaine penicillin i.m. daily for 3 wk with 500 mg of probenecid orally every 6 h, then 2.4 million U of benzathine penicillin G i.m. weekly to total of 3 mo for late-stage disease; 80 mg of steroids orally daily for 1 mo and then taper

i.m., intramuscularly.

ACKNOWLEDGMENT

The contributions of A. Julianna Gulya, M.D., (the author of this chapter in the third edition) are acknowledged. Her exhaustive outline could not be improved on and has been left intact. Portions of her chapter are still current and these portions have been left unchanged by the present authors.

HIGHLIGHTS

- The cochlear aqueduct, internal auditory canal, and spiral modiolar vessels are all important routes of access to the labyrinth for pathogenic organisms.
- Bacterial meningitis is an important cause of sensorineural hearing loss; early institution of appropriate antibiotic and corticosteroid therapy may minimize the risk of hearing loss.
- Viral meningitis has not been implicated in sensorineural hearing loss.
- Fungal meningitis has been related to a retrocochlear hearing loss, which may be reversible in certain cases of cryptococcal meningitis.
- Cytomegalovirus is an important pathogen in the cause of antenatal infections associated with perinatal manifestations, including sensorineural hearing loss.
- Idiopathic sudden sensorineural hearing loss probably represents an acute viral cochlear labyrinthitis and may be reversible in certain cases by corticosteroid therapy.
- Acute labyrinthitis usually reflects acute virally related loss of labyrinthine function associated with isolated atrophy of the vestibular nerves.
- Delayed endolymphatic hydrops probably represents the long-term sequela of neurolabyrinthitis.

- Herpes zoster oticus is a disorder that arises from reactivation of a latent herpesvirus and predominantly involves the seventh and eighth cranial nerve trunks.
- Luetic otitis is an important element in the differential diagnosis of sudden hearing loss, fluctuating hearing loss, or episodic vertigo.

REFERENCES

1. Gulya AJ. Infections of the labyrinth. In: Bailey BJ, Calhoun KH, eds. *Head and neck surgery—otolaryngology,* 3rd ed. Lippincott Williams & Wilkins, 2001.
2. Linthicum FH Jr. Personal communication, May 2005.
3. Nadol JB Jr. Hearing loss as a sequela of meningitis. *Laryngoscope* 1978;88:739–755.
4. Woolley AL, Kirk KA, Neumann AM Jr, et al. Risk factors for hearing loss from meningitis in children: the Children's Hospital experience. *Arch Otolaryngol Head Neck Surg* 1999;125:509–514.
5. Vernon M. Meningitis and deafness: the problem, its physical, audiological, psychological, and educational manifestations in deaf children. *Laryngoscope* 1967;77:1856–1874.
6. Stutman HR, Marks MI. Bacterial meningitis in children: diagnosis and therapy. *Clin Pediatr* 1987;26:431–438.
7. Dodge PR, Davis H, Feigin RD, et al. Prospective evaluation of hearing impairment as a sequela of acute bacterial meningitis. *N Engl J Med* 1984;311:869–874.
8. Rosenhall U, Nylen O, Lindberg J, et al. Auditory function after haemophilus influenzae meningitis. *Acta Otolaryngol (Stock)* 1978; 85:243–247 .
9. Keane WM, Potsic WP, Rowe LD, et al. Meningitis and hearing loss in children. *Arch Otolaryngol Head Neck Surg* 1979;105:9–44.
10. Berlow SJ, Caldarelli DD, Matz GJ, et al. Bacterial meningitis and sensorineural hearing loss: a prospective investigation. *Laryngoscope* 1980;90:1445–1452 .
11. Finitzo-Hieber T, Simhadri R, Hieber JP. Abnormalities of the auditory brainstem response in post-meningitic infants and children. *Int J Pediatr Otorhinolaryngol* 1981;3:275–286.
12. Eisenberg LS, Luxford WM, Becher TS, et al. Electrical stimulation of the auditory system in children deafened by meningitis. *Otolaryngol Head Neck Surg* 1984;92:700–705.
13. Brookhouser PE, Auslander MC, Meskan ME. The pattern and stability of postmeningitic hearing loss in children. *Laryngoscope* 1988;98:940–948.
14. Wenger JD, Hightower AW, Facklam FF, et al. Bacterial meningitis in the United States 1986: a report of a multistate surveillance study. *J Infect Dis* 1986;162:1316–1323.
15. Schlech WF III, Ward JI, Band JD, et al. Bacterial meningitis in the United States, 1978-1981: the National Bacterial Meningitis Surveillance Study. *JAMA* 1985;253:1749–1754.
16. Blank AL, Davis GL, Van de Water TR, et al. Acute Streptococcus pneumoniae meningogenic labyrinthitis. *Arch Otolaryngol Head Neck Surg* 1994;120:1342–1346.
17. Kesser BW, Hashisaki OT, Spindel JH, et al. Time course of hearing loss in an animal model of pneumococcal meningitis *Otolaryngol Head Neck Surg* 1999;120:628–637.
18. Bhatt SM, Laurentano A, Cabellos C. Progression of hearing loss in experimental pneumococcal meningitis: correlation with cerebrospinal fluid cytochemistry. *J Infect Dis* 1993;167:675–683.
19. Odio CM, Faingezicht I, Paris M, et al. The beneficial effects of early dexamethasone administration in infants and children with bacterial meningitis. *N Engl J Med* 1991;324:1525–1531.
20. Tunkel AR, Wispelwey B, Scheld WM. Bacterial meningitis: recent advances in pathophysiology and treatment. *Ann Intern Med* 1990;112:610–623.
21. Kastenbauer S, Klein M, Koedel U, et al. Reactive nitrogen species contribute to blood-labyrinth barrier disruption in suppurative labyrinthitis complicating experimental pneumococcal meningitis in the rat. *Brain Res* 2001;904:208–217.
22. Klein M, Koedel U, Pfister H-W, et al. Meningitis-associated hearing loss: protection by adjunctive antioxidant therapy. *Ann Neurol* 2003;54:451–458.
23. Brodie HA, Thompson TC, Vassilian L. Induction of labyrinthitis ossificans after pneumococcal meningitis: an animal model. *Otolaryngol Head Neck Surg* 1998;118:15–21.
24. Novak MA, Fifer RC, Barkmier JC. Labyrinthine ossification after meningitis: its implications for cochlear implantation. *Otolaryngol Head Neck Surg* 1990;103:351–356.
25. Tinling SP, Colton J, Brodie HA. Location and timing of initial osteoid deposition in postmeningitic labyrinthitis ossificans determined by multiple fluorescent labels. *Laryngoscope* 2004;114: 675–680.
26. McIntyre PB, Berkey CS, King SM, et al. Dexamethasone as adjunctive therapy in bacterial meningitis. A meta-analysis of randomized clinical trials since 1988. *JAMA* 1997;278:925–931.
27. Moller K, Skinhoj P. Guidelines for managing acute bacterial meningitis: speed in diagnosis and treatment is essential. *BMJ* 2000;320:1290.
28. Arditi M, Mason EO Jr, Bradley JS, et al. Three-year multicenter surveillance of pneumococcal meningitis in children: clinical characteristics, and outcome related to penicillin susceptibility and dexamethasone use. *Pediatrics* 1998;102:1087–1097.
29. Hartnick CJ, Kim HY, Chute PM, et al. Preventing labyrinthitis ossificans: the role of steroids. *Arch Otolaryngol Head Neck Surg* 2001;127:180–183.
30. Winter AJ, Comis SD, Osborne MP, et al. A role for pneumolysin but not neuramidase in the hearing loss and cochlear damage induced by experimental pneumococcal meningitis in guinea pigs. *Infect Immunol* 1997;65:4411–4418.
31. Rappaport JM, Bhatt SM, Burkard RF, et al. Prevention of hearing loss in experimental pneumococcal meningitis by administration of dexamethasone and ketorolac. *J Infect Dis* 1999;179:264–268.
32. Braun JS, Novak R, Herzog KH, et al. Neuroprotection by a caspase inhibitor in acute bacterial meningitis. *Nat Med* 1999;5: 298–302.
33. Richardson MP, Williamson TJ, Reid A, et al. Otoacoustic emissions as a screening test for hearing impairment in children recovering from acute bacterial meningitis. *Pediatrics* 1998;102: 1364–1368.
34. Marx RD, Baer ST. Spontaneous recovery of profound postmeningitic hearing loss. *J Laryngol Otol* 2001;115:412–414.
35. Aso S, Gibson WPR. Surgical techniques for insertion of a multielectrode implant into a postmeningitic ossified cochlea. *Am J Otol* 1995;16:231–234.
36. Johnson MH, Hasenstab MS, Seicshnaydre MA, et al. CT of postmeningitic deafness: observations and predictive value for cochlear implants in children. *Am J Neuroradiol* 1995;16:103–109.
37. Muren C, Bredberg G. Postmeningitic labyrinthine ossification primarily affecting semicircular canals. *Eur Radiol* 1997;7: 208–213.
38. Schwab J, Ryan M. Varicella zoster meningitis in a previously immunized child. *Pediatrics* 2004;114:273–274.
39. Mayer J-M, Chevalier X, Albert E, et al. Reversible hearing loss in a patient with cryptococcosis. *Arch Otolaryngol Head Neck Surg* 1990;116:962–964.
40. Davis LE, Johnsson L-G. Viral infections of the inner ear: clinical, virologic, and pathologic studies in humans and animals. *Am J Otolaryngol* 1983;4:347–362.
41. Schuknecht HF. *Pathology of the ear,* 2nd ed. Philadelphia: Lea & Febiger, 1993.
42. Schuknecht HF. Neurolabyrinthitis: viral infections of the peripheral auditory and vestibular systems. In: Nomura Y, ed. *Hearing loss and dizziness.* Tokyo: Igaku-Shoin, 1985:1–15.
43. Wilson WR, Veltri RW, Laird N, et al. Viral and epidemiologic studies of idiopathic sudden hearing loss. *Otolaryngol Head Neck Surg* 1983;91:653–658.
44. Veltri RW, Wilson WR, Sprinkle PM, et al. The implication of viruses in idiopathic sudden hearing loss: primary infection or reactivation of latent viruses? *Otolaryngol Head Neck Surg* 1981;89: 137–141.
45. Vasama J-P, Linthicum FH Jr. Idiopathic sudden sensorineural hearing loss: temporal bone histopathologic study. *Ann Otol Rhinol Laryngol* 2000;109:527–532.

46. Stagno S. Cytomegalovirus. In Remington JS, Klein JO, eds. *Infectious diseases of the fetus and newborn infant*, 4th ed. Philadelphia: WB Saunders, 1995:312–353.

47. Britt WJ, Alford CA. Cytomegalovirus. In: Fields BN, Knipe DM, Howley PM, eds. *Fields virology*, 3rd ed. New York: Raven Press, 1996:2493–2523.

48. Demmler GJ. Infectious Diseases Society of America and Centers for Disease Control. Summary of workshop on surveillance for congenital cytomegalovirus disease. *Rev Infect Dis* 1991;13: 315–329.

49. Rivera LB, Boppana SB, Fowler KB, et al. Predictors of hearing loss in children with symptomatic congenital cytomegalovirus infection. *Pediatrics* 2002;110:762–767.

50. Fowler KB, Dahle AJ, Boppana SB, et al. Newborn hearing screening: will children with hearing loss caused by congenital cytomegalovirus infection be missed? *J Pediatr* 1999;135:60–64.

51. Fowler KB, McCollister FP, Dahle AJ, et al. Progressive and fluctuating sensorineural hearing loss in children with asymptomatic congenital cytomegalovirus infection. *J Pediatr* 1997;130: 624–630.

52. Boppana SB, Rivera LB, Fowler KB, et al. Viral load in infancy predicts outcome in children with congenital CMV infection. Presented at the 41st Interscience Conference on Antimicrobial Agents and Chemotherapy, December 16–19, 2001, Chicago.

53. Strauss M. A clinical pathologic study of hearing loss in congenital cytomegalovirus infection. *Laryngoscope* 1985;95:951–962.

54. Fukuda S, Keithley EM, Harris JP. Experimental cytomegalovirus infection: viremic spread to the inner ear. *Am J Otolaryngol* 1988; 9:135–141.

55. Bauer PW, Parizi-Robinson M, Roland PS, et al. Cytomegalovirus in the perilymphatic fluid. *Laryngoscope* 2005;115: 223–225.

56. Hamprecht K, Maschmann J, Vochem M, et al. Epidemiology of transmission of cytomegalovirus from mother to preterm infant by breastfeeding. *Lancet* 2001;357:513–518.

57. Vochem M, Hamprecht K, Jahn G, et al. Transmission of cytomegalovirus to preterm infants through breast milk. *Pediatr Infect Dis* 1998;17:53–58.

58. Vollmer B, Seibold-Weiger K, Schnitz-Salue C, et al. Postnatally acquired cytomegalovirus infection via breast milk: effects on hearing and development in preterm infants. *Pediatr Infect Dis J* 2004;23:322–327.

59. Whitley RJ, Cloud G, Gruber W, et al. Ganciclovir treatment of symptomatic congenital cytomegalovirus infection: results of a phase II study. *J Infect Dis* 1997;175:1080–1086.

60. Kimberlin DW, Lin C-Y, Sanchez PJ, et al. Effect of ganciclovir therapy on hearing in symptomatic congenital cytomegalovirus disease involving the central nervous system: a randomized controlled trial. *J Pediatr* 2003;143:16–25.

61. Katz SL. Rubella (German measles) In: Joklik WK, Willett HP, Amos DB, et al., eds. *Zinsser microbiology*, 19th ed. East Norwalk, CT: Appleton & Lange, 1988:839–841.

62. Merchant SN, Adam JC, Nadol JB Jr. Pathology and pathophysiology of idiopathic sudden sensorineural hearing loss. *Otol Neurotol* 2005;26:151–160.

63. Wilson WR, Byl FM, Laird N. The efficacy of steroids in the treatment of idiopathic sudden hearing loss. *Arch Otolaryngol* 1980; 106:772–776.

64. Gagnebin J, Maire R. Infection screening in sudden and progressive idiopathic sensorineural hearing loss: a retrospective study in 182 cases. *Otol Neurotol* 2002;23:160–162.

65. Tucci DL, Farmer JC Jr, Kitch RD, et al. Treatment of sudden sensorineural hearing loss with systemic steroids and valacyclovir. *Otol Neurotol* 2002;23:301–308.

66. Uri N, Doweck I, Cohen-Karem R, et al. Acyclovir in the treatment of idiopathic sudden sensorineural hearing loss. *Otolaryngol Head Neck Surg* 2003;128:544–549.

67. Westerlaker BO, Stokroos RJ, Dhooge IJM, et al. Treatment of idiopathic sudden sensorineural hearing loss with antiviral therapy: a prospective randomized double-blind clinical trial. *Ann Otol Rhinol Laryngol* 2003;112:993–1000.

68. Chandrasekhar SS. Intratympanic dexamethasone for sudden sensorineural hearing loss: clinical and laboratory evaluation. *Otol Neurotol* 2001;22:18–23.

69. Laird N, Wilson WR. Predicting recovery from idiopathic sudden hearing loss. *Am J Otolaryngol* 1983;4:161–164.

70. Slattery WH, Fisher LM, Iqbal Z, el al. Oral steroid regimen for idiopathic sudden sensorineural hearing loss. *Otolaryngol Head Neck Surg* 2005;132:5–10.

71. Baloh RW, Honrubia V. *Clinical neurophysiology of the vestibular system*, 3rd ed. New York: Oxford University Press, 2001.

72. Schuknecht HF, Kitamura K. Vestibular neuritis. *Ann Otol Rhinol Laryngol* 1981;90[Suppl 78]:1–19.

73. Fetter M, Dichgans J. Vestibular neuritis spares the inferior division of the vestibular nerve. *Brain* 1996;119:755–763.

74. Baloh RW. Vestibular neuritis. *N Engl J Med* 2003;348:1027–1032.

75. Peppard SB. Effect of drug therapy on compensation from vestibular injury. *Laryngoscope* 1986;96:878–898.

76. Marill KA, Walsh MJ, Nelson BK. Intravenous lorazepam versus dimenhydrinate for treatment of vertigo in the emergency department: a randomized clinical trial. *Ann Emerg Med* 2000;36: 310–319.

77. Irving C, Richman P, Kaiafas C, et al. Intramuscular droperidol versus intramuscular dimenhydrinate for the treatment of acute peripheral vertigo in the emergency department: a randomized clinical trial. *Acad Emerg Med* 2002;9:650–653.

78. Ariyasu L, Byl FM, Sprague MS, et al. The beneficial effect of methylprednisolone in acute vestibular vertigo. *Arch Otolaryngol Head Neck Surg* 1990;116:700–703.

79. Galazka AM, Robertson SE, Kraigher A. Mumps and mumps vaccine: a global review. *Bull WHO* 1999;77:3–14.

80. Wilson WR. The relationship of the herpesvirus family to sudden hearing loss: a prospective clinical study and literature review. *Laryngoscope* 1986;96:870–877.

81. Kuhweide R, Van de Steene V, Vlaminck S, et al. Ramsay Hunt syndrome: pathophysiology of cochleovestibular symptoms. *J Laryngol Otol* 2002;116:844–848.

82. Sweeney CJ, Gilden DH. Ramsay Hunt syndrome. *J Neurol Neurosurg Psychiatry* 2001;71:149–154.

83. Chandrasekhar SS, Connelly PE, Brahmbhatt SS, et al. Otologic and audiologic evaluation of human immunodeficiency virus-infected patients. *Am J Otolaryngol* 2000;21:1–9.

84. Real R, Thomas M, Gerwin JM. Sudden hearing loss and acquired immunodeficiency syndrome. *Otolaryngol Head Neck Surg* 1987; 10:410–412.

85. Darmstadt GL, Harris JP. Luetic hearing loss: clinical presentation, diagnosis, and treatment. *Am J Otolaryngol* 1989;97:410–421.

86. McNaghten AD, Wan PCT, Dworkin MS. Prevalence of hearing loss in a cohort of HIV-infected patients. *Arch Otolaryngol Head Neck Surg* 2001;127:1516–1518.

87. Michaels L, Soucek S, Liang J. The ear in the acquired immunodeficiency syndrome: I. Temporal bone histopathologic study. *Am J Otol* 1994;15:515–522.

88. Davis LE, Rarey KE, McLaren LC. Clinical viral infections and temporal bone histologic studies of patients with AIDS. *Otolaryngol Head Neck Surg* 1995;113:695–701.

89. Pappas DG Jr, Chandra Sekhar HK, Lim J, et al. Ultrastructural findings in the cochlea of AIDS cases. *Am J Otol* 1994;15: 456–465.

90. Pappas DG Jr, Roland JT Jr, Lim J, et al. Ultrastructural findings in the vestibular end-organs of AIDS cases. *Am J Otol* 1995; 16: 140–145.

91. Soucek S, Michaels L. The ear in acquired immunodeficiency syndrome: II. Clinical and audiologic investigation. *Am J Otol* 1996; 17:35–39.

92. Marra CM, Wechkin HA, Longstreth WT Jr, et al. Hearing loss and antiretroviral therapy in patients infected with HIV-1. *Arch Neurol* 1997;54:407–410.

93. Roland JT, Alexiades G, Jackman AH, et al. Cochlear implantation in human immunodeficiency virus-infected patients. *Otol Neurotol* 2003;24:892–895.

94. Marcus U. Gonorrhoe und Syphilis in Deutschland bis zum Jahr 2000. *Epidemiol Bull* 2001;Nr; 38:287–291.

95. Syphilis Facts. Division of STD prevention, Centers for Disease Control and Prevention, Atlanta, GA. Available at http://www.cdc.gov/nchstp/dstd/Syphilis_Facts.htm.

96. Zoller M, Wilson WR, Nadol JB Jr, et al. Detection of syphilitic hearing loss. *Arch Otolaryngol* 1978;104:63–65.

97. Lowhagen G-B, Rosenhall U, Andersson M, et al. Central nervous system involvement in early syphilis. *Acta Derm Venereol (Stockh)* 1983;63:530–535.

98. Nagasaki T, Watanabe Y, Aso S, et al. Electrocochleography in syphilitic hearing loss. *Acta Otolaryngol (Stockh)* 1993; 504[Suppl]:68–73.

99. Wilson WR, Zoller M. Electronystagmography in congenital and acquired syphilitic otitis. *Ann Otol Rhinol Laryngol* 1981;90:21–24.

100. Wicher K, Horowitz HW, Wicher V. Laboratory methods of diagnosis of syphilis for the beginning of the third millennium. *Microbes Infect* 1999;1:1035–1049.

101. Murphy FT, George R, Kubota K, et al. The use of Western blotting as the confirmatory test for syphilis in patients with rheumatic disease. *J Rheumatol* 1999;26:2448–2453.

102. 1998 Guidelines for treatment of sexually transmitted diseases. *MMWR Morb Mortal Wkly Rep* 1997;47:1.

103. Klemm E, Wollina U. Otosyphilis: report on six cases. *J Eur Acad Dermatol Venereol* 2004;18:429–434.

Noise-Induced Hearing Loss

147

Robert A. Dobie

Noise and aging are responsible for most cases of permanent hearing loss in the United States. Although not correctable by medical or surgical treatment, noise-induced hearing loss (NIHL) is preventable.

Otolaryngologists see patients with NIHL in many different contexts. A noise-exposed worker may be referred for preemployment examination, for evaluation of threshold shifts or other abnormalities detected by a hearing conservation program (HCP) at work, or for examination for compensation purposes at the end of his or her career. The otolaryngologist is expected to verify the existence and severity of the hearing loss, to render a differential diagnosis, to recommend treatment and rehabilitation, to counsel the worker, and to report to referring parties. Otolaryngologists also may be called on as consultants by employers designing HCPs or by attorneys involved in medicolegal and compensation disputes.

Patients with NIHL are also seen through the normal pathways of self-referral or physician referral. These patients often have occupational or nonoccupational exposures that are uncontrolled, and the otolaryngologist's duty then is to provide at least the rudiments of an HCP: periodic audiometry, hearing protectors, and counseling. Unfortunately, most people with NIHL do not see otolaryngologists; thus, we should encourage primary care physicians to use screening audiometry for noise-exposed patients (1).

The goal of this chapter is to provide the otolaryngologist with most of the information needed to meet these needs.

PATHOGENESIS

Pure-Tone Threshold Shifts

Temporary Threshold Shifts

Exposure to loud noise for seconds to hours may cause a temporary sensorineural hearing loss that recovers almost completely within 24 hours. The magnitude of this temporary threshold shift (TTS) can be predicted from the acoustic parameters of the noise: its intensity, spectrum (frequency content), and temporal pattern. Obviously, more intense sounds lead to larger shifts. Pure tones cause TTS that are greatest at and slightly above the frequencies of the exposure sounds. As might be expected, the frequencies that we hear best are also the frequencies most susceptible to TTS. (See Chapter 129 for a discussion of the effects of middle-ear mechanics and ear canal resonance on thresholds for different frequencies.) Because high-frequency sounds (e.g., a 4-kHz tone) are usually more hazardous than low-frequency sounds (e.g., a 500-Hz tone) of the same intensity, risk cannot be predicted from measurements of decibel sound pressure level (dB SPL) alone. To avoid the cumbersome necessity of assessing risk separately for each of several octave bands of noise, there is an international consensus that estimates of hazard for NIHL should be based on measurements of decibels on the A scale (dBA), which gives greater weight to those frequencies most hazardous to human hearing (1 to 5 kHz) and lesser weight to higher and lower frequencies.

The effect of temporal pattern is more complex. Up to a point, longer exposures lead to increased TTS, but interrupted exposures cause less TTS than continuous exposures with the same overall duration. Presumably, recovery takes place during the rest intervals.

Permanent Threshold Shift

After repeated exposures to noises that initially cause only TTS, a worker may experience threshold changes that do not recover. This is called noise-induced permanent threshold shift (NIPTS). In epidemiologic studies, for example, a researcher determines the NIPTS attributable to 10 years' exposure at 100 dBA by measuring the hearing threshold levels (HTLs) of the workers and then subtracting the amount of hearing loss to be expected on the basis of aging. The amount of NIPTS and the frequencies involved depend primarily on the acoustic parameters of the noise, as described previously for TTS. As with TTS, intermittency has a protective effect especially for low-frequency NIPTS (2,3).

The consensus of most experts is that NIPTS does not progress after cessation of the offending exposure. That consensus view has been challenged by a review of serial audiograms from the Framingham Heart Study, showing that middle-aged men who had 4-kHz notches (presumably due to noise exposure in most cases) experienced more threshold shift at 2 kHz in subsequent years than men whose audiograms were not notched (4). These data have been interpreted by some as suggesting that noise damages the cochlea in ways that do not become apparent until after the noise has stopped. Unfortunately, there was no documentation that the men with audiometric notches had actually been noise-exposed (or that those without notches had not). In addition, many if not most of these men were below retirement age at the times of their initial audiograms, and there was no documentation that their occupational and nonoccupational noise exposures (if any) had ceased.

Although the acoustic reflex evolved before firearms and industrial noise, it is probably protective against NIPTS, at least for frequencies below 2 kHz, where the acoustic reflex effectively attenuates sound. Borg and coworkers (5) have shown in experimental animals and in humans with Bell palsy that permanent threshold shift (PTS) and TTS increase dramatically for lower frequencies when the reflex is inactivated. The efferent innervation of the outer hair cells probably exerts a protective role as well; at least in guinea pigs, strong efferent function is correlated with resistance to NIHL (6).

We have already mentioned several explanations for the familiar 4-kHz notch (which can also be at 3 or 6 kHz): the greater sensitivity of the human ear to frequencies between 1 and 5 kHz, the protective effect of the acoustic reflex below 2 kHz, and the fact that intermittency is most protective for low frequencies. Recently, another reason has been added: outer hair cells at the base of the cochlea are especially susceptible to oxidative stress (7). However, a notch is not proof of NIHL and can be seen after head in-

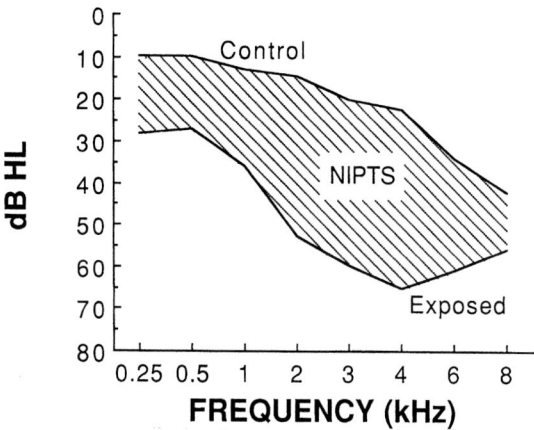

Figure 147.1 Median audiograms of retired jute weavers (exposed) and non–noise-exposed women of similar ages (control). Noise-induced permanent threshold shift is estimated by subtracting hearing threshold levels (HTLs) expected with aging from HTLs in the exposed group.

jury, after barotrauma, or even in the absence of any explanatory history.

In both TTS and PTS experiments in animals, the amount of threshold shift caused by a particular exposure can often be reduced by adding prior exposure at lower levels; this is called "toughening" or "conditioning" the ear (8). Clearly, inner ear injury and hearing loss are not simply related to the total amount of sound energy entering the ear.

A landmark cross-sectional study of the evolution of NIHL over a working career was reported by Taylor et al. (9), in a jute-weaving factory in which noise levels (over 100 dBA) had probably been constant for generations. Figure 147.1 shows the pattern of hearing loss found in retired female weavers compared with that of age-matched female controls who had had no hazardous occupational or nonoccupational noise exposure. The shaded area indicates the estimated median NIPTS; the greatest change was at 4 kHz. Figure 147.2 shows median NIPTS curves for varying lengths of employment in the mills. As many other studies have shown, when workers are exposed to typical

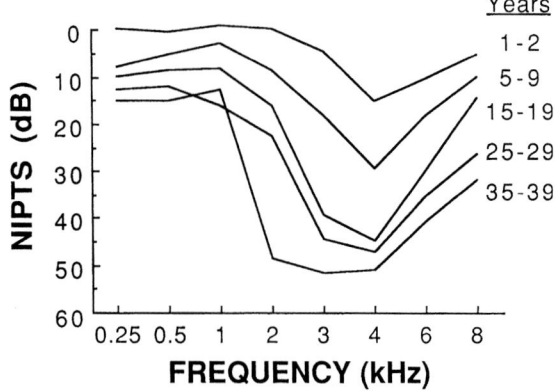

Figure 147.2 Median noise-induced permanent threshold shift as a function of audiometric frequency for different durations of exposure in jute-weaving mills (>100 dBA).

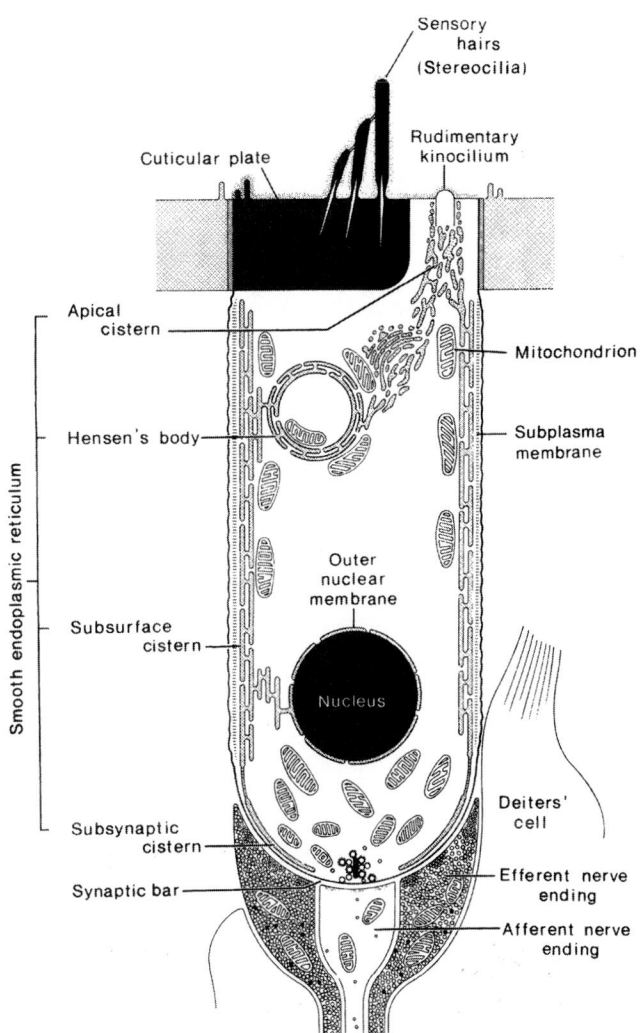

Figure 147.3 Diagrammatic cross section of a normal cochlea hair cell. (Redrawn after Lim DJ. Functional structure of the organ of Corti: a review. *Hearing Res* 1986;22:117, with permission.)

broad-spectrum industrial noise, the earliest changes are in the high frequencies (3 to 6 kHz). After about 10 years, loss in the high frequencies tends to plateau, but the loss continues to broaden gradually into lower frequencies.

Pathology

NIHL involves the organ of Corti, especially the hair cells (Fig. 147.3). The outer hair cells are much more susceptible to damage. It has been difficult to find anatomic correlates to TTS, but it appears that the stereocilia of the outer hair cells become less stiff and therefore respond poorly to stimulation. These floppy stereocilia may recover their normal mechanical properties and function normally again. With increasing intensity and duration of exposure sufficient to cause NIPTS, more severe damage is seen with fusion of adjacent stereocilia and loss of stereocilia. The primary site of injury appears to be the rootlets that connect the stereocilia with the top of the hair cell (10). As stereocilia are lost, the

hair cells themselves may die. As the severity of exposure increases, inner hair cells and supporting cells in the organ of Corti may be damaged (Fig. 147.4), and with severe hair cell loss, secondary neural degeneration is reflected in the auditory nerve and brainstem auditory nuclei.

Acoustic Trauma

A single exposure to a very intense short-duration sound can cause a permanent hearing loss not preceded by TTS. It is generally believed that in these instances sound mechanically damages the organ of Corti, tearing membranes, rupturing cells, and allowing perilymph and endolymph to mix. This is contrasted to the gradual loss of stereocilia and hair cells seen in NIHL, preceded by TTS, and usually attributed to metabolic processes. Acoustic trauma can produce losses that are more severe than those seen with NIHL, especially in the low frequencies. At extreme levels, such as with explosive or blast injury, even tympanic membrane or ossicular injury can occur, causing conductive or mixed hearing loss.

An important type of exposure that can create either NIHL or acoustic trauma is impulse noise (11). Impulses in the range of 0.2-ms duration have peak energy at 2 to 3 kHz, are therefore most hazardous to human hearing, and are typical of small arms gunfire. Such impulses, when above a critical level of 140 dB (peak), are considered potentially hazardous to human hearing (12).

Many industrial environments contain large amounts of impact noise, usually caused by collision of metal objects. These noises have high peaks and are often reverberant as well. Intense impact noises can cause acoustic trauma, but they are less likely than impulse noises to reach critical levels.

The levels at which continuous noise and tones (in contrast to impulses and impacts) cause acoustic trauma are not well defined. The earliest cordless telephones rang through the earpiece; if the person answering the phone failed to switch manually from "ring" to "talk" mode, the phone would ring directly into the ear with a 750- to 800-Hz tone at about 140 dB SPL. Dozens of cases of permanent hearing loss occurred from single-ring exposures, each probably less than 1 second in duration. At the other extreme, single 4-hour exposures below 110 dBA probably pose negligible risk of acoustic trauma (13).

Interactions

Aging

The nature of the interaction between NIPTS and age-related hearing changes has been the subject of considerable debate. Epidemiologic studies, such as those illustrated in Fig. 147.2, usually assume additivity; that is, the net hearing loss is the decibel sum of the threshold shifts from aging and from noise. When this question has been addressed explicitly, the bulk of evidence favors simple additivity.

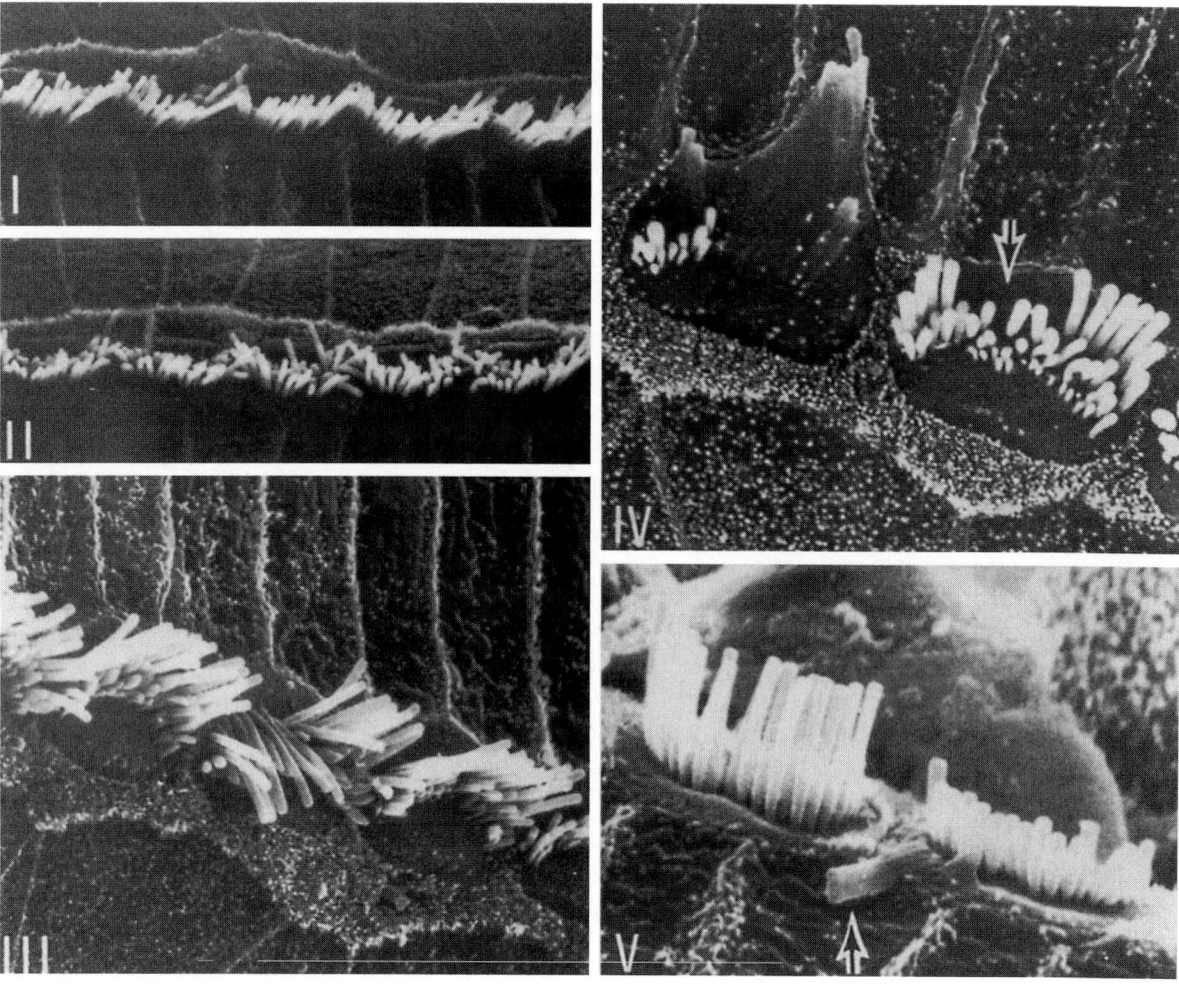

Figure 147.4   Scanning electron micrographs of cat inner hair cells that have been damaged by noise. (Redrawn after Liberman MC, Mulroy M. Acute and chronic effects of acoustic trauma: cochlear pathology and auditory nerve physiology. In: Hamernik RP, Henderson D, Salvi R, eds. *New perspectives on noise-induced hearing loss.* New York: Raven, 1982:122, with permission.)

For example, Macrae (14) showed that war veterans with NIHL developed about the expected amount of additional hearing loss, based on studies of age-related hearing loss, over the ensuing years. The American National Standards Institute (ANSI) supports the theory of additivity, with a small correction factor to be used when the total hearing loss exceeds 40 dB hearing loss (15).

Vibration

Czanto and Ligia (16) are among those who have shown that workers who develop "vibration-induced white finger" also develop excessive NIHL. This could mean that vibration interacts with noise to damage the ear, or that people who are susceptible to white finger (a peripheral vascular disorder) are also susceptible to NIHL.

Drugs and Chemicals

Humes (17) reviewed many studies and concluded that no substantial risk of hearing loss occurs from combining a noise exposure and an aminoglycoside drug when neither is present in sufficient amount to cause hearing loss on its own. Naturally, one would be reluctant to combine ototoxic drugs (primarily aminoglycosides and platinum-based antineoplastics) with hazardous noise exposures, but, with the probable exception of the newborn nursery where some borderline noise levels have been recorded, this is not a practical problem. The ototoxic drug most likely to be combined with industrial noise exposure is aspirin, but this causes a reversible hearing loss and has not been shown to potentiate or interact with NIHL.

Carbon monoxide (CO), xylene, styrene, and toluene have been reported to cause sensorineural hearing loss in rats. Workers exposed to toluene or xylene in addition to noise developed more hearing loss than those exposed to noise alone (18,19). Exposures in these studies, however, either were undocumented or were above Occupational Safety and Health Administration (OSHA) permissible time-weighted average exposures; thus, it is unclear whether exposures within OSHA regulations really cause hearing loss, either alone or by interacting with occupational noise.

On the other hand, a recent study (20) showed that styrene exposure below currently recommended values, plus noise, was associated with more hearing loss than noise exposure alone.

Susceptibility

Persons vary widely in the degree of TTS or PTS caused by noise exposures. Efforts to predict, measure, or explain these differences in susceptibility have generally been fruitless in humans. Men often display more hearing loss in noisy occupations than do women, but this may be due to different nonoccupational exposures (especially shooting) between the genders. Mice inherit susceptibility to both NIHL and age-related hearing loss (21,22); genetic tests or tests of efferent function (6) may someday permit prediction of human susceptibility to NIHL. In most experimental animals, there is a critical period in infancy, about the time of final maturation and innervation of the hair cells, in which susceptibility to NIHL is greater than at other times (23). If and when this happens in human infants is unclear.

Pathophysiology

Many investigators have wondered whether there was a vascular component to NIHL, but evidence has been conflicting. Cochlear blood flow has been shown to increase or decrease for long noise exposures, and it is unclear whether vascular disease increases susceptibility to NIHL (23).

Behavioral hearing tests in patients with NIHL can demonstrate deficits in speech recognition, in frequency and time resolution, and in other complex auditory tests. Otoacoustic emissions are predictably reduced or absent in NIHL. However, none of these tests has shown performance deficits specific to NIHL, and none has proved more useful than pure-tone threshold shifts for the early detection of NIHL.

EVALUATION AND DIAGNOSIS

Epidemiology

Hazardous noise exposure is common in our society. Table 147.1 shows the distribution of exposures in 19 industries believed by OSHA (in 1981) to contain most of the noisy workplaces in the United States (24). At least 5.1 million American workers were exposed at levels exceeding 85 dBA (massive job losses in manufacturing in the past 2 decades have almost certainly reduced those numbers). Hazardous nonoccupational exposure is probably more prevalent; the National Rifle Association estimates that 65 million Americans own guns (www.nraila.org, 2004), and many of them participate in hunting or target shooting. Significantly, firearms and occupational noise exposure often go together. The prevalence of handicapping NIHL in males has been estimated at 1.7% (25).

TABLE 147.1

NOISE EXPOSURE IN 19 U.S. INDUSTRIES (1981)[a]

Level (dBA)	Workers	Total (%)
<80	6,987,000	46.88
80–85	2,793,000	18.74
85–90	2,244,500	15.06
90–95	1,636,500	10.98
95–100	815,200	5.47
>100	427,700	2.87

[a]Machinery, transportation equipment, electrical machinery, fabricated metals, food, apparel, primary metals, textiles, printing and publishing, utilities, lumber and wood, rubber and plastics, stone and glass, chemicals, paper, furniture and textiles, petroleum and coal, tobacco, and leather.

Damage Risk Criteria

Animal research has been essential in describing the pathogenesis of NIHL and some of its features; however, the risk of human hearing loss with various exposures can be estimated only from epidemiologic studies. The results of many such studies measuring the hearing of noise-exposed workers have been generally consistent; good summaries and professional consensus statements can be found in publications by ANSI and OSHA (15,24).

Levels below about 80 dBA pose negligible risk to human hearing over a working lifetime. Above 85 dBA, risk grows rapidly for the high frequencies and more slowly for lower frequencies. Figure 147.5 shows the growth of NIPTS as a function of duration of employment for two frequencies (1 and 4 kHz) and two exposure levels (85 and 100 dBA) according to OSHA (24). Median threshold shifts are shown; half of all workers would show more shift and half would show less shift than indicated. No curve is plotted for 1 kHz at 85 dBA because less than 1 dB of shift is predicted even after 40 years. Note that at 4 kHz, NIPTS grows rapidly over the first 10 years and then reaches a plateau.

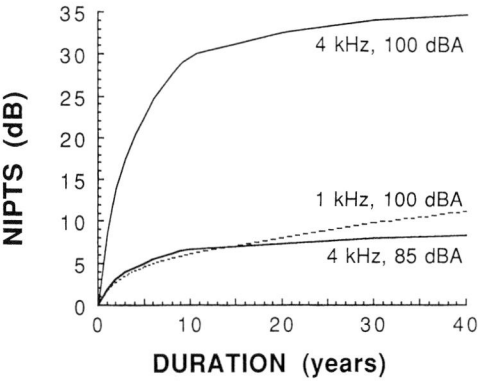

Figure 147.5 Median noise-induced permanent threshold shift as a function of exposure duration for 4 kHz (85 and 100 dBA) and 1 kHz (100 dBA).

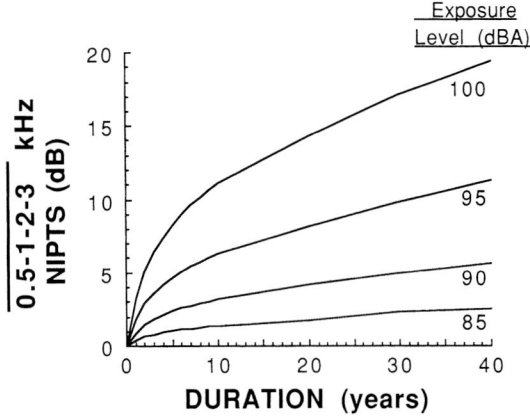

Figure 147.6 Median noise-induced permanent threshold shift for the pure-tone average (0.5, 1, 2, and 3 kHz) as a function of exposure duration, for different exposure levels (85 to 100 dBA).

For 1 kHz, growth is somewhat more gradual, but more than 50% of NIPTS is accrued in the first 10 years.

Similar NIPTS curves are shown in Fig. 147.6, using the pure-tone average (PTA) for 0.5, 1, 2, and 3 kHz [speech frequency average used in the American Medical Association (AMA) method of estimating "binaural hearing impairment"]. It is interesting to compare these curves with age-related permanent threshold shift (ARPTS) curves for men and women (Fig. 147.7), again for the 0.5, 1, 2, and 3 kHz PTA (15). ARPTS is an accelerating process (i.e., the rate of change of hearing loss increases with time), whereas NIPTS is a decelerating process (i.e., the rate of change decreases with time). This contrast can be helpful in determining the relative contribution of these two sources of hearing loss in individual cases.

Data like these can be used to estimate the median hearing loss for a population of workers with a given gender, age, duration, and level of exposure. The median expected hearing loss (0.5, 1, 2, and 3 kHz PTA) for 65-year-old men with 40 years of exposure at 90 dBA would be

about 20 dB (14 dB aging plus 6 dB NIPTS), using the data from Figs. 147.6 and 147.7. A greater loss than this prediction could be due to above-average susceptibility to aging or noise or both. One caveat: the data summarized in Fig. 147.7 represent highly screened individuals, excluding effects of otologic disease, audiometric anomalies, nonoccupational noise exposure, socioeconomic status, and so forth; more appropriate (unscreened) data are available (15) and should usually be used for medical-legal analysis (26).

Nonoccupational Exposures

The most important nonoccupational cause of NIHL is gunfire. Impulse levels from rifles and shotguns can reach 170 dB at the shooter's ear. The left ear of a right-handed shooter is at greater risk because the right ear is somewhat protected by the head shadow. Data from the interindustry noise study showed that men in nonnoisy jobs who reported hunting and shooting sustained hearing loss that was the equivalent of 20 years' occupational exposure at 89 dBA (27). Automobile airbags also produce very high impulse noise levels; they save lives but may cause acoustic trauma (28).

Exposures to leaf blowers, chain saws, and rock concerts can exceed 110 dBA. Very few people spend enough time in these exposures to cause NIPTS. The exception, of course, is occupational exposure; thus, professional gardeners, forestry workers, and rock musicians are at considerable risk. Nonetheless, it is not unreasonable to wear hearing protection even for occasional exposures at such levels. Personal cassette players are capable of producing dangerous noise levels, but most users choose levels well below 90 dBA. The most important risk of personal cassette players and radios is their use in a noisy work environment, where they can add to already-hazardous exposures.

Diagnosis of Noise-Induced Hearing Loss

In making a diagnosis of NIHL, the otolaryngologist must consider history, physical examination, audiometric findings (ideally over a period of many years), and sometimes the results of other tests. A history of occupational or nonoccupational noise exposure of hazardous intensity and duration should be sought. Noise exposure measurements from the workplace, if available, are most helpful. The history should document carefully all employment, including military service, with its often attendant noise exposure. Other etiologies of sensorineural hearing loss (heredity, ototoxicity, head injury, etc.) are primarily excluded by history. Physical examination excludes external ear and middle ear disorders and occasionally may detect cranial nerve or balance abnormalities that suggest an acoustic tumor.

The pure-tone audiogram in early cases usually shows a notch at 3, 4, or 6 kHz (not pathognomonic for NIHL); this notch is often lost over the years as loss becomes more

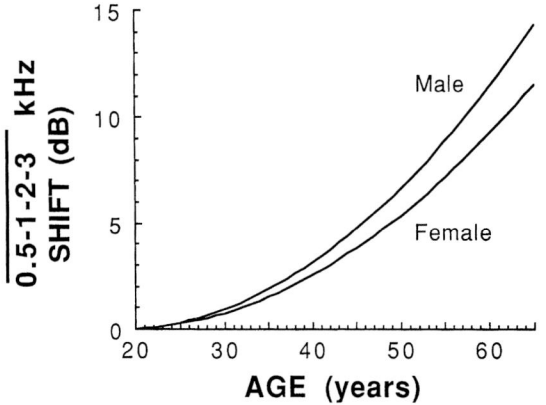

Figure 147.7 Median pure-tone average hearing changes (0.5, 1, 2, and 3 kHz) as a function of age for highly screened men and women.

severe and as aging changes are added to NIPTS. Pure-tone average asymmetries greater than about 15 dB suggest either another etiology or asymmetric exposures (29). Rifles and shotguns are the most common source for asymmetric NIHL. Most indoor factory environments are highly reverberant so that one ear rarely receives significantly more noise than the other. It is important to document whether hearing protectors have been used, what types are used, and when that use began.

A series of audiograms prior to employment and at intervals throughout a worker's career is most helpful. As suggested earlier, hearing loss that accelerates in middle age without any increase in noise exposure probably is due primarily to aging rather than to noise.

Laboratory and imaging tests are of no value in establishing the diagnosis of NIHL but occasionally are indicated to rule out other disorders, especially acoustic neuroma, when substantial asymmetries of hearing or other findings inconsistent with NIHL are present. The American College of Occupational and Environmental Medicine (30) has recently updated its policy statement on the diagnosis of NIHL (excerpted in Table 147.2).

Compensation

Otolaryngologists are frequently asked to evaluate workers for state workers compensation programs and for federal agencies such as the Veterans Administration and the Department of Labor. Compensation for NIHL varies widely, as do the formulas used for assessing hearing handicap (31).

Hearing handicap has been defined as a disadvantage "sufficient to affect the individual's efficiency in the activities of daily living," specifically, interference with speech communication (32). Whereas most of the acoustic power in speech is concentrated below 1000 Hz, most of the information content is in the higher frequencies. The typical patient with a handicapping degree of NIHL or age-related hearing loss can hear speech without difficulty because of the low-frequency power in vowel sounds but has difficulty discriminating among consonants because they are relatively high-frequency, low-intensity sounds. For example, *top* and *cop* may sound alike. These problems ultimately can lead to social withdrawal and isolation, depression, and a general reduction of quality of life. Depression also may be seen with tinnitus, which commonly accompanies NIHL.

In 1979, the American Academy of Otolaryngology-Head and Neck Surgery (AAO-HNS) revised their recommended method for evaluation of hearing handicap, which was subsequently accepted by the AMA (the AMA now uses the term "binaural hearing impairment" instead of "hearing handicap"). Most states have either adopted this method explicitly or have left the determination of hearing

---

TABLE 147.2

PRINCIPAL CHARACTERISTICS OF OCCUPATIONAL NOISE-INDUCED HEARING LOSS[a]

- It is always sensorineural, affecting the hair cells in the inner ear.
- Because most noise exposures are symmetric, the hearing loss is typically bilateral.
- Typically, the first sign of hearing loss due to noise exposure is a "notching" of the audiogram at 3000, 4000, or 6000 Hz, with recovery at 8000 Hz. This notching is in contrast to age-related loss, which also produces high-frequency hearing loss, but in a down-sloping pattern without recovery at 8000 Hz.
- Noise exposure alone usually does not produce a loss greater than 75 decibels (dB) in high frequencies, and 40 dB in lower frequencies. However, individuals with superimposed age-related losses may have hearing threshold levels in excess of these values.
- The rate of hearing loss due to chronic noise exposure is greatest during the first 10–15 years of exposure and decreases as the hearing threshold increases. This is in contrast to age-related hearing loss, which accelerates over time.
- Most scientific evidence indicates that previously noise-exposed ears are not more sensitive to future noise exposure and that hearing loss due to noise does not progress (in excess of what would be expected from the addition of age-related threshold shifts) once the exposure to noise is discontinued.
- In obtaining a history of noise exposure, the clinician should keep in mind that the risk of noise-induced hearing loss is considered to rise significantly with chronic exposures above 85 dBA for an 8-hour time-weighted average (TWA). In general, continuous noise exposure over the years is more damaging than interrupted exposure that permits the ear to have a rest period.

[a]Occupational noise-induced hearing loss, as opposed to occupational acoustic trauma, is hearing loss that develops slowly over a long period (several years) as the result of exposure to continuous or intermittent loud noise. Occupational acoustic trauma is a sudden change in hearing as a result of a single exposure to a sudden burst of sound, such as an explosive blast. The diagnosis of noise-induced hearing loss is made clinically by a medical professional and should include a study of the noise exposure history.

handicap to professional judgment. The AAO-HNS/AMA 1979 method (33) is based on several assumptions:

1. Hearing loss does not begin to be handicapping until the PTA at 0.5, 1, 2, and 3 kHz exceeds 25 dB HL.
2. Handicap grows at the rate of 1.5% per decibel of hearing loss beyond 25 dB.
3. Because unilateral deafness is only a mild handicap, the two ears should not be equally weighted. Specifically, a 5 to 1 weighting favoring the better ear is used.

The monaural impairment (MI) for each ear is first calculated from the four-frequency PTA:

$$MI = 1.5 \, (PTA - 25)$$

The binaural hearing impairment (BHI), ranging from 0% to 100%, is then calculated as a weighted average favoring the better ear:

$$BHI = [5 \, (MI_b) + (MI_w)]/6$$

where MI_b and MI_w represent the monaural impairment scores of the better and worse ears.

For example, consider a person whose thresholds are as follows:

Frequency	Right Ear	Left Ear
0.5 kHz	15 dB	20 dB
1 kHz	25 dB	40 dB
2 kHz	35 dB	60 dB
3 kHz	45 dB	80 dB

The right (better) ear PTA is $(15 + 25 + 35 + 45)/4 = 30$ dB. The better ear MI score is $(30 - 25)(1.5) = 7.5\%$.

The left (worse) ear PTA is $(20 + 40 + 60 + 80)/4 = 50$ dB. The worse ear MI score is $(50 - 25)(1.5) = 37.5\%$.

The BHI is $[5(7.5) + (37.5)]/6 = 12.5\%$.

Even when no other specific otologic disease is present, elevated HTLs in noise-exposed workers can usually be thought of as containing aging and noise-induced components. Age correction of audiograms is not appropriate for compensation assessment purposes. It is possible, however, to make reasonable estimates of the relative contributions of noise and aging, or of separate periods of noise exposure, in individual cases (13,34).

The physician's report of a compensation examination should be complete and concise, and, most importantly, should offer clear diagnostic conclusions based on clinical and scientific evidence with some explanation of the reasons for those conclusions. If a particular diagnosis is "more probable than not" (probability >50%), it can and should be stated as a "reasonable medical certainty"; this standard, which is typical for civil and workers' compensation cases, differs substantially from the "beyond a reasonable doubt" standard used in criminal trials. The AAO-HNS (34) has published guidelines for physicians' reports in such settings.

MANAGEMENT

Hearing Conservation

Since 1970, federal law has required most employers to prevent exposures exceeding 90 dBA for an 8-hour day. The detailed requirements for occupational HCPs, however, were not published until much later (35).

Many noise exposures are not steady state; the noise may fluctuate in intensity throughout the day. Other occupational exposures may be brief, as when a worker spends less than 1 hour a day in a particularly noisy part of the factory. Considerable controversy exists about how to handle such exposure variations, largely because there are only scanty epidemiologic data relating NIPTS to brief and varying exposures. If exposures containing equal sound energy were equally hazardous, one would adopt a trading rule in which the permissible exposure time would be cut in half for each 3-dB increase in exposure level (sound power, i.e., energy per unit time, doubles for each 3-dB increment). However, there is frequently a degree of intermittency in occupational noise exposures, thus reducing risk. For this reason, expert consensus led OSHA to adopt a 5-dB trading rule: a 4-hour exposure at 95 dBA and a 2-hour exposure at 100 dBA are considered equally as hazardous as an 8-hour exposure at 90 dBA. Each of these exposures would be considered to be 90 dBA "time-weighted average" (TWA: exposure level that if constant for 8 hours would be expected to pose the same risk of hearing loss as the briefer exposure in question). Time-intensity trading ends at 115 dBA: Above this level, OSHA permits only exposures of less than 1 second. This relationship between sound level and duration is shown in Table 147.3.

The maximum permissible exposure (without hearing protection) under OSHA regulations is 90 dBA TWA, but HCPs must be implemented for all workers whose exposures

TABLE 147.3
PERMISSIBLE NOISE EXPOSURES

Duration Per Day (hr)	Sound Level (dBA)
8	90
6	92
4	95
3	97
2	100
1.5	102
1	105
0.5	110
≤0.25	115

exceed 85 dBA TWA. Impulse noise exposure is limited to 140-dB peak level.

The essential components of an HCP are as follows:

- Noise exposure measurements
- Engineering or administrative controls to reduce exposure
- Periodic audiometry with follow-up and referral
- Use of personal hearing protection devices (HPDs)
- Education, motivation, and counseling

Measurements of noise exposure may be performed with sound level meters or devices called noise dosimeters, which attach to a worker's clothing and automatically compute his or her TWA exposure. Exposures that exceed permissible limits can be reduced by noise control or by reducing the time that employees spend in the noise. In situations in which neither engineering nor administrative controls can reduce exposures below 85 dBA TWA, a program of annual audiometry must be instituted. Although workplace audiometry is less reliable than clinical testing, PTA changes of 10 dB or more usually indicate real hearing changes (36). OSHA defines a standard threshold shift (STS) as a 10-dB or greater increase in threshold for the 2-, 3-, and 4-kHz average in either ear. Unfortunately, OSHA does not mandate otologic referral, even for large or asymmetric losses, although disorders other than NIHL are often found in such cases (37). Workers who demonstrate STS or who have exposures above 90 dBA TWA must use HPDs (earplugs, earmuffs).

Although the "noise reduction ratings" on the package labels of HPDs are typically 20 to 30 dB or even higher, these numbers reflect ideal fitting in laboratory conditions. Real-world attenuation values are much lower: On the average, premolded earplugs offer about 10 dB attenuation of A-weighted levels, formable foam plugs about 15 dB, and earmuffs about 20 dB. If worn only 4 hours out of a steady 8-hour noise exposure, no HPD can provide more than 5 dB of effective attenuation. Recently, there has been great interest in electronic noise cancellation headsets, which attempt to deliver a sound wave to the ear that is exactly out of phase with the ambient noise. These devices can effectively cancel out only low-frequency noises (up to about 500 Hz), and they can thus be quite helpful in environments where the noise is predominantly low-frequency, such as in private aviation. Unfortunately, the most hazardous spectral components for most occupational and recreational noises are well above 500 Hz; thus, noise cancellation has been of very little value in HCPs. In contrast, another type of electronic HPD has proved to be very useful in situations where the hazardous noise is only intermittent (such as recreational shooting): These "level-dependent" HPDs have an external microphone, an internal speaker, and circuitry that allows sounds below about 85 dB to pass into the ear while louder sounds are blocked.

The differences in protection afforded by various HPDs, when worn properly, are small compared with variations in protection that occur with improper or negligent use. The most important factors in choosing an HPD are proper fit and acceptance by the worker. Counseling and motivation are important. Many workers fear they will miss important communications or warning signals with HPDs in place. In fact, detection of such signals is usually not impaired. Speech and other signals need to be at a high level to be heard over industrial noise anyway, and with the HPD in place, both signal and noise are equally reduced. Some workers with high-frequency hearing loss perform more poorly than normal-hearing persons in detecting and discriminating signals in noise with HPDs in place (38); this problem can often be ameliorated by using HPDs with less high-frequency attenuation, which can usually provide adequate protection without making high-frequency signals inaudible.

Clinical Management

Many physicians have advocated treatments, usually based on vasodilatation or hemorheologic effects, for acute acoustic trauma. Considerable recovery of hearing is part of the natural history of such events, however, and no well-controlled studies have yet demonstrated benefit for any treatment, except in animals (not human patients) given antioxidants or other drugs prior to or during excessive noise exposure. This continues to be an active area of research, and future studies may yet show that drugs, vitamins, and/or nutritional supplements have a role in the treatment and prevention of NIHL (39,40). For example, the U.S. military is currently investigating the use of N-acetyl cysteine, a drug currently used as an antidote for acetaminophen overdose, as a protective and rescue drug for acoustic trauma.

Counseling to prevent further hearing loss is crucial. Workers who are not enrolled in occupational HCPs need to be scheduled for periodic monitoring audiometry and should be counseled regarding the appropriate use of HPDs. Hearing aids are helpful when hearing loss becomes handicapping, but of course they do not restore normal hearing.

Counseling hearing-impaired workers or their employers regarding fitness for continued safe and productive employment is extremely difficult. Factors to consider include not only the degree of hearing loss but also the acoustic environment at work, the communicative demands of the job, and nonauditory attributes of the worker, such as age, experience, linguistic background, and cognitive status (41).

NONAUDITORY EFFECTS

Loud noise interferes severely with speech communication at about the same levels at which hazard to hearing begins. This information can be useful in counseling and in assessing compensation claims. If a worker states that the workplace is noisy enough that he or she must speak very loudly or shout to converse at ordinary conversational distances, then, even in the absence of sound level measurements, it can be concluded that levels are probably over 80 dBA.

Other nonauditory effects of noise, including annoyance, sleep disturbance, and physiologic changes (in blood pressure, catecholamine secretion, and so on), are controversial. Certainly, annoyance and sleep disturbance may occur at levels far below any hazard for NIHL (42,43). An unwanted noise, such as a dripping faucet or a neighbor's party, even if quite faint, can be annoying and stressful. These effects are not due to the physical properties of the noise (intensity, spectrum, time) but to cognitive and psychological factors (44). It is impossible to predict these types of effects with a sound level meter. It is probably safe to say that most experts believe that no adverse long-term health effects of noise exposure have been demonstrated at exposures below those that could cause NIHL.

ACKNOWLEDGMENTS

Drs. Dixon Ward, William Melnick, Donald Henderson, and Jack Mills read earlier versions of the manuscript and made helpful suggestions. Michael Wilson prepared the figures; Julie Estrada and Mary Brown typed the original manuscript.

HIGHLIGHTS

- Noise-induced hearing loss, although not medically or surgically treatable, is the major preventable cause of hearing loss in the United States.
- NIPTS grows rapidly in the high frequencies (3 to 6 kHz) and then decelerates after about 10 years.
- After about 10 years at constant exposure levels, threshold shifts at lower frequencies (especially 2 kHz) begin to predominate.
- Within the organ of Corti, the outer hair cells are most susceptible to noise-induced damage.
- Workplace exposures below 80 dBA pose negligible risk to human hearing; exposures at levels above 85 dBA may cause significant noise-induced threshold shift.
- In contrast to noise-induced loss, age-related hearing loss is an accelerating process (rate of change increases with time).
- The most important nonoccupational cause of NIHL is gunfire.
- Federal regulations forbid occupational exposures over 90 dBA TWA (8-hour equivalent) without hearing protection but require HCPs for all workers whose exposures exceed 85 dBA TWA.
- The need to shout to converse in the workplace or a worker's complaint of temporary fullness, tinnitus, or muffled hearing after work usually indicates the presence of potentially hazardous noise levels.
- Diagnosis of NIHL should not be made on the basis of audiometric contour alone, but must include a careful history of occupational and nonoccupational noise exposure.

REFERENCES

1. Yueh B, Shapiro N, MacLean CH, et al. Screening and management of adult hearing loss in primary care. *JAMA* 2003; 289:1976–1985.
2. Bohne BA, Zahn SJ, Bozzay DG. Damage to the cochlea following interrupted exposure to low-frequency noise. *Ann Otol Rhinol Laryngol* 1985;94:122–128.
3. Sataloff J, Sataloff RT, Menduke H, et al. Intermittent exposure to noise: effects on hearing. *Ann Otol Rhinol Laryngol* 1983;92: 623–628.
4. Gates G, Schmid P, Kujawa S, et al. Longitudinal threshold changes in older men with audiometric notches. *Hearing Res* 2000;141:220–228.
5. Borg E, Nilsson R, Engström B. Effect of the acoustic reflex on inner ear damage induced by industrial noise. *Acta Otolaryngol* 1983;96:361–369.
6. Maison SF, Liberman MC. Predicting vulnerability to acoustic injury with a non-invasive assay of olivocochlear reflex strength. *J Neurosci* 2000;20:4701–4707.
7. Sha S, Taylor R, Forge A, et al. Differential vulnerability of basal and apical hair cells is based on intrinsic susceptibility to free radicals. *Hearing Res* 2001;155:1–8.
8. Niu X, Canlon B. Theories of sound conditioning. In Henderson D, ed. *Noise-induced hearing loss: basic mechanisms, prevention, and control.* London: NRN Publications, 2001.
9. Taylor W, Pearson J, Mair A. Study of noise and hearing in jute weaving. *J Acoust Soc Am* 1965;38:113–120.
10. Wang Y, Hirose K, Liberman M. Dynamics of noise-induced cellular injury and repair in the mouse cochlea. *J Assoc Res Otolaryngol* 2002;3:248–268.
11. Henderson D, Hamernik RP. Impulse noise: critical review. *J Acoust Soc Am* 1986;80:569–584.
12. McRobert H, Ward WD. Damage-risk criteria: the trading relation between intensity and the number of nonreverberant impulses. *J Acoust Soc Am* 1973;53:1297–1300.
13. Dobie RA. *Medical-legal evaluation of hearing loss,* 2nd ed. San Diego: Singular Publishing, 2001.
14. Macrae JH. Noise-induced hearing loss and presbyacusis. *Audiology* 1971;10:323–333.
15. American National Standards Institute. *Determination of occupational noise exposure and estimation of noise-induced hearing impairment.* ANSI-S3.44-1996. New York: Acoustical Society of America, 1996:27.
16. Czanto C, Ligia S. Correlation between vibration-induced white finger and hearing loss in miners. *J Occup Health* 1999;41: 232–237.
17. Humes LE. Noise-induced hearing loss as influenced by other agents and by some physical characteristics of the individual. *J Acoust Soc Am* 1984;76:1318–1329.
18. Cary R, Clarke S, Delic J. Effects of combined exposure to noise and toxic substances—critical review of the literature. *Ann Occup Hyg* 1997;41:455–465.
19. Sliwinska-Kowalska M, Zamyslowska-Szmytke E, Szymczak W, et al. Hearing loss among workers exposed to moderate concentrations of solvents. *Scand J Work Environ. Health* 2001;27: 335–342.
20. Morata T, Johnson A, Nylen P, et al. Audiometric findings in workers exposed to low levels of styrene and noise. *J Occup Environ Med* 2002;44:806–814.
21. Holme R, Steel K. Progressive hearing loss and increased susceptibility to noise-induced hearing loss in mice carrying a cdh23 but not a myo7a mutation. *J Assoc Res Otolaryngol* 2004;5:66–79.
22. Davis R, Kozel P, Erway L. Genetic influences in individual susceptibility to noise: a review. *Noise Health* 2003;5:19–28.
23. Saunders JC, Dear SP, Schneider ME. The anatomical consequences of acoustic injury: a review and tutorial. *J Acoust Soc Am* 1985;78:833–860.
24. Occupational Safety and Health Administration, US Department of Labor. Occupational noise exposure: hearing conservation amendment. *Fed Register* 1981:4078.
25. Phaneuf R, Hétu R. An epidemiological perspective of the causes of hearing loss among industrial workers. *J Otolaryngol* 1990;19(1):31–40.

26. Lutman ME, Davis AC. Distributions of hearing threshold levels in populations exposed to noise. In: Axelsson A, Borchgrevink H, Hamernik RP, et al., eds. *Scientific basis of noise-induced hearing loss.* New York: Thieme Medical, 1996.
27. Johnson DL, Riffle C. Effects of gunfire on the hearing level of selected individuals from the Inter-Industry Noise Study. *J Acoust Soc Am* 1982;72:1311–1314.
28. Yaremchuk K, Dobie RA. Otologic injuries from airbag deployment. *Otolaryngol Head Neck Surg* 2001;125:130–134.
29. Alberti PW, Symons F, Hyde ML. Occupational hearing loss: the significance of asymmetrical hearing thresholds. *Acta Otolaryngol* 1979;87:255–263.
30. ACOEM Noise and Hearing Conservation Committee. ACOEM evidence-based statement: Noise-induced hearing loss. *J Occup Med* 2003;45:579–581.
31. Dobie RA, Megerson SC. Workers' compensation. In: Berger EH, ed. *The noise manual,* rev. 5th ed. Fairfax, VA: American Industrial Hygiene Association, 2003.
32. American Academy of Otolaryngology—Head and Neck Surgery Foundation. *Guide for conservation of hearing in noise.* Washington, DC: American Academy of Otolaryngology—Head Neck Surgery Foundation, 1988.
33. American Medical Association (AMA). *Guides to the evaluation of permanent impairment,* 5th ed. Chicago: AMA Press, 2001.
34. American Academy of Otolaryngology—Head and Neck Surgery. *Evaluation of people reporting occupational hearing loss.* Alexandria, VA: American Academy of Otolaryngology—Head and Neck Surgery, 1998.
35. Occupational Safety and Heath Administration, US Department of Labor. Occupational noise exposure: hearing conservation amendment; final rule (anonymous). *Fed Register* 1983;48:9738.
36. Dobie RA. Reliability and validity of industrial audiometry: implications for hearing conservation program design (1983 Triological Society Thesis). *Laryngoscope* 1983;93:906–927.
37. Dobie RA, Archer RJ. Results of otologic referrals in an industrial hearing conservation program. *Otolaryngol Head Neck Surg* 1981; 89:294–301.
38. Abel SM, Kunov H, Pichora-Fuller MK, et al. Signal detection in industrial noise: effects of noise exposure history, hearing loss, and the use of ear protection. *Scand Audiol* 1985;14:161–173.
39. Kopke R, Coleman J, Liu J, et al. Enhancing intrinsic cochlear stress defenses to reduce noise-induced hearing loss. *Laryngoscope* 2002;112:1515–1532.
40. Le Prell CL, Dolan D, Schacht J, et al. Pathways for protection from noise-induced hearing loss. *Noise Health* 2003;5:1–17.
41. Dobie RA, VanHemel SB, eds. National Research Council. *Hearing loss: determining eligibility for social security benefits.* National Academy Press, Washington DC, 2004.
42. Raschke F. Arousals and aircraft noise: environmental disorders of sleep and health in terms of sleep medicine. *Noise Health* 2004;6:15–26.
43. Guski R. How to forecast community annoyance in planning noisy facilities. *Noise Health* 2004;6:59–64.
44. Ising H. Editorial. *Noise Health* 2004;6:1–2.

Ototoxicity

148

Rita M. Schuman   Gregory J. Matz

Drug-induced inner ear damage is a common finding in present-day medical practice. In many developing countries, where drugs such as the aminoglycosides are frequently prescribed to treat pneumonia, diarrhea, and tuberculosis, the incidence of ototoxicity is high (1). Physicians in practice need to recognize that ototoxic drugs can cause significant auditory and in many instances, poorly recognized, vestibular toxicity. Physicians therefore need to be cognizant of the many categories of drugs that produce ototoxicity.

Early examples of drug ototoxicity are arsenic, the salicylates, and quinine. Salicylates, for example, administered in doses in excess of 2,700 mg a day, once commonly used to treat arthritis, were found to cause a transient flat, bilateral sensorineural hearing loss and tinnitus. There has never been a case of permanent hearing loss following salicylate use in therapeutic drug dosing; however, most patients experience complete reversal within 2 to 3 days. Later, in the 1960s, thalidomide, a well-known drug used at that time and now known to cause amelia and phocomelia, was also discovered to cause aplasia of the inner ear.

The introduction of the first aminoglycoside, streptomycin, in 1944 by Waxman, who was awarded the Nobel prize for this discovery, heralded a new era of antibiotic therapy for the treatment of tuberculosis. Unfortunately, Hinshaw and Feldman at the Mayo Clinic described a significant number of patients with vestibular toxicity from this drug (2). A few years later, an analog of streptomycin, dihydrostreptomycin, was used in clinical practice with the hopes of reducing the streptomycin ototoxicity. Dihydrostreptomycin, however, was also shown to have an unacceptably high incidence of cochlear toxicity and was subsequently withdrawn from the market. Likewise, other early aminoglycosides, such as kanamycin and neomycin had unacceptably high rates of cochlear toxicity when used systemically and therefore are rarely used in that manner today. Later, a newer aminoglycoside, gentamicin, was shown to have about a 3% incidence of vestibular injury (3). Subsequent aminoglycosides such as netilmicin, tobramycin, and

amikacin were developed to reduce this incidence of toxicity. In fact, netilmicin has been found to be the least ototoxic of all of the aminoglycosides available (4).

Other considerations must include the cancer chemotherapeutic agents, such as cisplatin, which has been found to result in a moderate level of ototoxicity with resultant permanent bilateral hearing loss. Clinicians are also faced with a sporadic low incidence of ototoxicity with drugs such as vancomycin and the macrolides. Most studies in the literature regarding the ototoxicity of the macrolides have been found to be reversible. The mechanism by which these drugs are toxic is unknown. Finally, numerous case reports have also indicated that hydrocodone in combination with acetaminophen can cause a rapidly progressive sensorineural hearing loss. (5). The mechanism of toxicity at this time is unknown.

OTOTOXICTY OF OTOTOPICAL ANTIBIOTICS

It is well known that systemic administrations of aminoglycosides can cause both cochlear and vestibular toxicity. This naturally leads to the question of whether these drugs, which are used extensively to treat ear infections through topical administration to the middle ear, can cause ototoxicity. Animal data have been quite uniform in that almost all of the aminoglycoside antibiotics used in the middle ear as topical otic preparations are ototoxic (6). The use of aminoglycoside ototopical drops confined to the external auditory canal, however, presents little, if any, risk of ototoxicity.

Current review of the literature reveals documentation of a total of 54 cases of gentamicin vestibular toxicity from ototopical use in the middle ear or open mastoid cavity (7) (Table 148. 1). In addition, 24 of these patients developed an associated auditory toxicity. A review of the literature in the above cited study also included 11 patients who experienced auditory toxicity from the topical use of

TABLE 148.1

OTOTOXICITY OF OTOTOPICAL EAR DROPS

Drug	No. Cases	Ototoxicity Description
Gentamicin	54	All with vestibular loss and 24 with associated cochlear loss (8–12)
Neomycin/polymyxin	11	11 cases with auditory loss and 2 cases with vestibular loss (13–16)

neomycin-polymyxin-based eardrops. It was therefore recommended that when possible,

topical antibiotic preparations free of potential ototoxic side effects should be used in preference to ototopical preparations that have had the potential for ototoxic injury if the middle ear or mastoid are open (17). Aminoglycoside-containing antibiotic topical drops are not FDA approved for use in the middle ear or open mastoid cavity. Indeed, current labels contain warnings against the use of these drugs if the tympanic membrane is not intact. Although the evidence suggests that otologic damage from topical preparations with ototoxic potential is infrequent, the evidence also indicates that they offer no advantage over nonototoxic agents (17). If these ototoxic agents are considered, potentially ototoxic, antibiotic preparations should be used only in acutely infected ears and use should be discontinued shortly after the infection has resolved. Finally, if the clinician must use potentially ototoxic antibiotics in the middle ear or mastoid space, the patient or parents should be warned of the risk of ototoxicity (17).

OTOTOXICITY OF SYSTEMIC DRUGS

Table 148.2 lists the major classes of drugs that cause ototoxicity—the aminoglycoside antibiotics, the macrolides, loop diuretics, cisplatin, and the salicylates. These drugs are listed because they are commonly seen in otolaryngology consultation practice. There are currently no meta-analysis studies that evaluate ototoxicity for these drugs. Included in the bibliography are two reviews that include ototoxic evaluations for gentamicin and cisplatin in a large cohort of patients. Omitted for the sake of brevity in Table 148.2 are the low-incidence ototoxic drugs, such as chloroquine, which is rarely used in clinical practice in the United States.

For various reasons, the incidence of aminoglycoside ototoxicity in neonates and children is lower than adults (23). In children, it can be useful to obtain pretreatment audiograms to rule out preexisting hearing loss in patients who are to receive a course of aminoglycoside antibiotics. In the United States, that drug is usually gentamicin.

GENETICS OF OTOXICITY

It is well known that aminoglycosides are some of the most common ototoxic drugs causing acquired hearing loss. It was observed that many patients were developing hearing loss, despite the low dosages of aminoglycosides administered. It was also noted that certain families had an exceptionally high number of members with similar findings of aminoglycoside ototoxicity. Based on these observations and the ongoing research regarding the pathophysiology of hearing loss, it has been proposed that certain individuals may have a genetic predisposition or susceptibility to the ototoxic effects of certain drugs and in particular, the aminoglycosides (24).

Recent advances have identified that certain mutations in mitochondrial DNA are found to be associated with a number of hearing disorders, including ototoxicity. Mitochondrial DNA is a double-stranded molecule forming a closed circle. Replication and transcription occurs within the mitochondria, ultimately forming proteins involved with ATP synthesis and electron transport. This specific type of DNA is transmitted exclusively by the maternal line, equally affecting both male and female offspring.

In the early 1990s it was first discovered that a mutation at position 1555 in the nucleotides of the mitochondrial 12S ribosomal RNA was responsible for aminoglycoside toxicity in several Chinese families (25). It was also cited as a cause for a number of cases of nonsyndromic deafness in patients with no previous aminoglycoside exposure. Since that discovery, similar research has been conducted on numerous other families, as well as on sporadic patients with documented sensorineural hearing loss following the administration of intravenous aminoglycosides. These subsequent studies confirmed that these patients also had identical nucleotide mutations of their mitochondrial DNA. It has been proposed that the specific mutation creates another binding site for the aminoglycosides, thus increasing the patient's sensitivity to ototoxicity (26). Most of this work was conducted on an international basis, where severe infections such as tuberculosis more often require widespread use of intravenous aminoglycosides.

A large quantity of research continues in this area. As more becomes known about the genetics of hearing loss and the specific mutations that predispose patients to the ototoxic effects of some drugs, it may be possible to develop molecular tests to identify these patients prior to treatment. With that information, it may be possible to reduce the number of patients suffering from the toxicities of these antibiotics.

CHEMOPREVENTION OF OTOTOXICITY

In some instances, it may be necessary to use ototoxic drugs in order to effectively treat patients. In light of this fact, it is necessary to develop mechanisms by which it is

TABLE 148.2
DRUGS WITH OTOTOXICITY

	Incidence of Ototoxicity	Site of Injury	
The Aminoglycosides			
Gentamicin	2–3% incidence (3)	Cupula semicircular canal	Outer hair cell damage
			Loss of cochlear hair cells
		Cochlea	Type I hair cell loss of the cupula of the vestibular system
Kanamycin	High incidence of cochlear loss	Cochlea	Hair cell loss of cochlea
Neomycin	High incidence of cochlear loss	Cochlea	Hair cell loss of cochlea
	Use limited to topical application		
Tobramycin	3–4% incidence of vestibular loss	Cochlea	Hair cell loss of cochlea
	6% incidence of cochlear loss (3)		
Amikacin	14% incidence of cochlear loss (3)		Hair cell loss of cochlea
The macrolides			
Erythromycin	Causes transient cochlear loss		No reported temporal bone histopathology
	Permanent loss rare and dose related		
Azithromycin	Rare cases of transient hearing loss		
Antineoplastic agents			
Cisplatin	12–25% incidence of cochlear loss—dose dependent (18)	Cochlea	Hair cell loss of cochlea
			Degeneration of stria vascularis
			Decrease in ganglion cells (22)
Loop diuretics			
Furosemide	Less than 1% transient loss (19)	Cochlea	Abnormal stria vascularis
Ethacrynic acid	Rare incidence of ototoxicity	Cochlea	Abnormal stria vascularis (20)
		Semicircular canals	
	Cochlear loss can occur if used with an aminoglycoside (20)		
Salicylates			
Aspirin	Only transient hearing loss and tinnitus in doses over 2,700 mg/day		No reported temporal bone histopathology
Vancomycin	Can become ototoxic if used with aminoglycosides		
	Incidence of cochlear loss rare (21)		

possible to protect the inner ear from the toxicities of both the ototoxic intravenous antibiotics and the chemotherapeutic agents such as cisplatin. Some of the agents that have been proposed and studied include iron chelators (deferoxime) (27,28), antioxidants including L-N-acetyl cysteine (29), vitamin E, alpha-tocopherol (30–32), as well as the salicylates (33,34).

Recent research has demonstrated that administration of aminoglycosides causes the formation of an iron complex that is involved in the generation of free radicals, resulting in hair cell death and subsequent hearing loss (28). Based on this discovery, attempts have been made to use deferoxamine, an iron chelator, to help attenuate these toxic effects. Animal studies have been promising, but considerations must be taken so as to not alter the serum concentrations of the drugs, and a better understanding is needed of the side effects of administering iron chelators to patients and the potential of altering serum iron levels (27).

Cisplatin, a common chemotherapeutic agent used in head and neck cancer, is well known to cause bilateral, irreversible sensorineural hearing loss. Evidence suggests that glutathione reduction secondary to free radical production ultimately causes hair cell damage. Various chemoprotectants have been shown to exert antioxidant properties that ultimately reduce the ototoxic effects of cisplatin. Recent studies with vitamin E (31), L-N-Acetyl cysteine (29), and sodium thiosulfate (35) confirm this theory. Most of the research, however, has thus far been with animals. Further human studies must be done to truly know if these advances will be clinically significant and will ultimately reduce the ototoxic effects.

SUMMARY

One of the authors of this chapter (GJM) has written previously about the use of high-frequency audiometry (8 to 12 Hz) as a predictor of drug-induced ototoxicity (36). Although conventional audiometry may still have a role in monitoring patients exposed to ototoxic medications, high frequency testing is often problematic. It is an extremely difficult test to do for all practical purposes and is often not done clinically for that reason. Few centers perform pretreatment conventional audiograms from 0.25 Hz to 8 Hz when the two most common ototoxic drugs, gentamicin and cisplatin, are given. The authors are not aware of any outcome studies that demonstrate that pretreatment and post-treatment audiograms reduce the incidence of predicted ototoxicity. Some centers have found, however, that it may be beneficial to perform one pretreatment audiogram followed by serial audiograms, in addition to closely monitoring the serum drug levels of the ototoxic medications being administered. The use of vestibular testing both pretreatment and post-treatment for patients receiving long-term gentamicin is also difficult to do in the clinical setting. This is an important factor because gentamicin is mostly a vestibular toxic drug. Some centers do perform electronystagmography, rotational testing, and platform posturography in working up possible vestibular symptoms and have found these tests to be helpful.

It is now well known that the aminoglycoside antibiotics act synergistically with some drugs, thus increasing the incidence of ototoxicity. For example, the use of aminoglycoside antibiotics with loop diuretics can produce an unexpectedly high incidence of ototoxicity. This has been extensively documented in human case reports as well as in animal studies. Ethacrynic acid, an ototoxic loop diuretic, has been shown to increase the permeability of the stria vascularis, facilitating the diffusion of the aminoglycoside into the endolymph. Finally, it has been found that diuretics given prior to the administration of aminoglycosides are less damaging than if done in the reverse (37). Most recently noted is a similar response to aminoglycoside antibiotics and the use of metronidazole (38).

It is unclear at this time if antiviral and protease inhibitors are responsible for the anecdotal reporting of neurosensory hearing loss in patients with human immunodeficiency virus (39). Prospective studies are needed to confirm whether nucleoside analog reverse transcriptase inhibitor or antiviral agents cause hearing loss in this patient population. The use of chemoprevention measures as described in animal studies show promise, but so far no prospective clinical trials have

been performed and the authors are not aware of any medical centers with protocols to address this issue at this time.

The two most common ototoxic drugs given today in clinical practice are gentamicin and cisplatin. The patients selected in these groups are different. Gentamicin is normally monitored not by audiograms but by serum peak and trough levels. When gentamicin has to be given for long-term therapy (i.e., osteomyelitis), consideration has to be given to genetic testing to see if a patient is going to be more susceptible to ototoxic injury, thus giving the clinician the opportunity to obtain informed consent from the patient. Likewise, accurate dosing during chemotherapy has reduced the incidence of ototoxicity. Further research is necessary to determine if any of the chemopreventative agents will be successful in further animal and ultimately human trials to reduce the unfortunate toxicities of these necessary drugs.

HIGHLIGHTS

- Topical administration of ototoxic drugs may harm the cochlea.
- Cisplatin is associated with 12% to 25% incidence of hearing loss that is dose related.
- Predisposition to aminoglycoside-associated hearing loss may be genetically predetermined.
- Aminoglycoside antibiotics act synergistically with logs diuretics to produce unexpectedly high incidence of ototoxicity.

REFERENCES

1. *Chicago Tribune*, Nov. 24, 1988; sec 1:41.
2. Hinshaw HC, Feldman, WH. Streptomycin in the treatment of clinical tuberculosis—a preliminary report. *Proc Mayo Clin* 1945; 20:313–315.
3. Kahlmeter O, Dahlager JI. Aminoglycoside toxicity:a review of clinical studies between 1975–1982. *J Antimicrob Chemother* 1984;13 (Suppl A):9–22.
4. Kalkandelen S, Selimoglu E, Erdogas F, et al. Comparative cochlear toxicities of streptomycin, gentamicin, amikacin and netilmicin in guinea pigs. *J Intern Med Res* 2002;30:406–412.
5. Friedman RA, House JW. Profound hearing loss associated with hydrocodone/acetaminophen abuse. *Am J Otol* 2000;21: 188–191.
6. Roland PS, Ryback L, Hannley M, et al. Animal ototoxicity of topical antibiotics and the relevance to clinical treatment of human subjects. *Otolaryngol Head Neck Surg* 2004;13:S57–S78.
7. Matz G, Ryback L, Roland PS, et al. Ototoxicity of ototopical antibiotic drops in humans. *Otolaryngol Head Neck Surg* 2004;13:3: S79–S82.
8. Longridge NS. Topical gentamicin vestibular toxicity. *J Otolaryngol* 1999;23:444–446.
9. Lancaster JL, Mortimore S, McCormack M. Systemic absorption of gentamicin in the management of active mucosa chronic otitis media. *Clin Otolaryngol* 1999;24:435–439.
10. Marais J, Rutka JA. Ototoxicity of topical ear drops. *Clin Otolaryngol* 1998;23:360–367.
11. Bath AP, Walsh RM, Bance ML, et al. Ototoxicity of topical gentamicin preparation. *Laryngoscope* 1999;109:1088–1093.
12. Kaplan DM, Hehar SS, Bance ML. Intention ablation of vestibular function using commercially available topical gentamicin—betamethasone eardrops in patients with Ménière's disease: further evidence for topical eardrop ototoxicity. *Laryngoscope* 2002; 112:689–695.

13. Dumas G, Bessard G, Gavend M, et al. Risk of deafness following ototopical administration of aminoglycoside antibiotic. *Therapie* 1980;35: 357–363.

14. Linder TE, Zvickys S, Brandle P. Ototoxicity of ear drops: A clinical perspective. *Am J Otol* 1995;16:6537.

15. Lindo, Kristiansen B. Deafness after treatment with ear drops containing neomycin, gramicidin and dexamethasone. A case report. *ORL J Otorhinololaryngol Relat* 1986;48:52–54.

16. Rakover Y, Keywan K, Rosen G. Safety of topical ear drops containing antibiotics. *J Otolaryngol* 1997;26:194–196.

17. Roland PS, Stewart MG, Hannley M, et al. Consensus panel of role of potentially ototoxic antibiotics for topical middle ear use: introduction, methodology and recommendations. *Otolaryngol Head Neck Surg* 2004;13:S51–S56.

18. Simon THB, Dupuis W, Selle B, Berthold F. The incidence of hearing impairment after successful treatment of neuroblastoma. *Klin Padiatr* 2002;214:149–152.

19. Boston Collaborative Drug Surveillance Program. Drug-induced deafness. *JAMA* 1973;224:515.

20. Matz GJ. Ototoxic effects of ethacrynic acid in man and animals. *Laryngoscope* 1976;86:1065–1086.

21. Brummett RE, Fox KE, Jacobs F, et al. Augmented gentamicin ototoxicity induced by vancomycin in guinea pigs. *Arch Otolaryngol Head Neck Surg* 1990;116:61–64.

22. Hinojosa R, Riggs LC, Strauss M, et al. Temporal bone histopathology of cisplatin ototoxicity. *Am J Otol* 1995;16:731–740.

23. Siegel JD, McCraken GH. Aminoglycoside ototoxicity in children. In: *Aminoglycoside ototoxicity*. Boston: Little Brown, 1981:341–357.

24. Casano RA, Johnson DF, Byhovskya Y, et al. Inherited susceptibility to aminoglycoside ototoxicity: genetic heterogeneity and clinical implications. *Am J Otolaryngol* 1999;29:151–156.

25. Prezant TR, Agapian JV, Bohlman MC, et al. Mitochondrial ribosomal ARNA mutation associated with both antibiotic-induced and non-syndromic deafness. *Nat Genet* 1993;4:289–294.

26. Guan MX, Fischel-Ghodsian N, Attardi G. A biochemical basis for the inherited susceptibility to aminoglycoside ototoxicitiy. *Hum Mol Gen* 2000;9:1787–1793.

27. Conlon BJ, Perry BP, Smith DW. Attenuation of neomycin ototoxicity by iron chelation. *Laryngoscope* 1998;108:284–287.

28. Song BB, Anderson DJ, Schacht J. Protection from gentamicin ototoxicity by iron chelators in guinea pig in vivo. *J Pharm Exp Ther* 1997;282:369–377.

29. Feghali JG, Liu W, Van De Water TR, et al. L-n-acetyl-cysteine protection against cisplatin-induced auditory neuronal and hair cell toxicity. *Laryngoscope* 2001;111:1147–1155.

30. Fetone AR, Sergi B, Scarano E, et al. Protective effects of alpha-tocopherol against gentamicin-induced oto-vestibulo toxicity: an experimental study. *Acta Otolaryngol* 2003;123:192–197.

31. Kalkanis JG, Whitworth C, Rybak L. Vitamin E reduces cisplatin ototoxicity. *Laryngoscope* 2004;114:538–542.

32. Rybak L, Whitworth C, Somani S. Application of antioxidants and other agents to prevent cisplatin ototoxicity. *Laryngoscope* 1999;109:1740–1744.

33. Sha SH, Schact J. Salicylate attenuates gentamicin-induced ototoxicity. *Lab Invest* 1999;79:807–813.

34. Li G, Sha S, Zotova E, et el. Salicylate protects hearing and kidney function from cisplatin toxicity without compromising its on-colytic action. *Nature* 2002;82:585–596.

35. Muldoon LL, Pagel MA, Kroll RA, et al. Delayed administration of sodium thiosulfate in animal models reduces platinum ototoxicity without reduction of antitumor activity. *Clin Cancer Res* 2000;6:309–315.

36. Mowry HJ, Roeder JW, Matz GJ, Lerner SA. Auditory and vestibular assessment of patients receiving aminoglycosides. In: *Aminoglycoside ototoxicity*. Boston: Little Brown, 1981:249–254.

37. Brummett RE. Drug induced ototoxicity. *Drugs* 1980;19:412.

38. Riggs LC, Shofner WP, Shah AR, et al. Ototoxicity resulting from combined administration of metronidazole and gentamicin. *Am J Otol* 1999;20: 430–434.

39. Simdon J, Watters D, Bartlett S, Connick E. Ototoxicity associated with the use of nucleoside analog reverse transcriptase inhibitors: a report of 3 possible cases and review of the literature. *Clin Infect Dis* 2001;32:1623–1627.

Cerebellopontine Angle Tumors

149

Derald E. Brackmann   James V. Crawford   J. Douglas Green, Jr.

Cerebellopontine angle (CPA) tumors are a diverse group of tumors not infrequently encountered by the practicing otolaryngologist. A substantial fraction of an otolaryngologist's time is spent in the diagnostic evaluation of CPA tumors, which represent 10% of all intracranial tumors. CPA tumors are fatal without treatment (1). Vestibular schwannomas (acoustic neuromas) account for 78% of CPA tumors, and most of these originate on the vestibular branch of the eighth cranial nerve (2). A variety of other tumors may occur in this area, including meningiomas, other cranial nerve schwannomas, dermoid tumors, arachnoid cysts, lipomas, metastatic tumors, and vascular tumors.

Tumors of the CPA have figured prominently in the development of both diagnostic and surgical neurotology. Sir Charles Balance first achieved successful removal of a vestibular schwannoma in London in 1894, and in 1907 he reported that the patient was still alive, but had right-sided facial paralysis and right facial anesthesia (3,4). It remained for Harvey Cushing to describe the cerebellopontine angle syndrome in his 1917 monograph (5). He noted that the disease began with ipsilateral hearing loss and progressed to facial hypesthesia, hydrocephalus (headache and vomiting), and ultimately, if untreated, respiratory failure and death secondary to brainstem compression. Cushing (6) pioneered subtotal removal of these tumors, advocating bilateral suboccipital craniectomy for decompression. Dandy, however, was afraid of tumor recurrence, and advocated debulking followed by removal of the capsule by careful dissection from the brainstem using a suboccipital approach (7).

Walter Dandy built on Cushing's initial successes, lowering the operative mortality rate to 10% while achieving total tumor removal (7). The translabyrinthine approach was refined and resurrected by William House in the early 1960s, ushering in the modern era of CPA tumor surgery.

Using the microscope and a dental drill, Dr. House emphasized early identification and preservation of the facial nerve (8). He significantly reduced surgical mortality and also introduced the middle cranial fossa approach for vestibular schwannoma surgery (9,10).

ANATOMY

The CPA is an irregularly shaped potential space in the posterior fossa of the brain (11,12) (Fig. 149.1). The space is bound anteriorly by the posterior surface of the temporal bone and posteriorly by the anterior surface of the cerebellum. The medial boundary is formed by the inferior olive, and the superior boundary by the inferior border of the pons and cerebellar peduncle. The cerebellar tonsil forms the inferior border. The seventh and eighth cranial nerves course superiorly and laterally toward the internal auditory canal within this space, carrying with them a fine sheet of arachnoid tissue. Superiorly, the fifth nerve is visible, with the ninth, tenth, and eleventh nerves located inferiorly. Other important structures in this space are the flocculus, the lateral aperture of the fourth ventricle (foramen of Luschka), and the anterior inferior cerebellar artery. A loop of the anterior inferior cerebellar artery extends into the internal auditory canal in 40% of specimens. The labyrinthine artery is usually a branch of the anterior inferior cerebellar artery. This end artery supplies both the cochlea and the labyrinth.

The seventh and eighth nerves are encased in glial tissue throughout their intracranial course. Schwann cells surround these nerves beginning in the internal auditory canal, near the porus. The glial-schwann junction is also known as the Obersteiner-Redlich zone. The vestibular

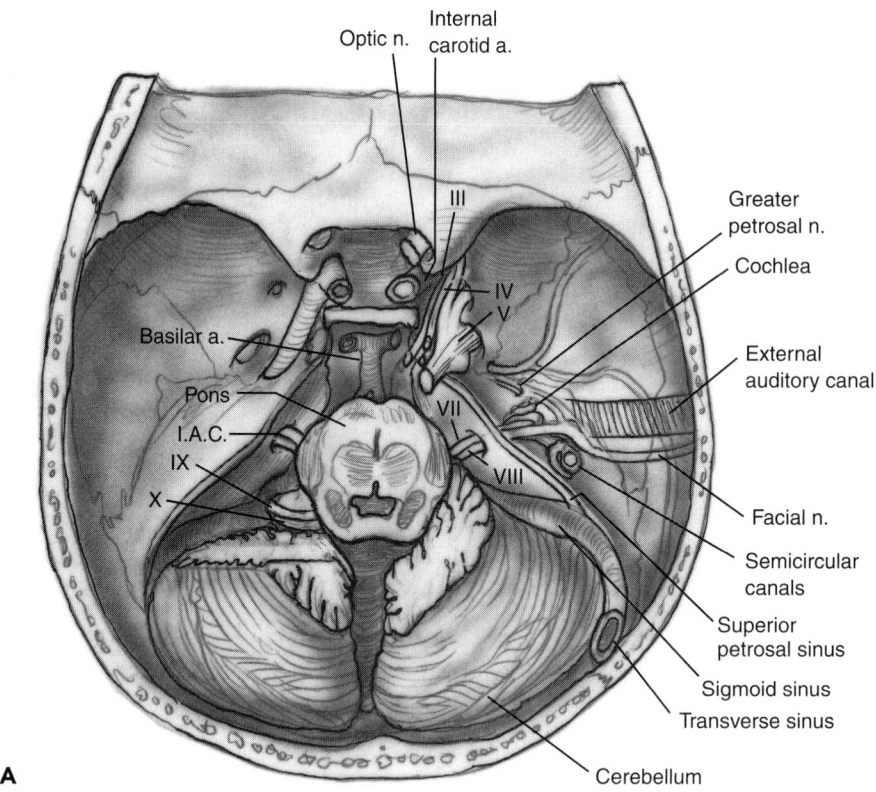

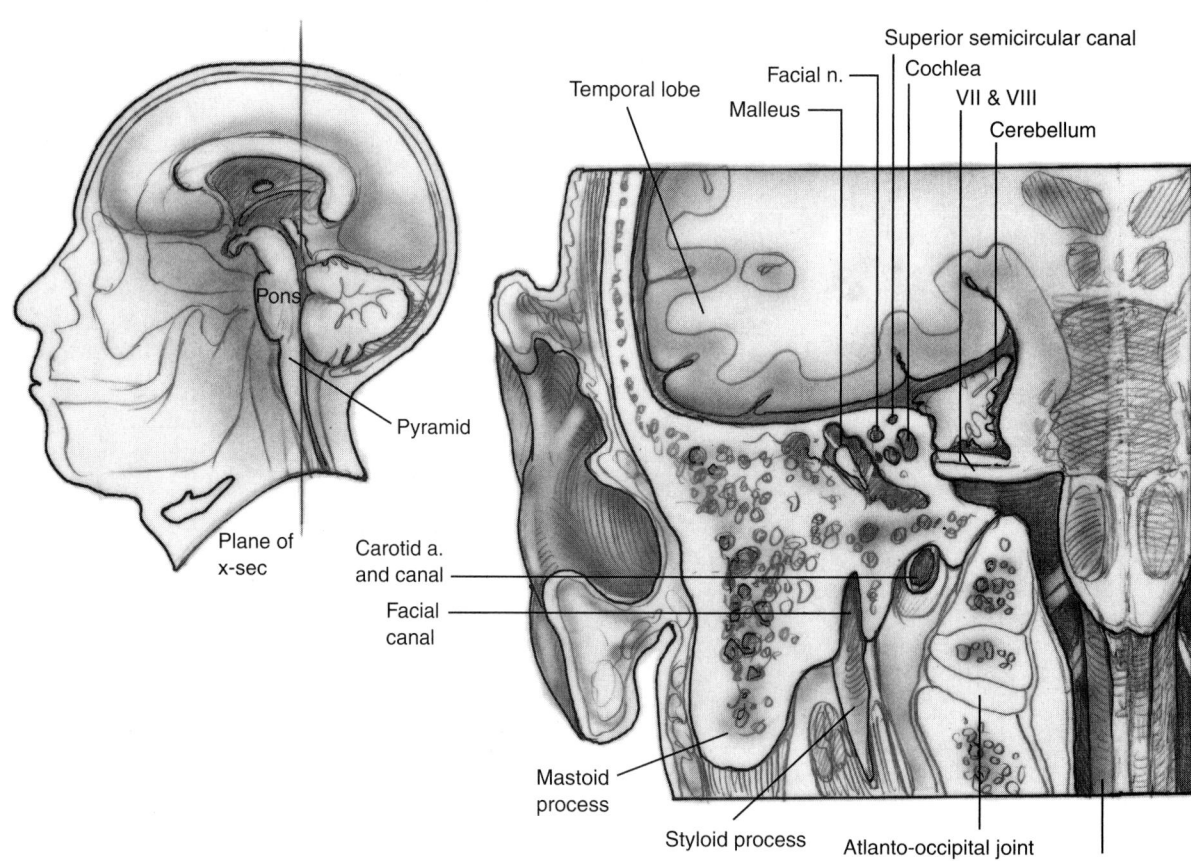

Figure 149.1 Coronal **(A)** and axial views **(B)** through the skull at the level of the internal auditory canals and cerebellopontine angles. *V*, trigeminal nerve; *VII*, facial nerve; *VIII*, cochleovestibular nerve; *IAC*, internal auditory canal.

ganglion (Scarpa ganglion) is located near the midportion of the internal auditory canal. The division of the eighth nerve into its vestibular and cochlear segments is variable and may occur within the subarachnoid space or in the medial segment of the internal auditory canal. The vestibular segment subsequently divides into the superior and inferior vestibular nerves, occupying the posterior half of the internal auditory canal. The cochlear nerve assumes an anteroinferior position within the internal auditory canal. The facial nerve courses into the anterosuperior portion of the internal auditory canal and is separated from the superior vestibular nerve by the Bill bar (vertical crest). The nerves occupying the superior half of the internal auditory canal (facial nerve and superior vestibular nerve) are separated from those occupying the inferior half of the internal auditory canal (cochlear nerve and inferior vestibular nerve) by the transverse crest.

VESTIBULAR SCHWANNOMAS

Epidemiology

The actual incidence of vestibular schwannomas has been difficult to determine accurately. Several autopsy series have shown the rate of occurrence to be 1.7% to 2.7% of undiagnosed and clinically silent vestibular schwannomas (13,14). A later review of one of these autopsy series found that the actual incidence was 0.8% rather than the 2.5% previously reported (13,15). However, even 0.8% is likely an overestimation of the true incidence of occult vestibular schwannoma. As imaging techniques have improved, smaller, asymptomatic tumors are being found on MRI obtained for nonotologic reasons. As a result, the incidence of acoustic neuromas has slightly increased over the past 15 years. One recent study found an incidence of 7 acoustic tumors per 10,000 MRIs obtained for nonotologic reasons (16). Epidemiologic studies have shown an annual incidence of 0.7 to 1.2 vestibular schwannoma per 100,000 population (17). Recently, a review of the national incidence of vestibular schwannomas in Denmark showed that the incidence truly has increased over the past several years and currently stands at approximately 1.3 vestibular schwannomas per 100,000 population (18).

Tumor Biology

Vestibular schwannomas arise from the vestibular segment of the eighth cranial nerve, with an equal frequency noted between the superior vestibular and the inferior vestibular nerves (19). A recent study from Japan suggested that about 85% of vestibular schwannomas arise from the inferior vestibular nerve, but that has not been our experience (20). They arise from Schwann cells, most commonly within the internal auditory canal (21). A long-standing misconception is that the tumors arise from the Obersteiner-Redlich zone (or the glial-schwann junction). In reality, most tumors

arise lateral to this zone in the area of Scarpa ganglion (22). Scarpa ganglion is the area with the greatest density of Schwann cells. Although vestibular schwannomas are commonly referred to as acoustic neuromas, this is a misnomer. They are not neuromas, and they rarely arise from the auditory, or acoustic, division of the eighth nerve. The more appropriate term is vestibular schwannoma. Schwannomas may occur rarely on the cochlear division of the eighth nerve. Cochlear schwannomas have a propensity for invasion into the cochlea (23).

Tremendous strides have been made in recent years in understanding the molecular genetics pertaining to vestibular schwannomas (21), which occur as a sporadic variety (95%). They also may occur bilaterally in cases of type 2 neurofibromatosis. Vestibular schwannomas in patients with type 2 neurofibromatosis (NF2) tend to occur in younger patients and in association with other intracranial meningiomas and spinal cord tumors. Two subtypes of NF2 are described: the Wishart subtype is more severe, and the Gardner subtype is less severe (24).

Mounting evidence points to a genetic defect on the long arm of chromosome 22 (chromosome 22q12) as the cause of the familial occurrence of type 2 neurofibromatosis (21). This autosomal-dominant condition has been hypothesized to occur because a tumor suppressor gene is absent in this location. It is thought that this tumor suppressor gene may be important in regulating proliferation of Schwann cells. Patients with type 2 neurofibromatosis are thought to be born without one allele of the tumor suppressor gene; when the other allele undergoes mutation, a relatively common event, vestibular schwannomas occur. It has been hypothesized that sporadic vestibular schwannomas occur as a result of two separate mutations at both alleles. More recent studies have shown that nearly all sporadic-type tumors have inactivation of the NF2 gene (25). The NF2 gene is a tumor suppressor gene. Therefore, when the gene product, Merlin/Schwannomin, is inactive, tumor growth occurs. Merlin appears to control cadherin-mediated cell-to-cell contact. Therefore, in its absence, cells lose the ability for contact-dependent growth arrest (26). Blood tests are now available to screen family members at risk for type 2 neurofibromatosis.

Biochemical factors also may play a significant role in the growth of vestibular schwannomas. It was recently demonstrated that vestibular schwannomas express neuregulin, which controls survival and proliferation of schwann cells, and its receptors, *erbB2* and *erbB3* (27). This would allow an autocrine loop for growth stimulation of schwann cells. Fibroblast growth factor (28), transforming growth factor β1 (29), platelet-derived growth factor, and vascular endothelial growth factor (30,31) all have been investigated and are thought to contribute to vestibular schwannoma proliferation. Several investigators have found that growth of vestibular schwannomas may accelerate during pregnancy (32). Although sex hormone receptors have been identified on vestibular schwannomas, recent studies have shown that they do not seem to affect the rate of tumor growth significantly, either during pregnancy or in a non-pregnant condition (33).

Clinical Manifestations

Symptoms

The medical history is a critical but often overlooked area of vestibular schwannoma diagnosis. The astute clinician should maintain a high degree of awareness for tumors in all patients with unilateral auditory or vestibular symptoms. Symptom progression in vestibular schwannomas is related to tumor size and growth (34). Intracanalicular tumors manifest hearing loss, tinnitus, and vestibular dysfunction (including vertigo). With tumor growth into the CPA, hearing loss worsens and dysequilibrium may be manifested. As the brainstem is compressed by further tumor growth, the fifth cranial nerve may become involved (midfacial hypesthesia). With further brainstem compression, hydrocephalus occurs, resulting in headache and visual loss. The clinician must keep in mind that atypical presentations for vestibular schwannomas are not infrequent, occurring in 15% to 20% of patients. These presentations have increased as more sensitive diagnostic testing has become available.

Cushing's 1917 monograph (5) on vestibular schwannomas remains pertinent today. Cushing stated, "The clinical diagnosis of an acoustic tumor can be made with reasonable assurance only when auditory manifestations definitely precede the evidences of other structures of the cerebellopontine angle." Unilateral hearing loss is present in more than 85% of patients with a vestibular schwannoma (35). Loss of speech discrimination out of proportion to hearing loss is most common. Patients frequently complain of distortion, which may be noted when they use the affected ear on the telephone.

Sudden sensorineural hearing loss will occur in up to 26% of patients with a vestibular schwannoma (35,36). A vestibular schwannoma will be found in 1% to 2.5% of patients who present with a sudden sensorineural hearing loss (SNHL) (37). Forty-eight percent of patients with a vestibular schwannoma has some recovery of hearing, so it is important to remember that recovery of hearing after a sudden SNHL does not eliminate the possibility of a vestibular schwannoma. When hearing preservation was attempted in patients with a sudden loss, there was no difference in hearing preservation between those who had suffered a sudden hearing loss and those who had not. Therefore, it is likely that the sudden hearing loss results from compression of the nerve, rather than vascular occlusion (37).

Tinnitus is the second most common presenting complaint and often precedes hearing loss. It has been found in 66% of patients with a vestibular schwannoma. It is typically described as a high-pitched ringing sound localized to the tumor ear (38). However, the tinnitus may vary from a "hissing" sound to other unusual pitches, and may even localize to the other ear. Some patients may even have tinnitus without subjective hearing loss. Therefore, unilateral tinnitus

should alert the clinician to the potential for a vestibular schwannoma.

Vestibular symptoms, although often present, are commonly described as only vague, transient lightheadedness that may be exacerbated by positional changes. Between 36% and 50% of patients describe symptoms of dysequilibrium as a result of the vestibular schwannoma (35,39). Less frequently, patients have episodes of true whirling vertigo; this has been found to be the presenting symptom in 27% of patients, but surprisingly, it primarily accompanies smaller tumors (39). Patients with vestibular schwannomas that have spread into the labyrinth may have symptoms identical to those of Ménière disease, most likely because of disruption of inner ear fluid dynamics.

Facial numbness most often occurs with larger tumors (tumors greater than 2 cm) and most frequently begins in the maxillary division of the trigeminal nerve. Typically, the corneal reflex will be absent prior to development of facial hypesthesia. Rarely, a patient presents with facial numbness (approximately 4%), leading to the diagnosis of a vestibular schwannoma (39). Facial weakness is rare with vestibular schwannomas and should alert the clinician to the possibility of another type of tumor within the CPA.

Ocular symptoms, also rare, may consist of decreased corneal reflex, nystagmus, diplopia or visual blurring. Nystagmus is frequently present and tends to beat toward the intact side. Visual blurring is rare, but when present is usually secondary to papilledema. Papilledema, untreated, may lead to optic atrophy, with loss of peripheral vision, tunnel vision, and eventual blindness. Papilledema is secondary to increased intracranial pressure, which is an unusual finding with current early diagnosis of vestibular schwannomas. Diplopia is extremely rare and is secondary to involvement of the sixth nerve. Symptoms of involvement of the lower cranial nerves are rare, consisting of dysphagia, hoarseness, and aspiration.

Symptoms of cerebellar involvement also may occur late in the course of the disease. They include incoordination, widely based gait, and a tendency to fall toward the affected side. Hydrocephalus may accompany a large tumor and is associated with severe headache and vomiting.

Signs

Any patient with unilateral auditory or vestibular symptoms should receive a thorough neurotologic examination. During otoscopic examination, the sensation of the posterior portion of the bony ear canal can be determined by palpation. Hitselberger sign, decreased sensation in the external auditory canal, occurs in acoustic tumors because the sensory branch of the seventh nerve is more sensitive to pressure than the motor portion of the nerve. Hence, even though facial weakness is seldom seen even with large tumors, this sign may be present even with a relatively small tumor.

The eyes are examined for nystagmus in all fields of gaze. Extraocular movements also are assessed. Facial sensation is checked for both pain (pinprick) and touch (cotton wisp). Corneal sensation can be evaluated by eliciting a blink reflex with a horse hair or a cotton wisp. The cornea is stimulated with the patient looking up and the examiner taking care not to let the patient see the stimulus coming or to feel it along the lower lid. The examiner asks the patient to clench the teeth, while he or she palpates, checks masseter and temporalis muscle function. Ophthalmoscopic examination is performed if other cranial nerve abnormalities are present or if visual changes are noted.

Facial movement is assessed by asking the patient to smile, wrinkle the nose, close the eyes, and raise the eyebrows. The patient's gag reflex is checked during examination of the oropharynx. The tongue is examined for atrophy or deviation during protrusion. The examiner asks the patient to shrug the shoulders and turn the head, while he or she applies resistance, assesses function of the sternocleidomastoid and trapezius muscles. Cerebellar function is checked while the patient performs heel-shin and finger-to-nose tests. The Romberg test and gait assessment also are performed. It is important to check the gait when the patient does not suspect he or she is being examined. Tests for dysmetria, fine motor movements, and tandem gait are performed if indicated.

Diagnostic Tests

Audiometric Testing

The retrocochlear test battery in audiology has changed significantly over the past 20 years. The original test battery contained tests such as the short increment sensitivity index, the alternate binaural loudness balance, threshold tone decay, etc. These tests have largely been replaced because of their rather poor sensitivity and specificity and the development of new tests. The standard test battery now includes basic pure-tone audiometry, speech discrimination scores, acoustic-reflex thresholds and acoustic-reflex decay, and auditory brainstem response (ABR) testing.

On pure-tone air and bone conduction testing, the patient who has a vestibular schwannoma typically has a \SNHL. Although any hearing loss configuration may be observed, a high-frequency SNHL is the most common pattern (65%), and it may be either a gradual slope or an abrupt configuration (40). It is important to know that 5% of patients have normal hearing (41).

The classic result on speech discrimination testing is a set of scores out of proportion with the pure-tone thresholds. For instance, a patient with mild SNHL and a vestibular schwannoma might understand only 50% of monosyllabic words presented at a comfortable listening level. A person who has a similar cochlear hearing loss should score above 80% correct; however, many patients with retrocochlear lesions score well on this test, so good scores should not be taken as evidence against the possibility of a vestibular schwannoma. The sensitivity of the test can be improved if additional speech discrimination scores are obtained at

higher presentation levels. The expected finding is that performance decreases significantly (20% to 30%) when the intensity of the speech signal is raised. This phenomenon, called rollover, can occur with cochlear losses but is more predominant with a retrocochlear lesion.

Acoustic reflex thresholds and acoustic reflex decay are evaluated with impedance, or admittance, testing. Reflex thresholds are obtained for pure tones of 500, 1,000, 2,000, and 4,000 Hz, and reflex decay is tested at 500 and 1,000 Hz. Reflex thresholds typically are either elevated (norms are available for given degrees of cochlear hearing loss for comparison) or absent in the patient with vestibular schwannoma. If a reflex is present, reflex decay can be measured by presenting the signal 10 dB above the reflex threshold for 10 seconds. If the contraction of the stapedial muscle cannot be maintained for at least half strength for the 10 seconds, the result of the test is a positive retrocochlear finding. Significantly increased or absent thresholds (in comparison with cochlear norms) or decay (or both) has a sensitivity of about 85% for detecting retrocochlear problems (40).

Electrophysiologic Testing

Auditory brainstem evoked response testing is the most sensitive and specific of the audiologic tests for detection of a vestibular schwannoma. Surface electrodes are applied at various locations on the head and ear, and electrical potentials are measured in response to broadband clicks of short duration (typically 100 msec). Between 1,000 and 2,000 clicks are presented (typical presentation rates are 7 to 20 per second), and a computer averages the responses over the first 10 msec after the signal presentation. After averaging, a series of five distinct waveforms is typically identified, with each succeeding waveform thought to represent neural activity at progressively higher auditory structures, beginning with the auditory nerve and reaching to the inferior colliculus in the brainstem. The latencies of each identifiable wave are calculated.

A variety of abnormalities may be seen in the auditory brainstem response (ABR) of patients with a vestibular schwannoma. The most common finding is to have all waves present, but to have an interaural difference in the latency of wave V, with a delay in the wave of more than 0.2 msec in the involved ear from the response in the uninvolved ear. This pattern is found in 40% to 60% of patients with vestibular schwannoma. In 20% to 30% of patients, there are no identifiable waveforms, a clearly abnormal finding if the patient does not have significant hearing loss in the higher frequencies (less than 60 dB hearing level). Another potential finding is that wave I is present (thought to represent initial firings of the auditory nerve), but all remaining waves, representing output from higher structures, are absent. Such a pattern occurs in 10% to 20% of patients who have vestibular schwannoma (42). Because the ABR is normal in 10% to 15% of patients, the sensitivity of the test is 85% to 90% (43). Earlier sensitivity estimates of ABR testing were around 95%, but this number appears to be decreasing because the sensitivity of radiographic imaging studies has improved, and smaller schwannomas are being detected. In general, the larger the vestibular schwannoma, the more likely the ABR is to be abnormal. The ABR test can be useful in predicting the size of the schwannoma, because a large mass with significant brainstem compression can cause a lengthened III–V interval on the contralateral side (44). More recently, a new ABR technique called stacked ABR appears to show improved sensitivity and specificity (45–47). With the improved radiographic imaging available today, we advocate the ABR as a screening test for patients in whom the possibility of a vestibular schwannoma is relatively low.

Vestibular Testing

Vestibular assessment of the patient with a suspected vestibular schwannoma always involves electronystagmography (ENG) and in some cases also may include computerized dynamic posturography and rotary chair testing. The ENG shows some abnormality in 70% to 90% of patients who have vestibular schwannoma (48), and the typical finding is unilateral weakness of the involved side on caloric testing. Because caloric testing assesses the function of only the horizontal (lateral) semicircular canal and, therefore, superior vestibular nerve function, tumors originating from the inferior vestibular nerve may be missed. In addition, as many as 50% of small tumors produce no abnormality on the ENG (49). It has been shown that 98% of vestibular schwannomas arising from the superior vestibular nerve will show a reduced caloric response, whereas only 60% of inferior nerve tumors will have a decreased response (50). As a result of these limitations, ENG is not recommended as a screening test for vestibular schwannoma.

Spontaneous nystagmus is frequently observed in patients with larger tumors and is relatively rare in smaller tumors. In small tumors, the nystagmus tends to have the characteristics of a peripheral labyrinthine dysfunction (fatiguing, horizontal), and in larger tumors, central characteristics are more common (vertical, nonfatiguing). As a rule, the nystagmus tends to beat away from the ear with the vestibular schwannoma (51).

Computerized dynamic posturography has shown a wide variety of responses in patients with vestibular schwannomas. Although performance is typically somewhat below normal, any pattern of results may be observed, from normal to free falls, on a number of the sensory conditions. Similarly, results of rotary chair testing are variable, and patients who have small tumors frequently have a normal response (52).

Imaging Studies

A vestibular schwannoma is definitively identified most commonly via an imaging study. The sensitivity of radiographic studies in diagnosing vestibular schwannomas has improved greatly over the past several years. Formerly,

plain film radiographs and polytomographs of the internal auditory canals were the mainstays of diagnosis. Bony erosion of the internal auditory canal was necessary for tumor diagnosis with these studies. The addition of iophendylate (Pantopaque®) to posterior fossa myelography improved the diagnostic accuracy, but the internal auditory canal was at times blocked by an arachnoid cyst or a loop of the anterior inferior cerebellar artery, yielding a false-positive imaging result.

The introduction of computed tomography (CT) in the 1970s allowed axial imaging with improved bone and soft tissue visualization. With the addition of intravenous iodinated contrast agent, 90% of vestibular schwannomas are enhanced, further improving the diagnostic accuracy of CT. Intracanalicular tumors and tumors extending less than 5 mm into the CPA frequently are missed with contrast-enhanced CT. One study has shown that CT is only 63% accurate in diagnosing vestibular schwannomas (53). The accuracy of the CT can be enhanced by the addition of air-contrast cisternography. The injection of 2 to 4 mL of oxygen into the subarachnoid space reveals a convex bulge of a mass at the porus of the internal auditory canal. Headaches are frequently noted in patients who have undergone air-contrast-enhanced CT.

Although the CT scan is excellent for demonstrating the bony anatomy of the temporal bone and internal auditory canal, soft-tissue resolution is less accurate unless intrathecal contrast or air CT cisternography is used. Magnetic resonance imaging (MRI) was introduced in the early 1980s and has become the gold standard for vestibular schwannoma diagnosis. MRI uses the interaction of magnetic fields and atomic nuclei to produce images. The seventh and eighth cranial nerves, as well as the cerebellum, brainstem, vasculature, and other structures, are well visualized on MRI (54).

The addition of gadolinium diethylenetriamine pentaacetic acid has further enhanced the diagnostic accuracy of MRI scanning (Fig. 149.2). Gadolinium is preferentially taken up into the vestibular schwannoma, allowing visualization of even very small tumors. It is important that gadolinium be used in all patients being examined for a vestibular schwannoma because it significantly enhances the diagnostic accuracy. On a gadolinium-enhanced study, vestibular schwannomas will enhance brightly on T1 or T2. On nonenhanced images, vestibular schwannomas remain isointense or slightly hypointense on T1 and are isointense on T2. We recommend MRI with gadolinium contrast for persons in whom there is a moderate-to-high degree of suspicion for vestibular schwannoma.

MRI can be performed in either the T1 setting (bright on fat density) or the T2 setting (bright on fluid density). Recent improvements in computer software, combined with the use of surface coils, have significantly improved resolution of the cerebrospinal fluid and inner ear fluids in the T2 setting. The seventh and eighth nerves can be visualized in relief in the internal auditory canal by T2 fast spin-echo MRI. This technique has been used to screen for

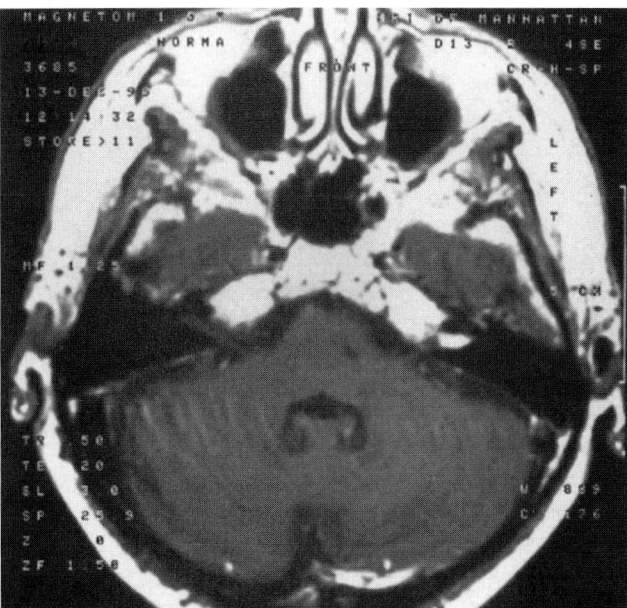

Figure 149.2 Magnetic resonance imaging with gadolinium showing intracanalicular vestibular schwannoma.

TABLE 149.1 ▉ 🄓 DIAGNOSIS
CEREBELLOPONTINE ANGLE TUMORS

Symptoms and signs
  Unilateral hearing loss
  Unilateral tinnitus
  Aural fullness
  Lightheadedness
  Facial hypesthesia
  Decreased corneal reflex

Audiometric and vestibular testing
  Pure-tone and speech discrimination audiometry
  Impedance audiometry
  Brainstem-evoked-response audiometry
  Electronystagmography

Radiographic imaging
  Magnetic resonance imaging (MRI): T2 fast spin-echo
    MRI with gadolinium
  Air-contrast cisternography computed tomography (CT)
  CT with contrast
  Plain film radiographs

vestibular schwannomas (55) (Fig. 149.3). Because the test can be performed without gadolinium contrast in a shorter imaging time, costs are reduced. It is used in some centers as a screen for retrocochlear pathology instead of ABR. However, abnormalities seen on fast spin-echo scans often require a standard thin-cut gadolinium-enhanced MRI for confirmation.

False negatives are rare with enhanced MRI, unless thick sections (≥10 mm) are used. False-positives are also rare, and most often associated with viral neuritis of the seventh or eighth nerve (56). These can usually be differentiated from vestibular schwannomas by the normal diameter of the neural complex. Also, it is important to include noncontrast images to differentiate other lesions that may enhance in the CPA that are not vestibular schwannomas (for example, globular region of bone marrow in a poorly pneumatized petrous apex).

The appearance of a CPA mass frequently calls for the differentiation between a vestibular schwannoma and a meningioma. A vestibular schwannoma tends to be centered on the internal auditory canal and has a globular appearance, causing an acute angle to be formed between the posterior face of the temporal bone and the tumor surface. The vestibular schwannoma generally extends into the internal auditory canal, giving an appearance often described as that of an ice cream cone. The internal auditory canal is frequently eroded by the tumor expansion. The tumor may have areas of cystic degeneration, and occasionally there is evidence of hemorrhage into the tumor (Table 149.1). Meningiomas, on the other hand, tend to be sessile and extend along the petrous ridge with an obtuse bone/tumor angle. They also typically have a "dural tail" of enhancement that extends along the periphery of the lesion. It is important to note that dural tails may occur with vestibular schwannomas (57). Meningiomas are typically isointense or mildly hypointense on T1, but vary from hypointense to hyperintense on T2. "En plaque" meningiomas are very flat and have a propensity for infiltrating the temporal bone (58).

Management

The management of vestibular schwannomas has been the source of considerable controversy for many years. With

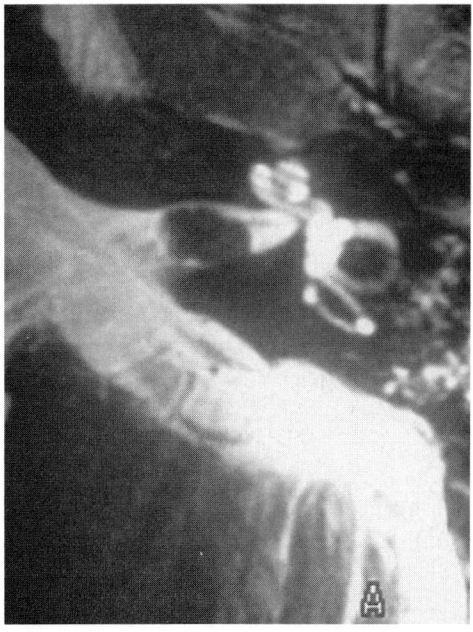

Figure 149.3 T2 fast spin-echo magnetic resonance image of an intracanalicular vestibular schwannoma. Note that nerves within the internal auditory canal can be delineated.

TABLE 149.2   ℞ TREATMENT
CEREBELLOPONTINE ANGLE TUMORS

Observation
Surgery
   Translabyrinthine approach
   Middle fossa approach
   Retrosigmoid-suboccipital approach
Stereotactic gamma irradiation

---

improvements in imaging studies, patients are presenting with hearing loss as their only symptom, and at times they are completely asymptomatic. The recent development of stereotactic radiosurgery provides another treatment option for patients and further fuels the controversy. When deciding how to manage a vestibular schwannoma, the surgeon should remember that the primary objective is to preserve life, bearing in mind the natural course of an untreated vestibular schwannoma. The second objective is preservation of facial nerve function. The third objective, when serviceable hearing exists preoperatively, is preservation of hearing within that serviceable level. A fourth goal, at our institution, is complete tumor removal (Table 149.2).

Observation

The growth rate of vestibular schwannomas varies greatly (59,60). A number of patients have been observed successfully for up to 10 years without appreciable change in symptoms (61). Weit et al. (62) promoted the "wait and scan" approach for small tumors in elderly patients. Studies that follow-up on this approach show significant variation (18,39,63). Growth rates vary from 1 mm to 2 mm per year, and one large study indicated that 82% of tumors followed for 3.8 years showed growth (63). Between 14% and 24% of patients watched will eventually go on to treatment (18).

Unfortunately, a single MRI scan does not predict long-term tumor growth. Elderly patients or those with serious medical disorders who have a small, slow-growing tumor and would be at high risk for general anesthesia are appropriate candidates for observation. Magnetic resonance imaging is repeated at 6 months and yearly thereafter. Long-standing hearing loss in the affected ear may reflect a slow growth rate in elderly patients (64). Biologic age does not necessarily equal chronologic age. Many elderly patients with a family history of longevity and who are in otherwise good health may be better suited for surgical removal (65). Age alone should not determine whether a patient is a candidate for surgical resection. Vestibular schwannomas in elderly patients can be removed with acceptably low rates of morbidity and mortality. Delaying surgery may mean that a larger tumor is removed from an older patient who may be in poorer health at a later stage of life. It is critical to take a long-term approach in deciding which patients are good candidates for tumor observation. Despite

a slow rate of tumor growth, a younger patient is better served by having a vestibular schwannoma removed because expected survival is long. Elderly patients who have large vestibular schwannomas should not be considered for observation given the potentially devastating effects of hydrocephalus in this population.

Surgery

Surgery is the primary treatment for patients with vestibular schwannomas. A team consisting of a neurosurgeon and a neurotologist who are familiar with surgery of the temporal bone and posterior fossa is critical for optimal removal of these tumors. Vestibular schwannomas are best removed at referral centers where anesthesia, nursing, and paramedical personnel are accustomed to working with these patients. Recent studies have shown that high-volume centers may have shorter length of stay and higher frequency of routine outcomes than lower volume centers (66,67). A variety of surgical approaches to vestibular schwannomas have been described that may be broadly divided into three categories. Critical to each of the approaches is the use of microsurgical technique with the operating microscope. In addition, intraoperative monitoring of the facial nerve should be routine during vestibular schwannoma surgery.

Each of the surgical approaches for vestibular schwannoma excision has inherent advantages and disadvantages. These advantages must be combined with the operative experience of the surgical team in deciding which approach is appropriate for a given tumor.

Translabyrinthine Approach

The translabyrinthine approach has several advantages that make it applicable to most vestibular schwannomas. It is the most direct route to the CPA and requires minimal cerebellar retraction. Identification of the facial nerve is possible in all cases within the temporal bone in an area undisturbed by the tumor. In addition, the fundus of the internal auditory canal is widely exposed so that the surgeon can ensure complete tumor removal in this area. Should the facial nerve be lost during tumor removal, the translabyrinthine approach offers the best opportunity for immediate repair by interposition nerve graft or through direct end-to-end anastamosis. We find that the recovery of patients from the translabyrinthine approach is quite rapid, with minimal pain and excellent facial nerve results.

The obvious disadvantage is that any residual hearing is sacrificed in the ear subjected to surgery. Most patients who have a vestibular schwannoma already have lost much of the hearing in the affected ear. The translabyrinthine approach may be used for tumors of all sizes. For patients who have good hearing (pure-tone average less than 30 dB and greater than 70% speech discrimination scores) and a tumor extending less than 2 cm into the CPA, we offer the

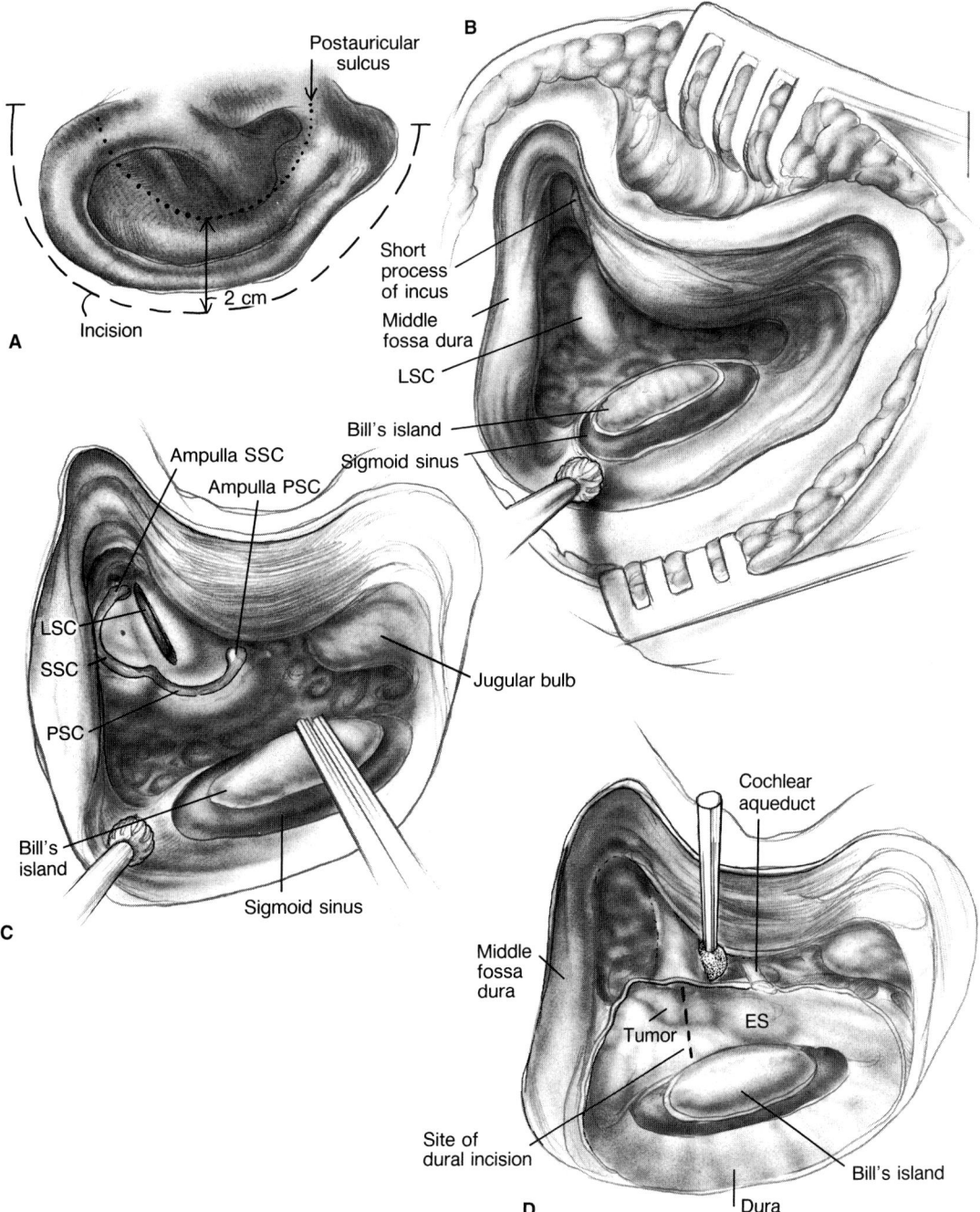

Figure 149.4 Translabyrinthine exposure. **A:** An incision is made 2 cm behind the postauricular sulcus. **B:** A complete simple mastoidectomy is performed. The sigmoid sinus is decompressed with a diamond bur. An island of bone over the dome of the sinus (Bill island) is preserved. **C:** Labyrinthectomy is begun. Bone in the sinodural angle is removed along the superior petrosal sinus. The semicircular canals are opened into the vestibule, and the ampulla of each semicircular canal and the subarcuate artery are identified as landmarks to assist the surgeon in outlining the internal auditory canal. **D:** The internal auditory canal is outlined inferiorly until the cochlear aqueduct is identified. *ES*, endolymphatic sac; *LSC*, lateral semicircular canal; *PSC*, posterior semicircular canal; *SSC*, superior semicircular canal.

option of a hearing preservation procedure. Other surgeons who use the translabyrinthine approach, however, do not believe that the small number of patients who ultimately will have their hearing saved is worth the additional risk involved in other approaches (68).

Technique

A postauricular incision is made 2 cm behind the postauricular sulcus (Fig. 149.4A). Complete mastoidectomy is done, with identification of the middle fossa dura, sigmoid sinus, lateral semicircular canal, fossa incudis, and facial nerve

(69). The sigmoid sinus is decompressed with a diamond bur, and care is taken to preserve an island of bone over the dome of the sinus (aka: "Bill island") (Fig. 149.4B).

A labyrinthectomy is begun by removal of bone in the sinodural angle along the horizontal semicircular canal. Each semicircular canal is then opened and followed into the vestibule, with care taken to identify the ampulla of each semicircular canal and the subarcuate artery (Fig. 149.4C). These landmarks guide the surgeon in outlining the internal auditory canal.

As bone is removed along the posterior fossa dura medial to the sigmoid sinus, the endolymphatic duct and sac are encountered. The inferior aspect of the internal auditory canal is identified first, with the surgeon cognizant of the variable location of the jugular bulb. By identifying the ampulla of the posterior semicircular canal, the surgeon is able to avoid injury to the jugular bulb. The bulb will always be located inferior to the ampulla of the posterior canal. Dissection proceeds inferiorly, using a diamond bur, until the jugular bulb is identified. This is the inferior extent of the dissection. Once the jugular bulb is identified, bone is removed around the inferior aspect of the internal auditory canal until the cochlear aqueduct is identified. The cochlear aqueduct is an important landmark for avoidance of injury to the ninth, tenth, and eleventh cranial nerves, which will be anterior and inferior to the cochlear duct. As the inferior edge of the internal canal is clearly identified, the posterior aspect of the canal is skeletonized until the superior edge of the internal canal is identified. Bone is then carefully removed between the middle fossa dura and the internal auditory canal. Once the medial portion of the canal is exposed for 270 degrees, the remaining piece of bone overlying the porus may be carefully removed. Laterally, the transverse crest should be identified at the fundus of the internal auditory canal. Superiorly, the Bill bar (vertical crest) is identified together with the labyrinthine portion of the facial nerve. At the conclusion of the dissection, the bone covering the middle and posterior cranial fossa dura is removed completely, along with the bone covering the entire posterior two thirds of the internal auditory canal (Fig. 149.4D).

The posterior fossa dura is opened inferior to and parallel to the superior petrosal sinus over the midportion of the internal auditory canal, around the porus acousticus, and in the internal auditory canal (Fig. 149.5A). Using the Bill bar as a guide, and with a fine hook, the surgeon separates the superior vestibular nerve from the facial nerve (Fig. 149.5B). If the tumor is smaller than 2 cm, debulking is unnecessary before it is separated from the facial nerve. If the tumor is larger, its posterior aspect is inspected to find an avascular area and to ensure that the facial nerve is located anteriorly in its customary position.

The capsule of the tumor is incised, and the tumor is gutted with the House-Urban dissector or ultrasonic aspiration (Fig. 149.5C). The remaining tumor, and its capsule, then can be separated from the facial nerve by using microinstrumen-

tation. Continuous facial nerve monitoring with auditory feedback is a tremendous asset in this portion of the dissection. At times, the facial nerve is not found in its usual location but is instead superior to the tumor. This situation is more common in a tumor originating from the inferior vestibular nerve. Often, the facial nerve will be widely spread out over the surface of the tumor, especially at the porus.

After tumor removal, meticulous hemostasis is achieved. The tensor tympani tendon is cut, and the eustachian tube opening is occluded with a hemostatic fabric (Surgicel™ NuKnit). The middle ear space is obliterated with muscle, and the dural defect is approximated with dural silk sutures (Fig. 149.5D). The remaining dural defect and the mastoid defect are then obliterated with strips of abdominal fat. A titanium mesh plate is placed over the defect in the temporal bone and secured with 4 titanium screws. The wound is closed in layers over the mesh. A mastoid dressing is applied.

Results

Initial attempts at removal of vestibular schwannomas were generally fatal (mortality rates of 80%). As surgical equipment, sterile technique, and surgical technique improved, so did mortality. In 1917 Cushing reported a mortality of 20%, and that had improved to 4% by 1931 (70). Prior to Dr. William House's initial efforts with the translabyrinthine approach, mortality in the state of California was approximately 40%. The most recent reports of outcomes for vestibular schwannoma surgery have shown mortalities of 0.2% to 0.1% (71–75). As expected, however, mortality associated with removal of small vestibular schwannomas was significantly less than that with removal of larger vestibular schwannomas.

The translabyrinthine approach has been criticized as inapplicable for large tumors. This belief most likely stems from lack of familiarity with the approach, because the view of the CPA is quite similar through either the retrosigmoid or the translabyrinthine approach. We have found that total tumor removal is possible in the overwhelming majority of patients undergoing surgery via this approach, regardless of tumor size (76). The inferior portion of the CPA, particularly in patients with an anteriorly positioned sigmoid and a high jugular bulb, is the main limitation of the translabyrinthine approach. A review by Shelton (77) revealed that the recurrence rate among 857 patients undergoing translabyrinthine tumor resection was 0.3% at an institution where complete tumor resection is the standard. Another review, by Thedinger et al. (78), found a 0.5% recurrence rate among 999 patients who underwent surgery primarily through the translabyrinthine approach. Important to the discussion of recurrence is to distinguish the amount of residual tumor left behind. At times, a small quantity of tumor may be adherent to the facial nerve, so that removal of the tumor places the facial nerve at risk. In these cases, a "near-total" excision may be performed. Near total implies that a less than 25-mm²- or greater than 2-mm-thick scrap of tumor remains. These fragments are visible on follow-up MRI in only 50% of cases and have been shown to have a 3% risk of recurrence

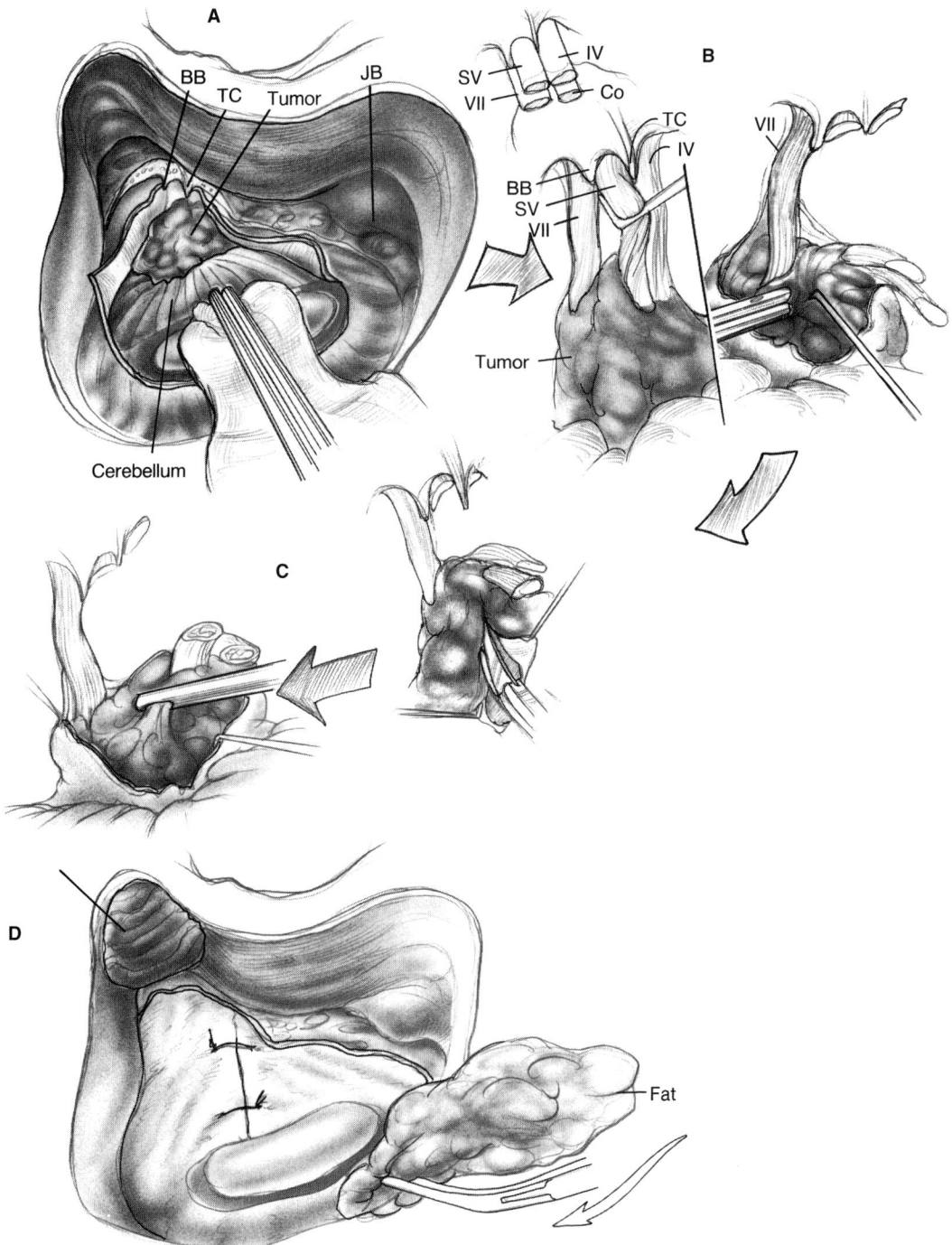

Figure 149.5 Tumor removal. **A:** The dura is opened inferior to and paralleling the superior petrosal sinus into the posterior fossa. **B:** With the Bill bar as a guide, the superior vestibular nerve is separated from the facial nerve with a fine hook. **C:** The capsule of the tumor is incised, and the tumor is gutted using the Urban dissector. **D:** The dura is closed with silk sutures, and the epitympanum is obliterated with muscle. The mastoid defect is filled with strips of abdominal fat. *BB*, the Bill bar; *TC*, transverse crest; *JB*, jugular bulb; *IV*, inferior vestibular nerve; *SV*, superior vestibular nerve; *Co*, cochlear nerve; *VII*, facial nerve.

(79,80). Other schools of thought favor a less aggressive approach and often perform a "sub-total" resection. A sub-total resection will leave a greater than 25-mm²- or greater than 2-mm-thick remnant. These remnants are often visible on follow-up MRI and have a much higher rate of recurrence—up to 10 times higher in most reports (79–81).

Rarely, complete tumor removal will not be possible because of persistent changes in the patient's vital signs during tumor resection. Cushing reflex is a bradycardia associated with hypertension, which occasionally occurs during resection of tumor from the brainstem. A similar situation arises, on occasion, as the tumor is dissected from the trigeminal nerve.

Facial nerve paralysis is by far the most debilitating complication of vestibular schwannoma removal. Anatomic preservation of the facial nerve has been possible with the translabyrinthine approach in 99% of patients, regardless of tumor size (71). Anatomic preservation of the facial nerve does not necessarily ensure postoperative facial function, because the nerve may be devascularized or traumatized to the extent that function will not return. In general, the immediate postoperative function is the best predictor of long-term facial nerve outcome. Falcioni et al. (82) found that the majority of their patients with immediate House-Brackmann (HB) grade VI facial paralysis returned to HB grade III by 1 year postsurgery. Other recent large series have confirmed that facial outcomes correlate with size of tumor at time of surgery. Facial nerve preservation (HB grades I to II) occurred in 97% to 100% of intracanilicular tumors, 92.5% to 95% of tumors less than 2 cm, and 63% of tumors greater than 2 cm (71,73,74). Another phenomenon, which occurs in patients with anatomically intact facial nerves and good immediate postoperative facial nerve results, is delayed facial nerve paralysis. This is defined as facial weakness developing more than 72 hours after surgery. The reported incidence varies but seems to be about 5% (83). A recent review found that 79% of these patients would return to the same HB grade they were in the immediate postoperative period by 1 year after surgery. Ninety-three percent will return to within one HB grade of their postoperative level. Greater delayed loss, in general, led to poorer recovery at one year.

Leakage of cerebrospinal fluid is the most common complication of vestibular schwannoma surgery. The incidence of cerebrospinal fluid (CSF) leak has seemed to plateau since the 1970s, despite variations in technique designed to reduce leakage. Some authors (72) report much lower leakage rates <3%). Most of these leaks occur through the incision, and when they occur, over-sewing the leakage point and application of a pressure dressing often resolves them. Cerebrospinal fluid rhinorrhea is sometimes noted. This may be elicited by asking the patient to lower the head between the knees for 3 minutes and observing for the fluid. Careful attention to the eustachian tube orifice, the dural closure, and to layering of abdominal fat into the wound in watertight fashion help significantly reduce the chance of rhinorrhea. If the cerebrospinal fluid leak presents as rhinorrhea, the initial management is placement of mastoid pressure dressing and a lumbar drain. The drain is left in place for 3 to 4 days. If the CSF leakage persists despite lumbar drainage, the patient is returned to the operating room for further obliteration of the eustachian tube and blind sac closure of the external auditory canal.

Meningitis is a rare complication of vestibular schwannoma surgery. Mental status changes, meningismus, or worsening postoperative headaches should alert the clinician to the possibility of meningitis. Changes in vital signs and, in particular, occurrence of fever may heighten suspicion. Culture-directed administration of antibiotics after lumbar puncture is started at an early stage and is critical in avoiding neurologic sequelae. The incidence of meningitis is higher in larger tumors. Not infrequently, meningitis proves to be aseptic. Meningitis occurs most often in patients with CSF leaks. Rare complications with this approach include sixth nerve palsy, vascular complications, lower cranial nerve paralysis, and cerebellar ataxia.

It was previously thought that the translabyrinthine approach precluded any preservation of hearing. Recent reports by McElveen et al. (84) suggest that the semicircular canals may be sealed with bone wax as they exit the vestibule, with hearing preserved in some patients. The most recent report found that serviceable hearing was preserved in 50% of patients using this approach.

Middle Fossa Approach

The middle cranial fossa approach for removal of vestibular schwannoma is unique because it has the potential for hearing preservation while allowing exposure of the lateral end of the internal auditory canal. This approach is limited to patients who have tumors that are less than 2 cm in greatest dimension, including the intracanalicular portion. The dissection is primarily extradural, decreasing the morbidity associated with the procedure. The facial nerve is identified at the lateral end of the internal auditory canal, so that the surgeon can establish a plane between the tumor and the facial nerve. Audiometrically, candidates for hearing preservation should have a 4 frequency PTA of less than or equal to 30 dB and a speech discrimination score of greater than or equal to 70%, although there are exceptions to these guidelines (85). Technical modifications developed by Brackmann et al. (86) to the middle fossa approach initially described by William House in 1961 (87) have significantly improved hearing results.

An extended middle fossa approach has been developed that allows attempted hearing preservation while removing tumors that extend into the CPA or toward the clivus. Hearing preservation in these patients is excellent, with 76% retaining serviceable hearing (88).

Several disadvantages make this a challenging approach for the surgical team. The surgeon must work around the facial nerve during tumor removal because the facial nerve is located in the superior portion of the internal auditory canal. The surgical procedure is technically more difficult than that in the translabyrinthine approach, and landmarks are sometimes absent on the floor of the middle cranial fossa.

Technique

The facial nerve and ABR are monitored throughout the case. With the surgeon seated at the head of the patient and the patient supine with the head turned away from the affected ear, an incision is made in the pretragal area. The incision extends superiorly and then curves posteriorly just above the auricle and makes a semicircular curve back toward the eyebrow. The completed incision resembles a

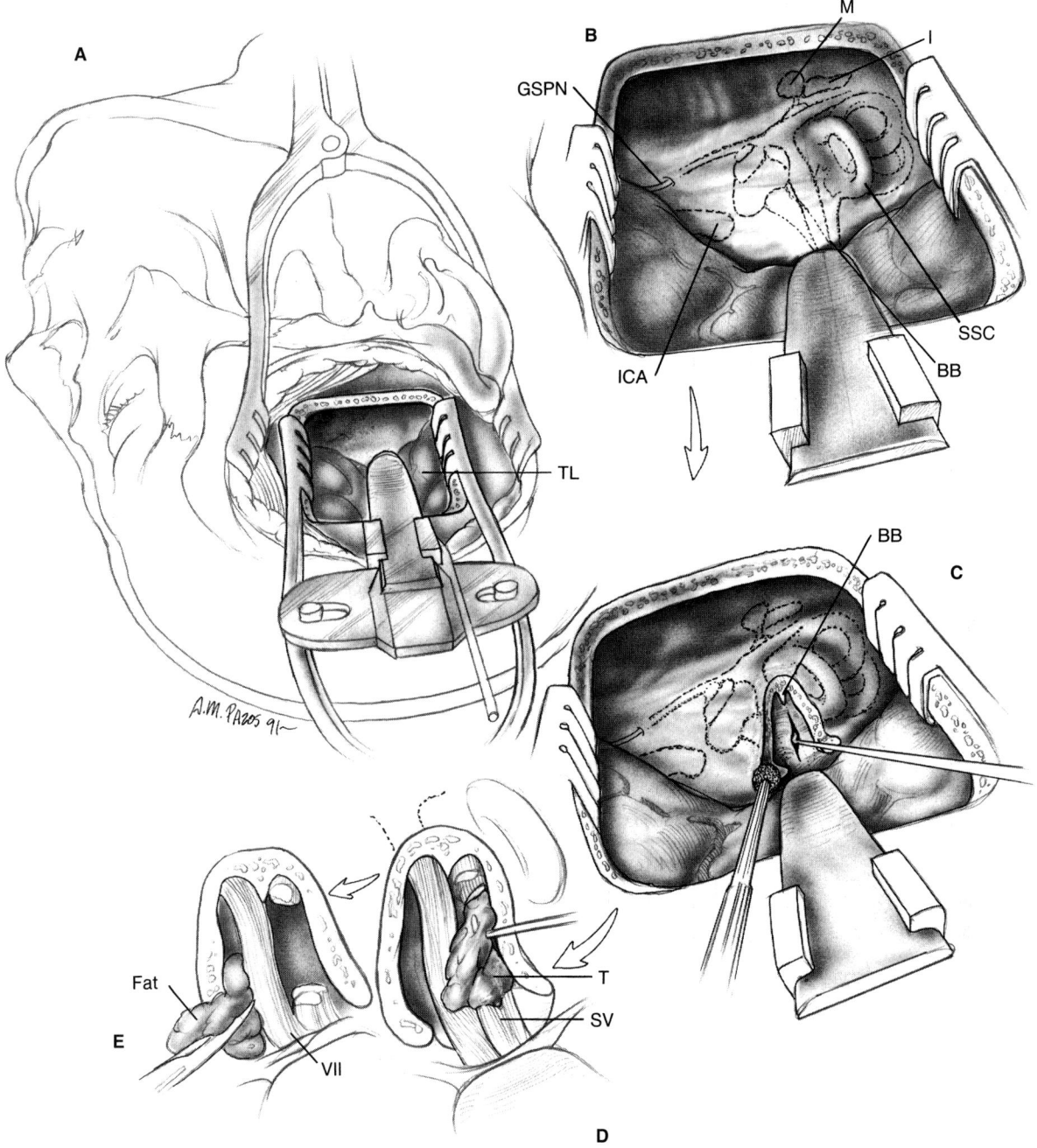

Figure 149.6 Middle fossa approach. **A** and **B:** The retractor is positioned so that the structures of the temporal bone can be identified. With the greater superficial petrosal nerve and the arcuate eminence as guides, bone removal is begun and the internal auditory canal is identified. **C:** The dura then can be incised away from the facial nerve under high magnification. **D:** Fine hooks are used to separate the superior vestibular nerve from the facial nerve. **E:** The internal auditory canal is filled with fat. *TL,* temporal lobe; *GSPN,* greater superficial petrosal nerve; *ICA,* internal carotid artery; *BB,* the Bill bar; *VII,* facial nerve; *SV,* superior vestibular nerve; *T,* tumor; *M,* malleus; *I,* incus; *SSC,* superior semicircular canal.

question mark. Dissection is carried down to the temporalis muscle, and a skin flap is raised superficial to the temporalis muscle. The temporalis muscle is then incised near its insertion with the base of the flap along the zygomatic arch. The temporalis muscle is elevated in a subperiosteal plane and retracted anteriorly. A temporal craniotomy is then made with a high-speed drill and continuous suction irrigation after outlining a 5 × 5-cm bone flap. The craniotomy is positioned so that two thirds of the flap is anterior to the external auditory canal (the more anterior, the better). The dura is then dissected from the floor of the middle cranial fossa until the arcuate eminence, the greater superficial petrosal nerve, and the "true" petrous ridge are identified (Fig. 149.6A). The middle meningeal artery is identified at the foramen spinosum and serves as the anterior limit of dissection. Posteriorly, the dura is elevated to the petrous ridge. A House-Urban retractor is inserted, and the blade of the retractor is placed over the posterior petrous ridge. It is important that this retractor be placed in line with the external auditory canal, bisecting an angle formed by the greater superficial petrosal nerve and the arcuate eminence (Fig. 149.6B).

Drilling is begun medially adjacent to the retractor blade and is carried down until the internal auditory canal is identified through the bone. Bone removal using the high-speed drill, with diamond burs, and continuous suction irrigation continues near the petrous ridge until the contents of the internal auditory canal are exposed for 270 degrees. The internal auditory canal then is followed laterally toward the fundus; progressively smaller burs are used with a tapering effect to expose the internal auditory canal only 90 degrees at the fundus, thus avoiding damage to the basal turn of the cochlea or the ampulla of the superior semicircular canal. Identification of the Bill bar at the entrance of the facial nerve into the fallopian canal marks the lateral limit of dissection. A recent review of the anatomy of the middle fossa defines the relatively narrow "safe zones" that exist around the structures of the inner ear (89). Without thorough dissection in the lateral portion of the canal, there is an area below the transverse crest that is not visible from the middle fossa (90).

The proximal labyrinthine portion of the facial nerve is decompressed about 3 mm to allow for any swelling that may occur as a result of trauma during dissection. The dura then can be incised posteriorly, away from the facial nerve, under high magnification (Fig. 149.6C). The fibers of the facial nerve are dissected free from the adherent portions of the tumor. The high magnification allows more precise dissection with fine hooks and scissors (Fig. 149.6D). A small tumor may require debulking of this portion at this time, with care taken to preserve all the vascular and neural structures. Tumor dissection then proceeds from medial to lateral off the cochlear nerve—a key for hearing preservation (86). The nerve of origin for the tumor at this point is cut, while the cochlear nerve and the other vestibular nerve are preserved.

After tumor removal is accomplished, a pledget of gel foam soaked with papaverine is placed onto the cochlear nerve in the internal auditory canal. The vasodilator effect increases cochlear blood flow. The dural defect is packed with a small amount of abdominal fat (Fig. 149.6E), the craniotomy flap is replaced and secured with titanium microplates, and the wound is closed in layers.

Results

Complete tumor removal, one of the major goals of surgery, was accomplished in 98% of patients undergoing the middle fossa approach for removal of a vestibular schwannoma in one large series (91). The other major goal of this approach is hearing preservation. Reported results vary

from 20% to 71%. A recent review of the long-term hearing results in a large group of patients who underwent middle fossa craniotomy for removal of vestibular schwannoma found hearing remained stable in 70% of patients, and the decline that were noted appeared to be symmetric with the unoperated ear (92). Long-term facial nerve outcomes have been shown to be similar between the middle fossa approach and the translabyrinthine approach (74,57). There is a slightly higher incidence of temporary immediate facial weakness associated with the middle fossa approach, likely because of the need for manipulation of the facial nerve to facilitate tumor removal. CSF leakage for the middle fossa is reported to be slightly less than that of either the retrosigmoid or the translabyrinthine approaches (72,75). The other complications associated with middle fossa craniotomy include meningitis, epidural or intracranial hemorrhage, seizures, and headaches. These are all rare and do not occur in any higher frequency than in the translabyrinthine approach.

Many studies have tried to determine preoperatively what characteristics would best predict hearing preservation in patients undergoing vestibular schwannoma surgery; however, results have varied significantly from study to study. A recent review of patients with serviceable hearing (pure-tone average less than 50 dB and speech discrimination scores greater than 50%—the 50/50 rule) and tumors less than 2 cm in greatest dimension found that serviceable hearing was maintained in 58.8%, and measurable hearing was preserved in 75.9% (93). Not all components of the ABR were beneficial in predicting outcome. Specifically, significantly better outcomes were found in patients with lower absolute intra-aural wave V latency and for lower absolute wave V values. A hypoactive response on preoperative ENG, indicating a superior vestibular nerve tumor, is also considered to be associated with a favorable prognosis for hearing preservation. There was no significant correlation between hearing preservation and ENG results, but there was a trend toward better outcomes in patients with hypoactive caloric responses (93).

Retrosigmoid-Suboccipital Approach

The suboccipital approach has been the traditional neurosurgical approach to the CPA. We have found this approach to be useful in patients with good preoperative hearing whose tumor is medially located within the internal auditory canal and protrudes 2 cm or less into the CPA. The advantage of this approach is the potential for hearing preservation and the ability to remove tumors of all sizes with the same approach. There is good visualization of the brainstem and lower cranial nerves through this approach.

This approach has several disadvantages, however. The potential for air embolism exists whenever the patient's head is higher than the chest. Some surgeons prefer to use the sitting position for the retrosigmoid approach, placing the patient at risk for this complication. The traditional position for the suboccipital approach has been the "park bench" position, in which the patient is semiprone. Some surgeons, including those at our institution, now perform this operation with the patient in the supine position. In addition, tumors spreading to the lateral one third of the internal auditory canal are difficult to remove without violating the vestibular labyrinth or the endolymphatic duct (94,95). It is believed that unrecognized injury to the endolymphatic duct may explain some of the long-term hearing deterioration seen in retrosigmoid removal. Also, because it is difficult to visualize the lateral portion of the internal auditory canal, it is not uncommon for a remnant of tumor to be left in the lateral portion of the internal auditory canal. As a result, there is a higher incidence of incomplete tumor removal and recurrence with the retrosigmoid approach. Another disadvantage to the suboccipital approach is the need for cerebellar retraction. Cerebellar flocculus compression can produce oculomotor abnormalities of pursuit, optokinetic gaze, and saccade (96). These abnormalities may contribute to the dysequilibrium noted after surgery. The biggest disadvantage of the retrosigmoid approach is the high incidence of postoperative headaches. Up to 54% of patients will report headaches after retrosigmoid removal of vestibular schwannoma, and approximately 10% report prolonged and disabling headaches (97).

Technique

With the patient in the supine position, the head is shaved like it would be for a translabyrinthine approach, but with 2 to 3 cm extra hair removed posteriorly. The skin is prepared with povidone-iodine, and draped in a sterile fashion. Intraoperative monitoring of the facial nerve and ABR is continued throughout the procedure. A curvilinear incision is made about 3 cm posterior to the postauricular sulcus, with the inferior portion of the incision curved slightly posteriorly. A limited mastoidectomy is performed to decompress the sigmoid sinus. Cauterization of the mastoid emissary vein is usually necessary.

The mastoidectomy drilling is carried down along the sigmoid sinus until it nears the jugular bulb. The sigmoid is also followed superiorly until the lateral sinus is identified. A 4-cm craniotomy is then made over the subocciput (Fig. 149.7A). The underlying dura is separated from the bone, and the bone flap is removed. The dura is incised in a semilunar fashion with the base of the dural flap positioned medially. Stay sutures are placed into the dura, the sigmoid sinus is reflected anteriorly, the cerebellum is gently retracted posteriorly, and dissection is carried medially to the cisterna lateralis (Fig. 149.7B). Cerebrospinal fluid egresses when this region is entered, and the cerebellum falls posteriorly. The dura over the posterior internal auditory canal then is incised down to the bone. Drilling with a diamond bur then is begun on the posterior lip of the internal auditory canal, which is skeletonized in 180 degrees of its circumference (Fig. 149.7C). The endolymphatic sac and duct are useful landmarks in this dissection because

the endolymphatic duct lies superficial to the posterior semicircular canal.

The tumor at this point must be debulked frequently with the House-Urban dissector or ultrasonic aspirator, with care taken initially to ensure that the facial nerve is not located on the posterior surface of the tumor. Tumor dissection begins medially near the brainstem and extends laterally. A plane must be developed between the seventh nerve and the tumor while facial nerve monitoring equipment is used to avoid injury to the nerve. Every effort should be made to avoid traction from lateral to medial, because the cochlear nerve at the modiolus is at great risk with this maneuver.

The bone edges should be sealed with wax. The dura over the cerebellum is sutured with a continuous running suture, and the bone flap is replaced in its original anatomic position and secured with titanium plates. The mastoid defect is obliterated with fat, and the suboccipital musculature is resutured in its original location. Soft tissues are approximated in layers, and a dry sterile dressing is applied.

Results

Recent results from centers where microsurgical removal of vestibular schwannomas is performed regularly show that mortality is low (less than 1%) with this approach (98). Complete tumor removal has varied, with most major centers reporting complete resection in more than 95% (99). Normal or near-normal facial nerve function also has varied, depending on preoperative tumor size, ranging from 58% to 93% in large series (99). Hearing preservation results have been difficult to interpret, because it is difficult to define a uniform group of patients in whom conservation of hearing has been attempted. Hearing preservation has ranged from 17% to 65% (100–102). A recent report, after comparing reported results from several institutions, found that hearing preservation in the same hearing class for middle fossa craniotomy occurred in 33% to 57% (median 48%), as opposed to a range of 0% to 68% (median 39%) for the retrosigmoid craniotomy. When comparing serviceable hearing preservation in patients with preoperative class A hearing, the middle fossa results ranged from 50% to 71% (median 69%) and the retrosigmoid results ranged from 17% to 88% (median 54%) (103). Cerebrospinal fluid leakage occurs in about 11% of patients. Tumor size and surgical approach have some small influence on the incidence of leakage. Retrosigmoid craniotomy has the highest leak rate, followed by translabyrinthine craniotomy. Middle fossa craniotomy has the lowest leakage rate. (74,104). Other complications, such as meningitis and postoperative hemorrhage, occur with similar frequency, regardless of the approach. Postoperative headaches, however, occur with much more frequency in the retrosigmoid approach. Headaches were initially thought to be caused by adherence between the nuchal musculature and the dura, but repair of the bone defect by either a cranioplasty or replacement of the bone flap has not

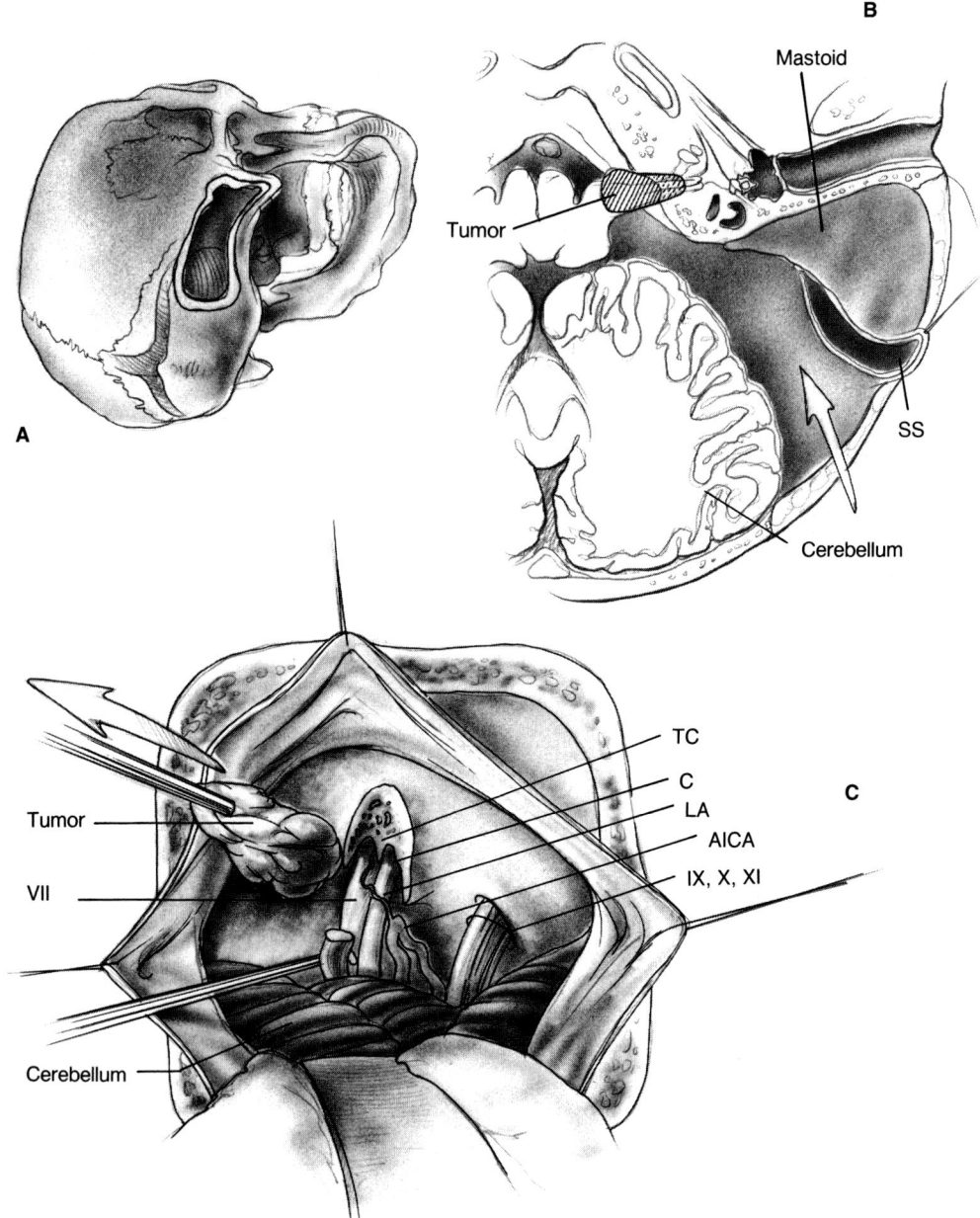

Figure 149.7 Retrosigmoid-suboccipital approach. **A:** A 3 cm craniotomy is made with the cutting bur, the sigmoid sinus serving as the anterior limit and the transverse sinus as the superior limit. A mastoidectomy with decompression of the sigmoid sinus also has been performed. **B** and **C:** The posterior lip of the internal auditory canal has been drilled away to expose the tumor and contents of the internal auditory canal. *SS,* sigmoid sinus; *TC,* transverse crest; *C,* cochlear nerve; *LA,* labyrinthine artery; *AICA,* anterior inferior cerebellar artery; *VII,* facial nerve; *IX,* glossopharyngeal nerve; *X,* vagal nerve; *XI,* spinal accessory nerve.

significantly reduced the incidence of headache. It is now thought that the headache may be caused by the bone dust from the intradural drilling of the internal auditory canal (97) (Tables 149.3 and 149.4)

Stereotactic Radiosurgery

"Stereotactic radiosurgery" is not truly surgical, but is a variation of radiation therapy. Leskell first introduced it in 1969 (105). The surgical moniker is derived from the fact

that only a selected area of tissue is addressed, as in surgery. This is accomplished by delivering multiple ionizing beams (gamma rays via a cobalt 60 source or photons via a cyclotron) of radiation to a specific intracranial target, delivered in a single treatment session. Unlike surgery, though, there is no removal or destruction of target tissue, so it is important to remember that the goal of radiosurgery is to stop tumor growth. Within the radiation therapy community, there are two distinct camps: the stereotactic radiosurgery

TABLE 149.3   EMERGENCIES AFTER TUMOR REMOVAL

Emergency	Management
Intracranial hemorrhage	Remove dressing and open wound, to allow rapid decompression of brainstem; move to operating room for control of hemorrhage.
Pneumocephalus	If unstable, emergency craniotomy to remove air; otherwise, discontinue lumbar drain and observe.
Meningitis	Lumbar puncture for culture and sensitivity; appropriate antibiotics intravenously; surgical closure of any cerebrospinal fluid leak.
Cerebrospinal fluid leak	Pressure dressing; if leak persists despite lumbar drain, surgical closure.

group and fractionated radiotherapy group. Fractionated radiotherapy differs in two ways: The source is often a linear accelerator, and the total dose is fractionated—meaning that it is delivered over several sessions. Both rely on computer modeling to determine the dose center—or isocenter—and the 50% isodose line, which is the periphery where the total dose delivered is one-half the total dose delivered to the isocenter. The 50% isodose line is currently set to be around 13 to 14 Gy. Radiosurgery claims the advantage of allowing more isocenters than are available with fractionated radiation therapy, thereby allowing better conformation of the target (106). The goal of both is to limit the dose and/or damage to surrounding structures, while maximizing delivery to the intended target. Overall, outcomes are very similar, regardless of the type of radiation used (106). Initial results using an 18-Gy dose showed high levels of tumor control but equally high incidence of injury to the trigeminal and facial nerves, and only very limited success (22%) with long-term hearing preservation. Oftentimes, the deficits developed in a delayed fashion, occurring several months to two years after treatment. As a result, radiotherapists lowered the total dose delivered to its current level.

Of concern is the finding that radiation doses six times more than the clinical maximum failed to eradicate schwannoma cells *in vitro* (107). Lee et al. (108) measured proliferating cell nuclear antigen (PCNA) in tumor cells from patients with tumors that were growing after radiosurgery.

TABLE 149.4   COMPLICATIONS CEREBELLOPONTINE ANGLE TUMORS

Sensorineural hearing loss
Facial nerve paralysis
Cerebrospinal fluid leak
Meningitis
Intracranial hemorrhage
Air embolism
Cerebellar ataxia
Headaches

They found that there was a lower proliferation potential in the tumors having undergone radiosurgery. They hypothesize that the radiation therapy led to apoptosis in the tumor cells that had the highest proliferation potential, and those cells that were dividing more slowly survived. This may also explain why there seems to be a period of several years between the time of radiation and continued growth. It also raises significant concern that the long-term results with the lower dose may be significantly worse. Earlier studies from the Karolinska Institute in Stockholm, Sweden, where the gamma knife was developed, found that 15% of tumors were larger at 1-year follow-up (109). Hearing was maintained in 22% of the patients who had useful pretreatment hearing, and some degree of facial weakness, frequently delayed, occurred in 17% of patients (110). Trigeminal dysfunction was noted in 19%. A second major series, from the University of Pittsburgh, showed only a 4% increase in tumor size 1 year after treatment (111). Useful hearing was preserved in about 33% of patients who had hearing before treatment, 21% developed facial nerve weakness, and 27% developed trigeminal nerve loss. A different study from the Mayo Clinic revealed that no patient had tumor progression at a mean follow-up of 16 months; however, the incidences of facial weakness and trigeminal neuropathy were 66.5% and 59%, respectively. Hearing was preserved in about 50% of the patients (112). These dismal results led to the reduction in total dose and improvement in the computer modeling. Recent studies have shown significantly better results in cranial nerve outcomes. However, there is debate regarding whether it is the improved tumor conformation achieved when using multiple isocenters, or whether it is the decreased dose that is yielding better cranial nerve outcomes. Foote et al. (105) found that regardless of the degree of conformation, or the number of isocenters, there were fewer cranial neuropathies when the maximum brainstem dose was lower. They also found that peripheral doses of less than 15 Gy yielded better cranial nerve outcomes. A recent study from Boston (113) using proton beam radiosurgery found that the incidence of facial nerve weakness was 8.9%, trigeminal function was decreased in 10.9%, and only 33% maintained serviceable hearing. Flickinger et al. (114) found that by using a reduced dose, they were able to reduce their facial neuropathy incidence to 1.1% and reduce their trigeminal neuropathy to 2.6%. Hearing was preserved in 74% of patients. All the radiation studies quote tumor control rates in the 96% to 98% range. Again, it is too early to tell what the long-term outcomes for tumor control will be, given that these are naturally slow-growing tumors, and the reduction in dose is a relatively recent phenomenon. Prolonged imbalance is unusual in patients undergoing microsurgery, but it is seen in up to 33% of patients treated with radiation (115). One possible explanation for this is that radiation leads to a decrease in vestibular function on the treated side, whereas microsurgery leads to complete loss of function due to sectioning of the vestibular nerve. Central compensation is more complete when the nerve is sectioned. Another complication that is more common after radiation than after microsurgery is hydrocephalus requiring shunting (105,113). Radiotherapy also has the unique risk of inducing malignancy in the irradiated field. Bari et al (116) reviewed four cases of malignancy that developed in radiated vestibular schwannomas. Sarcomas have also been found in the irradiated field, and there is a 1 per 2,000 risk of a malignancy developing up to 10 years after radiation (117).

Significant concerns have been raised about the results of surgery in patients who have had stereotactic irradiation for vestibular schwannomas. It is clear, at this point, that postirradiation tumor removal is more difficult and that there is more adherence and scaring between the facial nerve and/or the brainstem in these cases (118). Friedman et al. (R Friedman, D Brackmann, and W Hitselberger, unpublished data June 2005) recently reviewed the results of 44 patients who have presented to the House Ear Institute for treatment after failed radiotherapy. Forty-two percent of those patients were 1.5 to 3 years out from their radiation when they presented with tumor growth, 26% of them were greater than 4 years postirradiation. These radiation failures were randomly matched to patients who had not had radiation to compare outcomes. As a whole, the patients who had received radiation had poorer preoperative facial nerve function and poorer hearing thresholds. Postoperatively, the previously irradiated patients had poorer facial nerve outcomes at the first postoperative visit (46% grade VI in the irradiated group; 22% grade VI in the control group). The poorer outcomes were also present at 1-year follow-up, where only 52% of the radiated group had good facial function, whereas 72% of the controls did. Of note, there were more NF2 patients in the failure group than in the control group.

Microsurgery remains the treatment of choice for vestibular schwannomas. Stereotactic radiation has a role in treating patients with tumors less than 2 cm who are elderly or who are not good surgical candidates. It should be used with caution in patients with NF2. The effects of irradiation in NF2, where there is a known mutation in a growth control gene, is unpredictable. Rapid growth of

NF2 tumors following irradiation has been reported (119). Caution should also be used in younger patients because of the risk of growth even many years after radiation.

OTHER TUMORS OF THE CEREBELLOPONTINE ANGLE

Meningiomas

Meningiomas are the second most common tumor originating within the CPA, accounting for 3% of tumors in this region (120). The term *meningioma* was coined by Dr. Harvey Cushing (121), who in 1938 wrote a scholarly treatise outlining the histologic and anatomic classifications of meningiomas (122). Meningiomas tend to arise from the cap cells that collect in clusters around the tips of the arachnoid villi (123). These cap cells are most prevalent at dural venous sinuses and at the points from which the cranial nerves exit their respective foramina. Meningiomas are of two types, globular (more rounded), and en plaque (flat and sessile). The tumors do not metastasize, but tend to recur because of their propensity for bony invasion.

Symptoms of a meningioma are referable to the site of origin. Tumors arising within the internal auditory canal may produce symptoms identical to those of a vestibular schwannoma. Because most tumors arise from the posterior surface of the petrous bone, they often do not enter the internal auditory canal and generally are larger than a vestibular schwannoma before causing hearing loss or vestibular symptoms. Tumors arising more inferiorly—in the sigmoid sinus or jugular bulb—may cause hoarseness, dysphagia, or tongue atrophy. Signs of a meningioma are commonly related to the eye. Spontaneous nystagmus is seen, frequently along with facial hypesthesia and gait ataxia (124).

Patients who have meningiomas generally have better hearing than patients with comparably sized vestibular schwannomas. The audiometric findings, however, may be indistinguishable from those with a vestibular schwannoma. Pure-tone averages and speech discrimination scores are consistent with retrocochlear disease. In addition, ABR is normal in 25% of patients with meningiomas (125).

Specific radiographic differences usually allow the clinician to differentiate a vestibular schwannoma from a meningioma. On CT scans, meningiomas have a more dense appearance and generally are homogeneous in taking up contrast medium. Vestibular schwannomas usually are nonhomogeneous because of areas of central necrosis. A CT scan frequently shows evidence of hyperostosis with a meningioma, and occasionally calcification is noted within the tumor. Meningiomas generally appear as a sessile mass with a broad base that is not centered on the internal auditory canal. There is no widening of the internal auditory canal on either CT scanning or MRI. MRI shows a dural tail in 50% to 72% of patients who have a meningioma (Fig. 149.8). Meningiomas often have a "washed

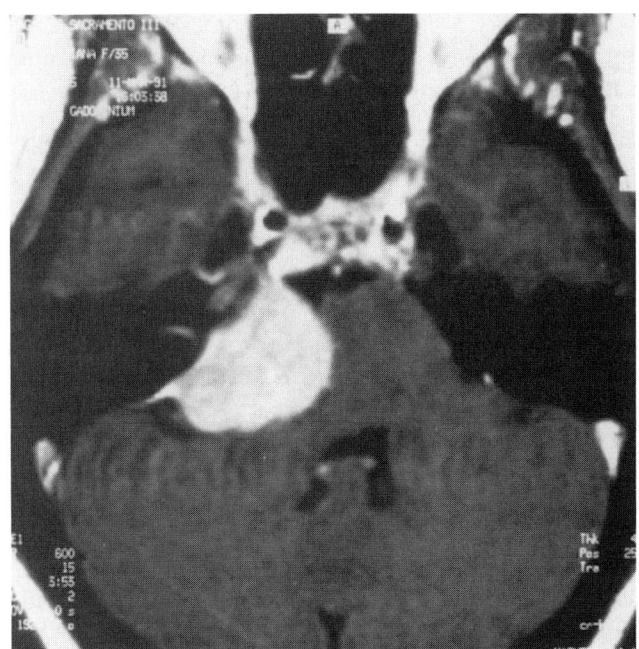

Figure 149.8 Magnetic resonance image of a large meningioma on the posterior face of the temporal bone. Note the broad-based appearance of this homogeneous tumor and the characteristic dural tail extending laterally. This tumor was removed by an extended middle fossa approach.

out" appearance because of vascularity, yielding a less bright image than that of a vestibular schwannoma.

Several histologic subtypes of meningiomas have been suggested. One widely used system characterizes these tumors as meningotheliomatous meningiomas (55%), fibrous meningiomas (15%), transitional meningiomas (25%), and angioblastic meningiomas (5%) (126). The transitional meningioma is a combination of the meningotheliomatous and the fibrous meningiomas. Psammoma bodies are abundant in the transitional meningioma. Transitional or fibrous meningiomas are more likely to exhibit calcium deposition within the tumor (127). Angioblastic meningiomas are the most aggressive tumors, with an increased rate of local recurrence. They also have a tendency to erode and infiltrate bone.

Surgical excision is the treatment of choice in patients who have a meningioma. The surgical procedure should be tailored to the location of the tumor as well as to the preoperative hearing level. In patients who have poor hearing and a meningioma in the CPA, the translabyrinthine approach has proved useful. In patients who have medial extension of the tumor to the internal auditory canal and onto the clivus, the transcochlear approach can be used. In the transcochlear approach, the greater superficial petrosal nerve is sectioned and the facial nerve is removed from the fallopian canal and transposed posteriorly (128). The cochlea then can be drilled away, allowing wide exposure anterior to the internal auditory canal. In some patients whose tumor extends into both the middle cranial fossa and the posterior cranial fossa, a combined petrosal approach has been used. In this approach, a middle fossa craniotomy is combined with one of several exposures into the posterior fossa to allow tumor removal in a single stage. The exposure into the posterior fossa can be tailored to the patient's preoperative hearing level. The sigmoid sinus, along with the superior petrosal sinus and the tentorium, may be sectioned for additional exposure. Excellent exposure is achieved into both the middle and the posterior cranial fossae through this approach. In patients who have good hearing preoperatively, the retrosigmoid approach has proved useful and may permit hearing conservation. In patients who have small intracanalicular meningiomas, the middle cranial fossa approach can be used. In patients who have larger tumors extending into the more superior portion of the CPA, the extended middle cranial fossa approach may prove helpful. This approach provides the opportunity for hearing conservation and complete tumor removal.

Removal of these vascular tumors often is associated with significant blood loss. Care should be taken not to damage cranial nerves or vascular structures to the brainstem when control of bleeding is attempted. Because these lesions tend to recur, complete excision, including a rim of normal dura, is necessary. Some investigators advocate removal of bone underlying the meningioma because meningiomas tend to infiltrate the underlying bone.

The morbidity associated with meningioma removal is greater than that with vestibular schwannomas and should be considered in the decision on management. Meningiomas are somewhat sensitive to radiation therapy. Elderly patients or patients who have severe medical conditions may be candidates for observation. Recent attempts have been made to treat meningiomas with stereotactic radiosurgery, but long-term results of this treatment are not available.

Facial Nerve Schwannomas

Schwannomas of the facial nerve are histologically identical to vestibular schwannomas and may occur anywhere along the course of the facial nerve. However, they are rarely isolated to the internal auditory canal, and generally have some involvement of the geniculate ganglion. They frequently have "skip lesions" and involve nonadjacent portions of the facial nerve. They may be manifested by unilateral hearing loss, tinnitus, and vestibular symptoms when they arise within the internal auditory canal. When the tumor is distal to the geniculate, it may fill the middle ear and present with aural fullness and a conductive hearing loss. Rarely, hemifacial spasm suggests a facial schwannoma. Facial nerve function is generally not impaired until the tumor is quite large. Audiometric findings are often similar to those of a vestibular schwannoma, making differentiation difficult. Impedance testing may show that the ipsilateral acoustic reflex is absent because of the involvement of the motor fibers of the facial nerve.

The contralateral reflex may be absent if the eighth nerve is involved. Auditory brainstem response testing usually yields the same results as an acoustic tumor (129). Electroneuronography may suggest a facial neuroma when a reduced response is found; however, we have seen patients with normal electroneuronographic findings who had facial nerve schwannomas. Magnetic resonance imaging is the method of choice in diagnosing a facial nerve schwannoma. In some cases, a cerebellopontine mass extends into the internal auditory canal through the fallopian canal to the geniculate ganglion with a mass in the middle cranial fossa. This appearance is highly suggestive of a facial nerve schwannoma.

The initial treatment of choice is observation, looking for either tumor growth or loss of facial function. Once either of these occurs, surgical resection with insertion of a cable nerve graft is the treatment of choice. However, the senior author has several patients who were managed by facial nerve decompression when facial weakness began to develop, and have now been followed many years without any further decrease in facial function. The translabyrinthine approach is used most commonly for tumor removal. Because differentiation of a vestibular schwannoma from a facial schwannoma may be impossible, we always inform patients in the preoperative discussion that resection of the facial nerve and a nerve graft may prove necessary (130).

Epidermoids

An epidermoid is a slow-growing lesion that may arise either within the temporal bone or in the CPA. Hemifacial spasm is a common early distinguishing feature, and progressive facial paralysis is frequently noted. Hearing loss, vertigo, ataxia, and paralysis of the fifth and sixth cranial nerves also may be presenting symptoms. These lesions are thought to arise from epithelial rests within the temporal bone. Physiologically, they are identical to cholesteatomas of the middle ear. Classically, they have been associated with a poor speech discrimination score relative to the pure tones, greater than that with a vestibular schwannoma. An extremely bright T2 signal on MRI is generally seen. Epidermoids of the CPA are usually treated surgically; however, the operation is difficult because of the propensity of the tumor to infiltrate between cranial nerves and blood vessels. The epidermoid tends to adhere to the structures in the brainstem, so that complete surgical removal is difficult.

Other Cranial Nerve Schwannomas

Any of the cranial nerves of the posterior fossa may give rise to a schwannoma. The symptoms of dysfunction are related to the nerve of origin and location. A schwannoma of the trigeminal nerve characteristically produces unilateral facial hypesthesia, and the Meckel cave is enlarged on CT scans. When the ninth, tenth, and eleventh cranial nerves are affected by a schwannoma, a jugular foramen syndrome is often produced, including dysphagia, hoarseness, and shoulder weakness. A mass extending down into the parapharyngeal space or into the posterior fossa may be seen. Schwannomas of the twelfth nerve usually cause hemiatrophy of the tongue and enlargement of the hypoglossal canal on CT scans.

Vascular Tumors

Several vascular tumors may occur in the CPA (131). A glomus jugulare tumor may spread into the cerebellopontine region from the temporal bone. Other vascular tumors, such as hemangiomas and hemangioblastomas, may occur primarily within this area. Glomus jugulare tumors are nonchromaffin paragangliomas that arise from chemoreceptor cells alongside the ninth and tenth cranial nerves in the jugular bulb. They commonly are manifested by pulsatile tinnitus. When they have spread to the posterior fossa, a jugular foramen syndrome with paralysis to the ninth, tenth, and eleventh nerves is usually present. CT studies show a characteristic irregular destruction of the jugular foramen, and MRI shows the classic "salt and pepper" pattern associated with glomous tumors. The treatment is surgical excision through the infratemporal fossa approach (132).

Hemangiomas are benign hamartomatous tumors that originate from blood vessels. They often arise in the geniculate ganglion and are announced by a slowly progressive facial paralysis. A honeycomb appearance of the bone surrounding the geniculate ganglion is characteristic. They also may originate in the internal auditory canal, producing symptoms typical of a vestibular schwannoma. Treatment is surgical excision by the middle fossa approach. Because of their intimate association with the facial nerve (133), facial grafting of the nerve is usually necessary.

Miscellaneous Cerebellopontine Angle Tumors

Arachnoid cysts are thin-walled sacs containing cerebrospinal fluid. They develop from adhesions within the arachnoid of the internal auditory canal. Cholesterol granuloma of the petrous apex may spread into the posterior fossa when it becomes large. It results from occlusion of the air cells in the petrous apex, and hemorrhage into the air cells causes the foreign body reaction and granuloma formation. These tumors show characteristically bright T1 and T2 images on MRI. Treatment of these cystic lesions is by drainage through a retrosigmoid approach for an arachnoid cyst and an infralabyrinthine or infracochlear approach for petrous apex cholesterol granuloma (134).

Various embryonic tumors, including dermoid tumors, teratomas, and chordomas, may develop in the CPA. Lipomas of the CPA may occur as hamartomatous lesions. They may be densely adherent to the brainstem and show a fat density on MRI.

Primary axial tumors of the central nervous system are rare. They generally develop in the brainstem or cerebellum and include hemangioblastomas, gliomas, and medulloblastomas. Treatment of these unusual tumors is surgical, with the approach determined by location of the tumor and amount of residual hearing.

Malignant tumors of the CPA are quite rare, but chondrosarcomas, malignant choroid plexus papillomas, and metastatic tumors have been encountered. Among patients with metastatic tumors in the temporal bone, breast cancer is most common in women, and prostate or lung cancer is most common in men. Facial paralysis with a rapidly growing lesion is most commonly seen. Lumbar puncture should be considered for cerebrospinal fluid cytology in these patients. Treatment is usually nonsurgical after an open biopsy to establish the diagnosis.

HIGHLIGHTS

- Vestibular schwannomas are the most common tumors occurring in the CPA and require a significant amount of diagnostic effort by the practicing otolaryngologist.
- Vestibular schwannomas in type 2 neurofibromatosis are thought to be caused by the absence of a tumor suppressor gene on the long arm of chromosome 22.
- Unexplained unilateral otologic or vestibular symptoms should prompt an evaluation to rule out a pathologic condition in the CPA.
- With improved radiographic imaging techniques, the tumor is being diagnosed in a greater percentage of patients without symptoms, or with atypical symptoms.
- Magnetic resonance imaging with gadolinium contrast allows for detection of very small vestibular schwannomas and now is the definitive procedure for the diagnosis of a vestibular schwannoma.
- In general, vestibular schwannomas are best treated by surgical excision, with the surgical approach tailored to preoperative hearing, tumor size and location, experience of the surgical team, and patient desires.
- Vestibular schwannomas vary greatly in growth rate, and the duration of symptoms is frequently correlated with tumor growth rate.
- The goals of vestibular schwannoma resection are, in order of importance: to preserve life, to avoid serious neurologic sequelae, to totally excise the tumor, to preserve facial nerve function, and to preserve hearing.
- It is possible to occlude the semicircular canals in the translabyrinthine approach and potentially save hearing.
- The advantages of the translabyrinthine approach for vestibular schwannoma surgery are that the CPA is approached directly, the facial nerve can be identified away from the tumor, cerebellar retraction is minimal, the fundus of the internal auditory canal is widely exposed, and the potential exists for facial nerve repair if necessary.

REFERENCES

1. Cushing H. *Intracranial tumours: notes upon a series of two thousand verified cases with surgical-mortality percentages pertaining thereto.* Springfield, IL: Charles C Thomas Publisher, 1932.
2. Revilla AG. Differential diagnosis of tumors at the cerebellopontine recess. *Bull Johns Hopkins Hosp* 1948;83:187–212.
3. House WF. A history of acoustic tumor surgery: 1800–1900, early history. In: House WF, Luetje CM, eds. *Acoustic tumors.* Vol. 1. Baltimore: University Park Press, 1979:3–8.
4. Rosenberg SI. Natural history of acoustic neuromas. *Laryngoscope* 2000;110:497–508.
5. Cushing H. *Tumors of the nervus acusticus and the syndrome of the cerebellopontine angle.* (Reprint of the 1917 edition.) New York: Hafner, 1963.
6. House WF. A history of acoustic tumor surgery: 1900–1917, the Cushing era. In: House WF, Luetje CM, eds. *Acoustic tumors.* Vol. 1. Baltimore: University Park Press, 1979:9–23.
7. Dandy WE. An operation for the total removal of cerebellopontine (acoustic) tumors. *Surg Gynecol Obstet* 1925;41:129–148.
8. House WF. Report of cases: monographtranstemporal bone microsurgical removal of acoustic neuromas. *Arch Otolaryngol* 1964; 80:617–667.
9. Glasscock ME III, Steenerson RL. A history of acoustic tumor surgery: 1961–present. In: House WF, Luetje CM, eds. *Acoustic tumors.* Vol. 1. Baltimore: University Park Press, 1979:33–41.
10. House WF. Exposure of the internal auditory canal and its contents through the middle cranial fossa. *Laryngoscope* 1961;71: 1363–1385.
11. Lang J. Clinical anatomy of the cerebellopontine angle and internal acoustic meatus. *Adv Otorhinolaryngol* 1984;34:8–24.
12. Hollinshead WH. *Anatomy for surgeons.* New York: Hoeber-Harper, 1954:67–87.
13. Hardy M, Crowe SJ. Early asymptomatic acoustic tumor: report of 6 cases. *Arch Surg* 1936;32:292–301.
14. Eckermeier LS, Sorenson GD, McGavran MH. Histopathology of 30 non-operated acoustic schwannomas. *Arch Otorhinolaryngol* 1979;222:1.
15. Leonard JR, Talbot ML. Asymptomatic acoustic neurilomoma. *Arch Otolaryngol* 1970;91:117–124.
16. Anderson TD, Loevner LA, Bigelow DC, et al. Prevalence of unsuspected acoustic neuroma found by magnetic resonance imaging. *Otolaryngol Head Neck Surg* 2000;122:643–646.
17. Tos M, Thomsen J, Charabi S. Incidence of acoustic neuromas. *Ear Nose Throat J* 1992;71:391–393.
18. Tos M, Stangerup S, Caye-Thomasen P, et al. What is the real incidence of vestibular schwannoma? *Arch Otolaryngol Head Neck Surg* 2004;130:216–220.
19. Clemis JD, Ballad WJ, Baggot PJ, et al. Relative frequency of inferior vestibular schwannoma. *Arch Otolaryngol Head Neck Surg* 1986;112:190–194.
20. Komatsuzaki A, Tsunoda A. Nerve of origin of the acoustic neuroma. *J Laryngol Otol* 2001;115:376–379.
21. Lanser MJ, Sussman SA, Frazer K. Epidemiology, pathogenesis, and genetics of acoustic tumors. *Otolaryngol Clin North Am* 1992;25:499–520.
22. Xenellis JE, Linthicum FH. On the myth of the glial/schwann junction (Obersteiner-Redlich zone): origin of vestibular nerve schwannomas. *Otol Neurotol* 2003;24:1.
23. Neff BA, Willcox TO, Sataloff RT. Intralabyrinthine schwannomas. *Otol Neurotol* 2003;24:299–307.
24. Brackmann DE, Fayad JN, Slattery WH, et al. Early and proactive management of vestibular schwannomas in neurofibromatosis type 2. *Neurosurgery* 2001;49(2):274–283.
25. Evans DGR. Molecular biology of skullbase lesions. In: Baguley D, Ramsden R, Moffat D, eds. *Fourth International Conference on Vestibular Schwannoma and Other CPA Lesions. Immediate Proceedings LTD.* Suffolk, United Kingdom: Bungray, 2003:89.
26. Lallemand D, Curto M, Saotome I, et al. NF2 deficiency promotes tumorigenesis and metastasis by destabilizing adherens junctions. *Genes Dev* 2003;17:1090–1100.
27. Hansen MR, Linthicum FH. Expression of neuregulin and activation of erbB receptors in vestibular schwannomas:

possible autocrine loop stimulation. *Otol Neurotol* 2004;25: 155–159.

28. Murphy PR, Myal Y, Sato Y, et al. Elevated expression of basic fibroblast growth factor messenger ribonucleic acid in acoustic neuromas. *Mol Endocrinol* 1989;3:225–231.

29. Diensthuber M, Brandis A, Lenarz T, et al. Co-expression of transforming growth factor-β1 and glial cell line derived neurotrophic factor in vestibular schwannomas. *Otol Neurotol* 2004;25:359–365.

30. Cayé-Thomasen P, Baandrup L, Jacobsen GK, et al. Immunohistochemical demonstration of vascular endothelial growth factor in vestibular schwannomas correlates to tumor growth rate. *Laryngoscope* 2003;113:2129–2134.

31. Brieger J, Bedavanija A, Lehr H, et al. Expression of angiogenic growth factors in acoustic neuroma. *Acta Otolaryngol* 2003;123: 1040–1045.

32. Hall JG. Possible maternal and hormonal factors in neurofibromatosis. *Adv Neurol* 1981;29:125–131.

33. Beatty CW, Scheithauer BW, Katzmann JA, et al. Acoustic schwannoma and pregnancy: a DNA flow cytometric, steroid hormone receptor, and proliferation marker study. *Laryngoscope* 1995;105: 693–700.

34. Selesnick SH, Jackler RK. Clinical manifestations and audiologic diagnosis of acoustic neuromas. *Otolaryngol Clin North Am* 1992; 25:521–551.

35. Selesnick SH, Jackler RK, Pitts LW. The changing clinical presentation of acoustic tumors in the MRI era. *Laryngoscope* 1993;103: 431–436.

36. Higgs WA. Sudden deafness as the presenting symptom of acoustic neurinoma. *Arch Otolaryngol* 1973;98:73–76.

37. Friedman RA, Kesser BW, Slattery WH, et al. Hearing preservation in patients with vestibular schwannomas with sudden sensorineural hearing loss. *Otolaryngol Head Neck Surg* 2001;125: 544–551.

38. Fahy C, Nikolopoulos TP, O'Donoghue GM. Acoustic neuroma surgery and tinnitus. *Eur Arch Otorhinolaryngol* 2002;259:299–301.

39. Hoistad DL, Melnik G, Mamioglu B, eet al. Update on conservative management of acoustic neuroma. *Otol Neurotol* 2001;22: 682–685.

40. Johnson EW. Results of auditory tests in acoustic tumor patients. In: House WF, Luetje CM, eds. *Acoustic tumors.* Vol. 1. Baltimore: University Park Press, 1979:209–224.

41. Beck HJ, Beatty CW, Harner SG, eet al. Acoustic neuromas with normal pure tone hearing levels. *Otolaryngol Head Neck Surg* 1986;94:96–103.

42. Musiek FE, Josey AF, Glasscock ME III. Auditory brain-stem response in patients with acoustic neuromas: wave presence and absence. *Arch Otolaryngol Head Neck Surg* 1986;112:186–189.

43. Wilson DF, Hodgson RS, Gustafson MF, et al. The sensitivity of auditory brainstem response testing in small acoustic neuromas. *Laryngoscope* 1992;102:961–964.

44. Moffat DA, Baguley DM, Hardy DG, et al. Contralateral auditory brainstem response abnormalities in acoustic neuroma. *J Laryngol Otol* 1989;103:835–838.

45. Kevanishvili Z. The detection of small acoustic tumors: the stacked derived-band ABR procedure. *Am J Otol* 2000;21:148–151.

46. Don M, Masuda A, Nelson R, et al. Successful detection of small acoustic tumors using the stacked derived-band auditory brain stem response amplitude. *Am J Otol* 1997;18:608–621.

47. Philibert B, Durrant JD, Ferber-Viart C, et al. Stacked tone-burst-evoked auditory brainstem response (ABR): preliminary findings. *Int J Audiol* 2003;42:71–81.

48. Jenkins HA. Long-term adaptive changes of the vestibulo-ocular reflex in patients following acoustic neuroma surgery. *Laryngoscope* 1985;95:1224–1234.

49. Nedzelski JM, Schessel DA, Pfleiderer A, et al. Conservative management of acoustic neuromas. *Otolaryngol Clin North Am* 1992; 25:691–705.

50. Linthicum FH. Electronystagmography findings in patients with acoustic tumors. *Semin Hear* 1983;4:47–53.

51. Smith IM, Turnbull LW, Sellar RJ, et al. A modified screening protocol for the diagnosis of acoustic neuromas. *Clin Otolaryngol* 1990;15:167–171.

52. Moretz WH Jr, Orchik DJ, Shea JJ Jr, et al. Low-frequency harmonic acceleration in the evaluation of patients with intracanalicular and cerebellopontine angle tumors. *Otolaryngol Head Neck Surg* 1986; 95:324–332.

53. Welling DB, Glasscock ME III, Woods CI, et al. Acoustic neuroma: a cost-effective approach. *Otolaryngol Head Neck Surg* 1990;103: 364–370.

54. House JW, Waluch V, Jackler RK. Magnetic resonance imaging in acoustic neuroma diagnosis. *Ann Otol Rhinol Laryngol* 1986;95: 16–20.

55. Shelton C, Harnsberger HR, Allen R, et al. Fast spin echo magnetic resonance imaging: clinical application in screening for acoustic neuroma. *Otolaryngol Head Neck Surg* 1996;114:71–76.

56. Lhuillier FM, Doyon DL, Halimi PM, et al. Magnetic resonance imaging of acoustic neuromas: pitfalls and differential diagnosis. *Neuroradiology* 1992;34:144–149.

57. Paz-Fumagalli R, Daniels DL, Millen SJ, et al. Dural "tail" associated with an acoustic schwannoma in MR imaging with gadopentetate dimeglumine. *AJNR Am J Neuroradiol* 1991;12:1206.

58. Russell DS, Rubenstein LJ. *Pathology of tumors of the nervous system,* 5th ed. Baltimore: Williams & Wilkins, 1989.

59. Deen HG, Ebersold MJ, Harner SG, et al. Conservative management of acoustic neuroma—an outcome study. *Neurosurgery* 1996;39:260–264.

60. Strasnick B, Glasscock ME III, Haynes D, et al. The natural history of untreated acoustic neuromas. *Laryngoscope* 1994;104:1115–1119.

61. Nedzelski JM, Canter RJ, Kassel EE, et al. Is no treatment good treatment in the management of acoustic neuromas in the elderly? *Laryngoscope* 1986;96:825–829.

62. Weit RJ, Young NM, Monsell EM, et al. Age considerations in acoustic neuroma surgery: the horns of dilemma. *Am J Otol* 1989;10:177–180.

63. Charabi S, Mirko T, Thomsen J, et al. Vestibular schwannoma growthlong term results. *Acta Otolaryngol* 2000; suppl 543:7–10.

64. Charabi S, Thomsen J, Mantoni M, et al. Acoustic neuroma (vestibular schwannoma): growth and surgical and nonsurgical consequences of the wait-and-see policy. *Otolaryngol Head Neck Surg* 1995;113:5–14.

65. Ramsay HA, Luxford WM. Treatment of acoustic tumors in elderly patients: is surgery warranted? *J Laryngol Otol* 1993;107: 295–297.

66. Slattery WH, Schwartz MS, Fisher LM, et al. Acoustic neuroma surgical cost and outcome by hospital volume in California. *Otolaryngol Head Neck Surg* 2004;130:726–735.

67. Barker FG, Carter BS, Ojemann RG, et al. Surgical excision of acoustic neuroma: patient outcome and provider caseload. *Laryngoscope* 2003;113:1332–1343.

68. Tos M, Thomsen J, Harmsen A. Is preservation of hearing in acoustic neuroma worthwhile? *Acta Otolaryngol Suppl* 1988;452: 57–68.

69. Day JD, Chen DA, Arriaga M. Translabyrinthine approach for acoustic neuroma. *Neurosurgery* 2004;54:391–396.

70. Cushing H. The acoustic tumors. In: *Intracranial tumors.* Springfield, IL: Charles C Thomas, 1932:85–92.

71. Kaylie DM, Gilbert E, Horgan MA, et al. Acoustic neuroma surgery outcomes. *Otol Neurotol* 2001;22:686–689.

72. Sanna M, Abdelkader T, Russo A, et al. Perioperative complications in acoustic neuroma (vestibular schwannoma) surgery. *Otol Neurotol* 2004;25:379–386.

73. Darrouzet V, Martel J, Enée V, et al. Vestibular schwannoma surgery outcomes: our multidisciplinary experience in 400 cases over 17 years. *Laryngoscope* 2004;114:681–688.

74. Wiet RJ, Mamioglu B, Odom L, et al. Long-term results of the first 500 cases of acoustic neuroma surgery. *Otolaryngol Head Neck Surg* 2001;124:645–651.

75. Slattery WH, Francis S, House CC. Perioperative morbidity of acoustic neuroma surgery. *Otol Neurotol* 2001;22:895–902.

76. Mamikoglu B, Wiet RJ, Esquivel CR. Translabyrinthine approach for the management of large and giant vestibular schwannomas. *Otol Neurotol* 2002;23:224–227.

77. Shelton C. Unilateral acoustic tumors: how often do they recur after translabyrinthine removal? *Laryngoscope* 1995;105: 958–966.

78. Thedinger BA, Glasscock ME III, Cueva RA, et al. Postoperative radiographic evaluation after acoustic neuroma and glomus jugulare tumor removal. *Laryngoscope* 1992;102:261–266.

79. Pace-Balzan A, Ley RH, Ramsden RT, et al. Growth characteristics of acoustic neuromas with particular reference to the fate of capsule fragments remaining after tumor removal: implications for patient management. In: Tos M, Thomsen J, eds. *Proceedings of the first international conference on acoustic neuroma.* Amsterdam: Kugler. 1992:701–703.

80. Bloch D, Oghalai JS, Jackler RK, et al. The role of less than complete resection of acoustic neuroma. *Otolaryngol Head Neck Surg* 2004;130:104–112.

81. Kemink JL, Tucci SA, Graham MD. Near-total and subtotal resection of acoustic neuroma. In: Tos M, Thomsen J, eds. *Proceedings of the first international conference on acoustic neuroma.* Amsterdam: Kugler, 1992:697–700.

82. Falcioni M, Agarwal M, Taibah A, et al. Total facial paralysis after vestibular schwannoma surgery: probability of regaining normal function. *Ann Otol Rhinol Laryngol* 2004;113:706–710.

83. Grant GA, Rostomily RR, Kim K, et al. Delayed facial palsy after resection of vestibular schwannoma. *J Neurosurg* 2002;97:93–96.

84. Magliulo G, Parrotto D, Stasolla A, et al. Modified translabyrinthine approach and hearing preservation. *Laryngoscope* 2004;114:1133–1138.

85. Friedman RA, Kesser B, Brackmann DE, et al. Long-term hearing preservation after middle fossa removal of vestibular schwannoma. *Otolaryngol Head Neck Surg* 2003;129:660–665.

86. Brackmann DE, House JR III, Hitselberger WE. Technical modifications to the middle fossa craniotomy approach in removal of acoustic neuromas. *Am J Otol* 1994;15:614–619.

87. House WF. Surgical exposure of the internal auditory canal and its contents through the middle cranial fossa. *Laryngoscope* 1961;71:163.

88. Shen T, Friedman RA, Brackmann DE, Slattery WH, Hitselberger WE, et al. The evolution of surgical approaches for posterior fossa meningiomas. *Otol Neurotol* 2004;25:394–397.

89. Sennaroglu L, Slattery WH. Petrous anatomy for middle fossa approach. *Laryngoscope* 2003;113:332–342.

90. Driscoll CL, Jackler RK, Pitts LH, et al. Is the entire fundus of the internal auditory canal visible during the middle fossa approach for acoustic neuroma? *Am J Otol* 2000;21:382–388.

91. Shelton C, Brackmann DE, House WF, et al. Middle fossa acoustic tumor surgery: results in 106 cases. *Laryngoscope* 1989;99:405–408.

92. Friedman RA, Kesser B, Brackmann DE, et al. Long-term hearing preservation after middle fossa removal of vestibular schwannoma. *Otolaryngol Head Neck Surg* 2003;129:660–665.

93. Brackmann DE, Owens RM, Friedman RA, et al. Prognostic factors for hearing preservation in vestibular schwannoma surgery. *Am J Otol* 2000;21:417–424.

94. Blevins NH, Jackler RK. Exposure of the lateral extremity of the internal auditory canal through the retrosigmoid approach: a radioanatomic study. *Otolaryngol Head Neck Surg* 1994;111:81–90.

95. Sulman CG, Vecchiotti MA, Semaan MT, et al. Endolymphatic duct violation during retrosigmoid dissection of the internal auditory canal: a human temporal bone radiograph study. *Laryngoscope* 2004;114:1936–1940.

96. Kim HH, Johnston R, Wiet RJ, et al. Long-term effects of cerebellar retraction in the microsurgical resection of vestibular schwannomas. *Laryngoscope* 2004;114:323–326.

97. Jackson CG, McGrew BM, Forest JA, et al. Comparison of postoperative headache after retrosigmoid approach: vestibular nerve section versus vestibular schwannoma resection. *Am J Otol* 2000;21:412–416.

98. Harner SG, Beatty CW, Ebersold MJ. Retrosigmoid removal of acoustic neuroma: experience 1978–1988. *Otolaryngol Head Neck Surg* 1990;103:40–45.

99. Ebersold MJ, Harner SG, Beatty CW, et al. Current results of the retrosigmoid approach to acoustic neurinoma. *J Neurosurg* 1992;76:901–909.

100. Kemink JL, La Rouere MJ, Kileny PR, et al. Hearing preservation following suboccipital removal of acoustic neuromas. *Laryngoscope* 1990;100:597–602.

101. Baldwin DL, King TT, Morrison AW. Hearing conservation in acoustic neuroma surgery via the posterior fossa. *J Laryngol Otol* 1990;104:463–467.

102. Fischer G, Fischer C, Remond J. Hearing preservation in acoustic neurinoma surgery. *J Neurosurg* 1992;76:910–917.

103. Mangham CA. Retrosigmoid versus middle fossa surgery for small vestibular schwannomas. *Laryngoscope* 2004;114:1455–1461.

104. Becker SS, Jackler RK, Pitts LH. Cerebrospinal fluid leak after acoustic neuroma surgery: a comparison of the translabyrinthine, middle fossa, and retrosigmoid approaches. *Otol Neurotol* 2003;24:107–112.

105. Foote KD, Friedman WA, Buatti JM, et al. Analysis of risk factors associated with radiosurgery for vestibular schwannoma. *J Neurosurg* 2001;95:440–449.

106. Linskey ME. Stereotactic radiosurgery versus stereotactic radiotherapy for patients with vestibular schwannoma: a Leskell Gamma Knife Society 2000 debate. *J Neurosurg* 2000;93(suppl 3):90–95.

107. Anniko M, Arndt J, Noren G. The human acoustic neurinoma in organ culture. II. Tissue changes after gamma irradiation. *Acta Otolaryngol (Stockh)* 1981;91:223–235.

108. Lee F, Linthicum F, Hung G. Proliferation potential in recurrent gamma knife radiosurgery versus microsurgery. *Laryngoscope* 2002;112:948–950.

109. Noren G, Greitz D, Hirsch A, et al. Gamma knife radiosurgery in acoustic neurinomas. In: Tos M, Thomsen J, eds. *Proceedings of the first international conference on acoustic neuroma.* Amsterdam: Kugler, 1992:289–292.

110. Hirsch A, Noren G, Anderson H. Audiologic findings after stereotactic radiosurgery in nine cases of acoustic neurinomas. *Acta Otolaryngol (Stockh)* 1979;88:155–160.

111. Lunsford LD, Linskey ME. Stereotactic radiosurgery in the treatment of patients with acoustic tumors. *Otolaryngol Clin North Am* 1992;25:471–491.

112. Foote RL, Coffey RJ, Swanson JW, et al. Stereotactic radiosurgery using the gamma knife for acoustic neuromas. *Int J Radiat Oncol Biol Phys* 1995;32:1153–1160.

113. Weber DC, Chan AW, Bussiere MR, et al. Proton beam radiosurgery for vestibular schwannoma: tumor control and cranial nerve toxicity. *Neurosurgery* 2003;53:577–588.

114. Flickinger JC, Kondziolka D, Niranjan A, et al. Results of acoustic neuroma radiosurgery: an analysis of 5 years experience using current methods. *J Neurosurgery* 2001;94:1–6.

115. Roland PS, Eston D. Stereotactic radiosurgery for acoustic tumors. *Otolaryngol Clin North Am* 2002;35:343–355.

116. Bari ME, Forster DM, Kemeny AA, et al. Malignancy in vestibular schwannoma. Report of a case with central neurofibromatosis, treated by both stereotactic radiosurgery and surgical excision, with a review of the literature. *Br J Neurosurg* 2002;16:284–289.

117. Thomsen J, Mirz F, Wetke R, et al. Intracranial sarcoma in a patient with neurofibromatosis type 2 treated with gamma knife radiosurgery for vestibular schwannoma. *Am J Otol* 2000;21:364–370.

118. Slattery WH III, Brackmann DE. Results of surgery following stereotactic irradiation for acoustic neuromas. *Am J Otol* 1995;16:315–319.

119. Ho SY, Kveton JF. Rapid growth of acoustic neuromas after stereotactic radiotherapy in type 2 neurofibromatosis. *Ear Nose Throat J* 2002;81:831–833.

120. Brackmann DE, Gherini SG. Differential diagnosis of skull base neoplasms involving the posterior fossa. In: Cummings CW, ed. *Otolaryngology-head and neck surgery.* Vol. 4. St. Louis: CV Mosby, 1986:3421–3436.

121. Cushing H. The meningiomas (dural endotheliomas): their source and favoured seats of origin. *Brain* 1922;45:282–316.

122. Cushing H, Eisenhardt L. *Meningiomas, their classification, regional behavior, life history and surgical end results.* Springfield, IL: Charles C Thomas, 1938.

123. Guthrie BL, Ebersold MJ, Scheithauer BW. Neoplasms of the intracranial meninges. In: Youmans JR, ed. *Neurological surgery: a comprehensive reference guide to the diagnosis and management of neurosurgical problems,* 3rd ed. Vol. 5. Philadelphia: WB Saunders, 1990:3250–3315.

124. Granick MS, Martuza RL, Parker SW, et al. Cerebellopontine angle meningiomas: clinical manifestations and diagnosis. *Ann Otol Rhinol Laryngol* 1985;94:34–38.

125. Selters WA, Brackmann DE. Acoustic tumor detection with brain stem electric response audiometry. *Arch Otolaryngol* 1977;103: 181–187.

126. Russell DS, Rubinstein LJ. *Pathology of tumours of the nervous system*, 4th ed. Baltimore: Williams & Wilkins, 1977.

127. Vassilouthis J, Ambrose J. Computerized tomography scanning appearances of intracranial meningiomas: an attempt to predict the histological features. *J Neurosurg* 1979;50:320–327.

128. House WF. Transcochlear approach to the petrous apex and clivus. *Trans Am Acad Ophthalmol Otolaryngol* 1977;84:927–931.

129. Brackmann DE, House JW, Selters W. Auditory brain stem responses in facial nerve neuroma diagnosis. In: Graham MD, House WF, eds. *Disorders of the facial nerve: anatomy, diagnosis, and management.* New York: Raven, 1981:87.

130. Barrs DM, Brackmann DE, Hitselberger WE. Facial nerve anastomosis in the cerebellopontine angle: a review of 24 cases. *Am J Otol* 1984;5:269–272.

131. Brackmann DE, Bartels LJ. Rare tumors of the cerebellopontine angle. *Otolaryngol Head Neck Surg* 1980;88:555–559.

132. Fisch U. Infratemporal fossa approach to tumours of the temporal bone and base of the skull. *J Laryngol Otol* 1978;92:949–967.

133. Shelton C, Brackmann DE, Lo WW, et al. Intratemporal facial nerve hemangiomas. *Otolaryngol Head Neck Surg* 1991;104: 116–121.

134. Giddings NA, Brackmann DE, Kwartler JA. Transcanal infracochlear approach to the petrous apex. *Otolaryngol Head Neck Surg* 1991;104:29–36.

Sudden Sensory Hearing Loss

150

George T. Hashisaki

Sudden hearing loss is often a startling and unsettling experience for the patient. If the loss is severe, the absence of hearing can be particularly bothersome. Fortunately, the vast majority of cases of sudden hearing loss are unilateral, and the prognosis for some recovery of hearing is good. For an unlucky few, the hearing loss can be bilateral and totally devastating.

Dilemmas in diagnosis make formulating a rational treatment plan for sudden hearing loss an elusive process. Patients stricken with sudden hearing loss are often frightened and desperate for a cure. There is an emotional burden carried by the physician to provide some definitive assistance. Because sudden hearing loss is a symptom common to many diseases, sifting through the myriad possibilities is a frustrating task.

DEFINITION

Sudden hearing loss is a deceptively simple term, yet the concept defies strict definition. Various investigators have put forth definitions based on the severity, time course, and frequency spectrum of the loss, as well as specific audiometric criteria. The most commonly used definition is a 30 decibel (dB) loss over three contiguous frequencies occurring within 3 days. Abrupt and rapidly progressive losses have both been encompassed under a single definition. Awakening with a hearing loss, hearing loss noted over a few days, selective low- or high-frequency loss, and distortions in speech perception have all been classified as sudden hearing losses. Taking a broad-minded view, let us consider any noticeable and measurable loss of hearing function—pitch or speech perception—occurring over a matter of minutes to days as a sudden hearing loss. Also,

sudden hearing loss encompasses definite etiologies as well as idiopathic causes.

EPIDEMIOLOGY

Estimates of the annual incidence of sudden sensory hearing loss range from 5 to 20 cases per 100,000 persons (1). Likely, there is an equal distribution of female-to-male cases. Cumulative data from several studies show a slight male preponderance at 53% (1,530/2,864) (1–7); however, another large study of 1,220 patients noted a slight female preponderance, without specifying numbers (8). Gender does not seem to be a risk factor.

Several studies have not delineated right versus left ears affected, other than to state an equal distribution. Curiously, from combined study data, hearing loss affected more left ears (824/1,503 = 55%) (1–4,6,9). An equal distribution between ears would be expected. Bilateral sudden hearing loss occurs in about 1% to 2% of cases (2–4,6,8,9).

Sudden hearing loss occurs in all age groups, but fewer cases are reported in children or the elderly (1,4,5). Middle-aged and young adults experience similar incidence rates (1,4,5,8). The median age at presentation ranges from 40 to 54 years (2–5,7).

DIFFERENTIAL DIAGNOSIS

Sudden hearing loss can be subdivided into categories of defined causes and idiopathic sudden sensory hearing loss (ISSHL). Defined causes of sudden sensory hearing loss are varied and uncommon (Table 150.1). Most cases of sudden sensory hearing loss are idiopathic.

TABLE 150.1

DIFFERENTIAL DIAGNOSIS IN SUDDEN HEARING LOSS

Category	Etiology
Infection	Bacterial
	Meningitis
	Labyrinthitis
	Syphilis
	Viral
	Mumps
	Cytomegalovirus
Inflammation	Autoimmune
	Cogan syndrome
	Systemic lupus erythematosus
	Multiple sclerosis
Trauma	Temporal bone fracture
	Acoustic trauma
	Perilymph fistula
Tumor	Cerebellopontine angle tumor
	Temporal bone metastasis
	Carcinomatous meningitis
Toxins	Aminoglycosides
	Aspirin
Vascular	Thromboembolism
	Macroglobulinemia
	Sickle-cell disease
	S/P coronary bypass graft surgery

Three main theories exist to explain idiopathic sudden sensory hearing loss: viral infection, vascular compromise, and intracochlear membrane rupture. There is additional evidence to support a fourth explanation: immune inner ear disease. With sudden hearing loss as a symptom, a disease process could involve any of these theoretical possibilities. Each theory may explain a number of episodes of sudden sensory hearing loss.

VIRAL INFECTION

Considerable circumstantial evidence implicates viral infection as one cause of ISSHL. From studies of patients with ISSHL, this trail of evidence can be traced from reports of a high prevalence of a recent viral type of illness, through evidence of recent viral seroconversion, to temporal bone histopathology. The weakest of these links is the associated history of a recent viral illness. Noncontrolled studies report that 17% to 33% of patients recall a recent viral illness (2,8). Lest those numbers seem significant, 25% of healthy patients visiting an otolaryngology clinic had experienced a potential viral illness within a month preceding the visit (10).

Wilson provided good evidence of viral seroconversion by comparing patients experiencing ISSHL with control patients. Rates of seroconversion for the herpesvirus family were significantly higher in the sudden-hearing-loss

population (11). Finally, temporal bone histopathologic studies of patients who experienced ISSHL found damage in the cochlea consistent with viral injuries (12–15). Loss of hair cells and supporting cells, atrophy of the tectorial membrane, atrophy of the stria vascularis, and neuronal loss were seen; these patterns were similar to findings in documented cases of mumps-, measles-, and maternal rubella–related hearing loss. Viral infection can be implicated as a cause of ISSHL, but it cannot as yet be proved.

VASCULAR COMPROMISE

The cochlea derives its blood supply from the labyrinthine artery, with no collateral vasculature. Cochlear function is exquisitely sensitive to changes in blood supply (16). Thus, vascular compromise of the cochlea caused by thrombosis, embolus, reduced blood flow, or vasospasm would seem a likely etiology for ISSHL. The abrupt or rapid time course in sudden hearing loss correlates well with a vascular event. A reduction in oxygenation of the cochlea is the likely consequence of alterations in cochlear blood flow. Alterations in perilymph oxygen tension have been measured in response to changes in systemic blood pressure or intravascular carbon dioxide partial pressure (P_{CO_2}) (17).

Histologic evidence of cochlear damage following occlusion of the labyrinthine vessels was documented in temporal bone studies in both animals and humans (15,18). Intracochlear hemorrhage was noted as an early development; subsequently, fibrosis and ossification of the cochlea evolved.

INTRACOCHLEAR MEMBRANE RUPTURE

Thin membranes separate the inner ear from the middle ear, and within the cochlea, delicate membranes separate the perilymphatic and endolymphatic spaces. Rupture of either or both sets of membranes theoretically could produce a sensory hearing loss. A leak of perilymph fluid into the middle ear via the round window or oval window has been postulated to produce hearing loss by creating a state of relative endolymphatic hydrops or by producing intracochlear membrane breaks. Rupture of intracochlear membranes would allow mixing of perilymph and endolymph, effectively altering the endocochlear potential. Simmons (19) favored the theory of intracochlear membrane rupture, as did Goodhill and Harris (20); histologic evidence was documented by Gussen (21).

IMMUNE INNER-EAR DISEASE

Sensorineural hearing loss (SNHL) induced by an autoimmune process has gained greater acceptance since the concept was introduced in 1979 by McCabe (22). Progressive sensorineural loss is seen with this condition. Whether or not sudden hearing loss occurs with autoimmune inner ear disease is unclear, but immunologic activity in the cochlea is supported by greater and greater evidence. The association of hearing loss in Cogan syndrome, systemic lupus erythematosus, and other autoimmune rheumatologic disorders has been well documented.

EVALUATION

Patient evaluation should proceed promptly and expeditiously. Early presentation to a physician and early institution of treatment improve the prognosis for hearing recovery (1,2,4,8). A diligent search for a treatable or defined cause of the sudden hearing loss is an immediate goal. Information about the onset, time course, associated symptoms, and recent activities may give helpful clues. Reviewing the past medical history, especially risk factors for hearing loss, is necessary. All medications, including over-the-counter products, must be delineated. A thorough head and neck examination, with special attention to the otologic and neurologic examination, is a requisite. Pneumotoscopy, in search of a fistula sign, should be included.

A complete audiometric evaluation, including pure-tone and speech tests and immittance (tympanometry and acoustic reflex) tests, is mandatory. Auditory brainstem response (ABR) and otoacoustic emissions (OAE) testing may provide additional information regarding the integrity of the auditory system. The presence of measurable otoacoustic emissions indicates preservation of some outer hair cell function. The ABR reflects function of the retrocochlear neural pathways. The ABR and OAE results also may assist in diagnosing a functional hearing loss. Vestibular tests are obtained when indicated by the history and physical examination.

An exhaustive set of laboratory tests would be overwhelmingly costly. One approach is to obtain those laboratory tests for which the results may influence the treatment plans (Table 150.2). At some point during the evaluation and treatment process, an imaging study of the internal auditory canal (IAC) and cerebellopontine angle (CPA) is advised. Approximately 0.8% to 4% of patients with ISSHL have been diagnosed with IAC or CPA tumors (1,2,8,23–26). A magnetic resonance imaging (MRI) scan with gadolinium diethylentriamine pentaacidic acid (DPTA) is the gold standard test for diagnosing CPA masses; alternatively, an ABR (if hearing levels permit) could be used as a screening test. In addition, MRI scanning can demonstrate evidence of demyelination, intracochlear hemorrhage, or vascular abnormalities (24–27). In younger patients, for whom there is only a small possibility of a vestibular schwannoma but a greater possibility of an anatomic abnormality, a non-contrast temporal bone computed tomography (CT) scan could be obtained. Anatomic defects such as cochlear dys-

TABLE 150.2

LABORATORY TESTS IN SUDDEN HEARING LOSS

Test	Purpose
CBC with differential	Polycythemia, leukemia, thrombocytosis
Sedimentation rate, ESR	Screen for autoimmune or inflammatory disease; follow with ANA or 68 kD Ab test
FTA-Abs or MHA-TP	Antibody test, *Treponema pallidum*, congenital or acquired
Coagulation studies	Coagulopathy (if indicated, by history)
Thyroid function tests	Hypothyroidism (if indicated, by history)
Imaging study	Retrocochlear evaluation, MS, intracochlear hemorrhage

68 kD Ab, 68 kiloDalton antibody; ANA, antinuclear antibody; CBC, complete blood count; ESR, erythrocyte sedimentation rate; FTA-Abs, fluorescent treponemal antibody-absorption test; MHA-TP, micro-hemagglutination—*Treponema pallidum*; MS, multiple sclerosis.

plasia, Mondini malformation, or an enlarged vestibular aqueduct might account for a sudden hearing loss (28).

TREATMENT

The treatment regimens for ISSHL are legion, and this diversity reflects both the different etiologies that may cause sudden hearing loss and the uncertainty in diagnosis. The therapies can be grouped by mechanism of action: (a) vasodilators, (b) rheologic agents, (c) antiinflammatory agents, (d) antiviral agents, (e) diuretics, (f) triiodobenzoic acid derivatives, and (g) surgery.

Vasodilators

Theoretically, vasodilators improve the blood supply to the cochlea, reversing hypoxia. Histamine, nicotinic acid, papaverine, procaine, niacin, and carbogen have been used in attempts to improve cochlear blood flow. Carbogen (5% carbon dioxide and 95% oxygen) inhalation has been shown to increase perilymph oxygen tension (17,29).

Rheologic Agents

Altering blood viscosity to improve blood flow and oxygen delivery has been the theory behind the use of low-molecular-weight dextrans, pentoxifylline, and the anticoagulants heparin and warfarin. Dextrans cause a hypervolemic hemodilution and affect Factor VIII, both effects influencing blood flow. Pentoxifylline allows greater platelet deformability, and anticoagulants interfere with the coagulation cascade.

Antiinflammatory Agents

Corticosteroids are the primary antiinflammatory agents used to treat ISSHL. The mechanism of action of corticosteroids in sudden hearing loss is unknown, although reduction of cochlea and auditory nerve inflammation is the presumed pathway.

Antiviral Agents

Acyclovir and amantadine have had limited use in treating ISSHL, presuming a viral etiology. Famciclovir and valacyclovir are newer agents, similar in structure and activity to acyclovir. Both of these medications have a three-times-daily dosing schedule, as compared to the five-times-daily schedule for acyclovir.

Diuretics

Under the assumption that some episodes of ISSHL are secondary to cochlear endolymphatic hydrops, diuretic therapy has been used as treatment. As in Ménière disease, the mechanism of action for diuretics in sudden hearing loss is not understood.

Triiodobenzoic Acid Derivatives

These agents are thought to affect the stria vascularis and assist in maintaining the endocochlear potential (7). Diatrizoate meglumine, an angiographic contrast agent, is the most commonly used derivative of triiodobenzoic acid.

Surgery

Repair of oval and round window perilymph fistulae has been used in cases of ISSHL associated with a positive fistula test or a history of recent trauma or barotrauma. Perilymph leaks could produce sudden hearing loss in accordance with the intracochlear membrane rupture theory. Alternatively, low perilymph pressure caused by a fistula could produce a state of relative cochlear endolymphatic hydrops.

RESULTS

Recovery rates for sudden sensory hearing loss are generally good. Published spontaneous recovery rates range from 47% to 63%, combining categories of complete and good or partial recovery (4,30,31). Mattox and Simmons defined complete recovery as a pure-tone average (PTA) less than 10 dB or equaling the uninvolved ear, and good recovery as a PTA less than 40 dB or more than 50 dB improvement from the initial audiogram (4). The recovery rate for these two groups was 63%. For Wilson et al. (30), complete recovery was defined as recovery to within 10 dB of the prehearing loss speech reception threshold (SRT) or

PTA. Partial recovery was defined as recovery to within 50% of the prehearing loss SRT or PTA. The unaffected ear was used to establish preexisting hearing levels for the involved ear. Fifty-two patients who had follow-up without treatment had a 58% spontaneous recovery rate. When combined with the placebo group in their study, the spontaneous recovery rate was 47%. Chen et al. (31) found similar rates of spontaneous recovery in their untreated patients, using either the criteria of Mattox and Simmons (4) or Wilson et al. (30).

A review of outcomes for the various therapeutic regimens gives conflicting results. With differences in inclusion criteria, exclusion criteria, recovery criteria, and duration of follow-up, comparisons between studies are difficult. Many studies lack control patients. Selection bias could influence measured outcomes; tertiary referral centers might accrue a different profile of patients than other practices, with some patients having a longer duration of symptoms or more severe hearing losses.

Several studies using vasodilator therapy as a component of treatment failed to show significant differences from placebo (3,10); however, Fetterman et al. (2) reported their best recovery results: 63% improved a PTA greater than 10 dB or speech discrimination greater than 15% when treatment included vasodilators. Based on controlled studies, little data support vasodilator therapy.

Studies including low-molecular-weight dextrans or pentoxifylline did not demonstrate recovery rates better than placebo (6,9,32). Redleaf et al. (7) reported 64% of patients improving, however. They also used diatrizoate therapy, and there was no placebo arm in the study.

Corticosteroid therapy has shown widely varying outcomes. Published recovery rates range from 41% to 61% (1–3,9,30,31). Wilson et al. (30) did demonstrate a significant improvement, finding 61% improved on oral steroids compared with a 32% improvement rate on placebo. They stratified their patient groups by audiometric patterns and determined that hearing losses between 40 and 90 dB responded better to steroid therapy; 78% in this severe loss group improved. Chen et al. also found a significant benefit with oral steroids in a study of 318 patients (31). They found the greatest magnitude of improvement in patients with greater than 60 dB PTA hearing loss, citing a "floor effect" limiting the degree of improvement in mild hearing losses. Because of the "floor effect," a benefit of oral steroids might be present in those with mild hearing loss, but the effect could not be proven.

Transtympanic steroid application has theoretical benefits of a high delivery concentration to the inner ear and low systemic concentrations. Several studies have addressed the efficacy of transtympanic steroid treatment, but because of differences in delivery technique, corticosteroid, dose, and dosing schedule, direct comparisons are difficult (33–35). Using a transtympanic injection of dexamethasone, Chandrasekhar found that 8 of 11 ears treated had some hearing improvement. The mean SRT improved by 9 dB and the mean speech discrimination or word recognition score improved from 61.5% to 77.3% (33). Kopke et al. placed a microcatheter into the round window niche through a tympanomeatal flap and perfused the niche with methylprednisolone. For 6 patients treated within 4 weeks of the onset of the hearing loss, all experienced some hearing return. The mean PTA improved 50.8 dB, and the mean word recognition score improved from 1.3% to 62.2% (34). Gianoli and Li applied topical steroids through a ventilation tube in the tympanic membrane. Hearing improvement was seen in 44% (10 of 23 patients) (35). Applying dexamethasone through a porous wick placed inside a ventilation tube, Light and Silverstein found a 10 dB improvement in PTA for 23% and a 15% improvement in speech discrimination for 35% in a study of 48 patients. For the patients experiencing a hearing improvement, the mean PTA improved 43% and the mean speech discrimination score (SDS)/word recognition score (WRS) improved 51% (36). Clearly, a large, randomizied, prospective, blinded study is warranted for this treatment.

Given the theoretical implication of viral infection as a cause of ISSHL, the use of antiviral therapy for ISSHL is a logical extension. A multicenter, randomized, prospective, double-blind trial comparing prednisolone against prednisolone and acyclovir did not show a significant beneficial effect of acyclovir (37). The study size was not large, having 22 patients in each arm of therapy. In patients treated with corticosteroids alone, 80% demonstrated at least a 10-dB PTA improvement. Tucci et al. (38) did not find a significant benefit from the addition of valacyclovir to concurrent oral prednisone therapy in a larger multicenter, randomized, prospective trial. Two additional studies found no benefit from the addition of antiviral antimicrobial therapy (39,40).

Two studies using diatrizoate were reviewed. Wilkins et al. (9) found no significant difference in recovery using diatrizoate in a multidrug regimen, compared with spontaneous recovery rates (4,30). Redleaf et al. (7), using diatrizoate and dextran, reported a beneficial effect: 64% of patients had improvement. Interestingly, using the hearing recovery criteria of Wilkins et al. (9), recalculated data from the Redleaf study indicated only a 36% recovery rate to a classification of complete or good.

Controversy regarding the results of surgical repair of perilymphatic fistulae continues. A universal standard for positive identification of a fistula has not been achieved. Without uniform standards, outcomes of surgical repair are difficult to compare.

Prognostic factors affecting outcome also have been postulated. The associated symptoms of vertigo or imbalance seem to portend a lower recovery rate (1,8,9,30). Two studies, in addition, found severe vertigo associated with more cases of high-frequency or profound hearing loss (4,5). This association could be explained anatomically by the close proximity of the basal turn of the cochlea to the vestibule (5). Patient age also may impact recovery, although there are less consistent data across studies. The youngest and the oldest patients may have lower recovery rates.

CONCLUSIONS

Sudden sensory hearing loss remains a puzzling affliction. Given the rate of spontaneous recovery, the prognosis for some hearing recovery is good. It is likely that selection bias affects most studies of ISSHL; patients with sudden hearing loss and spontaneous recovery within a few days probably will not seek medical evaluation. The true spontaneous recovery rate is unknown.

Treatment should be based on a rational approach. Should no definite or treatable etiology be found, the treatment regimen is dictated by the most likely factors involved. Remembering that the medications used in treatment of sudden sensory hearing loss have potential side effects and the dictum, "Do no harm," the physician and patient must agree on the best course of action.

HIGHLIGHTS

- Sudden sensory hearing loss occurs at an annual incidence of 5 to 20 cases per 100,000 population. Some cases resolve spontaneously and medical attention is not pursued; therefore, the true incidence rate may be higher.
- The prognosis for some recovery of the hearing loss is good. The spontaneous recovery rate may be as high as 63%.
- There are three generally accepted theories for the pathogenesis of sudden hearing loss. Viral infection, vascular compromise, and intracochlear membrane breaks are thought to explain most episodes of sudden hearing loss. A fourth entity, autoimmune inner ear disease, also may add to the number of cases.
- The evaluation of patients with sudden hearing loss should include a thorough history and physical examination. A diligent search for treatable causes of the hearing loss is very important. Laboratory tests can be useful for this purpose.
- Because 0.8% to 4% of patients presenting with sudden sensory hearing loss may have a CPA mass, a retrocochlear evaluation using MRI with gadolinium or ABR is warranted.
- Many treatment regimens for ISSHL exist, and the rationale behind any particular therapy employed should be understood.
- There is no single treatment of choice for ISSHL. Many diseases produce sudden hearing loss, and the treatment should be directed toward the most likely causes.

REFERENCES

1. Byl FM. Sudden hearing loss: eight years experience and suggested prognostic table. *Laryngoscope* 1984;94:647–661.
2. Fetterman BL, Saunders JE, Luxford WM. Prognosis and treatment of sudden sensorineural hearing loss. *Am J Otol* 1996;17:529–536.
3. Grandis JR, Hirsch BE, Wagener MM. Treatment of idiopathic sudden sensorineural hearing loss. *Am J Otol* 1993;14:183–188.
4. Mattox DE, Simmons FB. Natural history of sudden sensorineural hearing loss. *Ann Otol Rhinol Laryngol* 1977;86:463–480.

5. Nakashima T, Yanagita N. Outcome of sudden deafness with and without vertigo. *Laryngoscope* 1993;103:1145–1149.

6. Probst R, Tschopp K, Ludin E. A randomized, double-blind, placebo-controlled study of dextran/pentoxifylline medication in acute acoustic trauma and sudden hearing loss. *Acta Otolaryngol (Stockh)* 1992;112:435–443.

7. Redleaf M, Bauer CA, Gantz BJ. Diatrizoate and dextran treatment of sudden sensorineural hearing loss. *Am J Otol* 1995;16:295–303.

8. Shaia FT, Sheehy JL. Sudden sensori-neural hearing impairment: a report of 1,220 cases. *Laryngoscope* 1976;86:389–398.

9. Wilkins SA, Mattox DE, Lyles A. Evaluation of a "shotgun" regimen for sudden hearing loss. *Otolaryngol Head Neck Surg* 1987;97:474–480.

10. Mattox DE, Lyles A. Idiopathic sudden sensorineural hearing loss. *Am J Otol* 1989;10:242–247.

11. Wilson WR. The relationship of the herpesvirus family to sudden hearing loss: a prospective clinical study and literature review. *Laryngoscope* 1986;96:870–877.

12. Khetarpal U, Nadol JB, Glynn RJ. Idiopathic sudden sensorineural hearing loss and postnatal viral labyrinthitis: a statistical comparison of temporal bone findings. *Ann Otol Rhinol Laryngol* 1990;99:969–976.

13. Vasama JP, Linthicum FH Jr. Idiopathic sudden sensorineural hearing loss: temporal bone histopathologic study. *Ann Otol Rhinol Laryngol* 2000;109:527–532.

14. Schuknecht HF, Donovan ED. The pathology of idiopathic sudden sensorineural hearing loss. *Arch Otorhinolaryngol* 1986;243:1–15.

15. Yoon TH, Paparella MM, Schachern PA. Histopathology of sudden hearing loss. *Laryngoscope* 1990;100:707–715.

16. Perlman H, Kimura R, Fernandez C. Experiments on temporary obstruction of the internal auditory artery. *Laryngoscope* 1959;69:591–612.

17. Fisch U. Management of sudden deafness. *Otolaryngol Head Neck Surg* 1983;91:3–8.

18. Belal A. Pathology of vascular sensorineural hearing impairment. *Laryngoscope* 1980;90:1831–1839.

19. Simmons FB. Theory of membrane breaks and sudden hearing loss. *Arch Otolaryngol* 1968;88:67–74.

20. Goodhill V, Harris I. Sudden hearing loss syndromes. In: Goodhill V, ed. *Ear diseases, dizziness, and deafness.* Hagerstown MD: Harper & Row, 1979:664–681.

21. Gussen R. Sudden hearing loss associated with cochlear membrane rupture. *Arch Otolaryngol* 1981;107:598–600.

22. McCabe BF. Autoimmune sensorineural hearing loss. *Ann Otol Rhinol Laryngol* 1979;88:585–589.

23. Aslan A, De Donato G, Balyan FR, et al. Clinical observations on coexistence of sudden hearing loss and vestibular schwannoma. *Otolaryngol Head Neck Surg* 1997;117:580–582.

24. Schick B, Brors D, Koch O, et al. Magnetic resonance imaging in patients with sudden hearing loss, tinnitus and vertigo. *Otol Neurotol* 2001;22:808–812.

25. Fitzgerald DC, Mark AS. Sudden hearing loss: frequency of abnormal findings on contrast-enhanced MR studies. *AJNR: Am J Neuroradiol* 1998;19:1433–1436.

26. Aarnisalo AA, Suoranta H, Ylikoski J. Magnetic resonance imaging findings in the auditory pathway of patients with sudden deafness. *Otol Neurotol* 2004;25:245–249.

27. Shinohara S, Yamamoto E, Saiwai S, et al. Clinical features of sudden hearing loss associated with a high signal in the labyrinth on unenhanced T1-weighted magnetic resonance imaging. *Eur Arch Otorhinolaryngol* 2000;257:480–484.

28. Jackler RK, De La Cruz A. The large vestibular aqueduct syndrome. *Laryngoscope* 1989;99:1238–1243.

29. Rahko T, Kotti V. Comparison of carbogen inhalation and intravenous heparin infusion therapies in idiopathic sudden sensorineural hearing loss. *Acta Otolaryngol (Stockh)* Suppl 1997;529:86–87.

30. Wilson WR, Byl FM, Laird N. The efficacy of steroids in the treatment of idiopathic sudden hearing loss. *Arch Otolaryngol* 1980;106:772–776.

31. Chen CY, Halpin C, Rauch SD. Oral steroid treatment of sudden sensorineural hearing loss: a ten year retrospective analysis. *Otol Neurotol* 2003;24:728–733.

32. Samim E, Kilic R, Ozdek A, et al. Combined treatment of sudden sensorineural hearing loss with steroid, dextran and piracetam: experience with 68 cases. *Eur Arch Otorhinolaryngol* 2004;261:187–190.

33. Chandrasekhar SS. Intratympanic dexamethasone for sudden sensorineural hearing loss: clinical and laboratory evaluation. *Otol Neurotol* 2001;22:18–23.

34. Kopke RD, Hoffer ME, Wester D, et al. Targeted topical steroid therapy in sudden sensorineural hearing loss. *Otol Neurotol* 2001;22:475–479.

35. Gianoli GJ, Li JC. Transtympanic steroids for treatment of sudden hearing loss. *Otolaryngol Head Neck Surg* 2001;125:142–146.

36. Light JP, Silverstein H. Transtympanic perfusion: indications and limitations. *Curr Opin Otolaryngol Head Neck Surg* 2004;12:378–383.

37. Stokroos RJ, Albers FWJ, Tenvergert EM. Antiviral treatment of idiopathic sudden sensorineural hearing loss: a prospective, randomized, double-blind clinical trial. *Acta Otolaryngol (Stockh)* 1998;118:488–495.

38. Tucci DL, Farmer JC Jr., Kitch RD, et al. Treatment of sudden sensorineural hearing loss with systemic steroids and valacyclovir. *Otol Neurotol* 2002;23:301–308.

39. Westerlaken BO, Stokroos RJ, Dhooge IJ, et al. Treatment of idiopathic sudden sensorineural hearing loss with antiviral therapy: a prospective, randomized, double-blind clinical trial. *Ann Otol Rhinol Laryngol* 2003;112:993–1000.

40. Uri N, Doweck I, Cohen-Kerem R, et al. Acyclovir in the treatment of idiopathic sudden sensorineural hearing loss. *Otolaryngol Head Neck Surg* 2003;128:544–549.

Tinnitus

Alexander J. Schleuning Jr.[†]   *"Baker" Y. Shi*
William H. Martin

Tinnitus is the perception of noise in the absence of an acoustic stimulus. It can occur as a pure tone or as multiple tones and can be high pitched, low pitched, ringing, buzzing, roaring, clicking, hissing, rough, pulsatile, or steady. Because it is a complex symptom and not a disease, successful management requires thorough evaluation and appropriate application of management tools and strategies.

Forty to sixty million people in the United States experience tinnitus, although almost the entire population has had this symptom at some time. Ten to twelve million people have severe or troubling symptoms. Tinnitus is most prevalent between the ages of 40 and 70 and more often in men than women. It occasionally occurs in children. Tinnitus can be defined as objective or subjective.

OBJECTIVE TINNITUS

If a person has objective tinnitus, which is audible to the physician or another person or has a pulsating character, certain conditions are suspected. The differential diagnosis includes vascular abnormalities, eustachian tube abnormalities, and tympanic muscle problems (Table 151.1).

Vascular Abnormalities

Tinnitus related to vascular abnormalities is usually a soft, rushing, pulsatile sound, which is synchronous with the heartbeat. The diagnosis often can be made by the patient's observation of an increasing rate with exercise. This form is experienced by fewer than 10% of patients who have tinnitus. An audible bruit is heard in only a small proportion of these patients. The causes include arteriovenous shunts, arterial bruits, and venous hums.

Arteriovenous Shunts

Arteriovenous shunts may be intracranial or preauricular, congenital or acquired. They may or may not be associated with decreased hearing, depending on their origin.

Congenital Arteriovenous Malformations

Interconnections between the occipital artery and the transverse sinus, the internal carotid and the vertebral vessels, or the middle meningeal artery and the greater superficial petrosal artery all have been reported. Diagnosis is by exclusion and by magnetic resonance imaging (MRI) or angiography. Rarely is the symptom severe enough to merit therapy, but, if necessary, selective embolization or ligation constitutes accepted treatment.

Acquired Arteriovenous Shunts

The most common acquired tinnitus secondary to arteriovenous shunting is caused by a glomus tympanicum or glomus jugulare tumor. This tinnitus also is described as a soft or blowing sound, and it is often associated with diminished hearing. The lesion may be visible on examination as a reddish blue mass behind the tympanic membrane. If adjacent to the drum, the pulsatile nature is detected on positive pressure. Large tumors may affect adjacent nerves, including ninth, tenth, and twelfth cranial nerves. The diagnosis is made by computed tomography (CT) of the middle ear, demonstrating erosion of the caroticojugular spine, or by appearance of the lesion lying within the middle ear space.

Arterial Bruits

Arterial bruits are detected in aberrant carotid positions or are transmitted from the carotid or prevertebral vessels. Other types of arterial bruits are those coming from vascular loops within the internal auditory meatus pressing on the eighth cranial nerve. In these cases, diagnosis generally

[†]Deceased.

TABLE 151.1

VASCULAR ABNORMALITIES CAUSING OBJECTIVE TINNITUS

Arteriovenous shunts
  Congenital arteriovenous malformations
  Acquired arteriovenous shunt
  Glomus jugulare
  Glomus tympanum
Arterial bruits
  High-riding carotid artery
  Carotid stenosis
  Vascular loop
  Persistent stapedial artery
Venous hums
  Dehiscent jugular bulb
  Hypertension
  Transverse sinus obstruction
Patulous eustachian tube
  Palatal myoclonus
  Idiopathic stapedial muscle spasm

is made by air-contrast CT, MRI, or magnetic resonance angiography (MRA). Recently, advances in the technique of MRA have obviated the usual need for angiography. In rare instances, angiography still is required. The greatest difficulty in treating arterial bruits is making the decision about whether advanced studies are needed. A carotid bruit with a pulsatile tinnitus merits treatment, including endarterectomy. Other vascular lesions causing arterial bruits may be benefited by arterial ligation, embolization, or vascular decompression.

Venous Hums

Venous hums can be heard in patients who have hypertension or abnormal high placement of the jugular bulb. The tinnitus of a dehiscent jugular bulb often gives a soft, low-pitched venous hum, which can be altered by head position, activity, or pressure over the jugular vein. The tumor may be confused with a glomus jugulare in its transtympanic appearance. The diagnosis is based on CT evaluation. The tinnitus is commonly unilateral. An audible venous hum may be the result of partial occlusion or narrowing of the transverse sinus. The usual site of obstruction is at or near the transverse sinus/sigmoid sinus junction and is usually the result of ingrowth of arachnoid granulation, which creates turbulence and affects the blood flow. MRA or magnetic resonance venography (MRV) usually can define the abnormality. Treatment is fraught with great risk, however, and there is no defined specific management.

Patulous Eustachian Tube

Patients who have patulous eustachian tubes often complain of tinnitus, usually described as an ocean roar in the ear. The sound generally is synchronous with nasal respira-

tion. The symptoms are usually absent on arising but rapidly occur thereafter. Symptoms are diminished or alleviated by lying down. Placing the head in a dependent position may relieve the symptoms and is a useful diagnostic clue. Tympanography may be helpful for diagnosis by having the patient breathe sharply or quickly through his or her nose while being tested. Fluttering motion of the tympanic membrane associated with respiration is diagnostic. Patients also may complain of some reverberation and have abnormal awareness of their own voice (i.e., autophony). In the past, treatment included caustics to the nasopharynx, mucosal irritants, saturated solution of potassium iodide, and Teflon or Gelfoam injections around the torus tubarius. Development of this symptom frequently is associated with a significant postpartum, cancer-associated, or dietary weight loss. It occurs frequently in patients who have had radiation therapy involving the nasopharynx.

Palatomyoclonus

The myoclonus form of tinnitus is described as an irregular clicking sound heard within the ear. The sound is rapid (40 to 200 beats per minute) and occurs intermittently. It is caused by the mucous membranes of the eustachian tube snapping together in response to the movement of the palatal musculature. Additional symptoms include fullness in the ear and some distortion of hearing. Patients frequently give histories of muscle spasm resulting in post-occipital headache and temporomandibular joint pain. Symptoms increase during periods of stress.

Generally, the diagnosis is made by observation or hearing the clicking using a Toynbee tube. The tympanogram may be useful by recording movement synchronous with the contractions. Electromyographic studies of the palatal musculature may be necessary to confirm the diagnosis. The differential diagnosis for palatal myoclonus includes idiopathic stapedial muscle spasm. Multiple sclerosis, cerebral vascular disorders, and tumor must be excluded because they can cause similar symptoms.

Treatment relies on medication, including muscle relaxants (e.g., clonazepam, diazepam). Botulinum toxin injection into the active muscle has been of help in severe cases. Only rarely is surgery indicated.

Idiopathic Stapedial Muscle Spasm

This rough rumbling or crackling noise of idiopathic stapedial muscle spasm may be accentuated by external sound (e.g., water faucets, musical tones, certain voices). Diagnosis can be made on examination if tympanic membrane movement is synchronous with the noise. The diagnosis usually is based only on the patient's history. Treatment has consisted of division of the stapedius muscle and the tensor tympani muscle, which abolishes the symptoms, but this procedure is rarely required. Occasionally, muscle relaxants (e.g., diazepam) may relieve this symptom. Patients should be advised to avoid stimulants such as nicotine, coffee, and decongestants (1).

SUBJECTIVE TINNITUS

Subjective tinnitus is more common than objective tinnitus. Almost all persons experience tinnitus at some time. Two large-scale studies of tinnitus conducted in the United Kingdom, one by the National Study of Hearing and another by the United Kingdom Office of Population Census Surveys, demonstrated that 35% to 45% of the population experienced tinnitus of some type and duration. Eight percent of the population had some major sleep difficulty secondary to tinnitus, and 0.5% considered that their lives were significantly altered by their symptoms. In our own specialty clinic, 73% of the patients had sleep difficulty secondary to tinnitus, and 22% reported that the tinnitus interfered with their overall enjoyment of life. Although subjective tinnitus is complicated by an inability to obtain an absolutely objective measure, estimates of its severity can be made using severity indices. The symptoms of tinnitus can be likened to headache with multiple causes. It may be caused by abnormal conditions in the cochlea, the cochlear nerve, the ascending auditory pathway, or the auditory cortex. It has been postulated that the cochlear hair cells injured by noise or head trauma may discharge repetitively, stimulating nerve fibers to discharge synchronously in a way that the central auditory system cannot discriminate from actual sound. In the central nervous system or in the auditory pathways, there is the suggestion that spontaneous activity within individual auditory nerve fibers also may be synchronized because of injury or metabolic abnormality, resulting in tinnitus. It is also possible that hyperactivity in the nuclei of the ascending auditory pathways may stimulate the auditory cortex in a similar manner. An alternate theory proposes that injury to cochlear integrity from any cause reduces the suppressive influence of the central nervous system, allowing increased neuronal activity higher in the auditory system.

Medical Evaluation

In obtaining complete histories of tinnitus patients, several etiologic factors are prominent. These are classified as otologic, cardiovascular, metabolic, neurologic, pharmacologic, dental, and psychological factors (Table 151.2). In the following discussion, the incidences reported were derived from a study of patients referred to a large tinnitus clinic. They reflect only those patients who had more severe and troubling symptoms and not the more common or mild complaints seen in the general population.

Otologic Factors

The largest number of patients with tinnitus appears to have a history of noise exposure or are experiencing presbycusis.

TABLE 151.2

ETIOLOGIC FACTORS IN SUBJECTIVE TINNITUS

Otologic factors
  Presbycusis
  Noise-induced hearing loss
Ménière disease
  Otosclerosis
Metabolic function
  Hypothyroidism
  Hyperthyroidism
  Hyperlipidemia
  Zinc deficiency
  Vitamin deficiency
Neurologic abnormalities
  Skull fracture or closed head trauma
  Whiplash injury
  Multiple sclerosis
  Meningitic effects
Pharmacologic factors
  Aspirin compounds
  Nonsteroidal antiinflammatory drugs
  Aminoglycosides
  Heavy metals
Dental factors
  Temporomandibular joint syndrome
Psychological factors
  Depression
  Anxiety

In both instances, there is a high-frequency neurosensory hearing loss. Seventy-five percent of patients have a 30+ dB hearing loss from 3 to 8 kHz. This hearing loss is the single most consistent factor in patients with tinnitus. Generally, the pitch of the tinnitus occupies the region of the greatest hearing deficit or the most abrupt loss.

A variety of other otologic disorders appear to accentuate or cause tinnitus, especially Ménière disease, in which almost all patients complain of the symptom; however, only 4% of these patients have severe and intractable symptoms that are unresolved by any form of management. Three percent of patients had severe tinnitus secondary to prolonged otitis, and 2% had recurrent labyrinthitis. Although most patients with otosclerosis have tinnitus, only 4% said it was significant. Dizziness commonly is associated with tinnitus. Thirty-five percent of patients were dizzy at least part of the time, and a smaller percentage were dizzy all of the time. This rate of dizziness is higher than in the standard population for the respective age groups, and the symptom should be considered in the workup.

Cardiovascular Factors

Cardiovascular problems frequently are associated with tinnitus. Thirty percent of patients with severe symptoms had one or more cardiovascular complaints. The high incidence of cardiovascular disease is consistent with the age group (older than the age of 60 years), but it is still likely that hypertension is a major factor in the onset or severity of the patient's disease. Twenty-two percent of the patients who had tinnitus in our study had significant hypertension, and more than 1% related specific cardiovascular incidents to the onset of their complaint. Secondary vascular disorders must be excluded in evaluating these patients. These conditions include anemia (i.e., tinnitus secondary to increased cardiovascular output) and extensive arteriosclerosis, in which tinnitus tends to be objective and pulsatile.

Metabolic Function

Thyroid dysfunction can be associated with tinnitus. Hyperthyroidism, by increasing cardiac output, can cause a pulsatile or rushing noise. Hypothyroidism also has caused this complaint. It is severe in about 4% of this population. Hyperlipidemia is reported increasingly as a factor in tinnitus, particularly in association with fluctuating neurosensory hearing loss and associated dizziness. Vitamin A or B deficiency has been described as causing tinnitus.

Neurologic Disease

Nine percent of patients who had disabling tinnitus report that it was the result of major head trauma, often in conjunction with other factors, such as hearing loss. Trauma generally included a skull fracture or closed head injury. Seven percent of patients had tinnitus initiated by whiplash injury or cervical trauma, suggesting that abnormal proprioceptive input from nerve fibers in the neck and shoulders, or possibly brainstem injuries, are a factor. Tinnitus after whiplash injury usually occurs 7 to 10 days after the accident, and the appearance of tinnitus immediately after head trauma without clearly defined ear abnormalities or vestibular disease is uncommon. Therefore, the physician must be careful in assigning a causal relationship to this injury.

Past meningitis may be the cause of tinnitus. Multiple sclerosis also can have severe tinnitus in its constellation of symptoms.

Pharmacologic Factors

Five percent of patients relate the onset of significant tinnitus to initiation of or changes in pharmacologic therapy. All classes of medication are considered possible causes of tinnitus, but the main groups that are frequently incriminated are listed in Table 151.3. These include antiinflammatories, antibiotics, and antidepressants.

Aspirin and aspirin-containing compounds were identified as the most common inciting medications. As little as 600 to 1,000 mg per day of aspirin can create symptoms.

TABLE 151.3
MEDICATIONS THAT CAUSE OR ACCENTUATE TINNITUS

Aspirin and aspirin-containing compounds
 Percodan
 Darvon
 Bufferin
 Ecotrin
Aminoglycoside antibiotics
 Gentamicin
 Kanamycin
 Neomycin
 Streptomycin
 Tobramycin
Amikacin
Nonsteroidal antiinflammatory drugs
 Fenoprofen
 Ibuprofen
 Indomethacin
 Ketoprofen
 Naproxen
 Phenylbutazone
 Sulindac
 Tolmetin
Heterocycline antidepressants
 Amitriptyline
 Amoxapine
 Desipramine
 Doxepin
 Imipramine
 Maprotiline
 Nortriptyline
 Protriptyline
 Trazodone
 Trimipramine

Aspirin-containing medications, such as Percodan, Darvon, Bufferin, or Ecotrin, often are overlooked as possible causes of tinnitus. The effect of these drugs is similar to aspirin, although not as severe. Some antibiotics, chiefly the aminoglycosides, cause tinnitus. It occurs in most cases of antibiotics used concurrently with diuretics. Quinine-containing compounds and the synthetic analogues can elevate the severity of tinnitus.

Mercury, arsenic, lead, and other heavy metals in high doses can cause symptoms. A thorough history and alteration of medications are essential components in treating patients with this complaint.

Dental Abnormalities

Temporomandibular joint disorders and dental abnormalities must be considered in taking the general history, in the physical examination, and in devising a treatment course for tinnitus. Forty-five percent of patients with severe tinnitus describe active temporomandibular joint problems at some time. A smaller, but significant, percentage of patients who have severe tinnitus describe it as concurrent with an increase in the severity of their temporomandibular joint complaints. Bruxism, malalignment, and joint pain are other common complaints. The tinnitus is generally low pitched, rough, and associated with a feeling of fullness in the ear.

Psychological Factors

Psychological factors play a major role. Stress often increases the perception of tinnitus severity, and depression frequently accentuates the complaint. In some cases, the tinnitus itself may be the cause of the psychological disorder. Sixteen percent of the population with tinnitus admitted to depression. Seventy percent of patients seen in our specialty clinic admitted experiencing depression some time during their lives. Some studies concluded that 20% to 50% of patients were clinically depressed, and about half the depressed patients had a long history of depression before the onset of tinnitus. There is undoubtedly a significant population in whom depression plays a major role and for whom treatment must be appropriately directed as part of the tinnitus management program.

Examination and Tests

After obtaining a complete history on the tinnitus patient, a thorough medical evaluation is conducted. All patients should have blood pressure recordings from both arms, and routine studies should include audiometric evaluation (e.g., air, bone, speech discrimination). Laboratory studies should include hematocrit and fluorescent treponemal antibody absorption tests. If a patient presents with a straightforward and simple etiologic cause (e.g., bilateral high-frequency hearing loss secondary to acoustic trauma), the laboratory workup is complete at this point. With any suggestion of medical or metabolic abnormalities, however, blood chemistries, thyroid studies, a lipid battery, and other appropriate tests should be undertaken. With unilateral hearing loss, additional audiologic and radiologic studies may be necessary to exclude posterior fossa tumors. Most neoplasms and anomalies are best seen on bone algorithm CT studies. For patients with nonpulsatile tinnitus, MRI is the study of choice to exclude a vestibular schwannoma or other neoplasm of the cerebellopontine angle cistern (2).

Unilateral tinnitus also presents a different problem, and posterior fossa lesions must be excluded. The diagnostic workup for the unilateral tinnitus is similar to that for unilateral hearing loss. Only if there is an unambiguous cause of the unilateral symptom can a full workup be ignored.

Treatment

Figure 151.1 summarizes principles in tinnitus management. Any reversible otologic or medical disorder must be treated. If symptoms are mild, several guidelines should be observed. The physician should discuss with the patient the etiologic factors and status of the complaint. It is important not to exacerbate the patient's preoccupation with their complaint by creating unnecessary fear as to the cause of their tinnitus. The majority of tinnitus cases resolve spontaneously, but if the tinnitus persists, several management options are available (3). Generally, 25% of all patients improve significantly after its onset, 50% are improved to some degree, and the remaining 25% remain unchanged; a very small portion have progressive symptoms. The patient should avoid chocolate, coffee, tea, cola, or other caffeine-containing beverages or medications. Fifty-four percent of patients with severe tinnitus took excessive amounts of caffeinated beverages daily. The patient also should stop smoking.

Medications should be reevaluated, with specific avoidance of aspirin-containing compounds, nonsteroidal anti-inflammatory drugs, or other implicated medications. The patient should avoid disturbing noise, use noise protection, and employ home-masking techniques, which includes music at night or the radio tuned between the FM stations at a level of "white noise" that masks out the tinnitus. A bedside masker also can be recommended. In patients who have depression or anxiety, psychological testing and evaluation are advisable, which allows the physician to have the patient's emotional status reviewed before additional treatment and to tailor medications to the results.

These actions usually prove successful in managing most patients with tinnitus; however, if the cause cannot be reversed and general treatment is insufficient, a more extensive evaluation is required. Evaluation at a tinnitus clinic is useful.

Tinnitus Program

In attempting to treat patients disabled by their symptoms, measurement of the tinnitus is important. Four aspects of tinnitus are measured in the standard tinnitus program: pitch, loudness, minimum masking level, and residual inhibition (4,5). Additional psychobehavioral measures, such as Tinnitus Handicap Inventory (THI), have recently been advocated by researchers as useful tools in gauging tinnitus severity and its impact on patient's life (6).

Specific Treatment Regimens

On the basis of the evaluation of tinnitus, a sequence of management techniques can be outlined for the patient with symptoms unresolved by simpler treatment. These techniques include masking, stress management, medications, electrical stimulation, and surgery.

Masking

Masking can take several routes, including hearing aids, tinnitus instruments, and maskers. It relies on the principle

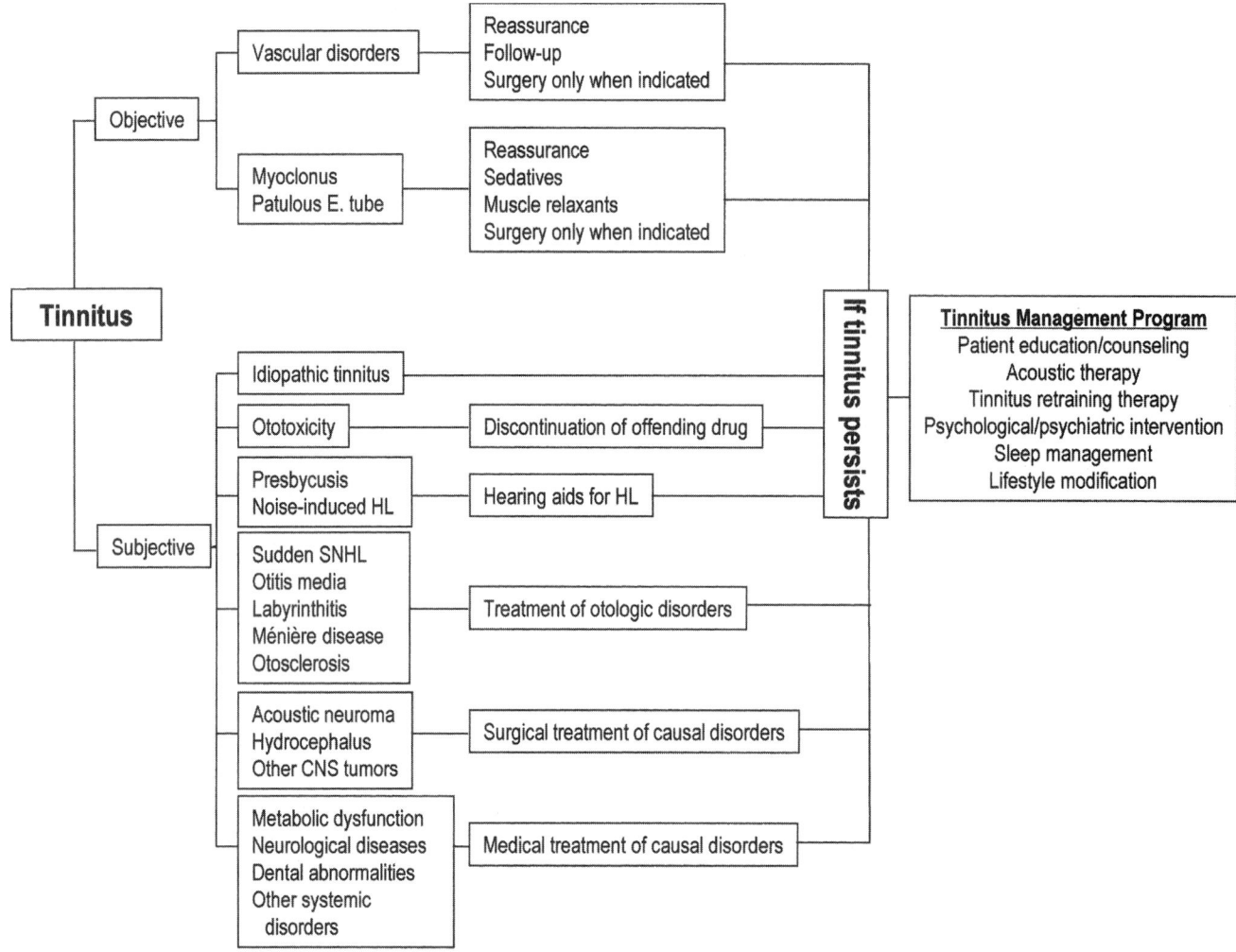

Figure 151.1   Management of tinnitus.

that an external noise can cover the sound internally generated by the patient. The minimal masking level provides some indication as to whether masking can be used successfully for patients. If the minimal masking level is at the 2- or 3-dB sensation level, masking has a good chance for success. If the minimal masking level is at the 10- to 15-dB sensation level, the success of masking is doubtful (7).

Masking is only a substitute for the tinnitus and not a cure. The patient should understand the limit of its usefulness before the trial of masking devices. Only 20% of patients with tinnitus require evaluation for masking, and in this group of severe tinnitus sufferers, 60% can benefit from some means of masking.

Hearing Aid

A hearing aid is the simplest means of direct masking in patients with hearing loss, and it can be a first-trial device. The increased sound from the hearing aid masks the offending sound and decreases the annoyance of the tinnitus perceived by the patient. Although hearing aids are useful in masking tinnitus, only 25% of patients are relieved by this method alone; 55% have symptoms that can be masked with the use of the tinnitus instrument if the symptoms are disabling.

Tinnitus Instrument

The tinnitus instrument is a combination of hearing aid and masking device in a single case. The masker is a device capable of producing a sound from 1500 to 8000 Hz, with a volume potential from 45 to 90 dB. This combination device, which looks similar to a hearing aid, more adequately masks the tinnitus of most patients who receive masking as treatment. The hearing aid and masker have different volume controls and can be adjusted for patient comfort. An advantage of this device is the ability to modify the input of the hearing aid and the masking device independently. At night or in quiet situations in which the tinnitus is severe, the masking sound can be increased without altering or using the hearing aid. In patients in whom the tinnitus can be masked, 55% can obtain significant long-term benefit from a tinnitus instrument.

Masker

The masker generally is limited to patients with normal or near-normal hearing. Few patients fall into this group, and only a third find the device helpful; however, it is worthwhile to try a masker because little else is successful in treating this population. Extended use of tinnitus instruments or maskers has not demonstrated any long-term effect on hearing threshold or discrimination, nor have these devices adversely affected the tinnitus.

Habituation of Tinnitus

Overall tolerance of tinnitus generally increases over time. Initial tinnitus maskability is a significant predictor of distress at later follow-ups (8).

Over the past several years, some investigators have directed attention to habituation therapy or tinnitus retraining therapy. In this technique, the patient is stimulated with broad-band noise up to 16 hours a day. The level of noise or masking initially presented is quite low and is increased progressively until it is audible to the patient but does not mask the patient's tinnitus. Over a period of months (10 to 18 months), the patient may become unaware of, or untroubled by, the tinnitus (9,10). Initial results are encouraging, and further study is being conducted (11).

Cognitive Behavioral Therapy

In many patients, stress or depression is a major factor in the intensity and severity of their complaints. Personality studies of tinnitus patients indicate a high incidence of abnormal psychological patterns and patterns of neuroses and depression (12). Patients who fall into this category benefit from attempts to modify their behavior. Although this therapy is generally not curative, tinnitus-related distress has been shown to decrease in many patients who receive cognitive behavioral therapy (8). Antidepressants and antianxiety medications are often given in association with counseling and psychological therapy.

Biofeedback is used extensively for stress reduction management as well. Its benefit for patients with severe tinnitus has been demonstrated but requires close cooperation of patient, physician, therapist, and psychologist (13).

Medications

Drugs are capable of increasing or decreasing tinnitus, but because the mechanism that causes tinnitus is not clearly understood, it is not generally possible to select a drug rationally to control it. Few drugs have been tested appropriately for their effects on tinnitus. The only medications that have proved useful have been drugs that affect the emotional status of patients through anxiety reduction, improved sleep pattern, and antidepressant effect (14). Alprazolam in its use as an antianxiety medication has

provided relief for about 50% of patients (15). Nortriptyline has provided relief for a majority of patients felt to suffer from depression (16). Gabapentin (Neurontin) and melatonin are drugs that have recently been studied for their effects on tinnitus. Preliminary studies suggest that they may provide symptom improvement in some patients, especially those with high severity scores and significant sleep difficulties (17,18). Other medications that have proved useful have been those that provide the patient with uninterrupted sleep. It should be noted that Food and Drug Administration (FDA) has not approved any medications specifically for the purpose of treating tinnitus.

Electromagnetic Stimulation

Electrical stimulation as treatment of tinnitus remains investigational. Transcutaneous, promontory, and round-window stimulation of the cochlea offer possible treatment for the future (19). The initial results of electrical stimulation have not been encouraging. Hopes have been based on reports that 50% to 90% of cochlear implant patients stated that their tinnitus was better with the device functioning and that only 11% found it worse with the use of the implant. Transcranial magnetic stimulation has also been shown to suppress tinnitus. In one report, this was followed by implant of an extradural electrode in the primary auditory area under the guidance of fMRI to produce lasting tinnitus suppression (20). Our experience with deep brain stimulation on tinnitus showed that nearly half of patients reported relief from tinnitus when the stimulator was turned on (21,22). In general, electromagnetic stimulation for tinnitus is experimental. Further studies are needed to establish its efficacy and safety.

Surgery

Surgery for associated otologic conditions (e.g., otosclerosis, chronic ear disease) can be helpful in alleviating tinnitus. Moreover, reports of tinnitus suppression with cochlear implants have been encouraging. Auditory nerve section has not proved consistently useful, even in patients who merit such treatment. Microvascular decompression has been reported to be helpful in some patients whose angiographic studies suggest contact between the anterointerior cerebellar artery (AICA) and the auditory nerve. This involves separating the AICA from the eighth cranial nerve in the cerebellopontine angle (23). Only limited number of cases has been reported. Overall, surgery currently has a very limited role in treating subjective tinnitus.

Alternative Medicine

Many herbal supplements have been advertised as effective in treating tinnitus. Few of these substances have been systematically studied, except maybe for *Ginkgo biloba*, which was shown to be no better than placebo in a double-blind study involving more than 1,000 patients (24). St. John's wort may help tinnitus patients through its antidepressant effects, but serious concerns exist regarding its interactions with several conventional drugs (25).

The role of acupuncture in tinnitus patients is still controversial. Although unblinded studies have suggested positive results, they have not been reproduced in blinded studies (26).

TINNITUS IN THE HEARING PERSON

Patients who have tinnitus but who hear normally remain a troubling and challenging group to treat. Often these patients suffer from hyperacusis as well. The cause is obscure, and these patients appear most affected by the least measurable matched loudness of tinnitus. They have severe associated sound intolerance and are disabled by normally tolerable noise levels. They also hear sounds not generally considered disturbing, such as fluorescent lights or refrigerator noise. Masking in this group is generally not tolerated. Medications hold the greatest hope. Antidepressants, particularly nortriptyline but also Triavil and fluoxetine (Prozac), as well as other antidepressants, have been of some benefit. Noise avoidance, noise protection, and strict avoidance of stimulants are necessary. Psychological evaluation and counseling are frequently required.

One other group of patients that has been particularly difficult to treat includes patients who have total loss of hearing or severe profound unilateral loss of hearing. These are the ones least affected by any of the treatments presently provided.

CONCLUSION

Because many etiologic factors have not been clearly identified, continued research holds the clue to management of this large group of patients. Improved techniques of objectively recording and testing patients need to be devised, and the interrelations of medical, psychological, and otologic factors must be specified.

HIGHLIGHTS

- Otologic factors are the most common underlying cause of subjective tinnitus; 75% of patients have a 30+ dB high-frequency hearing loss.
- Nine percent of patients with tinnitus have had major head trauma.
- The most frequent pharmacologic causes of tinnitus are the antiinflammatory drugs. About 10% of patients with tinnitus have symptoms related to medications.
- Forty-five percent of patients with severe tinnitus have at one time had active temporomandibular joint symptoms.
- Depression is common in patients with tinnitus, but it is not always clear whether the depression is primary or secondary.

- Only 25% of patients describe an increase in tinnitus over time. Most express some improvement.
- Objective measurements of tinnitus are made by pitch masking, loudness matching, determining minimal masking levels, and assessing residual inhibition.
- Although hearing aids are useful in masking tinnitus, only 25% of patients with significant tinnitus are relieved by this method alone. Fifty-five percent have symptoms that can be masked with the use of the tinnitus instrument if the symptoms are disabling.
- In patients with high stress levels, trials of antidepressants, amitriptyline, or perphenazine-amitriptyline combinations are helpful.
- The antianxiety drug alprazolam (Xanax) holds some promise for patients with sleep problems secondary to tinnitus. It tends to lessen the extent of the tinnitus and is useful in normal-hearing persons with this complaint.

REFERENCES

1. Lusk R, Babin R. Tensor tympanic and masseter muscle synkinesis. *Otolaryngol Head Neck Surg* 1985;93:555–558.
2. Weissman JL, Hirsch BE. Imaging of tinnitus: a review. *Radiology* 2000;216:342–349.
3. Noell CA, Meyerhoff WL. Tinnitus. Diagnosis and treatment of this elusive symptom. *Geriatrics* 2003;58:28–34.
4. Goodwin PE, Johnson RM. The loudness of tinnitus. *Acta Otolaryngol* 1980;90:353–359.
5. Henry JA, Meikle MB. Psychoacoustic measures of tinnitus. *J Am Acad Audiol* 2000;11:138–155.
6. Berry JA, Gold SL, Frederick EA, et al. Patient-based outcomes in patients with primary tinnitus undergoing tinnitus retraining therapy. *Arch Otolaryngol Head Neck Surg* 2002;128:1153–1157.
7. Johnson R, Griest S, Pren L, et al. A tinnitus masking program: efficiency and safety. *Hearing J* 1989;42:18–25.
8. Andersson G, Vretblad P, Larsen HC, et al. Longitudinal follow-up of tinnitus complaints. *Arch Otolaryngol Head Neck Surg* 2001;127:175–179.
9. Jastreboff PJ. Instrumentation and tinnitus, a neurophysiologic approach. *Heavy Instrument* 1994;45:7–9.
10. Jastreboff PH, Jastreboff MM. Tinnitus retraining therapy (TRT) as a method for treatment of tinnitus and hyperacusis in patients. *J Am Acad Audiol* 2000;11:162–177.
11. McKenny CJ, Hazell JWP, Graham RL. An evaluation of the TRT method. In: Hazell J, ed. *Proceedings of the Sixth International Tinnitus Seminar.* Bungay, England: RefineCatch, 1999:99–105.
12. Folmer RL, Griest SE, Meikle MB, et al. Tinnitus severity, loudness and depression. *Otolaryngol Head Neck Surg* 1999;121:48–51.
13. House J, Miller L, House RR. Severe tinnitus: treatment with biofeedback training transactions. *Am Ophthalmol Otolaryngol* 1976;89:697–703.
14. Brummett R. Drugs for and against tinnitus. *Hearing J* 1989;42:34–37.
15. Johnson RM, Brummett R, Schleuning A. Use of alprazolam for relief of tinnitus. *Arch Otolaryngol Head Neck Surg* 1991;119:842–845.
16. Dobie RA, Sullivan MD, Katon WJ, et al. Antidepressant treatment of tinnitus patients. *Acta Otolaryngol (Stockh)* 1992;112:242–247.
17. Zapp JJ. Gabapentin for the treatment of tinnitus: a case report. *Ear Nose Throat J* 2001;80:114–116.
18. Rosenberg SI, Silverstein H, Rowan PT, et al. Effect of melatonin on tinnitus. *Laryngoscope* 1998;108:305–310.
19. Hazell JW, Meerton LE, Ryan R. Electrical tinnitus suppression. *Hearing J* 1989;22:26–33.
20. De Ridder D, De Mulder G, Walsh V, et al. Magnetic and electrical stimulation of the auditory cortex for intractable tinnitus. Case report. *J Neurosurg* 2004;100:560–564.
21. Martin WH, Shi Y. Deep brain stimulation effects on hearing function and tinnitus In: Hazell J, ed. *Proceedings of the Sixth International*

Tinnitus Seminar. London: The Tinnitus and Hyperacusis Centre, 1999:68–72.

22. Shi Y, Martin WH. Deep brain stimulation—a new treatment for tinnitus? In: Hazell J, ed. *Proceedings of the Sixth International Tinnitus Seminar.* London: The Tinnitus and Hyperacusis Centre, 1999:578–580.

23. Okamura T, Kurokawa Y, Ikeda N, et al. Microvascular decompression for cochlear symptoms. *J Neurosurg* 2000;93:421–426.

24. Drew S. Davies E. Effectiveness of Ginkgo biloba in treating tinnitus: double blind, placebo controlled trial. *BMJ* 2001;322:73–75.

25. Ernst E. The risk-benefit profile of commonly used herbal therapies: ginkgo, St. John's wort, ginseng, Echinacea, saw palmetto, and kava. *Ann Intern Med* 2002;136:42–53.

26. Park J, White AR, Ernst E. Efficacy of acupuncture as a treatment for tinnitus: a systematic review. *Arch Otolaryngol Head Neck Surg* 2000;126:489–492.

Autoimmune Inner Ear Disease

152

Jeffrey P. Harris

Over the past 20 years, we have witnessed the development of an entirely new field of otology: immune-mediated sensorineural hearing loss (SNHL). Its importance stems from the fact that the inner ear is subject to the influences of immune response, inflammation, and autoimmunity, and through the effects of these conditions on the inner ear, hearing loss can occur. Most importantly, though, is the recognition that if detected early enough, hearing loss, once thought to be progressive and irreversible, can be restored through appropriate and judicious use of immunosuppressive drugs.

This chapter explores the basic fundamentals of inner ear immune responses and their relationship to clinical disease. There is no doubt that our understanding of these responses will improve and that new, more effective and less toxic treatments will be developed.

THE INNER EAR IMMUNE RESPONSE

The central nervous system (CNS) and the inner ear, by extension, originally were thought to be immunoprivileged sites through the actions of the blood-brain barrier and blood-labyrinthine barrier, respectively. It is now known that the inner ear, as well as the CNS, is capable of mounting an immune response (1,2).

The sequence of events that constitute this immune response in the inner ear were well characterized recently. In the normal resting state, the inner ear contains immunoglobulin and the endolymphatic sac contains immunocompetent cells. Immunoglobulin crosses the blood-labyrinthine barrier and is present in perilymph at a level of 1/1,000 the concentration found in serum. There is an increased concentration of immunoglobulin relative to the

levels in the CNS, possibly due to the water-resorptive properties of the endolymphatic sac. Levels of immunoglobulin G (IgG) appear to predominate, with lesser amounts of IgM and IgA present. This immunoglobulin-rich environment protects the inner ear from pathogens by its roles in neutralization, opsonization, and complement fixation. The two latter functions require the actions of immunocompetent cells in conjunction with immunoglobulin. The normal cochlea contains no discernible cells; on the other hand, the endolymphatic sac has been shown to contain a full array of immunocompetent cells within the endolymphatic sac: helper and suppressor classes of T cells, macrophages, and B cells bearing IgM, IgG, and IgA. Furthermore, the endolymphatic sac is in close approximation to lymphatics that appear to drain into the jugular vein and possibly into retropharyngeal lymph node chains, thus demonstrating all of the components and evidence to support the endolymphatic sac as the originating site for a local immune response.

Presumably, for local immune responses to be generated in the inner ear, antigen must gain access to the immunocompetent cells in the endolymphatic sac. We and others have shown that antigen, namely horseradish peroxidase (HRP), does diffuse to the endolymphatic sac after scala tympani injection. Through diffusion studies, its pathways can be traced and suggest movement through perilymph and the perisaccular tissues, as opposed to movement in the endolymphatic space. Furthermore, the concentrated staining of the spiral ligament with HRP reaction product in this study also supports the hypothesis that perilymph is resorbed from the inner ear by the spiral ligament and its dense network of small venules (3). The importance of the endolymphatic sac in initiating an immune response is supported by the evidence of phagocytosed antigen in macrophages of the endolymphatic sac lumen within hours of injection; no labeled cells appeared in the cochlea during the study period. By 72 hours following the HRP challenge, the cochlea, vestibule, and endolymphatic sac were cleared completely of HRP (3). This was also seen in a previous study in which keyhole limpet hemocyanin (KLH), a potent stimulator of cellular immunity, was used to investigate the development of inner ear immunocompetent cells. Both macrophages with phagocytosed antigen and T-helper cells appeared in the endolymphatic sac before they appeared in the cochlea. Hence, antigen quickly reaches the endolymphatic sac, and this appears to be the initial site of the immune response.

Antigen challenge of the inner ear has predictable consequences. Direct challenge of the perilymph with KLH results in an anti-KLH antibody increase in the perilymph, which peaks between 4 and 7 weeks, and is not caused by increased vascular permeability, serum contamination during the sampling process, or cerebrospinal fluid (CSF) contributions via the cochlear aqueduct. Numerous plasma cells are noted in the scala tympani and endolymphatic sac during the response (Fig. 152.1). An important aspect of the timing and magnitude of this response is the animal's immunization status. When a systemically KLH-sensitized animal receives inner ear challenge with KLH, the secondary humoral immune response is faster, peaking at 2 weeks, and larger, tenfold larger than the primary response. This finding suggests the egress of KLH-specific plasma cells from the circulation during the response. An increase in anti-KLH antibody also was seen after direct inoculation of the endolymphatic sac. Cellular infiltrates in and around the sac were deemed responsible for the increase in antibody in the perilymph of the cochlea in this study, again suggesting the importance of this structure in modulating the inner ear immune response during challenge (Fig. 152.2). Secretion of antigen-specific antibody is a mechanism of immune response used by the inner ear that occurs relatively late in the response and is greatly modified by previous immunization status. Previous

immunization, therefore, undoubtedly has an effect on the final outcome of an inner ear immune response.

In a series of experiments, the central role of the endolymphatic sac in inner-ear immune responses was established. Challenge of the cochlea with KLH in systemically immunized animals following endolymphatic sac obliteration resulted in markedly reduced perilymph antibody levels and cellular infiltrates in the cochlea, compared with controls. In addition, this effect was not secondary to surgical trauma. Furthermore, direct KLH challenge of the endolymphatic sac resulted in increased levels of perilymph antibody, and this response was abrogated by prior endolymphatic duct obstruction. Hence, the endolymphatic sac appears to be crucial in antigen processing and appears to be the site from which perilymph antibody emanates.

Models of the immune response in vivo as well as in vitro established the role of numerous chemicals elaborated by cells involved in the immune response as important mediators of the inflammatory event. A host of cytokines, namely interleukins, interferons, and tumor necrosis factors, as well as growth factors, have been characterized. Interleukin-2 (IL-2) and transforming growth factor-β (TGF-β) have been studied with respect to the inner ear inflammatory response. IL-2 is regarded as an early mediator and is released by T-helper cells on stimulation from IL-1, a lymphokine released by activated macrophages. IL-2 is believed to have myriad functions: activation of T-helper, T-cytotoxic, and T-suppressor cells; activation of B cells; enhancement of natural killer activity; chemoattraction for polymorphonuclear cells, monocytes, and lymphocytes; and immunoregulation for prevention of autoimmune disease. IL-2 is not present in perilymph in the resting state, but it is a component of the inner-ear immune response. Following inner-ear challenge of the scala tympani with KLH, IL-2 was measurable at 6 hours, peaked at 18 hours, and declined over 5 days. The time frame of this response suggests that the lymphokine is generated by T cells residing in the endolymphatic sac and that it plays a

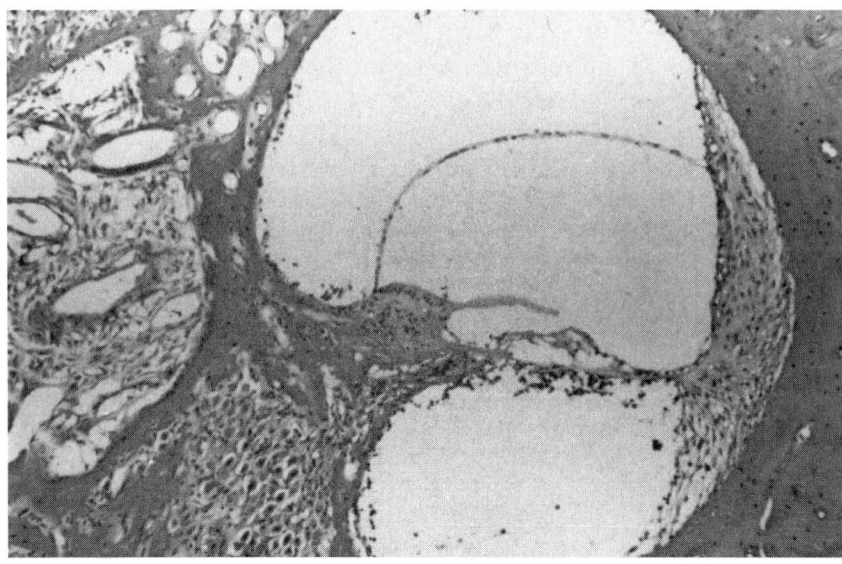

Figure 152.1 Experimental inner ear immune response to an antigen challenge (keyhole limpet hemocyanin) of the endolymphatic sac in guinea pigs. Note development of endolymphatic hydrops.

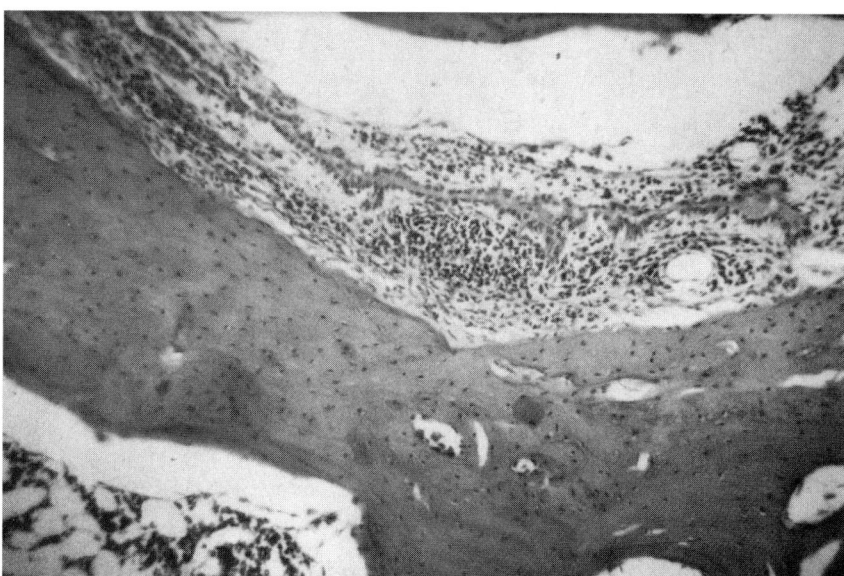

Figure 152.2 Secondary inner ear immune response centered around the endolymphatic sac resulting in hydrops. Note infiltrating lymphocytes, plasma cells, and macrophages in the perisaccular connective tissue.

comparable role in the inner ear, as noted in other inflammatory sites. The early egress of polymorphonuclear leukocytes and lesser amounts of monocytes and lymphocytes in this study may be secondary to the actions of IL-2, because this is one of its roles elsewhere in the body. TGF-β also has been identified as a mediator in the inner ear immune response. Following scala tympani challenge with KLH, leukocytes within the scala tympani and scala vestibuli were labeled with messenger RNA probes to TGF-β_1. This label was detected at 1 day, peaked at 3 days, and had decreased by 1 week (4). Its role in inflammation appears to be a combination of proinflammatory and negative feedback molecules. TGF-β has been purported to be chemoattractant for monocytes, T cells, and neutrophils while increasing levels of IL-1, IL-6, and platelet-derived growth factor. TGF-β also interferes with the IL-2 response, deactivates macrophages, and inhibits production of interferon-α and tumor necrosis fac-

tor (TNF-α). Our laboratory has recently demonstrated TNF-α and IL-1β-labeled cells released within 3 hours of antigen challenge, and IL-6 expressed later. This reaction in the inner ear is a chain of responses, with cytokines and growth factors all playing important roles.

Despite the importance of the endolymphatic sac in contributing immunocompetent cells and inflammatory mediators to the inner ear immune response, the inner ear also receives systemic immune cells for protection against viral and bacterial antigens. Both KLH challenge and viral inoculation of the inner ear cause massive cellular infiltration in both the scala tympani and, to a lesser extent, the scala vestibuli. The spiral modiolar vein (SMV) appears to play a key role in this cellular infiltration (5) (Figs. 152.3 and 152.4). Egress of lymphocytes from the circulation into lymph nodes has long been known to occur at specialized postcapillary venules, which have a unique mor-

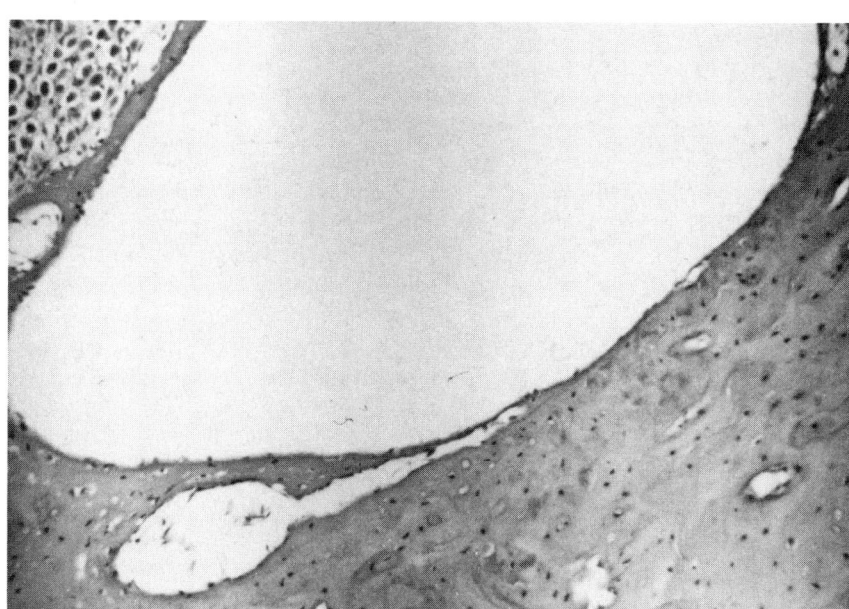

Figure 152.3 Spiral modiolar vein, with its collecting venule, along the scala tympani in a normal control guinea pig.

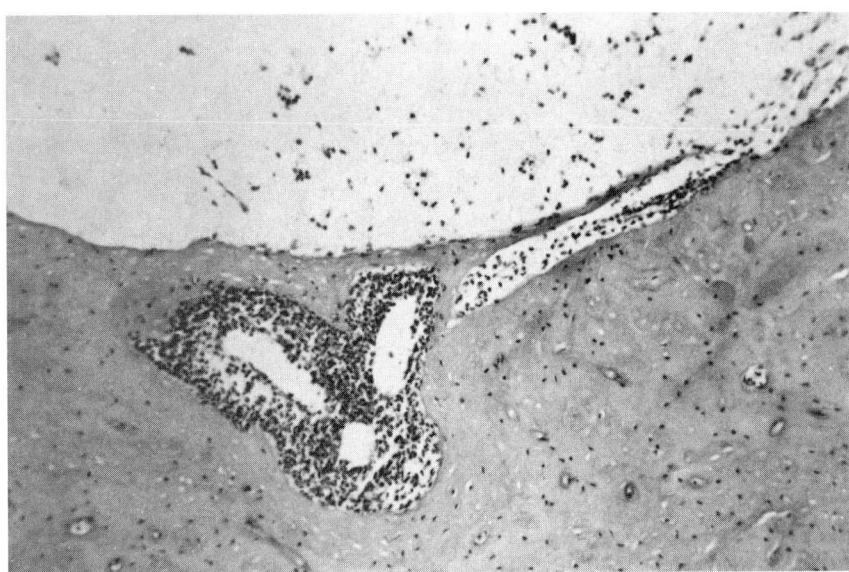

Figure 152.4 Spiral modiolar vein, with its collecting venule, in an animal undergoing inner ear immune response. Note the perivascular infiltration and cells streaming into the scala tympani from the systemic circulation.

phology and histochemistry, earning them the name high endothelial venules (HEVs). Somewhat surprisingly, the SMV has been shown to undergo an HEV-like transformation during the inflammatory response. This transformation consists of endothelial cells with large nuclei and increased cytoplasm and is present at day 2 following inner-ear inoculation of virus and continues to progress to day 6. In addition, lymphocytes can be seen adherent to and within the vascular wall (6). Hence, HEV-like morphology apparently can be acquired during an acute inflammatory condition in the cochlea. At least one adhesion molecule, intercellular adhesion molecule-1 (ICAM-1), has been demonstrated in the SMV and collecting venules in the acute phase of inner ear inflammation (7). Intercellular adhesion molecule-1 is expressed in HEVs of humans, mice, and rats and is involved in the interactions between leukocytes and endothelial cells and ultimate extravasation of cells. In a study of KLH-induced inner ear inflammation in rats, staining for ICAM-1 was found within 6 hours postchallenge on the epithelium of SMVs and collecting venules, reaching a maximum by day 2 and then fading gradually. In contrast, cellular extravasation peaked between days 3 and 7 in the cochlea. ICAM-1 also was found at 12 and 24 hours on the epithelium of the endolymphatic sac and perisaccular region, whereas cellular infiltration lagged by 2 to 3 days (7). These HEV-like changes seen in the SMV coincide with the expression of adhesion molecules such as ICAM-1 and the recruitment of systemic immunocompetent cells into the scala tympani.

The type and timing of cells that enter the cochlea also have been characterized. Macrophages and granulocytes are observed as early as 6 hours postchallenge in the cochlea and endolymphatic sac and rapidly increase thereafter. T-helper cells gradually increase in the endolymphatic sac, peaking at 2 to 3 weeks; their presence in the cochlea is noted on day 1 and continues to increase. Increased levels of T-suppressor cells are not detected in the cochlea or endolymphatic sac until 3 weeks postchallenge. Additionally,

immunoglobulin-bearing cells are seen early in the response. IgG cells are seen in the endolymphatic sac by day 1, and IgM follows shortly after with an increase on day 2. IgA cells do not appear until 3 weeks postchallenge. Inflammatory cells in the endolymphatic sac and cochlea continue to proliferate in situ during the response, and active proliferation is noted a full 6 weeks after challenge, suggesting a relatively weak immunoregulatory mechanism of the inner ear despite the aforementioned infiltration of T-suppressor cells. The actual quantities of cells derived from endolymphatic sac proliferation versus extravasation is unknown; however, the pattern of increase in cellular constituents is consistent with the roles proposed for each class. The early response of polymorphonucleocytes results in antigen clearing, and the egress of macrophages allows antigen processing and presentation. T-helper cells also arrive early, presumably to potentiate or regulate the response and accentuate the development of arriving B cells into immunoglobulin-secreting plasma cells. The late appearance of T-suppressor cells would be consistent with the proposed function as an immune down-regulator.

Concomitant with this cellular proliferation is a steady increase in extracellular matrix. Both suppurative and sterile labyrinthitis are known to result in the formation of a dense extracellular matrix and eventual ossification in the cochlea (8,9). The cells responsible for this outcome are now coming to light. Ki-67 immunoassay has revealed that by day 1 postchallenge, fibroblast and endosteal cells lining the scala tympani are proliferating. The numbers of these cells continue to increase, and signs of their proliferation are still present 6 weeks postchallenge. Fibrotic tissue becomes visible for the first time at 1 week, and ossification can be seen by 3 weeks (10). Ossification of the normally fluid-filled cochlear scalae is a common result of inner-ear inflammation. A variety of insults can result in labyrinthitis ossificans, including purulent labyrinthitis (8), sterile labyrinthitis, advanced otosclerosis, autoimmune inner ear disease, temporal bone trauma, labyrinthectomy, meningitis (11,12), vascular occlusion, and cochlear implantation. The inner ear seems particularly incapable of clearing this extracellular matrix during an immune response, which over time results in osteoneogenesis. The endosteal cells lining the scala tympani now appear to be a key component in this chain of events. According to Taguchi et al., the role of IL-6 in bone remodeling and in diseases such as osteogenesis is central (13), and according to Guillen et al. (14), IL-6 most likely interacts with parathyroid hormone-related protein.

Unfortunately, this elaborate chain of events, intended to protect the inner ear against pathogens, often can lead to hearing loss. Early studies on the effect of virally induced labyrinthitis revealed severe hearing loss in animals not previously exposed to the pathogen. A full 70% of these seronegative animals had profound elevations of the cochlear microphonic (CM) and eighth nerve N1 compound action potential (CAP) thresholds. Further research revealed that the immune response may be partially responsible for the negative effect on hearing. Investigation of the inner ear histopathology following virally induced labyrinthitis resulted in consistent findings of degeneration in the organ of Corti, stria vascularis, and spiral ganglion with mild endolymphatic hydrops (15). What argues for the role of the immune system in this damage is the fact that a variety of viruses can infect the inner ear at different sites and cell types, yet degeneration of these same structures appears to occur irrespective of the site of viral infection (15). In addition, negative effects on histopathology and hearing have been found with both virally induced and sterile labyrinthitis, and the amount of damage was associated with the magnitude of the immune response. KLH systemic sensitization prior to secondary inner ear challenge resulted in a much larger antibody response, greater histopathology, and more significant hearing loss as evidenced by CM and CAP, compared with animals receiving only primary inner ear challenge. Thus, the more robust immune response appears to result in greater damage to the inner ear. How the immune response damages the aforementioned structures is currently being elucidated. The apparent lack of clearing of the extracellular matrix and subsequent ossification appear to be due in part to activation of the endosteal cells (10). The degeneration of the spiral ganglion appears to be independent of this ossification, but the mechanism is not yet understood (9). The degeneration of the stria vascularis in these models presumably is a secondary event. Although these cells never express viral antigens in our cytomegalovirus labyrinthitis model, the damage is likely caused by edema resulting from the egress of cells in the downstream venules, creating venous stasis and eventually capillary stasis in the strial vessels. The danger of an inflammatory response in the inner ear therefore seems analogous to infections with pathogens at other sites in the body. Pneumonia results in scarring and fibrosis secondary to immune system intervention, immunocompetent cells destroy healthy bone around an osteomyelitis, and inflammatory infiltrates cause increased intracranial pressure in meningitis. Unfortunately, the inner ear seems particularly sensitive and incapable of controlling the deleterious effects of an inflammatory response.

EXPERIMENTAL PARADIGMS

Understanding the mechanisms of immunopathology in the inner ear should direct our efforts toward prevention of this immune-mediated damage. As previously mentioned, several studies revealed that interference with the predictable order of events is possible. As also mentioned, the normal cochlea contains no observable immunocompetent cells, whereas the endolymphatic sac appears to contain the cells necessary to initiate an immune response. Several studies support the importance of the endolymphatic sac in this function. Direct inoculation of the endolymphatic sac with guinea pig cytomegalovirus (GPCMV) in animals with systemic immunity to GPCMV resulted in marked inflammatory cell infiltration in the region of the sac and mild endolymphatic hydrops but no hearing loss or viral antigen production. Thus, the sac can protect the inner ear structures, but it does so at the expense of some damage to itself. Further evidence of the detrimental effects of the immune response on the inner ear comes from Darmstadt et al. It was demonstrated that immunosuppression with cyclophosphamide prior to GPCMV inoculation into the scala tympani actually reduced the amount of hearing loss as measured by CAP thresholds compared with controls. The amount of GPCMV antigen detected in the cochleas did not correlate with the CAP thresholds; however, the greater the inflammatory response to GPCMV in the cochlea, the higher the CAP threshold and thus the greater the hearing loss. The inflammatory response to GPCMV may be more important than the direct cytopathic effects of the virus in producing SNHL in GPCMV-induced labyrinthitis. As previously noted, the expression of ICAM-1 in the SMV and its collecting ducts increases during inflammation and undoubtedly has effects on cell trafficking (7). A modest decrease in this trafficking was accomplished with the use of monoclonal antibodies to ICAM-1 during inner ear inflammation. Despite this decrease in cellular infiltrates, anti-ICAM-1–treated animals did not show sparing of hearing compared with controls. Because of the modest decrease in cellular infiltrates, lymphokines or other adhesion molecules yet to be described in the inner ear must play a major role. Thus, from these experiments, we have been able to determine that inner ear inflammation can be manipulated by interfering with both the afferent and efferent limbs of the immune response and in doing so not only provide an increased understanding of the pathogenesis of many inner ear diseases but also help to open new avenues of treatment. An important off-shoot of the inner ear's immunologic response to antigen and viruses may have some influence on the future of gene transfer to the inner ear. It has been shown that viral vectors used to transfer DNA, such as vectors employing adenovirus, provoke a host inner ear immune response that

2252 Section IX: Otology

may limit their usefulness in advancing this important field of molecular genetics. The fact that these vectors provoke an immune response within the inner ear further substantiates the functional importance of this host defense mechanism.

ANIMAL MODELS OF AUTOIMMUNE INNER EAR DISEASE

There have been many animal studies in AIED in an attempt to find an ideal animal model that demonstrates the complex pathogenesis of this disease.

One type of animal model is based on immunization with native type 2 collagen. Yoo et al. (16) used female Lewis rats, immunizing the animals with either bovine and chick type 2 collagen or bovine type 1 collagen. In rats immunized with type 2 collagen, ABR recordings demonstrated decreased amplitudes and delayed latencies, but rats immunized with type 1 collagen did not show this. The investigators then immunized other animals (e.g., guinea pigs, rats, chinchillas) with purified bovine and chicken type 2 collagen, and found otospongiotic changes in structures such as the external auditory canal and the osseous labyrinth. Degeneration of spiral ganglion cells, and atrophic changes of the cochlear nerve, organ of Corti, and stria vascularis were found in the inner ear. All animals also developed endolymphatic hydrops, hearing loss, and vestibular dysfunction. Harris et al. (17) used the same protocol with Wistar-Furth rats divided into short-term (1 to 3 months) and long-term (9 to 11 months) groups, and found that all animals showed significant serum and perilymph antibody titers to type 2 collagen. Even though four animals developed spontaneous otitis media, none of the animals developed hearing loss. Thus, these findings did not support the role of type 2 collagen as a putative antigen in inner ear disease.

Beickert (18) was one of the first to develop an animal model for AIED using homologous inner ear tissue in guinea pigs. Though lesions within the cochlea were found histologically, there was no evidence of cellular or humoral immune responses. In later experiments using homologous cochlear tissue in complete Freund's adjuvant (CFA) in guinea pigs, Terayama and Sasaki (19) found alterations in the Preyer reflex and cochlear histopathology, but no immunological event. Based on these early studies, Harris immunized guinea pigs with homologous and bovine inner ear homogenate, and demonstrated cochlear lesions in all animals and hearing loss in 32% of the animals. There was no correlation, however, between the degree of hearing loss and either serum antibody titers or histologic changes (20). Yamanobe and Harris (21) later showed the presence of cellular infiltrate in the inner ear of guinea pigs after labyrinthitis was induced by subcutaneous injection of bovine inner-ear antigen in CFA. Hearing loss developed at day 7 and continued to regress after 4 weeks. In another study, Gloddek et al. (22) immunized inbred Lewis rats with heterologous inner ear tissue, and the re-

sulting inner-ear-specific T cells were later transferred into naive rats, which produced labyrinthitis. Though these experiments support the role of T cells in the pathogenesis of AIED, this study did not include electrophysiologic testing, and the specific antigens involved in the initiation and progression of the disease were not characterized.

Another animal model for AIED uses autoimmune mouse strains such as MRL/lpr and C3H/lpr because of the animals' ability to develop spontaneous deafness (23,24,25), thus suggesting the immune system's role in the pathogenesis of hearing loss. The lpr gene is an autosomal recessive mutation causing lymphoproliferation and autoimmunity in the mice. The lymphoid hyperplasia is characterized by Thy-1+ and CD4+ T cells that secrete B-cell growth factors. MRL/lpr and C3H/lpr are ideal models for systemic lupus erythematosus because immune complex renal disease develops from anti-DNA antibodies that appear early in life and from elevated serum immune complexes and cryoglobulins (26,27). Trune (28) has shown that these animals have circulating antibodies against vessels in the stria vascularis, and the endothelial cell tight junctions that make up the stria blood-labyrinth barrier break down and cause cochlear dysfunction (24). Trune et al. (29) later demonstrated that this dysfunction can be reversed with glucocorticoid therapy. These findings suggest that the immune system has a central role in the etiopathogenesis of hearing loss in these mice. Ruckenstein (30,31) recently challenged these studies by questioning whether the hearing loss is caused by an immunological event, or by genetic or metabolic abnormalities.

Another autoimmune mouse strain, NZB/kl, demonstrates spontaneous hearing loss at high auditory frequencies. Studies with the NZB/kl mouse have shown deposition of IgG on the capillary wall of the stria vascularis, and that this damage to the stria vascularis caused the hearing loss (32,33). Though this hearing loss is part of a systemic autoimmune disease and is not an ideal model for AIED, it still demonstrates the importance of the immune system in inner ear pathology.

AUTOIMMUNE IMMUNOPATHOLOGY

In addition to the damage incurred during an immune response to invading pathogens, the inner ear also may suffer insults from autoimmune phenomena. The three primary mechanisms for autoimmune disease are autoantibodies against tissue antigens, deposition of antigen–antibody immune complexes in tissue, and infiltration and destruction of tissue by specific cytotoxic T cells. There is evidence that the inner ear can be affected in a variety of non–organ-specific autoimmune diseases. Polyarteritis nodosa has been associated, albeit rarely, with cochlear injury. Although SNHL may be a rare complication of the disease, hearing loss may be the only presenting symptom, and histopathologic analysis has revealed ischemic changes as the likely etiology. Likewise, Wegener granulomatosis has been associated with both middle and inner ear pathology. The improvement of some patients who have SNHL with prednisone therapy underscores the autoimmune/inflammatory nature of the disease. Otologic manifestations also have been seen with systemic lupus erythematosus, including chronic otitis media with necrotizing vasculitis and progressive SNHL or disequilibrium. Although otologic pathology has been reported in patients with rheumatoid arthritis, no temporal bone studies have been reported, and the relationship of rheumatoid arthritis to inner ear disease has not been confirmed. Cogan syndrome, characterized by interstitial keratitis and vestibuloauditory dysfunction, may blur the distinction between non–organ-specific and organ-specific autoimmune disease. The syndrome is thought to be a hypersensitivity response to one or more infectious agents associated with vasculitis, yet lymphocyte transformation on exposure of the patient's lymphocytes to corneal antigen and inner ear antigen has been reported, suggesting possible specific autoimmunity. This evidence of specific autoimmunity directed against the eye and ear may merely be a secondary result of the nonspecific vasculitis.

Evidence exists that the inner ear may be a site of organ-specific autoimmunity. Lehnhardt in 1958 suggested that cases of bilateral deafness were caused by anticochlear antibodies, and McCabe in 1979 reestablished this hypothesis as a line of inquiry. Anticollagen type 2 antibody has received considerable attention as an animal model of autoimmune inner ear disease (AIED). Several investigators have found extensive damage to inner-ear structures and some hearing loss following initiation of type 2 collagen autoimmunity (34); however, others have not found damage. Initiation of autoimmune inner ear dysfunction has been accomplished with exposure of animals to heterologous cochlear tissue (35), with 32% of animals showing significant hearing loss in one study. Interestingly, despite the species of animal used in the study, analysis of sera from the hearing-impaired animals by Western blot revealed an antibody against an inner-ear antigenic epitope with a molecular weight of approximately 68,000 daltons (35,36). Even more compelling is the finding that some patients (33%) with progressive SNHL show evidence of this same 68,000-dalton anti–inner ear antibody in their serum on Western blot (36) (Fig. 152.5). This observation was confirmed by Moscicki in 1990 (37) in 11 patients who demonstrated this antibody on Western blot analysis and whose hearing improved with immunosuppressive therapy. In a more recent controlled clinical trial, this group found that 89% of patients who had active and progressive bilateral SNHL had antibodies to 68-kd inner ear antigen, whereas patients who had inactive disease were antibody negative. Additionally, of the anti-68-kd–positive patients, 75% responded to steroids, compared with 18% who were 68-kd antibody negative, suggesting the assay's value in predictive response to therapy. Humoral autoantibodies also are implicated as a cause of autoimmune SNHL by studies that showed immunofluorescent labeling following incubation of serum from patients with suspected autoimmune

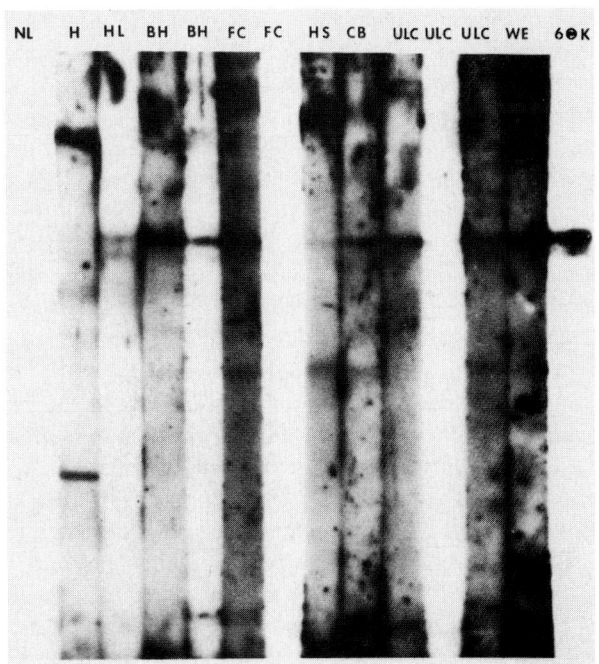

Figure 152.5 Western blot radioimmunoassay of several patients and animals suspected of autoimmune inner ear disease (*AIED*). Note heavy labeling at 68-kd molecular weight. *NL*, normal guinea pig (*g.p.*) serum; *H*, guinea pig immunized with inner ear antigen with maintained hearing; *HL*, hearing loss animal; *BH*, patient with AIED; *BH adjacent lane*, patient after immunosuppressive therapy; *FC*, patient with AIED; *FC adjacent lane*, cerebrospinal fluid from patient; *HS*, patient with active, progressive sensorineural hearing loss (*SNHL*); *CB, WE*, patients with Cogan syndrome; *ULC*, patients with ulcerative colitis and no hearing loss; *68K*, guinea pig immunized with 68-kd inner ear antigen. (Reprinted from Soliman AM. Type II collagen-induced inner ear disease: critical evaluation of the guinea pig model. *Am J Otol* 1990;11:27, with permission.)

SNHL onto sections of nonrelated, healthy human temporal bones. Unfortunately, interpretation of these results remains difficult because antigen degradation does occur with prolonged decalcification and human leukocyte antigen (HLA) differences between the patients and the cadavers may account for the labeling. Alternately, some investigators propose tests of cell-mediated immunity, particularly the lymphocyte transformation test, as a predictor of autoimmune inner ear disease. It may be that the combination of both tests may identify the most difficult cases to treat and the patients whose hearing is most jeopardized by the illness. Recently 82 patients were evaluated at the University of Washington for autoimmune inner-ear disease in whom Lyme titer, sedimentation rate, C-reactive protein, C1q binding assay, antineutrophil cytoplasmic antibody, treponemal pallidum microhemagglutination assay, anticardiolipin antibody, and Western blot for HSP-70 were obtained. These investigators reported that the Western blot test for HSP-70 was the best test for predicting steroid responsiveness. They found that the sensitivity was low at 42% of all patients tested but the specificity was high at 90%, leading to a positive predictive value of 91% (38). In another report, Berrettini et al. (39) found in a group of 13

2254	Section IX: Otology

patients a positive result for HSP-70 in 53.8%. Each of the three patients who responded to steroids had a positive Western blot result. In another study, Kosaka and Yamanobe examined sera of 195 patients with SNHL or vertigo by Western blot with bovine inner ear antigen. Patients with moderate to severe hearing loss showed positive reactions against 33- to 35-kd antigen (26%), 42-kd antigen (27%), and 68-kd antigen (71.5%). More recently, by immunizing mice intrasplenically with guinea pig inner ear tissue, investigators were able to create a monoclonal antibody directed at inner ear–supporting cells in guinea pigs. This monoclonal antibody, termed *KHRI-3*, was then purified and injected into the cochlea of guinea pigs, resulting in the majority of injected guinea pigs demonstrating substantial degrees of hearing loss. The targets of these monoclonal antibodies were identified among the supporting cells within the inner ear and against an antigen with a molecular weight of approximately 68,000–70,000 Daltons. Further research has suggested that the target may in fact be a choline transport channel, termed *choline transporter like protein-2 (CTL-2)* (40,41). Furthermore, the sera taken from patients with probable AIED and injected into guinea pigs was found to bind to the same inner ear–supporting cells as did the monoclonal antibody KHRI-3 just described. Investigators concluded that "these findings are highly suggestive that those human antibodies are also pathogenic" (40). This evidence, as well as the animal models of AIED developed earlier, argue strongly that at least a subset of patients with AIED, have antibody-mediated immunity as the mechanism of their inner ear damage. The Western blot assay, therefore, has gained acceptance as the most specific of the tests developed and is now recommended as the initial serologic test to help identify this condition. It is available commercially through Otoimmune Diagnostics, Inc, (Buffalo, New York; subsidiary of Immco Diagnostics, www.otoimmune.com) although this assay utilizes the inducible form of HSP-70, which appears to cross-react with the 68 kD antigen. As of this date the KHRI-3 monoclonal antibody assay has not become commercially available (2).

There has also been recent work that suggests that delayed hypersensitivity responses may also play a regulatory role in AIED. Evidence of type IV–mediated T cell damage to inner ear tissues has been reported in an animal model. The inner ear proteins cochlin and β-tectorin were used to immunize mice with resultant hearing loss demonstrated after 5 weeks. Flow cytometry was used to verify CD4+ cell activation. These investigators went on to isolate these CD4+ cells and inject them into naïve mice. These injected mice developed significant hearing loss 6 weeks after these T cells were transferred (42), suggesting an etiologic role of these cells in immune-mediated sensorineural hearing loss. Therefore, despite the difficulty in proving the presence and mechanism of organ-specific autoimmunity in the inner ear, the profound response of some patients with rapidly progressive SNHL to immunosuppressives and the clear existence of otologic pathology in some non–organ-specific autoimmune diseases support this as a clinical entity.

TREATMENT

Given the serious outcome in autoimmune inner-ear disease (AIED) patients who are left untreated or who have a significant delay in their treatment once the condition is identified, attempts at establishing the presumptive diagnosis are important. High-dose prednisone is the mainstay of treatment for this condition. Early institution of 60 mg of prednisone daily for about a month is now widely used, because short-term or lower dose long-term therapy has either been ineffective or fraught with the risk of relapse. Prednisone then is tapered slowly if a positive response to therapy is obtained. If during the taper, hearing suddenly falls, reinstitution of high-dose prednisone is mandated. One sensitive predictor of imminent relapse can be the appearance of loud tinnitus in one or both ears. If patients show steroid responsiveness but attempts at their taper result in relapse, the addition of a cytotoxic drug should be considered. The most widely used of these agents are MTX and cyclophosphamide (Cytoxan). MTX has the advantage of being less toxic and has fewer long-term hematopoietic risks, such as the development of neoplasia. In a retrospective study of 25 patients with AIED who were treated with MTX, Sismanis et al. (43) reported that 70% had improved hearing and 80% showed improvement of vestibular symptoms.

In an open-labeled prospective study of prednisone followed by MTX in AIED patients, Matteson et al. (44) reported that 11 of 17 (65%) patients improved, 2 (12%) worsened, and 4 (23%) remained the same compared with pretreatment hearing (44). Unfortunately, this positive effect did not exclude the possible benefits that the prior prednisone therapy had on the outcome.

Recently, a multi-institutional clinical trial was completed comparing the efficacy of MTX and prednisone with prednisone alone for the management of AIED. After one month of high-dose prednisone, 67 of the 116 (58%) patients enrolled in the trial demonstrated hearing improvement (45). These patients were then randomized to either MTX or placebo, along with an 18-week taper of prednisone. It was found that MTX was no more effective than placebo in maintaining the hearing improvement achieved with prednisone ($p = 0.30$).

If MTX is used, it should be given as an oral dose 7.5 to 20 mg weekly with folic acid (46,47). The patient should be monitored closely for toxicity with complete blood count, platelets, blood urea nitrogen, creatinine, liver function tests, and urinalysis. We should remember that the prednisone-sparing effects of MTX may take 1 to 2 months to achieve; therefore, prednisone should be maintained until such effects are obtained. It also should be stated that if high-dose prednisone has not been effective in restoring hearing, it is unlikely that MTX will offer additional efficacy. Therefore, for patients with severe hearing losses, positive 68-kd Western blots, and nonresponsiveness to prednisone or MTX therapy, consideration should be given to cyclophosphamide. At oral dosages of 1 to 2 mg/kg/day taken each morning with liberal amounts of fluid, the risk of hemorrhagic cystitis or drug effects on the bladder can be minimized. Again, appropriate monitoring of peripheral blood counts is required. Cytoxan should not be administered to children, and the risk of permanent sterility should be outlined. If, on the other hand, no response to high-dose prednisone is achieved, and the patient is 68-kd Western blot negative, it may be futile to continue potentially toxic drugs with little evidence for AIED as the etiology. As this field continues to evolve, there are no hard and fast rules, and a practitioner may be justified in trying cytotoxic drugs on an empiric basis because unrelenting progressive deafness is a serious handicap for a previously normal hearing person. Luetje (48) recommends plasmapheresis for difficult-to-manage patients, and this can be a useful adjunct to the aforementioned immunosuppressive drugs.

A number of newer agents aimed at modulating the immune response have been introduced for AIED. One example is etanercept, a TNF-α blocking agent. In a retrospective study of 12 patients with AIED, Rahman et al. (49) utilized etanercept on all patients and found that they either did not respond to conventional treatment or had significant side effects from that treatment before enrolled in the trial. Eleven of the 12 patients had improvement or stabilization of hearing and tinnitus. Furthermore, 7 of 8 (88%) who also had vertigo, and 8 of 9 (89%) who had aural fullness, also had improvement of these symptoms. Despite this favorable report, initial results from a recently concluded double-blind placebo-controlled trial with etanercept by Cohen et al. (50) failed to demonstrate significant hearing protection.

SUMMARY

We have reviewed the events of an inner ear immune response. The perilymph contains antibody, presumably derived from the systemic circulation and CSF, which would allow for neutralization and help with opsonization and complement fixation. The endolymphatic sac contains immunocompetent cells capable of processing and presenting viral or bacterial antigen, potentiating the immune response, attacking the invaders directly or attacking infected cells, and developing immunoglobulin responses in situ. The early release of mediators such as IL-2 likely emanate from the endolymphatic sac and result in potentiation and regulation of the response and may assist in changes in the SMV, including expression of ICAM-1, which aid in the egress of immune cells from the systemic circulation. Polymorphonuclear cells arrive first, followed by T cells and B cells, with secretion of specific antibody as a relatively

late event. Concomitant with the increase in cellular constituents is the formation of a dense extracellular matrix. The inner ear appears to have remarkable difficulty in clearing this matrix, ultimately resulting in ossification. The immune response is unfortunately deleterious to the inner ear, resulting in degeneration of the organ of Corti, stria vascularis, and spiral ganglion. Hearing loss is consistently seen following sterile- and virally induced labyrinthitis.

The inner ear also appears to be a target for autoimmune disease. Although inner-ear damage has been described as part of non–organ-specific autoimmune disease, specific disease against the inner ear is also likely. Experimental paradigms have allowed alterations of both the afferent and efferent limbs of this response, ultimately with the goal of altering the course of the response and the subsequent damage in patients.

Treatment modalities can be quite effective if this condition is recognized early in its course. As further studies of these patients are undertaken, more specific diagnostic methods may be developed so that we are not left to rely on empirical treatment for the presumptive diagnosis of this disorder, and even more effective and less toxic treatments should emerge.

HIGHLIGHTS

- It is now known that the inner ear as well as the CNS is capable of mounting an immune response.
- Understanding the mechanisms of immunopathology in the inner ear should direct our efforts to prevention of the immune-mediated damage.
- The three primary mechanisms for autoimmune disease are autoantibodies against tissue antigens, deposition of antigen–antibody immune complexes in tissue, and infiltration and destruction of tissue by specific cytotoxic T cells.
- Early institution of 60 mg of prednisone daily for about 1 month is now widely used, because short-term or lower dose long-term therapy has either been ineffective or fraught with the risk of relapse.
- At this writing, a multi-institutional clinical trial has been initiated to compare the efficacy of MTX and prednisone versus prednisone alone for the management of autoimmune ear disease.
- The inner ear appears to be a target for autoimmune disease. Although inner-ear damage has been described as part of non–organ-specific autoimmune disease, specific disease against the inner ear is also likely.
- A sensitive laboratory marker of this disease (Western blot anti–68-kd immunoassay) appears to have been developed and should aid in identifying treatable patients.

REFERENCES

1. Harris JP, Heydt BA, Keithley EM, et al. Immunopathology of the inner ear: an update. In: Berstein JM, Henderson D, eds. *Recent*

advances in immunological diseases of the ear. New York: New York Academy of Science, 1997:166–178.

2. Harris JP, Moscicki R, Hughes GB. Immunologic disorders of the inner ear. In: Hughes GB, Pensak M, eds. *Clinical otology.* New York: Thieme, 1997:381–391.

3. Yeo SW, Gottschlich S, Harris JP, et al. Antigen diffusion from the perilymphatic space of the cochlea. *Laryngoscope* 1995;105:623.

4. Yeo SW, Ryan AF. Transforming growth factor-β mRNA expression in the rat cochlea during experimental immune labyrinthitis. In: Mogi G, Veldman J, Kawauchi H, eds. *Immunobiology in otorhinolaryngology—progress of a decade.* Amsterdam: Kugler, 1994:181–188.

5. Harris JP, Fukuda S, Keithley E. Spiral modiolar vein: its importance in inner ear inflammation. *Acta Otolaryngol* 1990;110:357.

6. Stearns GS, Keithley E, Harris JP. Development of high endothelial venule–like characteristics in the spiral modiolar vein induced by viral labyrinthitis. *Laryngoscope* 1993;103:890.

7. Suzuki M, Harris JP. Expression of intercellular adhesion molecule-1 during inner ear inflammation. *Ann Otol Rhinol Laryngol* 1995;104:69–75.

8. Paparella MM, Sugiura S. The pathology of suppurative labyrinthitis. *Ann Otol* 1967;76:554.

9. Keithley E, Harris JP. Late sequelae of cochlear infection. *Laryngoscope* 1996;106:341.

10. Chen MC, Keithley E, Harris JP. Immunohistochemical identification of dividing cells in an inflammatory inner ear model using Ki-67 monoclonal antibody. Proceedings of the mid-winter meeting of the ARO, St. Petersburg, Florida, 1997:82.

11. Balkany T, Gantz BJ, Stenerson RL, et al. Systematic approach to electrode insertion in the ossified cochlea. *Otolaryngol Head Neck Surg* 1996;114:4.

12. Nadol JB. Histological considerations in implant patients. *Arch Otolaryngol* 1994;110:160.

13. Taguchi Y, Yamamoto M, Yamate T, et al. Interleukin-6-type cytokines stimulate mesenchymal progenitor differentiation toward the osteoblastic lineage. *Proc Assoc Am Physicians* 1998;110:559.

14. Guillen C, Martinez P, de Gortazar AR, et al. Both N- and C-terminal domains of parathyroid hormone-related protein increase interleukin-6 by nuclear factor-kappa B activation in osteoblastic cells. *J Biol Chem* 2002;277(31):28,109–28,117.

15. Keithley E, Woolf NK, Harris JP. Development of morphological and physiological changes in the cochlea induced by cytomegalovirus. *Laryngoscope* 1989;99:409.

16. Yoo TJ, Tomoda K, Stuart JM, et al. Type II collagen-induced autoimmune sensorineural hearing loss and vestibular dysfunction in rats. *Ann Otol Rhinol Laryngol* 1983;92(3 Pt 1):267–271.

17. JP Harris, Woolf NK, Ryan AF. A reexamination of experimental type II collagen autoimmunity: Middle and inner ear morphology and function. *Ann Otol Rhinol Laryngol* 1986;95:176–180.

18. Beickert P. Aur frage der empfindungsschwerhorigkeit und autoallergie. *Z Laryngol Rhinol Otol* 1961;40:837.

19. Terayama Y, Sasaki Y. Studies on experimental allergic (isoimmune) labyrinthitis in guinea pig cochlea to detect autoantibodies in inner ear disorders. *Arch Otorhinolaryngol* 1963;58:49.

20. Harris JP. Experimental autoimmune sensorineural hearing loss. *Laryngoscope* 1987;97:63–76.

21. Yamanobe S, Harris JP. Spontaneous remission in experimental autoimmune labyrinthitis. *Ann Otol Rhinol Laryngol* 1992;101(12):1007–1014.

22. Gloddek B, Gloddek J, Arnold W. Induction of an inner-ear-specific autoreactive T-cell line for the diagnostic evaluation of an autoimmune disease of the inner ear. *Ann NY Acad Sci* 1997;830:266–276.

23. Kusakari C, Hozawa K, Koike S, et al. MRL/MP-lpr/lpr mouse as a model of immune-induced sensorineural hearing loss. *Ann Otol Rhinol Laryngol Suppl* 1992;157:82–86.

24. Lin DW, Trune DR. Breakdown of stria vascularis blood-labyrinth barrier in C3H/lpr autoimmune disease mice. *Otolaryngol Head Neck Surg* 1997;117(5):530–534.

25. Ruckenstein MJ, Milburn M, Hu L. Strial dysfunction in the MRL-Fas mouse. *Otolaryngol Head Neck Surg* 1999;121(4):452–456.

26. Theofilopoulos AN, Prud'Homme GJ, Dixon FJ. Autoimmune aspects of systemic lupus erythematosus. *Concepts Immunopathol* 1985;1:190–218.

27. Kyogoku M, Nose M, Sawai T, et al. Immunopathology of murine lupus—overview, SL/Ni and MRL/Mp-lpr/lpr-. *Prog Clin Biol Res* 1987;229:95–130.

28. Trune DR. Cochlear immunoglobulin in the C3H/lpr mouse model for autoimmune hearing loss. *Otolaryngol Head Neck Surg* 1997;117(5):504–508.

29. Trune DR, Wobig RJ, Kempton JB, et al. Steroid treatment improves cochlear function in the MRL.MpJ-Fas(lpr) autoimmune mouse. *Hear Res* 1999;137(1–2):160–166.

30. Ruckenstein MJ, Hu L. Antibody deposition in the stria vascularis of the MRL-Fas(lpr) mouse. *Hear Res* 1999;127(1–2):137–142.

31. Ruckenstein MJ, Keithley EM, Bennett T, et al. Ultrastructural pathology in the stria vascularis of the MRL-Fasl(lpr) mouse. *Hear Res* 1999;131(1–2):22–28.

32. Tago C, Yanagita N. Cochlear and renal pathology in the autoimmune strain mouse. *Ann Otol Rhinol Laryngol Suppl* 1992;157:87–91.

33. Nariuchi H, Sone M, Tago C, et al. Mechanisms of hearing disturbance in an autoimmune model mouse NZB/kl. *Acta Otolaryngol Suppl* 1994;514:127–131.

34. Soliman AM. Type II collagen-induced inner ear disease: critical evaluation of the guinea pig model. *Am J Otol* 1990;11:27.

35. Orozco CR, Niparko JK, Richardson BC, et al. Experimental model of immune-mediated hearing loss using cross-species immunization. *Laryngoscope* 1990;100:941.

36. Harris JP, Sharp P. Inner ear autoantibodies in patients with rapidly progressive sensorineural hearing loss. *Laryngoscope* 1990;97:63.

37. Moscicki RA, San Martin JE, Quintero CH, et al. Serum antibody to inner ear proteins in patients with progressive hearing loss. *JAMA* 1994;272:611–616.

38. Hirose K, Wener MH, Duckert LG. Utility of laboratory testing in autoimmune inner ear disease. *Laryngoscope* 1999;109:1749–1754.

39. Berrettini S, Ravecca F, Bruschini L, et al. Progressive sensorineural hearing loss: immunologic etiology. *Acta Otorhinolaryngol Ital* 1999; 18(4 Suppl 59):42–50.

40. Nair TS, Prieskorn DM, Miller JM, et al. In vivo binding and hearing loss after intracochlear infusion of KHRI-3 antibody. *Hear Res* 1997;107:93–101.

41. Nair TS, Kozma KE, Hoefling NL, et al. Identification and characterization of choline transporter-like protein 2, an inner ear glycoprotein of 68 and 72 kDa that is the target of antibody-induced hearing loss. *J Neurosci* 2004;24:1772–1779.

42. Solares CA, Edling AE, Johnson JM, et al. Murine autoimmune hearing loss mediated by CD4+ T cells specific for inner ear peptides. *J Clin Invest* 2004;113:1210–1217.

43. Sismanis A, Wise CM, Johnson GD. Methotrexate management of immune-mediated cochleovestibular disorders. *Otolaryngol Head Neck Surg* 1997;116(2):146–152.

44. Matteson EL, Fabry DA, Facer GW, et al. Open trial of methotrexate as treatment for autoimmune hearing loss. *Arthritis Rheum* 2001;45(2):146–150.

45. Harris JP, Weisman MH, Derebery JM, et al. Treatment of corticosteroid-responsive autoimmune inner ear disease with methotrexate. *JAMA* 2003;290:1875–1883.

46. Sismanis A, Wise CM, Johnson GD. Methotrexate management of immune-mediated cochleovestibular disorders. *Otolaryngol Head Neck Surg* 1997;116:146.

47. Sismanis A, Thompson T, Willis HE. Methotrexate therapy for autoimmune hearing loss: a preliminary report. *Laryngoscope* 1994;104(part 1):932–934.

48. Luetje CM. Theoretical and practical implications for plasmapheresis in autoimmune inner ear disease. *Laryngoscope* 1989;99:1137–1146.

49. Rahman MU, Poe DS, Choi HK. Etanercept therapy for immune-mediated cochleovestibular disorders: preliminary results in a pilot study. *Otol Neurotol* 2001;22(5):619–624.

50. Cohen SB, Shoup A, Weisman M, et al. Etanercept treatment of autoimmune inner ear disease: results of a pilot placebo-controlled study. *Otol Neurotol* 2005;26(5):903–907.

Aging and the Auditory and Vestibular System

153

Peter S. Roland   Ravi N. Samy

The geriatric population is the fastest growing segment of the population of all industrialized nations, including the United States. As life expectancy increases and healthcare costs rise, the medical profession will be challenged to provide cost-effective quality care. Aging affects every system and organ in the body; it does not spare the auditory or vestibular systems but instead causes presbycusis and presbyastasis, respectively. Compounding these problems, the elderly suffer concomitant age-related declines in the immune, musculoskeletal, visual, proprioceptive, cardiovascular, and central nervous systems. As otolaryngologists, we impact on our patients' longevity and quality of life.

Between 25 and 50% of the elderly suffer sufficient hearing loss, which degrades their quality of life. Loss of hearing negatively affects social interaction, leading to progressive isolation and withdrawal. Although hearing loss in the geriatric population is often due to presbycusis, other causes should always be sought.

Dix states that dizziness is the most common presenting complaint in patients 75 years or older; it typically affects more women than men. Balance disturbances contribute to functional declines in the elderly. Postural stability involves the complex integration of the visual, proprioceptive, somatosensory, and vestibular signals. Pathology in any of these systems can cause dizziness. The end result of this can be the occurrence of falls. Falls are the sixth leading cause of death in patients over 75 years of age. They cause over 200,000 hip, vertebral, skull, and extremity fractures yearly in Americans over 65 years of age. Dizziness is directly associated with 7% of falls.

A large number of disorders can cause dizziness, sometimes making the diagnosis laborious and difficult. However, 90% of the causes of dizziness can be placed in 1 of 7 categories (Table 153.1). One study of dizziness among the elderly identified a cardiovascular cause in 28%, peripheral vestibular disorder in 18%, central neurologic disorder in 14%, more than one diagnosis in 18%, and no identifiable cause in 22%.

AGE-RELATED CHANGES IN THE AUDITORY AND VESTIBULAR SYSTEMS

Anatomic changes that affect hearing and balance occur because of physiologic aging. One such example involves the production of cerumen. Cerumen consists of desquamated epithelium mixed with the sebum produced from sebaceous glands and the watery secretions of modified apocrine sweat glands. Modified apocrine sweat glands atrophy with age. Without the watery component, cerumen becomes drier, harder, and less likely to be moved out the external auditory canal (EAC) by the canal's normal transport and cleansing mechanism. The tragi hairs found in adult males become coarser, larger, and more prominent with age. Their presence can prevent the natural dislodgement of cerumen from the EAC, contributing to the increased incidence of cerumen impaction in the elderly male.

Arthritic changes in the diarthrodial joints of the ossicles are universal after age 70. These changes do not appear to produce any effect on hearing, however. Schuknecht identified four categories of presbycusis based on clinical and histopathologic changes within the cochlea:

1. Sensory: epithelial atrophy with loss of sensory cells and the supporting cells of the organ of Corti. Progressive hair cell reduction begins at about age 40.
2. Neural: a reduction in the number of functioning cochlear neurons. Of the 35,500 cochlea neurons at

TABLE 153.1

ETIOLOGY OF "DIZZINESS"

Peripheral vestibular disorders
Cardiovascular disorders
Multisensory dizziness
Brainstem cerebrovascular disease
Neurologic disorders
Psychiatric disease
Hyperventilation syndrome

birth, Schuknecht has estimated that 2,100 neurons are lost each decade. When reduction has reached 50% or more of the normal neuronal population, hearing loss develops.

3. Strial: atrophy of the stria vascularis. A loss of 30% or more of strial tissue can result in hearing loss.

4. Conductive: alterations of the basilar membrane produce stiffening. The precise nature of these changes is partially hypothesized on the basis of conductive loss that remains otherwise unexplained.

Although this classification is interesting, each of the four changes may be found to various degrees in any one individual subject; consequently, the audiograms of elderly individuals rarely conform to these classic patterns (Table 153.2).

Age-related anatomic and physiologic changes to the vestibular system also have been described. This has been demonstrated by differences in caloric responses, including low-frequency, low-amplitude changes and a reduced duration of nystagmus. Degenerative changes of the otoconia and reduction in hair cells in the semicircular canals (cristae ampullares) and otolithic organs (saccule and utricle) become more marked as age increases. Age-related degeneration of neural elements in Scarpa ganglia and the vestibular nerves has been demonstrated. These specialized neural cells cannot undergo replication or renewal. Briner et al. have also stated that the number of neurons in the vestibular system decreases with age. Decreased cell counts in the temporal lobes and cerebellum associated with aging, increased time required for information processing in the brain, and possibly increased transmission in the central auditory pathways have all been identified.

AUDITORY DYSFUNCTION

All of the usual cases of hearing loss can affect the elderly (Table 153.3). These disorders are addressed elsewhere in this textbook. With the exception of conductive loss associated with aging as described by Schuknecht, conductive hearing loss in the elderly population will have the same differential diagnosis as in younger individuals. Cerumen impaction is a more frequent cause than in other populations, as described earlier.

PRESBYCUSIS

The auditory system's durability is determined by genetic resistance and the physical stress imposed (Fig. 153.1). Genetically mediated hearing loss can be difficult to distinguish from presbycusis. The ability to differentiate hearing loss caused by defective genetic material is increasing as the types and tests of chromosomal abnormalities are identified. In any given individual, though, it is difficult to determine what component of the hearing loss is due to inherent genetic determination and what component is a consequence of stresses imposed, such as acoustic trauma, viral infections, otologic diseases, vascular diseases, and ototoxic medications. Multiple variables have been evaluated that contribute to hearing loss associated with aging (Table 153.4).

A well-documented phenomenon in elderly subjects is the disproportionate deterioration of speech discrimination for any given pure-tone threshold shift (Fig. 153.2). Tests of central auditory processing include time-compressed speech (word rate per min) and overlapping or interruption of words. These tests suggest that older patients have poorer speech discrimination than younger patients because of changes in central auditory processing. Decreased neuronal populations contribute to this phenomenon, as well. Elderly patients demonstrate prolonged latencies and reduced amplitudes on the auditory brainstem response.

AUDITORY REHABILITATION

Increasing awareness of the prevalence of presbycusis is important, as those with hearing loss tend to be more socially withdrawn and isolated. Patients tend to become frustrated, as do those trying to communicate with them. The main treatment for presbycusis is amplification. Cochlear implantation is an option for some, depending on the severity of the hearing loss. Assistive listening devices (such as FM systems, speaker phones, etc.) can also

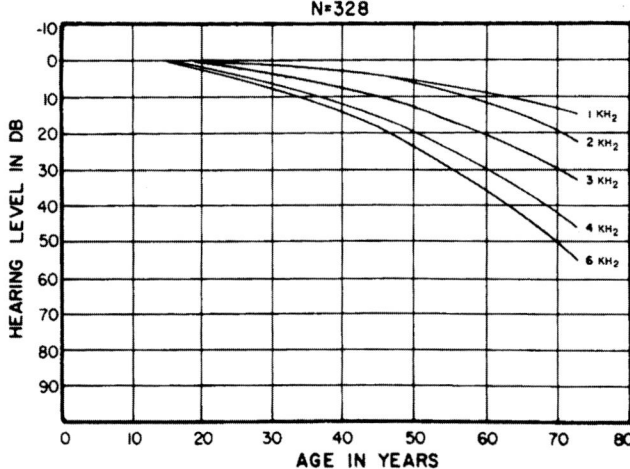

Figure 153.1 Hearing levels as a function of age. Hearing threshold shifts from 1 to 6 kHz. The pure-tone hearing levels (thresholds) increase with age, especially in the higher frequencies.

TABLE 153.2

CAUSES OF BILATERALLY SYMMETRIC SENSORINEURAL HEARING LOSS[a]

Disorder	Characteristics	Diagnosis	Treatment

Ménière disease	Episodic attacks of fluctuant SNHL, vertigo, tinnitus, aural fullness or pressure; bilateral in 20% to 30% of cases	History of typical attacks with symptom-free intervals; hearing loss involves low tones initially and later all frequencies; rule out neurosyphilis	Medical
			  Diuretics and low-salt diet
			Surgical
			  Decompression or shunt of endolymphatic sac; section of vestibular nerve

Luetic hearing loss (late-acquired syphilis)	Often bilateral SNHL with no characteristic audiometric pattern; speech discrimination score often worse than would be predicted on basis of pure-tone thresholds; often associated with vestibular symptoms; may mimic Ménière disease	Positive FTA-ABS test, with or without clinical history of syphilis	Penicillin and oral steroids
Paget disease	Slowly progressive SNHL and CHL; SNHL worse in high frequencies; maximum CHL of 20 to 30 dB at 500 Hz	Skeletal deformities of skull and long bones of extremities, elevated serum alkaline phosphatase and urinary hydroxyproline	Calcitonin
Hypothyroidism	Slowly progressive SNHL affecting all frequencies daily	Usual clinical stigmata of hypothyroidism; decreased serum T_4	Desiccated thyroid or synthetic mixture of T_4 and T_3
Ototoxic drugs	Hearing loss with or without vestibular dysfunction following treatment with known ototoxic drug	History	None
Hereditary progressive SNHL	Progressive SNHL beginning at earlier age than expected for presbycusis; possible positive family history	Family history	None
Noise-induced hearing loss	History of prolonged exposure to loud continuous noise or brief exposure to loud impulse noise	History; characteristic audiogram with maximum hearing loss at 4,000 Hz; may not be distinguishable from presbycusis	None; use of ear protectors may prevent further loss from noise exposure
Head trauma	Severe head injury often resulting in loss of consciousness and bilateral temporal bone fractures	History	None
Cochlear otosclerosis and far-advanced clinical otosclerosis	Far-advanced clinical otosclerosis (stapedial fixation) and cochlear otosclerosis; SNHLmay appear on audiogram as severe to profound SNHL; patient will have good speech modulation (unlike in profound SNHL) and will be wearing or will have worn a bone conduction hearing aid; possibly a family history of otosclerosis	History is suggestive but surgical exploration of stapes footplate is diagnostic and therapeutic; post-stapedectomy patient may be able to wear ear-level hearing aid with good results	Stapedectomy, sodium fluoride

SNHL, sensorineural hearing loss; FTA-ABS test, fluorescent treponemal antibody test; CHL, conductive hearing loss; Hz, hertz (cycles per second); dB, decibel (arbitrary unit of sound intensity).
[a]The hearing loss from any of these diseases may be improved with hearing aids unless it is of such a degree that hearing aids will be inadequate or unsatisfactory. Individuals with bilateral profound SNHL may be candidates for cochlear implant and should be evaluated by an otologist to determine their suitability for such a device.

be of aid. Patient should be taught to increase the signal-to-noise ratio of their surroundings, by reducing the ambient-/-background noise in a room and having someone look directly at them.

The effective use of hearing instruments and cochlear implants is made more complicated in the elderly by commonly associated deficits. Unfortunately, only about 30% of patients who can benefit from hearing aids actually have used them. Decreased vision, cosmetic concerns (feeling "old"), manual dexterity loss, and reduced mobility can make physically removing and adjusting these devices difficult. The financial costs and willingness to wear

TABLE 153.3
FACTORS CONTRIBUTING TO AGE-RELATED HEARING LOSS

Microvascular disease resulting in diminished profusion and hypoxia of labyrinthine hair cells and neurons
Effects of diet; in animals, free radical formation increases hearing loss
Noise exposure
Drug effects
Cigarette smoking

TABLE 153.4
CLINICAL MANIFESTATIONS OF PATHOLOGIC CHANGES WITHIN THE COCHLEA

Cochlear hair cell loss progresses the high-frequency hearing loss with speech discrimination preserved in the initial phases.
Neuronal loss: a nonprecipitous, generalized loss of pure-tone thresholds with speech discrimination impaired out of proportion to the threshold shift.
Atrophy of the stria: flat hearing loss with good preservation of speech discrimination.
Mechanical (cochlear conductive): gradually sloping high frequency hearing loss with speech discrimination impaired proportionate to the pure tone threshold shift.

the devices can be detriments. Cognitive deterioration and memory loss can seriously affect the elderly person's ability to extract maximum utility from hearing aids or cochlear implants. Technological advances include semi-implantable hearing aids, which may avoid some of the problems stated earlier.

VESTIBULAR DYSFUNCTION

The key to the evaluation of any patient with dizziness is a detailed description in the patient's own words of the sensation experienced. The subjective character of the dizziness can be classified into four broad categories (Table 153.5):

1. Vertigo (illusion of motion)
2. Presyncope
3. Dysequilibrium
4. Nonspecific (often psychological disorders)

The time course of the patient's symptoms can provide important clues to diagnosis. At the simplest level, one can distinguish between episodic or continuous symptoms. It

is helpful to elicit the temporal component of individual attacks as well as the entire course of the disorder:

1. Less than 1 minute: episodes of acute, rotational vertigo lasting less than 1 minute are most commonly associated with disorders of the peripheral vestibular system, such as benign paroxysmal positional vertigo (BPPV).
2. Less than 1 hour: Vertigo lasting a few minutes to an hour or two can be secondary to Ménière disease, transient cerebral hypoperfusion, migraine headaches, or phobic/anxiety disorders.
3. Several hours to 24 hours: This type of dizziness also suggests migraine headaches or Ménière disease. Viral or vascular labyrinthitis usually presents with acute rotational vertigo of several days' duration, with gradual improvement.

HISTORY AND PHYSICAL EXAMINATION

Before making a diagnosis in an elderly patient, the otologist needs to perform a thorough history and physical ex-

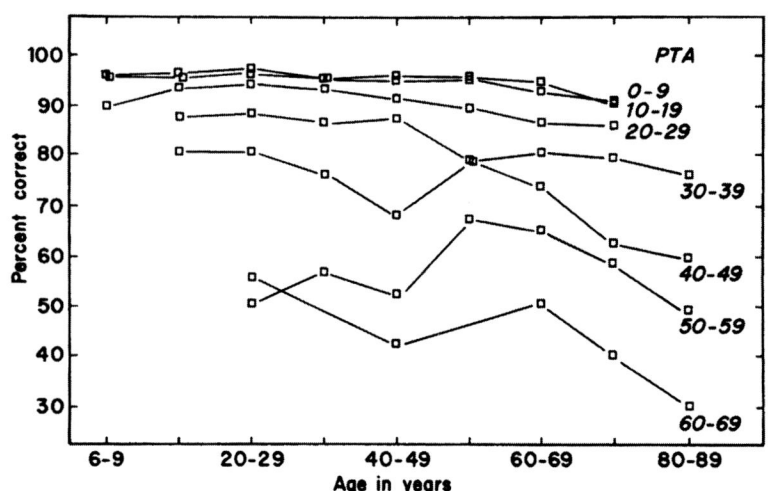

Figure 153.2 Prior to pure-tone hearing loss, the percentage of correct responses for speech discrimination decreases with increasing age. *PTA*, pure-tone average.

TABLE 153.5

TYPES OF DIZZINESS

Category	Sensation	Diagnosis
Vertigo	Illusion of motion, either linear or rotating (patient or environment)	Vestibular disturbance attributable to peripheral (BPPV, labyrinthitis) or central (brainstem, cerebellar) disease Cardiovascular disease
Presyncope	Impending faint	Diffuse cerebral ischemia attributable to vasovagal response, cardiac disease, or metabolic disorders
Dysequilibrium	Impaired balance and gaze	Impaired motor control due to neuromuscular disease, severe bilateral vestibular disease, stroke, multisensory deficits, or medications
Nonspecific	Light-headedness, "confusion," "wooziness," "foggy-headedness"	Often psychological disorders (anxiety, depression, panic), hyperventilation

amination. Presbystasis and presbycusis are diagnoses of exclusion; other pathologies must be ruled out. Associated otologic symptoms discussed with the patient include hearing loss, tinnitus, aural fullness, otorrhea, and otalgia. Patients also need to be asked about a history of significant noise exposure/trauma (e.g., loud music, gunfire, etc.), prior otologic/head and neck surgery, and a family history of hearing loss. Because of a high incidence of systemic illnesses in the elderly population, a detailed past medical and surgical history is obtained; one should delve after the presence of neurologic or ophthalmologic diseases, which can create symptoms of dizziness. Also, seek information about systemic disorders that interfere with cerebral blood supply that may produce vertigo due to either focal brainstem involvement or diffuse cerebral ischemia. Cardiac abnormalities (e.g., arrhythmia, valvular regurgitation/stenosis) can cause presyncopal episodes. Assess for systemic illnesses such as diabetes mellitus, hypothyroidism, human immunodeficiency virus (HIV) infection, and sexually transmitted diseases. The patient should be counseled on following with his primary care physician for the above conditions and to meet Centers for Disease Control (CDC) guidelines for screening tests and immunizations. If the patient presents with complaints of dizziness, he or she should be asked about a prior history of falls and whether driving or not.

A thorough history of prescription, nonprescription, and alternative medications is assessed. A social history is critical and should include an assessment of alcohol, caffeine, salt, tobacco, and illicit drug use. Cardiovascular drugs such as diuretics, beta-blockers, and vasodilators may produce presyncope and orthostatic symptomatology. Ototoxic drugs (e.g., aminoglycosides such as gentamicin) typically cause

disequilibrium and oscillopsia. Alcohol can cause postural hypotension resulting in presyncope. Psychiatric medications, muscle relaxants, and anticonvulsants also have been associated with disequilibrium (Table 153.6). It is believed that the more medications a geriatric patient is taking, the greater the chance of dizziness being present.

A complete neurologic examination should be performed and an evaluation made that is directed specifically at the otologic system. Otomicroscopic exam is done to rule out middle ear disease, cholesteatoma, or temporal bone tumors. A head and neck exam is done to rule out a concomitant otolaryngologic abnormality. A directed systemic (cardiovascular) examination may also be performed. Dix-Hallpike testing with Frenzel lenses should be performed. Drachman advocates the use of the Dizziness Simulation Battery in the office evaluation of dizziness (Table 153.7). The patient is asked to identify which of eight different maneuvers most closely reproduces a patient's dizziness. This test battery includes an assessment of hyperventilation, orthostatic hypotension, peripheral vestibulopathy, carotid sinus simulation, and multisensory disorders. The elderly patient with complaints of vertigo may suffer from all of the disorders that characterize the younger patient (e.g., BPPV, acute labyrinthitis, and Ménière disease) but more often typically has a multifactorial aspect to his or her symptoms.

Cerebrovascular insufficiency caused by ischemia of the labyrinth or central vestibular nuclei may result in episodes of acute vertigo associated with focal neurologic deficits such as dysphagia, hemiparesis, dysarthria, headache, or blurred vision. The diagnosis is clinically based and includes the presence of focal neurologic deficits. It can arise as a consequence of reduced flow caused by arterioscle-

TABLE 153.6		
MEDICATIONS THAT CAN PRODUCE OR EXACERBATE BALANCE DISTURBANCE		
Drug Class	**Type of Dizziness**	**Mechanism**
Alcohol	Unsteady gaze, positional vertigo	Cerebellar and vestibular dysfunction
Sedatives, anxiolytics	Nonspecific lightheadedness	Central nervous system depression
Antihypertensives	Presyncope	Orthostatic hypotension
Antiepileptics	Dysequilibrium	Cerebellar dysfunction
Aminoglycosides	Dysequilibrium, oscillopsia	Labyrinthine hair cell damage

rotic disease in the vertebrobasilar system, or it can arise as a consequence of compression of the vertebral arteries from cervical osteoarthritis. Positional vertigo is common among the elderly.

A brainstem stroke may present as paroxymal vertigo with unremitting nausea and vomiting, but a brief neurologic examination typically will uncover other neurologic deficits. Even so, patients are occasionally released from the emergency department with an inaccurate diagnosis because the patient may only be aware of the fact that even small, brief head movements precipitate overwhelming vertigo, nausea, and vomiting. He may be unaware of the other neurologic deficits produced by the infarct.

Orthostatic hypotension occurs only when the patient assumes the standing position from the supine or sitting positions. By strict criteria, orthostatic hypotension requires a 20 mm Hg decrease in systolic pressure or a 10 mm Hg reduction in diastolic pressure 2 minutes after standing. The sensitivity and specificity of this test has been debated. Many patients have subjective dysequilibrium, vertigo, and presyncope without ever meeting the strict definitional criteria. A cardiologist may perform tilt-table testing if the di-

agnosis is still suspected. Postural hypotension arises from pooling of blood in the lower extremities because of decreased tone. The chronic use of antihypertensive agents, prolonged bed rest, and autonomic dysfunction can all produce orthostatic hypotension. Vasovagal attacks (faints) may be induced when strong emotions activate the brainstem medullary vasodepressor centers. Vagal hyperactivity causes a decreased cardiac output, leading to a decrease in cerebral blood flow. Decreased cardiac output because of arrhythmia, congestive heart failure, myocardial infarction, and valvular disease (such as aortic stenosis) may lead to the presyncopal type of lightheadedness.

Bilateral symmetric vestibular loss results in persistent unsteadiness. This type of imbalance is typically worse in the dark, when visual cues are not available to help compensate for the loss. Bilateral vestibulopathy can arise from ototoxic drug exposure but also occurs as an idiopathic degenerative disorder. Proprioceptive and somatosensory loss can produce dysequilibrium that is worse in the dark. It is often secondary to peripheral neuropathy (common in patients with diabetes mellitus or renal failure). Osteoarthritis of the cervical spine may cause disequilibrium due to spinal stenosis with spinal cord compression. Such patients often demonstrate bowel and bladder dysfunction. Degenerative disease of the cervical spine may also produce a sense of disequilibrium and imbalance because of altered proprioceptive feedback from muscle stretch receptors and position sense receptors in the muscle and joints of the cervical spine.

Lesions of the frontal lobes or basal ganglia cause disequilibrium often associated with weakness, rigidity, or tremor. Cerebellar lesions cause severe disequilibrium with or without visual cues and are often associated with visible nystagmus, a wide-based gait, and truncal ataxia. Parkinson disease, common among the elderly, produces characteristic postural and motor abnormalities, resulting in a festinating gait. These patients usually stand in a posture of flexion with the thoracic spine bent forward and the head bent down. With forward locomotion, the patient takes short, shuffling steps that become successively more rapid, and the patient may fall without assistance. This disturbance of posture and motor control often re-

TABLE 153.7
DIZZINESS SIMULATION BATTERY

Cardiovascular
Orthostatic blood pressure testing
Potentiated Valsalva maneuver (produces presyncope)
Carotid sinus stimulation

Vestibular
Dix-Hallpike maneuver (only produces vertigo in patients with positioning vertigo)
Barany rotation (stimulates horizontal semicircular canals, producing vertigo in anyone who retains some vestibular function)

Multisensory
Walk and turn
Seated head turn

Psychiatric
Hyperventilation (30 seconds)

sults in disequilibrium. The postural instability typically does not repond to levodopa.

Multisensory impairments are due to impaired physiologic function in several systems simultaneously and are more common in the elderly than in the young. Modest disturbances in each of these symptoms may synergize to produce postural instability and disequilibrium out of proportion to the individual deficits. Subjects with multisensory impairments typically present with a sense of disequilibrium during standing or walking. Multidisciplinary care involving the geriatric specialist, cardiologist, neurologist, vestibular physical therapist, and ophthalmologist can be warranted.

Hyperventilation is often a consequence of anxiety or phobic disorders. Diffuse cerebral ischemia results from constriction of the cerebral vasculature caused by decreased carbon dioxide content in the blood. Anxiety and panic disorders, adjustment reactions, and depressive disorders are the most common diagnoses. Such patients often describe a chronic feeling of "wooziness." Two mechanisms have been proposed by Sloane: (a) Patients with underlying primary psychological disorders may be more susceptible to impairment by diseases affecting neurosensory systems, and (b) dizziness symptoms themselves impair function and may cause secondary psychological problems. Management consists of treating the appropriate underlying disorder when present.

DIAGNOSTIC EVALUATION

In straightforward cases (e.g., posterior canal BPPV), the diagnosis is easily determined by a careful and detailed history and physical examination. An audiogram is a relatively inexpensive but useful screening tool. In patients with vague symptoms, complicating histories, and significant comorbidities, detailed testing is required. This may include electronystagmography (ENG) or videonystagmography (VNG), rotary chair testing, auditory brainstem response (ABR), electrocochleography (ECochG), and posturography. Radiologic studies (CT and/or MRI scans) can be ordered as deemed necessary. These different tests are discussed further in detail elsewhere in this book.

MANAGEMENT

A sensation of imbalance and a fear of falling lead to a greater level of inactivity and social isolation, worsening the quality of life in a group of people who may have already lost spouses, friends, and other social support because of their age. When possible, treatment is directed at the underlying cause of the dizziness, as described under those conditions. Sometimes, however, the only available option is nonspecific therapy directed at symptom control. In general, medical therapy for patients with an acute loss of vestibular function is aimed at controlling the acute vestibular and autonomic symptoms. Five main classes of drugs are used: antihistamines (e.g., meclizine), phenothiazines (e.g., promethazine), anticholinergics (e.g., scopolamine), 5HT3 antagonists (e.g., ondansetron), and benzodiazepines (e.g., diazepam). All drugs should be administered sparingly and for short durations (1 to 2 weeks) because they can cause a reduction in central nervous system (CNS) compensation. Meclizine is typically administered in doses of 12.5 to 25 mg orally three times per day as needed for acute, peripheral vertigo of long duration. Benzodiazepines (usually diazepam at 2.5 to 7.5 mg daily in divided doses) suppress vestibular output of the vestibular nuclei.

Benzodiazepines are the most effective vestibular suppressants. 5HT3 antagonists may be helpful if nausea and/or vomiting are prominent symptoms. However, there is no evidence of 5HT3 receptors within the vestibular system. Phenothiazines can be administered rectally if nausea and/or vomiting does not allow oral intake of medications. All medication should be used cautiously in the elderly, to avoid CNS side effects. Many of these classes of drugs share the same side effect profile. Antihistamines, phenothiazines, and anticholinergics all share the propensity to produce sedation, dysphoria, and disorientation. If combination therapy is used, care is taken to avoid synergy of side effects. Many geriatric patients are already taking drugs with anticholinergic or sedative side effects. The interaction of vestibular suppressants with these medications is carefully considered.

Vestibular rehabilitation has been an effective therapy for more than 50 years. In addition, it can be used in conjunction with other types of physical therapy and exercise. Many of the problems associated with aging may be due primarily to inactivity. It is thought that some of the aging process itself can be slowed by exercising and physical activity. Vestibular rehabilitation involves specific habituation exercises designed to enhance the normal adaptive mechanisms in the CNS. The benefits of vestibular rehabilitation are not affected by a patient's age. The goal in these patients is fall prevention. One in three elderly people living in the community fall each year; hospital or nursing home patients fall two times more often. Vestibular symptoms precede falls in more than 50% of these patients. Program strategies vary depending on the patient's primary problem, but they are aimed at stabilizing gaze and posture, improving CNS adaptation, conditioning, and providing emotional and psychological support. The principal components of effective vestibular rehabilitation include gaze stabilization, balance retraining, and desensitization. Each aspect is addressed separately using different exercises.

Gaze stabilization exercises promote vestibular adaptation through exercises that stimulate the vestibulo-ocular reflex (VOR). Balance retraining starts with activities that progressively decrease the patient's base of support and progress to gaze exercises performed on varied surfaces (e.g., stairs, foam, balance beams). The balance system is challenged by having patients attempt to walk through crowded hallways. Strengthening exercises are prescribed to improve muscle strength and flexibility. Given the buoyancy of water, swimming pool exercises provide a safe environment in which the elderly can exercise. Repetitive head and arm movements designed to promote vertigo and unsteadiness in a safe and predictable environment enhance the CNS adaptive mechanisms. These exercises are repeated until they are no longer tolerated. Over a 6- to 8-week course, the number of repetitions is slowly increased. Vestibular rehabilitation is administered by a physical therapist with special expertise in treating vestibular disorders in the elderly. These rehabilitation strategies are effective in positional vertigo and to compensate for sudden loss of vestibular function (after recovery from an acute attack and after vegetative symptoms have disappeared). These exercises also provide improvement in patients with multisensory deficits.

ABLATIVE THERAPY

Patients who continue to suffer from incapacitating, lifestyle-limiting dizziness despite maximum medical therapy may be candidates for chemical or surgical ablative therapy, such as labyrinthectomy or vestibular nerve section. This therapy needs to be undertaken cautiously, however, particularly in the elderly. Recovery from unilateral loss of vestibular function is felt to be slower and less complete in the geriatric population.

SUMMARY

More than 12.5 million people over the age of 65 in the United States are thought to be significantly affected by dizziness or balance disturbances. Dizziness is the most common presenting complaint in patients over 75 years of age. The majority of the geriatric population with dizziness has multifactorial causes; it is important that one be familiar with the differential diagnosis, evaluation, and potentially multidisciplinary management of these disorders. It is inappropriate to attribute symptoms such as dizziness to the aging process alone; a complete evaluation must be performed. The otologist should be prepared to make referrals to a neurologist, audiologist, cardiologist, ophthalmologist, or psychiatrist and work in conjunction with the primary care physician to provide a full evaluation and comprehensive care.

HIGHLIGHTS

- Aging produces changes in the auditory and vestibular system that result in loss of function.
- Alterations in the physiology of the EAC lead to a dramatically increased incidence of cerumen impaction in the elderly.
- Presbycusis is multifactorial.
- Presbycusis is a diagnosis of exclusion; other cases should be sought.
- Elderly subjects with presbycusis may have degradation of speech discrimination out of proportion to pure-tone loss.
- Amplification and cochlear implantation can significantly improve the quality of life for elderly patients.
- Dizziness is the most common presenting complaint in patients over 75 years of age.
- A specific cause of dizziness and vertigo can be found in 85% of elderly patients.
- The differential diagnosis of balance disturbance in the elderly can often be rapidly narrowed by determining if they complain of symptoms of true vertigo, presyncope, chronic disequilibrium, or of nonspecific complaints.

SUGGESTED READINGS

Briner W, Linthicum FH, Gadre AK. Three dimensional structure of the human vestibular complex. *J Vestib Res* 1991;1:339–345.

Dix MR. Rehabilitation of vertigo. In: Dix MR, Hood JD, eds. *Vertigo.* New York: Wiley, 1984:467–479.

Eaton DA, Roland PS. Dizziness in the older adult. Parts 1 and 2. *Geriatrics* 2003 Apr:58(4).

Kennedy R and Clemis DJ. The geriatric auditory and vestibular systems. *Otolaryngol Clin North Am* 1990;23(6):1075–1080.

Lalwani AK. Vertigo, disequilibrium, and imbalance with aging. In: Jackler RK, Brackmann DE, eds. *Neurotology,* 2nd ed. Philadelphia: Mosby, 2005. 533–539.

LeBlanc KE, Bond TK. Exercise and aging. *Resid Staff Physician.* August 2004;50(8):34–39.

Moncada LV. Diagnosis and treatment of falls in the elderly. *Resid Staff Physician.* August 2004;50(8):28–33.

Roland PS, Eaton D, Meyerhoff WL. Aging in the auditory and vestibular system. *Otolaryngol Head Neck Surg* 2001;153:1941.

Rubenstein LZ, Josephson KR. The epidemiology of falls and syncope. *Clin Geriatr Med* 2002;18:141–158.

Schuknecht HF. *Pathology of the ear,* 2nd ed. Philadelphia: Lea & Febiger, 1993.

Sloane P, Hartman M, Mitchell M. Psychological factors associated with chronic dizziness in patients aged 60 and older. *J Am Geriatr Soc* 1994;42:847–852.

Sloane PD. Evaluation and management of dizziness in the older patient. *Clin Geriatr Med* 1996;12:785–801.

Whitney SL, Wrisley DM, Marchetti GF, et. al. The effect of age on vestibular rehabilitation outcomes. *Laryngoscope* 2002;112(10):1785–1790.

Cochlear Implants and Other Implantable Auditory Prostheses

154

Richard T. Miyamoto   *Karen Iler Kirk*

The electrically generated sensation of hearing has been extensively studied since Djourno and Eyries (1) first described direct excitation of the auditory nerve in 1957. Devices of increasing sophistication have secured a permanent role for cochlear implants in the management of selected children and adults with severe-to-profound hearing loss. Cochlear implants seek to replace a nonfunctional inner-ear hair-cell transducer system by converting mechanical sound energy into electrical signals that can be delivered to the cochlear nerve in profoundly deaf patients. The essential components of a cochlear implant system are as follows:

- A microphone, which picks up acoustic information and converts it to electrical signals;
- An externally worn speech processor that processes the signal according to a predefined strategy;
- A surgically implanted electrode array that is in the cochlea near the auditory nerve.

The processed signal is amplified and compressed to match the narrow electrical dynamic range of the ear. The typical response range of a deaf ear to electrical stimulation is on the order of only 10 to 20 dB, even less in the high frequencies. Transmission of the electrical signal across the skin from the external unit to the implanted electrode array most commonly is accomplished by the use of electromagnetic induction or radio frequency transmission. The critical residual neural elements stimulated appear to be the spiral ganglion cells or axons. Damaged or missing hair cells of the cochlea are bypassed (2).

COCHLEAR IMPLANT SYSTEMS

Multichannel, multi-electrode cochlear implant systems are designed to take advantage of the tonotopic organization of the cochlea. The incoming speech signal is filtered into a number of frequency bands, each corresponding to a given electrode in the array. Thus, multichannel cochlear implant systems use place coding to transfer spectral information in the speech signal as well as encoding the durational and intensity cues of speech. Several commercially available cochlear implant systems have received U.S. Food and Drug Administration (FDA) approval for use in adults and children.

Nucleus 24 Cochlear Implant System

Two of the FDA-approved implants, the Nucleus 22-channel system (3) and the Nucleus 24 cochlear implant system, are manufactured by Cochlear Corporation. The Nucleus 22-channel cochlear implant was the first multichannel cochlear implant to receive FDA approval for use in both adults and children and it has been used in more patients than any other cochlear implant system worldwide.

Early speech processing strategies (F0F2 and F0F1F2) used with the Nucleus 22-channel cochlear implant used feature-extraction schemes that conveyed information about key speech features such as the amplitude and frequency of vowel formants and the fundamental frequency of voiced sounds. The third generation speech processing strategy used in the Nucleus 22 device was the Mulitpeak (MPEAK) strategy. MPEAK encoded additional high-frequency information by stimulating two of three more basal fixed electrodes; the goal was to provide additional information that would yield improved consonant recognition scores. The most recent speech processing strategy offered in the Nucleus 22 channel cochlear implant system is the Spectral Peak (SPEAK) strategy, described below.

The Nucleus 24-channel cochlear implant system received FDA approval for use in adults and children in 1998. The Nucleus 24 electrode array contains 22 intracochlear electrodes and two extracochlear ground electrodes that permit up to 20 channels of information. It offers three speech-processing strategies. The first two, SPEAK (4) and Advanced Combination Encoder Strategy (ACE) (5), dynamically represent the dominant frequency and intensity characteristics (spectral peaks) of the speech signal by sequentially stimulating multiple electrodes with high-rate digital pulses. They differ in the number of spectral peaks identified per cycle (6 to 10 for SPEAK vs 8 to 12 for ACE) and in stimulation rate (ACE uses a faster stimulation rate than SPEAK). The third strategy, Continuous Interleaved Sampling (CIS) (6,7), filters the incoming sound into a small number of fixed frequency bands (between 8 and 12) and modulates one interleaved pulse train per frequency band with the envelope amplitude of each filter output. Thus, fine temporal details in the speech signal are preserved in the CIS strategy. All three programming strategies are offered in both a body-worn and a behind-the-ear speech processor.

Clarion Cochlear Implant System

The third commercially available device is the Clarion multichannel cochlear implant system (8–10). Early generations of this cochlear implant system received FDA approval for use in adults and children in 1996 and 1997, respectively. The newest version of the Clarion cochlear implant system is the Hi Resolution (HiRes) Bionic Ear. The system architecture is built around 16 independently controllable output circuits that drive 16 focusing intracochlear electrode contacts. HiRes divides the acoustic spectrum into 16 channels of frequency information, and the spectrum is processed across all channels at stimulation rates greater than 80,000 pulses per second. The Clarion cochlear implant system can stimulate the electrodes either non-simultaneously (using CIS) or simultaneously or in a variety of combinations (11). Thus, the programming audiologist can control the pattern of stimulation in the cochlea to permit up to 31 "virtual" channels (11). Both body-worn and behind-the-ear speech processors are available for users of the Clarion cochlear implant system.

Med-El Cochlear Implant System

The Med-El Combi 40+ cochlear implant system received FDA approval for use in adults and children in 2001. The Combi 40+ system uses an electrode array containing 12 electrode pairs that can be inserted deep into the apical regions of the cochlea (11,12). Two sequential, non-simultaneous, speech-processing strategies are available. The CIS+ is similar to CIS as implemented in the Nucleus device (11). The Med-El device also offers an *n-of-m* strategy similar to ACE that allows the programming audiologist to specify the number of spectral peaks (*n*) and the number of bandpass filters (*m*). Both body-worn and behind-the-ear speech processors are available.

New Developments in Cochlear Implant Design

Both Cochlear Corporation Ltd. and Advanced Bionics Corporation, Inc., manufacturers of the Nucleus and Clarion cochlear implants, respectively, have introduced new designs in the internal electrode array used with their speech processors. The Nucleus Contour electrode array and the Clarion HiFocus electrode array are both designed to more closely approximate the modiolar wall of the cochlea. Because the spiral ganglion cells are thought to be the sites stimulated by cochlear implants, this positioning may improve spatial specificity of stimulation and reduce the current needed to drive the electrodes (13). (However, because of a suspected relation to meningitis, the Clarion positioner has been withdrawn from the market.)

PATIENT SELECTION

Adults

Cochlear implantation was limited initially to postlingually deafened adults who received no benefit from hearing aids and had no possibility of worsening residual hearing. This population, particularly those with a recent onset of deafness, has been the most readily identifiable beneficiary of cochlear implants. A period of auditory experience adequate to develop normal speech perception, speech production, and language skills before the onset of deafness is an invaluable prerequisite. Experience gained with this initial cochlear implant population served to establish expected performance limits (14).

Table 154.1 presents the current cochlear implant candidacy criteria for adults. Adult candidacy criteria are based

---

TABLE 154.1

ADULT CANDIDACY CRITERIA FOR COCHLEAR IMPLANTATION

$\geq$ 18 years of age
Bilateral severe-to-profound hearing loss
Minimal benefit from conventional hearing aids (typically defined as sentence recognition scores < 40%–50% correct in the best aided condition)
No medical contraindications

primarily on aided speech recognition abilities. No upper age limit is used in the selection process as long as the patient's health will permit an elective surgical procedure. Cochlear implantation is appropriate if other selection criteria are met and the patient's general health permits an elective surgical procedure under general anesthesia. In a survey of Nucleus 22-channel cochlear implant recipients over the age of 65 years, Horn and McMahon (15) showed that elderly cochlear implant patients obtained benefits that were similar to those obtained by younger adult patients with the same device.

As indicated in Table 154.1, adult candidacy criteria now include adults with severe-to-profound hearing loss who derive some limited benefit from conventional hearing aids. Implantation of an ear with any residual, aidable hearing carries the risk that the implanted ear could be made worse than that ear with a hearing aid. Current investigations are testing the hypotheses that an ear with some residual hearing may have a better neuronal population, increasing the likelihood of superior performance with a cochlear implant, especially with more complex multichannel stimulation.

It should be noted that adults with prelingual hearing loss generally are not considered good candidates for cochlear implantation (16). However, prelinguistically deafened adults who have followed an aural/oral educational approach may receive significant benefit.

Children

Cochlear implantation in the pediatric population is a complex process that superimposes advanced technology upon existing rehabilitation and educational programs for deaf children. In contrast to adults, both prelingually and postlingually deafened children are candidates for cochlear implantation. As a result of several rigorous clinical trials evaluating safety and efficacy, a trend toward earlier cochlear implantation and implantation in children with more residual hearing has emerged. Current FDA guidelines permit implantation of children as young as 12 months of age.

Candidacy criteria differ according to the age of the patient being considered. Pediatric candidacy criteria are presented in Table 154.2.

One significant demographic factor affecting speech and language development in children with hearing loss is the age at which appropriate intervention is provided (17,18). Early auditory experience is critical for the development of neural connections in the peripheral and central auditory pathways. Animal studies indicate that early auditory deprivation causes a lack of maturation or degeneration of the auditory cortex (19,20). Restoration of hearing through cochlear implantation can mitigate the effects of auditory deprivation in animals, but only if it occurs during early sensitive periods in development (20,21). Data from humans also suggest the existence of a critical period for electrical stimulation of the auditory cortex in children with profound deafness. For example, the latency of the cortical evoked potential wave P1 is age-appropriate in children implanted by 3.5 years (22) but significantly delayed in children implanted at later ages (22,23). Sharma et al. (22) suggest that the central auditory system of young deaf children is maximally plastic during this early time window.

Prerequisites to early implantation include the early identification of hearing loss and the determination of hearing aid benefit in very young children (24). With the advent of universal newborn hearing screening, the average age at identification has dropped from 18 to 24 months to 2 months of age (25,26). This has mandated a reevaluation of the lower age limit appropriate for cochlear implantation, and more children than ever before now are being considered for cochlear implants near the time of their first birthday. In an attempt to ameliorate the detrimental effects of early auditory deprivation, several children have been implanted between the ages of 6 and 12 months. In fact, approximately 140 children in the United States have received a cochlear implant prior to their first birthday (27).

Because the development of speech perception, speech production, and language competence normally begins at

TABLE 154.2

PEDIATRIC CANDIDACY CRITERIA FOR COCHLEAR IMPLANTATION

Children Aged 12 mo to 24 mo	Children Aged 25 mo to 17 y, 11 mo
Bilateral profound hearing loss	Bilateral severe-to-profound hearing loss
Lack of auditory skills development and minimal hearing aid benefit (documented by parent questionnaire)	Lack of auditory skills development and minimal hearing aid benefit (word recognition scores < 30% correct)
No medical contraindications	No medical contraindications
Enrollment in a therapy of education program emphasizing auditory development	Enrollment in a therapy of education program emphasizing auditory development

a very early age, implantation in very young congenitally or neonatally deafened children may have substantial advantages. Early implantation may be particularly important when the etiology of deafness is meningitis, because progressive intracochlear ossification can occur and preclude standard electrode insertion. A relatively short window of time exists during which this advancing process can be circumvented.

Implanting very young children remains controversial because the audiologic assessment, surgical intervention, and postimplant management in this population can be challenging. Profound deafness must be substantiated and the inability to benefit from conventional hearing aids demonstrated. This can be difficult to determine in young children with limited language abilities. For very young children, parental questionnaires commonly are used to assess amplification benefit.

Because cochlear implantation involves an elective surgical procedure performed under a general anesthetic, it is imperative that an experienced pediatric anesthesiologist be an integral part of the surgical team. There may be a slightly greater anesthetic risk in children younger than 1 year of age (28). Special consideration must be given to the small dimensions of the temporal bone and to potential problems from postoperative temporal bone growth. In addition, the high incidence of otitis media in children under the age of 2 years might compromise the biosafety of cochlear implants. Nonetheless, extension of implant candidacy to the 6-to-12 months age group is feasible on an anatomic basis. The cochlea is adult size at birth, and by 1 year of age, the facial recess and mastoid antrum, which provide access to the middle ear for electrode placement, are adequately developed (29).

CLASSIFICATION OF COCHLEAR IMPLANT RECIPIENTS

Cochlear implant recipients can be loosely divided into three main categories, which significantly affect the anticipated outcomes when this technology is applied.

Postlingually Deafened Adults and Children

Patients who become deaf at or after age 5 years generally are classified as *postlingually* deafened. Even though these patients have developed many aspects of spoken language before the onset of their deafness, they frequently demonstrate rapid deterioration in the intelligibility of their speech once they lose access to auditory input and feedback. Implantation soon after the onset of deafness potentially can ameliorate this rapid deterioration in speech production and perception abilities. A postlingual onset of deafness is an infrequent occurrence in the pediatric population. If this were to be the only category for which cochlear implants

positively impacted deaf children, there would be limited applicability for this technology in children.

Congenitally or Early Deafened Children

Congenital or *early-acquired* deafness is the most frequently encountered type of profound sensorineural hearing loss in children. The acquisition of oral communication skills can be a difficult process for these children. However, with early implantation and appropriate habilitation, many children in this category are developing spoken language. Although considerable outcome variability exists, the most successful pediatric cochlear implant recipients demonstrate age-appropriate speech and language skills.

Congenitally or Early Deafened Adolescents and Adults

When cochlear implantation is considered in adolescence or young adulthood for a patient who has had little or no experience with sound because of congenital or early-onset deafness, caution must be exercised because this group has not demonstrated high levels of success with electrical stimulation of the auditory system.

AUDIOLOGIC ASSESSMENT

The audiologic evaluation is the primary means of determining suitability for cochlear implantation. Audiologic evaluations should be conducted in both an unaided condition and with appropriately fit conventional amplification. Thus, all potential candidates must have completed a period of experience with a properly fit hearing aid, preferably coupled with training in an appropriate aural rehabilitation program. The audiologic evaluation includes measurement of pure tone thresholds along with word and sentence recognition testing. Aided speech recognition scores are the primary audiologic determinant of cochlear implant candidacy. For very young children or those with limited language abilities, parent questionnaires are used to determine hearing aid benefit.

MEDICAL ASSESSMENT

The medical assessment includes the otologic history and physical examination. Radiologic evaluation of the cochlea is performed to determine whether the cochlea is present and patent and to identify congenital deformities of the cochlea. High-resolution, thin-section computed tomography (CT) scanning of the cochlea remains the imaging technique of choice (30). Usually, CT scanning can demonstrate intracochlear bone formation caused by labyrinthitis ossificans; however, when soft-tissue obliteration occurs following sclerosing labyrinthitis, CT may not image the obstruction. In these cases, T2-weighted magnetic resonance imaging (MRI) is an effective adjunctive procedure providing additional information regarding cochlear patency. The endolymph/perilymph signal may be lost in sclerosing labyrinthitis. Intracochlear ossification is not a contraindication to cochlear implantation, but can limit the type and insertion depth of the electrode array that can be introduced into the cochlea. Congenital malformations of the cochlea, likewise, are not contraindications to cochlear implantation. Cochlear dysplasia has been reported to occur in approximately 20% of children with congenital sensorineural hearing loss (31). Several reports of successful implantations in children with inner-ear malformations have been published (32–40). A thin cribriform area between the modiolus and a widened internal auditory canal is often observed (41) and is believed to be the route of egress of cerebrospinal fluid (CSF) when it occurs during surgery or postoperatively. A CSF gusher was reported in several cases. Temporal-bone dysplasia also may be associated with an anomalous facial nerve, which may increase the surgical risk.

The precise etiology for the deafness cannot always be determined but is identified whenever possible; however, stimulable auditory neural elements are nearly always present regardless of cause of deafness (42). Two exceptions are the *Michel deformity*, in which there is a congenital agenesis of the cochlea, and the *small internal auditory canal syndrome*, in which the cochlear nerve may be congenitally absent.

Routine otoscopic evaluation of the tympanic membrane is performed. An otologically stable condition should be present prior to considering implantation. The ear proposed for cochlear implantation must be free of infection, and the tympanic membrane must be intact. If these conditions are not met, medical or surgical treatment before implantation is required. The management of middle-ear effusions in children who are under consideration for cochlear implantation or who already have a cochlear implant deserves special consideration. Conventional antibiotic treatment usually accomplishes this goal, but when it does not, treatment by myringotomy and insertion of tympanostomy tubes may be required. Removal of the tube several weeks before cochlear implantation usually results in a healed, intact tympanic membrane. When an effusion occurs in an ear with a cochlear implant, no treatment is required as long as the effusion remains uninfected. Chronic otitis media, with or without cholesteatoma, must be resolved before implantation; this is accomplished with conventional otologic treatments. Prior ear surgery that has resulted in a mastoid cavity does not contraindicate cochlear implantation, but this situation may require mastoid obliteration with closure of the external auditory canal or reconstruction of the posterior bony ear canal.

PSYCHOLOGICAL ASSESSMENT

Psychological testing is performed for exclusionary reasons to identify subjects who have organic brain dysfunction, mental retardation, undetected psychosis, or unrealistic expectations. Valuable information related to the family dynamics and other factors in the patient's milieu that may affect implant acceptance and performance are assessed.

SURGICAL IMPLANTATION

Cochlear implantation in both children and adults requires meticulous attention to the delicate tissues and small dimensions. Skin incisions are designed to provide access to the mastoid process and coverage of the external portion of the implant package while preserving the blood supply of the postauricular skin. The incision used at the Indiana University Medical Center has eliminated the need to develop a large postauricular flap (Fig. 154.1). The inferior extent of the incision is made well posterior to the mastoid tip to preserve the branches of the postauricular artery. From here the incision is directed posterior-superiorly. In children, the incision incorporates the temporalis muscle to give added thickness. A subperiosteal pocket is created for positioning the

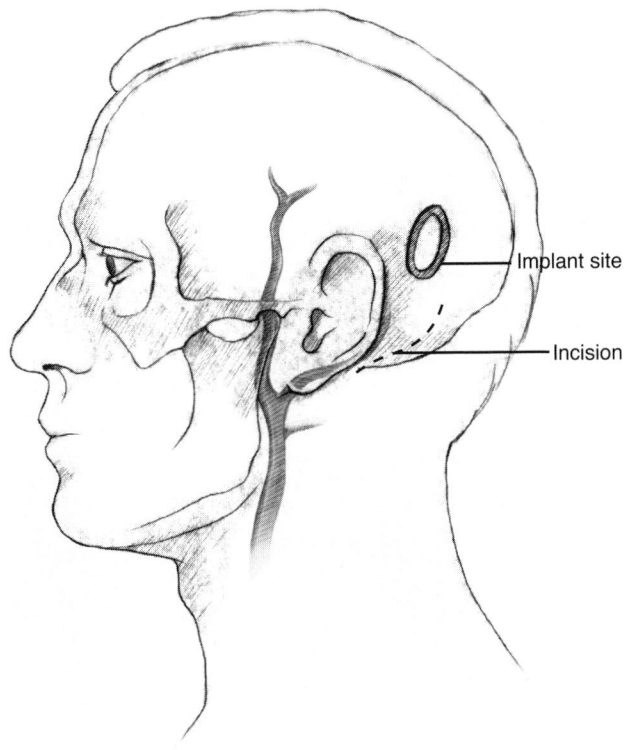

Figure 154.1 Incision and implant site for cochlear implantation.

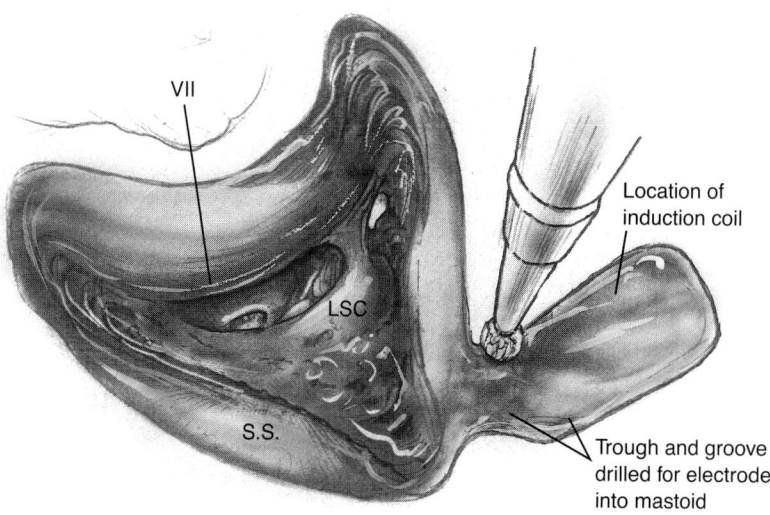

Figure 154.2 Location of induction coil. Trough and groove drilled for electrode implantation into mastoid.

implant induction coil (Fig. 154.2). A bone well tailored to the device being implanted is created, and the induction coil is fixed to the cortex with a fixation suture or periosteal flaps.

Following development of the skin incision, a mastoidectomy is performed. The horizontal semicircular canal is identified in the depths of the mastoid antrum, and the short process of the incus is identified in the fossa incudis. The facial recess is opened using the fossa incudis as an initial landmark. The facial recess is a triangular area bound by (a) the fossa incudis superiorly, (b) the chorda tympani nerve laterally and anteriorly, and (c) the facial nerve medially and posteriorly. The facial nerve usually can be visualized through the bone without exposing it. The round window niche is visualized through the facial recess about 2 mm inferior to the stapes (Fig. 154.3; Fig. 154.4). Occasionally, the round window niche is posteriorly positioned and is not well visualized through the facial recess or is obscured by ossification. Particularly in these situations, it is important

not to be misdirected by hypotympanic air cells. Entry into the scala tympani is accomplished best through a cochleostomy created anterior and inferior to the annulus of the round window membrane (Fig. 154.5; Fig. 154.6). A small fenestra slightly larger than the electrode to be implanted (usually 0.5 mm) is developed. A small diamond burr is used to "blue line" the endosteum of the scala tympani, and the endosteal membrane is removed by using small picks. This approach bypasses the hook area of the scala tympani, allowing direct insertion of the active electrode array. After insertion of the active electrode array, the cochleostomy area is sealed with small pieces of fascia.

Special Surgical Considerations

In cases of cochlear dysplasia, a CSF gusher may be encountered. The senior author prefers to enter the cochlea through a small fenestra and tightly pack the electrode at

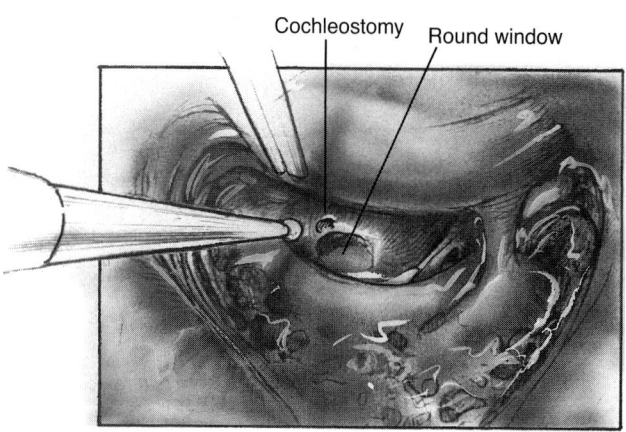

Figure 154.3 The facial recess is bounded by the fossa incudis superiorly, the chorda tympani nerve laterally and anteriorly, and the facial nerve medially and posteriorly. A cochleostomy is created anterior and inferior to the round window.

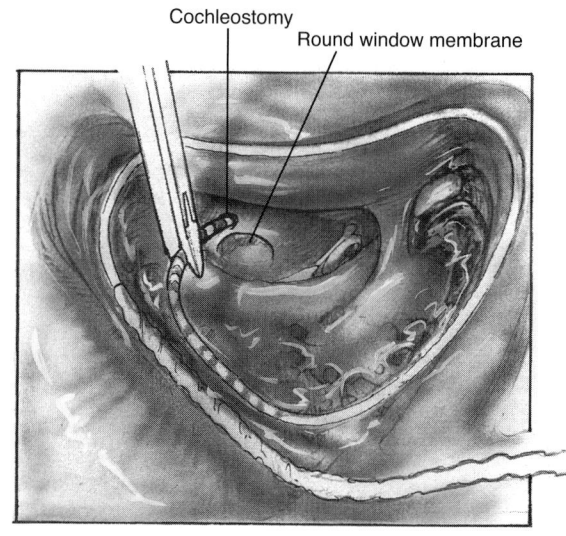

Figure 154.4 Electrode introduced into the basal end of the cochlea.

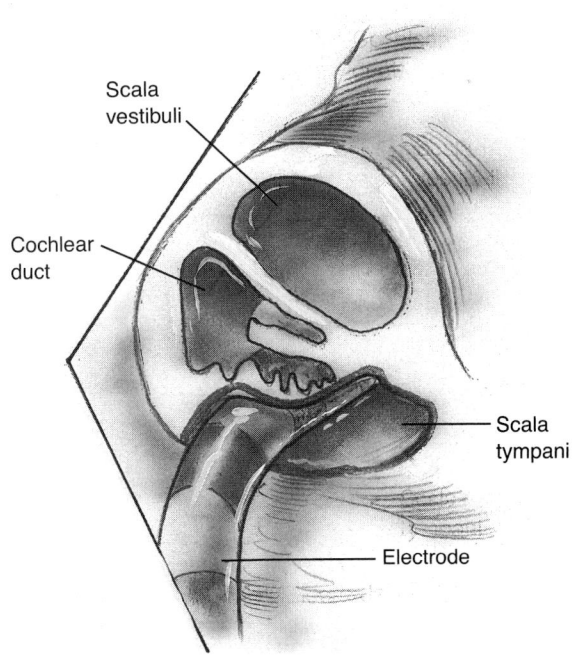

Figure 154.5 Electrode in scala tympani (cross section of basal turn on cochlea).

the cochleostomy with fascia. The flow of the CSF has been successfully controlled in this way. In patients who have severe malformations of the labyrinth, the facial nerve may follow an aberrant course. In these cases, the most direct access to a common cavity deformity may be by a transmastoid labyrinthotomy approach. The otic capsule is opened posterosuperior to the second genu of the facial nerve, and the common cavity is entered directly. Several patients have been treated in this way with no vestibular side effects (43).

In cases of cochlear ossification, our prior preference was to drill open the basal turn and to create a tunnel approximately 6 mm long and partially insert a Nucleus electrode. This allows implantation of 10 to 12 active electrodes, which has yielded satisfactory results. More recently, we have used the split electrode arrays (Med-El device; Nucleus, manufactured by Cochlear Corporation). One electrode is inserted as above and the other array is placed through a second cochleostomy created just anterior to the oval window. Gantz and colleagues (44) described an extensive drill-out procedure to gain access to the upper basal turn. Steenerson and co-workers (45) described insertion of the active electrode into the scala vestibuli in cases of cochlear ossification. Although this procedure has merit, the scala vestibuli is frequently ossified when the scala tympani is completely obliterated.

Complications

Complications have been infrequent with cochlear implant surgery and can be largely avoided by careful preoperative planning and meticulous surgical technique. Among the most commonly encountered problems are those associated with the incision and postauricular flap and facial nerve injury (46,47). Using the incision we describe, we have experienced only one flap breakdown in our pediatric cochlear implant population. (This occurred several years postoperatively after head trauma.) We experienced one transient delayed facial paresis and one CSF gusher in a child with a Mondini deformity (48). Several additional patients with the large vestibular aqueduct syndrome have also had gushers (49).

Because children are more susceptible to otitis media than adults, justifiable concern has been expressed that a middle-ear infection could cause an implanted device to

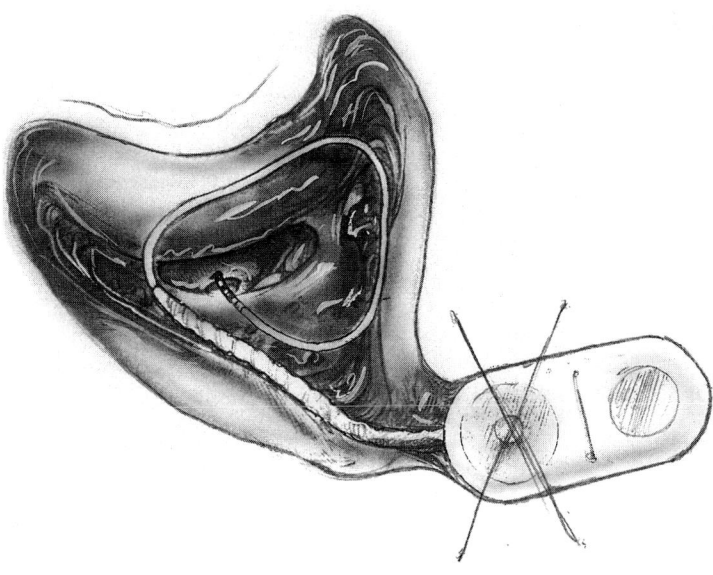

Figure 154.6 Receiver-stimulator with redundant loop of electrode in mastoid.

become an infected foreign body, requiring its removal. Two children in our series experienced a delayed mastoiditis (several years after the implant surgery) resulting in a postauricular abscess. These cases were treated by incision and drainage and intravenous antibiotics without the need to remove the implant. Of even greater concern is that infection might extend along the electrode into the inner ear, resulting in a serious otogenic complication, such as meningitis or further degeneration of the central auditory system. To date, although the incidence of otitis media in children who have received cochlear implants parallels that seen in the general pediatric population, no serious complications related to otitis media have occurred in our patients.

Meningitis in Cochlear Implant Recipients

During the early experience with cochlear implants, postimplantation meningitis was extremely rare. However, in the spring of 2002, a sudden increase in the number of postimplantation meningitis cases was reported in both Europe and North America. Identified risk factors related to the increased incidence of meningitis include young age, cochlear dysplasia, temporal bone abnormalities, and the use of a two-part electrode system. These observations lead to the voluntary withdrawal from the market of the Clarion implant devices, which incorporated a positioner (a wedge inserted next to the implanted electrode to facilitate transmission of the electrical signal by pushing the electrode against the medial wall of the cochlea). The importance of carefully packing the cochleostomy site with a soft tissue seal to prevent bacteria from entering the inner ear and intracranial spaces has been reemphasized (50,51). The FDA has emphasized the importance of vaccination against meningitis as a preventative measure in all children with cochlear implants. These children should be monitored and treated promptly for any bacterial infections after receiving the implant (52).

CLINICAL RESULTS

Cochlear implants are an established therapeutic option for selected deaf adults and children. There remains a wide range of performance with current implant systems, however. Some cochlear implant recipients can communicate without the benefit of lipreading and are able to communicate on the telephone without a telephone code, whereas others use their implants primarily to reestablish environmental contact and enhance their speech-reading abilities. This variation in performance levels is thought to relate to biologic and cognitive factors. It would be expected that poor auditory nerve survival or atrophic central auditory systems would correlate with poor performance,

whereas a more intact auditory nervous system should permit better results, given a well-designed and fitted cochlear prosthesis (53).

Adult Outcomes

The majority of adult cochlear implant recipients did not become profoundly deaf until after they had acquired speech and language skills. Thus, although their ability to understand speech through listening alone is severely impaired, they have little or no impairment in their speech production skills (11). Postlingually deafened adults must learn to use the auditory signal provided by a cochlear implant to access mental representations of speech established with normal auditory input. Early generations of cochlear implant systems provided limited auditory-only speech understanding (54,55). However, the technological advances in cochlear implant design have yielded ever-increasing levels of spoken word recognition in this population over the last 20 years (56–60).

Current generations of cochlear implant systems yield similar results despite the differences in electrode design and speech processing strategies across devices (11). On average, users of all three devices obtain at least some open-set speech understanding (61). Average auditory-only word recognition scores of approximately 35% to 45% correct and sentence recognition scores of approximately 65% to 80% correct have been reported for users of the Nucleus cochlear implant system with the SPEAK processing strategy (58,62), for users of the Clarion device with the CIS processing strategy or the Simultaneous Analog Stimulation strategy (59), and for users of the Med-El device with the CIS processing strategy (63). Compared with the results obtained with previous generations of cochlear implants, adults who use the current devices achieve higher word recognition skills and acquire those skills at a faster rate. Many adults now demonstrate substantial speech understanding as early as three months following cochlear implantation (64). However, there remains a great deal of variability in performance. Some adults are unable to understand any speech through listening alone, whereas others can communicate successfully on the telephone. As Wilson and colleagues point out (65), a number of within-subject factors also contribute to successful cochlear implant use. Two such factors are age at implantation and duration of deafness (64,66–70). Specifically, patients who are implanted at a young age and have a shorter period of auditory deprivation are more likely to achieve good outcomes. The findings regarding other predictive factors have been less conclusive. For example, Gantz et al. (55) found that measures of cognitive ability were not associated with patient performance, whereas Cohen et al. (67) reported that measures of IQ were significantly associated with good speech perception skills. Other factors that have been found to significantly correlate with adult outcomes include lipreading ability (67,68) and degree of residual hearing (44,68,71).

Pediatric Outcomes

Postlingually deafened adults and children use the information transmitted by a cochlear implant to access previously stored representations of spoken language. However, the majority of children who receive cochlear implants have congenital or prelingually acquired hearing loss. These children must use the sound provided by a cochlear implant to acquire speech perception, speech production, and spoken language skills. Furthermore, because young children have limited linguistic skills and attention spans, the assessment of performance in this population can be quite challenging. To effectively evaluate the communication benefits of cochlear implant use in children, a battery of tests that are developmentally and linguistically appropriate should be employed. (See Geers et al. [72,73] for a review of these issues.)

Over the last decade, advances in the design and implementation of cochlear implant systems and changes in candidacy criteria have led to large improvements in spoken language benefits obtained by children following cochlear implantation. Today, the expectations for speech and language development in children who receive a cochlear implant are higher than ever before (74).

Spoken Word Recognition

The majority of children who use current generations of cochlear implant technology are able to understand at least some speech through listening alone on tests of isolated word or sentence recognition (75–82), and many demonstrate substantial speech understanding (82,83). For example, Geers reported average auditory-only word recognition scores of 50% correct in a group of 181 children implanted by 5 years of age and tested at 8 to 9 years of age. When the stimuli were presented using both auditory and visual information, word recognition scores increased to 80% words correct. Tyler and colleagues (77) examined sentence recognition performance in a group of children with congenitally or early-acquired deafness; their performance was compared with that of a group of adults with postlingual deafness. They found that 60% of the adults and 70% of the children could correctly identify at least half of the sentences presented. Tyler et al. concluded that children with early onset of deafness could develop spoken language processing skills that are similar to those of adults who had the benefit of acquiring language using normal auditory input. However, in contrast to postlingually deafened adults, children continue to develop speech perception and spoken word recognition abilities over a relatively long time course (84).

A number of demographic factors have been shown to influence performance results in children with cochlear implants. There is a great deal of evidence that earlier implantation yields superior cochlear implant performance in children (83–88). Although the critical period for implantation of congenitally or prelingually deafened children has not been determined (89), preliminary evidence suggests that implantation prior to age 2 or 3 years may yield improved results (83,90–92). Finally, the variables of communication mode and/or unaided residual hearing also influence speech perception performance (93–96). Superior speech understanding often is demonstrated by children who use oral communication (82,83,97) and those who have more residual hearing prior to implantation (98–100). This has led to some controversy regarding whether to implant the better or the poorer hearing ear (94,101).

Speech Production and Language Outcomes

Improvements in speech perception are the most direct benefit of cochlear implantation. However, if children with cochlear implants are to succeed in the hearing world, they must also acquire intelligible speech and their surrounding linguistic system. The speech production and language abilities of children with cochlear implants improve significantly over time (89,102–106), and on average, exceed those of their age- and hearing-matched peers with hearing aids (104,105,107). Speech intelligibility and spoken language acquisition are significantly correlated with the development of auditory skills (103,108). Although a great deal of variability exists, following implantation the best pediatric cochlear implant users demonstrate highly intelligible speech (109) and develop language abilities at a rate similar to their normally hearing peers (106). These superior performers usually are implanted at a young age (83,110) and/or are educated in programs that emphasize oral-aural development (103,111,112).

CONCLUSIONS

Cochlear implant technology and candidacy criteria have evolved greatly over the last 20 years. Today, patients with severe-to-profound deafness and those as young as 12 months of age may be implanted. With earlier implantation and improved cochlear implant systems come continued increases in the benefits of cochlear implantation. Although wide variability exists, most postlingually deafened adults with cochlear implants achieve auditory-only word recognition and communicate very effectively when auditory cues are combined with lipreading. The best adult recipients can converse fluently without lipreading cues. In children, cochlear implants have been shown to promote the development of speaking and listening skills and the development of a spoken language system beyond what previously could be achieved with hearing aids. Children who are implanted at a young age and use oral communication have the best prognosis for developing intelligible speech and age appropriate language abilities.

OTHER IMPLANTABLE HEARING DEVICES

A substantial body of research has been performed to develop implantable hearing devices (IHDs) that couple with the ossicular chain in the middle ear, eliminating the requirement of acoustic coupling via the ear canal. This provides IHDs several potential advantages over conventional hearing aids: (1) elimination of acoustic feedback; (2) a wider frequency response; (3) elimination of a tight-fitting external ear canal mold; and (4) improved perception of the auditory signal.

Implantable hearing devices vibrate the ossicular chain by electromagnetic or piezoelectric means. An implanted magnet coupled to the ossicular chain is driven by an electromagnetic field generated by an induction coil. A number of innovative designs are currently in various stages of development (113-117). At the time of this report only two devices, the Vibrant Soundbridge and the Direct System, have completed FDA investigations and are available for commercial distribution.

Vibrant Soundbridge

The Vibrant Soundbridge (formerly Symphonix Devices, now Med-El) consists of two components: (1) A surgically implanted internal receiver that includes the floating mass

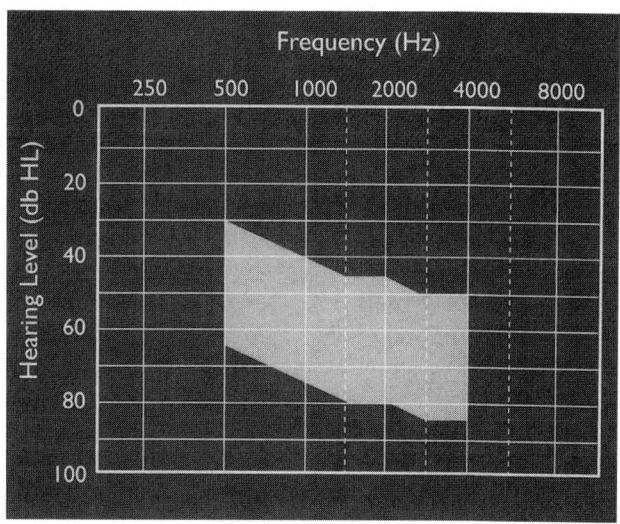

Figure 154.8 Range of moderate sensorineural hearing loss appropriate for Vibrant Soundbridge.

transducer, which is crimped onto the long process of the incus; and (2) the external processor, which picks up sound from the environment and transmits the signal to the implanted receiver. The implant is positioned through a mastoid-facial recess approach (Fig. 154.7).

The Vibrant Soundbridge is appropriate for a limited range of moderate sensorineural hearing loss. Speech discrimination must be at least 50%. The Soundbridge is not appropriate for conductive hearing loss or retrocochlear hearing loss. A stable middle ear should be present and the tympanic membrane must be intact. During the phase III FDA study of the Vibrant Soundbridge, an average functional gain of 10 to 15 dB across the frequency spectrum was reported. Aided speech recognition scores with the Soundbridge and conventional hearing aids were comparable (118). The floating mass transducer loading of the incus did not have a clinically significant effect on hearing (Fig. 154.8) (119).

Direct System

The Direct System (SOUNDTEC, Inc., Oklahoma City) consists of a neodymium-iron-boron (Nd-Fe-Bo) magnet that is implanted at the incudostapedial joint via a transcanal procedure (120). An external processor produces an electromagnetic field that sets the implanted magnet into motion. The Direct System produced an improvement in average functional gain of 10 to 15 dB for all tested frequencies lower than 6 Hz. There was no significant change in average residual hearing (121).

ACKNOWLEDGMENTS

This work was supported in part by NIH NIDCD grants RO1 DC00064, RO1 DC00423, and by Psi Iota Xi.

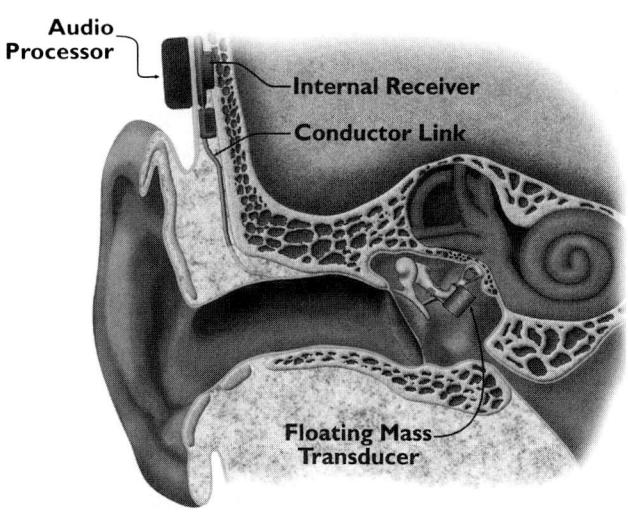

Figure 154.7 Vibrant Soundbridge with floating mass transducer attached to long process of incus.

HIGHLIGHTS

- Multichannel cochlear implants can provide salient information regarding all three dimensions of sound: intensity, timing, and frequency.
- Postlinguistically deafened adults, particularly those with a recent onset of deafness, are the most predictable beneficiaries of cochlear implants.
- Prelinguistically deafened adults as a group have not performed well with cochlear implants. However, selected prelinguistically deafened adults who have followed an oral program have benefited.
- Ossified or congenitally deformed cochleas (i.e., Mondini deformity) do not contraindicate cochlear implantation.
- A detailed hearing-aid trial with training is required to compare hearing-aid performance with that expected with a cochlear implant.
- The standard surgical approach is through the mastoid and facial recess, providing access to the round window.
- In children, the educational setting must provide an auditory environment but the communication mode may be total communication, auditory/aural, or cued speech.
- Detailed longitudinal studies are now clearly demonstrating improvements in speech perception, speech production, and language development in prelingually deafened children.

REFERENCES

1. Djourno A, Eyries C. Prothese auditive par excitation electrique a distance du nerf sensoriel a l'aide d'un bobinage inclus a demeure. *Presse Med* 1957;35:14.
2. Gates GA, Miyamoto RT. Cochlear implants. *N Engl J Med* 2003;349:421–423.
3. Clark GM, Tong YC, Dowell RC, et al. A multiple-channel cochlear implant: an evaluation using nonsense syllables. *Ann Otol Rhinol Laryngol* 1981;90:227–230.
4. Skinner MW, Clark GM, Whitford LA, et al. Evaluation of a new spectral peak (SPEAK) strategy for the Nucleus 22 channel cochlear implant system. *Am J Otol* 1994;15:15–27.
5. Staller S, Arcaroli J, Parkinson A, et al. Pediatric outcomes with the Nucleus 24 Contour: North American clinical trials. *Ann Otol Rhinol Laryngol* 2002;111:56–61.
6. Wilson BS, Lawson DT, Finley CC, et al. Coding strategies for multichannel cochlear prostheses. *Am J Otol* 1991;12:56–61.
7. Wilson BS. Strategies for representing speech information with cochlear implants. In: Niparko JK, Kirk KI, Robbins AM, et al, eds. *Cochlear implants: principles and practices.* Philadelphia: Lippincott Williams & Wilkins, 2000:129–170.
8. Schindler RA, Kessler DK. The UCSF/Storz cochlear implant: patient performance. *Am J Otol* 1987;8:247–255.
9. Schindler RA, Kessler DK. Clarion cochlear implant: phase I investigational results. *Am J Otol* 1993;14:263–272.
10. Kessler DK, Schindler RA. Progress with a multistrategy cochlear system: the Clarion. In: Hochmair-Desoyer IJ, Hochmair ES, eds. *Advances in cochlear implants.* Wein: Manz; 1994:354–362.
11. American Speech-Language-Hearing Association. Technical report: cochlear implants, *ASHA* 2003;(Suppl 24):1–35.
12. Gstoettner WK, Baumgartner WD, Franz P, et al. Cochlear implant deep insertion surgery. *Laryngoscope* 1997;107:544–546.
13. Wilson BS. Cochlear implant technology. In: Niparko JK, Kirk KI, Robbins AM, et al, eds. *Cochlear implants: principles and practices.* Philadelphia: Lippincott Williams & Wilkins, 2000:109–127.
14. Berliner KI. Selection of cochlear implant patients. In: Schindler RA, Merzenich MM, eds. *Cochlear implants.* New York: Raven Press, 1985:395.
15. Horn KL, McMahon NB. Functional use of the Nucleus 22-channel cochlear implant in the elderly. *Laryngoscope* 1991;101:284.
16. Waltzman SB, Cohen NL. Implantation of patients with prelingual long-term deafness. *Ann Otol Rhinol Laryngol* 1999;108:84–87.
17. Yoshinaga-Itano C. Efficacy of early identification and intervention. *Semin Hear* 1998;16:115–120.
18. Yoshinaga-Itano C, Sedey A, Coulter DK, et al. Language of early- and later-identified children with hearing loss. *Pediatrics* 1998;102:1161–1171.
19. Kral A, Hartmann R, Tillien J, et al. Congenital auditory deprivation reduces synaptic activity within the auditory cortex in a layer-specific manner. *Cereb Cortex* 2000;10:714–726.
20. Kral A, Hartmann R, Tillien J, et al. Delayed maturation and sensitive periods in the auditory cortex. *Audiol Neurootol* 2001;6:346–362.
21. Kral A, Hartmann R, Tillien J, et al. Hearing after congenital deafness: Central auditory plasticity and sensory deprivation. *Cereb Cortex* 2002;12:797–807.
22. Sharma A, Dorman MF, Spahr AJ. A sensitive period for the development of the central auditory system in children with cochlear implants: implications for age of implantation. *Ear Hear* 2002;23:532–539.
23. Ponton C, Don M, Eggermont J, et al. Maturation of human cortical auditory function: differences between normal-hearing children and children with cochlear implants. *Ear Hear* 1996;17:430–437.
24. Rizer F, Burkey J. Cochlear implantation in the very young child. *Otolaryngol Clin North Am* 1999;36:1117–1125.
25. Yoshinaga-Itano C. Benefits of early intervention for children with hearing loss. *Otolaryngol Clin North Am* 1999;32:1089–1102.
26. Yoshinaga-Itano C, Coulter DK, Thompson V. The Colorado Newborn Hearing Screening Project: effects on speech and language development for children with hearing loss. *J Perinatol* 2000;20:S132–S137.
27. Luxford W. Cochlear implantation in infants younger than 12 months of age. In: *VIII International Symposium on Cochlear Implants*, Indianapolis. Philadelphia, Elsevier, 2004.
28. Young NM. Infant cochlear implantation and anesthetic risk. *Ann Otol Rhinol Laryngol* 2002;111:49–51.
29. Lenarz T. Cochlear implantations in children under the age of two years. In: Honjo I, Takahashi H, eds. Cochlear implant and related sciences update. *Advances in Otorhinolaryngology*, Vol. 52. Basel: Karger, 1997:204–210.
30. Yune HY, Miyamoto RT. Medical imaging in cochlear implant candidates. *Am J Otol* 1991;12:11–17.
31. Jensen J. Tomography of the inner ear in deaf children. Radiological demonstration of two cases with the Mondini malformation. *J Laryngol Otol* 1967;81:27–35.
32. Mangabeira-Albernaz PL. The Mondini dysplasia: from early diagnosis to cochlear implant. *Acta Oto-Laryngologica* 1983;95:627–631.
33. Miyamoto RT, McConkey AJ, Myres WA, et al. Cochlear implantation in the Mondini inner ear malformation. *Am J Otol* 1986;7: 258–261.
34. Jackler RK, Luxford WM, House WF. Sound detection with the cochlear implant in five ears of four children with congenital malformations of the cochlea. *Laryngoscope* 1987;97:15–17.
35. Silverstein H, Smouha E, Morgan N. Multichannel cochlear implantation in a patient with bilateral Mondini deformities. *Am J Otol* 1988;9:451–455.
36. Tucci DL, Telian SA. Cochlear implantation in patients with cochlear malformations. *Arch Otolaryngol Head Neck Surg* 1995;121:833–838.
37. Buchman CA, Copeland BJ, Yu KK, et al. Cochlear implantation in children with congenital inner ear malformations. *Laryngoscope* 2004;114:309–316.
38. Beltrame MA, Bonfioloi MA, Frau GN. Cochlear implant in inner ear malformation. *Adv Otorhinolaryngol* 2000;57:113–119.
39. McElveen JT, Carrasco VN, Miyamoto RT, et al. Cochlear implantation in common cavity malformation using a transmastoid labyrinthotomy approach. *Laryngoscope* 1997;107:1032–1036.
40. Woolley AD, Jenison V, Stroer BS, et al. Cochlear implantation in children with inner ear malformations. *Ann Otol Rhinol Laryngol* 1998;107:492–500.
41. Schuknecht HF. Mondini dysplasia: a clinical and pathological study. *Ann Otol Rhinol Laryngol* 1980;89:1–23.
42. Hinojosa R, Marion M. Histopathology of profound sensorineural deafness. *Ann N Y Acad Sci* 1983;405:459–484.

43. McElveen JT Jr., Carrasco VN, Miyamoto RT, et al. Cochlear implantation in common cavity malformations using a transmastoid labyrinthotomy approach. *Laryngoscope* 1997;107:1032–1036.

44. Gantz BJ, McCabe BF, Tyler RS. Use of multichannel cochlear implants in obstructed and obliterated cochleas. *Otolaryngol Head Neck Surg* 1988;98:72–81.

45. Steenerson RL, Gary LB, Wynens MS. Scala vestibuli cochlear implantations for labyrinthine ossification. *Am J Otol* 1990;11:360–363.

46. Hoffman RA, Cohen NL. Complications of cochlear implant surgery. *Ann Otol Rhinol Laryngol* 1995;104:420–422.

47. Am Mylanus E, Van Den Broek P. Clinical results in paediatric cochlear implantation. *Cochlear Implants International* 2003;4:137–147.

48. Miyamoto RT, Young M, Myres WA, et al. Complications of pediatric cochlear implantation. *Eur Arch Otolaryngol* 1996;253:1–4.

49. Miyamoto RT, Bichey BG, Wynne MK, et al. Cochlear implantation with large vestibular aqueduct syndrome. *Laryngoscope* 2002:1178–1182.

50. Cohen NL, Roland JT Jr, Marrinan M. Meningitis in cochlear implant recipients: the North American experience. *Otol Neurotol* 2004;25:275–281.

51. O'Donoghue G, Balkany T, Cohen N, et al. Meningitis and cochlear implantation. *Otol Neurotol* 2002;23:823–824.

52. Reefhuis J, Honein MA, Whitney C, et al. Risk of bacterial meningitis in children with cochlear implants. *N Engl J Med* 2003;349:435–445.

53. Kessler DK, Loeb GE, Barker MJ. Distribution of speech recognition results with the Clarion cochlear prosthesis. *Ann Otol Rhinol Laryngol* 1995;104:283–285.

54. Dowell RC, Mecklenburg DJ, Clark GM. Speech recognition for 40 patients receiving multichannel cochlear implants. *Arch Otolaryngol* 1986;112:1054–1059.

55. Gantz B, Tyler RS, Abbas PJ, et al. Evaluation of five different cochlear implant designs: audiologic assessment and predictors of performance. *Laryngoscope* 1988;98:1100–1106.

56. Helms W, Westhofen M, Doring W, et al. Comparison of the TEMPO+ ear-level speech processor and the cis pro+ body-worn processor in adult Med-El cochlear implant users. *ORL J Otorhinolaryngol Relat Spec* 2001;63:31–40.

57. Holden LK, Skinner MW, Holden TA. Speech recognition with the MPEAK and SPEAK speech-coding strategies of the nucleus cochlear implant. *Otolaryngol Head Neck Surg* 1997;116:163–167.

58. Staller SJ, Menapace C, Domico E, et al. Speech perception abilities of adult and pediatric Nucleus implant recipients using Spectral Peak (SPEAK) coding strategy. *Otolaryngol Head Neck Surg* 1997;117:236–242.

59. Osberger MJ, Fisher L. New directions in speech processing: patient performance with simultaneous analog stimulation. *Ann Otol Rhinol Laryngol* 2001;109:70–73.

60. Parkinson AJ, Tyler RS, Woodworth GG, et al. A within-subject comparison of adult patients using the Nucleus F0F1F2 and F0F1F2B3B4B5 speech processing strategies. *J Speech Lang Hear Res* 1996;39:261–277.

61. Balkany T, Hodges A, Luntz M. Update on cochlear implantation. *Otolaryngol Clin North Am* 1996;29:227–289.

62. Hodges AV, Villasuso E, Balkany T, et al. Hearing results with deep insertion of cochlear implant electrodes. *Am J Otol* 1999;20:53–56.

63. Helms J, Muller J, Schon F, et al. Evaluation of performance with the Combi 40 cochlear implant in adults: a multicentric clinical study. *ORL J Otorhinolaryngol Relat Spec* 1997;59:23–35.

64. Geier LL, Fisher LM, Barker EJ, et al. The effect of long-term deafness on speech recognition in postlingually deafened adult Clarion cochlear implant users. *Ann Otol Rhinol Laryngol* 1999;108:80–83.

65. Wilson BS, Lawson DS, Finley CC, et al. Importance of patient and processor variables in determining outcomes with cochlear implants. *J Speech Hear Res* 1993;36:373–379.

66. Blamey PJ, Pyman BC, Clark GM, et al. Factors predicting postoperative sentence scores in postlingually deaf adult cochlear implant patients. *Ann Otol Rhinol Laryngol* 1992;101:342–348.

67. Cohen NL, Waltzman SB, Fisher SG, et al. A prospective, randomized study of cochlear implants. *N Engl J Med* 1993;328:233–237.

68. Gantz B, Woodworth G, Knutson JF, et al. Multivariate predictors of audiological success with multichannel cochlear implants. *Ann Otol Rhinol Laryngol* 1993;102:909–916.

69. Battmer RD, Gupta SP, Allum-Mecklenburg DJ, et al. Factors influencing cochlear implant perceptual performance in 132 adults. *Ann Otol Rhinol Laryngol* 1995;166:185–187.

70. Shipp D, Nedzelski J, Chen J, et al. Prognostic indicators of speech recognition performance in postlinguistically deafened adult cochlear implant users. In: Honjo I, Takahashi H, eds. *Advances in otorhinolaryngology: cochlear implant and related sciences update*. Basel: Karger, 1997:74–77.

71. Rubinstein JT, Miller CA. How do cochlear prostheses work? *Curr Opin Neurobiol* 1999;9:399–404.

72. Kirk KI, Diefendorf AO, Pisoni DB, et al. Assessing speech perception in children. In: Mendel L, Danhauer J, eds. *Audiological evaluation and management and speech perception training*. San Diego: Singular Publishing Group, 1997:101–132.

73. Kirk KI. Challenges in the clinical investigation of cochlear implant outcomes. In: Niparko JK, Kirk KI, Mellon NK, et al, eds. *Cochlear implants: principles and practices*. Philadelphia: Lippincott Williams & Wilkins, 2000:225–259.

74. Moog JS. Changing expectations for children with cochlear implants. *Ann Otol Rhinol Laryngol* 2002;111:138–142.

75. Cohen MH, Waltzman SB, Roland JT Jr, et al. Early results using the Nucleus C124M in children. *Am J Otol* 1999;20:198–204.

76. Osberger MJ, Zimmerman-Phillips S, Barker M, et al. Clinical trials of the Clarion cochlear implant in children. *Ann Otol Rhinol Laryngol* 1999;108:88–92.

77. Tyler RS, Rubenstein JT, Teagle H, et al. Prelingually deafened children can perform as well as postlingually deaf adults using cochlear implants. *Cochlear Implants International* 2000;1:39–44.

78. Young NM, Carrasco VN, Grohne KM, et al. Speech perception of young children using Nucleus 22-channel or Clarion cochlear implants. *Ann Otol Rhinol Laryngol* 1999;108:99–103.

79. Eisenberg LS, Kirk KI, Martinez AS, et al. Communication abilities of children with aided residual hearing: Comparison with cochlear implant users. *Arch Otolaryngol Head Neck Surg* 2004;130:563–569.

80. Kirk KI, Hay-McCutcheon M, Sehgal ST, et al. Speech perception in children with cochlear implants: effects of lexical difficulty, talker variability and word length. *Ann Otol Rhinol Laryngol* 2000;109:79–81.

81. Geers A, Brenner C. Speech perception results: audition and lipreading enhancement. *Volta Review* 1994;96:97–108.

82. Geers AE, Brenner C, Davidson L. Factors associated with development of speech perception skills in children implanted by age five. *Ear Hear* 2003;24:24S–35S.

83. Kirk KI, Miyamoto RT, Ying EA, et al. Cochlear implantation in young children: effects of age at implantation and communication mode. *Volta Review* 2002;102(monograph):127–144.

84. Fryauf-Bertschy H, Tyler RS, Kelsay, et al. Cochlear implant use by prelingually deafened children: the influences of age at implant and length of device use. *J Speech Lang Hear Res* 1997;40:183–199.

85. Miyamoto RT, Kirk KI, Robbins AM, et al. Speech perception and speech intelligibility in children with multichannel cochlear implants. In: Honjo I, Takahashi H, eds. *Advances in otorhinolaryngology: cochlear implant and related sciences update*. Basel: Karger, 1997:198–203.

86. Nikolopoulos TP, O'Donoghue GM, Archbold SM. Age at implantation: its importance in pediatric cochlear implantation. *Laryngoscope* 1999;109:595–599.

87. Lenarz T, Illg A, Lesinki-Schiedat A, et al. Cochlear implantation in children under the age of two: the MHH experience with the Clarion cochlear implant. *Ann Otol Rhinol Laryngol* 1999;108:44–49.

88. Illg A, Lesinki-Schiedat A, von der Haar-Heise S, et al. Speech perception results for children implanted with the Clarion cochlear implant at the Medical University of Hannover. *Ann Otol Rhinol Laryngol* 1999;108:93–98.

89. Brackett D, Zara CV. Communication outcomes related to early implantation. *Am J Otol* 1998;19:453–459.

90. Waltzman S, Cohen N, Shapiro W. Effects of cochlear implantation on the young deaf child. In: Uziel A, Mondain M, eds. *Advances in otorhinolaryngology*. Basel: Karger, 1995:125–128.

91. Waltzman S, Cohen NL, Gomolin R, et al. Perception and production results in children implanted between two and five years of

age. In: Honjo I, Takahashi H, eds. *Advances in otorhinolaryngology: cochlear implant and related sciences update.* Basel: Karger, 1997:177–180.

92. Waltzman SB, Cohen NL. Cochlear implantation in children younger than 2 years old. *Am J Otol* 1998;19:158–162.

93. Cowan RS, DelDot J, Barker EJ, et al. Speech perception results for children with implants with different levels of preoperative residual hearing. *Am J Otol* 1997;18:125–126.

94. Zwolan TA, Zimmerman-Phillips S, Ashbaugh CJ, et al. Cochlear implantation of children with minimal open-set speech recognition skills. *Ear Hear* 1997;18:240–251.

95. Osberger MJ, Fisher LM. Preoperative predictors of postoperative implant performance in children. *Ann Otol Rhino Laryngol* 2000; (Suppl 185).

96. Hodges AV, Ash MD, Balkany TJ, et al. Speech perception results in children with cochlear implants: contributing factors. *Otolaryngol Head Neck Surg* 1999;121:31–34.

97. Kirk KI, Pisoni DB, Miyamoto RT. Lexical discrimination by children with cochlear implants: effects of age at implantation and communication mode. In: Waltzman SB, Cohen NL, eds. *Cochlear implants.* New York: Thieme; 2000:252–254.

98. Gantz B, Rubenstein J, Tyler R, et al. Long-term results of cochlear implants in children with residual hearing. *Ann Otol Rhinol Laryngol* 2000;109:33–36.

99. Holt RF, Kirk KI, Eisenberg LS, et al. Spoken word recognition development in children with residual hearing using cochlear implants and hearing aids in opposite ears. *Ear Hear* 2005,(4 Suppl):82S–91S.

100. Osberger MJ, Fisher LM. Preoperative predictors of postoperative implant performance in children. *Ann Otol Rhinol Laryngol* 2000;185:44–46.

101. Reubenstein JT, Miller CA. How do cochlear prostheses work? *Curr Opin Neurobiol* 1999;9:399–404.

102. Allen MC, Nikolopoulos TP, O'Donoghue GM. Speech intelligibility in children after cochlear implantation. *Am J Otol* 1998;19:742–746.

103. Moog JS, Geers A. Speech and language acquisition in young children after cochlear implantation. *Otolaryngol Clin North Am* 1999;32:1127–1141.

104. Svirsky MA. Speech intelligibility of pediatric cochlear implant users and hearing aid users. In: Waltzman SB, Cohen NL, eds. *Cochlear implants.* New York: Thieme, 2000:312–314.

105. Svirsky MA, Robbins AM, Kirk KI, et al. Language development in profoundly deaf children with cochlear implants. *Psych Sci* 2000;11:153–158.

106. Svirsky MA, Chute PM, Green J, et al. Language development in children who are prelingually deaf who have used SPEAK or CIS stimulation strategies since initial stimulation. *Volta Review* 2002;102(4):199–213.

107. Tomblin B, Spencer LJ, Flock S, et al. A comparison of language achievement in children with cochlear implants and children using hearing aids. *J Speech Lang Hear Res* 1999;42: 497–511.

108. Pisoni DB, Svirsky MA, Kirk KI, et al. Looking at the "stars": a first report on the intercorrelations among measures of speech perception, intelligibility and language development in pediatric cochlear implant users. *Research on spoken language processing progress report,* no 21. Speech Research Laboratory. Bloomington, IN: Indiana University, 1996–1997.

109. Tobey EA, Geers AE, Brenner C, et al. Factors associated with the development of speech production skills in children implanted by age five. *Ear Hear* 2003;24:36S–45S.

110. Connor CM, Hieber S, Arts HA, et al. Speech, vocabulary, and the education of children using cochlear implants: oral or total communication? *J Speech Lang Hear Res* 2000;43:1185–1204.

111. Chin SB, Kaiser CL. Measurement of articulation in pediatric users of cochlear implants. *Volta Review* 2002;102(4):145–156.

112. Geers A, Nicholas J, Sedey A. Language skills of children with early cochlear implantation. *Ear Hear* 2003;24:46S–58S.

113. Maniglia AJ. Implantable hearing devices: state of the art. *Otolaryngol Clin North Am* 1989;22:175–200.

114. Fredrickson JM, Coticchia JM, Khosla S. Ongoing investigations into an implantable electromagnetic hearing aid for moderate to severe sensorineural hearing loss. *Otolaryngol Clin North Am* 1995;28:107–120.

115. Yanagihara N, Gyo K, Hinoshira Y. Partially implantable hearing aid using piezoelectric ceramic ossicular vibrator: results of the implant operation and assessment of the hearing afforded by the device. *Otolaryngol Clin North Am* 1995;28:85–97.

116. Kartush JM, Tos M. Electromagnetic ossicular augmentation device. *Otolaryngol Clin North Am* 1995;28:155–172.

117. Hough JVD, Bryce GE, Baker RS, et al. Implantable hearing devices for mild to moderately severe hearing loss. In: Bailey BJ, ed. *Head and neck surgery: otolaryngology.* Philadelphia: JB Lippincott, 1998:2225–2232.

118. Luetje C, Brackmann DE, Balkany TJ. Phase III clinical trial results with the Vibrant Soundbridge implantable middle ear hearing device: a prospective controlled multicenter study. *Otolaryngol Head Neck Surg* 2002;126:97.

119. Snik FM, Cremers WR. The effect of the "floating mass transducer" in the middle ear on hearing sensitivity. *Am J Otol* 2000; 21:42.

120. Hough JVD, Dyer RK Jr, Matthews P. Early clinical results: SOUNDTEC implantable hearing device phase II study. *Laryngoscope* 2001;111:1.

121. Roland PS, Shoup AG, Shea MC, et al. Verification of improved patient outcomes with a partially implantable hearing aid: the SOUNDTEC Direct hearing system. *Laryngoscope* 2001;111:1682–1686.

155

Hearing Aids and Assistive Listening Devices

Todd A. Ricketts   *Albert R. DeChicchis*   *Fred H. Bess*

Sensorineural hearing loss is a disability affecting an estimated 28 million, or approximately 1 in 10, Americans (1). Because noise exposure and aging are the leading causes of sensorineural hearing loss in adults, coupled with continued predictions of increased life expectancy, it is assumed that prevalence of hearing loss can only be expected to increase. Adults over the age of 65 already make up approximately 65% of the total population of individuals with hearing loss. People with sensorineural hearing loss suffer not only from a lack of sensitivity to sound, but also commonly complain of problems with speech understanding, particularly if the speech is presented in a background of noise.

The negative consequences of hearing loss involve not only a reduction in hearing sensitivity (impairment), but also activity limitations and participation restrictions as defined by the World Health Organization's International Classification of Functioning, Disability, and Health (2). It is clear that reductions in activity and participation can negatively impact an individual's quality of life. Several studies (three are cited here) have documented the relationship between adult-onset hearing loss and psychosocial problems such as social isolation, depression, anxiety, loneliness, and lessened self-efficacy and mastery (3–5). Even younger adults with mild hearing loss report a variety of psychosocial problems affecting everyday life (6). In addition, family, friends, and coworkers may experience frustration, impatience, anger, pity, and/or guilt when interacting with a person having hearing loss. Poor general health and reduced mobility have been associated with significant sensorineural hearing loss (7).

Although sensorineural hearing loss certainly presents difficulties and challenges for adult patients, the impact on the young child can be devastating. The presence of significant hearing loss prior to the development of speech and language places hearing-impaired children at particular risk, and the potential delays in speech and language development and the subsequent difficulties in learning cannot be overemphasized. The problems that hearing-impaired children may face with development of speech and language skills are only exacerbated by late identification and greater severity of hearing loss (8).

It is readily apparent that habilitation and rehabilitation services have the potential for considerable positive impact on the quality of life of individuals with hearing impairment. The process of audiologic rehabilitation, the cornerstone of which is the use of amplification, is aimed at optimizing the individual's auditory activities and minimizing any participation restrictions (9). The use of hearing aids has been shown to be an effective means of improving speech understanding over unaided listening, and to provide significant improvements in quality of life (5). For many individuals the rehabilitation process may include assistive listening devices, cochlear implants, or tactile and/or visual aids. These devices may be used in lieu of, or in addition to, hearing aids. In any case, device intervention must be coupled with counseling, communication training, and, in some cases, environmental modifications in the framework of a total audiologic rehabilitation approach (9).

This chapter reviews the current state of hearing aids and other personal amplification systems used by those who are hearing impaired. The discussion focuses on the function, use, and types of hearing aids; electroacoustic properties of hearing aids; the selection and evaluation process; and orientation to hearing aids and assistive listening devices.

HEARING AID FUNCTION

The purpose of any amplification device is to increase the magnitude of an acoustic signal at its output compared to that same signal at the instrument's input. The basic properties of a hearing aid correspond to those of a simple amplifier. A hearing aid is also called an *electroacoustic device* because it takes an acoustic signal, such as speech, and converts it to an electric signal before the amplification stage. Through amplification, hearing aids increase the audibility of sounds, including speech, for hearing-impaired listeners.

Figure 155.1 shows a simplified diagram of a basic, analogue hearing aid. The microphone receives the input signal, causing its diaphragm to vibrate. The vibratory motion alters the resistive properties in the microphone, thereby generating an electric signal. The electric signal is then sent to the amplifier, where it is enlarged. In the final stage, the amplified signal is directed to a tiny loudspeaker, called a receiver, where the electric signal is converted back to an acoustic signal and then delivered to the ear. Thus, in its most basic form, a hearing aid is composed of a microphone, an amplifier, and a receiver. Sounds in the environment are thus converted to electric events, increased in amplitude, transduced back into acoustic information, and delivered to the ear for auditory processing.

Although all hearing aids provide amplification to sound, the manner by which they process or control incoming signals differs. In the American market, hearing aids generally fall into one of three general categories: (1) nonprogrammable analogue devices, (2) digitally programmable analogue systems, and (3) digital signal processing (DSP) devices. For many years, analogue hearing aids were the only instruments available. These analogue systems provide a constant analysis of the incoming signal and, thereby, constantly modify the input stimulus. By the mid 1980s, improvements in hearing aid technology led to the development of digitally programmable analogue hearing aids. Digitally programmable analogue systems use analogue processing, but, in contrast to the more traditional analogue devices, these instruments program the hearing aid response characteristics into digital memory, and control the analogue circuit digitally. In many instances, programmable systems offer the hearing-impaired individual a variety of user memories, and different channels of signal processing, from which several different hearing aid responses may be selected depending on the listening demands. In addition to having more access to different processing strategies, programmable instruments allow for more precision in electroacoustic adjustments, and flexibility in adjusting gain and output as changes in hearing sensitivity occurs.

The most recent advances in hearing aid processing technology have centered on the use of DSP. The first two modern digital hearing aids arrived in 1993. Since then, manufacturers have quickly embraced this new technology and digital hearing aid market share has grown to more than 50% of all hearing aids sold in the United States. It is expected that all hearing aids will be digital in the near future. Digital hearing aids use many of the same microphones and receivers used by analogue instruments, but differ in that they represent sound as a string of numbers (referred to as analog-to-digital conversion or "digitizing") for signal processing. The sound can then be manipulated by DSP, which simply refers to applying mathematical algorithms to this string of numbers. All digital hearing aids then convert the new string of numbers back into sound (referred to as digital-to-analog conversion). In the most basic digital hearing aids the DSP ("math") is relatively simple, increasing the level of sound at some frequencies more than others and keeping sounds from being too loud. That is, the outcome of their operation is similar to traditional analogue hearing aids (albeit with much more fine control). The main advantage in these basic digital hearing aids is that they can be fit more easily and accurately to an individual hearing loss, and they can be made smaller and more cheaply than comparable analogue instruments. It is important to note that most listeners will notice little, if any, difference between these simple digital hearing aids and the best nondigital (analog) hearing aids. Current digital hearing aids, however, do have significant

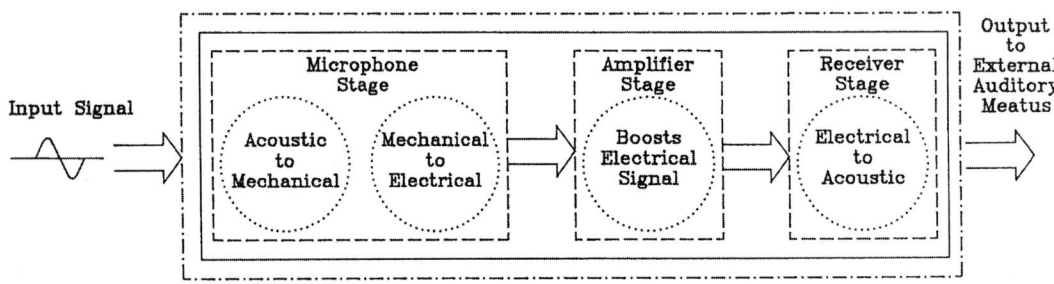

Figure 155.1 Basic components of a hearing aid system.

advantages. These advantages are related to complex signal processing that is not possible in traditional analogue hearing aids (10–12), as discussed later in this chapter.

Regardless of whether analogue or digital signal processing is implemented, amplification (gain) in hearing aids can be applied to incoming acoustic signals in either a linear or nonlinear (compressive or expansive) fashion. In linear amplification systems a direct relationship is maintained between the signal input and the output; thus, as the signal input increases, the amplified output increases by an equal amount, and the input/output function reflects a slope of 1.0 over the majority of the operating range. In contrast, nonlinear hearing aids produce an input/output function having a slope of other than 1.0. That is, nonlinear hearing aids vary gain through amplitude compression (decreasing gain with increasing input intensity levels) and/or amplitude expansion (decreasing gain with decreasing input intensity levels) so that sound level at the output of the hearing aid remains both audible and comfortable, over a broad range of input intensity levels. Expansion is a relatively new processing scheme for hearing aids, and is only available in digital hearing aids. This processing is used mainly to reduce the output intensity level of low-intensity microphone noise and annoying environmental sounds. A complete discussion of hearing aid compression is beyond the scope of this chapter; for a comprehensive review the interested reader is referred to the work of Souza (13). Briefly, compression is most useful for those individuals who have a reduced dynamic range of hearing in comparison to those with normal hearing [i.e., a small range between their threshold for hearing and their threshold of discomfort (TD)]. Some reduction in the dynamic range of hearing is present in nearly all individuals with sensorineural hearing loss (14). Compression can take many forms, but generally is categorized by its activation threshold (kneepoint) and desired effect. It should be pointed out that all compression hearing aids function as linear devices for sound intensity levels below their specified compression threshold (CT). Compression hearing aids with high activation thresholds (often called compression limiting) are used to limit the maximum output level from a hearing aid, while providing linear amplification for most speech input levels. In contrast, compression hearing aids with low CT (including wide dynamic range compression, WDRC, and automatic volume control, AVC) provide nonlinear amplification for most, or sometimes all, speech intensity levels.

Digital and analogue hearing aids are also both capable of taking advantage of advanced microphone technology to improve speech understanding in noise. Individuals with hearing impairment continue to have particular difficulty in background noise, especially if the background "noise" is the speech of other talkers. Data suggest that 25% of individuals, who own hearing aids but do not wear them, cite poor performance in background noise as the reason for hearing aid rejection (15). The signal-to-noise

ratio (SNR) is the primary factor that affects speech understanding in noise. The SNR quantifies the degree to which the signal of interest is audible above the interfering noise at any given moment. In order to improve an individual's speech intelligibility in noise, the SNR must be improved. Data suggest that hearing-impaired individuals require significantly more positive SNRs for equivalent speech recognition performance when compared to listeners with normal hearing. A large number of hearing aids use omnidirectional microphones. In general, omnidirectional hearing aids do not improve SNR in comparison to the unaided ear, and in some cases, SNR is made worse by amplification (16). In contrast, directional microphone hearing aids incorporate multiple microphones (or microphone ports) to allow for improved SNR based on the spatial location of the signal of interest (front hemisphere) relative to unwanted signals (usually in the rear hemisphere). The amount of attenuation provided by a typical pair of directional hearing aids worn by an average listener is shown in Figure 155.2. This can be contrasted to an omnidirectional hearing aid that reveals similar sensitivity to sound arriving at all angles. The resulting improvement in SNR relative to omnidirectional hearing aid fittings can lead to improved speech intelligibility in noisy environments. To date, directional microphones remain one of the only consistently effective methods for improving SNR across a broad range of noisy environments for the hearing aid wearer.

Directional hearing aids operate by taking advantage of timing differences between sounds arriving at the front and rear microphone ports. Because these timing differences are crucial for proper operation of a directional microphone, the directional SNR advantage will only be present when there is spatial separation between the signal of interest and the competing noise. Any factor that decreases the amount of spatial separation will reduce the directional effect.

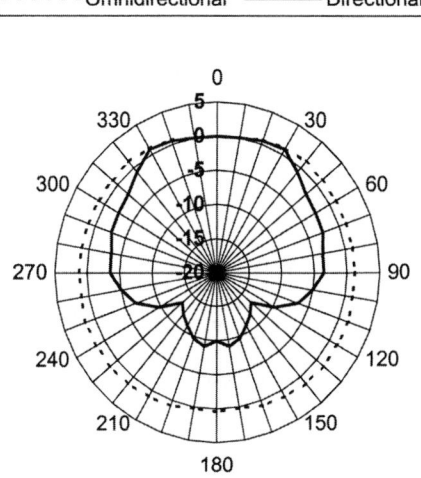

Figure 155.2 Relative attenuation as a function of angle provided to a typical hearing aid wearer fit bilaterally with omnidirectional and directional behind-the-ear style hearing aids.

Consequently, the effectiveness of these instruments is reduced with increased levels of reflected (as opposed to direct) sound energy, such as the case in reverberant environments and environments for which the signal of interest is located at great distance (e.g., when seated near the rear of an auditorium) (17,18). Although a variety of factors affect the performance of directional hearing aids (16,19,20), these instruments have been shown to be effective at improving speech intelligibility in noise across a number of simulated and real-world listening environments (16–18, 21). The SNR improvement provided by the current generation of directional hearing aids ranges from approximately 3 to 5 dB in average real-world environments, and can approach 7 to 8 dB in some listening situations (16). Full-time use of directional hearing aids is not recommended, however; hearing aids capable of both directional and omnidirectional processing are usually recommended (21). Automatic directional technology may be useful for patients who cannot make appropriate switching decisions, though no data are yet available that support the efficacy of this technology. Due in part to published reports of improved speech intelligibility in noise, and improved technology that allowed for the use of directional microphones in increasingly smaller hearing aid styles, the use of directional microphones in hearing aids has expanded significantly in recent years.

The use of microphone arrays for input into hearing aids and other devices such as cochlear implants has also increased. Microphone arrays, sometimes called beamformers, use multiple microphones for improved performance in noise over standard directional microphones. Microphone arrays, though showing significantly more SNR benefit than traditional directional microphones, are generally advocated for individuals with severe-to-profound hearing loss due to a few disadvantages. The main disadvantage of most current microphone arrays over traditional directional microphones relates to cosmetics. The use of multiple microphones, each separated in space, results in devices that are usually in excess of 3 or 4 inches in length. These size constraints do not generally allow for microphone arrays to be used in ear-level devices. Instead, the array is usually fixed to eyeglasses or worn around the neck. Currently there is at least one exception to this general rule. Specifically, one manufacturer has introduced a three-microphone array in a behind-the-ear (BTE) style hearing aid, which has been shown to enhance speech recognition performance in noise for listeners with hearing impairment (22).

Digital Signal Processing–Based Features

As a result of the introduction of DSP in hearing aids, there is currently extensive growth in the number of new sound processing schemes aimed at improved speech recognition, sound quality, and comfort in these devices. For example, DSP has allowed for the application of increasingly

complex methods of intensity-specific gain control. This includes the first use of amplitude expansion in hearing aids, and very complex, frequency-specific amplitude compression amplification schemes. These techniques generally increase the ease with which patient audibility for speech can be maximized. Several other signal-processing schemes have also been implemented into digital hearing aids, including digital noise reduction and digital feedback control.

Digital noise reduction (DNR) schemes generally decrease gain in frequency ranges in which speech is not detected. Detection of speech is usually based on the presence of amplitude modulations or co-modulations (11). Many implementations of DNR may improve sound quality and/or comfort (23,24). One implementation of DNR has shown improved speech recognition in steady-state noise in the laboratory, while another configuration has shown decreased performance under the same laboratory conditions (25). It is important to note that although DNR processing is recommended for enhancement of sound quality and listening comfort, most implementations will not impact speech recognition (11). Further, none of the DNR systems to date have been shown to positively impact speech recognition in the more common situation in which the background noise is amplitude modulated (varies in amplitude). Finally, not all implementations of DNR are equivalent, and data specific to individual implementations must be evaluated prior to selection.

Digital Feedback Suppression (DFS) systems can allow for increased gain under constant coupling constraints (e.g., the same hearing aid shell and vent size). Some DFS processing can substantially benefit users who experience occasional feedback, such as that associated with jaw movement and/or being close to objects. Some versions of this technology can also be used to allow for a larger air channel into the ear (vent) to improve the sound quality of the hearing aid wearer's own voice (26). That is, it can reduce the "it sounds like my head is in a barrel" effect commonly referred to as the "occlusion effect." DFS systems operate using a variety of techniques including notch filtering, cancellation, and phase shifting. Concern has been expressed related to a reduction in audibility for some implementations. A general recommendation for DFS processing cannot yet be made; however, specific systems are recommended that yield at least equivalent speech recognition performance in the presence of reduced occlusion and/or feedback.

STYLES AND TYPES OF HEARING AIDS

Although hearing aids may have similar internal components, they are available in many shapes and sizes (Fig. 155.3). The advantages and disadvantages of each of these styles are listed in Table 155.1. For the past half-century, improvements in technology allowed manufacturers to

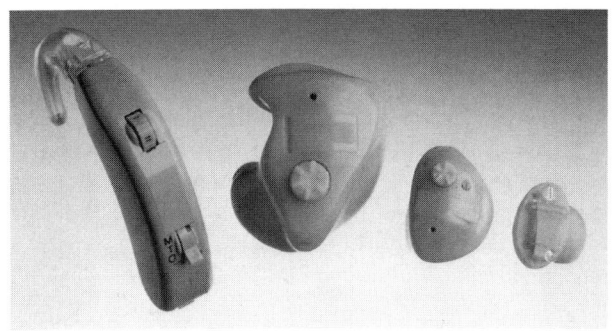

Figure 155.3 Hearing aids are classified into four basic types: (1) behind-the-ear (BTE), (2) in-the-ear (ITE), (3) in-the-canal (ITC), and (4) completely-in-the-ear. (Photo courtesy of Siemens Hearing Instruments, Inc.)

reduce the size of hearing aids and still maintain the power output and frequency response necessary to amplify the most severe hearing impairments. As such, these technological advances have rendered the previously worn body aids, where the hearing aid components were enclosed in a case that was attached to the clothing, and eyeglass hearing aids, which included the hearing aid in the temple of the eyeglasses, virtually obsolete.

By the mid-1970s, most people were wearing behind-the-ear (BTE) models. The BTE instrument offered several advantages over its body-worn counterpart. In addition to the cosmetic appeal of its relatively small size, the BTE models eliminated the body baffle effect created when the hearing aid was worn on the torso, which increased amplification in the frequency region below 800 Hz and caused a decrease in amplification for the frequencies from 1000 to 2500 Hz. The BTE instrument also eliminated the noise produced from clothes rubbing against the microphone and the problems associated with the body-worn aid's cords.

As advances in electronic circuitry continued, manufacturers were able to reduce further the size of the hearing aid and began developing custom hearing aids. Custom instruments include in-the-ear (ITE), in-the-canal (ITC),

TABLE 155.1
ADVANTAGES AND DISADVANTAGES OF HEARING AIDS BY TYPE

Type of Hearing Aid	Advantages	Disadvantages
Behind-the-ear	Range of power sufficient to reach severe and profound hearing loss. Allows adequate space to accommodate gain, output, and frequency response controls on analogue instruments for adjustment by dispenser. Allows for placement of directional microphone.	In cases of severe or profound hearing loss, earmold must fit snugly in the ear canal to eliminate feedback problems. May be slightly more difficult to place on ear in cases of manual dexterity problems. For those with small pinnae, particularly small children and infants, accessory devices may need to be considered to hold in place. However, custom instruments are inappropriate for small children and infants due to frequent changes in ear size and geometry.
In-the-ear	Cosmetically appealing. Placement of microphone takes advantage of pinna and concha effects enhancing amplification in the high frequencies. Microphone placement improves sound source localization as head is moved. May be easier to insert because only one component is involved. Allows for placement of directional microphone.	Because of close proximity of microphone and receiver, the amount of real ear gain may be limited because of feedback problems, especially in cases of severe profound high-frequency hearing loss.
In-the-canal	More cosmetically appealing because it fits almost entirely in the ear canal. Microphone placement takes advantage of pinna and concha effects boosting gain in the high frequencies. Microphone placement improves localization to sound source as head is moved.	Amount of gain is sufficient for no more than moderate hearing loss. Due to small size and small battery, may be difficult to handle for individuals with manual dexterity problems. Small size of instrument limits the number of output/response controls in analogue instruments. Venting options limited. Deep placement precludes use of directional microphone.
Completely-in-the-canal	Most cosmetically appealing because canal hearing aid is not visible when placed in the ear. Its deep insertion potentially takes full advantage of pinna and concha effects, boosts real ear gain (especially) in the high frequencies) and reduces occlusion effect.	Amount of gain is sufficient for no more than moderate hearing loss. Due to small battery, may be difficult to handle for individuals with manual dexterity problems. Small size of instrument limits the number of output/response controls in analogue instruments. Deep placement precludes use of directional microphone. Venting options very limited. Deep tight fit requires precision, and is not possible on all patients due to ear geometry.

and completely-in-the-canal (CIC) hearing aids. These instruments differ from other styles as they are usually packaged into a custom-made shell or casing. During the 1980s the percentage of people purchasing ITE, ITC, and CIC hearing aids grew quickly from 34% in 1980 to approximately 80% of total hearing aid sales in 1990. Since that time, the sales of the different hearing aid styles have remained relatively stable at this level. The principal reason for the increase in the popularity of custom instruments during that time span, as well as their current popularity, was one of cosmetics. The slightly larger ITE model fits entirely in the outer ear, filling the concha. The smaller ITC model fits almost exclusively in the ear canal and generally does not extend beyond the tragus. This placement gives the user the additional benefits of the normal acoustics provided by the pinna, and increases gain in the high frequencies because the microphone is located at the entrance to the ear canal. Pinna acoustics are also important in providing sound localization cues and some natural directional effect (greater sensitivity to sounds originating in front rather than behind the listener). The CIC hearing aid fits more deeply into the ear canal than any of the aforementioned instruments. This recessed placement has the potential for maximizing pinna and concha effects, which can result in even greater high-frequency gain and reduced occlusion when compared to other hearing aid styles (27). In order to obtain maximum acoustic benefits from CIC instruments, certain fitting criteria must be met, including the distance of the lateral end of the hearing aid from the meatal opening, and the distance of the medial end of the hearing aid from the tympanic membrane (27). These constraints make the true CIC fitting in the absence of discomfort unattainable for many hearing aid wearers. Consequently, it is common to fit the CIC style as if it were an ITC model, eliminating some of the advantages attributed to the CIC style.

Another type of instrument, referred to as contralateral routing of signal (CROS), is designed for patients with no usable hearing in one ear and normal hearing or a minimal hearing loss in the other ear. In the CROS system, a microphone is located on the impaired side and transmitted to the good ear via an open earmold or a polyethylene tube. The microphone and receiver may be coupled by a wire that runs around the back of the neck (or through the eyeglasses), or the signal may be transmitted in a wireless mode via radio frequencies. Hence, the wearer can use the good ear to hear signals from the impaired side. The BTE style accounts for the majority of CROS hearing aids currently available. Of the few eyeglass hearing aids still dispensed, the majority implement CROS amplification.

Listening conditions change throughout the day, and the CROS aid is beneficial for people who cannot always control the direction of the sound reaching their ears. These aids are more successful in some instances than others. For example, people with minimal hearing impairment in the better ear are more likely to purchase this instrument than

those with normal hearing. In these cases in which amplification is provided to the better ear in addition to contralateral routing of signal, the instruments are often referred to as BiCROS. CROS hearing aid fittings are often not successful unless the user is quite motivated to hear sounds arriving from both sides equally. The inconvenience of using two devices, poor sound quality, and poor cosmetics are often cited as reasons for rejection of CROS amplification. Successful users often report a critical communication need in an environment in which they are surrounded by important speakers. To alleviate some of these problems, a transcranial CROS fitting is sometimes attempted. Successful transcranial CROS intervention usually implements a single deep-fitting custom instrument (usually a CIC or BTE style), which is fitted to the ear without hearing. The deep fit can allow for mechanical coupling between the hearing aid shell and the bony portion of the ear canal. The mechanical coupling, when combined with high levels of hearing aid output, allows for transmission of sound to the contralateral cochlea through both bone conduction and air conduction (traveling around the head). Many users are not candidates for transcranial CROS because they find the resulting fitting uncomfortable or even painful, so appropriate screening must occur.

For some individuals, the use of conventional amplification devices (i.e., BTE, ITE, ITC) is precluded by medical conditions. For example, a hearing aid or earmold placed in the ear may exacerbate an existing ear problem or result in the recurrence of a pathologic condition. Under such circumstances, users must consider an alternative device such as a bone-conduction aid. With bone conduction hearing aids, a bone-conduction receiver is placed on the mastoid and held in position by a headband. A small wire connects the bone oscillator to a BTE hearing aid. With a bone-conduction device, the cochlea is stimulated in the same way as it is during bone-conduction threshold assessments. Unfortunately, more energy is required to stimulate the ear by bone conduction; consequently, this device can be used only with milder sensorineural hearing losses. Bone conduction hearing aids are most appropriate for listeners with hearing loss that is either entirely or mostly conductive in nature.

Somewhat more recently, bone-anchored hearing aids (such as the Baha) were introduced for listeners with primarily conductive hearing loss and listeners with medical conditions precluding the use of conventional amplification (28). The Enific Medical Systems Baha received U.S. Food and Drug Administration (FDA) approval for implantation in adults aged 18 years and older in January 1997; at the time of this writing, it remains the only FDA-approved bone-anchored hearing aid still available. In this percutaneous device, the hearing aid transducer is coupled to a titanium screw located in the upper mastoid region of the temporal bone via a titanium abutment screw that protrudes through the skin. Both an "all-in-one" ear level and a body-worn style are currently marketed. Data suggest the Baha can lead to a significant decrease in handicap, as well as an enhanced perception of general well being and disease-specific quality of life when compared to pre-treatment across a range of conductive hearing loss etiologies (29–31). Most recently, Baha fittings have been advocated for rehabilitation of unilateral hearing loss in lieu of traditional CROS amplification. Some support for this intervention exists, and data suggest the Baha can improve speech recognition in some listeners with unilateral hearing loss and reveal some advantages in terms of improved hearing aid benefit when compared to traditional CROS fittings (32).

In recent years, a second class of surgically implantable hearing aids referred to as middle ear implants (MEI) has been developed. MEIs are advocated for individuals with pure sensorineural and some types of mixed hearing loss. Current MEIs use piezoelectric, electromagnetic, or electromechanical principles to drive an output transducer mounted on the ossicular chain. Due to the small size of the piezoelectric crystal, some of these devices are entirely implanted, whereas only the output transducer is implanted in the current generation of electromagnetic and electromechanical devices. The use of MEIs for listeners with sensorineural hearing loss, in lieu of conventional amplification, stems from claims of improved fidelity, as well as reports of the elimination of feedback and the occlusion effect in listeners fit with these devices (28). Given advances in sound fidelity and reduced occlusion in digital air conduction hearing aids, one of the strongest reasons for fitting these instruments appears to be improved cosmetics (28). The future of MEIs is at this point uncertain, as at least two of the original five manufacturers have stopped pursuit of this technology.

ELECTROACOUSTIC CHARACTERISTICS OF HEARING AIDS

The fundamental purpose of a hearing aid is to provide sufficient acoustic information to allow the hearing-impaired person to maximize his or her communication skills. Several electroacoustic parameters are used to describe the performance of hearing aids. The American National Standards Institute (ANSI) has developed standards so that different hearing aids can be compared across clinics. The ANSI standard requires that these electroacoustic properties be measured in either an anechoic chamber or a specially designed test box containing absorbent material sufficient to reduce background noises. Electroacoustic measurements are accomplished by directing the output of a hearing aid into a 2-cm^3 coupler (a hard-walled cavity with a volume of 2 cm^3). The most recent standard, ANSI S3.22-1996, added methods for measuring gain in compression instruments, tests for induction coil sensitivity, equivalent input noise tests, and some changes in terminology. The three most important characteristics associated with the ANSI standard continue to be gain, output

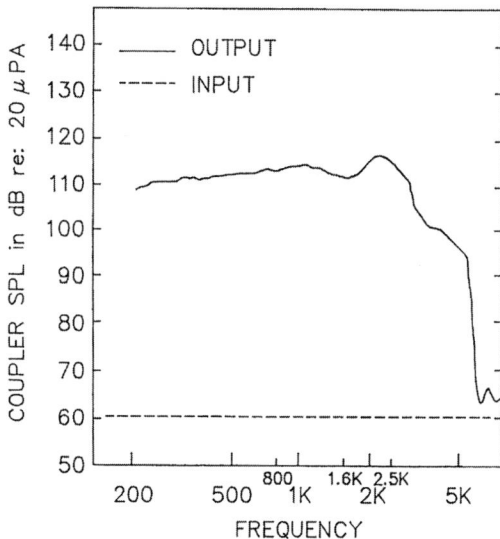

Figure 155.4 Illustration of hearing aid gain. The output curve represents the frequency response of a hearing aid for a 60-dB input.

sound pressure level with a 90-dB input (OSPL90), and frequency response.

The *gain* of a hearing aid reflects the difference in the output of the instrument relative to its input (Fig. 155.4). This measurement is obtained by presenting frequency-specific input signals of fixed (usually 50 or 60 dB) sound pressure level (SPL) to the microphone, then measuring the resultant output SPL. For example, assume that a 2,000-Hz tone is presented at an input level of 60 dB SPL and the measured output is 110 dB SPL. The gain of the hearing aid at this frequency is 50 dB. By definition, gain will vary as a function of input intensity level in nonlinear hearing instruments (those using compression and/or expansion). As a result, gain is measured using several different input levels during evaluation of these devices.

Gain can be represented in different ways. *Full-on gain* reflects the amount of amplification achieved when the volume control is adjusted to its maximum position. ANSI recommends that the hearing-aid gain be measured across the frequencies 1,000, 1,600, and 2,500 Hz, and refers to this measurement as the high-frequency average or the high-frequency full-on gain. *Reference test gain* describes the amount of amplification obtained when the volume control is adjusted such that the average gain at 1,000, 1,600, and 2,500 Hz is 17 dB below the OSPL90 or full on if the hearing aid has mild gain. Another gain measurement is referred to as *use gain* or *as-worn gain*. In this instance, the gain is measured with the volume control adjusted to its normal use position. This output gives a more realistic indication of the amount of gain the aid provides for the patient.

The *OSPL90* of the hearing aid yields the maximum amount of amplification provided by the instrument. As the input level to a hearing aid increases, the output level

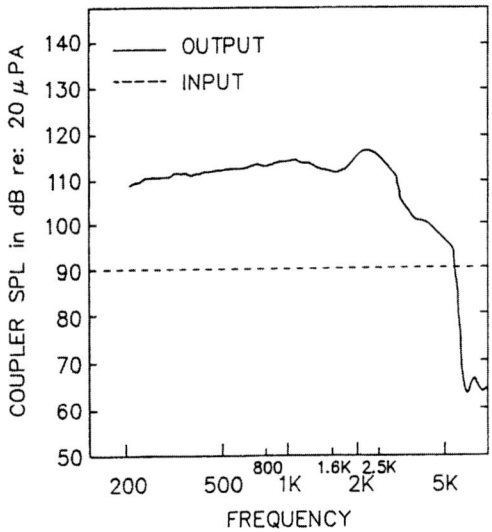

Figure 155.5   Output SPL with a 90-dB input SPL (OSPL90).

also increases up to a certain point, above which further increases in input do not affect the change in output. When this occurs, the hearing aid is said to have been driven into saturation. The OSPL90 of a hearing aid (Fig. 155.5) is obtained by delivering a 90-dB input signal from the loudspeaker in the test chamber to the microphone input of the hearing aid and measuring the overall output of the instrument across test frequencies.

The *frequency response* of a hearing aid describes the gain of a hearing aid across a range of frequencies. The range of frequencies for which a hearing aid offers amplification is limited. The aid's frequency response is determined by measuring its reference test gain. From that average, 20 dB are subtracted and a line is drawn parallel to the abscissa until it intersects the low-frequency end of the curve and the high-frequency end. These two cutoff points then represent the aid's frequency response.

Output Limiting

Hearing aid output does not become problematic until it exceeds an individual's threshold of discomfort (TD) (also referred to as loudness discomfort level, LDL). TDs represent the maximum sound level that the patient will voluntarily listen to for any length of time. Those with sensorineural hearing loss often have trouble tolerating loud sound. The range between sound that is just detectable, and that which produces discomfort (referred to as the dynamic range of hearing), is often much smaller in the hearing-impaired listener than for the person with normal hearing. As a result, consideration must be given to the overall output of the hearing aid, because it is very important to provide amplification lower than the patient's TD.

Data generally support measurement of the TD of individual listeners and the setting of the maximum hearing

aid output (OSPL90) so that it does not exceed TD, to minimize chances of auditory discomfort in the real world (33). Hearing aids employ various methods to limit output to a level at or below the individual patient's TD. Linear amplification systems limit hearing-aid output through a process called peak clipping (PC). PC hearing aids provide linear output until the hearing aid is incapable of reproducing the signal input, at which time the signal peaks are clipped. The primary disadvantage of this approach to output limiting is that it introduces harmonic and intermodulation distortion. In contrast, compression methods are preferred for output limitation because they can be used to provide output limitation while reducing distortion in comparison to PC methods.

HEARING AID CANDIDACY

Several factors must be included in selecting candidates for amplification (Table 155.2). Historically, decisions regarding the necessity for amplification have been governed by the amount of hearing impairment experienced by the listener, as determined by a careful audiologic evaluation. Even when a mild hearing loss is present, a certain degree of hearing difficulty is encountered, especially under difficult listening conditions such as background noise. The need for amplification increases, however, as the degree of hearing loss increases. Patients who reveal the greatest improvements in speech recognition from amplification are those who demonstrate a moderate to moderately severe hearing loss. This is because they must wear amplification almost all the time, and their ability to understand conversational speech, although reduced, is often good enough that the additional acoustic cues rendered by the hearing aid improve speech understanding appreciably. On the other hand, those with a mild hearing loss will likely reveal the greatest benefit under adverse listening conditions (e.g., in noise, when visual cues are obscured). At the other end of this spectrum are those with a severe to profound hearing loss. Their need for amplification is greatest, but because of poor word recognition skills, they derive the least improvement in speech recognition from amplification.

Nevertheless, all of these patients may be considered good candidates for a hearing aid. Despite the relationship between speech recognition improvements resulting from amplification and degree of hearing loss, numerous investigations have revealed that an individual's hearing aid satisfaction, perceived hearing aid benefit and performance, as well as reduction of hearing aid handicap are *not* significantly correlated with degree of hearing loss. Often, the person's work performance is significantly affected by even a mild hearing impairment. Significant problems can also arise in a child's development when even a minimal or unilateral hearing loss is present (34). Those with more severe hearing loss may find the hearing aid to be beneficial

TABLE 155.2

CONSIDERATIONS IN SELECTING HEARING AID CANDIDATES

- The first step in any hearing aid selection process is to determine the degree and type of hearing loss and determine the need for medical intervention.
- Secondly, how does the hearing loss impact on the individual's daily activities?
- Hearing loss of 25–35 dB HL may only be needed on a part-time basis (e.g., meetings or conferences for adults and educational environments for children), or a full-time basis.
- For those with moderate hearing loss (41–55 dB HL) communication is more difficult, particularly at distances of more than 4 feet, and amplification should be considered for many social and work-related environments.
- Individuals with hearing loss greater than 55–70 dB HL find communication with others very difficult without the use of amplification.
- For hearing losses greater than 70 dB HL, hearing aids are indispensable.
- What is the patient's word recognition ability?
- Are there any difficulties with loudness tolerance?
- Acceptance of hearing loss. Denial of the hearing problem reduces the motivation to wear the instrument and lessens the acknowledged benefit derived.
- Patient motivation. When an individual is not motivated toward the use of a hearing aid, the chances of achieving a successful hearing aid fitting is diminished. Counseling may improve the patient's attitude.
- Patient expectations. If expectations are too high the patient should be counseled appropriately so that the end result does not reduce the enthusiasm for wearing the instrument.

dB HL, decibels hearing level.

from a safety standpoint, even though they receive only minimal help with speech communication. In short, the audiometric data alone should not be the sole determining factor in deciding a patient's hearing-aid candidacy. Rather, assessment of hearing aid candidacy and the selection of hearing aid features should be based on a thorough assessment of the listener's communication and hearing needs.

Two other factors to consider are the patient's motivation toward hearing-aid use, and his or her acceptance of the hearing loss. Frequently, a patient seeks a hearing evaluation at the urging of a spouse or other family member. These patients do not always believe they have a hearing problem; consequently, their motivation to pursue amplification may be low. Sometimes, appropriate counseling can improve motivation, but if it cannot, the chances of obtaining a successful fitting are reduced. Others with hearing impairment simply deny the existence of the problem. The reason for this denial is unclear, but it could be due to the stigma long associated with hearing aids. For some, wearing a hearing aid is a sign of aging or an acknowledgement of a disability.

The overriding goal of fitting hearing aids is to provide sound amplification in an attempt to improve the quality of life of hearing-impaired individuals. The extent to which this is accomplished will depend on the complex interaction between the benefit provided by the hearing aid, and the individual patient's personality, motivation, and expectations (35). Consequently, the success of any hearing aid fitting must be judged not only by improvements yielded in speech recognition, but also by measures of the individual patient's perceptions of hearing aid benefit, performance, satisfaction, and/or "reduction of handicap."

MONAURAL OR BILATERAL AMPLIFICATION

Once it has been determined that an individual is a candidate for a hearing aid, the clinician must decide whether to recommend one or two hearing aids. Historically, there was some controversy concerning the benefits of bilateral over monaural amplification, but the present view is to fit bilaterally unless contraindicated. Subjectively, those who wear two hearing aids often indicate that they find speech easier to understand, especially in noisy listening conditions. Such impressions are not surprising when we consider the positive implications of binaural hearing, including localization of sound as well as "release from masking" (36). Release from masking (binaural squelch) refers to improved speech intelligibility in noise when listening binaurally due to the phase differences of the signal and noise occurring between the two ears. Another advantage to a second hearing aid is improved sound localization because the microphone is placed close to each ear. Bilateral amplification also eliminates the head shadow effects, which reduce the high-frequency cues necessary for hearing many consonants. Furthermore, the use of a second hearing aid results in an increase in the loudness of the sound due to binaural summation. In general, data support the use of bilateral amplification in listeners with reasonably symmetrical hearing loss. Ear symmetry cannot be used as a single deciding factor, however, because bilateral amplification may be beneficial in some cases even when there is a severe threshold asymmetry. Determinations of bilateral versus monaural fitting instead must be made on an individual basis.

SELECTING HEARING AIDS

The methods for selecting and evaluating amplification have undergone considerable change over the years. Rather than simply determining the appropriate hearing aid gain, hearing aid features such as directional microphones, DNR, DFS, and so forth, also must be considered. Currently, the most defensible hearing aid selection procedure is based on a thorough assessment of the listener's communication needs. This assessment should be followed by appropriate selection of hearing aid gain and output processing, as well as other features, which best address the individual patient's communication needs. The target populations for some hearing aid features were discussed above; however, a thorough discussion of assessment of communication needs and selection of features is far beyond the scope of this chapter. In brief, assessment of communication needs for the purpose of hearing aid selection may include, but is not limited to, assessment of hearing thresholds and threshold of discomfort; middle ear function; ear canal shape, geometry, and movement; speech recognition in quiet; threshold speech recognition in noise; hearing aid expectations; perceived hearing handicap; and specific listening environments in which the patient experiences difficulty.

Along with the selection of the optimal hearing aid style and features, the clinician must select the appropriate gain and output processing. It is assumed that specific goals and rationales underlie all hearing aid fittings. Selection of hearing aid gain and output generally are based on validated hearing aid fitting rationales. Several prescriptive methods have been proposed, and are being used in many hearing clinics throughout the United States and abroad. With the increased use of nonlinear gain (compression and expansion) in hearing aids, procedures designed to fit a range of amplified speech levels into the residual dynamic range of hearing have been developed (37,38). Generally, these procedures are based on their counterparts that were developed for fitting linear amplification. As opposed to the traditional fitting procedures that provide only a single gain target, these nonlinear methods provide multiple, frequency- and intensity-specific gain or output targets for different input levels of speech (e.g., soft, average, and loud speech intensities). The individual nonlinear fitting procedures are based on goals ranging from "restoration of normal loudness impression" to "making speech equally loud and comfortable across frequency bands, while attempting to maximize intelligibility." In addition to these fitting methods, several hearing aid manufacturers have developed fitting prescriptions specific to their own products. Usually proprietary in nature, these methods are often based on similar philosophies to those of existing methods. In some cases the manufacturer's product-specific methods are simply modifications of existing fitting schemes. Use of manufacturer-based prescriptive methods in lieu of more general prescriptive procedures does not appear warranted except in cases with supporting validation data.

VERIFICATION

To appropriately fit the hearing aid, verification of appropriate gain, output, and other features must be completed first. The fitting and verification procedure is viewed as a process rather than an event, which culminates in the optimal fitting for the individual patient. Verification procedures also serve as a benchmark against which future hearing aid changes can be compared. Verification procedures are based on validated hearing aid fitting rationales as described above. Hearing aid fitting and verification procedures are expected to yield a comfortable fit of a hearing aid, including all desired features.

The preferred method for verification of gain and output includes measurement of the hearing-aid output characteristics from within the ear canal using miniature probe microphones to obtain a representation of the "real ear" as opposed to the 2-cm^3 gain. One of the real-ear responses obtained is called *real ear insertion gain* or REIG (Fig. 155.6). REIG represents the SPL differences at the eardrum that occur with a functioning hearing aid and earmold in place (*top curve*) compared to that developed in an unaided ear canal (*lower curve*). Measurements such as these not only reflect the output SPL and frequency response of the hearing

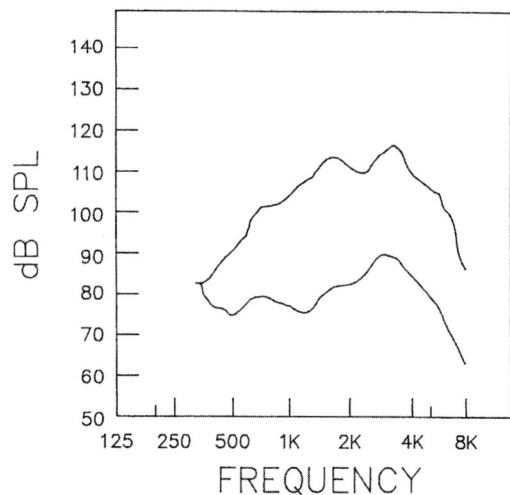

Figure 155.6   Insertion gain (obtained with probe microphone) with hearing aid and earmold (top curve) and with no hearing aid (lower curve).

aid, but also account for the combined effects of head diffraction and pinna, concha, and ear canal resonance.

Probe-tube microphone measurements employing an insertion gain protocol are not the preferred procedure for verifying electroacoustic characteristics of hearing instruments in children. Instead, verification using a probe-tube microphone measure of hearing aid output is advocated. As with the REIG method, a probe microphone measurement is made with the hearing aid in the child's ear while sound is presented through a loudspeaker at several intensity levels (i.e., soft, moderate, loud). The resulting real ear aided response (REAR) can be compared to thresholds and TDs (measured or age-appropriate estimation) converted to SPL, providing a direct measurement of audibility. The REAR method can also be used in lieu of the REIG method with adult patients. Probe microphone measures of real-ear hearing aid performance are usually not possible in young children. With younger children hearing aid performance in the ear can be assessed by applying measured, or age appropriate average, real ear coupler difference (RECD) values. In addition to probe microphone methods, aided soundfield threshold measurements may be useful for the evaluation of audibility of soft sounds. Soundfield methods are generally not recommended for verifying electroacoustic characteristics of hearing instruments for several reasons, including (1) relatively time consuming nature, (2) poor frequency resolution, (3) poor test-retest reliability, and (4) the fact that misleading information may be obtained in cases of severe to profound hearing loss, minimal, or mild loss. In addition, soundfield measures may provide misleading results in hearing aids implementing nonlinear signal processing, digital noise reduction, or automatic feedback reduction.

Special care must be taken when selecting appropriate test signals for probe microphone measures to ensure accurate electroacoustic verification. The test signal should adequately represent the frequency, intensity, and temporal aspects of speech. Investigations have illustrated that various advanced signal processing interacts with the test signal. The most accurate representation of the hearing aid's response will be through the use of a speech-like signal or by turning off signal processing during testing that attempts to reduce output for nonspeech test signals (38, 39).

VALIDATION AND ORIENTATION

Once the hearing aid has been fitted, the patient must be followed closely to ensure that he or she is deriving maximum benefits from the instrument. The purpose of orientation is to explain to the patient how to operate the hearing aid, maintain it in good working order, and use it successfully. Counseling the patient regarding hearing-aid use and adjusting to the newly restored sound is crucial to acceptance of the device. Usually an evaluation period of

1 month accompanies the purchase of the device. During this time, periodic visits with the audiologist give the patient a chance to express satisfaction or dissatisfaction with the aid so that adjustments can be made. Frequently, the patient has too high an expectation of what the hearing aid can do. Careful counseling and further instruction regarding different listening strategies may prove helpful. During the fitting and follow-up sessions, validation testing should also be completed. Such testing allows the clinician to formally assess hearing aid benefit, use, satisfaction, reduction of handicap, and so forth. The results of this testing should also be used to optimize hearing aid adjustments and counseling.

ASSISTIVE LISTENING DEVICES

A chapter on hearing aids would not be complete without a discussion of assistive listening devices (ALDs). Full-time hearing-aid use is not always beneficial or even necessary for many hearing-impaired individuals, especially those with very mild impairments. Hearing-impaired listeners are continually faced with different listening situations but typically have three types of communication needs: interpersonal communication and enjoyment of media; telecommunications; and signals such as wake-up alarms, fire alarms, and telephones. The personal hearing aid sometimes does not meet all of these needs adequately; consequently, ALDs have been developed to enhance listening. One factor that differentiates many ALDs from hearing aids is that they were developed for a specific listening situation. This includes ALDs designed as warning and wake-up devices (e.g., amplified and flashing alarms), television and radio amplifiers (hardwired, infrared, FM), and amplified telephones, to name a few (40).

As noted previously, hearing-impaired listeners often have significant difficulty understanding speech in noisy environments. In many cases the negative impact of poor SNR may reduce or even eliminate the hearing aid benefit, even in the case of hearing aids using directional microphones. Some ALDs have been designed specifically to aid listening in noisy situations. In some cases these devices have been shown to improve the SNR at ear level by as much as 15 to 20 dB in moderate noise and reverberation. There are several ALD systems designed to aid the user under a variety of adverse listening conditions. The following section briefly reviews some of the more common systems.

FM Wireless System

The FM system offers distinct advantages over the personal hearing aid and creates a better listening condition for the user. Its primary advantage is that it affords an acceptable SNR for speech understanding. These devices have been shown to improve speech perception in noise, reading/spelling ability, behavior, psychosocial function, on-task

TABLE 155.3

SUMMARY OF ACCESSORY AMPLIFICATION DEVICES

Input	Device	Description	Advantages	Disadvantages
Telephone	Internal telephone amplifier	Volume control installed by phone company in telephone receiver	Volume control easily adjusted; good range in gain; clear signal	Telephone usage restricted to modified phone; monthly fee; not available on all styles of phones
	External telephone amplifier	Hearing aid telecoil	A personal hearing aid can be used if aid equipped with circuit; adjustable volume control (can also be used with induction-loop systems)	Strength not always dependable; does not work on all phone styles
		Small device attaches to phone earpiece (used without hearing aid induction coil)	Portable; adjustable volume control; inexpensive; one-time expense	Battery operated; alignment problems
		Amplifier snaps on to earpiece (operates in conjunction with hearing aid induction coil)	Portable; adjustable gain control; provides extra power when used with hearing aid telecoil; versatile (some models can also be used as a television and radio amplifier)	Battery operated; alignment problems; relatively expensive
		Loudspeaker	Option for persons who have trouble manipulating T-switch or holding the receiver to aid for any length of time (provides extra gain without feedback problems when used in addition to one's personal hearing aid)	Limits phone usage to the modified phone
Television	Amplifier without a direct connection to source	Induction loop TV/radio kit: Kit includes materials for setting up an induction loop system in home or office (components can also be purchased separately from local TV/radio stores)	Mobility around room; improved signal/noise ratio	Trouble and expense of setting up; must have aid with T-switch; unable to hear environmental sound
		Radio with TV band	Good quality; can be used as radio	Fairly expensive
Radio	Same options as TV			
Tape recorder	Same options as TV and radio			
Signaling devices	Telephone signal amplifier	Suction cup attaches to surface of phone or doorbell, produces a loud tone	Allows individual to hear phone signal at some distance	Battery operated
	High-intensity doorbell	Large doorbell which provides much greater intensity than standard bells or chimes	Alerts person from some distance away	Installation

behaviors, and psycho-educational achievement in children (41). These devices have also been shown to effectively improve speech intelligibility in noisy environments in adults, though they are more commonly used with children in the educational system. Traditionally, the talker wears a transmitter/microphone around the neck, and a frequency-modulated signal is broadcast to an FM receiver unit worn by the listener. External receivers coupled to personal earmolds, earphones, or Walkman-type receivers are often used with these units. The receiver can also provide environmental microphones that allow for person-to-person communication, self-monitoring, and general auditory awareness of the environment. The environmental microphones also allow the unit to be used as a personal hearing aid when the FM signal is unavailable. The receiver includes internal frequency adjustments and power controls, thus making it adaptable to a wider range of individual needs.

Several techniques have been developed for dovetailing the personal hearing aid to an FM system. This concept evolved from an effort to maintain the electroacoustic-response parameters of the personal aid while at the same time providing the advantages of an improved SNR. The two most common ways to couple the FM system to the personal hearing aid are to use electrical coupling (often in the form of a snap-on "boot") or to use an inductive loop arrangement. In electrical coupling, the output voltage of the FM receiver is delivered directly to the personal hearing aid. With such an arrangement, several possible operational modes are usually available: FM only, personal hearing aid only, or a combination of the two inputs. In inductive coupling, a neck-worn induction loop is dovetailed to the FM receiver. The FM signal, sometimes mixed with an environmental signal within the FM receiver (FM mode and environmental microphone combined), is converted to an electromagnetic field via a wire loop around the listener's head. The personal hearing aid is worn in a telecoil position, thereby inductively coupling the hearing aid to the FM receiver/mini-loop combination. When the hearing aid is switched to the telecoil position, the listener's input is limited to auditory signals transduced by the FM transmitter. As an alternative to the neck-worn induction loop, a loop system may be installed for the entire classroom. Room loop systems are being used more commonly, particularly in preschool classrooms for deaf and hard-of-hearing children (41).

Soundfield Systems

Soundfield systems are designed to deliver the speech signal through a loudspeaker placed strategically in classroom environments. These systems are advantageous in that they can provide improved SNR in the classroom, which is beneficial for those children with minimal hearing loss as well as for those whose hearing loss has not been identified. Careful placement of the soundfield system loudspeakers is crucial in order to optimize benefit. Instruction of the classroom teachers about the importance of loudspeaker location may also be beneficial. For the interested reader, Crandell and Smaldino provide a review this system and other classroom ALDs (41).

Infrared Systems

In infrared systems, signals are transmitted via infrared light. These systems have become very common in public facilities (e.g., auditoriums, courtrooms) and are also used with televisions throughout the country. With this device,

the talker uses an FM microphone/transmitter, and an FM receiver is attached to the infrared transmitter. The talker's speech is converted from an acoustic signal to an electric signal, and then modulated into a radio frequency carrier wave by the FM microphone/transmitter. This signal is received by an infrared transmitter that modulates it into infrared light frequencies emitted from radiators. Several light-emitting radiators are usually placed throughout the room for uniform distribution. The modulated infrared light is then picked up by a receiver and demodulated before it enters the hearing aid. The microphone may be hard-wired to the infrared transmitter, eliminating the need for the initial FM transmission from the talker.

Other Assistive Listening Devices

Other devices that may be useful to a hearing-impaired listener are listed in Table 155.3. Two of the more common purposes for ALDs are using the telephone and listening to TV or radio. For many hearing-impaired people, the telephone is difficult to use without special amplification assistance such as a telecoil or a telephone amplifier. Unfortunately, many of the personal hearing aids sold today are not equipped with a telecoil. Several telephone handsets have been developed that can easily be attached to the phone and amplify the auditory signal by 15 to 30 dB.

Several systems are available to help the hearing-impaired listen to TV or radio. Some of these systems include a direct auditory input (a small microphone near the TV or radio speaker is hard-wired to the personal hearing aid) and wireless systems such as infrared and FM.

Finally, it is important to consider alerting devices that can be of assistance to many moderately to severely impaired people who wish to remain independent. Numerous devices have been developed to alert the hearing-impaired person to such signals as telephone rings, a baby's cries, doorbells, and smoke alarms. These alerting devices monitor sounds with a microphone and a hard-wired connection or an inductive pickup. The most common alerting stimuli include visual (bright lights or strobes) or tactile (vibration or airstream).

HIGHLIGHTS

- Hearing loss is common. Hearing impairment affects both functional health status and psychosocial well being. The primary rehabilitative measure for the hearing-impaired is a personal hearing aid or an assistive listening device.
- A basic hearing aid consists of a microphone, an amplifier, and a receiver.
- Hearing aids can be classified into the following styles: body-worn, behind-the-ear, eyeglasses, in-the-ear, in-the-canal, and completely-in-the-canal.
- The most popular hearing aids sold today are in-the-ear, in-the-canal, and completely-in-the-canal models.

- The use of digitally programmable and DSP hearing aids employing sophisticated algorithms is growing, already encompassing more than half of the total hearing aids dispensed.
- The use of directional microphones in hearing aids is experiencing resurgence as one of the only methods of significantly improving SNR in hearing aids.
- The three most common electroacoustic measures used to indicate the performance of a hearing aid are gain, frequency response, and saturation sound pressure level.
- Hearing loss is not the only criterion used for the selection of a hearing aid. Other important factors include the patient's work setting or profession, motivation, and acceptance of the hearing loss. A comprehensive assessment of the patient's communication needs is necessary for selection of optimal amplification.
- Bilateral amplification is generally recommended over monaural amplification.
- Appropriate hearing aid verification and validation procedures are necessary to quantify the appropriateness and success of the amplification intervention.
- Orientation to the device is an important component of fitting the hearing aid. The patient must learn to use the aid appropriately to gain maximum benefit. Often users or their significant others have too high an expectation; careful counseling becomes necessary.
- Assistive listening devices are valuable. Such items as FM systems, infrared systems, systems for radio and television, and alerting devices improve the quality of life for many hearing-impaired listeners.

REFERENCES

1. Lucas JW, Schiller JS, Benson V. Summary health statistics for U.S. adults: National Health Interview Survey, 2001. *Vital Health Stat 10* 2004;(218):1–134.
2. World Health Organization. *International classification of functioning, disability and health (ICF)*. Geneva: World Health Organization; 2001.
3. Campbell VA, Crews JE, Moriarty DG, et al. Surveillance for sensory impairment, activity limitation, and health-related quality of life among older adults—United States, 1993–1997. *MMWR CDC Surveill Summ* 1999;17;48(8):131–156.
4. Kramer SE, Kapteyn TS, Kuik DJ, et al. The association of hearing impairment and chronic diseases with psychosocial health status in older age. *J Aging Health* 2002;14(1):122–137.
5. Jackson PL. A psychosocial and economic profile of the hearing impaired and deaf. In: Hull RH, ed. *Aural rehabilitation: serving children and adults,* 3rd ed. San Diego: Singular; 1997.
6. Newman CW, Jacobson GP, Hug GA, et al. Perceived hearing handicap of patients with unilateral or mild hearing loss. *Ann Otol Rhinol Laryngol* 1997;106(3):210–214.
7. Mulrow CD, Aguilar C, Endicott JE, et al. Quality of life changes and hearing impairment: results of a randomized trial. *Ann Intern Med* 1990;113:188.
8. Tye-Murray N. Speech, language, and literacy development. In: Danhauer JL, ed. *Foundations of aural rehabilitation*. San Diego: Singular; 1998.
9. Kiessling J, Pichora-Fuller M, Gatehouse S, et al. Candidature for and delivery of audiological services: special needs of older people. *Int J Audiol* 2003;42(suppl 2):2S92–101.
10. Ricketts TA. Digital hearing aids: current "state-of-the-art." *ASHA Leader* 2001;6(14):8, 11.
11. Chung K. Challenges and recent developments in hearing aids. Part I. Speech understanding in noise, microphone technologies and noise reduction algorithms. *Trends Amplif* 2004;8(3):83–124.
12. Chung K. Challenges and recent developments in hearing aids. Part II. Feedback and occlusion effect reduction strategies, laser shell manufacturing processes, and other signal processing technologies. *Trends Amplif* 2004;8(4):125–164.
13. Souza PE. Effects of compression on speech acoustics, intelligibility, and sound quality. *Trends Amplif* 2002;6(4):131–165.
14. Plomp R. Noise, amplification, and compression: considerations of three main issues in hearing aid design. *Ear Hear* 1994;15(1):2–12.
15. Kochkin S, MarkeTrak V. "Why my hearing aids are in the drawer": The consumers' perspective. *Hear J* 2000;53(2):34–42.
16. Ricketts TA, Dittberner AB. Directional amplification for improved signal-to-noise ratio: strategies, measurement, and limitations. In: M. Valente, ed. *Strategies for selecting and verifying hearing aid fittings*, 2nd ed. New York: Thieme Medical Publishers; 2002: 274–346.
17. Ricketts TA. Impact of noise source configuration on directional hearing aid benefit and performance. *Ear Hear* 2000;21(3):194–205.
18. Ricketts TA, Hornsby BWY. Distance and reverberation effects on directional benefit. *Ear Hear* 2003;24(6):472–484.
19. Ricketts TA, Lindley G, Henry P. Impact of compression and hearing aid style on directional hearing aid benefit and performance. *Ear Hear* 2001;22(4):348–361.
20. Ricketts TA, Henry P. Gain equalization in directional hearing aids. *Am J Audiol* 2002;11(1):29–41.
21. Ricketts TA, Henry P, Gnewikow D. Full time directional versus user selectable microphone modes in hearing aids. *Ear Hear* 2003;24(5):424–439.
22. Bentler RA, Palmer C, Dittberner AB. Hearing-in-noise: comparison of listeners with normal and (aided) impaired hearing. *J Am Acad Audiol* 2004;15(3):216–225.
23. Ricketts TA, Hornsby BWY. Sound quality measures for speech in noise through a commercial hearing aid implementing digital noise reduction. *J Am Acad Audiol* 2005;16(5):270–277.
24. Boymans M, Dreschler WA. Field trials using a digital hearing aid with active noise reduction and dual-microphone directionality. *Audiology* 2000;39(5):260–268.
25. Galster J, Ricketts T. The effects of digital noise reduction time constants on speech recognition in noise. Paper presented at: International Hearing Aid Research Conference, August 26–29, 2004, Lake Tahoe, CA.
26. Kuk FK. Perceptual consequences of vents in hearing aids. *Br J Audiol* 1991;25:163–169.
27. Chasin M. The acoustic advantages of CIC hearing aids. *Hear J* 1994;47:13–17.
28. Chasin M, Westerkull P, Kroll K, et al. Bone anchored and middle ear implant hearing aids. *Trends Amplif* 2002;6(2):31–84.
29. Dutt SN, McDermott AL, Jelbert A, et al. The Glasgow benefit inventory in the evaluation of patient satisfaction with the bone-anchored hearing aid: quality of life issues. *J Laryngol Otol Suppl* 2002;28:7–14.
30. Hol MK, Spath MA, Krabbe PF, et al. The bone-anchored hearing aid: quality-of-life assessment. *Arch Otolaryngol Head Neck Surg* 2004;130(4):394–399.
31. McLarnon CM, Davison T, Johnson IJ. Bone-anchored hearing aid: comparison of benefit by patient subgroups. *Laryngoscope* 2004;114(5):942–944.
32. Hol MK, Bosman AJ, Snik AF, et al. Bone-anchored hearing aid in unilateral inner ear deafness: a study of 20 patients. *Audiol Neurootol* 2004;13;9(5):274–281.
33. Munro KJ, Patel RK. Are clinical measurements of uncomfortable loudness levels a valid indicator of real-world auditory discomfort? *Br J Audiol* 1998;32(5):287–293.
34. Tharpe AM, Bess FH. Minimal, progressive, and fluctuating hearing losses in children. Characteristics, identification, and management. *Pediatr Clin North Am* 1999;46(1):65–78.
35. Wong LL, Hickson L, McPherson B. Hearing aid satisfaction: what does research from the past 20 years say? *Trends Amplif* 2003;7(4):117–161.
36. Holmes AE. Bilateral amplification for the elderly: are two aids better than one? *Int J Audiol* 2003;42(suppl 2):2S63–7.

37. Dillon H. NAL-NL1: a new prescriptive fitting procedure for nonlinear hearing aids. *Hear J* 1999;52(4):10–17.
38. Cornelisse L, Seewald R, Jamieson D. Wide-dynamic-range compression hearing aids: the DSL [i/o] approach. *Hearing J* 1994; 47(10):23–29.
39. Scollie SD, Seewald RC. Evaluation of electroacoustic test signals I: comparison with amplified speech. *Ear Hear* 2002;23(5):477–487.
40. Lesner SA. Candidacy and management of assistive listening devices: special needs of the elderly. *Int J Audiol* 2003;42(suppl 2): 2S68–76.
41. Crandell C, Smaldino J. Classroom acoustics and amplification. In: Valente M, Roeser R, Hosford-Dunn H, eds. *Audiology. Volume II: Treatment.* New York: Thieme Medical Publishers; 2000.

Peripheral Vestibular Disorders

156

Carol A. Bauer   *Horst R. Konrad*

Dizziness is an extremely common symptom that affects more than 90 million people each year in the United States (1). In 1991, nearly 5.5 million outpatient visits involved evaluation of vertigo and imbalance (2). Severe dizziness can be incapacitating, resulting in decreased productivity and impaired quality of life. The proportion of patients with dizziness resulting from a peripheral vestibular disorder is not well known. Peripheral disorders are more likely to occur among persons younger than 50 years. Disturbances in central balance function are more common among older age groups. Particularly in the elderly patient with dizziness, a combination of peripheral and central dysfunction can occur (3). The symptom of dizziness increases in frequency with age (4). Among persons older than 75 years, balance disorders are the most common reason for visiting primary care physicians (5).

Peripheral vestibular disorders can result in symptoms of dizziness, vertigo, and imbalance in several ways. The presenting signs and symptoms are dictated by the anatomic and physiologic characteristics of the labyrinthine receptors and the central vestibular pathways. Under normal conditions there is symmetric tonic afferent activity from each vestibular nerve to the corresponding vestibular nucleus in the brainstem. Stimuli such as head turning or changes in head position with respect to gravity result, respectively, in movement of the endolymph within the semicircular canals or a shift in the otoconia within the utricle and saccule. These events are detected by the vestibular sensory epithelium and are reflected in either an increase or decrease in the tonic neural activity within each vestibular nerve (6). The physiologic reflex response to a change in head orientation is to move the eyes in an equal and opposite direction thus maintaining visual stability and focus during head movement. This response is the vestibuloocular reflex (VOR). The sensory structures within the left and right vestibular labyrinths work in tandem. When head movement or a change in head position causes a change in vestibular afferent activity, afferent activity from one vestibular nerve increases and activity from the opposite vestibular nerve decreases.

The signs and symptoms of peripheral vestibular disorders can result from a change in the sensitivity of the vestibular receptors to gravity (linear acceleration) and head movement (angular acceleration), an abnormal asymmetry in central vestibular activity, or a change in the gain of the VOR (ratio of eye movement to head movement amplitude). Signs and symptoms also depend on the timing and severity of the injury to the vestibular periphery. Vestibular injuries can be sudden, progressive, fluctuating, unilateral, or bilateral in nature. The rate of progression of the lesion, the degree or extent of injury, and the time course of central compensation will determine the presenting signs and symptoms. Central compensation is the normal recovery process that occurs soon after an injury to the peripheral vestibular system. The severity of signs and symptoms associated with peripheral vestibular injury are minimized through the process of central compensation. This process requires an intact and functional cerebellum integrated with the central vestibular pathways. The process is stimulated and facilitated by active head movement under visual conditions.

SIGNS AND SYMPTOMS

Unilateral Disorders of Sudden Onset

The causes of sudden-onset unilateral vestibular dysfunction include infectious (viral neuronitis; bacterial labyrinthitis;

Ramsey-Hunt syndrome), traumatic (temporal bone fracture), iatrogenic (labyrinthectomy, vestibular nerve section), and idiopathic etiologies (Ménière disease). In addition, labyrinthine damage can occur from exposure to ototoxic agents (gentamicin), vascular injury, and labyrinthine fistulae (7).

A lesion involving one labyrinth reduces the afferent activity from the affected side to the ipsilateral vestibular nucleus. There is a consequent reduction of activity within the reflex pathways between the vestibular brainstem and the oculomotor, cerebellar, and spinal-postural systems. In the acute stage, this asymmetry is interpreted centrally as movement (vertigo); the reduction in tonic activity to the oculomotor nuclei causes nystagmus; and the altered vestibulospinal and cerebellar activity is perceived as a sensation of falling. If the right labyrinth is affected, slow eye movements are to the right (fast-phase nystagmus to the left). There is also evidence of altered vestibulospinal activity (past-pointing, Romberg sign, rotation on the Fukuda stepping test). The severity of the symptoms depends on the extent of labyrinthine injury and the degree of central compensation that has occurred. When there is severe loss of function, changes in vestibular nucleus activity affect other brainstem nuclei, and nausea, vomiting, sweating, and bradycardia may occur.

Immediately after injury, nystagmus is present in all positions of gaze. It is suppressed by visual fixation, increases when gaze is directed away from the lesion, and decreases when gaze is toward the lesion. Nystagmus gradually disappears but can be present in the absence of visual fixation for a longer period of time. The vegetative symptoms of nausea and vomiting diminish over time. The rate of recovery from peripheral injury is directly related to activity level and is decreased with advanced age. Vestibulosuppressive medications also decrease the rate and extent of recovery from peripheral injury.

Bilateral Vestibular Lesions

Bilateral vestibular lesions result in a symmetric decrease in the tonic activity from each labyrinth to the brainstem. The primary symptoms are caused by reduction in vestibular sensitivity to head movement and gravitational position resulting in VOR inaccuracy. The smooth pursuit and optokinetic systems are not affected by labyrinthine disease and can maintain visual focus during low-velocity head movement. An accurately tuned VOR is necessary to maintain visual acuity during rapid head movement. Without an intact VOR, quick head movements cause a slip of the visual field on the retina, and visual acuity degrades. When vestibular function is normal the gain of the VOR is close to one. When bilateral vestibular input is inadequate to maintain accurate gain of the VOR, patients report visual disturbance and light-headedness. Blurry vision and disequilibrium are prominent with rapid head movement or when visual input is limited.

Cerebellar compensation mechanisms are needed for adjusting the gain of the VOR in response to altered labyrinth sensitivity. Symptoms of a partial bilateral loss usually resolve in a few days. Cerebellar compensation cannot accommodate total or near total loss of bilateral vestibular function, and patients have severe visual disturbances with head movement (oscillopsia). The causes of sudden-onset bilateral disorders include ototoxicity, meningitic labyrinthitis, and bilateral temporal bone trauma.

Unilateral Lesions of Gradual Onset

The causes of gradual-onset unilateral disorders include eighth-nerve neoplasia and degenerative and autoimmune disease. Lesions of gradual onset may not produce severe symptoms because the VOR is continuously monitored and adjusted to maintain accurate compensatory eye movements in response to head movement. Asymmetric responses are adjusted in the brainstem by mechanisms that are not completely known but that require commissural fibers between the vestibular nuclei (8). Gain of the VOR is adjusted by the lateral cerebellum (nodulus and flocculus) (9). If the lesion progresses slowly enough, as with acoustic neuroma, vestibular symptoms can be so mild as to be imperceptible. It is not uncommon for vestibular symptoms of acoustic neuroma to occur only when the lesion is large enough to cause brainstem compression or to compromise the blood supply to the peripheral labyrinth and cause a sudden decrease in unilateral vestibular function. Caloric testing, however, can show a decreased response on the side of the lesion when the tumor affects the superior vestibular nerve.

Bilateral Lesions of Gradual Onset

Bilateral lesions of gradual onset cause few symptoms because of the existence of cerebellar compensatory mechanisms within the nodulus and flocculus. Symptoms occur when there is a total or near-total loss of vestibular sensitivity. Symptoms of visual disturbance, light-headedness, and oscillopsia are prominent. Examples of gradual-onset bilateral disorders are aging, ototoxicity, autoimmune disease, syphilis, and degenerative disorders.

Fluctuating or Recurrent Symptoms

Unilateral intermittent disorders such as hydrops, benign paroxysmal positional vertigo, and dehiscence of the superior semicircular canal (10) present as intermittent episodes of vestibular dysfunction. When the sensitivity of the vestibular system changes episodically, as in Ménière disease or endolymphatic hydrops, the central nervous system does not have time to compensate for each episode of peripheral vestibular injury. Each attack is a sudden loss of vestibular function, and the symptoms last for a few hours or days. Recurrent episodes of injury to the labyrinth, as in

Ménière disease, eventually cause loss of vestibular sensitivity on the affected side and cessation of vestibular symptoms. Other causes of recurrent vestibular injury or stimulation can resolve spontaneously or persist until appropriately managed. Perilymph fistula, benign paroxysmal positional vertigo, and superior semicircular canal dehiscence syndrome are examples of recurrent unilateral vestibular disease that cause intermittent vestibular symptoms. Autoimmune disorders can affect one or both ears and can be gradually progressive or can cause fluctuating symptoms. Tertiary or congenital syphilis causes vestibular damage through lymphocytic infiltration, vasculitis, and hydrops, usually with fluctuating vestibular symptoms and eventually with bilateral loss of vestibular function.

DIAGNOSIS

Accurate diagnosis is critical in the treatment of patients with peripheral vestibular disorders. The history and physical examination are the most important evaluation tools available to astute clinicians in evaluating the patient with vertigo (Fig. 156.1). The clinical evaluation should determine the

onset and time course of events (acute, progressive, duration, frequency), a description of the symptoms (spinning, lightheadedness, imbalance, blurry vision), any associated symptoms (hearing loss, aural fullness, otorhea, otalgia, facial paralysis, headache, photophobia, nausea, vomiting), precipitating and alleviating factors, and relevant risk factors (head trauma, cerebrovascular disease, autoimmune disease). The status of other sensory systems critical for balance (vision, proprioception), the integrity of the central nervous system, and the integrity of compensatory mechanisms also must be evaluated. Compensation will be significantly affected by the use of certain prescription and nonprescription medications, and a thorough review is necessary.

The physical examination includes a complete head and neck examination, cranial nerve assessment, oculomotor evaluation with and without Frenzel glasses, and observation of gait and posture. The otologic examination includes pneumatic otoscopy and audiometry. Spontaneous nystagmus is carefully described in terms of type, degree, and the effect of visual fixation.

The presence of positional nystagmus and associated vertigo is assessed with Dix-Hallpike maneuvers. Pneumatic

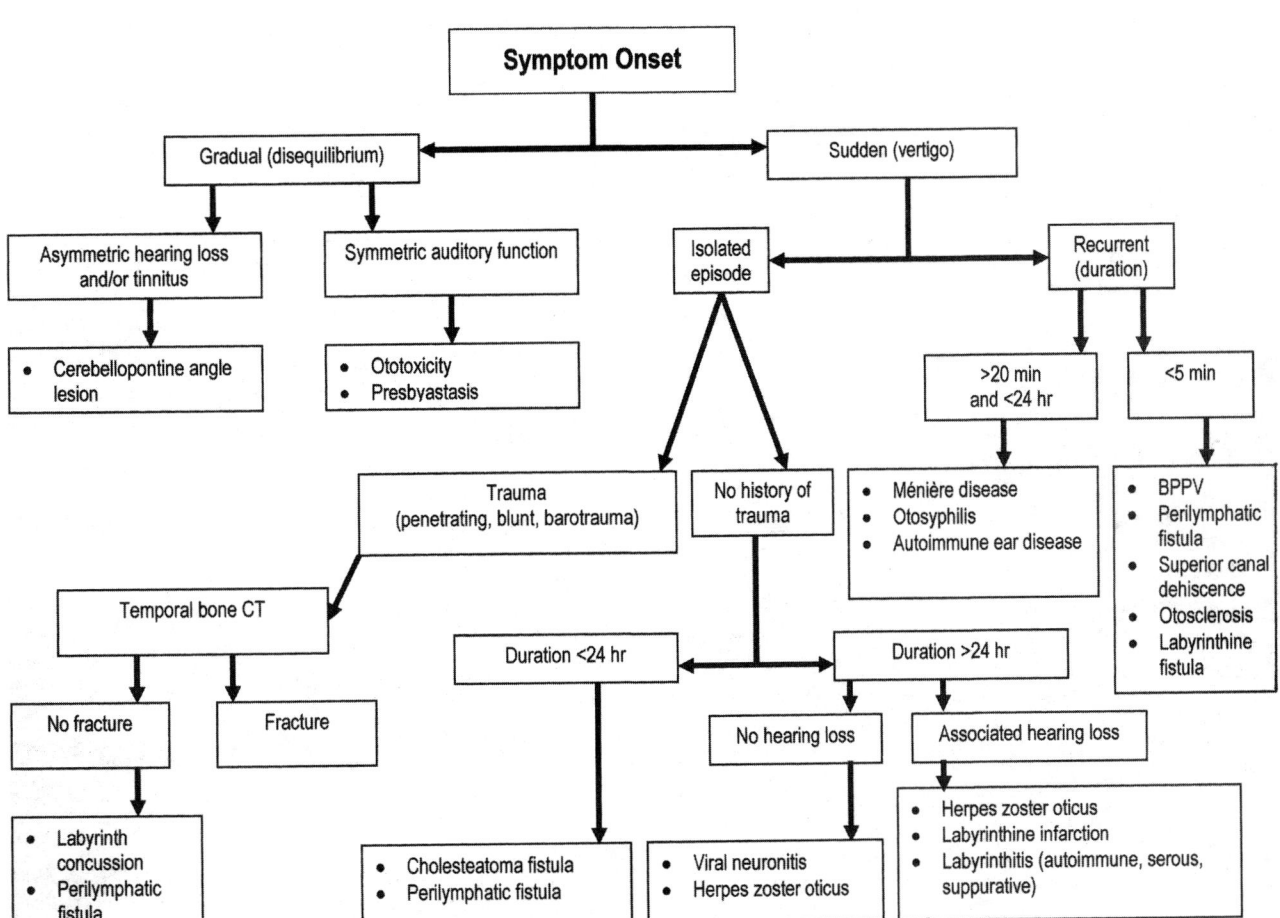

Figure 156.1 Symptoms of peripheral vestibular disorders.

otoscopy with positive and negative pressure and Frenzel glasses is used to assess Hennebert sign (vertigo and abnormal eye movements with positive or negative pressure in the ear canal with an intact tympanic membrane). Examination for the Tullio phenomenon with Frenzel glasses is performed if superior canal dehiscence is suspected (10). Clinical evidence of unilateral vestibular loss includes spontaneous nystagmus and refixation saccades during the head-thrust test (11). During the head-thrust test, the examiner briskly moves the patient's head to one side while the patient is directed to maintain visual fixation on the examiner's face. If there is unilateral vestibular weakness and inadequate VOR in one direction, the patient performs a refixation saccade after the head thrust to maintain visual fixation on the target. Clinical evidence of bilateral vestibular loss can be detected with the dynamic visual acuity test (12). This test is also useful in the assessment of recovery of function after therapy (13). The patient is asked to read the lowest line on a Snellen chart with the head stationary and then again during 2-Hz head oscillation. Patients with bilateral vestibular loss have visual blurring during head oscillation and lose three or more lines of acuity on the Snellen chart.

Patients with a history of visual impairment undergo evaluation of the eyes, vision, and visual fields. Because the visual system is directly involved in balance, impaired vison can contribute to balance symptoms and delay recovery after loss of vestibular function. Other special maneuvers performed during the examination are post–headshake nystagmus testing, hyperventilation-induced vertigo and nystagmus, and head-on-body rotation to evaluate cervical vertigo (14).

Vestibular function tests assess the labyrinth, vestibular-ocular control systems, postural control, and gait. The electronystagmography (ENG) is a battery of tests of vestibular function that includes evaluation of spontaneous and gaze-evoked nystagmus with and without visual fixation, positional testing, caloric response of the lateral semicircular canals, and rotational chair testing. Studies of eye movement include smooth pursuit and the optokinetic, saccade, and vestibuloocular reflexes. A variety of tests are available for evaluating the vestibulospinal system and postural control. These tests evaluate visual vestibular interaction, gait stability, and postural reflexes under different sensory conditions. A recent addition to the vestibular test battery is the vestibular evoked myogenic potential (VEMP) measurement. The VEMP assesses the function of structures not assessed by the standard battery of vestibular tests, the saccule and inferior vestibular nerve. This test is analogous to the auditory brainstem response (ABR) test in assessing a neural reflex arc. An acoustic signal is used to stimulate the saccule; the reflex arc spans the inferior vestibular nerve, vestibular nuclei, and vestibulospinal tract with output detected as a change in the sternocleidomastoid muscle potential (15). Potential applications of the VEMP include evaluation of superior canal dehiscence,

vestibular schwannoma, and early detection of Ménière disease (16).

If the findings at clinical evaluation and electronystagmography suggest disorders of the middle ear, mastoid, or internal auditory canal, then computed tomography or magnetic resonance imaging is indicated to establish the location of the lesion. Computed tomography is indicated if cholesteatoma or other disorders that destroy bone are suspected. Magnetic resonance imaging with gadolinium enhancement is indicated for evaluation of retrocochlear causes of vertigo. Focused evaluations limited to the temporal bone are cost effective for assessing the labyrinth and cerebellopontine angles but can miss signs of small-vessel atherosclerosis, demyelinating disorders, or neoplasms of the cerebrum or cerebellum.

A complete evaluation addresses etiologic diagnosis and the site of the lesion. In addition, the integrity of the central nervous system is assessed and the level of disability is ascertained. A social evaluation is performed to assess the work and home environments and family and community resources. Many other disorders frequently coexist with vestibular disorders, including migraine, acrophobia (fear of heights), agoraphobia (fear of crowds), and increased motion sensitivity. The patient's level of motivation and any associated litigation related to the vestibular injury are also evaluated. These factors can necessitate independent treatment or affect the successful management of the vestibular symptoms.

TREATMENT

The management goal for peripheral vestibular disorders is to decrease the severity of symptoms and restore function (Fig. 156.2). Treatment options include vestibulosuppressive medication, ablative surgery, chemical labyrinthectomy, and rehabilitation. Therapy for some disorders is aimed at the lesion itself; this is particularly important in the management of chronic otitis media, cholesteatoma, or bacterial labyrinthitis. Emergency operative intervention and antibiotic therapy are considered when chronic infection causes vertigo. Selection of treatment is dictated by the specific diagnosis, the frequency and duration of symptoms, and patient characteristics and needs.

Initial management goals for disorders that cause sudden loss of unilateral vestibular function are relief of the acute vestibular and autonomic symptoms. This is accomplished with intravenous, oral, or transdermal medications. Diazepam 5 to 10 mg intravenously slowly over several minutes will reduce the vertigo, nausea, and vomiting of severe unilateral loss of vestibular function. This drug is best used to manage vestibular neuronitis, posttraumatic loss of vestibular function, labyrinthitis, or severe episodic vertigo (17). Vestibular sedatives are contraindicated during active evaluation of the patient for central nervous system disease or head injury.

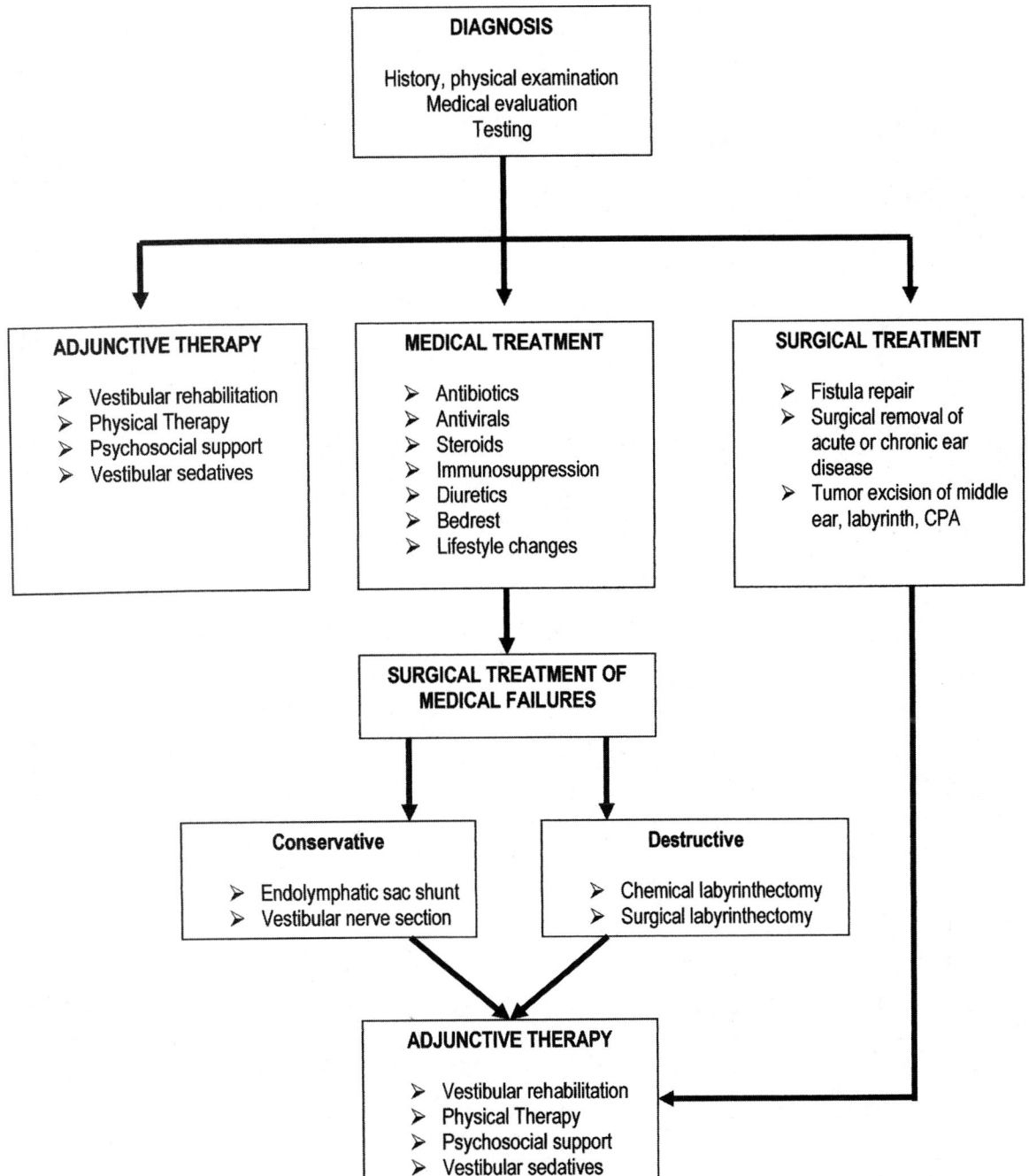

Figure 156.2 Management of peripheral vestibular disorders.

After the severe symptoms of acute vestibular injury have resolved, movement exercises must be started to rehabilitate remaining function (18,19). The goals of vestibular rehabilitation are to promote compensation for peripheral vestibular injury by altering the gain of the VOR (adaptation) and to develop substitution strategies to maintain balance. There is a critical period of 72 hours or less after which rehabilitation is less efficacious and complete recovery is less likely. Effective vestibular rehabilitation requires early initiation of active head movement with visual stimulation. Both visual and neck reflexes can be used to compensate for loss of

vestibular function. Oral vestibulosuppressive medications, such as meclizine or transdermal scopolamine, are useful during acute attacks, but doses are reduced and discontinued as soon as possible to minimize suppression of compensation.

Vestibular disease that is progressive or fluctuating poses the most common treatment problem. Degenerative labyrinthine disorders are best managed with minimal use of vestibulosuppressive medication during periods of rapid change in function. The same is true of episodic vertigo from vestibular hydrops (Ménière disease). As soon as the severe vertigo ends, vestibular suppressants are discontinued, and rehabilitation exercises are instituted.

The episodic vertigo of vestibular hydrops can be managed in many ways. Most patients with Ménière disease respond to a decrease in dietary salt intake and administration of diuretics. The rationale for this treatment is to reduce endolymph pressure. Some cases of Ménière syndrome are immune mediated and are successfully managed with immunotherapy and dietary elimination of food allergens (20). If the hydrops cannot be controlled or is end-stage disease, then symptomatic control can be achieved with the application of intratympanic gentamicin (21).

Patients who do not respond to treatment and continue to have incapacitating vertigo may need definitive surgical treatment. Options include shunting operations, vestibular neurectomy, and ablative procedures. Ablation of labyrinthine function has a high rate of success in relieving symptoms of episodic vertigo. Ablative procedures should be used with caution in elderly patients with poor central compensation and in patients at risk for bilateral loss of vestibular function.

Systemic administration of streptomycin to achieve a chemical labryinthectomy has been used to treat patients with bilateral Ménière disease, disease in an only hearing ear, or poor surgical candidates. Streptomycin is given intramuscularly twice a day while vestibular function is monitored with caloric tests. When caloric responses decrease, treatment is stopped. Caloric responses are used to measure the low-frequency portion of the dynamic range of the vestibular system. Streptomycin appears to ablate this area first while sparing higher frequency sensitivity, which is more important in physiologic head movement. Titration of streptomycin against the caloric response may relieve episodic vertigo without producing oscillopsia.

The technique of surgical labyrinthectomy can be performed by several routes. The procedure is used to treat patients who have incapacitating episodic vertigo but no useful hearing in the affected ear. The result is a loss of vestibular function and destruction of any residual hearing. Labyrinthectomy can be performed through the ear canal. If the oval or round windows are not clearly in view when the annulus and tympanic membrane are displaced anteriorly, a small amount of superior posterior ear canal bone is removed with curettes or a microdrill. After positive identification of the facial nerve in the middle ear, the stapes is removed and the bone between the oval and round window is removed with a microdrill. Portions of the membranous labyrinth can be removed with pick, hook, and suction device. A piece of gel foam sponge impregnated with streptomycin can be placed in the resulting space. Fascia or muscle tissue can be used for packing.

Removal of the vestibular labyrinth can also be accomplished through the transmastoid approach. After complete simple mastoidectomy, the facial nerve is identified and the horizontal canal removed. The superior and posterior canals are opened, and the vestibule with utricle and saccule is exposed and removed. Comparative efficacy in symptom relief between ablative labyrinthectomy and vestibular nerve section is still debated (22,23).

Surgery for superior canal dehiscence syndrome has been advocated as treatment for incapacitating symptoms associated with the disorder. The dehiscent semicircular canal is exposed using a middle cranial fossa approach, and either occluded with bone dust or resurfaced using fascia and bone. There is some controversy regarding the prevalence of symptomatic canal dehiscence and indications for surgery for this disorder are not yet well-established (24).

Positional vertigo of the benign paroxysmal type (BPPV) is one of the most common presenting causes of episodic vertigo among all age groups. A normal cupula of the semicircular canal is neutrally buoyant with respect to endolymph. The cupula becomes sensitive to gravity and produces all the signs and symptoms of cupular deflection when otoconial debris either adhere to the crista (cupulolithiasis) or become free-floating within a semicircular canal (canalithiasis). Clinical and histologic evidence indicates that both cupulolithiasis and canalithiasis can cause positional vertigo. The posterior canal is most commonly affected by canalithiasis although involvement of alternate canals can occur (25). Although BPPV increases in incidence with age, the diagnosis is frequently unrecognized in the elderly (3). The BPPV may present as an isolated vestibular dysfunction, or in association with other vestibulopathies (26) or ischemic vasculitis (27). Particle repositioning manuevers are highly successful in treating this benign but potentially incapacitating disorder (28,29). Surgery for incapacitating positional vertigo has been advocated. In cases unresponsive to particle repositioning maneuvers, occlusion of the posterior semicircular canal lumen with bone dust or sectioning the posterior canal ampullary nerve usually is effective (30).

Vestibular Rehabilitation

For many years, clinicians have expressed dissatisfaction with suppressive medication, decompressive surgery, and ablative surgery for the management of vertigo caused by peripheral disorders. Suppressive medications can reduce compensation to vestibular injury and have significant side effects, including drowsiness, dry eyes, and dry mouth. The results of decompressive surgery are not universally favorable, and ablative surgery can cause loss of hearing or necessitate intracranial operations with the attendant risk of cerebrospinal fluid leak, meningitis, and facial nerve injury.

Vestibular rehabilitation has been used in England since the 1930s and in continental Europe, the United States, and other countries since the 1940s. It has been most effective for the rehabilitation of patients with sudden loss of vestibular function or positional vertigo (31). Vestibular therapy can improve symptoms from vertigo of unknown causation and also improve general balance conditioning in the elderly (32). Vestibular rehabilitation frequently is adjunctive to other therapy (after use of suppressive medication in the acute postinjury phase) or after ablative surgery. In these situations, the exercises must include head movements in conjunction with active visual fixation and must be started soon after injury. Head movements that produce the greatest symptoms of disequilibrium often are the most effective in the rehabilitation process (33).

It is important to examine the patient carefully before recommending vestibular exercises to ensure that the disorder is not life threatening or easily managed by other means. In many cases, however, exercises are the best way to manage the condition, particularly when the patient has sudden loss of vestibular function, degeneration of vestibular function (unilateral or bilateral), or positional vertigo. There is increasing evidence that home treatment programs can be effective in facilitating vestibular habituation (33,34). Refractory symptoms may benefit from formal vestibular rehabilitation exercises conducted under the supervision of a physical therapist.

Vestibular rehabilitation encompasses a variety of techniques designed to improve the symptoms of vestibular hypofunction, decrease disability, and improve function. Vestibular rehabilitation treatment programs are initiated after a complete assessment of the patient's deficits, general physical condition, and functional limitations. Deficits in multiple sensory modalities can impede improvement and treatment plans must be designed to accommodate visual and proprioceptive disorders that complicate vestibular dysfunction. The assessment should determine the degree of static and dynamic postural stability as well as abnormalities of gait.

Vestibular rehabilitation programs rely on several mechanisms to promote recovery of function. Vestibular adaptation is responsible for the long-term changes that occur in the vestibular reflex arcs in response to changes in vestibular input. Altered gain in the vestibulo-ocular and vestibulospinal reflexes occurs after peripheral vestibular injury, and recovery of functional gain in these systems is promoted by active head and body movement combined with visual input. Various rehabilitation programs of graduated exercise are available for the management of patients with vestibular dysfunction. The programs incorporate structured movements of the head and neck combined with visual tracking and balance tasks that are environmentally contextual. The excercises are performed daily, and can be initiated during an inpatient or outpatient evaluation.

HIGHLIGHTS

- Peripheral vestibular disorders cause signs and symptoms by producing asymmetric input to the brain, altering the sensitivity of the receptors, and changing a rotational receptor to a gravity receptor.
- Symptoms depend on the rate of progression of the disorder and whether the disorder is constant or fluctuating and unilateral or bilateral.

- Dizziness is an extremely common symptom. Peripheral causes are more common in early life, central or combined peripheral and central in later life.
- Unilateral lesions produce spontaneous nystagmus with slow phase toward the side of the lesion.
- The rate of recovery from a peripheral lesion is improved with head movement with visual function.
- Patients who have absent responses to caloric stimulation may have residual vestibular function, particularly for high frequencies.
- With bilateral loss of vestibular function, patients often report visual disturbances during head motion rather than vertigo.
- One reason symptoms are so disturbing in disorders that cause episodic vestibular dysfunction is that the compensatory mechanisms do not have time to occur.
- Among diagnostic methods, history and physical examination are most important in evaluating patients with vertigo.
- Vertigo during bacterial otitis or mastoiditis is a serious symptom that suggests the need for emergency treatment.
- Management of vertigo of peripheral origin can necessitate use of vestibulosuppressive medications during the acute phase, ablative surgical therapy for severe fluctuating vertigo, and rehabilitative therapy for persistent or movement-provoked vertigo.

REFERENCES

1. Task Force on the National Strategic Research Plan. *Balance and the vestibular system.* Bethesda, MD: National Institutes of Health; 1989.
2. *Vital and Health Statistics, The National Ambulatory Medical Care Survey, 1991 Summary,* National Health Survey, Series 13, No. 116, DHHS Publication No. (PHS) 94-1777, May 1994:21. See Table R.
3. Oghalai JS, Manolidis S, Barth JL, et al. Unrecognized benign paroxysmal positional vertigo in elderly patients. *Otolaryngol Head Neck Surg* 2000;122(5):630–634.
4. Baloh RW. Vertigo in older people. *Curr Treat Options Neurol* 2000;2(1):81–89.
5. Sloane PD, Coeytaux RR, Beck RS, et al. Dizziness: state of the science. *Ann Intern Med* 2001 May 1;134(9 Pt 2):823–832.
6. Fernandez C, Goldberg JM. Physiology of peripheral neurons innervating semicircular canals of the squirrel monkey, II: response to sinusoidal stimulation and dynamics of peripheral vestibular system. *J Neurophysiol* 1971;34:661–675.
7. Minor LB. Labyrinthine fistulae: pathobiology and management. *Curr Opin Otolaryngol Head Neck Surg* 2003;11(5):340–346.
8. Precht W. Characteristics of vestibular neurons after acute and chronic labyrinthine destruction. In: Kornhuber HH, ed. *Vestibular system: handbook of sensory physiology.* Vol VI. Berlin: Springer; 1974:451.
9. Jeannerod M, Courjon JH, Flandrin JM, et al. Supravestibular control of vestibular compensation after hemilabyrinthectomy in the cat. In: Flohr H, Precht W, eds. *Lesion-induced neuronal plasticity in sensorimotor Systems.* Berlin: Springer; 1981:208.
10. Minor LB. Superior canal dehiscence syndrome. *Am J Otol* 2000;21:9–19.
11. Halmagyi GM, Curthoys IS, Cremer PD, et al. The human horizontal vestibulo-ocular reflex in response to high-acceleration stimulation before and after unilateral vestibular neurectomy. *Exp Brain Res* 1990;81:479–490.
12. Baloh RW, Honrubia V. *Clinical neurophysiology of the vestibular system.* Philadelphia: FA Davis; 1990.

13. Herdman SJ, Schubert MC, Das VE, et al. Recovery of dynamic visual acuity in unilateral vestibular hypofunction. *Arch Otolaryngol Head Neck Surg* 2003;129(8):819–824.
14. Wrisley DM, Sparto PJ, Whitney SL, et al. Cervicogenic dizziness: a review of diagnosis and treatment. *J Orthop Sports Phys Ther* 2000;30(12):755–766.
15. Robertson DD, Ireland DJ. Vestibular evoked myogenic potentials. *J Otolaryngol* 1995;243:3–8.
16. Shojaku H, Takemori S, Kobahashi K, et al. Clinical usefulness of glyceraol vestibular-evoked myogenic potentials: preliminary report. *Acta Otolaryngol Suppl* 2001;545:65–68.
17. Hain TC, Uddin M. Pharmacological treatment of vertigo. *CNS Drugs* 2003;17(2):85–100.
18. Norre MD. Vestibular habituation training: exercise treatment for vertigo based upon the habituation effect. *Otolaryngol Head Neck Surg* 1989;101:14.
19. Cohen HS, Kimball KT. Decreased ataxia and improved balance after vestibular rehabilitation. *Otolaryngol Head Neck Surg* 2004; 130(4):418–425.
20. Derebery MJ. Allergic management of Meniere's disease: an outcome study. *Otolaryngol Head Neck Surg* 2000;122:174–182.
21. Diamond C, O'Connell DA, Hornig JD, et al. Systematic review of intratympanic gentamicin in Meniere's disease. *J Otolaryngol* 2003;32(6):351–361.
22. Badke MB, Pyle GM, Shea T, et al. Outcomes in vestibular ablative prodecures. *Otol Neurotol* 2002;23(4):504–509.
23. Eisenman DJ, Speers R, Telian SA. Labyrinthectomy versus vestibular neurectomy. long-term physiologic and clinical outcomes. *Otol Neurotol* 2001;22(4):539–548.
24. Williamson RA, Vrabec JT, Coker NJ, et al. Coronal computed tomography prevalence of superior semicircular canal dehiscence. *Otolaryngol Head Neck Surg* 2003;129(5):481–489.
25. Honrubia V, Baloh RW, Harris M, et al. Paroxysmal positional vertigo syndrome. *Am J Otol* 199;20:465–470.
26. Karlburg M, Hall K, Quickert N, et al. What inner ear diseases cause benign paroxysmal positional vertigo? *Acta Otolaryngol* 2000;120(3):380–385.
27. Amor-Dorado JC, Llorca J, Costa-Ribas C, et al. Giant cell arteritis: a new association with benign paroxysmal positional vertigo. *Laryngoscope* 2004;114:1420–1425.
28. Woodworth BA, Gillespie MB, Lambert PR. The canalith repositioning procedure for benign positional vertigo: a meta-analysis. *Laryngoscope* 2004;114(7):1143–1146.
29. Herdman SJ. Treatment of benign paroxysmal positional vertigo. *Phys Ther* 1990;70:381–388.
30. Agrawal SK, Parnes LS. Human experience with canal plugging. *Ann N Y Acad Sci* 2001;942:300–305.
31. Gauchard GC, Gangloff P, Jeandel C, et al. Physical activity improves gaze and posture control in the elderly. *Neurosci Res* 2003;45(4):409–417.
32. Whitney SL, Rossi MM. Efficacy of vestibular rehabilitation. *Otolaryngol Clin North Am* 2000;33(3):659–672.
33. Yardley L, Donovan-Hall M, Smith HE, et al. Effectiveness of primary care-based vestibular rehabilitation for chronic dizziness. *Ann Intern Med* 2004;141(8):598–605.
34. Cohen HS, Kimball KT. Increased independence and decreased vertigo after vestibular rehabilitation. *Otolaryngol Head Neck Surg* 2003;128:60–70.

Central Vestibulopathy

157

C. Y. Joseph Chang   *Arun K. Gadre*

The term "central vestibular disorder" includes those pathologies occurring central to the labyrinth and vestibular nerve. Essentially, a central vestibular disorder implies the presence of an abnormal processing of normal peripheral vestibular sensory inputs by the central nervous system (CNS). There are various CNS conditions that are known to cause specific vestibular symptoms. These include migraine, vertebrobasilar insufficiency, multiple sclerosis, and cerebellopontine angle tumors. There are other conditions that are thought to produce vestibular symptoms, but the exact symptom complex associated with these disorders remains controversial. These include vascular loop compression, the Chiari malformations, and many others.

Our ability to understand and treat patients with vestibular abnormalities has been difficult for the following reasons. First, the term *vestibulopathy* can have different meanings for different individuals. For example, some may consider that vestibulopathies include only those conditions related to the labyrinth, vestibular nerve, or vestibular nuclei, whereas others may consider a more broad interpretation, including all patients with symptoms of vertigo, lightheadedness, and imbalance. Second, although many vestibular disorders are well defined, in many others, the pathophysiology, symptom complex, and natural history are not well defined. Furthermore, there are a substantial number of patients who exhibit vestibular symptoms but for whom a definitive diagnosis is not clear. Third, there are few definitive tests that rule in or rule out various vestibular disorders, and we are forced to rely largely on patient history and physical findings alone to determine a diagnosis. These factors confound our efforts to obtain a comprehensive understanding of vestibular disorders and to provide meaningful care to our patients. They also confound our efforts to understand the results of clinical studies, especially those concerning a disease entity in which diagnostic criteria are not well established. The syndrome of vascular loop compression is an example.

Estimates on the incidence of central etiologies in the population of patients with the complaint of dizziness are 10% to 20%. The incidence of central vestibulopathy in all patients presenting to a particular dizziness clinic was 13% (1). These figures may be underestimates or overestimates for the following reason. The differentiation between central and peripheral disorders is typically made based on patient symptoms, physical findings, and vestibular testing. Unless the findings are quite characteristic, there are no definitive confirmatory tests that can make the final distinction between a central and peripheral disorder. For example, there is no specific test that will confirm the presence of vestibular neuronitis, labyrinthitis, and many other syndromes, but the diagnosis is relatively clear in many cases based on clinical presentation and physical findings. Abnormalities found on electrocochleography have been associated with endolymphatic hydrops, but its sensitivity and specificity are unknown. There are a significant number of patients with vestibular findings not consistent with a peripheral disorder that is likely under-reported. Despite the many unknown factors in central vestibular disorders, this chapter will attempt to provide a rational course for work-up and treatment of these disorders.

PATHOPHYSIOLOGY

A detailed discussion on physiology and pathophysiology of the vestibular system is beyond the scope of this chapter (see Chapter 130). The reader is referred to Baloh and Honrubia (2) and Brandt (3) for a more comprehensive review. Briefly, the vestibular system is designed to keep the subject's body properly referenced in space and with respect to gravity. To this end, there are various sensory systems, including the labyrinth, proprioceptive organs, and visual system, that provide information to the central processor, which includes not only the vestibular

2304 Section IX: Otology

nuclei and cerebellum, but also numerous neural pathways within the brainstem. The exact functions of many of these pathways likely remain to be discovered, although the nature of some of the rudimentary processing information has been studied (4). Damage to any of these central processor units can cause vestibular dysfunction with resultant associated symptoms. The known types of central vestibular abnormalities are summarized in Table 157.1.

Remarkably, despite permanent damage to some parts of the central processor, the vestibular system can recover much of its overall effectiveness. This phenomenon is termed central compensation, and its exact mechanism is unknown. Central compensation appears to be hastened by repeated stimulation of the vestibular system. Central compensation is also the mechanism by which individuals with static peripheral vestibular lesions such as loss of unilateral labyrinthine function recover their balance function and become asymptomatic. Central compensation is not effective in the recovery from fluctuating peripheral vestibular dysfunction such as in Ménière disease.

DIAGNOSIS

In general, the history is of critical importance, because the physical findings and vestibular testing in most cases can only provide supportive information (5). Specifically, unless examination or testing reveals a specific finding such as the geotropic nystagmus of benign paroxysmal positional vertigo, the results are usually not pathognomonic of any single vestibular disorder.

TABLE 157.1

MAJOR TYPES OF CENTRAL VESTIBULAR ABNORMALITIES

Abnormality	Proposed cause	Clinical manifestation or finding
Vestibular cortex		
Thalamus	Simple partial seizures	Vestibular epilepsy
	Paramedian thalamic infarction	Ocular tilt reaction (OTR)
	Hemorrhage	Thalamic astasia
	Posterolateral thalamic lesions	
Vestibulocerebellum		
Flocculus	Disinhibition of vertical VOR in pitch	Downbeat nystagmus, vertigo
Nodulus		Positional downbeat nystagmus
Vestibular nuclei	Inappropriate canal-otolith interaction?	Central positional vertigo or nystagmus
Vestibulocerebellar loop?	Inappropriate canal-otolith interaction?	
Brainstem		
Mesodiencephalic	Tone imbalance of VOR in roll	Ocular tilt reaction
	Tone imbalance of vertical VOR in pitch	Upbeat nystagmus and vertigo
Pontomedullary	Transversally spreading ephaptic axonal activation	Paroxysmal dysarthria/ataxia in multiple sclerosis
	Vestibular nerve root plaque in M.S. or lacunar infarction	Pseudo "vestibular neuritis"
	Graviceptive pathway lesion with tone imbalance of VOR in roll	Ocular tilt reaction
	Tone imbalance of VOR in pitch	Downbeat nystagmus/vertigo
Medullary	Tone imbalance of VOR in pitch	Upbeat nystagmus/vertigo
	Vestibular nuclei lesion?	Paroxysmal vertigo evoked by lateral gaze or head position
Brainstem and cerebellum	AICA or PICA infarction with ischemia of superior labyrinth, vestibular nerve, vestibular nuclei	Pseudo "vestibular neuritis"
	Ischemic lesion-induced deviation of subjective vertical	Lateropulsion in Wallenberg syndrome
	Hereditary, metabolic?	Familial periodic vertigo
	Viral	Encephalitis with predominant vertigo
	Viral	Epidemic vertigo

[a]VOR, vestibuloocular reflux; AICA, anterior inferior cerebellar artery; PICA, posterior inferior cerebellar artery.
Adapted from Black FO, Pesznecker SC, Grimm RJ. Central vestibular disorders. In: *Head and Neck Surgery—Otolarynogology*, 2nd ed. Bailey BJ, ed. Philadelphia: Lippincott-Raven Publishers, 1998, with permission.

In interviewing a patient with dizziness, the physician should be cognizant of the various peripheral etiologies of vestibular dysfunction. A diagnosis of central vestibular disorder should be suspected if the patient's history is not consistent with any peripheral disorder (6). In general, the patient with central vestibulopathy will have dysequilibrium rather than vertigo, a longer duration of symptoms with gradual onset, and minimal vegetative symptoms such as nausea and vomiting, but there are many exceptions. The presence of neurologic symptoms such as visual aura, sensory and motor disturbances, and headaches increases the chances that a central disorder is present. There will be a substantial number of patients with a central vestibular disorder, however, who initially exhibit few symptoms that can identify it as a central disorder.

The physical examination should again focus on the presence of vestibular findings that are not consistent with a purely peripheral disorder. The presence of nystagmus that is not characteristic of a unilateral labyrinthine abnormality (unidirectional horizontal nystagmus) or semicircular canal pathology (geotropic or ageotropic rotatory nystagmus) should be sought. There are specific physical findings that are characteristic of central disorders, including nystagmus that is direction-changing, not suppressed by visual fixation, down-beating, up-beating, or dysconjugate, and abnormalities of smooth pursuit, saccades, and optokinetic nystagmus. Table 157.2 summarizes characteristics of nystagmus usually associated with central disorders. One must keep in mind that central disorders can cause nystagmus that typically occurs with peripheral disorders (7,8). The patient with central vestibulopathy may in some cases exhibit no nystagmus.

The patient's balance should be evaluated. Tests for evaluation of balance include gait; tandem gait; Romberg; and modified Romberg with feet in tandem, standing on foam with eyes open, with eyes closed, and with dome over the patient's face (the so called foam and dome test). The principle of this test is to challenge the balance system by decreasing afferent inputs from proprioception and vision. It must be kept in mind that balance abnormalities can occur with both peripheral and central vestibular pathologies. Signs of cerebellar dysfunction such as dysmetria on finger-to-nose testing, heel-shin testing, and dysdiadochokinesia

are quite characteristic of a central problem. Similarly, the presence of cranial nerve dysfunction (excluding the vestibulocochlear nerve or peripheral facial nerve), sensory and motor strength disturbances, coordination abnormalities, and mental status changes are characteristic of a central lesion. Vestibular function testing such as electronystagmography (ENG) can be helpful if it detects nystagmus characteristic of a central vestibulopathy, or if the smooth pursuit, saccades, or optokinetic nystagmus is abnormal (9). The absence of these findings does not rule out the presence of a central vestibular disorder.

Imaging studies such as computed tomography (CT) of the brain with contrast or magnetic resonance imaging (MRI) should be performed if a central vestibulopathy is suspected. MRI has largely supplanted CT in recent years. MRI can detect intracranial tumors, hemorrhage, craniovertebral junction anomalies such as the Chiari malformations, plaques from demyelinating diseases, and other findings (10–12). The absence of abnormalities on scanning does not rule out the presence of a central vestibular disorder. Other imaging studies such as magnetic resonance angiography (MRA) (13) and angiography should be ordered if a vascular etiology is suspected.

CENTRAL VESTIBULAR DISORDERS

A detailed discussion on the plethora of central vestibular disorders is beyond the scope of this chapter. Many of these syndromes are summarized in Table 157.3, and the treatments are summarized in Table 157.4. This section will describe the most common central etiologies of dizziness: migraine, vascular, cerebellar/Chiari malformation, and multiple sclerosis (1,14).

Migraine

Migraine is considered a vascular syndrome caused by serial constriction and dilation of intracranial blood vessels (15). The estimated incidence of headaches caused by migraine is variable. Reports have ranged from 6% of men and 15% to 18% of women in one study (16), to 15% to 20% in men, 23% to 29% in women, and 5% in children (17). There is a clear female preponderance in the majority of studies. Migraine headaches are subclassified into migraine with and without aura. Clinical characteristics of the aura associated with migraine are shown in Table 157.5. The visual symptoms are the most common component of the aura, followed by paresthesias, which is characterized by numbness, tingling, or both, affecting the upper or lower extremities, face, and occasionally the trunk. Less frequent symptoms of aura include olfactory and auditory hallucinations, weakness, speech difficulties, and dizziness.

The vestibular symptoms associated with migraine include motion intolerance, episodic vertigo, and dysequilibrium (15,18–22). These symptoms typically occur

TABLE 157.2

CHARACTERISTICS OF NYSTAGMUS USUALLY ASSOCIATED WITH CENTRAL ETIOLOGIES

Direction	Vertical, horizontal, or torsional
Direction-changing	Yes
Associated nausea	Minimal
Suppression by visual fixation	Minimal
Latency	None
Fatigue	None

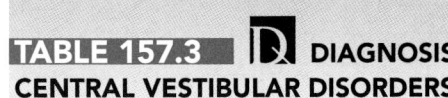

TABLE 157.3 | DIAGNOSIS

CENTRAL VESTIBULAR DISORDERS

Manifestation/Diagnosis	Diagnostic Aids
Degenerative	
Age-related degenerative disease	Progressive dysequilibrium
	Gait hesitancy
	Difficulty moving in darkness or on uneven surfaces
	Presbycusis
	"Visual or somatosensory dependence" SOT pattern on CDP
Infectious	
Otitic meningitis, encephalitis, epidural abscess, etc.	History of chronic ear disease with an ear that suddenly stops draining
	Recent acute mastoiditis
	CNS meningeal signs
	Lethargy
	Fever
	Elevated WBC with left shift
	Abnormal lumber puncture
Epidemic vertigo	Abscess on MRI/CT
Congenital syphilis (lues)	Antecedent viral infection
	Positive FTA-ABS (VDRL not as reliable)
	Reduced caloric and VOR responses
	Bilateral sensorineural hearing loss
	Stigmata of lues: Hutchinson teeth, frontal bossing, saddle nose, etc.
	May look like bilateral Ménière early in disease
Circulatory	
Vertebrobasilar insufficiency	Four D's: dizziness, diplopia, dysphasia, drop attacks (occurring episodically)
	May also include vision loss, hallucinations, ataxia, headache, weakness, perioral numbness
	Neurologic examination normal between attacks
	Cerebral angiogram may be abnormal
Wallenberg syndrome (lateral medullary infarction)	Acute-onset vertigo, N&V, ipsilateral facial pain, dysphagia, diplopia, dysphonia
	Ipsilateral Horner syndrome
	Facial, palatal, and pharyngeal numbness or paresis
	Spontaneous nystagmus
	Abnormal OTR
	Lateropulsion
Cerebellar hemorrhage	Abnormal cerebral angiogram
	CT/MRI may show wedge-shaped infarct
	Acute-onset vertigo with N&V
	Severe ataxia, inability to stand
	Headache and severe nuchal rigidity
	Gaze paresis
	Spontaneous or gaze-evoked nystagmus
	Abnormal CT/MRI scan: hemorrhage, hydrocephalus, brainstem compression
	Rapid deterioration if not treated
Autoimmune	
Cogan syndrome	Nonsyphilitic interstitial keratitis
	Fluctuating, progressive unilateral or bilateral deafness
	Spontaneous nystagmus
	Episodic vertigo
	Ataxia
Acute cerebellar syndrome	Dysarthria
Structural	
Arnold–Chiari malformation	Progressive unsteadiness and gait deterioration
	Oscillopsia
	Downbeat nystagmus
	Lower cranial nerve palsies
	Symptoms worsen with Valsalva
	CT/MRI may show hydrocephalus and/or tonsillar herniation
	Bilateral abductor paralysis if severe

(continued)

TABLE 157.3

(continued)

Manifestation/diagnosis	Diagnostic aids
Hydrocephalus	Altered mentation, lethargy, retardation
	Ataxia and dysequilibrium
	Clinical signs of increased intracranial pressure
	CT/MRI shows dilated ventricles
Systemic	
Multiple sclerosis	Vertigo, nystagmus
	Ataxia, impaired position and vibratory sense
	Optic neuritis
	Abnormal ABR and/or middle ear muscle reflexes
	Abnormal tests of central auditory function
	Demyelinated plaques ("bright spots") on MRI
	Abnormally elevated CSF globulin
Parkinson disease	Tetrad of symptoms: impairment of postural control, abnormal postural reflexes,
	Atypical muscle stiffness, muscle inflexibility
	Intention tremor
	Mechanical speech impairment
Carcinomatous	
Primary	Vertigo, hearing loss, local pain, facial paresis/palsy
	Visible tumor: tumor middle ear or external canal, mastoid swelling, etc.
	Otorrhea resistant to treatment
Secondary (metastatic)	Vertigo, imbalance, ataxia
	Facial paresis/palsy
	Hearing loss or deafness
	Reduced vestibular function
	Primary cancer elsewhere in body
Inherited	
Waardenburg syndrome	Bilateral moderate-to-profound sensorineural hearing loss
	Secondary endolymphatic hydrops with vertigo, tinnitus, aural fullness, etc.
	Physical stigmata: widened intercanthal distance, white forelock, heterochromia irides, flat nasal bridge, etc.
	Others affected in same family (dominant inheritance)
Huntington disease	Motor disturbances: chorea, bradykinesia, ataxia
	Abnormal dynamic posturography
Familial periodic vertigo	Episodic ataxia, vertigo
	Family history
	Responds to acetazolamide
Other	
Toxin exposure	Varies according to toxin: may include vertigo, nausea and vomiting, hearing loss, tinnitus, ataxia
Motion sickness	N&V, pallor, diaphoresis on exposure to motion
	May have symptoms when exposed to motion in visual periphery
Vestibular epilepsy	Abnormal EEG

SOT, sensory organization trial; CDP, computerized dynamic posturography; WBC, white blood cell count; MRI, magnetic resonance imaging; CT, computed tomography; FTA-ABS, fluorescent treponemal antibody absorption; VDRL, Venereal Disease Research Laboratory; VOR, vestibuloocular reflux; N&V, nausea and vomiting; OTR, ocular tilt reaction; CSF, cerebrospinal fluid; ABR, auditory brainstem response; EEG, electroencephalogram.
Adapted from Black FO, Pesznecker SC, Grimm RJ. Central vestibular disorders. In: *Head and neck surgery—otolaryngology*, 2nd ed. Bailey BJ, ed. Philadelphia:Lippincott-Raven Publishers, 1998, with permission.

prior to the migraine headache, during the aura phase. In some cases, the vestibular symptoms are not associated in time with the headaches. In other cases, the patient may no longer have migraine headaches, or may only have a family history of migraines. Therefore, migraine-related vestibulopathy should be suspected in patients with a personal or family history of migraine headaches, even if the patient does not experience headaches presently.

Episodic vertigo occurs in about 30% to 40% of patients with migrainous headaches, but only 10% of patients who have vestibular migraine also have headaches at the time of their vertigo attack. The vertigo can last from several minutes to several hours. Dysequilibrium is the most common vestibular complaint (75%). It is often exacerbated by head or body motion and can last from several minutes to several days. In some cases, the sensation is

TABLE 157.4 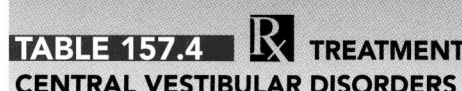 TREATMENT
CENTRAL VESTIBULAR DISORDERS

Manifestation/diagnosis	Treatments/alternatives
Degenerative	
Age-related degenerative disease	Specialized physical therapy
	Instruction in safety measures
	Environmental modifications
Infectious	
Otitic meningitis, encephalitis, epidural abscess, etc.	Culture and sensitivity
	Appropriate antibiotics
	Emergency surgical decompression of abscess (avoid acute decompression if ICP is high)
Epidemic vertigo	Supportive treatment (resolves spontaneously)
Congenital syphilis (lues)	High-dose penicillin: 20 million units i.v./day for 10–14 days
	Steroids: prednisolone 80–100 mg/day for 10–14 days, then taper (may need q.o.d. maintenance to prevent hearing loss progression)
	Maintenance steroids as required
Circulatory	
Vertebrobasilar insufficiency	Prophylactic antiplatelet drugs (ASA 300–600 mg/q.d. or b.i.d.)
	Severe cases: systemic anticoagulation with heparin, followed by maintenance warfarin therapy and monitoring of blood-clotting times
Wallenberg syndrome (lateral medullary infarction)	Symptomatic treatment
	Antiplatelet drugs (e.g., aspirin)
Cerebellar hemorrhage	Stat surgical decompression
	Supportive treatment
Autoimmune	
Cogan syndrome	High-dose steroids: prednisone 100 mg qd × 10–14 days, then tapered off and followed with maintenance dose (may require additional immunosuppression)
Acute cerebellar syndrome	Rehabilitation of hearing loss/deafness
Structural	
Arnold–Chiari malformation	Subocciptal craniotomy and decompression
Hydrocephalus	Short term: solute dehydration, aspiration of excess CSF (lumbar puncture)
	Long term: surgical shunting of CSF
Systemic	
Multiple sclerosis	ACTH, interferon, and other medications
	Symptomatic treatment
Parkinson disease	Levodopa
	Physical therapy and environmental modifications
	Stereotactic surgery: pallidotomy
Carcinomatous	
Primary	Local excision
	Chemotherapy, radiation therapy, etc.
	Symptomatic treatment
Secondary (metastatic)	Local excision
	Chemotherapy, radiation therapy, etc.
	Symptomatic treatment
Inherited	
Waardenburg syndrome	Symptomatic treatment of secondary hydrops
	Rehabilitation for hearing loss/deafness
	Genetic counseling
Huntington disease	Genetic counseling
Familial periodic vertigo	Acetazolamide
Other	
Toxin exposure	Removal of toxin
	Chelation (in some cases)
Motion sickness	Symptomatic treatment
	Prophylaxis prior to exposure: scopolamine patches, Dramamine, etc.
	Gradual, repeated exposure
Vestibular epilepsy	Anticonvulsant drugs
	Symptomatic treatment
	Control fluctuating peripheral disorder, if present

ICP, intracranial pressure; i.v., intravenous; q.o.d., every other day; ASA, aspirin; q.d., every day; b.i.d., twice a day; stat, immediately; CSF, cerebrospinal fluid; ACTH, adrenocorticotropic hormone.
Adapted from Black FO, Pesznecker SC, Grimm RJ. Central vestibular disorders. In: *Head and neck surgery— otolaryngology*, 2nd ed. Bailey BJ, ed. Philadelphia: Lippincott–Raven Publishers, 1998.

TABLE 157.5

CHARACTERISTICS OF THE AURA COMPONENT OF MIGRAINE (DESCENDING ORDER OF FREQUENCY)

1. Scotomata, or blind spots
2. Teichopsia, or fortification spectra, a zigzag pattern in the visual field resembling a fort
3. Flashing (photopsia) or colored lights
4. Paresthesia

present constantly (18). Interestingly, a study comparing the incidence of episodic vertigo vs. dysequilibrium in patients with tension headaches vs. migraine headaches showed no difference in incidence of dysequilibrium (28% in migraine, 22% in tension). There was a significantly higher incidence of episodic vertigo in the migraine group (27% in migraine, 8% in tension) (19). It is clear that there continues to be some controversy regarding the exact nature of vestibular symptoms associated with migraine, and it is important to have a systematic appraisal of these patients (23).

Migraine-related vestibulopathy is not associated with any specific findings on ENG or rotational testing. Abnormal ENG findings can include unilateral or bilateral caloric weakness, spontaneous nystagmus, positional nystagmus, direction-changing nystagmus, and directional preponderance. The most common abnormality on rotational testing is directional preponderance. The majority of patients have no abnormalities on ENG or rotational testing (15,18,19). Interestingly, the prevalence of ENG abnormalities is similar between migraine patients with and without vestibular symptoms (24). The vestibular pathophysiology is likely present in a significant number of patients with migraine, but the vestibular symptoms occur either intermittently or do not occur in all migraine patients with abnormalities of the vestibular system.

Fluctuating hearing loss of the Ménière type has been reported to occur in a small number of patients with migraine. This association is somewhat obfuscated by the possible pathophysiologic relation between migraine and Ménière disease (25). The exact nature of this relationship is not clear, but there are some data to suggest that the incidence of migraine is relatively high in patients with Ménière disease (26). Although hearing loss and tinnitus are reported to occur in patients with migraine, the most common auditory complaint is phonophobia, or aversion to loud noise (18,20,21).

There are several variants of migraine-related vestibulopathy that deserve mention. The first is basilar migraine, which was initially described by Bickerstaff (27). It consists of headache preceded by an aura with symptoms attributable to dysfunction in the distribution of the basilar artery. These symptoms of aura include scintillating scotomata, transient blindness, vertigo, paresthesias, slurred speech, ataxia, tinnitus, diplopia, loss of consciousness,

motor weakness, and hearing loss (28). The other variant is benign paroxysmal vertigo of childhood, which was initially described by Basser (29). He presented several children with spells consisting of fright, crying, staggering, pallor, diaphoresis, and vomiting. Some of these children reported a sensation consistent with vertigo. These spells lasted several seconds to a few minutes and resolved completely. These symptoms can recur over time but usually resolve completely by 7 or 8 years of age. Based on longitudinal studies showing that a substantial number of these children develop migraine headaches, benign positional nystagmus of childhood likely represents early manifestations of migraine (30).

Treatment options for migraine-related vestibulopathy include medical management and vestibular physical therapy. (For a more detailed review of the subject of medical management of vestibular disorders, please refer to Chapter 158.) It is important to determine if there are any dietary triggers, such as tyramine-containing foods, alcohol, or caffeine, associated with the vertigo and/or headaches, and if so, to eliminate them. Hypoglycemia is also known to trigger migraine and should be avoided. Treatment of the acute vertigo attacks should include agents to treat nausea, such as promethazine, and vestibular suppressants such as diazepam, lorazepam, and meclizine. Other medical treatments include prophylactic drugs against the onset of migraine headaches. These medications also appear to have some activity in preventing the onset of vestibular symptoms (18). Such medications include beta-blockers, calcium channel blockers, anticonvulsants and tricyclic antidepressants. Drugs such as amitriptyline and imipramine are effective, but because of their cholinergic side effects these have been largely replaced by secondary amines such as desipramine and nortriptyline (31). When beta-blockers such as propranolol are used, they are administered in high doses and can cause impotence in men, bronchospasm, and heart failure. Verapamil and flunarizine, which are calcium channel blockers, also have a role in the management of the condition. In Europe, the calcium channel blocker cinnarizine has been used for several years for migraine vestibulopathy and Ménière disease. It has a good safety profile and its cardiac action is 1/70 that of verapamil, but it is currently not available in the United States. The use of long-acting benzodiazepines such as clonazepam for prophylactic use in improving balance function has been suggested based on anecdotal reports of efficacy.

The medications used to control headaches once they occur, such as non-steroidal anti-inflammatory agents, are not thought to be useful in the treatment of vestibular symptoms (20). A recent study, however, showed a correlation between a medication's efficacy in controlling headaches and alleviation of vertigo attacks; sumatriptan, a headache-abortive medication, was most efficacious (32). Again, there remains controversy regarding treatment of this disorder.

Many of the patients with migraine vestibulopathy complain of chronic dysequilibrium. Medications that suppress vestibular function are not indicated for this condition. Although there is little data on the use of vestibular rehabilitation therapy (14), this form of intervention makes the most sense in treating the movement-associated dysequilibrium of migraine-related vestibulopathy (18). In fact, a recent study by Wrisley et al. (33) showed that vestibular physical therapy over several months does improve the vestibular symptoms of migraine patients.

Vertebrobasilar Insufficiency

Ischemic disease of the posterior circulation can cause varying degrees of dysfunction, from transient ischemic attacks (TIA) to infarctions. Many, but not all, of these patients have risk factors for cerebrovascular accidents (CVA) such as hypertension, heart disease, diabetes, and carotid artery disease. The central nervous system symptoms associated with infarctions of the posterior inferior cerebellar artery (PICA), known as Wallenberg syndrome or lateral medullary syndrome, and of the anterior inferior cerebellar artery (AICA) are readily recognized. They are sudden in onset and reflect the regions of the brainstem affected by transient ischemia attacks or infarction. TIAs are also thought to cause unmistakable central symptoms, but this has become more controversial recently, as described later in this section.

Vertebrobasilar pathology–causing infarctions in the distribution of PICA cause a constellation of symptoms recognized as Wallenberg syndrome. Typical symptoms include acute vertigo, ipsilateral lateral pulsion, ipsilateral facial pain, diplopia, dysphagia, dysarthria, and hoarseness. Physical findings include ipsilateral Horner syndrome; ipsilateral loss of pain and temperature sensation on the face; contralateral loss of pain and temperature sensation on the trunk and extremities; ipsilateral paralysis of the palate, pharynx, and larynx; ipsilateral abducens palsy; ipsilateral facial palsy; ipsilateral dysmetria, dysrhythmia, and dysdiadochokinesia; and spontaneous nystagmus (34). Infarctions in the AICA territory causes similar findings without the Horner syndrome and abducens palsy but with additional symptoms of hearing loss and tinnitus (35). The territories of AICA and PICA vary significantly among individuals, so the clinical findings will often be combinations of the these deficits, regardless of which vessel is involved.

TABLE 157.6
SYMPTOMS ASSOCIATED WITH TRANSIENT VERTEBROBASILAR INSUFFICIENCY

Visual changes, such as diplopia, hallucinations, visual field defects
Weakness of the extremities
Paresthesias
Headache
Confusion
Loss of consciousness
Drop attacks

The diagnosis of posterior circulation infarct is confirmed with MRI, and if necessary, with angiography. The treatment options in the acute setting are limited to providing supportive and symptomatic care, and providing antiplatelet medications. The use of anticoagulant and thrombolytic agents remains controversial (36). Vestibular suppressants can be administered to control vertigo in the acute setting, but should be tapered as soon as possible to avoid slowing the pace of central compensation. Although little data exist on the role of vestibular physical therapy for treatment of this condition, some patients have been noted to have improvement in their balance function after such treatment (14,37,38).

The syndrome of transient vertebrobasilar insufficiency is essentially a TIA of the posterior circulation. Patients may have risk factors for CVA such as hypertension, heart disease, diabetes, and carotid artery disease. Vertebrobasilar insufficiency is thought to present in most cases with distinctly central clinical findings that are listed in Table 157.6. The classic presentation is acute vertigo of abrupt onset, lasting several minutes and usually associated with nausea and vomiting. In some cases, the patient may not have vertigo, but instead a chronic sense of lightheadedness and dysequilibrium that has been persistent for several months (39). The clinical presentation has been described as quite variable. In some cases, the vertigo episodes occur without associated neurologic symptoms (40). In many of these patients, however, the associated neurologic symptoms occur later either together with vertigo, or as isolated events. Patients with chronic dysequilibrium without vertigo usually experience the neurologic symptoms in an episodic fashion. There may be hearing loss that is episodic or permanent.

Other than the presence of a vestibular dysfunction, mainly in the form of balance dysfunction, there are no specific physical findings that are diagnostic of transient ischemia of the vertebrobasilar circulation. ENG may show a unilateral paresis and various patterns of nystagmus, but a "normal" ENG does not rule out this condition. Posturography may again show a deficit in balance but is not specific. MRI and MRA may be considered to detect evidence of chronic ischemic changes in the brainstem parenchyma or vessel patency abnormalities, but these again could be negative (39). Transcranial Doppler studies performed on patients suspected of having vertebrobasilar insufficiency as a cause of dizziness have shown abnormalities in cerebral perfusion, but again, it is not diagnostic of this condition (41).

The treatment for vertebrobasilar insufficiency consists of alleviating the underlying pathology. The possible etiologies of this condition include atherosclerotic vessel disease, hypercoagulability, and hyperviscosity. The most common treatment regimen used is antiplatelet agents such as aspirin, dipyridamole, and pentoxifylline (39). There is very little data regarding efficacy of these agents in controlling vestibular symptoms. Anticoagulation is usually not considered unless the patient is suspected to be undergoing a stroke in evolution. The underlying risk factors such as diabetes, hypertension, hypercholesterolemia, and hyperlipidemia are treated. The chronic dysequilibrium usually improves with vestibular physical therapy.

The accepted treatment of acute ischemic stroke is emergency administration of intravenous tissue plasminogen activator (tPA) within three hours of stroke onset (42). This treatment modality results in a significant reduction in disease-related morbidity. Acute thrombolytic treatment is contraindicated in patients with hemorrhagic stroke and other bleeding risks. There was a 6.4% rate of intracranial hemorrhage associated with intravenous administration of t-PA (42).

The posterior circulation ischemia differs quite considerably from anterior circulation ischemia with regard to the time window for therapy and morbidity and mortality. The prognosis for acute basilar artery occlusion is generally poor, with mortality rates being as high as 80% to 90% (43). Although alertness and motor function preservation are positive indicators for outcome, negative indicators include coma, quadriplegia, need for ventilator support, and severe hypertension. The prognosis is worse with a more proximal location of the occlusion. In addition, the presence of minimal-to-absent collateral circulation such as an absent posterior communicating vessel portends a poorer prognosis. Recanalization of the vessel was associated with a significant decrease in mortality (46% in the recanalized group, as opposed to 92% in the nonrecanalized group) in a large series of 51 patients (44). Distal basilar artery occlusion is more likely to be embolic and respond to therapy, whereas midbasilar and proximal occlusion are associated with a thrombotic stroke mechanism, and stenosis often remains after recanalization is successful.

Unlike the striatum and cerebral cortex, the brainstem is relatively resistant to ischemia. Therefore, recanalization occurring up to 24 hours after stroke onset can reverse clinical effects in some cases. For this reason, the argument has been made for more aggressive management of posterior circulation thrombosis with thrombolytic treatments to be administered up to 24 hours after a posterior circulation stroke. (45)

Cerebellar infarctions are uncommon. They occur as a result of vascular disease in the distributions of PICA and the superior cerebellar artery (SCA) that perfuse various areas of the cerebellum. The acute vestibular symptoms consist of primarily vertigo and unsteadiness. Associated signs and symptoms can occur and consist of headache, clumsiness, ataxia, dysmetria, dysarthria, and lateropulsion (46,47). When nystagmus is present, it is usually in a horizontal direction, although vertical nystagmus occurs in a minority of cases (47). Since the vertigo can be exacerbated by positional changes, this condition can sometimes be mistaken for a peripheral vestibulopathy. It is important not to miss the diagnosis of cerebellar infarctions, because the natural course of the disease can include development of cerebellar edema and significant posterior fossa mass effect. Patients with this condition can die if surgical decompression is not performed promptly. Patients with infarctions in the PICA territory are at highest risk for developing this serious complication (47).

Craniovertebral Junction Disorders: Chiari Malformation

The Chiari malformation consists of an abnormal inferior displacement of the cerebellum and brainstem through the foramen magnum. The condition is categorized according to the degree of herniation of cerebellar and brainstem structures (Table 157.7). The various associated symptoms are thought to arise as a result of compression of the brainstem, spinal cord, and cerebellum, and stretching of the lower cranial nerves. A noncommunicating hydrocephalus can also occur. The condition can cause functional disruption of the motor and sensory tracts, cranial nerve nuclei, cerebellum, and lower cranial nerves.

The type II malformation, known as the Arnold–Chiari malformation, is the most common and usually presents during early childhood. It is often associated with

---

TABLE 157.7

CLASSIFICATION OF CHIARI MALFORMATIONS

Type I	Protrusion of cerebellar tonsils
Type II	Protrusion of cerebellar vermis, lower pons, and medulla (Arnold–Chiari malformation)
Type III	Herniation of cerebellum, forming a high cervical meningocele
Type IV	Cerebellar hypoplasia, generally not classified as a Chiari malformation now (variant of Dandy–Walker syndrome)

myelomeningocele, spina bifida, and hydrocephalus. Typical findings include a dissociated sensory loss, consisting of loss of pain and temperature sensation with relative sparing of vibratory sense and proprioception; lower cranial nerve dysfunction such as bilateral vocal cord paralysis; weakness; and ataxia. The type III malformation can cause similar but more advanced symptoms.

The type I Chiari malformation has been a topic of considerable controversy. The characteristic presenting symptoms have been reported in several large series (48,49) and include headache or head and neck pain (60% to 69%), including nuchal headache and facial pain, weakness of the extremities (42% to 56%), sensory complaints (52% to 60%), and unsteadiness (40%). Less data are available on specifics of auditory and vestibular impairments in patients with the type I Chiari malformation. There are numerous case reports describing such patients with unilateral or bilateral hearing loss, tinnitus, vertigo, and dysequilibrium (50–53). Rydell and Pulec (54) reported on series of 130 patients with the type I Chiari malformation and reported cochleovestibular complaints in 22%. On ENG, unilateral caloric weakness and spontaneous nystagmus have been noted, but these findings are not present in all patients. Some patients exhibit down-beating nystagmus characteristic of cerebellar vermis lesions (53,55,56).

Currently, the diagnostic modality of choice is MRI. The sagittal view is most helpful in determining first whether there is any herniation of posterior fossa structures through the foramen magnum, and second, the severity of the herniation. The presence of hydrocephalus, posterior fossa cysts, and myelocele can also be determined. The sensitivity of MRI has become somewhat problematic, as completely asymptomatic patients can be found to have mild herniation of cerebellar tonsils. A difficulty in diagnosis occurs in patients who complain mainly of dizziness, whether it consists of episodic vertigo or chronic dysequilibrium, without associated cerebellar, brainstem, or cranial nerve findings, but with MRI evidence of a Chiari I malformation. Unless specific physical or ENG findings consistent with a craniovertebral junction abnormality is detected, it is difficult to establish the abnormal radiologic finding as the etiology of the patient's symptoms, because the MRI findings could simply be incidental.

The establishment of a proper diagnosis in these cases is critical, because the main treatment option consists of a major surgical procedure: surgical decompression of the foramen magnum with or without cervical laminectomy. Ventriculoperitoneal shunting may also be needed if hydrocephalus remains unresolved. The efficacy of treatment regarding controlling general symptoms of Chiari I malformation such as pain and sensorimotor symptoms has been reported in large series. Roughly half of patients who undergo surgical treatment improve over long-term follow-up (48,49,57,58). The results of surgical treatment for control of vestibular symptoms is less clear. There are case

reports that show significant improvement in such patients (53), but some report no improvement of vestibular symptoms despite reduction of occipital headaches (52).

OTHER CRANIOVERTEBRAL JUNCTION ANOMALIES

There are several craniovertebral junction abnormalities that can cause symptoms similar to the Chiari malformations. These include basilar impression, assimilation of the atlas, and atlantoaxial dislocation. These conditions cause mainly spinal cord compression and not vestibular symptoms, but they will be discussed briefly.

Basilar impression refers to a condition in which the occipital bone around the foramen magnum deforms to cause a posterior and superior displacement of the odontoid process. The condition is associated with Paget disease, rheumatoid arthritis, osteomalacia, osteogenesis imperfecta, and rickets. Assimilation of the atlas refers to a bony union between the atlas and skull base. This condition is associated with posterior displacement of the odontoid. The most common cause is Klippel-Feil syndrome. Atlantoaxial dislocation refers to instability of the atlantoaxial joint, usually as a result of an abnormality of the transverse ligaments that normally stabilize this region. When the patient's head is flexed or extended, the odontoid can compress the spinal cord. There are multiple congenital etiologies of this condition, including Down syndrome, Hurler syndrome, Morquio syndrome, and achondroplastic dwarfism. Acquired etiologies include rheumatoid arthritis, retropharyngeal abscess, tuberculosis, and osteomyelitis. Treatments for these conditions consist of surgical stabilization as well as decompression of the odontoid process as needed (59).

Multiple Sclerosis

Multiple sclerosis is a multifocal demyelinating disease affecting the central nervous system. It typically presents during the third to fourth decade of life, and there is a female preponderance. It is thought to be the result of an immunologic disturbance that causes periodic demyelinization in various areas of the central nervous system, most commonly involving the supratentorial white matter in the periventricular region. Plaques, or areas of demyelinization, develop, disrupting signal conduction and leading to acute symptoms. A certain amount of remyelinization occurs during the healing process, allowing many of the acute symptoms of the disease to resolve. The plaques usually recur, however, and often in different areas. Since the demyelinization can occur anywhere within the central nervous system, multiple sclerosis can cause a myriad of symptoms. The clinical course consists of multiple exacerbations followed by remissions.

Blurred vision caused by optic neuritis is a common initial symptom of multiple sclerosis. Other symptoms include diplopia, weakness, sensory disturbance, clumsiness, and ataxia. The key to diagnosis is clinical involvement of multiple sites within the central nervous system as well as the characteristic waxing and waning clinical course over time. The presence of internuclear ophthalmoplegia is a strong supporting sign, as few other conditions result in this abnormality. Imaging studies such as MRI can show plaques within the white matter during symptomatic periods, but it can appear normal during remissions. Cerebrospinal fluid analysis can show elevation of immunoglobulin G levels (60). Hearing loss has been reported by patients with multiple sclerosis (61), but it is unclear if this is a common result of the disease process.

The vestibular symptoms are quite variable and range from episodic vertigo, a sense of lightheadedness, and imbalance. Although dizziness is not a common initial complaint of patients with multiple sclerosis, up to 50% of patients eventually develop some type of vestibular symptoms (59). The physical findings are nonspecific and can include abnormalities in balance, cerebellar function, and presence of spontaneous or positional nystagmus. Patients who are in the early stages of the disease often show subtle abnormalities, and there may not be many objective signs. In a series of ten such patients, most patients were found to exhibit abnormalities on ENG, but there was no specific pattern. Four patients showed non-direction-changing positional nystagmus, one showed a directional preponderance, three showed abnormal smooth pursuit, and one showed a unilateral weakness. On platform posturography, eight of the ten patients showed abnormalities (60).

Treatment options for patients with multiple sclerosis have been limited. The standard treatments for exacerbations of multiple sclerosis include high-dose steroids, methotrexate, azathioprine, cyclophosphamide. Drugs under study for treatment include statins, mycophenolate mofetil, various monoclonal antibodies (e.g., alemtuzumab, daclizumab, natalizumab, and rituximab), antibiotics and antivirals, and the pregnancy hormone estriol (62). The treatment for the vestibular symptoms is mostly supportive, including vestibular suppression for acute vertigo and vestibular therapy for balance dysfunction. Whether these interventions lead to any long-term benefit is unclear.

Tumors

The most common intracranial neoplasm that can cause vestibular symptoms is vestibular schwannoma (Fig. 157.1) (63,64). Although they are less common, meningiomas of the cerebellopontine angle can also lead to vestibular symptoms (65). Vestibular complaints such as episodic vertigo, positional vertigo, and dysequilibrium usually occur when the tumor is small. The tumor's effect on the vestibular

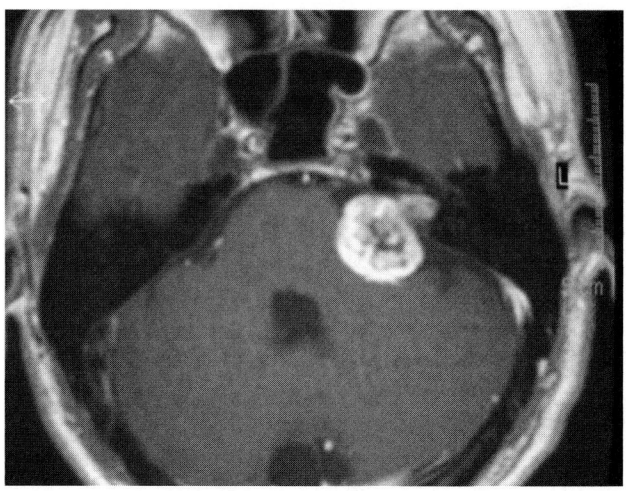

Figure 157.1 MRI with gadolinium showing moderate-size left vestibular schwannoma.

system is thought to be related to direct compression of the vestibular nerve or disruption of the vestibular blood supply. As the tumor grows, the vestibular function on the ipsilateral side diminishes and vestibular symptoms become less common as central compensation for the static loss of a labyrinthine function occurs. When the tumor enlarges to the point of causing significant compression of the brainstem and cerebellum, dysmetria, truncal ataxia, and dysequilibrium can occur (63). Brun nystagmus, which consists of a combination of a fine, horizontal, lateral nystagmus on contralateral gaze and a coarse, horizontal, lateral nystagmus on ipsilateral gaze, can occur in some cases of very large tumors. The fine nystagmus is thought to be related to dysfunction of the vestibular nerve and inner ear, whereas the coarse nystagmus is thought to be related to cerebellar dysfunction.

The treatment of the tumor by surgical excision often results in a vestibulopathy attributable to acute peripheral deafferentation, which usually improves spontaneously or with the help of vestibular physical therapy (66). There is very little information regarding the efficacy of the tumor resection in relieving the preoperative symptoms of vertigo, but it is assumed that the complete vestibular deafferentation that usually occurs during tumor resection is helpful in the long term. The information regarding control of preoperative dysequilibrium is also quite limited, but there are indications that the problem persists even after tumor resection. Two separate studies showed a significant correlation between the presence of dysequilibrium preoperatively and postoperatively (67,68). This may mean that in these patients, the vestibulopathy present prior to surgical treatment may still be present after surgery. The effect of stereotactic radiotherapy on vestibulopathy because of vestibular schwannomas is largely unknown (69).

Miscellaneous Central Vestibular Disorders

Several other conditions merit brief discussion. These include vestibulopathies caused by vascular loop compression syndromes, and seizure disorders.

The role of vascular loop compression of the eighth cranial nerve continues to be controversial. Vascular compression has been established as a legitimate cause of other cranial nerves, such as the trigeminal, facial, and glossopharyngeal nerves. For example, surgical decompression of vascular loops on the trigeminal nerve is considered an efficacious treatment option for trigeminal neuralgia (70). Vascular compression of the eighth cranial nerve as a cause of dizziness, hearing loss, and tinnitus has remained in question for various reasons. First, vascular loops are present in proximity or in contact with the eighth cranial nerve in many patients who have no cochleovestibular complaints and are in fact considered normal anatomic findings (71). Second, the diagnostic studies to demonstrate the presence of a pathologic vascular loop compression and to identify the pathologic side have remained unproven. These include air-contrast CT (72), auditory brainstem response (ABR) testing (73), and audiometry. Third, the symptomatology related to this disorder is quite variable and includes vertigo and/or dysequilibrium and motion intolerance, occurring either constantly or in attacks (73). Motion intolerance appears to be the most prominent symptom (72,73). The surgical outcomes of the primary treatment modality, craniotomy for vascular decompression, are difficult to assess because it is usually not clear if the patient population studied has the abnormality in question. Despite the skepticism regarding vascular compression as an etiology of cochleovestibular symptoms, there is a limited amount of histopathologic evidence to suggest that this syndrome exists (74,75). Because the primary treatment option for this syndrome is an intracranial procedure, it is critical to ensure that a confirmatory diagnostic test be available prior to subjecting patients to treatment. Until a widely accepted diagnostic test for the presence of vascular compression of the eighth cranial nerve becomes available, decompression surgery for dizziness will likely remain controversial.

Seizure disorder has been considered a rare cause of dizziness and vertigo (76). There is a syncopal type of syndrome experienced by up to 70% of patients with epilepsy, but only a small percentage of epileptic patients are thought to develop vertigo as a result of their seizure disorder (77). The vestibular symptoms when they occur consist mainly of brief episodes of dysequilibrium and/or vertigo. In one study, 23% of these patients had experienced generalized seizures at the time of presentation. In some patients, other symptoms consistent with seizure disorder, such as "absences," depersonalization, and others, occurred, usually not at the same time as the episodes of dizziness (76). Treatment with antiseizure medications will often alleviate or even eliminate the vestibular symptoms.

Very little information regarding the long-term natural history or treatment results of vestibular symptoms related to seizure disorder exists.

HIGHLIGHTS

- Central vestibular disorders represent a heterogeneous and large group of disorders affecting the central nervous system.
- A number of central disorders are recognized as causes of vestibular symptoms. The more common include migraine, vertebrobasilar insufficiency, multiple sclerosis, intracranial neoplasms, and several others.
- Some central disorders are thought to cause vestibular symptoms but remain controversial for various reasons, including disagreement about presenting symptoms, physical findings, and diagnostic testing, and even doubt about whether the particular syndrome exists. These disorders include vascular compression of the cochleovestibular nerve and Chiari malformation.
- The presenting symptoms for central vestibular disorders, even for the well-established syndromes, can be quite variable and can include vertigo, dysequilibrium, or sense of lightheadedness, occurring either episodically or constantly. Certain symptoms, such as lateropulsion are more specific for central disorders, but these are not present in most cases.
- There are specific physical findings that are characteristic of central disorders, including nystagmus that is direction-changing, not suppressed by visual fixation, downbeating, up-beating, or dysconjugate, abnormalities of smooth pursuit, saccades, and optokinetic nystagmus, and presence of dysmetria. These findings are not present in all patients with central vestibular disorder.
- The presence of other symptoms and findings consistent with a central nervous system abnormality can be helpful in rendering a diagnosis. Examples of this include Wallenberg syndrome, migraine, cerebellar infarctions, and multiple sclerosis. Patients presenting early in the course of disease may have only subtle associated central findings, however.
- Treatment options include interventions to reverse the underlying disease process, if available. Otherwise, treatments include vestibular suppressants for vertigo symptoms and vestibular physical therapy for dysequilibrium.
- Vestibulopathy of central origin can be the manifestation of an underlying intracranial disorder that may require urgent treatment. For example, intracranial neoplasm may require resection or radiation, and vertebrobasilar or cerebellar ischemia and infarcts may require urgent supportive care with or without emergent surgical decompression.

REFERENCES

1. Bath AP, Walsh RM, Ranalli P, et al. Experience from a multidisciplinary "dizzy" clinic. *Am J Otol* 2000, 21:92–97.
2. Baloh RW, Honrubia V. *Clinical neurophysiology of the vestibular system.* 2nd ed. Philadelphia: FA Davis, 1990:1–301.

3. Brandt TH. *Vertigo: its multisensory syndromes.* London: Springer-Verlag, 1991:1–24, 87–134, 173–185.
4. Goldberg JM, Minor LB, Fernandez C. The functional organization of the vestibular labyrinth and of some of its central pathways. In: Hwang JC, Daunton NG, Wilson VJ, eds. *Basic and applied aspects of vestibular function.* Hong Kong: Hong Kong University Press, 1988:3–12.
5. Solomon D. Distinguishing and treating causes of central vertigo. *Otolaryngol Clin North Am* 2000;33:579–602.
6. Baloh RW. Vertigo. *Lancet* 1998;352:1841–1846.
7. Sakata E, Ohtsu K, Itoh Y. Positional nystagmus of benign paroxysmal type (BPPN) due to cerebellar vermis lesions. Pseudo-BPPN. *Acta Otolaryngol Suppl* 1991; 481:254–257.
8. Buttner U, Helmchen C, Brandt T. Diagnostic criteria for central versus peripheral positioning nystagmus and vertigo: a review. *Acta Otolaryngol* 1999;119:1–5.
9. Kumar A, Valvassori G. An algorithm for neurotologic disorders. *Neurol Clin* 1984;2:779–796.
10. Inui H, Kitaoku Y, Yoneyama K, et al. MR-angiographic findings of patients with central vestibular disorders. *Acta Otolaryngol Suppl* 1998;533:51–56.
11. Miura M, Naito Y, Naito E, et al. Usefulness of magnetic resonance imaging in diagnosing vertebro-basilar insufficiency. *Acta Otolaryngol Suppl* 1997;528:91–93.
12. Casselman JW, Kuhweide R, Dehaene I, et al. Magnetic resonance examination of the inner ear and cerebellopontine angle in patients with vertigo and/or abnormal findings at vestibular testing. *Acta Otolaryngol Suppl* 1994;513:15–27.
13. Welsh LW, Welsh JJ, Jaffe SC, et al. Evaluation of the vestibular system by magnetic resonance angiography. *Laryngoscope* 1996;106:1138–1143.
14. Furman JM, Whitney SL. Central causes of dizziness. *Phys Ther* 2000;80:179–187.
15. Cutrer FM, Baloh RW. Migraine-associated dizziness. *Headache* 1992;32:300–304.
16. Lipton RB, Stewart WF. Prevalence and impact of migraine. *Neurol Clin* 1997;15:1–13.
17. Waters WE, O'Connor PJ. Prevalence of migraine. *J Neurol Neurosurg Psychiatry* 1975;38:613–616.
18. Cass SP, Furman JM, Ankerstjerne K, et al. Migraine-related vestibulopathy. *Ann Otol Rhinol Laryngol* 1997;106:182–189.
19. Kayan A, Hood JD. Neuro-otological manifestations of migraine. *Brain* 1984;107(pt 4):1123–1142.
20. Baloh RW. Neurotology of migraine. *Headache* 1997;37(10):615–621.
21. Parker W. Migraine and the vestibular system in adults. *Am J Otol* 1991;12:25–34.
22. Harker LA, Rassekh C. Migraine equivalent as a cause of episodic vertigo. *Laryngoscope* 1988;98:160–164.
23. Furman JM, Marcus DA, Balaban CD. Migrainous vertigo: development of a pathogenetic model and structured diagnostic interview. *Curr Opin Neurol* 2003;16:5–13.
24. Bir LS, Ardic FN, Kara CO, et al. Migraine patients with or without vertigo: comparison of clinical and electronystagmographic findings. *J Otolaryngol* 2003;32:234–238.
25. Neuhauser H, Lempert T. Vertigo and dizziness related to migraine: a diagnostic challenge. *Cephalalgia* 2004;24:83–91.
26. Radtke A, Lempert T, Gresty MA, et al. Migraine and Meniere's disease: is there a link? *Neurology* 2002;59:1700–1704.
27. Bickerstaff ER. Basilar artery migraine. *Lancet* 1961;1:15–17.
28. Harker LA, Rassekh CH. Episodic vertigo in basilar artery migraine. *Otolaryngol Head Neck Surg* 1987;96:239–250.
29. Basser LS. Benign paroxysmal vertigo of childhood. *Brain* 1964;87:141–152.
30. Lanzi G, Balottin U, Fazzi E, et al. Benign paroxysmal vertigo of childhood: a long-term follow-up. *Cephalalgia* 1994;14:458–460.
31. Hain TC, Uddin M. Pharmacological treatment of vertigo. *CNS Drugs* 2003;17:85–100.
32. Bikhazi P, Jackson C, Ruckenstein MJ. Efficacy of antimigrainous therapy in the treatment of migraine-associated dizziness. *Am J Otol* 1997;18:350–354.
33. Wrisley DM, Whitney SL, Furman JM. Vestibular rehabilitation outcomes in patients with a history of migraine. *Otol Neurotol* 2002;23:483–487.
34. Sacco RL, Freddo L, Bello JA, et al. Wallenberg's lateral medullary syndrome. Clinical-magnetic resonance imaging correlations. *Arch Neurol* 1993;50:609–614.
35. Amarenco P, Rosengart A, DeWitt LD, et al. Anterior inferior cerebellar artery territory infarcts. Mechanisms and clinical features. *Arch Neurol* 1993;50:154–161.
36. Becker KJ. Vertebrobasilar ischemia. *New Horiz* 1997;5:305–315.
37. Telian SA, Shepard NT, Smith-Wheelock M, et al. Habituation therapy for chronic vestibular dysfunction: Preliminary results. *Otolaryngol Head Neck Surg* 1990;103:89–95.
38. Cowand JL, Wrisley DM, Walker M, et al. Efficacy of vestibular rehabilitation. *Otolaryngol Head Neck Surg* 1998;118:49–54.
39. Keim RJ. William F. House Lecture. Neurotologic manifestations of microvascular hypoperfusion. *Am J Otol* 1995; 16:34–38.
40. Baloh RW. Vertebrobasilar insufficiency and stroke. *Otolaryngol Head Neck Surg* 1995;112:114–117.
41. Rubin AM, Gerard G, Bork C, et al. Central dizziness associated with cerebral blood flow disorders. *Am J Otol* 1994;15:625–633.
42. The National Institute of Neurological Disorders and Stroke rt-PA Stroke Study Group. Tissue plasminogen activator for acute ischemic stroke. *N Engl J Med* 1995;333:1581–1587.
43. Ferbert A, Bruckmann H, Drummen R. Clinical features of proven basilar artery occlusion. *Stroke* 1990;21:1135–1142.
44. Brandt T, Pessin MS, Kwan ES, et al. Survival with basilar artery occlusion. *Cerebrovascular Disease* 1995;5:182–187.
45. Cross DT III, Moran CJ, Akins PT, et al. Collateral circulation and outcome after basilar artery thrombolysis. *AJNR Am J Neuroradiol* 1998; 19(Sep. 8):1557–1563.
46. Amarenco P, Kase CS, Rosengart A, et al. Very small (border zone) cerebellar infarcts. Distribution, causes, mechanisms and clinical features. *Brain* 1993;116(pt 1):161–186.
47. Kase CS, Norrving B, Levine SR, et al. Cerebellar infarction. Clinical and anatomic observations in 66 cases. *Stroke* 1993;24:76–83.
48. Eisenstat DD, Bernstein M, Fleming JF, et al. Chiari malformation in adults: a review of 40 cases. *Can J Neurol Sci* 1986;13:221–228.
49. Paul KS, Lye RH, Strang FA, et al. Arnold-Chiari malformation. Review of 71 cases. *J Neurosurg* 1983;58:183–187.
50. Ahmmed AU, Mackenzie I, Das VK, et al. Audio-vestibular manifestations of Chiari malformation and outcome of surgical decompression: a case report. *J Laryngol Otol* 1996;110:1060–1064.
51. Cammalleri R, D'Amelio M, Gangitano M, et al. Monosymptomatic presentation of type I Arnold-Chiari malformation: report of two cases. *Ital J Neurol Sci* 1994;15:57–60.
52. Albers FW, Ingels KJ. Otoneurological manifestations in Chiari-I malformation. *J Laryngol Otol* 1993;107:441–443.
53. Chait GE, Barber HO. Arnold-Chiari malformation—some otoneurological features. *J Otolaryngol* 1979;8:65–70.
54. Rydell RE, Pulec JL. Arnold-Chiari malformation. Neuro-otologic symptoms. *Arch Otolaryngol* 1971;94:8–12.
55. Longridge NS, Mallinson AI. Arnold-Chiari malformation and the otolaryngologist: place of magnetic resonance imaging and electronystagmography. *Laryngoscope* 1985;95:335–339.
56. Pedersen RA, Troost BT, Abel LA, et al. Intermittent downbeat nystagmus and oscillopsia reversed by suboccipital craniectomy. *Neurology* 1980;30:1239–1242.
57. Levy WJ, Mason L, Hahn JF. Chiari malformation presenting in adults: a surgical experience in 127 cases. *Neurosurgery* 1983;12:377–390.
58. Dyste GN, Menezes AH, VanGilder JC. Symptomatic Chiari malformations. An analysis of presentation, management, and long-term outcome. *J Neurosurg* 1989;71:159–168.
59. Baloh RW, Harker LA. Central vestibular system disorders. In: Cummings CW, ed. *Otolaryngology—head and neck surgery,* 2nd ed. St. Louis, MO: Mosby, 1993:3177–3198.
60. Williams NP, Roland PS, Yellin W. Vestibular evaluation in patients with early multiple sclerosis. *Am J Otol* 1997;18:93–100.
61. Daugherty WT, Lederman RJ, Nodar RH, et al. Hearing loss in multiple sclerosis. *Arch Neurol* 1983;40:33–35.
62. Rizvi SA, Bashir K. Other therapy options and future strategies for treating patients with multiple sclerosis. *Neurology* 2004;63(12 suppl 6):S47–S54.
63. Matthies C, Samii M. Management of 1000 vestibular schwannomas (acoustic neuromas): clinical presentation. *Neurosurgery* 1997;40:1–9.

64. Mathew GD, Facer GW, Suh KW, et al. Symptoms, findings, and methods of diagnosis in patients with acoustic neuroma. *Laryngoscope* 1978;88:1893–1903.

65. Granick MS, Martuza RL, Parker SW, et al. Cerebellopontine angle meningiomas: clinical manifestations and diagnosis. *Ann Otol Rhinol Laryngol* 1985;94(1 pt 1):34–38.

66. Herdman SJ, Clendaniel RA, Mattox DE, et al. Vestibular adaptation exercises and recovery: acute stage after acoustic neuroma resection. *Otolaryngol Head Neck Surg* 1995;113:77–87.

67. El-Kashlan HK, Shepard NT, Arts HA, et al. Disability from vestibular symptoms after acoustic neuroma resection. *Am J Otol* 1998;19:104–111.

68. Driscoll CL, Lynn SG, Harner SG, et al. Preoperative identification of patients at risk of developing persistent dysequilibrium after acoustic neuroma removal. *Am J Otol* 1998;19:491–495.

69. Chang CYJ, Kamerer DB. Stereotactic radiosurgery for acoustic neuromas. In: House WF, Luetje C, Doyle KJ, eds. *Acoustic tumors: diagnosis and management*, 2nd ed. San Diego: Singular Publishing Group, 1997;309–346.

70. Lovely TJ, Jannetta PJ. Microvascular decompression for trigeminal neuralgia. Surgical technique and long-term results. *Neurosurg Clin N Am* 1997;8(1):11–29.

71. Mazzoni A, Hansen CC. Surgical anatomy of the arteries of the internal auditory canal. *Arch Otolaryngol* 1970;91:128–135.

72. McCabe BF, Gantz BJ. Vascular loop as a cause of incapacitating dizziness. *Am J Otol* 1989;10:117–120.

73. Moller MB, Moller AR, Jannetta PJ, et al. Diagnosis and surgical treatment of disabling positional vertigo. *J Neurosurg* 1986;64:21–28.

74. Herzog JA, Bailey S, Meyer J. Vascular loops of the internal auditory canal: a diagnostic dilemma. *Am J Otol* 1997;18:26–31.

75. Pulec JL, Patterson MJ. Vestibular nerve pathology in cases of intractable vertigo: an electronmicroscopic study. *Am J Otol* 1997;18:475–483.

76. Kogeorgos J, Scott DF, Swash M. Epileptic dizziness. *Br Med J (Clin Res Ed)* 1981;282:687–689.

77. Hughes JR, Drachman DA. Dizziness, epilepsy and the EEG. *Dis Nerv Syst* 1977;38:431–435.

Medical Management of Vestibular Disorders and Vestibular Rehabilitation

158

P. Ashley Wackym   Tammy S. Schumacher-Monfre

Over the past three decades, the diagnosis and management of peripheral and central vestibular disorders have evolved dramatically. Consequently, it is rare that a patient requires surgical intervention (1); however, a clear understanding of the pathophysiology and the scientific basis of medical treatment will help ensure appropriate management of these patients. The neuro-otologist commonly encounters three peripheral vestibular disorders: benign paroxysmal positional vertigo (BPPV), Ménière's disease, and vestibular neuronitis (neuritis), and one central disorder: vestibular migraine. Therefore, the medical management of these disorders will be emphasized. Additional disorders are amenable to medical management, and many of these will be addressed.

Pharmacotherapy of vertigo can be divided into two general categories: specific and symptomatic. Specific therapies include antibiotics for bacterial or syphilitic labyrinthitis, anticoagulants for vertebrobasilar insufficiency, and diuretics for Ménière's disease. Whenever possible, treatment should be directed at the underlying disorder. In the majority of cases, however, symptomatic treatment is combined with the specific therapy (e.g., viral vestibular neuronitis) or is the only therapy available.

Common causes and mechanisms of dizziness are outlined in Table 158.1. Tables 158.2 and 158.3 distinguish the common peripheral causes of vertigo from the common central etiologies. The diagnosis, pathophysiology, and treatment of most of these disorders are presented throughout several chapters in this section of the book; therefore, the focus of this chapter will be on medical management and the scientific rationale for each strategy.

The peripheral causes of vestibular dysfunction (Table 158.2) are presumed to be restricted anatomically to structures associated with the membranous labyrinth, peripheral branches of the vestibular nerve, Scarpa ganglion, and the vestibular nerve root. The central causes of vestibular dysfunction, though, compromise central vestibular circuits that mediate vestibular influences on posture (via vestibulo-spinal and vestibulo-collic pathways), control of gaze (via vestibulo-ocular and vestibulo-collic pathways), and autonomic functions. Unlike the peripheral vestibular system, which may be viewed strictly as sensors of linear and angular acceleration of the head, however, central vestibular pathways are multimodal neural circuits that integrate a variety of sensory and motor signals related to balance, posture, and eye movements. The vestibular nuclei are the primary central target of the vestibular nerve.

Other sites that receive primary afferents from the vestibular nerve include several other brainstem nuclei [abducens nucleus, nucleus prepositus hypoglossi, cochlear nuclei (probably from the sacculus), external cuneate nucleus and reticular formation]. Since the vestibular nerve terminates only in the ipsilateral brainstem, integration of information from coplanar pairs of peripheral vestibular end-organs(e.g., left and right lateral canal cristae, left superior and right posterior canal cristae, and left posterior and right superior canal cristae) is mediated by commissural connections. In addition to these vestibular inputs, the vestibular nuclei receive proprioceptive, visual (optic flow), and premotor/motor signals from different levels of the neuraxis (including cerebral cortex)

TABLE 158.1
COMMON CAUSES AND MECHANISMS OF DIZZINESS

Symptom	Causes	Mechanisms
Vertigo	Benign positional vertigo, labyrinthitis, vestibular neuronitis, Ménière's disease, vestibular migraine, otosyphilis, superior semicircular canal dehiscence syndrome, vertebrobasilar insufficiency, multiple sclerosis, brainstem or cerebellar infarction	Imbalance of tonic vestibular signals
Presyncopal light-headedness	Hyperventilation associated with panic disorders or chronic anxiety, postural hypotension, congestive heart failure, diffuse cerebrovascular disease	Diffuse ischemia of the brain
Dysequilibrium	Ototoxic drugs, peripheral neuropathy, presbystasis, autoimmune inner ear disease, genetic vestibular hair cell loss, cerebellar atrophy, cerebellar infarction, posterior fossa tumors, meningitides	Symmetric vestibular loss, proprioceptive loss, cerebellar damage
Visual distortion	New refractive prescription; cataract surgery with lens implant; ototoxic drugs; extraocular muscle dysfunction; multiple sclerosis; cranial nerve III, IV, or VI dysfunction; corneal disease	Visual and vestibular input mismatch
Multisensory dizziness	Psychophysiologic dizziness, diabetes mellitus, systemic vasculitis, adverse drug reaction, aging	Integrative dysfunction involving visual, proprioceptive, and/or vestibular systems

TABLE 158.2
COMMON PERIPHERAL CAUSES OF VERTIGO

Benign positional vertigo
Ménière's disease
Vestibular neuronitis (neuritis)
Post-traumatic
    Endolymphatic hydrops
    Labyrinthine concussion
Drug-induced toxicity
    Minocycline
    Phenytoin
    Quinidine
    Gentamicin
    Streptomycin
Other
    Bacterial labyrinthitis
    Viral labyrinthitis
    Tumors
    Otosclerosis
    Vasculitides

TABLE 158.3
COMMON CENTRAL CAUSES OF VERTIGO

Brainstem lesions
    Arteriovenous malformation (AVM)
    Tumor
    Trauma
Demyelinating disease
    Multiple sclerosis
Infarction or ischemia
    Vestibular migraine
    Brainstem
    Cerebellum
    Vertebrobasilar insufficiency
Hereditary disorders
    Spinocerebellar disease
Posterior fossa lesion
    Acoustic neuroma
    Meningioma
    Arachnoid cyst
    Metastatic tumor
    Other cerebellopontine angle tumor
    Arnold–Chiari malformation

that are related to postural and ocular control. One consequence of the polymodal inputs to these circuits may be the ability to use other sensory information to compensate for peripheral vestibularinjury.

Specific cell groups (or circuits) within the vestibular nuclei then contribute directly to vestibulospinal, vestibulo-ocular, vestibulo-collic, and vestibulo-autonomic pathways. The activity of each of these functional circuits within the vestibular nuclei is modulated by specific cerebellar circuits in the flocculonodular lobe, the vermis of the posterior lobe, and the anterior lobe. Classical clinical and anatomic evidence indicate that each of these cerebellar regions contribute to different vestibular motor functions. For example, flocculonodular lobe dysfunction has a primary impact on eye movements, whereas anterior lobe degeneration (e.g., alcoholic cerebellar degeneration) impacts predominantly on postural control. Cerebellar regions related to autonomic control have also been identified [for review see Balaban (2)]. Each of these larger cerebellar regions, though, is subdivided into smaller circuitry units (zones) that appear to directly influence specific vestibular nucleus output pathways. For example, there is a small region (zone) in the cerebellar flocculus that contributes to the control of eye movements in the plane of the horizontal semicircular canal by connections with the vestibular nuclei.

The direct cerebellar connections to the vestibular nuclei appear to be important for coordination and continual recalibration of motor responses to vestibular stimulation. Climbing fiber input from the inferior olive appears to play a critical role in these functions. The climbing fibers are believed to provide a "sensorimotor error signal" to cerebellar Purkinje cells, which may alter the responsiveness of the Purkinje cells to parallel fiber inputs via a mechanism termed "long-term depression," to achieve a rapid correction of function.

One important feature of central vestibular circuitry is its ability to compensate for peripheral injury. Although the phenomenon is well known, the mechanisms of compensation are poorly understood. The present evidence suggests that behavioral compensation involves synaptic plasticity in both the brainstem and the cerebellum. Two factors in compensation appear to be of particular relevance clinically. First, the stability of the vestibular dysfunction has an obvious impact on the efficacy of compensation. Stable, predictable dysfunction (e.g., vestibular nerve section) provides a baseline of dysfunction as a target for compensation. Conversely, compensation for fluctuating hypo- or hyperactivity (e.g., Ménière's disease) is expected to be ineffective because baseline function is unpredictable or unstable. Second, the functional status of the central nervous system, attributable to either age-related or organic changes, is an important consideration. For example, individuals with preexisting cerebellar damage may show decreased compensatory capability (1,3,4).

AUTONOMIC DYSFUNCTION, ANXIETY, AND PANIC ATTACKS: VESTIBULAR CIRCUITRY

Every clinician managing patients with vestibular disorders, as well as astronauts experiencing the rapid changes of vestibular input encountered during the various stages of space flight, are well aware of the marked autonomic dysfunction that is associated with these alterations of vestibular input (2,5). These signs and symptoms of nausea, vomiting, and pallor, as well as changes in respiration and circulation, are clinically apparent; however, the fundamental basis for these responses have only recently been elucidated via anatomic studies that have identified a network of vestibulo-autonomic projections in the brainstem of rabbits, rats, and cats (2).

The finding that vestibular nuclear and secondary visceral projections converge in the parabrachial nucleus (and other brainstem regions) provides important insights into potential neural substrates for phenomena such as respiratory, cardiovascular, and gastrointestinal (emetic) responses to vestibular stimulation, motion sickness, and autonomic responses to altered gravitational environments. In particular, these findings provide a potential neurologic basis for the close relationship between vestibular dysfunction and anxiety disorders with agoraphobia (2).

Anxiety, panic attacks, and agoraphobia are also commonly associated with vestibular dysfunction (2,6,7). In 1945, Sir Terrence Cawthorne described the terror that patients with acute vestibular injury may experience. Other clinicians have identified specific situations involving changes in spatial orientation that elicit symptoms of anxiety and panic. In 1947, Levy and O'Leary coined the term *street neurosis* to describe the anxiety that some patients develop after an acute vestibular attack. In 1975, McCabe observed the "supermarket syndrome" in patients with Ménière's disease and characterized these patients as experiencing an intolerance to looking back and forth along aisles and up and down shelves. Patients with vestibular deficits who are visually or proprioceptively dependent may have symptoms of imbalance, discomfort, anxiety, or phobic avoidance when in situations with inadequate visual or proprioceptive balance cues. Furman and Jacob have termed this situational specificity *space and motion discomfort*. These unpleasant manifestations of discomfort may also be considered "referred signs and symptoms" from vestibular pathways to visceral sites, and may serve as eliciting or reinforcing stimuli for conditioned avoidance of potentially dangerous situations (2,6,7). The diagnostic category "Space and Motion Phobia" develops when situational distress significantly impairs a patient's normal activities, particularly by avoidance behaviors that reduce vestibular discomfort (6,7). The neurologic linkage model has been proposed to explain the association of vestibular disorders and autonomic dysfunction, anxiety, panic attacks, and agoraphobia (2). The linkage appears to be mediated by (a) ascending vestibular pathways involving the parabrachial nucleus, amygdala, and infralimbic cortex; (b) noradrenergic pathways; and (c) serotonergic pathways. The consequences of this intimate neurologic linkage between vestibular function, autonomic regulation, and affective status are of great practical importance to the clinician. In particular, it is important to consider a multifactorial treatment plan to address the pathogenic mechanisms, obtain symptomatic relief from vertigo and nausea, facilitate vestibular compensation, and address emergent anxiety and depression of individual patients. The symptomatic pharmacotherapy of vestibular dysfunction is discussed later in this chapter; however, low doses of diazepam (2 mg orally t.i.d. prn), or lorazepam (0.5 mg orally t.i.d. prn) are useful in managing the associated symptoms of autonomic dysfunction, anxiety, panic attacks, and agoraphobia. For symptoms that occur more consistently, clonazepam (0.25 mg b.i.d. to t.i.d.) should be considered. Adjunctive techniques, particularly stress-reduction methods, such as biofeedback, hypnosis, and yoga, can likewise prove helpful in reducing these symptoms.

SPECIFIC PHARMACOTHERAPY

Specific forms of pharmacotherapy are directed toward reversing the proven or presumed pathophysiologic mechanisms responsible for disorders associated with vestibular dysfunction. Examples of such interventional schemes are outlined in Table 158.4.

TABLE 158.4   Rx   **TREATMENT**

SPECIFIC PHARMACOTHERAPY OF VESTIBULAR DISORDERS

Peripheral vestibular disorders
  Ménière's disease
    Low-sodium diet (1 to 1.5 gm Na⁺/day)
    Diuretic
      Triamterene and hydrochlorothiazide (Dyazide)
      Acetazolamide (Diamox)
      Hydrochlorothiazide
    Vasodilator
      Isosorbide dinitrate
      Niacin
      Papaverine
      Nylidrin
      Histamine
      Betahistine
      Cinnarizine
    Aminoglycosides
      Gentamicin (transtympanic)
      Streptomycin (IM or selective perfusion)
    Steroids
      Dexamethasone (transtympanic)
  Otosyphilis
    Penicillin (IV, IM), amoxicillin (PO)

TABLE 158.4   Rx
(continued)

      Doxycycline, tetracycline, erythromycin (for penicillin allergy)
      Steroids
    Viral neurolabyrinthitis (including vestibular neuronitis)
      Antiviral agents
        Acyclovir (Zovirex)
        Famciclovir (Famvir)
        Valaciclovir (Valtrex)
      Steroids
Central vestibular disorders
  Vertebrobasilar insufficiency
    Antiplatelet therapy
      Aspirin
      Ticlopidine
      Pentoxifylline
    Anticoagulation (reserve for impending stroke)
      Heparin
      Warfarin
    Postinfarction syndromes
      Dihydroergocristine, dihydroergocriptine
      Flunarizine
      Gangliosides
      Free radical scavengers
      21-aminosteroids
      Amphetamine
  Vestibular migraine
    Migraine abortive therapy (not used in basilar artery migraine)
      Ergotamine tartrate
      Sumatriptin
    Migraine prophylaxis
      Nortriptyline or imipramine
      Verelan PM
      Cinnarizine
      Propranolol (first-line agent for children)
      Neurontin
      Flunarizine
      Methysergide
  Psychophysiologic dizziness (associated with panic attacks)
    Antidepressants
      Imipramine
      Desimpramine
      Nortriptyline
    Tranquilizers
      Alprazolam
      Diazepam
      Lorazepam
    Monoamine oxidase inhibitors
      Phenelzine
  Familial ataxia syndromes
    Acetazolamide (Diamox)

Ménière's Disease

Medical therapy of Ménière's disease includes dietary modification, physiotherapy, psychologic support, and pharmacologic intervention. Diuretic therapy and salt restriction have long been considered to be the mainstay of medical intervention for endolymphatic hydrops, based on the assumption that these drugs can affect fluid balance within the inner ear and lead to a depletion of endolymph (1,4). Thiazide diuretics have been a popular form of such specific pharmacotherapy for Ménière's disease. These agents enhance excretion of sodium, chloride, and water by interfering with absorption of sodium ions across the epithelium of the cortical-diluting segment of the nephron. Other electrolyte effects include enhanced potassium, magnesium, phosphate, bromide, and iodide excretion. Long-term therapy produces decreased calcium excretion and hypocalciuria.

Prolonged thiazide diuretic therapy can be associated with metabolic alkalosis with hypokalemia and hypochloremia. A potassium-sparing diuretic such as triameterene or spironolactone is often used in conjunction with thiazides to offset potassium loss (e.g., triamterene and hydrochlorothiazide). Thiazides can induce hyperglycemia and exacerbate diabetes mellitus. Other potential adverse reactions include hyperuricemia and orthostatic hypotension. These agents may exacerbate preexisting renal or hepatic insufficiency.

Carbonic anhydrase inhibitors (e.g., acetazolamide) decrease sodium–hydrogen exchange in the renal tubule. These agents are used to decrease intraocular pressure in patients with glaucoma by reducing the formation of aqueous humor, and the analogy drawn between this disease state and Ménière's disease has led to the trial of these agents for treatment of endolymphatic hydrops. In addition, they are capable of decreasing CSF production by up to 50%. These diuretic agents increase excretion of bicarbonate, sodium, and potassium. Reduction of plasma bicarbonate can produce mild metabolic acidosis with chronic therapy. Rarely, hyperglycemia is exacerbated in patients with diabetes mellitus. Possible adverse effects include nephrocalcinosis, hyperhidrosis, distal paraesthesia, and gastrointestinal disturbance. Lip and distal paraesthesias may resolve with continued use or with decreasing the dosage; however, these symptoms, if tolerated by the patient, do not represent a contraindication to continued use. Particular caution should be taken in prescribing acetazolamide to patients with a previous history of nephrolithiasis, especially if the kidney stones were shown to be calcium oxalate. If a trial of acetazolamide therapy in such a patient is necessary, a 24-hour urine collection should be followed by analysis of calcium, oxalate, and citrate. If the patient demonstrates hypocitruria, which can be a consequence of metabolic acidosis induced by acetazolamide, administration of acetazolamide should be terminated, as hypocituria can induce calcium oxalate nephrolithiasis.

Vasodilators have been used for the treatment of Ménière disease, based on the hypothesis that the pathogenesis of endolymphatic hydrops results from ischemia of the stria vascularis. Such agents include niacin, papaverine, nylidrin, isosorbide dinitrate, intravenous histamine, and the oral histamine agonist betahistine. These agents have direct effect on vascular smooth muscle, producing vasodilation. Isosorbide dinitrate principally affects the venous system, whereas histamine causes vasodilation of small blood vessels and capillaries. Betahistine has also been shown to exert a direct inhibitory effect on polysynaptic neurons within the vestibular nuclei, independent of changes produced in cerebral blood flow; however, it should be noted that the FDA has withdrawn approval for betahistine (SERC) because of inconclusive efficacy data. The most common adverse reactions to these agents include flushing, headache, and hypotension.

The literature contains many anecdotal reports and uncontrolled studies reporting apparent beneficial effects of specific pharmacotherapy in patients suffering from Ménière's disease. Ruckenstein and colleagues (8) critically reviewed this literature in 1991 and concluded that nonspecific vestibular suppressants are the only medications that have been shown to alleviate vertigo associated with Ménière's disease. Three small double-blind studies showed short-term beneficial effects of betahistine, but this may be secondary to a nonspecific CNS suppression rather than a direct effect on cochlear blood flow, as previously described. Thus, no studies demonstrated definitive beneficial effects of vasodilator therapy in reversing endolymphatic hydrops.

Chemical Labyrinthectomy

Compliance with medical management (daily sodium restriction to 1,500 mg/day plus dyazide q.d. to b.i.d.) results in acceptable control of signs and symptoms in most patients; however, approximately 10% of patients reach a point where the symptoms are so severe that an operation or aminoglycoside treatment should be considered (1). Henceforward in this chapter, we will consider the aminoglycoside vestibulotoxic treatments to be included under the term *chemical labyrinthectomy*. When considering vestibular surgery or chemical labyrinthectomy, it is often useful to have the patient with Ménière's disease consult a dietitian in order to optimize the medical management prior to undertaking this course. From the standpoint of the severity of symptoms, the most appropriate group for surgical or chemical labyrinthectomy treatment include patients who cannot work, drive, make secure travel plans, or take care of a family. Candidates may also include those who are managing to carry out these activities only with great effort because they are highly motivated to do so (AAO-HNS functional levels 4, 5, and 6) (9). An endolymphatic sac procedure may be considered in some cases at AAO-HNS functional level 3, whereby there is no disability or immediate threat of disability, but there is disruption of daily activities because of the attacks of vertigo.

The overall goal of any treatment of vestibular disorders is to help make patients as functional and comfortable as possible. The operational goals are to control episodic vertigo and to avoid or minimize treatment-associated disequilibrium and hearing loss. The primary technical goal of chemical labyrinthectomy is complete unilateral vestibular ablation (1). The most common difficult problem to manage after any vestibular destructive surgery (vestibular neurectomy, labyrinthectomy, or aminoglycoside treatment) is persistent, troublesome disequilibrium, and this complication occurs in 20% of cases (1). Nearly all patients will experience vertigo and disequilibrium immediately after surgical labyrinthectomy or vestibular neurectomy. With aminoglycoside treatments, the disequilibrium begins when the chemical labyrinthectomy effect occurs. This effect typically occurs at least four days after the commencement of treatment.

Patients report symptoms of acute unilateral peripheral vestibular loss, including an acute sensation of rotational vertigo, imbalance, a tendency to fall toward the affected side, and intolerance to rapid head movement. They usually experience autonomic dysfunction (e.g., nausea and diaphoresis), as well as anxiety and general malaise. These symptoms improve spontaneously such that most patients are able to return to full activities by 6 to 8 weeks after labrinthectomy (1).

Patients treated with intramuscular aminoglycosides or those with a pretreatment contralateral vestibular deficit may also experience oscillopsia. This symptom is a bobbing of the visual field on ambulation. Patients will report that they have trouble reading street signs while driving or riding in a car, or difficulty reading labels as they move down the aisle of a store. Oscillopsia is a manifestation of reduction of vestibulo-ocular reflex caused by a loss of vestibular sensation. Oscillopsia usually improves in time, possibly because of central nervous system compensation or tolerance by the patient.

In nearly all instances, early postoperative disequilibrium will gradually resolve following ambulation of the patient, and additional treatment is not needed. If disequilibrium persists or occurs later following chemical labyrinthectomy, vestibular exercises or formal vestibular rehabilitation are usually helpful in improving balance function and comfort of movement.

Interest in intratympanic aminoglycoside (ITAG) as an alternative to endolymphatic sac surgery and vestibular neurectomy has increased in recent years. A key advantage is that ITAG can be a nonsurgical office procedure. Nevertheless, ITAG is, at present, an imprecise treatment, difficult to control, and in at least one current form of drug delivery, appears to be associated with a 10% rate of deafness in the treated ear [reviewed in Wu and Minor (10) and Cohen-Kerem et al. (3)]. Nonetheless, vertigo can be relieved in 90% of cases. Other protocols may be associated with a lower rate of deafness. ITAG has a place in the treatment of Ménière's disease, but the optimal treatment protocol and the boundaries of its exact role remain to be defined. Since 1998, when the second edition of this textbook was published, most otologists have greatly decreased the frequency with which they perform ITAG because of the risk of hearing loss. A recent longitudinal study of ITAG administration in 31 Ménière's disease patients reported a markedly reduced rate of profound hearing loss, however (10). In this study, Wu and Minor reported profound hearing loss in only one patient (3%). In addition, hearing improvement was seen in 5 (16%), unchanged in 21 (65%), and worse in 5 (16%). Vertigo was controlled in 90% of the patients. Their protocol

involves a single ITAG administration (26.7 mg/mL gentamicin, 0.4 mL typically injected), 30 minutes of solution contact with the round window, and subsequent removal of the residual gentamicin via aspiration. Minor's protocol now involves a single ITAG injection, and additional treatments are only administered if episodes of vertigo have persisted at the time of follow-up examination 3 weeks after injection.

Aminoglycosides do not seem to be concentrated in cochlear fluids, but the elimination half-life increases with chronic administration, suggesting sequestration of the drug by hair cells. Amikacin, dihydrostreptomycin, and kanamycin are primarily cochleotoxic, whereas gentamicin and streptomycin are primarily vestibulotoxic. At high doses, streptomycin is also cochleotoxic. For example, streptomycin, 25 mg/kg/day, administered systematically to cats resulted in loss of vestibular hair cells only, but at 100 mg/kg/day, both vestibular and cochlear hair cells were lost. Bioprotective mechanisms to avoid ototoxicity have recently been reviewed by Rybak and Kelley (11).

The hair cells of the cristae, the maculae, and the cochlea degenerate to different degrees following the administration of aminoglycosides. The primary vestibular neurons, the cochlear nuclei, and the vestibular nuclei are not directly affected, even at high doses. The basal turn of the cochlea is the region most susceptible to permanent loss of hair cells, resulting in an initial loss of high-frequency hearing. Although the mechanisms of this differential toxicity are incompletely understood, several contributing factors have been identified, including the route of administration, dose variables, and the specific aminoglycoside used.

Damage to vestibular dark cells, which are thought to play a role in the production of endolymph, has been reported following administration of doses of aminoglycoside below the threshold for damage to hair cells. An attractive hypothesis is that the impaired function of dark cells would be beneficial in Ménière's disease because decreased production of endolymph would affect the fluid homeostasis of the inner ear.

Preparation of Gentamicin Solution
Gentamicin solution may be used either as a stock solution of 40 mg/mL with a pH of about 5.4, or it may be buffered to a pH of 6.4 to reduce the discomfort associated with intratympanic injection. One method to prepare the buffered solution is as follows (1): 1.5 mL of gentamicin solution (40 mg/mL) is injected into a sterile 5-mL vial. A 0.6-M-sodium-bicarbonate-per-liter solution is prepared by combining 2 mL of 8.4% sodium bicarbonate and 1.36 mL of sterile water in a 5-mL sterile vial. Add 0.5 mL of the 0.6-M-sodium-bicarbonate solution to the sterile vial containing 1.5 mL of gentamicin to form 2 mL of a solution of gentamicin (30 mg/mL, pH 6.4) ready for injection.

Injection Technique
The patient should be comfortably positioned in the standard otologic position for examination under the

operating microscope, supine with the head turned away from the ear to be treated. In this position, the eustachian tube will be uppermost, to avoid dependent drainage of the gentamicin solution out of the middle ear. This position is maintained for 30 minutes following the injection, and the patient is instructed not to swallow or clear the middle ear during this period; providing a cup for gentle expectoration during this period helps accomplish this goal. Topical application of phenol to a small injection site on the surface of the tympanic membrane provides anesthesia, and the gentamicin is injected in the middle ear using a tuberculin syringe and a 27- or 25-gauge spinal needle. Typically, about 0.5 mL of solution fills the middle ear. The residual gentamicin is aspirated from the middle ear after 30 minutes of contact with the round window.

Administration Protocols

Numerous administration protocols have been described and a recent meta-analysis has been published (3). Nedzelski and colleagues had patients administer gentamicin intratympanically three times a day via a tympanostomy tube and a small flexible tubing for 4 days. The protocol introduced by Beck and Schmidt advocates a once-daily regimen until the earliest sign of ototoxicity is observed. With this schedule, 1 to 12 doses are given, with a mean of 4 to 6 doses. A number of other investigators use a dosing regimen that titrates the administration of ITAG using patient response measured by caloric response, audiometric function, and patient symptoms. The rationale is to reduce the risk of hearing loss while maintaining control of vertigo by giving less medication per dose and extending the time of treatment, with repeated applications as necessary. A second intratympanic injection of approximately 0.5 mL of gentamicin, 30 mg/mL, pH 6.4, is given 3 weeks after the first if vertigo is not controlled or recurs. Based on the far lower rate of profound hearing loss seen with the protocol developed by Minor (3% compared to 10%), however, it is anticipated that scheduled repeated injections will become less common.

Selective chemical vestibulectomy had also been utilized as an alternative to vestibular nerve section for refractory cases of unilateral Ménière's disease. Historically, a tuberculin syringe was used to introduce 2.5 µg to 25 µg of streptomycin in solution (25 µg/mL) through a fenestration in the horizontal semicircular canal. A multi-institution trial of this technique reported hearing loss in 68% of 47 patients undergoing labyrinthotomy with streptomycin infusion (12).

Parenteral streptomycin has been used successfully to manage cases of refractory bilateral Ménière's disease. Therapy is titrated to preserve some vestibular function. This method has helped to avoid post-treatment disequilibrium and oscillopsia associated with complete bilateral vestibular ablation. Total streptomycin dose varies from 5 g to 70 g in patients undergoing titration therapy, with a mean dose of approximately 25 g administered to achieve the desired endpoint. Langman and associates (13) improved or completely relieved episodic vertigo in 16 of 19 patients (84%) undergoing titration therapy for bilateral Ménière's disease. Persistent severe post-treatment disequilibrium occurred in three patients (16%), whereas changes in hearing were independent of the effect of streptomycin.

Intratympanic Dexamethasone

An emerging management technique for recalcitrant Ménière disease is the intratympanic injection of dexamethosone, and Doyle et al. have recently reviewed this topic (14). The technical aspects are identical to that described in the ITAG section discussed earlier. The senior author injects dexamethasone (24 mg/mL) and allows the patient to remain supine with the affected ear uppermost for 20 to 30 minutes. The procedure is performed three times, 1 week apart. Other authors have used single-dose applications via an exploratory tympanotomy followed by application, in the round window niche, of dexamethasone 8 mg, in hyaluronan on an absorbable gelatin sponge. A retrospective study of the latter approach in 21 ears of 19 patients was reported by Arriaga and Goldman (15). They found that a single application of dexamethasone/hyaluronan solution did not produce dramatic short-term hearing improvement in patients with endolymphatic hydrops; however, there were improvements reported—as much as a 38-dB gain in PTA and 38% gain in the speech discrimination score. This single patient's gain was tempered by 3 ears that experienced deterioration after treatment. Conservative performance of intratympanic dexamethasone is appropriate; however, there remain patients failing medical therapy who may benefit from this technique prior to a more aggressive surgical option being undertaken. Long-term controlled clinical trials remain to be completed; these will determine the efficacy of this treatment modality.

Otosyphilis

A presumptive diagnosis of otosyphilis is made in the patient with unexplained cochleovestibular dysfunction and positive fluorescent treponemal antibody absorption (FTA-ABS). Penicillin and steroids have been the primary treatment modalities. Although previous studies have shown benefit of intramuscular penicillin therapy (16), other studies have demonstrated that the intramuscular route of parenteral therapy fails to achieve treponemicidal levels in cerebrospinal fluid (CSF). For intramuscular therapy, treatment with 2.4 million units of benzathine penicillin weekly for three successive weeks constitutes minimal therapy. Other authors advocate extending therapy for as long as one year. New outpatient treatment regimens that include probenecid promise to achieve antitreponemal drug levels in the CSF. Probenecid increases the half-life and facilitates CSF penetration of penicillin derivative antibiotics. These regimens include 1.8 million units of intramuscular procaine penicillin G daily or 1 g oral amoxicillin six times daily, in combination with probenecid 500 mg four times daily.

For patients receiving intravenous therapy, 10 million units of penicillin G per day is administered in divided doses for 10 days, followed by 2.4 million units of intramuscular benzathine penicillin per week for 2 additional weeks. For patients with neurosyphilis, documented by a positive CSF Venereal Disease Research Laboratory slide test, (VDRL) 24 million units of penicillin G per day is administered intravenously for 14 days, followed by a 2-week course of benzathine penicillin and an 8-week course of high-dose oral amoxicillin. Patients with documented penicillin allergy receive 500 mg of tetracycline or erythromycin four times per day for 30 days. Alternatively, doxycycline (200 mg/day for 15 to 20 days) may improve patient compliance, as it is dosed twice a day and may be taken with food.

Many studies demonstrate enhanced efficacy when penicillin is combined with steroid therapy. Although dose recommendations vary, prednisone 40 to 60 mg/day for 2 weeks is accepted as minimal therapy. Therapy is continued for 4 weeks in patients who respond and is subsequently tapered according to patient symptomatology. Patients receiving prolonged therapy should be placed on an alternate-day regimen to minimize adrenal suppression. Absolute and relative contraindications to steroid therapy include hypersensitivity to corticosteroids, severe osteoporosis, brittle diabetes mellitus, peptic ulcer disease, diverticulitis, hypothyroidism, cirrhosis, thromboembolic disorders, and psychiatric illness. Because glucocorticoid therapy can reactivate tuberculosis, chemoprophylaxis should be used for patients with a history of active tuberculosis.

Seventy-five percent of patients undergoing antibiotic therapy for secondary syphilis will experience an acute, febrile reaction known as the Jarisch-Herxheimer reaction. The reaction typically begins within 4 hours after treatment is commenced and is manifest by fever and flu-like symptoms. This reaction is probably related to release of endotoxin from killed spirochetes or an allergic reaction to treponemal breakdown products. Symptoms typically subside within 24 hours after instituting therapy and seldom require interruption of therapy. Patients should be informed of this syndrome, though, because some will experience a transient exacerbation of cochleovestibular symptoms. Administration of prednisone for 24 hours prior to the initiation of antibiotic therapy reduces the febrile component of this reaction.

Penicillin and steroid therapy has been reported to improve vertigo in 58% to 86% of patients with symptoms secondary to otosyphilis. This compares favorably to patients with hearing loss, of which only 31% improve with treatment. Patients with disabling tinnitus or vertigo should undergo such therapy regardless of the duration of symptoms, as there is a reasonably high likelihood of improvement. Patients with isolated, long-standing hearing loss without fluctuation, however, are less likely to respond to therapy (16).

Migraine

Since the time of writing this chapter for the first edition, much has been learned about vestibular migraine (17–19). Likewise, there has been a much greater recognition of the frequency of occurrence of this disorder in both adults and children. It is a remarkably common disorder and no doubt represents many of the "atypical Ménière's disease" patients described in the past. Migraine has long been considered a vascular disorder, with vasodilation responsible for the headache and vasoconstriction responsible for the neurologic symptoms. Basilar artery migraine produces symptoms related to those areas of the central nervous system supplied by the posterior circulation. Serotonergic and central vestibular pathways may also be involved in migraine-associated vertigo and vertiginous auras, however (2). Approximately 30% to 40% of patients with classic migraine experience true vertigo. Other patients can present with vertigo without concomitant headache; this is referred to as a migraine equivalent. In fact, only 10% of patients with vestibular migraine also have headaches. This disease also occurs in children; however, unfortunately, the misnomer "benign positional vertigo of childhood" has been assigned to the condition by the neurology community.

Prophylactic therapy is indicated for those patients whose lives are being impacted by the recurrent vertigo associated with vestibular migraine, as all successful regimens have potentially troublesome side effects (17). The most common indication for prophylaxis is frequent migraine, with symptoms occurring more frequently than two episodes per month for 3 successive months. Interestingly, adults with vestibular migraine more often respond to tricyclic antidepressants or calcium channel blockers than to beta-blockers. Conversely, children with vestibular migraine respond to beta-blockers extremely well. Empiric therapy with the most commonly used agent may need to be followed with a change in class of medication until symptoms are controlled. Once symptoms are controlled with prophylactic therapy for 6 months, patients are weaned from their medication. If this is tolerated, then retreatment is necessary only if symptoms recur. Sometimes it is necessary to resume treatment with the prophylactic agent for another 3 to 6 months before attempting to wean the medication. Rarely, ongoing therapy is necessary, and this decision is guided by the patient's clinical features. Very often, children with vestibular migraine cease to have this disorder as they approach puberty. Dietary counseling is important, as tyramine- and caffeine-containing foods such as blue cheese, red wine, grape juice, chocolate, and tomatoes may serve as triggers for the migraine attacks. Likewise, excessive caffeinated beverage consumption, fatigue, stress, and skipping meals may induce vestibular migraine attacks in some patients.

Tricyclic antidepressants may be useful adjuncts for prophylaxis of migraine associated with panic attacks. For years, the tertiary amine antidepressants, such as amitriptyline and imipramine, have been used. Though effective, such medications have adverse anticholinergic side effects such as constipation, tachycardia, blurred vision, cognitive impairment, and orthostatic hypotension (17). These side effects can be detrimental, especially with the elderly population. As individuals age, there are decreased physiologic changes impacting pharmacotherapeutics. The specific changes involve water volume, cardiac output, circulatory blood flow, baroreceptor activity, gastric acid, gastric pH, intestinal absorption, hepatic blood flow and function, hepatic enzymatic functions, kidney efficiency, renal blood flow and general function, and visual acuity. New forms of tricyclics called secondary amines (such as desipramine or nortriptyline) have decreased side effects and are effective in the treatment of migraines. For this reason, the secondary amines are the tricyclics of choice. It should be noted, however, that if patients have significant reflux disease or problems with weight gain, tricyclics should be used with caution.

Beta-blockers, calcium antagonists, anticonvulsants, and tricyclic antidepressants are currently the most widely used agents for prophylaxis of migraine (17). Propranolol is normally used in a high-dose range (80 to 240 mg/day) and can produce significant side effects, including fatigue, bronchospasm, congestive heart failure, and male impotence. Calcium antagonists such as flunarizine (10-mg dose at night) or verapamil (240 to 320 mg/day) have been beneficial. Side effects, however, include sedation, weight gain, depression, and extrapyramidal disorders. When choosing a calcium channel blocker to treat vestibular migraine in adults, the authors usually begin treatment with Verelan PM 100 mg each night. This medication is a sustained-release formulation, and the dose is increased after 3 to 4 weeks if the symptoms have not come under control. A calcium channel blocker widely used in Europe and Asia for the treatment of vestibular migraine, and other vestibular disorders, is cinnarizine (Stugeron); however, it is presently not available in the United States. Despite the legal and safety questions associated with this practice, review of online resources suggests that this medication can be purchased and shipped to the United States. In addition to the calcium channel blocking properties, it also has an antihistamine function, thereby acting as a nonspecific vestibular suppressant, minimizing the vestibular-associated autonomic dysfunction. Recent studies also identify valproic acid (Depakene) and divalproex sodium (Depakote) as medications for the prophylactic treatment of migraines. The recommended starting dose is 250 mg twice daily, though some patients may need to titrate to 1,000 mg/day. Please note that anticonvulsants are contraindicated in individuals with liver function impairments.

Although infrequently used in vestibular migraine, ergotamine tartrate has been the drug of choice for aborting migraine symptoms for many years. It is a vasoconstrictive agent that stimulates alpha adrenoceptors and acts as a serotonin antagonist. It also inhibits free uptake of monoamines and sensitizes vascular smooth muscle to sympathetic stimulation. This agent is contraindicated in patients with sepsis or local infection, liver disease, and vascular disease. It should be used with caution in patients with hypertension or peptic ulcer disease. Usual dosage is 2 mg orally or as a rectal suppository, followed by additional 1-mg doses every half hour for 2 or 3 additional doses, if necessary. Frequent use of ergotamine can lead to rebound headaches.

Although sumatriptan (Imitrex) should not be used to treat vestibular migraine, it is a common parenterally administered vasoconstrictor that is an effective form of abortive treatment for nonbasilar artery migraine. It is a selective agonist for 5-hydroxytryptamine, a receptor found on the basilar artery and in the vasculature of the dura mater. It is administered as a 6-mg subcutaneous injection and relieves the headache associated with migraine within one hour in 70% of subjects. This agent should be used with caution in patients with hypertension, however, and it is contraindicated in patients with ischemic heart disease, as it may induce coronary vasospasm. Currently, sumatriptan is not recommended for patients with basilar migraine.

Vertebrobasilar Insufficiency

Approximately one third of transient ischemic attacks (TIAs) involve the territories of the vertebrobasilar system. These patients often manifest short-lived symptoms such as vertigo, diplopia, dysarthria, bilateral limb weakness, gait ataxia, variable and often bilateral sensory disturbance, and memory loss (20). Most often, patient history reveals that these signs and symptoms are exacerbated when abrupt changes in body position are made, specifically from a supine to a standing position. This can likewise occur when rapidly transitioning from a seated to standing position. This phenomenon is caused by venous pooling in the lower extremities and transient hypoperfusion of the brainstem caused by the compromised vertebrobasilar vasculature. Magnetic resonance angiography (MRA) has replaced traditional angiography in the diagnosis of vertebrobasilar insufficiency, and typically a tortuous and narrowed vasculature is seen. Antiplatelet therapy has been demonstrated as an effective treatment to reduce the incidence of stroke after TIA. This effect has been most clearly established for aspirin, which can reduce by half the risk for stroke after TIA (21–23).

Ticlopidine (Ticlid) is another platelet aggregate inhibitor that has been shown to have favorable effects on the risk for stroke after TIA, particularly for cases of vertebrobasilar insufficiency. This agent may be more effective than aspirin, reducing the risk for stroke by 48% compared to aspirin during the first year after TIA. This agent is associated with a risk of neutropenia that may be life-threatening, however, and therefore it should be reserved for patients who are intolerant to aspirin therapy. All patients on ticlopidine therapy should have a complete blood count (CBC) and white cell differential determination made at least once every 2 weeks through the first 3 months of therapy. Neutropenia reverses within 1 to 3 weeks after discontinuing treatment.

The efficacy of other compounds remains unproven. Dipyridamole (Persantine) and sulfinpyrazone (Anturane) confer no added benefit to aspirin therapy and are no longer recommended. Pentoxifylline (Trental) is a xanthine derivative that decreases blood viscosity and enhances microcirculation. This agent has been shown to enhance tissue oxygen levels in patients with peripheral vascular disease, and it may be useful for cases of vertebrobasilar insufficiency.

Full anticoagulation is typically reserved for patients with impending or evolving stroke. Occasionally, anticoagulants are used for tight stenosis of intracranial arteries, particularly if TIAs persist despite antiplatelet therapy. Therapy is commenced with continuous intravenous infusion of heparin to maintain a partial thromboplastin time that is 1.5 to 2.5 times normal. Subsequently, warfarin is added, and heparin is discontinued when the prothrombin time is elevated to 1.5 to 2.5 times normal.

More than 150 drugs have been reported to be of benefit to the recovery of patients who have suffered a stroke, but none has been proven to be effective by a careful clinical study. Glucocorticoids have been used extensively to limit cerebral edema, which may render viable brain sensitive to further ischemic damage. Clinical studies indicate that steroids are ineffective after ischemic infarction, however. Other commonly employed interventions, including osmotic and loop diuretics and hyperventilation, have not been subject to adequate clinical trial to confirm efficacy.

Several compounds are currently being investigated and may prove beneficial for recovery after acute stroke. Such agents include gangliosides, free radical scavengers, 21-aminosteroids, and amphetamine. Preliminary studies show that dihydroergocristine, an ergot alkaloid with potent dopaminergic activity, may reduce hypoxia-induced cerebral metabolic changes. The calcium channel antagonist flunarizine has been shown to protect the brain against neuronal damage in several models of cerebral ischemia. The ultimate utility of these agents in stroke patients awaits further clinical investigation.

Familial Ataxia Syndrome

Familial ataxia syndrome is a rare disorder with autosomal dominant inheritance that is manifest by recurrent episodes of vertigo and ataxia in several members of a family. Other prominent symptoms can include diplopia, dysarthria, tinnitus, and paraesthesia, but symptoms can vary considerably between families. Familial ataxia syndrome is one of the most treatable causes of chronic episodic vertigo. Acetazolamide, a carbonic anhydrase inhibitor diuretic, effectively prevents the episodic vertigo and ataxia. The mechanism of this action remains unclear. Systemic acetazolamide produces central nervous system acidosis by reducing serum lactate and pyruvate, but serum levels of lactate and pyruvate are normal in patients with this syndrome. The antihistamine dimenhydrinate, the benzodiazepine alprazolam, and the calcium antagonist flunarizine have been shown to be effective for symptomatic treatment of vertigo associated with the familial ataxia syndrome (24). Recently, mutations in the calcium channel gene CACNA1A have been demonstrated in patients suffering from episodic ataxia type 2 (25). This subtype of familial ataxia syndrome is characterized by episodic vertigo and ataxia.

Psychophysiologic Dizziness

Dizziness is associated with a wide range of psychiatric illnesses. Patients with anxiety disorders manifest by panic attacks are particularly susceptible to experiencing disequilibrium, often described as a feeling of imbalance or even a sensation of spinning inside the head. At present, the term "psychiatric dizziness" should be restricted to dizziness (a) that is a component of a recognized psychiatric syndrome and (b) that cannot be explained by clinical evidence of vestibular dysfunction (6,7). Psychiatric disorders associated with frequent complaints of dizziness include psychosis, abasia, depression, hysteria, panic disorder with agoraphobia, acrophobia, phobic postural vertigo, lightheadedness secondary to hyperventilation during panic, and the obsessive personality disorder. Patients with schizophrenia are more susceptible to motion sickness and show an increased incidence of abnormalities on vestibular testing. Administration of certain compounds, including lactate, caffeine, isoproterenol, yohimbine, and benzodiazepine antagonists, have been shown to elicit panic attacks in susceptible individuals. This evidence suggests that there may be an organic basis for the disequilibrium associated with psychophysiologic dizziness that would be amenable to specific pharmacotherapy.

Treatment of psychophysiologic dizziness relies on patient reassurance, psychotherapy, and pharmacotherapy Three classes of compounds have been shown to be effective in reducing the frequency of panic attacks. These agents include the benzodiazepines, tricyclic antidepressants, and monoamine oxidase inhibitors. Though clinically, all are effective, the side effects must be taken into consideration.

Benzodiazepines can have rebound symptoms following medication cessation. In addition, anxiety disorders are highly comorbid with depressive disorders and in fact can be exacerbated by benzodiazepines. Addictive tendencies also must be taken into consideration. Tricyclic antidepressants as mentioned earlier have high anticholinergic side effects. Safety becomes an issue in patient populations with coronary artery disease or cardiac dysrhythmias. Monoamine oxidase inhibitors have multiple food and drug interactions. In fact, they are contraindicated in populations with heart failure, pheochromocytoma, hypertension, liver disease, cardiovascular disease, seizure disorders, diabetes, and suicidal tendencies. Nevertheless, when used appropriately, these drugs can be highly effective.

Because of the numerous side effects of the previously stated compounds, a fourth class of drugs is presently under investigation. These include the selective serotonin reuptake inhibitors such as Prozac, Zoloft, Paxil, Luvox, and Celexa. Side effects such as agitation, headache, gastrointestinal upset, insomnia, and sexual dysfunction may occur. Formal analysis is pending at this time, although the preliminary data looks promising. It should be noted, however, that abrupt cessation results in the selective serotonin reuptake inhibitor discontinuation syndrome, which is associated with significant vestibular symptoms (26).

Future Perspectives

The pharmacotherapy of vertigo caused by other common causes of vestibular dysfunction currently relies on nonspecific suppression of symptoms. This is often the case because the underlying pathophysiology of many vestibular syndromes remains poorly understood. Current techniques of molecular biology promise to expand our understanding of both the physiology and pathophysiology of the human vestibular system. This knowledge may lead to the development of future forms of specific pharmacotherapy. For instance, cell and molecular biology techniques such as immunohistochemistry, in situ hybridization histochemistry, and immunoelectron microscopy have been used to identify neurotransmitters and receptors involved in modulation of primary afferent pathways in the vestibular neuroepithelium (5). These types of studies could lead to the development of pharmacotherapy aimed specifically at the vestibular end organ.

Vestibular neuronitis (neuritis) is an idiopathic form of acute unilateral vestibular paresis that is the third most common cause of vertigo. Current management relies on nonspecific treatment employing vestibular sedatives, physical therapy, and vestibular exercises (27). The epidemic occurrence of this condition, frequently following upper respiratory tract infections, suggests that viral infection of the vestibular nerve may explain the underlying pathophysiology of vestibular neuronitis. Histopathologically, degenerative changes in the vestibular nerve, Scarpa ganglion, vestibular neuroepithelium, and decreased synaptic density within the ipsilateral vestibular nuclei are consistent findings (28,29). Epidemiologic and serologic data suggest a viral etiology. The latent virus (e.g., herpes simplex virus) is thought to remain dormant within the vestibular primary afferent neurons (Scarpa ganglion). Identification of viral genomic DNA in the temporal bone of patients with vestibular neuronitis may lead to the development of new forms of such specific antiviral therapy. A few small studies appear to demonstrate the benefit of high-dose, intravenous acyclovir (Zovirax), which acts as a substrate for virus-specific thymidine kinase during DNA synthesis, in patients with Ramsay Hunt syndrome. In addition, the new so-called "pro-drugs," such as valciclovir (Valtrex) and famciclovir (Famvir) are available and have the advantage of achieving adequate therapeutic tissue levels via an oral route. Some of the herpes viruses (e.g., varicella-zoster

virus) require an intravenous route for acyclovir to reach tissue levels necessary to treat these infections. Likewise, the use of oral steroids would be appropriate in combination with an antiviral medication.

Gene transfer therapy is presently being developed for the treatment of peripheral hearing and balance disorders. One strategy, termed *in vivo* gene therapy, employs defective viral vectors to introduce a functional gene to replace a damaged gene within the inner ear. Several groups have successfully developed and introduced nonreplicating viral vectors, and other vehicles, into ganglion cells *in vitro* or directly into the cochlea *in vivo* (30). These methods will add an important weapon to our surgical armamentarium after more mechanisms of vestibular and auditory dysfunction are characterized at the molecular level.

SYMPTOMATIC PHARMACOTHERAPY

There are a number of commonly used antivertiginous medications that target symptomatic relief. The effectiveness of each drug has been determined empirically; however, it is difficult to predict which drug or combination of drugs will be most effective, since a patient may respond to one drug but not to others in the same class. Antivertigo drugs are typically classified by their chemical structure (e.g., diazepam is a benzodiazipine), behavioral properties (e.g., diazepam has sedative and anxiolytic properties), or mechanisms of action (e.g., benzodiazipines enhance inhibition via $GABA_A$ receptor–gated chloride channels). As a group, current antivertigo medications have multiple mechanisms of action, which include potentially efficacious actions that range from antagonism of muscarinic cholinergic, histaminergic, and monoaminergic transmission to calmodulin inhibition and blockade of voltage-gated calcium channels. It is also important to note that the direct effects of these drugs may also affect central neurotransmitter levels, which have the potential to affect vestibular pathways. For example, promethazine reduces dopamine turnover and increases noradrenaline turnover, dimenhydrinate reduces dopamine turnover, and meclizine has little effect on monoamine metabolism. Further, although flunarizine was characterized initially as a nonspecific Ca^{2+} channel and Na^+ channel blocker, other studies indicate that acute doses increase (31) and chronic treatment decreases extracellular striatal dopamine and metabolites (31) and that flunarizine administration inhibits dopamine uptake. Although there is ample evidence that monoaminergic, histaminergic, muscarinic cholinergic, and GABAergic mechanisms are present within the vestibular nuclei [Smith and Darlington (32)], there is inadequate evidence to implicate any specific central or peripheral sites with the efficacy of these medications. Four general classes of drugs are useful for treatment of vertigo and the associated autonomic symptoms of nausea and vomiting. The classes include anticholinergic agents, monoaminergic agents, antihistaminic agents, and anti-dopaminergic agents. Miscellaneous agents that are also effective include the benzodiazepine diazepam (Valium), the calcium antagonists flunarizine and cinnarizine, and the histaminic agent betahistine. Recent evidence has also favored the use of selective serotonin reuptake inhibitors (SSRI) and clonazepam, which are also particularly useful in minimizing the associated symptoms of anxiety and panic. Carvedilol, a beta-blocker that has found clinical applications for treatment of hypertension, has also been investigated as an agent for the symptomatic relief of vertigo.

Mechanism of Action

Numerous animal studies have documented that drugs with anticholinergic and monoaminergic activity diminish the excitability of neurons in the vestibular nucleus. Anticholinergic drugs suppress both the spontaneous firing rate and the response to vestibular nerve stimulation. Iontophoretically applied acetylcholine, methacholine, and carbamylcholine excite neurons in the medial and lateral vestibular nuclei, and this excitation is blocked with atropine. These observations suggest a cholinergic innervation on secondary vestibular neurons. In addition, cholinergic neurons in the nearby reticular formation project to the vestibular nuclei. Because muscarinic cholinergic mechanisms are distributed widely in the brain, however, actions at other levels of central vestibular pathways are also likely.

Drugs with significant antihistaminergic activity have long been used in treating vertigo and preventing motion sickness, yet little is known about their mechanism of action. More recent evidence further indicates that standard antihistaminergic antivertigo medications have significant antimuscarinic cholinergic activity in addition to antagonism of histamine H1 receptors. Since histamine excites neurons in the vestibular nuclei (33), it is expected that the combination of antihistaminergic and antimuscarinic actions of these drugs will depress activity in the vestibular nuclei. Appreciable histaminergic innervation is also present in brainstem autonomic regions and the parabrachial nucleus, so the antimotion sickness efficacy of these drugs may reflect actions at multiple levels in vestibulo-autonomic pathways.

Antagonism of dopamine D2 receptors, serotonin 5-HT2 receptors, and α1 adrenoreceptors are common features of antivertigo drugs with significant antiemetic actions. These drugs include the phenothiazines prochlorperazine (Compazine) and chlorpromazine (Thorazine) and the butyrophenones haloperidol (Haldol) and droperidol (Inapsine). The antiemetic actions are presumed to be due to effects at sites other than the vestibular nuclei. There are several potential direct actions on vestibular pathways, however. Because these drugs have antihistaminergic (H1) activity, they are expected to share actions with the "antihistaminergic" antivertigo drugs. Chlorpro-

mazine also has antimuscarinic activity and has been shown to depress the responsiveness of vestibular nucleus neurons. The possible actions of these drugs on noradrenergic and serotonergic transmission in the vestibular nuclei are more complex. For example, norepinephrine has been reported to increase and decrease the background activity of vestibular nucleus neurons, presumably via both α1 and α2 adrenoceptors. Because serotonin also has excitatory, inhibitory, and biphasic effects on different vestibular nucleus neurons, the precise mechanisms of action are unknown. The emergence of symptoms of a balance disorder after abrupt discontinuation of selective serotonin reuptake inhibitors (SSRI discontinuation syndrome) (26), however, indicates that serotoninergic mechanisms are perhaps a critical component of central vestibular neurochemistry. Clinically, it is important to note that extrapyramidal side effects of these medications result from their affinity for dopamine receptors.

Several tranquilizers are effective in suppressing vertigo. Diazepam (Valium) decreases the resting activity of vestibular nuclei neurons, possibly by decreasing another reticular facilitatory system. It also affects crossed vestibular and cerebellovestibular inhibitory transmission, and it decreases the production of CSF centrally.

Strategy in the Treatment of Vertigo

The choice of drug or drug combination is based on the known effects of each drug and on the severity and time course of symptoms. Prolonged severe vertigo is an extremely distressing symptom. The patient prefers to lie still with eyes closed in a quiet, dark room. In this setting, sedation is desirable, and the tranquilizing medications listed in Table 158.4 are most effective. Each of these drugs has significant side effects, however, and therefore must be used with caution. Parenteral diazepam, for example, can cause respiratory depression and hypotension and should be used only in a hospital, where emergency resuscitation equipment is available. If nausea and vomiting are severe, the antiemetic prochlorperazine can be combined with the antivertiginous medication.

The patient with chronic recurrent vertigo usually attempts to carry on normal activity, and therefore sedation is undesirable. Antihistaminic, monoaminergic, and anticholinergic medications are useful. Of the antihistamines, promethazine (Phenergan) has the most sedating effect and is therefore useful only when moderate sedation is desired. A combination of promethazine and the sympathomimetic ephedrine (25 mg of each) produces less sedation than promethazine alone and is more effective in relieving associated autonomic symptoms. Meclizine (Antivert), cyclizine (Marezine), dimenhydrinate (Dramamine), and scopolamine can be effective in treating mild episodes of vertigo.

Central compensation for peripheral vestibular dysfunction appears to involve changes in contributions of the intact labyrinth, utilization of alternate gravitoinertial sensory cues (vision, proprioception, somatosensation, and cardiovascular) and adoption of different strategies for performing movements. Since this process is a form of motor learning, it is essential that the patients return to normal activity to recalibrate central vestibular pathways. Viewed from this perspective, the combined sedative and antivertigo properties of medications for symptomatic relief require a therapeutic trade-off of acute relief at the expense of attenuating compensation. On the other hand, sympathomimetics and vestibular rehabilitation therapy can be added to facilitate the compensatory process.

Symptomatic management of positional vertigo is difficult because, although the vertigo is severe, it is short lived. To completely suppress these brief episodes, heavy sedation throughout the day would be required, which is usually unacceptable to the patient. The most common variety, benign paroxysmal positional vertigo, has a short duration (usually 30 seconds or less); however, some patients will complain of vestibular dysfunction lasting for much longer time intervals. This initial patient response can be extremely misleading, unless the otolaryngologist aggressively attempts to separate the episode of true vertigo from the autonomic dysfunction that follows. The severity of the autonomic dysfunction varies on an individual basis and may be severe with disabling imbalance and unsteadiness combined with nausea and diaphoresis. Other patients will experience mild true vertigo with movement in the plane of the involved semicircular canal. Very often the patient will identify this plane of rotation that elicits the vertigo and assiduously avoid this movement. Spontaneous remission occurs in more that 90% of patients within 6 months, although a small percentage do have recurrence. A simple explanation of the nature of the disorder and its favorable prognosis helps to relieve the patient's anxiety. Medications with mild sedative effects (e.g., diazepam, meclizine, or cyclizine) are useful when the episodes recur frequently, and to decrease the autonomic dysfunction that commonly impacts the patient's quality of life. Particle repositioning maneuvers and vestibular rehabilitation therapy are extremely effective in the treatment of benign positional vertigo (34). In rare cases of intractable benign positional vertigo, transection of the posterior ampullary nerve or plugging of the posterior semicircular canal has resulted in prompt remission of symptoms (1).

Prophylaxis of Motion Sickness

Generally, all antivertiginous medications targeting symptomatic relief are effective in treating and preventing motion sickness. The principal symptoms of motion sickness are malaise and nausea rather than vertigo, which may be considered as visceral referred symptoms of somatic origin. Tolerance develops after two or three days of constant stimulation, and prophylactic use of drugs several hours before travel is more effective than treatment of symptoms.

Oral or parenteral scopolamine was one of the first drugs used to treat motion sickness and was the first drug proved effective in its prevention. In the 1940s, controlled drug trials were carried out on military recruits during amphibious training, aviation training, and swing tests. A dose of 0.6 to 0.8 mg of scopolamine protected 50% of susceptible subjects for at least eight hours. Untoward effects (primarily drowsiness, dryness of the mouth, and blurred vision), however, limited the use of oral or parenteral scopolamine for motion sickness (35).

With the introduction and subsequent general use of antihistamines, particularly dimenhydrinate, scopolamine was neglected for many years. Interest in scopolamine was rekindled, in the form of transdermal scopolamine (Transderm Scop). With this delivery system, scopolamine is gradually released through a microporous polypropylene membrane contained in a patch that is placed on the skin behind the ear. A small dose (0.05 mg) is slowly released and absorbed over a 3-day period. Initial clinical trials indicate that transdermal scopolamine is effective in preventing motion sickness with minimal side effects, the main side effect being dryness of the mouth (35). The use of transdermal scopolamine for more than 3 consecutive days can result in withdrawal symptoms that mimic motion sickness, including dizziness, nausea, vomiting, and headache, upon discontinuation of therapy. To be effective, the patch must be in place several hours before exposure to motion.

Clinical trials of anti-motion sickness drugs under controlled laboratory conditions have shown that combinations of drugs are often more effective than any single drug (35). Particularly effective combinations have included scopolamine (0.6 mg), promethazine (25 mg) and dextroamphetamine (10 mg), and promethazine (25 mg) and ephedrine (25 mg). As in the treatment of vertigo, it is difficult to predict which drug or drugs will be most effective in preventing motion sickness in an individual. In controlled laboratory experiments, the responses of normal volunteers to the same drug or combination of drugs often vary greatly, even when identical motion stimuli are used.

HIGHLIGHTS

- It is rare that a patient requires surgical intervention for the treatment of peripheral and central vestibular disorders. Therefore, a clear understanding of the pathophysiology and the scientific basis of medical treatment will help ensure appropriate management.
- Marked autoimmune dysfunction is associated with alterations of vestibular input. Clinical signs and symptoms include nausea, vomiting, pallor, and changes in respiration and circulation.
- Anxiety, panic attacks, and agoraphobia are commonly associated with vestibular dysfunction. Acute vestibular injuries, as well as specific situations involving changes in spatial orientation, may elicit symptoms of anxiety and panic.

- Medical therapy of Ménière's disease includes dietary modification, physiotherapy, psychologic support, and pharmacologic intervention.
- Approximately 5% of patients with Ménière's disease will develop symptoms severe enough that operative or aminoglycoside treatment should be considered. The most common difficult problem to manage after any vestibular destructive surgery (vestibular neurectomy, labyrinthectomy, or aminoglycoside treatment) is persistent, troublesome dysequilibrium.
- A presumptive diagnosis of otosyphilis is made in the patient with unexplained cochleovestibular dysfunction and positive fluorescent treponemal antibody absorption. Penicillin and steroids have been the primary treatment modalities.
- Migraine has long been considered a vascular disorder, with vasodilation responsible for the headache and vasoconstriction responsible for the neurologic symptoms. Approximately 30% to 40% of patients with classic migraine experience true vertigo; other patients can present with vertigo without concomitant headache, referred to as a migraine equivalent
- Approximately one-third of transient ischemic attacks (TIAs) involve the territories of the vertebrobasilar system. TIA patients often manifest short-lived symptoms such as vertigo, diplopia, dysarthria, bilateral limb weakness, gait ataxia, variable and often bilateral sensory disturbance, and memory loss. Antiplatelet therapy (aspirin, in particular) has been shown to effectively reduce the incidence of stroke after TIA.
- Famial ataxia syndrome is a rare disorder with autosomal dominant inheritance that is manifest by recurrent epidoses of vertigo and ataxia in several members of a family. Other prominent symptoms can include diplopia, dysarthria, tinnitus, and paresthesia, but symptoms can vary considerably between families. Of the causes of chronic episodic vertigo, familial ataxia syndrome is one of the most treatable: acetazolamide, a carbonic anhydrase inhibitor diuretic, effectively prevents the episodic vertigo and ataxia.
- Dizziness is associated with a wide range of psychiatric illnesses. Patients with anxiety disorders manifested by panic attacks are particularly susceptible to experience dysequilibrium. Other disorders associated with frequent complaints of dizziness include psychosis, depression, hysteria, agoraphobia, acrophobia, phobic postural vertigo, and obsessive personality disorder. Treatment of psychophysiologic dizziness relies on patient reassurance, psychotherapy, and pharmacotherapy.
- Benign postural vertigo (BPV) is the most common peripheral vestibular disorder and is very effectively treated with vestibular rehabilitation. Advances have been made in the medical management of benign positional vertigo that have resulted in tremendously diminishing the number of patients with intractable BPV. The most commonly utilized single-treatment approach to BPV is the canalith reposition procedure.

REFERENCES

1. Wackym PA. Therapy—surgical alternatives. In: Goebel, JA ed. *Practical management of the dizzy patient.* Philadelphia: Lippincott Williams & Wilkins, 2000: 317–326.
2. Balaban CD. Projections from the parabrachial nucleus to the vestibular nuclei: potential substrates for autonomic and limbic influences on vestibular responses. *Brain Res* 2004;996(1):126–137.
3. Cohen-Kerem R, Kisilevsky V, Einarson TR, et al. Intratympanic gentamicin for Meniere's disease: a meta-analysis. *Laryngoscope* 2004;114(12):2085–2091.
4. Minor LB, Schessel DA, Carey JP. Meniere's disease. *Curr Opin Neurol* 2004;17(1):9–16.
5. Wackym PA, Balaban CD. Molecules, motion, and man. *Otolaryngol Head Neck Surg* 1998;118(3, pt2):S16–S24.
6. Furman JM, Balaban CD, Jacob RG. Interface between vestibular dysfunction and anxiety: more than just psychogenicity. *Otol Neurotol* 2001;22(3):426–427.
7. Furman JM, Jacob RG. A clinical taxonomy of dizziness and anxiety in the otoneurological setting. *J Anxiety Disord* 2001;15(1–2):9–26.
8. Ruckenstein MJ, Rutka JA, Hawke M. The treatment of Meniere's disease: Torok revisited. *Laryngoscope* 1991;101:211–218.
9. Committee on Hearing and Equilibrium. Committee on Hearing and Equilibrium guidelines for the diagnosis and evaluation of therapy in Ménière's disease. *Otolaryngol Head Neck Surg* 1995;113:176–178.
10. Wu IC, Minor LB. Long-term hearing outcome in patients receiving intratympanic gentamicin for Meniere's disease. *Laryngoscope* 2003;113(5):815–820.
11. Rybak LP, Kelly T. Ototoxicity: bioprotective mechanisms. *Curr Opin Otolaryngol Head Neck Surg* 2003;11(5):328–333.
12. Monsell EM, Shelton C, Anthony PF, et al. Labyrinthotomy with streptomycin infusion—early results of a multicenter study. *Am J Otol* 1992;13:416–422.
13. Langman AW, Kemink JL, Graham MD. Titration streptomycin therapy for bilateral Meniere's disease: follow-up report. *Ann Otol Rhinol Laryngol* 1990;99:923–926.
14. Doyle KJ, Bauch C, Battista R, et al. Intratympanic steroid treatment: a review. *Otol Neurotol* 2004;25(6):1034–1039.
15. Arriaga MA, Goldman S. Hearing results of intratympanic steroid treatment of endolymphatic hydrops. *Laryngoscope* 1998;108:1682–1685.
16. Smith ME, Canalis RF. Otologic manifestations of AIDS: the otosyphilis connection. *Laryngoscope* 1989;99:365–372.
17. Hain TC, Uddin M. Pharmacological treatment of vertigo. *CNS Drugs* 2003;17(2):85–100.
18. Marcus DA, Kapelewski C, Ruby TE, et al. Diagnosis of migrainous vertigo: validity of a structured interview. *Med Sci Monit* 2004;10(5):CR197–201.
19. Neuhauser H, Lempert T. Vertigo and dizziness related to migraine: a diagnostic challenge. *Cephalalgia* 2004;24(2):83–91.
20. Oas JG, Baloh RW. Vertigo and the anterior inferior cerebellar artery syndrome. *Neurology* 1992;42:2274–2279.
21. Albers GW. A review of published TIA treatment recommendations. *Neurology* 2004;62(8 suppl 6):S20–21.
22. Elkind MS. Secondary stroke prevention: review of clinical trials. *Clin Cardiol* 2004;27(5 suppl 2):II25–35.
23. Hankey GJ. Ongoing and planned trials of antiplatelet therapy in the acute and long-term management of patients with ischaemic brain syndromes: setting a new standard of care. *Cerebrovasc Dis* 2004;17 (suppl 3):11–16.
24. Sasaki O, Jen JC, Baloh RW, et al. Neurotological findings in a family with episodic ataxia. *J Neurol* 2003;250(3):373–375.
25. Baloh RW. Episodic vertigo: central nervous system causes. *Curr Opin Neurol* 2002;15(1):17–21.
26. Tamam L, Ozpoyraz N. Selective serotonin reuptake inhibitor discontinuation syndrome: a review. *Adv Ther* 2002;19(1):17–26.
27. Baloh RW. Clinical practice. Vestibular neuritis. *N Engl J Med* 2003;348(11):1027–1032.
28. Baloh RW, Lopez I, Ishiyama A, et al. Vestibular neuritis: clinical-pathologic correlation. *Otolaryngol Head Neck Surg* 1996;114:586–592.

29. Nadol JB Jr. Vestibular neuritis. *Otolaryngol Head Neck Surg* 1995;112:162–172.
30. Patel NP, Mhatre AN, Lalwani AK. Biological therapy for the inner ear. *Expert Opin Biol Ther* 2004;4(11):1811–1819.
31. Reiriz J, Ambrosio S, Cobos A, et al. Dopaminergic function in rat brain after oral administration of calcium-channel blockers or haloperidol: a microdialysis study. *J Neural Transm Gen Sect* 1994;95:195–207.
32. Smith PF, Darlington CL. Pharmacology of the vestibular system. *Baillieres Clin Neurol* 1994;3:467–484.
33. Wang JJ, Dutia MB. Effects of histamine and betahistine on rat medial vestibular nucleus neurones: possible mechanisms of action of anti-histiminergic drugs in vertigo and motion sickness. *Exp Brain Res* 1995;105:18–24.
34. Furman JM, Hain TC. "Do try this at home": self-treatment of BPPV. *Neurology* 2004;63(1):8–9.
35. Spinks AB, Wasiak J, Villanueva EV, et al. Scopolamine for preventing and treating motion sickness. *Cochrane Database Syst Rev* 2004;3:CD002851.

159

Surgical Management of Vestibular Disorders

Jeffrey T. Vrabec

Chapter 158 addressed the initial treatment of patients with vertigo caused by peripheral labyrinthine disorders. Medical management is successful in controlling symptoms for most patients with vestibular disorders. If medical management fails, however, surgical options are introduced for patients who feel disabled or severely incapacitated by recurrent episodes of vertigo.

Active unilateral peripheral vestibulopathy is the main disorder that can be managed surgically. When a peripheral labyrinthine disorder is quiescent but uncompensated, further observation or a vestibular rehabilitation program is considered. Bilateral dysfunction is a challenging clinical problem. In these cases, preservation of hearing is paramount, and the role of surgery is limited in favor of more conservative, pharmacologic intervention. Nonvestibular dizziness does not respond favorably to procedures designed to reduce or eliminate end-organ function. Severe central dysfunction is a contraindication to destructive labyrinthine operations. Other situations in which compensation can be impaired, such as poor vision, are relative contraindications to surgery.

The most common vestibular disorder necessitating surgery is Ménière's disease (1–3). The anatomic feature most commonly associated with Ménière's disease is endolymphatic hydrops. Therefore several of the surgical procedures discussed herein are designed for use only in the presence of hydrops. Deafferentation procedures such as vestibular nerve section (VNS) and labyrinthectomy are used for surgical management of both Ménière's disease and non-Ménière's vestibular dysfunction. Results are more favorable in Ménière's disease (1–3), perhaps because of enhanced ability to localize the site of the lesion and the affected side among patients with Ménière's dis-

ease. The emphasis herein is on proper patient selection and the strategy for intervention.

PREOPERATIVE ASSESSMENT

Possibly the most difficult task for surgeons is appropriate patient selection. The principal preoperative objectives are definition of the underlying disease, localization of the side of lesion, quantification of episodes of vertigo, and subjective and objective assessment of hearing. Insight into the extent of disability in relation to the patient's employment or prospects for such is paramount. The patient needs to understand fully the expected postoperative course and likely sequelae of surgery, such as residual disequilibrium.

The history often provides the most important information for diagnosis when a patient has vertigo. Onset of symptoms, duration of episodes, associated symptoms, timing of recurrent attacks, exacerbating factors, and temporal relation to a traumatic event are elicited for each patient. If constant imbalance is reported, a cause other than peripheral vestibulopathy is strongly considered. Common causes of unilateral peripheral vestibular dysfunction are outlined in Table 159.1. Although Ménière's disease is the most common diagnosis, it is important to exclude other causes. Endolymphatic hydrops can occur in conjunction with other inner ear disorders, such as otosyphilis. These disorders have a clinical presentation similar to that of Ménière's disease.

History and physical examination frequently help identify the affected side when a disorder is unilateral. The presence of tinnitus, aural pressure, hearing loss, or nystagmus characteristic of a peripheral disorder indicates which ear is affected. The most reliable indicators of the involved

TABLE 159.1 [D] DIAGNOSIS
DIFFERENTIAL DIAGNOSIS OF PERIPHERAL VESTIBULOPATHY

Ménière's disease
Trauma
Iatrogenic condition
Delayed endolymphatic hydrops
Chronic vestibular neuronitis
Labyrinthitis
   Cholesteatoma
   Chronic otitis media
   Viral infection
   Otosyphilis
Vascular insult
Autoimmune inner ear disease
Benign paroxysmal positional vertigo

side are associated sensorineural hearing loss and a unilateral decrease in vestibular response during caloric testing (4). Rotary chair testing and posturography are less helpful in localizing the side of a lesion.

Quantification of the severity of symptoms is necessary to compare treatment modalities. Guidelines for reporting results of therapy for Ménière's disease have been established by the Committee on Hearing and Equilibrium of the American Academy of Otolaryngology—Head and Neck Surgery (5). Four categories are used to define the accuracy of the diagnosis of Ménière's disease. Definite Ménière's disease requires two or more episodes of spontaneous rotational vertigo that last 20 minutes or longer, audiometrically documented hearing loss on at least one occasion, tinnitus or aural fullness in the affected ear, and other causes excluded. Certain Ménière's disease adds histopathologic confirmation to the definite criteria. Probable Ménière's disease is used when only one definitive episode of vertigo has occurred despite fulfillment of all other criteria in the definite category. Possible Ménière's disease applies to cochlear or vestibular variants of Ménière's disease when other causes have been excluded. Criteria for staging of hearing, functional status, and vertigo control are outlined in Tables 159.2 through 159.4.

TABLE 159.2
STAGING OF HEARING IN MÉNIÈRE DISEASE

Stage	Fourth-tone Pure-tone Average[a]
1	<26
2	26–40
3	41–70
4	>70

[a]Calculated as the mean of thresholds at 0.5, 1, 2, and 3 kHz from the patient's worst audiogram in the 6 months preceding treatment. These guidelines were designed only for certain and definite cases of Ménière's disease.

TABLE 159.3
FUNCTIONAL SCALE FOR MÉNIÈRE'S DISEASE

Level	Patient's Assessment of Current Status of Overall Function
1	No effect on activities.
2	I have to stop what I am doing during an attack but can resume activities when it has passed. I continue to work, drive, and engage in most activities I choose without restriction. I have made no changes in my activities to accommodate the dizziness.
3	I have to stop what I am doing during an attack but can resume activities when it has passed. I continue to work, drive, and engage in most activities I choose, but I have had to make changes in my activities to allow for the dizziness.
4	I am able to work, drive, travel, take care of my family, or engage in most essential activities, but I must exert a great deal of effort to do so. I must constantly make adjustments in my activities and budget my energy. I am barely making it.
5	I am unable to work, drive, or take care of my family. I am unable to do most of the active things I used to do. Even essential activities must be limited. I am disabled.
6	I have been disabled for 1 year or longer, or I receive compensation because of dizziness or balance problems.

These guidelines are intended for use in definite and certain cases. Probable, possible, and non-Ménière's cases can be reported with the same general guidelines but are specified as such and not mixed with data on definite and certain cases.

The status of the patient's hearing affects the choice of procedure and defines hearing preservation as a second objective. When the hearing is useful, labyrinth-destroying procedures are avoided. A number of factors are addressed to determine what constitutes useful hearing. The likelihood of contralateral disease is considered. For example, approximately one-third of patients with Ménière's disease eventually have involvement of the contralateral ear. With

TABLE 159.4
GUIDELINES FOR REPORTING VERTIGO CONTROL

Class	Numerical Score[a]
A	0 complete control of definitive spells
B	1–40
C	41–80
D	81–120
E	>120
F	Secondary treatment initiated because of vertigo

[a]Score calculated by means of dividing the number of definitive spells occurring 18 to 24 months after treatment by the number of spells in the 6 months immediately preceding treatment and multiplying by 100.

extended follow-up study, this figure approaches 50% (6). Friberg et al. (6) documented a mean pure-tone average in the affected ear of 50 dB to 60 dB after more than 9 years of follow-up evaluation and a mean speech discrimination score of approximately 50%.

For patients with fluctuating hearing loss, the best results of preoperative audiography are considered. Thresholds better than 70 dB and speech discrimination scores better than 20% warrant consideration of hearing preservation surgery. The ultimate decision about the usefulness of hearing rests with the patient. Surgical procedures on a patient's only hearing ear are avoided.

As a final prelude to planned surgery for vertigo, magnetic resonance imaging (MRI) of the brain with attention to the posterior fossa is performed to rule out a cerebellopontine angle tumor or brainstem lesion. In many cases, this study has been performed during a previous evaluation. Review of older images, however, can reveal insufficient detail about the internal auditory canal or that contrast material was not administered. If a question persists regarding the adequacy of a previous study, magnetic resonance imaging is repeated, and the images are reviewed by an experienced neuroradiologist.

SURGERY FOR BENIGN PAROXYSMAL POSITIONAL VERTIGO

A generally held belief is that benign paroxysmal positional vertigo (BPPV) is caused by accumulation of debris within the posterior semicircular canal (PSCC). The source of the debris is likely otoconia from a degenerating utricular macula. Otoconia have a density approximately 2.5 times greater than that of endolymph; thus particles in suspension tend to precipitate in the PSCC, the most dependent portion of the inner ear. Debate continues about whether the sediment remains free-floating or adheres to portions of the membranous labyrinth. Viral labyrinthitis, head trauma, and aging all predispose a patient to development of BPPV (7).

Epley (8) and Semont et al. (9) devised techniques for removal of this sediment by means of noninvasive exercises the authors call the *canalith repositioning procedure* and the *liberatory maneuver*, respectively. Each technique is based on the assumption that the debris can be moved to an asymptomatic region of the inner ear. Many studies have confirmed the usefulness of these approaches. Improvement of symptoms is achieved by nearly 90% of patients. Several series have included patients with prolonged or recurrent symptoms. Failure of one or both of these maneuvers after repeated trials is a prerequisite for surgical treatment of patients with BPPV.

Surgical procedures designed specifically to manage incapacitating symptoms of BPPV include singular neurectomy and PSCC occlusion. These procedures are designed to eliminate responses from the PSCC either by means of deafferentation (singular neurectomy) or by means of prevention of fluid movement through the posterior canal (occlusion). Patients considered candidates for surgery typically have had unrelenting or numerous recurrences of BPPV emanating from the same ear.

Singular neurectomy was initially described by Gacek, and he reports the most extensive individual experience with this operation (10). The singular nerve exits the lateral aspect of the internal auditory canal in the singular canal and courses inferiorly and posteriorly to the ampulla of the PSCC. The intermediate segment of the nerve is inferior–posterior to the round window niche. In this location, it is possible to sever the nerve without damaging the rest of the inner ear.

Several anatomic studies of the relation between the singular nerve and the round window niche have been conducted. The nerve can be lateral, medial, or directly inferior to the round window membrane. The most common location is lateral to the membrane in 50% of ears. The nerve is medial to the round window membrane in 14% to 27% of cases (11,12). In this instance, an attempt at transection entails risk of injury to the vestibule and basal turn of the cochlea. Results of anatomic studies suggest a high prevalence of surgically inaccessible singular nerves, but surgical reports rarely document difficulty in locating or sectioning the nerve.

The operation typically is performed through a transcanal approach. Removal of the inferior scutum will optimize visualization of the round window niche. The overhang of the round window niche must be taken down to view the nerve during transection. Resolution of positionally induced nystagmus is evident during an examination performed immediately after the operation. Most patients have spontaneous nystagmus, however, usually down beating, that persists for a few days.

Published rates of success of singular neurectomy in eliminating BPPV are close to 90% (10,13). Symptoms persist when the nerve cannot be unequivocally identified. Complications are few but include recurrent vertigo and sensorineural hearing loss. Vertigo can recur many years after the operation, and the adequacy of the neurotomy is questioned. Severe sensorineural hearing loss occurs among at least 5% of patients, as a consequence of either direct trauma to the inner ear or postoperative labyrinthitis. Lesser sensorineural losses occur among an additional 20% of patients. This procedure is extraordinarily difficult. Considerable practice in a temporal bone laboratory is advised for surgeons who want to perform this procedure.

Difficulty performing singular neurectomy stimulated development of PSCC occlusion as an alternative procedure. First described by Parnes and McClure (14), the procedure is based on the theory that elimination of endolymph flow in the canal prevents stimulation of the cupula with head motion. Observations of animal models have shown PSCC occlusion to have no effect on the sensitivity of the other vestibular end organs.

A transmastoid approach to the PSCC is used, this being much more familiar to most otologic surgeons than is dissection of the singular nerve. The PSCC is identified and blue-lined. The canal is opened with a footplate hook, and perilymph is wicked away. The lumen is occluded with autogenous tissue (fascia or bone paté) or bone wax. Alternative methods such as laser partitioning of the membranous labyrinth have been described; however, the adequacy of the occlusion with this technique is questioned. Failure to permanently occlude the canal has resulted in recurrence of symptoms.

The postoperative course can be marked by disequilibrium that persists for days to weeks. Most patients have transient sensorineural hearing loss, which usually resolves within 6 to 8 weeks of the operation. Sensorineural loss occurs among as many as 20% of patients, probably secondary to labyrinthitis. It ranges from mild high-frequency loss to anacusis. Series with long-term postoperative follow-up find complete resolution of symptoms nearly all cases and rare episodes of recurrent vertigo (15,16). Recurrent symptoms after singular neurectomy or PSCC occlusion would be amenable to formal vestibular nerve section. Additional data are necessary to determine which procedure entails the least overall risk to hearing.

OPERATIONS ON THE ENDOLYMPHATIC SAC (EXTERNAL SHUNTING)

Operations on the endolymphatic sac are performed primarily to manage vertigo caused by Ménière's disease. Originally promoted by Georges Portmann, opening the sac was thought to relieve high endolymphatic pressure. Later, Hallpike and Cairns, and Yamakawa independently identified dilatation of the endolymphatic space in cadavers of patients with Ménière's disease. This histopathologic finding seemed to provide support for Portmann's theory of endolymphatic hypertension. Temporal bone studies of patients with Ménière's disease have shown rupture of the intralabyrinthine membrane and fibrosis or obstruction of the endolymphatic, saccular, and utricular ducts. These findings led Schuknecht (17) to question the efficacy of sac surgery.

Numerous theories have been proposed to explain the cause of endolymphatic hydrops. These include infection, autoimmune dysfunction, vascular insufficiency, and altered production or reabsorption of endolymph. Theories also abound about the mechanism of action of sac procedures. Some experts believe they promote longitudinal flow of endolymph. Others believe endolymphatic hypertension is relieved. Others suggest changes in sac function occur after surgery, such as increased resorption of endolymph, altered secretion of proteins, or enhanced macrophage activity. The unknown therapeutic mechanism of sac surgery fuels the controversy about its role in the management of vertigo.

Several variations on the Portmann technique have been described. These include endolymphatic–subarachnoid shunting, sac decompression, sac excision, and use of endolymphatic–mastoid stents and unidirectional valves. The various techniques all have their proponents but rarely have they been studied in a randomized manner. Insight into the effects of modification of the technique is provided by retrospective analysis of an individual series. Brackmann and Nissen (18) compared shunting of endolymph to the mastoid with shunting to the subarachnoid space and found no difference in outcome. Huang and Lin (19) found little difference between decompression alone, saccotomy, and saccotomy with placement of an implant. Glasscock et al. (20) were unable to replicate the success of others with sac implants and abandoned sac surgery altogether. McKee et al. (21) summarized data from a number of reports and found that the mean success rate is near 75% regardless of technique.

No controlled studies have documented the efficacy of sac surgery, in part because of the difficulty in providing an appropriate control treatment. Evaluations of efficacy are based on nonsurgical controls and alternative surgical procedures. Bretlau et al. (22) performed a prospective, blinded comparison between endolymphatic sac decompression and mastoidectomy alone. The authors reviewed their results at intervals for as long as 9 years and found no difference in control of vertigo between the two groups. Welling and Nagaraja (23) reviewed the statistical methods of this study and recalculated the results at 1 year. They found that both treatment and control groups had marked reduction in vertigo 1 year after surgery, although the improvement was greater among the group that underwent active shunting. Thomsen et al. (24), colleagues of Bretlau et al. (22) later compared endolymphatic shunt placement with myringotomy and tube placement. This controlled study found no difference between the two procedures in vertigo control 1 year after surgery. Silverstein et al. (25) retrospectively reviewed the records of patients with Ménière's disease who were considered surgical candidates because of disabling vertigo. Each was offered endolymphatic sac surgery or vestibular nerve section. Those who declined surgical intervention were observed. Among the control patients, 57% had no vertigo after 2 years of follow-up evaluation and 71% had no vertigo at last follow-up contact; the follow-up period averaged 8.3 years. Among patients undergoing sac surgery, 40% had complete control after 2 years and 70% had complete control at last follow-up contact; the average follow-up period was 8.7 years. Among patients who underwent vestibular neurectomy, 93% had complete control 2 years after surgery. Although the results of none of these studies were conclusive, it appears that the benefit of sac surgery is limited in duration and that less invasive procedures can provide similar benefit.

The operation proceeds by means of a retroauricular incision and complete mastoidectomy. To facilitate exposure of the sac, the retrofacial air cells must be widely opened to the jugular bulb anteroinferiorly, facial nerve laterally, and PSCC superiorly. All bone is removed from the dura of the posterior fossa anterior to the sigmoid sinus. This often allows precise identification of the endolymphatic duct as it courses medially to the PSCC. The dura appears thickened in the region of the sac, because these two structures overlap. Once identified, the sac is opened, stented, or excised according to the surgeon's preference.

Endolymphatic sac surgery can be performed as an outpatient procedure, does not preclude further operative intervention, and carries little risk of iatrogenic hearing loss. Complete elimination of vertigo may be achieved by as many as 50% of patients, and improvement occurs among an additional 25%. Complications include total sensorineural hearing loss among less than 1% of patients. Mild-to-moderate losses occur among as many as 20% of patients, typically in the higher frequencies. This complication is thought to be caused by aggressive manipulation of the endolymphatic duct. Rare complications include conductive hearing loss caused by entrance of bone dust into the middle ear, facial nerve injury, cerebrospinal fluid (CSF) leak, or bleeding from injury to the sigmoid sinus or jugular bulb.

VESTIBULAR NERVE SECTION

Sectioning of the eighth cranial nerve for vertigo was initially described at the turn of the century. The hearing loss that resulted from total eighth nerve section and the frequent facial nerve dysfunction limited the popularity of this procedure. Use of selective VNS decreased the incidence of many of these complications. Dandy reported on more than 400 operations performed through posterior fossa craniotomy; vertigo was controlled for 90% of the patients. Facial nerve paralysis occurred among 7.5% of the patients, and VNS remained less popular than labyrinthectomy for control of intractable vertigo.

Renewed interest in vestibular neurectomy was incited by the introduction of the middle fossa approach by House in 1961. Glasscock, Fisch, and Garcia-Ibanez all confirmed the usefulness of this approach for selective VNS (3,21). The vestibular nerve also can be approached posteriorly through retrolabyrinthine or retrosigmoid craniotomy. Advocates of these approaches cite less need for brain retraction and ease of technique (2). Modern microsurgical techniques have decreased the incidence of complications that occurred earlier in the century and promoted greater use of selective vestibular neurectomy. The choice of approach is determined by the surgeon's preference. Familiarity with the relevant anatomic landmarks is of utmost importance.

Perioperative management is similar for all neurectomy procedures. The routine perioperative use of antibiotics and intraoperative monitoring of facial and cochlear nerve function are strongly suggested. Initial postoperative observation is conducted in an intensive care setting to monitor for

changes in neurologic status. Attention is given to prevention of postoperative hypertension. The patient can be transferred to a conventional nursing unit on the first or second day. The patient is observed for CSF leak and meningitis. Early walking with assistance is encouraged. The patient is discharged when he or she can walk unassisted.

Middle fossa VNS proceeds through a 4-cm by 4-cm temporal craniotomy centered slightly anteriorly to the external auditory canal. The middle fossa dura is elevated from posterior to anterior along the medial border of the petrous ridge. Temporal lobe elevation is maintained with a House middle fossa retractor. Methods to identify the internal auditory canal entail use of the greater superficial petrosal nerve, malleus head, and superior semicircular canal as the initial landmarks. Bone over the superior aspect of the internal auditory canal is removed to allow approximately 180 degrees of exposure. The dura is incised posteriorly to reduce risk of facial nerve injury. The superior and inferior vestibular nerves are sectioned laterally in the internal auditory canal. Care is taken to include the singular nerve. The facial and cochlear nerves are anterior. Once neurectomy is complete, a piece of muscle or fat is used to plug the dural opening. The temporal lobe is allowed to return to its normal position. Tacking sutures from the edges of the craniotomy to the dura limits the possibility of epidural hematoma.

Retrosigmoid and retrolabyrinthine operations begin with a postauricular incision placed farther posteriorly than in routine mastoid surgery. The retrosigmoid craniotomy is placed just posterior to the sigmoid sinus and inferior to the transverse sinus. Retrolabyrinthine craniotomy necessitates complete mastoidectomy and removal of bone posterior to the PSCC to a point 1 to 2 cm posterior to the sigmoid sinus. After dural incisions and release of CSF, the cerebellum can be gently displaced posteriorly, often without retraction. The sigmoid sinus can be retracted (anteriorly in retrosigmoid approaches, posteriorly in retrolabyrinthine approaches) to improve exposure of the porus acusticus. In this location, the vestibular portion of the eighth cranial nerve is superior to the cochlear portion. A cleavage plane is visible in approximately 75% of patients; existence of this plane allows separation of the two portions. Inability to define the cleavage plane may require removal of bone from the medial lip of the porus to expose the nerves farther laterally. An abdominal fat graft is used to obliterate the mastoid process and prevent CSF leak in the retrolabyrinthine area. The dura is more easily closed in the retrosigmoid approach, and a fat graft is unnecessary. Layered skin closure is followed by placement of a pressure dressing. Recent technical refinements to posterior fossa approaches include limiting the size of the craniotomy and use of endoscopes to improve visualization of the nerves in the medial aspect of the internal auditory canal (26).

The reported success rate of vestibular neurectomy varies with approach. In a series in which a middle fossa approach was used, complete elimination of vertigo was achieved by more than 90% of patients (1–3). With posterior approaches, complete elimination of vertigo was achieved by more than 80% of patients. If patients with substantial improvement in vertigo are included, the success rate for all approaches is more than 95%. The difference in outcome is probably explained by the greater likelihood of incomplete neurectomy when posterior approaches are used.

Complications most commonly associated with VNS include disequilibrium, headache, hearing loss, and CSF leak. Disequilibrium occurs among as many as one-third of patients. In most cases, this symptom does not limit activity, although a rare patient finds it debilitating. Incomplete or impaired central compensation is thought to cause persistent disequilibrium. Hearing loss as a direct consequence of surgery is uncommon. The magnitude of the loss ranges from isolated high-frequency threshold elevation to anacusis. Less common complications, occurring in less than 5% of cases, are wound infection, facial paralysis, and tinnitus. Rare complications unique to intracranial procedures include meningitis, intracranial hemorrhage, and stroke. Preventive measures, such as perioperative administration of antibiotics, diligent control of hypertension, and timely recognition of altered mental status limit the incidence and morbidity of these rare complications.

The incidence of specific complications varies according to the chosen approach. With the middle fossa approach, there is greater risk of facial nerve injury, which usually causes transient paralysis of the facial nerve. Injury to the labyrinthine artery may account for the greater incidence of total hearing loss. Memory disturbance has been described as a result of temporal lobe retraction. Retrolabyrinthine approaches are associated with a greater incidence of CSF leak (2,27). Conductive hearing loss can occur if bone dust enters the middle ear or if abdominal fat used to pack the mastoid process herniates into the epitympanum. Headache is most common with the retrosigmoid approach. The cause of the headaches is unclear. The incidence of headache is much greater if the medial portion of the internal auditory canal has been drilled out, allowing possible accumulation of bone dust within the posterior fossa (28).

LABYRINTHECTOMY

Destruction of the labyrinth is the final surgical option for management of vertigo. Milligan and Lake independently presented the first descriptions of labyrinthectomy in 1904. Both surgeons used a transmastoid approach (21). Lempert first described an endaural approach to labyrinthectomy that involved opening the vestibule through the oval window. Schuknecht and Cawthorne subsequently presented methods of transcanal labyrinthectomy. The translabyrinthine approach later was introduced for acoustic tumor surgery. Transmastoid labyrinthectomy

became an important preliminary step in more advanced temporal bone dissection and regained popularity for surgical control of vertigo.

Transcanal labyrinthectomy can be performed with local or general anesthesia. Surgery begins with development of a tympanomeatal flap. The incudostapedial joint is disarticulated, and the incus is removed. The stapedius tendon is divided, and the stapes is removed. The vestibule is drained of perilymph, which can induce vertigo. The oval window is enlarged with a drill or a curette to improve visibility and provide room to introduce additional instruments. The saccule can be removed easily under direct vision. The utricle is superior in the oval window, medial to the facial nerve. It is avulsed with a sweeping motion with a 3-mm right-angled hook. The hook is used to probe the ampullar ends of the semicircular canals. It is difficult to extract the canal ampullae, but severe damage can be caused by manipulation with the hook. Gelatin foam sponge soaked in an ototoxic medication can be packed into the vestibule.

The surgical objective of transmastoid labyrinthectomy is to completely excise all five end organs. The first step is complete mastoidectomy through a postauricular approach. It is important to visualize the facial nerve in the tympanic segment and at the second genu to avoid injury. The semicircular canals are defined by means of exenteration of the perilabyrinthine air cells. The lateral canal is entered on its superior aspect to minimize the risk of facial nerve injury. The superior canal is entered on its posterior aspect. The ampullae of these two canals are adjacent and are located superior to the vestibule. After these two structures are avulsed, the vestibule is enlarged medially and posteriorly to provide wide access for removal of the utricle and saccule (Figure 159.1). The lateral wall of the vestibule must be respected to avoid facial nerve injury. Vestibulotomy is carried further posteriorly, medially to the second genu, to identify the ampullar end of the posterior canal. This structure is removed. The wound is closed in layers and a mastoid dressing is placed.

The postoperative course after labyrinthectomy is independent of the operative approach. Vigorous horizontal nystagmus is present postoperatively and is accompanied by vertigo, which can be severe. Antiemetics and analgesics are prescribed as needed. A brief hospitalization is anticipated. Discharge depends on resumption of adequate oral intake and walking without assistance.

Excellent results have been obtained with both transmastoid and transcanal labyrinthectomy. In most series, there has been complete elimination of vertigo among more than 85% of patients and substantial improvement among an additional 10% (29,30). Proper technique is paramount in obtaining optimal results. The surgeon chooses a method that is familiar and efficient and that limits risk of complications.

More complete damage to the labyrinth may produce superior results. There are reported cases of persistent

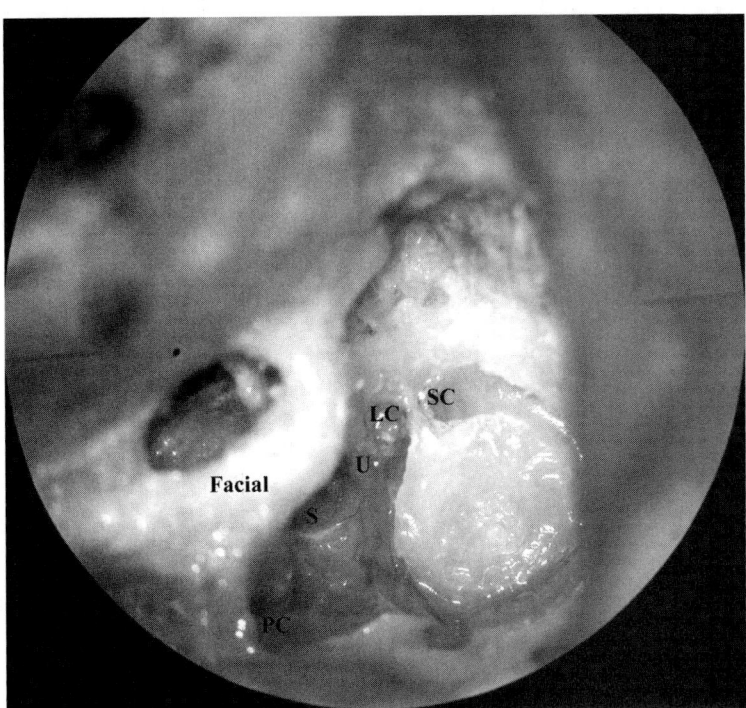

Figure 159.1 Identification of vestibular organs in transmastoid labyrinthectomy. Facial, facial nerve; *LC*, ampulla of lateral canal; *PC*, ampulla of posterior canal; *SC*, ampulla of superior canal; *S*, accule; *U*, utricle.

episodes of vertigo when residual end organs remain, and there have been reports of formation of traumatic neuroma (17). The perceived need for more complete labyrinthectomy has increased interest in the transmastoid approach. Some experts advocate translabyrinthine vestibular nerve section (TL-VNS) as the most definitive procedure. They argue that resection of the Scarpa ganglion further limits the tendency toward regeneration of the sectioned vestibular nerve endings. Clinical evidence supporting more aggressive labyrinthine destruction is scarce. Langman and Lindeman (31) retrospectively compared results of labyrinthectomy and TL-VNS. In their series, there was no difference between the two groups in control of vertigo.

Total loss of hearing is an expected consequence of labyrinthectomy, which limits its application to those with preoperative severe-to-profound hearing loss. There are fewer perioperative complications with labyrinthectomy than with VNS, although the incidence of postoperative disequilibrium is similar (32). Mild-to-moderate disequilibrium occurs among 30% of patients. Other complications, such as wound infection, hemorrhage, and facial nerve injury, are rare. If TL-VNS is being considered, the additional risks of CSF leak and meningitis associated with this procedure must be understood.

SUPERIOR CANAL DEHISCENCE SYNDROME

Minor (33) described a new vestibular disorder caused by a defect in the bony labyrinth—*superior canal dehiscence syndrome.* The most common symptom among these patients is disequilibrium or vertigo in response to loud sounds (Tullio phenomenon). Symptoms also are induced by changes in middle ear or intracranial pressure. Sneezing, coughing, Valsalva maneuvers, lifting, and autoinsufflation are among the activities that can produce symptoms. The existence of chronic disequilibrium and physical examination findings always suggest sound- or pressure-induced torsional nystagmus. The fast phase of nystagmus is directed toward the affected ear in response to sound or positive pressure. Audiometry frequently shows a mild conductive loss in the affected ear. Computed tomographic findings confirm the presence of dehiscence.

Carey et al. (34) studied the incidence of superior canal dehiscence in a series of human temporal bones. Complete dehiscence was found in 0.5% of specimens. Another 1.4% showed a bony covering less than 0.1 mm thick. Bilateral involvement was common. The site of dehiscence is on the medial aspect of the superior canal. The canal comes in contact with the superior petrosal sinus or, less commonly, the middle fossa dura. Examination of the temporal bones of infants showed that development of the bone covering the superior canal progresses from birth to 3 years of age. Altered postnatal bone development produces this anomaly. Caution must be exercised in interpreting temporal bone CT scans. A dehiscent-appearing superior canal may be seen in approximately 9% of temporal bone CT scans, because the thickness of the bone is beyond the limits of resolution (35). Therefore, clinical findings are the key to accurate diagnosis.

Patients are counseled to avoid the offending stimuli. Minor (33) found this suggestion effective in controlling symptoms for 10 of 17 patients. Debilitating symptoms are managed surgically. Minor (33) described both canal resurfacing and canal occlusion as surgical options. The procedure is performed through a middle fossa craniotomy. Elevation of the dura over the arcuate eminence is performed carefully to avoid damage to the membranous labyrinth. The canal defect is repaired with fascia and bone dust or sculpted cortical bone. An alternative is to occlude the lumen with bone paté or other equivalent material. The surgical management of this disorder is in development. Wider recognition of this syndrome and greater surgical experience will allow determination of the most effective operation.

PERILYMPH FISTULA

Few topics in otology are as controversial as perilymph fistula. Much of the controversy is attributable to incomplete understanding of the pathophysiologic mechanism of this disorder. *Perilymph fistula* is defined as abnormal patency between the inner and middle ear that allows flow of perilymph. A well-accepted mechanism for fistula production is temporal bone trauma. Subluxation or fracture of the stapes footplate and rupture of the round window membrane can occur in serious injuries. A less well-accepted postulate is that fistulae are caused by minor changes in middle ear or intracranial pressure, as with coughing or sneezing.

The only means of diagnosis of perilymph fistula is surgical exploration of the middle ear with visualization of a fluid leak in the oval or round window. This is a highly subjective process. Consider fluid accumulating in the oval window that covers the stapes footplate to a depth of 1 mm in 5 seconds. This translates to a rate of flow of approximately 1 μL/s. Precise localization of the source of fluid is obviously difficult. Factors complicating diagnosis include local injection passing into the middle ear, minor bleeding, and serous fluid that accumulates because of disruption of small adhesions in the oval window niche. One must be skeptical when a surgeon states unequivocally after visual inspection alone that fluid accumulating in the oval window at the rate of 1 μL or less per second is originating from the inner ear.

Further illustration of the difficulty in diagnosis is seen in the highly variable rates of fistula exploration, rate of abnormal findings at exploration, incidence of bilaterality, and recurrence rates among published studies (36). Even when criteria for diagnosis are standardized, the rate of exploration and percentage of abnormal results at exploration vary greatly among surgeons (37). Work to develop an accurate method to confirm the observed fluid is perilymph continues. Identification of a protein marker that occurs solely in perilymph is proposed as the ideal method of objective confirmation. β_2-Transferrin was initially touted as a reliable marker of the presence of perilymph. Subsequent study with perilymph extracted by means of labyrinthotomy showed the assay lacked adequate sensitivity (38).

Without objective evidence to confirm a fistula, it is impossible to determine the predictive value of the initial symptoms or audiometric, vestibular, or radiographic tests used for diagnosis. The sensitivity and specificity of individual diagnostic tests vary considerably among studies (39). The surgeon is rarely blinded to preoperative history and test data and has a predetermined opinion about the probability of finding a fistula. Thus a surgeon who usually finds a fistula reports highly sensitive test batteries, whereas a surgeon who rarely sees a fistula concludes the opposite. Surgeons who believe fistulae are common find more fistulae during surgical exploration (40).

Commonly reported symptoms of a perilymph fistula include aural pressure, disequilibrium exacerbated by exertion, and both conductive or sensorineural hearing loss. Symptoms can be fluctuating or progressive. A history of blunt, penetrating, or barometric trauma is expected. The Hennebert sign is frequently elicited at physical examination. Stapedectomy was associated with fistula formation in the 1960s. These fistulae were caused by a combination of prosthesis design and total footplate removal. Contemporary small fenestra stapedotomy techniques are not expected to cause fistulae (39). The probability of "spontaneous" fistula formation in a normally developed ear without previous trauma or surgery is exceedingly low.

The initial management of suspected fistula is bed rest. Some defects seal spontaneously. The time course of observation is arbitrary but is typically several weeks (40). Surgery is considered if symptoms are progressive and dizziness is debilitating. If surgical exploration is needed, a transtympanic endoscopic approach with only topical anesthesia is considered (41). This avoids the confounding effects of local infiltration anesthesia and surgical trauma induced by lifting a tympanomeatal flap. The oval and round windows are scrutinized for the presence of fluid. In the rare instance in which fluid is identified, a blood patch is placed. Indiscriminate patching of the oval and round windows is discouraged. One reason is that if Ménière's disease is diagnosed later, transtympanic instillation of gentamicin is impaired.

There is no uniform scale for reporting outcomes of fistula repair, making comparisons of studies difficult. Viewed collectively, vestibular symptoms are more likely to improve than hearing loss (40). The natural history of an untreated fistula cannot be determined, as there are no reports of surgically confirmed fistulas that were not repaired. Vestibular rehabilitation in patients with fistula symptoms produces results comparable with surgical repair, however (37). Complications of surgery are rare, but they include perforation of the tympanic membrane, dysgeusia, and conductive or sensorineural hearing loss.

PROCEDURES WITH LIMITED USEFULNESS

Over the years, many procedures have been described for management of vertigo caused by Ménière's disease (21). The proposed surgical objective has included establishment of an internal perilymph-endolymph shunt (Fick operation, Cody tack, cochleosacculotomy, otic-periotic shunt, cryosurgery), selective destruction of the labyrinth (ultrasound, cryosurgery), or elimination of negative middle ear pressure (tympanostomy tube placement). The reported results of these procedures in controlling vertigo often are remarkable. Closer scrutiny of the operations has tempered initial enthusiasm. Internal shunting procedures have been largely abandoned because of poor long-term results and unacceptable risk to hearing (42,43). Examination of temporal bones of animals subjected to ultrasound treatment showed no effect on the labyrinthine structures (17). Tympanostomy tube placement was in vogue in the 1960s as a treatment for Ménière's disease; however, vertigo control was found to be unreliable. Sporadic reports of efficacy continue to appear. The mechanism of action of tympanostomy tube placement is unknown.

SURGICAL PARADIGM

Selection of a surgical procedure depends on correct preoperative diagnosis. Nonsurgical forms of management are exhausted and contraindications to surgery are excluded. Procedures specific for BPPV, either singular neurectomy or PSCC occlusion, can be considered as the first option for this entity. Failure of these procedures can be followed by formal VNS. For patients without Ménière's disease, vestibular neurectomy or labyrinthectomy is recommended, depending on the status of the patient's hearing. For many of these patients, future involvement of the contralateral ear may not be an issue, possibly biasing the surgeon toward recommending labyrinthectomy when hearing is marginal.

Defining a paradigm for the care of patients with Ménière's disease is not as clear. Only one scenario lends itself to a simple decision; the patient's hearing is not fluctuating and is poorer than a speech reception threshold of 70 dB and a word recognition score of 20%. In this case, labyrinthectomy is advised. For all others, hearing conservation procedures are considered. Some experts advocate endolymphatic sac surgery as a first-line procedure whenever medical therapy fails. If this fails to control symptoms, revision shunt surgery or VNS can be offered. Other surgeons restrict surgical intervention to VNS, choosing instead to perform a more definitive procedure at the first operation. Transtympanic administration of gentamicin is becoming more popular for management of Ménière's disease. Because it is an outpatient procedure, it is an attractive option for patients considering surgery. Increasing use of this technique has reduced the number of all other surgical procedures performed for Ménière's disease.

New surgical techniques for the management of vertigo continue to be developed. Success will be determined with long-term follow-up study and accurate reporting of results. The pathophysiologic mechanism of many vestibular

disorders is uncertain. Greater insight into the mechanisms of disease will allow more effective and possibly less destructive procedures to be invented.

HIGHLIGHTS

- Surgical management of vertigo is considered for patients with incapacitating symptoms when conservative treatment has failed.
- Contraindications to surgery include central vestibular dysfunction, suspicion of impaired central compensation after surgery, bilateral vestibular dysfunction, and only hearing ear.
- The choice of surgical procedure depends on the underlying vestibulopathy, auditory acuity, concurrent illness, and patient's tolerance of complications.
- Elimination of episodes of vertigo with surgery is more successful among patients with Ménière's disease than among those with other forms of peripheral vestibulopathy.
- Surgical procedures appropriate for management of BPPV include singular neurectomy and PSCC occlusion.
- Reporting of results of surgery for Ménière's disease follows the guidelines established by the Committee on Hearing and Equilibrium of the American Academy of Otolaryngology—Head and Neck Surgery.

REFERENCES

1. Nguyen CD, Brackmann DE, Crane RT, et al. Retrolabyrinthine vestibular nerve section: evaluation of technical modification in 143 cases. *Am J Otol* 1992;13:328–332.
2. Glasscock ME III, Thedinger BA, Cueva RA, et al. An analysis of the retrolabyrinthine vs. retrosigmoid vestibular nerve section. *Otolaryngol Head Neck Surg* 1991;104:88–95.
3. Silverstein H, Wanamaker H, Flanzer J, et al. Vestibular neurectomy in the United States—1990. *Am J Otol* 1992;13:23–30.
4. Shone G, Kemink JL, Telian SA. Prognostic significance of hearing loss as a lateralizing indicator in the surgical treatment of vertigo. *J Laryngol Otol* 1991;105:618–620.
5. Committee on Hearing and Equilibrium guidelines for the diagnosis and evaluation of therapy in Meniere's disease. *Otolaryngol Head Neck Surg* 1995;113:181–185.
6. Friberg U, Stahle J, Svedberg A. The natural course of Meniere's disease. *Acta Otolaryngol Suppl (Stockh)* 1984;406:72–77.
7. Baloh RW, Honrubia V, Jacobson K. Benign positional vertigo: clinical and oculographic features in 240 cases. *Neurology* 1987;37:371–378.
8. Epley JM. The canalith repositioning procedure: for treatment of benign paroxysmal positional vertigo. *Otolaryngol Head Neck Surg* 1992;107:399–404.
9. Semont A, Freyss G, Vitte E. Curing the BPPV with a liberatory maneuver. *Adv Otorhinolaryngol* 1988;42:294–300.
10. Gacek RR, Gacek MR. Results of singular neurectomy in the posterior ampullary recess. *ORL J Otorhinolaryngol Relat Spec.* 2002;64:397–402.
11. Ohmichi T, Rutka J, Hawke M. Histopathologic consequences of surgical approaches to the singular nerve. *Laryngoscope* 1989;99:963–970.
12. Mills RP, Padgham ND, Vaughan-Jones RH. Surgical anatomy of the singular nerve. *Clin Otolaryngol* 1991;16:305–308.
13. Silverstein H, White DW. Wide surgical exposure for singular neurectomy in the treatment of benign positional vertigo. *Laryngoscope* 1990;100:701–706.

14. Parnes LS, McClure JA. Posterior semicircular canal occlusion in the normal hearing ear. *Otolaryngol Head Neck Surg* 1991; 104:52–57.

15. Agrawal SK, Parnes LS. Human experience with canal plugging. *Ann N Y Acad Sci* 2001;942:300–305.

16. Walsh RM, Bath AP, Cullen JR, et al. Long-term results of posterior semicircular canal occlusion for intractable benign paroxysmal positional vertigo. *Clin Otolaryngol* 1999;24:316–323.

17. Schuknecht HF. *Pathology of the ear,* 2nd ed. Philadelphia: Lea & Febiger, 1993:575–582.

18. Brackmann DE, Nissen RL. Meniere's disease: results of treatment with the endolymphatic subarachnoid shunt compared with the endolymphatic mastoid shunt. *Am J Otol* 1987;8:275–282.

19. Huang TS, Lin CC. Endolymphatic sac surgery for Meniere's disease: a composite study of 339 cases. *Laryngoscope* 1985;95: 1082–1086.

20. Glasscock ME III, Jackson CG, Poe DS, et al. What I think of sac surgery in 1989. *Am J Otol* 1989;10:230–233.

21. McKee GJ, Kerr AG, Toner JG, et al. Surgical control of vertigo in Meniere's disease. *Clin Otolaryngol* 1991;16:216–227.

22. Bretlau P, Thomsen J, Tos M, et al. Placebo effect in surgery for Meniere's disease: nine year follow-up. *Am J Otol* 1989;4: 259–261.

23. Welling DB, Nagaraja HN. Endolymphatic mastoid shunt: a reevaluation of efficacy. *Otolaryngol Head Neck Surg* 2000;122: 340–345.

24. Thomsen J, Bonding P, Becker B, et al. The non-specific effect of endolymphatic sac surgery in treatment of Meniere's disease: a prospective, randomized controlled study comparing "classic" endolymphatic sac surgery with the insertion of a ventilating tube in the tympanic membrane. *Acta Otolaryngol (Stockh)* 1998;118: 769–773.

25. Silverstein H, Smouha E, Jones R. Natural history vs. surgery for Meniere's disease. *Otolaryngol Head Neck Surg* 1989;100:6–16.

26. King WA, Wackym PA, Sen C, et al. Adjunctive use of endoscopy during posterior fossa surgery to treat cranial neuropathies. *Neurosurgery* 2001;49:108–115.

27. McKenna MJ, Nadol JB Jr, Ojemann RG, et al. Vestibular neurectomy: retrosigmoid-intracanalicular versus retrolabyrinthine approach. *Am J Otol* 1996;17:253–258.

28. Jackson CG, McGrew BM, Forest JA, et al. Comparison of postoperative headache after retrosigmoid approach: vestibular nerve section versus vestibular schwannoma resection. *Am J Otol* 2000; 21:412–416.

29. Kemink JL, Telian SA, Graham MD, et al. Transmastoid labyrinthectomy: reliable surgical management of vertigo. *Otolaryngol Head Neck Surg* 1989;101:5–10.

30. Gacek RR, Gacek MR. Comparison of labyrinthectomy and vestibular neurectomy in the control of vertigo. *Laryngoscope* 1996;106:225–230.

31. Langman AW, Lindeman RC. Surgery for vertigo in the nonserviceable hearing ear: transmastoid labyrinthectomy or translabyrinthine vestibular nerve section. *Laryngoscope* 1993;103: 1321–1325.

32. Eisenman DJ, Speers R, Telian SA. Labyrinthectomy versus vestibular neurectomy: long-term physiologic and clinical outcomes. *Otol Neurotol* 2001;22:539–548.

33. Minor LB. Superior canal dehiscence syndrome. *Am J Otol* 2000; 21:9–19.

34. Carey JP, Minor LB, Nager GT. Dehiscence or thinning of bone overlying the superior semicircular canal in a temporal bone survey. *Arch Otolaryngol Head Neck Surg* 2000;126:137–147.

35. Williamson RA, Vrabec JT, Coker NJ, et al. Coronal computed tomography prevalence of superior semicircular canal dehiscence. *Otolaryngol Head Neck Surg* 2003;129:481–489.

36. Bailey BJ, Vrabec JT. Victor Goodhill, MD, and perilymph fistula: reflecting on the man and the controversy. *Laryngoscope* 1997;107: 580–584.

37. Shepard NT, Telian SA, Niparko JK, et al. Platform pressure test in identification of perilymphatic fistula. *Am J Otol* 1992;13:49–54.

38. Buchman CA, Luxford WM, Hirsch BE, et al. Beta-2 transferrin assay in the identification of perilymph. *Am J Otol* 1999;20: 174–178.

39. Friedland DR, Wackym PA. A critical appraisal of spontaneous perilymphatic fistulas of the inner ear. *Am J Otol* 1999;20: 261–276.

40. House JW, Morris MS, Kramer SJ, et al. Perilymphatic fistula: Surgical experience in the United States. *Otolaryngol Head Neck Surg* 1991;105:51–59.

41. Poe DS, Bottrill ID. Comparison of endoscopic and surgical explorations for perilymphatic fistulas. *Am J Otol* 1994;15: 735–738.

42. Giddings NA, Shelton C, O'Leary MJ, et al. Cochleosacculotomy revisited: long-term results poorer than expected. *Arch Otolaryngol Head Neck Surg* 1991;117:1150–1152.

43. Jennings RP, Reams CL, Jacobson J, et al. Results of surgical treatment for Meniere's disease. *Otolaryngol Head Neck Surg* 1989;100: 195–199.

Facial Plastic and Reconstructive Surgery

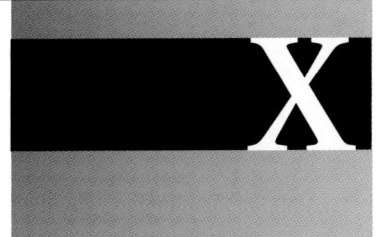

X

Grant S. Gillman   Dean M. Toriumi   Karen H. Calhoun

160

Grafts and Implants in Facial, Head, and Neck Surgery

G. Richard Holt

The biotechnology of implants in otolaryngology and head and neck surgery has expanded rapidly. Many of the technical discoveries have been made by workers in dentistry, orthopedics, and bioengineering.

CHARACTERISTICS OF IMPLANTS

Implant material is characterized by composition, strength, biodegradability, and resistance to stress and fatigue (1,2). The properties of bulk material, however, can differ from those of the implant surface at the tissue-implant interface because of surface alterations by design or physicochemical reaction. The materials and clinical applications for facial, head, and neck implants are summarized in Table 160.1.

Metallic Implants

Metallic devices can be composed of a single metal or an alloy of several metals. Alloys are developed to improve qualities of the original metal by adding other metals with characteristics that improve biocompatibility or mechanical attributes. The principal metals used in facial implants are titanium, stainless steel, and tantalum. Chromium, aluminum, cobalt, copper, nickel, and tungsten are included in alloys.

Metals are crystalline materials with well-defined, orderly, three-dimensional arrangements of atoms that form a microscopic lattice characteristic of each metal. The lattice can be modified by means of heating, cooling, hardening, or altering the physical properties of the metal to achieve a particular result. Lattice defects can modify the characteristics of the metal. Large structural defects can cause failure to withstand external stresses. Metallic biomaterials are characterized by elastic modulus, tensile strength, percentage elongation, compressive strength, shear strength and modulus, and strain. Stress is the ability of a material to withstand a given load per cross-sectional area. The material must be designed to meet the functional requirements of the dental or maxillofacial implant.

Stress versus strain curves are generated experimentally for implant materials. They provide information about the bulk material independent of shape or thickness. These can be used to predict the response of the material to mechanical forces on an implant in a particular use. The forces of shear, compression, tension, torsion, and bending must be considered in selection of a material for an implant. *In vitro* loading studies are performed to assess how a material responds to long-term wear. Most metals relax with time, and the relaxation can cause metal fatigue and implant failure. A relatively brittle metal, such as stainless steel, can function well initially but with long-term use can fail because of fatigue. All metals corrode when exposed to living tissue; the gradual result is failure of many metal implants. Stainless steel, an alloy of iron, chromium, nickel, molybdenum, and manganese, resists corrosion well. It can, however, undergo gradual plastic deformation.

Titanium and its alloys are among the most biocompatible metallic implants used today. Titanium is lightweight and corrosion resistant and has high tissue acceptance. It is

TABLE 160.1

FACIAL, HEAD, AND NECK IMPLANTS

Category	Biomaterial	Clinical Application
Metals and metallic alloys	Stainless steel	Sutures, fracture wires, reconstruction bars
	Cobalt alloys	Fracture fixation plates and screws
	Titanium and its alloys	Mandibular bone trays, osseointegrated implants, cranioplasty, orbital floor implants
	Platinum-iridium	Implantable electrodes
	Gold	Eyelid implant
Polymers	Polymethyl methacrylate	Cranioplasty, tissue adhesive
	Cyanoacrylate	Tissue adhesive
	Silicone elastomers	Soft-tissue augmentation, tissue expanders
	Polytetrafluoroethylene (PTFE)	Joint prosthesis covering, vocal cord injections
	Expanded PTFE	Soft-tissue augmentation, orbital floor implant
	Polyurethane	Artificial skin
	Dacron, nylon polyesters	Sutures, onlay mesh, mandibular trays
	High-density polyethylene, porous	Soft-tissue augmentation, temporo-mandibular prosthesis
Ceramics	Bioglass	Middle ear ossicular replacement
	Hydroxyapatite	Joint prosthesis covering, bone-conduction filler, bone augmentation
	Aluminum oxide	Cranioplasty, artificial ocular prostheses
Nonceramics	Hydroxyapatite cement	Bone filler, cranioplasty, bone conductive
Biologic materials	Polyglycolic acid	Sutures, implants
	Polylactic acid	Timed-release drug delivery, implants
	Collagen	Dermal augmentation, soft-tissue support
	Bone-stimulation proteins	Cartilage or bone induction
	Hyaluronic acid	Soft tissue filler
	Human acellular dermis	Soft tissue filler, augmentation

rather soft and when not anchored to bone can be deformed by loading forces. Used in mandibular reconstruction and for anchoring screws in facial applications, titanium performs well. Tantalum and vanadium have been use as bone trays for mandibular reconstruction, but the mechanical properties are not as good as those of titanium. Tantalum and vanadium are not strong, can fatigue rapidly, and must be removed after the mandible heals. Some metallic implants, such as stainless steel, have a better stress response than does bone. This can cause stress shielding of the bone and impede formation of new bone. Metal implants may have to be removed after the bone is stabilized to allow growth and development.

Ceramics

Ceramics have a microscopic lattice structure. Glass ceramics, on the other hand, have an amorphous atomic structure. Most biologic implants are glass ceramics—combinations of silicon dioxide (SiO_2) and crystalline lattice materials embedded in this glass. Glass ceramics are thermally resistant and can be used when thermal shock can occur. Glass ceramics last well in the body. They are well tolerated and biocompatible. Because of a peculiar grain size and distribution, however, glass ceramics are susceptible to cracking from stress concentration. Clinically, these

are considered brittle materials; they fracture rather than bend when subjected to excessive stress. This limits the use of glass ceramic implants in the head and neck to areas with minimal force loading, such as a tympanic ossicle.

Ceramics made with alumina compounds also are used in dental implants. The device is designed so the shape facilitates biomechanical stress application without fracture. Hydroxyapatite is another form of ceramic; it is characterized as bioreactive. It comes as a powder and is reconstituted as a paste for dental and bone replacement. Hydroxyapatite is resorbable and osteoconductive, and it increases bone density. It is composed of elements that exist in the ground substance of bone, that is, calcium and phosphorus. Hydroxyapatite can provide a substrate for osseointegration and osseoconduction when used as a bone replacement material for facial, head, and neck defects.

Hydroxyapatite cement (HAC), while similar to the solid form of hydroxyapatite, is actually a nonceramic that can be used as a paste to fill bony defects and as a bone augmentation material. Slow-setting HAC occurs in the presence of water, whereas fast-setting HAC requires a phosphate solution to hasten the process, reducing the setting time by at least half (8 to 10 minutes). This reduced set time can be clinically important when the cement is being utilized to fill a defect under soft tissue and needs to be confined to a specific space, not allowed to "creep." HAC is considered by many clinicians to be the biomaterial of choice for cranioplasty, especially in pediatric patients. Contact with the mucosa of paranasal sinuses is to be avoided, however.

Polymers

No synthetic implant material can exactly reproduce the biomechanical properties of bone. Ceramics and metals are stronger than human bone, and polymers are more flexible. Polymers are useful in implantation because the mechanical properties can be altered to suit the application. These properties are derived from the structural and chemical composition, which are related to length and cross-linking. Varying these two characteristics can produce a wide range of polymer properties, from soft and fragile to hard and brittle. The implant designer can choose a polymer that provides the characteristics needed for a particular situation.

The most commonly used medical polymers are polyurethanes, silicones, and polymethyl methacrylate. These polymers are reasonably strong and biocompatible. When supplied as porous fibers [polytetrafluoroethylene (PTFE), nylon, polylactic acid, and polyglycolic acid], these materials can be woven fabric as well as suture material. Expanded PTFE fabric [Gore-Tex (ePTFE)] has excellent biocompatibility when used for soft-tissue augmentation or vascular repair. Mechanical stresses on polymer implants usually are small. When used for mandibular replacement, a polymer is tested for the same mechanical tolerances as are metals, including tensile strength, modulus of elasticity, stress, and strain. Impact testing is important when a material is used for skull reconstruction. Internal defects that occur during molding and processing can cause cracks and implant failure.

Polymers are manufactured by means of thermoplastic molding (the material is formed in a heat-softened state in a mold) or by means of thermosetting (the insoluble polymers are cured by cross-linking). Suture material is formed by means of extrusion of the polymer through small holes in a die to produce a fiber thinned to the proper diameter before cooling. Used as a glue, polymethyl methacrylate, ethyl-2-cyanoacrylate, and butyl-2-cyanoacrylate produce histotoxic cellular reactions and an exothermic reaction. The use of polymer glues to stabilize implants is being evaluated.

Biologic Materials

Grafts of nonhuman biologic material and xenografts are considered implants because they often are used for tissue augmentation. Bovine collagen (injectable solution or sheets) is enzymatically modified to diminish cutaneous sensitivity reactions and to decrease resorption time. When the macrophage system of the host identifies this collagen as foreign, immunologic defenses form antibodies to the collagen. Because collagen is similar in many ways among species, this problem can be diminished but not eliminated with biochemical alteration of unique proteins. Synthesis of components of human dermal collagen and basement membrane, such as polyglycolic acid and polylactic acid, has produced suture and implant material that is slowly resorbed by means of acid hydrolysis. These materials do not induce the intense immunologic response of animal collagen. They also are used as the carriers of sustained-release drugs in implantable drug delivery systems.

Human acellular dermis matrix, harvested from cadavers, is utilized primarily as a soft tissue augmentation material for the face. It can also serve as a "filler" or "scaffolding" for repair of a nasal septal perforation, where this material is placed between opposing flaps of nasal mucosa; if exposed, it allows for reepithelialization on its surface. Foreign antigenicity of this human allograft is achieved by leaching out the cells; however, there are "ghost channels" of preexisting vascular structures that may serve to support revascularization of the tissue. There is a tendency of this biomaterial to resorb with time in some patients.

Biodegradable (resorbable) plates and screws are not dissimilar to certain biodegradable suture materials. These firm implants are generally composed of biosynthetic polymers and copolymers of polylactide and polyglycolide and are heat-malleable to fit the contour of the bony surface. They should be especially considered in pediatric fracture patients, where metallic plates can cause stress-shielding and loss of bone growth and remodeling capabilities.

Surface Properties of Implants

The surface of an implant can differ microscopically and macroscopically in appearance and reactivity from the bulk material. Titanium forms a titanium oxide layer on its surface as soon as it is exposed to air. This layer, approximately 10 nm thick, acts like a ceramic and helps produce excellent biocompatibility. The titanium oxide layer of the implant slowly thickens after implantation.

Various methods of surface texturing are being applied to implants to improve stability. For example, making ridges or pores on the surface by means of etching, or sputtering the surfaces, gives minute areas of surface relief. Surface relief has a critical size: too small, and there is ineffective surface area for protein matrix adsorption, but too large, and there are dead spaces not filled with the matrix necessary for cell adhesion.

Implant surface contamination during handling or processing can diminish tissue biocompatibility. When an implant fails, the surface must be analyzed to detect any contributing contamination. Proper surface preparation, especially with radiofrequency glow-discharge cleaning, can clear unwanted particles and chemicals. This increases free surface energy, exposes more ionic groups, and facilitates initial adsorption of protein matrix and formation of a substrate for cellular attachment. The interface between implant surface and body tissue is the most important factor determining biocompatibility. The fate of an implant depends on the events and processes taking place on its surface, and implant surface properties determine the host reaction.

Biocompatibility of Implants

Cells do not adhere directly to the surface of implanted synthetic materials. A substance in the extracellular matrix binds the cell to the surface. This substance is essential for initial cell adhesion and proliferation. The substrate needed varies with the type of cell. Well-differentiated cells, such as chondroblasts, osteoblasts, and epithelial cells, require substrate characteristics distinct from those needed by less differentiated cells, such as fibroblasts. Focal contacts represent adhesion sites to specific extracellular matrix proteins adsorbed on the implant surface. Focal contacts typically occur in low-motility cells, such as fibroblasts and epithelial cells. The composition of the substrate (the adsorbed layer of protein on the implant surface) is crucial for tight cellular adhesion. Proteins such as fibronectin, vitronectin, cold-insoluble globulin, and possibly proteoglycans provide the necessary substrate for this adhesion.

The extracellular matrix contains collagen, elastin, and fibronectin interwoven into a hydrated network of glycoaminoglycan chains. The glycoaminoglycan chains are long, negatively charged polysaccharide chains that link proteins to form giant proteoglycan molecules. Interaction with cell membrane receptors provides linkage for cellular attachment to adsorbed extracellular matrix on the surface of a biomaterial. Tissue cells do adhere to the implant surface—not directly but by means of a complex series of protein attachments.

When implants are placed in facial soft tissue, the primary tissue reaction includes protein adsorption and cellular attachment. The predominant cell attaching to the protein layer is the fibroblast. Within the first week, the fibroblast lays down immature collagen on the implant surface, or interstices. The usual response to a soft-tissue implant is production of a fibrous capsule or collagen fiber ingrowth, which secures the implant. A smooth implant such as silicone more often elicits dense capsule formation than does a porous implant. If an implant is too reactive, has surface contamination, or is biodegradable, the host-tissue response usually is aggressive macrophage activity, increased vascularity, breakdown of the overlying skin, and extrusion of the implant. The presence of inflammatory cells such as neutrophils and macrophages suggests poor tissue response to the implanted material.

After placement of an implant, protein adsorption occurs. As a hole is drilled into bone to receive the implant, the bone must not be heated to more than 45°C to 50°C, or osteoblasts die. An implant in bone induces a rapid host response. The first stage is formation of a small hematoma and a cascade of chemical breakdown products.

These substances act on blood vessels and attract cells from surrounding tissue. Because cortical bone is avascular, most blood products come from the marrow-containing spaces of the bone.

The second stage is tissue organization, regeneration, and repair. The duration is related to the extent of injury and implantation site geometry. Extracellular processes and cell functioning can be affected by soluble and insoluble particles from the implant and by the mechanical influence of the implant itself. The third stage of repair is remodeling, which affects the implant-host tissue interface and occurs over weeks or months. Appropriate stress levels must be imposed on the bone adjacent to the implant. Bone-binding intensity can be measured according to the shear or torque forces needed to produce failure. Bone is the main contributor to tensile strength of bonding; other tissues are less important. The basal lamina in contact with a bone implant contains type IV collagen, laminin, and proteoglycans. These constituents of the ground substance are deposited in or adjacent to the mineralized layer. Mineralization of the ground substance seems to be important for transmission of compression and for shear and tensile loads.

ASSESSMENT OF PATIENT NEEDS

Patients vary in suitability for treatment involving implantation. Most implants are used to manage bony or soft-tissue defects caused by trauma, tumor excision, or birth defects. Most patients with a history of irradiation of the proposed recipient sites are not good candidates for implants unless distant, nonirradiated tissues can be brought into the area. This often necessitates procedures with several stages and perioperative hyperbaric oxygen therapy for best results.

Before an implant is used, the patient's wound-healing potential and immunologic status are assessed. Patients with diabetes or hypertension, those who smoke heavily, or patients undergoing chemotherapy or taking immunosuppressive drugs are at risk of wound infection and implant extrusion. A history of sensitivity to any component of the implant must be sought. With metallic implants, difficulty in dosimetry is expected if further radiation therapy is planned.

When a young adult applies for a facial, head, or neck implant, the physician must ask about the person's usual physical activity level and sports participation. A common cause of implant loss is trauma, which causes hematoma formation, loosening of the implant, and extrusion. The patients must agree not to participate in contact sports or to delay implantation until the questionable activity is no longer a consideration. In the management of deformities attributable to ablative cancer surgery, it often is prudent to delay prosthetic implantation as long as 1 year after surgery. The patient is observed for an extended period after implantation for the development of residual or recurrent disease and for rejection of the implant.

There is a difference between implants for functional needs and for cosmetic indications. A functional implant is chosen to provide the best restoration and the lowest risk of complications. In cosmetic applications, emotional and psychologic development is considered as well. The condition of the recipient tissues is likely to be the limiting factor in functional cases, and psychologic factors count heavily in cosmetic implantation.

For osseous replacement or augmentation implants, radiologic assessment of the recipient area often is advisable. Conventional facial and skull radiographs are not sufficient for assessing the extent of osseous abnormality, and computed tomography (CT) is needed. Three-dimensional CT can be linked to a computer-aided design and fabrication system for precise manufacturing of the prosthesis (3). Magnetic resonance imaging is not as helpful for evaluation of osseous deformities as it is for soft-tissue assessment.

SURGICAL MANAGEMENT

Preoperative Counseling

If the patient is a candidate for an alloplastic or biologic implantation, the surgeon discusses the risks and complications associated with implantation. Foremost among these are infection, rejection, and extrusion of the implant. In the face, head, and neck, macromotion is possible unless the implant is firmly secured to the underlying tissue. Micromotion of an implant is expected and desirable, because the implant must closely simulate the characteristics of the host tissue. Autoimmune rejection is possible, but the usual causes of extrusion are trauma and infection. Most patients want improvement in function or appearance after surgical implantation, and they need reasonable expectations regarding outcome. I advise against showing photographs of patients who have undergone implantation because each case is unique. Rough drawings or photographs of the patient that have undergone computerized facial analysis are helpful as long as the patient understands that there is no expressed or implied guarantee of success.

Surgical Implantation

The ideal implant does not exist, but some possess many of the following qualities thought to be important:

Biocompatibility with host tissue
Noncarcinogenic nature
Simulation of the biomechanical features of the tissue it augments
Easy fabrication
Capability of being sterilized without degradation of essential properties
Capability of being resorbed or lack thereof depending on the tissue needs
Thorough investigation before use

Each region of the face, head, and neck requires an implant with unique properties. Each region is reviewed herein, but the specific surgical techniques are found elsewhere in this book and the medical literature. Table 160.2 summarizes site-specific selection of surgical implants.

Scalp

Little has been done in the development of scalp implants. Most scalp surgery is performed for hair replacement, and grafts or flaps are used. Autologous hair follicle unit implants are commonly used both for post-traumatic defects and for genetic baldness. Over the years, the size of the follicular grafts has decreased, and microfollicular grafts are now used, from 1 to 5 follicle units, thus allowing for better camouflage and filling in of the defect.

Silicone tissue expanders work well in the sustained expansion of skin for reconstruction after scalp loss. Expansion of the generally inelastic scalp requires 6 to 8 weeks to obtain a sufficient amount of expansion, depending on the size of the defect. Large, non-hair-bearing scalp defects can be excised, and expanded hair-bearing scalp can be advanced/rotated into the deficit. Attention must be given to hair growth direction and to maintaining the appropriate anterior hairline.

Skull

Cranioplasty with allopathic implants is one of the oldest head and neck procedures (4). Polymethyl methacrylate (PMMA), a common cranial implant, is formed from several monomers in the presence of a catalyst and can be molded to the defect before hardening (5). It can be drilled, sculpted, and secured to the surrounding bone. Its polymerization is exothermic, and the implant is sterile on hardening. Alloys of titanium and tantalum are available in plate or mesh-sheet form, and can be cut or bent as necessary. Because they deform slowly with external trauma, malleable metal implants for skull defects are likely to protect the brain, unlike polymethyl methacrylate, which is brittle and can fracture with trauma.

HAC can be utilized for cranioplasty defects, especially in children (6). Small defects can be molded in place, utilizing fast-setting HAC. For larger defects, computer-aided design/computer assisted manufacturing (CAD/CAM) of a larger HAC (or PMMA) can be preformed and placed into the defect with little alteration.

Ear and Temporal Bone

The best choice for prosthetic attachment to the head and face involves implantation of pure titanium fixtures into bone. These fixtures osseointegrate fully with bone before loading (7,8). They are attached to skin-penetrating abutments and linked with a gold bridgework that contains attachment magnets for the prosthesis. Similar implants can be used to anchor a hearing aid to the temporal bone for better sound transmission than is offered by a conventional

TABLE 160.2

SURGICAL IMPLANTS BY SITE

Site	Biomaterial	Clinical Application
Scalp	Silicone	Tissue expansion
Skull	Silicone, titanium tantalum, hydroxyapatite, polymethyl methacrylate	Cranioplasty
Ear	Silicone; porous, high-density polyethylene	Electrode covering
	Titanium	Osseointegrated implants
	Platinum-iridium	Cochlear electrodes
	Porous polyethylene	Auricular reconstruction
Orbit	Titanium	Osseointegrated implants
	Silicone hydroxyapatite, polytetrafluoroethylene (PTFE), expanded PTFE	Orbital volume
	Polycarbonate	Intraocular lens, artificial eye
	Methylcellular fiber silicone	Orbital floor fractures
Face	Expanded PTFE; carbon-PTFE; porous, high-density polyethylene; polyamide, hydroxyapatite	Soft-tissue and osseous augmentation
	Collagen	Dermal augmentation
	Human acellular dermis	Dermal augmentation
	Calcium-based hydroxyapatite	Soft tissue filler
	Hyaluronic acid derivatives	Soft tissue filler
Mandible	Dacron polyester, nylon, titanium alloy, tantalum alloy	Reconstruction tray
	Stainless steel	Reconstruction bar
	Titanium alloy	Miniplates and screws for trauma
	Titanium	Osseointegrated implants
	Silicone	Temporomandibular meniscus
	Hydroxyapatite	Bone conduction
	Silicone; expanded PTFE; carbon-PTFE; porous, high-density polyethylene; polyamide	Mentoplasty
Neck	Expanded PTFE	Vascular grafts and sutures
	Polyglycolic acid, polyglactin 910, polypropylene, stainless steel	Wound closure

bone-conduction hearing aid, particularly in congenital canal atresia and in postsurgical chronic tympanomastoiditis where a canal-dwelling ear piece causes recurrent drainage.

Cochlear implants contain stimulation electrodes inserted in the cochlea. They are made of platinum and iridium, two rare metals with high electrical conductance and minimal rectification at the electrode-tissue interface. They usually are coated with PTFE or silicone to diminish current loss into the tissues and to protect the electrode from corrosion.

Reconstruction for microtia has primarily utilized rib cartilage; it is easily accessible, can be carved and sculpted, has been shown to grow with the patient, and is an autologous biomaterial. There is a slight risk of pneumothorax, hypertrophic scar, or keloid, and it may not be properly placed in females where breast development has not yet occurred. Additionally, multiple stages of procedures are generally required to achieve a good result. However, rib cartilage is the gold standard for microtia repair.

Preformed porous polyethylene implants are utilized by some surgeons for a one- or two-stage reconstruction. This polymer implant must be covered by a temporo-parietal fascial flap, and the flap, in turn, covered by a thin, full-thickness skin graft. The immediate result is good, but the risk of complications is higher than with the rib graft—loss of the fascial flap, breakdown of the skin graft, hypertrophic scar of the scalp, and potential trauma caused by the firmness of the implant. Because the implant does not grow with the patient, sizing at a given age is problematic.

Orbit

Many surgeons use silicone sheets to support the orbital floor after an orbital blow-out fracture. The biocompatibility of this material is excellent, and if properly placed and sized, the implant has a low extrusion rate. For small fractures, thin sheets of methyl cellulose, such as Gelfilm, can be stacked and placed over the defect to serve as temporary support until scar tissue has formed and they are resorbed. Orbital volume in an enophthalmic orbit after trauma can

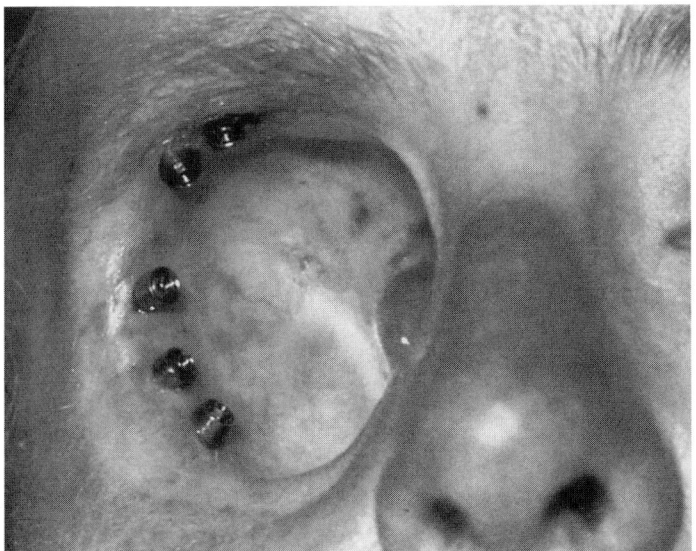
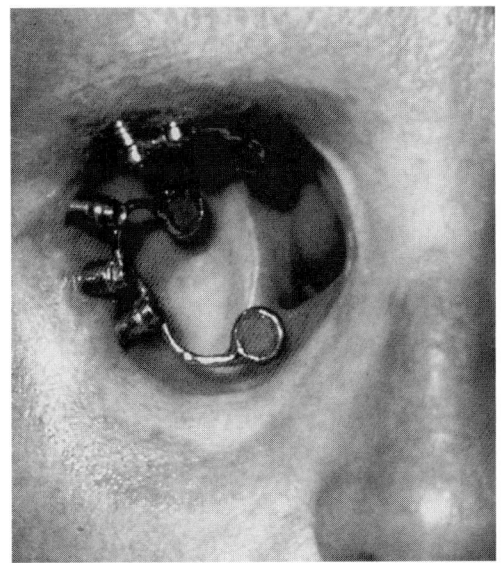
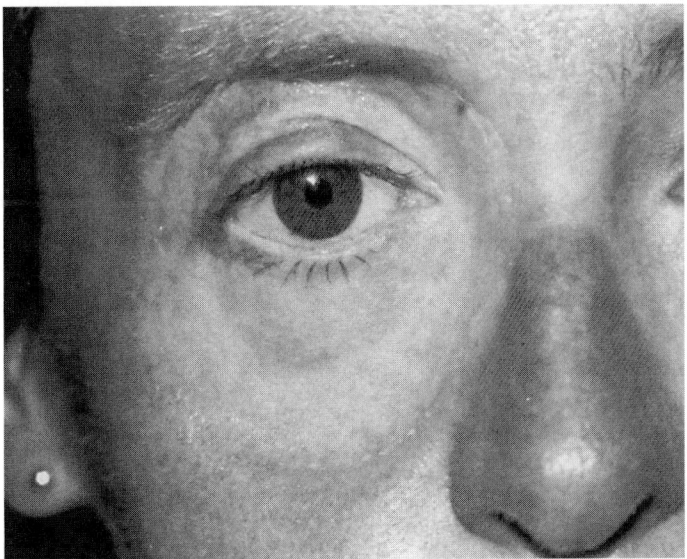

Figure 160.1 A: Right orbital defect in a female patient after orbital exenteration for tumor and implantation of titanium fixture. **B:** Implant bridgework in place with attached magnets. **C:** Magnetic attachment of the right orbital prosthesis secures it. (Courtesy of P.I. Branemark, MD, Branemark Implant Centers and The Institute for Experimental Biotechnology, Gothenberg, Sweden, and Stephen S. Parel, MD, The University of Texas Health Science Center, San Antonio, Texas.)

be replaced with bone grafts or with inert substances, such as PTFE or silicone beads and sheeting, a composite of vitreous aluminum oxide particles and PTFE (Proplast II), hydroxyapatite, or ePTFE fabric. Symmetric placement of the expanders, in consultation with an ophthalmologist, can diminish postoperative diplopia. Orbital osseointegrated implants have been used successfully to anchor prostheses after orbital exenteration (Fig. 160.1). Bone implants for patients who have undergone irradiation are less successful unless hyperbaric oxygen therapy is used.

Severe fractures of the orbital floor can be repaired with a size-altering titanium implant (9). The device is trimmed to the required size and is adjusted by means of bending to the required anatomic defect. The implant can be fixed to the orbital rim with self-tapping screws. Porous polyethylene preformed implants can also be utilized as a support for the orbital floor, either placed acutely or in a delayed reconstruction of a hyp/endophthalmic orbit. It is possible to

carve some of the polyethylene implant to fit the topography of the orbital defect.

Mesh implants made of polyglactin 910 can be used as a slowly resorbable replacement of the orbital floor (10). Soft-tissue pads (1 to 2 mm thick) made of ePTFE fabric can be used to repair posttraumatic hypophthalmos and for temporal augmentation. The rate of infection is low, the foreign-body reaction is minimal, and there is good incorporation into the tissues (11). This material is soft and pliable and easily contoured to the size and shape of the defect. Polyglactin 910 sutures can secure the implant to the medial and lateral orbit.

Artificial globe implants manufactured from new polymers such as polycarbonates can be designed and painted for a near-perfect match with the other eye. Intraocular lens implants also can be made of a polymer fabricated with a specific fixed focal length for patients who have undergone cataract extraction.

Gold and platinum weights are used successfully for rehabilitation of patients with facial paralysis. Use of weights can replace tarsorrhaphy in some cases. These rare metals are inert in tissue and well tolerated in the thin upper eyelid. Sutured to the tarsus muscle, a gold weight provides reversible surgical lowering of the eyelid (12). The proper weight is selected preoperatively from a "dummy" weight-sizing kit. The patient sits, and weights of varying sizes are taped to the eyelid until the desired lid position is achieved. The weight is sterilized and inserted under local anesthesia. It serves the purpose to help initiate a relaxation of the superior levator muscle of the upper eyelid, and to add to the graviational pull of the eyelid for closure.

Midfacial Augmentation

Augmentation of the malar region, the premaxilla, and the nasal dorsum sometimes is wanted. Although many surgeons prefer to use autogenous tissue such as cartilage or bone, alloplastic materials are being used with increasing success. Surgeons variously favor mesh(e.g., polyglactin 910, polyamide, and polyester) silicone rubber, porous PTFE or vitreous carbon fibers or aluminum oxide particles combined with PTFE, expanded PTFE mesh, and hydroxyapatite, such as BoneSource and Norian (13–15). Proplast I is black because of the presence of carbon fibers, and Proplast II is white because the carbon has been replaced by aluminum oxide particles. Each biomaterial has advantages and disadvantages related to fiber network, pore size, inflammatory response, and ability to be secured in place. Hydroxyapatite cements come in a thick paste form and can be molded and contoured as onlay grafts.

The least desirable materials are polyamide, such as Supramid, and polyester, such as Mersilene, fiber meshes because of relatively high extrusion and infection rates. Silicone rubber has excellent tissue biocompatibility, but it is prefabricated, allowing little opportunity for contouring. Silicone rubber also forms a fibrous connective tissue capsule that can be disrupted easily by external trauma.

In a fabric framework, such as ePTFE, which has a small pore size, tissue ingrowth occurs uniformly. Because of the 1- to 2-mm thickness of ePTFE, the fibroblasts can completely penetrate its depth, which is not always possible with the thicker porous implants such as Proplast and porous polyethylene such as MedPor. All of these materials can be cut and contoured to correct the defect (Fig. 160.2). Preformed ePTFE fabric chin and malar implants are available in addition to the facial augmentation sheets. Facial and lip augmentation can be performed safely with ePTFE fabric (16).

Although it is possible to place small implants subperiosteally, large, nonyielding implants placed beneath the periosteum can cause pressure resorption of the underlying bone. The use of alloplastic materials on the dorsum and tip of the nose is controversial. Hard silicone implants are used in Asia, but they have a high rate of extrusion. Some surgeons have had success with placing a silicone

implant on the nasal dorsum and autologous auricular cartilage grafts on the nasal tip and in the columella, which has reduced the previously reported high extrusion rate (17). Polyamide mesh has been used in augmentation of the dorsum of the nose but poses a high risk of infection and inflammation. Expanded PTFE fabric has been used successfully for augmentation of the tip of the nose (18). This graft seems to be easily tolerated by the thicker nasal dorsum tissues and, if secured to the periosteum, has a low rate of migration. It is soft and has a more "natural" feel than the more firm silicone. Human acellular dermis can be used as a nasal augmentation biomaterial, especially as a filler for defects when autologous cartilage is not readily available. There have been instances where it is totally resorbed, so one must be prepared for a second augmentation, should this occur. Successful immediate replacement of the alloplastic implant with autologous cartilage grafts has been reported and recommended (19).

Perioral and Facial

It has become increasingly important to some patients to have perioral and facial wrinkles reduced and the lips made more plump. Facial plastic surgeons utilize a number of alloplastic and biological materials to achieve these results. Human acellular dermis, expanded PTFE tubular implants, and autologous fat have been utilized for increasing the size and projection of the lips and to lessen the depth of the nasolabial folds. The tubular form of ePTFE seems to move freely with facial motions, albeit with some "awareness" by the patient of its presence (20). This alloplast may migrate with motion and time but can be removed relatively easy.

Fat injections, obtained from the submental region or abdomen, can also serve as a biological filler for these areas. Some initial erythema and reaction may result from the breakdown of the fatty acids, but usually the autologous graft is well tolerated. There may be some resorption, based on technique of harvest, so overinflation is generally observed.

Newer soft tissue fillers may have supplanted collagen injections for the purpose of wrinkle reduction and soft tissue augmentation. Calcium hydroxyapatite-based injectable implant can be used in most facial wrinkles, especially perioral and glabellar. Immediate pain on injection and short-term erythema have been reported (21). Other fillers include partially cross-linked hyaluronic acid and fully cross-linked hyaluron polymer. These filler last approximately 6 to 12 and 3 to 4 months, respectively. A cautious approach has been advocated in the widespread use of these filling agents until long-term data is available (22).

Mandible

The main source of bone for mandibular reconstruction is autogenous bone; a tray keeps grafts in position. Carrier trays are made of nylon, Dacron polyester, titanium, or tantalum. They are fabricated in the shape of the mandible

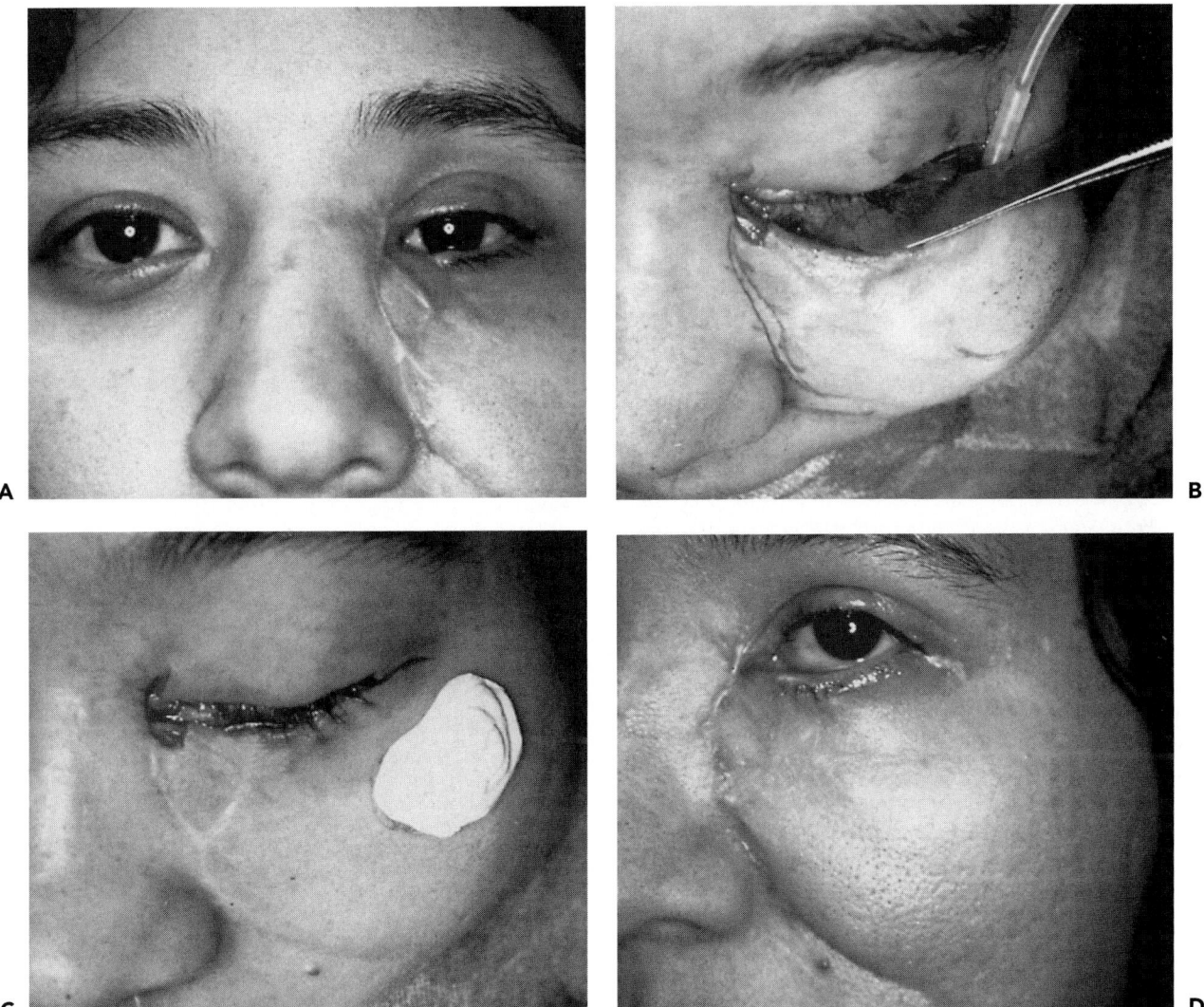

Figure 160.2   A: Woman with flattened left malar eminence after facial trauma. **B:** Rapid intraoperative expansion of tissue pocket to receive the implant. **C:** Layered ePTFE fabric implant is fitted to the left cheek. **D:** Augmented cheek 3 months after surgery.

and trimmed to resemble the missing segment. When the tray is filled with cancellous bone, new bone forms within it. The tray can be removed after sufficient bone has formed to withstand stress and load. Stainless steel or titanium reconstruction plates can be inserted after mandibulectomy to maintain spacing. These reconstruction bars are fixed with locking screws to the proximal and distal segments to minimize motion. They may be removed when a graft is placed. In some cases, the plate itself and a regional soft-tissue/muscle flap are adequate to support the bone grafts. Many mandibular reconstructions are performed using a free flap of bone and soft tissue, often including muscle, based on the mechanical requirements of the defect, and the feasibility of vascular anastomoses.

Repair of fractures of the the mandible and midface has been improved with miniplating and microplating systems in which a titanium alloy and self-tapping screws are used.

These plates can be left in place indefinitely except when the overlying skin is thin and the plates cause discomfort. These same screws and plates can be used to secure bone grafts and other implants to the facial bones. Resorbable fixation plates are becoming more comfortable an option for surgeons—they are typically composed of biodegradable materials, mainly polymers and co-polymers of polylactide and polyglycolide. They gradually lose their strength, enabling the underlying bone to begin to remodel with stress uptake. Their application is good in the uncomplicated mandibular fracture, in non-stress-bearing fracture locations (maxilla, frontal sinus, periorbit), and also in fixating suspension sutures (endoscopic brow lift). These resorbable plates can be heat-bent to the proper shape required using a thin metallic template as a guide.

The technology of osseointegrated intraoral implants has revolutionized the dental profession. Patients who could not previously wear dentures can do so with Branemark implants solidly anchored to the jaws. A single tooth, a partial denture, or a complete denture can be anchored in place with these fixtures. Fixtures can anchor augmentation bone grafts to the jaws and can be placed in a mandible reconstructed completely from autogenous cancellous bone or from a vascularized radius bone (23).

Mentoplasty implants are made from a variety of biomaterials—polymers (solid, gel, or mesh), carbon or aluminum oxide combined with PTFE, high-density porous polyethylene, and ePTFE fabric. As with other sites of facial augmentation, the implants are best placed extraperiosteally and secured to the periosteum by sutures. Both extraoral or intraoral insertions can be used, and both approaches seem to work well when placed by an experienced surgeon. Most surgeons tend to anchor the implant in the midline and use subperiosteal pockets to insert and secure the lateral arms of the implant. Patient satisfaction with ePTFE chin implants has been reported as high as 97% (24).

Hydroxyapatite has been used as a bone-conduction material to provide a nonorganic framework for ingrowth of osteoactive cells to correct small defects of the mandible and maxilla. The success of this approach varies. In the future, the material may function better if combined with osteoinductive intervention. Several replacement prostheses for the temporomandibular joint have been investigated, but a single best biomaterial has not emerged (25). Silicone sheeting has been a reasonable substitute for the meniscus in the joint, but the articulating surfaces of most implant prostheses have undergone wear and degradation.

Neck

In vascular surgery, the use of ePTFE patches has improved the results of carotid artery surgery for stenosis, primarily because of excellent biocompatibility with the hematogenous cellular and clotting factors and because it functions as a substrate for endothelial ingrowth. The silicone tracheoesophageal fistula prosthesis is a removable implant in the neck that has excellent surface properties in contact with aerodigestive tract secretions. A certain amount of fatigue and degradation occurs with this functional implant, and it must be replaced weekly. Use of tracheostomy tubes composed of highly surface-biocompatible silicone and PTFE with low-pressure polymer sheeting balloons have greatly reduced the complications of tracheal erosion and blockage of the tube lumen. Suture material for closure of neck wounds includes synthetic bioresorbable sutures such as polylactic acid or polyglactin 910; ePTFE vascular sutures; stainless steel skin staples; or polypropylene sutures, which also are hemocompatible for vascular repair. Use of these materials has decreased the incidence of wound breakdown and bleeding.

COMPLICATIONS AND EMERGENCIES

Bleeding, infection, trauma, mobility, and extrusion are the important complications of surgical implantation in the face, head, and neck. Malposition of the implant, overcorrection or undercorrection of the defect, patient dissatisfaction, and uninformed selection of implant material also affect outcome. These complications usually can be prevented through careful selection of both patient and implant. Preoperative counseling, meticulous surgical technique, and close follow-up evaluation all work toward good results.

If the implant site becomes infected, high doses of broad-spectrum antibiotics are prescribed, and hot compresses are applied. Most surgeons use perioperative antibiotic therapy, and all use aseptic surgical discipline. It is essential to prevent contamination of the implant before insertion (26). Impending extrusion or failure to control an infection necessitates immediate removal of the implant. Incorporation of antiseptic agents into the biomaterials can minimize the risk of infection (27).

Malposition of an implant necessitates a second operation to realign it. Undercorrection or overcorrection of a deformity is corrected only if the patient chooses to do so, without urging by the surgeon.

Some liquid implants have produced histotoxic effects or hypersensitivity reactions. Ethyl-2-cyanoacrylate, a short-chain cyanoacrylate derivative, activates severe cellular toxicity, but butyl-2-cyanoacrylate, a longer-chain derivative, has minimal histotoxic effects (28). If it is necessary to use a tissue glue for adhesion of one hard tissue to another, butyl-2-cranoacrylate is the better choice.

Another substance used widely for dermal augmentation is injectable bovine collagen. Hypersensitivity manifests as skin inflammation or gastrointestinal distress after eating beef. Each prospective patient is carefully evaluated for a history of hypersensitivity to beef products before treatment and is observed closely after collagen injections (29). A positive reaction to a skin test dose is an absolute contraindication to collagen injection. If a reaction occurs, it is managed medically with topical and systemic anti-inflammatory agents and local skin care. The injected tissue is removed surgically if the reaction cannot be controlled conservatively. Acellular human dermis is available in thin sheets and can be used for soft-tissue augmentation. It can be used safely in most previously irradiated fields (30,31).

If a vascular patch or area of revascularization begins bleeding, the patient is returned immediately to the operating room for repair of the leak. Few crises are worse than vascular emergencies in surgical implants in the face, head, and neck.

If a patient is dissatisfied with the results of a surgical implant, the surgeon reassures the patient until the swelling has subsided enough to gain an impression of the result. The patient-physician relationship is maintained with a

TABLE 160.3   C COMPLICATIONS

Complication	Prevention	Treatment
Infection	Perioperative antibiotics, aseptic technique	Antibiotics, hot compresses
Traumatic displacement	Patient education, implant stabilization	Surgical repositioning
Impending extrusion	Control of infection, immobilization of site	Removal of implant
Over- or undercorrection	Use of scans, photos, and measurements preoperatively	Revision according to patient's wishes
Malposition	Implant stabilization	Surgical repositioning
Bleeding	Meticulous hemostasis, compression	Surgical exploration
Patient dissatisfaction	Preoperative counseling, communication, and rapport	Reassurance and concern; revision if necessary

demeanor of concern, trust, and free communication. If the patient's dissatisfaction is justified, the surgeon can discuss the possibility of surgical revision. If the patient's concern is not justified, a second opinion from a respected colleague can defuse the situation. Whatever the conditions, the physician maintains a close and empathic relationship with the patient. Table 160.3 summarizes the complications and emergencies in the use of implants as well as prevention and management.

HIGHLIGHTS

- Metallic implants have excellent mechanical properties but can shield bone from stress. Implant removal after bone healing allows the bone to remodel in response to natural mechanical loading stresses.
- Hydroxyapatite is a bioreactive, nonorganic bone component. It is also a ceramic with bioreactive properties, can conduct osteogenetic cells into a bone defect, and can serve as a bone-conducting implant. It is slowly resorbed (demineralized) with time.
- Polymers have the widest application as implants because they have low reactivity in blood and tissues and have diverse mechanical properties and forms, depending on the fabrication method.
- Biologic materials such as collagen can continue to be antigenic even after structural enzymatic alteration. Safer biologic implants such as polyglycolic acid and polylactic acid are normal constituents of human skin and are slowly absorbed synthetics.
- The biocompatibility of an implant depends on initial tissue protein (fibronectin) adsorption to the implant surface and subsequent cell adherence through a network of intermediate glycosaminoglycan chains.
- Extracellular ground substance matrix adjacent to a bone implant must become mineralized to transmit compression and contend with sheer forces and tensile loads.

- A patient receiving a facial, head, or neck implant must not have previous sensitivity to any component of the implant. Whether the implant is functional or cosmetic, the patient must fully understand the goals and risks of the procedure and accept responsibility for protecting the implant.
- The proper implant for a particular site and tissue type matches the original tissue as closely as possible in biomechanics, texture, thickness, color, and biocompatibility.
- A good implant is biocompatible with host tissue, is noncarcinogenic, has similar biomechanical properties, is easily fabricated, can be sterilized without affecting intrinsic properties, is safe, and has been thoroughly investigated.
- Possible complications of surgical implants include infection, hypersensitivity, mobility, trauma, bleeding, malposition, overcorrection or undercorrection, extrusion, and patient dissatisfaction. Good communication and rapport with the patient assist in management of a complication.
- Resorbable implants are increasingly utilized for bony fixation, especially where a slow acquisition of stresses and strains will result in a positive bony reformation process.
- Facial fillers, including ePTFE, hyaluronic acid, collagen derivatives, and hydroxyapatite, may be helpful in reducing the depths of facial wrinkles, augmenting minor soft tissue defects, and increasing the bulk of the perioral region. They can be used effectively in conjunction with one another or facial implants.

REFERENCES

1. Holt GR. Physical characteristics and biocompatibility of implant materials. In: Glasgold AI, Silver FH, eds. *Applications of biomaterials in facial plastic surgery.* Boca Raton, FL: CRC Press, 1991:87.
2. Gosain AK, Persing JA. Biomaterials in the face: benefits and risks. *J Craniofac Surg* 1999;10:404–414.

3. Ousterhout DK, Zlotolow IM. Aesthetic improvement of the forehead utilizing methylmethacrylate onlay implants. *Aesthetic Plast Surg* 1990;14:281.

4. Donati L, Baruffaldi-Preis FW, DiLeo A, et al. Ten-year experience with craniofacial implants: clinical and experimental results. *Int Surg* 1997;82:325–331.

5. Gibbons KJ, Hicks WL Jr, Guterman LR. A technique for rigid fixation of methyl methacrylate cranioplasty: the vault-locking method. *Surg Neurol* 1999;52:310–315.

6. Magee WP Jr, Ajkay N, Freda N, et al. Use of fast-setting hydroxyapatite cement for secondary facial contouring. *Plast Reconstr Surg* 2003;114:289–297.

7. Holt GR, Parel SM, Branemark PI. Osseointegrated titanium implants. *Facial Plast Surg* 1986;3:113.

8. Arcuri MR, Rubenstein JT. Facial implants. *Dent Clin North Am* 1998;42:161–175.

9. Lo AK, Jackson IT, Ross JH. Severe orbital floor fractures: repair with a titanium implant. *Eur J Plast Surg* 1992;15:35–40.

10. Mauriello JA Jr, Wasserman B, Kraut R. Use of Vicryl mesh implant for repair of orbital floor fracture causing diplopia: a study of 28 patients over 5 years. *Ophthal Plast Reconstr Surg* 1993;9:191–195.

11. Fedok FG, van Kooten DW, Levin RJ. Temporal augmentation with a layered expanded polytetrafluoroethylene implant. *Otolaryngol Head Neck Surg* 1999;120:929–933.

12. Choi HY, Hong SE, Lew JM. Long-term comparison of a newly designed gold implant with the conventional implant in facial nerve paralysis. *Plast Reconstr Surg* 1999;104:1624–1634.

13. Friedman CD, Costantino PD, Takagi S, et al. BoneSource hydroxyapatite cement: a novel biomaterial for craniofacial skeletal tissue engineering and reconstruction. *J Biomed Mater Res* 1998;43:428–432.

14. Stelnicki EJ, Ousterhout DK. Hydroxyapatite paste (BoneSource) used as an onlay implant for supraorbital and malar augmentation. *J Craniofac Surg* 1997;8:367–372.

15. Goodman SB, Bauer TW, Carter D, et al. Norian SRS cement augmentation in hip fracture treatment: laboratory and initial clinical results. *Clin Orthop* 1998;348:42–50.

16. Robertson KM, Dyer WK 2nd. Expanded polytetrafluoroethylene (Gore-Tex) augmentation of deep nasolabial creases. *Arch Otolaryngol Head Neck Surg* 1999;125:456–461.

17. Ahn J, Honrado C, Horn C. Combined silicone and cartilage implants. *Arch Facial Plast Surg* 2004;6:120–123.

18. Waldman SR. Gore-Tex for augmentation of the nasal dorsum: a preliminary report. *Ann Plast Surg* 1991;26:520–525.

19. Raghavan U, Jones NS, Romo T III: Immediate autogenous cartilage grafts in rhinoplasty after alloplastic implant rejection. *Arch Facial Plast Surg* 2004;6:192–196.

20. Wall SJ, Adamson PA, Bailey D, et al.: Patient satisfaction with expanded polytetrafluoroethylene (Softform) implants to the perioral region. *Arch Facial Plast Surg* 2003;5:320–324.

21. Tzikas TL: Evaluation of the Radiance FN soft tissue filler for facial soft tissue augmentation. *Arch Facial Plast Surg* 2004;6:234–239.

22. Rohrich RJ, Rios JL, Fagien S: Role of new fillers in facial rejuvenation: a cautious outlook. *Plast Reconstr Surg* 2003;112:1899–1902.

23. Urken ML, Buchbinder D, Costantino PD, et al. Oromandibular reconstruction using microvascular composite flaps: report of 210 cases. *Arch Otolaryngol Head Neck Surg* 1998;124:46–55.

24. Godin M, Costa L, Romo T III, et al: Gore-Tex chin implants: a review of 324 cases. *Arch Facial Plast Surg* 2003;5:224–227.

25. 25. Stucker FJ Jr. Mentoplasty using rolled polyamide mesh. *Facial Plast Surg* 1986;3:107.

26. Holgers KM, Ljungh A. Cell surface characteristics of microbiological isolates from human percutaneous titanium implants in the head and neck. *Biomaterials* 1999;20:1319–1326.

27. Malaisrie SC, Malekzadeh S, Bedlingmaier JF. In vivo analysis of bacterial biofilm formation on facial plastic bioimplants. *Laryngoscope* 1998;108:1733–1738.

28. Toriumi DM, Raslan WF, Friedman M, et al. Histotoxicity of cyanoacrylate tissue adhesives. *Arch Otolaryngol Head Neck Surg* 1990;116:546.

29. Frank DH, Vakassein L, Fisher JC, et al. Human antibody response following multiple injections of bovine collagen. *Plast Reconstr Surg* 1991;87:1080.

30. Achauer BM, VanderKam VM, Celikoz B, et al. Augmentation of facial soft-tissue defects with Alloderm dermal graft. *Ann Plast Surg* 1998;41:503–507.

31. Dubin MG, Feldman M, Ibrahim HZ, et al. Allograft dermal implant (AlloDerm) in a previously irradiated field. *Laryngoscope* 2000;110:934–937.

Local Skin Flaps: Anatomy, Physiology, and General Types

Kevin A. Shumrick   **Jon B. Chadwell**   **Andrew C. Campbell**

The term *local skin flap* refers to flaps that are harvested adjacent (or very close) to the defect requiring reconstruction. Generally, they are rotated, advanced, or interpolated into the defect and rely on surrounding skin laxity for donor-site closure. In this day of free tissue transfer, local skin flaps remain the major tissue source for repair of defects following excision of facial malignancies or trauma. Advantages and disadvantages of local skin flaps are listed in Table 161.1.

VASCULAR ANATOMY

A flap's blood supply is the major determinant of its survival, and knowledge of the skin's circulation is crucial for success in designing flaps. Blood supply is also the basis for anatomically classifying the types of flaps used for facial reconstruction. Overall, there are three main types of flaps as determined by their blood supply: local or random-pattern flaps, axial-pattern flaps, and myocutaneous flaps.

To help understand these vascular classifications, a brief review of the total body circulation is in order. The first step toward supplying the skin with blood is the segmental blood vessels—large, named branches of the aorta that run below muscle masses and distribute blood to the rest of the body (these vessels form the basis for myocutaneous flaps) (Fig. 161.1). The segmental arteries give off perforating arteries that pass through the overlying muscles, giving off branches to supply blood to the muscle, and continue externally to the overlying subcutaneous tissues and skin. The overlying portion of skin supplied by a single perforating vessel is termed an *angiosome*. Adjacent angiosomes are interconnected by small choke vessels in the subdermis. There are two routes by which the perforating vessels may arrive at the skin: via direct cutaneous arteries, which run on top of muscles and send branches to the skin (these are the basis for axial-pattern flaps), and by simply passing through the muscle and subcutaneous tissue to anastomose with the overlying subdermal plexus (these are the basis of the random-pattern flaps). Local skin flaps are based on either a random-pattern or axial-pattern blood supply.

TABLE 161.1

LOCAL FLAPS

Advantages
　　Use local tissue with better donor site match
　　Most are one stage
　　Low donor site morbidity

Disadvantages
　　Random pattern blood supply with limited length
　　Donor site closure may distort surrounding structures
　　Not enough bulk for deep defects

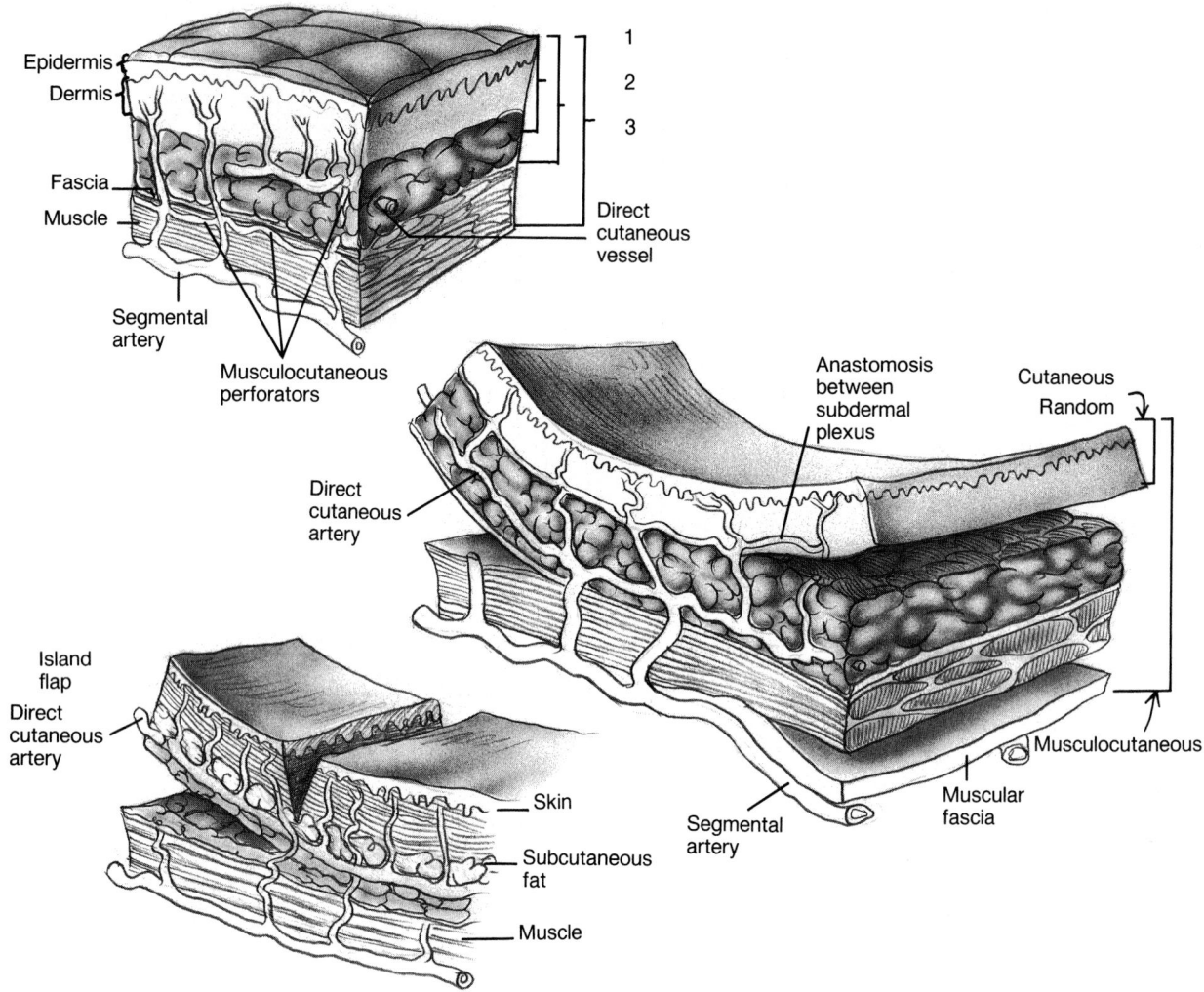

Figure 161.1 Generalized representation of the blood supply to the skin. Right side shows level and blood supply for various types of flaps. 1, Random-pattern flaps; 2, axial-pattern flaps; 3, myocutaneous flaps.

Random-Pattern Flaps

Based on the previous schema, it can be seen that random-pattern flaps do not have named arterial or venous vessels; instead, they rely on flow through the dermal and subdermal plexus, which eventually connects with perforating vessels at the base of the flap. Because most facial local skin flaps rely on a random-pattern blood supply, there are limits with regard to their length and width (Table 161.2).

Axial-Pattern Flaps

Axial-pattern flaps rely on a blood supply from named direct cutaneous arteries and veins running along the longitudinal axis of the flap (Table 161.3). These vessels course in the subcutaneous tissue superficial to the muscle, and the blood supply of the flap is considered secure for at least the length of these vessels. In addition, axial flaps may gain further length by incorporating a random-pattern portion of the flap distal to the termination of the axial vasculature.

The only local flap commonly considered to have an axial-pattern blood supply is the nasolabial flap, with its angular and infratrochlear vessels. Regional flaps with an axial blood supply are the deltopectoral, lateral forehead, and midline forehead flaps.

TABLE 161.2
CAUSES OF SKIN FLAP FAILURE

Extrinsic (to flap)
   Wound infection
   System hypotension
   Excessive tension
   Hematoma

Intrinsic
   Excessive flap length and random pattern blood supply
   Pharmacologic vasoconstriction (e.g., epinephrine, dopamine)
   Smoking
   Peripheral vascular disease

TABLE 161.3

AXIAL-PATTERN FLAPS

Flap	Blood Supply
Nasolabial flap	Angular
Median and paramedian forehead flaps	Supratrochlear
Lateral forehead flap	Superficial temporal
Deltapectoral flap	Perforating vessels of the internal mammary artery

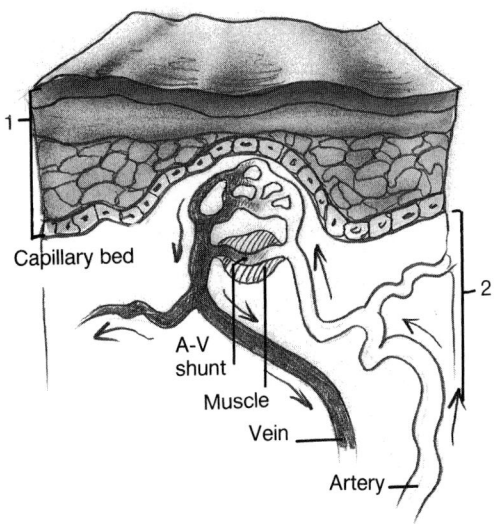

Figure 161.2 Blood supply to the skin, showing a capillary bed and aretriovenous (AV) shunt surrounded by smooth muscle. By varying the diameter of these shunts, changes in total skin blood flow can be accomplished, and theoretically, blood can bypass the capillary nutrient bed by preferentially traversing the AV shunt. It has been theorized that sympathetic denervation in acutely raised flaps causes dilation of these shunts with subsequent bypassing of the capillary beds. 1, Epidermis; 2, dermis.

Myocutaneous Flaps

Myocutaneous flaps are designed around a segmental artery and vein that run the length of the flap, sending perforating vessels to the overlying muscle and skin. The myocutaneous flap is raised as a unit (skin, subcutaneous tissue, muscle, and segmental vessels) and is limited only by the length of the vascular pedicle. Examples of myocutaneous flaps are the pectoralis major, trapezius, and latissimus dorsi flaps.

LOCAL FLAP PHYSIOLOGY

Most local flaps (the nasolabial being an exception) rely on a random-pattern blood supply. As mentioned, a random-pattern blood supply refers to the interconnecting anastomoses found within the dermis and subdermal plexus. These vessels are small-caliber, unnamed arterioles and venules, which respond to a different set of physiologic parameters from the general circulation. The survival of a local skin flap ultimately depends on adequate tissue perfusion, and a multitude of factors can influence blood supply to the skin and, therefore, affect flap survival. It appears that the skin receives much more blood than is required for basic nutrition. Skin perfusion may vary from 2 to 100 mL per minute per 100 g of tissue, although flow of only 1 to 2 mL per minute per 100 g of tissue will support a flap (1,2). This additional blood flow appears to be related to the skin's function as a thermal regulator and modifier of the total volume of circulating blood by changes in the skin's venous capacitance.

The circulatory system is designed to distribute blood (with its nutrients and oxygen) to all the cells in the body. To accomplish this, it starts with large volumes of blood in the aorta at a mean arterial pressure (MAP) of 90 to 100 mm Hg. The blood is then distributed through a succession of smaller and smaller vessels with a drop in pressure at each level. After traversing the segmental, perforating, and direct cutaneous arteries, the blood arrives at the precapillary distal arterioles with an MAP of 30 mm Hg. These arterioles have smooth muscles in their walls that relax or constrict, changing their resistance to flow, and can markedly alter cutaneous blood flow. In fact, arterial resistance is the primary determinant of the rate of cutaneous blood flow, whereas changes in venous capacitance determine the total amount of blood in the skin at any one moment.

Regulation of arterial resistance and venous capacity is under autonomic control via the central nervous system and its modulation of arteriovenous (AV) shunts. These AV shunts are ubiquitous precapillary communications between the arterial and venous circulations (Fig. 161.2). These AV shunts allow blood to bypass the capillary bed and, thus, function strictly as regulators of blood flow and not tissue nutrition. It is estimated that skin blood flow may vary by as much as 1,000-fold by varying the flow through these shunts (1). AV shunts are entirely innervated by the sympathetic nervous system. With an increase in sympathetic tone, the shunts narrow and total blood flow through the skin decreases. Conversely, if sympathetic tone decreases (or is interrupted surgically or pharmacologically), these shunts will open and total skin blood flow will increase. It has been speculated that with complete opening of these AV shunts, blood may be shunted away from the nutrient capillary bed and compromise the viability of the distal end of the flap. Riensch (3) performed a series of studies looking at local skin flap failure and presented convincing evidence that flaps undergoing necrosis (as determined by lack of fluorescein staining) actually have normal or even increased blood flow; however, the blood was felt to be preferentially passing through the AV shunts and bypassing the nutrient capillary bed.

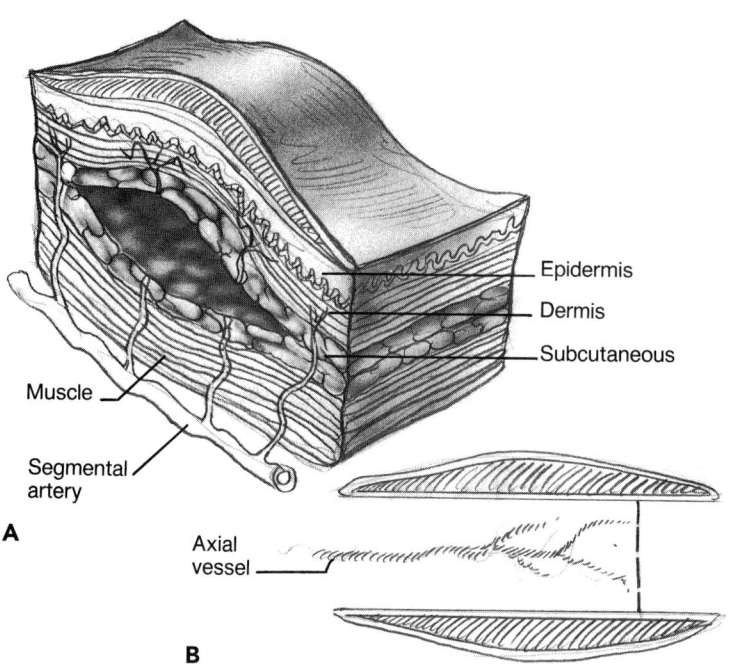

A

B

Figure 161.3 **A:** Cross section of the surgical delay procedure for a flap, showing interruption of the underlying musculocutaneous perforators as well as incising the margins of the flap. **B:** If a flap has an axial pattern (as illustrated by the axial vessel), then an additional random portion may be reliably included by incising the sides of the flap into the random-portion blood supply.

Length-to-Width Ratio

In the past, it was commonly believed that the surviving length of a local cutaneous flap could be increased by expanding its base. This theory held that a flap's surviving length was proportional to its width in a specific ratio (2). According to this theory, if a surgeon made the flap's base wide enough, a flap of almost any length could be obtained. It is now recognized that the length–width ratio is only a rough guideline, and it cannot be relied on as an absolute determinant of a flap's success. The length–width ratio fails because of the basic principle that the blood supply of a random-pattern pedicled flap originates from the nearest cutaneous arterial perforator, enters at the base of the flap, and perfuses it via the interconnecting dermal and subdermal plexi. The surviving length of a flap is determined by the perfusion pressure of the feeding vessels and the intravascular resistance. Increasing the width of a flap's base simply adds additional vessels, all with the same perfusion pressure facing similar resistance, and the surviving length of the flap will not be increased (2,4).

Delay Phenomenon

The delay phenomenon refers to the clinical observation that skin flaps that are partially incised and undermined but not transposed will survive to a consistently greater length when raised at a later date than a similar flap raised and transposed primarily. The exact mechanisms responsible for this increased length of flap survival have not been completely elucidated, but the most likely candidates are closure of AV shunts, increase in vessel caliber (particularly the choke vessels), increased vessel numbers with reorientation along the flap axis, and conditioning of the distal flap to tolerate ischemia (5–7). The most commonly cited

explanation for the delay phenomenon relates to the previously mentioned AV shunts. It has been speculated that by delaying a flap, the denervated AV shunts have time to narrow or close secondary to the development of autonomous tone from either regrowth of sympathetic nerves along the flap base or the development of sensitivity to circulating endogenous catecholamines. When the flap is then raised and transposed, the AV shunts remain closed, with no shunting of blood, and the flap survives to a greater length (3). Recently, animal studies have shown that the delay phenomenon effectively dilates preexisting choke vessels between adjacent perforators, thus capturing the adjacent angiosome and increasing the viable length of a flap (8,9). There are no conclusive data on the optimum timing for delaying a flap, but delays of 10 to 21 days are most common. It has also been noted that the beneficial effect of delaying a flap will be lost after 3 weeks to 3 months. The technique of delaying a flap is determined by the flap's blood supply. If the flap has a random-pattern blood supply with significant perforating vessels, the preferred technique is to make parallel incisions along the sides of the flap, leaving the ends connected (8,10) (Fig. 161.3). The sides of the flap must be incised and the flap must be undermined to disrupt the perforating vessels. The end of the flap is then incised at the time of transfer. If the flap has an axial-pattern blood supply with a direct cutaneous artery and vein, then simply incising the proposed margins of the flap is sufficient; undermining is not necessarily required.

SKIN BIOMECHANICS

When using local skin flaps, the surgeon must consider circulatory physiology and also the biomechanics of skin and the dynamics of how physiology and physical properties

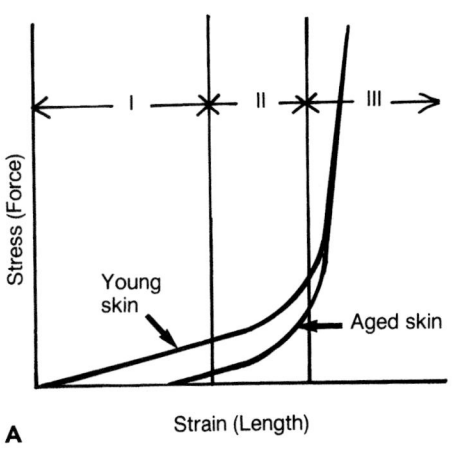

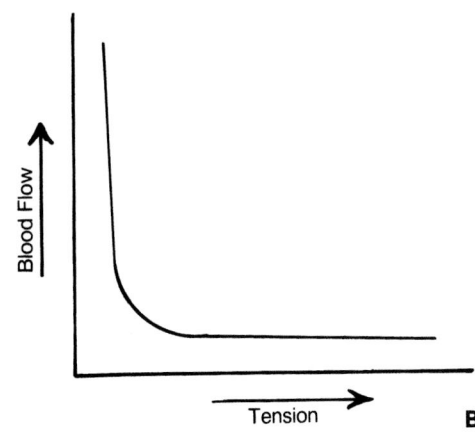

Figure 161.4 A: Stress/strain curve for young and aged human skin. Note that initially relatively little stress is accompanied by significant gains in length. With increasing length, however, there is a rapid increase in the amount of force required to gain small increments in length. (Adapted from Larrabee WF Jr, Sutton D. Biomechanics of advancement and rotation flaps. *Laryngoscope* 1981;91:726, with permission.) **B:** Inverse relationship between blood flow and tension. (Adapted from Gaboriau HP, et al. Skin anatomy and flap physiology. *Otolaryngol Clin North Am* 2001;34:555, with permission.)

interact. Local skin flaps rely on the fact that skin is elastic and tissue may be borrowed from one area to close a defect in another area, using skin elasticity to close the donor site. If performed correctly, this borrowing of tissue allows a surgeon to obtain the best aesthetic and functional results by optimal distribution of available materials. The skin's elasticity is largely determined by its collagen and elastin content. With stretching, the skin is, at first, easily deformed. This early phase of stretching is controlled by the elastin fibers. With continued stretching, collagen fibers start to align themselves along the direction of force, and the force required for comparable changes in length increases. When the collagen fibers have been completely oriented with the deforming force, additional tension produces little movement (11–15). (Fig. 161.4A).

Tension placed on a flap can have significant implications with regard to its viability, particularly when extensive undermining has been performed and a significant length of the flap relies on a random-pattern blood supply. Larrabee et al. (16) have shown that blood flow in a flap is inversely proportional to the tension placed across it (Fig. 161.4B). He found that the decreased blood flow with tension was not significant in short flaps but became the deciding factor with regard to ultimate flap survival in larger flaps.

Skin is a dynamic organ that can adapt to forces applied to it through its viscoelastic properties. Two manifestations of this adaptability are skin creep and stress relaxation. Skin creep refers to the clinically observed phenomenon that a flap placed under sudden constant tension more than 5 to 15 minutes will exhibit an additional increase in length beyond the original stretch. This is thought to be attributable to the deformation of the dermal framework fibers and extrusion of fluid from the dermis. Stress relaxation occurs in skin placed under constant tension over days to weeks, with the skin adapting by increasing its volume to relieve the stress. Stress relaxation is the principle

that allows tissue expansion or serial excision of lesions. The exact mechanism of stress relaxation is still under debate but appears to be a combination of permanent stretching of the skin proteins (collagen, elastin, and so forth) and increased cellularity. Relaxed skin tension lines (RSTL) run perpendicular to the lines of maximum extensibility (Fig. 161.5). They indicate the most favorable orientation of defects or incisions to obtain maximum skin

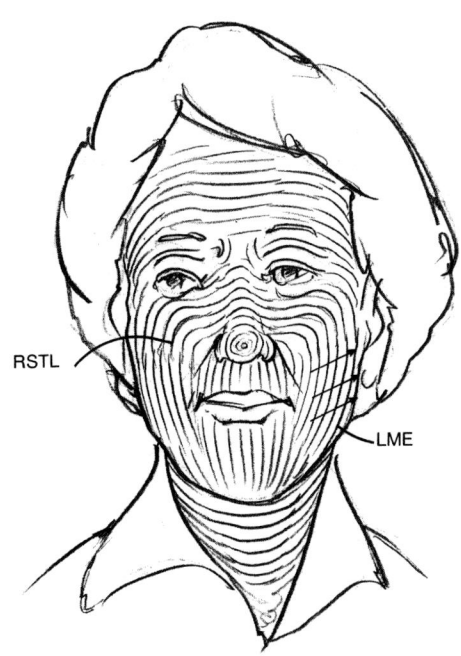

Figure 161.5 Relaxed skin tension lines (RSTL) of the face. Notice that the lines of maximum extensibility (LME) generally run perpendicular to the RSTLs. This is an important concept: An incision placed along the RSTLs will have the greatest chance for camouflage and will give the maximum amount of tissue for closure.

mobilization (with the least tension) for closure, as well as ensuring the least tension on the wound to prevent scar widening. Also, because wrinkles and creases tend to correspond to or parallel RSTLs, orienting the scar parallel with the RSTLs produces maximum scar camouflage. If possible, orient incisions with RSTLs, or in the case of flaps, plan the closure of the donor site so that it parallels the RSTLs.

SKIN FLAP FAILURE

A variety of factors may cause a skin flap to fail, with necrosis of all or part of the flap. The most common cause of flap failure is vascular insufficiency caused by an excessively long flap (with a random blood supply) or excessive tension. Pharmacologic agents causing vasoconstriction (such as nicotine, epinephrine, and dopamine) may also affect viability. In fact, some surgeons advocate delaying flaps in smokers because of the high incidence of flap failures in these patients. Conversely, pharmacologic agents such as buflomedil, pentoxifylline, nicotinic acid, and nicotinamide have been shown to increase skin flap survival in animals; however, no agent has thus far been experimentally shown to be beneficial in humans (17,18). Hematomas underlying a flap have been implicated as a cause of flap necrosis. There appear to be two ways a hematoma can cause necrosis. First, simple pressure from the hematoma causes increased wound tension and pressure on feeding vessels. Second, there appears to be a direct toxic effect from the hematoma breakdown products that contributes to flap necrosis; this probably is caused by

vasoconstriction from compounds in the hematoma (19). A seroma can also affect a flap in a similar manner; therefore, all large flaps or flaps requiring significant undermining should be drained. Experimentally, fibrin glue has been shown to decrease wound drainage in animals, thus, possibly eliminating the need for closed suction drainage in some cases (20). Factors such as diabetes, hypertension, infection, and compression of the flap pedicle can also affect flap viability and must be controlled.

TYPES OF LOCAL SKIN FLAPS

There are two basic types of local flaps (each with a number of variants): flaps that involve rotation about a fixed point to reach a defect and flaps that advance directly into the defect.

Rotation Flaps

True Rotation Flaps
A true rotation flap is semicircular and rotates in an arc, usually with a back cut or Z-plasty at the base to take care of redundant tissue (Fig. 161.6). Because of its broad base, its vascularity is reliable. Overzealous removal of the standing cutaneous deformity at its base, however, may compromise this vascularity, and, thus, a second-stage removal of the deformity may be necessary (21).

Transposition Flaps
Transposition flaps rotate about a fixed point into the defect, usually with an area of intact skin between the donor

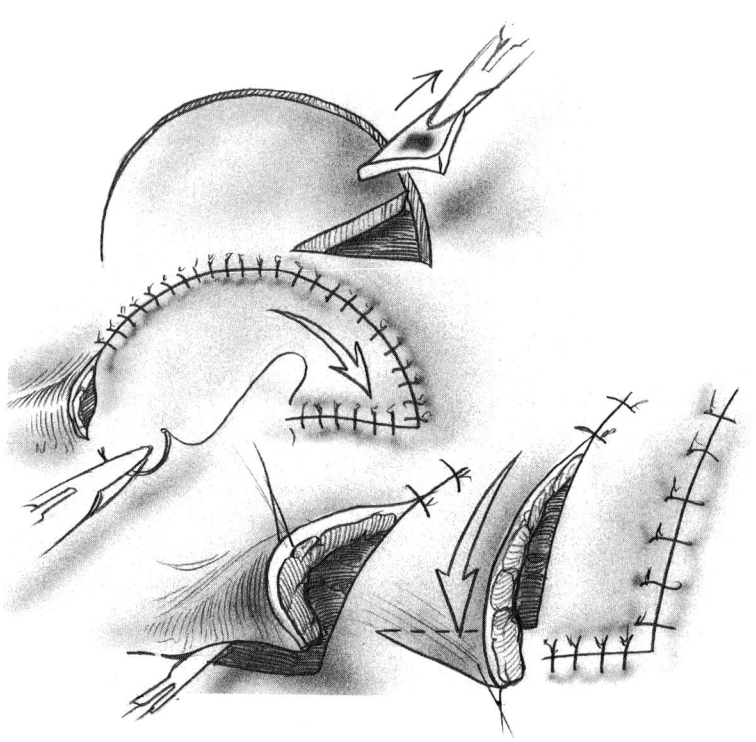

Figure 161.6 A true rotation flap designed in a semicircular fashion and advanced to fill the defect. There is usually a dog-ear at the base of the donor site that requires some adjustment via excision of a Burow triangle.

site and defect. Examples of transposition flaps are rhomboid flaps, bilobed flaps, and nasolabial flaps. In an interpolated flap, the donor site is separated from the recipient site, and the flap's pedicle must then pass over or under the intervening tissue to reach the recipient site. Examples of interpolated flaps are subcutaneous island flaps or nasolabial flaps that are transposed to the recipient site and allowed to pick up a blood supply; the pedicle is excised as a second-stage procedure when a blood supply has been established.

Rhomboid Flaps

Rhomboid flaps are rotation flaps that are probably the most commonly used local flaps on the face. The classic rhomboid flap is designed to fit a rhombic defect with two 60-degree and two 120-degree angles. For each rhomboid defect, four possible flap orientations may be used for closure (Fig. 161.7). A rhomboid flap is developed by extending a perpendicular line from the 120-degree angle that is equal in length to the diameter of the defect. A back cut is then performed in such a way as to create a 60-degree angle paralleling the margin of the defect and is extended for a distance equal to the length of one side of the defect. The flap is then transposed into the defect, and the donor site is closed on itself. A major advantage of the rhomboid flap is that the main area of tension is across the closure of the donor site, sparing any compromise of the flap tip (Fig. 161.7E).

Dufourmental Flaps

A variant of the rhomboid flap is the Dufourmental flap, which may be used for defects that do not correspond to the classic 60- to 120-degree dimensions. In the Dufourmental flap, imaginary lines are extended from the diameter of the defect and one of the defect sides (Fig. 161.8A). The angle created by these two lines is then bisected by a line that is the same length as a side of the defect. A back cut is then made that runs parallel to the long axis of the defect and that is the same length as one side of the defect. This flap is then rotated into position and closed in the same fashion as a standard rhomboid flap (Fig. 161.8B). The Dufourmental flap is more complicated than the standard rhomboid flap and requires experience for optimum results, but it allows the surgeon to handle a wider variety of defects without having to convert them to classic rhomboid defects.

Bilobed Flaps

Bilobed flaps are basically double rotation flaps in tandem with a single pedicle. The principle of the bilobed flap is to use skin laxity to distribute the tension over two flaps and donor sites, allowing closure of a defect with two rotation flaps of smaller size. The first flap is designed to be as long as the defect, somewhat narrower, and angled at about 90 degrees. The second flap is smaller than the first flap and again angled at roughly 90 degrees. When these flaps are incised and transposed, the donor site of the second flap closes primarily, and the bilobed flaps fill the remaining defects through local skin laxity (Fig. 161.9). Bilobed flaps are generally thought to work best on the nose, where tissue may be borrowed from the perinasal area (22–25). The disadvantages of bilobed flaps are the complexity of the scar and their tendency to pincushion.

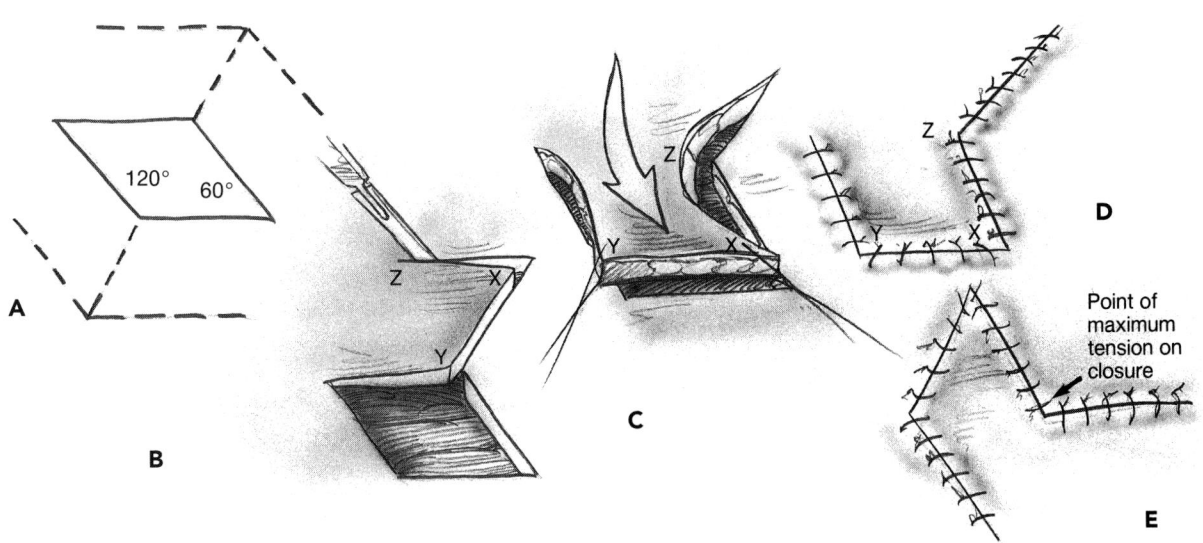

Figure 161.7 A: Classic rhomboid defect with 60-degree and 120-degree angles. Notice that there are four possible rhomboid flaps for each rhomboid defect (dotted lines). **B, C, D:** The flap is incised and rotated into position. **E:** Final closure. The point of maximum tension is on the donor site closure, not on the flap itself.

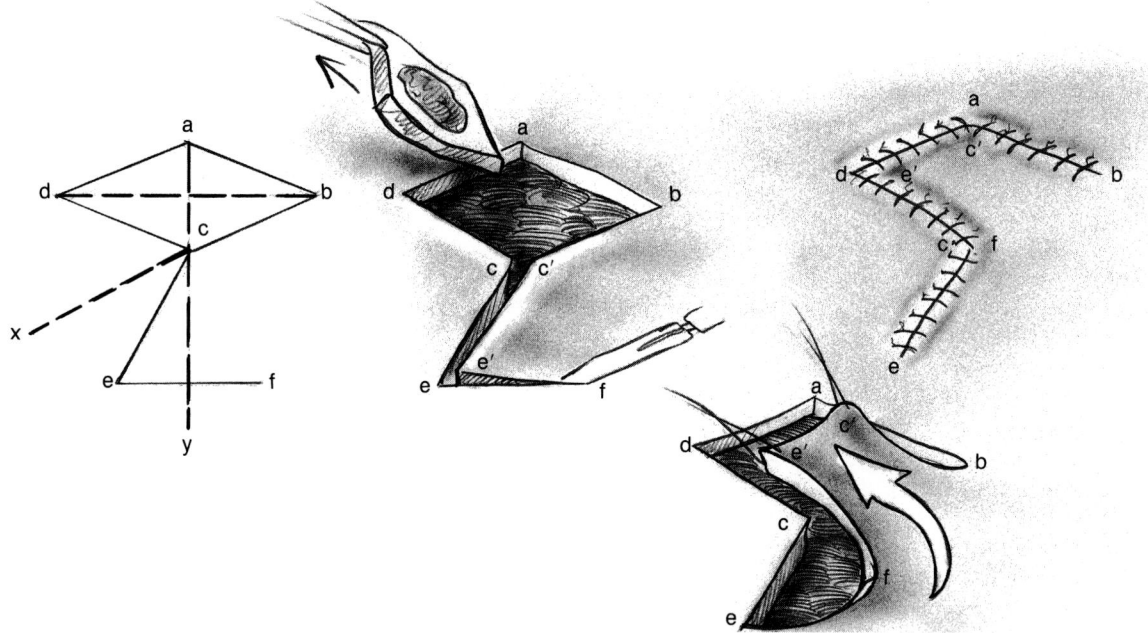

Figure 161.8 Dufourmental flap used for defects that do not confirm to the classic 60- to 120-degree rhomboid defects. In this flap, imaginary lines are extended from the diameter of the defect (y) and one of the defect's sides (x). These two lines are then bisected by a line the same length as the side of the defect (e). A back cut is then made that runs parallel to the long axis of the defect (f). The flap is then elevated and rotated into position just as for a classic rhomboid flap.

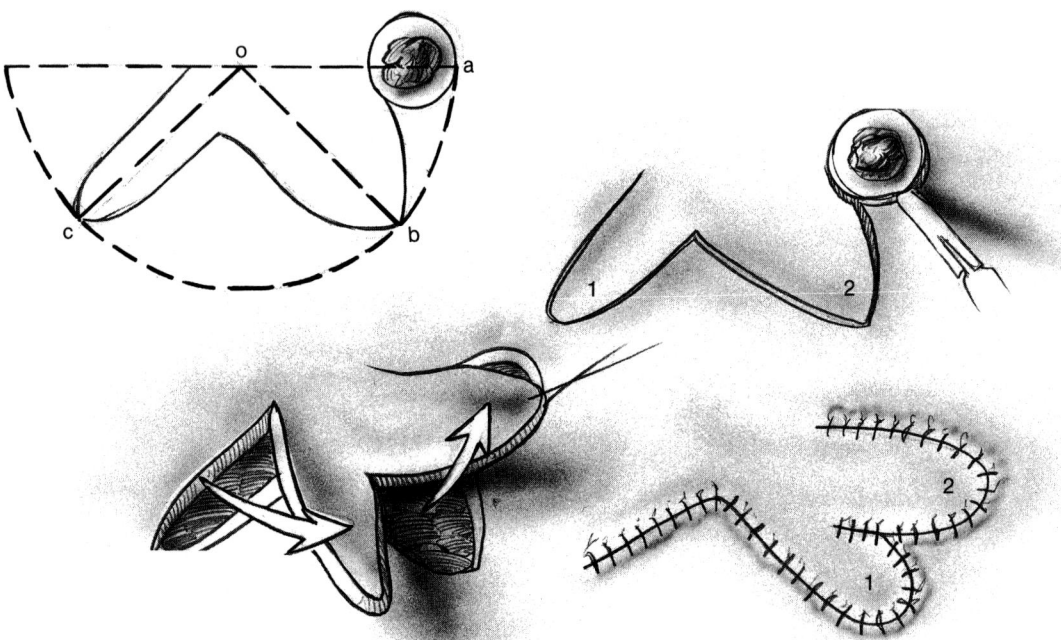

Figure 161.9 Design and execution of a bilobed flap. The bilobed flap works on the principle of distributing tissue and tension over two rotation flaps, connected by a single base, instead of one. The donor site for flap 1 closes primarily, and flap 1 is then used to close the donor site for flap 2. Flap 2 is used to close the original defect. Each flap is rotated about 90 degrees, with the total rotation accomplishing about 180 degrees.

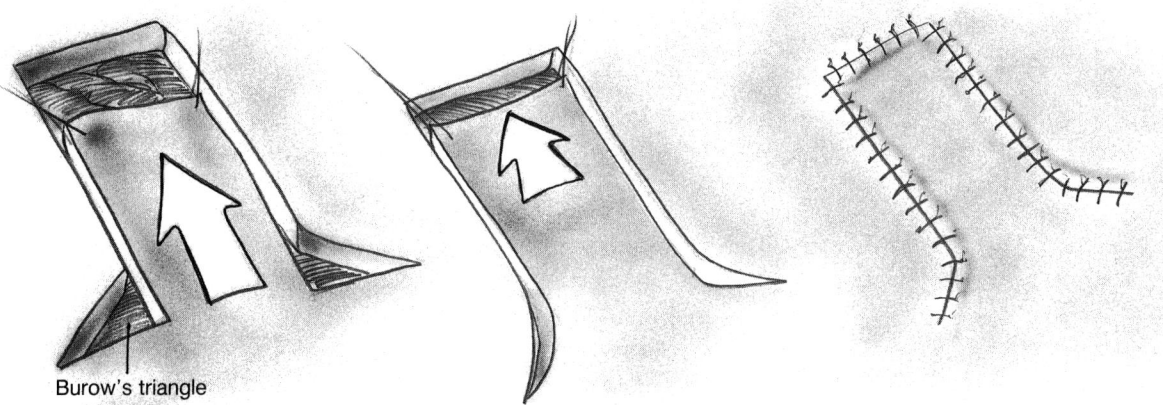

Burow's triangle

Figure 161.10 A monopedicle advancement flap is incised, undermined, and advanced to fill the defect. Redundant tissue at the base of the flap is handled by excising a Burow triangle.

Advancement Flaps

The primary motion of an advancement flap is a straight line from the donor site to the defect without rotation or lateral movement. Strictly speaking, primary closure of a fusiform or elliptical defect involves undermining and advancing two flaps adjacent to the defect. There are three commonly recognized variants of advancement flaps. Monopedicle advancement flaps are usually rectangular and move forward into a defect from one side of the defect (Fig. 161.10). Bipedicle advancement flaps advance from both sides of the defect (these are particularly useful for lips and forehead) (Fig. 161.11). Both monopedicle and bipedicle flaps usually require back cuts at the flap base to prevent tissue bunching. Often, Burow triangles need to be excised to completely smooth the skin. V-Y flaps are created by converting a V-shaped incision into a Y-shaped closure, advancing the central portion of skin into the defect (Fig. 161.12). V-Y flaps have the advantage of preserving

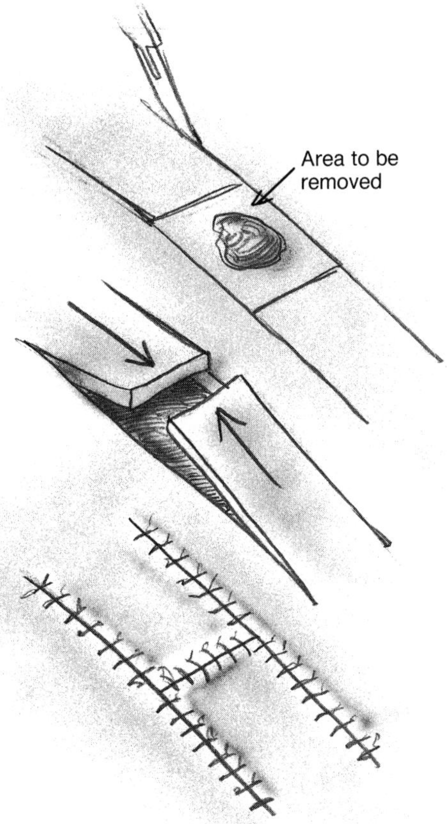

Area to be removed

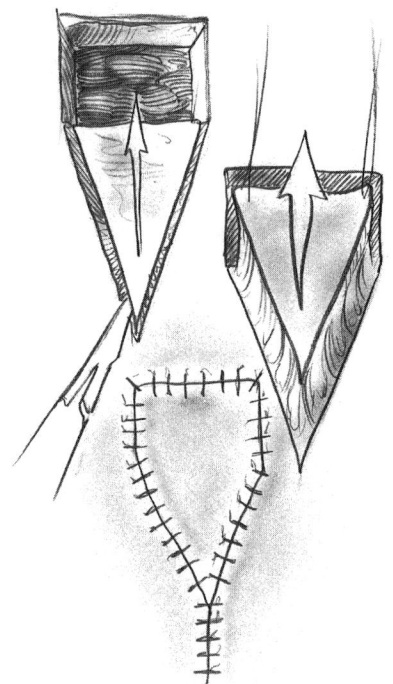

Figure 161.11 Bipedicle advancement flaps used to close a defect. They are particularly useful in areas such as the upper lip and forehead region.

Figure 161.12 V-Y advancement flap. A V-shaped incision is made on either side of a portion of tissue, and the tissue is advanced into the defect with primary closure of the donor site. Thus, a V-shaped incision is converted into a Y-shaped donor site.

the underlying subcutaneous circulation, thus, preventing pincushioning edema by providing adequate venous and lymphatic drainage (26,27).

Hinge Flaps

Cutaneous hinge flaps, also known as "trapdoor," "turn-in," or "turn-down" flaps are used to provide internal lining for a facial defect requiring both an internal and external lining. The flap is based at the edge of the defect and undermined in the subcutaneous plane. It is then reflected into the defect with the surface now lining the internal defect. A second flap or graft is then used to cover the donor defect. The disadvantages of the hinge flap include its limited blood supply and its need for a second flap or graft. It is a relatively simple technique to provide coverage for full-thickness nasal defects, however.

HIGHLIGHTS

- Local flaps remain the principal source of tissue for the repair of facial defects. They offer a superior tissue match and a single-stage procedure and do not disrupt underlying nerves or muscle function.
- Flaps are classified on the basis of their blood supply; there are three main types: random-pattern, axial-pattern, and myocutaneous. Random-pattern flaps rely on the dermal and subdermal plexus, whereas axial-pattern flaps receive their blood supply from named subcutaneous arteries and veins running superficial to the underlying muscle. Myocutaneous flaps are designed around a segmental artery and vein that run the length of the flap, sending perforating vessels through the muscle and up to the overlying skin. Most local facial flaps have a random-pattern blood supply. The blood supply to the skin is highly variable and is modified via the autonomic (sympathetic) control of precapillary arteriovenous shunts.
- Blood that preferentially passes through arteriovenous (AV) shunts, bypassing the nutrient capillary bed, is thought by many to be a major cause of local flap failure.
- The length-to-width ratio is an outdated concept. Its advocates believed that by increasing the width of a flap's base, the flap's surviving length could be indefinitely increased. However, a flap's surviving length is determined by the perfusion pressure of the feeding vessels and intravascular resistance. Making a flap wider only adds additional vessels, with the same perfusion pressure, and thus does not increase the surviving length of the flap.
- The delay phenomenon refers to the clinically observed fact that local flaps that are partially incised and undermined, but not transposed, have better survival when eventually raised than do similar flaps raised and transposed primarily. The exact mechanism for this increased survival is unclear but appears to be attributable to increased directional blood flow along the axis of the flap caused by dilatation of existing choke vessels as well as neovascularization.
- Blood flow in a flap is inversely proportional to the tension placed along its long axis.
- The most common intrinsic causes of local flap failure are excessive length or excessive tension, causing vascular insufficiency.
- Stress relaxation occurs in skin placed under constant tension over days to weeks and results in increased volume through stretching of the skin proteins, as well as increased cellularity.
- The most common extrinsic factors causing local flap failure are underlying hematomas, infection, diabetes, hypertension, and compression of the flap pedicle.

REFERENCES

1. Gullane PJ, Henneman H. *Regional flaps in the head and neck*. Self-instructional package. Washington DC: American Academy of Otolaryngology—Head and Neck Surgery, 1982.
2. Daniel RK. The anatomy and hemodynamics of the cutaneous circulation and the influence of skin flap design. In: Myers MB, Grabb WC, eds. *Skin flaps*. Boston: Little, Brown, 1975:111–143.
3. Reinsch JF. The pathophysiology of skin flap circulation. *Plast Reconstr Surg* 1975;54:585–598.
4. Milton SH. Pedicled skin flaps: the fallacy of the length/width ratio. *Br J Surg* 1970;57:502–508.
5. Myers MB. Attempts to augment survival in skin flaps: mechanism of the delay phenomenon. In: Myers MB, Grabb WC, eds. *Skin flaps*. Boston: Little Brown, 1975:65–69.
6. McFarlane RM, Heagg FC, Radin S, et al. A study of the delay phenomena in experimental pedicle flaps. *Plast Reconstr Surg* 1965;35:245–262.
7. Myers MB, Chery G, Milton S. Tissue gas levels as an index of the adequacy of circulation: the relation between ischemia and the development of collateral circulation. *Surgery* 1972;71:15–21.
8. Callegari PR, Taylor GI, Caddy CM, et al. An anatomic review of the delay phenomenon: I. Experimental studies. *Plast Reconstr Surg* 1992;89:397–407.
9. Cederna PS, Chang P, Pittet-Cuenod BM, et al. The effect of the delay phenomenon on the vascularity of rabbit abdominal cutaneous island flaps. *Plast Reconstr Surg* 1997;99:183–193.
10. Taylor GI, Corlett RJ, Caddy CM, et al. An anatomic review of the delay phenomenon: II. Clinical applications. *Plast Reconstr Surg* 1992;89:408–416.
11. Larrabee WF Jr. Design of local skin flaps. *Otolaryngol Clin North Am* 1990;23:899–923.
12. Larrabee WF Jr. A finite element model of skin deformation. I. Biomechanics of skin and soft tissue: a review. *Laryngoscope* 1986;96:399–405.
13. Larrabee WF Jr, Sutton D. The biomechanics of advancement and rotation flaps. *Laryngoscope* 1981;91:726–734.
14. Larrabee WF Jr, Sutton D. Variation of skin stress-strain curves with undermining. *Surg Forum* 1981;32:553–555.
15. Gaboriau HP, Murakami CS. Skin anatomy and flap physiology. *Otolaryngol Clin North Am* 2001;34:555–569. Review.
16. Larrabee WF Jr, Holloway GA Jr, Sutton D. Wound tension and blood flow in skin flaps. *Ann Otol Rhinol Laryngol* 1984;93:112–115.
17. Galla TJ, Saetzler RK, Hammersen F, et al. Increase in skin-flap survival by the vasoactive drug buflomedil. *Plast Reconstr Surg* 1991;87:130–136.
18. Im MJ, Hoopes JE. Improved skin flap survival with nicotinic acid and nicotinamide in rats. *J Surg Res* 1989;47:453–455.
19. Mulliken JB, Healey NA. Pathogenesis of skin flap necrosis from an underlying hematoma. *Plast Reconstr Surg* 1979;63:540–545.

20. Bold EL, Wanamaker JR, Zins JE, et al. The use of fibrin glue in the healing of skin flaps. *Am J Otolaryngol* 1996;17:27–30.
21. Baker SR. Local cutaneous flaps. *Otolaryngol Clin North Am* 1994;27:139–159.
22. Jackson IT. *Local flaps in head and neck reconstruction.* St. Louis: Mosby, 1985.
23. McGregor JC, Soutar DS. A critical assessment of the bilobed flap. *Br J Plast Surg* 1981;34:197–205.
24. Aasi SZ, Leffell DJ. Bilobed transposition flap. *Dermatol Clin* 2005;23:55–64.
25. Cook JL. A review of the bilobed flaps design with particular emphasis on the minimization of alar displacement. *Dermatol Surg* 2000; 26:354–362.
26. Kalus R, Zamora S. Aesthetic considerations in facial reconstructive surgery: the V-Y flap revisited. *Aesthetic Plast Surg* 1996; 20:83–86.
27. Andradedes PR, Calderon W, Leniz P, et al. Geometric analysis of the V-Y Advancement flap and its clinical applications. *Plast Reconstr Surg* 2005;115:1582–1590.

Microvascular Free Flaps in Head and Neck Reconstruction

Douglas B. Chepeha   *Theodoros N. Teknos*

Microvascular free-tissue transfer was introduced as a technique that allowed reconstruction of defects that could not otherwise be reconstructed. The viability of the revascularized tissue and the long operating time were initial concerns. During the 1980s, use of regional pedicled flaps (pectoralis, trapezius, latissimus dorsi) overshadowed microvascular free-tissue transfer. Regional flaps were technically much easier, required only one surgical team, and supplied nonirradiated tissue. Microvascular reconstruction continued to evolve. More flap sites were described each year, and the versatility of each site was explored and expanded. More surgeons were trained in microvascular techniques, and these surgeons became increasingly adept. As microvascular surgery became more widespread, it became clear that these transfers were reliable (95% to 98%) and represented only a 4- to 6-hour increase in operating time (1).

Controversy still exists about whether microvascular reconstruction is functionally superior to pedicled reconstruction of comparable defects. Intuition suggests that revascularized free-tissue transfer is functionally superior because it allows the reconstructive surgeon to customize reconstruction of defects of the head and neck. Free flaps can be designed to provide epithelium, subcutaneous tissue, muscle, nerve, and bone in proportions that closely resemble the missing tissue.

If microvascular reconstruction is functionally superior, is it cost effective? Several studies have suggested that use of pectoralis flaps are associated with longer hospital stays and higher complication rates than free-tissue transfer in comparable primary reconstructions (2). This suggests that the costs of longer operating times associated with free-tissue transfer may be offset by the longer hospitalizations associated with pedicled transfer.

The drive for reconstructive surgeons to provide the best functional and aesthetic reconstruction for their patients made revascularized free-tissue transfer the mainstay of head and neck reconstruction in the 1990s. Much research still has to be done to establish the value and exact place of these sophisticated reconstructive techniques in the various defects encountered in the head and neck.

This chapter is divided into two sections. The first section is an introduction to free-tissue transfers commonly used in head and neck reconstruction (Table 162.1). Each flap is described in terms of design and use, anatomic characteristics, anatomic variations, potential morbidity, technical considerations, preoperative considerations, and postoperative management. The second section is an introduction approach to commonly encountered defects of the head and neck.

FASCIAL AND FASCIOCUTANEOUS FLAPS

Radial Forearm Flap

Flap Description

The radial forearm free flap is a thin fasciocutaneous flap based on the radial artery and its venae comitantes and the

TABLE 162.1

MICROVASCULAR FREE SOFT-TISSUE FLAP SELECTION IN HEAD AND NECK RECONSTRUCTION

Flap	Quality	Advantages	Disadvantages
Radial forearm	Thin, pliable	Versatility, ease	Limited bulk, skin-graft donor site
Lateral arm	Moderately thin	Primary closure of donor site	Small-caliber pedicle
Lateral thigh	Moderately thick	Large surface area of tissue, long pedicle	Challenging harvest
Anterolateral thigh	Thin, pliable	Long pedicle, large cutaneous component	Muscle associated with musculocutaneous component
Temporoparietal fascia	Ultrathin	Can be transferred as pedicle flap	Challenging harvest, limited pedicle length
Rectus	Bulky	Versatility, ease of harvest	Risk of ventral hernia
Latissimus dorsi	Moderate bulk	Large surface area, ease of harvest	Lateral decubitus position
Gracilis	Thin muscle	Can be separated into functional units	Limited tissue available

cephalic vein (Fig. 162.1). This flap can be transferred as a composite flap that contains vascularized bone, vascularized tendon, the brachioradialis muscle, and vascularized nerve. The skin of the entire forearm, from the antecubital fossa to the flexor crease of the wrist, can be harvested. The vascular pedicle is long (20 cm) and the artery is 2 to 2.5 mm in diameter. The radial forearm free flap is a source of well-vascularized, thin, pliable skin with the potential for sensory reinnervation. It can be used to reconstruct small (<60 mm) to moderate volume (<200 cm^2) defects. The flap can be folded to facilitate sophisticated reconstructions and is a souce of a small amount of vascularized bone. This flap is used most often in reconstruction of the oral cavity and base of the tongue, partial and circumferential recon-

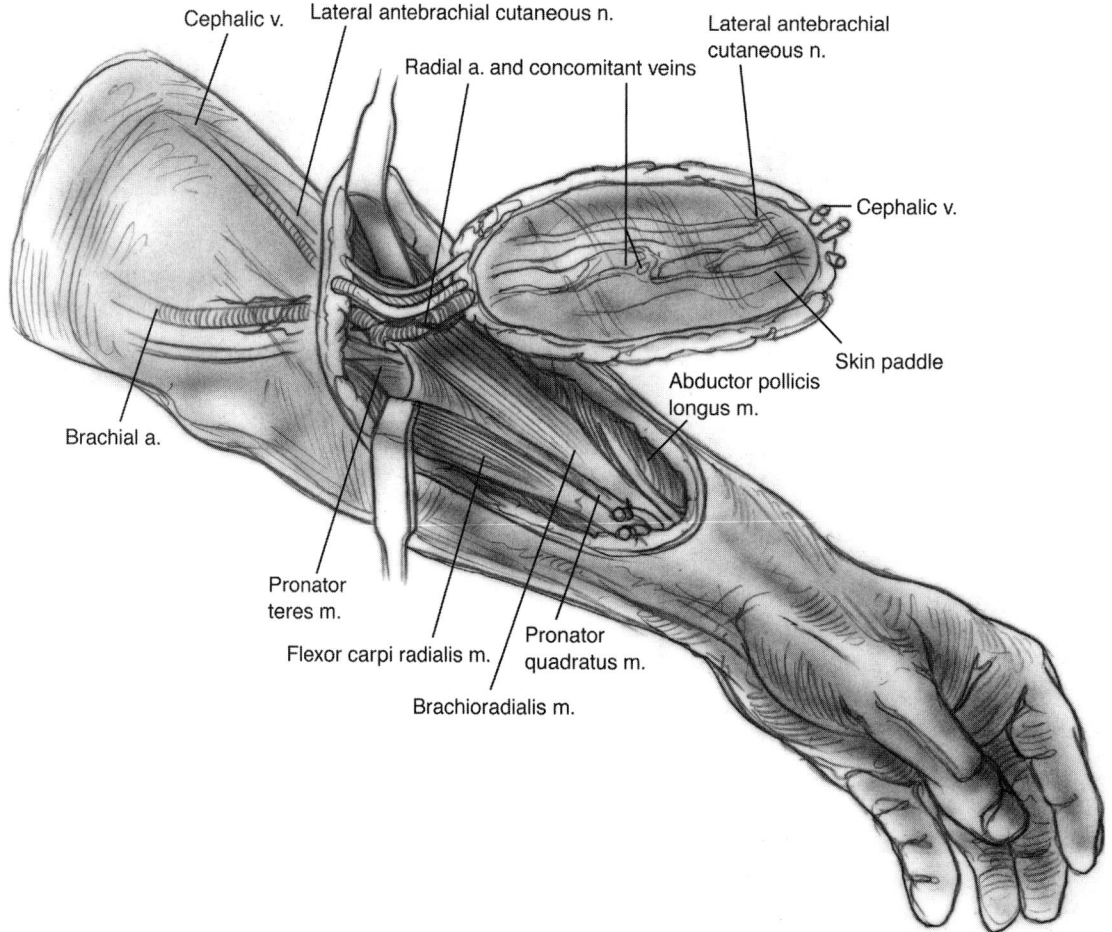

Figure 162.1 Lateral view shows left lateral forearm. The flap axis is slightly medial to the radial artery, and the flap is positioned to include the cephalic vein over the extensor compartment. Nutrient branches to the radius are immediately deep to the brachioradialis tendon. The superficial branch of the radial nerve is preserved in dissection of this flap.

struction of the pharynx, and reconstruction of the soft palate. It also can be used to manage cutaneous defects of the eye, lip, neck, and scalp. When transferred as a fascial flap, the radial forearm free flap can be used to manage soft-tissue defects and defects of the base of the skull, particularly for a previously treated patient, and local pericranial flaps are not available (3). When the flap is transferred as an osteocutaneous flap, a segment of radius 10 to 12 cm long and as much as 40% of its circumference can be harvested with overlying fascia and skin. This flap is useful for reconstruction of small-volume bone and soft-tissue defects of the face, such as the periorbital tissues, particularly if the patient has undergone or is to undergo radiation therapy (4). The disadvantages of use of the radial osteocutaneous flap are the limited amount of bone available and the risk of pathologic fracture of the radius.

Neurovascular Pedicle

The radial artery, with its two venae comitantes courses in the lateral intermuscular septum and has several fascial branches in the forearm (5). This fascial plexus supplies most of the skin in the forearm. The length of the arterial pedicle is limited by the radial recurrent artery, which is the first major branch of the radial artery after its takeoff from the brachial artery. The flap has a deep venous supply through the paired venae comitantes and the larger superficial veins, such as the cephalic vein. Numerous connections exist between the venae comitantes and the superficial venous system; these vessels provide excellent venous drainage of this flap. If necessary, and if proper testing of the venous drainage of the flap is conducted after elevation, it usually is possible to drain the flap through the superficial system alone. It is nearly always possible to drain the flap through the venae comitantes alone. The lateral antebrachial cutaneous nerve is the primary sensory nerve to the territory of forearm skin most commonly harvested. This nerve typically courses close to the cephalic vein in the upper forearm. When sensory reinnervation is needed, this nerve can be easily anastomosed to the recipient sensory nerve.

Anatomic Variations

The greatest concern in harvest of the radial forearm flap is the integrity of the ulnar arterial supply to the hand through the palmar arches. The combination of two concurrent arterial variations, an incomplete superficial palmar arch, and a lack of communication between the superficial and deep palmar arches puts the vascular supply of the thumb and index finger in jeopardy (6). This anomaly can be detected with an Allen test. This test involves assessment of capillary refill of the thumb and index finger with the radial artery occluded. The patient is asked to clench his or her fist. The examiner uses digital pressure to occlude the radial and ulnar arteries at the wrist. The patient opens the hand to approximately 10 degrees of flexion, the examiner releases the ulnar artery, and capillary refill is assessed. If there is uncertainty about digital blood flow during capillary refill assessment, Doppler assessment of the digital artery is performed, and the results are definitive.

Potential Morbidity

Often the donor site cannot be closed primarily, and a skin graft is necessary, which can be unsightly. Poor take of the skin graft can be caused by inadequate immobilization of the hand or failure to preserve the paratenon over the flexor tendons. Radial osteocutaneous flaps are limited by risk of fracture of the radius and a detrimental effect on supination, wrist flexion, grip strength, and pinch strength (7).

Technical Considerations

The design of a radial forearm flap begins with an outline of the path of the dominant subcutaneous veins and the palpable pulse of the radial artery. The flap is oriented over the radial artery and cephalic vein. It is preferable not to elevate the flap over the ulnar artery. Additional subcutaneous tissue can be incorporated into the flap when needed. During flap harvest, the paratenon over the flexor tendons is preserved to facilitate skin graft healing. If necessary, the flexor tendons can be covered with turnover muscle flaps to improve the donor-site bed for skin grafting.

Preoperative Considerations

Accurate performance of an Allen test is the most important consideration in avoiding the catastrophic complication of ischemia of the hand. When the Allen test results are equivocal, the opposite hand or an alternative flap is selected. When the patient has had an indwelling radial artery catheter, it is prudent to select another donor site.

Postoperative Management

After a fasciocutaneous flap, the forearm and wrist are immobilized with a volar splint with the wrist in the position of function for 6 to 7 days. Then a removable volar plastic splint is used for an additional 3 to 5 weeks until the skin graph is healed over the donor site. After an osseocutaneous flap, the elbow and wrist are immobilized with a full arm cast with the hand in the positon of function. This cast is left on for 4 weeks, then the wrist is immobilized with a forearm cast, and this is left on for an additional 2 weeks. The patient is encouraged to use the arm throughout the casting period. The underlying philosophy is to allow time for reshaping of the load lines in the radial bone. Any limb with circumferential dressing needs to be closely observed in the immediate postoperative period for signs of vascular insufficiency.

Lateral Arm Flap

Flap Description

The lateral arm flap is a moderately thin fasciocutaneous flap that can be reinnervated for cutaneous sensation with the posterior cutaneous nerve of the arm (8). Unlike the procedure for radial forearm flap, the donor site usually can be closed primarily when the width of harvested skin is limited to 6 to 8 cm, or one-third the circumference of the arm. Larger flaps have been harvested and necessitate that a skin graft be placed over the donor site. The flap can be harvested as a fascial flap and is a good source of vascularized tissue for augmentation of subcutaneous defects caused by lateral temporal bone resection or total parotidectomy (9). The flap can include the posterior cutaneous nerve of the forearm for use as a vascularized nerve graft. The application of the lateral arm flap is affected by the body mass index of the patient and the placement of the flap. In patients with a lower body mass index (BMI), the lateral arm can be used for low-volume oral cavity, low-volume oropharyngeal, and low-volume cutaneous defects. In patients with higher BMI, the latereal arm flap can be used for higher volume base of tongue, lateral oropharynx including the parapharyngeal space, anterior oral glossectomy, lateral temporal bone, parotid and mid facial defects (10). The thickness of the flap can be varied with flap placement, as the skin over the lateral epicondyle is much thinner than the skin over the mid upper arm. When estimating volume, it is important to remember that the subcutaneous tissue over the deltoid is more prone to long-term atrophy than the subcutaneous tissue over the mid lateral arm. Many of the applications of the lateral arm flap have been supplanted by the anterolateral thigh flap because of its larger, longer pedicle and ease of primary closure. In situations where estimation of volume is critical, the lateral arm may be a better choice than an anteroleteral thigh because of the unpredictable volume of muscle that may be included in an anterolateral thigh flap.

Neurovascular Pedicle

The vascular supply of the lateral arm flap is based on the terminal branch of the profunda brachii artery and the posterior radial collateral artery and its venae comitantes, which travel with the radial nerve in the spiral groove of the humerus. The blood supply to the skin is derived from four to five septocutaneous perforators that arise from the posterior radial collateral artery in the lateral intermuscular septum. In the region of the deltoid insertion, where the posterior radial collateral artery enters the lateral intermuscular septum, the artery has an average diameter of 1.55 mm (range: 1.25 to 1.75 mm) and a maximum pedicle length with additional dissection of 8 to 10 cm (11). Additional pedicle length and caliber can be obtained by means of extending the dissection proximally between the lateral and long heads of the triceps muscle. The muscular branches from the radial nerve to the triceps muscle must be identified and preserved when this approach is used. In practice, it is difficult to obtain more than 4 to 5 cm of pedicle length without detaching a large amount of triceps and risking damage to the motor branches to the triceps muscle. To accommodate the fairly short pedicle, the flap can be moved to a more distal location over the lateral epicondyle. A second superficial venous system incorporates the cephalic vein but is rarely used in practice. Two sensory nerves are encountered

during elevation of the flap; each arises from the proximal portion of the radial nerve. The nomenclature of these sensory nerves is confusing. The nerve that supplies sensation to the skin of the lateral arm flap is the posterior cutaneous nerve of the arm (also called the lower lateral cutaneous nerve of the arm and the inferior lateral brachial cutaneous nerve). The posterior cutaneous nerve of the forearm (also called the posterior antebrachial cutaneous nerve) runs through the lateral arm flap to the forearm and can be used as a vascularized nerve graft. A variable area of cutaneous anesthesia over the mid extensor surface of the forearm results.

Anatomic Variations

Unlike the radial forearm flap, the lateral arm flap does not affect the circulation to the distal portion of the arm. The profunda brachii artery can be interrupted without ischemic sequelae. The incidence of duplication of the profunda brachii artery ranges from 4% to 12% in different series.

Potential Morbidity

The radial nerve, which lies in the spiral groove of the humerus, is identified and protected from injury during flap harvest. Postoperative radial nerve palsy has been attributed to constrictive dressings or tight wound closure. Use of split-thickness skin grafts is preferable to exceedingly tight primary closure.

Technical Considerations

The lateral intermuscular septum is approximately 1 cm posterior to a line drawn from the insertion of the deltoid muscle and the lateral epicondyle. The central axis of the flap design is based on the intermuscular septum (Fig. 162.2). Preservation of the occipital artery as it crosses the internal jugular vein helps reduce the challenges with pedicle length and size match in lateral reconstructions.

Preoperative Considerations

The thickness of the flap is assessed by means of palpation. The flap thins and becomes more pliable the more distally it is positioned on the upper arm. By means of measurement, one can determine the width of cutaneous paddle that can be harvested and closed primarily (one-third the circumference of the upper arm).

Postoperative Management

The donor site usually can be closed primarily with minimal undermining. A suction drain is recommended. If a skin graft is used, a volar slab is fashioned and the donor site is managed in a manner similar to the radial forearm donor site.

Lateral Thigh Flap

Flap Description

The lateral thigh flap was popularized by Hayden (12), who found it useful in head and neck reconstruction. For

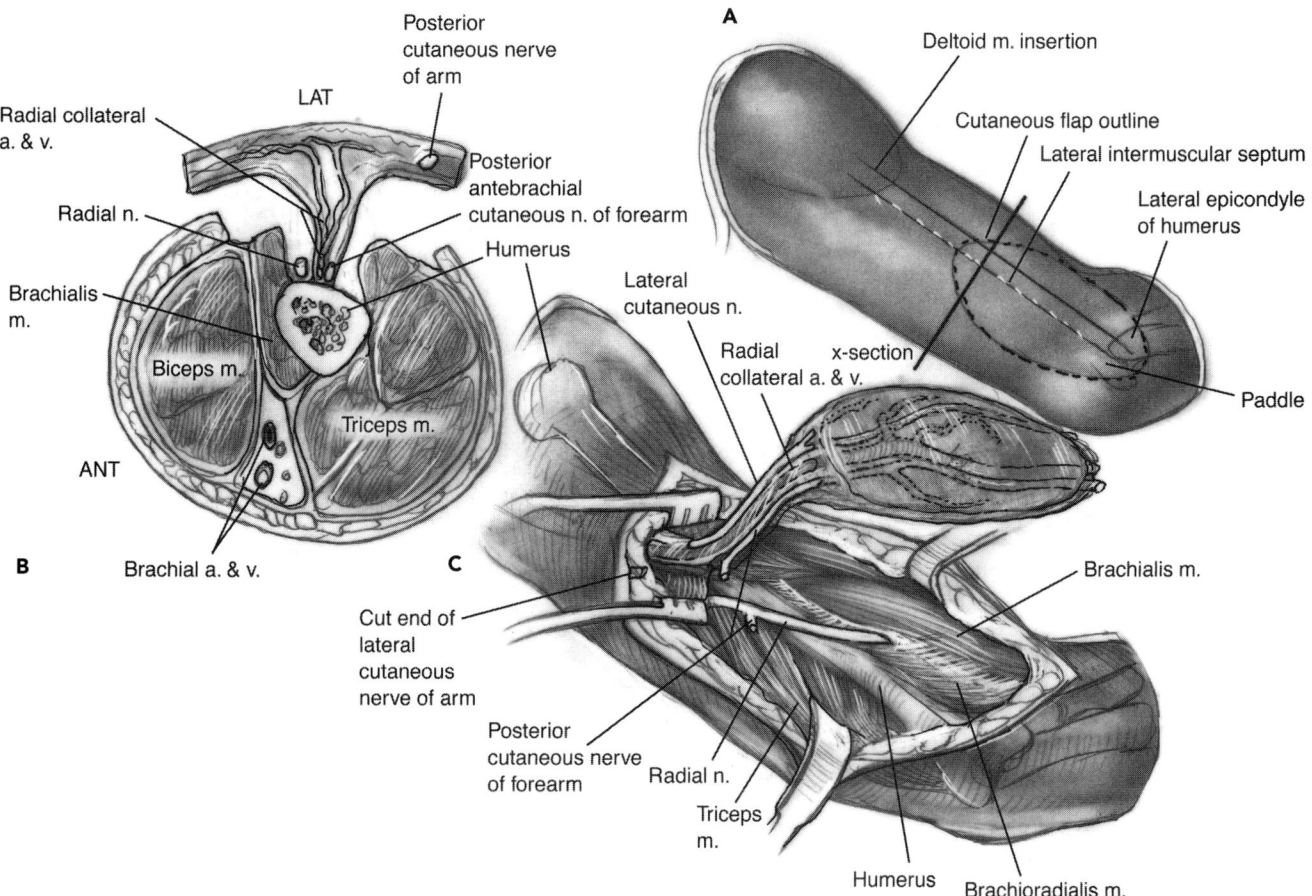

Figure 162.2 A: The flap is marked over the lateral epicondyle and 1 cm dorsal to a line drawn from the tip of the deltoid muscle to the lateral epicondyle. This position maximizes pedicle length and centers the flap over the lateral intermuscular septum. **B:** Cross section shows upper arm at the level shown in A. The lateral arm flap is elevated but still attached by the intermuscular septum to the humerus. At this level, the posterior cutaneous nerve of the arm is in the subcutaneous fat, whereas the posterior cutaneous nerve of the forearm still is in the intermuscular septum. **C:** Lateral view shows lateral arm flap, with the pedicle still in continuity. The radial nerve crosses the humerus and enters the cleft between the brachialis and the brachioradialis muscles.

selected patients with favorable body habitus, this donor site provides a large surface area of expendable tissue with an adequate vascular pedicle. Flaps as large as 25 × 14 cm have been transferred successfully (13). This fasciocutaneous flap ranges from thin to moderately thick, depending on the patient's body habitus. This flap is most useful for intraoral and pharyngeal reconstruction. With reinnervation, it is possible to restore sensation to the cutaneous portion of the flap through use of the lateral femoral cutaneous nerve. This flap is technically challenging and has been supplanted by the anterolateal thigh flap, which is technically easier to harvest and has a long vascular pedicle.

Anterolateral Thigh Flap

Flap Description

The anterolateral thigh flap is a septocutaneous or musculocutaneous flap based on the descending branch of the lateral circumflex femoral artery and its associated venea comitantes. This flap can be harvested with any of the structures supplied by the common pedicle of the lateral femoral circumflex vessels. The flap can include the tensor fascial lata, vastus lateralis, and/or the rectus femoris. The flap can be harvested as large as 20 × 15 cm. The skin is thin and pliable in most males, whereas in females, this flap can be thicker, depending on the pattern of fat deposition in the thigh. The anterolateral thigh flap has become one of the workhorse flaps for soft-tissue reconstruction in the head and neck. It has many of the same characteristics as a radial forearm flap, such as thin pliable skin and a long vascular pedicle. The anterolateral thigh flap is larger and usually has slightly more subcutansous tissue than a radial forearm flap and as a result has been nicknamed its "big brother." The nerves for sensation are the anterior femoral cutaneous and the lateral femoral cutaneous and run axially in the flap. The applications for this flap include face, neck, full-thickness buccal, hemiglossectomy, subtotal

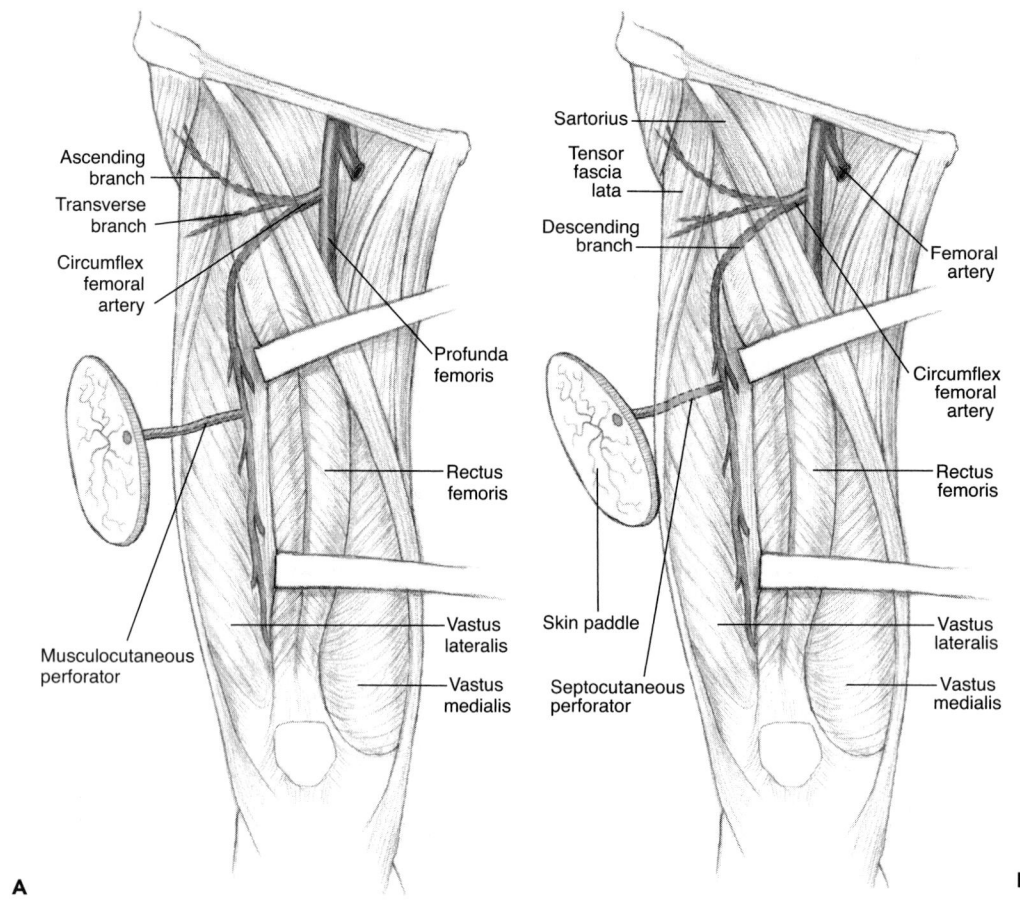

Figure 162.3   A: Type I vertical musculocutaneous perforator, which is the most common variant.
B: Type III septocutaneous perforator.

glossectomy, oropharynx, total pharyngeal, and skull base defects (14). The donor site is closed primarily when the flap is less than 9 cm in width. The disadvantage is the variable pedicle, which makes the volume of the flap unpredictable. A musculocutaneous pedicle may require inclusion of the larger portion of vastus lateralis, which will involute over the first year and can negatively impact volume-sensitive reconstructions. A perforator-based flap is an alternative, but the dissection is tedious and the free-tissue transfer becomes less reliable.

Neurovascular Pedicle
The pedicle is located on a line drawn from the anterior superior iliac spine to the lateral edge of the patella. The perforators are usually at the junction of the upper and middle thirds of the line. A Doppler probe is used to locate the perforators.

Anatomic Variations
There are four patterns of vascular supply to the skin paddle (15). There are two musculocutaneous types, the vertical musculocutaneous (50%) and the horizontal musculocuta-

neous (30%), and two septocutaneous types, the vertical septocutaneous (15%) and the horizontal septocutaneous (5%) (Figure 162.3A and B).

Potential Morbidity
There is little morbidity reported, even with harvest of large portions of the vastus lateralis. With more long-term follow-up, morbidity will become better defined.

Technical Considerations
There is wide variablility in the amount of muscle that needs to be harvested with a musculocutaneous perforator flap. The pedicle is first identified with the medial incision, but the perforators are identified with the lateral incision as they pass through the vastus lateralis into the skin paddle. Once the perforators are identified, a strip of muscle is harvested that incorporates these musculocutaneous perforators.

Preoperative Considerations
A history of vasculopathy with bypass grafts is a contraindication. For some reconstructions, a larger muscle component

may not be desirable. If a large muscle component is not desirable, an alternative site should be prepped out in the event the musculocutaneous perforators require a large muscle component. Perforator-based flaps are possible in patients with a large muscle component but are tedious and have a slightly higher failure rate.

Postoperative Management

The site can usually be closed primarily after the muscles have been approximated over a suction drain. Little rehabilitation is needed other than ambulation.

Temporoparietal Fascial Flap

Flap Description

The temporoparietal fascial flap has gained popularity in reconstruction of defects of the head and neck. In head and neck reconstruction, the fascia is most commonly transferred as a pedicled flap, but it also can be used as a free flap when the arc of rotation is inadequate. The temporoparietal fascial flap is ultrathin, highly vascular, pliable, and durable.

The flap can be transferred independently or in combination with skin. The temporoparietal fascial flap can be harvested with dimensions of 17 × 14 cm, with extensive scalp undermining. The thickness of the flap ranges from 2 to 4 mm. As a free-tissue transfer, this flap has highly specialized uses for hemilaryngeal reconstruction, or a low-volume cutaneous reconstruction when the forearm sites are not available. Most often, it is used as a rotational flap in the midface, upper face, skull base, or lateral temporal bone to cover bone, support dural closure, or support calvarial bone grafts.

Neurovascular Pedicle

The temporoparietal scalp consists of five distinct layers (Fig. 162.4A). The temporoparietal fascia is deep to the skin and subcutaneous tissue, to which it is firmly bound. The temporoparietal fascia is superficial to the temporalis muscular fascia, which envelops the muscle. Above the superior temporal line, the temporoparietal fascia becomes the galea aponeurotica (16). The superficial temporal artery and vein, which supply this flap and travel within the temporoparietal

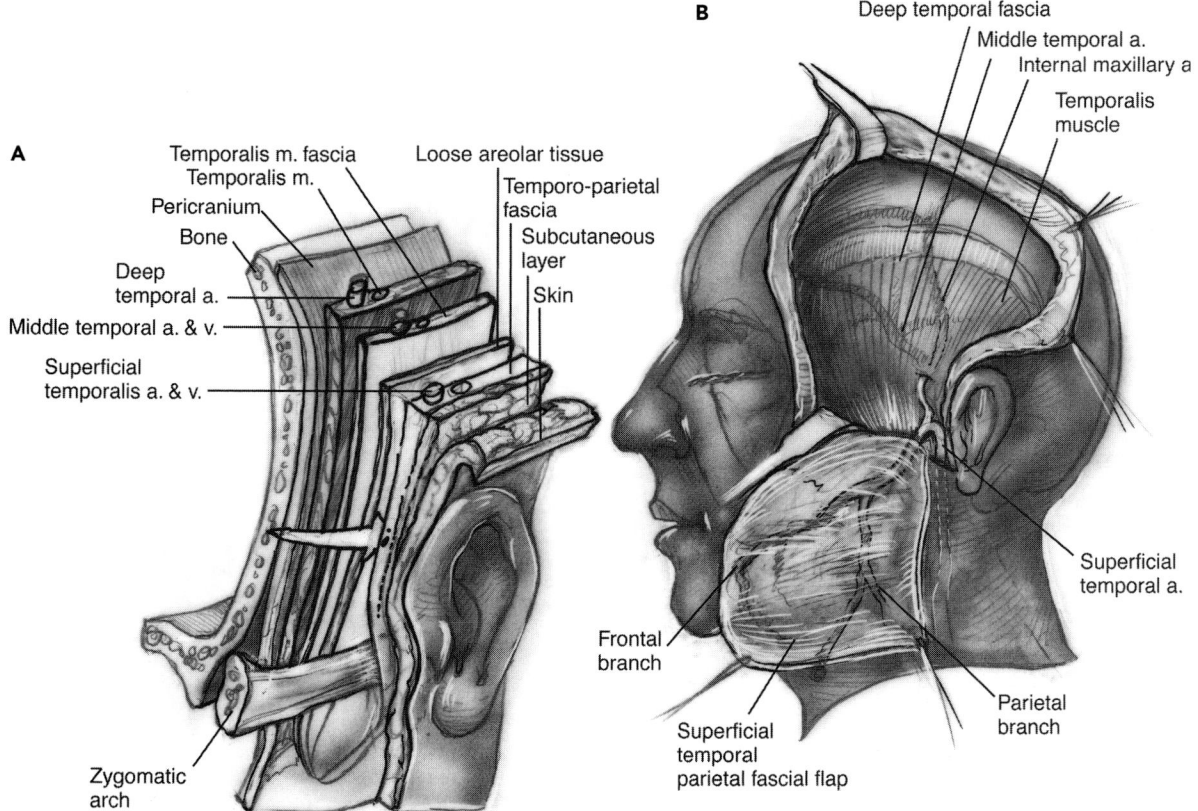

Figure 162.4 A: Cross section shows layers of the temporal scalp, superficial temporal space, and temporal skull. The superficial side of the temporoparietal facial flap is intimately associated with the subcutaneous fat of the scalp. The superficial dissection is started inferiorly just below the level of the hair follicles. As it proceeds superiorly, dissection becomes more difficult. *Arrow* denotes the deep side of the temporoparietal flap. **B:** Lateral view of the head with the temporoparietal flap folded inferiorly shows the vascular anatomic features. Dissection of the deep layer of the flap is in loose areolar tissue and is much more straightforward than is superficial dissection. Superficial dissection is completed before deep dissection.

fascial layer, are best isolated approximately 3 cm superior to the root of the helix, where the vessels branch into frontal and parietal divisions. The flap is most commonly based on the parietal branch. The base is centered over the middle third of the superior auricular helix. The frontal branch of the superficial temporal artery is routinely ligated 3 to 4 cm distal to its separation from the parietal branch to avoid injury to the frontal branch of the facial nerve. The middle temporal artery arises from the proximal superficial temporal artery at the level of the zygomatic arch and supplies the temporalis muscular fascia. If the middle temporal artery is included, a two-layered fascial flap can be raised on a single vascular pedicle (Fig. 162.4B).

Anatomic Variations

The superficial temporal artery consistently divides into two branches 3 cm above the root of the helix. Tracing the course of the posterior parietal branch with Doppler sonography ensures that the planned territory of the temporoparietal fascial flap is well vascularized.

Potential Morbidity

The anterior dissection of the flap is limited by the course of the frontal branch of the facial nerve, which also is in the temporoparietal fascia. Secondary alopecia can be caused by injury to the hair follicles by dissection that is too superficial. The venous pedicle can course with the artery or can course 2 to 3 cm posteriorly. Both the artery and vein must be included within the confines of the flap.

Technical Considerations

To harvest the temporoparietal fascial flap, a vertical incision is made from the root of the helix to the superior temporal line if a wider flap is required. A V-shaped extension at the superior limit of the incision facilitates exposure. The superficial aspect of the flap must be dissected first in a plane just below the hair follicles. The deep side of the flap is a layer of loose areolar tissue that separates the temporoparietal fascia from the temporalis muscular fascia and allows straightforward dissection. The caudal extension of the pedicle dissection is limited by the location of the main trunk of the facial nerve.

Preoperative Considerations

Prior neck or parotid surgery, previous bicoronal incision, and external carotid embolization are relative contraindications to use of a temporoparietal fascial flap. Preoperative Doppler assessment of the patency and location of the pedicle is necessary.

Postoperative Management

Meticulous hemostasis with bipolar cautery that avoids injury to the hair follicles. The site can be primarily closed over suction drainage.

MUSCLE AND MUSCULOCUTANEOUS FLAPS

Rectus Abdominis Flap

Flap Description

The rectus abdominis flap has assumed an important role in head and neck reconstruction because it is easy to harvest, has a long vascular pedicle, and is extremely reliable. The area of skin harvested with a single rectus muscle encompasses a substantial portion of the abdomen and lower chest. One can include the entire muscle or only a small portion in the paraumbilical region, where the dominant perforators are located. For patients with excessive amounts of subcutaneous tissue in the anterior abdominal wall, a thinner flap can be harvested by means of skin grafting the muscle. This flap is used to reconstruct high-volume defects such as total glossectomy defects, skull base defects, and large cutaneous defects. At present, this flap is one of the best alternatives for total glossectomy defects because the rectus fascia can be sutured to the mandible to maintain the tongue mound in a position to obliterate the oral cavity. The rectus fascia can also be used to suspend the larynx. For patients with little subcutaneous tissue, the rectus abdominis flap can be used to manage moderate-volume defects such as hemiglossectomy and lateral temporal defects. In hemiglossectomy defects where the management of the reconstructed volume is critical to long-term function, a perforator-based rectus flap may be preferable. The disadvantages of this flap are poor color match to facial skin and a tendency to become ptotic. The versatility of the rectus abdominis flap, based on the deep inferior epigastric system of vessels, is shown in Fig. 162.5. The most commonly used configuration of the rectus flap is the transverse rectus abdominus myocutaneous (TRAM) flap, which is used for breast reconstruction. This configuration can be quite useful in the head and neck, particularly when large volumes of tissue are required in low-BMI patients or when cosmesis is an issue (for example, a young, low-BMI patient with a large tongue defect).

Neurovascular Pedicle

The rectus abdominis muscle has two dominant vascular pedicles, the deep superior epigastric artery and vein and the deep inferior epigastric artery and vein. The two systems connect above the umbilicus through a system of small-caliber vessels called *choke vessels* (17). When it is used for head and neck reconstruction, the rectus abdominis flap is based on the deep inferior epigastric system because of a larger pedicle size (the deep inferior epigastric artery is an average of 3 to 4 mm in diameter) and because the musculocutaneous perforators are direct branches of the deep inferior epigastric artery and vein and can supply a much larger territory of skin. The flap can be reinnervated

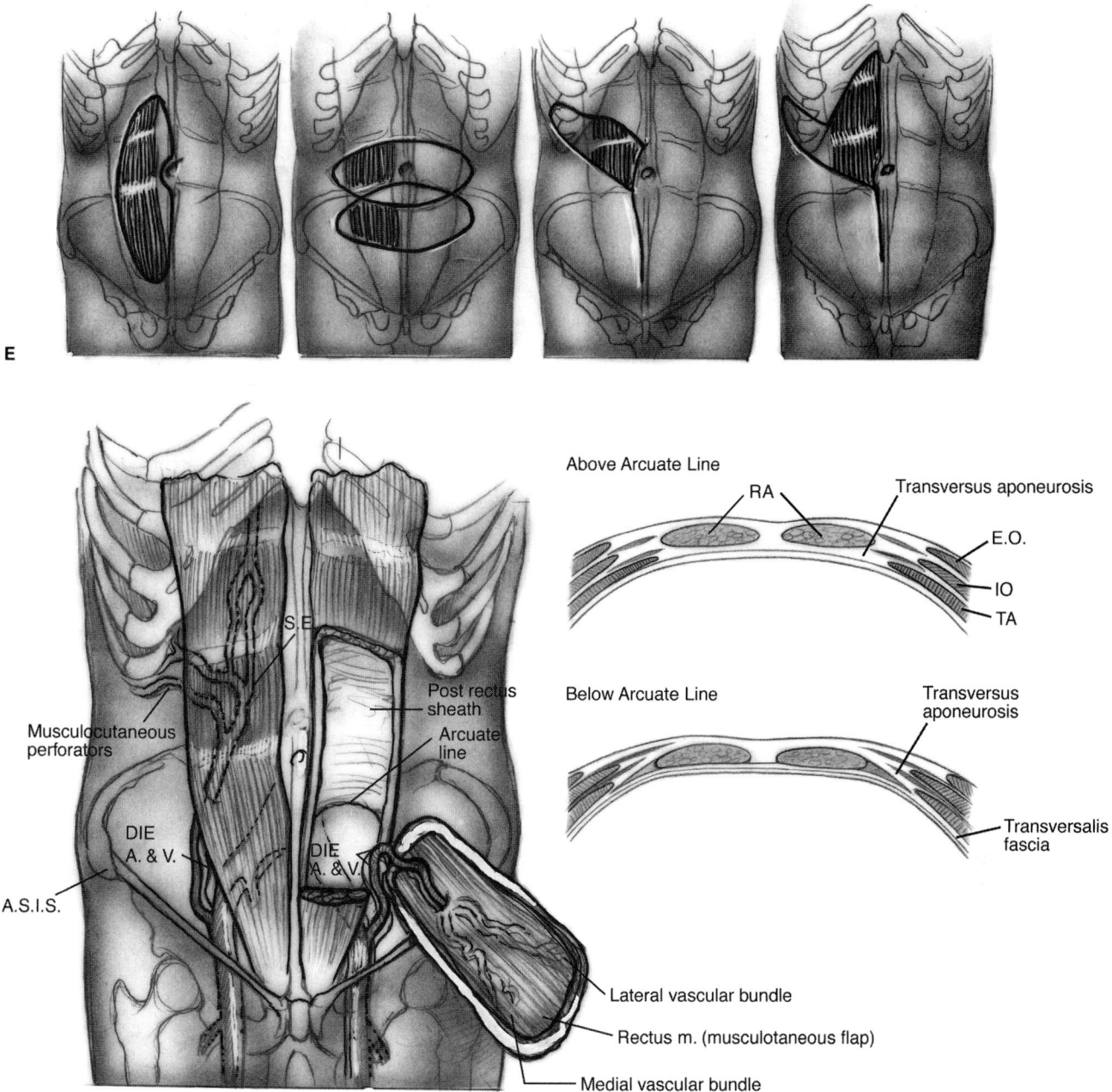

Figure 162.5 Versatility of the rectus abdominis flap. **A:** Vertical rectus flap. **B:** Middle and lower transverse rectus abdominis flaps. **C:** Thoracoumbilical rectus flap. **D:** Combined thoracoumbilical and vertical rectus flap. **E:** The abdominal wall with the left rectus muscle reflected inferiorly to expose the arcuate line. The layers of the rectus sheath are visible above and below the arcuate line.

with any of the lower six intercostal nerves, which supply segmental innervation to the rectus abdominis muscle and sensory supply to the overlying skin. The segmental sensory innervation of this flap makes it difficult to perform effective sensory reinnervation.

Anatomic Variations

Few variations of the deep inferior epigastric artery and vein have been described. Sometimes the pedicle courses an unusually long distance along the lateral aspect of the muscle before taking a medial intramuscular route.

Potential Morbidity

Removal of the rectus abdominis on one side with a portion of the overlying fascia can weaken the anterior abdominal wall and predispose the patient to ventral herniation or midline bulge. Primary closure with a 0.0 monofilament Prolene on a taper needle will decrease the likelihood of a hernia.

Technical Considerations

Understanding the anatomic characteristics of the fascial envelope is perhaps more critical for rectus abdominis flaps than it is for any other flap (Fig. 162.5E). Prevention of herniation depends on restoring the integrity of the abdominal wall through effective closure of the fascial layers. An important transition occurs in the posterior sheath at the arcuate line, which is approximately at the level of the anterior superior iliac spine. Above the arcuate line, the posterior sheath is composed of contributions from the aponeuroses of the transversus abdominis and internal oblique muscles. Below the arcuate line, the aponeurotic extensions of all three muscle layers contribute to the anterior rectus sheath. The posterior sheath is composed only of transversalis fascia. The posterior rectus sheath is sufficient to prevent abdominal herniation or bulge above the arcuate line, although most surgeons reinforce this closure with closure of the anterior rectus sheath. Below the arcuate line, the anterior sheath must be reapproximated to prevent abdominal herniation. The donor site can nearly always be closed primarily.

Preoperative Considerations

Preoperative assessment must include a careful history and physical examination of the abdomen to ensure that previous surgical procedures do not interfere with flap harvest. Rectus abdominis flaps may have to be avoided in patients who have undergone inguinal herniorrhaphy or appendectomy because there can be scarring in the region of pedicle dissection. A preoperative angiogram may be required in select patient where preexisting hernia or diastasis recti can complicate donor-site closure and militate against use of this flap. Vascular surgery, such as an aortofemoral bypass are contraindications to this flap.

Postoperative Management

Ileus can occur in the early postoperative period. Vigorous exercise that involves the abdomen is avoided for 6 weeks postoperatively.

Latissimus Dorsi Flap

Flap Description

A latissimus dorsi flap can be used for head and neck reconstruction as either a pedicled flap or a free flap. When the availability of a recipient vessel is in question, such as after radical neck dissection, this flap can be rotated onto the recipient site as a pedicled flap. When recipient vessels are available, the advantages of transferring the latissimus dorsi flap in a free-tissue transfer are as follows: There is more flexibility in flap positioning; the cutaneous portion of the flap can be centered over the vascular pedicle; the flap can be inset more superiorly, as for scalp reconstruction; and there is less risk of pedicle kinking. When the flap is transferred as muscle alone, the latissimus dorsi muscle atrophies

to a thickness of approximately 4 mm. This makes it ideal for scalp reconstruction, but poor for large-volume defects. In the setting of massive scalp defects that require the entire muscle, the elevation of the latissimus can be staged. The staging procedure is performed by elevating the distal portion of the latissimus muscle and placing clips on five or six of the segmental, paravertebral, intercostal perforators that supply the second and third angiosome. The latissimus flap is definitively elevated 3 weeks later. For large-volume defects or large cutaneous neck defects, the latissimus dorsi muscle is transferred in a musculocutaneous flap. Attempts have been made to provide mobility of the mound in total glossectomy reconstruction by reinnervating the latissimus dorsi muscle with the hypoglossal nerve.

Neurovascular Pedicle

The thoracodorsal vessels arise from the subscapular vessels, which are branches of the third portion of the axillary artery and vein. The average diameter of the artery at its origin is 2.7 mm (range, 1.5 to 4.0 mm); the diameter of the vein is 3.4 mm (range, 1.5 to 4.5 mm); the average length of the pedicle is 9.3 cm (range, 6.0 to 16.5 cm). One of the many appealing features of this flap is the length of the vascular pedicle. The thoracodorsal nerve provides motor innervation to the latissimus dorsi muscle. The thoracodorsal nerve usually crosses the axillary vessels approximately 3 cm proximal to the subscapular artery and vein.

Anatomic Variations

The arterial supply and venous drainage of the latissimus dorsi flap have a number of anatomic variations, but none precludes elevation of the flap or compromises pedicle length. The anatomic variations involve independent origin of the thoracodorsal vein or the thoracodorsal artery from the axillary artery or vein. When the origins are separated, the subscapular artery arises proximally in the axilla by an average of 4.2 cm (18).

Potential Morbidity

Marginal flap necrosis can occur, but the cause is likely that the skin paddle was designed to be over the more distal aspect of the muscle (19). There is little morbidity except when a pectoralis muscle flap has been elevated on the ipsilateral side.

Technical Considerations

The patient must be carefully positioned on a beanbag in a semidecubitus position. With the patient in a 15-degree semidecubitus position, the flap can be harvested simultaneously with the resection of the primary lesion. The anterior border of the latissimus dorsi muscle is along a line between the midpoint of the axilla and a point midway between the anterior superior iliac spine and the posterior superior iliac spine. The thoracodorsal artery and vein enter the undersurface of the muscle 8 to 10 cm below the

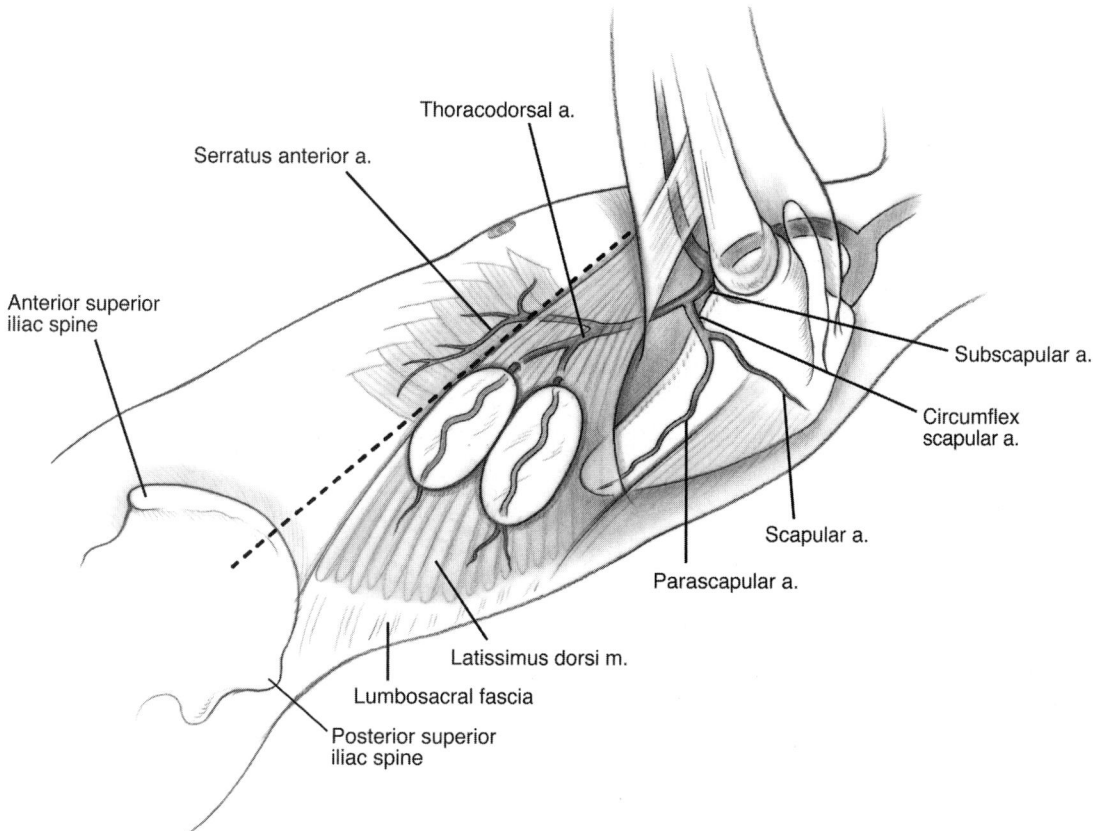

Figure 162.6 Left flank with the patient in the lateral decubitus position. The medial and lateral branches of the thoracodorsal artery are visible at the anterior edge of the muscle. The distal muscle can be used if a delay procedure that involves dividing the paraspinous perforators is performed 2 to 3 weeks before harvest. Additional pedicle length can be obtained if the circumflex scapular artery is divided.

midpoint of the axilla. The vascular branches to the serratus anterior muscle are ligated during flap harvest. The surgeon can harvest either a limited amount of latissimus dorsi muscle under the skin or the entire muscle, depending on reconstructive demands. It is possible to design a two-paddle perforator-based flap on the medial and lateral branches of the thoracodorsal vessels (Fig. 162.6). It is also possible to elevate a perforator-based latissimus flap based on the lateral branch of the thoracodorsal artery. The advantages are harvest of a small volume of latissimus muscle, preservation of the innervation of the latissimus muscle from the medial branch of the long thorassic nerve, and better control of the reconstructed volume, as there is little muscle present in the flap that will undergo atrophy, and presumably, there will be less deficit in shoulder function.

Preoperative Considerations
Previous axillary lymph node dissection is a relative contraindication to the use of the latissimus dorsi flap. Preoperative angiography has been advocated in this setting to assess the patency of the thoracodorsal vessels.

Postoperative Management
Suction drains must be placed and left in place for several days postoperatively because of the high incidence of seroma that occurs with use of with the latissimus dorsi flap.

Gracilis Flap

Flap Description
This thin muscle flap from the medial thigh was introduced by Harii et al. (20), in 1976 and was subsequently popularized as a muscle-only flap for dynamic facial reanimation. The primary use of the gracilis muscle in the head and neck has been facial reanimation, in which the muscle is both revascularized and reinnervated to restore contractile activity. To restore synchronous mimetic movement when the proximal stump of the facial nerve is not available, a two-stage procedure is performed with a cross-face sural nerve graft at the initial stage. The Tinel sign is used to monitor the progression of axonal growth across the face, which usually takes 9 to 12 months after initial transfer. When the examination shows that the distal end of the sural graft has viable axons, the free muscle is transferred, revascularized, and reinnervated to the stump of the cross-face nerve graft. The advantages of this flap

for facial reanimation are its neuromuscular structure, long vascular pedicle, and ease of dissection.

Neurovascular Pedicle

The dominant pedicle of the gracilis flap is the terminal branch of the adductor artery, which arises from the profunda femoris artery and runs a circuitous course between the adductor longus muscle anteriorly and the adductor brevis and magnus muscles posteriorly before entering the gracilis at the junction of the upper third and lower two thirds. The point of entrance of the vascular pedicle into the muscle is consistently between 8 and 10 cm inferior to the pubic tubercle. The artery to the gracilis is accompanied by two venae comitantes, which either join or drain separately into the profunda femoris vein. The caliber of the artery usually is 2 mm, and the caliber of the venae comitantes measures 1.5 to 2.5 mm. The motor supply to the gracilis muscle is the anterior branch of the obturator nerve, which enters the muscle in an oblique course approximately 2 to 3 cm cephalic to the entry point of the vascular pedicle (18).

Anatomic Variations

The main variability of the gracilis flap is the blood supply to the overlying skin rather than the vascular or nerve supply to the muscle. Yousif et al. (21) described variations in which there were no musculocutaneous perforators from the gracilis muscle, and most of the skin supply was from septocutaneous vessels or from the inferior branch of the superior external pudendal artery.

Technical Considerations

The branching pattern of the anterior division of the obturator nerve allows separation of the gracilis muscle into at least two functional muscular units. To minimize the bulk of muscle transferred, a single neuromuscular unit can be transferred that innervates the anterior portion of the muscle. The skin paddle, when needed, can be oriented longitudinally over the gracilis muscle. An alternative transverse orientation has been described. In either case, the cutaneous paddle must be centered over the dominant musculocutaneous perforator, which is 8 to 10 cm distal to the pubic tubercle (Fig. 162.7).

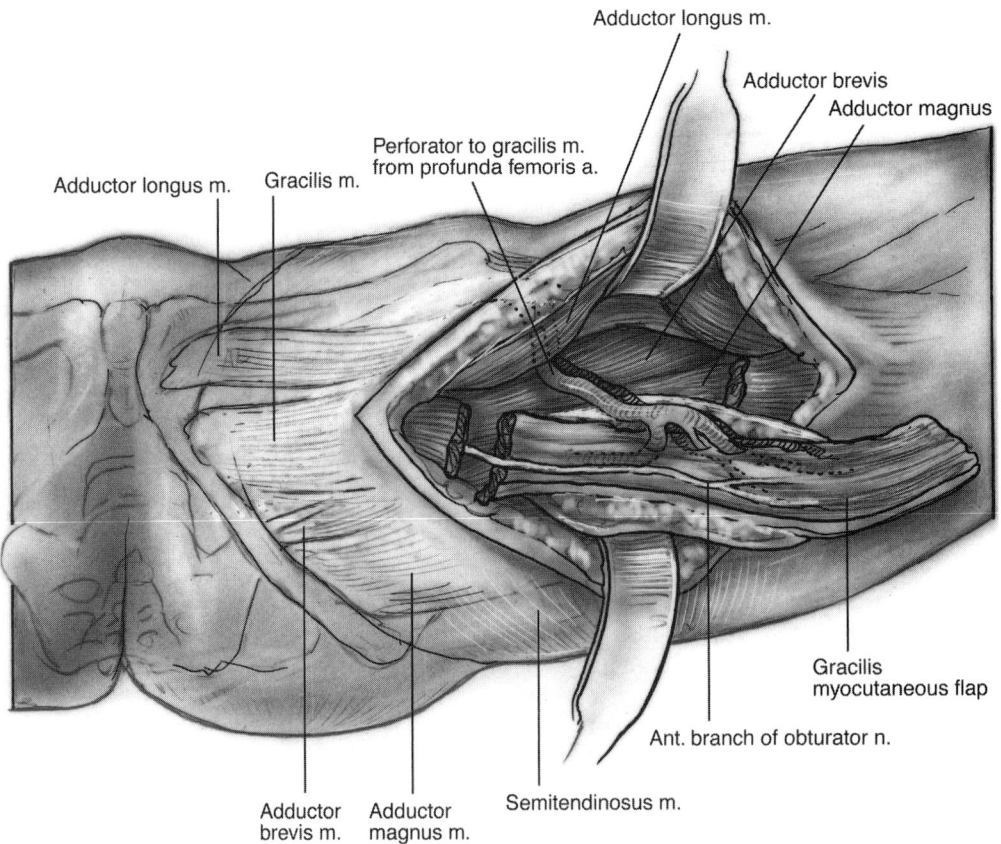

Figure 162.7 The inner thigh of the left leg with a musculocutaneous gracilis flap dissected and only attached by its pedicle. The patient is positioned with the knee flexed and the hip externally rotated. With the knee flexed, the anterior edge of the gracilis muscle is marked with a line from the adductor tubercle to the tibial tubercle. The pedicle inserts on this line approximately 8 to 10 cm from the adductor tubercle.

COMPOSITE FREE FLAPS

Fibular Osteocutaneous Flap

Flap Description

The free fibular graft was first described by Taylor et al. in 1975 (22) for long bone replacement after trauma or cancer. Hidalgo (23) first described the free fibular flap for mandibular reconstruction in 1989. The fibula provides the longest possible segment of revascularized bone (25 cm) and has the thinnest associated skin paddle. Because of the small volume of the skin paddle, large-volume soft-tissue defects may require a second revascularized flap. Although the fibula can span nearly any mandibular defect, it lacks the diameter to reconstruct many dentulous mandibles. Unless adjunctive procedures, such as onlay bone grafting or vertical distraction osteogenesis, are performed, it lacks the cross-sectional diameter to reliably fix osseointegrated implants for implant bone prosthesis. The fibula is also useful for infrastructure (oral palate) maxillary reconstruction because of its long-pedicle, thin, associated skin paddle and small-caliber bone bone stock (24). The flap is amenable to a two-team approach because of the distance between the harvest site and the head and neck area.

Neurovascular Pedicle

The peroneal artery and vein provide the primary blood supply to the fibular osteocutaneous flap. Preoperative angiography or magnetic resonance angiography are recommended to ensure adequate arterial supply to the foot when the peroneal artery is sacrificed. Sensation can be variably restored when the lateral sural cutaneous nerve is used. The branches, once they supply the skin paddle, can be multiple, small, and tedious to dissect. The peroneal communicating branch can be harvested as a vascularized nerve graft to bridge the gap in the inferior alveolar to mental nerve to restore lower lip sensation.

Anatomic Variations

Much has been reported on the reliability of the blood supply to the skin (25). The perforators that supply the skin can course entirely through the posterior intermuscular septum as septocutaneous perforators or can travel as musculocutaneous perforators through the flexor hallucis longus and soleus muscles. A cuff of flexor hallucis longus and soleus should be included in the flap harvest (Fig. 162.8A). In 5% to 10% of cases, the blood supply to the skin paddle is inadequate.

Technical Considerations

When preoperative evaluation shows that either fibula is a suitable donor site, the donor site is chosen on the basis of ease of insetting. If the skin paddle is to be placed intraorally, the flap is harvested from the leg contralateral to the side of the inset and the recipient vessels in the neck. The flap is centered over the posterior intermuscular septum, which is anterior to the soleus muscle and posterior to the peroneus muscle (Fig. 162.8B and C). A Doppler flowmeter is used to identify cutaneous perforators along the posterior septum in the 15 to 25 cm range. Schusterman et al. determined that the greatest number of cutaneous perforators is present in this region (25). Shifting the skin paddle distally increases pedicle length. Flap elevation usually is performed with a thigh tourniquet inflated to 300 mm Hg. In the event that the skin paddle is inadequately perfused, a second soft-tissue donor site, which is usually the radial forearm site, is prepared.

Potential Morbidity

A variety of donor-site complications have been reported, including rolling out of the ankle, cold intolerance, and edema. Elevation and closure are important. The motor nerve to the lateral compartment will be exposed when the peroneal muscles are dissected from their origin on the fibula. It is not technically challenging to avoid this nerve, but knowledge of its location will facilitate indentification and preservation. When reapproximating the muscles after elevation of the fibula, it is important to not injure the nerve supply to the lateral compartment and to reapproximate the flexor hallucis at an anatomic length, so that it can effectively flex the toe. An 8-cm segment of fibula is preserved both proximally and distally to protect the common peroneal nerve proximally and to ensure stability of the ankle joint distally. A skin graft sometimes is needed for closure of the donor defect and is preferable to closure under excessive tension.

Preoperative Considerations

Assessment of the vasculature to the foot is essential before fibular transfer. MRI angiography has supplanted conventional angiography in most cases. A history of lower-extremity fracture, joint replacement, and bypass grafting directs the surgeon away from a particular extremity. Careful physical examination of the lower extremity for peripheral edema or non-healing ulcers is advisable in selection of the donor site because diseases related to peripheal vascular compromise and peripheral neuropathy such as diabetes may direct the surgeon to alternative donor sites.

Postoperative Management

Distal pulses in the foot are monitored as closely, as are the flap pulses to avoid the complication of vascular insufficiency to the foot, which can be caused by excessively tight closure or dressings. A prefabricated walking boot is fit in the operating room. It is left in position for 6 to 7 days to facilitate healing of the skin graft. Then the dressing is changed daily and the patient wears the boot for another 3 to 5 weeks to allow complete healing of the skin graft and to control pain. Ambulation is initiated with

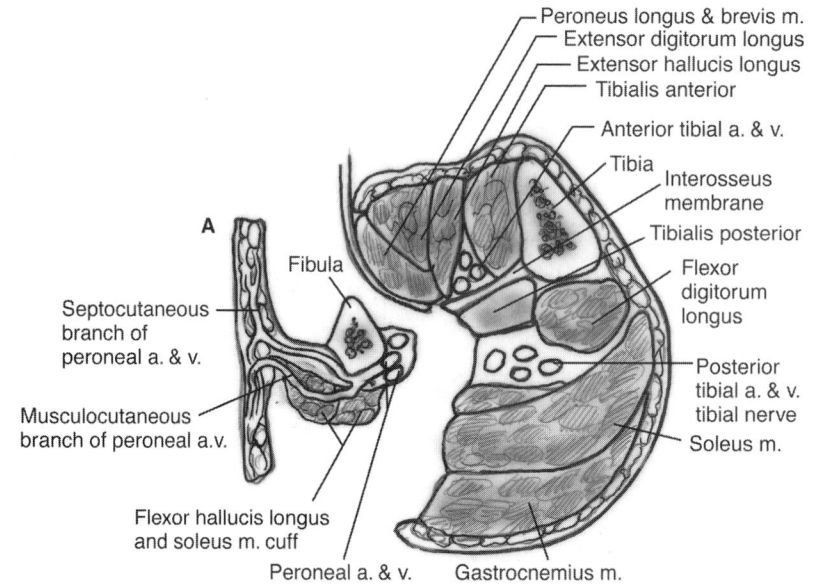

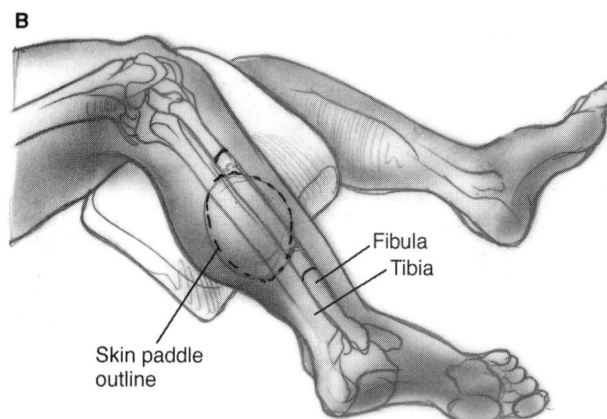

Figure 162.8 **A:** Cross-section of the leg shows the fibula flap is elevated and that both musculocutaneous and septocutaneous perforators course from the peroneal artery to the skin paddle. **B:** The flap is marked on the lateral aspect of the right leg. The cutaneous paddle is marked along the posterior intermuscular septum, which is visible when the foot is flexed and inverted. Dominant cutaneous perforators can be located with a Doppler flowmeter before the flap is elevated (10 to 25 cm distal to the fibular head). The presence of septocutaneous perforators can be confirmed after the cutaneous portion of the flap over the lateral compartment is elevated. **C:** Flap detached from the vascular pedicle with the soleus muscle still attached for illustrative purposes. The anterior approach to this flap is useful for obtaining a wide cuff of flexor hallucis and soleus muscles to encompass the musculocutaneous perforators.

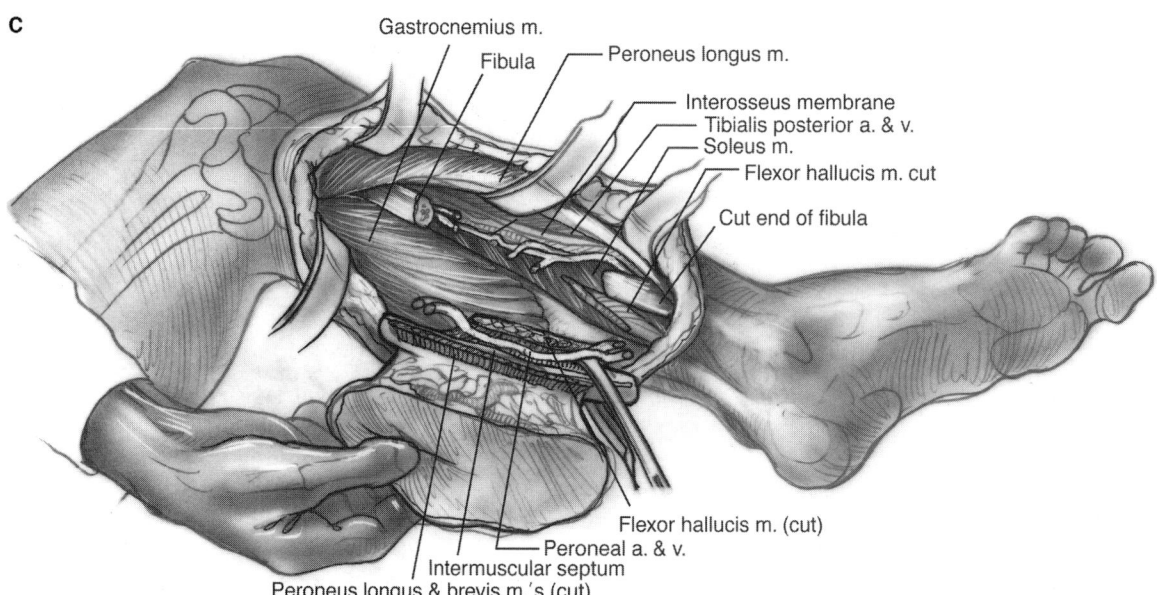

partial weight bearing on the third postoperative day, with the assistance of physical therapy and a walker. Full weight bearing with the assistance of a walker or a cane can take place on postoperative day five.

Osteocutaneous and Osteomusculocutaneous Iliac Crest Flaps

Flap Description

The iliac crest flap can be harvested as an osseous, osseomyous, or an osseomyocutaneous flap. The pedicle is 5 to 6 cm long and can be lengthened if the segment of iliac crest is harvested at a more distal site. The original descriptions of the flap (22,26) were for mandibular reconstruction. Up to 16 cm of bone can be harvested. When harvested as an osseous flap, it is ideal for segmental mandibular defects with very limited soft-tissue component, such as those associated with odontogenic lesions. When harvested as a myosseous flap, it is ideal for segmental mandibular and maxillary defects with limited associated soft-tissue defects. The osseomyocutaneous is excellent for combined external skin defects. The skin paddle does not rotate easily into the oral cavity. If there is a large soft-tissue component combined with a segmental mandibular defect, the scapula flap or two flaps may be a better alternative. The iliac crest is also the best flap for retention of osseointegrated implants, as it has the largest cross-sectional area when compared to a fibula or scapula flap. The iliac crest is not the most commonly used osseous flap in oromandibular reconstruction because oral cavity defects usually involve intraoral soft tissue of the tongue, cheek, or palate and would require a second flap in addition to the iliac crest flap. The associated donor site morbidity is greater than either the fibula or the scapula.

Neurovascular Pedicle

The deep circumflex iliac artery arises from the lateral aspect of the external iliac artery, approximately 1 to 2 cm cephalic to the inguinal ligament. The ascending branch of the deep circumflex iliac artery supplies the internal oblique muscle in 80% of the cases. The remaining patients have multiple smaller branches supplying the internal oblique from the deep circumflex iliac artery (DCIA). This vascular pattern does not prevent use of the internal oblique muscle. The deep circumflex iliac vein usually is composed of two paired venae comitantes, which merge a variable distance lateral to the external iliac vein. The caliber of the deep circumflex iliac artery is 2 to 3 mm. That of the deep circumflex iliac vein ranges from 3 to 5 mm. There is no easily identifiable sensory component.

Potential Morbidity

Herniation of the abdominal wall can occur in the postoperative period. Meticulous, layered closure of the abdominal wall is essential to prevent ventral hernia. The transversus abdominis muscle is approximated to the cut edge of the iliacus muscle. This layer can be reinforced by means of placing drill holes into the cut edge of the iliac bone through which sutures are placed to reinforce the deep layer of closure. The next layer of closure approximates the external oblique muscle and aponeurosis to the tensor fascia lata and gluteus medius muscles. To decrease the likelihood of direct herniation, the internal oblique muscle is retained in a position inferior to the anterior superior iliac spine. This triangle of muscle is closed back to the lateral rectus sheath; 2.0 or 0.0 polypropylene is used, and a figure-of-eight suture is placed for each layer of this closure. The iliac crest osseomyocutaneous flap has robust blood supply to the bone and internal oblique muscle, but problems can occur with the blood supply to the skin. The skin is supplied by perforators from the deep circumflex iliac artery. The perforators can be easily sheared as they pass through all three layers of the abdominal wall.

Technical Considerations

The skin paddle is centered on an axis drawn from the anterior superior iliac spine to the inferior tip of the scapula (Fig. 162.9). Along this line, the zone of cutaneous perforators starts approximately 9 cm from the anterior superior iliac spine. The perforators are about 2.5 cm medial to the edge of the iliac crest. A generous cuff of external oblique, internal oblique, and transversus abdominis layers must be preserved as the cutaneous perforators course through these layers. This produces a bulky, relatively immobile skin paddle. The skin must not be rotated independently of the bone, to avoid twisting or stretching the cutaneous perforators.

Preoperative Considerations

Evidence of ventral herniation or previous inguinal herniorrhaphy can lead the surgeon to select an alternative donor site. If the patient has severe peripheral vascular disease, the surgeon needs to be sure that iliac artery bypass grafting has not been performed. If bypass grafting has not been performed, angiography of the deep circumflex iliac artery is performed to ensure vessel patency.

Postoperative Management

Progressive mobilization begins on the third postoperative day. On the fifth postoperative day, the patient can walk with a walker and progress to a cane and independent walking, as tolerated. Rigorous abdominal exercise is avoided for 3 months.

Fasciocutaneous and Osteofasciocutaneous Scapular and Parascapular Flaps

Flap Description

The unique features that make the scapular system of flaps so useful for head and neck reconstruction include the long length and caliber of the vascular pedicle; the abundant surface area of relatively thin skin that can be transferred; the separation of the soft-tissue and bone flaps,

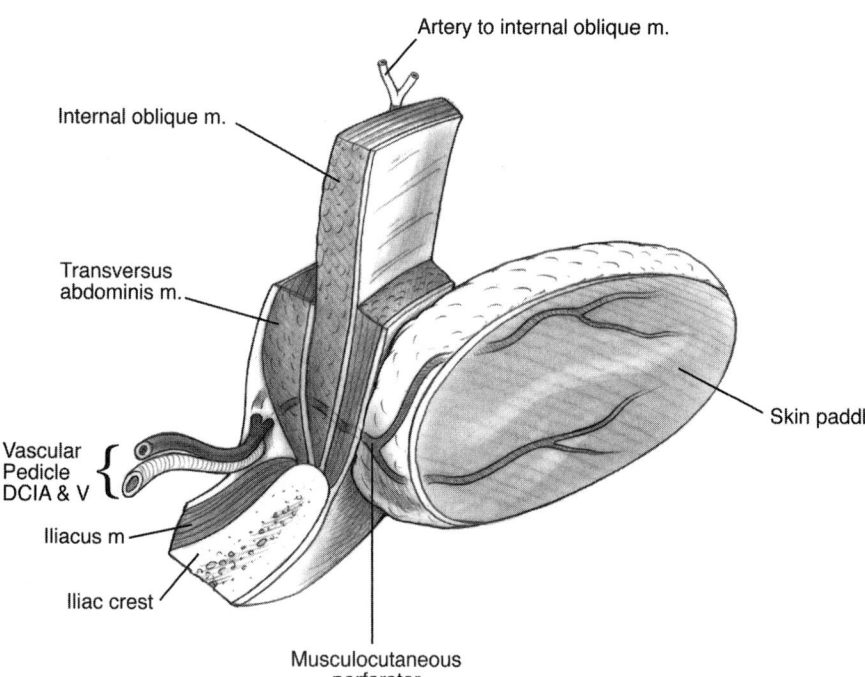

Artery to internal oblique m.

Internal oblique m.

Transversus
abdominis m.

Vascular
Pedicle
DCIA & V

Iliacus m

Iliac crest

Musculocutaneous
perforator

Skin paddle

Figure 162.9 Vascular anatomic features of the iliac crest flap. The deep circumflex iliac artery (*DCIA*) courses in the superior aspect of the iliacus muscle. After it gives off the the ascending branch, the DCIA runs in the groove between the iliacus and transversus abdominis muscles before penetrating the transversus abdominis muscle and passing over the pelvic brim near the posterior superior iliac spine. The bone must be cut low enough to include the pedicle. The ascending branch can be identified on the undersurface of the internal oblique muscle and dissected proximally to help identify the DCIA. *DCIV*, Deep circumflex iliac vein.

which provides the most freedom for three-dimensional insetting; and the ability to combine the scapular flap with the latissimus dorsi and the serratus anterior muscles, with or without overlying skin. This flexibility allows closure of complex orofacial defects (22). Up to 10 cm of bone, harvested from the lateral aspect of the scapula below the glenoid fossa, can be reliably transferred. The bone stock is variable and may be inadequate for the placement of osseointegrated implants for the purpose of mandibular rehabilitation. The fasciocutaneous flap is an excellent source of well-vascularized, moderately thin, hairless skin. The circumflex scapular artery has two cutaneous branches, which can supply two cutaneous flaps. The horizontally oriented scapular flap is based on the transverse cutaneous branch, and the vertically oriented parascapular flap is based on the descending cutaneous branch (27) (Fig. 162.10). The scapular flap is used most often to manage complex composite midfacial or oromandibular defects. A variation that is being used with increasing frequency is the scapular tip flap. This flap is a latissimis dorsi flap that is harvested with the scapular tip that is supplied by several branches from the thoracodorsal artery. This variation has a long vascular pedicle, supplies the entire scapular tip, and is useful for complex multisurfaced, high-volume midface and combined orbital reconstructions. This flap can be considered a latissimis osseomyocutaneous flap and can be combined with any variation of the scapular flap.

Neurovascular Pedicle

The parent vessels of the scapular flap are the subscapular artery and vein, which arise from the third part of the axillary artery and vein. The circumflex scapular artery and vein emerge from the triangular space defined by the teres

major and teres minor muscles and the long head of the triceps muscle. The circumflex scapular artery is accompanied by paired venae comitantes, which usually join the thoracodorsal vein before entering the axillary vein. The average diameter of the circumflex scapular artery at its takeoff from the subscapular artery is 4 mm. At its origin from the axillary artery, the subscapular artery has an average diameter of 6 mm. When the circumflex scapular artery is harvested at its takeoff from the subscapular vessels, the fasciocutaneous flap has a pedicle length of 4 to 6 cm. Although a maximum pedicle length of 11 to 14 cm has been extensively quoted in the literature, in pratice the length is much closer to 8 cm. The latissimus dorsi musculocutaneous flap, the scapular tip, and a portion of the serratus anterior muscle can be carried by the same vascular pedicle. When both the latissimus and scapular flaps are elevated, this flap can be referred to as a "mega" flap.

Anatomic Variations

There are five anatomic variations, but they are of little clinical consequence. The most common pattern is a single subscapular artery and a single subscapular vein supplying both the scapula and the latissimis flap. One of the variations is a duplicated circumflex artery. Of the remaining variations three, all are related to separate origins of the vein or artery for each of the two flaps.

Potential Morbidity

Morbidity of the brachial plexus can be caused by lateral decubitus positioning during flap harvest. If the patient is positioned fully decubitus, an axillary roll is needed, as is careful attention to arm positioning. Scapular osteotomy must stay 1 cm inferior to the glenoid fossa to avoid injury

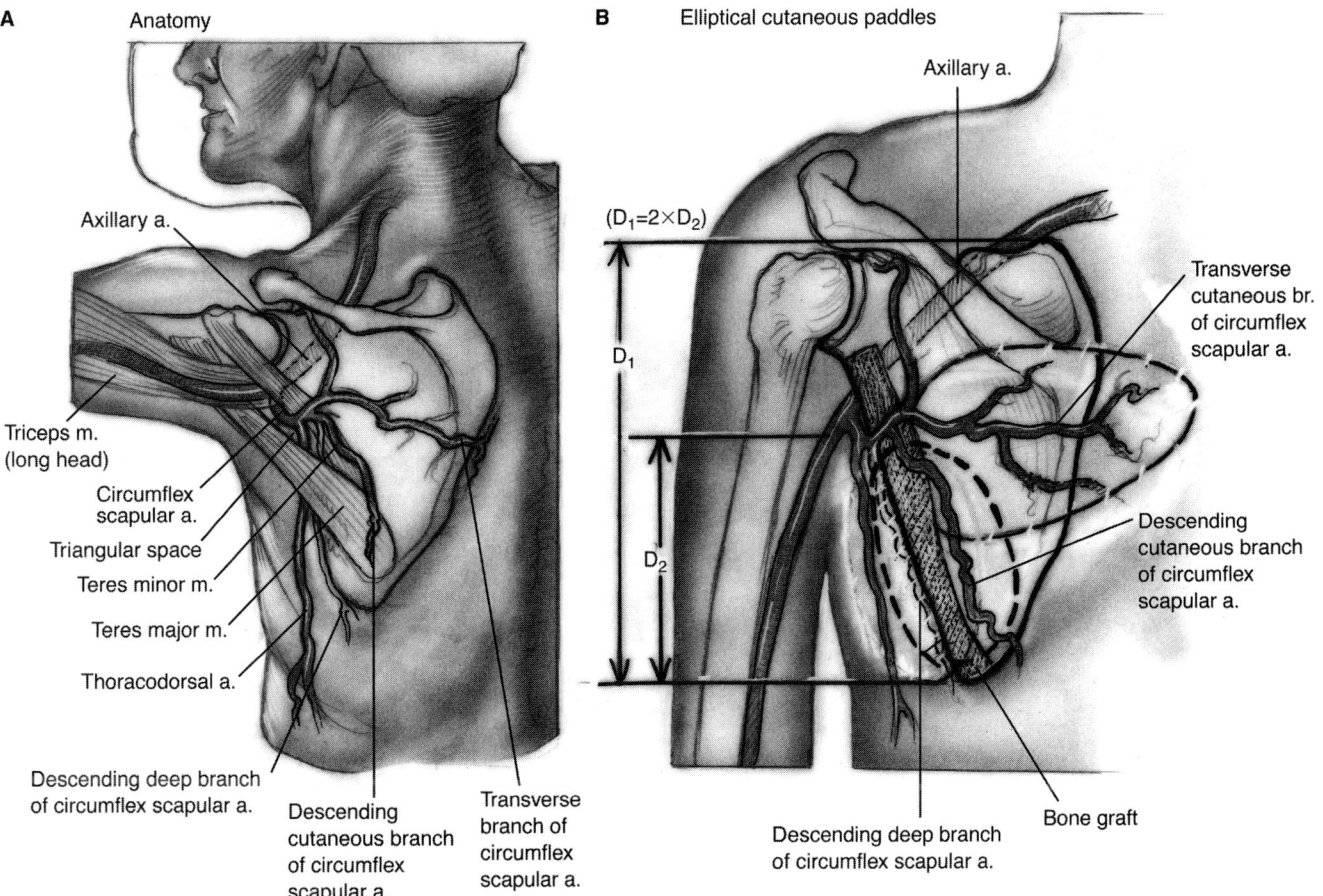

A Anatomy

Axillary a.

Triceps m.
(long head)

Circumflex
scapular a.

Triangular space

Teres minor m.

Teres major m.

Thoracodorsal a.

Descending deep branch
of circumflex scapular a.

Descending
cutaneous branch
of circumflex
scapular a.

Transverse
branch of
circumflex
scapular a.

B Elliptical cutaneous paddles

Axillary a.

$(D_1 = 2 \times D_2)$

D_1

D_2

Transverse
cutaneous br.
of circumflex
scapular a.

Descending
cutaneous branch
of circumflex
scapular a.

Descending deep branch
of circumflex scapular a.

Bone graft

Figure 162.10   A: Vascular anatomic features of the left scapula. The subscapular artery sends the circumflex scapular branch through the triangular space to the scapular flap. The muscles that define the triangular space are palpated and marked preoperatively. The soft triangle is best approached by means of dissection over the teres major muscle at the lateral boarder of the scapula. Once the triangular space is located, the teres minor muscle can be retracted superiorly, and the pedicle can be dissected through the axillary space. **B:** The triangular space also can be located by means of marking the midpoint of the lateral aspect of the scapula. Three of the possible scapular paddles and their vascular supply are outlined. The deep branch is intimately associated with the lateral border of the scapula, which it supplies. If a bone flap is to be included, care is taken not to injure the deep branch after dissection of the cutaneous flaps.

to the joint space. Harvest of the scapular osteocutaneous flap necessitates detachment of the teres major, teres minor, subscapularis, and infraspinatus, which can cause shoulder weakness and limited range of motion. These muscles must be meticulously reapproximated.

Technical Considerations
To make two-team surgery easier, the patient can be placed in a 15-degree decubitus position with the assistance of a beanbag. Flap harvesting is technically more difficult than it is when the patient is in a 15-degree decubitus position, but the benefit is reduction in total operative time. A separate axillary incision can be helpful in dissecting the pedicle to the axillary artery and vein. If the bone of the scapula is elevated, the teres major, subscapularis, and latissimus dorsi muscles are reattached to the scapula with 2.0 or 0.0 polypropylene. Care is taken not to injure the motor nerve supply to the teres major muscle during flap elevation.

Modified Kirchmeyer sutures can be useful for optimizing reapproximation of the cut end of the teres major muscle to the scapula.

Preoperative Considerations
Previous axillary node, dissection, shoulder reconstruction or prior shoulder dislocation is a contraindication to the use of fasciocutaneous and osteofasciocutaneous scapular and parascapular flaps.

Postoperative Management
If the scapular skin paddle is raised without bone, shoulder pain is minimized by immobilization for 3 or 4 days, followed by active range of motion exercises. If an osseocutaneous scapular flap has been raised, the shoulder is immobilized for 5 days to allow healing and pain resolution. A physical therapy program that includes active and passive range of motion is begun.

VISCERAL FLAPS

Jejunum

Flap Description

The free jejunal autograft has been successful in reconstruction of circumferential pharyngoesophageal defects (28). The diameter of the jejunum is a good match with the cervical esophagus and maintains an ideal mucosal surface for food bolus transit. In one series, (29) jejunal free-flap reconstruction of circumferential defects of the pharyngoesophagus was accomplished with low mortality (5%) and early functional restoration in terms of swallowing. The graft is harvested by a general surgeon in a simultaneous two-team approach.

Neurovascular Pedicle

Transilluminating the mesentery facilitates selection of a segment of intestine with sufficient arborization from a single mesenteric artery and vein to supply the graft (Fig. 162.11). The second arcade of the jejunum usually is best for pharyngeal reconstruction.

Potential Morbidity

Stricture of the upper or lower anastomosis occurs in about 10% of free jejunal transfers and responds well to dilation. This rate of stricture is lower than that encountered when tubed cutaneous flaps are used. Despite the lower stricture rate and relative ease of inset, the jejunum can have long-term functional problems. The peristalsis of the jejunum produces functional obstruction during swallowing, a wet voice among patients who speak by means of

tracheoesophageal puncture, and dysgeusia from the succus entericus. The long-term functional problems can be nearly eliminated with postoperative radiation therapy. This reconstruction is optimal for a planned combined surgery followed by radiation therapy.

Technical Considerations

A suture is placed at the proximal end of the graft at harvest to ensure isoperistaltic reconstruction of the pharyngoesophagus. Any redundancy of the jejunal segment is avoided to prevent dysphagia. The proximal end of the jejunum can be divided along the antimesenteric border to facilitate closure to the tongue base. The distal end of the jejunum is anastomosed in an end-to-end manner to the stump of cervical esophagus. To break up the circumferential scar, a lock-and-key type of closure can be made by means of vertical incision of the cervical esophagus. Postoperative monitoring is facilitated by exteriorizing a monitoring segment of the jejunum. This segment is based on the same mesenteric arcade as the rest of the flap (30). This segment can be observed for peristalsis and evaluated directly with a Doppler probe.

Preoperative Considerations

Extension of disease into the proximal thoracic esophagus is an absolute indication for esophagectomy and gastric pull-up. Several donor-site factors point the surgeon toward an alternative method of reconstruction. These include presence of ascites, chronic intestinal diseases such as Crohn disease, and previous extensive abdominal surgery or intraperitoneal sepsis. Patients with limited pulmonary reserve are at increased risk of morbidity after laparotomy.

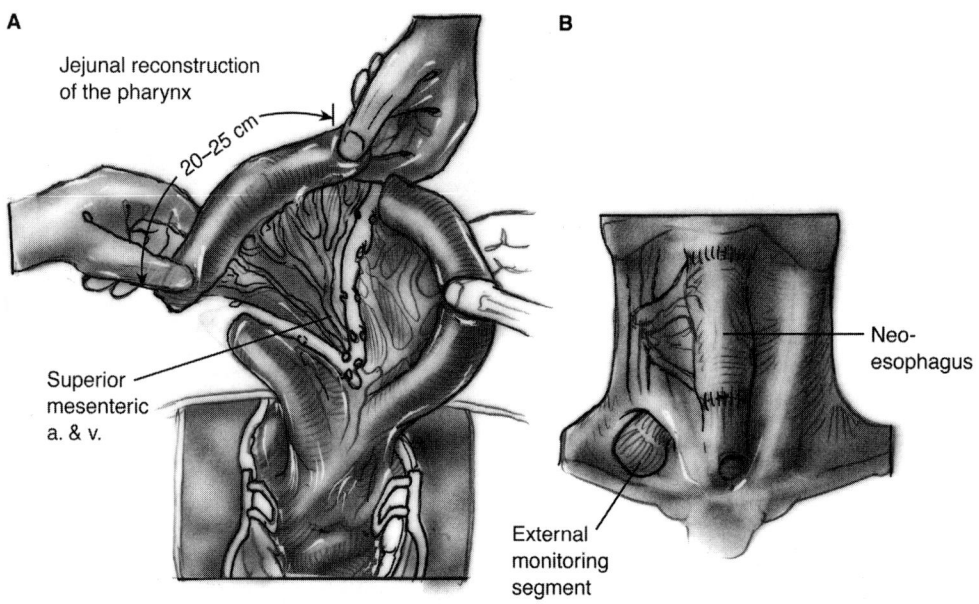

Figure 162.11   A: Segment of proximal jejunum of sufficient length supplied by a single arcade. **B:** The jejunum is shown as a segmental reconstruction of a total pharyngeal defect with a monitoring segment. The jejunum is inset under a minor degree of tension to reduce dysphagia.

Postoperative Management

The external monitoring segment of jejunum is removed at the bedside on postoperative day seven by means of suture ligation of its mesentery.

Omentum and Gastroomentum

Flap Description

The greater omentum is a double layer of peritoneum that hangs like a sheet from its main attachments to the greater curvature of the stomach and transverse colon (Fig. 162.12). The blood supply to this structure arises from the right and left gastroepiploic vessels, which course in the cephalic edge of the omentum, where it attaches to the stomach (31). The omental free flap has a variety of uses in head and neck reconstruction, including coverage of large scalp defects, repair of extensive midfacial defects with coverage of split rib or calvarial grafts, management of osteoradionecrosis and osteomyelitis in the head and neck region, and facial contouring. Gastroomental free flaps can be used for oral or pharyngeal defects; omentum is used to provide carotid coverage. The surgeon must carefully weigh the functional and aesthetic benefits of this flap against the risks of an intra-abdominal procedure.

Neurovascular Pedicle

The right gastroepiploic artery is more favorable for supplying omental flaps. The diameter of the right gastroepiploic artery ranges from 1.5 to 3.0 mm.

Potential Morbidity

A wide range of intra-abdominal complications can occur after harvest of a gastroomental free flap. The most serious is gastric leak with peritonitis and intra-abdominal abscess formation. Gastric outlet obstruction can occur if the mucosal flap is too large or is placed too close to the pylorus.

Preoperative Considerations

A history of gastric outlet obstruction or peptic ulcer disease is a contraindication to this procedure.

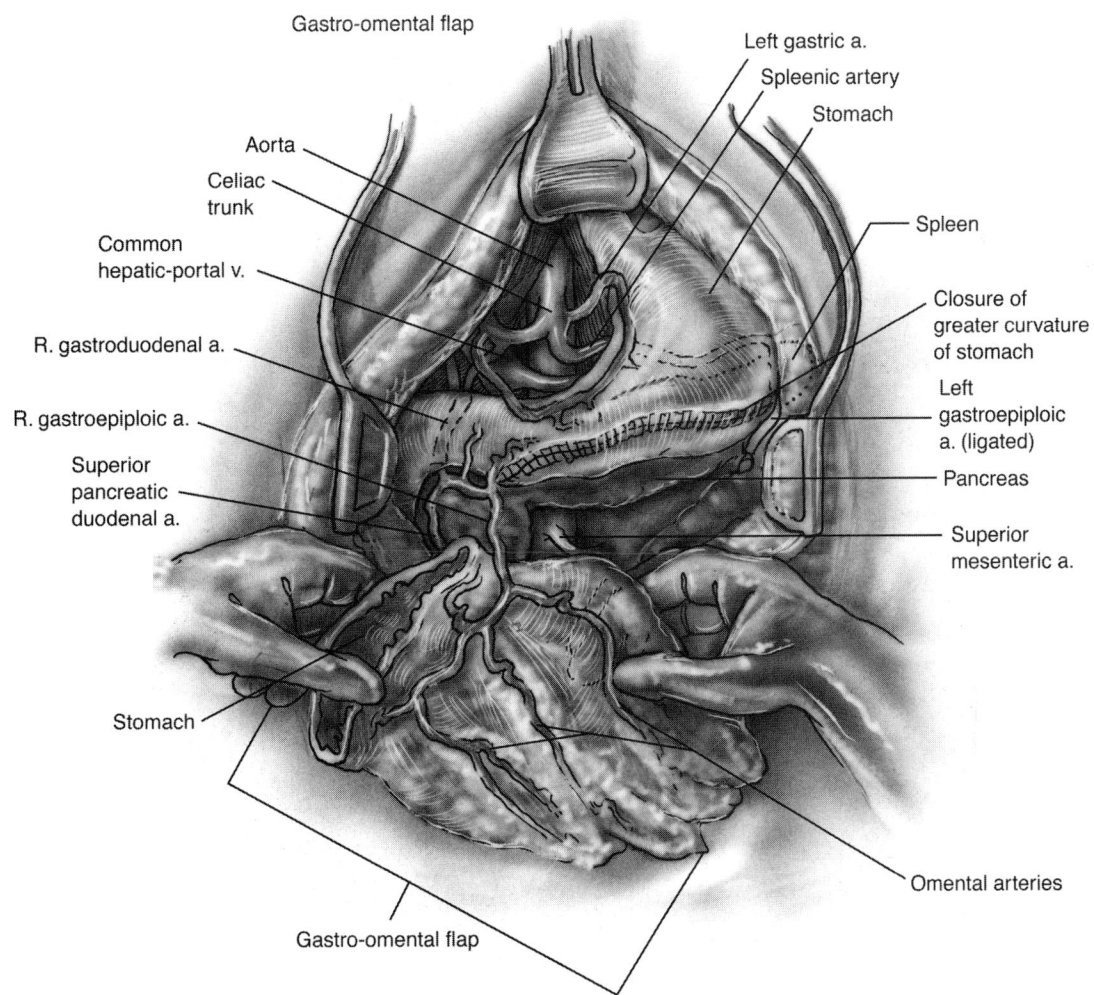

Figure 162.12 Gastroomental flap completely elevated from the greater curvature of the stomach.

MICROVASCULAR RECONSTRUCTIVE APPROACHES TO DEFECTS IN THE HEAD AND NECK

When reviewing various reconstructive approaches in the literature, it can be difficult to interpret results within a study or compare results between studies because there is no universally adopted system for coding head and neck defects. An effort has been made to classify defects on the basis of loss of epithelium, bone, nerves, and supporting musculature (32).

Pharyngoesophageal Defects

Pharyngoesophageal defects are classified according to circumferential involvement (partial, near total, and total) and whether the esophagus or a large portion of the oropharynx was included in the resection. Also important in determining the optimal reconstruction is consideration of the mechanism of postoperative voice production (tracheoesophageal puncture versus electrolarynx) and the use of postoperative radiation therapy.

Partial pharyngoesophageal defects are defects in which approximately 50% of the pharynx has been sacrificed, such as one piriform fossa and 50% of the posterior pharyngeal wall, and primary closure cannot be performed without high risk of pharyngeal stenosis. Near-total pharyngoesophageal defects are defects in which only a thin strip of pharynx (1 cm) remains. Total pharyngeal defects are those in which there is complete absence of a segment of the pharyngoesophagus and is the defect in which free-tissue transfer has had the greatest impact.

Partial and near-total pharyngeal defects can be reconstructed with either pedicled regional flaps or free-tissue transfer. The following factors are taken into account to assist in decision making: (a) There must be adequate vascular access for a free-tissue transfer. (b) If a modified radical or radical neck dissection has been performed and carotid protection is believed beneficial, a pedicled regional flap such as a pectoralis or latissimus dorsi flap can be used so that the muscle can be laid over the great vessels. (c) If there is a total or near total defect and the regional flaps are thicker than 2 cm, use a free-tissue transfer that is thinner than 2 cm.

For total pharyngoesophageal defects, four types of reconstructions are considered; these include a gastric transposition (this is a pedicled flap), colon interposition, free-tissue jejunal transfer, and large free fasciocutaneous transfers such as radial forearm or an anterolateral thigh. The majority of total pharyngeal reconstructions can be performed with a free jejunal or free fascial free-tissue transfer. If the defect extends into the mediastinum, preoperative consultation with a thorasic surgeon and planning of a colon interposition flap is appropriate. Gastric transpositions are no longer the best reconstructive option because they do not remain well vascularized when extended up into the oropharynx and are associated with significant reflux.

The jejunal flap was once the technique most commonly used to reconstruct total pharyngoesophageal defects. The shortcomings are a wet voice, especially if the patient does not undergo postoperative radiation therapy, and dysphagia from autonomous peristalsis, halitosis, and difficulty with reconstructing more extensive oropharyngeal defects. Fasciocutaneous flaps (radial forearm, anterolateral thigh) are replacing the jejunum as the reconstructive option of choice. These flaps can provide better voice, less dysphagia, and less donor-site morbidity than does jejunum. There has been difficulty with stricture formation with radial forearm flaps. Insertion of a salivary bypass tube at the time of surgery nearly ameliorates this coplication (33).

In the situation of surgical salvage after failure of chemoradiation therapy, the fistula rate with primary hypopharyngeal closure is high. Use of fasciocutaneous free-tissue transfer for support of primary closure of hypopharyngeal defects decreased the fistula rate to 20% in a small case series (34). It seems reasonable to support primary hypopharyngeal closure with vascularized tissue to reduce wound complications and length of hospital stay.

Oral Cavity and Oropharyngeal Defects

In the oral cavity and oropharynx, microvascular reconstruction has improved function and reduced complications of the tongue and mandible (3). The sensate radial forearm flap has become the workhorse of low-volume, soft-tissue oral cavity reconstruction; the sensate lateral arm flap is an alternative for slightly larger volume defects. Reconstruction of associated mandibular bony defects can compromise soft-tissue reconstruction because the soft tissue associated with free revascularized bone flaps is not as versatile as a sensate radial forearm flap. When the functional results are likely to be compromised by use of the soft-tissue component of an osseous flap, two flaps can be used. A sensate soft-tissue flap and an osseous flap can be combined to optimize speech, swallowing, and cosmetic results. An example is an angle-to-angle mandibular defect combined with two-thirds anterior glossectomy. A fibular flap can be used for bony reconstruction, and a lateral arm flap or anterolateral thigh flap can be used for the glossectomy reconstruction. In the repair of larger soft-tissue defects that include the entire tongue, musculocutaneous flaps such as the rectus and latissimus dorsi flaps are used.

The principles of oral cavity reconstruction are to obtain watertight closure; maintain mobility; provide sensation, including cable grafting of segmentally resected sensory nerves; maintain the volume of the resected tissue; maintain oral competence; and prevent medically significant aspiration. The radial forearm flap is uniquely suited to reconstruction of the oral cavity when there is remaining functional tongue. It is a thin, supple flap of ample size to provide mobility. The antebrachial cutaneous nerve can be used to innervate the flap and provide cable grafts for the inferior alveolar or lingual nerves. De-epithelialized segments can be used to contour the flap to restore the original contour of the defect (35).

In total glossectomy defects, the muscle of a rectus or latissimus flap is used to reconstruct the floor of the mouth, and a large volume of subcutaneous tissue is made into a mound to allow contact between the flap and the remaining sensate mucosa in the oral cavity. If a laryngectomy has not been performed, the hyoid bone must be resuspended to the mandible to help prevent aspiration.

Complex full-thickness defects (defects that include oral mucosa in continuity with external skin) usually are encountered in conjunction with mandibular defects. These defects can be closed with an osteomusculocutaneous iliac crest flap, a multipaddled osteocutaneous scapula, or a combination of a soft-tissue flap and an osteocutaneous fibular flap.

Midfacial Defects

Midfacial defects traditionally have been managed with a prosthesis. Revascularized free-tissue transfer has been valuable in reconstructing the maxilla to maintain midfacial projection in the premaxillary, zygomatic, and infraorbital regions. It also has been useful in providing soft tissue to the cheek and orbit. The principles of midfacial reconstruction are to restore the contour and projection of the midface, to facilitate rehabilitation of an occlusal surface in the upper jaw, to provide oronasal separation, to close the orbit or provide a platform for prosthetic rehabilitation of the eye, and to maintain a functioning lacrimal system if the globe is intact. Use of a hard-palate obturator is an excellent approach to a maxillectomy defect, and that is limited to the ipsilateral secondary palate. When evaluating a patient for reconstruction of the midface, it is important to consider how a prosthesis can act in concert with free-tissue transfer to optimize the functional and aesthetic results.

It is helpful to classify defects involving the maxilla. These defects can be categorized first by dividing them into infrastructure (oral palate) and combined infrastructure and suprastructure defects (oral palate, maxillary buttresses, orbital rim, and orbit). Infrastructure (oral palate) defects are uncommon and can be approached with a wide variety of techniques. Combined infrastructure and suprastructure defects can be subdivided as follows: (a) maxillectomy with intact orbital rim, (b) maxillectomy including the infraorbital rim, (c) maxillectomy including the infraorbital rim and orbital contents, and (d) composite defects, which can include any of the other defects combined with facial skin. The principles to be addressed are midfacial projection in the area of the infraorbital rim, orbital floor support, oral-nasal separation, and a stable platform for mastication.

Maxillectomy defects with intact orbital rim are effectively reconstructed with an obturator. The obturator provides adequate oronasal separation and a stable platform for mastication. Maxillectomy defects including infraorbital rim are best reconstructed with free-tissue transfer, either alone or in concert with a prosthesis. An effective approach is an osseocutaneous forearm flap for infraorbital rim reconstruction and orbital floor support in combination with a prosthesis. An osseocutaneous flap, such as an iliac crest, fibular, or scapular flap, in combination with osseointegrated implants, has become a more frequently used approach to avoid an obturator.

Maxillectomy defects including the infraorbital rim and orbital contents are much larger volume defects. The principles to be addressed are the same as those for defects with an intact orbital rim with the additional issue of volume requirement in the orbit. A osseocutaneous scapular flap alone or an osseocutaneous radial forearm flap in combination with a maxillary prosthesis is used. Orbital prostheses usually are not accommodated in the primary reconstruction. A closed orbit is considered cosmetically superior (4).

The composite maxillectomy defect is complex. The osseocutaneous scapular flap has been most useful in the management of this defect. The osteocutaneous radial forearm is a distant second because of the small volume of bone stock and donor-site morbidity. The scapula has adequate bone stock to recontour most maxillary defects, the soft tissue can be positioned independently from the bone, and there is ample subcutaneous tissue to recontour the cheek and fill the orbit as needed. The scapular tip flap with its long pedicle, the latissimus for internal lining, and the scapula for external lining is a variation with a high level of utility.

Defects of the Base of the Skull

Microvascular reconstruction has been a key factor in facilitating skull-base surgery. The rectus flap has been used because of its bulk, long vascular pedicle (if the rectus muscle is included as part of the pedicle length), ability to make multiple skin islands by means of de-epithelialization, and ease of patient positioning and ability to perform primary closure at the donor site. The disadvantage of use of a rectus flap is poor color match and a tendency toward ptosis. These cosmetic limitations have decreased the use of the rectus flap in favor of osseocutaneous flaps. Bone defects associated with skull-base defects frequently are reconstructed with split calvarial bone or hydroxyapatite compounds. Any area of bony projection is reconstructed with vascularized bone if the patient has undergone or plans to undergo radiation therapy.

The principles of skull-base reconstruction are to support the dural closure (separation of the cranial cavity from the upper aerodigestive tract), provide carotid coverage, obliterate dead space, support nonvascularized bone reconstruction, and restore calvarial and facial contour. The defects can be anterior or lateral defects. Anterior defects that include the orbit and maxilla are best reconstructed with a large-volume flap such as an osseocutaneous scapular flap or a rectus flap as a distant second choice. Anterior defects with an intact maxilla that cannot be reconstructed with local flaps can be reconstructed with a scapular fasciocutaneous or a partially de-epithelialized radial forearm flap. Lateral skull-base defects are best reconstructed with a scapular flap, lateral arm flap, or thick anterolateral thigh flap. These flaps have better color match and a tendency not to become ptotic. Difficulties with patient positioning, however, have decreased the frequency of use of the scapular flap. As in the management of midfacial defects, careful consideration of the effect of free-tissue transfer on future prosthetic reconstruction is important to obtain the best functional and aesthetic results.

External Soft-Tissue Defects

Revascularized free-tissue transfer is useful in the management of massive cutaneous defects of the scalp or skin that cannot be reconstructed with local tissue or when reconstruction with a regional pedicled rotational flap gives suboptimal cosmetic results. The optimal flap for reconstruction is based on the site of the defect. For defects of the face and neck, the scapular flap and lateral arm flap are used because they have an adequate amount of subcutaneous tissue to allow contouring, and the contour is stable and does not become ptotic. The anterolateral thigh is being used more as an alternative. Further investigation is needed to determine its tendency to become ptotic. For scalp defects, the latissimus dorsi muscle with a split-thickness skin graft is used because it is thin, is tightly adherent to the skull, and easily allows fitting of a wig. Any calvarial defects are recontoured at primary reconstruction because any calvarial irregularity becomes obvious as the latissimus dorsi flap atrophies. For forehead defects, a radial forearm flap is used most often, although the color match is poor. The principles of reconstruction of large soft-tissue defects are to provide coverage of critical structures (large vessels, dura, or cranial nerves), restore the skeletal contour with split calvarial bone or hydroxyapatite paste, restore soft-tissue contour, allow fitting of a wig as appropriate, and obtain optimal color match.

HIGHLIGHTS

- Revascularized free-tissue transfer is a reliable and cost-effective approach to head and neck reconstruction.
- The evolution of microvascular free-tissue transfer has advanced head and neck reconstruction. The technique enables the surgeon to perform exacting and sophisticated reconstruction and primary resection in a single stage.
- Free-tissue transfer is most useful for management of sophisticated oromandibular reconstruction, total pharyngeal defects, complex midfacial defects, skull-base defects, and large, external soft-tissue defects of the head and neck.

- The advantages of free-tissue transfer are reliability, vascularity, abundant supply of high-quality tissue, potential for sensory and motor reinnervation, and inset into a heavily irradiated bed if necessary.
- The disadvantages of free-tissue transfer are complexity, need for special instrumentation and training, increased operating time, and involvement of two surgical teams.
- Radial forearm free-tissue transfer has become the workhorse of head and neck reconstruction because the flap is reliable, thin, pliable, and sensate and can be contoured to the defect.
- Musculocutaneous free-tissue transfers are more bulky than fasciocutaneous flaps. The flaps are used for management of larger soft-tissue defects, such as those caused by total glossectomy or of large skull-base defects.
- Selection of the osteocutaneous flap to be used for reconstruction depends on many factors, including vascular anatomic features, vessel quality, available bone, versatility of the soft tissue, donor-site morbidity, and feasibility of simultaneous two-team surgery.
- There is no ideal osteocutaneous flap for the management of combined bone and large volume soft-tissue defects.
- Pharyngoesophageal reconstruction requires careful preoperative assessment of extent of the tumor, consideration of method of voice rehabilitation, and the planning of radiation therapy before the reconstruction and surgical team can be chosen.
- When evaluating a patient for midfacial or skull-base free-tissue transfer, it is important to consider the integration of prosthetics to obtain the optimal functional and aesthetic results.

REFERENCES

1. Schusterman MA, Horndeski G. Analysis of the morbidity associated with immediate microvascular reconstruction in head and neck cancer patients. *Head Neck* 1991;13(1):51–55.
2. Chepeha DB, et al.. Pectoralis major myocutaneous flap vs revascularized free-tissue transfer: complications, gastrostomy tube dependence, and hospitalization. *Arch Otolaryngol Head Neck Surg* 2004;130(2):181–186.
3. Chepeha DB, Wang SJ, Marentette LJ, et al. Radial forearm free-tissue transfer reduces complications in salvage skull base surgery. *Otolaryngol Head Neck Surg* 2004;131(6):958–963.
4. Chepeha DB, Wang SJ, Marentette LJ, et al. Restoration of the orbital aesthetic subunit in complex midface defects. *Laryngoscope* 2004;114(10):1706–1713.
5. Urken ML. Radial forearm. In: ML Urken, ML Cheney, MJ Sullivan, et al., eds. *Atlas of regional and free flaps for head and neck reconstruction.* New York: Raven Press, 1995:155.
6. Funk GF, Valentino J, McCulloch TM, et al. Anomalies of forearm vascular anatomy encountered during elevation of the radial forearm flap. *Head Neck* 1995;17(4):284–292.
7. Richardson D, Fisher SE, Vaughan ED, et al., Radial forearm flap donor-site complications and morbidity: a prospective study [see comment]. *Plast Reconstr Surg,* 1997;99(1):109–115.
8. Sullivan MJ, Carroll WR, Kuriloff DB. Lateral arm free flap in head and neck reconstruction. *Arch Otolaryngol Head Neck Surg* 1992;118(10):1095–1101.
9. Teknos TN, Nussenbaum B, Bradford CR, et al., Reconstruction of complex parotidectomy defects using the lateral arm free tissue transfer. *Otolaryngol Head Neck Surg* 2003;129(3):183–191.

10. Civantos FJ Jr, Burkey, B, Lu FL, et al., Lateral arm microvascular flap in head and neck reconstruction. *Arch Otolaryngol Head Neck Surg* 1997; 123(8):830–836.

11. Rivet D, Buffet M, Martin D, et al., The lateral arm flap: an anatomic study. *J ReconstrMicrosurg* 1987;3(2):121–132.

12. Hayden RE, Deschler DG. Lateral thigh free flap for head and neck reconstruction. *Laryngoscope* 1999;109(9):1490–1494.

13. Wei FC, Jain V, Celik N, et al., Have we found an ideal soft-tissue flap? An experience with 672 anterolateral thigh flaps.[see comment]. *Plast Reconstr Surg* 2002;109(7):2219–2226(discussion 2227–2230).

14. Lueg EA. The anterolateral thigh flap: radial forearm's "big brother" for extensive soft tissue head and neck defects. *Arch Otolaryngol Head Neck Surg* 2004;130(7):813–818.

15. Shieh SJ, Chiu HY, Yu JC, et al. Free anterolateral thigh flap for reconstruction of head and neck defects following cancer ablation. *Plast Reconstr Surg* 2000;105(7):2349–2357(discussion 2358–2360).

16. Cheney ML, Varvares MA, Nadol JB Jr. The temporoparietal fascial flap in head and neck reconstruction. *Arch Otolaryngol Head Neck Surg* 1993;119(6):618–623.

17. Taylor GI, Palmer JH. The vascular territories (angiosomes) of the body: experimental study and clinical applications. *Br J Plast Surg* 1987;40(2):113–141.

18. Strauch B, Yu H. *Atlas of microvascular surgery: anatomy and operative approaches.* New York: Thieme Medical Publishers, 1993:560.

19. Earley MJ, Green MF, Milling MA, A critical appraisal of the use of free flaps in primary reconstruction of combined scalp and calvarial cancer defects. *Br J Plast Surg* 1990;43(3):283–289.

20. Harii K, Ohmori K, Torii S. Free gracilis muscle transplantation, with microneurovascular anastomoses for the treatment of facial paralysis. A preliminary report. *Plast Reconstr Surg* 1976;57(2):133–143.

21. Yousif NJ, Matloub HS, Kolachalam R, et al. The transverse gracilis musculocutaneous flap. [see comment]. *Ann Plast Surg* 1992;29(6):482–490.

22. Taylor GI, Miller GD, Ham FJ. The free vascularized bone graft. A clinical extension of microvascular techniques. *Plast Reconstr Surg* 1975;55(5):533–544.

23. Hidalgo DA. Fibula free flap: a new method of mandible reconstruction. *Plast Reconstr Surg* 1989;84(1):71–79.

24. Futran ND, Wadsworth JT, Villaret D, et al., Midface reconstruction with the fibula free flap. *Arch Otolaryngol Head Neck Surg* 2002;128(2):161–166.

25. Schusterman MA, Reece GP, Miller MJ, et al. The osteocutaneous free fibula flap: is the skin paddle reliable? *Plast Reconstr Surg* 1992;90(5):787–793(discussion 794–798).

26. Urken ML, Vickery C, Weinberg H, et al., The internal oblique-iliac crest osseomyocutaneous free flap in oromandibular reconstruction. Report of 20 cases. *Arch Otolaryngol Head Neck Surg* 1989;115(3):339–349.

27. Sullivan MJ, Baker SR, Crompton, R, et al., Free scapular osteocutaneous flap for mandibular reconstruction. *Arch Otolaryngol Head Neck Surg* 1989; 115(11):1334–1340.

28. Carlson GW, Schusterman MA, Guillamondegui OM. Total reconstruction of the hypopharynx and cervical esophagus: a 20-year experience. *Ann Plast Surg* 1992;29(5):408–412.

29. Bradford CR, Esclamado RM, Carroll WR, et al. Analysis of recurrence, complications, and functional results with free jejunal flaps. *Head Neck* 1994;16(2):149–154.

30. Bradford CR, Esclamado RM, Carroll WR. Monitoring of revascularized jejunal autografts. *Arch Otolaryngol Head Neck Surg* 1992; 118(10):1042–1044.

31. Urken. Free omentum and gastro-omentum. In: ML Urken, ML Cheney, MJ Sullivan, et al., eds. *Atlas of regional and free flaps for head and neck reconstruction.* New York: Raven Press, 1995: 321–328.

32. Urken ML, Weinberg H, Vickery C, et al. Oromandibular reconstruction using microvascular composite free flaps. Report of 71 cases and a new classification scheme for bony, soft-tissue, and neurologic defects. *Arch Otolaryngol Head Neck Surg* 1991; 117(7):733–744.

33. Varvares MA, Cheney ML, Gliklich RE, et al. Use of the radial forearm fasciocutaneous free flap and montgomery salivary bypass tube for pharyngoesophageal reconstruction. *Head Neck* 2000;22(5):463–468.

34. Teknos TN, Myers LL, Bradford CR, et al. Free tissue reconstruction of the hypopharynx after organ preservation therapy: analysis of wound complications. *Laryngoscope* 2001;111(7):1192–1196.

35. Urken ML, Moscoso JF, Lawson W, et al. A systematic approach to functional reconstruction of the oral cavity following partial and total glossectomy. *Arch Otolaryngol Head Neck Surg* 1994; 120(6):589–601.

Surgical Reconstruction after Mohs Surgery and Tissue Expansion

163

Karen H. Calhoun   *William W. Shockley*

This chapter deals with the options available for reconstruction of cutaneous defects of the face, scalp, and neck. First we give you guidelines for deciding whether secondary intention healing, a skin graft, or a local flap is most appropriate for a given defect. Then we detail the specifics of choosing which local or locoregional flap will work best. Finally, we talk about special options for defects of unique facial features, including the lips, nose, eyelids, eyebrows, ears, and scalp.

HOW TO START?

When a patient is initially seen with a facial (or neck or scalp) defect, your first task is to describe the defect:

Measure it.
How many centimeters is it in diameter?
Is it oval or elliptical?
How deep is it?
    Just through the skin to the subcutaneous fat?
    All the way to the muscle fascia?
Is the muscle intact? Partially resected?
Is bone or cartilage exposed?
If so, is it bare or covered with perichondrium or periosteum?
What anatomic subunit does it occupy?
    Does it involve more than one subunit?
If the defect resulted from excision of a skin cancer, are the margins free of tumor?

WHAT TYPE OF RECONSTRUCTION?

The choices for reconstruction are secondary intention healing, direct (primary) closure of the original skin defect, closure of the defect after excision of additional skin, skin graft, or a local flap (adjacent tissue transfer) (Table 163.1).

Secondary Intention Healing

Small (<1 cm in diameter) defects limited to the medial canthal area usually heal better by secondary intention than with skin grafts or flaps, most of which become bulky, later requiring revision (Fig. 163.1). The other reasons for choosing secondary intention healing are multiple comorbidities, making further surgery risky or inconvenient (anticoagulation that cannot be discontinued, etc.), or patient preference ("I don't want ANY more surgery").

Forehead defects also heal fairly nicely by secondary intention healing. Secondary intention healing of defects involving the free edge of the lips, nasal ala, or eyelids can result in notching or retraction, with the potential of oral incompetence, nasal obstruction, or exposure keratitis leading to blindness. Secondary intention healing of a defect within the hair-bearing scalp leads to an area of alopecia. For other facial locations, a wide variation exists in the quality of an individual's skin and the amount of hypertrophic scarring.

TABLE 163.1

CHOICES FOR RECONSTRUCTION

Choice	Advantages	Disadvantages
Secondary intention healing	No further surgery required	(1) Requires days or weeks of daily dressing changes (2) May be unattractive, central hypertrophic scarring (3) Contraction may distort adjacent structures
Skin graft	Technically quick and easy	(1) Requires an additional surgical site for skin-graft harvest (2) Potentially poor match in skin color, texture, and level
Direct closure of skin defect	(1) Technically straightforward (2) Usually good appearance outcome	Appropriate only for an elliptical defect with long axis oriented along relaxed skin lines
Direct closure of skin defect after excision of additional skin	Usually good appearance outcome	Requires excision of additional normal skin
Local flap	Usually very good appearance outcome	(1) Technical design and execution more challenging (2) Creates additional scars (3) Potential for greater reconstructive challenge if flap fails

Skin Grafting

For most small facial defects, if a graft is appropriate, a full-thickness skin graft is used. Occasionally, for a very large defect, a split-thickness skin graft is appropriate.

Skin grafts often result in a cosmetic result that is less satisfactory than that with local flaps. Reasons for choosing skin grafting include patient preference, selected anatomic areas where skin grafting usually results in good appearance (lateral nasal sidewall), and comorbidities demanding the shortest possible and least complex surgical procedure.

The use of a skin graft on a deep defect, such as one into or through the facial musculature, results in a "divot" or contour defect. A local skin flap usually results in a better appearance for such defects. When cartilage or bone is exposed, a skin graft *can* be used only *if* perichondrium or periosteum is intact. Skin grafts *do not* survive on bare cartilage or bare bone. Grafts on bone or cartilage also will result in significant contour defects. Vascularized tissue must be used to cover bare cartilage or bone.

Rarely, when no other good reconstructive choice exists, multiple small "punch" excisions of cartilage or decortication of bone will permit through-growth of granulation tissue, either permitting secondary intention healing or making a healthy bed for skin grafting.

Skin-graft donor sites should be carefully chosen for good camouflage or unobtrusive appearance. Common sites include supraclavicular and postauricular skin. Other good facial choices include preauricular skin, melolabial folds, and upper eyelids. The caveat with these locations is *not* to create noticeable facial asymmetry. When a large amount of skin is required for grafting, consider taking half of the skin from each side (i.e., half from each upper eyelid, or half from each preauricular area).

Direct Closure of Skin Defect

Defects suitable for direct closure are uncommon but technically easy to close with good-appearance outcome when

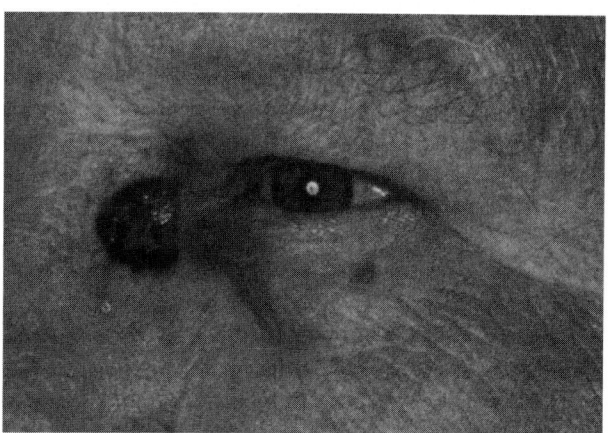

Figure 163.1 This type of defect in the medial canthal area usually does very well with secondary intention healing.

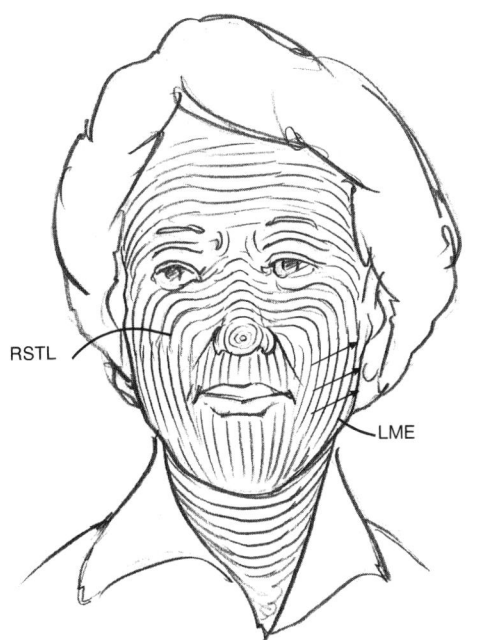

Figure 163.2 This shows the relaxed skin-tension lines running perpendicular to the underlying muscle.

recognized. An example would be a horizontal elliptical defect in the midforehead. Note that the long axis of the ellipse is oriented *along* relaxed skin-tension lines (Fig. 163.2). When you encounter such a favorable defect, cosmetic results after closure are enhanced by wide undermining and layered closure.

Direct Closure of Skin Defect after Additional Skin Excision

We encounter more or less circular skin defects more often than elliptical defects. Excising additional normal skin permits turning this defect into an ellipse with long-axis orientation along relaxed skin-tension lines. When this option is available, it is usually the best choice for closure. Common examples include defects located along the melolabial fold or small defects on the upper lip.

Local Skin Flaps

If none of the preceding options meets your patient's needs, the next step will be deciding *which* local skin flap will provide the best functional and appearance outcome. The two most important factors in your decision are the anatomic subunit(s) involved and the amount and location of surrounding skin potentially available to be moved.

Anatomic Subunit

Decide which anatomic subunit the skin defect occupies. Estimate the approximate percentage of the subunit the defect composes. If the defect occupies more than one subunit, consider each separately. In some circumstances, if the defect takes up more than 60% or 70% of the subunit, the final cos-

metic result may be better if you excise the remaining normal skin in that subunit. Reconstructing the subunit as a whole may avoid conspicuous scars crossing anatomic subunits.

Potentially Available Skin

Consider the location of the anatomic unit. Determine approximately how *much* skin is potentially available for reconstruction in *what location* of the area around the defect. Determine whether closure of the *secondary* defect will cause distortion of facial landmarks. The cheeks, temple, forehead, and neck are typically areas from which skin can be borrowed. The location of nondistortable facial landmarks also should be considered. including eyebrows, eyelids, nasal ala, lips, pinnae, and hairline.

Specific Flaps

Note

This simplest of flaps is used to repair a round defect by using tissue immediately adjacent to the defect. It can be used when available skin is found on any side of the defect. It is designed so that transfer of the flap assists in closure of the donor site (Fig. 163.3).

Rhomboid

The versatile rhomboid flap is used for repair of a rhomboid-shaped defect. The rhomboid had two 60-degree angles and two 120-degree angles. Although this sounds like an esoteric shape, many round, oval, or square or rectangular defects can be *converted* to a rhomboid with minimal excision of normal skin (Fig. 163.4).

Each rhomboid defect has four potential flap designs. This must be remembered in those circumstances in which a circular defect is being converted to a rhomboid defect. In these cases, the orientation of the "new" rhomboid defect will affect the donor-site choices. The rhomboid flap is designed by extending a line along the short axis of the flap. At a distance from the point, equal to the distance between points, two lines are drawn. One is up, and one is down, paralleling and equal in length to the defect side. This results in four potential flaps. Depending on the location of the defect, one of these options is usually clearly the best option, based on available skin and minimizing distortion of facial landmarks like the eyebrow or the nasal ala. Rhomboid flap design virtually closes the donor-site defect

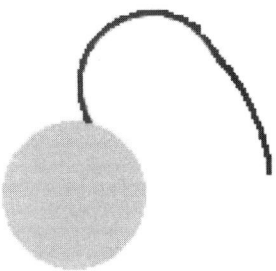

Figure 163.3 A note flap.

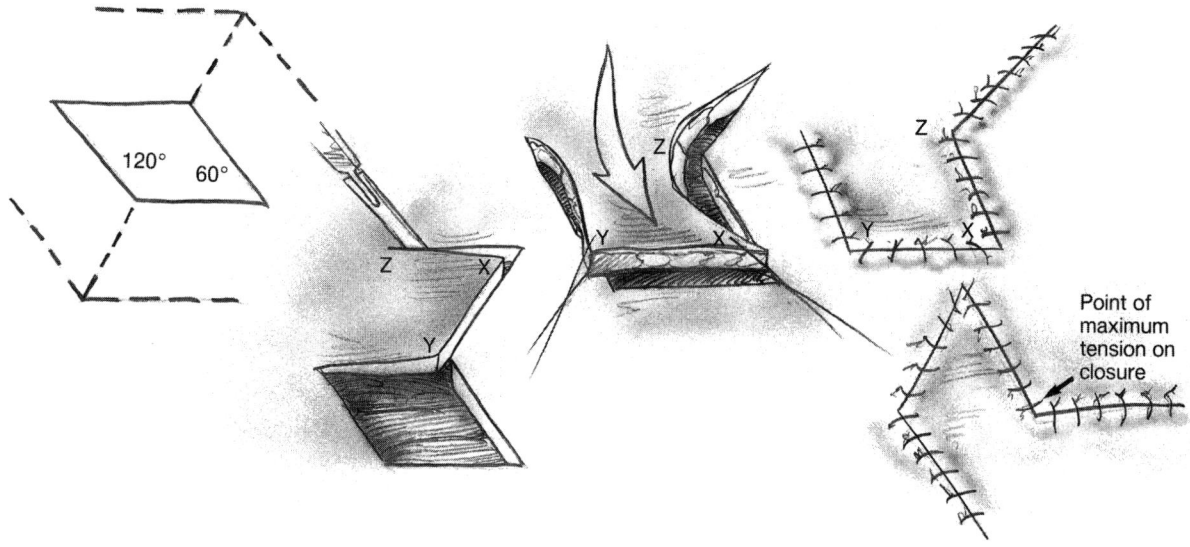

Figure 163.4 The design of a rhomboid skin flap.

with transfer of the flap to the original defect. The pivot point is shown on this diagram.

Triple Rhomboid

This flap design considers a circle to be made up of three 120-degree rhomboids. For each of these rhomboids, a separate rhomboid flap is designed. It is critical that the final leg of each flap be *all* clockwise or *all* counterclockwise! The final scar looks a bit like a drunken spider.

Bilobed

The bilobed flap "robs Peter to pay Paul." It is most useful in areas like the nasal tip, where a note flap is potentially useful, but borrowing tissue in a vertical direction results

in an undesirable consequence such as nasal alar retraction. Adding a second lobe to the flap permits you essentially to transfer the borrowing to a vertical direction, where the skin is more plentiful, and no undesirable consequence results.

Several ways exist to design a bilobed flap. Most involve making the first flap about the same size as the defect and creating the second flap slightly smaller, placed with its long axis at about 90 degrees to the long axis of the first flap (Fig. 163.5)

A-to-T

The A-to-T flap closure repairs an isosceles triangle–shaped defect (the "A"), resulting in an inverted "T" scar. It is most

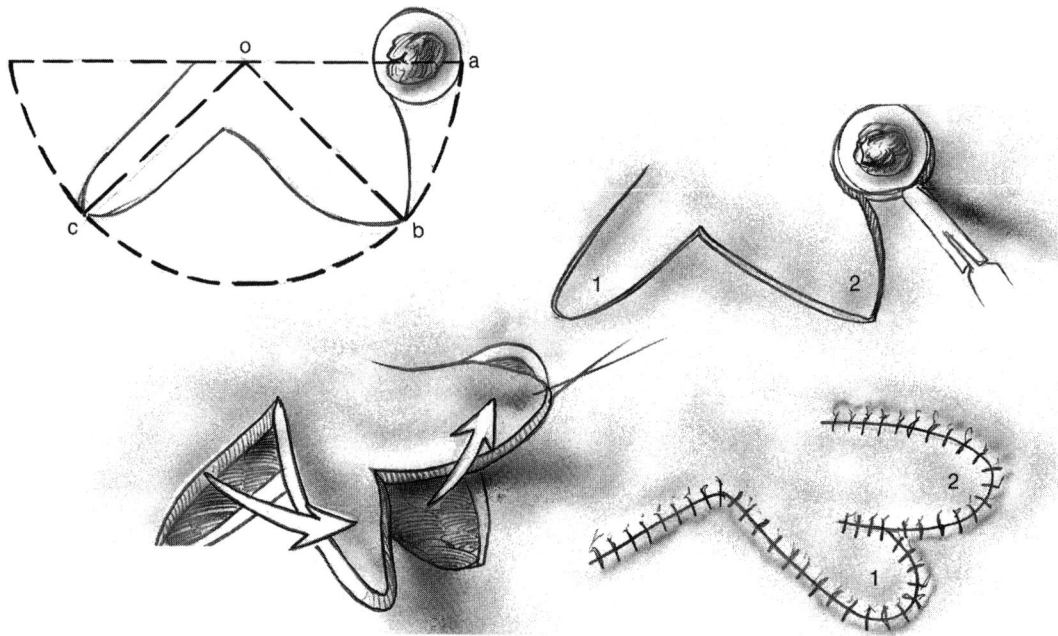

Figure 163.5 The design of a bilobed flap.

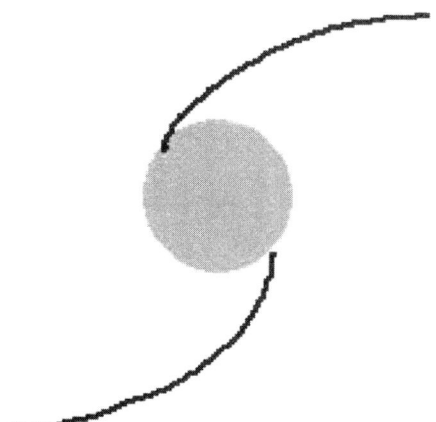

Figure 163.6   The design of an O-to-Z flap.

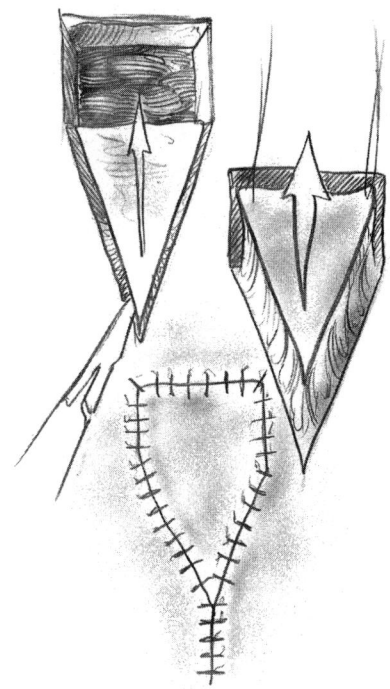

Figure 163.7   The design of a V-to-Y flap.

useful for any roundish or squareish defect immediately adjacent to a long landmark (eyebrow, hairline) in which the horizontal portion of the T can be camouflaged.

An A-to-T flap is designed by first choosing the long part of the scar, usually camouflaged in the hairline (a horizontal forehead wrinkle, etc.). This is centered to the defect. A small triangle encompassing the defect is drawn with arms of equal length, the third side sitting on the long part. Frequently, a Burow triangle is required on the ends of the long incision, on the opposite side from the triangle around the defect.

O-to-Z

An O-to-Z flap is most useful for repairing circular defects (the "O") for which donor tissue is available on both sides of the defect. The resulting scar is an "S" or lazy "Z."

The O-to-Z flap is designed so that two lazy curves start at opposite sides of the defect, 180 degrees apart, and curve away from the defect in opposite directions. The points of these two flaps thus created are brought together to form a Z-shaped scar (7) (Fig. 163.6).

V-to-Y

The V-to-Y island flap works best with "borrowable" skin on one side of the defect, yet this potentially available skin cannot be markedly narrowed. Unlike the flaps described earlier, this flap is *subcutaneously* pedicled. This means that the entire perimeter of the flap is incised, but it is only partially undermined. Although either end of the flap may be undermined to allow some forward movement, a generous subcutaneous pedicle must be left intact to preserve sufficient blood supply to the flap (Fig. 163.7).

The V-to-Y flap is designed by drawing a long V with the top based on the defect. The long arms of the V are incised through the full thickness of the skin. Very careful undermining of the edges is carried out sufficiently to move the top of the flap to meet the opposite edge of the defect. The apex of the V is closed to itself, creating the long-standing leg of the Y-shaped resulting scar (Fig. 163.8).

Subcutaneously Pedicled Island Flap

This flap is used for a round defect that has no immediately adjacent useable tissue. A circle about the same size as the defect is drawn, and the skin is incised for the entire circumference. A subcutaneous tunnel is developed between the flap circle and the defect, just beneath the skin. A second tunnel is then developed between the subcutaneous tissue and the muscle fascia. This leaves a skin flap pedicled on subcutaneous tissue. The skin flap is passed through the tunnel to fill in the defect and is sutured in place.

Over time, as this approximately-round suture line contracts, the flap often "pooches up" to become bulky. One technique that helps prevent this is the use of two to four mini-Z-plasties at the time the original flap is sewn in place. This also can be used after bulkiness has developed, as a remedial fix.

Overview

Seldom does only one good flap-reconstruction option exist. Your job as the reconstructive surgeon is to consider all possible options and choose the one that seems likely to give the best result for a particular patient, considering the patient's age, skin laxity, comorbidities, and degree of potential functional impairment (1).

Specific Locations

Several anatomically complex facial areas where specific functional considerations must be considered in additional to appearance outcome.

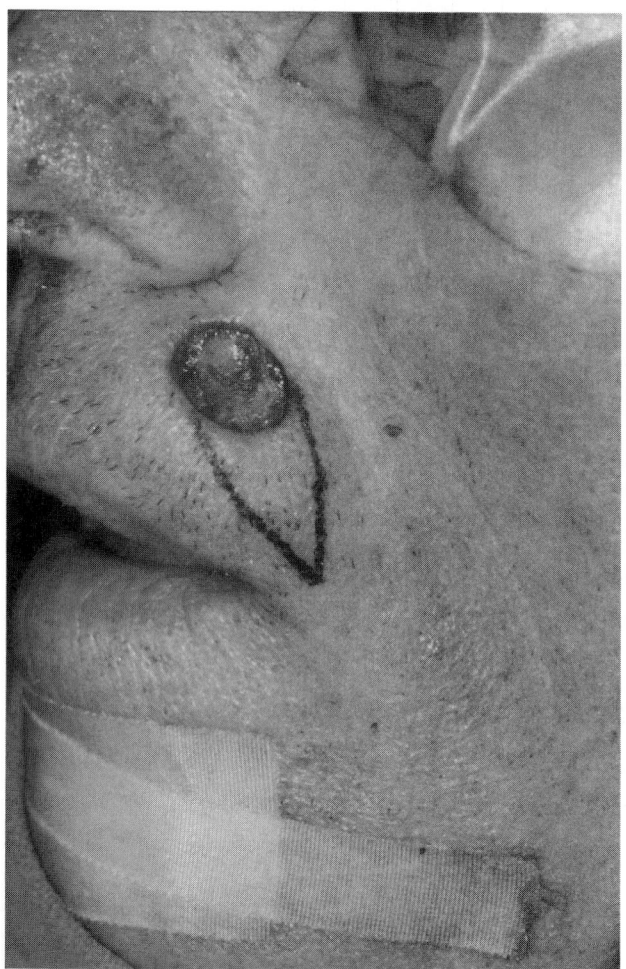 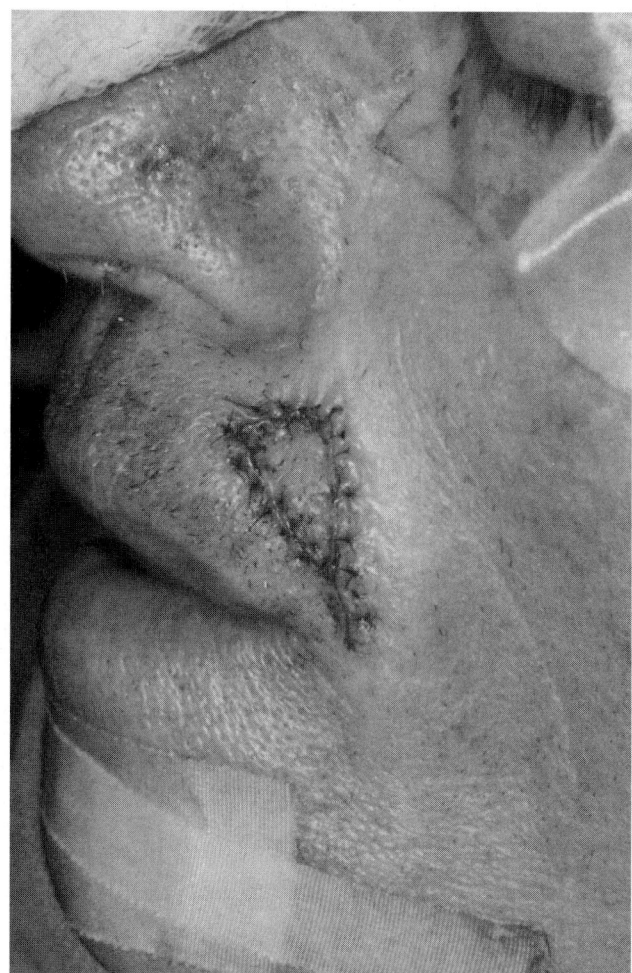

A   B

Figure 163.8 **A:** Left upper lip defect with planned V-Y advancement flap. **B:** Flap advanced into position.

Lip

The skin of the lip overlies the muscular ring of the orbicularis oris. Relaxed skin-tension lines are radial to the oral opening (think "smoker's wrinkles"). Most small (>1.2-cm diameter) lip defects, whether skin-only or full thickness (skin–muscle–mucosa) can be repaired by transforming them into ellipses with the long axes along the relaxed skin-tension lines.

Matching the vermilion edges and white roll is crucial for good cosmesis. Although the borders seem obvious under normal circumstances, once the blanching after the vasoconstriction of the local anesthetic occurs, it may not be obvious at all. In our experience, the best way to tell accurately the boundary between skin and vermilion is to wet the tissue lightly. The skin appears more matte in finish, and the vermilion, shinier. Another method is to mark the vermilion–cutaneous junction before injection of local anesthesia.

Defects of up to a third of the lower lip may be closable primarily, depending on the individual's anatomy. Because the symmetry of the upper lip is so apparent, it is critical to try to maintain this feature. This may mean a defect involv-

ing half of the lateral subunit of the upper lip may be best repaired with a Webster perialar crescentic advancement flap (Fig. 163.9) or, if full thickness, a lipswitch (Abbe) flap from the central lower lip (Fig.163.10). For larger lower lip defects, an Estlander (lateral lip switch) flap, Gilles fan flap, or Karapandzic flap (which carries with it its own neurovascular bundle) will be better options.

If insufficient tissue remains in the "ring" of the orbicularis oris (i.e., if "closing" the ring will result in microstomia), tissue from the cheek, neck, or distant areas (radial artery forearm flap) must be considered.

Nose

See Chapters 165, 170, and 173.

Eyelid

The eyelid is composed of the anterior lamella and the posterior lamella. The anterior lamella is the skin and orbicularis muscle. The posterior lamella is conjunctiva, tarsus, and (depending on the location on the eyelid), Muller and levator muscles, the levator aponeurosis, the orbital septum, or a combination of these. Defects involving the

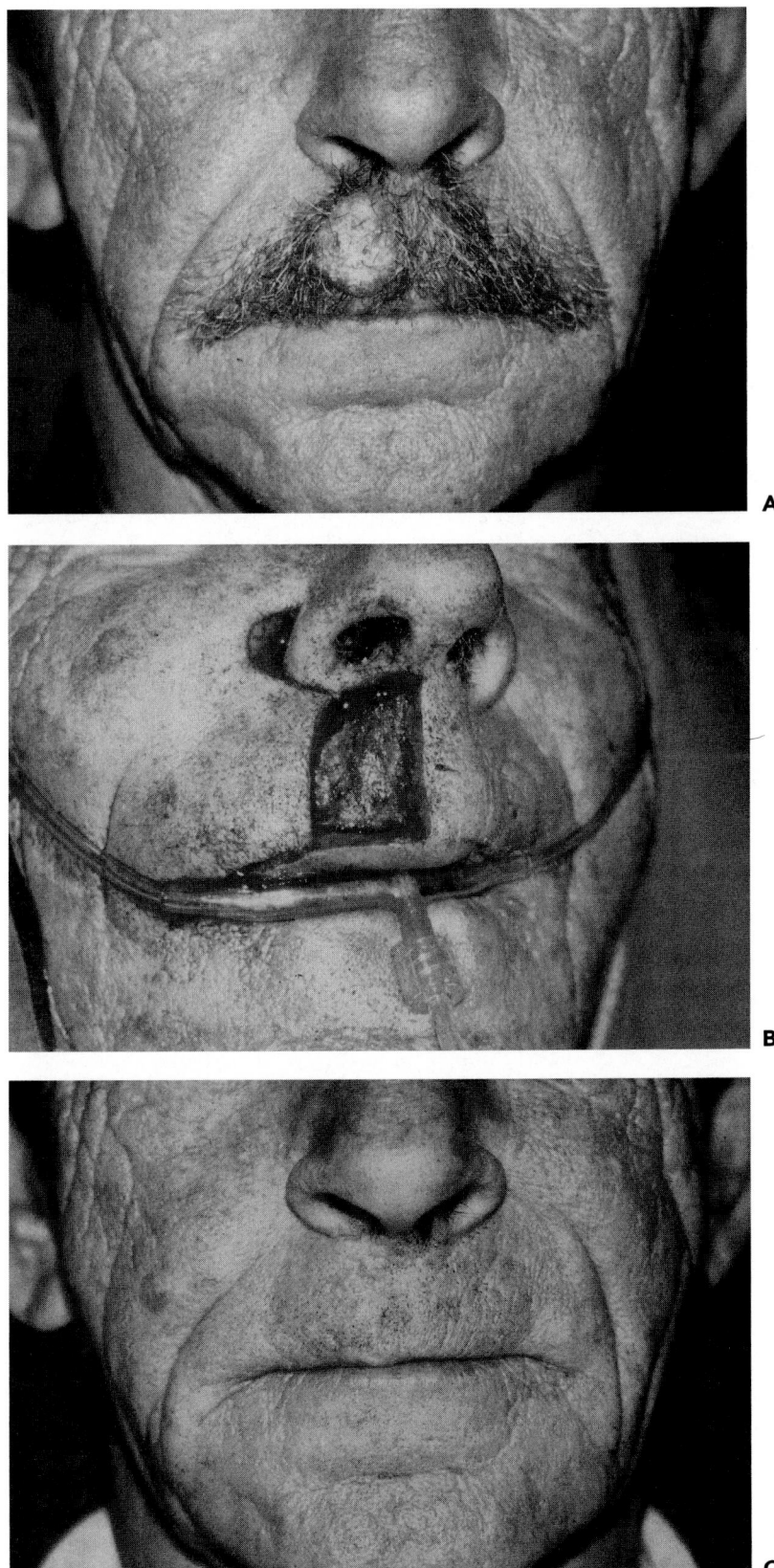

Figure 163.9 **A:** Patient with keratoacanthoma, right upper lip. **B:** Defect after excision of lesion with negative frozen sections. Note that excision was carried to boundaries or aesthetic units. Lip advancement flap design with perialar crescentic excision of skin to allow advancement of flap. **C:** Result 2 months after surgery.

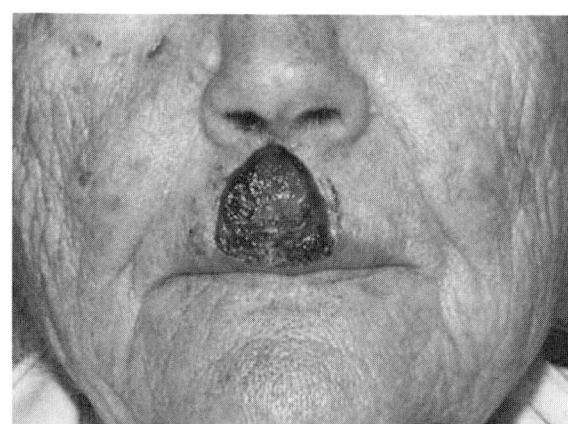
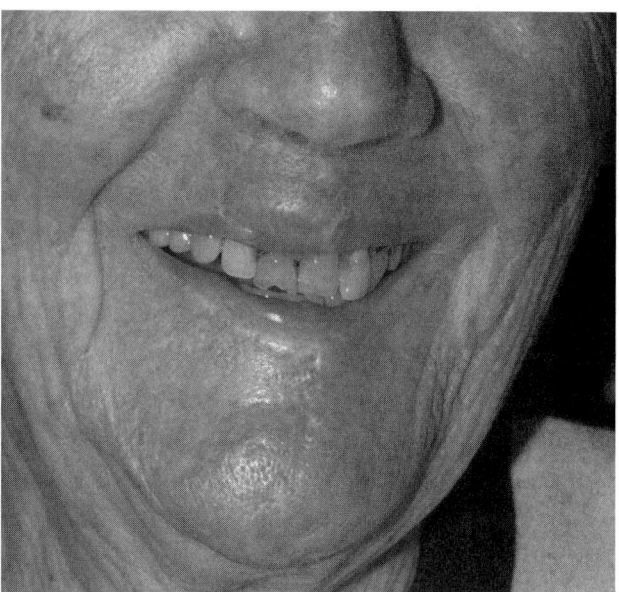

Figure 163.10   A: Central lip defect. **B:** After repair with a lip-switch flap from the center lower lip.

eyelid require careful analysis. Numerous reconstructive options are available, but these must be tailored to the extent of the defect (8). Small skin-only defects of the upper and lower lid can be treated with skin grafting (Fig. 163.11). Full-thickness defects of less than a fourth of the lid (upper or lower) can usually be closed primarily (layered closure). A rotation flap using lateral orbital skin can be used for larger defects (upper and lower lid), lined with a mucosal graft if needed. For major defects of the lower eyelid, a cheek transposition flap may work well (Fig. 163.12). For a still larger defect (subtotal or larger) of the upper eyelid, a pedicled flap of skin, muscle, and conjunctiva from the lower eyelid (pedicled through the lower eyelid) is transferred, leaving the lower-lid margin in its normal anatomic position. This type of flap does obstruct vision until it is divided and inset at 6 to 8 weeks. A subtotal defect of the lower lid is usually repaired with a skin-rotation flap from the lateral orbital area/upper cheek. These can be lined with a mucosal graft. A cartilage graft can be used to replace the tarsus if required.

Pinna

Skin-only defects that do not expose bare cartilage (i.e., have at least perichondrium at the bottom of the wound) do well with full-thickness skin grafting. Small full-thickness (skin–cartilage–skin) defects on the helical rim can be closed by converting the defect to a wedge or star (1.0 cm or smaller defect). Larger helical-rim defects (up to 2.5 cm) are nicely closed by helical rim advancement flaps (Fig. 163.13). Skin-only defects in the concha can be repaired well with full-thickness skin grafts. These can be put on top of cartilage if the perichondrium is intact. If bare cartilage occurs in the concha, one can excise the entire conchal cartilage and graft skin on the underlying soft tissue. Alternately, a posteriorly

pedicled postauricular flap can be passed through a slit in the posterior skin and positioned to cover the conchal area. "Cookie bite" defects usually require staged reconstruction, with cartilage graft from the opposite concha or from rib cartilage. A postauricular skin flap covers the attached cartilage at the first stage, with skin-flap division and insetting, and full-thickness skin graft to the resulting harvest-site defect, at the second stage.

Scalp

Scalp tissue is less elastic than facial skin, so flap planning must take this into account. One excellent choice for a vertex defect is the triple rhomboid flap (Fig. 163.14).

For a large defect, if periosteum is intact, skin grafting is an option. Scalp-rotation flaps will work well for some large defects (Fig. 163.15). More-massive defects will require free flap reconstruction by using a large flat muscle free flap such as latissimus dorsi or a fasciocutaneous flap such as the radial forearm flap. Omentum has also been used successfully.

If only bare bone is found, decortication (removal of the outer calvarial bone with an otologic cutting burr) will be followed by granulation tissue and satisfactory secondary intention healing (Fig. 163.16). Last, placement of tissue expanders can "create" enough new skin to allow later primary closure. If expanders are placed *through* the defect, a minimum of 3 weeks should pass before any expansion, to avoid extrusion. Alternately, the expanders can be placed via smaller lateral incisions, and expansion can begin sooner.

Tissue Expansion

Tissue expansion is a technique designed to "create additional skin" to cover large defects. An expander (similar to

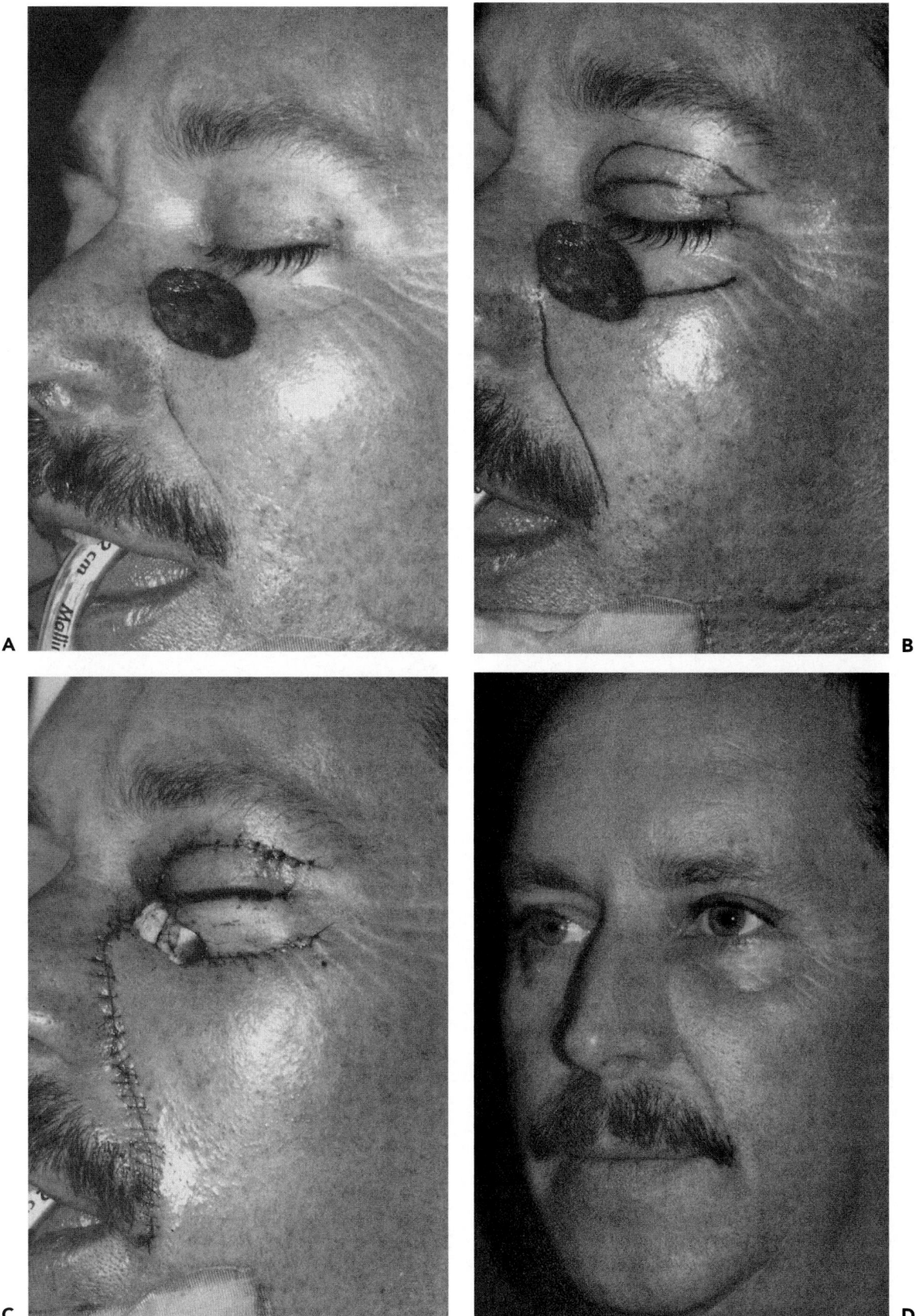

Figure 163.11   A: Eyelid and cheek defect after excision of basal cell carcinoma. **B:** Proposed cheek advancement flap with full-thickness skin graft from upper eyelid. **C:** Flap advanced into position with skin graft for eyelid portion of defect. Bolster in place. **D:** Results 6 months after surgery.

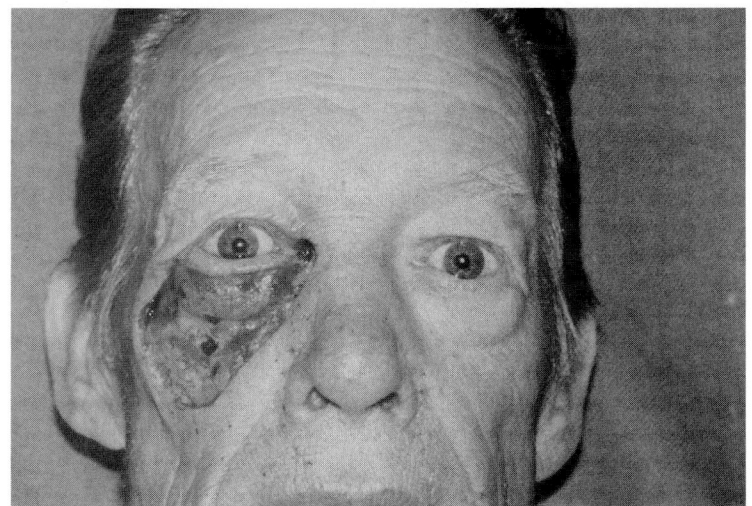

A

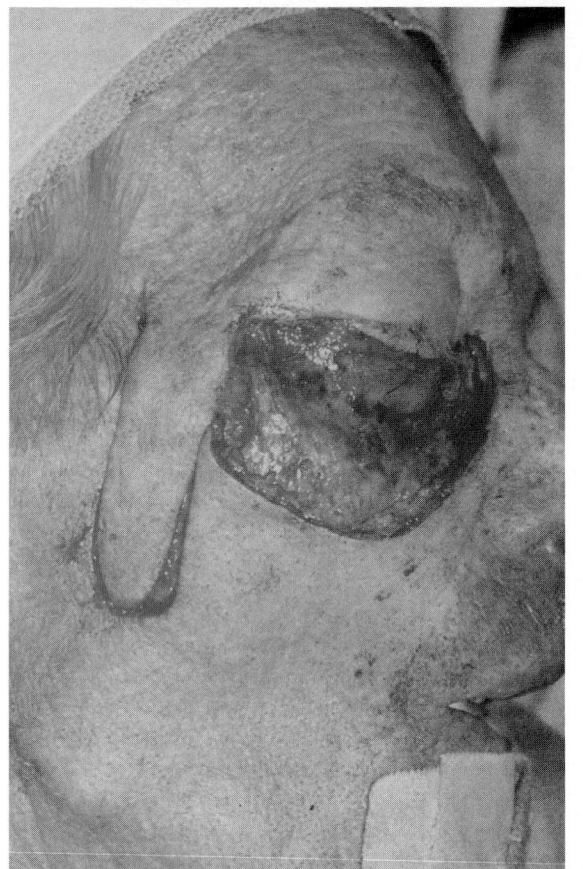

B

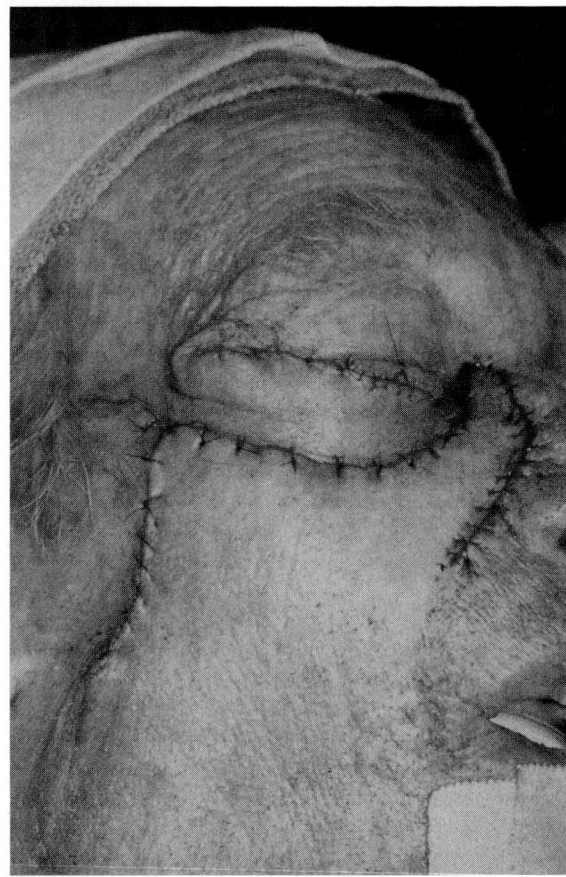

C

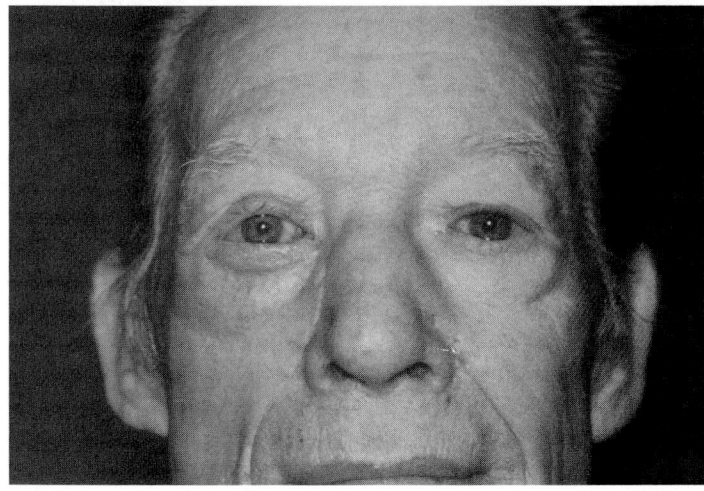

D

Figure 163.12 A: Defect involving lower eyelid and upper cheek. **B:** Superiorly based transposition flap planned for reconstruction of eyelid defect. **C:** Cheek advancement rotation flap in position, along with transposition flap. **D:** Result 9 months after surgery.

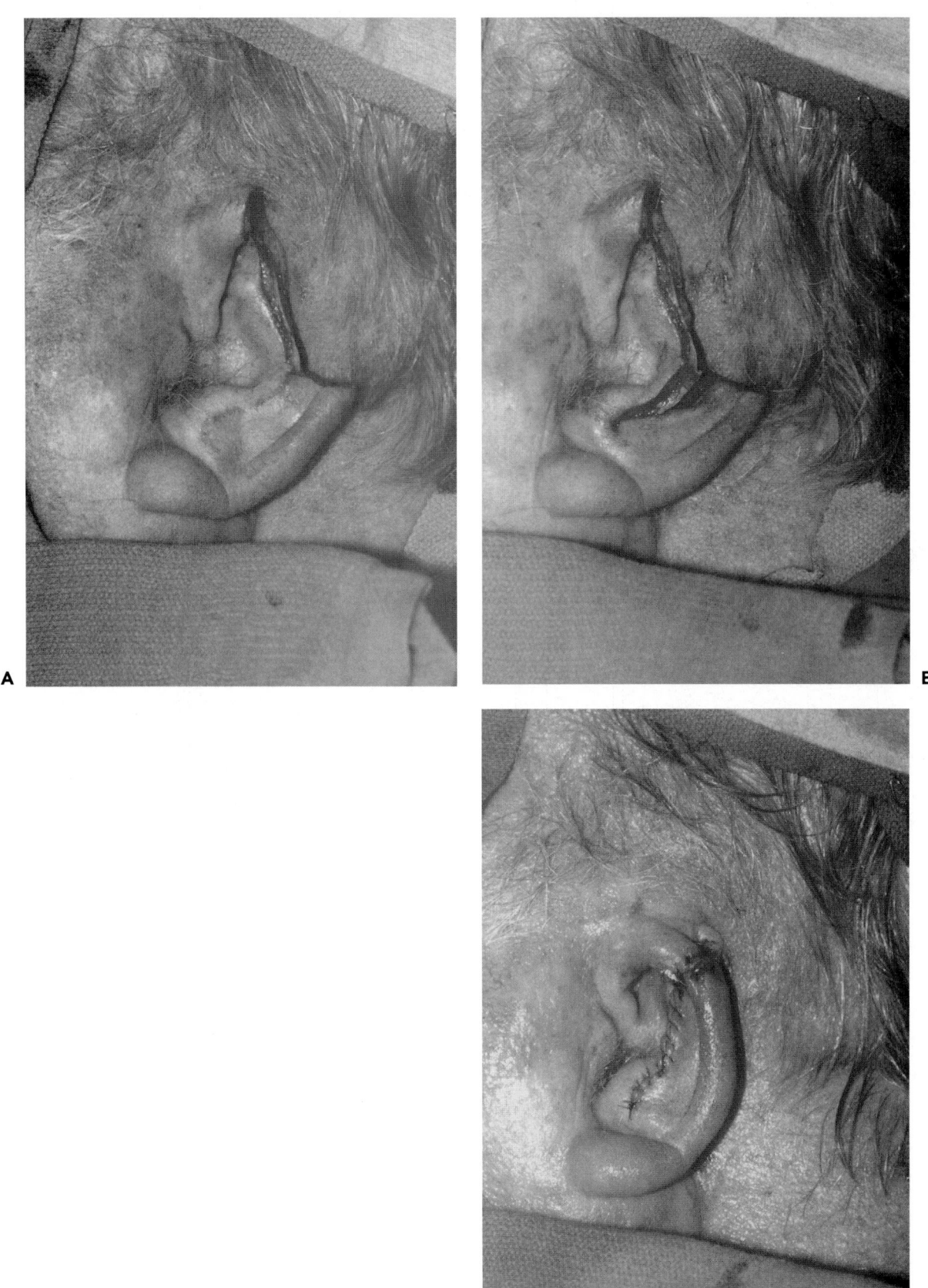

Figure 163.13   A: Defect of the left pinna after excision of squamous cell carcinoma. **B:** Planned chondrocutaneous advancement flap. **C:** Flap sutured into position. (See also Color Plate 60.)

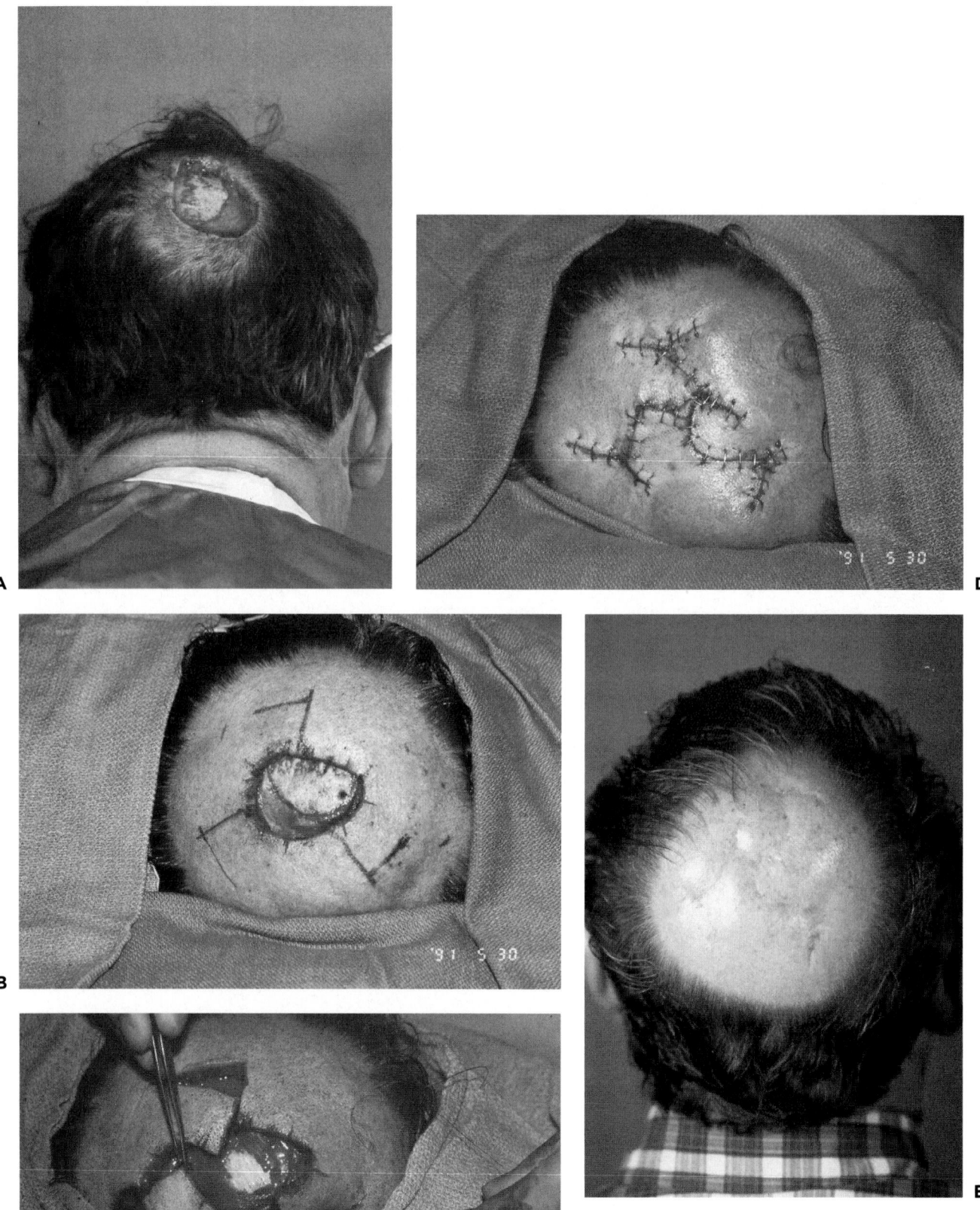

Figure 163.14 **A:** Defect in vertex of scalp after excision of basal cell cancer. **B:** Triple rhomboid flap designed. **C:** Intraoperatively during flap creation and transfer. **D:** Immediately after surgery. **E:** Six months after surgery. (See also Color Plate 61.)

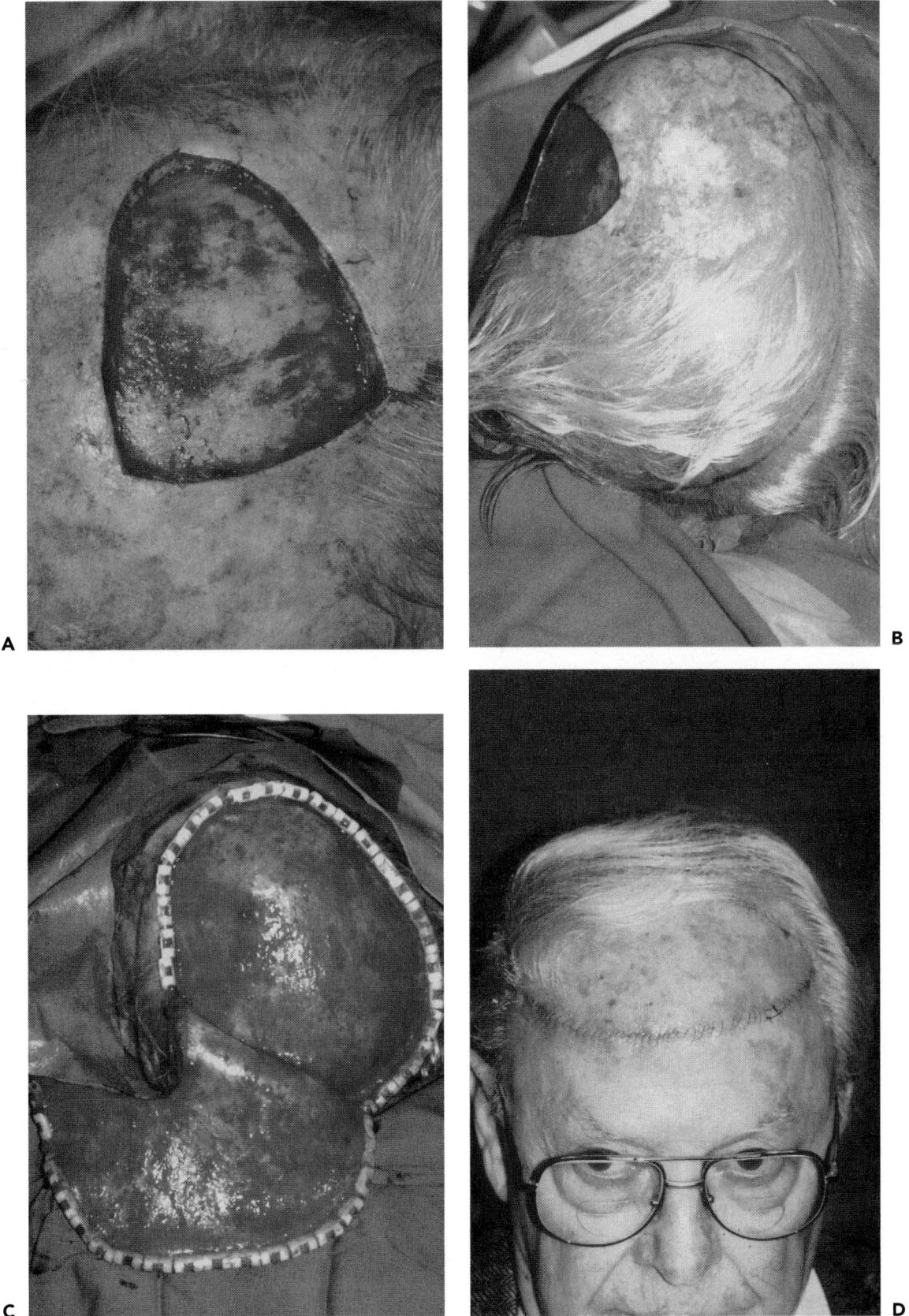

Figure 163.15   A: Left temporoparietal scalp defect. 6 × 7 cm. **B:** Defect shown with planned scalp rotation flap. **C:** Scalp rotation flap after elevation. **D:** Result 1 week after surgery. Note closure of defect in left temporoparietal region.

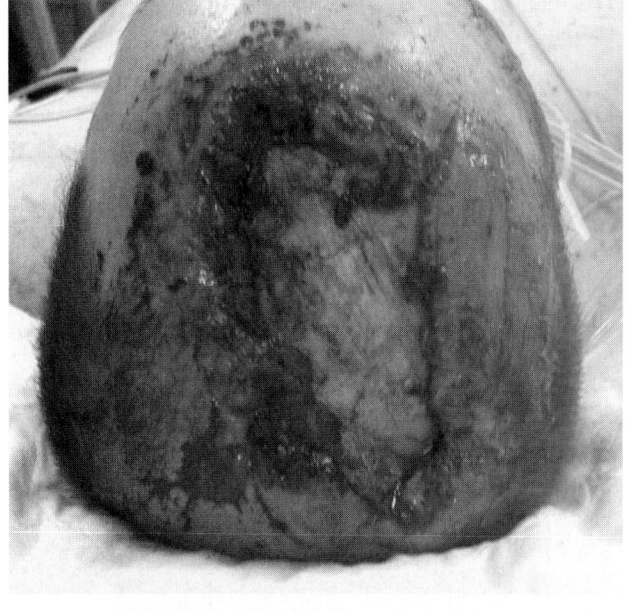

A

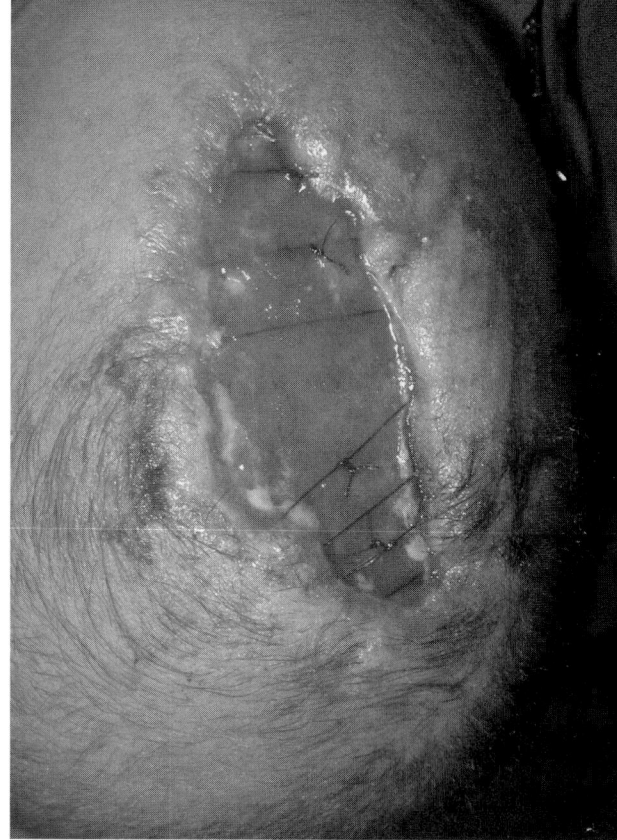

B

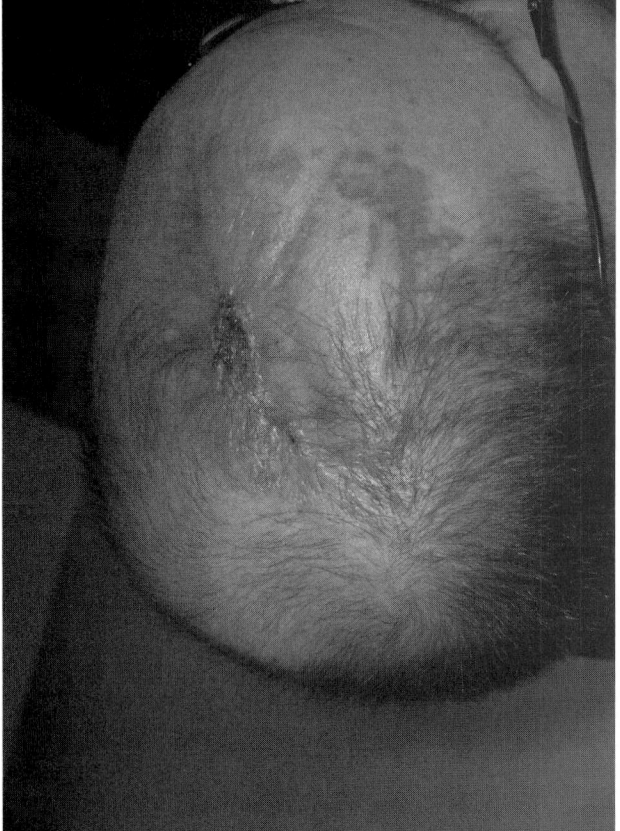

C

Figure 163.16 **A:** Scalp defect with exposed bone and embedded "road" material. **B:** Defect during healing after superficial bone decortication. Note healthy granulation tissue covering the defect. **C:** At 3 months, almost completely healed.

a deflated balloon) is placed under the skin adjacent to the area of defect. It is attached to an injection port, which is placed nearby, connected to the expander by small tubing. Once the incision used for placement is well healed (usually 2 to 3 weeks), inflation of the expander is begun. Fluid is injected into the injection port to the limit of tolerance of the overlying tissue. Usually this is performed weekly,

resulting in slow expansion of the overlying skin (akin to the expansion of a pregnant woman's abdominal skin to accommodate a growing fetus). The additional skin created this way is used for defect coverage (9).

The advantage of tissue expansion is to allow a defect to be repaired with adjacent skin of the same color, texture, and thickness. This skin brings its own innervation and blood supply. The disadvantage is that, especially during the latter phases of expansion, a tissue expander on the face, neck, or scalp can be hard to disguise, giving the patient the temporary appearance of an "alien."

In the head and neck, a rectangular tissue expander is most often used. The base of the expander should be approximately the size of the defect or slightly larger. In this area of the body, expanders are usually placed subcutaneously, although submuscular or other placements are possible. The incisions used for developing the placement pocket and inserting the expander are carefully designed to be used during the later reconstructive procedure. Endoscopic pocket development and endoscopically assisted expander placement can aid in keeping the incision(s) small.

Before placement, the expander is filled with saline, and then all fluid is withdrawn. As the fluid is withdrawn, the surgeon carefully smooths out all ridges and aggregations of the plastic, making the surface of the expander as smooth as possible. Once expansion has begun, ridges can turn into sharp edges, leading to expander extrusion.

The injection port is usually connected to the expander by small tubing and is placed remote from the expander by 4 to 15 cm. Experience has shown that an expander placed over a bony surface such as the mastoid tip or forehead is more likely to extrude. The injection port is usually about 1.5 cm in diameter, with a "bubble" of plastic, backed by a small metal plate. The metal plate acts as a "stop" for the needle while injecting, preventing the needle from going through and out the back of the expansion port.

Typically, a wait of about 3 weeks is required between tissue-expander placement and beginning expansion. If the expander is placed endoscopically, or otherwise via a very small incision with minimal undermining, expansion can begin sooner.

Sterile saline suitable for injection is used to fill the expander. Some practitioners add an antibiotic to the fill solution in an attempt to minimize infection. Expansion is usually carried out weekly, because this is most convenient for outpatients. Faster expansion can be obtained with twice weekly or 3 times weekly expansion.

Expanders are classified by their total expected expanded volume. Keep a record of how much fill is injected each week, so the total volume of fluid used for expansion is known. Most expanders tolerate expansion well beyond their rated volume.

Tissue expansion is carried out as fast as possible without causing complications. During each filling, the physician watches the skin overlying the expander, looking for blanching, and continually inquires about the patient's discomfort level. If maximally tolerated discomfort appears before skin blanching, withdraw a few milliliters of fluid so that patient-discomfort level decreases. If blanching occurs first, this indicates compromise of the microcirculation of the skin overlying the expander. Fluid is withdrawn until the blanching disappears. If the rate of expansion is limited by the patient's discomfort, but

blanching has not yet occurred, it is sometimes worthwhile to allow the patient to sit quietly for 15 to 20 minutes, and then attempt to add some additional fluid.

The most common complication of tissue expansion is discomfort during expansion. Even with prudent expansion, flap-tissue necrosis, hematoma, seroma, or infection can occur. Expander extrusion and flap failure are the most severe complications, sometimes necessitating beginning again with a new reconstructive plan (10). On occasion, enough expansion occurs to go ahead with reconstruction (ahead of schedule) at the same time that the extruding tissue expander is removed.

When it is time to use the flap, the planned excision is made, and the expander and injection port are removed. The surgeon will find a thick greyish capsule between the expander and the overlying tissue. This capsule has an excellent blood supply. It is sometimes possible to dissect sharply between the capsule and the overlying soft tissue, using the capsule itself as an additional vascularized flap that can be skin grafted.

It is always a surprise how much the tissue seems to shrink once the expander is removed. If time is not of the essence, waiting 2 to 3 weeks after the final expansion injection seems to minimize the apparent shrinkage. The expanded skin is deployed as a flap, as designed during the preoperative planning period.

COMPLICATIONS

Unfortunately, not every facial skin–defect repair is followed by a smooth postoperative course and an excellent functional and cosmetic outcome.

Intraoperative

Arterial Insufficiency

The most common intraoperative problem we have seen is a subtle arterial insufficiency that becomes apparent when suturing a flap into its new position. A faint crease appears across the flap, and the skin is definitely paler distal to this crease. When this occurs, it will usually be followed by death of the distal flap unless remedial action is taken.

The simplest action is to undo several skin sutures. If this relieves the tension sufficiently, leave these areas open to be closed several days later in the office. Occasionally it is necessary to undo most of the sutures, or even to replace the flap back into its original (donor) site before this pallor resolves. Use of warm compresses and topical papaverine (especially if this is an axial flap) may be helpful. It is permissible to delay such a flap by leaving the flap in its original anatomic position for a few days, dressing the wound, and suturing the flap into the defect several days later.

Venous Congestion

Because the arteries have thicker walls and a greater flow-pressure head, they are less vulnerable to problems caused by bending or kinking. If the arterial supply is adequate, but venous drainage is a problem, the flap will begin to take on a violet or bluish color. Pricking the skin with a needle results in immediate enthusiastic flow of dark blood, and the flap skin becomes visibly pinker. If the venous congestion persists, small stab incisions can be performed with an 11 scalpel blade. Continued bleeding from these can be encouraged during the postoperative period by gently opening them with a sterile needle or rubbing the crust with a heparin/saline-soaked gauze. Finally, a leech or two may serve a similar function and may be more acceptable to the patient who is tired of being bothered with needles or gauze-rubbing. Remember that a patient receiving leech therapy also must receive antibiotic coverage.

Perioperative

Epidermolysis

Epidermolysis is a vesiculation of the superficial layer of the epidermis. Treated with local wound care only, this phenomenon has virtually no impact on the long-term cosmetic outcome of the flap.

Cellulitis

Persistent or increasing redness of the skin of the flap and adjacent area can be cellulitis or sometimes a topical sensitivity to neomycin. If such redness occurs, any neomycin-containing topical medication should be discontinued, and an oral antibiotic started or adjusted. Any frank pus is cultured with the intent of using sensitivity information, when available, to direct antibiotic therapy, replacing the initial empiric choice.

Full-Thickness Skin Loss

The sight that really makes a reconstructive surgeon's heart sink is the black leathery appearance of full-thickness skin loss. If this is *dry*, akin to dry gangrene, leave it alone. It functions as a wound dressing while skin from secondary intention healing creeps in from the edges, eventually lifting this eschar. See the patient weekly, and trim any loose eschar. Generally speaking, however, the less intervention, the better.

Long Term

Bulky Flap

Some bulkiness will settle down with time, especially with daily firm massage. For flaps that do not respond to this conservative treatment, tightening the superficial skin with one or more dermabrasions can markedly improve the appearance. Other alternatives are using a 2-mm liposuction cannula (which works more by inducing fibrosis than by actual fat removal) or actually incising part of the flap perimeter, and lifting and debulking the flap directly. Judicial use of triamcinolone injections may also diminish excessive subcutaneous tissue.

As mentioned earlier, if contraction of a circumferential scar contributes to the bulkiness, a series of mini Z-plasties around the perimeter scar can ameliorate this.

Inverted Scar

This is a scar the depths of which lie below the level of the surrounding skin. If dermabrasion can be carried out on the skin in the depths, this will improve the appearance. If the scar is too low for this, good results can be obtained by first dermabrading the surrounding area and then excising the 1 to 2 mm of scar, permitting this to heal by secondary intention. Excision of the scar, undermining of the adjacent skin, and layered plastic closure (using vertical mattress sutures) also may be a viable option.

Hypertrophic Scar

Early hypertrophic scarring can often be resolved by daily firm massage (with or without topical steroids). The next level of treatment is topical sheeting—either steroid-impregnated tape (Cordran) or silicone sheeting. For needle-tolerant adults, steroid injections are highly effective (Kenalog, 10 to 20 mg/mL) and can be repeated q2 to 4 weeks.

Once frank mature keloids develop, laser or surgical excision is usually needed.

Specific Scar Locations

Lateral ectropion often resolves with firm massage. Rarely, increasing local soft tissue with skin grafting and cartilage and mucosal grafting is needed. Untreated lateral ectropion can lead to exposure keratitis and, potentially, blindness.

Medial ectropion causes epiphora (by pulling the inferior punctum away from the globe) as well as exposure keratitis. If this does not resolve with conservative treatment, correction can be attained with release of the lower lid. A full-thickness skin graft is used to reconstruct the defect. The use of a vertical traction suture (Frost suture) during the initial phase of healing is mandatory.

Lip notching can cause a "sneering" appearance, as well as leading to oral incompetence (drooling, articulation problems). Often excision of the "notched" area with reapposition solves the problem.

Nasal alar notching or retraction usually requires bringing in additional tissue. Most commonly, correction involves internal nasal placement of an elliptical composite (skin–cartilage) graft.

Similarly, helical rim notching of the pinna is treatable by excision of the scar or defect with reapproximation.

CONCLUSION

Repair of facial defects is planned to restore any functional compromise (especially defects involving the lips, eyelid, and nose). The next focus is cosmetic appearance, in which the aim is for the defect to look as normal as possible.

Local tissue flaps usually yield the best color, texture, and contour match. Under certain circumstances, tissue expansion may be required for the best possible flap design and especially should be considered for large scalp defects. Occasionally, secondary intention healing or skin grafting is a preferable choice, as outlined in this chapter.

- Arterial insufficiency, often due to vessel kinking with flap transposition, can be managed by replacing the flap into its original anatomic position, delaying transfer for several days.
- Epidermolysis, or death of the superficial epidermis, does not usually have a bad effect on the final cosmetic outcome of a flap.

HIGHLIGHTS

- Begin with analysis of the defect: What tissues are missing? Which aesthetic units are affected?
- Skin grafts are most suitable for shallow defects. Decision about where to harvest a skin graft should include aesthetic considerations.
- Secondary intention healing on the face can have unpredictable scarring. It yields the most consistent results in the medial canthal area and other areas overlying bone.
- When considering which local flap to use, note which local tissue is easily available, and which nearby landmarks you want to avoid distorting.
- A subcutaneously pedicled flap is usually chosen only when no other local flap is suitable.
- On the lips, the best scars are oriented radially (not always vertically).
- For a full-thickness eyelid defect, the anterior and posterior lamellas usually require separate reconstruction.
- Skin on the scalp does not stretch as much as facial skin.

REFERENCES

1. Calhoun KH, Seikaly H, Quinn FB. Teaching paradigm for decision making in facial skin defect reconstructions. *Arch Otolaryngol Head Neck Surg* 1998;124:60–66.
2. Mobley S. Bilobed flap design in nasal reconstruction. *Ear Nose Throat J* 2004;83:26–27.
3. Dinehart SM. The rhombic bilobed flap for nasal reconstruction. *Dermatol Surg* 2001;27:501–504.
4. Tramier H. Simple method of designing a bilobed flap. *Plast Reconstr Surg* 2000;105:2633–2634.
5. Cook JL. A review of the bilobed flap's design with particular emphasis on the minimization of alar displacement. *Dermatol Surg* 2000;26:354–362.
6. Stevens CR, Tan L, Kassir R, et al. Biomechanics of A-to-T Flap Design. *Laryngoscope* 1999;109:113–117.
7. Buckingham ED, Quinn FB, Calhoun KH. Optimal design of O-to-Z flaps for closure of facial skin defects. *Arch Facial Plast Surg* 2003;5:92–95.
8. Jewett BS, Shockley WW. Reconstructive options for periocular defects. *Otolaryngol Clin North Am* 2001;34(3):601–625.
9. Hudson DA. Maximising the use of tissue expanded flaps. *Br J Plast Surg* 2003;56:784–790.
10. Cunha M, Nakamoto HA, Herson MR, et al. Tissue expander complications in plastic surgery: a 10-year experience. *Rev Hosp Clin Fac Med Sao Paulo* 2002;57:93–97.

164

Scar Camouflage

Marcelo Hochman   *Ricardo A. Beas*

SCAR ANALYSIS

The healing of a wound results in a scar. The appearance of the scar depends on the wounding mechanism, wound location, wound tension, initial treatment, infection, and dehiscence.

Classification of Scars

Hypertrophic scars
Keloids
Striae distensae
Atrophic scars
Pigmented scars

The surgeon's goal is to make the scar less noticeable. It is necessary that the patient have realistic expectations of the outcome. The physician's responsibility is to inform the patient that elimination of scars is virtually impossible, but that improvement often is possible. On maturation, an ideal scar is level with the surrounding skin, is of good color match, is narrow, is parallel to or lies within favorable skin-tension lines, is located either at the periphery of the face or at a transition between two cosmetic subunits, and lacks obvious straight lines (1). A desirable scar is something that may be undetected by the layperson. Not every scar benefits from revision. In such cases, the patient may benefit from counseling.

Causes of unfavorable scar formation can be genetic, iatrogenic, circumstantial, or idiopathic (2). In scar revision, timing is paramount. Patients traditionally were counseled to wait 6 to 12 months before revision. It is known, however, that early revision with realignment of the scar can accelerate its maturation (3). Healing wounds incorporate high fibroblastic activity; thus dermabrasion can be beneficial as early as 6 weeks after wounding. A convincing argument also can be made for early revision of scars that are obviously poorly aligned or that interfere with function.

SCAR CAMOUFLAGE TECHNIQUES

Staged procedures involving different techniques often are needed. The techniques are shown in Table 164.1. The indications, advantages, and disadvantages of each method are as follows.

Excisional Techniques

Scars due to trauma are haphazard; those made by a surgeon must be planned. The best camouflage is obtained when incisions lie within margins of orifices (nose, mouth, ear, or eye); parallel to or in relaxed skin-tension lines; at the junction of facial aesthetic units; or in a location that can be covered with hair (4) (Fig. 164.1).

Fusiform Excision
The simplest technique used to correct scars that are too wide or that have misaligned edges is fusiform excision. The technique is useful, however, only when the scar lies in a favorable position. The scar is excised elliptically with opposing angles of 30 degrees or less. An essential concept in all scar revision is preservation of the deep scar and subcutaneous layers. These help to efface the closure and contribute to new wound strength. It makes no sense to remove an entire scar that the body will have to reproduce. Only when the deep scar tissue contributes to the deformity is it excised. The surgeon must follow natural curving contours or relaxed tension lines with the ellipse to avoid making a straight-line scar (Fig. 164.2). After undermining, the wound is repaired with careful dermal approximation and equalization of the edges. If the angles are between 30 and 60 degrees, M-plasty closes the wound without tension and with minimal normal tissue removal. Lesions that cannot be removed with opposing angles of less than 60 degrees are poorly suited for fusiform excision.

TABLE 164.1

TECHNIQUES OF SCAR REVISION AND CAMOUFLAGE

Excisional techniques
  Incision placement
  Fusiform excision
  Shave excision
  Scar repositioning
  Serial partial excision
Irregularization techniques
  Z-plasty
  W-plasty
  Geometric broken-line closure
  Dermabrasion, laser resurfacing
  Fillers
Adjunctive techniques
  Steroids
  Dressings, medications
  Cosmetics

Shave Excision

Scars that are acceptably narrow but have contours elevated a few millimeters above the surrounding skin can be improved by means of shave excision. Scars with uneven wound edges or small standing cones can be similarly revised. With a thin scalpel or flexible razor blade, the scar is tangentially shaved down to skin level. Care is taken to preserve intact dermis. Healing occurs by means of reepithelialization.

Scar Repositioning

A scar can be objectionable simply because of its location. Small scars that lie close to a relaxed skin-tension line can be repositioned by means of excision. Typical examples include transferring a scar from the cheek into the nasolabial crease or from the exposed forehead into the hairline. This often involves sacrifice of tissue between the scar and the desirable site. The surgeon must be sure that repositioning does not cause greater deformity.

Serial Partial Excision

When the size and elasticity of a scar prohibit one-stage excision and closure without distortion of nearby normal structures, serial excision can be performed. This technique involves excising part of the scar and advancing the adjacent skin in sequential procedures. The normal skin is

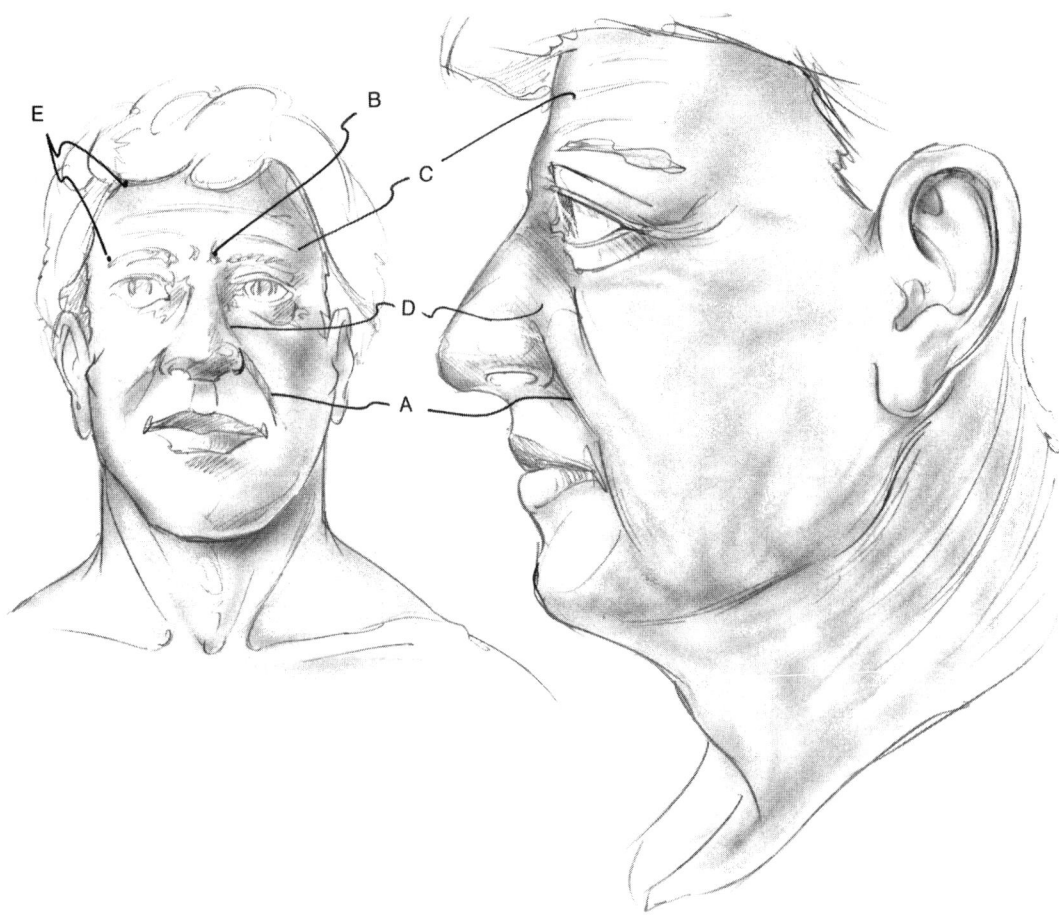

Figure 164.1 Sites for placement of elective incisions that can aid in scar camouflage. *A,* Nasolabial crease; *B,* glabellar furrows; *C,* horizontal forehead creases; *D,* junction of anatomic units (ear and cheek, nose and cheek); *E,* hairline. These and others become more obvious on an aged face.

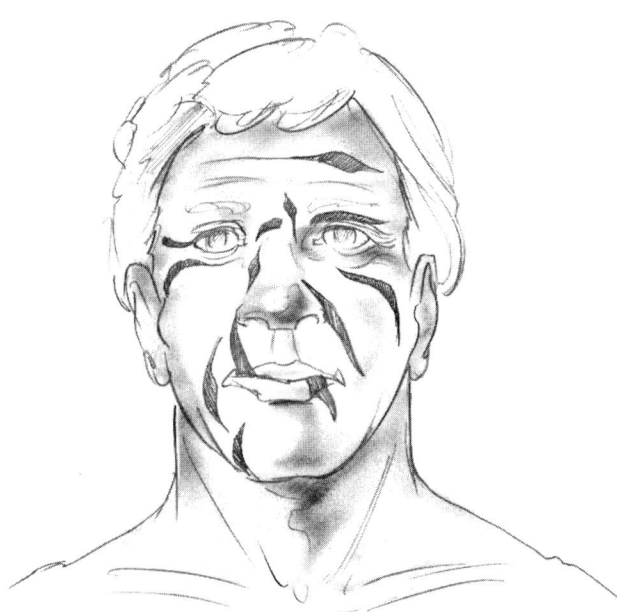

Figure 164.2 Examples of ideal placement of fusiform excision in contour lines or relaxed skin-tension lines for improved scar appearance.

undermined and stretched in stages to fill the area of resected scar until all of the scar is excised. How rapidly this is achieved depends on the size of the scar and the elasticity of the adjacent skin. An older patient with more redundant skin may need fewer procedures than may a younger patient. With the use of tissue expanders, total removal of large areas of scarred tissue is possible with relatively fewer intervening steps.

Scar Irregularization

Long, straight scars are perceived as unnatural and conspicuous, even though the quality of the scar is acceptable.

The same can be said of scars that bridge natural concavities and produce a webbed appearance or scars that cross adjacent aesthetic units. For these, the surgeon uses techniques that break up the scar line.

Z-Plasty

The first reference to Z-plasty was by Denonvilliers in 1856 (5). Through transposition of triangular skin flaps, Z-plasty lengthens the scar and changes its direction. It is particularly helpful in the management of scars that cross important relaxed skin-tension lines, distort anatomic landmarks, or make bands or webs across concavities. By spreading the forces on a given point in several directions, Z-plasty helps to minimize distortions caused by the strong contractile forces of wound healing.

The classic Z-plasty has two 60-degree angles and three limbs of equal length (Fig. 164.3) (6,7). Undermining the two flaps made by incising these limbs and transposing them theoretically increases the length of the scar by 75%. The actual amount of lengthening depends on the elasticity and availability of the surrounding skin. The ideal flap thickness is located between the subdermal plexus and the subcutaneous fatty tissue. The increase in length from rotated Z-plasty triangles varies with the angle between the central and peripheral limbs. Angles less than 30 degrees can cause necrosis of the tip of the flap. Angles greater than 75 degrees can cause redundant standing cones (Fig. 164.4).

Every Z-plasty has four possible designs for the lateral limbs. Correctly designed Z-plasty uses lateral limbs that parallel the relaxed skin-tension line of interest. The ends of the lateral limbs must lie precisely in the line where the new central limb is to be placed. The angles can be varied and made unequal to ensure that the limbs falls in the desired position. Several Z-plasties can be used in tandem around the curve of a trapdoor deformity. This method

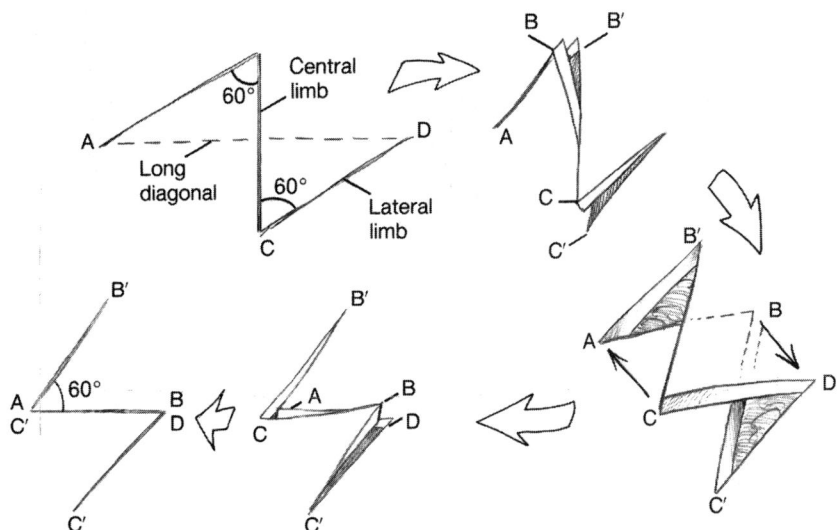

Figure 164.3 Classic equal-angle 60-degree Z-plasty.

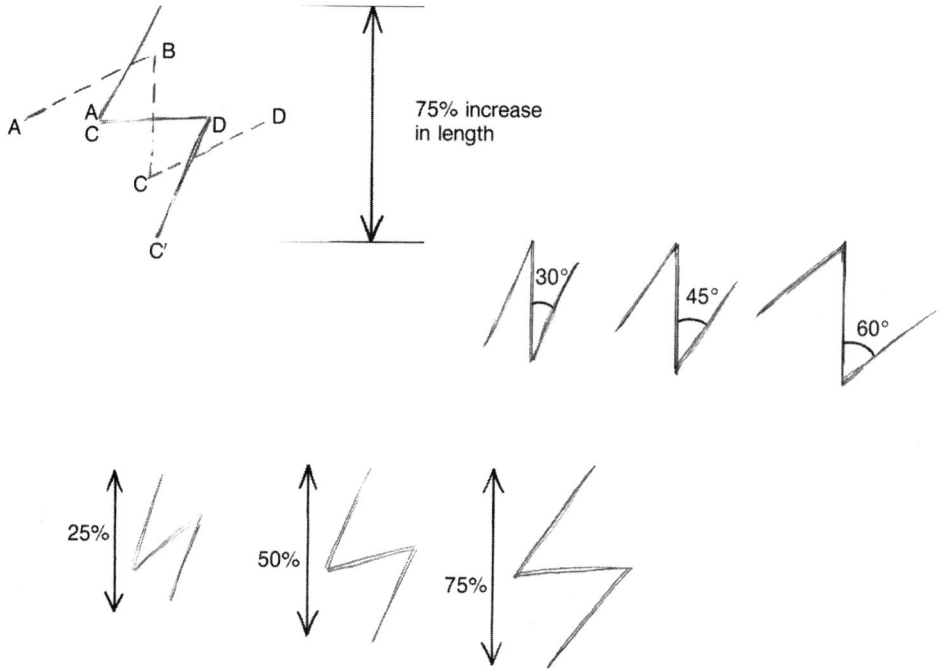

Figure 164.4 Rotated Z-plasty. Larger angles increase length.

allows interdigitation of flap and surrounding skin. Less lateral distortion is obtained with several Z-plasties rather than one large Z-plasty centered on the scar. This is important around the medial canthus, where changes measuring a millimeter can be functionally and cosmetically important. The surgeon must weigh the versatility and benefits of Z-plasty against the fact that it necessitates two extra incisions, and subsequent scars, to correct one scar (8,9).

W-Plasty

Running W-plasty is useful around areas of convex curvature, such as along the mandibular border, antihelical fold, or dorsum of the nasal. A vertical forehead scar sometimes is amenable to revision with this technique. The advantages of W-plasty over Z-plasty are that segments with shorter limbs are used, and the technique does not cause overall lengthening of the scar. W-plasty rarely is performed with a single W; rather, consecutive small triangles of skin are excised on

each side of the scar, and the resultant triangular flaps are imbricated. As many of the component incisions as possible are placed parallel to relaxed skin-tension lines (Fig. 164.5). Intermingling of small scars and normal tissue camouflages the site. The usefulness of W-plasty is limited on broad, flat surfaces such as the cheek, because the result is a predictable, regularly irregular scar that is somewhat conspicuous. Most scars once revised by means of W-plasty are now better served with the geometric broken-line technique (10).

Geometric Broken-Line Closure

Geometric broken-line closure is a scar-excision technique that involves disruption of the linearity of a scar. The technique consists of irregular geometric patterns with a mirror-image pattern on the opposite side of the excision (Fig. 164.6). The triangles, rectangles, and squares are no longer than 6 mm in any dimension. Figures smaller than 3 mm tend to be too small to close, and those greater than

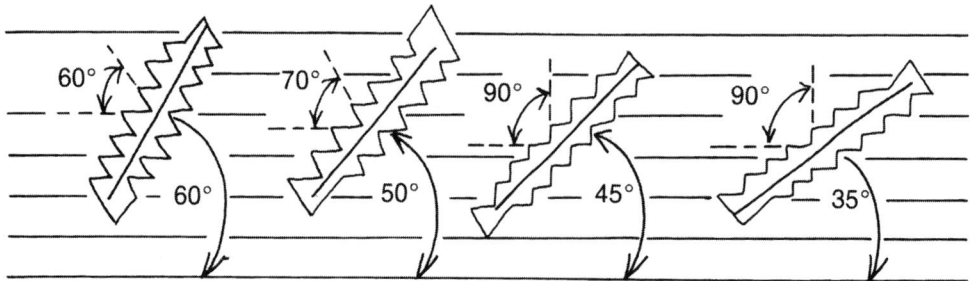

Figure 164.5 Stair W-plasty on scars inclined from 60 to 35 degrees. As scar inclination decreases, the degree of the angles is increased so that as many of the segments as possible follow relaxed skin-tension lines.

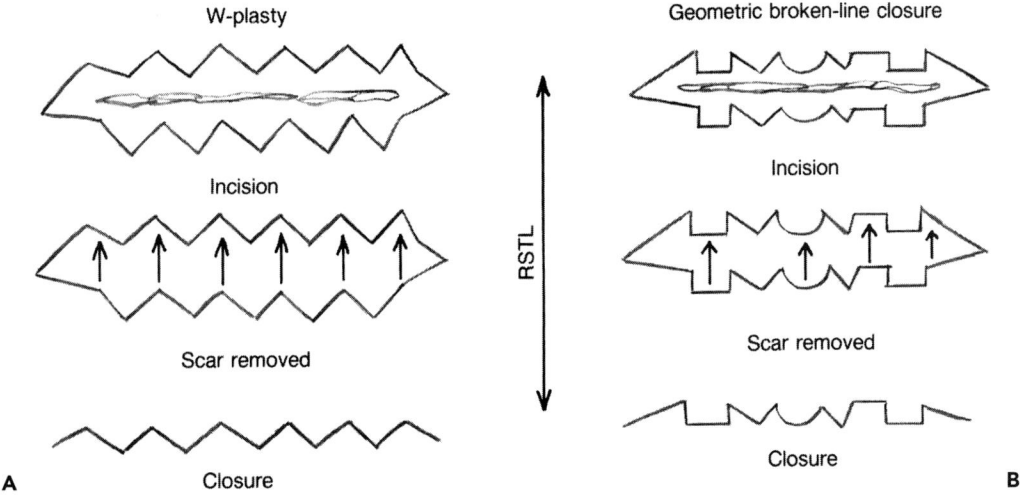

Figure 164.6   A: W-plasty produces an irregular scar through interposed triangular figures, making the scar less noticeable. **B:** Geometric broken line produces irregularity in a more unpredictable pattern to enhance camouflage.

7 mm tend to be too visible individually to effect camouflage. After careful dermal and subcutaneous closure, the epidermis typically is sutured with running locking stitch of rapidly absorbing catgut (Fig. 164.7). Although it is time-consuming to perform, geometric broken-line closure is the best technique for most long, unbroken facial scars. Camouflage can be improved with dermabrasion 6 weeks after closure (11).

Dermabrasion and Laser Resurfacing

The purpose of dermabrasion is to level the skin and promote reepithelialization with new collagen production. The result is blending and smoothing of the revised scar. Acne scarring, rhinophyma, and facial rhytids also are managed with this technique. It is critical to injure only the papillary dermis. This preserves the adnexal structures, which, along with the wound edge, are the source of epidermal cells for migration across the abraded surface.

Abrading into the reticular dermis, marked by the appearance of parallel short white fibers and adnexal structures, greatly increases the risk of adverse scarring. If fat is seen, the reticular dermis has been penetrated. Collagen remodeling in the dermis occurs and is important for tightening of the skin. This is particularly important for correction of actinic changes but is less well understood for scars.

Dermabrasion is performed with a high-speed rotating diamond fraise or wire brush. The dermabrader is moved at a right angle to the direction of wheel rotation. Otherwise loss of control can occur, and the dermabrader can advance in the direction of wheel rotation (Fig. 164.8). Local regional anesthesia can be supplemented with intravenous sedation. A topical refrigerant to freeze the skin is useful on broad, soft surfaces such as the cheek and interbrow area. Freezing the skin to a rigid state maintains the surface of the skin with minimal traction. Care is taken to avoid freezing over bony prominences and in areas of very thin skin. The areas of dermabrasion overlap

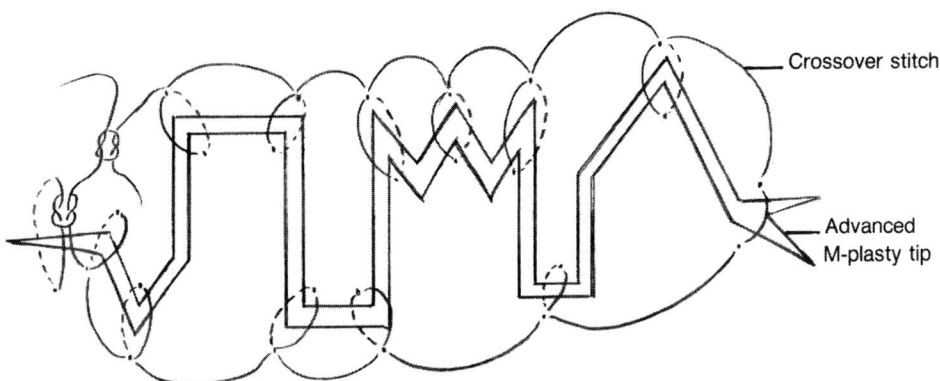

Figure 164.7   Closure of the geometric broken line with a running locking stitch of rapidly absorbing catgut placed at a geometric corner. Dermal interrupted sutures of absorbable material have been placed in key positions.

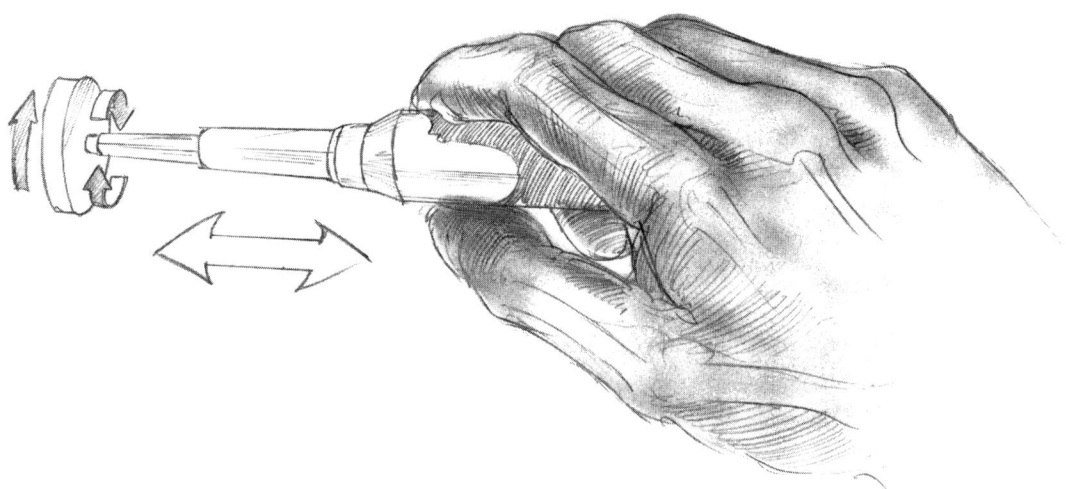

Figure 164.8 The dermabrader is moved at a right angle to the direction of wheel rotation to minimize the risk of uncontrolled advancement of the wheel.

each other, and the periphery is feathered to blend into the surrounding skin.

A high-energy ultrapulsed carbon dioxide laser can be used for the same indications as is traditional dermabrasion. The CO_2 laser wavelength is selectively absorbed by water in the target tissue cells. The principles behind remodeling of the epidermis and dermis appear to be the same as those for dermabrasion. Judging the depth of dermal destruction seems to be more accurate with a laser because the procedure is bloodless, and immediate visual assessment of the change in surface irregularities and dermal tightening is possible. More recently, the use of short- and long-pulsed erbium lasers in conjunction with CO_2 laser resurfacing has been shown to reduce the area of thermal damage. Laser resurfacing has opened the door to treating the periocular skin, which is not readily amenable to traditional dermabrasion.

Patient selection is important for laser or mechanical abrasion. The risk of pigment inconsistency is higher among dark-skinned patients. A history of vitiligo, collagen vascular disease, and hypertrophic or keloid scar formation as well as active herpes simplex can increase the risk of unfavorable results. Antiviral medications especially are important for laser resurfacing and should be administered 2 to 3 days before and 7 to 10 days after the procedure for every patient regardless of previous experience with herpes labialis. Concurrent use of oral contraceptives can precipitate *melasma*, a type of hyperpigmentation usually involving the forehead and cheeks. When this reticulated, mottled, brownish coloration occurs during pregnancy, it is called *chloasma*. Either of these conditions alerts the surgeon to the possibility of blotchy pigmentation changes as a result of resurfacing. A delay of at least 6 months to 1 year after discontinuation of use of 13-*cis*-retinoic acid is prudent, because scarring has been reported after earlier dermabrasion

(12). A history of Raynaud phenomenon or cold urticaria is sought if the use of a skin refrigerant is planned during the procedure.

Milia (small epidermal cysts) are not uncommon after dermabrasion. Most respond to mild abrasive cleansers, but persistent milia can be unroofed with a scalpel blade to release the trapped epidermal element. Milia can be minimized and postoperative healing facilitated if the wound is covered with ointment or a semiocclusive dressing until epithelial resurfacing has occurred, usually within the first week.

It is common to touch up a revised scar with spot dermabrasion until the optimal result is obtained. Because erythema and sensitivity to sunlight persist for a few months, protection from ultraviolet radiation is important to prevent pigmentation problems (13,14).

Nonablative Laser Systems

Most of the nonablative laser systems used today emit light within the infrared portion of the electromagnetic spectrum (1,000 to 1,500 nm). At these wavelengths, absorption by superficial water-containing tissue is relatively weak, thereby effecting deeper tissue penetration. Nonablative laser resurfacing induces collagen remodeling by creation of a dermal wound without disruption of the epidermis. Nonablative laser skin remodeling is in its infancy and, although several systems have been shown to effect improvement in rhytides and atrophic scars, they still do not approximate the improvement typically seen after ablative laser treatment.

Hypopigmentation

Hypopigmented areas can be camouflaged with cosmetics. If a more permanent solution is desired, cultured epithelial autografts, laser or dermabrasion with thin skin grafting, or dermal micrografts can be used (15–19).

Hyperpigmentation

Successful treatment of pigmented scars often requires the use of a pigmented-specific laser, including any number of Q-switched (nanosecond) systems [e.g., 510-nm pulsed dye, 532-nm Nd:YAG, or potassium titanyl phosphate (KTP), 694-nm ruby, 755-nm alexandrite, 1,064-nm Nd:YAG].

Depressed Scars

Resurfacing can be helpful in blending depressed scars with the surrounding tissue levels. (Deeper or more isolated depressions can be filled in with fat grafts, dermal-fat grafts, collagen, or synthetic materials) (20).

Fillers

An ideal injectable soft tissue filler is one that is inexpensive, easy to use, biocompatible, nonpyrogenic, nontoxic, noncarcinogenic, nonallergenic, nonimmunogenic, and nonmigratory, and one with long-lasting effects (21,22).

Current biologic implants include autologous, allogeneic, and xenogeneic materials, such as bovine collagen, autologous collagen, allogeneic collagen, autologous fibroblasts, autologous fat, gelatin matrix, hyaluronic acid gels, preserved particulate fascia lata, and micronized allogeneic dermis (23–25). Although these implants are biocompatible, reabsorption and lack of permanency are their main disadvantages. The alloplastic injectable soft tissue fillers can provide permanent soft tissue augmentation, which is the major advantage over biologic implants. However, when problems arise, the permanence of these implants can be a distinct disadvantage because they are difficult to remove.

ADJUNCTIVE TECHNIQUES

Although proper choice of technique, careful execution, and meticulous closure are necessary for good results, several adjunctive measures can be used to optimize the outcome.

Steroids

Corticosteroids can be used either to manage hypertrophic scars or keloids or to prevent their formation or recurrence after surgery. Injection into small flaps is useful when persistent fullness detracts from the cosmetic result. Intralesional injection of triamcinolone acetonide at various time intervals is administered intradermally, transdermally by using a gun (Dermajet), or at the dermal–subcutaneous junction (26,27). Injection into fat can cause atrophy. The concentration used varies from 10 to 40 mg/mL. Higher

concentrations, however, are more likely to cause local side effects. A few reports of blindness have been made after facial percutaneous injection of steroids (28). Topical steroids are effective only on superficial wounds such as those made by dermabrasion (29).

Silicone Sheets and Gels

Silicone sheets or gels can be used alone or combined with laser therapy to aid the resolution of hypertrophic scars (30,31). The most prevalent theory has focused on the ability of silicone occlusive dressings to increase hydration of the stratum corneum (32).

Mechanical Forces

Pressure and massage aid in resolution of hypertrophic scars (33,34).

Dressings, Medications, and Cosmetics

Apart from being a mechanical barrier to contamination, dressings are important in optimizing results. The initial strength of the wound depends on the suture materials used in closure. Additional support and immobilization are gained with reinforced tape strips. The strips are particularly helpful on the face, where constant mimetic motion can disrupt the healing wound at the microscopic level.

Topical antibiotic or pure petrolatum ointment used on sutured wounds minimizes crusting and retards bacterial contamination. Wounds that heal by means of epithelial resurfacing, such as dermabrasion or shave excision, heal faster if kept moist because the epithelium seeks a plane of migration with a critical humidity (35).

Patients often apply retinoids, vitamin preparations, and over-the-counter emollients. Although the efficacy of these preparations in scar revision is not well documented, they do not seem to affect healing adversely. Patients may want to use them and benefit from a sense that they are actively participating in the therapeutic plan. A professional cosmetician can be helpful during the healing stages of induration and erythema. Scars that cannot be further improved surgically and remain unsightly can be masked with cosmetics. Hair styling can camouflage some scars, and the patient needs to be aware of these techniques (1).

COMPLICATIONS

A systematic approach to scar analysis, incision placement, and choice of technique improves the results of scar revision and camouflage (Fig. 164.9). The key to success is correct preoperative analysis of the problem. Inappropriately placed Z-plasty can cause as much distortion as a traumatic wound. Fusiform excision oriented perpendicular to the relaxed skin-tension lines

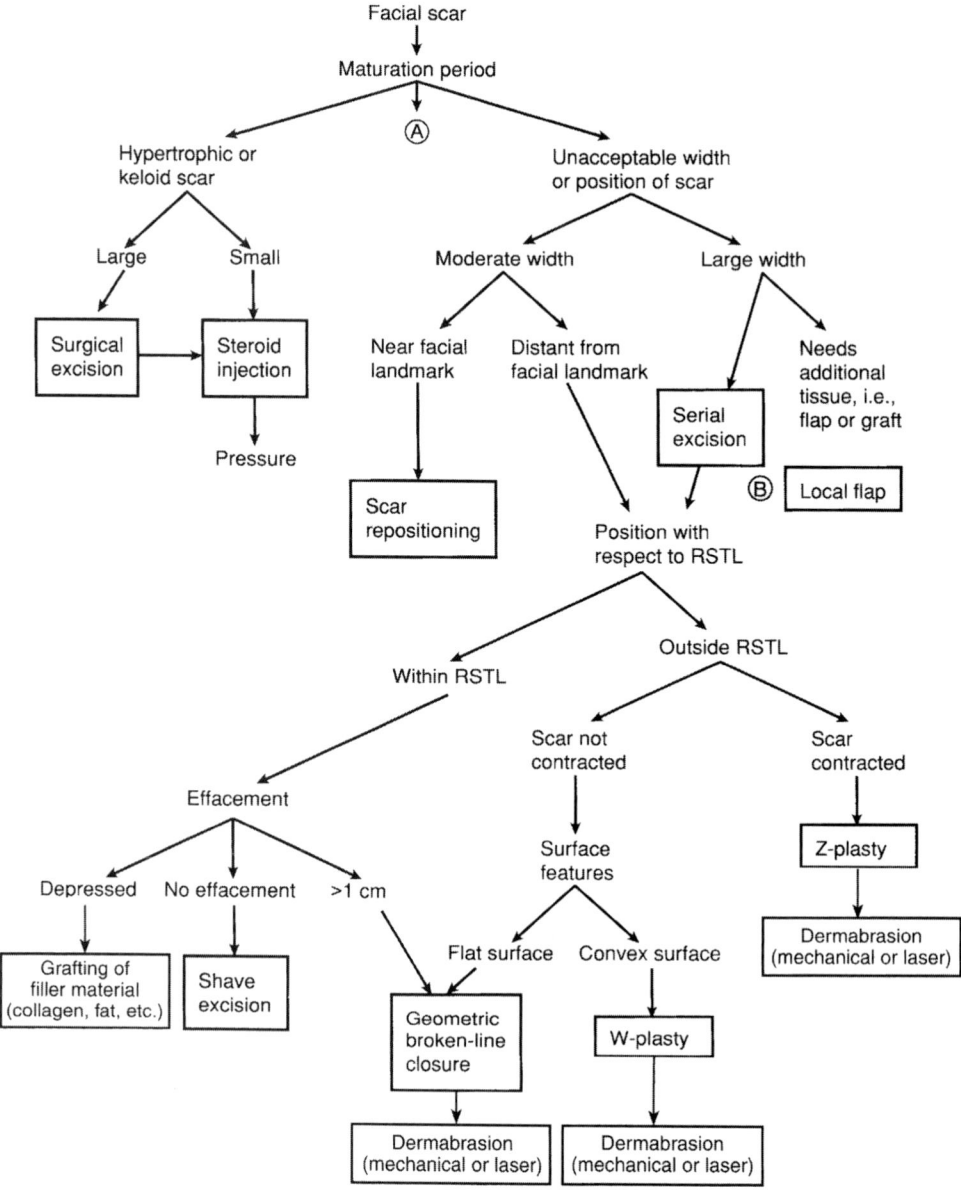

Figure 164.9   Scheme for scar analysis and preoperative planning essential for effective scar revision. (Modified from Thomas JR, Mechlin DC. Scar revision. In: Holt GR, Mattox DE, Gates GA, eds. *Decision making in otolaryngology.* Toronto: BC Decker, 1984:104, with permission.)

yields poor results no matter how carefully it is executed. Postoperative wound care with ointment, reinforcing dressings, and steroids can enhance a correctly oriented simple excision. Preoperative laser evaluation should include a basic medical history including documentation of medications and allergies. A history of abnormal scarring, excessive sun exposure, allergic or inflammatory conditions, herpes simplex virus outbreaks, immune disorders, or previous cosmetic procedures within the involved area should also be ascertained. Proper pretreatment education and close physician follow-up, in addition to a carefully executed postoperative wound-care regimen, helps to reduce morbidity and allows potential problems to be recognized and addressed early.

HIGHLIGHTS

- The ideal scar is flat and level with the surrounding skin, of good color match, narrow, parallel to or within favorable skin-tension lines, and curved, without long unbroken segments.
- The best camouflage is obtained when incisions are designed to lie parallel to or in relaxed skin-tension lines, at the junction of facial aesthetic units, within margins of orifices, or at the edge of a hairline.
- Attempting to improve a scar that at maturity is already optimal can be disastrous.
- Although the vagaries of wound healing can produce an unfavorable scar, the optimal location can be chosen for an elective surgical scar.

■ Early revision is indicated for scars that are malpositioned or poorly aligned or that interfere with function.

■ The traditional 6- to 12-month wait before revision often is unnecessary and can be detrimental.

■ Staged procedures often are necessary to obtain optimal results. The surgeon and patient must recognize that the process is slow and painstaking.

■ Deep scar and subcutaneous tissues always are preserved during scar revision because they help efface the closure and contribute to the strength of the wound. It makes no sense to remove tissue that the body needs to reproduce. Deep scar tissue is removed only if it contributes to deformity.

■ Straight scars are conspicuous even if the quality of the scar is acceptable.

■ Z-plasty spreads the forces on a point over several directions. It minimizes distortions produced by contractile forces during healing. This procedure is useful when wounds cross relaxed skin-tension lines, distort anatomic landmarks, or produce bands across concavities.

■ W-plasty is useful around areas of convex curvature such as the mandibular border, antihelical fold, or dorsum of the nose.

■ Geometric broken-line closure is the best technique for most long, unbroken scars that cross the face.

■ In dermabrasion or laser resurfacing, it is critical to effect superficial injury only into the papillary dermis. This preserves the adnexal structures responsible for reepithelialization.

■ Wounds epithelialize more quickly in a moist environment. Topical ointment helps maintain critical humidity and provides antibacterial protection.

■ Professional assistance in camouflage with cosmetics and hair styling is not to be overlooked during the healing stages of induration and erythema or for scars that cannot be improved surgically.

REFERENCES

1. Thomas JR, Holt GR, eds. *Facial scars: incision, revision and camouflage.* St. Louis: Mosby, 1989.
2. Moran ML. Scar revision. *Otolaryngol Clin North Am* 2001; 34(4):767–780, vi.
3. Borges AF. Principles of scar camouflage. *Facial Plast Surg* 1984; 1:226.
4. Tardy ME, Thomas JR, Paschow MS. The camouflage of cutaneous scars. *Ear Nose Throat J* 1981;60:61.
5. Denonvilliers CP. Blepharoplastie. *Bull Soc Chir Paris* 1856; 7:243.
6. Rohrich RJ, Zbar RI. A simplified algorithm for the use of Z-plasty. *Plast Reconstr Surg* 1999;103:1513–1517.
7. Da-Yuan C. Mathematical principle of planar Z-plasty. *Plast Reconstr Surg* 2000;105:105–108.
8. Bernstein L. Z-plasty in head and neck surgery. *Arch Otolaryngol* 1969;89:36.
9. Furnas DW, Fischer GW. The Z-plasty: biomechanics and mathematics. *Br J Plast Surg* 1971;24:144.
10. Borges AF. Improvement of antitension-line scar by the "W-plastic" operation. *Br J Plast Surg* 1959;12:29.
11. Davidson TM, Webster RD. *Scar revision.* Charleston, SC: American Academy of Otolaryngology–Head Neck Surgury Foundation, 1987.
12. Stegman SS. Avoid dermabrasion soon after Accutane therapy. *Schoch Lett* 1984;34:44.
13. Hinman CD, Maibach H. Effects of air exposure and occlusion on skin wounds. *Nature* 1963;200:377.
14. Farrior RT. Dermabrasion in facial surgery. *Laryngoscope* 1985; 95:534.
15. Chen YR, Yeow VK. Cleft lip scar camouflage using dermal micrografts. *Plast Reconstr Surg* 1999;103:1250–1253.
16. Bernstein LJ, Kauvar AN, Grossman MC, et al. Scar resurfacing with high-energy, short-pulsed and flashscanning carbon dioxide lasers. *Dermatol Surg* 1998;24:101–107.
17. Alster TS, Lewis AB, Rosenbach A. Laser scar revision: comparison of CO_2 laser vaporization with and without simultaneous pulsed dye laser treatment. *Dermatol Surg* 1998;24:1299–1302.
18. Acikel C, Ulkur E, Guler MM. Treatment of burn scar depigmentation by carbon dioxide laser-assisted dermabrasion and thin skin grafting. *Plast Reconstr Surg* 2000;105:1973–1978.
19. Stoner ML, Wood FM. The treatment of hypopigmented lesions with cultured epithelial autograft. *J Burn Care Rehabil* 2000;21: 50–54.
20. De Benito J, Fernandez I, Nanda V. Treatment of depressed scars with a dissecting cannula and an autologous fat graft. *Aesthetic Plast Surg* 1999;23:367–370.
21. Fagien S. Facial soft tissue augmentation with injectable autologous and allogeneic human tissue collagen matrix (autologen and dermalogen). *Plast Reconstr Surg* 2000;105:362–373.
22. Mak K, Toriumi D. Injectable filler materials for soft tissue augmentation. *Otolaryngol Clin North Am* 1994;27:211–222.
23. Klein AW. Skin filling, collagen and other injectables of the skin. *Dermatol Clin* 2001;19(3):491–508, ix. Review
24. Jankovic J, Hallet M, eds. *Therapy with botulinum toxin.* New York: Marcel Dekker, 1994.
25. Wallace DG, McPherson JJ, Ellingsworth LE, et al., Injectable collagen for tissue augmentation. In: Nimni ME, ed. *Collagen, Vol. III. Biotechnology.* Boca Raton: CRC Press, 1988:117–144.
26. Funcik T, Hochman M. The effect of intradermal corticosteroids on skin flap edema. *Arch Otolaryngol Head Neck Surg* 1995;121:654.
27. Morris DE, Wu L, Zhao LL, et al. Acute and chronic animal models for excessive dermal scarring: quantitative studies. *Plast Reconstr Surg* 1997;100:674–681.
28. Shafir R, Cohen M, Gur E. Blindness as a complication of subcutaneous nasal steroid injection. *Plast Reconstr Surg* 1999;104: 1180–1184.
29. Dannenberg AM. The anti-inflammatory effects of glucocorticoids: a brief review of the literature. *Inflammation* 1979;3:329.
30. Suetak T, Sasai S, Zhen YX, et al. Effects of silicone gel sheet on the stratum corneum hydration. *Br J Plast Surg* 2000;53: 503–507.
31. Wittenberg GP, Fabian BG, Bogomilsky JL, et al. Prospective single-blinded, randomized, controlled study to assess the efficacy of the 585-nm flashlamp-pumped pulsed-dye laser and silicone gel sheeting in hypertrophic scar treatment. *Arch Dermatol* 1999;135: 1049–1055.
32. Baum TM, Busuito MJ. Use of a glycerin-based gel sheeting in scar management. *Adv Wound Care* 1998;11:40–43.
33. Costa AM, Peyrol S, Porto LC, et al. Mechanical forces induce scar remodeling: study in non-pressure-treated versus pressure-treated hypertrophic scars. *Am J Pathol* 1999;155:1671–1679.
34. Patino O, Novick C, Merlo A, et al. Massage in hypertrophic scars. *J Burn Care Rehabil* 1999;20:267–271.
35. Eaglestein WH. Experiences with biosynthetic dressings. *J Am Acad Dermatol* 1985;12:434.

Nasal Restoration with Flaps and Grafts

165

Stephen S. Park

The practice of nasal restoration has evolved significantly from early, rudimentary attempts to provide covering for large nasal defects. In contemporary nasal reconstruction, surgeons combine a mastery of aesthetics and surgical techniques, to create a nose that is visually inconspicuous and functionally stable, for the life of the patient. Ancient methods focused on using soft tissue to cover the cavity, with little regard for the intrinsic contours of the nose or structural framework. Nasal reconstruction in the twenty-first century has raised the bar to a level where the new nose may go unnoticed by the casual observer, nasal function returns to the baseline, and the patient integrates back into society without undue self-consciousness.

HISTORY OF NASAL RECONSTRUCTION

The history of nasal reconstruction dates back to antiquity when, during the fourth Egyptian dynasty (2575–2467 B.C.), prostheses were molded for the deceased, because "only those without physical disfigurement would enter the Kingdom of Osiris" (1). Reconstruction came into greater demand with the rise of nasal mutilation as a common form of humiliation or punishment. Around 1500 B.C., when Prince Lakshmana of India deliberately amputated the nose of Lady Surpunakha, King Ravana arranged for the reconstruction of Lady Surpanakha's nose by his physicians, documenting one of the earliest accounts of nasal restoration in human history (2,3). *Sushruta Samhita*, an ancient Indian Sanskrit written during the Vedic period (600–1000 B.C.), describes nasal reconstruction as performed by a caste of Indian potters, using cheek tissue to cover the nasal defect (4). Early descriptions of using forehead tissue to repair a nasal defect exists in writings by the

Kangiara family from 1440 A.D. (5). Despite the long history with this type of reconstruction, very little international exchange occurred because of the lack of maritime commerce and communication between Europe and Asia during that period. In the sixteenth century, Gusparo Tagliacozzi described his success with a two-staged method of nasal reconstruction using a pedicled, cutaneous flap from the upper arm, based on the brachial vessels. This was followed by attempts with pedicled flaps from other individuals, especially slaves. Outcomes became discouraging and further progression was shortly abandoned.

In 1794, the first description of the Indian forehead flap in the English language was published in the *Madroas Gazette* and later reproduced in *Gentleman's Magazine* (6). Joseph Carpue, an English general surgeon, is credited with the introduction of this forehead flap to the Western world when he described his experience with two successful Indian forehead flaps for nasal reconstruction (7). Subsequently, the classic forehead flap for nasal reconstruction became widespread throughout the globe and the standard method of repair during the early nineteenth century. This "classic" Indian median forehead flap was based on bilateral supratrochlear arteries with a wide pedicle that could not extend beyond the level of the brows. The wide base limited the rotation and length of the forehead flap. This limitation became more evident when it was recognized that intranasal lining left to heal by second intention resulted in significant distortion, contracture, and nasal obstruction.

Pedicled flaps moved slowly to the United States; the first American reports of forehead flaps for nasal reconstructions are from the 1940s (8,9). These early flaps were traditional "median" forehead flaps with wide pedicle bases capturing both supratrochlear vessels. Kazanjian and

Converse believed that the paired arteries were needed to adequately perfuse the forehead flap. Because of the limited length of this early median forehead flap, many variations were described, largely aimed at mobilizing more tissue with greater flap length: "Gillies' up-and-down flap" (10), "New's sickle flap" (11), "Converse's scalping flap" (12), and the "Washio flap" (13). In spite of the variety of flaps attempted, none have stood the test of time primarily because of the poor quality of scalp skin in contrast to forehead skin and the significant donor site morbidity.

Millard repopularized the paramedian flap with a "seagull" design for resurfacing the nose (14–17). The primary advantage of this paramedian flap was the narrow pedicle base, which allowed for an improved arc of rotation. The inferior reach of the flap could be further extended by basing the pedicle below the level of the brow. This design created less narrowing of the brows in contrast to the original "median" forehead flap. Millard also noted that the supratrochlear artery traveled in a plane between the skin and frontalis muscle, and, consequently, the frontalis muscle could be selectively trimmed off the undersurface of the flap without jeopardizing flap vascularity. Gary Burget and Fred Menick have since refined these concepts of the paramedian forehead flap design and have brought nasal reconstruction to its higher standards (18).

ETIOLOGY OF NASAL DEFECTS

Defects of the nose arise from a large array of causes and, in many circumstances, it is worthwhile to consider the specific etiology, as it may impact the method of repair. The nose is the most common site for *de novo* cutaneous malignancies. Basal-cell carcinomas predominate, and there are histologic subtypes with varying degrees of aggressiveness. The nodular subtype is most common, as characterized by a circumscribed growth pattern, and carries the most favorable prognosis. Aggressive histologic subtypes, such as the morphea form or infiltrating, can develop small nest patterns and are more likely to involve the internal lining or to recur following surgical excision. These latter subtypes are best treated with Mohs surgery. Squamous cell carcinoma is the second most common type and also behaves aggressively, with a greater incidence of regional metastasis. Melanoma is the most serious skin tumor, warranting an aggressive surgical intervention. Recurrent skin tumors or tumors that have been previously irradiated have a less predictable vascular anatomy, which may impact flap design and closure options. Vascular and adnexal tumors of the nose are less common but often warrant more aggressive treatment plans. Sharp trauma to the nose. such as a windshield injury, is another etiology for a nasal defect, which is often repaired immediately and completely. Animal or human bites are grossly contaminated, and a delay in repair is often advocated. This dogma arises from experience with extremity injuries; however, the face is characterized by such a robust vascularity that immediate repair will often be successful.

NASAL ANATOMY

A firm understanding of the normal nasal anatomy is a natural prerequisite for a high-quality nasal reconstruction. The biomechanics of covering flaps, the importance of a firm framework, and the anatomic basis for internal lining repair, are imperative concepts as one proceeds through the algorithm of reparative options.

The *external nasal skin* is variable at different areas of the nose, being thick at the nasion and tip, and extremely thin along the rhinion. The thin epithelial sleeve along the alar rim and nasal facets make these areas especially vulnerable to notching and contour irregularities following reconstruction.

There are four layers of *soft tissue* between the skin and the nasal skeleton—the superficial fatty panniculus, fibromuscular layer, deep fatty layer, and, finally, the periosteum or perichondrium. The superficial fatty panniculus is located immediately below the skin and consists of adipose tissue with interlacing vertical fibrous septi coursing from the deep dermis to the underlying fibromuscular layer. The fibromuscular layer contains the intrinsic nasal musculature and the nasal subcutaneous muscular aponeurotic system, which is a continuation of the facial aponeurotic system. The deep fatty layer located between the subcutaneous muscular aponeurotic system and the thin covering of the nasal skeleton contains the major superficial blood vessels and nerves. The periosteum of the nasal bones extends over the upper lateral cartilages and fuses with the periosteum of the piriform process laterally (19). Perichondrium covers the nasal cartilages, and dense fibrous interconnections can be found between the paired tip cartilages. Between the framework and the deep fatty layer is a plane of loose areolar tissue that is free of fibrous septae, making it an ideal plane for dissection and elevation of the soft-tissue envelope.

The *nasal musculature* of the nose is well defined, with greatest activity along the junction of the upper lateral and alar cartilages (20). This allows for muscular dilation and stenting of the functionally critical nasal valve area. All nasal musculature is innervated by the zygomaticotemporal division of the facial nerve (21).

The nasal *blood supply* is via a predictable and consistent network of named vessels through both the internal and external carotid systems. The angular artery branches from the facial artery and is a discrete landmark along the nasofacial junction. Feeder vessels off the angular artery perforate the levator labii superioris and provide the vascular basis for the design of melolabial flaps. A medial branch of the angular artery, the lateral nasal artery, supplies the lateral surface of the caudal nose. This lateral nasal artery courses in the sulcus between the ala and nasal sidewall and is covered by the levator labii superioris alaeque nasi. It arborizes multiple times to enter the subdermal plexus covering the nostril and cheek. The dorsal nasal artery, a branch of the ophthalmic artery, pierces the orbital septum above the medial palpebral ligament and travels along the side of the nose to anastomose with the lateral nasal artery. The dorsal nasal artery provides a rich axial blood supply to the dorsal nasal skin, and serves as the main arterial contributor to dorsal nasal flaps. The columella and tip are supplied by the columellar arteries, branches of the superior labial artery. The external nasal branch of the anterior ethmoidal artery, a branch of the ophthalmic artery, pierces bone on the medial wall of the orbit at the point where the lamina papyracea of the ethmoid bone articulates with the orbital portion of the frontal bone (frontoethmoid suture). The vessel enters the ethmoid sinuses to supply the mucosa and sends branches to the superior aspect of the nasal cavity. The external nasal branch of the anterior ethmoidal artery emerges between the nasal bone and the upper lateral cartilage to supply the skin covering the nasal dorsum and tip. The venous drainage of the external nose is through corresponding vessels, leading into the facial vein, the pterygoid plexus, and the valveless ophthalmic veins.

The *intranasal mucosa* has a similar number of named vessels. The septal branch of the superior labial artery is a dominant feeder to the septal mucosa. In fact, a flap of the entire septal mucosa, back to the sphenoid sinus, can be based on this single vessel. The anterior and posterior ethmoidal vessels supply the superior portion of the septum. Terminal branches of the anterior ethmoidal artery cover the dorsal nasal septum, a critical region for the swinging septal flaps used for internal lining and structure. Terminal branches of the sphenopalatine artery supply the posterior septum and posterior lateral nasal wall. The vasculature of the intranasal lining is the anatomic basis of mucosal flaps used for major nasal reconstruction.

The *sensory nerve* supply of the nasal skin is via the ophthalmic and maxillary divisions of the fifth cranial nerve. Branches of the supratrochlear and infratrochlear nerves supply the skin covering the radix, rhinion, and cephalic portion of the nasal sidewalls. The external nasal branch of the anterior ethmoidal nerve supplies the skin over the caudal half of the nose. The infraorbital nerve provides sensory branches to the skin of the lateral aspect of the nose.

The *structural framework* of the nose is composed of the paired nasal bones to the upper third, the nasal septum and upper lateral cartilages to the middle vault, and the paired lower lateral cartilages within the nasal tip. Dorsal support to the middle vault is primarily achieved through the rigidity of the cartilaginous septum, and to a lesser extent, the paired upper lateral cartilages. Their fusion at the midline is important clinically because of the tendency for the upper lateral cartilages to progressively contract intranasally and lead to obstruction. If a disarticulation be-

tween the septum and upper lateral cartilages occurs, the middle vault should be diligently reconstructed.

The tip is supported by the overall size and strength of the lower lateral cartilages, their ligamentous attachments to the caudal septum, the scroll with the upper lateral cartilages, and the adherence to the overlying soft tissue. Each lower lateral cartilage is subdivided into medial, intermediate, and lateral crura. The shape, length, and angulation of the intermediate crura determine the external morphology of the tip lobule and the position of the tip defining point. Disruption or weakening of the lateral crus predisposes to alar retraction and notching, an important consideration in nasal reconstruction when these structures may have been compromised. Laterally, small sesamoid cartilages are interconnected by a dense, fibrous connective tissue.

The *alar lobule and nasal sidewall* is a functionally pivotal area of the nose that is not often highlighted during rhinoplasty discussions but has a critical role during reconstructive surgery. This *keystone* region is located between the lateral border of the lower lateral cartilage and the bony piriform aperture. Externally, it corresponds to the supra-alar crease and is the most common location for a clinically significant, dynamic valve collapse. Beneath the skin, the area consists of a firm, fibrous-fatty aponeurosis, an occasional sesamoid cartilage, and a portion of the transverse nasalis muscle. Typically, this histologic architecture provides sufficient rigidity to prevent collapse during inspiration. If compromised, nasal function will be impaired unless it is aggressively restored with liberal grafting in a nonanatomic fashion. The *internal nasal valve* is a distinct area defined by the dorsal septum medially, upper lateral cartilage superolaterally, and the head of the inferior turbinate inferomedially. The *external nasal valve* is the cross-sectional area under the alar lobule proper. It does not entirely correlate with the lateral crus of the lower lateral cartilages. The alar rim does not have cartilage within it, and collapse or notching can readily occur. To avoid this, structural grafts to the alar rim are often needed. The junction between the ala and cheek forms an acute angle and is difficult to reconstruct; most repairs heal with gradual effacement of that alar-facial angle and may become increasingly conspicuous. If at all possible, one should try to preserve the alar-facial junction and keep incisions slightly onto the nose. The *limen vestibule* is the junction between the internal nasal lining and the stratified squamous epithelium of the nose. It does not lie at the inferior-most border of the alar lobule but rather slightly intranasally, within the vestibule. Reconstruction of full-thickness defects of the alar rim should keep this in mind and allow the resurfacing flap to roll inward before suturing to the internal lining flap.

There is a *bony piriform platform* that surrounds the nose, and its role in tissue support is often poorly appreciated. The nasal sil, anterior nasal spine, and medial maxilla (including the frontal process of the maxilla), provide an essential stage for the nose, and resection of these structures will require a separate repair, such as with a split calvarial bone graft. Failure to rebuild this platform will often result in a soft-tissue collapse and facial asymmetry.

DEFECT ANALYSIS

Analyzing a given defect and arriving at the ideal method of repair is a challenging and rewarding exercise. On occasion, the "correct" flap will be intuitive, as it appears to define itself. At other times, however, it can be a creative dilemma as one struggles to visualize the incisions, flap transfer, surrounding vectors of tension, and final scars. This mental challenge requires a dynamic, three-dimensional image of the nasal repair. At times, it is worthwhile to have a structured algorithm for defect analysis. Although it does not necessarily define the ideal flap, it can be very useful in avoiding errors in design. In particular, the line of questioning can guide one away from creating disfiguring mistakes such as eyelid retraction or an unnatural hairline. Once flaps are elevated and transposition is attempted, the reconstruction is committed; this is clearly not the time to discover a gross design flaw.

For every cutaneous defect, there are six questions that are reviewed prior to the first incision (Table 165.1):

1. *Immobile structures.* What surrounding landmarks must not come under any tension during flap transposition, such as the eye lid, alar margin, or upper lip? It does not necessarily mean that tissue cannot be recruited from that region but rather, adequate structure must be available in the area to fully support the adjacent flap. A common example is a cheek flap that jeopardizes lower-eyelid retraction and is vertically supported with anchors to the infraorbital rim. For the nose, there are three "immobile structures:" the alar rim, nasal tip symmetry, and lateral nasal wall. The immobility of the lateral nasal wall is perpendicular to the cutaneous plane, in the third dimension, where collapse and functional compromise can occur with rotation flaps over that area.
2. *Area of recruitment.* Given which surrounding areas are "immobile," from where can tissue be recruited without distorting those areas? Also, in what direction do the lines of maximal extensibility exist and how can the flap be designed to slide parallel with them?
3. *Facial lines.* There are numerous descriptions of facial lines that can assist with flap selection and design. Langer

lines were first described by Langer in 1961 as a recommendation for orienting elliptical skin excisions (19). Circular defects in postmortem patients became elliptical as rigor mortis ensued and these lines were mapped throughout the body. Clinical practice has shown that these lines do not always orient along lines for optimal healing. Relaxed skin tension lines (RSTLs) more accurately reflect the intrinsic tension within the dermis while at rest. Wounds heal under less tension when oriented along them and they can usually assist with flap design. Lines of minimal tension (also known as skin creases) are defined by the repeated contraction of the underlying muscle as they permanently orient elastin and collagen fibers within the dermis. These lines usually run parallel with the RSTLs but the supratip, glabella, and lateral canthal regions are in conflict. It is usually recommended to incise along lines of minimal tension over RSTLs.

The other "facial lines" that exist in the face are those created by the borders of *aesthetic units,* and the subunits of the nose. The principle of aesthetic units is based on the fact that the human eye can only perceive things as a series of block images, thus our inability to scan a horizon without a saccadic motion. The face, or nose, is visualized as a discrete set of block images that are put together subconsciously and interpreted as a single image. These images are defined by predictable reflections of light, natural creases, and undulations in cutaneous topography. The nose has subunits defined as the nasal tip, dorsum, columella, paired ala, sidewalls, and soft-tissue facets (Fig. 165.1). Scars that are

<table>
<tr><td colspan="2">**TABLE 165.1**</td></tr>
<tr><td colspan="2">**DEFECT ANALYSIS**</td></tr>
<tr><td>1. Immobile structures</td></tr>
<tr><td>2. Area of recruitment</td></tr>
<tr><td>3. Facial lines</td></tr>
<tr><td>4. Resultant scars</td></tr>
<tr><td>5. Nasal function</td></tr>
<tr><td>6. Depth</td></tr>
</table>

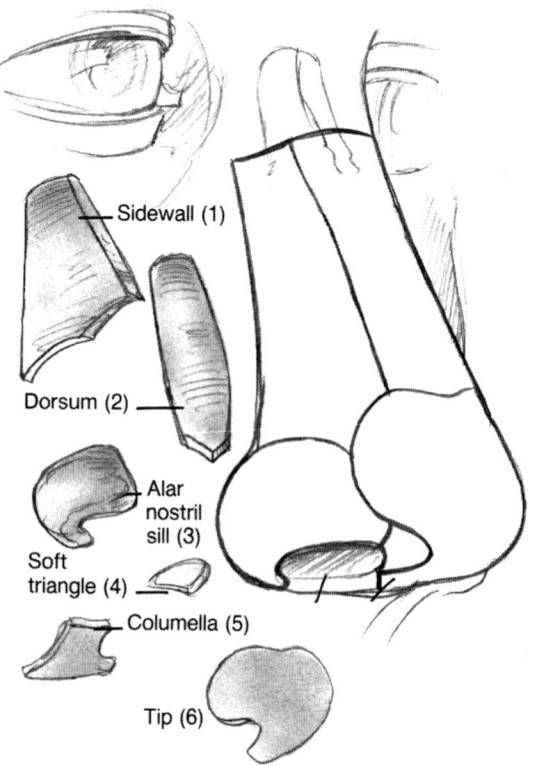

Figure 165.1 Nasal aesthetic subunits.

strategically placed at the border of two units will be less conspicuous than those resting within one. In order to achieve this, one usually has to modify the size/shape of the original cutaneous defect. The aesthetic subunits may require modifications with some patient groups who have other unique nasal characteristics. At times, a patient may have a significant transition from one skin type to another within the nose, such as individuals with rosacea or a rhinophyma (20).

4. *Resultant Scars*. The final question in this algorithm is anticipating the final scars for each proposed flap and how they relate to preexisting facial lines. At times, this exercise is not intuitive, such as the resultant scars of a rhombic flap. This question forces the surgeon to try different orientations of flap design that might yield more favorable scars while still abiding by the previous tenets of immobile structures and area of recruitment.

5. *Function*. During the defect analysis, one of the essential considerations is the *location* in terms of function and potential lateral wall collapse. A cutaneous defect involving the critical area along the supra-alar crease will place the nasal airway at jeopardy even if the original defect does not violate native cartilage. This critical "red zone" must alert the reconstructive surgeon of the need for structural reinforcement in the form of cartilage grafting. Anatomically, it corresponds to the fibroareolar tissue immediately lateral to the lateral crus of the lower lateral cartilage and is distinct from the precise *internal* and *external nasal valves*. Similarly sized defects along the dorsum or upper third do not have the associated functional concerns.

6. *Depth*. Assessing the depth of the nasal defect is important to determine if any structural cartilage or bone is missing and to explore the internal nasal lining. Any violation of the intranasal mucosa must be recognized preoperatively, as it will alter the reconstructive plan significantly; all missing lining must be meticulously repaired prior to grafting and resurfacing. Failure to do so will risk contracture, lumen stenosis, graft exposure and resorption, and alar notching.

SMALL CUTANEOUS DEFECTS

Cutaneous defects of the nose can be found in a variety of sizes, depths, and shapes. Intuitively, the smaller ones should be more straightforward in terms of repair, but that is often not the case. Whereas large defects have a limited number of options, those less than 1.5 cm can be repaired with an array of flaps and grafts, often creating a greater intellectual challenge. Furthermore, patient expectations are generally higher with small lesions, and even small irregularities that often plague these repairs can be problematic, such as alar base asymmetry, notching, conspicuous scars, pincushioning, or valve collapse.

Pertinent Anatomy

Nasal topography during reconstruction is often discussed in terms of aesthetic subunits, but since smaller defects frequently involve only small portions of an individual site, it is more practical to discuss the defect in terms of the upper, middle and lower thirds of the nose. The *upper third* has relatively thin skin except for the nasion region, where the subcutaneous tissue is much more prominent. The lateral borders are adjacent to the medial canthus and represent *immobile* regions that cannot be distorted, especially from contracture during second intention healing. The area of recruitment is primarily from the glabella and, to a lesser extent, from the nasal dorsum. There is little functional concern with defects in this zone.

The *middle third* of the nose has skin that is thin medially but thicker laterally. Whereas the upper lateral cartilages support the medial portion of this zone, the lateral aspect has support only from fibroareolar tissue without native cartilage. Tissue can be recruited from multiple directions, but any vertical vector must be minimal, as alar or tip elevation can quickly occur. Functional implications are important along the lateral aspect of the middle vault, even if no native cartilage has been violated. The lateral nasal artery is found immediately cephalad to the supra-alar crease and is the basis for many local flaps of the nose.

The *lower third* of the nose consists of the nasal tip, alar lobule, columella, and soft-tissue triangle. The skin is typically thicker and more sebaceous, leading to less favorable wound healing. Most defects of this region are repaired with tissue recruited from the middle vault, but great care must go into flap design and the subsequent vectors of tension. This zone is significant for its free alar margin and the fact that small degrees of wound contracture may lead to retraction and gross alar base asymmetries. The supra-alar crease and alar–facial junction are important natural landmarks that should be preserved or recreated. The alar lobule proper does not contain native cartilage, and disruption to this area predisposes to a dynamic external nasal valve collapse. Consequently, nonanatomic cartilage grafting is essential to prevent alar rim retraction and collapse.

SELECTION OF GRAFTS AND FLAPS

At times, the simplest method of repair is also the preferred one in terms of optimal aesthetic results. Second intention healing, skin and composite grafts, and local flaps all enter the algorithm for repair of such defects, and proper selection becomes the cornerstone for a successful outcome (Table 165.2). Individuals with a large nose, prominent hump, or broad nasal tip can have their nose reduced slightly, and it will not only create more tissue for recruitment but also reduce the relative size of the defect. For many marginal defects, this maneuver can allow the transition from a more elaborate repair to a simpler one with local flaps.

TABLE 165.2

COMMON RECONSTRUCTIVE OPTIONS FOR SMALL CUTANEOUS DEFECTS

Upper 1/3	1. Full thickness skin graft
	2. Local transposition flaps
	3. Second intention
Middle 1/3	1. Bilobe transposition flap
	1. Primary closure (midline)
	2. Full-thickness skin graft
	3. Single-stage forehead flap
Lower 1/3	1. Bilobe transposition flap
	1. Composite graft (alar rim, columella)
	1. Primary closure (midline, broad tip)
	2. Interpolated melolabial flap (ala, columella)
	3. Full-thickness skin graft—delayed

Upper Third

Smaller defects in this zone are readily repaired with either a full-thickness skin graft or by second-intention healing. Those larger than 1.5 cm can be resurfaced with a sliding glabellar or Reiger flap (21). Other transposition flaps recruited from the forehead and middle third of the nose are less common alternatives.

Middle Third

Small midline defects are often amenable to primary closure with wide undermining, and this represents the first option for optimal repair. This method will leave a vertically oriented central scar with tension evenly distributed, thus maintaining nasal symmetry. Small transposition flaps (rhombic, bilobe, rotation) are frequently utilized and represent another workhorse repair for this region. Skin grafts can blend in well with the thin skin of this zone, but even small contour depressions are difficult to disguise, as their shadows often remain conspicuous. If a cartilage graft is needed along the lateral wall, a vascularized resurfacing flap is needed. Those larger than 1.5 cm often require a more elaborate flap.

Lower Third

Precise midline defects are ideally suited for primary closure, particularly when the premorbid nasal tip is somewhat bulbous and can afford to be narrowed. A bilobe flap is often utilized for defects of the nasal tip, allowing the tension to be distributed more widely and at an adequate distance from the free alar margin. The alar lobule is often repaired with composite grafts, restoring structure and covering simultaneously. Smaller defects limited to the supra-alar crease can do well through second-intention healing, but moderately sized defects will jeopardize nasal patency. The single-stage melolabial flap can also be used; however, the supra-alar crease is often obliterated and leaves the

appearance of asymmetry. A two-stage, interpolated melolabial flap is preferable for larger defects of the alar lobule, especially when cartilage grafts have been placed and the aesthetic unit completed. Small, full-thickness defects involving the alar margin are best repaired with a three-layered composite graft from the ear, whereas larger ones require a multilayered reconstruction involving the internal lining, structural framework, and resurfacing. The columella is characterized by a very narrow column of thin skin and lends itself well to small composite and skin grafts. For larger columellar defects, structural grafting along with a pedicled melolabial flap is most often used. The soft-tissue triangle defect is ideally restored by allowing second-intention healing to occur with a natural-appearing web.

TECHNIQUES FOR GRAFTS AND FLAPS

Second-intention Healing

Local wound care is the most important aspect when selecting this method of repair. Keeping the wound bed moist and preventing the development of a dry eschar will encourage the most prompt and favorable healing. Cytotoxic agents, especially hydrogen peroxide, should be avoided. A *guiding suture* can be employed in a similar fashion to the purse-string closures used for large defects on the scalp and face. This guiding suture partially closes a small defect and allows the remainder to heal secondarily. The greatest utility of this suture is for small defects along the alar rim. The suture can be placed horizontally, thus converting the circular defect into a vertical elliptical shape, which resists the vertical contracture that will ensue. The suture itself will often notch the alar rim inferiorly slightly, but it contracts to a normal position during healing. The suture is removed after 2 to 3 weeks. This technique will allow more defects to be managed in a conservative fashion.

Skin and Composite Grafts

Superficial defects can be immediately repaired with full thickness skin grafts and do quite nicely (Table 165.3). For deeper defects, or those exposing bare cartilage, it may be

TABLE 165.3

PEARLS FOR SKIN AND COMPOSITE GRAFTS

1. Consider delay.
2. Square wound borders.
3. Bevel edges towards defect.
4. Minimize "pie crusts."
5. Small perforations through cartilage for larger composite grafts can help.

prudent to delay the repair for 7 to 10 days allowing a layer of granulation tissue to accumulate within the recipient bed. This enhances vascularity and fills in the depression, thereby improving surface contour. The defect shape is modified, in order to create straight lines with square corners, rather than leaving a circular defect. The entire aesthetic subunit is not necessarily completed. Wound margins are beveled toward the center of the defect in order to smooth the transition between graft and the native nasal skin. Skin grafts can be harvested from the supraclavicular, periauricular, and melolabial areas. Graft thickness is modified following harvest to best match the surrounding skin texture, especially along the nasal tip, where thicker skin is found. Small "pie crusts" can be cut into the graft to allow the egress of serous fluid, recognizing that these perforations often become discolored and remain noticeable. A bolster dressing is rarely needed on the nose as long as small tacking sutures are placed to maintain close apposition between the graft and recipient bed.

A two- or three-layered composite graft is usually taken from the ear—either the root of the helix, the conchal bowl, or the triangular fossa. Anterior auricular skin is tightly adhered to auricular cartilage and has a good success rate. The shape of the cartilage is usually concave toward the skin, and although this shape can be unfavorable for external resurfacing, it is ideal for internal lining. The auricular donor site is closed primarily with little distortion. Excising cartilage from the apices of the donor site can avoid the "cookie bite" deformity to the ear. The composite graft must be securely attached to the nose, often with through-and-through sutures or a small bolster. These grafts are ideally suited for defects along the alar rim and columella (Fig. 165.2). Many composite grafts will appear moderately dusky for a week but will usually recover during the ensuing days. Larger grafts may undergo a degree of epidermolysis, which will lead to a less favorable color and texture match. Three-layered composite grafts are kept less than 1.5 cm because the sole blood supply is from the peripheral margin. Two-layered composite grafts, on the other hand, can be designed larger because the nourishing bed is the entire surface area of the graft. When utilizing these larger, two-layered composite grafts, one can excise several small, 2-mm punch holes through the cartilage only, taking care not to puncture the overlying skin. These small perforations will allow granulation tissue to penetrate the cartilage and nourish the epithelial covering.

Primary Closure

Primary closure with wide undermining is an excellent option for many small cutaneous nasal defects, especially those located in the precise midline of the lower two thirds of the nose and when the tip is modestly wide or bulbous to begin with. Lateral undermining over the perichondrium, and deep to the nasal superficial musculoaponeurotic system (SMAS) layer, is essential. The elliptical design requires that the vertical extensions extend further superiorly and inferiorly than the traditional 30-degree apices, in order to avoid an asymmetric narrowing of the nose. Failure to do so will narrow the nose at the site of the original defect but leave the supratip or infratip segments disproportionately wide. Common rhinoplasty maneuvers, such as an interdomal suture and cephalic trim, are frequently utilized concomitantly, in order to narrow the tip, reduce wound tension, and facilitate primary closure (Fig. 165.3). Defects that are off midline will leave a paramedian vertical scar and may create nasal asymmetry because of uneven recruitment and tension.

Rhombic Flap

The design of the classic Limberg rhombic flap was originally described in 1946 and remains a versatile flap with predictable scars and vectors of tension (22). Because the resultant scar crosses all aesthetic units, it is difficult to orient the flaps such that scars are maximally camouflaged. In order to minimize wound tension, however, flaps are specifically designed such that the vectors of tension parallel those lines of maximal tissue recruitment. In the nose, this laxity is usually from the lateral nasal wall and medial cheek. In addition, an inferiorly based flap tends to have fewer problems with postoperative congestion and edema.

Bilobe Flap

The bilobe flap is widely used for small nasal defects because it allows one to distribute tensions further from the primary defect, thus controlling the degree of tension along the alar margin. Whereas early designs utilized a 180-degree arch of rotation, contemporary methods have narrowed this angle in order to minimize the standing cutaneous deformity (23). Common sequelae to these flaps include postoperative edema and "pin-cushioning," which can arise from several factors: (a) the curvilinear scars of the flap design will undergo natural contraction and, as they shorten, tend to bunch and lift the skin paddle of the flap; (b) a bilobe is relatively wide with respect to its pedicle, predisposing to congestion; and (c) a plane of scar tissue will form beneath the flap and further impede lymphatic egress. In an attempt to minimize these effects, certain modifications of the bilobe can be employed. By decreasing the arc of rotation to 90 degrees, the size of the standing cutaneous deformity and the overall width of the flap are decreased. The primary flap should be aggressively debulked, removing all muscle and a majority of the subcutaneous fat. When possible, an inferiorly based flap design will be more favorable, as it permits lymphatic drainage. The entire nose is widely undermined, creating a more even plane of scar and contracture. Finally, the apex of the secondary flap can be left as a triangle rather than trimming it, leaving a sharp corner that contracts less. Wound edges along a bilobe often become inverted and

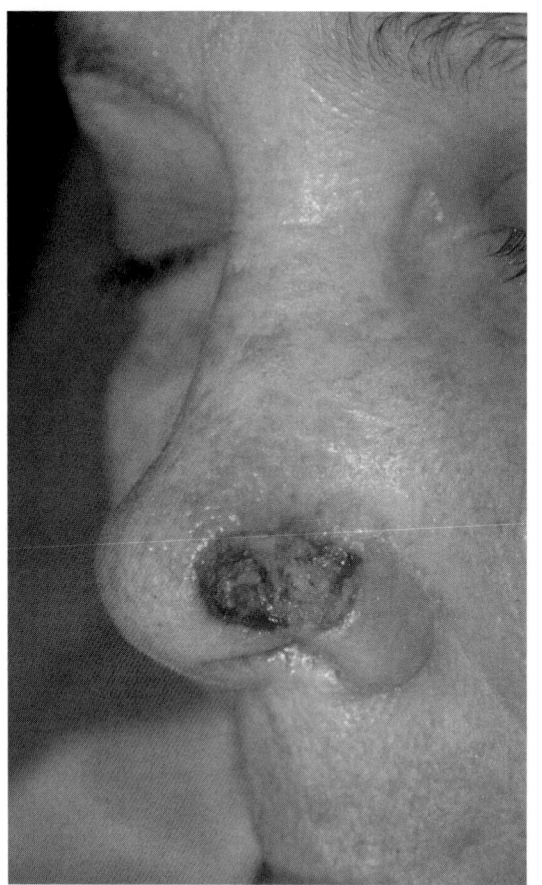

A

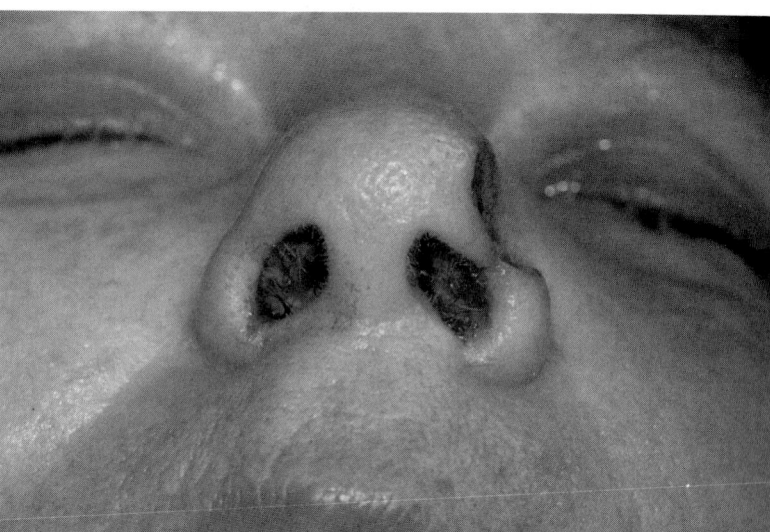

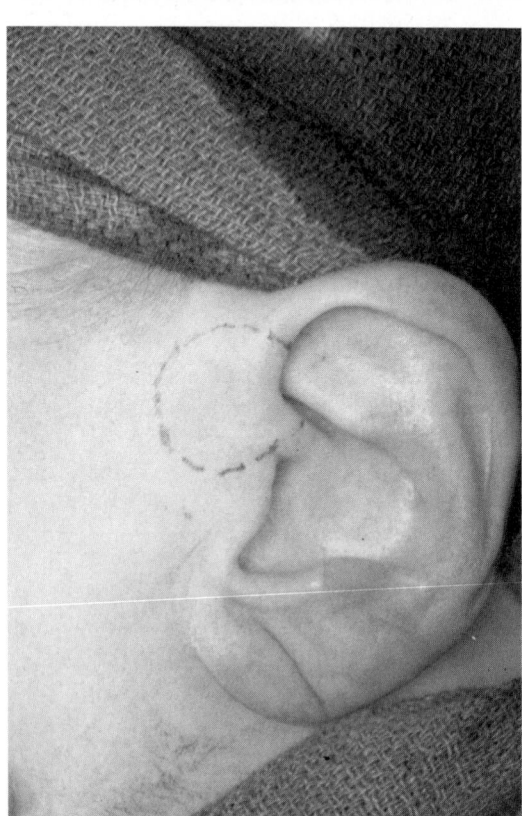

C

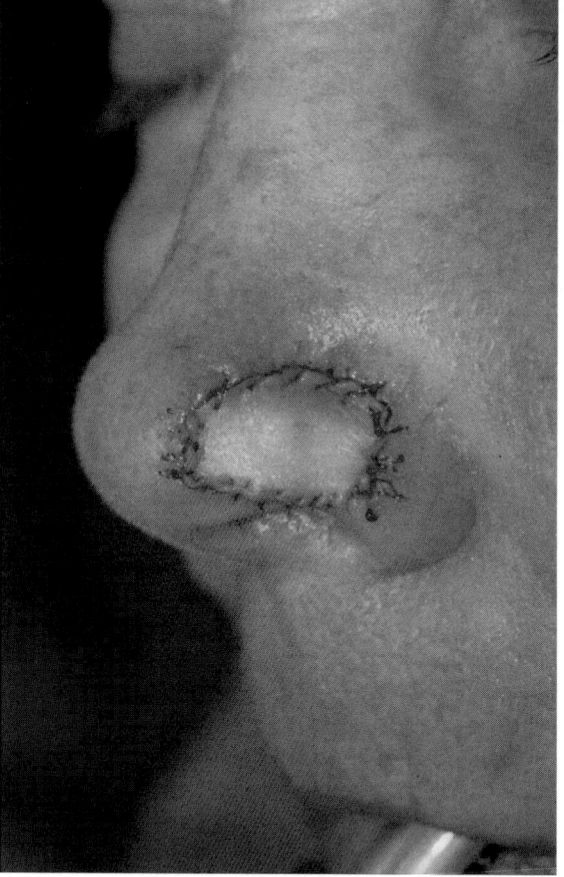

D

Figure 165.2   Composite graft. **A:** Defect involving left alar and tip, oblique view. **B:** Base view. **C:** Composite graft from left ear. **D:** Graft secured in defect.

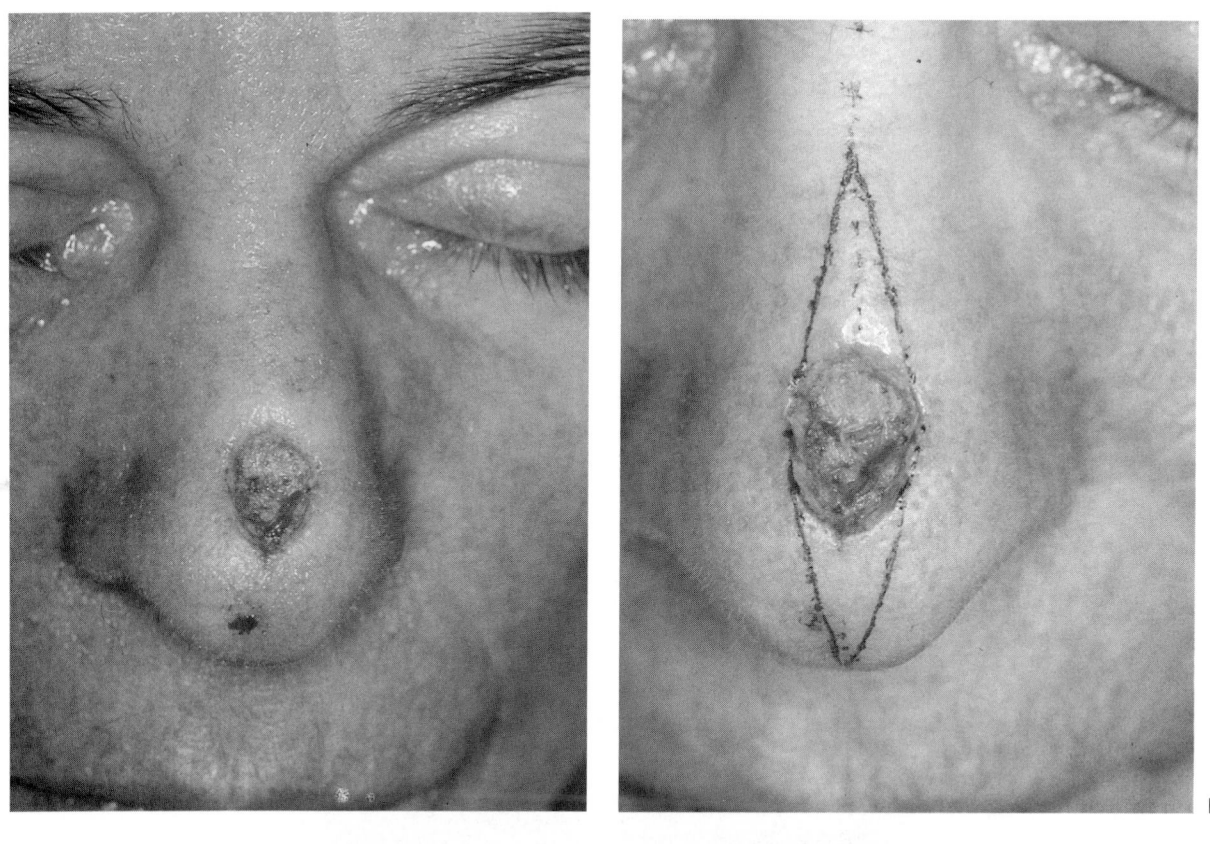

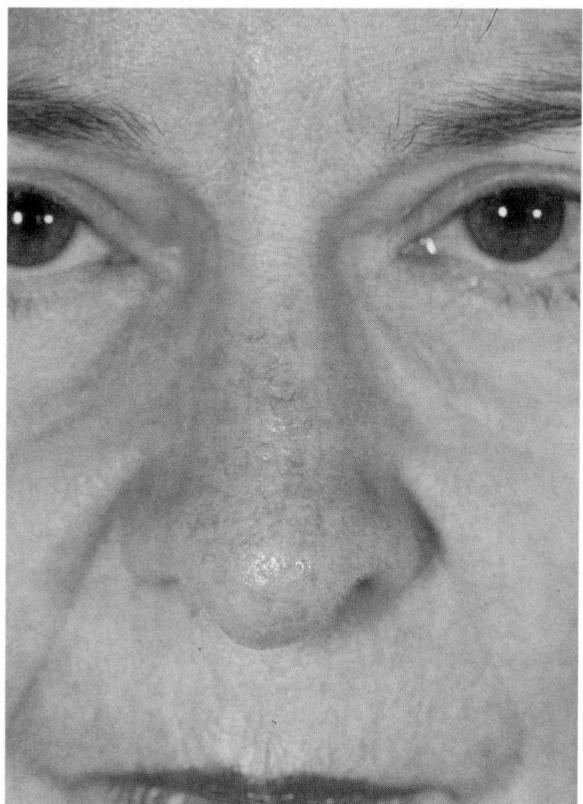

Figure 165.3   **A:** Midline defect of nasal tip. **B:** Elliptical excision with primary closure with bilateral advancement flaps. **C:** Nine-month postoperative view.

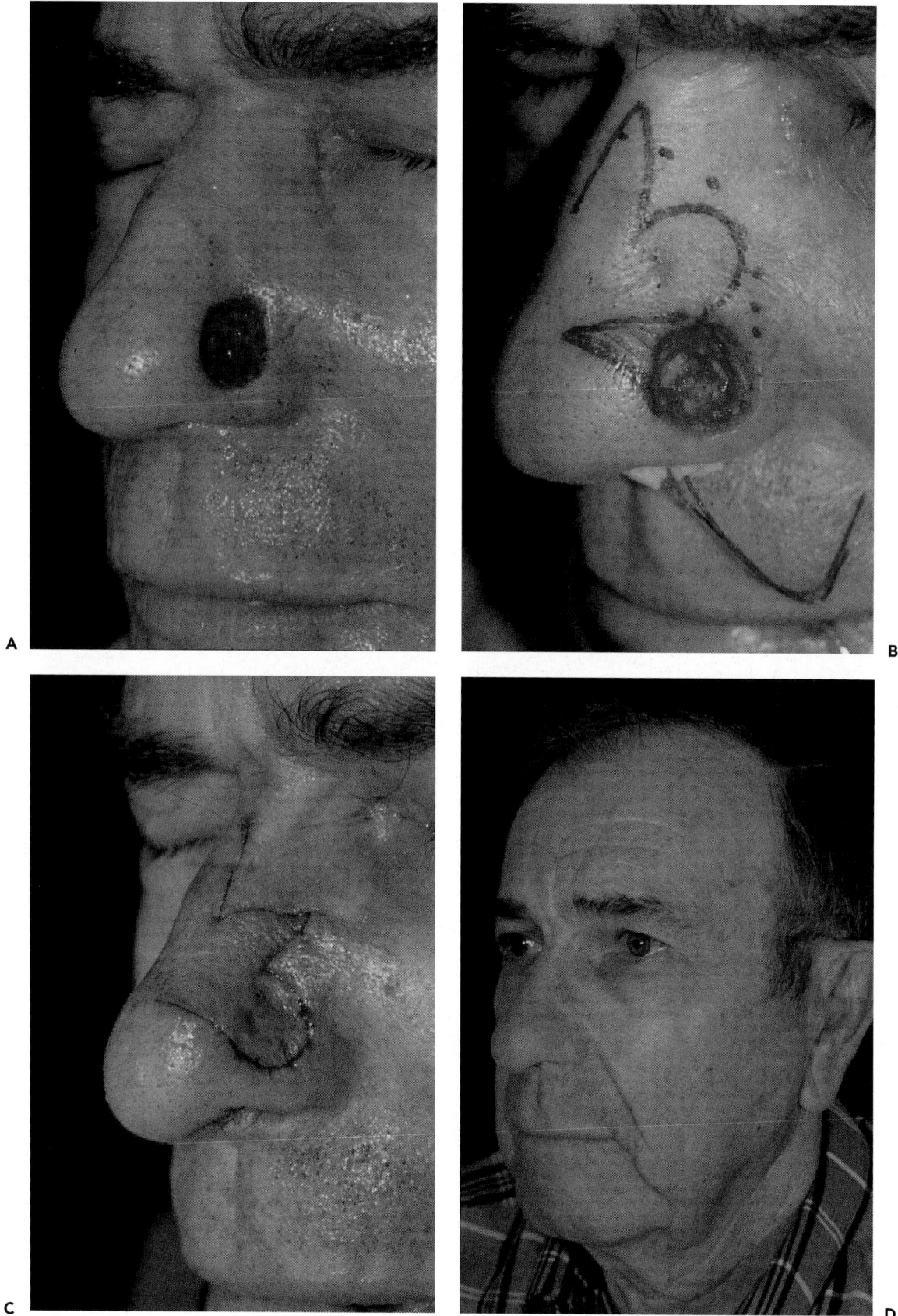

Figure 165.4   Nasal bilobe flap. **A:** Cutaneous defect of left ala and sidewall. **B:** Bilobe flap design. **C:** Flap transposed with preservation of a triangular flap. **D:** Six-month postoperative view.

depressed. Great effort must be made to maximize skin eversion during closure with meticulous subdermal sutures. It is often possible to orient the flap such that one limb of the primary flap and the straight line from the secondary flap closure are indiscreet. One can place the Burrow triangle from the primary flap along the supra-alar crease or orient the secondary flap vertically, such that the closure of this donor site parallels the borders of aesthetic subunits (Fig. 165.4). The vector of tension from a bilobe is often counterintuitive in that there is an inferior force that can push the alar rim inferiorly. The flap may need to be trimmed in order to pull the rim cephalad. Because of the natural convexity of the nose, the pivot point of a bilobe also has a third-dimensional vector that is perpendicular to the plane of the flap and impinges on the airway. Most bilobes designed with the pedicle based laterally along the keystone area will compromise the valve and will require a prophylactic sidewall batten graft. Those based medially, on the other hand, tend to be more functionally forgiving, and may even serve to pull the sidewall open.

Reiger Flap

The Reiger flap utilizes glabellar skin based on a unilateral medial brow/supratrochlear region. The donor site is closed primarily as the glabellar and dorsal nasal skin is advanced and rotated caudally. It is ideally suited for defects of the upper two thirds. For lower-third defects, it is a moderately large flap that often leaves some alar base asymmetry as well as unnatural nasal creases.

Melolabial Flap

The interpolated melolabial flap is designed with a distinct pedicle based superiorly through the perforators off the angular artery. The skin paddle is located on the medial cheek area and will have an excellent match to the normal nasal skin (Fig. 165.5). The flap is initially elevated in the subdermal plane, becoming progressively thicker as it ascends superiorly into the pedicle proper. The skin paddle must be kept thin with only a layer of subdermal fat. The pivot point for the pedicle is located along the nasal facial groove and, although the skin incisions are narrowed superiorly to facilitate rotation, the subcutaneous portion remains thick and bulky. The vascular basis of this flap is via perforators within the subcutaneous fat and levator labii superioris, not the skin itself. After the flap is transferred, the melolabial fold is re-created with medial advancement of the cheek. Pedicle division is performed after a three-week interval to allow for neovascularization from the recipient bed into the skin paddle. The stump of the pedicle is usually excised and donor site closed primarily, leaving a single scar along the nasofacial junction. This is done at the expense of creating subtle facial asymmetry along the melolabial folds. Alternatively, the pedicle can be returned to the midface, although this will create two vertical scars,

one being in the cheek facial unit. The melolabial flap is ideally suited for smaller defects of the alar lobule and columella. It can be extended to the nasal sidewall and nasal tip. It brings vascularized tissue that can cover a cartilage graft. By being based on the cheek, it avoids the functional handicap created by a forehead flap pedicle, such as with eye glasses.

LARGE CUTANEOUS DEFECTS

Preoperative Considerations

Most large-skin defects are addressed with more elaborate, interpolated flaps, but on occasion less invasive options can still represent the most practical means of repair. There are individual considerations that might discourage a more aggressive procedure. Advanced age, significant small-vessel disease, previous radiation therapy, and overall patient health all might preclude a lengthy and more involved surgical intervention. A large skin graft to the nose may represent the most practical repair for select patients, and, at times, the outcomes can be surprisingly satisfactory. In addition, individual patient expectations and postoperative cooperation should be clearly defined. Although the optimal aesthetic outcome is often the surgeon's goal, patient needs may be quite different, with a much lower cosmetic concern and greater priority toward a speedy recuperation. The logistical inconveniences to the patient, especially with a staged procedure such as an interpolated forehead flap, must be appreciated. The pedicle will often preclude the use of eye glasses, rigorous work outdoors (which many of these patients may do), and many public positions of employment, for example, waiters, receptionists, and so on.

Simultaneously, when selecting a simpler alternative for short-term convenience purposes, it is important to communicate the aesthetic and functional sacrifices that are being made. A month of inconvenience may be small when that considering the result of the nasal restoration is life long. This too must be clearly communicated. A majority of the larger nasal defects occur on a more elderly population, and one certainly needs to develop a feel for their surgical candidacy, level of support, and emotional expectations. For some individuals, a simpler covering such as a full-thickness skin graft will meet their needs as long as they do not develop significant nasal obstruction. On the other hand, there are many senescent patients who remain socially active and are entirely deserving of the optimal repair. Even patients in their eighth and ninth decade of life may have an additional life expectancy of greater than 10 years, and an aesthetic and functional repair will be borne for many meaningful years. This is especially true when weighing the total additional time and morbidity consumed by the more elaborate repair versus the simpler one; a forehead flap brings only a few additional weeks of recovery. The subtotal and total nasal reconstructions require a period of

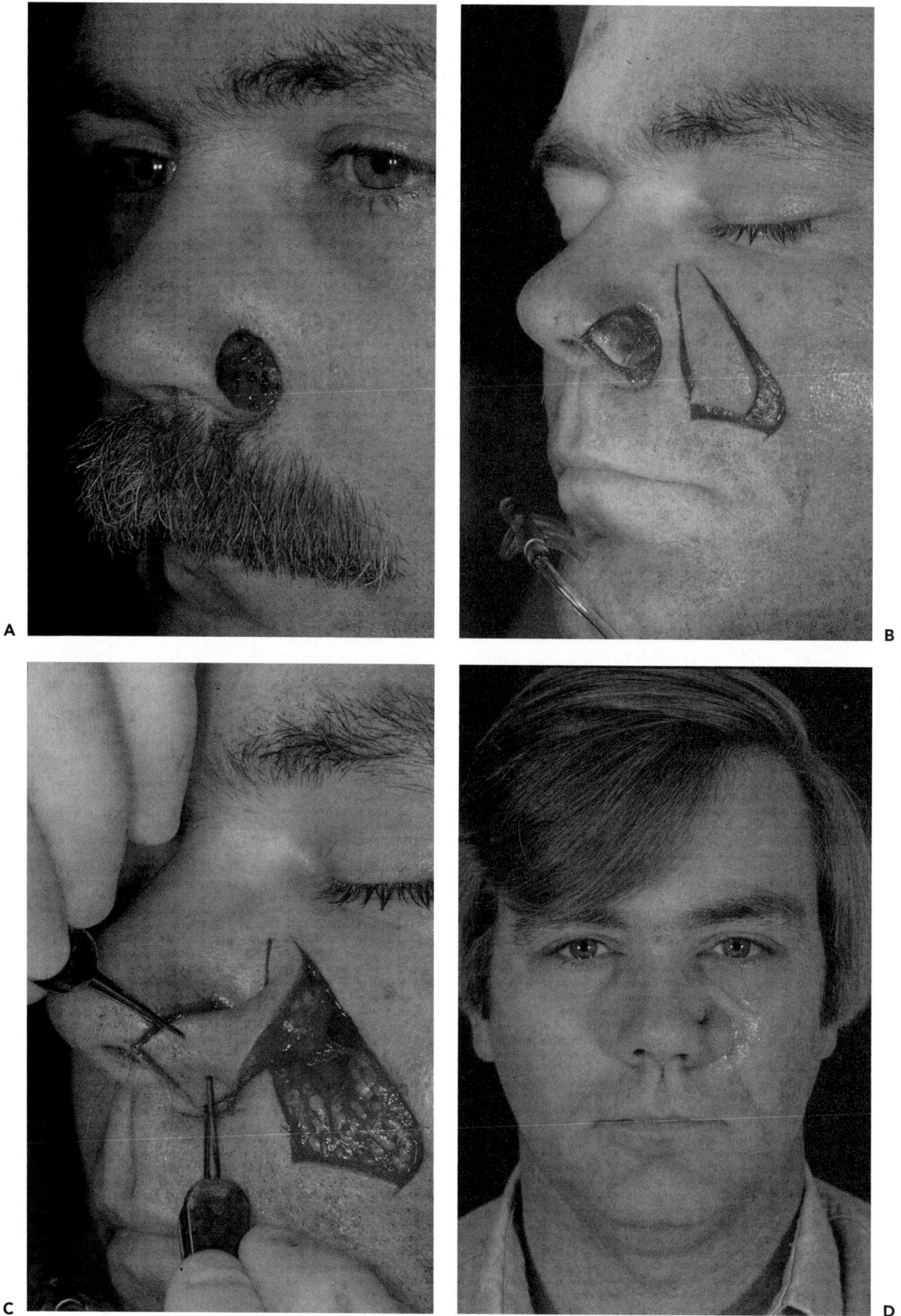

Figure 165.5   A–G: Melolabial flap.

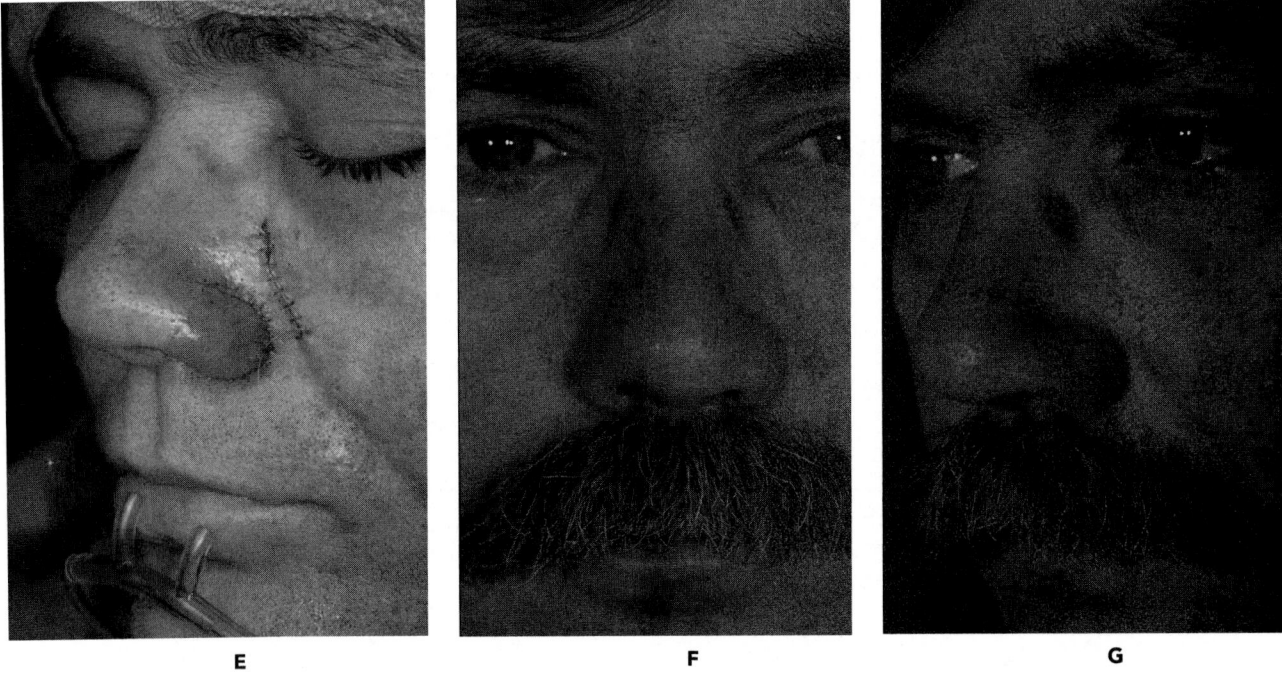

E   F   G

Figure 165.5 *(continued)*

significant convalescence, irrespective of age. The chronologic age of most patients has only a minor role in the decision making for a major nasal restoration.

Forehead Flap

The most common method of nasal resurfacing for large
(>1.5 cm) defects is with the forehead flap. Despite its ancient origins, this flap remains the major workhorse, as it
fulfills many of the criteria for the ideal facial flap. There is
an excellent match in color and skin texture and sufficient
donor skin to resurface the entire nose. This flap is dependable and robust, leaves an acceptable donor site morbidity, and is, in short, the gold standard for contemporary
major nasal restoration. Several pearls should be borne in
mind during repair with a forehead flap (Table 165.4).

Defect Preparation
The nasal aesthetic subunits are drawn directly on the nose
at the onset of surgery, irrespective of the preexisting nasal

TABLE 165.4
PEARLS FOR A FOREHEAD FLAP

1. Analyze defect shape and subunits involved.
2. Create precise 3-D template.
3. Aggressive thinning of skin paddle.
4. Narrow pedicle base (less than 1.5 cm).
5. Consider functional grafting or sutures.
6. Thin upper flap during pedicle division.

defect. Although the general topography is similar from
nose to nose, each individual has intrinsic variations of
their nose that must be recognized. This is especially true
when there is marked dorsal asymmetry or ethnic variations. As the subunits are defined on the nose, great attention is made to preserving the sharp corners at the border
of each subunit. There is a tendency to round the corners
during each of the stages of repair, from drawing the subunits to creating a flap that fits the modified defect. Based
on the size and shape of the cutaneous defect, it is then
usually modified to complete the corresponding aesthetic
subunit such that the resultant scars lay along the borders
of these subunits. This invariably involves enlarging the existing defect. This principle is applied liberally yet not exclusively. When only a small portion of a given subunit is
involved (usually <10%), it may be more practical to
modify the shape by enlarging the adjacent subunit and
thereby minimize excessive resection of normal tissue. This
is especially true when the additional subunit will significantly lengthen or widen the skin paddle of the forehead
flap. Another exception to the aesthetic subunit principle
is a midline vertical scar of the upper two thirds of the
nose; although this bisects the dorsal subunit, the casual
observer also sees the face and nose as two halves, and a
vertical line between them can remain inconspicuous.

Asian patients, although rarely afflicted with cutaneous
malignancies, have a nasal topography slightly different
from most occidentals, particularly in terms of dorsal and
tip projection, and the subunit principle should reflect
that (24). Their nose tends to be proportionally smaller,

and there may not be sufficient nasal skin to cover even defects less than 1.5 cm. Under these circumstances, one may need to complete the aesthetic subunits and resurface with a regional flap from the forehead.

The *nasal-facial junction* lies more medial on the "nose" than first impression, and it is one of the sacred borders that should not be crossed. The cheek flap should be brought up to the junction and suspended to the periosteum of the piriform aperture, and even to the bone itself if necessary. Crossing the aesthetic border often creates a degree of facial asymmetry and becomes more conspicuous.

Preexisting nasal deformities can influence the surgical outcome and should be recognized with consideration for adjustment during defect preparation. Aesthetic units are defined, in large part, by the reflections of light that arise from contour changes. A twisted nose will have asymmetric and irregular subunits that do not support the aesthetic subunit principle as well, and one might consider correcting the deformity and restoring symmetry and balance to the nose. It can be an opportune time to straighten the dorsum with osteotomies, reduce a prominent hump, or refine a broad and amorphous nasal tip. Through the combination of traditional cosmetic rhinoplasty maneuvers and basic reconstructive tenets, the surgical outcome can be enhanced.

The *depth of the defect* (and the associated subunits) is always taken down to the perichondrium of the cartilaginous framework, even if the primary defect is more superficial. This allows one to shape the exposed cartilages with sutures and conservative resections. Moreover, the forehead flap is often plagued with being too thick and increasing the depth of the nasal defect will allow a better contour match between the nose and the flap. The additional resection will also only improve the recurrence rate from the original Mohs surgery. It has been suggested that for high-risk individuals, the adjacent subunits be analyzed for occult cutaneous malignancies, as the skin has been exposed to the same degree of actinic injury (25).

Template

A precise template is made of the final cutaneous defect utilizing the aluminum package from a suture. This can be somewhat laborious but is imperative to get an accurate, three-dimensional map of the defect and corresponding skin paddle. One can use the contralateral side as a reference to ensure nasal symmetry. Care is taken to cut straight edges and crisp corners of this template, which is then transferred to the forehead for an accurate tracing. The vertical position of the template is determined by measuring from the medical aspect of the brow down to the nasal defect, recognizing that the length-limiting point is not always the most inferior aspect of the wound but may be the proximal, contralateral corner. The template design has no wasted skin from the forehead as it is an accurate replica of the nasal defect; all incisions are made along the internal margin of the markings. Murrell et al. have described the

application of a three-dimensional pattern using Aquaplast (WFR/Aquaplast Corporation, Wyckoff, New Jersey) to transfer a more aesthetically precise template (26). Once the template has conformed to the contour of the patient's nose, it is converted to a two-dimensional tracing for the forehead.

Anatomic Basis

The blood supply to the forehead flap is primarily through the supratrochlear artery. This artery is a terminal branch of the ophthalmic, from the internal carotid system. It exists from the supratrochlear notch or, less frequently, foramen, and courses superiorly between the corrugator muscle deep and the orbicularis oculi muscle superficially, finally piercing the orbicularis roughly 1.5 cm above the notch. The artery then anastomoses extensively with the contralateral supratrochlear and ipsilateral supraorbital vessels. The forehead vessels have a dependable axial pattern in the vertical direction, running immediately superficial to the frontalis muscles, and give this flap an axial pattern vascular basis in addition to the named pedicle artery. The pedicle is centered on the supratrochlear vessel but has more than that artery supplying it; the driving anatomic basis for this flap is the robust perfusion pressure located along the medial brow area. The terminal branch of the angular artery supplies the pedicle base and is a major contributor to the arterial supply of the forehead flap. Silicone rubber casts were created from a forehead flap after cannulation of the facial artery alone, that is, no fixative was injected in the internal carotid system. This demonstrated the extensive network of collateral vessels in the medial brow region and a significant perfusion into a forehead flap without flow from the supratrochlear artery (Fig. 165.6) (27).

Midline vs Paramedian

The skin paddle of the forehead flap can be placed in the paramedian position, immediately centered on the supratrochlear artery. This has the advantage of incorporating much of the artery within the pedicle and, in theory, improves flap viability. Some individuals have a low "widow's peak," and the paramedian design can avoid it. The skin paddle can also be placed in the precise midline, creating a "midline forehead flap," with some discrete advantages (28). The pedicle is still based on a *unilateral* medial brow area, but it diverts obliquely to course in the middle of the forehead. This pedicle design will not incorporate as much of the supratrochlear artery, but the vertical axial pattern of the subdermal plexus remains. The advantage of this design is that the resultant scar will be in the exact midline of the forehead, rather than paramedian. Like the aesthetic subunits of the nose, the face is also visually divided into two halves. The midline vertical scar, despite being perpendicular to the horizontal forehead furrows, is often quite inconspicuous. There is also a natural divergence of the frontalis muscle in the superior forehead, allowing for better scar camouflage, because forehead furrows often do not

Doppler confirmation or localization of the supratrochlear artery is rarely needed, especially because the perfusion pressure and extensive collateralization is a major driving factor. The notch of the supratrochlear vessels can usually be palpated and the skin pedicle is centered there. One can include a cuff of periosteum at the base of the pedicle. This serves to give the flap a small amount of additional length. It also provides some rigidity to the pedicle base.

The base of the pedicle should not exceed 1.3 cm, which provides ample vascularity yet does not strangulate the pedicle or hinder the flap rotation. Most flaps can be narrowed to closer to 1 cm at the proximal end. The pedicle can also be extended into the brow for additional length.

Skin Paddle Elevation and Thinning

One of the common problems with the forehead flap of years past was excessive bulk, often sacrificing normal nasal form for fear of compromising viability. One of the greatest modifications and advancements made with the forehead flap may be the realization that the skin paddle can, and should, be thinned aggressively during the initial stage (Fig. 165.8). In most cases, the distal skin paddle of the forehead flap is elevated in the subcutaneous plane rather than the subgaleal one, lifting the flap off the frontalis muscle. The galea (frontalis muscle and fascia) is left down on the forehead during this initial flap elevation. After 2 to 3 cm, the plane of elevation drops to the avascular subgaleal layer and continues effortlessly. Once the flap is up, additional thinning is performed to match the intrinsic variations of normal nasal skin thickness. Axial, subdermal vessels are often encountered within the galea during this process, and the thinning can continue around them without sacrificing the vessels themselves. With healthy patients, the flap thinning will continue to the subdermal layer, and fluctuate slightly to best match the variability in native skin thickness (e.g. tip skin vs columella). The proximal skin paddle and entire pedicle is elevated in the subgaleal layer. Additional thinning of the skin flap is accomplished during pedicle division. Leaving the frontalis on the forehead has the distinct advantage if the donor site cannot be closed primarily. Second-intention healing will proceed much more rapidly over the galea.

An exception to this style of elevation is in smokers or others with small vessel disease. For these high-risk situations, the skin paddle and pedicle is elevated in the bulky subgaleal layer and transferred en bloc. An *intermediate stage* is used to thin the flap (discussed later).

Donor Site

A great majority of forehead defects less than 3.5 cm can be repaired primarily through wide undermining out to the temple areas. Deep sutures must be through the galeal layer in order to ensure sufficient strength; it is often necessary to place all the deep sutures prior to closure and tying of sutures. The standing cutaneous deformity at the supe-

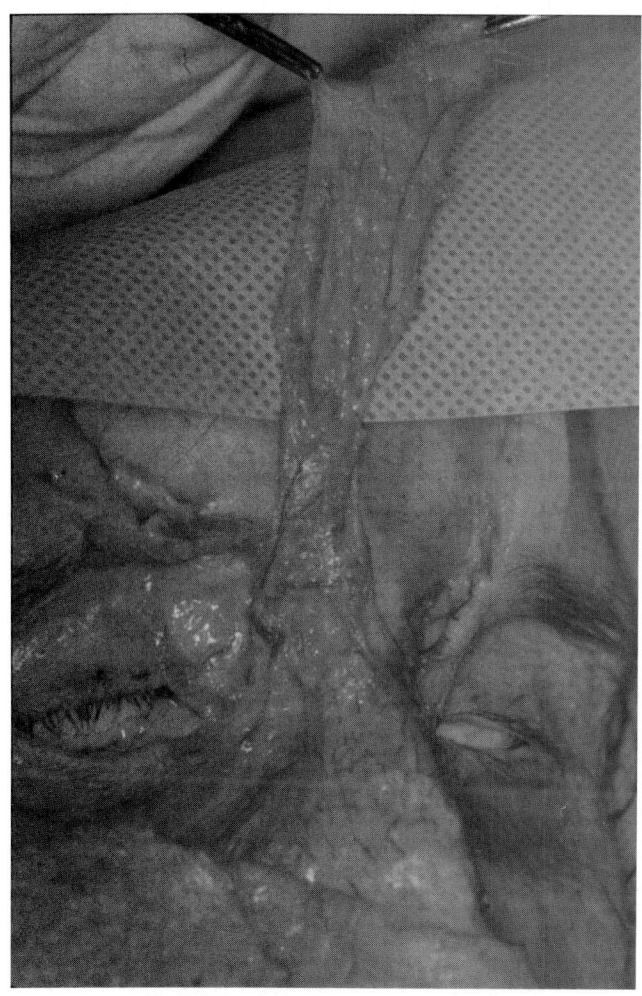

Figure 165.6 Cadaveric perfusion of facial artery without perfusion from supratrochlear vessel.

cross from side to side. In addition, the oblique pedicle design allows a slightly longer reach as compared with the straight paramedian flap (Fig. 165.7).

Pedicle Design

It was originally thought that the forehead flap pedicle needed to be wide enough to capture both supratrochlear vessels in order to survive. It has later been shown that this forehead flap can be raised off only a single supratrochlear artery and that the pedicle can be safely narrowed to 1.5 cm without jeopardizing viability (14,15,16,17). The pedicle for the flap can be based either ipsilateral or contralateral to the nasal defect (assuming it is not midline). Each has its unique advantages. The ipsilateral pedicle is closer to the defect and permits a shorter pedicle distance, which can be very advantageous in people with a relatively low hairline. The contralateral pedicle has a longer reach but less rotational arc, thus reducing the amount of twisting that occurs at the pedicle base and possibly improving venous return from the flap. All else being equal, the contralateral flap is safer and more robust.

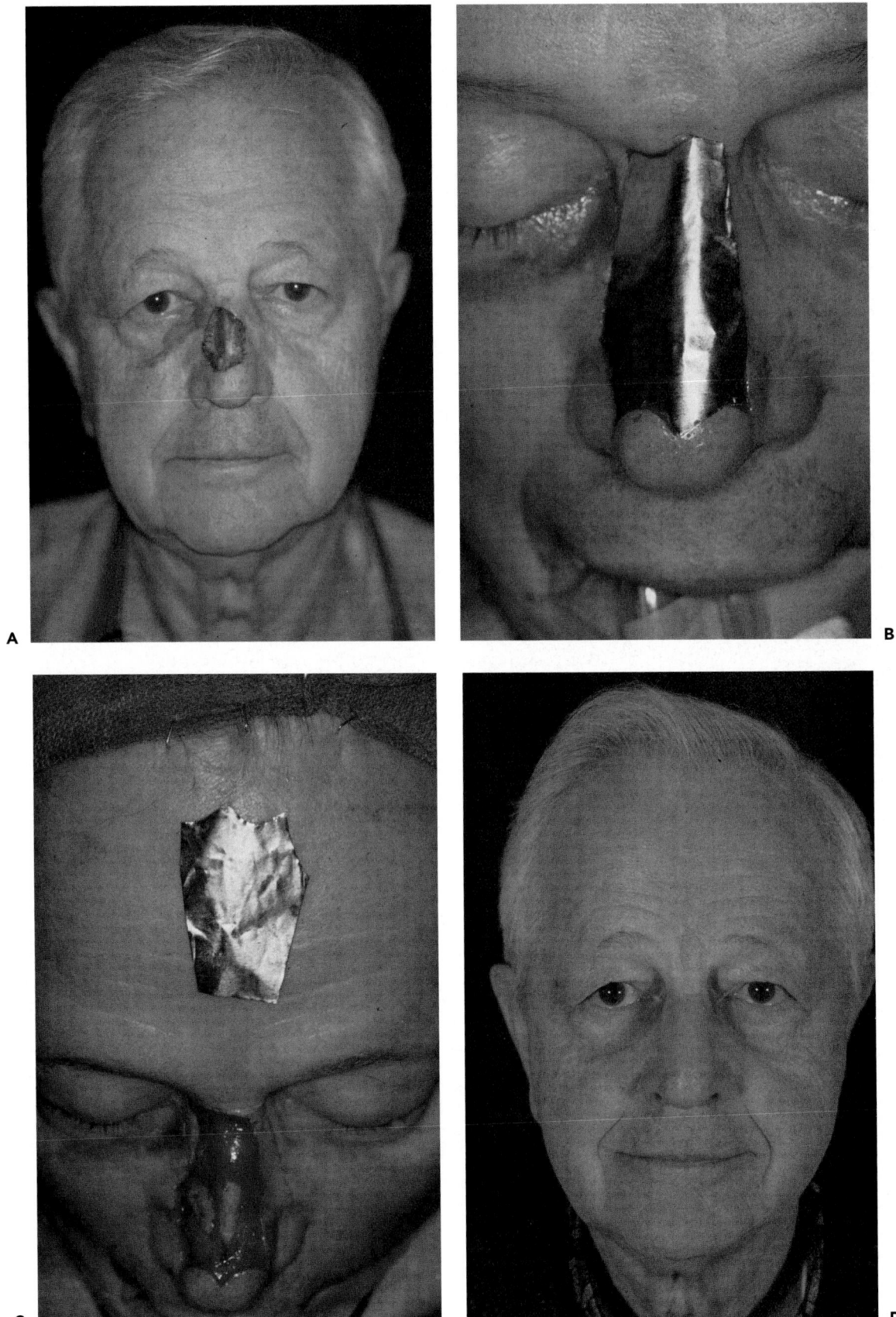

Figure 165.7   A: Nasal defect anterior view. **B:** Template of nasal defect. **C:** Template transferred to precise midline. **D:** Postoperative view, noting preservation of bilateral forehead furrows.

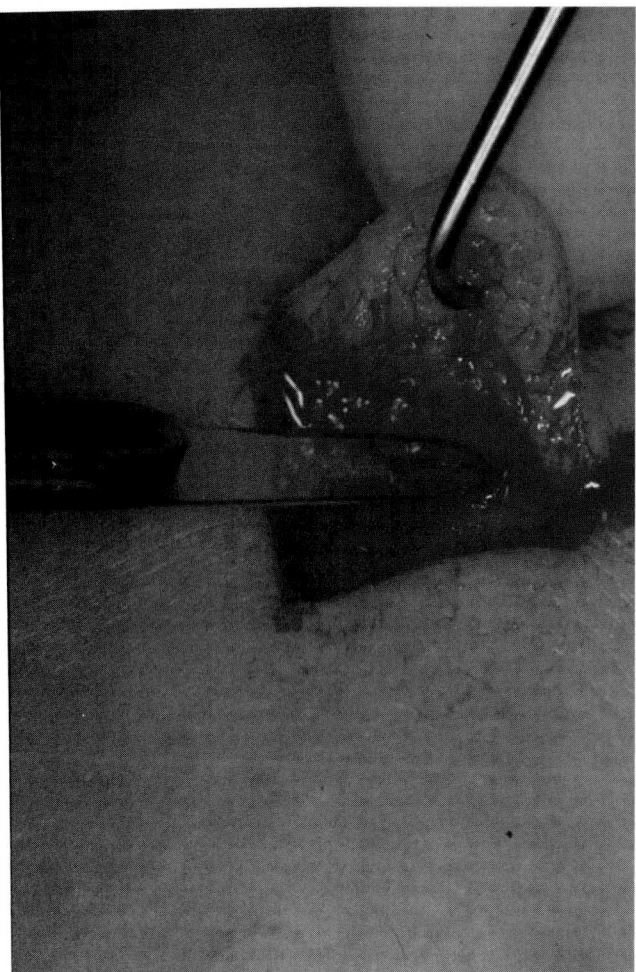

Figure 165.8 It is important to aggressively thin the forehead flap prior to inset

rior border is directly excised in a vertical fashion with the incision extending into the frontal hair. Alternatively, the forehead can be mobilized and closed in an "O to T" fashion with a horizontal limb at the hairline. Like a trichophytic browlift, this can be closed in a running "W-plasty" to further camouflage the scar.

For wider defects, vertical galeatomies may allow additional recruitment from the sides. Any remaining defect on the forehead is allowed to heal by second intention. The resultant scar following wound contracture will generally be superior to other options, especially with the galea down. A skin graft will allow that area to heal quickly but generally remains more noticeable. Tissue expansion has been described as an alternative for the tight forehead or the low hairline (29). Although this does create an abundant amount of tissue and permit primary closure following wide forehead flaps, the expanded skin is less favorable in terms of flap physiology. Some flap contracture will occur, even following direct excision of the expander capsule, and will compromise the final nasal form.

Pedicle Division

The pedicle is the obligatory nutrient supply for the skin paddle until sufficient neovascularization occurs from the recipient bed into the flap itself. Vascular in-growth is predictable and is driven, in part, by the ischemic gradient between the nasal defect and the distal flap (30). There is probably sufficient support for the flap after a 10-day period, but a 3-week interval is allowed to lapse to ensure greater fibroblast development, increased tensile strength, and adequate adherence of the flap to the nose. The pedicle is divided transversely, a few millimeters above the original nasal defect. Undermining proceeds in a superior-to-inferior direction, immediately under the dermal plane, to roughly halfway down the skin paddle. One can leave the subcutaneous portion of the pedicle intact, thus allowing it to provide countertraction as the skin is undermined. The bulk of the subcutaneous tissue is then removed while tapering the inferior border to smooth the transition. It is imperative to debulk this portion of the flap and allow the flap to conform to the normal nasal topography. The edges of the original nasal defect are carefully freshened and corners are squared off. Over the preceding three weeks, the border of the defect will have contracted and started to reepithelialize.

The superior stump of the pedicle is then trimmed accordingly and inset back into the glabellar area. There is a tendency for this portion of the pedicle to thicken and pincushion. Aggressive thinning of the underlying muscle will help minimize this. It is essential to restore symmetry to the eyebrows, as the pedicle side tends to be pulled inferiorly. After the medial brow is resuspended, the new standing cutaneous deformities can be directly excised. One often extends the excision up the forehead for about 2 cm, as that portion of the scar tends to be inverted and unfavorable. This arises because the original forehead flap pedicle often has a wide frontalis portion and the closure is deficient of subcutaneous bulk. On occasion, one can dermabrade some of the scars of the nose or the forehead at this relatively early stage (Fig. 165.9).

Intermediate Stage—Forehead Flap

In higher risk individuals such as smokers, the original forehead flap is transposed as a composite of skin and frontalis muscle without preliminary flap thinning. As an *intermediate stage*, the skin paddle is elevated from laterally as a bipedicled flap, attached at the medial brow proximally and the nasal tip distally. The flap is then thinned and sculpted to the appropriate level to restore nasal form (Fig. 165.10). An additional 3 weeks are allowed to pass before the final pedicle division is performed. While this methodology leaves the pedicle intact for 6 weeks, the inconvenience is justified by improved flap viability and better outcomes within a high-risk patient group.

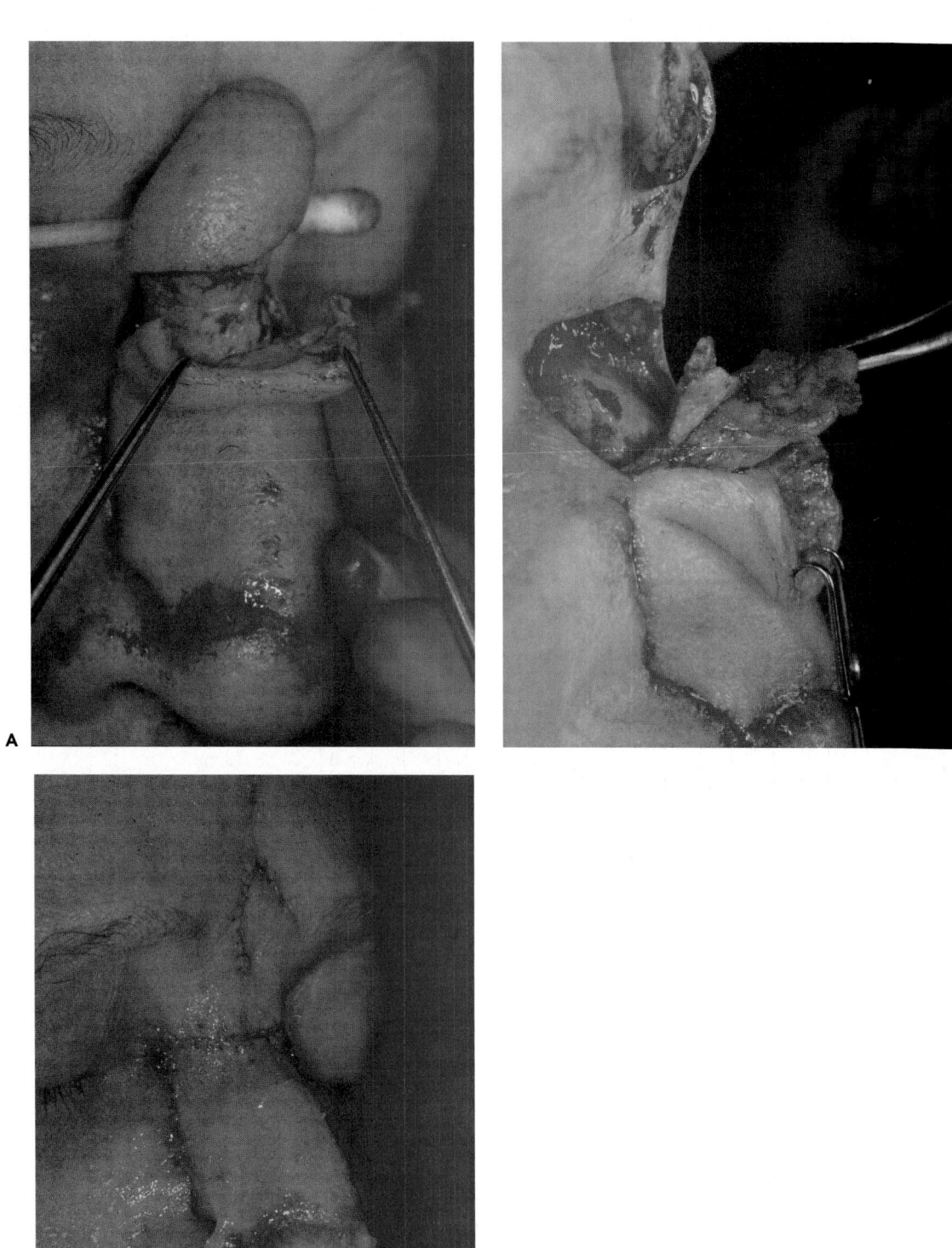

Figure 165.9 Pedicle division. **A:** Skin elevated with subcutaneous portion providing countertraction. **B:** Debulking subcutaneous portion. **C:** Pedicle inset with attention to brow symmetry.

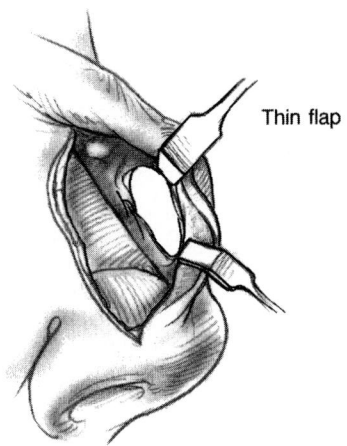

Figure 165.10 Intermediate stage with debulking.

Single-stage Forehead Flap

The single-stage forehead flap (Table 165.5) utilizes a deep-ithelialized pedicle and was originally described by Converse in 1963 as a modified median forehead flap based on both supratrochlear vessels (31). It had problems with a limited arc of rotation and flap congestion and was subsequently abandoned. Utilizing what is known today about the robust vascularity of the contemporary forehead flap, one can create a single-stage, island forehead flap based on a *unilateral* medial brow area (32). This single-stage flap has a similar anatomic basis as the conventional, interpolated forehead flap but does not require a pedicle division. The advantages of accomplishing a major nasal resurfacing in a single stage can be tremendous for those patients in whom the pedicle and need for a second surgery create a hardship that is difficult to overcome. The vascularity from a subcutaneous pedicle is, however, more tenuous, and this type of forehead flap should be avoided in high-risk individuals, for example, smokers, small vessel disease, diabetes, hypertension.

Both a unilateral supratrochlear artery and the rich collateral supply from the angular artery provide the perfusion pressure that supports the skin paddle. It should be based on the contralateral side to avoid excessive torsion on the pedicle. This flap is converted to an island flap as the glabellar skin is carefully dissected off the pedicle. Tremendous care must be taken to avoid inadvertent changes in plane during this stage because pedicle amputation is the result. The glabellar skin is undermined

TABLE 165.5
PEARLS FOR THE SINGLE-STAGE FOREHEAD FLAP

1. Select patient carefully.
2. Create adequate room under glabellar skin.
3. Fill forehead depression with procerus and frontalis muscles.
4. Watch for flap congestion.

widely, and the resultant tunnel is connected to the defect of the nose. Portions of the procerus muscle can be resected in order to create sufficient room to accommodate the pedicle without compression and congestion. The flap is then tunneled under the intact glabellar skin and the skin paddle delivered into the nasal defect and closed in the usual fashion. The donor site is closed primarily, often incorporating a W-plasty inferiorly that parallels the natural glabellar furrows. There is a soft-tissue void where the subcutaneous pedicle was originally located, and portions of the frontalis muscles can be mobilized to fill this depression and improve glabellar contour. This flap works best for nasal defects limited to the upper two thirds of the nose; nasal tip and alar defects require a lengthier forehead flap and may not remain viable (Fig. 165.11).

STRUCTURAL SUPPORT AND GRAFTING

In addition to the cross-sectional area of a nasal defect, it is imperative to determine its depth and location in terms of its impact on nasal function and form. Many small and superficial defects of the lower third of the nose are repaired with composite grafts, thus providing a covering and support simultaneously. Larger and more complex defects usually require separate support grafting and an independent resurfacing flap. Structural grafting is placed for two primary reasons: first, to provide rigidity to the sidewall or dorsum, thus preventing collapse and nasal obstruction, and second, to create or maintain form, especially along the alar rim and tip.

Nasal Function

New onset nasal obstruction can compromise an otherwise excellent surgical outcome and be the source of significant patient dissatisfaction. Predicting those lesions that will lead to nasal obstruction is important and is influenced not only by the defect's depth but also by its location. When the depth is such that native structural support has been removed (e.g., a portion of the lateral crus), the defect will uniformly require reconstruction with some form of cartilaginous grafting. An exception is small defects of the nasal bones, albeit rare, as an isolated finding. Lesions located over the alar lobule or nasal sidewall are particularly prone to collapse and subsequent nasal obstruction at the level of the internal and external nasal valves. There is a critical area located at the junction of the two anatomic valves, corresponding to the supra-alar crease externally, and the area lateral to the lateral crus internally. There may be an isolated sesamoid cartilage within the characteristically firm, fibro-fatty aponeurosis between the lateral crus and the bony piriform aperture. In this area, even small defects that violate the fibroareolar tissues will tend to collapse, especially following local transposition flaps. Therefore, it is not solely the size of the

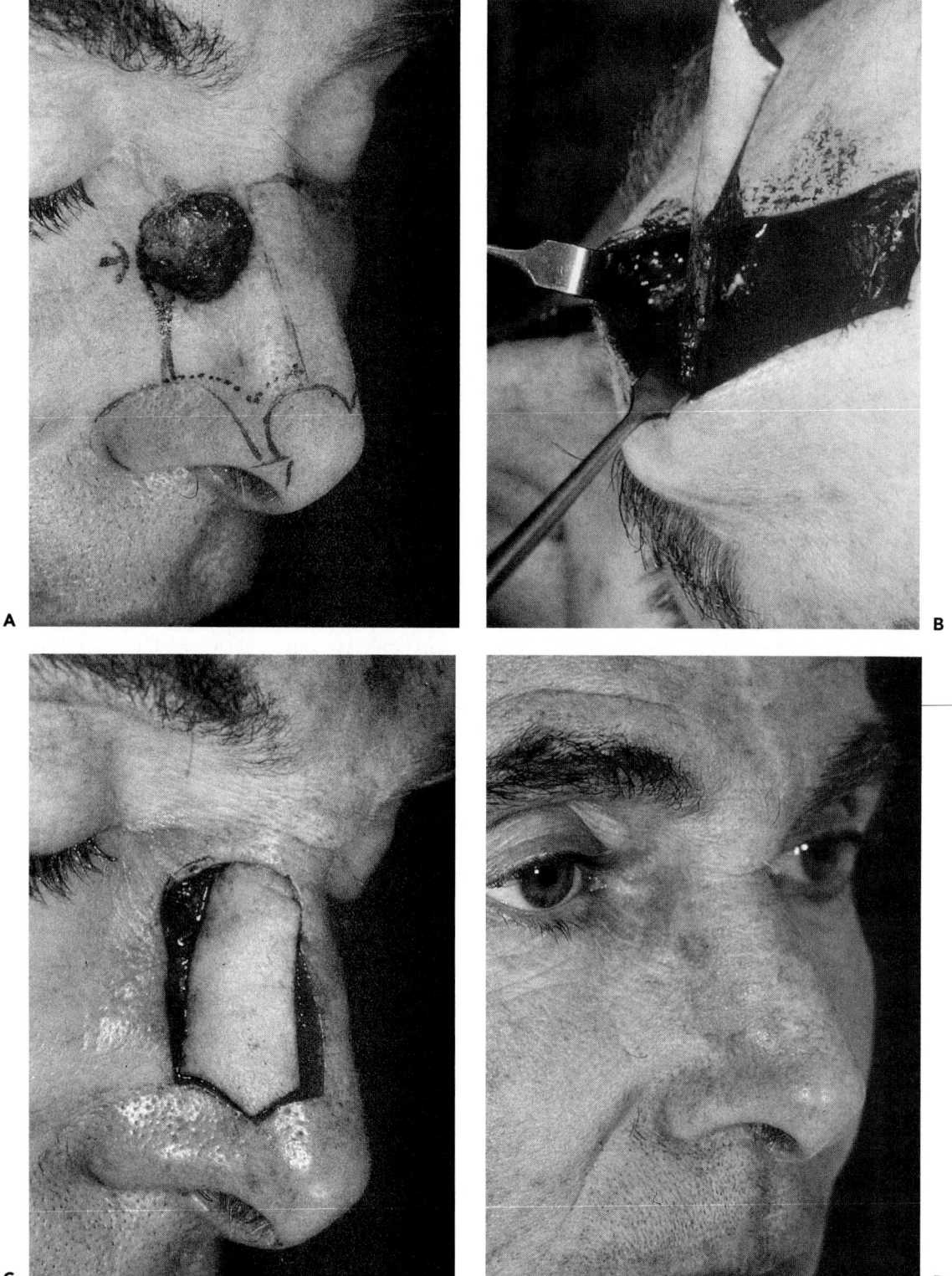

Figure 165.11   Single-stage forehead flap. **A:** Right nasal defect involving sidewall and cheek. **B:** Single-stage forehead flap elevated on subcutaneous pedicle. **C:** Flap transferred under intact glabellar skin. **D:** One-year postoperative view.

defect but the depth that may be the indication for structural grafting. Lesions within the ala or sidewall often require a repair that involves some rigidity. Straight septal cartilage works well for support to the lateral nasal wall of the middle vault, and conchal cartilage is most often used for the alar lobule.

One can enhance nasal airflow by placement of a *flaring suture* across the upper lateral cartilages (33). The middle nasal vault is often exposed during nasal reconstruction and subject to contractile forces. Because of the concavity over the dorsum, this can lead to subtle pinching of the middle third of the nose and some degree of narrowing at the internal valve. The flaring suture placed across the dorsum serves to hold open the upper lateral cartilages during the healing process and support the airway. A long-lasting suture is placed as a horizontal mattress across each upper lateral cartilage, with the dorsal septum serving as a fulcrum. As the suture is tightened, the upper lateral cartilages will flare upward and outward, thus opening the internal nasal valve (Fig. 165.12). This can be placed during any nasal reconstruction where the upper lateral cartilages become exposed, even with smaller procedures such as a bilobe flap.

Grafting for Form

The alar rim is one of the free margins that represent an "immobile landmark" during the defect analysis stage. Normal wound healing and contracture will tend to pull the alar rim up and create a notch deformity; preserving alar base symmetry is one of the greater challenges in nasal restoration. Any defect that encroaches on the free margin of the ala will require some form of structural support to resist the powerful wound contracture that ensues. The curve found along the inferior conchal bowl conforms well to the natural shape and curl of the alar lobule. Grafts may also be placed at the nasal tip to improve definition and form. Many of the common tip grafts used in aesthetic rhinoplasty can be employed here with equal success. Because the covering flap tends to be thicker, one can exaggerate this grafting with minimal risk of creating an unnatural "unitip." Traditional shield or cap grafts should be sutured secured to the underlying structure. Grafts to the tip can also serve to stabilize the junction of a reconstructed framework, such as the union between alar rim grafts and the midline support (e.g. columella). Bridging the junction of cartilage grafts creates substantial more stability than a primary, end-to-end union of grafts alone.

Large lesions may remove portions of the midline dorsal support, and its reconstruction can be more complex. Unlike a dorsal augmentation during the correction of a saddle nose deformity, this reconstruction must bring sufficient rigidity to support the cutaneous and *intranasal* dorsum. This can be accomplished by one of three mechanisms: septal cartilage, cantilevered split calvarial bone, or costal cartilage grafting. Some complex nasal lesions extend

on to the cheek, not only cutaneously but in terms of structure as well. If portions of the premaxilla or lateral bony piriform aperture have been resected, they must be individually repaired in order to recreate a solid platform for the nose. Failure to do so will lead to progressive collapse of the nose. The bony aperture of the nose is an essential foundation upon which other structural grafts and flaps can be added (Fig. 165.13).

Techniques for Grafting

The *middle vault and sidewall* areas are ideally reconstructed with straight *septal cartilage*. This material is readily available and should be long enough to rest on the bony piriform aperture laterally and reach the midline dorsum. The *alar lobule* is best supported by autogenous *conchal cartilage* from the ear, but it must be carefully sculpted. It can be harvested through either the anterior or posterior approaches with little risk of creating significant donor site morbidity. Like septal cartilage, the conchal cartilage graft must be sufficiently long to rest on the bony, medial buttress and extend up to the existing cartilages, or close to the midline. Small discs of cartilage grafts will tend to fall intranasally and not function as the batten that is needed. These cartilage grafts are placed in small subcutaneous pockets laterally, but only blunt dissection should be performed in this area in order to minimize risk of injury to the lateral nasal artery. The medial border is firmly anchored to the tip cartilages in an overlapping manner. The superior margin of the graft should be slightly more medial than the inferior margin, forcing the plane of the graft to mimic the contour of the lobule and create a supra-alar crease. In order to maintain the vertical height of the alar rim, one should ensure that the caudal border of the graft is positioned sufficiently inferior, anticipating the vertical contractile force of wound healing. Grafts are suture-secured to the intranasal lining with through-and-through sutures, thus pulling open the airway under the graft. The natural curvature of the cartilage holds the airway patent, even slightly over corrected. The ala will also feel unnaturally firm with respect to the contralateral side, but this is anticipated and unavoidable (Fig. 165.14).

Dorsal reconstruction can be achieved through a *composite septal flap*, pivoted out of the nose with a hinge along the anterior nasal spine. A full thickness incision is created through the nasal septum, along the dorsum superiorly, vertically posteriorly, and off the maxillary crest inferiorly. This mobilizes the septum as a composite flap composed of cartilage and bilateral mucosal flaps, rotated anteriorly, bringing structure and internal lining simultaneously. A small wedge of septal cartilage should be excised at the posterior septal angle to facilitate the outward pivot. It is imperative for the septal branch of the anterior septal artery be intact, as it is the primary blood supply to the flap. Each vessel can support the entire ipsilateral septal mucosa

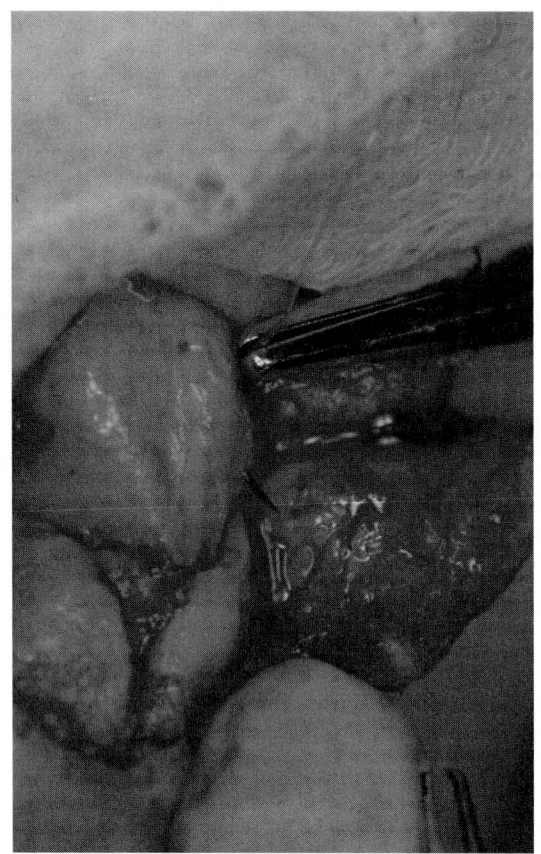

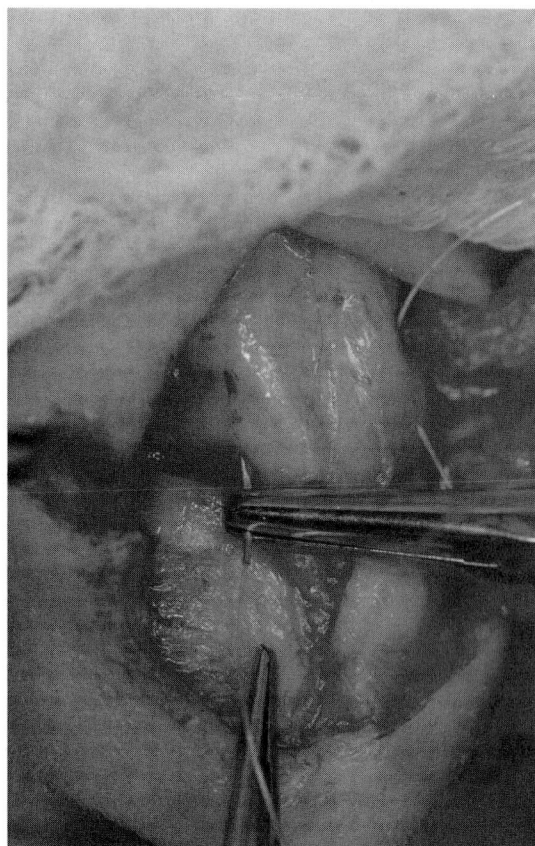

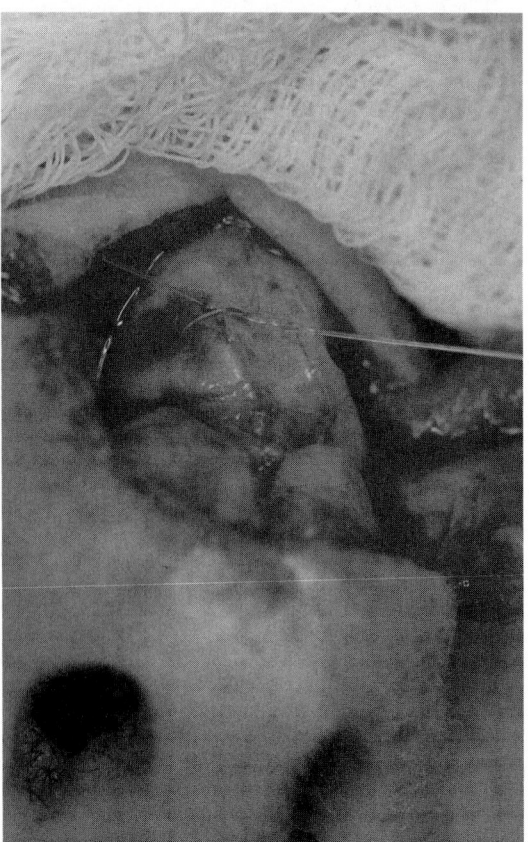

Figure 165.12 **A:** Flaring suture passed through left lateral cartilage. **B:** Through right upper lateral cartilage. **C:** Tied across nasal dorsum to flare internal nasal valve.

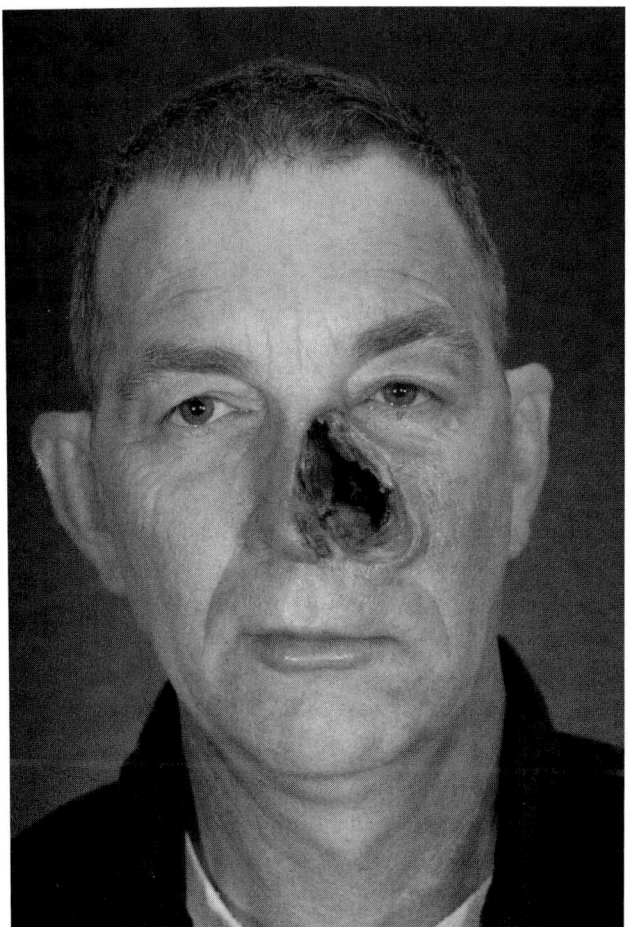 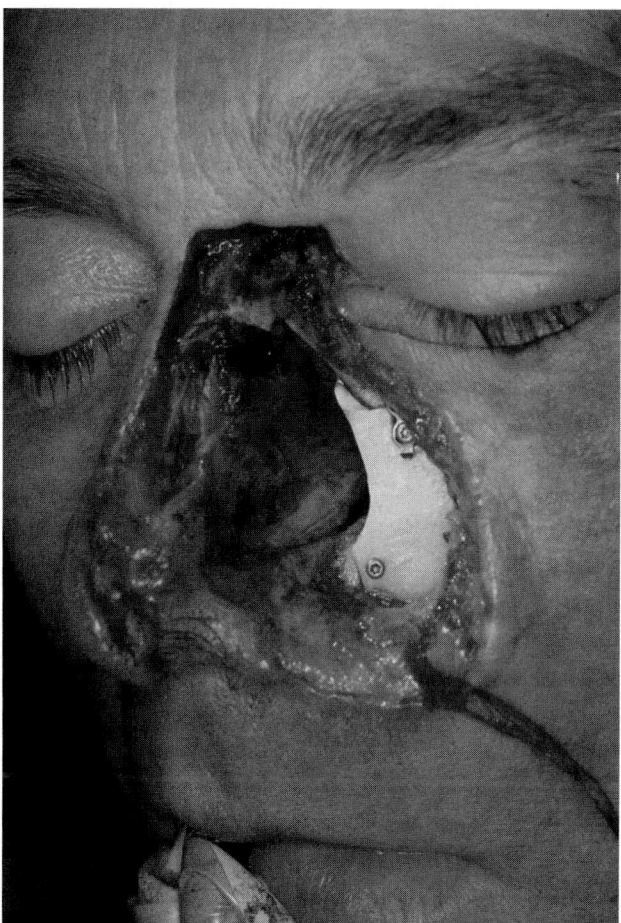

Figure 165.13 **A:** Large left heminasal and cheek defect involving maxilla. **B:** Split calvarial bone to reconstruct medial buttress.

and underlying cartilage. Once the composite flap is rotated outward, it is secured with permanent sutures to the residual dorsum and the anterior nasal spine. Septal splints may be useful to provide additional support during the healing phase, reducing the risk of lateral displacement and nasal obstruction. By necessity, this three-layered septal composite flap will leave behind a permanent septal perforation. Although this adds to the convalescence, only rarely is it symptomatic after healing. This technique works well for reconstruction of complex and full-thickness defects of the dorsum, tip, and columella (Fig. 165.15).

Costal cartilage and *split calvarial bone* are excellent structural grafts for total dorsal reconstruction. Nasal defects of this magnitude are usually associated with deficiencies of internal lining, which will always require an independent reconstruction. Cartilage can be harvested from either the seventh, eighth, or ninth rib. Most skin incisions do not need to exceed 4 cm and the rectus abdominus muscle can be split rather than transected, thus reducing the postoperative pain. A straight portion of the rib should be harvested and only the precise central core utilized for graft-

ing, as eccentric portions of a rib graft will progressively warp. Graft resorption, displacement, and *in situ* warping, are the more common complications that can arise. Split calvarial bone is similarly abundant and generally harvested from the straight parietal region of the skull. Its edges are carefully beveled with a drill, and it may be secured at the nasion with a lag screw technique. Both calvarial bone and costal cartilage will leave the nose feeling unnaturally rigid and immobile. It should be supported at the caudal end with an extended columellar strut graft and laterally with conchal cartilage grafts. This lateral support is essential to reduce inward collapse as well as camouflage the lateral borders of the dorsal reconstruction graft.

INTERNAL LINING DEFICITS

The complexity of a nasal defect is dictated as much by its depth as by its overall size. Violation of the internal lining of the nose is one of the major variables that elevates the level of sophistication of the repair. Early efforts at internal

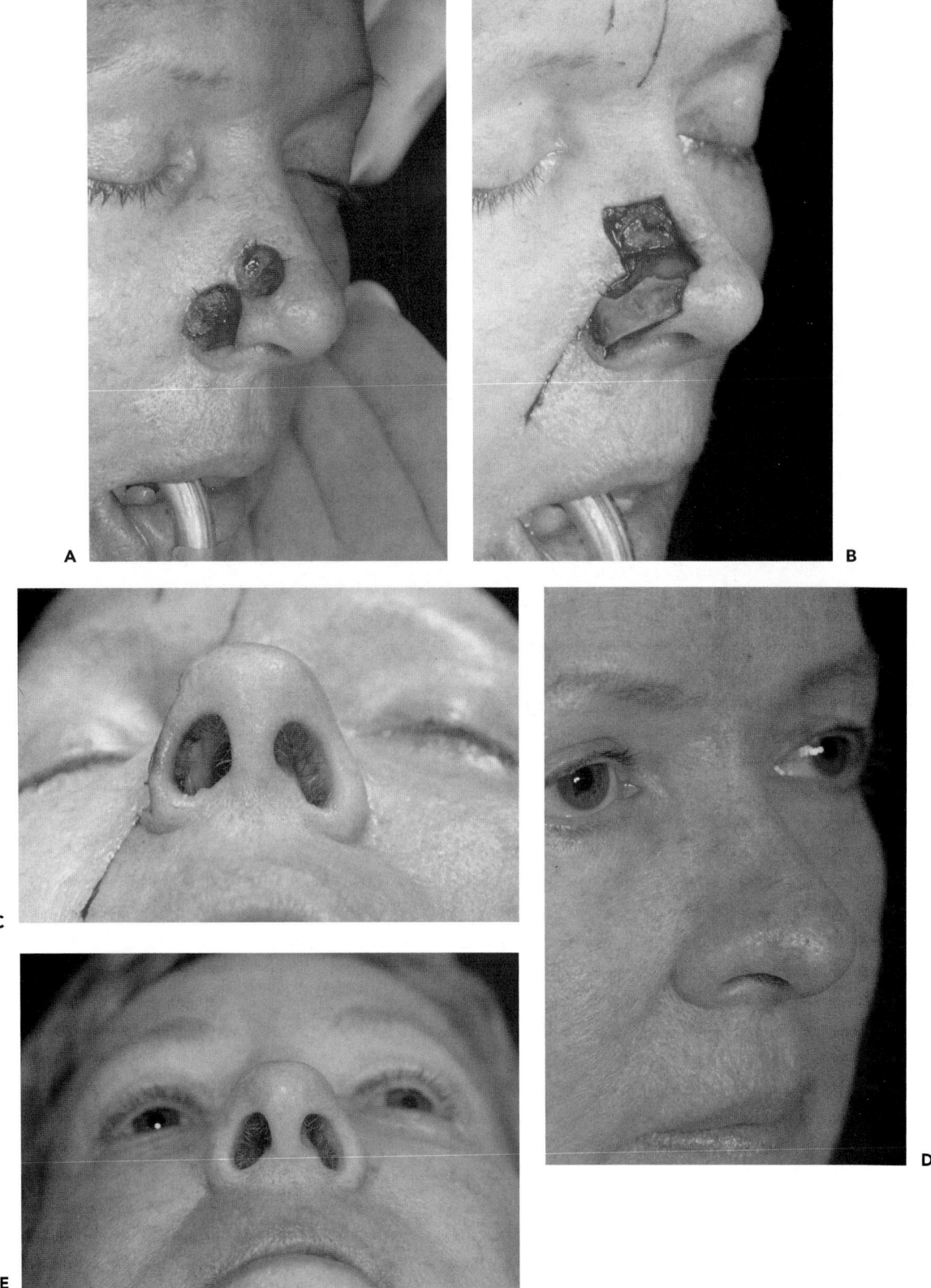

Figure 165.14   Alar batten graft. **A:** Nasal defects of right ala and sidewall. **B:** Conchal cartilage batten graft in non-anatomic position. **C:** Base view demonstrating vestibular support and patency. **D:** One-year postoperative, oblique view showing alar rim contour. **E:** Base view.

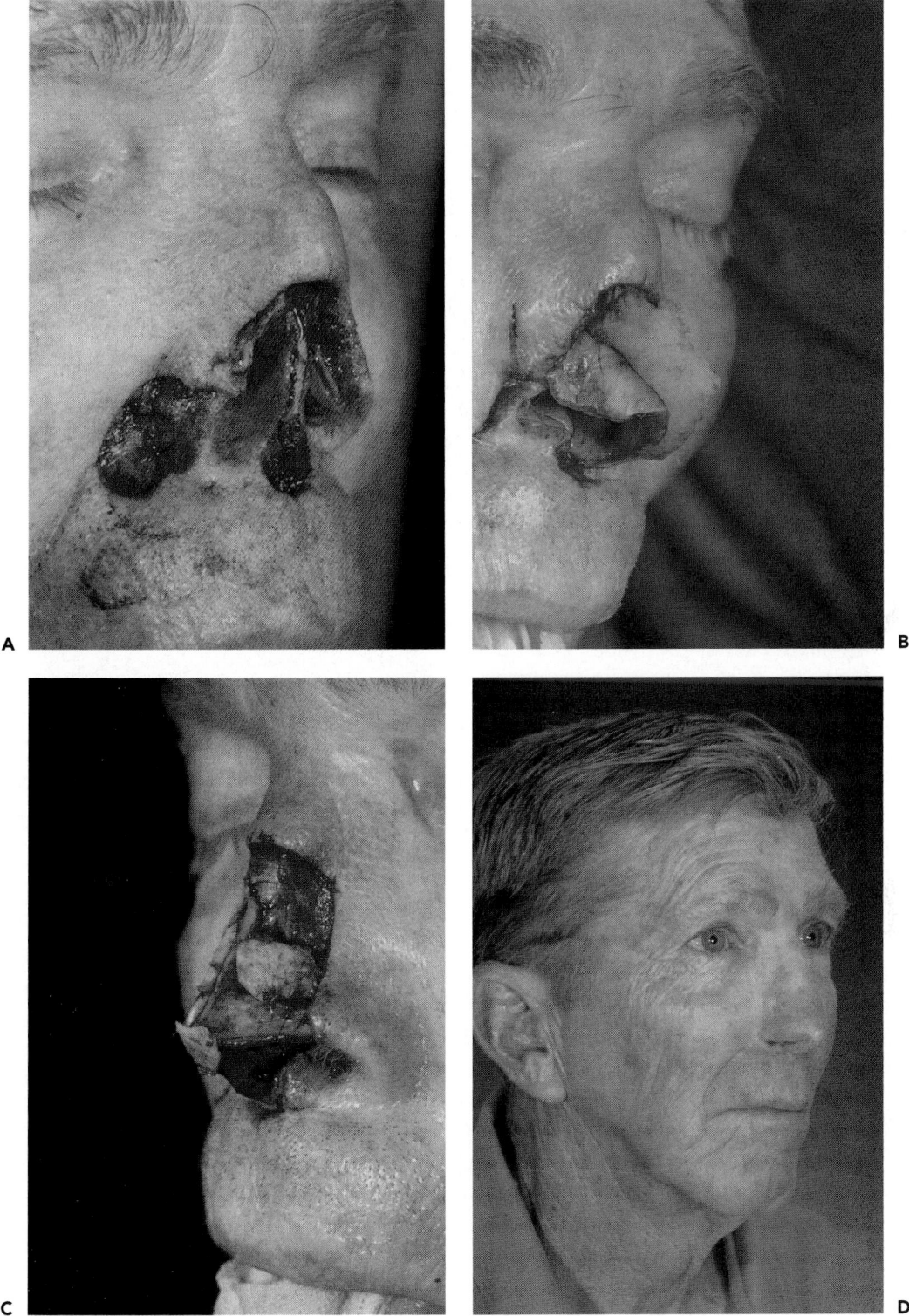

Figure 165.15 **A:** Full-thickness nasal defect. **B:** Nasal septum pivoted externally along posterior septal angle. **C:** Dorsal reconstruction with septum and conchal cartilage grafting. **D:** One-year postoperative view showing adequate dorsal support.

lining repair failed because of flap necrosis or excessive rigidity, in which the lining dictated the nose morphology rather than conformed to it. A preliminary stage of placing grafts and internal lining to the forehead flap also failed because of its lack of flexibility after the flap was transposed. It can be tempting to disregard the lining as one focuses on form and resurfacing, especially because the immediate result will not be affected, but the long-term outcome will be uniformly unfavorable. The purpose of a meticulous repair of all lining defects is twofold: First, a vascularized internal covering is needed for structural grafts (e.g. conchal cartilage batten grafts), and, second, second-intention healing of intranasal areas will lead to alar notching and cicatricial stenosis, progressing to a compromise of form and function. Consequently, even small perforations of the intranasal mucosa must be addressed in some form. Not infrequently, many options for lining repair have been eliminated by the nature of the defect, and one must proceed down an algorithm to alternative techniques. For this reason, it is imperative that one becomes facile with a number of grafts and flaps for the internal lining prior to embarking on a reconstruction of this complexity. Being able to predict the involvement of intranasal mucosa is difficult but can be useful. Certain subtypes of cutaneous malignancies are characterized by their aggressive growth patterns and propensity to extend via small isolated nests of cells beyond the gross margins, e.g. morpheaform BCCA. It is prudent to recognize this propensity for intranasal involvement and plan the excision and reconstruction accordingly, including the incorporation of Mohs micrographic surgery and anticipation of a full-thickness nasal defect. In addition, one should bear in mind that the intranasal defect represents the surgical margin for the cutaneous malignancy, and close follow-up of this area is imperative. This is most accurately performed with nasal endoscopes, common to the otolaryngologist.

Very small perforation of the internal lining can be often closed primarily with a single catgut suture. It is best to close the deficit vertically rather than horizontally, in order to minimize the propensity to retract the alar rim. Larger defects will require a flap or graft and can be defined based on their tissue origin (Table 165.6). Selecting the proper internal lining flap is challenging and often based on the location of the defect; many grafts and flaps are limited to either the middle third or lower third of the nose (Table 165.7). Only rarely is an internal lining repair needed within the upper third of the nose.

Grafts

Full-thickness skin grafts require a vascularized recipient bed, and, as such, will rarely be utilized for internal lining repair because of the concomitant need for structural grafts. An exception might be along the upper one half of the nose, where collapse and contracture are much less of a concern. Many times, second-intention healing will suffice

---

TABLE 165.6

OPTIONS FOR REPAIR OF INTERNAL LINING DEFECTS

1. Primary closure
2. Grafts
   a. Skin
   b. Composite
3. Cutaneous epithelial flaps
   a. Folded, distal resurfacing flap
   b. Nasal epithelial "turn-in" flap
   c. Second cutaneous flap
4. Intranasal flaps
   a. Ipsilateral septal mucosa flap
   b. Contralateral swinging composite flap
   c. Bipedicled "bucket handle" flap
   d. Inferior turbinate flap
5. Pericranial flap
6. Distant microvascular flap

---

in this area. Grafts from the hard palate have more intrinsic rigidity and may be applied for intermediate size defects.

A composite graft of skin and cartilage from the ear is extremely versatile and can be liberally applied to full thickness nasal defects. It may be the technique of choice for lining deficits of the distal one third of the nose, especially the alar lobule, because it brings a thin epithelium to an area that is normally stratified squamous epithelium, and includes a structural graft that forms well to the natural contour of the ala. Small defects of the alar rim and soft tissue facet can be repaired with a composite graft harvested from the root of the helix, utilizing the skin on the inner surface of the helix, within the concha cymba. Larger defects that involve the alar lobule are best reconstructed with a composite graft from the conchal bowl. The donor site can often be closed primarily with minimal auricular deformity. Alternatively, a full-thickness skin graft can be secured to the donor site. In

---

TABLE 165.7

INTERNAL LINING REPAIR

Middle vault
1. Contralateral, swinging composite septal flap
2. Epithelial "turn-in" flap
3. Inferior turbinate flap

Distal $^1/_3$/alar lobule
1. Ipsilateral septal mucosal flap
2. Composite graft from ear
3. Bipedicled "bucket handle" flap
4. Folded distal resurfacing flap (forehead flap)

Columella
1. Composite graft
2. Septal mucosal flaps
3. Folded distal resurfacing flap (melolabial flap)

both cases, the skin portion of the graft is closely adhered to the cartilage with little intervening fat, thus making it an excellent option for composite grafts. The graft should be firmly secured to the undersurface of the resurfacing flap, entirely obliterating any potential dead space that might arise. A through-and-through bolster is very effective for this purpose (Fig. 165.16).

Cutaneous Epithelium

Cutaneous epithelium is an additional source for internal lining repair and has some distinct advantages. Large amounts of tissue can be mobilized to the nose with little or no morbidity (e.g., the epithelial "turn-in" flap). Earlier concerns regarding the nonphysiologic nature of this flap (i.e., bringing keratinizing epithelium to the intranasal space), has not borne out to be problematic. Desquamation, odor, or crusting has not been a major complaint for these patients. There is additional thickness and bulk to this type of flap, and it is important to thin the skin paddle aggressively prior to transposition. Nasal obstruction from a thick flap is difficult to correct secondarily. Perhaps the greatest concern is the mobilization of sun-exposed and potentially actinically injured skin to within the nose, especially considering the high nature of recurrence of metachronous lesions. The intranasal examination postoperatively is best performed by the otolaryngologist and with a nasal endoscope.

A *second epithelial flap* can be elevated and mobilized intranasally for internal lining repair. Common sites include a separate melolabial flap or second forehead flap. These are not only associated with extra morbidity but also utilize a precious resource for possible future needs. Distant tissue through microvascular transfer is a more dramatic means of bringing lining to within the nose. It should be viewed as a preliminary step requiring numerous stages for thinning and sculpting (34).

The *distal portion of the primary resurfacing flap* can be folded on itself to wrap around a cartilage graft and provide internal coverage. This utilizes cutaneous epithelium and is subject to the same guidelines in terms of risk of transferring actinically injured skin. There is often no additional morbidity associated with this technique because it may represent the portion of the flap that would be excised during removal of the standing cutaneous deformity that arises from the flap. The skin paddle should be thinned aggressively. Moreover, this portion of the forehead flap may include the frontal hair and have to be trimmed regularly. There is concern over the vascularity of this distal part of the flap, particularly after folding it on itself, but the robust nature of vascular perfusion appears to be adequate. Perhaps the greatest shortcoming has to do with the free margin of the ala. Although the intranasal lumen may be functionally adequate, the alar rim often takes on an unnaturally thick and straight appearance when using this method. This option is not used as often as others for internal lining repair.

The *epithelial "turn-in" flap* is a versatile flap for internal defects limited to the lower half of the nose (35). It utilizes the cutaneous epithelium from the upper nose and turns it in 180 degrees, so that it faces intranasally. Elevation begins superiorly in the subdermal plane and descends deeper as one proceeds inferiorly in order to create a flap with a healthy subcutaneous pedicle. The pedicle base requires careful dissection in order to avoid amputation and often leaves an area of bulk and fullness to the external nose. The ideal defect has the intranasal edge in close proximity to the skin edge, allowing for primary edge-to-edge approximation. One must closely survey the quality of the skin prior to elevation and transfer. In some cases, this method of internal lining repair comes at no cost of additional morbidity; at times, the "turn-in" flap represents skin that would be discarded during the completion of the nasal aesthetic subunits. It has the advantage of not disrupting the native intranasal mucosa, which can greatly accelerate recovery. It is limited in terms of the amount of skin available and is best suited for small internal defects of the lower nose only (Fig. 165.17).

Intranasal Tissue

It is ideal to replace tissue with like tissue, and intranasal mucosa has several options that provide a thin, pliable, robust, and physiologic lining for the full-thickness nasal defect. The *inferior turbinate mucosal flap* provides a modest amount of mucosa without major donor site morbidity and can be an excellent flap for defects involving the middle or lower thirds of the nose (36). It is rare for a primary cutaneous malignancy to invade so far posteriorly that it disrupts the head of the inferior turbinate. Mesenchymal tumors of the lateral nasal wall, on the other hand, can extend posteriorly to involve the turbinates or even maxillary sinus. The inferior turbinate flap is based anteriorly on its head and is best elevated by first extracting the entire turbinate, including bone, as a flap based anteriorly. The conchal bone is then dissected off and the mucosal flap mobilized to fill the lining defect as an interpolated flap. The pedicle is usually quite short and does not necessarily require revision.

The *bipedicled "bucket-handle" mucosal flap* is an excellent option for relatively small lining defects along the alar lobule. It utilizes intranasal mucosa immediately above the defect and hinges it inferiorly as a flap based medially and laterally. The septal artery territory does not dependably extend to this portion of the internal lining, and the lateral pedicle must be maintained. Any contribution from the ethmoid system is severed by the flap design. Wide undermining is critical in order to allow complete mobilization inferiorly without superior traction. A relaxing incision can be created with an angled beaver knife. The extent of undermining should be to the nasal bones, where the secondary donor site defect is allowed

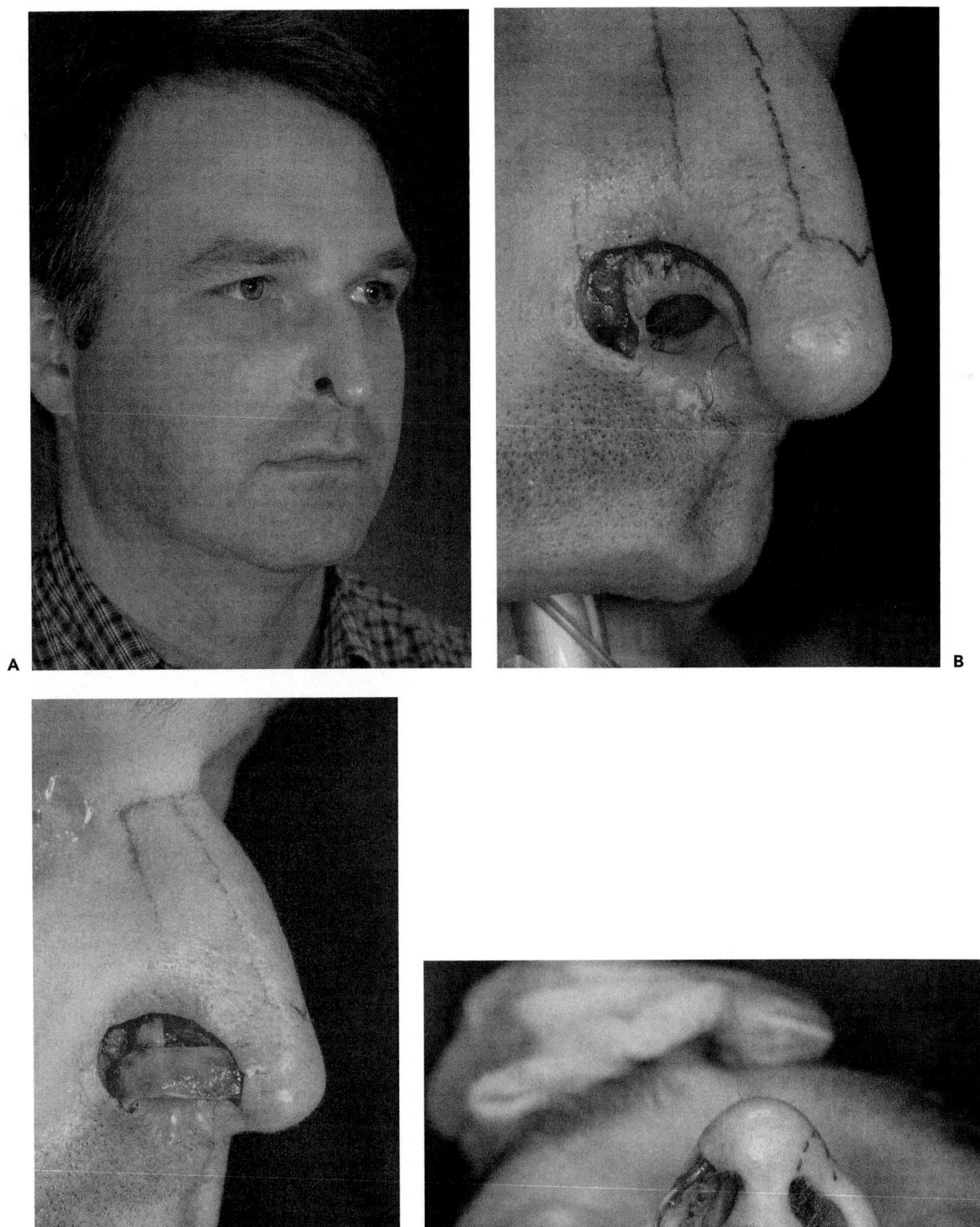

Figure 165.16   Composite graft. **A:** Full-thickness defect of right ala . **B:** Superior skin margin excised . **C:** Auricular composite graft. **D:** Base view demonstrating patency and support.

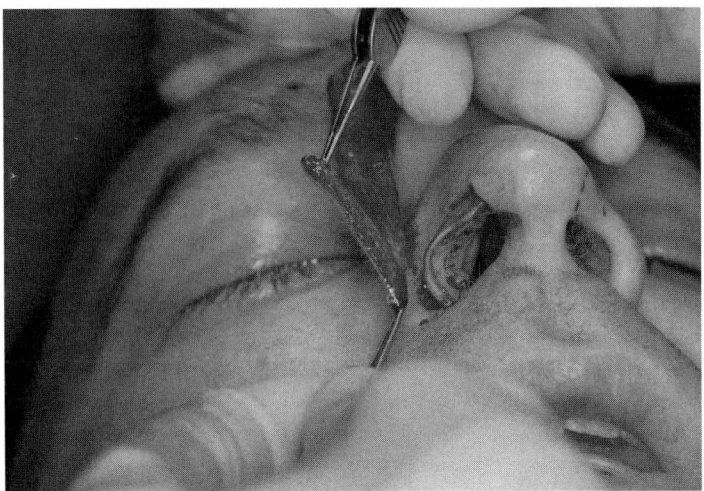

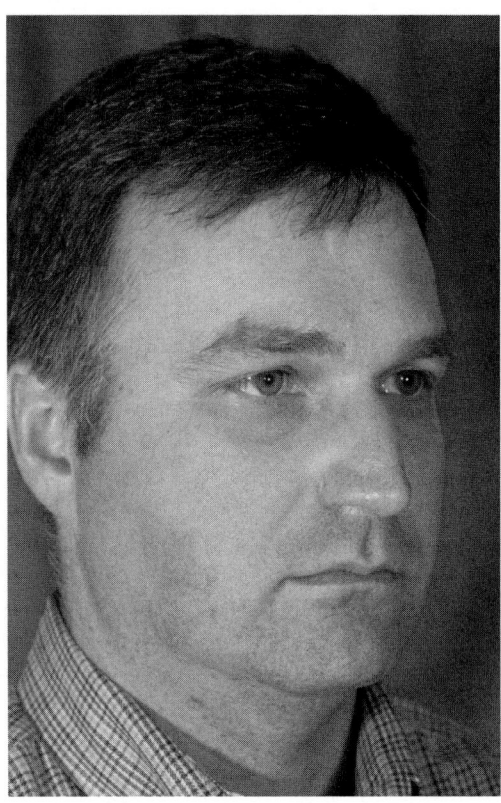

E   **F**

Figure 165.16 *(continued)*   **E:** Forehead flap transferred. **F:** One-year postoperative view.

to heal by second intention. Placing a skin graft to this location is an alternative, but rarely necessary. Any superior retraction will inevitably pull the free alar margin and compromise the alar base symmetry.

The contralateral septal mucosa can be used via a *swinging, composite septal flap*, based on the dorsal septum and the branches of the anterior ethmoid artery. It is an excellent means of providing both intranasal lining and cartilaginous framework to the middle third of the nose. It does not have sufficient size to provide structural framework to the alar lobule. The cartilage is typically straight and can also assist with dorsal support to that area as it rests on the bony ledge of the piriform aperture. The ipsilateral septal mucosa is elevated off the septal cartilage and preserved. A full-thickness incision is then made through the septum, creating a swinging door of cartilage and contralateral septal mucosa, based on a hinge along the dorsum. The cartilage rests lateral to the bony ledge, but the mucosa is sewn directly to the internal lining margin. There is a tendency for the flap to swing back medially, and this is resisted by securing the cartilage to the lateral bone. The ipsilateral septal mucosa can be used for alar lining for larger defects or can be replaced to fill the resultant septal perforation. Often, this area will break down and a perforation will recur.

The ipsilateral, septal mucosa flap is a workhorse for larger and complex internal lining defects of the nose. First described by Millard in 1967 (15), it is a thin and dependable flap based on the septal branch of the superior labial artery. The entire septal mu-

cosa is lifted off the cartilage and mobilized to line the lower two thirds of the nose. Tremendous care should be observed to stay in the correct subperichondrial plane, especially if there coexists septal spurs or fractures. The pedicle to this mucosal flap may cross the nasal valve and cause nasal obstruction. This can be divided at a subsequent stage. A large septal perforation will often develop but is only rarely symptomatic. The only prerequisite for this flap is the preservation of the anterior/inferior portion of the septum and the nasal sill, as this functions as the flap base.

Pericranial Flap

The pericranial flap is a thin and versatile flap often used by neurosurgeons for anterior cranial defects. It can also be elevated for internal nasal lining and transferred as part of the forehead flap. The pericranium should be covered with a skin or mucosal graft because, although epithelialization will occur eventually, wound contracture and desiccated cartilage may present problems. The forehead flap can be elevated full thickness (i.e., with the periosteum of the forehead), then split longitudinally to excise the frontalis muscle and create a bifid flap that encapsulates the cartilage grafts of the nose. The pericranium is based on the same pedicle as the forehead flap. It can be dunked intranasally during the pedicle division at 3 weeks.

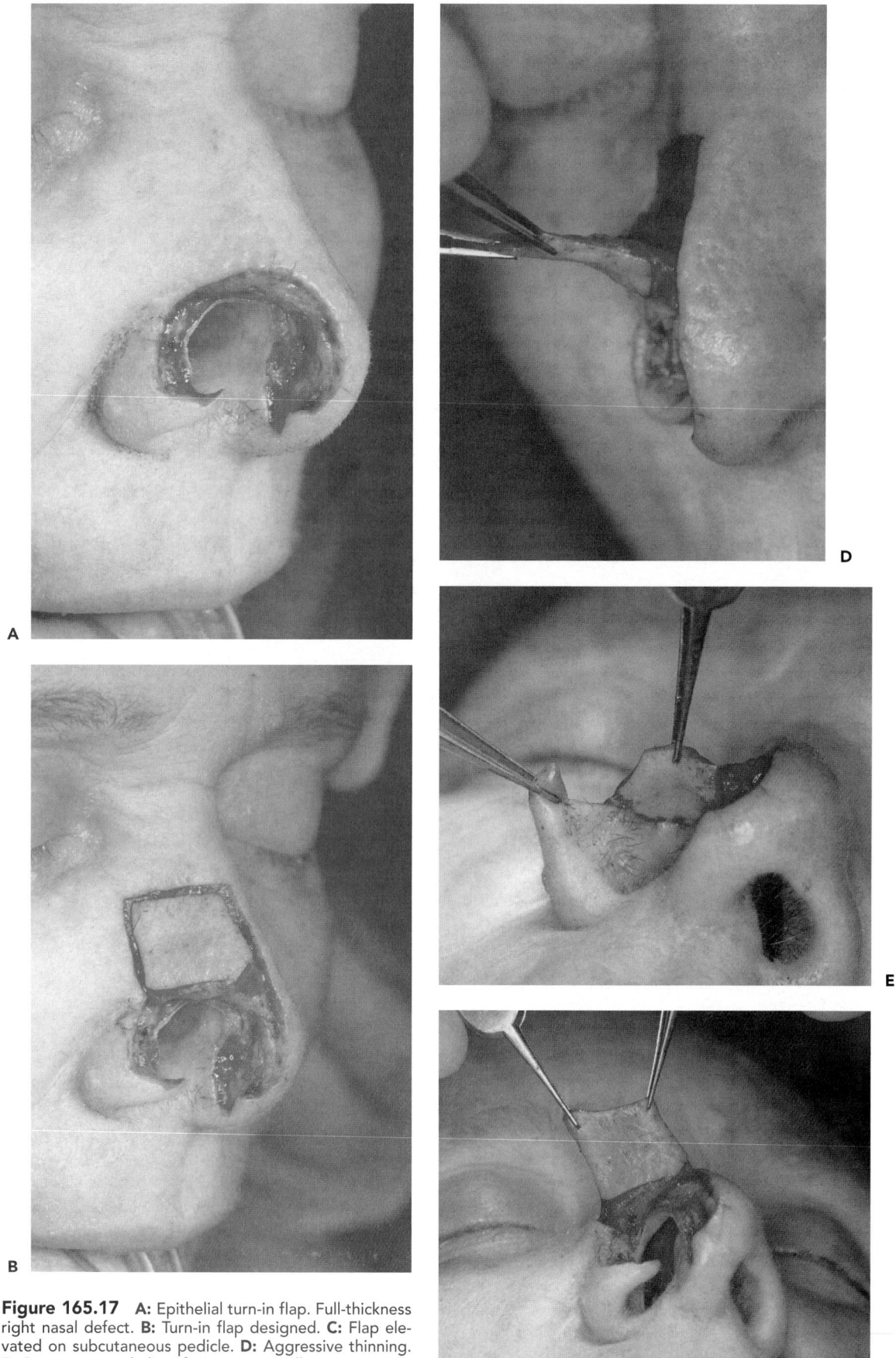

Figure 165.17   **A:** Epithelial turn-in flap. Full-thickness right nasal defect. **B:** Turn-in flap designed. **C:** Flap elevated on subcutaneous pedicle. **D:** Aggressive thinning. **E:** Cutaneous epithelium facing intranasally.

CONCLUSION

Nasal restoration in the twenty-first century has reached a new milestone that has brought together centuries of experiences, lessons, errors, and rewards. The bar has been set and it is nothing less than a restoration of normal function and social acceptance. The aesthetic expectations of both minor and major nasal repair include symmetry, natural contour, excellent color and texture match, and a final product that remains inconspicuous to the casual observer. The major tenets that have been realized today include the wide application of the subunit principle, liberal and nonanatomic cartilage grafting (for form and function), and addressing each of the three layers of the nose independently. The robust nature of the forehead flap has expanded its applications and lifted the outcomes of major nasal resurfacing. Anticipating resultant scars and vectors of tension are the subtle nuances of local flaps that ensure a pleasing result. The next dimension will expand on the physiology of wound healing, improving predictability, and controlling outcomes.

HIGHLIGHTS

- Using a reconstructive algorithm can assist with flap selection and avoiding pitfalls.
- Alar base symmetry must be preserved with small flaps.
- Wide use of the aesthetic subunit principle can improve results.
- The forehead flap is a robust flap that remains the workhorse for resurfacing.
- Complex defects must address each of the three layers of the nose independently.
- Nasal function is paramount and usually addressed with nonanatomic, cartilage grafts secured to the lateral nasal wall.
- All internal lining defects must be specifically repaired.

REFERENCES

1. Conroy B. The history of facial prostheses. *Clin Plast Surg* 1983; 10:689–707.
2. Almast S. History and evolution of the Indian method of rhinoplasty. In: Sanvenero-Rosselli G, ed. *Transactions of the fourth International congress of Plastic and Reconstructive Surgery.* (Rome, 1967) Amsterdam: Excerpta Medica Foundation, 1969:49.
3. Antia NH, Daver BM. Reconstructive surgery for nasal defects. *Clin Plast Surg* 1981;8(3):535–563.
4. Sushruta S. *The Sushruta Samhita.* English translation based on original Sanskrit text. Kaviraj Kunja Lal Bhishagratna, ed. Bose, Calcutta: Kaviraj Kunja Lal Bhishagratna, 1907–1916.
5. Antia NH, Daver BM. Reconstructive surgery for nasal defects. *Clin Plast Surg* 1981;8:535–563.
6. "BL." Letter to the Editor. *Gentleman's Magazine*, London, October 1794:891. Reprinted in: *Plast Recon Surg* 1969;44:67–69.
7. Carpue J. An account of two successful operations for restoring a lost nose from the integuments of the forehead. London: Longman, Hurst, Reese, Orme and Brown Publishers, 1816. Reprinted in: *Plast Reconstr Surg* 1969;44:175–185.
8. Kazanjian VH. The repair of nasal defects with the median forehead flap primary closure of the forehead wound. *Surg Gynecol Obstet* 1946;83:27–32.
9. Converse JM. New forehead flap for nasal reconstruction. *Proc R Soc Med* 1942;35:811–815.
10. Gilles HD. Experiences with the tubed pedicle flaps. *Surg Gynecol Obstet* 1935;60:291–293.
11. New GB. Sickle flaps for nasal reconstruction. *Surg Gynecol Obstet* 1945;80:497–499.
12. Converse, JM. Reconstruction of the nose by the scalping flap technique. *Surg Clin North Am* 1959;39:335–364.
13. Washio H. Retroauricular temporal flap. *Plast Reconstr Surg* 1969; 43:162–165.
14. Millard DR. Total reconstructive rhinoplasty and a missing link. *Plast Reconstr Surg* 1966;37:167–170.
15. Millard DR. Hemirhinoplasty. *Plast Reconstr Surg* 1967;40:440–445.
16. Millard DR. Reconstructive rhinoplasty for the lower half of the nose. *Plast Reconstr Surg* 1974;53:133–138.
17. Millard DR. Reconstructive rhinoplasty for the lower two-thirds of the nose. *Plast Reconstr Surg* 1976;57:722–728.
18. Burget GC, Menick FJ. *Aesthetic reconstruction of the nose.* St. Louis: Mosby–Year Book, 1994:1–600.
19. Langer C. Zur anatomie und physiologie der haut. *Sitzungsb Acad Wissensch* 1861;45:223–229.
20. Singh DJ, Bartlett SP. Aesthetic considerations in nasal reconstruction and the role of modified nasal subunits. *Plast Recon Surg* 2003;111(2):639–648.
21. Reiger RA. A local flap for repair of the nasal tip. *Plast Reconstr Surg* 1967;40:147–149.
22. Limberg AA. *Mathematical principles of local plastic procedures on the surface of the human body.* Leningrad: In-government Publishing House for medical literature (Medgiz), 1946.
23. Zitelli JA. The bilobed flap for nasal reconstruction. *Arch Dermatol* 1989;125:957.
24. Yotsuyanagi T, Yamashita K, Uroshidate S, et al. Nasal reconstruction based on aesthetic subunits in Orientals. *Plast Reconstr Surg* 2000;106(1):36–44.
25. Lang PG, Duncan IM, Hochman M. Occurrence of subclinical tumor in excised facial subunits. *Arch Facial Plast Surg* 2004;6: 158–161.
26. Murrell GL, Burger GC. Aesthetically precise templates for nasal reconstruction using a new material. *Plast Reconstr Surg* 2003; 1855–1861.
27. Park SS. Reconstruction of nasal defects larger than 1.5 cm in diameter. *Laryngoscope* 2000;110(8):1241–1250.
28. Tardy ME, Sykes J, Kron T. The precise midline forehead flap. *Clin Plast Surg* 1985;12:481.
29. Adamson JE. Nasal reconstruction with the expanded forehead flap. *Plast Recon Surg.* 1988;81(1):12–20.
30. Park SS, Rodeheaver G, Levine PA. Role of ischemic gradient on neovascularization of interpolated skin flaps. *Arch Otolaryngol Head Neck Surg* 1996:122(8):886–889.
31. Converse JM, Wood-Smith D: Experiences with the forehead island flap with a subcutaneous pedicle. *Plast Reconstr Surg* 1963; 31:521–527.
32. Park, SS. Single stage forehead flap: An alternative with advantages. *Arch Facial Plastic Surg.* 2002:4;32–36.
33. Park SS. The flaring suture to augment the repair of the dysfunctional nasal valve. *Plastic Reconstr Surg.* 1998:101(4):1120–1122.
34. Moore EJ, Strome SA, Kasperbauer JL., et al. Vascularized radial forearm free tissue for lining in nasal reconstruction. *Laryngoscope* 113(12):2078–2085, 2003.
35. Park SS, Cook TA, Wang TD. The epithelial "turn-in" flap in nasal reconstruction. *Arch Otolaryngol Head Neck Surg* 1995:121; 1122–1127.
36. Murakami CS, Kriet D, Ierokomos AP. Nasal reconstruction using the inferior turbinate mucosal flap. *Arch Facial Plast Surg* 1999; 13:97–110.

166

Surgery for Exophthalmos

G. Richard Holt   Jean Edwards Holt   Randal A. Otto

Exophthalmos is a condition of altered thyroid metabolism that causes protein depositions within the extraocular muscles, increasing their bulk as much as tenfold. The infiltration of lymphocytes, plasma cells, mast cells, and macrophages, especially in the extraocular muscles and retrobulbar structures, is related to abnormal antibody-receptor site complexes in these tissues. The T lymphocyte appears to be the primary culprit in this abnormal autoimmune response. It is also known as Graves ophthalmopathy, thyroid orbitopathy, and dysthyroid orbitopathy (1).

Because of the fixed volume of approximately 30 mL of the orbit, expansion of the cross-sectional diameter of the extraocular muscles is manifested by an outward movement of the globe, with anterior protrusion of the mobile, although compartmentalized, orbital fat. The globe effectively decompresses itself by this protrusion in the only available outlet, the anterior orbit. For an increase in soft-tissue volume of 5 mL in a dysthyroid orbit, a 16% increase in volume, the globe becomes approximately 4 to 5 mm proptotic.

In addition to thickening of the muscles, fat herniation, and proptosis, upper and lower eyelid retraction and divergence of gaze is also present (Fig. 166.1). This retraction is caused by fibrosis of the lid retractor muscles, and it further accentuates the globe proptosis by creating a widened interpalpebral distance. Except in acute cases of exophthalmos, the eyelids can close sufficiently to protect the cornea because of the strong overcompensation of the orbicularis oculi muscles and the Bell phenomenon of globe rotation superiorly. Although more than 50% of patients with Graves disease have eye symptoms, only about 5% are severe enough to warrant intervention.

PATIENT EVALUATION

Because exophthalmos is caused by hyperthyroidism, there are no solid epidemiologic or demographic markers, such as those seen in the endemic hypothyroidism of the Midwest because of iodine-poor soils. Some patients complain of the symptoms of hyperthyroidism, including heat and cold intolerance, weight loss, and emotionally and physically hyperactive states. For other patients, exophthalmos may be the only indication of the disease. Any patient with unilateral or bilateral exophthalmos should be presumed to have thyroid disease. Most patients with Graves disease are initially evaluated by a medical specialist rather than a head and neck surgeon, but it is important to understand the evaluation of the dysthyroid patient. Most tests are repeated in the preoperative assessment for stability of the disease and for comparison with baseline test results.

In the acute stages of Graves disease, the values are characteristically increased for total triiodothyronine and free triiodothyronine, total thyroxine and free thyroxine, reverse triiodothyronine thyroid uptake, clearance and release of iodine 131, and serum assays of thyrotropin-releasing hormone and thyroid-stimulating immunoglobulin. After medical ablation with iodine 131 and thyroxine replacement, these values should return to normal, although thyrotropin-releasing hormone and thyroid-stimulating immunoglobulin may remain mildly elevated despite an euthyroid status. The assay for long-acting thyroid-stimulating hormone may be performed at special reference laboratories and is helpful for marginal cases. These tests are particularly indicated because of the lag time in developing ophthalmopathy as the hyperthyroid state recesses clinically.

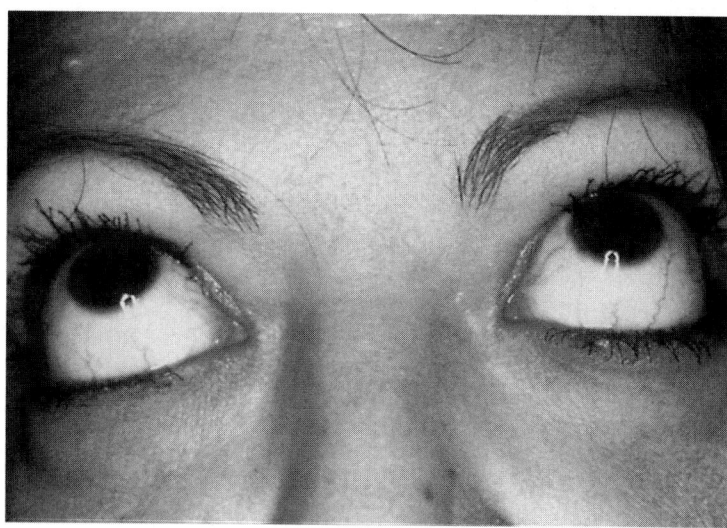

Figure 166.1 Patient with exophthalmos, divergent gaze on extreme gaze, and eyelid retraction seen in dysthyroid ophthalmopathy.

Ultrasound of the orbit can help confirm the suspicion of orbital thyroid disease detected on physical examination. This test can demonstrate a thickening of all extraocular muscles, especially the medial, lateral, and inferior recti. The edematous soft tissues strike a characteristic response pattern to the reflected ultrasound signal. In the hands of an experienced technician, this test can be diagnostic, but for most clinicians, computed tomography (CT) or magnetic resonance imaging (MRI) provides the best anatomic diagnosis. On both scans, the pathognomonic enlargement of the recti muscles can be readily identified. The scans are required to rule out any other pathologic condition of the orbit, either etiologic or concomitant, especially in the unilateral case of exophthalmos. MRI measurement of T2 relaxation time is a useful technique for detecting eye muscle edema in patients with exophthalmos. If such inflammatory edema is found, appropriate medical therapy can be initiated. Those patients with increased mean T2 relaxation times are more likely to respond to antiinflammatory therapy (2). If, however, there is no prolonged T2 relaxation time, the patient may be a candidate for an orbital decompression. If considering surgical decompression, the scans should include the paranasal sinuses. Infectious, allergic, or inflammatory conditions of the sinuses may disallow surgery unless adequately resolved preoperatively. Other deformities (e.g., hypoplastic maxillary sinus) should be identified before developing the surgical plan because alternatives to inferior decompression may need to be considered.

The physical examination can confirm the upper and lower lid retraction, proptosis, and other physical signs of hyperthyroidism. If the patient is not euthyroid, the physician may notice tachycardia, sweating, hyperactivity, and anxiety during the examination. A particularly revealing physical sign is a hyperemia over the lateral rectus muscles (Fig. 166.2). This is pathognomonic for thyroidal eye disease. A complete ophthalmologic examination and a head and neck evaluation should be performed, giving particular attention to the thyroid status. Using Hertel exophthalmometry, the amount of globe protrusion can be measured, quantifying the problem for preoperative and postoperative comparison and identifying the severity of the condition. A patient with exophthalmos and a mass in the thyroid gland may have a hyperfunctioning nodule, which should be evaluated by scanning techniques and fine-needle aspiration. A complete guide to the evaluation of the patient with a thyroid mass may be found in Chapter 114. Active hyperthyroid status requires control before considering surgery for exophthalmos. Table 166.1 summarizes the preoperative evaluation for exophthalmos.

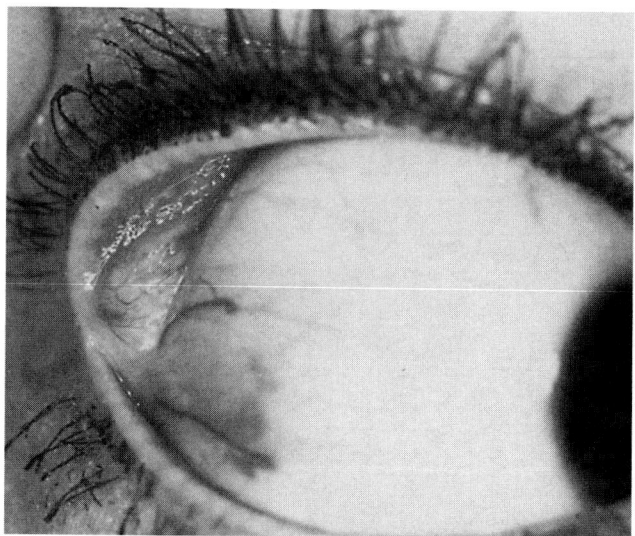

Figure 166.2 Characteristic finding of hyperemia along the lateral rectus muscle in dysthyroid ophthalmopathy.

TABLE 166.1

PREOPERATIVE ASSESSMENT FOR EXOPHTHALMOS

General physical examination
Complete head and neck examination
Laboratory assays
  Serum T3, T4
  Thyroid-stimulating immunoglobulin
  Thyroid-stimulating hormone
  Thyrotropin-releasing hormone
  Long-acting thyroid-stimulating hormone
  T_3 suppression test
Radiographic evaluation
  Orbital ultrasound
  Computed tomography
  Magnetic resonance imaging
  Thyroid scan
Ophthalmologic evaluation
  Hertel exophthalmometry
  Indirect ophthalmoscopy
  Visual-evoked potentials
  Visual acuity
  Visual fields
  Extraocular muscle function
  Intraocular pressure
  Schirmer test

DIFFERENTIAL DIAGNOSIS

The most common differential diagnosis to consider in bilateral exophthalmos is pseudotumor cerebri. This ill-defined condition causes soft-tissue edema within the orbit and can give rise to exophthalmos characterized as mild to severe. CT or MRI can show generalized edema of the soft tissues, occasionally including areas of the brain, but no specific enlargement of the extraocular muscles that is so characteristic of thyroid-induced exophthalmos. The use of high-dose steroids in pseudotumor cerebri usually improves the proptosis, often within 24 to 48 hours. If acute, the cornea should be protected by taping, ointment, and a moisture shield until the steroids have begun to improve the problem. If not responsive to this medical treatment, decompression of the orbit may be required.

Lymphoma of the orbit can produce proptosis and greatly resemble thyroid-induced exophthalmos. The patient with lymphoma is usually elderly, but the pseudotumor cerebri patient is more likely to be a teenaged or young woman. With lymphoma, there is a more localized mass seen on the scan, usually near the apex, and the proptosis may be acentric. Thyroid exophthalmopathy is usually centric. A complete examination may reveal lymphadenopathy in other lymph-bearing areas. Ultrasonography of the orbit in qualified hands may differentiate between a mass due to lymphoma and to thyroid disease. A localized mass suspected of being lymphoma requires a tissue biopsy by transconjunctival needle aspiration or by orbitotomy for tissue diagnosis.

Other space-occupying masses, such as metastatic tumor, vascular anomaly, neurofibroma, and retinoblastoma, can cause unilateral proptosis and must be accounted for in the complete evaluation of an orbital mass. In these cases, the patients are to be euthyroid before treatment.

Congenital shallowness of the orbits produces an obvious unilateral or bilateral exophthalmos. The facial growth should be allowed to continue as long as the corneas continue to be adequately moistened with a blink and closure at night. A decompression procedure can be considered in the early teens of such a patient if necessary, although cosmesis is the general indication. Orbital reconstruction is also used in the craniofacial reconstruction of severe facial deformities (e.g., Apert syndrome and Crouzon disease).

MANAGEMENT

Except in acute and progressive thyroid exophthalmos, the disease is self-limited in most patients. In some patients, it can be documented by visual field testing that the vision progressively becomes tunneled and limited, making restoration of vision, and not cosmesis, the prime concern. Before thyroid disease was fully understood and thyroidectomy for Graves disease was undertaken, the natural history was progression to blindness because of corneal exposure or optic neuropathy.

All patients with dysthyroid ophthalmopathy require complete endocrinologic evaluation and management of their hyperthyroidism. The medical management of Graves disease usually centers on suppression of thyroid activity through subtotal thyroidectomy, iodine 131 ablation, or exogenous thyroid hormone. After euthyroid status has been achieved for at least 6 months, the orbital status usually stabilizes, and the subsequent need for surgical intervention can be established. However, 1% to 2% of patients develop acute deterioration of their orbital status, usually in the form of decreased visual acuity or field defects due to optic neuropathy. The treatment of choice is administration of 80 to 120 mg of prednisone daily for as long as 14 days. If the visual dysfunction does not improve or if prolonged use of oral steroids is required to maintain visual acuity, decompression is indicated. The use of cyclophosphamide and plasmapheresis for acute optic neuropathy remains questionable and cannot be recommended as proven therapy. Adjunctive treatment for exposure keratitis and conjunctivitis includes the use of ocular lubricants and artificial tears, moisture chambers, and taping retracted eyelids if possible.

Exophthalmos persists in approximately 5% of patients with thyroid dysfunction, even after they become euthyroid. For the patient wishing to discuss the possibility of surgery for exophthalmos, the surgeon must review the complete records of the past diagnosis and medical treatment and obtain evidence of the current euthyroid status of the patient. The patient's ophthalmologic findings should be reviewed with the patient's ophthalmologist and a conclusion reached by the team of internist, ophthalmologist, and head and neck surgeon about the advisability of recommending surgery. Low-dose radiation therapy has been used successfully, but there is a risk to the lens and the optic nerve with this technique. The team should consult a radiation therapist with experience in treating exophthalmos.

Preoperative counseling for exophthalmos surgery is best done using a model of the skull and precise charts of eyelid and orbital anatomy. These aids greatly enhance the surgeon's ability to explain the procedures and potential risks, and they allow the patient to understand the procedure and ask questions. The major counseling issues center on risks of vision motility disorders and failure to achieve a satisfactory result. Although the risk to vision is low, the globe is already under tension from the exophthalmic state, and undue or prolonged globe retraction during orbital decompression can cause optic nerve or retinal injury. Retrobulbar hematoma from bleeding caused by the surgical approach is an emergency that can lead to blindness. The decompression procedures themselves can lead to epistaxis, damage to the infraorbital nerve, scarring of skin incisions, and infection. Surgeons should openly discuss these potential complications and their experience with the procedure. What is reported in national studies may not reflect the results of particular surgeons; results may be better or worse in their hands. In general, the more advanced the exophthalmos, the more extensive the surgery required to gain even modest improvement, and very few patients are completely satisfied with the initial procedure.

SURGICAL TREATMENT

Surgical management is considered for two stages of dysthyroid exophthalmos (3). In the acute or subacute stage, steroids are used to resolve or improve visual disturbances caused by optic neuropathy. If the patient fails to regain visual acuity or if steroids are required for long-term maintenance, surgical decompression is indicated. In the late stage, when palpebral retraction, exophthalmos, or oculomotor involvement is seen, cosmetic decompression is indicated, but only after eye findings have been stable for at least 6 months.

The usual functional indications for surgical decompression are decreasing visual acuity, visual field defects, abnormal visual-evoked potentials, and disk edema. The indications are related primarily to optic neuropathy. These patients are usually older, have less proptosis, and have a shorter duration of eye disease than patients operated on for nonfunctional findings. With patients who have significant lid retraction, corneal exposure with keratitis not responsive to conservative medical management is another indication for decompression. In general, decompression of the orbit precedes strabismus surgery for diplopia, which precedes lid-lengthening procedures for lid retraction.

Several factors correlate well with the reduction in proptosis by surgical decompression: the percentage increase in orbital volume after surgery, the absolute increase in orbital

volume, and the degree of "stiffness" of the orbital tissues preoperatively. The first two of these variables are inversely correlated with the third. Orbital stiffness is the loss of resilience of orbital tissues and the increase in adherence between orbital tissue planes. Other factors may play a role in the final result obtained from decompression, including the anterior orbital aperture, the resistance of the orbital septum, and pressure changes in the orbit. Progressive exophthalmos may result in a marked cosmetic abnormality. Because it commonly affects young adult to middle-aged women, the orbital appearance can become a significant social and psychologic problem (4). Improvement of the cosmetic aspect of this disorder is becoming recognized as a valid indication for orbital decompression, as long as the patient understands the inherent risks to vision.

Orbital Decompression

In 1911, Dollinger was the first to publish a report on the decompression of the orbit for Graves disease, using the Kronlein approach to the lateral orbit. Other surgeons are credited with the advocacy for other types of decompression, including Naffziger (superior), Hisch and Urbanek (inferior), Sewell (medial), and Walsh and Ogura for combined medial and inferior decompression (Fig. 166.3). We prefer to describe the various decompression procedures by their anatomic location (e.g., medial orbit) rather than by their eponyms. Anatomic nomenclature better describes the procedure and is easier to remember.

Three-wall decompression, which has recently become popular, uses approaches to the medial, inferior, and lateral orbital walls (5–7). Other surgeons prefer a medial and inferior approach only because they believe an inferior approach has the potential for extraocular muscle imbalance,

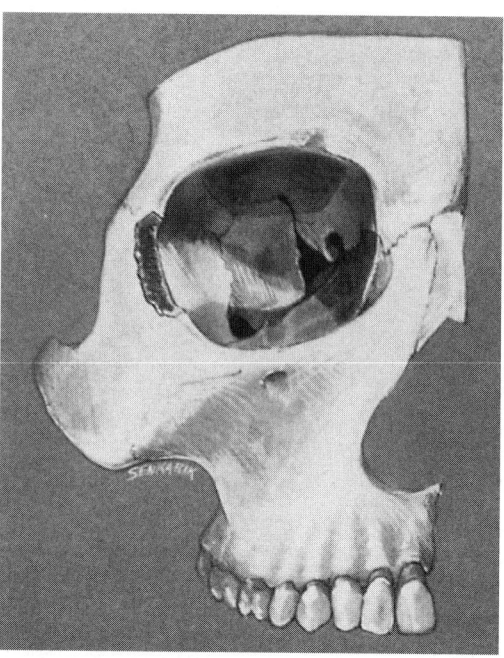

Figure 166.3 Sites of decompression of the orbit: medial, inferior, lateral, and superior.

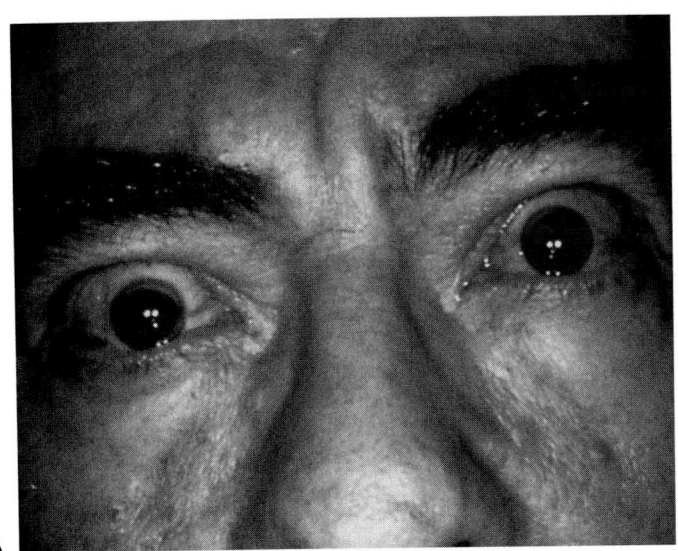
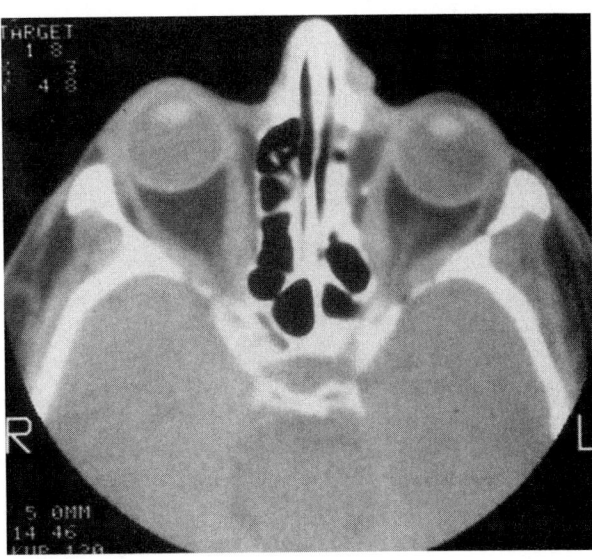

Figure 166.4 **A:** A 50-year-old man with eye findings of Graves disease. **B:** Computed tomography demonstrates thickening of the medial and lateral rectus muscles.

hypoophthalmia, infraorbital nerve damage, and maxillary sinusitis. Figures 166.4 through 166.11 depict a three-wall decompression in a patient with optic neuropathy and eyelid retraction. Some authors refer to orbital decompression as orbital expansion. (For further information regarding orbital decompression, see the companion to this textbook, the *Atlas of Head and Neck Surgery–Otolaryngology,* Second Edition, Chapter 162, by Scott Manning.)

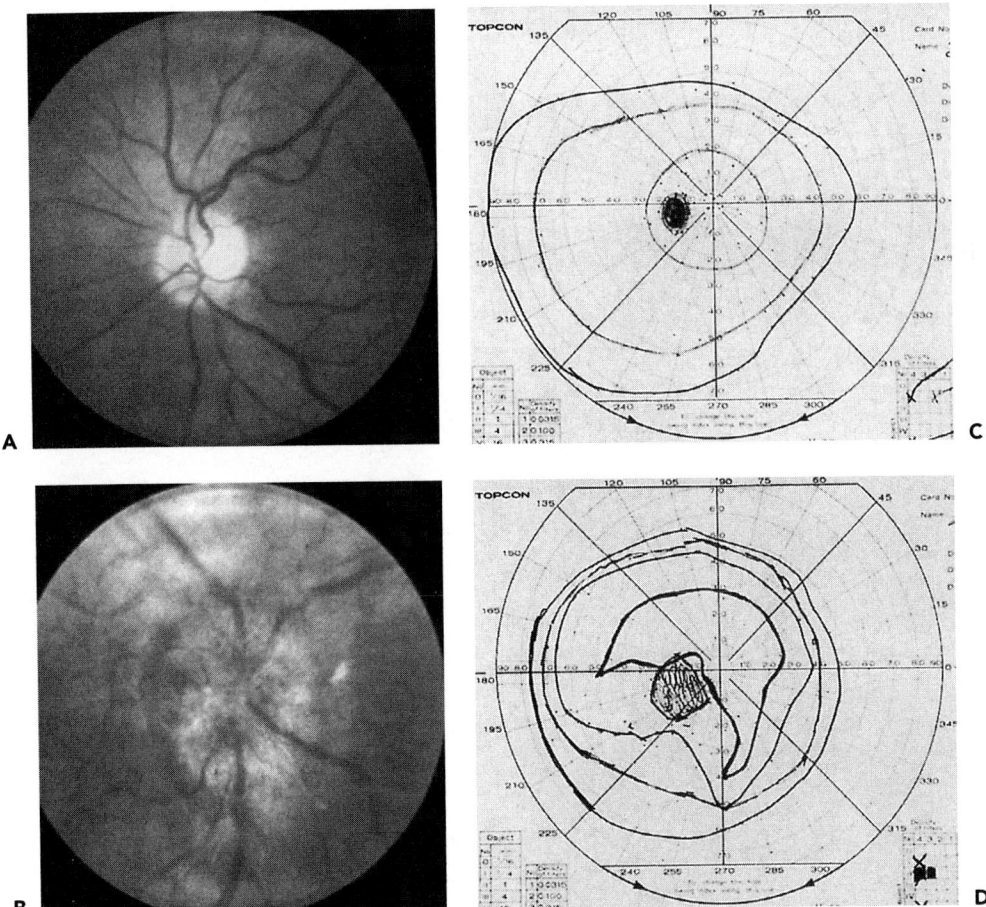

Figure 166.5 **(A, right)** and **(B, left)** fundus photos demonstrate characteristic disk findings in left optic neuropathy. **C** and **D:** Left visual field changes progressed over 1 year, until decompression of the orbit was required.

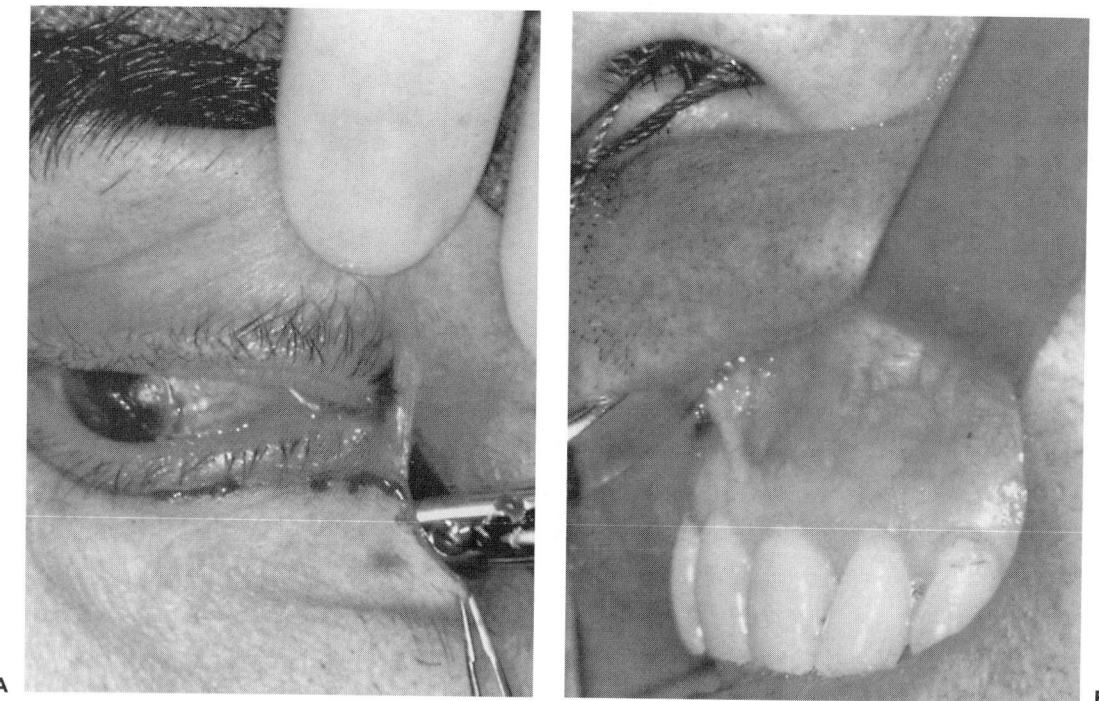

Figure 166.6 A subciliary incision **(A)** and Caldwell-Luc approach **(B)** for inferior orbital decompression.

Medial Orbital Decompression

Medial orbital decompression can be approached through the standard external ethmoidectomy incision or through a coronal forehead approach, which is used to expose the frontal sinus or used in a craniofacial anomaly recon-struction. If the standard ethmoidectomy incision is used, it is best to outline the incision as a "lazy S" or a "gull wing" to prevent web contraction of the resulting scar. The coronal approach should also be considered in cosmetic decompression in female patients and young adults.

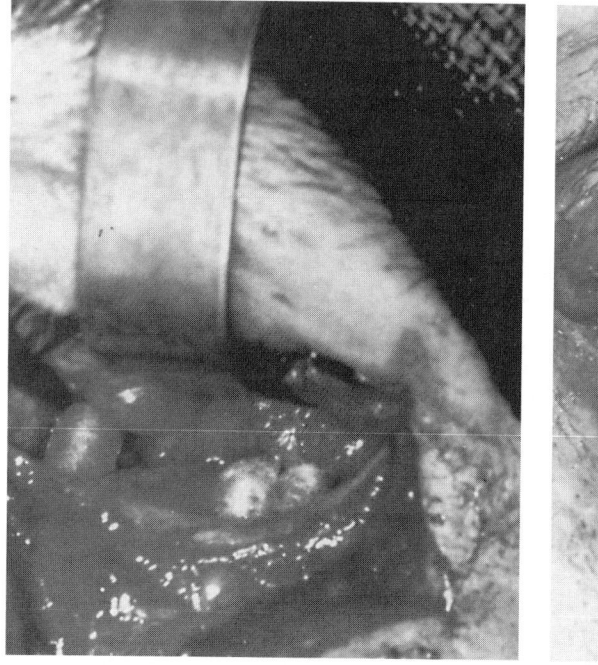
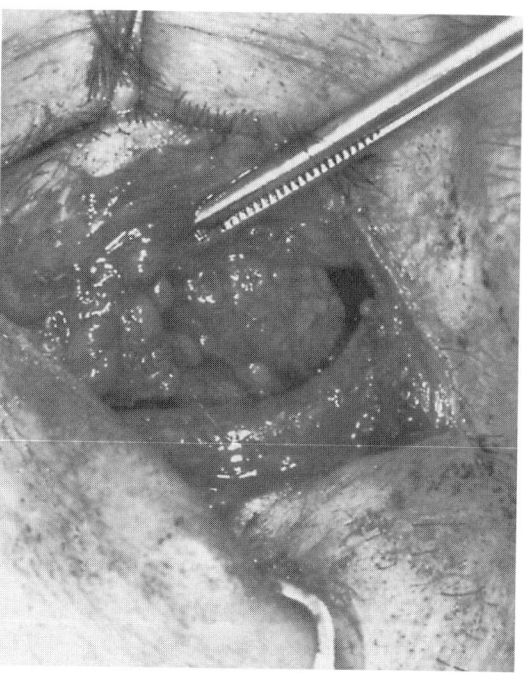

Figure 166.7 **A:** After decompression of the left orbital floor, the cotton swabs protrude into the defects medial and lateral to the infraorbital nerve. **B:** After opening the periosteum, the orbital fat is gently teased into the defects.

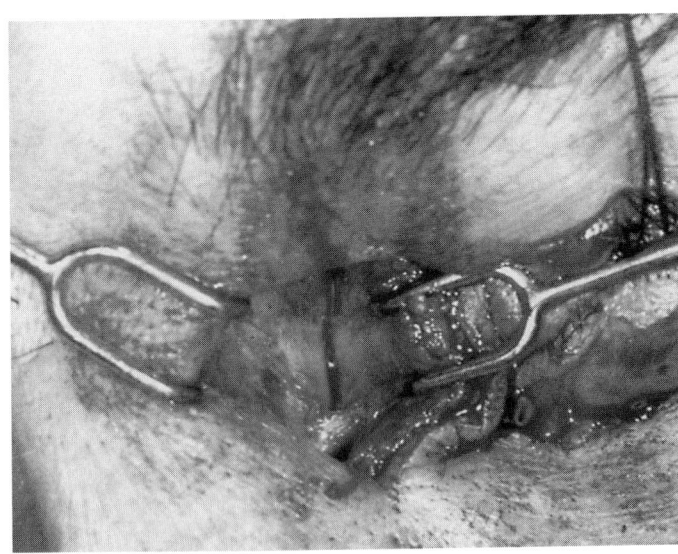 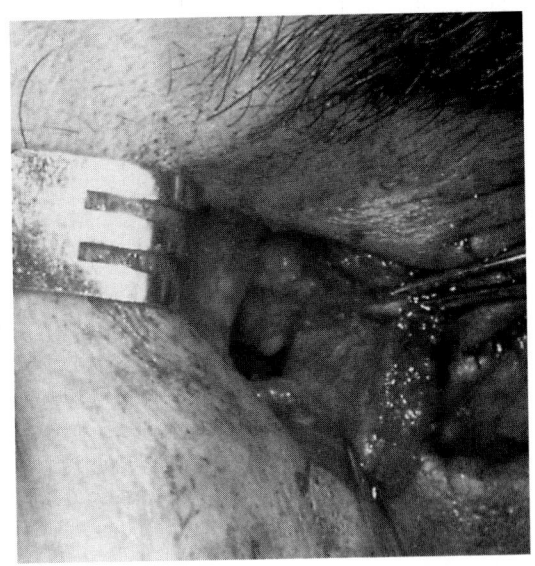

Figure 166.8 A: Standard external ethmoidectomy incision for medial orbital decompression. **B:** After decompression, the orbital fat herniates into the sinus defect.

With the standard ethmoidectomy approach, the medial canthal tendon is displaced laterally by elevating the periosteum over the anterior lacrimal crest. The lacrimal sac is elevated out of its fossa and retracted laterally with a Sewell retractor. The anterior and posterior ethmoid arteries are identified and ligated with small stainless steel vascular clips. The anterior artery is divided for exposure, but the posterior artery is left intact for orientation; the ethmoidectomy is carried posteriorly only to this landmark. The two arteries also serve as a reminder of the superior level of the fovea ethmoidalis and the cribriform plate.

Beginning at the lacrimal fossa, a complete ethmoidectomy is performed, but without the characteristic surgical widening of the middle meatus. All mucosa-bearing septae

are removed to lessen the subsequent risk of mucopyocele formation. The posterior ethmoid cells are exenterated as far back as the posterior ethmoid plate, but care is taken to avoid any injury to the optic nerve in the region of the optic foramen or by excessive traction on the globe and nerve during the decompression. Especially if there is optic neuropathy and even for cosmetic decompression, the optic nerve may be quite fragile.

When the coronal incision is used, the medial canthal tendon is left intact, and the ethmoidectomy is carried out from above. This is a different approach from the one most otolaryngologists use, and care must be taken to remain oriented with respect to the arteries and the fovea. This approach carries the greater potential risk of injury to the lacrimal sac and

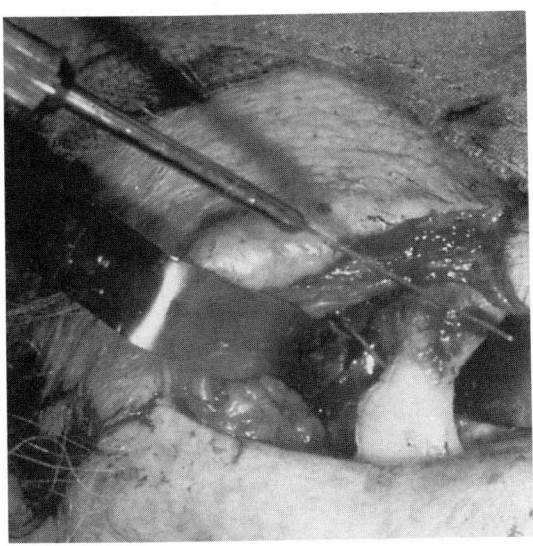 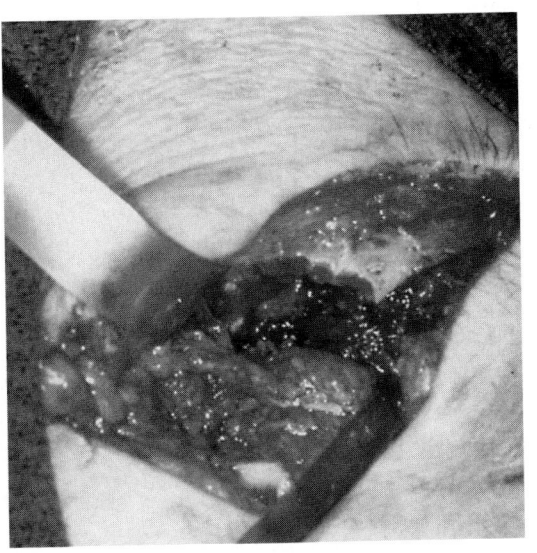

Figure 166.9 A: Right lateral orbitotomy through a curvilinear incision, exposing and removing the lateral orbital rim. **B:** Herniation of the orbital fat through the defect created into the temporal fossa.

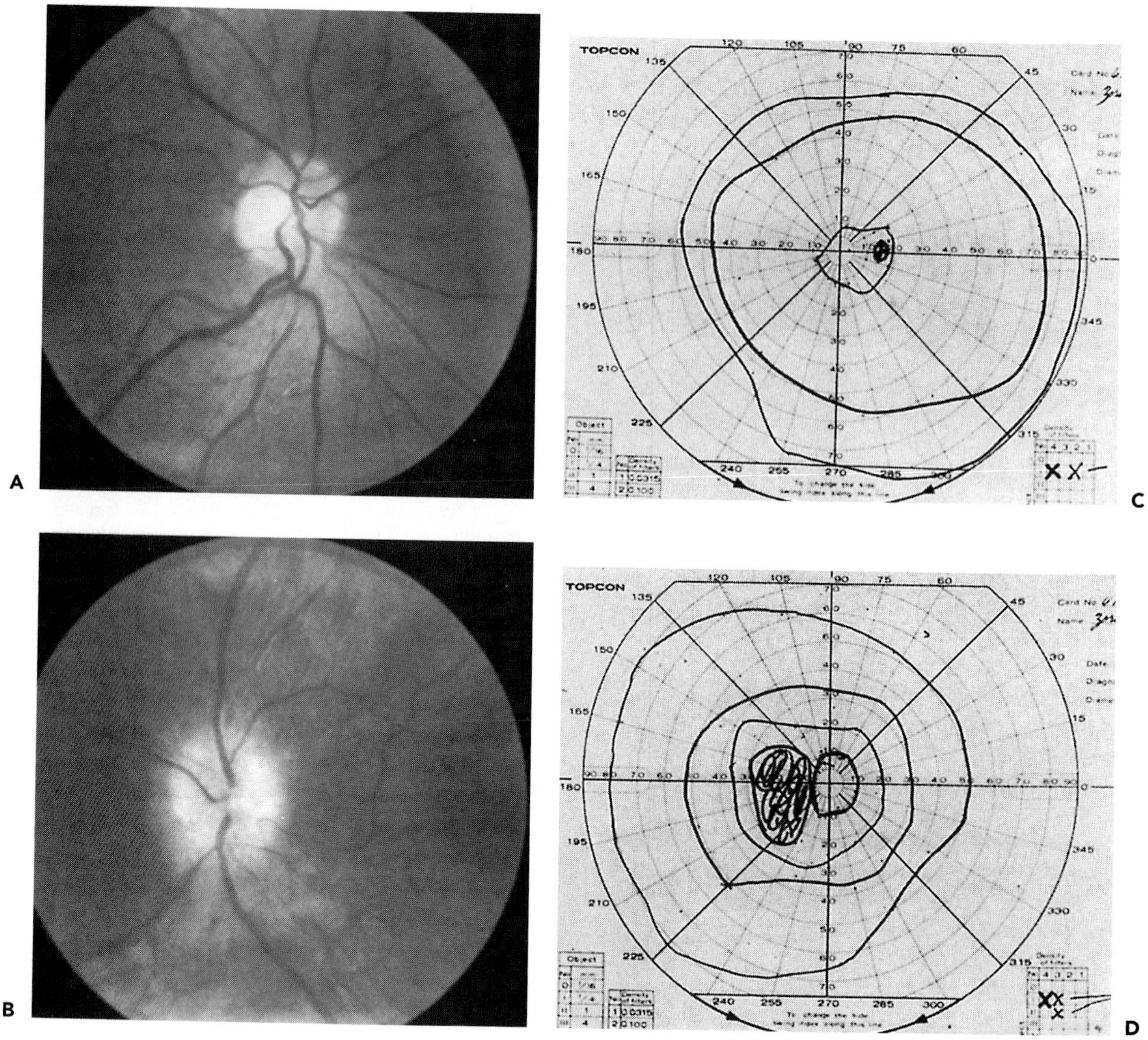

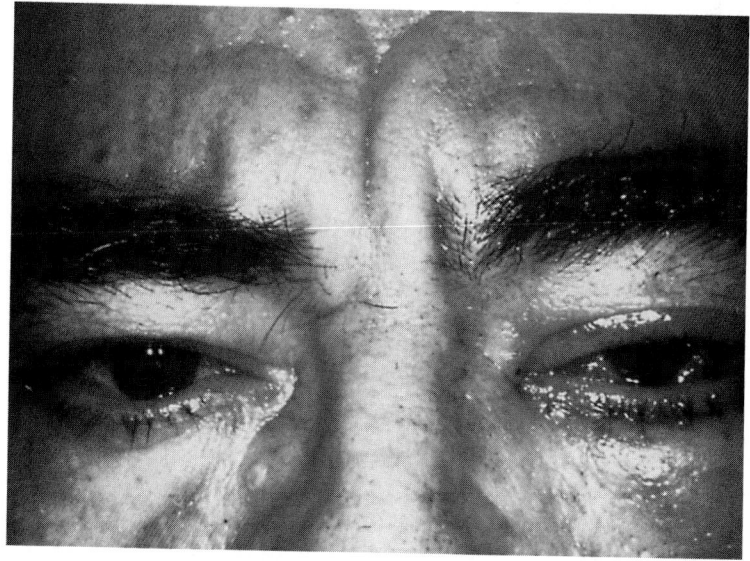

Figure 166.10 **(A, right)** and **(B, left)** fundus photographs show improvement of the swelling of the left optic disk after decompression. **(C, right)** and **(D, left)** visual fields show improvement in the field of vision.

Figure 166.11 Postoperative appearance of the patient after three-wall decompression surgery.

insertion of the trochlea because of the need for wider periosteal undermining to achieve adequate exposure.

After the ethmoidectomy is accomplished, the medial orbital periosteum is incised longitudinally with the axis of the orbit or in an H-shaped outline, allowing the orbital fat to herniate through the keriosteal defect into the ethmoidectomy cavity. The fat may be gently teased out of the orbit with forceps, but care should be taken not to injure the medial rectus muscle or to start any bleeding that might cause a retrobulbar hematoma. The incisions are closed in the standard fashion, usually with Penrose drains for short-term operative site drainage.

Inferior Orbital Decompression

Inferior orbital decompression effectively creates a large orbital floor blow-out fracture but spares injury to the infraorbital nerve. We prefer to approach the orbital floor through a subciliary eyelid incision and a Caldwell-Luc maxillary antrotomy. Although it is feasible to remove the orbital floor from either approach, we believe the combined approach allows safe visualization of the floor through the orbital exposure while removing the bone from the antrotomy. A transconjunctival eyelid excision can be substituted for the subciliary incision, but few head and neck surgeons have experience with this approach.

A skin-muscle flap is elevated in the lower eyelid and the orbital rim visualized. After incising the periosteum over the rim, it is elevated from the orbital floor by approximately 4 cm. After a wide antrostomy is performed by means of the Caldwell-Luc incision, the mucoperiosteum is removed from the roof of the maxillary sinus. The course of the infraorbital nerve is identified, and using a periosteal elevator or small osteotome, the bone medial and lateral to the nerve is carefully fractured. Using Takahashi forceps and a back-biting rongeur placed in the antrostomy, the remainder of the bone of the floor is removed. It is important to remove this bone under direct visualization so that inadvertent injury of the globe, muscles, or optic nerve is avoided.

It is evident when enough bone has been removed from the orbital floor because the thin, easily removable bone becomes thicker and denser as the surgeon reaches the posterior extent of the orbit. In general, a 3-cm anteroposterior range for bone removal is safe. Medially, the bone can be removed to the lacrimal fossa, and laterally it can removed to the thick bone of the zygoma.

After creating as large a defect as possible or necessary, the periorbita is carefully incised longitudinally to allow the orbital fat to herniate into the defect and into the maxillary sinus. This must be done carefully because it is possible to injure the inferior rectus and inferior oblique muscle or even the globe if the surgeon is not cautious. Gentle spreading of the periosteal incisions with a hemostat and teasing of the fat out through these defects can also be performed.

After the decompression, forced duction testing can be performed on the globe to ensure that the muscles of the inferior orbit are not hindered in their action by entrapment from a bony protuberance. The fat herniates into the two defects on either side of the infraorbital nerve, but the nerve courses across the defect and somewhat limits the amount of herniation that can take place.

It is important to provide an adequate drainage or ventilation orifice for the maxillary sinus by enlarging its middle meatal ostium or by creating a new nasal antrostomy. Only light packing, such as a Penrose drain, should be placed in the sinus through the opening into the nose, and the sinus should be irrigated free of blood and debris before closing the Caldwell-Luc incision, to decrease the likelihood of perioperative contamination. The eyelid incision should be closed only with closure of the orbital rim periosteum and the eyelid skin, without any intervening soft-tissue sutures. This can decrease the chance for ectropion formation. As with all decompression procedures associated with the paranasal sinuses, perioperative antibiotic prophylaxis is prudent. Combined antral and ethmoid decompression has been shown to produce over 5 mm of mean reduction of proptosis (7). Using an inferior decompression via a transconjunctival approach alone and a lateral canthotomy for exposure, one might anticipate approximately a 3.5-mm mean reduction. When performed for worsening vision, at least 25% of patients will improve.

Lateral Orbital Decompression

The lateral approach can be made through a variety of incisions, including a coronal direct rim incision or through an extended lateral canthotomy. We prefer the direct lateral orbital incision because it does not alter the shape of the lateral palpebral angle as the lateral canthotomy incision can, nor is it as extensive as the coronal forehead flap, in which injury to the temporal branch of the facial nerve can occur. The direct lateral orbit incision can be made as an extension of the subciliary incision into a smile wrinkle line when the two types of decompression are used concomitantly. The lateral canthotomy incision is used more frequently for a lateral orbitotomy approach to the posterior orbit, for which extensive retraction on the globe may be necessary. The surgeon should be able to visualize the globe; therefore, release of the eyelids with a canthotomy can be advantageous.

After the periosteum over the lateral orbital rim is exposed, it is incised widely directly over the rim. The periosteum is elevated from the orbital side and the infratemporal fossa side of the lateral orbit for approximately 3.0 to 3.5 cm posteriorly.

For acute decompressions in which there is a need for an extensive increase in orbital volume, or if it is not necessary to maintain the continuity of the lateral orbital rim for cosmetic purposes, the lateral rim can be removed by drill, osteotome, or saw and discarded. This facilitates the extensive removal of lateral orbital bone posterior to the rim. In the usual case, however, it is desirable to maintain the continuity of the rim postoperatively; the rim can be cut and mobilized, but with its attachment to the periosteum maintained intact for later replacement into its proper position. With the duckbill rongeurs, as much of the lateral orbital bone as possible can be removed, until the thick bone of the skull base is encountered. An approximately 2.5- to 3.5-cm-diameter circle of bone is removed. Alternatively, the operating drill with mastoid cutting burs and irrigation may be used, but the globe must be protected by a malleable retractor. Prolonged retraction must not be placed on the globe because the intraocular pressure and degree of optic nerve fragility may already be high.

As with the other sites of decompression, the periorbita is incised and the orbital fat gently teased out to protrude into the newly created space. The lateral extension of the orbital fat is limited by the position of the temporalis muscle, and as in maxillary sinus decompression, the fat extrusion is not extensive.

The orbital rim fragment, still attached to the periosteum, can be replaced and wired into position. Alternatively, microplates can be used for fixation, but in our experience, they are more symptomatic for the patient in the late postoperative course. The wound can be drained with a Penrose drain brought out through the incision.

Endoscopic Intranasal Decompression

Introduced by Kennedy et al. in 1990, endoscopic medial orbital decompression has now emerged as a viable, minimally invasive option in the treatment of thyroid ophthalmopathy (8). This technique can potentially reduce morbidity by obviating the need for cutaneous or gingival incisions, eliminating the dysaesthesia associated with nerve trauma (which may occur with external ethmoidectomies/Caldwell-Luc approaches) and avoid the discomfort associated with packing in Caldwell-Luc patients. In many cases, a lateral orbital decompression is also performed to augment the volumetric expansion of the orbit, which will be addressed in a separate section of this chapter.

When evaluating patients for possible endoscopic decompression, close attention to the clinical and radiographic assessment is necessary to determine the ultimate appropriateness of this approach for a given patient (9,10). Important features to note include any history of facial trauma, previous sinus disease, or sinus surgery. Likewise, a history of complications arising from sinus disease, such as orbital abscesses, are particularly pertinent. If the patient is atopic, determining which season is less problematic can be helpful in determining the best time to consider scheduling the patient's surgery (11,12). Review also the ophthalmologist's report and determine the urgency of the surgery. Patients with histories of corneal ulceration, severe exposure keratitis refractory to treatment, or optic nerve compromise may necessitate an emergent surgery; others

may be less urgent. Closely review the past medical and surgical history of the patient. Particularly pertinent are histories of any medications that may be associated with increased bleeding. Such medications are appropriately withheld during the entire perioperative period. Extremely rarely does one perform decompressions under local or monitored anesthesia care (MAC) anesthesia; however, any history of claustrophobia, back pain, or back surgery in the patient will result in a recommendation of a general anesthetic to the patient.

During patient examination, assess the degree of eye discomfort. Evaluate for clinical indicators of dacrocystitis and sinus pathology. On nasal endoscopy, examine the nasal anatomy, including the anatomy of the septum and lateral nasal wall. Occasionally, severely deviated septal deflections may require correction at the time of decompression, but this has been rare in our experience. If nasal polyps or mucopurulence is present, this will need to be addressed, and perhaps resolved, prior to performing the endoscopic decompression surgery. On occasion, it is possible to perform endoscopic sinus surgery for sinus disease simultaneously with endoscopic orbital decompression surgery, but generally one should be prepared to separate the two procedures. In those cases where it is elected to treat both simultaneously, one should be very selective, aggressively treat preoperatively with antibiotics, and inform the patient that you may choose to abort the orbital decompression if active persistent infection is encountered. Once the active sinus disease has been addressed, then can the decompression stage of the procedure be performed.

Close evaluation of the sinus CT, in both the axial and coronal planes is critical. When reviewing the radiographic studies, not only assess for evidence of sinus pathology, but also examine closely the relationship of the lamina papyracea to the uncinate anteriorly; its thickness, particularly as it transitions to the floor of the orbit; the presence of Haller cells; and the thickness of the posterior aspect of the nasolacrimal duct, which potentially might be injured with anterior expansion of the maxillary sinus antrostomy. Superiorly, evaluate closely for evidence of potential "hazards" in the fovea ethmoidalis, which may take the form of dehiscences, thick ethmoid partitions intersecting with thin roof sections (thus promoting fractures in the skull base with forceful removal of bone from the cavity). Posteriorly, inspect the CT closely for evidence of extensive pneumatization of the ethmoids adjacent to the optic nerve (also known as Onodi cells), the relationship of the ethmoids to the sphenoid and again the thickness of the lamina, particularly at the junction of the posterior ethmoids and sphenoid, where the optic nerve comes into close approximation.

When scheduling the surgery, it is wise to offer to perform bilateral surgery when indicated and consistent with the patient's desires. If staged, one should first select the side most severely affected.

On the day of surgery, the patient is positioned and prepped as typical for endoscopic sinus surgery with the exception of the addition of tarsorrhaphy stitches or clear corneal protectors to be placed for additional eye protection. Occasionally, image guidance is employed and can be helpful—but is not routinely required. Meticulous nasal injections are placed prior to prepping the patient, as is our tradition with all endoscopic sinus surgery, to allow adequate time for the vasoconstrictor properties to take effect. The uncinate is then removed, generally using a ball tip probe to elevate and a back biter or microdebrider to excise. If the preoperative scans reveal the uncinate to be parodoxically bent and in close approximation to a thin lamina papyracea, our preference is to us the backbiter to avoid inadvertent periorbital violation. One then performs a total ethmoidectomy and meticulously removes all partitions, to completely expose the lamina papyracea. Once completely exposed, the lamina can be gently fractured with a frier or caudal elevator and teased free of the periorbita without violation of the periorbita. Oftentimes this becomes more difficult anteriorly as you encounter the lacrimal bone, which can be predicted by your preoperative evaluation of the CT scans in this area. Occasionally, the backbiter may be necessary to remove the posterior portion of the lacrimal bone. Again, care should be exercised so as not to inadvertently injure the lacrimal apparatus. Review of the CT in this area will allow the surgeon to anticipate the thickness of the bone surrounding the lacrimal duct. If bleeding is encountered during this portion of the procedure, simple placement of cottonoids saturated with a vasoconstrictor into the cavity for a few minutes generally suffices to secure a very dry surgical field, which is paramount for the next step. Once the periorbita is sufficiently exposed and the field is dry, the periorbita is incised. Although theoretically it makes sense to open the periorbita from posterior to anterior to prevent the herniation of orbital fat prematurely into the field, practically it is less of a problem than anticipated. Indeed, many surgeons often now use a Bellucci scissor to "nick" the periorbita anteriorly, then place one blade of the scissor inside the periorbita, the other outside the periorbita and then cut posteriorly. Care is taken not to injure the medial rectus, which may be in close proximity to the periorbita. The most anterior extreme of the cut in the periorbita is sometimes the more difficult. Here a sickle knife or small miniscetomy knife can be useful. The surgeon can also extend the periorbita incisions superiorly and inferiorly to promote herniation of the orbital fat. To encourage herniation, gently massage the globe while simultaneously teasing out the orbital fat with a ball-tip probe. Initially there was a concern that this may be made more difficult in patients having received previous orbital irradiation, but this has not been the case. Once complete, recheck the maxillary antrostomy, which generally has previously been slightly enlarged anteriorly and inferiorly, to ensure that it will not become obstructed by the herniated orbital fat. A gelfilm stent is then placed into the antrostomy and a small amount of bactroban ointment into the cavity.

Postoperative management includes the standard instructions for endoscopic sinus surgery, with a particular stressing of the instruction for the patient not to blow the nose and to sneeze with the mouth open, to prevent air entering into the orbit.

Although, theoretically, the risks of CSF leak, retrobulbar hemorrhage, dacrocystitis, secondary sinusitis, orbital cellulites, and rectus muscle injury all exist, thus far we have not experienced any such events. Although the patients do experience considerable discomfort with some of the lateral orbital decompression procedures, they experience minimal to no discomfort from the endoscopic components. The average reduction in proptosis generally will range from 2 mm to slightly less than 4 mm.

Other Interventional Treatment

High-dose (80 to 120 mg) daily prednisone for 14 days is recommended for decreasing visual acuity or constructing visual fields initially. If the steroid therapy fails to improve the vision or high doses are required to maintain vision, the patient must be considered a candidate for decompression. Cytotoxic and immunosuppressive drugs like cyclophosphamide and cyclosporine have been used experimentally to alter the autoimmune aspect of the disease, but the side effects and complications of these drugs are high, and long-term efficacy in a large study group has not been seen. Therefore, their use is not considered standard treatment. Plasmapheresis has been attempted but was successful only when combined with high-dose steroid therapy.

External beam radiation therapy has its proponents for use in dysthyroid exophthalmos. It is not likely to be successful in acute or subacute cases of visual loss because of the inherent edema that occurs in the early days of radiation therapy, which can worsen the orbital problem. However, for the late sequelae of stable dysthyroid ophthalmopathy, it may be considered as a reasonable alternative to surgery, although its results are usually not as dramatic. Usually 200 cGy of fractionated photon radiation is administered over 2 weeks. For most treated patients, the condition responds favorably by stabilizing or improving, but rarely does the exophthalmos resolve. The patients who undergo radiation therapy should be chosen carefully because if they also require surgical decompression, the intraorbital scarring and increased vascularity from the irradiation can make the surgery more difficult and increase the risk of complications.

Treatment Decisions

Table 166.2 depicts the treatment options for dysthyroid exophthalmos. Nonsurgical treatment is initiated usually by the endocrinologist, internist, and ophthalmologist as they attempt to improve deteriorating visual acuity or constricting visual fields. The otolaryngologist–head and neck surgeon is consulted for functional surgical decompression if the medical therapy does not resolve the loss of vision or if the ophthalmopathy becomes stable and cosmetic decompression is indicated. For mild (i.e., 2 to 3 mm) exophthalmos, any of the three decompression approaches may be

TABLE 166.2	
TREATMENT: DYSTHYROID EXOPHTHALMOS	
Therapy	**Indications**
Nonsurgical treatment	
High-dose steroids	Rapid visual deterioration
Immunosuppressive agents (cyclophosphamide, cyclosporine)	Experimental
Radiation therapy (200 cGy)	Slowly progressive visual loss
Surgical treatment	
Medial decompression	Mild exophthalmos (2–3 mm)
Lateral decompression	Mild exophthalmos
Inferior decompression	Mild to moderate exophthalmos
Superior decompression	Congenital orbitopathy
Two-wall decompression	Moderate exophthalmos (3–5 mm)
Three-wall decompression	Severe exophthalmos (5–7 mm)
Endoscopic medial decompression	Only by experienced endoscopist
Eyelid retraction surgery	Widened palpebral fissure and exposure
Strabismus surgery	Diplopia

used, and factors such as postoperative scars, preexisting sinus disease, and desires of the patient should be taken into consideration. We believe that for moderate exophthalmos, the inferior decompression alone may be sufficient, and the cosmesis of the subciliary incision is excellent, although a combination of two walls for decompression (i.e., medial and lateral) can also suffice. For severe exophthalmos (i.e., 5 to 7 mm), a three-wall decompression is indicated. The maximal improvement in proptosis from this combined surgery is about 5 to 7 mm.

After healing and stabilization of the orbital decompression procedure(s), additional surgery for retraction of the eyelids may be performed (4). For slight upper eyelid retraction, resection of Müller muscle can help. For greater retraction, insertion of Gore-Tex grafts, fascia, banked sclera, or cartilage can lengthen the eyelids after transecting the eyelid retractors. After orbital decompression and eyelid retraction procedures are performed, strabismus surgery for residual diplopia can be planned. These surgeries are best performed by or in conjunction with an ophthalmologist experienced in oculoplastic surgery. Strabismus surgery is usually performed after the globes have settled into their new positions postoperatively and after the lid retractors have been cut and the eyelids lengthened.

COMPLICATIONS

Untreated disease, medical treatment, and surgery for dysthyroid ophthalmopathy have associated complications. If the disease is allowed to progress unchecked, some patients develop progressive optic neuropathy, which can cause blindness. Others develop only the widely retracted eyelids, stiffness of the orbital tissues, and exophthalmos. If there is significant eyelid retraction and exophthalmos, exposure of the cornea, ulcerations, and subsequent endophthalmitis

can occur, and the globe can be lost to infection. Many patients have only a mild form of the disease, but others develop various degrees of diplopia. It is the preservation of sight and function to which the treatment is directed (13).

The major complication of medical management is the failure to recognize when it is not sufficient treatment and to delay surgery. The decision to decompress the orbit may be postponed while medical therapy is used, but vision may continue to deteriorate while on steroids. If the steroids are used too long, the patient can become steroid dependent and require a tapered release from the medication. Other complications from steroids include gastric ulcer and perforation, irritable personality, failure to heal wounds well, and reactivation of previously dormant infections. If cyclophosphamide or cyclosporine is used, serious suppression of the immune system can occur, and the complications can be worse than the disease being treated. Radiation therapy with inadequate protective shielding can cause cataracts, pituitary suppression, and optic fibrosis. If surgery is performed after irradiation, more bleeding and scar tissue can be encountered, and the increased stiffness of the orbit can diminish the outcome of decompression.

The function and cosmesis of approximately 75% of patients stabilize or improve after surgical decompression of the dysthyroid orbit. Some degree of diplopia may be experienced by as many as 50% of these patients preoperatively and postoperatively, but this incidence can be decreased somewhat by early recognition of the progressive orbital disease and careful decompression (11). Postoperative muscle imbalance may be significantly reduced by complete removal of the inferior periorbita, which precludes the formation of fibrotic bonds with the extraocular muscles. It is also likely that taking great care in teasing the orbital fat into the decompressed area can help to lessen this possibility.

Corneal abrasion after decompression surgery can occur because the cornea is not protected with a corneal shield

TABLE 166.3   COMPLICATIONS
ORBITAL DECOMPRESSION

Complication	Prevention	Treatment
Corneal abrasion	Scleral protector, Frost suture, lubrication	Topical antibiotics, patch or shield eye
Optic nerve compromise	Gentle and short retraction	Canthotomy and release of pressure
Retrobulbar hematoma	Careful periorbita incisions and separation, no aspirin before surgery	Bipolar cautery, evacuation of hematoma, globe massage, diuretics
Muscle injury	Careful spreading of tissue, awareness of anatomy	Strabismus surgery
Ectropion	One-layer closure of eyelid (skin only)	Massage, release of scar tissue, possible skin graft
Infection	Perioperative antibiotics, prophylaxis during upper respiratory infection	Antibiotics
Infraorbital nerve injury	Careful removal of adjacent bone, gentle retraction	Time, steroid injection, neurolysis if dysesthetic
Retinal vascular occlusion	Careful selection of surgical candidates, gentle retraction	Ophthalmologic consultation is needed

during surgery or by using a Frost suture through the lower eyelid, with closure of the lower eyelid over the cornea during surgery. If the eyelids are too stiff and retracted, a scleral shield and frequent irrigations of balanced salt solution should be helpful in preventing an ulcer. However, it is important to visualize the pupil periodically during the decompression with whatever corneal protective technique is used because excessive traction on the globe and optic nerve is heralded by a dilating pupil. Additional injury to an already compromised optic nerve can occur from retracting the globe too long and too hard during the decompression procedures. The eyeball must be retracted for only short periods and then allowed to "breathe" to reduce the stresses on the vasculature and intraocular pressure. Failure to do so could result in a blind eye. Retrobulbar hematoma formation from bleeding in the fat pad after incising the periorbita and teasing out the fat can also cause blindness. It is important to irrigate the wound after the decompression and to identify and cauterize any bleeding in the adipose tissues, taking great care not to cauterize too close to a muscle or the optic nerve. Bipolar cautery is preferred because its current is not carried into the tissues adjacent to the optic nerve.

Injury to the infraorbital nerve during the inferior decompression procedure is not uncommon, and at least temporary neuropraxia occurs in most cases. The patient should be apprised preoperatively of the risk of nerve injury, including neuroma formation and dysesthesia. Postoperative steroid injections may improve a dysthetic nerve, but only time can improve neurapraxia. Ectropion after a lower eyelid subciliary incision is usually transient and responds to time and gentle massage. If it worsens with time, it is probably due to an injudicious closure of the tarsal plate to the deeper soft tissues or periosteum, and it requires release, perhaps when the eyelid retraction surgery is performed.

Retinal hemorrhage is observed rarely after decompression, and it occurs almost exclusively in diabetic patients. With extensive decompression into the ethmoid and maxillary sinuses, there is a chance for an orbital cellulitis or abscess if significant sinusitis occurs and involves the relatively unprotected orbital tissues. Early use of antibiotics for purulent rhinorrhea appears to be justified to prevent this complication. Orbital infection can especially be a risk in a patient with a history of recurrent sinusitis or sinus disease. Table 166.3 summarizes the potential complications and their prevention or treatment.

EMERGENCIES

Retrobulbar hematoma, retinal vascular occlusion, and corneal ulcer are the major sight-threatening emergencies associated with orbital decompression procedures.

Postoperative retrobulbar hematoma is treated by opening the skin incisions in the emergency or operating room, evacuating the hematoma, irrigating clots in the wound, bipolar cauterization of bleeding vessels, and adequate drainage of the wound.

Retinal vascular occlusion and corneal ulcer are serious vision-threatening conditions and should be managed on an emergent basis by the patient's ophthalmologist, although no delay in receiving care should be allowed. Retinal vascular occlusion is usually related to increased intraocular pressure, which is due to edema of the orbit, excessive retraction, or retrobulbar hematoma. It cannot always be reversed by the ophthalmologist, and despite heroic efforts, blindness can result. The patient should be cautioned after discharge from the hospital to seek immediate care for increasing pain in the eye or for decreasing vision.

Although most emergencies occur while the patient is still hospitalized, later incidents are possible, especially with corneal ulcer caused by exposure. Late complications should be anticipated, and the patient should be discharged with the appropriate lubricants, artificial tears, and instructions on taping the eye shut if necessary. Remind the patient that prevention is easier than treating an emergency.

HIGHLIGHTS

- Dysthyroid ophthalmopathy occurs to some degree in approximately 50% of patients with Graves disease.
- About 5% of patients with Graves disease develop a vision-threatening orbital process that requires medical or surgical management.
- Enlargement of the extraocular muscles, edema of the orbital soft tissues, and retraction of the eyelids lead to the common appearance of exophthalmos in dysthyroid disease.
- Optic neuropathy, leading to decreasing visual acuity and constrictive visual fields, and exposure keratitis are the most common reasons for urgent medical or surgical care.
- Acute visual loss is best treated initially by administering 80 to 120 mg of prednisone daily for 14 days.
- If steroid therapy does not improve the vision or is required for more than 2 weeks to maintain vision, surgical decompression is indicated.
- Surgical therapy for cosmetic improvement of exophthalmos and eyelid retraction includes, in sequence, orbital decompression, release of eyelid retraction, insertion of filler grafts, and strabismus surgery.
- Mild exophthalmos can be improved by medial, inferior, or lateral decompression; moderate exophthalmos by medial and inferior or inferior and lateral; and severe exophthalmos by medial, inferior, and lateral decompressions. Superior decompression is rarely used.
- Postoperative complications include retinal vascular occlusion, blindness, diplopia, failure to adequately correct the exophthalmos, retrobulbar hematoma, corneal ulceration, and infraorbital nerve hyperesthesia.
- The emergencies of vascular occlusion and corneal ulceration are best managed by an ophthalmologist.
- In lieu of or in addition to orbital decompression, fat excision can be performed to reduce soft-tissue crowding. Levator lengthening can be performed at the same time.
- Endoscopic ethmoid and medial orbital floor removal can be accomplished safely if careful attention is paid to protecting the ethmoid arteries, the lacrimal sac, and the medial rectus muscles.

REFERENCES

1. Scott IH, Siatkowski MR. Thyroid eye disease. *Semin Otolaryngol* 1999;14:52–61.
2. Ohnishi T, Noguchi S, Murakami N, et al. Extraocular muscles in Graves' ophthalmopathy: usefulness of T2 relaxation time measurements. *Radiology* 1994;190:857–862.
3. Morax S, Hurbli T. Choice of surgical treatment for Graves' disease. *J Craniomaxillofac Surg* 1987;15:174.
4. Lyons CJ, Rootman J. Orbital decompression for disfiguring exophthalmos in thyroid orbitopathy. *Ophthalmology* 1994;101:223–230.
5. Mourits MP, Koornneef L, Wiersinga WM, et al. Orbital decompression for Graves' ophthalmopathy by inferomedial, by inferomedial plus lateral, and by coronal approach. *Ophthalmology* 1990;97:636.
6. Wilson WB, Manke WF. Orbital decompression in Graves' disease: the predictability of reduction of proptosis. *Arch Ophthalmol* 1991;109:343.
7. Weisman RA, Osguthorpe JD. Orbital decompression in Graves' disease. *Arch Otolaryngol Head Neck Surg* 1994;120:831–834.
8. Kennedy DW, Goodstein ML, Miller NR, et al. Endoscopic transnasal orbital decompression. *Arch Otolaryngol Head Neck Surg* 1990;116:275.
9. Asaria RH, Koay B, Elston JS, et al. Endoscopic orbital decompression for thyroid eye disease. *Eye* 1998;12(Pt 6):990–995.
10. Metson R, Dollow RL, Shore JW. Endoscopic orbital decompression. *Laryngoscope* 1994;104:950–957.
11. Trokel S, Kazim M, Moore S. Orbital fat removal: decompression for Graves' orbitopathy. *Ophthalmology* 1993;100:674–682.
12. Adenis JP, Robert PY, Lasudry JG, et al. Treatment of proptosis with fat removal orbital decompression in Graves' ophthalmopathy. *Eur J Ophthalmol* 1998;8:246–252.
13. Ulualp SO, Massaro BM, Toohill RJ. Course of proptosis in patients with Graves' disease after endoscopic orbital decompression. *Laryngoscope* 1999;109:1217–1222.

Facial Reanimation

167

Steve Parnes   *Rami Batniji*

The facial nerve is responsible for emotional and voluntary facial expression, protection of the eye, lacrimation, oral competence, salivation, taste, and sensation. The patient presenting with facial paralysis has suffered an event that is devastating both cosmetically and functionally. Although numerous reanimation techniques have been developed to rectify this problem, it is imperative that the surgeon embarks upon extensive preoperative counseling with regard to realistic expectations with the patient prior to intervention.

Reanimation of the paralyzed face falls into two categories: dynamic and static techniques. Dynamic techniques include primary facial grafting, cable nerve grafts, crossed nerve anastomoses, and regional or microneurovascular free flaps. Static reanimation techniques include rhytidectomy, brow lift, and facial suspension using a variety of materials as slings, such as fascia lata, polytetrafluoroethylene, acellular dermal allograft, or a multivectored suture suspension technique (1). The cause of the facial paralysis, type of injury and its location, and the anticipated duration of paralysis contribute to the selection of the appropriate reanimation method.

ANATOMY

To perform reanimation procedures, the surgeon must have a thorough knowledge of the anatomy of the facial nerve. It originates within the pons and then exits between the olive and the inferior cerebellar peduncle. There, it forms the 12- to 14-mm intracranial portion within the cerebellopontine angle (Fig. 167.1). The facial nerve then enters the temporal bone, where it is confined within a bony conduit. As it enters the internal meatus, the facial nerve lies medial to the eighth cranial nerve. Within 10 mm, it reaches the lateral end of the meatus superior to the crista transversalis and anterior to the vertical crista (Bill bar). As it exits the internal auditory canal, the nerve curves gradually in an anterior direction around the basal turn of the cochlea; it then enters the intratemporal portion for 2 to 4 mm (the narrowest portion). At the geniculate ganglion, the greater superficial petrosal nerve leaves anteriorly, whereas the nerve itself makes a 40- to 80-degree turn (the external or first genu) and courses posteriorly and slightly inferiorly 11 mm across the tympanic cavity. This horizontal course lies superior to the fossula at the vestibular fenestra (oval window). As it leaves the oval window niche, the facial nerve makes the second genu, passing anteriorly and caudal to the lateral semicircular canal. It then passes lateral to the sinus tympani and stapedius muscle to form the vertical (mastoid) portion within the temporal bone. At the end of this 13-mm segment, it exits from the stylomastoid foramen, where it becomes the extracranial segment, first innervating the posterior belly of the digastric muscle and then, at 15 to 20 mm, entering the parotid gland. There is divides at the pes anserinus into its two main branches, the temporofacial and cervicofacial branches. Terminal ramifications of these branches to the temporal, zygomatic, buccal, mandibular, and cervical regions are variable (Fig. 167.2). The nerve fibers travel in groups of fascicles (which vary according to level) surrounded by three types of connective tissue: endoneurium, perineurium, and epineurium. The structure of the fascicles varies considerably throughout the course of the nerve; for this reason, direct repair of the fascicles is not feasible and may even be counterproductive (2).

GENERAL CONSIDERATIONS

Prior to surgical intervention, it is important to elucidate both the etiology and the anticipated duration of the facial paralysis. For example, those patients with facial paralysis with anticipated spontaneous recovery should be observed rather than operated on. Furthermore, the prognosis of the patient may also dictate the method of reanimation; those patients with a limited life expectancy may benefit from an immediate but less cosmetically acceptable result.

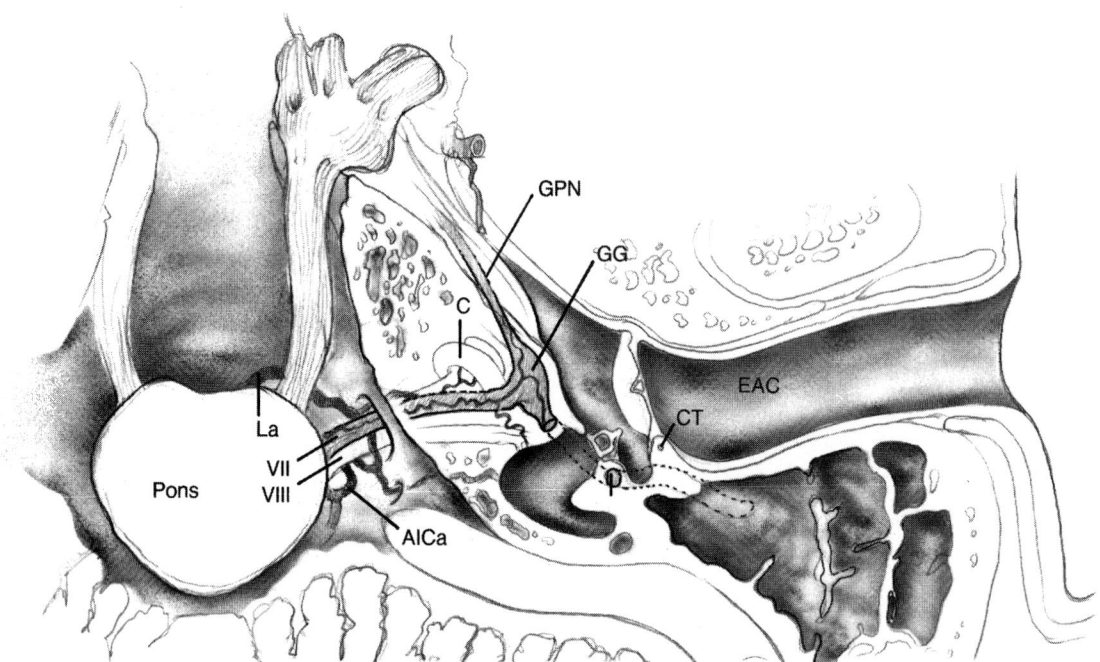

Figure 167.1 Superior view of the intracranial, meatal, labyrinthine, and tympanic segments of the facial nerve. *AICa*, anterior inferior cerebellar artery; *C*, cochlea; *CT*, chorda tympani; *EAC*, external auditory canal; *GG*, geniculate ganglion; *GPN*, greater petrossal nerve; *La*, labyrinthine artery.

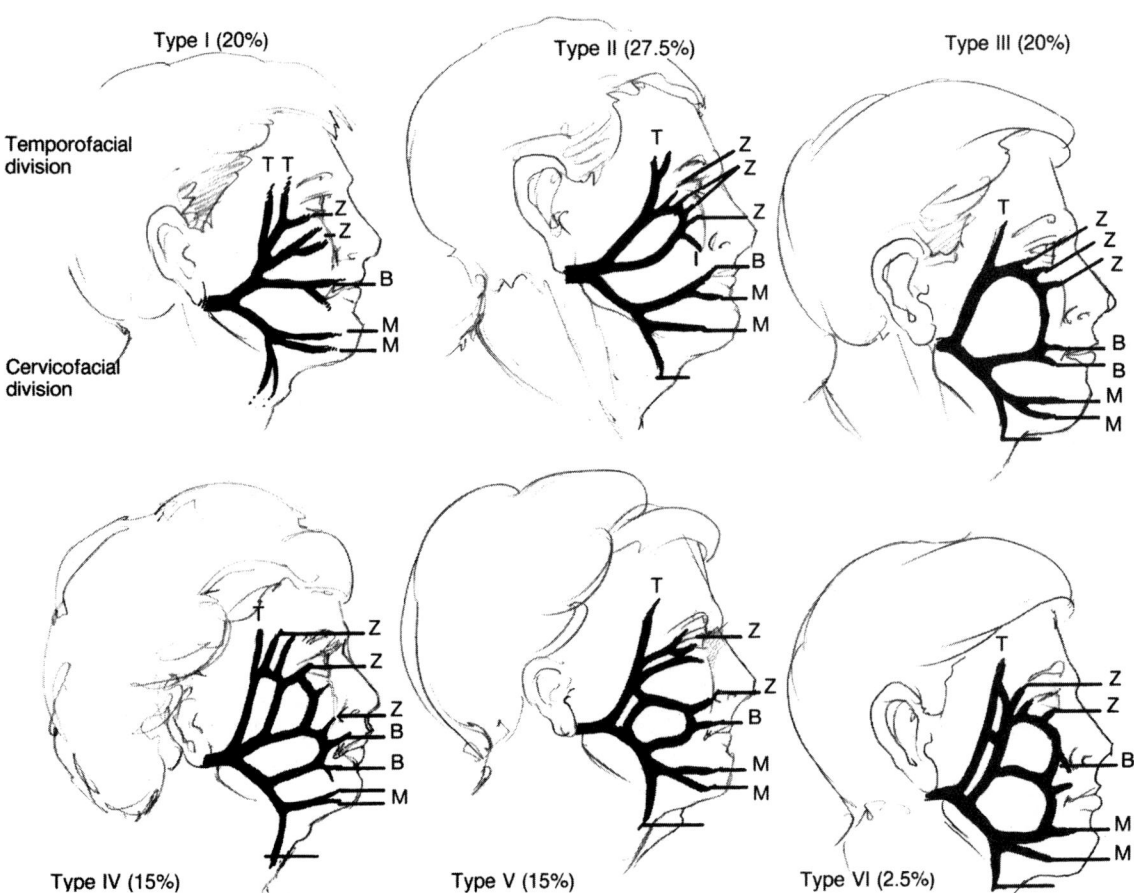

Figure 167.2 Terminal branches of the facial nerve, demonstrating its variability. *B*, buccal; *M*, mandibular; *T*, temporal; *Z*, zygomatic.

Ophthalmologic consequences of facial paralysis include exposure keratitis and corneal ulceration, leading to decreasing visual acuity and blindness. Treatment of the paralytic eye begins with regular ocular lubrication with artificial tear drops 5 to 10 times daily and ophthalmic ointment nightly. Other adjunctive measures include taping or a moisture chamber; both techniques should be used in conjunction with drops and ointment.

While there are many modes of physical therapy rehabilitation for patients with facial paralysis, the most promising technique is facial neuromuscular reeducation using surface electromyography (3). In addition, steroid therapy coupled with antiviral therapy has shown benefit in patients with facial paralysis secondary to Bell palsy (4).

The duration of facial paralysis determines the choices of technique, because the neural techniques depend heavily on the survival of the motor endplates. These techniques are not used after paralysis has been present for 3 or more years. If there is any doubt whether the integrity of the facial nerve is disrupted, a waiting period of at least 12 months should elapse before attempting surgical interruption that may result in irreversible damage to the facial nerve (5). An electronystagmogram (ENG) to detect motor unit potentials or a muscle biopsy to demonstrate viable motor endplates may also be utilized.

TECHNIQUES

Facial Nerve Anastomosis

When the facial nerve has been disrupted, usually because of trauma, benign tumors, or an iatrogenic condition, it is important to reapproximate the nerve without tension. Therefore, it may be necessary to reroute the nerve within the temporal bone or release it in the area of the parotid gland to afford additional length. Barrs reviewed the literature regarding the optimal time for facial nerve anastomosis and concluded that the best results are attained with early repair (6). Wallerian degeneration takes approximately 3 days to manifest; therefore, the surgeon can stimulate the distal end of the nerve for assistance in identification prior to the development of degeneration. If this is impossible, as in cases of massive trauma when the patient is unstable, then within 30 days is acceptable. During this time, there is maximum axoplasmic flow, particularly within the 3- to 4-week period, so that the nerve has the best physiologic opportunity to regenerate.

The surgeon should use magnification with either loupes or microscope. The nerve endings are freshened, and then sutures of 8-0 nylon or smaller are applied, with two of three sutures applied to the epineurium (Fig. 167.3). If the injury occurs in the temporal bone, sutures are unnecessary; rather, placing the ends in contact is satisfactory (Fig. 167.4). Fibrin glue and other tissue adhesives appear to offer no benefit; trophic factors and polyglycolic acid conduits have shown equivocal results (7).

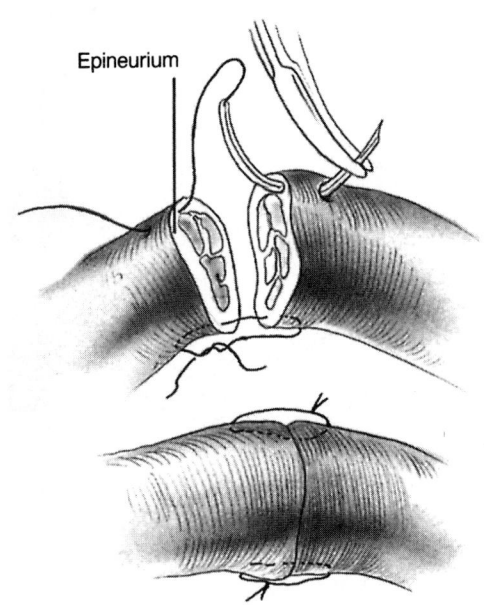

Figure 167.3 Direct facial-facial anastomosis using two 8-0 nylon sutures through the epineurium.

Some authors have advocated a perineural repair; however, it has been shown that spatial orientation is not maintained throughout the nerve, and, therefore, this technique has been abandoned in favor of an epineural repair (8).

A nerve injury involving one of the major branches should be repaired in similar fashion. As a rule of thumb, however, if a plumb line is dropped from the lateral canthus and the injury is distal to this line, it is usually unnecessary to repair the injury. Spontaneous recovery will generally occur without surgical intervention (Fig. 167.5) (9).

Facial Nerve Repair with Grafts

Interposition facial nerve grafting is used when the proximal and distal ends of the nerve cannot be coapted without tension. If less than 10 cm is required, then the greater auricular nerve serves as an excellent graft. It is easily identified by the following technique: draw an imaginary line between the mastoid tip and angle of the mandible; the nerve usually bisects this distance perpendicular to the line, lying on the superficial surface of the sternocleidomastoid muscle (Fig. 167.6). If more length is required, the sural cutaneous nerve can be harvested by making an incision on the lateral aspect of the leg. The nerve is 1 to 2 cm lateral to the saphenous vein, medial and posterior to the lateral malleous of the ankle (Fig. 167.7). According to the method of Fisch and Lanser, two branches are used: one to the upper and one to the lower branch of the facial nerve. Furthermore, they recommend clipping the branches of the digastric muscle, the retroauricular muscle, the platysma, and most of the buccal branches. In doing so, regeneration is directed to the more important upper

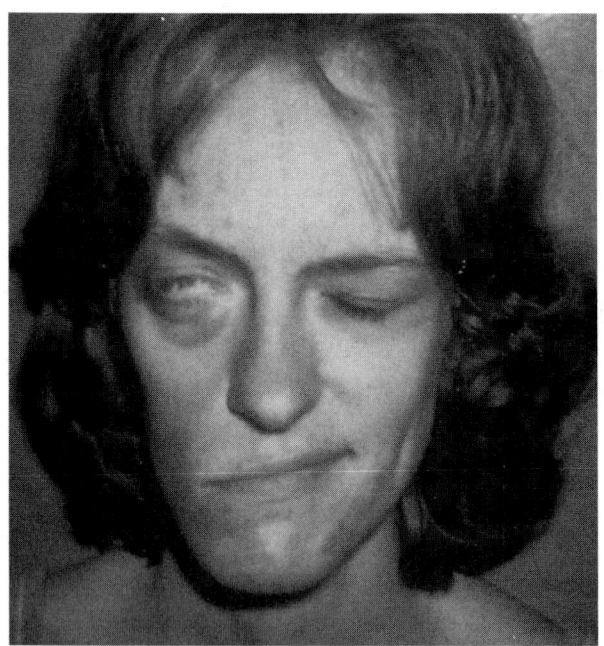

A

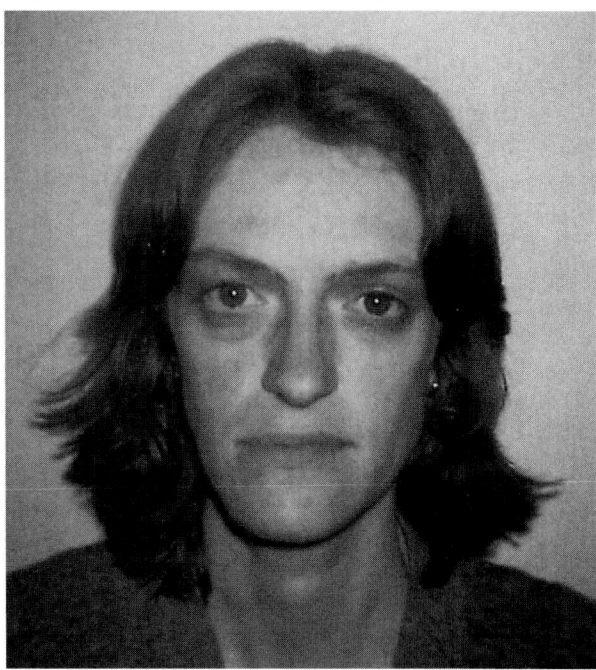

B

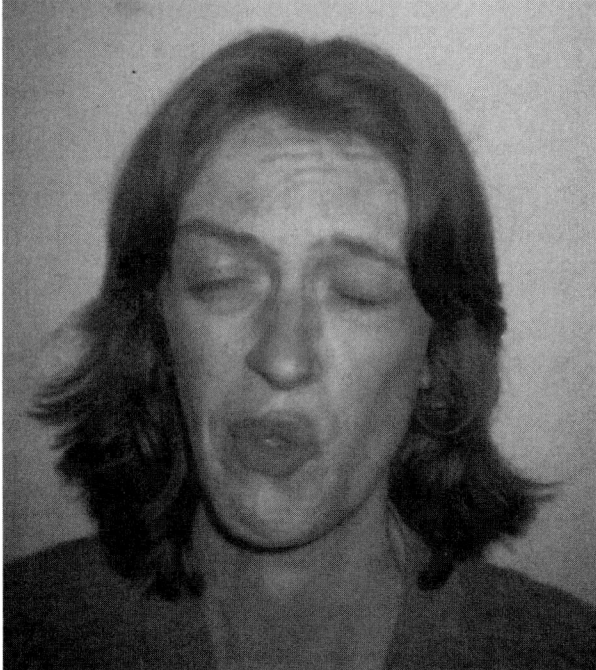

C

Figure 167.4 **A:** Right facial paralysis after injury to facial nerve within the mastoid. **B:** Two years after direct anastomosis. Patient in repose with good symmetry. **C:** Excellent eye closure and mobility of the mouth with slight asymmetry.

and lower regions of the face while minimizing mass movement in the midface (10).

Crossover Technique

There are basically three crossover techniques: hypoglossal to facial, spinal accessory to facial, and facial to facial. These techniques, of which the hypoglossal to facial is the most popular, remain a dependable and effective treatment of facial paralysis in the following conditions: irreversible facial nerve injury, intact mimetic function, intact motor endplate function, intact proximal donor nerve, and

intact distal facial nerve (11). This technique is most effective if performed prior to atrophy of the facial musculature and distal facial nerve. Indeed, most clinical studies have shown that crossover procedures performed within a year of facial paralysis are successful (12).

Advantages of this technique include low degree of technical difficulty, relative short time to movement (4 to 6 months), one anastomotic suture line, and motion that can resemble mimetic function with practice. Disadvantages include donor site morbidity with paralysis of the ipsilateral tongue in the case of hypoglossal-to-facial crossover, and some degree of mass movement. To minimize the mass

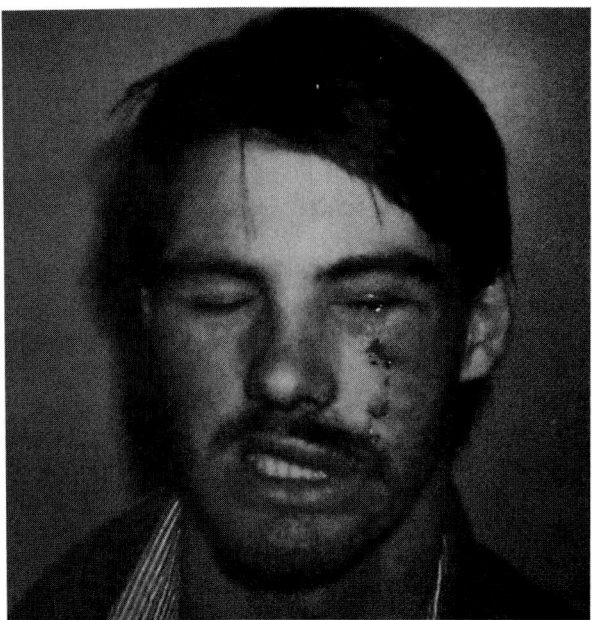

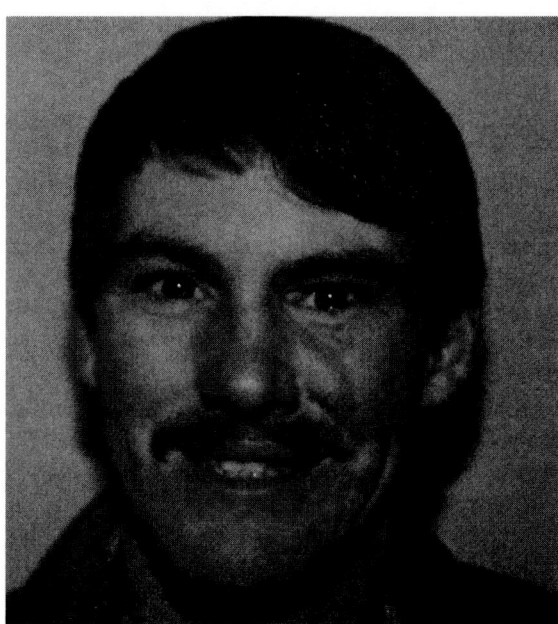

Figure 167.5 **A:** Patient suffering chainsaw injury to face with severance of buccal branch. **B:** Two years after repair of laceration without facial nerve repair. Patient demonstrates excellent recovery of function.

movement, or synkinesis, some authors advocate the use of this technique in only one of the major branches. Also, the judicious use of botulinum toxin has improved the results (13).

Only the hypoglossal to facial crossover is discussed in detail. The spinal accessory to facial crossover results in significant disability; however, use of the branch to the sternocleidomastoid muscle rather than the entire spinal accessory nerve may decrease the morbidity (14). In some authors' hands, the facial-to-facial anastomosis has been successful, but the results are often inconsistent, and more

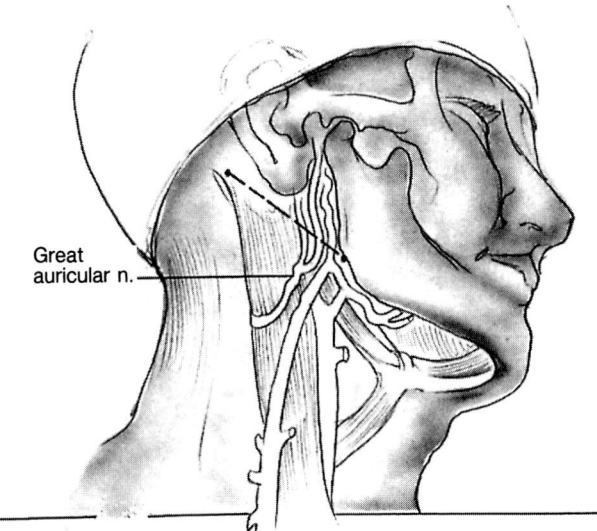

Figure 167.6 Greater auricular nerve located superficial to the sternocleidomastoid perpendicular to a line drawn between the mastoid and the angle of the mandible.

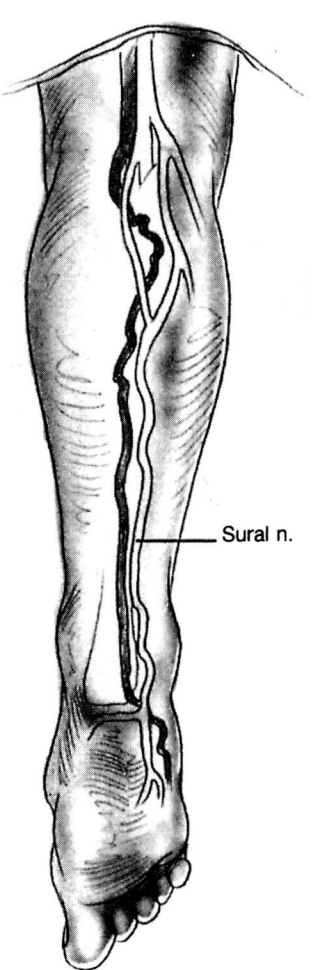

Figure 167.7 Sural nerve located just lateral to the saphenous vein and medial and posterior to the lateral malleolus of the ankle.

sophisticated free muscle flaps or a second donor nerve is usually required in conjunction with this technique to improve results.

In performing the hypoglossal to facial anastomosis, the two nerves are almost always long enough to preclude exposure of the facial nerve within the temporal bone; therefore, the facial nerve is transected as it exits the stylomastoid foramen. Therefore, to identify the facial nerve, the surgeon proceeds with a parotidectomy via a modified Blair incision. Once the appropriate flaps are elevated, the anterior border of the sternocleidomastoid foramen is identified and separated from the parotid gland. The cartilaginous auditory canal is then skeletonized and further delineated to identify the so-called pointer. Then, with visualization and palpation, the facial nerve can be identified as it exits the stylomastoid foramen, usually several millimeters inferior to the pointer. By palpating the mastoid tip and styloid process, the precise location of the facial nerve can be determined. The facial nerve is then isolated from surrounding tissue up to the pes anserinus; if further mobilization or length of the facial nerve is needed, then the dissection can be carried up to the two major branches of the facial nerve.

The hypoglossal nerve is then identified inferior to the digastric muscle and confirmed with a nerve stimulator. The hypoglossal nerve is then isolated from surrounding tissue distally toward the tongue. Then, the hypoglossal nerve is transected as distally as possible and sutured directly to the main trunk of the facial nerve using techniques similar to those of direct anastomosis (Figs. 167.8 and 167.9). Some authors recommend splitting the nerve to reduce the degree of hemiglossal atrophy.

Muscle Transposition Techniques

Regional muscle transfer using temporalis and masseter muscles have been described (15). Temporalis transfer has been used more frequently than masseter transfer. Also, dual system reanimation produces the most successful outcomes, with temporalis transfer for the lower face rehabilitation and gold weight implant for upper eyelid rehabilitation (16).

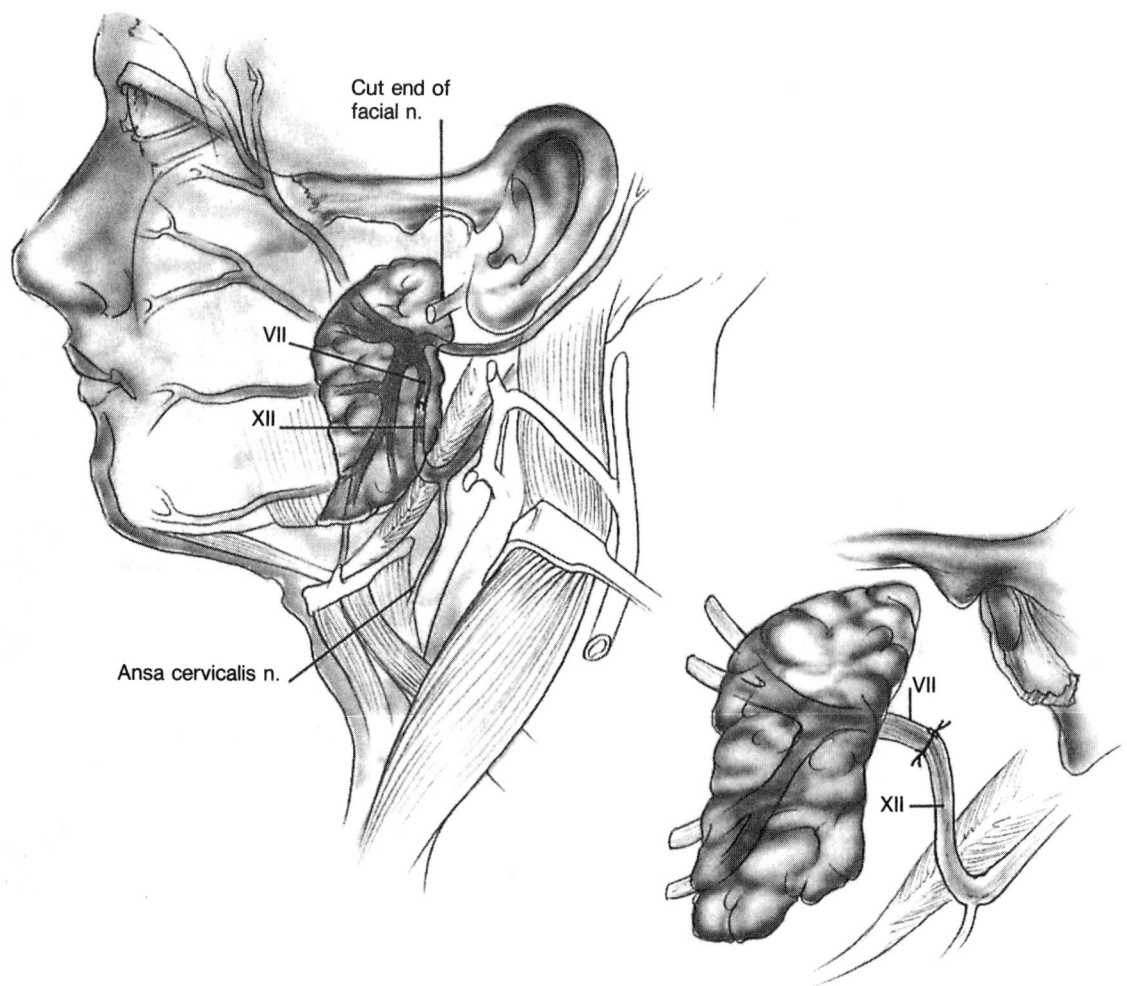

Figure 167.8 Nerve crossover using the proximal trunk of the hypoglossal nerve to the distal trunk of the facial nerve.

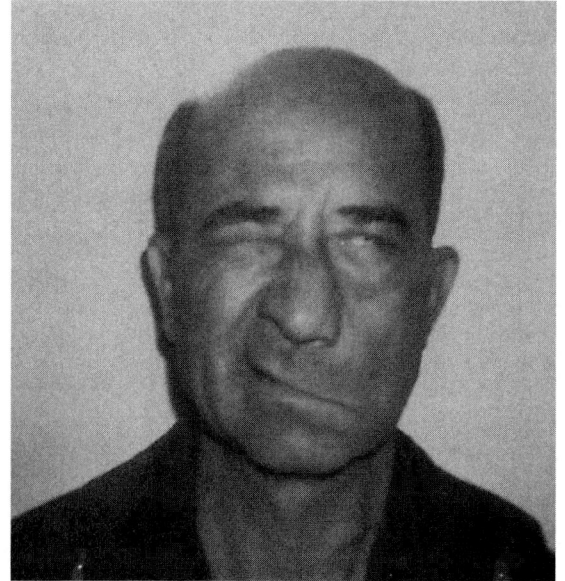

A

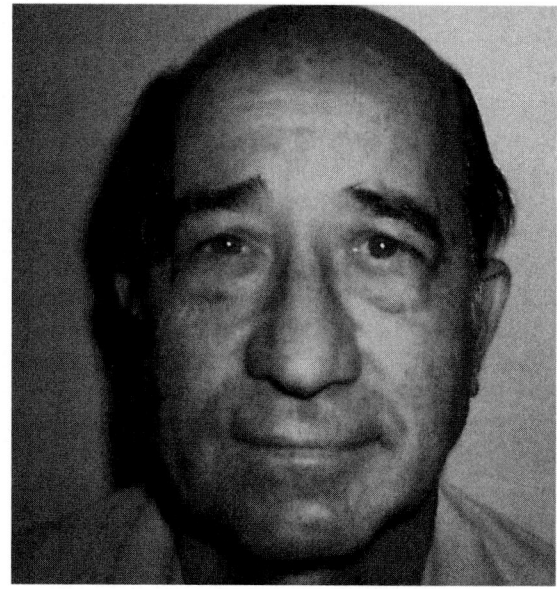

B

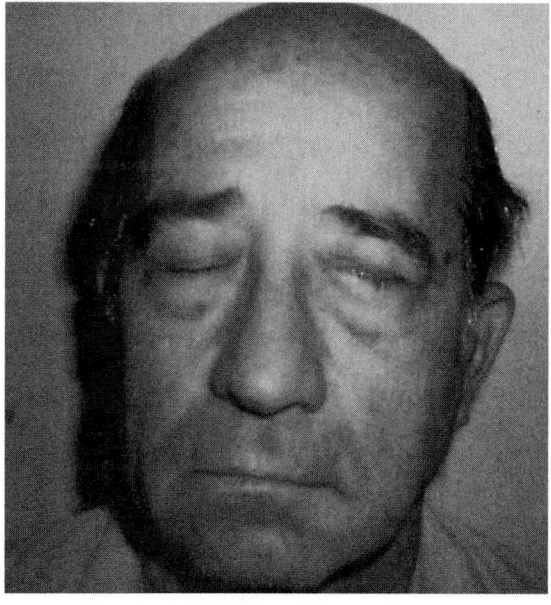

C

Figure 167.9 **A:** Patient with right facial paralysis after resection of acoustic neuroma and loss of facial nerve. **B:** One year after VII–XII crossover, patient demonstrates symmetric smile. **C:** Excellent eye closure without mass movement.

Muscle transposition techniques are used in several instances: (a) when neural techniques are unsuitable because there is no longer an intact facial neuromuscular system due to absence, such as in a congenital facial paralysis (Möbius syndrome); (b) when there is a loss of motor endplates from longstanding facial nerve interruption for at least 3 years; or (c) when other cranial nerves are sacrificed, thus eliminating crossover technique as a viable option.

The temporalis is a fan-shaped muscle radiating from the narrow coronoid process of the mandible to the broad temporal fossa of the temporal bone. The temporalis muscle is used for reanimation of the corner of the mouth. The temporalis muscle and fascia are exposed by making an incision in the preauricular crease and extending it into the superior temporal line (Fig. 167.10). The plane of dissec-

tion is above the superficial muscular aponeurotic system to avoid facial nerve injury. After obtaining wide exposure of the temporalis muscle, an incision is made down to the periosteum, elevating muscle fibers. Traditionally, one of the major criticisms of temporalis transfer is the bulge of muscle over the zygomatic arch. As a result, most authors now recommend transfer of only the middle third of the muscle (17). A large tunnel is made over the zygomatic arch. A second incision is made in the vermilion border at the oral commissure to expose the orbicularis muscle. The edge of the muscle is then attached to the orbicularis muscle with permanent 2-0 suture and is pulled up superiorly and laterally in an overcorrected position. In some patients, a temporoparietal fascial flap may be rotated in the temporalis fossa to fill the defect created by the harvested muscle. The vermilion incision can be closed with 4-0

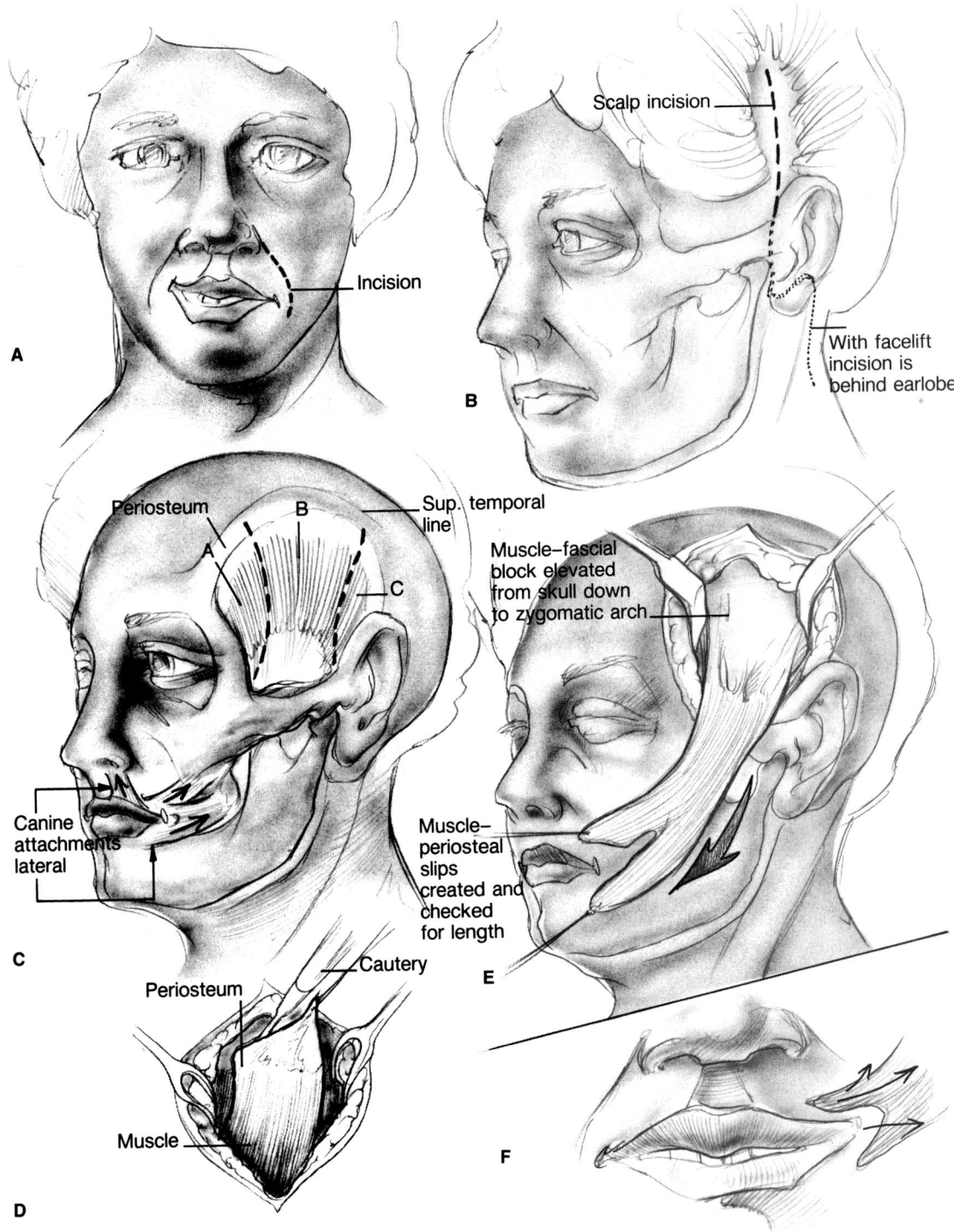

Figure 167.10   A–F: Procedure for temoralis muscle transposition.

chromic and running 6-0 nylon; the preauricular incision is closed with 3-0 chromic and running 6-0 nylon. The dressing includes Steri-strips to continue pulling the corner of the mouth up for overcorrection (Fig. 167.11).

The masseter muscle technique is used when the temporalis muscle is unavailable because of either resection or reconstruction, such as a temporal bone resection. In addition, this technique may be a surgeon's preference because a large facial incision can be avoided in the intraoral application. The disadvantage is that there is less muscle to use and the vector force of the muscle is more horizontal, thus providing less superior angulation to the corner of the

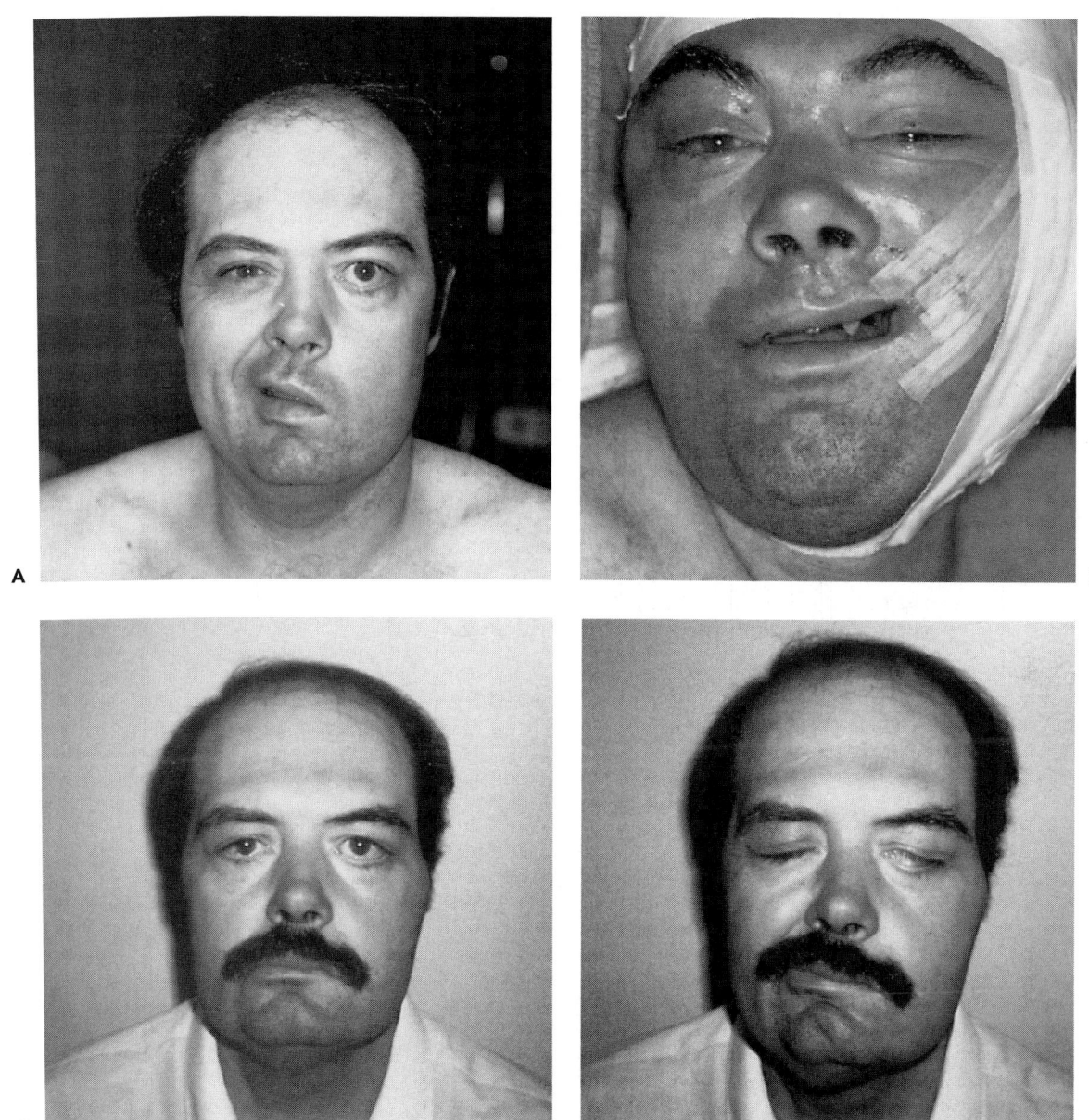

Figure 167.11   **A:** Right facial paralysis after resection of glomus jugulare that involved the facial nerve. **B:** Patient undergoing temporalis muscle fascia transfer. Note overcorrection and Steri-strips applied to maintain this position. **C:** One year after surgery, patient in repose with excellent symmetry. **D:** Patient attempting to smile, with minimal movement and slight asymmetry.

mouth. In the intraoral approach, the muscle is exposed by making a large incision in the gingival mucosa along the sulcus of the mandible (Fig. 167.12). The muscle is exposed by creating a plane between the mucosa and the muscle and then freed immediately by raising the muscle off the mandible with periosteal elevators. Once the muscle is freed medially and laterally, it is detached from its insertion at the inferolateral edge of the mandible with a curved right-angle scissors. It is important that this vertical incision of the muscle is not extended too far superiorly or posteriorly, or the nerve supply to the muscle could be

jeopardized. The anterior half is then split again to fashion two slips of muscle; ultimately, these slips will be tunneled into the small external incisions made along the vermilion border. These external incisions, each measuring 1 cm, are placed in the lateral inferior lip, half the distance between the melolabial line in the upper lip and the vermilion border. A lateral tunnel is then created with a sharp scissors in a plane just above the masseteric fascia and medial to the soft tissues of the face. Two clamps are then passed through the lip incisions to the intraoral area to grasp the slips of masseter muscle, guiding them into place. The

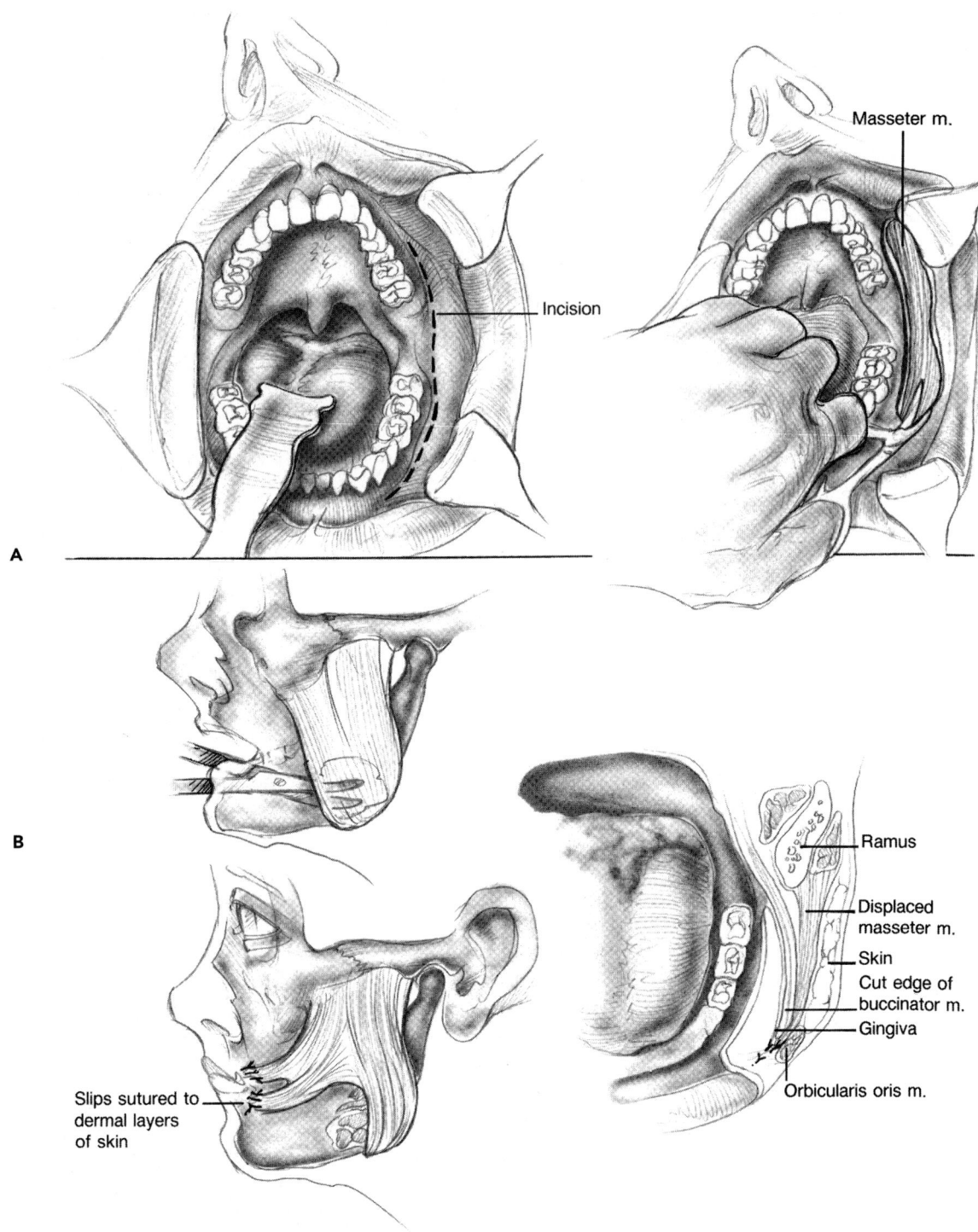

Figure 167.12   A: Intraoral approach to harvest the masseter muscle for transfer. Incision is made along the gingival sulcus. **B:** One muscle is exposed; curved scissors are used to transect the muscle in midportion. **C:** Two slips of muscle are attached to the dermal layers of the skin for over-correction of smile.

muscles are then fixed to the lips and commissure, pulling upward and laterally to overcorrect. The lips and muscles are secured in place with permanent sutures directly into the deep dermal layers of the skin. The wounds are closed. The dressing contains Steri-strips to support the overcorrection (Fig. 167.11).

An alternative approach to the masseter muscle includes an extraoral approach via a rhytidectomy incision or modified Blair incision, usually in conjunction with another procedure. Modifications of the masseter transposition would be the position of a fascial sling, harvested from the fascial lata of the thigh. In this case, a sling is passed around the anterior half of the muscle and the ends are sutured to the orbicularis oris muscle in front of the nasolabial fold with the other end sutured to the lower lip and oral commissure; 5 to 8 mm of restored motion can be obtained at a right angle to the muscle contraction. The advantage of this method is that it is less invasive and easier to perform.

ANCILLARY PROCEDURES

Ancillary procedures include the facial plastic techniques (rhytidectomy, blepharoplasty, brow lift, and midface lift), the prosthetic implants (spring and gold implants), and canthopexy and lid-tightening techniques. Although these techniques have indications similar to the transposition techniques, these ancillary procedures can be used as supplements to the transposition technique, particularly to protect the eye during the interval while facial recovery is anticipated. This is particularly true as an alternative to tarsorrhaphy, which has been the standard of care in patients who have facial nerve preservation but in whom recovery is not expected for several months to a year. It is most commonly used in a patient who has had a cerebellopontine angle tumor resected and in whom the fifth and seventh nerves are preserved but are transiently not functioning.

The rhytidectomy, blepharoplasty, and brow lift are discussed in detail in other chapters in this text. Certain principles of the brow lift are worth mentioning here, however. Brow ptosis caused by unilateral facial paralysis is usually corrected with a direct brow lift; however, a supraciliary scar is needed. Although endoscopic brow suspension provides an alternative technique, this requires special equipment, expertise, and decreased durability and symmetry. Botulinum toxin injections provide a "chemical brow lift" without the need for surgery; yet several injections are needed (18). More recently, a minimally invasive brow suspension has been proposed for the treatment of brow ptosis secondary to unilateral facial paralysis with promising results (19).

The use of prosthetics, particularly gold and spring implants, has proven useful in the rehabilitation of the eye following facial paralysis. Prior to surgical intervention, a complete eye examination should include assessment of visual acuity, lower lid laxity by the snap test, tear production with a Schirmer test, lacrimal excretory system with a Jones test, and measurement of the margin gap, which is the distance between the borders of the upper and lower eyelids on closure.

Implantation of gold weights within 30 days of paralysis is as effective for the management of paralytic lagophthalmos as delayed implantation and is not associated with higher complication rates. Early implantation of gold weights should be considered in all patients with paralytic lagophthalmos (20).

Several techniques have been described regarding upper lid weight implantation for paralytic lagophthalmos, including a retrograde, postlevator aponeurosis technique (21). The following is a brief description of the senior author's technique: a small incision is made several millimeters above the upper eyelid margin. Sharp scissors are used to expose the tarsal plate. Prefabricated gold implants are used; generally 1 to 1.2 grams will suffice. Recent reports demonstrate success with platinum implants, which are smaller, because of their higher density compared to gold, and have been used with success (22). With the tarsal plate exposed, 8-0 nylon is used to secure the implant in place. The wound is closed in two layers. If there is anticipated incomplete closure, a millerectomy may be performed prior to the placement of the implant (Fig. 167.13).

If there is poor levator action, a spring implant may prove more efficacious. The enhanced palpebral spring requires tightening of the levator and is technically more challenging than gold weight implant and has a high extrusion rate (23).

The lid margin may be incomplete following gold weight implantation of the upper lid; this is often related to coexisting ectropion of the lower lid, which is treated with lateral canthopexy (24). Treatment of the paralytic lower eyelid with ectropion includes tarsorrhaphy, lateral canthal suspension, periocular placement of silicone or fascia lata slings, and retractor lysis combined with lower lid stenting with the use of free autogenous tarsal, auricular cartilage, or hard palate mucosal grafts. If ectropion of the lower lid results in eversion of the inferior punctum, one may consider a medial canthoplasty to reposition the inferior punctum.

Paralytic midfacial ptosis superimposed on age-related midfacial sag and lower lid laxity may aggravate paralytic lower lid ectropion and retraction. Indeed, Elner et al. (25) recently reported on midfacial elevation as a safe and effective adjunct in the treatment of lower eyelid retraction in chronic facial palsy.

The senior author prefers the lateral tarsal strip procedure to treat patients with great laxity of the lower eyelid with resulting ectropion. This relatively simple technique is started by first performing a lateral canthotomy and then

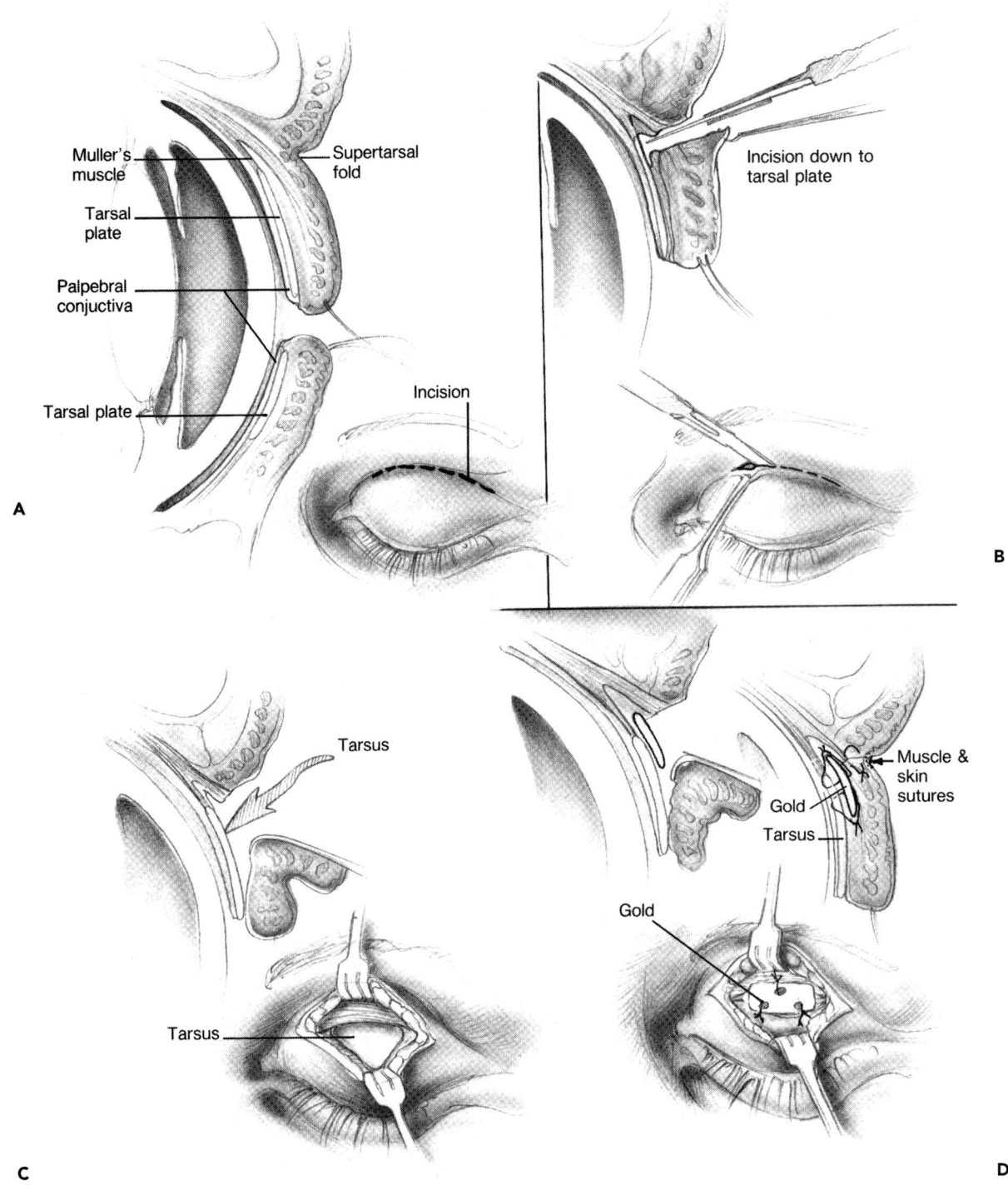

Figure 167.13 Gold implant technique for upper eyelid closure. **A:** Incision is made several centimeters above the upper eyelid. **B:** With a sharp instrument, the tarsal plate is identified. **C:** The gold implant is sutured in place, straddling the tarsal plate and slightly posterior to it. **D:** Lateral view, showing the position of the gold implant in the upper eyelid.

dividing the lateral portion of the lower eyelid into musculocutaneous and tarsoconjunctival layers. The tarsoconjunctival layer is grasped with a skin hook, and the conjunctiva over this is abraded with a sharp blade to promote adherence and avoid formation of epithelial deposits. The resulting tarsal strip is then sutured to the periosteum of the inner aspect of the orbital rim laterally to shorten and elevate the lower eyelid. The resultant excess tissue of the musculocutaneous layer is removed and then closed with mild chromic (Fig. 167.14).

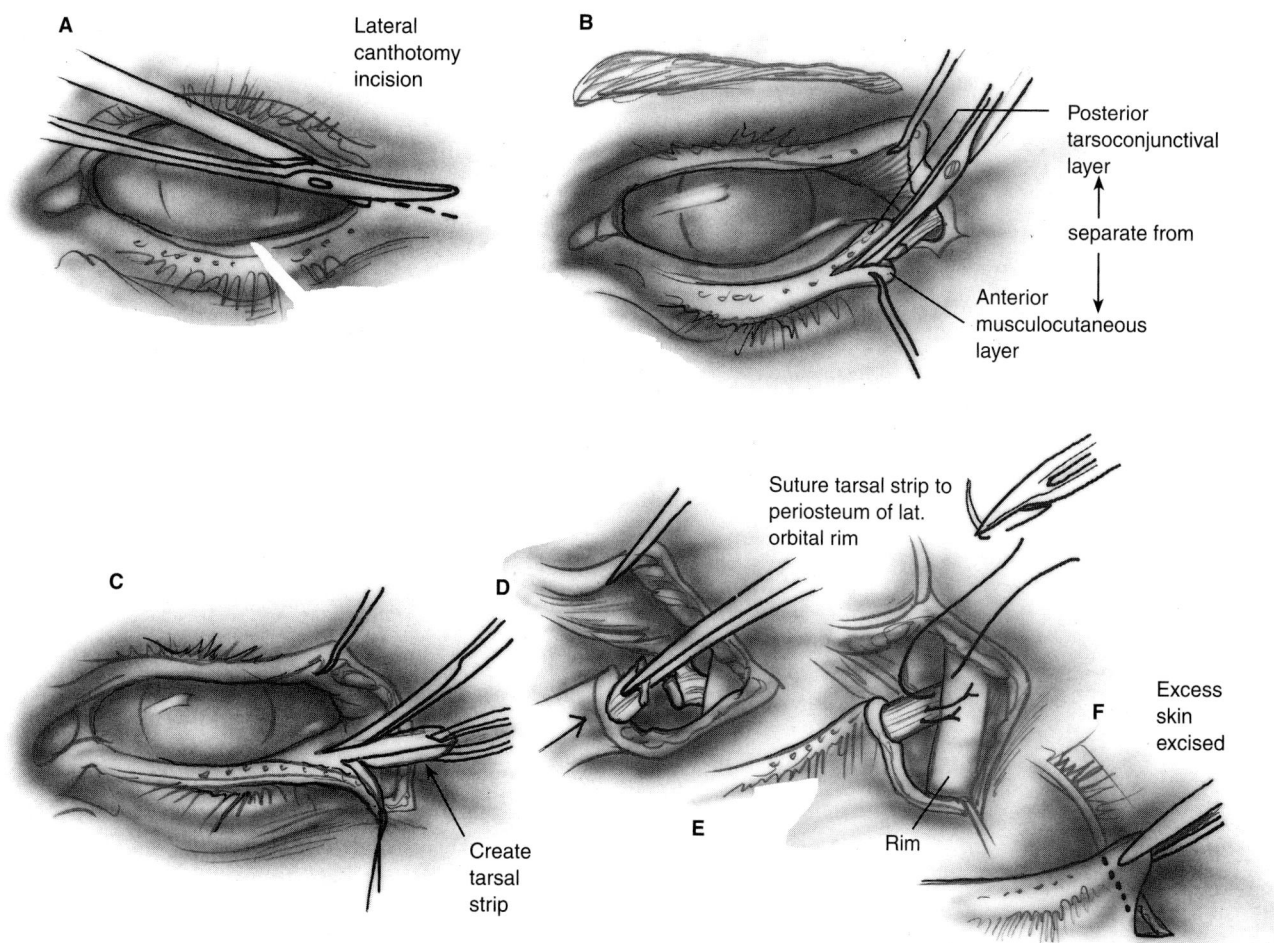

Figure 167.14 Lateral tarsal strip procedure for ectropion of the lower lid. **A:** Lateral canthotomy incision. **B:** Division of the lateral aspect of the lower lid into an anterior musculocutaneous layer and posterior tarsal conjunctival layer. **C:** Tarsal strip grasped with skin hook. **D:** Tarsal strip positioned inside the lateral rim of the orbit, which has been exposed. **E:** Tarsal strip sutured to periosteum inside of lateral orbital rim. **F:** Excess skin excised and wound closed.

FREE MUSCLE FLAPS

Harii et al. first was the first to report on the use of microneurovascular techniques to transfer free gracilis muscle for the treatment of facial paralysis (26). Indications for the use of free muscle flaps such as the gracilis, serratus anterior, latissimus dorsi, or extensor digitorum brevis are the same as for muscle transfers. Additionally, the gracilis muscle has been used as a compound flap to include a skin paddle for repair of skin defects with good results (27).

The procedures often require two stages: A nerve graft is harvested and attached to the opposite normal side and then, 6 to 9 months later, a free muscle flap with its neurovascular bundle intact is anastomosed with the appropriate nerve and vessels for reanimation. Nutrient vessels for the gracilis muscle are not particularly long; therefore the gracilis muscle is best utilized when the superficial temporal and/or facial vessels are available. Otherwise, the latissimus dorsi pedicle is long enough to reach vessels in the upper neck (28). A one-stage procedure using the abductor hallucis muscle and latissimus dorsi have also been performed. The results have been good to excellent, but the procedures are technically difficult and should be performed only by experienced surgeons with extensive knowledge of microvascular techniques.

CONCLUSION

When the patient presents with a total facial paralysis, particularly when the nerve has been totally disrupted, it is impossible to effect total restoration with a natural spontaneous expression, full motor power, and perfect congruent movement. The techniques described, however, can provide marked cosmetic and functional improvement. As these procedures evolve, the patients with total facial paralysis will be afforded the possibility of leading normal lives without the stigma of facial disfigurement.

HIGHLIGHTS

- The patient with facial paralysis has both obvious cosmetic and significant functional defects affecting mastication, speech production, and eye protection.
- Total unilateral facial paralysis may be managed using direct facial nerve anastomosis, an interpositional graft, anastomosis to other motor nerves, dynamic musculofascial transposition, static musculofascial transposition, or a facial plastic procedure.
- Patient counseling is crucial when total transection of the main trunk has occurred. Such patients will suffer some impairment of mimetic expression, mastication, eye protection, and articulation; none of these patients will achieve 100% functional restoration.
- The goal of facial reanimation is to improve the patient's facial muscle functions (facial tone and expression, eye protection, mastication, and articulation).
- The facial nerve fibers travel in groups of fascicles that vary with the region of the nerve. Fascicular perineural suturing techniques, once popular with some surgeons, have not been shown to be more effective than epineural suture repair.
- Nerve techniques are indicated in patients with a duration of facial paralysis of less than 2 years. The patient will not have complete restoration and probably will have some mass motion and synkinesis.
- If the patient's paralysis lasts longer than 2 years or if there are no intact proximal and distal nerve sites, a muscle transposition, either temporalis or masseter, should be used. Although these are dynamic techniques, the results are less than ideal.
- The best functional results can be achieved when facial nerve anastomosis can be performed. The optimal timing for this procedure is as soon as possible after the injury.
- The second-best functional results can be obtained using facial nerve repair with a graft. Grafting prevents excessive tension at the anastomosis. The great auricular nerve and the sural nerve are used most commonly.
- There are three crossover techniques: hypoglossal to facial, spinal accessory to facial, and facial to facial (contralateral side). Acoustic neuroma excision is a common etiology for these patients. Some restoration usually results, but the outcome is often unpredictable.
- Muscle transposition techniques are used when the facial neuromuscular system (congenital facial paralysis) is not intact or there is loss of motor function (longstanding facial paralysis). The temporalis muscle is usually used, but the masseter muscle is an option.
- The highest priority in facial nerve paralysis is to protect the eye from the effects of drying. Techniques used include tarsorrhaphy, canthopexy, tarsal strip, and gold weights and springs.
- Free muscle flaps (gracilis, serratus anterior, extensor digitorum brevis, abductor hallucis) can be used for similar indications as for other muscle transfer procedures.

REFERENCES

1. Alex JC, Nguyen DB. Multivectored suture suspension. *Arch Facial Plast Surg* 2004;6:197–201.
2. Parnes SM. The facial nerve. In: Jahn AF, Santos-Sacchi J, eds. *Physiology of the ear.* New York: Raven, 1988:125.
3. Vanswearingen JM, Brach JS. Validation of a treatment based classification system for individuals with facial neuromotor disorders. *Phys Ther* 1998;78:678–689.
4. Axelsson S, Lindberg S, Stjernquist-Desatnik A. Outcome of treatment with valacyclovir and prednisone in patients with Bell's palsy. *Ann Otol Rhinol Laryngol* 2003;112:197–201.
5. May M. *Facial paralysis: rehabilitation techniques.* New York: Thieme Medical Publishers, 2003.
6. Barrs DM. Facial nerve trauma: optimal timing for repair. *Laryngoscope* 1991;101:835–848.
7. Weber RA, Breidenbach WC, Brown RE, et al. A randomized prospective study of polyglycolic acid conduits for digital nerve reconstruction in humans. *Plast Reconstr Surg* 2000;106:1036–1045.
8. Parnes SM. The facial nerve. In: Jahn AF, Santos-Sacchi J, eds. *Physiology of the ear.* New York: Raven Press, 1988:125.
9. May M, Sobol S, Mester S. Managing segmental facial nerve injuries by surgical repair. *Laryngoscope* 1990;100:1062.
10. Fisch U, Esslen E. The surgical treatment of facial hyperkinesias. *Arch Otolaryngol* 1972;95:400–405.
11. Koh KS, Kim JK, Kim CJ, et al. Hypoglossal-facial crossover in facial nerve palsy: pure end to side anastomosis technique. *Br J Plast Surg* 2002;55:25–31.
12. Burgess LPA, Goode RL. Total facial paralysis. In: Burgess LPA, Goode RL, eds. *Reanimation of the paralyzed face.* New York: Thieme Medical Publishers, 1994:11–26.
13. De Maio M. Use of botulinum toxin in facial paralysis. *J Cosmet Laser Ther* 2003;5:216–217.
14. Griebie MS, Huff JS. Selective role of partial XI–VII anastomosis in facial reanimation. *Laryngoscope* 1998;108:1664–1668.
15. Croxson GR, Quinn MJ, Coulson SE. Temporalis muscle transfer for facial paralysis: a further refinement. *Facial Plast Surg* 2000;16:351–356.
16. Casler JD, Conley J. Simultaneous "dual system" rehabilitation in the treatment of facial paralysis. *Arch Otolaryngol Head Neck Surg* 1990;116:199–203.
17. Sherris DA. Refinement in reanimation of the lower face. *Arch Facial Plast Surg* 2004;6:49–53.
18. Frankel AS, Kamer FM. Chemical browlift. *Arch Otolaryngol Head Neck Surg* 1998;124:321–323.
19. Constantino PD, Hiltzik DH, Moche J, et al. Minimally invasive brow suspension for facial paralysis. *Arch Facial Plast Surg* 2003;5: 171–174.
20. Snyder MC, Johnson PJ, Moore GF, Ogren FP. Early versus late gold weight implantation for rehabilitation of the paralyzed eyelid. *Laryngoscope* 2001;111:2109–2113.
21. Kao CH, Moe KS. Retrograde weight implantation for correction of lagophthalmos. *Laryngoscope* 2004;114:1570–1575.
22. Berghaus A, Neumann K, Schrom T. The platinum chain: a new upper-lid implant for facial palsy. *Arch Facial Plast Surg* 2003;5: 166–170.
23. Levine RE, Shapiro JP. Reanimation of the paralyzed eyelid with the enhanced palpebral spring or the gold weight: modern replacements for tarsorrhaphy. *Facial Plast Surg* 2000;16:325–336.
24. Nakazawa H, Kikuchi Y, Honda T, et al. Treatment of paralytic lagopthalmos by loading the lid with a gold plate and lateral canthopexy. *Scand J Plast Reconstr Surg Hand Surg* 2004;38:140–144.
25. Elner VM, Mauffray RO, Fante RG, et al. Comprehensive midfacial elevation for ocular complications of facial nerve palsy. *Arch Facial Plast Surg* 2003;5:427–433.
26. Harii K, Ohmori K, Torii S. Free gracilis muscle transplantation, with microneurovascular anastomoses for the treatment of facial paralysis. *Plast Reconstr Surg* 1976;57:133
27. Chuang DC, Mardini S, Lin S, et al. Free proximal gracilis muscle and its skin paddle compound flap transplantation for complex facial paralysis. *Plast Reconstr Surg* 2004;113:126–132.
28. Takushima A, Harii K, Asato H, et al. Neurovascular free-muscle transfer for the treatment of established facial paralysis following ablative surgery in the parotid region. *Plast Reconstr Surg* 2004; 113:1563–1572.

168

Facial Analysis and Preoperative Evaluation

Karen H. Calhoun   *Kweon I. Stambaugh*

PREOPERATIVE ASSESSMENT

Establishing a Relationship

The facial plastic surgeon has two important tasks during the preoperative period. The first is establishing a good relationship with the patient, including assessment of psychological stability and motivations for surgery. The second is objective analysis of the patient's appearance, with meticulous surgical planning.

The initial interview provides the surgeon time to explore the patient's thoughts and desires and to educate the patient. Taking the time to educate the patient about details of the perioperative experience and reasonable outcome expectations yields a calmer and, ultimately, more satisfied patient. In some cases, the surgeon may discover information leading to turning down a particular patient for surgery (1). This investment of time in relationship building goes a long way toward preventing malpractice claims (2).

The patient's medical history may reveal conditions or medications that affect the safety of the proposed elective cosmetic surgery. Review by the patient's primary care provider may be advisable for those with questionable medical status. Formal psychological assessment is rarely necessary for patients requesting aesthetic surgery, but should be considered when the surgeon is uncertain about the advisability of surgery.

Patient Selection: Concept of Deformity

Our self-image is affected by the opinions and reactions of others. Today's society idolizes youthful beauty, and many seek ways to achieve or preserve this ideal to maintain their self-image (3). In our society, wanting to change one's appearance is considered sufficient indication for surgery. A patient requesting surgery to achieve or maintain youthful beauty is no longer labeled vain. Most patients seeking surgical improvement of appearance are psychologically stable and have realistic surgical expectations (4).

Usually, patient and the surgeon share a perception of "deformity" and the correction needed. Some patients, however, have a self-image including perception of a deformity not obvious to others. A patient seeking surgical correction of such a self-visualized deformity should be carefully considered. Surgical correction has the potential to promote positive changes in self-esteem and image (5). On the rare occasion that a dramatic difference is present between the patient's perceived self-image and the surgeon's observation, further counseling and perhaps psychological evaluation are prudent. A patient with "body dysmorphic disorder" can become preoccupied with a minor or imagined defect (6). Attempting a surgical solution may result in a problem patient (7).

Preoperative Interviews

The primary goal of the preoperative interview is establishing good communication between the surgeon and the patient. A common-sense approach to selecting candidates for surgery greatly reduces the chance of encountering an unhappy or problem patient (8) (Fig. 168.1).

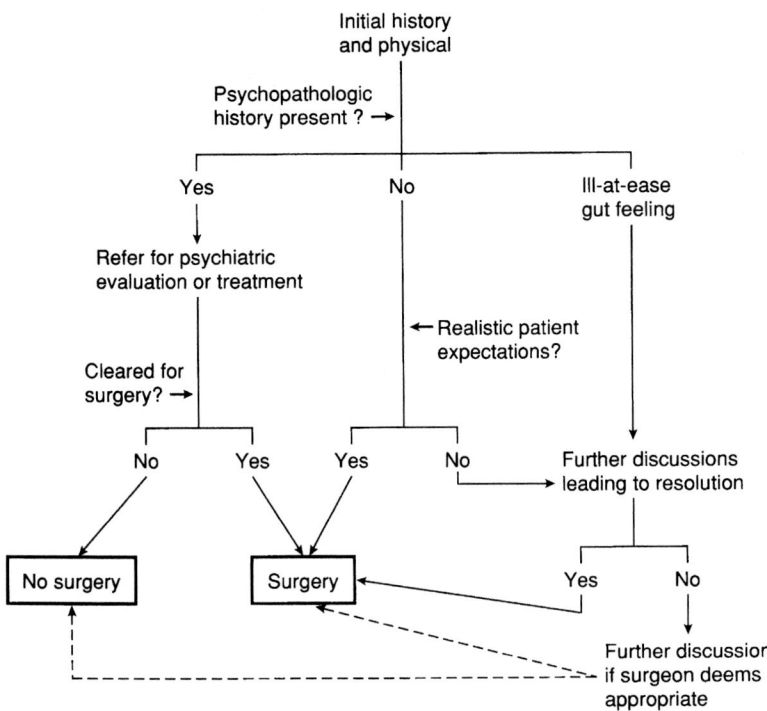

Figure 168.1 Preoperative evaluation for the patient seeking aesthetic facial surgery.

The surgeon seeks to understand:

1. What are the patient's expectations?
2. Are the expectations realistic and reasonable?
3. Can the expectations be fulfilled?
4. Can the patient be satisfied?

First, the surgeon must understand the patient's self-image and the surgical correction desired. Some patients are hesitant to express all their desires, preferring for the surgeon to decide what corrections are desirable. Such patients must be educated to awareness that a decision for elective aesthetic surgery is a cooperative effort. The patient can benefit from understanding the surgeon's perception of the problem, surgical possibilities, and expected outcome.

The surgeon's next task is to decide whether the patient's expectations about surgical outcomes are realistic. During the preoperative discussion, the surgeon develops a feeling for how the patient will view the outcome and whether the patient's expectations are reasonable. The 50-year old patient expecting to look again as she or he did at age 20, or the shy person expecting to become extroverted after surgery are doomed to disappointment. Such a patient often blames the surgeon for the disappointment. Educating the patient about what is and is not possible will save the surgeon and patient from postoperative disappointment. Mac-Gregor (9) observed that the patient's ability to accept the surgical result is highly correlated with the degree to which the patient has been prepared. A disappointed postsurgical patient may claim breach of contract, believing that the surgeon did not provide what was promised.

Unless the surgeon is confident that the patient can be satisfied with the surgical outcome, the patient should not undergo surgery. Accurate prediction of surgical outcome requires a surgeon's realistic assessment of his or her own capabilities. Venturing beyond one's technical skills increases the probability of an unfortunate result and an unhappy patient.

The experienced surgeon also develops a wariness for the patient who creates a sense of uneasiness, a feeling that "perhaps I should not operate on this patient." Situations that may raise caution flags include history of having sued another physician, comments made by the patient degrading another surgeon, extreme demands on the office workers, or evidence of the patient having gone from doctor to doctor. Such patients should be scheduled for additional preoperative meetings, possible psychological evaluation, and may ultimately be turned down for surgery.

Having a family member or close friend present during preoperative discussions further facilitates a good relationship and creates a well-informed support person for the patient. Because patients often suffer from selective amnesia or absorb only what they choose to hear, the family member can assist by recalling what was said during the interviews. Having a family member present also gives the surgeon insight into family functioning. This facilitates working with the patient and family throughout the planned operation and recovery period.

Computer Imaging

Computer imaging that allows the surgeon to demonstrate possible surgical outcomes to the patient is a double-edged tool. As a marketing tool, it permits the patient to understand what may be aesthetically possible, but it does so without regard for the limitations of tissue, healing, or surgical technique. Use of computer imaging requires additional time with the patient, which can foster development of better rapport. Conversely, the "implied promise" of a certain outcome, coupled with the commonly "selective" memory during preoperative counseling, may lead the patient to disregard the surgeon's disclaimer that the imaging process shows possibilities, not promises (10). Lawsuits currently in the courts center around this particular issue.

PSYCHOPATHOLOGY IN THE AESTHETIC PATIENT

Mere decades ago, patients seeking aesthetic surgery were assumed to have deep psychological issues. In 1960, Jacobson et al. (11) suggested that most cosmetic surgery patients required psychiatric evaluation because of the high rate of psychiatric problems in this group. Meyer et al. (12) reported that motivation for aesthetic surgery was partly driven by sexual identification conflicts, particularly the sexual symbolism of the nose. Meerloo (13) warned of latent depressions precipitated by rhytidectomy.

Today, with the widespread acceptance of purposeful appearance improvement through surgery, psychopathology among those seeking cosmetic surgery is similar to that in the general population. Nevertheless, some psychological diagnoses are helpful for the surgeon to recognize preoperatively. Although few of these diagnoses are absolute contraindications to surgery, foreknowledge of such a diagnosis will allow the surgeon to tailor her or his preoperative counseling and postoperative care to address the patient's likely concerns.

Depression

Traditionally, patients with history of depression were rejected for facial cosmetic surgery, as it was feared surgery would trigger deeper postoperative depression (14). One 1960 study identified four evenly divided groups of patients with postoperative depression: early transient, late transient, early prolonged, and late prolonged. Only the late-onset prolonged group, whose depression appeared 2 to 3 weeks postoperatively, had a causal relation between surgery and depression. The Minnesota Multiphasic Personality Inventory showed these patients to be passive-dependent personalities desiring care. They found the immediate postoperative period ideally satisfying, with caring and nurturing by others. Later, as this sought-after support waned, the patients realized that surgery had not fulfilled their unreasonable expectations, and became more depressed.

We now know that almost half of aesthetic surgery patients display clinically apparent postoperative depression, even with a good outcome (14,15). In the past, fear of precipitating depression resulted in preoperative psychiatric

evaluation of many patients. As cultural norms have evolved, the level of concern about physical appearance that would once have been deemed psychologically abnormal has come to seem normal, and it is the rare patient who is required to undergo preoperative psychiatric evaluation.

A preoperative diagnosis of depression is not an absolute contraindication to surgery, but the surgeon should realize that a risk exists of the depression intensifying. Despite preoperative depression, these patients can undergo aesthetic surgery without intensification of psychologic symptoms, but should undergo preoperative psychiatric evaluation (16). Best outcomes occur with care coordination between the surgeon and the psychiatrist.

Psychosis/Schizophrenia

Psychotic patients have often been rejected by aesthetic facial surgeons but may be reasonable surgical candidates (16,17). The schizophrenic patient is not at higher risk for further psychiatric illness due to facial aesthetic surgery, nor is the surgeon at increased risk, legally or physically. Such patients may experience improvement of the psychologic status after aesthetic surgery (15,17). Despite reports that most schizophrenic patients are not high risks, surgeons remain reluctant to operate on them. A thorough evaluation by and close cooperation with a psychiatric colleague is recommended before operating on such a patient.

The paranoid schizophrenic, however, is a potentially dangerous patient. At least one surgeon has been killed by such a patient who was unhappy with the results of his cosmetic procedure (18). Patients with frank schizophrenic psychosis or paranoid psychosis are a definite risk for themselves and the surgeon and should be avoided.

Neurotic patients were once considered unfavorable candidates for facial aesthetic surgery (19) but actually make excellent cosmetic surgery candidates. They require support, understanding, and patience from the surgeon, the time-honored tenets of a good doctor–patient relationship. Answering questions, explaining details, and spending time caring for the patient are usually rewarded.

I remember a neurotic patient who underwent upper and lower facial rejuvenative procedures. During each preoperative and postoperative visit, she asked many questions, mostly repetitive. She asked questions about seemingly trivial matters. This type of patient gradually frazzles a surgeon's nerves. However, remembering the rule that hand holding is better than confrontation in these situations, I answered the questions as diplomatically as possible. Ultimately, she was a very satisfied patient after her anxieties were put to rest.

The neurotic patient is reassured by the surgeon's sincere concern and understanding. I tell patients preoperatively that I look more critically at their postoperative results than they do. I educate them preoperatively about the expected postoperative visits to assess healing progress.

They understand before surgery that revisions or touch-up procedures will not take place until at least 6 months after surgery, to allow wound healing. Establishing such ground rules preoperatively initiates a good rapport with the patient.

Personality Disorder

Personality disorders are the most common psychopathology among patients seeking cosmetic surgery, and these manipulative patients can be difficult to handle (16,20). They are poorer candidates for aesthetic surgery, often exhibiting body dysmorphism (20). A California study of malpractice cases involving plastic surgeons found a predominance of borderline personality, with patient idealization of the surgeon at the initial contact degenerating into a contentious relationship (20).

Surgeons dealing with these patients often experience aggravation, frustration, and impatience. Unlike the neurotic patient who requires gentle treatment, the personality disorder patient must be handled firmly, sometimes requiring an almost patronizing manner. After the doctor–patient relationship is established and the patient knows that no manipulation can occur, the patient either cooperates or seeks another surgeon (16). In either case, the problem is solved, and the work can begin.

MINIMAL DEFORMITY PATIENTS

One definition of aesthetic or cosmetic surgery is surgery to correct defects that the average prudent observer considers within normal range (21,22). Surgeons were traditionally warned to avoid patients seeking surgery for minimal deformities (23). More recently, however, it has been found that most patients with minimal defects van be very satisfied after surgical correction. They can be very demanding, as they focus on minute details (29) and require a lot of "hand-holding" by the surgeon and staff.

Surgeons must trust their gut feelings. Patients with whom the surgeon cannot establish a comfortable relationship, despite additional office visits, should be referred for evaluation or turned away. If the patient refuses the offer of a referral for psychologic evaluation, the surgeon has the choice of politely rejecting the patient or accepting the patient and at the same time accepting a higher risk of postoperative problems.

PATIENT DISSATISFACTION

The patient's perception of a successful outcome is influenced by many factors, including the surgeon's reaction. Surgeon honesty is mandatory, but no dishonesty exists in expressing satisfaction with the surgical results. The surgeon's experience with expectations at various staging of healing allows her or him to counsel and reassure the patient, especially during the early postoperative period.

Preoperatively, the surgeon lays the groundwork for dealing with patient concerns and dissatisfactions in the postoperative period. The joint decision between surgeon and patient about the surgical procedure should leave the surgeon feeling confident of an agreement between parties. Not doing this creates ample room for postoperative misunderstanding. Building a relationship among the patient, family, and surgeon, important in this phase of building the doctor–patient relationship, is an important part of preoperative counseling, with welcoming of relevant and constructive suggestions from the patient and family. Studies show that a lack of rapport between the surgeon and patient is a major factor leading to more than 50% of malpractice suits (24). Any postoperative problem should be discussed immediately. When a patient points out a problem or concern, often the surgeon's knee-jerk response is defensive and silencing. The surgeon may not be happy with the surgical outcome, may feel guilty, or may not want to listen to complaints about his or her work. A smarter choice it to listen to the patient, encouraging him or her to discuss it thoroughly. A patient needs to express his or her distress about problems (16). Active compassionate listening reassures the patient and conveys the surgeon's concern for the patient's worries.

At first, it does not matter whether the surgeon agrees that a problem exists. The patient believes a problem is present and feels only hurt or distrust if the surgeon denies it or tries to explain it away (12). If the problem is one that will resolve with time or one that has been expected, the patient should be reassured. If a true problem concerns the surgeon also, being candid it the best choice. The surgeon should convey sincere concern, explain how the problem will be rectified. Allowing the patient to know that both parties are in agreement about the problem assures the patient, and the surgeon remains in control. This is important because the patient first chose the surgeon because the patient had confidence in the surgeon's abilities. The patient maintains that confidence as long as the surgeon maintains control.

Most small defects and even some of the major deviations resolve or improve significantly with time (25). This is the time to demonstrate support for the patient and not to put up a defensive barrier. The patient wants the surgeon's understanding and answers (15). The good surgeon–patient rapport established before surgery holds the surgeon in good stead during such conflict resolution after surgery. The wise surgeon continues to cultivate the relationship while the problem is being solved.

It is the surgeon's responsibility to determine unrealistic patient expectations before surgery. It is not appropriate to point this out to the patient who has just discovered an undesirable result, because this is invariably interpreted as defensive posturing. Instead, the surgeon should allow the patient to vent frustration or anger. Afterward, it is the surgeon's turn to explain to the patient what is and is not a problem and what can and cannot be done about it. The patient is reassured by knowing that the surgeon will be working with the patient to resolve the defect.

The issue of unreasonable expectations should be directly addressed and an understanding reached between the surgeon and the patient before any agreement to perform surgery. Accepting the challenge to perform the surgery with full knowledge that the patient has an unreasonable expectation is unwise.

FACIAL ANALYSIS

Attractiveness and beauty are important concepts in plastic surgery, but difficult to characterize objectively. It is especially difficult in the face, where beauty occurs by a combination of facial features and balance rather than a specific attribute. A primary objective for facial plastic surgeons is identifying and improving aesthetically undesirable qualities and proportions, as defined by the patient's desires and our cultural norms. Understanding the combination of characteristics composing the aesthetic "ideal" is an essential foundation for facial cosmetic surgeons. Although seasoned facial plastic surgeons often rely on their subjective aesthetic sense, residents and fellows do not have the advantage of these years of experience. Quantitative methods for developing aesthetic judgment and evaluating surgical results are therefore valuable educational tools.

History

The identification of aesthetic facial qualities began with ancient civilizations such as those of the Egyptians and Greeks, who captured their ideals of beauty in art. Subsequently, Greek artists and philosophers began analyzing their perceptions of beauty and establishing standards for ideal facial proportions. The classical Greek canons of facial balance influenced anatomic scholars of the Renaissance period, and many of these, with modifications, are still embraced as the basic foundations for aesthetic facial analysis today. The Greeks, followed by Leonardo da Vinci in the 15th century, advanced the notion of facial harmony existing when the proportions of the upper, middle, and lower facial thirds were roughly equal.

Further anatomic studies have equated facial aesthetics with mathematical formulas and ratios the better to quantify ideal facial relationships. Ricketts (26) supported the Greek concept that facial balance and attractiveness are related to the repetition of proportions throughout the face. The ideal or "divine" proportion is the mathematical ratio of 1:1.618 (phi), which was believed to be the rate of mathematical progression most pleasing to the eye. The ratio refers to the point along a line at which the ratio of the smaller portion to the larger portion is the same as the ratio of the larger portion to the original line (Fig. 168.2) (27).

$$A \quad B \quad C \qquad \frac{AB}{BC} = \frac{AC}{AB} = 1.618(\phi)$$

Figure 168.2 When the ratio of the long segment to the short segment (*AB/BC*) is the same as the ratio of the whole line to the long segment (*AC/AB*), the ratio is equivalent to the divine ratio, phi (1.618). (Adapted from Ricketts RM. Divine proportions in facial esthetics. *Clin Plast Surg* 1982;9:401–422, with permission.)

Farkas et al. (28) performed detailed anthropometric studies of different ethnic populations to assess the validity of the classical Greek canons for beauty and determined multiple "normal" values for various facial proportions. Absolute numeric values, of course, are less important than the relationships and harmony among various aesthetic units. Measurement and memorization of multiple normal values are cumbersome and quickly become impractical for everyday use by aesthetic surgeons.

Modern science has defined beauty as a biologic and cross-cultural concept of attractiveness. In one study (29), infants prefered looking at faces adults perceived as aesthetically pleasing. Other studies (30) note a preference for symmetry in facial architecture (31,32). Another (33) found that test subjects preferred a composite of attractive faces to a composite of average faces, which was true across ethnic boundaries. Qualities found attractive in females included high cheekbones, a thinner jaw, large eyes, and a shorter vertical third of the face. Ethnic differences in aesthetic ideals, however, must be considered during facial analysis to avoid inappropriate "westernization" of ethnic features (34–38).

DEFINING TERMS

Anatomic landmarks are used for analysis of facial characteristics (Fig. 168.3). On the frontal view of the face, the trichion (Tn) marks the superior margin of the forehead, at the frontal hairline. The nasion (N) is the depression at the root of the nose corresponding to the nasofrontal suture. The radix (R) is the root of the nose, part of the continuous curve descending from the superior orbital brow to the lateral nasal wall. The subnasale (Sn) is the junction of the columella and the upper lip at the nasal base. The mucocutaneous junctions of the upper and lower lips are called the superior and inferior vermilion border (Vs and Vi). The stomion (St) is the embrasure of the lips. The menton (M) is the lower border of the soft-tissue contour of the chin.

On lateral view, the glabella (G) is the most prominent point in the midsagittal plane of the forehead. The rhinion (Rh) is the junction of the bony and cartilaginous nasal dorsum, usually the point of maximal prominence of the nasal dorsum. The tip-defining point (Tp) is the anteriormost projection of the nasal tip, corresponding to the dome of the lower lateral cartilages. The columellar point (Cm) is the anteriormost soft-tissue point of the nasal columella. Laterally, the alar crease (A) is the most posterior aspect of the nose. On the chin, the mentolabial sulcus

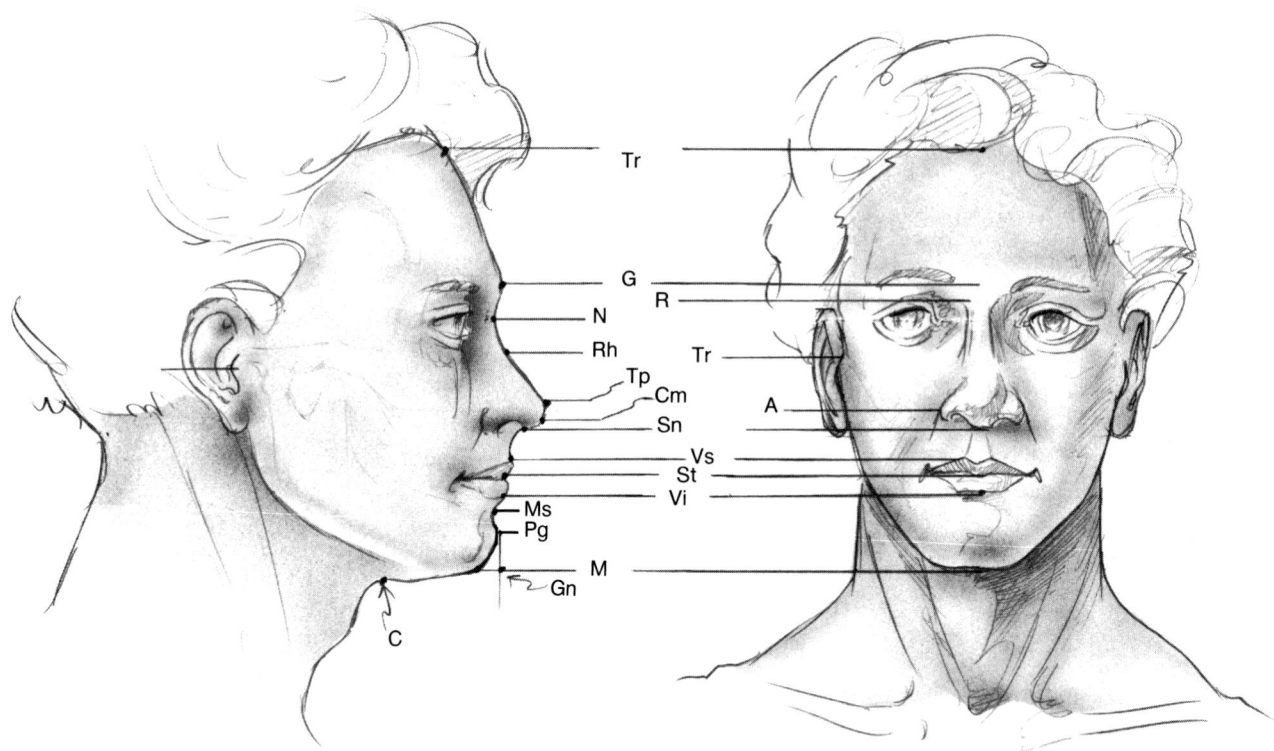

Figure 168.3 Basic anatomic landmarks for facial analysis. See text for explanation.

(Ms) is the point of depression between the lower lip and chin, and the pogonion (P) represents the most prominent anterior projection of the chin. The gnathion (Gn) is a point derived from determining the junction of the line tangent to the pogonion and the line tangent to the menton. The cervical point (C) is the junction of the line tangent to the anterior margin of the neck and the line tan-gent to the menton. Finally, the tragion (Tr) is the point at the supratragal notch of the ear.

Many reference planes and angles have been developed to qualify and define interfacial relations on profile view (Fig. 168.4). The nasofrontal angle (NFA) measures the obtuse angle at the nasion, formed by lines through the glabella and the nasal dorsum (G-N-Tp). The nasofacial

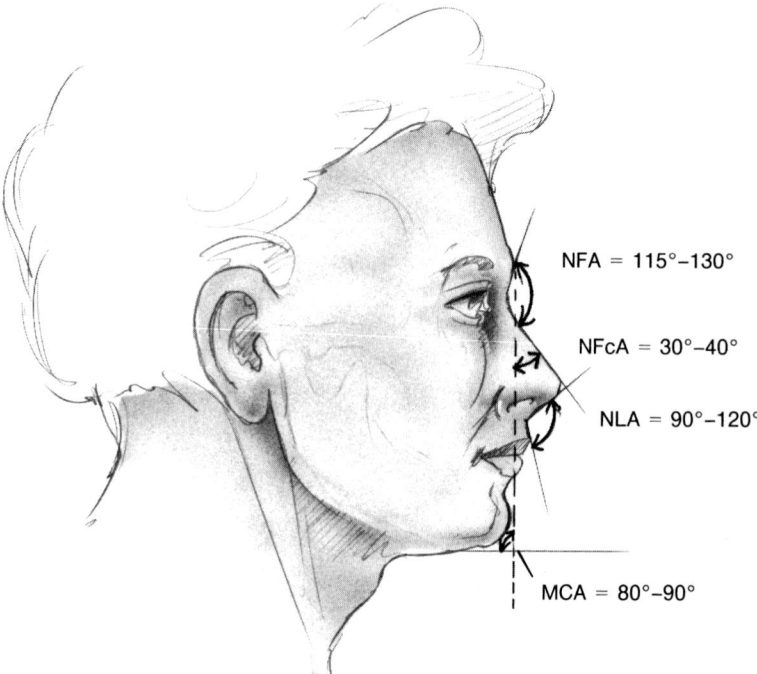

Figure 168.4 Profile angles for facial analysis. See text for explanation.

angle (NFcA) measures the angle of inclination of the nasal dorsum from the anterior face. The nasolabial angle (NLA) measures the inclination between the nasal columella and upper lip (Cm-Sn-Vs). The mentocervical angle (MCA) measures the angle at the gnathion (Pg-Gn-M). The Frank-fort horizontal is a reference line that is used primarily for cephalometric analysis. It is drawn from the superior margin of the external auditory canal on lateral radiographs to the inferior border of the infraorbital rim. For ease of reproducibility using lateral patient photographs, a true horizontal line that is drawn through the tragion is more frequently used by aesthetic surgeons.

General Facial Assessment

The simplest methods of facial analysis, using soft-tissue landmarks, are fraught with inaccuracy, but they are easiest to remember and are therefore the most practical for the beginning surgeon. Basic tenets of facial analysis include assessment for overall symmetry and proportion of the face. The major aesthetic masses of the facial architecture are considered both individually and in relation to the rest of the face. These include the forehead, eyes, nose, lips, cheeks, and jawline. In addition, the ears, neck, and dental occlusal relations should be considered. Each of these separate features affects the aesthetic impact of the others, and therefore the relations between them can be evaluated to quantify better the aesthetic ideal.

On the frontal view, the symmetry of the face is assessed about the vertical midline, and the width-to-length ratio of the face should approximate a 3:4 ratio. Further assessment of symmetry and proportion can be accomplished by dividing the face into fifths vertically, with each fifth approximating one eye width (Fig. 168.5).

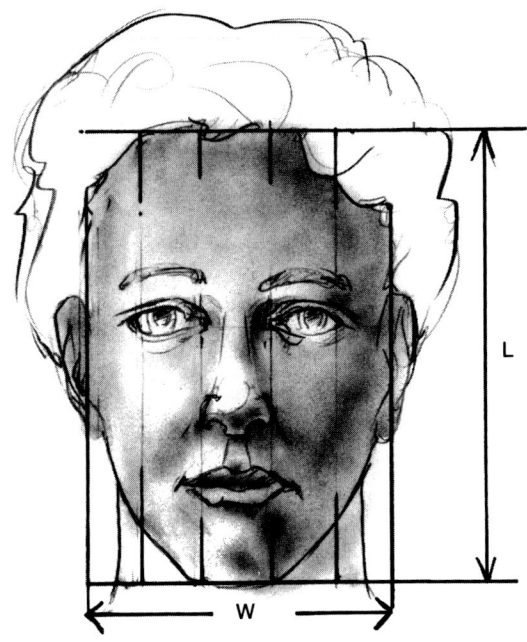

Figure 168.5 Ideal frontal symmetry and proportion. The width-to-length ratio should approximate 3:4.

Facial height is evaluated by dividing the face into thirds horizontally, with the upper third extending from trichion to glabella, the middle third from glabella to subnasale, and the lower third from subnasale to menton. Because the trichion is variable because of receding of the hairline in some men, the upper extent of frontalis muscle movement also can be used to mark the upper facial third. The lower face also can be divided into thirds, with the upper lip length from subnasale to stomion equaling one third and the lower lip and chin encompassing two thirds (Fig. 168.6).

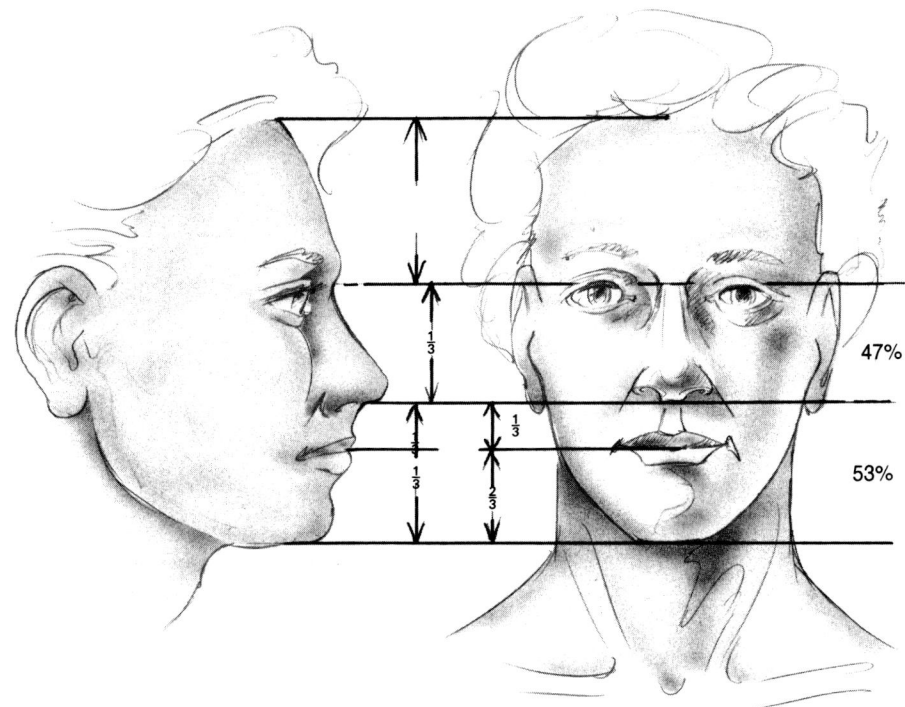

Figure 168.6 The facial thirds: trichion to glabella, glabella to subnasale, subnasale to menton. The lower face also is divided into thirds: The upper lip from subnasale to stomion is one third, and the lower lip and chin is two thirds. The face from nasion to subnasale is 47% and from subnasale to menton is 53% of the total height from nasion to menton. (From Powell N, Humphries B. *Proportions of the aesthetic face.* New York: Thieme-Stratton, 1984, with permission.)

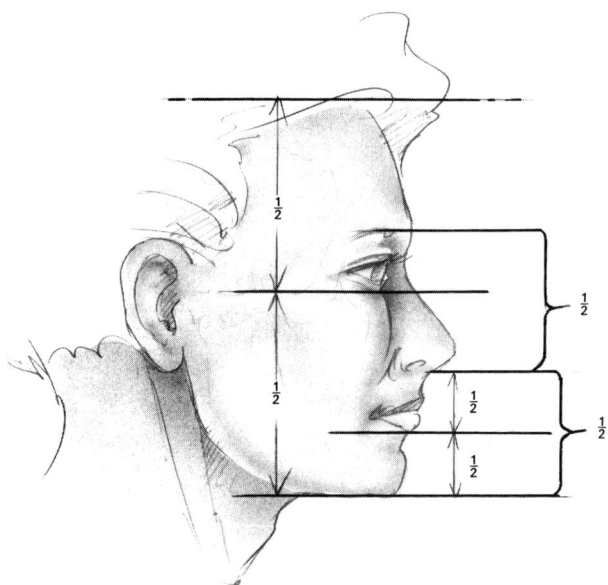

Figure 168.7 An alternate method of estimating vertical proportion. The eyes should rest on a horizontal line dividing the face in half. The subnasale should lie halfway between the brow and menton, and the lower vermilion should be halfway between the subnasale and menton.

An alternative method for quickly assessing vertical height involves dividing the face in half horizontally. The eyes should lie on this line. The subnasale should be on a line drawn halfway between the eyebrow and chin, and the lower-lip vermilion border should lie on a line halfway between the subnasale and chin (Fig. 168.7).

On profile view, the face is assessed for degree of convexity. Ideally, the anterior facial plane visualized from the forehead to the chin is straight. It may be convex, with a sloping forehead and retrusive chin, or concave, with a retrusive maxilla, as in a "dish-face" deformity. Gonzales-Ulloa (39) defined the aesthetic profile in relation to a line perpendicular to the Frankfort horizontal passing through the nasion. The outline of the midforehead, subnasale, upper and lower lips, and pogonion should rest on this line (Fig. 168.4).

Forehead

The basic anatomy of the forehead is seldom altered surgically, so it is a good reference point from which to assess the remainder of the face. The forehead makes up the upper third of the face, extending from the trichion to the glabella and superior aspect of the eyebrows laterally. The degree of prominence of the glabella and supraorbital ridge varies by sex. Males have more supraorbital bossing than is desirable in females, who have a more gradual curvature of the upper facial third. Although the forehead may vary in contour, it should be consistent with the rest of the face. A protruding forehead calls more attention to a retrusive chin, and vice versa.

The most important characteristic of the forehead from the surgical standpoint is the NFA. The vertex of the angle

corresponds to the nasion (G-N-Tp). The position of the NFA vertex may vary vertically to effect changes in the nasal length. Ideally, the vertex of the NFA should be located on a horizontal plane level with the superior limbus of the eye. It may, however, be located anywhere between the supraciliary ridge and the medial canthus. Surgically advancing the NFA superiorly will effectively lengthen the nose. The degree of angulation of the NFA should range from 120 to 135 degrees. Deepening of the angle at surgery will make the angle less obtuse and will alter the dorsal nasal profile such that nasal projection is effectively increased.

Eyes

The periorbital region includes the eyebrows, the upper and lower lids, and the globe itself. The size, shape, position, and symmetry of the individual components should be assessed, as well as their relation to the remaining face. Although the position of the orbit itself is seldom changed, except in some of the major craniofacial abnormalities, the contour of the lids and position of the brows may be altered. The interocular, or intercanthal, distance should be approximately equal to the width of one eye, the interpalpebral distance. An alternative method to determine the optimal intercanthal distance is to measure the interpupillary distance (40). Ideally, the intercanthal distance equals to the interpupillary distance (Fig. 168.8).

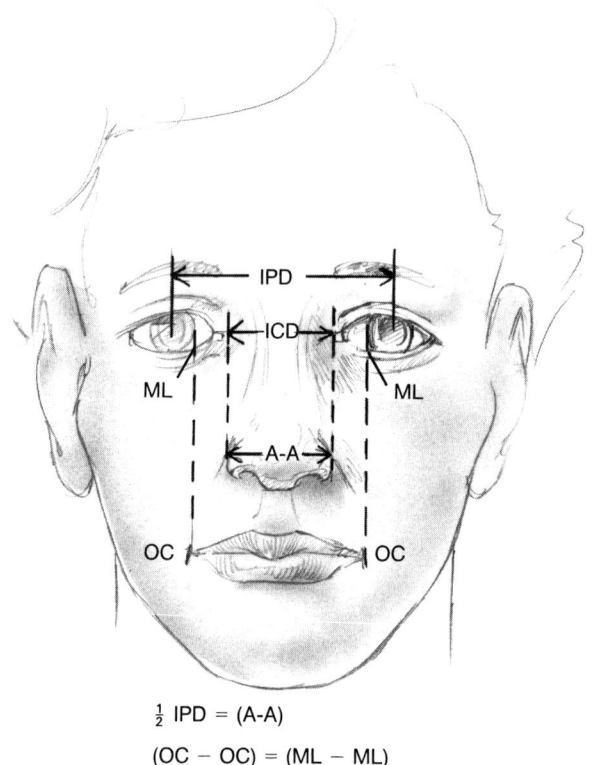

$\frac{1}{2}$ IPD = (A-A)

(OC − OC) = (ML − ML)

Figure 168.8 The alar–alar distance (*A-A*) should equal the intercanthal distance (*ICD*) or half the interpupillary distance (*IPD*). The lateral oral commissure (*OC*) should lie on a vertical line tangent to the medial limbus (*ML*) of the eye. An oblique line parallel to the lateral brow should parallel the vermilion border of the upper lip.

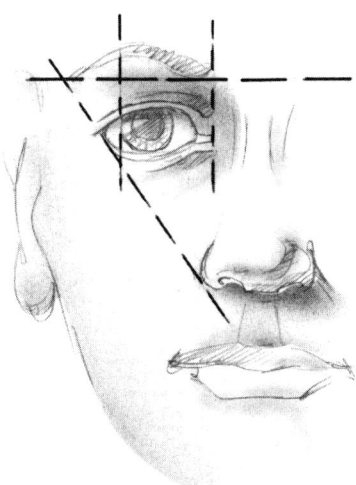

Figure 168.9 The brow should begin along a vertical line tangent to the medial canthus and reach its maximal arch along a vertical line tangent to the lateral limbus. The lateral brow should stop at an oblique line through the alar–facial junction and the lateral canthus. (Adapted from Brennan GH. Correction of the ptotic brow. *Otolaryngol Clin North Am* 1980;13:265–273, with permission.)

In the white patient, the intercanthal distance should also equal the interalar width of the nasal base. The average intercanthal distance is 30 to 35 mm, whereas the average interpupillary distance is 60 to 70 mm.

Brow shape and position vary by sex. The female brow is positioned above the supraorbital rim, with a higher arch, and the male brow is positioned directly over or slightly inferior to the supraorbital rim, with little arch (41). The medial and lateral ends of the brow lie on a horizontal line, and the medial brow begins at the vertical line through the lateral alar crease and the medial canthus (Fig. 168.9). The location of the maximal brow arch should lie on a vertical line tangent to the lateral limbus of the iris, at the junction of the middle third and lateral third of the brow.

The upper eyelid should cover 2 to 3 mm of the superior iris, whereas the lower lid usually lies within 1 to 2 mm of the inferior limbus. The upper lid is larger and more rounded than the lower lid. The oblique line tangent to the lateral lid margin of the upper lid should parallel a line tangent to the superior vermilion border (Fig. 168.9). The junction of the medial and middle thirds of the upper lid marks its most superior point, whereas the junction of the middle and lateral thirds marks the most inferior point of the lower lid. The distance from lash line to lid crease on the upper lid varies from 7 to 15 mm in the non-Asian patient.

Nose

The nose is the most prominent aesthetic mass of the face, certainly of the facial profile, because it is the most anteriorly projecting feature on lateral view. As well, it is positioned in the midline on frontal view, so that nasal asymmetries are readily apparent. Because the nose is the aesthetic mass most frequently altered by plastic surgery, much has been written to define the aesthetic proportions of the nose and its relation to the rest of the face. The overall shape and proportions of the face, as well as the body habitus of the patient, affect the ideal proportions of the nasal characteristics. A long thin nose on a short wide face would seem disproportionate; likewise, a short wide nose would not be desirable on a thin tall individual with a long face.

On frontal view, nasal characteristics to consider include nasal width, symmetry, and the presence of any dorsal nasal curvature or deviation. Desirable nasal width from alar groove to alar groove has been described as equaling 70% of the nasal length from nasion to tip-defining point. Wider interalar distances are acceptable in Asian and black patients.

Nasal Profile

Nasal parameters to consider on profile view include the overall contour of the nasal profile, the projection and rotation of the nasal tip, and the nasal length. The extent of protrusion of the rhinion from the anterior facial plane determines the degree of apparent nasal "hump" or sloop deformity. Ideally, the dorsal nasal profile should be relatively straight, although a slight prominence at the rhinion is acceptable. Fullness in the supratip region causes a polly-beak deformity.

Tip projection is the extent of protrusion of the nasal tip from the anterior facial plane, especially as seen on lateral view of the face. Rotation is the degree of inclination of the NLA. The NLA has its vertex at the subnasale and is formed by the intersection of a line tangent to the columellar point through the subnasale (Cm-Sn), with a line drawn from the subnasale to the upper vermilion border (Sn-Vs) (Fig. 168.4). The NLA usually measures 90 to 105 degrees in males and 100 to 120 degrees in females. Usually, more rotation is acceptable in shorter individuals than in taller ones. Length is defined as the distance along the dorsum of the nose from nasion to tip-defining point. All three parameters interact such that increasing the rotation effectively increases the projection but decreases the nasal length (42) (Fig. 168.10).

Tip Projection

Although most authors agree on the accuracy of the aforementioned methods for assessing rotation and length of the nose, various methods have been proposed for defining and measuring nasal tip projection. Actual measurement of projection may begin from the subnasale, the alar-facial groove, or a line drawn through the nasion or glabella, depending on the method chosen. Because much controversy exists regarding the optimal method for directly measuring nasal tip projection, the NFcA is frequently used to evaluate indirectly the degree of tip projection. Brown and McDowell (43) determined the NFcA by intersecting a line drawn from the glabella to the pogonion,

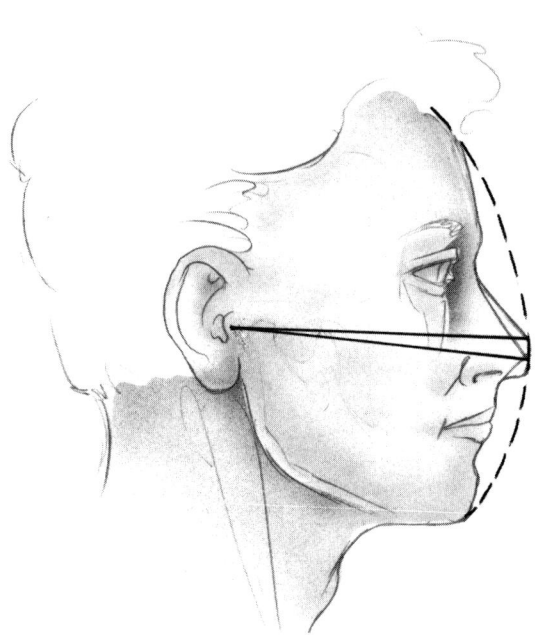

Figure 168.10 The apparent projection of the nose increases with increased rotation, whereas the apparent length decreases with increased rotation. (Adapted from Simons RL. Nasal tip projection, ptosis and supratip thickening. *J Ear Nose Throat* 1982;61: 452–455, with permission.)

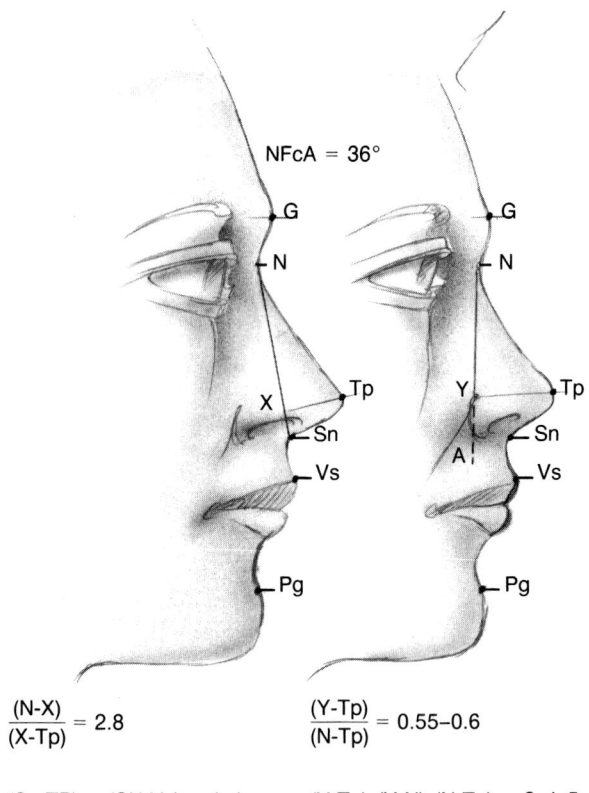

$$\frac{(N\text{-}X)}{(X\text{-}Tp)} = 2.8 \qquad\qquad \frac{(Y\text{-}Tp)}{(N\text{-}Tp)} = 0.55\text{--}0.6$$

$$(Sn\text{-}TP) = (SN\text{-}Vs) = 1\!:\!1 \qquad (Y\text{-}Tp)\!:\!(Y\text{-}N)\!:\!(N\text{-}Tp) = 3\!:\!4\!:\!5$$

Figure 168.11 Assessment of nasal projection. **A:** The Powell and Humphries (11) tip projection–to–nasal height ratio. By using a line from nasion (*N*) to subnasale (*Sn*), the ratio of projection (*X-Tp*) to height (from *N-X*) should be 2.8:1. Simons (13) suggested that the projection (*Sn-Tp*) should equal upper lip length (*Sn-Vs*). **B:** The Goode method. Projection-to-length ratio should equal 0.55 to 0.6:1. Crumley and Lancer (12) described a right triangle with projection to height (from *N-A*) to length equaling 3:4:5.

with a line tangent to the nasal dorsum (Fig. 168.4). It is widely accepted in the literature that the NFA is optimal at 36 degrees.

The ideal relation between tip projection and nasal height is defined by Powell and Humphries (44) as a 2.8:1 ratio (Fig. 168.11), where height is measured from nasion to subnasale, and tip projection is measured by a line drawn perpendicular to the first line through the tip-defining point. This method, however, disregards the effect of alar length on apparent tip projection.

Goode's method of assessing tip projection takes into account the distance from the alar groove to the tip and relates this measurement of tip projection to the length of the nasal dorsum. A right triangle is created by drawing lines from the nasion to the alar-facial groove; a second line perpendicular to this through the tip-defining point, which measures tip projection; and a line from the nasion to the tip, which measures nasal length. With this method, the ideal ratio of tip projection to nasal length is 0.55 to 0.6:1. This method is taken one step further by Crumley and Lancer (45), who defined the relation of tip projection, nasal length, and vertical height as a right triangle whose sides have a 3:4:5 ratio. With these parameters, the NFA will approximate the ideal 36 degrees (Fig. 168.11).

The simplest method of assessing tip projection is that of Simons (46), who relates projection, as measured from the tip-defining point to the subnasale, to the length of

the upper lip, as measured from the subnasale to the vermilion border. He suggested that tip projection and the length of the upper lip should be approximately equal (Fig. 168.11). Although this can be used to get a quick estimate of ideal tip projection, especially in the operating room, considerable variability exists in upper lip length, making this an unpredictable rule for assessment of tip projection.

Nasal Base

As visualized on base view, the nose should have the appearance of an equilateral triangle, with the columella dividing it into two right triangles (47). The columella-to-lobule ratio should approximate 2:1, and the lobular width should equal 75% of the entire nasal base width (Fig. 168.12). The nostrils should be slightly pear shaped, with the widest portion toward the nasal base. On lateral view of the base, the ala-to-lobule ratio should be 1:1, and there should be 2 to 4 mm of columellar show.

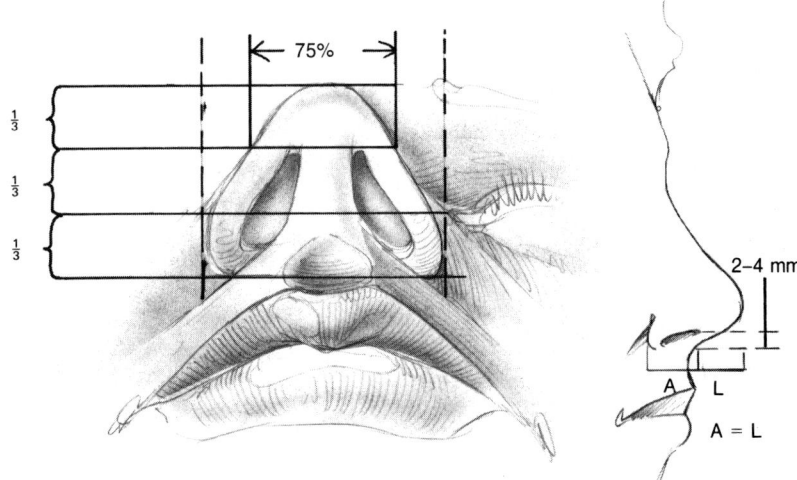

Figure 168.12 The width of the nasal lobule should be 75% of the width of the nasal base. The lobule-to-columella ratio should be 1:2. On lateral view, the ala-to-lobule ratio should be 1:1, and there should be 2 to 4 mm of columellar show.

Malar Region

The prominence of the malar bones is essential to the attractiveness of the face. On frontal view, the face is widest at the level of the zygomatic arches. Two prominent highlights should be evident on frontal view of the cheeks: the malar eminence anterolaterally and the zygomaticus, which is the most prominent point on the zygomatic arch posteriorly. The degree of prominence is related to both the underlying bony structure and the overlying soft tissue. The prominence of the malar eminence is highlighted by the inferior hollow of the cheek at the anterior border of the masseter. On frontal view, the prominence should lie within the space formed between lines drawn from the nasal ala to the tragus and from the oral commissure to the lateral canthus (48).

Chin and Neck

Although the chin itself extends from the mentolabial sulcus to the menton, any alterations in the chin will affect the lower lip and neck profile, so they are generally considered together. As noted previously, the ratio of the chin and lower lip length to that of the upper lip should be 2:1. Protrusion or retrusion of the chin is assessed on the profile view and is most easily estimated by dropping a vertical line from the lower vermilion border of the lip. This line should be tangent to the pogonion in males and up to 2 to 3 mm anterior to the pogonion in females. The mentolabial sulcus should lie 4 mm posterior to a vertical line drawn from the lower vermilion border to the pogonion. In evaluating the chin and lips, the state of the dental occlusion must be considered, including the inclination of the incisors and the relation of the dental arches.

The neck length from menton to suprasternal notch should be approximately half of the head height from vertex to menton. The relation of the neck to the chin was evaluated by Legan and Burstone (49) with the lower face–throat angle. The vertex of this angle is at the gnathion and

is formed by the intersection of a line from subnasale to pogonion (Sn-Gn), with a line tangent to the menton through the cervical point (Gn-C). The ratio of the vertical height Sn-Gn to horizontal depth Gn-C is used to evaluate the balance between the lower facial third and the submental depth (Fig. 168.13). Because this angle does not define the position of the chin and neck in relation to the upper face, Powell and Humphries (44) used the MCA to

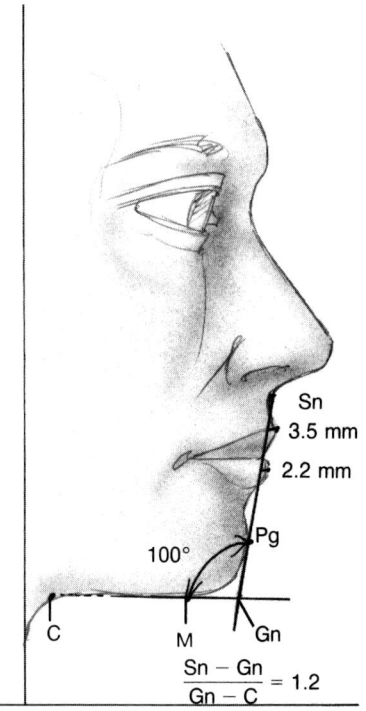

Figure 168.13 The most anterior point of the upper lip should be 3.5 mm, and that of the lower lip should be 2.2 mm, from the Sn-Pg line. Legan and Burstone (16) described the lower face–throat angle (Sn-Gn-C), which should be 100 degrees. The lower facial height (Sn-Gn) to depth (Gn-C) ratio should equal 1.2:1.

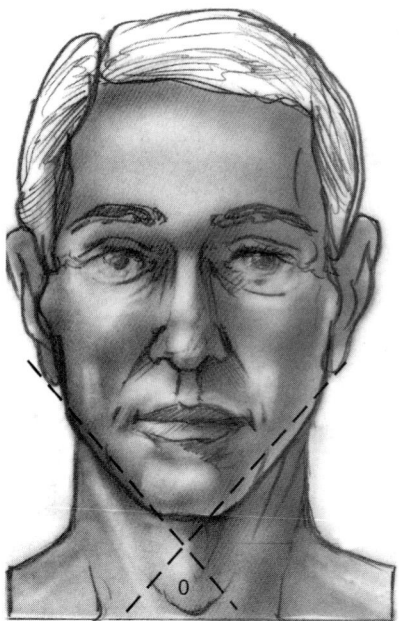
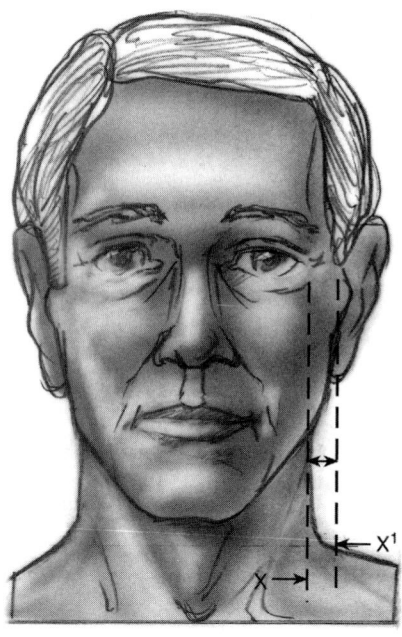

Figure 168.14 The lines of mandibular divergence and the degree of soft-tissue gonion projection compared with the lateral neck projection, bizygomatic width, and bitemporal width.

define the ideal chin-to-neck relation based on the facial profile. The vertex of this angle is at the intersection of a line drawn from glabella to pogonion, with a line drawn through the cervical point and menton (Fig. 168.4).

Jawline and Mandibular Angle

The importance of the jawline, and particularly the posterior jawline, has been frequently overlooked in discussions of facial harmony and aesthetics. The inferior border of the face must complement the chin and other facial features already discussed. Assessment of the jawline should include an evaluation of its contour and symmetry and its relation to facial width as defined by the bizygomatic and bitemporal widths. Ideally, the lines of mandibular divergence should form straight lines from soft-tissue menton to soft-tissue gonion (Fig. 168.14). The projection of the soft-tissue gonion on frontal view should exceed the lateral tissue plane of the neck by 12 to 18 mm (50). In addition, the bizygomatic width should be greater than the bitemporal width, which should exceed the bigonial width. A tangent line connecting the lateral contour of the zygoma to the soft-tissue gonion should form an angle of 5 to 10 degrees with the true vertical. On lateral view, the mandibular angle should be well defined, with proportionate ramus height and ramus-to-body transition

Lips

Any evaluation of the lips has to take into consideration the relation between the lips and the chin, nasal base, premaxilla, and dental occlusion. Abnormalities of these structures will affect the position of the lips. The vertical length of the upper lip from subnasale to stomion should

equal one third of the lower facial third, whereas the lower lip and chin from stomion to menton should compose two thirds of the lower facial third. On lateral view, the upper lip is somewhat fuller than the lower lip and should protrude just slightly anterior to it. The horizontal position of the lip can be evaluated by measuring the distance from a line drawn from subnasale to pogonion (Sn-Pg) (51). Both lips should be anterior to this line, with the upper lip protruding 3.5 mm and the lower lip protruding 2.2 mm (Fig. 168.13).

On frontal view, the lateral aspect of the oral commissures should lie along a vertical line tangent to the medial limbus of the iris (Fig. 168.8). The interlabial gap and the degree of incisor exposure at rest are important in the evaluation of vertical face height. The upper lip and lower lip should just meet with the teeth in occlusion and the lips relaxed, with no more than a 3-mm interlabial gap. No more than 2 mm of the maxillary incisal edge should show with the lips in repose, and no more than two thirds of the maxillary incisor should be exposed on full smile (52). Gingival show on smiling is undesirable.

Ears

The location and orientation of the auricle become especially important when dealing with reconstruction of congenital microtia or after traumatic loss of the ear but are also of consideration for patients with prominauris. Superiorly, the top of the helix should be on a horizontal line with the lateral eyebrow. The inferior attachment of the ear lobe should be at the level of the alar–facial junction. The width-to-length ratio should be approximately 0.6:1. On lateral view, the longitudinal axis of the ear is posteriorly inclined approximately 20 degrees off the vertical (53). Likewise, the angle of protrusion of the ear from the posterior scalp should approximate 20 degrees.

Dental Occlusion

Angle's classification of dental occlusion describes the horizontal relation of the two dental arches. Because this relation affects the contour of the face, a basic understanding is essential for the facial plastic surgeon. These classifications are easiest to remember by referencing the relation of the mandible to the maxilla. Dental relations are classified as mesial (toward the midline of the dental arch), distal (away from the midline of the dental arch),

buccal (toward the cheek), and lingual (toward the tongue). Class I is normal occlusion defined as having the mesiobuccal cusp of the maxillary first molar in occlusion with the buccal groove of the mandibular first molar (Fig. 168.15). If the mandible is retrusive in relation to the maxilla (retrognathic), class II occlusion exists. In this case, the buccal groove of the mandibular first molar will lie distal to the mesiobuccal cusp of the maxillary first molar. If the mandible is protrusive relative to the maxilla (prognathic), then class III occlusion exists. In this case, the buccal groove of the mandibular first molar will lie mesial to the mesiobuccal cusp of the maxillary first molar.

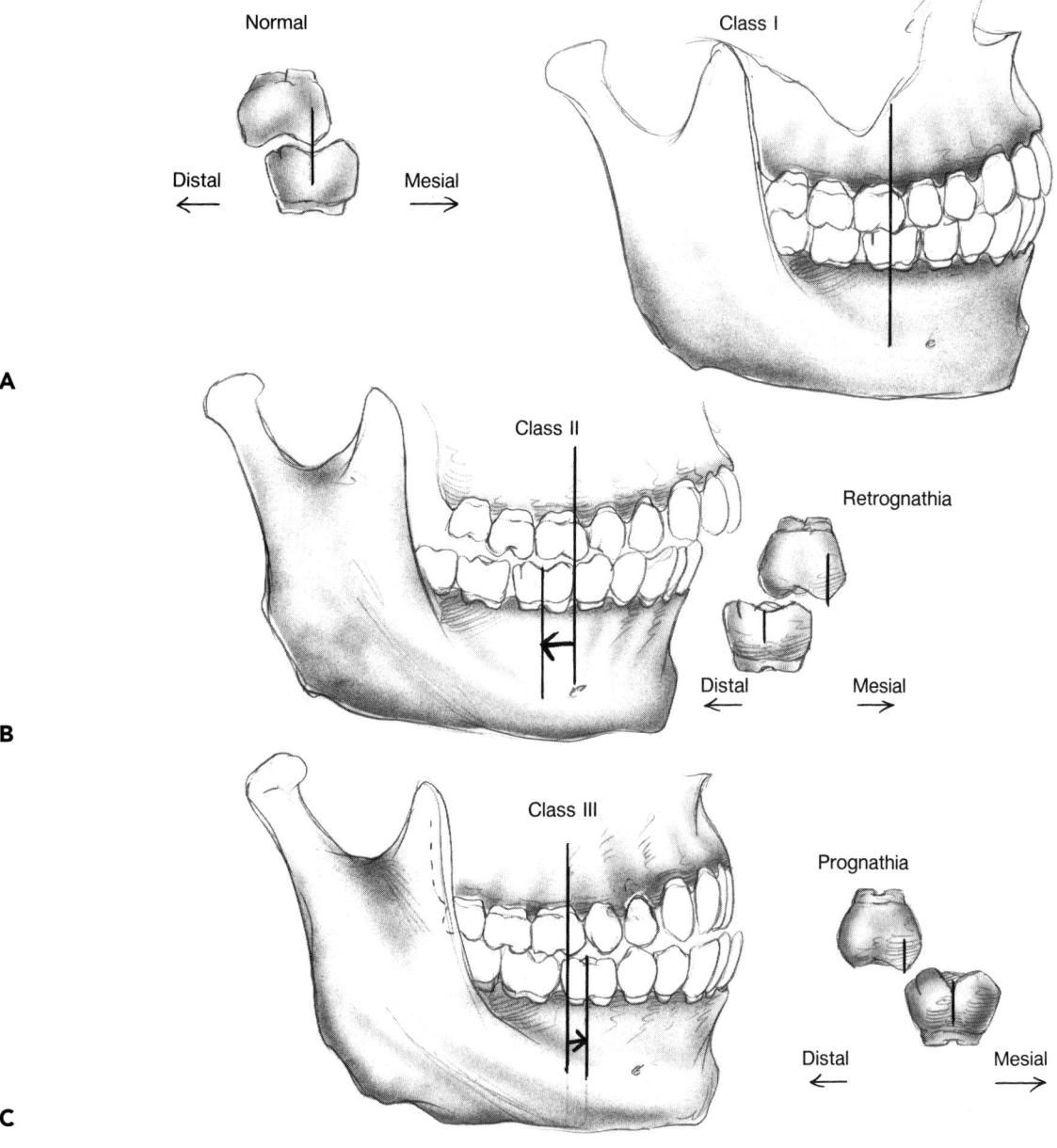

Figure 168.15   The first molar relations in Angle's classifications of occlusion (see text for explanation). **A:** Class I occlusion (orthognathic). **B:** Class II occlusion (retrognathic). **C:** Class III occlusion (prognathic).

Methods of Facial Analysis

Cephalometrics

Orthodontists and oral maxillofacial surgeons have favored the use of cephalometric analysis to plan treatment and evaluate their results. This method involves measurement of the maxillary, mandibular, and dental relations on tracings of bony and soft tissues on lateral radiographs of the face and skull base. A cephalostat is used to hold the head in a fixed reproducible position to take the radiographs. Once obtained, soft-tissue and skeletal landmarks are traced to plot multiple points, lines, and angles, which are then used to evaluate the anterior–posterior position of the jaws and teeth in reference to the cranium and each other. Six major relations have been described (54): maxilla to cranium, mandible to cranium, maxilla to mandible, maxillary teeth to maxilla, mandibular teeth to mandible, and maxillary teeth to mandibular teeth. Numerous systems of cephalometric analysis have been proposed; each incorporates a set of reference values for the assorted linear and angular measurements. Although the various measurements required in this method are elaborate and somewhat time consuming and labor intensive, it is an excellent method for evaluating craniofacial and orthognathic relations.

Photometrics

Direct consideration of soft-tissue proportions on facial photographs, as opposed to radiographic craniofacial relations, is the method preferred by most facial plastic surgeons. Soft-tissue thicknesses vary depending on the area of the face. In addition, postsurgical skeletal repositioning is not absolutely correlated to a similar change in the overlying soft-tissue contour. Because facial plastic surgeons routinely use photographs and video images to document patient findings and surgical results, it is convenient to use these images to assess facial proportions and compare the pre- and postoperative results. Similar to cephalometrics, multiple angles and ratios between the aesthetic units are calculated based on the photographic profile. Only a few soft-tissue analysis systems are discussed. An excellent summary of several cephalometric and photometric analysis systems can be found in Powell and Humphries (11).

Select Analysis Systems

Peck and Peck (55) described a useful lateral photometric method (Fig. 168.16). Nasal, maxillary, and mandibular angles are measured to establish vertical proportions. The vertex for these angles is at the tragion (Tr), and lines are drawn to the nasion (Tr-N), the tip-defining point (Tr-Tp), the superior vermilion border (Tr-Vs), and the pogonion (Tr-Pg). The nasal angle evaluates vertical nasal height from nasion to nasal tip (N-Tr-Tp), the maxillary angle evaluates maxillary height from nasal tip to the upper lip (Tp-Tr-Vs), and the mandibular angle evaluates the mandibular height from the upper lip to the pogonion (Vs-Tr-Pg). Normal values for these angles and other ratios discussed are included in Table 168.1.

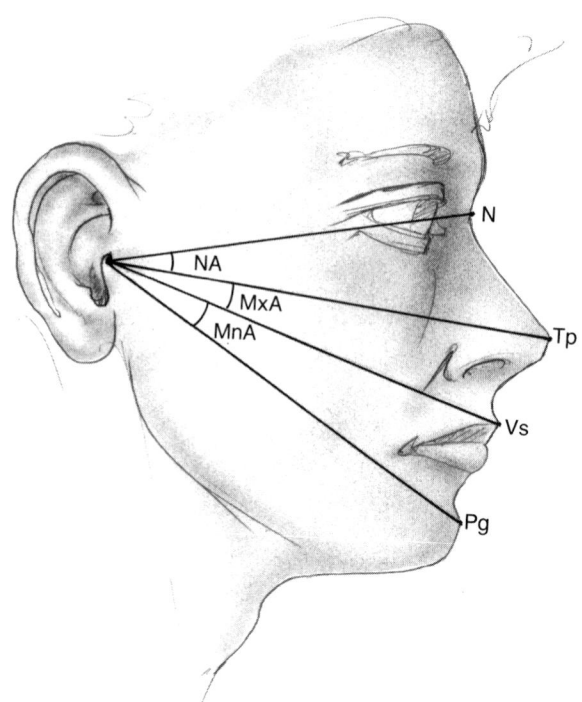

Figure 168.16 The facial angles of Peck and Peck (22). The nasal angle, maxillary angle, and mandibular angles are used to assess facial proportions.

TABLE 168.1

NORMAL VALUES FOR FACIAL ANALYSIS

Vertical facial height [Powell and Humphries (11)]
Nasal height ratio (N-Sn): 47%
Lower facial height ratio (Sn-Gn): 53%
Facial convexity angle (G-Sn, Sn-Pg): 8–16 degrees (12 degrees)

Aesthetic triangle [Powell and Humphries (11)]
Nasofrontal angle (G-N-Tp): 115–130 degrees
Nasofacial angle (G-Pg, N-Tp): 30–40 degrees (36 degrees)
Nasomental angle (N-Tp-Pg): 120–132 degrees
Mentocervical angle (G-Pg, M-C): 80–95 degrees

Facial proportions [Peck and Peck (22)]
Nasal angle (N-Tr-Tp): 20–27 degrees
Maxillary angle (Tp-Tr-Vs): 12–17 degrees
Mandibular angle (Vs-Tr-Pg): 14–20 degrees
Nasal projection (Goode ratio, A-Tp/N-Tp): 0.55–0.6:1
Nasal projection (Powell ratio, Sn-Tp/N-Sn): 2.8:1
Nasolabial angle (Cm-Sn-Vs): 90–120 degrees
Alar-lobule ratio: 1:1
Nasal width = interocular distance = $^1/_2$ interpupillary distance: 30–35 mm
Lower facial third ratio (Sn-St/St-M): 0.5:1
Horizontal projection upper lip (from Sn-Pg): 3.5 mm
Horizontal projection lower lip (from Sn-Pg): 2.2 mm
Mentolabial sulcus (from Sn-Pg): 4.0 mm
Interlabial gap: 0–3 mm
Lower face–throat ratio: 1.2:1

N, nasion; Sn, subnasale; Gn, gnathion; G, glabella; Pg, pogonion; Tp, tip-defining point; M, menton; C, cervical point; Tr, tragion; Vs, superior vermilion border; A, alar crease; Cm, columellar point; St, stomion.

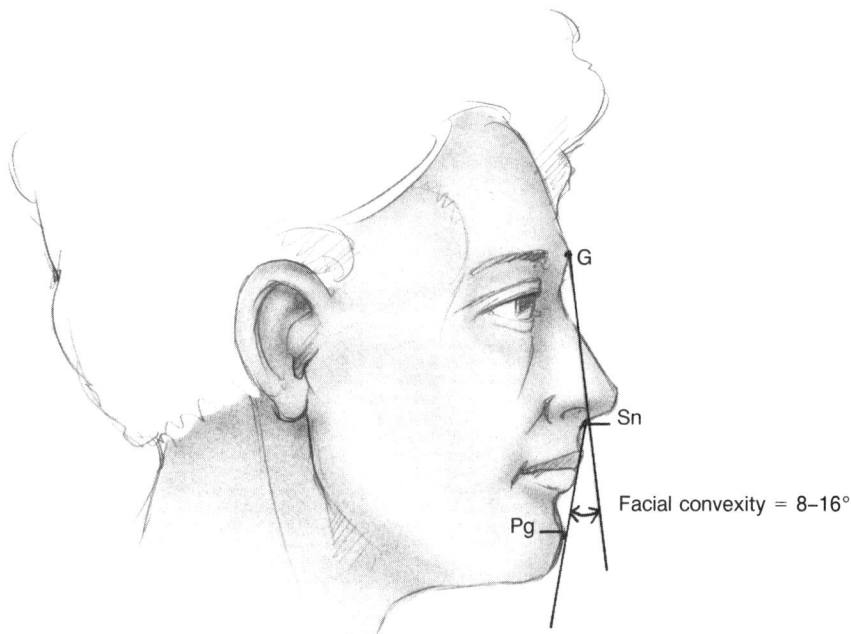

Figure 168.17 The angle of facial convexity of Legan and Burstone (16).

Legan and Burstone (49) used soft-tissue cephalometric analysis to evaluate the degree of facial convexity (Fig. 168.17). The angle of facial convexity is formed by the line drawn through the glabella and subnasale (G-Sn) and the line from the subnasale to pogonion (Sn-Pg). To determine the relative horizontal position of the mid and lower face, a line is dropped perpendicular to the horizontal from the glabella (G). The horizontal distance of the subnasale (Sn) from this line is an indication of maxillary protrusion or retrusion. As well, the horizontal distance of the pogonion (Pg) from this line is an estimate of the degree of mandibular prognathism or retrognathism.

Powell and Humphries (44) contributed their concept of the aesthetic triangle to facial analysis. The important angles in this system are the NFA, NFcA, nasomental angle (NMA), and the MCA. The NMA has its vertex at the nasal tip and is formed by lines drawn from nasion to the tip (N-Tp) and from tip to pogonion (Tp-Pg). Again, the NFcA is formed by the intersection of the G-Pg line with the line tangent to the nasal dorsum, and the MCA is formed by the intersection of the G-Pg line with the M-C line. These angles are used to define the relation of all five major aesthetic masses of the face with reference to the stable forehead and each other (Fig. 168.18).

CONCLUSION

Surgeons can no longer follow the past warnings cautioning that every male patient seeking aesthetic surgery or every rhinoplasty patient should be psychologically evaluated. Most patients seeking aesthetic surgery are well informed about the procedures they seek, and few have hidden motivations. Patients with underlying psychopathology do exist,

and the facial cosmetic surgeon must identify these patients preoperatively. Patients who elicit a negative gut feeling in the surgeon should always be further evaluated.

The best approach to the concerned or dissatisfied postoperative patient is listening. When an actual problem exists, the surgeon should reassure and outline plans for remediation.

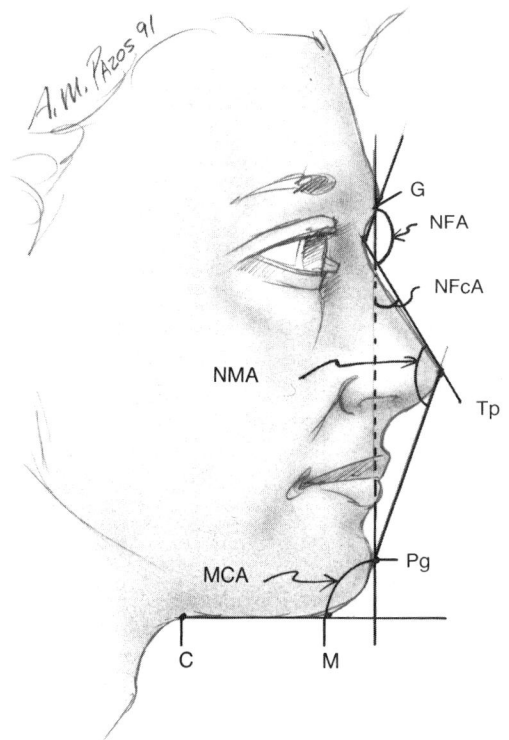

Figure 168.18 The aesthetic triangle of Powell and Humphries (11). Normal values are given in Table 168.1.

Objective analysis of facial balance and proportion is an essential part of preoperative planning before facial plastic surgery. It is important for training surgeons to become practiced at stepwise analysis of facial symmetry and proportion. Overall facial symmetry should be assessed initially, and any existing asymmetries should be pointed out to the patient preoperatively. Before evaluating facial proportions, dental occlusal relations should be considered, including Angle's classification and bite, to identify major occlusal abnormalities. Assessment of vertical facial proportions on frontal and lateral view can then be evaluated by using the rule of facial thirds (Fig. 168.4). Profile analysis is carried out by looking at the horizontal relation of the aesthetic masses to the anterior facial line (G-Pg). The profile can also be assessed by using the angle of facial convexity. Interfacial proportions can subsequently be evaluated by calculating the angles of the aesthetic triangles—the NFA, NFcA, NMA, and MCA angles—and/or the angles of Peck—nasal, maxillary, and mandibular angles.

Separate evaluation of the individual aesthetic masses should include the forehead, eyes, nose, malar region, chin, and jawline, in addition to the lips, neck, and ears. Frontal nasal analysis should include nasal width at the dorsum and base and evaluation of any dorsal curvature or deviation. The nasal base width should approximate the intercanthal distance, and the intercanthal distance should be approximately half of the interpupillary distance. On profile nasal analysis, an assessment of the nasal profile contour, the nasal length, the degree of rotation and the NLA, and the extent of nasal projection are important. Remember that apparent length and projection vary with rotation when planning surgical alterations.

Optimal chin position can be estimated by dropping a vertical line from the lower vermilion. Exact assessment of chin position in relation to the facial profile can be made by determining the MCA or lower face–throat angle. The ratio of the lower facial height to cervical depth also is helpful in evaluating chin projection. The projection of the jawline should be evaluated in relation to the cheeks, the temples, and the lateral neck projection. As well, the line and contour of the mandibular divergence line can be determined on frontal view. Profile analysis of the lips should include the relation to the nasal spine and chin and to the dental occlusion and bite. In the vertical dimension, the upper lip length to lower lip and chin ratio should be 0.5:1. The horizontal lip position can be evaluated by measuring the distance of each lip from the Sn-Pg line.

These measurements can be somewhat cumbersome when carried out by hand on tracings of radiographs or photographs, which discourages the use of in-depth facial analysis on all but the most complicated cases. Fortunately, recent applications of video-analysis computers have made the measurement of the multiple lines, angles, and ratios required for facial analysis much easier and more easily adaptable to routine clinical use. As well, further advances in three-dimensional analysis are on the horizon.

HIGHLIGHTS

- Properly selecting patients for facial plastic surgery is essential to preventing unhappy patients. The surgeon must understand the patient's expectations, whether they are reasonable, and decide whether the surgeon can deliver what the patient expects.
- The concept of facial deformity has changed over the years and is often different from patient to patient or between patient and doctor.
- Approximately half of cosmetic surgery patients display clinically apparent postoperative depression without serious consequences. Schizophrenia is not a contraindication to surgery, but paranoid schizophrenia is. Patients with psychiatric problems need preoperative evaluations, and the surgeon must work closely with the therapist if the operation is to be performed.
- Neurotic patients are usually reasonable candidates for facial aesthetic surgery, but require more support, understanding, and patience from the surgeon than do other patients.
- No matter how excellent the surgeon is, unhappy patients will appear. By listening, the surgeon is neither admitting guilt nor allowing the patient to take control. Allowing the patient to express concerns shows the patient that the surgeon cares. This is an important step in conflict resolution.
- A system of objective measurements rather than subjective assessment is important for presurgical planning. Thorough facial analysis allows the facial plastic surgeon to identify and define specific facial disproportions. Once this is accomplished, accurate determination of surgical goals and the successful correction of those deformities more easily follows.
- Overall facial symmetry should be assessed. Any preexisting asymmetries should be noted and pointed out to the patient. Vertical facial proportions should be assessed on frontal and lateral view by using the rule of facial thirds or the ratio of nasal height to lower facial height (47% N-Sn, 53% Sn-Gn). Abnormalities in the dental occlusal relations should be identified.
- Profile analysis begins with evaluating the horizontal positions of the important aesthetic masses in relation to each other and the anterior facial line and measuring the angle of facial convexity. An evaluation of the interfacial proportions involves calculating the angles of the aesthetic triangle (11) or the facial angles of Peck and Peck (22). The aesthetic triangle angles include the NFA, NFcA, NMA, and MCA. The angles of Peck include the nasal, maxillary, and mandibular angles.
- Evaluation of the individual aesthetic masses should include the forehead, eyes, nose, malar region, chin, and jawline, as well as the lips, neck, and ears.
- Nasal analysis should include profile analysis of the nasal length, tip projection, and rotation and frontal evaluation of any dorsal curvature or deviation, the width of the dorsum, nasal base, and a comparison with the intercanthal distance. Analysis of the lips should include assessment of their relation to the nasal spine, chin, and dentition on profile view. On frontal view, the upper lip

length to lower lip and chin length should be 1:2. Horizontal chin position can be measured by the MCA and the lower face–throat angle. An estimate of the ideal position can be obtained by dropping a vertical line from the lower vermilion. The jawline should be evaluated for its lateral projection and the linearity of its divergence on frontal view, as well as the proportion and contour of the angle and ramus-to-body configuration.

REFERENCES

1. Grossbart TA, Sarwer DB. Psychosocial issues and their relevance to the cosmetic surgery patient. *Semin Cutan Med Surg* 2003;22: 136–147.
2. Maksud DP, Anderson RC. Psychological dimensions of aesthetic surgery: essentials for nurses. *Plast Surg Nurs* 1995;15:137.
3. Sarwer DB, Grossbard TA, Didie ER. Beauty and society. *Semin Cutan Med Surg* 2003;22:79–92.
4. Hilhorst MT. Philosophical pitfalls in cosmetic surgery: a case of rhinoplasty during adolescence. *J Med Ethics: Med Human* 2002; 28:61–65.
5. Pruzinsky T. Psychological factors in cosmetic plastic surgery: recent developments in patient care. *Plast Surg Nurs* 1993;13:64–69.
6. Hasan JS. Psychological issues in cosmetic surgery: a functional overview. *Ann Plast Surg* 2000; 44:89–96.
7. Phillips KA. Body dysmorphic disorder: the distress of imagined ugliness. *Am J Psychiatry* 1991;148:1138.
8. Honigman RJ, Phillips KA, Castle DH. A review of psychosocial outcomes for patients seeking cosmetic surgery. *Plast Reconstr Surg* 2004;113:1229–1237
9. MacGregor FC. Social and psychologic considerations in aesthetic plastic surgery: old trends and new. In: Rees TD, ed. *Aesthetic plastic surgery*. Philadelphia: WB Saunders, 1980:29–39.
10. Thomas JR, Freeman MS, Remmler DJ, et al. Analysis of patient response to preoperative computerized video imaging. *Arch Otolaryngol Head Neck Surg* 1989;115:793.
11. Jacobson WE, Edgerton MT, Meyer E, et al. Psychiatric evaluation of male patients seeking cosmetic surgery. *Plast Reconstr Surg* 1960;26:356.
12 Meyer E, Jacobson WE, Edgerton MT, et al. Motivational patterns in patients seeking elective plastic surgery: women who seek rhinoplasty. *Psychosom Med* 1960;22:193.
13. Meerloo JA. The fate of one's face. *Psychiatry Q* 1956;30:31.
14. Goin MK, Burgoyne RW, Goin JM, et al. A prospective psychological study of 50 female face lift patients. *Plast Reconstr Surg* 1980;65:436.
15. Pertschuk M. Psychosocial considerations in interface surgery. *Clin Plast Surg* 1991;18:11.
16. Wright MR. Management of patient dissatisfaction with results of cosmetic procedures. *Arch Otolaryngol* 1980;106:466.
17. Hinderer UT. Dr. Vasquez Anon's last lesson. *Aesthet Plast Surg* 1978;2:375.
18. Housman SB. Psychological aspects of plastic surgery. In: McCarthy JG, ed. *Plastic surgery*. Philadelphia: WB Saunders, 1990:113–138.
19. Hill G, Silver AG. Psychodynamic and aesthetic motivations for plastic surgery. *Psychosom Med* 1950;12:345.
20. Napoleon A. The presentation of personalities in plastic surgery. *Ann Plast Surg* 1993;31:193.
21. Goin MK, Goin JM. Psychological effects of aesthetic facial surgery. *Adv Psychosom Med* 1986;15:84.
22. Meyer E, Knorr NJ. Psychiatric aspects of plastic surgery. In: Converse J, ed. *Reconstructive plastic surgery*. Philadelphia: WB Saunders, 1977:549–564.
23. Schweitzer I. The psychiatric assessment of the patient requesting facial surgery. *Aust NZ J Psychiatry* 1989;23:249.
24. Wengle HP. The psychology of cosmetic surgery: old problems in patient selection seen in a new way. Part II. *Ann Plast Surg* 1986;6:487–493.
25. Goin JM, Goin MK. *Changing the body: psychological effects of plastic surgery*. Baltimore: Williams & Wilkins, 1981.
26. Ricketts RM. Divine proportions in facial esthetics. *Clin Plast Surg* 1982;9:401–422.
27. Adamson PA,Galli SK. Modern concepts of beauty. *Curr Opin Otolaryngol Head Neck Surg* 2003;11:295–300.
28. Farkas LG, Hreczko TA, Kolar JC, et al. Vertical and horizontal proportions of the face in young adult North American caucasians: revision of neoclassical canons. *Plast Reconstr Surg* 1985;7:328–338.
29. Langlois JH, Roggman LA, Casey RJ, et al. Infant preferences for attractive faces. *Dev Psychol* 1987;23:363–369.
30. Enquist M, Arak A. Symmetry, beauty, and evolution. *Nature* 1994;372:169–172.
31. Penton Voak IS, Jones BC, Little AC, et al. Symmetry, sexual dimorphism in facial proportions and male facial attractiveness. *Proc R Soc Lond* 2001;268:1617–1623.
32. Pearson DC, Adamson PA. The ideal nasal profile: rhinoplasty patients vs the general public. *Arch Facial Plast Surg* 2004;6: 257–262.
33. Perrett DI, May KA, Yoshikawa S. Facial shapes and judgements of female attractiveness. *Nature* 1994;368:239–242.
34. Porter JP, Lee JI. Facial Analysis: maintaining ethnic balance. *Facial Plast Surg Clin North Am* 2003;10:343–349.
35. Erbay EF, Caniklioglu CM. Soft tissue profile in Anatolian Turkish adults: Part II: comparison of different soft tissue analyses in the evaluation of beauty. *Am J Orthod Dentofac Orthop* 2002;121: 65–72.
36. Yehezkel S, Turley PK. Changes in the African American female profile as depicted in fashion magazines during the 20th century. *Am J Orthod Dentofac Orthop* 2004;125:407–417.
37. Choe KS, Sclafani AP, Litner JA, et al. The Korean American Woman's face: anthropometric measurements and quantitative analysis of facial aesthetics. *Facial Plast Surg* 2004;6:244–252.
38. Porter JP. The average African American male face. *Arch Facial Plast Surg* 2004;6:78–81.
39. Gonzales-Ulloa M. Quantitative principles in cosmetic surgery of the face (profile-plasty). *Plast Reconstr Surg* 1962;29:186–198.
40. Holt GR, Holt JE. Nasoethmoid complex fractures. *Otolaryngol Clin North Am* 1985;18:89.
41. Brennan GH. Correction of the ptotic brow. *Otolaryngol Clin North Am* 1980;13:265–273.
42. Simons RL. Nasal tip projection, ptosis and supratip thickening. *J Ear Nose Throat* 1982;61:452–455.
43. Brown JB, McDowell F. *Plastic surgery of the nose*. St. Louis: Mosby, 1951:30–34.
44. Powell N, Humphries B. *Proportions of the aesthetic face*. New York: Thieme-Stratton, 1984.
45. Crumley RL, Lancer R. Quantitative analysis of nasal tip projection. *Laryngoscope* 1988;98:202–208.
46. Simons RL. Adjunctive measures in rhinoplasty. *Otolaryngol Clin North Am* 1975;8:717–742.
47. Bernstein L. Esthetics in rhinoplasty. *Otolaryngol Clin North Am* 1975;8:705–715.
48. Binder WJ, Schoenrock LD, Terino EO. Augmentation of the malar-submalar/midface. *Facial Plast Surg Clin North Am* 1994;2: 265–283.
49. Legan H, Burstone C. Soft-tissue cephalometric analysis for orthognathic surgery. *J Oral Surg* 1980;38:744–751.
50. Taylor CO, Teenier TJ. Evaluation and augmentation of the mandibular angle region. *Facial Plast Surg Clin North Am* 1994;2:329–337
51 Burstone CJ. Lip posture and its significance in treatment planning. *Am J Orthod* 1967;53:262–284.
52. Vig KD, Ellis E. Diagnosis and treatment planning for the surgical-orthodontic patient. *Clin Plast Surg* 1989;16:645–658.
53. Tolleth H. Artistic anatomy, dimensions, and proportions of the external ear. *Clin Plast Surg* 1978;5:337.
54. Khouw FE, Proffitt WR, White RP. Cephalometric evaluation of patients with dentofacial disharmonies requiring surgical correction. *Oral Surg* 1970;29:789.
55. Peck H, Peck S. A concept of facial aesthetics. *Angle Orthod* 1970;40:284–317.

Pictorial Documentation: Traditional Photography and Digital Imaging

169

Samuel M. Lam

Pictorial documentation, whether film or digital based, serves multiple important purposes for the head and neck surgeon: medicolegal documentation, physician–patient communication, lay and professional education, and physician self-education. In particular, the subfield of facial plastic and reconstructive surgery relies heavily on the need for standardized photographs for all of these reasons. Accordingly, this chapter focuses on the principles of good medical photography that relate, for the most part, to cosmetic and reconstructive facial surgery. Nevertheless, all the topics discussed can be easily applied across the broad spectrum of head and neck surgery, as indicated. The emerging, and arguably now well-established, role of digital photography also is reviewed in depth and contrasted against traditional 35-mm photography to help the surgeon decide which format is better suited for his or her practice.

PRINCIPLES OF PHOTOGRAPHY

Rather than divide this section into 35-mm film and digital photography, the basic fundamental tenets that underscore good photography are universally applicable and can be discussed without reference to a chosen format. The primary spotlight will remain on good pre- and postoperative portrait photography, as this subject represents one of the most challenging and vital for the surgeon to undertake correctly. However, some practical tips on quality intraoperative photographs also are outlined.

Informed Consent

Respect for a patient's privacy is of paramount importance for both ethical and legal grounds. Use of patient photography for media or educational purposes should always be preceded with a thorough and explicit written consent. For instance, now with the rise of the Internet as a ubiquitous medium, consent forms should reflect every medium in which the surgeon intends to use the photographs, including print, television, in-office, Internet, etc. The surgeon also can state that the photograph will be used only for educational purposes and restrict the use of those photographs explicitly to scientific lectures or scientific articles or both. Further, the patient may be offered the option to camouflage his or her identity by blackening out the eyes, using only one angle of view, or cropping the image in a certain prescribed way—all of which should be stated clearly in the consent and with which the surgeon should comply. The surgeon also should guarantee in the consent that the patient's name and identity will not be further revealed unless otherwise stipulated by the patient (e.g., as a testimonial).

Standardization

For a photograph to carry any meaningful significance, the photographs must be standardized in the following manner: same photographic media, equipment, and settings; consistent patient positioning and absence of distracting elements (makeup, jewelry, hairstyle); and identical lighting and background. Besides these considerations, the same photographer (physician or staff member) should try to take all of the photographs because slight individual interpretation of these rules can lead to dissimilar photographic results. Before taking the postoperative images, the photographer also should review the preoperative images and then alter the necessary parameters to match the preoperative photographs. For example, if the preoperative oblique view shows that the patient is turned too far laterally, the photographer should try to match the same patient positioning (albeit less than ideal) so that the postoperative image can be meaningfully compared.

Standardized Equipment

Whether the physician ultimately decides to use film or digital media in his or her practice, the same camera should be used for all "before-and-after" photographs to ensure exact reproducibility in the photographic image. In addition, the same camera lens and camera settings (aperture, shutter speed, and exposure values) should be maintained, as any slight deviation can cause a quite obvious disparity in color, contrast, and shadowing. If the surgeon is using film, the exact same film stock also should be used [i.e., the brand, film speed, and type, color reversal (slide, transparency) versus negative, must be preserved].

Standardized Patient Positioning and Related Information

Proper patient positioning is the most demanding aspect of achieving reproducible photographic images. The same camera-to-subject distance must be maintained: this objective can be attained by placing the patient's stool and the camera over prescribed markings on the floor (Fig. 169.1). By using a fixed lens (i.e., a lens that has no "zoom" capacity), the physician also can minimize any distortion and variability caused by altering the focal distance. The Frankfort Horizontal Plane also must be observed: the line that runs from the supratragal point through the inferior orbital rim defines the horizontal plane of the image (Fig. 169.2A–C). The Frankfort Horizontal Plane should be respected in the frontal, oblique, and lateral views. The basal view that is mandatory for rhinoplasty, malar augmentation, and midfacial trauma is defined by aligning the tip of the nose with the infrabrow line (Fig. 169.2D). On the oblique view, the patient should also be turned to a certain angle by one of two methods: (a) align the inner canthus of the eye with the oral commissure, or (b) align the nasal tip with the malar eminence (Fig. 169.2B). Whichever method is chosen, the surgeon should attempt

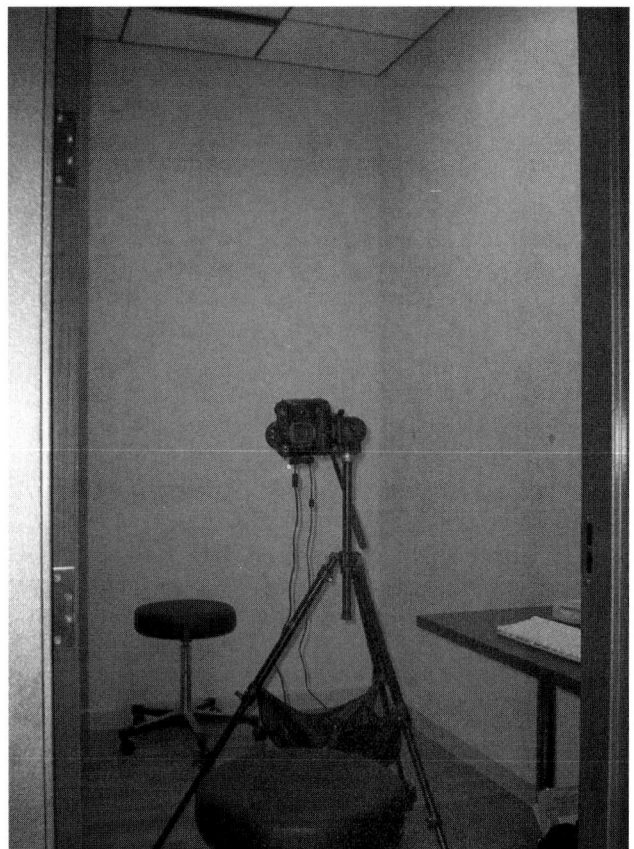

Figure 169.1 Standardized photography requires a dedicated photography room where all pre- and postoperative photographs are taken. A rotating stool with a low back or no back is used to rotate the patient's entire body to the prescribed angle for each view. The digital camera is mounted on a tripod with a quick-release head that can easily adjust from a vertical to a horizontal frame position. In turn, the tripod rests on a rolling dolly to facilitate maneuverability. Markers have been placed on the wall to guide the patient in how far to rotate the body in the oblique and lateral positions. In this setup, the back leg of the patient's stool contacts the wall, and the tripod's center frame is aligned with the edge of the computer table to maintain a standardized camera-to-subject distance. (If flash photography is used, the patient should not be so close to the wall, to avoid harsh background shadows.) The back wall is painted a light blue as a neutral background color.

to rely on the same method for all images. Another reliable technique to ensure that the patient turns to the correct angle each time is to place markers on the wall that indicate where the patient should turn and face for an oblique and lateral view. When turning to the oblique and lateral positions, the patient should rotate the entire body in alignment with the face and not just turn the head to those positions, which creates neck distortion, especially in the lateral view. A rotating stool with a low back (that does not enter the frame of the image) is ideal for this goal.

One of the most common errors encountered is patient positioning with the neck tilted upward and extended, especially in the more mature patient who wants to reduce the appearance of unwanted neck-tissue redundancy. In addition to distortion of the neck, over- or underrotation

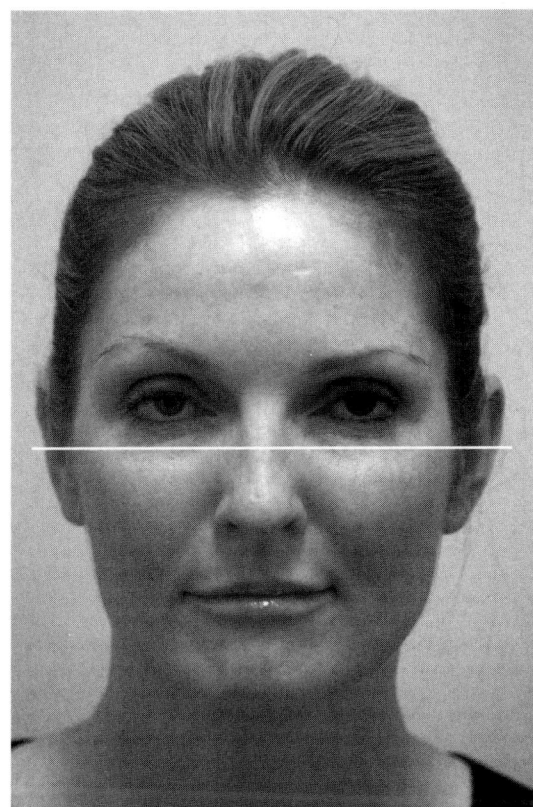
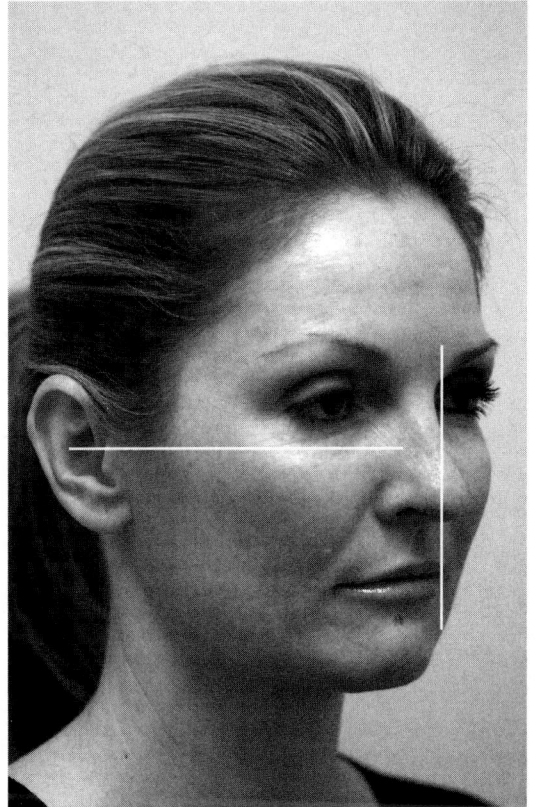
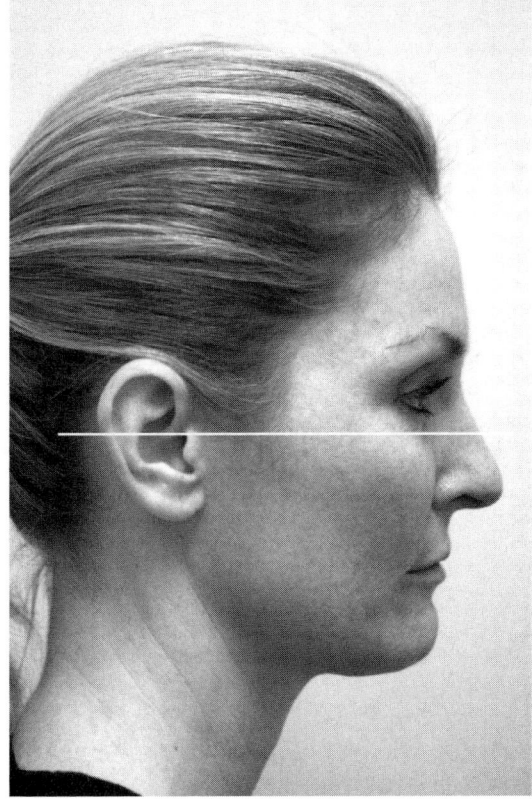
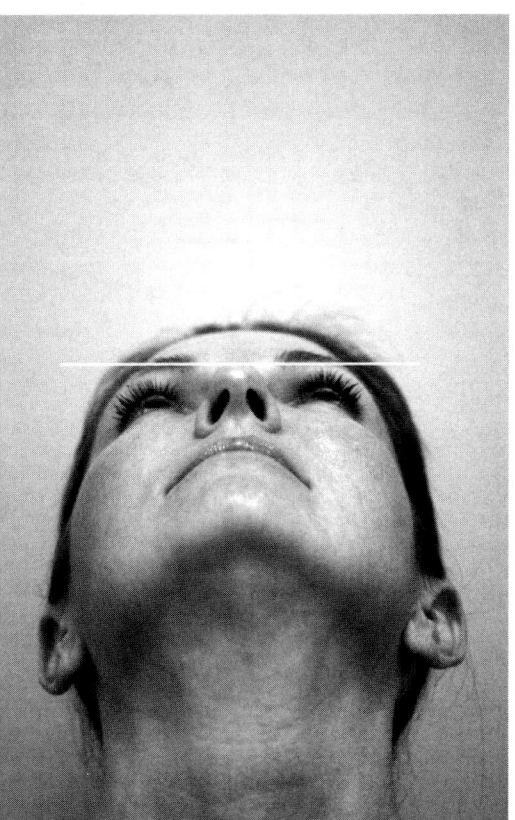

Figure 169.2 Standardized photographic views that show **(A)** frontal, **(B)** right oblique, **(C)** right lateral, and **(D)** basal of the patient. The horizontal lines drawn in **A–C** indicate the Frankfort Horizontal Plane that runs through the supratragal point and the inferior orbital rim, which should be respected. The horizontal line in **D** shows the alignment of the nasal tip with the infrabrow line. The vertical line in **B** shows the alignment of the nasal tip with the malar eminence.

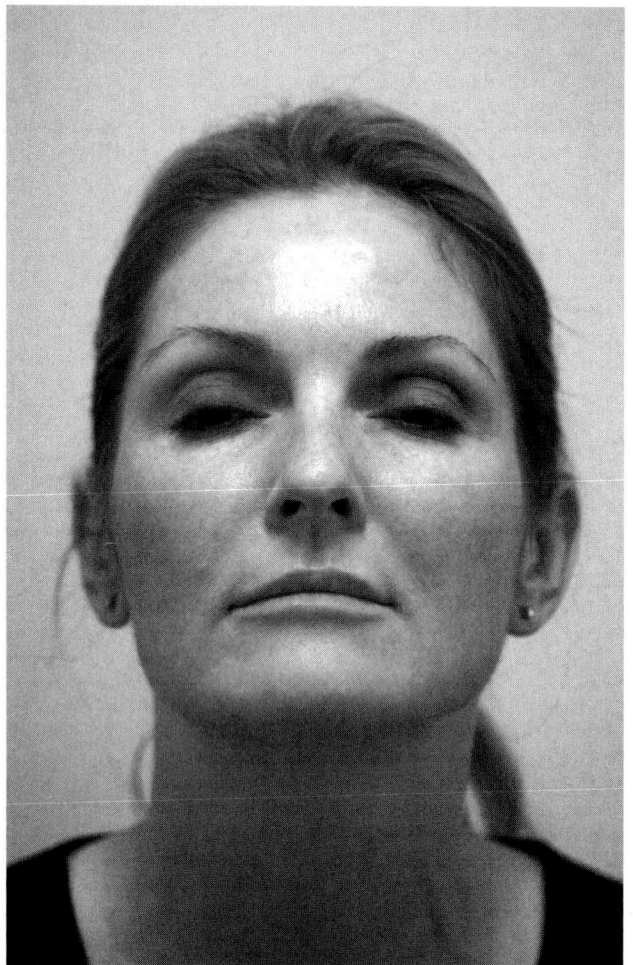 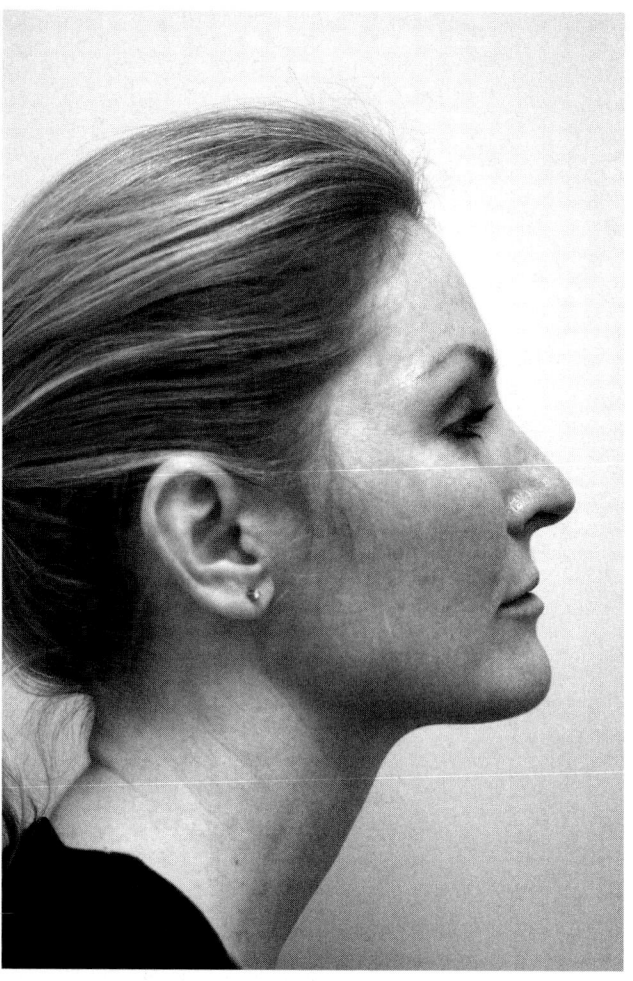

A   B

Figure 169.3 Poor patient positioning is shown with the neck overrotated and extended, which leads to distortion of the neck as well as the nose.

of the neck can cause the nose to appear erroneously rotated or derotated, respectively, and would compromise any photography for rhinoplasty (Fig. 169.3). Patients also may reflexively attempt to lift their brows if they have significant brow ptosis, making the pre- and postoperative result for browlift or upper blepharoplasty less meaningful. If the patient exhibits this behavior, the photographer should ask that the patient close his or her eyes forcefully and slowly open them until they appear fully open. This maneuver will help break the unwitting contribution of the frontalis muscle. The patient also may instinctively smile when posing for a photograph, so the photographer should gently remind the patient that no facial expression should be displayed.

Each type of planned surgical procedure mandates a different set of standardized positions with or without additional optional views (Table 169.1) (1). Besides patient positioning, distracting elements from jewelry, makeup, clothing, and hairstyling should be minimized. All obstructive jewelry (e.g., necklaces and pendulous earrings) should

be removed. Turtlenecks and high-necked collars also can obstruct a straightforward view of the neck and should be pulled down or folded inward to enhance effective communication. All eyeglasses should be removed regardless of what facial surgery is being contemplated. Hairstyling ideally should be pulled back to show an unobstructed view of the eyes, nose, ears, lips, and neck and to be reduced to an unobtrusive element. Shorter hairstyles that do not interfere with any of the major facial features and the neck can be left alone or swept behind the helix of the ear as needed. All makeup should be removed, especially if any dermatologic resurfacing or scar revision is planned.

Lighting and Background

Lighting also is a critical element that should be standardized. Ambient lighting can be used alone or combined with fill lights or flash strobes. If the ambient lighting is too strong and casts a heavy shadow over the patient's facial features, then balanced fill lighting can be used to soften these harsh shadows. Hot lights positioned at 45 degrees in front

TABLE 169.1

RECOMMENDED STANDARDIZED PHOTOGRAPHIC VIEWS FOR SPECIFIC FACIAL PROCEDURES

Procedure	Standardized Views
Botulinum toxin (Botox)	Frontal; frontal smiling: frontal frowning: frontal brow elevation (All photographs are taken before the first session, regardless of what areas will be treated, to enhance patient dialogue should the patient complain, as well as to reduce the need for further photography if the patient desires other areas treated during future sessions.)
Rhinoplasty	Frontal; basal; L/R oblique; L/R lateral; $\pm$ dorsal (head tilted down for a crooked nose) $\pm$ smiling laterally (If the patient has an active depressor septi muscle that alters the nasal tip position during animation.)
Blepharoplasty/Browlift	Frontal; L/R oblique; L/R lateral; closeup (May also take with eyes closed and upward gaze)
Rhytidectomy	Frontal; L/R oblique; L/R lateral
Otoplasty	Frontal; L/R oblique; L/R lateral; posterior; R/L lateral closeup (Remember to tie long hair back in a bun and/or wear a headband to lift away obstructing hair.)
Malar augmentation	Frontal; L/R oblique; L/R lateral; basal
Hair transplant	Frontal; L/R oblique; L/R lateral; posterior; posterior with head tilted back; frontal with head tilted down $\pm$ closeup of anterior/lateral hairline (When photographing the hair, the hair should be styled in a standardized fashion and "comb-overs" eliminated.)
Lip augmentation	Frontal; L/R oblique; L/R lateral; closeup mouth (Remember to remove lipstick, lip liners, and other makeup that can interfere with reproducible photography.)
Scar revision	Frontal; L/R oblique; L/R lateral; closeup (Consider reducing the exposure value to highlight the scar)

on both sides of the patient can be further softened by aiming the lights away toward reflective umbrellas. A "kicker" light placed behind the patient can fill in any remaining shadows cast by the two forward-placed 45-degree lamps and slaved to go off when the camera's shutter is depressed (Fig. 169.4). Placing the patient an appropriate distance away (~2 feet) from the rear wall also can minimize unwanted shadows. Generally, an on-camera flash tends to cause excessive highlights and shadows and a "washed-out" appearance to skin tones, but experimentation will determine the best balance of lighting for a particular room and camera. Rather than use fill lights or strobes, the ambient lighting and the camera's aperture/exposure can be adjusted to achieve the desired lighting objective. Furthermore, the ambient room lighting can be altered to match the color spectrum (e.g., daylight balanced) of the film used or the settings of the camera so that, for example, a green cast from fluorescent lights may be avoided. If shadows and highlights are desired to accentuate a scar or other contour irregularity (e.g., prominent nasolabial lines for correction with a soft-tissue filler), then the balanced fill lights (if used) should be turned off. In addition, the exposure value can be reduced to draw out the intended feature. Obviously, the same settings should be used for the postoperative views.

The background also should be uniform and light in color. Ideally, a powder-blue background is preferred. Too dark a background can swallow the facial features and should be avoided. Rather than hanging a blue drape behind the patient, a smooth wall can be painted the desired blue, as a wall will remain flat and wrinkle free. Again, using the exact same room with the same lighting will aid in achieving reproducible results. Conversely, carrying a portable blue background material from room to room to photograph the patient will most likely lead to subtle, if not obvious, inconsistencies in the photography. If a wall is to be painted blue, it may be wise to record the exact shade of blue, or corresponding numeric code, so that if the physician should have to relocate the photography room in the future, the same blue color can be precisely reproduced.

Intraoperative Photography

Although good pre- and postoperative photography remains the core of this section, proper techniques for superior intraoperative photography should be mentioned herein. Intraoperative photographs can be used to document medicolegally what transpired in the operating theater

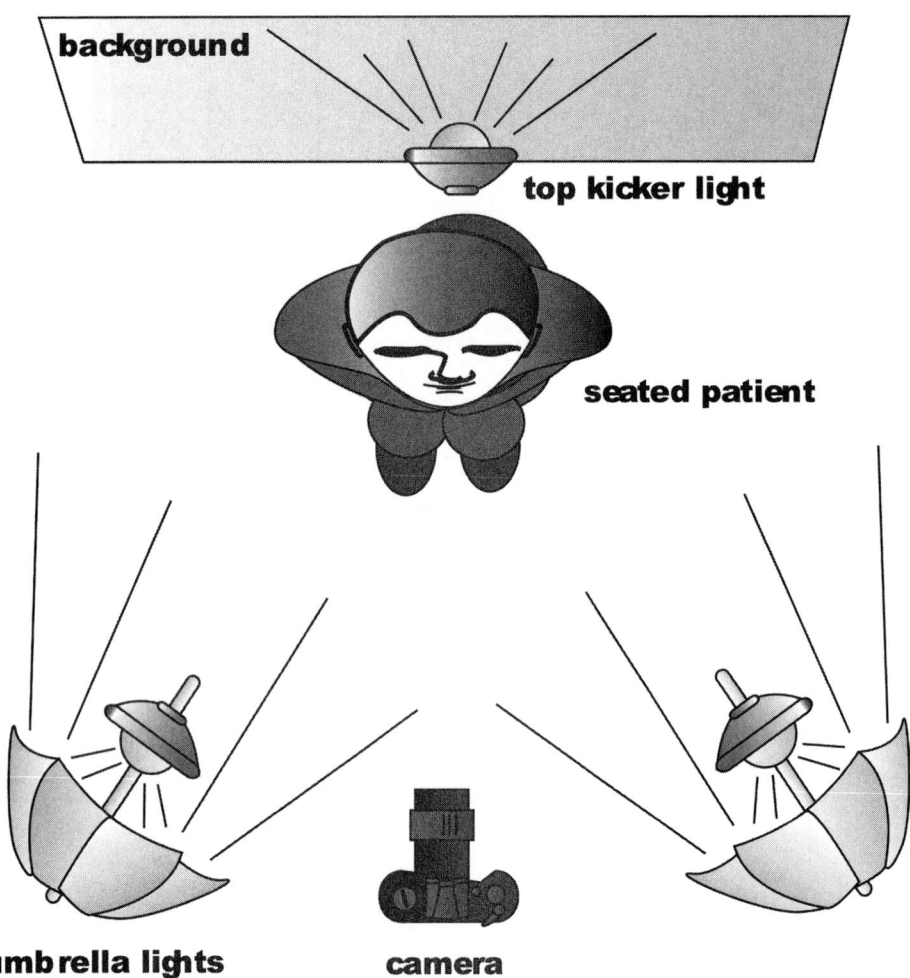

Figure 169.4 Standardized lighting is very important for good photography. If the ambient lighting is insufficient or casts very harsh shadows, fill lights can be used to soften the shadows. Ideally, two lights placed at 45-degree angles in front of the patient can be softened with the use of reflective umbrellas, and a "kicker" light that illuminates the background can be positioned above and behind the patient. These lights can be triggered to strobe as a slave unit when the camera's shutter is depressed or remain constantly on, to be turned off after the photographic session is over. (Illustration by Samuel A. Lam, M.D.)

but primarily serve as an educational tool for other training surgeons or as part of a didactic presentation in a scientific forum. A few basic techniques that have evolved from practical experience should be mentioned to help the surgeon achieve excellent results.

First, when taking any intraoperative photograph, care should be exercised to remove all bloodstains both on the patient's tissues and on the surgeon's gloves, as these elements that may appear inconspicuous through the lens become glaringly obtrusive when the final photograph is viewed. If sequential photographs are taken to document the stepwise approach to a procedure, the same angle should be maintained to enhance the clarity of communication. If a removed specimen is to be photographed, a ruler should be placed adjacent to it to provide dimensional understanding of the specimen. A metallic ruler can often cast a glare and obscure the legibility of the measurements: instead, a black ruler with white measurement markings minimizes glare and is ideal, albeit possibly difficult to procure.

Although a ring flash mount may provide uniform intraoral or other facial illumination, another method may serve as a better option. The intraoperative room lights are turned off, and only two dedicated overhead, directional lights are positioned at 45-degree angles to the specific facial feature that the surgeon wants to highlight. The camera is set to spot meter off of the subject so that the surrounding background fades to a uniform black. The wrinkled blue background of a surgical gown or other drape held behind the subject always looks unprofessional and distracting. The described technique should be practiced with a particular camera's settings until the correct exposure is established (2).

TRADITIONAL PHOTOGRAPHY

Traditional, 35-mm film photography remains the "gold standard" by which the quality of digital photography is judged. The following section discusses the various equipment needs for 35-mm photography: many of the components discussed for 35-mm photography also apply to digital imaging, as camera body and lens designs for digital imaging have often been based on original 35-mm models.

Camera

Camera models can be divided into two basic types: point-and-shoot and single-lens reflex (SLR). Point-and-shoot cameras typically have the lens and body sold as one compact unit and are convenient for nonprofessional purposes like vacation photographs in which portability is a priority. SLR cameras are higher-end models that usually consist only of the camera body with the lens (which can be interchanged with lenses of other focal lengths as needed) sold separately. Besides higher production quality that is characteristically associated with an SLR camera, this kind of camera also benefits from the absence of parallax error. An SLR camera avoids this distortion because the image seen through the viewfinder exactly matches what the film plate will be exposed to, as a mirror that transmits the image through the lens to the viewfinder is displaced to expose the film plate when the shutter is depressed.

With the increased availability of digital products, prices for 35-mm SLR cameras have plummeted. Nevertheless, many of the very advanced features that appear on an SLR camera are excessive for clinical photography (e.g., high rate of frames taken per second, manual controls). A basic SLR camera body that will accommodate high-quality lenses is sufficient for clinical use.

Data Back

An optional feature that may be worth purchasing for an SLR-type camera body is a data back, which usually replaces the hinged door on the back side of the camera used for film exchange. The data back provides the capacity of recording time and date onto the exposed film, which may serve as a useful tool for memory recall, photographic organization, and legal documentation. Digital cameras, conversely, do not require this feature, as the time, date, and other information are recorded with each image automatically.

Viewfinder Grid

The standard unmarked viewfinder can be replaced in many camera models with one that has vertical and horizontal markings on it. These marks help guide the photographer when following the guidelines enumerated in Figure 169.1 for good photography (e.g., the Frankfort Horizontal Plane). (Electronic, on-demand grids come equipped on some high-end digital camera models that replicate this feature.)

Lens

A well-crafted, aspherical lens that attaches to an SLR camera is the most critical element to attain distortion-free, high-quality photographs, and commensurate funds should be allocated for its purchase. A reputable manufacturer (e.g., Nikkor or Zeiss) is a reliable indicator for the quality of a fabricated lens. Besides quality of the lens, the right lens for the right purpose should be chosen. For 35-mm portrait photography, a 105-mm macro lens will provide photographic images without shape distortion like a disproportionately magnified nose and reduced ears in a fish-eye look that may be present with other focal lengths.

Camera Settings: Aperture and Shutter Speed

Basic photography terminology is not reviewed in depth herein, but a simplified strategy using proper camera settings is suggested for clinical implementation. Four basic types of settings exist for most advanced SLR cameras: automatic, aperture priority, shutter priority, and manual. Automatic mode functions by allowing the camera's onboard computer to decide both aperture and shutter speeds. Although intuitively attractive, the automatic feature may permit unintended variability. Manual mode allows absolute photographic control but can be burdensome and yield poorly exposed photographs in less than professional hands. Aperture priority allows the photographer to adjust the aperture setting while the camera's onboard computer automatically alters the shutter speed to achieve the ideal exposure, given the ambient conditions; shutter priority allows the converse (i.e., control of the shutter speed while the computer adjusts the aperture automatically). Clinically, aperture priority is typically the preferred mode of choice, as different apertures permit the surgeon control of varying degrees of depth of field (i.e., what percentage of a photograph will remain in focus). The smaller aperture (that correlates with a higher numeric "f"-stop) yields greater depth of field. The physician is encouraged to experiment with different aperture settings to determine the ideal depth of field—one that does not require an excessively long shutter speed, which can in turn lead to camera shake and a resultant blurred photographic image.

Tripod

Speaking of camera shake, a tripod on which a camera can be mounted promotes a stable platform for portrait photography. For intraoperative use, setting up and using a tripod can be overly taxing and also violate the sterile surgical field. If a tripod is to be used for portrait photography, several tripod features are worth acquiring. A quick-release feature on the tripod head permits the camera to be rapidly removed and taken free hand as needed. An easily adjustable tripod neck that allows rotation of the camera to achieve horizontal and vertical framing is also an important feature. Finally, wheels that can be mounted to the base of the tripod afford easy maneuverability so that the tripod can be positioned without having to lift and relocate it.

Film

Although traditional film-based photography may be divided into 35-mm, medium-, and large-format film types, 35 mm has remained the mainstay of practical clinical photography, with the latter two types relegated to nonmedical, artistic endeavors. The 35-mm film may be purchased either as negative or transparency (reversal) stock. Generally, the latter has been preferred for several reasons. Slide film produces accurate skin tones, is relatively inexpensive, is easy to project for scientific and patient communication, requires little storage space, and can have good archival preservation. Generally, if sufficient lighting is present, then a fine-grain film like 25- or 64-speed film is preferred for the high quality of the image and reproducibility of that quality when enlarged (3). If the physician prefers to remain in a film-based medium, it would be advised to consider using a digital camera or a Polaroid for immediate feedback and to ensure that the necessary image has been obtained. Use of a digital camera or Polaroid or both facilitates immediate patient dialogue that would otherwise be deferred because of processing time of slide film.

DIGITAL PHOTOGRAPHY

A few years ago, digital photography was in a nascent stage of development, and chapters described digital imaging only briefly as a tentative alternative. Today, digital photography has made rapid technologic strides and is challenging 35-mm photography for its many benefits: no consumable costs of film, instant image feedback, capacity for digital morphing, no physical storage space, no processing time or expense, and easy reproducibility and backup. Nevertheless, the initial setup cost for digital photography can be quite high because of the associated hardware requirements (e.g., computer, cables, software, storage). Today, most offices already use computers, so little additional hardware expenditure is typically required. Moreover, the cost of technology is rapidly tumbling, and the lack of consumables will offset initial outlay very rapidly, unless every photograph is printed, for instance, on expensive inkjet paper. The primary criticism leveled against digital photography in the past concerned the purported dubious image quality as compared with the gold standard of 35-mm film. However, that argument is truly obsolete with the increase of 12-megapixel cameras and beyond. No accurate comparison can be made between a digital pixel and the silver-halide grain of film, but this argument really borders on arcane academic banter and lacks any practical clinical import. This section discusses input devices [digital cameras and scanners (to convert 35-mm images over to digital)]; image processing and storage (compression, archiving, and morphing); and output devices (printers and projectors) (4).

Input Devices

Cameras

Like 35-mm film cameras, digital cameras may be broadly classified as point-and-shoot and SLR type models (Fig. 169.5). Because of an SLR digital camera's expense, many consumers purchase a point-and-shoot digital model. Like 35-mm cameras, an SLR digital camera can offer higher image quality and flexibility. Often, an SLR digital model will accommodate traditional 35-mm lenses, which can greatly save expense for the owner of these same lenses. Obviously, a high-quality, aspherical lens achieves commensurate value as in 35-mm photography. However, unlike that in traditional 35-mm film photography, the digital camera body contributes significantly to image quality, in terms of pixel resolution, color variation, dynamic range (i.e., the ability to capture the broad spectrum of bright whites to dark blacks), and light sensitivity. For these reasons, as mentioned for SLR cameras, it is imperative that

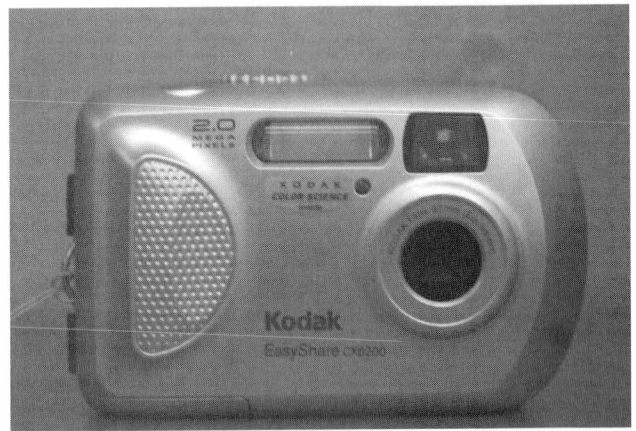
A

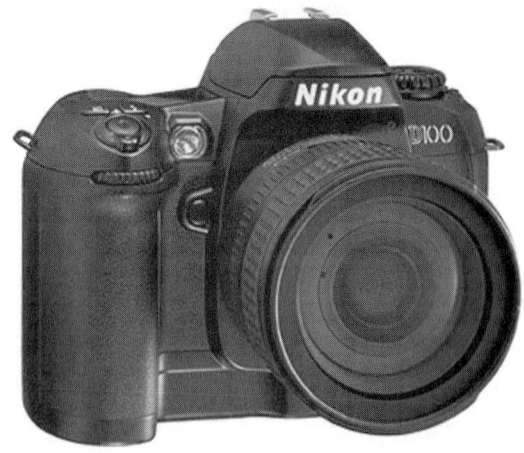
B

Figure 169.5 Like 35-mm cameras, digital cameras can be classified as point-and-shoot (**A**) and as single-lens reflex (SLR) models (**B**). Unlike in 35-mm photography, the digital camera body can be as important as the quality of the lens in obtaining superlative photographic results. In general, digital SLR models have better build-out quality, but the prospective consumer should always evaluate objective reviews before any purchase.

the same digital camera and lens (not to mention the same lighting and studio) be used to attain consistent photographic results. Unlike 35-mm film in which a 105-mm macro-type lens provides a distortion-free image in portrait photography, various lenses may provide a true 1:1 image for a particular digital camera based on the size of the CCD (charge-coupled device) or CMOS (complementary metal-oxide semiconductor), which would be analogous to the 35-mm film plate. The prospective consumer should ask the manufacturer of the SLR digital camera which focal-length lens will provide a distortion-free 1:1 image for that specific camera model. Because film is not used, ISO or ASA ratings that describe the light sensitivity of a particular film stock are not applicable for digital cameras. Nevertheless, as most consumers are familiar with what an ISO/ASA rating means, some digital cameras have adopted this terminology to describe the light sensitivity of a CCD/CMOS, with standard digital models having an ISO rating of between 50 and 200 and higher-end cameras, over 400. Depth of field also can be different for a specific f-stop, as compared with a traditional 35-mm setup. Generally, a smaller numeric f-stop (i.e., wider aperture) will yield a greater depth of field than in a 35-mm equivalent. Despite these differences, many of the principles outlined for good photography and basic equipment parallel those discussed for 35-mm photography.

Scanners

Scanners are used to convert a 35-mm library or select printed images into the digital medium. Basically two types exist: flatbed and film scanners. The former consists of a specialized camera housed below a clear glass panel with a hard, opaque cover that scans an image in a linear fashion to convert it into a digital version. The flatbed scanner benefits from versatility (ability to scan multiple media, like photographs, tables, graphs, text, and—with the right adapter—even transparency or negative film) and economy (a relatively low cost). Film scanners are dedicated to scanning only slides or negatives and can do so often very quickly and at a higher resolution. Unfortunately, they also tend to cost considerably more. Sophisticated image-correction software to repair damaged and faded slides also is featured in some high-end film scanners, as with the Nikon's series of film scanners.

Four parameters define a scanner's ultimate output quality: optical resolution, bit depth, color accuracy, and optical density. Optical resolution simply refers to the number of pixels per inch (ppi) and can be achieved by a straightforward pixel-per-pixel output or manipulated by a process known as *interpolation*, which can prove to be inferior. Most scanners offer an optical resolution between 300 and 4,800 ppi and an interpolated resolution of 0 to 1,900 ppi. Generally, 300-ppi scanning is sufficient for printed materials, whereas a 72-ppi resolution is adequate for web or monitor display. Bit depth refers to the maximal number of colors that each pixel of an image can dis-

play. This numeric value is expressed as the exponential power of 2. For instance, a 1-bit image has two colors (2^1), like black and white. Although most monitors only output 24-bit images (i.e., 2^{24}, or 16.7 million colors), scanners can exceed this value and be 30, 36, or even 42 bits. These higher bits are not superfluous, however; the added data undergo a selection process for the best bits of color information to yield a 24-bit output product. Color accuracy refers to the scanner's ability to reproduce faithfully the original photographic image's colors. The International Color Consortium (ICC) measures this accuracy with the "Delta E" value. Good Delta E values fall below 10, whereas poorer figures exceed 30. Finally, the optical density (OD) usually is a descriptor only on higher-end models and denotes the brightness that a scanner can capture. OD is expressed in a logarithmic fashion so that a scanner with a 3.6 D (or OD) will have 10 times the brightness of one with a mere 2.8 D. If a scanner does not list an OD, the rating probably falls between 2.8 and 3.0. It is recommended to have a minimum of 3.2 D for transparencies and 3.4 D for negatives.

Image Retrieval, Storage, and Morphing

Compression

Compression refers to the mathematical algorithm used to reduce an image's overall size and therefore necessary memory allocation. Although many competing compression formats exist, the two most popular and relevant for clinical utility are TIFF (Tagged Image File Format) and JPEG (Joint Photographic Experts Group). TIFF represents a "lossless" compression, in which no loss in image resolution occurs after the image is compressed. Unfortunately, due to the smaller compression ratio (typically 2:1 or 3:1), file sizes can be quite large, on the order of several megabytes. JPEG images are "lossy" images that lose some quality (usually undetectable to the human eye) when compressed with reduction in file size from 10:1 to 300:1. Clearly, the more the file is compressed, the greater the loss in quality. Interestingly, every time a JPEG image is cropped or altered in any way and then saved, additional loss of image quality is incurred. If the image will be manipulated numerous times, it may be wise to work from a TIFF image and then convert to JPEG on the final edit.

Editing and Morphing

One of the complaints about digital imaging concerns the ability to "doctor" or alter an image unethically. This charge is a bit misguided because 35-mm film also can be digitally altered and returned to its original format. Further, some editing software, like Canfield Scientific's Mirror system, has a built-in authentication process to detect altered images. What constitutes ethical editing? Color balancing and fine adjustment of hues and brightness, just as if you had sent film to a processing laboratory, should be considered proper. Further, cropping extraneous elements in an image, so long as the image integrity has not been undermined, should be deemed acceptable as well. These powerful tools underscore the strengths of the digital format. Intentional editing, or morphing, allows alteration of a digital image so that the surgeon can communicate with the patient an intended aesthetic result. Care should be taken to avoid over promising and to remind the patient the shortcomings in accuracy of a digitally morphed image. Morphing can be particularly effective when demonstrating to a patient the change in nasal profile or change in the neck and chin region, or both, for two principal reasons. First, the patient rarely if ever sees himself or herself from the side view. Second, the soft tissues are contrasted against a blue background, making image alterations relatively straightforward (as compared with moving skin over skin in a frontal view).

Archiving

The lack of physical space that a digital library occupies also is an undeniable benefit. However, the physician would be wise to select a good archiving program early so that the growing catalog of digital images can be easily organized and subsequently retrieved. The two basic types of archiving software are browser and catalog. Browser-type software permits simple retrieval of graphic images and is usually bundled free with purchased digital cameras. Conversely, catalog software often permits more sophisticated handling of many file types (text, graphic, video, and audio) and can attach metadata to a file. *Metadata* refers to the descriptive text that can be attached to a file to facilitate its retrieval (e.g., "Susan Smith," "Crooked Nose"). It is often easier to maintain the alphanumeric name that a camera assigns to an image (e.g., DSC_1789.jpg) and simply attach descriptive metadata to it. When organizing patient's images in a hierarchical folder, placement of the year, followed by the month, and then the day (e.g., 2005-11-6 for November 6, 2005) is preferred so that chronologic order is maintained.

Storage

Digital imaging permits infinite backup without the considerable expense associated with copying film transparencies or negatives. Backing up data should occur on a daily or weekly basis, and data should be stored both on premises and off site to ensure maximal protection. Many options exist for data storage including magnetic drives, magnetic-optical drives, optical drives, tape drives, and hard drives. Generally, tape and magnetic media are preferred for large storage backups, whereas optical media are better suited for smaller file-to-file storage.

Output Devices

Printers

Three principal types of printers exist for photographic reproduction: inkjet, dye-sublimation, and color laser. Inkjet printers compose the majority of printer sales and can provide high-quality print resolution. They function by spraying small amounts of ink onto the paper in halftones that are layered on top of one another. Parameters that define a high-quality printer are as follows: printer resolution expressed in dots per inch (dpi), with a good printer having upwards of 1,440 dpi; the number of color inkwells (three being a relatively low number, and six being a favorable number); and the size of the ink droplets (3 to 4 pL is superior to 6 to 18 pL). Lightfastness refers to the printer's capacity to produce an image that retains color and avoids unfavorable color shifts over time, with some recent models being able to exceed 100 years in lightfastness. Dye-sublimation printers, or dye-subs, work by depositing vaporized ink lifted from a colored ribbon onto a specialized paper to achieve a more continuous-toned print. Unfortunately, these printers are more expensive and can print only a predetermined size (e.g., 5 × 7 or 8 × 10 inches). Paper costs also can exceed those of quality inkjet paper. Color laser printers can produce high-quality images at a faster rate than can inkjet printers. In addition, consumable costs can be lower, and machines are more durable. However, initial cost outlay for a laser printer can be considerably higher than that for a standard inkjet. Office volume and cost expenditure will dictate which printer is best suited for the job. The one major limitation that still faces the conversion of on-screen to printed digital images concerns color correction. Many digital images are created in RGB (red–green–blue) mode that is native to computer monitors. However, printers work in CMYK [cyan, magenta, yellow, and black (the "key" color)] mode. The translation from one color scheme to another can cause some color mismatch. Details for color correction lie beyond the scope of this chapter.

Projectors

Scientific, marketing, and business conferences have attested to the advent of the digital revolution: increasingly, digital projectors are preferred to traditional slide projectors for effective communication. The ability to embed animation and video footage during a digital presentation has made the digital format an unquestionably superior medium of communication. The different types of projectors that are available today include cathode ray tubes (CRTs), liquid crystal displays (LCDs), digital light projectors (DLPs), and plasma display panels (PDPs). CRT projectors deliver a strictly analog signal, as compared with all of the other aforementioned types. Despite this fact, some proponents of CRTs argue that they provide as good if not superior image quality to their digital counterparts. LCD projectors may be divided into higher-quality polysilicon types and standard active-matrix styles. DLPs rely on micromirrors and have been cited to produce brighter images and have superior video capacity. However, LCDs have been thought to have better color contrast and saturation. Plasma screens work by combining pixels with CRT phosphors.

Several specific parameters should be sought when evaluating a projector's utility. Clearly, portability is important for someone seeking this option. Native resolution comes in VGA (640 × 480), SVGA (800 × 600), XGA (1,024 × 768), SXGA (1,280 × 1,024), and UXGA (1,600 × 1,200). CRTs do not have a native resolution and are deemed resolution independent, which means that they do not need to be matched to a monitor's resolution. Conversely, digital projectors should be matched to a monitor's resolution as precisely as possible. If several computers are intended for use with one projector, then the projector should be matched to the computer monitor with the highest resolution. The minimum of a SVGA projector should be acquired for straightforward graphic presentations, but an SXGA is preferable. A projector's brightness is measured in ANSI lumens with a minimum of 300 to 500 ANSI recommended for dimly lit rooms and 1,000 ANSI for a well-lit room. For an auditorium, at least 1,500 ANSI should be sought. The contrast ratio that describes the range of brightest whites to darkest blacks is also a valuable feature, with a range of 100:1 (low) to 2,000:1 (high). Zoom lenses permit image size adjustment without the burden of having to move the unit. Digital keystone correction adjusts the image to reduce distortions that arise from aiming the projector at the wall from an angle. Lamp life can range from 40 to 40,000 hours, with the majority falling between 1,000 and 2,000 hours. Lamp replacement can be expensive, so this factor should also be integrated into the choice of a projector.

CLOSING THOUGHTS AND THE FUTURE

Good photographic principles should be adhered to whether working in 35-mm or digital photography. Photographic documentation should always be obtained in any cosmetic or reconstructive endeavor but also may serve as a reliable tool for other types of head and neck surgical procedures on an individual case-by-case basis. The rise of digital photography has transformed the landscape of scientific and professional communication. As technology continues to evolve, digital photography will most likely entirely supplant analog 35-mm film. The next edition of this chapter will probably bear the shorter title "Pictorial Documentation: Digital Imaging."

HIGHLIGHTS

■ Other than the photographer and the subject, only four elements are required to take a photograph: camera body, lens, film, and lighting. For digital imaging, a memory card replaces film. A computer with sufficient RAM and hard-drive space, image management software, and a memory card reader also is required to record a digital image.

■ An SLR camera with a high-resolution 80- to 105-mm macro lens affords the proper perspective in facial photography. A digital camera with 2 to 3 million pixel resolution and the same "35-mm equivalent" lens parameters is preferable. Proper exposure of film may be ensured through standard settings (f-stop and shutter speed) that can be predetermined and set for a given unchanging lighting situation.

■ Lighting can be the single most important component of the process. Three types of light sources are commonly used in medical photography: the ring flash for deep-cavity photos, dual strobe-flash units attached to the camera, and dual stationary studio lighting.

■ A medium-blue background is commonly used for both still photography and digital imaging. Other popular colors include gray, light tan, and light blue.

■ Obtaining proper consent for photography and the use of photographs should be standard practice. The consent should allow the patient to select or reject all potential uses of the photos and should be prepared consistent with respective state law.

■ Consistency in photographic technique is paramount in medical pictorial documentation. Standardized and precise photographic records are required for realistic comparison of preoperative and postoperative results.

■ Each photographic view should follow an established standard so that reliable facial landmarks lie in consistent positions.

■ The commitment to detail in patient positioning for each photograph is a salient component in ensuring quality images. Great attention should be directed to ensuring a leveled Frankfort horizontal line. The photographer must not allow chin thrusting or tilting of the head. The hair should be pulled back from the face and distracting jewelry and makeup removed.

■ An organized system of archiving and storing photos is helpful for easy retrieval. This is greatly facilitated with the use of digital images and image-management software.

REFERENCES

1. Kontis TC. Photography in facial plastic surgery. In: Papel L Jr, ed. *Facial plastic and reconstructive surgery,* 2nd ed. New York: Thieme Medical Publishers, 2002:116–124.
2. Williams EF, Lam SM. *Comprehensive facial rejuvenation: a practical and systematic guide to surgical management of the aging face.* Philadelphia: Lippincott Williams & Wilkins, 2004.
3. Tardy ME. *Principles of photography in facial plastic surgery.* New York: Thieme Medical Publishers, 1992.
4. Lam SM. Digital imaging in the plastic surgical practice. *Int J Cosm Surg Aesthetic Dermatol* 2002:199–212.

Surgical Anatomy of the Nose

170

David W. Kim   *Ted Mau*

GENERAL PRINCIPLES

Success in rhinoplasty depends on the surgeon's ability to create favorable functional and cosmetic changes to the nose. The operation is difficult for a number of reasons: noses are complex, three-dimensional, highly variable structures; most maneuvers attempt to alter a framework that has inherent resistance to manipulation; and the changes that are created are often subtle and subject to relentless postoperative forces of scar contracture. To overcome these challenges, the surgeon must have the ability to analyze a nose and match its variations to underlying structural correlates. Techniques may then be chosen to alter these structures into an optimal form while maintaining support and function. Finally, the maneuvers must be executed with meticulous precision. In rhinoplasty, these steps of diagnosis, selection of technique, and execution are possible only with a clear understanding of the complex anatomy.

This chapter describes sequentially the anatomy of the different regions and components of the nose. Infinite variations of these regions exist and may be the result of differences in ethnicity, gender, age, trauma, congenital deformity, or prior surgery. The unique structural characteristics of each nose underlie each individual's external appearance and may motivate that person to seek surgery. Whether or not these variations should be classified as variant anatomy is a semantic question, but because of this huge diversity, it is problematic to designate a "normal" archetypal anatomy toward which rhinoplasty surgery should aspire.

Each section in this chapter begins with general anatomic concepts, detailing the orientations and relations that are most commonly encountered. Subsequently, "variations" from normal anatomy are discussed, particularly as they pertain to rhinoplasty. A separate section focuses on the structural architecture of the nose, emphasizing how the various individual anatomic elements integrate into a stable unit. Although the chapter emphasizes anatomy predominantly, discussions on rhinoplasty philosophy, analysis, technique, and complications are included where germane.

SURFACE ANATOMY

Discussion of the surface anatomy of the nose begins within the larger contextual framework of the face. In general, the nose occupies the central horizontal third of the face, from the glabella to the subnasale, and central vertical fifth, between the medial canthi. Variations of nasal dimension and position may cause the nose to extend outside of these confines. These divergences may draw attention to the nose and may therefore be a patient's motivation to undergo rhinoplasty. Directional references and topographic landmarks are illustrated in Figures 170.1 through 170.5.

Subunits

The external topography of the nose is divided into six subunits. These consist of the nasal dorsum, sidewalls, tip, columella, ala/sill, and soft triangles (Fig. 170.6). These areas are defined by the shadows and highlights cast by incident light. Human visual processing depends on these light–dark contrasts to form a perception of the nose. The subunits do not necessarily have sharply defined boundaries and do not mirror exactly the underlying anatomic

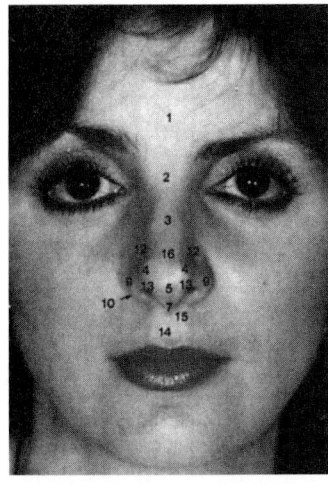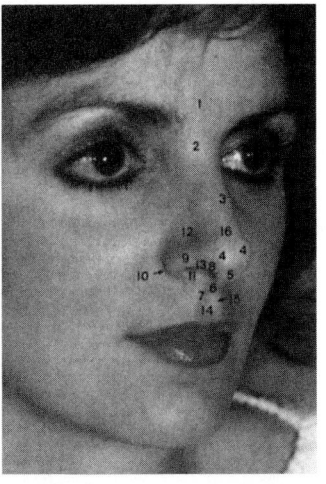

Figure 170.1 Topographic key landmarks and accepted designations for **(A)** frontal and **(B)** oblique views of the nose. 1, Glabella; 2, nasion, nasofrontal angle; 3, rhinion (osseocartilaginous junction); 4, tip-defining point; 5, infratip lobule; 6, columella; 7, columella-labial junction; 8, facet; 9, alar sidewall; 10, alar–facial junction; 11, medial crural footplate; 12, supraalar crease; 13, alar margin; 14, philtrum; 15, philtral crest; 16, supratip dorsum. (From Tardy ME. *Surgical anatomy of the nose.* New York: Raven Press, 1990, with permission.)

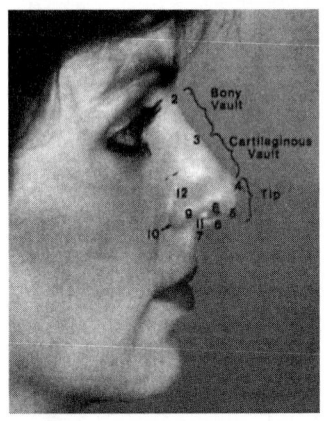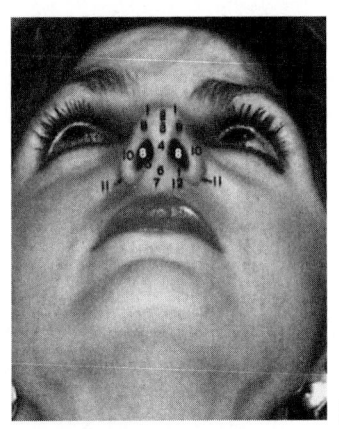

Figure 170.2 A: Topographic key landmarks and accepted designations for lateral view of the nose. 1, Glabella; 2, nasion (nasofrontal junction); 3, rhinion (osseocartilaginous junction); 4, tip-defining point; 5, infratip lobule; 6, columella; 7, columella-labial junction; 8, facet; 9, alar lobule; 10, alar–facial junction; 11, medial crural footplate. **B:** Topographic key landmarks and accepted designations for basal view of the nose. 1, tip-defining point; 2, interdomal area, alar lobule; 3, infratip lobule; 4, columella; 5, medial crural footplate; 6, columella–labial junction; 7, philtrum; 8, nostril aperture; 9, facet; 10, alar sidewall; 11, alar–facial junction; 12, nostril sill. (From Tardy ME. *Surgical anatomy of the nose.* New York: Raven Press, 1990, with permission.)

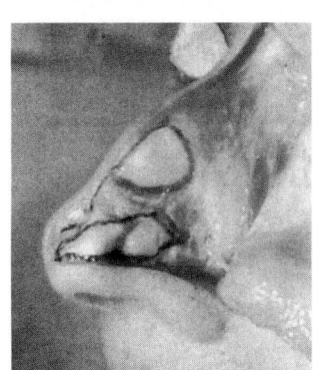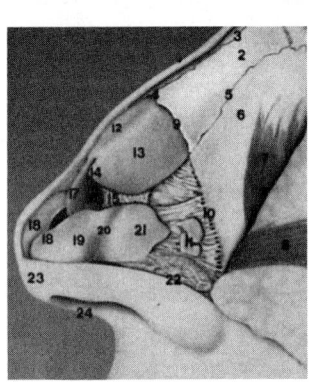

Figure 170.3 Key anatomic landmarks **(A)** and standard terminology **(B)** for lateral view of fresh cadaver dissection of nose. 1, Nasofrontal suture line; 2, nasal bone; 3, intranasal suture line; 4, osseocartilaginous junction (rhinion); 5, nasomaxillary suture line; 6, ascending process of maxilla; 7, levator labii superioris muscle; 8, transverse nasalis muscle; 9, cephalic portion of upper lateral cartilage (articulates to undersurface of nasal bone); 10, piriform margin; 11, sesamoid cartilages; 12, cartilaginous dorsum; 13, upper lateral cartilage; 14, caudal free margin of upper lateral cartilage; 15, intercartilaginous ligament; 16, quadrangular cartilage; 17, anterior septal angle; 18, tip-defining point alar cartilage; 19, lateral crus of alar cartilage; 20, concavity ("hinge") of lateral crus; 21, lateral aspect of lateral crus; 22, alar lobule; 23, infratip lobule; 24, columella. (From Tardy ME. *Surgical anatomy of the nose.* New York: Raven Press, 1990, with permission.)

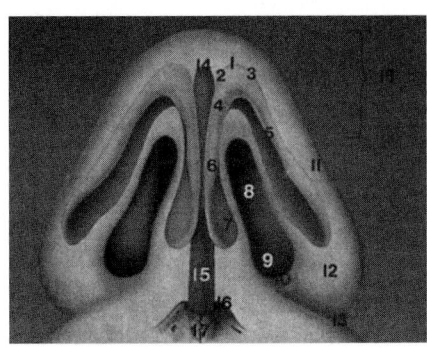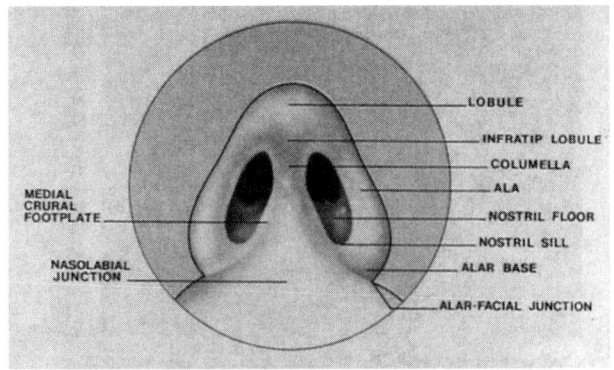

Figure 170.4 Additional anatomic landmarks **(A)** and standard nasal terminology of base of nose **(B)**. 1, Apex of alar cartilage; 2, medial genu; 3, lateral genu; 4, transitional segment; 5, lateral crus; 6, medial crus; 7, medial crural footplate; 8, nostril aperture; 9, nostril floor; 10, nostril sill; 11, lateral alar sidewall; 12, alar lobule; 13, alar–facial junction; 14, anterior septal angle; 15, caudal septum; 16, maxillary crest; 17, nasal spine; 18, infratip lobule. (From Tardy ME. *Surgical anatomy of the nose.* New York: Raven Press, 1990, with permission.)

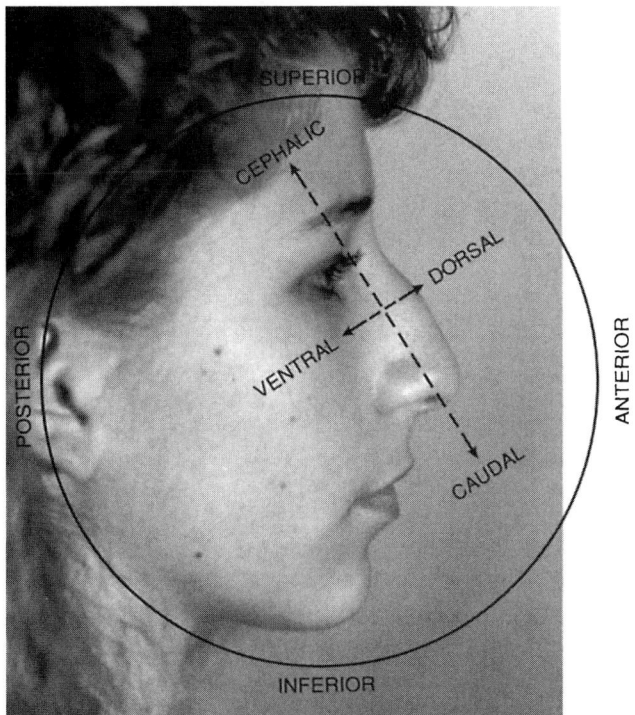

Figure 170.5 Preferred directional references applied to the nose. Note that the axes shift to lie oriented to the nasal dorsal line.

Topography

A discussion of surgical anatomy must begin with the external topography that surgery aims to alter. A detailed discussion of aesthetic facial analysis is found in Chapter 168. What follows is a limited discussion of nasal analysis and definitions of terms with specific relevance to rhinoplasty anatomy. Correlation of nasal topography to underlying structural anatomy are introduced—details of this anatomy are discussed in greater depth in subsequent sections.

On frontal view, a gentle, unbroken curve should appear from the lateral brow to the nasal tip on each side of the nose (Fig. 170.1A). These *brow-tip aesthetic lines* should follow the normal changes of nasal width: wider cephalad at the brow/nasal root transition, narrower in the middle vault, and wider again at the tip. An irregular brow–tip aesthetic line may be correlated to bony and cartilaginous vault irregularities through palpation and close inspection with a light placed above the patient to enhance shadowing. When the upper cartilaginous vault is overly narrow, the curvature of these brow–tip lines is exaggerated.

General tip shape may be determined from the frontal and base views (e.g., bulbous, deviated, wide, amorphous, asymmetrical). The unique features of tip shape are determined by the endless variations of form, dimension, and position of the lower lateral cartilages (LLCs) and surrounding structures. Inference about the thickness of the nasal skin may be made from inspection of the contour of the tip. A tip with sharp features reflects underlying structures transmitting through thin skin. A smooth, bulbous tip is likely covered by thick skin.

The base view also provides information about the shape and size of the columella, alar base, nostrils, and infratip lobule (Figs. 170.2B and 170.4). In most noses, the frontal and base views reveal a triangular shape of the nose in which the nasal base (interface of nose and face) is wider than the tip and dorsal line. The triangularity of the tip depends on the presence of an unbroken line from a

structures. Nonetheless, it is crucial for the nasal surgeon to identify them in preoperative assessment, particularly in external nasal reconstruction. During reconstruction, effort should be made to place scars within subunit borders whenever possible, as the human eye is more apt to discern a scar that traverses across a subunit than one that outlines it. This may require a surgeon to resect and replace an entire subunit (or subunits) involved, rather than replace only the primary defect, even if this requires removal of areas of healthy tissue. Tissue of a similar thickness, color, and consistency should be used to reconstruct these defects.

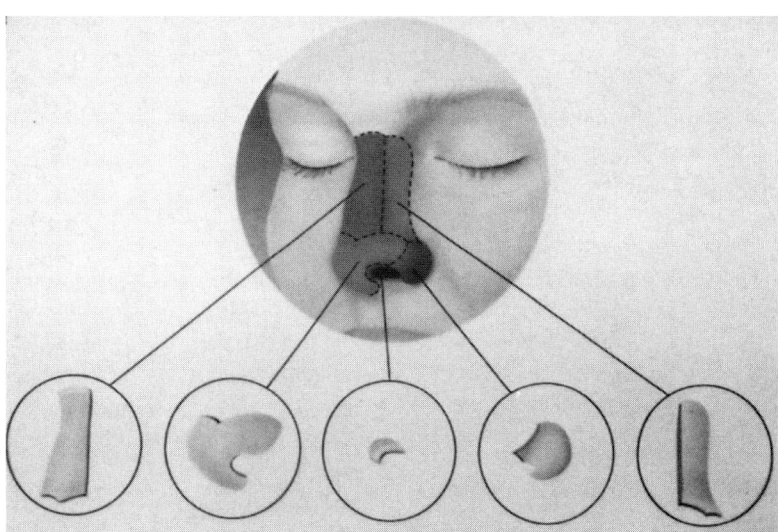

Figure 170.6 Aesthetic topographic subunits of the nasal surface. From left to right: dorsum, tip/columella, soft-tissue triangle, alar lobule, and sidewall. The columella may be considered a separate distinct subunit. (From Tardy ME. *Surgical anatomy of the nose*. New York: Raven Press, 1990, with permission.)

narrower nasal tip to a wider nasal base. Poor structural support along this line will manifest as alar pinching or concavity of the alar margins on frontal and base views. When the base is excessively narrow or the tip overly wide, a square or trapezoidal shape instead of triangular configuration is present (1). The width of the infratip lobule reflects the underlying shape of the intermediate crura of the LLCs. Asymmetry in the columella may be caused by asymmetries of the shape or trajectory of the medial crura, deflection of the caudal edge of the cartilaginous septum, or both. The lateral flaring of the alar lobules is only indirectly determined by the shape and strength of the lateral crura of the LLCs, as the lobules themselves are composed of soft tissue only and are caudal to the lateral crura.

On lateral view, several important external landmarks may be identified (Fig. 170.2A). The nasion is the most concave point at the nasofrontal angle and corresponds anatomically to the midline of the nasofrontal suture. This angle is determined by the height of the radix, the most cephalic portion of the nasal dorsum, and the slope of the forehead. An average nasofrontal angle measures 120 degrees in the Caucasian nose. The vertical position of the nasion marks the nasal starting point and is typically between the supratarsal crease and the upper eyelid margin. The rhinion corresponds to the osseous–cartilaginous junction and often marks the location of a dorsal hump. Proceeding caudally, the presence or absence of a supratip breakpoint depends on the dorsal height of the cartilaginous septum and the projection of the domal region of the LLCs. The tip-defining point, or the pronasale, is the most anterior projection of the nose. The overall projection and rotation of the nasal tip may be assessed by using Goode's method, in which the nasal-tip projection (from the alar crease to the tip-defining point) is divided by nasal length (from nasion to tip-defining point). According to Goode, the normal value should be 0.55. The nasolabial angle in men is typically between 90 and 95 degrees, and in women, between 95 and 105 degrees. This angle may be affected by variations of the size and shape of the upper lip and premaxillary bone. Therefore the nasolabial angle does not always reflect the degree of tip rotation. The lateral view of the ideal nostril is oval-shaped, with 2 to 4 mm of the columella visible beneath the alar rim.

Variant Anatomy

Because the nose is a three-dimensional structure that is viewed in whole, the topographic dimensions of one area have an optical effect on the appearance of other areas. This is critical during rhinoplasty, as surgical changes to one region or parameter of the nose create the illusion of change to another. Examples as they pertain to external nasal topography follow.

Dorsal Height

The overall height of the nasal dorsum is determined predominantly by the size and development of the highly vari-able cartilaginous and osseous nasal septum. In general, an increased overall projection of the dorsum on the lateral view corresponds to a narrower appearance on the frontal view. Conversely, a low nasal bridge creates a wider-appearing nose from the front. This is explained by the concept that one looks down the apex of a triangle when observing a nose from the front. In a nose with a high dorsum, the side walls are subject to more shadowing, and the apex of the triangle appears narrower. In a nose with a low bridge, the cross-sectional triangular geometry of the nose is flattened, or if surgical hump reduction has occurred, it is truncated into a trapezoid. With less shadowing of the side walls, the nose appears wider on frontal view. Local differences in dorsal height create other illusions. In a normal profile, the radix, mid-dorsum, supratip, and nasal tip are linear or nearly colinear. Because our eyes are accustomed to this norm, deviations from these relations create certain optical illusions. For instance, the presence of a mid-dorsal convexity creates an illusion of an underrotated nasal tip, irrespective of absolute tip position. A dorsal concavity, in contrast, creates a perception of increased tip rotation and a shorter nose. Before the surgeon commits to making true alterations of tip position, the effects of dorsal height and its modification must be carefully weighed.

Radix and Nasofrontal Angle

Variations in radix height have an effect on numerous aesthetic nasal parameters such as the nasal starting point, nasofrontal angle, overall dorsal profile, and apparent intercanthal distance. A low radix, as commonly seen in individuals of African or Asian descent, creates an illusion of increased intercanthal distance (see earlier explanation). If associated with tip underprojection, a low radix may create an appearance of a dorsal hump. Correction of this appearance may be accomplished with augmentation of the radix and increasing tip projection instead of reduction of the dorsum to the level of the low radix (Fig. 170.7). Maintaining a higher dorsum offers the advantages of a narrower appearance on front view and avoidance of an open-roof deformity associated with hump reduction. A high radix, in contrast, creates an appearance of decreased intercanthal distance. When excessive height at the radix blunts the nasofrontal angle, the distinction between the nose and forehead may be blurred, creating the illusion of a longer nose. This is particularly true in the presence of a posteriorly sloping forehead. Because of the abundant overlying soft tissue in this area, reduction of osseous height at the radix does not transmit well to overall profile reduction. Conversely, a more acute nasofrontal angle creates an illusion of a shorter nose, independent of the actual vertical position of the nasal starting point.

Nasolabial Angle

The nasolabial angle, formed by the upper lip and columella, is widely used as a metric for the degree of rotation of the nasal tip. This region, however, is composed of nu-

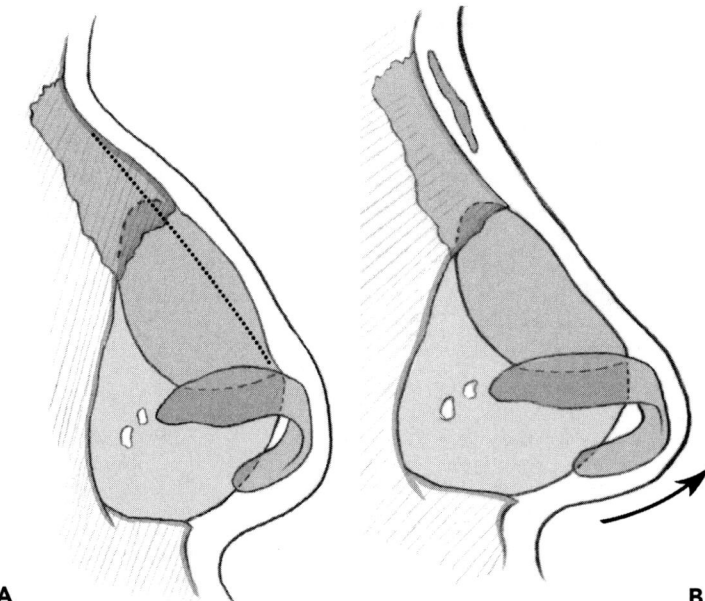

Figure 170.7 **A:** Profile view of a nose with a true dorsal hump in the region of the rhinion. Correction may involve reduction of the hump. **B:** Nose with a relative dorsal convexity due to a low radix and an underprojected nasal tip. Correction might involve elevating of the radix with a graft and increasing tip projection. Final external dorsal contour is similar in both examples.

merous anatomic components with a high degree of variation, and in reality may not accurately reflect the overall degree of nasal-tip rotation. Fullness in this area may be caused by an overdeveloped quadrangular cartilage in the area of the posterior septal angle, a prominent nasal spine and premaxillary bone, or tenting of the soft tissue in a projecting nose. These variations create a more obtuse angle, irrespective of the true rotational position of the nasal tip. However, even if the true rotational position of

the tip is not changed, an increased nasolabial angle creates an illusion of increased tip rotation. Conversely, when these structures are less developed or retrusive, a relative deficiency on the nasolabial angle may be present, leading to a perception of counterrotation (Fig. 170.8).

Alar–Columellar Relation

With alar retraction or a dependent caudal edge of the cartilaginous septum, excessive columellar height is visible

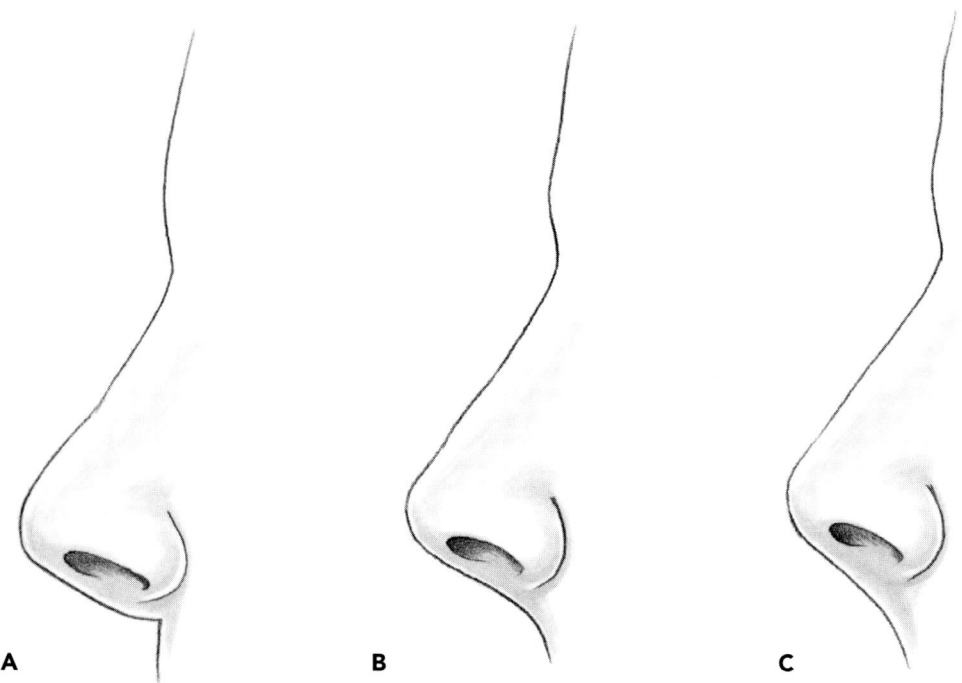

Figure 170.8 Lateral view of three noses with identical tip position. **A:** Relative deficiency of tissue at the nasolabial area and an acute nasolabial angle creates an illusion of underrotation of the tip. **B:** Nose with a moderate nasolabial angle. **C:** Fullness at the nasolabial area with an obtuse nasolabial angle creates an illusion of increased tip rotation.

on the lateral view. This hanging columella may create an illusion of a ptotic nasal tip, even when tip position is normal. In contrast, a retracted caudal septum or a low alar margin may lead to a relative lack of columellar show and an associated illusion of increased tip rotation. The size, position, and interrelations of the medial crura, caudal septum, lateral crura, and alar soft tissue determine these variations.

SKIN–SOFT TISSUE ENVELOPE

The nose is constructed of a skeletal framework onto which a skin–soft tissue envelope (SSTE) is draped. Although the framework is the subject of most surgical techniques, the appearance of the nose is determined by the manner in which the SSTE drapes over the modified skeleton. An understanding of the composition of the SSTE and its variant anatomy guides the surgeon in choosing appropriate techniques for successful surgery.

Skin

The skin of the nose varies in thickness depending on its location. The skin is thickest at the nasion and thinnest at the rhinion (2). From the rhinion, the skin becomes progressively thicker as it descends along the dorsum to the tip, where a large number of sebaceous glands reside. The skin becomes thin again at the most caudal aspect of the nose along the alar margin and columella.

Understanding skin-thickness variation along the dorsum aids the rhinoplasty surgeon in performing dorsal hump reduction. Because the skin is thinnest at the rhinion, a straight external profile requires a small relative convexity to remain in this region. If the dorsum is reduced so that a straight skeletal profile results, a slight concavity at the mid-dorsum is likely to result after skin redraping (3). This may create a cartilaginous polybeak, in which the supratip dorsum projects above the plane of the dorsum cephalad to it. To avoid this, hump reduction should be carried out incrementally, with verification of the effect of each pass on external contour through the SSTE.

Subcutaneous Tissue

The subcutaneous layer of the nose is made up of the superficial fatty layer, the fibromuscular layer, the deep fatty layer, and the periosteum or perichondrium. The superficial fatty layer is directly connected to the dermis. The fibromuscular layer comprises the nasal subcutaneous muscular aponeurotic system (SMAS) (4). The nasal SMAS is in continuity with the SMAS of the rest of the face and encases and interconnects the mimetic muscles of the nose. The deep fatty layer contains the neurovascular system of the soft-tissue envelope. Dissection in the avascular plane between the deep fatty layer and the perichondrium and periosteum is met with little mechanical resistance or bleeding and results in the least postoperative scarring and contraction.

Muscles

The mimetic muscles of the nose reside within the SMAS. They are divided into four groups (5; Table 170.1). The *elevator* muscles shorten the nose and dilate the nostrils; the *depressor* muscles lengthen the nose and dilate the nostrils, the *compressor* muscles lengthen the nose and narrow the nostrils; and the *minor dilator* muscles widen the nostrils. In addition to these individual functions, the muscles work synergistically to alter the shape of the nasal tip, alae, and dorsum. For example, simultaneous contraction of the levator labii superioris and the depressor septi nasi may depress the nasal tip, "round-up" the supratip area, and lengthen the nose (6). The muscles, particularly the dilator naris (7), also serve to maintain the tone of the nostrils during inspiration, as illustrated in the patient with ipsilateral facial nerve paralysis with unilateral alar collapse (8). Dissection in the sub-SMAS layer of the soft-tissue envelope allows the surgeon to avoid the nervous supply to the nasal muscles.

Although most rhinoplasty techniques do not directly address nasal muscles, division of the depressor septi nasi may correct drooping of the nasal tip and shortening of the upper lip during facial animation. The small, paired muscle that originates at the anterior nasal spine and inserts onto the medial crura footplates may be addressed through simple division (6), muscular release and plication (9), or dissection and transposition of the muscle (10). In selected patients, these techniques may reduce gingival show and nasal-tip descent during smiling, elevate the nasal tip, and elongate the upper lip in the resting state.

Arterial Supply

The superficial vascular supply to the external nose derives from both the external and internal carotid systems. The

TABLE 170.1
INVESTING NASAL MUSCULATURE

Elevator muscles
  Procerus
  Levator labii-superioris alaeque nasi
  Anomalous nasi
Depressor muscles
  Alar nasalis
  Depressor septi nasi
Compressor muscles
  Transverse nasalis
  Compressor narium minor
Minor dilator muscles
  Dilator naris anterior

facial artery branches into the angular artery and the superior labial artery. The lateral nasal branch of the angular artery supplies the lateral surface of the caudal nose. Branches of the superior labial artery supply the nasal sill and the base of the columella. The columellar artery, a branch of the superior labial artery, is often encountered in the transcolumellar incision used in the external rhinoplasty approach. The septal branches of the superior labial artery enter the nose on each side of the nasal spine and form the major blood supply to the anterior septum. Large septal mucosal flaps may be pedicled on the nasal spine area with these branches for reconstructive purposes.

The dorsal nasal artery, an external branch of the ophthalmic artery, anastomoses with the lateral nasal branch of the angular artery, forming an axial arterial network for the dorsal nasal skin. Arterial supply to the nasal tip derives from branches of the anterior ethmoid and angular arteries. The external nasal branch of the anterior ethmoid artery perforates the transverse nasalis muscle of the nasal sidewall and descends toward the nasal tip. The lateral nasal branch of the angular artery sends off branches from the ala anteriorly toward the nasal tip. The vascular plexus to which these arteries contribute resides predominantly in the adipose layer just deep to the SMAS. Remaining in the plane just above the perichondrium and periosteum during dissection minimizes injury to these vessels.

Sensory Nerve Supply

Sensation to the external nasal skin is supplied by branches of the ophthalmic and maxillary divisions of the trigeminal nerve. Twigs from the supratrochlear and infratrochlear branches of the ophthalmic nerve supply sensation to the skin of the radix, the rhinion, and the cephalic portion of the nasal side walls (11). The external nasal branch of the anterior ethmoidal nerve supplies the skin over the dorsum of the caudal nose down to and including the nasal tip. This branch emerges between the caudal edge of the nasal bone and the upper lateral cartilage (ULC) and courses in the SMAS layer. Injury to this nerve during intercartilaginous or cartilage-splitting incisions can result in tip numbness (11). Branches of the infraorbital nerve provide sensation to the side of the lower half of the nose and the lateral vestibule. The nasopalatine nerve, a branch of V2 that enters the nose through the incisive foramen, provides the major sensory supply to the posterior two thirds of the nasal septal mucosa, maxillary gingiva, and anterior palatal mucosa. This nerve may be injured during surgery involving the maxillary crest or nasal floor and can result in temporary numbness near the incisors (12).

Inner Lining

The nasal vestibule is lined with keratinizing squamous epithelium. The surfaces of the nasal cavities, with the exception of the superior olfactory epithelium, are covered by ciliated stratified or pseudostratified respiratory epithelium (13). Because of its high vascularity, the vestibular epithelium and intranasal mucosa are excellent sources of local flaps for reconstruction of the inning lining in full-thickness nasal defects. In such procedures, a free cartilage graft is often used to rebuild structure for the nose. The rich vascular intranasal lining flap nourishes the cartilage graft from its undersurface. Common inner lining donor sites are the nasal septum or nasal vestibule. These flaps are discussed in more detail in Chapter 165. During routine rhinoplasty, care must be taken to preserve vestibular skin in the internal nasal valve area to avoid web formation and nasal valve stenosis (14).

Variant Anatomy

Thickness of the SSTE varies with ethnicity, age, and gender. Noses with thin, less sebaceous skin assume a shape that closely matches the underlying cartilaginous and osseous structure. In contrast, the underlying nasal architecture does not accurately transmit through the soft-tissue envelope in thicker-skinned noses. These concepts are critical in rhinoplasty.

In the thick-skinned individual, modifications of the underlying framework, particularly reductive alterations, may not result in significant changes in external appearance because of poor redraping of the overlying SSTE. In these patients, the surgeon should consider augmenting areas of relative deficiency to create a framework that pushes and stretches the thick SSTE into a desirable shape. In such cases, overall proportion of the nose becomes more important than absolute size. Because a thick SSTE cannot conform onto the underlying structure after reduction, scar tissue may fill the resulting void. An example is the soft-tissue/scar polybeak that results after aggressive supratip hump reduction in a thick-skinned individual. Little to no external lowering of the supratip convexity occurs as the cartilaginous hump is simply replaced by scar beneath a noncompliant SSTE.

In patients with thin skin, even small irregularities of the underlying structure may become evident after surgery as the soft tissue envelope redrapes very closely to the framework below. In these cases, care must be taken to camouflage grafts, edges of bone and cartilage, and any other contour irregularities. Graft must be placed in a precise manner, and any edges that may transmit through the skin should be beveled or crushed to blend seamlessly into surrounding structures. Soft-tissue or crushed cartilage onlay grafts may aid in camouflaging irregularities.

SKELETAL FRAMEWORK

The skeletal framework of the nose may be divided into thirds, the upper third consisting of the osseous vault; the middle third consisting of the upper cartilaginous vault;

and the lower third consisting of the lower cartilaginous vault. The nasal septum, consisting of a bony and a cartilaginous portion, provides support in all three sections and divides the nasal cavity into two lateral halves. In this section, these structures are discussed individually, with an emphasis on anatomic forms and their variations. In a later section, the interrelations of these bodies as they pertain to nasal structural mechanics are discussed.

Septum

The nasal septum is a sagittal midline structure that divides the nose into two cavities and provides structural support to the osseous and cartilaginous vaults (15). The septum is divided into a cephalic–posterior osseous septum, composed of the perpendicular plate of the ethmoid and the vomer, and a caudal–anterior cartilaginous septum, consisting of the quadrangular cartilage.

The perpendicular plate of the ethmoid forms the dorsal aspect of the osseous septum. Its superior attachment consists of the frontal bone and its nasal spine anteriorly and the cribriform plate posteriorly. Anterosuperiorly, it articulates with the inward projection of the nasal bones in the midline. Anteroinferiorly, it borders the quadrangular cartilage, and posteroinferiorly, it borders the vomer. The thickness of the perpendicular plate of the ethmoid varies considerably, and it is rarely pneumatized. Because it is attached to the cribriform plate, aggressive lateral force high on the osseous septum may lead to fracture of the skull base and resultant cerebrospinal fluid leak or olfactory bulb injury.

The vomer, one of the bones that make up the skull, is shaped like the keel of a boat. In a midsagittal view of the skull, its superior edge forms a line connecting the sphenoid sinus to the anterior nasal spine. Superiorly, the vomer articulates with the perpendicular plate of the ethmoid. Inferiorly, it attaches to the midline nasal crest of the palatine bone posteriorly and the maxilla anteriorly. Anterior to its articulation with the vomer, the maxillary crest forms a groove into which the quadrangular cartilage sits. The posterior free edge of the vomer forms the posterior border of the choanae.

The quadrangular cartilage comprises the cartilaginous septum. This structure rests within a groove in the nasal spine and maxillary crest inferior to it. This ventral surface is typically thickened in comparison to the remainder of the structure. Dorsally, the quadrangular cartilage forms the contour of the nasal bridge externally. The ULCs articulate with the cephalic aspect of the quadrangular cartilage, forming the dorsum of the central third of the nose. The most caudal portion of the cartilage extends anterior to the nasal spine and is the least rigid portion (Fig. 170.9). Three angles may be identified at the caudal edge of the septum (Fig. 170.10). The anterior septal angle is usually the most anterior projection of the septum and forms the transition between the dorsal and caudal components of the sup-

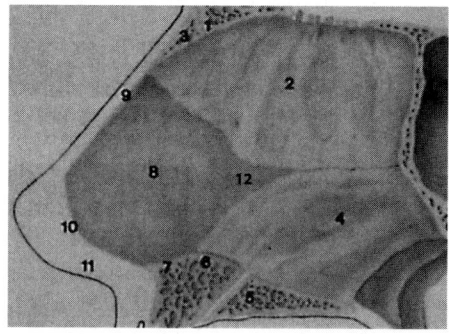

Figure 170.9 Anatomy of the typical nasal septum. 1, Nasal process and frontal bone; 2, perpendicular plate of ethmoid bone; 3, nasal bone; 4, vomer bone; 5, palatine bone; 6, maxillary crest; 7, nasal spine; 8, quadrangular cartilage; 9, upper lateral cartilage; 10, caudal margin quadrangular cartilage; 11, membranous septum. 12, posterior projection of "tongue" of quadrangular cartilage (variable length) (From Tardy ME. *Surgical anatomy of the nose.* New York: Raven Press, 1990, with permission.)

portive cartilaginous septal L-strut. The domal regions of the LLCs are in intimate proximity and typically project beyond the anterior septal angle, creating the external topography of the nasal tip. Because of this relation, deviations of the anterior septal angle may cause distortions of nasal-tip position. The posterior septal angle is located at the quadrangular cartilage articulation with the anterior nasal spine. The intermediate septal angle lies between the anterior and posterior septal angles.

The membranous septum is the soft-tissue continuation of the cartilaginous septum. Consisting of a central layer of subcutaneous areolar tissue between vestibular skin on each side, the membranous septum bridges the caudal edge of the cartilaginous septum to the medial crura and columella. Contained within it are the ligamentous attachments of the medial crura to the caudal septum. Because of a lack of cartilage, it is mobile and displaces easily with manipulation of the columella.

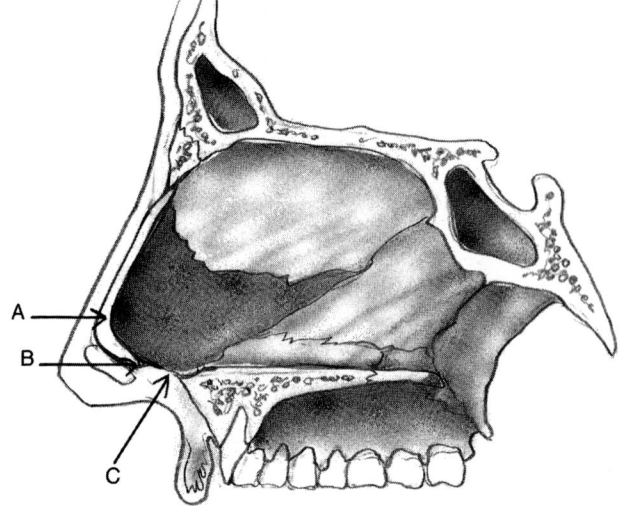

Figure 170.10 *Arrows,* The three anatomic angles composing the caudal aspect of the nasal quadrangular cartilage. *A,* Anterior septal angle. *B,* Midseptal angle. *C,* Posterior septal angle.

The septum is lined with an inner layer of perichondrium or periosteum covered by an outer layer of mucosa. The two layers of septal lining are closely attached and together contain the vascular and nervous supply to the septum. Separation of the mucoperichondrium from the underlying cartilage, as may occur in traumatic or postsurgical septal hematoma, may lead to ischemic necrosis of the affected septum and result in a perforation or a saddle-nose deformity. When portions of septal cartilage or bone are removed during surgery, the lining flaps from each side of the septum are left to readhere and scar. Thus during septal surgery, perforations may also result after opposing bilateral mucosal tears are created. Because the perichondrial and periosteal layers bear the majority of the biomechanical strength of the septal lining, the surgeon must remain deep to these layers during flap dissection, to maximize strength of the resulting lining flaps and reduce the risk of perforation. If the flap elevation occurs in a submucosal plane, the perichondrium or periosteum may be inadvertently resected with the septal cartilage and bone, leaving only the relatively weak mucosa, and increasing the risk of perforation (16).

Variant Anatomy

Differences in the size and development of the nasal septum account for many of the functional and aesthetic variations in the nose. Because the septum is attached to the cartilages that determine nasal shape (LLCs and ULCs), its overgrowth may lead to excessive projection of these structures. In these situations, the septum pulls the cartilaginous elements of the nose under tension—the underpinnings of the so-called tension-nose deformity. Such noses are characterized by a high cartilaginous dorsum, a tip-defining point that is determined by a projecting anterior septal angle (instead of the domal angle of the LLC), and a low-hanging columella that is created by a prominent caudal septal border. In such patients, conservative trimming of the septum may be necessary to create a less-conspicuous profile.

An inverse relation exists between the sizes of the cartilaginous septum and osseous septum. Patients with short nasal bones and long ULCs tend to have a greater abundance of quadrangular cartilage and less vomer and ethmoid plate. The opposite is true in noses with long nasal bones and short ULCs. This relation may help the rhinoplasty surgeon predict how much septal cartilage will be available for graft harvesting before surgery.

The septum rarely exists in a true midsagittal plane. Deviations from the midline have both functional and cosmetic implications. Particularly along the floor of the nasal airway, deviations may cause considerable airway obstruction. Most often, a combination of cartilaginous and osseous deformities contributes to the obstruction. Surgical treatment may require removing or repositioning these deviated skeletal elements. After trauma in particular, portions of the septum may be jagged and angulated. Meticulous elevation of the septal lining from these structures is required before their removal to prevent septal perfora-

tion. Uncorrected deviations of the perpendicular plate of the ethmoid and vomer may result in persistent posterior airway obstruction after septal surgery.

Deviations of the caudal and dorsal edge of the septum have cosmetic implications in addition to functional effects. From the rhinion to the anterior nasal spine, septal deviations may translate to visible external deformities. Deviation of the mid-dorsal septum, anterior septal angle, midcaudal septum, and posterior septal angle may lead to a crooked nose deformity at the upper cartilaginous vault, the nasal tip, the columella, or the columellar base, respectively. These irregularities may originate from a traumatic event. However, the septum will eventually develop an inherent memory to its new shape and position. Thus the correction of a severely crooked nose may require repositioning or replacing these septal elements (17).

Osseous Vault

The osseous vault is a pyramidal structure that, together with the bony septum, provides the principal structural support for the nose. It consists of the frontal process of the maxilla and the paired nasal bones. The cephalic portion of the osseous vault articulates with the frontal bone at the nasofrontal suture line. The superior portion of the nasal bones rests on the nasal spine of the frontal bone and also derives midline support from the perpendicular plate of the ethmoid. Caudally, the free edge of the osseous vault forms the superior portion of the pyriform aperture. The caudal edge is joined by a connective tissue to the upper cartilaginous vault in the keystone area.

Each nasal bone may be thought of as an elongated quadrangle, with its lateral long edge articulating with the frontal process of the maxilla and its medial long edge articulating in the midline with its contralateral partner. The cephalic edge at the nasofrontal suture line is narrow, whereas the free caudal edge is wider. The nasal bones are thick cephalically at the nasofrontal suture line and thin progressively toward the free caudal edge. Most traumatic nasal fractures occur in the caudal, more projecting portion of the nasal bones where they are the thinnest.

The bony pyramid of the osseous vault may be mobilized with osteotomies during rhinoplasty. Medial osteotomies disconnect the two halves of the osseous vault so each may be moved independently, and lateral osteotomies free the anterior sidewall of the osseous vault from its attachment to the rest of the frontal process of the maxilla. The lateral osteotomy is made on the frontal process of the maxilla and preserves the nasomaxillary suture line. A wide range of height, length, and width of the osseous vault occurs, and this should be taken into account in the planning of osteotomies.

Variant Anatomy

The overall thickness of the nasal bones varies by age, gender, and ethnicity. As elsewhere in the body, the nasal bones are subject to age-related osteopenia and may become thinner and more fragile over time, particularly in women. Such individuals are particularly prone to nasal fractures, even with moderate-energy trauma. After such injuries, it may take these patients longer to reach stable osseous union, potentially prolonging the time window in which closed nasal reduction may be performed. Surgical osteotomies should be performed cautiously in noses with thin, fragile bone, as a higher risk exists of creating overly mobile, free-floating osseous segments. In contrast, patients with thick, rigid nasal bones may be relatively resistant to nasal fractures, may heal rapidly after fractures occur, and may require greater force to create adequate osteotomies during surgery. Often in rhinoplasty, the goal is to create a modest narrowing of the osseous vault. This may be accomplished through a controlled back-fracture of the bridge of bone that remains between the cephalic termination of the medial and lateral osteotomies. In patients with thick bone, this osseous bridge may resist back-fracture. In such cases, the area of intact bone may be weakened before back-fracture through a transcutaneous bridging osteotomy. By using a 2-mm osteotome, a series of small perforations may be made through the bone through a single entry point in the skin.

Variations in the width and medial–lateral position of the nasal bones may be hereditary or acquired. Hereditary variations are more likely to manifest as a symmetrical but unusually narrow or wide osseous vault. Gross asymmetries are more likely to be acquired traumatic injuries. In many cases, these are injuries incurred very early in life or even during the birth process. Correction of these deformities typically requires repositioning of the nasal bones through surgical osteotomies. The lateral osteotomies should lie lateral to the bony deformity so that it may be incorporated into the segment of mobilized bone. In cases in which the nasal bone has a very convex, concave, or irregular topography, the bone may need to be mobilized in more than one segment to correct the contour irregularities. In such situations, an intermediate osteotomy may be necessary between the medial and lateral osteotomies. When several osteotomies are needed, they are performed medial to lateral so that the cuts are always made on stable bone. The distance of osteotomies needed to mobilize the nasal bones is dictated by their length, which is also highly variable.

Upper Cartilaginous Vault

The upper cartilaginous vault consists of the paired, shield-like ULCs that are fused in the midline to the dorsal edge of the cartilaginous septum. The septum and the ULCs are fused early in embryonic development and form a single structural unit in this area (18). Although the cartilaginous septum provides support to the ULCs at their midline dorsal fusion, the nasal bones provides the majority of reinforcement to the ULCs at their cephalic margin, the key-

stone area. Here, the ULCs overlap the caudal border of the osseous vault, extending cephalad under the bony arch for a distance of up to 11 mm. This attachment is critical in maintaining the structural integrity of the nasal framework. Vigorous downward force on the ULCs can lead to their dislocation from the nasal bones, a deformity that causes collapse of the upper cartilaginous vault. Because the nasal bones stabilize the ULCs at their cephalic aspect, the upper cartilaginous vault is less rigid and more mobile caudally.

The upper cartilaginous vault is wider cephalically where the ULCs take on a more horizontal course as they articulate with the septum. The arch of the ULCs closely follows the arch of the nasal bones in this region. Caudally, the ULCs slope more acutely away from the dorsal septum, creating a narrower dorsal line. At their caudal-most aspect, a free edge of the ULCs may diverge away laterally from the septum. This relatively narrow area of the upper cartilaginous vault corresponds intranasally to the internal nasal valve area, the region with the greatest nasal airway resistance. These regional variations are easily visualized on cross sections (Fig. 170.11).

Along with the cartilaginous septum, the ULCs determine the appearance of the middle third of the nose. The transition between these structures should be smooth and unbroken. Surgical alterations in this area, such as with hump reduction or spreader grafting, should result in a smooth, co-planar dorsal surface.

Variant Anatomy

The distance from nasion to rhinion defines the cephalic–caudal length of the osseous vault. The upper cartilaginous vault refers to the area of the nose from rhinion to the caudal edge of the ULCs. Despite their common nomenclature of upper and middle thirds of the nose, the lengths of these regions rarely occupy exactly one third of total nasal length. The lengths of the osseous vault and upper cartilaginous vault have an inverse relation. That is, individuals with long nasal bones have a short upper cartilaginous vault and vice versa. The length of the upper cartilaginous vault typically corresponds to the length of the quadrangular septal cartilage. Thus the presence of long nasal bones and a short upper cartilaginous vault should alert the surgeon that a relative deficiency of septal cartilage may be present.

The relative lengths of these areas have significant implications on the supportive mechanism of the internal nasal valve. Patients with long nasal bones and short ULCs tend to have more support of the internal valve area because of a greater contribution of the rigid support provided by the nasal bones. In contrast, long ULCs have less rigid osseous support and are therefore more prone to collapse, particularly at their caudal aspect in the area of the internal nasal valve (Fig. 170.12). Individuals with preexisting narrowing in this region may already have nasal valve insufficiency or collapse of the ULC during inspiration. These patients are predisposed to develop postrhino-

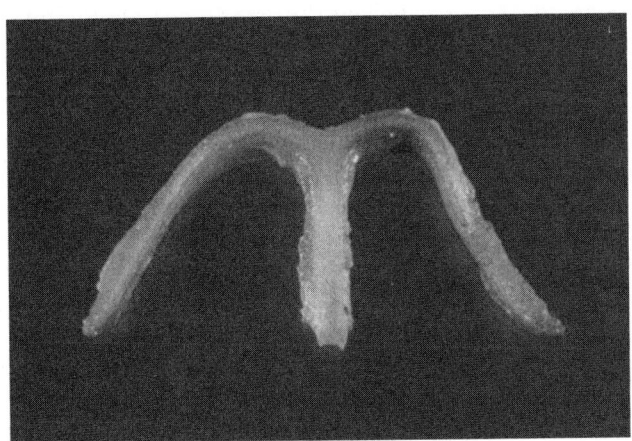
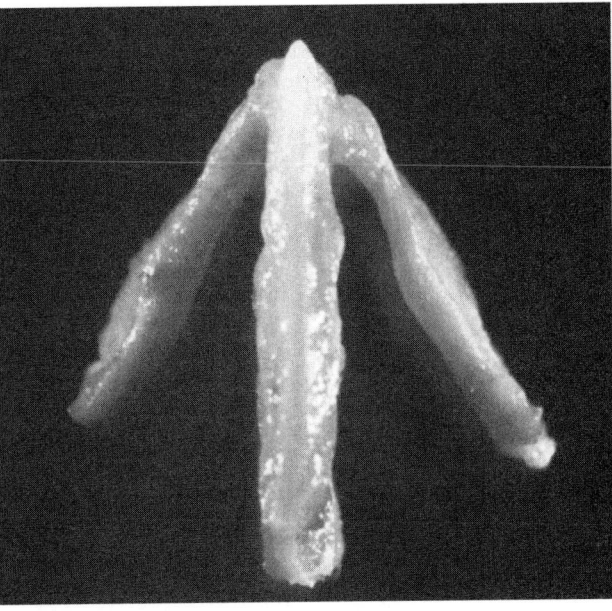

A   **B**

Figure 170.11   A: Cross section of the upper cartilaginous vault just below the rhinion. The broad arch of the upper lateral cartilages closely follows the caudal margin of the nasal bones in this region. **B:** Further caudal in the area of the internal nasal valve, the structures are more flexible and a much narrower relation exists between the upper lateral cartilages and nasal septum. (Photograph courtesy of Dean Toriumi.)

plasty nasal obstruction after dorsal hump reduction. In such cases, the articulation of the ULCs and septum is resected with the hump, leaving the ULCs unsupported along the dorsum. Ensuing inferomedial collapse of the ULCs occurs, leading to internal valve narrowing, medial pinching of the central area of the dorsal line, and the inverted-V deformity, in which cephalic ULC collapse reveals the outline of the V-shaped caudal border of the nasal bones. To prevent such complications, the ULC should be

resupported onto the septum with a technique such as spreader grafting.

Lower Cartilaginous Vault

The key elements in the lower cartilaginous vault are the paired lower lateral (or alar) cartilages. Perhaps more than anywhere else in the nose, endless anatomic variations and divergences are found between individuals in these

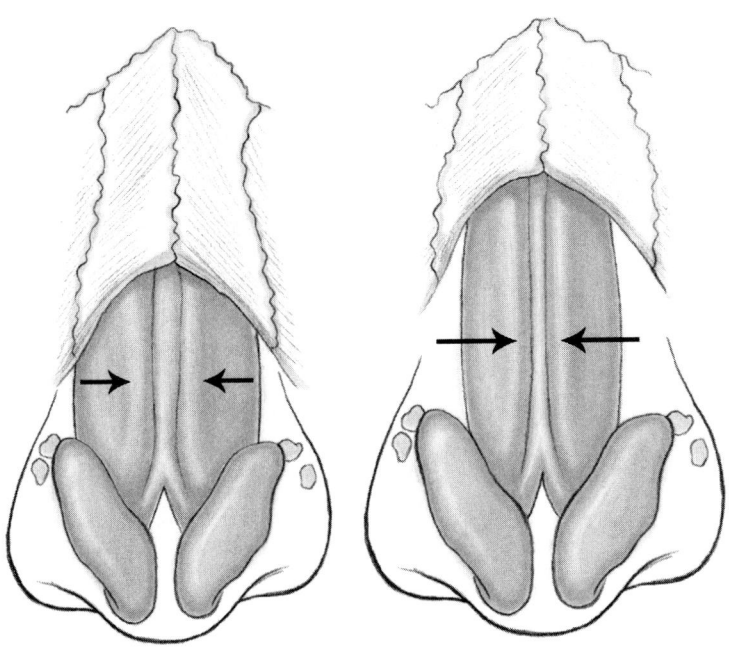

A   **B**

Figure 170.12   A: Long nasal bones create more stabilization of the caudal cartilaginous elements of the nose with less tendency for inferomedial collapse of the upper lateral cartilages with inspiration or with scarring after hump reduction. **B:** Short nasal bones and a long upper cartilaginous vault may cause narrowing of the upper lateral cartilages after they are separated from the nasal septum following hump reduction. Restabilization with spreader grafts may prevent this complication in such patients.

structures. However, the extent to which the LLCs determine the shape and configuration of the nasal tip and base is variable, depending on the thickness of the SSTE and the tensile and compressive forces imparted to these areas by the attachments to the surrounding fixed structures of the nasal septum, pyriform aperture, ULCs, and nasal bones. Nonetheless, surgical modifications of the nasal tip and base in rhinoplasty almost always involve some modification to the shape or position of the LLCs.

With the septum, the LLCs provide support to the nasal tip. Each LLC may be considered in three sections: the medial crus, the intermediate crus, and the lateral crus. The three areas are not necessarily distinct anatomic entities, but transition from one to the next through a series of bends and undulations in the continuous roll of cartilage. These myriad turns and divergences create the nuances of this structure, which then form the unique external topography of each nasal tip. Two distinct angles, however, are fairly consistent in most noses and consequently are generally conceptualized as transition points that separate the three crura: the lateral genu and the medial genu (Fig. 170.4A). The subsequent discussion covers the general anatomy of each subsite of the lower lateral crura. The more commonly encountered variant anatomy is then discussed. The role of the LLCs as they pertain to mechanical stabilization of the nose is discussed subsequently.

The Medial Crus

With their connection to the caudal septum, the medial crura form the structural support of the columella. The width of the LLCs is narrowest in this region and may be as little as 4 to 5 mm. Each medial crus may be divided into an anterior columellar segment and a posterior footplate segment. On base view, each columellar segment parallels its contralateral counterpart and is connected to it and the caudal septum by fibrous tissue. The footplate segment flares posterolaterally and contributes to the normal widening of the columella at its base or pedestal. On the lateral or base view of an ideal Caucasian nose, the anterior limit of the medial crus corresponds to the columellar–lobular junction at the apex of the nostril (Fig. 170.4).

Variant Anatomy

Variation in the length and shape of the medial crus affects the appearance of the nasal base and position of the nasal tip (19). A short medial crus results in a short columella and a small anteroposterior dimension of the nostril. This tends to result in deficient nasal tip projection and a small nostril–lobular ratio. A long medial crus that extends anteriorly beyond the apex of the nostril creates a flat, projecting nasal tip. Endless variations exists in the degree of symmetry, curvature, flare, and smoothness of these structures. The intervening soft tissue between the columellar segments may camouflage irregularities, but a thin SSTE may lead to a bifid appearance of the columella. In general, the goals during

surgery are to place the medial crura into a symmetrical, midline position. Fixation sutures to resecure the medial crura are a reliable technique to this end, but care must be taken to maintain a normal relation between the crura and surrounding structures. For instance, the medial crura should be bound together only at their cephalic borders to retain the natural flare of the caudal edges so as to maintain adequate columellar width (11). Even a small degree of malposition of the medial crura may have significant impact on nasal-tip rotation, projection, columellar show, and nasolabial angle. Fixation, therefore, must be executed with enormous forethought and meticulous technique.

The width of the individual medial crura and their distance from each other determine the width of the columella. In some cases, the normal flare of the posterior medial crura (footplates) is exaggerated, leading to a wide columellar base, which may compromise airflow at the nostril aperture. Caudally positioned medial crura may result from excessive cartilaginous width, lax ligamentous attachments to the caudal septum (wide membranous septum), or caudal overgrowth of the septum, which tensions the medial crura downward. Particularly in the presence of retracted nasal ala, low medial crura will lead to excessive columellar show. Such patients may complain that their nostrils are too conspicuous. Surgical correction usually involves elevating or trimming the caudal margin of the medial crura.

The Intermediate Crus

Also called the domal segments, the intermediate crura bridge the medial and lateral crura, extending from the medial genu to the lateral genu. This structure represents the transition from the convergent and divergent portions of the paired LLCs. The region of the lateral genu is often the anteriormost projecting point of the LLC and may correspond topographically to the tip-defining point. In this region, the intermediate crus may narrow abruptly, rendering it susceptible to transection during surgery. The angle formed between the two intermediate crura as they flare away from each other laterally is termed the angle of divergence (Fig. 170.13). The ideal angle is approximately

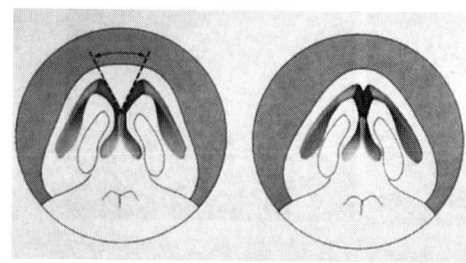

Figure 170.13 The intermediate crura bridge the lateral and medial crura of the lower lateral cartilages. The angle of divergence is shown on the left. If the intermediate crura are widely bifurcated, a broad trapezoid appearance of the tip results, as shown on the left. If the intermediate crura are closely opposed, a triangular appearance results, as shown on the right.

60 degrees and provides a natural-appearing width to the infratip lobule as it transitions from the columella to the nasal tip on frontal or basal views. The intermediate crura also diverge from the medial crura in a cephalic direction by approximately 50 degrees. Externally on lateral view, this bend corresponds to the columellar–lobular angle, dividing the nasal base into the infratip lobule anteriorly and columella posteriorly—the basis of the double break.

Variant Anatomy

Variations in the length and curvature of the intermediate crura and the degree of angulation at the medial and lateral genua determine the shape of the infratip lobule on frontal and basal views. Gentle turns at the genua and a smooth convex curvature of the intermediate crus produce a convex domal segment. A broad and flat intermediate crura with angulated connections at the genua result in a "boxy" configuration. If the intermediate crura are concave, a "double dome" segment is created (2). Variation in the angle of divergence also will affect the shape of the tip lobule. A narrow angle of divergence results in a narrow lobule and creates a more triangular appearance to the tip on base view. An angle of divergence approaching 90 degrees produces a boxy tip that appears trapezoidal on base view. These variations in the cartilage configuration may not be reflected in the shape of the tip lobule if overlying skin is thick (Fig. 170.13).

Excessive thickness or convexity of the intermediate crura in the cephalic–caudal dimension may manifest externally as bulging of the infratip lobule. On lateral view, the tip may appear rounded, transitioning to the infratip lobule with one unbroken curve, rather than as a distinct normal double break.

The Lateral Crus

The lateral crus extends from the lateral genu of the LLC posteriorly. Normally, it assumes a gentle convex shape and parallels the alar rim for its medial half, then flattens and turns posterosuperiorly for its lateral portion, ending short of the pyriform aperture. It generally becomes wider as it leaves the lateral genu, and then narrows again toward its lateral termination. It is typically the broadest portion of the LLC. Although a centimeter in width is a reasonable estimate of average width, tremendous variation exists (20).

A portion of the medial cephalic borders of the lateral crura may overlap. In this region, the LLCs may be connected to each other and to the caudal border of the ULC by fibrous tissue. The connection to the ULCs are often reinforced by overlapping segments of cartilage. This scroll area is highly variable and may be thickened in comparison to other parts of the LLC (Fig. 170.14).

Variant Anatomy

The variations of lateral crus anatomy are too numerous to detail (20), but some of the more commonly seen variations are discussed herein. Variations in the width and curvature of the lateral crura greatly influence the appearance of the tip and ala. The widest portion of the lateral crus may vary from 7 to 15 mm (20). Broad convex lateral crura impart a bulbous, amorphous appearance to the tip. The concept is similar to the relation of dorsal height and the appearance of width discussed earlier. In a normal nose, the relative narrowness at the nasal tip/domes and the relative width at the alar base create a visual contrast that makes the tip look appropriately distinct and refined. If the transition from the tip to base is characterized by widely

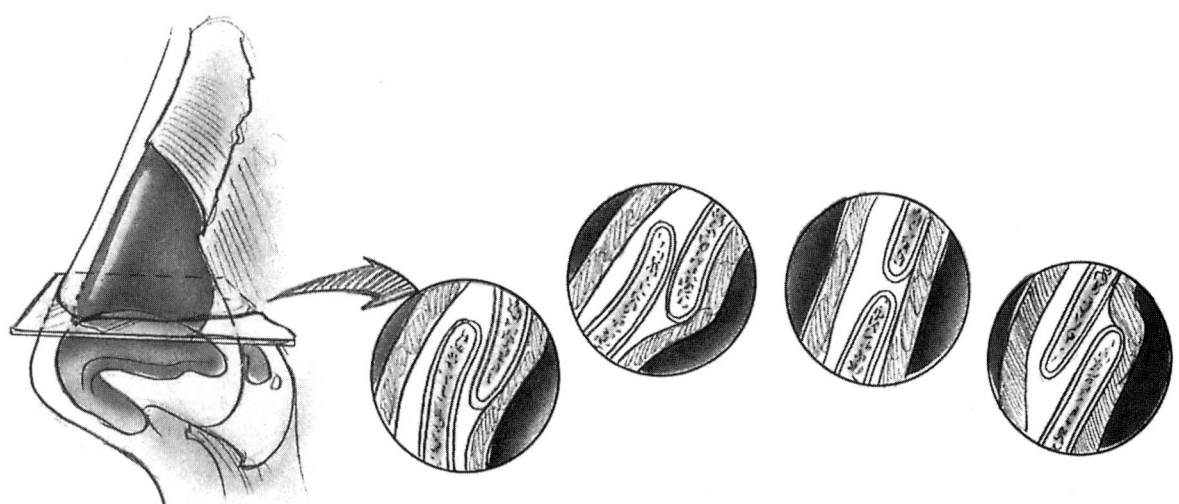

Figure 170.14 A variety of anatomic relations between the cephalic margin of the lower lateral cartilage and the caudal margin of the upper lateral cartilage is found in dissection of cadaver specimens. As individuals age, the intimate relation between the cartilages may be lost. (From Tardy ME. *Surgical anatomy of the nose*. New York: Raven Press, 1990, with permission.)

curving lateral crura and nasal ala, this contrast is indistinct, creating the appearance of a wide nose. Correction of such a deformity may require techniques to straighten the overly curved lateral crura, such as suture modification or structural grafting. Aggressive techniques that focus only on narrowing the domes themselves and ignore the convexity of the lateral crura may result in no improvement of the appearance of the tip while incurring structural and cosmetic complications.

Less commonly, the LLCs may be concave as they diverge away from the domes. Externally, this may manifest as a hollow, sunken appearance at the alar lobule with an exaggerated supra-alar crease. If severe, the concavity may narrow the nasal vestibule, impairing nasal airflow. Surgical correction may require structural onlay or underlay grafting, resection and graft replacement of the concave segment, or simply flipping over the concave segment through excision, inversion, and suture fixation.

The strength and thickness of the intermediate and lateral crura determine much of the inherent support of the nasal tip. Stronger cartilage is more resistant to alteration and may result in visible or palpable deformities after surgery. The surgeon must remember Tardy's admonition of the risks of bossae formation after excisional techniques to narrow the tip in patients who possess the triad of tip bifidity, thin skin, and strong LLCs. In such situations, the thick edges of cartilage gradually become apparent through the thin skin envelope as contracture distorts the disrupted tip structures. Modification through suture techniques with avoidance of LLC division is less likely to lead to bossae formation in such patients.

As discussed, the medial aspect of the cephalic border of the lateral crura may overlap for a variable distance. This degree of overlap depends on the overall cephalocaudal position of the lateral crura. In extreme cases, the trajectory of the upper border of the lateral crura is actually straight cephalad, each edge overlapping with the other in the midline over the dorsal septum. In such noses, the lateral crura may diverge from the midline only near its lateral termination. External deformities may be discernable in such patients, particularly in those with thin skin. The classic description is the parenthesis deformity, so named because the bulky outline on frontal view created by the cephalically positioned lateral crura looks as if it is framed by two parentheses on either side of the supratip—"( )". A high dorsum at the supratip on the lateral view in such patients may be misdiagnosed as overdevelopment of the quadrangular cartilage in this region when it may be caused by the overriding cephalic lateral crura. Lowering the dorsum in such patients may require trimming of the cephalic margin of the lateral crura or suture repositioning of the lateral crura instead of dorsal septal excision, the conventional approach to profile reduction. Another consequence of cephalic lateral crura is the resultant decrease in support to the alar margin. With the lateral crus angled further cephalad, less structural reinforcement is provided to the caudal alar rim, predisposing patients to alar pinching or external nasal valve insufficiency.

Another variation of the lateral crus that may affect nasal airflow is inward (medial) recurvature of its lateral terminus. In some patients, this creates a visible or palpable mass in the lateral nasal vestibule, potentially impairing nasal airflow. In other cases, the deformity may not be apparent until after other rhinoplasty maneuvers have caused medialization of the lateral nasal wall, such as dome narrowing or tip-projecting maneuvers. Correction may involve simple excision of this portion of the lateral crus if it is caused by overly long, redundant cartilage. Repositioning the area with a stiff underlay graft may be needed in other situations.

Asymmetries of the lateral crura may create tip irregularities and contour deformities. When these asymmetries are severe, they may create tip deviation, even in the presence of a midline caudal septum.

NASAL BASE

The main structures of the nasal base are the paired nasal alae, the nasal sills, the soft triangles, and the columella. These structures form a continuous ring around each of the nares or nostrils, the external openings of the nasal cavities. The normal Caucasian nostril should be oval, with a vertical axis less than 45 degrees from the columella and a nostril-to-infratip lobule ratio of 2:1. Ethnic differences account for significant divergences from these values.

The *nasal ala* is the most lateral winglike portion of the nostril (21). The main body of the alar lobule is devoid of cartilaginous structure and consists of fibroareolar tissue. Because of this, the shape of the alar lobule is not typically sculpted directly in rhinoplasty. However, cartilaginous elements frame the nasal ala, and their modification alters its shape. The lateral crus of the LLC sweeps over the superomedial portion of the ala. The sesamoid cartilages are located in the soft tissue overlying the pyriform aperture above the ala. Their number is variable, with zero to five cartilaginous bodies present. Interlaced with collagen and fibrous tissue, these accessory cartilages form the sesamoid complex, the connection between the mobile termination of the lateral crus to the rigid pyriform aperture rim.

The insertion of the nasal ala to the face at the junction of the lip and cheek subunits determines the width of the nasal base. Interalar width refers to the horizontal distance from one alar crease to the other. The overall width of the nostrils is also affected by the alar flare, as defined by the degree of bowing of the ala above its insertion. The insertion to the face is three-dimensional, paralleling the curved alar crease that frames the nostrils laterally. Along with the position of the columella, the vertical position of the alar insertion determines the degree of columellar show.

The *nasal sill* is the soft-tissue continuation of the ala as it curves medially to join the columella at the nasal spine. It represents the floor of the nostril and is generally wider in those individuals with a large interalar width. Inadvertent injury to the thin skin in this area may lead to visible scar or contraction leading to stenosis of the nostril.

The *soft triangle* is a small base-up triangular subunit bordering the columella medially, the ala laterally, and apex of the nostril anteriorly. This area is unique in that it contains minimal subcutaneous tissue. The external nasal skin folds directly onto the internal vestibular skin, spanning across the genua of the LLC. Because of the lack of subdermal support, this delicate skin is prone to scar contracture if violated. Cicatrix in this area can also lead to reduction in the cross-sectional area of the nostril.

The *columella* is made up of the paired medial crura, which are bound together with fibrous attachments and covered with a skin envelope continuous with the membranous septum. In most individuals, the columella is fairly mobile, limited only by the attachments of the medial crura to the relatively fixed caudal border of the cartilaginous septum. The shape of the columella is determined by the paired medial crura and the most caudal edge of the cartilaginous septum. Distortions of the columella on base view often result from a deviated caudal tip of the septum, which may be easily revealed with side-to-side manipulation.

Variant Anatomy

The alar base represents one of the most highly variable regions of the nose. Width of the alar insertion is rarely within the confines of the medial canthi, as widely described, even in the leptorrhine Caucasian nose. Overall nasal alar width results from the combination of interalar width and alar flare. Patients of Asian and African descent are more likely to have greater alar base width, alar flare, a shorter columella, and more horizontally oriented nostrils. These external differences are ascribable to underlying variations of structural anatomy: weaker, flatter LLCs; thick SSTE; and deficiency of the premaxilla and nasal spine (22). Thickness of the alar wall is also inconstant and reflects the amount of subcutaneous fatty fibroareolar tissue. These variations account for a wide range of nostril orientations and resultant deviation from the "normal" nostril-to-infratip lobule ratio of 2:1. Farkas (23) categorizes the variants of nostril position into seven types ranging from vertical to horizontal.

It is crucial that the rhinoplasty surgeon precisely diagnose the cause of a wide alar base before surgery. Some individuals have a wide interalar distance associated with wide nasal sills as the predominant cause. Correction of such a deformity might require segmental excision and closure of a portion of the nasal sills or suture technique to narrow the sills. Other patients may have a normal alar insertion with normal interalar distance, but excessive alar flare. Reduction of the ala above the insertion would then be indicated. Reduction of the sill without addressing the alar side walls in such patients may actually lead to an exaggeration of the flare, as the ala are forced to curve more acutely. Many patients have components of both an increased interalar width and alar flare, requiring treatment of both the sill area as well as the alar side walls.

In addition, the internal and external circumferences of the nostrils must be considered so that the geometry of the excision may be appropriately adjusted. Some individuals have a normal or even small inner nostril circumference, but have an overall wide alar base because of thick alar walls. Such individuals benefit from a triangular or trapezoidal wedge excision such that more tissue is excised from the external rim of the nostril than is removed from the inner circumference. In extreme cases, the alar side wall itself may be debulked and thinned through an alar rim incision.

MECHANICS AND STABILITY

Structural Elements and Relations

Considerations regarding the mechanical stability of the nose are too often overlooked in rhinoplasty. Compromise to the structures and relations that maintain the nose's architecture leads to long-term complications impairing both function and cosmesis. In this section, the regional anatomy of the nose is revisited as it pertains to the mechanical stabilization of the nose. Also discussed are several conceptual models, some of them co-opted from engineering principles, which are commonly invoked to help surgeons conceptualize the elements of nasal structural stability.

The stability of the nose derives from the strength and resiliency of its complex anatomic elements and their various interconnections. Three echelons of support may be conceptualized, each contributing various degrees of stabilization. First, the osseous framework, including the nasal bones, pyriform aperture, osseous septum, and nasal floor, provides the rigid foundation onto which the cartilaginous and soft-tissue elements are built. Second, the rigid quadrangular cartilage, which is fixated to bone along its ventral and cephalic borders, directly supports the upper and lower cartilaginous vaults. And third, the intrinsic architectures of the LLCs, ULCs, and associated soft tissue, which are all supported by the osseous and septal foundations, provide much of the stability of the nasal tip and base. The extent to which these regions exert support to the nose depends on the region of the nose. Cephalad, the nasal bones and osseous septum provide nearly all of the rigid support. The middle third of the nose is supported by the nasal bones cephalically and by the quadrangular cartilage, which serves as a pillar beneath. The nasal tip and base area, farthest removed from the osseous framework, is the most flexible and dynamic region and depends most on the support of the cartilaginous buttressing of the caudal septum and the inherent strength of the LLCs.

Cantilever Concept

Sheen (19) has described the nasal skeleton as a cantilever, in which the osseous vault is a stable extension of the skull. Like a cantilever, the upper cartilaginous vault projects as a beam, supported cephalically through the thick fibrous attachment of the keystone area, and carries the load of the dependent aspects of the nose along its length and at its distal end. The strength of this support depends on the length and thickness of the nasal bones. Longer bones impart more caudal support. The fusion of the osseous vault and the upper cartilaginous vault with the dorsal edge of the septum forms this structural I-beam that extends from the nasion toward the nasal tip. This complex forms the basis of dorsal support for the nose. Disruption of the connections between the nasal bones or of the ULCs or both to the septum greatly weakens the central support provided by the I-beam. This occurs during hump reduction in which the medial septal support element for the ULCs is resected. The ULCs then must rely only on the cephalic attachments to the nasal bones for support. Unless this medial support is reestablished, for example with spreader grafts, the ULCs may collapse inferomedially, creating pinching, internal valve compromise, and the inverted-V.

Role of the Nasal Septum

The nasal septum supports the cantilever from its undersurface much as a support wall holds up a roof. Particularly at its caudal aspect, the quadrangular cartilage, functioning as a pillar, carries much of the burden of nasal-tip support in most noses. Because the quadrangular cartilage is inherently rigid and sits firmly in an osseous foundation from the nasal spine along the maxillary crest and up the osseous septum to the nasal bones, it provides significant stabilization to the nose. The combination of the cantilevering dorsal element and the buttressing caudal element forms the basis of the L-shaped strut—the most structurally important aspect of the quadrangular cartilage. Compromise to the dorsal component leads to a saddle-nose deformity with ventral collapse of the upper cartilaginous vault. The classic example of this is quadrangular cartilage resorption after an untreated septal hematoma. Compromise to the caudal component may lead to nasal-tip ptosis, particularly in the presence of weak medial crura. Traumatic or iatrogenic injury is most often the cause. This is shown in studies in which removal of the cartilaginous septum in cadavers has been shown to result in a significant loss in nasal-tip projection (24). For these reasons, it is critical to maintain structural integrity of the L-strut during surgery. Although conventional teaching emphasizes the need to maintain an uninterrupted 1.5-cm-wide dorsal–caudal strut, malposition or deformity

of the strut itself may be the cause of external deformities, particularly in the crooked nose. Correction of these problems may mandate the use of techniques that modify the septum and may require repositioning, camouflaging, or reconstruction of the L-strut itself (17).

Ligamentous Attachments

The nasal bones and the quadrangular cartilage serve as the rigid support structures of the nose. The more mobile caudal elements are reinforced onto these foundations through a network of fibrous adhesions. Although termed "ligaments," these connections do not conform to the strict definition of an attachment between an osseous origin and insertion. Rather, they bind the cartilaginous structures to each other, to the nasal septum, and to the pyriform aperture. Numerous histologic and cadaver studies have been conducted in an attempt to better characterize the nature of this tissue. Although the characteristics of these attachments are variably reported, most authors believe they impart a variable degree of structural stabilization to the nose, and in particular, the nasal tip. The ligamentous systems most commonly described are discussed later: the attachments between the ULCs and lateral crura, the intercrural ligaments, the attachments between the lateral crura and pyriform aperture, and the connection between the ULCs and nasal bones at the keystone region (discussed earlier).

The area of overlap between the caudal aspect of the ULCs and the cephalic margin of the lateral crura is commonly referred to as the *scroll region*, owing to the interlocking curved cartilaginous elements. In reality, the relation between these structures is highly variable. In the most common orientation, the upper borders of the lateral crura overlap above the ULCs. It is thought that the extent of recurvature of the ULC is determined by the tension exerted onto its cephalic margin as it is driven cephalad during fetal development (25). The angle of curvature may range from slight (less than 45 degrees) to complete (180 degrees). Other orientations exist with various relations between the cartilaginous structures (Fig. 170.14). Irrespective of the particular orientation, the cartilages are bound together within the scroll region by fibrous tissue, also described as the "intercartilaginous ligament" (26). This articulation forms a hinge mechanism around which the nasal tip is suspended and can flex (27). With advancing age, the intimate relation between the ULCs and the lateral crura may be lost as these ligamentous connections relax and the nasal tip settles caudally. In such cases, a diastasis between the upper and lower cartilaginous vaults may be present instead of a normal thickened scroll area.

The intercrural ligament, also termed "the ligamentous sling" (28), binds the medial aspect of the lateral crura, the intermediate crura, and the medial crura to each other. This ligamentous structure is thought to pull the paired

LLCs into the midline. It is widely believed that fibrous attachments connect this ligament to the caudal margin of the septum in the region of the medial crura, providing additional tip support at the base of the nose (29). Other cadaver studies, however, dispute the existence of such connections. The contribution of the intercrural ligament in overall tip support, however, is fairly clear. After division of the intercrural ligament, nasal-tip support is decreased by 25% to 35%, as measured by tensigrometry (30). These studies highlight the need to restore the integrity of these attachments after they are disrupted during surgery, to prevent postoperative loss of tip support. An effective means to this end is through stabilization of the tip at the nasal base. Such techniques involve suture stabilization of the medial and intermediate crura to a stable midline foundation, such as a long nasal septum, a nasal septal caudal extension graft, or a columellar strut (1).

The connection between the lateral crura and the pyriform aperture consists of collagen fibers arranged irregularly with muscular fibers interspersed (31). This connection, which in some individuals contains embedded sesamoid cartilages, also is called the *sesamoid complex or the lateral crural complex*.

Nasal-Tip Support: Tripod Concept

The nasal tip is a complex structure whose integrity is maintained by an interrelated network of supporting mechanisms made up of both the tip cartilages and the ligaments that connect them. One classic model used for understanding nasal-tip support and dynamics is the tripod analogy (32). The apex of the tripod is the nasal tip, with each of the lateral crura extending cephalolaterally to form two legs of the tripod, and the conjoined medial crura together forming the third leg. Modification of the limbs of the tripod results in changes in nasal-tip position. Shortening the limbs results in a loss of tip projection, whereas lengthening increases projection. Tip rotation increases as a result of either truncating the lateral limbs or extending the medial limb. The opposite maneuvers lead to decreased tip rotation. Although the tripod concept is useful to conceptualize these dynamic consequences of crural modification, the analogy falls short as a model for tip structural support. Unlike a true tripod, the LLCs do not rest on a stable surface. Rather, their "feet" are tethered by ligamentous connections to the osseous rim of the pyriform aperture and nasal spine, whereas the apex is tensioned anteriorly and cephalad by the intercrural ligament and the scroll (33). Thus the nasal-tip tripod is a dynamic unit that is suspended and supported by its rigid surrounding structures (Fig. 170.15).

Nasal-Tip Support: Tardy Classification

In his classic description of nasal-tip support, Tardy includes three major and six minor mechanisms (Table 170.2),

TABLE 170.2
TIP-SUPPORT MECHANISMS

Major
  Size, shape, and resilience of the medial and lateral crura
  Medial crural footplate attachment to the caudal border of the quadrangular cartilage
  Attachment of the upper lateral cartilages (caudal border) to the alar cartilages (cephalic border)
Minor[a]
  Ligamentous sling spanning the paired domes of the alar cartilages
  Cartilaginous septal dorsum
  Sesamoid complex extending the support of the lateral crura to the pyriform aperture
  Attachment of the alar cartilages to the overlying skin and musculature
  Nasal spine
  Membranous septum

[a]On occasion, because of extreme anatomic variability, a "minor" tip support may assume the importance of one of the more major supports.

each of which imparts variable degrees of support depending on individual anatomy (6). The three major mechanisms are the size, shape, thickness, and strength of the medial and lateral crura; the attachment of the medial crural footplate to the caudal border of the quadrangular cartilage; and the attachment of the caudal border of the ULCs to the cephalic border of the LLCs. The minor tip-support mechanisms are thought to augment the major ones. The classification into major and minor groups was based on clinical experience rather than on one specific structural model. Tardy advocates assessment of tip recoil through digital palpation to determine the relative importance of the various tip-support mechanisms in a given patient.

Nasal-Tip Support: Other Models

Other schema of nasal tip–support mechanisms have been reported. Based on multiple cadaver dissections, Janeke and Wright (28) proposed that the tip support is based on the fibrous connection between the ULCs and LLCs; the connection between the lateral crus to the pyriform aperture; the interdomal ligament between the paired domes of the LLCs; and the attachment of the medial crus to the caudal septum (28). Two of these are considered major tip-support mechanisms in the Tardy classification. The importance of the interdomal ligament, classified as a minor mechanism by Tardy, also is echoed by other authors who concluded that this intercrural ligament is a major tip-support mechanism and should be reconstructed during open rhinoplasty (29,34). Conversely, other authors believe that the attachment of the medial crural footplates to the septum, a major mechanism in the Tardy classification, plays only a small role in the stability of the nasal tip (33). This is supported by histologic studies of cadaveric noses showing the lack of defined attachments in this area (18,28,31).

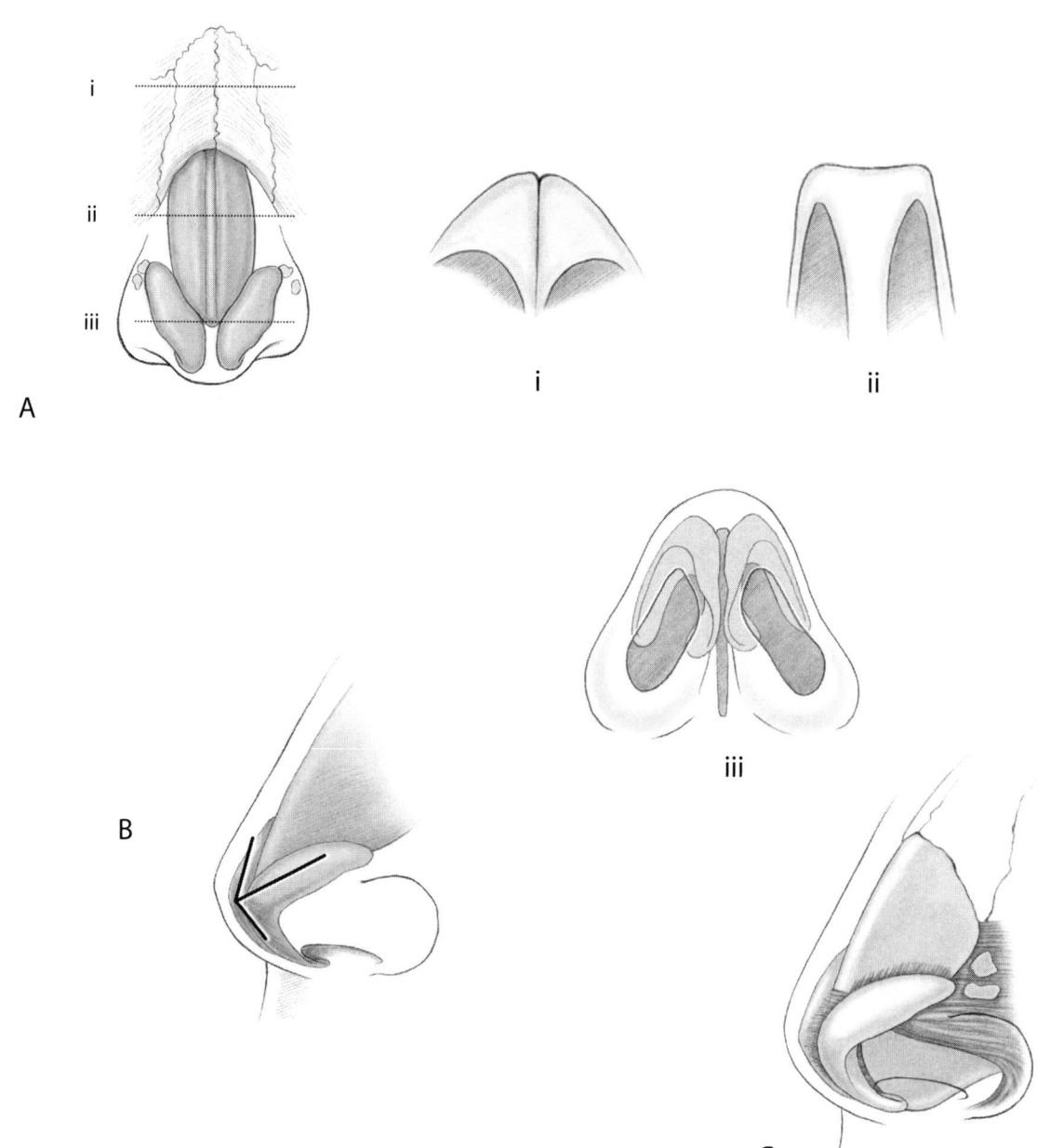

Figure 170.15 Various support mechanisms of the nose. **A:** The nasal septum functions as a supporting wall that reinforces the dorsal elements of the nose. (i) Cross section through osseous vault, (ii) upper cartilaginous vault, (iii) and nasal base. **B:** The two lateral crura and the conjoined medial crura create a nasal-tip tripod, a model useful for understanding nasal-tip dynamics. The degree to which the inherent strength of these structures contributes to nasal-tip support varies significantly from individual to individual. **C:** The network of ligamentous attachments reinforce and interconnect the skeletal elements of the nose. The upper lateral cartilages are connected firmly to the undersurface of the nasal bones, forming a cantilever-like support for the dorsum. The nasal tip and base are stabilized through ligamentous attachments between the lateral crura and upper lateral cartilage, the lateral crura and pyriform aperture, and between the two dorsal regions of each lower lateral cartilage.

Tardy points out that minor mechanisms become major contributors (and vice versa) in certain individuals depending on their particular anatomy.

Several of the ligamentous tip-support structures have been examined in histologic detail in fresh cadaveric noses, and the results are consistent with the macroscopic findings from dissections and from clinical experience. For example, the fibrous connection between the ULCs and LLCs is shown to consist of dense collagen fibers running in the same direction and anchored firmly to each cartilage (4,7,31). This meets the histologic criteria of a true ligament.

The concept of the nasal tip as a dynamic structure is carried further in the tensegrity model of nasal-tip support as proposed by Dyer (33). Applying an engineering and architectural concept to the nasal skeleton, Dyer proposed that the nasal tip may be thought of as a tensegrity structure, in which stability derives from the distribution of mechanical stress throughout all its components. Such a structure is self-stabilizing, consisting of an equilibrium of compressive and tensile elements. In the nasal tip, the LLCs and the cartilaginous septum are the compression-bearing members, and the fibrous, ligamentous connections are tension-bearing members. The nasal-tip structure is thus viewed as an integrated structure in which disruption of one element affects the stability of the whole. Although it is difficult to test this description of nasal-tip support scientifically, it is a useful concept that has already been applied to rhinoplasty techniques (33).

Areas of Structural Void

Two areas of the nose devoid of cartilaginous support are particularly susceptible to collapse in certain patients. First, the lateral nasal wall that is lateral (and often cephalad) to the termination of the lateral crura and medial to the pyriform aperture is prone to dynamic collapse with inspiration. This area corresponds intranasally to the internal valve area and may require reinforcement with graft such as alar batten grafts. In the normal state, this area is supported by the dilator naris and nasalis muscles (7). A second area is the alar margin, particularly lateral to the point at which the lateral crura diverge cephalically. In patients with projecting, thin noses, the alar margins are susceptible to collapse and resultant external valve narrowing.

In summary, the stability of the nasal skeleton derives from its rigid elements, the nasal bones, pyriform aperture, and nasal septum. The dynamic caudal structures, the nasal tip and base, are stabilized largely through the lower lateral crural attachments to these anchoring structures through networks of interconnecting fibrous tissue or ligaments. The means of support may be conceptualized both as a cantilevering mechanism from the nasal bones and ULCs cephalically and a pillar-like support from the septum ventrally. Although the inherent strength and resiliency of the LLCs create a dynamic tripod and provide form and some support to the nasal tip, a significant loss of tip support is incurred if the attachments of the tripod to the surrounding rigid structures are violated. In rhinoplasty, it is therefore imperative to reconstitute tip support through methods such as suture stabilization of the medial and intermediate crura to a stable midline foundation to prevent postoperative tip instability.

Variant Anatomy

The infinite variations of form are evident in the different structural orientations encountered in different noses. As Tardy reminds us, the relative role of any of the structural component of the nose differs from person to person. For example, individuals with long, broad nasal bones are more apt to have greater stability imparted to upper cartilaginous vault and to the caudal elements of the nasal tip and base. Within the tip itself, thicker, more developed

cartilage provides greater strength and has a larger role in structural support than in someone with weak, thin cartilages. These differences are important to remember when choosing rhinoplasty techniques. For instance, one traditional method to decrease projection of the tip is simply to perform a full transfixion incision and an intercartilaginous incision. Because this incision violates many of the anchoring ligamentous attachments of the tip tripod, the nasal tip may settle toward the face, thus reducing overall projection. However, in a nose in which the medial crura are long and broad, their inherent strength and resiliency may prevent the tip from moving. Methods that reposition and fixate the tip structures to stable surrounding structures are more reliable, reducing the unpredictability of results based on patient variant anatomy (1).

FUNCTIONAL VALVULAR ANATOMY

Internal Nasal Valve

The internal nasal valve area is the narrowest portion of the nasal passage. It is framed superolaterally by the caudal border of the ULC, medially by the septum, inferiorly by the floor of the pyriform aperture, and posteriorly by the head of the inferior turbinate (35). The *internal nasal valve,* formed by the caudal border of the ULC and the septum, is a specific slitlike structure within the internal nasal valve area and is often the narrowest region of the internal valve area. The angle formed by the attachment of the ULCs to the septum is 10 to 15 degrees in the Caucasian nose and wider in the African or Asian nose. If this angle is less than 10 degrees, the patient will likely experience nasal obstruction because of the collapse of the internal valve on inspiration.

External Nasal Valve

The external nasal valve consists of the nare and the nasal vestibule. The nasal vestibule is the space just inside the external nare and is the compartment caudal to the internal valve area. The vestibule is bordered medially by the septum and columella and laterally by the alar sidewalls. The vestibule contains vibrissae, or nasal hair, on a fold of skin under the lateral crus. Functioning as a coarse filter for inspired air, the vibrissae also serve a resistive purpose to slow the inspired air current and directing it posteriorly into the nasal cavity (36).

The internal and external nasal valves are dynamic structures that function together to deliver a smooth air current to the nasal cavities for humidification. During normal, quiet inspiration, the nasal valves change little in their cross-sectional areas. On deep inspiration, the nostrils flare to increase the diameter of the external valve. With increased airflow, the intraluminal pressure in the internal valve area decreases according to the Bernoulli principle. The tendency for the valve to collapse, however, is counterbalanced by the resistance of its cartilaginous structure to deformation, as well as by isometric contraction of the alar dilator muscles to keep the lumen open. In normal nasal function, the cross-sectional area of the internal valve should be relatively unchanged during inspiration (37). Valvular collapse that occurs only during forced inspiration can be considered physiologic and does not usually require surgical correction (14).

Certain variants of normal nasal anatomy predispose people to nasal obstruction. Individuals with a narrow upper cartilaginous vault tend to have a more acute angle in the internal nasal valve and may be more susceptible to nasal obstruction, even in the resting state. Poiseuille's law states that the rate of air flow is directly proportional to the fourth power of the radius of the conduit. Therefore even miniscule differences in airway size may have significant clinical effects. Individuals with weak ULCs or lateral nasal walls or both may have more collapse of the internal valve area during inspiration. Preexisting or traumatic septal deviation in the internal valve area also can narrow the valve and cause nasal obstruction. Collapse of the external valve on deep inspiration can result from insufficient support of the alar rim and alar lobule. Patients predisposed to such collapse have particular features that should alert the rhinoplasty surgeon: short nasal bones and a long upper cartilaginous vault (discussed earlier); narrow, projecting noses; slitlike nostrils; exaggerated supraalar creases; visible pinching of the lateral wall with inspiration; thin cartilages and thin skin; and cephalically positioned lateral crura, which provide minimal support to the alar margins (38).

ETHNIC VARIATIONS

Three broad nasal morphology types have been used to describe ethnic variations. The *leptorrhine* ("tall and thin") nose is associated with Caucasian or Indo-European descent. The leptorrhine nose has served as the basis of aesthetic ideal in Western culture, and the specific nasal-analysis parameters associated with this ideal are discussed elsewhere in this textbook. Because it is the most extensively studied in modern nasal analysis, it also inevitably becomes the reference point for comparison when studying noses of different ethnicities. Only recently have non-Caucasian standards of nasal analysis been developed for specific ethnic groups.

The *platyrrhine* ("broad and flat") nose is associated with African descent. It is characterized by very thick skin, a low radix, a short dorsum, a bulbous and underprojected tip, and flared nostrils. An analysis of the African-American female nose shows that compared with the Caucasian standard for nasal analysis, the columella-to-lobule ratio is decreased, and the alar width relative to the intercanthal distance is increased. With regard to the bulbous and underprojected tip, cadaver studies in African-American males have demonstrated that the dimensions of the lateral crura are not significantly different from those of the Caucasian nose (39). However, the smallest cartilages were found among noses of the African subtype, and the largest were found in the Afro-Caucasian and Afro-Indian subtypes. This variability may underscore the effect of racial mingling on the canonic platyrrhine nose.

The *mesorrhine* ("intermediate") nose has features intermediate between the leptorrhine nose and the platyrrhine nose. The "typical" Asian or Latino nose is commonly regarded as mesorrhine, with a low radix, variable anterior dorsal projection, rounded and underprojected tip, and rounded nostrils. Note that considerable variation exists in this group. An individual from Northern China or Japan is likely to have a mesorrhine nose with strong leptorrhine characteristics, whereas another from Southeast Asia will likely share more platyrrhine features.

Generalized characteristics of the canonic nasal morphology types are listed in Table 170.3 (40–42).

Any discussion of rhinoplasty for the "non-Caucasian nose" is by its nature flawed. It is overly simplistic to classify a non-Caucasian nose as an "ethnic" nose to which "ethnic rhinoplasty" principles apply. Two noses from two different ethnic backgrounds are likely to be as different from each other as they are from a Caucasian nose. In addition, as may be expected from studies of the Caucasian nose, significant variations in facial features are found within any given ethnic group, for example, as documented in African-American women (43). Intragroup differences may be as great as intergroup differences. For

TABLE 170.3			
GENERAL NASAL CHARACTERISTICS BY MORPHOLOGY			
	Platyrrhine	**Mesorrhine**	**Leptorrhine**
Skin type	Very thick	Moderately thick	Thin
Dorsum	Short, wide, concave	Short, wide	Long, narrow
Radix	Low	Low	High
Nasal bones	Short	Short	Long
Nasal tip	Bulbous, underprojected	Rounded, underprojected	Projected
Columella	Short	Short	Long
Nasal alar width	Wide	Intermediate	Relatively narrow
Ala	Prominent flaring	Variable	Modest flaring

instance, Latinos with Caribbean ancestry are more likely to have platyrrhine noses, whereas those of Central and South American descent have more leptorrhine noses (44). It would be incorrect to apply ethnic group characteristics blindly to an individual patient based on his or her background alone. Nevertheless, an awareness of the global differences between ethnic nasal morphologies will make a rhinoplasty surgeon more sensitive to the needs of all patients in preserving desired ethnic characteristics.

CONCLUSIONS

The nose is a dynamic and inconstant structure, its anatomy varying from individual to individual. The anatomic principles and support mechanisms described in this chapter are not intended to be inflexible rules applicable to all patients. Rather, they are meant to be guidelines with which any one individual's anatomy may be assessed to understand his or her tissue characteristics, structural dynamics, and anatomic features. Selection of the appropriate surgical techniques should begin with an accurate assessment of the individual anatomy. Only then will the rhinoplasty surgeon maximize the likelihood of achieving the intended aesthetic and functional result.

HIGHLIGHTS

- Altering the topographic dimensions of one region of the nose may have a significant visual impact on the appearance of another region.
- Modifications to the underlying nasal skeleton are less accurately transmitted through a thick SSTE, particularly when they are reductive. Even small contour changes or irregularities may transmit clearly through a thin SSTE.
- An inverse relation exists between the lengths of the nasal bones and upper cartilaginous vault. Long nasal bones provide greater stabilization to the ULCs and other caudal elements of the nose than do short nasal bones.
- The tremendous variation in the size, position, shape, and contour of the LLCs accounts for much of the diversity of nasal-tip form and support.
- The structural support of the nose is provided by the osseous framework, nasal septum, and the ligamentous network that attaches the cartilaginous elements to these foundations and to each other.
- Certain anatomic variations predispose patients to destabilization and valvular insufficiency after rhinoplasty: short nasal bones, narrow projecting noses, deep supraalar creases, inspiratory pinching of the lateral wall, and cephalic LLCs.
- An understanding of individual variant nasal anatomy and the features of nasal morphology that exist for different ethnicities allow the rhinoplasty surgeon to tailor treatment for each patient's unique needs.

REFERENCES

1. Kim DW, Toriumi DM. Open rhinoplasty. In: Behrbohm H, Tardy ME, eds. *Essentials of septorhinoplasty.* New York: Thieme, 2004.
2. Lessard ML, Daniel RK. Surgical anatomy of septorhinoplasty. *Arch Otolaryngol* 1985;111:25–29.
3. Bernstein L. Surgical anatomy in rhinoplasty. *Otolaryngol Clin North Am* 1975;8:549–558.
4. Letourneau A, Daniel RK. The superficial musculoaponeurotic system of the nose. *Plast Reconstr Surg* 1988;82:48–57.
5. Griesman BL. Muscles and cartilages of the nose from the standpoint of typical rhinoplasty. *Arch Otolaryngol* 1944;39:334.
6. Tardy ME, Brown RJ. *Surgical anatomy of the nose.* New York: Raven Press, 1990.
7. Bruintjes TD, van Olphen AF, Hillen B, et al. A functional anatomic study of the relationship of the nasal cartilages and muscles to the nasal valve area. *Laryngoscope* 1998;108:1025–1032.
8. May M, West JW, Hinderer KH. Nasal obstruction from facial palsy. *Arch Otolaryngol* 1977;103:389–391.
9. De Souza Pinto EB. Relationship between tip nasal muscles and the short upper lip. *Aesthetic Plast Surg* 2003;27:381–387.
10. Rohrich RJ, Huynh B, Muzaffar AR, et al. Importance of the depressor septi nasi muscle in rhinoplasty: anatomic study and clinical application. *Plast Reconstr Surg* 2000;105:376–383.
11. Oneal RM, Beil RJ Jr, Schlesinger J. Surgical anatomy of the nose. *Clin Plast Surg* 1996;23:195–222.
12. Filippi A, Pohl Y, Tekin U. Sensory disorders after separation of the nasopalatine nerve during removal of palatal displaced canines: prospective investigation. *Br J Oral Maxillofac Surg* 1999;37:134–136.
13. Paparella MM, Shumrick DA, eds. *Otolaryngology,* 2nd ed. Philadelphia: Saunders, 1980.
14. Goode RL. Surgery of the incompetent nasal valve. *Laryngoscope* 1985;95:546–555.
15. Beeson WH. The nasal septum. *Otolaryngol Clin North Am* 1987;20:743–767.
16. Kim DW, Toriumi DM. The biomechanical strength of human nasal septal lining: a comparison of the constituent layers. Presented at the American Academy of Otolaryngology—Head and Neck Surgery Fall Meeting. New York: September 21, 2004.
17. Kim DW, Toriumi DM. Management of the post-traumatic nose: the twisted nose deformity and saddle nose deformity. *Facial Plast Clin North Am* 2004;12:111–132.
18. Daniel RK, Letourneau A. Rhinoplasty: nasal anatomy. *Ann Plast Surg* 1988;20:5–13.
19. Sheen JH, Sheen AP. *Aesthetic Rhinoplasty,* 2nd ed. St. Louis: Quality Medical Publishing, 1998.
20. Zelnik J, Gingrass RP. Anatomy of the alar cartilage. *Plast Reconstr Surg* 1979;64:650–653.
21. Lanza DC, Kennedy DW, Koltai PJ. Applied nasal anatomy & embryology. *Ear Nose Throat J* 1991;70:416–422.
22. Brissett AE, Sherris DA. Changing the nostril shape. *Facial Plast Clin North Am* 2000;8:433–445.
23. Farkas LG, Hreczko TA, Deutsch CK. Objective assessment of standard nostril types: a morphometric study. *Ann Plast Surg* 1983;11:381–389.
24. Adams WP Jr, Rohrich RJ, Hollier LH, et al. Anatomic basis and clinical implications for nasal tip support in open versus closed rhinoplasty. *Plast Reconstr Surg* 1999;103:255–261.
25. Drumheller GW. Topology of the lateral nasal cartilages: the anatomical relationship of the lateral nasal to the greater alar cartilage, lateral crus. *Anat Rec* 1973;176:321–327.
26. Dion MC, Jafek BW, Tobin CE. The anatomy of the nose: external support. *Arch Otolaryngol* 1978;104:145–150.
27. Adamson PA, Morrow TA. The nasal hinge. *Otolaryngol Head Neck Surg* 1994;111:219–231.
28. Janeke JB, Wright WK. Studies on the support of the nasal tip. *Arch Otolaryngol* 1971;93:458–464.
29. McCollough EG, Mangat D. Systematic approach to correction of the nasal tip in rhinoplasty. *Arch Otolaryngol* 1981;107:12–16.
30. Beaty MM, Dyer WK 2nd, Shawl MW. The quantification of surgical changes in nasal tip support. *Arch Facial Plast Surg* 2002;4:82–91.
31. Han SK, Lee DG, Kim JB, et al. An anatomic study of nasal tip supporting structures. *Ann Plast Surg* 2004;52:134–139.

32. Anderson JR. The dynamics of rhinoplasty. In: Bustamante GA, ed. *Proceedings of the Ninth International Congress in Otorhinolaryngology*. Amsterdam: Excerpta Medica, 1969. Excerpta Medica, International Congress Series, No. 206:708–710.

33. Dyer WK 2nd. Nasal tip support and its surgical modification. *Facial Plast Surg Clin North Am* 2004;12:1–13.

34. Johnson CM, Toriumi DM. *Open structure rhinoplasty*. Philadelphia: WB Saunders, 1990.

35. Kasperbauer JL, Kern EB. Nasal valve physiology: implications in nasal surgery. *Otolaryngol Clin North Am* 1987;20:699–719.

36. Cottle MH. Structures and function of the nasal vestibule. *Arch Otolaryngol Head Neck Surg* 1955;62:173.

37. Cole P. The four components of the nasal valve. *Am J Rhinol* 2003;17:107–110.

38. Constantian MB. Four common anatomic variants that predispose to unfavorable rhinoplasty results: a study based on 150 consecutive secondary rhinoplasties. *Plast Reconstr Surg* 2000;105: 316–331.

39. Ofodile FA, James EA. Anatomy of alar cartilages in blacks. *Plast Reconstr Surg* 1997;100:699–703.

40. Papel ID, Capone RB. Facial proportions and esthetic ideals. In: Behrbohm H, Tardy ME, eds. *Essentials of septorhinoplasty*. Stuttgart: Thieme, 2004:65–74.

41. Rohrich RJ, Muzaffar AR. Rhinoplasty in the African-American patient. *Plast Reconstr Surg* 2003;111:1322–1339.

42. Ofodile FA. Nasal bones and pyriform apertures in blacks. *Ann Plast Surg* 1994;32:21–26.

43. Porter JP, Olson KL. Analysis of the African American female nose. *Plast Reconstr Surg* 2003;111:620–626.

44. Milgrim LM, Lawson W, Cohen AF. Anthropometric analysis of the female Latino nose: revised aesthetic concepts and their surgical implications. *Arch Otolaryngol Head Neck Surg* 1996;122: 1079–1086.

Introduction to Rhinoplasty

171

Gregory J. Renner

Rhinoplasty is the general name for any surgical procedure that modifies the shape or restores the tissues of the nose for the purpose of improving function, appearance, or both. Septoplasty is the name given to any surgical correction that is done to the nasal septum. When surgery involves both the septum and any part of the nasal dorsum, the procedure is commonly referred to as a septorhinoplasty. The most common functional nasal problem is airway obstruction (see Chapter 23). Aesthetic deformity of the nose may be of congenital origin, acquired through trauma or other insult or a consequence of aging. Typical aesthetic problems include presence of a high dorsal "hump," a broad or otherwise poorly shaped nasal tip, or a deviation from the normal symmetrical, midline shape of the nose.

INITIAL EVALUATION AND CONSULTATION

Initially, the surgeon must perform a thorough assessment of the patient's desires and the reasons for wanting nasal surgery. It is critical that this be done thoroughly. The patient should be asked to describe in detail what he or she likes and dislikes about the shape and function of the nose. It is often helpful to have the patient view himself or herself in a mirror and point out exactly what defects are perceived to be there. Often there are differences in what the patient perceives to be a problem and what the surgeon would consider to be a problem. The surgeon must try to clearly determine what the patient desires and then determine if it is possible and if it is appropriate for that to be accomplished. It can be a problem when the patient is not able to express well exactly what he or she wants done

and, more so, if the patient has unrealistic expectations of what can or is likely to be achieved with the surgery. Although it is proper for the surgeon to make suggestions, it is important that every significant change that will be made be found acceptable and agreed to by the patient before it is done. As much as possible, the surgeon and patient must develop a similar plan for any nasal surgery.

Examination

Evaluation usually starts with a careful look at the overall external shape of the nose (see Chapters 168 and 170). All features need to be assessed. The surgeon must have a good understanding of the various intricacies of shape that comprise the "normal" nose. The surgeon must also have a good understanding for what variations are normal and should be allowed for different nasal features. The range of standards for each patient will necessarily vary with considerations for age, sex, and ethnicity. The nose must be examined from every conceivable angle as one attempts to judge the quality and desirability of its shape.

A specific determination should be made whether the nose is both straight or is deviated in some way. Determination should be made whether it is situated correctly in the center of the face and whether it is proportionate to the other facial features of that person (Fig. 171.1A,B). The surgeon must then assess whether the nose, in general, and all of its parts are of appropriate length, width, and projection. Each distinct feature should be evaluated, with particular attention given to the general nasal profile; the nasofrontal angle; the nasolabial angle; the rotation and projection of the nasal tip; and the width and general shape of the nasal base, tip, alae, and upper nasal parts (Fig. 171.2). Appreciation for the

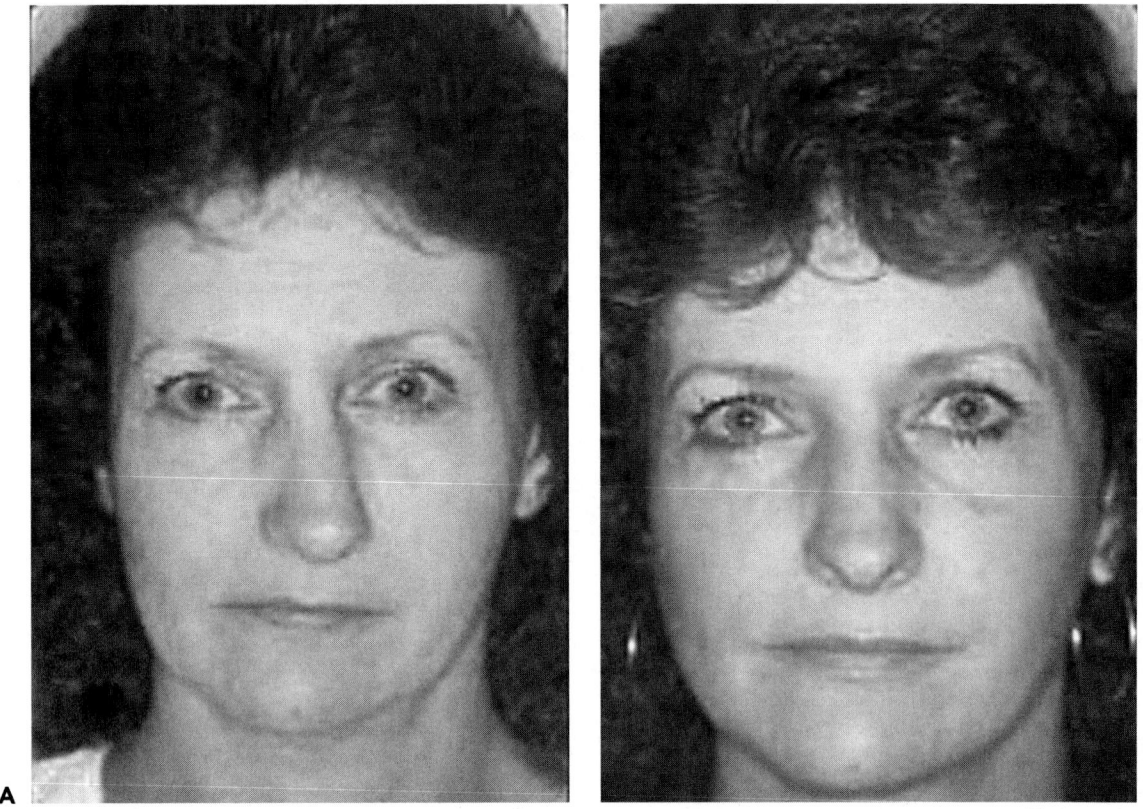

A   B

Figure 171.1   A: Patient with severe nasal deviation. **B:** Later postoperative result after attempted straightening of the nose. Although the nose is reasonably straightened, there is still a faint favor to the left. This can be made more obvious when compared against other facial asymmetries. The surgeon must be aware that photographers will often align a frontal view with the nose more so than the face in general. For surgical purposes, exacting and reproducible standardization of views is important.

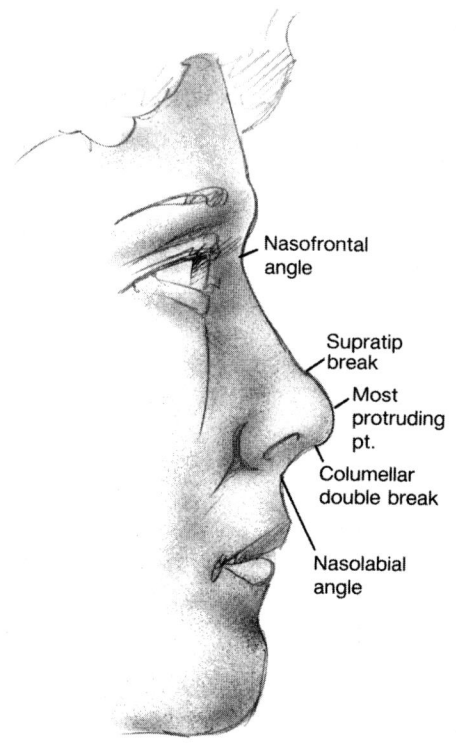

Nasofrontal
angle

Supratip
break

Most
protruding
pt.

Columellar
double break

Nasolabial
angle

Figure 171.2   A generally pleasing Caucasian nasal profile. Tip rotation will tend to settle with age.

relative thickness and other characteristics of the skin and subcutaneous tissues is also important, because it may be more difficult to effect a desired change beneath skin that is thicker or more sebaceous (Fig. 171.3).

Evaluation of the nasal tip is particularly important. A very detailed appreciation of its shape and position is required. All features should be looked at in detail to assess what is desirable and what is not and what would be amenable to surgical correction. The shape, thickness, and strength of the lower lateral cartilages should be studied along with analysis of how they relate to the nasal septum and upper lateral cartilage complex. The quality of nasal tip support should be studied carefully. As considerations are made for potential surgical alterations in the tip, strong consideration should be made for how each maneuver would potentially affect its support over time. Again, it is necessary to consider how characteristics of the nasal skin would affect what one seeks to accomplish with surgical maneuvers to the tip region.

A determination of adequacy of the nasal airway is very important. This should begin with having the patient simply breathe through the nose while observing the ease with which it is done. An evaluation of the nasal vestibule on both sides should be done both in passive manner and then with the aid of a nasal speculum. It is expected that

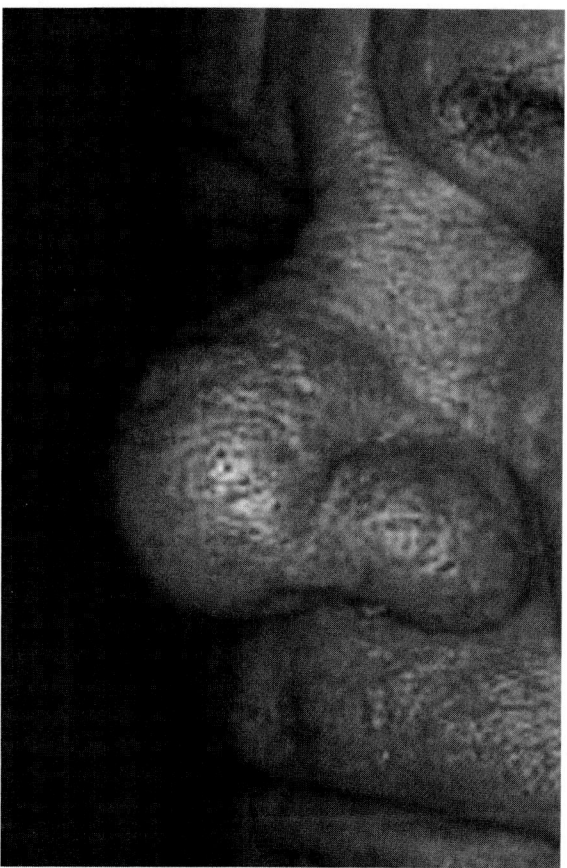

Figure 171.3 Thick, sebaceous skin in this patient will mask any subtle changes made in his tip cartilages and poses a greater demand for good and lasting cartilage support.

the patient will breathe better with the nasal vestibule held open. The surgeon must be able to assess whether the vestibular airway is adequate when the speculum is not holding it open. Issues such as ptosis of the nasal tip and collapsing of the lateral crura of the lower lateral cartilage(s) must be recognized (Fig. 171.4).

The region of smallest diameter in the normal nose is at its entrance, which many refer to as the "anterior nasal

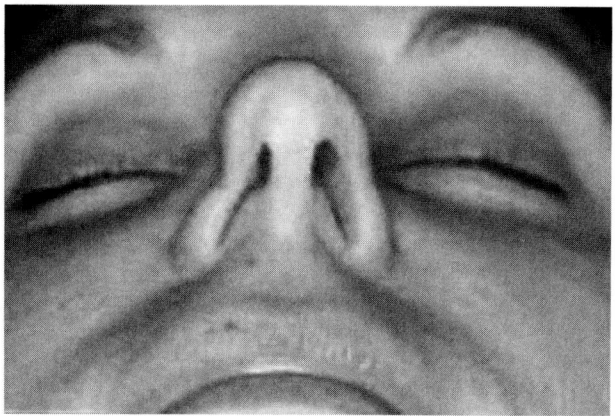

Figure 171.4 With deeper inspiration, the right nasal ala shows a partial collapsing. This must be noted and considered prior to any nasal surgery.

valve." Unfortunately in the literature there is some ambiguity as to exactly what structures constitute the anterior nasal valve. Some limit this definition to the site that is bounded medially by the nasal septum, superiorly and laterally by the caudal margin of the upper lateral cartilage, and more laterally by the anterior portion of the inferior nasal turbinate. Others consider this to constitute an "internal" portion of the anterior nasal valve and that the structures of the nasal vestibule immediately anterior to this point constitute an "external" portion of the valve, bounded medially by the nasal columella and laterally by the lateral crura of the lower lateral cartilage.

Assessment should be made of the entire nasal airway on each side. Examination of the nasal airway may be improved with use of a decongesting nasal spray that reduces swelling of the turbinates. This simple maneuver can enhance the quality of the nasal examination significantly and help in the determination of whether medical or surgical treatment would be more appropriate. In the normal nasal airway the surgeon, with proper illumination, should be able to visualize all the way into the nasopharynx and be able to appreciate the soft palate and posterior wall. In some patients, the use of either flexible or rigid fiberoptic nasal endoscopy, under topical anesthetization, may yield useful information, particularly when there are septal deviations, polyps, or other pathologies that obscure visualization of deeper portions of the nasal cavity. Occasionally it is necessary to perform a more complete examination of the nasopharynx to be certain that there are no problems there as well.

Once the surgeon has made assessment of what potential changes are seen as possible or desirable, it is necessary to determine how compatible such a plan would be with the desires and expectations of the patient. As much as possible the surgeon must develop a deep understanding of what things the patient truly hopes to gain with the surgery. In some cases, the patient may have very unrealistic expectations. It is the duty of the surgeon to help make the patient understand, as well as possible, just what real limitations may be present in any given situation. The surgeon should not feel obligated to make a commitment to do surgery based on the initial patient encounter. If there are issues that need to be better clarified, it can sometimes be very helpful to arrange for one or more later follow-up encounters, which may prove useful in establishing a better physician-patient understanding and rapport.

The potential benefits and risks of all maneuvers that are to be considered should be carefully explained to the patient. It is important to explain how the process of healing will evolve and what the consequences of the surgery could be both in the short term and over the course of many years. Issues that need to be discussed include possible bleeding, infection, intranasal scarring, inadequate corrections, palpable or visible irregularities, tissue necrosis, unsatisfactory cosmetic outcome, and even unusual outcomes such as cerebrospinal fluid (CSF) leakage, meningitis, and death. Although one does have to advise the patient of the potential for significant problems, they should be discussed in a factual manner that does not create misconception or unnecessary fear. It is important that the surgeon obtain a reasonably complete general medical history and at least pertinent physical examination to help determine whether there are any other issues that would have to be addressed or that would make the patient a less suitable surgical candidate.

The patient should be advised of what to expect in both the early and later phases of recovery. Patients are generally more accepting of postoperative edema, bruising, and discomfort when they have prepared for these in advance. They should be prepared for the possibility of black eyes in the first week or two and for the possibility that there could be difficulties with wearing of eyeglasses for a time. The patient should be prepared for issues of bleeding, nasal hygiene, and wound management. They should be encouraged to use cold compresses to the midface for the first 12 to 48 hours. Elevation of the head can also help reduce paranasal edema in the first week or more. Even if they are not actually used, it is best to explain to all patients that nasal packing could be placed for as much as several days and that they would typically cause some discomfort and impede nasal breathing while present. The anticipated or potential use of both dorsal and intranasal splints should also be discussed in detail. The patient should be advised of what to expect with later removal of any nasal packing or splint.

The patient should always be advised that all of the desired changes may not be fully accomplished with the first surgery and that there is at least some possibility that a later additional procedure may be found necessary. They should be advised that edema will tend to mask some of the surgical changes for a time. It would be proper to discuss what expenses might be incurred with any additional procedure. (Many surgeons do not charge an additional fee for minor revisions.)

A series of preoperative photographs is obtained either at the initial consultation or at some other time prior to the surgery (see Chapter 169). Sometimes these may be used to help the patient to better visualize what problems are present and what changes to anticipate with the procedure. Some physicians make use of computer-generated imaging to help in planning the surgery and some will use these to help show patients what type of changes are being sought. If alterations are made to any photograph or computer image, it must be clearly disclaimed that these are intended aims and not necessarily the exact results that the patient can be promised with their surgery.

In review of the patient's history it must be determined whether they are on any medication or dietary supplement that could interfere with normal blood clotting. The patient should be asked specifically if they take any aspirin or other nonsteroidal antiinflammatory medication. There will be less tendency for both intraoperative and postoperative bleeding if the patient can refrain from using any of these for at least 2 weeks prior to the surgery. If the patient is on coumadin or other anticoagulant therapy it must be first determined whether the surgery should be done at all

TABLE 171.1
INITIAL CONSULTATION AND DIAGNOSIS

Chief complaint
Nasal obstruction, dissatisfaction with nasal appearance, or both

Nasal obstruction
Right side, left side, or both
Continuous or intermittent
History of injury
Sinusitis, nasal polyps
Rhinitis, seasonal allergy
Mouth breathing, snoring

Medications
Topical nasal medications
Systemic decongestants, antihistamines, steroids
Anticoagulants, aspirin products, other NSAIDs
Accutane
Cocaine, other illicit drugs

Medical history
History of previous nasal or sinus surgery
Hypertension, diabetes
Bleeding disorder (personal and family history)
Immune deficiency
Any connective tissue disease (i.e., Wegener granulomatosis, relapsing polychondritis, etc.)
Tobacco use, alcohol
Pregnancy (date of LMP)

Appearance
Patient's perception of nasal deformity
Physician's assessment of deformity

LMP, last menstrual period; NSAIDs, nonsteroidal antiinflammatory drugs.

and, if so, then how best to wean from the medicine to some safer level for the perioperative interval. The patient should be asked to discontinue use of any dietary supplement that could interfere with normal blood clotting for at least a week or more prior to the surgery. Detailed instruction on what foods, liquids, and medicines should otherwise be taken in the 24 hours prior to surgery should be done with the patient and perhaps even written out to minimize any later confusion. The initial consultation should include all issues indicated in Table 171.1.

SURGICAL PLANNING

The keys to a successful rhinoplasty are careful study of the patient and all photoimages and meticulous surgical planning. The surgeon should have a very clear idea of what steps will most likely be taken to accomplish the desired tasks, recognizing that in some cases an adjustment to the plan may become necessary, depending on what is encountered at the time of surgery. Each step that is taken should be for very specific reasons. If the goal is to narrow the tip, the surgeon should go into the surgery with a fairly clear idea of what actual surgical maneuvers would likely be required to accomplish that task.

TABLE 171.2
TREATMENT PLANNING

1. Determine very specifically patient's goals and expectations for surgery.
2. Explore patient's motivations for surgery.
3. Take photographs and perform detailed anatomic analysis (some may use computer imaging).
4. Discuss financial arrangements.
5. Decide on method of anesthesia.
6. Obtain informed consent.
7. Determine suitability for surgery with history and examination.
8. Do preoperative teaching (surgical experience postoperative care, and long-term healing).

In planning, the surgeon should perform the operation several times in his or her own mind before the surgery. Experience is very important in rhinoplasty. One can maximize learning from all cases by maintaining a very detailed record of exactly what steps were taken to perform each operation, review this record as one sees the patient in follow-up, and continue to follow each patient carefully for a period of at least several years (ideally throughout one's life). Postoperative photographs should be taken at regular intervals and compared with those taken earlier to note all favorable or unfavorable changes. It is generally agreed that the real result from a rhinoplasty is not really known until 6 months to a year have passed, when nearly all edema is gone and the effects of fibrosis have pretty well maximized. The surgeon must always be aware that the nose will continue to change to some degree throughout the patient's life and that changes made at the surgery can sometimes have a significant influence on this.

An outline for proper treatment planning is given in Table 171.2.

ANESTHESIA

Rhinoplasty is done either under local or general anesthesia. The patient should be presented with the option for either of these, although many surgeons have a strong favor for one or the other. Many feel that local anesthesia with intravenous sedation offers less risk, a little less tendency for bleeding, quicker recovery, and less cost. If the patient is in generally good health, the risk of general anesthesia, administered by a capable specialist, is in most cases very low and is favored by many surgeons and patients. Even when general anesthesia is used, local anesthetic solution is normally injected into the soft tissues of the nose, allowing a lighter plane of general anesthesia, greater local vasoconstriction, and less intraoperative bleeding, which affords greater visualization. As with any surgical procedure, pulse and blood pressure should be monitored throughout the case. The airway must be maintained and protected, particularly when an endotracheal tube is not placed. Continuous electrocardiography and pulse oximetry is strongly

recommended. Proper emergency resuscitative drugs and equipment must be readily available, along with an adequately trained nurse or other medical personnel.

Most rhinoplasty surgeons use a combination of topical and injected local anesthetic and vasoconstrictive medications during surgery. Lidocaine is the injected local anesthetic most commonly used, in concentrations of 0.5% to 2.0%. Epinephrine is the vasoconstrictive agent and added to the solution to achieve a concentration of usually 1:100,000 or 1:200,000 epinephrine. The maximum dose of lidocaine without epinephrine is 4.5 mg/kg (2 mg/lb) and about 300 mg for an average adult (1–4). The maximum dose of lidocaine with epinephrine is 7 mg/kg (3.5 mg/lb) and about 500 mg for an average adult (1–3). Recommendations in children are less. Smaller doses are desirable to limit tissue distortion from the injection and to minimize the chances for adverse reaction to the injected medications. The concentration of the solution affects the length of the local anesthesia: 0.5% lidocaine tends to last for about 1 hour if used alone and about 2 hours if used with epinephrine; 1% lidocaine tends to last about 1.5 hours when used alone and about 3.5 hours when used with epinephrine (3).

Several medications are commonly used to induce local vasoconstriction. Many surgeons begin their nasal preparation with intranasal sprays of a vasoconstrictive and decongestive agent such as oxymetazoline. These effects are enhanced with use of injected epinephrine with the local anesthesia. A number of surgeons still prefer the vasoconstrictive and anesthetic properties of cocaine, which can be administered in either liquid or powdered form. Cocaine is available commercially in a 4% concentration, with a maximum dose generally considered to be about 5 mL for an average size adult. In the powdered or crystal form the maximum dose is variously considered to be between 150 and 200 mg for an average adult (1–3). Liquid preparatory medications may be applied to the nasal mucosa with multiple cotton pledgets that are first soaked in the agent and then left in the nose for a short time before making the first incision. Powered cocaine may be applied with dry cotton swabs (with cotton wound loosely so that it can actually pick up the crystals well). Lidocaine with epinephrine tends to be effective for about 2 to 3 hours, oxymetazoline for about 8 to 12 hours, and cocaine for about 2 hours (3).

Injection of the local anesthesia is typically done with a 25- or 27-gauge needle, with preference for smaller size. What pattern to inject is left to surgeon preference. All parts of the nose that are to be opened should be injected. Injections throughout the nasal dorsum should be done in the subcutaneous plane and immediately superficial to the nasal skeleton. Some surgeons prefer to make all injections of the nasal dorsum via the nasal vestibule, whereas others prefer injections directly through the dorsal nasal skin. Injections within the nose should be made deep in the soft tissues on both sides of the septum, with care taken to avoid lacerating the septal cartilage. The nasal columella should be injected and any location within the nose where an incision will be placed, particularly about the nasal vestibules. Injections should be made along the planned course for any osteotomy, with infiltration done along the outer surface in all cases and along the inner surface in at least cases done under local anesthesia. The nasal tip should be injected well, but without causing undo distortion. Normally a total of 8 to 15 mL of 1% lidocaine with 1:100,000 epinephrine is used. To a limited extent, massage can help to disperse some of the subcutaneous local anesthesia. The cotton pledgets that were removed to allow the local injections may again be placed into the nasal cavities and allowed to remain in place for as much as 10 to 15 minutes to optimize the vasoconstrictive effects.

OVERVIEW OF SURGERY

The three major areas of surgical change during a septo-rhinoplasty are the septum, the nasal tip, and the nasal dorsum. Surgical techniques for straightening of the nasal septum are described in the chapter on nasal obstruction (see Chapter 23). In most cases, surgery to the nasal septum is done first because it affords a straightening of the central structure of the nose, which then allows for more exacting correction to the other nasal parts.

The order with which surgery to the other nasal parts is done depends on surgeon preference and, more importantly, the degree to which a change in one part may affect changes made in another. A logical approach would be to do any correction of the nasal dorsum while other parts are still stable. Lateral osteotomies would be done next to properly correct the width and overall shape of the nasal dorsum. Although in some cases it may be done earlier in the scheme, refinement of the nasal tip is often best done when all other nasal parts are in their corrected positions so that tip adjustment can be more exacting. The surgeon will have to choose if this is the preferred order or if some other plan of steps would be more appropriate for that particular case.

Major intraoperative emergencies are not common but must be anticipated, with a plan and system in place that is ready and able to respond appropriately (Table 171.3).

Incisions

There are a variety of incisions that can be used to gain access to the septum, the tip, or the nasal dorsum, with each having its own particular advantages and limitations. The surgeon must choose the incision(s) that allows adequate exposure with a minimum of adverse consequence. Approach to the septum is most often done via either the endonasal hemitransfixion incision or by extending exposure from an external rhinotomy incision (Figs. 171.5 and 171.6). With either approach, it is best to limit scarring within the membranous columella and respect the fibrous attachments of the lower lateral cartilage complex. With some controversy, this author generally favors approaching the septum through a hemitransfixion incision, even when an external rhinotomy inci-

TABLE 171.3
INTRAOPERATIVE EMERGENCIES: RHINOPLASTY

Excessive bleeding
Pack and wait 2–10 minutes.
Ensure that patient is not hypertensive.
Locate specific bleeding point and cauterize or tie.
Apply sponges with vasoconstrictive agent.
Use microfibrillar collagen.
Pack firmly and abort procedure.

Medication toxicity
Cease administration of additional pain or sedative medications.
Give naloxone if appropriate.
Treat arrhythmias, blood pressure problems per ACLS protocols.
Airway support as appropriate.

Restless patient (local anesthesia)
Ensure adequate oxygenation.
Consider drug toxicity.
Administer more local anesthesia if believed inadequate and not toxic.
Give additional pain, sedative medication if considered appropriate.
Change to general anesthesia or abort procedure.

ACLS, advanced cardiac life support.

sion is used to access the tip and nasal dorsum. Access to the columella, the medial crura, and the premaxilla is readily available via the hemitransfixion incision. Use of a complete transfixion incision is usually discouraged because it causes disruption to the fibrous attachments between the base portion of the medial crura and the nasal septum, producing a reduction in tip projection, unless it is corrected for. Approach to the septum via an external rhinotomy incision requires separation of the upper lateral cartilages from the upper margin of the septum and commonly also some separation of the medial crura of the lower lateral cartilages.

Access to the dorsum can be achieved via either anterior endonasal or external rhinotomy incisions. With the endonasal approach, access to the dorsum is made with either a unilateral or bilateral intercartilaginous incision. In this setting, the hemitransfixion incision is converted to a full transfixion incision in its upper half only, which allows continuity with the intercartilaginous incision on both sides. Connecting the two with a high transfixion incision also allows a greater release of the soft tissues from the caudal portion of the nasal dorsum. In variation of the intercartilaginous incision, the surgeon may choose to make an incision a measured degree more anterior and directly through the lower lateral cartilage on both sides with intention to resect the cephalic portion of the cartilage (intracartilaginous or transcartilaginous incision, Fig. 171.7).

Connection of the cephalic margin of the lower lateral cartilages to the caudal margin of the upper lateral cartilages is normally found to be with some form of scrolled and interlocking edges. As the two are separated, soft tissue of the nasal dorsum is carefully elevated in the plane

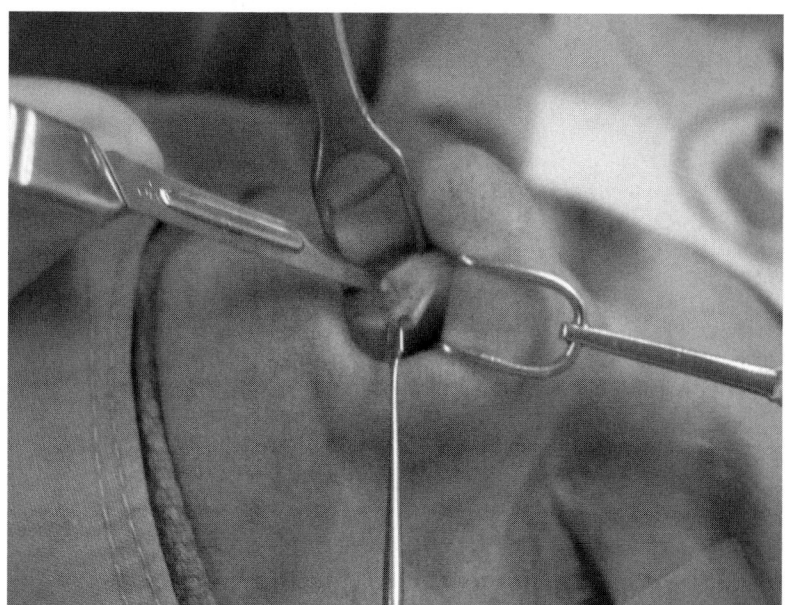

Figure 171.5 A typical endonasal hemitransfixion incision. The incision is made along the caudal margin of the septum and not in the membranous columella. After the incision is made, scraping over the distal septum with the knife blade held in beveled fashion allows easy exposure through the perichondrial layer.

immediately superficial to the upper lateral cartilage on each side (Fig. 171.11). Staying close to the cartilage will tend to result in less bleeding. With use of a periosteal elevator, the soft tissues can then be raised from the bony portion of the nasal dorsum as desired. In general, it is best to only elevate that amount of soft tissue from the bony dorsum that is truly necessary to accomplish any given task. Leaving soft tissue attachments, at least laterally, can help stabilize the nasal bones somewhat when osteotomies are performed.

Endonasal access to the lower lateral cartilages can be accomplished by adding a second incision along the caudal margin of the lower lateral cartilage on both sides (Fig. 171.7). With parallel incisions placed at the cephalic and caudal margins of the lower lateral cartilages, either can be pulled out to some degree through the anterior incision on each side in what is referred to as a cartilage "delivery" technique (Fig. 171.8).

The external rhinotomy incision is made as an irregular line across the middle or upper third of the anterior sur-

face of the nasal columella. It is recommended not to make a straight-line incision horizontally across the columella so that a notching effect does not occur with later scar contracture. Although various broken-line patterns can be used, most surgeons favor a horizontal incision that is broken up with a small, raised triangle in its center (referred to by many as a "gull wing" incision, Figs. 171.6 and 171.7). The incision is carried upward on both sides along the caudal margin of the medial crura of the upper lateral cartilage. The incision is continued on both sides along the caudal margin of the lateral crura and referred to as an anterior marginal incision. With the external rhinotomy or so-called "open" approach, visualization and access to the nasal tip is greater (Fig. 171.9A,B). The lower lateral cartilages do not have to be pulled into view with instrumentation. Placement of sutures or grafts in the nasal tip region can be done with greater ease and in some cases greater precision as well. With the external rhinotomy approach, the relationship of the lower lateral cartilage complex can be more easily appreciated as it relates to the upper lateral cartilages and caudal margin of the septum. Use of the external rhinotomy incision does, however, result in greater and longer lasting edema of the nasal tip and to at least temporary sensory impairment of the tip region.

Nasal Tip Surgery

Details of surgical changes in the nasal tip region are discussed in Chapter 173. The surgeon's goal is to create an aesthetically pleasing nasal tip that sits well with respect to other structures of the nose and midface. Typical tasks are to adjust projection and/or rotation of the tip, improve definition of the tip, provide better tip support, and adjust any asymmetries or other fine details of tip shape (Fig. 171.10A,B). In some cases, the aim of surgery could also be to strengthen or otherwise modify structures of

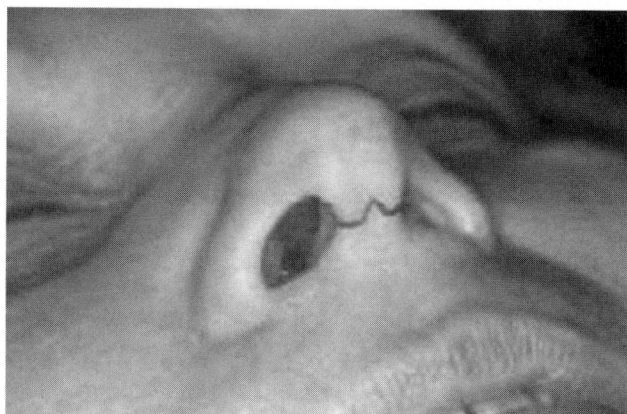

Figure 171.6 Typical external portion of anterior rhinotomy incision.

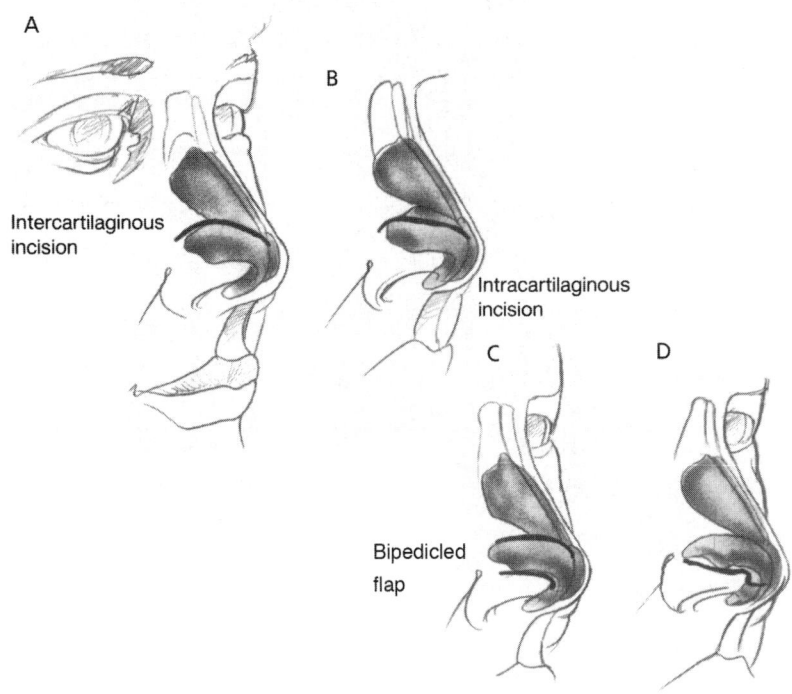

Figure 171.7 **A:** The intercartilaginous incision is made between the cephalic margin of the lower lateral cartilage and caudal margin of the upper lateral cartilage. **B:** The intracartilaginous (transcartilaginous) incision is made at a specifically chosen site transversely through the lateral crura of the lower lateral cartilage, normally with intent to resect the cartilage segment cephalic to the cut. **C:** The bipedicled flap is made with an intercartilaginous incision and a second incision placed along the caudal margin of the lower lateral cartilage. **D:** The incision for an external approach involves placement of a broken-line transverse incision across the anterior surface of the columella, combined with an anterior marginal incision on both sides.

the distal nose to improve the nasal airway with batten grafts or other procedures. It is very important that the surgeon give strong consideration to the potential long-term consequences of any cartilage resection or repositioning in the distal portion of the nose. Overresection of cartilages should be avoided very carefully. While working for good cosmesis, ensuring good long-term support is strongly advised.

Surgery of the Dorsum

There are four principle reasons for directing surgery to the nasal dorsum: removal of a dorsal hump, straighten-

ing of the nasal dorsum, adjusting the width of the upper nose, and augmentation for deficiency of the nasal dorsum.

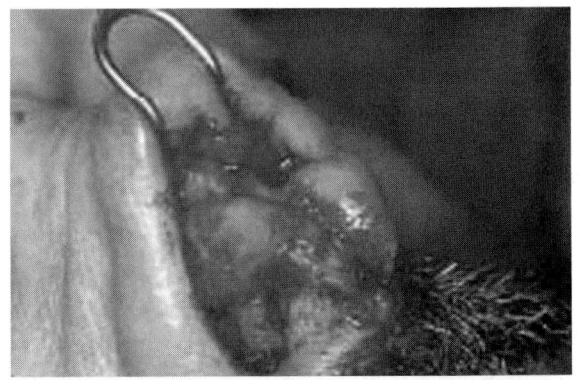

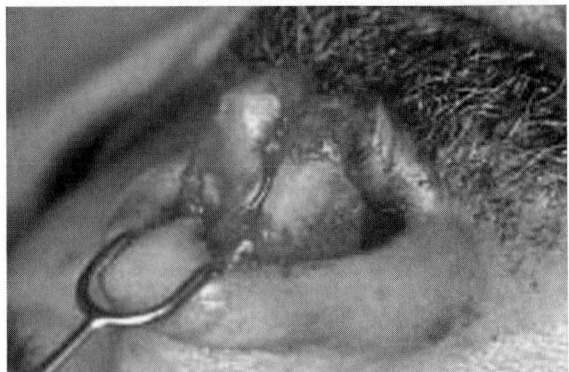

Figure 171.9 **A** and **B:** Examples of exposure to nasal tip afforded with external (open) rhinotomy approach.

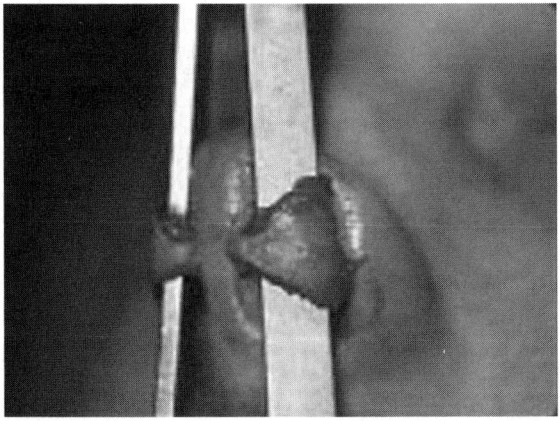

Figure 171.8 Example of bipedicled flap on both sides with delivery of lower lateral cartilages through anterior marginal incision sites.

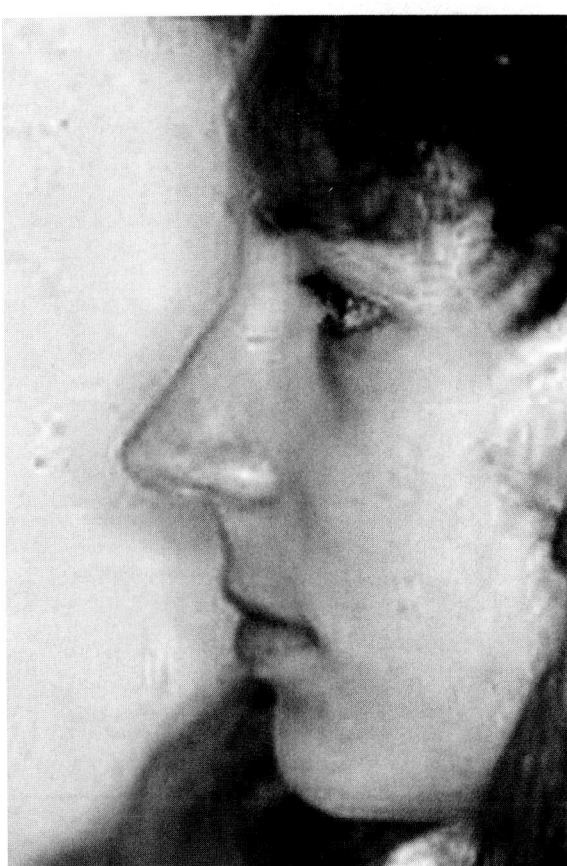
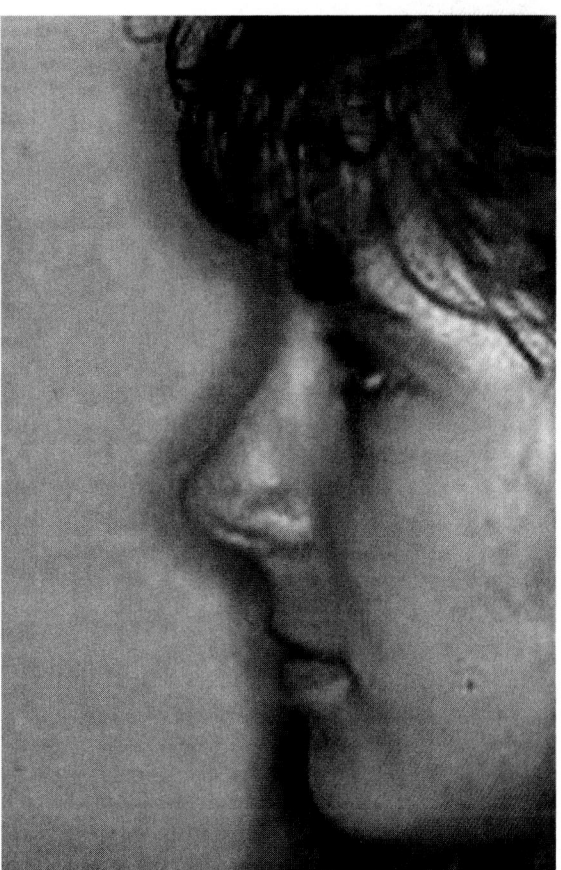

A   B

Figure 171.10 **A** and **B:** Preoperative and 10-month postoperative photos of young woman who had undergone surgery to straighten her nose and had very slight reduction of her dorsum with deprojection of the nasal tip.

Hump Reduction

When examining a perceived overprojection of the nasal dorsum, one must determine if there is an actual overgrowth of midnasal skeletal tissue or an underprojection of the more distal portion of the nasal septum (Fig. 171.11A,B). In most cases, overprojection will typically involve the nasal bones primarily, but the uppermost portion of the cartilaginous nasal dorsum will normally also be involved to some extent. In general, the dorsal profile of a cosmetically ideal nose appears as a relatively straight line from the nasofrontal angle to the supratip region with a slight projection of the nasal tip (Fig. 171.10).

The nasofrontal angle should ideally lie at about the level of the upper tarsal crease. Appreciable deviations from this are not common. In some patients, the nasofrontal angle may be slightly higher, lower, or more deep-set, any of which could create a perceived cosmetic deformity. A high-set angle tends to produce a relatively strong nasal profile. The need to resect bone from this region is infrequent and can be technically difficult. When the nasofrontal angle is unusually low-set or deep, the nose may appear to be somewhat flat in its upper portion. When augmentation is felt necessary in the nasofrontal angle, it is generally done with placement of some type of graft or implant material, with a common source being tissue from a resected hump.

Although fine tuning of the nasal tip is often done last, it is often helpful to correct undesirable projection or rotation of the nasal tip prior to removal of a dorsal hump so that a more exact planing of the nasal dorsum can be accomplished best. Most surgeons will carefully trim down the cartilaginous portion of the dorsum to a more desired level before they address removal of the overprojected portion of the nasal bones. This resection may be done either with a knife or scissors, depending on one's preference. Resection with the knife can allow for a more gradual or incremental resection. Care should be taken to avoid over resection of the medial portion of the upper lateral cartilage on either side, as what is left will need to respan the open defect that is made. Because the overlying soft tissue in the middle portion of the nose tends to be thinner, it is advised to leave a slight skeletal convexity in the midnasal dorsum to accommodate for this or the final nasal profile could have a slightly "scooped-out" appearance (Fig. 171.12). A common error in rhinoplasty is to leave the distal portion of the cartilaginous dorsum a little high, which is one of the causes for pollybeak deformity.

Correction of a small dorsal hump or other irregularity may be best done with use of a rasp. Rasps are designed either with the sharp edge of their teeth arranged to scrape away bone with either a "push" maneuver or in opposite direction to allow bone scraping with a "pull"

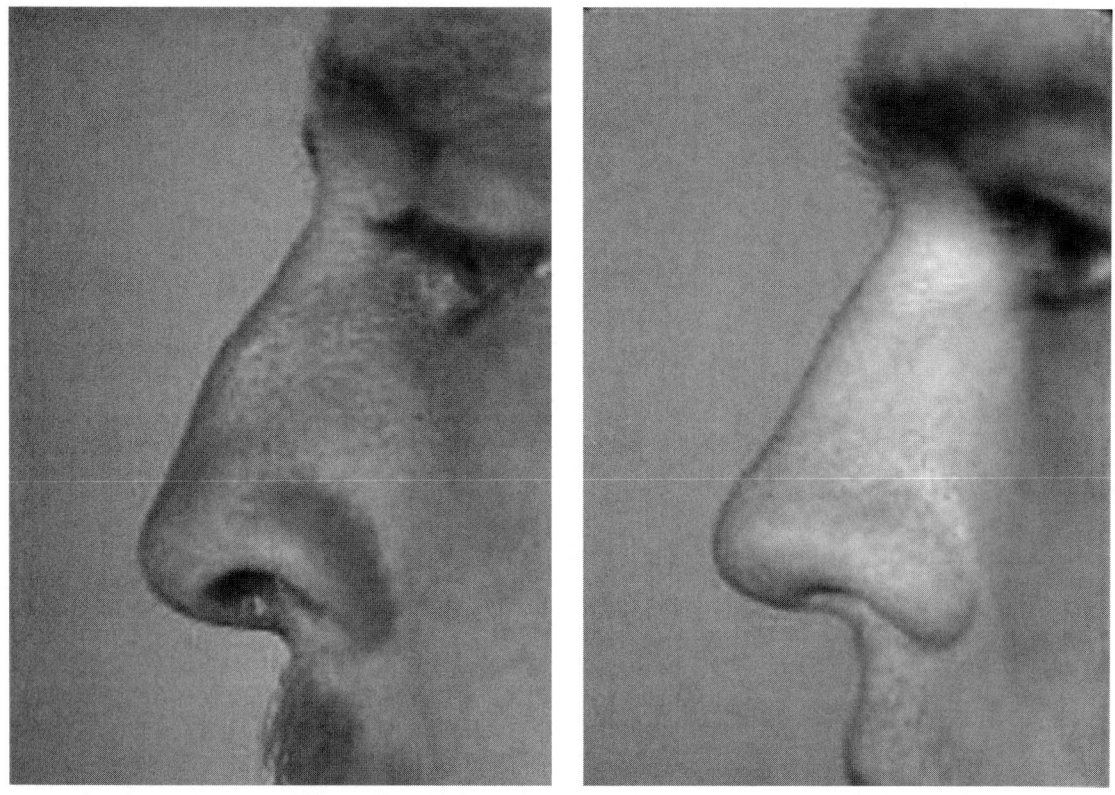

Figure 171.11   A: Patient with typical overprojection (hump) of the bony and cartilaginous dorsum. **B:** Patient with appearance of slight hump made at least in part by early-life dislocation of nasal septum that causes a slight deficiency in what would likely have been the projection of the more distal portion of his nose. Note that the columellar length is also a little short.

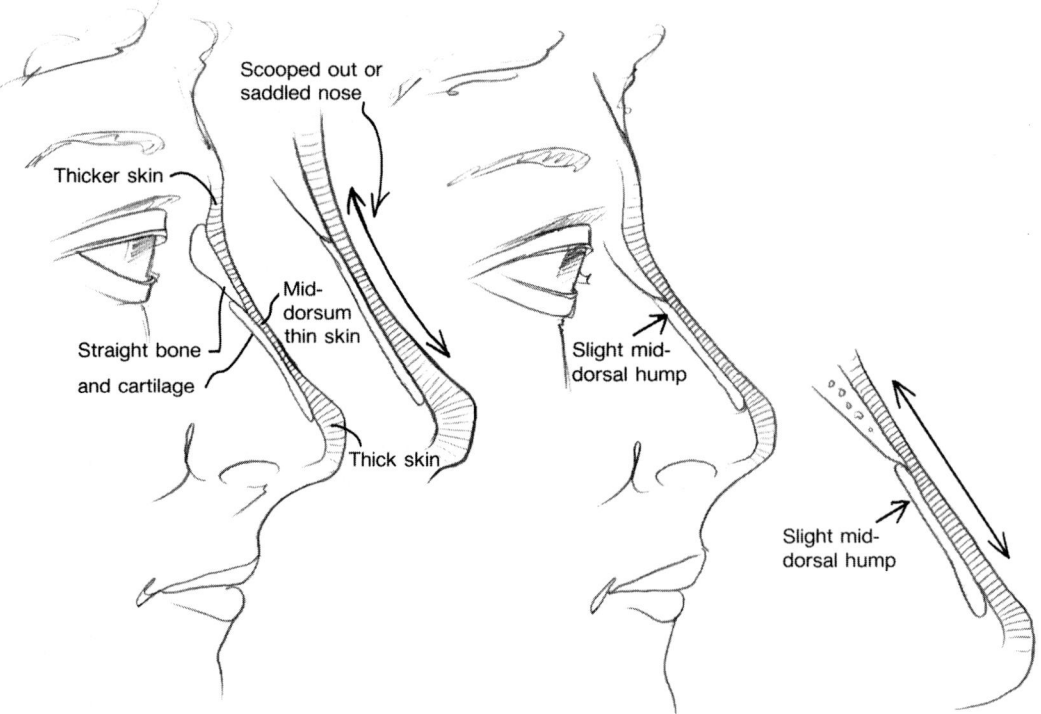

Figure 171.12   Soft tissues of the nasal dorsum tend to be thinner in the midnose region. Accommodation for this should be made when removing a dorsal skeletal hump so that the reconstructed dorsum does not later develop a scooped-out appearance after healing has matured.

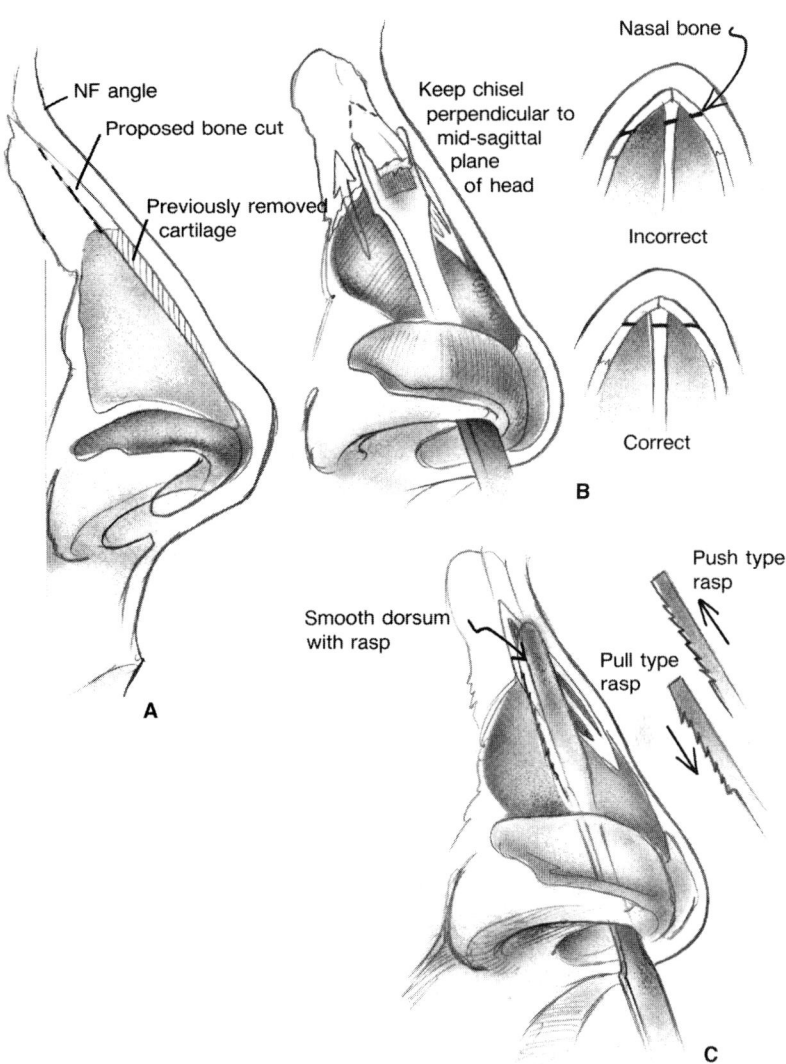

Figure 171.13 **A:** Usually the cartilaginous portion of the dorsum is resected first. **B:** The overprojected bone is then resected, being careful not to resect too much. **C:** Illustration of both push and pull type rasps.

maneuver (Fig. 171.13). Some argue that there is less possibility that a bone fragment could become avulsed with use of the pushing type rasp; however, pulling action is a more natural hand maneuver and is preferred by most. Rasping is typically done with repeated gentle, quick motions. Rasps are much more efficient if they are kept sharp.

Larger humps are usually removed with a broad osteotome (Fig. 171.13). In contrast to a chisel, which has a bevel on only one side of its blade, an osteotome has an edge that is beveled on both sides, which allows the instrument to continue in a reasonably straight fashion as it is passed through bone. The osteotome is placed at the caudal margin of the bony hump, typically at the level that has already been established with the earlier cartilage resection. With use of a small hammer and repeated gentle tapping, the osteotome is then advanced superiorly toward the nasofrontal angle. Special care must be taken when using the osteotome so that one does not remove too much bone and create a skeletal deficiency in the bony dorsum. The osteotome also must not be allowed to en-

gage deeper into the bony dorsum as it is advanced superiorly. In general, the osteotome should be kept level as it is passed so that an even amount of bone is resected on each side, unless there is reason to do differently. With hump removal in the patient with a crooked nose or large hump, special consideration should be made for how much skeletal tissue should be removed on each side so that a deficiency is not encountered as the remaining skeletal walls are later brought together to reshape the dorsum (Fig. 171.14). It is also important in hump reduction that one consider issues of age, sex, and ethnicity because all of these can have bearing on what amount of hump removal is appropriate for a particular patient Fig. 171.15A,B).

There are times when it can be difficult to smoothly terminate the cephalic end of the hump resection with the osteotome. One method of dealing with this is to direct a 2-mm osteotome directly through the skin at the midline near the nasofrontal angle and perform a transverse scoring of the bone on each side. This will then help predetermine the exact location for the osteotomy fracture, much like the scoring of glass before it is cut.

Pre-hump removal

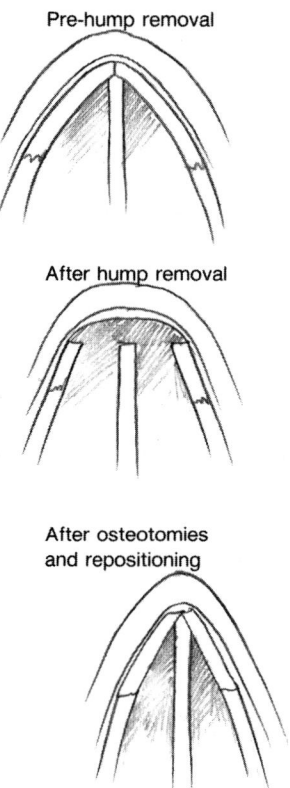

After hump removal

After osteotomies
and repositioning

Figure 171.14 Removal of bone from the nasal dorsum usually results in a discontinuity of the nasal bones from the septum, creating an "open sky" deformity. After performing osteotomies, the bones are then tilted inward to close this dorsal skeletal defect. One must be careful to avoid resecting too much of the nasal bone on either side so that they can easily reach to the septum as they are repositioned.

After the hump has been removed, the bone edges are smoothed with a gentle rasping maneuver. Most rasping should be done prior to performing lateral osteotomies so that the bony edges can be made smooth. A refined trimming may then be required in the area of the bony-cartilaginous junction to make sure this area is smooth and well-tailored.

Medial and Lateral Osteotomies

After the hump has been removed, the nose has an open deformity until the remaining lateral nasal walls are fractured and tilted inward to restore the skeletal continuity of the nasal dorsum. What remains of the nasal bones must be disconnected from the maxilla on both sides so that they can be tilted inward to close the open roof deformity after hump removal (Fig. 171.14). Medial osteotomies are bony cuts made to separate the medial margin of the nasal bones from the nasal septum (Fig. 171.16). Lateral osteotomies are bony cuts made principally along the course of the naso-maxillary junction that separate the bones of the nose from the maxilla on each side. In some cases, an "intermediate" osteotomy may be made vertically somewhere midway

between the medial and lateral osteotomies when there is significant irregularity to the contour of the nasal bone.

Osteotomes come in a wide variety of shapes and sizes (Fig. 171.17). Although most are straight, some are made with a gentle curve. Most are designed with a rectangular head, with sizes ranging from 2 mm to more than 2 cm. Some are made with a projecting guard on one or both corners that serves as a palpable marker to help keep easier track of the osteotome as it is passed. Because the guard is typically wider, it can also be used to help hold the blade in correct position even without the use of palpation. Osteotomes also are designed with a variety of shapes and features in their handle portion. Some surgeons will use a specially designed Stephen's knife or other small elevator to first create a subperiosteal tunnel along the course for the lateral osteotomy, particularly if they are to use a guarded osteotome, so that there will be less soft tissue tearing. A double-guarded type is designed for removal of the bony hump (Fig. 171.13). Many surgeons prefer to use unguarded osteotomes, choosing a width that can make the bone cut and still be detected by palpation as they are passed. The trend has been to use osteotomes of narrower size, with intent to minimize disruption of the soft tissues that lie adjacent to the bone. The use of narrower osteotomes requires a little more skill but does serve to lessen bleeding, swelling, and tendency for the cut bones to be too loose or mobile. Osteotomes perform much better if they are kept sharp.

The medial osteotomy is normally performed first. If there has been no hump removal, the osteotome is placed at the caudal margin of the nasal bone, immediately lateral to the septum on the side that is to be cut (Fig. 171.16). The osteotome can be placed directly over an intact upper lateral cartilage and engages the nasal bone by simply pushing down on the cartilage slightly. Correct positioning is monitored by detecting the side of the septum with the osteotome. As the osteotome is advanced upward, the cut is made with a gradual outward angulation to a desired point. In some cases when a large hump has been removed, there may be not need for a medial osteotomy. In cases in which old fractures are present, one may find it possible to pass the osteotome with a gentle pressure and avoid the hammer tapping. When an extending medial osteotomy is made after hump resection, it is important to avoid creating a point of angulation that could interfere with easy inward tilting of the nasal bone ("rocker deformity").

The lateral osteotomy begins above the floor of the piriform aperture, immediately lateral to the anterior end of the inferior nasal turbinate. If the lateral osteotomy is started at a lower point, there could be improper narrowing of the anterior nasal valve, causing airway obstruction (Figs. 171.18 and 171.19). After selecting the beginning point the osteotome is advanced forward a short distance, engaging the bone of the lateral nasal wall. With hammer-assisted tapping the osteotome is then advanced superiorly

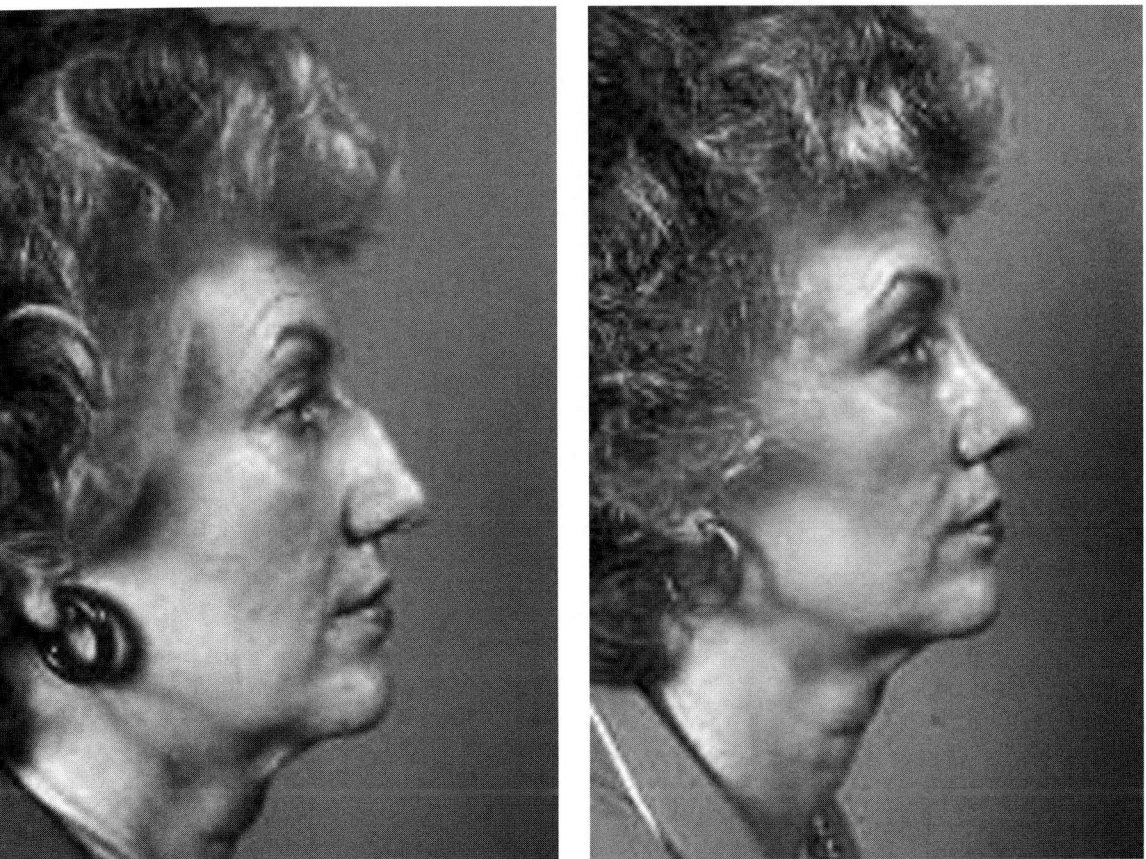

Figure 171.15   A and **B:** It is appropriate that removal of a dorsal hump in this elderly woman be conservative. Any intended cephalic rotation of her nasal tip should also be more conservative to keep her appearance more appropriate for her age.

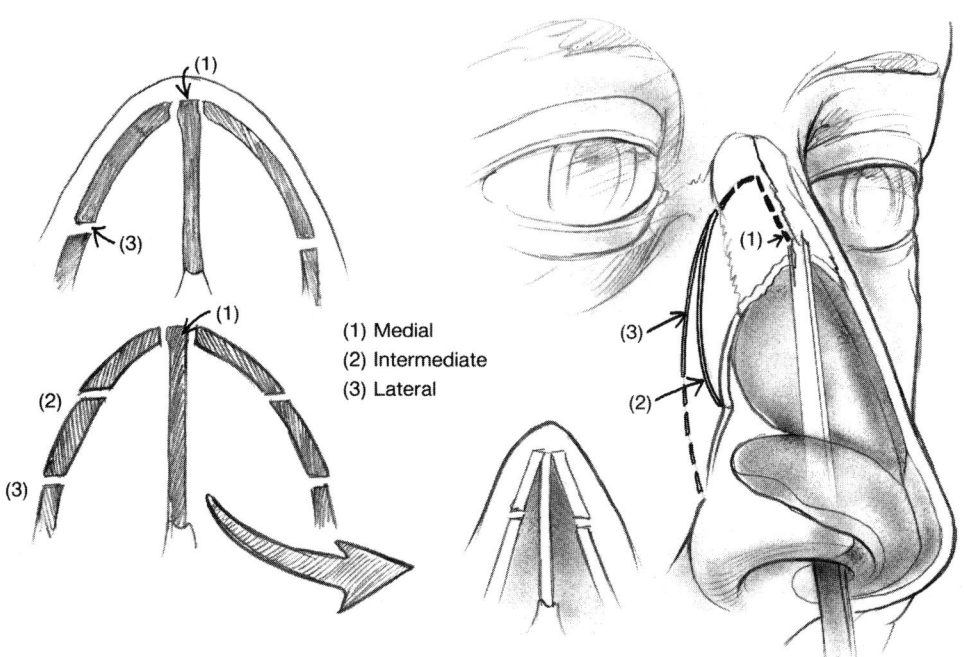

(1) Medial
(2) Intermediate
(3) Lateral

Figure 171.16   Illustration of sites for medial, intermediate, and lateral osteotomies. The caudal origin site for the lateral osteotomy must be placed too low so that the airway does not become obstructed as the bones are repositioned (Figs. 171.18 and 171.19).

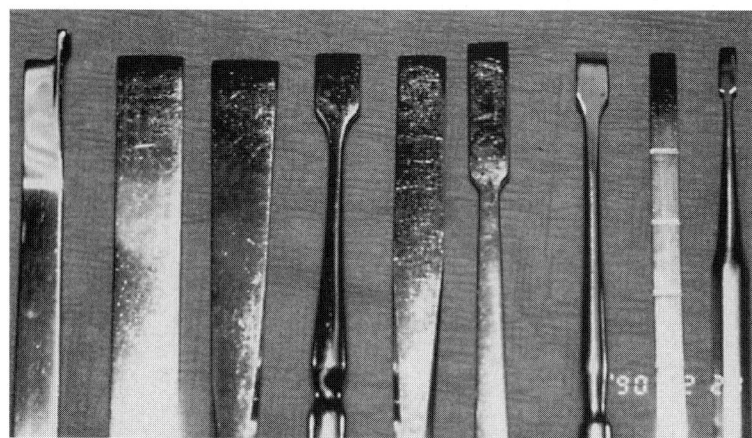

Figure 171.17 Examples of a variety of osteotomes.

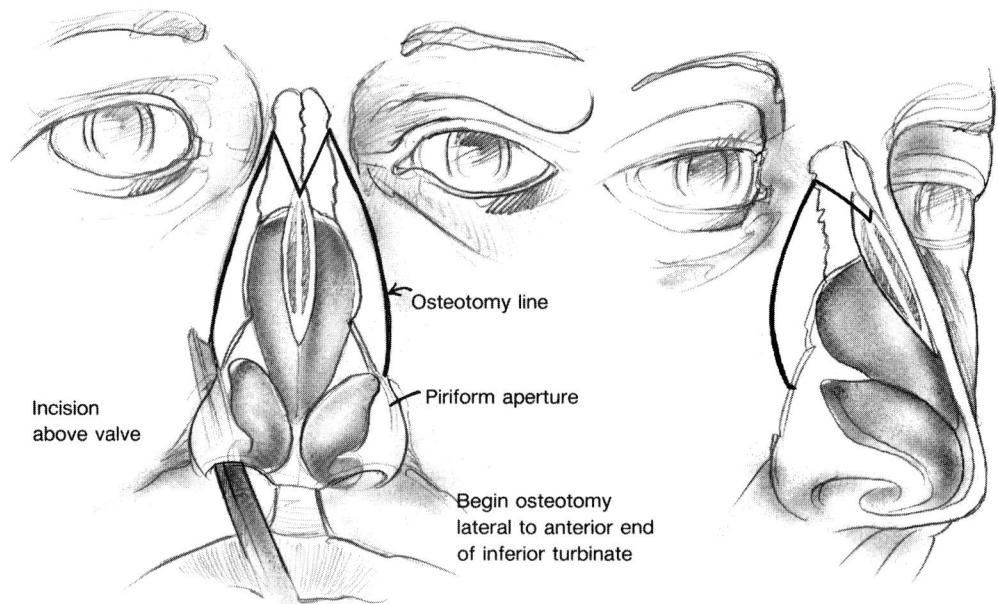

Osteotomy line

Piriform aperture

Incision
above valve

Begin osteotomy
lateral to anterior end
of inferior turbinate

Figure 171.18 Illustration of medial and lateral osteotomies. Orientation of the medial osteotomy may need to be more sagittal from the cephalic portion of the hump reduction site to avoid creation of a "rocker" situation as the nasal bones are tilted medially.

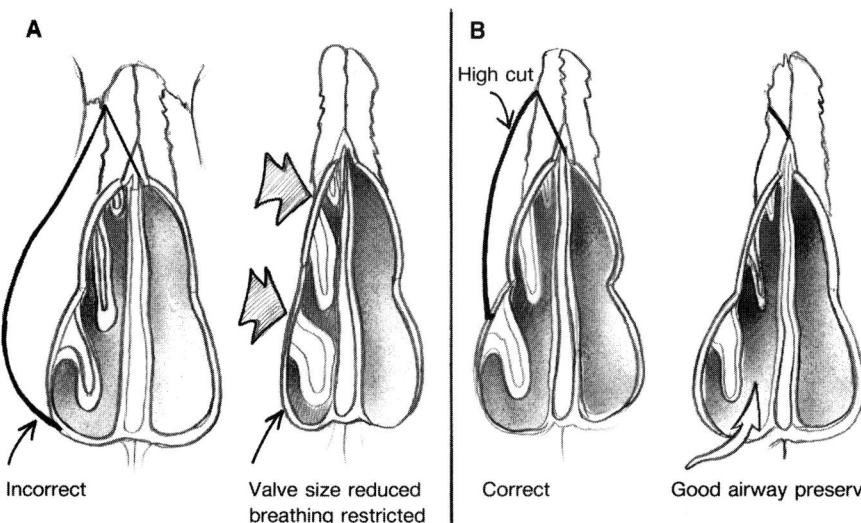

A

B

High cut

Incorrect

Valve size reduced
breathing restricted

Correct

Good airway preserved

Figure 171.19 A: If the lateral osteotomy is begun too low along the piriform aperture, medialization of the bone can cause an obstruction of this portion of the nasal airway. **B:** Beginning the osteotomy at a higher point allows for medial tilting of the bone without clinical compromise to the airway.

along the course of the nasomaxillary sulcus. At a desired point, the osteotomy is turned gradually so that it becomes connected to the medial osteotomy. The point at which the lateral osteotomy should be turned upward will vary somewhat depending on the shape of the nasal bone and the need for release. If desired, one could draw an outline for the proposed lateral osteotomy with a skin-marking pen. One should understand that the fracture produced by the osteotome actually precedes the instrument for a short distance. As one nears the end of the lateral osteotomy, it is generally helpful to complete the fracture with a prying motion of the osteotome, because this maneuver minimizes further trauma and allows a better periosteal attachment, which may help prevent hypermobility of the nasal bone fragment.

If the lateral osteotomy is placed too medially on the nasal bone, a "stair-step" line may be visible on the side of the nose after the fragment has been moved. If the lateral osteotomy is placed too laterally onto the maxilla, it may allow the fragment to fall inward to some degree. One can usually detect engagement onto the maxilla during the osteotomy by sudden change to a more dull sound with continued tapping on the osteotome. One must avoid leaving an incomplete or "greenstick" type of fracture, because this may allow the bone fragment to either not move fully or to move back to its original position when pressure is removed.

Injury to the lacrimal apparatus should not occur with a properly designed lateral osteotomy. One can normally feel the anterior portion of the lacrimal crest and easily avoid this structure. In a cadaver study, Thomas and Griner (5) has shown that lateral osteotomies, performed by either an experienced or novice surgeon, averaged approximately 7 mm from the lacrimal crest, with the closest being 4 mm.

If an intermediate osteotomy is to be done, it is best to make it after the medial osteotomy and before the lateral

osteotomy so that the nasal bone is not too unstable. Access is normally gained from the dorsal nasal exposure. After all osteotomies are completed the nasal bones are adjusted into better position and wound closure is begun.

Prior to closure it is advised that the surgeon carefully drape all overlying soft tissues into their normal anatomic position and then perform a detailed survey to check for any skeletal or soft tissue irregularities. A useful maneuver is for the surgeon to moisten the index finger of his or her glove and carefully palpate along the nasal dorsum. This "wet touch" allows for a very easy and smooth motion and significantly increases the ability of one to detect subtle subcutaneous irregularities in the nasal dorsum.

Table 171.4 lists a number of perioperative considerations.

Closure and Splinting

Intranasal incision sites are closed with interrupted absorbable sutures, usually 4-0 chromic. Closure of an external rhinotomy incision is commonly done with 6-0 nylon sutures that are removed in approximately 5 days. This closure could be done with small, fast-absorbing gut sutures. In some cases, one or more buried sutures may also be used in external rhinotomy closure, if desired. Reapproximation of the mucoperichondrial flaps of the nasal septum is greatly facilitated by use of a quilting suture that is passed back and forth through the septum multiple times, preferably in a very random pattern. Again 4-0 chromic suture works well for this. Depending on how one places the sutures, they can actually help hold a repositioned septal cartilage in an adjusted position. I favor making one or more passes directly over the maxillary crest. The placement of two or more transseptal quilting sutures very near the caudal margin of the septum can serve to also prevent posterior migration of a columellar graft.

TABLE 171.4
OTHER PERIOPERATIVE PROBLEMS

Excess bone or cartilage removal	Replace removed tissue or use other augmentation
Laceration of skin	Meticulous repair with 6-0 or 7-0 sutures
Cartilage disruption	Careful suture repair (figure-of-8 suture technique or application of overlapping support graft can help stabilize)
Palpable irregularity	Gentle rasping Place tissue graft (crushed cartilage, fascia, etc.) or "sheet" product such as Gelfilm
Regional swelling, ecchymosis	Minimize volume of injections: use massage to help spread Handle tissue gently Minimize tissue elevations Use small osteotomes Maintain elevation of head Apply cold compresses

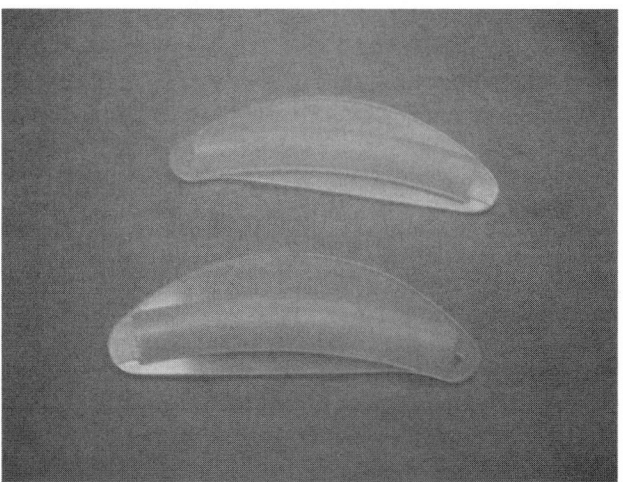

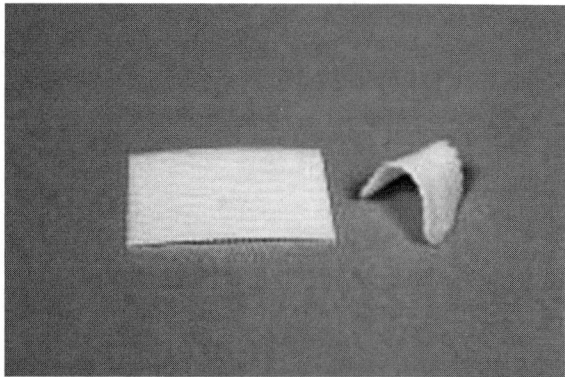

Figure 171.20 Example of silastic intranasal splints. These have a semicircular airway tubing that help allow better breathing with the splints in place and can serve also as a spacer to help hold the airway open in the early course of healing. They may be of added help when there has been attempted outfracture of the inferior nasal turbinates.

Figure 171.21 Example of thermoplastic external nasal splint. The splint can first be cut to desired shape and softened by placing it in hot water. It can then be applied over micropore tape on the nasal dorsum, to which it will stick if applied while still tacky.

Filling the nasal cavities with intranasal packs tends to be very bothersome to the patient and should only be done in extreme situations. The use of soft silastic intranasal splints, although still a source of irritation, is normally better tolerated. I favor use of silastic splints that have a semicircular tube on one side (Fig. 171.20). If kept patent, this tube then allows for some degree of nasal breathing and in some cases can also serve as a spacer to help hold open the airway or prevent excessive medial displacement of the fractured nasal bones. To prevent posterior displacement and potential aspiration, the intranasal splints should be loosely held together with a single transseptal suture such as 3-0 nylon. Some favor use of commercially available silastic splints that have magnets to help hold them together on both sides of the septum; however, it is wise to further secure their placement with either a single transseptal suture or with a tie that is secured loosely anterior to the nasal columella. Intranasal splints may be left in place anywhere from a few days to two or more weeks, as felt best. If they are kept for an extended time, it is advisable to see the patient periodically to help clear any crusting and monitor for any sign of pending erosion of the septal mucosa.

The application of an external nasal splint can serve to both provide some support for the adjustments to the nasal skeleton and restrict the amount of postoperative edema that would otherwise develop in the early postoperative interval. The skin is first cleaned of all blood and then coated with either tincture of benzoin or Mastisol to increase adhesiveness. Micropore paper tape or Steri-Strips are cut to match the shape of the nose and then applied in an overlapping fashion from the supratip region to the nasofrontal angle. If additional temporary support is desired

for the nasal tip, a narrow tape strip may be carefully draped about this structure, pulled upward slightly and secured to the tapes covering the nasal dorsum. Care must be taken to be sure that taping about the nasal tip does not become too tight and risk necrosis.

Once taping has been done most surgeons will choose to apply an external nasal splint for a period of normally 1 to 2 weeks. A plaster splint may be fabricated but is messy to apply, particularly if the patient is recumbent and material is likely to run off of the splint and into the eyes. Malleable aluminum splints with foam undersurface are commercially available and favored by many surgeons. A thermoplastic (Aquaplast) splint is very easy to apply and can be shaped very well to each particular nose (Fig. 171.21). This material comes as a semirigid plastic material that can be easily cut to desired shape and size, softened with warm water, and then stiffened again after it has been applied very exactly over the nasal dorsum.

As the patient is leaving the operating room, a folded or cut gauze sponge may be taped over the nares to collect any light bleeding or drainage from the nose. This "drip pad" may then be changed as necessary over the next 12 to 24 hours at the patient's convenience.

POSTOPERATIVE CARE

After the surgery, the patient should lie quietly for a time with the head elevated about 30 degrees. Cool compresses may be applied over the eyelids and paranasal region off and on over the next 12 to 24 hours as tolerated or convenient. The surgeon should prescribe an appropriate analgesic medication and give careful instructions on postoperative pain management. In some cases, a prophylactic antibiotic may also be prescribed for a time. The patient should be instructed to avoid lifting and other strenuous activity for a period of at least 2 to 3 weeks.

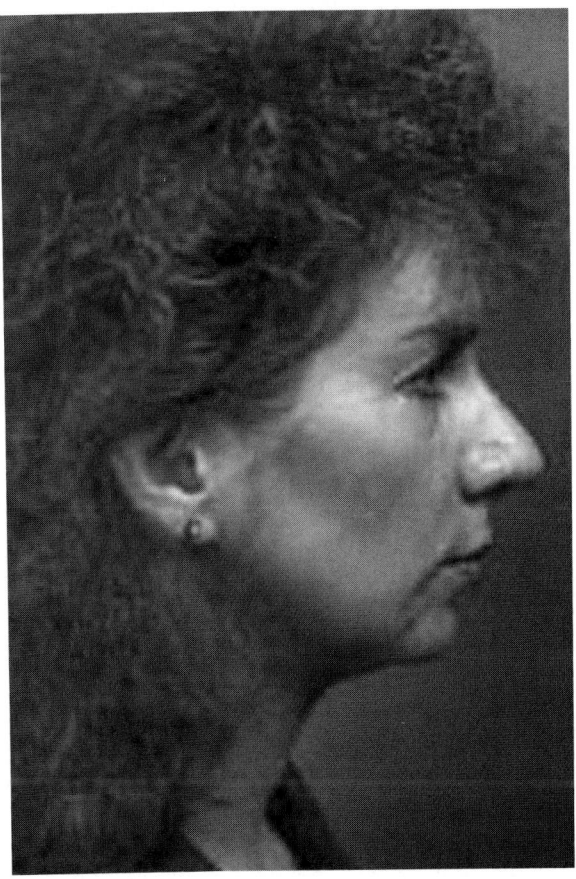 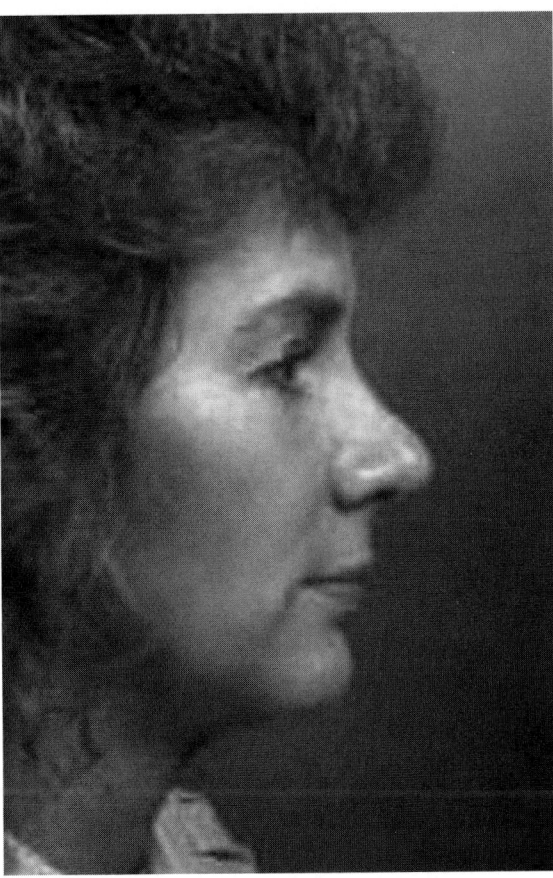

A   B

Figure 171.22 **A** and **B**: Young woman who has undergone a rhinoplasty for straightening of the nose and slight change of the dorsum and simultaneous placement of a chin implant which does a great deal to improve the perceived relative proportion of her nose.

ADJUNCTIVE PROCEDURES

The surgeon must realize that the nose is but one feature of the face and that disproportions of other parts may affect the way in which the nose is perceived by others (see Chapter 168). There are situations in which surgery to other facial parts will have an influence on the appearance of the nose. Occasionally, surgery to modify the relative position of the chin or other part will add to the overall result that is desired with rhinoplasty (Fig. 171.22A,B).

HIGHLIGHTS

- It is necessary to fully understand the patient's desires and motivations for surgery.
- The surgeon must determine what anatomic problems are present that adversely affect either function or appearance.
- The surgeon must determine exactly what should be done to attempt appropriate correction for each problem.
- Any unrealistic expectation must be identified and discussed openly.

- It must be decided if the patient is an appropriate candidate for surgery, considering both psychological and medical issues.
- The experience for both patient and surgeon will be better if good preoperative instruction is given.
- The plan for anesthesia must be appropriate.
- Adequate vasoconstriction is very important to allow ease of surgery and safety for patient.
- The surgeon must choose which surgical approach will provide adequate exposure and minimal adverse consequence for the patient.
- Reduction of a hump should be conservative and appropriate. Better to undercorrect than overcorrect and create a new deformity. Incremental reduction may be helpful.
- Nasal skin is thinnest in the central region of the nose. Accommodation must be made for this in hump reduction.
- Thickness of skin should be considered when planning for alterations in nasal tip cartilages.
- Medial osteotomy should be done first. Intermediate osteotomy, if any, should be done second. Lateral osteotomy should be done last.

- Lateral osteotomy should begin at about the level of the anterior attachment of the inferior turbinate. Starting the osteotomy too low along the piriform aperture can cause narrowing in this region and obstruction of the airway.
- One should always give consideration to the long-term effects of all incisions, tissue resections, and other issues related to the nasal surgery.
- The surgeon should consider how issues of age, race, and sex should influence the goals for surgery.
- One should consider how the nose relates to other features of the face.

REFERENCES

1. *Physicians' desk reference.* Montdale, NJ: Thompson PDR, 2002 and 2003. (Newer editions do not include this information.)
2. Fletcher M. Anesthesia in facial plastic surgery. In: Papel ID, ed. *Facial plastic and reconstructive surgery,* 2nd ed. New York, Thieme, 2002;145–152.
3. Calhoun KH. Introduction to rhinoplasty. In Bailey BJ, ed. *Head & neck surgery–otolaryngology.* Philadelphia, JB Lippincott, 1993;2113–2127.
4. Clinical Pharmacology. Gold Standard. 2005. Available at http://cp.gsm.com.
5. Thomas JR, Griner N. The relationship of lateral osteotomies in rhinoplasty to the lacrimal drainage system. *Otolaryngol Head Neck Surg* 1986;94:362–367.

Management of the Upper Two Thirds of the Nose

172

Randolph B. Capone   *Ira D. Papel*

Of all the aesthetic facial units, the nose plays perhaps the most important role in facial proportion and harmony. A single unpaired structure occupying the midface, it serves to balance the facial thirds and fifths as well as those aesthetic units surrounding it. Seemingly small changes after rhinoplasty or traumatic injury frequently affect dramatic changes in nasal appearance. The nose is not, however, only an aesthetic structure but also a respiratory and olfactory organ. This duality of nasal form and function mandates that rhinoplasty must enhance nasal appearance and optimize the nasal airway. It is essential, therefore, that the nasal surgeon have a detailed understanding of nasal anatomy and physiology, and a thorough grasp of the many interventions available in rhinoplasty. In this chapter, we discuss these issues with regard to management of the upper two thirds of the nose, that is, the bony and cartilaginous vaults.

ANATOMY

The upper two thirds of the nose contains the dorsum and sidewall aesthetic subunits, whereas the tip, columella, soft tissue triangles, and alae constitute the lower third of the nose (Fig. 172.1) (1). Topographically, the upper two thirds of the nose is that portion from the *nasion* to the level of the alar groove (Fig. 172.2), where the nasion is defined as the most posterior point along the curve from the glabella to the nasal dorsum. The *radix* is the region of the nasal dorsum that defines the contour of the paired nasal bones from the glabella toward the nasal tip.

Skin and Subcutaneous Tissue

The skin overlying the upper nasal two thirds has variable thickness. Relatively thick at the nasion (2 to 5 mm), it becomes thin and mobile over the dorsum (3.2 mm), thinnest at the rhinion (2 to 2.2 mm), and gradually thickens again, becoming sebaceous toward the tip (5 mm) (2). This variability is important in planning the dorsal profile because creation of a straight skeletal profile will not likely create a straight postoperative profile. When edema diminishes, the surgeon may find that the rhinion has been over-resected if no allowance for skin thickness was considered during surgery.

Beneath the skin is a thin fibrous layer designated the nasal superficial musculoaponeurotic system (SMAS) (3). Analogous to the facial SMAS, the nasal SMAS encompasses the nasal musculature and is located immediately superficial to the periosteum and perichondrium. Dissection just below the nasal SMAS provides a less traumatic and easier dissection plane during rhinoplasty, with preservation of nasal vasculature, nerves, and lymphatics that lie within the skin-soft tissue envelope (4).

Nasal Bones and Upper Lateral Cartilages

Deep to the nasal SMAS are the paired nasal bones and upper lateral cartilages. The nasal bones fuse with the frontal bone approximately 11 mm superior to the intercanthal line and are on average 2.5 cm in length (5). This length can be quite variable and represents a significant

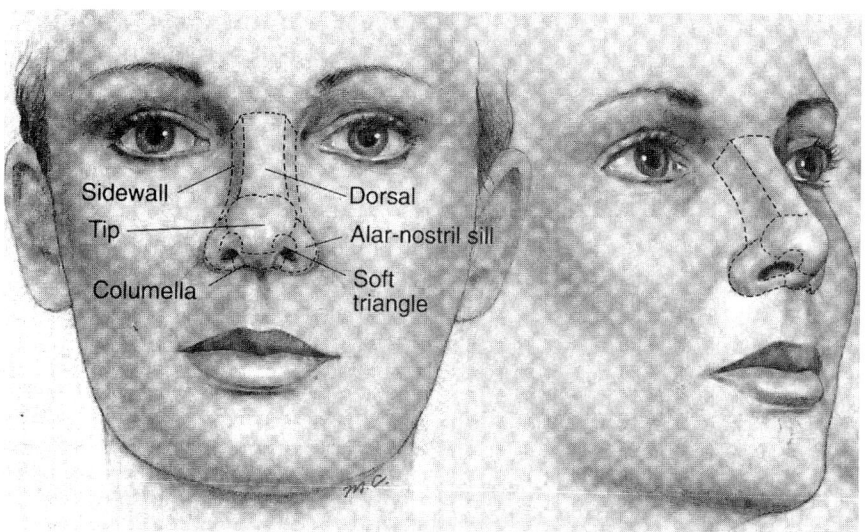

Figure 172.1 Nasal aesthetic subunits. (From Burget GC, Menick FJ. *Aesthetic reconstruction of the nose*. St. Louis: Mosby, 1994:7, with permission.)

risk factor for airway compromise after rhinoplasty (6). The caudal margin of the nasal bones overlaps the cephalic margin of the upper lateral cartilages, which in turn interlock with the paired lower lateral cartilages at the *scroll* (Fig. 172.3). Each of these connections is an important structural component that contributes to nasal integrity and support.

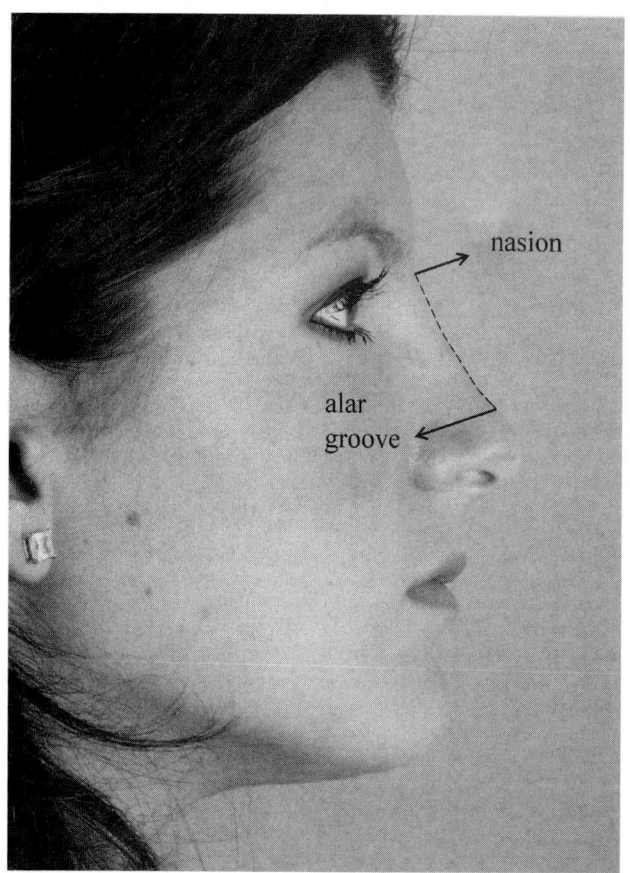

Figure 172.2 Upper nasal two thirds: nasion to alar groove.

Laterally, the caudal margin of the nasal bones and the anterior margin of the ascending processes of the maxilla form the *pyriform aperture*. The lateral margin of the upper lateral cartilages fuses with dense connective tissue, and the medial margin fuses with the septum superiorly but separates and is mobile inferiorly. Mucosa is tightly adherent to the internal surface of the cartilages and is continuous with the lining of the septum and lateral nasal wall.

The caudal margin of the upper lateral cartilage, the anterior head of the inferior turbinate, the proximate septum, and floor of the nose define the borders of the *internal nasal valve*. The angle between the upper lateral cartilages and the septum is the *nasal valve angle*, normally 10 to 20 degrees. The nasal valve typically has a cross-sectional area of 55 to 83 mm^2 and represents the site of greatest nasal resistance. It is the primary airflow-limiting segment of the nasal cavity (7).

The Bony and Cartilaginous Vaults

The upper nasal two thirds can be thought of as two contiguous arches, or vaults—a superior *bony vault* and an inferior *cartilaginous vault*. The nasal bones and the paired ascending processes of the maxilla comprise the bony vault, and the cartilaginous vault is composed of the upper lateral cartilages and the cartilaginous dorsal septum. The region of transition of the bony vault to the cartilaginous vault is known as the *rhinion*. The soft tissue linkage that occurs at the rhinion is comprised of upper lateral cartilage perichondrium that inserts on the undersurface of the paired nasal bones. This union allows for motion of the inferior vault relative to the superior vault.

As the name implies, nasal vaults are critical for support, distribution of forces, maintenance of dorsal height, and maintenance of nasal projection. As with any arch, the most essential support element occurs at the keystone. The nasal *keystone area* is the convergence of the caudal margin

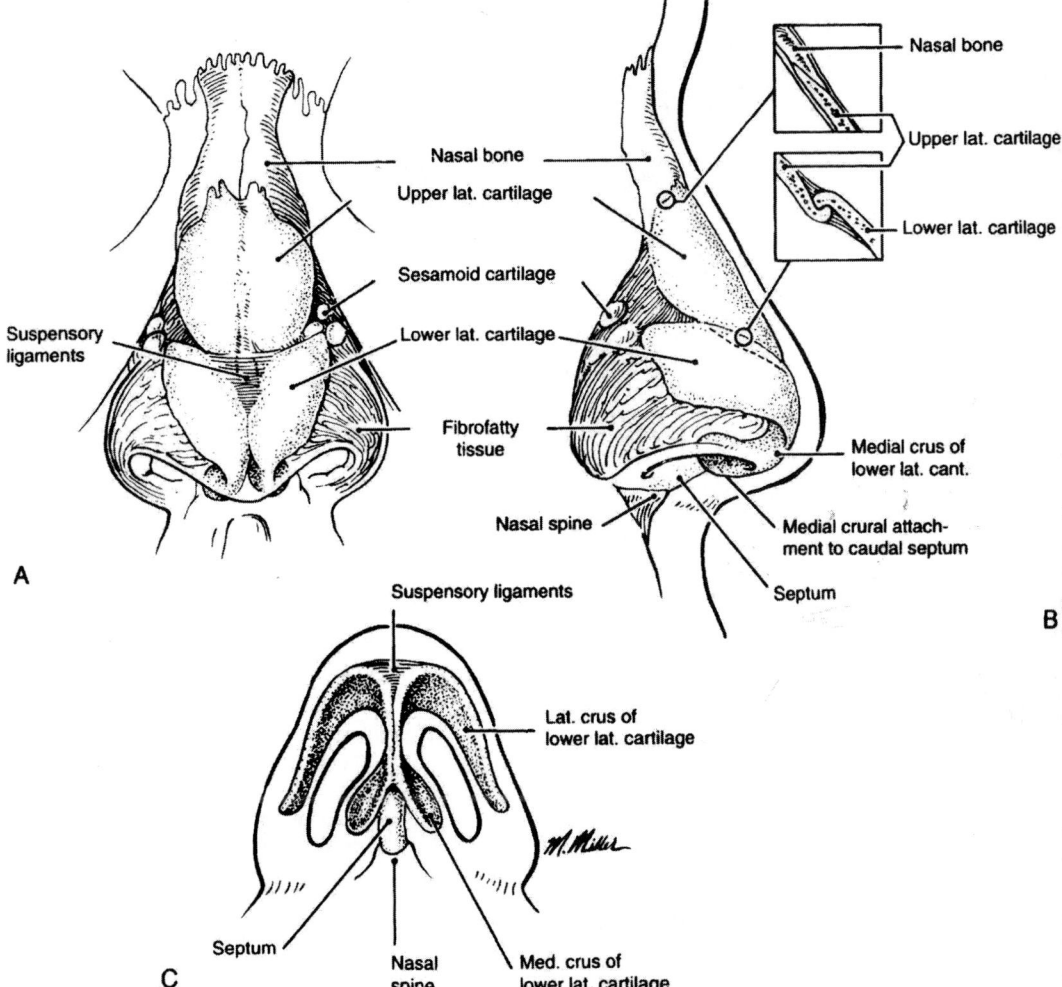

Figure 172.3 Anatomic relationships of the nasal bones, upper lateral cartilages, and lower lateral cartilages. (Modified from Papel ID. Management of the middle vault. In: Papel ID, ed. *Facial plastic and reconstructive surgery*, 2nd ed. Stuttgart: Thieme, 2002:408, with permission.)

of the nasal bones, the perpendicular plate of the ethmoid bone, the cephalic margin of the upper lateral cartilages, and the cartilaginous septum. Understanding this area is critical during planning and execution of osteotomies so as to effect a change without disruption of important support mechanisms.

NASAL ANALYSIS

The face is a complex set of surfaces with tremendous variability. The goal of facial analysis is to provide a consistent framework to compare pre- and postoperative results despite this variability. Nowhere is this more important than in rhinoplasty. Every rhinoplasty candidate should have high-quality six-view photography to facilitate analysis. In addition, an additional chin-down view is especially useful in evaluation of patients with nasal vault deformity (Fig. 172.4).

Aesthetic Angles

Analysis of the nasal aesthetic angles reveals the importance of the dorsum in evaluation of the rhinoplasty patient. Of the five facial aesthetic angles, three are determined using the geometry of the nasal dorsum: the nasofacial, the nasofrontal, and the nasomental angles. The *nasofacial angle* is the angle prescribed by the intersection of the facial plane (glabella to pogonion) and a line tangent to the nasal dorsum. Ideally, it is 36 to 40 degrees. The *nasofrontal angle* is determined by the intersection of the line connecting the nasion and glabella and the nasal dorsum tangent, ideally 115 to 130 degrees. Lastly, the *nasomental angle* is determined by the intersection of the line connecting the tip-defining point to the pogonion and the nasal dorsum tangent. The ideal nasomental angle is 120 to 132 degrees. Each of these angles should be carefully considered during the examination and photographic evaluation of the rhinoplasty candidate.

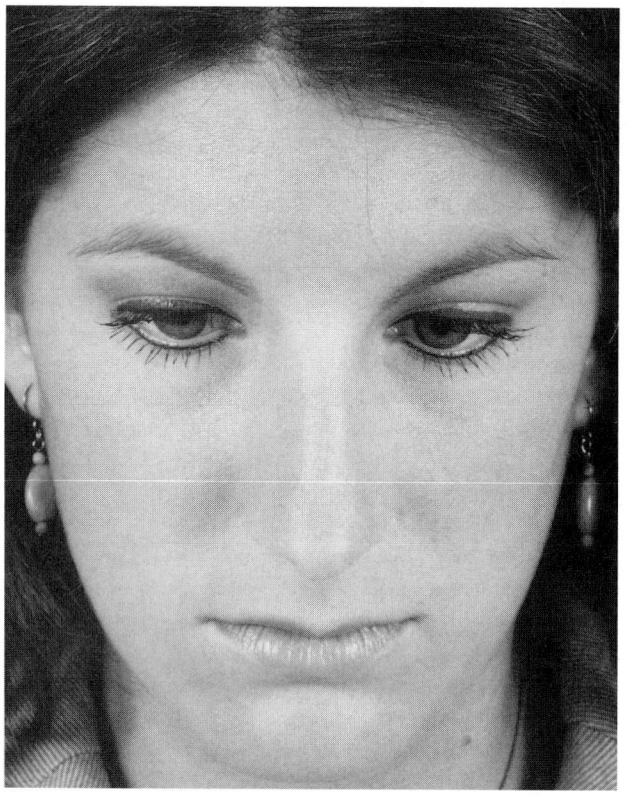

Figure 172.4 The chin down view of nasal dorsum is useful to detect the presence of subtle radix contour irregularities or asymmetry.

Nasal Length

Leonardo da Vinci introduced the practice of dividing the face into equal vertical thirds and horizontal fifths for the purpose of facial analysis. Later modified by Powell and Humphreys (8), this serves as the basis for modern-day facial analysis. A method more specific to nasal analysis, however, divides the lower face into two parts using the nasion, subnasale, and menton as landmarks (9). Using this method, nasal length (nasion to subnasale) should be three fourths the distance from the subnasale to the menton (Fig. 172.5).

Nasal Width and Radix Contours

On frontal view, nasal width should increase along its length, with a minima occurring at the intercanthal line. Maximal nasal width occurs at the alae and should equal one-fifth the width of the face. The upper nasal contour should follow a gentle curve from the medial eyebrow to the ipsilateral tip-defining point. Any irregularities in this contour will quickly be noted as different from the contralateral side, thereby contributing to asymmetry and an unsightly appearance. The pair of these curves, known as *radix contours,* is highlighted by the nasal light reflex and should be symmetric (Fig. 172.6).

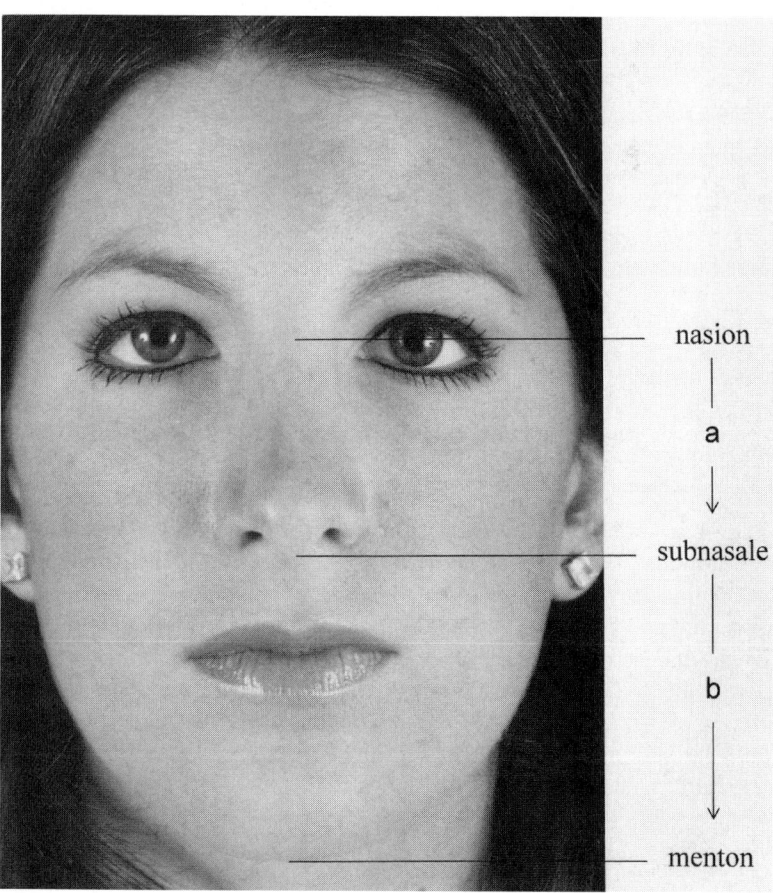

nasion

a

subnasale

b

menton

Figure 172.5 Determination of nasal length using the nasion, subnasale, and menton: ideally a = $^3/_4$ b.

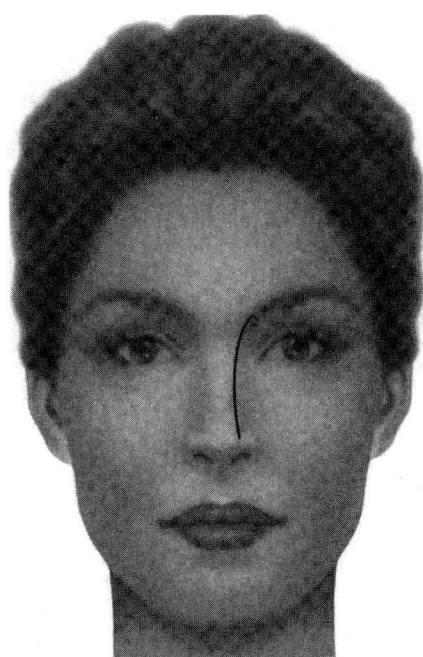

Figure 172.6 Radix lines. (From Orten SS, Hilger PA. Facial analysis of the rhinoplasty patient. In: Papel ID, ed. *Facial plastic and reconstructive surgery*, 2nd ed. Stuttgart: Thieme, 2002:361, with permission.)

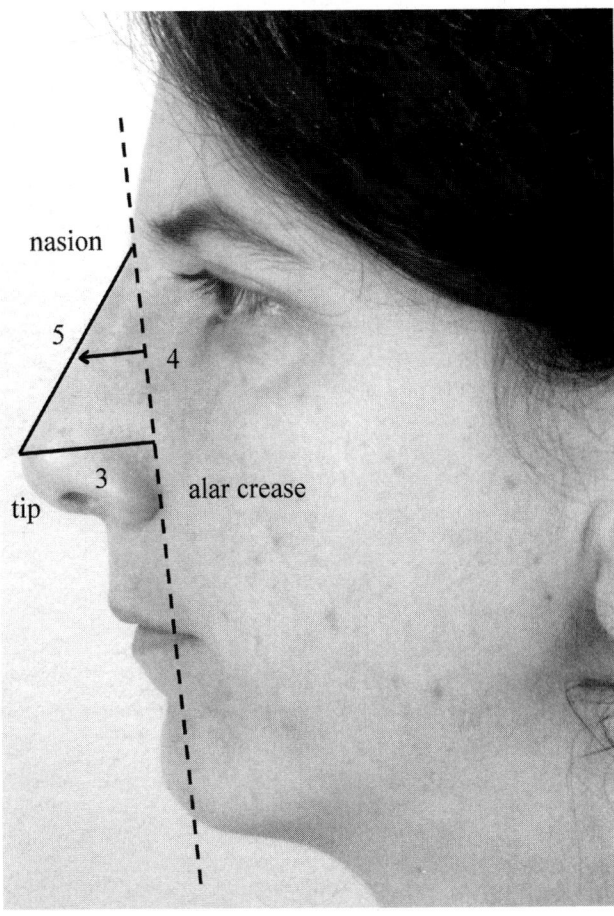

Figure 172.7 Determination of ideal dorsal projection using Crumley's tip projection analysis. At any point along the dorsum, the ratio of dorsal projection to the distance from the nasion should equal 3/5 (0.6).

Dorsal Projection

The nose projects anteriorly from the face, with its forward thrust orthogonal to the facial plane and parallel to the midsagittal plane. Quantification of nasal projection is a critical component of the rhinoplastic evaluation, yet of the many methods previously described, none specifically address *dorsal projection* (i.e., dorsal height) (10–12). Determination of proper tip projection using Crumley's method, however, utilizes the geometry of the 3:4:5 triangle; that is, projection of the nasal tip should equal three-fifths (0.6) the length from the nasion to the tip-defining point. This method can be used simultaneously to yield the ideal dorsal projection at any point along the dorsum, because the proportions of a 3:4:5 triangle are constant (Fig. 172.7). If dorsal projection exceeds this limit (0.6), it is indicative of the presence of a dorsal hump. Because a slight dorsal concavity can be attractive, dorsal projection just less than this limit is allowable, but a significantly lower measurement would be indicative of a saddle-nose deformity.

DEFECTS OF THE NASAL VAULTS

Bony Vault Defects

Most deformities involving the bony vault arise from blunt trauma (Table 172.1). Fractured nasal bones can be comminuted and/or displaced, often resulting in an unsightly twist, depression, spur, or hump. Frequently, the skin overlying the bony dorsum is lacerated causing additional deformity by the presence of cicatrix and adherence of the dermis to the nasal bone periosteum. Severe fractures such as nasoorbital ethmoid (NOE) fractures are often quite disfiguring due to retrodisplacement of the nasal bones, deprojection and flattening of the nasal dorsum, and shortening of the nose. The resultant telescopic defect is often associated with traumatic telecanthus due to the

TABLE 172.1	
NASAL VAULT DEFECTS	
Dorsal hump	
Deep nasion	Curvatures
Saddle nose	Pollybeak
Asymmetric nasal bones	Bony prominences
Short/long nasal bones	Rocker deformity
Wide/narrow bony pyramid	Open roof deformity
Depressions	Inverted versus deformity
Twists	
Partial/total rhinectomy (nasal cancer, gunshot wound)	

disruption of the medial canthal tendon insertion on the nasal bones. Trauma involving the bony vault does not typically cause functional deficit, unless the keystone area, the septum, or the middle vault is also affected. Less common causes of upper vault deformity include prior rhinoplasty, neoplasia, and congenital anomalies (13,14).

Cartilaginous Vault Defects

Deformity of the middle nasal vault can be more complex than that of the bony vault because it is frequently accompanied by internal nasal deformity contributing to airway compromise. The internal nasal valve occurs near the junction of the upper lateral cartilages and the dorsal septum and is often weakened or narrowed subsequent to trauma affecting the middle vault. Furthermore, the soft tissue nature of the middle vault makes it susceptible to deformity caused by other etiologies, including unrecognized birth trauma, infections, inflammatory diseases, or autoimmune processes (15–17).

Treatment of the middle vault in rhinoplasty was for many years considered little more than removal of a hump deformity. In the 1980s, however, surgeons began to describe numerous long-term complications of this limited approach, including the inverted-V deformity, nasal valve collapse, open roof deformity, and pollybeak deformity. As a result, rhinoplasty techniques were modified to avoid these problems (18,19).

MANAGEMENT OF THE CARTILAGINOUS VAULT

Surgical correction of the middle vault involves correction of existing deformities, while ever mindful of additional deformity prevention. When certain risk factors are present, such as short nasal bones, weak upper lateral cartilages, thin skin, narrow bony pyramid, or previous trauma or surgery, preventative action may be required utilizing cartilage grafting, precise structural realignment, and fixation of nasal valve structures.

Correction of middle vault starts with septoplasty. The old saying "as the septum goes, so goes the nose" indicates the importance of straightening the central strut of the nose. With the goal of making the dorsal septum as straight as possible, the open approach is often used. Accessing the septum from above via the separation of the medial crura of the lower lateral cartilages allows better exposure than the traditional endonasal approach (20). Further separation of the upper lateral cartilages from the dorsal septum results in maximal septal exposure. The deviated portions of the quadrangular cartilage and perpendicular plate of the ethmoid bone are removed, making sure that 1 cm dorsal and caudal struts are maintained. Wide mucoperichondrial elevation, weakening incisions, wedge excisions, and sutured struts are adjuncts useful in straightening the deviated septum (21).

Spreader grafts are probably the next most common corrective modality used for middle vault rehabilitation. First described by Sheen and Sheen (22), these rectangular cartilage grafts are placed between the junctions of the upper lateral cartilages and septum to widen and stabilize the nasal valve. Spreader grafts not only lateralize the upper lateral cartilages but also strengthen the middle vault to resist the inward motion on inspiration associated with Bernoulli's principle. They can be placed either through open or closed rhinoplasty techniques but are easier to stabilize with direct sutures via the open approach. Septal cartilage is the most frequently used grafting material, but auricular cartilage may be used if septum is not available. Spreader grafts can also be used for aesthetic purposes. For patients with unilateral middle vault depressions, a single spreader graft can elevate and lateralize the upper lateral cartilage to restore symmetry.

In many revision rhinoplasty cases involving middle vault pathology, separation of the septum and upper lateral cartilages has occurred due to prior hump removal. There is usually fibrous connective tissue present instead of the native cartilaginous junction. Therefore, preservation of the mucoperichondrium and creation of a pocket for graft placement through the open approach is usually preferred. If the upper lateral cartilages are fused with the septum in the internal nasal valve area, sharp dissection with an elevator will preserve the mucoperichondrium and maintain stability. In cases in which the upper lateral cartilages have been almost completely resected, conchal cartilage onlay grafts may be needed in addition to spreader grafts to augment lateral support or camouflage depressions. The grafts are carved, aligned, and fixed into position with 5-0 PDS (Polydiaxonone, Ethicon, Sommerville, NJ) mattress sutures. Most spreader grafts are 1.5 to 2.5 cm in length and 1 to 3 mm in width. In general, the grafts should run along the dorsal septum from below the bony-cartilaginous junction to the anterior septal angle. In severe cases, the grafts may be layered to provide additional bulk. Grafts of unequal width may also be used to correct asymmetries in the middle vault. Spreader grafts can also be used as internal splints to help straighten a caudal septal deflection. The technique of spreader graft placement and fixation is demonstrated in Figs. 172.8 to 172.11. Placement of spreader grafts is greatly facilitated by placement of a 30-gauge needle through the cartilage complex while suturing.

A corollary to spreader grafting that deserves mention is reverse spreader grafting. This technique can be useful in patients with an overly broad middle vault, minimal nasal obstruction, and no nasal valve collapse. In these cases, patients can benefit from reduction of the horizontal width of the cartilaginous dorsum, which can be thought of as the reverse of spreader grafts (23).

Additional methods to augment the function of the nasal valve involve the placement of alar batten grafts, butterfly grafts, and various suture methods. Schlosser and

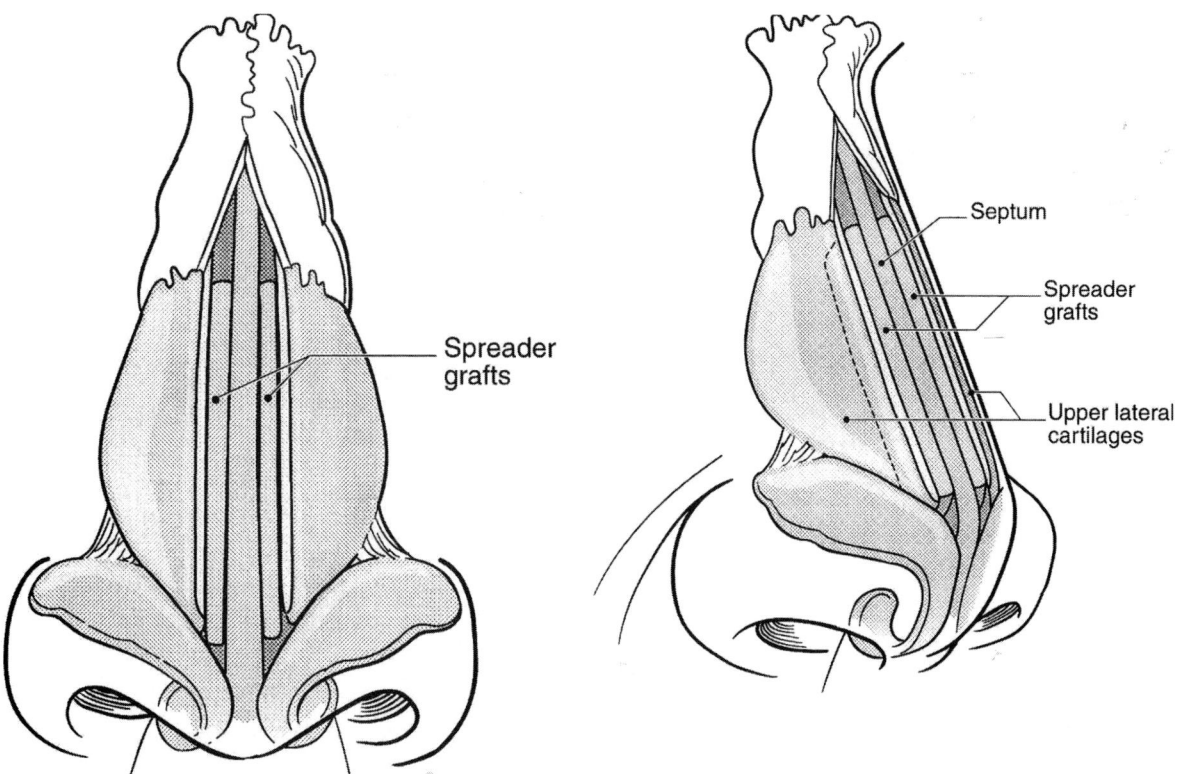

Figure 172.8 Placement of spreader grafts between septum and upper lateral cartilages. (From Papel ID. Management of the middle vault. In: Papel ID, ed. *Facial plastic and reconstructive surgery*, 2nd ed. Stuttgart: Thieme, 2002:409, with permission.)

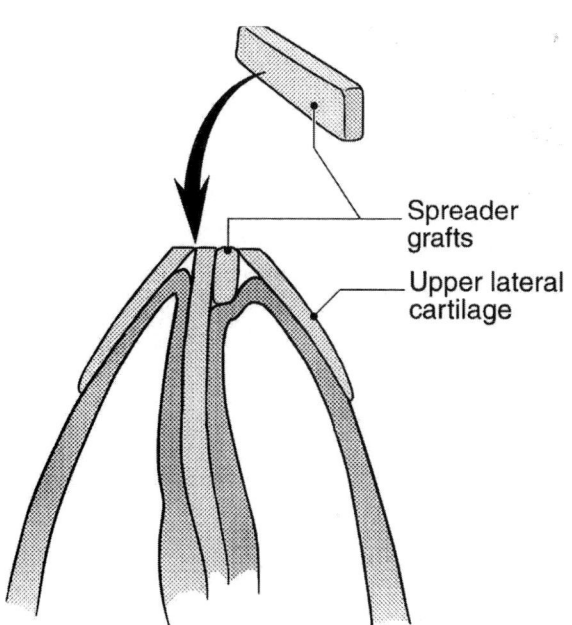

Figure 172.9 Placement of spreader graft lateralizes and elevates the upper lateral cartilage, widening the middle vault. (From Papel ID. Management of the middle vault. In: Papel ID, ed. *Facial plastic and reconstructive surgery*, 2nd ed. Thieme, 2002:409, Fig. 35-5, with permission.)

Park (24) described the use of 5-0 clear nylon flaring sutures that span the upper lateral cartilages and septum horizontally. Tightening the suture theoretically increases the angle of the internal nasal valve and therefore improves nasal airflow. Their study indicated that flaring sutures used concomitantly with spreader grafts increase airflow more than the use of spreader grafts alone. Other suture techniques such as tip-lifting sutures, or valve maneuvers like internal valve M-plasty or lateral crural J-flap, can also be useful adjuncts but are outside the scope of this chapter.

Patients with saddle-nose deformity frequently have middle vault collapse without soft tissue support, commonly due to a large septal perforation. Fixation of a dorsal graft helps to enhance dorsal projection, support the soft tissues, and restore the integrity of the nasal valve. Calvarial bone secured with a lag screw or rib cartilage secured with sutures have been very useful in these patients (25,26). In addition, dorsal calvarial grafts can serve as anchors for other reconstructive grafts (27). In some cases, the use of crushed cartilage or Alloderm (LifeCell Corp., Branchburg, NJ) over the dorsum and graft material can help smooth an irregular profile.

The pollybeak deformity is a complex nasal deformity with multiple etiologies that deserves special mention. It represents a *relative* underprojection of the nasal tip with regard to the projection of the dorsum. This can occur if

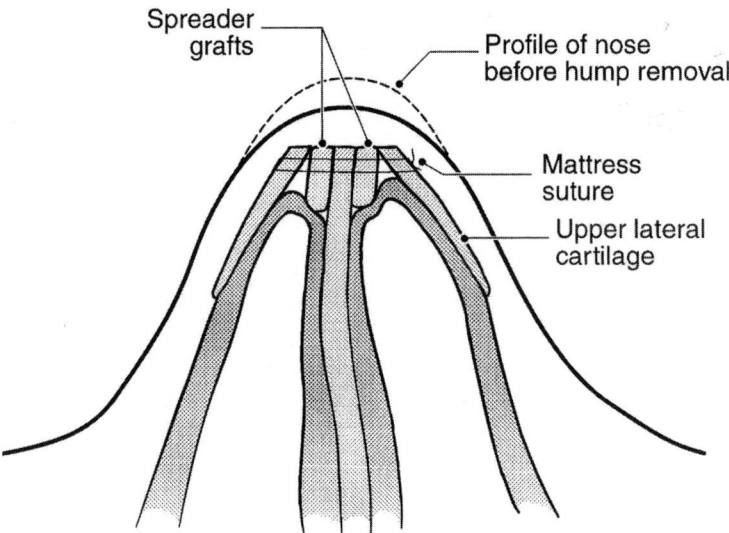

Figure 172.10 Spreader grafts in place and fixed with mattress sutures. The original dorsal height is identified. (From Papel ID. Management of the middle vault. In: Papel ID, ed. *Facial plastic and reconstructive surgery,* 2nd ed. Stuttgart: Thieme, 2002:409, with permission.)

tip projection is aesthetically correct but the dorsum is overprojected (a "dorsal pollybeak"), or if dorsal projection is aesthetically correct but the tip is underprojected (a "tip pollybeak"). The pollybeak deformity can occur naturally, or as the result of prior rhinoplasty. An iatrogenic dorsal pollybeak is frequently caused by insufficient lowering of the dorsum, whereas an iatrogenic tip pollybeak is frequently caused by disruption of tip support without reconstitution, over reduction of tip projection, or inappropriate de-rotation of the tip. As such, there are different management strategies for the pollybeak, depending on the nature of the deformity. The important point is that the rhinoplasty surgeon recognizes the importance of the

critical relation between tip projection and dorsal projection during rhinoplasty.

MANAGEMENT OF THE BONY VAULT

Deformity of the upper nasal vault represents a challenge to the rhinoplasty surgeon, requiring thorough preoperative evaluation and careful surgical technique to manage. Improper or incomplete treatment of the bony vault may lead to suboptimal results, including persistence of existing defects or the creation of new ones. The presence of iatrogenic deformities listed in Table 172.1 bear witness to

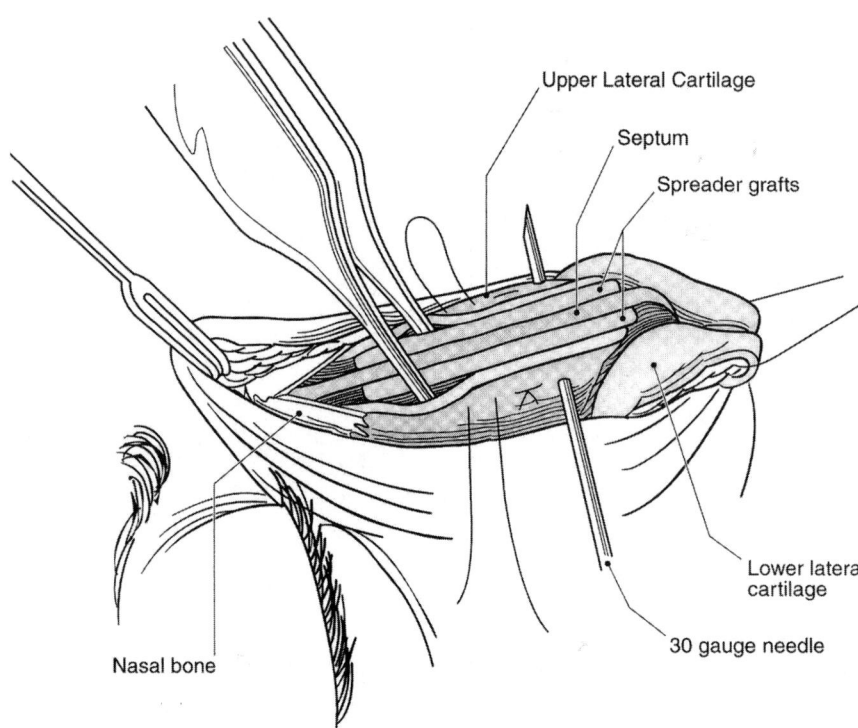

Figure 172.11 Demonstration of mattress suture fixation and use of 30-gauge needle for stabilization. (From Papel ID. Management of the middle vault. In: Papel ID, ed. *Facial plastic and reconstructive surgery,* 2nd ed. Stuttgart: Thieme, 2002:409, Fig. 35-7, with permission.)

this. Surgical treatment of the bony vault should aim to accomplish the following: (a) establishment of appropriate dorsal projection, (b) creation of a smooth dorsal contour free of bony irregularity, (c) correction of nasal width, and (d) straightening of the crooked nose.

Techniques used to accomplish these aims include hump reduction, osteotomies, and grafting.

Hump Reduction

John Orland Roe (1848 to 1915) provided the modern age with the first account of dorsal defect correction in 1891 (Fig. 172.12) (28). Regional dorsal overprojection is managed with wide soft tissue envelope elevation and the removal of portions of the nasal bones. This can be done either through an open or closed approach. Adequate exposure must be balanced with the maintenance of soft tissue support, and it must be remembered that the upper lateral cartilages insert deep to the caudal margin of the nasal bones. Care must be taken not to disarticulate this union. The best way to avoid this is to elevate the nasal bone periosteum using a Joseph elevator 1 to 2 mm superior to the rhinion (29). Bone removal is subsequently accomplished with a double-guarded osteotome or a carbide tungsten pull rasp, depending on the amount of bone to be removed. After sharp incision of the cartilaginous component, large humps typically require removal with the osteotome. Care should be taken to follow the planned trajectory and not make an oblique cut by straying laterally or canting the osteotome (Fig. 172.13). Refinements can then be performed by rasping just off midline in a slightly oblique manner so as not to avulse the upper lateral cartilages (30).

Osteotomies

Osteotomies have evolved greatly since the time of Jacques Joseph (1865 to 1934), one of the rhinoplasty pioneers who touted their importance (31). Early techniques were

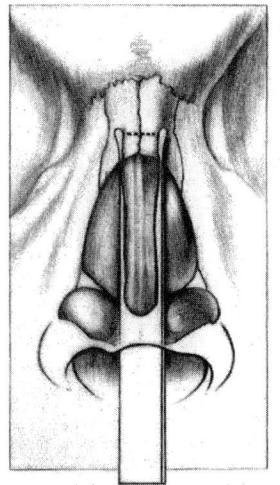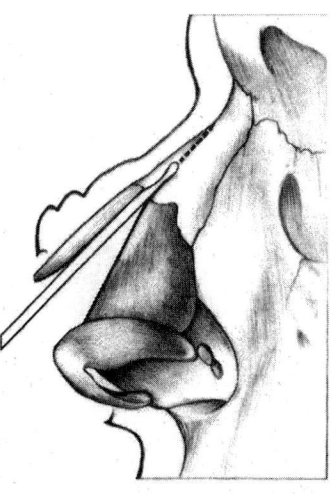

Figure 172.13   Removal of dorsal excess. (From Mostafour SP, Murakami CS, Larrabee WF Jr. Management of the bony nasal vault. In: Papel ID, ed. *Facial plastic and reconstructive surgery,* 2nd ed. Stuttgart: Thieme, 2002:403, with permission.)

fraught with nasal airway compromise largely due to a trajectory that caused wide disruption of periosteum and release of lower lateral cartilage lateral suspensory ligaments. Modifications have led to the emergence of modern techniques that place equal importance on preservation of the nasal airway and aesthetic improvement, in accord with the dual tenet of the rhinoplasty operation (32,33).

Osteotomies can be performed laterally, medially, or intermediately. Lateral osteotomies should be limited to the thin bone of the pyriform aperture, lateral to the anterior margin of the ascending maxillary processes. If too far lateral, the thick bone at the nasofacial transition will be encountered, rather than the average 2.5 mm thickness typically encountered along the osteotomy path (34).

Lateral osteotomies can be linear or perforating, internal or external. The ideal trajectory is described as "high–low–high," which indicates the antero-posterior position on the nasal pyramid. A standard lateral osteotomy is a linear, internal cut that is initiated with a mucosal stab incision made just lateral to the anterior face of the inferior turbinate. The curved guarded 4-mm osteotome is placed into the incision on the margin of the pyriform aperture, at about a 45-degree angle to the facial plane, or roughly perpendicular to the face of the aperture (Fig. 172.14). Preservation of the inferior segment of the pyriform maintains the lateral suspensory ligaments and width important for the nasal airway. Soon after the initial cut, the osteotome should be transitioned roughly parallel to the facial plane and directed toward the medial canthal area. The osteotomy should then curve anteriorly and superiorly to terminate at the level of the medial canthus, midway between the dorsal line and the medial canthus. The telltale sound of the osteotome meeting the thicker frontal bone is indicative of the proper stopping point. If the osteotomy extends superior to the medial canthus, there is greater risk

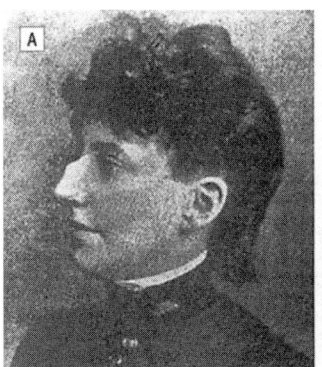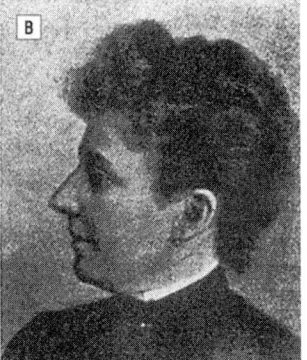

Figure 172.12   John Orlando Roe patient: before **(A)** and after **(B)** dorsal hump removal (1891). (From Lam SM. John Orlando Roe: father of aesthetic rhinoplasty. *Arch Facial Plast Surg* 2002;4:122–123, with permission.)

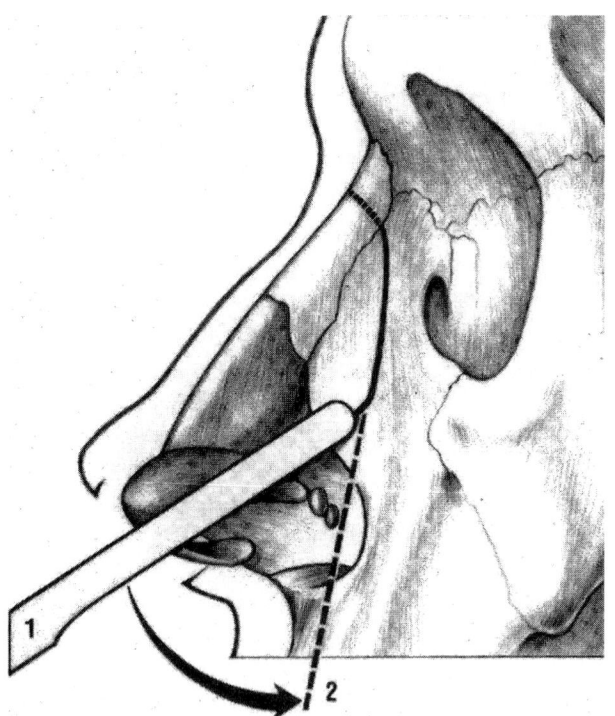

Figure 172.14 The lateral osteotomy is initiated at the anterior face of the inferior turbinate, initially perpendicular to the plane of the pyriform aperture (position 1). The osteotomy is then transitioned (position 2) and carried to the medial canthal area. (From Mostafour SP, Murakami CS, Larrabee WF Jr. Management of the bony nasal vault. In: Papel ID, ed. *Facial plastic and reconstructive surgery*, 2nd ed. Stuttgart: Thieme, 2002:404, with permission.)

of creating a rocker deformity, which occurs when the nasal bone inferior to the osteotomy sinks relative to the bone superior to the cut. The osteotomy is completed with pronation and medialization of the osteotome, causing back-fracture across the superior aspect of the nasal bone. Elevation of the periosteum in this vicinity liberates the nasal bones from the soft tissue envelope, allowing the osteotomized bone to heal free of the influence of soft tissue contracture. If the back-fracture is incomplete or inadequate, it can be augmented percutaneously using a 2-mm osteotome. Alternatively, the entire back-fracture can be completed percutaneously.

Perforating lateral osteotomies can be performed either internally (transnasally) or externally (percutaneously). The perforating technique is the ideal method to complete an exact osteotomy with minimal trauma. It is preferred when maintenance of support is critical, such as in revision rhinoplasty or short nasal bones, because there is far less disruption of periosteal support and the intact periosteum stabilizes and splints the mobilized segments, enhancing precise healing (35,36). A series of perforations are made at fixed intervals along the desired fracture trajectory and then completed with minimal manual manipulation. The intranasal perforating osteotomy is useful to widen the pyriform aperture by displacing the bones laterally (37).

Medial and intermediate osteotomies should be used judiciously; however, they can be essential when the pyriform is very thick, the nose is significantly deviated, or a very large nose needs to be reduced. Both medial and intermediate osteotomies are usually performed transnasally with a 3-mm osteotome. Medial osteotomies are initiated on the medial aspect of the caudal margin of the nasal bones near the septum. This is very near the keystone area of the nasal vaults so considerable care must be taken. The percutaneous perforation technique can be used to perform medial osteotomies to further ensure preservation of the keystone. The trajectory of the fracture is superolateral, meeting with the back-fracture of the previously performed lateral osteotomy. If further correction is needed, intermediate osteotomies can also be performed. The intermediate osteotomy is also initiated on the caudal margin of the nasal bones, intermediate to the medial and lateral osteotomies. The trajectory should parallel the lateral osteotomy and meet with the superior back-fracture. Because intermediate osteotomies are difficult to execute if the lateral bone has already been mobilized, they are best performed prior to lateral osteotomies.

Grafts

Contemporary grafts useful in treatment of the bony vault include radix grafts, onlay grafts, and anchored bone grafts. Radix grafts serve to increase the projection of the nasofrontal trough, correcting the excessively deep nasion. If septal or auricular cartilage is readily accessible, it can be used either as a single morselized piece or multiple fragments sutured together as a plumping graft (38). The graft is placed either superficial or deep to the nasal bone periosteum and held in place by the overlying skin envelope. Although Alloderm can also be used as a radix graft, it is perhaps more useful as a dorsal onlay graft to camouflage small irregularities as well as to add height. When significant bony defects are present, as after cancer resection or NOE telescoping nasal deformity, calvarial bone grafts may be required to reconstruct the upper vault. These grafts are cantilevered off the frontal bone and anchored precisely with titanium screws.

CONCLUSION

Facial aesthetics and attractiveness rely in large part on the appearance of the nose. Deformities affecting the nasal vaults are distinct and independent from those affecting the nasal tip and contribute not only to unsightly appearance but also to improper nasal function. Building on the past experience of prior rhinoplasty surgeons, surgical techniques dealing with nasal vault deformities have evolved, ever mindful that restoration of proper anatomic vault relations significantly enhances the appearance of the nose and nasal function. The contemporary rhinoplasty surgeon must be facile with analysis and management of the bony and cartilaginous nasal vaults that comprise the upper two thirds of the nose and be able to integrate this into management of the nasal tip for successful performance of the rhinoplasty operation.

HIGHLIGHTS

- The internal nasal valve is near the junction of the upper lateral cartilages and the dorsal septum.
- Spreader grafts between the upper lateral cartilages and septum may widen and stabilize the valve.
- The valve may also be augmented with batten grafts, butterfly grafts, and suture methods.
- Pollybeak deformity is a relative under projection of the nasal tip relative to the dorsum.
- Upper vault deformity is managed with hump reduction, osteotomies, and grafting
- The insertion of the upper lateral cartilages on the caudal margin of the nasal bones must not be disarticulated.

REFERENCES

1. Burget GC, Menick FJ. *Aesthetic reconstruction of the nose.* St. Louis: Mosby, 1994.
2. Behrbohm H. Preoperative management. In: Behrbohm H, Tardy ME Jr, eds. *Essentials of septorhinoplasty: philosophy, approaches, techniques.* Stuttgart: Thieme, 2004:89–106.
3. Mitz V, Peyronie M. The superficial musculo-aponeurotic system in the parotid and cheek area. *Plast Reconstr Surg* 1976;58:80.
4. Tardy ME, Brown RJ. *Surgical anatomy of the nose.* New York: Raven Press, 1995.
5. Oneal RM, Beil RJ Jr, Schlesinger J. Surgical anatomy of the nose. *Otolaryngol Clin North Am* 1999;32:145–181.
6. Guryon B. Nasal osteotomy and airway changes. *Plast Reconstr Surg* 1998;102:856–860; discussion 861–863.
7. Papel ID Management of the middle vault. In: Papel ID, ed. *Facial plastic and reconstructive surgery,* 2nd ed. Stuttgart: Thieme, 2002: 407–413.
8. Powell N, Humphreys B. *Proportions of the aesthetic face.* New York: Thieme-Stratton, 1984.
9. Papel IP, Capone RB. Facial proportions and esthetic ideals. In: Behrbohm H, Tardy ME Jr, eds. *Essentials of septorhinoplasty: philosophy, approaches, techniques.* Stuttgart: Thieme, 2004:65–74.
10. Simons R. Nasal tip projection, ptosis, and supratip thickening. *Ear Nose Throat J* 1982;61:44.
11. Crumley R. Quantitative analysis of nasal tip projection. *Laryngoscope* 1988;98:202–208.
12. Baum S. Introduction. *Ear Nose Throat J* 1982;61:426.
13. Dingman RO, Natvig P. The deviated nose. *Clin Plast Surg* 1977; 4:145–152.
14. Vuyk HD. A review of practical guidelines for correction of the deviated, asymmetric nose. *Rhinology* 2000;38:72–78.
15. Verwoerd CDA, Verwoerd-Verhoef HL. Developmental aspects of the deviated nose. *Facial Plastic Surgery* 1989;6:95.
16. Fernandez-Vozmediano JM, Armario Hita JC, Gonzales Cabrerizo A. Rhinoscleroma in three siblings. *Pediatr Dermatol* 2004;21: 134–138.
17. Pirsig W, Pentz S, Lenders H. Repair of saddle nose deformity in Wegener's granulomatosis and ectodermal dysplasia. *Rhinology* 1993;31(2):69–72.
18. Sheen JH. Spreader graft: a method of reconstructing the roof of the middle nasal vault following rhinoplasty. *Plast Reconstr Surg* 1984;73:230–237.
19. Toriumi DM, Johnson CM. Open structure rhinoplasty: featured technical points and long-term follow-up. *Fac Plast Clin North Am* 1993;1:1–22.
20. TerKonda RP, Sykes JM. Repairing the twisted nose. *Otolaryngol Clin North Am* 1999;32:53–64.
21. Foda MTF. The role of septal surgery in management of the deviated nose. *Plast Reconstr Surg* 2005;115:406–415.
22. Sheen JH, Sheen AP. *Aesthetic rhinoplasty.* St. Louis: CV Mosby, 1987.
23. Thomas JR, Prendiville S. Overly wide cartilaginous middle vault. *Facial Plast Surg Clin North Am* 2004;12:107–110.
24. Schlosser RJ, Park SS. Surgery for the dysfunctional nasal valve. *Arch Fac Plast Surg* 1999;1:105–110.
25. Frodel JL, Marentette LJ, Quatela VC, Weinstein GS. Calvarial bone graft harvest: techniques, considerations, and morbidity. *Arch Otolaryngol Head Neck Surg* 1993;119:17–23.
26. Quatela VC, Jacono AA. Structural grafting in rhinoplasty. *Arch Facial Plast Surg* 2002;18:223–232.
27. Papel ID. Augmentation rhinoplasty utilizing cranial bone grafts. *Md Med J* 1991;40:479–483.
28. Lam SM. John Orlando Roe: father of aesthetic rhinoplasty. *Arch Facial Plast Surg* 2002;4:122–123.
29. Larrabee WF Jr. Open rhinoplasty and the upper third of the nose. *Facial Plast Surg Clin North Am* 1993;1:26.
30. Mostafour SP, Murakami CS, Larrabee WF Jr. Management of the bony nasal vault. In: Papel ID, ed. *Facial plastic and reconstructive surgery,* 2nd ed. Thieme: 2002:402–406.
31. Aufricht G. Joseph's rhinoplasty with some modifications. *Surg Clin North Am* 1971;51:299–316.
32. Webster RC, Davidson RC, Smith RC. Curved lateral osteotomy for airway protection in rhinoplasty. *Arch Otolaryngol* 1977;103: 454–458.
33. Thomas JR, Griner NR, Remmler DJ. Steps for a safer method of osteotomies in rhinoplasty. *Laryngoscope* 1987;97:746–747.
34. Larrabee WF Jr, Murakami CS. Osteotomy techniques to correct posttraumatic deviation of the nasal pyramid: a technical note. *J Craniomaxillofac Trauma* 2000;6:A–E.
35. Tardy ME Jr. Contemporary rhinoplasty: principles and philosophy. In: Behrbohm H, Tardy ME Jr, eds. *Essentials of septorhinoplasty: philosophy, approaches, techniques.* Stuttgart: Thieme, 2004: 37–63.
36. Rohrich RJ, Minoli JJ, Adams WP, et al. The lateral nasal osteotomy in rhinoplasty: an anatomic endoscopic comparison of the external versus internal approach. *Plast Reconstr Surg* 1997;99: 1309–1313.
37. Byrne PJ, Walsh WE, Hilger PA. The use of inside-out lateral osteotomy to improve outcome in rhinoplasty. *Arch Facial Plast Surg* 2003;5:251–255.

Nasal Tip Surgery

Grant S. Hamilton III   **Dean M. Toriumi**

Rhinoplasty is a complex operation that requires precise analysis, a thoughtful operative plan, and meticulous execution. Unique to rhinoplasty is the need for a three-dimensional vision of the attractive nasal tip. The key to successful nasal tip surgery is the ability to create that desired shape.

Most primary rhinoplasty patients have a large nose and would like to have it made smaller. Historically, rhinoplasty techniques have emphasized excision and removal of tissue to achieve that goal. Recently, however, this philosophy has shifted as some reductive techniques have been correlated with poor long-term functional and aesthetic results. Whereas excision tends to weaken the supporting framework of the nose, the structural approach emphasizes reinforcement of the bony and cartilaginous components so that they may better withstand the relentless and insidious forces of scar contracture in the soft tissue envelope. For example, narrowing of the nasal tip by resecting lateral crural cartilage tends to result in supra-alar pinching, alar retraction, lateral nasal wall weakness, and collapse of the nasal valve. Removal of a dorsal hump without reconstitution of the attachment between the upper lateral cartilages and the septum often leads to middle vault collapse, airway obstruction, and an inverted V deformity. Excessive resection of tip cartilage in a thick-skinned patient with a big nose is likely to create a poorly supported, ptotic, "bag of skin" that lacks definition and airway support. These pitfalls are not necessarily the result of poor technique. Rather, inadequate assessment, diagnosis, and surgical judgment are often to blame. If the rhinoplasty surgeon has an understanding of the long-term consequences of weakening the nose, many of these unfortunate sequelae can be avoided.

ANALYSIS AND DIAGNOSIS

Analysis of the tip, which is only one component of the nasal examination, is not undertaken in isolation. For the sake of brevity, this chapter focuses only on the contribution of the tip to the form and function of the nose. The reader is encouraged to consult another source (Chapter 170) for a thorough overview of nasal analysis.

Before undertaking an intelligent analysis of the nasal tip, it is imperative to have a mastery of nasal anatomy as well as a clear understanding of the ideal contours and relationships of the nose (Figs. 173.1–173.6). When evaluating the tip, the surgeon should attempt to visualize the underlying structures by inspecting the skin. The first step is to try to quantify the thickness of the skin envelope. Most surgeons classify patients into thin, medium, and thick skin categories. This can be estimated by inspection and palpation of the skin by rolling it between the thumb and index finger. When assessing skin thickness, freckles are a reliable indicator of thin skin (1). Thick skin tends to be more sebaceous and have thick nostril rims.

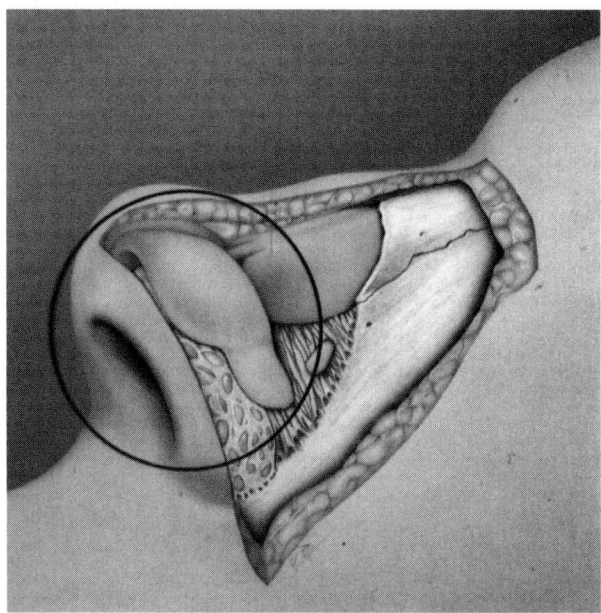

Figure 173.1 Anatomic structures of the nasal tip.

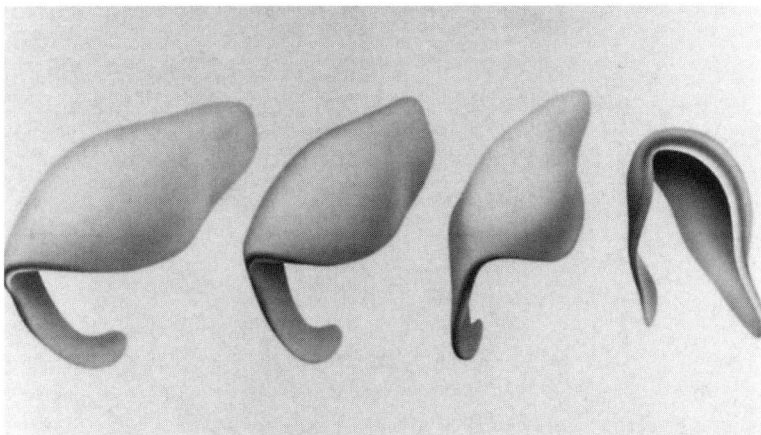

Figure 173.2 Typical alar cartilage anatomy from four separate views.

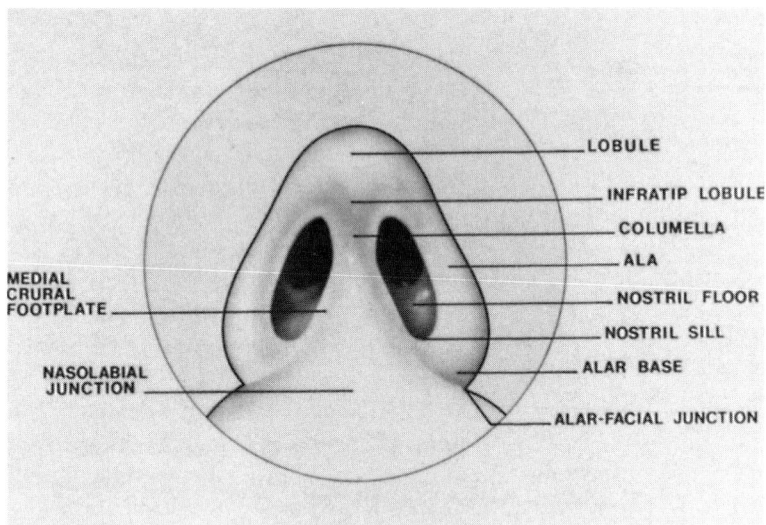

Figure 173.3 Anatomy and nomenclature of the nasal tip viewed from the basal aspect.

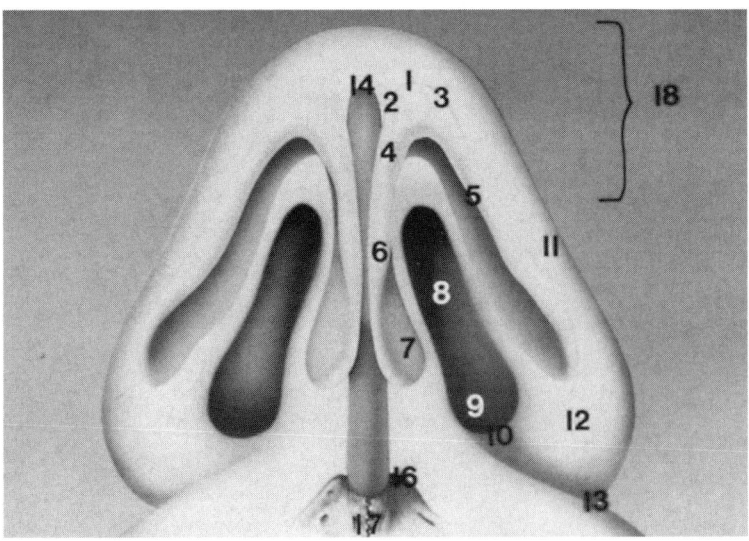

Figure 173.4 Further anatomy of the nasal tip from the basal view, with indicated nomenclature. *1*, Apex of alar cartilage; *2*, medial angle of dome; *3*, lateral angle of dome; *4*, alar cartilage transitional segment, intermediate crus; *5*, lateral crus alar cartilage; *6*, medial crus alar cartilage; *7*, medial crural footplate; *8*, nostril aperture; *9*, nostril floor; *10*, nostril sill; *11*, lateral alar sidewall; *12*, alar lobule; *13*, alar-facial junction; *14*, anterior septal angle; *15*, caudal septum; *16*, maxillary crest; *17*, nasal spine; *18*, infratip lobule.

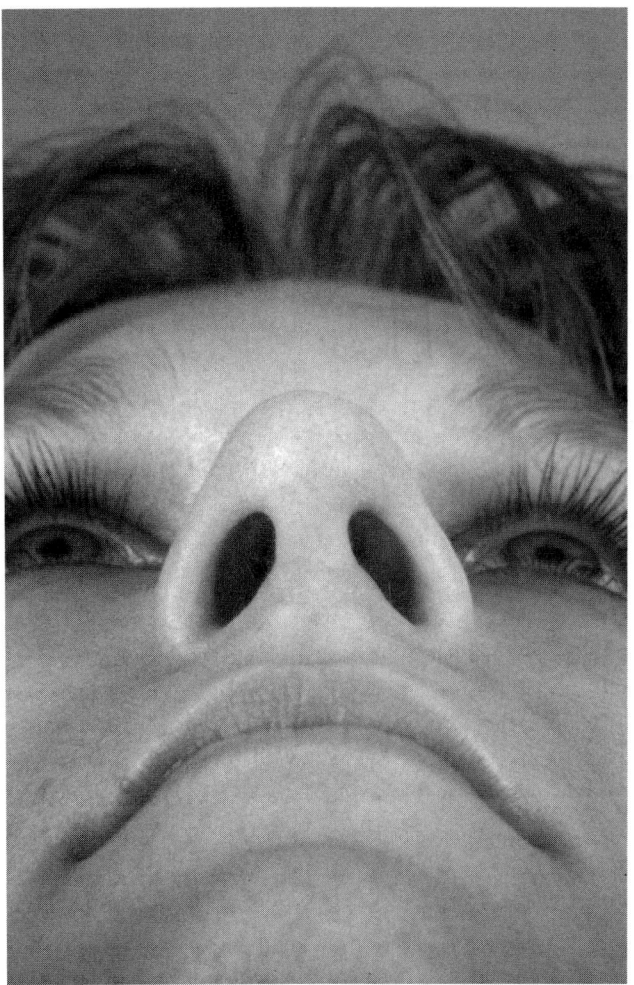

Figure 173.5 Ideal nasal tip contour. Note the triangular base view with an uninterrupted arch from alar rim to tip to alar rim.

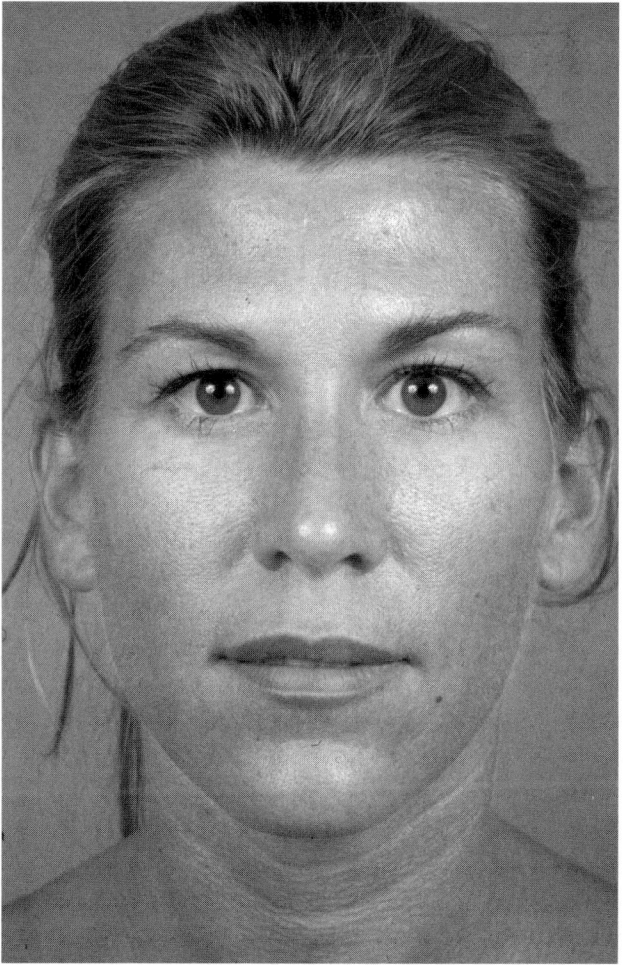

Figure 173.6 Ideal nasal tip contour with a smooth transition between the tip lobule and the well-supported nasal sidewall without bulbousness or pinching.

Understanding the implications of skin thickness should radically alter the surgical plan with an emphasis on long-term results. Thin-skinned patients require a high degree of precision and symmetry without sharp edges of bone or cartilage, lest they be visible shortly after surgery. Thin-skinned patients should also be advised that they have a greater risk of developing small, visible asymmetries than patients with thicker skin. Conversely, they will enjoy a more rapid course of healing than their thick-skinned counterparts. Thick-skinned patients, on the other hand, have fewer surgical options than those with thin skin. It is critical that the surgeon not promise a result that is impossible to attain. For example, thick-skinned patients often request a more refined tip. Although a bulbous tip can be improved, a thick-skinned nose will not have defined soft triangles or a "chiseled" appearance postoperatively, despite the surgeon's efforts. Many thick-skinned patients also have large noses and want them made smaller. Because a thick skin envelope will not contract to any significant degree, it is a mistake to expect that cartilage resection alone will refine the contour of the tip and result in a

smaller nose. Counsel these patients that, although their tip can be refined, it often needs to be projected into their thick skin envelope to achieve that definition. Otherwise, they risk having a loose, ptotic, poorly supported tip that is unlikely to satisfy them. Too many patients with thick skin undergo multiple revisions wherein the revising surgeon attempts to trim "just a little bit more," which only exacerbates the problem (Fig. 173.7).

Palpation of the tip and its ability to recoil when depressed can identify weak lower lateral cartilages or a low anterior septal angle (Fig. 173.8). The septum can also be palpated by placing the tip of the thumb and index finger in each of the nasal vestibules. This maneuver facilitates recognition of a weak or deviated caudal septum (1).

Evaluation of the tip must include assessment of the tip supporting structures (Fig. 173.9). Anderson's tripod model of the nasal tip clarified the dynamics of altering tip support (2). In it, the conjoined medial crura represent one leg of the tripod and the lateral crura the other two. Tip position, therefore, is a consequence of the combined forces of the three legs of the tripod. This model illustrates the

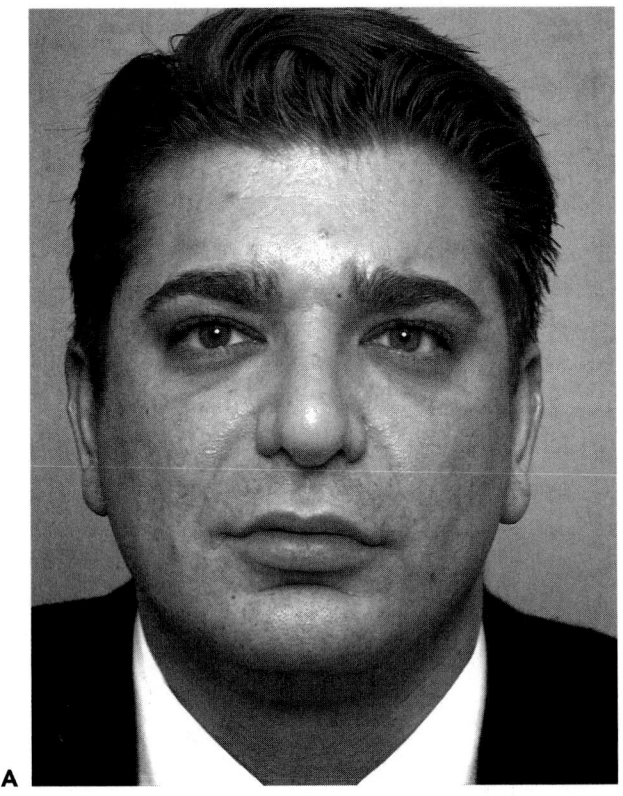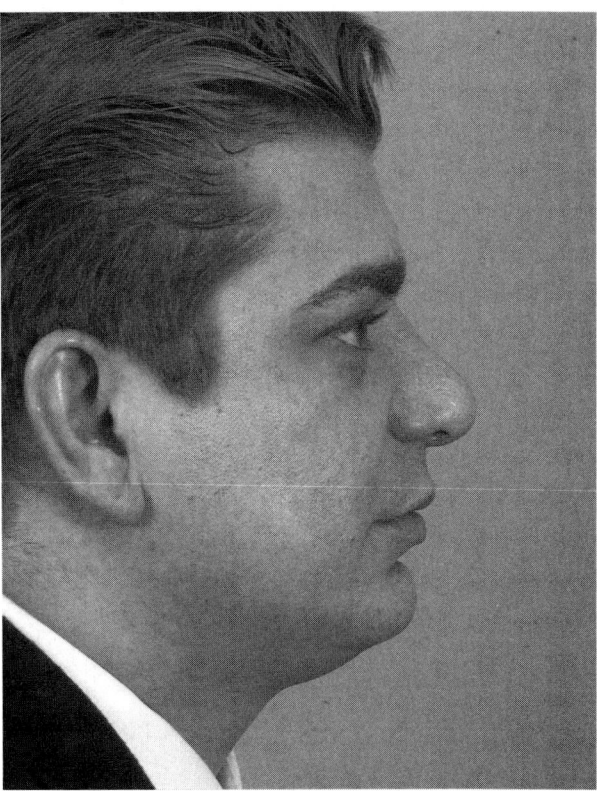

A **B**

Figure 173.7   This patient had a bulbous tip and thick skin. After several reductive procedures, the tip is poorly supported and unrefined.

variable contributions of the medial and lateral crural length when assessing projection, rotation, and the columella-labial angle.

The medial crura should be inspected by looking at the nasal base. Medial crural length has several surgical implications. Short medial crura provide little tip support and will require reinforcement to prevent postoperative deprojection and counter rotation. If the surgeon intends to

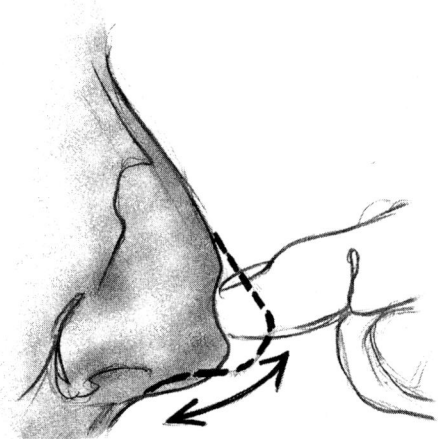

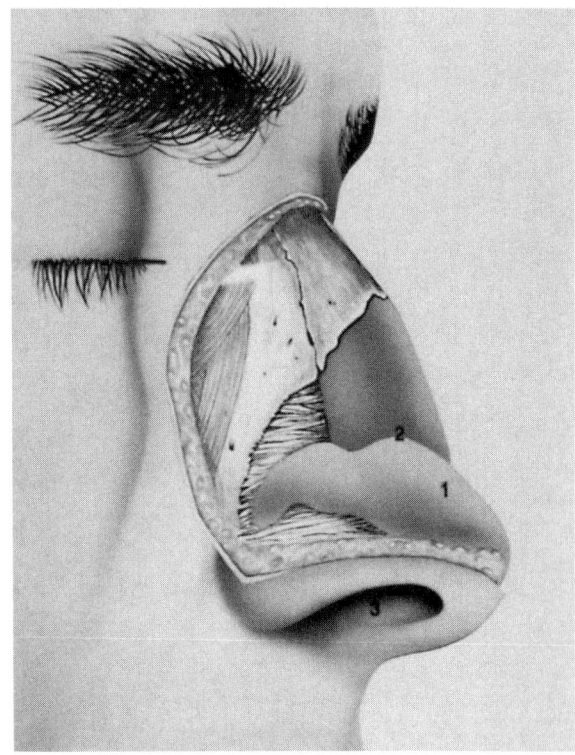

Figure 173.8   Demonstration of finger palpation of the recoil mechanism of the nasal tip. The relative resistance to deformity demonstrated by the nasal tip provides a useful indication of the integrity of nasal tip support mechanisms.

Figure 173.9   The three major tip supports of the nose, including (1) the strength, size, and shape of the alar cartilages; (2) the attachment of the caudal margin of the upper lateral cartilage to the cephalic margin of the alar cartilage; and (3) the medial crural footplate attachment to the caudal septum.

rotate the tip by performing a cephalic trim of the lateral crura, the poor support of short medial crura will preclude any meaningful cephalic rotation. Similarly, long medial crura may provide excellent tip support, but if the nose needs to be deprojected, techniques such as a full transfixion incision will have minimal impact. These long crura will likely need to be divided and overlapped to deproject the nose. In general, desired changes in rotation or projection will be hindered by long, strong cartilages that lie ahead of the intended tip movement or weak ones that are behind. Any deficiencies in these major tip support mechanisms need to be addressed at the time of surgery.

Assessment of tip projection must be undertaken in the context of the entire profile. The nasofrontal angle, depth of the radix, and chin all affect the appearance of nasal projection (Fig. 173.10). When examining an abnormally projected nose, the surgeon must identify where in the nose the projection is distorted. For instance, in an over-projected nose, the medial crura may be excessively long, the domes may be too tall, or the anterior septal angle may be too anteriorly positioned. Similarly, short medial and lateral crura, a low anterior septal angle, flat domes, or a hypoplastic premaxilla can result in an under-projected nose. Sometimes these factors occur in combination. Therefore, although recognizing that a nose is over- or under-projected is an important first step; the appropriate treatment options are widely divergent depending on the reason for the deformity. Unless the surgeon can identify these subtleties, good results are only a product of chance.

Tip deformities and nasal obstruction can also be a result of irregularities in the shape and rigidity of the lower lateral cartilages. Two important and frequently overlooked tip deformities are cephalically positioned lateral crura and internal curvature of the lateral crura. Cephalically positioned lateral crura are often the cause of a dynamic airway obstruction because of poor support of the lateral nasal wall. A hypermobile nasal sidewall is susceptible to collapse on inspiration, which narrows the internal nasal valve. Aesthetically, cephalic positioning of the lateral crura often appears as a bulbous tip with an attendant

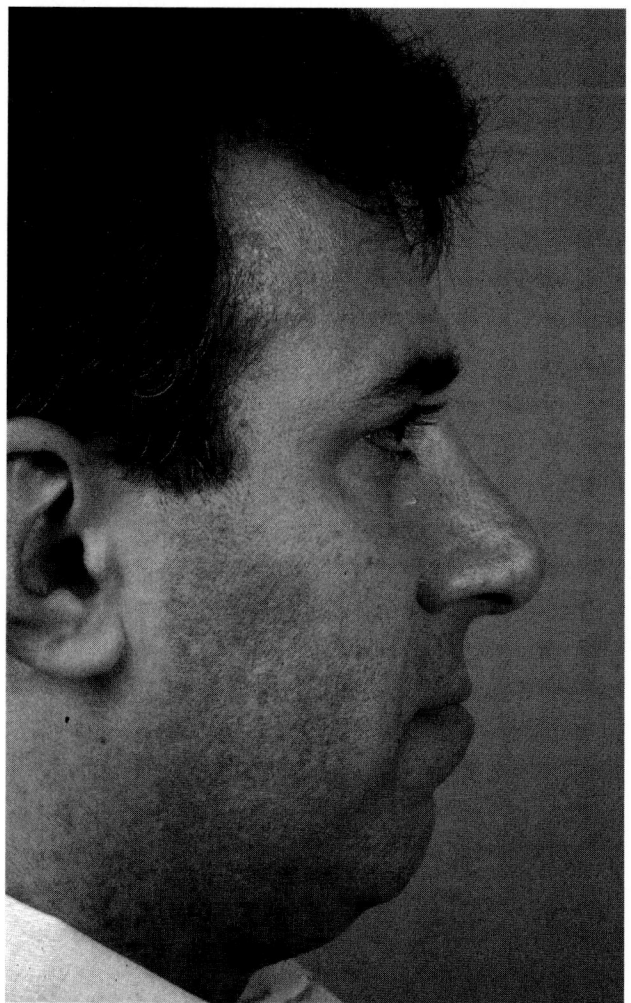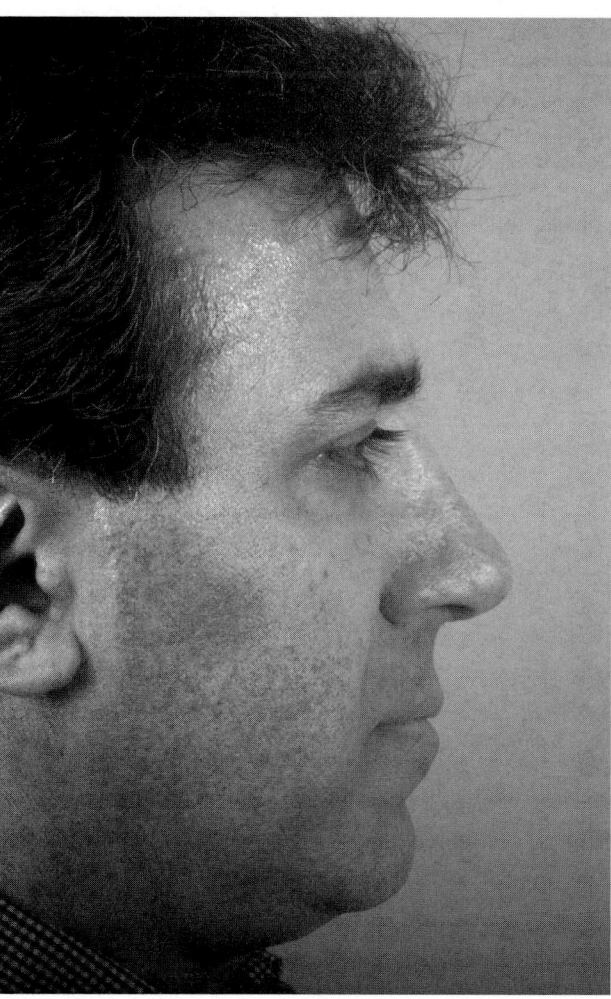

A   B

Figure 173.10 Demonstration of the value of chin augmentation associated with nasal tip surgery when microgenia accompanies the nasal deformity. **A:** Before surgery. **B:** After surgery.

pollybeak deformity. The lateral crura may also be internally recurvate. This, too, diminishes lateral wall support and can cause a static obstruction. Before formulating a plan for operating on the nasal tip, the surgeon must first accurately analyze the underlying structure that is responsible for the patient's deformity.

PREOPERATIVE PLANNING

Standardized photography is mandatory for any surgeon committed to learning from experience. It also allows the surgeon to communicate more effectively with the patient about the goals and techniques of the planned operation. Computer imaging software permits morphing or side-by-side evaluation of the preoperative and planned postoperative states. In addition, many surgeons print the manipulated images to use as a guide during surgery.

In the operating room, it is helpful to mark the patient before injecting local anesthetic (Fig. 173.11). The distort-

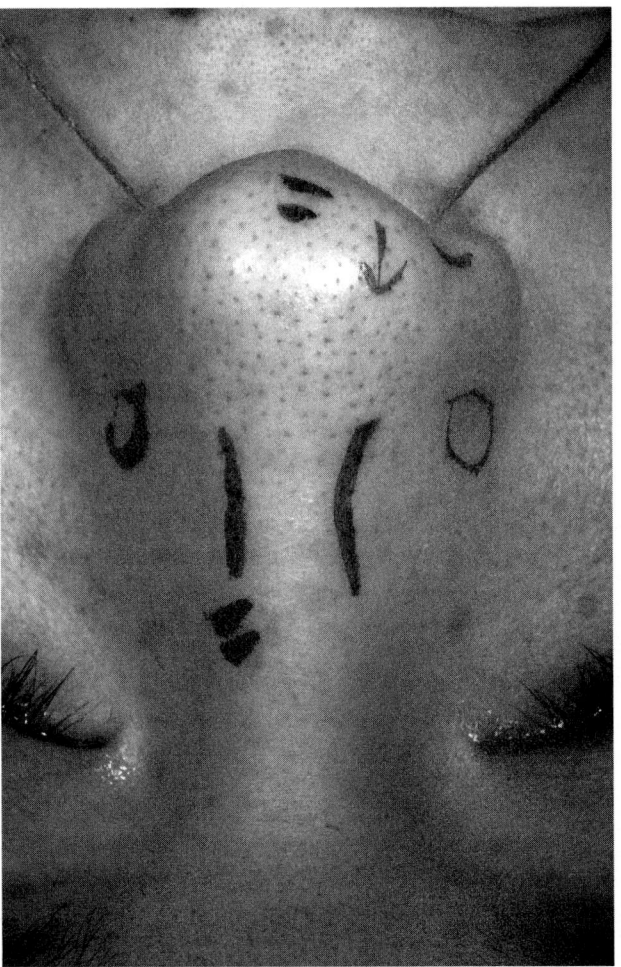

Figure 173.11 Preoperative topographic markings on the nasal surface are often useful in planning skeletal changes in nasal tip surgery.

ing effects of local anesthesia and intraoperative edema can mask many of the asymmetries and contour irregularities that should be addressed by the surgery.

SURGICAL TECHNIQUES

Controlling Nasal Tip Projection

The long-term effects of scar contracture in the operated nose cannot be over emphasized. If the surgeon can create a tip support structure that can withstand a lifetime of scar contracture, then projection of the tip will be preserved. The hallmark of a tip that is poorly supported is the pollybeak deformity. When the tip deprojects postoperatively, the tip–supratip relationship is reversed. The ideally concave supratip break becomes an unattractive convexity. This tempts some surgeons to over-resect the septum in order to prevent this deformity. This, however, also results in an unnatural outcome where the dorsum appears "scooped out." Tip projection is also critical in patients with thick skin. Thick nasal skin will not contract and redrape as favorably as thinner skin will. If a thick-skinned patient desires a more refined tip, it is imperative that the structure of the nose be "projected into" the thick soft tissue envelope (Fig. 173.12). These examples serve to illustrate the importance of controlling tip projection. When the surgeon can ensure that the tip is adequately supported, the dorsum can be left high. This benefits the patient by creating a narrower looking nose on the frontal view. Precise, predictable control of tip projection removes much of the guesswork from rhinoplasty.

Historically, passionate debate has existed about the relative merits of the endonasal and open approaches to rhinoplasty. Much of the controversy has dissipated as surgeons have come to understand that both approaches are best used complementarily. Although endonasal techniques are appropriate for many patients, the open, structural approach has the benefit of permitting greater freedom in tip placement (Fig. 173.13). When operating endonasally, most surgeons set tip position first and then adjust the upper two thirds of the nose to fall in line. Sometimes this is an aesthetic compromise that is a result of having a more limited set of options for placing the tip. Structural techniques allow the tip to be adequately projected and, therefore, allow the surgeon to keep the dorsum high with a lower incidence of postoperative loss of tip projection.

Stabilizing the Nasal Base

Before meaningful changes can be made to the tip lobule, the surgeon must create a stable foundation at the nasal base. Specific maneuvers that can be used to stabilize the medial crura include suture fixation of the medial crura to the caudal septum or caudal extension graft,

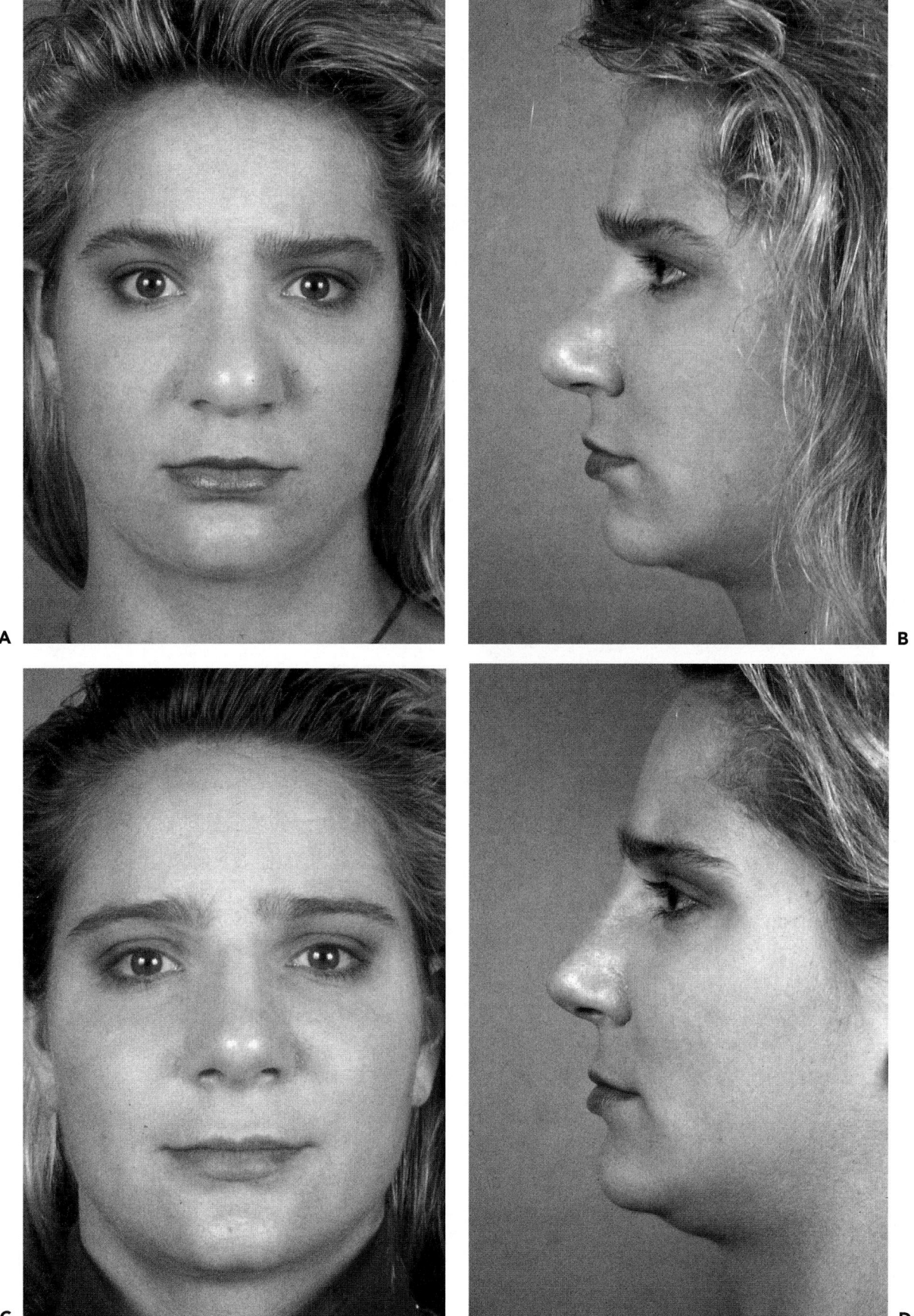

Figure 173.12 This patient also has a bulbous nose and thick skin. **A, B:** Before. **C, D:** After projecting the tip structures into the thick skin to achieve definition and refinement.

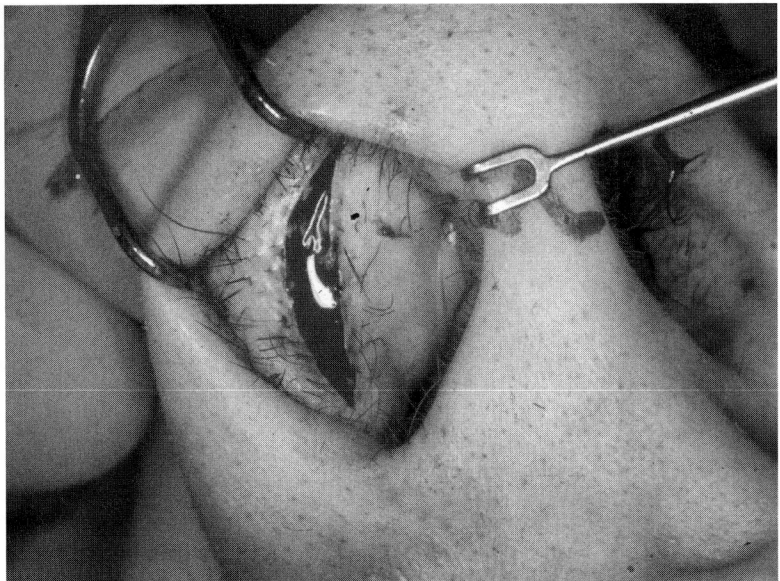

A

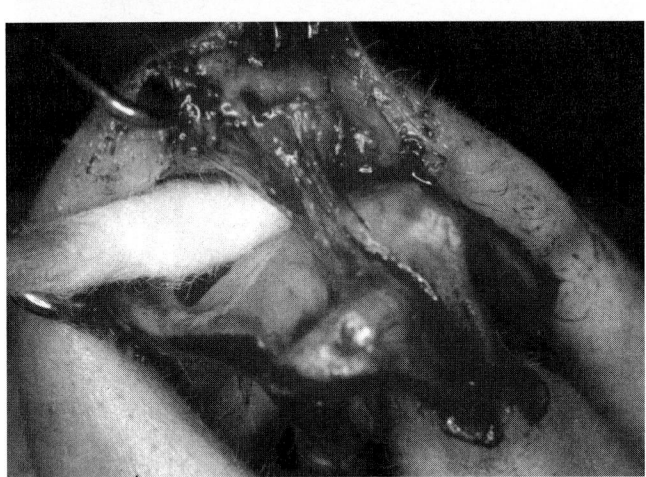

B

Figure 173.13 The external approach to nasal tip surgery. **A:** Transcolumellar and marginal incisions. **B:** Exposure of tip structures via the external approach.

a sutured-in-place columellar strut, or an extended columellar strut. Patients who have a hanging columella and an overly long caudal septum are good candidates for fixation of the medial crura to the septum. This is done by dissecting between the medial crura to provide access to the septum. A septoplasty is easily performed through this approach by elevating bilateral mucoperichondrial flaps. The medial crura are then positioned on the caudal septum in a tongue-in-groove manner with a 4-0 chromic mattress suture (Fig. 173.14). Once the tip position is satisfactory, a 5-0 polydioxanone (PDS) suture is passed through the medial surfaces of the medial crura and the septum. A 4-0 plain gut suture on a Keith needle is then used to quilt the septal mucoperichondrial flaps and redistribute any excess mucosa. Bunching of the mucosa is a potential pitfall in patients with an

over-projected tip or hanging columella. Careful reapproximation of the flaps nearly always precludes the need to resect mucosa or vestibular skin, however. Fixation of the medial crura in this manner provides excellent support for the nasal tip. It also affords precise control of the tip projection, rotation, and alar–columella relationship without having to excise mucosa or estimate the amount of postoperative tip settling. This maneuver is suited to patients with a tension-nose deformity, overprojected tip, underprojected tip, or hanging columella. If using this technique, the surgeon must avoid creating a retracted columella, obtuse columella-labial angle, or over-rotated nose. These pitfalls can be avoided by restricting this technique to those patients who have an inappropriately long caudal septum that would otherwise need to be resected.

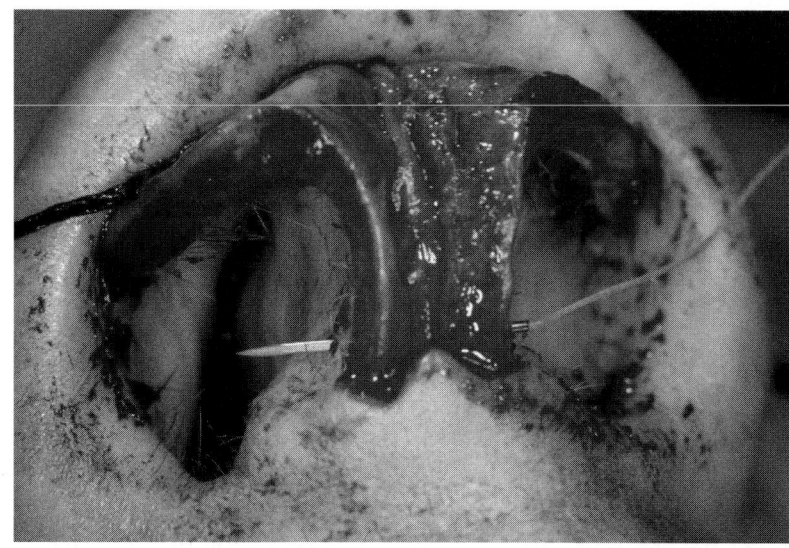

Figure 173.14 Repositioning the medial crura to set tip position and stabilize the nasal base.

Alternately, a caudal extension graft can be used to create a septum long enough to bind to the medial crura in the midline (3). This is a graft that typically overlaps the caudal septum and allows suture fixation of the medial crura to stabilize the nasal base (Fig. 173.15). Occasionally, if the septum is in the midline and the nasal airway would be compromised by overlapping with the septum, the graft can be attached inline with the caudal margin with several figure-of-eight sutures and splinting cartilage grafts (Fig. 173.16). Another suture through the periosteum of the anterior nasal spine will greatly improve the sturdiness of an inline graft. Regardless of the technique used, the caudal margin of the graft should be in the midline.

Orientation of the caudal extension graft is an important detail in its placement. If the graft is trapezoidal and has its longer edge posteriorly, it will help to open an acute nasolabial angle. A longer anterior edge will counter rotate the tip. A rectangular graft is helpful in correcting a retracted columella.

If the medial crura are in good position but are buckled or warped, a columellar strut can be placed (4). A columellar strut should be 5 to 12 mm in length and 3 to 6 mm wide. Ideally, a strut is less than 3 mm thick. It is placed by dissecting a pocket between the medial crura and suturing it in the midline. The strut should not extend to the nasal spine because this can lead to clicking if it slides from side to side. A floating strut will not increase projection but will support the medial crura in their contribution to a stable nasal base.

In contrast to a floating columellar strut, an extended columellar strut is beneficial to use in patients with an underprojected tip caused by poor tip support. The extended columellar strut is usually attached to the anterior nasal spine periosteum and is carved from costal cartilage. Sometimes, a notch can be carved in the posterior end of the graft to accept the nasal spine to reinforce its midline placement. Similarly, an extended strut can interdigitate with a premaxillary graft. This is especially helpful

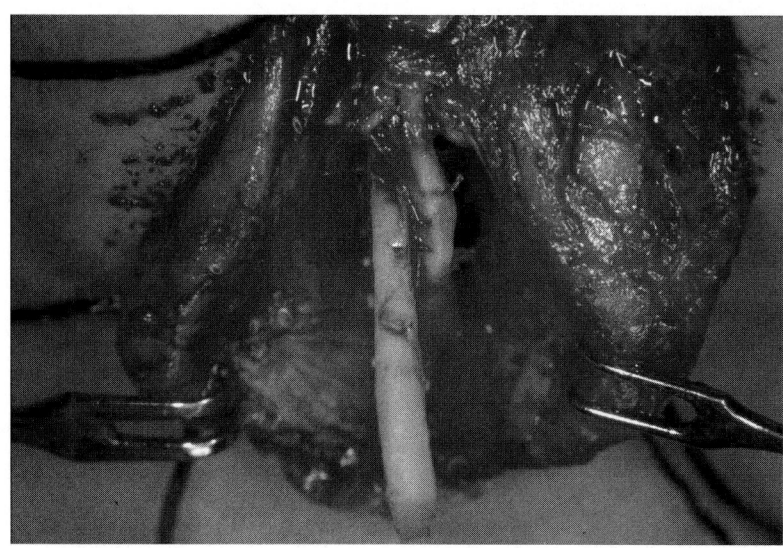

Figure 173.15 Anterior view of a caudal extension graft.

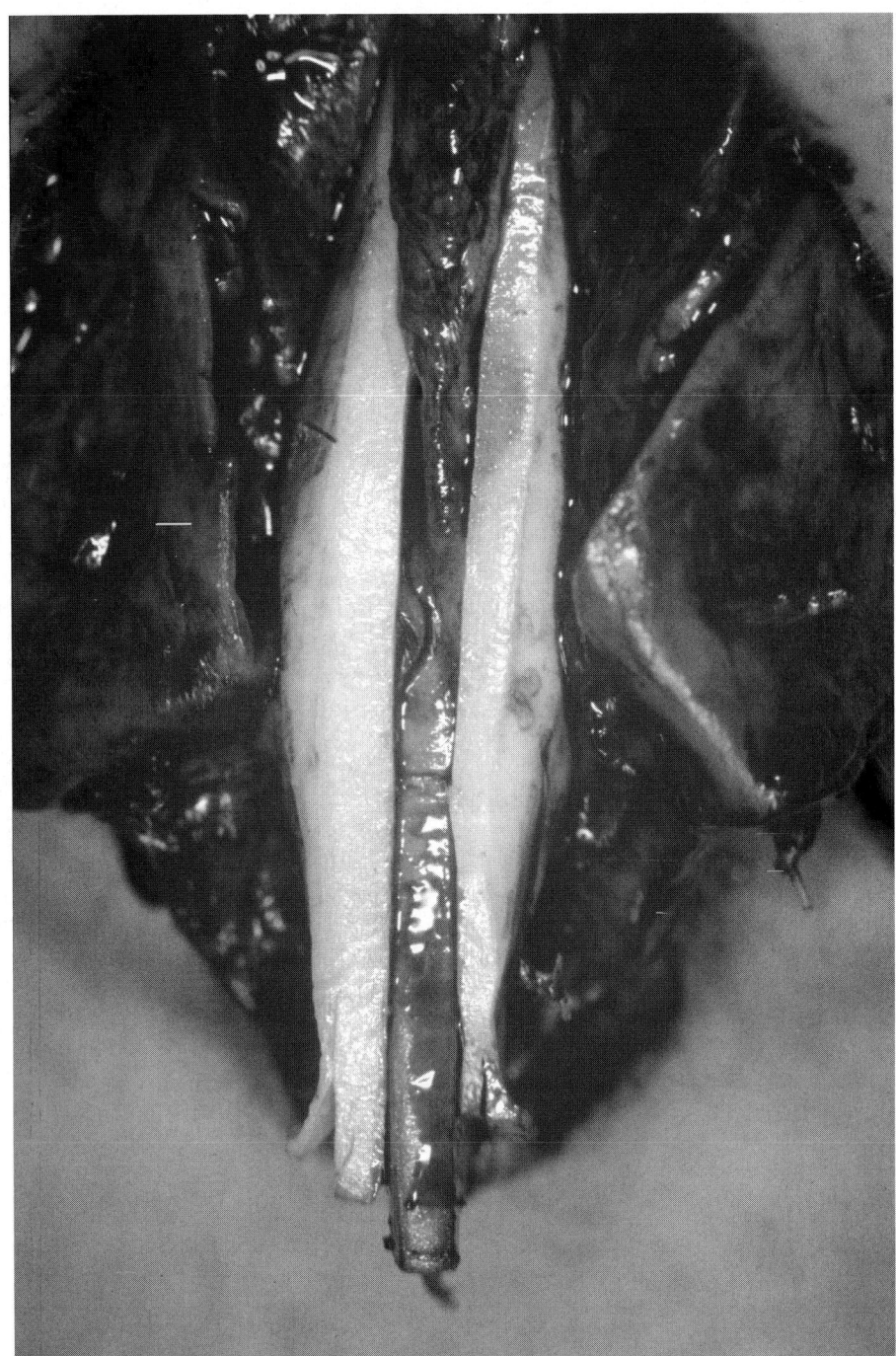

Figure 173.16   Inline caudal extension graft with splinting cartilage grafts.

in patients whose poor projection is a result of inadequate tip support and a deficient premaxilla, such as those with a cleft lip nasal deformity. As is the case with the caudal extension graft, the medial crura can be advanced anteriorly and fixed in a more projected position. Often, the soft tissue over the anterior nasal spine needs to be dissected free to permit advancement of the nasal base. This also has the effect of softening the nasolabial angle.

Nasal Tip Surgery

Once a solid foundation has been created at the nasal base, the tip can be modified. Following is a brief overview of some common structural techniques for improving the aesthetic contour and proportions of the nasal tip.

When the tip is underprojected in the lobule, a dome-binding suture or shield graft is good technique for

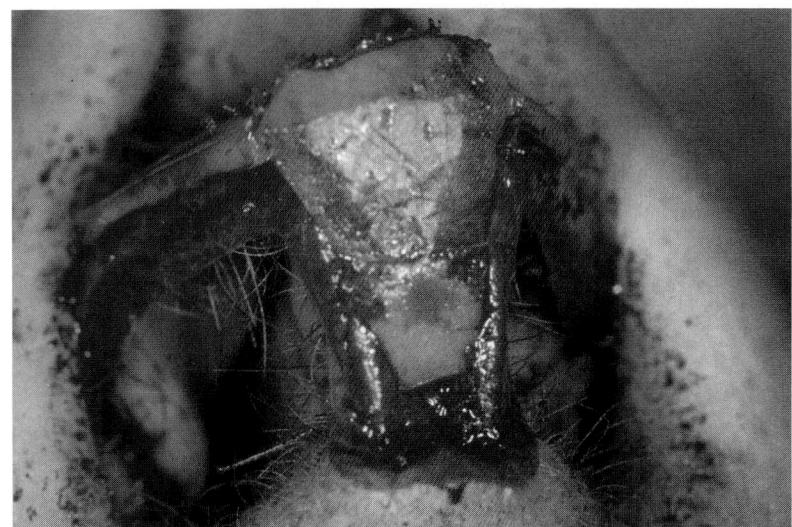

Figure 173.17 Shield graft affixed to the medial crura.

increasing projection without altering the nasal base (4). Dome-binding sutures will narrow and project the domes. These are discussed in more detail later in the chapter. A shield graft is attached to the medial crura in the infratip lobule (Fig. 173.17). The posterior edge should have a shallow bevel to allow the contour of the graft to blend with the caudal edge of the medial crura. Because the purpose of the graft is to push into the tip skin to increase projection, no matter how much the anterior edge is beveled, a risk exists of the graft being visible after surgery. Because of this, the authors avoid using shield grafts in thin-skinned patients (5). Although thick-skinned patients are tolerant of shield grafts, medium-skinned patients should have some sort of camouflage of the leading edge. Perichondrium and fascia are excellent materials for softening the contours of a shield graft. Several layers can be used to prevent visibility of the graft in the long term. A buttress or cap graft is another method for camouflaging a shield graft

(4,5). This graft is a small rectangle of cartilage that is sutured to the cephalic edge of the shield and stabilizes it while providing a smoother transition between the shield and the domes.

Sometimes the lateral crura are so misshapen or over-resected that lateral crural grafts are appropriate for reconstruction (4,5). Lateral crural grafts are also a good way to camouflage a shield graft that projects more than 3 mm above the domes, whether or not the lateral crura need structural reinforcement. These grafts create a transitional structure that bridges a shield graft to the lateral crura and simultaneously provides lateral support to the tip (Fig. 173.18). Lateral crural grafts are sutured to the anterolateral margin of a shield graft with a 5-0 PDS suture. A 6-0 Monocryl suture is placed laterally to secure the lateral crural graft to the existing lateral crus. A mattress suture of 4-0 chromic adds additional fixation support. It is best to place the knot, which can be large, inside the vestibule.

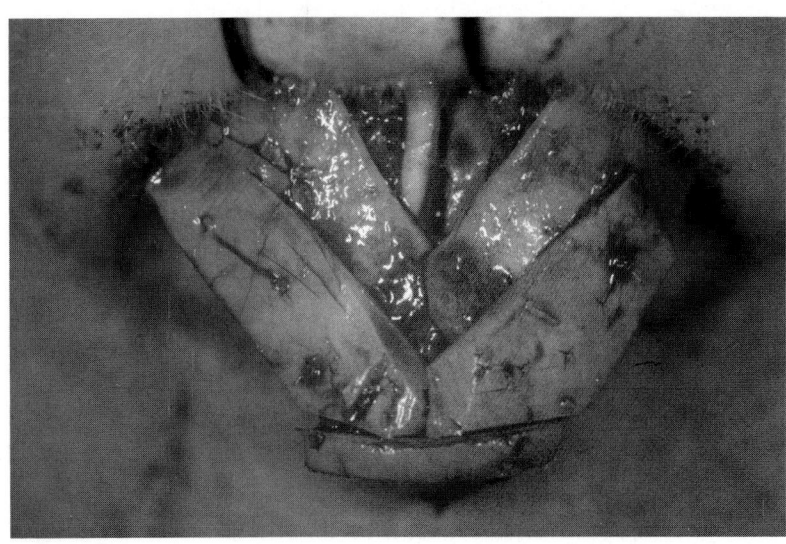

Figure 173.18 Lateral crural grafts conjoined with a shield graft.

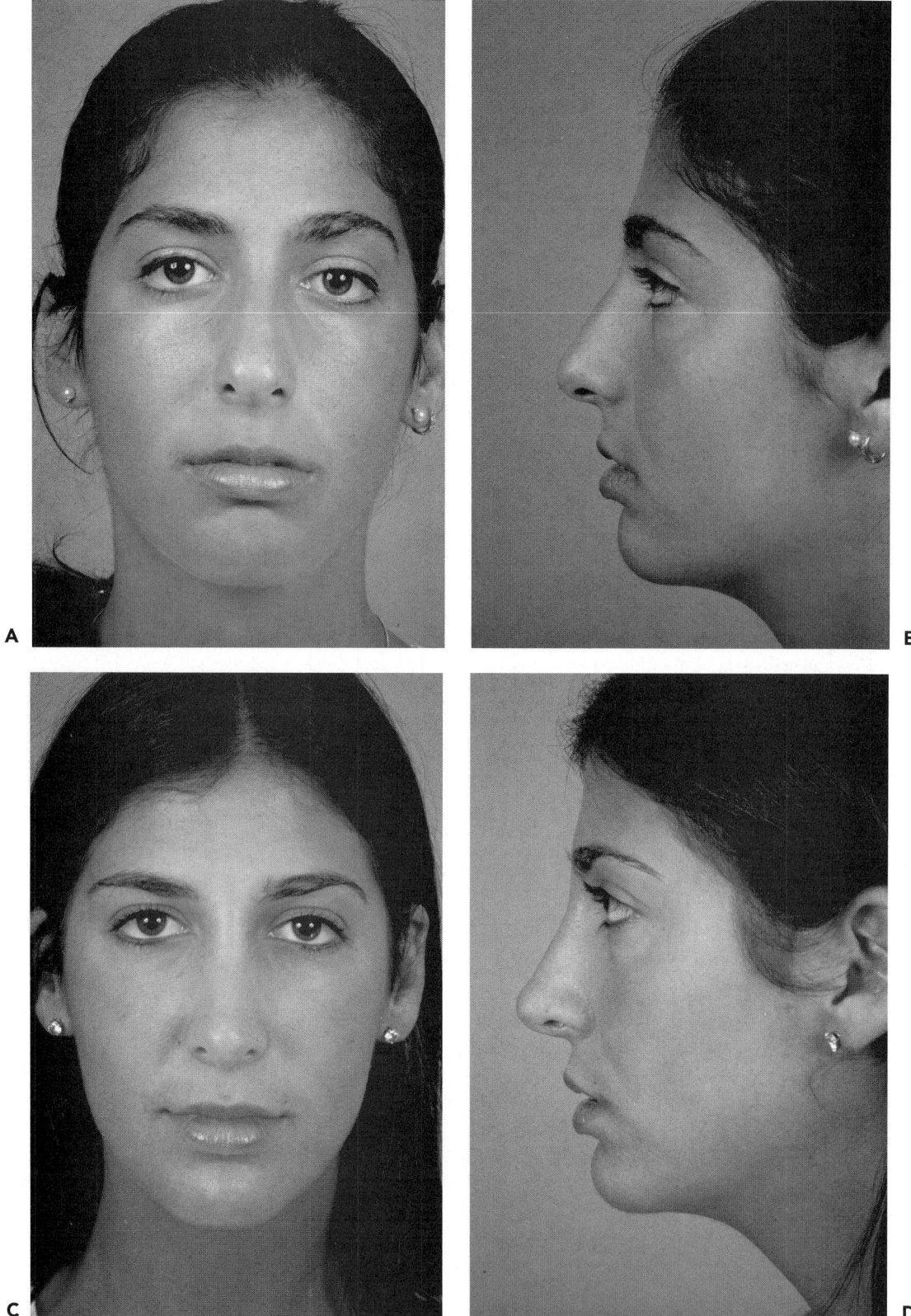

Figure 173.19   Bulbous tip **A, B:** Before lateral crural strut grafts and (**C, D,**) after procedure.

The lateral crura can also be augmented by placing grafts in a pocket between them and the vestibular skin. These lateral crura strut grafts can be used to accomplish several goals (6). They are useful in flattening lateral crura that are bulbous or internally recurvate (Fig. 173.19). When the lateral crura are of an appropriate length but lack the stiffness for appropriate lateral wall support, lateral crura strut grafts are a good reconstructive option. Lateral crura strut grafts are usually created from stiffer cartilage from the septum or rib. Their length depends on the needs of the graft. Longer grafts are used when counter rotating the nose so that they project into the dome to move it to a more caudal position. These grafts are typically 3 to 4 mm wide and 1 to 2 mm thick. Local anesthetic should be injected to hydrodissect the plane beneath the lateral crus. Several minutes after injection, a pocket can be dissected from the cephalic margin of the lateral crus between the cartilage and the vestibular skin. The graft is then placed in the pocket and affixed with several 5-0 clear nylon mattress sutures with the knots placed above the lateral crus.

Lateral crural strut grafts are often performed with a cephalic trim of the lateral crura (Fig. 173.20). The cephalic trim can also be performed independently as a maneuver to decrease the bulk in the supratip area. The cephalic trim should be performed medially because this is the area that contributes to a bulbous tip. Trimming laterally will have little effect on the tip and will only weaken the nasal sidewall. When reinforcing the lateral crura with strut grafts, more of the lateral crura can be removed without compromising the support of the nose.

Often there is a lack of support lateral to the tip in the alar margin. This disruption of the favorable triangular shape of the base creates shadows that make the tip appear to be separate from the alae (Fig. 173.21). The cause of poor support in this area can be cephalic positioning of the lateral crura or prior tip modifications. Alar rim grafts can be used to correct this pinched look (7). These are narrow cartilage grafts that are usually 5 to 8 mm in length, 2 to 3 mm in width, and 1 to 2 mm thick. They are placed in pockets in the caudal aspect of the marginal incision (Fig. 173.22). Alar rim grafts should be softer than other grafts because they are susceptible to becoming visible medially if they extend into the tip. The cartilage resected from a cephalic trim of the upper lateral cartilages makes excellent

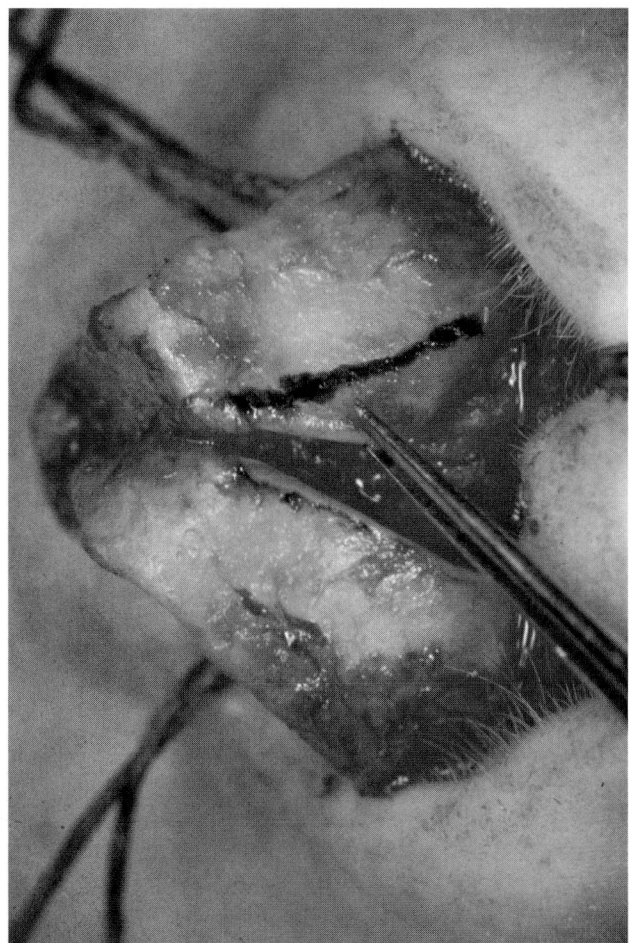

Figure 173.20 Medial-cephalic reduction of the alar cartilages, maintaining a generous residual complete strip.

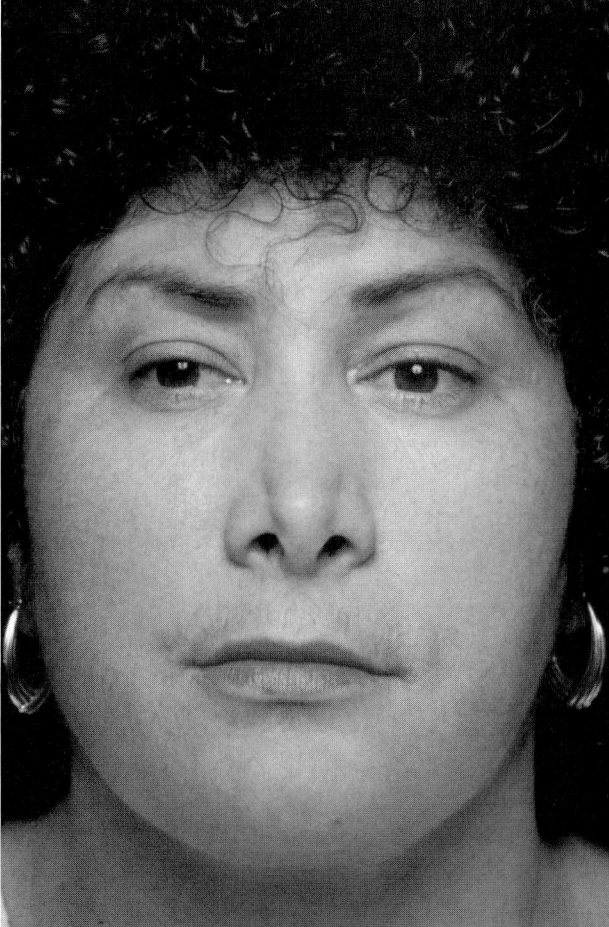

Figure 173.21 Example of alar rim and supraalar pinching as a result of weakening the nose.

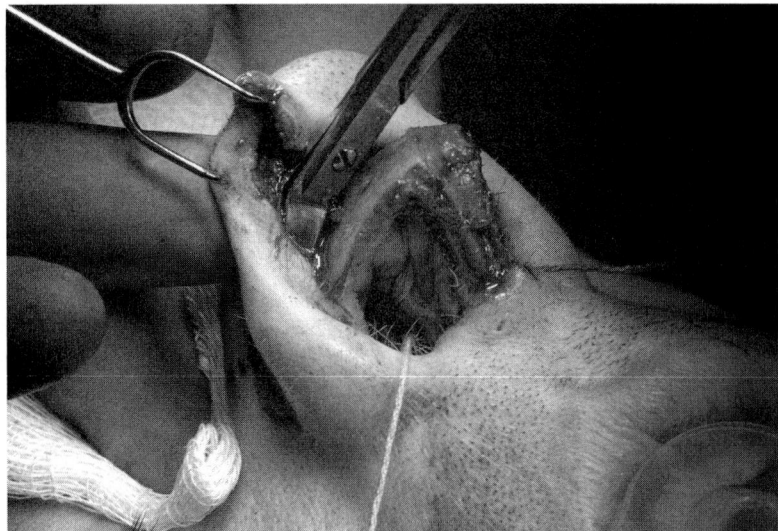

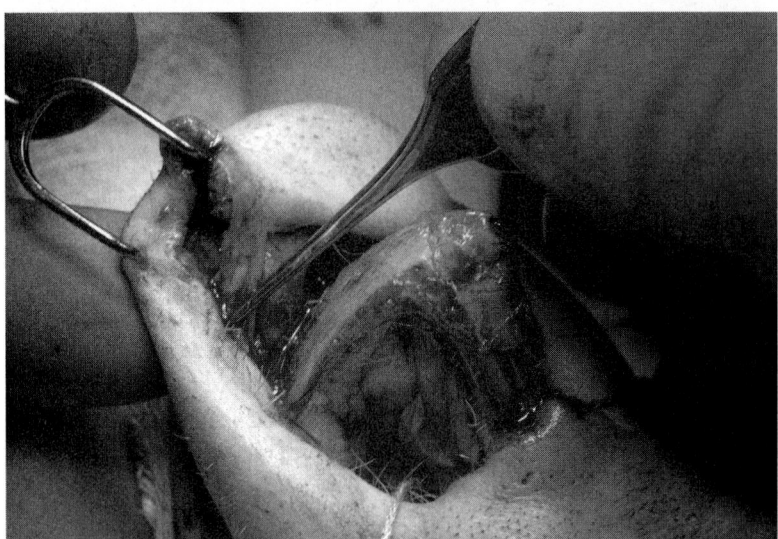

Figure 173.22 Proper insertion of alar rim grafts. (See also Color Plate 62.)

rim grafts. After placing the grafts in the pockets, they are fixed with 6-0 Monocryl suture at the medial aspect. The area medial to the suture should be gently morselized with a Brown-Adson forceps to further minimize the likelihood of graft visibility. Grafts that are too stiff also tend to be visible and sometimes palpable. Alar rim grafts are also an effective way to correct external valve collapse.

The importance of tip cartilage camouflage cannot be over emphasized. Although postoperative edema can be present for years after surgery, the surgeon should anticipate that eventually the edema will resolve and potentially reveal the underlying structure of the tip. Perichondrium from an auricular or costal cartilage graft is an excellent material for covering tip grafts (Fig. 173.23). Patients should be warned that the use of perichondrium will result in prolonged postoperative edema in the tip. In thin-skinned patients, this is favorable and should be described to patients as such. Once the postoperative edema resolves, the tip will have a soft, natural contour.

Suture modification is a safe way to alter tip contour in a nondestructive manner (8,9). A bulbous tip can be improved by placing a dome-binding suture to narrow the domes and flatten the bulbous lateral crura (Fig. 173.24). Sometimes, a dome suture can cause an undesirable concavity lateral to the suture, which can be a result of improper suture placement, tension, or the patient's unique anatomy. This lateral deformity of the lateral crus can be improved with a lateral crural strut graft. Dome division is a more aggressive method for managing the bulbous tip and should be limited to patients with thick skin.

Surgery of the nasal tip is a challenging endeavor and fraught with pitfalls. The surgeon must understand that the operated nose is a dynamic structure that changes throughout the life of the patient. It is imperative, therefore, that the surgical plan encompasses every effort to ensure an acceptable long-term result, sometimes at the expense of a rapid decrease in postoperative swelling.

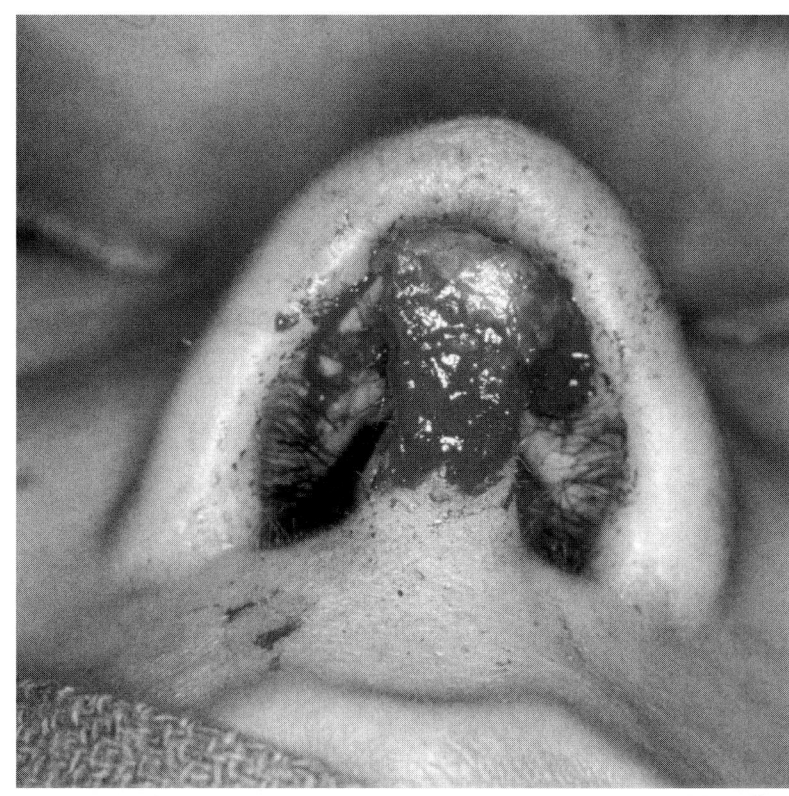

Figure 173.23 Perichondrium covering nasal tip grafts to prevent postoperative graft visibility. (See also Color Plate 63.)

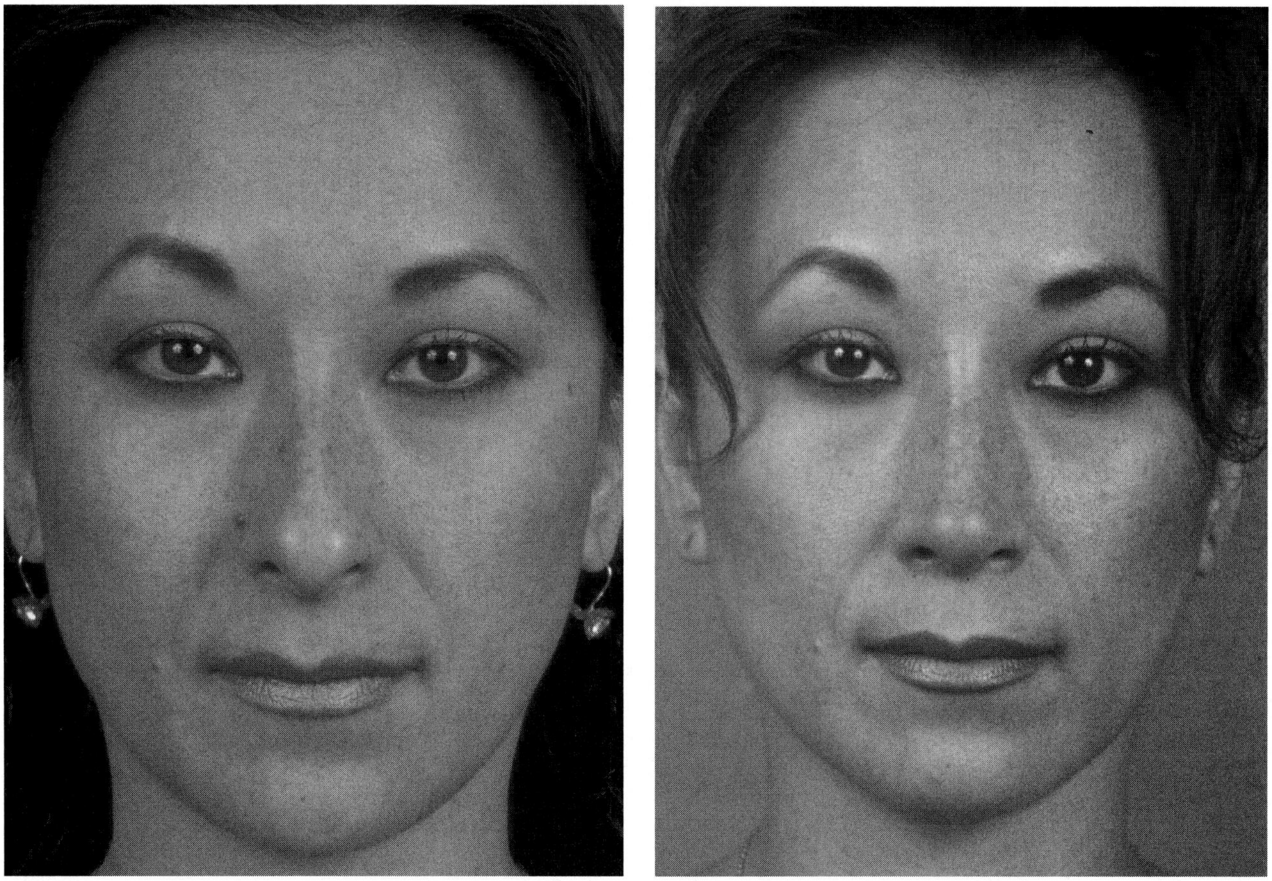

A   B

Figure 173.24 Narrowing of the tip with dome-binding sutures (A) before and (B) after procedure.

HIGHLIGHTS

- Removal of structurally supportive tissue weakens the nose.
- Structural principles can ensure that the healing nose can withstand the relentless and insidious forces of scar contracture.
- Accurate analysis and diagnosis are the foundation of a successful rhinoplasty.
- Thick-skinned patients are treated significantly differently than thin-skinned patients.
- Thick-skinned patients often need their tip structures projected into the skin-soft tissue envelope.
- Thin-skinned patients benefit from preservation of dome continuity and need extensive soft-tissue camouflage of any cartilage grafts to prevent them from becoming visible.
- The tripod model provides the basis for understanding changes in rotation and projection.
- Care should be taken not to compromise the structure of the nasal sidewall, because this will adversely affect breathing.
- Before making any meaningful changes to the tip, first stabilize the nasal base.
- The structural approach to rhinoplasty emphasizes reinforcement of the tip cartilages by careful augmentation with cartilage grafts.
- Perichondrium and fascia are valuable materials for tip graft camouflage.
- Suture techniques are another nondestructive method of altering tip shape.
- Patients must understand that their noses will change over many years as the forces of scar contracture act on the supportive structures.

REFERENCES

1. Tardy ME. *Rhinoplasty: The art and the science.* Philadelphia: W.B. Saunders, 1996.
2. Anderson JR. The dynamics of rhinoplasty. *In Proceedings of the Ninth International Congress of Otolaryngology.* Exerpta Medica International Congress Series, No. 206. Amsterdam, Exerpta Medica, 1969:708–710.
3. Toriumi DM. Caudal extension graft for correction of the retracted columella. *Op Tech Otolaryngol Head Neck Surg* 1995;6:311–318.
4. Johnson CM, Toriumi DM. *Open structure rhinoplasty.* Philadelphia: WB Saunders, 1989;1:1–22.
5. Toriumi DM, Johnson CM. Open structure rhinoplasty: featured technical points and long-term follow-up. *Facial Plastic Surgery Clinics of North America* 1993;1:1–22.
6. Gunter JP, Friedman RM. Lateral crural strut graft: technique and clinical applications in rhinoplasty. *Plast Reconstr Surg* 1997;99:943–955.
7. Rohrich RJ, Raniere Jr J, Ha RY. The alar contour graft: correction and prevention of alar rim deformities in rhinoplasty. *Plast Reconstr Surg* 2002;109(7):2495–2505.
8. Tebbetts JB. Shaping and positioning the nasal tip without structural disruption. *Plastic Reconstr Surg* 1994;94:61–77.
9. Toriumi DM, Tardy ME. Cartilage suturing techniques for correction of nasal tip deformities. *Op Tech Otolaryngol Head Neck Surg* 1995;6:265–273.

Management of the Post-Traumatic Nasal Deformity

174

Benjamin C. Marcus   Tom D. Wang

The nose is one of the most prominent and defining features of the face. When the nasal contour is in harmony with the face, the patient's eyes become the focus of attention. Conversely, a nose that is overly large, asymmetric, or deformed will draw the viewer's attention. The nose is the most commonly injured of the facial bones because of it prominence and the minimal quantity of force required to induce fracture (1). In addition to its aesthetic qualities, the nose has essential functional elements that are dependent on its intrinsic architecture. As the entry point for inspiration, the nose must warm, humidify, and effectively deliver inspired air to the lower airway. Traumatic nasal injury both alters the cosmetic nasal appearance and can significantly alter nasal function as well. When assessing blunt nasal trauma, both functional and aesthetic consequences must be considered

BACKGROUND

Nasal trauma is a relatively common injury. In maxillofacial injuries, the nose is the most commonly injured aspect of the face. Nasal bone fractures make up 39% to 45% of all facial fractures (2). Males suffer nasal trauma about twice as often as their female counterparts (3). Additionally, the highest incidence occurs for those in the 15 to 30 year age range (4). Although significant numbers of pediatric and elderly facial injuries occur, the cause of these is most often accidental. Conversely, most common nasal

fractures occur during altercations, sporting activities, and to a lesser extent motor vehicle and other accidents (5). The advent of supplemental restraint devices (e.g., airbags) had been thought to reduce the incidence of facial fractures. Interestingly, recent studies (6) have demonstrated no significant reduction of blunt nasal trauma or nasal bone fracture when the crash vehicle has been equipped with airbags.

ANATOMY

The appearance of the nose is directly related to its underlying architecture. Bony, cartilaginous, and soft tissue elements combine to create a unique feature (Fig. 174.1). The bony framework is pyramidal in shape. The paired nasal bones articulate with the nasal process of the frontal bone superiorly and the ascending process of the maxilla laterally. The nasal bone complex is thickest at its caudal border and thinner cephalically. The paired nasal cartilages include the upper and lower laterals. The upper lateral or triangular cartilages articulate with the caudal edge of the nasal bones and with the septum medially. Their integrity is partly responsible for the patency of the internal nasal valve. The lower lateral or alar cartilage is responsible for the size and shape of the nasal tip. The soft tissue envelope of the nose is loosely attached to the cartilaginous and bony scaffold. All arterial, venous, and nervous structures lie in the superficial plane.

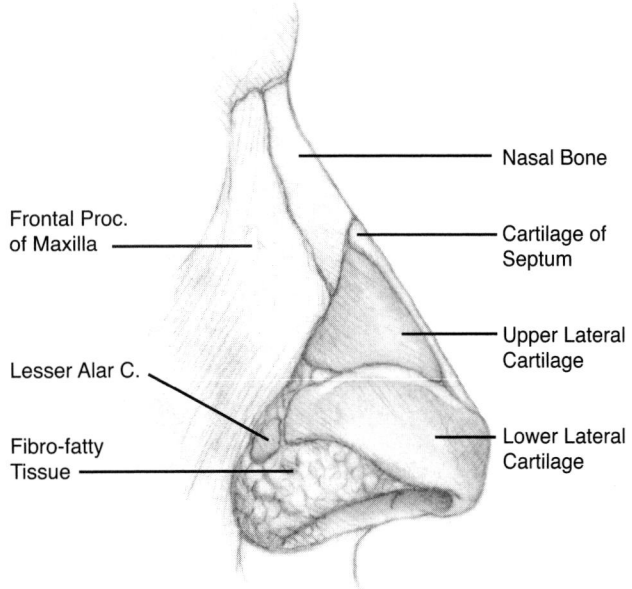

Figure 174.1 The cartilaginous anatomy of the nose. Paired upper lateral and lower lateral cartilage help define the nasal contour.

The nasal septum (Fig. 174.2) has cartilaginous and bony components. The anterior component consists of the quadrangular cartilage and the membranous septum. The inferior septum articulates with the maxillary crest. Posteriorly, the cartilaginous septum articulates inferoposterior with the vomer superiorposterior with perpendicular plate of the ethmoid.

The blood supply of the external nose includes the lateral branch of the angular artery, the dorsal nasal artery,

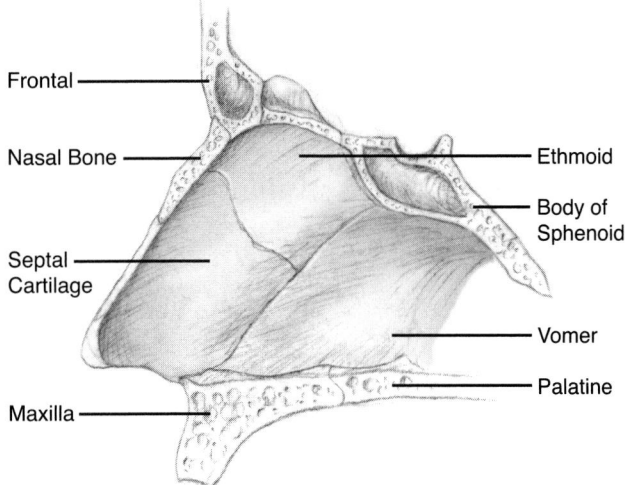

Figure 174.2 A sagital view of the nose, demonstrating the contributions of the quadrangular cartilage, vomer, and perpendicular plate of the ethmoid to the nasal septum.

the external nasal artery, and the infraorbital artery. Venous drainage is through the angular and ophthalmic veins. The sensory innervation of the external nose is supplied from the supratrochlear, infratrochlear, and infraorbital nerves. The nasal septum is supplied by the sphenopalatine, anterior and posterior ethmoidal, and facial arteries. The nasal septum derives sensation via the anterior ethmoidal nerve and maxillary branches of the sphenopalatine ganglion.

PATHOGENESIS

Facial bones create an intricate system of defense for the contents of the cranial vault. These buttresses that are in the horizontal and vertical planes serve to absorb and distribute force when it is applied to the face. Although the mandible and frontal bar can absorb large degrees of force, the midface, and especially, the nose is much weaker (Fig. 174.3). To prevent the transmission of force from the nasal region to the skull base, the nasal bones and septum have "crumple zones" that serve to absorb most of the applied force.

In addition to damage to the nasal bones, midface injury also often results in septal injury. The cartilaginous septum is essentially stabilized in three-point fixation via its attachments to the nasal dorsum, the bony septum, and maxillary crest. Differences in cartilage thickness also result in areas of differential strength. Verwoerd (7) described the pathogenesis of septal fractures by identifying these areas of structural importance. This study demonstrated that the dorsal posterior, inferior, and caudal segments of the septum have the thickest cartilage. The central portion of the quadrangular cartilage is the thinnest. The structural support, therefore, is based on the stronger posterior septum. After nasal trauma, septal fractures are most commonly seen at the caudal-inferior, cephalic-dorsal, and central septum. Other authors have correlated subtypes of septal fractures with the type of nasal bone injury. Using physical examination and computed tomography (CT), Rhee et al. (8) demonstrated that specific vectors of force produced predictable septal fracture patterns. A lateral blow to the nasal pyramid produced a C-shaped fracture displaced to the contralateral side. A force directed in the anterior–posterior axis creates a septal spur at the inferior caudal septum (Fig. 174.4).

The supporting forces on the cartilaginous septum are normally counterbalanced. After fracture, the internal stresses on the quadrangular cartilage are unlocked and unbalanced. Fry (9) demonstrated that distortion of the septum continues unless these internal stressing forces are balanced. Furthermore, nonrepaired septal fractures will continue to distract the nasal bones in the direction of the septal injury (10).

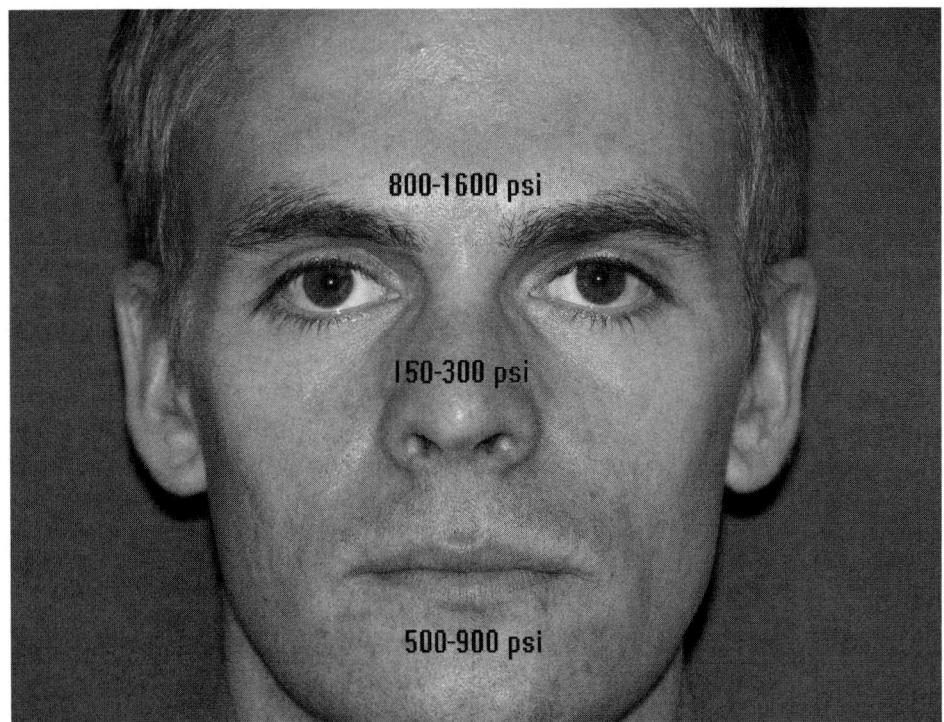

Figure 174.3   The amount of force (pounds per square inch) required to fracture the facial bones.

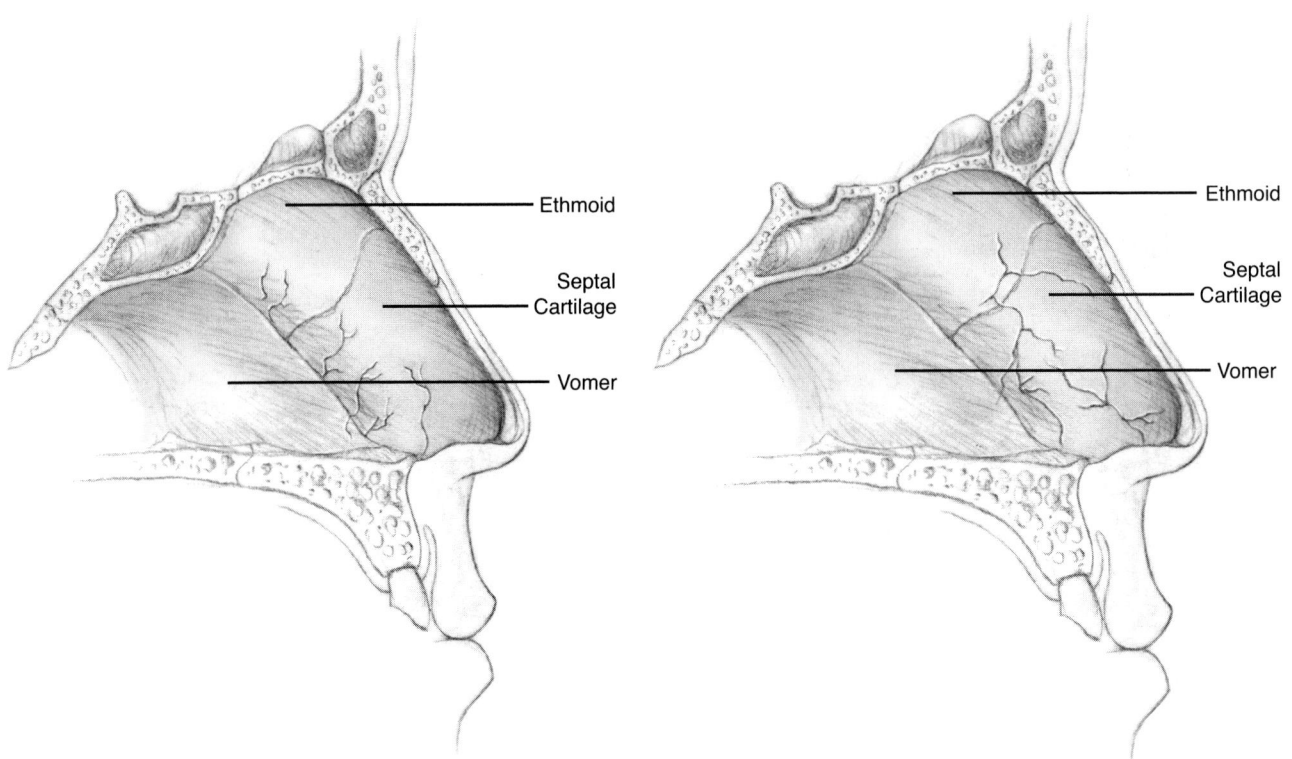

Figure 174.4   A sagital view of the nasal septum. The two most common fracture patterns are depicted. **A:** The fracture from a low-velocity impact. **B:** The fracture from a high-velocity impact.

PATIENT ASSESSMENT

The patient encounter begins with a thorough history of the injury. Special care is taken to elucidate the injury mechanism. High-energy midface trauma must be evaluated in a different fashion from isolated nasal trauma. Similarly, the magnitude and nature of force imparted to the midface can help predict the extent of injury to the nasal bones. In addition to the mechanism of injury, a series of postinjury symptoms should be thoroughly documented. New onset nasal obstruction can represent multiple postinjury pathologies, including septal hematoma, septal fracture, or an internal nasal valve injury. A history of epistaxis can indicate a loss of mucosal integrity. Although less common with isolated nasal trauma, injury to adjacent structures should be evaluated during the initial history. Specifically, a history of visual changes (e.g., diplopia, altered acuity, or gaze restriction) warrants an ophthalmologic evaluation. A suggestion of malocclusion or intraoral lacerations promotes a more thorough evaluation for more extensive midfacial fractures. Any neurologic symptoms (e.g., loss of consciousness) suggest possible intracranial pathology.

After documentation of the nasal trauma is complete, a full medical history should be obtained. Pertinent findings would include a history of seasonal or perennial rhinitis, chronic sinusitis, nasal polyposis, or previous hyposmia. Any previous nasal surgery should be documented. A medication history should focus on drugs with an anticoagulation profile (e.g., aspirin, warfarin, and clopidogrel). Other medications of interest include nasal steroids and nasal decongestants (e.g., pseudoephedrine).

The physical examination of the patient, if possible, should begin with an examination of a preinjury photograph. For the adult patient population, the driver's license photograph will usually suffice. Specific attention should be paid to preexisting lateral displacement of the nasal dorsum, dorsal humps, or any other facial asymmetry. The subsequent physical examination must be meticulous and ordered. A full head and neck examination should be performed focusing lastly on the nasal injury. Special attention should be paid to findings that indicate other traumatic injuries. The nasal examination begins with external visualization. Lacerations are documented for later repair. The upper third is examined for altered bony anatomy. The middle and lower vaults are then inspected for deviation from the midline. Careful external palpation is the used to evaluate for depressed bony fragments and integrity of the upper lateral cartilages. Palpation of the tip may reveal deviation of the caudal septum and indicate degree of remaining tip support.

The internal examination is best performed in two stages. An initial examination without topic decongestants and anesthesia is useful to understand the baseline mucosal status. The preliminary anterior rhinoscopy is started with a Vienna nasal speculum. The subsequent internal examination requires anesthesia. The patient is placed in a comfortable powered chair. Using a headlight, the examiner administers the anesthesia. The authors prefer the topical application of 4% cocaine with nasal pledgets. This provides both topical anesthesia and decongestion. This can be combined with bilateral infraorbital nerve blocks (Fig 174.5) for excellent overall anesthesia. Other methods of topical anesthesia

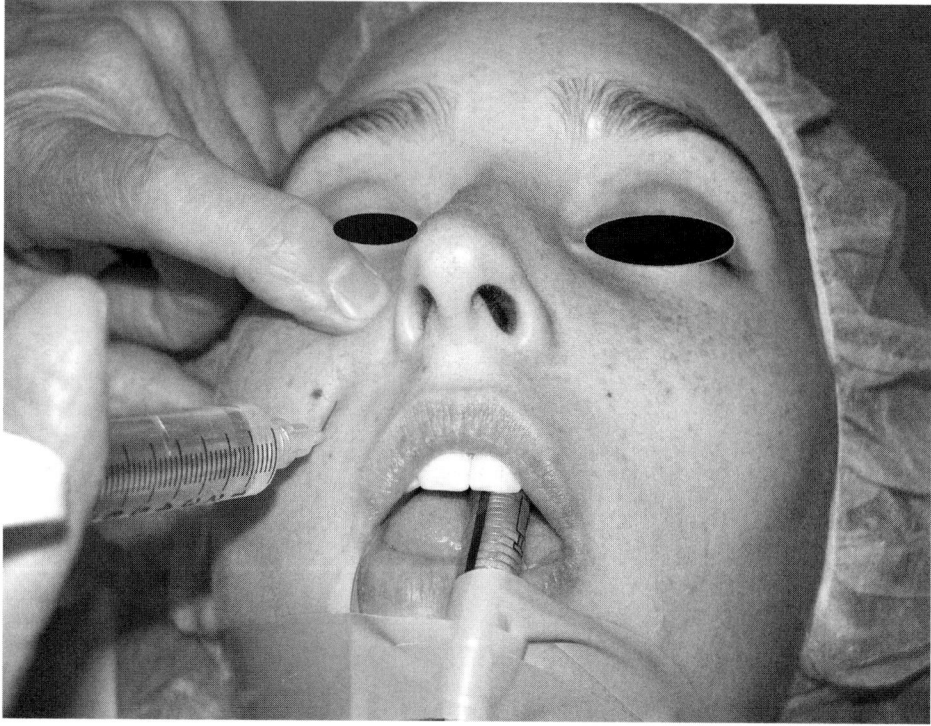

Figure 174.5   Location for an infraorbital nerve block.

include the use of aerosolized medications, either alone or in combination. Other authors have had success using combinations of tetracaine and oxymetazoline (11), as well as lidocaine and phenylephrine (12).

After adequate anesthesia, a systematic intranasal examination is essential. This is ideally performed in combination with either a 2.7-mm rigid or a 3-mm flexible endoscope. A global survey is the initial maneuver, with careful attention to the presence of septal hematoma and the integrity of the nasal mucosa. Septal lacerations should increase the suggestion of a septal fracture. Once the survey is completed bilaterally, the remainder of the examination is systematically carried out in an anterior to posterior, caudal to cephalic manner. The examination can be completed in three passes of the endoscope. The initial pass enters the nasal vestibule and proceeds posterior to the choanae. Structures observed include the inferior turbinate, the inferior cartilaginous septum, maxillary crest, and the bony cartilaginous septal junction. The second starts at the caudal septum and proceeds posterior and cephalic. The internal nasal valve, the main body of the quadrangular cartilage, and the middle meatus are inspected. The final pass of the endoscope proceeds posterior along the dorsal border of the septum. High dorsal septal deflection may be detected during this portion of the examination.

Adjunctive imaging studies use is somewhat controversial. Historically, patients with midface trauma were further evaluated with plain film radiographs. The routine use of plain films has been shown to be unnecessary for the effective diagnosis of isolated nasal fractures (13). A radiographically apparent nasal bone fracture may have little clinical relevance. Conversely, an unrecognized septal fracture may have significant aesthetic ramifications, despite a normal plain film study. The authors, therefore, do not routinely obtain plain film studies. The exception is in the patient with severe midface or pan-facial trauma. Here, the use of CT is routine. In this patient population, the clinical examination can be obscured by the associated injuries. Imaging in this patient population may identify otherwise missed nasal bone injuries (14). (Fig. 174.6)

CLASSIFICATION

A number of classification systems for blunt nasal trauma exist. On the whole, these are most useful for accurate communication and cataloging of injury. Nasal bone fractures have been classified by Harrison et al. (4) in four distinct patterns based on cadaver impact data. Pollock et al. (15) also utilized experimental nasal trauma studies to define nasal injuries into three distinct nasal zones. Injuries were classified by lower, middle, and upper nasal vaults. Rhee et al. (8) present a grading system based on CT findings for both nasal bone and septal injuries. Bony injuries are graded from 1 to 3. This represents a spectrum from nondisplaced to comminuted fractures. The septal grading

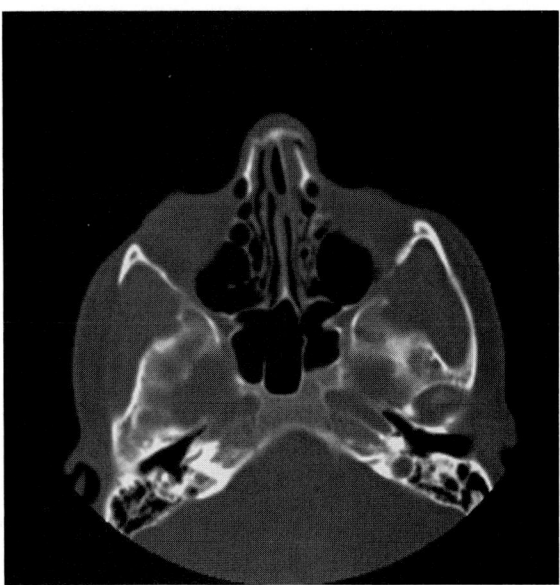

Figure 174.6 An axial computed tomography (CT) scan demonstrating bilateral nasal fracture with a left-sided impaction.

system stretches between grades 0 to 4. Theses grades describe progression from a straight septum to one that has lateralized and touches the nasal sidewall. Rohrich and Adams (35) propose an alternative grading system that describes five levels of nasal injury. Type 1 is a simple unilateral fracture; type 2 is bilateral; type 3 is comminuted. The most important distinction is with type 4 fractures that have an associated septal injury. Finally, type 5 fractures are nasoorbitoethmoid (NOE) fractures. Each of these individual grading systems is useful when used in a consistent fashion among the members of the facial trauma team. A standardized method for describing the nasal injury facilitates the proper workup and treatment plan.

MANAGEMENT

Initial patient contact for blunt nasal trauma can occur in the emergency department. The physician may be required to treat acute epistaxis before further evaluation and treatment can proceed. As stated, the proper treatment of epistaxis requires that the patient can be examined with the necessary tools. Proper lighting, suction, and adjunctive tools should be assembled before beginning the examination. As opposed to isolated nasal hemorrhage, epistaxis with suspected nasal fracture requires rapid resolution so that further examination and treatment can be pursued. Traditional treatments as digital pressure can be useful for minor bleeding. Interestingly, Teymoortash et al. (16) have shown that the use of ice packs does little to alter nasal blood flow or reduce epistaxis. Although nasal packing, especially by an otolaryngologist, (17) is effective, these methods limit further effective examination. Novel hemostatic agents such as octyl cyanoacrylate (18) and fibrin glue (19) have been used effectively to produce rapid hemostasis without the bulk of intranasal packing.

After initial stabilization and subsequent identification of the patient's injuries, establish a timeline of treatment. The immediate postinjury edema and ecchymosis often mask important anatomic deformities. The use of oral steroids (e.g., methylprednisolone) has been shown to facilitate reduction of facial edema (20,21). The authors prefer to reassess patients 3 to 5 days after the initial nasal trauma. Unless medically contraindicated, a brief course of oral steroids (e.g., a methylprednisolone dose-pack) is usually prescribed. With reduction of postinjury edema, a careful assessment of both functional and cosmetic changes can be obtained. For functional deficits (e.g., new onset nasal obstruction) most patients will be amenable to surgical intervention. Patients with major postinjury cosmetic deformities are also usually enthusiastic about repair. Subsets of patients wish, however, to delay surgical intervention. Modest deformities that are often apparent to the physician may be inconsequential to the patient. Unless the patient's condition has the potential for future complications (e.g., septal hematoma), the decision for surgery ultimately rests with the patient. Emergent intervention for patients with septal hematoma or abscess is detailed in the *Complications* section, beginning on p. 2591.

If the patient desires a surgical intervention, the proper time for that maneuver must then be determined. If the patient is to have a closed reduction, the authors prefer to wait until the patient is approximately 3 to 5 days postinjury. This will allow for the maximal reduction of injury-related edema and still allow for a facile reduction of the fractured segments. Multiple investigators cite that their best results are achieved with early intervention. Ridder et al. (22) have shown similar findings with their series of 96 fractures treated with closed reduction (23). Conversely, Fernandes (24) demonstrated satisfactory closed reduction results with treatment delays up to 30 days. It is our belief that if a patient presents further than 10 days out from injury, alternative procedures must be considered. In these cases, optimal results from a formal septorhinoplasty are best achieved after an interval of 10 to 12 weeks from the original injury.

Closed reductions can be accomplished with local or general anesthesia. Depending on physician and patient preference, the procedure can be performed in the operating room, clinic treatment room, or in the emergency ward. Newton and White (25) report that 90% of their patients who had closed reduction found it less painful than a dental filling procedure. Rajapakse et al. (26) reviewed their series of 197 nasal fractures that were treated with closed reduction. Interestingly, a significant number of patients stated that if they were to refracture their nose, they would prefer general anesthesia. Despite this patient preference, the investigators found no significant difference in patient satisfaction with the results of their reduction. Although not statistically significant, the study also demonstrated that patients who had closed reduction with local anesthetic proceeded on to further surgery in greater proportion. In further study, Courtney et al. (27) demonstrated that patients who had a closed reduction under general anesthetic often went on to have a more involved procedure during that anesthetic. Patients were far more likely to have rhinoplasty maneuvers such as detachment of the upper lateral cartilages, dorsal hump reduction, or acute osteotomies. In contrast, patients who had their treatment under local anesthesia most often were treated only with closed reduction. In this same cohort, the patients treated with local anesthesia were significantly more likely to have a revision procedure. If excluding revision procedure as a complication, neither study demonstrated any significant difference in intraoperative or perioperative complications.

Although the choice of anesthetic should be made by the patient in concert with the treating physician, certain strong indications exist for the use of general anesthetic. Patients who are 16 years or younger are best treated with a general anesthetic in the controlled setting of the operating room. If the patient has sustained significant concurrent injuries (e.g., polytrauma), management will also be facilitated by anesthesia monitoring. Patients who have significant epistaxis that poses a risk to their airway should also be treated in the most conservative manner.

The use of preprocedure antibiotics for blunt nasal trauma is not routine. If a nasal bone fracture is open or involves exposed cartilage, it is prudent to initiate antimicrobial coverage for staphylococcus and other skin flora. Because of the risk for septal abscess (28), patients who present with a septal hematoma should also be started promptly on antibiotics after adequate incision and drainage. Although patients who have required nasal packing were traditionally started on antibiotics to prevent or decrease the incidence of toxic shock syndrome (TSS), this presumption has been called into question. Keller et al. (29) have illustrated that patients may be susceptible to TSS regardless of antibiotic use. Furthermore, analysis of nasal flora after use of prophylactic antibiotics demonstrated no significant decrease in levels of *Staphylococcus aureus* (30). Because of the overall low incidence of toxic shock syndrome with nasal packing, however, it is difficult to fully ascertain the usefulness of prophylactic antibiotics. For this reason, the authors recommend the continued use of antibiotic prophylaxis for the duration of nasal packing.

Much controversy surrounds the methodology of nasal fracture reduction. For many years, the standard therapy has been a simple closed reduction. Reference to closed reduction can be found as early as the medical literature of 14th century Anatolia (31). In many cases, closed reduction will produce an outcome that is satisfactory to the patient and the surgeon. Multiple case series demonstrate up to a 90% satisfaction with the postprocedure results (32). For many facial plastic surgeons, any deformity that is not addressed by the initial closed reduction can be managed at a secondary definitive rhinoplasty. This, of course, is delayed 10 to 12 weeks after the initial injury.

A growing body of literature demonstrates that a more aggressive initial approach to the nasal injury can provide a more controlled surgical outcome. Rhee et al. (8) performed a complete direct visualization of the septum in each of 52 patients with a simple nasal bone fracture. Interestingly, 96% of these patients were found to have septal fractures. Of the patients, 78% had septal fractures that were designated severe and, therefore, were repaired. Although the authors found maxillofacial CT scans to be helpful in identifying septal fractures, the severity of the septal injury could not be correlated to the CT findings. The most predictive finding for septal fracture was the discovery of mucoperichondrial tears on physical examination.

The possibility of unrecognized septal injury has been postulated to account for up to 30% of patients who have an unfavorable result from closed reduction alone (33). In a very large case series of 756 patients Murray et al. (34) found that nearly 41% of their patients had an unsatisfactory result if a septal injury was not addressed. In response to these results, Rohrich and Adams (35) developed an algorithm to assist in the management of septal injury. The classification system is detailed earlier within this chapter. In brief, any nasal fracture that has an associated septal injury is addressed with septal repositioning or reconstruction. In their series of 110 patients, acute septal manipulation resulted in a revision rate of only 10%.

The addition of maneuvers to address the acutely injured septum has arguably improved the outcomes in treating acute nasal fractures. Staffel (36) has suggested an alternative algorithm that includes multiple rhinoplasty procedures in the acute setting. This open reduction protocol is a step-wise treatment plan that relies on visual inspection to determine the endpoint for acute manipulation. The procedure is initiated with a standard closed reduction. An acute septoplasty is added if the preoperative examination indicates septal injury. Completion osteotomies (i.e., medial and lateral) are initiated as the next intervention. The next step-wise procedure in this protocol is the release of the septum from the upper lateral cartilages. Staffel believes that if a patient has a preinjury twist to the nasal dorsum, the detachment of the upper lateral cartilages is always added to the procedure. If this series of interventions does not produce a satisfactory cosmetic result, Staffel will then acutely fracture the perpendicular plate of the ethmoid. Ultimately, if the repositioning of the nasal pyramid cannot be accomplished, a series of camouflage grafts are then used to create an acceptable nasal contour. With this protocol, Staffel (36) demonstrated a significant improvement in his postoperative cosmetic results when compared with his own patients who were treated with a closed reduction protocol alone. Although patient satisfaction was not evaluated, only 2 of 76 patients in this

study required revision surgery. The open reduction protocol as outlined by Staffel (36) represents the most aggressive end of nasal trauma management. For a subset of patients who represent the most complicated examples of nasal trauma, however, a patient benefit is found with this algorithm.

Multiple circumstances can lead to a delayed repair of nasal trauma. Patients who have significant concurrent injuries (e.g., intracranial hemorrhage) may not be able to undergo a procedure within a week of their trauma. Other patients may simply have a delayed entry to the health care system. In any circumstance in which a patient presents more than 7 days after an original injury, the repair must be postponed. We prefer to allow a minimal interval of 12 weeks to pass before undertaking a formal septorhinoplasty. Secondary repair of nasal trauma requires that the surgeon reconstruct the nature of the acute injury. It is not sufficient to recognize the cosmetic deformity. Proper surgical planning includes an assessment of bony injury, septal displacement, and nasal valve competence. Once all elements of the prior injury have been catalogued, a proper plan can be formulated for the rhinoplasty, which often includes medial osteotomies, lateral osteotomies, and septal work. Additional rhinoplastic maneuvers can be added as necessary to restore the preinjury cosmesis.

Pediatric Management

Blunt nasal trauma in the pediatric population is a relatively uncommon event. Most injuries that do occur happen in the context of sporting activity. The major impediment to accurate treatment is difficulty in obtaining a complete examination. One review documents that in a major treatment center 80% of the pediatric nasal trauma patients received a radiographic study, whereas only 20% were formally examined by an otolaryngologist (37). The accurate diagnosis of nasal pathology, including septal injury, is essential for effective treatment. Children who can tolerate intranasal administration can be given topical anesthesia and decongestant in a liquid format. For children who are unable to cooperate with the examination, consider the use of a sedation protocol. Many centers have an anesthesia or emergency department team that will facilitate this for the otolaryngologist (38).

After an adequate examination, the pediatric patient is best treated using general anesthesia in the operating room setting. In this population, most nasal fractures can be treated with a closed reduction. If septal injury is detected, it should be repaired with the goal of retaining the maximal amount of septal cartilage. Repositioning, rather than resection, is the goal with this patient group. Patients without nasal fracture, but with suspected septal hematoma, should also be evaluated in the operating room. Standard incision and drainage with subsequent packing is accomplished with much greater success in this setting.

TECHNIQUE

After the decisions regarding timing and method of nasal fracture repair, actual repair begins. Of utmost importance is the application of anesthesia. Regardless if general or local anesthesia with sedation is used, certain preoperative maneuvers remain constant.

The nose is initially prepared with a topical decongestant and vasoconstrictive agent. Multiple preparations are available. Many authors use oxymetazoline Multiple cocaine preparations are available as well. The most common is a 4% liquid. The cocaine solution is best applied with the use of cotton pledgets. Other authors prefer the use of purified cocaine crystals (personal communication). When using the purified crystals, its application is facilitated by the use of cottonoid applicators. The applicators are used to paint the cocaine paste along the mucosal surfaces of the septum and turbinates. One cottonoid is placed at the anterior ethmoid artery, a second at the middle meatus, and the third along the inferior turbinate in the region of the sphenopalatine artery (Fig. 174.7). Most practitioners then inject local anesthesia. The use of lidocaine is most common, with concentrations varying from 0.5% to 2%. The inclusion of epinephrine at a ratio of 1:100,000 is also standard. The authors prefer a 50:50 mixture of 0.5% bupivacaine and 1% lidocaine, with a total concentration of 1:100,000 epinephrine. If the procedure

is to occur without general anesthesia, 10% by volume of an 8.4% bicarbonate solution is included in the mixture. This mixture produces an excellent rapid-onset anesthesia with successful longer tern analgesia. Bilateral infraorbital nerve blocks facilitate lateral nasal manipulation. Further injection of the septum, dorsum, and tip can be added if procedures are anticipated in these areas (Fig. 174.8).

The closed reduction of a nasal fracture relies on the disimpaction of the in-fractured nasal bones. A variety of instruments have been created for this purpose. The three most commonly used instruments include the Boies elevator, and Asch and Walsham forceps (Fig. 174.9). The Asch forceps were originally designed for septal realignment, but have been used by many surgeons for nasal bone repositioning. Whether the Asch or Walsham forceps are used, the technique is similar. One tine is placed intranasally on the side of the fracture. The second tine is externally placed. The fractured segment is then grasped between the tines and simultaneously disimpacted and reduced (Fig. 174.10). The external tine is often padded to reduce soft tissue trauma. Great care must be taken when using these instruments because intranasal mucosal damage can commonly occur. The Boies elevator can also be used effectively, but with much less soft tissue trauma. The elevator is placed intranasally and gently advanced to underlay the nasal dorsum. The elevator is lifted dorsally to disimpact the segment and rotated gently to

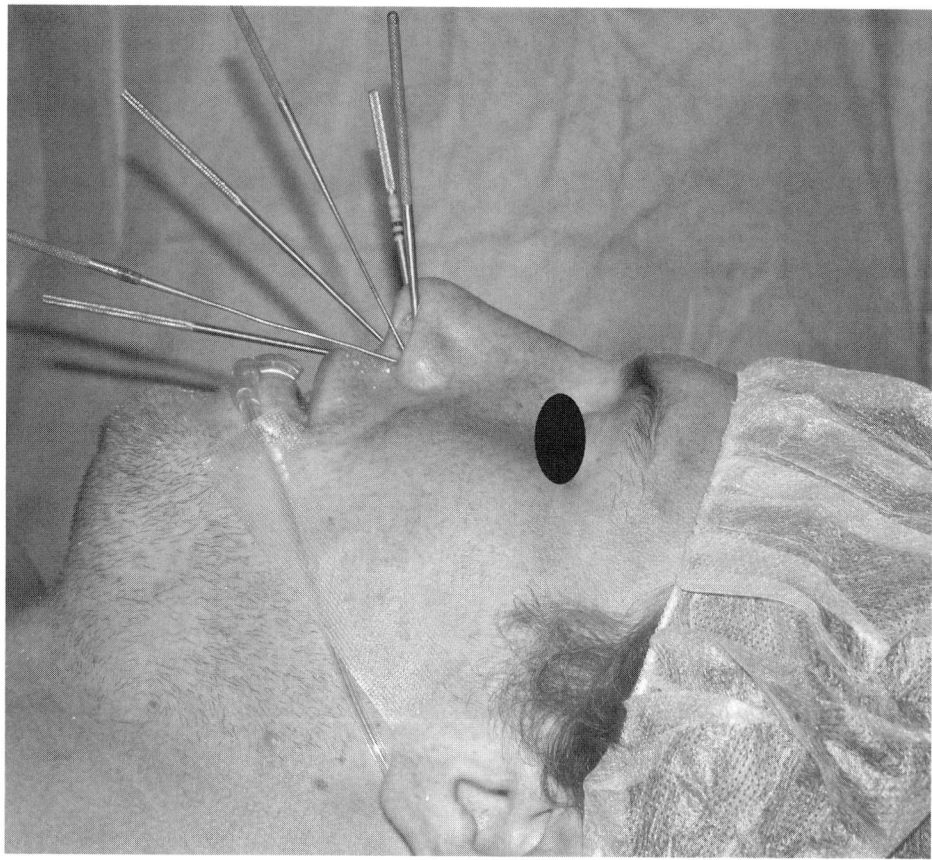

Figure 174.7 Proper placement of cotton-tip applicators for achieving nasal local anesthesia.

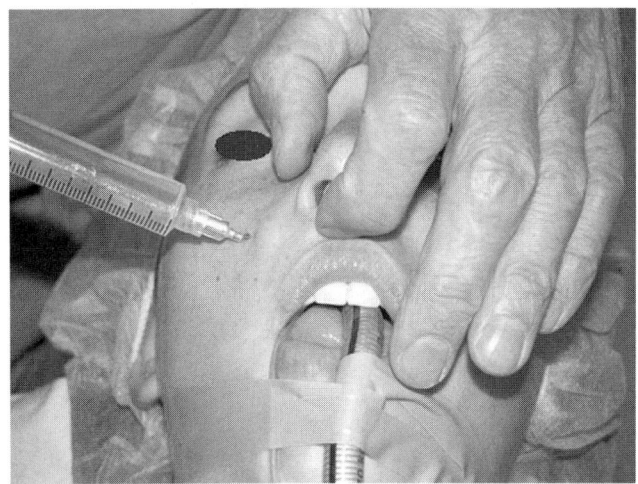

A

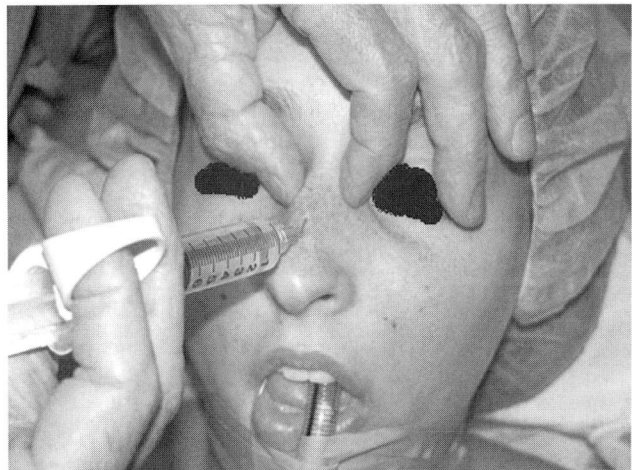

B

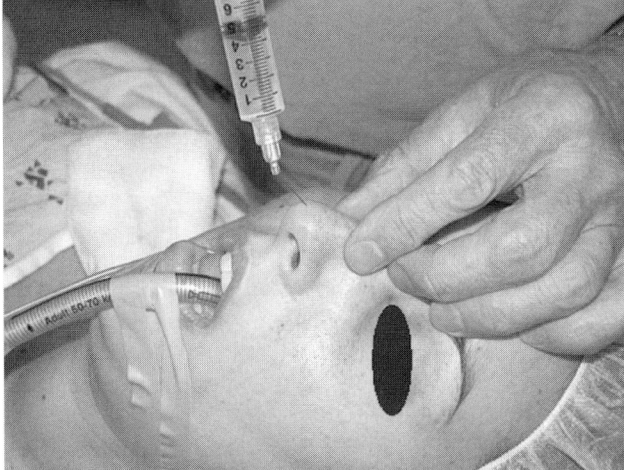

C

Figure 174.8 Locations for injection of local anesthesia. **A:** Nasal sidewall. **B:** Nasal dorsum. **C:** Nasal tip.

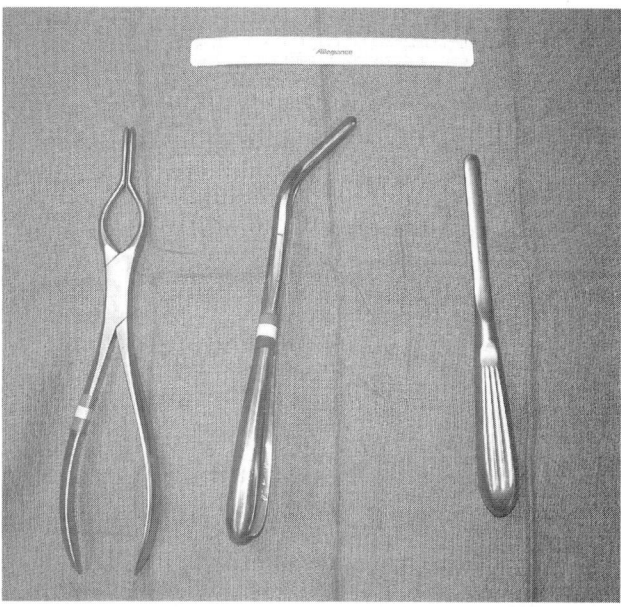

Figure 174.9 Three common tools for closed reduction of nasal bones and septum: the Walsham and Asch forceps, and Boies elevator.

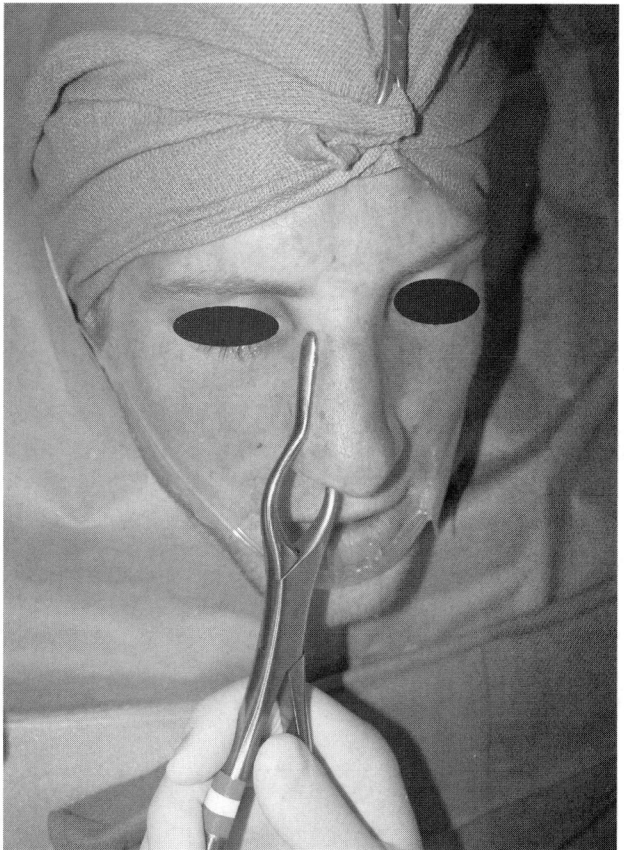

Figure 174.10 Closed reduction technique using the Walsham forceps.

return the nasal bone to its anatomic location (Fig. 174.11). These maneuvers will prove effective if the nasal septum if not fractured (Fig. 174.12). Should concurrent septal pathology exist, it should be addressed before the nasal bone reduction.

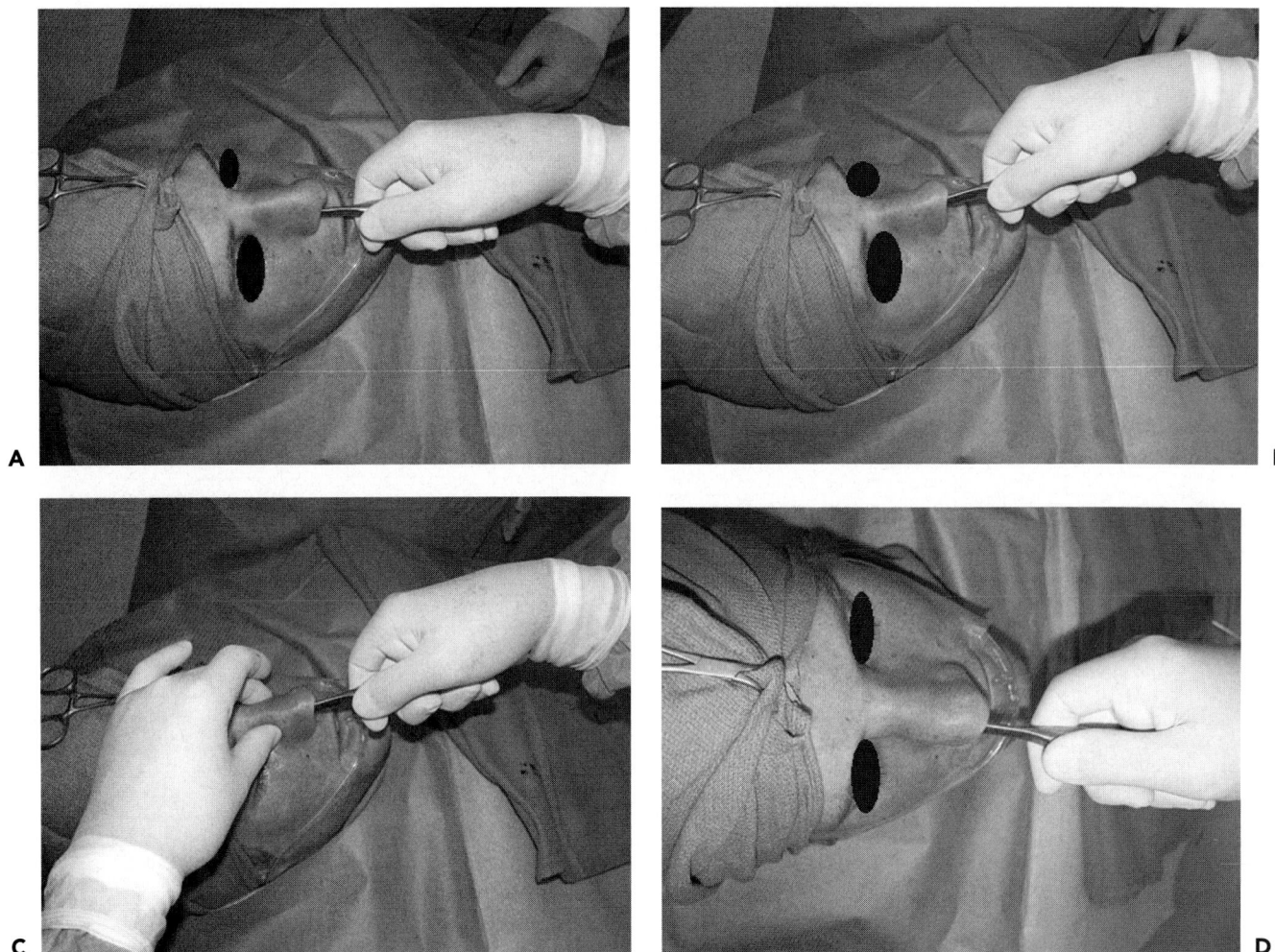

Figure 174.11   Closed reduction technique using the Boies elevator. **A:** Intranasal placement of the elevator. **B:** Careful force applied in the anterior direction. **C:** Nasal bone fragment is disimpacted. **D:** Fragment is reduced to its anatomic position.

Septal displacement, as detected on physical examination, can represent the dislocation or fracture of the nasal septum. In the case of displacement of the septum from the vomer or maxillary crest, the Boies elevator can be used to return the septum to its anatomic location (Fig. 174.13). If the septum cannot be reduced or has been fractured, more aggressive techniques are required. Repair of septal fracture is best addressed via a hemi-transfixion incision. After raising these flaps, the septal fragments can be reduced under direct vision. Difficult to reduce segments can be secured with a septal batten graft (39). Disruption to the septum, which results in an irreducible fracture, leaves the physician with several options: (a) the minimal area of deflection can be resected. (b) If a large area of the septum is involved, the segment can be removed en bloc, morselized, or scored to remove contour and then replaced within the mucoperichondrial pocket. (c) For the most complicated septal injuries, the entire cartilaginous septum can be explanted

(40), refashioned to a dorsal and caudal strut, then transplanted back to the patient (Fig. 174.14).

If a patient has a preexisting contour deformity in the middle third of the nose or if the septum remains misaligned despite repair, the upper lateral cartilage can be detached. This maneuver can be accomplished from either an endonasal or open rhinoplasty approach. During an open procedure, the upper lateral cartilages can be directly dissected from the septum at their dorsal attachments. If mucoperichondrial flaps have been elevated, the cartilage can be separated from the septum by a continuation of the dissection from inferior to dorsally. During an endonasal procedure, the surgeon can again approach the upper lateral cartilage from the dorsal approach via an intercartilaginous incision if the soft tissue envelope has been elevated (41). Alternatively, if the dorsum will not addressed during the procedure, the upper lateral cartilage can be disengaged from the septum directly from the inferior approach. This

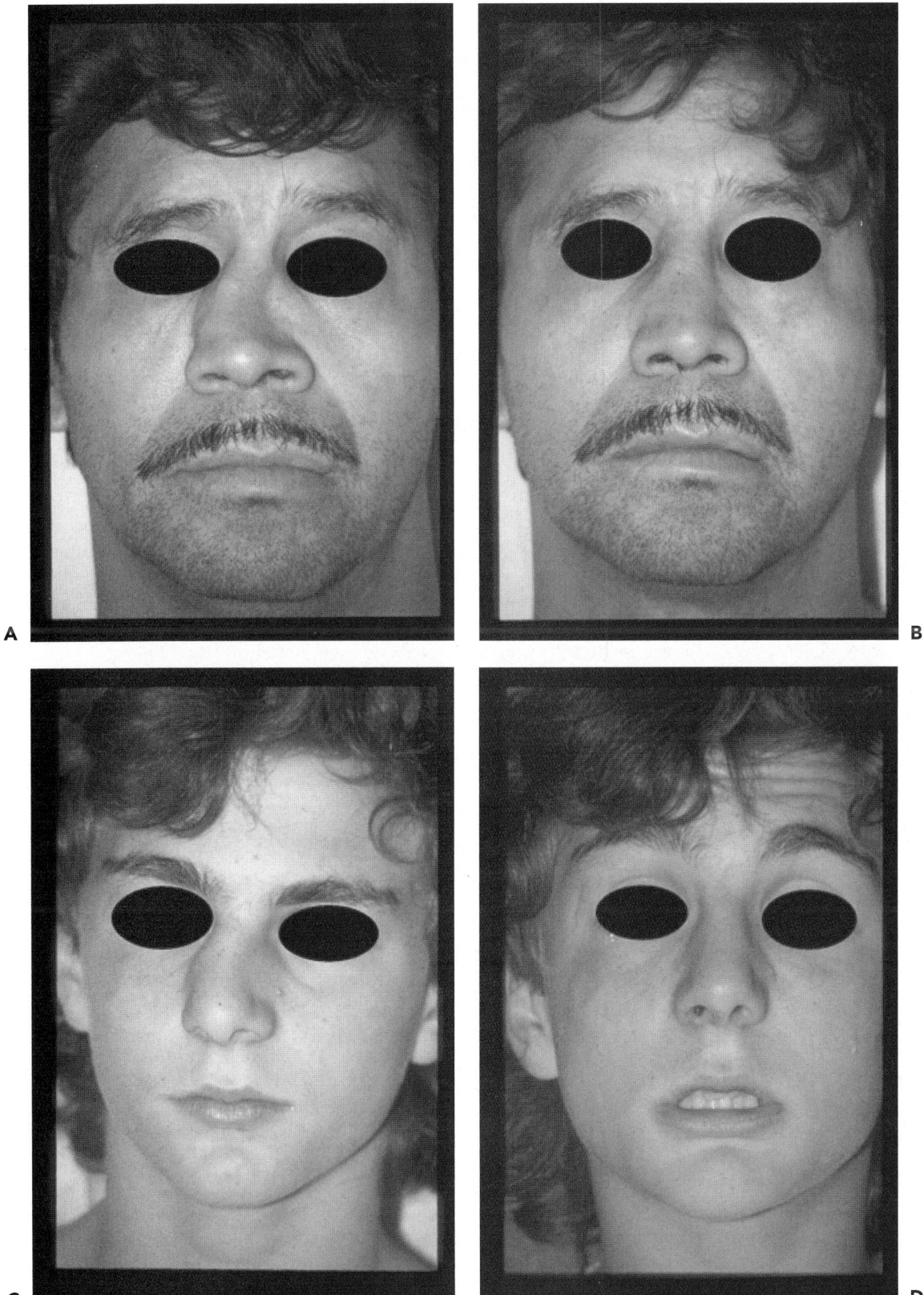

Figure 174.12   Two cases of blunt nasal trauma. **A:** Septal and nasal bone fracture with resultant nasal deformity. **B:** Immediately after closed reduction. **C:** Blunt nasal trauma resulting in nasal bone fracture with displacement of nasal septum. **D:** Immediately after closed reduction.

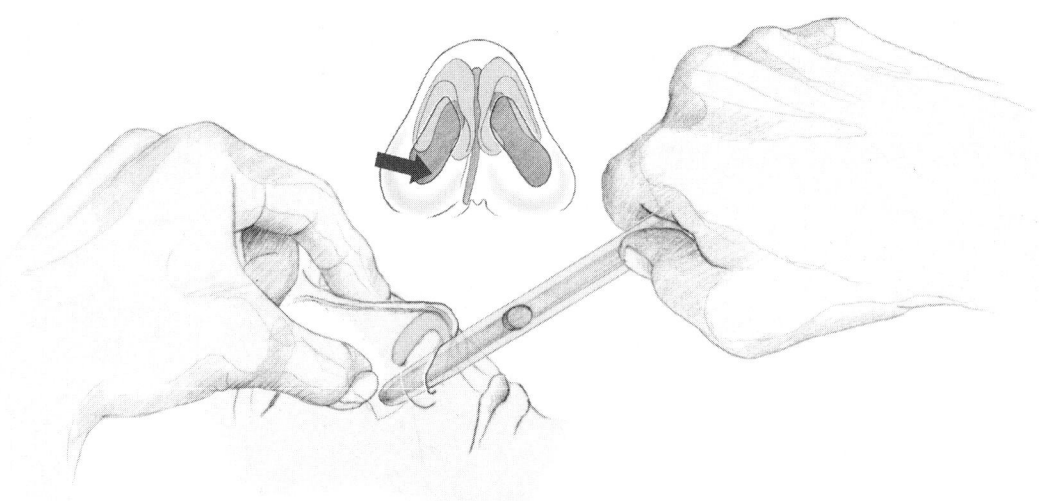

Figure 174.13   Technique of reducing the nasal septum when it has been displaced from the maxillary crest.

can be performed in a mucosal-sparing fashion or "postage-stamped" directly through the nasal mucosa. Regardless of technique, after bony and septal reduction with upper lateral release, most nasal fractures will be adequately treated.

Use of completion osteotomies in the acute treatment of nasal trauma is controversial. Many surgeons will reserve this maneuver for a secondary rhinoplasty in the nonacute setting (42). Staffel (36) and others have advocated the use of completion osteotomies when incomplete reduction of nasal bone fractures cannot be accomplished. In the setting of acute nasal trauma, the potential exists for preexisting damage to the periosteum. When the trauma of a continuous lateral osteotomy is included, concern arises for the stability of the repositioned fragment (43). If acute osteotomies must be performed, consider percutaneous or "inside-out" micro-osteotomies to minimize periosteal trauma (44). For lateral osteotomy, the authors prefer the use of a 3-mm or 4-mm straight guarded osteotome. The guard can be used to facilitate tactile location of the blade and to ensure accuracy of bony cuts. Alternatively, the senior author has used the guarded aspect of the osteotome intranasally. Anecdotally, this has served to create controlled mucosal lacerations that allow fluid egress and appear to minimize postoperative ecchymosis.

With high-velocity nasal trauma, the surgeon may have to deal with comminution of the nasal bones that will not properly reduce with the use of standard techniques. For these patients, an open technique can be considered. If the patient has an open nasal fracture, the soft tissue laceration can serve as the access to the bony fragments. Alternatively, an external transverse incision at the nasofrontal angle will provide excellent access to the nasal dorsum. The coronal incision will also allow direct visualization of the fractured segments and prevent a facial scar. Another approach that will create wide exposure without facial incisions is the

midface degloving technique (45). A disadvantage of this technique is the postprocedure nasal deprojection that occurs secondary to the full septal transfixion incision that the technique requires. Once exposed, the comminuted fragments can be wired (46), sutured (47), or internally fixated with titanium miniplates (48).

Place a nasal dressing when all corrective maneuvers have been completed. A wide variety of materials exist for both internal and external nasal splinting. Initially, most surgeons apply a tape dressing to the nose. This serves to help eliminate dead space and protect the underlying skin from the external casting material. The cast, regardless of material, protects the repositioned nasal bones, lessens postoperative edema, and reminds the patient to be cautious of the recently manipulated nose. Traditional cast material includes plaster of Paris (49), thermoplastic resin (50), and premade foam splints (Fig. 174.15). No significant postoperative advantage has been demonstrated within this group of materials. The surgeon's familiarity and product availability often determine cast choice. Recently, fiberglass resin has been adapted to create fast-setting nasal casts (51). The resin sets quickly and does not require temperature manipulation. It is possible, therefore, that its rapid application could assist in minimizing edema after nasal manipulation. In contradistinction, Camirand et al. (52) recommend no external dressing. In their series of more than 800 primary and secondary rhinoplasties, they report no early displacement of nasal bones.

Internal nasal packing is usually not required. If a reduced nasal bone is unstable, a wedge of absorbable packing (e.g., Gelfoam) can be used to splint the fragment in place. Alternatively, a standard sponge pack can be used. Nasal tampons that have an embedded airway are best for patient comfort. Nasal packing is highly recommended if a septal hematoma has been treated or if significant postoperative bleeding occurs.

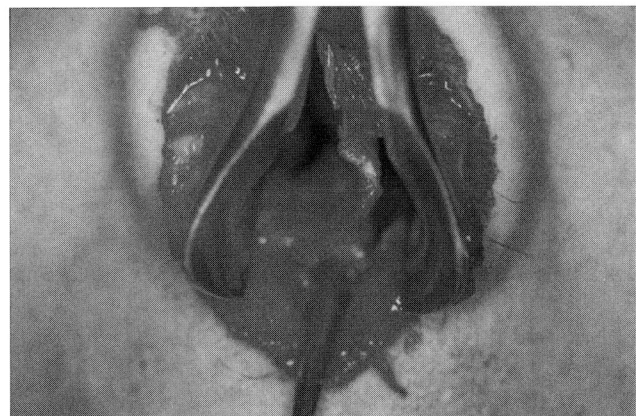
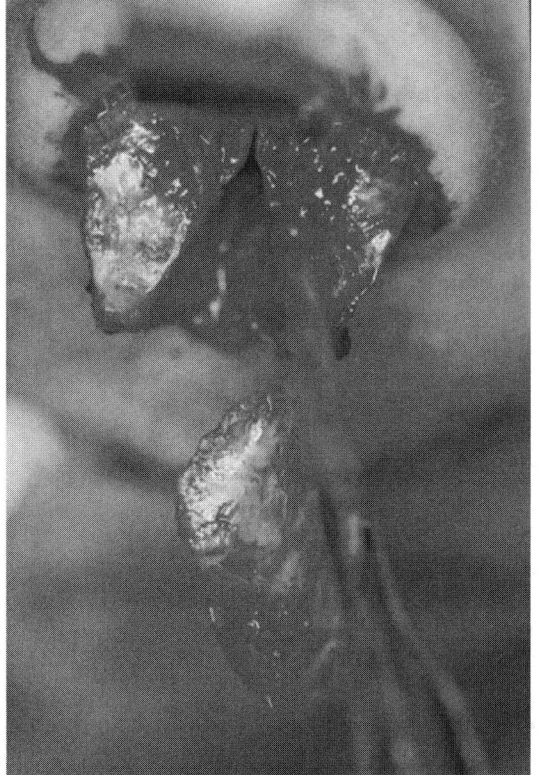
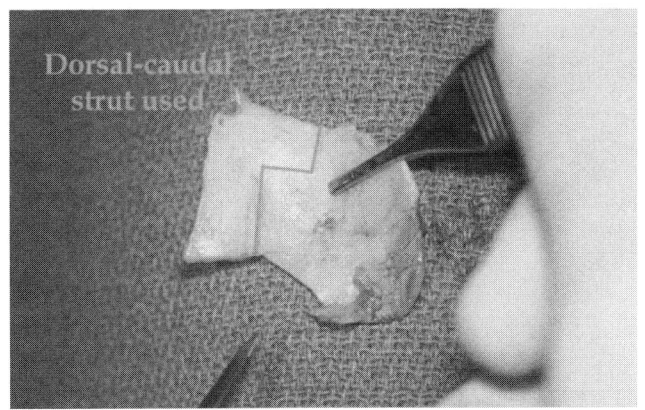
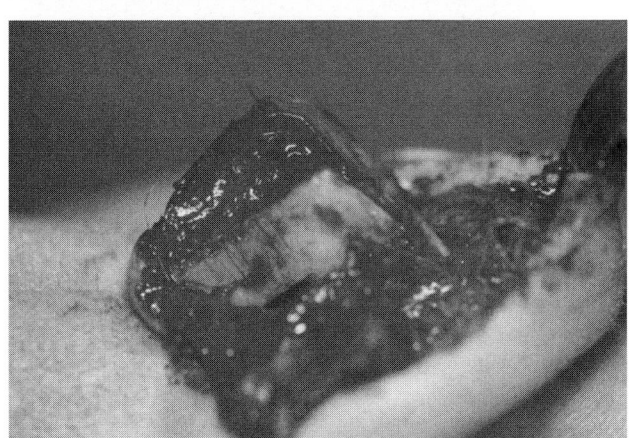

Figure 174.14   Technique of septal transplant. **A:** Exposure of nasal septum via open septorhino-plasty. **B:** Harvest of cartilaginous septum. **C:** Creation of an L-shaped dorsal-caudal strut. **D:** Replacement and fixation of the refashioned septum.

COMPLICATIONS

Blunt nasal trauma has a broad horizon for postinjury complications. Significant problems can occur in the immediate postinjury phase and in months to years after the incident. For acute complications, the initial physical examination and assessment is the essential window of time to identify potential problems.

A septal hematoma requires prompt intervention. Septal hematoma can be observed as an abnormal thickening of the septum. A septum that exceeds the standard width of 2 mm to 4 mm should suggest a hematoma. In addition to the septal thickening often a deep red or blue discoloration will be noted. Although best diagnosed with a physical examination, common symptoms of septal hematoma include nasal obstruction (95%), pain (50%), fever, and occasional nonspecific rhinorrhea (53). Treatment of the hematoma is incision and drainage. When the hematoma is bilateral, the mucoperichondrial incisions should be made so that they do not overlap and create a potential for later septal perforation. After adequate drainage, a compressive nasal pack should be used to prevent recurrence. Expedited treatment of a septal hematoma is important to prevent secondary nasal deformities.

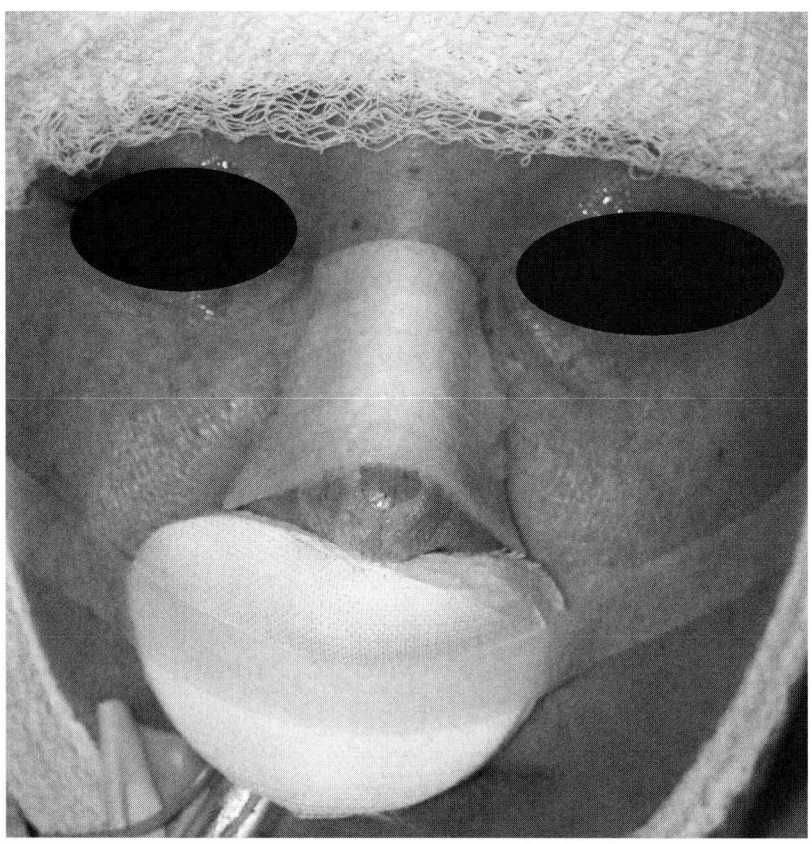

Figure 174.15 The Aquaplast thermoplastic splint.

An untreated hematoma can lead to devitalization of septal cartilage, necrosis, and saddle-nose deformity (54).

The untreated septal hematoma can also lead to a septal abscess. The pooled blood acts as an excellent culture medium. Although rare, most abscesses will reveal *S. aureus* or *Streptococcus pneumonia* (55). Treatment consists of incision and drainage, nasal packing, and appropriate broad-spectrum antibiotics. A devastating complication of septal abscess, if left untreated, is secondary meningitis. This can occur secondary to retrograde bacteremia via the emissary veins (56).

Even with adequate diagnosis and treatment of nasal injuries, the ultimate cosmetic result may be unacceptable to the patient or physician. A formal rhinoplasty or a revision septorhinoplasty must be considered one of the ultimate risks of treating blunt nasal trauma. As stated, revision rates range from 10% to 40%, depending on the initial treatment used. Proper patient counseling includes educating the patient of this possible eventuality.

by the injury itself. All nasal fractures are not the same. Recognition of injury to the septum, upper lateral cartilages, and other supporting structures allows complete treatment of the nasal injury. When blunt nasal trauma is addressed in this step-wise manner, secondary nasal deformity and revision rhinoplasty can be greatly reduced.

HIGHLIGHTS

- The history of the mechanism of injury is an important component of the evaluation.
- Assessment of the preinjury status of the nose may avoid future difficulty.
- Proper lighting, suction, instrumentation, and assistance are essential during emergency management of nasal trauma.
- Also consider and rule out concurrent injury.
- A septum wider than 2 mm to 4 mm may represent a hematoma.

CONCLUSIONS

Management of blunt nasal trauma requires a careful, step-wise approach to ensure proper treatment and excellent long-term outcomes. Treatment begins with the acute stabilization of the injury followed by a detailed physical examination. Medical and surgical management is then dictated

REFERENCES

1. Wang TD, Facer GW, Kern EB. Nasal fractures. In: Gates GA, ed. *Current therapy in otolaryngology: head and neck surgery*, Vol. 4. Philadelphia: BC Decker, 1990:105–109.
2. Doerr, T. Nasal fractures. In: Cummings CW, ed. *Otolaryngology head and neck surgery*. Baltimore: Mosby, 1998:Chapter 46.
3. Dickson MG, Sharp DT. A prospective study of nasal fractures. *J Laryngol Otol* 1996;100:543–546.

4. Harrison DH. Nasal injuries: their pathogenesis and treatment. *Br J Plast Surg* 1979;32:57–64

5. Hussain K, Wijetunge DB, Grubnic S, et al. A comprehensive analysis of craniofacial trauma. *Journal of Trauma-Injury Infection & Critical Care* 1995;36(1):34–47.

6. Simoni P, Ostendorf R, Cox AJ 3rd. Effect of air bags and restraining devices on the pattern of facial fractures in motor vehicle crashes. *Arch Facial Plast Surg* 2003;5(1):113–115.

7. Verwoerd, CD. Present day treatment of nasal fractures: closed versus open reduction. *Facial Plastic Surgery* 1992;8(4):220–223.

8. Rhee SC, Kim YK, Cha JH, et al. Septal fracture in simple nasal bone fracture. *Plast Reconstr Surg* 2004;113(1):45–52.

9. Fry HJ. The interlocked stresses of articular cartilage. *Br J Plast Surg* 1974;27(4):363–364.

10. Wexler MR. Reconstructive surgery of the injured nose. *Otolaryngol Clin North Am* 1975;8(3):663–677.

11. Renner GJ. Management of nasal fracture. *Otolaryngol Clin North Am* 1971;24:195–213.

12. Cara DM, Norris AM, Neale LJ. Pain during awake nasal intubation after topical cocaine or phenylephrine/lidocaine. *Anesthesia* 2003;58(8):777–780.

13. Logan M, O'Driscoll K, Masterson J. The utility of nasal bone radiographs in nasal trauma. *Clin Radiol* 1994;49:192–194.

14. DeMarino DP, Steiner E, Poster RB. Three-dimensional computed tomography in maxillofacial trauma. *Arch Otolaryngol Head Neck Surg* 1986;112(2):146–150.

15. Pollock RA. Nasal trauma: pathomechanics and surgical management of acute injuries. *Clin Plast Surg* 1992;19:133–147.

16. Teymoortash A, Sesterhenn A, Kress R, et al. Efficacy of ice packs in the management of epistaxis. *Clin Otolaryngol* 2003;28(6):545–547.

17. Evans AS, Young D, Adamson R. Is the nasal tampon a suitable treatment for epistaxis in Accident & Emergency? A comparison of outcomes for ENT and A&E packed patients. *J Laryngol Otol* 2004;118(1):12–14.

18. Singer AJ, McClain SA, Katz A. A porcine epistaxis model: hemostatic effects of octyl cyanoacrylate. *Otolaryngol Head Neck Surg* 2004;130(5):553–557.

19. Walshe P. The use of fibrin glue to arrest epistaxis in the presence of a coagulopathy. *Laryngoscope* 2002;112(6):1126–1128.

20. Weber CR, Griffin JM. Evaluation of dexamethasone for reducing postoperative edema and inflammatory response after orthognathic surgery. *J Oral Maxillofac Surg* 1994;52(1):35–39.

21. Habal MB. Prevention of postoperative facial edema with steroids after facial surgery. *Aesthetic Plast Surg* 1985;9(2):69–71.

22. Ridder GJ, Boedeker CC, Fradis M, et al. Technique and timing for closed reduction of isolated nasal fractures: a retrospective study. *Ear Nose Throat J* 2002;81(1):49–54.

23. Murray JA, Maran AG, Mackenzie IJ, et al. Open vs. closed reduction of the fractured nose. *Arch Otolaryngol* 1984;110(12):797–802.

24. Fernandes SV. Nasal fractures: the taming of the shrewd. *Laryngoscope* 2004;114(3):587–592.

25. Newton CR, White PS. Nasal manipulation with intravenous sedation. Is it an acceptable and effective treatment? *Rhinology* 1998;13:491–494

26. Rajapakse Y, Courtney M, Bialostocki A, et al. Nasal fractures: a study comparing local and general anesthesia techniques. *Aust NZ J Surg* 2003;36:114–116.

27. Courtney MJ, Rajapakse Y, Duncan G, et al. Nasal fracture manipulation: a comparative study of general and local anesthesia techniques. *Clin Otolaryngol* 2003;28:472–475

28. Lopez MA, Liu JH, Hartley BE, et al. Septal hematoma and abscess after nasal trauma. *Clin Pediatr* 2003;39(10):609–610.

29. Keller JL, Evan KE, Wetmore RF. Toxic shock syndrome after closed reduction of a nasal fracture. *Otolaryngol Head Neck Surg* 1999;120(4):569–570.

30. Jacobson JA, Stevens MH, Kasworm EM. Evaluation of single-dose cefazolin prophylaxis for toxic shock syndrome. *Arch Otolaryngol Head Neck Surg* 1988;114(3):326–327.

31. Koc A, Erginoglu U, Karaaslan O. Otorhinolaryngological procedures in the fifteenth century in Anatolia. *Ann Otol Rhinol Laryngol* 2004;113(5):414–417.

32. Illum P. Long-term results after treatment of nasal fractures. *J Laryngol Otol* 1986;100(3):273–277.

33. Waldron J, Mitchell DB, Ford G. Reduction of fractured nasal bones; local versus general anesthesia. *Clin Otolaryngol* 1989; 14(4):357–359.

34. Murray JA, Maran AG. The treatment of nasal injuries by manipulation. *J Laryngol Otol* 1980;94(12):1405–1410.

35. Rohrich RJ, Adams Jr WP. Nasal fracture management: minimizing secondary nasal deformities. *Plast Reconstr Surg* 2000;106(2): 266–273.

36. Staffel JG. Optimizing treatment of nasal fractures. *Laryngoscope* 2002;112(10):1709–1719.

37. Alvarez H, Osorio J, De Diego JI, et al. Sequelae after nasal septum injuries in children. *Auris Nasus Larynx* 2000;27(4):339–342.

38. Brown L, Denmark TK, Wittlake WA, et al. Procedural sedation use in the ED: management of pediatric ear and nose foreign bodies. *Am J Emerg Med* 2004;22(4):310–314.

39. Byrd HS, Salomon J, Flood J. Correction of the crooked nose. *Plast Reconstr Surg* 1998;102(6):2148.

40. Riechelmann H, Rettinger G. Three-step reconstruction of complex saddle nose deformities. *Arch Otolaryngol Head Neck Surg* 2004;130(3):334–338.

41. Teller DC. Anatomy of a rhinoplasty: emphasis on the middle third of the nose. *Facial Plastic Surgery* 1997;13(4):241–252.

42. Murakami CS, Larrabee WF. Comparison of osteotomy techniques in the treatment of nasal fractures. *Facial Plast Surg* 1992; 8:209–219.

43. Gryskiewicz JM, Gryskiewicz KM. Nasal osteotomies: a clinical comparison of the perforating methods versus the continuous technique. *Plast Reconstr Surg* 2004;113(5):1445–1456.

44. Byrne PJ, Walsh WE, Hilger PA. The use of "inside-out" lateral osteotomies to improve outcome in rhinoplasty. *Arch Facial Plast Surg* 2003;5(3):251–255.

45. Cultrara A, Turk JB, Har-El G. Midfacial degloving approach for repair of naso-orbital-ethmoid and midfacial fractures. *Arch Facial Plast Surg* 2004;6(2):133–135.

46. Kurihara K, Kim K. Open reduction and interfragment wire fixation of comminuted nasal fractures. *Ann Plast Surg* 1990;24(2): 179–185.

47. Renner GJ. Management of nasal fractures. *Otolaryngol Clin North Am* 1991;24(1):195–213.

48. Sargent LA, Rogers GF. Nasoethmoid orbital fractures: diagnosis and management. *J Craniomaxillofac Trauma* 1999;5(1):19–27.

49. Webster RC, Smith RC, Barrera A, et al. External splinting of the nose. *Laryngoscope* 1983;93:1615–1616.

50. Cunningham MW, Yousif NJ, Sanger JR, et al. Aquaplast for nasal splinting. *Ann Plast Surg* 1984;13:357–358.`

51. Ahn MS, Maas CS, Monhian N. A novel, conformable, rapidly setting nasal splint material: results of a prospective study. *Arch Facial Plast Surg* 2003;5(2):189–192.

52. Camirand A, Doucet J, Harris J. Nose surgery (rhinoplasty) without external immobilization and without internal packing: a review of 812 cases. *Aesthetic Plast Surg* 1998;22(4):245–252.

53. Canty PA, Berkowitz RG. Hematoma and abscess of the nasal septum in children. *Arch Otolaryngol Head Neck Surg* 1996;122: 1373–1376.

54. Wilson SW, Milward TM. Delayed diagnosis of septal haematoma and consequent nasal deformity. *Injury* 1994;25(10):685–686.

55. Lopez MA, Liu JH, Hartley BE, et al. Septal hematoma and abscess after nasal trauma. *Clin Pediatr* 2000;39(10):609–610.

56. Eavey RD, Malekzakeh M, Wright HT Jr. Bacterial meningitis secondary to abscess of the nasal septum. *Pediatrics* 1977;60(1): 102–104.

Secondary Rhinoplasty

175

Stephen W. Perkins   Shervin Naderi

Despite new cosmetic procedures and techniques developed throughout the last several decades, rhinoplasty remains one of the most challenging and rewarding surgeries performed by facial plastic surgeons. It is an operation that can dramatically alter the appearance of a patient and detract from the undue attention the nose draws in the center of the face. With good results, it can bestow confidence on young and old alike. With poor outcome, the patient can become withdrawn, self-conscious, and even depressed. It remains one of the most common cosmetic procedures sought by both men and women. It is an operation done on almost all age groups and walks of life.

Rhinoplasty is an operation that takes years to learn well and a lifetime to attempt to perfect. Its aesthetic and functional outcomes go hand in hand, which must be well understood by the surgeon to result in a happy patient. The progressively evolving surgical result must be closely studied even years later to witness and learn from surgical decisions and maneuvers made pre- and intraoperatively. The "Gunter-like" diagram is a valuable tool in this self-evaluation and self-improvement by each surgeon.

Proper aesthetic facial analysis provides the first challenge to the rhinoplasty surgeon. In an operation where millimeters determine outcome, the ideal surgical result relies on appropriate presurgical planning. The second challenge for the rhinoplasty surgeon is the three-dimensional aspect of the nasal bony and cartilaginous architecture. Each surgical maneuver aimed at manipulating a certain view of the nose results in changes in multiple other nasal views as well. The soft tissue envelope and its "shrink wrapping" over time provide the third and most unpredictable challenge to the rhinoplasty surgeon. Although traditionally the 1-year postoperative result is deemed the rhinoplasty's final result by surgeons and patients, because of the continual soft tissue changes over time, the final results must be reevaluated even 10 to 20 or more years later.

These factors are what a rhinoplasty surgeon considers when operating on a "virgin" or primary nose. Because of a variety of reasons, however, a surgeon may need to operate on a nose that has been operated on previously, either by the same surgeon or another. Often, this is the third or fourth operation, making the term "revision rhinoplasty" possibly more descriptive than the commonly used term, "secondary rhinoplasty." A variety of reasons contribute to the need for revision rhinoplasty. These include, but are not limited to, poor surgical planning, improper technique, underresection, or, more commonly, overzealous reduction rhinoplasty, very thick or very thin nasal soft tissue envelope, insufficient nasal framework, unpredictable healing, inadequate surgeon and patient preoperative communication, unrealistic patient expectations, or traumatic injury to the previously operated nose.

Revision rhinoplasty introduces a new series of challenges for the facial plastic surgeon. Variable degree of scarring, loss of nasal support mechanisms because of aggressive reduction rhinoplasty, and lack of adequate septal cartilage for rebuilding are only some of the obstacles a surgeon can face venturing back into a previously operated nose. The use of auricular cartilage or other suitable building blocks [e.g., rib cartilage, irradiated cartilage, GORE S.A.M. (Gore-Tex subcutaneous augmentation material), AlloDerm (or other acellular tissue) and other alternatives to autogenous septal cartilage] are also more common than in primary rhinoplasty. Even in secondary rhinoplasty, however, allografts should be used as an alternative rather than a substitute for the more preferential autografts (1). A graft material not commonly used but worth consideration is an autologous dermal graft, especially for patients concerned about the potential of prions and other small infectious particles possibly associated with cadaveric tissue (3).

Preoperative planning, including in-office patient examination and counseling, is a crucial investment of time. We cannot stress the importance of "imaging" enough. This is an opportunity for the surgeon and patient to visually communicate their respective goals for the operation. This technology also allows the surgeon to show the possible limitations of the operation with respect to each patient's anatomy through the use of morphing software. The office consult also provides a forum for the discussion of possible implant choices. The recovery room is not the ideal place to inform a patient that he or she now has a foreign or cadaveric implant if this possibility had not been previously addressed with the patient. Yet each patient has to be aware that it is usually after entering the nose that the surgeon can properly evaluate what was previously done and what further needs to be done to correct the problem. The columellar incision must also be mentioned to the patient. Frequently, major revisions, especially of the lobule, necessitate an external approach, whereas other problems can be approached through an endonasal technique for pocket grafting, alar retraction correction, or dorsal refinement.

The problems requiring revision rhinoplasty can be categorized in relation to the anatomic site as well as the types of aesthetic and functional defects commonly seen. Common areas to address include the pyramid, lobule, and airway. Most of these issues can be attributed to errors of omission or errors of commission. We define errors of omission as those maneuvers that needed to be done and were not done in the previous surgery. On the contrary, errors of commission are those maneuvers that were not necessary in the previous surgery or were done too aggressively, leaving the nose usually destabilized with an overoperated appearance. In this chapter, we present the most common reasons for revision rhinoplasty in our practice and offer some time-tested solutions.

ERRORS OF OMISSION

Errors of omission most commonly include inadequate tip refinement, dorsal hump reduction, or pyramid narrowing. A nose that is still overprojected or underrotated is yet another example of this error. These problems are easy to address and require completion of the maneuvers that were either done too conservatively in the previous operation or not done at all (Fig. 175.1).

Here and elsewhere throughout this chapter is noted that the first step in correction of any nasal deformity, whether primary or revision is the appropriate diagnosis of the internal structural variations leading to the external aesthetic or functional abnormality. As in any area of medicine and surgery, diagnosis is the initial crucial step. The good rhinoplasty surgeon studies each nose, diagnoses the problem, and offers a tailored solution. Much too frequently, surgeons learn a "standard" rhinoplasty operation and apply the same series of maneuvers to each nose, regardless of the problem at hand and the subtle individual variations in anatomy. Without the appropriate diagnosis, the proper surgery cannot be carried out.

The Overprojected Tip

Multiple causes of an overprojected tip exist and, hence, multiple techniques for addressing this problem. These include excess length of the caudal septum, long lower lateral cartilages, a "hanging" or underrotated tip giving the appearance of overprojection, and previously excessive augmentative use of tip grafts. It is crucial to realize the aesthetic relationship between tip projection and rotation and how each surgical maneuver can affect one or both. Our first choice for deprojection is a complete transfixation incision to disrupt nasal tip support mechanisms. The second maneuver would be appropriate resection of the caudal septum. If further deprojection is needed, the Lipsett technique is used and we use 6.0 polydioxanone (PDS) for this purpose. This technique involves transection of the medial crus of the lower lateral cartilage somewhere between its upper and middle third followed by overlapping and suturing to shorten the medial crus of the lower lateral cartilage. In addition to deprojection, this maneuver also creates derotation. Although usually done bilaterally, the Lipsett technique can be done unilaterally to correct tip asymmetries. The original description by Lipsett (3) did not include suture stabilization, but given the contracture caused by healing, we believe suturing allows for more predictable results.

The Underrotated Tip

To increase tip rotation, an inverted triangular wedge of caudal septum can be resected. This will also decrease projection, as hinted above, and must be taken into account. Lateral crural flap is also a useful technique, which provides deprojection as well as rotation. This technique involves elevation of vestibular skin and mucosa at the lateral crus of the lower lateral cartilage somewhere between the middle and lateral third followed by division, overlay, and suture stabilization using 5.0 Monocryl. Our technique is a modification of the one described by Kridel in 1991 (4).

Furthermore, it is important to understand that cephalic trim allows for rotation, which is enhanced by domal sutures. Proper placement of a columellar strut also pushes on the medial crus of the lower lateral cartilages and enhances rotation as well as providing support to the tip. More dramatic tip rotation can be achieved by releasing connections between the lower lateral cartilages (LLC) and the caudal and dorsal septum and resuturing the LLC in a more rotated position.

ERRORS OF COMMISSION

Errors of commission are the more common problems encountered in our practice. It is not uncommon to find a mixture of problems that combine errors of omission and

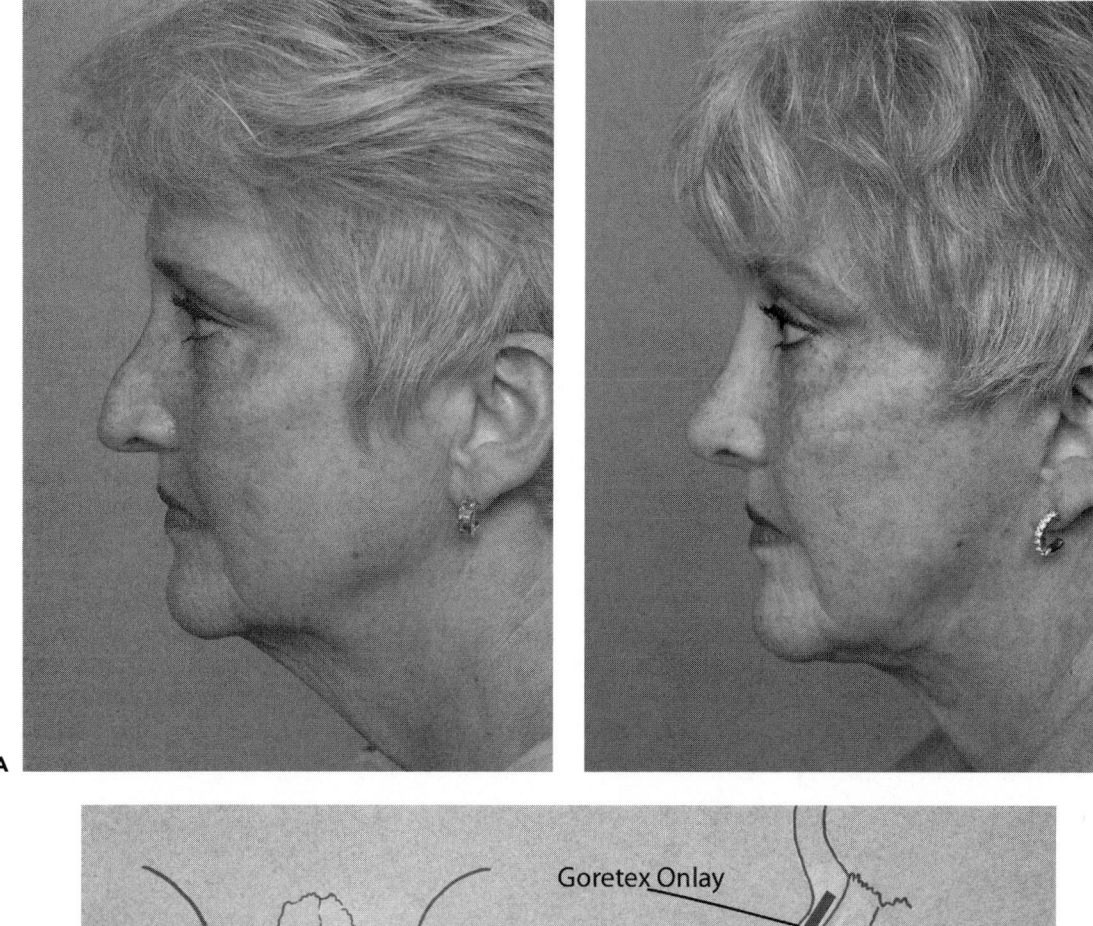

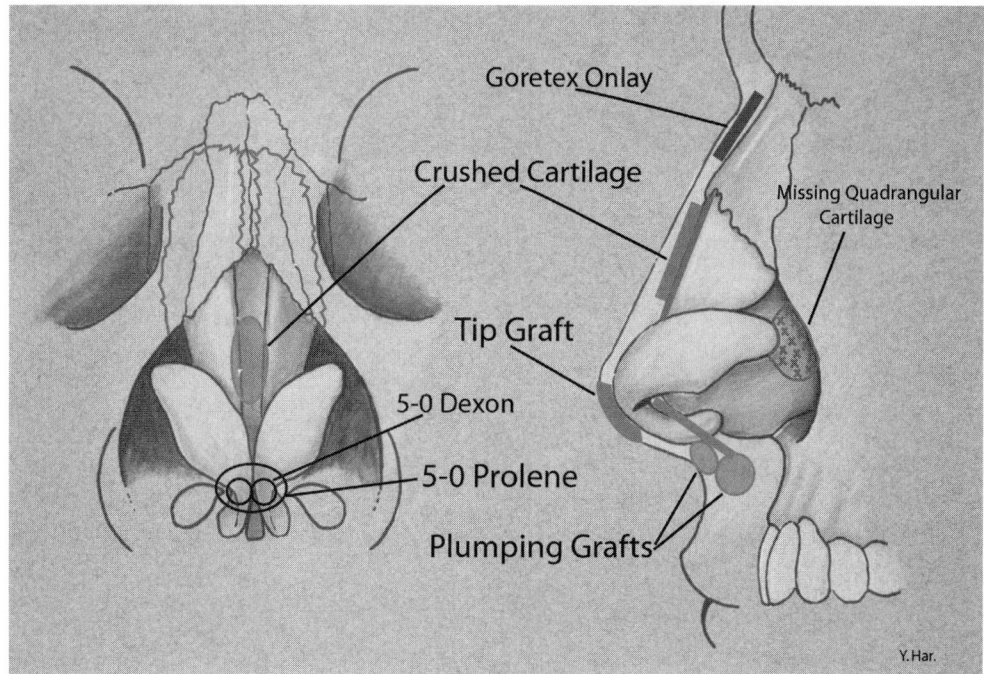

Figure 175.1   Errors of omission. **A–C:** Polly-beak deformity caused by underresection of cartilaginous dorsum. Dorsal cartilaginous middle vault lowered followed by placement of crushed cartilage for camouflage. Also note radix graft.

errors of commission. Many of these problems result from a combination of factors commonly involving aggressive reduction rhinoplasty with destabilization of the nose as well as inadequate resection in certain areas making the proper diagnosis challenging. For example, a nose with saddle deformity can be caused by overresection of the bony dorsum, underresection of the cartilaginous supratip, or both.

Pyramid Abnormalities or Irregularities

Pyramid problems usually encountered in this part of the nose include dorsal ridges or visible "humps," which commonly show up after several months, when the nasal edema has subsided, highlighting irregularities that were not addressed initially, or grafts placed intraoperatively that now show through migration or through thin skin not recognized previously. Treatment of such problems is straightforward and can be done through an endonasal approach, with direct shaving of cartilage or use of rasps in addition to crushed cartilage as camouflage "onlay." Here, thin strips of GORE S.A.M, AlloDerm, or other noncellular dermal matrix, can also be used in a patient with thin skin

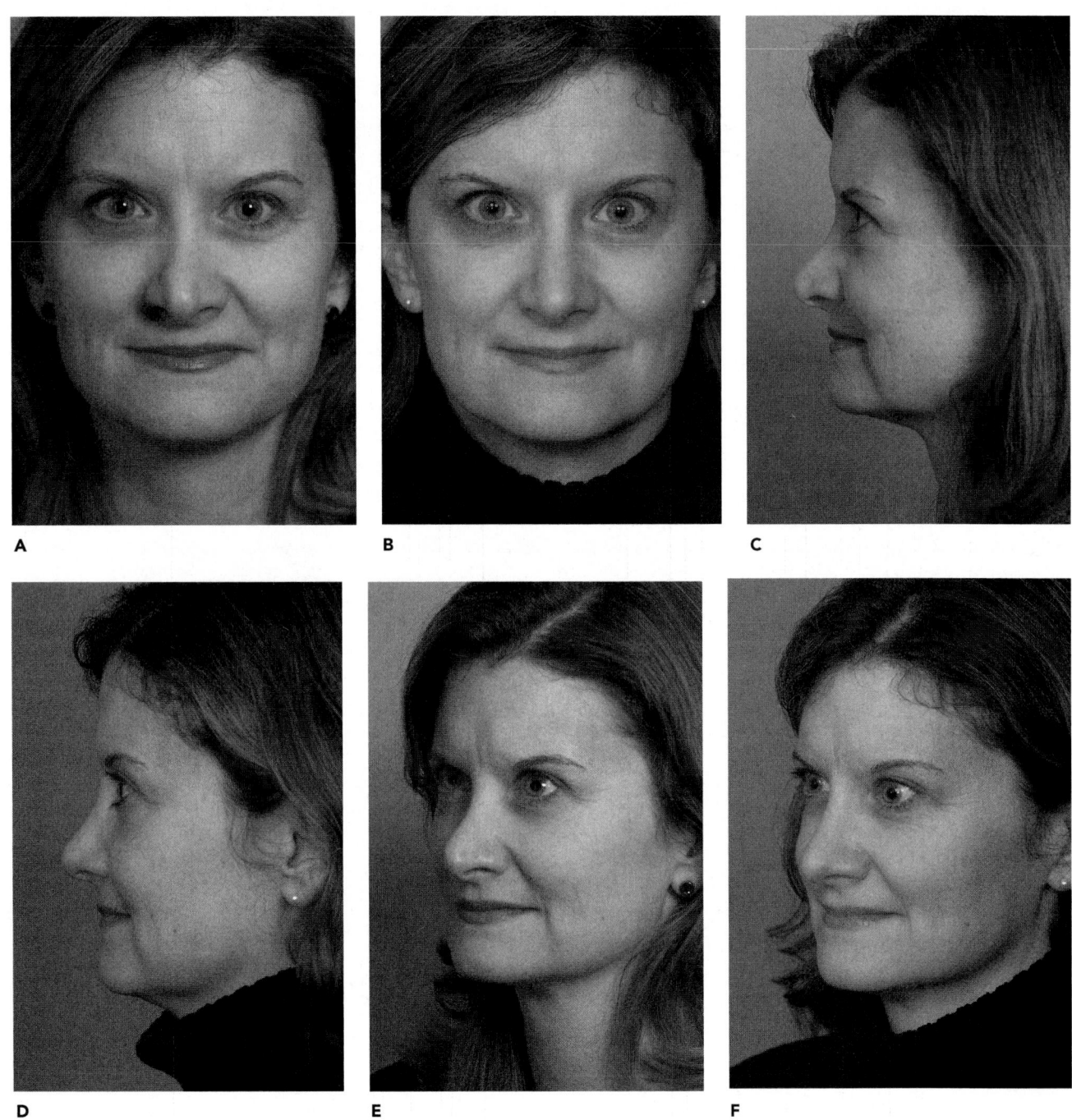

Figure 175.2   A–G: Saddle-nose deformity with narrow dorsum and tip asymmetry. Use of multiple grafts, including septal and auricular cartilage as well as AlloDerm.

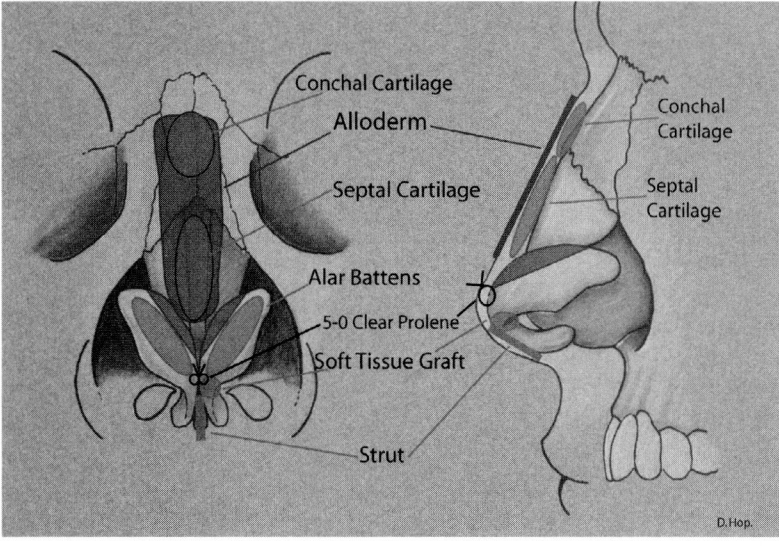

G

Figure 175.2 (*continued*)

for camouflage and thickening. Nasal fibro fatty tissue or soft tissue is also an invaluable contouring tool found usually in abundance in the form of scar in a previously operated nose.

Improper width or asymmetric nasal bones are the next common dorsal abnormalities requiring attention. The flared nasal bones or wide dorsum is easy to correct with osteotomies. A combination of medial fading osteotomies and lateral osteotomies is the most common technique used by the rhinoplasty surgeon to narrow the nasal width. A nose previously treated with osteotomies can often be remanipulated using firm bimanual pressure.

Treatment of the overly narrow dorsum, as well as "open roof" deformity, dictates the use of spreader grafts or onlay grafts (Figs. 175.2 and 175.3). This deformity is commonly the result of upper lateral cartilage retraction, which usually can be prevented by judicious dorsal height reduction with identification of different bony and cartilaginous components, and stepwise reduction of each offending component as well as identification of the need for spreader grafts during the primary operation. Rohrich et al. (5) has described this technique in a five-step method. We prefer meticulous separation of the upper lateral cartilages from the dorsal septum followed by placement of fashioned spreader grafts. Two 30-gauge needles can be used to hold the grafts in place while 5.0 Monocryl sutures are used in a mattress fashion to secure the grafts. Crushed or morsalized cartilage grafts can be also used for dorsal width augmentation and camouflage. In the event no cartilage is available, GORE S.A.M. or AlloDerm can be substituted for this purpose. Proper osteotomies are also crucial in closing an open roof deformity in a nose with

previous bony dorsal hump reduction where the surgeon failed to bring the nasal bones together.

Occasionally, a double, or intermediate, combined with a lateral osteotomy, or even an external transverse root osteotomy is necessary to correct a deviated or crooked nasal pyramid. It has been shown that the puncture sites for external osteotomies are cosmetically well accepted (6).

Treatment of the deviated nose is one of the most challenging aspects of nasal surgery. Often the bony skeleton requires multiple osteotomies, as mentioned earlier, but proper correction requires evaluation of the cartilaginous framework as well. Middle vault straightening is crucial to straightening the nose. Correction of asymmetries here with reduction, augmentation, or spanning sutures may be necessary. The proper correction of a "crooked" pyramid may also require evaluation of the septum's contribution to the deformity with resultant septoplasty and septal cartilage scoring. In certain revision noses, this may only be feasible through an external approach from above. Unilateral spreader grafts are also viable options in straightening the crooked nose, as are onlay grafts (Figs. 175.2 and 175.3).

The correction of the pyramid also includes evaluation of pyramid height. An overly resected dorsum will contribute to a saddle deformity, whereas an underresected cartilaginous dorsum will result in a "polly-beak" deformity (Fig. 175.1). Furthermore, a combination of overresection of the bony dorsum along with an underresection of the cartilaginous dorsum and possible supratip scar tissue will result in a polly-beak deformity. Each of these esthetic problems are addressed by proper evaluation and diagnosis followed by

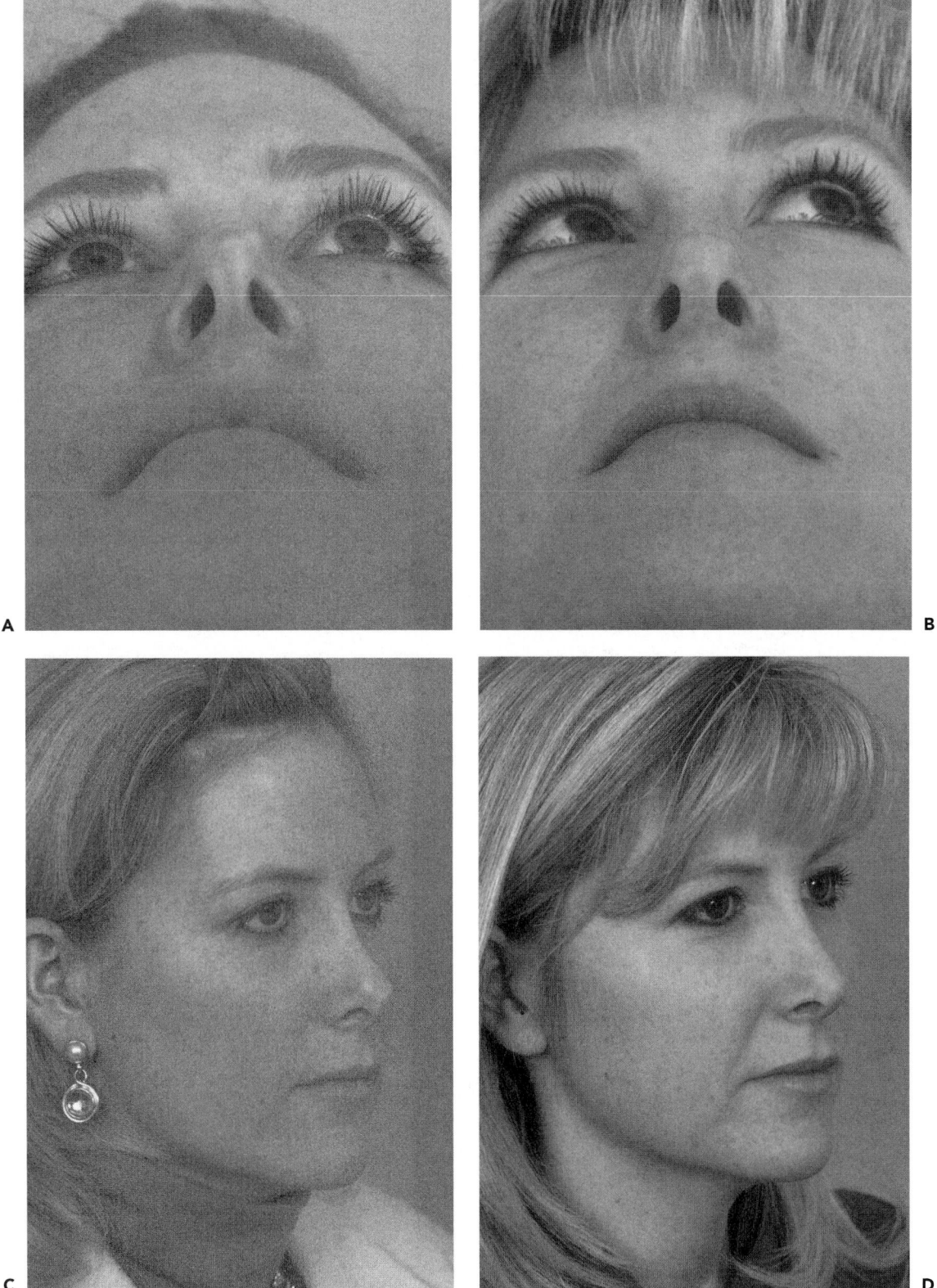

Figure 175.3   A–H: Collapsed right midvault corrected with right spreader graft. Tip bosses with asymmetry corrected with conchal cartilage alar strut grafts and double layer tip graft. Alar retraction corrected with composite conchal cartilage grafts. Dorsal saddle-nose deformity corrected with cartilage onlay.

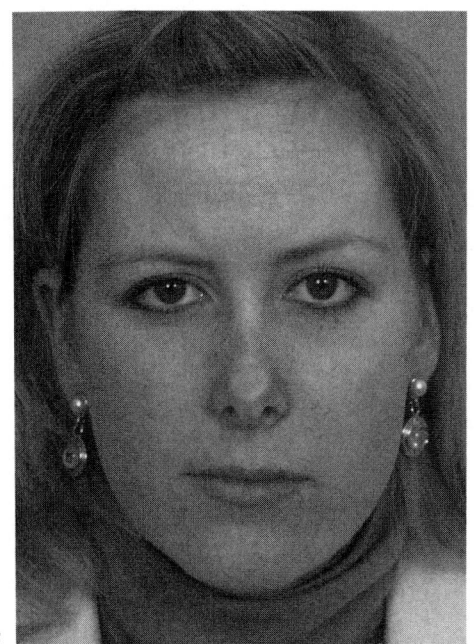

E

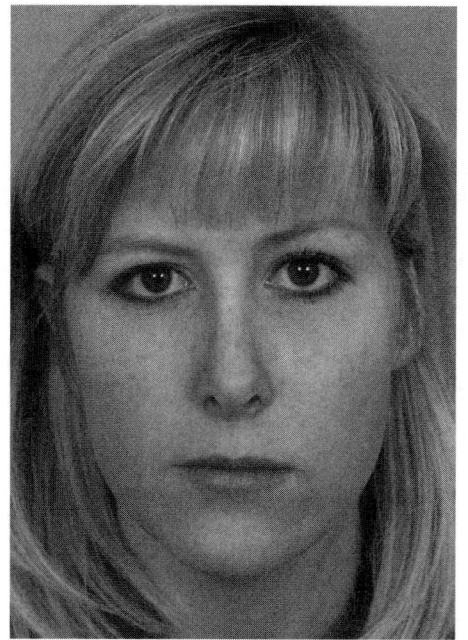

F

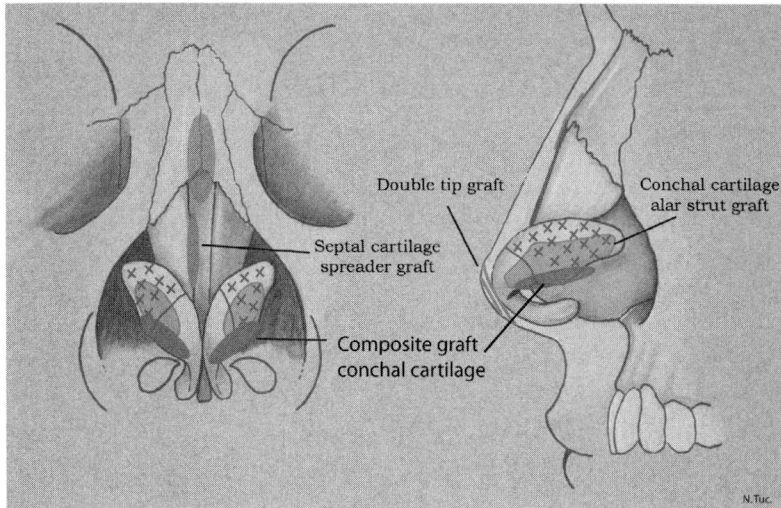

G

Double tip graft

Conchal cartilage alar strut graft

Septal cartilage spreader graft

Composite graft conchal cartilage

N.Tuc.

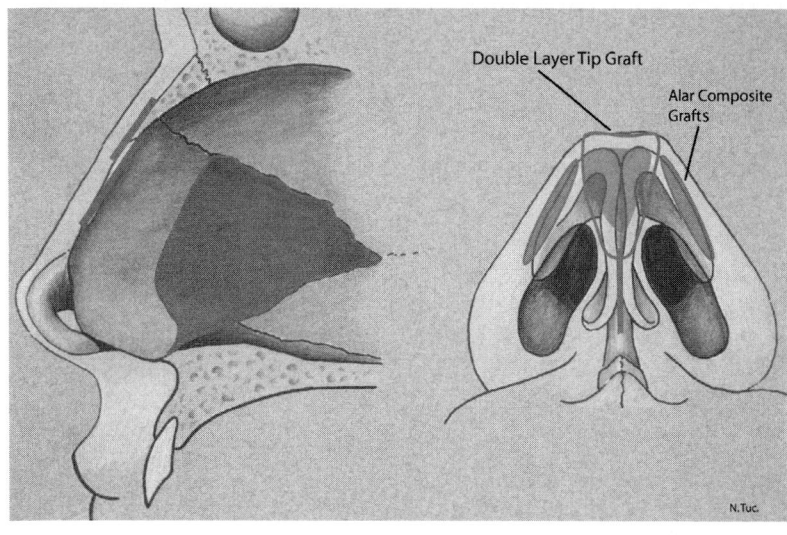

H

Double Layer Tip Graft

Alar Composite Grafts

N.Tuc.

Figure 175.3 (*continued*)

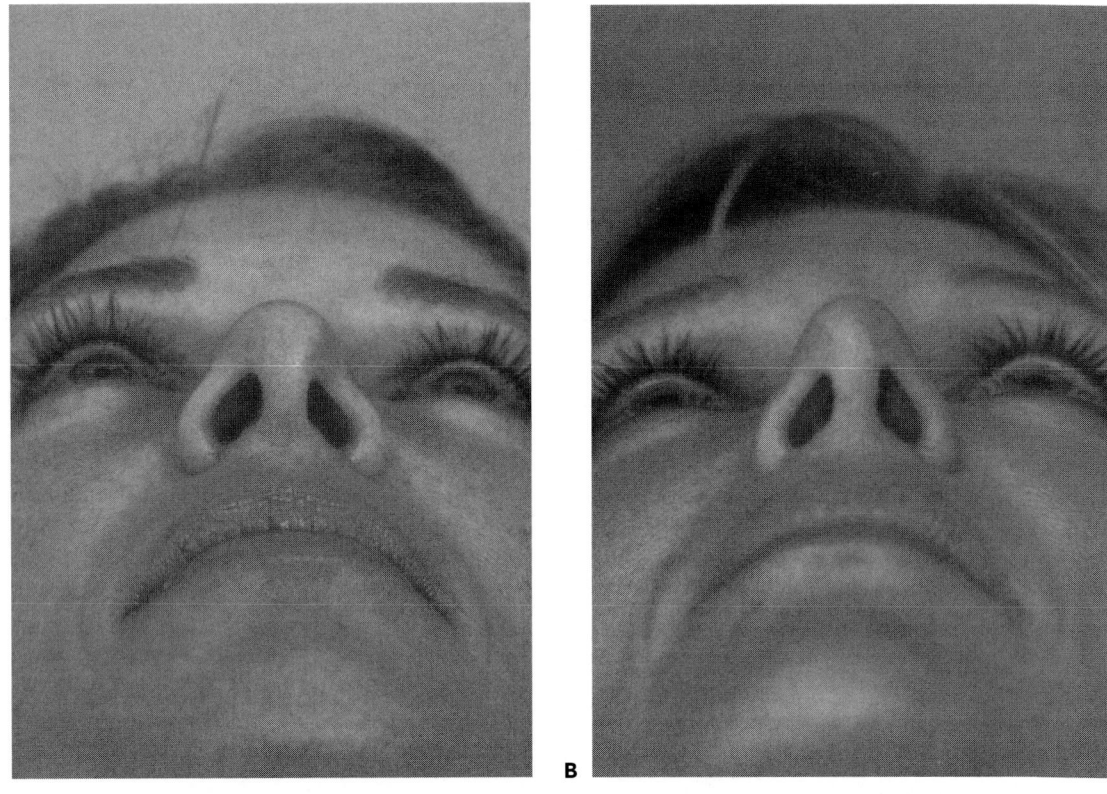

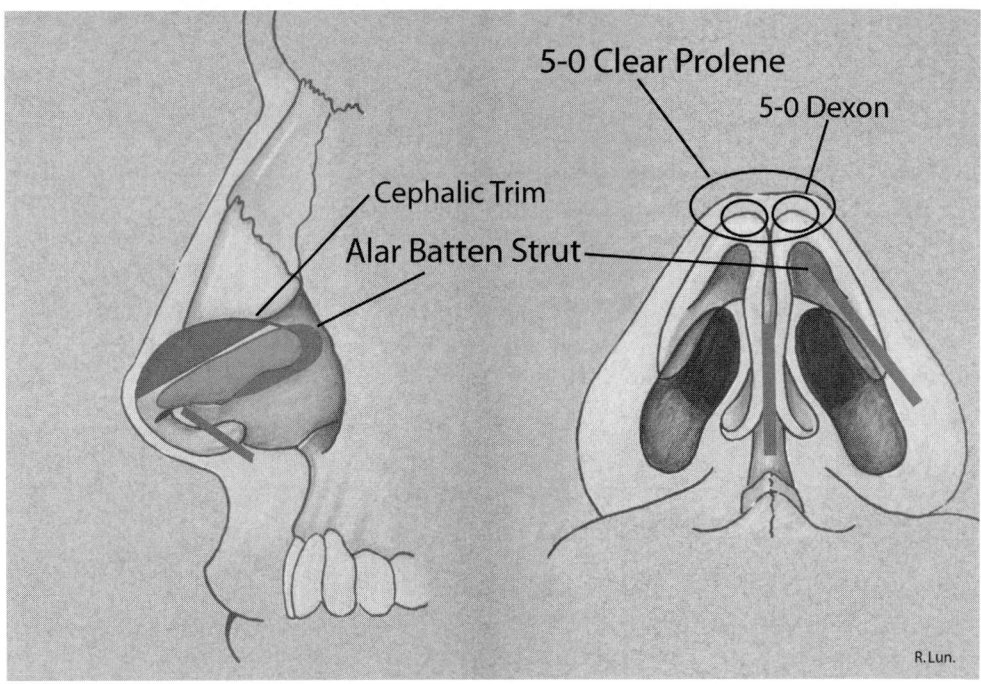

Figure 175.4   A–C: Errors of commission. Collapsed left ala caused by overresection of left lower lateral cartilage corrected with alar strut graft.

correction of the problem and aesthetic alignment of the dorsum in relation to tip and supratip height. In-office steroid injections may be necessary to reduce supratip scarring and hypertrophy (7).

The saddle nose will require augmentation with cartilage, alloplastic material, or both. Occasionally, the dorsal septum must also be augmented, especially in cases of excessive septal resection or septal necrosis. In severe cases, rib cartilage is our preferred choice, although multiple layers of auricular cartilage wrapped in AlloDerm or Merselene mesh can also be used. Alternatively, GORE S.A.M. is an acceptable, easily available choice.

A more serious and more common pyramid abnormality, as mentioned earlier, is the "open roof" deformity caused by collapse or retractions of the upper lateral cartilages. This problem can be addressed with a variety of techniques, including the use of spreader grafts, dorsal onlay grafts, and osteotomies.

Our indication for the use of spreader grafts are (a) unilateral asymmetry with in-fracture or inward curvature of one upper lateral cartilage; (b) bilateral inward curvature of upper lateral cartilages with "hour glass" appearance; (c) extremely narrow pyramid with tall middorsal hump and thin skin; and (d) prevention of late contracture deformity at the upper lateral cartilage–bony junction.

Lobule Abnormalities

Some lobular problems can be addressed through an endonasal approach with precise pocket grafting. Other more severe abnormalities necessitate an external columellar approach.

Alar Collapse or Retraction

Alar collapse or retractions are caused by weakness of the ala secondary to lack of cartilaginous support or scaffolding in this area. In a patient presenting for revision rhinoplasty, this defect may have been congenital and unrecognized by the primary surgeon or iatrogenic as a result of the previous surgery. These defects can be corrected through an endonasal technique. For alar collapse, cartilage grafts can be placed through a marginal incision in a precise pocket as an alar batten (Fig. 175.4). This maneuver also helps with symptoms of nasal airway obstruction caused by external valve collapse. Alar retractions of significance require composite auricular cartilage grafts obtained through an anterior approach from the cymba concha and secured in place with 5.0 plain gut suture. Bolsters are not necessary. The harvested composite graft is placed on the vestibular side of the ala to replace missing or contracted vestibular skin or mucosa, as well as provide cartilaginous support at the point of maximal retraction. Our technique for graft harvest, which is similar to that described by Constantian (8), differs from his in that we are usually able to close the defect primarily by extending the incision at the concha cymba inferiorly along the antihelix with undermining of the concha skin enabling tension-free closure.

More severe alar collapse causing a "pinched" tip appearance usually results from buckling of the lateral alar crus, aggressive cephalic trims, lateral division or rim strips, or total removal of the lateral crus. These problems necessitate providing support in the form of alar strut grafts. These are placed underneath the lateral crus of the

lower lateral cartilages and in an open approach can be secured using absorbable sutures (Figs. 175.5 and 175.6). Alternatively, the graft can be the only cartilage in this area used to rebuild the lateral crus because of a total resection. The ultimate goal is a nasal base that is triangular in shape with good alar support.

Lobular Reconstruction and the "Short Nose"

Major lobular reconstruction is a challenging problem that requires an external columellar incision with careful study of the underlying problems. Problems to be addressed are asymmetries of tip and ala, unusual bosses, alar-columellar disproportions, rotation, and projection. A variety of reasons exist for the development of bosses and each problem needs to be evaluated fully and treatment individualized (9). Areas that need to be resolved often include loss of tip support, or tip underprojection or overrotation. Iatrogenic causes of a "short nose" include overresection of caudal septum, overshortening of upper lateral cartilages, overrotation or resection of alar cartilages, overresection of dorsum, loss of nasal septum, or stunt of growth from previous surgical maneuvers in younger patients.

If the nose is not overtaken by scar tissue and if adequate tip cartilage is in place, then techniques used in primary rhinoplasty can also be used here (e.g., lateral crural steal or modifications of the Goldman tip technique for tip projection) (10,11). These techniques involve borrowing cartilage from the more lateral portions of the lower lateral cartilages to augment the dome and provide enhanced projection. Often given the findings encountered in a revision nose such as hostile scar tissue and inadequate lower lateral cartilages, the best approach, however, is the "back-to-basics" approach. This involves rebuilding of the cartilaginous support scaffolding of the nose from the ground up (Fig. 175.6; Fig. 175.7). The rhinoplasty surgeon must be comfortable with nasal anatomy and be able to use septal, auricular, or rib cartilage in addition to other materials to recreate the tip architecture. Once the major support mechanisms are restored, fine-tuning can be done with a variety of grafts or minor reductive shaves or augmentative onlays and grafts. Dorsal augmentation, infratip lobule grafts, single- and double-layer shield grafts, "cap" grafts, Peck grafts, "blocking" grafts, and excision of posterior caudal septal angle, to name a few, are all techniques that must be learned well and considered in such situations. In more severe cases, the dynamic adjustable rotation tip (DART) technique with the use of spreader grafts or a dorsal onlay graft combined with a columellar strut in a cantilever technique may be a viable option (12) (Fig. 175.8). In yet more radical situations, the use of GORE S.A.M. and other synthetic material may be required. We do not use calvarial bone. Occasionally, in a severely retracted nose, the limiting factor will be the pliability of the skin and soft tissue envelope. In some cases, the surgeon can discuss with the patient the possible need for total nasal reconstruction with the use of paramedian forehead flaps.

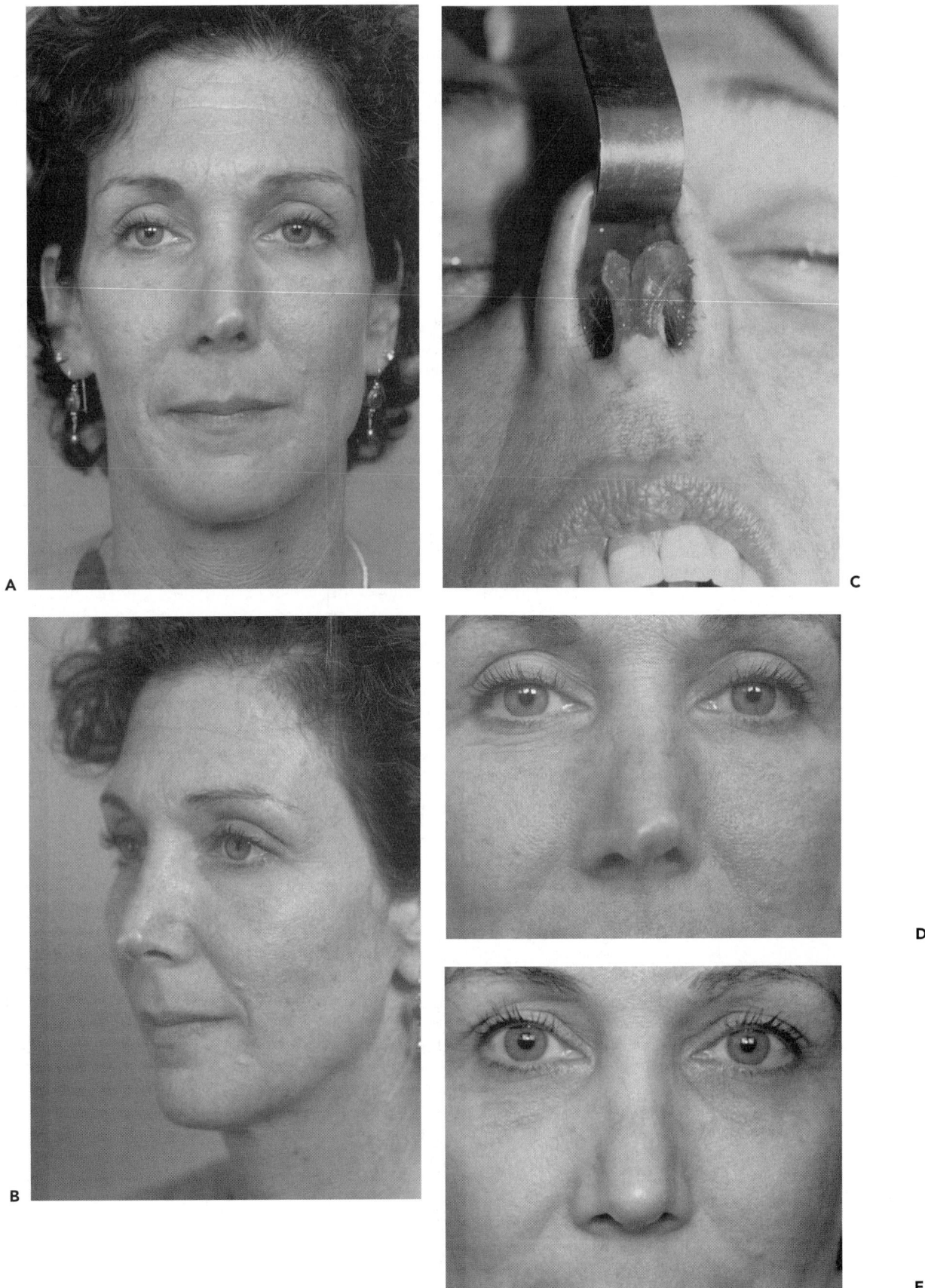

Figure 175.5   A–E: Severe tip asymmetry caused by overresection of lower lateral cartilages with dome division.

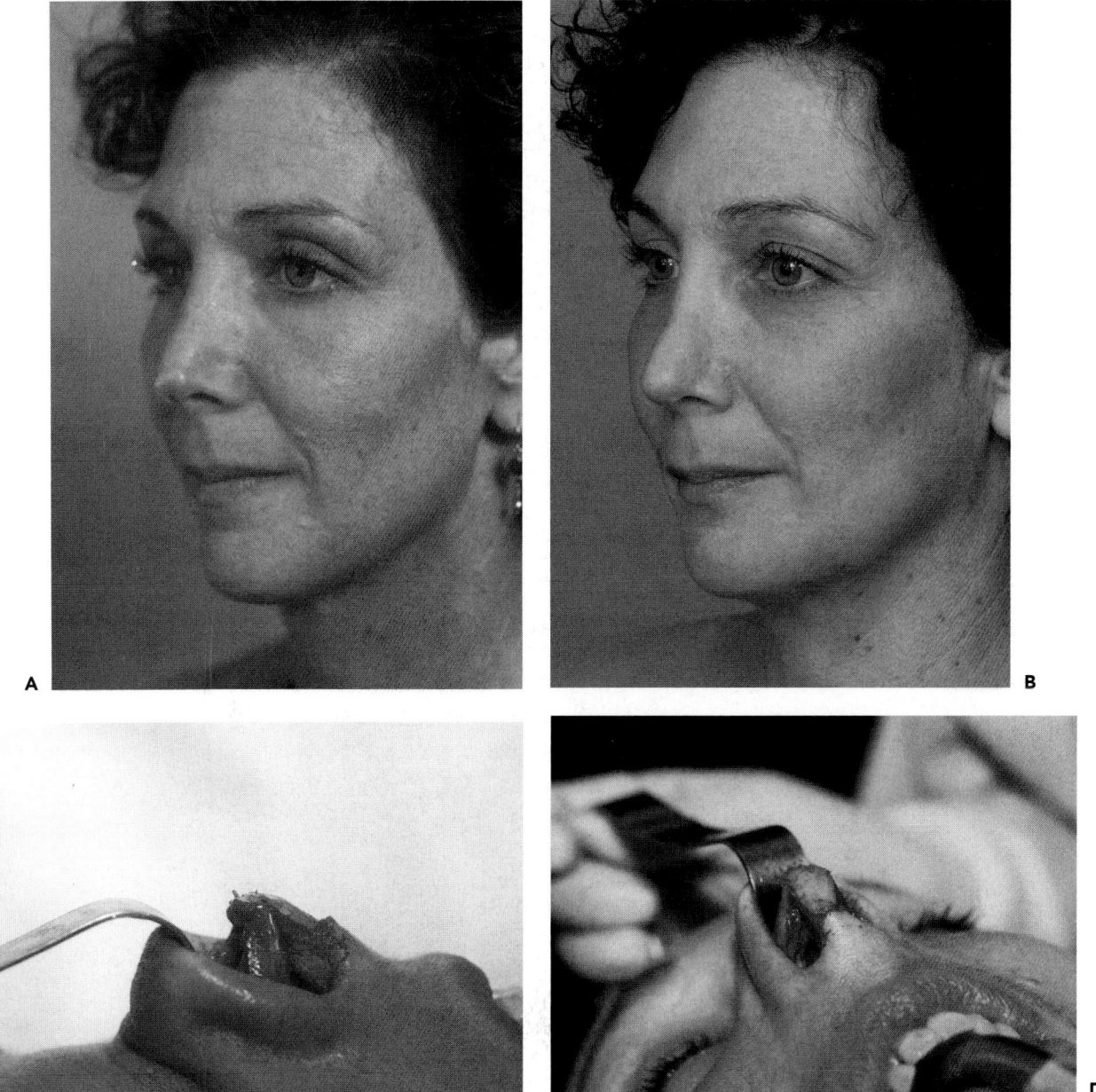

Figure 175.6   A–F: Total lobular reconstruction. Use of bilateral alar strut grafts, columellar strut graft, and tip graft to rebuild the tip cartilage architecture. (*continues*)

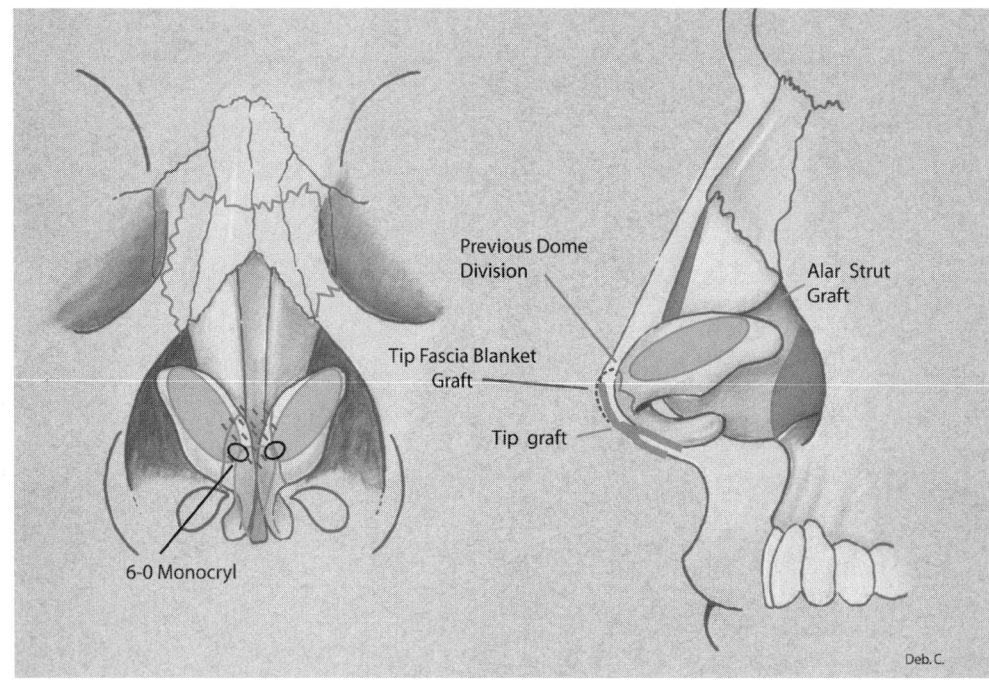

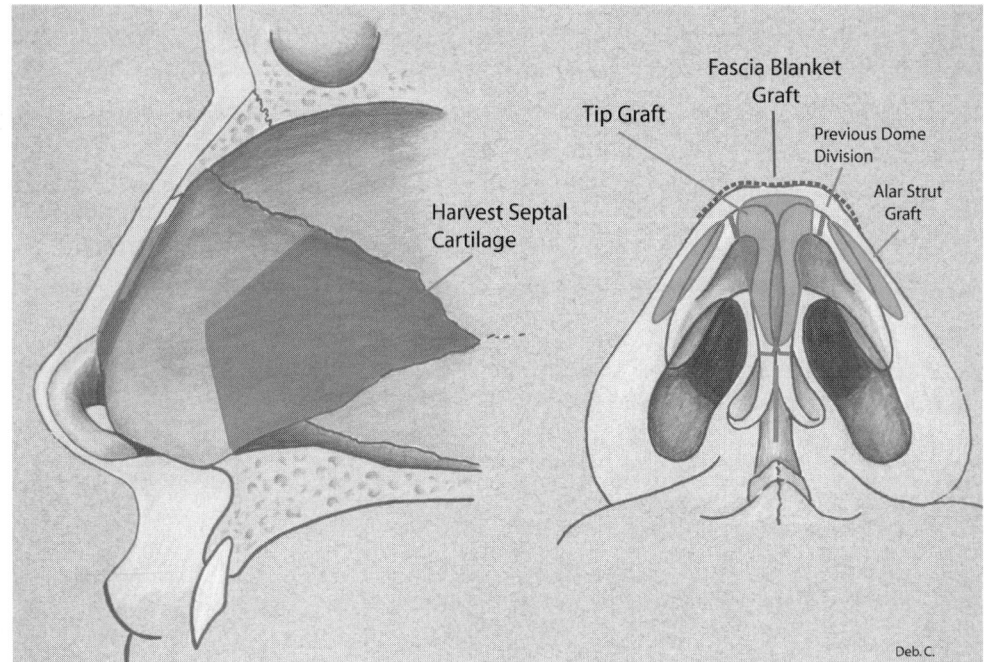

Figure 175.6 (*continued*)

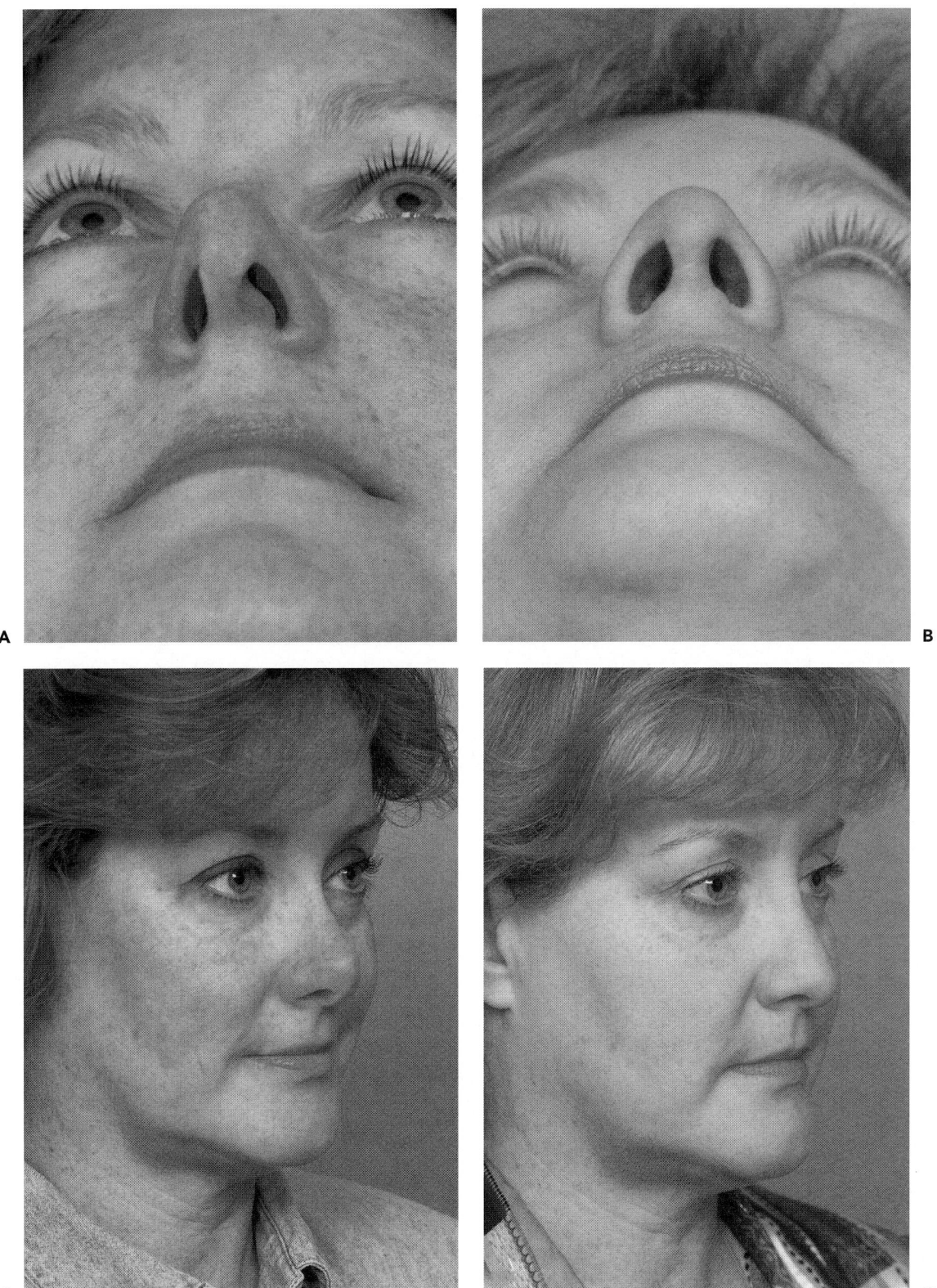

Figure 175.7 A–F: Complete lobular reconstruction with "back-to-basics" approach. Rebuilding the tip cartilages from the "ground up." (*continues*)

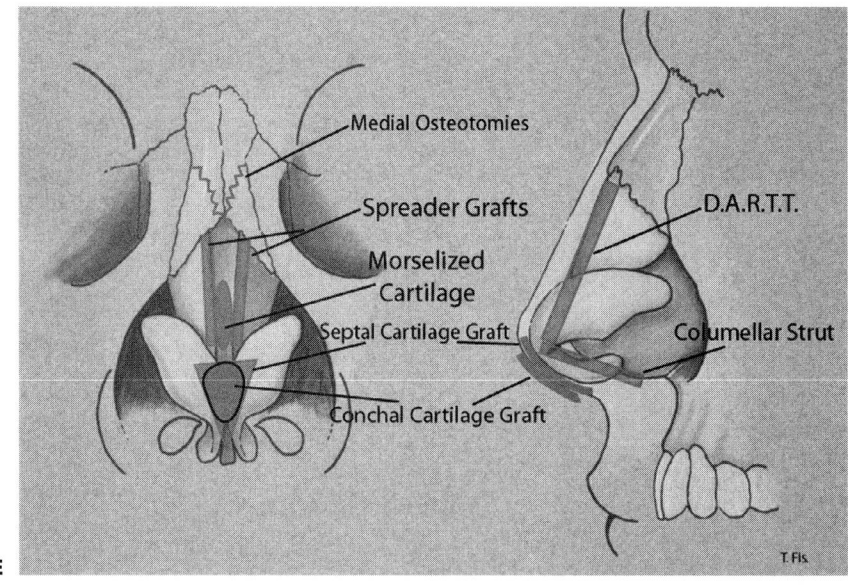

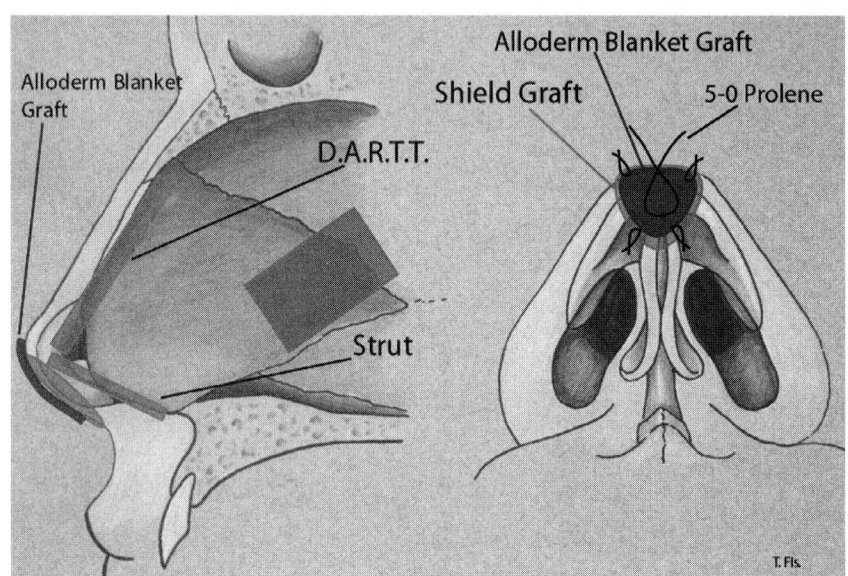

Figure 175.7 (continued)

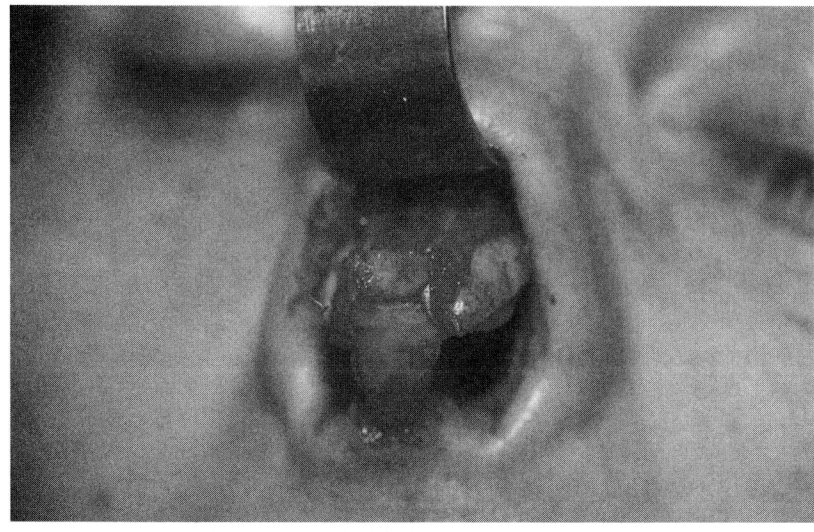

Figure 175.8 Short nose with overrotated tip, narrow dorsum, and tip asymmetry corrected with multiple grafts.

SUMMARY

Entering a previously operated nose brings with it a long list of challenges and the satisfaction of completing an often mentally tasking procedure. The first requirement for success is the proper diagnosis of the aesthetic and functional problem at hand. Minute cartilage, bony, and soft tissue asymmetries will show up down the line and will bother the patient and the surgeon and, hence, must be addressed intraoperatively. Although diagnosis is the first step, each surgeon must have a variety of techniques available to address each diagnosed problem. With such a combination approach and respect for the nasal tissue, good operative results can be expected.

Many of the techniques discussed here are commonly used in the complicated primary rhinoplasty as well. What each facial plastic surgeon must be able to rely on is the back-to-basics approach. When all else fails, do not be afraid to take the nose, the scar tissue, and whatever remnant cartilage apart and build from the ground up. This is the essence of being able to properly revise a previously operated nose.

Also, make all the minor adjustments needed as you see them at the time of the operation. Chances are if some minor detail bothered you during the case but you "let it go," with time and resolution of edema, this annoyance will be further highlighted and may distract you and the patient from appreciating an otherwise great surgical result.

HIGHLIGHTS

- Revision rhinoplasty is challenging surgery, and results are less predictable than in primary rhinoplasty.
- Successful revision rhinoplasty depends on an accurate and specific diagnosis using anatomic and aesthetic classification of the deformities.
- Bosses are knoblike irregularities of the tip cartilage that cause asymmetry. These deformities are corrected by shaving the cartilage on the more prominent side or by augmenting the cartilage on the deficient side to create a more pleasing appearance.
- Pinching is usually caused by overresection of the lateral crus of the lower lateral cartilage, causing nasal valve collapse and nasal obstruction. This is corrected by reinforcing the deficient area with a batten of auricular or septal cartilage.
- Alar retraction is usually caused by excessive resection of cartilage and vestibular skin. It is corrected using a composite graft of auricular cartilage and skin, replacing the "unrolled" vestibular skin, which then becomes part of the external nasal alar skin.

- Columellar retraction can be caused by congenital, traumatic, or surgical factors. The deficiency of caudal septal cartilage is replaced with septal or auricular cartilage or, if the membrane is also deficient, a composite skin-cartilage graft.
- Polly-beak deformity is excessive fullness of the supratip region. Correction of this deformity depends on accurate diagnosis of the cause and can include waiting for further scar remodeling, steroid injection, additional reduction of cartilaginous septum, removal of thick scar tissue, augmentation of the bony pyramid, or augmentation of the lower lateral cartilage.
- Midnasal asymmetry can be congenital but is commonly caused by traumatic subluxation of the attachment of the upper lateral cartilage to the nasal bone. Correction can be made by using a cartilage onlay graft to camouflage the asymmetric area of depression.
- Saddle-nose deformity is a concave appearance of the nasal dorsum. In postrhinoplasty patients, this is usually caused by overly aggressive resection of the bone or cartilage of the dorsum. Repair of this defect usually requires cartilage grafting.

REFERENCES

1. Rokade AV, Hughes K. Outcome of GORE-TEX implants in augmentation rhinoplasty. *Otolaryngol Head Neck Surg* 2004;131(2):81.
2. Erdogan B, Tuncel A, Adanali G, et al. Augmentation rhinoplasty with dermal graft and review of the literature. *Plast Reconstr Surg* 2003;111(6):2060–2068.
3. Lipsett E. A new approach to surgery of the lower cartilaginous vault. *Arch Otolaryngol* 1959;70:42–47.
4. Kridel RW, Konior RJ. Controlled nasal tip rotation via the lateral crural overlay technique. *Arch Otolaryngol Head Neck Surg* 1991;117(4):411–415.
5. Rohrich RJ, Muzaffar AR, Janis JE. Component dorsal hump reduction: the importance of maintaining dorsal aesthetic lines in rhinoplasty. *Plast Reconstr Surg* 2004;114(5):1298–1308.
6. Hinton AE, Hung T, Daya H, et al. Visibility of puncture sites after external osteotomy in rhinoplastic surgery. *Arch Facial Plast Surg* 2003;5:408–411.
7. Hanasono MM, Kridel RWH, Pastorek NJ, et al. Correction of the soft tissue pollybeak using triamcinolone injection. *Arch Facial Plast Surg* 2002;4:26–30.
8. Constantin MB. Indications and use of composite grafts in 100 consecutive secondary and tertiary rhinoplasty patients: introduction of the axial orientation. *Plast Reconstr Surg* 2002;110(4):1116–1133.
9. Kridel RWH, Yoon PJ, Koch J. Prevention and correction of nasal tip bossae in rhinoplasty. *Arch Facial Plast Surg* 2003;5:416–422.
10. Kridel RW, Konior RJ, Shumrick KA, et al. Advances in nasal tip surgery. The lateral crural steal. *Arch Otolaryngol Head Neck Surg* 1989;115(10):1206–1212.
11. Goldman IB. The importance of the mesial crura in nasal-tip reconstruction. *Arch Otolaryngol Head Neck Surg* 1957;65:143–147.
12. Dyer WK 2nd, Yune ME. Structural grafting in rhinoplasty. *Facial Plast Surg* 1997;13(4):269–277.

Blepharoplasty

176

Norman J. Pastorek   *Andres Bustillo*

The ideal upper eyelid and brow in women includes a relatively full brow positioned medially at the orbital rim, centrally just at or slightly above the orbital rim, and laterally above the orbital rim. The entire brow should form a gentle arch or should be slightly flat at the center. The lid crease is usually present less than 10 mm above the lid margin. The sulcus below the superior orbital rim should not actually define the bony margin. Laterally, the youthful appearing eye has no hooding of the skin at or beyond the orbital margin and the central lid is free of skin redundancy. The medial upper lid appears concave or flat, never convex. The surgeon should have a general aesthetic sense of the ideal upper eyelid to discuss the subject intelligently with patients. Besides keeping up to date on the current medical literature, it may be valuable to follow the fashion media as well.

A baggy lower lid has always been considered unattractive. The fullness of the orbicularis just beneath the lid margin, a natural look in childhood and early youth, is different from the progressive hypertrophy of the pretarsal orbicularis that can accompany age. Fullness or bagginess beneath the preseptal orbicularis is always unattractive in the adult lower lid and gives the appearance of fatigue or even dissipation. This fullness can be secondary to fat pseudoherniation or preseptal orbicularis muscle swag. Any contribution secondary to fluid retention must be ruled out.

EVALUATION

Evaluation of the patient presenting for blepharoplasty must include both motivational and medical history; examination of both the upper lid-brow complex and the lower lids; and a discussion of the surgical options, the preoperative preparation, the postoperative care and course, and possible problems and complications. Preoperative photographs are taken. Table 176.1 summarizes the diagnosis and evaluation.

Motivational History

As in all aesthetic surgery evaluation, determining the reason a patient is seeking surgery is important. The ideal patient for blepharoplasty has a family history of baggy lids and a relatively long-term desire for reversal of a progressively deteriorating lid appearance. The ideal patient is seeking surgery for self-improvement or would like to maintain or advance in a public-oriented career position and is realistic about the expected result. The patient who appears for aesthetic surgery consultation on a sudden decision is always asked to come for another consultation later to ensure that the decision is reliable. Patients with psychiatric history should have proper consultation and clearance before scheduling surgery. No patient should expect external-world changes as a result of the surgery. A change in the course of a relationship, career, or other goal should never be dependent on the outcome of the surgery.

Many patients presenting for blepharoplasty have had full and heavy upper lids all their lives, even as children. The surgeon will be creating an entirely new look to the

TABLE 176.1   **DIAGNOSIS**
BLEPHAROPLASTY

Complaint of baggy eyelids (progressive)
Positive family history
No allergic, fluid retention, or metabolic etiology
Strong motivation for cosmetic change
Absent or progressive loss of upper lid crease secondary
    to skin redundancy
Upper medial fat pocket herniation
Hooding of lateral upper skin
Herniation of fat into lower lid
Lower lid skin redundancy
Check for lagophthalmos, lower lid laxity, vision loss,
    dry-eye syndrome, ptosis of lacrimal gland, ptosis of eyebrows

patient's face, not one that the patient remembers from the past. It is important that the new look is clearly explained and demonstrated before surgery in this case, especially to a spouse or significant other.

Medical History

Any medical condition that would preclude elective surgery contraindicates blepharoplasty. Care must be taken to evaluate any condition that might be aggravated by the vasoconstrictors in local anesthesia. Many of the newer psychotropic medications can change a patient's normal reactivity to sympathomimetic amines. Any medical problem that causes fluid retention should be controlled before surgery. A few patients have a combination of blepharochalasis and fluid retention of the lower lids. These patients will have persistent lower lid morning edema for several weeks postoperatively. As the scar tissue matures in the lower lids, the edema will resolve. An ophthalmic history is critical. Obvious ophthalmic problems must be dealt with by an ophthalmologist. A patient with full-blown dry-eye syndrome should not have blepharoplasty. The most important problem in this aspect is the occult dry-eye syndrome. Even conservative upper lid blepharoplasty can result in upper lid closure failure, exposing the cornea to drying and bringing an occult dry-eye syndrome into obvious dry-eye syndrome with severe consequences. In these patients, a minimal upper lid skin excision can be done in the patient with severe upper lid skin redundancy to relieve the pressure sensation of the skin weighing on the eyelashes. Any preoperative history of tearing, burning, use of artificial tears, or stinging pain at night requires a full dry-eye evaluation.

A near-field vision test can easily be incorporated into the patient's history form as a reading test with each eye covered in turn. A previous blepharoplasty history is significant in that a secondary procedure must be very conservative to avoid lagophthalmos or significant scleral show.

SURGICAL ANATOMY

The orbicularis muscle is intimately attached to lid skin. It is divided by location into a muscular ring superficial to the tarsus (pretarsal orbicularis) and to the orbital septum (preseptal orbicularis), and an outer muscular ring that extends under the eyebrow and over the inferior orbital rim (orbicularis). The orbital septum is separated from the overlying orbicularis muscle by areolar tissue. The orbital septum is contiguous with the tarsal plates, both having a simular embryonic origin. The orbital septum attaches peripherally to the orbital rim and, with the tarsal plates, forms a diaphragm protecting the orbital contents. The orbital fat compartments, which pseudoherniate in some persons on a hereditary basis, occupy two spaces in the upper lid and three spaces in the lower lid. In the upper lid, the central and medial compartments are divided by the superior oblique muscle. In the lower lid, the central and medial compartments are separated by the inferior oblique muscle. The central and lateral compartments are separated by a fascial sling. The floor of the fat compartments in the upper lid is formed by the levator aponeurosis. The levator aponeurosis attaches to the superior tarsal plate and functions to elevate the lid. In the lower lid, the lower lid retractors attach to the inferior tarsal plate. The lateral canthal ligament inserts into the lateral orbital rim just behind the orbital tubercle. The inferior and superior preseptal orbicularis muscles blend together laterally over the orbital tubercle as the lateral palpebral raphe.

Evaluation of the Upper Lid–Brow Complex

The brow position is all important in considering the aesthetic position of the upper lids. Brows tend to descend from their normal position (as indicated for the ideal position) as the patient ages; however, the brow can be very low at any age. If a substantial amount of upper lid skin redundancy is actually infrabrow skin, the surgeon must be aware that removing this apparent skin redundancy can depress the brow further. The best aesthetic result can be obtained by surgically repositioning the eyebrow into a normal relationship with the superior orbital rim. This can be done by a coronal, hairline, endoscopic, midforehead, or direct brow lift. For the patient with brow ptosis who does not want brow repositioning, the upper lid blepharoplasty must always be a compromise operation, and the patient must understand this. The surgeon must understand that ideal brow position relative to the superior orbital rim is relative. The position is influenced by individual tastes. Whereas a difference of opinion can exist between the patient and surgeon, the patient's desire is always paramount.

Significant unilateral brow ptosis, when present in repose, can be corrected by a midforehead brow lift if forehead rhytids are present. An upper lid blepharoplasty in the presence of an uncorrected unilateral ptosis will make the brow problem more obvious. The elements that can be altered in blepharoplasty include the skin, orbicularis oculi muscle, and fat pseudoherniation. Occasionally, a ptotic lacrimal gland must be repositioned; rarely, an infrabrow fat pad must be excised; and exceedingly rarely, a lateral superior orbital rim bone segment must be removed to improve the overall appearance of the eye. In the evaluation, the surgeon anticipates the amount of skin that must be excised, with special attention to the presence of lateral hooding. The amount of medial and central fat is estimated. The presence of a ptotic lacrimal gland is noted. If, when the lateral upper lid skin is elevated, a bulge is noted in the superior lateral upper lid, then a ptotic gland is suspected. The position of the eyelid crease at the superior tarsal margin is measured as the distance from the lid margin. Orbicularis oculi muscle hypertrophy or redundancy is determined.

Skin type is especially important in upper lid blepharoplasty. The thin-skinned older patient usually requires a conservative resection of fat from the central compartment and a conservative resection of orbicularis oculi muscle as well to avoid a hollow look in the central upper lid sulcus just below the superior orbital rim. Conversely, the patient with heavy skin, especially the younger patient with thick skin who has never had a discernible upper eye crease, requires a more aggressive surgical approach. Surgical creation of a sculptured eyelid in thicker skinned patients requires excision of considerable skin, fat, orbicularis oculi muscle, and possibly a lateral extension of the skin excision. It is important to note the symmetry or asymmetry of the palpebral fissures and to make the patient aware of any unilateral lid ptosis that may be causing asymmetry. A 1- to 2-mm lid ptosis usually is not corrected in an aesthetic surgical procedure. The patient is usually unaware of the minimal palpebral inequality. Demonstrating this palpebral fissure inequality to the patient preoperatively is important. Recent onset of ptosis bears investigation: It may result from opposite-side exophthalmos or same-side Horner syndrome. Finally, it is important to determine whether any degree of lagophthalmos (incomplete eye closure) exists in either eye. Some degree of lagophthalmos is usually present in patients who have had previous blepharoplasty, but it also can be present after even minor lid injuries in youth. The presence of lagophthalmos dictates a conservative blepharoplasty. Although unilateral seventh-nerve weakness is uncommon, the strength of both lids should be tested against pressure to rule it out. It is also important to test for the presence of Bell phenomenon. In a patient with an absent Bell phenomenon, any postoperative lagophthalmos can be especially devastating because the central cornea would be exposed.

Evaluation of the Lower Lid

The lower lid is examined to determine the type of surgical approach to be used to achieve the optimal result. The simplest approach is the transconjunctival. The transconjuctival blepharoplasty, however, is used only in cases of fat psuedoherniation and either absent or very minimal redundant skin or lax orbicularis muscle. This procedure is used mostly in younger patients with early signs of baggy lid secondary to heritary fat psuedoherniation. The very minimal associated skin redundancy (1 to 2 mm) can be treated with the CO_2 or other laser technology or with a "skin pinch" approach in the subciliary line at the time of the transconjuctival blepharoplasty. When fat psuedoherniation is accompanied by skin redundancy and muscle swag, an external subciliary incision allows for either a skin flap alone or a skin-muscle flap to control the skin,

muscle, and fat problems. The skin flap has a very limited usefulness aside from minimal skin redraping. Today, most isolated skin excess can be controlled with the CO_2 or other types laser modalities. Newer intense pulse light technology can also be used to control minimal lower lid skin redundancy. The most useful approach to the aging lower eyelid is the skin-muscle flap. The incorporation of an orbicularis suspension suture with the skin-muscle flap allows for a powerful tightening of the entire lower lid. The relationship of the limbus to the lower lid margin should be noted. Any preoperative scleral show should be viewed by the patient. It is most important to measure the strength of the orbicularis oculi muscle and tension of the lid. Opening the lid with gentle force while the patient is holding the lids tightly closed gives an impression of the strength of the seventh nerve. Occasionally, unilateral seventh nerve weakness is present in the orbicularis oculi muscle. Pulling the lower lid away from the globe and then quickly releasing it allows the surgeon to determine the lid strength or laxity (snap test) (Fig. 176.1). The lid should spring quickly to contact the globe without the influence of blinking. If the lid does not snap back to touch the globe but remains away from the globe until the patient blinks, a lid-shortening procedure is indicated. This procedure is beyond the scope of the chapter.

The lower bony orbital margin is palpated to determine to what extent, if any, the bony margin is contributing to the lower lid appearance. The presence and extent of malar or cheek bags are noted. These edematous skin conditions

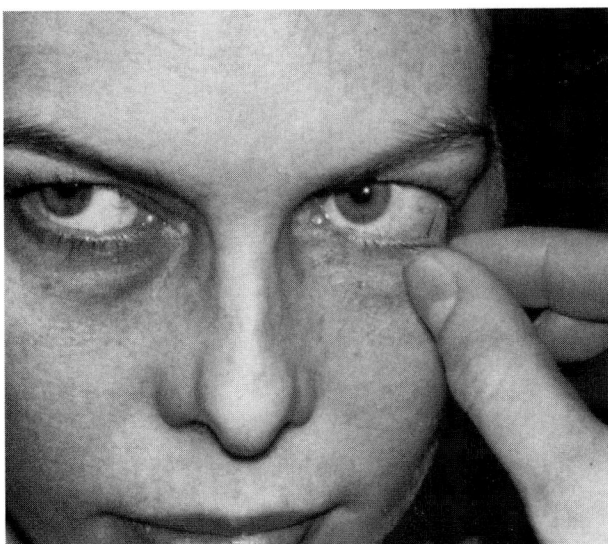

Figure 176.1 The lower lid is tested for tension strength by grasping the lower lid skin, pulling the lid slightly away from the globe, and releasing it. The normal lid should snap back quickly against the globe. Having the patient look down while performing this maneuver tests the ultimate lid tension. A slow return indicates caution with skin excision and the possible need for a horizontal lid-shortening procedure. No return or a very slow return may contraindicate aesthetic blepharoplasty.

can result from fluid retention or the presence of a palpebromalar raphe. This condition is distinct from fat herniation and is present below the orbital rim away from the lid itself over the malar eminence. This malar bag is difficult to treat and may not be entirely eliminated even with placement of the suspension suture.

In both the upper and lower lids, note the presence of any skin lesions (e.g., syringoma, trichoepithelioma, hyperplastic sebaceous glands, papilloma, or xanthoma). These may or may not be excised at the same time as blepharoplasty. Removal of these lesions is separate from the blepharoplasty procedure for the surgeon. The lesions are seen as part of the problem for the patient.

At this point, after a complete examination of the lower lids, a decision is made to approach the lower lids via a suspension skin-muscle flap or via a transconjunctival incision. The older patient with large fat pseudoherniation, significant redundant skin, and prominent orbicularis muscle swags is an obvious case for skin-muscle flap because this approach allows for adequate skin removal and tightening of the loose muscle and skin with a suspension suture. The younger patient with smooth skin, moderate fat pseudoherniation, and no muscle swag is an obvious candidate for transconjunctival blepharoplasty because no need is seen to remove skin or tighten the muscle. Since the advent of the CO_2 resurfacing laser and other laser skin tightening technologies, the indications for transconjunctival blepharoplasty have expanded. It is possible both to smooth fine wrinkles and to tighten the lower lid skin to some degree with the other modalities, lessening the need for the skin-muscle flap procedurein patients who have 1 to 2 mm of estimated skin laxity. Beyond 3 mm of skin laxity, it is probably best to use the skin-muscle flap. By pushing the skin-tightening features of the laser, the risk is increased that scleral show, ectropion, or scarring might occur because of tissue contraction. Also, overuse of the CO_2 laser can result in thinning of the skin which, in the long term, can *produce* fine rhytids. The subciliary scar of skin-muscle blepharoplasty has never been an aesthetic problem. Using the transconjunctival approach simply to avoid this scar would be a mistake. The skin-muscle procedure does take longer than the transconjunctival approach, but it remains a reliable method to tighten the loose lid skin and muscle. Expediency in lower lid blepharoplasty should be a minor factor in surgical judgment. The patient should be aware of the surgical plan and should understand the reason for a particular approach.

Malar bags (skin wrinkling or edema extending over the malar complex) may not be entirely removed with blepharoplasty and may keep the same appearance. Lateral orbital rhytids beyond the orbital rim probably will not be affected at all by blepharoplasty, but can be helped to some extent by laser resurfacing and the use of botulinum neurotoxin injections.

PHOTOGRAPHY

As with any aesthetic surgical procedure, preoperative photographic documentation is imperative. It can be done by a professional photographer or by the surgeon. Photographs must be standardized. The usual views include a full face at a ratio of 1:10, followed by close-up lid views at a ratio of 1:5 or 1:4. These close-up views are frontal eyes open, frontal gaze upward, frontal eyes closed, both obliques, and both laterals. For a detailed discussion of photodocumentation, see Chapter 169.

PREPARATION FOR SURGERY

The decision to perform blepharoplasty is based on favorable psychological, general medical, and lid examinations. The patient's expectations should coincide with what is possible surgically. All patients are prepared for surgery with an in-depth, preoperative discussion about what is expected of the patient before surgery, what the operation will be like, what the normal postoperative course will be, and what problems and complications can occur.

All medications that interfere with blood coagulation must be avoided for 2 weeks before surgery. This includes aspirin, nonsteroidal antiinflammatory drugs, vitamin E, and anticoagulant herbal preparations, especially gingko, gensing, grape seed oil, and garlic capsules. Alcohol should be avoided for approximately 4 days before surgery. Any postoperative physical activity, especially sports and excersize programs that can interfere with the surgical result, are discussed. Financial arrangements and the surgeon's payment policies are discussed.

THE OPERATION

Anesthesia

Most blepharoplasty surgery can be performed satisfactorily with the patient under local anesthesia as an outpatient or ambulatory procedure using preoperative and intraoperative sedation and analgesia. Lidocaine (2% with 1:100,000 epinephrine) buffered with sodium bicarbonate (8.4% in a ratio of 10 mL lidocaine and 1 mL bicarbonate) is used for local anesthesia. About 1 mL is infiltrated into the eyelid skin with a 1.5-inch 25- or 27-gauge needle. At least 10 minutes must elapse before the incision to allow for adequate vasoconstriction. If all four lids are being done under local anesthesia, it may be advisable to mix bupivacaine 0.25% in equal amounts with the lidocaine solution to provide for a prolonged anesthesia of the lids. If a transconjunctival approach is planned for the lower lids, tetracaine 0.25% drops are used in the inferior conjunctival cul de sac before injection. The transconjunctival injection is best done with a 30-gauge needle. Of all the tissues of the face, the eyelids maintain anesthesia for the shortest period. If all four lids are anesthetized at the same time, sensation may return before the final lid is completed. It is advisable to first anesthetize the upper lids and the lower lids later as the upper lids are completed. Optimal anesthesia then will be present as each lid is operated. The needle is *always* held in a direction parallel to the eyelid. This eliminates the possibility of the patient ever moving upward into a needle directed vertically to the eyelid.

Surgical Marking

Surgical marking of the upper lids begins with a thorough removal of all skin oils with alcohol. A fine-line surgical pen is used to demarcate the upper lid crease. Easily seen in a bright light, this is the upper anatomic boundary of the tarsal plate. The line should be at least 8 mm above the upper lid margin. If it is less than 8 mm, then the skin mark is placed above the natural crease at a distance of 8 to

10 mm. The lid creases are usually symmetric; any asymmetry is adjusted so that the two planned lid creases are symmetric and 8 to 10 mm above the margin. The line is carried medially to include all the crêped skin into the sulcus into the nasal junction. Laterally, the line is carried to the sulcus between the lateral orbital rim and lid. If hooding is seen of the skin lateral to this point, the drawn line angles slightly upward (Fig. 176.2).

When the patient is in a supine position, the weight of the forehead and scalp displaces the eyebrows superiorly. To estimate upper lid skin removal correctly, the brow is pushed gently downward with the thumb and forefinger. The redundant skin is grasped gently with forceps. The lower blade is at the already marked lid crease, and the upper blade is in the region of the maximal estimated excision (Fig. 176.3A). With forceps blade closure, the upper lid margin should not elevate. This amount of skin excision allows for cosmetic enhancement but not for lagophthalmos. The skin is marked at several points, and the

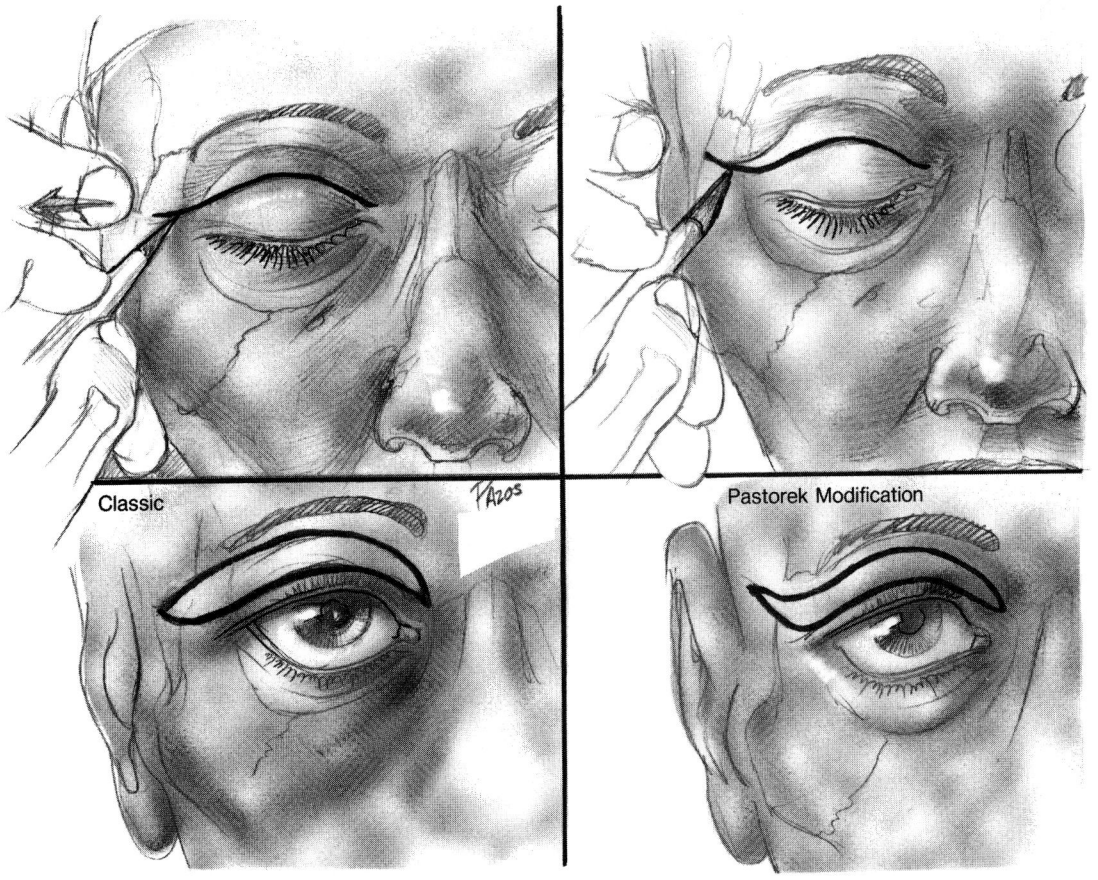

A   **B**

Figure 176.2   A: The classic extension of the upper lid skin excision is in a horizontal line carried laterally at the orbital rim. This line classically was placed in a lateral rhytid (crow's foot). This extension, however, often made a fine lateral rhytid permanent and more obvious and also had the effect of pulling the lateral brow downward. **B:** By curving the lateral skin excision upward into the space between the lateral canthus and the lateral eyebrow, the wound can be camouflaged by cosmetics. The other major advantage is that natural tethering, which is present close to the lateral brow, prevents the downward pull of the brow.

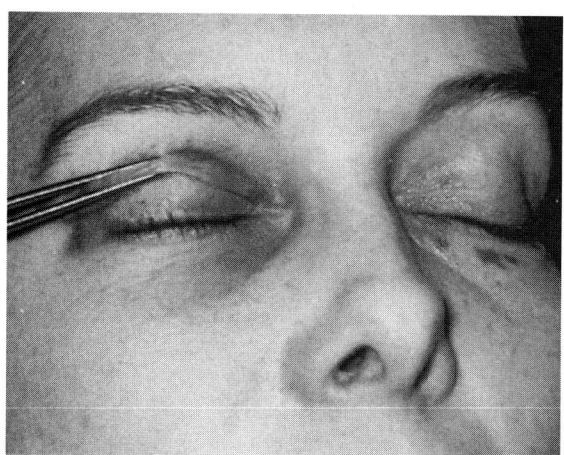
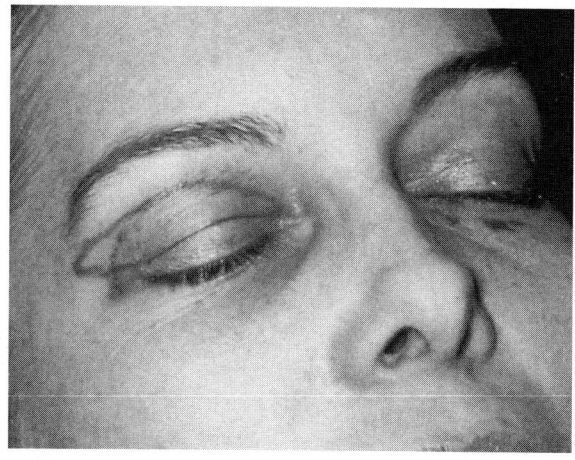

A

B

Figure 176.3 **A:** Estimating the amount of upper lid skin excision. As the redundant skin is drawn together with a forceps, the upper lid margin should not elevate. **B:** The redundant skin is completely marked. The amount of excision that extends beyond the orbital rim is indicated with the patient's eyes closed.

points are connected into a line. The lateral extent of the skin excision is determined by the amount of lateral hooded skin. The skin excision must incorporate all lateral hooding (Fig. 176.3B). If necessary, the incision can be carried 1 cm or more past the orbital margin. The direction of the final scar should be planned to lie between the lateral brow and the lateral canthus. In this position, the scar can be camouflaged by eye shadow makeup in the immediate postoperative period.

The medial skin redundancy should always be underestimated slightly if the patient has a large medial fat compartment. The defect caused by the excision of a large fat compartment is likely to create a subcutaneous dead space. If slightly less skin is removed, the skin can drape into the defect rather than tenting over the defect at the time of closure. Medial tenting of skin is a cause for hypertrophic scarring postoperatively. Both medially and laterally, the skin excision lines should meet at 30-degree angles.

If a skin-muscle flap is planned, the lower lid is marked at the lateral lid at a point 2.5 mm below the lid margin and just at the lateral canthus. The entire incision medial to the point continues along at 2.5 mm below the lid margin in the subciliary crease to the lacrimal puncta. Lateral to this point, the incision breaks to become horizontal just as it crosses the orbital rim. The incision should not angle downward laterally.

Upper Lid

It is customary to complete both upper lid procedures before beginning surgery on the lower lids. The initial incision is made across the lower limb of the planned skin excision in a single sweep while holding the lid skin taut, followed by a skin incision of the upper limb. The skin excision is completed by separating the skin from the orbicularis muscle with a curved Stevens scissors. Next, the orbic-

ularis muscle is excised in all but the most thin-skinned patients. The muscle excision removes a central trough of orbicularis muscle along the path of the skin excision (Fig. 176.4A). The depth of the excision is to the orbital septum. In the upper lid, the central fat compartment is the easiest to remove initially. A large amount of central fat can completely obscure the medial fat compartment. The orbital septum is opened sharply and the fat is teased into the wound. Only fat that easily flows into the wound is removed. The fat is infiltrated with local anesthetic, clamped, and excised. The stump is cauterized with hot tip or electrocautery to eliminate bleeding once the clamp is released. The use of an electocautery under local anesthesisa can cause pain even if the fat is injected with xylocaine.

The medial compartment usually requires some gentle exploration, especially in cases of a small amount of fat. If the medial fat compartment is identified as an aesthetic problem preoperatively, it must be sought at the time of surgery. Gentle pressure on the globe usually makes its location obvious. The central and medial fat compartments are separated by the superior oblique oculi muscle. This muscle is rarely observed, but it is wise to look for it before clamping the medial fat.

Theoretically, a lateral fat compartment should not be present in the upper lid; sometimes in a patient with larger amounts of fat, a lateral compartment is found overlying the lacrimal gland (Fig. 176.4B and C). If a ptotic lacrimal gland is identified, a 6-0 polypropylene suture needle is used to carefully pick up the gland capsule. The needle is the used to pick up the periosteum of the orbital roof just behind the orbital rim. As the knot is pulled tight, the gland advances upward into its normal position. Polypropylene 6-0 is recommended for wound closure. It is a reliable suture that will not leave suture marks, even if left in place for more than the usual 3 to 4 days. The most tension in the upper lid closure occurs laterally. This portion of the wound

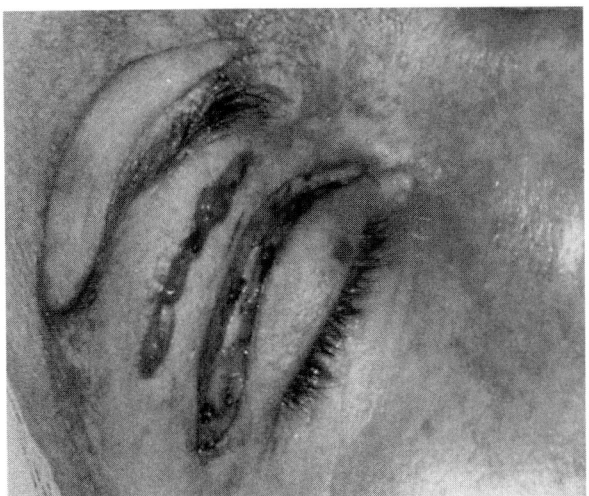

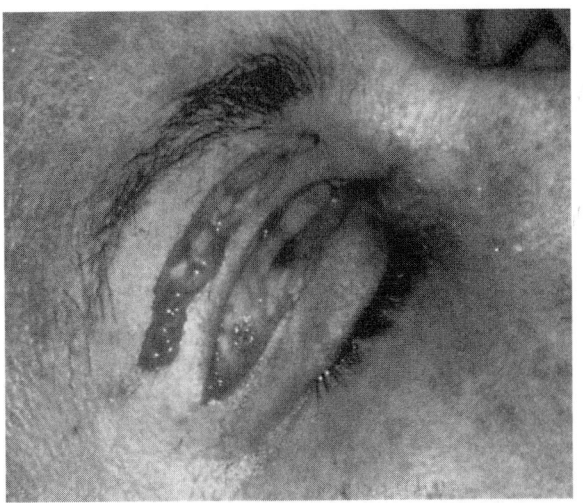

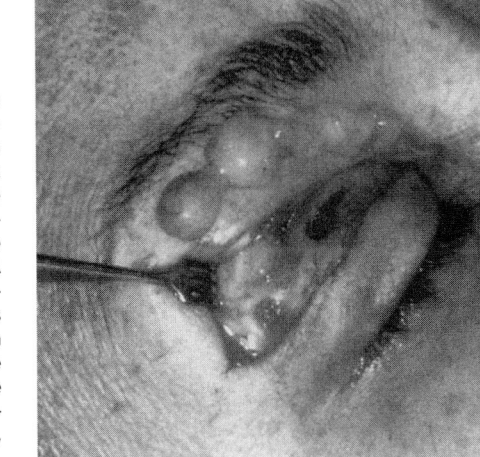

Figure 176.4 **A:** A strip of orbicularis oculi muscle has been excised down to the orbital septum. This muscle excision is variable. In the thin-skinned older eyelid, sometimes no muscle is removed, whereas in the heavy lid with thick skin, the muscle is often hypertrophic, requiring considerable excision. The purpose of the muscle excision is to define better the lid crease by allowing scarring at the wound closure to the region of the superior border of the tarsal plate. **B:** A large amount of hypertrophic orbicularis oculi muscle requires excision down to the orbital septum. **C:** Large amounts of pseudoherniated fat have been excised. In this patient, a lateral fat compartment was present over the area of the lacrimal gland. The gland is displaced by the retractor. If the gland is ptotic, it must be reattached to the orbital roof periosteum by a polypropylene suture. If it is not resuspended, it will be palpable as a subcutaneous nodule.

is closed with interrupted simple sutures (Fig. 176.5). The rest of the wound is closed with a subcuticular suture, beginning medially and continuing laterally. It is unnecessary to knot the ends of the subcuticular suture. To alleviate any tension in the lateral portion of the wound, this area can be taped at the conclusion of the procedure. If any redundancy still exists medially, small triangles of skin can be excised above and below the closure line. The triangle's base is at the initial incision. Usually, these excisions do not require closure, but paper tape can be used if necessary.

Lower Lid

Skin-Muscle Flap Approach

The lower lid incision is made with a small sharp blade at the lateral canthal mark 2.5 mm below the lid margin in the subciliary crease. The initial incision is through the skin and measures about 6 to 7 mm. A small, straight, sharp scissors then is used to carry the subcutaneous incision medially to the puncta (Fig. 176.6). A small skin flap then is developed for about 3 mm to expose and preserve

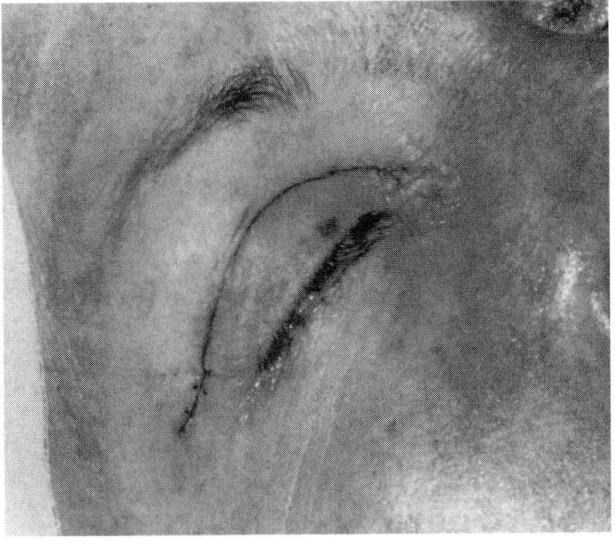

Figure 176.5 The surgical wound is closed laterally with individual polypropylene sutures because this is the area of maximal tension in eyelid wound closure. The remainder of the wound, centrally and medially, is closed with a subcuticular polypropylene suture.

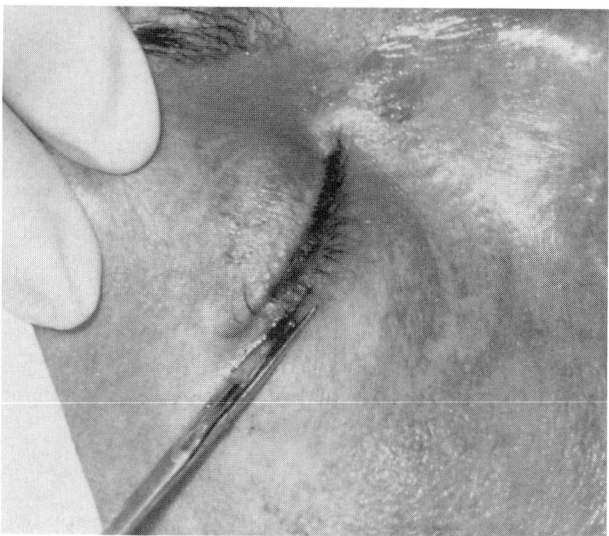

Figure 176.6   The lower lid is marked for a distance of less than 1 cm at the lateral canthus. This line parallels the orbital margin and is 2.5 mm below the margin. The skin incision is made over the skin marking. The remainder of the lower lid incision is made with a small straight sharp scissors. The incision is carried to the lacrimal puncta.

the pretarsal fibers of the orbicularis oculi muscle (Fig. 176.7). By preserving this pretarsal sling, the lid will have more immediate tension response after surgery, reducing the possibility of scleral show or ectropion. A curved Stevens scissors then is used to separate the preseptal and pretarsal muscle to the puncta. This incision stays above the orbital septum. Blunt dissection with a cotton-tipped applicator sweeps the preseptal orbicularis muscle away from the orbital septum to the orbital rim exposing the lateral, central, and medial fat compartments (Fig. 176.8A).

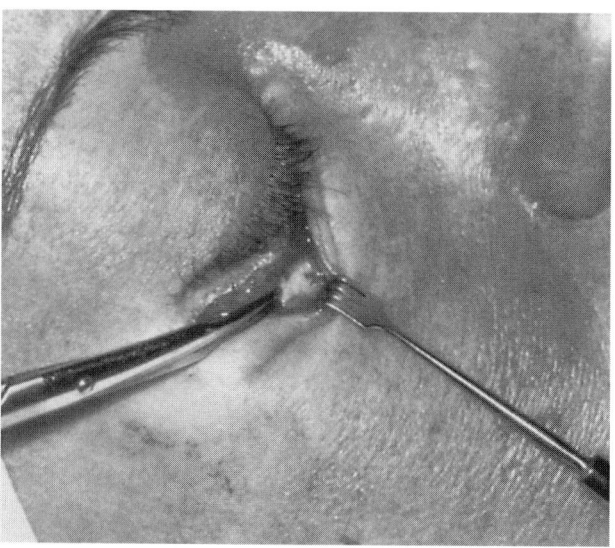

Figure 176.7   A skin flap is developed for 3 to 4 mm. This skin flap allows the pretarsal orbicularis oculi muscle to remain intact along the entire lid margin, providing an active muscle sling for lid support immediately and lessening the possibility of scleral show and ectropion.

Fat removal is begun laterally. The orbital septum over the lateral fat compartment is very dense and is separated from the central fat compartment by a fascial barrier (Fig. 176.8B). Local anesthetic infiltration into this fat, clamping, excision, and cautery are the same as for the upper lid. The central compartment fat pad is usually the most obvious and the easiest to remove in the lower lid (Fig. 176.8C). The medial fat compartment, which is more elusive, usually contains more fat than is obvious from the patient's supine position. In this compartment, it is usually necessary to tease the fat from the orbit somewhat more aggressively than the central or lateral compartments (Fig. 176.9).

Before clamping the medial fat pocket, the inferior oblique muscle should be observed. In contrast to the situation in the upper lid, this muscular structure is almost always visible and should be found before clamping to avoid injury to the muscle. The fat in this location is also more dense and vascular than in the other compartments of the lower lid. Hemostasis here must be absolute to avoid a bleeding medial fat stump that could retract back into the orbit. The fat excision in the lower lid should leave the orbital rim exposed 1 mm. This depth of fat excision provides a good aesthetic result with no depression along the inferior orbital rim. If the preoperative examination revealed a tear trough deformity (i.e., a deep sulcus along the medial eyelid–bony orbital rim junction), the surgeon should consider a fat repositioning procedure. Fat repositioning will either partially, or less frequently, entirely efface the depth of the tear trough. The neccessity of repositioning is made before surgery. The orbital septum in incised at the inferior orbital rim (arcus marginalis). The fat is teased into the wound. The medial orbicularis muscle is then elevated away from the medial one third of the infraorbital bone. Care is taken not to injure the infraorbital nerve. If the periosteum is left intact, it is possible to suture the fat down into the depths of the tear trough. The authors have found that simply moving the fat down onto the anterior face of the maxilla beneath the elevated orbicularis muscle is sufficient to efface the tear trough. Some surgeons have advocated placing a trancutaneous suture through the repositioned orbital fat. If central compartment fat is removed so that it lies just 1 mm below the rim, the transitional area between lid and bony rim should be smooth.

The suspension suture in the lateral orbicularis will prevent a depression in the lateral eyelid-lateral orbital rim junction. Before beginning closure, the lateral fat compartment is inspected again to determine whether additional fat should be removed. Also, the area beneath the fascial barrier separating the lateral and medial compartments occasionally sequesters a small amount of the central compartment fat. This area should be inspected if additional fat needs to be removed.

Once fat removal, or repositioning, and hemostasis are complete, the skin-muscle flap is draped superiorly. Skin excision is done with a straight Stevens scissors while the patient is looking upward with the mouth open (Fig. 176.10).

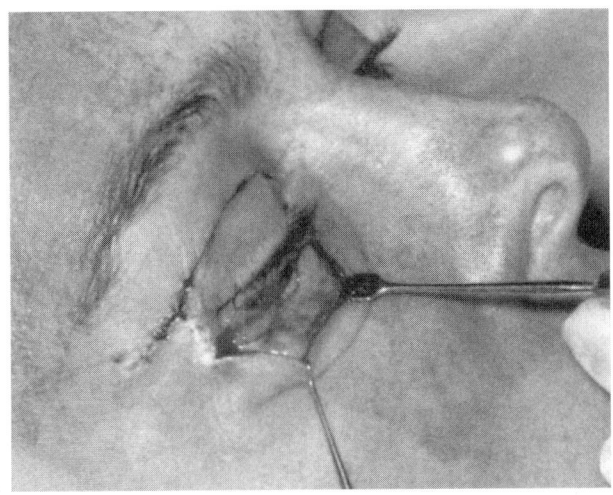

A

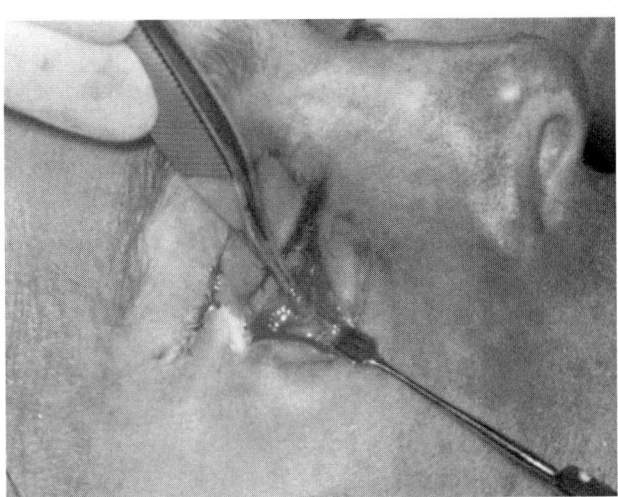

B

Figure 176.8 **A:** The skin-muscle flap is elevated down to the inferior orbital rim. Festooning of the muscle or extreme skin redundancy dictates that the skin-muscle flap is extended further inferiorly. In such situations, the surgeon should note that a blood vessel accompanies the eyelid nerve branch from the infraorbital nerve. When cut, this muscle bleeds vigorously. Cautery of the vessel invariably affects the sensory nerve, producing hypesthesia in the lower lid that can be prolonged. **B:** The lateral fat pocket lies high against the junction of the lower orbital rim and the lateral rim. It is divided from the middle compartment by a fascial barrier. The orbital septum is heaviest in the lateral region. The fat pocket, once encountered and drawn into the wound, can cause deep pain, which must be alleviated by a local anesthesia injection. The thickness of the orbital septum can camouflage the lateral fat pocket. If the lateral fat pocket was identified as a problem during the preoperative evaluation, it must be sought at surgery. **C:** The central fat compartment is the most obvious and must be removed to a level at least 2 mm below the orbital margin to produce an aesthetic effect. Removal of fat is accomplished by first injecting a small amount of local anesthesia to prevent pain when the hemostat is applied. A small cuff of fat must be left on the clamp to allow application of the hot-tipped cautery.

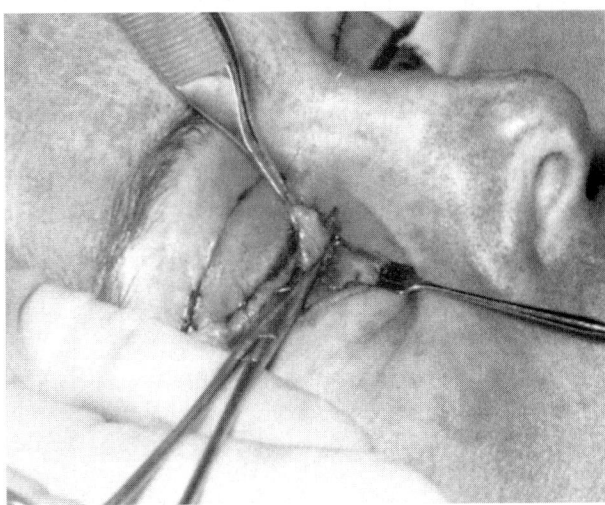

C

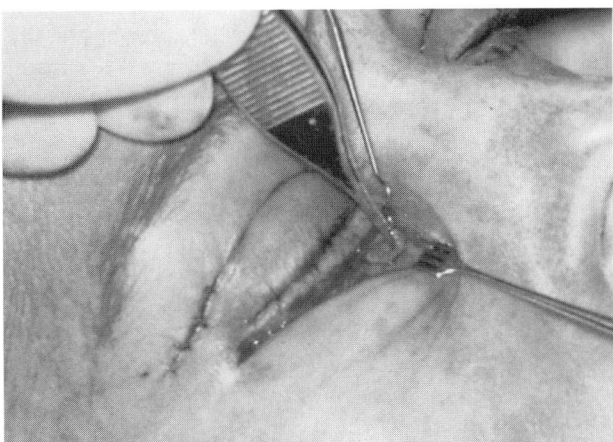

Figure 176.9 The medial fat pocket is teased into the wound after the orbital septum is opened. The inferior oblique muscle must be observed while the medial fat pocket is being clamped to ensure that no injury occurs to the muscle. If the patient has a tear trough deformity (a deep depression at the maxillary–medial lid junction), the fat is repositioned rather than excised. A pocket is developed by firmly elevating the medial orbicularis muscle from its firm attachment to the medal maxilla. The fat is released by an arcus marginalis incision and positioned beneath the muscle. It can be secured with a 6-0 polydioxanone suture (PDS), but this has not been found to be absolutely necessary for the fat to remain in the new postion.

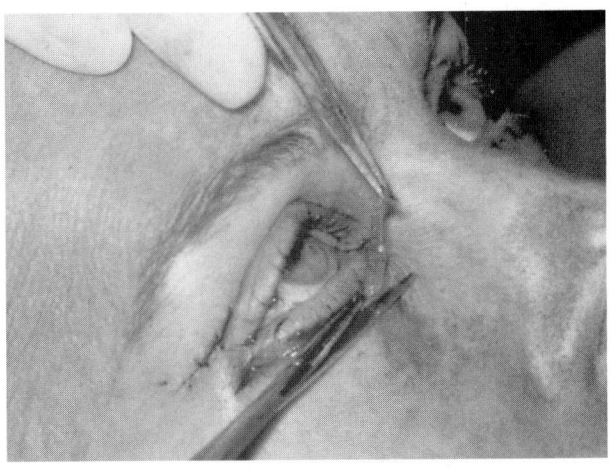

Figure 176.10 The amount of redundant lower lid skin to be removed is gauged while having the patient look upward with the mouth open. If the amount of skin to be removed leaves the two skin edges in complete opposition, little possibility of scleral show or ectropion exists. The patient and surgeon may believe that not enough skin was removed. If slightly more skin is excised, the lid can be supported by a suspension suture to ensure an appropriate lid level and obtain maximal skin tightness.

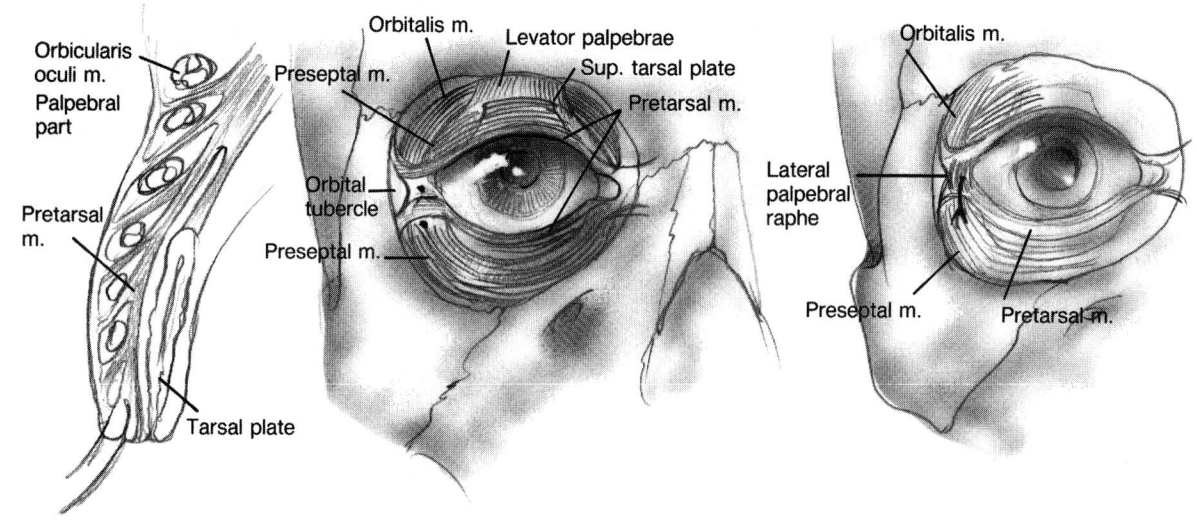

Figure 176.11 A: This view shows the orbicularis muscle reflected off the orbital rim and the two areas that are encompassed by the needle and suture for the suspension suture (*arrow*). *1*, The periosteum over the orbital tubercle; *2*, the preseptal orbicularis muscle. **B:** The direction of the suspension suture must be vertical.

This maneuver places maximal tension on the lower lid, providing a guide for the safe excision of skin and muscle. To ensure that no downward pull occurs on the lower lid, no wound gap should exist after excision with the patient looking upward with the mouth open. This can be achieved under general anesthesia by making sure the limbus is covered by the lower lid margin by at least 1mm. This minimal safe excision, however, can leave some patients with some skin redundancy. To allow further excision of skin, to prevent scleral show, and to draw the lateral skin upward, a lid suspension suture is used after excision of skin (Fig. 176.11A). The lid suspension suture is placed between the lateral orbicularis oculi muscle in the skin-muscle flap and the lateral orbital periosteum (Fig. 176.11B). The most appropriate suture is a clear 5-0 polypropylene. The suture is placed in a vertical direction so that the lid is pulled neither laterally nor medially. It is a buried suture placed so that when tied, the knot will be directed downward. The suture is placed so no purchase occurs on the subcutaneous tissue and, hence, no indentation of the lid skin at the point of suture.

Once these suspension sutures are placed, the wound is closed with a simple running 6-0 polypropylene suture (Fig. 176.12). Multiple surgical tapes are used to suspend the lid laterally and resist the downward pull on the postoperative lid. Figure 176.13 shows preoperative and postoperative views of one patient after upper lid blepharoplasty and lower lid skin-muscle blepharoplasty. Table 176.2 summarizes the procedures.

Transconjunctival Approach

After the application of tetracaine drops to the lower lid and scleral conjunctiva, lidocaine (2% with epinephrine 1:100,000) is injected into the subconjunctival space along the inferior margin of the tarsal plate from the puncta medially to the lateral canthus (Fig. 176.14). The lower lid is also injected subcutaneously as if a skin-muscle flap is to be done. The subcutaneous injection provides increased relaxation of the orbicularis muscle for improved visualization of the orbital fat. It also provides anesthesia if the lower lid skin is to be laser resurfaced or if a pinch of skin is to be removed.

The procedure begins with an incision through the conjunctiva along the inferior tarsal border and through the attached inferior lid retractors (Fig. 176.15). Because of the vascularity of the arcuate vessels in this area, it is essential the incision is made with a fine electrodissection needle, such as the Colorado pediatric microdissection. The fine needle does minimal damage to the tear glands in the conjuctiva. Two sutures of silk or polyester fiber are placed

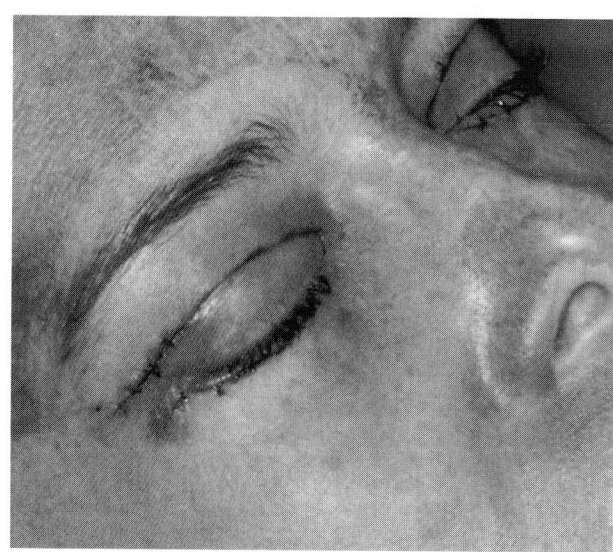

Figure 176.12 The immediate postoperative appearance of the upper and lower lid skin-muscle flap blepharoplasty.

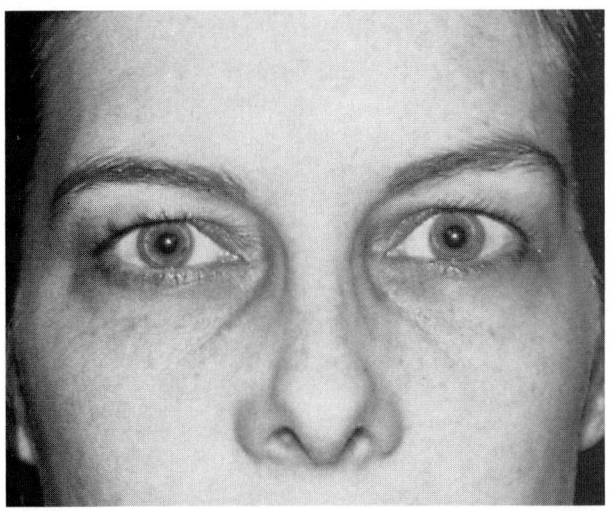

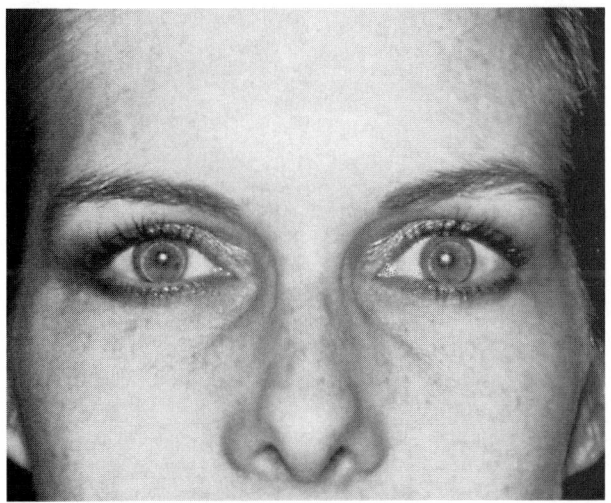

A

B

Figure 176.13 **A:** Preoperative frontal view of upper and lower lid skin-muscle blepharoplasty in a woman 29 years of age. **B:** Postoperative view.

through the proximal conjunctiva at the incision line approximately at the location of the medial and lateral limbus margin. These sutures are draped over the patient's forehead and frontal area (Fig. 176.16).

TABLE 176.2 ℞ **TREATMENT**

BLEPHAROPLASTY

Upper lid
Excision of redundant skin
Orbicularis muscle
Herniated fat

Lower lid
Excision of skin redundancy
Orbicularis muscle (if required)
Herniated fat
Postoperative cold compresses
Limitation of physical activity
Preoperative and postoperative avoidance of anticoagulants
Suture removal 3–4 days postoperative

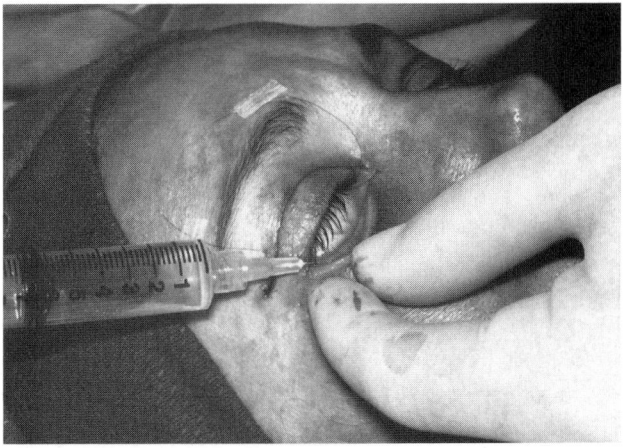

Figure 176.14 After application of tetracaine drops to the conjunctiva, the subconjunctival space is infiltrated with lidocaine (2% with epinephrine) along the inferior tarsal border from the puncta medially to the area of the lateral canthus.

Hemostats applied to the suture ends act as a gentle weight, pulling the proximal conjunctiva over the cornea. The dissection is now immediately over the orbital septum and under the orbicularis muscle. Firm blunt dissection separates the orbicularis away from the orbital septum down to the orbital rim. At this point, the exposure is identical to the presentation afforded by the skin-muscle flap after separating the flap from the orbital septum. Each of the three fat pseudohernias is opened as with the skin-muscle flap and resected sharply after clamping (Fig. 176.17). Fat is removed to 1 mm below the orbital margin. A hot tip or electrocautery is used on the fat stumps. The orbital septum is not repaired. The lid is grasped and elevated superiorly and released. Gentle compression of the globe will reveal any pulsation of orbital fat irregularity and provide a

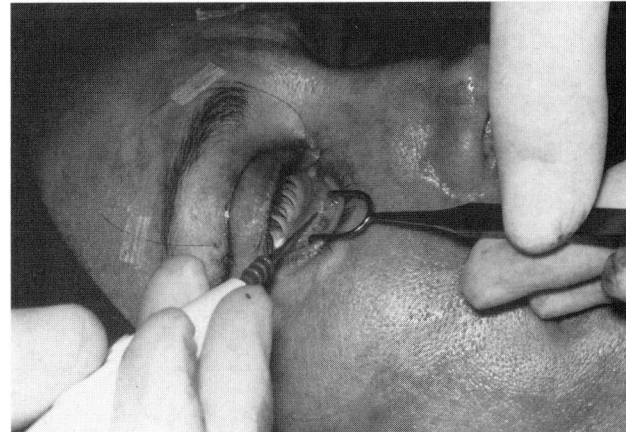

Figure 176.15 The initial incision in the conjunctiva is made with a fine guarded electrocautery needle. The arcuate vessels immediately beneath the conjunctiva will bleed profusely if this incision is made without the use of electrocautery. The incision is made quickly to avoid dissipating heat into the adjacent conjunctiva. The tear glands in this conjunctiva are valuable and necessary for the protective tear film. Destruction of these glands has led to dry eye by using the wider destructive swath that can be caused by a CO_2 laser used for this incision.

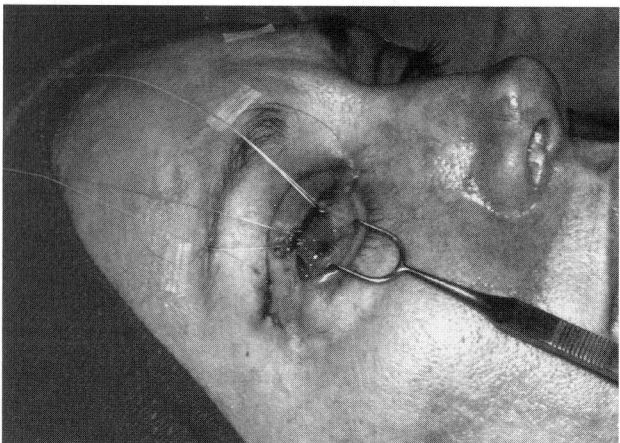

Figure 176.16 A pair of sutures placed through the proximal side of the conjunctival incision are used to drape the conjunctiva over the cornea. The sutures are clamped with a hemostat to give weight to the suture retraction. A corneal shell also can be used.

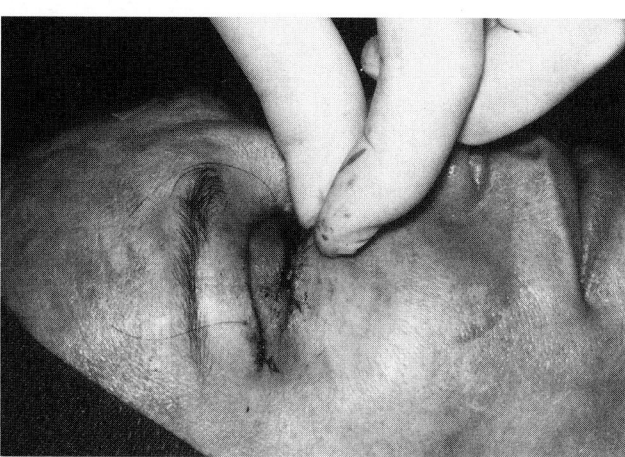

Figure 176.19 At completion of the procedure, the lid is elevated as far superiorly as possible and released, ensuring that the edges of the conjunctival incision are in close apposition. No sutures are required in the incision. Sutures can be contraindicated because they will irritate the sclera or cornea or cause granulation.

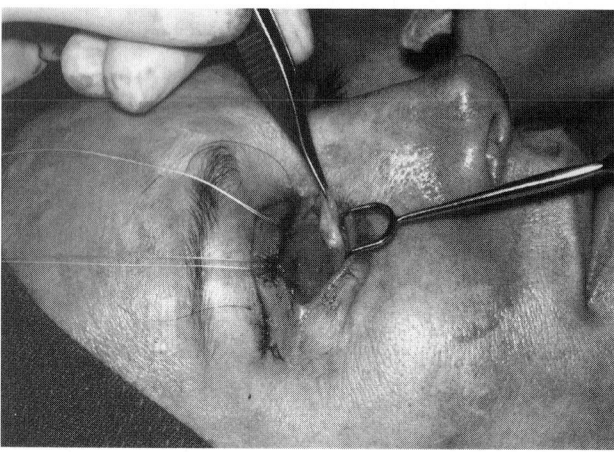

Figure 176.17 After the incision through the inferior lid retractors, blunt dissection is used to separate the orbicularis muscle away from the orbital septum, down to the orbital rim. The orbicularis muscle is retracted with a blunt double-pronged hook. Exposure at this point is exactly the same as that with a skin-muscle flap. The fat pseudohernias are removed from the lateral, central, and medial compartments in the same fashion as with the skin-muscle flap.

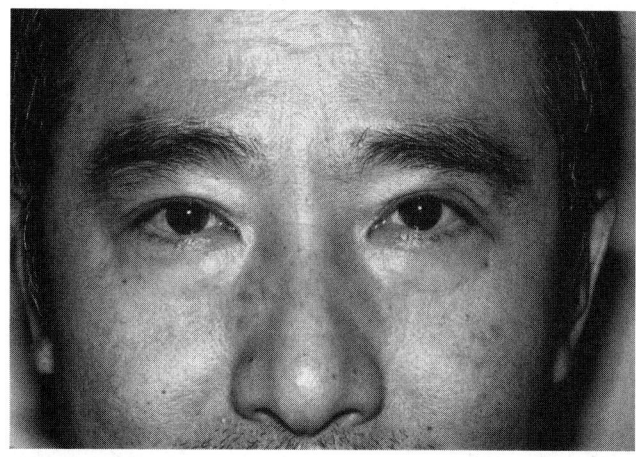

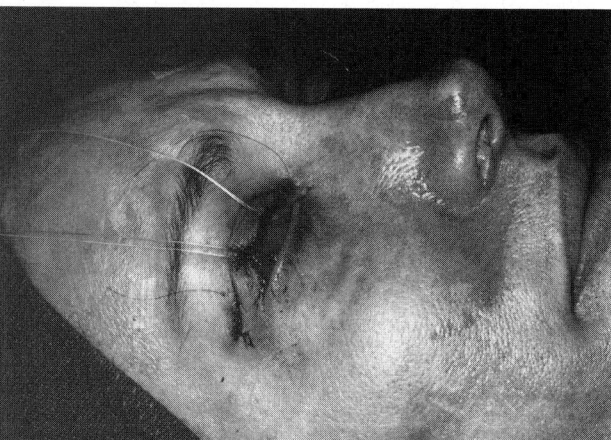

Figure 176.18 After fat removal, the lower lid skin is redraped in its normal position. With gentle pressure on the globe, nuances of additional fat can be detected as they pulse outward beneath the lid skin and muscle. Any additional fat then is carefully removed.

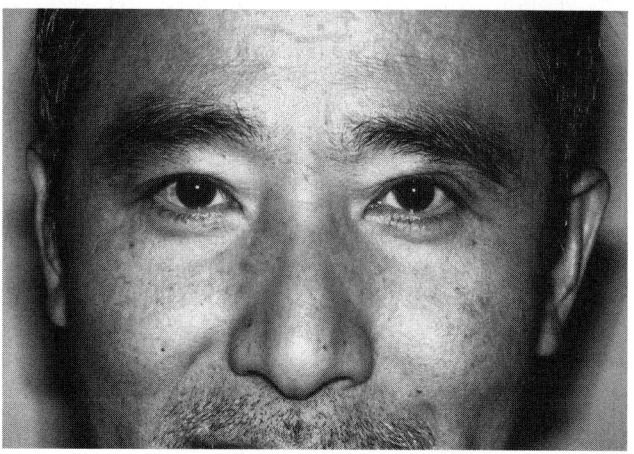

Figure 176.20 **A:** A man 48 years of age with massive familial lower lid pseudoherniation of fat. **B:** Postoperative view of the patient after transconjunctival lower lid blepharoplasty.

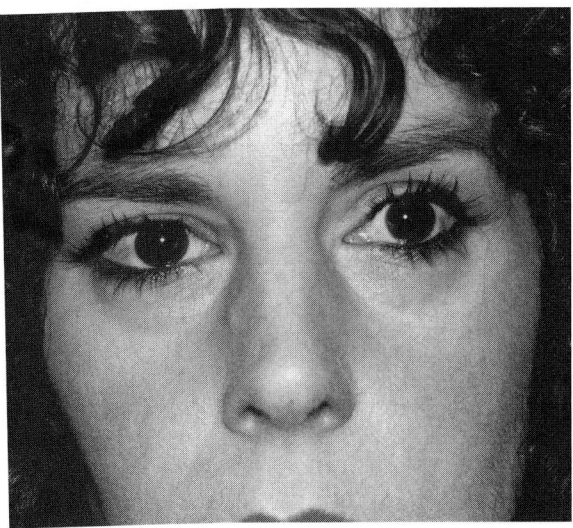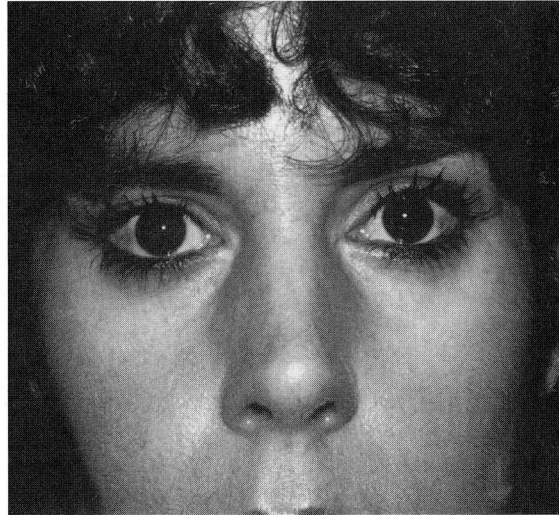

Figure 176.21   A: A woman 35 years of age with marked lower lid familial blepharochalasis. **B:** Postoperative view after lower lid transconjunctival blepharoplasty.

guide to any additional subtle fat removal (Fig. 176.18). As in the skin-muscle flap procedure descibed above, the medial fat can be repositioned beneath the medial orbitalis muscle to efface any tear trough deformity. The retraction sutures then are cut, and the lid is again draped superiorly to ensure that the transconjunctival incision lies in approximation (Fig. 176.19). Sutures are not required to close the transconjunctival incision. If any laser resurfacing is planned, it can be done just before removing the retraction sutures so that the benefit of corneal protection is continued during laser use. Skin removal with the pinch technique is done after releasing the traction sutures.

Several quarter-inch surgical tape strips are used laterally to help support the lid during the stage of continued anesthesia effect and later while the lid is heavy with post-surgical edema. Figures 176.20 and 176.21 demonstrate preoperative and postoperative views of patients who have had transconjunctival lower lid blepharoplasty. Both patients had remarkable orbital pseudoherniation of fat without any fine-skin wrinkling or skin laxity preoperatively. At the conclusion of the transconjunctival blepharoplasty in a patient with fine wrinkling or minimal skin laxity, a CO_2 skin resurfacing procedure can be done immediately to smooth and tighten the skin. The skin resurfacing also can be done at a later date if fine wrinkling becomes apparent in the proximal postoperative period.

POSTOPERATIVE CARE

No bandages are used on the lower lids, but the eyes are covered by cold compresses. The wounds are lubricated with an antibiotic ointment. The patient should remain quiet for the remainder of the day of surgery. The cold compresses are used continuously. Pain is usually minimal; acetaminophen with codeine is usually adequate for pain relief. Looking

downward for the next 24 hours is forbidden because the downward gaze could allow the skin-muscle flap to slide inferiorly over the underlying orbicularis septum. Occasionally, after transconjunctival lower lid blepharoplasty, the patient will notice a temporary lower lid elevation, which is caused by the transection of the lower lid retractors away from their attachment to the inferior tarsal plate. It is common to note slight bleeding from the transconjunctival incision, which is seen as a drop of blood on the lower lid margin. The bleeding is entirely self-limited.

Only sedentary activities are allowed until the sutures are removed on the third or fourth postoperative day. It is usually advisable to retape the lateral upper wound for 2 to 3 days more to prevent even minimal wound separation. Eye makeup can be used on the sixth postoperative day. Mild physical activities can resume on the tenth postoperative day. Contact lenses can be safely used at 9 to 10 days postoperatively.

COMPLICATIONS

Complications and emergencies are listed in Tables 176.3 and 176.4.

Hematoma

Hematoma is rare after upper lid blepharoplasty, but is more common after lower lid blepharoplasty. Unilateral swelling and discoloration immediately postoperatively should raise the question of hematoma that should be differentiated from ecchymosis, which would appear dark but soft; hematoma has a palpable firmness. The wound is reopened, the bleeding vessel cauterized, and the wound closed. Meticulous hemostasis during surgery is the best preventative of hematoma. Because the transconjunctival

TABLE 176.3	COMPLICATIONS
BLEPHAROPLASTY	

Severe cutaneous ecchymosis
Hematoma
Subconjunctival ecchymosis
Chemosis
Lagophthalmos
Scleral show
Ectropion
Pigmented, wide, too-low scars
Loss of vision
Dry-eye syndrome

incisions are not closed, any bleeding has an immediate escape path. Hematoma risk in the procedure is greatly diminished.

Subconjunctival Ecchymosis

Subconjunctival ecchymosis is unusual, and its cause in seemingly routine cases remains unexplained. It is far more frightening to the patient than to the surgeon. It always resolves completely in 3 weeks or more, and reassuring the patient is important. Medical therapy to speed the resolution is usually unsuccessful.

Chemosis

Chemosis is usually related to lower lid blepharoplasty. It can occur with or without the use of suspension sutures. Either it resolves quickly (several days) or it will remain for up to 6 weeks. When it is present, the gelatinous conjunctiva holds the lid away from the orbit, making the eye look almost proptotic or as though the palpebral fissure on the affected side is wider. The patient must be reassured that this condition is temporary and always resolves satisfactorily. If it is present beyond 2 weeks, a steriod ophthalmic drop is recommended.

Lagophthalmos

Lagophthalmos can be present for a short time after upper lid blepharoplasty. It is usually mild and can cause minor tearing and burning. The use of artificial tears or ointments usually alleviates the symptoms until full healing occurs. Severe lagophthalmos usually occurs after secondary upper lid blepharoplasty when an inexperienced surgeon overestimates the amount of skin excision or when a forehead lift

TABLE 176.4	EMERGENCIES
BLEPHAROPLASTY	

Progressive hematoma
Severe dry-eye syndrome
Vision loss

and upper blepharoplasty are performed simultaneously. Conservatism in upper lid blepharoplasty is important.

Ectropion

Scleral show is possible after lower lid blepharoplasty, even with conservative or no skin excision. Postoperative squint exercises and upward massage usually reverse this problem. Ectropion occurs when an obvious shortening of the lid accompanies a too-generous skin excision. It also can occur when a horizontal lid laxity exists preoperatively but is not identified. In the latter condition, a horizontal lid-shortening procedure is required. Occasionally, ectropion will occur from a downward displacement of the skin-muscle flap. In this condition, the lid appears to be "stuck" when the patient attempts an upward gaze. A simple releasing incision, which elevates the skin-muscle flap and redrapes it, may resolve this problem.

Poor Scars

Obvious scars in the lateral upper lid wound can occur when wound separation occurs at the time of suture removal and is not recognized or when sun exposure occurs in the immediate postoperative period to pigment the wound. In either case, a small secondary excision and repair may be necessary. Poor medial upper lid scars are always caused by excessive skin excision in the face of a large medial fat compartment. Scars result when the wound is repaired over a large dead space. These scars can be treated by injecting very small amounts of triamcinolone (10 mg/mL).

Loss of Vision

Most reported cases of visual loss follow hematoma formation after lower lid or lower and upper lid blepharoplasty. Hypertension, old age, anticoagulant medication, and metabolic diseases are often present as cofactors. In the case of a hematoma, rapid decompression of a progressing retrobulbar hematoma is essential to preserve vision.

HIGHLIGHTS

- Successful blepharoplasty depends on the surgeon's understanding of the interplay of the aesthetic components contributing to the appearance of the eye region and to the face as a whole.
- Preoperative medical screening of the patient desiring blepharoplasty should include evaluation of medical problems that might be aggravated by medications required in the perioperative period and an ophthalmic history, including dry-eye symptoms and a near-field vision test.
- Evaluation of the brow area includes consideration of brow position with respect to the bony superior orbital rim, bilateral brow symmetry, brow shape, and hair distribution.

- Evaluation of the upper eyelid includes skin condition (thin or thick), palpebral fissure position, presence of orbicularis muscle hypertrophy, fat pseudoherniation, superior orbital rim bone position, lacrimal gland position, existing lagophthalmos, and presence of Bell phenomenon.
- Evaluation of the lower eyelid includes skin condition, presence of skin crêpiness, pigmentation, festooning, fat pseudoherniation, inferior orbital rim position, and lid laxity.
- Preblepharoplasty photography ideally includes a full-face view at 1:10 ratio and closeup eyelid views at a 1:4 or 1:5 ratio in frontal, eyes open, frontal gaze upward, frontal eyes closed, both obliques, and both lateral views.
- Preoperative surgical marking of the eyelids is performed with a surgical pen with the patient in a supine position. Depressing the brow mimics the upright position.
- In the lower lid, the transconjunctival approach is selected for those with a predominance of fat with minimal skin redundancy and muscle swag. The subciliary incision and skin-muscle flap is chosen for patients in whom remarkable skin redundancy and muscle hypertrophy are of as much concern as the amount of fat. After transconjunctival blepharoplasty, laser resurfacing can both smooth the crêped skin and diminish a small amount of skin redundancy.
- During fat removal from the eyelid compartments, only fat that flows easily into the wound is removed; fat is never pulled forcefully from deeper within the orbit. Before removal, the fat is infiltrated with local anesthetic and clamped. After removal, the stump is cauterized to eliminate bleeding before the clamp is released. Slightly more aggressive fat removal is required from the lower lid's medial compartment. The inferior oblique muscle should be located before clamping fat to avoid injury to the muscle. Fat repositioning is considered when a tear trough deformity exists.
- Complications of blepharoplasty include hematoma (rare on the upper lid, more common on the lower lid), subconjunctival ecchymosis, chemosis, lagophthalmos, ectropion, poor scars, and loss of vision (thought to be secondary to retrobulbar hematoma formation).

BIBLIOGRAPHY

Baker SR. Orbital fat preservation in lower lid blepharoplasty. *Arch Facial Plast Surg* 1999;1:33–37.

Castanares S. Anatomy for a blepharoplasty. *Plast Reconstr Surg* 1974; 53:587.

Castanares S. Blepharoplasty for herniated infraorbital fat: anatomical basis for a new approach. *Plast Reconstr Surg* 1951;8:46.

Fagien S. Reducing the incidence of dry eye symptoms after blepharoplasty. *Aesthetic Surg J* 2004;24:464–468.

Freidman WH. Surgical anatomy of the orbit. In: Tardy E, ed. *Facial plastic surgery*. Vol. 4. New York: Thieme Medical Publishers, 1987:475.

Groth MJ. Transconjunctival lower blepharoplasty. *Facial Plast Surg Clin* 1998;6(1):59–70

Heppler RS, et al. The occurrence of blindness in association with blepharoplasty. *Plast Reconstr Surg* 1976;57:233.

Honrado CP, Pastorek N. Longterm results of lower-lid suspension blepharoplasty: a 30 year experience. *Arch Facial Plast Surg* 2004; 6(3):150–154.

Jelks GW, Jelks EB. Preoperative evaluation of the blepharoplasty patient: bypassing the pitfalls. *Clin Plastic Surg* 1993;20:213–223.

McCord CD, et al. Lateral canthal tightening. *Plast Reconstr Surg* 2003; 112(1):222–237.

McCurdy JA. Upper blepharoplasty in the asian patient: "the double eyelid" operation. *Facial Plast Surg Clin* 2002;10(4):351–368.

Millman A, et al. The septal-myocutaneous flap in blepharoplasty. *Ophthalmol Plast Reconstr Surg* 1997;13:2.

Murakami CS, Plant RL. Complications of blepharoplasty surgery. *Facial Plastic Surg* 1994;10:214–224.

Papel ID. Muscle suspension blepharoplasty. *Facial Plastic Surg* 1994; 10:1447–1449.

Pastorek N. Blepharoplasty update. *Facial Plast Surg Clin* 2002; 10(1):23–27

Pastorek N. *Blepharoplasty. Self-instructional package*, 3rd ed. Alexandra, VA: American Academy of Otolaryngology-Head and Neck Surgery, 1994.

Pastorek N. Upper lid blepharoplasty. *Facial Plast Surg* 1996;12: 157–169.

Patipa M. The evaluation and management of lower eyelid retraction following cosmetic surgery. *Plast Reconstr Surg* 2000;106(2): 438–453.

Perkins SW, Dyer WK II, Simo F. Transconjunctival approach to lower lid blepharoplasty. Experience, indications, and technique in 300 patients. *Arch Otolaryngol Head Neck Surg* 1994;120:172–177.

Rees TD, Jelks GW. Blepharoplasty and the dry eye syndrome. *Plast Reconstr Surg* 1981;28:249.

Smith B, Nesi FA. The complications of cosmetic blepharoplasty. *Ophthalmology* 1978;85:726.

Zide BM, Jelks GW, eds. *Surgical Anatomy of the Orbit*. New York: Raven Press, 1985.

The Aging Face (Rhytidectomy)

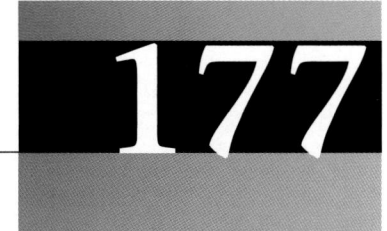

Russell W. H. Kridel   *Peyman Soliemanzadeh*

The term rhytidectomy is derived from the Greek for removal of wrinkle. The present day rhytidectomy procedure is much more a resuspension of the facial soft tissues with skin removal rather than wrinkle excision. We are witness to a steady evolution of technical and anatomic advances producing a new generation of facelifts. Presently, we continue to evaluate these newer techniques in search of the ideal procedure that will give our patients a long-term, natural correction with rapid recovery and few complications.

Patients with aging faces requesting consultation for a facelift generally seek a youthful, more rested appearance. These patients have a well-developed self-image and do not want to look otherwise. Rather, they desire a natural appearing result that turns back the hands of time to a more youthful version of themselves. For the surgeon, the goal is to determine what physical characteristics of the face are contributing to the impression of aging, which stigmata are reversible, and by what means. Ideally, the surgeon brings to this consultation a thorough understanding of the processes that lead to an aged appearance and is familiar with a wide variety of medical and surgical interventions appropriate for addressing the clinical problem. As with all elective facial plastic surgery, it is imperative for the surgeon to achieve a balanced, harmonious result. The patient who presents with an interest in facelift who also has brow ptosis and four quadrant dermatochalasis can be poorly served if the incongruity is not discussed before proceeding with the surgery. Moreover, these patients often will be left with more stigmata of a lifted appearance should they only address the lower face because of this incongruity. For these reasons, in addition to the facelift, it is important to discuss the potential benefits of browlift, blepharoplasty, laser resurfacing, and adjunctive procedures (e.g., soft tissue fillers, Botox injection, or implant placement). Whereas these components can individually or in various combinations contribute toward improvement of the aging face, this chapter focuses on the anatomy and development of the present day rhytidectomy.

PHYSIOLOGY OF THE AGING FACE

To understand the present day rhytidectomy procedure, the surgeon must have full knowledge of both the underlying surgical anatomy and the aging physiology of the face that leads patients to seek rejuvenation surgery. In general, the aging face presents five landmarks that are points of interest to patients and surgeons alike. These areas include (a) the jowl, (b) the deepened nasolabial folds and lateral perioral jowling, (c) platysma muscle banding and submental fullness in the neck region, (d) orbicularis oculi muscle and malar fat pad ptosis, and (e) aging skin itself (Fig. 177.1A).

In youth, the facial skin is maintained in normal anatomic position by retaining "ligaments" that run from deep facial structures to the dermis itself (1). With aging, attenuation of these "ligamentous" supports then results in malar soft tissue descent. The result of this descent is not only deepening of the melolabial folds but also jowling of the platysma muscle and soft tissue between the masseteric and mandibular ligaments at the jawline. Moreover, this descent of the malar fat pad along with ptosis of the orbicularis oculi also results in hollowing in the infraorbital region. Finally, loss of platysma muscle tone results in anterior banding and the classically pictured "turkey gobbler" neck (2) (Fig. 177.1B).

Separate from the described underlying soft tissue changes, the surgeon must note the cumulative effects of

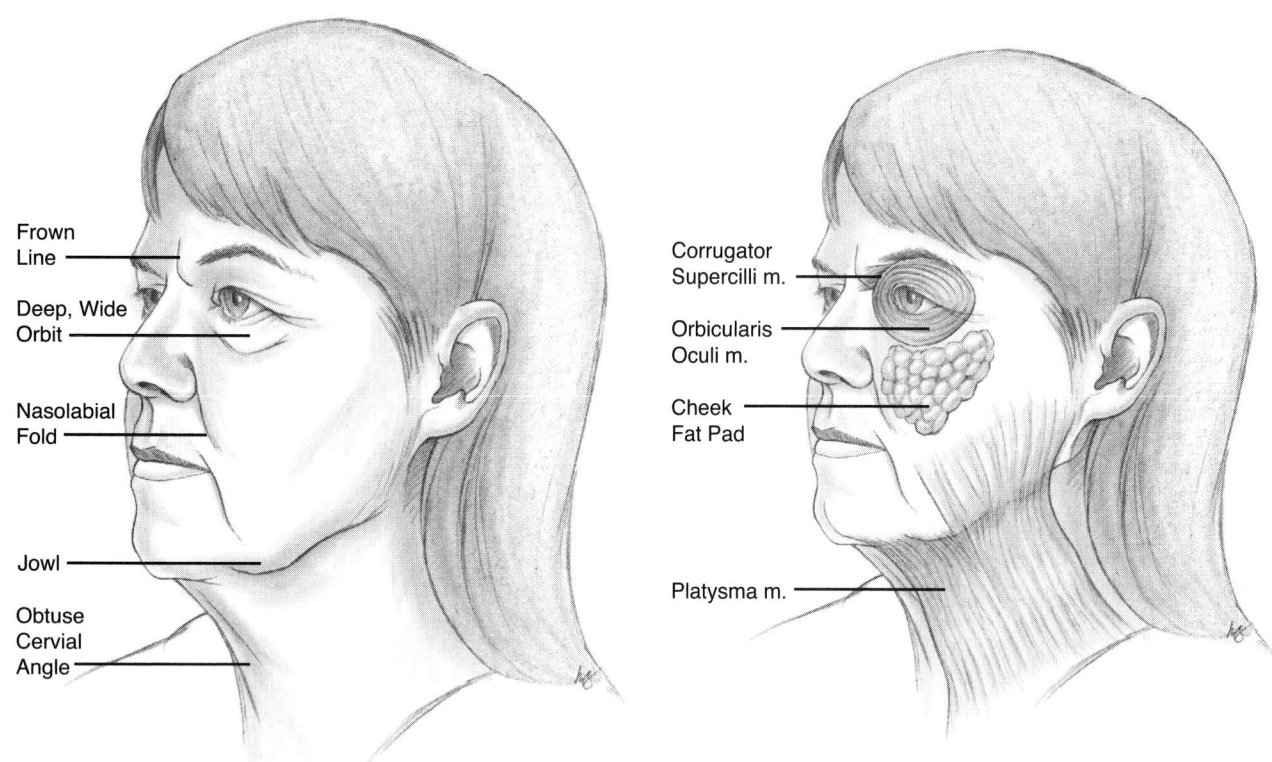

Frown Line

Deep, Wide Orbit

Nasolabial Fold

Jowl

Obtuse Cervial Angle

Corrugator Supercilli m.

Orbicularis Oculi m.

Cheek Fat Pad

Platysma m.

A   **B**

Figure 177.1 **A:** Topographic changes seen in the face with aging. **B:** Underlying soft tissue and muscular changes seen in the aging face. (Adapted from Zimbler MS, Kokoska MS, Thomas JR. Anatomy and pathophysiology of facial aging. *Facial Plast Surg Clin N Am.* 2001;9:179–187.)

the inherent aging process coupled with the effects of environmental exposure on the skin itself. Although a comprehensive review of the changes associated with aging skin is beyond the scope of this chapter, it is important for the surgeon to have a fundamental understanding of these changes. In this regard, it is convenient to think of skin aging in terms of intrinsic and extrinsic factors, although in reality it is difficult to separate these concepts (3). Intrinsic aging refers to the natural effects of time and is generally characterized by tissue atrophy and reduction in skin cellular and protein components. In fact, chronologically aged skin has reduced epidermal thickness, flattening of the dermal–epidermal junction, atrophy of the dermis, and a general decline in a variety of cell populations, including melanocytes and Langerhans' cells (4). This epidermal thinning then makes the skin more susceptible to damage from shearing-type forces (3). Moreover, Yousif and Mendelson (5) showed how habitual facial expressions lead to coarse skin wrinkling and deep folds (5). Kligman et al. (6), however, noted that no histologic features distinguish the various types of wrinkles from the surrounding skin (6). They noted, instead, that a configurational change results from mechanical stress acting on lax, excessive skin, especially in actinically damaged regions.

On the other hand, photoaged epidermis is characterized by striking variability: in its thickness, with alternating areas of atrophy and hyperplasia; in pigmentation, with alternating lentigenes and depigmented areas; in the degree of nuclear atypia; and in orderliness of keratinocytes maturation (7). In the past, sun-damaged epidermis was thought to be characterized by a reduction in structural elements, leading to skin wrinkling. In fact, the most striking feature of photodamaged skin is the presence of large quantities of thickened, poorly organized, degraded elastic fibers that degenerate into an amorphous mass (8). The result is aged skin that does not retain moisture and loosens and hangs. The ground substance component of the dermal connective tissue matrix is greatly increased. In the dermal cell population, photodamaged skin shows numerous, hyperplastic fibroblasts and abundant, partially degranulated mast cells, which result in a chronic low-grade inflammation termed "heliodermatitis." Finally, photodamaged skin shows extensive changes in the microcirculation, which can affect flap viability.

Overall, the aging face can be viewed as a coupling of redistributed ptotic underlying soft tissue with overlying skin changes. Together, these changes combine to contribute to the overall impression of the aging face. For most patients with aging faces, this means that facial rejuvenation will necessitate the surgeon concentrating on five points of interest: (a) The jowl, (b) the deepened melolabial folds, (c) the neck, (d) the malar region, and (e) the skin itself.

SURICAL ANATOMY

The past 20 years have brought about numerous improvements in facelift surgery. These new advances have largely come about through better understanding of anatomy and of how the aging process alters these anatomic components throughout the face and neck. Certain salient points of the facial anatomy for rhytidectomy, including vascular supply, details of the superficial musculoaponeurotic system (SMAS) and its relation to the facial nerve, as well as the presence of retaining "ligaments," are described here.

The facial skin is supplied by branches of the external carotid artery. Specifically, the superficial temporal artery, facial artery, transverse facial artery, and infraorbital artery anastamose with one another in the subdermal plexus. The subcutaneous flap is based solely on the subdermal plexus, which is supplied by muscular cutaneous arteries arising from branches of the facial and infraorbital arteries. The standard subcutaneous and SMAS two-layered facelift, however, effectively divides the skin from its underlying perforating branches. A recent study comparing the vascular anatomy of basic skin flaps in the subcutaneous and SMAS rhytidectomy, the composite rhytidectomy, and the subperiosteal rhytidectomy, not surprisingly, found that the best blood supply was found in subperiosteal dissection, whereas the most tenuous supply was in the subcutaneous flap (9). Other than smokers and those patients with small vessel disease, one must consider that each of these techniques has been used for many years with minimal low-flap perfusion rate complications (2).

Perhaps the first, and most important, development in the evolution toward the present day rhytidectomy was the description of the SMAS. In fact, whereas the precise boundaries of the SMAS continue to be a source of debate, the significance of this fascial layer in relation to present day rhytidectomy is unquestionable. The SMAS, which is a fibromuscular fascial layer, invests and interlinks the muscles of facial expression. Moreover, in this function, it maintains consistent relationships with the facial nerve and major vessels within the facial region. For the operating surgeon, mastery of these relationships and planes of dissection, therefore, are critical (10).

The regional variations found in the relationship between the SMAS and the neurovascular structures are most profound when examining the SMAS and the facial nerve above versus below the zygoma (11). Specifically, in the temporal region above the zygoma, the superficial temporal artery and frontal branch course through the SMAS (also called temporoparietal fascia). Below the zygoma, the SMAS fans out over the parotid gland and then above the masseter muscle before it surrounds the facial mimetic muscles. In the lower face, therefore, the facial nerve branches are always deep to the SMAS and innervate the facial mimetic muscles on their undersurface (Fig. 177.2). It should be noted, however, that even in the deep plane and composite lifts, the dissection medial to the zygomati-

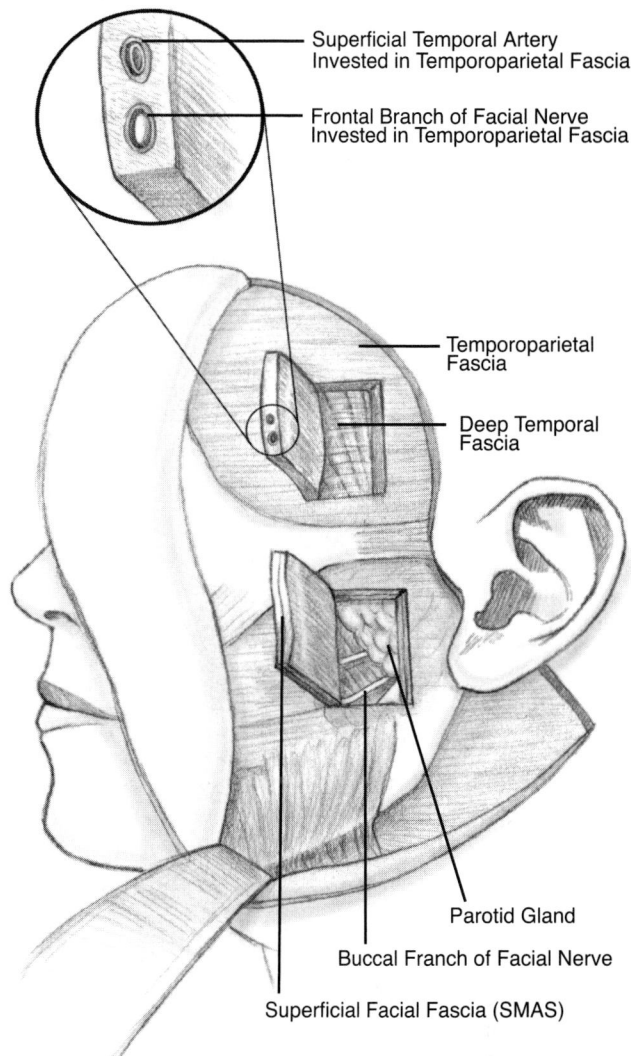

Figure 177.2 In the temporal region, above the zygoma, the frontal nerve branch travels through the superficial musculoaponeurotic system (SMAS). In the lower face, below the zygoma, the facial nerve branches lie deep to the SMAS and innervate the facial mimetic muscles from their deep surface. (Adapted from Stuzin JM. The relationship of the superficial and deep facial fascias: relevance to rhytidectomy and aging. *Plast Reconstr Surg* 1992;89(3):441–449.)

cus major and minor is actually above the SMAS because the SMAS thins out over this region. Moreover, it should be noted that a significant, distinct myofascial layer superficial to the parotid fascia is not always clinically apparent. In fact, Jost and Levet (12) have suggested that the SMAS overlying the parotid includes what we have otherwise distinguished as the parotid fascia.

Finally, as previously alluded, the SMAS has been noted to have a number of "ligamentous" supports that make it adherent at specific points to the overlying dermis and underlying muscular or osseous attachments. Specifically, four ligaments support the soft tissues of the cheek: (a) The parotidomasseteric ligament, (b) the platysmal auricular ligament, (c) the zygomatic ligament (McGregor patch),

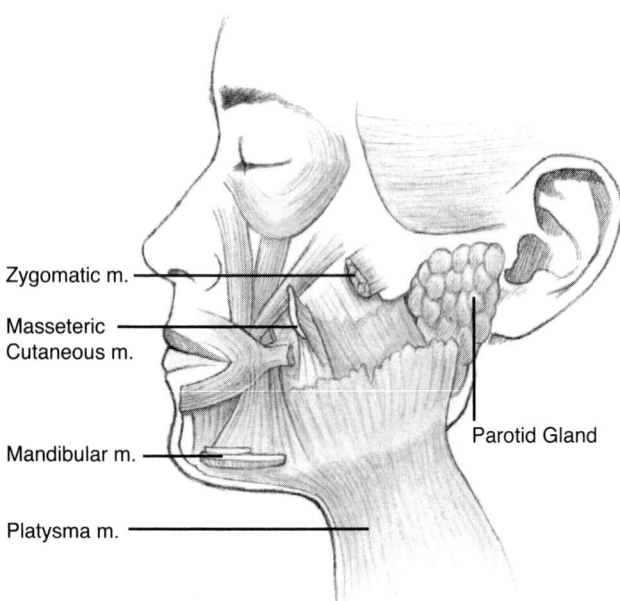

Zygomatic m.

Masseteric
Cutaneous m.

Mandibular m.

Platysma m.

Parotid Gland

Figure 177.3 The four retaining ligaments of the cheeks.

and (d) the mandibular ligaments (Fig. 177.3). Although not true ligaments, these fascial condensations are especially important in the deep plane and composite rhytidectomy (13). Release of these ligaments, however, must be undertaken with extreme caution because branches of the facial nerve are in close proximity.

SURGICAL EVOLUTION

A steady evolution of anatomically derived technical advances has occurred in the rhytidectomy procedure since the early days of simple skin flap advancement. The first major contribution to advance facelifting was provided by Skoog. Sometime in the mid 1960s, Skoog began to elevate a "complex morphologic unit" in the cervical region and advance it posteriorly (14). It was observed that this "two-layered shift" of the cervical fascia corrected the anterior banding of the neck and the redundant skin of the cervical region. Skoog, subsequently followed this with his description in 1974 of his technique of superficial rhytidectomy of the face and neck based on a subfascial dissection. The new era in facelift surgery had begun (15–17).

In 1976, Mitz and Peyronie (18) defined the "complex morphologic unit" referred to by Skoog as the superficial musculoaponeurotic system. The SMAS lift approach, which then became vogue, was a significant step in the evolution of the present day rhytidectomy. Some surgeons, in pursuit of the ideal lift, however, still found the results of the SMAS lift to be short lived and complicated by perioperative problems. Moreover, the SMAS lift did not appear to sufficiently address the ptotic midface and melolabial fold region. Lemmon and Hamra (19) then presented their

observation that the anatomic restoration of the SMAS in the face was more lasting, but that platysma muscle advancement in the cervical region did not produce a similar result. Submentoplasties, cervical lipectomies, platysmaplasty, along with the new generation deep plane, composite, and subperiosteal lifts were expounded.

To date, it is uncertain what percentage of surgeons is now doing the extended sub-SMAS lifts versus the traditional SMAS plication or imbrication techniques. Moreover, questions remain to the superiority of the results that are achieved in the deep plane versus plication techniques. In fact, whereas anecdotal reports abound to this effect, it will be difficult to conduct a study that definitively answers this and a whole host of other questions. Baker (20) and Kamer (21) maintain reservations regarding the superiority of the results from the deep plane lifts, especially when these "implied benefits" are weighed in relation to the added risks to the facial nerve. Baker and Conley (22) note that a review of the world literature in 1979 found an incidence of 0.01% permanent facial nerve injury. He then notes that the published articles on the new deep dissection techniques raise concern because they report a relatively high incidence of facial weakness in the hands of extremely qualified surgeons. He questions what happens when these procedures are attempted by less-experienced surgeons. Time and experience are still needed before we will know if the added work and increased potential risk for complication are worth the improved aesthetic results.

ASSESSING CANDIDACY

With an understanding of the physiologic and anatomic changes that present with facial aging, the surgeon is ready to determine whether the patient is a candidate for facial rejuvenation surgery, in general, and rhytidectomy, in particular. This evaluation includes surgical, medical, and psychological components.

The surgical criterion to be addressed is whether rhytidectomy will create physical changes in the patient's face that will contribute meaningfully to a more youthful appearance. In making this determination, it is helpful to divide the stigmata of facial aging into two categories: those that are improved by repositioning of facial tissues and those that require changes in the structure of the tissues themselves. The first category would include ptosis in the jowl, submentum, and anterior neck leading to a disruption of the ideal youthful contours of the jawline, cervicomental angle, and neck, respectively. These are the primary areas improved by rhytidectomy. Malar ptosis will be modestly improved as well.

On the other hand, intrinsic changes in the tissues themselves are not well addressed by rhytidectomy. As noted earlier, concomitant with the ptosis described above, aging brings about many changes in the skin itself. Fine lines and deeply etched wrinkles in the skin are the grossly visible correlate of crevices in the dermis and subcutaneous tissues formed over time as a result of actinic damage, senescence of connective tissues, and habitual facial expressions. These cosmetic defects will be minimally improved, at best, by rhytidectomy. Instead, they can be addressed more directly by resurfacing techniques, including both chemical and laser exfoliation. In the situation in which such intrinsic properties of the skin comprise a significant portion of the aesthetic problem, the patient should be encouraged to consider skin resurfacing as an adjunct or, in some cases, an alternative to rhytidectomy.

Once the surgeon has determined that a rhytidectomy will address the patient's aesthetic concerns appropriately, it is imperative to assess medical candidacy for the procedure. Most patients who seek cosmetic surgery are in good health, so medical contraindications to the proposed procedure rarely exist. Vigilance is essential to avoid disaster. Facelift candidates—people who feel young inside and want their outward appearance to mirror that vitality—are exactly the same people who tend to minimize medical complaints and can even forget to relate serious medical problems, unless questioned directly. Significant bleeding diatheses and American Society of Anesthesiologists (ASA) class IV or V, in which a patient has a dangerously compromising medical condition, should be considered absolute medical contraindications to rhytidectomy. A patient in ASA class III, in which a medical condition impairs the patient's activities to some degree, should be approached with great caution. The severity of the condition and its potential impact on the safe conduct of the operation should be explored in detail. Conditions that can adversely affect healing, including uncontrolled diabetes, diseases requiring chronic steroid therapy, or connective tissue abnormalities such as the Ehlers-Danlos syndrome, should be considered strong relative contraindications to facelift surgery. Consultation with the primary care physician may be necessary to coordinate prescription medication regimens and facilitate the management of relevant medical conditions.

On the other hand, no age limitations exist for facelift surgery, and age should not be a reason to deny surgery if the patient is in otherwise good health. A healthy patient in his or her late 70s or early 80s may have 15 or 20 more years of quality life ahead, and the desire to have an improved appearance is indeed valid.

Finally, but not least important, an accurate assessment of the patient's psychological status is central to determining patient candidacy. The surgeon should determine patient motivation and attempt to ascertain whether the patient might fail to view a successful surgical outcome favorably or might react inappropriately to any aspect of the surgery. A thorough discussion of the patient's goals and objectives should provide important clues to that patient's psychological profile (23). Although many patients are unaware of exactly what surgery can and cannot accomplish, others have clearly unreasonable expectations, which can include looking exactly as they did 10 or 20 years ago, having surgery without scars, requesting an unnaturally tight lift, or attempting to obtain promises and guarantees. Patients who are excessively occupied with minute flaws also may be poor surgical candidates. Moreover, patients who have recently had a major change in their personal status (e.g., the death of a loved one or divorce) may be subject to depression or psychological unevenness and require special care.

PREOPERATIVE EVALUATION AND PLANNING

General Considerations

Once a patient is deemed an appropriate candidate for rhytidectomy, that patient needs to be educated clearly before surgery. The patient must understand that rhytidectomy helps with excessive skin and jowling and provides for redraping of the skin, but it does not change the quality of the skin itself. If fine or deep rhytids are present preoperatively, they will be present postoperatively as soon as the swelling goes down. In patients with severely sundamaged skin, full-face deep chemical peeling with phenol solution or CO_2 laser resurfacing is often necessary as an adjunct, which can be done several weeks after the initial facelift surgery. If significant rhytids are limited to the perioral or periorbital areas, these cosmetic units can be safely peeled or removed by laser simultaneously with the rhytidectomy as long as these areas are not undermined during the procedure.

To assess further the overall improvement possible with rhytidectomy, the underlying structure of the face must be critically evaluated. Patients who had a good bony structure of the cheekbones, chin, and jaw during their youth will have the best results, because redraping of skin will help to highlight these attractive bony structures. Therefore, patients who have a thinner, angular face and good bony definition are generally much better candidates than patients with rounder faces, low cheekbones, or a short mandible (Figs. 177.4–177.6)

Adjunctive chin and submalar cheek augmentation may be necessary in conjunction with a facelift to achieve the desired result. Patients who have a retrusive chin cannot get desired cervicomental definition without a chin implant, even after a facelift. Also, because the aging process sometimes causes a hollow cheek deformity from atrophy of soft tissue and fat with ptosis of the fat pads, older patients sometimes require submalar augmentation or resupport of the fat pads simultaneously with the facelift. Redraping the skin alone will not replace soft tissue cheek hollowness.

As the underlying structures of the face dictate the aesthetic results possible above the jawline, those in the neck

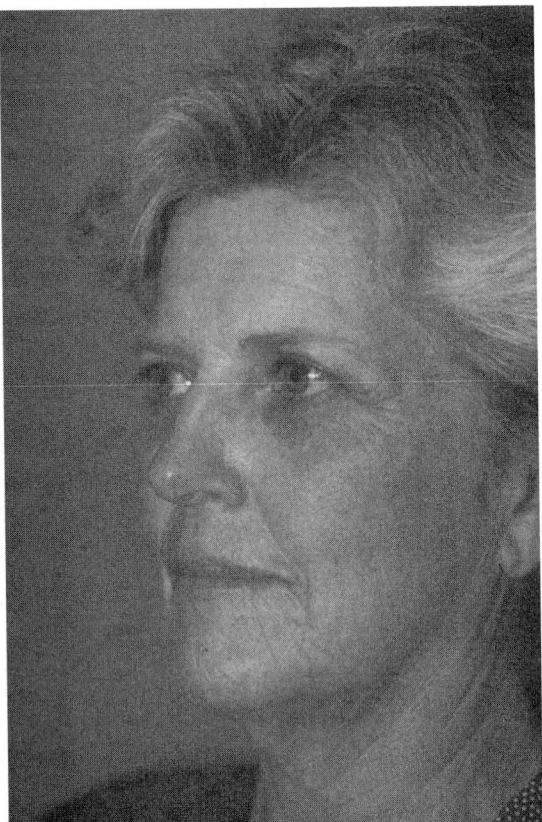

Figure 177.4 Excellent candidate for a facelift: little fat, good bone structure, and not too much skin.

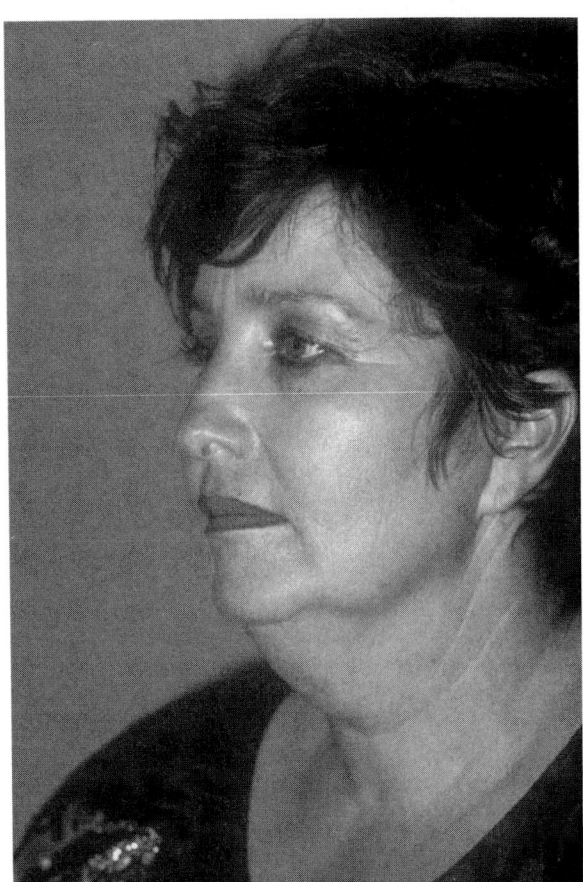

Figure 177.6 A less-than-ideal candidate for a facelift: excessive skin and fat and rounded, bony contours.

similarly limit the outcome there. In particular, the position of the hyoid bone relative to the mandible varies from patient to patient. This relationship defines the course of the suprahyoid musculature of the floor of the mouth and delimits the maximal improvement possible in the cervicomental angle. A relatively high and posterior hyoid is ideal, allowing maximal elevation of the submental contour and the greatest definition between the submentum and neck in profile. A relatively low and anterior hyoid limits the possible improvement in this area to a predictable degree. It is mandatory, therefore, that hyoid position be assessed and its effects on the possible outcome discussed with the patient in a way that is easily understood. We have found the use of diagrams illustrating hyoid position to be helpful in our practice (Fig. 177.7).

A full evaluation of the facial nerve and muscles should be done preoperatively, particularly noting any asymmetries, especially around the mouth. Sometimes, patients have asymmetric smiles or inadvertently elevate the brow. Static asymmetries may be present as well, ranging from minor unilateral cheek or jowl fullness to generalized asymmetry as in hemifacial microsomias. Any asymmetry should be documented, photographed, and discussed with the patient before surgery, or the patient may attribute the asymmetry to the surgery (24). Further, it gives the surgeon the opportunity to point out that minor asymmetry is

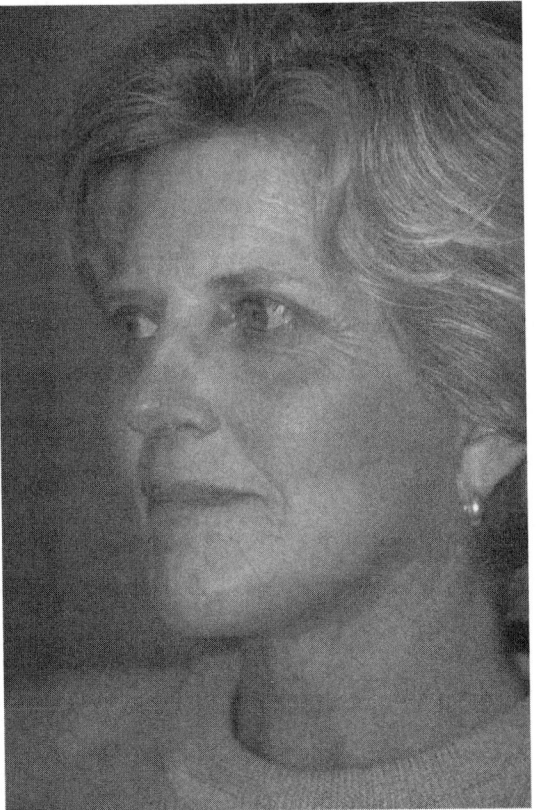

Figure 177.5 Postoperative views of same patient after facelift and upper eyelid blepharoplasty.

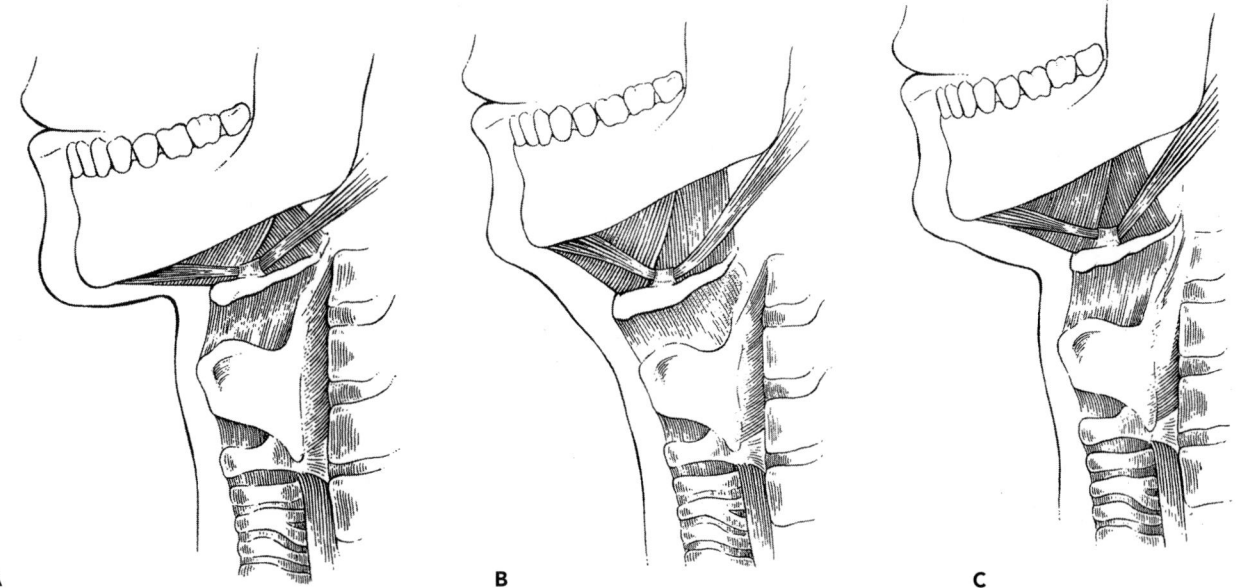

Figure 177.7 Schematic representation of the limits of improvement in the cervicomental contour imposed by the underlying hyoid bone and suprahyoid musculature. A high posterior hyoid bone is most favorable for facelifting **(A)**, and a low anterior hyoid bone is least favorable **(B)**; most patients fall somewhere in between **(C)**. (Reprinted from Conley, J. *Face-lift operation.* Springfield, IL: Charles C. Thomas, 1968:40–41, with permission.)

normal and that perfect symmetry cannot be a surgical goal. The surgeon also should note any traumatic facial and neck lacerations, sites of previous biopsies, acne scars, facial or neck scars, subcutaneous depressions, surface irregularities, and focal lesions.

Generally, the older patient who presents with voluminous sagging skin or the patient with a fat face and neck would not be as good a candidate as the thinner patient 40 to 50 years of age because postoperative skin draping with such excess is less satisfactory, especially if elastosis is present. Such patients should be advised that, for a better result, a tuck procedure may be necessary 6 months to 1 year after all the retraction has occurred from the original facelift (25). If liposis is limited to the submental area, the patient will be a better candidate than one who has a full, rounded face with fat throughout. Liposuction in conjunction with a facelift exerts its maximal effect in the submental area.

Similarly, if a patient contemplates a weight loss of more than 10 pounds, it may be better to postpone surgery until afterward. We discourage patients who have a history of repeated weight gain and loss from considering facelift surgery because repeated stretching of the facial skin can cause a premature return of skin laxity.

Men seek a facelift operation less commonly than women, but several clinical distinctions are relevant to a facelift between the two that merit consideration. In general, female facelift patients have better aesthetic results than male patients, although men seem to have less stringent expectations and are more satisfied with overall improvement. Female facelift patients are often very particular about any kind of asymmetry, wrinkle, or bulge that is left, or any result that does not return them to the way they were many years ago. This is an interesting difference, because in rhinoplasty surgery men are generally much more particular than women. Not as good a result is achieved in the male facelift patient, however, probably because of the thickness of the skin, secondary to beard formation. Men often have much larger parotid glands than women and, therefore, will still have a full-cheek appearance postoperatively, contributing to a less aesthetic result. Much excessive skin may mask parotid masses, and the parotid glands should be palpated for any masses preoperatively. Other considerations are relevant to incision placement, and these gender differences will be discussed below in the section on incision planning.

Smoking history is also particularly relevant. Rees and Aston (26) noted that smokers have 12 times more risk of skin slough than nonsmokers, possibly secondary to vasoconstriction, and also have a higher incidence of hematoma formation. Postoperative coughing can contribute to this complication. Smoking has long-term effects on the skin that cannot be erased by simple cessation perioperatively. If the patient stops smoking for 1 month before and after surgery, however, many complications associated with smoking can be limited. Even with smoking cessation 1 month before surgery, superficial epidermolysis in the preauricular area is not infrequent. Moreover, these patients very likely would be better candidates for a deep plane facelift to limit these possible complications.

Patients with a history of excessive alcohol intake may have characteristic nutritional or liver deficiencies that can lead to poor surgical healing. They also may be uncooperative in the perioperative period, when alcohol consumption is not allowed. Be alert for physical findings associated with excessive alcohol use and hepatic insufficiency.

A prior facelift or other neck surgery can complicate the proposed procedure. The placement and quality of prior facelift incisions should be noted and discussed with the patient. Although it may be desirable to revise scars at the time of surgery, often "the die is cast," and improved camouflaging may not be possible. Additionally, it may be useful to explore the patient's attitude toward the prior surgery. If the patient was dissatisfied with the result, the surgeon should proceed with caution. The patient may have been unhappy with a poor result, or may just be difficult to please, even with a technically sound job. Dissection also can be more difficult in a secondary surgery. Some surgeons have reported, particularly in these revision cases, that a deep plane facelift sometimes allows for better planes of dissection. The surgeon must be honest with himself or herself and with the patient about the ability to improve the aesthetic result. Any prior neck surgery or irradiation might also adversely affect the ease of dissection and progress of healing or, as in the case of neck dissection, might expose deep neck structures to catastrophic injury. Incorporating these considerations into the surgical plan will help avoid a grave outcome.

PREOPERATIVE PREPARATION

Full-disclosure, informed consent for surgery and photographs are obtained. The patient is given a packet that includes preoperative and postoperative instructions and a description of what to expect during recovery. Having the patient fill all prescriptions in advance serves two purposes: It removes the distraction of a rushed visit to the pharmacy for the patient and caretakers in the early postoperative period when even simple things can be difficult. Also, it allows the patient to take antibiotics the night before surgery to assist in preventing infection and it provides the patient with sedatives should sleep be difficult the night before surgery.

The patient is urged to stop smoking 1 month before surgery. All medications containing aspirin, steroids, nonsteroidal anti-inflammatory agents, vitamin E, as well as all herbal medications should be discontinued at least 2 weeks before surgery. If there is a history consistent with a bleeding diathesis, however tenuous, preoperative bleeding time, platelet count, prothrombin time (PT), partial thromboplastin time (PTT), or other coagulation studies should be ordered. The goal is to avoid hematoma, the most common complication of rhytidectomy.

SURGICAL PLANNING

Successful facelift surgery is achieved through thoughtful planning and execution of every aspect of the procedure (27). The amount of actual skin excised, the tightness and completeness of the lift in the cheeks, the ability to contour and resuspend the neck, the smoothness of the submental region, and the degree to which the incisions can be camouflaged all are important considerations in achieving a natural, nonoperative appearance. Rhytidectomy is an operation of compromises.

Anesthesia

We prefer to perform facelifts with the patient under general anesthesia in a hospital ambulatory setting or outpatient surgical center (28). Most of our patients prefer the idea of complete somnolence and amnesia and are relieved of any anxiety concerning positional discomfort or surgical pain. An anesthesiologist's presence permits monitoring of the patient's vital signs and status and allows the surgeon to concentrate on the events in the operative field. Communicating any special needs with the anesthesia professionals greatly facilitates the entire operative and postoperative course. The draped endotracheal tube can be moved side to side and does not interfere with the procedure. The anesthesia team strives for rapid, effective anesthesia with a smooth and deep emergence phase coupled with a relatively rapid recovery. Smooth extubation must be guaranteed, because bucking on the endotracheal tube can predispose the patient to hematoma formation. No long-acting muscle relaxing agents are permitted, to allow proper facial nerve intraoperative monitoring. We prefer to have the patient emerge from anesthesia after the dressing is in place, which seems to facilitate dressing placement and allows optimal gentle pressure on the skin flaps to decrease further the risk of hematoma formation.

Marking

Markings are first applied to the patient in a sitting position to delineate the location and amount of excess fat, sagging and laxity of the skin, acquired position of the jowl area, and the degree of platysma muscle banding and loss of cervicomental definition. While sitting, natural gravitational forces give a more accurate picture of the signs of facial and neck aging than might be seen with the patient supine. Moreover, marking while the patient is upright helps to prevent judgmental errors regarding the amount of fat removal, the degree of laxity, and the amount of suspension required (29). Vertical platysma muscle bands are identified and similarly highlighted. Weak platysma muscle bands can be seen best with the patient upright. The patient is asked to jut the lower jaw forward and to grimace, which more easily demonstrates the platysma muscle bands. Other important anatomic landmarks to be marked include the anterior borders of the sternocleidomastoid muscles, the submental crease, the region of jowl formation, the mandible angle, the inferior mandibular border, and the geniomandibular groove.

Incisions

Although much recent literature on rhytidectomy describes techniques for improving the quality of the facelift, far less attention has been devoted on detailing how to avoid visible incision lines (30). In fact, although patients present with an interest in facial rejuvenation, rarely would they pursue these goals at the price of visible incision lines.

Several factors can influence incision location, but we have found that the most important variable is an appreciation for the importance of preserving the temporal hair tuft and the posterior hairline in the female patient. The temporal region is key because a poorly designed and executed incision in this area can lead to temporal alopecia (Fig. 177.8). Descriptions of many of the classic facelifts include a vertical preauricular incision that enters the temporal scalp posterior to the sideburn hair, and then angles forward in a curvilinear fashion. The redraping of the ante-

rior facial skin into the temporal sideburn then creates an area of hair loss. This obvious, unwanted sequel of facelift surgery results from lifting and removing the natural temporal hair tuft. It is especially apparent in patients requiring a relatively large amount of skin removal from this region, who postoperatively may already have thin, light-colored hair and a high tuft. No salvage facelift procedure, however, can improve this complication, which is remedied by hair flaps or follicular unit hair transplantation.

To avoid this problem, we use a temporal hair tuft sparing incision (30) (Fig. 177.9). The incision begins horizontally no higher than the level of the supraauricular crease (*B*, segment c-d). As it extends horizontally, the incision has a vertical limb (segment b-c) followed by an anteroinferior limb (segment a-b) to accommodate any excessive skin reduction and prevent tissue coning. To avoid visibility of this incision, the angle of the first horizontal portion closest to the ear is designed to bevel across the hair follicles; thus, even if no hair exists below this line, the hair follicles above will grow through the advanced lower facial skin flap and hide the scar. The more anterior vertical hair tuft (segment b-c) and then horizontal limb are made parallel to the hair follicles to avoid alopecia (Fig. 177.10). For each segment of this temporal incision, attention must be paid to the direction of beveling.

Several alternatives for the posterior occipital incision must also be carefully considered. Whereas an incision along the inferior edge of the postauricular hairline completely preserves the existing hairline and simplifies redraping, postoperative widening of the scar or potential tissue loss makes this choice less desirable and requires the patient to wear the hair longer to camouflage the scars. Moreover, these patients can no longer wear their hair up because of the conspicuous scars.

Incisions that curve high into the postauricular area are completely hidden; however, potential flap necrosis and derangement of the hairline call for a compromise regarding posterior incision placement. We prefer a horizontal incision that extends posteriorly into the hair from slightly below the midconchal region. In placing this incision, we take into consideration the spacing from the ear to the beginning of the posterior hairline. The incision extends about 5 cm and angles inferiorly at the distal end to reduce the potential cutaneous cone (dog-ear) after flap rotation. This incision allows for an anterior vector during redraping to maximize the amount of hairline that is preserved. With experience, these postoperative posterior hairlines look full and natural. Respect and consideration for the patient's existing hairline and hair-bearing tissues pay great dividends in terms of patient satisfaction.

Additional factors regarding incision placement involve differences between incision done in men and in women, especially in the preauricular limb, but also in the earlobe and postauricular areas (31). Before surgery, we advise male patients that afterward they may need to shave

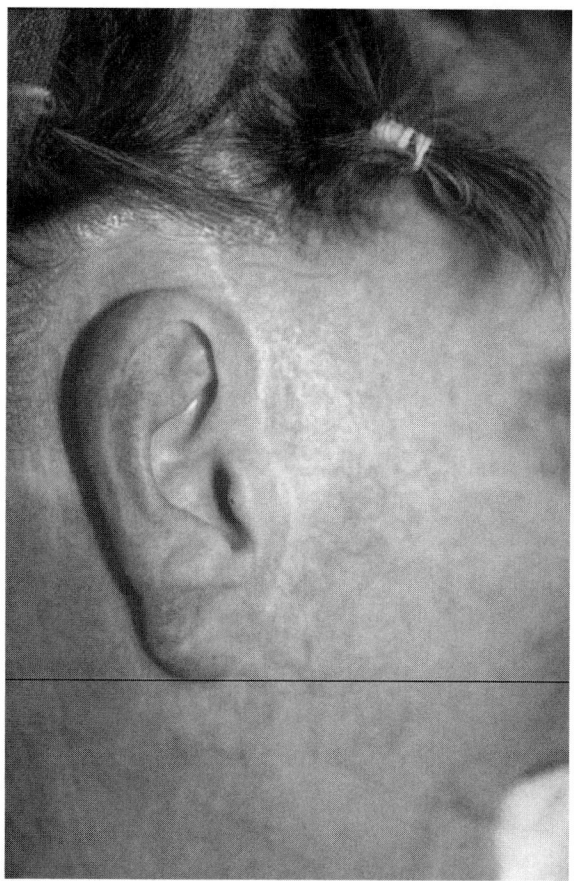

Figure 177.8 This patient had a facelift performed elsewhere, with improperly placed incisions that caused temporal alopecia and a pixie ear deformity.

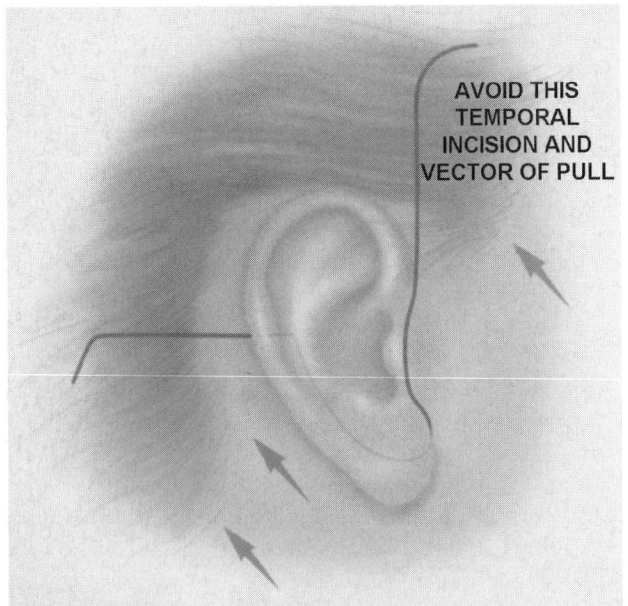

A

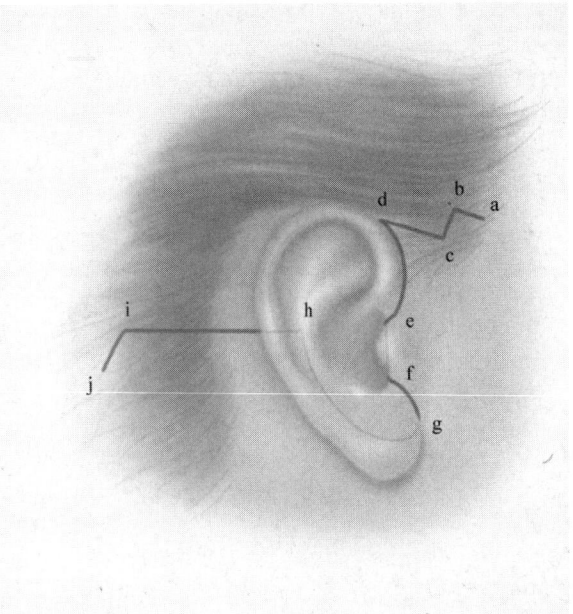

B

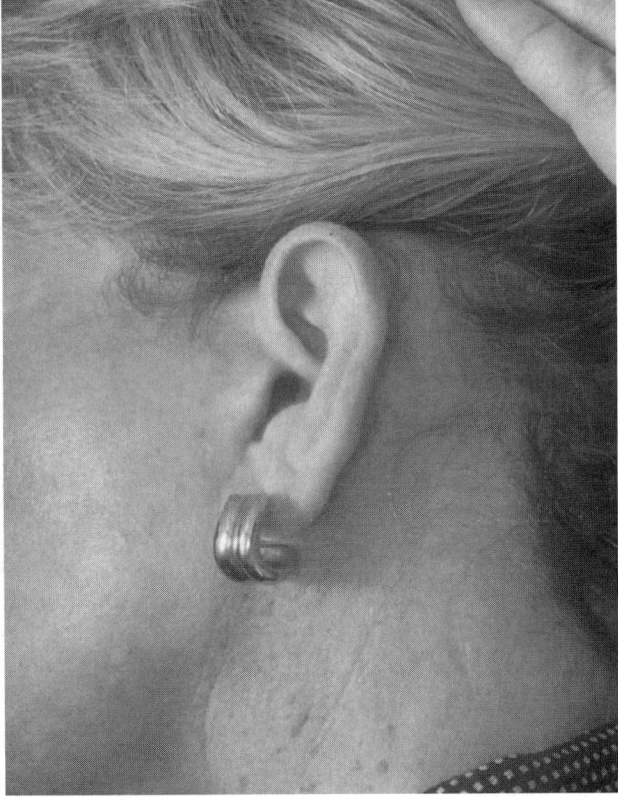

C

Figure 177.9 **A:** Schema of a typical female facelift incision performed elsewhere; the temporal portion of this incision should be avoided in women because skin excision after a posterosuperior pull leads to loss of the temporal hair tuft. **B:** Schema of our incision with various segments labeled. **C:** Postoperative result of a typical patient with our incision showing no temporal hair tuft loss and well-concealed pre- and postauricular incisions. (Reprinted from Kridel, RWH. Techniques for inconspicuous face lift scars. *Arch Facial Plast Surg.* 2003;5:323–333, with permission.)

behind the ear, depending on the degree of lift, because beard skin that is elevated and tailored after suspension rhytidectomy can become relocated to the postauricular area. We also advise men that their anterior temporal hair tuft generally will be thinner in width and density as the beard is advanced cephalad and slightly posterior. Some surgeons advocate a preauricular crease incision in men so that hair-bearing, bearded skin is not brought onto the car-

tilaginous tragus (Fig. 177.11). In those patients who prefer a retrotragal incision, we attempt to inactivate the hair follicles that will abut the tragus or the immediate preauricular area by using the cautery unit on the hair follicle bulbs. Moreover, we inform them that they may need postoperative electrolysis to remove hair in this region.

Native earlobe position, angulation, and relative size are noted and discussed preoperatively. The incision

Hair at edge of incision

Advanced face lift
flap at surgery

Hair camouflaging
incision

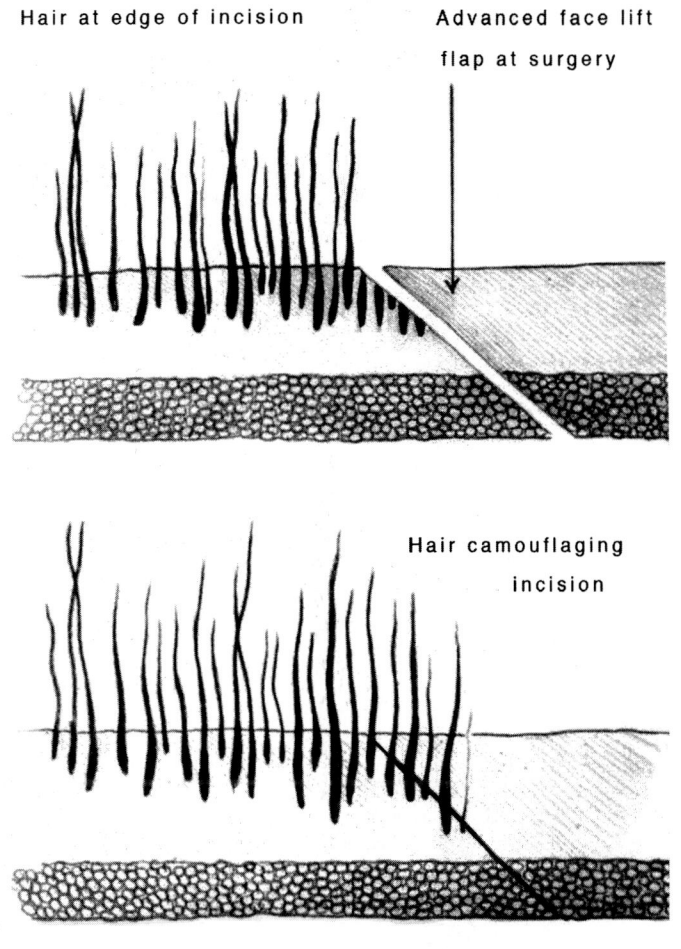

A

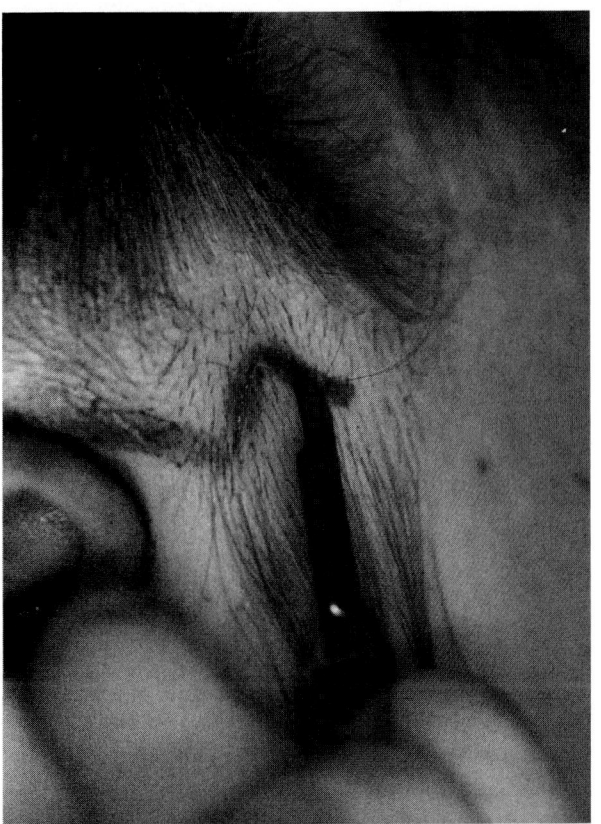

B

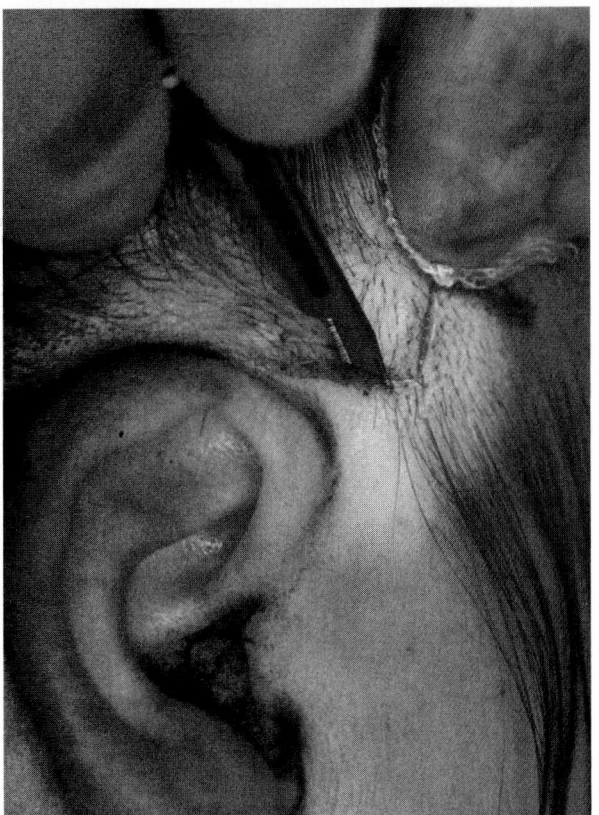

C

Figure 177.10 A: Beveling of an incision *perpendicular* to hair
shafts allows hair to grow through the advanced skin flap. B: Beveling
of incision *parallel* to hair shafts when hair remains on the inferior skin
flap, even after excision of excess skin. C: Intraoperative view of incision beveled *perpendicular* to hair follicles. (Reprinted from Kridel,
RWH. Techniques for inconspicuous face lift scars. *Arch Facial Plast
Surg* 2003;5:323–333, with permission.)

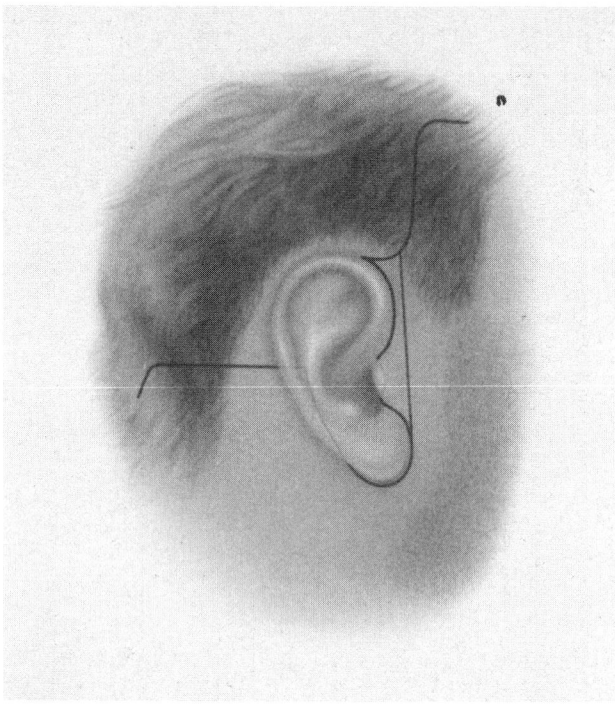

Figure 177.11 Schema of two options for male facelift incision. Note a cuff of non–hair-bearing skin is left around the lobule and the postauricular incision is placed in the sulcus and not onto the concha, as in women, to prevent men from having to shave in these areas. (Reprinted from Kridel, RWH. Techniques for inconspicuous face lift scars. *Arch Facial Plast Surg* 2003;5:323–333, with permission.)

around the earlobe is at the inferior attachment, except in the male patient, where a margin of non–hair-bearing skin is preserved so that beard hair does not abut the lobe postoperatively.

OPERATIVE STAGE

The classic, now outdated, facelift procedure involved only the development of facial skin flaps and the redistribution and excision of excess skin (9). Undermining of the skin in the single-layer skin flap is usually extensive. This older technique is effective; however, the single-layer skin closure often places greater tension on the tissues and results in wider scarring or possible tissue loss. Theoretically, the skin-only, long-flap facelift may not be as long-lasting and could predispose to an increased risk of postoperative bleeding.

Contemporary facial plastic surgeons use either the concept of the two-layer cervicofacial rhytidectomy with suspension of the SMAS or the extended sub-SMAS or deep plane rhytidectomy (32). As discussed, although many surgeons feel that the deep plane lift gives more long-lasting results and decreases the incidence of hematomas, no definitive studies yet confirm these findings. In fact, whereas one study attempted to compare

"deep plane vs. superficial musculoaponeurotic system plication" facelifts, many questions remain unanswered (33,34). We will provide a brief descriptive outline of both procedures.

In both the SMAS and sub-SMAS rhytidectomy, surgeons have incorporated the use of suction-assisted lipectomy and platysmaplasty (29,35,36). The two-layer SMAS suspension technique and liposuction has numerous advantages. Open liposuction under direct surgical vision permanently removes fat cells and recontours difficult facial areas (e.g., jowl and periparotid gland). To gain the maximal improvement in the neck, most patients should have platysmaplasty at the time of facelift. Most patients who are candidates for a facelift also have ptosis of the anterior platysma muscle, which causes banding. This problem is best handled by low division of the offending bands and resection of the excess muscle under direct vision. Also, unlike the musculature of the face, the platysma muscle of the neck is naturally dehiscent in the midline, with only a tenuous fascial connection between the paired muscles. In the absence of midline platysmal plication, SMAS suspension pulls the anterior margins of the platysma muscle laterally, actually weakening support for the submental fat. Plication of the anterior margins resists this lateral migration and allows suspension to strengthen submental support and enhance recontouring of the neck. Finally, in most patients, a significant proportion of the excess submental fat is actually in the anatomic submental triangle, deep to the platysma muscle, and therefore not accessible by closed liposuction. In these cases, the platysmaplasty approach allows access to this area, with direct open lipectomy. It has been our experience that the addition of routine platysmaplasty to rhytidectomy has both enhanced results in the neck and increased the duration of the aesthetic improvement (see Fig. 177.19).

Flap Elevation

After appropriate marking of the patient and initiation of general and infiltrative anesthesia, the procedure is begun in the submental area. A horizontal incision 1.5 cm long is made in the submental crease. Sharp dissection is used to start a plane just below the dermis. Next, a double lumen blunt-tipped liposuction cannula is advanced radially to form an even subcutaneous pocket in the submental/cervical region. Then the cannula is advanced, with the lumen toward the deep tissues at all times, in a back-and-forth fashion. Fat is suctioned from the previously delineated areas. Dissection is facilitated by tenting the skin upward and using a rapid motion, which avoids suctioning in the same area for too long. Using the "pinch and roll" technique (i.e., palpation of the skin between the thumb and forefingers), ensure that no excessive fat deposits are inadvertently omitted during this part of the procedure. Liposuction is carried inferiorly over the hyoid and toward the thyroid notch, then laterally to overlap the anterior border

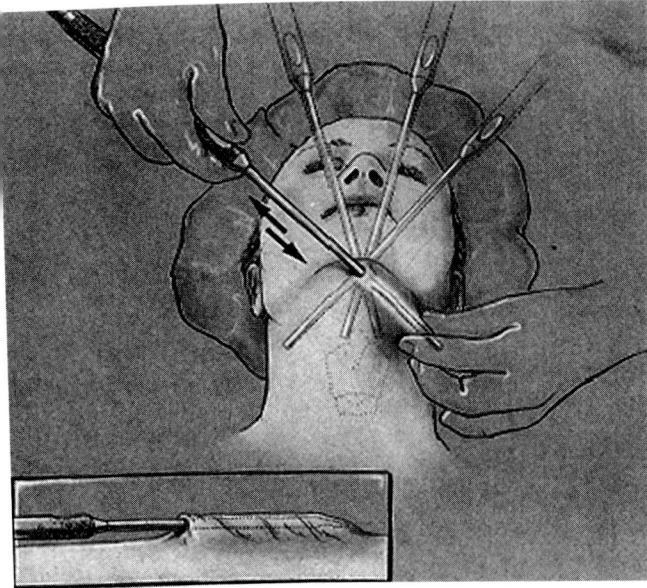

Figure 177.12 The direction of submental liposuction in a fan-like configuration.

of the sternocleidomastoid muscles, and then superiorly to the dependent portion of jowl formation and the edge of the mandibular border (Fig. 177.12).

The submental, subcutaneous pocket is inspected with the assistance of a fiberoptic headlight and a modified Converse retractor looking for individual neurovascular septations and controlling any rare bleeding points by suction cautery. The anterior borders of the platysma muscle are then identified and a small amount of horizontal sectioning of the platysma muscle is done at the level of the thyroid notch. The anterior borders of the platysma muscle are then reapproximated in the midline, using a corset platysmaplasty of 2-0 Ethibond suture. At all times, the vector of force is medial and superior. The plication is at least to the level of the hyoid bone, however, care is taken to avoid excessive tightening, which can result in a central band.

The submental incision is left open until the end of the lift to provide access for inspection and further cautery needed. Only after both flaps have been elevated, trimmed, and sewn into place should the submental incision be closed. We prefer a layered closure, using 5-0 chromic for the subcutaneous layer and 6-0 Prolene in a running, locking manner for the skin.

Next, beginning on one side, the previously delineated incision is made. Dissection is started occipitally and the skin flap begun using facelift scissors. With the scissors tips pointed upward, a gliding motion is used to develop the skin flap (Fig. 177.13). The skin may be densely adherent to the sternocleidomastoid fascia, and meticulous dissection in this area serves to elevate the flap without injury to the greater auricular nerve. The earlobe is dissected completely free and the skin mobilized over the tragus with

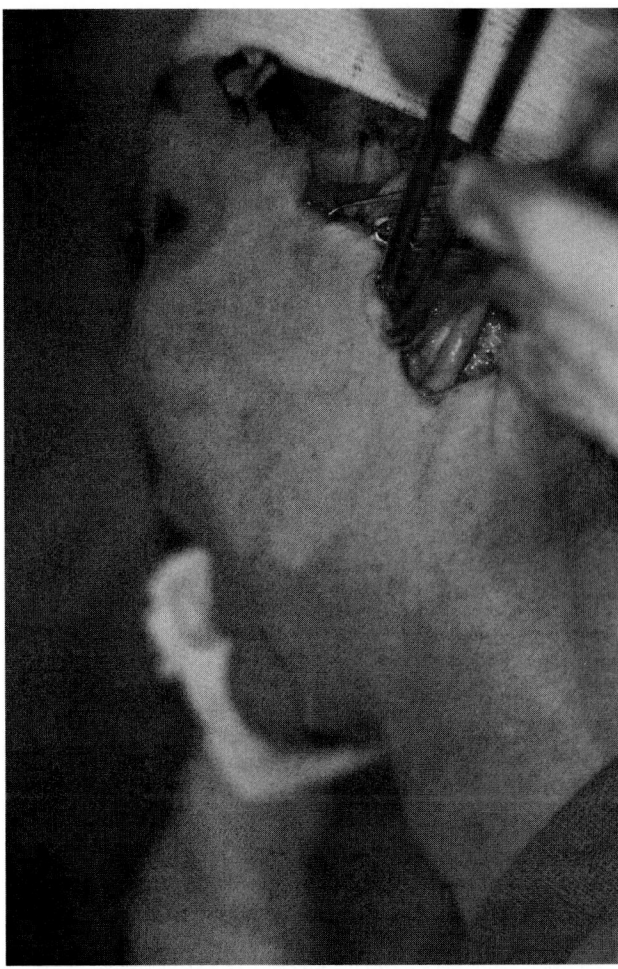

Figure 177.13 Intraoperative use of facelift scissors, with the skin retracted. Notice the tips of the curved scissors can be seen.

small iris or serrated dissecting scissors. Because the temporal incision is placed to preserve the hair tuft, the plane of dissection should not be as deep as the temporalis fascia, but rather just under the hair follicles. Superficial flap elevation in this region avoids injury to the frontal branch of the facial nerve, which crosses the zygomatic arch at this point.

We usually develop a long flap in the neck and connect broadly with the submental preplatysmal dissection to allow optimal redraping of neck skin. Fat deposits are removed gently under direct visualization, and facial contouring is inspected for uniformity and desired appearance. The area is irrigated with saline and the dissection examined for hemostasis. Bleeding is controlled with bipolar cautery to avoid facial nerve or skin flap injury.

Superficial Musculoaponeurotic System Suspension

After flap elevation, direct surgical management of the SMAS fascia is performed. SMAS suspension is the foundation on which the longevity, safety, and aesthetically pleasing result is built. SMAS suspension permits tension-free closure of the incision by transferring the strength and support of the facelift rejuvenation to the deeper structures and tissues. SMAS suspension can be achieved by several different methods (37–40).

Imbrication techniques involve direct incision, resection, or undermining of the SMAS fascia with the reapproximation or overlap of the cut SMAS fascia edges. With imbrication methods, the SMAS is usually identified and incised within the region anterior to the tragus and below the earlobe, overlying the deeper parotid fascia. Many surgeons undermine a separate SMAS fascia layer and resect excess tissue after advancement and redraping. Proper suture placement buries each knot to prevent suture splitting. An alternative imbrication technique involves excising a segmental portion of SMAS and resuspending the anterior cut layer without additional undermining. Increased sharp dissection associated with imbrication techniques increases the risks of bleeding, nerve injury, and skin slough. In patients with wide, chubby faces, imbrication tends to flatten the region overlying the parotid gland and, therefore, offers some advantages in early surgical definition of this region.

Plication techniques for SMAS suspension avoid direct cutting and undermining of the SMAS layer. Fold the SMAS fascia on itself and secure the newly folded tissues with permanent buried sutures. Because SMAS plication involves less dissection and surgical time, the potentially decreased risks are thought to offer some significant advantage over imbrication.

With either technique, SMAS suspension lifts and resupports the attached skin layer and reduces the amount of potential cavity space created during flap elevation. The question of which technique is better in terms of long-term results and decreased morbidity is controversial. Webster et al. (41) studied imbrication versus plication by performing each method on opposite sides of the face. By taking exact measurements and confirming the findings on fresh cadaver dissections, they concluded that no objective benefit favored imbrication over plication during the surgical procedure. Subsequent studies failed to demonstrate any long-term advantages either. Because imbrication theoretically involves a greater chance for surgical morbidity, we prefer plication for SMAS suspension.

The direction of forces applied to the SMAS layer by sutures is important, and specific vector patterns are used routinely. Plication is done by tugging on the SMAS fascia in a bidirectional vector. Before placing any sutures, the effect of each tug on the face and neck should be noted and the desirable sites secured with 2-0 nonabsorbable sutures. Braided sutures are used to provide knot security without multiple ties, which can otherwise lead to palpable suture knots. Multiple buried sutures are placed along each vector to avoid relying on only one suture. The first suspension vector generally runs from the angle of the mandible to the fascia near the superior mastoid cortex. Suturing at this

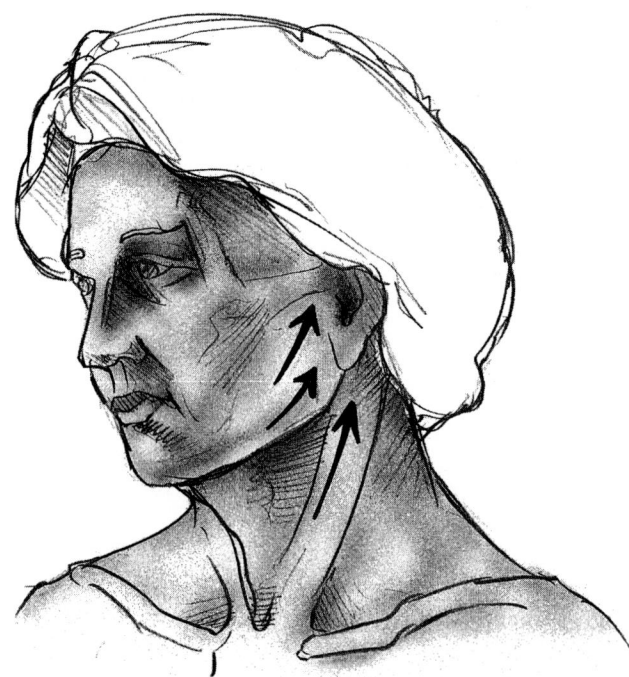

Figure 177.14   *Arrows* indicate the direction of pull for a superficial musculoaponeurotic system (SMAS) plication.

point affects the cervicomental angle and the angular bony contour of the mandible, which define a smooth jawline and neck. Attention then turns to the second vector, which originates in the SMAS of the cheek and mandibular ramus near the anterior border of the parotid gland. The SMAS here is extended with a more superior than posterior vector toward the preauricular sulcus and tragus. Finally, the third vector extends from the posterior border of the cervical platysma muscle in a predominantly superior direction to the sternocleidomastoid fascia in the region of the mastoid tip. Additional sutures are placed, where required, for even, firm plication.

The overall direction of pull remains superior and only partially posterior (Fig. 177.14). A pull that is too posterior creates a distinctly unattractive and artificial appearance. Posterior lifts tend to widen and flatten the oral commissure, resulting in a disproportionately large mouth. This common complication stems from the often mistaken assumption that SMAS suspension will correct or improve the nasolabial folds. In fact, SMAS suspension alone can deepen the melolabial groove. The standard rhytidectomy with SMAS suspension often fails to improve the nasolabial fold to a significant extent. The SMAS inserts on the mimetic muscles of the face (18). In the perioral area, these include the platysma muscle and the same lip retractors and elevators discussed previously. SMAS suspension, therefore, results in further lateral and superior displacement of the perioral soft tissues, which are densely attached to the mimetic musculature with relatively little effect on the malar soft tissues, which at best are associated

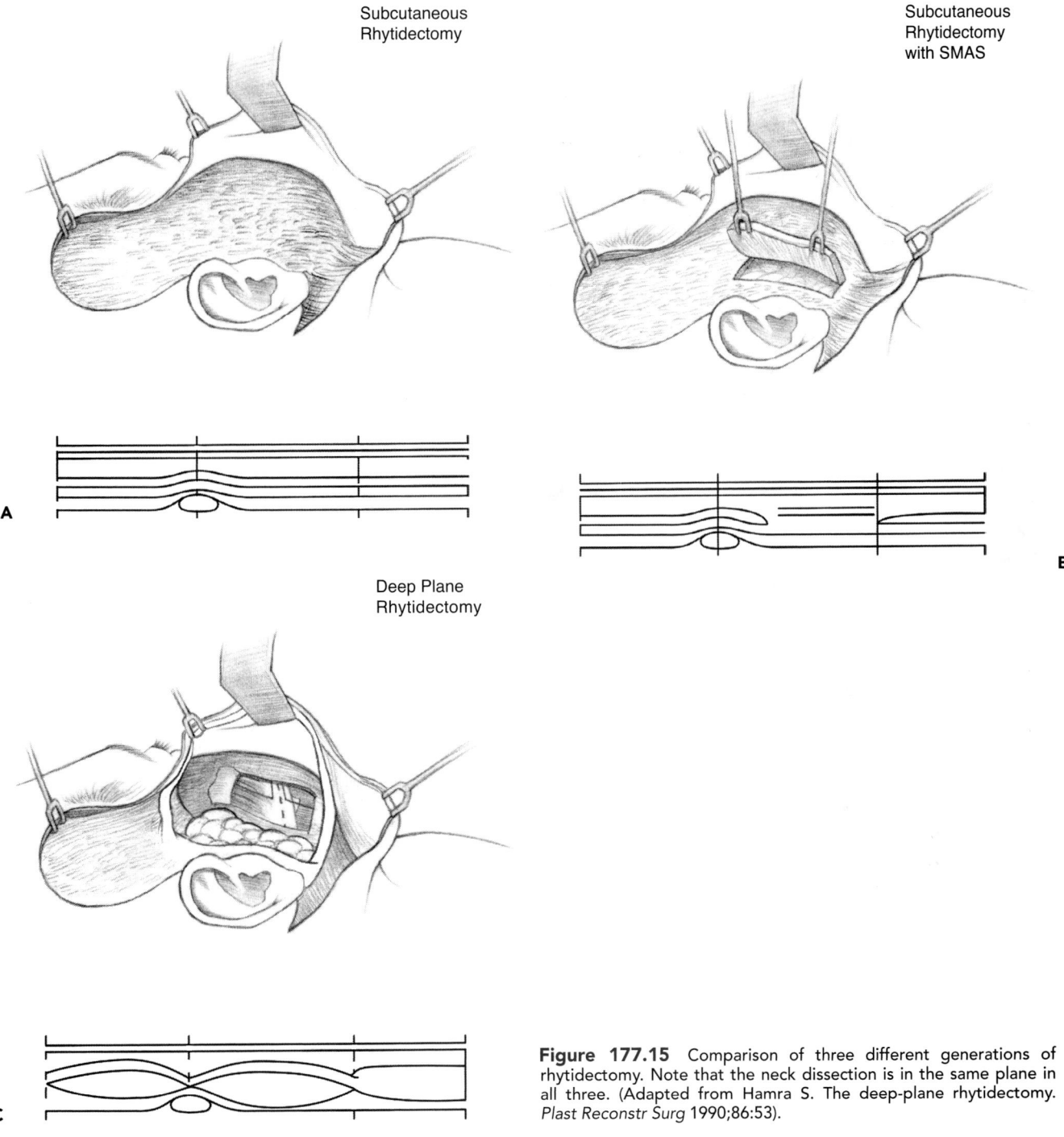

Subcutaneous
Rhytidectomy

Subcutaneous
Rhytidectomy
with SMAS

Deep Plane
Rhytidectomy

A

B

C

Figure 177.15 Comparison of three different generations of rhytidectomy. Note that the neck dissection is in the same plane in all three. (Adapted from Hamra S. The deep-plane rhytidectomy. *Plast Reconstr Surg* 1990;86:53).

only weakly with the muscular plane. In isolation, then, the act of SMAS suspension theoretically would deepen the nasolabial fold even further. That it does not seem to deepen in practice likely results from the excision of excess skin performed after SMAS suspension. The greater amount of skin excised, the more improvement in the fold. Because of preoperative skin laxity, it is generally possible to excise sufficient skin to result in a small net improvement in the fold without closing under undue skin tension and predisposing to skin slough or scar widening.

It should be noted, however, that suture placement, application of tension, removal, and redraping of skin are so individually variable that different surgeons will find widely disparate results while using the same overall technique.

Deep Plane Lift

The SMAS suspension facelift is a highly effective operation. With appropriate case selection and planning, both patient and surgeon can expect a technically sound surgery to produce very satisfactory results. Cosmetic surgeons and their patients, however, are very demanding. Innovative surgeons, therefore, have continued to attempt to improve the SMAS plication facelift by doing deep plane or sub-SMAS facelifts (21,42–44).

Patient and surgeon dissatisfaction with generally accepted facelift techniques primarily have been related to the nasolabial fold, the inconsistency in achieving long-term results, and perioperative complications. Deep dissection rhytidectomies are aimed primarily at improving the nasolabial fold to a greater extent than is possible using the widely accepted SMAS suspension techniques. Of the various techniques that have been reported (42–44), the deep plane or the more recent composite rhytidectomy of Hamra has attracted the most interest. The key distinctions of deep plane rhytidectomy relative to the SMAS plication procedure described in detail are discussed below, noting the theoretical advantages and disadvantages.

The deep plane rhytidectomy, in fact, is carried out at three different planes, depending on the area of the face and neck being dissected (21,43) (Fig. 177.15). Neck dissection (inferior to the jawline) is preplatysmal and is connected subcutaneously with the contralateral dissection. A platysmaplasty with submental lipectomy is performed. In this area, the operation is similar to that already described.

Lower face dissection is carried out in a sub-SMAS plane, in contradistinction to the subcutaneous plane described previously, but similar to most SMAS imbrication techniques. One significant point of difference with established techniques is that the sub-SMAS dissection is carried out anterior to the parotid gland where the buccal and marginal branches of the facial nerve may be encountered. A second distinction is that the subcutaneous plane is developed only minimally so that the bulk of the elevated flap contains SMAS along with the skin and subcutaneous fat.

Finally, midface dissection is done over the malar eminences into the central face. This dissection is much more extensive than in other SMAS suspension techniques. The subcutaneous plane is maintained initially for 2 to 3 cm anterior to the tragus, presumably to avoid injury to the frontal branch of the facial nerve. A thick flap then is developed anteriorly, with dissection immediately superficial to the orbicularis and zygomaticus muscles. No other motor nerve branches should be encountered in this plane, because they enter the muscles from their deep surface (45). The two facial dissection planes are bluntly connected to create a large, thick flap. Excess skin is excised after the flap is resuspended under tension at the SMAS level (43).

The major theoretical advantage of this and similar procedures is that the malar fat and skin can be elevated and resuspended, and the nasolabial fold can be undermined, allowing for its effacement. Additionally, the facelift flap is maintained as a "myocutaneous" flap (43) consisting of platysma muscle, SMAS, and the superficial tissues, pur-

portedly allowing increased viability and closure under greater tension than is possible with standard procedures. Further possible advantages include a decrease in hematomas because of a more avascular dissection plane and a decrease in skin slough because of the theoretically increased viability. The major theoretical disadvantage of the deep plane dissections is the increased exposure to the facial nerve in the lower face with the concomitant possibility of injury. Moreover, patients with deep rhytids or acne scarring also find improved results from SMAS suspension with an extended skin flap, which can stretch the skin itself more directly. Because of the widespread interest in this procedure, it is important to evaluate these potential advantages and disadvantages critically.

If ptotic subcutaneous fat in the malar region is a significant contributor to a prominent nasolabial fold, improvement could occur in the nasolabial fold with infrazygomatic undermining, as described by Hamra and others (42,43,46). This fat is not to be confused with the buccal fat pad (of Bichat), which gives the cheek most of its fullness, but lies at a deeper plane in intimate association with the facial nerve. On the other hand, anatomic studies of the nasolabial fold demonstrate that it usually consists of little more than skin excess (18,47). In this case, it would seem that only skin resection, and not deep tissue repositioning, is used to attain significant improvement in this area. Because the current SMAS suspension procedures usually do not involve undermining medial to the malar eminence, the deep plane procedures, as described, should have some advantage in malar skin redraping and resection.

As for theoretically improved viability with the deeper plane of dissection, this depends on the vascular anatomy of the flap. For the deep plane facelift flap to be a true fasciocutaneous flap of the SMAS based on the facial artery, as asserted, there must be multiple small perforators from the SMAS to the overlying skin, with only the distal few centimeters immediately anterior to the pinna left random, because this area is undermined subcutaneously. At least one recent study of the vascular anatomy of the face calls this interpretation into question (46). The authors have observed many small perforators from the facial system in the medial face but only a few perforators in the transverse facial and posterior auricular distributions. Abundant small perforators from the facial system via the SMAS fascia are not described. Indeed, subcutaneous facelift dissection results in little bleeding above the jawline and in front of the ear, except for the transection of the transverse facial perforators, which are divided in the deep plane dissection as well. These observations suggest the possibility that both the classic and deep plane facelift flaps are similarly viable large random flaps. As skin slough is a relatively rare complication, extensive experience with deep plane facelifting will be required before reliable empiric judgments can be made.

A much lower incidence of hematoma (~1%) relative to the classic procedure (8%) is reported for the deep plane procedure (43), providing some indirect evidence that the dissection is more avascular. Given that dissection in the neck for both procedures is in a similar plane, only the incidence of facial hematoma is likely to be lower. It may be, however, that neck hematomas can be reduced as well by remaining strictly in the preplatysmal plane as recommended by Hamra (43), rather than hugging the subcutaneous tissues, as described above, regardless of whether a deep plane or a more standard SMAS suspension procedure is performed.

In most SMAS suspension procedures practiced today, the facial nerve is well protected. As long as SMAS undermining is not carried forward of the anterior margin of the parotid gland, the nerve is shielded by the gland parenchyma. Anterior to the gland, the nerve courses within the buccal fat pad deep to the SMAS and, therefore, is exposed to injury by SMAS undermining in this area. In a similar vein, dissection that remains meticulously superficial to the zygomatic arch will protect its innervation; however, the branches to the lower orbicularis are more superficial (the orbicularis lies in a plane superficial to the zygomatic arch) and can be vulnerable to injury by dissection over the malar eminence if care is not exercised to remain strictly superficial to the orbicularis as well (45). Both areas are manipulated by the deep plane lifting techniques, which therefore carry theoretically greater risks of nerve injury. A working estimate of the incidence of temporary weakness in deep plane facelift can be obtained by combining cases from several recent reports (43,48,49). These authors report a total of 23 cases of temporary paralysis in 638 deep plane rhytidectomies, for an estimated incidence of 3.6%. By contrast, a classic review of facial nerve injury in more standard rhytidectomy revealed 50 cases of paralysis in 6,500 rhytidectomies, for an incidence of 0.8%. Seven of these cases were permanent (22). Although no cases of permanent paralysis have yet been reported for deep plane rhytidectomy, it would seem reasonable that the incidence would be correspondingly higher.

Flap Closure

Drains

Many surgeons elect not to drain their standard facelift flaps and reserve drains for excessively long procedures or for those in which less than perfect hemostasis was achieved (50). An argument can be made for omitting drains because the percentage of early seroma and hematoma formation is low, and no one has been able to demonstrate that either open or closed suction drainage systems prevent hematoma.

We, nevertheless, favor the use of closed suction drainage for our patients having a facelift. We have noted great improvement in early skin flap adherence to the deeper layers of dissection because the drains actively re-

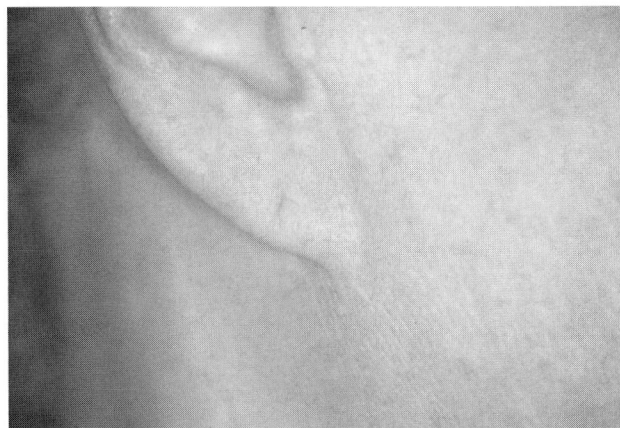

Figure 177.16 Pixie ear or satyr ear deformity caused by excessive skin excision or tension at the ear lobe.

move small amounts of fluid. Our patients have reported much less discomfort with suction drains than without them, perhaps because no fluid pressure builds up beneath the flap. A 14 French Blake flat, perforated drain is placed through a separate posterior stab incision. Aspiration via a bulb suction device continues until the first postoperative day or longer, on rare occasions. A fluffy pressure dressing is still used to support the face and neck and ensure uniform, gentle pressure on the flap.

Earlobe and Tragus

Special attention is given to the flap closure in the area of the earlobe and tragus to prevent postoperative sequelae often associated with these structures. An elongated earlobe directly attached to the facial cheek skin, known as the pixie or satyr earlobe, is a common complication. (Fig. 177.16). Other problems include earlobes that are too pendulous and scars visible below the earlobe.

Prevention is by far the best management of these difficulties. During closure, a generous amount of perilobular flap skin needs to be left around the earlobe. Additionally, the skin flap can be fixed to the SMAS or mastoid fascia superiorly. We have seen consistently pleasing earlobes in our patients by adhering to the following principles. The earlobe complex is dissected completely free from the skin and subcutaneous tissue, rendering it completely mobile. After the initial perilobular flap cut is made before SMAS plication, we seldom alter this incision length (Fig. 177.17). Before closure, the earlobe shape is preserved by a horizontal mattress-type suture of 5-0 polypropylene, as described by Clyde Litton (personal communication, Washington, DC, 1986) (Fig. 177.18). This suture suspends the earlobe superiorly, maintains a normal crease, and prevents the lobe from being pulled downward. The inferior edge of the earlobe is attached to the skin flap by a separate individual polypropylene suture.

The tragus shape and projection are similarly affected by flap closure techniques when a posttragal incision is used.

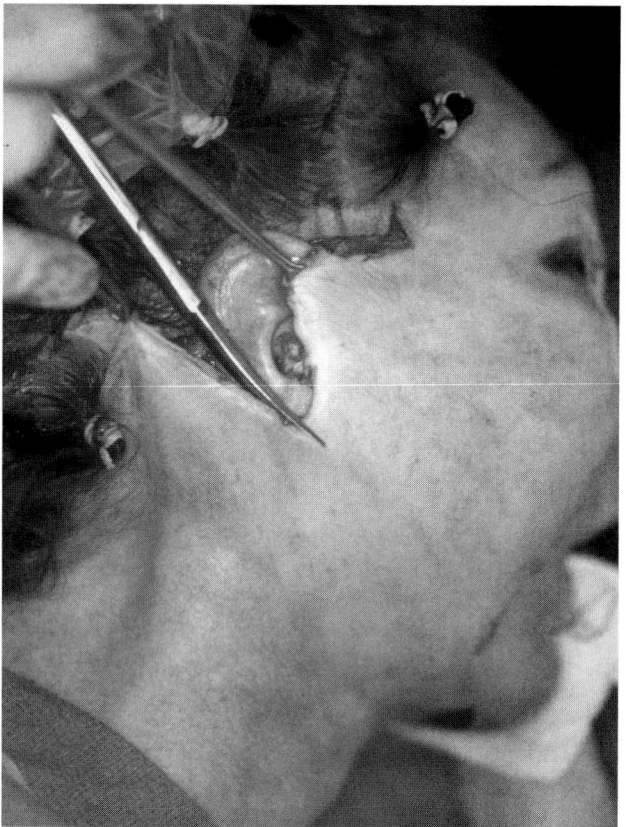

Figure 177.17 Intraoperative photograph, before plication, showing the perilobular flap cut to set the lobule.

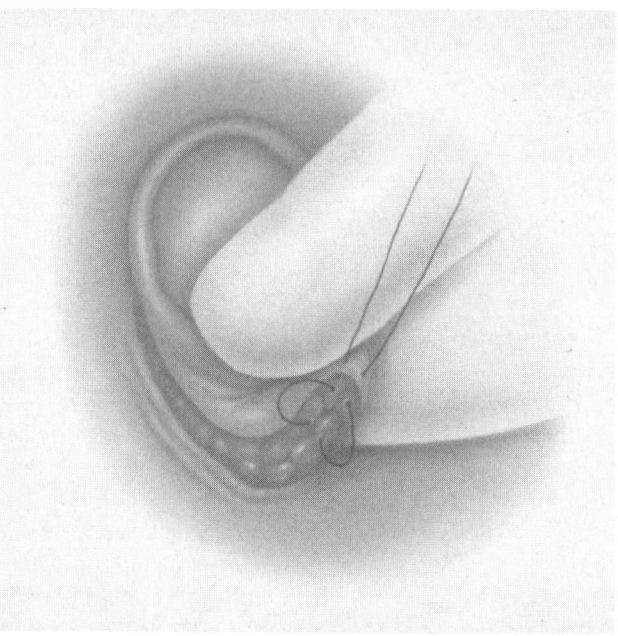

Figure 177.18 To further prevent tethering of the lobule, a mattress stitch with 5-0 polypropylene is placed at the free cut edge of the lobule and secured to the underlying tissues (Clyde Litton, oral communication, 1986). (Reprinted from Kridel, RWH. Techniques for inconspicuous face lift scars. *Arch Facial Plast Surg* 2003;5:323–333, with permission.)

Common postsurgical tragal deformities include blunting, irregularity, and anteriorly dislocated cartilage. Blunting is prevented with a pretragal deep polydioxanone (PDS) suture. Moreover, in addition to defatting the skin overlying the tragus, the flap in this area is trimmed to leave a generous portion of extra skin that sufficiently covers the tragal cartilage without tension. This segment is sutured to the canal portion of the tragal skin with individual 5-0 plain gut sutures, taking care to avoid needle entry into the cartilaginous tragus.

Wound Closure

The postauricular flap and the temporal region have been trimmed and the incision approximated in these areas by using skin staples. Wound-edge eversion is helpful to fine-line incision healing. We oppose the skin edges with a lightly run, locking suture of 5-0 plain gut, even in areas that have been stapled. This hemostatic-type stitch also ensures an airtight flap closure, which allows the suction drain to function more effectively. This extra attention to wound eversion also seems to improve the appearance of the incisions.

POSTOPERATIVE CARE

The patient should be given detailed typewritten postoperative instructions before the surgery to allow the patient and family to read the instructions in detail and ask questions before surgery. After surgery, the patient and family are informed again of problems that might arise and instructed to call the physician for any questions.

We use a large, bulky dressing right after surgery, partly to discourage turning of the head, which can lead to hematoma formation. Patients often complain that their bandage is too tight right after surgery, which usually indicates that they are feeling the tightening of the lift and the bandage. If a compressive dressing is used, a vertical incision can be made in the midline of the dressing at the inferior border to offer relief, but patients must be ready to accept a feeling of tightness.

Postoperative orders are geared toward keeping the patient calm and as pain free as possible. Increased pain leads to increased blood pressure, which can increase the likelihood of complications. Likewise, a full bladder after a long procedure can increase blood pressure.

The surgeon should check on the patient the night of surgery. Any unilateral pain that is unrelenting and unresponsive to routine pain medication should alert the physician to possible hematoma formation and must be addressed as soon as possible. The patient also should be seen on the first postoperative day; drains are usually removed at this time, depending on the amount of drainage noted. Before releasing the tension of the bandage and removing the drains, fluffs are held over the area from which the drains are going to be removed, and pressure is applied. Pressure is maintained in those areas until a new bandage can be reapplied. This step helps to keep down the flaps and prevent hematoma or seroma formation. Before placing the new dressing on the first postoperative day, antibiotic ointment or cream is applied on all incisions (we prefer gentamicin cream), making sure to apply some at the external auditory canal to prevent any *Pseudomonas* organisms from the external canal contaminating the incisions.

Usually by the second or third postoperative day, the large, bulky dressing can be totally removed, and an elasticized facial sling can be used. This helps the skin flap to maintain close contact with the subcutaneous tissue and provides faster revascularization and even contraction. It is important to pad the ears because these elasticized bandages can rub the thin skin of the pinna and thus cause irritation.

Usually at the fifth postoperative day, a few of the anterior preauricular stitches are removed and the patient's hair is washed in a shampoo sink in the office. Patients are cautioned not to use hair dryers in the immediate postoperative period because some numbness of the periauricular and scalp areas will be present, possibly causing patients to burn the skin with the hair dryer because of lack of sensation.

Over ensuing visits, all the sutures are removed and the incisions examined under the microscope, especially in the hair-bearing areas to check for ingrown hairs, which can occur up to several months after surgery. After performing beveled incisions, this step also ensures that the hair will actually grow through the incision for camouflage. Often hairs become trapped and need help to come through the advanced flap.

Almost all patients have significant swelling or bruising postoperatively, and often this is difficult for the patient to accept. Gentle reassurance is the key in the first postoperative weeks. As Goin and Goin (51) pointed out, if everything has gone well and the results are good, it is important for the physician to tell the patient so. Patients do not know how they should look and whether things were done well unless the doctor says so. Patients often forget what they looked like before surgery. For that reason, giving them prints of their preoperative photographs at the first or second postoperative visit is extremely helpful. This allows patients to compare their preoperative and postoperative conditions.

COMPLICATIONS

Nerve Injury

Facial nerve injury is a rare complication, with a reported incidence of between 0.4% and 2.6% (24,52–54). The motor nerve branch most vulnerable to direct, technical

injury is the frontal branch of the zygomatic–temporal division of the facial nerve. This is because of its superficial location as it traverses the midportion of the zygomatic arch (Fig. 177.19). We avoid deep plane dissection entirely in the region superior to the arch and anterior to the temporal hairline to negate the risk of frontal nerve branch injury. Anatomic considerations are important for the marginal mandibular nerve and buccal nerve divisions as well. Marginal nerve injury results in an asymmetrically oriented smile with a higher position of the lower lip on the affected side because of unopposed action of the opposite depressor lip musculature (Fig. 177.20). Platysma muscle transection and excessive SMAS traction in the region near the angle of the mandible and inferior mandibular border can result in marginal nerve paralysis. Buccal motor nerve branches are injured with aggressive dissection medial to the anterior border of the parotid gland. An asymmetric flattening of the midfacial contour can accompany buccal division injury.

Total facial nerve injury is extremely rare. If it is seen postoperatively and complete nerve transection is doubtful, consider a concomitant Bell palsy (52). Transient paralysis of one or more facial nerve branches often is related to local action imposed by infiltrative anesthesia. Any prolonged paresis merits additional investigation and should not be attributed to the lidocaine effect. Additional causes of facial nerve injury include thermal injury by

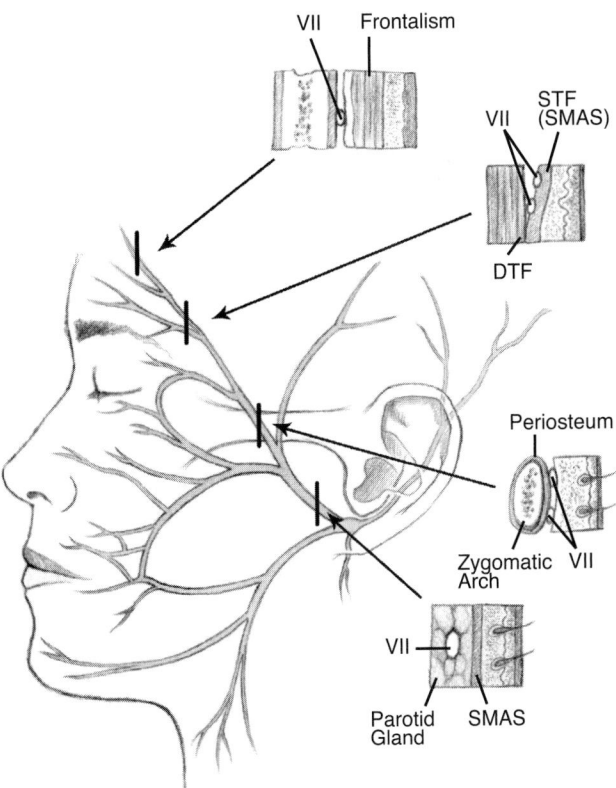

Figure 177.19 The frontal branch of the facial nerve at different locations in its course.

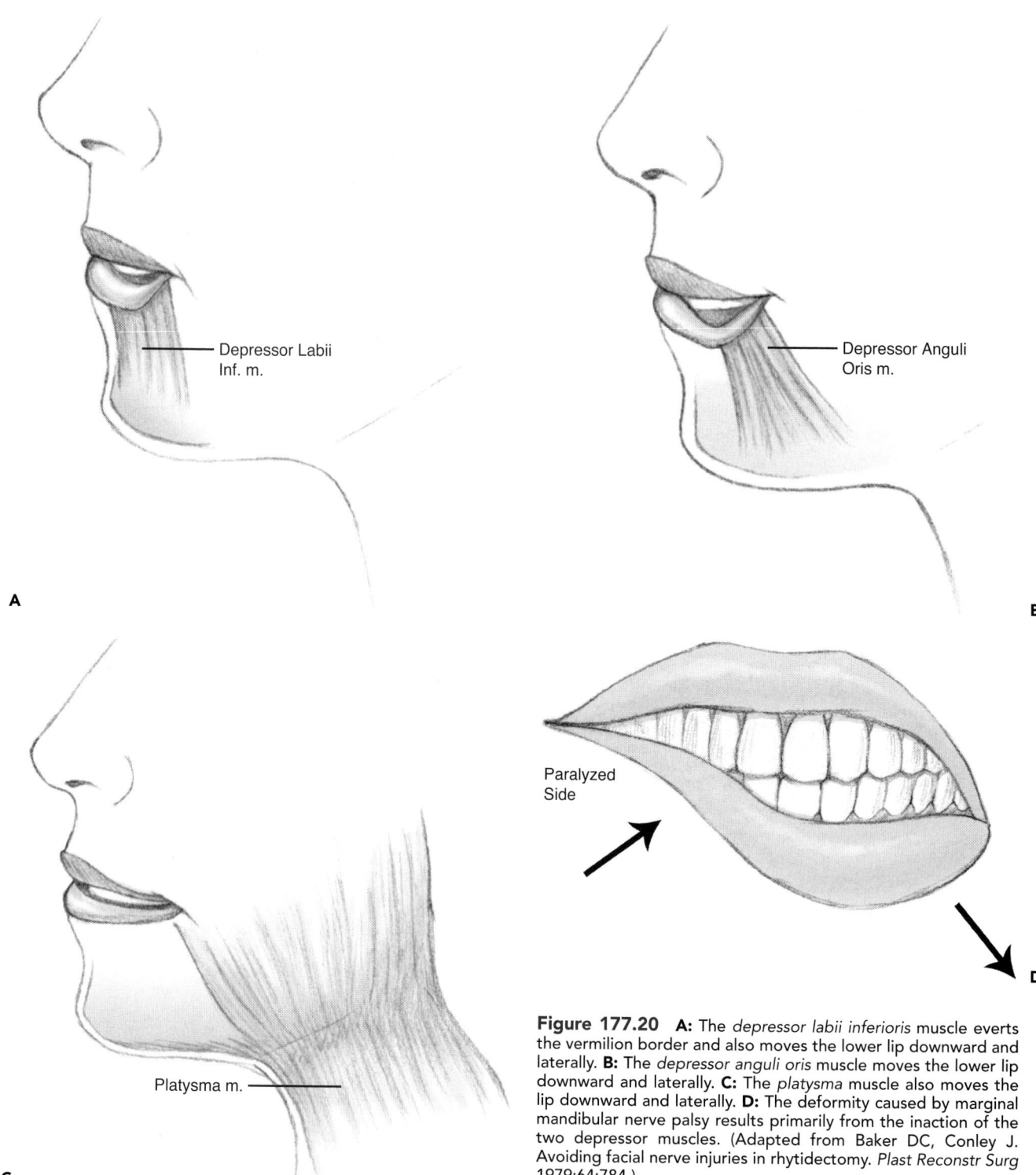

Figure 177.20 **A:** The *depressor labii inferioris* muscle everts the vermilion border and also moves the lower lip downward and laterally. **B:** The *depressor anguli oris* muscle moves the lower lip downward and laterally. **C:** The *platysma* muscle also moves the lip downward and laterally. **D:** The deformity caused by marginal mandibular nerve palsy results primarily from the inaction of the two depressor muscles. (Adapted from Baker DC, Conley J. Avoiding facial nerve injuries in rhytidectomy. *Plast Reconstr Surg* 1979;64:784.)

electrocoagulation; crush or pinch injuries caused by instrumentation or deep suture ligature; excessive SMAS traction; inflammation or infection; pressure from hematoma formation; and distortion, fibrosis, and scarring from previous facelift surgery (52).

The most commonly injured nerve is the sensory greater auricular nerve because of its intimate association with the firm fascia surrounding the sternocleidomastoid muscle

(54,55). Often, the skin flap is adherent in this area and sharp dissection or traction can injure the nerve, resulting in permanent sensory deficit of the ear and periauricular skin.

Hematoma

With a reported incidence as high as 8.5%, hematoma formation remains the most common and feared complication of facelift surgery (50,52,55). Expanding hematomas require immediate reoperation to control the bleeding source and to evacuate and drain the newly dissected skin flaps. Rapid filling of a suction drain reservoir is a sign of bleeding that must be investigated. Smaller or delayed hematomas can be managed with serial needle aspiration and pressure dressings. Patient complaints of pain, swelling, or firmness of the buccal region and ecchymosis, especially if unilateral, necessitate immediate inspection of the skin flaps. Intraoral inspection revealing mucosal ecchymosis often signals a hematoma that can be hidden by the external bandage.

Techniques that seem to reduce the incidence of hematoma formation include careful attention to intraoperative hemostasis, closed suction drainage, shorter skin flaps, and two-layer or deep plane facelift technique. Unrecognized and improperly treated, hematomas result in skin necrosis, infection, prolonged ecchymosis, alopecia, subcutaneous nodules and skin puckering, and scar contracture.

Incision Problems

Tension on the suture line and skin flaps is the key danger to any facelift procedure that otherwise may have been executed flawlessly. Careful preparation, incision placement, SMAS suspension, and accurate skin flap redraping without tension minimize incision complications. Preventing tension on skin incisions is the best way to avoid unattractive wide scars, skin slough, and hypertrophic scarring.

Cyanotic changes precede skin necrosis, but sometimes can be reversed by increasing the oxygen tension to the skin flap. Often, removing a few key sutures is helpful. A skin gap can granulate in, but dead skin is irreplaceable. If skin slough occurs, spontaneous demarcation with expectant management may limit the extent of tissue loss (56). Superficial débridement and topical antibiotic ointment can be done to clean the wound and begin the process of reepithelialization.

Active, hypertrophic scars respond to serial injections of triamcinolone at 3- to 4-week intervals. New silastic or silicone sheeting may also prove useful. Direct excision of residual hypertrophic scars or a widened incision is delayed until after considerable skin relaxation and healing.

Prevention of structural deformities such as the satyr earlobe, blunted and anteriorly dislocated tragus, elevated temporal hairline, and conspicuous incisions already have been thoroughly discussed. Chondritis of the tragus, external auditory canal, and auricle may occur and can result in structural deformity. Suspected chondritis often responds to ciprofloxacin or other antipseudomonal and antistaphylococcal antibiotics. Creation of bloody culture media in the ear canal can be avoided by occluding the canal before surgery with an iodine-soaked cotton ball. No sutures are placed through tragal cartilage, thereby preventing the direct introduction of organisms into the cartilage.

Other incision problems include ingrown hairs, which can establish a nidus of infection and inflammation. During each postoperative visit, ingrown hairs are identified by magnified inspection of the incision and then removed. Occasionally, buried permanent sutures used in SMAS suspension find their way to the skin surface. Removing sutures that have extruded after a long follow-up should create no difficulty for the patient. Rarely, persistent hemosiderin deposits are visible beneath the skin and require cosmetic cover.

Alopecia

Other than poorly planned incisions, tension seems to be the main cause of postoperative alopecia. Some loss can be transient and result from temporary shock to the hair follicles, which can exhibit recovery in about 3 months. Many series report an incidence ranging from 0.20% to 1.8% (50).

In cases of permanent hair loss, single follicular unit hair transplantation or excision of the bare area with tissue advancement may be necessary (Fig. 177.21). Larger areas of alopecia may also require tissue expansion with hair flap rearrangement for aesthetic, full-density hair coverage.

Unsatisfactory Results

Despite our best intentions, plans, and efforts, some patients may be unhappy because of real or perceived unsatisfactory results. Remember, the patient may not always be as critical of the outcome as is the surgeon. We consider it inappropriate to impose our desires for near perfection on a patient who otherwise may be perfectly happy with the degree of improvement. On the other hand, mutual concerns over acquired asymmetries, incomplete lifts, persistent facial irregularities, or general unsatisfactory results are best acknowledged openly, with plans made for further correction, if possible. Of course, facelift surgery does not arrest the aging process, and the need for minor tuck-up procedures should not be considered a complication of facelift surgery. This is especially true in older patients whose skin has lost its elasticity and patients with heavy neck who require a lot of fat removal. In fact, some surgeons believe in planned, sequential rhytidectomy and address this issue in the preoperative assessment (25,55).

FINAL WORD

The dictum "above all else, do no harm" is of paramount importance in elective aesthetic facial surgery and should be heard loudly in every surgeon's ear while planning and performing facial rejuvenation surgery. Functional, permanent, or disfiguring complications can be particularly

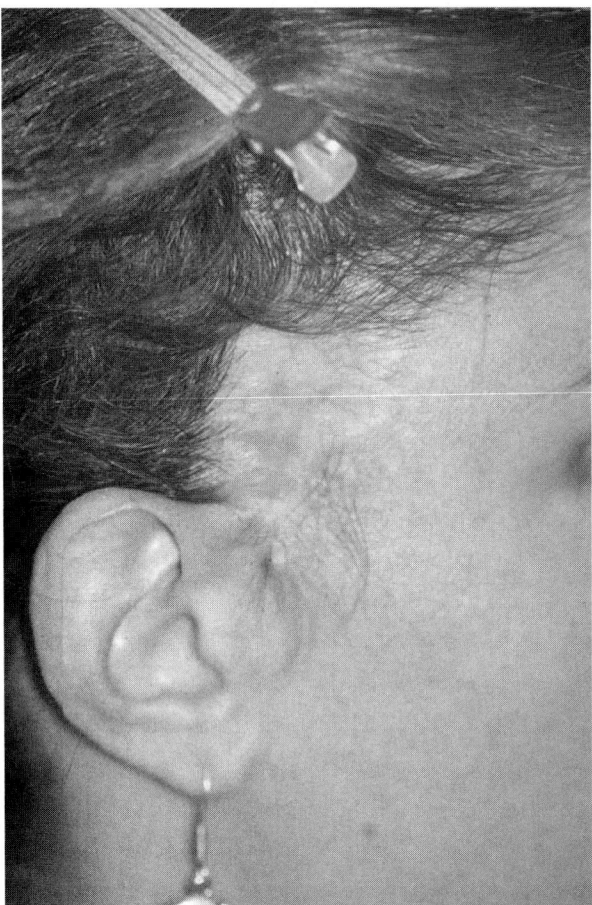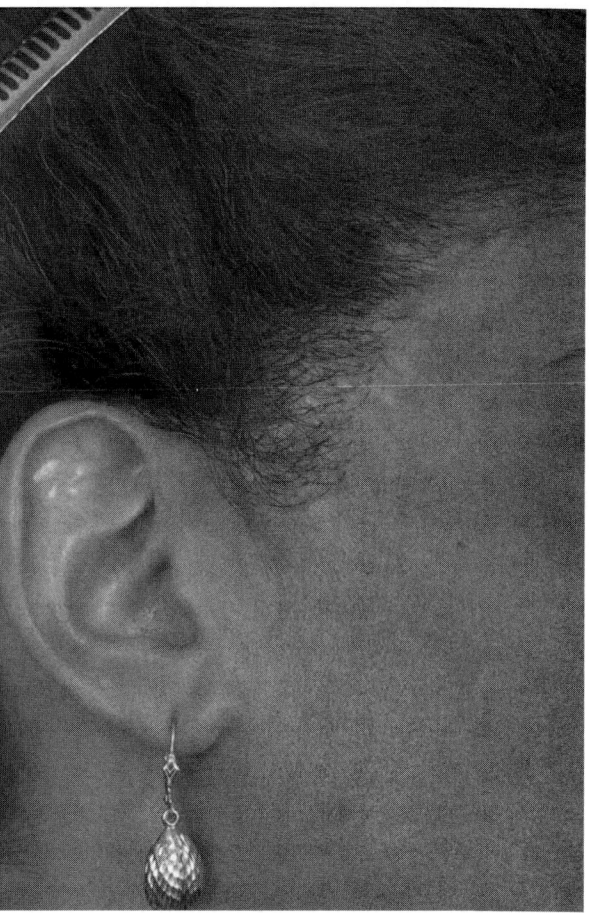

A   B

Figure 177.21 **A:** Preoperative photograph of a patient with temporal alopecia secondary to scarring. **B:** Postoperative result following tissue expansion, scalp advancement, scar excision, and two sessions of microfollicular-unit hair transplantation. (Reprinted from Kridel, RWH. Techniques for inconspicuous face lift scars. *Arch Facial Plast Surg* 2003;5:323–333, with permission).

devastating to patients who were not ill but simply wanted to look and feel better about themselves. Honesty and integrity must characterize the relationship between the surgeon and patient, and patient education is important to that relationship.

The deep plane techniques have led surgeons to think more rigorously about facial anatomy and the goals of rhytidectomy. Ultimately, many of these techniques can be incorporated into standard rhytidectomy practice. Until that time, however, continued critical assessment of the benefits and risks of these procedures is needed, and caution is urged for surgeons contemplating deep dissection in the medial face.

HIGHLIGHTS

■ The ideal patient for facelift surgery is mid 40 to 50 years of age and in good general health; has a strong jawline, chin, and cheekbones; and a high posterior hyoid bone, a relatively thin neck and face, and minimal photoaging of the skin.

■ Rhytidectomy mainly corrects jowl ptosis and cervicomental angle blunting. If creases and wrinkles of the skin contribute to the aged appearance, consider chemoexfoliation or laser resurfacing as an adjunct procedure. Periorbital and perioral resurfacing can be done safely at the same sitting as rhytidectomy.

■ The "facelift" is truly only a cheek and neck lift, and often ptosis of other facial regions also contributes to the aged appearance. Blepharoplasty, forehead lift, and other rejuvenation surgery should be considered at the same sitting as the facelift. Final facelift results depend on a good, strong bony framework; augmentation of the cheekbones, submalar areas, and chin also may be necessary.

■ To assess whether a patient's expectations are realistic, ensure that improvement and not perfection is the mutual goal, that the patient does not expect to look exactly as she or he did many years ago, and that the patient understands that a facelift is surgery, with inherent risks and possible complications.

■ Thorough preoperative evaluation of the patient's medical condition is mandatory. Because smoking greatly increases the risk of skin slough, smokers should be operated on cautiously. Medical conditions that predispose to abnormal bleeding (e.g., coagulopathies, severe hypertension, hepatic or renal disease), if not correctable preoperatively, are contraindications to rhytidectomy.

- Incisions must be planned differently for men and women. Preserving the anterior hair tuft is the key in women. In men, a preauricular incision is preferable, with maintenance of a hair-free border around the ear and under the lobule to prevent beard hair from annoying the patient postoperatively.

- In a SMAS-suspension rhytidectomy, the pull should be mainly superior, with only a slight posterior vector to counter the chronic effects of gravity. All tension should be carried by this layer, with the skin closed under no tension at all. Too much skin tension can lead to skin slough, increased telangiectasias, or a widened scar.

- Submental liposuction and platysmaplasty have enhanced the degree and duration of improvement in submental contour over SMAS-plication rhytidectomy alone.

- Hematoma is the most common complication of rhytidectomy. Because this and most other complications are most likely to occur in the immediate postoperative period, vigilance for symptoms and signs of impending problems is mandatory. Meticulous long-term follow-up care will help ensure an optimal result.

- Prominent nasolabial folds are a source of concern for patients and surgeons alike, and improvement with standard rhytidectomy is limited. Deep plane rhytidectomy offers some promise as a means of improving this area, but the cosmetic benefit has not yet been clearly established, and the theoretical risk of injury to the facial nerve is greater than with standard techniques. Caution is urged for surgeons contemplating deep plane approaches to the medial face.

REFERENCES

1. Furnas DW. The retaining ligaments of the cheeks. *Plast Reconstr Surg* 1989;83:11.
2. Sherris DA, Larrabee WF. Anatomic considerations in rhytidectomy. *Facial Plast Surg* 1996;12(3):215.
3. Weiss JS, Swanson NA. Baker S. Anatomy and physiology of aging skin. In: Krause CJ, ed. *Aesthetic facial surgery.* Philadelphia: JB Lippincott, 1991:461.
4. Bhawan J, Andersen W, Lee J, et al. Photoaging versus intrinsic aging: a morphologic assessment of facial skin. *J Cutan Pathol* 1995;22:154.
5. Yousif, NJ, Mendelson BC. Anatomy of the midface. *Clin Plast Surg* 1995;22:227.
6. Kligman AM, Zheng P, Lavker RM. The anatomy and pathogenesis of wrinkles. *Br J Dermatol* 1985;113:37.
7. Gilchrest, BA. Skin aging and photoaging: An overview. *J Am Acad Dermatol* 1989;21:610.
8. Kligman LH. Photoaging: manifestations, prevention, and treatment. *Dermatol Clin* 1986;4(3):517.
9. Kabaker SS. Kridel RWH, Krugman ME, et al. Tissue expansion in the treatment of alopecia. *Arch Otolaryngol Head Neck Surg* 1986;112:720.
10. Larrabee WF, Henderson JL. Face lift: the anatomic basis for a safe, long-lasting procedure. *Facial Plast Surg* 2000;16(3):239.
11. Stuzin JM, Baker TJ, Gordon HL. The relationship of the superficial and deep facial fascias: relevance to rhytidectomy and aging. *Plast Reconstr Surg* 1992;89(3):441.
12. Jost G, Levet Y. Parotid fascia and face lifting: a critical evaluation of the SMAS concept. *Plast Reconstr Surg* 1984;74:42.
13. Quatela VC, Sabini P. Techniques in deep plane face lifting. *Facial Plast Surg Clin N Am* 2000;8(2):193.
14. Lemmon ML. Superficial fascia rhytidectomy: a restoration of the SMAS with control of the cervicomental angle. *Clin Plast Surg* 1983;10(3):449.
15. Owsley JQ. Platysma-fascia rhytidectomy. *Plast Reconstr Surg* 1977;60:843.
16. Lemmon ML, Hamra ST. Skoog rhytidectomy: a five year experience with 577 patients. *Plast Reconstr Surg* 1980;65:283.
17. Aston SJ. Platysma-SMAS cervicofacial rhytidoplasty. *Clin Plast Surg* 1983;10:507.
18. Mitz V, Peyronie M. The superficial musculoaponeurotic system (SMAS) in the parotid and cheek area. *Plast Reconstr Surg* 1976;58:80.
19. Webster RC, Smith RC, Smith KF. Facelift. Part I: Extent of undermining of skin flaps. *Head Neck Surg* 1983;5:525.
20. Baker DC. Deep dissection rhytidectomy: a plea for caution. *Plast Reconstr Surg* 1994; 93:1498.
21. Kamer FM. One hundred consecutive deep-plane face-lifts. *Arch Otolaryngol Head Neck Surg* 1996;122:17.
22. Baker DC, Conley J. Avoiding facial nerve injuries in rhytidectomy. *Plast Reconstr Surg* 1979;64:781.
23. Tobin HA. Patient motivations and expectations. In: Krause CJ, ed. *Aesthetic facial surgery.* Philadelphia: JB Lippincott, 1991:469.
24. Baker DC. Anatomy and injuries of the facial nerve in cervicofacial rhytidectomy. In: Kaye BI. Gradinger GP, eds. *Symposium on problems and complications in aesthetic plastic surgery of the face.* St. Louis: Mosby, 1984:150.
25. Kamer FM, Sequential rhytidectomy and the two-stage concept. *Otolaryngol Clin North Am* 1980:13:305.
26. Rees TD, Aston SJ. Complications of rhytidectomy. *Clin Plast Surg* 1978;5:109.
27. Webster RC, Davidson TM, White ME, et al. Conservative facelift surgery. *Arch Otolaryngol* 1976:102:657.
28. Colton JJ, Beekhuis GJ. Anesthesia for facial cosmetic surgery. In: Krause CJ. ed. *Aesthetic facial surgery.* Philadelphia: JB Lippincott, 1991:503.
29. Kridel RWH, Konior RJ, Buchwach KA. Suction lipectomy. In: Krause CJ, ed. *Aesthetic facial surgery.* Philadelphia: JB Lippincott, 1991.
30. Kridel RWH, Liu ES. Techniques for creating inconspicuous face-lift scars: avoiding visible incisions and loss of temporal hair. *Arch Facial Plast Surg* 2003;5:325.
31. Webster RC, Fanous N, Smith RC. Male and female facelift incisions. *Arch Otolaryngol* 1982:108:299.
32. McCollough EG, Perkins SW, Langsdon PR. SASMAS suspension rhytidectomy: rationale and long-term experience. *Arch Otolaryngol Head Neck Surg* 1989;115:228.
33. Becker FF, Bassichis BA. Deep plane facelift vs. superficial musculoaponeurotic system plication face- lift. A comparative study. *Arch Facial Plast Surg.* 2004;6:8.
34. Baker SR. Is deep plane face lift better than superficial musculoaponeurotic system plication facelift? *Arch Facial Plast Surg.* 2004;6:8.
35. McCollough EG. Facelifting in the nineties: selecting the appropriate technique. In: Stuker FJ, ed. *Plastic and reconstructive surgery of the head and neck.* Philadelphia: BC Decker, 1991:165.
36. Feldman LJ. Corset platysmaplasty. *Plast Reconstr Surg* 1990;85:333.
37. Webster RC, Smith RC, Smith KF. Facelift. Part II: Etiology of platysma cording and its relationship to treatment. *Head Neck Surg* 1983;6:590.
38. Webster RC, Smith RC, Smith KE. Facelift. Part III: plication of the superficial musculoaponeurotic system. *Head Neck Surg* 1983; 6:696.
39. Webster RC, Smith RC, Smith KF. Facelift. Part IV: Use of superficial musculoaponeurotic system suspending sutures. *Head Neck Surg* 1984;6:780.
40. Webster RC, Smith RC. Smith KF. Facelift. Part V: Suspending sutures for platysma cording. *Head Neck Surg* 1984:6:870.

41. Webster RC, Smith RC, Papsidero MJ, et al. Comparison of SMAS plication with SMAS imbrication in facelifting. *Laryngoscope* 1982;92:901.

42. Hamra S. The deep-plane rhytidectomy. *Plast Reconstr Surg* 1990; 86:53.

43. Hamra ST. Composite rhytidectomy. *Plast Reconstr Surg* 1992; 90:1.

44. Ramirez OM. The subperiosteal rhytidectomy: the third-generation face-lift. *Ann Plast Surg* 1992;28:218.

45. Freilinger G, Gruber H, Happak WE, et al. Surgical anatomy of the mimic muscle system and the facial nerve: importance for reconstruction and aesthetic surgery. *Plast Reconstr Surg* 1987;80: 686.

46. Whetzel TP. Mathes SJ. Arterial anatomy of the face: analysis of vascular territories and perforating cutaneous vessels. *Plast Reconstr Surg* 1992;89:591.

47. Zutlerey J. Anatomic variations of the nasolabial fold. *Plast Reconstr Surg* 1992;89:225.

48. Barton Jr FE. Rhytidectomy and the nasolabial fold. *Plast Reconstr Surg* 1992;90:601.

49. Mendelson BC. Correction of the nasolabial fold: extended SMAS dissection with periosteal fixation. *Plast Reconstr Surg* 1992:89: 822.

50. Kridel RWH, Aguilar EA, Wright WK. Complications of rhytidectomy. *Ear Nose Throat J* 1985;64:44.

51. Goin JM, Goin MK. *Changing the body: psychological effects of plastic surgery.* Baltimore: Williams & Wilkins, 1981.

52. Guerrero-Santos J. Complications of the neck lift. In: Kaye BL, Gradinger GP, eds. *Symposium on problems and complications in aesthetic plastic surgery of the face.* St. Louis: Mosby, 1984:274.

53. Castanares S. Facial nerve paralysis coincident with, or subsequent to, rhytidectomy. *Plast Reconstr Surg* 1974;54:637.

54. Thomas JR. Complications of aesthetic surgery. In: Johns ME, ed. *Complications in otolaryngology–head and neck surgery.* Philadelphia, Toronto: BC Decker, 1986:281.

55. Anderson JR. The tuck-up operation: a new technique of secondary rhytidectomy. *Arch Otolaryngol* 1975:101:739.

56. Berman WE. Rhytidectomy. In: Krause CJ, ed. *Aesthetic facial surgery.* Philadelphia: JB Lippincott, 1991:513.

The Aging Neck

178

Edwin F. Williams III   Allison T. Pontius

The typical appearance of the aging neck is caused by a constellation of changes associated with both heredity and the aging process. Each patient will demonstrate different anatomic components contributing to the overall appearance of an aging neckline. The anatomic factors that contribute to an ideal cervical contour include a strong chin, a distinct mandibular border, a cervicomental angle of 90 degrees, a visible subhyoid bone depression, a gentle indentation at the thyroid notch, and visible anterior borders of the sternocleidomastoid muscles (1) (Fig. 178.1). Obtaining these ideal contours should be the goal of any surgical correction of the aging neck. To achieve these goals, however, the surgeon must carefully and systematically analyze each patient to determine the anatomic abnormalities that need to be addressed. An individualized approach ensures that specific deformities are clearly delineated so a youthful and graceful neckline may be restored.

ANATOMY

The aging process exerts an impact on each anatomic element of the cervical region to varying degrees in each patient. Additionally, some patients also display hereditary abnormalities contributing to an unfavorable cervical contour, including a low-positioned hyoid bone, poor chin projection, and a congenital collection of submental fat. As stated, each element of the contributing anatomy should be delineated preoperatively and sequentially addressed in the surgical correction to provide an optimal aesthetic outcome. The anatomic areas to be addressed include skin, fat, platysma muscle, chin position, and other unfavorable anatomy (low hyoid bone position, ptotic submandibular glands, overdeveloped suprahyoid bone musculature) (2).

Skin

With time, collagen and elastin fibers degenerate so the overlying skin no longer adheres to the soft tissue contours of the neck. The skin becomes redundant and sags, leading to the development of horizontal cervical rhytids and effacement of the cervicomental angle.

Fat

Fat deposition in the neck can be congenital or acquired. Three areas where fat accumulation is typically seen are (a) a supraplatysmal layer diffusely distributed throughout the cervical region; (b) a submental fat collection, which is usually subplatysmal and overlies the mylohoid muscle between the anterior bellies of the digastric muscles; and (c) facial fat contributing to a ptotic jowl and loss of the definition of the inferior mandibular border.

Platysma Muscle

The platysma muscle is a paired muscle that is innervated by the cervical branch of the seventh cranial nerve. It originates from the fascia of the pectoralis major and deltoid muscles and ascends in the neck to insert on the inferior border of the mandible (Fig. 178.2). In 30% of the population, the fibers of the platysma muscle decussate in the midline (3). The "turkey gobbler" deformity is caused by a laxity in the platysma muscle that does not decussate in the midline. Laterally, the posterior border of the platysma muscle ends in front of the sternocleidomastoid muscle. As the platysma muscle is followed superiorly to the mandible, the medial fibers insert into the periosteum to stabilize one end of the muscle during contraction. The central fibers blend intimately with the risorius muscle. The posterior third of the platysma muscle sweeps up over the mandible to course anteriorly and fuse with the superficial musculoaponeurotic system (SMAS). The cervical skin receives part of its blood supply from perforating vessels arising from the platysma muscle. These vessels and thick fibrous septa coursing through the subcutaneous fat anchor the dermis to the superficial cervical fascia and platysma muscle.

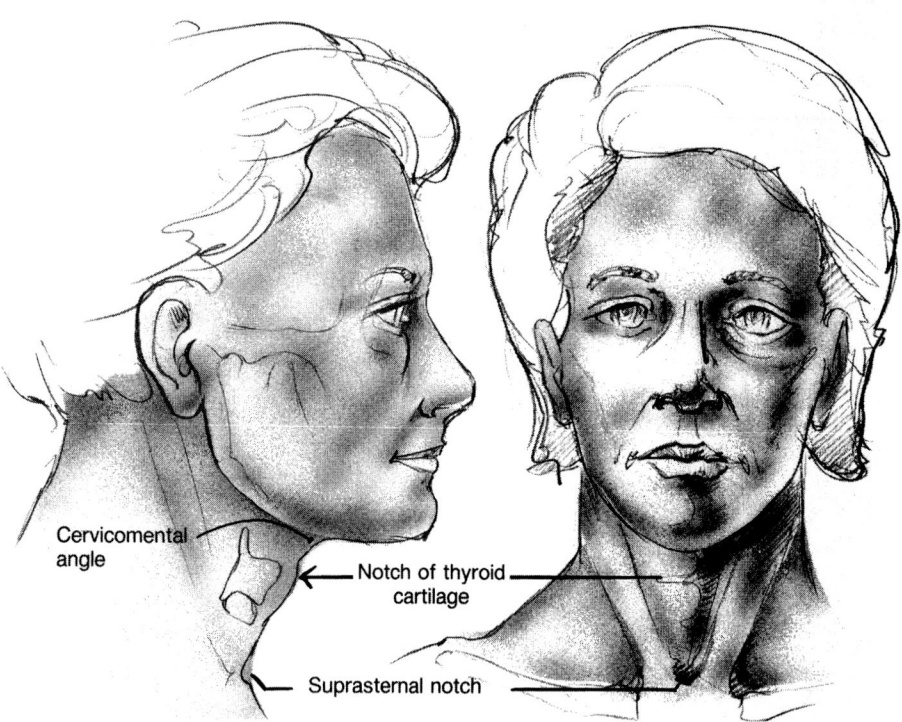

Figure 178.1 The anatomic factors that contribute to an ideal cervical contour include a strong chin, a distinct mandibular border, a cervicomental angle of 90 degrees, a visible subhyoid bone depression, a gentle indentation at the thyroid notch, and visible anterior borders of the sternocleidomastoid muscles.

The platysma muscle functions to stabilize the chest muscles against the jaw during heavy lifting. It also provides a layer of protection over vital structures of the neck. It is a somewhat vestigial structure in humans, representing a remnant of the panniculus carnosus muscle that forms a continuous subcutaneous layer in lower mammals (4).

With aging, the platysma muscle becomes atrophic and falls toward the midline. First, convexity occurs in the submental region; then, as the muscle loses tone, it forms the pathognomonic anterior banding of the aged neck. On profile, the apex of the cervicomental angle is blunted by the anterior border of the muscle as it runs diagonally from the mandible to the lower neck. Loss of the platysmal muscle sling allows ptosis of the underlying cervical contents (4).

Chin Position

An appropriately projected chin is prerequisite for an optimal aesthetic cervical contour. Ideally, in a patient with Angle's class I occlusion, the pogonion (the most anterior projecting point of the chin) should touch a line dropped vertically from the vermillion border of the lower lip on profile view. It is aesthetically acceptable in women if the chin is slightly posterior to this line; however, in men, this line should be tangent to the pogonion (5) (Fig. 178.3). The chin contour is determined by the shape and position of the mandible, as well as the overlying soft tissues, in the case of chin ptosis. A weak chin, or microgenia, is most commonly congenital; however, senile absorption of alveolar bone should also be considered in the older patient.

Mandibular hypoplasia is an acquired condition secondary to varying degrees of bony resorption of the mandible. With aging, specific progressive soft tissue atrophy and bone reduction occur in the region between the chin and jowl. This resulting groove has been termed "the prejowl sulcus" (5). Mandibular hypoplasia should not be confused with retrognathia. Patients with retrognathia demonstrate Angle's class II occlusion and are optimally treated with a bony advancement technique (e.g.,

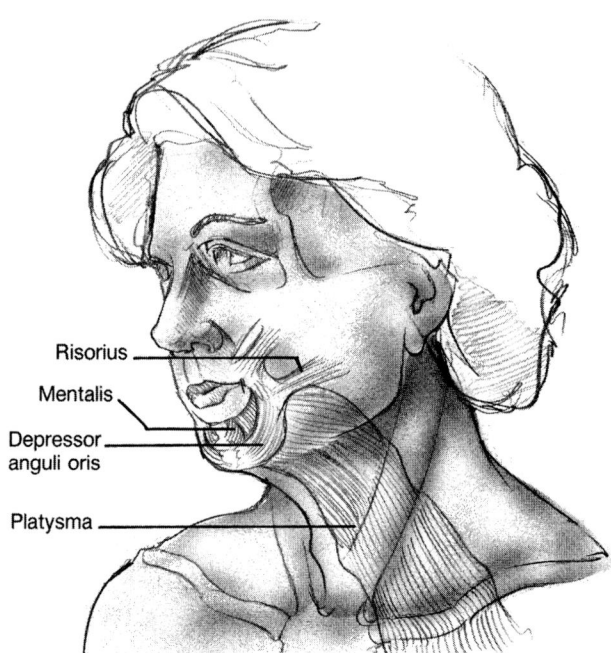

Figure 178.2 The platysma muscle ascends in the neck to blend with the superficial musculoaponeurotic system (SMAS).

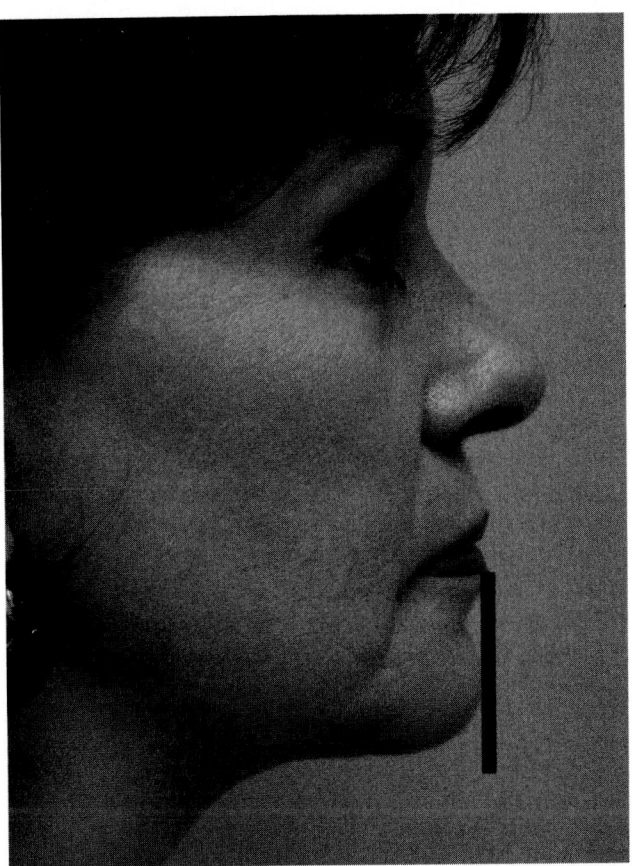

Figure 178.3 The anterior-most projection of the chin (pogonion) should touch a line dropped vertically from the vermillion border of the lower lip on profile view.

a sagittal-split osteotomy), whereas patients with microgenia or mandibular hypoplasia are better treated with alloplastic augmentation.

Unfavorable Anatomy

The hyoid bone supports the floor of the mouth as it is suspended by the digastric, mylohyoid, stylohyoid, and tongue musculature. Ideally, it should be at the level of the fourth cervical vertebrae (6). A hyoid bone that is in a relatively inferior position in the neck causes the suprahyoid musculature to course in a more vertical direction, blunting the angle between the chin and neck (7). A low hyoid bone position is a major limiting factor in the optimal rejuvenation of the cervical region.

Submandibular gland ptosis is commonly seen with aging, which is identified as two bulges at the anterior edge of the submandibular triangle. Diagnosis is confirmed by palpation of the gland's cobblestoned surface. The position of the glands should be elucidated preoperatively for both patient counseling and surgical planning.

Overdevelopment of the suprahyoid bone musculature, especially the digastric muscles, can also lead to fullness of the submental region. Identification is facilitated by having the patient flex the neck with the mouth closed (2).

CLASSIFICATION AND EVALUATION

Dedo's preoperative classification of the neck (8), which is used below, is a useful tool to help delineate the anatomic features contributing to a particular patient's pathology and to help guide targeted surgical intervention (Fig. 178.4).

A patient with a class I neck is typically a younger patient who has minimal, if any, deformity, which may or may not require surgical intervention. A patient with class I neck should ideally wait until more of an aesthetic problem develops, because any intervention at this time is essentially prophylactic. An "S-lift," a limited rhytidectomy with an incision that extends only under the ear lobule in a lazy-S configuration, may provide enough exposure for dissection and adequate skin excision (9) (Fig. 178.5). Intervention at this time may not yield dramatic results, but it will delay facial ptosis while maintaining the present contour for 4 to 5 years (4).

The class II patient has skin laxity, only without significant fat or muscle pathology. Treatment of these patients typically requires a standard cervicofacial rhytidectomy.

A class III deformity is caused by excessive cervical liposis. Liposuction is the treatment of choice for these patients. In patients with good skin elasticity, liposuction alone may be sufficient if minimal skin laxity is present. The mild dermal injury inflicted by the liposuction cannula promotes contraction of the overlying skin (10), thus obviating the need for skin excision in patients with good skin elasticity. If, however, a large accumulation of fat is present, especially in patients with poor skin elasticity, liposuction alone can lead to poor redraping and contraction of the anterior cervical skin, causing postoperative "rippling" and other deformities (7). The early fourth decade appears to be a transition time when skin elasticity decreases and liposuction alone can result in less than optimal results. Patients in this age group are typically better candidates for a rhytidectomy in conjunction with submental liposuction with anterior platysmaplasty. According to Kamer and Minoli (11), the combination of suction lipectomy and rhytidectomy predisposes the patient to the development of postoperative platysmal banding, even if anterior platysmal banding is not clinically evident preoperatively. Anterior platysmaplasty, therefore, is suggested when performing liposuction and rhytidectomy concurrently to avoid the untoward sequela of postoperative platysmal banding.

The class IV patient has a pathologic platysma muscle either in repose or on voluntary contraction. It can be diagnosed in the thin neck as anterior platysma banding; however, in patients with submental adiposity or redundant anterior cervical skin, it may not be readily apparent that the platysma muscle is contributing to the deformity.

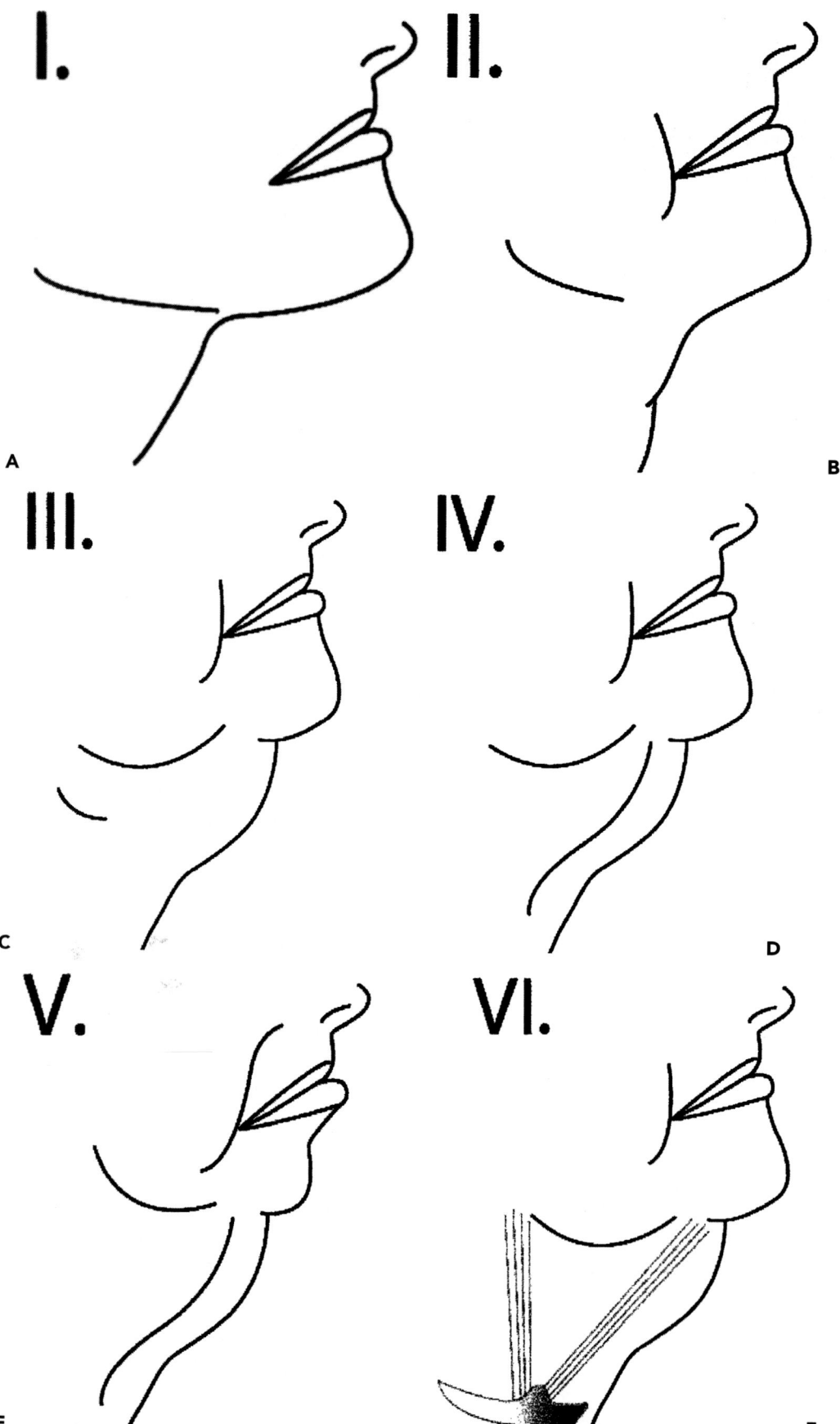

Figure 178.4 Dedo classification of cervical abnormalities: **A:** Class I deformity describes only minimal cosmetic deformity. **B:** Class II deformity describes only skin laxity. **C:** Class III deformity refers to the excessive submandibular and submental adipose. **D:** Class IV deformity refers to anterior banding of the platysma. **E:** Class V deformity describes the condition of microgenia or retrognathia. **F:** Class VI deformity describes a low-positioned hyoid bone.

The "S" Lift

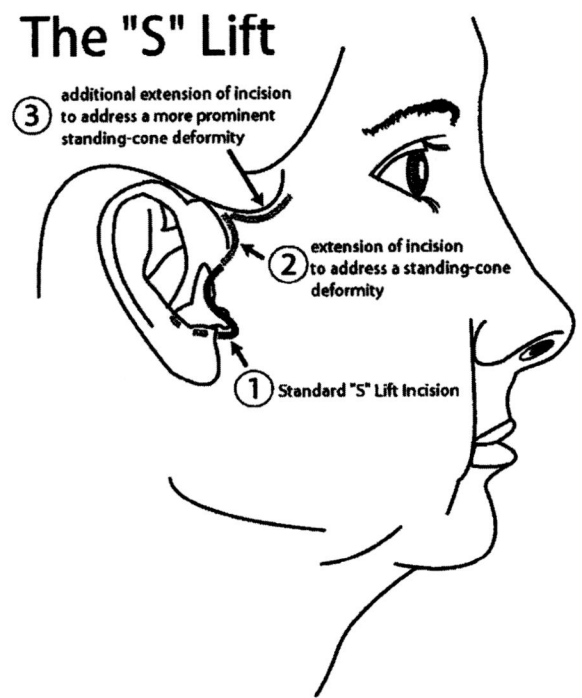

Figure 178.5 The configuration of the incision resembles an S-shape. The abbreviated length is suitable for younger patients who do not have significant skin redundancy but only some incipient jowling. To address a standing-cone ("dog-ear") deformity that may arise, the anterior skin incision can be extended up to (or all the way around) the temporal tuft, as needed.

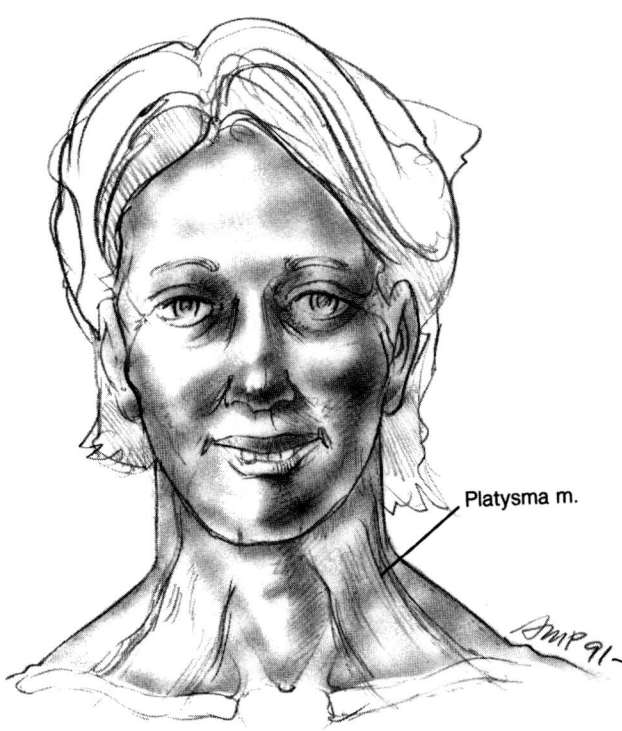

Figure 178.6 The medial and lateral borders of the platysma muscle can be better delineated by having the patient grimace with the teeth clenched.

In this case, diagnosis is facilitated by having the patient grimace with the teeth clenched to delineate the medial and lateral borders of the muscle (Fig. 178.6). These patients need anterior platysmaplasty to correct the deformity.

In the original Dedo classification (8), the class V patient has a weak mandibular projection from a congenital or acquired retrognathia. The term microgenia, however, may be more appropriate to describe most of these patients. Although, the terms retrognathia and microgenia have been used interchangeably in the scientific literature, each word denotes a different condition. Retrognathia refers to an Angle's class II occlusion in which the hypoplastic and retruded mandible leads to an overbite and dental malocclusion. Microgenia simply refers to an underprojected chin, independent of occlusal considerations (9). Retrognathia is typically corrected with mandibular osteotomies and bony advancement, whereas microgenia is corrected with alloplastic chin augmentation. It should be noted, however, that it is acceptable in certain patients with *mild* retrognathia to perform chin augmentation instead of pursuing the more aggressive treatment with bony advancement. By evaluating the patient's occlusion and distinguishing between true retrognathia and microgenia, the appropriate treatment can be offered to the patient to optimize the aesthetic outcome.

A class VI patient has an inferiorly positioned hyoid bone that creates an obtuse cervicomental angle. Diagnosis is made by palpating the hyoid bone and evaluating its relationship to the mandible and clavicles. The hyoid bone should reside at the level of the fourth cervical vertebra (6). A low-positioned hyoid bone is a major limiting factor in optimal aesthetic correction of the aging neck unless more aggressive surgical treatment is undertaken.

TREATMENT

After careful analysis of each anatomic factor contributing to the individual patient's deformity, a targeted surgical treatment plan can be instituted (Table 178.1). It should be noted that a weak chin can be a compounding factor in any of the classification groups. In addition to treating the soft tissue abnormalities, therefore, an alloplastic chin implant can also be used in any patient with evidence of microgenia. Again, in patients with significant retrognathia, chin augmentation alone may not give optimal aesthetic results and bony advancement techniques should be considered.

In young patients with minimal deformity (class I), the most prudent course of action would be simply to wait before any surgical intervention is offered. The improvement gained at this time would be minimal; however, intervention may delay soft tissue ptosis from developing as quickly. In the fastidious patient with realistic expectations, a limited

TABLE 178.1	
TARGETED SURGICAL TREATMENT PLAN	
Modified Dedo Classification	**Treatment Options**
Class I (minimal deformity)	• No surgical intervention • "S-lift" • ±Chin augmentation
Class II (laxity of cervical skin)	• Rhytidectomy • ±Chin augmentation
Class III (excess fat)	• Cervical liposuction • ±Anterior platysmaplasty • ±Rhytidectomy (for skin laxity) • ±Chin augmentation
Class IV (platysmal banding)	• Rhytidectomy (with anterior platysmaplasty) • ±Submental liposuction • ±Chin augmentation
Class V (microgenia or retrognathia)	• Chin augmentation (microgenia) • Bony osteotomy and advancement (retrognathia)
Class VI (low hyoid or other unfavorable anatomy)	• Treat soft-tissue abnormalities with standard techniques (with realistic expectations given anatomical limitations) • ±Division of suprahyoid musculature from mandible • ±Gor-Tex cervical sling • ±Mastoid-to-mastoid suture sling • ±Partial excision of anterior digastric muscles • ±Chin augmentation

rhytidectomy (S-lift) can be considered (Fig. 178.5). This approach allows a limited SMAS suspension and excision of skin without committing the patient to a standard rhytidectomy.

In patients with redundant skin of the cervical region (class II), a standard rhytidectomy is generally considered the treatment of choice. To remove excess skin and to efface jowling along the inferior mandibular border, an SMAS imbrication technique is used to provide long-lasting improvement of the contour of the lower one third of the face and neck.

In patients demonstrating isolated fat accumulation (class III), cervical liposuction is the procedure of choice. In the younger patient with good skin elasticity and no platysmal pathology, liposuction can be performed as an isolated procedure. If platysmal banding is noted, however, a formal submentoplasty (submental liposuction and anterior platysmaplasty) is performed (see *Surgical Technique: Submentoplasty*). Recent reports have suggested that other liposuction techniques (e.g., tumescent, liposhaving, ultrasound-assisted) are superior to traditional liposuction. The tumescent technique, which has been applied with success

for body liposuction, is less than ideal for the cervicofacial region because the distortion engendered renders assessment difficult and the persistent edema that arises is an unwarranted drawback. The risk of third space volume shifts further compounds the problem with the tumescent method. Although safety and efficacy of treatment with the liposhaver has been documented in a multi-institutional review (12), the device's ability to cut through muscle and other soft tissue (including blood vessels and nerves) creates the potential for significant complications. The ultrasound method suffers from the attendant risk of increased thermal injury (if internally applied) and neural and cutaneous flap injury. These adverse outcomes are not definitively established because no controlled studies exist, but they remain of concern nevertheless. In essence, these additional technologies have not proved themselves more useful or beneficial than traditional liposuction, even in experienced hands.

Class IV patients are those with platysmal abnormalities (e.g., muscle ptosis, atrophy, and midline banding). These patients are best served with a rhytidectomy and anterior platysmaplasty. The combination of SMAS suspension rhytidectomy and anterior platysmaplasty creates a "cervical corset" to support the underlying soft tissues. Additionally, if excess fat is also apparent, submental liposuction can be performed in conjunction with the above procedures.

Class V patients are those with microgenia or retrognathia. As above, a weak chin may be seen in conjunction with other soft tissue abnormalities and should be treated appropriately after determining the occlusal status.

Class VI patients are those with a low-positioned hyoid bone. Additionally, in this category, other unfavorable anatomy are considered: anterior digastric muscle hypertrophy and submandibular gland ptosis. Preoperatively, these patients should understand the limitations of their particular anatomy so they have a realistic expectation of the outcome. They should be treated appropriately with standard methods; however, more aggressive techniques may be considered to optimize the aesthetic outcome. In a series of 16 patients with a low-positioned hyoid, Guyuron (13) demonstrated notable aesthetic improvement in cervicomental contour in all 16 patients treated with transection of the suprahyoid musculature (anterior belly of the digastric, geniohyoid, and mylohyoid) from the inferior border of the mandible. Cephalometric tracings confirmed a statistically significant elevation of the hyoid bone and no patients had evidence of postoperative difficulty with mandibular movement or swallowing.

To treat digastric muscle hypertrophy, up to 75% of the anterior bellies of the digastric muscles can be excised by tangential shaving (4). Suturing of the anterior bellies of the digastric muscles has been reported as a method to eliminate a submental concavity after lipectomy, but not as a method to alter hyoid bone position (4). In an anatomic study by Prendiville et al. (14) the addition of a mastoid-to-mastoid suture sling, as described by Giampapa and DiBernardo (15), produced significant changes in the cervicomental angle and the sternum-to-cervicomental distance. The effect appeared to result from cephalic repositioning of the cervicomental angle without elevation of the hyoid bone. The technique involves placement of two horizontal mattress sutures in the mastoid periosteum and interlocked in the midline. They are placed in a preplatysmal plane after the completion of all other cervical procedures (Fig. 178.7).

Another option for treatment of the obtuse cervicomental angle in those with unfavorable anatomy is placement of an ePTFE (Gore-Tex) sling. As with the mastoid-to-mastoid sutures, the ePTFE sling extends in a preplatysmal plane between the mastoid periosteum bilaterally. A submental incision is used to guide the sling across to the opposing side. The preferred size of the sling is 2 × 30 cm and it must be prestretched by the surgeon before placement. After placement, it is secured with several buried CV-4 ePTFE (Gore-Tex) sutures to the mastoid periosteum (Fig. 178.8). The ePTFE sling is typically reserved for the fastidious patient having a secondary rhytidectomy who accepts an alloplastic implant and the possible postoperative sequel of a sensation of neck tightness.

Ptotic submandibular glands, which are commonly seen in elderly patients, represent a limitation to optimal aesthetic outcome. Surgical removal or reduction is certainly

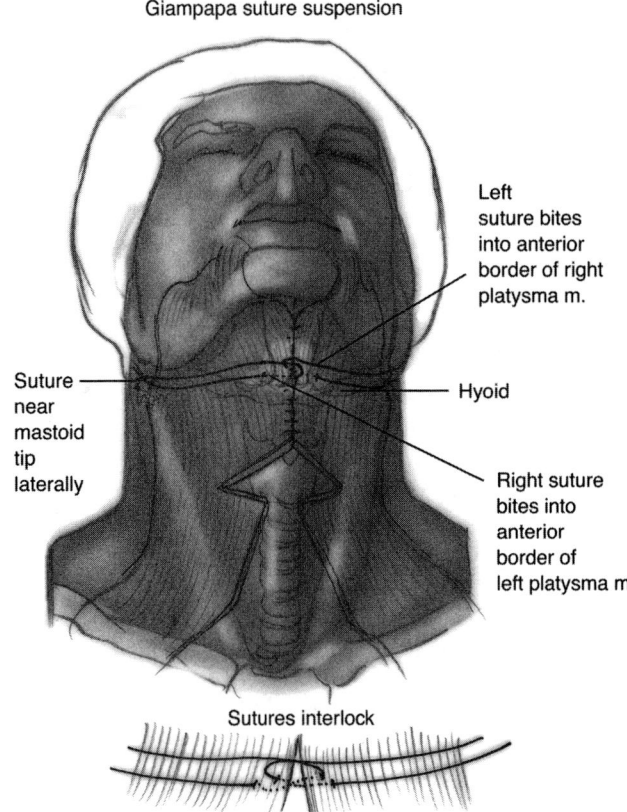

Figure 178.7 The Giampapa suture suspension of the neck involves placement of two horizontal mattress sutures in the mastoid periosteum and interlocked in the midline in a preplatysmal plane.

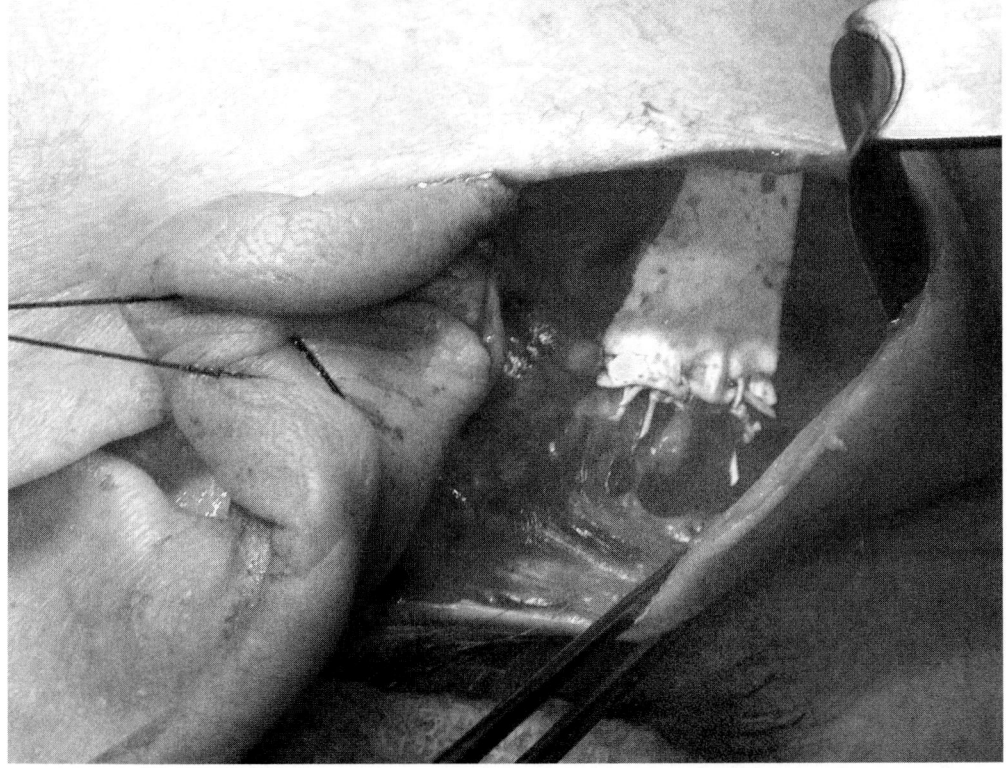

Figure 178.8 After the ePTFE sling has been prestretched, it is secured with several buried sutures to the mastoid periosteum and then passed through the submental incision to the opposite side.

beyond the scope of aesthetic surgery; however, by creating a well-supported "cervical corset" with SMAS suspension and anterior platysmaplasty, the ptotic glands will be elevated to a more favorable position.

Surgical Technique: Submentoplasty (Submental Liposuction and Anterior Platysmaplasty)

The submentoplasty (9) is always performed at the outset before a rhytidectomy, because the approximated anterior border of the platysma muscle is difficult to unite after the lateral pull of the rhytidectomy has been completed. Similarly, submental liposuction always precedes anterior platysmaplasty because the removal of adipose and the concomitant undermining permit visualization of the skeletonized platysma. Chin augmentation should follow the submentoplasty and precede the rhytidectomy, because the submentoplasty incision is used as a point of entry for chin implantation. Further, vigorous submentoplasty can disturb the position of the implant if done after chin augmentation.

The submentoplasty begins with a straight incision about 1 to 2 mm posterior to the submental crease that extends typically 2 cm in breadth (Fig. 178.9). The incision should fall slightly posterior to the submental crease because placement of the incision directly in the crease will deepen over time so that the line may become conspicuous.

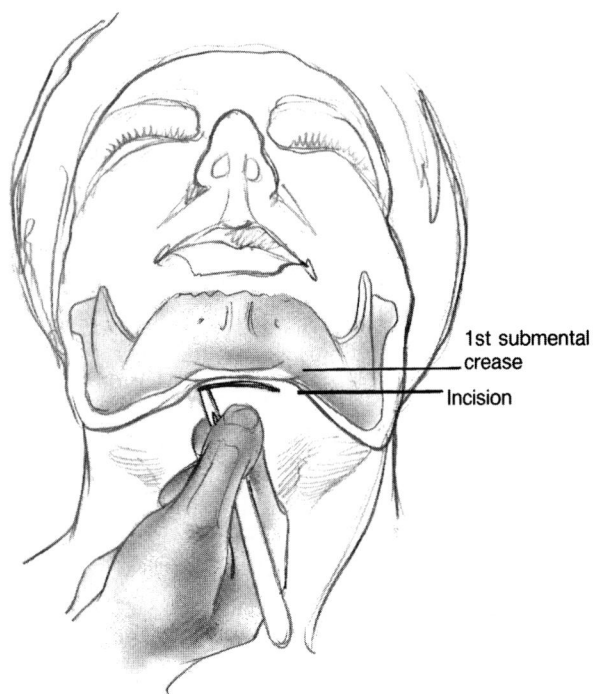

Figure 178.9   The submental incision is placed just behind (1 to 2 mm) the submental crease. If chin augmentation is to be performed, the incision should be placed even further posteriorly (4 to 5 mm behind the crease) to prevent a conspicuous postoperative scar.

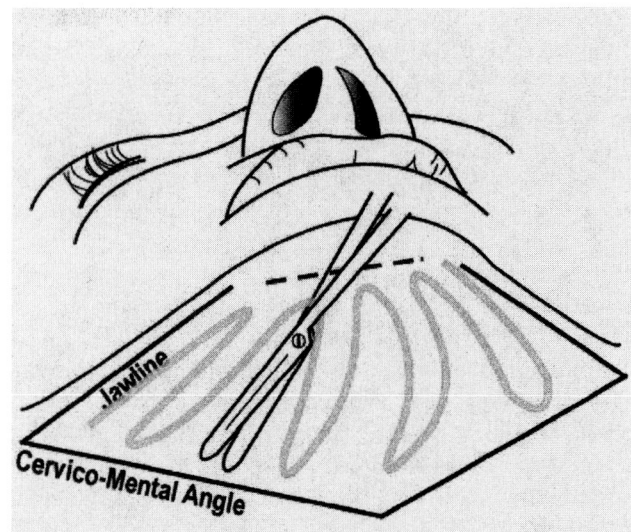

Figure 178.10   Wide undermining of the flap is performed from just inferior to the jaw line (1 to 2 cm below) across the submental region to the contralateral jaw line using a pair of Metzenbaum scissors in the subcutaneous plane.

Additionally, if chin augmentation is to be performed, the incision should be placed even further posteriorly (4–5 mm) from the submental crease. This is necessary because, following placement of the chin alloplast, the anterior portion of the incision has the tendency to move cephalically, potentially creating a visible incision near the inferior edge of the mandible.

After the initial incision through the skin, wide double-hooked retractors are placed in the superior and inferior aspects of the wounds for proper tension and retraction. The assistant retracts the superior flap while the surgeon retracts the inferior flap. The surgeon then performs wide undermining of the flap from just inferior to the jaw line (1–2 cm below) across the submental region to the contralateral jaw line using a pair of Metzenbaum scissors in the subcutaneous plane (Fig. 178.10). Dissection should not pass directly over the jaw line in order to minimize risk of injury to the marginal mandibular nerve. Although the nerve should be protected under the platysma muscle in most cases, an attenuated or dehiscent platysmal layer may predispose the nerve to inadvertent harm. The depth of dissection should leave approximately a 3- to 4-mm thick skin subcutaneous flap to avoid an uneven contour that may develop after liposuctioning and to ensure vascularity to the overlying skin flap. The lateral extent of the undermining should be to the anterior borders of the sternocleidomastoid muscle bilaterally.

After the submental region has been widely undermined, a liposuction cannula can be introduced with the aperature *always* facing deep, away from the flap, to avoid the development of an irregular skin contour from suctioning the overlying flap. Furthermore, the vascular supply of

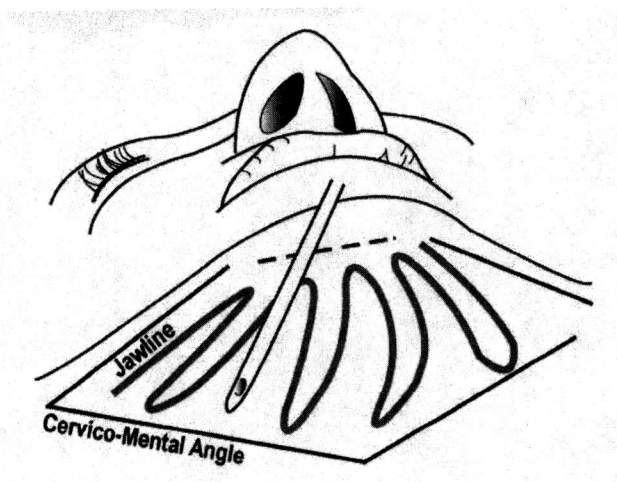

Figure 178.11 The liposuction cannula should be evenly passed over the entire expance of the undermined submental region.

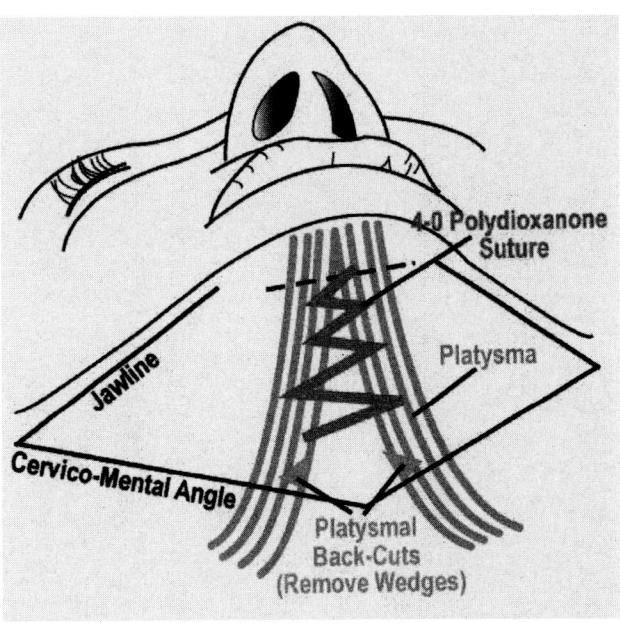

Figure 178.12 After exposure of the anterior platysmal borders, the free edges are approximated with 4-0 polydioxanone suture in a running, nonlocking fashion. The suture should be started approximately at the thyroid notch or cervicomental angle, immediately superior to the platysmal back-cuts.

the flap emanates from its deep surface, and liposuction under the flap can lead to vascular compromise. The liposuction canister pressure should be set at 29 mm Hg before initiating the procedure. The surgeon should ensure that the instrument is evenly passed over the entire expanse of the undermined submental region, with perhaps additional treatment centrally where a greater adipose deposit may be observed (Fig. 178.11). Open, direct lipectomy is not routinely used because it has potential to leave an uneven contour or, even worse, a "cobra deformity." Conservative central lipectomy, however, can be used as an adjunct in select cases. First, a central lipectomy can be done to remove discrete adipose pockets that remain in the midline after a broad liposuction has been carried out. Second, a central lipectomy may be required to visualize the anterior platysmal bands obscured by exuberant fat deposition.

The platysmaplasty can be undertaken after the liposuction has exposed the anterior platysmal border. With headlight illumination and a Converse retractor, the surgeon should properly visualize the anterior terminal fibers of the platysma muscle. If the platysma muscle appears to be obscured by a wealth of overlying adipose, a selective lipectomy can be performed with scissor dissection or with the liposuction cannula, as mentioned. The surgeon may elect to resect a narrow strip along the anterior border of the platysma muscle to promote better adherence. Although the efficacy of this step has not been rigorously validated, the authors routinely undertake it unless the platysma muscle is determined to be minimally redundant and the consequent tension of closure would be too great if additional platysmal resection is performed. If the platysmal borders appear widely separated, which would preclude a relaxed closure, then sufficient undermining is done to facilitate closure. Significant subplatysmal dissection, however, increases both the likelihood of poorly controlled and visualized hemorrhage and the risk to the marginal mandibular branch of the facial nerve. Before the platysma muscle can be approximated, the inferior extent of the platysmal closure should be identified (the cervicomental angle, typically located at the thyroid notch). Small (1–2 cm) back-cuts with Metzenbaum scissors into each side of the platysma muscle at this level are executed for two reasons: (a) tension of the closure can effectively be reduced, and (b) the neck profile appears more natural with a graduated break at the cervicomental angle. After the platysmal borders have been properly exposed and dissected, then approximate the anterior free edges with 4-0 polydioxanone, or equivalent, suture in a running, nonlocking fashion (Fig. 178.12). The suture should not be tied very tightly to avoid the complication of a bunched appearance in this area after resolution of edema. To reiterate, the suture should be started approximately at the level of the thyroid notch, immediately superior to the platysmal back-cuts, and proceed in a superior direction. If a chin implant is not planned, then the submental incision is closed with a 6-0 running, locking polypropylene suture.

The pre- and postoperative photographs of a patient who had cervical liposuction–submentoplasty and SMAS imbrication rhytidectomy demonstrate effacement of the jowls and the creation of a cervicomental angle of 90 degrees (Fig. 178.13).

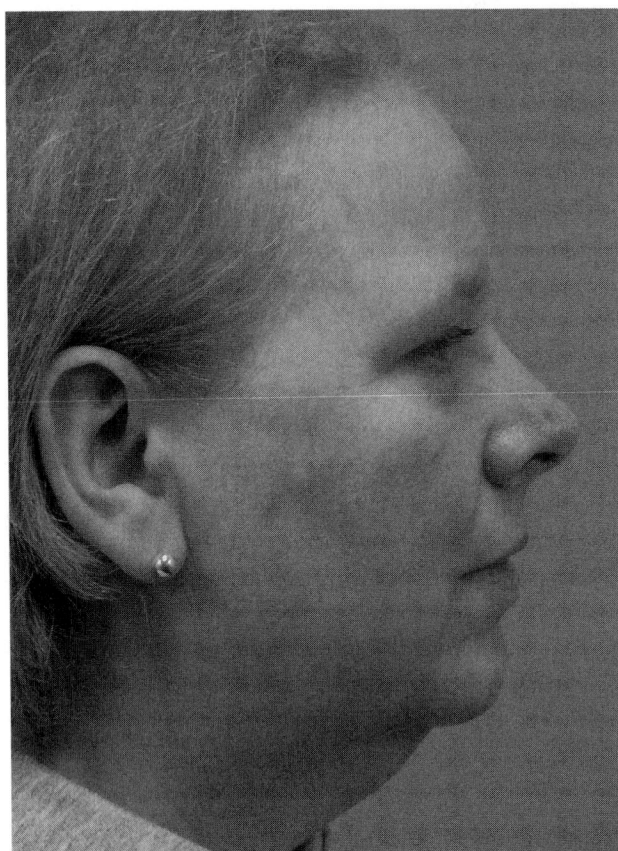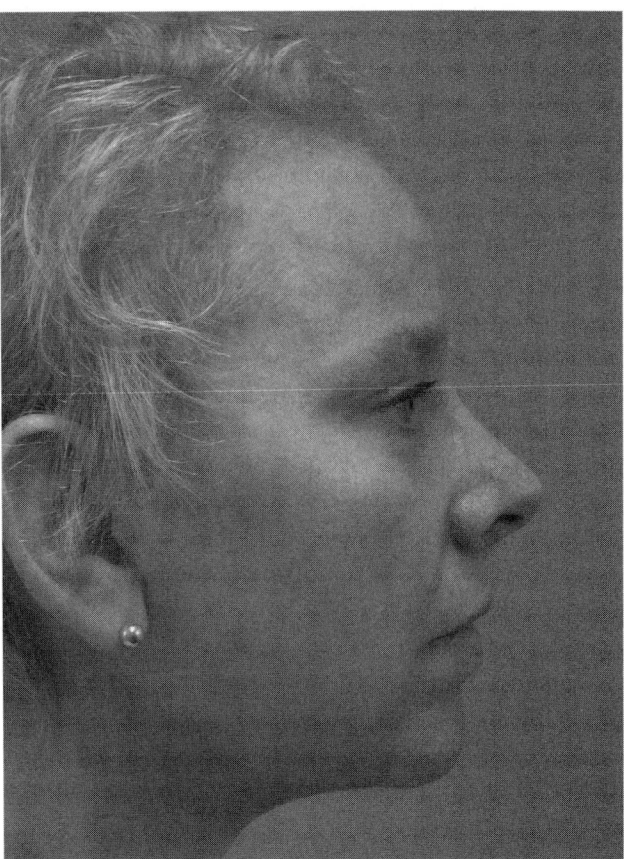

A   B

Figure 178.13 A,B: The pre- and postoperative photographs of a patient who had cervical liposuction–submentoplasty and superficial musculoaponeurotic system (SMAS) imbrication rhytidectomy demonstrate effacement of the jowls and creation of a cervicomental angle of 90 degrees.

COMPLICATIONS AND MANAGEMENT

Early Complications

Early complications following submental liposuction and anterior platysmaplasty include hematoma, seroma, sialocele, infection, contour irregularity, and injury to the marginal mandibular branch of the facial nerve. Hematoma, seroma, or sialocele is seen in less than 1% of patients when liposuction is used as a primary procedure (16). Sialocele is more commonly seen when liposuction is performed over the parotid gland bed in association with a rhytidectomy. Treatment for a sialocele includes pressure dressings, anticholinergics, and repeat aspiration or drainage. A seroma is a collection of serous fluid that occurs in the submental region. These are best treated with needle aspiration and placement of a pressure dressing to prevent reaccumulation.

A large, expanding hematoma is an emergency and the patient should be returned to the operating room for wound exploration, irrigation, and control of all bleeding sites. Smaller hematomas can be managed in the office setting. A limited hematoma discovered on the first postoperative day can be treated by direct aspiration with an 18-gauge needle or by using a gauze sponge to roll out the blood through a small stab incision over the area of concern. A discrete collection discovered somewhat later may require 7 to 10 days to liquefy before it can be aspirated. Persistence of a hematoma predisposes the patient to infection and skin flap necrosis. Because blood is an excellent culture medium, all patients with a hematoma should be placed on a prophylactic antibiotic regimen.

Ideally, the best treatment for a hematoma is prevention. In the preoperative phase, the patient's blood pressure should be well controlled. All preoperative medications that could compromise effective coagulation must be ceased for a period of 2 weeks pre- and 2 weeks postoperatively, including prescription medications (e.g., naproxen, warfarin), over-the-counter medications (e.g., aspirin, ibuprofen), herbal medications (e.g., St. John's wort, gingko biloba), vitamin E, and alcohol. In all circumstances, a male patient requires the surgeon to be at an increased level of attention, given the richer vascularity that the hair-bearing skin of the lower face exhibits and the concomitant risk of hematoma formation.

Infections are rare, occurring in less than 1% of patients (16). Most surgeons, however, elect to put their patients on a prophylactic antibiotic regimen despite the lack of scientific evidence to support their use. An alloplastic implant (e.g., chin implant or ePTFE sling) can be a source for infection. If an abscess develops at the site of implantation, it is almost assured that the implant will require removal. Removal of the implant with reinsertion later when the infection has subsided is the best treatment policy. At the first sign of an infection, a dose of intravenous antibiotics is administered to ensure immediate, proper therapeutic levels, followed by a full regimen of broad-spectrum oral antibiotics until the infection clears.

Early contour irregularities following cervical liposuction are the rule rather than the exception. Most resolve as healing progresses and edema lessens. Patients should be reassured during the first several weeks postoperatively that irregularities generally smooth out with time. Permanent contour irregularities are discussed later in the chapter.

Permanent injury to the marginal mandibular branch of the facial nerve is rare, as long as the surgeon remains superficial to the platysma muscle. Temporary paresis can occur with aggressive liposuction in a patient with an attenuated, thin platysma muscle, which typically resolves within 6 months.

Late Complications

Late complications include scarring, platysmal banding, and irregular neck contour. Hypertrophic or wide scars are rarely seen in the submental incision, but are more commonly seen with rhytidectomy incisions secondary to excessive tension on the skin closure. Additionally, patients with Fitzpatrick skin types V or VI are more susceptible to the development of hypertrophic scars and keloids. Management should include injection of the scars with triamcinolone (10 mg/mL) at 3- to 4-week intervals until improvement is noted. More frequent injections carry the risk of dermal atrophy and hypopigmentation. Additionally, the pulsed dye laser has been shown to be a useful adjunct (9). If the scar persists despite these measures, scar revision may be considered after a 12 month interval.

Platysmal banding, which can occur postoperatively, most commonly occurs secondary to unrecognized, and therefore untreated, preoperative platysmal banding. This is most commonly seen in patients with submental obesity and redundant skin (17). To avoid the complication, preoperative recognition is essential. Platysmal banding can be treated primarily, or secondarily, with anterior platysmaplasty.

An irregular neck contour can result from direct, sharp lipectomy, or from an uneven liposuction technique. Especially in the immediate submental region, overzealous excision of fat can produce a central concavity. A "cobra deformity" describes the situation in which a patient has a central submental concavity from overzealous fat removal in combination with prominent platysmal bands, resembling a cobra about to strike. This deformity is even more pronounced when the anterior borders of the platysma

muscle are not united following central lipectomy (11). Irregularities can be prevented by widely undermining the cervical skin with a 3- to 4-mm layer of fat remaining attached to the overlying dermis and by gauging the thickness of this layer with bimanual palpation during liposuction. Additionally, to avoid further irregularities, the surgeon must make sure the aperture of the liposuction cannula is always facing *away* from the dermis.

Even in the best of hands, neck irregularities still occur. If necessary, small localized depressions can be treated with a soft tissue filler (e.g., autologous fat); however, large depressions may require placement of dermal graft materials (i.e., cadaveric acellular dermis) for correction (16). Again, prevention is the best treatment.

HIGHLIGHTS

- The anatomic factors that contribute to an ideal cervical contour include a strong chin, a distinct mandibular border, a cervicomental angle of 90 degrees, a visible subhyoid bone depression, a gentle indentation at the thyroid notch, and visible anterior borders of the sternocleidomastoid muscles.
- Several anatomic elements contribute to the appearance of an aging neck, including skin, fat, platysma muscle, chin projection, and hyoid bone position.
- Each anatomic element contributing to the deformity should be delineated preoperatively and sequentially addressed to provide an optimal aesthetic outcome.
- A classification system can be used to categorize patients and to target treatment to their specific needs (Table 178.1).
- The rhytidectomy and submentoplasty procedures are the cornerstones of treating the aging neck.
- Early complications of surgery on the aging neck include hematoma, seroma, sialocele, infection, contour irregularity, and injury to the marginal mandibular branch of the facial nerve.
- Late complications include scarring, platysmal banding, and irregular neck contour.

REFERENCES

1. Ellenbogen R, Karlin JV. Visual criteria for success in restoring the youthful neck. *Plast Reconstr Surg* 1980;66:826.
2. Dayan SH, Bagal A, Tardy Jr ME. Targeted solutions in submentoplasty. *Facial Plast Surg* 2001;17:141–149.
3. Cardoso de Castro C. The anatomy of the platysma muscle. *Plast Reconstr Surg* 1980;66:680–688.
4. Dedo DD. The aging neck. In: Bailey BJ, ed. *Head and neck surgery—otolaryngology*, 2nd ed. Philadelphia: Lippincott-Raven, 1998: 2717–2732.
5. Koch RJ, Hanasono MM. Aesthetic facial analysis. In: Papel IR, ed. *Facial plastic and reconstructive surgery*, 2nd ed. New York: Thieme Medical Publishers, 2002:135–144.
6. Conley J. *Facelift operation.* Springfield: Charles C Thomas, 1960:39.
7. Kamer FM, Pieper PG. Surgical treatment of the aging neck. *Facial Plast Surg* 2001;17:123–128.
8. Dedo D. A preoperative classification of the neck for cervicofacial rhytidectomy. *Laryngoscope* 1980;90:1984.

Section X: Facial Plastic and Reconstructive Surgery

9. Lam SM, Williams EF, III. Lower facial rejuvenation. In: Williams EF III, Lam SM, eds. *Comprehensive facial rejuvenation: a practical and systematic guide to surgical management of the aging face.* Philadelphia: Lippincott, Williams & Wilkins, 2004:105–151.

10. Adamson PA, Cormier R, Tropper GJ, et al. Cervicofacial liposuction results and controversies. *J Otolaryngol* 1990;19:267–273.

11. Kamer FM, Minoli JJ. Postoperative platysmal band deformity. *Arch Otolaryngol Head Neck Surg* 1993;119:193–196.

12. Becker DG, Cook TA, Wang TD, et al. A 3-year multi-institutional experience with the liposhaver. *Arch Facial Plast Surg* 1999;1:171–176.

13. Guyuron B. Problem neck, hyoid bone, and submental myotomy. *Plast Reconstr Surg* 1992;90:830–837.

14. Prendiville S, Kokoska MS, Hollenbeak CS, et al. A comparative study of surgical techniques on the cervicomental angle in human cadavers. *Arch Facial Plast Surg* 2002;4:236–242.

15. Giampapa VC, DiBernardo BE. Neck recontouring with suture suspension and liposuction: an alternative for the early rhytidectomy candidate. *Aesthetic Plast Surg* 1995;19:217–223.

16. Kridel RWH, Kelly PE. Liposuction of the face and neck: the art of facial sculpture. In: Papel ID, ed. *Facial plastic and reconstructive surgery*, 2nd ed. New York: Thieme Medical Publishers, 2002:196–222.

17. Ahn MS, Kabaker SS. Complications of facelifting. *Facial Plast Surg Clinics North Am* 2000;8:211–221.

The Aging Forehead

179

Peter A. Adamson   Ravi Dahiya

As the demand for cosmetic surgery increases, so increases the expectation for substantial improvement in surgical results. Management of the periocular region is an integral part of facial rejuvenation, as the eyes are central in interpersonal communication. For many patients, blepharoplasty alone is not sufficient to rejuvenate the eyes and thereby the face. Uncorrected ptosis of the eyebrows conveys fatigue, age, and even anger. Facelifting procedures and blepharoplasty clearly do not address this aesthetic subunit adequately. This shortcoming has been the impetus for the increasing use of forehead rejuvenation procedures and for the efforts to improve the surgical technique. The forehead lift now plays an essential role in providing a harmonious rejuvenation to patients with aging that includes the upper one third of the face.

HISTORY

Lexer (1,2) purportedly performed the first classic forehead lift as early as 1906 but did not describe it until 1931. Passot (3) was the first to publish his experience with the forehead lift in 1919. He described elliptical excisions in the temporal region as well as within forehead rhytids. Over the next several decades, the literature was limited to small series of minor modifications to the previously described techniques. In 1965, Vinas (4) described several clinical insights into the anatomy and treatment of the aging forehead that remain salient today. He noted the difference between static and dynamic rhytids and realized that treatment for the two types also would differ. Vinas also astutely described the need to free adhesions over the orbital rims to mobilize and elevate the eyebrows adequately. Brennan in 1978 (1,2) provided a review of previous procedures and modifications. Pitanguy (5) presented one of the largest series of forehead lifts in 1981, which included insights into technique as well as a record of complication rates. Adamson et al. (6) in 1992 reviewed

modifications of the coronal forehead lift including the pretrichial incision. 1992 also was the year when Isse (7) first presented the endoscopic forehead lift. This technique has had several proposed variations since then, mainly regarding the means of fixation of the mobilized soft tissues of the forehead and eyebrows. Initially the endoscopic approach was widely accepted with great enthusiasm, but more recently, the results of this approach have elicited greater criticism. The next several years will likely reveal the appropriate role of the endoscopic forehead lift in the armamentarium of the cosmetic surgeons.

FOREHEAD ANATOMY

The bony anatomy is defined primarily by the supraorbital ridges, which form the upper boundary of the orbit and separate the midface from the forehead. In men, the supraorbital rim is more prominent in its lateral third, and a convexity of the upper forehead may occur in association with prominent frontal bossing over the frontal sinus. Women tend to have a smoother, continuous curve from the supraorbital rim to the upper forehead because of the lack of frontal bossing and a less prominent supraorbital rim (8).

Blood supply laterally is through the superficial temporal artery, a branch of the external carotid artery. The zygomaticotemporal artery, a branch of the superficial temporal artery, is present at the lateral orbital margin, which occupies the subcutaneous plane in the preauricular region. Medially, the supraorbital artery arises from the supraorbital foramen, about 2.5 cm lateral to the midline. The supratrochlear artery arises medial to this. Both vessels are branches of the ophthalmic artery, a branch of the internal carotid system (Fig. 179.1). Sensory nerve supply is via the supraorbital and supratrochlear nerves, which are branches of the trigeminal nerve (V1). They exit as multiple branches from the supraorbital and frontal foramina, respectively, and provide sensation to the entire central

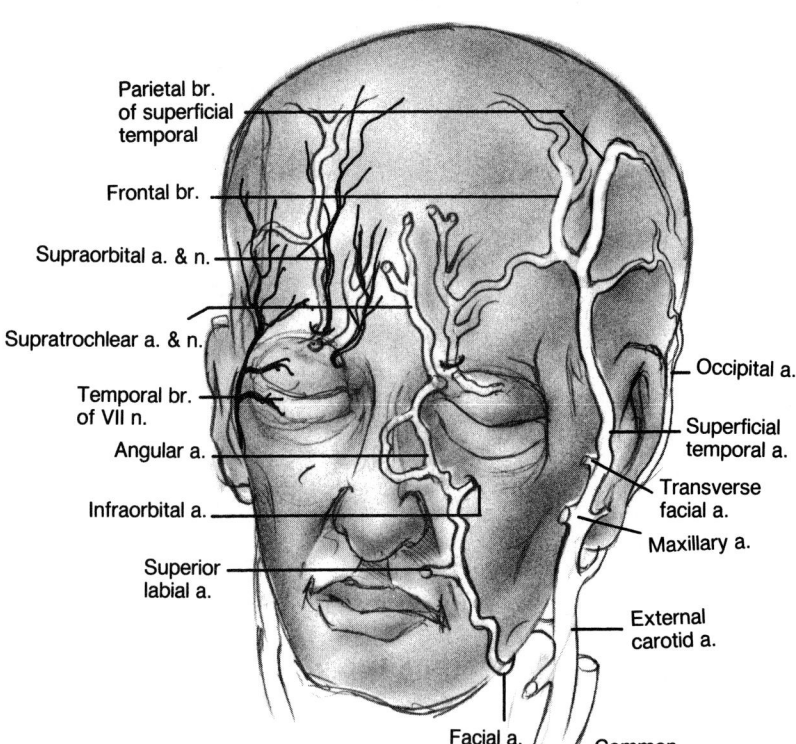

Parietal br. of superficial temporal

Frontal br.

Supraorbital a. & n.

Supratrochlear a. & n.

Temporal br. of VII n.

Angular a.

Infraorbital a.

Superior labial a.

Facial a.

Common carotid a.

External carotid a.

Maxillary a.

Transverse facial a.

Superficial temporal a.

Occipital a.

Figure 179.1 Vessels and nerves of the forehead. The major arterial and sensory innervation is through the supraorbital vessels and nerves. They arise about 2.5 cm from the midline. The temporal branch of the facial nerve is the most functionally significant.

forehead. The lacrimal (V1), zygomaticofacial (V2), zygomaticotemporal nerves (V2), and auriculotemporal (V3) nerves supply lateral forehead sensation. The facial nerve arises from a point about 1.5 cm below the external auditory canal, and the temporal branch runs obliquely superomedially to the forehead region. Its course is about 1 cm lateral to the lateral eyebrow, and it becomes superficial in the region of the hair-bearing and non–hair-bearing skin. A recent cadaver study by Quatela et al. (9) demonstrated that the course of the temporal branch can reliably be predicted by its relation to what is known as the cephalic or sentinel vein, running just superficial to this vessel. This branch innervates the forehead musculature from its undersurface.

The layers of skin in the forehead can be remembered easily by the mnemonic "scalp." The skin is superficial to the subcutaneous tissue, which in turn overlies the aponeurosis and frontalis muscle. Beneath this is loose areolar tissue overlying the pericranium (Fig. 179.2). The galea aponeurotica, also known as the epicranial aponeurosis, attaches to the superior nuchal line of the occipital bone and is only loosely adherent to the underlying pericranium by virtue of the loose areolar tissue, which allows mobility of the scalp. The galea splits to enclose the frontalis muscles and extends over the temporal fascia to attach to the zygomatic arches. The posterior sheath of the galea aponeurotica extends to the eyebrow region. Inferior to this, in the same plane, is the orbital septum of the eyelid. Superficial to the posterior galeal sheath is the eyebrow

fat pad. This contributes to eyebrow mobility, especially in the lateral brow. Individual variations in thickness and extent of the brow fat pad may be found. In some persons, it may extend inferiorly into the suborbicularis preseptal plane in the eyelid to become the lateral "preseptal fat"

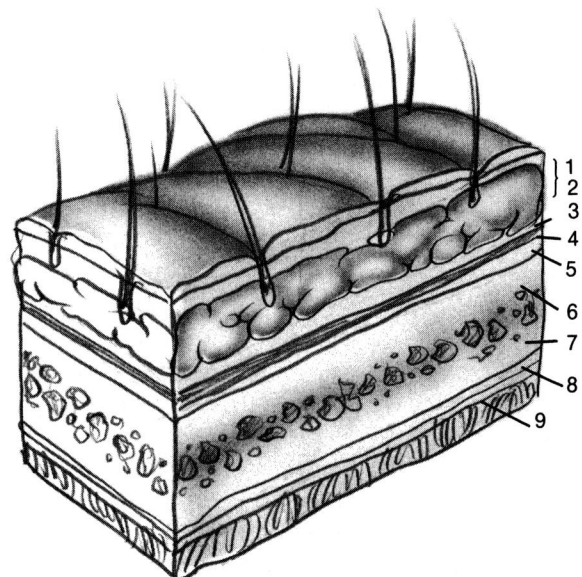

Figure 179.2 Forehead skin. Scalp refers to the layers of the forehead skin. *1*, Skin; *2*, subcutaneous tissue; *3*, epicranial aponeurosis (galea and frontalis m.); *4*, lax areolar tissue; *5*, pericranium; *6*, outer table; *7*, inner table; *8*, dura mater; *9*, arachnoid.

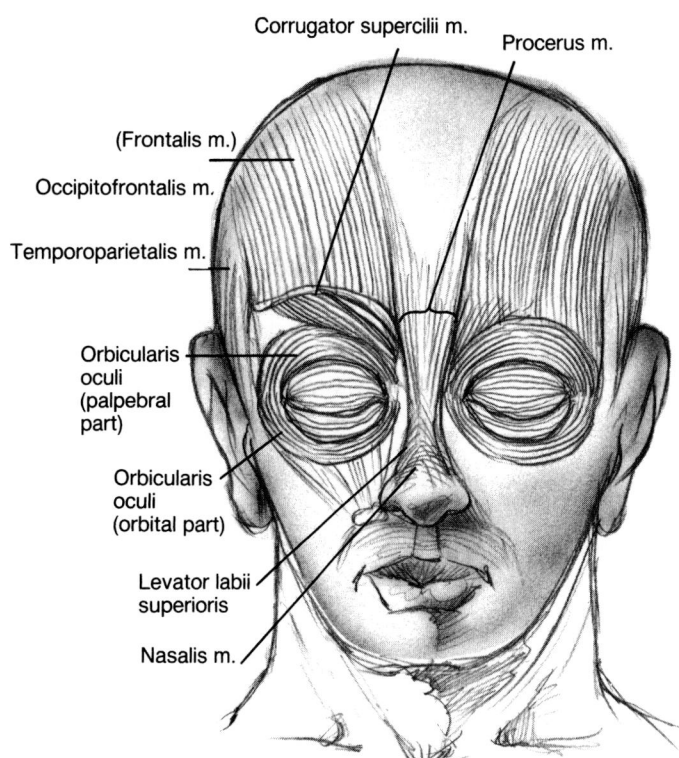

Corrugator supercilii m.

Procerus m.

(Frontalis m.)

Occipitofrontalis m.

Temporoparietalis m.

Orbicularis oculi (palpebral part)

Orbicularis oculi (orbital part)

Levator labii superioris

Nasalis m.

Figure 179.3 Forehead muscles. Forehead muscle activity causes the development of the rhytids associated with aging. The frontalis muscle produces horizontal forehead rhytids, the corrugator supercilius muscle vertical glabellar rhytids, and the procerus muscle horizontal glabellar rhytids.

seen in blepharoplasty. Superficially, the galea is attached to the skin by firm fibrous superficial fascia.

The frontalis muscle, which is paired bilaterally, attaches inferiorly to the supraorbital dermis and interdigitates with the orbicularis oculi muscle, the skin of the eyebrows, and the root of the nose (Fig. 179.3). It also blends with the corrugator supercilii muscles and procerus muscle medially. Although it has no bony attachments, its action is to raise the eyebrows through these interdigitations, which is how horizontal forehead rhytids are formed. The corrugator supercilii muscles arise from the bone over the medial aspect of the supraorbital arch and pass obliquely deep to the frontalis and orbicularis muscles to insert by interdigitation with these muscles throughout the medial half of the eyebrow. Their action is to draw the eyebrows medially.

The procerus is a pyramid-shaped muscle that arises from the fascia over the nasal bones and upper lateral cartilages to insert in the skin between the eyebrows and interdigitate with the corrugator supercilii muscles. Its action is to draw the medial edge of the eyebrow downward. The orbicularis oculi, an oval muscle surrounding the orbit, consists of three distinct bands that blend into the medial and lateral canthal tendons. These bands form the orbital, preseptal, and pretarsal divisions. The orbital division, which interdigitates with the frontalis muscle, originates from the medial orbital rims between the supraorbital arch and the infraorbital foramen. The muscle is a sphincter for the eye, but with forcible closure, the eyebrows also are pulled downward.

PHYSIOLOGY OF AGING

In youth, the forehead, temple, and glabella are unfurrowed. The hairline is irregularly irregular, and no evidence appears of male pattern baldness or thinning hair in women. Of particular importance is the relation of the thicker infrabrow skin with the upper eyelid skin. In youth, the higher brow position allows the contour of the lateral supraorbital rim to be well demarcated and, below this, the upper eyelid cleft to be apparent.

With aging, the upper third of the face undergoes several changes (Fig. 179.4). Loss of skin elasticity, decreased bulk of subcutaneous tissue, and increased skull bone resorption is seen. As a result of the effects of gravity, sagging or ptosis of the forehead, glabella, temple, and eyebrows occurs, initially in the region of the lateral third of the eyebrow, resulting in skin redundancy in the infrabrow and upper eyelid and hooding of the skin. A superolateral visual field defect may result in more pronounced cases. With ptosis, crow's feet develop in the temple region, and horizontal furrows develop in the glabella in association with redundant skin in the medial canthal region. This "closed eye" appearance is often associated with sadness, fatigue, anger, and unacceptable aesthetics.

With descent of the eyebrows, the patient tends to increase frontalis muscle activity to elevate the brows dynamically, especially when communicating or looking in the mirror. With time, the initially superficial and transient rhytids become deeper and permanent, as the fascia

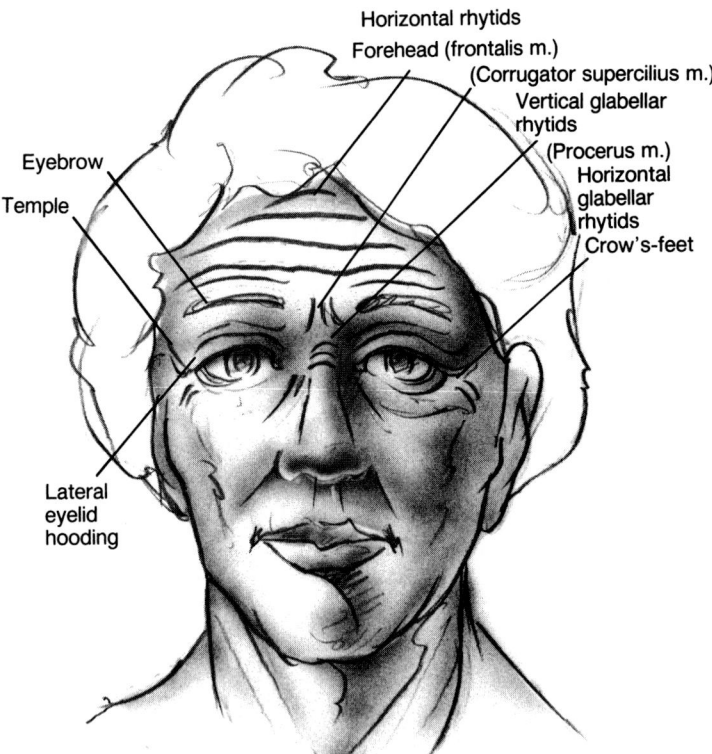

Figure 179.4 Physiology of aging. Ptosis initially occurs at the lateral brow but eventually involves the entire brow and forehead. Rhytids are caused by voluntary and involuntary muscle activity.

contracts and causes a permanent skin crease, even when the muscle is at rest. Squinting requires activity of the corrugator supercilius muscle and the progressive development of vertical and oblique rhytids in the medial eyebrow region. Activity of the procerus muscle to elevate the ptotic glabella results in the progressive development of horizontal rhytids. Ptosis of the nasal tip also occurs with aging but is more likely related to loss of soft-tissue support in the premaxillary region rather than to loss of support from the forehead and glabellar structures.

Every person has unique facial expressions, and thus each develops a unique pattern of upper facial rhytids and eyebrow position. The patient's skin type, history of sun exposure, smoking habits, and other factors also affect the facial parameters associated with aging.

FOREHEAD AESTHETICS

Eyebrow position is usually considered the key landmark in determining the aesthetic configuration of the upper third of the face (10,11). The medial end of the eyebrow should have a club-head configuration and should be in line with a vertical line drawn through the ala of the nose. It arches superolaterally above the supraorbital rim to its apex between vertical lines drawn from the lateral limbus and lateral canthus. It then tapers into a handle shape to end laterally at an oblique line drawn through the ala of the nose and the lateral canthus. The medial and lateral

ends of the eyebrows should be on a horizontal line. In men, the brow is more commonly at the level of the supraorbital rim and does not arch as high as that in women. Eyebrow hairs may extend in an inferior, lateral, or superior direction and are usually much thicker in men. By today's standards, a lower, thicker brow still may be considered attractive in women, depending on its harmony with their overall facial aesthetics. The brow, medial orbital rim, and nasal bones should approximate a Y-shaped configuration in women and a T-shaped configuration in men.

ASSESSMENT

Each patient must specify his or her particular concerns if the appropriate procedure is to be chosen. This is especially important when considering forehead rejuvenation. For instance, many patients request an upper blepharoplasty to correct hooding when the ideal procedure may well be one to elevate ptotic brows. Other patients are more concerned about aging of the lower face, as most people usually elevate their eyebrows unconsciously when looking in the mirror or having photographs taken and therefore do not recognize the degree of forehead and brow ptosis normally present. Evaluate patients with their facial muscles in repose, preferably as they look in a mirror. Elicit a previous history of upper blepharoplasty, which may produce a relative lack of upper-eyelid skin for lifting procedures, or a history of dry-eye problems. Patients who have previous alopecia may be at an increased risk for surgical hair-follicle shock. The coronal forehead lift may be performed in men who have no indications that they will develop male-pattern baldness and are fully informed of the incision. Increasing numbers of male and female patients also may consider hair transplants in conjunction with a forehead lift, thus allowing expanded use of a pretrichial incision.

Routine investigations before any forehead procedure include an ophthalmology examination. Specifically indicated are visual acuity, visual fields for superolateral defects, and the Schirmer test to rule out dry-eye conditions. Photographic documentation is done, and standard physical examination and investigations appropriate for each patient are ordered. The following are characteristics of the upper face that must be assessed before recommending the ideal surgical procedure.

Ptosis

Aging results in brow, forehead, glabellar, and temple ptosis. The surgeon must differentiate between lateral eyelid hooding that is a result of upper-eyelid skin redundancy and that due to ptosis of the eyebrow. Frontalis contraction must be eliminated by complete patient relaxation to eliminate pseudoelevation of the eyebrows. In patients who have eyebrow ptosis, upper blepharoplasty usually will correct upper-eyelid hooding only partially and will not elevate the ptotic eyebrow. Younger patients who have ptotic brows and upper-eyelid hooding and no other signs of upper facial aging often see greater improvement with a forehead lift rather than upper-eyelid blepharoplasty. Furthermore, aggressive upper-eyelid blepharoplasty may result in further brow ptosis and short-upper-lid syndrome. Correction of glabellar ptosis also may improve skin elasticity and rhytids in the upper half of the nose significantly, thus improving nasal appearance, even though the nasal tip may not have its degree of rotation changed. Correction of temple ptosis improves lateral canthal crow's feet.

The effects of the forehead/brow lift may be demonstrated to the patient by gently elevating the forehead in the midline and laterally. The degree of surgical brow elevation required can be assessed by having the patient actively elevate the eyebrows while the surgeon holds a ruler at a predetermined landmark on the brow. In this way, the ideal amount of brow elevation can be determined, allowing for a degree of stretch-back.

Rhytids

Noting the forehead, glabellar, and temple rhytids along with the relative degree of activity of the upper facial muscles with mimetic expression helps to determine the extent of myoplasty required for the involved muscles. Rhytids are more pronounced in older patients who have subcuta-

neous atrophy, and thus the actions of the muscles are transmitted more directly to the skin.

Hairline Patterns

Women who have a medium- or low-forehead hairline are candidates for the standard coronal or endoscopic forehead lift. Those with higher hairlines may need to style their hair over the forehead to camouflage the high hairline that may result from a standard coronal lift. Conversely, such patients might benefit from a trichophytic lift, which not only maintains their hairline position but also reduces the vertical height of their high forehead. Men may be candidates for a standard coronal lift if they are not expected to develop male-pattern baldness and they are fully informed of the incision. Men and women who are undergoing or willing to undergo hair transplants may be candidates for a trichophytic lift, although these are very rarely required. Minigrafts or micrografts may be all that is required for scar camouflage. This also is true of women with thinning hair and in whom a trichophytic lift is relatively contraindicated otherwise. The direction of the eyebrow hairs may determine whether a direct brow lift is advisable. Men in whom the hair grows superiorly and women with thicker eyebrows will be better able to camouflage the scar from a direct eyebrow lift.

Skin Type

Fair- and thin-skinned patients usually heal with more ideal scars than do those with darker and thicker or sebaceous skin. Women tend to scar better than males. Older patients, because of their skin elasticity, often have finer scars than do younger patients.

Asymmetries

Note both passive and dynamic asymmetries of the eyebrows. Dynamic eyebrow asymmetries should not be altered surgically. Passive asymmetries are not usually corrected unless it is the patient's expressed wish, as this may alter the patient's unique facial characteristics. Even so, the coronal forehead lift and its modifications are usually unsuccessful in correcting eyebrow asymmetries because of their distance from the eyebrows. Direct eyebrow or midforehead eyebrow lifts are more successful if such correction is desired. Patients who have hyperdynamic forehead-muscle activity, resulting from efforts to correct marked degrees of brow ptosis or as a characteristic feature of their facial expression, may need more aggressive myoplasties to decrease this degree of activity and minimize recurrence of forehead and glabellar rhytids. The clinical assessment and photographic documentation must be performed with the patient's facial muscles in repose.

Bony Contour

Women who have a prominent supraorbital rim and excessive forehead bossing may appear masculinized. They may benefit from bone reduction of the supraorbital rim or methyl methacrylate augmentation in association with a coronal forehead lift (8).

DIFFERENTIAL DIAGNOSIS

Coronal forehead lifting and brow lifting will have no effect on the eyes other than to improve brow position and lateral hooding. Conversely, upper blepharoplasty will not alter eyebrow position and, if aggressive skin resection is carried out, may cause further lateral eyebrow ptosis. The lateral infrabrow skin cannot be excised in upper blepharoplasty, and thus minimal improvement may be achieved in the patient seeking correction of lateral hooding with an upper blepharoplasty rather than with some form of eyebrow lift. Patients should be advised that rejuvenation surgery will "turn the clock back" but will not stop the aging process. The patient's specific concerns in conjunction with full facial assessment must be addressed: this is the only way the correct procedures can be chosen. Patients seeking a facelift should be advised that it will not alter the appearance of the upper face.

MANAGEMENT

Aging takes place at a unique pace for each person. Significant factors affecting the speed of aging include genetic predisposition, sun exposure, and smoking. No one can determine at what pace a person will age in the future or the exact degree of rejuvenation a patient will achieve with any given procedure. Patients can be shown in the mirror the results that might be achieved and photographs of other patients to get a general idea of the degree of improvement possible. Surgery may not always be indicated; other methods may be used to correct a specific defect that is of great concern to the patient or to temporize until the patient is a better candidate for surgery. Other such methods include the following:

1. Sun avoidance and protection will prevent photodamage to the skin and help prevent squinting and thus decrease vertical glabellar rhytids.
2. Judicious use of cosmetics may camouflage forehead rhytids.
3. Retin-A cream may increase the vascularity of the skin and the organization of collagen bundles and may thicken the skin, resulting in a more youthful overall appearance and improvement in fine rhytids. It does not improve deeper furrows. Chemical peels will provide a greater effect.

4. Styling the hair over the forehead will camouflage rhytids, although it usually cannot camouflage brow ptosis.
5. Fillers such as collagen or hyaluronic acid–based products may be used selectively for temporary effect in forehead rhytids or furrows and crows feet.
6. Eyeglasses may camouflage both brow ptosis and glabellar rhytids.
7. Botulinum toxin (Botox) injections can provide several months of muscle paralysis with partial effacement of furrows.

Surgical procedures other than those to rejuvenate the upper face may improve the patient's overall appearance and occasionally offer greater benefits than a forehead procedure. In patients who have reasonable eyebrow position and minimal forehead rhytids, lateral hooding with fat ptosis of the upper eyelids may be better corrected with an upper blepharoplasty. Patients who have significant jowling or cervicofacial ptosis may benefit more from cervicofacial liposuction and rhytidectomy. It is important to think in terms of surgery in regional aesthetic units and what will be of most benefit for the patient.

All patients should be counseled that the goal is improvement, not perfection. Rejuvenation is achieved, but aging continues. Patients will appear younger than if they had not had the surgery but in time will redevelop most of the same features that were improved by the surgery. They must be aware that a specific result, a perfect result, or a no-risk procedure cannot be guaranteed. Each procedure will have specific effects, and patients must be aware of what will and will not be achieved with the procedures they choose. Specifically, patients should be counseled about the general and local complications associated with the procedures they are contemplating, outlining the preoperative, postoperative, and surgical protocols in detail. Literature with instructions and advice about the surgery should be given to the patient, because a well-informed patient can choose the procedure that has the highest likelihood of success for him or her. Of primary importance in forehead-rejuvenation procedures are the patient's specific goals, the hairline changes involved, and the acceptability of scar placement.

SURGICAL PROCEDURE AND TECHNIQUE

The choice of surgical procedure for rejuvenation of the upper face can be considered within three surgical groups: the coronal forehead lift and its modifications (Fig. 179.5), the direct brow lift and its modifications (Fig. 179.6), and the endoscopic forehead lift. The indications and surgical technique for each of these follow.

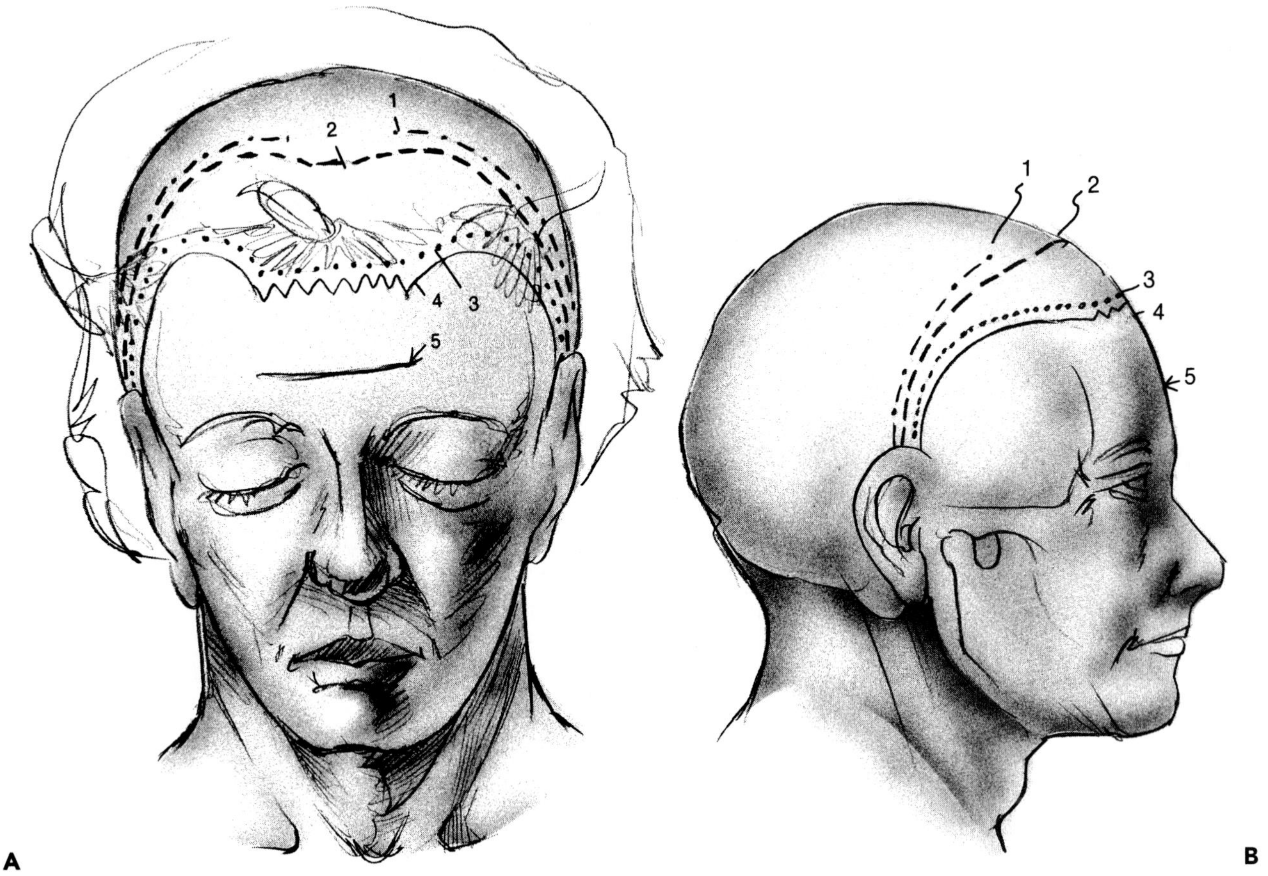

Figure 179.5 The coronal incision is the standard incision. Modifications may be made depending on the patient's hairline, degree of ptosis, rhytids, skin type, asymmetries, sex, and personal preference. **A:** Frontal view. **B:** Lateral view. *1,* Bilateral (temporal); *2,* coronal (forehead); *3,* trichophytic; *4,* pretrichial; *5,* midforehead.

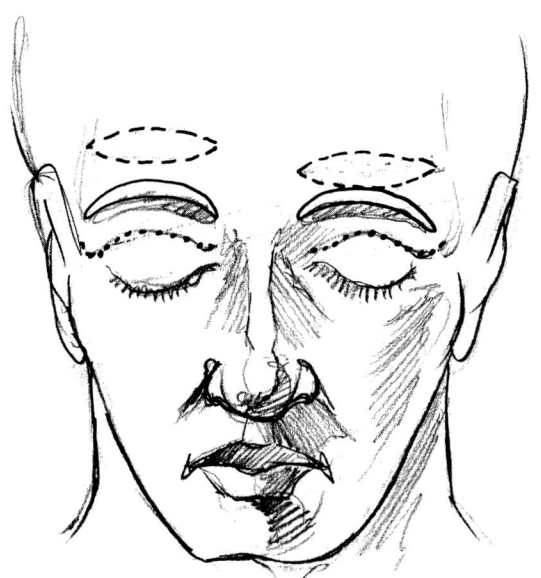

Figure 179.6 The direct brow lift (*solid lines*) is the standard incision. More recent modifications, such as the indirect brow lift (*dashes*) and browpexy (*dots*), can be useful in selected patients.

Coronal Forehead Lift

The standard coronal forehead lift and its modifications are arguably the procedures of choice for rejuvenation of the upper face. The coronal lift is especially useful for patients who have both generalized ptosis and rhytids of the upper face and a normal or low hairline (Fig. 179.7). Relative contraindications include men with male-pattern baldness and women with high hairlines. The tricophytic forehead lift is ideal for these patients with a high hairline. These lifts are not useful to correct brow asymmetries. Advantages of the open lifts are the well-concealed incision behind and in the hairline and superb exposure of the forehead muscles, allowing accurate and extensive myoplasty. They allow the surgeon to address all the major deformities caused by upper facial aging. The disadvantages include elevation of the frontal hairline, although this is an advantage in patients with a low frontal hairline. Other disadvantages include the temporary, and occasionally permanent, hypesthesia or paresthesia posterior to the incision line. The wide undermining increases the risk for hematoma, and tension on the wound closure may predispose to temporary or permanent hair loss.

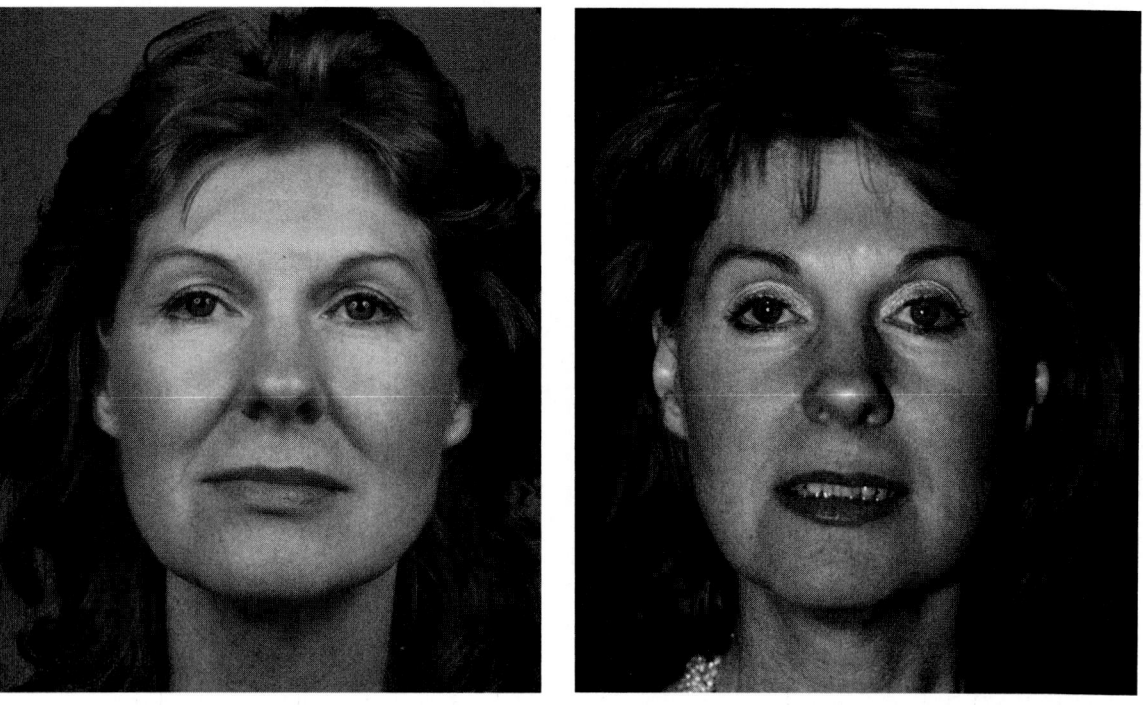

Figure 179.7   A: A 51-year-old woman with moderate eyebrow ptosis, mild forehead rhytids, and normal hairline. **B:** Same woman 2.5 years after a coronal forehead lift, four-lid blepharoplasty, and cervicofacial rhytidectomy.

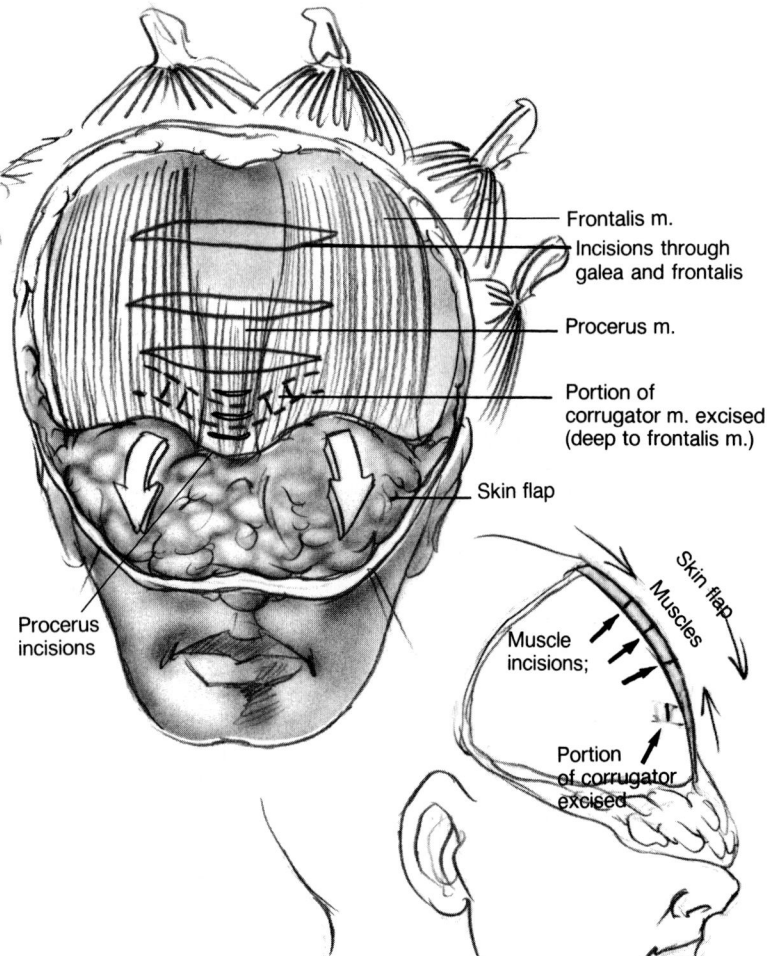

Frontalis m.

Incisions through galea and frontalis

Procerus m.

Portion of corrugator m. excised (deep to frontalis m.)

Skin flap

Procerus incisions

Muscle incisions;

Portion of corrugator excised.

Skin flap

Muscles

Figure 179.8 The coronal incision is beveled parallel to the shafts of the hair follicles. The flap is elevated over the supraorbital margins and to the zygoma. A portion of the corrugator supercilius is excised, and the procerus and frontalis are incised.

Technique

The procedure is done under local intravenous sedation anesthesia unless multiple other procedures also are being performed (6,12). A curvilinear incision about 4 to 6 cm posterior to the anterior hairline is marked, and a thin strip of hair removed along the incision line. Local infiltration anesthesia of lidocaine 1% with epinephrine 1:100,000 and bupivacaine 0.5% with epinephrine 1:200,000 mixed in equal parts is used initially to effect a regional block at the supratrochlear and supraorbital nerves. Next, a ring block is completed by following the supraorbital margins, the zygomas, and the scalp at the incision site. Infiltration is completed in the subgaleal plane beneath the entire area of the flap to be elevated. Time must be allowed for vasoconstriction.

The coronal incision is beveled parallel to the shafts of the hair follicles, usually obliquely anterior at the midline and becoming more horizontal or even obliquely posterior in the temple region (Fig. 179.8). The flap is elevated with broad scalpel sweeps in the subgaleal plane, abetting this action with firm upward traction on the flap. The pericranium is kept intact and moistened with saline gauze. Premonitory vessels may be seen coursing superiorly from the supraorbital vessels about 2 to 3 cm superior to their origin. Scalpel dissection is carried inferiorly to about 1 cm above the supraorbital rims. Dissection laterally must be carried down to the zygoma; this is most safely done with the blade handle and gentle blunt dissection just above the temporalis fascia.

Blunt interfibrillar scissor dissection is done to identify and free the corrugator muscles from the supratrochlear and supraorbital nerves and vessels, which are multiple and course around the muscle. The flap is dissected over the supraorbital rims, but not so far as to expose orbital fat. In this way, the brow is freed so that it may be elevated above the supraorbital rims. The muscle is cauterized with bipolar cautery at two points about 1 cm apart, and the central portion excised. Any bleeding is meticulously controlled with bipolar cautery, taking care not to injure any nerves. The procerus in the midline is identified and incised horizontally by using unipolar cautery. The frontalis muscle is identified in the flap, and the unipolar cautery is used to incise the frontalis muscle and galea immediately deep to the transverse forehead creases. Cauterization is maintained medial to the pupils bilaterally to prevent injury to the temporal branch of the facial nerve and also to preserve some natural forehead movement through the action of the frontalis muscle laterally. Excision rather than incision of the procerus and frontalis muscles may lead to contour irregularities of the glabella and forehead.

The temporalis branch of the facial nerve is at risk in the region between the brow and the temporal hairline as it traverses this area superomedially. The nerve is deep within the parotid gland but becomes superficial in the

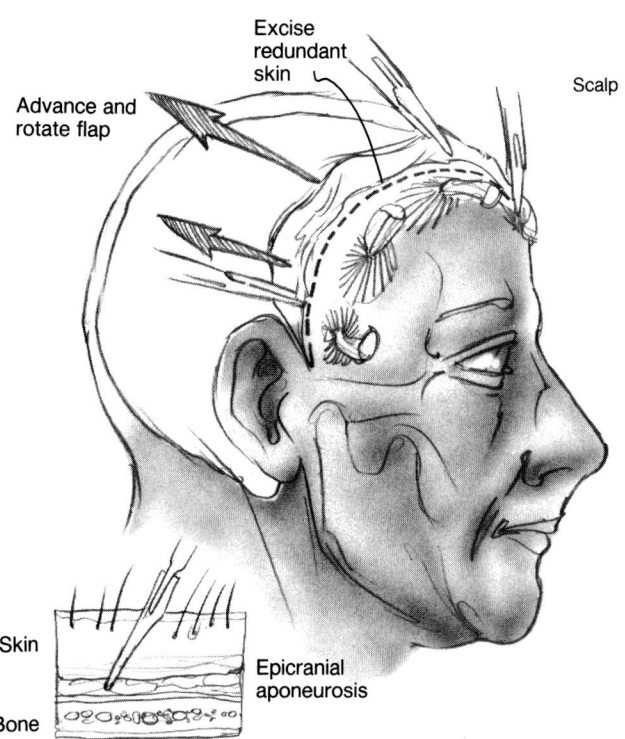

Figure 179.9 The flap is advanced and rotated in a superior and posterior direction, and the appropriate portion of redundant skin is excised parallel to the hair follicles.

subdermal fat as it crosses the zygomatic arch. It then courses deeply again to pierce the frontalis muscle about 1 cm from the lateral canthus. Therefore, the frontalis muscle must not be divided in this region between the eyebrow and the temporal hairline. Absolute hemostasis is secured, paying special attention to superficial temporal artery branches in the supraauricular region. The galeal vessels are cauterized, avoiding bleeding vessels in the subcutaneous tissue so as not to damage hair follicles.

Advancement and rotation of the flap are done in a superior and posterior direction, and the appropriate portion of redundant skin parallel to the hair follicles is excised (Fig. 179.9). This amount can be determined by assessing the amount of brow elevation required and then increasing this by about 5 mm to allow for stretch-back. Usually, about 12 to 18 mm of skin can be excised. Obviously, this amount will vary with each patient, and a conservative excision is indicated to prevent an overelevated and scared look. More skin may be excised from the central or temporal region, depending on the desired correction. The excision usually is extended laterally to 1 to 2 cm above the anterior helical root. A suction drain is placed through a separate stab incision in the temple; the galea is closed by using interrupted and inverted polyglycolic acid sutures, and the skin, with staples.

A light dressing then is applied. Ophthalmic drops and ointment are prescribed for any indications of corneal exposure. The dressing and drain are removed on the first postoperative day, and surgical staples, on day 7 and day 9.

Brow Lift and Upper Blepharoplasty

A special relation exists between forehead or brow lifting and upper blepharoplasty. Temporary lagophthalmos for several days is common after forehead or brow lifting, and a concomitant upper blepharoplasty will increase the degree and duration of lagophthalmos. The brow lift should be performed first, as a more accurate assessment of the degree of eyelid skin to be excised then can be made. Conservative skin excision is advisable. If no skin must be removed, redundant upper-eyelid fat can be excised through a standard excision just above the tarsal plate. Take care not to injure the insertion of the levator aponeurosis.

The eyelid margin should not be above midpupil after surgery and usually closes within 7 to 10 days. Aggressive postoperative ocular lubrication is necessary until full closure of the palpebral fissure occurs.

Eyelid skin can be stored as a graft for up to 3 weeks and used as a full-thickness donor graft to its original site if eyelid closure is unsatisfactory. Patients are advised that a touch-up excision of upper-eyelid skin can be performed 9 to 12 months later if necessary.

Patients who have had a previous upper blepharoplasty and require correction of eyebrow ptosis may be candidates for any of the forehead or brow-lifting procedures; however, the surgeon must be careful to assess the degree of redundant upper-eyelid skin, the status of the tear film, and the amount of skin excised for elevation. Conservativism is advised.

Bilateral Temple Lift

This procedure has essentially the same incision as the coronal forehead lift, except that the incision is carried from just above the anterior helical root up to the mid-pupillary line, but it does not extend completely across the midline scalp (Fig. 179.5). The incision is beveled parallel to the hair follicles, and a subgaleal dissection is carried out with blunt and sharp scissor dissection down over the supraorbital margin and to the zygoma inferiorly. The temple flap is redraped superolaterally, and the redundant skin excised; it is usually about 10 mm at its widest. The galea is closed with 3-0 polyglycolic antitension sutures, and the skin, with surgical staples. No drain is usually placed.

This procedure is indicated in men or women who have primarily lateral eyebrow ptosis and upper eyelid hooding. It is advantageous in that it does not elevate the central hairline, as does the full coronal forehead lift and, because of the scar position, can be used in both men and women; however, it does not allow myoplasty procedures in the forehead, and its somewhat confined exposure for elevation makes it difficult to control any bleeding vessels at the supraorbital margin. Although it appears to offer good intermediate-term results, it does not appear to offer the longer-lasting results seen with the coronal forehead lift.

Pretrichial Lift

In this modification of the coronal forehead lift, the incision temporally remains the same but is brought anteriorly in the widow's-peak region. It then follows a gently sinuous course just at or behind the anterior hairline or, alternatively, as a W-plasty with limbs about 5.5 mm long and 55-degree angles that interdigitate with the anterior hairline follicles (Fig. 179.5). The forehead flap is elevated as for the coronal lift, and myoplasty of forehead rhytids and correction of ptosis is done.

The primary indication for the pretrichial forehead lift is for women who have a high hairline and long vertical height to the forehead (Fig. 179.10). This procedure then offers all the advantages of the coronal forehead lift but does not raise the anterior hairline to an unaesthetically high level. Furthermore, resection of the redundant forehead skin reduces the vertical height of the forehead, and this often is an aesthetic improvement. It is best used in women who have thick hair and are prepared to wear their hair forward to camouflage the scar (Fig. 179.11). It can be used in men who are undergoing or who are willing to undergo hair transplants to camouflage the scar further. Having said this, the incision usually heals very well, especially in lighter-skinned individuals, and rarely needs camouflage.

The advantage of the pretrichial lift is that it allows the same wide access to the forehead musculature as the coronal lift and thus allows correction of all the components of the aging forehead. Disadvantages include the necessity for meticulous technique to obtain the finest possible scar and the possibility of postoperative scar camouflage being required. A broader area of anesthesia occurs, usually permanent to some degree in most patients, posterior to the incision. This is larger than that seen with the coronal forehead lift because of lack of additional sensory innervation from the posterior scalp nerves.

Trichophytic Forehead Lift

The tricophytic incision is currently the preferred technique when an open approach is chosen. This incision is a modification of the pretrichial incision; it is placed at the anterior hairline but is better camouflaged because hair follicles regrow through the scar (Fig. 179.12)(13,14). It is indicated for women with high foreheads and hairlines and may be considered in men who do not have male-pattern baldness or who would agree to hair transplants should this occur (Fig. 179.13).

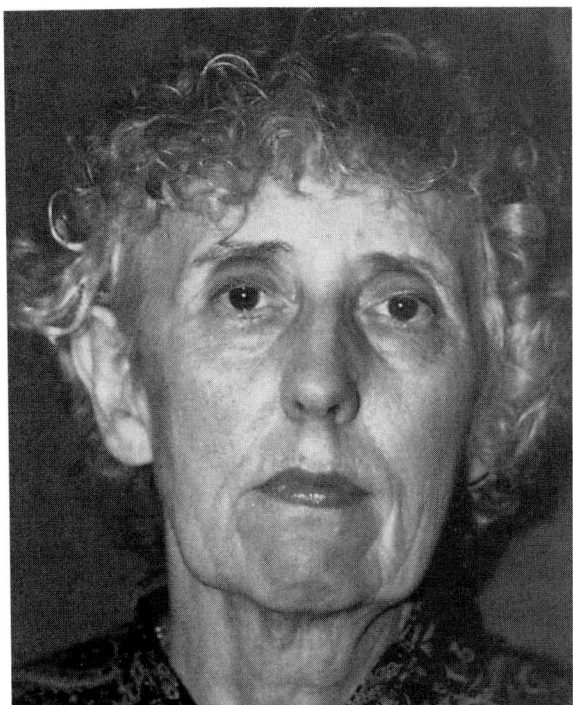
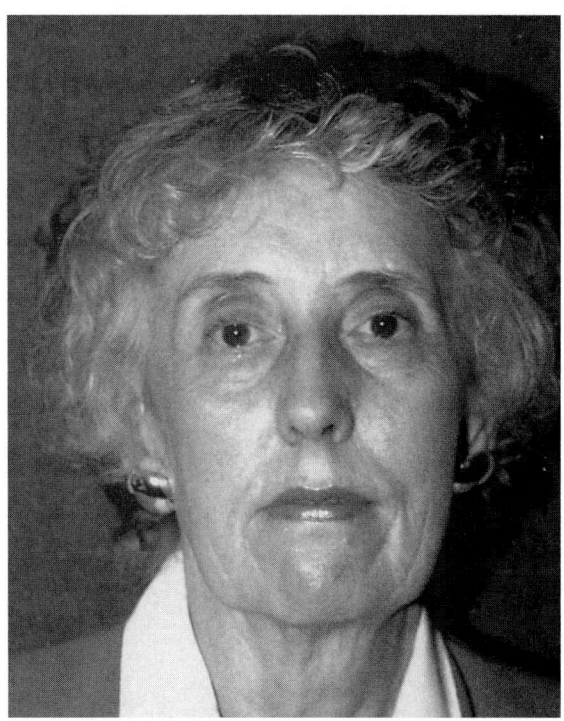

A   B

Figure 179.10 **A:** A 62-year-old woman with moderate eyebrow ptosis, forehead rhytids, and a high forehead. **B:** Six months after a pretrichial forehead lift.

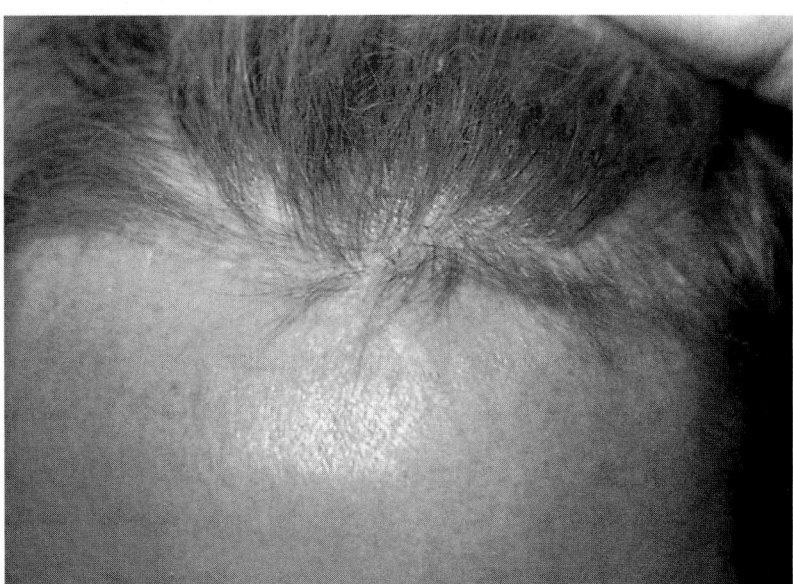

Figure 179.11 Anterior forehead hairline 3 months after W-plasty pretrichial incision in a woman.

The incision is an irregular beveled incision made just posterior to the anterior hairline (Fig. 179.5). The superficial aspect of the incision is placed perpendicular to the hair shafts and is extended down through the epidermis only. Then it is beveled from posterior to anterior through the dermis and subcutaneous tissues to the subgaleal plane. This effectively deepithelializes about 2 mm of the leading edge of the posterior or hair-bearing flap and preserves the underlying hair follicles, although their shafts

are excised. After the myoplasty procedures and redraping of the forehead flap, the redundant skin is excised from the non–hair-bearing flap in a beveled fashion to allow the edge of the forehead flap to appose accurately the opposite bevel of the deepithelialized portion of the posterior hair-bearing flap. Galeal sutures again are used for antitension, and the wound is closed with a running 6-0 nylon suture along the forehead skin junction and with staples within the hair-bearing scalp, taking care to prevent damage to

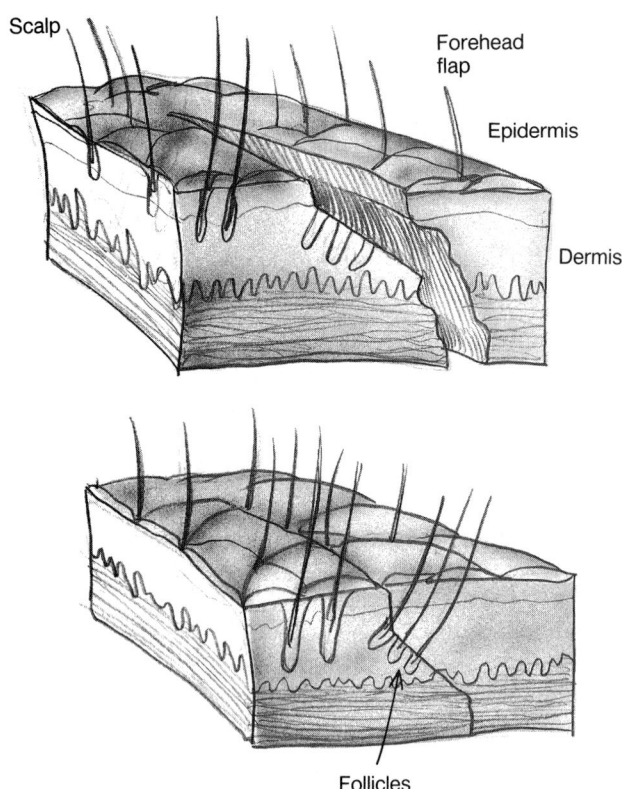

Figure 179.12 A: The trichophytic incision is an irregular beveled incision made just posterior to the anterior hairline. **B:** The follicles below the deepithelialized portion of the flap will produce hair growth through the scar.

hair follicles. With further hair growth from the hair follicles below the deepithelialized portion of the posterior flap, follicles will grow through the scar itself, thus improving camouflage.

The trichophytic incision has the advantage of providing an improved scar but again requires meticulous execution to achieve the desired result. Inaccurate incision placement or wound tension causing strangulation of the hair-follicle vasculature will compromise the result. This incision has become the preferred hairline incision. The scar heals so well that most patients can wear their hair back without scar camouflage.

Midforehead Lift

The midforehead lift, when performed in the central forehead, can be considered a modification of the coronal forehead lift because the dissection can be carried into the subgaleal plane, and myoplasty is possible (15,16). The incision is placed in a central midforehead crease, and subcutaneous rather than subgaleal elevation is performed down to the supraorbital margins (Fig. 179.5). This preserves the sensory supply of the forehead, which otherwise would be lost if the midforehead incision were deepened to the subgaleal plane. Access to the corrugator supercilii and procerus muscles is possible by developing a central subgaleal flap inferiorly. Myoplasty can be done if indicated, and the frontalis muscle can be divided between the supraorbital nerves. This approach does not permit the same extent of forehead muscle myoplasty as that in the coronal forehead lift. The inferior flap is redraped superiorly, and the redundant skin is excised to correct ptosis of the glabella and medial eyebrows. If the excision is extended laterally in the subcutaneous plane, some degree of elevation of the lateral eyebrows also can be achieved. In such cases, the procedure is comparable to that of the indirect brow lift or midforehead brow lift. This procedure is indicated in patients who have significant

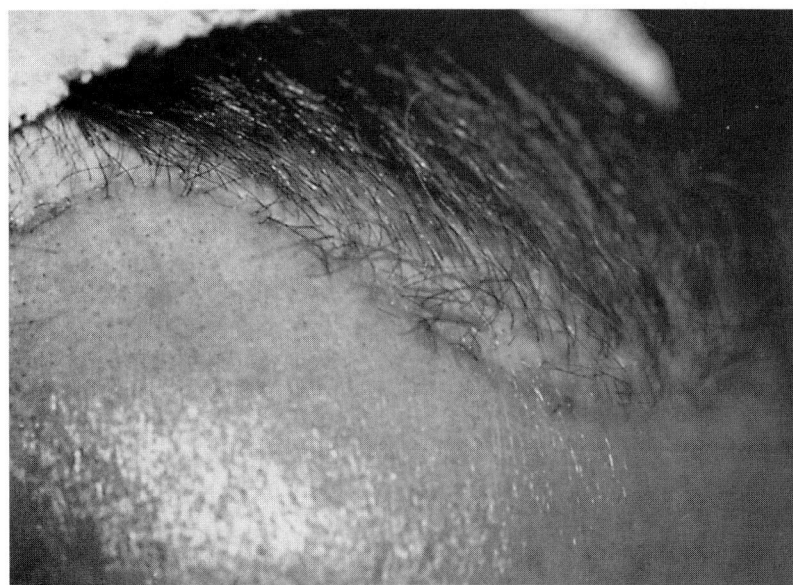

Figure 179.13 Temporal and anterior hairline of a man 3 months after a trichophytic forehead lift. Hair can be seen growing through the incision. By 6 months, this scar becomes almost imperceptible.

forehead rhytids in which the scar can be camouflaged, such as men in whom a coronal forehead lift is contraindicated. It is a possible but less desirable option for a woman with a high hairline who does not wish a trichophytic lift (Fig. 179.14). This procedure is advantageous because of the closer and more direct approach to the glabella, and it does not distort the hairline. It also allows myoplasty, but it does not offer improvement to the lateral brow region or upper forehead. Its major disadvantage is a potentially unsatisfactory scar and an inability to have a satisfactory lateral brow elevation; this is minimized by making the scar irregular rather than symmetrical, as it follows the crease line.

Direct Brow Lift

The standard direct brow lift consists of selective excision of skin directly above the eyebrows, combined with suspension of the orbicularis oculi muscle to the periosteum (Fig. 179.15) (17,18). This procedure is indicated primarily for men with bushy eyebrows and occasional women patients who are not candidates for a coronal or a trichophytic forehead lift (Fig. 179.16). Because of the direct approach, it may be more useful than a coronal lift to correct brow asymmetries and also can be more effective to correct marked ptosis of the lateral eyebrow. It can be used unilaterally to improve facial-nerve paresis functionally. It is relatively contraindicated in patients who have thin, light-colored eyebrows and patients who have thick sebaceous skin that may not scar well.

Technique

The inferior incision for the direct brow lift is placed just within the most superior growth of fine eyebrow hairs. It should not extend medial to the medial aspect of the eyebrow, as poor glabellar scarring will result. The incision should be carried lateral to the lateral eyebrow and extended horizontally in a gentle arc but not superiorly. The superior incision is carried in a gentle arch superiorly from its medial aspect to reach a high point between the lateral limbus and lateral canthus and then gently curved inferiorly to complete the excision. The superior incision defines the new position of the eyebrow, and the point of maximal height will determine the degree of masculinity (apex more medial toward the lateral limbus) or femininity (apex more lateral toward the lateral canthus) of the ultimate brow appearance. The skin is excised down to the subcutaneous plane, taking care not to injure the frontalis muscle or the supratrochlear and supraorbital nerves medially. Usually, a maximum of 10 to 12 mm of skin is excised. Minimal undermining is done inferiorly, taking care not to injure the hair follicles, with 1 to 1.5 cm of undermining in the subcutaneous plane superiorly. Four or five permanent 4-0 Mersilene sutures are placed through the orbicularis muscle at the level of the supraorbital margin;

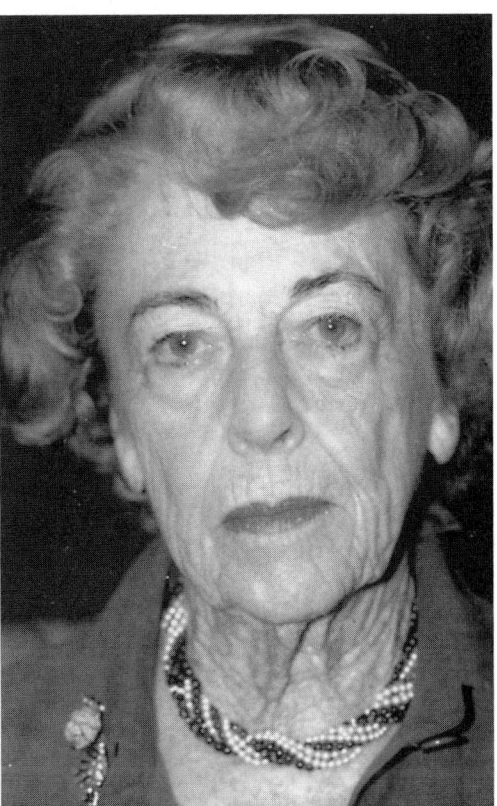

A

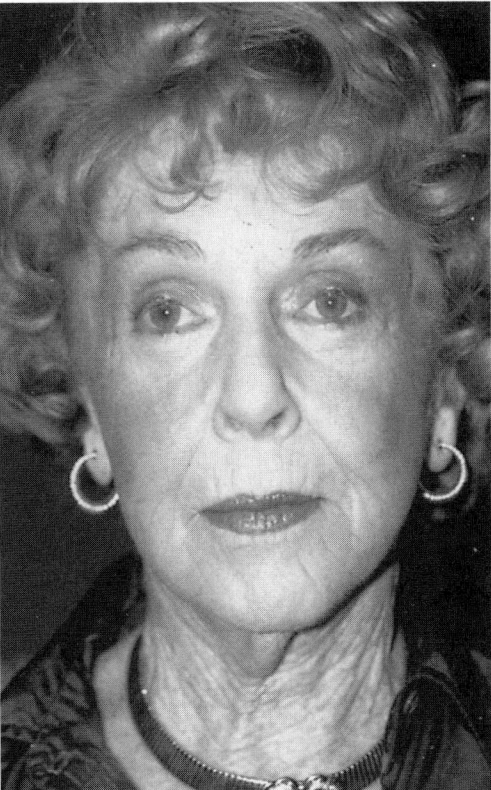

B

Figure 179.14 A: Elderly woman with moderately marked eyebrow ptosis and forehead rhytids and high anterior hairline. **B:** After midforehead lift, four-lid blepharoplasty, and cervicofacial rhytidectomy. (Photograph courtesy of C. M. Johnson, Jr., MD.)

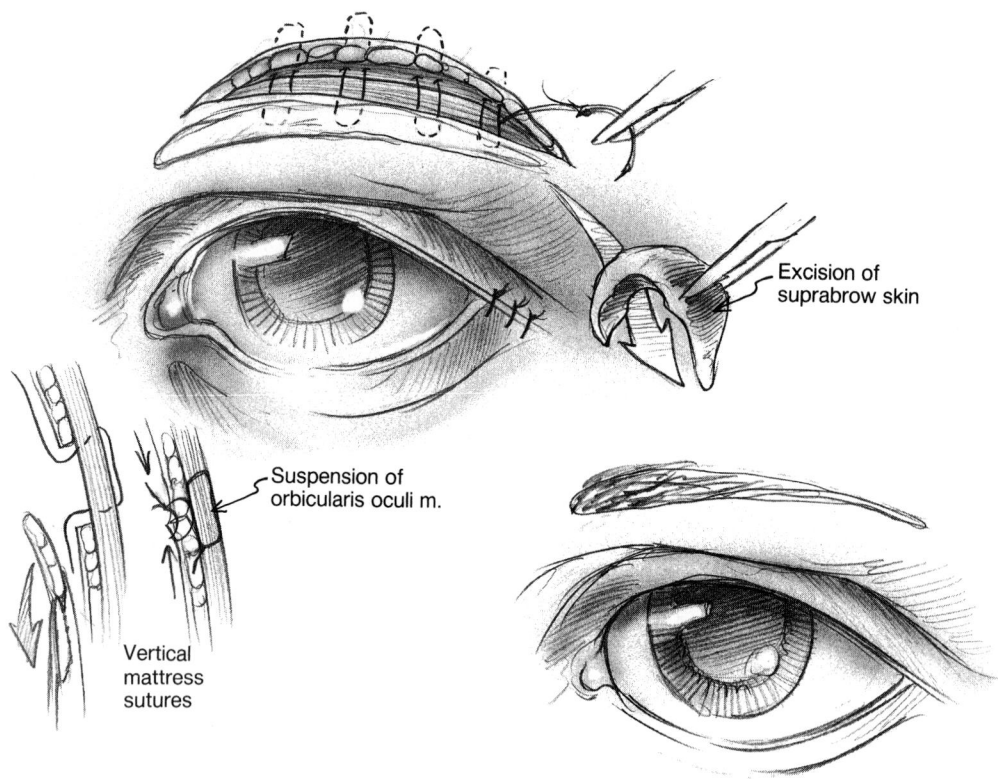

Figure 179.15 Excision of suprabrow skin and suspension of the orbicularis oculi muscle produces direct elevation of the eyebrow.

then this suspension suture is secured to the periosteum at the level of the superior incision. This latter suture is placed in a horizontal fashion to decrease the risk of injury to branches of the facial nerve. The apical suture is placed first, followed by those medially and laterally. Vertical mattress 5-0 nylon sutures are used for closure and to obtain maximal skin eversion. The sutures are removed on day 4, and light laser abrasion is done if indicated 6 to 12 weeks postoperatively.

Advantages of direct brow lifting include a long-lasting lift as a result of the excellent orbicularis muscle suspension that can be achieved. It is the best technique to correct brow asymmetries or unilateral brow ptosis secondary to facial-nerve paresis. More precise positioning of the eyebrow can be obtained than with the more distant coronal lifting, and less dissection is required than for coronal lifting. A significant disadvantage is the eyebrow scar, especially in patients who have sebaceous skin or those with thin brows or in whom meticulous technique is not applied. If the incision is not beveled parallel to the hair follicles, the superior aspect of the eyebrow may be lost in time, giving the appearance that the scar has migrated superiorly. Direct brow lifting has no effect on forehead, glabellar, or temple ptosis and cannot be used to improve forehead or glabellar rhytids. Prominent forehead rhytids may be distorted, giving an unnatural appearance.

Indirect Brow Lift

The indirect brow lift has been associated with the midforehead lift by some authors, and others have called it the midforehead brow lift (10,16). It is essentially the same procedure as the direct brow lift, but the skin excision is performed bilaterally at some distance above the eyebrow in the forehead. The indirect brow lift is indicated in patients with marked or asymmetrical brow ptosis and forehead furrows and those in whom a coronal forehead lift is contraindicated. The patient's skin type must be satisfactory, and the patient must be advised fully about the resultant scar. Men who have male-pattern baldness or women who have thin and light hair with a high hairline are potential candidates.

The surgical approach is similar to that for the direct brow lift, except the inferior incision is placed in a deep rhytid at a distance above the brow, and the superior incision is arched above this. This differs from the midforehead lift, in which the redundant skin is excised from below the initial crease incision rather than above. Undermining the inferior forehead flap must be maintained in the subcutaneous plane down to the supraorbital rims so as not to interfere with sensory or motor innervation. In most cases, the orbicularis muscle is suspended, as described for the direct brow lift.

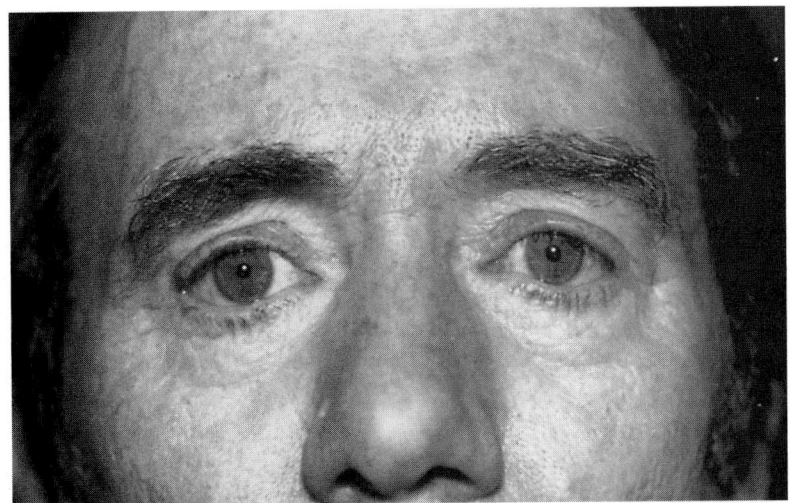

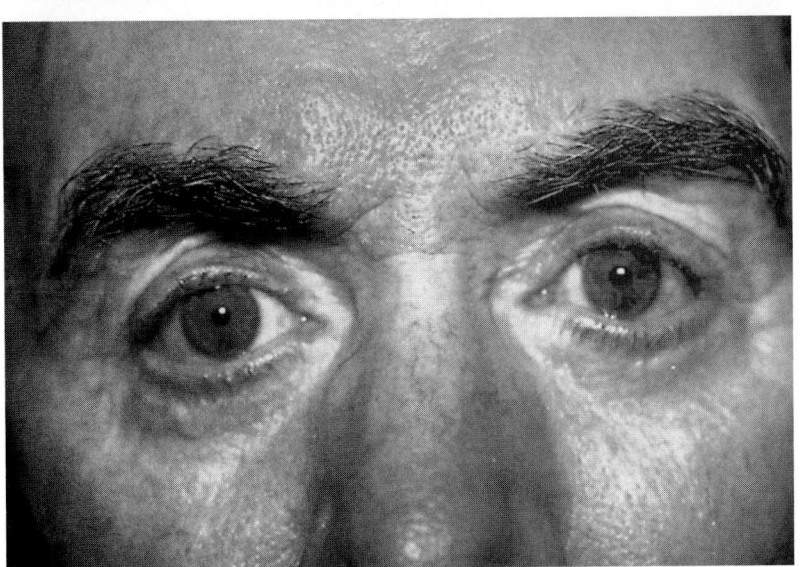

Figure 179.16   A: 53-year-old man with marked eyebrow ptosis, bushy eyebrows, and male-pattern baldness. **B:** Three years after direct eyebrow lift and four-lid blepharoplasty.

Advantages of the indirect lift include its ability to conceal the forehead incision within a skin crease and at the same time achieve a relatively proximal suspension for the eyebrow, thus leading to a long-lasting and precise elevation. Depending on the location and extent of the skin excision, the shape of the brow also can be configured as desired. Disadvantages include its relatively selective use: It may be indicated in patients who have significant rhytids and skin that will heal well and who are not candidates for a coronal forehead lift.

Browpexy

This procedure is unique in that it is performed through an infrabrow rather than a suprabrow incision (11). It therefore can be used in association with upper blepharoplasty and may negate the need for suprabrow procedures. This procedure may be indicated in the younger woman who is primarily concerned about fullness or puffiness in the lateral portion of the upper eyelids. Other indications are women with mild to moderate eyebrow ptosis and a flatter, androgynous eyebrow appearance. Lateral prominence in the infrabrow region due to a prominent supraorbital margin or brow fat pad also may be improved with this technique. It is particularly useful in association with upper blepharoplasty. Relative contraindications include patients who have severe brow ptosis or more generalized signs of aging of the upper face.

The browplasty is performed first through an upper blepharoplasty incision. Preoperatively, the supraorbital vessels and nerves, which are identified by palpation at their exit from the supraorbital notch, and the location of the lateral brow fullness, should be marked. Dissection is extended superiorly 1 to 1.5 cm above the superior and lateral orbital rim in the submuscular plane just deep to the orbicularis oculi muscle. The redundant brow fat pad can be seen overlying the orbital margin; it is removed from the region of the central third of the superior orbital margin laterally as far as the frontozygomatic suture. The fat pad is excised in an elliptical fashion measuring about 1 to 1.5 cm in vertical dimension and tapering nasally and temporally. The underlying periosteum is left intact to prevent adhesions. If brow elevation is not required, the blepharoplasty is completed in standard fashion.

In patients requiring elevation of the central and lateral eyebrow, browpexy is performed to elevate and suspend the brow above the supraorbital margin. The eyebrow position can be fixed superiorly by using two or three permanent 4-0 Mersilene sutures. Each suture is placed transcutaneously at the level of the infrabrow hairs into the subbrow space and then passed through the periosteum 1 cm above the supraorbital rim. It then is secured through the subeyebrow tissue at the level of the original transcutaneous suture. With tightening of the suture, the eyebrow will be elevated an appropriate amount above the supraorbital margin after the original transcutaneous suture end is drawn through the skin. The placement and tension of each suture can be used to obtain the configuration of the eyebrow and degree of elevation desired. The blepharoplasty procedure then is completed, removing redundant fat and upper-eyelid skin.

Advantages of this technique include the single eyelid incision, which is also compatible with that made for upper blepharoplasty. It allows brow elevation with a more minimal procedure than a coronal forehead lift and allows direct access for trimming the lateral eyebrow fat pad; however, its use is restricted to patients who have only mild to moderate eyebrow ptosis, and the exposure is more difficult compared with direct eyebrow lifting. Removing the eyebrow fat pad transects the cutaneous nerves, resulting in brow anesthesia for several months over this region. Injury to the supraorbital vessels or nerves could result in heavy bleeding or forehead anesthesia. If the suspension suture is placed through the preseptal orbicularis muscle, postoperative dimpling of the thinner eyelid skin and lagophthalmos may occur secondary to eyelid tethering. Inadequate correction of brow ptosis also has been reported.

Endoscopic Forehead Lift

Endoscopic forehead-lifting techniques allow correction of brow ptosis and reduction of forehead and glabellar rhytids (19–24). The indications for this technique are identical to those for the conventional coronal approaches (Fig. 179.17). Direct endoscopic visualization affords the ability to identify and preserve the supraorbital and supratrochlear neu-

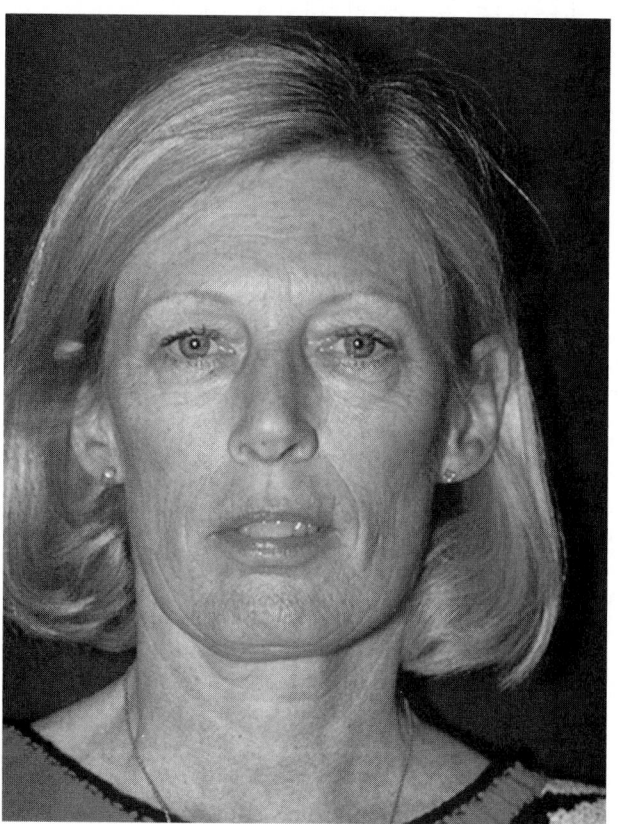 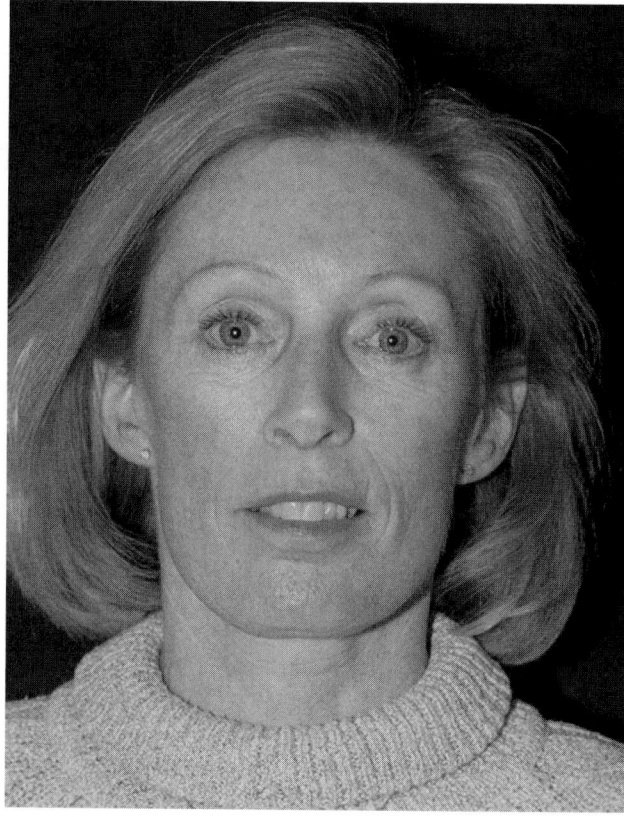

A **B**

Figure 179.17 **A:** A 59-year-old woman with moderate brow ptosis, moderately marked forehead and glabellar rhytids, and moderately high forehead. **B:** The patient 3 years after endoscopic forehead lift, four-lid blepharoplasty, and deep plane face and neck lift..

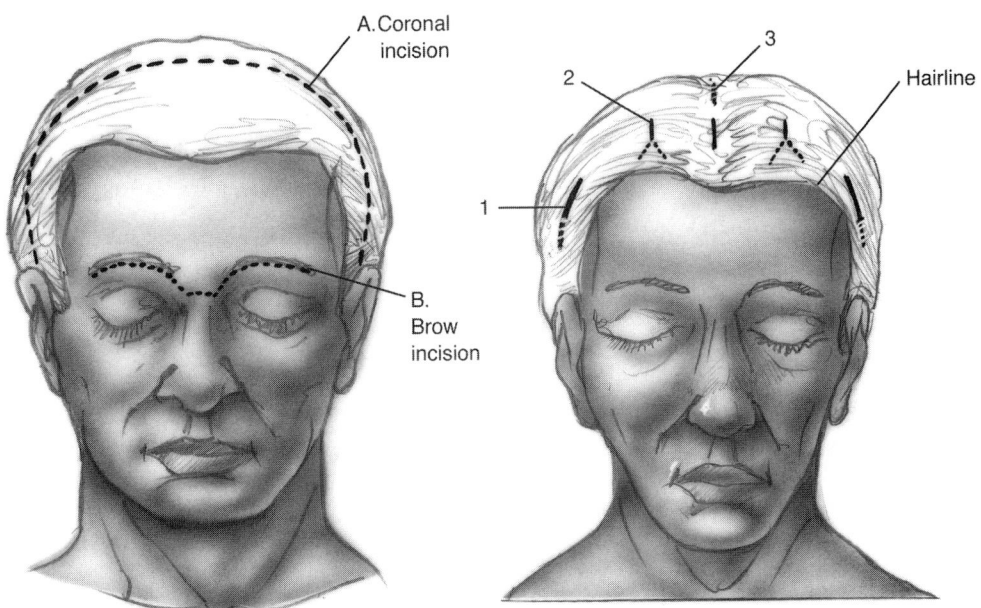

Figure 179.18 The standard endoscopic forehead lift incisions (*solid lines*) are placed 1 cm posterior to the hairline and may vary with surgeon preference. *1,* The temporal incisions may be extended to increase exposure (*dashed lines*). *2,* Y to V advancement flaps (*dashes*) will allow for skin excision. *3,* A central posterior vertex incision (*dashes*) provides exposure for miniplate placement.

rovascular bundles (25), although no more clearly than with the direct approach. Sensory neuropathy and scarring are decreased further because of incision size reduction, change in incision placement, and lack of skin excision (19,25). The most favorable result can be obtained in the thin-skinned white patient with glabellar rhytids, minimal brow ptosis, and minimal skin redundancy (20). Relative contraindications include women with high hairlines, male-pattern baldness, and Asians and American Indians who have tight, thick skin and extensive bony attachments (22).

Advantages of the endoscopic approach include smaller incisions, decreased incidence of sensory neuropathy and alopecia, less bleeding, and a faster recovery period (19–22,25). Disadvantages involve the need for specialized training and experience with endoscopic techniques, increased intraoperative time, the need for external fixation, and the need for confirmation of long-term lift results (20–22).

Preoperatively, the location of the supraorbital and supratrochlear neurovascular bundles is identified and marked. The amount of skin advancement to provide an adequate brow lift, usually 10 to 16 mm, is determined and marked with the patient sitting and supine (19). Glabellar and forehead furrows to be addressed also are marked.

This procedure may be performed with the patient under either general anesthesia or local anesthesia with intravenous sedation, depending on patient and surgeon preferences. Local infiltration with lidocaine 1% with epinephrine 1:100,000 and bupivicaine 0.5% with epinephrine

1:200,000 mixed in equal parts is used in a coronal distribution to provide vasoconstriction before the incision.

The standard endoscopic forehead lift is performed with three to six incisions, which are about 2 cm long (Fig. 179.18). A midline sagittal incision, bilateral paramedian incisions at the level of the midbrow, and bilateral coronal temporal incisions parallel to the hair follicles are placed 1 to 1.5 cm posterior to the hairline. The location of these incisions will vary with surgeon preference. Glabellar rhytid reduction without correction of brow ptosis may be performed without the use of the temporal incisions (24). Y- to V-advancement flaps can be designed at the incision line if skin excision is desired. The forehead elevation is initiated by extending the vertical incisions through the pericranium. The dissection proceeds in the subperiosteal plane, which, because of its decreased vascularity, permits superior visualization. Wide subperiosteal undermining of the scalp is performed in a blind fashion with a periosteal elevator, anteriorly to a level 2 cm above the supraorbital rims inferiorly and the temporal lines laterally, and posteriorly to the nuchal line. The supraorbital dissection is performed under direct endoscopic visualization. A 4-mm 30-degree scope is introduced into the central incision, and a small endoscopic elevator is used in the paramedian incisions (Fig. 179.19). The supraorbital and supratrochlear nerves are identified and preserved by using blunt dissection with the endoscopic scissors. The dissection is extended inferiorly over the orbital rims and onto the nasion.

The temporal incisions are extended through the temporoparietal fascia, preserving the superficial layer of the

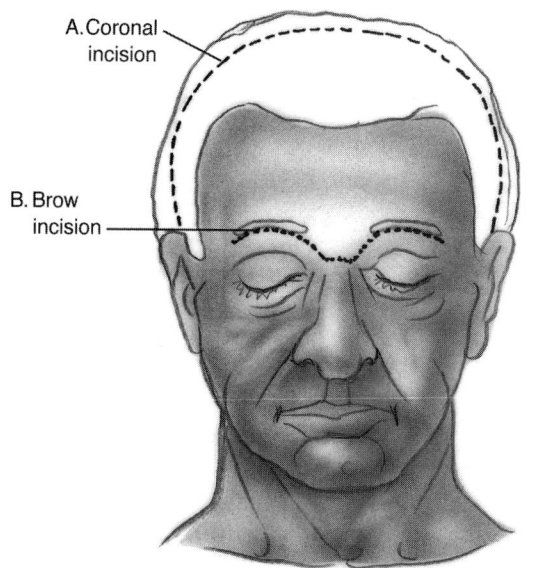

A. Coronal incision

B. Brow incision

Figure 179.19 The supraorbital dissection is performed with the 4-mm 30-degree scope in the central incision and a small endoscopic elevator in the paramedian incisions.

deep temporal fascia. The endoscope and the endoscopic periosteal elevator are used to dissect the lateral orbital rim region inferiorly to the zygomatic arch. The fused fascial planes of the galea, temporoparietal fascia, deep temporal fascia, and periosteum, which insert on the temporal line, are released with sharp dissection. A zygomaticotemporal vein may be encountered 5 to 10 mm lateral to the zygomaticofrontal suture (19,20).

Transverse releasing incisions are made through the periosteum along the supraorbital margin to allow forehead flap advancement. The corrugator and procerus muscles are divided by using the endoscopic scissors. Frontalis muscle division, although not routinely performed, may be performed between the supraorbital neurovascular bundles. Hemostasis is obtained with cauterization.

Flap suspension and fixation are performed after advancement of the flap to predetermined levels. Several different flap-fixation techniques are described in the literature, which include the following: (a) skin staples and taping, (b) microscrew placement in the paramedian incisions of the anterior flap and fixation with skin staples posterior to the microscrew (25), (c) suspension sutures with cortical microscrew fixation (16), (d) nylon suspension sutures with fixation to a posterior vertex titanium miniplate, (e) sutures secured through cortical bone tunnels, (f) absorbable screws and cortical anchors (Endotine Coapt Systems, Palo Alto, CA), and (g) fibrin glue. A surgeon's experience or preference may determine to some degree the method of fixation used. Recent studies, though, will help confirm or deny the scientific merit of some of these techniques. More specifically, fixation methods that

rely on temporary means of fixations such as fibrin glue or removable transcutaneous screws are likely to be ineffective according to recent studies examining the time frame for periosteal adhesion. Perhaps the best study on the subject by Scalfani et al. (26,27) demonstrated that approximately a minimum of 6 weeks is required for adhesion between the cranium and overlying periosteum. Thus, short-term fixation is unlikely to be adequate to maintain brow elevation. Suture fixation to a microscrew in the anterior flap incision is frequently used. Lateral forehead and brow suspension is obtained with superolateral flap advancement followed by fixation with 2.0 polydioxanone (PDS) sutures from the temporoparietal fascia to the superficial layer of the deep temporal fascia. A subperiosteal drain may be placed. The scalp incisions are closed with surgical staples. A pressure dressing is applied. The screws are removed on postoperative day 10 in the office.

The incidence of postoperative scarring, alopecia, and sensory neuropathy may be decreased in comparison with those after the standard coronal lift. All other complications are similar to standard forehead-lifting techniques. The amount of forehead lifting that can be achieved and maintained has yet to be consistently confirmed. Although endoscopic forehead-lifting techniques offer distinct advantages, longer-term studies are needed to assess whether the results are comparable to those of the coronal procedures.

COMPLICATIONS

Upper facial rejuvenation procedures may be performed with the patient under neuroleptic anesthesia if performed alone or under general anesthesia with more extensive facial rejuvenation procedures. The potential complications associated with any general anesthesia or surgery are present.

Diagnosis of the deformities present in the upper face poses a greater challenge for the surgeon than does that for the lower face. As such, the surgeon must specifically identify both the patient's concerns and the signs of aging that may be corrected by surgery. Such accurate diagnosis will lead to the choice of the most appropriate procedure. Patients must understand exactly what can and cannot be achieved with any given procedure, and their expectations must be realistic. Otherwise, they may be dissatisfied with a satisfactory surgical result. Specific potential complications are discussed in the following sections (28,29).

Bleeding

Significant bleeding is rare but may be encountered from the superficial temporal artery in the coronal, pretrichial, or trichytic lifts or from the supratrochlear or supraorbital arteries in any of these procedures. In the lateral canthal region, bleeding may occur from the zygomaticotemporal artery. Absolute hemostasis with bipolar cautery is recommended. Heavy bleeding can occur from the scalp itself in the coronal forehead lift. We do not use Raney clips but believe that the vasoconstriction achieved with epinephrine in the local infiltration anesthetic is most important. Scalp vessels in the galeal plane should be cauterized, taking care to avoid hair follicles.

Sensory Nerve Injury

Temporary hypesthesia or occasionally hyperesthesia may occur because of irritation of the supratrochlear and supraorbital nerves during flap elevation over the supraorbital margin. Permanent hypesthesia or anesthesia centrally just posterior to the coronal lift incision, up to 2 cm in diameter, is not uncommon. This is usually of no concern to patients, although they should be advised of this preoperatively. The pretrichial or trichophytic lift will cause a larger area of hypesthesia posterior to the incision line. The browplasty procedure results in temporary hypesthesia over the lateral eyebrow margin for several months.

Motor Nerve Injury

The frontal branch of the facial nerve is at risk primarily in the zygomatic region, probably as much from the infiltration anesthesia as from surgical dissection. To decrease the risk of injury to this nerve laterally, the central forehead incision of the frontalis muscle should be kept between the pupils. If sharp hooks are used, they must be placed and removed judiciously, especially in the temporal region.

Lagophthalmos

It is most unlikely that lagophthalmos will occur when any of the forehead-lifting procedures is used alone. In the case of either a previous or concurrent upper blepharoplasty, however, it is important to be conservative in excising forehead skin or suspending the eyebrows to prevent inadequate upper eyelid closure, corneal exposure, and possible corneal scarring with visual loss. Inaccurate placement of the suspension sutures through the orbicularis oculi muscle in the browpexy procedure may cause temporary lagophthalmos. In most cases, the gradual resolution of the overcorrected forehead or eyebrows associated with lifting procedures results in resolution of initial mild lagophthalmos. Patient compliance in using ophthalmic drops and ointment must be obtained in these early phases.

Scar Widening

Scar widening most often occurs in the temporal region, probably as a result of the oblique nature of the hair follicles and inaccurate beveling of the initial or excisional

incisions in the coronal forehead lift. Excess tension or excess electrocauterization also may contribute to loss of scalp follicles.

Alopecia

Patients may presume that they are experiencing hair loss if all hair trimmed during surgery is not combed out. True thinning resulting from follicle shock is unusual and often is preceded by a history of alopecia. If a secondary coronal lift is performed with the second incision posterior to the first, hair loss may occur between the two incisions.

Infection

Infection is rare. Its incidence is increased after hematoma development in diabetic patients and in those who have protracted surgery. Patients are covered with a single dose of a broad-spectrum antibiotic (cefazolin) 1 hour before surgery. Irrigation of the wound with antibiotic solution can be done if indicated. Treatment consists of incision and drainage and intravenous or oral antibiotics where indicated. If permanent sutures are used for the galeal closure, splitting occasionally may occur.

EMERGENCIES

Hematoma

A rapidly expanding hematoma under a forehead flap could compromise vascularity of the flap or at least predispose to significant hair loss. Bleeding to cause this problem most commonly occurs from branches of the superficial temporal artery at the superior helical root but also could occur from the supraorbital or supratrochlear arteries. Immediate elevation of the flap with exploration and cauterization of bleeding sites should be done and a suction drain placed. Intravenous and then oral antibiotics are given to decrease the risk of subsequent infection. A smaller, localized hematoma, as in the glabella or associated with a direct brow lift, may be managed satisfactorily by using incision and drainage, followed by a compression dressing. This is repeated daily until no further recurrence of the hematoma is seen.

Corneal Ulceration

Corneal ulceration is most likely to occur in association with a coronal or direct brow lift performed at the same time as an upper blepharoplasty or if the latter was performed previously. Early recognition of exposure due to lagophthalmos is mandatory. Management includes ophthalmic drops and ointment and an eye shield or a tarsorrhaphy if necessary. Early ophthalmologic consultation is indicated.

Nerve Injury

Partial and temporary sensory nerve injuries are not rare when any manipulation is carried out in the region of the supraorbital and supratrochlear nerves. Expectant observation is the rule. Frontal nerve injury resulting in partial or complete paralysis of the nerve also requires only hopeful observation; however, firm patient reassurance and frequent follow-up are required in view of the cosmetic nature of these procedures. Should function not return within 3 weeks, nerve studies are performed to confirm the integrity of the nerve and to reassure the patient and surgeon. Long-term management of any residual deformity would include direct brow lifting on the affected side to improve asymmetry in repose.

Adjuvant treatments also are an important aspect of rejuvenating the upper one third of the face. Botox has clearly changed how this region is addressed, as it provides excellent effacement of dynamic rhytids and, thus, reduces the need to be as aggressive about performing surgical myoplasty. Filler materials based on hyaluronic acid provide a longer-lasting option to patients than did collagen, and future materials will likely continue to extend the duration of the efficacy of fillers. Finally, resurfacing techniques, whether they be chemical, laser, or light based (i.e., intense pulsed light), provide a solution to the finer rhytids of the skin. Skin resurfacing serves to be synergistic with the effects of surgical treatments to the forehead. As resurfacing modalities continue to improve, so will the final results we will be able to deliver to our patients.

DISCUSSION

The past few years have seen a tremendous increase in interest in rejuvenation of the upper face. The coronal forehead lift and direct brow lift have undergone numerous modifications to achieve more natural and superior results. This increase in surgical options mandates more accurate attention to deformity diagnosis and procedure selection. Some techniques are specific to a given indication, such as the use of the direct browlift in a patient with unilateral forehead/eyebrow paralysis. Nonetheless, although clearly many approaches and techniques are used, the most frequently used types of forehead lift by the senior author are the tricophytic and endoscopic lifts. The discussion at national meetings and literature for a period in the 1990s suggested the decline and likely end to the use of open procedures with replacement by the endoscopic approach. LaFarriere and Perkins (30,31) summarized their experience with the endoscopic brow lift as compared with open forehead lifts by concluding that no difference in the results is apparent. However, more recent analysis of long-term results suggests that the answer is not so clear. Both a national survey and a study by Baker (32,33) reviewing the results of 21 New York surgeons demonstrated complication rates that were closer to those of the open procedures than previously reported. These studies also revealed that the aesthetic outcomes of the endoscopic lift also were not thought to be as favorable as previously described. A trend toward the increasing use of open approaches and a decline of the endoscopic approach are apparent (32,33). This is not meant to suggest a condemnation of the endoscopic forehead lift, as both approaches have valuable roles in the treatment of the aging forehead. However, it is an acknowledgement that each patient must be assessed as an individual, taking into account the hairline, skin type, degree of rhytids, brow position, and the individual's aesthetic goals before a surgical treatment can be recommended.

HIGHLIGHTS

- The eyebrow is the key landmark in forehead aesthetics. Its passive and dynamic characteristics, gender differences, and changes with aging are important factors in selecting the appropriate rejuvenation procedure.
- The major lifting procedures for upper facial rejuventation are the coronal forehead lift, endoscopic forehead lift, and the direct eyebrow lift. Modifications of each have specific indications.
- Accurate diagnosis of each patient's specific complaints and findings is needed so that the correct procedure can be chosen.
- The resultant scars should be explained in detail so that the patient can help choose the ideal procedure.
- The complete ophthalmologic examination is required for patients who had previous upper blepharoplasty or in whom an upper blepharoplasty is to be performed concomitant with forehead or brow lifting. Specific attention to dry-eye problems and conservative surgery are indicated.
- All incisions must be made to maintain hair follicle integrity, avoiding the first branch of the trigeminal nerve and the frontal branch of the facial nerve.
- For long-lasting results, elevation of the forehead flap over the supraorbital margin and galeal suspension are required. In direct brow-lifting procedures and their modifications, the orbicularis oculi muscle must be suspended to the periosteum.
- To maintain a smooth forehead contour, incise rather than excise the procerus and frontalis muscles.
- When redraping, overcorrect to allow the inevitable stretch-back.
- Forehead procedures may be indicated in patients who are not usually considered candidates, including young women who have premature ptosis of the eyebrows and men who do not have male-pattern baldness or are candidates for hair transplants.

REFERENCES

1. Brennan HG. The frontal lift. *Arch Otolaryngol* 1978;104(1): 26–30.
2. Brennan HG. The forehead lift. *Otolaryngol Clin North Am* 1980; 13(2):209–223.
3. Paul MD. The evolution of the brow lift in aesthetic plastic surgery. *Plast Reconstr Surg* 2001;108:5 1409–1424
4. Vinas JC. Plan de la ritidoplastia y zona tabu. In: *Transactions of the 4th Brasilian Congress on Plastic Surgery. Porte Alegre, Brazil, Oct. 5–8,* 1965:32.
5. Pitanguy I. Indications for treatment of frontal and glabellar wrinkles in an analysis of 3404 consecutive cases of rhytidectomy. *Plast Reconstr Surg* 1981;67(2):157–168.
6. Adamson PA, Cormier R, McGraw BL. The coronal forehead lift: modifications and results. *J Otolaryngol* 1992;21(1):25–29.
7. Isse NG. Endoscopic forehead lift. Presented at the Annual Meeting of the Los Angeles County Society of Plastic Surgeons. Los Angeles, September 12, 1992.
8. Ousterhout DK. Feminization of the forehead: contour changing to improve female aesthetics. *Plast Reconstr Surg* 1987;79(5): 701–713.
9. Sabini P, Wayne I, Quatela VC. Anatomical guides to precisely localize the frontal branch of the facial nerve. *Arch Facial Plast Surg* 2003;5(2):150–152.
10. Cook TA, Brownrigg PJ, Wang TD, et al. The versatile mid-forehead brow lift. *Arch Otolaryngol Head Neck Surg* 1989;115(2): 163–168.
11. McCord CD, Doxanas MT. Browplasty and browpexy: an adjunct to blepharoplasty. *Plast Reconstr Surg* 1990;86(2):248–254.
12. Adamson PA. The forehead lift: refinements in surgical technique. *J Otolaryngol* 1986;15(2):89–93.
13. Fleming RW, Mayer TG. Scalp flaps: reconstruction of the unfavorable result in hair replacement surgery. *Head Neck Surg* 1985; 7(4):315–331.
14. Kerth JD, Toriumi DM. Management of the aging forehead. *Arch Otolaryngol Head Neck Surg* 1990;116(10):1137–1147.
15. Brennan HG, Rafaty FM. Mid-forehead incisions in treatment of the aging face. *Arch Otolaryngol Head Neck Surg* 1982;108(11): 732–734.
16. Johnson CM Jr, Waldman SR. Mid-forehead lift. *Arch Otolaryngol Head Neck Surg* 1983;109(3):155–159.
17. Brennan HG. Correction of the ptotic brow. *Otolaryngol Clin North Am* 1980;13(2):265–273.
18. Jarchow RC. Direct browplasty. *South Med J* 1987;80(5):597–600.
19. Core GB, Vasconez L, Graham HD. Endoscopic browlift. *Clin Plast Surg* 1995;22:619–631.
20. Graham HD III, Core GB. Endoscopic forehead lifting using fixation sutures. *Tech Otolaryngol Head Neck Surg* 1995;8:245–252.
21. Isse NG. Endoscopic facial rejuvenation: endoforehead, the functional lift: case reports. *Aesthetic Plast Surg* 1994;18:21–29.
22. Ramirez OM. Endoscopic techniques in facial rejuvenation: an overview. Part I. *Aesthetic Plast Surg* 1994;18:141–147.
23. Vasconez LO, Core GB, Gamboa-Bobadilla M, et al. Endoscopic techniques in coronal brow lifting. *Plast Reconstr Surg* 1994;94: 788–793.
24. Hamas RS. Reducing the subconscious frown by endoscopic resection of the corrugator muscles. *Aesthetic Plast Surg* 1995;19: 21–25.
25. Miller PJ, Wang TD, Cook TA. Rejuvenation of the aging forehead and brow. *Facial Plast Surg* 1996;12:147–155.
26. Sclafani AP, Fozo MS, Romo T III, et al. Strength and histological characteristics of periosteal fixation to bone after elevation. *Arch Facial Plast Surg* 2003;5:63–66.
27. Romo T III, Sclafani AP, Yung RT, et al. Endoscopic forehead-plasty: a histologic comparison of periosteal refixation after endoscopic versus bicoronal lift. *Plast Reconstr Surg* 2000;105: 1111–1117.
28. Adamson PA, Johnson CM Jr, Anderson JR, et al. The forehead lift: a review. *Arch Otolaryngol Head Neck Surg* 1985;111(5): 325–329.
29. Beeson WH, McCollough EG. Complications of the forehead lift. *Ear Nose Throat J* 1985;64(12):575–583.
30. Puig CM, LaFerriere KA. A retrospective comparison of open and endoscopic brow-lifts. *Arch Facial Plast Surg* 2002;4(4): 221–225.
31. Dayan SH, Perkins SW, Vartanian AJ, et al. The forehead lift: endoscopic versus coronal approaches. *Aesthetic Plast Surg* 2001; 25(1):35–39.
32. Chiu ES, Baker DC. Endoscopic brow lift: a retrospective review of 628 consecutive cases over 5 years. *Plast Reconstr Surg* 2003; 112:628–633.
33. Elkwood A, Matarasso A, Rankin M, et al. National plastic surgery survey: brow lifting techniques and complications. *Plast Reconstr Surg* 2001;108(7): 2143–2150.

Congenital Auricular Malformation

180

Eugenio A. Aguilar III

The analysis of auricular malformations requires a comprehensive knowledge base to select the proper correction. Incomplete study has led to disastrous results, and the plastic surgeon should be well aware of the many surgical procedures that exist before undertaking one. This chapter covers ear deformities ranging from simple protruding ears to major congenital deformities. The single most important ingredient for a successful outcome is the surgical experience of the surgeon. Adequate reading and meticulous attention to detail will lead to the best possible outcome. In addition, the plastic surgeon should realize that the care of the patient with an ear deformity may necessitate a team approach that includes an otologist, psychiatrist, audiologist, and radiologist. The family deserves a coordinated approach and should know the total plan at the outset.

PROTRUDING EARS

Protruding ears are a fairly common defect that many plastic surgeons are called on to correct. An extensive array of choices is available, and every plastic surgeon should know at least one technique that can be used to achieve reliable results. It takes a combination of art and technical skill to deliver the best results consistently. Although the diagnosis of protruding ears is usually made simply based on sight, the surgeon needs certain information to make a decision regarding intervention. The normal angle between the ear and the head should be between 15 and 25 to 30 degrees (1). Usually, an angle greater than 30 degrees makes the decision to operate much easier. Other less noticeable defects require knowledge of the anatomy of the ear. Sometimes the angle of the ear is less than 30 degrees, but some

particular anatomic feature makes the ear offensive to the family or patient.

Anatomy and Embryology

Topographic landmarks in a normal ear are shown in Figure 180.1. Of particular importance are the helix, superior crus, inferior crus, scapha, and antihelix, as well as the cymba conchae and the cavum conchae, the two structures that make up the entire conchal bowl.

The development of the auricle is first seen in the 5-week-old embryo. The auricle begins as six mesenchymal proliferations at the dorsal ends of the first and second pharyngeal arches surrounding the first pharyngeal cleft. Initially, the external ear is located in the lower neck. As the mandible develops, the ear ascends to the side of the head at the level of the eyes. The most common thinking (Fig. 180.2) is that the six hillocks correlate directly with the tragus, helix, cymbum, scapha, antihelix, and antitragus (2).

Intrinsic and extrinsic musculature is associated with each ear. The intrinsic muscles are the major and minor helixes, the tragus, the antitragus, the transverse, and the oblique. The external muscles include the anterior auricularis, superior auricularis, and posterior auricularis.

The auricle receives its blood supply from three arteries: the superficial temporal, the posterior auricular, and the occipital. The venous system involves the posterior auricular, external jugular, superficial temporal, and retromandibular veins. The lymphatics of the ear drain anteriorly to the parotid lymph nodes and posteriorly to the cervical lymph nodes. The innervation of the auricle is via cranial nerve VII, with the temporal branch supplying the anterior and superior auricularis muscles, and the posterior auricular branch

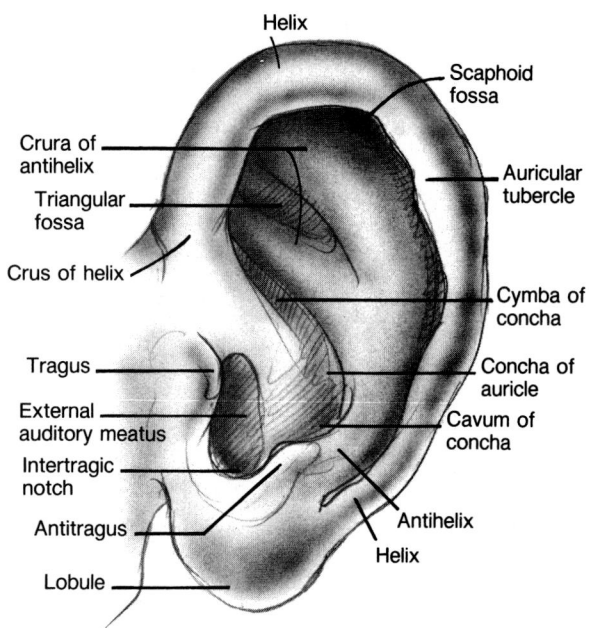

Figure 180.1 Anatomy of the auricle.

supplying the posterior auricularis muscles. The sensory innervation is primarily from the lesser occipital nerve, the mastoid branch of the lesser occipital nerve, the greater auricular nerve (C2, C3), and the auricular temporal nerve. The Arnold nerve, a branch of cranial nerve X, supplies the concha.

A normal auricle and its dimensions are shown in Figure 180.3. The vertical axis of the auricle is thought to be inclined about 20 degrees posteriorly. The vertical height is usually equal to the distance between the lateral orbital rim and the root of the helix at the level of the brow (~6 cm). The width should be about 55% of the length, and usually the helical rim protrudes 1 to 2 cm from the skull; the angle of protrusion should be between 21 and 30 degrees. The superior aspect of the ear is usually level with the brow (3).

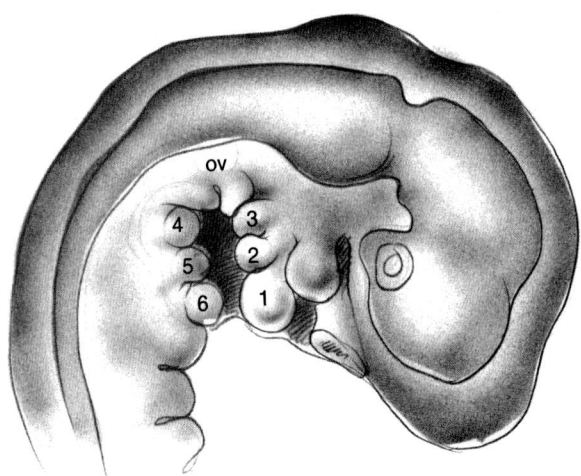

Figure 180.2 Auricle in 5-week human embryo develops from six hillocks.

Preoperative Evaluation

When the dimensions of the patient's auricle differ from these rules of thumb, an auricular deformity exists that may require surgical intervention. To achieve the most normal-looking ear possible through surgery, several significant auricular landmarks must be considered.

The ear will usually have a poor antihelical fold and overdeveloped concha. Often the scapha will be abnormally formed, with an obvious lack of a superior and an inferior crus surrounding the fossa triangularis. In addition, the helix may be abnormal in both definition and curvature.

The usual goal of the operation is to achieve some reduction of the auricle, bringing it to within the 15- to 25-degree range while maintaining normal appearance and curvature of the auricular components. The helical curve should remain gentle after surgery, with no unusual breaks or pinching effects. It also may be necessary to reduce an overlarge conchal bowl during the surgery. The helical rim should be evaluated after the surgery, and its height from the mastoid skin documented. The middle third of the helix should measure 14 to 16 mm, and the superior third, 16 to 18 mm.

The preoperative evaluation always should include several good photographs. In addition to the frontal view, adequate documentation should include oblique, lateral, and rear views. Both ears should be compared and evaluated with regard to at least three basic criteria: the thickness and stiffness of the cartilage and the symmetry of one ear compared with the other. Darwinian tubercles should be noted, as should any other preauricular tags that may exist.

The surgeon will want to develop a checklist such as that in Table 180.1. This will be extremely helpful during the preoperative evaluation and will ensure that no important details are missed. This information should be discussed fully with the patient and family to clarify any points of uncertainty. The more involved the patient is in helping to plan the surgical procedure, the more likely it is that the necessary postoperative care will be implemented properly. Otoplasty is best begun before the child starts school, between ages 5 and 6 years, when the child is old enough to withstand the necessary postoperative manipulations.

Emphasizing the importance of making ear reconstruction a family affair, Eavey (4) counsels parents about the condition as well as techniques to correct the ear. He also outlines research efforts that are being conducted in the arena of tissue engineering.

In a study of 92 pediatric patients, Eavey (4) observed that children with microtia and significant auricular malformation require global attention to early family guidance, expected and unexpected hearing loss, language development, associated medical conditions, and both auricular and otologic reconstruction issues.

In 1999, Wang (5) advocated the use of early prosthetic treatment as psychologically beneficial to children who have an ear defect resulting from congenital malformation and described procedures to confirm locations of

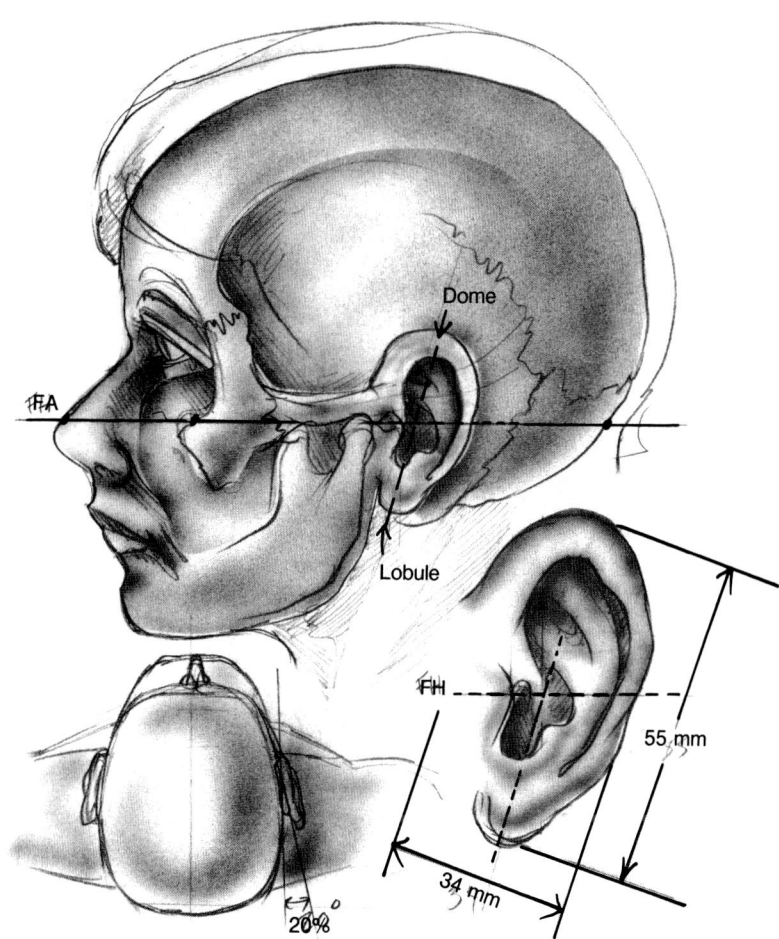

Figure 180.3 Normal ear, with average dimensions for a 6-year-old child.

craniofacial auricular implants by using computed tomographic (CT) scan information. The procedures also can be applied to children and adults to identify locations for auricular implant placement—a method that ensures precise locations for implant placement and a better prosthodontic prognosis for auricular defect patients.

Surgical Techniques

Mustarde Technique

The Mustarde technique (Fig. 180.4) involves placing several horizontal mattress sutures (usually Ethibon or Ticron) along the scapha in a curved line to create an antihelical sulcus. This technique has several advantages. A normal-appearing antihelical fold can be created, and when placed correctly, the sutures hold indefinitely. Even an inexperienced surgeon can expect excellent results. Most surgeons tend to forget that a Mustarde suture also can be used to create a more than adequate superior or inferior crus.

Problems can be expected if the sutures are incorrectly placed. They could become noticeable or could erode through the postauricular skin. If they fail to maintain the proper curve of the antihelical fold, a second operation

may be required. Simply using a Mustarde technique is not usually enough for most otoplasties, because work must be done in the conchal bowl area as well.

Converse Technique

The Converse technique (Fig. 180.5) is somewhat more complicated and can be executed only by an experienced surgeon (1). An island of cartilage is created that sets anterior to the rest of the conchal cartilage. This cartilage produces a normal-appearing fold, with no sharp edges on the corrected antihelix. The advantages of this technique are that it allows more permanent retraction of the auricle and is a potentially more permanent correction of the antihelix. In addition, because the island itself is not sutured, the curvature of the antihelix is gentle.

Farrior Technique

The Farrior technique (Fig. 180.6) also requires an experienced surgeon (6). The incisions are made through the cartilage on the conchal rim only; then longitudinal wedges are removed at the level of the superior crus and the future antihelical fold. An incision then is made through the cartilage at the level of the antihelical fold, creating an island similar to that of the Converse technique. The island

TABLE 180.1	DIAGNOSIS
OTOPLASTY	

Deformity criteria
Angle between ear and head, 25 to 30 degrees or greater
Dimensions different from normal auricle
Vertical axis—about 20 degrees posteriorly
Vertical height—about 6 cm
Width—about 55% of length
Helical rim—1- to 2-cm protrusion from skull
Angle protrusion—21 to 30 degrees
Superior aspect—usually level with brow
Other anatomy that makes ear offensive to family or patient
One or more significant auricular landmarks of deformity
Very poor antihelical fold
Overdeveloped concha
Abnormally formed scapha
Obvious lack of superior and inferior crus surrounding fossa
   triangularis

Comparative criteria
Thickness of scaphal cartilage
Stiffness of scaphal cartilage
Symmetry of two ears
Darwinian tubercles
Other preauricular tags

Documentary photographs
Frontal view
Oblique view
Rear view

widens from the inferior to the superior. This technique produces a more gentle bend of the antihelix.

Pitanguy Technique

The Pitanguy technique (Fig. 180.7) uses a smaller island flap and a conchal setback suture (1). It is appropriate for use with patients who have only a small amount of antihelical cartilage. Again, this technique requires an experienced surgeon.

Furnas Technique

The Furnas conchal mastoid suture technique (Fig. 180.8) is an important procedure for reducing a conchal bowl, part of any successful otoplasty procedure. When it is too large, an island can be taken out of the conchal bowl to narrow it and to allow the proximal portion to lie firmly against the mastoid. The Furnas technique should always be used in conjunction with a conchal-reducing technique. This technique helps to retract the auricle permanently. If the suture is placed too far anteriorly on the mastoid, it has been thought to cause some forward buckling of the conchal bowl at the os of the external canal, causing partial closure of the canal. To avoid narrowing the external auditory canal, it is important to remember to place the mastoid end of the conchal mastoid suture as far posterior as possible. These five otoplasty techniques are summarized in Table 180.2.

Complications and Emergencies

Four major complications can occur after otoplasty (Table 180.3). The most feared complication is chondritis. The most common complication is inadequate correction, and patients and their families should be alerted to this possibility. A secondary operation may be required within a year, even when the initial otoplasty has been performed by a well-trained surgeon. A hematoma is probably the easiest problem to detect and is often revealed during the first postoperative examination. Simple drainage should prevent any untoward results.

Another complication is the "telephone ear" deformity, which is caused by too much flexion of the antihelix at a level equal to the mid-portion of the ear and inadequate flexion at the superior and inferior poles. This problem can be prevented by repeatedly checking the tension on all sutures during surgery. Reverse telephone ear can occur

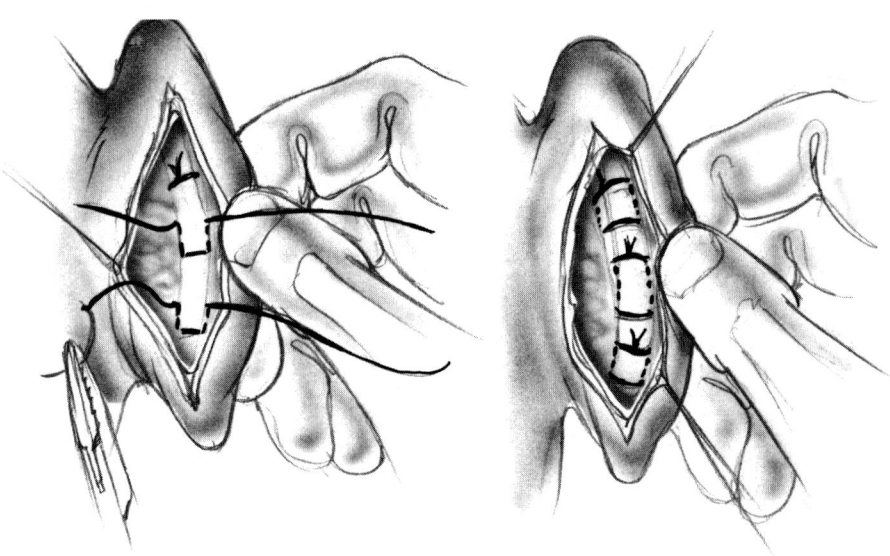

A   B

Figure 180.4 Technique of Mustarde. **A:** Marking antihelical fold with methylene blue. **B:** Placing horizontal mattress sutures.

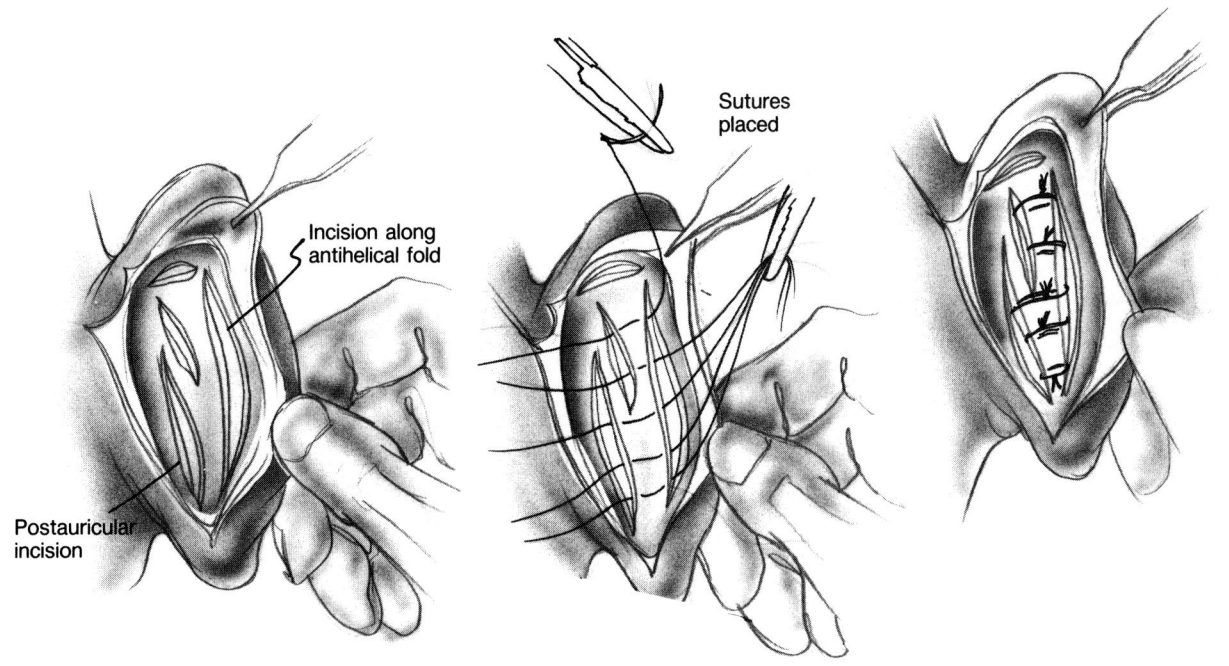

Sutures
placed
Incision along
antihelical fold
Postauricular
incision
A
B

Figure 180.5 Converse technique of otoplasty. **A:** Postauricular incision and incision along antihelical fold. **B:** Sutures along antihelix.

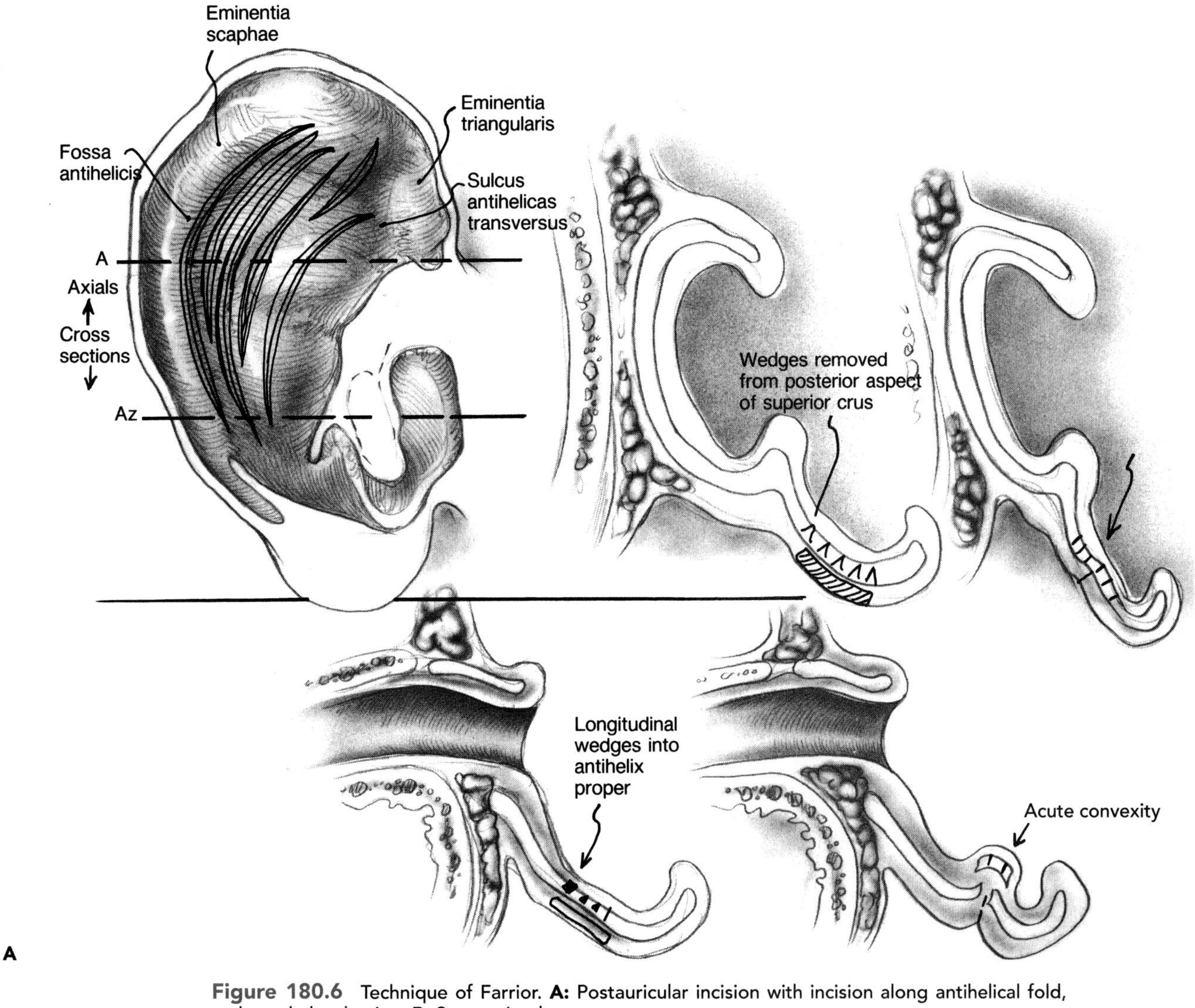

Eminentia
scaphae
Eminentia
triangularis
Fossa
antihelicis
Sulcus
antihelicas
transversus
A
Axials
Cross
sections
Az
Wedges removed
from posterior aspect
of superior crus
Longitudinal
wedges into
antihelix
proper
Acute convexity
A

Figure 180.6 Technique of Farrior. **A:** Postauricular incision with incision along antihelical fold, and conchal reduction. **B:** Sutures in place.

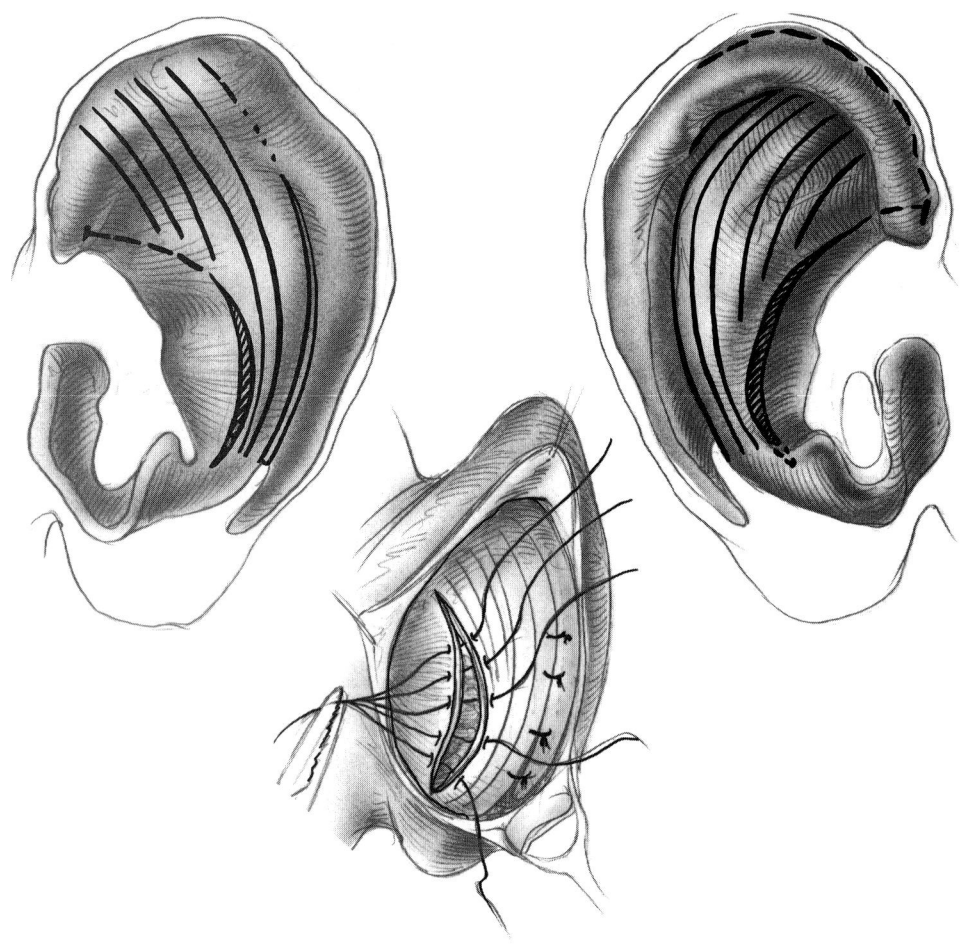

B

Figure 180.6 *(continued)*

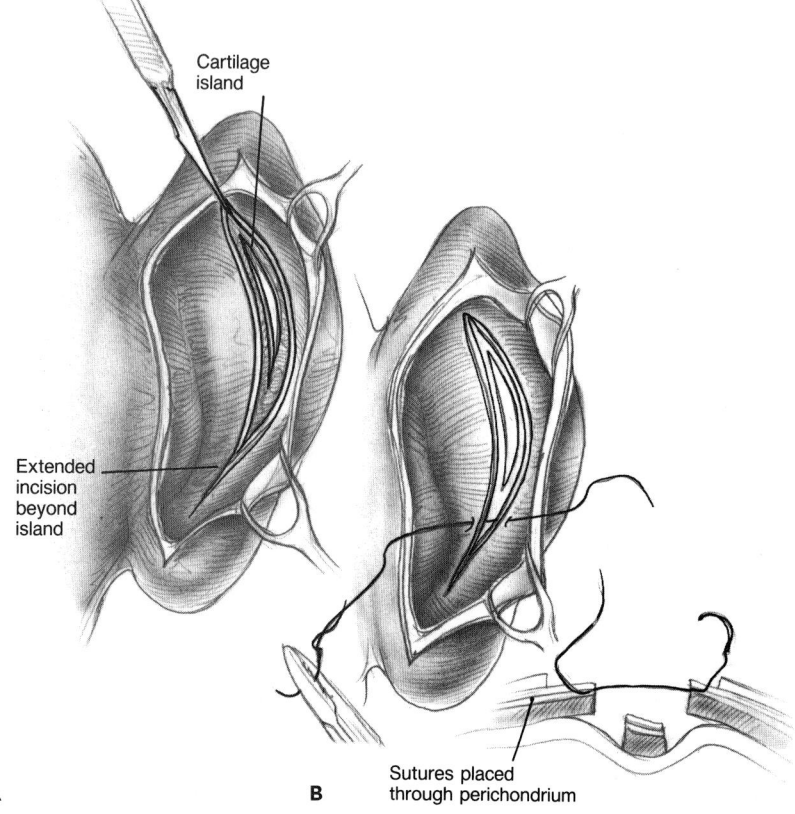

Cartilage
island

Extended
incision
beyond
island

Sutures placed
through perichondrium

A   **B**

Figure 180.7 Technique of Pitanguy. **A:** Post-auricular incision and creation of antihelical island flap. **B:** Conchal reduction sutures and sutures around island flap.

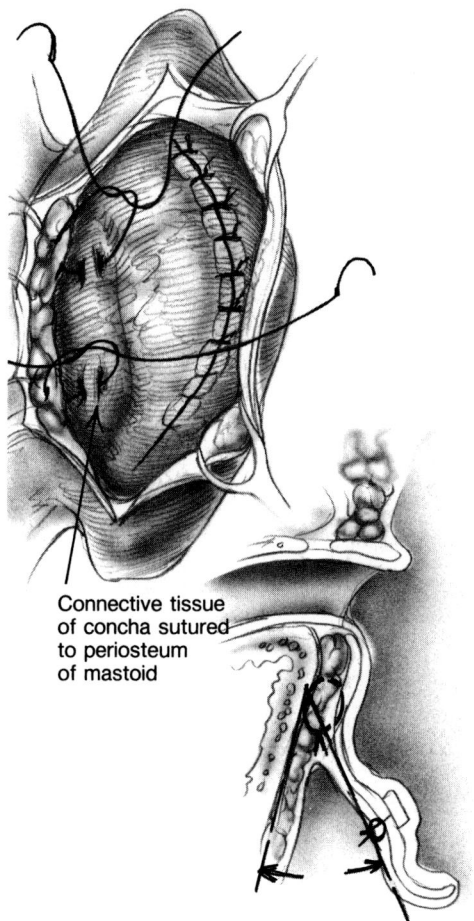

Figure 180.8   Conchal mastoid suture of Furnas.

Connective tissue of concha sutured to periosteum of mastoid

from overzealous tightening of the superior and inferior third of the ear. Significant infection of the cartilage after an otoplasty can cause permanent, devastating changes in the anatomy of the auricle. It can create defects for which no viable solution exists.

For clinical indicators for plastic repair of the external ear, see Table 180.4.

CONGENITAL MALFORMATIONS

The next greatest area of auricular conditions that necessitate surgical intervention are the congenital malformations, and external ear deformities exist in 1% of births today.

Correcting a major congenital malformation of the auricle tests the plastic surgeon's skill. The definition of microtia has been the subject of numerous publications, as clinicians have attempted to define the different grades that exist. This section focuses on the grades of microtia for which surgeons can initiate surgical reconstruction with a high degree of success.

Tanzer (7,8) in 1959 published the first article on auricular reconstruction by using autogenous rib cartilage. In 1966, Cronin (9) popularized the use of silicone rubber (Silastic) as an implant material to reconstruct auricles. Brent (10),

TABLE 180.2 ℞ TREATMENT OTOPLASTY

Mustarde technique
Advantages
   Very normal-appearing antihelical fold can be created, which su tures can hold indefinitely.
   Sutures also can be used to create good superior or inferior crus.
   Inexperienced surgeons can use this technique successfully.
Disadvantages
   Incorrectly placed sutures will cause problems.
   Technique is not applicable for work in conchal bowl area.

Converse technique
Advantages
   Island of cartilage with normal-appearing fold can be created.
   More permanent retraction of auricle is facilitated.
   Gently curved and potentially more permanent correction of antihelix is permitted.
Disadvantage
   Experienced surgeon must perform.

Farrior technique
Advantage
   Bend of antihelix is gentle.
Disadvantage
   Experienced surgeon must perform.

Pitanguy technique
Advantage
   Patient can have small amount of antihelical cartilage.
Disadvantage
   Experienced surgeon must perform.

Furna conchal mastoid suture technique
Advantage
   Permanent retraction of auricle is facilitated.
Disadvantage
   Partial closure of os of external canal occurs.

who first reported his work in 1974, today is considered the world's foremost authority on auricular reconstruction.

Classification

In 1988, Aguilar and Jahrsdoerfer (11) amended the 1926 grading system of Marx, and in 1996, Aguilar (12) reaffirmed this concise classification for congenital ear malformations.

TABLE 180.3 POTENTIAL COMPLICATIONS AND EMERGENCIES OTOPLASTY

Complications
Chondritis (most feared)
Inadequate correction (most common)
Hematoma (easiest to detect)
Emergencies
Acute infection
Hematoma

TABLE 180.4

CLINICAL INDICATORS FOR PLASTIC REPAIR: EXTERNAL EAR

Strategy
Indicators (one of the following):
    Congenital or traumatic amputation, defect, or deformity
    Reconstruction following resection of benign or malignant
      tumor
Laboratory tests (as indicated)
Other tests (as indicated)
Type of anesthesia (as indicated)
Location of service (as indicated)
Process
Criteria for discharge
Recovery from anesthesia
No bleeding
Outcome
Results
Adequacy of resection margin
Treatment plan for malignant disease if found
Follow-up
Wound healing
Cosmetic result
Evidence of recurrence
Counseling of patient regarding disease process

The American Academy of Otolaryngology–Head and Neck Surgery and the American Society for Head and Neck Surgery have published clinical indicators for surgical procedures. These clinical indicators are educational statements that have been drafted to assist surgeons in their practice and to promote discussion. These indicators are not practice guidelines nor do they represent standards of practice with which individuals must conform.

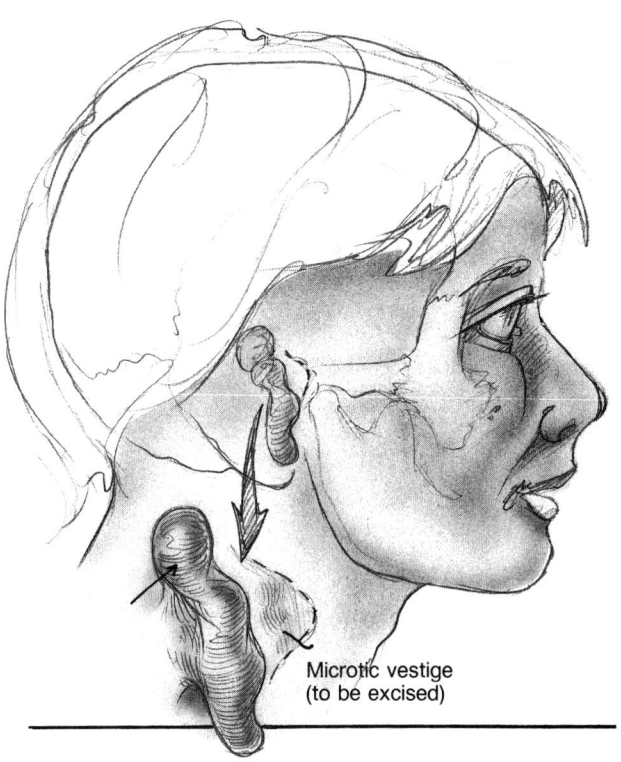

Figure 180.9   Grade III microtia.

Grade I is a normal ear. Grade II has some of the auricular framework present, but obvious deformities are present. Grade III is the standard "peanut ear" deformity, which encompasses anotia (Marx's grade IV) (Fig. 180.9).

The concomitant atresia complicates the classification schemes, yet many try to include them: Altmann in 1955 (the first schema based on the temporal bone itself, looking at the status of the canal, tympanic bone, drum, and ossicles), and Lapchenko in 1967 and Gill in 1969 both set up a four-tier scale, examining the degree of middle-ear and external canal development and the presence of ossicular abnormality. He noted that Gill also incorporated into this system the degree of pneumatization of the mastoid, because this seemed to predict the relative success of operative interventions. Ombredonne, Nager, and Colman each sought to establish simplified and clinically practical systems based on Altmann's original, but these were inconsistent at predicting outcome in those cases of major aplasia or group II anomalies.

Fernandez said that Jahrsdoerfer's 1992 system is a grading scale for selecting patients that would most likely benefit from attempts at repair of their atresia. He commended this scale for its "predictive power." Furthermore, Jahrsdoerfer's system is not subject to interobserver bias, and it allows a quantitative analysis of the temporal bone

and those structures deemed vital to the success of an operation. This scale, based on temporal bone CT findings, assesses nine different parameters that area used in making the determination of candidacy for surgery. Of note, Fernandez said, is that the stapes and oval window complex account for 3 of 10 points possible. Other parameters include the middle ear cleft, facial nerve position, status of the ossicles and round window, and pneumatization of the mastoid. Scores of 6 through 10 range from marginal to excellent candidates for surgery, whereas a score of 5 or less usually points to a poor outcome.

In 1977, Tanzer (13) proposed a clinical classification of auricular defects that has been well documented in virtually all articles that have since been published:

1. Anotia
2. Complete hypoplasia (microtia)
    A. With atresia of the external auditory canal
    B. Without atresia of the external auditory canal
3. Hypoplasia of the middle third of the auricle
4. Hypoplasia of the superior third of the auricle
    A. Constricted (cup and lop) ear
    B. Cryptotia
    C. Hypoplasia of entire superior third
5. Prominent ear

In 1974, Rogers (14) published a similar classification that divided defects into four groups:

1. Macrotia
2. Lop ear

TABLE 180.5

WEERDA'S COMBINED CLASSIFICATION OF AURICULAR DEFECTS, INCLUDING SURGICAL RECOMMENDATIONS

1. *First-degree dysplasia.* Average definition: most structures of a normal auricle are recognizable (minor deformities). Surgical definition: reconstruction normally does not require the use of additional skin or cartilage.
   A. Macrotia
   B. Protruding ears (synonyms: prominent ears, bat ears)
   C. Cryptotia [synonyms: pocket ear, group IV B (Tanzer)]
   D. Absence of upper helix
   E. Small deformities: absence of the tragus, satyr ear, darwinian tubercle, additional folds (Stahl ear)
   F. Colobomata (synonyms: clefts, transverse coloboma)
   G. Lobule deformities [pixed lobule, macrolobule, absence of lobule, lobule colobomata (bifid lobule)]
   H. Cup ear deformities
      i. Type I: cupped upper portion of the helix, hypertrophic concha, reduced height [synonyms: lidding helix, constricted helix, group IV A (Tanzer), lop ear, minor (mild or moderate) cupping]
      ii. Type II: more severe lopping of the upper pole of the ear; rib cartilage is used as support when a short ear must be expanded or the auricular cartilage is limp

2. *Second-degree dysplasia.* Average definition: some structures of a normal auricle are recognizable. Surgical definition: partial reconstruction requires the use of some additional skin and cartilage. Synonym: second-degree microtia (Marx).
   A. Cup ear deformity, type III: the severe cup ear deformity is malformed in all dimensions [synonyms: cockleshell ear, constricted helix, group IV (Tanzer), snail-shell ear]
   B. Mini-ear

3. *Third-degree dysplasia.* Average definition: none of the structures of a normal auricle are recognizable. Surgical definition: total reconstruction requires the use of skin and large amounts of cartilage. Synonyms: complete hypoplasia group II, peanut ear, third-degree microtia (Marx); normally concomitant congenital atresia is found
   A. Unilateral: one ear is normal; no middle ear reconstruction is performed on any child; auricle reconstruction is begun at age 5 or 6 years
   B. Bilateral: bone-conduction hearing aid before the first birthday; middle ear surgery at age 4 years without transposition of the vestige; bilateral reconstruction of the auricle at age 5 or 6 years
   C. Anotia

3. Cup ear
4. Prominent ear

Weerda (15), from Europe, in 1988 combined all of the classifications into a concise document. Definitions proposed by Marx and Tanzer and modified by Rogers (16) were presented. This system included surgical guidance for each classification (Table 180.5). These recommendations can be questioned, however, and alternatives exist. For bilateral microtia, a bone-conduction hearing aid can be placed at birth. In addition, even in bilateral cases, middle-ear surgery can follow the first two stages of auricular reconstruction rather than being the first procedure (17). Guidelines for diagnosis are listed in Table 180.6.

Surgical Reconstruction of Auricular Deformities

In cases of congenital microtia and concomitant atresia, complete coordination should exist between the otologist and the plastic surgeon. Aguilar in 1996 (12) presented the concept of the integrated auricular reconstruction protocol (IARP). As shown in Table 180.7, microtia repair is accomplished in five stages. The work of the plastic surgeon should be performed first, and the operation should be staged to facilitate total reconstruction of the microtia–atresia complex.

TABLE 180.6 DIAGNOSIS

CONGENITAL MALFORMATION OF THE AURICLE

Age of patient
Grade of deformity
Size of cartilage
Atresia present
Otologic evaluation
Photographs

TABLE 180.7 **Rx** **TREATMENT**
CONGENITAL MALFORMATION
OF THE AURICLE

Stage	Treatment
I	Auricular reconstruction (creation of a cartilaginous framework with autogenous rib cartilage)
II	Lobule transposition
III	Atresia repair (by otologist)
IV	Tragal construction
V	Auricular elevation

Despite advances made in technique and imaging in recent decades, it is still hard for experienced surgeons to agree on several key issues: the prime time for timing of surgery in general, when to operate on cases of unilateral atresia, and the operability of cases with severe craniofacial malformations. Most agree that the earliest age to proceed is 4 to 5 years, thus allowing time for adequate mastoid and middle-ear pneumatization and increasing patient compliance with postoperative care. Most clinicians think that surgery should be instigated earlier in cases of unilateral atresia with evidence of cholesteatoma, infection, or with very thin atresia plates. Opinions differ in regard to cases of grade II and III unilateral atresia in patients with normal hearing in the other ear. Jahrsdoerfer thinks that the benefit of binaural hearing exceeds the risk of facial nerve injury and other complications. De la Cruz also favors early operations on unilateral atresias if CT findings point to a favorable outcome.

Correction of microtia usually should begin at the age of about 6 years, especially for unilateral cases, and the best material is autogenous costal cartilage. By this age, sufficient cartilage is present to permit surgical reconstruction, and the patient is psychologically able to manage the necessary postoperative care. Bilateral microtia and atresia cases can be started at an earlier age, but only if sufficient cartilage exists to form a new ear. Historically, use of other sources for the framework has failed. Neither irradiated cartilage nor Silastic has stood the test of time: irradiated cartilage reabsorbs, and Silastic tends to extrude with time. Furthermore, Silastic implants are notorious for their inability to withstand trauma.

In 1997, Williams et al. (18) reported on the use of polyethylene (Medpor) implants in auricular reconstruction. These can be used to support skin grafts when used to reconstruct defects in auricular cartilage. Studied in an animal model, it was concluded that these implants are well tolerated as replacements for native cartilage in auricular reconstruction. Polyethylene implants tolerated wound exposure as early as 4 days after implantation and showed the ability to heal by secondary intention and to support skin grafts. Authors surmised that this is because of the extent of fibrovascular ingrowth from surrounding tissue, which allows the material to act more like native tissue and less like a foreign body in this setting.

At the University of Antwerp (Wilrijk) in the year 2000, Somers (19), at a Politzer Society Meeting, described major breakthroughs in reconstructive surgery of the auricle, opening new possibilities in the rehabilitation of patients with an absent auricle. Somers reported on clinicians who had adopted 33 bone-anchored prostheses and performed 22 total auricular reconstructions. These clinicians reported that the surgery for an episthesis, as long as the surgeon takes into consideration the conditions of osseointegration, is easy and has no major risks. Patients were satisfied with the prosthesis and wear it all day. For the total auricular repair, mainly in major congenital malformations, two techniques were used: the Brent technique followed by the Nagata technique. The Brent technique was found to be safe with good results, but the modification by Nagata had two more advantages: a reduction of the operative stages from four to two and a better definition of the relief of structures as the antihelix, crus anterior and posterior, and antitragus tragus. More experience saw the results of total auricular reconstructions improve considerably. The surgeons recommended centralization of this type of complex surgery.

Surgical Planning and Treatment

Preoperative planning should include photographs of the patient. Most important is the proper preparation of the template. In unilateral cases, the template is based on the patient's contralateral ear; in bilateral cases, the model is made from the mother's ear. The site of implantation of the cartilage framework on the side of the head should be properly measured to avoid malpositioning of the ear.

If radiologic examination has not already been done, it should be ordered before surgery. A high-resolution CT scan of the temporal bones should be obtained. Although a CT scan is unnecessary for the microtia, it does provide information to the surgical team. As a team, the plastic surgeon and the otologist can describe the entire course of the planned reconstruction to the family and the patient before any surgical procedures are undertaken.

The auricular reconstruction (Figs. 180.10 to 180.12) is undertaken during stage I. Note that the dissection of the cartilage is extraperichondrial, and no stripping of perichondrium is done at any point during rib harvesting. Stainless-steel 5-0 wire is used to anchor the eighth rib to the sixth and seventh rib complex. This technique is essentially the one popularized by Brent (20), and when performed by trained surgeons, it produces reliable results. The most common complication that can occur from this stage I procedure is atelectasis; other complications include

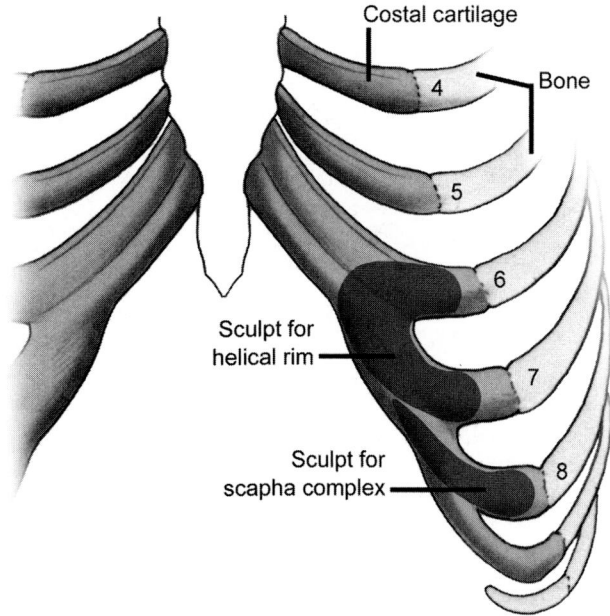

Figure 180.10   Harvesting costal cartilage of ribs 6, 7, and 8.

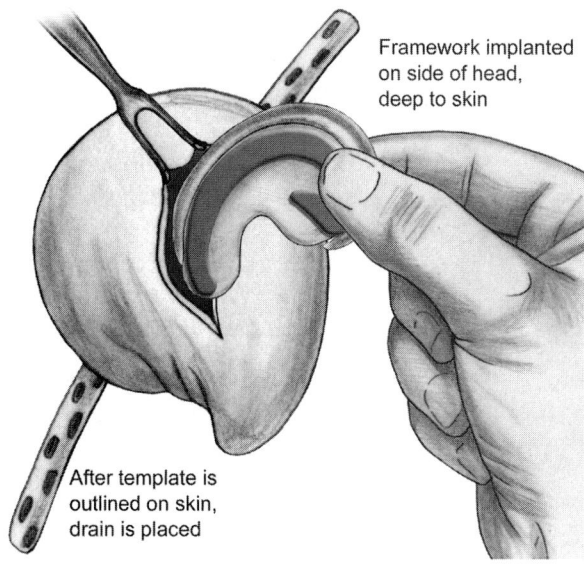

Figure 180.12   Implanting framework on side of head.

pleural tear (not a true complication unless not appreciated intraoperatively), pneumothorax, pneumomediastinum, chest wall aberration, hypertrophic scarring, and pneumonia.

Stage II involves lobule transposition and is shown in Figures 180.13 and 180.14 (Fig. 180.14 depicts the peanut ear). To avoid protrusion of the lobule, the incision on the back of the ear should be fairly high. The inferiorly based pedicle flap is quite thin; thus great care should be taken in its handling.

Stage III, atresia repair by the otologist, should be undertaken after the first two stages of repair by the plastic surgeon. The temporal bone remnant is in only one location; thus, the opening to that remnant can be made in only one location on the overlying skin. Therefore, it is quite easy to manipulate the framework and line it up where the otologist has drilled the canal. If the otologist drills the canal first, as a stage I procedure, the complication rate is much higher, and it is more difficult to place a cartilage framework around an external canal. Moreover, the amount of scar and the possible compromise to blood flow make complications harder to avoid. The maneuvering of the framework into the proper position on the side of the head is shown in Figures 180.15 and 180.16.

Stage IV, tragal construction, is shown in Figures 180.17 to 180.21. The composite cartilage is taken from

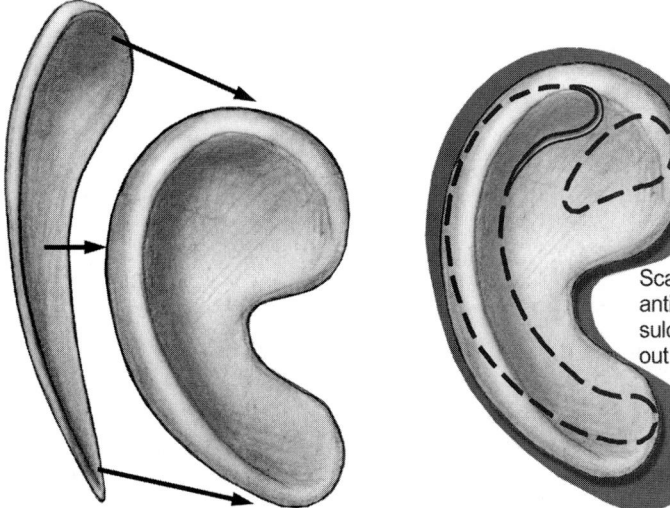

Figure 180.11 Sculpting cartilage to form framework.

Costal cartilage from 8th rib

Costal cartilage from 6th and 7th ribs

Sculpt 6th and 7th cartilage using template

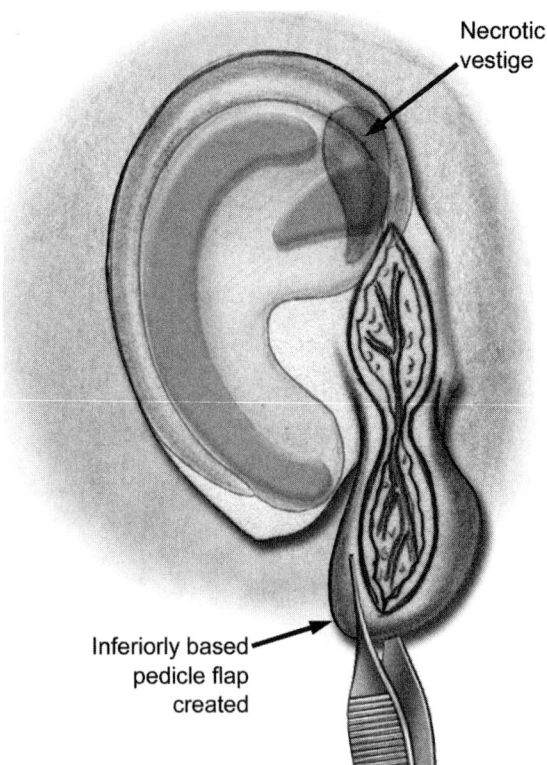

Figure 180.13 Creating inferiorly based pedicle flap.

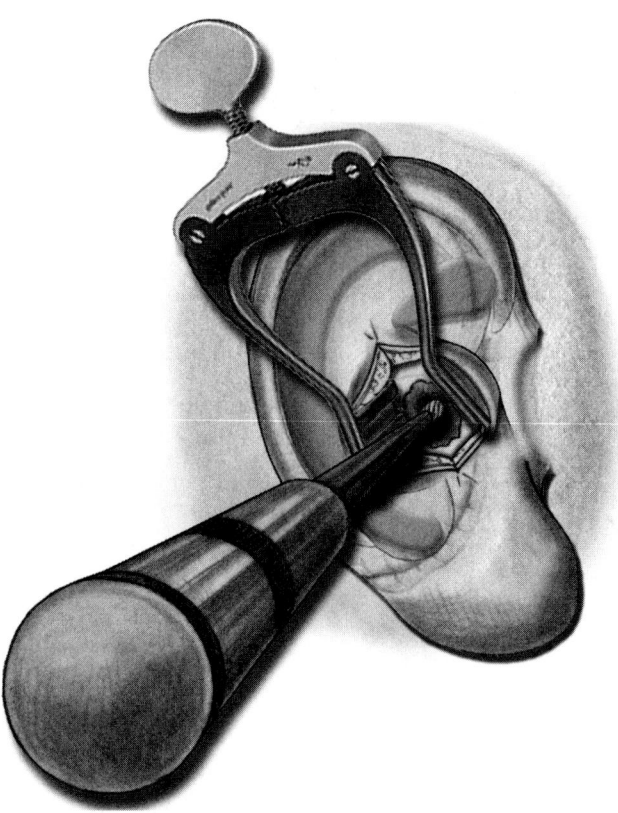

Figure 180.15 Drill-out of temporal bone, creating canal.

the opposite side. Auricular elevation, stage V, is shown in Figures 180.22 and 180.23. The reconstructed ear is shown in Figure 180.24.

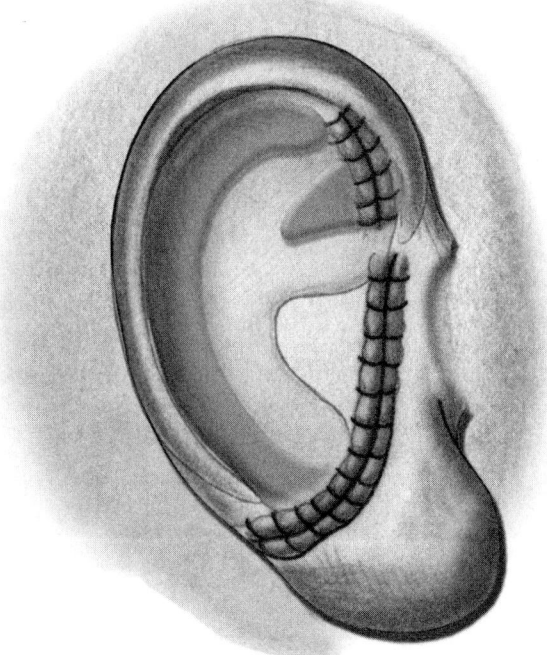

Figure 180.14 Transposing flap into framework.

Complications

Complications are possible during the surgical reconstruction, as listed in Table 180.8. Placement of the cartilage graft places severe strain on the overlying skin, which can cause skin necrosis. Skin necrosis of 1 to 2 mm can be treated by the application of ointment and careful observation until closure occurs. If the necrosis is greater than 5 mm, the proper course is closure with a pedicled temporal-parietal fascia flap and skin graft. Infection can result in reabsorption of cartilage, with improper placement of the framework. Any grafting procedure always involves the risk of graft loss. Finally, the possibility of keloid formation is higher when the graft is harvested from the abdomen or the buttocks. Potential emergencies are listed in Table 180.9.

TABLE 180.8 C COMPLICATIONS CONGENITAL MALFORMATION OF THE AURICLE

Skin necrosis overlying cartilage framework
Chondritis
Reabsorption
Malposition of auricle implant
Tissue breakdown of skin graft or of posterior aspect of ear
Keloiding of donor incision site or skin-graft areas

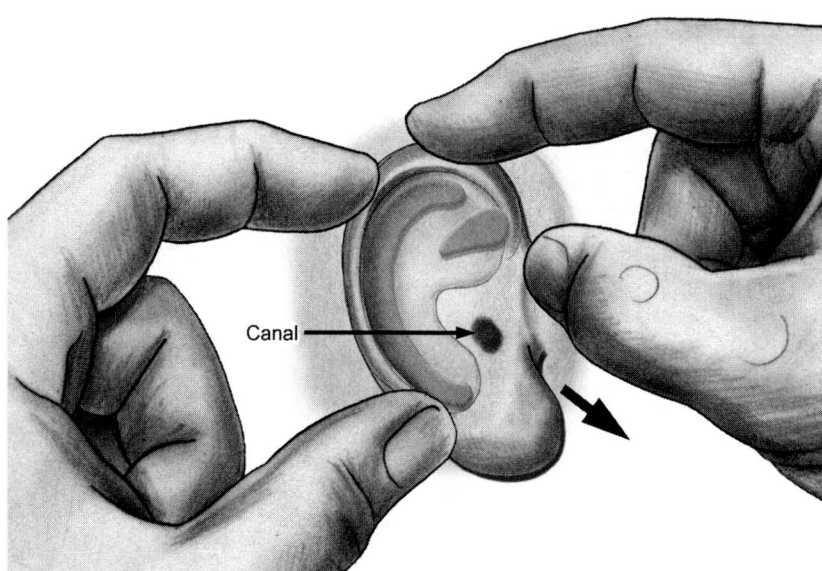

Figure 180.16 Maneuvering framework into proper position around ear canal.

Canal

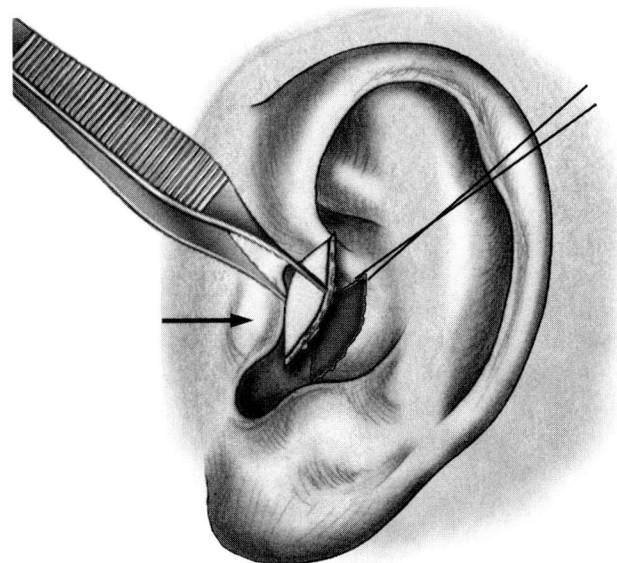

Figure 180.17 Harvesting composite graft.

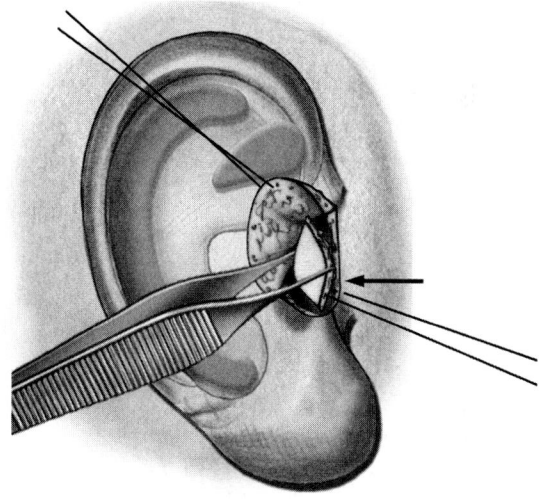

Figure 180.19 Placing composite graft and suturing anterior limb.

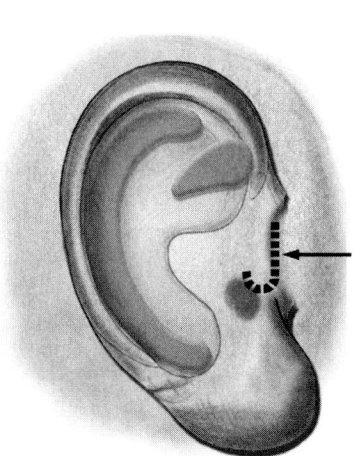

Figure 180.18 J-type incision with anterior skin elevation.

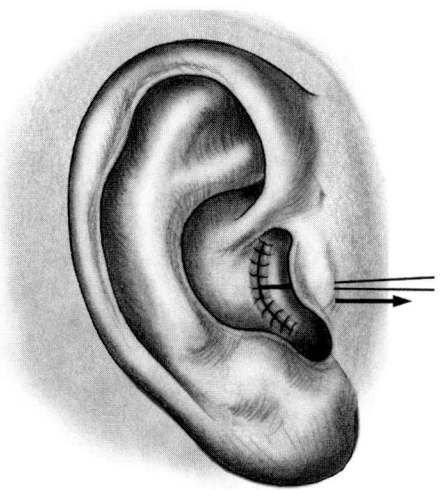

Figure 180.20 Pull-up suture in place with tension.

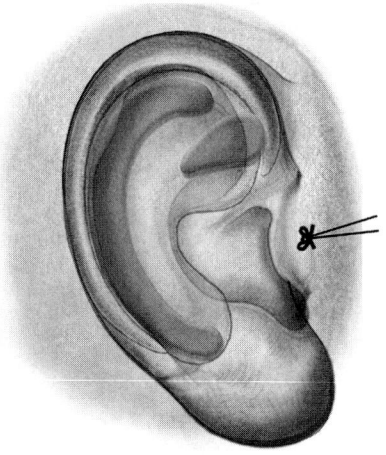

Figure 180.21 Skin graft in place posteriorly.

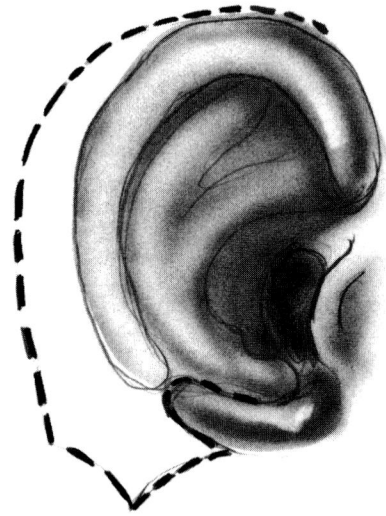

Figure 180.22 Incision in postauricular area.

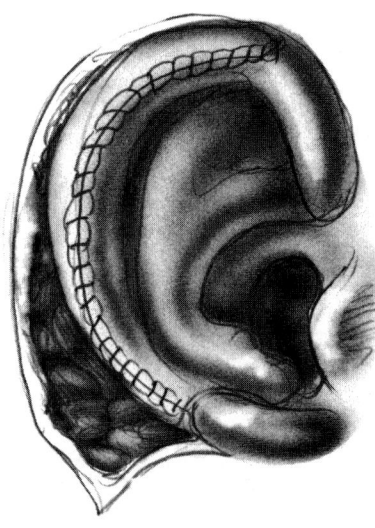

Figure 180.23 Elevating auricle and covering back with split-thickness skin graft.

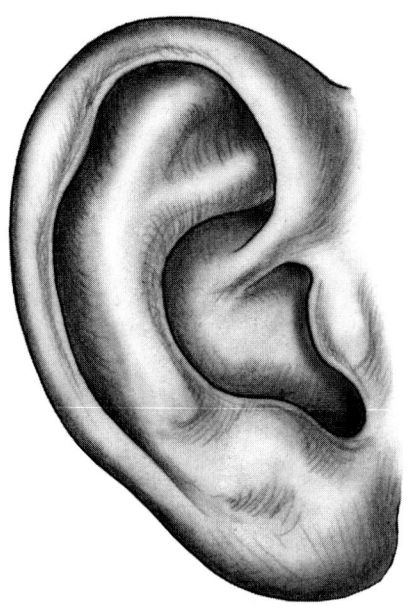

Figure 180.24 Reconstructed ear.

CONCLUSION

The surgery to correct auricular protrusion is more complicated than it looks. With each of the techniques described, complications can occur, even in the hands of experienced surgeons. The surgery always requires postoperative evaluations, and often the surgeon will not be totally satisfied. Therefore, performing this surgery requires a commitment to continuing education and additional experience. Surgical correction of congenital microtia requires commitment by the plastic surgeon, who should be performing more than 5 to 10 operations per year to maintain proficiency. The team approach, as described in this chapter, is invaluable to the families; failure to offer this approach is a significant disservice to the patient.

The future of auricular reconstruction must include the ever-burgeoning field of tissue engineering. The nexus of cell-growth biology and cell-scaffolding technology is rapidly changing the landscape of surgical options. The

TABLE 180.9 EMERGENCIES
CONGENITAL MALFORMATION OF THE AURICLE

Stage	Emergency
I	Pneumothorax; pneumomediastinum, severe skin necrosis
II	Lobule necrosis
III	None
IV and V	Chondritis

technology still has to overcome issues such as tissue rejection and integrity of form.

RECENT LITERATURE

Beahm (21,22) published a significant review of all facets dealing with auricular reconstruction, and this makes excellent review material for any student of auricular reconstruction.

Thorn et al. (23) gave an excellent strategy for deciding which patients are the best candidates for autologous reconstruction and which patients are the best candidates for prosthetic devices.

Park (24) wrote a significant article dealing with the use of tissue expanders placed subfascially and using a standard two-flap method for microtia repair. This is a significant contribution in that it is a different way of thinking about the problem. Park (25) further published an article on the use of an omental free flap in reconstruction of the ear in the devascularized temporoparietal region.

Finally, Han (26) describes experience using osseointegrated implants in children. These articles should be added to the reading list of all interested in this field.

HIGHLIGHTS

- The decision to correct protruding ears is based on the angle of the auricle (>30 degrees) and on other specific anatomic defects of the auricle.
- The helical rim should be 14 to 18 mm above the mastoid skin at the middle and superior thirds.
- The vertical axis of the auricle should be inclined about 20 degrees posteriorly.
- A detailed checklist is extremely helpful during the preoperative evaluation.
- The best age to perform the otoplasty surgery is 5 or 6 years.
- Mustarde sutures are horizontal mattress sutures used to create an antihelical fold.
- The Furnas technique must be used with caution. The conchal mastoid suture must be directed posteriorly to avoid narrowing the external auditory canal.
- The most feared complication is chondritis, which should be treated with extensive antibiotic therapy.
- Each patient should be seen on the first postoperative day to allow early intervention for hematoma or infection.
- Every patient and family should be informed of all risks and made aware that a second procedure may be required later (within a year).
- Every surgeon should learn multiple approaches to otoplasty to be able to offer each patient the best chance for success.
- Autogenous cartilage is best because no rejection and limited reabsorption occur.

- Materials such as Silastic and irradiated cartilage are less than satisfactory alternatives to autogenous cartilage.
- Auricular reconstruction should be performed before atresia repair to preserve the integrity of the skin and the blood supply. Atresia repair should be performed after the plastic surgery, because this allows the movement of the framework to the proper site.
- Age 6 years is appropriate for unilateral microtia correction, both psychologically and anatomically.
- The framework can be maneuvered to align the meatus and the canal.
- The total reconstruction concept is important. A surgical team should be available to handle both the microtia and the atresia.
- For best results, cooperation with the otologist should exist in the staging of the repair.
- Surgeons performing auricular reconstruction should ensure that the cooperating otologist has completed the necessary audiologic evaluations.
- Each surgeon undertaking auricular reconstruction should be committed to this surgery, performing more than 5 to 10 operations per year.

REFERENCES

1. Pitanguy I, Flemming I. Plastic operations on the auricle. In: Naumann HH, ed. *Head and neck surgery.* Philadelphia: WB Saunders, 1982.
2. Gulya AJ. Developmental anatomy of the ear. In: Glascock ME III, Shambaugh GE Jr, eds. *Surgery of the ear,* 3rd ed. Philadelphia: WB Saunders, 1990:5–33.
3. Farkas LG. Anthropometry of normal and anomalous ears. *Clin Plast Surg* 1978;5:401.
4. Eavey RD. Microtia and significant auricular malformation: ninety-two pediatric patients. *Arch Otolaryngol Head Neck Surg* 1995; 121:57–62.
5. Wang R. Presurgical confirmation of craniofacial implant locations in children requiring implant-retained auricular prosthesis. *J Prosthet Dent* 1999;81:492.
6. Farrior RT. Modified cartilage incisions in otoplasty. *Facial Plast Surg* 1985;2:109.
7. Tanzer RC. Total reconstruction of the external ear. *Plast Reconstr Surg* 1959;23:1.
8. Tanzer RC. Correction of microtia with autogenous costal cartilage. In: Tanzer R, Edgerton M, eds. *Symposium on reconstruction of the auricle,* Vol 10. St. Louis: CV Mosby, 1974:46–57.
9. Cronin TD. Use of a Silastic frame for total and subtotal reconstruction of the external ear: preliminary report. *Plast Reconstr Surg* 1966;37:399.
10. Brent B. Ear reconstruction with an expansible framework of autogenous rib cartilage. *Plast Reconstr Surg* 1974;53:619.
11. Aguilar EA III, Jahrsdoerfer RA. The surgical repair of congenital microtia and atresia. *Arch Otolaryngol Head Neck Surg* 1988; 98:600.
12. Aguilar EA III. Auricular reconstruction of congenital microtia (grade III). *Laryngoscope* 1996;106(suppl 82):1–26.
13. Tanzer RC. Congenital deformities of the auriele. In: Converse JM, ed. *Reconstructive plastic surgery.* 2nd ed, Vol 3. Philadelphia: WB Saunders, 1977:1671–1719.
14. Rogers B. Anatomy, embryology and classification of auricular deformities. In: Tanzer R, Edgerton M, eds. *Symposium on reconstruction of the auricle,* Vol 10. St. Louis: CV Mosby, 1974:3–11.
15. Weerda H. Classification of congenital deformities of the auricle. *Facial Plast Surg* 1988;5:385.
16. Rogers B. Microtic, lop, cup and protruding ears. *Plast Reconstr Surg* 1968;41:208.

17. Aguilar EA III. Classification of auricular congenital deformities. In: Papel ID, Nachlas NE, eds. *Facial plastic and reconstructive surgery.* St. Louis: Mosby Year Book, 1992:532–534.

18. Williams JD, Romo T III, Sclafani AP, et al. Polyethylene implants in auricular reconstruction. *Arch Otol Head Neck Surg* 1997; 123:578–583.

19. Somers HT. Politzer Meeting Abstract. St. Augustinus Hospital, University of Antwerp, April 17, 2000.

20. Brent B. Auricular repair with autogenous rib cartilage grafts: two decades of experience with 600 cases. *Plast Reconstr Surg* 1992; 90:355–374.

21. Beahm EK. Auricular reconstruction for microtia: Part I.: anatomy, embryology, and clinical evaluation. *Plast Reconstr Surg* 2002;109(7):2473–2482.

22. Beahm EK. Auricular reconstruction for microtia: Part II. surgical techniques. *Plast Reconstr Surg* 2002;110(1):234–249.

23. Thorne CH, Brecht LE, Bradley JP, et al. Auricular reconstruction: indications for autogenous and prosthetic techniques. *Plast Reconstr Surg* 2001;107(5):1241–1252.

24. Park C. Subfascial expansion and expanded two-flap method for microtia reconstruction. *Plast Reconstr Surg* 2000;106(7);1473–1487.

25. Park C. Total ear reconstruction in the devascularized temporoparietal region, II: use of the omental free flap. *Plast Reconstr Surg* 2003;III(4):1391–1397.

26. Han K. Osseointegrated alloplastic ear reconstruction with the implant-carrying plate system in children. *Plast Reconstr Surg* 2002;109(2):496–503.

181

Chin and Malar Augmentation

William E. Silver   Anurag Agarwal

Genioplasty or alteration of the chin is a common procedure. It is frequently done in conjunction with rhinoplasty but can be performed separately. Augmentation of the malar prominence also is becoming increasingly popular. This chapter discusses augmentation of the chin and the cheeks, including what constitutes a proper chin line or projection and a proper cheek protrusion and the steps to correct predictably any nonaesthetic findings or deformities of these areas (Table 181.1). These deformities and their corrections are discussed as though no problem exists with dental occlusion; orthognathic surgery is discussed elsewhere in this textbook.

CHIN AUGMENTATION

Evaluation of the Chin

To determine the appropriate chin projection, a method should be adopted that is reproducible, meets the aesthetic lines of the face, and most important, is easy to perform (Table 181.2). A common and easy method uses a line perpendicular to the Frankfort horizontal line intersecting the vermilion border of the lower lip. The chin should approach this perpendicular line (Fig. 181.1). For conservative degrees of augmentation, the chin will come short of this line.

The following methods are more difficult to reproduce, calculate, and use clinically (1):

1. Legan angle (Fig. 181.2): the angle contained by lines from the glabella to the subnasale and the subnasale to the soft-tissue pogonion. This should be 12 ± 4 degrees for appropriate chin projection.

2. Merrifield Z angle (Fig. 181.3): created by the Frankfort horizontal line and a line connecting the soft-tissue pogonion and the most anterior part of the lip. The Z angle should be 80 ± 5 degrees.

3. Gonzales-Ulloa (Fig. 181.4): determines chin projection based on a line perpendicular to the Frankfort horizontal line that intersects the nasion. The chin should approximate this line. Options for management of chin deficiencies are listed in Table 181.3.

Other preoperative considerations include the presence of a "geniomandibular groove," chin–soft-tissue ptosis ("witch's chin"), or vertical microgenia. The geniomandibular groove is identified as a depression along the mandibular border, just anterior to the jowl fat pad. In patients with deep grooves, use of an extended chin implant may be prudent to avoid accentuating the grooves with a standard implant.

As noted by Frodel and Sykes (2), chin–soft-tissue ptosis is caused by loosening of the attachments of chin musculature, including the mentalis and depressor labii inferior muscles. Failure to recognize inferior descent of the chin–soft tissue pad before chin augmentation will lead to a persistent and potentially accentuated "witch's chin" postoperatively. A technique to correct chin–soft-tissue ptosis is to remove the dependent excess fat through the submental incision, followed by excision of any redundant skin.

An assessment of the vertical height of the chin and the position of the labiomental fold will allow one to choose the appropriate procedure. Chin augmentation in a patient with vertical microgenia may excessively deepen the labiomental groove. Zide (3) has cautioned against alloplastic augmentation in female patients with a high labiomental fold, as this may enlarge the entire lower third of the face

TABLE 181.1

EVALUATION OF THE CHIN AND MALAR AREAS

Deficiency of chin or malar projection with secondary disharmony according to predetermined facial proportions

Effects of the proposed changes or enhancement of the patient's overall facial aesthetics

Determination of the adjunctive procedures to accomplish desired results such as facelift, rhinoplasty, liposuction

Overall facial features, including dental occlusion, skin texture, anatomic proportions, prior facial trauma, and emotional stability

TABLE 181.2   DIAGNOSIS

CHIN DEFICIENCIES

Methods of evaluating proportional chin projection
    Legan angle
    Merrifield Z-angle
    Gonzales-Ullao zero meridian
Relation of bony projection and final aesthetic soft-tissue projection
Simplest method to evaluate chin projection
    Perpendicular line to the Frankfort horizontal line at the vermilion/cutaneous lower lip border

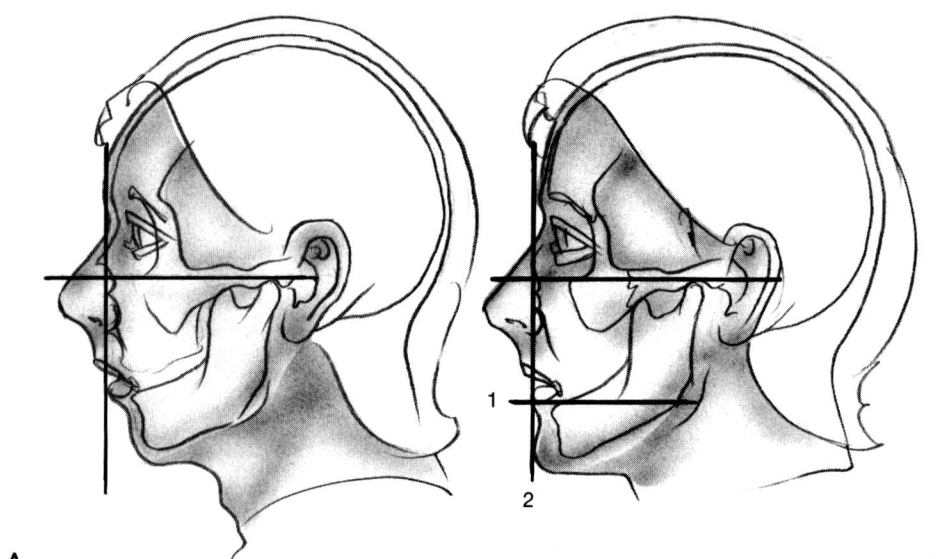

A   B

Figure 181.1   Silver's chin soft-tissue assessment. **A:** Preoperative view. **B:** Postoperative view. *1*, Line parallel to Frankfort horizontal line, which intersects the vermilion cutaneous border of the lower lip; *2*, drop perpendicular from (*1*). Chin should be at or slightly behind (*2*).

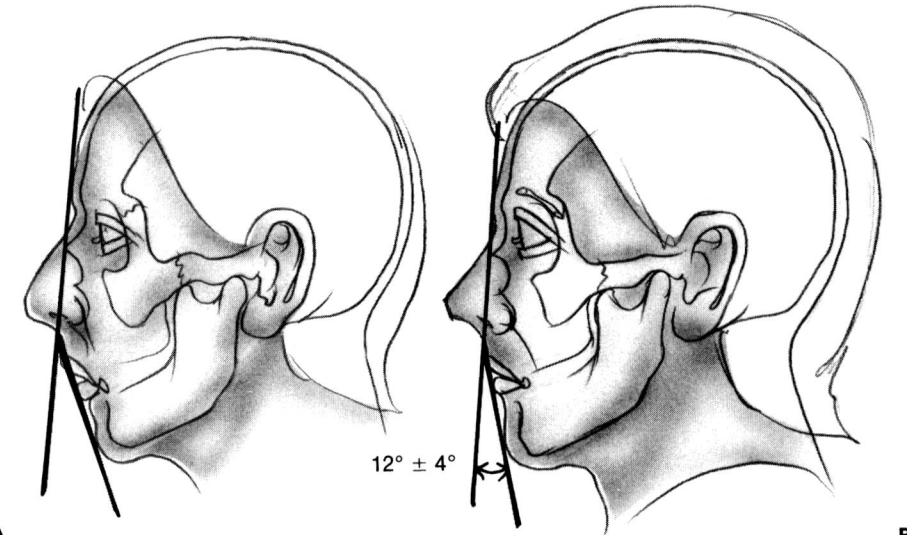

12° ± 4°

A   B

Figure 181.2   Legan angle. **A:** Preoperative view. **B:** Postoperative view. *1*, Glabella to subnasale; *2*, subnasale to soft-tissue pogonion. Angle created by (*1*) and (*2*) is 12 ± 4 degrees.

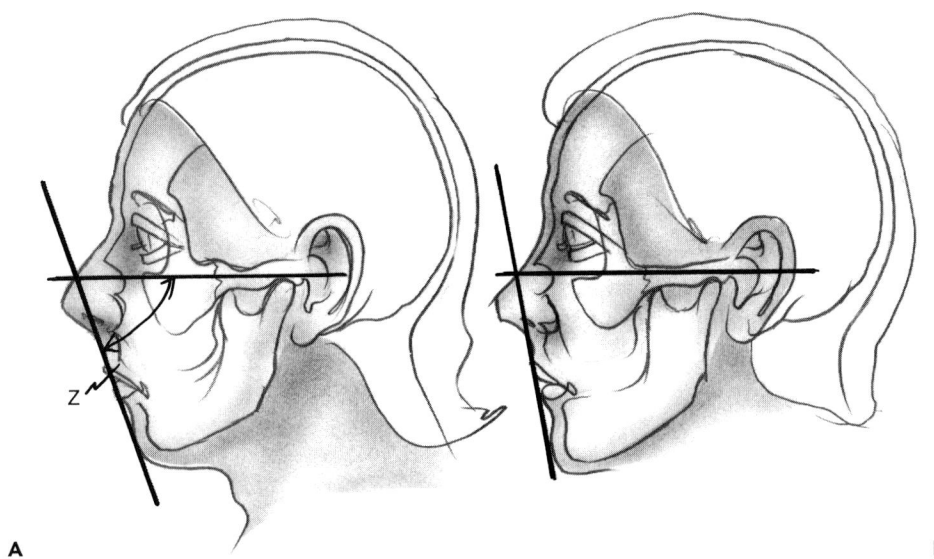

A   **B**

Figure 181.3 Merrifield Z angle. **A:** Preoperative view. **B:** Postoperative view. *1*, Frankfort horizontal line; *2*, line intersecting soft-tissue pogonion. Z angle is 80 ± 5 degrees.

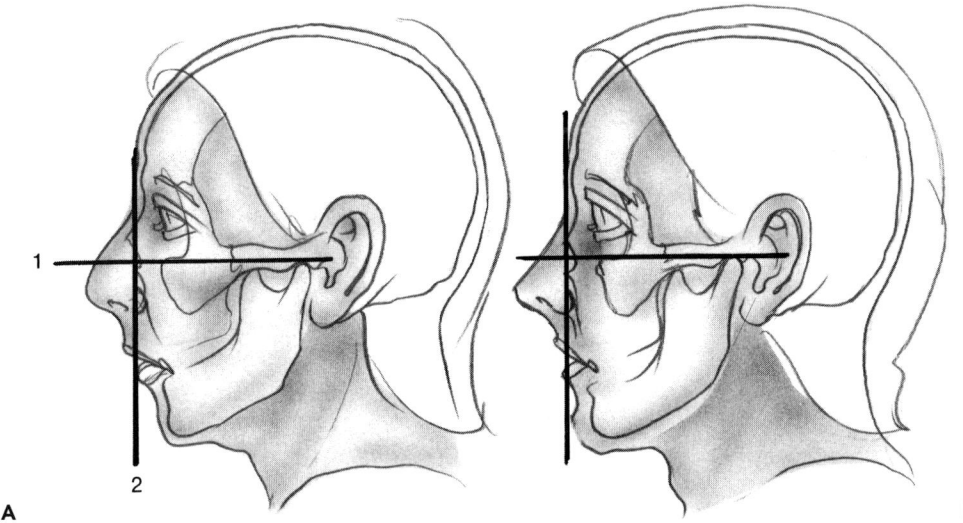

A   **B**

Figure 181.4 Zero meridian of Gonzales-Ulloa. **A:** Preoperative view. **B:** Postoperative view. *1*, Frankfort horizontal line; *2*, perpendicular from nasion to (*1*). Chin should be at or just behind (*2*).

TABLE 181.3   ℞   TREATMENT
CHIN DEFICIENCIES

Alloplasts vs. sliding genioplasty
   Alloplasts: simpler, removable, fewer complications
   Sliding genioplasty: useful in asymmetric jaws and extreme microgenia
Intraoral vs. extraoral alloplast placement
   Intraoral
     Bothersome suture lines
     Anterior geniobuccal sulcus scar contracture
   Extraoral
     External scar
     Subperiosteal placement of implant is desirable
Various alloplastic materials and shapes are available commercially; Silastic is most commonly used. Final soft-tissue augmentation represents 70% of implant width.

TABLE 181.4

CONTRAINDICATIONS TO CHIN IMPLANTS

Severe periodontal disease
Extreme microgenia
Excess or insufficient vertical mandibular height
Labial incompetence with chin dimpling and strain (9)

postoperatively in a masculine fashion. In these patients, a sliding genioplasty with the orientation of the osteotomies tailored to the individual's anatomic variations should be considered.

Contraindications to alloplastic chin augmentation are listed in Table 181.4.

Chin Implants

When the decision has been made to augment the chin, two choices exist: a sliding genioplasty or an implant. When the choice is made for the implant, the surgeon must consider the type and size of the implant and the surgical approach (intraoral or extraoral). The most common alloplastic implant is solid silicone, either soft or firm. Other types of implants include reinforced expanded polytetrafluoroethylene (e-PTFE) made by W.L. Gore, porous polyethylene made by Porex, and Mersilene mesh. In a review of 324 cases of Gortex chin implants, Godin et al. (4) found reinforced e-PTFE implants to be easily inserted, well tolerated by the tissues, and free of any bony resorption. Only two (0.62%) of 324 implants became infected and were ultimately removed. A manufactured silicone liquid–filled implant is no longer used because of the concern of possible leakage.

Mersilene mesh is a nonabsorbable polyester fiber sheet with large pores that allow tissue ingrowth. Gross et al. (5) reviewed their 14-year experience using Mersilene mesh chin implantation on 264 patients. The results show an infection rate of only 0.8% and no incidents of absorption, rejection, or extrusion. The only disadvantages are the extra time and technical expertise required to craft the implants.

At present, we prefer a customized firm Silastic implant made by Implantech (Fig. 181.5). It has a cleft made into

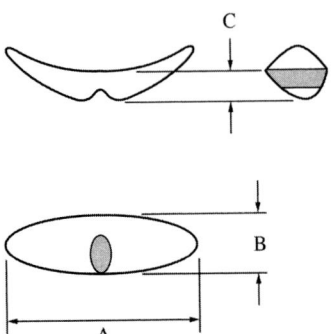

Figure 181.5 Silver Silastic chin implant by Implantech.

the exact anterior center of the implant, a blue line demarcating the vertical center on the posterior surface, extremely fine tapered lateral margins, and a slight concavity on the posterior surface. The purpose of this design is to be inserted into a very small opening in the skin or the mucosa. With the slight concave posterior surface, it tends to conform to the underlying bone. The blue line helps to center the implant under direct vision when only a small portion of the implant is visible through the incision. The cleft on the anterior surface allows the surgeon to palpate the center of the implant after the incision has been closed to ensure that when the final pressure dressing is applied, the implant has remained in the midline position. In addition, this anterior cleft enables one to determine clinically by means of palpation whether the implant becomes dislocated to one side many months later. Sometimes, many months later, a patient may complain of an asymmetry of the implant. This small cleft makes it much easier to determine whether the implant has dislodged or the mandible is slightly asymmetrical. We strongly recommend that if a porous implant or a mesh implant is used, the interstices of the implant should be pressure loaded with antibiotic solution. We use 300 mg of clindamycin per 15 mL of saline. Clindamycin is the antibiotic of choice because of the extremely low sensitivity or allergic reaction. Many other implants are available through various vendors.

McGhan Silastic implants are available in small, medium, and large sizes. The size and shape of the implant to be used are based on how much chin augmentation is needed anteriorly and laterally. Kent (6) determined that after implant placement, a 70% gain in soft-tissue projection is found. Thus a 10-mm implant would yield a 7-mm soft-tissue increase. The gain is reduced because of a small amount of implant settling, bone resorption, and soft-tissue compression. Actual soft-tissue augmentation stabilizes in 2 years at 70% of implant thickness. If a sliding genioplasty is used, about a 70% to 97% gain in soft tissue is seen, which stabilizes after 2 years (7).

We use the following method to determine the size of the implant needed to obtain the desired results. First, the face is placed in a profile position held in the horizontal position (the Frankfort horizontal line is parallel to the ground). A vertical line is then dropped from the inferior vermilion border perpendicular to the Frankfort horizontal line. The ideal chin position should approximate that line. The distance from the preoperative position to the proposed position then is multiplied by 1.4 to determine the thickness of the implant. This parameter can vary from patient to patient; therefore, the surgeon must rely on aesthetic judgement to set the final chin projection. It is always safer to underaugment slightly to avoid deformity.

Next, the surgical approach must be considered. Intraoral insertion has the advantage over extraoral insertion in that no external scars are present, but it has the disadvantages of intraoral contamination, suture-line irritation, a larger incision line, the inability to stabilize the implant internally, and the potential for labial incompetence if the mentalis muscle is disrupted. The external approach can be made through a very inconspicuous and small submental crease incision, which avoids irritation of the intraoral sutures and potential contamination. A 10- to 15-mm incision is generally sufficient to accommodate implant placement and allows the implant to be suture stabilized to the periosteum. Often the implant is inserted at the time of liposuction in the neck area, either as an isolated procedure or with a facelift, and the same incision can be used for both procedures.

Operative Procedure

The patient flexes the neck to locate the submental crease, which is marked. Then, with the patient under monitored anesthesia care or general anesthesia, a half-and-half mixture of 2% lidocaine with epinephrine 1:100,000 and 0.5% bupivacaine with epinephrine is infiltrated in the area of the mental nerve, the incision line, and the soft tissues of the chin. The bupivacaine is used for two reasons. First, if the chin augmentation is performed in conjunction with a rhinoplasty, the chin surgery is performed first, and minimal to no feeling of the chin area exists during the rhinoplasty. Second, the anesthesia of the chin area should be present at the conclusion of the rhinoplasty so that the pressure dressing can be placed without discomfort.

A skin incision 10 to 15 mm long then is made. The incision is deepened through the subcutaneous fat layer and muscle layer down to the periosteum. The periosteum is sharply cut with a no. 15 blade for 2.5 cm and elevated with a Joseph elevator superiorly in the midline up to the mid-portion of the mandible. Care should be taken not to disrupt the anterogingivobuccal sulcus. If this periosteal elevation is carried too high, the implant could rise and shallow out or obliterate the sulcus and change the position of the anterior projection and even interfere with the natural smile. To keep the implant from rising too superiorly, a suture can be placed into the inferior side of the periosteum and then into the implant.

To elevate and extend the subperiosteal envelope laterally, a Pennington elevator can be used. The surgeon must know the location of the mental foramen to avoid injuring the mental nerve on lateral dissection. This elevation can be done under direct vision by using a Senn or similar retractor if desired. Hemostasis is maintained with bipolar cautery.

The implant should have a deep anterior central groove and a vertical central line so that the surgeon can see through the incision when the implant is centered and can palpate externally after the incision is closed and when the dressing is about to be applied. This also can serve as a guide after the swelling has resolved to determine whether any implant displacement has occurred. This central groove does not show externally and can be felt only with careful palpation. The implant is inserted by retracting the periosteum with a Senn retractor and placing one end into

the subperiosteal pocket slightly more than halfway beyond the midline and bending the implant so that the other end can be inserted under the other side of the periosteal envelope. The implant then is moved back and forth until the deep groove is centered in the midline, as seen through the submental incision.

The closure is performed in two layers. First, the periosteum is closed with three interrupted 3-0 chromic sutures, followed by skin closure with locking 6-0 nylon or 5-0 fast-absorbing plain catgut suture. If an intraoral incision is used, a vertical incision is made through the anterior gingivobuccal frenulum. The incision is carried through the muscle down to the periosteum. The incision is retracted horizontally (laterally), and the periosteum is exposed and cut in a horizontal direction. It is elevated with a Pennington elevator until the desired subperiosteal pocket is made. The implant is inserted as described earlier, but this incision is closed by first closing muscle with 3-0 chromic and then mucosa with 3-0 chromic sutures.

The dressing is applied in three layers. The first is 0.5-inch paper tape, alternating from the superior to inferior arch, compressing the soft tissue around the implant. Then a strip of 2-inch Elastoplast with a horizontal slit is placed over the chin with the implant protruding through the slit, followed by another layer of 0.5-inch paper tape. The dressing stays on for 4 to 5 days, and the sutures are removed when the dressing comes off.

Complications

Complications of chin implants are rare (Table 181.5). For the most part, all complications are reversible by removing the implant. The following steps are taken to prevent complications:

1. Use of preoperative antibiotics
2. Washing implants and gloves of all powder or oils
3. Making the superiosteal pocket only as big as necessary to accept the implant
4. Suturing the implant to the periosteum
5. Selecting the implant size preoperatively and carefully

Displaced Implant
The implant may slide too far superiorly and obliterate the anterior gingival–lip sulcus, resulting in an abnormal

---

TABLE 181.5 **COMPLICATIONS**
CHIN IMPLANTS

Displaced implant
Infection or tissue reaction
Bony resorption
Improper size selection
Mental nerve injury
Hypertrophic scar

smile; the patient is often aware of this problem. Treatment is to remove the implant and pull it inferiorly, placing it over the pogonion and suturing it in place to the periosteum.

The implant also can slide to one side or can be displaced inferiorly on one side and superiorly on the other side. In these situations, the implant must be removed and replaced in the subperiosteal pocket appropriately and sutured to the periosteum. Yaremchuk (8) advocates screw fixation of the implant, which prevented any implant migration in his series of 46 patients. The choice of suture fixation or screw fixation is a matter of surgeon preference.

Infection or Tissue Reaction

Infection is extremely rare. If inflammation is present around the implant, it is often a sterile reaction, either related to particles of powder from the surgeon's glove or just a foreign-body reaction to the implant. In the rare situation in which the surrounding tissue is infected, a culture is obtained, and a course of appropriate antibiotics is given empirically. If the reaction does not resolve within 10 days, the implant is removed, and 8 weeks should elapse before attempting to reinsert it. If a microporous implant is used, it should be removed without delay. Another isolated, unrelated complication concerns development of an apical tooth abscess of one of the lower incisors. This could set up a delayed (many years later) reaction that will cause the tissue around the implant to become infected. The treatment is to remove the implant, have the tooth problem corrected, and then wait for the appropriate time to reinsert the implant.

Bony Resorption

Bony resorption occurs in almost all alloplastic implants, whether they are placed supraperiosteally or subperiosteally. The real question is whether the resorption will cause any problem to the underlying teeth. Although bony absorption is self-limiting in the vast majority of patients, Matarasso et al. (9) identified a subset of patients who may be at risk for extensive, clinically significant bony erosion with Silastic implants. These patients all had preoperative labial incompetence with resultant mentalis muscle hyperactivity, manifested by strain and chin-skin dimpling. The more common problem with bony resorption is a decrease in projection when the implant moves posteriorly into the mandible. We have seen this occur after many years in several cases, but without any dental sequelae.

We place the implant subperiosteally; however, some researchers claim that inserting the implant above the periosteum may reduce the possibility of cortical resorption beneath the implant. From a practical point of view and from many years of experience using both methods, we find no difference. Another method that has been de-scribed is to incise the periosteum on either side of the midline, insert the implant under the periosteum laterally, and leave it over the periosteum in the midline. We have not found this technique to show any clinical benefit.

Improper Size Selection

Implant size should be determined preoperatively, as discussed; however, as the wound heals, the surgeon may notice that more projection would be better or that the implant is too large. The treatment is to remove the implant and reinsert the appropriate size. The surgeon should wait at least 3 months before making that decision to see what swelling and tissue reaction will actually do to the appearance. In choosing a Silastic implant, it is better to use a smaller one than a larger one, because the capsule around the implant tends to increase the projection with time. This may be an advantage for considering the reinforced e-PTFE, because a true capsule does not develop around the porous e-PTFE.

Mental Nerve Injury

We have not seen this rare complication, but lateral dissection conceivably could cause this injury. It is more common in a degloving procedure when performing a sliding genioplasty. The greater areas of dissection when using the longer tapered implants theoretically place the nerve at greater risk. The mental nerve must always be kept in mind when performing an augmentation mentoplasty.

Hypertrophic Scar

The possibility of a scar should always be mentioned to the patient before surgery, but the use of a small incision, well placed and accurately closed in two layers (platysma and subcutaneous tissue in one layer and skin separately) with fine skin sutures, should avert such a problem. In rare situations, the scar may need to be excised and re-closed.

SLIDING GENIOPLASTY

Chin augmentation with the sliding genioplasty is a much more formidable procedure; however, it has the advantage of using the patient's own tissue. It also can be used to decrease the vertical height of the chin if necessary by tapering the bone incision downward or more posteriorly (10). Its disadvantages include an increased surgical time, a longer healing time, a risk of injury of the anterior teeth and membranes around the chin and lip area, and loss of lip competence (poor reapproximation of the mentalis muscle). Sliding genioplasty should be considered in patients with excess or insufficient vertical mandibular height, extreme microgenia, hemifacial atrophy or mandibular asymmetry, and failed alloplastic chin augmentation. This part of the discussion addresses patients who have acceptable

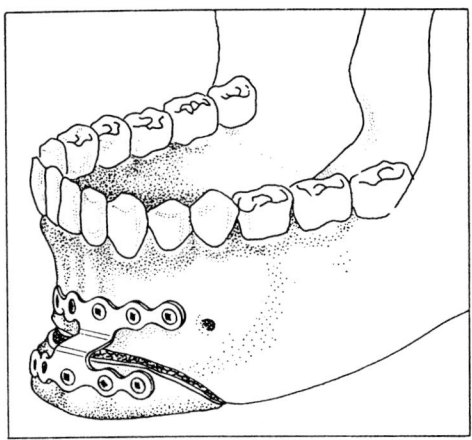

Figure 181.6 Smith Genioplasty plate by KLS Martin.

occlusion but a contour deficit of the chin. Cephalometric analysis of bony and soft tissue as well as panorex radiographs aid in preoperative determination of the type of genioplasty required. They will also show the position of the dental roots.

The basic technique of sliding genioplasty is as follows (11,12). An incision is made anterior to the gingivobuccal sulcus and extends just laterally to the cuspid teeth. The incision is carried to the mandible, passing through the orbicularis and mentalis muscles, which are later carefully reapproximated. The periosteum is elevated inferiorly and laterally, and the mental foramina identified. Suprahyoid muscles and lingual periosteum remain attached medially, providing blood supply to the bone segment. A midline vertical groove is made with a small cutting burr. We prefer the Smith genioplasty plate with 2-mm screws, made by KLS Martin (Fig. 181.6). The most common H plate sizes are 3, 5, or 7 mm. An H plate is used to reapproximate the mandible after the portion is advanced. An osteotomy is made below the cuspid apices and mental foramina at an appropriate angle. If only advancement is to be accomplished, then the osteotomy should be made below the apices of the teeth and in a line parallel to the dentition of the lower jaw. The inferior segment is advanced and held in place with a four-screw cross-plate that is preshaped to allow for the exact millimeter of advancement that was determined preoperatively. The incision is closed in two layers, taking care to reapproximate the mentalis muscle to avoid lip incompetence. A pressure dressing is applied to support the lip.

Variations of the technique are well discussed by Hinds (10). These variations can reduce or augment vertical height and address asymmetry.

Alloplastic augmentation and sliding genioplasty are not mutually exclusive procedures. In some instances, combining these techniques will achieve the desired results. For example, if after performing a sliding genioplasty, the chin contour is still deficient, an implant can be added to yield an enhanced contour.

TABLE 181.6	**D** DIAGNOSIS

MALAR AREA DEFICIENCIES

Flattened and recessed melolabial folds that may give a sad or tired look
Malar prominence that falls more than 5 mm posterior to the nasolabial groove
Increased fullness may give a youthful, bright facial appearance

MALAR AUGMENTATION

The malar region can add to or detract from the overall aesthetic appearance of the face (Table 181.6) (13). Fullness of the malar region gives a youthful appearance to an older face, because it tends to decrease the depth of the melolabial lines and provides a happier, decisive look to the face. Indications for malar implants are as follows:

1. Lack of malar prominence
2. As an adjunct to facelift surgery if patient has deepened melolabial folds
3. Accentuation of the malar prominence, creating a more pleasing aesthetic appearance
4. Asymmetry of the malar prominence from congenital deformity, surgical resection, or incomplete reduction of malar fracture

Evaluation

Determining when to add bulk to the malar area is related more to aesthetic appreciation than to an actual measurement, but a general rule can be applied. In our experience, when the malar prominence falls more than 5 mm posterior to the nasolabial groove on a true lateral projection, a deficiency of the malar area exists (Fig. 181.7). To determine the malar area to augment, one of us (W.E.S.) developed the Silver malar prominence triangle, determined by examining more than 100 photographs of models' faces and making a composite drawing of a triangle over the most prominent area of the malar region. Within the malar prominence triangle, the implant is placed to create an appropriately tapered (shaped) malar region. Placement of the malar implant is determined as follows (Fig. 181.8):

1. Drop a vertical line from the lateral canthus.
2. Draw a horizontal line bisecting the upper lip. The intersection of lines 1 and 2 forms point A.
3. Reflect a line from point A to the medial canthal area.
4. Reflect a line laterally from point A, creating the same angle as created in step 3.
5. Draw a horizontal Frankfort line.

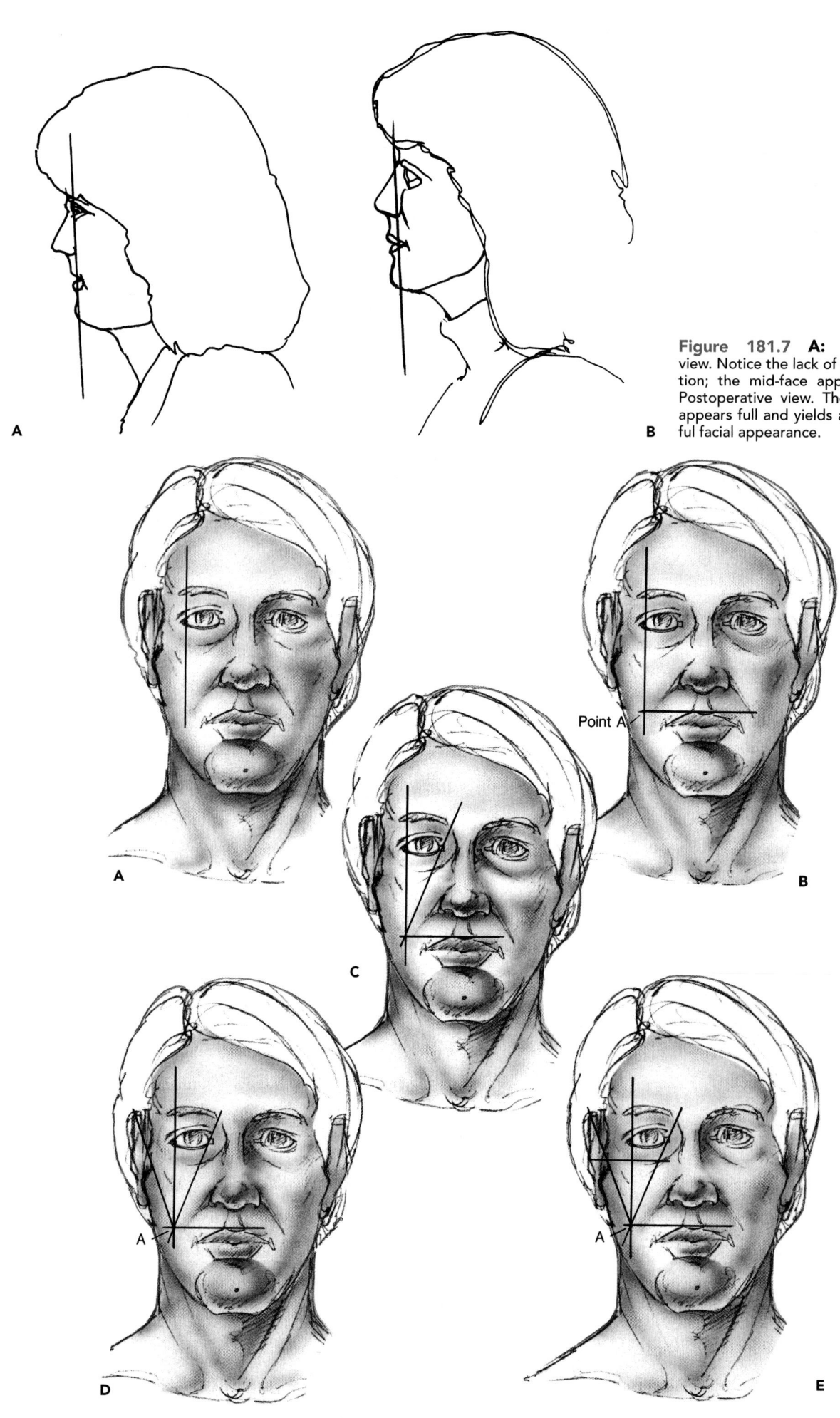

Figure 181.7 A: Preoperative view. Notice the lack of malar projection; the mid-face appears flat. **B:** Postoperative view. The malar area appears full and yields a soft, youthful facial appearance.

A

B

Point A

C

A
D

A
E

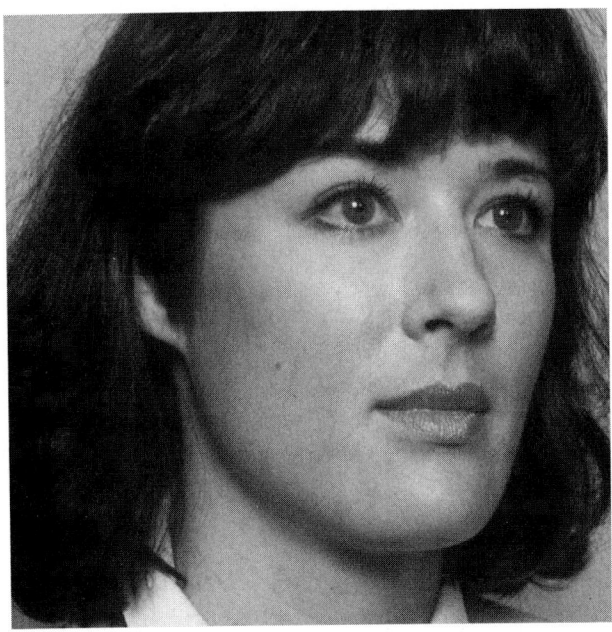
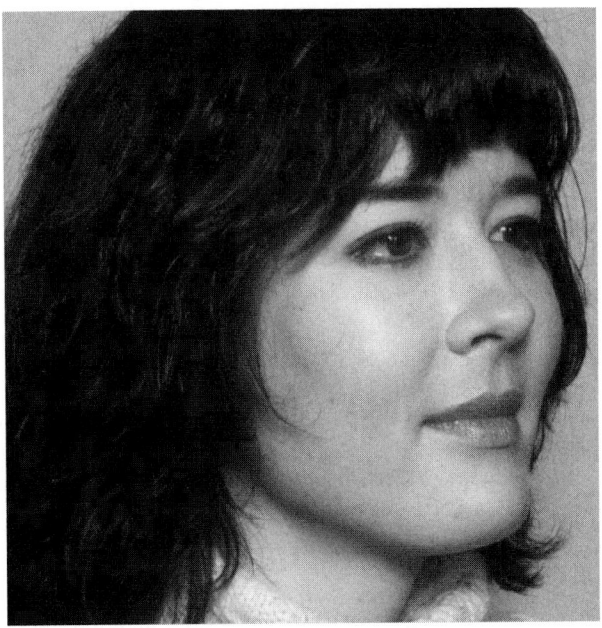

Figure 181.9   Young model who desired more fullness of her cheekbones. A: Preoperative view: nonprominent malar bone. B: Postoperative view shows fullness of cheek.

6. The area contained within the large triangular area represents the malar prominence triangle and the area to be augmented by the malar implant with lateral tapering of the implant.

The tail of the malar implant follows out into and slightly beyond the upper outer angle of the malar prominence triangle. The Frankfort horizontal line is several millimeters above the superior limit of augmentation to avoid infraorbital nerve injury. The implant tapers from the central area to create a natural convexity, simulating a natural malar prominence. Figures 181.9 through 181.17 show preoperative and postoperative views of patients.

Implant Selection

Our recommended implant material in the past had been a carefully designed implant made by Novamed from Proplast-HA (Table 181.7), but Novamed has stopped production of this implant in the United States. Therefore, we currently use a Silastic implant manufactured by Spectrum Designs Medical for McGhan Medical Corporation (Fig. 181.18). It is teardrop shaped and has holes in the posterior portion. These holes are used to thread a silk tie through to hold the implant in position for 24 hours after insertion. The implant with the closest properties to the

Proplast HA implant on the market today is the preformed reinforced e-PTFE implant manufactured by W.L. Gore. This implant was introduced in December 1996 and has become quite popular. It conforms easily and stays in position without slipping. Tissue ingrowth tends to keep it in position.

Silastic
Advantages
The Silastic implant, such as the McGhan implant, can be inserted into a smaller pocket. An infection around the implant can be treated with the implant in place. It can be used over a malar bone (maxillary sinus) that has been fractured with less concern for future infection from sinus infection contamination.

TABLE 181.7 ℞ TREATMENT MALAR DEFICIENCIES

Malar prominence triangle for positioning malar implant; preformed Silastic malar implants are most commonly used
Antibiotic implant loading required for porous implants, systemic antibiotics required perioperatively for all implants
Canine fossa intraoral insertion and subperiosteal dissection
Watertight two-layer closure of muscle and mucosa

Figure 181.8   Constructing Silver's malar prominence triangle. **A:** Drop a vertical line from the lateral canthus. **B:** Draw a horizontal line bisecting the upper lip. The intersection of these lines forms point A. **C:** Reflect a line from point A to the medial canthal area. **D:** Reflect a line laterally from point A, creating the same angle as created in (**C**). **E:** Draw a horizontal Frankfort line. The area contained within the large triangle represents the malar prominence triangle and the area to be augmented by the malar implant with lateral tapering of the implant.

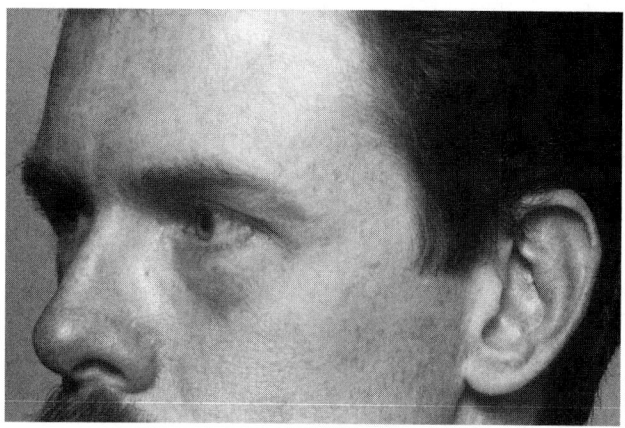 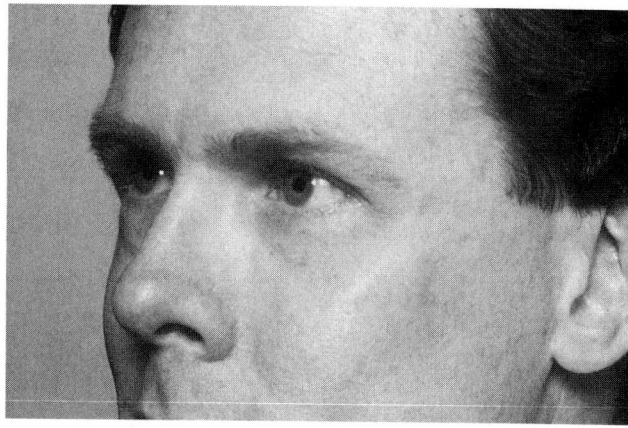

Figure 181.10 Patient with flattened, withdrawn look. **A:** Preoperative view: flattened malar prominence. **B:** Postoperative view: malar prominence accentuates facial sharpness.

Disadvantages

Silastic malar implants tend not to stay in their original position and must be anchored with a suture at initial insertion. It also forms a surrounding capsule that may be palpated easily as the surgical site matures.

Reinforced Expanded Polytetrafluoroethylene
Advantages

This e-PTFE forms no capsule and has good tissue fixation secondary to its porosity. The design of the implant with its thinly tapered tail provides a nice aesthetic transition from implant to zygomatic arch.

Disadvantages

If an infection in the immediate area of the implant from surrounding tissue, such as a tooth or previously fractured infected sinus, should develop, then the microporous implants must be removed. A large pocket must be formed for insertion.

Porous Polyethylene
Advantages

The porous polyethylene implant has an average pore size that ranges from 100 to 250 μm. This allows excellent tissue ingrowth. This material is biocompatible, and minimal

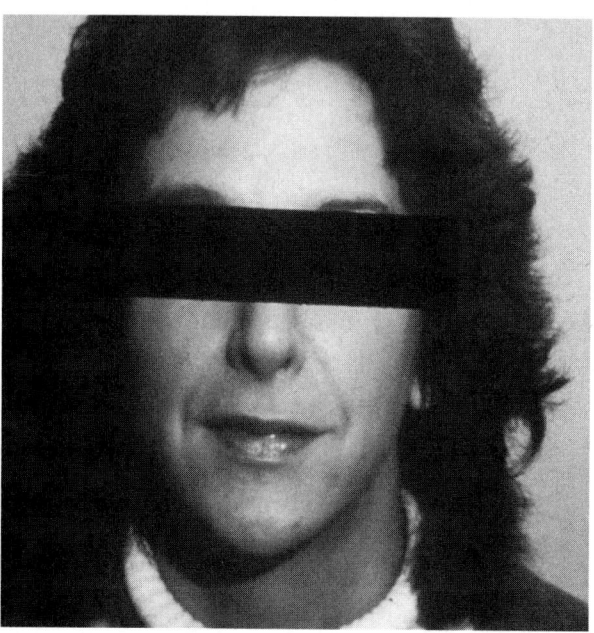 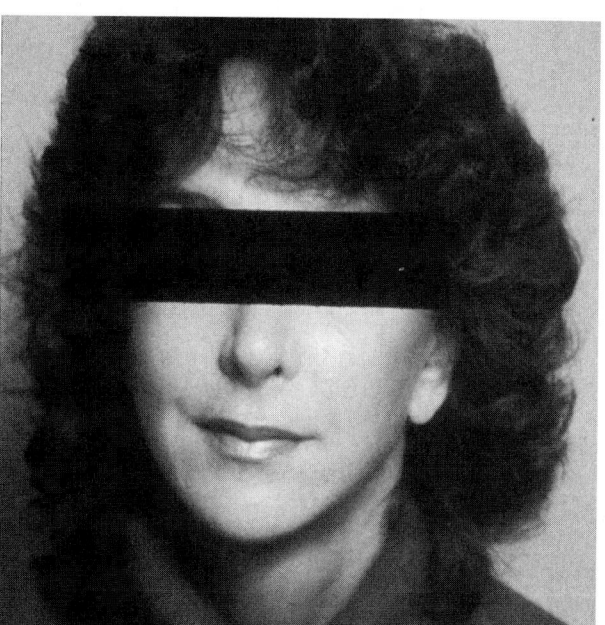

Figure 181.11 Facelift patient with deep melolabial folds; combined facelift and malar implants. **A:** Preoperative view: facelift with flat malar prominence and deep melolabial folds. **B:** Postoperative view: facelift with insertion of cheek implants. Melolabial folds are now shallow.

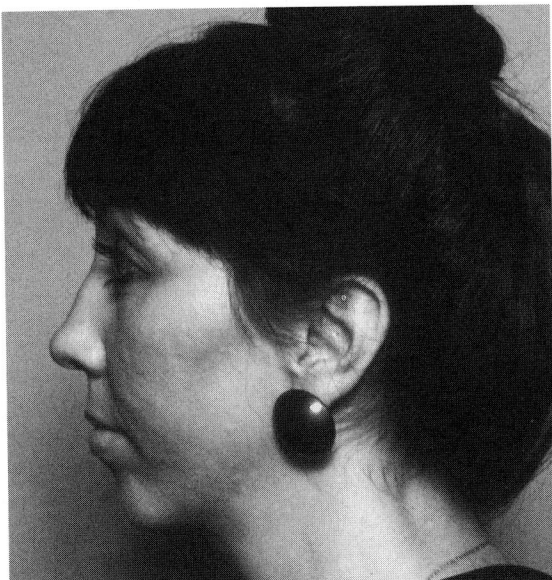
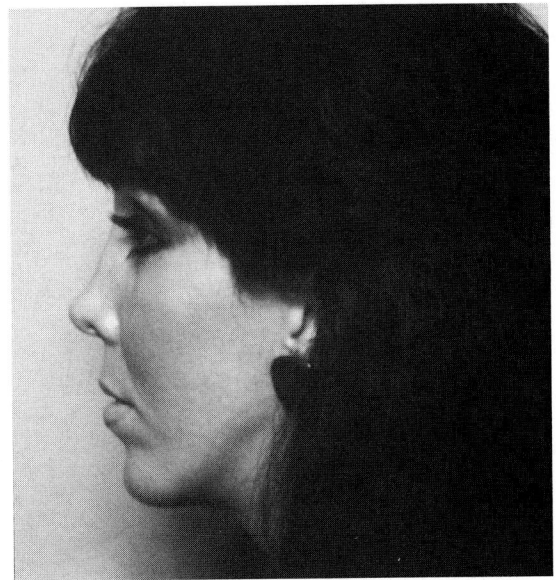

Figure 181.12 This patient had a facelift, rhinoplasty, chin augmentation, and malar implants. **A:** Preoperative view: patient with flattened malar prominence and receding chin. **B:** Postoperative view: facelift with chin implant and cheek implant. Notice the malar prominence and strong chin with shallow melolabial fold. (See also Color Plate 64.)

soft-tissue reaction has been identified with this implant. Bony resorption has been reported to be less with this implant (14). It also can be slightly molded at the operating room table if the surgeon has access to very hot, sterile water.

Disadvantages

It is not as flexible as the Silastic or reinforced e-PTFE. Custom shape and sizing may be a little more difficult. As with other porous implants, if infection develops, the implant must be removed.

Operative Procedure

The intraoral incision is 3 cm in length and is placed just inferior and slightly anterior to the parotid duct. The incision is carried through mucosa and muscle with a no. 15 blade or needle-point unipolar cutting cautery down to the periosteum. Then the periosteum is cut and elevated with an endobrow elevator. The elevation is superior and lateral over the malar and zygoma. The location of the orbital rim and the infraorbital nerve must be kept in mind to avoid

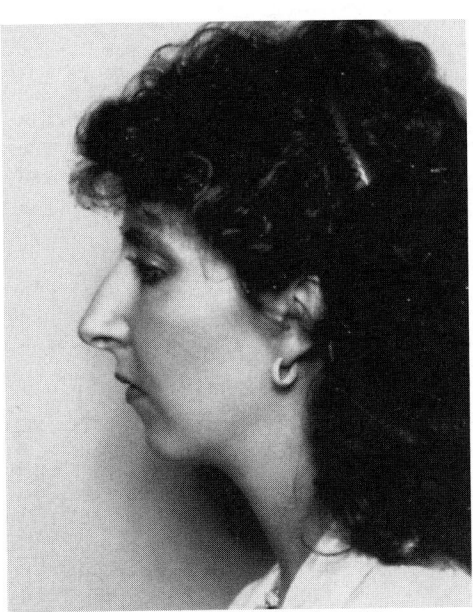
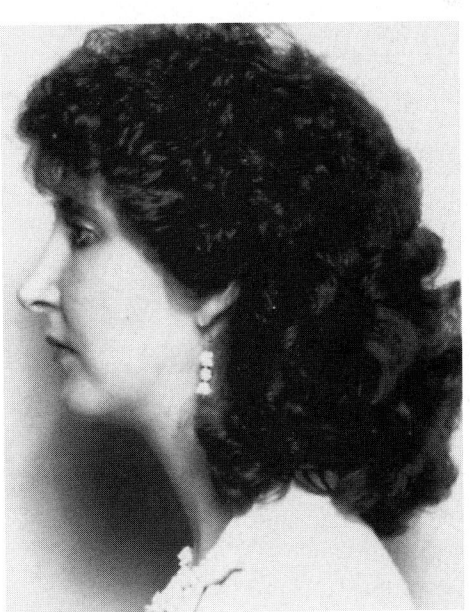

Figure 181.13 This patient had chin augmentation and rhinoplasty. **A:** Preoperative view: patient with a nasal dorsal hump and a hypoplastic mandible. **B:** Postoperative view: rhinoplasty with chin implant.

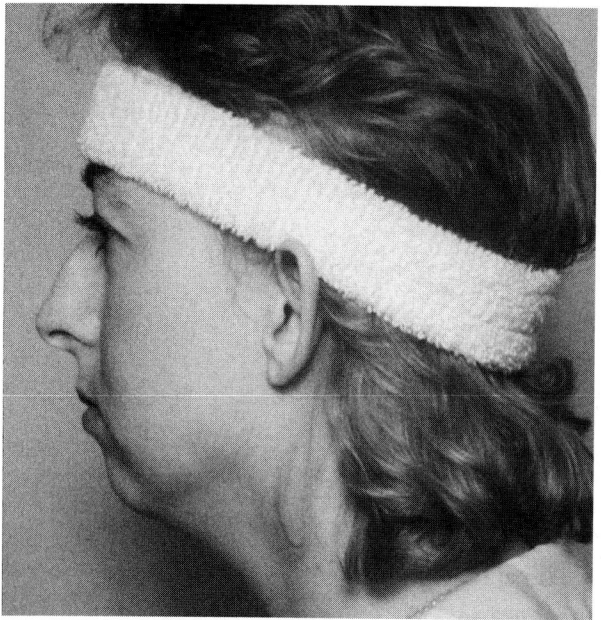
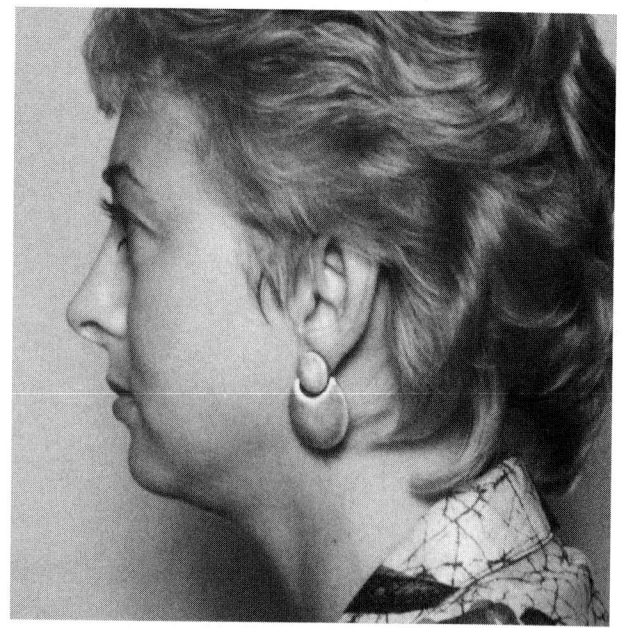

Figure 181.14   This patient had chin augmentation and rhinoplasty. **A:** Preoperative view: nasal dorsal hump and a hypoplastic mandible. **B:** Postoperative view: rhinoplasty with chin implant.

injury to the infraorbital nerve. The pocket must be large enough to allow implant placement. As long as the dissection is under the periosteum or close to the zygomatic arch, the seventh nerve is not in danger of injury. Bleeding is usually minimal, and hemostasis is maintained with the bipolar cautery.

Various sizers then are used to select the proper size implant. The implant is selected and prepared for insertion. If a porous implant is used, it should be pressure loaded with clindamycin and saline (600 mg clindamycin and 30 mL normal saline). The pressure loading is performed with a 50-mL syringe, alternating positive and negative pressure to displace the antibiotic/saline solution into the interstices of the implant (15). The implant then is inserted under an Army-Navy retractor. Care is taken not to compress the implant. After the prominent portion of the

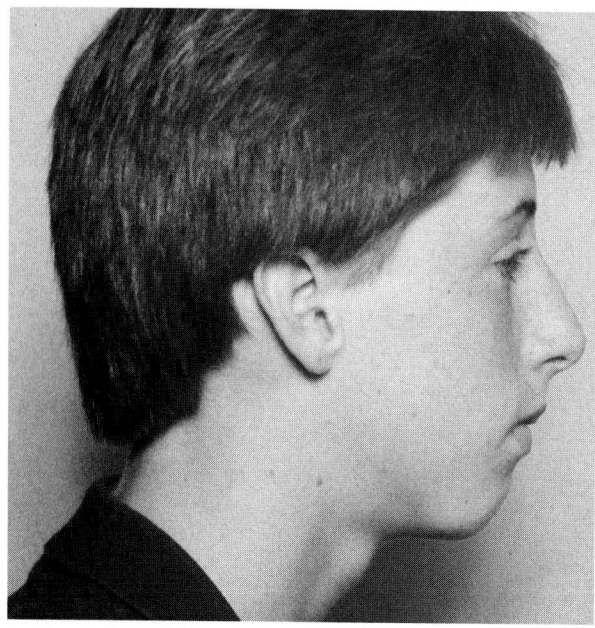
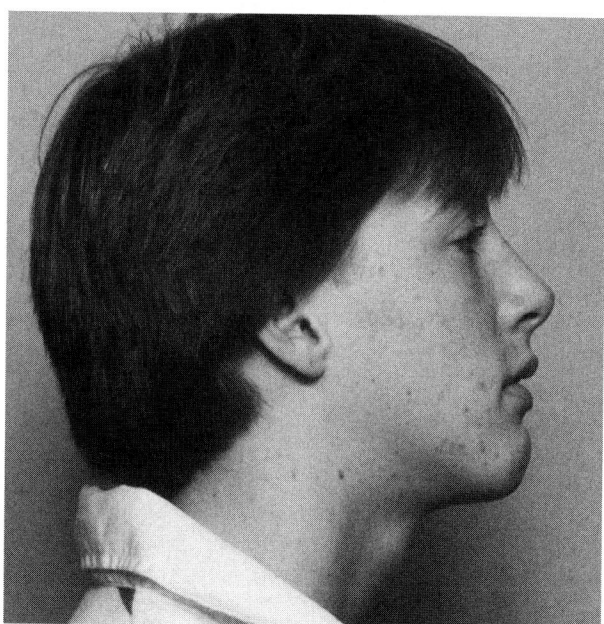

Figure 181.15   This patient had genioplasty and rhinoplasty. **A:** Preoperative view. **B:** Postoperative view.

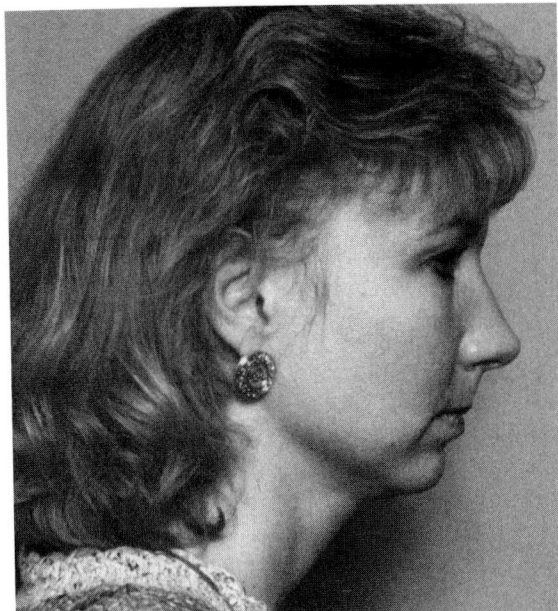 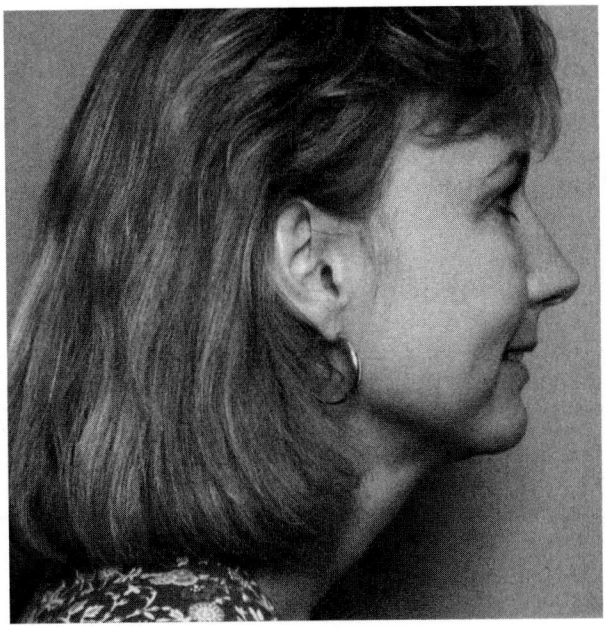

Figure 181.16 Chin augmentation alone. **A:** Preoperative view: hypoplastic mandible makes the nose appear prominent. **B:** Postoperative view: chin implant. The nose appears to be in better proportion to the rest of the face. (See also Color Plate 65.)

implant is in the position corresponding to the prominent area on the cheek previously drawn on the skin, the retractor is removed. With slight pressure, the incision then is approximated and is closed in two layers of 3-0 chromic suture material. If a Silastic malar implant is used, a sizer is inserted to determine the correct size implant (i.e., no. 1, 2, 3, or 4). After selection of the implant, a silk suture is applied to the most lateral portion of the implant and passed through a long Staymen needle or a wire passer, which is passed into the most superolateral part of the pocket and then passed into the hairline. The implant then is pulled and pushed into the appropriate position. The suture is tied over a bolster and left in place for 3 days to stabilize the implant. The incision is closed as described earlier. Ice packs are applied for the next several hours. Antibiotics are given postoperatively for 4 days, and 1 g of cephalothin is given intravenously 30 minutes before insertion of the implants.

Complications

Complications include a malpositioned implant, an implant too large or too small, infection secondary to sinus or tooth infection, asymmetrical implants, a local tissue reaction (rejection), an expanding or infected capsule, and implant exposure (Table 181.8).

A malpositioned implant must be surgically removed and replaced. If no inflammation exists around the implant, it can be removed, reimpregnated with antibiotic (clindamycin), and reinserted. The same procedure would be followed if the implant were too big: it would be removed, reduced, and replaced. If using a porous implant, all connective tissue must be completely freed from around the entire implant before trying to remove it. This differs from a Silastic implant, which slips out easily once the capsule is opened. If the capsule surrounding a Silastic implant becomes so large as to cause asymmetry of the malar prominence, then a capsulotomy is performed, followed by insertion of a smaller implant.

In the case of an asymmetrical malar prominence, a larger implant can be used on one side than on the other. If additional augmentation is needed, a small additional amount of e-PTFE can be added to the implant after it has healed by placing a disk of the e-PTFE superficial to the original implant.

If an infection develops around a porous implant, the implant must be removed, and the source of the infection determined and treated. A new implant should not be reinserted for 6 to 8 weeks. If the infection is a communication

TABLE 181.8 **C** COMPLICATIONS
MALAR IMPLANTS

Implant malposition
Infection or tissue reaction
Infraorbital nerve injury

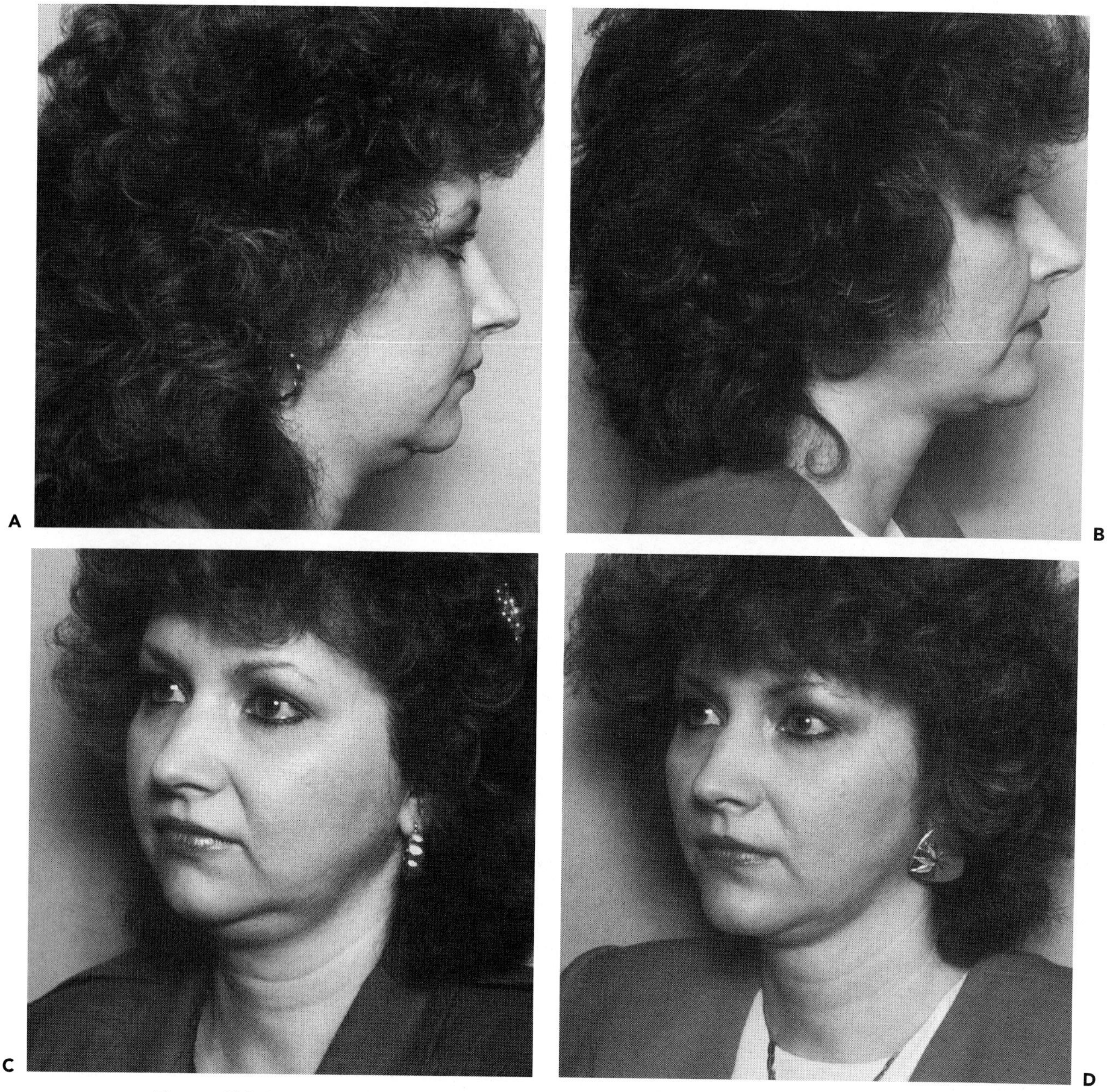

Figure 181.17 Chin augmentation and lipectomy. **A:** Preoperative view: hypoplastic mandible and fullness of fatty tissue in submental area. **B:** Postoperative view: liposuction and insertion of chin implant. Notice the more acute cervical mental angle.

from the anterior wall of the maxillary sinus, the new implant should be Silastic, a nonporous implant.

If the implant used is Silastic and it becomes infected, a short course of antibiotics may be used. If no improvement is seen in 4 to 5 days, the implant should be removed. The area is allowed to heal, and the implant can be reinserted 6 to 8 weeks later.

If exposure of a Silastic implant occurs intraorally, the implant must be removed, the size adjusted, and reinsertion performed. In the case of a porous implant, the implant must be removed and replaced with a new one because of the risk of bacterial invasion into the implant interstices, which, if it occurs, cannot be eradicated with

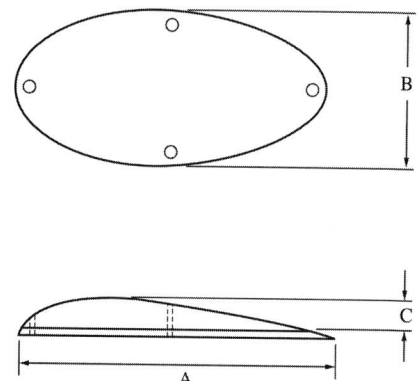

Figure 181.18 Silastic extended malar implant.

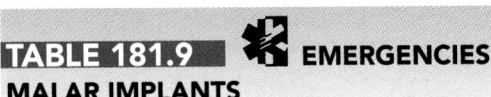

TABLE 181.9 EMERGENCIES

MALAR IMPLANTS

Infection
Implant extrusion

- The malar prominence triangle was created to help surgeons place the implant properly. Malar implants can be made of preformed porous material or silicone.
- Complications of malar implants are a malpositioned implant, exposure of the implant, an implant too large or too small, and an infection around the implant.

antibiotics (Table 181.9). If the maxillary sinus has been fractured, a porous implant should not be used but rather only a solid silicone implant.

HIGHLIGHTS

- Ideal chin projection can be determined by using a perpendicular line to the Frankfort horizontal line, intersecting the lower lip vermilion border.
- A solid silicone implant is an excellent choice for chin augmentation, inserted through an external submental incision. Submental placement is preferred. A two-layer closure is needed, followed by a pressure dressing.
- Complications of chin implants are displaced implant, infection or tissue reaction, periosteal resorption, improper size selection, mental nerve injury, and hypertrophic scar.
- Sliding genioplasty is an alternative to a chin implant but is technically more difficult. It should be considered in patients with insufficient vertical mandibular height, mandibular asymmetry, or failed alloplastic chin implant.
- Malar implants are used to increase the fullness of the malar area. This decreases the depth of the melolabial fold and gives a decisive look.
- Indications for malar implants are deep melolabial folds, a flattened malar prominence, asymmetry of the malar prominence, and as an adjunct to facelifts.

REFERENCES

1. Powell N. *Proportions of the aesthetic face.* New York: Thieme Medical, 1984:41.
2. Frodel J, Sykes J. Chin augmentation/genioplasty: Chin deformities in the aging patient. *Facial Plast Surg* 1996;12(3):279–283.
3. Zide B, Pfeifer T, Longaker M. Chin sugery, I: Augmentation: The allures and the alerts. *Plast Reconstr Surg* 1999;104(6):1843–1862.
4. Godin M, Costa L, Romo T, et al. Gore-Tex chin implants. *Arch Facial Plast Surg* 2003;5:224–227.
5. Gross E, et al. Mersilene mesh chin augmentation. *Arch Facial Plast Surg* 1999;1:183–190.
6. Kent J. Chin and zygomaticomaxillary zugmentation with proplast. *J Oral Surg* 1981;39:912.
7. Park H, Ellis E. A retrospective study of advancement genioplasty. *Oral Surg Oral Med Oral Pathol* 1989;67:487.
8. Yaremchuk M. Improving aesthetic outcomes after alloplastic chin augmentation. *Plast Reconstr Surg* 2003;112(5):1422–1432.
9. Matarasso A, Elias A, Elias R. Labial incompetence: A marker for progressive bone resorption in Silastic chin augmentation. *Plast Reconstr Surg* 1996;98(6):1007–1014.
10. Hinds E. Genioplasty: The versatility of horizontal osteotomy. *J Oral Surg* 1969;27:690.
11. Steed D. Surgery of the chin. In: Holt R, Bailey R, eds. *Surgery in the mandible.* New York: Thieme Medical, 1987:117.
12. Epker B, Wolford L. *Dentofacial deformities.* St. Louis: CV Mosby, 1980:119.
13. Binder W. Submalar augmentation: A procedure to enhance rhytidectomy. *Ann Plast Surg* 1990;24:200.
14. Golshani S, Zhoa Z, Prasad G. Applications of Medpor porous polyethylene in facial augmentation. *Am J Cosmetic Surg* 1994;11:105–109.
15. Goldberg J, Silver W. Antibiotic pressure loading of PTFE facial implants: An adjunct to perioperative antibiotics. Presented at the American Academy of Facial and Plastic Reconstructive Surgery, Fall Meeting, 1996.

Chemical Peeling

J. Gregory Staffel

History assures us that the struggle against aging skin is as inevitable as it is pervasive. Medicine has played a role in this struggle in part by taking advantage of the skin's unique ability to generate a healthier version of itself after limited surface injury. Controlled wounding of the skin, which stimulates a more youthful appearance, may be performed by mechanical (dermabrasion), thermal (laser), or chemical means. This chapter deals with the limited destruction and regeneration of skin by application of certain chemicals, a process known as chemical peeling and also referred to as chemexfoliation.

PHOTODAMAGE

The most common indication for chemical peeling is photodamage. This occurs when skin is exposed to ultraviolet (UV) light in the form of sunlight (or tanning beds). Histologic changes include a thickened stratum corneum, a thinned stratum spinosum, disorganized epidermal maturation, irregular melanin dispersion, decreased dermal collagen, decreased dermal glycosaminoglycans, and disorganized dermal elastin. Malignant transformation may also eventually occur. Clinically, the skin becomes rough, sallow, wrinkled, and mottled.

Topical Therapy

Prevention is the best treatment for photodamage, and patients should use sun precautions including sunscreens that block both UVA and UVB rays. Topical therapy starts with tretinoin (Retin-A, Renova). Originally used for acne treatment, patients undergoing long-term therapy noted improvement in their fine wrinkles, eventually causing the media to label this an "antiwrinkle cream." Prolonged use of tretinoin has been shown to thin the stratum corneum; thicken the stratum spinosum; disperse melanin; restore order to keratinocyte maturation; and cause deposition of new collagen, elastin, and blood vessels. This decreases fine wrinkles, evens pigmentation, and smoothes the skin. Because it can be drying, tretinoin has been mixed with a moisturizer and marketed as Renova. Tretinoin can also cause sun sensitivity and is classed as pregnancy category C.

Alpha hydroxy acids at the appropriate concentrations and pH have similar, although less dramatic, effects. They work well in combination with tretinoin and are often less irritating. These acids in lower doses are used in many over-the-counter products. Hydroquinone inhibits tyrosinase, an enzyme used in the production of melanin. Similar compounds include kojic acid and azelaic acid. These are used in cases of uneven pigmentation and melasma.

Concomitant use of tretinoin, an alpha hydroxy acid, and a melanin synthesis inhibitor forms the basis for topical skin therapy, but long-term compliance is an issue in our time-pressed society. When topical therapy has reached the limit of its effectiveness in treating photodamage, actinic preneoplasia, or melasma, a chemical peel may be indicated (1).

CHEMICAL PEELING

Chemical peeling involves the controlled wounding of skin to a desired level with the subsequent regeneration of a more youthful appearance. Destruction of the stratum corneum leaves the regenerated skin feeling smoother. Wounding down to the epidermal basement membrane (where the melanocytes and melanosomes lie) leaves the healed skin lighter and more evenly pigmented. Destruction through the papillary dermis to the upper-reticular dermis results in smoothing and lightening of the skin and in deposition of new collagen, elastin, and glycosaminoglycans with subsequent reduction in fine wrinkles. Wounding to the mid-reticular dermis will stimulate deposition of significant amounts of new collagen, causing even more pronounced wrinkle reduction. Destruction deep to the middle layer of the reticular dermis can cause new collagen formation to become so exuberant and disorganized that the result is a scar.

Chemical peels are classified by the depth of expected histologic necrosis. Usually, peels are called superficial (involving the epidermis), medium (through the papillary dermis and to the upper-reticular dermis), and deep (to the mid-reticular dermis). Upper-reticular dermal peels are referred to as medium depth by some authors and deep by others (2,3). The depth of a peel is affected and can be controlled by multiple factors including the chemicals used, their concentration, the technique of application, the condition of the skin, and individual patient sensitivity.

Superficial Chemical Peels

The most superficial form of a chemical peel involves only the stratum corneum. Various acids may be used to remove the stratum corneum. The most popular is probably glycolic acid. At low concentrations this may be applied to the face for a few minutes and then washed off with water or "neutralized" with a sodium bicarbonate solution. The patient has a slight stinging sensation and may have a slight flush. Patients like that their skin feels smoother, it has a nice glow afterward, and there is no "down time." These peels are often performed repeatedly on a weekly, biweekly, or monthly basis. Other compounds that may be used include Jessner solution (lactic acid, salicylic acid, and resorcinol 14% wt./vol., respectively, in ethanol), resorcinol, or 10% trichloroacetic acid (TCA). Peels that include the entire stratum corneum and go further toward the basement membrane may cause a light desquamation over the ensuing 2–3 days. These peels may be performed with slightly higher concentrations of glycolic acid, a few more coats of Jessner solution, or a slightly stronger concentration of TCA.

Medium-Depth Chemical Peels

A medium-depth chemical peel extends through the basement membrane and may extend through the papillary dermis to the upper-reticular dermis. Because a medium-depth peel extends beyond the basement membrane where the melanocytes and melanosomes lie it usually will lighten the skin and even out pigmentary changes. New collagen may also be formed so that fine wrinkles are improved. The amount of new collagen deposited depends on the depth of the peel and on individual patient response.

Scarring may occur with any subepidermal wound, although it remains somewhat unpredictable and poorly understood. Peels performed with concentrations of TCA higher than 40% may have a higher incidence of scarring (2–4). For this reason some authors have tried to augment the effect of 35% TCA in the papillary and upper-reticular dermis by pretreating the skin with either Jessner solution (as described by Monheit) (4), glycolic acid (as described by Coleman) (5), or solid CO_2 (as described by Brody) (3). The idea is to disrupt the epidermis to allow deeper penetration by the TCA while minimizing the risk of scarring. These peels have proved to be effective and popular. The Obagi "blue peel" involves the combination of a proprietary yucca plant extract and some blue coloring with TCA and falls into this same category of medium-depth peeling.

Most authors pretreat patients for several weeks with tretinoin (Retin-A) and possibly hydroquinone and a glycolic acid product prior to a medium-depth peel. Pretreatment with tretinoin may even the peel and speed reepithelialization, although actively irritated skin should not be peeled. After a medium-depth peel usually the skin will turn dark brown and then exfoliate in 4–7 days. Afterward, the new skin is quite pink. Usually a patient is socially

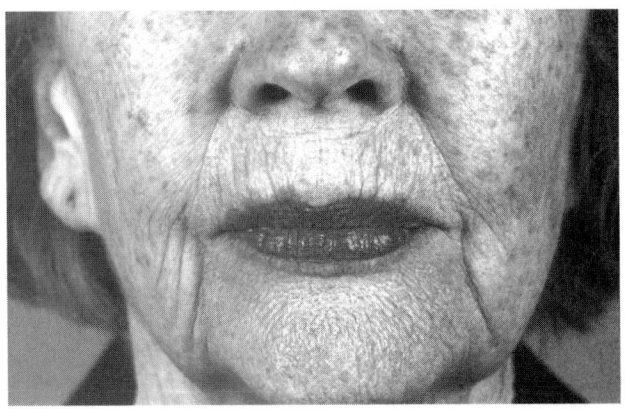 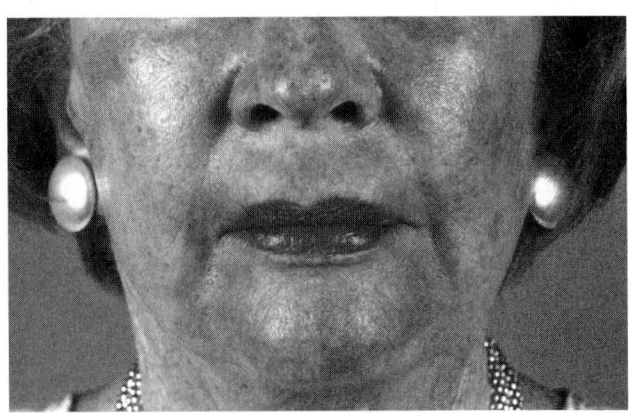

Figure 182A.1 This patient underwent a revision facelift. The perioral wrinkles were treated with wire-brush dermabrasion by hand. The cheeks were treated with a Jessner 35% TCA (trichloroacetic acid) peel. **A:** Preoperative. **B:** One month postoperative. Photographs courtesy of J. Gregory Staffel, MD.

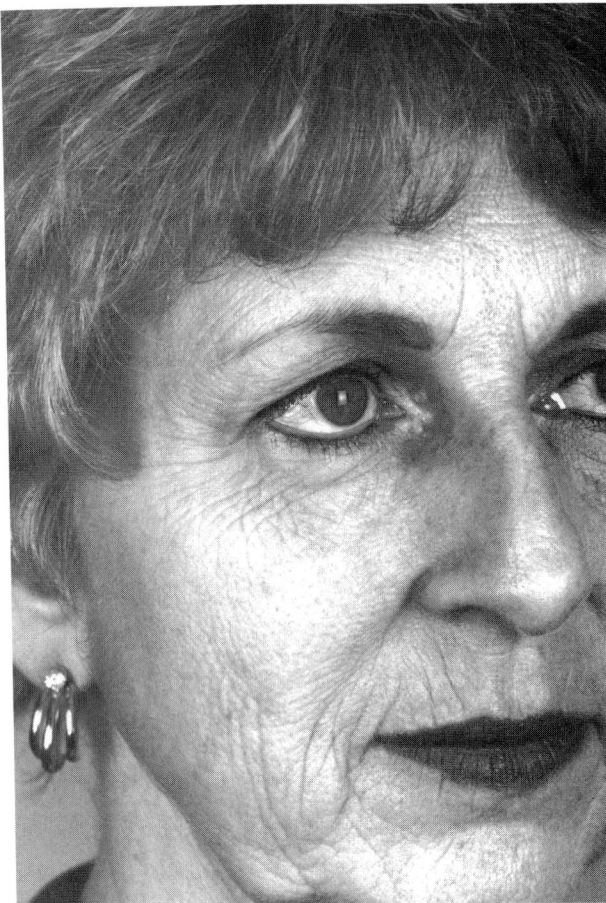
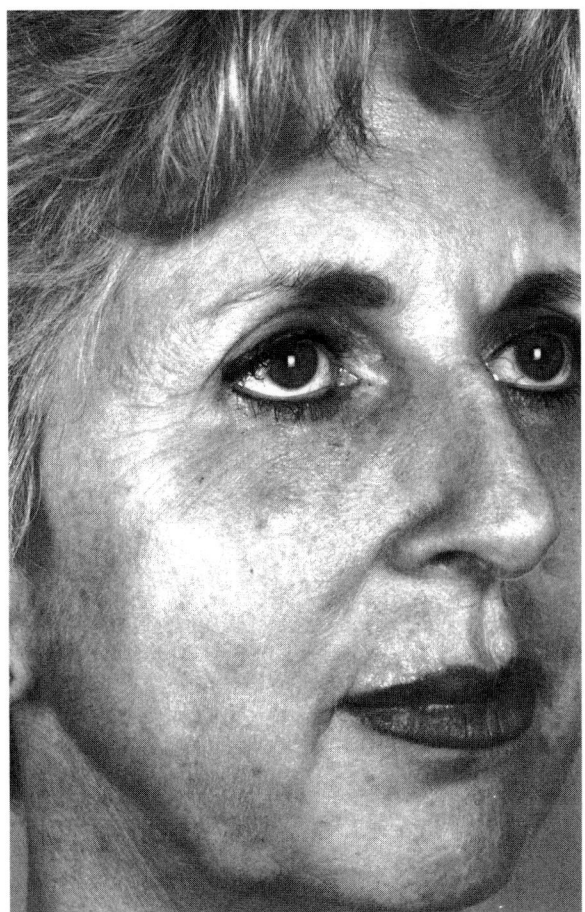

A   B

Figure 182A.2 This patient underwent a facial peel with 33% phenol and 1.1% croton oil. **A:** Preoperative. **B:** Three months postoperative. Upper blepharoplasty also performed. Photographs courtesy of J. Gregory Staffel, MD.

incapacitated for about 7 days after a medium peel, maybe longer if they do not want to wear makeup (Fig. 182A.1).

Deep Chemical Peels

Deep chemical peels usually extend to the mid-reticular dermis. The standard deep peel is the Baker-Gordon peel. This consists of a "classic" formula of 3 cc of 88% phenol, 2 cc of water, 8 drops of Septisol, and 3 drops of croton oil, representing roughly a mixture of phenol 49% and croton oil 2.1%. Phenol and water are nonmiscible, and the solution must be agitated prior to application. It is applied with cotton-tipped applicators to one section of the degreased face at a time. Slow application to regional subunits limits systemic absorption of phenol, preventing arrhythmias. The frosting is immediate and long-lasting. Some occlude the peel with tape, others with petrolatum ointment, whereas others use no occlusion. The swelling is intense after this peel as the epithelium releases over the first couple of days. Reepithelialization takes more than a week, with ointment being applied constantly and with serous exudate being washed off by the patient at intervals of 2–3 hours. The skin

is very red after this peel and eventually fades over months. Some hypopigmentation is an expected sequela of this peel, varying in degree by patient. Because the peel goes down into the reticular dermis, new collagen formation is robust and long-lasting. Fine and deep wrinkles respond well (Fig. 182A.2 and Table 182A.1).

FACTORS AFFECTING THE DEPTH OF A PEEL

Agent and Concentration

The agent and concentration used are two of the biggest factors affecting the depth of a chemical peel. Usually, superficial peels are performed with glycolic acid or TCA 10–20%. Jessner solution by itself will also give a superficial peel. Medium-depth peels are usually performed with TCA 25–35%, often used in combination with Jessner solution, glycolic acid, or solid CO_2. Some classify an 88% phenol peel as medium in depth, whereas others contend that if this is rubbed long enough, it will yield a deep peel.

TABLE 182A.1

INDICATION AND DEPTH OF PEELS

Level	Layer	Indications (Photodamage, Dyschromias, and Acne)	Agent (Depth is technique and patient dependent as well.)
Very superficial	Stratum corneum	Rough texture Scaly skin	Resorcinol 20–30% × 2–20 min., Jessner, CO_2, Retin-A, 5-FU (fluorouracil), alpha hydroxy acids, TCA 10–20%, glycolic acid 30–50% × 1–2 min
Superficial	Basement membrane (basal cell layer)	Some lentigines Epidermal melasma Acne	TCA 10–30%
Medium	Papillary dermis to upper-reticular dermis	Ephelides Senile and solar lentigines Melasma Postinflammatory hyperpigmentation Actinic keratoses Epidermal premalignant neoplasia	Jessner + 35% TCA CO_2 + 35% TCA 70% glycolic acid + 35% TCA TCA 35–50% Glycolic acid 70% Phenol–croton oil (Hetter variations) Phenol 88%
Deep	To mid-reticular dermis	Above plus Deep and fine rhytids	Phenol–croton oil 49%/2.1% (Baker–Gordon) occluded or unoccluded Phenol–croton oil 33%/1.1% (one of Hetter's formulas)

TCA, trichloroacetic acid.

Deeper peels may be achieved with phenol–croton oil preparations including a standard Baker-Gordon formula. Hetter has modified the Baker-Gordon formula and technique to yield a range of depths (6–9).

Condition of Skin

Recently irritated skin will react more strongly to a peel. This includes patients who have had recent facial waxing, depilation, electrolysis, or facial surgery. If the skin is irritated or actively exfoliating from tretinoin pretreatment, then it may be stopped several days before the peel. Some pretreat with tretinoin prior to phenol–croton oil peels and others do not.

Technique

Prepeel Degreasing
Before most peels the skin is degreased using a sponge with alcohol or acetone. If the sponge is vigorously rubbed over the skin, it may remove a significant amount of the stratum corneum, allowing deeper penetration.

Applicator
Peeling agents may be applied using various methods including a paint brush, cotton swabs, makeup-type sponges, 2 × 2 sponges, and rectal swabs.

Rubbing
With some peels the agent is rubbed on until the appropriate amount of frosting of the skin is noted. The harder and longer one rubs, the deeper the peel will go.

Time
The longer an agent is in contact with the skin, the deeper it may be expected to penetrate up to a point. This is especially true with glycolic acid.

Occlusion
Phenol–croton oil peels may be occluded with either tape or petrolatum ointment. Some believe this deepens the peel.

Individual Sensitivity

Patient response to peels can be generalized to an extent, but each person's response to a peel is unique. The same peel performed in the same way on two patients with similar skin types may yield somewhat different results. Thus, some patients' wrinkles respond well to medium-depth TCA peeling, whereas other patients' do not. Some patients will develop scarring with a peel, whereas others will not. In fact, the response can be so variable that in the past some authors recommended performing a test patch on an unobtrusive area prior to performing a peel. This has been abandoned because the test patches were not predictive.

AFTERCARE

For superficial peels aftercare consists simply of avoiding the sun and any other skin irritants. Medium-depth peels will cause significant exfoliation. Ointment may be used to keep the skin lubricated during this time. The most important aspect of care after a medium-depth peel is for the patient not to grab, pick, scratch, or help the dead skin to peel in any way. The shedding epidermis should be allowed to "release" on its own. If it is pulled off, it may leave a scar. When the underlying epithelium is adequately healed, the superficial layers will release.

Deeper chemical peels require more intensive care. If the peel has been occluded with tape, then usually the physician will remove this in 1 to 2 days. There is a tremendous amount of exudate after a deeper peel, which forms crusts on the skin if allowed to dry. For this reason patients are instructed to use some type of bland ointment on the skin as often as every 2 hours during the first several days. Neomycin-containing ointments are to be avoided because the incidence of topical sensitivity is high. It is often easiest for patients to wash their face and apply the ointment in the shower. Care is intense for the first several days. Eventually the epithelium will regrow and prevent the transudation of serum. Once this occurs there is no more crusting and ointment use may be curtailed.

The healed skin will be sensitive to sunlight, and appropriate precautions should be taken for several months. Sunlight may also induce hyperpigmentation. Makeup may be needed to camouflage redness for several months after a deeper peel. Hydroquinone may be required after reepithelialization to prevent hyperpigmentation.

COMPLICATIONS

See Tables 182A.2 and 182A.3.

Infection

Bacterial (*Staphylococcus aureus*, *Streptococcus*, *Pseudomonas*), herpetic, and fungal (*Candida*) infections are possible after medium and deep peels. Both phenol and TCA are bacterici-

TABLE 182A.2   COMPLICATIONS CHEMICAL PEELING

Prolonged erythema/pruritus
Hyperpigmentation or hypopigmentation
Infection
Scarring
Poor physician–patient relationship
Cardiac, renal, hepatic toxicity

TABLE 182A.3   RELATED EMERGENCIES CHEMICAL PEELING

Emergency	Treatment
Arrhythmia	Prehydrate, stop phenol application, supportive
Spill	Flush eyes if necessary, solution in reserve
Infection	Culture and treat, aggressive wound care
Scar	Topical/injected steroids, topical silicone, pulsed-dye laser

dal, and almost all bacterial and fungal infections are the result of suboptimal postoperative wound care by the patient. Some authors give prophylactic antiviral medications to all patients, whereas others limit prophylaxis to patients with a history of herpes labialis. Postoperative antibiotics may be given for medium and deep peels as well. Occasionally dilute vinegar washes are recommended to lower the pH to a level intolerable to *Pseudomonas*. Any wound that is not healing properly should undergo bacterial, viral, and fungal cultures with subsequent antimicrobial therapy. Extremely rare infectious complications include toxic shock syndrome (3).

Hyperpigmentation

The Fitzpatrick system classifies skin based on the typical response at 24 hours and 1 week after exposure to an early summer sun (Table 182A.4) (10). Postinflammatory hyperpigmentation is more likely with darker (Fitzpatrick IV–VI) skin. This can be treated with hydroquinone for several weeks before the peel and several months after reepithelialization is complete. This is often combined with tretinoin, an alpha hydroxy acid, and a mild steroid cream. Because the sun stimulates melanin production, it is to be avoided both before and after a peel, and sunscreens must be used during this time. Estrogen-containing compounds and pregnancy can exacerbate hyperpigmentation. In recalcitrant cases, repeeling is an option. Nevi may also turn darker with peeling.

Hypopigmentation

Hypopigmentation may occur after deep peeling and is not undesirable in limited amounts. Hypopigmentation is more common with phenol–croton oil peels than with TCA peels. If it does occur, the contrast between peeled and nonpeeled skin is more apparent in darker skin (Fitzpatrick IV–VI) and very light, freckled skin (Fitzpatrick I). Feathering of the peel at the edges can help camouflage the transition. Carbon dioxide laser resurfacing was initially felt to cause less hypopigmentation than peeling, but long-term follow-up has dampened the initial enthusiasm for this concept.

TABLE 182A.4
FITZPATRICK CLASSIFICATION

Skin Type	Color	Reaction at 24 hr	Result at 1 Week
I	White	Painful burn	No tan
II	White	Painful burn	Light tan
III	White	Slightly tender burn	Moderate tan
IV	White	No burn	Good tan
V	Brown	Almost never	Tan
VI	Black	Never	Tan

After their first exposure to 45–60 min of noontime sun in early summer:
"How painful is your burn at 24 hours?"
"How much tan will you develop in 1 week?"

Scarring

Scarring is poorly understood, but it can be aggravated by a postoperative infection leading to delayed healing. Any nonhealing areas are immediately cultured, and appropriate therapy is instituted. Areas of delayed healing may benefit from artificial wound dressings.

Predisposition to scarring may include recent or subsequent treatment with isotretinoin (Accutane). Waiting ranges of 6 months to 2 years after therapy and prior to performing a peel have been reported. Scarring has also been reported when isotretinoin treatment was started several months after a peeled or dermabraded area has already healed (3). Previously radiated skin and recent facial surgery may also predispose to scarring. Any history of facial keloids should be taken into consideration. Skin should not be concomitantly undermined and deeply peeled. Phenol–croton oil peels may be safely performed on the lower lids, however, after a transconjunctival lower blepharoplasty.

For unknown reasons certain locations are more prone to scarring. The area along the lower border of the mandible extending back to the angle of the mandible seems to be a bit more prone to scarring with TCA. The area just beside and around the mouth seems to be a bit more prone to scarring with phenol–croton oil peels. The neck should not be peeled deeply because it has a much lower density of appendages, which serve as reservoirs of skin cells that regenerate new epidermis.

A persistent area of redness in an area that is otherwise healing well is considered an incipient hypertrophic scar. Topical steroids and topical silicone are instituted. Steroid injections and pulsed-dye laser therapy may also be appropriate.

Prolonged Redness

Prolonged erythema and intermittent flushing with emotional or environmental changes may occur based on individual response. This resolves with time, but it might inconvenience the patient who is unwilling to wear makeup (11).

Persistent Wrinkles

Persistent wrinkles are not a complication—they are sequelae of which the patient should be informed prior to the peel. Pigment, wrinkles, and texture all respond differently in different patients.

Miscellaneous Complications

Phenol toxicity may cause arrhythmias, and for this reason phenol peels are performed slowly and by regional units while the patient is kept well-hydrated to promote excretion of the phenol and its metabolites. This also requires adequate kidney and liver function, which are evaluated along with an electrocardiogram prior to a full-face phenol-containing peel. Patients are monitored during and after a full-face peel containing phenol. Laryngeal edema responding to warm mist has been reported after a phenol–croton oil peel. Contact dermatitis may occur during the healing phase, especially on exposure to neomycin-containing ointments. Acne may flare. Milia may be unroofed as needed. Textural changes in the skin may require further treatment (3).

SPECIAL CONSIDERATIONS

Certain issues are unique to chemical peeling. The ultimate outcome of the peel depends heavily on patient cooperation. Patients who are not compliant should be avoided, as should patients who are psychiatrically unstable. Preparation of the chemicals to be used should be precise and well-documented. Commercial preparations of TCA, Jessner solution, and glycolic acid are inexpensive, are well standardized, and avoid inherent mixing errors. Drop size in mixing croton oil–containing solutions is important and should be standardized (see later). Solution containers should be kept away from the patient during the peeling process. The eyes should be meticulously avoided, and preparations should be made for immediate irrigation should any peeling agent be inadvertently introduced. Small medicine cups are easily turned over, especially on unstable Mayo stands. Peeling solution may be placed in a small, closed, plastic bottle that allows agitation and may be opened to introduce cotton-tipped applicators or to pour out solution. Phenol–croton oil solutions are usually mixed just prior to a peel. One way to avoid the need for remixing in case of a spill is to prepare enough solution for two peels and keep one solution in reserve while performing the peel.

Patients who have undergone a medium or deep peel have a frightening appearance afterward and a relatively prolonged postoperative course. Comments by well-meaning family and friends may plant seeds of distrust that can blossom into litigation. Peel patients should be psychologically stable, compliant, willing to stay out of the sun, and willing to wear makeup after the peel. Good patient communication and documentation are important.

MYTHS AND MISPERCEPTIONS

Previous dogma has held that phenol in higher concentration stops its own penetration by coagulating the protein in the skin and that croton oil was a relatively minor component of the peeling formula. Hetter has disproved the paradoxical penetration of phenol dogma and has shown that croton oil is important enough in determining the predicted depth of a peel that drop size should be standardized. Based on Hetter's experience some have simply decreased the number of drops from 3 to 2 (or 1) in the classic Baker-Gordon formula, keeping other variables the same to produce a lighter peel (12). Published reports of the results of this technique are awaited. As a bit of trivia, many authors attribute the Baker-Gordon formula to Baker's first article, but in fact the first two formulas published in 1961 and 1962 are quite different from the "classic" one published first by Batstone and Millard in 1968 and then by Baker and Gordon in 1971 (13–16).

WHERE PEELING FITS IN

Skin resurfacing may be performed by mechanical (dermabrasion), thermal (laser), or chemical means. Experience has shown that acne scars usually respond better to dermabrasion and laser resurfacing than to chemical peeling (17). Although many peel the upper lip, wire-brush dermabrasion performed by hand can also be very effective. However, peeling is effective for dyschromias, and many maintain that nothing has been shown to be better than a classic Baker peel for deep rhytids. Varying the phenol and

croton oil concentration has introduced more control over the depth of these peels, much as using combinations of modalities has allowed more control with the medium-depth techniques. Lasers continue to evolve but thus far are still cumbersome, are expensive, and have not yet been shown to be better than chemical peeling for many patients with photodamage and dyschromias.

HIGHLIGHTS

- Peeling is for photodamage, premalignant changes, and dyschromias.
- The patient should be stable, compliant, and willing to wear makeup and avoid the sun.
- Avoid recently irritated skin, recent Accutane therapy, and undermined skin (deep peels).
- Take spill precautions and have reserve solutions premixed.
- Early, aggressive treatment of infection and scars.

REFERENCES

1. Rubin MG. *Manual of chemical peels, superficial and medium depth.* Philadelphia: J.B. Lippincott, 1995.
2. Halaas YP. Medium depth peels. *Facial Plast Surg Clin North Am* 2004;297–303.
3. Brody HJ. *Chemical peeling and resurfacing.* St. Louis: Mosby, 1997.
4. Monheit GD. The Jessner's-trichloroacetic acid peel; an enhanced medium-depth chemical peel. *Dermatol Clin* 1995;13(2):277–283.
5. Coleman WP, Futrell JM. The glycolic acid trichloroacetic acid peel. *J Dermatol Surg Oncol* 1994;20:76–80.
6. Hetter GP. An examination of the phenol–croton oil peel: part I. Dissecting the formula. *Plast Reconstr Surg* 2000;105:227–239.
7. Hetter GP. An examination of the phenol–croton oil peel: part II. The lay peelers and their croton oil formulas. *Plast Reconstr Surg* 2000;105:240–251.
8. Hetter GP. An examination of the phenol–croton oil peel: part III. The plastic surgeons' role. *Plast Reconstr Surg* 2000;105:752–763.
9. Hetter GP. An examination of the phenol–croton oil peel: part IV. Face peel with different concentrations of phenol and croton oil. *Plast Reconstr Surg* 2000;105:1061–1087.
10. Fitzpatrick TB. The validity and practicality of sun-reactive skin types I through VI. *Arch Dermatol* 1988;124:869–871.
11. Maloney BP, Millman B, Monheit G, et al. The etiology of prolonged erythema after chemical peel. *Dermatol Surg* 1988;24:337–341.
12. Mendelsohn JE. Update on chemical peels. *Otolaryngol Clin North Am* 2002;35(1):55–72.
13. Baker TJ, Gordon HL. The ablation of rhitides by chemical means; a preliminary report. *J Fla Med Assoc* 1961;48:451–454.
14. Baker TJ. Chemical face peeling and rhytidectomy. *Plast Reconstr Surg* 1962;29:199–207.
15. Batstone JH, Millard DR. An endorsement of facial chemosurgery. *Br J Plast Surg* 1968;21:193–199.
16. Baker TJ, Gordon HL. Chemical face peeling and dermabrasion. *Surg Clin North Am* 1971;51:387–401
17. Lawrence N, Brody H, Alt T. Chemical Peeling. In: Coleman WP, Hanke CW, Alt TH, et al., eds. *Cosmetic surgery of the skin.* St. Louis: Mosby; 1997:85–111.

Laser Skin Resurfacing

Paul J. Carniol

There are currently 75 million baby boomers—adults born between 1946 and 1964. Their impact on the economy in general and facial plastic surgery in particular is significant. Baby boomers increasingly are looking for ways to maintain their youthful appearance and achieve facial skin rejuvenation. Some of these adults are unhappy with the appearance of their acne scars. Others express growing concerns that wrinkles, skin damage, and aging changes in facial appearance are negatively affecting their personal and professional lives. As these trends continue during the next decade, the public will insist on new, effective, and safe technology for skin rejuvenation. To meet these needs, a proliferation of new technology is likely to result, and evaluating skin rejuvenation technology outcomes will become increasingly challenging. This will continue to be the case until there is a single technology that yields desirable results for most patients.

Available skin rejuvenation technologies fall into the following categories: ablative lasers, nonablative lasers, fractionated laser, intense pulsed light, and radiofrequency devices. Lasers for treatment of wrinkles and acne scars are considered ablative, resurfacing, and nonablative lasers. When using a laser or other device for skin rejuvenation it is important to follow all of the proper safety precautions.

LASER SAFETY

Skin rejuvenation lasers fall under the Federal Laser Product Performance Standard as Class IV devices. These lasers can be hazardous to the eyes and skin. There is a risk of injury from a direct laser beam as well as a reflected laser beam. Furthermore, there is an associated risk of fire. The current standards for laser safety are described in detail in other publications (1,2).

Before using a laser it is important that all personnel and the patient have the proper protective eyewear in place. Any windows in the room in which the laser is used must be covered to prevent any accidental eye injury. Furthermore, there should be a sign outside the room that describes the laser in use including the laser wavelength. Protective eyewear should also be available outside the laser room. The eyewear should be designed to prevent injury from the laser wavelength(s). The optical density (OD) of the eyewear and the wavelength that it protects against should be marked on the eyewear. The OD is an inverse exponential measure. Thus if the OD is marked as five, then only one ten-thousandth of the energy at the indicated wavelength will get through the protective lenses. It is important to try to avoid a direct laser eye injury because the lenses may not be completely protective. When using a laser on the face it is best for the patient to wear metallic, nonreflective protective eye shields. Laser safety standards were developed and revised by the Laser Institute of America (Orlando, FL) Accredited Standards Committee (of which I am a member). These standards currently are being reviewed by the American National Standards Institute.

RESURFACING LASERS

Currently there are two main types of ablative resurfacing lasers: the carbon dioxide (10,600-nm) and the erbium: YAG (2,940-nm) laser. Each of these laser wavelengths is absorbed by water. Water is the chromophore for these lasers. The ablative lasers work by a process that is known as photothermolysis. The laser's energy is absorbed by the water component of the tissues. A high-energy fluence results in rapidly heating the intracellular water to 100°C. Once this occurs, the water boils and the cell is vaporized. The greater the percentage of water content in the tissue, the greater the resurfacing laser absorption by that tissue.

The effect of the resurfacing laser on the tissue varies with the absorption coefficient. This absorption coefficient of water for the erbium laser is 10 times the absorption coefficient for the carbon dioxide laser. This means that the energy from the erbium laser is absorbed 10 times greater than the carbon dioxide laser.

Because there is a lower absorption with the carbon dioxide laser, the intracellular water heating is slower and there is greater heat spread to the adjacent tissues. This results in greater adjacent tissue injury. Associated with this is a slower recovery and longer redness after carbon dioxide laser treatment than after erbium laser treatment. However, this adjacent thermal injury also has a greater stimulating effect on collagen production. The carbon dioxide laser is also hemostatic. This contrasts with the erbium laser that is not hemostatic.

The carbon dioxide laser also produces thermally induced tissue tightening (3). The amount of tightening varies and is not predictable. This tightening is an added benefit for many areas of facial resurfacing. However, when resurfacing eyelids this must be taken into consideration because there is a risk of postresurfacing ectropion.

The substance that absorbs the laser energy is called chromophore. These resurfacing laser wavelengths have one clinically significant chromophore: water. Other lasers such as the 532- and 595-nm vascular lasers have more than one competing chromophore. For those vascular lasers the chromophores are both oxyhemoglobin and melanin. When lasers with these wavelengths are used for treating vascular lesions, the presence of competing chromophore, melanin, makes treating the vascular lesions more difficult. The undesirable absorption by melanin when treating vascular lesions can result in postlaser dyschromia.

These resurfacing lasers are used to perform a limited and controlled skin ablation. In this process, the top layers of the skin are removed to reduce rhytids, actinic changes, superficial lesions, and acne scars based on two mechanisms: first, by vaporization, they remove or decrease the undesired pathology, then they give additional benefit by stimulating neocollagen production with healing. The greater the adjacent tissue thermal injury, the greater the production of neocollagen.

Resurfacing lasers are quite effective in reducing rhytids and acne scars. In one series of 31 patients wrinkle depth was reduced an average of 91% 6 weeks after the procedure. This wrinkle reduction persisted 2 years after treatment, with a mean wrinkle reduction of 87% (4).

Most surgeons use either a carbon dioxide or an erbium laser. However, it has also been shown that additional laser resurfacing with an erbium laser facilitates recovery from carbon dioxide laser resurfacing. This is performed not to increase the depth of the resurfacing but to remove some of the residual debris and adjacent thermally injured tissues. It is postulated that in this way the inflammatory response associated with healing is reduced.

Although these lasers are effective in reducing rhytids and acne scars, they have decreased in popularity over

TABLE 182B.1

FITZPATRICK SKIN TYPE CLASSIFICATION

Skin Type	Reaction to Sun Exposure	Skin Pigment
I	Burns, never tans	White, pale
II	Typically burns, may develop light tan	Thite
III	Tans, may burn	White, brown or hazel eyes
IV	Tans, rarely burns	White, darker skin
V	Tans	Light brown
VI	Tans	Dark brown

several years. This may be the result of patients not desiring to have pinkness potentially for weeks after laser resurfacing. In one series of patients who had undergone laser resurfacing, 88% of patients considered the results very good. However even with this result, 77% of the patients stated that they would not be willing to have another laser resurfacing procedure (5).

When evaluating patients for laser resurfacing it is important to consider their skin type. The Fitzpatrick skin classification system (Table 182B.1) has six levels and is based on the reaction of the patient's skin to sun exposure. The lowest skin type has a white-pale appearance, whereas the highest skin type has dark-brown pigmentation. The higher the skin type, the greater the chance of developing dyschromia after laser resurfacing. Because of the higher risk of postresurfacing dyschromia and the potential difficulty in correcting this problem, the author does not perform resurfacing in patients with Fitzpatrick skin types IV, V, or VI.

The issue of the long recovery and the greater potential for complications (6) associated with deeper resurfacing led to one-pass superficial resurfacing with the carbon dioxide laser or superficial resurfacing with the erbium laser (7). In a study comparing these two lasers for superficial resurfacing it was demonstrated that for equal depths of resurfacing, there were equivalent results with modest rhytid improvement, and on immediate histologic evaluation there were equivalent thermal injury and fibroplasias (8).

Cervical skin is different than facial skin. It has fewer pilosebaceous units. Healing after laser resurfacing relies on the pilosebaceous units. Therefore, it is not surprising that there is a greater incidence of healing problems and scarring after cervical laser resurfacing. In one series (9) in which 10 patients had cervical laser resurfacing, four patients developed hypopigmentation and three patients had scarring. Another study reported on a trial of single-pass carbon dioxide laser cervical resurfacing to try to reduce the rate of complications. In this study none of the patients had an improvement in their wrinkles. Three patients had mild patchy hypopigmentation of the lower neck (10). Considering the risks involved, I do not perform carbon dioxide laser resurfacing of the cervical region. The erbium laser has also been used for cervical resurfacing. In a series of 25 consecutive patients treated with the laser there was a 51% satisfaction rating. However, one patient had erythema that lasted for 6 months after the procedure and another patient had spotty hypopigmentation with some limited areas of atrophic scarring (9). Even with the reported 51% patient satisfaction rating, I do not perform this procedure on cervical skin because I consider the significant complication rate too high for my patients.

RADIOFREQUENCY RESURFACING

Radiofrequency resurfacing is used to treat epidermal and dermal pathology (11,12). This process is named coblation. It uses radiofrequency current to create ionized plasma that breaks the molecular bonds between adjacent cells (Visage, Arthrocare Corp., Sunnyvale, CA). I have used this device to treat epidermal and superficial papillary dermal pathology. It can be used to treat superficial rhytids and lesions. Care must be taken when performing this procedure to keep the radiofrequency bipolar electrode in contact with the tissues. If it is lifted and a gap is formed, there can be unwanted arcing of the radiofrequency current. Immediately after treatment, the skin displays a pale appearance; shortly afterward, it turns a pink color. This pinkness resolves in 1 to 3 weeks. Postinflammatory-type hyperpigmentation can develop as part of the healing process (12). A case of hypertrophic scarring has also been reported (12).

NONABLATIVE AND OTHER TECHNOLOGY

There are several lasers and radiofrequency technology that have been used for nonablative treatment. The technology or techniques selected will vary depending on the pathology being treated and the patient's goals. Whereas the carbon dioxide laser can simultaneously treat problems in the epidermis and the papillary dermis, the nonablative technologies usually treat only one problem. Therefore the first issue is to identify the location and type of pathology. Then the treatment is designed to address the pathology. This is important to optimize the potential for improvement. For example, a nonablative laser that stimulates collagen production in the papillary dermis is not going to improve the epidermal surface changes associated with photoaging.

When evaluating skin, besides wrinkling, assess whether there are any lentigines or telangiectasias. If present, it is important to treat these as well as the wrinkles or scars to achieve a satisfactory improvement (Fig. 182B.1).

Of note, when evaluating the results of nonablative skin rejuvenation, an increase in collagen on histologic evaluation may not correspond with an observable improvement in the appearance of the facial skin and patient satisfaction (13).

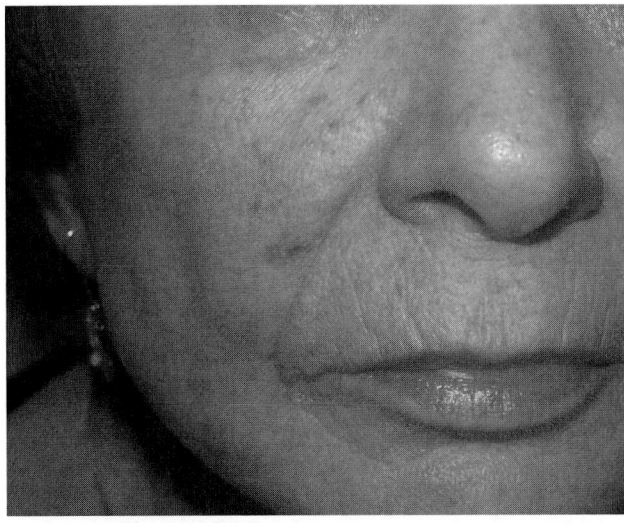

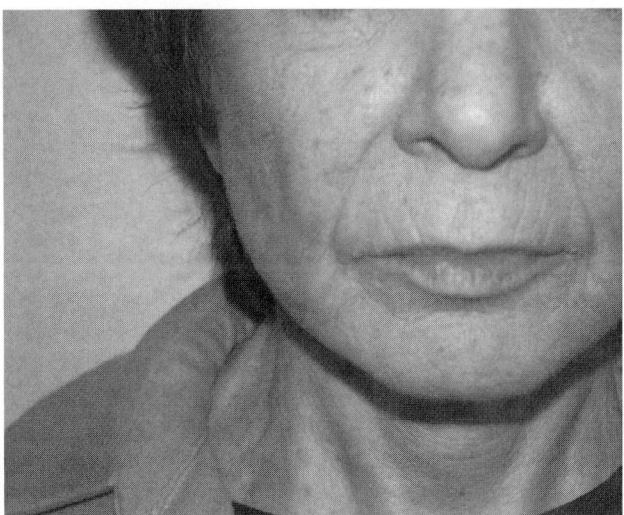

Figure 182B.1   A: This lady was unhappy with the pigmented lesion adjacent to her right nasolabial fold. Before initiating treatment, a small incisional biopsy was taken to ensure it was a benign lentiginous lesion. **B:** Once this was confirmed it was treated with a long-pulse 532-nm laser (DioLite, VariLite, Iridex, Mountainview, CA).

INTENSE PULSED LIGHT

Intense pulsed light (IPL) has been used to treat the superficial changes associated with facial photoaging. The IPL is absorbed by melanin, hemoglobin, and sebaceous glands (14). As such it can be used to treat pigmentary and vascular skin changes as well as provide some smoothing of the skin surface (14). Different mechanisms of action have been proposed for IPL. This includes using heat energy to stimulate dermal fibroblasts to make collagen (15). It has also been hypothesized that IPL may improve the appearance of the skin by decreasing Demodex or by inducing cytokine production (16).

When using IPL it is important to wear proper eye protection and to adjust the IPL settings based on the patient's skin type.

532-NM AND 1,064-NM LASERS FOR NONABLATIVE SKIN REJUVENATION

The 532-nm diode laser has been used alone and in combination with the 1,064-nm laser for nonablative skin rejuvenation. The 532-nm laser is primarily used to treat facial vascular and pigmented lesions. In one nonablative rejuvenation half-face study, 7 patients were given a series of 4 treatments. Of the patients, 71% had a 25% improvement (17). Another study used the 532-nm laser and the 1,064-nm laser for sequential treatments. Four months after treatment there was an average improvement of 30–31% depending on the regimen. The necessary improvements included uneven pigmentation, solar-induced erythema, telangiectasia, and fine solar–induced rhytids. Improvements in skin texture and skin laxity were observed (18).

The 1,064-nm laser has also been used for nonablative skin rejuvenation. In one study using a 50-millisecond pulse width, 7 weekly treatments were performed at 1- to 4-week intervals. As with many of the nonablative modalities, the observed improvements occurred gradually during the course of the treatments. At the completion of the study there was improvement in wrinkles, skin roughness, and skin laxity and an overall improvement in the skin appearance (19).

1320-NM DERMAL COLLAGEN-STIMULATING LASER

The current nonablative collagen-stimulating lasers are designed to exert their effects in the dermal layer. The goal of these lasers is to heat the dermis and induce neocollagen formation. The 1,320-nm laser (CoolTouch) was the first one to become widely available. This laser gives three 300-microsecond pulses at 100 Hz. The total fluence can be adjusted. To decrease the effect on the epidermis the laser has a dynamic cooling spray device that provides prelaser or postlaser epidermal cooling. Tetrafluoroethane is used in the coolant spray. The laser handpiece also has an incorporated thermal sensor. To avoid epidermal injury the goal is to keep the skin surface temperature between 40°C and 49°C and to heat the superficial papillary dermis to 60° to −70°C.

To minimize pain associated with the procedure, topical anesthetic is recommended. Usually patients have some transient redness after treatment; this lasts from 1 to 4 hours. Because this laser exerts its effects on the dermal layer, two authors have recommended sequentially combining it with treatments for the epidermal layer (20,21) to enhance visible results.

1450-NM DERMAL COLLAGEN-STIMULATING LASER

The 1,450-nm mid-infrared laser uses a series of laser pulses interspersed with coolant pulses to heat the papillary dermis and thereby stimulate neocollagen formation. It exerts most of its effects at a depth of 150 to 400 μ in the papillary dermis. In one study the 1,450-nm mid-infrared laser was found to be more effective than the cooling alone for treating rhytids (22).

This laser has also been used to reduce active acne lesions (23). In one study involving this laser for treatment of acne scars, four treatments were sequentially combined with trichloroacetic acid peels. In this study readily visible improvements were achieved (24) (Fig. 182B.2).

Thermage is a radiofrequency device that is used to perform skin tightening (Thermage, Inc, Hayward, CA). Ra-

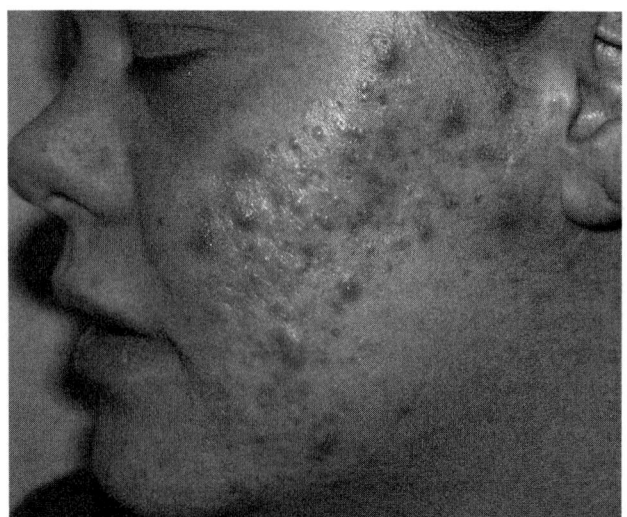
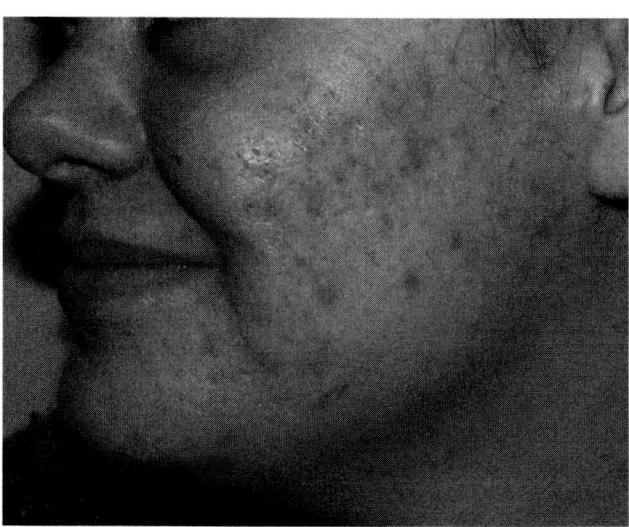

Figure 182B.2 A: This patient had significant acne and acne scarring. **B:** After four treatments with the 1450-nm laser (Smoothbeam, Candela Laser, Wayland, MA) she had a significant improvement in her facial acne and a reduction in her acne scarring. (See also Color Plate 66.)

diofrequency energy is used to heat the dermis and superficial subcutaneous tissue to induce collagen contracture. This device does not change the appearance of the skin, so it should not be used for treatment of wrinkles or scars. As with many technologies, the results can vary. It also has some associated risks. The procedure does not replace facelift-type procedures; instead, it serves as a nonsurgical alternative that offers a more limited result. Multiple authors have reported on these results (25–28).

The latest new technology is fractionated laser therapy (Reliant Technology, Palo Alto, CA) for treatment of photoaging changes. This device uses a 1,550-nm laser to create multiple thermal wounds separated by unaffected tissues, 200 to 300 μ apart. Each wound is 50 to 70 μ in diameter. Approximately 2000 separate wounds are created per square centimeter. This is designed to allow rapid healing and reepithelialization from the adjacent tissues. Topical anesthesia is necessary for this procedure. Several treatments may be necessary to achieve the optimal result. The long-pulse 532-nm laser can also be used with a scanner to provide uniform laser beam spacing for fractionated laser therapy.

HIGHLIGHTS

- When evaluating a patient for laser resurfacing, consider skin type. Pigmented skin is more likely to develop dyschromia.
- When using radiofrequency to treat superficial rhytids and skin lesions, avoid unwanted arcing.
- When using intense pulsed light to treat pigmentary and vascular changes, always provide eye protection for patient and staff.

REFERENCES

1. Beeson WH. Laser Safety. In: Carniol PJ, ed. *Laser skin rejuvenation.* Philadelphia: Lippincott-Raven Publishers, 1998:49–64.
2. Gilmore J, Clark P, Carniol P. Laser Safety. In: Carniol PJ, ed. *Facial surgery. facial rejuvenation.* New York: Wiley-Liss, 2000: 263–280.
3. Fitzpatrick RE. CO_2 laser resurfacing. *Dermatol Clin* 2001;19(3): 443–451.
4. Bisson MA, Grover R, Grobbelaar AO. Long-term results of facial rejuvenation by carbon dioxide laser resurfacing using a quantitative method of assessment. *Br J Plast Surg* 2002;55(8):652–656.
5. Trelles MA, Pardo L, Ayliffe P, et al. Patients' answers to a postoperative questionnaire related to laser resurfacing. *Facial Plast Surg* 2001;17(3):187–192.
6. Bridenstine JB, Carniol PJ. Managing postresurfacing complications. In: Carniol PJ, ed. *Laser skin rejuvenation.* Philadelphia: Lippincott-Raven Publishers, 1998:243–260.
7. Ruiz-Esparza J. One-pass carbon dioxide laser resurfacing. in facial surgery. In: Carniol PJ, ed. *Facial rejuvenation.* New York: Wiley-Liss, 2000:305–312.
8. Ross EV, Miller C, Meehan K, et al. One-pass CO_2 versus multiple-pass ER:YAG laser resurfacing in the treatment of rhytids: a comparison side-by-side study of pulsed CO_2 and ER:YAG lasers. *Dermatol Surg* 2001 Aug;27(8):709–715.
9. Goldman MP, Rostan EF, Fitzpatrick RE. Laser rejuvenation of the photodamaged Neck. *Am J Cosmetic Surg* 2002;19(1):21–27.
10. Fitzpatrick RE, Goldman MP, Sripracha-Anunt S. Resurfacing of photodamaged skin on the neck with an UltraPulse® carbon dioxide laser. *Lasers Surg Med* 2001;28(2):145–149.
11. Carruthers A. Coblation for facial resurfacing. In: Carniol PJ, ed. *Facial rejuvenation.* New York: Wiley-Liss, 2000:413–428.
12. Carniol PJ, Maas CS. Bipolar radiofrequency resurfacing. *Facial Plast Surg Clin North Am* 2001;9:337–342.
13. Sadick SM. A structural approach to nonablative rejuvenation. *Cosmetic Dermatol* 2002;15:39–43.
14. Goldberg DJ, Cutler KB. Non-ablative treatment of rhytides with intense pulse light. *Lasers Surg Med* 1999;25:229–236.
15. Prieto VP, Saddick NS, Shea C. effects of intense pulsed light on sun-damaged human skin: routine and ultrastructural analysis. *Lasers Surg Med* 2002;30:82–85.
16. Trelles MA, Allones I, Luna R. Facial rejuvenation with a non-ablative 1320nm Nd:YAG laser. *Dermatol Surg* 2001;27:111–116.
17. Carniol PJ, Farley S, Friedman A. Long-pulse 532-nm diode laser for nonablative facial skin rejuvenation. *Arch Facial Plast Surg* 2003;5:511–513.
18. Tan MH, Dover JS, Hsu TS, et al. Clinical evaluation of enhanced nonablative skin rejuvenation using a combination of a 532 and a 1,064 nm laser. *Lasers Surg Med* 2004;34:439–445.
19. Dyan SH, Vartanian J, Menaker G, et al. Nonablative laser resurfacing using the long-pulse (1064-nm) Nd:YAG laser. *Arch Facial Plast Surg* 2003;5:310–315.
20. Levy JL, Trelles M, Lagarde JM, et al. Treatment of wrinkles with the nonablative 1,320-nm Nd:YAG laser. *Ann Plast Surg* 2001;47(5): 482–488.
21. Chan HH, Lam LK, Wong DS, et al. Use of 1320 nm Nd:YAG laser for wrinkle reduction and the treatment of atrophic acne scarring in Asians. *Lasers Surg Med* 2004;34(2):98–103.
22. Goldberg DJ, Rogachefsky AS, Silapunt S. Non-ablative laser treatment of facial rhytids: A comparison of 1450-nm diode laser treatment with dynamic cooling as opposed to treatment with dynamic cooling alone. *Lasers Surg Med* 2002;30:79–81.
23. Paithankar DY, Ross EV, Saleh BA, et al. Acne treatment with a 1450 nm wavelength laser and cryogen spray cooling. *Lasers Surg Med* 2002;31:106–114.
24. Carniol PJ, Vynatheya J, Carniol E. Evaluation of acne scar treatment with a 1450-nm midinfrared laser and 30% trichloroacetic acid peels. *Arch Facial Plast Surg* 2005;7:251–255.
25. Koch RJ. Radiofrequency nonablative tissue tightening. *Facial Plast Surg Clin Am* 2004;12(3):339–346.
26. Fritz M, Counters JT, Zelickson BD. Radiofrequency treatment for middle and lower face laxity. *Arch Facial Plast Surg* 2004;6(6): 370–373.
27. Nahm WK, Su TT, Rotunda AM, et al. Objective changes in brow position, superior palpebral crease, peak angle of the eyebrow, and jowl surface area after volumetric radiofrequency treatments to half of the face. *Dermatol Surg* 2004;30(6):922–928.
28. Alster TS, Tanzi E. Improvement of neck and cheek laxity with a nonablative radiofrequency device: a lifting experience. *Dermatol Surg* 2004;30(4 Pt 1):503–507.

Management of Benign Facial Lesions

Fred F. Shahan   Karen J. Johnson   John A. Zitelli   Henry H. Roenigk, Jr.

Successful management of facial lesions depends on accurate diagnosis, knowledge of natural history, and use of a specific appropriate treatment. A functional classification scheme, together with history and physical examination, allows narrowing of diagnostic possibilities. Most benign facial lesions are noninflammatory, including various tumors, cysts, and melanocytic lesions (Table 183.1). Important exceptions include specific infectious, degenerative, and metabolic conditions that clinically appear and behave as inflammatory disorders (e.g., verruca, molluscum contagiosum). "Benign" facial lesions can signal serious systemic diseases (Tables 183.2–183.4).

HISTORY AND PHYSICAL EXAMINATION

Important questions to ask relate to duration of lesion, family history, fluctuation in size or drainage of any material, rapidity of onset, pain (e.g., leiomyomas are often spontaneously painful), and associated physical findings (e.g., tuberous sclerosis). Inspection and palpation are aided by adequate lighting or side lighting. Diascopy (pressing a clear microscope slide over the lesion to determine whether it is blood-filled—that is, of vascular origin) also is useful. The lesion is classified by depth (epidermal, dermal, or subcutaneous) and other characteristics (cystic versus solid; tenderness; color; texture; mobility; surface features, such as smooth or verrucous; presence of a central punctum), distribution and arrangement of lesions, and associated inflammation.

EPIDERMAL LESIONS

Epidermal lesions are most common, including seborrheic keratosis, actinic keratosis, comedones, milia, cutaneous horn, and epidermal cysts (1–5).

Actinic keratosis (or solar or senile keratosis) is composed of small, usually multiple erythematous lesions on sun-exposed areas, such as the face, exposed scalp, and dorsum of the hands. They have a rough, adherent scale and are more easily felt than seen. Actinic keratosis can develop into squamous cell carcinoma (10% to 20%), which usually does not metastasize. The lifetime risk of squamous cell carcinoma in an individual with actinic keratosis has been estimated to be 6% to 10% (6,7).

An analogous lesion to an actinic keratoses, actinic cheilitis (Fig. 183.1; see also Color Plate 67), occurs on the lip's vermilion border. It presents with hyperkeratosis, erosions, and a dull opaqueness.

Cutaneous horns (Fig. 183.2; see also Color Plate 68) are hyperkeratotic conical lesions whose height is at least half their largest diameter. Various types of lesions may be present at their bases (actinic keratosis, verruca, squamous cell carcinoma, seborrheic keratosis, and rarely trichilemmoma or basal cell carcinoma). Cutaneous horns require adequate removal so their bases can be examined histopathologically (8).

Seborrheic keratoses have brownish-black, verrucous papules or plaques with a "stuck-on" appearance, reflecting their epidermal origin. The sign of Leser-Trélat, the abrupt appearance or explosive expansion in size and number of

TABLE 183.1

CLASSIFICATION OF BENIGN FACIAL LESIONS

Inflammatory lesions
  Xanthelasma
  Molluscum
  Verruca

Noninflammatory lesions
  Epidermal tumors and cysts
    Seborrheic keratosis
    Epidermal cyst
    Milia
    Dermoid cyst
    Actinic keratosis
    Keratoacanthoma
    Comedones
    Cutaneous horn
  Skin appendage tumors
    Trichofolliculoma
    Trichoepithelioma
    Pilomatricoma
    Trichilemmoma
    Nevus sebaceous
    Sebaceous hyperplasia/rhinophyma
    Hidrocystoma
    Syringoma

Non–skin-appendage tumors
  Vascular
    Hemangiomas (capillary, cavernous, flammeus)
    Angiomas
    Telangiectasias
    Pyogenic granuloma
    Venous lake
  Fibrous
    Soft fibroma (skin tag)
    Fibrous papule
    Adenoma sebaceum (angiofibroma)
    Hypertrophic scar/keloid
  Neural
    Neurofibroma
  Fatty/muscular/osseous
    Lipoma
    Multiple milliary osteomas
    Leiomyomas
    Melanocytic lesions
    Nevi
    Lentigines
    Ephelides (freckles)
    Nevus of Ota
    Blue nevus
    Spitz nevus

TABLE 183.2

DIFFERENTIAL DIAGNOSIS OF SYNDROMES ASSOCIATED WITH MULTIPLE BENIGN FACIAL LESIONS

Disease	Onset	Cutaneous Features	Systemic Features
Neurofibromatosis	Variable to adulthood, 7 types	Neurofibromas Cafe-au-lait macules Axiliary freckling	Multiple skeletal, endocrine, and neurologic abnormalities, increased incidence of malignancy (Wilms, CNS/PNS rhabdomyosarcoma, leukemia)
Tuberous sclerosis	Variable (early childhood to young adult life)	Angiofibromas (adenoma sebaceum, shagreen patches, periungual fibromas, ash leaf white macules)	Mental retardation, epilepsy, multiple organ hamartomas (eye, kidney, heart)
Gardner syndrome	May first appear at age 7–10, 50% display syndrome by age 20	Multiple epidermal cysts	Malignant degeneration (40%), osteomas of facial bones, fibromas, lipomas, leiomyomas of stomach or ileum
Muit-Torre syndrome	Variable	Sebaceous tumors of skin (most are adenomas) with or without keratoacanthomas (often very large)	Visceral neoplasms (often multiple, especially GI, larnyx, endometrium)
Cowden disease	Variable	Multiple trichilemmomas, gingival fibromatosis	Greatly increased risk of breast carcinoma, thyroid adenomas and carcinomas
Multiple endocrine neoplasia (type 2b)	Early childhood	Neuromas of oral and nasal mucosa, upper GI tract and conjunctiva, lentigines, "blubbery" lips	Increased risk for medullary thyroid carcinoma, pheochromocytoma, marfanoid habitus, kyphoscoliosis

CNS, central nervous system; PNS, peripheral nervous system; GI, gastrointestinal.

TABLE 183.3

HEREDITARY TELANGIECTATIC SYNDROMES

Disease	Onset	Cutaneous Features	Systemic Features
Rothmund-Thomson syndrome	3 mo to 2 yr	Telangiectasias, mottled pigmentation and atrophy (poikiloderma) of face, arms, legs, buttocks	Moderate dwarfism, sparse hair, cataracts, photosensitivity
Bloom syndrome	Infancy	Erythema and telangiectasias of butterfly area of face, forehead, ears, lids, hands, and forearms	Dwarfism, photosensitivity
Cockayne syndrome	Second year	Erythema and mottled pigmented scarring of butterfly area of face	Physical and mental retardation, loss of subcutaneous fat on face, Mickey Mouse ears
Hereditary hemorrhagic telangiectasia	Childhood	Punctate or linear telangiectasias of face, lips, ears, conjunctiva, upper trunk, arms	Mucosal hemorrhage
Ataxia-telangiectasia	3–5 years	Linear telangiectasias of conjunctiva, eyelids, ears, cheeks	Dwarfism, ataxia

A differential diagnosis also includes the collagen vascular diseases and liver diseases.
Modified from Champion RH, Burton JL, Burns AD, et al., eds. *Rook's textbook of dermatology*, 6th ed. London: Blackwell, 1998, with permission.

TABLE 183.4

SYNDROMES WITH MULTIPLE MELANOCYTIC LESIONS

Disease	Onset	Cutaneous Features	Systemic Features
Neurofibromatosis	See Table 183.1	See Table 183.1	See Table 183.1
Albright syndrome	Melanotic macules appear soon after birth	Melanotic patches (unilateral)	Polyostotic fibrous dysplasia, precocious puberty, endocrine dysfunctions
Peutz-Jeghers	Hyperpigmented macules are usually present at birth or early childhood	Melanotic macules of lips and oral mucosa	Degeneration (2%–3%) of granulosa cell tumors in females (20%), increased association of duodenal cancer
LEOPARD syndrome	Lentigines appear in infancy and increase in numbers	Multiple lentigines	Ocular hypertelorism, pulmonary (Moynahan syndrome) stenosis, abnormalities of genitalia, growth restriction, deafness (neural)
Lamb syndrome	—	Facial and genital lentigines, mucocutaneous myxomas, blue nevi	Atrial myxomas
Name syndrome	—	Nevi, myxoid neurofibromata, freckling (ephelides)	Atrial myxoma
Centrofacial lentiginosis	Lentigines appear in first years of life	Mid-facial freckling, sacral hypertrichosis, fusion of eyebrows	High arched palate, missing upper incisors, seizures, mental retardation, scoliosis, spina bifida
Cronkhite-Canada syndrome	—	Melanotic macules on face, extremities, alopecia, onychodystrophy, hyperpigmentation	Gastrointestinal polyposis

LEOPARD: lentigines, electrocardiographic abnormalities, ocular hypertelorism, pulmonary stenosis, abnormal genitalia, retardation of growth, deafness.

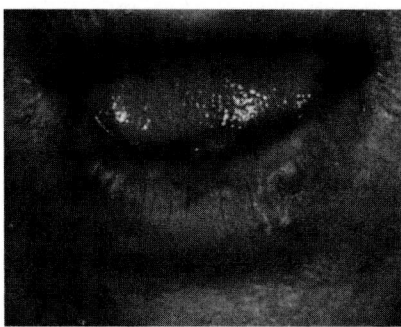

Figure 183.1 Actinic cheilitis. (Reprinted from McKee P, du-Vivier A. *Atlas of clinical dermatology.* London: Gower, 1986, with permission.) (See also Color Plate 67.)

multiple seborrheic keratoses, especially if accompanied by pruritus, has been implicated as a cutaneous marker of internal malignancy (9,10). In black patients, they may appear on the face as multiple brown to black papules over the cheeks, called dermatosis papulosa nigra.

Epidermal cysts are often compressible and may have visible puncta. If they have been inflamed, they may be fixed to surrounding tissue. It may be difficult to tell epidermal cysts from lipomas or neurofibromas. Lipomas are soft and often lobulated, lack puncta, and are movable against overlying skin. Neurofibromas similarly lack puncta and often display "button-holing" (described later).

Milia are small, yellowish-white, 1- to 2-mm papules. Primary milia develop spontaneously, commonly in newborns and people who are predisposed to them. Secondary milia may develop from trauma, from subepidermal blistering diseases, in areas of topical corticosteroid–induced atrophy, or postdermabrasion. In the latter case, the milia are probably a proliferative postinjury epithelial response.

Comedones superficially resemble milia but occur in specific situations. Open comedones (blackheads) are small (1- to 2-mm) papular lesions with a central black plug. They are usually multiple, occurring with acne vulgaris or

actinically damaged skin. Closed comedones (whiteheads) are 1- to 2-mm white lesions seen with acne vulgaris. Histologically, comedones are dilated cystic hair follicles filled with keratinous and lipoid material.

SKIN-APPENDAGE TUMORS

Skin-appendage tumors have diverse clinical presentations. They are common on the face and scalp because of the numerous appendageal structures there.

Many facial appendage tumors are small skin-colored papules. Trichofolliculomas occur in adults as solitary facial lesions. They have a central pore with a white woollike tuft of hair, a diagnostic feature.

Trichoepitheliomas are also small, flesh-colored papules. They are solitary or multiple. Multiple lesions are autosomal dominant, first appearing in childhood, with the number of lesions gradually increasing. Multiple trichoepitheliomas cluster around the central face and can occur with cylindromas, another benign appendage tumor often occurring on the scalp. These can grow together, resembling a turban (turban tumor). At times, trichoepitheliomas can be confused with basal cell carcinomas, both clinically and pathologically.

Trichilemmomas are small, pink to brown facial papules, in solitary and multiple forms. The multiple form can be a feature of the multiple hamartoma syndrome or Cowden disease, an autosomal-dominant genodermatosis associated with a high incidence of neoplasms (both benign and malignant) of the breast and thyroid, which occur in up to two-thirds of patients (11). Multiple trichilemmomas occur in all patients with Cowden disease and precede development of breast cancer, allowing identification of women at risk. These lesions appear nonspecific or can resemble small verrucae. In Cowden disease, oral lesions appear as 1- to 3-mm skin-colored papules that can assume a subtle cobblestone appearance or be so extensive that they involve the entire oral cavity, including the tongue.

Sebaceous hyperplasia is a common papular lesion occurring in older people. It is composed of 2- to 3-mm yellow to orange lobulated papules with a slight central umbilication. They can be solitary or multiple, commonly on the forehead and nose (highest number of sebaceous glands). They are enlargements of normal sebaceous glands. They also can occur with cyclosporine use and can be a feature of acne rosacea (rhinophyma) (Fig.183.3; also see Color Plate 69).

Syringomas are small, flesh-colored to translucent papules that are intraepidermal eccrine duct adenomas. A syringoma may occur at any site on the body but are prone to occur in the periorbital area, especially the eyelids. Syringomas often have a predilection for apocrine areas (axillae, vulva) or eruptive forms on the trunk or in dermatomal patterns. The lesions are removed from women more commonly than men, although it is not entirely clear that this represents a gender predilection rather than biopsy selection bias resulting from cosmetic or social factors.

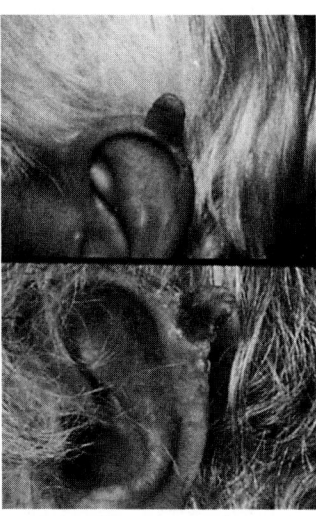

Figure 183.2 Cutaneous horn. (Reprinted from McKee P, du-Vivier A. *Atlas of clinical dermatology.* London: Gower, 1986, with permission.) (See also Color Plate 68.)

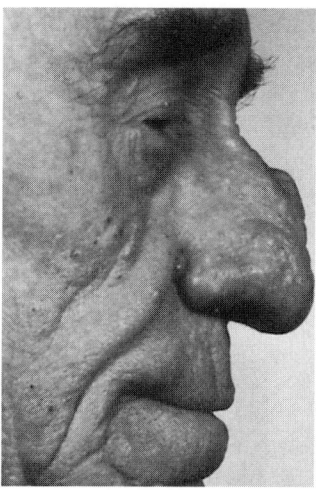

Figure 183.3 Rhinophyma. (Reprinted from McKee P, duVivier A. *Atlas of clinical dermatology.* London: Gower, 1986, with permission.) (See also Color Plate 69.)

Hidrocystomas are small, uncommon cystic periorbital lesions, most commonly seen on the eyelid margin. They are 2 to 15 mm in diameter, with a translucent bluish quality. Apocrine hidrocystomas are larger and solitary, whereas eccrine hidrocystomas are smaller and multiple.

Pilomatricomas (Fig. 183.4 see also Color Plate 70) are tumors typified by follicular matrical cornification, usually presenting as a solitary, hard, deep-seated nodule, usually on the face or upper extremities. The nodules may have a faint bluish-red color and are sharply demarcated, ranging in diameter from 0.5 to 3.0 cm. They are common in children and young adults.

Nevus sebaceus (Jadassohn nevus; Fig. 183.5; see also Color Plate 71) is a hamartoma that exhibits follicular, sebaceous, and apocrine malformation to varying degrees(12). The lesion is a congenital lesion presenting as a solitary, often linear, slightly raised, orange-yellow hairless plaque on the scalp or face. Its morphologic appearance changes with the activity of underlying sebaceous glands by becoming more verrucous and nodular at puberty. It is

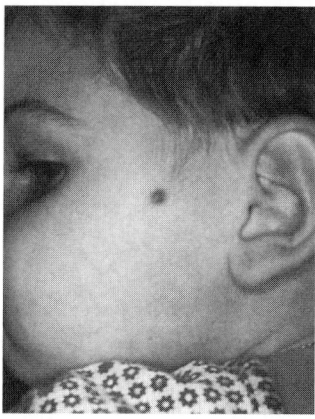

Figure 183.4 Pilomatricoma. (Reprinted from McKee P, duVivier A. *Atlas of clinical dermatology.* London: Gower, 1986, with permission.) (See also Color Plate 70.)

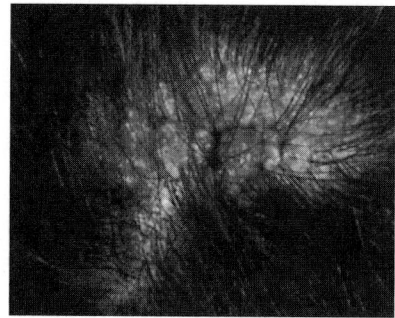

Figure 183.5 Nevus sebaceus. (Reprinted from McKee P, duVivier A. *Atlas of clinical dermatology.* London: Gower, 1986, with permission.) (See also Color Plate 71.)

well-established that nevus sebaceus may develop secondary adnexal neoplasms, most commonly benign but sometimes malignant. Trichoblastoma and syringocystadenoma papilliferum are the most commonly found benign neoplasm, whereas basal cell carcinoma is found in less than 1% of the cases (13–15). Patients rarely have extensive nevus sebaceus plaques with an associated neurocutaneous syndrome (epilepsy, mental retardation, skeletal deformities).

NON–SKIN-APPENDAGE TUMORS

Lesions derived from non–skin-appendage elements include vascular, fibrous, neural, fatty, muscular, and osseous tissues (1–4).

Vascular Tumors

Cherry angiomas are a very common, benign vascular proliferation found on most adults. They are bright-red, dome-shaped papules, 2 to 4 mm in diameter, most commonly found on the trunk and extremities. Patients usually bring these to the attention of the physician when they are chronically traumatized or cosmetically undesirable.

Vascular malformations include capillary malformations (port-wine stain), venous malformations (cavernous hemangioma), lymphatic malformations (lymangioma, lymphangioma circumscriptum, cystic hygroma), and arteriovenous malformations. It is important therapeutically and prognostically to distinguish among these. Port-wine stains (capillary malformation) are often present at birth as large, flat, pink, well-demarcated patches that demonstrate a growth pattern that parallels the growth of the child. With age, the affected skin develops a more pronounced red color, thickens, and becomes more nodular. Various syndromes are associated with capillary malformations. Sturge-Weber syndrome is a sporadic neurologic disorder in which a facial capillary malformation (usually V1 distribution of the trigeminal nerve) is associated with ipsilateral ocular and leptomeningeal anomalies. When capillary malformations occur on an extremity, a progressive overgrowth of the affected extremity may occur

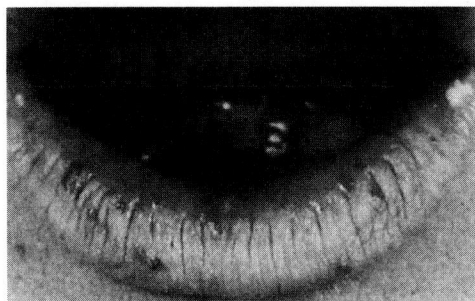

Figure 183.6 Osler-Rendu-Weber disease (hereditary hemorrhagic telangiectasia). (Reprinted from McKee P, duVivier A. *Atlas of clinical dermatology.* London: Gower, 1986, with permission.)

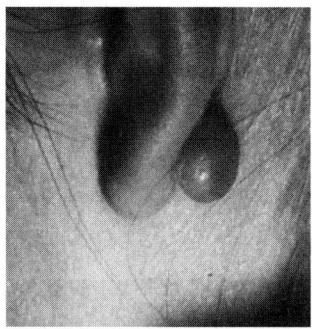

Figure 183.7 Keloid. (Reprinted from McKee P, duVivier A. *Atlas of clinical dermatology.* London: Gower, 1986, with permission.) (See also Color Plate 72.)

with underlying osteohypertrophy and arteriovenous fistulae, which is known as Klippel-Trenaunay syndrome.

Capillary hemangiomas are more common in females and premature infants. They appear between the third and fifth weeks of life, grow for several months to 1 year, and then regress. Of capillary hemangiomas, 70% regress by age 7 years. Ultimately, only 6% are cosmetically problematic. Histologically, there is vascular endothelial cell proliferation.

The most common acquired hemangioma is a pyogenic granuloma, often found on the face and extremities. It is a rapidly growing, friable, solitary red papule or polyp that frequently ulcerates and easily bleeds. Pyogenic granulomas are often precipitated by minor trauma or pregnancy.

The second major group of vascular lesions of the face are the ectasias, or dilatations of blood vessels (not new vessel growth). These include telangiectasias and venous lakes. Most are acquired or may have syndromal features (Table 183.3).

Facial telangiectasias are extremely common and consist of dilated capillaries that appear as tiny, red, cutaneous vessels that blanch when pressure is applied. Telangiectasias may present in a linear pattern or spiderlike with a central feeding vessel and radiating dilated vessels. These lesions occur with conditions such as rosacea, scleroderma, dermatomyositis, radiation dermatitis, chronic alcoholism, liver disease, pregnancy, childhood, Osler-Rendu-Weber disease (Figure 183.6), carcinoid syndrome, idiopathic telangiectasia (generalized essential telangiectasia), or actinic skin degeneration.

Venous lakes are deep-blue cutaneous nodules usually on the lips, ears, or face. Histologically, they are dilated venules in the dermis that blanch with compression.

Fibrous Tumors

Facial fibrous tissue tumors include skin tags, fibrous papules, adenoma sebaceum, hypertrophic scars, and keloids. A skin tag (soft fibroma) is the most common fibrous lesion. These are small (1- to 2-mm), smooth, filiform, flesh-colored growths commonly located around the

eyes or on the neck. They are usually multiple, distinguished from verrucae by their smooth surface. Skin tags occur elsewhere on the body (particularly the inguinal folds and axillae) and can occur as large, solitary, baglike structures on the lower trunk.

Fibrous papules are solitary, dome-shaped, flesh-colored papules located on the central face of adults, most commonly the nasal ala and alar crease. These can clinically simulate intradermal nevi, adnexal tumors, or basal cell carcinomas. Sampling biopsies are often done to exclude a basal cell carcinoma. Otherwise, these lesions are benign and do not require further treatment unless it is of cosmetic concern to the patient.

Hypertrophic scars can be confused with keloids. Both are red, raised, smooth, and shiny, but hypertrophic scars remain within the injury area, whereas keloids (Figure 183.7; see also Color Plate 72) extend beyond the original injury site. Hypertrophic scars flatten over time, and keloids proliferate. There is familial and racial predilection (darker skin pigmentation) for keloid formation. Hypertrophic scars develop after wound infection or in certain anatomic locations (deltoid, angle of mandible, sternum). Keloids are uncommon on the face, even in keloid-forming individuals with the exception of the ears.

Adenoma sebaceum (Fig. 183.8; see also Color Plate 73) is an uncommon but characteristic feature of tuberous scle-

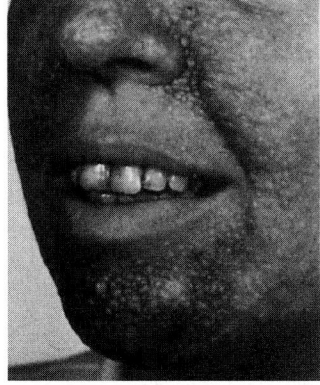

Figure 183.8 Adenoma sebaceum. (Reprinted from McKee P, duVivier A. *Atlas of clinical dermatology.* London: Gower, 1986, with permission.) (See also Color Plate 73.)

rosis. Adenoma sebaceum, mental retardation, and epilepsy form the classic triad of this dominantly inherited neurocutaneous syndrome. Adenoma sebaceum is a misnomer because these growths are not adenomas nor are they sebaceous. These growths are actually angiofibromas. They are numerous small, reddish, smooth papules symmetrically distributed around the nose, cheeks, and chin, sparing the upper lip. They first appear in late childhood, so they are a late sign of tuberous sclerosis.

Fatty/Muscular Tumors

Tumors of fatty, muscular, and osseous tissue occasionally occur on the face (1–5). The most common are lipomas. Clinically, lipomas are single or multiple, soft, rounded, lobulated growths that are freely movable against the overlying skin. These collections of mature fat cells with a thin connective tissue capsule must be differentiated from other soft, round growths such as neurofibromas and epidermal cysts.

Leiomyomas occur less commonly on the face (Fig. 183.9; see also Color Plate 74). These small, firm, reddish-brown nodules arise from erector pili hair follicle smooth muscle. They are often multiple, arranged in a group or line, and painful.

Neural Tumors

Neurofibromas are benign nerve sheath tumors that can develop as solitary lesions or as multiple lesions as part of neurofibromatosis (NF1) (von Recklinghausen disease). Solitary neurofibromas are soft flesh-colored tumors that resemble normal nevocytic nevi. They may become pedunculated. When pressed, the tumor easily invaginates through a small skin opening (button-hole sign). Subcutaneous neurofibromas are either deep, firm, discrete nodules or, more characteristically, large, flabby, plexiform neuromas that feel like a bag of worms. The plexiform neurofibroma is especially important because it is considered

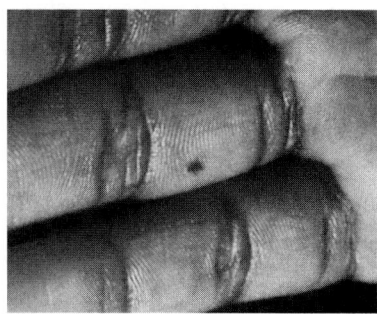

Figure 183.10   Junctional nevus. (From the Institute for Dermatologic Communication and Education, 1976, with permission.)

pathognomonic of neurofibromatosis and requires proper patient management (16).

Melanocytic Tumors

Melanocytic nevi contain intraepidermal or dermal collections of nevus cells or both (1–5).

Melanocytic nevi are congenital or acquired and described by their histologic location of the nevus cells within the skin as either junctional, compound, or intradermal. Very few nevi are present at birth; therefore, most nevi are acquired and follow a specific life cycle. Most nevi appear in childhood, adolescence, or early adulthood, with few new nevi developing past middle adulthood. As age increases, the number of nevi progressively decreases. They pass through successive stages of junctional, compound, and intradermal development. Most nevi in children are junctional; in older adults, most nevi are intradermal.

Nevus appearance corresponds with histology. Junctional nevi (Fig. 183.10) are flat and pigmented; dermal nevi (Fig. 183.11) are flesh colored and dome shaped or

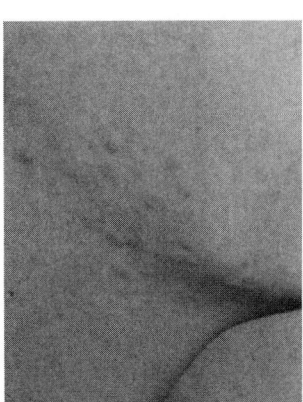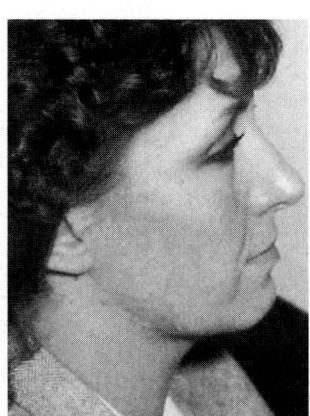

Figure 183.9   Multiple leiomyomas. (Reprinted from McKee P, duVivier A. *Atlas of clinical dermatology.* London: Gower, 1986, with permission.) (See also Color Plate 74.)

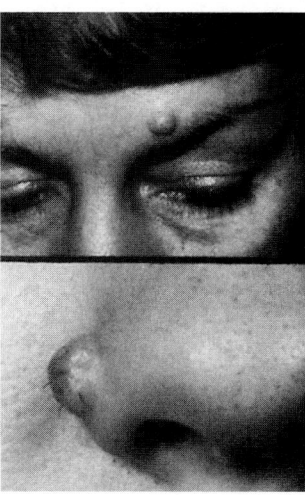

Figure 183.11   Dermal nevi. (Reprinted from McKee P, duVivier A. *Atlas of clinical dermatology.* London: Gower, 1986, with permission.)

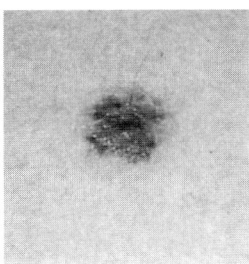

Figure 183.12 Compound nevus. (Reprinted from McKee P, duVivier A. *Atlas of clinical dermatology*. London: Gower, 1986, with permission.)

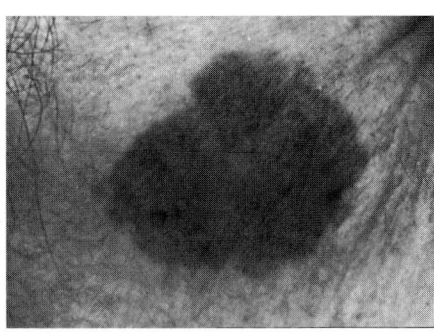

Figure 183.14 Lentigo senilis. (Reprinted from McKee P, du-Vivier A. *Atlas of clinical dermatology*. London: Gower, 1986, with permission.) (See also Color Plate 75.)

pedunculated; compound nevi (Fig. 183.12) are in between. Congenital nevi are larger than acquired nevi, are pigmented and slightly elevated, and may have increased hair. Compared with acquired nevi, they have deeper nevus cell extension into dermis, distribution of nevus cells near cutaneous appendages, and extension of nevus cells between collagen bundles. Giant congenital nevi have an increased risk for malignant transformation (17,18), whereas small- and medium-sized congenital nevi have little or no increased risk for developing into melanoma.

Spitz nevus (epithelioid and spindle cell nevus) is a rare type of melanocytic nevus (Fig. 183.13). It is a solitary, well-circumscribed, dome-shaped papule or nodule varying in color from pink to tan to brown. Their size varies from about 2 mm to about 2 cm, and they occur on the face and extremities of children and young adults. Although benign, it can resemble malignant melanoma histologically and may require treatment as melanoma unless a definitive distinction of benign versus malignant can be assured by the pathologist.

The principal tumors of epidermal melanocytes are freckles (ephelides) and lentigines. These flat, pigmented lesions are distinct from seborrheic keratoses or junctional nevi, which they resemble. Actinically induced lentigines are lentigo senilis (Fig.183.14; see also Color Plate 75), whereas randomly occurring ones are lentigo simplex. Most facial lesions are lentigo senilis. They are light to

dark-brown flat lesions, 5 to 20 mm in diameter or larger. Most are benign, but occasionally on the face they are confused with malignant lesions such as lentigo maligna or melanoma *in situ*. Other features distinguishing lentigines from freckles are onset later in life, lack of seasonal variation, and larger size. Psoralen and ultraviolet A photochemotherapy lentigines are lesions precipitated by ultraviolet A phototherapy with psoralen. Freckles, in contrast, are easily recognized as small, brown, scattered macules occurring on sun-exposed areas of fair-skinned people. They have no malignant potential, darken in response to sunlight, and develop in childhood. Multiple facial lentigines are a prominent feature of numerous syndromes (Table 183.4).

The main facial dermal melanocytic lesions are benign intradermal and compound nevi, as described earlier. Other less common lesions include nevus of Ota and common blue nevus. Nevus of Ota is a unilateral blue to brown pigmented patch involving the skin of the periorbital, temple, forehead, or malar areas that occurs predominantly in dark-skinned races. Usually, the ipsilateral sclerae (Fig. 183.15) is involved, and occasionally the conjunctiva, cornea, retina, and oral and nasal mucosa are

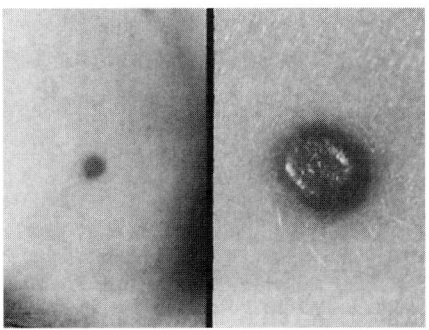

Figure 183.13 Spitz nevus. (Reprinted from McKee P, duVivier A. *Atlas of clinical dermatology*. London: Gower, 1986, with permission.)

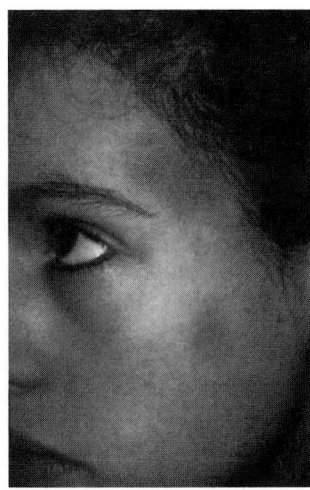

Figure 183.15 Nevus of Ota. (Reprinted from McKee P, du-Vivier A. *Atlas of clinical dermatology*. London: Gower, 1986, with permission.)

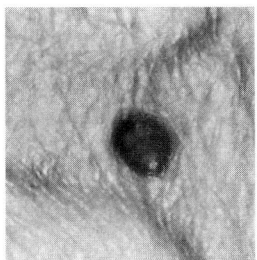

Figure 183.16   Blue nevus. (Reprinted from McKee P, duVivier A. *Atlas of clinical dermatology*. London: Gower, 1986, with permission.) (See also Color Plate 76.)

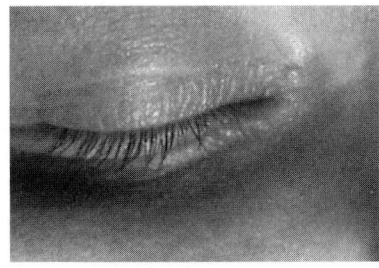

Figure 183.18   Molluscum contagiosum. (From the American Academy of Dermatology, 1977, with permission.)

involved. Nevus of Ota has two times of onset: early childhood before the age of 1 year and around puberty. Malignancies arising in nevi of Ota are rare but when present do not adhere to the typical ABCD rules of melanoma (19). Several cases of primary malignant melanoma of the choroid, orbit, iris, chiasma, and meninges have developed in association with nevus of Ota that exhibited eye involvement (20).

Common blue nevi are small (<1 cm), smooth, dome-shaped papules (Fig. 183.16; see also Color Plate 76) with a characteristic blue appearance as a result of the presence of deep intradermal melanin pigment that is viewed through intact skin (Tyndall effect). The lesions may appear anywhere, but about 50% of cases are found on the dorsa of the hands and feet.

Infectious Lesions

Warts (verruca vulgaris) are composed of intraepidermal lesions resulting from local infection with the human papilloma virus (1–5). They occur at any age, are spread by local contact or autoinoculation, have an unpredictable course, and are usually asymptomatic. They are more common and resistant to treatment in patients who are immunocompromised.

There are more than 100 genotypes of human papilloma virus, including common, filiform, plantar (including mosaic), flat, and anogenital warts. They have an irregularly corrugated (verrucous) surface, with pinpoint black

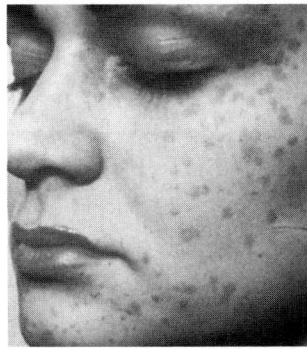

Figure 183.17   Flat warts. (Reprinted from McKee P, duVivier A. *Atlas of clinical dermatology*. London: Gower, 1986, with permission.)

dots of thrombosed capillaries. On mucosal surfaces, they may be smooth-surfaced papules or on flexible, pedunculated stalks.

Common warts are firm, sessile papulonodular growths, uncommon on the face. Filiform warts, common on the face, are taglike protuberances resembling skin tags. Flat warts (Fig. 183.17) also are common on the face, particularly in young women, and can be missed if not viewed with side lighting. They are slightly elevated, light-brown, 1- to 5-mm grouped discrete lesions.

Molluscum contagiosum (Fig. 183.18) is a cutaneous infection caused by a poxvirus. It produces shiny, flesh-colored to pink, dome-shaped, firm papules with central umbilication. It is spread by local contact or autoinoculation and is common in children, sexually active young adults, and individuals who are immunocompromised. When central umbilication is not apparent, they resemble milia or closed comedones. In patients who are immunocompromised, these lesions can form large crateriform and plaquelike lesions involving large areas of the face. Molluscum lesions have a central expressible inclusion, which can confirm the diagnosis. In patients who are immunocompromised, disseminated deep fungal infections (e.g., *Cryptococcus*) are also part of the differential diagnosis.

LABORATORY STUDIES

Most dermatologic diagnoses can be made by inspection or skin biopsy (shave, punch, or excision) (2,21,22). A shave biopsy uses a scalpel blade to shave the lesion flush with, or slightly below, the surrounding skin (Fig. 183.19). This biopsy contains epidermis and a small amount of dermis, so it is appropriate for pathology in those layers, such as actinic keratosis, verruca, benign nevi, trichoepithelioma, or trichofolliculoma. A full-thickness skin biopsy (punch or excisional) is used for pathology in the deep dermis (pilomatricoma) or when entire architecture is required for accurate diagnosis (Spitz nevus). Punch biopsies are performed using a 2- to 8-mm circular sharp blade on a handle (Fig. 183.20). It is pressed firmly against the skin and twisted back and forth to penetrate the full thickness of the

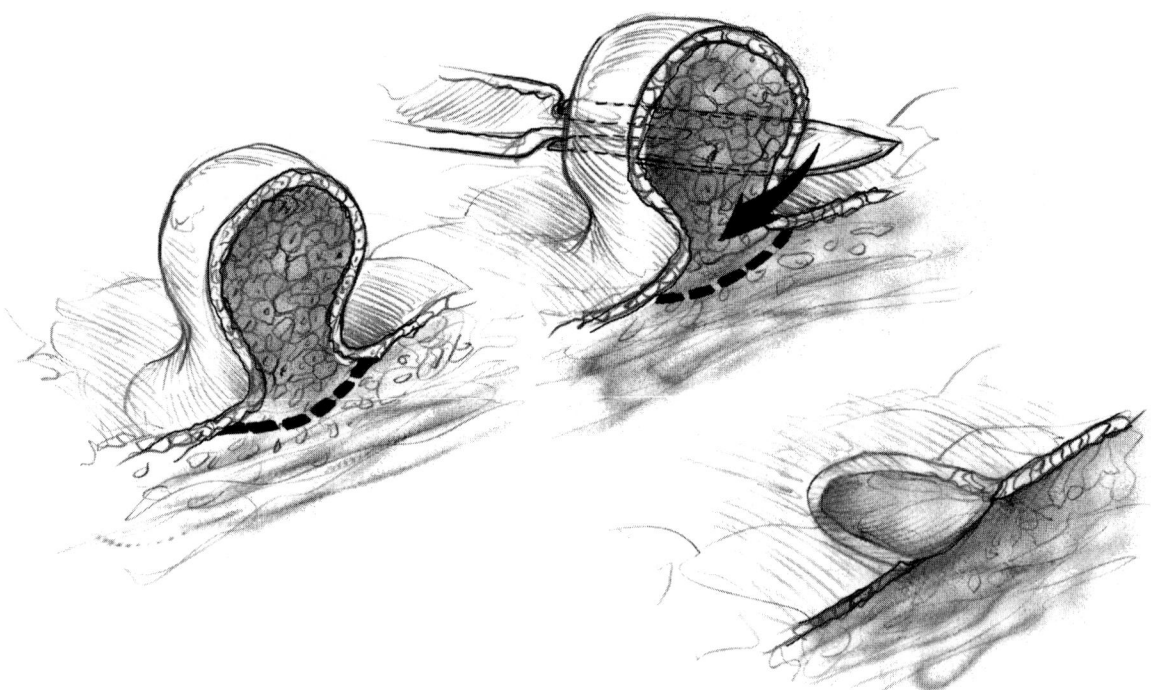

Figure 183.19   Shave biopsy.

skin (Fig. 183.21). These are used to diagnose inflammatory conditions or small tumors. For larger lesions, an excisional biopsy is performed. This is used if carcinoma is suspected or the pathologic process involves the fatty layer.

THERAPEUTIC CONSIDERATIONS: TECHNIQUES AND INSTRUMENTATION

Dermal Curette

The dermal curette is a small instrument with a semi-sharp round to oval blade of variable size (2 to 10 mm) (Fig. 183.22). This allows the surgeon to distinguish between normal and diseased collagen because the semi-sharp blade

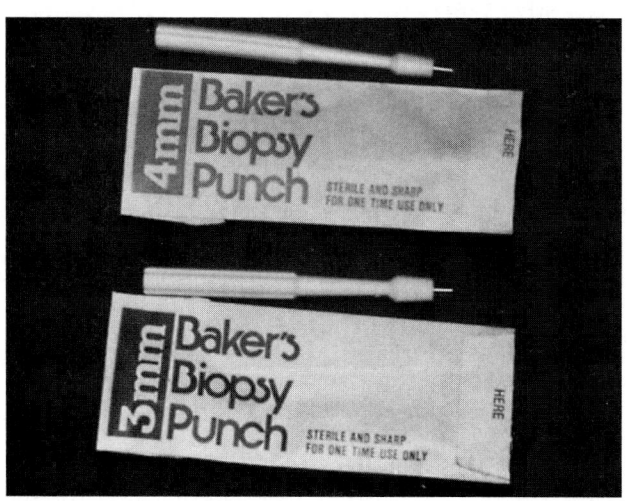

Figure 183.20   Punches (3 and 4 mm).

will not normally cut through normal collagen. Dermal curettes also are used to remove superficial epidermal lesions, which may be scraped off the skin's surface (seborrheic keratosis, warts) (Fig. 183.23). The instrument is easy and safe to use, but some experience is needed for the surgeon to distinguish reliably between diseased and normal dermal tissue.

Electrosurgery

In electrosurgery, rapidly oscillating electrical fields destroy tissue thermally and mechanically. A monopolar device (e.g., Hyfrecator) requires no grounding plate and results in superficial tissue destruction; a bipolar device requires a grounding plate and causes deeper tissue destruction. Either can be used for electrodesiccation. For electrosurgery, the needle tip is touched to tissue, destroying a deep sphere of tissue. For electrofulguration, the tip is held near the lesion, and a spark jumps from needle tip to tissue, destroying a broad superficial arc of tissue. Figure 183.24 shows electrofulguration with curettage to remove a xanthelasma. Electrosurgery is fast with minimal bleeding, but healing by second intent takes 2 to 3 weeks, there is no tissue for histologic examination, and there can be excessive scarring from thermal damage. Electrosurgery is often used with a dermal curette to define lesion margin or to remove tissue as it is destroyed. Complications include combustion of nondry alcohol-treated skin and interruption of certain cardiac pacemakers.

Cryotherapy

In cryotherapy, a cryogen (usually liquid nitrogen) destroys tissue. Freezing causes formation of extracellular and intracellular ice crystals, resulting in cell-membrane damage.

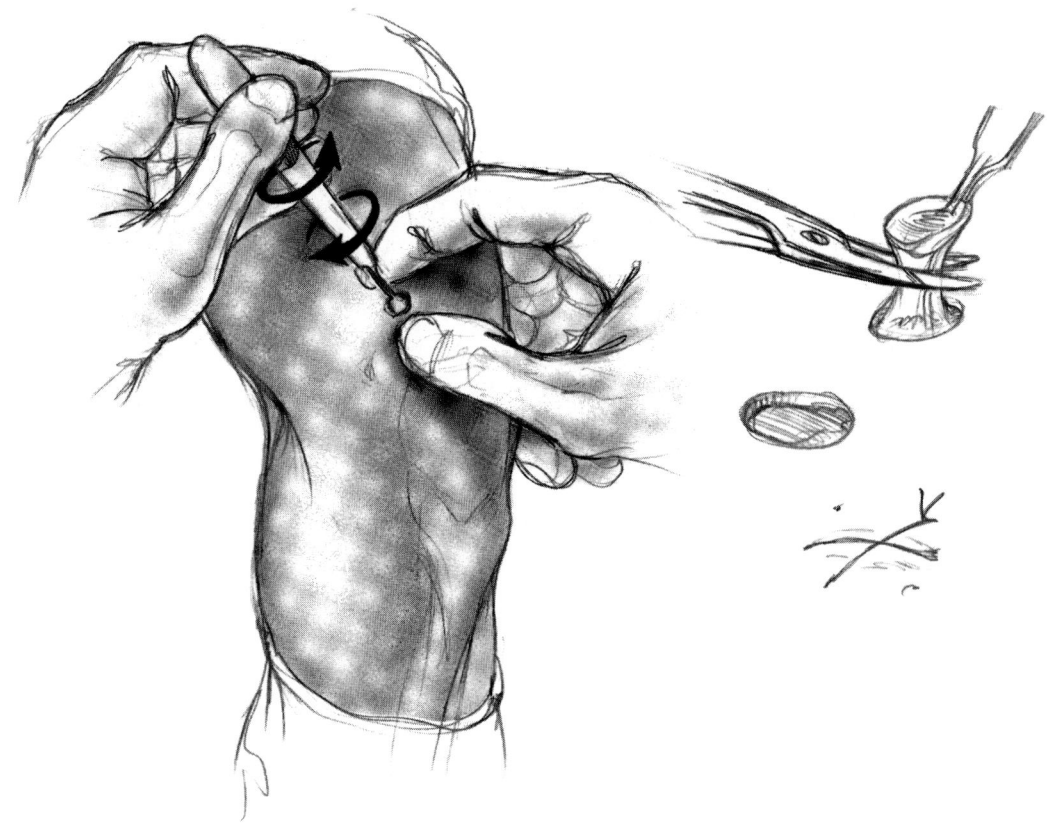

Figure 183.21   Punch biopsy technique.

Most cell damage occurs during thaw, when electrolyte concentrations become abnormal. Rapid freezing followed by slow thawing is most lethal to cells, with melanocytes being the most susceptible to injury. Tissue destruction is determined by the volume of cryogen applied, the duration of exposure, and the technique used.

A commonly used cryogen is liquid nitrogen, which is the coldest (−196°C) and most versatile agent. Common techniques of application include the cotton-tipped applicator, which is the easiest to learn but evaporates rapidly, necessitating frequent redipping. Spray can also be applied quickly to several lesions but requires skill to direct the cryogen to the specific lesion.

Intralesional Corticosteroid Therapy

Corticosteroid therapy, topical or intralesional, is used to treat inflammatory conditions. Intralesional steroids offer a more concentrated and sustained effect than topical steroids but have more side effects, such as atrophy (usually reversible in 12 months or more) or hypopigmentation (in darker-pigmented skin). Significant systemic absorption can occur when more than 20 mg are injected in a single session or at frequent intervals (Table 183.5).

Intralesional steroids are often used to soften or reduce the size of keloids or hypertrophic scars (10 to 40 mg/mL), repeated every 2 to 3 weeks to minimize systemic toxicity. Intralesional steroid injections also are used after laser or scalpel excision to prevent or reduce recurrence of keloid formation. Intralesional steroids are also used for acne cysts and inflamed epidermal cysts (2.5 to 5.0 mg/mL).

Chemical Peeling

Chemical peeling (chemexfoliation) improves skin quality and texture by applying exfoliants. This causes a variable depth of epidermal and dermal injury that, on healing, has thicker dermal collagen and, in some cases, increased dermal glycosaminoglycans and restoration of elastic fibers

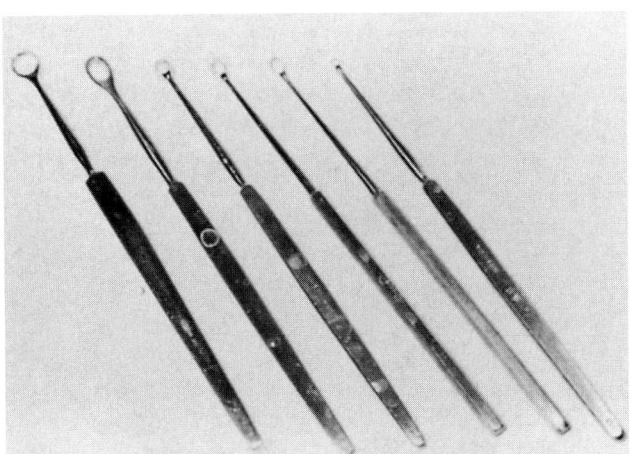

Figure 183.22   Curettes of various sizes.

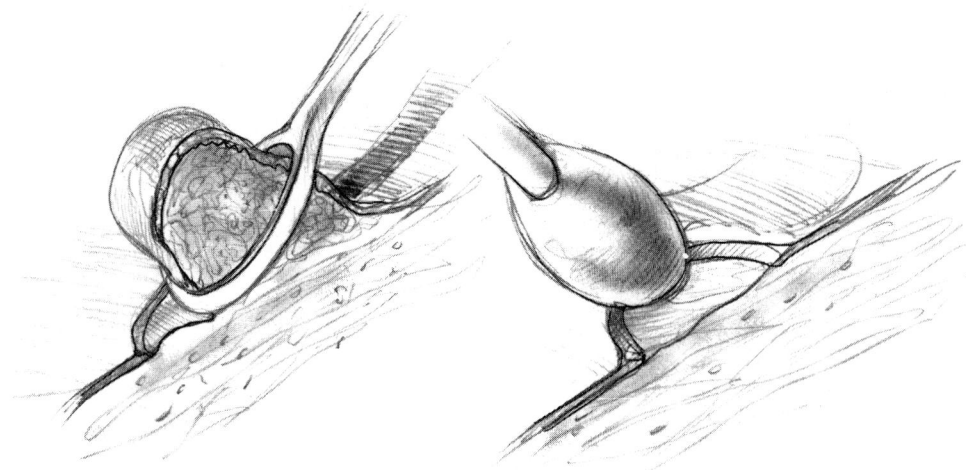

Figure 183.23 Curettage of a seborrheic keratosis.

in actinically damaged skin. Various peeling agents and combinations have been used, including trichloroacetic acid, phenol, resorcinol, salicylic acid, and more recently lactic and glycolic acid, each with different properties and depth of penetration. Phenol has a significant risk profile and the potential for systemic toxicity (Table 183.6).

Dermabrasion

Dermabrasion is an abrading procedure performed on skin to remove superficial lesions. Initially used to treat acne scars, more recently it has been applied to many cutaneous lesions (Table 183.7). Dermabrasion is performed with a motor-driven instrument with an abrading piece at the end. The abraders (commonly wire brush or diamond

fraise) come in various sizes, shapes, and degrees of coarseness.

Competent dermabrasion requires a high level of skill. One must control precisely the depth of the abrasion because prominent scarring occurs if abrasion penetrates reticular dermis. Dermabrasion has similar complications to chemical peeling (Table 183.6). Dermabrasion results can be more predictable than chemical peeling because the extent of wounding can be more precisely controlled.

Laser Surgery

The properties of lasers that make them useful in treating facial lesions (Table 183.8) are precise margination, good control of destruction depth, good hemostasis, decreased

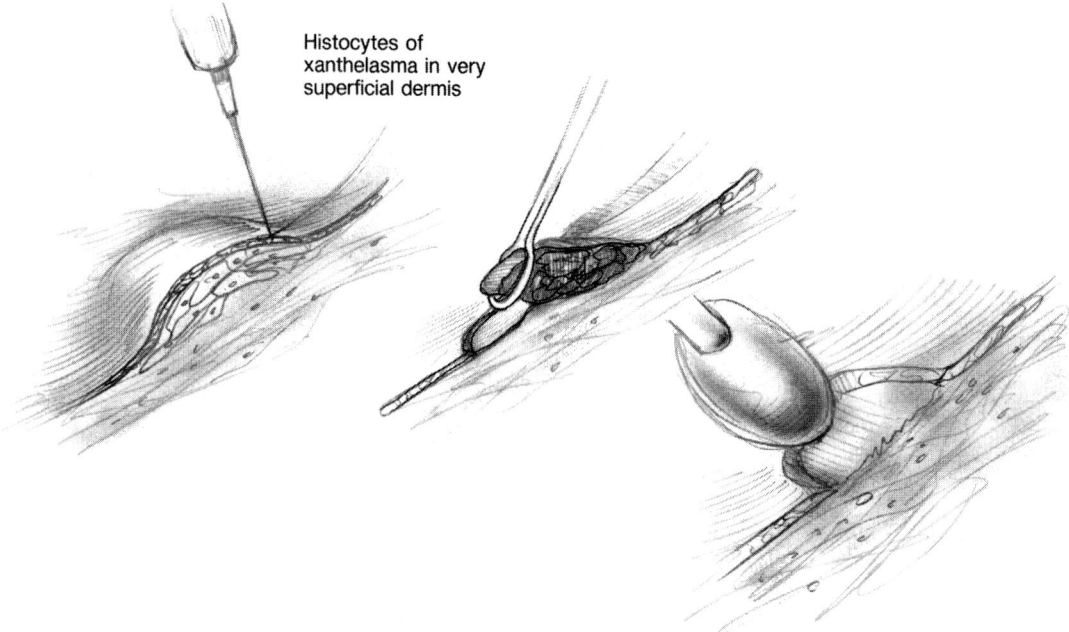

Histocytes of xanthelasma in very superficial dermis

Figure 183.24 Electrofulguration and curettage of a lesion of xanthelasma.

TABLE 183.5
SIDE EFFECTS OF INTRALESIONAL CORTICOSTEROIDS

Local side effects
Atrophy
Striae, stellate pseudoscars
Telangiectasia, purpura, erythema
Hypopigmentation
Impaired wound healing
Exacerbation of cutaneous infections

Systemic side effects
Cardiovascular effects: hypertension
Central nervous system effects: mood alterations, psychosis, pseudotumor cerebri
Endocrine effects: hypothalamic–pituitary–adrenal axis suppression, hirsutism, menstrual irregularities, truncal obesity, moon facies, buffalo hump
Gastrointestinal effects: peptic ulcer, pancreatitis
Hepatic effects: diabetes mellitus
Hematologic effects: lymphopenia, monocytopenia, neutrophilia
Immunologic effects: opportunistic infections
Musculoskeletal effects: osteoporosis, aseptic necrosis of femoral or humeral heads, myopathy
Ophthalmic effects: glaucoma, cataracts (posterior subcapsular)
Renal effects: sodium and fluid retention, hypokalemic alkalosis

Modified from Bondi E, ed. *Dermatology: diagnosis and therapy.* Norwalk, CT: Appleton & Lange, 1991:346, with permission.

postoperative pain, and target specificity (23). Lasers emit coherent light at specific wavelengths peculiar to the lasing material. This light energy is selectively absorbed by specific skin structures (chromophores) and converted into thermal energy, damaging the tissues. Thermal damage to surrounding tissues can be further reduced by pulsing the laser emission (selective photothermolysis).

Hemostatic Agents

Hemostatic agents are used to control bleeding from removal of superficial cutaneous lesions, which usually results in capillary or venous bleeding.

Monsel solution (ferric subsulfate) is a protein coagulant that is very effective but carries the slight risk of permanent discoloration from iron pigment deposition. Aluminum chloride (20%) is the most commonly used hemostatic agent. It is a colorless but less effective when

TABLE 183.6   COMPLICATIONS
CHEMICAL PEELING DERMABRASION

Pigmentary abnormalities (especially in dark-skinned patients)
Increased sun sensitivity
Hypertrophic scarring (especially over jawline, nasal bridge)
Reactivation or dissemination of herpes simplex
Persistent erythema
Milia

TABLE 183.7
ENTITIES TREATED WITH DERMABRASION

Acne, active
Acne rosacea
Actinically damaged skin
Adenoma sebaceum
Age- and sun-related wrinkle lines
Angiofibromas of tuberous sclerosis
Basal cell carcinoma (superficial type)
Chloasma
Chronic radiation dermatitis
Darier disease
Dermatitis papillaris capilliti
Favre-Racouchot syndrome
Fox-Fordyce
Freckles
Hair transplantation (elevated recipient sites)
Hemangioma
Keratoacanthoma
Leg ulcer
Lentigines
Lichen amyloidosis
Lichenified dermatoses
Molluscum contagiosum
Multiple pigmented nevi
Nevus flammeus
Verrucous
Multiple seborrheic keratoses
Multiple trichoepitheliomas
Neurotic excoriations
Nevi
   —Congenital pigmented nevi
   —Linear epidermal
Porokeratosis of Mibelli
Pseudofolliculitis barbae
Rhinophyma
Scars
   —Early operative
   —Keloids
   —Postacne
   —Traumatic
   —Smallpox or chickenpox
Scleromyxedema
Striae distensae
Syringocystadenoma papilliferum
Syringoma
Systemic lupus erythematosus
Tattoos
   —Amateur (India ink)
   —Blast (gunpowder)
   —Professional
Vitiligo
Telangiectasia
Xanthelasma
Xeroderma pigmentosum

compared to Monsel solution. Silver nitrate comes conveniently in a stick form or solution but is less effective than Monsel solution or aluminum chloride and can stain skin. It is useful in treating granulation tissue.

All chemical cauterants must be applied to a dry field so there is contact between the bleeding dermal bed and the

TABLE 183.8		
LASERS USED IN THE MANAGEMENT OF FACIAL SKIN LESIONS		
Laser	**Wavelength**	**Indications**
Argon (continuous)	488, 514 (blue-green)	Telangiectasias, thick PWS in adults, lentigines and ephelides
Argon-pumped tunable dye (continuous)	504–690 (green-yellow-red)	Telangiectasias, thick PWS in adults, lentigines and ephelides
Flashlamp-pumped dye (short-pulsed)	510 (green)	Lentigines and ephelides
Copper vapor/bromide (quasicontinuous)	511 (green)	Lentigines and ephelides
Krypton (continuous)	521,531 (green)	Lentigines and ephelides
KTP (quasicontinuous)	531 (green)	Telangiectasias, thick PWS in adults, lentigines and ephelides
Frequency-doubled Q-switched Nd:YAG (pulsed)	532 (green)	Lentigines and ephelides
Krypton (continuous)	568 (yellow)	Telangiectasias, thick PWS in adults
Copper vapor/bromide (quasicontinuous)	578 (yellow)	Telangiectasias, thick PWS in adults
Flashlamp-pumped dye (long-pulsed)	585 (yellow)	Flat PWS in children, telangiectasias, hypertrophic scars
Q-switched ruby (pulsed)	694 (red)	Lentigines, ephelides, blue nevus, nevus of Ota
Q-switched alexandrite (pulsed)	755 (near infrared)	Lentigines, ephelides, blue nevus, nevus of Ota
Q-Switched Nd: YAG (pulsed)	1,064 (infrared)	Blue nevus, nevus of Ota
Carbon dioxide (continuous, pulsed, super/ultrapulsed)	1,060 (infrared)	Rhinophyma, trichoepithelioma, syringoma, angiofibroma, keloids, xanthelasma, scars and rhytides

PWS, port-wine stain.

coagulant. These agents sting when used without local anesthetic.

TREATMENT OF SPECIFIC LESIONS

Seborrheic Keratosis

Seborrheic keratosis lesions are removed by dermal curette or by tangential excision with a scalpel, literally scraped off the skin's surface. If there are numerous lesions, cryotherapy or CO_2 laser can be used. Dermatosis papulosa nigra is treated with light electrodesiccation using fine-tipped cautery needles, then curettage.

Actinic Keratosis

Actinic keratosis lesions usually are treated with cryotherapy. Multiple lesions may require several sessions or alternative therapies, including dermabrasion, chemical peeling, topical 5-fluorouracil (Efudex, Fluoroplex), or topical imiquimod. 5-Fluorouracil comes in concentrations of 1% to 5% and is applied to the face twice daily for 3 weeks. A brisk inflammatory response develops in affected areas. Healing occurs over 6 to 8 weeks and is accelerated by the use of topical corticosteroids. Results are excellent but not

permanent, with retreatment often necessary in 2 to 3 years. Imiquimod 5% cream was approved in 2004 for the treatment of actinic keratosis of the face or scalp. Whether administered as monotherapy or adjunctive therapy, topical therapies provide the opportunity to effectively manage actinic keratosis and will likely emerge as an important tool for health care providers (24).

Cutaneous Horns

Cutaneous horns are completely removed (shave or punch technique) so the base can be examined histologically. Usually an actinic keratosis is found, so it is reasonable to curette and electrodesiccate the base lightly after lesion removal. If a squamous cell or basal cell carcinoma is confirmed by histologic examination, a wider excision is performed.

Epidermal Cysts

Small inflamed cysts occur with acne vulgaris and are treated with intralesional steroids in concentrations of 2 to 5 mg/mL. This results in complete resolution in 3 to 5 days, with a low incidence of recurrence. The injection may cause temporary dermal atrophy, which resolves in 6 to 12 months.

Infected cysts are generally large and of longer duration than small acne-associated cysts. They are tender with surrounding erythema. These are best treated with systemic antibiotics, especially those with additional antiinflammatory effects such as tetracycline and erythromycin. For tense and severely inflamed lesions, incision, drainage, culture, and sensitivity determination should be performed, and the treated lesions should be packed with iodoform gauze. Antibiotics against *Staphylococcus aureus* are empirically started. Surgical therapy is deferred for 4 to 6 weeks after infection because infection thins the cyst wall and dermal collagen, making the procedure difficult and increasing the chances of infection spreading. Intralesional steroids should not be used on infected cysts.

The treatment of noninfected, noninflamed cysts is surgical, with complete cyst wall removal (to prevent recurrence). Freely mobile cysts have little connection with the overlying epidermis and are easily removed. Injection of local anesthetics between the cyst wall and surrounding tissues (hydrodissection) facilitates surgical removal.

If the cyst is firmly adherent to the surrounding tissues, the entire cyst and surrounding fibrous tissue are excised. The use of a punch biopsy instead of an ellipse may provide an opening large enough to remove the cyst with excellent cosmetic results. Epidermal cysts that are freely or partially mobile may be removed through incisions at distant sites where cosmetic factors are overriding (e.g., a mucosal approach to remove a lip cyst or an incision in the hairline to remove a nearby forehead cyst).

Complications include infection, bleeding, and dehiscence and are usually a result of poor technique. If the cyst wall ruptures with spillage of keratinous material, the area is irrigated with normal saline and all recognizable keratinous debris is removed. Necrosis of overlying skin once a cyst is removed usually occurs when a large cyst has been removed, resulting in large dead space with overlying epidermis. To avoid necrosis, all underlying dead space is removed and tension at the skin edges is minimized. Any redundant skin that may occur in cyst surgery is excised.

Milia

A milia is treated by incising its roof and extracting its keratinous core with a milia comedo extractor. No local anesthetic is required. This technique also may be used for large closed comedones. Smaller closed comedones and open comedones (blackheads) are treated with topical retinoic acid (Retin-A).

Trichofolliculomas

Trichofolliculomas are removed by shaving, punch excision with suturing, or vaporization with a CO_2 laser.

Trichoepitheliomas

Solitary trichoepitheliomas are removed the same way as trichofolliculomas. However, distinction of basal cell carcinoma and solitary trichoepithelioma is difficult both clinically and pathologically. Multiple trichoepitheliomas are removed with dermabrasion and CO_2 laser with excellent results.

Pilomatricomas

Pilomatricomas, deep-seated nodules, require surgical excision in most cases.

Trichilemmomas

Solitary lesions of trichilemmoma are treated as trichofolliculomas. Multiple lesions can be treated with dermabrasion.

Nevus Sebaceus

A nevus sebaceus lesion is sometimes completely excised because it has malignant potential; however, its risk for malignancy is low. It also may be followed for changes of malignancy and treated at a later date if necessary.

Sebaceous Hyperplasia

Sebaceous hyperplasia lesions are treated with cryotherapy or light electrodesiccation with fine-tipped cautery needles.

Rhinophyma

Rhinophyma is treated with electrosurgery, dermabrasion, and argon or CO_2 laser. Excessive sebaceous tissue is excised and the nose is sculpted to its predisease shape. Dermabrasion and CO_2 laser allow the surgeon to sculpt with control and precision, the latter maintaining a relatively bloodless field. Regardless of technique, results are usually excellent. Removing tissue below the pilosebaceous apparatus results in an unattractive, unnaturally smooth, poreless scar.

Hidrocystoma

The hidrocystoma cyst is surgically excised if necessary for cosmetic reasons. Simple incision and drainage result in recurrence.

Syringoma

Syringomas usually present as multiple lesions; therefore, surgical excision is usually not feasible. Dermabrasion and superficial CO_2 laser offer fair results on those selected lesions that are more cosmetically concerning to the patient. Electrodesiccation is sometimes sufficient.

Hemangiomas

Most capillary hemangiomas resolve spontaneously, so treatment is usually not necessary. Exceptions are hemangiomas that ulcerate, encroach on a vital structure (nose, eyes, mouth), or are frequently traumatized (buttock, foot). For these, medical therapy (prednisone and interferon-alpha) or intralesional corticosteroids are used. A nevus flammeus (port-wine stain) is treated with tunable dye lasers or, more recently, copper vapor, krypton, or flashlamp-pumped pulsed-dye lasers (Table 183.8). Complications are uncommon with these techniques, with occasional hypopigmentation or skin texture alterations. Scarring and tissue induration are rare. Lesions in dark-skinned patients lighten less than others because epidermal melanin causes some absorption of the laser light.

Pyogenic Granuloma

Pyogenic granulomas are treated aggressively because recurrence is common if excision is incomplete. Shave removal with electrosurgery of the base is simple and effective, as is elliptical excision. Ablation with a CO_2 laser, argon laser, dye laser, or copper vapor laser is also effective.

Telangiectasias

Telangiectasias can be treated simply with electrodesiccation using fine cautery needles (epilating needles). The lowest possible setting on a Hyfrecator or Bovie is used to avoid scarring. Telangiectasias also can be treated with laser therapy (argon, argon-pumped tunable dye, copper vapor, krypton, frequency-doubled Nd:YAG, or flashlamp-pumped pulsed dye). Sclerotherapy (injection of sclerosing agent into the telangiectasia) can be used, but there is the potential of introducing some sclerosant into the cavernous sinus or deep venous drainage of the head and neck, causing potentially grave complications (e.g., blindness, cavernous sinus thrombosis).

Spider Angiomas

Spider angiomas are treated similarly to telangiectasias. In electrosurgery, the needle is placed into the central punctum of the spider angioma. Lesions can recur, so additional treatment may be needed.

Venous Lakes

Small lesions of venous lakes are treated by excision or electrodesiccation. Larger lesions are treated with laser therapy (argon, dye, or copper vapor).

Skin Tags

Skin tags can be snipped off at the base with a sharp curved iris scissors. Local anesthetic is generally not required. Electrodesiccation also can be used.

Fibrous Papule

For a fibrous papule, simple shave excision produces an acceptable cosmetic result and is preferable to superficial destruction methods (CO_2 laser, electrosurgery), which do not permit histologic examination.

Adenoma Sebaceus

Adenoma sebaceus lesions are treated with dermabrasion, CO_2 laser, or argon laser. The argon produces excellent cosmetic results, particularly in patients who have lightly pigmented skin.

Hypertrophic Scars and Keloids

Hypertrophic scars and keloids are managed with intralesional steroids; dermabrasion; pressure; or, most recently, silicone gel matrix. Several treatment strategies often are combined in hopes of better treatment outcomes. Many hypertrophic scars flatten over time. However, long-term results of all treatment options for keloids are poor. Results in the literature are difficult to interpret because most lack long-term follow-up (at least 2 years) and histopathologic criteria to confirm that the lesions are keloids and not hypertrophic scars.

Neurofibromas

Neurofibromas can be excised, CO_2 vaporized, shaved, or removed with electrosurgical cutting current to the base. If the entire lesion is not removed, however, it will regrow slowly. Multiple facial lesions can be dermabraded or excised by CO_2 laser.

Lipomas

Small lipomas can be removed through a small stab incision in the overlying skin. Some lipomas extend insidiously beyond their clinical borders and lie deep to fascia or within muscle. These need to be sharply dissected from surrounding tissue. Giant lipomas may be removed by liposuction. The liposuction cannula is inserted via a small incision. Some lipomas have multiple fibrous septae, requiring careful scissor dissection. Beware of lipomas on the forehead because they often are located beneath the frontalis muscle (subgaleal lipomas). Attempts at excision are frustrating unless the surgeon knows to look in this deeper plane.

Leiomyomas

Leiomyomas are best treated with simple excision.

Melanocytic Nevi

With melanocytic nevi, we are discussing benign nevi, not congenital or dysplastic nevi. Benign nevi can be intradermal, compound, or junctional and can be partly or completely removed. Except for junctional nevi, most nevi are elevated and can be removed by shave technique. This leaves a recurrence risk from residual nevus cells of 10% to 20%. A small hypopigmented area usually results. When a nevus is recurrent, histopathologic interpretation of these often shows atypical or pleomorphic-appearing cells, which can be difficult to distinguish from melanoma (pseudomelanoma).

Two other problems occurring after a shave excision are a depressed scar or peripheral lipping. Depression occurs if local anesthetic infiltration raises the lesion above the skin surface and is avoided by allowing the anesthetic to diffuse out of the lesion before shaving it off. Lipping results if the nevus is not removed flush with surrounding skin because of variable shear forces during shaving. Hemostasis is achieved with aluminum chloride. Monsel solution can hinder histopathologic interpretation of a recurrent nevus because its ferrous subsulfate can be misconstrued as melanin pigment within dermal macrophages.

The second method of removing nevi is complete excision of the lesion. This is necessary for flat nevi. The incision is placed in relaxed skin tension lines. Spot dermabrasion of the scar after 4 to 6 weeks improves the cosmetic result. Complete excision provides a specimen for histologic examination and minimizes recurrence risk.

Spitz Nevi

Spitz nevi are excised for histopathologic examination. This is important because they can resemble malignant melanoma microscopically and the pathologist relies on architectural features lost in a shave biopsy.

Blue Nevi

Simple blue nevi are removed with shave technique or excision. Larger lesions that look like blue nevi are best excised for complete histopathologic examination. Nevi of Ota have been treated successfully with Q-switched Nd:YAG and ruby lasers.

Lentigines and Ephelides

Lentigines and ephelides respond to similar therapy and are similar pathologic processes. For just a few lesions, cryotherapy is probably the easiest treatment. Laser therapy (ruby, alexandrite, pulsed dye, krypton, copper vapor, or frequency-doubled Nd:YAG) is also successful (Table 183.8). For widespread multiple lesions, chemexfoliation is best. A wide variety of agents has been used: retinoic acid, trichloroacetic acid, and alpha hydroxy (glycolic) acids. Retinoic acid carries the fewest risks and is started at low strength (0.025% cream) to minimize irritant effects.

Molluscum Contagiosum

Small numbers of lesions respond well to curettage, cryotherapy, or daily application of topical imiquimod. In patients who are immunocompromised, lesions may

number in the thousands and become thick, verrucous, and refractory to treatment. Most recently, chemical peeling with trichloroacetic acid and retinoic acid has been used successfully.

Verrucae

Common and filiform varieties respond well to cryotherapy and electrodesiccation and curettage, although recurrences are common. Flat warts (usually multiple and superficial) respond well to chemexfoliation with retinoic acid or trichloroacetic acid as well as to cryotherapy or topical imiquimod. Harsh keratolytics (e.g., salicylic acid) and blistering agents should not be used in treating facial verrucae because they may lead to scarring.

HIGHLIGHTS

- A classification scheme helps narrow the diagnostic possibilities.
- Seemingly benign facial lesions may be a sign of serious systemic disease.
- Biopsy is the most valuable laboratory aid for diagnosing skin lesions.
- Cosmetic outcomes are important in treating benign facial lesions.
- The risks of all facial surgery should be described to the patient in detail preoperatively.

REFERENCES

1. Freedberg IM, Eisen AZ, Wolff K, et al., eds. *Fitzpatrick's dermatology in general medicine*, 6th ed. New York: McGraw-Hill, 2003.
2. Arndt KA, Leboit PE, Robinson JK, et al., eds. *Cutaneous medicine and surgery*. Philadelphia: WB Saunders, 1996.
3. Champion RH, Burton JL, Burns AD, et al., eds. *Rook's textbook of dermatology*, 6th ed. London: Blackwell Scientific, 1998.
4. Elder DE, Elenitsas R, Jaworsky C, eds. *Lever's histopathology of the skin*, 8th ed. Philadelphia: Lippincott-Raven, 1997.
5. Bolognia JL, Jorizzo JL, Rapini RP. *Dermatology*. London, New York: Mosby, 2003.
6. Salasche SJ. Epidemiology of actinic keratoses and squamous cell carcinoma. *J Am Acad Dermatol* 2000;42:S4–S7.
7. Glogau RG. The risk of progression to invasive disease. *J Am Acad Dermatol* 2000;42:S23–S24.
8. Bondeson J. Everard Home, John Hunter, and cutaneous horns: a historical review. *Am J Dermatopathol* 2001;23:362–369.
9. Vielhauer V, Herzinger T, Korting HC. The sign of Leser-Trélat: a paraneoplastic cutaneous syndrome that facilitates early diagnosis of occult cancer. *Eur J Med Res* 2000;5:512–516.
10. Heaphy MR Jr, Millns JL, Schroeter AL. The sign of Leser-Trélat in a case of adenocarcinoma of the lung. *J Am Acad Dermatol* 2000;43:386–390.
11. Eng C. Will the real Coden syndrome please stand up: revised diagnostic criteria. *J Med Genet* 2000;37:828–830.
12. Prioleau PG, Santa Cruz DJ. Sebaceous gland neoplasia. *J Cutan Pathol* 1984;11:396–414.
13. Jaqueti G, Requena L, Sanchez Yus E. Trichoblastoma is the most common neoplasm developed in nevus sebaceus of Jadassohn: a clinicopathologic study of a series of 155 cases. *Am J Dermatopathol* 2000;22:108–118.
14. Cribier B, Grosshans E. Tumor of the follicular infundibulum: a clinicopathologic study. *J Am Acad Dermatol* 1995;33:979–984.

15. Cribier B, Scrivener Y, Grosshans E. Tumors arising in nevus sebaceus: A study of 596 cases. *J Am Acad Dermatol* 2000;42:263–268.

16. Scheithauer BW, Woodruff JM, Erlandson RA. Tumors of the peripheral nervous system. In: *Atlas of Tumor Pathology*, Third series, Fascicle 24. Washington, DC: Armed Forces Institute of Pathology, 1999:1–415.

17. DeDavid M, Orlow SJ, Provost N, et al. A study of large congenital melanocytic nevi and associated malignant melanomas: review of cases in the New York University Registry and the world literature. *J Am Acad Dermatol* 1997;36:409–415.

18. Marghoob AA, Schoenbach SP, Kopf AW, et al. Large congenital melanocytic nevi and the risk for the development of malignant melanoma. A prospective study. *Arch Dermatol* 1996;132:170–175.

19. Patel BC, Egan CA, Lucius RW, et al. Cutaneous malignant melanoma in oculodermal melanocytosis (nevus of Ota): report of a case and review of the literature. *J Am Acad Dermatol* 1998;38:862.

20. Teekhasaenee C, Ritch R, Rutnin U, et al. Ocular findings in oculodermal melanocytosis. *Arch Ophthalmol* 1990;108:1114.

21. Roenigk RK, Roenigk HH Jr, eds. *Dermatologic surgery: principles and practice*. New York: Marcel Dekker, 1996.

22. Bennett RG. *Fundamentals of cutaneous surgery*. St. Louis: Mosby, 1988.

23. Wheeland RG. Clinical uses of lasers in dermatology. *Lasers Surg Med* 1995;16:2.

24. Jorizzo JL. Current and novel treatment options for actinic keratosis. *J Cutan Med Surg* 2004;8(suppl)3:13–21.

Management of Alopecia

Benjamin A. Bassichis   **Raymond J. Konior**

Burns, traction, dermatitis, autoimmune disease, neoplasms, radiation exposure, and chemotherapy all can cause hair loss in humans (Table 184.1). The most common type of hair loss in men and women, however, is androgenetic alopecia (AGA), also known as male pattern baldness (MPB). This form of alopecia affects scalp follicles with a genetic potential to androgen inhibition, resulting in the conversion of susceptible terminal hairs to vellus hairs. The hair follicles most likely to demonstrate AGA are in the frontotemporal and the crown regions of the scalp. Several different surgical options are available for restoring hair growth on a balding scalp. The procedure of choice for any given individual will depend on many factors. These include (a) patient's age, (b) degree of baldness, (c) density within the donor region, (d) contrast characteristics of the hair and skin, and (e) patient expectations.

A classification system for MPB is essential for planning and comparing the results of different surgical procedures. The Norwood system, the one most often used, organizes MPB into seven categories, ranging from class I (minimal frontotemporal recession) to class VII (a very narrow,

TABLE 184.1
ETIOLOGY OF ALOPECIA

Androgenic alopecia (male pattern baldness)
Autoimmune disease
Burns
Chemotherapy
Dermatologic disorders (e.g., psoriasis)
Neoplasms
Radiation exposure
Traction

TABLE 184.2 ℞
TREATMENT—ANDROGENETIC ALOPECIA

Extensive scalp reduction
Finasteride (Propecia)
Flaps
Hair-bearing autografts:
   Follicular unit grafts
   Micrografts
   Minigrafts
   Scalp reduction
   Standard circular grafts
Minoxidil (Rogaine)
Tissue expansion

horseshoe-shaped band of hair in the temporal and low occipital regions) (1). Table 184.2 lists treatment options for MPB.

MEDICAL TREATMENT OF ANDROGENETIC ALOPECIA

Attempts to medically manage MPB are nothing new. Hippocrates, in about 400 B.C., prescribed several concoctions composed of animal and plant products to treat baldness.

Ideally, the medical treatment of AGA should be directed against dihydrotestosterone (DHT), the active agent involved in MPB. Finasteride (Propecia), which has been used for years to manage prostate hypertrophy, has been more recently approved by the U.S. Food and Drug Administration (FDA) for the treatment of MPB. Finasteride is a competitive and specific inhibitor of type II 5α-reductase, an intracellular enzyme that converts the androgen testosterone into DHT. Two distinct 5α-reductase isozymes are found in humans. The type II 5α-reductase isozyme is primarily found in the prostate, seminal vesicles, epididymides, and hair follicles. Finasteride has no affinity for androgen receptors but works by blocking the peripheral conversion of testosterone to DHT. Using the recommended dose of 1 mg/day, finasteride produces statistically significant increased hair counts in men with mild-to-moderate degrees of androgenetic alopecia. Systemic therapy that reduces or interferes with androgen levels enough to stop hair loss has the potential to reduce libido and sexual potency, making this form of treatment unacceptable to some men. Drug-related sexual adverse experiences resulting in discontinuation of therapy have been reported in 1.2% of patients on finasteride versus 0.9% of patients on placebo (2,3).

Minoxidil (Rogaine) was the first drug approved by the FDA for the medical management of MPB. This drug, which traditionally had been used to treat resistant hypertension, was noted to occasionally produce hypertrichosis as a side effect of oral therapy in adults. Minoxidil functions as a potassium channel opener and vasodilator. Currently, the dosages available are 2% and 5% formulations. In men, the 5% minoxidil solution demonstrates a significant advantage over treatment with the 2% solution (4). The mechanism by which minoxidil works to stimulate hair growth remains unclear. In addition, Minoxidil does not have any known effect on the production, excretion, or interactions of human androgens. Most, if not all, hair transplant surgeons recommend the use of minoxidil and/or finasteride to the majority of their patients (5).

SURGICAL TREATMENT OF ALOPECIA

Hairline Design

The most important goal of hair-replacement surgery is to restore aesthetic balance to the face by recreating a natural, age-appropriate frontal hairline and part. The surgically restored hair should be easy to maintain and should not require extraordinary hairstyles for camouflage.

The mature male hairline usually demonstrates distinct triangular region bilaterally at the junction of the frontal and the temporal hair (Fig. 184.1). These frontotemporal triangles are formed by recession of the frontal hairline superiorly and the temporal hairline posteriorly. The ultimate goal of surgical hair restoration is to recreate the natural frontotemporal triangles, where the frontal hairline side is created from transplanted hair and the lateral side consists of the naturally receding temporal fringe (6).

A natural frontal hairline is convex, with the central portion positioned slightly inferior to the frontotemporal triangle region. The apex of the frontotemporal triangle marks the lateral aspect of a natural hairline. Regardless of

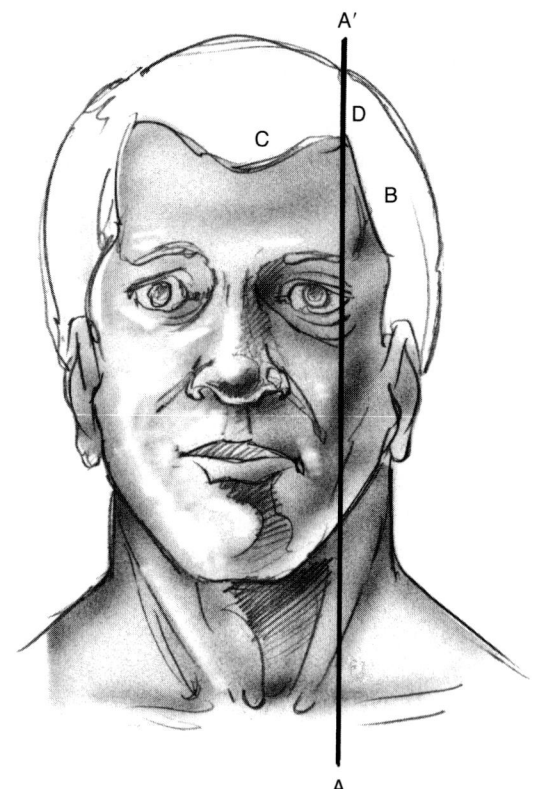

Figure 184.1 The frontotemporal triangle (*BCD*) is defined by the frontal and the temporal hairlines. When planning surgical restoration of the frontal hairline, the apex of the triangle is designed to fall on a vertical line (*AA'*) that intersects the lateral canthus.

the extent of hairline recession, the apex is designed to fall on a vertical line drawn upward from the lateral canthus of the eye. Because the temporal hairline intersects the lateral extent of the frontal hairline, advanced temporal recessions require a more posterior frontal hairline. Any attempt to fill a large frontotemporal triangle as a means of compensating for advanced temporal recessions will result in an unnatural hairline and part. Scalp reductions can be considered for raising the temporal hairline in those patients with a low-lying superior temporal fringe.

Patient Evaluation

During the first consultation, the patient should receive a thorough physical evaluation and an explanation of the surgical options available. The physician must understand the patient's motivations and expectations regarding hair-restoration surgery. Patients who seem emotionally labile may require a psychiatric assessment to evaluate their true motivations, but most patients requesting hair replacement do not have emotional problems; they simply would prefer not to be bald.

Several factors determine what procedure, if any, is appropriate for restoring an alopecic scalp. It is not uncommon for the patient to expect more than can be accomplished with the donor area available. The major reason for rejecting a patient is an inadequate supply of donor hair relative to the patient's final goals.

The ideal patient is one with enough donor hair to completely fill all current or potential areas of alopecia. The younger the patient, the more conservative the physician must be in estimating the donor hair present and establishing a long-term treatment plan. An accurate assessment of the donor area is required to prevent moving follicles at risk for future alopecia into cosmetically important areas on the scalp, because any future hair loss in those transplanted follicles will result in exposed scars over the scalp. In younger patients whose final hair-loss patterns cannot be determined, the physician should try to delay hair restoration until the physician is secure with the availability of donor hair.

Low-density donor hair may be a contraindication to hair transplantation. Patients with fewer than eight hairs in a 4-mm diameter circular area tend to be poor candidates for hair transplantation, unless they are willing to accept very thin hair density from the transplantation procedures. Age is not a contraindication to hair transplantation. Older patients generally have well-established patterns of alopecia that allow a more reliable assessment of the donor area.

Hair color, skin color, and hair texture are important factors in surgical hair restoration. A sharp contrast between the hair and the skin may result in an unnatural-appearing hairline. This is especially true if transplantation is performed with grafts that contain more than one follicle-unit, such as large minigrafts or standard 4-mm circular punch grafts. The best hair colors for surgical hair restoration in light-skinned patients are white, salt-and-pepper, and blond. Patients with dark skin and dark hair and those with wiry hair generally are good candidates for hair restoration. Naturally curly hair appears thicker than straight hair, thereby enhancing the results of most hair-replacement procedures.

FEMALE PATTERN HAIR LOSS

In hair restoration, men constitute more than 90% of the patients seeking treatment. As techniques in surgical management continue to improve and public awareness of high patient satisfaction increases, however, there are increasing numbers of women undergoing treatment for hair loss. The approach to female pattern hair loss is much different than male pattern baldness, as only 10% of women have an androgenic hair loss pattern. Therefore, the overwhelming majority of women have hair loss for variety of other reasons, such as hormonal and autoimmune.

The workup involves recognizing the enormous psychological toll hair loss takes on a woman and using appropriate sensitivity when treating women with hair loss. Referral to an endocrinologist is usually part of the workup. Minoxidil 2% solution has been effective in treating female pattern hair loss. Increased dosages of 5% minoxidil have caused unacceptable rates of facial hypertrichosis to occur. Finasteride has not been shown to have benefit in women. Surgical hair restoration remains the only permanent treatment for hair loss in women. The same principles of adequate donor area and advanced transplantation techniques lead to better outcomes (7).

ANESTHESIA

Because most patients require multiple procedures, an adequate comfort level is essential to maintaining motivation for completion of the entire restoration process. Local anesthesia is sufficient for most hair-restoration procedures, but general anesthesia is occasionally necessary for extensive scalp reductions or flap procedures.

A preoperative sedative is commonly given before the injection of local anesthesia. Regional frontal, occipital, and temporal nerve blocks using 1% lidocaine with 1:100,000 epinephrine are performed before performing a wide-field, circumferential scalp block. This technique anesthetizes the entire hair-bearing scalp.

AUTOGRAFT HAIR TRANSPLANTATION

Okuda (8), a Japanese dermatologist, is generally regarded as the first to describe the successful use of full-thickness hair-bearing autografts for correcting alopecia of the scalp, eyebrow, and mustache areas. Hair transplantation using punch grafts was introduced in the United States in 1959 by Orentreich (9). He coined the term *donor dominance* to describe the fact that autografts maintain characteristics of the donor tissue when transplanted into other regions of the body. Patients followed for more than 30 years continue to demonstrate persistent hair growth following punch-graft hair transplantation (10).

Donor Site

The donor site is that portion of the scalp that contains permanent hair dense enough to permit the harvesting of graft material. This area is usually found on the sides and the back of the head and is limited anteriorly by a vertical line through the external auditory canal. The superior border of the safe donor area in the mid-occipital region is generally located beneath a horizontal line that intersects the superior attachment of the auricles to the scalp.

The ideal harvesting method for hair transplantation uses a multiblade knife to simultaneously remove several parallel strips of scalp from the donor region (11). The space between the scalpel blades on this device can be adjusted to allow the harvesting of different strip widths. Most often, the donor strips measure 1.5 to 3.0 mm in width; the exact dimensions depend on what size grafts the surgeon requires for the recipient site. Usually a total width of no more than 1 cm is removed from the donor site, to minimize tension following closure of the wound site.

Some patients' follicles exhibit tremendous directional variations throughout the donor scalp region. In these cases, the multiblade parallel-strip harvesting technique increases the risk of marginal follicular loss secondary to direct follicle transection. To minimize this situation, the preferred harvesting method for patients with multidirectional follicle growth at the donor site involves removing a single strip of donor scalp, usually about 1 cm wide. Using a single scalpel blade to incise the scalp, these donor sites are obtained with particular care in ensuring the blade is parallel to the angle of follicular growth.

Before harvesting grafts, the hair along the donor site is trimmed to about 3 mm. Saline is then infiltrated into the donor site to tense the mobile scalp skin. Donor site turgidity minimizes the soft-tissue distortion that results from pressure generated by the scalpel as it cuts the scalp. Failure to tense the scalp predisposes to irregularly shaped strips and follicular transection. The scalpel blades must be parallel the hair follicles to produce an excellent-quality strip. Strip margins are routinely examined during harvesting for evidence of tissue distortion or follicle damage. Poor strip quality may require additional saline infiltration into the surrounding tissues or better alignment of the scalpel blades with the existing hair shafts. The donor strips are removed by incising the subfollicular fat just beneath the base of the follicles. The donor site is sutured closed with a running 4-0 nylon suture. A tension-free closure is mandatory to prevent follicular necrosis and a wide scar along the donor site incision line.

Follicular unit extraction is similar to the older punch extraction technique but uses smaller punches. The purpose of this technique is to avoid the longer incisions, which may widen over time. The proponents of this technique also claim there is less pain and chance of scarring. The disadvantages are that the tiny punches use a relatively "blind" technique, which requires a great amount of attention to proper angling. The technique is mentioned here, as it may have a role in cases that involve smaller graft numbers or in patients who are fearful of any visible scarring in the donor area (12).

The donor site strips are examined using magnification, and any transected hair shafts are removed from the edges. Excess subcutaneous fat is trimmed, taking care to leave about 2 mm of fat below the matrix zone of the hair follicles. The strips are then placed flat on a sterile, back-lit cutting surface. Individual grafts are made by using a scalpel blade to cut the strips parallel to the path of the embedded follicles. Follicular units used in the hairline should be trimmed to create a teardrop-shaped graft. This method allows for improved density and decreased potential for pitting and graft trauma (13). Different sized grafts can be developed by adjusting the width of the cuts being made

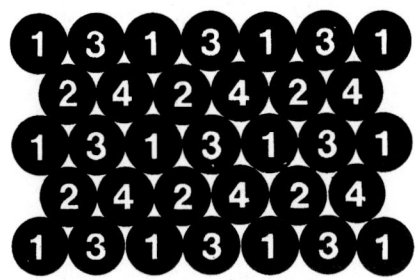

Figure 184.2 Autograft hair transplantation is commonly performed in four sessions; a typical grafting sequence is shown. Precise spacing is required during each session to establish maximum hair density and to maintain adequate circulation around the newly placed grafts.

along the donor strips. Microscopic dissection techniques are preferred to assure the highest quality, most natural-appearing grafts.

Recipient Site

Most alopecic areas can be filled with dense-appearing hair using two to four transplant sessions. Grafts are inserted into the recipient site using holes made with either a trephine punch or slits from a scalpel blade. The grafts are spaced evenly apart from each other, taking care to preserve an intact, circumferential bridge of skin between adjacent grafts. This is necessary to maintain adequate circulation around each graft (Fig. 184.2). To maintain a natural hair-growth pattern, the original hair direction and exit angle from the scalp are followed when cutting the recipient site slits or holes. Consistent angling is required throughout all graft sessions to prevent transecting previously transplanted follicles. The hair along the frontal hairline is directed anteriorly at approximately a 10-to-15-degree angle. As the placement of slits extends laterally toward the temple, the hairline is pointed more inferiorly toward the ear and leaves the scalp at a very flat angle.

Modern hair transplantation techniques favor using one of two methods to achieve both density and refinement within the transplanted hairline regions: (a) the exclusive use of follicular unit grafts (14); and (b) combinations of minigrafts and micrografts (15). A follicular unit is a microscopic cluster of closely united follicles. Each cluster of related follicles maintains a microscopically anatomic separation from adjacent follicle unit clusters. A follicle unit usually contains one to four hairs. Follicular unit transplantation requires the use of an operating microscope for optimal graft preparation. The frontal hairline is composed of single hair follicular units, with 2 to 4 hair follicular units placed more posteriorly. Microscopic assistance is not used with minigraft and micrograft techniques. Minigrafts contain three to eight hairs, whereas micrografts have only one or two hairs. Micrografts are commonly used to refine the outer perimeter of the transplanted recipient site, especially along the anterior aspect of the frontal hairline. Micrografts soften the transition zone between the bald forehead skin and the transplanted frontal hairline (16). Minigrafts, because of their larger size, are used to create higher density hair, more posteriorly within the recipient site.

Transplantation of the crown requires re-creation of a natural whorl. The center of the whorl usually begins in the middle of the crown's lower quadrant adjacent to the part side. The grafts are angled to mimic a natural whorl, where hair radiates around the predetermined central point.

It is recommended that at least 4 months pass between subsequent transplant sessions. Hair does not grow for an average of 3 months after a transplant session. Therefore, the surgeon should wait 4 months before planning further transplant sessions to evaluate the hair growth from the previous sessions. The surgeon can then examine the quantity and quality of the new hair growth before placing additional grafts. Waiting to see new hair growth also allows the surgeon to precisely and completely fill the spaces left between the edges of the previously placed grafts. Crusts form on the grafts soon after surgery, and the grafted hairs shed in about 1 to 2 weeks postprocedure. The freshly transplanted grafts enter a telogen effluvium phase and lose their preexistent hair over the subsequent 2 to 6 weeks. New hair begins to grow about 10 to 16 weeks after surgery and grows at the normal rate of 1/2 to 1 inch per month. Occasionally, the new hair will appear coarser than the original hair.

Sequelae and Complications

Table 184.3 lists complications of hair-restoration surgery. Most patients experience little discomfort after hair transplantation and require nothing more than acetaminophen with codeine. Severe forehead edema occasionally develops postoperatively; however, this swelling is temporary and may be controlled with postoperative steroids (e.g., Medrol Dosepak).

Keloidal healing is rare. If any questions regarding a patient's predisposition remain after a thorough preoperative history, a single test graft can be performed at the margin of the fringe. This graft should be observed for 3 to 4

TABLE 184.3 COMPLICATIONS HAIR-RESTORATION SURGERY

Arteriovenous fistula
Hematoma
Infection
Necrosis
Poor hairline design
Scarring
Telogen

months before scheduling any further transplants. Graft elevation above the surrounding recipient site (cobblestoning) occurs when grafts are not trimmed properly or when there is a size discrepancy between the graft and the recipient opening. Elevated grafts are corrected by shaving the raised epidermal surface parallel to the normal adjacent scalp with a scalpel blade.

Tissue necrosis at the donor site is rare and usually results from overaggressive harvesting techniques. Wide scars occur when excessive tension is used to close the donor site. Infections following hair transplants occur in less than 1% of patients. Bleeding is unusual and is usually controlled with firm pressure. Arteriovenous fistulae are rare after transplantation and often resolve spontaneously within 3 to 6 months. Direct steroid injection, suture ligation, or complete excision is required for persistent lesions or progressive enlargement.

SCALP REDUCTION

Scalp reductions are used to excise bald skin from the crown and central scalp regions. The hair-bearing scalp is undermined and advanced superiorly to cover the excision site. The inherent flexibility of the scalp determines the success or failure of this technique. Patients with extremely flexible scalps may undergo a tremendous excision of bald scalp in a single operation, whereas patients with very tight scalps realize minimal benefit following a standard scalp reduction. This technique is most useful for reducing crown alopecia in patients with Norwood class IV to VI MPB.

Several scalp reduction patterns have been described (17) (Fig. 184.3). The sagittal midline pattern is the easiest to perform, but it creates a central scar over the vertex of the head and a slot that extends into the midoccipital hair-bearing scalp. Although more time consuming, a Y-pattern reduction can be used in place of the sagittal midline pattern to excise crown alopecia without creating a slotlike deformity at the occipital hairline. A variety of other reduction designs, including C, J, S, and lateral crescent-shaped patterns, use laterally placed scars along the fringe of the bald area to reduce crown alopecia without causing unnatural slot formations in the occipital scalp. Lateral patterns, however, are more difficult to perform than midline patterns, and they produce more central scalp hypesthesia.

Most scalp reductions are performed in a prone position using local anesthesia with intravenous sedation. Skin incisions are carried down through the galea aponeurotica, taking care to bevel the scalpel to avoid transecting adjacent hair follicles. A subgaleal dissection is extended inferiorly to the superior attachment of the auricle and to the nuchal ridge. The surgeon can overlap the undermined scalp to estimate a safe excision margin. This technique prevents overexcising the scalp and reduces the potential for excessive incision line tension. The overlapping bald

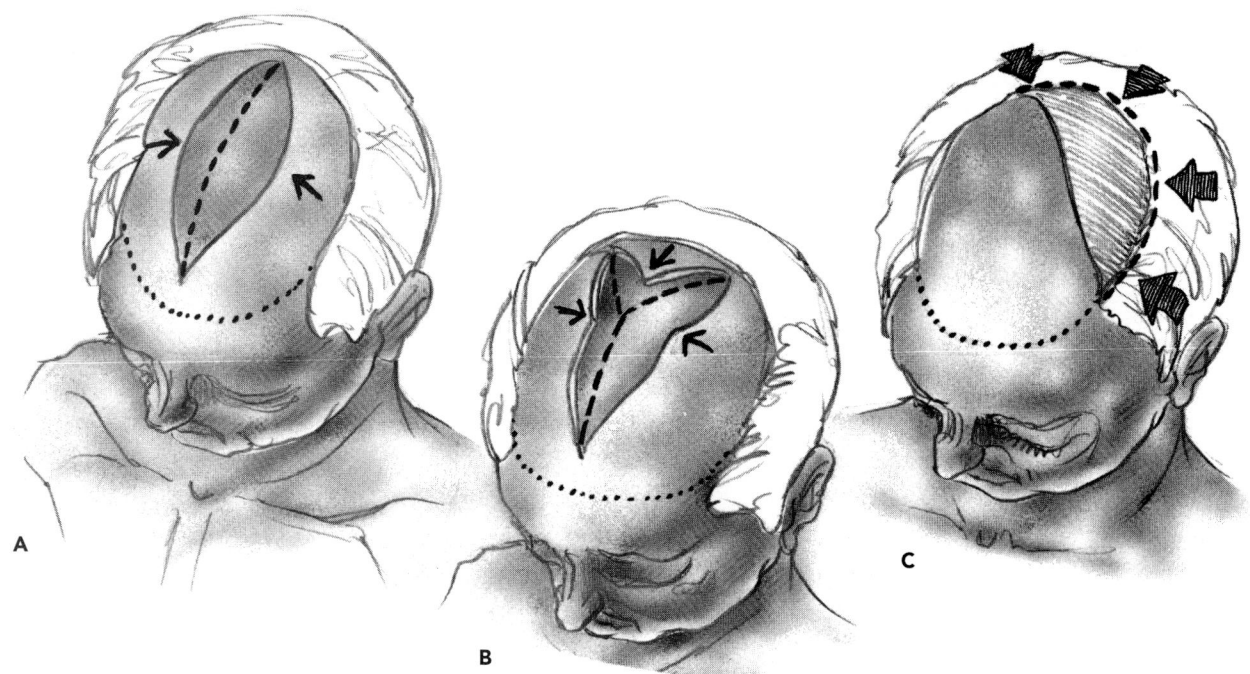

Figure 184.3 Common scalp reduction patterns. **A:** Midline sagittal ellipse. **B:** Y pattern. **C:** Lateral crescent.

skin is excised with a scalpel, and the scalp is closed in two layers. A secure galea aponeurotica closure is required to minimize incision line tension.

Few complications occur with standard scalp reductions. Occasionally, a deep suture reaction results in suture extrusion and open wounds along the incision line on the scalp. Suture removal and local wound care remedy this situation. Postoperative bleeding, infection, dehiscence, and permanent hair loss are unusual complications. Graft transplantation is usually required to camouflage the mid-scalp and crown scars that are produced following a scalp reduction. A poorly executed scalp reduction can produce an unnatural hair direction if the inferiorly directed temporal hairline is pulled too far superiorly to the midline of the scalp.

Extensive Scalp Reductions

Extensive scalp reductions were popularized by Brandy, who described the bilateral occipitoparietal (BOP) flap and the bitemporal (BT) flap (18,19). The BOP flap and BT flap differ significantly from standard scalp reductions with respect to the tremendous degree of undermining that is performed to elevate the scalp from the skull. These procedures were designed to eliminate alopecia in the crown and vertex regions for patients with Norwood class IV to VI baldness. As with standard scalp reduction procedures, extensive scalp reductions do not provide hair in the frontal region. A frontal hairline is usually created with mi-crografts and minigrafts after the reduction procedures.

Most patients with Norwood class IV to VI hair loss can be treated with two or three procedures, depending on the degree of scalp flexibility present. The BOP and BT flaps each allow the excision of about 7 cm of bald skin as measured from ear to ear. In most patients, the BOP flap is performed first, followed by a BT flap 2 to 3 months later. In patients with less scalp flexibility, two BOP flaps may be required before performing a BT flap. The BT flap is used as a primary procedure in patients with hair loss limited to the central mid-scalp.

Extensive scalp reductions require staged ligation of the occipital vessels 2 to 6 weeks before the actual reduction procedure. Ligation delays the large flap created with this technique and decreases the risk of postoperative scalp necrosis. Occipital artery ligation is performed through a 1-cm vertical incision over the nuchal ridge.

Both procedures require precise identification of the superficial temporal arteries (STAs). The incision for the BOP flap begins anterior to the STAs in the temporal hairline region (Fig. 184.4). The incision is carried through the temporal hair anterior to the STAs, maintaining an appropriate bevel to preserve hair follicles. The incision turns at the superior temporal hairline and follows the entire fringe of the temporoparietal and occipital regions. A similar incision is performed on the contralateral side to create a horseshoe-shaped incision over the top of the scalp. Undermining is carried inferiorly to the auricle, extending onto the posterior surface of the conchal cartilage. The skin overlying the mastoid process is elevated in a superficial subcutaneous plane. Elevation of the occipital scalp extends

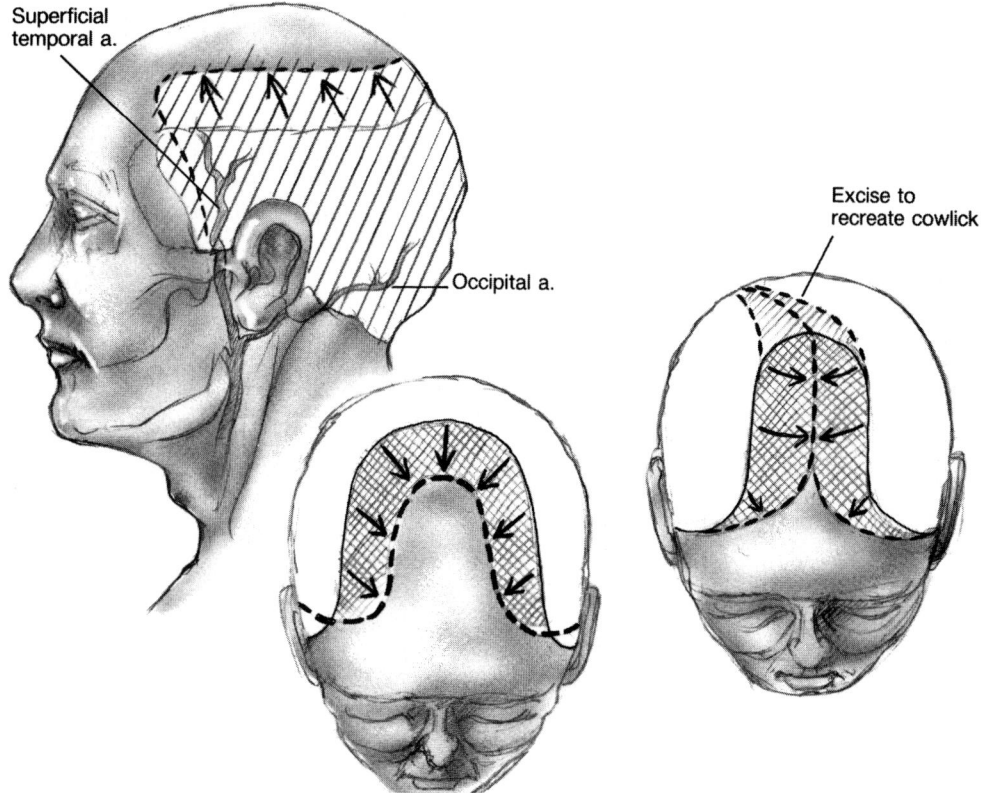

Figure 184.4 Extensive scalp reduction. Extensive scalp reductions differ from standard reductions by requiring staged ligation of the occipital vessels 2 to 6 weeks before flap advancement (*left*). This technique requires wide undermining (*cross-hatched area*) for flap advancement. The hair-bearing bilateral occipitoparietal flap is advanced superomedially and anteriorly to replace a horseshoe-shaped bald area (*cross-hatched area*) adjacent to the donor fringe (*center*). A bitemporal flap is usually performed after a BOP flap to remove the remaining mid-scalp bald region (*cross-hatched area*). The incision lines veer into the hair-bearing occipital scalp to recreate a natural whorl (*right*).

inferiorly by dividing the fibrous attachments of the occipitalis muscle and the galea aponeurotica along the nuchal ridge. Additional undermining is carried inferiorly to the nape of the neck in a plane that divides the fascia from the superficial surface of the trapezius muscle, thereby mobilizing the entire hair-bearing portion of the scalp. The BOP flap is then advanced anteriorly and superomedially, and the overlapped bald skin is excised from the top of the head. The skin is closed in two layers, similar to a standard scalp reduction.

The BT flap procedure is performed 2 to 3 months after the BOP flap when the scalp has regained its elasticity. If the BT flap is performed as an isolated procedure, the occipital vessels are ligated 2 to 6 weeks preoperatively. A BT flap uses incisions similar to a BOP flap, except in the occipital region, where the incision lines veer laterally into the occipital hairline to recreate a cowlick. After undermining the scalp, the skin is advanced superomedially and anteriorly to cover the remaining bald portions of the central and occipital scalp.

Although the BOP and BT flaps restore hair over the mid-scalp and crown regions, these procedures are associated with more complications than are standard scalp reductions. Both procedures create a large advancement flap at the expense of transecting key vascular connections. The reduced blood supply inherent to these large flaps can result in temporary telogen. There is a definite risk of necrosis with an extensive scalp reduction; however, it is uncommon, following planned ligation of the occipital vessels. Other complications include widening of the mid-scalp scar, visible scar formation in the anterior temporal incision line, and thinning hair density within the donor scalp regions. Unacceptable scars are corrected with minigraft or micrograft hair transplants directly into the scar lines. The surgeon must carefully examine the patient preoperatively for signs of thinning in the anterior temporal region. If the incision line is placed too far anteriorly, progressive temporal alopecia will eventually result in a clearly exposed scar line (20).

TISSUE EXPANSION

Scalp tissue expansion redistributes hair follicles in the donor area over a larger surface area on the stretched scalp

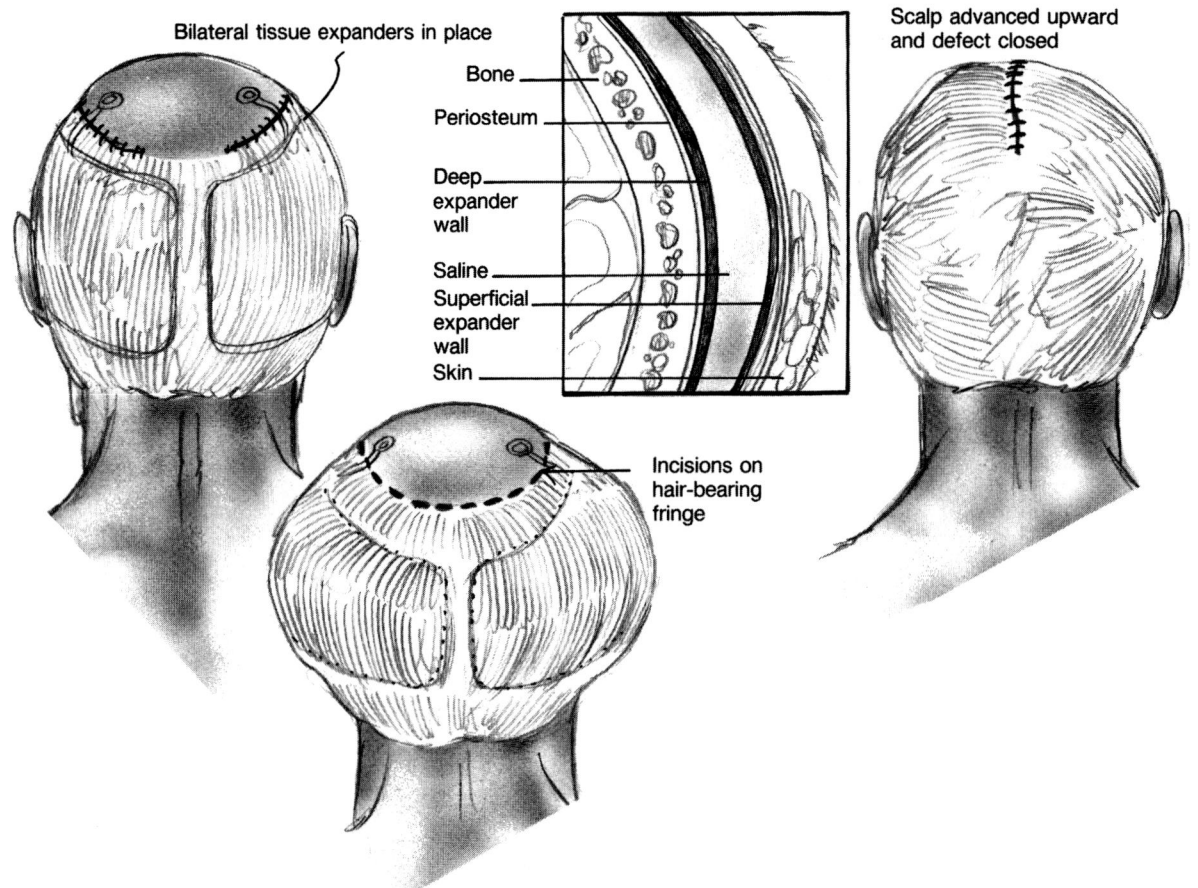

Figure 184.5 Tissue expansion for treating crown and mid-scalp baldness. Tissue expanders are placed bilaterally through incisions (*dashed lines*) along the balding fringe (*left*). After the expansion process is complete, incisions are made along the hair-bearing fringe, and the bald skin on the crown and mid-scalp is removed (*center*). The expanded hair-bearing scalp is advanced upward to close the defect (*right*).

(21). This technique has been successfully performed in patients with hair loss secondary to trauma, burns, neoplasms, and MPB. Various tissue expanders that allow the surgeon to customize the expansion process for any given area of the scalp are available. This modality is especially useful in patients with MPB who would benefit from a hair-bearing flap or a scalp reduction but are limited by poor scalp flexibility. Tissue expansion enables the surgeon to remove large areas of bald skin without changing the hair color or texture. It is a relatively rapid technique that has few complications when properly performed. The disadvantages include the need for repeated injections to expand the scalp, the pain associated with the injections, and the temporary cosmetic deformity that results with progressive tissue expansion.

Tissue expansion can be used to provide a relatively rapid restoration of hair-bearing skin over the crown and mid-scalp regions in patients with Norwood class IV to VI MPB and poor scalp flexibility. Scalp expanders are designed to expand the entire temporoparietal and occipital donor regions. This technique does not provide hair coverage in the frontal region, however. In patients with coexis-

tent frontal baldness, standard transplant techniques or a modified transposition flap are used after the expansion procedure is completed.

The expanders are placed through incisions along the temporoparietal and occipital fringe (Fig. 184.5). The hair-bearing scalp is mobilized inferiorly to the superior attachment of the auricle and to the nuchal ridge. Remote injection ports are used to prevent accidental puncture of the tissue expander during the inflation process. The expanders are placed flat against the skull, and the injection ports are placed in a separate pocket under the alopecic mid-scalp region. About 30 mL of sterile saline is injected into the expanders immediately after skin closure to eliminate dead space.

Tissue expansion begins 2 to 3 weeks postoperatively. The expanders are injected two or three times a week, depending on the patient's pain tolerance during the injection process. Each expander is injected with sterile saline using a 25-gauge needle until the pain threshold is just reached. Each filling session requires about 30 to 60 mL of sterile saline. If pain is a problem, the patient can take a mild analgesic before the injection sessions. The expanders are gradually filled to capacity (500 to 800 mL) over 6 to 8 weeks. Expansion is finished when the cumulative tissue gain across the domes of the expanded tissue exceeds the width of the alopecic defect.

Excision of bald scalp begins by partially deflating the expanders. A horseshoe-shaped incision beginning at the apex of the planned frontotemporal triangle is made superior to the hair-bearing fringe. The expanders are removed, and the expanded scalp is moved superiorly. If additional advancement is required, the capsule is incised inferiorly, and additional undermining is performed. The overlapped bald skin is excised from the top of the head, and the hair-bearing flaps are brought together in the midline.

Complications of tissue expansion include infection, hematoma, exposure of the implant, and implant failure. Proper technique and the use of preoperative and postoperative antibiotics minimize the potential for these complications.

JURI FLAP

The Juri flap is a pedicled transposition flap based on the STA for surgical restoration of the frontal hairline (22). A single flap is used for frontal hairline restoration in patients with hair loss limited to the frontal region. In suitable candidates with more advanced balding over the top of the head, two flaps and a scalp reduction can be staged to provide about 12 cm of dense hair in the frontal and mid-scalp regions.

The Juri flap requires four stages for completion. The first stage begins with designing a hairline and the flap (Fig. 184.6). The STA is identified by Doppler ultrasonography about 3 cm above the root of the helix. The flap is 4 cm wide and has the STA located in the central portion of the base. The base begins posteriorly about 3 cm above the root of the helix and inclines 35 to 45 degrees in an anterior and superior direction. The flap is arched superiorly

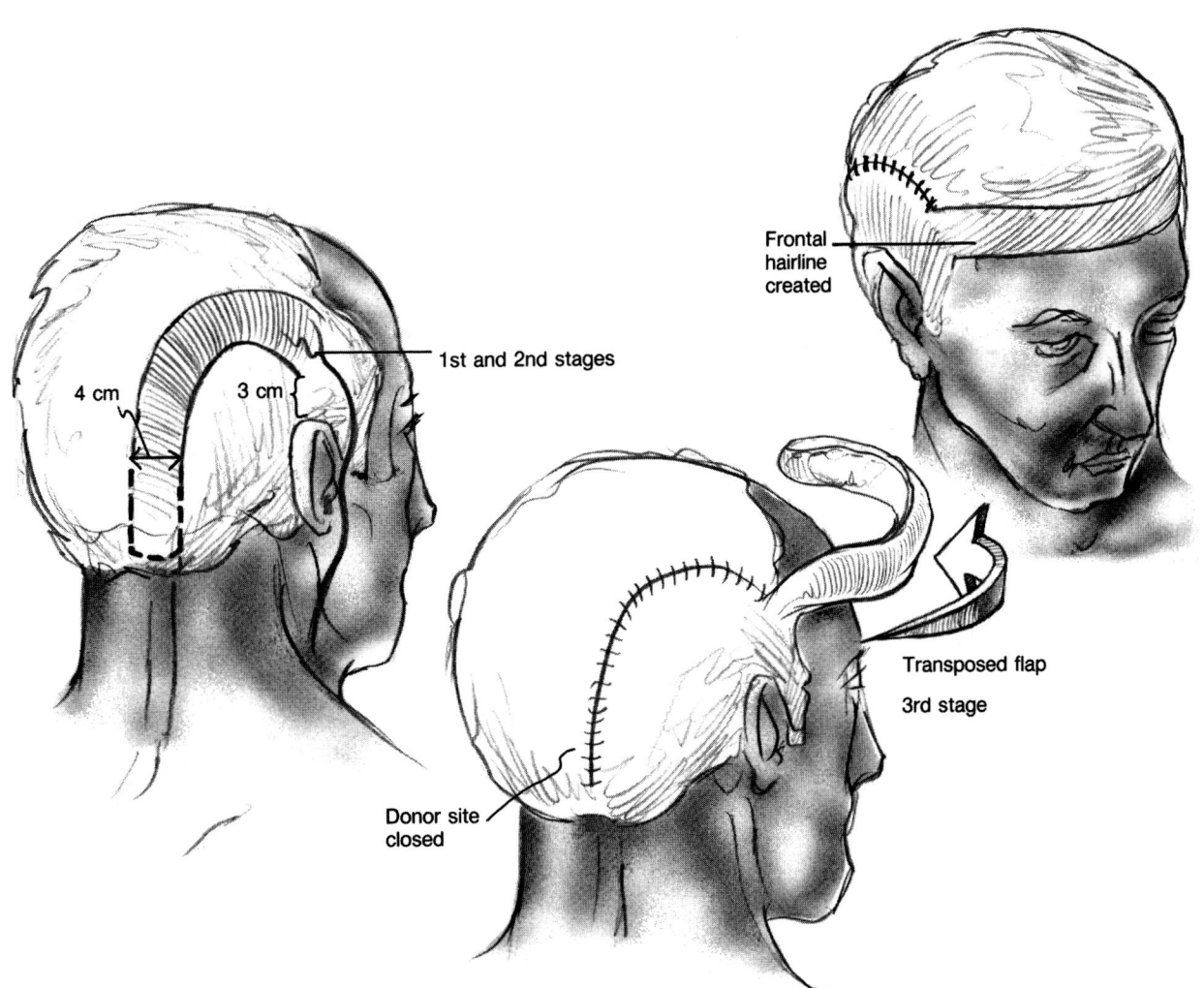

Figure 184.6 The Juri flap. The temporal and parietal portions of the flap are incised during the first stage (*solid lines*). The second stage involves mobilizing the tail of the flap in the occipital region (*dashed lines*) (*left*). The donor site is closed, and the flap is transposed during the third stage (*center*). The flap is designed to recreate the frontal hairline (*right*).

into the temporal scalp and gently turned posteriorly and inferiorly into the parietal and occipital regions, taking care not to cross the midline or to extend into any areas having the potential for future hair loss. The flap length is determined by measuring the distance from the base of the flap across to the distal end of the frontal hairline. About 4 cm is added to accommodate the "dog ear" that forms when the flap is transposed.

The first two procedures are performed using a local anesthetic. To prevent flap necrosis, epinephrine is never used near the base or the tail of the flap. The first stage consists of incising the proximal three-fourths of the flap through the galea aponeurotica, with attention to maintaining an angle that preserves hair follicles. The flap is not elevated during this stage. One week later, the tail of the flap is incised and elevated to the level of the previous week's incision lines. The occipital vascular plexus is cauterized or ligated and the flap then laid down without entering the region of the prior week's procedure.

The flap is transposed 1 week after the second delay procedure, most often under general anesthesia. The flap is elevated in a subgaleal plane and carefully inspected for adequate circulation at the distal end. A beveled incision is made across the planned anterior hairline, and the scalp is widely undermined in a subgaleal plane superior and inferior to the flap donor site. Homeostasis is checked, and the donor site is closed in layers.

After the donor site is closed, the flap is transposed to lie across the frontal region. A 1-mm strip of epidermis is removed from the frontal edge of the flap with fine forceps and tenotomy scissors. This maneuver allows the surgeon to bury a small strip of dermis along the hairline aspect of the flap below the forehead skin. As hair grows along the de-epithelialized strip, it will exit through the overlying forehead skin and incision line, thereby helping to camouflage the frontal scar. The frontal incision line is carefully sutured together. Any overlapping bald skin posterior to the flap is then excised, taking care to avoid tension along the incision line.

Any dog ear that forms at the transposition site is revised 6 weeks after rotating the flap. The flap is cut directly across the dog ear. Limited incisions are made adjacent to this cut along the anterior and posterior margins of the flap. The base of the flap is rotated posteriorly, thus restoring natural hair directionality over the entire temporal scalp. The hairline side of the cut flap is then turned posteriorly to recreate a frontotemporal triangle that is symmetric with the contralateral side. Overlapping bald skin posterior to the flap is excised to accommodate proper flap positioning.

If needed, a second flap is placed 4 cm posterior to the first flap 2 to 3 months after restoration of the frontal hairline. The bald space between the two flaps is excised 2 to 3 months later, resulting in 12 cm of dense hair coverage over the anterior scalp.

One sequela of the Juri flap is the posteriorly oriented frontal hair that results after flap transformation. Severe complications including scalp necrosis and permanent hair loss are more common with flap procedures than with other forms of hair-restoration surgery. These problems are unusual in patients with normal scalp circulation; however, patients with a history of extensive donor graft harvesting over the flap's donor site are especially prone to these complications. Poor hairline design, wide scars, infection, and hematoma are other possible complications of frontal flap hairline restoration (23).

HIGHLIGHTS

- Androgenetic alopecia, commonly referred to as male pattern baldness, is the most common cause of hair loss in adults.
- Many surgical options are available to manage all but the most severe cases of alopecia.
- Currently, topically applied minoxidil (Rogaine) and oral finasteride (Propecia) are the only medications approved by the FDA for the medical management of hair loss in humans.
- The term *donor dominance* refers to the fact that hair-bearing autografts maintain characteristics of the donor tissue when transplanted into other regions of the body.
- In the past, standard punch-graft techniques were often criticized for producing unnatural, artificial-appearing hairlines, especially in patients with straight dark hair and light skin color. Technical advances with follicular unit transplant, as well as minigraft and micrograft hair transplants allow the reconstruction of natural, nonsurgical-appearing frontal hairlines.
- Various scalp reduction techniques are available to reduce crown baldness, offering hope for patients with advanced alopecia who want to attain natural hair restoration over the entire scalp.
- Tissue expansion permits the effective removal and restoration of large alopecic regions in patients with tight, inflexible scalps.
- For patients desiring maximum hair density, the Juri flap is another tested option for completely restoring the frontal hairline.

REFERENCES

1. Norwood OT, Shiell RC. *Hair transplant surgery,* 2nd ed. Springfield, IL: Charles C Thomas, 1984.
2. Kaufman KD. Long term (5-year) multinational experience with finasteride 1 mg in the treatment of men with androgenetic alopecia. *Eur J Dermatol* 2002;12:38–49.
3. Whiting DA, Olsen EA, Savin R, et al. Efficacy and tolerability of finasteride 1 mg in men aged 41 to 60 years with male pattern hair loss. *Eur J Dermatol* 2003;12:150–160.
4. Olsen EA, Dunlap MD, Funicella T, et al. A randomized clinical trial of 5% topical minoxidil versus 2% topical minoxidil and placebo in the treatment of androgenetic alopecia in men. *J Am Acad Dermatol* 2002;47:377–385.
5. Avram MR, Cole JP, Gandelman M, et al. The potential role of minoxidil in the hair transplantation setting. *Dermatol Surg* 2002;28:894–900.

6. Shapiro R. Creating a natural hairline in one session using a systematic approach and modern principles of hairline design. *Int J Cosmetic Surg Aesthetic Dermatol* 2001;3(2):89–99.

7. Epstein JS. The treatment of female pattern hair loss and other applications of surgical hair restoration in women. *Facial Plast Surg Clin N Am* 2004;12:241–247.

8. Okuda S. Clinical and experimental studies of transplantation of living hairs. *Jpn J Dermatol Urol* 1939;46:135–138.

9. Orentreich N. Autografts in alopecias and other selected dermatological conditions. *Ann NY Acad Sci* 1959;83:463.

10. Orentreich D, Orentreich N. Androgenetic alopecia and its treatment. In: Unger W, Nordstrom R, eds. *Hair Transplantation*. New York: Marcel Dekker Inc, 1988:1.

11. Buchwach KA. Standard grafts, minigrafts, and micrografts: their use in hair transplantation. *Facial Plast Surg Clin North Am* 1994;2:149.

12. Rassman WR, Bernstein RM, McLellanR, et al. Follicular unit extraction: minimally invasive surgery for hair transplantation. *Dermatol Surg* 2002;28(8):720–728.

13. Shapiro R. Principles and techniques used to create a natural hairline in surgical hair restoration. *Facial Plast Surg Clin N Am* 2004;12:201–217.

14. Bernstein RM, Rassman WR. The logic of follicular unit transplantation. *Dermatol Clin* 1999;17:277.

15. Konior RJ. Current concepts in hair transplantation. Operative techniques. *Otolaryngol Head Neck Surg* 1995;6:257.

16. Marritt E. Single hair transplantation for hairline refinement: a practical solution. *J Dermatol Surg Oncol* 1984;10:962.

17. Unger MG. Scalp reduction. *Facial Plast Surg Clin N Am* 1994;2:163.

18. Brandy DA. The bilateral occipitoparietal flap. *J Dermatol Surg Oncol* 1986;12:1062.

19. Brandy DA. The Brandy bitemporal flap. *Am J Cosmetic Surg* 1986;3:12.

20. Marritt E, Konior RJ. Patient selection, candidacy, and treatment plan for hair replacement surgery. *Facial Plast Surg Clin N Am* 1994;2:111.

21. Konior RJ. Tissue expansion in scalp surgery. *Facial Plast Surg Clin N Am* 1994;2:203.

22. Juri J. Use of parieto-occipital flaps in the surgical treatment of baldness. *Plast Reconstr Surg* 1975;55:456.

23. Epstein JS, Kabaker SS. Scalp flaps in the treatment of baldness, long-term results. *Dermatol Surg* 1996;22(1):45–50.

Cosmetic Uses of Botox and Injectable Fillers

185

Grant S. Gillman   Julio F. Gallo

The use of botulinum toxin A (Botox) and injectable fillers, either alone or in combination, has proven over time to be an effective, minimally invasive and extremely popular treatment option for facial wrinkles. Whereas Botox injections are best used to eliminate or soften certain *dynamic* facial lines (wrinkles that appear with active contraction of the facial muscles) by selectively weakening the underlying muscles, the fillers as a group are generally used to help efface facial wrinkles or creases that are apparent even *at rest*. In that sense, Botox can be thought of as *preventing* selected facial wrinkles from developing or deepening, whereas the injectable fillers are used for the treatment of *already established* rhytids. In many cases, the combination of the two might yield a better result than either product alone.

Although the risk/benefit ratio for these products is extremely favorable, familiarity with the actions, indications, contraindications, and treatment expectations, and proper patient selection, is vital to maximizing patient satisfaction and minimizing complications. Knowledge of the regional anatomy and proper technique are an equally important part of the foundation on which successful use of these products is built.

REGIONAL ANATOMY

For the most common cosmetic applications of Botox, one must understand the relevant muscular anatomy of the forehead, glabella, brow, periorbital and perioral regions, and neck (Fig. 185.1).

Horizontal forehead rhytids are caused by repeated contraction of the frontalis muscle—the sole elevator of the brow. In general, there is a midline separation between the two frontalis muscles, and the vertical contraction of those muscles elevates the brow and scalp, leading to the formation of transverse lines in the forehead. The frontalis originates from the galea aponeurotica superiorly and interdigitates with the brow depressors inferiorly.

Brow elevation by the frontalis muscles is opposed by the brow depressors, which include the procerus, corrugator supercilii, orbicularis oculi, and depressor supercilii (the fibers of the orbicularis below the medial brow). The procerus muscle originates inferiorly from the lower nasal bones in the midline and runs vertically to blend with the frontalis and insert in the soft tissue between the brows. Contraction of the procerus is what creates the transverse crease at the root of the nose.

The paired corrugator supercilii muscles originate deep to the frontalis and orbicularis near the medial supraorbital ridge, where the frontal and nasal bones meet, and passes superolaterally to insert in the skin and subcutaneous tissue just above the mid-brow. Contraction of the corrugator muscles is what accounts for the vertical glabellar lines between the brows (the "frown" lines).

The orbicularis oculi consists of two parts—the orbital (the outermost portion) and the palpebral (preseptal and pretarsal portions). The muscle broadly encircles the orbit,

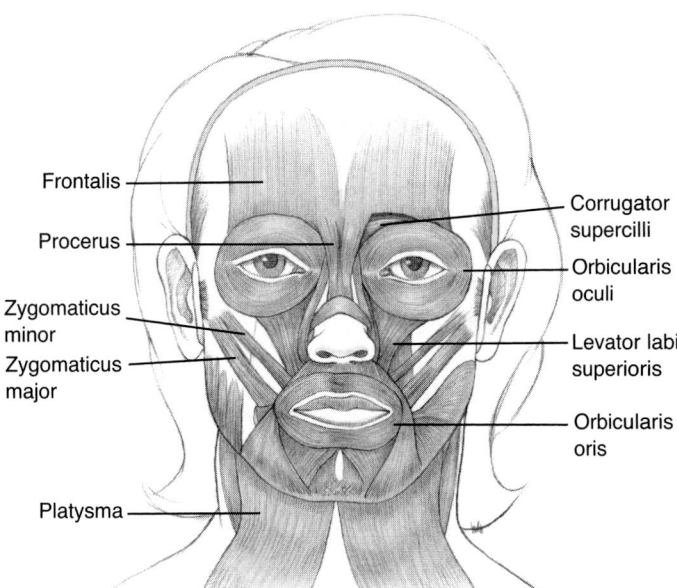

Figure 185.1   Facial musculature.

interdigitating with the corrugator muscle medially and superiorly and the frontalis muscle superiorly. Contraction of the orbital portion of the muscle is what leads to the formation of lateral orbital rhytids or "crow's feet." Some of the medial fibers of the orbicularis oculi known as the depressor supercilii insert into the skin below the medial eyebrow and act as medial brow depressors.

The orbicularis oris muscle encircles the mouth and functions both as an oral sphincter and to protrude the lips. Its fibers merge with the depressor anguli oris and the risorius muscles lateral to the oral commissure and the zygomaticus major and minor superiorly. Contraction of the orbicularis oculi will result in the fine vertical rhytids that radiate around the upper and lower lips.

The platysma muscle is responsible for horizontal neck creases and vertical bands in the neck. It originates from the fascia overlying the upper chest and clavicle and extends superiorly to insert on the lower mandible and mentum medially, and blend with the perioral muscles centrally. More posteriorly and superiorly, the platysma is continuous with the SMAS in the lower two thirds of the face.

BOTOX

Mechanism of Action

Botulinum toxin A is a potent neurotoxin that is produced by the anaerobic bacterium Clostridium botulinum. This organism produces eight antigenically distinct toxins, seven of which are neuroparalytics. The toxin produces a temporary chemical denervation by inhibiting the release of acetylcholine from the presynaptic neuron at the motor endplates of voluntary muscle.

The paralysis that follows is temporary in nature because chemodenervation is followed initially by the growth and sprouting of new axonal collaterals, which establish new connections at the motor end plate. At about 3 months, neural transmission through the original nerve terminal is reestablished, and the collateral axons regress (1). This correlates with clinical recovery of function typically in the 3-to-4-month range.

Indications and Contraindications

Botox is currently approved by the Food and Drug Administration (FDA) for use in cervical dystonia, strabismus, and blepharospasm and for the temporary improvement in vertical glabellar rhytids caused by the action of the corrugator and procerus muscles. Although technically "off-label," the clinical use of Botox has expanded widely to include the treatment of many other conditions, including other facial hyperkinetic lines, migraine headaches, hyperhidrosis, bruxism, Frey syndrome, muscle tension dysphonia, torticollis, and bilateral masseteric hypertrophy.

The use of Botox is contraindicated in individuals with preexisting neuromuscular disorders (e.g., myasthenia gravis, amyotrophic lateral sclerosis, Eaton-Lambert syndrome) and those with an albumin allergy. Use in pregnant women or lactating mothers is not recommended, as there is no safety data regarding use in such circumstances.

Cosmetic Applications of Botox

Commercially available botulinum toxin A (Botox; Allergan; Irvine, CA) is supplied in a crystalline form as 100-unit vials. Dilution with 2.5 mL of preservative-free normal saline yields a concentration of 4 units per 0.1 ml. The volume of dilution (and hence the concentration) can vary with the clinician's preference, but high concentration–low volume injections will help minimize unwanted dispersion of the Botox to surrounding tissues. According to the product information, once reconstituted, the toxin should be used within 4 hours, although many clinicians have refrigerated any unused toxin for up to 30 days (2). Following injection, the onset of muscle weakness generally occurs between 2 to 5 days, and should last on average 3 to 4 months before full recovery is noted.

Although there are many potential applications for the use of Botox, as noted earlier, this chapter will review only the most common uses for improving facial aesthetics—the treatment of glabellar rhytids ("frown lines"), transverse forehead rhytids, lateral periorbital rhytids ("crow's feet"), the adjustment of brow contour and position (the "chemical" browlift), the treatment of platysmal banding in the neck, and vertical upper lip rhytids.

Glabellar Rhytids

Glabellar rhytids include the vertical "frown" lines produced by contraction of the corrugator supercilii muscles, as well as the transverse crease at the nasion produced by contraction of the procerus. The procerus is injected with 4 to 5 units of Botox, in the region of the nasion at the intersection of two lines, each of which extends from the medial brow to the opposite medial canthus. Each corrugator muscle is injected with 4 to 8 units of Botox, into the belly of the muscle, above the medial brow, roughly in line with the medial canthus, and 4 units further laterally along the muscle, staying medial to the mid-pupillary line (Fig. 185.2). The latter two injections should always be at or above a transverse line drawn though the mid-eyebrow and above the superior orbital rim, to minimize the chance of diffusion into the levator palpebrae of the upper lid, which could result in a transient eyelid ptosis (3).

Transverse Forehead Rhytids

Because the frontalis muscle is the only elevator of the brow, isolated treatment of horizontal forehead lines must be done with some consideration. In the patient with heavy glabellar rhytids or a very low brow, one should assume that the brow depressors are quite strong and active, in which case isolated treatment of the frontalis may cause or further aggravate brow ptosis. In such cases, concomitant treatment of the brow depressors (corrugators, procerus) should be discussed with the patient.

Effective treatment of the transverse forehead rhytids involves subcutaneous or intramuscular injections into the frontalis, in a relatively uniform grid-like fashion across the forehead (Fig. 185.2). Typically 2 units per injection site will suffice, and 8 to 10 injections (for a total of 16 to 20 units) will yield a favorable result. Care is taken to stay a minimum of 1 to 1.5 cm above the brow for all injections, to minimize the risk of eyebrow ptosis.

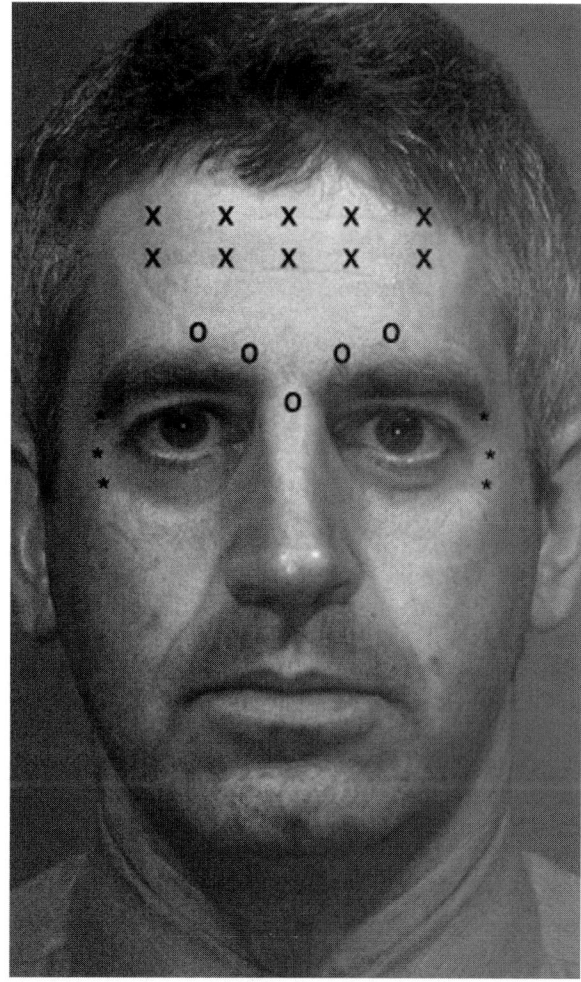

Figure 185.2 Typical injection points for transverse forehead rhytids (*X*), glabellar rhytids (*O*), and lateral periorbital rhytids (asterisk). (See also Color Plate 77.)

Lateral Periorbital Rhytids

Lateral periorbital rhytids ("crow's feet") result from repeated contraction of the lateral portion of the orbicularis oculi. Because the muscle is very thin and superficial, subdermal injections are sufficiently deep. Injections should also be at least 1.5 cm lateral to the lateral canthus and 1 cm outside the lateral orbital rim, to minimize the chance of any diffusion through the lid into the levator palpebrae superioris, which could result in a temporary upper eyelid ptosis. Treatment of the crow's feet is best avoided in anyone with a preexisting upper eyelid ptosis, lagophthalmos, or upper facial palsy.

Having the patient smile or squint will help identify the specific area or lines in need of treatment. Multiple serial injections are then used, typically two to four, perpendicular to the muscle and just outside the orbital rim (Fig. 185.2). Two to four units are injected per site, depending on the distribution of the lines and the activity of the underlying orbicularis oculi.

Adjustment of Brow Position and Contour (the "Chemical Browlift")

At least to some degree, brow position is felt to be the result of an equilibrium reached between the action of the brow elevator (the frontalis), and the action of the brow depressors (the corrugator, procerus, orbicularis oculi, and the depressor supercilii) (4,5). As such, selective weakening of the brow depressors with Botox A, either medially or laterally, may result in a modest (several-millimeter) "pharmacologic" brow lift.

Elevation of the entire brow will require attention to both the medial and the lateral brow depressors. Frequently, however, elevation of only one end of the brow or the other might be desired (more commonly the lateral), in which case it suffices to address those muscles only. For elevation of the medial brow, treatment of the corrugators and procerus (as previously described) as well as the depressor supercilii is required. The latter muscle is treated with an injection of 2 to 4 units just below and just lateral to the medial head of the brow, taking care to remain outside the orbital rim to avoid unwanted diffusion into adjacent muscles. Elevation of the lateral brow requires a subdermal injection of the orbicularis oculi muscle just below the eyebrow lateral to the high point of the brow, once again remaining outside the orbital rim. One to three injections may be required, with a total of 4 to 10 units of Botox.

Platysmal Banding

Administration of Botox to platysmal bands can be a useful adjunct in the treatment of the senescent neck (6). Best results are seen with mild to moderate banding (7), and the changes are most appreciable with dynamic contraction of the platysma than at rest.

Having the patient contract the muscle will best demonstrate the platysmal bands, which are then grasped and injected with 5 units of Botox at multiple sites each 1 to 1.5 cm apart, from below the jawline to the lower neck. Typically each band will receive a total of 15 units, with treatment of 2 to 4 bands, totaling 30 to 60 units. Caution must be exercised to avoid excessive doses and to inject into the muscle but not deep into it to avoid dysphagia and neck weakness.

Vertical Lip Rhytids

Very low doses of Botox injected into the upper lip can help efface or soften vertical upper lip lines. This treatment may be an alternative to perioral chemical peels or laser resurfacing, and can be used alone or in combination with injectable fillers. In order to avoid problems with oral incompetence, the injections are kept very superficial (subdermal) and very small doses are used initially. Nonetheless, professional public speakers and wind instrument musicians may not be ideal candidates for this treatment.

Four evenly spaced injections of 1 to 2 units each are given across the upper lip at or immediately above the vermilion border. Starting with the lower doses and increasing if necessary is most prudent. In addition to reducing the depth of apparent vertical lip lines, some degree of lip eversion is also frequently noted.

Botox Complications

As noted earlier, the safety profile of Botox A when used in cosmetic applications is quite favorable. Sound knowledge of the regional anatomy, attention to proper doses and technique, and the use of high concentration–low volume dilutions all help minimize the incidence of unwanted side effects. Furthermore, since the effect of Botox is a temporary one, so too are the complications. There have been no deaths reported or adverse long-term effects from the cosmetic use of Botox (8).

Medications that might potentiate the activity of Botox include aminoglycosides, cyclosporins, neuromuscular blockers, calcium channel blockers, quinidine, magnesium sulfate, and D-penicillamine.

General sequellae of Botox injections include pain, erythema and bruising at the injection site, headache, flu-like symptoms, malaise, and fatigue. Aside from injection-related discomfort, erythema, and perhaps bruising, the others are much less common.

Site-specific complications should be infrequent if suitable consideration is paid to technical detail. The most significant complication of glabellar or lateral periorbital injections is upper eyelid ptosis. This results from migration of the injected Botox deep to the orbital septum, where it may affect the levator palpebrae superioris of the upper eyelid. Staying outside the orbital rim with all injections (as indicated earlier) should prevent this complication from developing. Upper eyelid ptosis can develop up to 1 week after injections and usually resolves within 2 to 6 weeks. Should it develop, ptosis can be treated with alpha-adrenergic ophthalmic drops, such as Iopidine 0.5% (apraclonidine, Alcon Laboratories, Fort Worth, TX) or Phenylephrine 2.5% (Myfrin 2.5%, Alcon Labs), both of which stimulate Mueller's muscle to help elevate the eyelid margin (9). The typical dose is 1 to 2 drops 3 times daily until the ptosis resolves. Injection of the crow's feet can also result in diplopia by affecting the lateral rectus, which is why it is important to stay 1 cm outside the lateral orbital rim at all times.

Treatment of transverse forehead rhytids can result in brow ptosis, which is best avoided by staying at least 1 to 1.5 cm above the brow. Older patients, those with a low-set brow, and those with very active brow depressors are at greatest risk. Brow ptosis can be alleviated, if necessary, by secondary treatment of the brow depressors.

Injection of the platysmal bands may affect the larynx and hypopharynx if too deep, resulting in dysphagia or hoarseness, or the sternocleidomastoid muscle if too far lateral, which can cause neck weakness. Staying superficial and avoiding excessive dosing is critical. Dietary modification (soft foods, liquid diet) and metoclopramide hydrocholoride may be necessary for severe dysphagia (9).

Lip weakness or oral incompetence may result from perioral use of Botox. Prevention is most important and requires use of very low doses initially, together with superficial placement as noted earlier.

Resistance to Botox may result from the formation of neutralizing antibodies. This is generally associated with repeated use of high doses (more than 300 units) and is relatively uncommon with the lower doses used for cosmetic applications (10).

Finally, patient dissatisfaction may result from either over-treatment or under-treatment, and unmet or unrealistic expectations. Proper patient selection, education, and counseling, together with consistent procedural skills will help limit the number of unhappy patients.

SOFT-TISSUE AUGMENTATION

The use of injectable materials for soft tissue augmentation has a long history, dating to Neuber in 1893 when he harvested fat from the arm and injected it into a patient's facial defects (11).

Since that time, many other materials have been developed in the search for a filler substance to correct facial scarring from trauma and acne, static rhytids and augmentation of the lips, and melolabial folds.

In the early part of the 1900s, paraffin injection became popular. This treatment quickly fell out of favor, however, and became secondary to repeated granulomatous-type reactions resulting in paraffinomas. In the 1940s to 1950s, silicone was introduced. Long-term studies with this material indicated that it resulted in granulomatous reactions and scarring, however. In the 1970s, Stanford researchers experimented with animal- and human-derived collagen, as implantable materials that eventually led to the introduction of bovine collagen, which is still in use today (12).

In recent years, research in this area remains intense because of patient demand and the industry's search for the ideal filler. Patient demand in this area is high because injectable fillers offer distinct advantage over surgical procedures. Injections can be performed on an outpatient basis, with minimal or no recovery time. Occasionally, mild erythema or induration can persist for 48 to 72 hours. Certain defects are more easily corrected with contour filling rather than with surgical intervention. Likewise, the short-term cost to the patient is less.

The ideal filler has yet to be found, however. It would have to be easy to use and biocompatible, avoiding risks of allergic reactions, immunogenic toxicity, or carcinogenicity. It would also be inexpensive and have an inexhaustible source. Furthermore, the material would have to be well tolerated and accepted by the host, so that long-term correction could be achieved.

In general, most of the currently available materials are made to be injected into the dermis. The dermis is the middle layer of the integument, composed of viscoelastic tissue lying between the epidermis and the subcutaneous tissue. The predominant cell type in this layer is the fibroblast, which secretes the cellular matrix of collagen type I and elastin. These are embedded in a gel-like ground substance of glycosaminoglycans (primarily hyaluronic acid), which bind water, maintaining skin turgor. Collagen fibers provide tensile strength, whereas the elastin is responsible for elastic recoil (13).

The discussion of dermal fillers that follows is not exhaustive, and there are many more products under investigation that may eventually prove to be more effective. Currently used dermal fillers can be divided into the following categories: xenografts (donor and recipient are different species), autografts (donor and recipient are the same individual), homografts (donor and recipient are same species), and synthetic materials.

Xenografts

Bovine Collagen

Bovine collagen is the most widely used dermal filler and has the longest track record. It is the gold standard to which other fillers are compared. Three types of bovine collagen are commercially available: Zyderm I, Zyderm II, and Zyplast (INAMED Aesthetics, Santa Barbara, CA) are all derivatives of enzyme-digested bovine collagen—primarily type I—suspended in phosphate-buffered saline and lidocaine. During the preparation, antigenicity is reduced by pepsin proteolysis (14).

Zyderm I contains 35 mg/mL of collagen and was approved by the FDA in 1981. Because of significant resorption, Zyderm II was introduced containing 65 mg/ml of collagen and was approved by the FDA in 1983. On the other hand, Zyplast contains 35 mg/mL of collagen, cross-linked with glutaraldehyde to make the material less susceptible to enzymatic degradation and resorption. Zyderm is recommended for superficial, mild-to-moderate wrinkles such as the glabellar creases, periorbital crow's feet, and perioral rhytids, and the material should be place in the upper dermis. Because of early resorption with this material, overcorrection is recommended. Conversely, Zyplast is injected into the deeper reticular dermis, and because it is more resistant to resorption, overcorrection is not needed.

A significant disadvantage of bovine collagen is the risk of a hypersensitivity reaction displayed as induration, erythema, pruritus, and tenderness at the injection site. Skin testing for allergic sensitivity is therefore required before definitive use. About 3% to 4% of patients undergoing skin testing will display a hypersensitivity reaction (15,16). Although a majority of patients will show a reaction to skin testing in the first week, about 20% to 30 % will display a delayed reaction for which it is necessary to examine the injection site 4 to 6 weeks later. In addition to a hypersensitivity reaction, bovine collagen injections can result in tissue necrosis (17), foreign body reactions (18), and infrequent systemic reactions, such as headache, nausea, and arthralgias.

Hyaluronic Acid Products (Hylaform, Restylane)

Hyaluronic acid is a macromolecule composed of repeating disaccharide units in the family of glycosaminoglycans. This is one of the major components of the extracellular matrix in the dermis. Because it has the ability to bind 1,000 times its volume in water, hyaluronic acid confers a certain amount of turgor to the skin by affecting dermal volume and compressibility (19). Hyaluronic acid is unique in that it is identical in all species. Therefore, its derivatives should not be antigenic across species. The injected product is degraded locally and then metabolized by the liver into carbon dioxide and water.

There are currently two forms of injectable hyaluronic acid available: Hylaform (Biomatrix, Inc., Ridgefield, NJ) and Restylane (Q-Med, Uppsala, Sweden). Hylaform is a purified animal product made from rooster combs. This is an extremely pure gel, and the processing removes any remaining avian proteins. There have been few reports of any local or systemic reactions (20). In one study, 60% of rhytids showed some degree of correction 18 months after injection (21).

Restylane is derived from laboratory fermentation of bacterial cultures of equine streptococci. The material is processed, heat stabilized, and packaged in disposable syringes of 0.7 cc (20 mg/mL) and 1.0 cc (20 mg/mL). Restylane is a viscous clear gel that is injected into the mid-dermis to effect correction of mild to moderate wrinkles (Fig. 185.3). Although Perlane is not yet available in the United States, it is a more highly concentrated formulation of hyaluronic acid and is indicated for deeper folds and wrinkles. Because the hyaluronic acid attracts water once injected, it tends to maintain its volume, and overcorrection is not required. Multiple series of patients indicate that the correction achieved with these products can last anywhere from 8 to 9 months (22–24).

Although the current product is highly purified there are still minute amounts of associated proteins (25). Since hyaluronic acid is identical across species, the manufacturers do not recommend skin testing prior to injection. In multiple studies (26–28), there were a few cases of localized hypersensitivity resulting in local erythema and induration resolving in 4 to 20 weeks. Overall risk of an allergic reaction was less than 1 percent.

Autografts

Autologous Fat

Autologous fat has the longest history of use since Neuber (11) first injected it in 1893. The interest in autologous fat transplantation has vacillated over the years because of the variability in results. Some investigators report that between

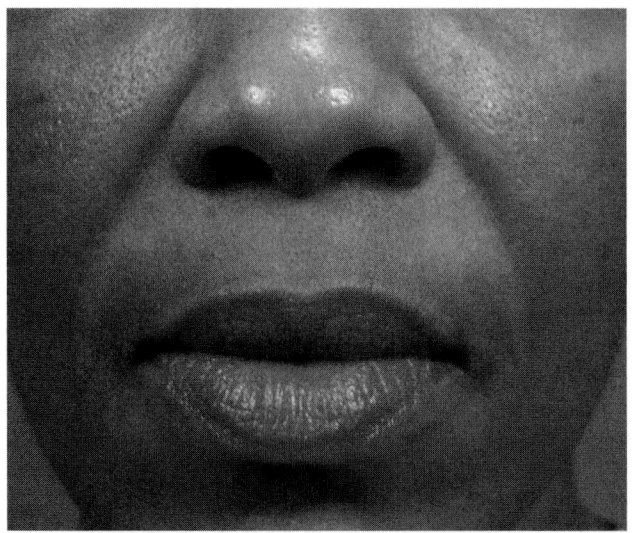

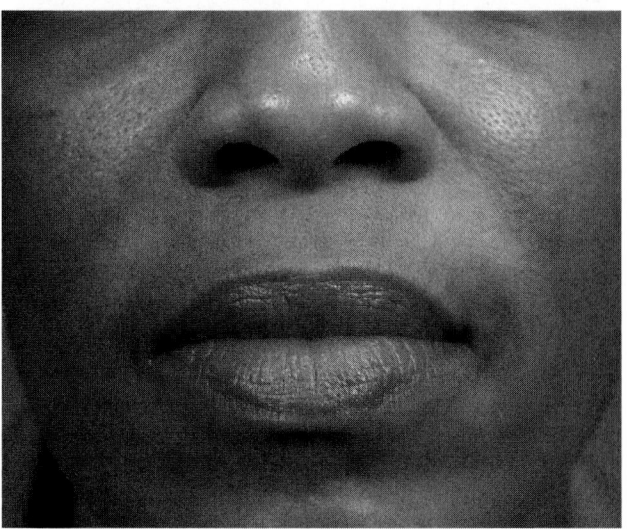

Figure 185.3 Before (**A**) and after (**B**) Restylane injections to melolabial creases.

30% and 60% of the injected fat will be resorbed (29). Since the advent of liposuction in the 1970s, however, interest in fat transplantation has increased. Some authors such as Coleman (30) recommend injection of small amounts of fat in subcutaneous tunnels to maximize the amount of blood flow to the transplanted fat, thus increasing its chance of survival. Likewise, the fat has to be treated gently, with minimal syringe pressure during harvesting, while using large bore cannulas.

To date, there is no universally accepted method for the harvesting, processing, and reinjection of autologous fat, and often results are not reproducible. The advantage of fat transplantation is the large amounts available in the human body, and because it is autologous, it negates the concern for allergic reactions and biocompatibility. This also creates a donor site with its own set of complications, however. In addition, fat grafting has the disadvantage of having an unpredictable resorption rate.

Isolagen

Isolagen (Isolagen Technologies, Houston, TX) was introduced in the mid 1990s as a way to inject patients with their own fibroblasts, the cells responsible for production of the extra cellular matrix. In this way, the problems of allergic reactions and nonbiocompatibility could be avoided. The process of manufacturing the Isolagen begins with a 3-mm punch of skin harvested from the patient's postauricular area. The specimen is sent to the Isolagen laboratories, where it is cultured *in vitro*, together with growth factors, to produce an amount of living fibroblasts. The syringe with the fibroblasts is then returned by overnight mail to the doctor's office for injection into the patient the following day. Several treatments are required to achieve the desired correction. Although Isolagen may have some benefits, the expense, time factor in production, and need for precise coordination between manufacturer, doctor, and patient make it somewhat impractical.

Nonetheless, initial studies with the product showed encouraging results. At 6 months time, histological analysis of the injection site showed integration of the fibroblasts into the dermal matrix without inflammation (31). The FDA has this product on hold pending further studies because of the growth factors used in production.

Homografts

CosmoDerm and CosmoPlast

With the approval of both CosmoDerm and CosmoPlast (INAMED Aesthetics, Santa Barbara, CA) by the FDA in March 2003, the use of injectable collagen replacements was taken to a new level. Previous bovine collagen requires skin testing, and the risk of allergic or hypersensitivity reactions still exists. Because these products are derived from bioengineered human fibroblasts, no pretesting is required. The cell lines used for production are grown in a bioreactor in the presence of cell medium. The extracellular collagen is collected, processed, and purified. Both CosmoDerm and CosmoPlast contain 35 mg/mL of purified human collagen in lidocaine. However, the latter is cross-linked with glutaraldehyde, which presumably delays the biodegradation of the product by collagenase. CosmoDerm is indicated for superficial lines and wrinkles, whereas CosmoPlast is better able to treat deeper grooves and scars. These products are longer lasting than bovine collagen, however; on average, they will last for 3 to 6 months. Once again, although these products are an improvement over the previously available bovine products, they are by no means ideal. In fact, some authors prefer to use this in combination with other products to obtain a cosmetically pleasing result (e.g., combining the use of hyaluronic acid products and human-based collagen products to provide fullness, definition, and support to the lips.)

Alloderm

AlloDerm (LifeCell Corp, Branchburg, NJ) is an acellular, freeze-dried dermal graft processed from human cadaver dermis. It is available in sheets as AlloDerm and in an injectable form under the trade name Cymetra (micronized AlloDerm). The freeze-drying process removes all the cells, leaving collagen IV and VII and elastin. AlloDerm integrates rapidly into the surrounding tissue, showing neovascularization by the patient's own blood supply. No skin testing is required for either product.

AlloDerm requires rehydration of the sheet of tissue to be used, along with proper cutting and sizing, however. Cymetra requires rehydration with lidocaine prior to injection, which can take up to 10 minutes. No long-term studies are yet available.

Synthetic Materials

Silicone

Silicone is composed of long chains of polymerized dimethylsiloxane. The technique of microdroplet injection was popularized by Webster (32), and Orentreich and Orentreich (33). With this technique small amounts of medical-grade liquid silicone are injected into the subdermis 1 mm apart. Care is taken not to overcorrect, as part of the augmentation is created by the body's fibrous encapsulation of the silicone over the ensuing weeks. Although Webster (32) reported a long-term follow-up with a series of 524 patients with good results and few complications, others have reported a long list of local and systemic complications. These reactions range from chronic inflammation, migration, extrusion ulceration, and skin necrosis to granulomatous hepatitis, pulmonary embolism, and silicone pneumonitis (34–36). In 1991, the FDA declared the use of injectable silicone illegal. With the recent approval of injectable silicone in ophthalmology for retinal detachments, however, the off-label use for soft-tissue augmentation has been revived.

Artecoll

Artecoll (Rofil Medical, Breda, The Netherlands) is a combination of a xenograft and a synthetic material. It is composed of 30 to 40 micron spheres of polymethyl methacrylate (PMMA) suspended in 3.5 % bovine collagen. Theoretically, as the collagen resorbs over a period of months, the PMMA spheres become encapsulated by fibrous tissue, ensuring a constant augmentation (37). This material needs to be injected into the subdermis; otherwise, a persistent painful nodule may persist. Also, skin testing is required because of the presence of bovine antigens, as previously discussed. Proponents (37) of Artecoll cite that improper injection can lead to complications. According to Lemperle, most of their patients received satisfactory results when the material was used properly. Others, however, have reported multiple foreign body granulamatous reactions, resulting in poor results, increased morbidity, and scarring (38). The FDA has not yet approved Artecoll for use in the United States, but studies are under way.

Radiesse

Radiesse (Bioform, Franksville, WI) is composed of 35% synthetic, spherical, 25- to 45-micron particles of calcium hydroxyapatite suspended in a gel containing water, glycerin, and sodium carboxymethylcellulose. Standard Radiance has particles ranging in size from 75 to 125 microns and is FDA approved for laryngeal augmentation, radiological soft-tissue marking, and filling or dental augmentation. Because the particle size of Radiesse is smaller, it can be injected through a narrow needle and can be used to augment melolabial folds, marionette lines, glabellar creases, and lips (Fig. 185.4). Occasionally, injections into the lips can produce palpable painful nodules. These are easily excised, however. In a series of 90 patients, Tzikas (39) found over-

all patient satisfaction at 88% at 6 months. Radiesse is not yet approved by the FDA for cosmetic usage.

CONCLUSION

Although no ideal filler is yet available, intense research continues in this area of facial plastic surgery. There are many choices offered on the market that can fulfill patients' needs. It is necessary to stay informed on the current materials in order to better inform patients to make appropriate choices. Often, two or more of the products used in combination offer the best results. Likewise, it is not uncommon to combine Botox Cosmetic in the upper third of the face and fillers in the melolabial folds, marionette lines, and perioral region to obtain a refreshed and rejuvenated appearance.

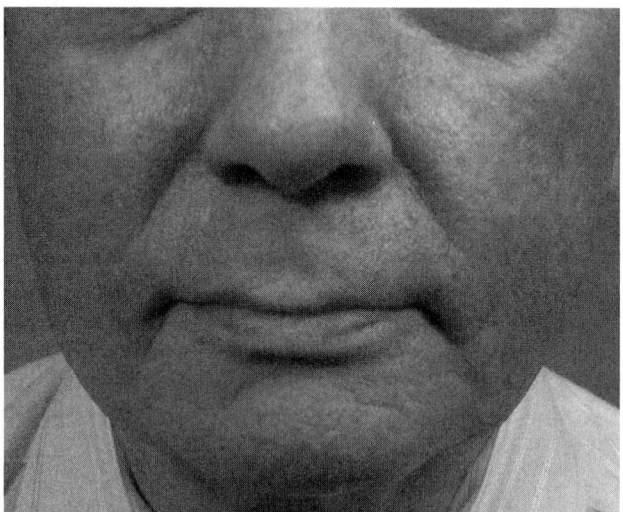
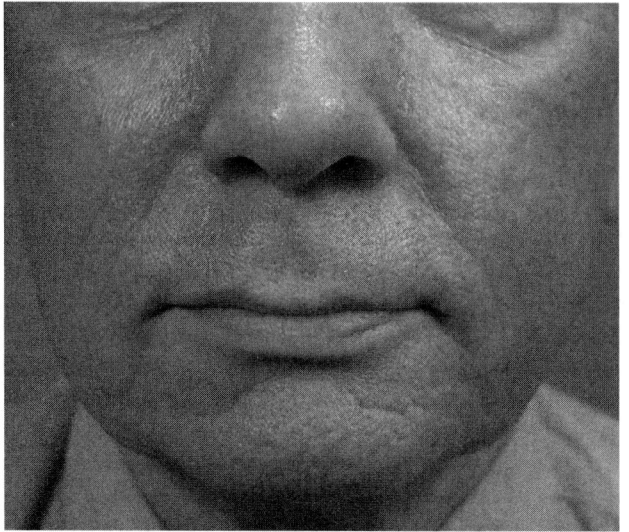

Figure 185.4 Before (**A**) and after (**B**) Radiesse injections to melolabial creases and marionette lines.

HIGHLIGHTS

- Botox is used in the treatment of dynamic facial rhytids to prevent them from either developing or deepening.
- Botox works by temporarily inhibiting presynaptic release of acetylcholine at the motor end plate. Its use is contraindicated in those with neuromuscular disease and albumin allergy.
- Familiarity with regional facial anatomy, proper technique, and the use of high concentration–low volume dilutions will minimize the risk of adverse outcome with Botox.
- Injectable fillers are used for soft tissue augmentation to add contour and volume. They are commonly used for camouflage of established facial rhytids and scars, and for lip augmentation.
- A great variety of injectable dermal fillers is available. Proper selection will depend on region, patient preference, and hypersensitivities. When hypersensitivity reactions are an issue (bovine collagen, Artecoll), skin testing is required prior to use.

REFERENCES

1. Alderson K, Holds JB, Anderson RL. Botulinum-induced alteration of nerve-muscle interactions in the human orbicularis oculi following treatment for blepharospasm. *Neurology* 1991; 41: 1800–1805.
2. Klein AW. Dilution and storage of botulinum toxin. *Dermatol Surg* 1998;24:1179–1180.
3. Macdonald MR, Spiegel JH, Raven RB, et al. An anatomical approach to glabellar rhytids. *Arch Otolaryngol Head Neck Surg* 1998;124:1315–1320.
4. Frankel AS, Kamer RM. Chemical browlift. *Arch Otolaryngol Head Neck Surg* 1998;124:321–323.
5. Ahn MS, Catten M, Maas CS. Temporal brow lift using botulinum toxin A. *Plast Reconstr Surg* 2000;105:1129–1135.
6. Brandt FS, Bellman B. Cosmetic use of botulinum A exotoxin for the aging neck. *Dermatol Surg* 1998;24:1232–1234.
7. Matarasso A, Matarasso SI, Brandt FS, et al. Botulinum A exotoxin for the management of platysmal bands. *Plast Reconstr Surg* 1999;103:645–652.

8. Blitzer A, Binder WJ, Boyd JB, et al. *Management of facial lines and wrinkles.* Philadelphia: Lippincott Williams & Wilkins, 2000.
9. Klein AW. Complications, adverse reactions, and insights with the use of botulinum toxin. *Dermatol Surg* 2003;29:549–556.
10. Vartanian AJ, Dayan SD. Complications of botulinim toxin A use in facial rejuvenation. *Facial Plast Surg Clin N Am* 2003; 11:483–492.
11. Neuber F. Fettransplantation. *Chir Kongr Verhandl Dsch Gesellch Chir* 22;66:1893.
12. Klein A, Elson M. The history of substances for soft tissue augmentation. *Dermatol Surg* 26(12);1096:2000.
13. Parker F. Structure and function of the skin. In: Orkin M, Mailbach HI, Dahl MV, eds. *Dermatology.* San Matteo, CA: Appleton and Lange, 1991:1–14.
14. Wallace DG, McPherson JJ, Ellingsworth LE, et al. Injectable collagen for tissue augmentation. In: Nimni ME, ed. *Collagen,* Vol 3. Boca Raton, FL: CRC Press, 1988:117–144.
15. Framer FM, Churukium MM. Clinical use of injectable collagen: a three-year retrospective review. *Arch Otolaryngol* 1984;110:93–98.
16. Cooperman LS, Mackinnon V, Bechler G, et al. Injectable collagen: a six-year clinical investigation. *Aesthetic Plast Surg* 1985; 9:145–151.
17. Hanke CW, Hingley HR, Jolivette DM, et al. Abscess formation and local necrosis after treatment with Zyderm or Zyplast collagen implant. *J Am Acad Dermatol* 1991;25:319–326.
18. Overholt MA, Tschar JA, Font RL. Granulomatous reaction to collagen implant: light and electron microscopic observations. *Cutis* 1993;51:95–98.
19. Haake A, Holbrook K: The structure and development of the skin. In: Freeberg I, Eisen A, Wolff K, et al., eds. *Fitzpatrick's dermatology in general medicine,* 5th ed. New York: McGraw Hill, 1999:89.
20. Melton JL, Hanke CN. Soft tissue augmentation. In: Roegnik RK, Roegnik HH, eds. *Dermatologic surgery, principles and practice.* New York: Marcel Dekker, 1996:1077.
21. Piacquadio D. Cross-linked hyaluronic acid as a soft tissue augmentation material: a preliminary assessment. In: Elson ML, ed. *Evaluation and Treatment of the Aging Face.* New York: Springer-Verlag, 1995:30.
22. Bosquet MT, Agerup B. Restylane lip implantation: European experience. *Oper Tech Oculoplastic Orbital Reconstr Surg* 1999;2:172–176.
23. Cantisano-Zilkha M, Bosniak S. Hyaluronic acid gel injections for facial rejuvenation: a 3-year clinical experience. *Operat Tech Oculoplast Orbital Reconstr Surg* 1999;2:177–181.
24. Duranti F, Salti G, Bovanti B, et al. Injectable hyaluronic acid gel for soft tissue augmentation: a clinical and histologic study. *Dermatol Surg* 1998;24:1317–1325.
25. Manna F, Dentini M, Desideri P, et al. Comparative chemical evaluation of two commercially available derivatives of hyaluronic acid used for soft tissue augmentation. *J Eur Acad Dermatol* 1999;13:183–192.
26. Lupton JR, Alster TS. Cutaneous hypersensitivity reaction to injectable hyaluronic acid gel. *Dermatol Surg* 2000;26:135–137.
27. Lowe NJ, Maxwell CA, Lowe P, et al. Hyaluronic acid skin fillers: adverse reactions and skin testing. *J Am Acad Dermatol* 2001; 45(6):930–933.
28. Friedman PM, Mafong EA, Kauvar AN, et al. Safety data of injectable nonanimal stabilized hyaluronic acid gel for soft tissue augmentation. *Dermatol Surg* 2002;28(6):491–494.
29. Chajchir A, Benzaquen I. Fat-grafting injection for soft-tissue augmentation. *Plast Reconstr Surg* 1989;84:921–934.
30. Coleman SR. Facial contouring with lipostructure. *Clin Plast Surg* 1997;24(2):347–367.
31. Watson D, Keller GS, Lacombe V, et al. Autologous fibroblasts for treatment of facial rhytids and dermal depressions. *Arch Facial Plast Surg* 1999;1:165–170.
32. Webster RC, Fuleihan NS, Gaunt JM, et al. Injectable silicone for small augmentations: twenty year experience in humans. *Am J Cosmet Surg* 1984;1(4):1–10.
33. Orentreich DS, Orentreich N. Injectable fluid silicone. In: Roegnik RK, Roegnik HH, eds. *Dermatologic surgery principles and practice.* New York: Marcel Dekker, 1989:1349–1395.
34. Ellenbogen R, Ellenbogen R, Rubin L. Injectable fluid silicone therapy: human morbidity and mortality. *JAMA* 1975;234:308–309.
35. Ficarra G, Mosqueda-Taylor A, Carlos R. Silicone granuloma of the facial tissues: a report of seven cases. *Oral Surg Oral Med Oral Pathol Oral Radiol Endod* 2002;94(1):65–73.
36. Pearl RM, Laub DR, Kaplan EN. Complications following silicone injections for augmentation of the contours of the face. *Plast Reconstr Surg* 1978;61:888–891.
37. Lemperle G, Hazan-Gauthier N, Lemperle M. PMMA microspheres for skin and soft-tissue augmentation. Part II: clinical investigations. *Plast Reconstr Surg* 1995;96:627–634.
38. Rudolph CM, Soyer HP, Schuller-Petrovic S, et al. Foreign body granulomas due to injectable aesthetic micro-implants. *Am J Surg Pathol* 1999;23(1):113–117.
39. Tzikas TL. Evaluation of the radiance FN soft tissue filler for facial soft tissue augmentation. *Arch Facial Plast Surg* 2004;6:234–239.

186

Rejuvenation of the Midface

Edwin F. Williams III   *Allison T. Pontius*

Recent major advancements in comprehensive facial rejuvenation have focused on management of midfacial aging. In attempts to avoid the "face-lifted" appearance of years past, multiple innovative techniques to rejuvenate the midface have evolved. The key common denominator behind these techniques is the principle of lifting the descended soft tissue in a primarily vertical vector, as opposed to the primarily lateral vector of the traditional facelift. Multiple techniques have been ingeniously created to address the aging midface; however, by the mere nature of so many approaches, we can see that no one technique has prevailed. Although the nasolabial region remains a challenge to correct by any current technique, we advocate a reliable, effective, and safe approach that provides comprehensive rejuvenation of the midface, lateral brow and jawline.

With age, the convex contour of a youthful face is lost as the malar fat pad descends in an inferomedial direction, leaving in its wake a hollowed appearance to the lower eyelids, a skeletonized infraorbital rim, a prominent nasojugal fold, deepening of the nasolabial fold, and a pronounced labiomandibular fold with jowling (Fig. 186.1). Unfortunately, the changes seen with midfacial aging are not adequately addressed by traditional rhytidectomy alone.

Over the past 15 years, multiple surgical techniques to address the midface have been introduced, including the deep-plane rhytidectomy (1), the composite rhytidectomy (2), the transblepharoplasty subperiosteal midface lift with (3) or without (4) formal canthoplasty, the transblepharoplasty endoscopic subperiosteal midface lift (5), direct suspension of the malar fat pad with sutures (6,7), the transmalar subperiosteal midface lift (8), and the percutaneous technique of malar fat pad elevation (9), among others (10–15). The current concept is to address the brow and midface as a single unit, providing comprehensive rejuvenation to the upper two thirds of the face. In addition, in appropriate candidates, the brow/midface lift is also combined with a SMAS rhytidectomy to provide complete facial rejuvenation. The key to a successful operation is to weigh the advantages of performing each technique against the limitations and potential risks of the procedures.

The operation is performed through a minimal-incision brow-lift approach that relies on tactile feedback (the "smart-hand" technique) without the use of endoscopic guidance. The midface dissection and elevation is, however, performed under direct visualization through a temporoparietal incision with the use of appropriate retraction and headlight illumination. This technique has been performed in more than 650 patients over a 9-year period by the senior author and was found to be safe, reliable, and effective (16).

Potential sequelae or complications associated with midface lifting include temporary or permanent injury to the temporal, zygomatic, or buccal branches of the facial nerve, decreased sensation over the malar region, lateral canthal distortion, lower lid malposition, temporal wasting, incisional alopecia, and prolonged postoperative edema (17–19). With judicious patient selection, attention to the appropriate surgical planes, and gentle handling of tissues, however, the incidence of these morbidities have decreased to very reasonable levels.

ANATOMY

Knowledge of the surgical anatomy of the temporal and midface region is essential to perform safe and effective brow and midface surgery. Dissection during the brow and midface lift occurs in multiple anatomic planes, and

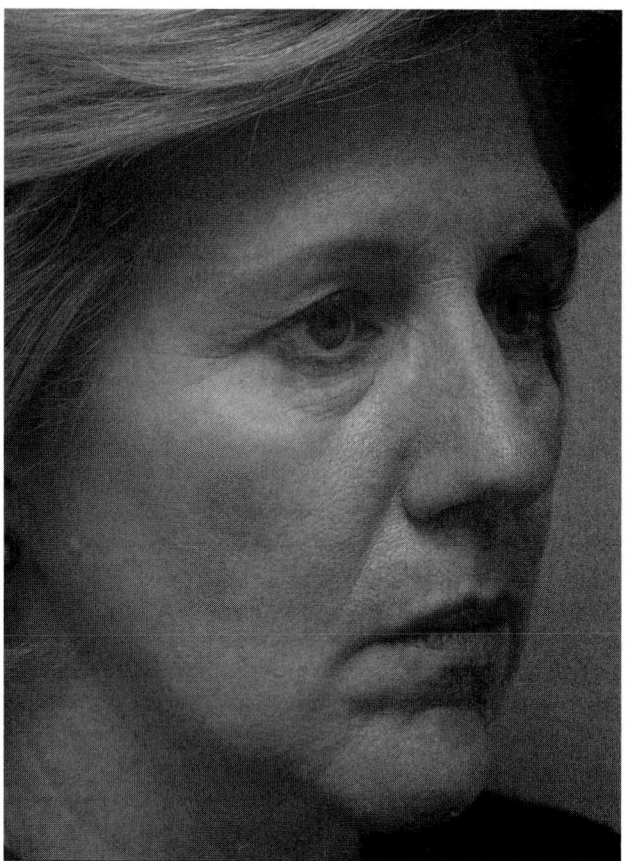

Figure 186.1 Characteristic findings seen with aging include a hollowed appearance to the lower eyelids, a skeletonized infraorbital rim, a prominent nasojugal fold, deepening of the nasolabial fold, and a pronounced labiomandibular fold with jowling.

taches to the superior edge of the zygomatic arch laterally, and the deep layer of the deep temporal fascia attaches medially. Underneath the deep layer of the deep temporal fascia lies the deep temporal fat pad. Overzealous dissection causing injury to the deep temporal fat pad carries the risk of developing postoperative temporal wasting (20).

The malar fat pad is triangular in shape, with its base at the nasolabial fold and its apex at the malar eminence. It is situated between the skin and the SMAS. It is loosely adherent to the SMAS and firmly attached to the skin. In detailed anatomic and histologic studies, Mendelson, et al. (21–22) described the surgical anatomy of the midface and the ligamentous attachments of the lower lid and the lateral canthus. Through an understanding of these attachments, we can see how gravitational forces acting on the midface against these fixed attachments creates the typical findings seen in an aging midface and lateral brow. In youth, the midface is characterized by a malar fat pad seated over the zygomatic arch, with its upper border covering the orbital part of the orbicularis oculi and its inferior border located along the nasolabial fold (23). With age, the malar fat pad descends over the SMAS in an inferomedial direction, causing an apparent increase in the apparent length of the lower eyelid and an increased prominence of the nasolabial and labiomandibular folds (Fig. 186.3). Correction of this deformity requires resuspension of the malar fat pad in a primarily vertical vector, with a slight 15-degree posterior angulation.

awareness of pertinent vital structures within these planes is crucial (Fig. 186.2).

The superficial temporal fascia is also referred to as the temporoparietal fascia (TPF) and is located deep to the subcutaneous fat of the temporal region. The TPF is continuous medially with the galea and is continuous inferiorly with the superficial musculoaponeurotic system (SMAS) of the lower face. The temporal branch of the facial nerve lies within the TPF. Immediately deep to the TPF is the true temporalis fascia. All dissection in this region takes places immediately superficial to the true temporalis fascia and deep to the TPF, in order to avoid injury to the temporal branch of the facial nerve. The temporal branch of the facial nerve crosses the zygomatic arch halfway between the lateral canthus and the root of the auricular helix within the TPF. The true temporal fascia splits at the level of the supraorbital ridge to become the superficial layer of the deep temporal fascia and the deep layer of the deep temporal fascia, between which lies the superficial temporal fat pad. Once the supraorbital margin is traversed, the superficial fat pad is gently entered, as dissection proceeds toward the zygomatic arch. The superficial layer of the deep temporal fascia at-

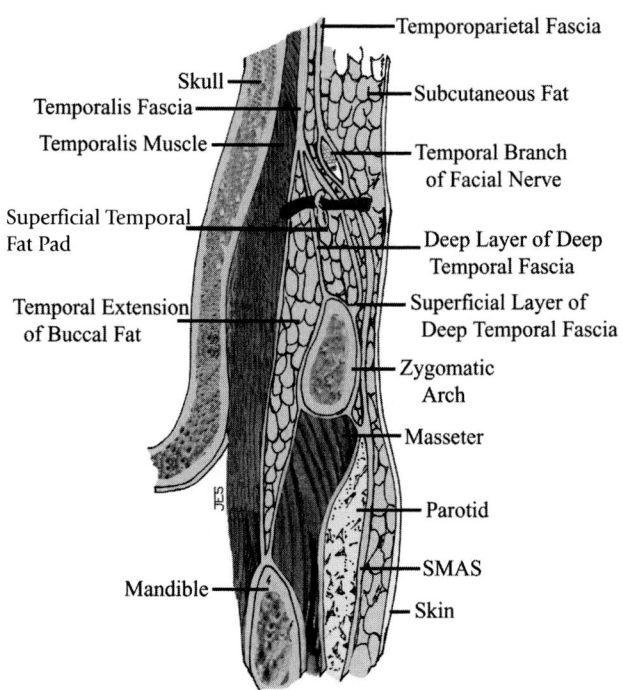

Figure 186.2 Anatomy of the temporal region. (Courtesy of Jesse Ellis Smith, MD)

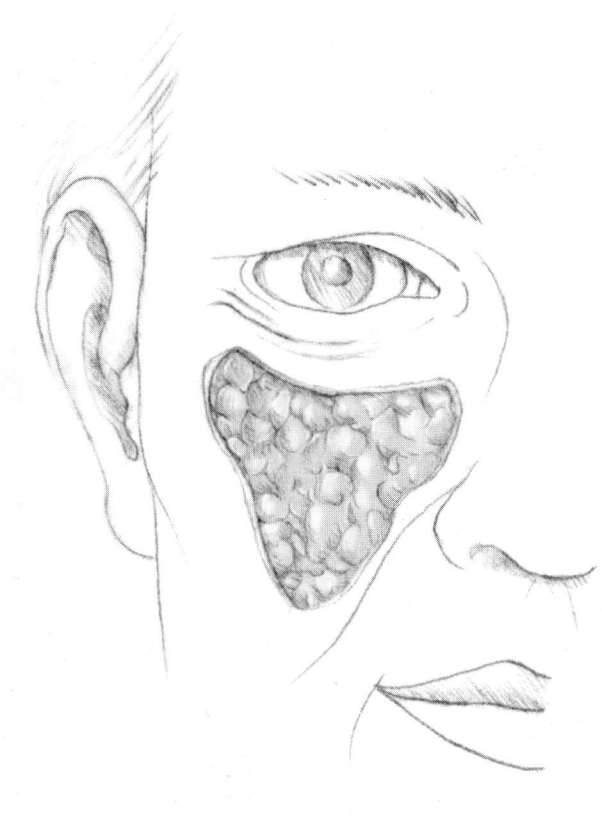

Figure 186.3 Inferomedial ptosis of the malar fat pad creates the appearance of an elongated lower eyelid and an increased prominence of the nasolabial fold and labiomandibular folds.

INDICATIONS

Any patient undergoing a browlift procedure should be considered as a candidate for a concomitant midface lift. The lateral brow region and the midface age in concert, and correction of one while overlooking the other, will lead to less than optimal rejuvenation for the patient. The procedures are carried out through the same incisions, with minimal additional morbidity. This is especially true in the younger patients (40 to 50 years old), who have evidence of lateral brow and midface descent but may not yet be candidates for a traditional rhytidectomy. In patients with significant aging in the lower face and neck, however, the extended midface lift can be performed with a concurrent rhytidectomy. In addition, the extended midface lift can be performed in conjunction with resurfacing procedures without risk to the vascularity of the overlying flap, given the subperiosteal plane of dissection.

SURGICAL TECHNIQUE

Five standard endoscopic browlift incisions are marked out, with one situated in the midline, two located lateral to midline in the paramedian position (approximately at the lateral canthus) just posterior to the hairline, and two additional, longer incisions located more temporally, also camouflaged by the hairline and extending over a 4-cm distance above the helical crus and over the temporalis muscle and fascia (24).

If a transconjunctival lower-lid blepharoplasty is entertained, then this procedure should be undertaken before brow and midfacial suspension. After midfacial elevation, the lower lid becomes extremely taut, restricting ease of transconjunctival entry into the lid. Conversely, an upper-lid blepharoplasty should be deferred until the brow and midface are appropriately elevated, so an accurate assessment of residual cutaneous redundancy can be made.

First, the midline brow incision is made extending through the periosteum. A small, sharp, flat periosteal elevator is used to dissect subperiosteally for a distance of a few centimeters circumferentially around the incision site. Posterior elevation is limited to approximately 4 to 5 cm, as more extensive dissection toward the occiput provides limited additional benefit in transposition of the brow upward. A larger, sharp, flat periosteal elevator that reduces the risk of injury to the periosteum is then introduced to elevate the central pocket down to the orbital rim in order to release the arcus marginalis, but no aggressive dissection of the glabellar musculature is undertaken.

After the surgical maneuvers have been completed through the midline-brow incision, the same technique of subperiosteal dissection is carried out via the two paramedian ports. Again, the sharp, flat periosteal elevator is used to carry out blind dissection down to the arcus marginalis for proper periosteal release at the orbital rim. The elevator is handled only in an upward, gentle lifting motion when the elevator tip approaches a 1- to 2-cm distance above the supraorbital notch, though, in order to avoid any paresthesias or neuropraxias that may ensue from violating the supraorbital neurovascular bundle. With proper wound retraction using wide, double-pronged hooks, a hand drill outfitted with a 1.5-mm-wide × 6-mm-long drill bit is used to enter the outer calvarial table at 30 degrees (to the horizontal) and joined with an opposing entry of the drill in order to form a bone tunnel through which the brow-fixating suture may be passed at the end of the case (Figure 186.4). The bone tunnel should be made in the posterior aspect of the incision because suspension of the brow upward will cover the bone tunnel if the tunnel is created too anteriorly relative to the incision.

The longer, lateral temporo-parietal incisions are then addressed. Dissection is carried down through the TPF so that a proper tissue plane may be achieved between the TPF and the true temporalis fascia, to avoid injury to the temporal branch of the facial nerve. The incision should be situated approximately 1 cm behind the hairline, to lie over the temporalis muscle, and not more posteriorly, to avoid transection of the superficial temporal artery and to minimize the long trajectory of dissection needed to reach the

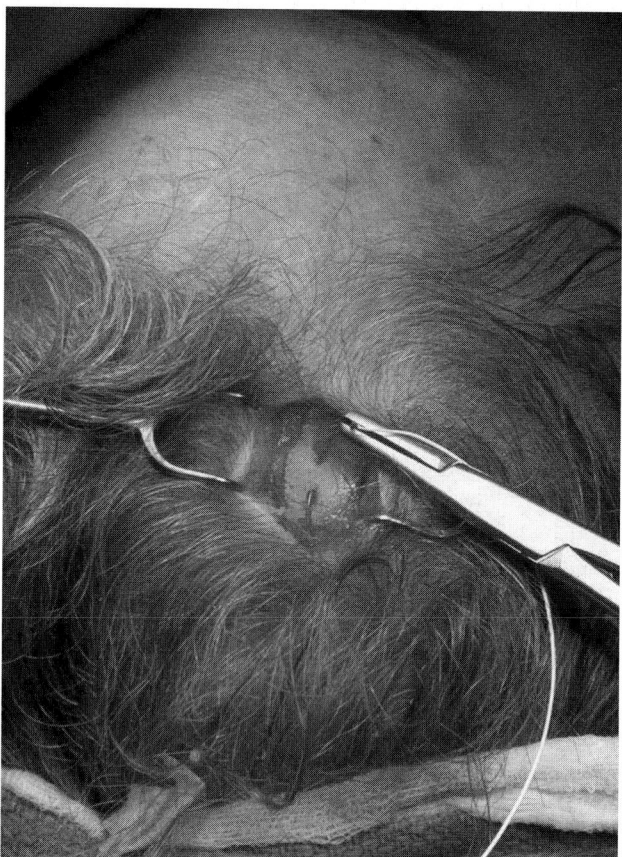

Figure 186.4 A bone tunnel is created through the outer calvarial table to secure the suspension suture for the brow elevation.

midface (Fig. 186.5). Initial dissection is performed with a large, blunt elevator over the true temporalis fascia, and then the larger, flat periosteal elevator is used to break the conjoined tendon of the temporalis muscle that divided the central and lateral pockets.

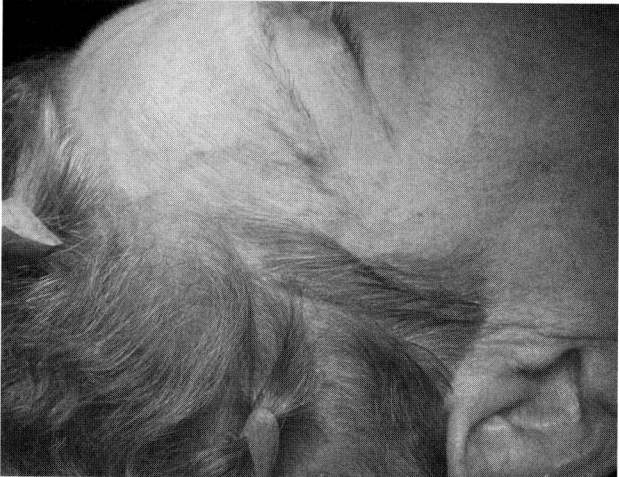

Figure 186.5 The temporoparietal incision is approximately 4 cm long and is placed 1 cm behind the hairline to lie over the temporalis muscle.

Under direct vision with a headlight and a Converse retractor, dissection is taken downward to the orbital rim with the small, sharp periosteal elevator, carefully looking for the presence of the sentinel vein. If the vein lies in the direct path between the upper and midface, then it may be skeletonized and cauterized with a bipolar device and transected with scissors in order to permit entry into the midface. Injudicious cautery of the sentinel vein, especially if the bipolar cautery tips are aimed superficially, may jeopardize the temporal branch of the facial nerve. The arcus marginalis is then released from the superolateral orbital rim near the lateral canthus with the periosteal elevator. The assistant places a finger along the lateral margin of the orbital rim to limit the surgeon's dissection and to avoid excessive release of periosteum from the lateral canthus. This 1-cm cuff of periosteum around the lateral canthus, the lateral orbital thickening (22), is retained to avoid undesirable lateral-canthal elevation or distortion.

Again, under direct view, the large, sharp periosteal elevator is guided downward to gently enter the superficial temporal fat pad and then to release the periosteal attachments overlying the zygomatic arch itself. This technique allows direct access to the midfacial structures. Next, an angled periosteal elevator is used to continue dissection inferiorly over the malar eminence to release the zygomaticus major and minor muscular attachments and the malar fat pad from the underlying zygomatic and maxillary bone. The dissection proceeds inferiorly over the masseter muscle until all midfacial structures are adequately released (Fig. 186.6). A CV-3 suture (Gore-Tex, WL Gore and Associates, Flagstaff, AZ) is passed through the temporalis fascia and muscle just antero-inferior to the temporoparietal incision and then passed through the malar fat pad with a long needle driver. The suture is pulled superiorly, to test if sufficient release of the midfacial tissues has been achieved. If not, then further dissection medially and inferiorly is carried out until appropriate release of the midface is observed. The paramedian suture on the same side is

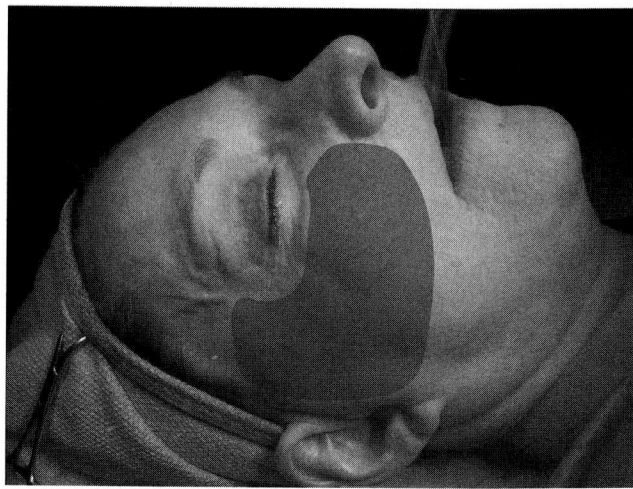

Figure 186.6 Extent of undermining.

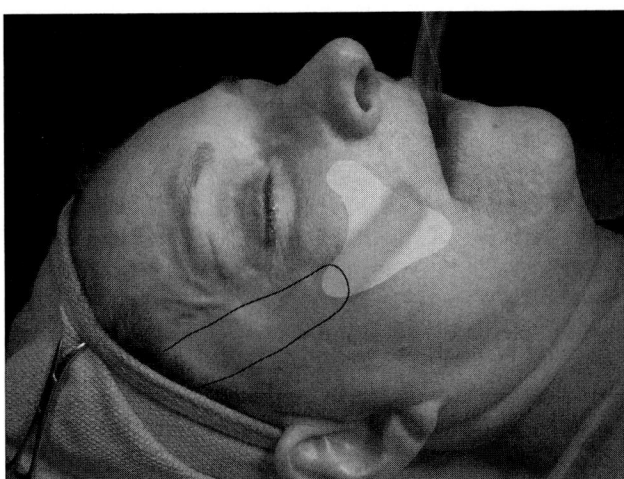

Figure 186.7 A suture is placed in the ptotic malar fat pad and zygomaticus major muscle.

tied down before the suture in the malar fat pad is fastened superiorly to the temporalis fascia. The paramedian suture is fixated first, in order to relieve any tension on the suture that elevates the midface and to permit better brow positioning by suspending the most superior suture initially. A CV-3 suture (Gore-Tex, WL Gore and Associates, Flagstaff, AZ) is used to secure the overlying frontalis muscle through the bone tunnel in the paramedian incision. After the paramedian suspension has been completed and the incision closed, the surgeon should return to the lateral temporal incision to suspend the already distally placed suture through the malar fat pad to the proximal temporalis muscle and fascia at the incision site. The vector of suspension should be essentially vertically oriented (with approximately 15 degrees of posterior angulation), and the suture through the malar fat pad should be situated more laterally over the malar prominence—both of which minimize untoward distortion of the lateral canthus (Figures 186.7 and 186.8). Next, the TPF just anterior to the temporoparietal incision is sutured to the temporalis muscle and fascia with the CV-3 suture (Gore-Tex, WL Gore and Associates, Flagstaff, AZ) to pull the overlying brow and soft tissue superolaterally. This suture placement is undertaken twice. All incisions are closed with surgical clips. Bacitracin ointment is applied to the external incisions, and a pressure dressing is fashioned into place.

POSTOPERATIVE CARE

The patient is seen on postoperative day one, and the wounds are inspected and cleaned with peroxide. A lighter dressing is applied that the patient will remove on the following day. The patient returns on postoperative day 6, and the surgical staples are removed at that time (Figure 186.9A–F).

COMPLICATIONS

Problems associated with rejuvenation of the upper and midface can be minimized with meticulous attention to proper tissue handling and to the proper plane of dissection. Asymmetry in brow elevation may be noted by the patient postoperatively; however, this is most commonly secondary to an unnoticed preoperative asymmetry. It is critical in the preoperative assessment that any preexisting brow and/or facial asymmetries are pointed out to the patient, as it may not be possible to completely correct their underlying asymmetry with surgery.

Most concerning to patient and surgeon alike is the postoperative development of a motor or sensory nerve deficit. The most common causes for this outcome include excessive retraction on the temporoparietal flap, dissection in an improper plane in the temporoparietal region (temporal branch injury) or midfacial region (zygomatic or buccal branch injury), injudicious use of bipolar cautery in the region of the cephalic vessel (25), and injury during the midface dissection. Additionally, aggressive midfacial dissection medially toward the nasolabial sulcus has been associated with a greater likelihood for buccal-branch paresis. In more than 650 cases, the senior author has encountered 9 cases of temporal branch and 2 cases of buccal branch neuropraxias that all completely resolved within a 6-month timeframe. However, one additional case of temporal branch palsy has failed to resolve in 12 months and is now considered permanent. In addition, one case of permanent, unilateral cranial nerve V2 (infraorbital nerve) paresthesia has also been encountered (16). Management includes expectant care, with frequent visits to provide reassurance during the postoperative course. If indicated, ocular lubrication may be necessary.

Incisional alopecia and unfavorable scars on the scalp can be minimized by proper handling of tissues and

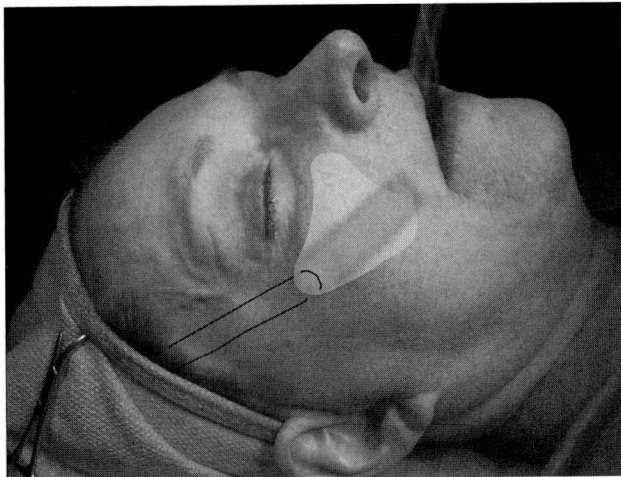

Figure 186.8 After securing the suture to the temporalis fascia, the descended midface structures are elevated to a more youthful position.

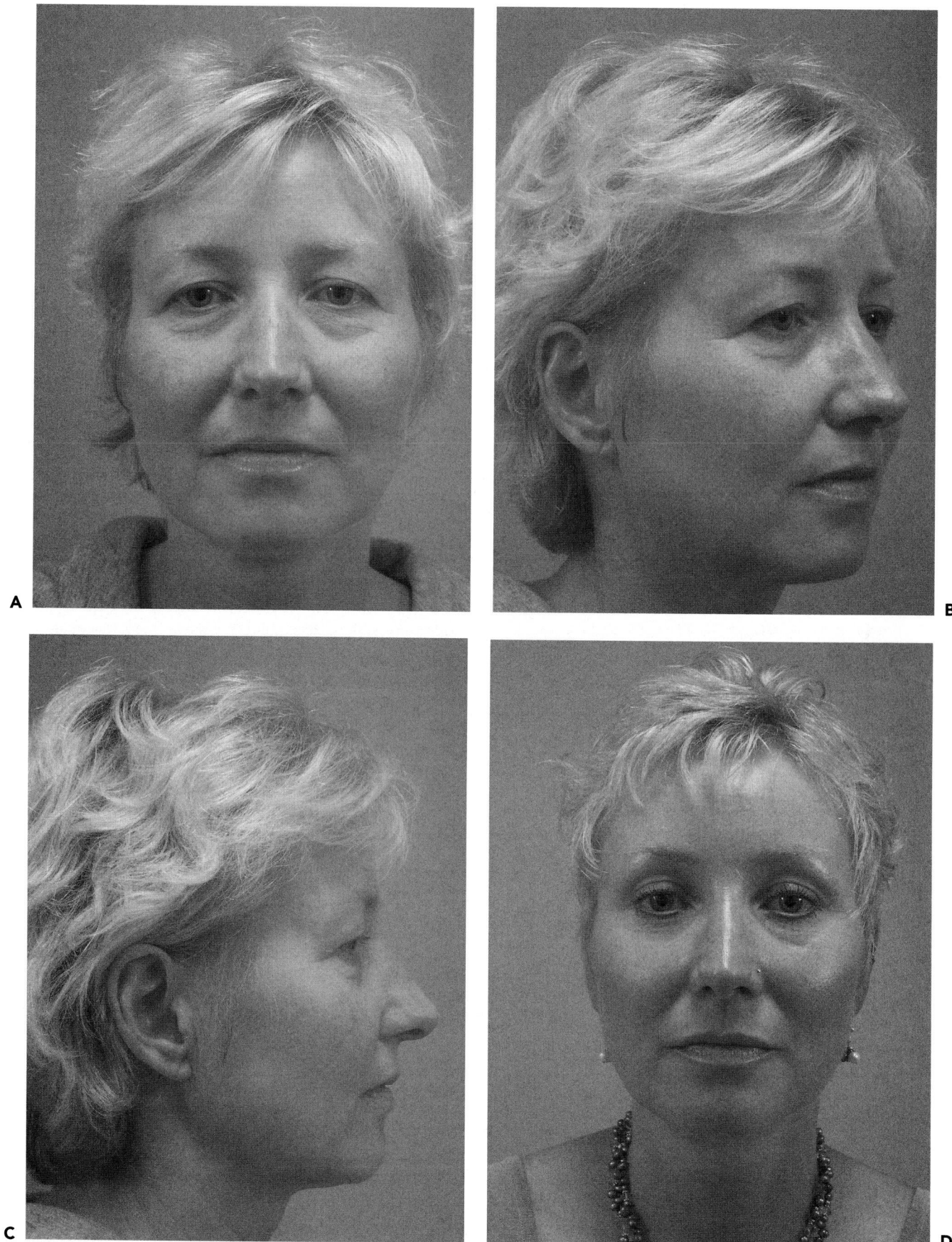

Figure 186.9   Pre- and postoperative views of a patient after undergoing a midface lift.

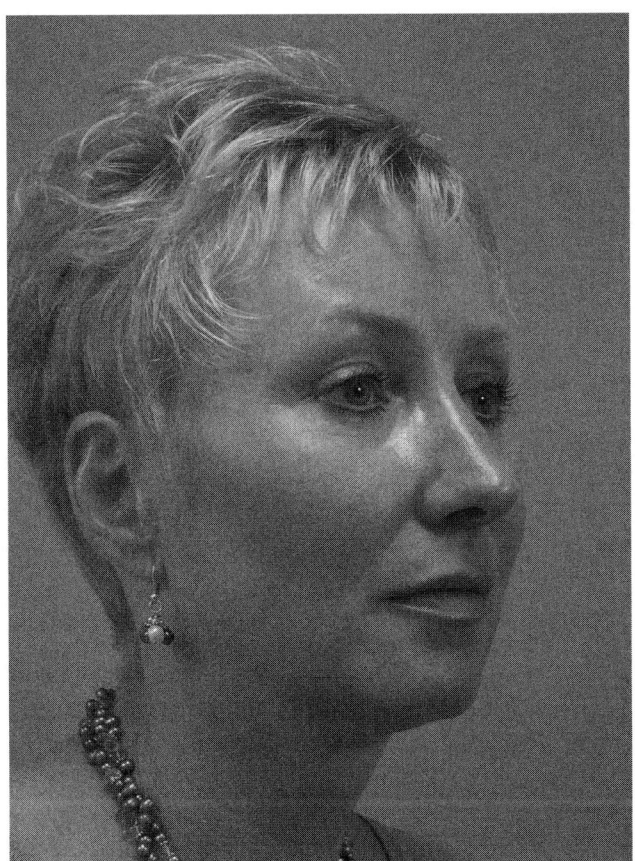
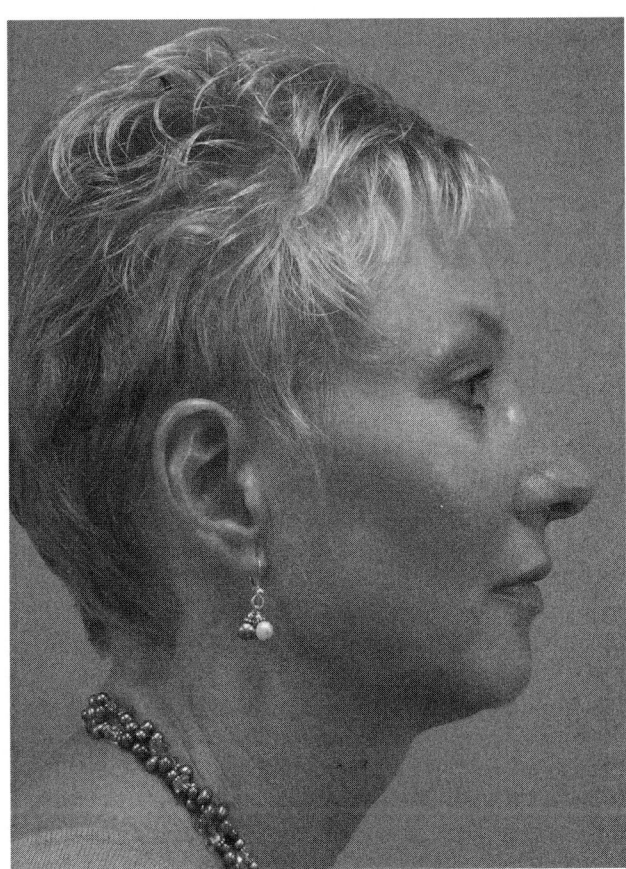

E

F

Figure 186.9 (*continued*)

attention to avoiding transection of the hair follicles by beveling the knife blade according to the direction of hair growth. For the three medial incisions, the knife blade should be perpendicular to the scalp, and it should be beveled posteroanteriorly for the two temporal incisions. In addition, excessive monopolar cautery should be minimized at the wound edges and undue tension on wound closure should be avoided. Following modification of the brow suspension technique from a screw suspension to a bone-tunnel technique, we have seen no further evidence of incision alopecia or unfavorable scarring. This is thought to be due to the fact that the screw held the brow suspended by the skin rather than by the frontalis muscle causing a compression alopecia.

LIMITATIONS

As alluded to in the introduction, multiple procedures to rejuvenate the midface have been developed over the years. What has been discovered is that there is no perfect procedure that is without its own set of limitations. One of the limitations of the minimal-incision brow-lift approach to the midface, as in the majority of midface techniques, is the modest improvement seen in the region of the na-

solabial fold. The senior author critically reviewed a random group of 100 patients who underwent the procedure (with 6 to 50 months of follow-up) by assessing midface elevation in three facial zones by three independent evaluators. Zone I represented the malar/infraorbital complex; zone II, the nasolabial fold; and zone III, the jawline (Fig. 186.10). The zones were rated on a scale from 0 to 2 (0, no improvement; 1, mild improvement; and 2, marked improvement). The evaluators found that the majority of patients (70%) had marked improvement in zone I (30% with mild improvement and 0% with no improvement), 30% of the patients had marked improvement in zone III (50% with mild improvement and 20% with no improvement), and only 4% of the patients had marked improvement in zone II, the nasolabial fold (60% with mild improvement and 36% with no improvement) (16). This correlates with conclusions drawn by Hamra (26) after critically reviewing his long-term results (with a minimum 10-year follow-up) of patients on whom he performed a deep-plane facelift. He found that the results with malar fat repositioning at 1 to 2 years post-operatively were successful, but the long-term results showed a failure of the early improvement, manifested by a recurrence of the nasolabial folds. He concluded that only direct excision of the nasolabial folds provides permanent correction.

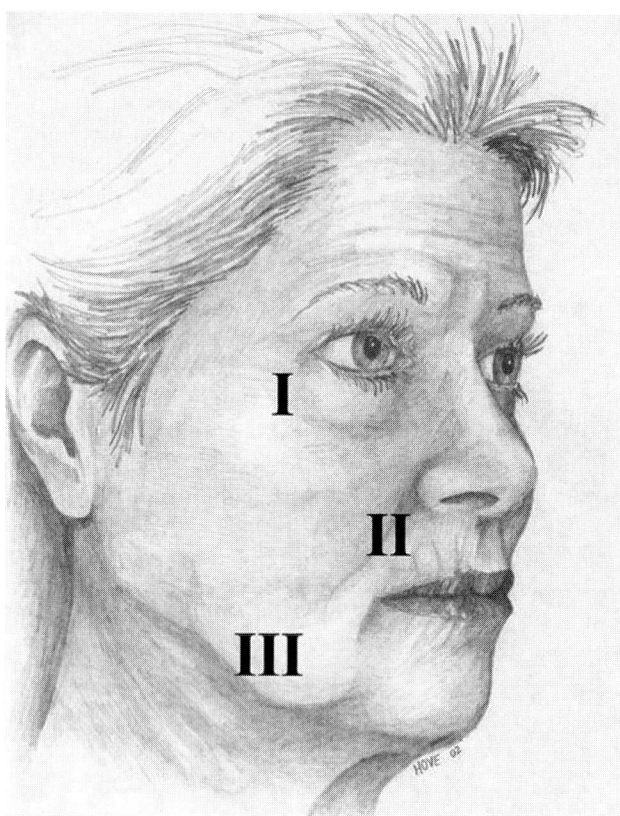

Figure 186.10 The three facial zones: Zone I represents the malar/infraorbital complex; zone II, the nasolabial fold; and zone III, the jawline. (Courtesy of Christopher Hove, MD.)

HIGHLIGHTS

■ The aging midface demonstrates a hollowed appearance to the lower eyelids, a skeletonized infraorbital rim, a prominent nasojugal fold, deepening of the nasolabial fold, and a pronounced labiomandibular fold with jowling.

■ To correct midface aging and to avoid the "face-lifted" appearance, the primary vector of suspension should be in a vertical direction.

■ The midface lift via a minimal-incision brow-lift approach provides rejuvenation to the upper two-thirds of the face by effectively targeting midface soft-tissue descent and lateral brow ptosis. These procedures can be performed alone or in conjunction with traditional rhytidectomy to provide comprehensive facial rejuvenation.

■ Complications can be minimized by careful attention to the relevant anatomy of the region, adherence to dissection in proper tissue planes, and careful handling of tissues.

■ The major limitation of the procedure is the difficulty in providing long-term correction of the nasolabial fold; however, consistent use of this technique in appropriately selected patients will provide the surgeon and patient with significant benefits and a low risk of complications.

REFERENCES

1. Hamra ST. The deep-plane rhytidectomy. *Plast Reconstr Surg* 1990;86:53–61.
2. Hamra ST. Composite rhytidectomy. *Plast Reconstr Surg* 1992; 90:1–13.
3. Hester TR Jr., Codner MA, McCord CD. The "centrofacial" approach for correction of facial aging using the transblepharoplasty subperiosteal cheek lift. *Aesthetic Surg Q* 1996;16:51.
4. Gunter JP, Hackney FL. A simplified transblepharoplasty subperiosteal cheek lift. *Plast Reconstr Surg* 1999;103:2029–2041.
5. Williams JV. Transblepharoplasty endoscopic subperiosteal midface lift. *Plast Reconstr Surg* 2002;110:1769–1777.
6. Owsley JQ. Lifting the malar fat pad for correction of prominent nasolabial folds. *Plast Reconstr Surg* 1993;91:463–474.
7. Byrd HS, Andochick SE. The deep temporal lift: a multiplanar, lateral brow, temporal and upper facelift. *Plast Reconstr Surg* 1996;97:928–937.
8. Finger ER. A 5-year study of the transmalar subperiosteal midface lift with minimal skin and superficial musculoaponeurotic system dissection: a durable, natural-appearing lift with less surgery and recovery time. *Plast Reconstr Surg* 2001;107:1273–1284.
9. Keller GS, Namazie A, Blackwell K, et al. Elevation of the malar fat pad with a percutaneous technique *Arch Facial Plast Surg* 2002;4:20–25.
10. Quatela VC, Jacono AA. The extended centrolateral endoscopic midface lift. *Facial Plast Surg* 2003;19:199–207.
11. Ramirez OM. Three-dimensional endoscopic midface enhancement: a personal quest for the ideal cheek rejuvenation. *Plast Reconstr Surg* 2002;109:329–340.
12. Byrd HS, Burt JD. Achieving aesthetic balance in the brow, eyelids, and midface. *Plast Reconstr Surg* 2002;110:926–933.
13. De Cordier BC, de la Torre JI, Al-Kakeem MS, et al. Rejuvenation of the midface by elevating the malar fat pad: review of technique, cases, and complications. *Plast Reconstr Surg* 2002; 110:1526–1540.
14. Scalfani AP. The multivectorial subperiosteal midface lift. *Facial Plast Surg* 2001;17:29–36.
15. Dempsey PD, Oneal RM, Izenberg PH. Subperiosteal brow and midface lifts. *Aesthet Plast Surg* 1995;19:59–68.
16. Williams EF III, Vargas H, Dahiya R, et al. Midfacial rejuvenation via a minimal-incision brow-lift approach. *Arch Facial Plast Surg* 2003;9:470–478.
17. Kaye B. A subperiosteal approach as an improved concept for correction of the aging face. *Plast Reconstr Surg* 1988;82:393–398.
18. Psillakis JF, Rumlay TO, Comargo A. Subperiosteal approach as an improved concept for correction of the aging face. *Plast Reconstr Surg* 1988;82(3):383–394.
19. Maillard GF, Cornette de St Cyr B, Scheflan M. The subperiosteal bicoronal approach to total facelifting: the DMAS—deep musculoaponeurotic system. *Aesthet Plast Surg* 1991;15:285–289.
20. Quatela VC, Graham D III, Sabini P. Rejuvenation of the brow and midface. In: Papel ID et al., eds. *Facial plastic and reconstructive surgery*. New York: Thieme Medical Publishers, 2002:171–184.
21. Mendelson BC, Muzaffar AR, Adams WP Jr. Surgical anatomy of the midcheek and malar mounds. *Plast Reconstr Surg* 2002;110(3): 885–896.
22. Muzaffar AR, Mendelson BC, Adams WP Jr. Surgical anatomy of the ligamentous attachments of the lower lid and lateral canthus. *Plast Reconstr Surg* 2002;110(3):873–884.
23. Yousif NJ, Mendelson BC. Anatomy of the midface. *Clin Plast Surg* 1995;22:227–240.
24. Williams EF III, Lam SM. Upper and midfacial rejuvenation. In: Williams EF III and Lam SM, eds. *Comprehensive facial rejuvenation: a practical and systematic guide to surgical management of the aging face*. Philadelphia: Lippincott Williams & Wilkins, 2004: 54–104.
25. Trinei FA, Januszkiewicz J, Nahai F. The sentinel vein: an important reference point for surgery in the temporal region. *Plast Reconstr Surg* 1998;101:27–32.
26. Hamra ST. A study of the long-term effect of malar fat repositioning in face lift surgery: short-term success but long-term failure. *Plast Reconstr Surg* 2002;110:940–951.

Miscellaneous

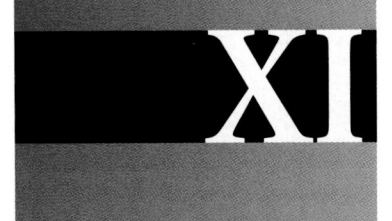

Byron J. Bailey   *Shawn D. Newlands*

Medical Ethics Rounds

187

Sharen J. Knudsen   Byron J. Bailey

The physician–patient relationship is recognized as fundamentally important to the patient's well-being. Society expects this relationship to have a fiduciary quality characterized by trust, beneficence, confidentiality, and patient advocacy. In exchange for holding the physician to a higher standard, society rewards physicians financially and with high social status. When the physician–patient relationship is ruptured, intense public outrage follows.

This chapter examines the challenges to the physician–patient relationship that face us today. Although many physicians are bewildered by the changes in this relationship, others welcome opportunities to forge meaningful relationships with patients. We have an array of technically sophisticated diagnostic and therapeutic modalities to offer patients, but we must now decide when the use of expensive and often invasive techniques is beneficial.

NEW CHALLENGES IN MEDICAL ETHICS

The formal process of medical training emphasizes mastering technical procedures and accumulating a medical database. Training in ethics receives less attention, and the student is likely to regard ethical training as peripheral. In practice, however, ethical and legal issues can be central to the delivery of patient care because patients and society expect physicians to practice with technical proficiency and at the same time to identify and respond to important ethical issues (1).

The need to make life-and-death decisions often comes unexpectedly. When problems have not been thought out in advance, the ability to make reasoned choices is diminished. Alternately, the prepared physician is aware of current key issues, such as these:

■ Must physicians always prolong life?
■ Does cutting costs mean cutting corners?
■ Who controls patient care?

■ How much should physicians tell patients?
■ When should physicians break confidentiality?
■ Is "legal" equivalent to "ethical"?

Answers to these questions are not found easily nor are they universal. Yet to be an ethical advocate for the patient, the physician must stay abreast of current issues and must participate in the ongoing dialogue. Societal cues, institutional guidelines, and the emergence of hospital ethics committees can ease the burden of making weighty decisions at the bedside.

Case histories provide an excellent teaching substrate for the study of ethical and medicolegal issues. The following cases illustrate various ethical dilemmas and are designed to provoke further questions and thought; they do not provide a complete analysis. All vignettes are fictitious, but they are all taken directly from our own clinical experiences.

Principles of Medical Ethics

The following statements are from the American Medical Association's Code of Medical Ethics (1).

1. A physician shall be dedicated to providing competent medical service with compassion and respect for human dignity.
2. A physician shall deal honestly with patients and colleagues, and strive to expose those physicians deficient in character or competence, or who engage in fraud or deception.
3. A physician shall respect the law and recognize a responsibility to seek changes in those requirements that are contrary to the best interests of the patient.
4. A physician shall respect the rights of patients, of colleagues, and of other health professionals, and shall safeguard patient confidences within the constraints of the law.
5. A physician shall continue to study, apply, and advance scientific knowledge; make relevant information avail-

able to patients, colleagues, and the public; obtain consultation; and use the talent of other health professionals when indicated.

6. A physician shall, in the provision of appropriate patient care, except in emergencies, be free to choose whom to serve, with whom to associate, and the environment in which to provide medical services.

7. A physician shall recognize a responsibility to participate in activities contributing to an improved community.

CASE HISTORY 1: DEALING WITH MEDICAL ERRORS

You have operated inadvertently on the left ear when the consent has been given for stapedectomy on the right ear. Both ears show some conductive hearing loss, but the deficit is worse on the right. During the surgery, you find a congenitally malformed incus that has a tenuous fibrous connection with the stapes capitulum; you elect to repair it with an ossicular chain prosthesis. The operation goes well, and you expect an excellent result. What is the best way to tell the patient that you operated on the wrong ear?

The fallibility of physicians is a reality. A quick search of a litigation database shows that at least 30 cases have occurred involving operative procedures on the wrong ear; in fact, one of the first tort cases involved an operation on the wrong ear. In a survey of 400 physicians regarding their attitudes toward medical mistakes, 43% of respondents reported that they always tell the patient of mistakes; 48% said they sometimes tell (2). A strong caution came from the respondents: "Don't think mistakes can't happen in your practice; they will."

In this particular case, the surgeon may offer to operate on the other ear and waive the fee. The physician was negligent, but with a good outcome; establishing that the patient was actually harmed would be difficult. The patient may be so delighted with a good hearing result that forgiveness for the mistake is offered freely. How would the same patient feel if the surgeon tried to cover up the mistake or refused to admit the error up front?

The Institute of Medicine (IOM) has issued a thoughtful report on the subject of medical errors in the United States (3). The IOM estimates that nearly 100,000 unnecessary deaths occur in this country every year because of errors made by healthcare providers. This has stimulated a marked upgrading of the systems for reporting errors and reengineering medical care settings in order to reduce the number of such adverse events (4). Each of us must shoulder the individual responsibility to make our offices, clinics, and hospitals safer for our patients.

Physicians who do not admit errors, who use evasive language (with words such as inadvertent or misadventure), or who withhold information selectively will eventually lose the confidence of their patients. The risk is that pa-

tients will discover errors on their own and sue. The defense will have difficulty exonerating a physician once an element of deception has been introduced.

CASE HISTORY 2: END OF LIFE/WITHHOLDING LIFE-SAVING MEASURES

A 46-year-old alcoholic man with hoarseness is found to have a large, nearly obstructing hypopharyngeal tumor. He requires emergent tracheotomy, for which he volunteers consent. Postoperatively, he writes this note: "I am sane, and if my time comes for me to go . . . let me go. Anyone who tries to keep me alive on a machine I will follow into Hell." Further communications indicate that he does not want to be kept alive by artificial means or undergo cardiopulmonary resuscitation. He has not yet accepted treatment for the cancer. This man has no living relatives or surrogate; he is a medically indigent adult and is a social derelict.

Following tracheotomy, the patient develops delirium tremens and is near death. He has no further opportunity to sign a natural death directive, since his deteriorating condition has rendered him incompetent to make decisions. Without treatment, his cancer will surely kill him; with treatment, the chance of survival is less than 20%. Treatment carries a high likelihood of complications, prolonged hospital convalescence, and permanent social dependency.

Do you resuscitate the man? Is there such a thing as a slow code? The patient has not had an opportunity to explore treatment options for his stage IV disease. He has no family members to confirm his wishes or to speak on his behalf. Should you proceed with treatment? The man is indigent and the cost of his care is borne by society. Is he entitled to a prolonged stay in an intensive care setting?

Many issues arise in this case. One issue is the "do not resuscitate" order, which the patient has expressed clearly but has not formalized by a Patient's Directive to Physicians or by a living will. Some states have enacted the Durable Power of Attorney for Health Care, making it possible for another person to act as a legally authorized representative to make healthcare decisions on the patient's behalf. The chief value of these documents is that they carry clear legal authority for a surrogate to advocate the patient's preferences. In the absence of such authority, the court must appoint a guardian. Hospital-based ethics committees may be helpful in determining a sound course of action in conjunction with the guardian. Many of the serious questions that need rapid answers in cancer care can be foreseen and resolved in advance.

Finally, the patient's socioeconomic status is relevant. The patient's claim to health care is great but not unlimited. A collective society, desirous of an equitable distribution of healthcare resources, provides an extrinsic factor in the determination of individual patient care. Traditional medical care ignores such pressures and focuses only on the patient's needs, regardless of socioeconomic status. Frank and Davidson (5) write, "Some would argue that any socioeconomic constraints should derive from institutional or governmental decisions and should be consistent for all persons." Others argue that great caution must be exercised when societal considerations influence decisions at the level of the individual. There is consensus that the physician must serve the patient's interest and that limitations should be placed by the collective actions of society through the instrument of government. Physicians must remember the tragic historic precedents in which the lines became blurred between the notion that some lives were not worth living and the decision that some lives should be terminated (6).

End-of-life care presents some of the most frequent and most challenging dilemmas. One study of the key issues encountered focused on the topics that are most important to our patients (7). Quality of end-of-life care must address adequately the following five domains:

1. Adequate management of pain and other symptoms
2. Avoiding the inappropriate prolongation of dying
3. Achieving a sense of control for patients in their last days
4. Relieving loved ones of the burden of making decisions
5. Strengthening the patients' relationship with their families

Today's complex medical dilemmas involve a mixture of confusion and uncertainty based on conflicting guidelines drawn from medical traditions, ethics, law, religion, economics, and philosophy. Dissenting opinions abound, depending on the perspectives and backgrounds of different observers. Most medical decisions result in some expenditure of resources. These resources are finite; they are also inadequate to meet the needs of all who suffer. How society and its specific agents (physicians) set priorities for medical resource allocation will be a major topic during the next decade. Ethicists will be important guides through these minefields.

CASE HISTORY 3: EXPERT WITNESS TESTIMONY

You are being defended in a malpractice case that you believe has little merit. Your outrage is understandable when you discover that the expert witness for the plaintiff will be a physician who has earned the unenviable reputation of being an itinerant testifier. How can you protect yourself against such courtroom tactics?

When physicians think of an expert, the image comes to mind of a leading investigator in the field who is respected for special knowledge of a problem and who renders an opinion about a particular diagnosis and management strategy. We might envision testimony that is much like the case discussions in the *New England Journal of Medicine*.

The opinions of the expert should be based on an objective interpretation of the available data and should represent the best interpretation by that person.

The adversarial process of jurisprudence, however, generates a different picture of the medical expert. Courts have wide latitude in determining who qualifies as a medical expert, because legislatures do not define precise qualifications. The expert is expected to support the position of either the plaintiff or the defendant. Most courts adhere to Rule 702 of the Federal Rules of Evidence for guidance on the admissibility of expert testimony. Rule 702 states that expert testimony is admissible if "it assists the trier of fact to understand the evidence or determine a fact in issue." This is a more liberal interpretation of what constitutes expert testimony than the previous Frye rule, which stipulated that the expert must identify the field involved in the case and demonstrate that the theory proposed is generally accepted by members of that field.

Brokers of expert testimony provide, for a fee, physicians available for witness duty. This practice is entirely legal, but even the American Bar Association has issued an opinion that these brokering activities raise "substantial ethical problems." It is unethical for an expert to receive a contingency fee.

As for the problem of the itinerant testifier, the most effective tactic is to discredit the "expert" during the legal proceedings. This can be done through careful questioning by the defense attorney: Has the expert personally treated this particular condition recently? Has the expert personally performed the operative procedure? What were the results? What data support a different course of action than that taken by the defendant, and are these anecdotal or based on fact? Past testimony given by the itinerant testifier can be exposed during a trial. Repositories of testimony have been compiled by various professional societies. Previous testimony by the expert on a similar matter may restrict expert opinion or invite the possibility of perjury if the present testimony espouses opinions diametrically opposed to those given under oath in a different yet similar case.

The epidemic of medical litigation has profoundly influenced the contemporary practice of our specialty. Table 187.1 shows the types of allegations and their frequency in a surgical specialty, based on a study by the American College of Surgeons. Defensive medicine increases the annual cost of medical care; like the large annual professional liability premiums, these costs are ultimately paid by patients. Unfortunately, neither expense adds to the quality of care received by those who are suffering. Physicians tend to recoil from any involvement with the legal system, but two factors must be kept in mind: If no courts were available for the redress of grievances, the only alternative would be violent revenge.

The simple truth is that our legal system cannot function properly without our involvement as experts in medical practice standards. When we do become involved, it

TABLE 187.1

ALLEGATIONS IN PROFESSIONAL LIABILITY CLAIMS

Type	Number (%)
Improperly performed procedure or procedure not performed	127 (65.1)
Error in diagnosis or failure to diagnose	37 (19.0)
Failure to instruct or communicate information	12 (6.2)
Medication error	10 (5.1)
Performed when not indicated or contraindicated	8 (4.1)
Wrong patient or wrong body part	1 (0.5)
Total[a]	195

[a]Ten cases did not have an allegation that could be coded.

Reprinted from Nora PF, Karnell LH. Liability pilot survey examines claims, expert witnesses. *Am Coll Surg Bull* 1990;75:17, with permission.

is our task to support good medical practices and to oppose bad medical practices. At the same time, we are demonstrating to a skeptical public that we are putting the best interests of our patients above all other considerations (8).

The American system of adversarial justice guarantees that plaintiffs and defendants will be represented in court by advocates who are loyal to the party who hires and pays them. Therein lies the problem when paid expert witnesses join the legal contest, and this forms the basis for a need to develop guidelines that will produce testimony that results in a fair conclusion to the trial (9).

Expert witness testimony has legal protection as long as it is defensible on the basis of supporting publications, is consistent with prior testimony of the expert, and is not false, deceptive, or misleading. Most judges will require that expert witnesses meet several common sense standards:

1. They have current and substantial experience in the area of their testimony.
2. They testify honestly in regard to the scientific and medical facts.
3. They be familiar with the prevailing standards of practice (10).

CASE HISTORY 4: PATIENT CONFIDENTIALITY

You have a self-employed patient who is seropositive for the human immunodeficiency virus (HIV) and needs surgery. He is healthy except for recurrent sinus infections caused by a deviated septum and nasal polyposis. His internist believes this may be a source for a potentially lethal infection. Since his condition was diagnosed 2 years ago, he has been careful to conceal it from his insurance carrier. The patient entreats you not to tell the hospital personnel, for fear that his insurance carrier will drop his coverage if his HIV-seropositive condition is discovered. Do you perform the sinus surgery? Do you tell other hospital personnel? Do you document on the chart his HIV-seropositive status?

Some would argue that physicians should treat all patients as though they were seropositive. Most surgeons use universal precautions on all patients. Yet surgeons sustain needle sticks despite the best precautions. Some gloves are found to contain small holes even before use. Furthermore, it is impossible to ensure that healthcare workers, from surgeon to housekeeper, will not be exposed to the AIDS virus as a result of the surgery. Most agree that elective surgery should not be performed on an HIV-positive patient. If the operation is not elective, is the surgeon obligated to operate on this man? The American Medical Association (AMA) is on record as saying that a patient's HIV status, in and of itself, does not provide ethical grounds for refusing treatment. Surgeons argue, however, that those who are pushing for invasive interventions are not the practitioners taking the risk. The risk to healthcare workers must be weighed against the benefit to the AIDS patient; surgery is indicated only when there are clear indications that the surgical intervention will outweigh the risks.

The physician must inform other hospital personnel of the patient's HIV status because of the imperative to protect those who might be exposed. One method would be to imply but never document the diagnosis and require blood and body fluid precautions. Another would be to document the diagnosis but instruct the patient not to release confidential medical records. Above all, healthcare workers should be aware that the public health is served if patients with contagious diseases visit physicians and get treatment. Confidentiality encourages the reticent patient to seek medical attention.

CASE HISTORY 5: INAPPROPRIATE PATIENT REQUESTS

A patient asks you to prevaricate, distorting facts concerning the degree of sinus disease and nasal obstruction so that her septorhinoplasty will be covered by insurance. Without question, the procedure is for cosmesis only. She discloses that another surgeon will honor this request. How should you respond?

This is a straightforward case of deception. In this instance, the surgeon has several options:

- Go along with the patient's request.
- Reassess the patient specifically for nasal dysfunction secondary to deformity and submit this as justification for surgery.
- Decline the request completely and offer to work out a payment plan agreeable to the patient.
- Refer the patient to the other surgeon.

Selecting the best option requires assessing the risks and benefits associated with each. Simple compliance with the request to lie carries with it the risks of being caught, of pursuing a patient–physician relationship based on deception, and of being exposed to the local medical community as one who is inclined to stray from the truth. Although the risks involved with this option may prove to be exaggerated, the consequences of a bad outcome may be very grave.

Sometimes a patient requests that records be modified to establish eligibility for reimbursement. Some patients do this naively, in the belief that such a "little white lie" does no harm to anyone. Other patients comment that they have paid high premiums for years and have never filed a claim, expressing a form of financially based rationalization that they find logical. Some rationalize that other patients do this sort of thing—and may even cite examples.

Most patients respond reasonably to a sympathetic explanation of why it is unethical and illegal to falsify medical records to obtain reimbursement under any circumstances. Patients who leave your office in search of an unethical surgeon are exercising the most foolish form of poor judgment; such patients will not represent a significant loss to the practice you are building.

CASE HISTORY 6: CORPORATE GIFTS

A sales representative from a large pharmaceutical company has invited you and your two partners on a complimentary fishing trip in the Caribbean. Although you would love to go, you are concerned about the ethics of this type of product promotion. Your partners express annoyance, countering that this gift will in no way influence your medical judgment. Besides, they argue, millions of dollars are spent in this manner, and why should you decline when another physician will surely accept the invitation? Are your concerns valid?

Absolutely! A recent position paper by the American College of Physicians (11) states the following policy: "Gifts, hospitality, or subsidies offered to physicians by the pharmaceutical industry ought not to be accepted if acceptance might influence or appear to others to influence the objectivity of clinical judgment." As a useful criterion in determining acceptable activities and relationships, physicians should ask themselves if they would be willing to have these arrangements generally known.

In the contemporary corporate patterns of medical practice, physicians may be invited to participate in arrangements that appear to place personal financial gain ahead of the best interests of the patients we serve. A recent publication prepared by the Ethics Committee of the American Academy of Otolaryngology—Head and Neck Surgery offers helpful insights in dealing with these complex issues (12).

Recent studies have shown that many physicians have a rather permissive view concerning acceptance of gifts from pharmaceutical companies (13,14). Younger physicians and house staff are more likely to believe that these promotional activities will not influence their patient care decisions than are more senior physicians and the public. There is a consensus among professional societies, ethicists, and many leaders in medicine that these are serious ethical challenges, especially concerning the targeting of high-volume prescribers and busiest physicians, and the excessive monetary value of some of the gifts, trips, and money they receive from drug companies (15).

CASE HISTORY 7: SEXUAL BOUNDARIES

As consenting adults, you and the office manager of your large group practice become romantically involved. After a brief affair, things cool between you, and the affair ends amicably. What, if any, is your risk of litigation for sexual abuse?

The answer to this question is more complex than the parties involved probably imagine. A sexual harassment complaint is worrisome to every employer. The Equal Employment Opportunity Commission defines sexual harassment as any "verbal or physical conduct of a sexual nature [that] has the purpose or effect of unreasonably interfering with an individual's work performance or creating an intimidating hostile or offensive working environment." Federal laws apply to businesses with 15 or more employees, but several states have laws that cover smaller operations. A behavior merely meant to be friendly can be illegal under the broad interpretations that current law allows.

A landmark Supreme Court decision in 1986 illustrates this point well (16). In the case of Vinson v. Meritor Savings Bank, a suit was brought against the bank by a woman who had a sexual relationship with her supervisor. During the 4 years she worked in the bank, she never complained about harassment. She was promoted consistently and left the position of her own accord. The suit did not claim monetary loss; instead, she successfully argued that she should receive monetary compensation for emotional damage. The Supreme Court decision recognized sexual harassment as a form of sexual discrimination. The "hostile" environment created by the supervisor's actions was declared illegal, despite the fact that the woman did not lose her job or suffer monetary loss.

Substantial nonmonetary damages can result from sexual harassment charges, as well. Claims against an employer for sexual harassment are a matter of public record and may surface in the local newspaper. The local or county medical society or hospital board may require a formal hearing, and loss of privileges could result. Insurance carriers may balk at covering the expense of legal defense, settlement, or payment of damages, because sexual harassment is considered an intentional act specifically excluded by most policies.

A related problem concerns the sexual boundaries between physicians and their patients. The guidelines' prohibiting sexual contact between physicians and patients is founded on ethical arguments that these relationships violate the principles of respect for patient autonomy and beneficence. It is proposed that in addition, there is an argument based on virtue—namely that physicians should honor the professional virtues of self-effacement and self-sacrifice and see them as barriers preventing sexual contact with patients (17).

Often, the defense for these relationships is the statement that they are consensual. This argument tends to fail in courts and in the decisions of state licensing boards because of the "power imbalance" in the doctor–patient relationship. Most patients have some degree of vulnerability, and physicians must never exploit that aspect of those who have come seeking help. Medical practice is a high privilege, not a right (18).

Most of us have sworn an oath to serve the sick and to abstain from mischief and corruption, including seduction of patients. The good news is that a recent report from the Oregon Board of Medical Examiners indicates that a program of public and physician education on this subject led to a reduction in the number of complaints of sexual misconduct in that state (19).

CASE HISTORY 8: THE IMPAIRED PHYSICIAN

You live in a small community where the actions of local physicians are highly visible. One of your surgical colleagues has become intoxicated at social events on more than one occasion. Your suspicion that this problem with alcohol is more than social drinking is confirmed when you assist during an emergency procedure. The physician smells of alcohol, makes unreasonable technical errors, and demonstrates impaired judgment. Ancillary personnel, concerned about this behavior, ask you to "do something."

What responsibility do you, the assisting physician, have to report this behavior? To whom is such a report given? Should you inform the patient? What is your liability as a codefendant if litigation is initiated for a bad outcome?

The issue of substance abuse is not new, but it is particularly painful when a fellow physician is involved. The duty to report such behavior to an appropriate body and to urge the impaired colleague to seek treatment is clearly

stated by the AMA's Council on Ethical and Judicial Affairs. What is not stated is the difficulty in confronting the impaired physician, in collecting credible evidence, and in determining the appropriate body to review such evidence. The issues of confidentiality and treatment are collateral to the central issue of substance abuse but are of utmost importance in resolving the problem. The appropriate body is usually the State Board of Medical Examiners or state or county medical societies, not the patient or the patient's family. Measures are taken to preclude discovery of the reporting physician, and confidentiality is preserved until the final actions of the board are taken.

Because the surgery was emergency and not elective, there is good reason to believe that a jury would hold you blameless for the actions of the impaired physician provided you could demonstrate that you did in fact report to the appropriate bodies the danger posed by this physician to the public. If you did not charge for the services, you might be covered by the Good Samaritan laws. Furthermore, your lawyer could claim that the outcome could have been much worse had you not been present to assist.

In this case, the actions of the impaired surgeon also put the hospital at risk for litigation. The medical staff is responsible for the granting of privileges, and the appropriate members of the hospital staff must be informed. It is probable that a thorough investigation will produce a body of findings that are substantiated by affidavits from those who have witnessed questionable behavior. The range of sanctions includes a long list of options, from medical license revocation, suspension, or restriction, down to less severe punishments, such as reprimand, limitation of clinical privileges, or the requirement for supervision of medical practice.

Reporting an impaired physician may be difficult when the questionable behavior is noted by a competitor. You should anticipate the need for documentation if the charges are serious, especially if a patient has suffered an injury at the physician's hands. That each of us has a responsibility to deal with impaired physicians is an inescapable fact of life. We owe it to our patients, to our colleagues, and to the profession to come forward with the relevant facts and work to initiate a program of rehabilitation for the involved physician (20).

The impaired physician has certain rights, also. The right of presumed innocence until proven guilty and the right to due process and fairness must be built into the investigation. In the case of drugs and alcohol, rehabilitation is the centerpiece of recovery from the period of impairment.

CONCLUSION

In this chapter, we have provided an overview of the ethical and legal concepts encountered most frequently in clinical practice. The interfaces between medicine, ethics, and the law are shifting constantly, but their importance increases each year (21).

REFERENCES

1. Code of Medical Ethics: Current opinions with annotations. 1996 American Medical Association. http://www.ama-assn.org/ethic/ceja/pome.htm.
2. Gray J. Should you tell the patient when you mess up? *Med Econ* 1990;23:135.
3. Kohn LT, Corrigan JM, Donaldson MS, eds. *To Err Is Human. Building a safer health system.* Washington, DC: National Academy Press, 1999.
4. Singer PA. Medical ethics—clinical review: recent advances. *Br Med J* 2000;321(7256):282–285.
5. Frank H, Davidson T. Ethical dilemmas in head and neck cancer. *Head Neck* 1989;1:22.
6. Boyd K. What can medical ethics learn from history? *J Med Ethics* 1995;21:197.
7. Singer PA, Martin DK, Kelner M. Quality end-of-life care: patients' perspectives. *JAMA* 1999;281(2):163–168.
8. Casler J. Medical legal ethics. *Otolaryngol Head Neck Surg* 1996;115:250.
9. Runkle D. Biomedical scientists and physicians as experts in federal courts. *Acad Med* 2001;76(8):762–763.
10. Rohrich RJ. The expert witness in plastic surgery: criteria and obligations. *Plast Reconstr Surg* 2003;111(6):2051–2052.
11. Position paper, American College of Physicians. Physicians and the pharmaceutical industry. *Ann Intern Med* 1990;112:625.
12. Ethics Committee of the American Academy of Otolaryngology—Head and Neck Surgery. Commercial relationships (Chapter 8). *AAO-HNS Foundation Ethics Committee report to the membership of the American Academy of Otolaryngology—Head and Neck Surgery* (available upon request to the AAO-HNS, One Prince Street, Alexandria, VA). 1996;115:220.
13. Gibbons RV, Landry FJ, Blouch DL, et al. A comparison of physicians' and patients' attitudes toward pharmaceutical industry gifts. *J Gen Intern Med.* 1998;13:151–154.
14. Steinman MA, Shlipak MG, McPhee SJ. Of principles and pens: attitudes and practices of medicine house staff toward pharmaceutical industry promotions. *Am J Med* 2001;110:551–557.
15. Brett AS, Burr W, Moloo J. Are gifts from pharmaceutical companies ethically problematic?: a survey of physicians. *Arch Intern Med* 2003;163(18):2213–2218.
16. Gorn S. Little things that can get you sued for sexual harassment. *Med Econ* 1990; 20(August):131.
17. McCullough LB, Chervenak FA, Coverdale JH. Education: ethically justified guidelines for defining sexual boundaries between obstetricians-gynecologists and their patients. *Am J Obstet Gynecol* 1996;175(2):496–500.
18. Legal brief—Patient protection laws and the issue of consensual sexual relationships with physicians. *CMAJ* 2004;170(1):34–35.
19. Enbom JA, Parshley P, Kollath J. A follow-up evaluation of sexual misconduct complaints: The Oregon Board of Medical Examiners, 1998 through 2002. *Am J Obstet Gynecol* 2004;190(6):1642–1653.
20. Ethics Committee of the American Academy of Otolaryngology—Head and Neck Surgery. The impaired physician (Chapter 7). *AAO-HNS Foundation Ethics Committee report to the membership of the American Academy of Otolaryngology—Head and Neck Surgery* (available upon request to the AAO-HNS, One Prince Street, Alexandria, VA). 1996;115:213.
21. Bailey BJ, ed. *Head & neck Surgery—otolaryngology,* 3rd ed. Philadelphia: Lippincott Williams & Wilkins, 2001.

Eponyms in Otolaryngology

188

Kim R. Jones   Harold C. Pillsbury III

Eponyms are valuable in medical conversation because of their ability to describe succinctly complex combinations of symptoms and physical examination findings. They often serve as useful tools in written and verbal communication among physicians. Eponyms are important as well in reminding us of important medical pioneers, upon whose figurative shoulders we are able to move to higher levels of clinical practice. We offer this collection of eponyms as an opportunity to refresh past knowledge and to expand your repertoire of terminology.

Abrikossoff tumor   A benign neoplasm that may occur in a variety of visceral, mucosal, and cutaneous sites but is most frequently seen in the tongue. It usually presents as a small, firm, circumscribed nodule. Excision is the treatment of choice. It is also known as a *granular cell tumor.*

Ackerman tumor   Another name for *verrucous carcinoma.*

Albright syndrome   Characterized by polyostotic fibrous dysplasia. Scattered melanotic macular spots and, in females, precocious puberty also are typical. The bony lesions may occasionally occur in single bones; therefore, this syndrome should be in the differential diagnosis of any patient presenting with a bony lesion in the face or jaw.

Alexander syndrome   The least severe type of inner ear dysplasia. The cochlear duct and basilar turn of the cochlea are usually the only structures affected, resulting in a high-frequency, rather than a total, hearing loss.

Alport syndrome   An autosomal-dominant syndrome that consists of progressive glomerulonephritis (usually starting in the mid-teens) and progressive sensorineural hearing loss. The auditory deficit is symmetric, worse in the high frequencies, and primarily due to a loss of hair cells.

Apert syndrome   A rare craniofacial disorder occasionally seen by the otolaryngologist because of the associated hypoplastic maxilla or cleft palate (25%). Some of these patients reportedly have a conductive hearing loss secondary to stapes footplate fixation.

Arnold nerve   The auricular branch of the vagus. It arises from the jugular ganglion, passes through the temporal bone via the mastoid canaliculus, and exits the skull through the tympanomastoid fissure. It supplies the skin of the posterior external canal and posterior auricle.

Ascher syndrome   A rare, possibly autosomal-dominant disorder. Manifestations are a loss of elasticity in the skin of the eyelids (blepharochalasis), goiter, and edema and thickening of the gingivobuccal mucosa, which gives the appearance of double lips.

Avellis syndrome   One of a number of syndromes caused by thrombosis of the vertebral artery. The nucleus ambiguus and the spinothalamic tract are affected, often with involvement of the bulbar nucleus of the spinal accessory nerve. This results in an ipsilateral paralysis of the soft palate, pharynx, and larynx, with loss of pain and temperature sensation on the contralateral trunk and extremities. See also *Babinski-Nageotte syndrome* and *Cestan-Chenais syndrome.*

Babinski-Nageotte syndrome   Thought to be caused by multiple infarcts in the distribution of the vertebral artery. Almost any cranial nerve may be affected; the most common motor deficits are paralysis of the ipsilateral pharynx, larynx, soft palate, and sometimes tongue. Possible sensory deficits include loss of taste and loss of pain and temperature sensation around the face. Horner syndrome also may be present.

Baelz syndrome   Characterized by onset in childhood or early adolescence of thickening of the lower lip and hyperplasia of the minor salivary glands in this region. Papules sometimes form at the duct openings, and saliva can be easily expressed. Some forms may predispose toward an increased risk of squamous cell cancer.

Bárány syndrome   A combination of unilateral headache in the back of the head, periodic ipsilateral deafness (alternating with periods of unaffected hearing), vertigo, and tinnitus. It is also known as *Bárány benign positional vertigo*.

Barre-Lieou syndrome   Consisting of sharp pain beginning in the neck and radiating up to the occiput and then forward. It is most common in patients between 40 and 60 years of age. Pain is usually on one side and aggravated by certain movements of the head. Sensory disturbances, including vertigo, tinnitus, and cloudy vision, may accompany the pain. The cause is not known. It is also known as *cervical migraine*.

Barrett esophagitis   Replacement of the squamous epithelium of the distal esophagus by columnar epithelium, similar to that which lines the stomach. The most common cause is chronic gastroesophageal reflux, and 2% to 5% of cases may progress to adenocarcinoma.

Bartholin duct   The major duct of the sublingual gland. It is formed by the confluence of several of the more anterior small sublingual ducts (ducts of Rivinus) and empties into the submandibular duct. It is variably present in humans.

Battle sign   Ecchymosis over the mastoid process. It is indicative of a temporal bone or posterior fossa fracture.

Behçet syndrome   Classically, a symptom complex consisting of oral ulcers, genital ulcers, and iritis. The oral lesions can be extensive and may be the initial manifestation of the disease. It is seen most frequently in young adults in Japan and in Mediterranean countries. The cause is unknown; both viral and immune-complex etiologies have been proposed.

Besnier-Boeck-Schaumann syndrome   Eponym for systemic sarcoid.

Bezold abscess   A subperiosteal abscess of the temporal bone, most commonly found in the region just anterior to the mastoid tip. The cause is usually a mastoiditis with extravasation through the inner bony table into the digastric fossa.

Boerhaave syndrome   Spontaneous rupture of the esophagus, usually due to severe vomiting.

Bogorad syndrome   Profuse lacrimation during eating. It is usually the result of faulty regeneration of autonomic nerves after facial trauma, with parasympathetic fibers originally intended for the salivary glands going to the lacrimal gland instead. It is also known as *syndrome of crocodile tears*.

Bohn nodules   See *Epstein pearls*.

Bonnet syndrome   A combination of tic douloureux and Horner syndrome.

Bourneville-Pringle syndrome   Eponym for tuberous sclerosis, a neurocutaneous disease characterized by epilepsy, mental retardation, and adenoma sebaceum of the face and oral mucosa.

Bowen disease   A variant of squamous cell cancer characterized by a full-thickness dysplasia of the epidermis. It is by definition noninvasive, but it can progress to invasive carcinoma. It appears as a red, scaly patch in sun-exposed areas, and it can be confused with psoriasis.

Brissaud-Marie syndrome   Unilateral paralysis or spasm of the tongue and lips of a hysteric nature.

Brown sign   Blanching of a red or blue mass in the tympanic membrane when air pressure is applied by pneumootoscopy. It is indicative of a glomus tympanicum tumor.

Brown vertical retraction syndrome   A congenital or acquired pseudoparesis of the inferior oblique muscle, whereby the eye cannot be elevated beyond mid-gaze. The congenital form is thought to be due to a congenitally shortened superior oblique tendon, whereas the acquired syndrome may be due to either recent trauma (e.g., orbital fracture with entrapment) or previous trauma with formation of adhesions.

Broyle ligament   Anterior commissure ligament of the larynx.

Brunner abscess   Abscess of the posterior floor of the mouth.

Burckhardt dermatitis   An eruption of the external ear. It consists of red papules and vesicles that appear after exposure to sunlight. The rash usually resolves spontaneously.

Burton line   A sign of lead intoxication. It is a dark line a few millimeters in width that follows the margins of the gingiva. It is caused by the deposition of insoluble lead sulfide in the capillary endothelial cells and histiocytes. Burton line is not seen in edentulous patients.

Cannon nevus   An autosomal-dominant disorder characterized by extensive white lesions of the oral mucosa. The mucosa appears thickened, deeply folded, and spongy. The lesions are asymptomatic and may be found from the newborn period until adolescence. The nevi are generally asymptomatic and do not require treatment.

Carhart notch   An apparent loss of bone conduction sensitivity seen between 2,000 and 4,000 Hz in patients with otosclerosis. It is thought to be due to the fact that when the mastoid bone is vibrated, the ossicular chain vibrates slightly out of phase, causing a relative movement of the stapes footplate to the cochlea. In otosclerosis, this does not occur because of footplate fixation. Why the effect is most strongly seen between 2,000 and 4,000 Hz is not known.

Cestan-Chenais syndrome   Paralysis of the soft palate, pharynx, and larynx caused by occlusion of the vertebral artery. The point of blockage is below the origin of the posteroinferior cerebellar artery. Ipsilateral cerebellar asynergia and Horner syndrome are also present. Contralateral hemiplegia and diminished proprioception and tactile sensation occur.

Chédiak-Higashi syndrome   An autosomal-recessive syndrome of granulocyte defects, partial albinism, photophobia, and abnormalities in platelet and coagulation function. Patients may present to the otolaryngologist because of recurrent periodontal disease and oral ulcers.

Chvostek sign   A facial twitch obtained by tapping the distribution of the facial nerve. It is indicative of hypocalcemia.

Cogan syndrome   Typically a sudden onset of interstitial keratitis and vestibuloauditory symptoms, usually in young persons but sometimes in the elderly. Patients report blurring of vision, orbital pain, vertigo, and tinnitus. The symptoms may progress quickly to blindness and deafness, followed by resolution and later relapse. Treatment currently consists of steroids.

Collet-Sicard syndrome   Unilateral paralysis of cranial nerves IX, X, XI, and XII. The most common cause is an extradural tumor in the posterior fossa, but there have been reports of the syndrome occurring from compression at the skull base from tumors of the deep lobe of the parotid. Vocal cord paralysis may be the presenting symptom.

Costen syndrome   A symptom complex consisting of pain in the temporomandibular joint (TMJ) area, the side of the head, and the tongue, with tinnitus and vertigo. It is thought to be due to TMJ disease, but the mechanism has not been elucidated.

Cowden syndrome   An unusual disorder whose primary ear-nose-throat manifestation is a warty, pebbly enlargement of the gingiva and sometimes the oral mucosa. Patients with this disease also may have thyroid goiters or adenomas, gastrointestinal polyps, and fibrocystic breast disease. They are at increased risk for malignancies in all of these areas.

Crouzon disease   Characterized by hypertelorism, a hypoplastic mandible, and downward-sloping palpebral fissures. It is a craniofacial disorder also known as *craniofacial dysostosis*. It is caused by premature closure of the cranial bones. Treatment is surgical.

Curtius syndrome   Hypertrophy of an entire side of the body or of a single part. When it occurs in the face, it is known as *congenital hemifacial hypertrophy*.

Dandy syndrome   Oscillopsia caused by bilateral loss of vestibular function, usually as the result of bilateral labyrinthectomy.

Darier disease (keratosis follicularis)   Multiple erythematous, crusted papules distributed over the face and body. These may be particularly troublesome in the external ear canal. White, ragged papules also may be present in the oral cavity.

Dejean syndrome   Characterized by exophthalmos, diplopia, superior maxillary pain, and numbness along the route of the trigeminal nerve. It is classically caused by a nasal tumor that traverses the pterygopalatine fossa and invades the floor of the orbit.

DiGeorge syndrome   Defective development of the third and fourth pharyngeal pouches, most frequently manifesting as partial or total agenesis of the thymus and parathyroids. Abnormal development of the heart, aortic arch, mandible, external ear, and philtrum also may be present. The most common presenting sign is hypocalcemia in the neonatal period.

Eagle syndrome   Elongation of the styloid process or ossification of the stylohyoid ligament, causing recurrent nonspecific throat discomfort, foreign body sensation, dysphagia, or facial pain. The only effective treatment is surgical shortening of the styloid process.

Ebner, gustatory glands of   Minor salivary glands in the posterior part of the tongue near the circumvallate papillae.

Epstein pearls   Multiple small white nodules on the palate and oral mucosa of newborns. Histologically, they are composed of concentric layers of keratin. No treatment is needed, because they disappear spontaneously within a few months.

Escherich sign   Action of protrusion of the lips caused by percussion of the inner surface of the lips or tongue. It is seen in hypoparathyroidism.

Fordyce disease   A developmental anomaly characterized by enlarged, ectopic sebaceous glands (Fordyce spots) in the oral mucosa. These glands appear as numerous small yellowish white granules.

Foville syndrome   Ipsilateral paralysis of cranial nerves VI and VII and contralateral hemiplegia. The syndrome is usually caused by an infarct near the brainstem nuclei of the affected nerves and damages the motor pathways as they pass through this area before decussating.

Frey syndrome   Also known as *auriculotemporal syndrome*. In the normal person, the sweat glands are innervated by sympathetic nerve fibers. During a parotidectomy, these fibers are severed as the anterior skin flap is raised. The parasympathetic fibers from the auriculotemporal nerve also lose their site of innervation when the parotid is removed, and so it is thought that these fibers grow into the severed axonal sheaths of the sympathetic nerves to provide an aberrant innervation of the sweat glands. Thus, when a stimulus for salivary flow occurs, sweating over the anterior skin flap area also occurs.

Garcin syndrome   Consists of motor and sensory deficits involving cranial nerves III through XI. Garcin syndrome can be caused by basilar skull fracture with hemorrhage, basal meningitis, cavernous sinus thrombosis, or tumors of the parapharyngeal space. It is also known as *hemipolyneuropathy*.

Gardner syndrome   Characterized first usually by multiple osteomas that develop in the skull and facial bones, including the mandible. It is an autosomal-dominant disease; other symptoms include multiple epidermoid cysts of the skin and polyposis of the colon and rectum. There is a tendency for these polyps to become malignant.

Goldenhar syndrome   Characterized by underdevelopment that may involve the mandible, external ear, orbit, and facial muscles. In addition, another manifestation may be hemivertebrae of the vertebral column. It is probably a variant of hemifacial microsomia, one of the more common congenital syndromes of the first and second arches.

Gradenigo syndrome   Suppurative otitis followed by pain in the distribution of the ophthalmic branch of the trigeminal nerve and paralysis of the abducens nerve. Originally caused by an extradural abscess involving the petrous bone, this syndrome is now more commonly caused by a tumor at the petrous apex, such as a cholesteatoma, meningioma, or other tumor. It is also known as *petrous apex syndrome.*

Griesinger sign   Pain, redness, and swelling of the tip of the mastoid, indicative of thrombophlebitis of the sigmoid sinus with involvement of the mastoid emissary veins.

Grisel disease   Atlantoaxial dislocation secondary to infection. Symptoms are severe neck pain and rigidity; Grisel disease has been reported to follow a tonsillectomy or severe nasopharyngeal infection.

Hallermann-Streiff syndrome   Significant for its associated hypoplastic mandible. Other features are brachycephaly, a characteristic beaklike nose (parrot nose), and hypotrichosis.

Hennebert sign   In the presence of a normal tympanic membrane, changes in pneumatic pressure produce nystagmus (Positive Fistula Test). The nystagmus is more marked upon application of negative pressure. This sign is present with congenital syphilis and is believed to be due to an excessively mobile footplate or to be caused by motion of the saccule mediated by fibrosis between the footplate and the saccule.

Hollander syndrome   A rare syndrome in which congenital deafness (presumably due to cochlear abnormalities) is linked to the appearance of a goiter in the third decade of life. Thyroid function tests are normal, but biopsy of thyroid tissue shows a partial defect in thyroxine biosynthesis.

Horner syndrome   Characterized by ptosis, miosis, and anhidrosis due to loss of the cervical sympathetic nerves.

Horton neuralgia   An autonomic nervous system disorder also known as *cluster headache.* Patients have unilateral headaches centered behind or close to the eye, along with ipsilateral nasal congestion, suffusion of the eye, and increased lacrimation. Attacks may occur daily for several weeks, then disappear for months or years until another series (cluster) begins.

Hutchinson teeth   Characterized by small and widely spaced teeth (especially the upper incisors) with notches on their biting surfaces. Only permanent, rather than deciduous, teeth are affected. It is a characteristic sign of congenital syphilis.

Jacobson nerve   The tympanic branch of the ninth cranial nerve. It supplies sensory fibers to the mucosa of the middle ear; running with it are preganglionic parasympathetic fibers that leave the middle ear as the lesser superficial petrosal nerve to eventually innervate the parotid. These fibers are cut in an attempt to relieve the gustatory sweating seen in Frey syndrome.

Jacod syndrome   Consists of progressive ophthalmoplegia, usually starting with paralysis of the oculomotor nerve. This is accompanied or followed by hypesthesia in the distribution of the ophthalmic branch of the trigeminal nerve, exophthalmos, and finally involvement of the optic nerve itself. It is caused by a middle cranial fossa tumor that compresses the nerves near the apex of the orbit. It is also called *orbital apex syndrome.*

Kallmann syndrome   Consists of hypogonadism secondary to lack of gonadotropins, and anosmia due to agenesis of the olfactory bulbs. It is dominant with variable penetrance. The male-to-female ratio is 3:1.

Kiesselbach plexus or area   An area in the anterior septum in which the capillaries merge. It is often the site of anterior epistaxis. It also has been referred to as *Little area.*

Koplik spots   Pale round spots on the oral mucosa and conjunctiva that are seen in the beginning stages of measles.

Körner septum   A remnant of the petrosquamous suture line, which may persist as a plate of bone separating the superficial (squamous) group of mastoid air cells from the deeper (petrous) cells.

Krause nodes   Lymph nodes in the region of the jugular foramen.

Kussmaul disease   Salivary duct obstruction caused by fibromucinous plugs. It occurs in dehydrated patients.

Langer lines   Tension lines in the skin.

Lermoyez syndrome   Characterized by attacks of tinnitus and deafness followed by a bout of vertigo that surprisingly relieves the vestibuloacoustic symptoms. It is similar to Ménière disease. The symptoms in Lermoyez syndrome tend to occur in younger patients than Ménière disease does, and unlike the latter, gradually resolve over time with no permanent hearing loss.

Lillie-Crowe test   Used to diagnose unilateral lateral sinus occlusion. Digital compression of the opposite internal jugular vein causes the retinal veins to dilate, because the major venous outflow tracts on both sides are now blocked.

Little area See *Kiesselbach plexus.*

Louis-Bar syndrome Characterized by ataxia during early childhood and also possibly telangiectasias of the orbit, face, or neck. It is better known as *ataxia-telangiectasia.* Affected patients also have a lack of immunoglobulin A and often have recurrent pulmonary and sinus infections.

Ludwig angina A rapidly spreading infection of the submandibular, sublingual, and submental spaces. It produces swelling and elevation of the tongue and a brawny induration of the floor of the mouth. It is a diffuse infection, with little or no abscess formation. Its major danger is airway obstruction, and patients may require a tracheostomy until the swelling subsides. The cause of Ludwig angina is usually an odontogenic infection, with streptococci and oral anaerobes being the most common pathogens. Treatment is by antibiotics and drainage of any area of fluctuance.

Luschka pouch The pharyngeal bursa. See *Tornwaldt cyst.*

Maffucci syndrome Characterized by cavernous hemangiomas of the head and neck. Affected patients also have multiple endochondromas, with shortening of the involved bones. Twenty percent to 40% of patients have malignant degeneration of one or more endochondromas into chondrosarcoma.

Marcus Gunn phenomenon Usually a congenital condition, consisting of unilateral ptosis of the eyelid with opening of the eye during movements of the mandible. The cause is unknown.

Marcus Gunn syndrome (jaw winking syndrome) Usually an acquired condition following abnormal regeneration of the facial nerve. There is associated movement between the orbicularis oculi and the muscles around the mouth, often resulting in elevation of the upper eyelid when the mouth is open and ptosis when the mouth is closed.

Marjolin ulcer A squamous cell carcinoma that arises at the site of an old burn scar, often 20 to 40 years after the initial burn. It is often locally aggressive and metastasizes early.

Meckel cartilage The embryonic cartilage from which the mandible, incus, and malleus are derived.

Meckel cave A diverticulum of dura and arachnoidea encephali mater that lies on the anterolateral surface of the petrous ridge in the middle cranial fossa and contains the trigeminal ganglion.

Meckel ganglion Sphenopalatine ganglion.

Melkersson-Rosenthal syndrome Characterized by manifestations in childhood or early adolescence as recurring attacks of unilateral or bilateral facial paralysis with concomitant swelling of the lips and tongue. Affected patients also have a fissured tongue that becomes more prominent with age. It is an autosomal-dominant disease with variable penetrance. The cause is unknown.

Michel aplasia Total lack of development of the inner ear. Middle ear structures may or may not be present. The external ear and canal are usually normal in appearance.

Mikulicz disease Bilateral, recurrent swelling of the lacrimal and salivary glands, usually as a manifestation of some other systemic disease, such as lymphocytosis or tuberculosis. Pathology shows a diffuse lymphocytic infiltrate.

Millard-Gubler syndrome Ipsilateral paralysis of the abducens and facial nerves with contralateral hemiplegia of the extremities. It is caused by a lesion in the ventral part of the pons (either infarction or tumor) that damages the cranial nerve roots and the adjacent pyramidal tract.

Möbius syndrome Congenital facial paralysis (usually bilateral) with paralysis of the abducens nerve and sometimes other oculomotor nerves. Pathologically the few cases studied have usually shown hypoplasia of the involved brainstem nuclei.

Mondini dysplasia Malformation of the middle and apical cochlea, vestibule, and endolymphatic system. Children with this defect present with a significant sensorineural hearing loss and a predisposition to perilymph fistulae and meningitis.

Morgagni, sinus of A defect between the upper edge of the superior constrictor muscle and the buccopharyngeal fascia through which the eustachian tube passes.

Morgagni, ventricle of The invagination of mucosa between the false cords and the true cords in the larynx. It extends laterally as the laryngeal sinus. It also separates the quadrangular membrane superiorly from the conus elasticus inferiorly.

Nager syndrome Characterized by facies similar to those seen with Treacher Collins syndrome. Affected patients also present with preaxial upper limb defects, microtia, atresia of the external auditory canals, and malformation of the ossicles. Conductive and mixed hearing losses may occur. The inheritance pattern has not been determined, because most cases are sporadic. Also known as *acrofacial dysostosis.*

Neurofibromatosis (von Recklinghausen disease) It is primarily of interest to the otolaryngologist because of neurofibromatosis type II (familial acoustic neuroma).

Nothnagel syndrome A combination of ipsilateral third nerve palsy and contralateral cerebellar ataxia. It is caused by tumors of the mid-brain involving the area around the red nucleus, through which fibers of the third nerve pass. The most common cause is a pineal body tumor.

Oliver sign A pulling sensation felt in the larynx and trachea due to an aortic arch aneurysm. It is most evident when the head is extended.

Ondine curse Failure of respiratory drive, especially during sleep. Most cases present within a few hours of birth, and other neurologic abnormalities are present in approximately 50% of cases. Treatment is tracheostomy with mechanical ventilation at night, although bilateral phrenic pacing has been used successfully in some patients.

Ortner syndrome   A rare cause of hoarseness in infants with congenital cardiac disease. Compression of the left recurrent laryngeal nerve between the aorta and a dilated pulmonary artery results in paralysis of the left vocal cord.

Osler-Weber-Rendu disease (hereditary hemorrhagic telangiectasia)   Characterized by punctate hemangiomas usually developing around puberty and commonly seen in the oral and nasal mucosa and tongue. Other common sites include the gastrointestinal tract, bladder, and liver. It is an autosomal-dominant disease well known to otolaryngologists.

Pancoast syndrome   Shoulder pain radiating down the distribution of the ulnar nerve of the arm, caused by local extension of a tumor in the apex of the lung that eventually invades the brachial plexus. Horner syndrome, indicating involvement of the cervical sympathetic chain, also may be present.

Parinaud syndrome   Bilateral palsy of the third and fourth nerves, leading to decreased upward gaze and ptosis. It is caused by compression of the nuclei of the third and fourth nerves in the tectum and may be due to an astrocytoma, meningioma, or tumor of the pineal body.

Passavant ridge   A horizontal mucosal fold across the posterior pharynx that is the point of contact by the soft palate when the nasopharynx is closed during the act of swallowing. Whether this is an active or passive fold is still unresolved.

Paterson-Brown-Kelly syndrome   See *Plummer-Vinson syndrome.*

Pendred syndrome   An autosomal-recessive syndrome consisting of a bilateral congenital sensorineural hearing loss and the appearance of a goiter years later in mid-childhood. T4 levels are usually low to absent, and a perchlorate test is diagnostic. The hearing loss is nonreversible.

Peutz-Jeghers syndrome   An autosomal-dominant disorder whose two main components are benign polyps of the intestinal tract and mucocutaneous melanotic macules. The latter bring these patients to the attention of the otolaryngologist and may appear at any time from infancy to adulthood. The macules are most common around the facial orifices (perioral, perinasal, periorbital) and on the buccal mucosa. This syndrome is not to be confused with Gardner syndrome, in which the intestinal polyps tend to become malignant.

Pierre Robin syndrome   Consists of glossoptosis, micrognathia, and cleft palate. There is no sex predilection. The cause is believed to be arrested intrauterine development; the syndrome may occur as an isolated triad or as part of a larger constellation of defects. Affected infants often present with choking and aspiration, presumably due to the hypoplastic mandible and glossoptosis. A tracheostomy may help, and if the child lives beyond infancy, mandibular growth accelerates so that a relatively normal profile and normal oral function are present by about 5 years of age.

Plummer-Vinson syndrome   Characterized by pale skin, dysphagia, atrophy of the tongue papillae, and sometimes oral leukoplakia or angular cheilosis, found almost exclusively in middle-aged women. This condition is primarily due to an iron-deficiency anemia, with a deficiency of vitamins and protein apparently also playing a role. The dysphagia is attributed to the formation of an esophageal web, although how or why the web is formed is unknown. There also may be an increased risk of postcricoid cancer in these patients. Treatment is iron supplementation. It is also known as *sideroblastic dysphagia.*

Prussak space   The upper tympanic recess, bounded by the pars flaccida laterally, the neck of the malleus medially, the lateral mallear ligament superiorly, and the lateral process of the malleus inferiorly. Because it has only small openings anteriorly and posteriorly, it can be a common site for loculated middle-ear infections.

Raeder syndrome   Characterized by severe unilateral orbital pain with accompanying miosis and ptosis, but not anhidrosis. Paralysis of one or more ocular nerves may be seen. It is also known as *incomplete Horner syndrome.*

Ramsay Hunt syndrome   Classically described as a unilateral otalgia and facial paralysis accompanied by a vesicular rash in the external ear. It is caused by a herpetic infection of the cranial nerves. Patients also can have a sensorineural hearing loss, vertigo, and tinnitus. There have been some reports of improvement in symptoms following treatment with oral acyclovir.

Rathke pouch   A diverticulum of mucosa that develops into the anterior lobe of the hypophysis and the pars intermedius. The path that this diverticulum takes during development may persist as the craniopharyngeal canal.

Riedel struma (Riedel thyroiditis)   An extremely rare form of chronic thyroiditis in which a fibrotic reaction of unknown etiology replaces most thyroid tissue and frequently extends out of the thyroid capsule to compress adjacent structures. Patients are usually middle-aged women and may present with a painless neck mass, dysphagia, or hoarseness.

Rivinus, ducts of   A dozen or more small salivary ducts that pass directly from the upper border of the sublingual gland to empty into the oral cavity. See also *Bartholin duct.*

Rouvier, node of   Lateral retropharyngeal node. It is a common target of metastases in nasopharyngeal carcinoma.

Santorini cartilage The small corniculate cartilage of the larynx, lying on top of the arytenoid cartilage.

Santorini fissures Fissures in the anterior bony external auditory canal leading to the parotid region.

Scarpa, foramen of The incisive foramen on the hard palate through which the nasopalatine nerve passes.

Scarpa ganglion The ganglion containing the cell bodies of the bipolar cells making up the vestibular nerve. It is located at the lateral end of the internal auditory canal.

Scheibe aplasia The most common type of cochlear dysplasia. The bony labyrinth is completely formed, as are the utricle and semicircular canals. The pars inferior (saccule and cochlear duct) are undifferentiated, and the membranous cochlea is malformed. Some low-frequency hearing may be present.

Sjögren syndrome (sicca syndrome) Defined by the presence of two or more of the following symptoms: dry eyes (keratoconjunctivitis sicca), dry mouth (xerostomia), painless swelling of the parotid glands, and polyarthritis. Most frequently seen in middle-aged women, its etiology is unknown, although an autoimmune cause is suspected.

Sluder headache A unilateral headache thought to be due to pressure on the middle turbinate by a nasal spur. Its diagnosis is confirmed if injection of local anesthetic at the point of contact relieves the headache.

Sluder neuralgia Similar to Horton neuralgia (cluster headache) and also known as *sphenopalatine neuralgia*. It is sometimes treated by vidian neurectomy.

Sturge-Weber syndrome Characterized by a unilateral port-wine stain somewhere within the distribution of the trigeminal nerve. It is apparently a defect of the mesodermal component of blood vessels and is further characterized by angioma of the leptomeninges, orbit, mouth, and nasal mucosa. Intracerebral calcifications seen on plain radiographs are diagnostic. Symptoms include seizures, hemiparesis, and glaucoma. There is no known treatment.

Tapia syndrome Characterized by wasting of the tongue, sternocleidomastoid, and trapezius, as well as a paralyzed vocal cord. It was first described in two bullfighters who were gored in the neck. Symptoms are caused by a lesion in the neck (usually traumatic) involving cranial nerves X, XI, and XII below the level of the inferior ganglion of nerve X. The syndrome also may be caused by a tumor in the deep lobe of the parotid.

Tolosa-Hunt syndrome Unilateral retroorbital pain and ophthalmoplegia, which may be either steadily progressive or recurrent. It is thought to be due to inflammation of the cavernous sinus by any of several causes.

Tornwaldt cyst A cyst that arises from the pharyngeal bursa (pouch of Luschka). Its location is in the midline of the posterior nasopharynx, surrounded by adenoid tissue. It can become infected and present as a nasopharyngeal mass.

Treacher Collins syndrome Characterized in children by a severely hypoplastic mandible. Infants sometimes require tracheostomy because of lack of anterior support of the tongue. Other features of the syndrome are antimongoloid palpebral fissures, defects of the external ear, auditory canal, and ossicles, and occasionally, cleft palate. It is also known as *mandibulofacial dysostosis*.

Trotter syndrome (sinus of Morgagni syndrome) May be seen with tumors of the nasopharynx that block the eustachian tube and produce a conductive hearing loss secondary to middle-ear fluid. Other symptoms may be pain in the distribution of the ophthalmic branch of the trigeminal nerve, decreased mobility of the soft palate, and possibly trismus.

Trousseau sign Tetany caused by a tourniquet placed around the arm of a patient with hypocalcemia.

Tullio phenomenon Said to be present when a loud noise precipitates vertigo. It can be present with congenital syphilis or a perilymph fistula. The tympanic membrane and ossicular chain must be intact with a mobile footplate.

Turner syndrome/Gonadal dysgenesis syndrome The phenotype is always female, and the karyotype is usually XO. Signs and symptoms include growth retardation, webbed neck, primary amenorrhea, lack of secondary sex characteristics, cardiac abnormalities, and ocular problems. Treatment is estrogen replacement.

Usher syndrome Characterized by a multitude of progressive sensory deficits, including retinitis pigmentosa and anosmia. The mechanism is postulated to be degeneration of both central pathways and neuroectodermal tissue at the sensory end-organ. Usher syndrome is one of the more common causes of congenital sensorineural deafness.

Vail syndrome A unilateral, nocturnal pain in the nose, face, and eye along with rhinorrhea and symptoms of sinusitis. It is postulated to be due to irritation of the vidian nerve secondary to sphenoid sinusitis. It is also known as *vidian neuralgia*.

Vernet syndrome Another jugular foramen syndrome with involvement of cranial nerves IX, X, and XI. It may be due to trauma, an aneurysm, a tumor, or other conditions.

Vidian nerve Also called the *nerve of the pterygoid canal*. It is formed by the union of the greater and deep petrosal nerves. It is sometimes sectioned in an attempt to control severe vasomotor rhinitis.

Villaret syndrome Similar to Vernet syndrome, with the addition of the deficits associated with Horner syndrome, indicating involvement of the cervical sympathetic chain. This syndrome suggests a lesion distal to the jugular foramen, usually in the retrostyloid area.

Waardenburg syndrome A well-known cause of sensorineural hearing loss, which may be present at birth or develop later in life. The loss is thought to be due to atrophy of the stria vascularis and organ of Corti and ranges from almost total to moderate, with preservation of the high frequencies. Other manifestations of the syndrome include hypertelorism and partial albinism, the latter often expressed as a characteristic white forelock.

Wallenberg syndrome Characterized by vertigo, nystagmus, nausea and vomiting, Horner syndrome, dysphagia, dysphonia, falling to the side of the lesion, and loss of pain and temperature sense on the ipsilateral face and contralateral side below the neck. It is caused by thrombosis of the posteroinferior cerebellar artery, leading to ischemia of the ipsilateral brainstem. Wallenberg syndrome is also known as *lateral medullary syndrome*.

Weber syndrome Classic symptoms of damage to the oculomotor nerve at its emergence from the mid-brain, combined with damage to the adjacent pyramidal tract prior to its decussation. In addition there is ipsilateral paralysis of cranial nerve III and contralateral paralysis of the extremities, face, and tongue.

Wildervack (cervico-oculo-acoustic) syndrome A congenital syndrome seen primarily in females, presenting at birth with a mixed hearing loss, a short, webbed neck with fused cervical vertebrae, and bilateral abducens palsy. It is similar to Klippel-Feil syndrome.

Winkler disease (chondrodermatitis nodularis chronica helicis) A disease of the helix of the ear, seen primarily in men over 40 years of age. It presents as one or more painful nodules. Pathologically, both the skin and the perichondrium are involved. Treatment is surgical excision, with recurrences common.

Wrisberg cartilage A small cuneiform cartilage of the larynx located in the aryepiglottic fold.

Wrisberg nerve The nonmotor root of the facial nerve, consisting of sensory and parasympathetic fibers. It may travel separately from the motor portion until well into the internal auditory canal. Also called the *nervus intermedius*.

Overview of Alternative Medicine

189

Benjamin F. Asher

The burgeoning interest in nontraditional or unconventional therapies among Americans was uncovered by Eisenberg et al. in their now landmark survey (1). The survey of 1,539 adults revealed that one out of every three respondents utilized an unconventional therapy. Furthermore, 75% of these individuals had not informed their personal physician of their practice. It was estimated from the survey that 13.7 billion dollars are spent annually on these treatments. In a follow-up study, Eisenberg et al. found that use of alternative therapies had increased from 33.8% in 1990 to 42.1% in 1997 (2). Estimated expenditures increased 45.2% between 1990 and 1997, with a total expenditure now estimated at 21.2 billion dollars (2). In another survey, Astin found that patients choose alternative medicine not because of a dissatisfaction with conventional medicine but because these alternatives are more congruent with their philosophical orientation toward health and life (3). This groundswell of interest in alternative medicine among the general population is permeating the medical establishment, resulting in courses in medical schools, the creation of research centers, and numerous publications of research studies and reviews in the medical literature (4).

Alternative therapies are available through various licensed and unlicensed providers, including naturopaths, chiropractors, acupuncturists and medical doctors who practice traditional Chinese medicine, homeopaths, osteopaths, massage therapists, mind/body practitioners (e.g., hypnotherapists, rebirthers, guided imagery therapists), and holistic allopathic physicians. The surge of interest in this area can be monitored in the lay press, where articles on the subject appear almost daily; at bookstores, where literally hundreds of new titles are appearing; and on the Internet, where there is a multiplicity of web sites devoted to this subject. Most medical schools have introduced courses on alternative medicine. Several peer-reviewed journals are now devoted to alternative and complementary medicine. Some states now require insurance companies to cover alternative therapies. And, the National Institutes of Health (NIH) has created a National Center for Complementary and Alternative Medicine to promote research in the field.

As the use of alternative therapies has become more accepted in the mainstream of conventional medicine, there is now a need to redefine what is considered "alternative." Attempts at redefining this have led to the terms *complementary, holistic, non-traditional,* and *integrative.* Each term has a different meaning but none is completely satisfactory. *Alternative* implies that the therapy is utilized as a substitute for conventional practices. However, this is often not the case, and thus the concept of complementary medicine arose. *Complementary* implies that the therapy works in conjunction with a conventional approach, but that the complementary approach does not stand on its own. *Non-traditional* as a term is relativistic in nature. Approaches considered non-traditional in western culture, such as acupuncture and traditional Chinese medicine, are regarded as conventional in much of the world. The term *holistic* refers to a style of medical practice that considers the totality of the patient: a complete physical, mental, emotional, and spiritual perspective. The holistic approach is well illustrated in many current cancer treatment programs where a patient may participate in talk therapy groups, or have massage or prayer added to their course of physical treatment. However, holism does not refer to the underlying theory of pathophysiology. Allopathic physicians may be quite holistic and an alternative practitioner may not be holistic at all. The most recent term to emerge—*integrative medicine*—attempts to blend all of the above concepts. As noted by Snyderman and Weil, "It calls for the restoration of the focus of medicine on health and healing and emphasizes the centrality of the physician-patient relationship" (5). It assumes that practitioners have a basic understanding of all of the various conventional and unconventional therapies available and in what situations they may enhance each other. The term implies that all options will then be considered, from a holistic perspective, in devising an individual course of treatment. Therapies may or may not complement each other. A specific unconventional approach or a specific conventional approach may be the best and only therapy required. The term *integrative medicine* may become the preferred term because it is the most inclusive. However, for the purposes of this chapter, to avoid any confusion, the term *alternative therapies* will be used.

The purpose of this chapter is to give the otolaryngologist—head and neck surgeon an overview of the most prevalent alternative medical models and to present some of the alternative treatments for common otolaryngologic problems. It should be noted that the scientific evidence supporting these treatment modalities is evolving. Some have been shown to be efficacious, some merit further research, some may be ineffective but benign, and some are clearly dangerous. This chapter describes the underlying philosophies of various alternative/complementary systems in medicine. Where it is available, research will be presented. In discussing these therapies, they are in no way being advocated. It is apparent, though, that people will utilize alternative therapies regardless of their scientific validity. Because so many patients are seeking this type of care and so few are informing their physicians, it is incumbent upon the physician to be informed about the subject of alternative medicine. Having a basic understanding of the most commonly utilized alternative medical practices will improve physician-patient communication and allow us to better serve our patients.

NATUROPATHIC MEDICINE

Naturopathic medicine finds its roots in ancient medical practices, but as a form of medicine it was brought to the United States in the late 19th century by Benedict Lust, who was schooled in the practice of hydrotherapy. He founded the first college of naturopathy in New York City. Naturopaths today are rather an eclectic group of practitioners. The scope of their practice includes homeopathy, manipulation, Ayurveda, nutritional medicine, naturopathic obstetrics, botanical medicine, and minor surgery. Naturopathic education consists of four years at one of three colleges of naturopathy in the United States. Graduates receive a Doctor of Naturopathy degree (ND). Naturopaths are formally licensed in at least 11 states, but many naturopaths practice in states without formal licensure. Fundamental to the practice of naturopathy is the concept of *vitalism*. The philosophy of vitalism is based on the concept that life is too well organized to be explained simply as a complex assemblage of physical and chemical reactions. The whole is greater than the sum of the parts, and the body has the ability to heal itself. At a conference in the late 1980s, six unifying principals of naturopathy were established, as follows:

1. *Vis Medicatrix Naturae* (the healing power of nature).
2. Treat the whole person.
3. *Primum No Nocere* (first do no harm).
4. *Tolle Causam* (identify and treat the cause).
5. Prevention is the best cure.
6. *Docere* (doctor as teacher).

Because the practice of naturopathic medicine remains eclectic, naturopathic treatments fall into several categories: nutrition, diet, and botanicals. Some naturopaths also utilize homeopathic remedies for these disorders, but homeopathy will be dealt with as a separate subject.

Based upon a study by Nsouli et al., IgE-mediated food allergy has assumed a major role in the naturopathic treatment of both acute and chronic otitis media (6). Although this study has many design weaknesses, it is quoted often in the naturopathic literature. In this study, 104 nonrandomized unselected patients with both recurrent acute otitis media and chronic otitis media with effusion were evaluated with skin prick testing, radioallergosorbent testing (RAST), and food challenge; 78% of these patients had specific food allergies. With a 16-week elimination diet, 86% of the middle ear effusions improved. Then, 70 of these patients received a non-double-blinded food challenge, and 94% of the effusions recurred.

Pizzorno and Murray in their *Textbook of Natural Medicine* suggest the following treatment for acute otitis media: beta carotene, vitamin C, zinc picolinate, bioflavonoids, evening primrose oil, and thymus extract (7). They also recommend the following botanicals: *Echinacea angustifolia*, *Hydrastis canadensis* (Goldenseal), and *Glycyrrhiza glabra* (liquorice). *Echinacea angustifolia*, Goldenseal, and thymus extract are all compounds that are thought to stimulate the immune system and improve immune function (8). Mullein flower and garlic in eardrops made with an olive oil base are often prescribed as an analgesic and antiinflammatory medication.

Sinusitis is understood by many naturopaths as a condition caused by the overproduction of mucus. According to naturopathic principles, mucus is thought to be overproduced when the bowels, kidneys, and skin are not properly eliminating waste material. Treatment addresses excess mucus production with diet, botanicals, and inhalation therapy. Types of dietary management include elimination of "mucogenic food," such as wheat and dairy, as well as adding foods that are "cleansing," such as hot lemon drinks, garlic, onions, and horseradish. A botanical prescription might include *Hydrastis canadensis* (Goldenseal). Other potential herbs for sinusitis include *Solidago virgaurea*, *Sambucus nigra*, *Echinacea*, and *Baptisia tinctoria*. Nutritional supplements for acute sinusitis include vitamin C, bioflavonoids, vitamin A, beta-carotene, zinc lozenges, and thymus extract. Steam inhalation treatment may also be prescribed. This may include compounds such as Benzoin, eucalyptus, peppermint, lavender, and pine oil. Saline nasal irrigation also may be utilized. One frequently prescribed method for nasal irrigation utilizes the Neti pot. This is a small porcelain pot with a narrow spout. Several other plastic devices for nasal irrigation are now on the market.

Shea butter placed on the upper lip is often used as a nasal decongestant. This butter is made from the seed of the Shea butter tree, *Butyrospermum parkii*, from Africa. One study found it to be effective as a nasal decongestant (9).

Naturopathic treatment of tonsillitis also attempts to improve immune function. Goldenseal and Echinacea are again given for immune support. Garlic is given for its purported anti-microbial properties.

Vitamin C, bioflavonoids, vitamin A, beta carotene, zinc lozenges, and thymus extract may be given as nutritional supplements.

Gingko biloba has been studied for tinnitus with conflicting reports. An initial French study was promising, but follow-up trials have been unable to replicate the results. The mechanism of action of Gingko is not completely known, but the main effects appear to be related to its properties as an antioxidant and vasodilator, and its ability to decrease blood viscosity (10–12).

Echinacea is perhaps one of the most popular herbs used for the prevention of upper respiratory infections, and it has been one of the most extensively studied (13). Three different species of Echinacea are commonly used; each is chemically different (*Echinacea purpurea*, *E. pallida*, and *E. angustifolia*). Multiple studies have shown conflicting results about the efficacy of Echinacea in the prevention and treatment of upper respiratory infections. Several meta-analyses and critical reviews have suggested that Echinacea may be effective for treating upper respiratory tract infections (13). The German Commission E Monographs published positive assessments for *E. purpurea* herb and *E. pallida* root. There were insufficient data for other preparations. A randomized double-blind placebo-controlled trial looking at efficacy of *E. angustifolia* vs. *E. purpurea* vs. placebo for the prevention of upper respiratory tract infections showed no statistically significant difference between placebo and herb (14). A well-designed double-blind study showed that Echinacea was ineffective in reducing the duration of upper respiratory infection symptoms in children (13). Another well-designed placebo-controlled trial of an Israeli proprietary supplement (Chizukit) containing Echinacea, propolis, and vitamin C found a statistically significant preventive effect in reducing the numbers of upper respiratory infections in children (15).

Various nutritional supplements have been shown to affect wound healing. Vitamin E diminishes platelet adhesion and in the laboratory has been shown to diminish wound healing. Vitamin A has a positive effect on wound healing and reverses the immune depression associated with injury, sepsis, and surgery. Bromelain, derived from the stem of the pineapple plant, has documented antiinflammatory activity and can be helpful in the resorption of hematomas (16).

ACUPUNCTURE AND TRADITIONAL CHINESE MEDICINE

Traditional Chinese medicine is thousands of years old and is rooted in Taoist philosophy. Fundamental to Chinese medicine are the concepts of Yin and Yang and Qi (pronounced *Chee*). *Yin* represents water, quiet, substance, and night, whereas *Yang* represents fire, noise, function, and day. The two are polar opposites, and there is a balance between these two forces in the body. *Qi* can be translated in many different ways, but it is fundamentally the vital energy throughout the body and the universe. Chinese medicine stresses the interaction between the individual's Qi and that of the natural environment. It is important to recognize that Chinese medicine considers the individual as a part of the entire universe, and that this relationship influences an individual's health. The language of Chinese medicine reflects this philosophy. Thus the five elements (wood, fire, earth, metal, and water), as well as other environmental factors (e.g., the wind, heat, humidity), are all integral factors considered in health and disease. When there is an imbalance of Yin and Yang, the body can be invaded and diseases can arise. Qi flows through specific channels in the body called *meridians*. Altering the flow of Qi can re-establish balance in the body, and health can be returned.

The acupuncturist assesses the individual's health through medical history and examination of the pulse and of the tongue. Traditional Chinese medicine identifies 28 different pulse qualities such as wiry, choppy, slippery, or deep floating. The tongue is examined for color, shape, and coating. Based on this information, the state of balance of the body is understood and a therapeutic plan is created. Needles may be placed in the appropriate acupuncture points to re-establish balance. Many practitioners also use traditional Chinese herbs; *moxibustion* (a very intense heat treatment focused on specific points); and massage treatments, including cupping, which utilizes a suction cup device.

Practitioners of acupuncture and Chinese medicine receive training in various ways. Physicians with an MD or DO degree can become certified acupuncturists through a program at the University of California at Los Angeles. Non-physicians can receive training at one of the many schools of acupuncture and traditional Chinese medicine throughout the United States. Acupuncturists are licensed in some states. Some states require certification, and some states do not regulate acupuncture practice at all.

Problematic to bridging conventional western medicine with traditional Chinese medicine is the completely different concept of the origins of disease. As an example, the traditional Chinese concept of the pathophysiology of otitis media is explained below.

Otitis Media

Otitis media is categorized as acute serous, acute suppurative, and chronic suppurative. "Acute serous otitis media results from external pathogenic wind, either in the form of an infection which spreads to the ear, or cold wind blowing on the ear; a damp pathogenic factor due to damp weather or too much swimming; or heat which affects the gall bladder channels." The treatment principle is to expel the wind and release the exterior, clear the heat, and resolve the toxicity (17).

"Acute suppurative otitis media is caused by invasion of external pathogenic wind-heat toxin, often originating in the respiratory tract, which rises up to the ear." The treatment principle is to clear the heat and bring down the dampness, resolve the toxicity, reduce the swelling, and alleviate the pain (18).

Chronic suppurative otitis media is the result of not cured or partially cured acute otitis media or because of severe weakening of the body from overwork or long-term disease. The treatment principle is to move the Qi in the ear and disperse the blockage, invigorate the blood, and expel the pathogenic factor (18).

Specific treatments for otitis media may include acupuncture, administering herbs that increase digestive fire, reducing intake of foods that form phlegm (i.e., dairy and sugar), and performing massage around the ears to improve drainage (*tui na*).

The NIH Consensus Development Panel on Acupuncture identified several areas with convincing evidence to support acupuncture therapy, including control of postoperative pain, chemotherapy-induced nausea and vomiting, and postoperative dental pain (19).

Several trials utilizing acupuncture for tinnitus have been done, with conflicting results. But perhaps the best placebo-controlled study showed no effect on noise-induced tinnitus (20).

In an unpublished case series by the author of this chapter, five patients with severe chronic sinusitis and nasal polyposis documented on computed tomography (CT) had no improvement when treated with traditional Chinese medicine and followed with post-treatment CT scans.

Tai Chi, a form of Chinese exercise, was found to be effective in improving patients with mild balance disturbance (21).

HOMEOPATHY

Homeopathy was developed in the late 1700s by Samuel Hahnemann, a German physician, who was frustrated by the failings of the then-current medical practices. Homeopathy is based on two fundamental principles, the law of similars and the law of infinitesimals. The *law of similars* states that like cures like (*similia similibus curantur*). A substance that causes symptoms in a healthy person will help cure those same symptoms in a sick person. Hahnemann developed this theory while experimenting with quinine. He noted that when he took quinine in high doses, it produced symptoms quite similar to malaria. He hypothesized that by giving a remedy that mimicked a patient's symptoms, the body's ability to fight the same symptom would be enhanced. The *law of infinitesimals* states that dilution of a remedy increases its potency. Homeopathic remedies undergo serial dilution and are vigorously shaken or succussed in between each dilution. Remedies may be diluted anywhere from a ratio of 1 to 10, to 1 to 1 billion, with the highest dilution containing no actual molecules of the remedy being the most potent (22).

There are two basic approaches in classical homeopathy, the complex or clinical approach and the isopathic approach. In the clinical approach, homeopathic remedies are applied to conventional allopathic disease classifications. The isopathic approach incorporates disease causes and biological processes into the homeopathic method. In the isopathic approach, homeopathic remedies are prepared from diseased tissues or secretions and given to the patient. An example would be a remedy that is prepared from infected skin, and then given to a patient with a similar skin infection. Homeopathy is used to treat both acute and chronic conditions. For an acute condition, such as a sore throat, the history and symptoms reviewed may be entirely problem centered. For a chronic condition, such as chronic sinusitis, however, the homeopath catalogs an extremely detailed history that includes not only localized symptoms but also general information such as tolerance to temperature, quality of sleep, appetite, sexual desire, an overall review of systems, levels of energy, emotional limitations, the quality of interpersonal relationships, and so forth. The homeopathic practitioner then matches a patient's symptoms to a specific remedy. Remedies are classified in the homeopathic *Materia Medica* by a detailed description of the symptoms that they provoke in high dosages. The U.S. Food and Drug Administration regulates homeopathic remedies. Homeopathic practitioners are usually medical doctors, doctors of osteopathy, naturopathic physicians, or chiropractors. In some states, homeopaths are certified homeopathic physicians with no doctoral degree. Homeopathic practice is regulated in many states. In some states, however, there are no regulations regarding homeopathic practice. Homeopathy is far more accepted in Europe. According to a survey conducted by the National Center for Homeopathy, 40% of Dutch, 39% of French, 20% of German, and up to 37% of British physicians use homeopathy.

Recent research has shown positive treatment associations in homeopathic treatment of seasonal allergic rhinitis (23) and influenza (24). A recent placebo-controlled study on homeopathic treatment of recurrent acute otitis media revealed a reduced duration of symptoms with homeopathic treatment, but the results were not statistically significant (25).

Another randomized double-blind controlled study showed that a proprietary homeopathic remedy (Vertigoheel) was as effective as betahistine hydrochloride in the treatment of patients with vertigo of various origins (26).

OSTEOPATHIC MEDICINE

Osteopathic medicine is no longer considered "alternative," as most osteopathic physicians now practice allopathic medicine. The primary difference between allopathic and osteopathic training is that osteopathic students receive additional training in manipulative medicine. This is why osteopaths and chiropractors have often been considered together. Only a small percentage of osteopathic physicians limit their practice to osteopathic manipulative medicine and many practice no manipulation at all.

Osteopathy was founded by Andrew Taylor Still in 1872 as an alternative for the crude allopathic practices of the mid to late 1800s. Dr. Still was an allopathic physician who was disaffected by conventional medicine after the death of his wife and children from "spinal meningitis." He quit practicing medicine after the Civil War, and he spent time observing the relationship between structure and function in the body. From his observations he developed osteopathic medicine. He believed that the action of muscles, ligaments, joint mechanics, joint surfaces, and joint motion all influenced the cardiovascular and nervous systems. He postulated a general theory that lesions, or disturbances of particular regions, of the spinal column resulted in disease (somatic dysfunction) in the organs that are fed by the nerve impulses coming from those areas (27).

In essence, the original concept of osteopathy held that

(a) With any human body there exists a constant tendency towards health. If this capacity is recognized, and if treatment takes its relevance into account, then prevention and normalization of disease processes is enhanced. (b) The structure of the body is reciprocally related to its function. By this it is meant that any change in structure will alter some aspect of function and converse any alteration and function will result in structural changes. (c) Health is the primary area to be studied in attempting to understand disease. (d) The musculoskeletal system, which incorporates the bones, ligaments, muscles, fascia, etc. forms a structure which, when disordered, may affect the function of other parts and systems of the body. This might be the result of irritation or abnormal response of the nerve and/or blood supply to these other organs or parts. (5) The body is subject to mechanical disorder and is therefore capable of mechanical correction. (27)

Osteopathic manipulative practice is quite varied. There are many techniques that attempt to restore normal physiologic

motion to areas in which motion is restricted or dysfunctional. Some of these techniques include high-velocity manipulative techniques, muscle energy techniques, massage, and cranial osteopathy. An offshoot of cranial osteopathy that is practiced by non-physicians is the Upledger Craniosacral Therapy, which has become very popular with many massage therapists and physical therapists. Of all the osteopathic manipulative therapies, cranial osteopathy is perhaps the most controversial and therefore the most *alternative*. William Garner Sutherland, a student of Dr. Still, developed cranial manipulation. Sutherland observed the internal bevel of the suture between the squama of the temporal bone and the greater wing of the sphenoid and the external bevel of the suture between the temporal bone and the inferior border of the parietal bone. He postulated that this type of joint was designed for motion. He further postulated that there were five types of intrinsic motion associated with the cranium, central nervous system, and sacrum: (a) the articular mobility of the cranial bony mechanism, (b) the articular mobility of the sacrum between the ilia, (c) the inherent mobility of the central nervous system, (d) the fluctuations of the cerebrospinal fluid, and (e) the inherent motion of the dural membranes. He called this the *primary respiratory mechanism*. He believed that restrictions in the mobility of this mechanism would result in various disease processes. Sutherland experimented on himself, utilizing mechanical devices to produce and correct distortions of his own cranium. He then applied these principles to his patients. The inherent motions of the cranial bones and the primary respiratory mechanism have now been well documented in osteopathic sources (28).

Practitioners of cranial osteopathy postulate that restrictions in the primary respiratory mechanism may result in conditions such as otitis media and sinusitis. Otitis media is believed to be the result of restriction of the normal physiologic motion of the temporal bones, thereby impeding eustachian tube function. Sinusitis is thought to result in part from restriction of motion of the bones of the midface, thereby impeding drainage of the sinuses. Therapy is directed at re-establishing normal physiologic motion to these areas through gentle manipulative techniques (28). A recent study evaluating the efficacy of osteopathic manipulative treatment (OMT) for recurrent acute otitis media suggested a potential benefit of OMT in the prevention of recurrent acute otitis media, and in the potential reduction of the need for ventilating tubes and reducing antibiotic therapy (29).

AYURVEDIC MEDICINE

Ayurvedic medicine was developed in ancient India. The word is derived from two Sanskrit roots, *ayur* (life) and *veda* (knowledge). Ayurvedic physicians were the first to perform plastic and reconstructive surgery. The forehead flap was initially described in the *Sushruta Samhita*, the ayurvedic textbook of surgery, circa 800 BCE.

Ayurvedic physicians (*vaidyas*) consider diseases to be an imbalance in an individual's constitution (*prakriti*). The psychosomatic temperament of the person, an individual's constitution, is determined by a particular combination of three qualities (*doshas*): *vata*, *pitta*, and *kapha*. There are seven combinations in all.

Ayurvedic physicians believe that in health the doshas are all balanced. Disease results when there is an imbalance. Ayurvedic diagnosis attempts to discover the types of imbalances present and therapy is directed toward re-balancing the doshas. Ayurvedic therapy includes cleansing, palliation, rejuvenation, and mental hygiene. A few techniques include diet, herbs, purgative, enemas, massage, and meditation (30).

Ayurvedic physicians in India receive formal medical training at an ayurvedic medical school. Practitioners of ayurvedic medicine in the United States, who have not trained in India, are trained at one of a few institutes of ayurvedic medicine in the United States. Ayurvedic training is also available at the naturopathic colleges. There is no specific licensure or certification for ayurvedic practitioners.

Although there are no studies validating the efficacy of ayurvedic treatments for otitis media and sinusitis, the following are treatment regimens that are often prescribed.

Otitis media is often seen as an imbalance (increase) of Pitta-Kapha. Treatment attempts to reduce Kapha. Garlic oil in the ear canal may be utilized. The herb *Berberis aritata* taken internally and as oil in the ear canal may also be given. Massage of the neck to improve lymphatic drainage is also prescribed.

Sinusitis is also a Pitta-Kapha imbalance. For acute sinusitis the treatment includes nasal lavage with a neti-pot. The herbs *Berberis aritata* and Neem may be taken internally or included in the lavage. Heat packs and hot pepper gargles may also be used. The evaluation for chronic sinusitis is much more complex. Factors such as poor digestion and poor liver function are taken into account. Treatment supports the immune system with the herb Amla, and improves digestion and reduces Kapha with ginger and an ayurvedic herbal preparation called Triphal. Herbal enemas may also be used.

CHIROPRACTIC MEDICINE

Chiropractic medicine was developed by Daniel David Palmer in 1895. Palmer postulated that the vitality of an individual is sustained by the normal functioning of the central nervous system. The function of the central nervous system is impaired by subluxations (misalignments) of the spinal column. He came to this conclusion after he realigned a bump on the back of his deaf janitor's neck and restored his hearing (31). The American Chiropractic Association defines chiropractic as "that science and art which utilizes the inherent recuperative powers of the body and the relationship between the musculoskeletal structures of the body, particularly the spinal column and the nervous system, in the restoration and the maintenance of health" (32).

Chiropractors manually adjust spinal vertebrae to re-establish motion in the vertebral column. They believe that this re-establishes normal functioning of the nervous system, which serves as a basis for an individual's health and well being. Among practitioners of chiropractic, there are some philosophical differences, which are reflected in the main chiropractic societies. The American Chiropractic Association is the largest society and reflects the views of most chiropractors. This philosophy of chiropractic holds that chiropractors may choose not only to practice spinal manipulation, but also may incorporate treatments such as counseling about nutrition, lifestyle, body mechanics, stress management, acupressure, soft tissue manipulation, and homeopathy. The conservative philosophy of Palmer is carried forth by the Federation of Straight Chiropractic Organizations. Members of this organization limit their practice to adjustments of the vertebral column. They believe in the "innate intelligence of the spinal column" and firmly believe that chiropractic adjustments should not be mixed with other types of therapy (32).

Chiropractic education requires four years of study. At least two years of college with specific basic science prerequisites are required prior to admission. Chiropractic students, like medical students, receive training in basic sciences such as anatomy, neuroscience, biochemistry, microbiology, and pathology, but they receive little training in pharmacology, general medicine, and surgery. The main focus of their clinical training is in chiropractic technique and philosophy, chiropractic diagnosis, neuromusculoskeletal diagnosis, and radiology. All chiropractic students are required to have at least 900 clinic hours in a college-operated clinic.

Passing the National Board of Chiropractors examination is required for licensure in most states.

Chiropractors are licensed in all states to adjust the spine and related structures. However, there are differences among states as to the types of adjunctive care that chiropractors are permitted to perform. As an example, some states only permit spinal adjustments and do not allow the dispensing of nutritional supplements or the ordering of blood tests, whereas other states allow chiropractors to administer non-prescription proprietary drugs, order diagnostic tests, and perform massage.

Most research on chiropractic has focused on the treatment of musculoskeletal problems. Chiropractic manipulation has been found to be effective for neck pain, back pain, and headaches (33). There have been no significant studies to date evaluating chiropractic for acute otitis media.

BODY WORK

Body work is a term to describe a variety of therapeutic modalities that incorporate hands-on healing (such as massage and/or body awareness). Although there is no research relating body work to the conditions discussed in this chapter, body work is perhaps the most popular adjunctive therapy. Therefore, it is being discussed to provide the otolaryngologist a familiarity with the most commonly used terms so that communication with patients may be facilitated.

Most hands-on therapists are licensed as massage practitioners. Although the licensure requirements of most states include between 500 and 1,500 hours of training, some states allow virtually anyone to call himself or herself a massage therapist. Massage therapist education usually includes anatomy and physiology courses, but the one- to two-year course of study has no educational prerequisites. The American Massage Therapy Association (AMTA) has a voluntary national certification program that requires passing written, verbal, and practical examinations. Members also have continuing education requirements. Although these practitioners do not consider themselves qualified to diagnose diseases or design a course of medical treatment, many believe that their techniques can enhance or assist the healing process.

Massage techniques vary from the vigorous kneading of muscles and deep tissue to a very gentle laying on of hands in which practitioners claim subtle energy flows from their hands to the patient. Specific styles include Swedish massage, Rolfing, Hellerwork, Shiatsu, acupressure, Lomi Lomi, Reiki, Reflexology, Polarity, and trigger-point therapy.

Many massage techniques, such as Trager work and Aston Patterning, incorporate body awareness. These techniques attempt to retrain the way an individual moves and maintains their body in space. Some approaches focus on body awareness and movement alone without hands-on techniques. Many of these movement approaches, such as the Feldenkrais method, The Alexander Technique, Pilates, and Gyrotonics, have their roots in dance. Because practitioners of body awareness and movement reeducation do not practice hands-on therapy, no licensure is required. However, these instructors are often certified by the organization through which they teach.

PSYCHONEUROIMMUNOLOGY

The field of mind-body medicine or *psychoneuroimmunology* investigates the inter-relationship between the mind and the body and disease. Research in this field is growing, especially in the areas of stress reduction and oncology. Stress reduction through various techniques has been shown to be efficacious for numerous problems including asthma, anxiety disorders, hypertension, heart disease, and depression (34).

CONCLUSION

This chapter has presented the most common alternative therapies that patients coming to an otolaryngologic practice may be utilizing. I have also discussed the rationale for

otolaryngologists becoming familiar with these therapies. Although a detailed discussion of each of these therapeutic modalities has not been possible, this overview of alternative treatments should give the practicing otolaryngologist some insight into the world of alternative medicine. By being informed about the therapies that many of our patients receive, communication with patients should be enhanced. This communication is the foundation of a solid physician-patient relationship.

> **HIGHLIGHTS**
>
> - Alternative therapies are used by more than 40% of Americans.
> - More than 75% of those who use alternative therapies *do not* inform their doctor.
> - Physicians must have a basic understanding of the alternative therapies available and understand how they may interact with conventional therapy.

REFERENCES

1. Eisenberg DM, Kessler RC, Foster C, et al. Unconventional medicine in the United States. *N Engl J Med* 1993;328:246–252.
2. Eisenberg DM, Davis RB, Ettner SL, et al. Trends in alternative medicine use in the United States, 1990–1997: results of a follow-up national survey. *JAMA* 1998;282:1569–1575.
3. Astin JA. Why patients use alternative medicine? *JAMA* 1998;279: 1548–1553.
4. Asher BF, Seidman M, Snyderman C. Complementary and alternative medicine in otolaryngology. *Laryngoscope* 2001;111: 1383–1389.
5. Snyderman R, Weil A. Integrative medicine: bringing medicine back to its roots. *Arch Intern Med* 2002;162:395–397.
6. Nsouli TM, Nsouli SM, Linde RE, et al. Role of food allergies in otitis media. *Ann Allergy* 1994;73:215–218.
7. Pizzorno J, Murray M, eds. *Textbook of natural medicine.* Seattle: John Bastyr College Publications; 1989:292–295.
8. Pizzorno J, et al, eds. *Encyclopedia of natural medicine.* Rocklin, CA: Prima; 1990:507–509.
9. Tella A. Preliminary studies on nasal decongestant activity from the seed of the shea butter tree, *Butyrospermum parkii. Br J Clin Pharmacol* 1979;7:495–497.
10. Meyer B. A multicenter randomized, double-blind drug versus placebo study of ginkgo biloba extract in the treatment of tinnitus. *Presse Med* 1986;15:1562–1564.
11. Holgers KM, Axelsson A, Pringle I. Ginkgo biloba extract for the treatment of tinnitus. *Audiology* 1994;33:85–92.
12. Wedel HV, Calero L, Walger M, et al. Soft laser/ginkgo therapy in chronic tinnitus. In: Rudert H, Werner JA, eds. *Lasers in otolaryngology, and in head and neck surgery. Advances in Otorhinolaryngology.* Vol 49. Basel: Karger; 1995:105–108.
13. Taylor J, Weber W, Standish L, et al. Efficacy and safety of Echinacea in treating upper respiratory tract infections in children. *JAMA* 2003;290:2824–2830.
14. Melchart D, Walther E, Linde K, et al. Echinacea root extracts for the prevention of upper respiratory tract infections. *JAMA* 1998;7: 541–545.
15. Cohen H, Versano I, Kahan E, et al. Effectiveness of an herbal preparation containing Echinacea, propolis, and vitamin C in preventing respiratory tract infections in children. *Arch Pediatr Adolesc Med* 2004;158:217–221.
16. Petry JJ. Surgically significant nutritional supplements. *Plast Reconstr Surg* 1996;97:233–240.
17. Scott J. *Acupuncture in the treatment of children.* London: Portland Press; 1980:201–209.

18. Scott J. *Natural medicine for children.* New York: Aron Books, 1990:120.
19. NIH Consensus Panel on Acupuncture. *JAMA* 1998;280:1518–1524.
20. Axelsson A, Andersson S, Gu LD. Acupuncture in the management of tinnitus: a placebo controlled study. *Audiology* 1994;33:351–360.
21. Hain TC, Fuller L, Weil L, et al. The effect of Tai Chi on balance. *Arch Otolaryngol Head Neck Surg* 1999;125:1191–1195.
22. Jonas W, Jacobs J. *Healing with homeopathy.* New York: Warner Books; 1996:1–120.
23. Reilly DT, Taylor MA, McSharry C, et al. Is homeopathy a placebo response? Controlled trial of homeopathic potency, with pollen in hayfever model. *Lancet* 1986;2(8512):881–886.
24. Ferly JP, Zmirou D, D'adhemar D, et al. A controlled evaluation of a homeopathic preparation in the treatment of influenza-like symptoms. *Br J Clin Pharmacol* 1989;27:329–335.
25. Jacobs J, Springer D, Crothers D. Homeopathic treatment of acute otitis media in children: a preliminary randomized placebo-controlled trial. *Pediatr Infect Dis J* 2001;20(2):177–183.
26. Weiser M, Strosser W, Klein P. Homeopathic vs. conventional treatment of vertigo: a randomized double-blind controlled clinical study. *Arch Otolaryngol Head Neck Surg* 1998;124:879–885.
27. Chaitow L. *Osteopathy: a complete health care system.* London: Thorsons Publishers Ltd; 1982:1–17.
28. Magoun H. *Osteopathy in the cranial field,* 3rd ed. Kirksville, MO: Journal Printing Co; 1976.
29. Mills M, Henley C, Barnes L, et al. The use of osteopathic manipulative treatment as adjuvant therapy in children with recurrent acute otitis media. *Arch Pediatr Adolesc Med* 2003;157:861–866.
30. Lad V. An introduction to ayurveda. *Ayurveda Today.* Spring 1994.
31. Marti J. *The alternative health medicine encyclopedia.* Detroit: Visible Ink Press; 1995.
32. Altman N. *Everybody's guide to chiropractic health care.* Los Angeles: JP Tarcher; 1990:1–111.
33. Kaptchuk T, Eisenberg DM. Chiropractic: origins, controversies, and contributions. *Arch Intern Med* 1998;158:2215–2224.
34. Kabat-Zinn J. *Full catastrophe living: using the wisdom of your body and mind to face stress, pain, and illness.* New York: Delta; 1990.

The Business of Medicine and Planning Your Future

190

Lee D. Eisenberg

As you progress through your residency, your main concern is learning about the field of otolaryngology–head and neck surgery. During residency, however, personal issues become more important, and financial planning and insurance needs are a constant. Deciding whether to do a fellowship, looking for employment, and starting up practice become significant concerns during the third and fourth years of training, but should be considered throughout. By the fourth year of training, you begin to think about your future in practice. Among the issues confronting you are decisions about where you want to live and the type of practice (solo, small or large group, single specialty, two specialties, academic) that interests you. Family considerations may be the most important factor in deciding where you finally settle down. As unusual as this chapter is for a textbook of otolaryngology, the hope is that it will help you begin to think, in a rational way, about your future.

What kind of planning assistance do you need? There are three individuals that are of importance: financial planner, accountant, and attorney. Your personal situation will determine when each of these individuals should be consulted in your planning.

FINANCIAL PLANNING AND INSURANCE

It is never too early to save for the future. Your needs will change with time, but your future financial security will not come by chance. Most people need to save for three major financial objectives: buying a home, funding children's education (www.savingforcollege.com), and planning for retirement. The types of investments you make are an individual decision, and many sources of advice are available. Brokerage or other financial planning firms can offer guidance and assist with planning, both for the near and far term.

The questions you need to ask yourself include the following:

1. How much money am I saving now?
2. If I continue to save as I have in the past, how much money will I have in 10 years?
3. Am I satisfied with my current savings plan?
4. Will I save systematically to reach my financial goals?

There are two ways to save: spend first and save, or save first and spend what is left. Of the two, the latter is the better choice. Saving should be at the top of one's priorities, but doing so requires discipline and planning.

Table 190.1 emphasizes the advantage of saving at an early age, showing the monthly investments required at different ages to accumulate $1,000,000 by age 65, assuming an 8% compounded rate of return. The benefits of starting to save early are evident.

Hiring a professional to help you with these issues will pay dividends in the long term. One should start by looking for someone with the Certified Financial Planner designation (1). In addition, family, friends, an accountant, or an attorney may be able to recommend a financial planner. Once you have developed a comfort level with the financial planner, you may develop a

TABLE 190.1
SAVING

Age when Investments Begin	Monthly Investments Required to Reach Goal at Age 65
25	$285
35	$667
45	$1,686
55	$5,430

life-long relationship, even if you live in a different part of the country.

Investment Philosophy

Surrounding yourself with a competent planner, accountant, and attorney as soon as possible will undoubtedly put you on the path toward financial independence.

Treat your investments like a business. Every business has a plan, which should be outlined on paper, and have a specific strategy. Rebalancing investment accounts annually is also a sound practice. The following is an example of a sound investment philosophy.

1. Seek expert guidance to create an overall plan.
2. Use your plan to help develop an overall long-term investment strategy.
3. Create a plan consistent with your risk tolerance, time horizon, and goals.
4. Determine a diversification strategy with this asset allocation analysis to meet your various investment needs.
5. Use professionally selected quality investments designed to match your asset allocation strategy.
6. Use annual rebalancing to remove emotion from decision-making.
7. Manage the impact of taxes and inflation.
8. Evaluate your plan relative to your long-term goals and benchmarks.
9. Resist the temptation to change your plan during up or down market movements.
10. Start early, invest regularly, and dollar cost average.

The many different options for investing include stocks, bonds, real estate, and mutual funds. Mutual funds often offer a safe, dependable way to invest for your future.

A *mutual fund* is a diversified investment company that invests on behalf of individuals and institutions that share common financial goals. Professional managers use this pool of money to buy a wide range of stocks, bonds, and/or money market instruments based on the objective of the fund. Mutual funds provide the following benefits:

- Full-time professional management
- Wide variety of investment objectives
- Automatic investment/withdrawal options
- Convenient way to invest and liquidate

- Broad diversification of assets
- Yearly tax information

Most physicians are not skilled investors, and seeking professional advice is the best way to ensure that your savings will grow over time.

Insurance Planning

As with financial planning, many resources are available to assist in determining your insurance needs. These can include insurance brokers, insurance agencies, and financial planning firms.

Although there are many insurance needs, the two that often require the most attention initially are *disability income insurance* and *life insurance*.

Disability Income Insurance

You often have insurance for your life, health, car, and home, but you need to insure your salary, as well. Most disability policies don't start paying benefits until at least 30 days from the date the insurer says you became unable to work. This means you have to be able to support yourself until then; therefore, savings play an important role. If you have a disability policy that has a 90-day waiting period, which is often much less expensive, your savings need to be that much greater to cover your expenses until the policy becomes effective.

There are two basic types of disability coverage: any occupation and own occupation. The former means that you are disabled only if you cannot work anywhere. The latter will give you benefits if you cannot work in your medical specialty. Own-occupation coverage is significantly more expensive and, for physicians, very difficult to obtain. If one can find such a policy, however, it may be worth the cost for "peace of mind."

The bottom line for physicians is to obtain disability coverage early, and purchase as much as you can afford. Premiums depend upon the amount of coverage and the waiting period before the insurance becomes effective, as mentioned above. Many disability income insurance carriers are limiting the amount of benefits for physicians. Understand what you have available to you through your employer, and then supplement this with an individual plan.

Lastly, consider the impact that taxes may have on your disability insurance. Understand how much benefit you would be receiving each month, after taxes, in the event you were unable to work for an extended time.

Life Insurance

As with disability, there are two basic types of life insurance: term and permanent (or whole life). Which form is more suitable for your needs is an individual decision. Brokers and agencies can offer advice, but you should remember that they might be biased in their opinions and suggestions. They make commissions on the policies they sell, and that may influence their recommendations. As in medicine, a second opinion may be appropriate.

Term insurance is exactly that: you pay a specific premium for a certain amount of coverage for a specified time, which may be up to 10, 15, 20, or in some cases 30 years. After that period of time, the policy may or may not be renewed at a higher rate. It is a "temporary" protection. Compare term insurance to renting an apartment: the out-of-pocket cost is generally lower than buying a house and having a mortgage; however, you build no equity, and the rent may very well go up over time.

In some ways, *whole life insurance* is a type of savings, in that the policyholder obtains some benefit of the investment that can increase the value of the policy over time (cash value). Permanent insurance is typically used for long-term estate planning needs because it provides protection that never expires. In addition, one may borrow against the cash value of the policy.

Your individual circumstances will determine the type and amount of life insurance you need. Factors to consider include how much debt you have accumulated (house, loans), future cost of education for children, and spousal and perhaps parental support.

The three most important questions to ask with respect to life insurance planning are as follows:

1. How much? Get the right amount. Remember, no beneficiary ever said "there was too much insurance" upon receiving a claim check. Insurance is not for the people who die; it is for the people you leave behind. Consider needs for covering a mortgage, future cost of college education, and income replacement.
2. What type? Get the right type—term or permanent or some combination of both.
3. What company? Start with AAA-rated carriers—several good ones are out there.

FELLOWSHIPS

Do you need a fellowship? Before making this decision, consider what your intent for practice is in the future. If you plan to enter the academic environment, a fellowship is almost essential. Full-time academic appointments are available directly from residency, but these are not common. Academic appointments will depend upon the needs of the institution and where you did your training

In the private practice setting, your desire to specialize in a specific area of otolaryngology may influence your decision. It will also depend upon the strengths and weaknesses in your training. Most otolaryngologists will refine their practice over time, and become more proficient in specific areas (e.g., sinus surgery) and decide not to do other procedures (e.g., head and neck cancer). Completing a fellowship does not necessarily limit your practice, but may influence your decision about practice areas

(e.g., neuro-otology, pediatrics). In many circumstances, the decision to do fellowship training is based on the desire to develop strength in a specific discipline that will eventually become the majority of your practice (e.g., facial plastics).

Where you do your fellowship will often depend upon exactly what you feel your needs are and what is available. Your attendings, both full time and clinical, will likely be your best source of information. As with all training, there will be different areas of strength and weaknesses within a fellowship. One area may better fit your interests and may be the deciding factor. As with residency applications, there may a matching process. If you are considering additional training, the beginning of your fourth year of otolaryngology residency is the time to start the process.

LIFESTYLE

Where you live, the type of practice chosen, and family considerations are the most important factors in ensuring your contentment in the future. Your earnings will not compensate for dissatisfaction or unhappiness.

There are basically three types of communities from which to choose: rural, suburban, and urban. Which community best fits your life will often depend upon on your interests, family needs, type of practice, and job availability. The last category may be the overriding factor, especially in the academic environment.

If you prefer small town living with less congestion and more outdoor recreation, then living in a large metropolitan area may not be appropriate. Your spouse may be offered a promotion, which requires a move to a new locale; this may well become the deciding factor. The desire to be close to family must also be taken into consideration. Finally, where the practice opportunities exist will influence the decision as well. Remember that the first place you live need not be the last. A change in environment or practice style may be important for everyone's happiness.

TYPE OF PRACTICE AND AVAILABILITY

The type of practice setting one has to choose from is quite variable: solo, group, single or multispecialty, staff model health maintenance organization (HMO), or academic. Most otolaryngologists still practice in a setting of one to three physicians. It is becoming much more difficult to be in solo practice, and this is especially true in larger metropolitan areas. Group practices vary widely. They may be single or multispecialty, and may consist of two physicians to more than 100 other physicians. Each situation is unique and affords different benefits. In solo practice, you are your own boss, but along with that comes the responsibility of running a business. In the group setting, there may a loss of some autonomy, but less administrative responsibility and better financial security. In the staff model HMO, all physicians are employees of the organization. Kaiser Permanente is the classic example. As you progress through residency, take the opportunity to observe and ask about the different practice types. The community you choose to live in will often have an effect on your decision.

After these considerations, finding the "right" opportunity available is the next step. Is there a need in the community? There are a number of resources with this information. One of the best is the American Academy of Otolaryngology–Head and Neck Surgery (AAOHNS), either *The Bulletin* or the Web site. At the annual meeting, there are also job listings located at the AAOHNS booth. Otolaryngology journals often have job advertisements, as well. Recruitment firms abound and will send you information on a regular basis, even after you have entered practice. Local contacts in the community, either where you trained or where you are from, can be of great help. If you are interested in a specific community, you can ask other physicians if there is a need. Talking to pediatricians, internists, and family practitioners may give you the best perspective.

If entering the academic environment, usually after a fellowship, your options may be limited by availability. Your faculty, either at your place of residency or fellowship, may be the best resource, but the AAOHNS and the various journals have this information as well.

You should begin to look for a practice at the end of the fourth year of residency or, if doing a fellowship, prior to finishing the fifth year. This will give you the opportunity to evaluate and interview at a more relaxed pace.

Interviewing the practice is an important step. Obviously, the physicians will want to get to know you, but you have the responsibility to know the practice.

Whether you interview in person or on the telephone (if the practice is at a distance), you should obtain the same basic information: an overall description of the practice such as areas of concentration, how many offices, ancillary services, hospital affiliations, call, whether there is an ambulatory surgery center, ages of other physicians in the practice, and salary and benefits. If someone has recently left the practice, ask why and, if possible, speak to that individual. This preliminary discussion will often determine whether you or the practice wishes to pursue an agreement. One of the best opportunities for initial contacts is at the AAOHNS annual meeting, and should be limited to two or three interviews on any given day.

When you visit the practice for the first time, that cost may often be borne by you. If invited back for more serious discussions, the practice should help defer some of those costs. At the second visit, your spouse should also come. At this visit you may wish to look at places to live, schools, employment opportunities for your spouse, and what activities the community has to offer. Contacting a

realtor in advance will often be of great help in these areas. As discussed previously, your family's happiness is imperative and those other considerations are important as well. Having dinner with the other physician(s) and their spouse(s) will be beneficial. They will not be your best friends, but you should feel comfortable. You should ask around the community, especially at the hospital(s)—the nursing staff is often a good source—about the reputation of the individual or group. Remember, this is a potentially lifelong commitment and you want and need all the information available to make an intelligent decision.

I always have one caveat about a practice: If a spouse of one of the other physicians is an employee, especially the office manager or in charge of billings and collections, I would seriously consider looking elsewhere. As hard as they try, it is impossible for them to be neutral. In addition, the office manager often acts as a buffer between the staff and the physician(s). You are an employee and as such may wish to have someone to talk to. If the office manager is a spouse, you and the staff may be hesitant to do so. On the financial side, the emphasis on collections may be influenced toward the physician whose spouse has this position. This is not to say that this arrangement may not work, but experience is that it often leads to difficulties within a practice and may eventually lead to its dissolution.

CONTRACTING ISSUES

One cannot overestimate the importance of seeking legal advice before entering into a contract with a prospective physician, medical group, or hospital. Any expense you incur would be far exceeded by the long-term problems that could arise without this advice. Your legal advisor should have expertise in the area of physician's contracting, and will very often be a lawyer at a large firm that has a healthcare law practice component. Finding the right attorney is critical, and very often a "word-of-mouth" recommendation may be invaluable. Speaking to a local attending physician may be a fine place to start, especially if he or she has had a good experience with an attorney.

Once you contact the attorney, it is fair for you to ask what the billing arrangement will be. The attorney should be able to advise you as to the approximate cost of the project. This cost could vary, depending upon the complexity of the task involved. The point to be aware of, however, is that you should understand exactly how you will be charged before retaining the lawyer.

Very often you will be presented with a contract to sign from the group or hospital. Obviously, before even considering signing this document, you should have it reviewed by the appropriate counsel. There are a multitude of issues that the contract will cover, some of which are infinitely more important than others. Some of the important issues are outlined in Table 190.2.

TABLE 190.2
CONTRACT ISSUES

Business Terms
1. Compensation
2. Bonus
3. Retirement plans
4. Insurance: malpractice; life; disability; and health
5. Other fringe benefits: dues; Board exam, books and journals, meetings, automobile, and telephone
6. Indemnification

Term of Contract
1. Length
2. Reasons for termination prior to expiration of contract
3. What happens on expiration?

Restrictive Covenants
1. Enforceability
2. Length of time: geographic limitations
3. Coordination with termination provisions

Ultimate Purchase of Interest in Practice
1. Pre-tax vs. post-tax dollars
2. Practice valuation
3. Stock purchase vs. salary offset
4. Accounts receivable
5. Shareholders agreement

As you can see, the number of issues involved in the contract can be overwhelming. However, it is critical that you understand some issues are much more important than others. Very often a young physician becomes preoccupied with a relatively insignificant issue in a contract. As an example, whether the practice you are considering being employed by will pay for your "beeper" may seem important, but in the larger scheme of things it is virtually irrelevant. Regarding these minor financial business points, the reality is that your comfort level with the group and with the more senior physicians will be more important than the written word of a contract. The contract, however, will control larger issues that would become the subject of litigation in the event of a disagreement. These are the issues outlined above, which should be resolved in the contract.

The first general area, dealing with the business terms of the contract, tends to need less input from an attorney than the others. Basically, before even contacting the attorney, you should understand what the accepted levels of compensation would be in the area of the country in which you will be practicing. Speaking with other physicians and consultants, and reading various journals should be of great assistance in this regard. You should have an understanding of your base compensation, as well as whether you will be receiving a bonus. If a bonus is being given, you should understand the methodology that will control the calculation of the bonus. You should have a clear understanding of the fringe benefits to which you will be entitled. Equally as important, you should understand

whether the group is asking you to *indemnify* them in the event they are sued for any action you have taken. For example, if you commit malpractice, and there is a judgment against you that exceeds the amount of your malpractice coverage, the contract may ask you to indemnify, or reimburse, the group for any economic damage they may incur. This is a dramatic remedy that the group may be asking for, and if you agree to it you should understand fully what type of liability you are being asked to assume.

The length of the contract, and what would occur at the end of this term, is a critical combination that must be reviewed together. Very often the contract will appear to last for a specific number of years, but in reality, it could be terminated much earlier for a multitude of reasons. For example, one provision in the contract may say that it is to last for 3 years. Another provision, however, may discuss reasons for termination, which could dictate that the contract end prior to the initial term of years that is listed. Reasons for earlier termination can vary from those that are generally defined as "for cause," to those that exist for reasons having nothing to do with cause. It is not uncommon for an employer to want to include a provision that allows the employer to terminate the contract "without cause," to ensure that the employer will be able to terminate a new employee who simply does not fit into the practice. In other words, the doctor may be a capable physician, but may clash with the patients and staff in a way that is very damaging to the practice. Because of this, there is often a provision in the contract that allows this type of termination "without cause," and you should be careful about this. Terminating a contract for "cause," on the other hand, is often determined by a more objective standard, such as a loss of a medical license, and is therefore somewhat of a lesser concern.

You then must carefully review what obligations you will assume once the contract terminates. Very often these contracts contain a "restrictive covenant" that precludes you from practicing in the general geographical area of the existing practice for a certain period. The enforceability of these restrictive covenants varies from state to state and should be reviewed by your attorney. The important point, however, is that you could be faced with an incredibly difficult situation if the termination provisions and the covenant are onerous. For example, if the contract was to last for 5 years, but you could be terminated "without cause" for virtually any reason during this period, you are potentially confronted with a dangerous situation if there is also a restrictive covenant. This could effectively mean that 1 day prior to the expiration of the term of years, you could be terminated for virtually no reason, and then still be subject to a restrictive covenant that precludes you from practicing in the geographical area where you have resided for the past 5 years. It seems unfair that a covenant should be held against you at that point if you are terminated for no substantive reason. Alternatively, it might not be unfair for the group to be able to terminate you "without cause" in the early part of the contract, to protect it against a situation where an employee simply does not fit into the general practice scheme. The critical point is that you should understand how these provisions interact with one another.

The final major area of the contract concerns what will occur if things actually work out and you become a partner or shareholder of the group. More often than not, your initial employment agreement will not deal with your ultimate purchase into the practice. These provisions become much more complicated than normal employment contract provisions, and could increase your legal fees significantly. Very often the medical group will not want to include these provisions in the initial contract because they may never actually come to pass. You should, however, have a general understanding as to what will occur regarding your ultimate partnership prospects, and how you will pay for this interest.

One major issue you may want to explore is whether you can purchase this interest with "pre-tax" rather than "post-tax" dollars. For example, if the purchase price is $250,000, and you are required to pay this amount to become a partner, you effectively will have to earn a significant amount more than this to "net" the necessary dollars involved after taking taxes into account. Thus, you might have to actually earn twice that amount, pay taxes on it, and then have enough funds available to make the purchase.

Alternatively, if you agree to simply receive lesser compensation, you will be able to buy into the practice without having to pay tax on the compensation you are foregoing. This could result in significant economic savings to you. However, such an arrangement must be drafted carefully because there are tax implications to both you and the practice, and the Internal Revenue Service is careful to review such arrangements. For this reason, consulting an attorney is critical from both the legal and economic point of view.

As you can see, the number of issues involved in the contract can be overwhelming. There are, however, the practical realities of joining a practice that simply seems "right" for you. This factor should not be overlooked, because often your initial "gut reaction" may determine your ultimate happiness with the group. Your initial impressions, combined with the issues set forth previously and the advice of your attorney, will help you decide what is important to you in deciding whether to sign any given contract.

As a general rule, contracting with a group is a much more flexible situation than entering into a contract with either a university or hospital. The latter types of contracts may involve issues such as office hours, research support, teaching responsibilities, and other departmental responsibilities that do not exist in the more normal business contract. However, as a general rule, the larger issues outlined earlier may be less negotiable than they would be when contracting with a more traditional, business-oriented medical group.

STARTING UP YOUR PRACTICE

In advance of starting in a new practice, whether solo or joining an existing group, there are things that need to be done in advance: state licensure, which can take 6 months; hospital privileges, which may precede licensure; telephone directory listing, for which you need to check the closing date for the following year (usually April or May); and HMO membership, which is not an easy task and may require licensure (1–5).

If you are entering solo practice, your requirements will be greater. At a minimum, you will need financing, office space, employees, billing and collections, letterhead, telephones, office furniture, medical equipment, and malpractice insurance. Your first employee is most important and, if possible, should be someone with experience. The local medical society may be of invaluable help. In addition, the AAOHNS, American Medical Association, and American College of Surgeons all have material on setting up a practice (5).

Once you begin, it is wise to find an accountant experienced with medical practices. When you are joining a practice, consider hiring a personal accountant, to avoid any possible conflicts.

ADVANCING YOUR PRACTICE

Now that you have "arrived," you need to meet and greet. Sending announcements, taking out newspaper advertisements, and using press releases is only the beginning.

Eat lunch at the hospital(s), walk through the emergency department, sit in the doctor's lounge, and introduce yourself to the nursing staff and the intensivist. Visit the offices of potential referring physicians. You may not always meet the physician, but at least introduce yourself to the office manager and staff, who often make suggestions to patients about specialists. Bring some "goodies" and remember to leave business cards.

Make yourself available for speaking engagements, including grand rounds, schools, senior citizen groups, and other organizations. Join the local medical society and let them know you are available as a speaker.

Finally, be aware of three attributes that can be invaluable to enhancing your practice: affability, communication, and availability.

Affability

Be nice. Seems trite, but being nice goes a long way.

Be early. In the office, this will allow you to review messages, answer some phone calls, discuss with the staff your schedule for the day, and permit you to start seeing patients on time. If you are more than 20 minutes behind schedule at any given time, offer an apology to the patient. This recognizes the fact that you have kept them waiting and often defuses their anger. In the circumstance where the delay is longer, have the office staff rearrange the schedule for that day. Offer the patients already in the office the opportunity to reschedule or return later that day. Those patients with later appointments should be telephoned to make changes. If you will be late to the office, the same scenario holds true. Patients appreciate this thoughtfulness.

In the operating room, *always* be there at least 15 minutes ahead of schedule. This will let the staff know that you are prompt. More importantly, it allows you to discuss your needs for the procedure(s) before you begin. This is especially true when you are new or performing an infrequent procedure at that hospital. When you are not the first case in the assigned room, it behooves you to call before leaving your office to find out the status of your case. This allows you to better plan your day, and again demonstrates to the OR staff that time is important to you.

Communication

Sending letters to referring physicians is an excellent method of teaching. The letters should be concise. Some physicians prefer to send a cover letter with a copy of the typewritten office notes. Either way, this keeps the referring physician informed of what you found and the planned work-up and treatment.

Occasionally a phone call to the referring physician, or at least to the office, is best (in addition to a letter). Such circumstances may include a same-day request by the referring physician for a patient to be seen, or if such a call will facilitate the care of the patient. Be judicious, as phone calls may be disruptive.

Availability

Evening and Saturday office hours have great appeal to patients. This is especially true with single parents or if both parents work. Friday afternoons are also beneficial. It is possible that you may be the only specialist available at that time. In addition, taking your own call as much as possible can be very helpful. Your patients and referring physicians will appreciate being able to contact you if the need arises.

The more accessible you are, the better it is for building your practice.

In this chapter, we have covered a great deal of material. This hopefully will act as a stimulus to begin thinking about your future and the planning that is required to make you and your family's life more fulfilling.

HIGHLIGHTS

- Family comes first.
- Saving early is important for your future.
- An attorney with medical contracting experience is a must.
- Where you start your practice is not dependent upon where you train.
- Affability and availability are practice builders.
- It is never too early to start saving.
- Family considerations are important in deciding where to practice.
- If you are not happy in a practice situation, do not hesitate to change.
- An attorney experienced in physician contracting is a must.

ACKNOWLEDGMENT

The author wishes to acknowledge the writing assistance of Jon P. Betlow, CFP, CLU, ChFC, Bleakley, Dwyer & Schwartz, LLC, in the Financial Planning and Insurance section, and Marc Berman, Cole, Schotz, Meisel, Forman & Leonard, PA in the Contracting Issues section.

WEB RESOURCES

savingforcollege, LLC. www.savingforcollege.com.
Certified Financial Planners Board of Standards, Inc. www.cfp.net/search.

REFERENCES

1. Coker R, Daigrepont J. *Starting a medical practice,* 2nd ed. Chicago: AMA Press; 2002.
2. Campen R. *Going into medical practice.* Malden, MA: Blackwell Science; 2001.
3. Lichstein D. *Preparing for medical practice.* Miami: Medmaster; 1998.
4. Sotile WM, Sotile MO. *The medical marriage: sustaining healthy relationships for physicians and their families,* 2nd ed. Chicago: AMA Press; 2001.
5. *Transition to practice.* Alexandria, VA: American Academy of Otolaryngology–Head and Neck Surgery; 2002.

Professionalism

191

Byron J. Bailey

Medical knowledge and skill and medical professionalism are the enduring foundations of successful medical practice. This oversimplification of the complex subject of medical professionalism introduces a topic of heated discussions, passionate editorials, and this chapter.

During the past four decades, medical knowledge has increased at an unprecedented rate, while medical professionalism has declined at an equally unprecedented rate. Although some will challenge that statement and insist that the medical profession has never been more successful in advancing its scientific base and more effective in curing disease, let me offer some background for the extreme concern about the "un-professionalizing" of medicine.

First, there are sound reasons why many medical societies, professional organizations, and hospitals have assigned a high priority to "professionalism" programs for their members and their workforce.

Second, in recent years medical school curricula and residency training have introduced required professionalism educational modules.

Third, it is no coincidence that the number of MEDLINE journal articles listed under the heading of "medical professionalism" is zero for the decade from 1966 to 1976 (the first 10 years of MEDLINE) while there are 98 articles on the same topic in the decade from 1994 to 2004.

Fourth, the largest medical specialty certifying board, the American Board of Internal Medicine, has launched an intensive program called "Project Professionalism." They summarized their increasing level of concern as follows: recent changes in the healthcare delivery system have resulted in "stress surges" that can have a negative impact on the professional behavior of physicians. This concern is sharpened as physician reimbursement changes, and health care is provided in a competitive environment of managed and prepaid care, which threatens to reduce the status of patients to commodities rather than people with an affliction.

Something important is happening here, at a time when our technology is advancing and our information base is exploding, as public opinion polls show that the level of trust of physicians by patients is dropping.

It is apparent that since the shift from a fee-for-service medical reimbursement system to managed care, the very nature of the doctor-patient relationship has changed and many patients have begun to doubt the altruism of physicians generally. That is to say that they no longer believe that physicians are putting patient interests above self-interest.

So, perhaps we are facing more than a professionalism problem. Maybe we have a professionalism crisis.

DEFINING PROFESSIONALISM AND ITS IMPORTANCE

Medical professionalism begins with a set of *beliefs*—your beliefs—about your patients, yourself, and the society in which you live.

You bring these beliefs to every patient encounter, and they are the basis for your attitudes toward specific clinical situations that arise in the outpatient area and the operating room. Your attitudes are then manifested in the final step in the process—your behaviors, which are ultimately either professional or unprofessional.

Defining professionalism is difficult. Many would say simply, "I can recognize it when I see it." Reasonably, then, we can suggest that the opposite behaviors, which have been called "unprofessionalism," though hard to define, can also be recognized when we see them in others, and occasionally in ourselves.

Physicians, and especially surgeons, tend to be perfectionists, but we usually resent criticism, especially any challenge regarding our level of professionalism. The fact is that everyone reading this chapter is a highly educated and highly motivated individual with a positive self-image.

We see ourselves as giving patients our best effort whenever we are with them, and we find it difficult to understand how patients might view us and our colleagues as unprofessional.

We need to step back and analyze some specific issues around medical professionalism objectively. We are guided in this analysis by reviewing the key points in the Medical Professionalism Project of the American Board of Internal Medicine (ABIM) (1).

"PROJECT PROFESSIONALISM"

The ABIM states that medical professionalism has four defining foundations.

1. *Physician accountability:* placing the needs of the patient first, commitment to scholarship, helping colleagues, and being responsive to societal needs.
2. *Humanistic qualities:* addressing patient needs with integrity, respect, compassion, responsibility, courtesy, and sensitivity.
3. *Physician impairment:* recognizing substandard performance in yourself or a colleague and intervening in cases of alcohol or substance abuse, depression, dementia, or other disorders.
4. *Professional ethics*: having a commitment to professional ethics that is expressed in the form of collegiality and moral and ethical behavior in all areas of our work—in teaching, research, and patient care.

We can summarize these foundations and define medical professionalism simply by stating that physicians must always serve the interests of patients above their own self-interest. This is *altruism* and it is the heart of medical professionalism.

Other concepts that complete our definition of medical professionalism and are central to the theme of this chapter are as follows:

1. *Excellence:* exceeding patient expectations and committing to the goal of lifelong learning.
2. *Duty:* committing to serve, even when it is inconvenient, dangerous, or unpopular.
3. *Honor* and *Integrity:* manifesting as being fair and truthful, keeping your word, and recognizing and avoiding conflicts of interest.
4. *Respect:* for patients and their families, colleagues and nurses, other healthcare workers, and trainees.

Let's illustrate these issues with a practical scenario that we all encounter in our career as a physician and see how it is enlightening about medical professionalism.

Would It Be Professional?

These are the sort of scenarios we deal with every day. We are continually balancing the demands of medicine against the demands of family and the important elements of our lives away from medicine.

It is the middle of the afternoon of your day in the office, and you are running about 30 minutes behind in your full list of scheduled appointments. You are feeling the pressure. Your nurse hands you two telephone messages.
1: A local pediatrician's wife is experiencing her second episode of tinnitus, decreased hearing, and severe nausea this month. The first episode lasted 6 hours and they didn't want to bother you with it, but this one is more severe and both he and his wife are quite upset and hope that you will see her this afternoon.
2: Your wife called to remind you that your 12-year-old daughter's award ceremony for her prize-winning essay is at 6 PM at her school. You would have been barely able to make it to the ceremony if you had been able to stay on time. Now you will be a half hour late (or more) if you don't add the pediatrician's wife to your appointment schedule; you'll probably miss your daughter's event entirely if you do add this patient.
What would you do?

The answers are not simple, nor are they easy. Of course, there are strategies and contingency plans that we should employ to assist us when these circumstances arise. For example, many physicians leave two or three appointment slots open at the end of their afternoon schedule so that urgent referrals can be seen without keeping the staff in the office beyond regular working hours.

Another strategy is to have an understanding with practice associates that you will be available to help them out in this sort of situation, and depend on their reciprocal help when you are overwhelmed.

ISSUES OF PROFESSIONALISM IN OUR ORGANIZATIONS

Medicine is a moral and ethical enterprise, and when we band together to form professional societies, these organizations should be moral and ethical as well: that is to say, they should serve the best interests of society while serving their physician members. As a reflection of each of us individually, our medical organizations should be held to high standards in their work.

Most of the professional organizations in our specialty are relatively young. Only a few are more than a century old, and most were formed to provide educational benefits to their members. Others were formed as elitist organizations whose limited membership served to recognize a small group of physicians who had made significant contributions to a particular subspecialty. As new subspecialties arose within otolaryngology, the physicians practicing in those fields joined together, not only for educational purposes, but additionally to promote the advancement of their economic interests. Issues related to reimbursement, coding and billing procedures, political issues, and turf battles with other specialties became important agenda items for all of our professional societies. The nature of our organizations underwent important changes during the second half of the 20th century, as serving the business needs of the membership was given a very high priority.

For example, one organization, the American Council of Otolaryngology, was founded in the 1960s for the express purpose of advancing the political and economic interests of its members. The organization subsequently merged with the American Academy of Otolaryngology–Head and Neck Surgery (AAOHNS) in 1981, and the AAOHNS, Inc. now promotes the socioeconomic interests of its members while the AAOHNS Foundation addresses their education.

Although it is reasonable for professional societies to serve all of the needs of those who join and pay dues, there are ethical tensions and compromises involved in some organizations' activities. Heavy public education activities and legislative lobbying efforts are quite expensive, and while they may benefit the membership financially, there is no revenue generated for the organization, and significant financial burdens can arise.

To be effective in the realm of socioeconomic and political competition, it is usually necessary to hire additional staff and consultants, and even lobbyists in some instances. Forming coalitions with other societies to increase their impact may lead organizations into expensive and occasionally compromising relationships. Success often breeds more success in the socioeconomic realm; for example, the AAOHNS membership now comprises most of the practicing specialists in the United States because the Academy is so successful in meeting all the needs of its members.

As the membership size grows in our various professional organizations, so does the volume of their requests for help and the efforts of the specialty society to meet those demands. And so does the size of the staff and the annual budget. The scope of activities ranges from the publication of manuals that help in setting up a practice, lobbying for Medicare reimbursement, relief from rising medical liability insurance premiums, and slowing the intrusion into medical practice by non-physicians. The list of activities is almost endless, leaving an organization looking for sources of revenue other than membership dues. Consequently, medical organizations have found willing corporate sponsors eager to support meeting costs, travel grants, high-profile and expensive meeting functions, and journal supplements on themes that address the area of their commercial products.

But doesn't this leave some of our professional societies in the position of walking a thin line? Once these corporate relationships have been forged, how far should a medical organization travel down that slippery slope, and just how difficult is it to know when the relationship has gone too far?

Should we assume that our corporate sponsors are simply good-hearted and like to show their good will through these grants? Maybe they just want to help us with our worthy projects and get a bit of name recognition when they provide these funds.

On the other hand (as attorneys like to say), maybe the studies that document the success of these sponsorships and gifts in the marketing program for specific products are valid. If corporate charity is more of an investment or marketing expense, many have urged caution and some have advocated the elimination of these highly visible sponsorships because of the damage they do to our professional image with the public (2).

In time, we will understand more clearly how far we should go with the commercialization of our professional organizations, but for now we would be wise (at the least) to acknowledge the risks involved. Our specialty societies are too important to allow them to be diminished by an excessive focus on revenue from corporate initiatives that are over the line of professional ethics.

A related question deserves our attention as well: how far should an organization go in advocating vigorously and publicly on behalf of its members, especially if the interests of the physicians are seen as self-serving? How important is it to society that physician's incomes be maintained at current levels or allowed to grow annually?

As an example, the efforts of the American Medical Association (AMA) during the 1960s to derail the creation of the Medicare program were quite visible and extremely forceful. When those efforts failed, the professional stature of the AMA was diminished in the eyes of the public, and today most non-physicians regard it as a doctors' labor union.

Pellegrino and Relman (3) urge adherence to guidelines that they feel would keep medical organizations on the moral high ground where the members like to stand. These societal guidelines include the following:

1. Medical associations should be viewed as working in the public interest.
2. Avoid the transition from professional society to labor union.
3. Avoid conflicts of interest (e.g., gifts from companies that sell medical products) and for-profit business ventures.
4. Society journals must be kept independent of editorial or problematic advertiser influence to remain credible.
5. Medical meetings should focus on the educational needs of the members and should not become medical bazaars.

Our societies must understand how important it is that they are perceived as acting in the public interest. It is essential for their survival that both the organizations and the individual members be seen as honoring the basic social contract (i.e., the patient comes first) if all are to keep their privileged place in society.

An example in practical terms would be for our organizations to lobby for greater access to medical care and containment of its cost. As Richmond and Eisenberg (4) point out, "The failure of the organized medical profession to deal with rising health expenditures is also important. Without proactive policies to define 'how much is enough' and to deal with the concerns of public officials, employers, and the public, it was inevitable that entrepreneurs would emerge and, especially through managed care, become dominant in determining how medicine is practiced and health policies are formulated."

Cruess et al. (5) observe that there are no easy answers to the needed re-emphasis of professionalism in our professional associations. Clearly, all physicians must assume greater responsibility for these societies and must insist they serve the best interests of the public as well as their members.

PROFESSIONALISM IN YOUR PRACTICE AND YOUR HOSPITAL

It doesn't take a wizard with a crystal ball to see the pitfalls in the future if we continue to stand by and watch the rise of managed care and the merchandising of medicine change our concept of who we are and what we do.

All of us must keep in mind that beyond the business of medicine there is something more valuable: the beliefs, attitudes, and behaviors of a professional. We must focus in our practices and hospitals on the key features of medicine as a profession, not as a business. The following are the features of a profession:

1. Expert knowledge,
2. Self-regulation, and
3. Placing the needs of our patients first (6).

The impact of market forces on physician practices and hospitals has been so formidable that it is now undermining the professionalism of former years. The pressure to control rising costs has incentivized the restriction of care. Physicians feel caught in the middle between the option to "do the right thing" for their patients or to do the smart business thing for the bottom line. Ludmerer (6) refers to this dilemma as the physician becoming a "double agent" purportedly serving the patient, but in fact, at times opting to limit patient care for the financial benefit of those who are seeking a healthy return on their investment.

So the time is ripe for a renewal of a "professionalism" emphasis in our hospitals and academic health centers, particularly the latter, because the next generation of physicians are in training in these centers and are watching their role models cope with these issues.

A large hospital is "a community of health care professionals dedicated to education, research, and patient care" where "professionalism is the standard of conduct" under the right conditions (7). It is a place where patients place

their lives in our hands, believing that we have set and maintained standards of competence and integrity; that is the basis for their trust in us and their faith that we will place their interests above our own, and that is the foundation of our contract with society.

So what are the guidelines, what should we be measuring, and how are we doing?

Our hospital has developed a Professionalism Charter (7) that provides some clear guidelines in terms of the professional responsibilities that are expected of us. These include the following 10-point contract for professions:

1. Commitment to professional competence: lifelong learning and maintaining the necessary knowledge and skills for high-quality performance.
2. Commitment to honesty: full disclosure, informed consent, and prompt reporting and analysis of errors.
3. Commitment to confidentiality: safeguarding personal and sensitive information.
4. Commitment to appropriate relations: protection of vulnerable and dependent individuals in clinical and research settings.
5. Commitment to improving quality: efforts to improve continuously in all spheres of professional activity.
6. Commitment to improve access: working to reduce the barriers that prevent so many from receiving needed care.
7. Commitment to just allocation of resources: cost-effective management of resources that are inadequate to meet all of the need.
8. Commitment to scientific knowledge: promoting the discovery, dissemination, and appropriate use of new knowledge.
9. Commitment to avoid conflicts of interest: recognizing, disclosing, and dealing swiftly with conflicts of interest.
10. Commitment to professional responsibilities: respect, teamwork, and self-regulation to uphold high standards of professionalism.

Of course, it's not a simple matter to put these commitments into practice. For example, there is a tremendously important conflict between putting the best interests of the patient first and point number 7, the commitment to just allocation of resources. Brennan points out that compromise in this area is inevitable (8). But when does compromise become the same as failing to be professional?

And putting the best interest of patients ahead of one's own best interest "does not accurately reflect a basic level of human nature: namely to act in one's own best interest," as pointed out by Wartman (9), who suggests that we compromise and try to find a congruence of interests that is more practical. But isn't that the basic problem: all too often there is no congruence of interests.

Or maybe Arnett (10) is right when he points out that in the ABIM Professionalism Charter, two of the three principles are in conflict with each other (individual rights and social justice) and two of the 10 responsibilities place the interests of others above those of the patient (public advocacy and just distribution of finite resources). He then expresses concerns that the agenda of those who developed the charter have gone beyond what's needed (a simple return to a code of patient-centered ethics), and insists that it goes too far.

At the same time, Haskell (11) feels that it doesn't go far enough, because it doesn't specifically address business integrity as it involves medical record documentation, coding, and billing. He argues that these areas are central to a new field he calls "healthcare ethics." So we are left with the dilemma of conducting a successful medical practice on a difficult and changing playing field. Perhaps no generation of physicians has faced such a daunting task as this generation of healers.

PROFESSIONALISM AND SURGEONS

We come to a key topic at this point, because as surgeons, we engage in a doctor-patient relationship of great intensity. Society grants us enormous privileges that carry a heavy responsibility and place special demands on us to put the best interests of our patients ahead of our own welfare. Indeed, we recognize that the level of trust our patients can place in us is one of the most important factors in determining the outcome of our procedures.

The American College of Surgeons (ACS) has been a leader in the movement to focus our attention once again on the professional origins of surgical practice. The ACS Task Force on Medical Professionalism has drafted a formal surgeon's code of Professional Conduct (12) that reaffirms our personal responsibility to:

1. Advocate for our patients' needs,
2. Disclose all therapeutic options,
3. Disclose and resolve any conflict of interest,
4. Respect patient vulnerability,
5. Disclose any adverse event or error,
6. Respect cultural and spiritual needs of patients,
7. Care for terminally ill patients,
8. Support the needs of patients families, and
9. Respect other healthcare professionals.

The ACS Task Force Report emphasizes that in addition to our doctor-patient relationships, we also have a social contract—a contract that holds us accountable to our communities and to society in general.

In this regard, as surgeons we must accept the responsibility to:

1. Provide the highest quality surgical care;
2. Value honesty, confidentiality, and altruism;
3. Pursue lifelong learning;
4. Maintain our competence;
5. Set, maintain, and enforce practice standards;
6. Improve care via outcomes assessment;
7. Provide public education;
8. Work to improve the health of the public;
9. Support the just distribution of healthcare resources;
10. Provide care to all, without regard to gender, race, disability, religion, social status, or the ability to pay; and
11. Participate in educational programs addressing professionalism.

The trust of our patients, and the privileges that we derive from our contract with society, are built on the foundation of professionalism. We must incorporate the elements outlined above into ourselves and into our behaviors as surgeons.

As Walter Lawrence, Jr., MD of the University of Virginia concluded recently in an article that provides an excellent institutional roadmap to address these issues (13), "Our experience has convinced the committee that the entire problem of professional behavior deserves our close scrutiny. As so many opposing forces participate in our healthcare and health education environment, surgeons must continue to vigilantly guard the values that have led us to our career choice."

Some authors have expressed reasons for optimism in the efforts to renew a strong focus on professionalism (5). They see positive signs of improvement and feel these are based on three fundamental reasons:

1. Faith in the democratic process and the important place held by organized medicine in this process.
2. Physicians no longer control the healthcare system; consequently, our behaviors and comments are seen as being more objective.
3. Society has a great need for our services and depends on us to manage their basic health problems; moreover, we want to be held in high regard by our patients. Therefore, we are highly motivated to raise society's perception of medical professionalism.

At this crucial time in the profession of medicine, when the traditional doctor-patient relationship has been victimized by marketplace forces and layers of bureaucracy, it behooves each of us, as surgeons, to shoulder our personal responsibility and to stand firmly in support of the principles of professionalism in our daily lives as surgeons.

REFERENCES

1. Brennan T, Blank L, Cohen J, et al. Members of the Medical Professionalism Project: ABIM Foundation. Medical professionalism in the new millennium: a physician charter [Perspective]. *Ann Intern Med* 2002;136(3):243–246.
2. Rothman DJ. Medical professionalism: focusing on the real issues [Sounding Board]. *N Engl J Med* 2000;342(17):1283–1286.
3. Pellegrino ED, Relman AS. Professional medical association: ethical and practical guidelines [Commentary]. *JAMA* 1999;282(10):984–986.
4. Richmond JB, Eisenberg L. Medical professionalism in society [correspondence]. *N Engl J Med* 2000;342(17):1288–1290.

5. Cruess RL, Cruess SR, Johnston SE. Renewing professionalism: an opportunity for medicine. *Acad Med* 1999;74(8): 878–884.

6. Ludmerer KM. Instilling professionalism in medical education [editorial]. *JAMA* 1999;282(9):881–882.

7. The University of Texas Medical Branch (UTMB) Professionalism Charter. 2003. Available at: http://www.utmb.edu/professionalism/activities/charter. Accessed January, 2006.

8. Brennan TA. Charter on medical professionalism: putting the charter into practice [Letters: Comments and Responses]. *Ann Intern Med* 2003;138(10):851.

9. Wartman SA. Charter on medical professionalism: putting the charter into practice. [Letters: Comments and Responses]. *Ann Intern Med* 2003;138(10): 854–855.

10. Arnett JC. Charter on medical professionalism: putting the charter into practice [Letters: Comments and Responses]. *Ann Intern Med* 2003;138(10):853.

11. Haskell CM. Charter on medical professionalism: putting the charter into practice [Letters: Comments and Responses]. *Ann Intern Med* 2003;138(10):852.

12. ACS Task Force on Professionalism. *Code of professional conduct.* Chicago, IL: American College of Surgeons; 2004.

13. Lawrence W. Is our level of professionalism where it should be? *Bull Am Coll Surg* June 2004;21–25.

Physician Communication Skills: An Essential Competency

192

Byron J. Bailey

We live in a time that has been called the "communication age." We communicate important information faster, more completely, and more widely than ever before in the history of civilization.

Physicians and other healthcare professionals have begun to focus their attention on the critical nature of communication skills in every aspect of their work. This chapter will discuss the medical communication skills that are important for a successful medical career. We will emphasize (a) verbal communication in the clinical setting, (b) presenting a medical talk to an audience, and (c) medical writing. Our purpose is to engage you, the reader, in our effort to bring you the best current knowledge in this field and to motivate you to improve your verbal communication and your medical writing.

Recently, the Accreditation Council for Graduate Medical Education (ACGME), the organization that accredits residency training in the United States, has designated skill in communication as one of the six essential competencies that must be demonstrated by all residents trained in this country.

WHY IS DOCTOR-PATIENT COMMUNICATION SO IMPORTANT?

Think back for a minute on your own life experiences as a patient or family member of a patient with a serious medical problem. What can you recall from your personal interaction with the doctor about the quality of the communication that was involved? Was it clear? Was it sympathetic? Were you told as much as you wanted to know? Do you remember the doctor being a good listener? Perhaps you even remember an early communication with your doctor that was a factor in your decision to become a physician.

Now think of one of your teachers or a colleague who is an outstanding medical communicator. What has given you the impression that they communicate well? Do you think they were born with that skill or did they learn it? Do outstanding verbal skills give you the impression that the person is also an outstanding and competent physician?

Interesting questions arise around the topic of communication skills. And yet, the bottom line question for many is "Why spend a lot of time and energy working to improve my communication skills—what's in it for me?"

That's a good question. Here's what I have found in the recent scientific literature: the five good reasons why doctor-patient communication is important:

1. *Patient satisfaction.* Recent studies have shown that communication skills are the single most important factor in patients' satisfaction with their care, and that patient satisfaction with care is the primary determinant in patients' decisions about which doctor they will select. This is a key issue in building a successful practice. Remember that it has been reported that a satisfied patient will tell, on average, three other patients about how pleased they were. On the other hand, patients who are dissatisfied with their encounter will tell, on average, 19 other individuals about their unpleasant experience.

2. Good communication skills are a factor in *better over-all outcomes* in patient care, while poor communication skills have a negative influence. For example, the study by Cegala (1) documents the role of improved communication with patients leading to increased compliance with physician recommendations and adherence to therapeutic plans.

3. Good communication skills increase efficiency in practice. We can cope with the demands of a busy practice by communicating clearly and effectively, even if we have less time available to spend with each patient. On several occasions, my patients have told me that they were extremely pleased with the care they received from a certain famous heart surgeon in our region who is known to spend less than a minute with each of his patients when he makes his postoperative rounds. They described how he took the time to explain how the surgery had gone and that he left them with the feeling that they were the most important patient of all those for whom he was caring. This is a clear example of mastery of the art of doctor-patient communication.

4. *Risk management.* Good communication skills correlate with a decreased probability of professional liability lawsuits. Recently, I listened to a well-educated, professional woman in our bridge group describe her encounter with a physician in another state who saw her while she was on vacation. The physician diagnosed the pain and swelling in her right calf as an infection and treated it with antibiotics. Several days later, when she was no better, she returned to the clinic and was seen by a second physician, who diagnosed thrombophlebitis and admitted her to the hospital for treatment. She improved slowly, and after a week she was discharged from the hospital. Several days later, the first physician (who missed the correct diagnosis) called her to inquire how she was doing and to express to her his sincere sympathy for all she had been through. The patient was extremely impressed by the phone call and the time the physician spent communicating with her. She expressed to the rest of us how much she wished that there were more caring physicians like him.

5. *Professional survival.* In some geographic regions, managed care organizations periodically survey patients in their plans, collect patient satisfaction data on individual physicians, and make this data available to other patients and to their employers. Similarly, patient satisfaction scores are included as key data in the managed care organization's decisions regarding which physicians to include or exclude from specialist panels.

CAN COMMUNICATION SKILLS BE TAUGHT?

Communicating well is a skill and a behavior that can be taught and learned, just as any other skill. There is growing interest in this area, as reflected in the curriculum in many medical schools.

Once it was felt that obtaining the history of a patient's illness was a fairly simple and straightforward exercise. Students were provided with a format to follow and basic lecture instructions regarding the facts to be obtained. However, evidence was gathered documenting that many students had difficulty with this approach as they moved from the patient-centered focus they were taught in the preclinical years to the disease-centered (biomedical) focus that is practiced in the clinical years of medical school and in residency (2). In many medical schools today, faculty are improving the preparation of students for clinical encounters by designing programs that emphasize student identification of doctor-patient communication problems and working with residents and faculty to develop appropriate solutions. This approach is more successful than lectures because it utilizes current theories of adult learning that have shown increased effectiveness in settings where the learner is more autonomous and self-motivated rather than responding to a set of instructions given by a teacher.

Exactly how to teach students and residents the finer points of communicating has drawn a lot of attention recently, because the "best practices" in this field are still being debated. Two thirds of medical schools currently teach communication skills, but the success of these efforts remains uncertain, especially as medical students move into residency and clinical practice (3). Sophisticated approaches have been taken to define specific communication competencies and design effective programs to move students to those competencies. An excellent collaborative example of this is the work done by the New York University School of Medicine, Case Western Reserve University School of Medicine, and the University of Massachusetts Medical School. Faculty from these three schools developed the Macy Model of tasks and skills that they propose as the best practices for the doctor-patient communication relationship. The details of the Macy Model are shown in Figure 192.1.

Using a performance-based, controlled evaluation of the Macy Model at three medical schools, the leaders of this initiative concluded that it is possible to teach communication skills effectively. The data collected also suggest that the model could be adapted to strengthen the communication skills of residents as well.

Documenting competent resident communication in various settings is no longer an elective matter. The Accreditation Council for Graduate Medical Education (ACGME) sets and enforces the standards for graduate medical education in the United States. The ACGME has developed a list of six competencies that must be addressed and documented for each resident in every specialty. In order for a training program to be accredited, there must be documentation that the residents are taught communication skills and that they have demonstrated "Interpersonal and communication skills that result in effective information exchange and teaming with patients, their families, and other health professionals" (4).

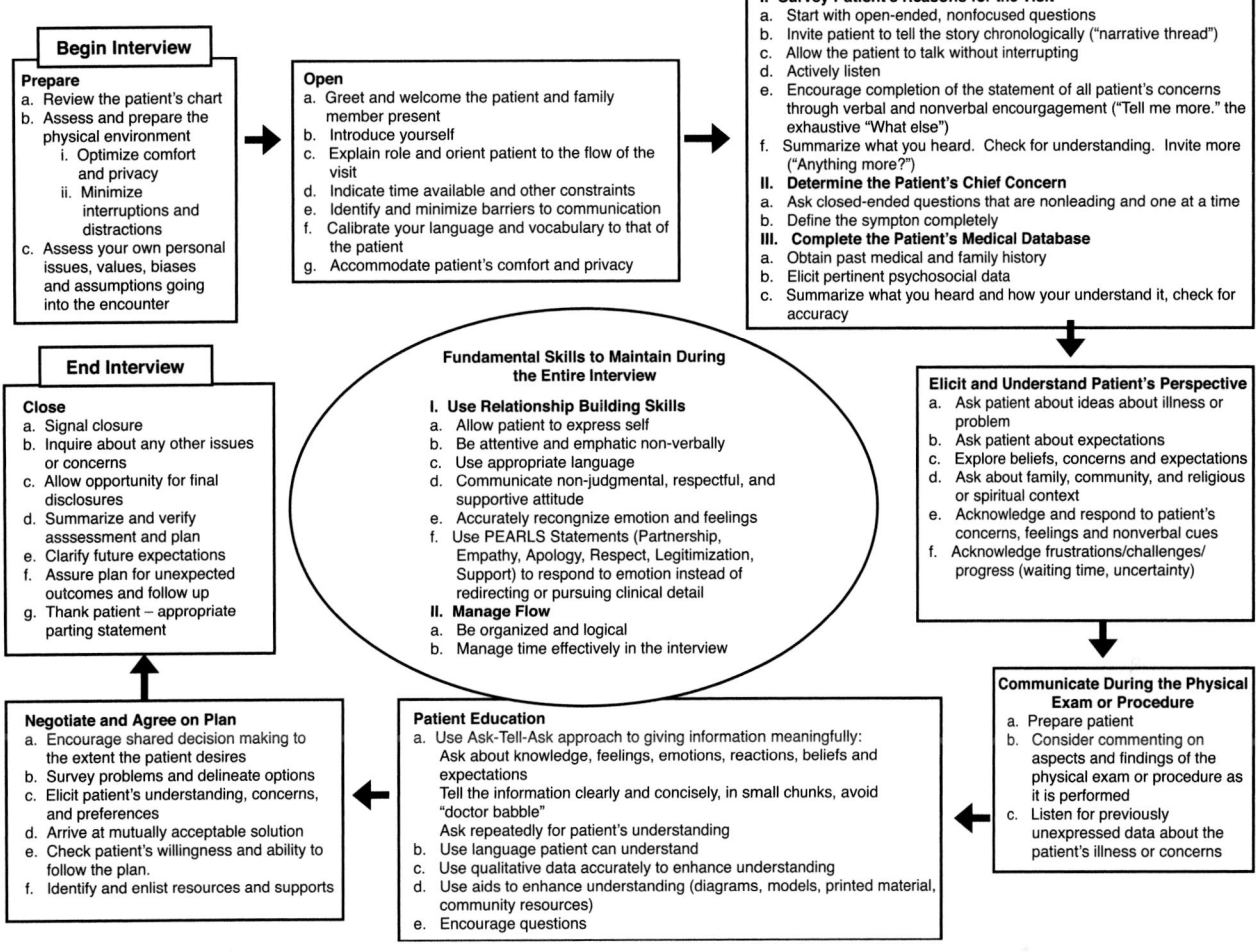

Figure 192.1 The Macy Model of tasks and skills that define best practices for the doctor-patient encounter. (From Kalet A, Pugnaire MP, Cole-Kelly K et al. Teaching communication in clinical clerkships: models from the Macy Initiative in health communications. *Acad Med* 2004;79:511–520.)

The ACGME allows flexibility in the methods of instruction and the tools used for evaluating resident competency in interpersonal and communication skills. The organization encourages innovative assessment tools and maintains examples of such instruments on its web page at www.acgme.org/outcome. Methodologies employed include the 360-Degree Evaluation Instrument, the Chart Stimulated Recall Oral Examination, the Global Rating of Live or Recorded Performance, and the Objective, Structured Clinical Examination (OSCE).

Among the most promising tools available to assess communication effectiveness is the 360-Degree Evaluation Instrument. It is a global rating evaluation that is completed by several categories of people who have had the opportunity to observe and interact with a resident in various settings and to assess performance of specific skills in a range of situations. The responders to this tool may include faculty, fellow residents, patients, and patients' families. The format includes questions and responses designed to assess how well the resident performs in key areas, including:

1. Creating and sustaining a therapeutic and ethical relationship with patients,
2. Effective listening skills,
3. Eliciting and sharing information
4. Effective nonverbal communication,
5. Writing skills, and
6. Working effectively with others.

The importance of strong, effective communication skills cannot be overemphasized. Communication is the only skill that provides a means for a physician to show that he/she possesses and effectively uses all the other key competencies such as medical knowledge, sound patient care, systems-based practice, and professionalism (5).

SPECIAL MEDICAL COMMUNICATION SITUATIONS

Imagine for a moment that you have just examined a very successful young professional in your community who comes to see you because of progressively increasing hoarseness. He is 35 years old, is married with three young children, and he smokes two packs of cigarettes per day. On fiberoptic laryngoscopy, you see an exophytic lesion involving the left true vocal fold and there is no vocal fold motion on that side.

Even though you don't have a tissue biopsy diagnosis, you are fairly certain from the appearance of the lesion that you are dealing with cancer, and it's not an early vocal cord carcinoma. *Practice the conversation* you would begin at that point as you remove the scope, turn to the patient, and begin to explain the situation.

Breaking the news to a patient about the diagnosis of cancer, or even "possible cancer" is a very tense and emotional communication. It carries a message of potential prolonged illness, loss of livelihood, possible pain, likely disability, and the threat of death. Here are some guidelines to keep in mind as you interact with this patient or with any other patient confronting a serious medical diagnosis:

1. Before the conversation, be sure that the patient brings a family member to the meeting. This type of discussion should always be face-to-face, and never over the phone or at a time when you are unprepared to deal with all of the demands of that situation.

2. Allow enough time for all the patient's questions to be answered. These discussions are best held before a lunch break or at the end of the day if they are in your office. They may run much longer than you planned.

3. Always present the same information and give the same thoughts about prognosis to both the patient and the patient's family.

4. Present the whole truth, but it is all right to be optimistic.

5. "I'm afraid that I have some bad news for you" is a reasonable way to begin the discussion. Remember that people will vary quite widely in their response to a diagnosis of cancer or another major illness. While you are talking about a medical issue, they are thinking about (a) their loss of control over their body and fact that it has betrayed them, (b) their loss of identity as a healthy person, and (c) their loss of relationships and roles in their life up to this point.

6. Listen carefully to the response that patients have to the news that you are giving them, and try to learn exactly what your words have meant to them.

7. Listen carefully for their comments about their religious beliefs, as these will frequently influence future discussions.

8. Be empathetic.

9. Don't take away the patient's hope.

10. Understand that the patient may not comprehend much of what you have said to him or her, and may not hear any of the conversation that follows after the word "cancer." This is an extremely loaded word that has the ability to jam all communications for some period of time after it enters the conversation.

LEARN TO LISTEN—IT'S IMPORTANT!

Some doctors seem to believe that the art of medical communication consists of self-training and practice to learn to speak clearly and professionally so that they will not possibly be misunderstood by their patients. Although that is a good start, it's only half of the task. It is equally important to learn how to *listen*.

Here's a key point about letting the patient tell you the story of their illness so that you can diagnose their problem accurately. Studies have shown that on average, doctors *interrupt* patients who are describing their complaint very early in the first interview. We're all pressed for time, but we should learn to allow patients to tell us what is important to them before we begin to question them.

Some other key points about listening are as follows:

1. Every patient comes to you with an agenda. Sometimes the agenda is short and simple; sometimes it is lengthy and convoluted. To get to the heart of patient problems and to establish the rapport that is necessary for successful treatment, we often have to spend a considerable amount of time pursuing the items on the patient's agenda. Listen to what they are saying and listen to what they are *not* saying as you take a careful history.

2. Remember that patients seldom return to doctors who don't take the time to listen to what they have to say.

3. Remember that you don't really know if the patient is hearing what you have to say, unless you listen to the questions they are asking and the comments they are making.

4. Videotaped interviews show that doctors interrupt their patients and redirect the communication to areas that they feel are more relevant after an average of 19 seconds of patient dialogue. Patients often have more than one agenda item, and it is better to allow them to express their entire agenda before you divert the information flow in another direction.

OVERCOMING BARRIERS TO OPTIMAL COMMUNICATION IN YOUR PRACTICE

There are many significant barriers to what we might define as ideal medical communication. Some of these barriers exist within patients and their families, and the most important of these are as follows:

1. Patients and their families frequently tend to steer conversations away from difficult or emotionally laden topics.
2. Shyness, confusion, and fear of death or disability.
3. Sometimes patients and their families are simply unable to accept bad news.
4. Patients and their families have a tendency to overestimate the probability of a cure in difficult situations. Television programs focusing on doctor-heroes tend to emphasize the happier outcomes.

5. Information obtained from the Internet and the news media may frequently confuse the patients and cause them to have difficulty hearing your message.

Other barriers to optimal medical communication may reside within some of us as physicians for various reasons, such as the following:

1. Physicians frequently fear causing pain with the bad news they have to convey.
2. Some physicians lack good communication skills.
3. Some doctors view death as an enemy to be defeated. When death or disability cannot be prevented, they take it personally and feel that they have failed as a physician.
4. Some physicians tend to anticipate a disagreeable response from patients or their family, and in order to avoid this they present a misleading picture of the patient's condition and prognosis for full recovery.
5. Some physicians fear the medical/legal consequences of the strong negative reactions that patients may have to bad news. Having to convey the probability of a negative outcome causes them to feel powerless and vulnerable, and results in communication that is less than candid.

SO YOU'RE GOING TO GIVE A MEDICAL TALK

Most doctors enjoy talking and have fairly good conversational skills. Most of us do pretty well discussing a patient care matter in a small group of healthcare professionals in the hospital. But everything changes when we think about standing before a group of 50 or several hundred people and giving a formal scientific talk.

In fact, surveys have shown that the fear of delivering a presentation to a large audience ranks higher on the anxiety scale than any other common fear. We are afraid that we will be too nervous to speak well, or that we will make a mistake and look foolish.

Whether you are preparing a Grand Rounds presentation, giving a talk to the hospital medical staff, or delivering an address to our national Academy of Otolaryngology–Head and Neck Surgery, there are a few simple rules to follow that will result in a positive experience for the speaker and the audience.

First, the BIG RULES:

1. Know your audience and know what they want and need.
2. Know your subject.
3. Organize your thoughts.
4. Speak clearly and concisely.
5. Use language that is natural and effective to connect with your audience.

I have found it helpful to begin by preparing an outline of the topic that I'm presenting. This helps to define a limited or focused segment of a larger topic so that the audience is able to focus on a manageable amount of information.

The next step is to research the subject very thoroughly. This supplements your knowledge and experience with the most current important new scientific information in the literature.

Then, it usually is necessary to eliminate the information that is not essential or is less important so that your presentation fits into the allotted time. At this point, it's a good idea to identify the six to ten points that you want to emphasize to your audience. These become the "take home" message that you build your talk around as you boil it down to the essentials.

Adult learning is based on providing information that the listener perceives as having practical value, using repetition to drive home the key points, and presenting it in a clear, interesting, and organized manner. Good visual material, vocal inflection, enthusiasm, gestures, eye contact, and emphasizing the real-life value of the information add value to your presentation (6).

Steve Sabol, the originator of the very successful National Football League Film Program, has said, "Tell me a fact and I'll learn, tell me a truth and I'll believe, but tell me a story and it will live in my heart forever." The most effective speakers are those who can tell the story of their message, and their ability to do this passes their knowledge on to us. We remember what they said because they boiled the story down to manageable size, they told us what they were going to tell us, then they told their story, and then they told us what the story meant.

Invariably, the master teachers know the subject, they are enthusiastic about the topic, and they have passed their knowledge and enthusiasm on to us.

NOW, YOU'RE GOING TO BE AN AUTHOR

Whether you are in private practice or in an academic setting, you must polish your writing skills. This is because the field of medical publishing provides an enormous opportunity for you to share your unique knowledge and experience with your colleagues. Well-regarded journals with rigorous peer review of manuscripts are the source for the best new information for managing patients. In academia the quality and number of publications in good journals are key elements in establishing your reputation and advancing your career. "Publish or perish" is as true a phrase today as it was a century ago.

Physicians in private practice gain satisfaction from publishing that adds luster to the challenges and rewards of patient care. As a general rule, there is a close correlation between those who lecture and write well, and successful clinical practice.

Based on the experience gained from 12 years as the editor of the *AMA Archives of Otolaryngology–Head and Neck*

Surgery and 10 years as editor of *The Laryngoscope*, I can state confidently that medical publishing is a dynamic field of great importance to those who write and those who read the important new scientific information in our journals. I want to provide you with some insight into the "best practices" and the pitfalls in preparing a successful manuscript. First, however, you must understand three important facts about the world of medical publishing.

- Number one: Medical journals are published as a commercial venture in almost every case. To be successful, journals must gain revenue by generating a product that has value for the readers in order to attract subscribers. No journal is large enough to publish all the good manuscripts it receives, because the cost of paper, printing, postage, and staff must be controlled. So, authors compete on the basis of manuscript quality and importance for the privilege of publishing.
- Number two: There are rigorous standards, set by the journal, in regard to literary quality, content validity, and scientific relevance. Authors must consider each of these areas thoughtfully if their work is to be accepted by a leading journal.
- Number three: The competition is stiff. Because editors receive more good manuscripts than they can publish, they rely on peer review by experts in the field to assist them in selecting work that has value to the readers. When preparing your manuscript, consider each word in the phrase *"important, new, scientific information"* very carefully, and if your report qualifies on all four counts, it will almost certainly be published.

Also, following the advice above will avoid the embarrassment of a review similar to one received recently by an author, which said, "Your manuscript provides new and important information. Unfortunately, the part that is new is not important and the part that is important is not new."

Journal quality comes directly from the peer review system. Authors should take seriously the reviewers' comments, as they are the key to improving your manuscript and moving it toward publication. Review the final draft of your paper very carefully yourself, and then have it reviewed by a critical colleague before you send it to an editor.

Important Steps in Preparing a Manuscript

Every medical publication begins with a study of some type. So, Rule 1 is to design properly a study that will test a hypothesis or answer an important question. You must put in the time and effort to design the study in such a way that when you begin to analyze the data and draw conclusions, they will withstand the challenges of the review process. Consult with a biostatistician *before* you begin to be certain that you are studying a phenomenon with a quantifiable outcome (e.g., decibels of hearing improvement; percentage of cancer patients surviving). Determine the size of the result of your intervention, and from this, derive the number of subjects that you must study to generate data that are statistically significant. Include an appropriate control group to deal with the placebo effect and chance, and select carefully the appropriate statistical tests to analyze your data. Don't make the serious mistake of waiting until the study is in progress to consult with a biostatistician.

Table 192.1 will be helpful as you organize the content of your manuscript.

TABLE 192.1
BEST PRACTICES AND PITFALLS IN MEDICAL WRITING

Best Practices	Pitfalls
1. Explain clearly the background, importance, methodology, and conclusions of your work	1. Assuming that readers have the same level of knowledge and interest in your topic as you have.
2. Write the entire manuscript yourself in almost every instance.	2. Allowing colleagues or corporate sponsors to write important sections.
3. Be objective in the analysis of your data and the writing of your manuscript	3. Getting carried away with the importance of your work and exaggerating its value or slanting your conclusions.
4. Publish the same message only once, even if you have added more patients.	4. Duplicate publications with the same message, especially with failure to cite your prior work.
5. Publish the entire study in one article so that readers get the whole story at once.	5. Fragmenting the same study into multiple articles (salami slicing) to get more on your CV.
6. Authorship rules must be followed carefully to avoid abuse of the term "author."	6. Adding individuals with insufficient participation in the study or writing of the article to the list of authors.

Who Is an Author (Who Is Not)

You would think that after several thousand years of writing, we might all agree on the use of the term "author." Unfortunately, that does not seem to be the case (7).

To be included in the list of authors, an individual must participate sufficiently in the preparation of the manuscript to deserve recognition and to take responsibility for defending its content. All authors must have been important in the concept and design of the study and the analysis and interpretation of the data. Authors must have been involved in the writing, revising, and final draft of the manuscript.

Examples of roles that do not qualify as authors are departmental chairs and lab supervisors who do not meet the above criteria. Those who have only provided resources, colleagues who have provided advice, or patient subjects may deserve acknowledgment, but do not meet the standards for authorship.

Provide a Clear Message

Conveying complex biomedical information is a challenging task. How often have you read a journal article and found that the author has left important questions unanswered?

As an author, you must address the following eight key areas with clarity in order to meet the standards for publications:

1. What is the *purpose* of your report?
2. What *research design* was used?
3. In what *setting* was the study performed?
4. Who were the *subjects*? How were they chosen? Exclusions?
5. Exactly what *intervention*?
6. How were results and *variables* measured?
7. What *observations* were made?
8. What *conclusions* do the data support?

Readers can track your work and even repeat it, if you have answered all eight questions in your manuscript.

Avoid excessive wordiness, don't ramble aimlessly over trivial details, don't speculate about conclusions not supported by your findings, and don't let bias creep into your study or your writing.

Your Abstract Is Very Important

Spend the time to write an excellent abstract. It may be the most important section of your manuscript, because it can pull a busy reader into the full content of your article when it is published. Most readers do not take the time to read every article in a journal, so the abstract should contain key information that is likely to catch the attention of readers.

Remember also, that the abstract may be all that appears in many electronic versions of your publication (e.g., MEDLINE). When clinicians and researchers conduct a literature search, they often scan a large number of abstracts, from which they select a smaller number of complete articles to review. The better your abstract, the more likely it is to be among those selected.

Most journals today require a *structured* abstract with specific sections, such as:

1. Objectives/Hypothesis
2. Study Design
3. Methods
4. Results
5. Conclusions

The Discussion Section Tells Your Story

After the Abstract, the Discussion section of your manuscript is the most likely element to be read by busy physicians. It is the place where you report your findings and put the information in perspective.

As you begin to write the "Discussion" section of your manuscript, it is a good idea to read very carefully what you have written up to that point. Your objective is to answer the basic questions you addressed in your study. Don't get bogged down in an extensive literature review or lengthy explanation of data that appeared earlier in the manuscript.

This is your opportunity to summarize the key findings from your study in the context of your introduction and within the framework of your methodology. The "Discussion" is the section where you put forward your strongest arguments for the validity of your work and where you emphasize why your results are new, different, and important to the reader. It is acceptable to speculate and offer opinions about the relevance and application of your findings, but you must have adequate data to support your views.

Avoid the following pitfalls in your "Discussion" section:

1. Don't let your enthusiasm distort your scientific objectivity.
2. Don't let your rhetoric go beyond your data. Excessive "selling" of your ideas can weaken your overall effort.
3. Report the limitations and weaknesses in your study along with the strengths.
4. Don't overlook any potential undisclosed conflict of interest that you or one of your co-authors might have.

It is helpful to have a clear and concise mental checklist as you begin to organize the first draft of your manuscript. Table 192.2 may be a helpful guide.

Lucente (8) summarized the topic of medical communication with clarity and elegance when he wrote,

> Our communications both reflect the functioning or our minds and influence our performance. Our ability to define, explore, and resolve clinically relevant problems develops as our communication skills improve, particularly as we develop the ability to organize thoughts precisely and present them clearly. The physician who is trained to

TABLE 192.2

ELEMENTS OF A MEDICAL MANUSCRIPT

Abstract:	• *Structured:* Objectives/Hypothesis, Study Design, Methods, Results, Conclusion • It must stand alone, contain your key message, and attract readers
Introduction/Objectives:	• State the problem, question, or hypothesis you are addressing • Set the stage, arouse interest • Convince the reader that the question is unanswered and important
Methods:	• Tell the reader exactly what you did • Clear, detailed, and understandable • Reader could repeat your work
Results:	• Tell what you found; use tables • No interpretation • No discussion
Discussion:	• Orderly, systematic, and thoughtful consideration of each finding • Present in the context of Introduction • Discuss in the framework of Methods • Argue for validity and importance • Clarify what is new and relevant
Conclusion:	• Emphasize a *few* points you want the reader to remember • No new information here • Not a summary • Be sure you have presented data that support your conclusions

organize material for subsequent communication will function more efficiently than one for whom organization is an afterthought. The physician who is able to use language precisely and economically will often function more effectively.

REFERENCES

1. Cegala DJ, Marinelli T, Post D. The effects of patient communication skills training on compliance. *Arch Fam Med* 2000;9(1):57–64.
2. Benbassat J, Baumal R. Teaching doctor-patient interviewing skills using an integrated learner and teacher-centered approach. *Am J Med Sci* 2003;322(6):349–357.
3. Kalet A, Pugnaire MP, Cole-Kelly K, et al. Teaching communication in clinical clerkships: models from the Macy Initiative in health communications. *Acad Med* 2004;79(6):511–520.
4. Program Requirements for Residency Education in Otolaryngology. Available online at; www.acgme.org. Accessed January 2006.
5. Raksha J, Ling FW, Jaeger J. Assessment of a 360-degree instrument to evaluate residents competency in interpersonal and communication skills. *Acad Med* 2004;79(5):458–463.
6. The Health Care Communication Group. *Writing, speaking and communication skills for health professionals.* New Haven, CT: Yale University Press; 2001.
7. Bailey BJ. What is an author? *Laryngoscope* 2000;110:1787–1788.
8. Lucente FE. *Preparing, presenting and evaluating medical communications. Continuing education program monograph series.* Rochester, MN: American Academy of Otolaryngology–Head and Neck Surgery Foundation; 1982.

Index

Note: Page numbers followed by *f* indicate figures; those followed by *t* indicate tables.

A

A-to-T flap, after Mohs surgery, 2396–2397
Abbe flap, in lip reconstruction, 1541*f*, 1543–1545, 1544*f*–1545*f*
Abdominal injuries, in trauma patients, 929–930
Abductor spasmodic dysphonia, laryngeal dysfunction and, 876–877
Abrasions, facial soft tissue, management of, 937
Abrikossoff tumor, 2789
Abscess(es)
    antimicrobial agents in, 64
    cerebral, 123
        in otitis media, 2047, 2050
        in rhinosinusitis, 500*f*, 501
    epidural, in rhinosinusitis, 500, 500*f*
    orbital, 495
    periosteal, transcaruncular drainage of, 499, 499*f*
    retropharyngeal, in pediatric patients, 1070, 1071*f*, 1072*f*
    septal. *See* Septal abscesses
    subdural
        in otitis media, 2048, 2051
        in rhinosinusitis, 500–501, 501*f*
    subperiosteal, in rhinosinusitis, 495, 496*f*
    vestibular, 616, 616*f*
Accent method, of voice therapy, 885
    common applications to voice disorders, 889*t*
Acetaminophen, 232–233
Achalasia, 760–761, 761*f*
Acid reflux disease, obstructive sleep apnea and, 654
Acinic cell carcinoma, salivary gland, 1519, 1520*f*
Ackerman tumor, 1731, 2789
Acne rosacea, 2734, 2735*f*
    treatment of, 2745
Acne scarring, 1420-nm dermal collagen stimulating laser in, 2728–2729, 2728*f*
Acoustic neuroma, 120–121, 1981–1982, 1981*f*, 1982*f*
    computed tomography in, 89
    removal of, facial nerve monitoring during, 1956

Acoustic reflectromety, in otitis media, 1270
Acoustic rhinometry, 315, 322
Acoustic stapedial reflex measurement, 1932–1933
Acquired immunodeficiency syndrome. *See also* Human immunodeficiency virus infection
    clinical manifestations of, 266–272
    defining and staging of, 266
    dermatologic conditions in, 267–268, 269*t*
        treatment of, 269*t*
    epidemiology of, 263–264
    historical background of, 263
    HIV virology and, 264–265
    larynx in, 271
    manifestations of, 263–275
    neck in, 271–272
    nose and paranasal sinuses in, 269–270
    oral cancer in, 1558
    oral cavity and pharynx in, 270–271
    otologic manifestations of, 268–269
    postexposure prophylaxis of, 273*t*, 274
    precautions for otolaryngologist, 273, 273*t*
    stomatitis due to, 598
    transmission of, occupational risk of, 272–274
Acral lentiginous melanoma, 1470. *See also* Malignant melanoma
Acrocephalosyndactyly, type I, 1376–1377, 1377*f*
Acromegaly, obstructive sleep apnea and, 653–654
Actinic cheilitis, 2731, 2734*f*
Actinic keratoses, 1459, 1459*f*, 2731
    treatment of, 2744
Actinomycosis, 186, 186*f*, 383–384, 384*f*, 627
Acupuncture, and traditional Chinese medicine, 2799–2800
Acyclovir
    in herpes simplex virus stomatitis, 580
    in varicella zoster virus stomatitis, 581
Addison disease, 162
Adductor spasmodic dysphonia, laryngeal dysfunction and, 876–877

Adeno-associated viral vectors, 1394
    in gene therapy, 1394
Adenocarcinoma
    ceruminous, 2013
    esophageal, 747, 748*f*, 766–767
    salivary gland, 1519–1520
        polymorphous low-grade, 1520
    sinonasal, 1483. *See also* Sinonasal tumors
Adenoid(s). *See also* Tonsil(s)
    anatomy, 1183–1184, 1184*f*, 1185*t*
    clinical evaluation, 1188–1189, 1192*t*
    diseases in, 1183
        clinical classification of, 1187–1188, 1187*t*
        complications of, 1195*t*
        management of, 1193–1194, 1193*t*
        pathogenesis of, 1187
    enlargement of, 1234*f*
    immunology of, 1187
    microbiology of, 1186–1187
    microorganisms commonly cultured from, 1186*t*
Adenoid cystic carcinoma, 2013
    lacrimal, 1509
    salivary gland, 541–542, 543*f*, 1519, 1519*f*
    sinonasal, 1483–1484. *See also* Sinonasal tumors
    tracheal, 1794–1795, 1794*t*
Adenoidectomy. *See also* Tonsillectomy
    complications of, 1195*t*
    controversies in, 1199
        certain indications for, 1199–1200
        efficacy for recurrent otitis media in children with tympanostomy tubes, 1204*t*
        elective indications for, 1202
            obstructive adenoids and adenoiditis, 1202–1203
            recurrent/chronic sinusitis, 1203
            with or without tonsillectomy, 1203
        recommendations for the clinician, 1206–1207, 1207*t*
    indications for, 1193*t*
    for otitis media prophylaxis, 1272–1273
Adenoiditis, acute, chronic, or recurrent acute, 1188, 1192*t*

Adenoma
  ceruminous, 2012–2013
  mediastinal, 1651
  of middle ear, 1970*f*
  parathyroid, 1647
    imaging of, 96
  pituitary. *See* Pituitary adenoma
  pleomorphic, 2013
    parotid surgery and, 561
      management of recurrences,
        561–562
    of salivary gland, 538, 539*f*
    of salivary glands, malignant
      variations of, 542–543
  salivary
    monomorphic, 1518
    pleomorphic, 1515–1516, 1517*t*
    sinonasal, 1483
  thyroid, 1632
Adenoma sebaceum, 2736–2737, 2736*f*
  treatment of, 2746
Adenomatoid odontogenic cyst,
  1575–1576
Adenomatous tumors, of middle ear,
  2014–2015
Adenotonsillar hypertrophy, in pediatric
  patients, 1074, 1075*f*
Adenotonsillar surgery, in children,
  1059–1060
Adenoviral vectors, in gene therapy,
  1392–1393, 1393*f*, 1394*f*
Adrenal gland
  anatomy and physiology of, 161
  dysfunction of, 162
Adrenal insufficiency, preoperative
  management of, 222
Adrenocortical insufficiency, 162
Adrenocorticotropic hormone,
  156–157, 157*f*
  deficiency of, 158
  excess secretion of, 158
Advancement flaps, 2363–2366, 2365*f*
Aerodigestive foreign bodies,
  1162–1163
  workup, 1163–1164, 1163*f*, 1164*f*
Aerodigestive tract. *See also under* Head
  and neck
  congenital anomalies of
    anatomy and physiology,
      1119–1120
    adult versus pediatric larynx, 1121*f*
    common types, 1122*t*
      esophagus, 1130–1131
      larynx
        glottis, 1126–1127
        subglottis, 1127–1128, 1128*f*
        supraglottis, 1126
      nose, 1124–1126
      oropharynx, 1126, 1127*f*
      trachea, 1128
      vascular, 1129–1130

evaluation and diagnosis, 1120–1122
  endoscopic evaluation, 1123–1124
    position of infant for,
      1125–1126*f*
  physical examination, 1122–1123
  radiologic examination, 1123
  fetal development of, 1120*f*
endoscopic evaluation of, 745–753
postoperative leaks in, dysphagia and,
  730, 731*f*
radiographic anatomy of, normal,
  722–723*f*, 724
radiographic examination of, 721–732
Agency for Healthcare Policy and
  Research, 1419
Aging. *See also* Elderly patients
  auditory and vestibular systems and,
    2257–2264
  biology of, 235–236
  cell-culture studies in, 235–236
  factors influencing, 2668
  hearing changes and, 238–239,
    2258–2263. *See also*
    Presbycusis
  hearing loss and, 2258–2263
  physiology of, 2665–2666, 2666*f*
  sense of taste and, 576
  theories of, 235–236
  of upper face, management of, 2668
  vision loss and, 128–129
  wound healing and, 207–208
Agnosia, olfactory, 293
Agoraphobia, vestibular dysfunction
  and, 2319
Air embolism
  as complication of mastoid surgery,
    2110
  following cranial-base surgery,
    1850–1851
  during otitis media surgery, 2053
Airflow, regulation of, larynx in, 699
Airway. *See also* Upper airway obstruction
  anatomy of, 693, 694*f*
    and function of, 693–702
    physiology of, and pathophysiology
      of, 1095–1098, 1096*f*, 1097*t*,
      1098*f*, 1099*f*
  assessment of, for induction of
    anesthesia, 152
  complex problems of, 771–783
    case report of, 779–780, 780*f*
    general considerations in, 771
    management methods in, 771–779,
      781*f*, 782*f*
    results of, 780–781
  congenital malformations of, 1056
  emergency management of, 788–790,
    799, 799*f*
  glottic obstruction of, in pediatric
    patients, 1066–1067, 1066*f*,
    1067*f*

imaging of, in children, 1063–1078
initial management, in bilateral vocal
  fold paralysis, 862–863
larynx and protection of, 821
nasal. *See* Nasal airway
normal, 1063, 1064*f*
securing of, for induction of
  anesthesia, 152–153
subglottic obstruction of, 1067–1069,
  1067*f*
supraglottic obstruction of,
  1065–1066, 1065*f*
trauma to, primary survey of,
  920–923, 921*f*, 922*f*
Airway management
  and anesthesia, 152–153
  in elderly patients, 244
  in lip cancer, 1548
  in stridor, 1109
Airway obstruction
  in pediatric patient, 1063–1069
  physiology of, 648–649, 649*f*
  after thyroidectomy, 1643–1644
Airway stents, upper airway obstruction,
  and use of, 812
Albright syndrome, 2789
Alcohol use/abuse
  fetal alcohol syndrome and, 1386,
    1386*f*
  oral cancer and, 1554, 1555
  surgery in, 233
Aldosterone, secretion of, 161, 162*f*
Alexander syndrome, 2789
Alexander's Law, 1919
Alfentanil, 148
Alimentary bypass, in chronic
  aspiration, 1113
Allergens, 338–339
Allergic angiitis granulomatosis, 176
Allergic rhinitis, 353
  clinical presentation of, 355–356
  history taking in, 356
  immunotherapy in, 360
  impact on asthma, 354*f*
  management of, guidelines for,
    361–362
  physical examination in, 356–357
  and rhinosinusitis, 407
  treatment of
    allergen avoidance in, 358
    pharmacotherapy for, 358–360,
      358*t*
  treatment plan for, 361*f*
Allergy
  antigen exposure in
    early response to, 339, 341*f*
    late response to, 339–341, 340*f*
  aspirin, 396–397
  to chemotherapeutic drugs, 1438,
    1438*t*
  development of, 338–339

diagnosis of, 347
food, otitis media and, 1267
immunology and, 335–349
immunotherapy in, 55
laryngitis and, 830t, 835
nasal polyps and, 397–398
neural component of, 341–342
therapy of, 347
vasculitides and, 176
Allergy testing, in rhinitis, 357–358
Alloderm, for soft-tissue augmentation, 2767
Alopecia
  androgenetic
    medical treatment of, 2749–2750
    surgical treatment of
      hairline design for, 2750, 2750f
      patient evaluation for, 2750–2751
    treatment of, 2749t
  etiology of, 2749t
  following forehead lift, 2681
  following rhytidectomy, 2647, 2648f
  hair transplantation in. See Hair transplantation
  Juri flap in, 2757–2758, 2757f
  management of, 2749–2759
    anesthesia for, 2751
  scalp reduction in. See Scalp reduction
  tissue expansion in, 2755–2757, 2756f
  in women, 2751
Alport syndrome, 50, 2789
  hearing loss in, 1305t, 1313
Alternative medicine, 2797–2804
  acupuncture and traditional Chinese, 2799–2800
  ayurvedic, 2801–2802
  body work, 2802–2803
  chiropractic, 2802
  homeopathy, 2800–2801
  naturopathic, 2798–2799
  osteopathic, 2801
  psychoneuroimmunology, 2803
Alveolar carcinoma, 1563–1564. See also Oral cancer
Alveolar nerve, inferior, nerve blocks of, 143
Alveolar rhabdomyosarcoma, in children, 1364–1366, 1364t, 1365t
Alveolus, of mandible, 961f
Amblyopia, 136–137
  definition of, 136
  detection of, 136–137
  treatment of, 137
Ameloblastic fibroma, 1577, 1577f
Ameloblastoma, 1574, 1575f
Amifostine, in xerostomia, 557–558
Amikacin, 60, 61
  ototoxicity of, 1298

Aminoglycosides, 60–61
  in aspiration, 1113
  laryngeal dysfunction and, 875
  ototoxicity of, 1298
Aminopenicillins, 58
Amiodarone, 225
Amoxicillin, 58
  for otitis media, 1270, 1271
  for prophylaxis, 1204t
Amoxicillin-clavulanate, 58
Amphotericin B, 420–421
Ampicillin, 58
Ampicillin-sulbactam (Unasyn), 58
Amplification, accessory devices providing, 2289–2291, 2290t
Amyloidosis, 192, 193f
  head and neck manifestations of, 192
  laryngitis and, 830t, 832
Amyotrophic lateral sclerosis, 115
  laryngeal dysfunction and, 872
Anaplastic thyroid carcinoma, 54
Anatomic stimulation, 74–76
Anesthesia
  airway management and, 152–153
  for alopecia management, 2751
  for blepharoplasty, 2614–2615
  emergencies associated with, 151t
  for endoscopic procedures, 153
    in children, 1102
  general, 144–147
  and intraoperative monitoring of facial nerve, 1954–1955
  local, 141–144
  monitoring of, 150–152
  in obstructive sleep apnea, 659–660
  in posttraumatic nasal deformity management, 2582–2583, 2582f, 2586, 2586f, 2587f
  for rhinoplasty, 2537–2538
  for rhytidectomy, 2634
  in turbinate hypertrophy, 328–329
Anesthesia machine, 150–151
Anesthesiology, 141–154
Anesthetic agents
  amide, 141
  ancillary, 147
  ester, 141
  inhalational, 144–146, 144t
  intravenous, 146–147, 146t
  local, 141–143, 142t
  nerve blocks, 143–144
  neurophysiologic effects of, 1830t
Aneurysmal bone cyst, of jaw, 1582
Angelman syndrome, 46
Angioedema, laryngitis and, 830t, 834–835
Angiofibroma
  juvenile, 448, 1075–1076, 1075f, 1815–1817, 1816f
    endoscopic surgery in, 450, 450f
    recurrence following, 451

epistaxis in, 507
nasopharyngeal, 441–442, 441f
Angiogenesis, vascular endothelial growth factor and, 100, 100t
Angiography, of salivary glands, 530
Angiolymphoid hyperplasia, 1823
Angiomas
  cherry, 2735
  spider, treatment of, 2746
Angiomatosis, bacillary, 183
  in HIV infection, 267
Angiosarcoma, 1819, 1819f
Angiotensin II, 161
Angle, of mandible, 961f
  dental occlusion, classification of, 961, 962f
  fracture
    management, 967–968
    treatment options, 965t
Animal bites, management of, 945–946
Animal-scratch disease, salivary glands and, 547–548
Ankylosis, of temporomandibular joint, 634
Anosmia, 292–293
  aging and, 292
  causes of, 293–296
  after sinus surgery, 489
Anoxia, perinatal, hearing loss and, 1299
Anterior neck dissection, 1596
Anterolateral thigh flap, 2373–2375, 2374f
Anti-IgE, in rhinitis, 360
Antibiotics. See also specific agents
  activity against target pathogens, 62t
  in acute rhinosinusitis, 413–415, 414t
  in frontal sinus fractures, 1011
  in herpes simplex virus stomatitis, 580
  in infections of deep spaces of neck, 665
  in intracranial complications of rhinosinusitis, 502
  in nasal polyps, 399
  in odontogenic infections, 629
  in orbital complications of rhinosinusitis, 497–498
  in otitis media, 2048, 2051
  in otosyphilis, 2324
  ototopical, ototoxicity of, 2201–2202, 2202t
  in recurrent aphthous stomatitis, 597
Antibodies, 1409–1410. See also Immunoglobulins
  monoclonal, 54, 54t, 1431–1432
    for extranodal lymphoma, 1624, 1624t, 1625–1626
Anticholinergic sprays, topical, in rhinitis, 360
Anticholinesterase agents, 150

Anticoagulants
   preoperative management in use of,
      218
   in thromboembolic disease, 220
Anticonvulsants, 251
Antidiuretic hormone, 156, 156f
   syndrome of inappropriate secretion
      of, 158, 222–223
Antifungal agents, 420–421, 423
Antigens
   in immune response, 1406–1408,
      1407f
   tumor cell, 1408–1409
Antihistamines
   in nasal polyps, 399
   in rhinitis, 358–359, 358t
Antiinflammatory agents, in sudden
      sensory hearing loss, 2234
Antimalarial agents, ototoxicity of, 1298
Antimicrobial agents, 57–61. See also
      specific types and agents
   in surgical prophylaxis, 64–65
   treatment strategies using, 61–64
Antimicrobial proteins, innate
      immunity and, 337
Antisense gene therapy, 1399
Antitussives, 1116
Antivertiginous medications,
      mechanism of action of, 2328
Antiviral agents, in sudden sensory
      hearing loss, 2234
Antral choanal polyp, 396
Antrostomy
   inferior meatal, complications of, 480
   middle meatal, complications of, 480
Anxiety, vestibular dysfunction and,
      2319
Apert syndrome, 1376–1377, 1377f,
      2789
Aphthous stomatitis, recurrent
   clinical features of, 596, 596f
   differential diagnosis of, 596–597
   etiology of, 596
   histopathology of, 596–597
   treatment of, 597
Apnea, after neck dissection, 1605
Apoptosis, in radiation therapy,
      1444–1445
APUDomas, 163
Arnold-Chiari malformations, laryngeal
      dysfunction and, 868, 870f
Arnold nerve, 2789
ARNSHL genes, in hearing loss,
      1304–1307, 1305t–1306t
Artecoll, for soft-tissue augmentation,
      2767–2768
Arterial dissection, headache in, 257
Arterial supply
   for central nervous system,
      1827–1828, 1828f
   to nose, 2517

Arteriosclerosis, ocular manifestations
      of, 138–139, 139t
Arteriovenous fistula, 1817, 1818f
Arteriovenous malformations, 1356
Artery(ies). See also Blood vessels
   anterior ethmoidal, ligation of, in
      epistaxis, 510–511
   maxillary
      embolization of, in posterior
         epistaxis, 512
      transantral ligation of, in epistaxis,
         513
   to salivary glands, 520
   sphenopalatine, endoscopic ligation
      of, in epistaxis, 511–512, 512f
Arthritis, rheumatoid. See Rheumatoid
      arthritis
Arthrocentesis, 631
   in disorders of temporomandibular
      joint, 636–637, 636f
Artificial larynx, following
      laryngectomy, 1779–1780
Arytenoidectomy
   endoscopic partial laser, 864
   endoscopic total laser, 864, 864f
Arytenoids
   adduction of, for unilateral vocal fold
      paralysis, 857–859
   larynx and, 817–819, 819
Ascher syndrome, 2789
Aspergillosis, 387
Aspiration
   aspirated materials in, 1111–1112
   cricopharyngeal myotomy in, 738,
      738t
   diagnosis of, 734t, 1112–1113
   differential diagnosis of, 1111t
   enhancement of glottic closure in,
      737
   etiology of, 733–734, 734f
   evaluation and diagnosis in, 735,
      735f, 1110–1112
   identification of, 733
   management of, 733–743, 741f,
      1113–1114
      alternative strategies in, 737t
      decision making in, 735–736
      initial, 736, 736f
      nonsurgical, 737
      surgical, 737, 739–741, 739f, 740f
      therapeutic options in, 736–741
   medialization thyroplasty in, 737,
      738t
   partial supraglottic closure in,
      738–739
   predisposing factors for, 1110, 1111t
   radiography and diagnostic studies
      in, 1112–1113
   in sensory loss, 735
   tracheostomy and, 735
Aspiration biopsy. See Biopsy

Aspirin, 217
   hypersensitivity to, 396–397
Aspirin-exacerbated respiratory
      disease
   aspirin sensitivity in, 396
   clinical presentation of, 396
   diagnosis of, 396–397
   pathophysiology of, 397
Assistive listening devices
   FM wireless system, 2289–2291
   hearing aids and, 2279–2293. See also
      Hearing aids
   infrared systems, 2291
   soundfield systems, 2291
Asthma, 396
   allergic rhinitis impact on, 354f
Astrocytoma, 120
Ataxia, in elderly patients, 239–240
Ataxia syndrome, familial, medical
      management of, 2326
Atazanavir, 266
Atelectasis, preoperative management
      of, 227
Atelectatic sinus, 436–437, 437f
Atenolol, 224
Atracurium, 150
Atresia
   aural. See Aural atresia
   auricular, 1055
   choanal. See Choanal atresia
   esophageal, tracheoesophageal fistula
      and, 1128, 1129f, 1130f
   supraglottic or glottic, laryngeal
      stenosis and, 1135
Atrophy
   multisystem, laryngeal dysfunction
      and, 871–872
      common voice therapy applications
         for, 889t
   severe vocal fold, aging and,
      appropriate voice therapy
      referrals for, 890
Atropine, 225
Audiogram, in otosclerosis, 2127–2129,
      2128f
Audiologic assessment. See also Hearing
      evaluation
   indications for, 1939
Audiologic test battery, 1927–1933
Audiometry. See also Hearing evaluation
   in otitis media, 1269–1270
   pure-tone, 1927–1930, 1928f
   speech, 1931
   in vestibular schwannomas, 2211
Auditory artery, internal, thrombosis of,
      119
Auditory brainstem responses,
      1933–1937, 1934f, 1935f,
      1944–1945
   testing of, 1281–1282
   in infant screening, 1279, 1289

Auditory canal
    external
        development of, 1871, 1872*f*
        embryology of, 2027
        imaging of, 1963–1967
        and pinna, neoplasms of,
            2010–2014
        stenosis of, as complication of
            temporal bone trauma, 2076
    internal
        lesions of, 1981–1984, 1981*f*,
            1982*f*, 1983*f*
        neoplasms of, 2020–2023
        stenosis of, following surgery for
            aural atresia, 2039
Auditory evoked responses, 1933–1937,
    1934*f*, 1935*f*
    cortical, 1936–1937
    recording options, 1951, 1951*t*
Auditory function, peripheral and
    central, assessment of,
    1927–1942
Auditory nerve, physiology of, 1891*f*,
    1893–1895, 1894*f*, 1895*f*,
    1896*f*
Auditory neuropathy, 1307
Auditory processing disorders,
    1286–1287
    assessment of, 1938–1939
    central auditory nervous system
        dysfunction and, 1938
    test battery, 1938–1939
Auditory prostheses, implantable,
    2265–2277
Auditory steady-state response, 1282,
    1902
Auditory system, and vestibular system,
    aging and, 2257–2264
Augmentin (amoxicillin-clavulanate),
    58
Aural atresia, congenital, 2027–2040
    audiometric evaluation in, 2029
    classification of, 2028–2029
    computed tomography in,
        2029–2030, 2031*f*, 2032*f*
    grading system for, 2032*t*
    medical management of, 2030
    patient evaluation in, 2029
    physical examination in, 2029–2030
    surgery for, 2030–2033
        complications of, 2038–2039
        facial nerve monitoring during,
            1957, 1957*t*
        findings in, 2037, 2037*f*
        hearing following, 2038
        meatoplasty in, 2036
        patient selection for, 2030–2031,
            2031*f*, 2032*f*
        skin grafting in, 2036–2037, 2036*f*
        technique of, 2033–2037, 2033*f*,
            2034*f*, 2035*f*, 2036*f*

        drilling canal in, 2033–2034,
            2033*f*, 2034*f*, 2035*f*
        incision in, 2033
        meatoplasty in, 2036
        middle ear surgery in, 2034,
            2035*f*
        ossicular chain exposure in, 2034,
            2035*f*
        skin grafting in, 2036–2037,
            2036*f*
        tympanic membrane grafting in,
            2035–2036
        timing of, 2031–2032
        unilateral and bilateral, repair of,
            2030
Aural immittance (impedance)
    measurement, 1931
Auricle(s)
    anatomy of, 1987, 1988*f*
    development of, 1870–1871, 1871*f*
        anomalies of, 1870–1871
    major malformation of, 2028–2029
    minor malformation of, 2029
Auricular hematoma, management of,
    943–944, 944*f*, 945*f*
Auricular nerve, great, anatomy of,
    518–519
Auriculotemporal nerve, anatomy of,
    519–520
Auriculotemporal syndrome, 555
Auto-titrating positive airway pressure
    device, in obstructive sleep
    apnea, 656
Autografts, for soft-tissue augmentation,
    2766–2767
Autoimmune disease, of salivary glands,
    in children, 1249
Autosomal dominant inheritance, 42*f*,
    43, 1371–1373, 1372*f*
Autosomal recessive inheritance, 42–43,
    42*f*, 1372*f*, 1373
Aveillis syndrome, 2789
Avelox (Moxifloxacin), 60
Avulsion injuries
    auricular, 943–944, 944*f*
    dental, 1345
    facial soft tissue, management of,
        939, 939*f*
Ayurvedic medicine, 2801–2802
Azelastine, 399
Azithromycin, 59, 183
Aztreonam (Azactam), 59

B
B cell(s), 344–345, 1406. *See also*
    Lymphocytes
    in head and neck cancer, 1410–1411
B-cell lymphoma, in children,
    1361–1363, 1362*t*
Bárány syndrome, 2790
Babinski-Nageotte syndrome, 119, 2789

Bacillary angiomatosis, 183
    in HIV infection, 267
Baclofen, 260
Bacterial infections, 183–187, 382–386
    pharyngitis due to, 603–606
Bacterial meningitis. *See* Meningitis,
    bacterial
Bacteroides sp., pediatric rhinosinusitis
    and, 1232, 1232*t*
Bactrim (trimethoprim-
    sulfamethoxazole), 61
Bactroban (mupirocin), 61
Baelz syndrome, 2790
Balance
    drug effects on, 2262*t*
    findings in common disorders, 1925*t*
    function tests of, 1917–1926, 1918*t*
Barbiturates, 146–147, 230
Bardach two-flap technique, for cleft
    lip, 1328
Barium swallow
    to demonstrate aspiration, 735, 735*f*
    modified, of upper aerodigestive
        tract, 722–723
Barre-Lieou syndrome, 2790
Barrett esophagitis, 746*f*, 747, 748, 2790
Bartholin duct, 2790
Basal cell carcinoma. *See* Skin cancer
Basal cell nevus syndrome, 1572
Basilar artery, infarction of, 118
Basilar impression, 2312
Basophils, 342–343
Battle sign, 2790
Baudet technique, 944*f*
Behavioral audiologic assessment,
    1279–1281
    in otitis media, 1269–1270
Behavioral observation audiometry,
    1269–1270, 1280
Behavioral therapy, in obstructive sleep
    apnea, 655
Behçet disease, 178–179, 2790
Bell palsy, 2147–2148
Belting, as vocal performance style, 898
Benedikt's syndrome, 119
Benign mixed tumor
    of lacrimal gland, 1508–1509, 1508*f*
    of salivary gland, 1515–1516
Benzodiazepines, 147, 230
Bernard cheiloplasty, Webster
    modification of, 1546–1547,
    1546*f*
Besnier-Boeck-Schaumann syndrome,
    2790
β-blockade therapy, preoperative, in
    cardiac abnormalities,
    223–224
β-lactam antibiotics, 59
Bezold abscess, 2790
Biaxin (Clarithromycin), 59
Bicoronal flap incision, 1495*f*

Bilobed flaps, 2363, 2364f
  in cutaneous nasal defects,
      2427–2431, 2430f
    after Mohs surgery, 2396, 2396f
Biologic materials, as implants, 2346t,
      2347
Biologic therapy, for head and neck
      cancer, 1431
Biopsy
  of bone marrow, in extranodal
      lymphoma, 1623
  image guidance for, 69–71
  of lip, 1537
  of lymph nodes
      indications for, 272, 272t
      in melanoma, 1472–1474
      in oral cancer, 1560
      sentinel node, 103–104, 1591
  of melanoma, 1471
  of N0 neck
      sentinel node, 1615, 1617–1618
      ultrasound-guided, 1614
  of olfactory system, 302
  of oral cavity, 1559, 1560
  of parathyroid, 1650
  of salivary gland, 558–559
      fine-needle aspiration, 1522
      surgical, 1523
  sentinel lymph node, 103–104
  of sinonasal tumors, 1486–1487
  of thyroid, 1636–1637
Birthmarks, vascular, 1353–1354, 1354f
Bisoprolol, 224
Bisphosphonates, 165
  in osteomyelitis, 626–627
Bites, animal and human, management
      of, 945–946
Bivalirudin, 218
Blastomycosis, 188, 386
  laryngitis and, 830
  South American, 188
Bleeding. See also Hemorrhage
  as complication of mastoid surgery, 2110
  intraoperative and postoperative,
      testing/management in,
      218–219
  from nose. See Epistaxis
  postoperative, in sinonasal tumor
      surgery, 1497–1498
Bleeding diatheses, epistaxis in, 507–508
Bleomycin, toxicity of, 1627
Blepharitis, 131
Blepharoplasty, 2611–2625, 2621t
  anesthesia for, 2614–2615
  complications of, 2623–2624, 2624t
  diagnosis for, 2611t
  in elderly patients, 243
  evaluation of lower lid for, 2613–2614,
      2613f
  evaluation of upper lid-brow complex
      for, 2612–2613

lower-lid
    skin-muscle flap approach for,
        2617–2620, 2618f, 2619f,
        2620f, 2621f
    transconjunctival approach for,
        2620–2623, 2621f, 2622f,
        2623f
  medical history taking for, 2612
  motivation for, 2611–2612
  patient evaluation for, 2611–2612
  photodocumentation for, 2614
  postoperative care following, 2623
  preparation for, 2614
  upper-lid, 2616–2617, 2617f
      and brow lift, surgical procedure
          for, 2672
      surgical marking for, 2615–2616,
          2615f, 2616f
Blindness. See Vision loss
Blood components, 216t
  preoperative transfusion of, 216–217
Blood dyscrasia, ocular manifestations
      of, 138
Blood flow, cerebral, 1829–1830
Blood loss, excessive, from
      mastoidectomy, 2053
Blood supply. See specific organs
Blood transfusions. See Transfusions
Blood vessels. See also Artery(ies);
      Vein(s)
  anomalies of
      causing tracheal compression, 1107,
          1107f, 1108f
      stridor in, 1107–1108
      tinnitus in, 2237–2238, 2238t
  of forehead, 2663–2664, 2664f
  injury to
      as complication of sinus surgery,
          489
      in penetrating neck trauma, 1024
  of nose, 505–507, 506f
Blowin fractures, in children, 1346
Blowout, jugular vein, after neck
      dissection, 1606
Blowout fractures, in children, 1347
Blue nevus, 2739, 2739f
  treatment of, 2747
Blue rubber bleb, 1356, 1356f
Body, of mandible, 961f
  fracture in
      management, 967, 968f
      treatment options, 965t
Body work, as alternative medicine,
      2802–2803
Boerhaave syndrome, 768–769, 769f,
      2790
Bogorad syndrome, 2790
Bohn syndrome, 2790
Bone(s)
  complications of, in rhinosinusitis,
      502–503, 503f

diseases of, otologic manifestations
      of, 2162–2164
  malignant tumors of, imaging of,
      445, 445f
  tumors of. See also specific types and
      sites
      imaging of, 443–445, 444f
Bone densitometry, in
      hyperparathyroidism, 1649
Bone healing, 1027–1028
  wound healing and, 210
Bone marrow biopsy, in extranodal
      lymphoma, 1623
Bonnet syndrome, 2790
Botox
  for brow adjustment, 2764
  complications associated with,
      2764–2765
  contraindications to, 2762
  cosmetic applications of, 2762–2763
  in glabellar rhytids, 2763, 2763f
  in gustatory sweating, 556–557
  indications for, 2762
  and injectable fillers, cosmetic uses
      of, 2761–2769
  laryngeal, for bilateral vocal fold
      paralysis, 863
  laryngeal site identification,
      electromyography and, 881
  in lateral periorbital rhytids, 2763,
      2763f
  mechanism of action of, 2762
  in parotid cysts, 557
  for platysmal banding, 2764
  in transverse forehead rhytids, 2763,
      2763f
  in vertical lip rhytids, 2764
Botryoid tumors, 2017
Bottle feeding, with cleft lip/cleft palate,
      1320
Botulism, laryngeal dysfunction and,
      875
Bourneville-Pringle syndrome, 2790
Bovine collagen, for soft-tissue
      augmentation, 2765–2766
Bowel disease, inflammatory, 389
Bowen disease, 1459, 2790
Brachytherapy, 1442–1443, 1443t. See
      also Radiation therapy
  in recurrent nasopharyngeal cancer,
      1665–1666, 1665f
Brain. See also under Central nervous
      system; Cerebral
  injury to, as complication of sinus
      surgery, 489
  metastases to, 121
  radiation effects on, 1452
  venous drainage system of,
      1828–1829, 1828f
Brain abscess, 123
  in otitis media, 2047, 2050

Brain herniation
  in cholesteatoma, 2091
  in otitis media, 2053
Brainstem, vestibular, 1913–1914, 1913f
Branchiootorenal syndrome, 1305t,
      1310, 1377–1378, 1378f
Breast feeding, with cleft lip/cleft palate,
      1320
Breathing. See also Respiration
  sleep-disordered. See Sleep-disordered
      breathing
  trauma and, primary survey of,
      923–924, 923f, 924f
Brissaud-Marie syndrome, 2790
Bronchiectasis, in Kartagener syndrome,
      1381
Bronchoscope
  for endotracheal intubation, 797
  pediatric, 153
  selection of, by age, 1101t
Bronchoscopy, virtual, 81
Brow(s)
  adjustment of, Botox for, 2764
  asymmetries of, forehead lift and,
      2667
Brow lift
  "chemical," 2764
  direct, 2675–2676, 2677f
    technique for, 2675–2676, 2676f
  incisions for, 2668, 2669f
  indirect, 2676–2677
  surgical procedure for, 2676–2677
  and upper blepharoplasty, surgical
      procedure for, 2672
Brown sign, 2790
Brown vertical retraction syndrome,
      2790
Broyle ligament, 2790
Brucellosis, 183
Brunner abscess, 2790
Buccal cancer, 1561–1562. See also Oral
      cancer
Buccal space, odontogenic infections of,
      618, 618f
Bulb press test, 484, 484f
Bulbar palsy, laryngeal dysfunction and,
      872
Bullard laryngoscope, 776–779, 778f,
      779f
Bullets
  cavitation effects of, 1017, 1017f
  rotational ballistics of, 1017, 1018f
Bullous pemphigoid
  pharyngitis in, 611
  stomatitis due to
    clinical features of, 588–589
    differential diagnosis of, 589
    etiology of, 588
    histopathology of, 589
    treatment of, 587–588t, 589
Bupivacaine, 142, 233

Buprenorphine, 148
Bupropion, in smoking replacement
      therapy, 280
Burckhardt dermatitis, 2790
Burkitt lymphoma. See also Lymphoma
  in children, 1361–1363, 1362t
  extranodal, treatment of, 1626
Burns
  chemical, ocular, 135–136
  evaluation and treatment, 946–947,
      947f
  laryngeal stenosis and, 1137
  laryngitis and, 834
  types of, 946
Burton line, 2790
Business, medical. See Medical practice,
      business aspects of
Butorphanol, 148
Buttress system, midface, 975

C
Caffeine, in migraine, 251
Calcifying epithelial odontogenic
      tumor, 1576
Calcitonin, 160, 165, 192
Calcium
  deficiency of, 165
    in thyroid surgery, 222
    after thyroidectomy, 1643–1644
  excess of, 164–165
Calcium carbonate, 222
Calcium gluconate, 222
  for hypocalcemia, after
      thyroidectomy, 1643–1644
Calcium metabolism, parathyroid
      glands and, 159–160, 160f
Calculi, salivary. See Sialolithiasis
Caldwell-Luc approach, indications for,
      365–366, 366t
Caldwell-Luc procedure
  complications of, 482, 489
  in sinusitis, 498
Caloric requirements, daily, 215
Calvaria, anatomy of, 3, 4f
Calvarial bone harvest, 1034f, 1035
Canalicular injuries, of eyelid, 942, 943f
Cancer. See Neoplasms and specific sites
      and types
Candidiasis
  angular, 595, 595f
  atrophic, 595, 595f
  esophageal, 748, 748f, 765
  hyperplastic, 595
  mucocutaneous, 595
  mucosal, in AIDS, 270
  pharyngeal, 608–609
  stomatitis due to
    clinical presentation of, 594–595,
      595f
    etiology of, 594
    histopathology of, 596

treatment of, 596
Canine space, odontogenic infections
      of, 617
Cannon nevus, 2790
CAPE-V (Consensus Auditory-
      Perceptual Evaluation of
      Voice), 825
Capillary hemangiomas, 2736
  orbital, 1502–1503
Capillary malformations, 1353–1354,
      1354f
Capnography, 151–152
Capravirine, 266
Capsaicin, 400
  in oral pain, 576
Carbamazepine, 260
Carbenicillin, 58
Carbon dioxide lasers, 2725–2726. See
      also Laser therapy
  for skin cancer, 1463–1464
Carbunculosis, 1998
Carcinoid tumors, 163
Carcinoma ex-pleomorphic adenoma,
      salivary gland, 1520, 1520f
Cardioembolism, 117
Cardiogenic shock, in trauma patients,
      925–926
Cardiovascular disorders
  β-blockade therapy and, 223–224
  obstructive sleep apnea and, 653
  postoperative, risk factors for, 223
  preoperative management of,
      223–225
Carhart notch, 2790
Carotid artery
  injury to, in temporal bone trauma,
      2076
  internal, balloon occlusion test of,
      1832, 1832t
  rupture of, otitis media and,
      2054–2055
Carotid artery dissection, 1600–1601
Carotid artery rupture, after neck
      dissection, 1606
Carotid body tumors, 1820–1823,
      1822f, 1823f
Carotid drill, in carotid artery injury,
      490t
Cartilage, nasal, for nasal
      reconstruction, 2441, 2444f
Cat-scratch disease, 183
Cataracts
  formation of, 129
  radiation-related, 1452, 1496t
Caustic ingestions
  clinical presentation, 1159, 1159f
  complications, 1161–1162, 1161f,
      1162t
  diagnosis/evaluation, 1159t
  endoscopic appearance of esophageal
      burns, 1160t

Caustic ingestions *(continued)*
  esophageal injuries from, 770,
      1157–1158
  laryngeal stenosis and, 1137
  treatment, 1159–1161, 1161*t*
Cavernous hemangioma, 1811–1812,
      1812*f*
  orbital, 1502
Cavernous sinus disease, 132, 132*f*
Cavernous sinus surgery, 1844–1845
Cavernous sinus thrombosis, 123
  in odontogenic infections, 624–625,
      625*f*
  in rhinosinusitis, 496
Cefaclor (Ceclor), 58–59
Cefazolin (Ancef, Kefzol), 58
Cefdinir (Omnicef), 58
Cefixime (Suprax), 59
Cefotaxime (Claforan), 59
Cefpodoxime proxetil (Vantin), 58
Cefprozil (Cefzil), 58–59
Ceftazidime (Fortaz), 59
Ceftibuten (Cedax), 59
Ceftriaxone (Rocephin), 59
Cefuroxime axetil (Ceftin), 58
Cell death, in radiation therapy,
      1444–1445
Cellulitis
  of lip, 616, 616*f*
  orbital, 123, 495, 496*f*
  preseptal, 493–495, 496*f*
Cemento-ossifying fibroma, of jaw,
      1579–1580, 1580*f*
Central auditory processing disorders,
      1286–1287
Central compartment dissection, 1596
Central giant cell lesion, of jaw,
      1580–1582, 1582*f*
Central nervous system. *See also* Brain
  arterial supply of, 1827–1828, 1828*f*
  auditory, 1892*f*, 1897–1902, 1900*f*
  infections of, headache in, 258–259
  taste disorders and, 575
  tumors of, 120–122
Central venous occlusion, headache in,
      257
Cephalalgia, trigeminal autonomic,
      253–255
Cephalexin (Keflex), 58
Cephalometric roentgenograms, in
      suspected sleep apnea,
      651–652
Cephalometrics, in facial analysis, 2494
Cephalosporins, 58–59
Ceramic implants, 2346–2347, 2346*t*
Cerebellar artery
  anterior inferior, infarction of, 118
  posterior inferior, infarction of, 118
  superior, infarction of, 118
Cerebellopontine angle
  anatomy of, 2207–2209, 2208*f*

lesions of, 1981–1984, 1981*f*, 1982*f*,
      1983*f*
  neoplasms of, 2020–2023
  tumors of, 2207–2230
    complications of, 2223*t*
    diagnosis of, 2213, 2213*t*
    facial nerve monitoring during,
        1956
    vascular, 2226
Cerebral edema
  after cranial-base surgery, 1850
  after neck dissection, 1605
Cerebral metastases, 121
Cerebrospinal fluid
  circulation of, 1829, 1829*f*
  evaluation of, for meningitis, 1847,
      1847*t*
  leakage of
    as complication of mastoid surgery,
        2109–2110
    postoperative, 1498
  production of, 1830
Cerebrospinal fluid fistula
  postoperative
    in cranial-base surgery, 1846–1849
    in sinus surgery, 487
    surgical management of, 1848–1849
  in temporal bone fracture, 2071–2075
  closure of, 2073–2075, 2074*f*
Cerebrospinal fluid pressure, low,
      headache in, 258
Cerebrospinal fluid rhinorrhea,
      endoscopic repair of,
      455–456
Cerebrovascular disease, 117–120
Cerebrovascular system, evaluation of,
      for cranial-base surgery,
      1831–1832, 1832*t*
Cervical contour, ideal, 2651, 2652*f*
Cervical nodes. *See* Lymph nodes
Cervical plexus, nerve block of,
      143–144
Cervical spine injuries, in trauma
      patients, 929*f*
Cervical vascular disorder, headache in,
      257–258
Cervico-oculo-acoustic syndrome, 2796
Cestan-Chenais syndrome, 119,
      2790–2791
Cetuximab, 1431
Chalazion, 131
CHARGE association, 44, 1378
Chédiak-Higashi syndrome, 2791
Cheek, cancer of, 1561. *See also* Oral
      cancer
Cheilitis, actinic, 2731, 2734*f*
Cheilitis granulomatosa, 1382
Cheiloplasty. *See* Lip(s), cancer of,
      surgery for
Chemical peeling, 2717–2723
  aftercare in, 2721

  agents for, 2718, 2719–2720
  in benign facial lesions, 2741–2742,
      2743*t*
  classification of, 2718
  complications of, 2721–2722, 2721*t*
  deep, 2719, 2719*f*
  depth of, factors affecting, 2719–2720
  emergencies associated with, 2721*t*,
      2722
  indications for, and depth of, 2720*t*
  individual sensitivity and, 2720–2721
  medium depth, 2718–2719
  in photodamage, 2717
  procedure for, 2717–2718
  special considerations for,
      2722–2723
  superficial, 2718, 2718*f*
  techniques for, 2720
Chemosensory systems, intranasal, 290
Chemosis, following blepharoplasty,
      2624
Chemotherapy. *See also specific cancers
      and agents*
  agents in
    classification of, 1427–1428, 1428*t*
    in standard regimens, 1430–1431
  clinical trials of, 1428–1429
  combination, 1428, 1432
  complications of, 1437–1438, 1437*t*,
      1438*t*
  oral, 1863–1864, 1863*t*
  efficacy of, 1428*t*
  determinants of, 1427
  for extranodal lymphoma,
      1624–1627
    complications of, 1627
  future directions for, 1438
  for hypopharyngeal cancer,
      1705–1706
  indications for, 1429
  induction (neoadjuvant),
      1435–1437, 1435*t*, 1436*t*
  for laryngeal cancer, 1773–1774
  for melanoma, 1476
  for nasopharyngeal cancer, 1664
  for oral cancer, 1560
  otolaryngologist's role in, 1428
  overview of, 1439
  postoperative adjuvant, 1434
  principles of, 1427–1428
  with radiation therapy, 1429,
      1433–1435, 1433*t*
  in resectable disease, 1435
  for salivary gland tumors, 1528
  for sinonasal cancer, 1488
  targeted, 1428
  in unresectable disease, 1433–1434
Cherry angiomas, 2735
Chiari malformation, 2311–2312, 2311*t*
Chickenpox, 580
Children. *See* Pediatric patients

Chin
  augmentation of, 2701–2707
    contraindications to, 2704t
    evaluation for, 2701–2704, 2702f,
      2702t, 2703f
    implants for, 2704–2705, 2704f
      complications of, 2705–2706,
        2705t
    operative procedure for, 2705
    with sliding genioplasty,
      2706–2707, 2707f
  deficiencies of, 2701
    diagnosis of, 2701, 2702t
    treatment of, 2701, 2703t
    evaluation of, 2701–2704, 2702f,
      2702t, 2703f
  and neck, assessment of, for plastic
    surgery of face, 2491–2492,
    2491f
  position of, 2652–2653, 2653f
Chinese medicine, traditional,
    acupuncture and, 2799–2800
Chiropractic medicine, 2802
Chlorambucil, for extranodal
    lymphoma, 1624–1627,
    1624t
Chloramphenicol (Chloromycetin), 60
Chloroma, orbital, 1504
Chloromycetin (Chloramphenicol), 59
Chloroquine, ototoxicity of, 1298
Chlorphenesin, 260
Choanal atresia, 1055, 1071–1073, 1074f
  airway obstruction and, 808
  nasal obstruction in, 313, 1087, 1088f
Cholesteatoma, 121, 1982, 1983f,
    2007–2009, 2081–2092, 2226
  acquired, 2081–2082
    imaging of, 1969–1970, 1969f
  as complication of temporal bone
    trauma, 2076
  complications of, and emergencies in,
    2089–2091, 2089t
  congenital, 1970–1971, 1982, 1983f,
    2008, 2081, 2082f
  diagnosis of, 2008
  of external ear, imaging of, 1964,
    1965f
  facial paralysis in, 2046
  incidence of, 2008
  lateral attic wall erosion, 2117–2119,
    2118f, 2119f
  morphologic appearance of, 2008
  pathogenesis of, 2082–2084, 2082t,
    2083f, 2084f
  preoperative evaluation of,
    2085–2088, 2087f
  prevention of, 2084–2085, 2087f
  sinus tympani retraction, 2117
  surgical anatomy of, 2084–2085,
    2084f, 2085f, 2086f, 2087f
  surgical goals of, 2087–2088, 2088f

  surgical management of, 2032–2033,
    2088–2089, 2088f, 2089t
  terminology associated with,
    2007–2008
  treatment of, 2008–2009
Cholesterol granuloma
  causes of, 2019
  diagnosis of, 2019
  imaging in, 1968–1969, 1969f
  of petrous apex, 2019
Chondritis, 1998
Chondrodermatitis nodularis chronica
    helicis, 2014, 2796
Chondrosarcoma
  imaging of, 445, 445f
  sinonasal, 1486. See also Sinonasal
    tumors
  of skull base, 2017–2018
CHOP regimen, for extranodal
    lymphoma, 1624–1627, 1624t
Chorda tympani
  damage to, taste phantoms and,
    575–576
  taste and, 569–570
  taste disorders and, 574–575
Chordoma, 121–122
  sinonasal, 1485. See also Sinonasal
    tumors
  of skull base, 2018
Choristoma, in middle ear, 2019
Choroidal melanoma, orbital invasion
    by, 1511
Chromosomal anomalies, 44
Chromosomes, 1303
Chronic lymphocytic thyroiditis, 1631
Churg-Strauss syndrome, 176, 381
Chvostek sign, 2791
Chylous fistula
  after neck dissection, 1604–1605
  postoperative, in oral cancer, 1566
Cicatricial pemphigoid
  laryngitis and, 830t, 833
  pharyngitis due to, 610–611
  stomatitis due to
    clinical features of, 586, 588f, 589f
    differential diagnosis of, 586
    etiology of, 586
    histopathology of, 586
    treatment of, 587–588t, 588
Cigarette smoking. See Tobacco use
Ciliary dyskinesia, 396
  primary, 315–316, 407
Ciprofloxacin (Cipro), 60
Circulation, in trauma patients, primary
    survey of, 924–926, 926f
Circulatory reflexes, larynx and, 700
Cisatracurium, 150
Cisplatin, 1428t, 1430
  in metastasis of nasopharyngeal
    cancer, 1668
  ototoxicity of, 1298

Clarithromycin (Biaxin), 59
Cleft lip/cleft palate, 1317–1334
  anatomic deformities in, 1320–1321
  bilateral cleft lip, 1320
  classification of, 1319–1320, 1319f
  embryology of, 1318–1320
  epidemiology of, 1317
  etiology of, 1317–1318, 1318t
  facial growth and, 1320
  feeding in, 1320
  genetics of, 1317–1318, 1318t
  incidence of, 1317–1318
  initial care in, 1320
  nursing care in, 1320
  parental education about, 1334
  prenatal diagnosis of, 1334
  psychosocial concerns in, 1320
  recurrence risk rates for, 1318t
  in Robin sequence, 1383
  surgery for, 1320–1333
    cleft lip repair in, 1322–1328
      bilateral, 1327–1328, 1327f
      unilateral, 1323–1327, 1324f, 1325f
    cleft palate repair in, 1328–1333
      bilateral, 1330, 1331f–1332f
      for clefts of secondary palate,
        1330–1333, 1332f, 1333f
      Furlow palatoplasty in,
        1330–1333, 1333f
      unilateral, 1328–1330,
        1329f–1330f
      Wardill-Kilner V-Y advancement
        in, 1330, 1332f
    lip adhesion in, 1321, 1322,
      1322f, 1323f
      bilateral, 1322, 1323f
      unilateral, 1322, 1322f
    prenatal, 1334
    sequencing and timing of,
      1321–1322
    taping prior to, 1321
  syndromic vs. nonsyndromic,
    1317–1318, 1318t
  team approach for, 1320
  unilateral cleft lip, 1320
Cleocin (Clindamycin), 59
Clindamycin (Cleocin), 59
Clinical data
  causality of
    analysis of, measurement scales for,
      21t
    assessment of, 20–21
  interpretation of
    questions for, 18–31, 19t
    study design for, 19t
  numerical, descriptive statistics and,
    22t, 23
  sampling population for, 27–29, 28f
  statistical significance of, versus
    clinical importance of, 25
  understanding of, 17–32

Clinical guidelines, 1419–1425. *See also* Clinical pathways
  evidence-based medicine and, 1420
  history of, 1419–1420
  Internet resources for, 1423*t*
  medicolegal aspects of, 1421
  outcome measures for, 1422
  purpose of, 1419
Clinical pathways
  creation of, 1420–1421
  definition of, 1420
  documentation of, 1421
  evidence-based medicine and, 1420
  flow charts of, 1420, 1421*f*
  format for, 1420–1421
  Gantt charts of, 1420
  in head and neck cancer, 1422–1425
    examples of, 1422
    Internet resources for, 1423*t*
    intraoperative, 1423–1424
    outpatient, 1422–1423
    perioperative, 1423–1424
    postoperative, 1424–1425
  history of, 1419–1420
  medicolegal aspects of, 1421
  outcome measures for, 1422
  overview of, 1425
  purpose of, 1419
  structure of, 1420–1421
Clinical-severity index, creation of, 34–35
Clinical studies
  results of, validity of, 25–27
  types of, 33
Clinical trials, 1428–1429
Clival tumors, surgery of, 1845
Clonidine, in smoking cessation therapy, 280–281
Clonidine-withdrawal syndrome, 224
Cloning, positional, 45
Clostridium botulinum, laryngeal dysfunction and, 875
Cluster headache, 253–255
  clinical features of, 254–255
  diagnostic criteria for, 254, 254*t*
  episodic, 254
  incidence of, 254
  treatment of, 255, 255*t*
Coagulation phase, of wound healing, 199
Cocaine, 142–143
  in hemorrhage during sinus surgery, 488
  midline granuloma and, 382
Coccidioidomycosis, 188, 386
Cochlea
  alterations of, in congenital cytomegalovirus, 2175
  anatomy of, 1887–1893, 1887*f*, 1888*f*, 1889*f*, 1890*f*, 1891*f*, 1892*f*

gross extracellular potentials in, 1890–1893, 1893*f*
  pathologic changes in, clinical manifestations of, 2260*t*
  transduction and, 1888–1889, 1892*f*, 1893*f*
Cochlear implants, 1975, 2265–2277
  for adolescents and adults, 2268
  for children, 1285–1286, 2267–2268, 2267*t*, 2273
    meningitis and, 1297, 2272
  Clarion, 2266
  clinical results of, 2272–2273
    in adults, 2272–2273
    in children, 2273
  design of, new developments in, 2266
  Med-El, 2266
  medical assessment for, 2268–2269
  Nucleus 24, 2265–2266
  patient selection for, 2266–2268, 2266*t*
  in postlingual deafness, 2268
  psychological assessment for, 2269
  speech production and language outcomes with, 2273
  spoken word recognition and, 2273
  surgical implantation of, 2269–2271, 2269*f*, 2270*f*
    complications of, 2271–2272
    meningitis following, 1297, 2272
Cochlear modifier, 1889
Cochlear nucleus, 1901, 1901*f*
Codeine, 232
Cogan syndrome, 179, 2791
Cognitive behavioral therapy, in tinnitus, 2243
Collagen
  bovine, for soft-tissue augmentation, 2765–2766
  lysis of, 203–204
  metabolism of, and wound healing, 202–204
  synthesis of, 202–203, 203*f*
  types of, 203*t*
Collagen vascular disease, ocular manifestations of, 137
Collet-Sicard syndrome, 120, 2791
Colon interposition, in cervical esophageal cancer, 1715, 1715*f*
Coma, otitis media and, 2054
Comedones, 2734
Comminuted fractures, 970–971
Common cavity deformity, 1971, 1972*f*
Comorbid conditions
  definition of, 35
  identification of, 35
Complement system, innate immunity and, 336–337
Complementary medicine, 2797

Composite grafts, in cutaneous nasal defects, 2426–2427, 2426*t*, 2428*f*
Compound nevi, 2738, 2738*f*
Computed tomography
  of acoustic neuroma, 89
  of allergic fungal rhinosinusitis, 424, 424*f*
  of angiofibroma of nasopharynx, 90
  of chronic rhinosinusitis, 411–412, 411*f*, 412*f*, 413
  of congenital aural atresia, 2029–2030, 2031*f*, 2032*f*
  coronal, of larynx, 93
  of cranial-base surgery, 1830
  before endoscopic sinus surgery, 464–466, 464*f*, 465*f*
  following middle ear surgery, 89
  of frontal sinus fractures, 1011
  of hypopharyngeal cancer, 1694
  for image-guided biopsy, 69, 69*f*
  for image-guided endoscopic sinus surgery, 71, 72*f*
  intraoperative, in maxillary/periorbital fractures, 992
  of juvenile angiofibroma, 450, 450*f*
  of laryngeal trauma, 950–952, 951*f*
  of larynx, 93
  of maxillary/periorbital fractures, 979, 980*t*
  of nasal obstruction, 322
  of nasal polyps, 394, 395*f*
  of nasopharyngeal cancer, 1659, 1660*f*
  of olfactory system, 301
  of orbital complications of rhinosinusitis, 497
  of parathyroid glands, 95–96
  of parotid glands, 563
  of salivary glands, 94, 528–529
  of sinuses, 90, 411–412, 411*f*, 412*f*, 429–430, 430*f*
  of soft tissue of neck, 91–92
  of temporal bone, 87–89, 1961, 1962*f*
  of thyroid gland, 95
Computer-assisted surgery, 439
  in maxillary/periorbital fractures, 991–992
Concha bullosa, nasal obstruction in, 313
Conditioned play audiometry, 1281, 1281*f*
Conductive hearing loss. *See also* Hearing loss
  vs. sensorineural hearing loss, 293
Condyle, mandibular, 961*f*
  fractures of, 964, 964*t*
    in children, 1338–1342, 1344, 1344*f*. *See also* Facial fractures, in children

management, 968–970, 970t
treatment options, 965t
Confidential voice therapy, 885–886
common applications to voice
disorders, 889t
Configuration, 1930
Conformal radiation therapy, 1443. *See
also* Radiation therapy
Congenital infections, hearing loss in,
1291–1295
Congenital malformations. *See also
specific sites and types*
of airway, 1056
auricular, 1055
definition of, 1374
formes frustes of, 1374
inheritance of, 1371–1374, 1372f,
1373f
midline nasal, 1056
of nares, 1055–1056
of neck, 1056–1057
of oral cavity, 1056
otolaryngologic, 49, 1371–1387. *See
also* Otolaryngologic
syndromes
Conjunctiva
lymphangioma of, 1503
trauma to, 134–135
Conjunctivitis, 131
Connective tissue disease(s), 169–179
autoantibody relations in, 170t
fibrinoid necrosis in, 169, 170f
mixed, 175–179
head and neck manifestations of,
176
Consensus Auditory-Perceptual Evaluation of Voice (CAPE-V), 825
Continuous positive airway pressure, in
obstructive sleep apnea,
656–657, 656f
Contract issues, in medical practice,
2808–2810, 2809t
Contrast agents, intravenous injection
of, contraindications to, 430
Contusions, facial soft tissue,
management of, 937
Conus elasticus, larynx and, 818
Cordotomy, transverse, for bilateral
vocal fold paralysis, 863, 863f
Cornea
trauma to, 134–135, 135f
ulceration of, due to forehead lift,
2681
Coronoid process, of mandible, 961f
Corporate gifts, acceptance of, case
illustrating, 2785
Cortical auditory evoked responses,
1936–1937
Corticosteroids, 178, 221
for adrenal suppression, 222, 222t
for benign facial lesions, 2741

controversies in use of, 910
for emergent vocal problem, 904
for hemangiomas, 1352
inhaled, laryngitis and, 830t, 835
intralesional, side effects of, 2743t
for lupus erythematosus stomatitis, 583
for management of scars and keloids,
2417
for nasal polyposis, 399
for rhinitis, 358t, 359–360
wound healing and, 207
Corticotropin, 156–157, 157f
Corticotropin-secreting tumors, 121
Cortisol, 161
Cosmetics, for scar camouflage, 2417
CosmoDerm, for soft-tissue
augmentation, 2767
CosmoPlast, for soft-tissue
augmentation, 2767
Costen syndrome, 2791
Cough
differential diagnosis of, 1115–1116
endoscopy in, 1115
evaluation of, 1114–1115
functions and phases of, 699
history and physical examination in,
1114
laboratory studies in, 1114–1115
management of, 1116
mechanics of, 1095–1097
Cowden syndrome, 2791
COX-2 inhibitors, platelet dysfunction
and, 217
COX-2 promoter, in gene therapy, 1396
Cranial anatomy, 3, 4f
Cranial autonomic ganglia, 111f
Cranial base
anatomy of, 456, 456f
anterior
anatomy of, 1834, 1834f
surgical approaches to, 1837–1839,
1838f, 1839f
endoscopic approaches to, 451–455
endoscopic transoral surgery of, 1845
foramina of, 1833t
middle
anatomy of, 1834–1836, 1835f,
1836f, 1837f
surgical approaches to, 1839–1843,
1840f, 1841f
neurophysiology of, 1829–1830
parasellar endoscopic approach to,
453–454
posterior
anatomy of, 1836
surgical approaches to, 1843
regions of, 1832
surgical approaches to, 1837t
transpterygoid approach to, 454–455
tumors of, 1831, 1832t
management of, 1837–1843

Cranial-base surgery, 1827–1852
adjuvant therapies in, 1845–1846
complications of, 1846–1850, 1846t
emergencies following, 1850–1851,
1850t
endoscopic endonasal
transsphenoidal, 1844
evaluation for, 1830–1832, 1831t
intraoperative monitoring in, 1830,
1831t
minimally invasive techniques for,
1843–1845
navigation systems for, 1843–1844
neuroanatomic considerations in,
1827–1829
surgical anatomy for, 1832–1837
Cranial fossae, anatomy of, 3–4
Cranial nerve(s), 112–114t
deficits of, following cranial-base
surgery, 1849
schwannomas of, 2226
taste and, 569, 570, 571f
Craniofacial dysostosis, 1378
Craniovertebral junction disorders,
2311–2314
Cribriform plate, 308
Cricoarytenoid joint
arthritis of, 172
larynx and, 818, 819
Cricohyoidoepiglottopexy, 1743. *See
also* Glottic and supraglottic
cancer, early, open surgery for
technique of, 1745–1750,
1746f–1752f
Cricohyoidopexy, 1743. *See also*
Glottic and supraglottic
cancer, early, open surgery for
technique of, 1745–1750,
1746f–1752f
Cricoid cartilage
laryngeal stenosis, and anterior split
of, 1140–1141, 1140f, 1140t
larynx and, 817–819
Cricopharyngeal achalasia, 242
dysphagia in, 728, 728f
Cricopharyngeal dysfunction,
esophageal symptoms in,
762–763, 762f
Cricopharyngeal myotomy, in
aspiration, 738, 738t, 1113
Cricopharyngeal sphincter, in
deglutition, 687, 687f
Cricothyroid muscle, voice production
and, 896, 898
Cricothyroidotomy, tracheotomy versus,
808–809, 809f, 809t
Cricothyrotomy, 788, 789f, 922f
Cricotracheal resection, for laryngeal
stenosis, 1142f, 1143
Cricotracheal separation, management
of, 956–957

Critical pathways. *See* Clinical pathways
Crohn disease, pharyngitis in, 609
Cross-lip flaps, 1541*f*, 1545–1546
Croup
  glottic obstruction in, 1066, 1067, 1067*f*
  management of, 64
  stridor in, 1108–1109
  upper airway obstruction and, 803
Crouzon syndrome, 1378–1379, 2791
Cryotherapy, in benign facial lesions, 2740–2741
Cryptococcosis, 188
Curare, 150
Curettage, 2740, 2742*t*
  with electrodesiccation, for skin cancer, 1462
Curettes, dermal, 2740, 2741*f*
Curtius syndrome, 2791
Cutaneous horns, 2731, 2734*f*
  treatment of, 2744
Cyanosis, in newborn, differential diagnosis of, 1099, 1100*t*
Cyclophosphamide, for extranodal lymphoma, 1624–1627, 1624*t*
Cyst(s)
  aneurysmal bone, of jaw, 1582
  brachial cleft, first arch, 550–551, 551*f*
  cholesterol, imaging in, 1968–1969, 1969*f*
  dentigerous, 1570–1571, 1570*f*
  dermoid. *See* Dermoid cysts
  epidermal, 2734
    treatment of, 2744–2745
  esophageal, 766
  Gorlin, 1572–1573
  incisive canal, 1573
  nasolacrimal duct, nasal obstruction in, 1087, 1088*f*
  nasopalatine duct, 1573
  odontogenic, 616, 616*f*, 1569–1573. *See also* Odontogenic cysts
  orbital, 1510, 1510*f*
  parotid, 550, 557
  periapical, 1569–1570, 1570*f*
  radicular, 1569–1570, 1570*f*
  retention, 435, 435*f*
  salivary gland, 536–538, 537*f*, 538*f*, 550–551, 550*t*
    in children, 1244
  sialo-odontogenic, 1572–1573, 1573*f*
  thyroglossal duct, 1630–1631
  vocal fold, 838
    appropriate voice therapy referrals for, 890
    common voice therapy applications for, 889*t*
Cystic fibrosis, 407
  nasal polyps in, 395
  otolaryngologic problems in, 1059

Cystic hygroma, 1071, 1073*f*, 1817, 1818*f*
Cytokines
  in gene therapy, 1399
  in head and neck cancer, 1411, 1412
  in immunotherapy, for head and neck cancer, 1413
  in wound healing, 204–206, 205*t*, 208
Cytomegalovirus esophagitis, 765
Cytomegalovirus infection
  congenital, 2174*t*
    hearing loss in, 1291–1292, 1291*t*, 1292*t*
    pharyngitis due to, 608

D

Dacryoadenitis, 1508
Dacryocystitis, 132–133
Dandy syndrome, 2791
Dapsone, 186
Darier disease, 2791
Data. *See* Clinical data
Deafness. *See* Hearing loss
Deafness dystonia syndrome, 1313
Débridement, as laceration treatment, 937*f*
Decongestants, in rhinitis, 358*t*, 359
Deformations, 1374. *See also* Otolaryngologic syndromes
Deglutition. *See also under* Swallow
  abnormal, assessment of, 725–726, 726*f*
  bolus characteristics and, 690
  coordination in, 689
  development and aging and, 690
  fiberoptic endoscopic evaluation of, 749–750
  flexible endoscopic evaluation of, 909–910
  function of, instrumental techniques for evaluation of, 704–710
  functional endoscopic evaluation of, 1112
  glottic closure in, 734
  mechanism of, anatomy of, in children and adults, 1098, 1099*f*
  normal physiology of, 724
  phases of, 724, 725*f*, 1674–1675
  physiology of, 734
  postural techniques to improve, 714–715, 714*t*
  posture and, 690
  pressure generation for, 687–689, 688*f*
  respiratory-swallow coordination and, 691
  sensory enhancement techniques to improve, 715–716
  six valves operating during, 685, 686*f*
  stages of, 1097–1098

  therapy procedures to improve, 716–718
  as three stage event, 703
  types of, 690–691
  upper esophageal sphincter relaxation in, 734
  value function for, 685–687, 686*f*, 687*f*
  voluntary control and, 690
Dejean syndrome, 2791
Delirium tremens, 233
Demeclocycline, 223
Demyelinating disorders, 107–109
Dendritic cells, 345, 1406–1408, 1407*f*, 1412–1413
Dental. *See also* Teeth
Dental implants, osseointegrated, 1861–1863, 1862*f*
Dental infections. *See* Odontogenic infections
Dental injuries
  in children, 1345
  in mandibular fractures, 970. *See also* Mandibular fractures
  radiation-induced, 1451, 1452
Dental numbering system, universal, 961, 962*f*
Dental occlusion
  classification of, 961, 962*f*
  evaluation of, for plastic surgery of face, 2493, 2493*f*
  following maxillary/periorbital fractures, 990–991
  incisal relationships and, 1035–1036, 1035*f*
Dental-sinus-orbital infections, in odontogenic infections, 625–626, 625*f*
Dentigerous cysts, 1570–1571, 1570*f*
Dentoalveolar fractures, in children, 1338–1342
  surgery of, 1345
Deoxyribonucleic acid (DNA). *See* DNA
Depression, facial cosmetic surgery and, 2483
Dermabrasion
  in benign facial lesions, 2742
  complications of, 2743*t*
  conditions treated with, 2743*t*
  for scar camouflage, 2415–2416, 2416*f*
Dermal curette, 2740, 2741*f*
Dermal nevi, 2737–2738, 2737*f*
Dermatitis, infectious eczematoid, 1998, 1999*f*
Dermatomyositis, 174–175
  laryngeal dysfunction in, 875
Dermatoses
  bullous, esophageal symptoms in, 766
  mimicking otitis externa, 1999–2000

Dermoid cysts, 2018–2019
  nasal, 1077, 1077f
    congenital development of,
        1218–1219, 1219–1220f
    clinical and pathologic features,
        1219–1220, 1221f,
        1224–1225t
    evaluation, 1223, 1224f
    surgical treatment, 1223–1226,
        1224f, 1225f
  orbital, 1510, 1510f
  temporal bone, 2018
Desflurane, 145
Desmopressin, 217, 223
Desquamative gingivitis, stomatitis due
    to, 581–582, 581f, 582f, 582t
Dexamethasone, in Ménière disease,
    2323
Dextrocardia, in Kartagener syndrome,
    1381
DFNB gene, in hearing loss,
    1304–1306, 1305t–1306t
Diabetes insipidus
  cause of, 222–223
  central hypothalamic, 158–159
  after cranial-base surgery, 1849–1850,
    1849t
  treatment of, 223
Diabetes mellitus
  ocular manifestations of, 138
  preoperative management of,
    220–221
  type 1, 163
  type 2, 163
Diabetic emergencies, 167
Diagnostic imaging. See Imaging and
    specific modalities
Diagnostic tests, statistical terms
    associated with, 23–24, 23t
Dialysis, preoperative, in chronic renal
    failure, 228–229
Diarrhea, antibiotic-associated, 228
Diazepam, 147, 230
Dicloxacillin, 57
Didanosine, 274
DiGeorge syndrome, 44, 2791
Digestive tract, upper, anatomy and
    physiology of, 685–692
Digital cameras
  applications in imaging, 76–80
  benefits of, 77–78, 78t
  limitations of, 78–80
  for photography of head and neck,
    77–80, 77f, 78f, 79f
Digital photography, for pictorial
    documentation, 2506–2509,
    2506f
Digoxin, 225
Diltiazem, 225
Diphtheroid infection, pharyngitis due
    to, 604–605

Diplopia, 130
  following sinus surgery, 486
Direct System implantable hearing
    device, 2274
Diskectomy, 631
Disodium etidronate, 192
Disomy, uniparental, 46
Disruptions, 1374–1375. See also
    Otolaryngologic syndromes
Diuretics
  ototoxicity of, 1298
  in sudden sensory hearing loss, 2234
Diverticulum(a), esophageal, 747, 747f,
    763–764, 765f
Dizziness. See also Vertigo; Vestibular
    disorders
  ablative therapy in, 2264
  causes and mechanisms of, 2317,
    2318t
  diagnostic evaluation in, 2263
  dizziness simulation battery and,
    2262t
  etiology of, 2257, 2258t
  management of, 2263–2264
  psychophysiologic, medical
    management of, 2326–2327
  types of, 2261t
DNA, 53, 1304
DNA microarrays, 99
Dobutamine, 227
Docetaxel, 1428t, 1430
Dominance traits, 1303
Dopamine, 227
Double aortic arch, congenital, 1129,
    1130f
Down syndrome, 44, 1379–1380,
    1379f
  hearing loss in, 1314, 1379
Doxorubicin
  for extranodal lymphoma,
    1624–1627, 1624t
  toxicity of, 1627
Doxycycline, in parotid cysts, 557
Drugs. See Medications
Dry-eye syndrome, 139
Duckbill voice prosthesis, following
    laryngectomy, 1781–1782,
    1782f
Dufourmental flaps, 2363, 2364f
Dural sinus thrombosis, imaging in,
    1967–1968, 1968f
Dysautonomia, familial, dysphagia in,
    728, 728f
Dysequilibrium, in elderly patients,
    239–240
Dysgeusia, 567, 573
  as complication of mastoid surgery,
    2109
Dyskinesia, laryngeal, stridor in, 1108
Dysmorphology. See Congenital
    malformations

Dysosmia, 293
  causes of, 296–297
Dysphagia. See also under Swallow
  clinical evaluation in, 703–710
  diseases causing, 726–731, 727f,
    728f, 729f, 730f, 731f
  evaluation of, 703–711
  management of, 713–719
  therapy considerations and, 718–719
  treatment of, compensatory
    procedures in, 713–716
Dysphonia, spasmodic
  appropriate voice therapy referrals for,
    890
  common voice therapy applications
    for, 889t
  laryngeal dysfunction and, 876–877
  surgery for, controversies in use of,
    914
Dysplasia, fibrous. See Fibrous dysplasia
Dysrhythmias, preoperative
    management of, 225
Dyssomnia, 647
Dystonia, 116
  laryngeal dysfunction and, 876–877

E

Eagle syndrome, 2791
Ear. See also Eustachian tube system;
    Hearing
  anatomy of, 2685–2686, 2686f
  auricular hematoma, management of,
    943–944, 944f, 945f
  average dimensions of, 2686, 2687f
  burns, management of, 947
  congenital malformations of, 1055,
    2685–2700, 2691–2696,
    2692f. See also
    Otolaryngologic syndromes
    classification of, 2691–2693, 2693t
    diagnosis of, 2693t
    surgical reconstruction of,
        2693–2696, 2694t
      complications of, 2696, 2696t
      emergencies associated with,
        2698t
      technique for, 2694–2696, 2695f,
        2696f, 2697f, 2698f
  development of, 1869–1881, 1870t,
    2027–2028, 2685, 2686f
    auricular, 1869–1871, 1871f
    control of, 1879–1880
    external and middle ear,
        1871–1873, 1872f, 1873f
    inner ear, 1875–1879, 1875f, 1876f
    ossicles, 1871, 1873
  disorders of
    gene therapy for, 1400, 1400f
    headache in, 259
  evaluation of, for plastic surgery of
    face, 2492–2493

Ear *(continued)*
external
anatomy and physiology of, 1883–1884, 1884*f*, 1987–1989, 1988*f*, 1989*f*
benign neoplasms of, imaging of, 1964–1965, 1965*f*
congenital anomalies of. *See also* Otolaryngologic syndromes imaging of, 1963–1964, 1964*f*
development of, 1871–1873, 1872*f*, 1873*f*
infections of. *See* Otitis externa
inflammatory diseases of, 1966–1967, 1966*f*
malignant neoplasms of, imaging of, 1965–1966, 1966*f*
plastic repair of, clinical indicators for, 2692*t*
sound pressure and, 1883–1884, 1884*f*
implants for, 2349–2350, 2350*t*. *See also* Cochlear implants
infections of. *See also under* Otitis
complications of, 122–124
facial paralysis with, 2054
inner
autoimmune disease of, 2247–2256
animal models of, 2252
immunopathology of, 2252–2254, 2253*f*
otologic manifestations of, 2162
treatment of, 2254–2255
congenital anomalies of, 1971–1972, 1971*f*, 1972*f*, 1973*f*, 1974*f*. *See also* Otolaryngologic syndromes
development of, 1875–1879, 1875*f*, 1876*f*
disorders of, gene therapy for, 1400, 1400*f*
gene delivery to, 1400, 1400*f*
immune disease of, sudden sensory hearing loss in, 2232–2233
immune response, 2247–2251, 2248*f*, 2249*f*, 2250*f*
immunopathology of, immune-mediated damage and, 2251–2252
inflammation and hemorrhage of, 1972–1973, 1974*f*, 1975*f*
maldevelopment of, 1873, 1877–1879, 1878*f*, 1878*t*, 1879*f*. *See also* Otolaryngologic syndromes
neoplasms of, 1973, 1975*f*, 1976*f*
tumors of, 1971–1975
and lateral skull base, neoplasms of, 2003–2025, 2004*t*, 2005*f*
malformations of. *See* Otolaryngologic syndromes

manifestations of systemic disease in, 2155–2167
middle
anatomy of, 1885
development of, 1052–1053, 1052*f*, 1053*f*
embryology of, 1871–1873, 1872*f*, 1873*f*, 2027–2028
function of, 1884–1887, 1885*f*, 1886*f*
imaging of, 1967–1971
infection of. *See* Otitis media
maldevelopment of, 1872–1873
neoplasms of, 2014–2019
surgery of
in aural atresia, 2034–2035
computed tomography following, 89
and temporal bone, trauma to, 2057–2079
tumors of, 1899*f*, 1970
nonlinear properties of, 1895–1897, 1898*f*
protruding, 2685–2691
surgical correction of. *See* Otoplasty
resection of, prosthetic rehabilitation in, 1861, 1861*f*
surgery of, facial nerve monitoring during, 1957
Ear tubes, for otitis media, 1272
Earlobe, and tragus, closure in area of, in rhytidectomy, 2643–2644, 2643*f*, 2644*f*
Eastlander flap, in lip reconstruction, 1541*f*, 1545, 1546*f*
Ebner, gustatory glands of, 2791
Ecchymosis, subconjunctival, following blepharoplasty, 2624
Ectopic thyroid, 1629–1630
Ectropion
following blepharoplasty, 2624
lateral tarsal strip procedure for, 2477, 2478*f*
Edema
cerebral
after cranial-base surgery, 1850
after neck dissection, 1605
facial, after neck dissection, 1605
pulmonary
acute, endotracheal intubation and, 798
preoperative management of, 227
Reinke
common voice therapy applications for, 889*t*
severe, appropriate voice therapy referrals for, 890
vocal fold, 840
Edentulous mandible fractures, 970, 972*f*
Edrophonium, 150

Eighth nerve monitoring, direct, 1947, 1947*f*, 1950, 1951
Elderly patients
airway management in, 244
benign and nonsquamous neoplasms in, 243
care of, knowledge for, 235
chronic conditions in, 236, 236*f*
dysequilibrium and ataxia in, 239–240
epidemiology and demography of, 236–237
facial fractures in, 244
facial plastic surgery in, 243–244
hearing loss in, 238–239, 2258–2263. *See also* Presbycusis
olfaction and gustation in, 240–241
otolaryngologic disorders in, 237, 237*t*
hospital stays in, 238*t*
peripheral nerves in, 242, 242*t*
presbyopia in, 128–129
presbyphagia in, 241–242
problems of activities of daily living in, 236, 236*f*
sinusitis and nasal symptoms in, 241, 241*t*
skin changes in, 244
squamous cell carcinoma in, 243
use of health-care system by, 236–237, 237*f*
voice disorders in, 239*t*, 240, 240*t*
Electrocochleography, 1936, 1936*f*, 1945–1947, 1946*f*
Electrodesiccation, with curettage, for skin cancer, 1462
Electroglottography, to improve deglutition, 718
Electrolarynx, following laryngectomy, 1779–1780
Electromagnetic stimulation, in tinnitus, 2243
Electromyography
in aspiration, 1112–1113
to assess deglutition, 707–708, 707*f*, 708*f*, 709*f*
evoked, for facial nerve monitoring, 1953–1954, 1954*f*
for facial nerve monitoring, 1953
laryngeal
bilateral vocal fold paralysis, 861–862
controversies in use of, 908–909
unilateral laryngeal paralysis, 854–855
abnormal tracing, 855*f*
classification of findings, 855*t*
vocal fold paralysis, 873*f*
laryngeal and pharyngeal muscles, 881*f*
technique, 879–881, 879*f*, 880*f*

surface electrode, to improve deglutition, 718
Electronystagmography, 1917–1921, 1918t
  bithermal caloric tests in, 1919–1920
  fistula test, 1920
  interpretation of, 1920t
  optokinetic system in, 1921
  positional and positioning tests in, 1919
  pursuit system in, 1920–1921
  saccadic system in, 1920
  spontaneous and gaze nystagmus and, 1918–1919
  system for recording eye movement, 1918, 1918f
Electrophysiologic testing
  in central auditory processing disorders, 1286, 1287t
  in vestibular schwannomas, 2211–2212
Electroporation, in viral gene transfer, 1396
Electrosurgery, in benign facial lesions, 2740, 2742f
Eliachar stent, in aspiration, 739, 739t
Embolism
  air
    as complication of mastoid surgery, 2110
    following cranial-base surgery, 1850–1851
    during otitis media surgery, 2053
  cardioembolism, 117
  pulmonary
    as complication of otitis media surgery, 2053
    preoperative, 220
Embryonal rhabdomyosarcoma, in children, 1364–1366, 1364t, 1365t
Emphysema, subcutaneous, as complication of sinus surgery, 487
Empyema, subdural, 122
Emtricitabine, 266
Encephalitis, herpes simplex, in infants, hearing loss in, 1294–1295
Encephalocele
  as complication of mastoid surgery, 2109
  nasal, congenital development of, 1219, 1220f
    clinical and pathologic features, 1221, 1222f, 1223, 1223f, 1224–1225t
    evaluation, 1223, 1224f
    surgical treatment, 1223–1226, 1224f, 1225f
End-of-life care, withholding life-saving measures and, case illustrating, 2782–2783

Endo-extralaryngeal suture lateralization, bilateral vocal fold paralysis and, 863
Endochondrial pseudocysts, auricular, 2014
Endocrine abnormalities, preoperative management of, 220–223
Endocrine emergencies, 164–167, 167t
Endocrine system, 155
  disorders of, 166–167, 166t, 167t
Endocrinology, 155–168
Endolymphatic hydrops, delayed, 2181
  treatment of, 2181t
Endolymphatic sac tumors, 1973, 1976f, 2015–2016
  bony invasion by, 2015
  clinical manifestations of, 2015
  diagnosis of, 2016
  extension of, 2015–2016
  resection of, 2016
Endolymphatic shunt, in surgery of mastoid, 2103–2104, 2105f
Endoscopes, for nasal endoscopy, 410, 410f
Endoscopic endonasal transsphenoidal surgery, 1844
Endoscopic forehead lift, 2678–2680, 2678f, 2679f, 2680f
Endoscopic procedures
  anesthesia for, 153
  complications of, 451
  in frontal sinus fracture management, 1013–1014, 1013f
  in maxillary/periorbital fractures, 991, 991f
Endoscopic sinus surgery, 437–439
  anesthesia for, 466, 466f, 467f
  extended frontal sinus procedures in, 474, 474f
  general principles of, 459–460, 460f, 461f
  history of, 459
  image guidance for, 71–73, 72f, 73f
  indications for, 461–462, 462f
  instrumentation for, 462–463
  intraoperative surgical navigation in, 474
  outcomes of, 470–472, 470f, 471f
  patient evaluation for, 463–464
  postoperative care following, 469–470
  preoperative evaluation for, 464–466, 464f, 465f
  revision, 472–474, 472f, 473f
  simulator for, 75–76, 75f
  technique for, 466–469, 467f, 468f, 469f
Endoscopic transoral surgery, of skull base, 1845
Endoscopy
  advances in, 80–82

diagnostic virtual endoscopy, 80, 80f
  virtual bronchoscopy, 81
aerodigestive tract, congenital anomalies of, evaluation and diagnosis, 1123–1124
  position of infant for, 1125–1126f
approaches for benign sinonasal tumors, 449–451, 449f
bent functional, outcomes for pediatric rhinosinusitis, 1235t
in cerebrospinal fluid rhinorrhea repair, 455–456
in cough, 1115
culture equipment for, 414, 414f
in evaluation of aspiration, 1112
in evaluation of upper aerodigestive tract, 745–753
fiberoptic. See Fiberoptic endoscopy
flexible, swallowing evaluation using, 909–910
functional, to evaluate swallowing, 1112
for laryngeal stenosis management, factors in failure with, 1139t
for malignant paranasal sinus tumors, 448–449
in management of neoplasms of nose and paranasal sinuses, 447–457
in mastoid surgery, 2103
nasal, 410–411, 411f
  in rhinitis, 357
in nasopharyngeal cancer, 1661–1662, 1661f
in neck surgery, 82
in otology, 81–82
partial laser arytenoidectomy using, 864
pediatric airway
  in caustic ingestions, 1160t
  for recurrent respiratory papillomatosis, 1172
pediatric microdebrider, for recurrent respiratory papillomatosis, 1176
staging of, image guidance and, 73–74
in stridor in child, 1101–1102
surgical adjuvants to, 81–82
total laser arytenoidectomy using, 864, 864f
upper airway obstruction and, 804
Endotracheal intubation, 153, 796–799
  bronchoscope for, 797
  complications of, 798–799, 798t, 816f
  in head trauma, 797
  history of, 796, 796t
  with large-bore laryngoscope, 797
  long-term, 798–799

Endotracheal intubation (continued)
  new tubes for, 797–798
  in oral cancer, 1565–1566
  techniques of, 796–798
Endotracheal tubes, 153
  advanced over introducer, 772–773,
      773f
Enfurtivide, 266
Enlarged vestibular aqueduct syndrome,
      1308, 1308f
Eosinophilic granuloma, 180,
      2016–2017
Eosinophils, 342
Ephelides, 2738
  treatment of, 2747
Epidermal cysts, 2734
  treatment of, 2744–2745
Epidermal growth factor, in wound
      healing, 204–205
Epidermal growth factor receptor
      (EGFR), 53–54
Epidermoids. See Cholesteatoma
Epidermolysis bullosa
  laryngitis and, 830t, 833
  pharyngitis in, 611
Epiglottis
  larynx and, 818
  soft palate, laryngeal neurologic
      disorders and, 868f
Epiglottitis
  chemical, caustic ingestions and,
      1158f
  diagnosis of, 1065, 1065f
  management of, 64
  stridor in, 1109
  upper airway obstruction and, 803
Epilepsy. See Seizures
Epinephrine, 142
  in hemorrhage during sinus surgery,
      488
Episcleritis, 131
Epistaxis, 505–514
  etiology of, 507–508, 507t
  exsanguinating, management of,
      508–510, 509f, 509t, 510t
  major, management of, 510–511
  management of, 508–513, 508t
  minor, management of, 508
Epstein-Barr virus
  in children, 1243
  pharyngitis due to, 607–608
Epstein pearls, 2791
Erbitux, 1431
Erbium lasers, 2725–2727
Erlotinib, 1431–1432
Erthromycins, 59
Erythema, following chemical peeling,
      2722
Erythema multiforme
  major, 592
  minor, 591–592

stomatitis due to
  clinical features of, 591
  etiology of, 591
Erythrocyte abnormalities, preoperative
      management of, 217
Erythroplasia, 1558–1559
Escherich sign, 2791
Eschmann endotracheal tube
      introducer, 772, 772f
  with Holinger laryngoscope, 772,
      772f
Esophageal cancer, 766–767,
      1711–1719
  adenocarcinoma, 747, 748f
  clinical presentation of, 1712
  complications of, 1717, 1717t
  diagnostic surgery in, 1712–1713
  emergencies in, 1717–1718, 1718t
  epidemiology of, 1711–1712
  evaluation of, 1712–1713, 1713t
  laboratory tests in, 1712
  management of, 1713–1717, 1713t
    advances in, 1718
    nonoperative, 1713–1715
    operative, 1714f, 1715–1717, 1715f,
      1716f
  staging of, 1713
Esophageal disorders, 755–770
  Barrett esophagitis, 746f, 747, 748
  benign neoplasms and cysts, 766, 766f
  carcinoma. See Esophageal cancer
  complications and emergencies
      associated with, 767–770, 768t
  cricopharyngeal dysfunction,
      762–763, 762f
  diagnosis of, 757–758, 757t
  diffuse esophageal spasm, 761–762,
      761f
  diverticula, 747, 747f, 763–764, 765f
  endoscopic examination in, 758, 758t
  esophageal candidiasis, 748, 748f
  esophageal motility, 760–764, 761f,
      762f, 763f
  esophageal webs and rings, 763, 763f
  hiatal hernia, 747, 748f
  laboratory tests in, 757–758
  manometric studies in, 758
  nutcracker esophagus, 762
  pH monitoring in, 758
  physical examination in, 756–757
  progressive systemic sclerosis, 762
  radiologic studies in, 758
  symptoms of, 756
  treatment of, 757t
Esophageal diverticula, 763–764, 765f
Esophageal injuries, penetrating, 1025
Esophageal obstruction, 769
Esophageal perforation, 768–769, 768t
Esophageal rupture, 768–769, 768t
Esophageal spasm, diffuse, 761–762,
      761f

Esophageal speech, following
      laryngectomy, 1780
Esophageal sphincter
  lower, 756
  upper, 756
Esophageal Tracheal Combitube, 774,
      775–776, 778f
Esophageal webs and rings, 763, 763f
Esophagitis
  causes of, 764, 766
  symptoms of, 764–765
  types of, 765–766
Esophagoscope, selection of, by age,
      1101t
Esophagoscopy
  transnasal, 745–749
    for assessment of esophageal
      motility, 747
    complications of, 749
    for diagnosis, 910
    esophagoscopes for, 746
    indications for, 748–749, 748f,
      749f
    insertion of esophagoscope for,
      745–746, 746f
    technique of, 746–747, 746f
  types of, compared, 758, 758t
Esophagus
  anatomy of, 755
  blood supply to, 755, 756t
  in caustic ingestions, 770
  cervical
    anatomy of, 1711
    cancer of. See Esophageal cancer
    physiology of, 1711
  congenital anomalies of, 1122t
    duplication, 1130
    hiatal hernia, 1131
  foreign body in, stridor in, 1069, 1070f
  functions of, 756
  hemorrhage of, 769
  infectious and inflammatory
      conditions of, 764–766
  nutcracker, 762
  physiology of, 755–756
  tracheoesophageal fistula and atresia
      of, 1128, 1129f, 1130f
Esotropia, 136
Essential tremor
  appropriate voice therapy referrals for,
      890
  common voice therapy applications
      for, 889t
  laryngeal dysfunction and, 877
Esthesioneuroblastoma
  endoscopic technique in, 452, 452f
  imaging of, 443, 443f
Ethacrynic acid, ototoxicity of, 1298
Ethical issues. See Medical ethics
Ethmoid sinuses. See also Sinus(es)
  anatomy of, 8, 307–309, 368

surgery of, 367–370
  complications of, 370
  indications for, 368
  operative technique for, 368–370,
    368f, 369f
  postoperative management in, 370
Ethmoidectomy
  external
    complications of, 481–482
    in sinusitis, 498
  intranasal, complications of, 481
  transantral, complications of, 481–482
Etomidate, 147
Eustachian tube
  development of, 1052–1053, 1052f
  patulous, tinnitus in, 2238
Eustachian tube system
  anatomy of, 1253–1255, 1254f
    infant versus adult, 1257–1258,
      1257t
    muscles, 1255–1257, 1255f, 1256f
  physiology of, 1258f
    pressure regulation function, 1258f,
      1261–1262
    protective and clearance functions,
      1258, 1258f
    model for, 1258–1261, 1258f,
      1259f, 1260f
Evidence-based medicine, 37–40, 1420
  appraisal of quality of evidence in,
    38–39
  asking answerable question in, 38
  evidence levels for studies in, 39
  grading of, 39, 39t
  integration of evidence with clinical
    experience, 39–40
  outcomes research and, 33–40
  results and recommendations in, 39
  search for best available evidence in,
    38
Evoked otoacoustic emissions testing,
  1289
Ewing sarcoma, 2018
Exercise programs, to prevent
  dysphagia, 719
Exercises, to improve deglutition,
  716–718
Exophthalmos, 2453, 2454f
  differential diagnosis of, 2455
  dysthyroid, treatment of, 2463–2464,
    2464t
  high-dose prednisone in, 2463
  management of, 2455–2456
  patient evaluation in, 2453–2454,
    2454f
  surgery for, 2453–2466
    emergencies associated with, 2465
    orbital decompression in. See
      Orbital decompression, for
      exophthalmos
  preoperative assessment for, 2455t

Exostoses
  of external auditory canal, 2013–2014
  of external ear, imaging of,
    1964–1965, 1965f
Exotropia, 136
Expectorants, 1116
Expert witness testimony, case
  illustrating, 2783–2784
Exposure(s)
  cranioorbital, 1036, 1036f
  facial, in facial trauma, 1036–1037,
    1036f, 1037f
Expressivity, phenotypic, 1374
External ear. See Ear, external
Extracellular matrix, major components
  of, 200t
Extravasation, of chemotherapeutic
  drugs, 1438, 1438t
Extremity injuries, in trauma patients,
  930–931
Eye
  anatomy of, 6, 6f
  in arteriosclerosis, 138–139, 139t
  assessment of, for plastic surgery of
    face, 2488–2489, 2488f,
    2489f
  in blood dyscrasia, 138
  care of, in facial paralysis, 2153
  in collagen vascular disease, 137
  congenital abnormalities of, 136
  in diabetes, 138
  in Graves disease, 137, 137f
  heterotropia of, 127, 127f
  in hypertension, 138–139, 139t
  injuries of
    from blunt trauma, 135
    burn, 135–136
    of cornea and conjunctiva,
      134–135
    examination of, 133–134
    history of, 133
    orbital, 134
    penetrating, 135
  in metastatic cancer, 138, 138f
  in neurologic disease, 137
  proptosis of, 127, 127f
  radiation effects on, 1452, 1494,
    1496t
  reactions to medications, 138
  red. See Red eye
  in systemic disease, 137–139
  in thyroid ophthalmopathy, 137
Eye examination, 125–128
  external inspection and pupil
    examination in, 126–127
  for intraocular pressure, 128
  for motility, 127–128, 127f
  for ocular trauma, 133–136
  ophthalmoscopic, 128
  for visual acuity, 125–126, 126t
Eyebrow. See Brow(s)

Eyelid
  abnormalities of, 130–131
  anatomy of, 4–5, 5f
  burns of, 947
  damage to, in maxillary/periorbital
    fractures, 988–989, 990f
  laceration of, 134
  lower, blepharoplasty of
    evaluation for, 2613–2614, 2613f
    skin-muscle flap approach for,
      2617–2620, 2618f, 2619f,
      2620f, 2621f
    transconjunctival approach for,
      2620–2623, 2621f, 2622f,
      2623f
  lymphangioma of, 1503
  skin flap for, after Mohs surgery,
    2398–2400, 2401f, 2402f
  soft tissue trauma, management of,
    941–943, 942f, 943f
  tumors of, 1511
  upper, blepharoplasty of, 2616–2617,
    2617f
    evaluation for, 2612–2613

F
Face
  abnormal growth of, as complication
    of sinus surgery, 489
  aging, 2771, 2772f
    physiology of, 2627–2628, 2628f
    rhytidectomy for. See Rhytidectomy
  analysis of
    normal values for, 2494t
    and preoperative evaluation,
      2481–2497
  anatomy of, 8–9, 9f
  benign lesions of
    classification of, 2732t
    epidermal, 2731–2734, 2734f
    history taking and physical
      examination in, 2731
    laboratory studies in, 2739–2740,
      2739f
    management of, 2731–2748
    syndromes associated with,
      differential diagnosis of, 2732t
    therapeutic considerations in,
      2740–2744
  blunt trauma to. See Facial fractures
  changing configuration with age,
    1049, 1050f
  complex trauma to. See also Facial
    fractures
    complications of, 1042, 1043t
    emergencies in, 1037–1038, 1038t
    plating in, 1027–1044
    soft tissue loss in, 1041–1042, 1042f
  fatty/muscular tumors of, 2737
  fibrous tumors of, 2736–2737
  infectious lesions of, 2739, 2739f

Face (continued)
　melanocytic tumors of, 2737–2739
　midportion of. See Midface
　minimal deformity of, facial cosmetic
　　　surgery and, 2484
　muscles of, 2761–2762, 2762f
　neural tumors of, 2737
　non–skin-appendage tumors of,
　　　2735–2739
　penetrating trauma to, 1017
　　complications of, 1020–1021, 1021t
　　gunshot wounds, 1019–1020, 1020f
　　management of
　　　general, 1018, 1019f
　　　specific, 1020
　　　staging of, 1018
　　shotgun injuries, 1018–1019, 1041,
　　　1042f
　　stab wounds, 1019
　plastic surgery of. See also specific
　　　procedures and structures
　　computer imaging for, 2482–2483
　　in elderly patients, 243–244
　　facial analysis for, 2485, 2485f
　　　anatomic landmarks in,
　　　　2485–2487, 2486f
　　　general, 2487–2493, 2487f, 2488f
　　　methods of, 2494–2495, 2494f,
　　　　2495f
　　patient dissatisfaction with,
　　　2484–2485
　　patient selection for, 2481
　　preoperative assessment for,
　　　2481–2483
　　preoperative interviews for,
　　　2481–2482, 2482f
　　psychopathology of patient and,
　　　2483–2484
　regional anatomy of, 2761–2762,
　　　2762f
　skeletal structure of, 1033–1034,
　　　1034f
　　and cranial skeleton, 1039, 1039f
　　reestablishment in reconstruction,
　　　1039–1040, 1040f
　skin-appendage tumors of,
　　　2734–2735
　surgical anatomy of, 2629–2630,
　　　2629f, 2630f
　temporal region of, anatomy of,
　　　2772, 2772f
　upper, aging of, management of,
　　　2668
　vascular tumors of, 2735–2736
Facial aesthetics, mathematical
　　　formulas and ratios for, 2485,
　　　2485f
Facial bone, fracture of, in penetrating
　　　facial trauma, 1020
Facial edema, after neck dissection,
　　　1605

Facial fractures
　in children, 1337–1347
　　condylar, 1344, 1344f
　　dentoalveolar, 1345
　　emergency management of, 1338
　　epidemiology of, 1337–1338
　　etiology of, 1338–1339
　　facial growth and, 1339–1340
　　mandibular arch, 1344–1345,
　　　1345f
　　maxillary, 1347
　　midface, 1345
　　nasal, 1342–1343
　　nasoethmoidal complex, 1346,
　　　1346f
　　orbital floor, 1346–1347
　　radiographic examination of,
　　　1338–1339
　　rigid fixation of, 1340–1342
　　surgical approaches in, 1340–1342
　　zygomaticomalar complex,
　　　1345–1346
　classification of, 1028, 1028f
　in elderly, 244
　incisions and exposure in,
　　　1036–1037, 1036f, 1037f
　panfacial, approach to, 1037–1041,
　　　1040f
　pathophysiology of, 1028–1029
　reduction of, 1033–1035, 1034f
　rigid fixation of
　　devices for, 1030
　　principles of, 1029–1030, 1029f,
　　　1030f
　　rationale for, 1029
Facial lacerations, 937, 939
　closing stellate wounds, 939f
　débridement and undermining of,
　　　937f
　suturing, 938f
　trapdoor, 938f
Facial muscles, 8, 9f
Facial nerve, 9, 9f, 108f
　abnormalities of, 2141
　　in aural atresia, 2028
　anatomy of, 518, 518f, 519f,
　　　2139–2140, 2140f, 2467,
　　　2468f
　　surgical, 2140–2141, 2140f, 2141f
　arterial supply to, 2141
　　in aural atresia, 2037
　development of, 1873–1875
　dissection of, with parotidectomy,
　　　559–560
　embryology of, 2028
　idiopathic paralysis of, 1977–1978,
　　　1979f
　imaging of, 1976–1978
　inflammation of, 1977–1978
　injury to, 552. See also Facial paralysis
　　management of, 940–941

　　during otologic surgery,
　　　management of, 2108–2109
　　in penetrating facial trauma, 1020
　　in rhytidectomy, 2645–2646, 2646f
　　in surgery for aural atresia, 2038
　　in temporal bone fracture,
　　　2065–2071
　　types of, 1952, 1952t
　intraoperative monitoring of,
　　　1951–1957
　　anesthesia and, 1954–1955
　　benefits and applications of,
　　　1956–1957
　　direct, 1954
　　history of, 1952
　　indications for, 1955–1956, 1955t
　　monitoring systems for, 1952–1954
　　objectives of, 1953t
　　in parotid surgery, 560, 1530
　locations of, 2645f
　maldevelopment of, 1874–1875,
　　　1874f
　neoplasms of, 1977
　normal vascular variants and,
　　　1978–1979, 1979f
　paralysis of. See Facial paralysis
　in parotidectomy
　　identification of, 1524, 1524t
　　injury of, 1528–1530
　　monitoring of, 560, 1530
　pathophysiology of, 2143–2147
　schwannomas of, 2020, 2225–2226
　taste and, 569
　topographical organization of, 2141
　tumors of skull base and, 2152–2153
Facial pain, 122
　anatomy and pathobiology of head
　　　and, 247–248
　atypical, 260–261
　cranial neuralgias and, 259–261
　extracranial patterns of referral and,
　　　248
　headache and, 247–261
Facial paralysis
　acute, 2139–2154
　　differential diagnosis of, 2143t
　assessment of, 2142t
　in children, 1058
　in cholesteatoma, 2090
　due to temporal bone fracture,
　　　2065–2071
　　facial nerve outcomes following,
　　　2067–2068, 2067t
　　facial nerve repair in, 2068–2071
　　management of, 2069–2071, 2070f
　due to trauma, 2149–2151, 2151f,
　　　2152f
　　management of injuries in, 2150t
　with ear infection, 2054
　electrophysiologic tests in,
　　　2145–2147, 2145t, 2146f

history taking in, 2142
laboratory studies in, 2143
in newborn, 2153
in otitis media, 2046, 2149
   treatment of, 2049–2050
physical examination in, 2142–2143
postoperative, 1528–1530
recovery from, classification of, 2144t
in salivary gland cancer, 1532
Facial reanimation, 2467–2480
   ancillary procedures in, 2477–2478,
      2478f, 2479f
   crossover technique for, 2470–2472,
      2472f, 2473f
   facial nerve anastomosis for, 2469,
      2469f, 2470f, 2471f
   facial nerve and, 2467, 2468f
   facial nerve repair with grafts,
      2469–2470, 2471f
   free muscle flaps in, 2479
   general considerations for,
      2467–2469
   muscle transposition techniques for,
      2470–2477, 2474f, 2475f,
      2476f
   techniques for, 2469–2477
Facial syndromes, 122
Facial translocation, for cranial-base
      surgery, 1841f, 1843
Facilitating techniques, in voice therapy,
      886
Facio-auriculo-vertebral sequence, 1314,
      1380–1381, 1380f
Factive (Gemifloxacin), 60
Famcyclovir
   in herpes simplex virus stomatitis,
      580
   in varicella zoster virus stomatitis,
      581
Fasciculus, solitary, 570
Fasciitis, synergistic necrotizing,
      622–623, 623f
Fat
   autologous, for soft-tissue
      augmentation, 2766
   deposition in neck, 2651
Fat pad, malar, 2772, 2773f
Fatty/muscular tumors, facial, 2737
Febrile neutropenia, chemotherapy-
      related, 1438t
Feeding, with cleft lip/cleft palate, 1320
Fellowships, medical practice and, 2807
Fentanyl, 148
Fetal alcohol syndrome, 1386, 1386f
Fetal wound healing, 208–209
Fever, postoperative
   causes of, 231, 231t
   evaluation of, 231
   treatment of, 231
Fiberoptic endoscopy, 706
   in swallowing evaluation, 749–751

with sensory testing, 706
   benefits of, 750–751
   technique/interpretation of, 750
Fiberoptic laryngoscopy, telescopic
      laryngology versus, 907
Fibrin glue, in wound healing, 208
Fibroblast growth factors, in wound
      healing, 205–206
Fibroma
   ameloblastic, 1577, 1577f
   ossifying, 191
      imaging of, 444
      of jaw, 1579–1580, 1580f
      sinonasal, 1485. See also Sinonasal
         tumors
Fibromyalgia
   definition of, 631, 632
   symptoms of, 632
   treatment of, 632
Fibroplasia phase, of wound healing,
      199
Fibrosarcoma
   sinonasal, 1485. See also Sinonasal
      tumors
   of temporal bone, 2018
Fibrosis, radiation, 1452
Fibrous dysplasia, 189–191, 190f
   differential diagnosis of, 191
   imaging of, 444, 444f
   of jaw, 1580, 1581f
   otologic manifestations of, 2164,
      2164f
   and Paget disease, compared, 191t
Fibrous histiocytoma, 180
Fibrous mass, of vocal fold, 838
   appropriate voice therapy referrals for,
      890
   common voice therapy applications
      for, 889t
Fibrous papules, 2736
   treatment of, 2746
Fibrous tumors, facial, 2736–2737
Fibular osteocutaneous flap,
      2381–2383, 2382f
Financial planning, medical practice
      and, 2805–2806
Finasteride (Propecia), 2749–2750
Fine-needle aspiration biopsy. See Biopsy
Fistula
   cerebrospinal fluid
      as complication of cranial-base
         surgery, 1846–1849
      as complication of sinus surgery,
         487
      as complication of temporal bone
         fracture, 2071–2075
         closure of, 2073–2075, 2074f
      postoperative, surgical management
         of, 1848–1849
   chylous, after neck dissection,
      1604–1605

dentocutaneous, 616–617, 617f
oroantral, 626
postoperative, in oral cancer, 1566
salivary, postoperative, 1530
Flail chest, from trauma, 929, 929f
Flaps. See also Skin flaps
   in lip reconstruction, 1543–1547,
      1543f–1547f
   microvascular free, 2369–2391, 2370t
      composite, 2381–2385
      fascial and fasciocutaneous,
         2369–2376
      muscle and musculocutaneous,
         2376–2380
      visceral, 2386–2387, 2386f
   in oral cavity reconstruction, 1560
Flavor, definition of, 568
Flexible fiberoptic laryngoscopy, in
      stridor in child, 1100, 1100f
Floor of mouth cancer, 1564. See also
      Oral cancer
Flow charts, of clinical pathways, 1420,
      1421f
Fluid management, in vocal therapy,
      884
Fluoroquinolones, 60
Fluoroscopy, of upper aerodigestive
      tract, 721
5-Fluorouracil, 1428t, 1430
Focal neurologic deficits, otitis media
      and, 2054
Follicle-stimulating hormone, 158
Follicular adenoma, thyroid, 1632
Follicular thyroid cancer, in children,
      1366–1367
Food allergy, otitis media and, 1267
Fordyce disease, 2791
Forehead
   aesthetics of, 2666
   aging, 2663–2683
   analysis of, for plastic surgery of face,
      2488
   anatomy of, 2663–2665, 2664f,
      2665f
   assessment of, 2666–2668
   transverse rhytids of, Botox injections
      in, 2763, 2763f
Forehead flaps, for nasal restoration,
      2433–2439, 2433t, 2435f,
      2436f, 2437f, 2438f, 2439f,
      2439t, 2440f
Forehead lift
   complications of, 2680–2681
   coronal
      advantages and disadvantages of,
         2669, 2670f
      contraindications to, 2669
      incision for, 2668, 2669f, 2670f
      technique for, 2670f, 2671–2672,
         2671f
   differential diagnosis for, 2668

Forehead lift (continued)
  endoscopic, 2678–2680, 2678f,
      2679f, 2680f
  history of, 2663
  midforehead, 2674–2675, 2675f
  pretrichial, 2672, 2673f
  trichophytic, 2672–2674, 2674f
Foreign bodies, 382
  aspiration of, 1111–1112
  esophageal, stridor from, 1069, 1070f
  nasal, 1073
Formaldehyde, inhaled, laryngitis and,
      830t
Formant regions, voice production and,
      897
Forme fruste, 1374
Formula feeding, with cleft lip/cleft
      palate, 1320
Fosphenytoin, 230
Foster-Kennedy syndrome, 120
Foville syndrome, 2791
Fraceschetti-Zwahlen-Klein syndrome,
      1384–1385, 1384f
Fractures. See specific types and sites
Fragile X syndrome, 46
Freckles, 2738
  treatment of, 2747
Freon, inhaled, laryngitis and, 830t
Frey syndrome, 122, 555, 1530–1531,
      1530f, 2791
Frontal bone fractures, in children,
      1338–1342. See also Facial
      fractures, in children
  surgery of, 1338
Frontal sinus
  ablation of, 375
  anatomy of, 309, 1009
  fractures of, 1009–1015
    antibiotic prophylaxis in, 1011
    biomechanics of, 1009–1010
    complications of, 1014–1015, 1014t
    endoscopic assistance in,
        1013–1014, 1013f
    epidemiology and etiology of, 1009
    evaluation of, 1010–1011
    frontonasal drainage and, 1014
    management of, 1009, 1010f,
        1011–1013, 1012f
    radiologic evaluation of, 1011
    treatment of, 1010f, 1011
  Lothrop procedure on, 375
  Lynch procedure on, 375
  management of, 1012f, 1013f
  surgery of, 373–375
    complications of, 375
    historical review of, 1011
    indications for, 374
    postoperative management in, 375
    techniques for, 374–375
Frontoethmoidectomy, external,
      374–375

Frostbite, 947
Frova Intubating Introducer, 773–774,
      775f
Functional aphonia
  common voice therapy applications
      for, 889t
  laryngeal dysfunction and, 878
Functional magnetic resonance
      imaging, 67
Fundamental frequency, in voice
      production, 897
Fundoplication, in aspiration, 1113
Fungal ball, sinus, 422–423
Fungal infections, 188, 386–387
  pharyngitis in, 608–609
Fungal infestation, saprophytic, 422
Fungal laryngitis, 830
Fungal rhinosinusitis, 417–428. See also
      Rhinosinusitis
Furlow palatoplasty, 1330–1333, 1333f
Furlow technique, for cleft lip, 1328
Furosemide, 227, 229, 400
  ototoxicity of, 1298
Furunculosis, 1998

G
Gabapentin, 260
Gadolinium-diethylenetriamine
      pentaacetic acid, 432
Gag, dysphagia and, 704
Gamma knife, in cranial-base surgery,
      1845–1846
Gantt charts, 1420
Garcin syndrome, 2791
Gardner syndrome, 2791–2792
Garel-Gignoux syndrome, 120
Gastric acid reflux, laryngeal stenosis
      and, 1137
Gastric injury, caustic, 1158f
Gastric pull-up and pharyngogastric
      anastomosis, in cervical
      esophageal cancer,
      1715–1717, 1716f
Gastroesophageal reflux
  complications of, 759
  diagnostic tests in, indications for,
      759, 759t
  dysphagia in, 726–727, 727f
  evaluation in, 759, 759t
  stridor in, 1108
  vs. laryngopharyngeal reflux,
      759–760, 760t, 833t
Gastrointestinal disorders, preoperative
      management of, 227–228
Gastroomentum, microvascular flaps
      of, 2387, 2387f
Gastrostomy, feeding, in chronic
      aspiration, 1113
Gatifloxacin (Tequin), 60
Gefitinib, 1431–1432
Gemifloxacin (Factive), 60

Gene array, and protein patterns, 101
Gene-directed, enzyme-prodrug
      therapy, 1398
Gene "libraries," 45
Gene products, in squamous cell
      carcinomas of head and neck,
      102, 102t
Gene targeting, strategies in, 48
Gene therapy, 1391–1401, 1438
  antisense, 1399
  cytokine, 1399
  ex vivo, 1391, 1392f
  gene transfer in, 1391, 1392f
  nonviral, 1395–1398
    promoters in, 1396
    targeting strategies in, 1396–1398,
        1398f
    viral vectors in, 1392–1395, 1398
  germ cell, 1391
  for head and neck cancer, 1400, 1400f
  immune response in, 1398–1399
  otologic, 1400, 1400f
  overview of, 1391–1392
  permanent, 1391–1392
  RNA interference, 1399
  somatic, 1391
  suicide, 1398
  therapeutic approaches in,
      1398–1399, 1398–1401
  transient, 1391
  in vivo, 1391, 1392f
Genetic anticipation, 46
Genetic disorders
  gene mapping for, 44–46
  management of patients with, 48–49
  molecular diagnosis of, 47–48, 47f, 47t
Genetic imprinting, 46
Genetic markers, in oral and head and
      neck cancers, 99–100
Genetic therapy, 48
Genetic transmission, patterns of, 42–44
Genetics, 41–51
  chromosomal anomalies and, 44
  nontraditional, 46
  of otolaryngologic disorders, 49–50
  principles of, 1303–1304
  transmission patterns in. See
      Inheritance
Genioglossus advancement,
      mandibular osteotomy with,
      662
Genioplasty, sliding, 2706–2707, 2707f
Genital herpes, fetal infection in,
      hearing loss and, 1294
Genotype, 42
Gentamicin, 58, 60, 61, 133
  in Ménière disease, 2322
  ototoxicity of, 1298
Geometric broken-line closure, for scar
      camouflage, 2414–2415,
      2415f

Germ cell gene therapy, 1391
Giant cell arteritis, 177–178, 178f
  headache in, 257–258
Giant cell reparative granuloma,
    388–389
Gingivitis, desquamative, stomatitis due
    to, 581–582, 581f, 582f, 582t
Gingivostomatitis, herpetic, 580, 606
GJB genes, in hearing loss, 1306–1307
Glabellar rhytids, Botox injections in,
    2763, 2763f
Glandular tumors
  of external auditory canal, 2012–2013
    histologic types of, 2012–2013
  of external ear
    diagnosis of, 2013
    treatment of, 2013
Glasgow coma scale, 926, 927t
Gliomas, 120
  nasal, congenital development of,
      1219, 1220–1221f
    clinical and pathologic features,
        1220–1221, 1224–1225t
    evaluation, 1223, 1224f
    surgical treatment, 1223–1226,
        1224f, 1225f
  optic nerve, 1505–1506, 1506f
Glomus jugulare, 1823
Glomus jugulare tumors, 121, 1980,
    1980f, 2006
Glomus tympanicum, 1970, 1970f
Glomus vagale tumor, 1821, 1823f
Glossopharyngeal nerve, 109f
  damage to, taste phantoms and, 576
  taste and, 569
  taste disorders and, 575
Glossopharyngeal neuralgias, 260
Glottic and supraglottic cancer,
      1768–1773
  advanced, treatment of, 1771–1773
  early, 1727–1741
    complications of, 1744t
    cricoarytenoid unit in, 1745, 1745f
    cricohyoidoepiglottopexy for,
        1722–1725
    cricohyoidopexy for, 1722–1725
    diagnosis of, 1728, 1729t, 1743t
    emergencies in, 1744t
    endoscopic treatment of,
        1722–1725
      in anterior commissure,
          1724–1725, 1724f
      glottic reconstruction after, 1725
      phonomicrosurgical, 1722
      subepithelial saline-epinephrine
          infusion into Reinke space in,
          1722, 1723f
      vertical partial laryngoscopy in,
          1723–1724
    invasive epidermoid, treatment of,
        1730

lymph node metastases in,
    1750–1751
  N0 neck in, 1750–1751
  open surgery for, 1743–1755
    for glottic cancer, 1751–1753
    indications for, 1751–1753
    postoperative care in, 1754
    preoperative planning of,
        1744–1745
    after radiation failure, 1753–1754
    for supraglottic cancer, 1753
    technique of, 1745–1750,
        1746f–1752f
    organ preservation in,
        1744–1745, 1745f
    radiation therapy for, 1721
    open surgery after, 1753–1754
  severe dysplasia and carcinoma in
      situ, 1729, 1730f
  staging of, 1744
  surgical management of,
        complications of, 1739, 1740
    treatment of, 1728–1738,
        1744–1745, 1744f, 1744t,
        1745f
    future directions in, 1753–1754
    verrucous, treatment of, 1731
  microinvasive, management of,
      1729–1730
Glottic closure reflex, 1097, 1098f
Glottic cycle, phonatory, 823f
Glottis, congenital anomalous conditions
    of, 1122t, 1126–1127
Glucocorticoids, 165. See also
    Corticosteroids
Goiter
  cervical, 1632
  nodular, 1632
  substernal, 1632, 1633t
  Goldenhar syndrome, 1380–1381,
      1380f, 2792
    hearing loss in, 1314, 1380
Gonadal dysgenesis syndrome, 2795
Gonorrhea, pharyngitis due to, 605
Gorlin cyst, 1572
Gorlin syndrome, 1572
Gout, 182–183, 549
  otologic manifestations of, 2162
Gracilis flap, 2379–2380, 2380f
Grade, Roughness, Breathiness,
    Asthenia, and Strain (GRBAS)
    scale, 825
Gradenigo syndrome, 2792
Grafts, in facial, head, and neck surgery,
    2345–2356
Granular cell myoblastoma, vs. oral
    cancer, 1557
Granulation tissue, 199
  extradural, in otitis media,
    2046–2047
  management of, 2050

management of laryngeal trauma
    and, 957t, 958
Granulocyte-macrophage colony-
    stimulation factor (GM-CSF),
    53
Granulocytic sarcoma, of orbit,
    1504–1505
Granulocytopenia, chemotherapy-
    related, 1438t
Granuloma
  giant cell reparative, 388–389
  midline, cocaine-induced, 382
  pyogenic, 181, 181f, 2736
    treatment of, 2746
  reparative, 181
  vocal fold, 840
  vocal-process, surgical controversies
    of, 910–911
Granulomatosis, Wegener, 176–177,
    177f, 380–381
Granulomatous disease, 179, 434
  laryngeal stenosis and, 1136–1137
  pharyngitis in, 609
  of salivary glands, 546–547
    in children, 1244
Graves disease
  ocular manifestations of, 137, 137f
  thyroid storm in, 165
GRBAS (Grade, Roughness, Breathiness,
    Asthenia, and Strain scale), 825
Griesinger sign, 2792
Grisel disease, 2792
Group B streptococcal disease, in
    children, hearing loss in, 1294
Growth and development
  abnormal. See Otolaryngologic
      syndromes
  patterns of, 1048–1055, 1048f, 1049f
Growth factors, in wound healing,
    204–206
Growth hormone, 155, 157–158
  deficiencies of, 158
  in wound healing, 206
Guillain-Barré syndrome, 116
Gum elastic bougie, 772, 772f
Gunshot wounds, facial, 1019–1020,
    1020f
Gustation, in elderly patients, 240–241
Gustatory sweating, 1530–1531, 1530f
  diagnosis of, 555–556
  prevention of, 556
  treatment of, 556–557

H

Haemophilus influenzae
  laryngitis due to, 829
  meningitis due to, in children,
      hearing loss in, 1296–1297
  rhinosinusitis due to, 1232, 1232t
Hair cells, of inner ear, regeneration of,
    gene therapy for, 1400, 1400f

Hair loss. *See* Alopecia
Hair transplantation, autograft
  donor site for, 2751–2752
  history of, 2751
  recipient site for, 2752–2753, 2752f
  sequelae and complications of, 2753,
    2753t
Hairline patterns, forehead lift and,
  2667
Hairy cell leukoplakia, 1558
  in AIDS, 270–271
Hallermann-Streiff syndrome, 2792
Hallgren syndrome, 1385
Halothane, 144–145
Hand-Schüller-Christian disease, 180,
  2017
Hansen disease. *See* Leprosy
Hard palate. *See* Palate
Harmonics, voice production and, 897
Hashimoto thyroiditis, 1631
Head and neck
  anatomy of
    facial pain and, 247–248
    surgical, 3–16
  movement of, 1905, 1906f
  pain-sensitive structures of, 248, 248t
  surgery of. *See also specific procedures
    and indications*
    pictorial documentation for,
      2499–2509. *See also*
      Photodocumentation
Head and neck cancer. *See also specific
  sites and types*
  in children
    lymphoma, 359–1363
    nasopharyngeal, 1367
    neuroblastoma, 1367
    sarcoma, 1364–1366
    thyroid, 1366–1367
  clinical pathways in, 1422–1425. *See
    also* Clinical pathways
  exogenous immunosuppressants and,
    1413
  immune response in, 1406–1413
    activation of, 1409
    cellular effectors in, 1410–1411
    cytokines in, 1411
    effector mechanisms in, 1409
    immunoglobulin structure and
      function in, 1409–1410, 1409f
    interferons in, 1411
    interleukins in, 1411–1413
    physiology of, 1406–1408, 1407f
    tumor cell antigens in, 1408–1409
  metastases in. *See* Metastases
  N0 neck in, 1560, 1566, 1611–1619.
    See also N0 neck
  orbital, 1501–1513. *See also* Orbital
    tumors
  radiation therapy for, 1441–1453. *See
    also* Radiation therapy

salivary gland, 1518–1532. *See also*
    Salivary gland disease
  treatment of
    biologic therapy in, 1431–1432
    chemotherapy in, 1427–1439. *See
      also* Chemotherapy *and
      specific cancers and agents*
    gene therapy in, 1399–1401. *See
      also* Gene therapy
    immunotherapy in, 1413–1414
    multidisciplinary approach in,
      1419, 1420t
    tumor biology in, 1403–1405
    clinical applications of, 1405–1406
Head trauma, 926–927, 927f
  intubation in, 797
  laryngeal dysfunction after, 872
  smell impairment in, 295
Headaches
  chronic daily, 252
  cluster. *See* Cluster headache
  cough, 256
  in cranial and cervical vascular
    disorder, 257–258
  diagnosis of, 249, 249t
  in disorders of face or cranial
    structures, 259
  epidemiology of, 247
  exertional, 256
  and facial pain, 247–261
  in head and neck trauma, 256–257
  and hematomas, 256–257
  hypnic, 256
  in intracranial hypertension, 258
  in low cerebrospinal fluid pressure,
    258
  migraine. *See* Migraine
  in nervous system infection, 258–259
  new-daily persistent, 256
  in nonvascular intracranial disorders,
    258–259
  otitis media and, 2054
  postcraniotomy, 257
  postoperative, 257
  primary, 248, 249–256
  in pseudotumor cerebri, 258
  secondary, 248, 256–261
  in sexual activity, 256
  sinus, 259
  Sluder, 2795
  stabbing, 256
  in temporomandibular disorders, 259
  tension-type, 250–251
    chronic, 252–253
    episodic, 252–253
  thunderclap, 256
    acute subarachnoid hemorrhage
      and, 257
Healing encounter, health status after,
  21f
Health insurance issues, 2806–2807

Hearing
  anatomy and physiology of,
    1883–1903
  development of, 1277
Hearing aids
  analogue, components of, 2280,
    2280f
  and assistive listening devices,
    2279–2293
  bone-anchored, 2284–2285
    in aural atresia, 2039
  candidates for, 2286–2287, 2287t
  for children, 1283–1285
  contralateral routing of signal type,
    2284
  digital signal processing, 2280–2281,
    2282
  directional
    attenuation provided by, 2281,
      2281f
    operation of, 2281–2282
  electroacoustic characteristics of,
    2285–2286, 2285f, 2286f
  functions of, 2280–2282
  gain and output of, 2285–2286,
    2285f, 2286f
    verification of, 2288–2289, 2288f
  microphone arrays for input into,
    2282
  middle ear implants, 2285
  output limiting by, 2286
  selection of, factors influencing, 2288
  styles and types of, 2282–2285, 2283f
    advantages and disadvantages of,
      2283t
  in subjective tinnitus, 2242
  use of one vs. two, 2287–2288
  validation and orientation in use of,
    2289
Hearing devices, implantable,
    2265–2277. *See also* Cochlear
    implants
Hearing evaluation
  after aural atresia surgery, 2038
  in children, 1277–1287, 1289–1291,
    1314–1315
    auditory brainstem response testing
      in, 1281–1282, 1289
    auditory steady-state response in,
      1282
    behavioral audiologic assessment
      in, 1279–1281
    behavioral observation audiometry
      in, 1269–1270, 1280
    behavioral testing in, 1280
    in central auditory processing
      disorders, 1286, 1287t
    conditioned play audiometry in,
      1281
    evoked otoacoustic emissions in,
      1289

genetic testing in, 1314–1315
history in, 1290
immitance testing in, 1280
in infants, 1277–1279, 1278t,
    1289, 1307
one-three-six rule for, 1314
in otitis media, 1269–1270, 1290,
    1290f
otoacoustic emission testing in,
    1282
overview of, 1287
pure-tone testing in, 1280
review of test results in,
    1282–1283, 1282f
speech testing in, 1280
team approach in, 1289–1290
visual reinforcement audiometry in,
    1269–1270, 1280–1281
indications for, 1939
in otosclerosis, 2127–2129, 2128f
Hearing handicap
evaluation of, 1930–1931, 1930t
permanent, definition of, 1930
Hearing impairment, permanent,
    definition of, 1930
Hearing loss
age-related, 128–129, 238–239,
    2258, 2258f, 2260f, 2260t
in AIDS, 269
in Alport syndrome, 1305t, 1313
assistive devices for. See also Hearing
    aids
in auditory neuropathy, 1307
after aural atresia surgery, 2039
in branchiootorenal syndrome,
    1305t, 1310, 1377–1378,
    1378f
in CHARGE association, 1378
in children
    amplification for, 1283–1286
    assistive devices for, 1285
    cochlear implants for, 1285–1286,
        1297
    drug-induced, 1297–1299, 1297t
    evaluation of. See Hearing
        evaluation, in children
    genetic, 1303–1315
        in autosomal dominant
            disorders, 1305t–1306t,
            1309–1312
        in autosomal recessive disorders,
            1304–1309
        in chromosomal disorders, 1314
        diagnosis of, 1306, 1307f,
            1314–1315
        genetic counseling for, 1315
        genetic principles and,
            1303–1304
        in mitochondrial disorders,
            1306t, 1313–1314, 1315
        in multifactorial disorders, 1314

in otolaryngologic syndromes,
    1375–1386. See also
    Otolaryngologic syndromes
overview of, 1315
in X-linked disorders, 1305t,
    1312–1314
management of, 1283–1287
otolaryngologists role in, 1286
sensorineural, 1289–1302
    epidemiology of, 1289
    etiology of, 1289–1300
    evaluation of, 1289–1291. See
        also Hearing evaluation, in
        children
    overview of, 1290–1291,
        1300–1302
speech and language development
    and, 1283, 1283t
cholesteatoma and, 2089
conductive, vs. sensorineural, 293
in congenital syphilis, 1293–1294
in congenital toxoplasmosis,
    1292–1293
in Crouzon syndrome, 1378–1379
in cytomegalovirus infection,
    1291–1292, 1291t, 1292t,
    2174–2175
in deafness dystonia syndrome, 1313
in Down syndrome, 1314, 1379
in elderly patients, 238–239,
    2258–2263
in enlarged vestibular aqueduct
    syndrome, 1308, 1308f
FM wireless system for, 2289–2291
in Goldenhar syndrome, 1314,
    1380–1381, 1380f
hearing aids for, 2279–2293. See also
    Hearing aids
hereditary, 49–50
idiopathic sudden sensorineural,
    2176–2177
infrared systems for, 2291
in Jervell and Lange-Nielsen
    syndrome, 1305t, 1307–1308
in Kartagener syndrome, 1381
in Kearnes-Sayre syndrome, 1314
in Klippel-Feil syndrome, 1313
level of impairment in, 2279
after mastoid surgery, 2109
in MELAS syndrome, 1314
in Melnick-Fraser syndrome,
    1377–1378, 1378f
in meningitis, 1296–1297, 2174t
in MERRF syndrome, 1314
in MIDD syndrome, 1314
in neonatal sepsis, 1294
in neurofibromatosis, 1310–1311
noise-induced. See Noise-induced
    hearing loss
nonsyndromic, 50
in Norrie disease, 1305t, 1312

in otitis media, 1269–1270, 1290,
    1290f
in otopalatodigital syndrome,
    1312–1313
in otosclerosis, 1311
in Paget disease, 191
in Pendred syndrome, 1305t, 1308
permanent, definition of, 1930
in rubella, 2175–2176
sensorineural
    causes of, 2259t
    in children, 1057–1058
    incidence of, 2279
    loudness and, 1895, 1897f
    symmetric, 2259t
    vs. conductive, 293
in Sildevanck syndrome, 1313
soundfield systems for, 2291
in Stickler syndrome, 1305t, 1311
sudden sensory, 2231–2236
    definition of, 2231
    differential diagnosis of,
        2231–2232, 2232t
    epidemiology of, 2231
    evaluation in, 2233
    in immune inner-ear disease,
        2232–2233
    in intracochlear membrane rupture,
        2232
    treatment of, 2233–2234
        results of, 2234–2235
    vascular compromise in, 2232
    in viral infection, 2232
in syphilis, 187
temporal bone trauma and,
    2075–2076
in Treacher Collins syndrome, 1306t,
    1311
in Turner syndrome, 1314
in Usher syndrome, 1306t,
    1308–1309
in Waardenburg syndrome, 49, 1305t,
    1311–1312, 1385–1386,
    1385f, 2795–2796
Heerfordt syndrome, 548
Hemangioendothelioma, Kaposi,
    1350–1351
Hemangiomas, 1349–1353, 1351f,
    1352f, 1811–1813
capillary, 2736
    orbital, 1502–1503
cavernous, 1811–1812, 1812f
    orbital, 1502
characteristics of, 1350t
classification of, 1811, 2009
congenital, 1127–1128, 1128f, 1350
diagnosis of, 1349–1350
facial nerve and, 2009
geniculate, 2009
incidence of, 1349
infantile, 1349–1350

Hemangiomas (continued)
life cycle of, 1349
lobular capillary, 181, 181f, 389
management of, 1352–1353
in PHACE syndrome, 1351–1352
retropharyngeal, 1071, 1073f
salivary gland, 541
subglottic, 1069, 1070f, 1090, 1091f, 1812, 1812f, 1813f
congenital, 1127–1128, 1128f
management of, 1352–1353
in PHACE syndrome, 1351–1352
stridor in, 1104, 1105f
treatment of, 1812–1813, 2009, 2746
Hemangiopericytoma, 1819, 2009
sinonasal, 1485–1486. See also Sinonasal tumors
Hematologic abnormalities, preoperative management of, 216–219
Hematoma
auricular, management of, 943–944, 944f, 945f
following blepharoplasty, 2623–2624
following cranial-base surgery, 1850
following forehead lift, 2681
following rhytidectomy, 2646–2647
following submentoplasty, 2660
headache and, 256–257
nasal septal, 327–328
orbital, sinus surgery and, 483
after thyroidectomy, 1643
Hemicrania, paroxysmal, 255
Hemicrania continua, 256
Hemifacial microsomia, 1380–1381, 1380f
Hemilaryngectomy, in early glottic carcinoma, 1731–1733
Hemoglobinopathies, preoperative management of, 217
Hemolytic streptococci
laryngitis and, 829
pediatric rhinosinusitis and, 1232, 1232t
Hemorrhage. See also Bleeding
acute subarachnoid, thunderclap headache and, 257
as complication of forehead surgery, 2680–2681
as complication of sinus surgery, 488
esophageal, 769
intracranial, 117
subarachnoid, 117
after thyroidectomy, 1642–1643
Hemostatic agents, in benign facial lesions, 2743–2744
Hemostatic disorders, 218t
preoperative management of, 217–218
Hennebert sign, 1294, 2792
Heparin, 217–218, 219
Hereditary telangiectasia, 2733t
hemorrhagic, 2736, 2736f, 2794

Hernia, hiatal, 747, 748f
congenital esophageal, 1131
Herpes esophagitis, 765
Herpes simplex encephalitis, in infants, hearing loss in, 1294–1295
Herpes simplex virus infection
of external auditory canal, 1999, 2155
pharyngeal, 606–607
diagnosis of, 607
stomatitis due to
clinical features of, 579–580, 580f
differential diagnosis of, 580
etiology of, 579
histopathology of, 580
treatment of, 580
Herpes virus vectors, 1395
Herpes zoster oticus, 1999, 2148–2149, 2180
Herpetic neuralgia, 260
Heterogeneity, 1304
Heterozygosity, 1303–1304
Hiatal hernia, 747, 748f
congenital esophageal, 1131
Hidrocystomas, 2735
Hinge flaps, 2366
Histiocytoma, fibrous, 180
Histiocytosis X. See Langerhans cell histiocytosis
Histoplasmosis, 188
laryngitis and, 830, 831f
Hoarseness, in AIDS, 271
Holinger laryngoscope, Eschmann endotracheal tube introducer with, 772, 772f
Holistic medicine, 2797
Hollander syndrome, 2792
Homeopathy, 2800–2801
Homografts, for soft-tissue augmentation, 2767
Homozygosity mapping, 45
Hordeolum, 130–131
Hormones. See under Endocrine
Horner syndrome, 122, 2007, 2792
Horton neuralgia, 2792
Hughlings Jackson syndrome, 119
Human bites, management of, 945–946
Human immunodeficiency virus
labyrinthitis associated with, 2182
life cycle of, 265f
properties of, 264–265
Human immunodeficiency virus infection. See also Acquired immunodeficiency syndrome
in children, viral sialadenitis and, 1243
clinical manifestations of, 266–272
external ear disease in, 2000
immune response in, 266
otologic manifestations of, 2159
pharyngitis in, 608

therapeutic targets for, 265–266
virology of, 264–265
Human papillomavirus, 1167–1168. See also Recurrent respiratory papillomatosis
oral cancer and, 1554–1555
skin cancer and, 1456
Hürthle cell adenoma, 1632
Hürthle cell carcinoma, 1633–1634
Hutchinson teeth, 2792
Hyalinizing trabecular adenoma, 1632
Hyaluronic acid products, for soft-tissue augmentation, 2766, 2766f
Hydration, for vocal therapy, 884
Hydrocephalus, otitic, in otitis media, 2047, 2050–2051
Hydrocortisone, 221
for adrenal suppression, 222, 222t
Hydrocystoma, treatment of, 2745
Hylaform, for soft-tissue augmentation, 2766
Hyoid bone, 817–819
anatomy of, 10, 11f
Hyoid myotomy, and suspension, in obstructive sleep apnea, 662–663
Hyperadrenocorticism, 162
Hyperaldosteronemia, 162
Hyperbilirubinemia, neonatal, hearing loss and, 1299
Hypercalcemic crisis, 164–165
Hyperglycemia, preoperative management of, 220
Hyperosmia, 293
causes of, 297
Hyperparathyroidism, 54–55, 1648–1650, 1648t
brown tumor of, 444–445, 445f
familial hypocalciuric, 55
Hyperpigmentation
following chemical peeling, 2721, 2722t
laser management of, 2417
Hyperplasia, primary chief cell, 1648
Hyperprolactinemia, 158–159
Hypersensitivity. See Allergy
Hypersensitivity vasculitides, 176
Hypertension
epistaxis in, 507
intracranial, headache in, 258
ocular manifestations of, 138–139, 139t
perioperative pharmacologic control of, 224, 224t
in pheochromocytomas, 163–164
preoperative management of, 224
Hypertrophic scars, 2736
treatment of, 2746
wound healing and, 211

Hypertrophy, turbinate. *See*
    Turbinate(s), hypertrophy of
Hypesthesia, as complication of sinus
    surgery, 489
Hypocalcemia, 165
    in thyroid surgery, 222
    after thyroidectomy, 1643
Hypogeusia. *See* Taste, loss/alteration of
Hypoglossal nerve, 110*f*
Hypopharyngeal cancer, 1691–1710
    diagnosis of
        history taking in, 1693, 1693*f*
        physical examination in,
            1693–1694
        radiology in, 1694
    emergency care in, 1708, 1708*t*
    molecular pathology of, 1696
    in neck region, management of,
        1704–1705
    pathology of, 1694–1696, 1694*t*
    patterns of spread of, 1694–1696,
        1695*t*
    postcricoid, 1704, 1707
    posterior wall, 1697–1700, 1697*f*,
        1698*f*, 1699*f*, 1700*f*, 1706
    prognosis in, 1704*t*, 1706–1707
    staging of, 1696
    T1 and T2 pyriform sinus cancer and,
        1700–1703, 1701*f*, 1702*f*,
        1703*f*, 1706–1707
    T3 and T4 pyriform sinus cancer and,
        1701*f*, 1702*f*, 1703–1704,
        1703*f*, 1706–1707
    treatment of, 1696–1706, 1706*t*
        chemotherapy in, 1437, 1705–1706
        radiation therapy in, 1696, 1696*t*,
            1705–1706
        surgery in, 1696–1705, 1697*f*,
            1698*f*, 1699*f*, 1700*f*, 1701*f*,
            1702*f*, 1703*f*
        complications of, 1708, 1708*t*
        reconstruction following,
            1707–1708
Hypopharynx
    anatomy of, 13, 1691–1692, 1691*f*,
        1692*f*
    foreign body in, 1065, 1065*f*
    obstruction of, respiratory distress in,
        1088–1089
Hypopigmentation
    camouflage of, 2416–2417
    following chemical peeling,
        2721–2722
Hyposmia, 292–296
    age-related, 292
    causes of, 293–296
Hypotension
    perioperative, pharmacologic control
        of, 225*t*
    postoperative, prevention of,
        224–225

Hypotheses, testing of, analytic statistics
    and, 24–25, 24*t*
Hypothyroidism, 158
    obstructive sleep apnea and, 653–654
    preoperative management of, 221
Hypovolemic shock, in trauma patients,
    924–925
Hypoxia
    perinatal, hearing loss and, 1299
    tumor cell, in radiation therapy,
        1446, 1446*f*, 1447*f*

I
Ibritumomab, for extranodal lymphoma,
    1624, 1624*t*, 1625
Idiopathic orbital inflammation,
    1509–1510, 1509*f*
Ileus, adynamic, postoperative
    management of, 228
Iliac crest flaps, osteocutaneous and
    osteomusculocutaneous,
    2383, 2384*f*
Image guidance
    for biopsy, 69–71
    description of, 68–69
    equipment for, 72*f*
    in otolaryngology, 68–74
    and staging endoscopy, 73–74
Imaging, 85–97. *See also specific*
        modalities
    in aspiration, 1112
    conventional, 86, 86*t*
    in cranial-base surgery, 1830–1832,
        1831*t*
    digital camera applications in, 76–80
    high-technology, 87, 88*t*
    in hypopharyngeal cancer, 1694
    modalities of, 86–87
    in odontogenic infections, 628
    in ophthalmology, 139
    in otolaryngology
        image guidance for, 68–74
        technology in, 67–83
    principles of, 85
IMC225, 1431
Imipenem, 59
Immune response, 335–336
    dendritic cells in, 1406–1408, 1407*f*,
        1412–1413
    in head and neck cancer, 1406–1413
    immunoglobulins in, 1409–1410,
        1409*f*
    in neonate, 1406, 1409
    physiology of, 1406–1408, 1407*f*
Immune system
    adaptive, 337–338
    cells of, 342–347
    innate, 336–337
Immunization
    for melanoma, 1475–1476
    for otitis media, 1272

for *Streptococcus pneumoniae*, in
    infants and children, 1059
Immunodeficiency, otitis media and,
    1266–1267
Immunoglobulins, 345–347
    IgA, 346
    IgD, 346
    IgE, 346–347
        development of, 339, 341*f*
    IgG, 346
    IgM, 346
    structure and function of, 1409–1410,
        1409*f*
Immunologic diseases, otologic
    manifestations of, 2159–2161
Immunology
    and allergy, 335–349
    geriatric, 242–243, 243*t*
Immunosuppression, laryngitis and, 832
Immunotherapy
    active, 1413
    adoptive, 1413
    allergen-specific, 347
    in allergy, 55
    for extranodal lymphoma, 1624,
        1624*t*, 1625–1626
    for head and neck cancer, 1413–1414
    in rhinitis, 360
Impacted tooth, dentigerous cyst and,
    1570–1571, 1570*f*
Implantable hearing devices,
    2265–2277
Implants
    biocompatibility of, 2348
    biologic materials as, 2346*t*, 2347
    bioresorbable, for
        maxillary/periorbital
        fractures, 991
    ceramic, 2346–2347, 2346*t*
    cochlear. *See* Cochlear implants
    dental, 1861–1863, 1862*f*
    in face, head, and neck, 2345–2356
        characteristics of, 2345–2348, 2346*t*
        complications and emergencies
            associated with, 2354–2355,
            2355*t*
        indications for, 2348–2349
        patient evaluation for, 2348–2349
        preoperative counseling for, 2349
        qualities needed for, 2349
        surgical management for,
            2349–2354
    metallic, 2345–2346, 2346*t*
    placement of, complications of, 628
    polymers as, 2346*t*, 2347
    surface properties of, 2347–2348
    visibility of, in maxillary/periorbital
        fractures, 990
In vitro testing, in rhinitis, 357
Incisions. *See also specific procedures and*
        approaches

Incisions (continued)
  in facial trauma, 1036–1037, 1036f, 1037f
  mandibular, 1036, 1037f
Incisive canal cyst, 1573
Increased intracranial pressure, headache in, 258
Infants. See also Pediatric patients
  hearing loss in. See also Hearing loss, in children
    screening for, 1277–1279, 1278t, 1289, 1307. See also Hearing evaluation, in children
Infections, 183–189. See also specific sites and types
  facial, 2739, 2739f
  "hygiene hypothesis" of, 338
  otolaryngologic, in children, 1058–1059
  otologic manifestations of, 2155–2159
Infectious mononucleosis, Epstein-Barr-associated
  atypical, 607–608
  clinical course of, 607–608
  diagnosis of, 607
  pharyngitis in, 607
  symptoms of, 607
Inflammatory bowel disease, 389
Inflammatory diseases, of unknown etiology, 377–380
Inflammatory phase, of wound healing, 199
Infratemporal bone, in sinonasal cancer, 1492
Infratemporal fossa, approaches to, 1840f, 1842–1843
Inhalation injuries, in trauma patients, 931
Inheritance. See also Genetics
  autosomal dominant, 42f, 43, 1371–1373, 1372f
  autosomal recessive, 42–43, 42f, 1372f, 1373
  expressivity and, 1374
  heterogeneity and, 1374
  maternal, 46
  multifactorial, 43–44
  penetrance in, 1373–1374
  pleiotropy and, 1374
  sex-linked, 42f, 43
  X-linked, 1372f, 1373
Injectable fillers, Botox and, cosmetic uses of, 2761–2769
Injection augmentation laryngoplasty. See also Laryngeal injectables
  lipoinjection, 913–914
  synthetic materials, 913
Inner ear. See Ear, inner
Innominate artery compression, 1130, 1131f

Inspiratory and expiratory pressure threshold training, in voice therapy, 886
  common applications to voice disorders, 889t
Instrumentation, for plates and screws, 1033
Insulin, preoperative, in diabetes mellitus, 220, 220t, 221
Insurance planning, medical practice and, 2806–2807
Integrative medicine, 2798
Intense pulsed light, for skin resurfacing, 2727
Intensity modulated radiation therapy, 1443, 1444f–1445f
Interarytenoidius muscle, voice production and, 896
Interferon(s)
  for hemangiomas, 1352, 1813
  immunosuppressive effects of, 1413
  in immunotherapy, for head and neck cancer, 1413
  for skin cancer, 1463, 1475, 1476
    melanoma, 1475, 1476
Interleukins
  in gene therapy, 1399
  for head and neck cancer, 1413–1414
Intermaxillary fixation, in children, 1345
Intracochlear membranes, rupture of, sudden sensory hearing loss in, 2232
Intracranial pressure, 1829
  increased, headache in, 258
Intraocular pressure, 128
Intraoperative monitoring, neurophysiologic, 1943–1960
  applications and benefits of, 1947–1951, 1949f, 1950f
  auditory system monitoring techniques, 1944–1947
  of facial nerve, 1951–1957
  of recurrent laryngeal nerve, 1643
Intraoral prosthetics, to improve deglutition, 715–716
Invasive fibrous thyroiditis, 1631–1632
Iressa, 1431–1432
Iridocyclitis, 131–132
Iris, melanoma of, orbital invasion by, 1511
Iritis, 131–132
Isolagen, for soft-tissue augmentation, 2767

J
Jackson vagus-accessory-hypoglossal paralysis, 119
Jacobson nerve, 2792
Jacood syndrome, 2792
Jadassohn nevus, 2735, 2735f

Jaundice, neonatal, hearing loss and, 1299
Jaw. See also Mandible; Maxilla
  aneurysmal bone cyst of, 1582
  central giant cell lesion of, 1580–1582, 1582f
  cysts of, 1569–1573
    nonodontogenic, 1571–1573
    odontogenic, 1569–1571. See also Odontogenic cysts
  fibrous dysplasia of, 1580, 1581f
  odontogenic tumors of, 1573–1577. See also Odontogenic tumors
  ossifying fibroma of, 1579–1580, 1580f
  osteoma of, 1578
  osteomochondroma of, 1578–1579, 1579f
  vascular malformations of, 1582–1583
Jaw winking syndrome, 2793
Jawline, assessment of, for plastic surgery of face, 2492, 2492f
Jejunal interposition graft, dysphagia and, 730, 730f
Jejunostomy, in chronic aspiration, 1113
Jejunum, microvascular flaps of, 2386–2387, 2386f
Jet ventilation stylet introducer, 773, 774f
Journal articles
  grandeur in, signs of, 18t
  interpretation of, 17–32
  worth reading, identification of, 17–18
Jugular vein blow-out, after neck dissection, 1606
Jugular vein thrombosis, 624, 624f
  after neck dissection, 1605–1606
Juguloparaganglioma, 1823
Junctional nevus, 2737, 2737f
Juri flap, in alopecia, 2757–2758, 2757f

K
Kallmann syndrome, 159, 2792
Kanamycin, 61
  ototoxicity of, 1298
Kaposi sarcoma, 1820
  in AIDS, 267–268, 268f, 270
  oral, 1558
Kaposiform hemangioendothelioma, 1350–1351. See also Hemangiomas
Karapandzic labioplasty, 1541f, 1543, 1543f, 1545
Kartagener syndrome, 49, 1381–1382
Kasabach-Merritt phenomenon, kaposiform hemangioendothelioma in, 1350–1351. See also Hemangiomas
Kawasaki disease, 179

Kearnes-Sayre syndrome, 1314
Keloids, 2736, 2736f
  treatment of, 2746
  wound healing and, 211
Keratinocyte growth factor, 53
Keratitis, 131
Keratoacanthoma, 1459–1460, 1459f
  of lip, 1538
Keratocysts, odontogenic, 1571–1572, 1571f
Keratoses
  actinic, 2731
    treatment of, 2744
  seborrheic, 2731–2734
    treatment of, 2744
  senile, 1459, 1459f
Keratosis follicularis, 2791
Keratosis obturans, imaging of, 1964, 1965f
Kernicterus, hearing loss and, 1299
Ketamine, 147
Ketek (Telithromycin), 59
Ketolides, 59
Kiesselbach plexus/area, 2792
Klack's solution, 171
Klebsiella pneumoniae, laryngitis and, 829
Klebsiella rhinoscleromatis, 832
Klippel-Feil syndrome, hearing loss in, 1313
Klippel-Trenaunay syndrome, 1356
Körner septum, 2792
Koplik spots, 2792
Krause nodes, 2792
Kussmaul disease, 2792

L
Labial arteries, 1535, 1536f
Labyrinth
  anatomy of, 2169–2170
  form and function of, 2169–2170
  infections of, 2169–2187
  injury of, in surgery for aural atresia, 2038
  membranous
    development of, 1875–1876, 1876f
    innervation of, development of, 1876–1877
  osseous, development of, 1877
  physiology of, 2169–2170
Labyrinthectomy
  chemical, in Ménière disease, 2321–2322
  in vestibular disorders, 2338–2339, 2339f
Labyrinthine fistula, as complication of cholesteatoma, 2089–2090
Labyrinthitis
  acute cochlear, and neuritis, 2176–2177
  acute vestibular, 2177–2179

  audiometric evaluation in, 2178
  differential diagnosis of, 2178
  treatment of, 2178–2179, 2178t
  in bacterial meningitis, hearing loss and, 1297
  hemorrhagic, 1972–1973, 1974f, 1975f
  in human immunodeficiency virus, 2182
  measles, 2179–2180, 2180t
  mumps, 2179, 2179t
  in otitis media
    diagnosis of, 2046
    treatment of, 2049–2050
  syphilitic, 2182–2184
  viral, 2173–2174
    perinatal, 2174
    postnatal, 2176
Lacerations, facial, 937, 939
  closing stellate wounds, 939f
  débridement and undermining of, 937f
  suturing, 938f
  trapdoor, 938f
Lacrimal glands/system, 5, 5f
  inflammation/infection of, 1508
  radiation injury of, 1452
  traumatic injuries of, management of, 941–943, 942f, 943f
  tumors of, 1508–1509, 1508f
  lymphoid, 1504, 1508
Lagophthalmos, 2681
  following blepharoplasty, 2624
  paralytic, weight implantation in, 2477, 2478f
Lambert-Eaton syndrome, laryngeal dysfunction and, 874–875
Lamina papyracea, 308
Lamina propria
  anatomy, 820
  benign lesions of, 838–839
Lamivudine, 274
Langer lines, 2792
Langerhans cell histiocytosis, 179–180
  incidence of, 180
  orbital involvement in, 1505
  organ systems involved in, 180
  otologic manifestations of, 2164–2165
  treatment of, 180
Language. See also Speech; Voice
  development of, 1057t
  production of, 897
Laryngeal cancer
  advanced, 1757–1777
    adjuvant radiation in, 1770
    chemotherapy and organ preservation in, 1773–1774
    complications of radiation in, 1775
    complications of surgery for, 1774–1775, 1775t

  diagnostic surgery in, 1764–1765
  differential diagnosis of, 1765
  emergency surgery in, 1775–1776, 1776t
  evaluation and diagnosis of, 1761–1765, 1763t
  history taking in, 1761–1762
  improving prognosis of, 1774
  multidisciplinary care in, 1765
  natural history of, 1765–1766
  patterns of spread of, 1759–1760, 1760f
  physical examination in, 1763
  staging of, 1760–1761, 1762t
  subglottic lesions in, 1773
  treatment of, 1766–1771, 1766t
  biology of, 1727–1728
  chemotherapy for, 1437
  epidemiology of, 1758
  glottic lesions in. See Glottic and supraglottic cancer
  lymphoma. See Lymphoma, extranodal
  metastasis to neck, 1767, 1767t
  supraglottic lesions in, 1768–1770, 1768t, 1769f, 1771. See also Glottic and supraglottic cancer
  treatment of, organ-preserving, 1436–1437
Laryngeal dyskinesia, stridor in, 1108
Laryngeal electromyography. See Electromyography, laryngeal
Laryngeal incompetence, management of, in aspiration, 1114
Laryngeal injectables, 857t. See also Injection augmentation laryngoplasty
  medialization laryngoplasty and, 857–859, 858f
Laryngeal mask airway, for extratracheal ventilation, 774, 776f, 777f
Laryngeal nerve(s)
  age-related changes in, 242, 242t
  severed recurrent, management of, 957
Laryngeal pacing, 864
Laryngeal separation, complications of, 739t
Laryngeal stenosis
  acquired
    postintubation, 1135–1136
    postoperative, 1136
  anatomy, pediatric versus adults, 1133
  complications, 1144
  congenital
    grading scale for, 1135t
    subglottic, 1127, 1134–1135
      histopathologic classification of, 1135t
    supraglottic or glottic atresia and, 1135

Laryngeal stenosis (continued)
  webs, 1135
  decision making, 1143
  differential diagnosis, 1137–1138,
      1138t
  emergencies, 1144–1145
  infectious or inflammatory, 1136–1137
  management
    endoscopic, factors in failure with,
        1139t
    medical therapy, 1138, 1139t
    natural history, 1138
    preoperative assessment, 1138
    surgical treatment, 1138–1140, 1139t
      anterior cricoid split, 1140–1141,
          1140f, 1140t
      cricotracheal resection, 1142f,
          1143
      laryngotracheal reconstruction–
          anterior and posterior
          cartilage grafts, 1143
      laryngotracheal reconstruction–
          anterior cartilage graft, 1141,
          1141f
      laryngotracheal reconstruction–
          posterior cartilage graft, 1141
      stenting options, 1143, 1144f
    in trauma, 957t, 958
  signs and symptoms of, 1133–1134,
      1134t
  subglottis, management of, 811
Laryngeal trauma, 949. See also Trauma
  complications, 957–958, 957t
  diagnosis and evaluation, 950t
    history, 950
    physical examination, 950
    radiologic evaluation, 950–952,
        951f
  injury groups, 958t
  management
    algorithm, 952, 952f
    cricotracheal separation, 956–957
    emergency care, 952–953, 953t
    grafting, 955
    medical treatment, 953–954
    severed recurrent laryngeal nerve,
        957
    stents, 955–956, 957f
    surgical treatment, 954–955, 954f,
        955f, 956f
    treatment decision making, 953,
        953t
  pathophysiology of, 949–950
  stenosis and, 1137
Laryngectomy
  near-total, 1769, 1769f
  open partial, in early glottic
      carcinoma, 1731,
      1732–1733f, 1734f
  operative defect following, anatomy
      of, 1779, 1780f

supracricoid partial, with
    cricohyoidopexy, 1768–1769,
    1769f
  supraglottic, 1768, 1769f
    partial, 1743
  tracheoesophageal puncture following.
      See Tracheoesophageal
      puncture
  vertical partial, in early glottic
      carcinoma, 1738, 1738f
    with laryngoplasty, 1731, 1733–1738,
        1735f, 1736f, 1737f
  voice rehabilitation after, 1779–1791
  voice restoration during, 1787, 1787f,
      1788f
Laryngitis, 829
  antimicrobial agents for, 64
  diagnosis, 830t
  immunologic defenses against, 835
  infectious, 830t
    bacterial, 829–830
    blastomycosis and, 830
    fungal, 830
    histoplasmosis and, 830, 831f
    immunocompromised host and,
        832
    leprosy and, 831
    scleroma and, 832
    syphilis and, 831
    tuberculosis and, 831
    viral, 829
  inflammatory (reactive), 830t
    allergies and, 835
    angioedema, 834–835
    inhaled steroids and, 835
    laryngopharyngeal reflux, 833–834
    radiation and, 835
    thermal injury, 834
    traumatic, 834
  relapsing polychondritis and, 833
  systemic diseases causing, 830t
    amyloidosis, 832
    cicatricial pemphigoid, 833
    epidermolysis bullosa, 833
    rheumatoid arthritis, 832
    sarcoidosis, 833
    systemic lupus erythematosus, 833
    Wegener granulomatosis, 832
Laryngology
  diagnostic controversies
    flexible endoscopic evaluation of
        swallowing, 909–910
    laryngeal electromyography,
        908–909
    laryngopharyngeal reflux diagnosis,
        909
    stroboscopy, 907–908
    telescopic versus fiberoptic, 907
    transnasal esophagoscopy, 910
  medical therapy controversies, 910
  surgical controversies

early carcinoma of vocal fold, 911
    injection augmentation
        laryngoplasty, 913–914
    laryngoplastic phonosurgery,
        911–912
    microlaryngeal surgery, 912–913
    office-based, 914
    Polytef (Teflon) use, 911
    spasmodic dysphonia, 914
    vocal-process granulomas, 910–911
  uses, 881, 881f
Laryngomalacia, 1126
  in infants, 1065–1066
  stridor in, 1089, 1089f
  stridor in, 1102–1103, 1104f
    exercise-induced, 1108
    in infants, 1089, 1089f
Laryngopharyngeal reflux, 830t
  controversies in diagnosis of, 909
  controversies in treatment of, 910
  gastroesophageal reflux versus, 833t
  laryngitis and, 833–834
  voice therapy and, 884
  vs. gastroesophageal reflux disease,
      759–760, 760t
Laryngoplastic phonosurgery. See also
      Medialization laryngoplasty
  controversies in use of, 911–912
Laryngoscope
  anterior commissure, 772, 773f
  flexible fiberoptic, 153
  Holinger, Eschmann endotracheal
      tube introducer with, 772,
      772f
  large-bore, endotracheal intubation
      with, 797
Laryngoscopy
  direct, 152
  fiberoptic, in obstructive sleep apnea,
      660
  flexible fiberoptic, in stridor in child,
      1100, 1100f
Laryngospasm
  airway obstruction in, 1090
  episodic paroxysmal, 878–879, 878f
Laryngotracheal injuries, in penetrating
      trauma, 1025
Laryngotracheal reconstruction
  with anterior and posterior cartilage
      grafts, for laryngeal stenosis,
      1143
  with anterior cartilage graft for
      laryngeal stenosis, 1141, 1141f
  with posterior cartilage graft for
      laryngeal stenosis, 1141
Laryngotracheal separation
  in aspiration, 739–741, 740t, 1114
  in endotracheal intubation, 798, 798f
Laryngotracheal stenosis, stridor in,
      1103–1104, 1105t
Laryngotracheobronchitis

glottic obstruction in, 1066, 1067, 1067*f*

stridor in, 1108–1109

upper airway obstruction and, 803

Larynx. *See also under* Laryngeal; Vocal fold(s); Voice

age-related changes in, 821

in AIDS, 271

airway protection and, 821

anatomy of, 13–14, 13*f*, 695–698, 695*f*, 696*f*, 1758–1759, 1758*f*, 1759*f*

in children vs. adults, 1053–1054, 1053*f*, 1054*f*, 1121*f*, 1133

framework, 817–819

membranous vocal fold, 820–821

muscles and nerves, 696–698, 697*f*, 819–820

normal, in infant, 1095, 1096*f*, 1097*f*

artificial, following laryngectomy, 1779–1780

circulatory reflexes and, 700

closure of, in laryngeal incompetence, 1114

congenital anomalies of, 1122*t*

glottis, 1126–1127

neonatal respiratory distress in, 1089–1090, 1090*f*, 1091*f*

subglottis, 1127–1128, 1128*f*

supraglottis, 1126

in deglutition, 686–687, 686*f*

imaging of, 92–93

lymphoma of. *See* Lymphoma, extranodal

mucosal cover of, 698, 698*f*

mucosal defenses of, 835

neurologic disorders, 867

anterior horn cell/motor neuron disease

amyotrophic lateral sclerosis, 872

bulbar palsy, 872

neuropathies, 873–874

poliomyelitis, 872

postpolio syndrome, 873

central nervous system disease, 867–872

Arnold-Chiari malformations, 868, 870*f*

closed head injury and, 872

multiple sclerosis, 868–869, 871*f*

Parkinson disease, 869–871

Parkinsonism plus syndromes, 871–872

stroke, 872

Wilson disease, 872

dystonia, 876

episodic paroxysmal laryngospasm, 878–879, 878*f*

essential tremor, 877

examinations for, 869*t*

functional aphonia, 878

miscellaneous, 877–878

muscle tension dysphonia, 878

myoclonus, 877

myopathic

dermatomyositis, 875

muscular dystrophies, 875

polymyositis, 875

at neuromuscular junction

aminoglycoside antibiotics, 875

Botox mechanism, 875

botulism, 875

Lambert-Eaton syndrome, 874–875

myasthenia gravis, 874

myasthenic syndrome, 874–875

paradoxical vocal fold motion disorder, 878–879, 878*f*

soft palate, epiglottis and, 868*f*

spasmodic dysphonia, 876–877

tic disorders, 877

phonation and, 700–701

respiration and, 698–700, 822

skeleton of, 695–696, 696*f*, 697*f*, 698*f*

voice and, 822–824, 823*f*

Laser(s)

532-nm and 1,064-nm, for nonablative skin rejuvenation, 2728

1320-nm dermal collagen stimulating, for nonablative skin rejuvenation, 2728

1420-nm dermal collagen stimulating, for nonablative skin resurfacing, 2728–2729, 2728*f*

carbon dioxide, 2725–2726

erbium, 2725–2727

precautions in use of, 139

resurfacing, 2725–2727

Laser-assisted uvulopalatoplasty, in snoring, 657, 658*f*

Laser therapy

for benign facial lesions, 2742–2743, 2744*t*

for capillary malformations, 1353–1354

in endoscopic arytenoidectomy

partial, 864

total, 864, 864*f*

for hemangiomas, 1352

for recurrent respiratory papillomatosis in children, 1174–1176

safety issues in, 2725

for skin cancer, 1463–1465, 1465*f*

skin resurfacing, 2725–2729

lasers for, 2725–2727

patient selection for, 2726, 2726*t*

for scar camouflage, 2415–2416

Lateral arm flap, 2371–2372, 2373*f*

Lateral cricoarytenoid muscle, voice production and, 896

Lateral neck dissection, 1596, 1597*f*

Lateral thigh flap, 2372–2373

Lateral thyroid tissue, 1630

Latissimus dorsi flap, 2378–2379, 2379*f*

Le Fort fractures, 977–978, 977*f*, 978*f*

in children, 1338–1342. *See also* Facial fractures

surgery of, 1347

Lee Silverman Voice Therapy, 870–871, 871*t*, 886

Legal issues, in standards of care, 1421

Leiomyoma(s)

of esophagus, 766, 766*f*

multiple, 2737, 2737*f*

treatment of, 2746

Leishmaniasis, 188–189, 387–388

Lemierre syndrome, 624, 624*f*

Lentigines, 2738

treatment of, 2747

Lentigo maligna, 1470

Lentigo senilis, 2738, 2738*f*

Lentivirus vectors, 1395

Leprosy, 185–186, 383

classification of, 609

histopathology of, 609

manifestations of, 186*t*

otologic manifestations of, 2158

pharyngitis in, 609

treatment of, 186, 609

Leptomeningeal disease, 1982–1984

Lermoyez syndrome, 2792

Lethargy/coma, otitis media and, 2054

Letterer-Siwe disease, 180, 2017

Leukemia

orbital involvement in, 1504–1505

temporal bone involvement in, 2010

Leukoplakia, 1558–1559

candidal, 595

hairy cell, 1558

in AIDS, 270–271

Leukotriene modifiers, in rhinitis, 360

Levo-bupivacaine, 142

Levofloxacin (Levaquin), 60

Lichen planus, stomatitis due to

clinical features of, 592–593, 593*f*

differential diagnosis of, 593–594

etiology of, 592

histopathology of, 593, 594*f*

treatment of, 593–594

Lidocaine, 141–142, 225

Lillie-Crowe test, 2792

Linezolid (Zyvox), 61

Lingual thyroid, 1629

Lingual tonsils, 1197

Lip(s). *See also under* Oral

anatomy and physiology of, 1535–1537, 1536*f*

biopsy of, 1537

cancer of, 1535–1548

airway management in, 1548

Lip(s) *(continued)*
  biologic behavior of, 1537
  clinical evaluation of, 1537–1538
  diagnosis of, 1537–1538, 1538*t*
  etiology of, 1537
  incidence of, 1535
  nodal metastases in, 1537,
    1539–1540
  nutrition in, 1548
  overview of, 1535, 1548
  radiation therapy for, 1538–1539
    complications of, 1548, 1548*t*
    risk factors for, 1537
  staging of, 1537
  surgery for, 1538–1548
    complications of, 1548, 1548*t*
    reconstructive, 1540–1547,
      1541*f*–1547*f*
    cellulitis of, 616, 616*f*
  cleft. *See* Cleft lip/cleft palate
  in deglutition, 685, 686*f*
  evaluation of, for plastic surgery of
    face, 2491*f*, 2492
  keratoacanthoma of, 1538
  premalignant lesions of, 1538
  skin flap of, after Mohs surgery, 2398,
    2399*f*, 2400*f*
  swelling of, in Melkersson-Rosenthal
    syndrome, 1382
  ulcers of, differential diagnosis of,
    1538
  vertical rhytids of, Botox in, 2764
Lipoma
  of cerebellopontine angle, 2023
  imaging of, 2023
  of internal auditory canal, 1982,
    1983*f*, 2023
  of salivary glands, 541, 541*f*
  treatment of, 2746
Liposarcoma, of salivary glands, 541
Liposome-based vectors, in gene
    therapy, 1396
Liposuction, submental, and anterior
    platysmaplasty, 2658–2659,
    2658*f*, 2659*f*, 2660*f*
  complications of, 2660–2661
Literature. *See also* Journal articles
  interpretation of, 17–32
Lithium, 165
Lithotripsy, in sialolithiasis, 558
Little area, 2793
Lobular capillary hemangioma, 181,
    181*f*, 389
Loracarbef (Lorabid), 58–59
Louis-Bar syndrome, 2793
LT receptor antagonists, 400
Ludwig angina, 619, 619*f*, 2793
Lung. *See under* Pulmonary
    complications
Lupus erythematosus
  discoid, 171

otologic manifestations of,
    2160–2161
stomatitis due to
  clinical features of, 582–583
  differential diagnosis of, 583,
    584–585*t*
  etiology of, 582
  histopathology of, 583
systemic, 169–171
  diagnostic criteria for, 170*t*
  head and neck manifestations of,
    170–171, 171*f*
  laryngitis and, 830*t*, 833
  treatment of, 171
Luschka pouch, 2793
Luteinizing hormone, 158
Lyme disease, otologic manifestations
    of, 2157–2158
Lymph node(s)
  salivary gland, 520
  sentinel, dissection of, in skin cancer,
    562
Lymph node biopsy
  indications for, 272, 272*t*
  in oral cancer, 1560
  sentinel node, 103–104, 1591
    of N0 neck, 1615, 1617–1618
    in oral cancer, 1560
Lymph node metastases. *See also* N0
    neck
  in early glottic/supraglottic cancer,
    1750–1751
  imaging of, 91
  in lip cancer, 1537, 1539–1540
  in melanoma, 1472–1474, 1476
    treatment of, 1476
  in oral cancer, 1560
  in sinonasal cancer, 1490
  in skin cancer, 1467
  in thyroid cancer, 1645
Lymphadenopathy
  in AIDS, 272
  in odontogenic infections, 627–628
  retropharyngeal, 1070, 1071*f*, 1072*f*
Lymphangioma, 1814–1815, 1815*f*
  orbital, 1503, 1502
  of salivary glands, 541
Lymphatic drainage
  of hypopharynx, 1692, 1692*f*
  of lips, 1535–1537, 1536*f*
  of oral cavity, 1552–1554, 1554*f*
  Lymphatic malformations, 1355
Lymphatic vessels, of neck, 15
Lymphocytes, 343–345
  B, 344–345, 1406
    in head and neck cancer, 1410–1411
  geriatric, 242–243
  in head and neck cancer, 1410–1411
  structure and function of, 1406–1408
  T, 343–344, 1406–1408, 1407*f*
    activation of, 242, 243*t*

in head and neck cancer, 1409,
    1410–1411
  tumor-infiltrating, for head and neck
    cancer, 1413, 1414
Lymphoepithelioma
  nasopharyngeal, treatment of, 1437
  oropharyngeal, treatment of,
    1678–1679
Lymphokines, in head and neck cancer,
    1411, 1412
Lymphoma
  in children
    Hodgkin, 1359–1361
    non-Hodgkin, 1361–1363
  extranodal, 1621–1627
    bone marrow biopsy in, 1623
    clinical assessment in, 1623
    clinical presentation of, 1621–1622
    diagnosis of, 1621
    evaluation in, 1622–1623
    future challenges in, 1627
    histologic classification of,
      1622–1623, 1622*t*
    history in, 1623
    HIV-related, 1626
    overview of, 1627
    physical examination in, 1623
    prognostic factors in, 1624
    sites of, 1621–1622
    staging of, 1623*t*
    treatment of, 1624–1627, 1624*t*
    complications of, 1627
  HIV-related
    extranodal, 1626. *See also*
      Lymphoma, extranodal
    oral, 1558
  non-Hodgkin, 443, 443*f*
    in children, 1361–1363
    oral, 1558
  orbital involvement in, 1503–1504
  oropharyngeal, treatment of, 1679
  salivary gland, 542–543, 1521
  sinonasal, 1486, 1621–1627. *See also*
      Sinonasal tumors
  temporal bone, 2009–2010
  thyroid, 621–627, 1634
  tumor lysis syndrome in, 1626

M

Macrolides, 59
  in chronic hypertrophic
    rhinosinusitis, 400
Macular degeneration, senile, 129
Maffucci syndrome, 1824, 2793
Magnesium, 225
  oral chelated, 251–252
Magnetic resonance imaging
  for cranial-base surgery, 1830–1831,
    1831*t*
  equipment for use with, 74*f*
  functional, 67

in headache diagnosis, 249
for image-guided biopsy, 70–71, 70f
for image-guided endoscopic sinus surgery, 72f
of larynx, 93
in nasopharyngeal cancer, 1659–1661
of olfactory system, 301–302
of paranasal sinuses, 90, 431–432, 431f, 432f
of parathyroid glands, 96
of parotid gland, 563
of salivary glands, 94, 529–530, 563
of soft tissue of neck, 91–92
of temporal bone, 87–89, 1961–1963, 1963f
in temporomandibular joint disorders, 635–637, 635f
of thyroid gland, 95
Magnetic resonance sialography, of parotid gland, 563
Magnetic resonance therapy unit, 70, 70f
Malar area, evaluation of, 2707–2709, 2708f
Malar augmentation
    complications of, 2713–2715, 2715t
    implant selection for, 2709–2711, 2709t, 2714f
    indications for, 2707, 2707t
    operative procedure for, 2711–2713
    preoperative and postoperative views of, 2709f, 2710f, 2711f, 2712f, 2713f, 2714f
    preoperative evaluation for, 2707–2709, 2708–2709f
Malar fat pad, 2772, 2773f
Malar region, assessment of, for plastic surgery of face, 2489–2490, 2490f
Malignant fibrous histiocytoma, 1558
Malignant hyperthermia, treatment of, 231–232, 232t
Malignant melanoma, 442–443, 1469–1478
    acral lentiginous, 1470
    biopsy for
        of lesion, 1471
        of lymph nodes, 1472–1474
    choroidal, orbital invasion by, 1511
    clinical presentation of, 1470
    desmoplastic, 1471
    diagnosis of, 1470–1471
    differential diagnosis of, 1470
    epidemiology of, 1469–1470
    evaluation in, 1470
    of external ear
        diagnosis of, 2012
        growth phase of, 2012
        incidence of, 2011
        treatment of, 2012
    growth of, 1470

lentigo maligna, 1470
metastases from
    to lymph nodes, 1472–1474
    to salivary glands, 1523
mucosal, 1471
nodular, 1470
nonpigmented, 1470
oral, 1558
overview of, 1477–1478
sinonasal, 1484. See also Sinonasal tumors
staging of, 1471–1474
subtypes of, 1470
superficial spreading, 1470
surveillance in, 1476–1477, 1477t
treatment of
    chemotherapy in, 1476
    interferon in, 1475
    lymphadenectomy in, 1474
    for metastases, 1476
    primary resection in, 1474
    radiation therapy in, 1474–1475
    tumor vaccine in, 1475–1476
Malignant otitis externa. See Otitis externa, necrotizing (malignant)
Malingering, olfactory disorders and, 302
Malleus-incus complex, in aural atresia, 2037, 2037f
Mallory-Weiss syndrome, 768
Malnutrition
    preoperative, 215–216
    protein-calorie, 215
    wound healing and, 207
Malocclusion. See also Dental occlusion
    following maxillary/periorbital fractures, 990–991
MALT system, anatomy of, 1183
Malta fever, 183
Mandible. See also Jaw
    anatomy of, 9–10, 9f, 961, 961f
    biomechanics of, 961–962
    chronic diffuse sclerosing osteomyelitis of, 626
    implants for, 2350t, 2352–2354
    intraoral approach to, 1036, 1037f
    osteoradionecrosis of, 1565
    prosthetic rehabilitation in, surgical techniques for, 1858, 1858f
    reconstruction of, following oropharyngeal surgery, 1686, 1686t
    tori of, 1577–1578, 1578f
Mandible advancement device, in obstructive sleep apnea, 656
Mandibular angle
    assessment of, for plastic surgery of face, 2492, 2492f
    plane of, 1019–1020, 1020f
Mandibular arch
    anatomic landmarks in, 1853–1854, 1854f

fractures of. See Mandibular fractures, arch
Mandibular fractures. See also Facial fractures
    arch, in children, 1338–1342, 1345f. See also Facial fractures, in children
        surgery of, 1344–1345
    classification, 962, 963f
    complications, 972, 972t
    emergencies, 972–973, 973t
    evaluation and diagnosis, 963t
        history, 962
        physical examination, 963–964, 964f
        radiographic evaluation, 964–965, 965f
    future considerations, 973
    management
        angle, 967–968
        body, 967, 968f
        closed reduction, 966
        condyle, 968–970, 970t
        general, 965–966, 965t
        open reduction, 966–967, 967f, 970t
        ramus, 968–970
        symphysis-parasymphysis, 967, 968f
    pediatric, 1338–1344, 1343f
    special considerations
        comminuted fractures, 970–971
        edentulous fractures, 970, 972f
        external fixation, 970, 971f
        hardware removal, 972
        pediatric fractures, 971–972
        teeth in line of fracture, 970
Mandibular hypoplasia, 2652–2653
Mandibular osteotomy, with genioglossus advancement, 662
Mandibular projection, neck anatomy and, 2652, 2653f
Mandibulectomy, for oral cancer, complications of, 1565
Mandibulofacial dysostosis, 1384–1385, 1384f
    hearing loss in, 1306t, 1311
Manometry, esophageal, 758
Manual circumlaryngeal techniques, in voice therapy, 886–887
    common applications to voice disorders, 889t
Marcus Gunn phenomenon, 2793
Marcus Gunn syndrome, 2793
Marjolin ulcer, 2793
Mast cell stabilizers, in rhinitis, 358t, 359
Mast cells, in allergic reactions, 338–339
Masticator space, lesions of, 536
Masticular space, odontogenic infections of, 620

Mastoid
  embryology of, 2027–2028
  imaging of, 1967–1971
  neoplasms of, 2014–2019
  obliteration of, 2102–2103
  surgery of, 2093–2111. *See also*
        Mastoidectomy
    complications of, 2108–2110, 2108*t*
    excessive blood loss from, 2053
    facial nerve monitoring during,
        1957
    history of, 2093
Mastoidectomy
  complete, 2097–2099, 2097*f*, 2098*f*,
        2099*f*
    with facial recess approach,
        2099–2100, 2099*f*
  incisions of, 2093–2095, 2094*f*,
        2095*f*
  indications for, 2094*t*
  intact canal (open), versus canal-wall-
        down (closed), 2100–2101,
        2100*t*
  radical, 2101
    modified, 2101–2102, 2101*f*
        Bondy procedure for, 2102
  simple, 2097
  surface landmarks for, 2095–2096,
        2096*f*
  technique of, 2093–2102
Mastoiditis
  antimicrobial therapy of, 64
  imaging in, 1967, 1967*f*, 1968*f*
  management of, 2048
  meningitis due to, 2051
  in otitis media, 2045–2046, 2051
Maternal inheritance, 46
Matrix-assisted laser desorption and
        ionization, 101
Matrix metalloproteinases, 102, 102*t*,
        103*t*
Maxilla. *See also* Jaw
  anatomy of, 9, 10*f*, 975–976, 1853,
        1854*f*
  prosthetic rehabilitation in, surgical
        techniques for, 1856–1857,
        1856*f*, 1857*f*
Maxillary arch, anatomic landmarks in,
        1853, 1854*f*
Maxillary/periorbital fractures, 975–993
  in children, 1338–1342. *See also*
        Facial fractures, in children
    surgery of, 1347
  complications of, 988–991, 989*t*,
        990*f*
  management of, 985–986, 985*f*
    extended access approaches in,
        980–981, 981*f*
    immediate reconstruction in, 980,
        980*t*
    maxillomandibular fixation in, 980

  principles of, 980–981
    stable internal fixation in, 981
    surgical techniques for, 981–988
  patient evaluation in, 979–980, 980*t*
  technical adjuvants in, 991–992
Maxillary sinus. *See also* Sinus(es)
  anatomy of, 8, 308
  Caldwell-Luc approach to, 365
    indications for, 365–366, 366*t*
  surgery of
    complications of, 367, 367*t*
    operative technique for, 366–367,
        367*f*
    postoperative management in, 367
  surgical anatomy of, 366–367
Maxillectomy
  inferior, 1493*f*
  medial, with lateral rhinotomy,
        1488*f*–1489*f*
  total, 1491*f*–1492*f*
  rehabilitation after, 1487
Maxillomandibular surgery, in
        obstructive sleep apnea, 662
McCune-Albright syndrome, 189
Measles, 2179–2180, 2180*t*
  hearing loss in, 1295
  otologic manifestations of,
        2156–2157
  pharyngitis due to, 607
Meatoplasty, 2103, 2104*f*
  in aural atresia, 2036
Mecamylamine, in smoking cessation
        therapy, 280–281
Mechanotransduction, basic physics of,
        1907–1908, 1908*f*
Medial maxillectomy, with lateral
        rhinotomy, 1488*f*–1489*f*
Medialization laryngoplasty
        techniques, 912
  for unilateral vocal fold paralysis,
        857–859, 858*f*
Mediastinal adenoma, 1652
Mediastinitis, 769
  descending necrotizing, 623–624,
        623*f*, 676–677, 676*f*
Medical data. *See* Clinical data
Medical errors, dealing with, case
        illustrating, 2782
Medical ethics, 2781–2788
  ethical dilemmas in, case histories
        illustrating, 2782–2786
  issues relevant to, physician
        awareness of, 2781
  new challenges in, 2781
  principles of, 2781–2782
Medical litigation, professional liability
        claims and, 2783–2784,
        2784*t*
Medical practice
  business aspects of
    advancing of practice, 2810–2811

    contracting issues in, 2808–2810,
        2809*t*
    fellowships and, 2807
    financial planning in, 2805–2806
    insurance and, 2806–2807
    lifestyle and, 2807
    starting of practice, 2810
    type and availability of practice,
        2807–2808
  communication in
    doctor-patient, 2819–2820, 2821*f*
    examples of, 2821–2822
    optimal, barriers to, 2822–2823
Medical professionalism. *See*
        Professionalism
Medical writing, 2823–2826. *See also*
        Journal articles
  best practices and pitfalls in, 2824*t*
  manuscript elements for, 2826*t*
  manuscript preparation and, 2824
Medications. *See also specific drugs and*
        indications
  balance disturbance due to, 2262*t*
  effects on taste, 576
  esophagitis due to, 766
  ocular toxicity of, 138
  ototoxic, 1297–1299, 1297*t*
  ototoxicity of, 2202, 2203*t*
  rhinitis due to, 354, 355*t*
  for scars, 2417
  tinnitus due to, 2243
Mediterranean fever, 183
Medullary thyroid cancer, 1645–1647
  in children, 1366–1367
Melanocytic lesions, multiple,
        syndromes with, 2733*t*
Melanocytic nevi, 2737–2738, 2737*f*,
        2738*f*. *See also* Nevus
  treatment of, 2746–2747
Melanoma. *See* Malignant melanoma
Melanotic schwannoma, 442, 442*f*
MELAS syndrome, hearing loss in, 1314
Melkersson-Rosenthal syndrome, 1382,
        2793
Melnick-Fraser syndrome, 1377–1378,
        1378*f*
Melolabial flap, in cutaneous nasal
        defects, 2431, 2432–2433*f*
Mendelsohn maneuver, to improve
        deglutition, 717–718
Ménière disease, 2333
  diagnosis of, accuracy of, 2334
  functional scale for, 2334*t*
  medical management of, 2320–2323
    administration protocols for, 2323
    chemical labyrinthectomy in,
        2321–2322
    gentamicin solution for, 2322
    injection technique in, 2322–2323
    intratympanic dexamethasone in,
        2323

staging of hearing in, 2334t
vertigo control in, reporting of, 2334t
Meningioma, 120, 1981–1982, 1982f,
    2224–2225
  clinical presentation of, 2022
  diagnosis of, 2022
  etiology of, 2021–2022
  histologic subtypes of, 2225
  orbital, 1506, 1511
  radiographic differences in,
      2224–2225, 2225f
  symptoms of, 2224
  temporal bone, 2021
  treatment of, 2022–2023, 2225
Meningitis, 122
  bacterial
    etiology of, 2170–2171
    evaluation and management of,
        2171–2173, 2173f
    follow-up protocol in, 2172, 2172f
    hearing loss in, 1296–1297, 2174t
    pathology of, 2171
  cerebrospinal fluid evaluation for,
      1847, 1847t
  in cochlear implant recipients, 2272
  as complication of rhinosinusitis,
      500
  due to mastoiditis, 2051
  following cranial-base surgery,
      1847–1848
  fungal, 2173
    hearing loss related to, 2174t
  in otitis media, 2047–2048, 2051
  types of, and causes of, 1847t
  viral, 2173
Meperidine, 232
Mepivacaine, 142
Merkel cartilage, 2793
Merkel cave, 2793
Merkel cell carcinoma, 2014
Merkel ganglion cave, 2793
MeroGel (bioresorbable nasal
    dressing), 1235, 1235f
Meropenem, 59
Merrem (imipenem and meropenem),
    59
MERRF syndrome, 1314
Mesenchymal tumors, orbital,
    1506–1508
Metabolic disorders, otologic
    manifestations of, 2162
Metabolically active tumors, 163–164
Metallic implants, 2345–2346, 2346t.
    See also Implants
Metalloproteinases, matrix, 102, 102t,
    103t
Metastases
  cerebral, 121
  from lip cancer, 1537
  lymph node. See Lymph node
      metastases

microscopic, 1427
  ocular, 138
  orbital, 1512
  from salivary gland tumors, 1532
Methimazole, 221
Methotrexate, 1428t, 1430
  toxicity of, 1627
Methylprednisolone, 222
Methysergide, 251
Metocurine, 150
Metoprolol, 223–224
Metronidazole, 60, 228
Michel aplasia, 1971, 1971f, 2793
Microarray technology, 99–100
Microbiology, of orbital complications
    of rhinosinusitis, 497, 498t
Microdeletion syndrome, 44
Micrographic surgery. See Mohs surgery
Microlaryngeal surgery, controversies in
    use of, 912–913
Microlaryngoscopy, using insufflation
    technique, 1102, 1102f
Microsomia, hemifacial, 1380–1381,
    1380f
Microtia, 1055
  Grade III, 2692, 2692f
Microvascular free flaps. See Flaps,
    microvascular
Microvascular reconstruction
    approaches, 2388–2390
Midbrain syndromes, 119
MIDD syndrome, hearing loss in, 1314
Middle ear. See Ear, middle
Midface. See also Face
  aging of, 2771, 2772f
  anatomy of, 975–977, 2771–2772,
      2772f
  augmentation of, implants for, 2350t,
      2352, 2353f
  defects of, microvascular reconstructive
      approaches to, 2389
  rejuvenation of, 2771–2778
    complications of, 2775–2777
    indications for, 2773
    limitations of, 2775–2777, 2778f
    postoperative care, 2775,
        2776–2777f
    surgical technique for, 2773–2775,
        2774f, 2775f
Midface fractures, 1338–1342
  in children. See Facial fractures, in
      children
  surgery of, 1345
Midforehead lift, 2674–2675, 2675f
Midline destructive disease, idiopathic,
    380
Midline granuloma syndrome, 380
Migraine, 249–252, 2305–2310
  aura in, 250–251, 2309t
  chronic daily headache and, 252
  disability assessment in, 251

familial hemiplegic, 249–250
  International Classification of
      Headache Disorders and,
      250, 250t
  medical management of, 2324–2325
  and sinus headache, 251
  treatment of, 2309–2310
    acute, 251, 252t
    preventive, 251–252, 253t
  trigeminovascular theory of, 249
  vestibular symptoms associated with,
      2305–2309
Mikulicz disease, 173, 2793
Milia, 2734
  treatment of, 2745
Millard-Gubler syndrome, 2793
Minoxidil (Rogaine), 2750
Mivacurium, 150
Mohs surgery
  for lip cancer, 1539
  local skin flaps after, 2395–2397,
      2395f, 2396f, 2397f
  secondary intention healing after,
      2393, 2394f, 2394t
  for skin cancer, 1463, 1464f, 1467
  skin defect after
    direct closure after additional
        excision, 2395
    direct closure of, 2394
    skin grafting following, 2394
    surgical reconstruction after
      choices for, 2394t
      complications of, 2407–2408
    and tissue expansion, surgical
        reconstruction after,
        2393–2409
Molluscum contagiosum, 2739, 2739f
  treatment of, 2747
Mondini cochlear deformity, 1971, 1972f
Mondini dysplasia, 2793
Monitoring, intraoperative. See
    Intraoperative monitoring
Monitoring devices, portable, in
    suspected sleep apnea, 652
Monoclonal antibodies, 54, 54t,
    1431–1432
  for extranodal lymphoma, 1624,
      1624t, 1625–1626
Monocytes, 343
Monokines, in head and neck cancer,
    1411, 1412
Monomorphic adenoma, of salivary
    glands, 1518
Montelukast, 400
Möbius syndrome, 1058, 2793
Moraxella catarrhalis, pediatric rhino-
    sinusitis and, 1232, 1232t
Morgagni sinus, 2793
Morgagni ventricle, 2793
Morphine, 148, 232
Motion sickness, prophylaxis of, 2329

Motor nerve, injury to, during forehead lift, 2681
Movement disorders, 116–117
Moxifloxacin (Avelox), 60
Mucocele
    computed tomography of, 436–437f
    magnetic resonance imaging of, 432, 432f
    orbital, 1511
    salivary gland, 551
Mucoepidermoid carcinoma, salivary gland, 541, 542f, 1518–1519, 1519f
Mucolytic agents, 1116
Mucopolysaccharidoses, otologic manifestations of, 2162
Mucormycosis, 386–387, 387f
Mucosa-associated lymphoid tissue (MALT) system, anatomy of, 1183
Mucosal thickening, clinical significance of, 433–434
Mucosal wound healing, 210
Mucositis, stomatitis due to, 597–598, 597f
Muller's maneuver, 321
Multifactorial inheritance, 43–44
Multiple endocrine neoplasia syndromes, 164, 164t
Multiple sclerosis, 107–109, 2312–2313
    laryngeal dysfunction and, 868–869, 871f
    treatment of, 2313
    vestibular symptoms associated with, 2313
Mumps, 1242, 2179
    hearing loss in, 1295
    otologic manifestations of, 2156
    temporal bone manifestations of, 2179
    treatment of, 2179t
Mupirocin (Bactroban), 61
Muscle(s)
    of face, 2761–2762, 2762f
    of forehead, 2665, 2665f
    of nose, 2516–2517, 2517t
Muscle fatigability, in myasthenia gravis, 109–115
Muscle relaxants, 148–150, 149t
Muscle tension dysphonia
    common voice therapy applications for, 889t
    laryngeal dysfunction and, 878
    primary versus secondary, appropriate voice therapy referrals for, 890
Muscular dystrophies, laryngeal dysfunction and, 875
Musculocutaneous lymph node syndrome, 179
Mutations, dynamic, 46, 46t

Myasthenia gravis, 109–115
    laryngeal dysfunction and, 874
Mycetoma, 434
Mycobacteria, 383
    nontuberculous, 185
Mycology, basic, 417–428
Mycoses, 188, 386–387
    pharyngitis in, 608–609
    saprophytic, 422
Myelitis, radiation-related, 1451
Myelopathy, radiation-related, 1452
Myiasis, 189, 387–388
Myoclonus, laryngeal dysfunction and, 877
Myoelastic aerodynamic theory of phonation, 822
Myositis, 174–175
    head and neck manifestations of, 175
    treatment of, 175
Myospherulosis, as complication of sinus surgery, 489
Myotomy
    cricopharyngeal, in aspiration, 738, 738t
    hyoid, and suspension, in obstructive sleep apnea, 662–663
Myotonic dystrophy type I, laryngeal dysfunction and, 875
Myringotomy
    with tube insertion, 1203, 1205t, 1272
    without tube insertion, 1203
Myxedema coma, 166–167
Myxomas, 2014

N
N0 neck
    in glottic cancer, 1750–1751
    management of, 1560, 1566, 1611–1619
        biopsy in
            sentinel node, 1615, 1617–1618
            ultrasound-guided, 1614
        controversies in, 1611–1612, 1615–1617
        elective treatment in, 1613–1615
            operative, 1612, 1615–1617
            radiation therapy, 1617
            vs. watchful waiting, 1612, 1616
        future directions in, 1617–1618
        imaging studies in, 1613–1615
        occult metastases and
            impact of, 1613
            incidence of, 1612–1613, 1612t, 1613t
            risk factors for, 1612, 1612t, 1618
        overview of, 1611–1612, 1618–1619
        selective treatment in, 1615
    occult metastases in, pathologic predictors of, 1618
    staging of, 1613

Nafcillin, 57–58
Nager syndrome, 2793
Nalbuphine, 148
Naloxone, 148
Narcotic agonists, 147–148
Narcotic antagonists, 147–148
Nares, congenital malformations of, 1055–1056
Nasal. See also Nose
Nasal airway resistance, 314–315
Nasal base
    stabilizing of, in nasal tip surgery, 2568–2570, 2571f, 2572f
    structures of, 2512f, 2524–2525
Nasal cancer. See Sinonasal tumors
Nasal cavity, anatomy of, 7, 7f
Nasal challenge, in rhinitis, 357–358
Nasal cytology, in rhinitis, 357
Nasal dorsum, surgery of
    for hump reduction, 2559, 2559f
    in rhinoplasty, 2540
Nasal fractures
    in children, 1005–1006, 1338–1343. See also Facial fractures, in children
        surgery of, 1343–1344
    complications of, 1006–1008, 1007t
    diagnosis of, 1000–1001, 1000f, 1000t
    emergency care of, 1007t, 1008
    nasofrontal-ethmoidal, 1006
    patterns of, 996–1000, 998f, 999f
    reduction of, 2584–2585
        closed, 1002–1003, 1003f
        open, 1003–1004, 1004f, 1005f
    treatment of
        delayed, 1004–1005
        general, 1001, 1002f
        goals of, 1001t
Nasal injuries
    history of, 2579
    management of, 944–945
    pathogenesis of, 2580, 2581f
Nasal obstruction
    in AIDS, 269–270
    anatomic causes of, 311–317
    in children, 1071–1073, 1073–1077, 1074f, 1075f, 1076f, 1077f
        evaluation and management of, 1087–1088, 1088f
    common causes of, 319, 320t
    differential diagnosis of, 320
    history taking in, 319–320
    investigations in, 321–322
    management of, 322–333, 322t
    orofacial development and, 807–808
    physical examination in, 320–321
Nasal polyposis, 313, 435–436, 436f
    chronic rhinosinusitis with, 394t
    clinical presentation of, 393–394, 394f
    computed tomography in, 394, 395f

conditions displaying, 393
in cystic fibrosis, 395
diagnosis of, 394
histology of, 395
incidence of, 393
pathophysiology of, and disease
     associations of, 395–397
in pediatric patients, 1073–1074, 1074f
surgical treatment of, 400–401
treatment of, 313
Nasal septum
anatomy of, 311, 311f, 2518–2520,
     2518f, 2519f
deviated
  causes of, 323
  septoplasty in. See Septoplasty
dislocation of, 996, 997f
fractures of, 997–998, 997f, 998f
hematoma of, 327–328
perforation of, 326–327, 326f, 327f,
     328f
role of, 2526
vascular anatomy of, 505, 506f
Nasal sinus, fractures of, 995–1008
Nasal surgery. See also Nose
in obstructive sleep apnea, 660
in snoring, 657–658
Nasal tip
anatomy of, 2563, 2563f, 2564f
ideal contour of, 2563, 2565f
position of, 2515, 2516f
projection of, assessment of, for
     plastic surgery of face,
     2489–2490, 2490f
ptosis of, nasal obstruction in, 321
support of, 2527–2529, 2528f
  Tardy classification of, 2527, 2527t
  tripod concept of, 2527
surgery of, 2563–2578
  analysis and diagnosis for,
     2563–2568, 2566f, 2567f
  controlling projection in, 2568,
     2569f, 2570f
  modification of tip in, 2572–2576,
     2573f, 2574f, 2575f, 2576f,
     2577f
  preoperative planning for, 2568,
     2568f
  in rhinoplasty, 2539, 2541f
  stabilizing nasal base in,
     2568–2570, 2571f, 2572f
  techniques for, 2568–2576
Nasal tumors. See Sinonasal tumors
Nasal valve
anatomy of, 311, 312f
collapse of, nasal obstruction in,
     312–313
obstruction of, 321, 330–332, 331t
  surgical technique in, 331–332,
     331f, 332f, 333f
  complications of, 331t, 332

results of, 332
physical examination of, 321
Nasal wall, lateral, anatomy of,
     307–309
Nasociliary neuralgia, 260
Nasoethmoidal complex
fractures of, in children, 1338–1342,
     1346f. See also Facial
     fractures, in children
surgery of, 1346
in panfacial fractures, 1041
Nasolacrimal duct, 478
cyst of, nasal obstruction in, 1087,
     1088f
injury to, during sinus surgery, 487
Nasopalatine duct cyst, 1573
Nasopharyngeal anatomy, 12, 12f
Nasopharyngeal angiofibroma,
     441–442, 441f
computed tomography in, 90
Nasopharyngeal cancer, 1657–1671
chemotherapy for, 1437
in children, 1367
clinical presentations of, 1658–1659
diagnosis of
  imaging studies in, 1659–1661,
     1660f
  serology in, 1659
distant metastasis of, management of,
     1668
histologic classification of,
     1657–1658, 1658f
histopathology of, 1657–1658
nonkeratinizing, 1658, 1658f
oncogenic factors in, 1657
persistent or recurrent, management
     of, 1664–1668
recurrent, management of, 1664–1668,
     1665f, 1666f, 1667f
rhabdomyosarcoma, 1076, 1076f
squamous cell, 1657, 1658f
staging of, 1662, 1662t, 1663t
treatment of
  chemotherapy in, 1663–1664
  follow-up, 1664
  radiotherapy in, 1662–1663
undifferentiated, 1658, 1658f
Nasopharyngectomy, in recurrent
     nasopharyngeal cancer,
     1666–1668, 1666f, 1667f
Nasotracheal intubation, 796–797
Natural killer cells, 336
Naturopathic medicine, 2798–2799
Neck. See also under Cervical
in advanced glottic carcinoma, 1773
in advanced laryngeal cancer, 1770
aging, 2651–2622
  anatomy of, 2651–2653, 2652f
  digastric muscle hypertrophy of,
     treatment of, 2656–2657,
     2657f

obtuse cervicomental angle of,
     treatment of, 2657, 2657f
  treatment of, 2655–2659, 2656t
    surgical technique for, 2658–2659,
       2658f, 2659f, 2660f
anatomy of, 1021, 1021f
  arterial supply, 15, 15f
  cervical triangles, 14, 14f
  inferior portion, 14–15, 14f
  lateral portion, 15
  lymphatic system, 15
  venous supply, 15, 16f
  visceral structures, 16, 16f
classification and evaluation of,
     2653–2655, 2654f, 2655f
congenital malformations of,
     1056–1057
deep spaces of
  above hyoid bone, 670–671
  anatomy of, 668–671, 669f, 670f,
     670t
  below hyoid bone, 670–671
  entire neck, 668–670
  infections of, 665–682
    bacteriology of, 671–672, 672t
    complications of, 675–677, 675t,
       676f
    diagnosis of, 672–674, 672t, 673f
    etiology of, 665
    management of, 674, 675f
    odontogenic, 620
    specific, 677–682, 678f
    spread of, fasciae and, 665–667,
       667f
fasciae of, 666–667, 668f
  spread of infection and, 665–667,
     667f
implants for, 2350t, 2354
injuries of, 927–928, 928f
  penetrating
    complications of, 1021, 1021t,
       1025
    diagnosis of, 1022, 1022t, 1023t
    entry zones for, 1021, 1022f
    management of, 1023–1025,
       1023f
    zone I injuries in, 1023–1024
    zone II injuries in, 1024
    zone III injuries in, 1024
manifestations of AIDS in, 271–272
metastasis of laryngeal cancer to,
     1767, 1767t
soft tissues of
  diagnostic imaging of, 91–92
  imaging of, 91–92
Neck dissection, 1585–1606
adjuvant therapy with, 1601–1602
air leaks after, 1603–1604
anatomy of, 1585–1589
  fascial compartment, 1588, 1588f
  lymphatics, 1588–1589, 1589f

Neck dissection (continued)
　marginal mandibular branch of
　　facial nerve, 1585–1586
　nerve to levator scapulae, 1587
　platysma muscle, 1585
　spinal accessory nerve, 1586–1587
　thoracic duct, 1587–1588
　vasculature, 1585, 1586f
　anterior, 1596
　apnea after, 1605
　biopsy for
　　fine-needle aspiration, 1591
　　sentinel node, 1591
　bleeding in, 1604
　blindness after, 1605
　carotid artery dissection in,
　　1600–1601
　carotid artery rupture after, 1606
　central compartment, 1596
　chylous fistula after, 1604–1605
　classification of, 1592, 1592t
　complications of, 1603–1606
　current controversies in, 1602–1603
　diagnostic evaluation for, 1590–1591,
　　1590t
　endoscopic, 82
　extended supraomohyoid, 1596,
　　1596f
　extent of, 1602
　facial/cerebral edema after, 1605
　imaging studies for, 1590–1591,
　　1590t
　incisions in, 1585, 1586f
　infection after, 1603
　jugular vein blow-out after, 1606
　jugular vein thrombosis after,
　　1605–1606
　lateral, 1596, 1597f
　overview of, 1606
　paratracheal, 1600
　physiology of, 1589–1590
　planned, after organ-preservation
　　surgery, 1602–1603
　posterolateral, 1596, 1597f
　radiation therapy after, 1602
　radical, 1592–1595, 1593f
　indications for, 1593
　　modified, 1593–1595, 1594f, 1595f
　　rationale for, 1593
　retropharyngeal, 1599–1600
　selective, 1595–1599
　　extended, 1599–1601
　　indications for, 1598–1599
　　rationale for, 1598
　　types of, 1596, 1596f, 1597f
　sequelae of, 1603
　staging and, 1591–1592
　upper mediastinal, 1600
Neck masses and cysts, congenital. See
　　also Oropharynx, congenital
　　anomalies of

clinical indicators, 1215t
complications, 1214t
diagnosis, 1214t
embryology, 1210t
emergencies, 1214t
of entire neck
　hemangiomas, 1214
　lymphatic malformations,
　　1213–1214, 1213f
lateral
　branchial anomalies, 1209–1211,
　　1210f, 1211f
　laryngoceles, 1211, 1211f
　pseudotumor of infancy, 1212
　thymic cysts, 1211
by location, 1209t
management algorithm, 1215f
midline
　dermoid cysts, 1212, 1212f
　plunging ranulas, 1212, 1213f
　teratomas, 1212–1213
　thyroglossal duct cysts, 1212
treatment, 1214t
Neck-tongue syndrome, 260
Necrolysis, toxic epidermal, 592
Necrotizing fasciitis, synergistic,
　　622–623, 623f
Necrotizing mediastinitis, descending,
　　623–624, 623f
Necrotizing sialometaplasia, 181
　vs. minor salivary gland tumor, 1523
Neisseria meningitidis infection, congeni-
　　tal, hearing loss in, 1296
Neomycin, 61
Neonatal sepsis, hearing loss in, 1294
Neonate
　facial paralysis in, 2153
　hearing loss in. See also Hearing loss,
　　in children
　　screening for, 1277–1278, 1289
　herpes simplex virus infection in,
　　hearing loss in, 1294–1295
　hyperbilirubinemia in, hearing loss
　　and, 1299
　immune response in, 1406, 1409
　stridor in, 1091–1092, 1092f
Neoplasms, 179–182. See also specific
　　sites and types
　benign and nonsquamous, in elderly
　　patients, 243
　of cell-specific origin, 2003–2010
　of ear and lateral skull base,
　　2003–2025, 2004t, 2005f
　imaging in, 440–445
　of internal auditory canal and cerebell-
　　opontine angle, 2020–2023
　of nose and paranasal sinuses,
　　endoscopic management of,
　　447–457
　of pinna and external auditory canal,
　　2010–2014

of salivary glands, 538–543
　in children
　　mesenchymal tumors, 1244–1246
　　malignant, 1246
　　solid tumors
　　　benign, 1247–1248
　　　epithelial, 1246–1247
　　　malignant, 1248–1249
Neostigmine, 150
Nephrotic syndrome, 192, 193f
Nerve blocks, 143–144
Nerve growth factor, 342
Nerve regeneration, in wound healing,
　　209–210, 210f
Nerve sheath tumors, imaging of, 92
Nervus intermedius
　damage to, taste phantoms and, 576
　taste disorders and, 575
Nervus intermedius neuralgia, 260
Neural tube formation, 1217, 1218f
Neuralgias, cranial, and facial pain,
　　259–261
Neurilemoma. See Schwannoma
Neuroblastoma, 1367
　olfactory, 1484–1485. See also
　　Sinonasal tumors
　imaging of, 443, 443f
Neurodegenerative diseases, smell
　　impairment in, 296
Neuroepithelium, 1908–1909, 1909f
Neurofibromas
　cervical, airway compromise in, 1071,
　　1074f
　facial, 2737
　treatment of, 2746
Neurofibromatosis, 2793
　hearing loss in, 1310–1311
　type 1, 1382, 1382f
　type 2, 1382–1383
Neurogenic sarcoma, sinonasal, 1485.
　　See also Sinonasal tumors
Neurogenic shock, in trauma patients,
　　925
Neuroimaging, of olfactory system,
　　301–302
Neurolabyrinthitis, 2176
Neurologic disorders
　laryngeal involvement in, 867
　　examinations for, 869t
　　hypokinetic, 867–872
　　　Arnold-Chiari malformations,
　　　868, 870f
　　　laryngeal dysfunction after closed
　　　head injury, 872
　　　multiple sclerosis, 868–869, 871f
　　　Parkinson disease, 869–871
　　　Parkinsonism plus syndromes,
　　　871–872
　　　stroke, 872
　　　Wilson disease, 872
　ocular involvement in, 137

Neurology, 107–124
Neuromuscular blocking agents, 148–150, 149*t*
  depolarizing, 149
  nondepolarizing, 149
Neuromuscular disorders, 109–116
Neurophysiologic intraoperative monitoring. *See* Intraoperative monitoring, neurophysiologic
Neurophysiologic monitor, ideal, characteristics of, 1944*t*
Neuropsychiatric problems, postoperative management of, 230
Neutropenia, febrile, chemotherapy-related, 1438*t*
Neutrophils, 342
Nevus
  basal cell, 1572
  blue, 2739, 2739*f*, 2747
    treatment of, 2747
  Cannon, 2790
  compound, 2738, 2738*f*
  dermal, 2737–2738, 2737*f*
  Jadassohn, 2735, 2735*f*
  junctional, 2737, 2737*f*
  malignant changes in, 1470
  melanocytic, 2737–2738, 2737*f*, 2738*f*, 2746–2747
    treatment of, 2746–2747
  of Ota, 2738–2739, 2738*f*
  Spitz, 2738, 2738*f*, 2747
Nevus basal cell carcinoma syndrome, 1572
Nevus flammeus, 1353–1354, 1354*f*, 1813
Nevus of Ota, 2738–2739, 2738*f*
Nevus sebaceus, 2735, 2735*f*
  treatment, 2745
Nicardipine, 224
Nicotine replacement therapy, 280
Nitroprusside, 224, 227
Nitrous oxide, 145–146
NK cells, in head and neck cancer, 1413–1414
Nocardia, 186
Nodal metastases. *See* Lymph node metastases
Nodular goiter, 1632
Nodular melanoma, 1470. *See also* Malignant melanoma
Nodules, vocal fold, 838
  common voice therapy applications for, 889*t*
Noise-induced hearing loss, 2189–2199
  acoustic trauma and, 2191
  age-related hearing changes and, 2191–2192
  in children, 1299
  clinical management of, 2197
  compensation and, 2195–2196

  diagnosis of, 2194–2195, 2195*t*
  drugs and chemicals and, 2192–2193
  epidemiology of, 2193–2194, 2193*f*, 2193*t*, 2194*f*
  hearing conservation and, 2196–2197, 2196*t*
  management in, 2196–2197, 2196*t*
  nonauditory effects of, 2197–2198
  pathogenesis of, 2189–2193
  pathology of, 2191, 2191*f*, 2192*f*
  pathophysiology of, 2193
  pure-tone threshold shifts in, 2189–2191, 2190*f*
Non-Hodgkin lymphoma. *See* Lymphoma
Non-traditional medicine, 2797
Nonsteroidal antiinflammatory drugs
  in headache, 259
  in lupus erythematosus stomatitis, 583–586
  in migraine, 251
  in recurrent aphthous stomatitis, 597
Norrie disease, hearing loss in, 1305*t*, 1312
Nose. *See also* Eustachian tube system; Nasal
  acquired immune response in, 316
  aesthetic angles of, 2553
  aesthetic subunits of, 2424, 2424*t*
  alar lobule and nasal sidewall of, 2423
  analysis of, 2553–2555, 2554*f*, 2555*f*
  anatomy of, 352, 995–996, 996*f*, 997*f*, 2422–2424, 2579–2580, 2580*f*
    surface, 2511–2515, 2512*f*, 2513*f*, 2514*f*, 2515*f*, 2516*f*
      subunits of, 2511–2513, 2513*f*
      topography and, 2513–2515, 2514*f*, 2515*f*, 2516*f*
    surgical, 2511–2532
    valvular, 2529–2530
    vascular, 505–507, 506*f*
  areas of structural void, 2527–2529, 2528*f*
  assessment of, for plastic surgery of face, 2489–2490, 2490*f*, 2491*f*
  blood supply to, 2422–2423, 2517
  bony piriform platform surrounding, 2423–2424
  bony vault defects of, 2555–2556, 2555*t*
    management of, 2558–2560, 2559*f*, 2560*f*
  cantilever concept of, 2526
  cartilaginous vault defects of, 2556
    management of, 2556–2558, 2557*f*, 2558*f*
  chemosensory systems of, 290
  congenital anomalies of, 1122*t*, 1217

  choanal atresia/stenosis, 1124–1125
  clinical and pathologic features, 1219–1221, 1219–1223*f*, 1223, 1224–1225*t*
  embryology, 1217–1219, 1218*f*, 1219–1220*f*
  evaluation, 1223, 1224*f*
  septal deformity, 1125–1126
  surgical treatment, 1223–1226, 1224*f*, 1225*f*
  contour of, nasal obstruction and, 320–321
  defects of
    analysis of, 2424–2425, 2424*t*
    etiology of, 2422
    large
      forehead flap in, 2433–2439, 2433*t*
      preoperative considerations in, 2431–2433
    small, 2425
      bilobed flap in, 2427–2431, 2430*f*
      grafts and flaps for, 2425–2431, 2426*t*
      melolabial flap in, 2431, 2432–2433*f*
      primary closure of, 2427, 2429*f*
      reconstructive options for, 2426*t*
      Reiger flap in, 2431
      rhomboid flap in, 2427
      second intention healing in, 2426
      skin and composite grafts in, 2426–2427, 2426*t*, 2428*f*
  diseases of
    complications of, 378*t*
    diagnosis of, 378*t*
    symptoms of, 378*t*
    treatment of, 379*t*
  dorsal, reconstruction of, with composite septal flap, 2441–2443, 2445*f*
  dorsal projection of, 2555, 2555*f*
  ethnic variations in, 2530–2531, 2530*t*
  external, anatomy of, 7, 7*f*
  function of, maintenance of, following nasal restoration with flaps and grafts, 2439–2441, 2442*f*
  grafting of
    for form, 2441, 2443*f*
    techniques of, 2441–2443, 2444*f*
  granulomatous and autoimmune diseases, 377–391
  injuries to, management of, 944–945
  inner lining of, 2517
  intermediate crus of, 2522–2523, 2522*f*
  internal lining defects of, repair of, 2443–2446, 2446*t*

Nose (continued)
cutaneous epithelium for, 2446–2447, 2450f
full-thickness skin grafts for, 2446–2447, 24482449f
intranasal tissue for, 2447–2449
pericranial flap for, 2449
intranasal mucosa of, 2423
lateral crus of, 2523–2524, 2523f
length of, 2554, 2554f
ligamentous attachments of, 2526–2527
lower cartilaginous vault of, 2521–2522
mechanics and stability of, 2525–2529
medial crus of, 2521–2522
musculature of, 2422
nerve supply to, 2517
obstructions in, orofacial development and, 807–808
osseous vault of, 2520
osteotomies of, 2559–2560, 2560f
pathophysiology of, 996–1000, 997f, 998f, 999f
physiology of, 314–317, 352–353
posttraumatic deformity of
in blunt trauma, management of, 2586–2587, 2589f
classification of, 2583
closed reduction of, 2584, 2586–2587, 2587f, 2588f, 2589f
initial stabilization of, 2584
management of, 2579–2593
anesthesia for, 2582–2583, 2582f, 2586, 2586f
complications of, 2591–2592
imaging studies for, 2583, 2583f
patient assessment for, 2582–2583
splinting in, 2590, 2592f
technique for, 2586–2590, 2586–2592f
in pediatric patient, 2585
septal injury in, management of, 2585, 2588, 2590f, 2591f
profile of, analysis of, for plastic surgery of face, 2489, 2490f
protection of, 315–317
reconstruction of
with flaps and grafts, 2421–2451
history of, 2421–2422
structural support and grafting for, 2439–2443, 2442t, 2443, 2444, 2445
resection of lesions of, prosthetic rehabilitation in, 1860, 1860f
sensory nerve supply of, 2423
skeletal framework of, 2518–2524
skin-soft tissue envelope of, 2516–2518
soft tissue of, 2422
structural framework of, 2423, 2525–2526
transnasal esophagoscopy, as diagnostic tool, 910
tumors of. See Sinonasal tumors
upper cartilaginous vault of, 2520–2521, 2521f
upper two thirds of
anatomy of, 2551–2553, 2552f
bones and lateral cartilage of, 2551–2552, 2553f
bony and cartilaginous vaults of, 2552–2553, 2553f
grafts in, 2560
management of, 2551–2561
skin and subcutaneous tissue of, 2551
width and radix contours of, 2554, 2555f
Nothnagel syndrome, 2793
Nutcracker esophagus, 762
Nutrition
preoperative, 215–216
wound healing and, 207
Nystagmus
gaze, assessment in, 1918–1919
in multiple sclerosis, 107
spontaneous, assessment in, 1918–1919

O
O-to-Z flap, after Mohs surgery, 2397, 2397f
Obesity, obstructive sleep apnea and, 654
Obstructive adenoid hyperplasia, 1188, 1192t
Obstructive sleep apnea. See Sleep apnea, obstructive
Obstructive tonsillar hyperplasia, 1188, 1192t
Occipital neuralgia, 260
Occlusion, dental. See Dental occlusion
Ochronosis, otologic manifestations of, 2162
Ocular trauma. See Eye, injuries of
Oculoauriculovertebral dysplasia, 1314, 1380–1381, 1380f
hearing loss in, 1314
Odontogenic cysts, 616, 616f, 1569–1573
adenomatoid, 1575–1576
calcifying (Gorlin), 1572
dentigerous, 1570–1571, 1570f
glandular, 1572–1573, 1573f
keratocysts, 1571–1572, 1571f
in nevus basal cell carcinoma syndrome, 1572
radicular, 1569–1570, 1570f
Odontogenic infections, 615–630
actinomycosis, 627
of canine space, 617
cavernous sinus thrombosis in, 624–625, 625f
classification of, 615–628
complications of, 627t
of deep neck, 620
dental-sinus-orbital infections in, 625–626, 625f
diagnosis of, 622t
diagnostic imaging in, 628
emergency, 627t
gas-forming, 623, 623f
localized, 616–617
lymphadenopathy in, 627–628
of masticular space, 620
microbiology of, 615
necrotizing, 622–623, 623f
oroantral fistula in, 626
orofacial, 617
of parapharyngeal space, 620–621, 620f, 621f
regional, 617–622
of retropharyngeal space, 621–622, 622f
septicemia, 627
of sublingual space, 618
of submandibular space, 618, 619f
of submental space, 618–619
treatment of, 625t, 628–629
vascular complications of, 624, 624f
Odontogenic tumors, 1573–1577
adenomatoid odontogenic cyst, 1575–1576, 1576f
ameloblastic fibroma, 1577, 1577f
ameloblastoma, 1574, 1575f
calcifying epithelial, 1576
myxoma, 1576–1577, 1577f
Pindborg, 1576
Odontomas, 1574
Odors, identification of, 567. See also Olfaction
Office-based laryngeal surgery, 914
OK-432, for lymphatic malformations, 1355
Older adults. See Elderly patients
Olfaction, 55
changes in, 292–296. See also Anosmia; Hyposmia
age-related, 240–241, 292
after sinus surgery, 489
evaluation of, 567
vs. taste, 567–568
Olfactory neuroblastoma, 1484–1485. See also Sinonasal tumors
imaging of, 443, 443f
Olfactory system, 289–305
anatomy and physiology of, 290–292
biopsies of, 302
disorders of, 292–297, 294–295t
clinical history in, 297–298

olfactory testing in, 299
physical examination in, 298–299
treatment of, 302–304
epithelium of, 290–292, 290f
evaluation of
electrophysiologic tests of, 300–301, 301f
neuropsychologic tests of, 301
psychophysical tests of, 299–300, 300f
tests in malingering, 302
neuroimaging of, 301–302
olfactory bulb of, 292
olfactory cortex and, 292
Oligonucleotides, 47
Oliver sign, 2793
Omentum, microvascular flaps of, 2387
Oncocytoma, salivary gland, 540–541, 540f, 1517
Oncology, 53–54
Ondine curse, 2793–2794
Ophthalmologic evaluation, 125–140
imaging in, 139
in maxillary/periorbital fractures, 979–980
pediatric, 136–137
Ophthalmoscopy, 128
Optic nerve
anatomy of, 455f
decompression of, 455
injury to, treatment of, 485, 485t, 486f
Optic nerve glioma, 1505–1506, 1506f
Optic nerve meningioma, 1506
Optic neuritis, 130, 130f, 260
in multiple sclerosis, 107
Optic neuropathy, nonarteritic ischemic, 139
Oral appliances, in obstructive sleep apnea, 656
Oral cancer. See also Oropharyngeal cancer
biological markers in, 1566
buccal, 1561–1562
diagnosis of, 1556–1559, 1556t
differential diagnosis of, 1557–1558
emergencies in, 1565–1566, 1565t
epidemiology of, 1554–1566
etiology of, 1554–1555
follow-up in, 1561t
future directions for, 1566
in HIV infection, 1558
imaging studies in, 1556–1557, 1557f
incidence of, 1554
Kaposi sarcoma, 1558
lymphoma, 1558
melanoma, 1558
nodal metastases in, 1560
overview of, 1566
pretreatment evaluation in, 1556, 1556t

prevention of, 1560, 1566
prognosis of, 1559
prophylactic cervical radiation for, 1560
recurrence of, 1566
signs and symptoms of, 1556
squamous cell, 1557
staging of, 1557, 1558t
survival in, 1554
treatment of
chemotherapy in, 1559–1560
complications of, 1564–1565, 1565t
N0 neck management in, 1560, 1566
radiation therapy in, 1559, 1560
reconstructive surgery in, 1560–1561
site-specific, 1561–1564
surgery in, 1561–1564
tumor thickness in, 1559
verrucous, 1559
Oral cavity
anatomy of, 1551–1554, 1552f–1555f, 1853–1854, 1854f
areas for support of prosthesis in, 1853–1854, 1854f
biopsy of, 1559
burns of, 947
cancer of. See Oral cancer
complications in, related to cancer therapy, 1863–1864, 1863t
congenital malformations of, 1056, 1122t
development of, 1053
disorders of, in HIV infection, 1558
evaluation of, 1854–1855, 1855f
hairy cell leukoplakia of, 1558
lymphoma of, 1558, 1679. See also Lymphoma, extranodal
manifestations of AIDS in, 270–271, 271t, 272t
microvascular reconstructive approaches to, 2388–2389
odontogenic cysts of, 1569–1573. See also Odontogenic cysts
and pharynx, six valves of, 685, 686f
precancerous lesions of, 1558–1559
structures of, anatomy of, 9–12, 10f, 11f, 12f
ulcers of, radiation-induced, 1565
Oral contrast agents, for examination of upper aerodigestive tract, 723–724
Oral mucosa, radiation injury of, 1451
Orbicularis oris muscle, 1535, 1536f
Orbit
abscess of, 495
anatomy of, 6, 6f, 976–977, 976f, 977f
complications of sinusitis and, 493

complications of
related to sinus surgery, 483–487
in rhinosinusitis, 493–499
implants for, 2350–2352, 2350t, 2351f
sinonasal tumor extension to, 1488–1490, 1511
outcome in, 1494t
surgery for, 1493f
Orbital apex syndrome, 123–124
Orbital cellulitis, 123, 495, 496f
Orbital decompression, for exophthalmos
approaches for, 2456, 2457f, 2458f, 2459f, 2460f
complications of, 2464–2465, 2465t
endoscopic intranasal, 2462–2463
inferior, 2461
lateral, 2461–2462
medial, 2458–2461
sites of, 2456, 2456f
Orbital exenteration, 1493f
prosthetic rehabilitation in, 1859f, 1860
Orbital fissure syndrome, superior, 123
Orbital fractures. See also Maxillary/periorbital fractures
floor, 979, 979f
in children, 1338–1342. See also Facial fractures, in children
surgery of, 1346–1347
repair of, in panfacial fractures, 1041
nasoethmoidal, 1006, 1007f
roof
in children, 1338–1342
surgery of, 1346
Orbital massage, 486f
Orbital pseudotumor, 1509–1510, 1509f
Orbital trauma, 134
Orbital tumors, 1501–1513
benign, 1501
in children, 1501
cystic, 1510, 1510f
granulocytic sarcoma, 1504–1505
hematopoietic, 1503–1505
in Langerhans cell histiocytosis, 1505
leukemic, 1504–1505
lymphoid, 1503–1504, 1504f
incidence of, 1501
inflammatory, 1509–1510, 1509f
lacrimal gland, 1508–1509
lymphoma, 621–627, 1503–1504, 1504f. See also Lymphoma, extranodal
mesenchymal, 1506–1508
fibrous dysplasia, 1507
osteoma, 1507–1508
osteosarcoma, 1508

Orbital tumors *(continued)*
  rhabdomyosarcoma, 1506–1507, 1507*f*
  metastatic, 1501, 1512, 1512*f*
  neural, 1505–1506
  meningioma, 1506, 1511
  optic nerve glioma, 1505–1506, 1506*f*
  schwannoma, 1505, 1505*f*
  overview of, 1501–1502, 1512–1513
  secondary, 1488–1490, 1493*f*, 1494*t*, 1501, 1510–1512, 1511
  signs and symptoms of, 1501, 1502*f*
  types of, 1501
  vascular, 1502–1503
    capillary hemangioma, 1502
    cavernous hemangioma, 1502
    lymphangioma, 1502
Orbital varices, 1503
Orbital vasculitis, 1509–1510
Orbital walls, reconstruction of, 986–988, 987*f*, 988*f*, 989*f*
Organ of Corti, hair cells of, 1888, 1890*f*, 1891*f*, 1891*t*
Oroantral fistula, 626
Orofacial development, nasal obstruction and, 807–808
Oropharyngeal cancer, 1673–1689. *See also* Oral cancer
  diagnosis of, 1676–1677, 1677*t*
    endoscopic staging in, 1677, 1677*t*
    history taking in, 1676
    physical examination in, 1676
    radiologic studies in, 1676–1677
  emergencies in, 1687, 1687*t*
  etiology of, 1675
  histopathology of, 1675
  natural history of, 1675–1676, 1676*t*
  prognosis in, 1687, 1687*t*
  surgery in, complications of, 1675
  treatment of, 1677–1682, 1678*t*
    complications of, 1686, 1687*t*
    follow-up after, 1687, 1687*t*
    new and developing, 1688
    nonsurgical, 1679
    for squamous cell carcinoma, 1677–1678, 1678*t*
    surgical, 1679–1682
      mandibular lingual release in, 1679–1680, 1680*f*
      reconstruction of defects following, 1683–1686, 1686*f*, 1686*t*
      transmandibular approaches for, 1680–1682, 1683*f*, 1684*f*, 1685*f*
      transoral approaches for, 1679
      transpharyngeal approaches for, 1680, 1681*f*, 1682*f*
Oropharyngeal defects, microvascular reconstructive approaches to, 2388–2389

Oropharyngeal swallow. *See* Deglutition
Oropharynx
  anatomy of, 12–13, 1673–1674, 1674*f*
  congenital anomalies of, 1122*t*
    masses and cysts, 1126, 1127*f*
    surgery for, 2388–2389
  obstruction of, respiratory distress in, 1088–1089
  physiology of, 1674–1675
Orotracheal intubation, 796
Ortner syndrome, 2794
OSI-774, 1431–1432
Osler-Weber-Rendu disease, 1824, 2736, 2736*f*, 2794. *See also* Telangiectasia, hereditary hemorrhagic
Ossicles
  in aural atresia, 2037, 2037*f*
  development of, 1872, 1873*f*
    abnormal, 1873
Ossicular chain, reconstruction of, 2113–2123
  intraoperative approach for, 2114
  postoperative care following, 2114
  preoperative assessment for, 2113–2114
  technical considerations for, 2119–2122, 2120*f*, 2121*f*, 2122*f*
Ossifying fibroma, 191
  imaging of, 444
  of jaw, 1579–1580, 1580*f*
Osteitis deformans. *See* Paget disease
Osteoarthritis, 633
Osteoarthrosis, 633
Osteogenesis imperfecta, 2129
  otologic manifestations of, 2162–2163, 2163*f*
Osteogenic sarcoma, 2018
  sinonasal, 1486
Osteoma
  of external ear, 2013
    imaging of, 1964–1965, 1965*f*
  of jaw, 1578
  sinonasal, 1485. *See also* Sinonasal tumors
Osteomochondroma, of jaw, 1578–1579, 1579*f*
Osteomyelitis, 122
  chronic diffuse sclerosing, of mandible, 626
  diagnosis of, 626
  predisposing factors in, 626
  treatment of, 626–627
Osteopathic medicine, 2801
Osteopetrosis, otologic manifestations of, 2163
Osteophytosis, dysphagia in, 727–728, 727*f*, 728*f*
Osteoradionecrosis, 207, 1451
  mandibular, 1565

Osteosarcoma, of orbit, 1508
Osteosclerosis, 1974, 1977*f*
Osteotomy
  mandibular, with genioglossus advancement, 662
  in upper two thirds of nose, 2559–2560, 2560*f*
Ostiomeatal complex, 408, 438, 438*f*, 439*f*
Otic capsule, development of, 1877
Otitis externa, 1966–1967, 1966*f*, 1987–2001, 1989–1994
  acute, 1989
  bacteriology of, 1990
  bullous, 1997
  chronic stage, 1989–1990, 1993
  complications of, 1993*t*, 1994*t*
  conditions related to, 1997–2000
  diagnosis of, 1992*t*
  differential diagnosis of, 1992
  granular, 1997–1998
  history taking in, 1990
  hypertrophic chronic, surgical management of, 1994, 1994*t*
  medical treatment of, 1992
  moderate stage, 1992–1993
  natural history of, 1992
  necrotizing (malignant), 1966, 1966*f*, 1994–1997
    clinical and radiographic findings in, 1994–1996, 1995*f*
    complications of, 1997*t*
    diagnosis of, 1994, 1995*t*
    medical treatment of, 1996, 1997*f*
    surgical treatment of, 1996–1997, 1997*t*
  physical examination in, 1990
  radiation-induced, 1997
  recalcitrant, 1993
  severe stage, 1993
  staging of, 1990–1991, 1990*f*, 1991*f*
Otitis media, 1058–1059, 1265–1274. *See also* Adenoidectomy; Tonsillectomy
  adenoidectomy for, 1272–1273
  after adenoidectomy versus adenotonsillectomy without tympanostomy tubes, 1205*t*
  amoxicillin in, 61
  anatomic factors in, 1267
  bacteriology of, 2044*t*
  brain abscess in, 2047
  cephalosporins in, 58
  chronic suppurative, 1204–1206
    antimicrobial therapy in, 64
    effectiveness of various treatments for, 1206*t*
    myringotomy with/without tympanostomy tubes, 1205*t*
  classification of, 1265

complications of, 122–124, 1273–1274, 1273t, 2041–2056, 2057t
evaluation and diagnosis of, 2041–2042
infratemporal and intracranial, diagnosis of, 2043–2045, 2043t, 2045t
management of, 2048–2051, 2052t
pathophysiology of, 2041
precursors to, 2041–2042, 2043t
related to surgery in, 2053
treatment-associated, 2051–2053, 2052t
definitions and terminology of, 1265
diagnosis of, 1268–1270, 1268t
effusion in, 1265
duration of, 1266, 1266f
emergent, 2053–2055, 2054t
epidemiology of, 1265–1266, 1266f
etiology of, 1267
extradural granulation tissue or abscess in, 2046–2047, 2050
facial paralysis in, 2046, 2050, 2054, 2149
hearing evaluation in, 1269–1270, 1290, 1290f
history in, 1268–1269
in HIV infection, 268–269
imaging in, 1967, 1967f
immunization for, 1272
labyrinthitis in, 2046, 2049–2050
in Langerhans cell histiocytosis, 180
mastoiditis in, 2045–2046, 2048
meningitis in, 2047–2048, 2051
microbiology of, 1268
myringotomy and tube insertion for, 64, 1272
otitis hydrocephalus in, 2047, 2050–2051
overview of, 1274
pathogenesis of, 1267, 1267f
pathophysiology of, 1267
Chinese medicine concept of, 2800
patterns of disease in, 2043–2048, 2043t
penicillins in, 58
petrositis in, 2046, 2048
physical examination in, 1269, 1270–1271
prevention of, 1204t, 1272–1273
radiation-related, 1452
recurrent, 1203–1204, 1265
adenoidectomy efficacy in children with tympanostomy tubes, 1204t
risk factors for, 1266–1267
sigmoid sinus thrombophlebitis in, 2047, 2050
signs and symptoms of, 1268–1269, 1269t

subdural abscess in, 2048, 2051
tonsillectomy for, 1272–1273
treatment of, 1270–1272
with tympanostomy tubes, 64
Otoacoustic emissions, 1889, 1896–1897, 1899f
clinical applications of, 1938t
in infant screening, 1279
measurement of, 1282, 1937–1938
equipment for, 1937, 1937f
Otodystrophies, 1974, 1977f
OTOF gene, in hearing loss, 1307
Otolaryngic genetics, 41–51
Otolaryngologic syndromes, 1055, 1371–1386, 2685–2700, 2691–2696, 2692f
Apert syndrome, 1376–1377, 1377f
associations in, 1375
brachio-oto-renal syndrome, 1377–1378, 1378f
CHARGE association, 1378
classification of, 1375–1376, 2691–2693, 2693t
Crouzon syndrome, 1378–1379
deformations in, 1374
diagnosis of, 2693t
disruptions, 1374–1375
Down syndrome, 1379–1380, 1379f
fetal alcohol syndrome, 1386, 1386f
formes frustes in, 1374
genetic counseling for, 1375
genetics of, 49–50
Goldenhar syndrome, 1314, 1380–1381, 1380f
heterogeneity of, 1374
history in, 1375
inheritance of, 1371–1374, 1372f, 1373f. See also Inheritance
Kartagener syndrome, 1381–1382
malformations in, 1374
Melkersson-Rosenthal syndrome, 1382
Melnick-Fraser syndrome, 1377–1378, 1378f
neurofibromatosis, 1382–1383, 1382f
physical examination in, 1375
practical approach to, 1375–1376
Robin sequence, 1383, 1383f
sequences in, 1375
Shprintzen syndrome, 1383–1384, 1384f
surgical reconstruction of, 2693–2696, 2694t
complications of, 2696, 2696t
emergencies associated with, 2698t
technique for, 2694–2696, 2695f, 2696f, 2697f, 2698f
Treacher Collins syndrome, 1384–1385, 1384f
Usher syndrome, 1385

Waardenburg syndrome, 1385–1386, 1385f
Otolaryngology
eponyms in, 2789–2796
geriatric, 235–245
imaging in, 68–74. See also Imaging
molecular, 53
outcomes research in, 36–37
pediatric, 1047–1061
Otolith organs, microanatomy and biophysics of, 1910–1912, 1911f, 1912f
Otologic conditions, in AIDS, 268–269
Otologic gene therapy, 1400, 1400f
Otologic implants, 1975, 1978f. See also Cochlear implants
Otology, endoscopy in, 81–82
Otomycosis, 1998–1999, 1999f
Otopalatodigitial syndrome, 1312–1313
Otoplasty
complications and emergencies associated with, 2688–2691, 2691f
diagnostic criteria for, 2688t
preoperative evaluation for, 2686–2687
surgical techniques for
Converse technique, 2687, 2689f
Farrior technique, 2687–2688, 2689–2690f
Furnas technique, 2688, 2691f
Mustarde technique, 2687, 2688f
Pitanguy technique, 2688, 2690f
Otosclerosis, 1311, 2125–2137
amplification in, 2129–2130
audiologic testing in, 2127–2129, 2128f
diagnosis of, 2129
differential diagnosis of, 2129
embryology of, 2125
epidemiology of, 2127
histology of, 2125–2126
history taking in, 2127
management of, 2129
medical management of, 2130
pathophysiology of, 2126–2127, 2126f
physical examination in, 2127
surgical management of, 2130
complications of, 2130t, 2136–2137
computed tomography following, 89
contraindications to, 2131
indications for, 2136t
patient counseling for, 2131–2132
patient selection for, 2130–2131
technique for, 2132–2136, 2132f, 2133f, 2134f
Otosyphilis, medical management of, 2323–2324
Ototoxicity, 1297–1299, 1297t, 2201–2205

Ototoxicity *(continued)*
chemoprevention of, 2202–2204
genetics of, 2202
of ototopical antibiotics, 2201–2202, 2202*t*
of systemic drugs, 2202, 2203*t*
Outcomes research
definition of, 33
and evidence-based medicine, 33–40
in otolaryngology, results from, 36–37
outcomes to be measured in, 35–36
quality of life measurements and, 35
steps in performing, 34–36
types of, 33*t*, 37
validity and, 35–36
Outer ear. *See* Ear, external
Oxazolidinones, 61
Oximetry, in suspected sleep apnea, 652
Oxygenation, monitoring of, in anesthesia, 151–152
Oxytocin, 156

P
Paclitaxel, 1428*t*, 1430
Paget disease, 190*f*, 191–192, 2129
differential diagnosis of, 191
head and neck manifestations of, 191
hearing loss in, 191
otologic manifestations of, 2163–2164, 2164*f*
radiographic findings in, 191–192
treatment of, 192
vs. fibrous dysplasia, 191*t*
Pain
facial. *See* Facial pain
headache. *See* Headaches
oral, treatment of, 576
postoperative, pharmacologic management of, 232–233, 232*t*
Palatal myoclonus, 116–117
Palatal surgery, in obstructive sleep apnea, 660–661
Palate
anatomy of, 9, 11*f*
cancer of, 1562–1563, 1562*f*. *See also* Oral cancer
cleft. *See* Cleft lip/cleft palate
fractured, management of, 984–985, 984*f*
soft
in deglutition, 686, 686*f*
pillar implants in, in snoring, 657
prosthetic rehabilitation in, surgical techniques for, 1857–1858, 1857*f*
radiofrequency tissue ablation of, in snoring, 657
tori of, 1577–1578, 1578*f*
Palatomyoclonus, tinnitus in, 2238
Palifermin, 53
Pancoast syndrome, 2794

Pancreas
dysfunction of, 163
physiology of, 163
Pancuronium, 150
Panic attacks, vestibular dysfunction and, 2319
Papillary thyroid cancer, 1632–1633
in children, 1366–1367
Papilloma
inverted
endoscopic approaches for, 449–450
imaging of, 441, 441*f*
sinonasal, 1482–1483, 1483*t*. *See also* Sinonasal tumors
squamous cell, 2014
voice therapy and, 890
Papillomatosis, laryngeal, recurrent respiratory, stridor in, 1105–1106, 1105*f*, 1106*f*
Paracoccidioidomycosis, 188
Paradoxical vocal fold motion disorder, 878–879, 878*f*
common voice therapy applications for, 889*t*
Paraganglioma(s), 1820, 1821*f*
of middle ear, 1970, 1970*f*
of temporal bone, 2003–2007
diagnosis of, 2006–2007
growth patterns of, 2006
incidence of, 2005–2006
as nonchromaffin paraganglia, 2003–2007
treatment of, 2007
vagal, 1823, 1824*f*
Paralysis
bilateral vocal fold
clinical presentation and evaluation, 860–862, 861*f*
clinical history, 860–861
direct microlaryngoscopy, 862, 862*f*
imaging, 861
laryngeal electromyography, 861–862
neurology and internal medicine workup, 861
palpation for mobility, 862
physical examination, 861
serology, 861
etiology, 859–860, 860*t*
non-surgical, 860*t*
management
initial, of airway, 862–863
long-term surgical solutions, 863–864, 863*f*, 864*f*
temporizing treatments, 863
unilateral vocal fold
etiology, 847, 848*f*, 849–850, 849*t*, 851*f*
surgical or iatrogenic, 849*t*

history
airway, 850–851
vocal inventory, 850
vocal quality and swallowing, 850
physical examination
general, 851–852
laryngeal, 852–854, 852*f*, 853*f*, 854*f*
surgical treatment
injection augmentation, 856–857, 857*t*, 858*f*
laryngeal framework, 857–859
treatment, 855–859
determining need for early intervention, 856
patient factors in, 856*t*
workup
imaging studies, 854–855
serology, 854
Paranasal sinuses. *See* Sinus(es)
Parapemphigus, pharyngitis in, 611
Parapharyngeal space, 670, 679*f*
anatomy of, 532–533
infections of, 678–679, 678*f*
odontogenic, 620–621, 620*f*, 621*f*
lesions of, 536
Parasitic infections, 188–189, 387–388
Parasomnia, 647
Parasympathetic nervous system, salivary glands and, 523–524, 523*f*
Parasymphysis, of mandible, 961*f*
fracture
management, 967, 968*f*
treatment options, 965*t*
Parathyroid cancer, 1653
Parathyroid gland(s), 1647–1653
adenoma of, 1647–1648
anatomy of, 16, 16*f*, 1647, 1650
benign lesions of, 1647–1650
calcium metabolism and, 159–160, 160*f*
congenital abnormalities of, 1647
disorders of, preoperative management of, 220–221, 221*t*
embryology of, 1647
hyperplasia of, 1647–1648
imaging of, 95–96
molecular biology of, 54–55
preoperative localization of, 1649–1650
in thyroidectomy
autotransplantation of, 1641
preservation of, 1640–1641
vascularization of, 1650
Parathyroid hormone, 155
hypersecretion of, 1648–1650
intraoperative measurement of, 1650
preoperative measurement of, 1649

Parathyroidectomy, 1650–1653
  for cancer, 1651
  endoscopic, 1652–1653
  failure of, 1651
  minimally invasive, 1652–1653
  for multigland disease, 1652
  postoperative care in, 1652
  preoperative workup for,
      1649–1650
  principles of, 1650
  technique for, 1650–1651
Paratracheal neck dissection, 1600
Parenchyma, laceration of, 552
Parenteral nutrition, preoperative,
    215–216
Paresthesia, as complication of sinus
    surgery, 489
Parinaud syndrome, 119, 2794
Parkes Weber syndrome, 1356
Parkinson disease
  common voice therapy applications
      for, 889t
  laryngeal dysfunction and, 869–871
  Lee Silverman Voice Therapy and,
      870–871, 871t
Parkinsonism plus syndromes
  common voice therapy applications
      for, 889t
  laryngeal dysfunction and, 871–872
Parotid duct(s)
  injury to
    management of, 941, 941f
    in penetrating facial trauma, 1020
    ligation of, and submandibular gland
        excision, in aspiration,
        1113–1114
Parotid gland. See also Salivary gland(s)
  in AIDS, 271–272
  anatomy of, 8, 9f, 517–518, 518f, 519f,
      530–532, 531–532f, 533f
  in cutaneous malignancies of face
      and scalp, 562
  cysts of, 550, 557
  hemangioma of, 1353
  hypertrophy of, 552
  imaging of, 562–564
  major masses of, fine-needle
      aspiration in, 558–559
  surgery of 1528–1531
    in benign mixed tumors, 560–561
    facial nerve identification/monitor-
        ing in, 1524, 1524t, 1530
    in metastasizing tumors, 561
    nerve dissection in, 559–560
    preoperative evaluation for, 558
    technique of, 1524, 1525f–1526f
    tumors of, 1515–1532, 1516t
Parotid masses, in AIDS, 271–272
Parotitis
  chronic recurrent, 545–546, 547f
  mumps, hearing loss in, 1295–1296

Passavant ridge, 2794
Paterson-Brown-Kelly syndrome, 2794
Pathology, diagnostic, trends in, 99–105
Patient care, guidelines for, 1419–1425.
    See also Clinical guidelines;
    Critical pathways
Patient confidentiality issues, case
    illustrating, 2784
Patient requests, inappropriate, case
    illustrating, 2784–2785
P15e, immunosuppressive effects of,
    1413
Pediatric patients
  aerodigestive foreign bodies,
      1162–1163
    workup, 1163–1164, 1163f, 1164f
  airway imaging in, 1063–1078
  bilateral choanal atresia in, upper
      airway obstruction and, 808,
      808f
  cancer in, 1359–1368
    lymphoma, 1359–1363
    nasopharyngeal, 1367
    neuroblastoma, 1367
    sarcoma, 1364–1366
    thyroid, 1366–1367
  caustic ingestions
    clinical presentation, 1159, 1159f
    complications, 1161–1162, 1161f,
        1162t
    diagnosis/evaluation, 1159t
    endoscopic appearance of
        esophageal burns, 1160t
    esophageal injuries from,
        1157–1158
    treatment, 1159–1161, 1161t
  congenital malformations in,
      1371–1387. See also
      Congenital malformations
  dental trauma in, 1345
  diagnostic audiologic assessment in,
      1939
  eustachian tube system anatomy in
      adults versus, 1257–1258,
      1257t
  facial fractures in, 1337–1347. See also
      Facial fractures, in children
  growth and development in,
      1048–1055, 1048f, 1049f
  hearing loss in, 1277–1287
    central auditory processing
        disorders and, 1286–1287
    evaluation for, 1277–1283. See also
        Hearing evaluation
    management of, 1283–1287. See
        also Hearing loss
    speech and language development
        and, 1283, 1283t
  laryngeal components in, 1133
  lymphoma, 1359–1363
  mandibular fractures, 971–972

nasal fractures in, 1005–1006
neck masses and cysts, congenital
  clinical indicators, 1215t
  complications, 1214t
  diagnosis, 1214t
  embryology, 1210t
  emergencies, 1214t
  of entire neck
    hemangiomas, 1214
    lymphatic malformations,
        1213–1214, 1213f
  lateral
    branchial anomalies, 1209–1211,
        1210f, 1211f
    laryngoceles, 1211, 1211f
    pseudotumor of infancy, 1212
    thymic cysts, 1211
  by location, 1209t
  management algorithm, 1215f
  midline
    dermoid cysts, 1212, 1212f
    plunging ranulas, 1212, 1213f
    teratomas, 1212–1213
    thyroglossal duct cysts, 1212
  treatment, 1214t
nose, congenital anomalies of, 1122t,
    1217
  choanal atresia/stenosis, 1124–1125
  clinical and pathologic features,
      1219–1221, 1219–1223f,
      1223, 1224–1225t
  embryology, 1217–1219, 1218f,
      1219–1220f
  evaluation, 1223, 1224f
  septal deformity, 1125–1126
  surgical treatment, 1223–1226,
      1224f, 1225f
ocular disorders in
  amblyopia, 136–137
  congenital abnormalities of, 136
  esotropia and, 136
  exotropia, 136
  pseudostrabismus, 136
  strabismus and, 136
orbital complications of sinusitis in,
    493–499
orbital tumors in, 1501
otitis media in, 1265–1274
otolaryngologic disorders in,
    1047–1061
  special issues in, 1060
otologic procedures in, facial nerve
    monitoring during, 1957
posttraumatic nasal deformity in,
    2585
recurrent respiratory papillomatosis,
    1167
  adjuvant treatment modalities,
      1177, 1179–1180, 1179t
  new horizons under investigation
      for, 1179t

Pediatric patients (continued)
  clinical features, 1170–1171
  epidemiology, 1169–1170
  etiology, 1167–1169, 1169f
  other considerations, 1172
  patient assessment
    airway endoscopy, 1172
    history, 1171–1172
    physical examination, 1172
  postoperative care, 1176
  preoperative planning, 1174
  staging, 1177, 1178f
  surgical management, 1172–1174,
    1173t
    CO$_2$ laser, 1174–1176
    endoscopic microdebrider, 1176
  transmission, 1170
  rhinosinusitis
    bacteriology, 1232, 1232t
    differential diagnosis, 1229, 1230t
    etiology, 1231–1232
    medical management, 1232–1233,
      1233t
    other diagnostic aids, 1230, 1230t,
      1231f
    physical examination, 1229–1230
    signs and symptoms, 1229, 1230t
    surgical management, 1233–1236,
      1234t, 1236f
      complications, 1236–1239,
        1237t, 1238f, 1239f
  salivary gland disease, 1241
    autoimmune conditions, 1249
    chronic inflammation, 1243–1244
    diagnosis and management, 1242t
    inflammatory conditions,
      1241–1243
    mesenchymal tumors, 1244–1246,
      1245t, 1246t
    sialorrhea, 1249–1251
    solid tumors, 1246–1249
    trauma, 1251
  salivary gland tumors in, 1515, 1516t,
    1517t
  sleep-disordered breathing in, 1079
    adult sleep-disordered breathing
      versus, 1081t
    complications, 1084
    diagnostic evaluation
      history, 1081
      laboratory evaluation, 1082–1083
      physical evaluation, 1081–1082,
        1082f
    epidemiology, 1079
    obstruction levels and types in,
      1083t
    pathophysiology, 1079–1080, 1080t
    syndromes and conditions
      associated with, 1083t
    treatment options, 1084
  soft tissue trauma, 936

  speech and language development in,
    hearing loss and, 1283, 1283t
  tracheotomy, 1147
    communication concerns, 1154
    complications, 1152–1153
    decannulation, 1154
    history, 1147–1148
    indications for, 1148t
    postoperative care
      home, 1152
      hospital, 1151–1152
    prolonged intubation versus, 1149
    technique, 1149–1150f, 1149–1151
    tubes for, 1153
  tracheotomy in, 790, 791f
  vascular lesions in, 1349–1357. See
    also Vascular lesions, in
    children
  vestibular testing of, 1924
Pedicled island flap, subcutaneous, after
    Mohs surgery, 2397, 2397f,
    2398f
Pemphigoids
  esophageal symptoms in, 766
  pharyngitis due to, 610–611
  stomatitis due to, 586–591
Pemphigus
  familial benign chronic, 610
  pharyngitis in, 610
  types of, 610
Pemphigus vulgaris, stomatitis due to
  clinical features of, 589–590, 590f
  etiology of, 589
  histopathology of, 590–591, 590f
  treatment of, 591
Pendred syndrome, 50, 1305t, 1308,
    2794
Penetrance, 1303
  of gene/trait, 1373–1374
Penetrating trauma, to larynx,
    pathophysiology of, 950
Penicillin(s), 57–58, 187
  anaphylaxis and, 57
  antipseudomonal, 58
  antistaphylococcal, 57–58
  augmented, 58
  in odontogenic infections, 629
  in otosyphilis, 2324
  in streptococcal pharyngitis, 604
Penicillin G, 186
Peptococci/peptostreptococci, pediatric
    rhinosinusitis and, 1232,
    1232t
Periapical cysts, 1569–1570, 1570f
Pericardiocentesis, for acute cardiac
    tamponade, 926f
Perichondritis, 1998
Pericoronitis, 617
Perilymph fistula, surgical management
    of, 2340
Perioral region, implants for, 2352

Periorbital fractures. See Maxillary/
    periorbital fractures
Periorbital rhytids, lateral, Botox
    injections in, 2763, 2763f
Peripheral nerves
  age-related changes in, 242, 242t
  taste loss or alteration and, 574–575
  taste system and, 569–570
Peritonsillar abscess, 1197
Peritonsillar space, 671
  infection of, 680–681
Personality disorder, facial cosmetic
    surgery and, 2484
Pertussis, pharyngitis due to, 605
Petrosa, surgery of, 2093–2111
Petrosal nerve, superficial, taste and,
    570
Petrositis
  diagnosis of, 2046
  imaging in, 1968
  management of, 2048
Petrous apex
  imaging of, 1967–1971
  surgical access to, 2105–2108, 2106f,
    2107f
Petrous apicectomy, 2105–2108, 2106f,
    2107f
Peutz-Jeghers syndrome, 2794
PFAPA, pharyngitis in, 611
PH monitoring, in esophageal
    disorders, 758
Pharyngeal pouches, dysphagia in, 729,
    729f
Pharyngitis, 601–613
  antibiotic treatment in, 63
  due to bacterial infections, 603–606
  due to fungal infections, 608–609
  due to integumentary disorders,
    610–611
  due to viral infections, 606–608
  in granulomatous diseases, 609
  idiopathic, 611–612
  radiation, 610
  reflux, 611
Pharyngoesophageal defects,
    microvascular reconstructive
    approaches to, 2388
Pharyngoesophagram, of upper
    aerodigestive tract, 722
Pharyngoplasty, transpalatal
    advancement, in obstructive
    sleep apnea, 661
Pharyngotonsillitis, noninfectious
    granulomatous, 609
Pharynx
  airway physiology of, 694–695
  anatomy of, 12–13, 12f, 601–603,
    602f, 693, 694f
  functions of, 693
  injuries of, in penetrating trauma,
    1025

manifestations of AIDS in, 270–271, 271t, 272t
pressure measurements of, to assess swallowing, 710
radiographic anatomy of, normal, 722–723f, 724
surgery of, postoperative strictures following, dysphagia and, 730, 731f
Phenobarbital, 230
Phenol peels. *See* Chemical peeling
Phenotypic expressivity, 1374
Phenoxybenzamine, 164
Phenytoin, 230, 260
Pheochromocytomas, 163
Phlebolith, 550
Phonation
    anatomy and physiology for, 895–896
    glottic cycle in, 823f
    myoelastic aerodynamic theory of, 822
    principles of, 897–898
    stretch and flow, in voice therapy, 888
        common applications to voice disorders, 889t
Phonation, vocal folds and, 700–701
Phonomicrosurgery, of vocal folds
    equipment for, 841–842
    overview, 840–841
    preoperative considerations, 841
    procedures, techniques, and methods, 842–845, 843f, 844f
Phonosurgery, laryngoplastic. *See also* Medialization laryngoplasty
    controversies in use of, 911–912
Photocoagulation
    for capillary malformations, 1353–1354
    for hemangiomas, 1352
Photodamage
    chemical peeling in. *See* Chemical peeling
    topical therapy in, 2717
Photodocumentation
    digital, 2506–2509, 2506f
    informed consent for, 2499
    intraoperative, 2503–2504
    principles of, 2499–2504
    standardization of, 2500–2503, 2500f, 2501f, 2502f, 2504f
    for specific procedures, 2502, 2503t
    traditional, 2504–2506
Photodynamic therapy, for skin cancer, 1462–1463
Photometrics, in facial analysis, 2494, 2494f
Physician, impaired, case illustrating, 2786
Pictorial documentation. *See* Photodocumentation

Pierre Robin syndrome, 2794
Pigmentation changes
    camouflage of, 2416–2417
    following chemical peeling, 2721, 2722t
    laser management of, 2417
Pilocarpine, in xerostomia, 557
Pilomatricoma(s), 2735, 2735f
    treatment of, 2745
Pilomatrixoma, 2014
Pindborg tumor, 1576
Pinna
    and external auditory canal, neoplasms of, 2010–2014
    skin flap for, after Mohs surgery, 2400, 2403f
Piperacillin, 58
Pitressin, 223
Pituitary
    cell types and secretory products of, 156, 156t
    dysfunction of, 158–159
    embryology and anatomy of, 155–156
    physiology of, 156–158
Pituitary adenoma, 121, 159
    preoperative management in, 222–223
Pituitary apoplexy, headache in, 257
Plasmacytoma
    extramedullary, of temporal bone, 2010
    sinonasal, 1486. *See also* Sinonasal tumors
    of temporal bone, 2010
Plastic surgery. *See* Face, plastic surgery of
Platelet abnormalities, preoperative management of, 217
Platelet-derived growth factor, in wound healing, 205
Platelet gels, autologous, in wound healing, 208
Plates, application of, 1032–1033, 1032t
    in complex facial trauma, 1027–1044
    instrumentation for, 1033
Platysma muscle, 2651–2652, 2652f
Platysmal banding, Botox for, 2764
Platysmaplasty, anterior, and submental liposuction, 2658–2659, 2658f, 2659f, 2660f
    complications of, 2660–2661
Play audiometry, 1281, 1281f
    in otitis media, 1270
Pleiotropy, 1374
Pleomorphic adenoma
    parotid surgery and, 561
        management of recurrences, 561–562
    of salivary glands, 538, 539f, 1515–1516, 1517t

malignant variations of, 542–543
    recurrence of, 1531
Plummer-Vinson syndrome, 2794
Pneumococcal meningitis, in children, hearing loss in, 1296–1297
Pneumoparotitis, 552
Pneumothorax, management in trauma patients, 923–924, 924f
Pocket principle, for auricular hematoma repair, 943–944, 944f
Poliomyelitis, 115
Polyarteritis nodosa, 176
    otologic manifestations of, 2161
Polychondritis, relapsing, 175, 381, 1998
    laryngitis and, 830t, 833
    otologic manifestations of, 2159–2160
Polymers, as implants, 2346t, 2347
Polymorphous low-grade adenocarcinoma, of salivary gland, 1520
Polymyalgia rheumatica, 177–178
Polymyositis, 174–175
    laryngeal dysfunction and, 875
Polyps
    antral choanal, 396
    nasal. *See* Nasal polyposis
    vocal fold, 838
        appropriate voice therapy referrals for, 890
        common voice therapy applications for, 889t
Polysomnography, in suspected sleep apnea, 652–653
Polytef, injection in paralyzed vocal fold, 911
Pontine branch
    lateral, infarction of, 118–119
    medial, infarction of, 118
    upper, infarction of, 119
Port-wine stains, 1353–1354, 1354f, 1813
Positional cloning, 45
Positioning devices, in obstructive sleep apnea, 656
Positive airway pressure devices, in obstructive sleep apnea, 656–657, 656f
Positron emission tomography, 67, 68f
    in nasopharyngeal cancer, 1660f, 1661
    of parotid gland, 563–564
    of soft tissue of neck, 92
Posterior cricoarytenoid muscle, voice production and, 896
Posterolateral neck dissection, 1596, 1597f
Postherpetic neuralgia, 260
Postural techniques, to improve swallow functioning, 714–715, 714t

Posture, deglutition and, 690
Posturography, dynamic, 1923–1924, 1923f, 1923t
Pott's puffy tumor, 122, 502, 503f
Prader-Willi syndrome, 46
Prednisone, 178, 222, 258
    for exophthalmos, 2463
    for extranodal lymphoma, 1624–1627, 1624t
    for hemangiomas, 1352
Pregnancy, alcohol abuse in, fetal alcohol syndrome and, 1386, 1386f
Preoperative management. *See under* Surgery
Presbycusis, 238–239, 2258–2263, 2258f, 2260f, 2260t
    assistive devices in, 239
    history and physical examination in, 2261–2263, 2262t
    rehabilitation in, 2258–2260
    types of, 238, 238t
Presbyopia, 128–129
Presbyphagia, 241–242
Pressure regulation, of eustachian tube system, 1258f, 1261–1262
Pretrichial lift, 2672, 2673f
Prevertebral and danger space, 670
    infections of, 678
Primary chief cell hyperplasia, 1648
Primaxin, 59
Professional voice
    anatomy and physiology for voice production, 895–896
    care of, 895
    pathophysiology, 900–901
    performance cancellation, 904
    performance styles, 898–900
    sound production principles, 897–898
    vocal difficulties
        evaluation, 901–902
        management
            acute care, 904
            general principles, 902–904
            surgical management
                indications, 904–905
                techniques, 905
Professionalism, 2813–2818
    communication skills and, 2819–2826
    defining foundations of, 2814
    in hospital, 2816–2817
    importance of, 2813–2814
    issues in professional organizations, 2814–2815
    for medical talk, 2823
    in medical writing, 2823–2826, 2824t, 2826t
    in practice, 2816–2817
    and surgeons, 2816–2817

Progressive bulbar palsy, laryngeal dysfunction and, 872
Progressive systemic sclerosis, esophageal symptoms in, 762
Prolactin, 158
Prolactinomas, 159
Promoters, in gene therapy, 1396
Propofol, 147
Propranolol, 164, 165, 251
    in migraine, 2325
Proptosis
    differential diagnosis of, 1501
    orbital tumors and, 1501, 1502t
Propylthiouracil, 165, 221
Prostheses
    intraoral, to improve deglutition, 715–716
    stapedial, 1975, 1978f
    voice
        duckbill, following laryngectomy, 1781–1782, 1782f
        low-pressure, following laryngectomy, 1782, 1783f
Prosthetic rehabilitation
    evidence-based, 1864
    of extraoral lesions, 1859–1861, 1859f, 1860f, 1861f
    in oral cavity, 1856–1858, 1857f, 1858f, 1859f
    principles of, and information for, 1855–1856
    surgical techniques to enhance, 1853–1865
Protein-calorie malnutrition, 215
Protein patterns, gene array and, 101
Prussak space, 2794
Pseudobulbar palsy, 115
    laryngeal dysfunction and, 872
Pseudoepiglottitis, dysphagia and, 730, 730f
Pseudomembranous colitis, 59
Pseudomonas aeruginosa, pediatric rhinosinusitis and, 1232, 1232t
Pseudostrabismus, 136
Pseudotumor cerebri, headache in, 258
Psychogenic dysphonia, laryngeal dysfunction and, 878
Psychoneuroimmunology, 2803
Psychosis, facial cosmetic surgery and, 2483–2484
Pterygopalatine fossa, 505
    in sinonasal cancer, 1490
    transpterygoid endoscopic approach to, 454–455
Ptosis, forehead lift and, 2667
Pulmonary complications
    of anesthesia and surgery, 226
    predisposing factors for, 226
Pulmonary disorders
    anesthesia choice in, 226

postoperative pulmonary insufficiency in, 226–227
    preoperative management of, 226–227
Pulmonary edema
    acute, endotracheal intubation and, 798
    preoperative management of, 227
Pulmonary embolism
    as complication of otitis media surgery, 2053
    preoperative, 220
Pulmonary insufficiency, postoperative, 226–227
Pulse oximetry, 151
Pulsed light, intense, for skin resurfacing, 2727
Punch biopsy, technique of, 2739–2740, 2741f
Punches, biopsy, 2739–2740, 2740f
Pupils, examination of, 126–127
Pyogenic granuloma, 181, 181f, 2736
    treatment of, 2746
Pyriform sinus, contralateral, dysphagia in, 729, 730f

Q

Quinine, ototoxicity of, 1298
Quinupristin and dalfopristin (Synercid), 61

R

Radial forearm flap, 2369–2371, 2370f
Radial forearm-palmaris longus flap, in lip reconstruction, 1547, 1547f
Radiation
    laryngeal stenosis and, 1137
    laryngitis and, 835
    wound healing and, 206–207
Radiation esophagitis, 765–766
Radiation fibrosis, 1452
Radiation injury, to salivary glands, 551
Radiation therapy, 1441–1453
    biology of, 1443–1449
    brachytherapy, 1442–1443, 1443t
    cell cycle effects in, 1446–1447
    cell death in, 1443–1444
    with chemotherapy, 1429, 1433–1435, 1433t
    complications of, 1451–1452, 1452t
        ocular, 1452, 1494, 1496t
    conformal, 1443
    dose fractionation in, 1446, 1446f
    dose-response relationship in, 1448–1449, 1448t, 1449f
    for early glottic/subglottic cancer, 172
    efficacy of, 1448–1449, 1448t, 1449f
    external beam, 1441–1442
        for exophthalmos, 2463
    for extranodal lymphoma, 1624–1627

complications of, 1627
for hypopharyngeal cancer, 1696,
1696f, 1705–1706
intensity-modulated, 1443,
1444f–1445f
in xerostomia, 558
for laryngeal cancer, 1770–1771
complications of, 1775
for lip cancer, 1538–1539
complications of, 1548, 1548t
for N0 neck, 1617
for nasopharyngeal cancer, 1664
for oral cancer, 1559
complications of, 1564–1565
prophylactic, 1560
oral complications of, 1863–1864,
1863t
osteonecrosis in, 1565
overview of, 1452–1453
palliative, 1449
physics of, 1441–1443
regimen selection for, 1449–1451
regression rates for, 1449
repair of sublethal injury in,
1445–1446
repopulation after, 1446–1447, 1449f
for salivary gland tumors, 1528
sensitivity to, 1448–1449, 1448t,
1449f
shrinking-field technique in, 1450,
1450f
for sinonasal cancer, 1487
for skin cancer, 1462
as sole therapy, 1450
with surgery, 1449, 1450–1451,
1450f, 1451t, 1452f
preoperative vs. postoperative, 1451
tumor cell hypoxia in, 1446, 1446f,
1447f
tumor size and, 1448–1449, 1448t
Radical neck dissection. See Neck
dissection
Radicular cysts, 1569–1570, 1570f
Radiesse, for soft-tissue augmentation,
2768, 2768f
Radioallergosorbent test, 357
Radiofrequency skin resurfacing, 2727
Radiography
plain-film, of salivary glands, 527,
528f
of salivary glands, 524
standard, of sinuses, 429, 430f
in suspected sleep apnea, 651
of upper aerodigestive tract, 721–732
Radioiodine ablation, after
thyroidectomy, 1644
Radiology, in stridor, 1100–1101
Radionuclide scanning
in aspiration, 1112
of salivary glands, 94, 530
of thyroid gland, 94

Radiosurgery, in cranial-base surgery,
1845–1846
Raeder syndrome, 2794
Ramsay Hunt syndrome, 2180, 2794
in AIDS, 267
Ramus, of mandible, 961f
fracture in
management, 968–970
treatment options, 965t
Rapacuronium, 150
Rathke pouch, 2794
Rectus abdominis flap, 2376–2378, 2377f
Recurrent laryngeal nerve, in thyroidectomy, injury of, 1643
Recurrent respiratory papillomatosis,
1167
adjuvant treatment modalities, 1177,
1179–1180, 1179t
new horizons under investigation
for, 1179t
clinical features, 1170–1171
epidemiology, 1169–1170
etiology, 1167–1169, 1169f
other considerations, 1172
patient assessment
airway endoscopy, 1172
history, 1171–1172
physical examination, 1172
postoperative care, 1176
preoperative planning, 1174
staging, 1177, 1178f
surgical management, 1172–1174,
1173t
CO$_2$ laser, 1174–1176
endoscopic microdebrider, 1176
transmission, 1170
Red cell abnormalities, preoperative
management of, 217
Red eye, 130–133
in conjunctivitis, episcleritis, and
scleritis, 131
in eyelid abnormalities and
blepharitis, 130–131
in iritis and iridocyclitis, 131–132
symptoms of, 132, 132t, 133t
treatment of, 132–133
Reflux
gastroesophageal. See
Gastroesophageal reflux
laryngopharyngeal. See
Laryngopharyngeal reflux
Reflux pharyngitis, 611
Refractive errors, 128
Reiger flap, in cutaneous nasal defects,
2431
Reinke edema
common voice therapy applications
for, 889t
severe, appropriate voice therapy
referrals for, 890
vocal fold, 840

Relapsing polychondritis. See
Polychondritis, relapsing
Remifentanil, 148
Remodeling phase, of wound healing,
201–202, 201f
Renal disease
chronic, 390
perioperative management of,
228–229
Renal failure
acute
perioperative management of, 229
postoperative causes of, 229
chronic
perioperative management of,
228–229
postoperative management in, 229
Renal toxicity, of chemotherapeutic
drugs, 1438
Reparative granuloma, 181
Resonant voice, in voice therapy, 887
common applications to voice
disorders, 889t
Respiration. See also Breathing
control of, larynx and sensory input
to, 699–700
larynx and, 822
nose and, 314–315
Respiratory disease, aspirin-exacerbated.
See Aspirin-exacerbated
respiratory disease
Respiratory distress
in child, signs and symptoms of, 1095
neonatal, 1087–1093
evaluation of nose in, 1087–1088,
1088f
Respiratory distress syndrome, adult,
227
Respiratory retraining, in voice therapy,
887–888, 889t
Respiratory-swallow coordination, in
deglutition, 691
Respirodeglutometry, to assess
deglutition, 708–710, 709f
Restylane, for soft-tissue augmentation,
2766, 2766f
Retention cysts, 435, 435f
Retinal arterial occlusion, central, 129
Retinal detachment, 129–130
Retinitis pigmentosa, in Usher syndrome,
1306t, 1308–1309, 1385
Retinoblastoma, orbital invasion by,
1511–1512
Retromolar trigone, cancer of, 1563. See
also Oral cancer
Retropharyngeal masses, in pediatric
patients, 1069–1071, 1071f,
1072f, 1073f, 1074f
Retropharyngeal neck dissection,
1599–1600. See also Neck
dissection

Retropharyngeal space, 668–670
  abscess of, 678
  odontogenic infections of, 621–622,
      622f
Retrovirus vectors, 1395
Rhabdomyosarcoma
  alveolar, 2017
  in children, 1364–1366, 1364t, 1365t
  of nasopharynx, 1076, 1076f
  of orbit, 1506–1507, 1507f
  pleomorphic, 2017
  sinonasal, 1485. See also Sinonasal
      tumors
Rheologic agents, in sudden sensory
      hearing loss, 2233
Rheumatic fever, 604, 604t
Rheumatoid arthritis, 171–172
  diagnosis of, 172
  head and neck manifestations of, 172
  laryngitis and, 830t, 832
  otologic manifestations of, 2161
  treatment of, 172
Rheumatologic lesions, of vocal folds,
      840
Rhinitis
  allergic. See Allergic rhinitis
  allergy testing in, 357–358
  burden of, 352
  clinical presentation of, 355–356
  definition of, 351
  diagnosis of, 356–358
  drug-induced, 354–355, 355t
  epidemiology of, 351–352
  hormonal, 354
  idiopathic (vasomotor), 354, 355t
  immunotherapy in, 360
  irritative-toxic (occupational), 354
  nasal endoscopy in, 357
  nonallergic, 354–355
    clinical presentation of, 356
    with eosinophilia, 355
  pathophysiology of, 353–355
  prevalence of, 351–352
  surgery in, 360–361
  treatment of
    allergen avoidance in, 358
    education in, 358
    pharmacotherapy for, 358–360,
        358t
Rhinomanometry, 314–315
  in nasal obstruction, 322
Rhinometry, acoustic, 315
  in nasal obstruction, 322
Rhinophyma, 2734, 2735f
  treatment of, 2745
Rhinoplasty, 2533–2550
  adjunctive procedures to, 2549, 2549f
  anesthesia for, 2537–2538
  closure and splinting in, 2547–2548,
      2548f
  in elderly patients, 243

evaluation and consultation for,
      2533–2536, 2536t
  examination for, 2533–2536, 2534f,
      2535f
  hump reduction in, 2541–2544,
      2542f, 2543f, 2544f
  incisions for, 2538–2539, 2539f, 2540f
  medial and lateral osteotomies in,
      2544–2547, 2544f, 2545f,
      2546f
  nasal tip surgery in, 2539, 2541f
  overview of surgery in, 2538–2548
  perioperative problems in, 2547t
  postoperative care after, 2548
  secondary, 2595–2609
    in errors of commission,
        2596–2603, 2598f,
        2600–2601f, 2602f, 2604f,
        2605–2606f, 2607–2608f
    in errors of omission, 2596, 2597f
    in lobule abnormalities, 2603,
        2604–2606f, 2607–2608f
    in overprojected tip, 2596
    in pyramid abnormalities,
        2598–2599f, 2598–2603,
        2600–2601f
    in underrotated tip, 2596
  surgery of dorsum in, 2540
  surgical planning for, 2536–2537,
      2537t
Rhinorrhea, cerebrospinal fluid,
      endoscopic repair of,
      455–456
Rhinoscleroma, 183–184, 382–383
Rhinoscopy, 321
Rhinosinusitis. See also Sinusitis
  acute
    pathophysiology of, 405–406, 406f,
        407t
    treatment of, 413–415, 414t
  allergic fungal
    "allergic mucin" in, 425
    culture of fungi in, 425
    diagnostic criteria for, 425–426
    history and physical examination
        in, 423–424
    immunologic testing in, 425
    radiology of, 424–425, 424f, 424t
    treatment of, 426
  bony complications of, 502–503, 503f
  chronic
    and allergic rhinitis, 407
    computed tomography in, 411–412,
        411f, 412f, 413
    costs of, 405
    diagnosis of, 409–412, 409t, 410t
    diagnostic correlates of, 413
    environmental factors in, 407–408
    eosinophilic, 396–398, 401t
    genetic/physiologic factors in,
        406–407

medical treatment of, 399–400
    with nasal polyposis, 394t
    pathophysiology of, 405–409
    staging systems for, 412, 412t
    structural factors in, 408–409
    treatment of, 415
      outcomes of, 415
      surgery in, 400–401
  complications of, 493–504
  eosinophilic chronic, 396–398
    therapeutic interventions for, 401t
  eosinophilic fungal, 426
  eosinophilic mucin, 398
  fungal, classification of, 417–426, 418t
  incidence of, 405
  intracranial complications of,
      499–502, 500f
    anatomic considerations in, 499
    classification of, 499–501
    microbiology of, 498t, 501
    treatment of, 502, 502t
  non-allergic fungal eosinophilic
      chronic, 398
  noneosinophilic chronic, 395–396
  nonpolypoid, 405–416
  orbital complications of, 493–499
    anatomic considerations and, 493
    classification of, 493, 494–495f,
        495t
    evaluation in, 496–497
    microbiology of, 497, 498t
    radiography in, 497
    treatment of, 497–499, 499f
  pediatric, 1059
    bacteriology, 1232, 1232t
    differential diagnosis, 1229, 1230t
    etiology, 1231–1232
    medical management, 1232–1233,
        1233t
    other diagnostic aids, 1230, 1230t,
        1231f
    physical examination, 1229–1230,
        1230t
    signs and symptoms, 1229, 1230t
    surgical management, 1234t
      adenoidectomy, 1233–1234
      antral lavage, 1234
      bent functional endoscopy,
          outcomes after, 1235t
      complications, 1237t
        frontal sinusitis and epidural
            abscess, 1237f, 1238f
        intracranial, 1238–1239
        orbital, 1236–1238, 1239f
      ethmoidectomy, 1235–1236
      guided imaging in, 1236f
      inferior meatal antrostomy, 1234
      middle meatal antrostomy, 1234
      nasal antral windows, 1234
  risk factors for, 407–408
  signs and symptoms of, 409, 409t

superantigen-induced eosinophilic
chronic, 398–399
Rhinosporidiosis, 188, 386
Rhomboid flaps, 2363, 2363*f*
in cutaneous nasal defects, 2427
after Mohs surgery, 2395–2396,
2395*f*, 2396*f*
Rhytidectomy, 2627–2650
anesthesia for, 2634
complications of, 2645–2647, 2648*f*
deep plane lift in, 2641–2643, 2641*f*
in elderly patients, 244
flap closure in, 2643
flap elevation for, 2638–2639, 2639*f*
incisions for, 2635–2638, 2635*f*,
2636*f*, 2637*f*, 2638*f*
problems associated with, 2647
operative procedures for, 2638–2644,
2639*f*, 2640*f*, 2641*f*, 2643*f*,
2644*f*
patient assessment for, 2630–2631
planning for, 2631–2634, 2633*f*
postoperative care in, 2644–2645
preoperative evaluation for, 2631,
2632*f*
preoperative preparation for, 2634
superficial musculoaponeurotic
system suspension for,
2639–2641, 2640*f*
surgical evolution of, 2630
surgical planning for, 2634–2638
Rhytids
forehead lift and, 2667
glabellar, Botox injections in, 2763,
2763*f*
lateral periorbital, Botox injections in,
2763, 2763*f*
transverse forehead, Botox injections
in, 2763, 2763*f*
vertical lip, Botox injections in, 2764
Riboflavin, 251–252
Ribonucleic acid. *See* RNA
Riedel struma, 2794
Riedel thyroiditis, 1631–1632, 2794
Rifampin, 61
Right aortic arch, congenital, 1130,
1131*f*
Rigid fixation, facial. *See* Facial
fractures, rigid fixation of
Rituximab, for extranodal lymphoma,
1624–1627, 1624*t*
Rivinus, ducts of, 2794
RNA, 53
RNA interference gene therapy, 1399
RNA microarrays, 99
Robin sequence, 1383, 1383*f*
Rocephin (Ceftriaxone), 59
Rocuronium, 150
Ropivacaine, 142
Rotary chair, to test balance,
1921–1922, 1921*f*

Rotation flaps
bilobed, 2363, 2364*f*
dufourmental, 2363, 2364*f*
rhomboid, 2363, 2363*f*
transposition, 2362–2363
true, 2362, 2362*f*
Rouvier, node of, 2794
Rubella
congenital, hearing loss in, 1295
hearing loss in, 2175–2176
Rubeola. *See* Measles

S
Saccharin test, 315
Saliva
antimicrobial activity provided by,
522
buffering system of, 521–522
flow rates of, 524
functions of, 521
production of, 522–523
Salivary fistula, postoperative, 1530
Salivary gland(s)
acute inflammatory lesions of,
545–546
anatomy of, 517, 518*f*, 530–533,
531–532*f*, 533*f*, 1515, 1523,
1524*f*, 1530*f*
arterial supply of, 519–520
autonomic innervation of, 523–524,
523*f*
biopsy of, 558–559
fine-needle aspiration, 1522
surgical, 523, 1523
chronic inflammatory disorders of,
546–547, 547*f*
cysts of, 536–538, 537*f*, 538*f*,
550–551, 550*t*
developmental anatomy of, 517, 518*f*
diagnostic imaging of, 527–530
dysfunction of, systemic and
exogenous sources of, 546,
546*t*
granulomatous diseases of, 546–547
imaging of, 93–94, 527–544, 543*t*
inflammatory disease of, 533–538
chronic, 534–535, 534*f*, 535*f*
lymphatic drainage of, 520
lymphoma of, 542–543, 1521. *See
also* Lymphoma, extranodal
major, 1515
minor, 1515
anatomy of, 521
nonneoplastic diseases of, 545–554
complications of, 553, 554*t*
physiology of, 521–524, 1515
primary tuberculosis of, 547–548
radiation injury of, 551, 1451
radiographic imaging of, 524
salivary flow rates and, 524
secretory process in, 522–523

secretory unit of, 522, 522*f*
venous drainage of, 520
Salivary gland disease, 442, 538–543,
1515–1532
benign, 538–541, 539*f*, 540*f*, 541*f*,
1515–1518
in children, 1247–1248
monomorphic adenoma, 1518
oncocytoma, 1517
pediatric, 1515
pleomorphic adenoma, 1515–1516,
1517*t*
Warthin tumor, 1516–1517, 1518*f*
in children, 1241, 1246–1249
autoimmune conditions, Sjögren
syndrome, 1249
benign, 1247–1248
chronic inflammation
cysts, 1244
granulomatous lesions, 1244
sialectasis, 1243
sialolithiasis, 1243–1244
diagnosis and management, 1242*t*
epithelial, 1246–1247
inflammatory conditions
acute bacterial sialadenitis,
1241–1242
neonatal sialadenitis, 1242
viral sialadenitis
Epstein-Barr virus, 1243
HIV and, 1243
mumps, 1242
malignant, 1248–1249
mesenchymal, 1244–1246, 1245*t*
malignant, 1246, 1246*t*
sialorrhea, 1249–1251
trauma, 1251
classification of, 1516*t*
clinical presentation of, 1521–1522
diagnosis and management of, 553*t*
controversies in, 555–565
differential diagnosis of, 1523, 1524*f*
epithelial, in children, 1246–1247
etiology of, 1521
of hard palate, 1562–1563
history in, 1521–1522
imaging of, 522–523
incidence of, 1515, 1516*t*, 1517*t*
of lip, 1538
location of, 1515, 1516*t*, 1517*t*
prognosis and, 1532
malignant, 541–543, 542*f*, 543*f*. *See
also* Oral cancer
acinic cell carcinoma, 1519, 1520*f*
adenocarcinoma, 1519–1520
polymorphous low-grade, 1520
adenoid cystic carcinoma, 1519,
1519*f*
carcinoma ex-pleomorphic
adenoma, 1520, 1520*f*
chemotherapy for, 1528

Salivary gland disease (continued)
 in children, 1248–1249
  lymphoma, 1521, 1621–1627. See
    also Lymphoma, extranodal
  mucoepidermoid carcinoma,
    1518–1519, 1519f
  pediatric, 1515, 1517t
  sarcoma, 1521, 1520
  squamous cell carcinoma, 1520–1521
  undifferentiated carcinoma, 1521,
    1520
 metastases from, 1532
 physical examination of, 1522
 prognosis of, 1531–1532, 1531t
 radiation therapy for, 1528
 recurrence of, 1531
 risk factors for, 1521
 staging of, 1523t
 surgery for, 1524–1528
  complications of, 1528–1531
  for minor gland tumors, 1528
  for parapharyngeal space tumors,
    1525, 1527f
  for parotid tumors, 1524,
    1525f–1526f, 1529–1531
  for submandibular tumors, 1528,
    1529f, 1531
  vs. oral cancer, 1557–1558
Salmon patch, 1353, 1354f
 in orbital lymphoma, 1504, 1504f
Sampling population, for clinical data,
  27–29, 28f
Santorini cartilage, 2795
Santorini fissures, 2795
Sarcoidosis, 181–182, 182f, 377–379,
  379f, 407
 diagnosis of, 182
 head and neck manifestations of, 182
 laryngitis and, 830t, 833
 natural history of, 182
 salivary gland involvement in, 548
 symptoms of, 377
Sarcoma. See also specific sites and types
 in children, 1364–1366
 granulocytic, of orbit, 1504–1505
 orbital, 1504–1505, 1506–1507
 salivary gland, 1521
 sinonasal, 1485. See also Sinonasal
   tumors
 of temporal bone, 2017
Scalp
 anatomy of, 3, 4f, 1833–1834
 cutaneous malignancies of, parotid
   gland in, 562
 implants for, 2349, 2350t
 layers of, 940f
 skin flap for, after Mohs surgery,
   2400, 2404f, 2405f
 wounds, 939–940
Scalp reduction, in alopecia,
   2753–2755, 2754f, 2755f

complications of, 2754
 extensive
  complications of, 2755
  ligation of vessels for, 2754
  technique of, 2754–2755, 2755f
 patterns for, 2753, 2754f
 technique of, 2753–2754
Scapular and parascapular flaps,
   fasciocutaneous and
   osteofasciocutaneous,
   2383–2385, 2385f
Scarlet fever, 604
Scarpa, foramen of, 2795
Scarpa ganglion, 2795
Scar(s)
 acne, 1420-nm dermal collagen
   stimulating laser in,
   2728–2729, 2728f
 camouflage of, 2411–2419
  complications of, 2417–2418
  dermabrasion for, 2415–2416, 2416f
  excisional techniques for,
    2411–2413, 2412f, 2413f
  laser resurfacing for, 2415–2416
  scar irregularization for,
    2413–2415, 2413f, 2414f,
    2415f
  soft tissue fillers for, 2417
  techniques of, 2411–2417
 classification of, 2411
 depressed, management of, 2417
 following blepharoplasty, 2624
 following chemical peeling, 2722
 hypertrophic, 2736
  treatment of, 2746
  wound healing and, 211
 revision of, scar analysis and
   preoperative planning for,
   2417–2418, 2418f
 widening of, following forehead lift,
   2681
Scheibe aplasia, 2795
Schizophrenia, facial cosmetic surgery
   and, 2483–2484
Schmidt syndrome, 119–120
School, hearing screening in, 1279
Schwannoma
 of cranial nerve, 2226
 of facial nerve, 2020, 2225–2226
 intralabyrinthine, 1973, 1975f
 melanotic, 442, 442f
 orbital, 1505, 1505f
 of temporal bone
  categories of, 2020
  development of, 2020
  diagnosis of, 2020–2021
  management of, 2021
 trigeminal, 2020
 vestibular. See Vestibular schwannoma
Scintigraphy
 to examine swallowing, 706–707

 radionuclide, in aspiration, 1112
Scleritis, 131
Scleroderma, 173–174
 esophageal symptoms in, 762
 head and neck manifestations of,
   174, 174f
 treatment of, 174
Scleroma, laryngitis and, 832
Scopolamine, in gustatory sweating, 556
Screening, hearing
 in infants, 1277–1278, 1277–1279,
   1278t, 1289, 1307
 in school-age children, 1279
Screw(s)
 application of, 1030–1033
  instrumentation for, 1033
  principles of, 1030–1031, 1031f
 lag, application of, 1031–1032, 1032f
Scrofula, 185
Scurvy, 202
Sebaceous hyperplasia, 2734
 treatment of, 2745
Seborrheic keratoses, 2731–2734
 treatment of, 2744
Secondary intention healing
 of cutaneous nasal defects, 2426
 after Mohs surgery, 2393, 2394f,
   2394t
Sedative agents, intravenous, 147
Seizures
 otitis media and, 2054
 postoperative
  causes of, 230
  in cranial-base surgery, 1851, 1851t
  management of, 230
 vestibular symptoms in, 2314
Sella turcica, transsphenoidal approach
   to, 1839–1842, 1840f
Sellar face, endoscopic surgical
   approach to, 453, 453f
Semicircular canals
 deformity of, 1971, 1972f
 dehiscence of, 1972, 1974f
 microanatomy and biophysics of,
   1909–1910, 1910f
Senile keratosis, 1459, 1459f
Sensorineural hearing loss. See Hearing
   loss
Sensory enhancement techniques, to
   improve deglutition, 715
Sensory loss, aspiration in, 735
Sensory-motor integration procedures,
   to improve deglutition,
   716–717
Sensory nerve, injury to, during
   forehead lift, 2681, 2682
Sentinel node biopsy, 103–104, 1591
 of N0 neck, 1615, 1617–1618
 in oral cancer, 1560
Sentinel node dissection, in skin cancer,
   562

Sepsis, neonatal, hearing loss in, 1294
Septal abscesses, 327
    management of, 327–328
Septal deviation, nasal obstruction in, 312
Septicemia, following oral-cavity instrumentation, 627
Septoplasty
    clinical indications for, 323, 323t
    complications of, 325, 326t
    endoscopic, 324–325, 324f, 325f
    incision for, 323–324, 323f, 324f
    operative procedure for, 323
    revision, 325
Septra (sulfamethoxazole plus trimethoprim), 61
Septum
    caudal deflection of, nasal obstruction in, 321
    nasal. See Nasal septum
Sevoflurane, 145
Sex-linked inheritance, 42f, 43
Sexual harassment, risk of litigation for, case illustrating, 2785–2786
Shaker exercise, to improve deglutition, 716
Shave biopsy, 2739, 2740f
Shingles, 580
Shock, in trauma patients
    cardiogenic, 925–926
    hypovolemic, 924–925
    neurogenic, 925
Short-lasting unilateral neuralgiform headache with conjunctival injection and tearing, 255–256
Shotgun injuries, facial, 1018–1019, 1041, 1042f
Shprintzen syndrome, 1383–1384, 1384f
Shunts and valves, for voice restoration following laryngectomy, 1780–1781, 1781f, 1782f
Sialadenitis, 534–535, 534f, 535f
    acute bacterial, in children, 1241–1242
    acute suppurative, 545–546, 553
    neonatal, 1242
Sialadenosis, 552
Sialectasis, in children, 1243
Sialo-odontogenic cysts, 1572–1573, 1573f
Sialography
    of parotid gland, 563
    of salivary glands, 527–528
Sialolithiasis, 536, 549–550, 558
    in children, 1243–1244
    complications of, 550, 550f, 553
    submandibular, 550, 550f
Sialometaplasia, necrotizing, 181, 552–553
    vs. minor salivary gland tumor, 1523

Sialorrhea
    in children, 1249–1251
    control of, in aspiration, 1113
Sicca syndrome, 172, 2795
Sigmoid sinus thrombophlebitis, in otitis media, 2047, 2050
Sildevanck syndrome, hearing loss in, 1313
Silicone
    for management of scars, 2417
    for soft-tissue augmentation, 2767
Simulation, anatomic and surgical, 74–76
Simulator, for endoscopic sinus surgery, 75–76, 75f
Singer's format, 897
Sinonasal tract
    anatomy of, 307–311, 310–311f
    embryology of, 307, 308f
    and external environment, 317
Sinonasal tumors, 1481–1498
    benign
        endoscopic approaches for, 449–451, 449f
        epithelial, 1482–1483
        nonepithelial, 1485
    biopsy of, 1486–1487
    chemotherapy for, 1488
    complications of, 1494–1497
        emergent, 1497–1498
        postoperative, 1494, 1495–1496
        skull base, 1496–1497
    diagnosis of, 447–448, 448t, 1481–1482, 1482t
    endoscopic management of, 447–457, 449f
        complications of, 451t
        emergencies in, 451t
    epidemiology of, 1481
    evaluation of, 1481–1486
    extension of
        to infratemporal fossa, 1492–1494
        to orbit, 1488–1490, 1494t, 1511
        to palate, 1562, 1562f
        to pterygopalatine fossa, 1490
        to skull base, 1492–1494
    imaging of, 440–441, 440f, 1481–1482
    lymphoma, 1486, 1621–1627. See also Lymphoma, extranodal
    malignant
        epithelial, 1483–1485
        nonepithelial, 1483t
        postoperative care in, 1487
    metastatic, 1486, 1490–1494
    pathology of, 1482–1486
    preoperative evaluation in, 447–448
    radiation therapy for, 1487–1488
        complications of, 1494–1495
    staging of, 1486, 1487t
    surgery for, 1486–1487

approaches in, 1488f–1490f, 1495f
complications of, 1494, 1495–1496
technique of, 1488f–1493f
types of, 1482–1486, 1483t
Sinus(es). See also under Sinonasal and specific sinuses; specific sinuses
    anatomy of, 8, 8f, 477–479, 479t
    atelectatic, 436–437, 437f
    computed tomography of, 411–412, 411f, 412f, 429–430, 430f
    development of, 1051–1052, 1051f, 1051t
    dimensions of, measurement of, 478, 478f
    disorders of
        complications of, 378t
        diagnosis of, 378t
        granulomatous and autoimmune, 377–391
        radiologic signs of, 87t
        smell impairment in, 295–296
        symptoms of, 378t
        treatment of, 379t
    evaluation of
        computed tomography in, 90
        plain radiography in, 89–90
    imaging of, 86, 86t
    magnetic resonance imaging of, 90, 431–432, 431f, 432f
    pathology of, 433–437
    standard radiography of, 429, 430f
    treatment complications in, 479–483, 480t
    tumors of. See also Sinonasal tumors
        diagnosis of, 447–448, 448t
        endoscopic management of, 447–457
        preoperative evaluation in, 447–448
Sinus fungal ball, 422
Sinus headache, 259
Sinus infections
    complications of, 122–124
    fungal, noninvasive, 422–426
Sinus obstruction, causes of, 409
Sinus of Morgagni syndrome, 2795
Sinus surgery
    complications of, 477–491, 480t
    endoscopic, 437–439
    external approaches in, 365–376
    frontal, with osteoplastic flap, complications of, 460–461
    frontal (endoscopic), complications of, 482–483
    image-guided endoscopic, complications of, 482–483
    orbital complications of, 483–487
    powered endoscopic, complications of, 482
Sinusitis. See also Rhinosinusitis
    acute, 433, 433f
        antimicrobial agents in, 62–63

Sinusitis (continued)
  allergic fungal, 434, 435f
  chronic, 433, 433f
    in AIDS, 269–270
  diagnostic criteria for, 251t
  geriatric, 241, 241t
  invasive fungal, 417–422, 434
    acute fulminant
      clinical presentation and
        diagnosis of, 418–419
      pathogenesis of, 420
      prognosis in, 421
      radiology of, 419–420
      treatment of, 420–421
    chronic
      clinical presentation of, 421
      diagnosis of, 421
      pathology of, 422
      radiology in, 422
      treatment and prognosis in, 422
    differential diagnosis of, 419t
    features of, 418, 418t
    granulomatous, 422
  in Kartagener syndrome, 1381, 1382
  orbital cellulitis in, 123
  postoperative, 1498
Sinusotomy, frontal, with or without
    osteoplastic flap, 375
Sistrunk procedure
  for thyroglossal duct cancer, 1631
  for thyroglossal duct cyst, 1630
Sjögren syndrome, 172–173, 382,
    533–534, 534f, 2795
  in children, 1249
  clinical manifestations of, 172, 173t,
    548, 548f
  head and neck manifestations of,
    173, 382
  laboratory findings in, 549
  symptoms of, 549
  treatment of, 173
Skin
  of aging neck, 2651
  in AIDS, 267–268, 269t, 270t
  biomechanics of, local skin flaps and,
    2360–2362, 2361f
  blood supply to, 2357, 2358f, 2359f
  changes in, age-related, 244
  of forehead, 2664–2665, 2664f, 2667
  nasal, 2516, 2551
  premalignant lesions of, 1458–1460,
    1459f
  tension lines of, of face, 2361–2362,
    2361f, 2395f
Skin-appendage tumors, 2734–2735
Skin cancer, 1455–1468, 2010–2011. See
    also Malignant melanoma
  anatomic location of, 1460, 1460t,
    1461f
  basal cell
    diagnosis of, 2010–2011

evaluation of, 1456
histopathology of, 1456, 1457f,
    1458f
incidence of, 2010
keratotic, 1457
treatment of, 2011
complications of, 1467, 1467t
epidemiology of, 1455
etiology of, 1455–1456
of eyelid, 1511
of face and scalp, parotid gland in,
    562
human papillomavirus and, 1456
metastases from
  nodal, 1467
  salivary, 1523
overview of, 1467–1468
premalignant lesions and,
    1458–1460, 1459f
prognosis of, 1460–1462
recurrent, 1460–1462
risk factors for, 1455–1456, 1460t
of scalp, 562
squamous cell
  evaluation of, 1457–1458
  histopathology of, 1458
TNM classification for, 1460, 1460t
treatment of, 1462–1466, 1466f
  cryosurgery in, 1462
  curettage with electrodesiccation in,
    1462
  excisional surgery in, 1463, 1467
  interferon-a in, 1463
  laser therapy in, 1463–1465, 1465f
  Mohs surgery in, 1463, 1464f, 1467
  palliative, 1464–1465
  photodynamic therapy in,
    1462–1463
  radiation therapy in, 1462
  reconstructive surgery in,
    1465–1466, 1466t
  results of, 1464t
  tumor behavior in, 1460
Skin disorders, radiation-related,
    1451–1452
Skin flaps. See also Flaps
  local
    advantages and disadvantages of,
      2357t
    anatomy, physiology, and types of,
      2357–2367
    axial-pattern, 2357, 2359t
    delay phenomenon and, 2360,
      2360f
    failure of, 2358t, 2362
    length-to-width ratio of, 2360
    after Mohs surgery, 2395–2397,
      2395f, 2396f, 2397f
    myocutaneous, 2359
    physiology of, 2359–2360, 2359f,
      2360f

random-pattern, 2357
skin biomechanics and,
    2360–2362, 2361f
types of, 2362–2366
vascular anatomy of, 2357–2359,
    2358f, 2359f
Skin grafts
  in aural atresia, technique for,
    2036–2037, 2036f
  in cutaneous nasal defects,
    2426–2427, 2426t
  following Mohs surgery, 2394
  healing of, 210–211
Skin rejuvenation, nonablative
  532-nm and 1064-nm lasers for, 2728
  1320-nm dermal collagen stimulating
    laser for, 2728
Skin resurfacing
  intense pulsed light for, 2727
  laser. See Laser therapy, skin
    resurfacing
  nonablative, 2727, 2727f
    1420-nm dermal collagen
      stimulating laser for,
      2728–2729, 2728f
  radiofrequency, 2727
Skin tags, treatment of, 2746
Skin testing, in rhinitis, 357
Skin type, classification of, 2726, 2726t
Skull. See also under Cranial
  bony lesions of, 189–192
  implants for, 2349, 2350t
  infant and adult, craniofacial skeletal
    comparison of, 1049, 1050f
Skull base
  defects of, microvascular
    reconstructive approaches to,
    2389–2390
  invasion of, in sinonasal cancer,
    1492–1494
  lateral
    and ear, neoplasms of, 2003–2025
    metastatic disease of, 2023
    surgery of, facial nerve monitoring
      during, 1956
    tumors of, facial nerve and,
      2152–2153
Skull-base complications, of sinonasal
    tumor surgery, 1496–1497
Sleep
  non-rapid eye movement, 646
  normal, 646–647
  physiology of, 646–647
  rapid eye movement, 646
Sleep apnea
  obstructive
    classification of, 648, 648t
    complications of surgery in, 660,
      660t
    definition of, 648
    diagnosis of, 651t

epidemiology of, 645–646
pharynx and, 694–695
preoperative medical evaluation in, 653–654
snoring and, 645–664
surgical emergencies in, 660, 660t
treatment of, 654–663, 659t
  indications for, 654–655
  nonsurgical, 655–656
  surgical, 658–663
  surgical treatment of snoring in, 656–658, 656f, 658f
suspected
  cephalometric roentgenograms in, 651–652
  clinical evaluation in, 649–653
  diagnostic studies in, 652
  history taking in, 649–650, 650f
  multiple sleep latency test in, 653
  physical examination in, 650–651
  polysomnography in, 652–653
  portable monitoring devices in, 652
  radiographic evaluation in, 651
Sleep architecture, normal, young adult, 646, 646t
Sleep-disordered breathing, 647
  in children, 1079
    complications, 1084
    diagnostic evaluation
      history, 1081
      laboratory evaluation, 1082–1083
      physical evaluation, 1081–1082, 1082f
    epidemiology, 1079
    obstruction levels and types in, 1083t
    pathophysiology, 1079–1080, 1080t
    syndromes and conditions associated with, 1083t
    treatment options, 1084
    vs. in adults, 1081t
Sleep disorder(s), obstructive, 647–648
  in children, 1059–1060
  mixed, 647, 648f
Sleep studies, upper airway obstruction and, 804
Sluder headache, 2795
Sluder neuralgia, 2795
Smell. See Olfaction
Smell Identification Test, 293
Smith-Magenis syndrome, 44
Smoking. See Tobacco use
Snoreplasty, in snoring, 657
Snoring
  classification of, 647
  nonapneic, treatment of, 657, 659t
  and obstructive sleep apnea, 645–664
  surgical treatment of, in obstructive sleep apnea, 658–2139, 658f, 660f
Sodium sulfacetamide, 132

Sodium valproate, 260
Soft palate. See also Palate
  in deglutition, 686, 686f
  pillar implants in, in snoring, 657
  prosthetic rehabilitation in, surgical techniques for, 1857–1858, 1857f
  radiofrequency tissue ablation of, in snoring, 657
Soft tissue
  augmentation of, 2765–2768
    autografts for, 2766–2767
    homografts for, 2767
    synthetic materials for, 2767–2768, 2768f
    xenografts for, 2765–2766, 2766f
  benign tumors originating in, 441–442, 441f, 442f
  bullet wound of, cavitation effects of, 1017, 1017f
  loss of, in complex facial trauma, 1041–1042, 1042f
  malignant tumors originating in, 442–443, 443f
  of neck, diagnostic imaging of, 91–92
  reconstruction of, following oropharyngeal surgery, 1685–1686, 1686f, 1686t
  subcutaneous, nasal, 2516, 2551
Soft-tissue defects, external, microvascular reconstructive approaches to, 2390
Soft tissue fillers, 2417
Soft tissue necrosis, radiation-related, 1451
Soft tissue sarcoma, in children, 1364–1366, 1364t, 1365t
Soft tissue trauma. See also Trauma
  etiology, 935
  evaluation, 935–936
  facial, emergency interventions for, 936t
  in pediatric patients, 936
  wound management, 936
    abrasions, 937
    animal and human bites, 945–946
    auricular, 943–944, 944f, 945f
    avulsion, 939, 939f
    complications, 945t
    contusions, 937
    eyelid and lacrimal system, 941–943, 942f, 943f
    facial, suturing principles for, 938f
    facial nerves, 940–941
    lacerations, 937, 937f, 939, 939f
    nasal, 944–945
    parotid duct, 941, 941f
    postoperative care, 945
    scalp wounds, 939–940, 940f
    suturing techniques, 938f
Solar keratosis, 1459, 1459f

Solvents, inhaled, laryngitis and, 830t
Somatic gene therapy, 1391
Somnolence syndrome, radiation-related, 1452
South American blastomycosis, 188
Spasmodic dysphonia
  appropriate voice therapy referrals for, 890
  common voice therapy applications for, 889t
  laryngeal dysfunction and, 876–877
  surgery for, controversies in use of, 914
Spectral envelope, voice production and, 897
Speech. See also Voice
  articulation and, 701
  control of, sensory input to, 701
  following laryngectomy. See Voice rehabilitation, after laryngectomy
  phonation and, 700–701
  production of, 897
  resonance and, 701
  upper airway and, 700–701
Speech threshold, 1931
Sphenoethmoidal recess, 438, 438f
Sphenoid sinus. See also Sinus(es)
  anatomy of, 8, 309–311, 370–371, 371f
  ostium of, 478–479
  pneumatization of, classification of, 370, 370f
  surgery of
    columellar flap modification in, 372f, 373
    complications of, 367t, 373, 374t
    transseptal approaches for, 371–373, 372f
Sphenoidotomy, complications of, 482
Sphenopalatine foramen, endoscopic approach to, 454–455, 454f
Spider angiomas, treatment of, 2746
Spinal accessory nerve, 110f
Spinal artery, anterior, infarction of, 118
Spinal injuries, in head trauma, 926–927
Spiramycin, for cytomegalovirus infection, in pregnancy, 1292, 1293
Spitz nevus, 2738, 2738f
  treatment of, 2747
Spondee words, 1931
Squamous cell carcinoma
  cutaneous. See Skin cancer
  ear and lateral skull base, 2011
  in elderly patients, 243
  orbital, 1511
  oropharyngeal, treatment of, 1677–1678, 1678t
  of pinna, 2011

Squamous cell carcinoma *(continued)*
  salivary gland, 542, 1520–1521
  tracheal, 1794–1795, 1794t
  treatment of, 2011
Squamous cell papilloma, 2014
Stab wounds, facial, 1019
Staging system, creation of, 34–35
Standards of care. *See* Clinical
      guidelines; Clinical pathways
Stapedectomy
  complications of, 2130t, 2136–2137
  facial nerve monitoring during, 1957
  indications for, 2136t
  patient counseling for, 2131–2132
  patient selection for, 2130–2131
  technique for, 2132–2136, 2132f,
      2133f, 2134f
Stapedial muscle spasm, tinnitus in,
      2238–2239
Stapedial reflex measurement, acoustic,
      1932–1933
Staphylococcal infection, pharyngitis
      due to, 604
Staphylococcus aureus infection
  in HIV disease, 267
  laryngitis in, 829
  pediatric rhinosinusitis in, 1232, 1232t
Statistical tests
  for related samples, 27, 27t, 28t
  results of, strength and consistency
      of, 30, 30t
  for valid analysis, 26–27, 26t, 27t
Status epilepticus, 230
  pharmacologic management of, 230,
      230t
Stavudine, 274
Stenosis. *See also* Laryngeal stenosis
  congenital choanal, 1124–1125
Stents
  airway, upper airway obstruction, and
      use of, 812
  laryngeal, 955–956, 957f
  laryngeal stenosis and, 1143, 1144f
Stereotactic radiotherapy
  in cranial-base surgery, 1845–1846
  for recurrent nasopharyngeal cancer,
      1665
  for vestibular schwannomas,
      2222–2224
Steroids. *See* Corticosteroids
Stevens-Johnson syndrome, 592
  pharyngitis in, 610
Stickler syndrome, hearing loss in,
      1305t, 1311
Stomach, caustic ingestions and, 1158f
Stomatitis, 579–599
  in desquamative gingivitis, 581–582,
      581f, 582f, 582t
  due to acquired immunodeficiency
      syndrome, 598
  due to candidiasis, 594–596

  due to erythema multiforme,
      591–592
  due to herpes simplex virus, 579–580
  due to lichen planus, 592–594
  due to lupus erythematosus,
      582–586, 584–585t
  due to mucositis, 597–598, 597f
  due to pemphigoids, 586–591
  due to varicella zoster virus, 580–581
  recurrent aphthous. *See* Aphthous
      stomatitis, recurrent
Stork bites, 1353–1354, 1354f
Strabismus, 136
Streptococcal infections
  complications of, 604
  pharyngitis due to, 603–606
Streptococcus pneumoniae
  laryngitis and, 829
  pediatric rhinosinusitis and, 1232,
      1232t
Streptococcus pneumoniae vaccination, in
      infants and children, 1059
Streptogramins, 61
Streptomycin, 61
  ototoxicity of, 1298
Stress ulcers
  preventive management of, 227–228
  treatment of, 228
Stretch and flow phonation, in voice
      therapy, 888, 889t
Stridor, 803
  in children, 1091–1092, 1092f, 1095,
      1096f, 1096t, 1097f
    complications of, 1109
    differential diagnosis of, 1102–1109,
      1103t
    history and physical examination
      in, 1098–1100, 1100f, 1100t
    radiology and special studies in,
      1100–1101
Stroboscopy, 824–825
  controversies in use of, 907–908, 908t
Stroke
  after carotid artery dissection, 1601
  due to thrombosis, 117–118
  laryngeal dysfunction and, 872
Sturge-Weber syndrome, 1356, 1824,
      2795
Sty, 130–131
Subarachnoid hemorrhage, 117
Subclavian artery, anomalous, 1129
Subdural abscess, in otitis media, 2048,
      2051
Subdural empyema, 122
Subglottic cancer, advanced, 1773
Subglottic hemangioma, 1127–1128,
      1128f
  management of, 1352–1353
  in PHACE syndrome, 1351–1352
Subglottic pressure, voice production
      and, 898

Subglottic stenosis
  congenital, 1127
  laryngeal trauma management and,
      957t, 958
  management of, 811
  postintubation, 1135–1136
  postoperative, 1136
  stridor in, 1104
Subglottis, posterior cleft, 1128
Sublingual glands. *See also* Salivary
      gland(s)
  anatomy of, 521, 521f, 533
  tumors of, 1515, 1516t
Sublingual space, odontogenic
      infections of, 618
Submandibular glands. *See also* Salivary
      gland(s)
  anatomy of, 11–12, 12f, 520–521,
      520f, 521f, 533
  excision of, and parotid duct ligation,
      in aspiration, 1113–1114
  tumors of, 1515, 1516t
    surgery for, 1528, 1529t
      complications of, 1531
      technique of, 1528, 1529f
Submandibular space, 670–671
  infections of, 679–680
  odontogenic infections of, 618, 619f
Submental space, odontogenic
      infections of, 618–619
Submentoplasty, 2658–2659, 2658f,
      2659f, 2660f
  complications of, 2660–2661
Succinylcholine, 149
Sufentanil, 148
Sulcus vocalis, 839–840
  appropriate referrals for, 890
  common voice therapy applications
      for, 889t
Sulfamethoxazole plus trimethoprim
      (Bactrim, Septra), 61
Sulfonamides, 61, 186
Sun exposure
  lip cancer and, 1537
  skin cancer and, 1455–1456
Superior canal dehiscence syndrome,
      surgical management of,
      2339–2340
Superior laryngeal nerve injury, in
      thyroidectomy, 1643
Superior laryngeal nerve paresis, 874
Superior orbital fissure syndrome,
      625–626, 625f
Suppurative sialadenitis, acute, 545–546
Supracricoid partial laryngectomy,
      1743, 1745–1750,
      1746f–1752f. *See also* Glottic
      and supraglottic cancer, early,
      open surgery for
Supraglottic cancer. *See* Glottic and
      supraglottic cancer

Supraglottic closure, partial, in aspiration, 738–739

Supraglottic partial laryngectomy, 1743, 1745–1750, 1746f–1752f. *See also* Glottic and supraglottic cancer, early, open surgery for

Supraglottic quadrangular membrane, larynx and, 818

Supraglottic vocal tract, voice production and, 897–898

Supraglottis, congenital anomalous conditions of, 1122t, 1126

Supraglottitis, 829–830
diagnosis of, 1065, 1065f
stridor in, 1109
upper airway obstruction and, 804

Supraomohyoid neck dissection, 1596, 1596f

Supraorbital rim fractures, in children, 1338–1342. *See also* Facial fractures, in children
surgery of, 1346

Surface-enhanced laser desorption/ionization, 101

Surgery. *See also specific indications*
computer-assisted, 439
evaluation of surgical margin for, 101
preoperative evaluation for, 215
preoperative malnutrition and, 215–216
prophylaxis for wound infections in, 64–65

Surgical stimulation, 74–76

Sutures/suturing
endo-extralaryngeal lateralization, for bilateral vocal fold paralysis and, 863
for facial soft tissue trauma, 938f

Swallow maneuvers, to improve deglutition, 717–718

Swallow study, videofluoroscope, in aspiration, 1112

Swallow therapy, 713

Swallowing. *See* Deglutition; Dysphagia

Sweating, gustatory, 555–557, 1530–1531, 1530f

Sympathetic nervous system, salivary glands and, 524

Symphysis, of mandible, 961f
fracture
management, 967, 968f
treatment options, 965t

Syndactyly, in Apert syndrome, 1377, 1377f

Syndrome of inappropriate antidiuretic hormone secretion, 158, 222–223
after cranial-base surgery, 1849t, 1850

Syndromes
definition of, 1374

otolaryngologic, 1375–1387. *See also* Otolaryngologic syndromes

Synechiae, after sinus surgery, 488–489

Synercid (quinupristin and dalfopristin), 61

Synkinesis, electromyography of vocal fold immobility, 881, 881f

Synthetic materials, for soft-tissue augmentation, 2767–2768

Syphilis, 186–187, 187f, 384–386, 385f
head and neck involvement in, 187
hearing loss in, 187
congenital, 1293–1294
laryngitis in, 831
otologic manifestations of, 2157
pharyngitis in, 605–606
serologic tests for, 606
tertiary, 606

Syphilitic labyrinthitis
etiology of, 2182–2183
evaluation in, 2183
incidence of, 2182
treatment of, 2183–2184, 2184t

Syringobulbia, 115

Syringoma, 2734
treatment of, 2745

Systemic lupus erythematosus. *See* Lupus erythematosus

Systemic sclerosis. *See* Scleroderma

T

T cells, 343–344, 1406–1408, 1407f. *See also* Lymphocytes
activation of, 242, 243t
in head and neck cancer, 1409, 1410–1411

Tachydysrhythmias, preoperative management of, 225

Tapia syndrome, 2795

Tarceva, 1431–1432

Tarsus, anatomy of, 4, 5f

Taste, 567–578
anatomy of, 568–570
cranial nerves and, 569, 570, 571f
evaluation of, 572–574
genetic variation in, 570–572
intensification of, 572
loss/alteration of, 567–578, 572, 574–575, 576–577
age-related, 576
in cancer, 576
causes of, 302–303
coping with, 577
cumulative, 575
diagnosis of, 572–574
drug-induced, 576
management of, 303
mixtures of, 567–568
peripheral nerves and, 569
quality coding, 568
sensations of, 567

stimuli, receptor sites and, 568
venous, 574
vs. olfaction, 567–568

Taste buds, 568

Taste nerves, interactions among, 570

Taste papillae, 568–569

Taste phantoms, 573–574
from peripheral nerve damage, 575–576

Technetium 99m sestamibi scan
in hyperparathyroidism, 1649
of parathyroid glands, 95

Technetium scan, of parotid gland, 563

Teeth. *See also under* Dental
evaluation of, for prosthetic rehabilitation, 1855, 1855f
Hutchinson, 2792
identification of, universal numbering system for, 1853, 1854f
impacted, dentigerous cysts and, 1570–1571, 1570f
infections of. *See* Odontogenic infections
injuries of
in children, 1345
in mandibular fractures, 970. *See also* Mandibular fractures
radiation-induced, 1452
numbering system for, 961
osseointegrated prosthetic, 1861–1863, 1862f

Teflon injection, in paralyzed vocal fold, 911

Telangiectasia, 1817–1819, 2736
hereditary, 2733t, 2794
hereditary hemorrhagic, 1824
epistaxis in, 508
management of, 513
treatment of, 2746

Telescope, for laryngology, fiberoptic laryngoscopy versus, 907

Telithromycin (Ketek), 59

Telomerase, 100

Telomeres, 100–101

Temple lift, bilateral, surgical procedure for, 2669f, 2672

Temporal arteritis, 177–178, 178f
headache in, 257–258

Temporal bone
computed tomography of, 87–89, 1961, 1962f
development of, 1052–1053, 1052f
diagnostic radiology of, 87, 88t
imaging of, 86, 86t, 1961–1985
implants for, 2349–2350, 2350t
magnetic resonance imaging of, 87–89, 1961–1963, 1963f
metastatic disease of, 2023
neoplasms of, 2014–2019
paragangliomas of, 2003–2007
trauma to, 1975–1976, 1978f

Temporal bone (*continued*)
    classification of, 2058–2060, 2060f, 2061f
    clinical evaluation in, 2060–2065, 2062f
    complications of, 2059t
    epidemiology of, 2057–2058, 2058f
    evaluation in, 2060–2065, 2062f, 2063f, 2064f
    management of, 2065–2076
        with middle ear trauma, 2057–2079
    pathophysiology of, 2058, 2059f
    radiographic evaluation in, 2063–2065, 2063f, 2064f
    vascular anomalies and diseases of, 1978–1981
    vascular neoplasms and, 1980, 1980f
Temporal space, masticular space, and anterior visceral space, 671
    infections of, 681
Temporomandibular joint
    ankylosis of, 634
    arthroscopy of, 637, 637f
    components of, 634f
    degenerative joint disease of, 633, 634
    disk displacement in, 632, 633f, 634f
    disorders of, 632–643
        arthrocentesis in, 636–637, 636f
        clicking in, 636
        headache in, 259
        imaging in, 635–637, 635f, 635t
        magnetic resonance imaging in, 635, 635f
        and surgery of, 637–643
        treatment of, 635–637, 635t
    inflammation of, 633–634
    injury to, in maxillary/periorbital fractures, 991
    internal derangements of, congenital and developmental, 634
    joint hypermobility in, 632
    physiology of, 631–632
    postoperative care of, 641
    reconstruction of, total joint prosthesis in, 640–641, 641f
    surgery of
        approaches in, 637, 637f
        complications of, 641t, 642t
        excision of disk in, 638f, 639
        harvesting cartilage in, 639, 639f
        intraarticular, options for, 638f, 639
        plate fixation in, 639–640, 640f
        techniques of, 637–641, 637f, 638f
Temporoparietal fascial flap, 2375–2376, 2375f
Tension pneumocephalus, postoperative, 1497
Tequin (Gatifloxacin), 60

Teratomas, of temporal bone, 2019
Tetanus, 116
Tetracycline(s), 60
    for parotid cysts, 557
Tetraiodothyronine, 161
Thoracic injuries, in trauma patients, 928–929, 929f
Thoracostomy, tube, in trauma patients, 923–924, 923f
Thrombocytopenia, chemotherapy-related, 1438t
Thromboembolic disease
    diagnosis of, 219
    management of, 220
    prevention of, 219
    pulmonary embolism in, 220
        as complication of otitis media surgery, 2053
        preoperative, 220
    risk factors for, 219
Thrombophlebitis, sigmoid sinus, in otitis media, 2047, 2050
Thrombosis
    cavernous sinus, 123
        in rhinosinusitis, 496
    jugular vein, 624, 624f
        after neck dissection, 1605–1606
    stroke due to, 117–118
    venous sinus, in rhinosinusitis, 501
Thrush. *See* Candidiasis
Thyroglossal duct cancer, 1631
Thyroglossal duct cysts, 1630–1631
Thyroid
    adenoma of, 1632
    anatomy of, 16, 16f, 1629–1630
    benign lesions of, 1631–1632
    biopsy of, 1636–1637
    congenital abnormalities of, 1629–1631
    disorders of, preoperative management of, 220–221, 221t
    ectopic, 1629–1630
    embryology of, 1629–1631
    imaging of, 94–95, 1635–1636
    lateral aberrant tissue of, 1630
    lingual, 1629
    neoplasms of, molecular differentiation of, 54
    physiology of, 160–161
    radioiodine ablation of, after thyroidectomy, 1644
Thyroid cancer
    anaplastic, 1634
    in children, 1366–1367
    diagnosis of, 1634–1636
    follicular, 1633
    Hürthle cell, 1633–1634
    imaging studies in, 1635–1636
    lymphoma, 621–627, 1634. *See also* Lymphoma, extranodal
    medullary, 1645–1647

    metastases in
        distant, 1645
        nodal, 1644–1645
    papillary, 1632–1633
    preoperative laryngoscopy for, 1634–1635
    prognostic factors in, 1644
    recurrent/persistent, 1644
    staging of, 1644
    surgery for, 1637–1645. *See also* Thyroidectomy
Thyroid cartilage
    in children vs. adults, 1054, 1055f
    fracture of, 954f
        surgical treatment for, 954
    larynx and, 817–819
Thyroid nodule, evaluation of, 1634–1636, 1635t
Thyroid ophthalmopathy, ocular manifestations of, 137
Thyroid-stimulating hormone, 157, 157f
    recombinant, 155
Thyroid storm, 165–166
    medical control of, 221–222, 221t
Thyroidarytenoid muscle, voice production and, 896
Thyroidectomy, 1637–1645
    airway obstruction after, 1644
    approach in, 1637
    complications of, 1642–1644
    endoscopic, 82
    extent of, 1642
    hematoma after, 1643
    hemorrhage after, 1642–1643
    hypocalcemia after, 1643–1644
    infection after, 1643
    lateral thyroid dissection in, 1638
    lymph node microdissection in, 1646
    for medullary cancer, 1646
    nerve infiltration/injury in, 1640
    parathyroid gland in
        autotransplantation of, 1641
        preservation of, 1640–1641, 1641f
        patient positioning and preparation for, 1637
    preoperative workup in, 1637
    radioiodine ablation after, 1644
    recurrent laryngeal nerve in, 1638–1639, 1638f–1641f
        injury of, 1643
    seroma after, 1643
    strap muscles in, 1637–1638
    superior laryngeal nerve injury in, 1643
Thyroiditis, 1631–1632
    chronic lymphocytic, 1631
    Hashimoto, 1631
    invasive fibrous, 1631–1632
    Riedel, 1631–1632, 2794
Thyrotoxic crisis. *See* Thyroid storm

Thyrotoxicosis, preoperative management of, 221
Tic disorders, laryngeal dysfunction and, 877
Ticarcillin, 58
Timolol, 251
Tinnitus, 2237–2245
  cognitive behavioral therapy in, 2243
  electromagnetic stimulation in, 2243
  habituation of, 2243
  in hearing person, 2243
  incidence of, 239, 239t
  medications and, 2243
  objective, 2237–2239
    vascular abnormalities causing, 2238t
    in palatomyoclonus, 2238
    in patulous eustachian tube, 2238
    in stapedial muscle spasm, 2238–2239
  subjective, 2239–2244
    cardiovascular factors in, 2239–2240
    dental abnormalities and, 2240–2241
    etiologic factors in, 2239t
    hearing aid in, 2242
    masking in, 2241–2242, 2243
    medical evaluation in, 2239, 2241
    metabolic function and, 2240
    in neurologic disease, 2240
    otologic factors in, 2239
    pharmacologic factors in, 2240, 2240t
    psychological factors in, 2241
    treatment of, 2241–2244, 2242f
  surgery in, 2243
Tinnitus instrument, 2242–2243
Tipranavir, 266
Tissue adhesives, in wound healing, 208
Tissue expansion
  in alopecia, 2755–2757, 2756f
  after Mohs surgery, 2400–2407
Tissue inhibitors of metalloproteinases, 102
Tobacco use
  background of, 277–286
  cessation of, 277–286
    after cancer diagnosis, 283–284
    patient satisfaction with counseling on, 282
    pharmacotherapy aids for, 280–282, 281t
    resources for, 279, 279t, 284
    stages of change and, 281–282
  clinical intervention in, 278–280, 278t
    effectiveness of, 282–284, 283t
    physician compliance with, 283, 283t
  laryngitis and, 830t

oral cancer and, 1554, 1555
  patterns of, 277
  varying with age, 277–278
Tobramycin, 60, 61, 133
  ototoxicity of, 1298
Toll-like receptors, 336
Tolosa-Hunt syndrome, 2795
Tomography. See Computed tomography
Tongue. See also under Oral
  anatomy of, 10, 11f, 1552, 1552f–1554f
  cancer of, 1564. See also Oral cancer
  in deglutition, 685–686, 686f
  prosthetic rehabilitation in, surgical techniques for, 1858, 1859f
  surgery of, in obstructive sleep apnea, 661–662
  taste alteration and, 572f, 574
  taste and, 568
  taste papillae of, 568–569
  tongue map of, 568–569
Tongue-hold maneuver, to improve deglutition, 718
Tongue-retaining device, in obstructive sleep apnea, 656
Tonsil(s). See also Adenoid(s)
  anatomy, 1184f, 1185–1186, 1185f, 1185t
  clinical evaluation, 1189–1191, 1190f, 1192t, 1193
    grading classification, 1191f
  disorders of, 1183
    clinical classification of, 1187–1188, 1187t
    complications of, 1195t
    management of, 1194–1197
    pathogenesis of, 1187
  immunology of, 1187
  lingual, 1197
  microbiology of, 1186–1187
  unilateral hyperplasia, 1197
Tonsillectomy. See also Adenoidectomy
  complications of, 1195t
  controversies in, 1199
    certain indications for, 1199–1200
    elective indications for
      chronic tonsillitis, 1201–1202, 1272–1273
      obstructive tonsils, 1202
      peritonsillar abscess, 1202
      recurrent tonsillitis, 1200–1201, 1201t
    recommendations for the clinician, 1206–1207, 1207t
  indications for, 1194t
  for otitis media prophylaxis, 1201–1202, 1272–1273
Tonsillitis
  acute, 1188, 1192t
  amoxicillin in, 63–64

chronic (persistent), 1188, 1192t
  recurrent acute, 1188, 1192t
Tonsilloadenoiditis, 63–64
Tooth. See Teeth
Topiramate, 251
Tori, 1577–1578, 1578f
Tornwaldt cyst, 2795
Tositumomab, for extranodal lymphoma, 1624, 1624t, 1625
Total parenteral nutrition, preoperative, 215–216
Toxic epidermal necrolysis, 592
Toxic shock, as complication of sinus surgery, 489
Toxoplasmosis, 189
  congenital, hearing loss in, 1292–1293
Trachea
  compression of, in vascular anomalies, 1107, 1107f, 1108f
  obstruction of, in pediatric patients, 1091, 1091f
  tumors of, 1793–1810
    airway management in, 1793–1794
    anesthetic technique in, 1796–1797
    classification of, 1794–1796, 1794t, 1795t
    diagnosis of, 1796, 1796t
    emergencies in, management of, 1794, 1794t
    primary, management results, 1801–1807
    radiologic evaluation of, 1793
    signs and symptoms of, 1796
    surgery in
      approach for, 1800f, 1801
      complications of, 1802, 1802t
      effects at resection margins, 1806, 1806t
      irradiation following, 1807–1808, 1808t
      long-term survival following, 1802–1805, 1803f, 1804f, 1805t, 1808–1809
      lymph node status following, 1806–1807, 1806t
      mortality associated with, 1802
      recurrence following, 1805–1806, 1806t, 1807
      technical features of, 1801–1802
      technique for, 1797–1801, 1797t, 1798f, 1799f, 1800f
      unresectable, 1801, 1801t
Trachea, congenital anomalies of, 1122t, 1128
  stenosis, 1130
Tracheal agenesis, 1128
Tracheitis, bacterial
  glottic obstruction in, 1066, 1067f
  stridor in, 1109

Tracheobronchoscopy, in office, 751–752
  equipment for, 751
  patient selection/indications for, 751
  practical considerations for, 752
  technique for, 751–752
  topical anesthesia for, 751
Tracheoesophageal diversion, in aspiration, 739, 740t
Tracheoesophageal fistula, 1128, 1129f, 1130f
Tracheoesophageal puncture, 1783–1784, 1784f
  dysfluent speech after, management of, 1786, 1786t
  emergencies associated with, 1789–1790, 1789t
  surgical technique of, 1785–1787, 1785f, 1786f
  voice failure after, 1784–1785, 1784t
  for voice restoration during laryngectomy, 1787–1789, 1788t, 1789f
Tracheomalacia, 1068, 1068f, 1069f, 1128
Tracheostomy. See also Tracheotomy
  and aspiration, 735
  for bilateral vocal fold paralysis, 863
    flap-type, 864
  indications for, 1148t
Tracheostomy tube, valving of, in aspiration, 736–737, 736f
Tracheotomy
  for aerodigestive foreign body, 1164f
  Björk flap in, 787, 788f
  complications of, 790–792, 790t, 792f
  cricothyroidotomy versus, 808–809, 809f, 809t
  elective, 786, 788f
  emergency, 787, 789f
  history of, 785, 785t
  indications for, 785–786, 786–787t
  and intubation, 785–801
  in laryngeal incompetence, 1114
  in obstructive sleep apnea, 663
  open versus percutaneous, 809–810, 810t
  pediatric, 790, 791f
    communication concerns, 1154
    complications, 1152–1153
    decannulation, 1154
    history, 1147–1148
    indications for, 1148t
    postoperative care
      home, 1152
      hospital, 1151–1152
    prolonged intubation versus, 1149
    technique, 1149–1150f, 1149–1151
    tubes for, 1153
  percutaneous dilational, 792–796

  advantages and disadvantages of, 794
  complications of, 794–795, 795t
  as controversial technique, 795–796
  history of, 792
  indications for, and contraindications to, 792–793, 793t
  patient selection for, 793t
  and standard tracheotomy, compared, 795
  technique of, 793–794, 794f
  techniques of, 786–788, 788f
  timing of, 810, 810f, 810t, 811f
Tracheotomy tubes, dysphagia and, 718
Transcribriform approach, to cranial base, 451–453, 452f
Transforming growth factors, in wound healing, 204
Transfusions
  complications of, 216–217
  preoperative, 216–217
Transnasal esophagoscopy, controversies as diagnostic tool, 910
Transposition flaps, 2362–2363
Transverse myelitis, radiation-related, 1451
Trapdoor fracture, in children, 1347
Trauma. See also Soft tissue trauma and specific sites and types
  principles of, 919
    definitive management, 931
    metabolic response, 920
    neuroendocrine response, 919–920
    otolaryngologist role, 931
    primary survey of
      airway, 920–923, 921f, 922f
      breathing, 923–924, 923f, 924f
      circulation and shock, 924–926
    secondary survey of, 926
      abdominal injuries, 929–930
      extremity injuries, 930–931
      head and spine injuries, 926–927, 927f
      inhalation injuries, 931
      neck injuries, 927–928, 928f
      thoracic injuries, 928–929, 929f
    treatment, 920
  salivary gland disease in children and, 1251
Traumatic brain injury, 926–927, 927f
  intubation in, 797
  laryngeal dysfunction after, 872
  smell impairment in, 295
Treacher Collins syndrome, 1384–1385, 1384f, 2795
  hearing loss in, 1306t, 1311, 1384
Tremor, 117. See also Essential tremor
Trephination, of frontal sinus, 374

Trichilemmomas, 2734
  treatment of, 2745
Trichoepitheliomas, 2734
  treatment of, 2745
Trichofolliculomas, treatment of, 2745
Trichophytic forehead lift, 2672–2674, 2674f
Trigeminal autonomic cephalalgia, 253–255
Trigeminal nerve, 108f
  anatomy of, 247–248
  nerve blocks of, 143
Trigeminal neuralgia, 259–260
Triiodobenzoic acid derivatives, in sudden sensory hearing loss, 2234
Triiodothyronine, 161
Trimethoprim-sulfamethoxazole, 61
Trinucleotide repeats, unstable, 46, 46t
Triptans, in migraine, 251, 252t
Trisomy 21, 44, 1379–1380, 1379f
  hearing loss in, 1314, 1379
Trotter syndrome, 2795
Trousseau sign, 2795
Tube feeding, preoperative, 215–216
Tuberculosis, 184–185
  diagnosis of, 184, 184f
  incidence of, 184
  laryngeal, 184–185, 831
  nasal, 383, 384f
  otologic manifestations of, 185, 2158–2159
  primary, of salivary glands, 547–548
  treatment of, 185
Tubocurarine, 150
Tubulization techniques, in nerve regeneration, 209, 210f
Tularemia, 187
Tullio phenomenon, 1294, 2795
Tumor-infiltrating lymphocytes, for head and neck cancer, 1413, 1414
Tumor lysis syndrome, in lymphoma, 1626
Tumors. See Cancer; Neoplasms and specific sites and types
Turbinate(s)
  hypertrophy of, 328–330
    reduction in
      anesthesia for, 328–329
      goals of, 328t
      radiofrequency-assisted, 330
      submucosal, 329, 329f
      submucosal microdebrider-assisted, 329–330
  inferior
    anatomy and function of, 311
    hypertrophy of, nasal obstruction in, 313
Turner syndrome, 44, 2795
  hearing loss in, 1314

Tympanic membrane
  development of, 1871
  grafting of, in aural atresia,
      2035–2036
  reconstruction of, 2113–2123
    intraoperative approach for, 2114
    postoperative care following, 2114
    preoperative assessment for,
        2113–2114
    technical considerations for,
        2114–2119, 2115*f*, 2116*f*,
        2117*f*, 2118*f*, 2119*f*
Tympanometry, 1931–1932, 1932*f*
  in otitis media, 1270
Tympanostomy tubes
  acute otitis media with, 64
  controversies about, 1199
  efficacy of, 1204*t*
  for otitis media, 1272–1723
  recommendations for the clinician,
      1206–1207, 1207*t*
  vs. myringotomy alone, 1205*t*
Tyrosine kinase inhibitors (TKI), 54, 54*t*

U
Uhtoff's phenomenon, in multiple
    sclerosis, 107
Ulcers
  contact, vocal fold, 840
  of lip, differential diagnosis of, 1538
  oral, radiation-induced, 1565
  stress
    preventive management of,
        227–228
    treatment of, 228
Ultrasound
  in biopsy, 69. *See also* Biopsy
  of larynx, 93
  of parathyroid glands, 95
  of salivary glands, 93–94, 530
  of soft tissue of neck, 91
  in swallowing evaluation, 1112
  of thyroid gland, 94–95
  in viral gene transfer, 1396
Unasyn (ampicillin-sulbactam), 58
Undulant fever, 183
Unilateral tonsil hyperplasia, 1197
Upper airway obstruction
  causes of, 805, 805*t*
  controversial topics
    airway stents for, 812
    bilateral choanal atresia in
        newborn infants, 808, 808*f*
    decannulation, 810–811
    nasal, orofacial development and,
        807–808
    subglottic stenosis management,
        811
    tracheotomy
      cricothyroidotomy versus,
          808–809, 809*f*, 809*t*

open versus percutaneous,
    809–810, 810*t*
  timing of, 810, 810*f*, 810*t*, 811*f*
evaluation
  diagnosis, 804–805, 804*f*, 804*t*
  signs and symptoms, 803–804
highlights, 812
management
  nonsurgical, 805–806
  surgical, 806–807, 806*t*,
      807*t*
physiology of, 648–649, 649*f*
Upper airway resistance syndrome,
    647–648
Upper mediastinal lymph node
    dissection, 1600
Upper respiratory infections, smell
    impairment in, 295
Usher syndrome, 1306*t*, 1308–1309,
    1385, 2795
  type 1, 49–50
Uveitis, 131
Uveomeningoencephalitic syndrome,
    otologic manifestations of,
    2161–2162
Uveoparotid fever, 548
Uvulopalatopharyngoplasty, 645
  contraindications to, 661
  in snoring, 656–657, 656*f*
Uvulopalatoplasty, laser-assisted, 645,
    661
  in snoring, 657, 658*f*

V
V-to-Y flap, after Mohs surgery, 2397,
    2397*f*, 2398*f*
Vaccines
  for melanoma, 1475–1476
  for otitis media, 1272
  for *Streptococcus pneumoniae*, in
      infants and children, 1059
Vagus-accessory syndrome, 119–120
Vagus nerve, 110*f*
Vail syndrome, 2795
Valproic acid, 251
Valsalva maneuver
  larynx and, 822
  vocal folds and, 699
Vancomycin, 60, 228
Varicella-zoster, otologic manifestations
    of, 2155–2156
Varicella zoster virus infection,
    2180–2181
  stomatitis due to
    clinical features of, 581
    etiology of, 580–581
    treatment of, 581
  treatment of, 2180–2181, 2181*t*
Varices, orbital, 1503
Vascular compromise, sudden sensory
    hearing loss in, 2232

Vascular emergencies, following cranial-
    base surgery, 1850
Vascular endothelial growth factor,
    angiogenesis and, 100, 100*t*
Vascular injuries, as complication of
    temporal bone trauma, 2076
Vascular lesions, in children,
    1349–1357
  hemangiomas, 1349–1353
Vascular lesions, vocal fold, 840
Vascular loop compression syndromes,
    2314
Vascular malformations, 1129–1130,
    1813–1814, 1814*f*
  arteriovenous, 1356
  in children, 1353–1356
    blue rubber bleb, 1356, 1356*f*
    capillary, 1353–1354, 1354*f*
    characteristics of, 1350*t*
    in Klippel-Trenaunay syndrome,
        1356
    overview of, 1357
    in Parkes Weber syndrome, 1356
    in Sturge-Weber syndrome, 1356
    venous, 1355–1356
  of jaw, 1582–1583
  venous, 1355–1356
Vascular tumors, 1811–1825, 1811*t*
  benign, 1811–1819
    localized, 1811–1817
  facial, 2735–2736
  generalized, 1817
  inflammatory, 1817–1819
  malignant, 1819–1823
  orbital, 1502–1503
Vasculitides, 176
  hypersensitivity, 176
Vasculitis, orbital, 1509–1510
Vasodilators, in sudden sensory hearing
    loss, 2233
Vasopressin, 156, 156*f*
Vectors, in gene therapy
  nonviral, 1395–1398
  viral, 1392–1395. *See also* Viral
      vectors
Vecuronium, 150
Veins. *See also* Blood vessels
  of brain, 1828–1829, 1828*f*
  of salivary glands, 520
Velocardiofacial syndrome, 44, 45*f*,
    1383–1384, 1384*f*
Velopharyngeal incompetence
  in pediatric patients, 1077
  in Shprintzen syndrome, 1383–1384
Velopharynx, in deglutition, 686, 686*f*
Venous lakes, 2736
  treatment of, 2746
Venous malformations, 1355–1356
Venous sinus thrombosis, in
    rhinosinusitis, 501
Venous taste, 574

Ventilation, monitoring of, in anesthesia, 151–152
Ventilation techniques, noninvasive, 799
Vermilionectomy, for cancer, 1539
    reconstruction after, 1540–1547, 1541f–1547f
Vernet syndrome, 120, 2795
Verrucae, 2739, 2739f
    treatment of, 2747
Verrucous carcinoma, oral, 1559
Vertebral artery, infarction of, 119
Vertebrobasilar insufficiency, 2310–2311
    medical management of, 2325–2326
    transient, symptoms of, 2310, 2310t
    treatment of, 2311
Vertigo. See also Dizziness; Vestibular disorders
    antivertiginous medications in, 2327–2328
    benign paroxysmal positional, surgery for, 2335–2336
    central causes of, 2317, 2318t
    control of, in Ménière disease, 2334t
    in multiple sclerosis, 107
    peripheral causes of, 2317, 2318t
    of peripheral origin. See Labyrinthitis, acute vestibular
    treatment of, 2328–2329
Vestibular abscess, 616, 616f
Vestibular aqueduct, enlarged, 1971, 1972f
Vestibular autorotation test, to test balance, 1922
Vestibular disorders, 2260–2261, 2261t
    age-related, 239, 240t
    central, 2303–2316
        diagnosis of, 2304–2305, 2306–2307t
        nystagmus and, 2305
        pathophysiology of, 2303–2304
        treatment of, 2308t
        types of, 2304t
    medical management of, 2317–2331
    peripheral, 2295–2302
        in bilateral lesions, 2296
            of gradual onset, 2296
        diagnosis of, 2297–2298
        differential diagnosis of, 2333, 2334t
        with fluctuating or recurrent symptoms, 2296–2297
        management of, 2298–2301, 2299f
        signs and symptoms of, 2295–2297
        in unilateral lesions
            of gradual onset, 2296
            of sudden onset, 2295–2296
        vestibular rehabilitation in, 2300–2301
    pharmacotherapy of, 2320–2329, 2320t

surgical management of, 2333–2342
    endolymphatic sac operations in, 2336–2337
    labyrinthectomy in, 2338–2339, 2339f
    preoperative assessment for, 2333–2335
    selection of procedure for, 2341
    vestibular nerve section in, 2337–2338
    vestibular circuitry and, 2319–2320
Vestibular evoked myogenic potentials, 1924
Vestibular injury, as complication of tympanomastoid surgery, 2109
Vestibular neuritis. See Labyrinthitis, acute vestibular
Vestibular schwannoma, 2313f. See also Acoustic neuroma
    clinical manifestations of, 2210–2211
    diagnostic tests in, 2211–2213
    epidemiology of, 2209
    management of, 2213–2214, 2214t
    observation of, 2214
    surgery for, 2214–2224, 2313
        emergencies after tumor removal, 2223t
        middle fossa approach for, 2218–2220, 2219f
        retrosigmoid-suboccipital approach for, 2220–2222, 2222f
        stereotactic radiosurgery as, 2222–2224
        translabyrinthine approach for, 2214–2218, 2215f, 2217f
    tumor biology in, 2209–2210
    vestibular symptoms in, 2313
Vestibular system
    afferents of, 1912–1913
    and auditory system, aging and, 2257–2264
    brainstem and, 1913–1914, 1913f
    central, compensation for injury, 2319
    disorders of. See Vestibular disorders
    function of, and anatomy of, 1905–1915
    gross anatomy of, 1905–1906
    movement of head and, 1905, 1906f
Vestibular testing, in vestibular schwannomas, 2212
Vestibulopathy, central. See Vestibular disorders, central
Vibrant Soundbridge implantable hearing device, 2274, 2274f
Videofluoroscopic swallow study, 704–706, 705f
    in aspiration, 1112
Videokymography, phonation and, 701
Videostroboscopy, phonation and, 701

Vidian nerve, 2795
Villaret syndrome, 120, 2007, 2795
Vincristine
    for extranodal lymphoma, 1624–1627, 1624t
    toxicity of, 1627
Viral infections. See also specific infections
    pharyngitis in, 606–608
    of salivary glands, 545
    sudden sensory hearing loss in, 2232
Viral vectors
    adeno-associated, 1394
    in gene therapy, 1392–1395
    herpes virus, 1395
    lentivirus, 1395
    replication-selective, 1398
    retrovirus, 1395
    targeting of, 1396–1398, 1397f
Virtual bronchoscopy, 81
Virtual endoscopy, 80, 80f
Vision loss, 128–130
    due to maxillary/periorbital fractures, 990
    following blepharoplasty, 2624
    gradual, 129
    after neck dissection, 1605
    pathological, 129–130
    physiological, 128–129
    after sinonasal tumor surgery, 1498
    after sinus surgery, 483–486
    sudden, 129–130
    transient, 130
    treatment of, 485t
Visual abnormalities, 128–130
Visual acuity, 125–126, 126t
    dynamic, assessment of, 1924–1925
    reduction in, otitis media and, 2055
Visual reinforcement audiometry, 1280–1281
    in otitis media, 1269–1270
Vitamin A deficiency, wound healing and, 207
Vitamin C deficiency, 202
    wound healing and, 207
Vitamin D, 160
Vocal cords. See also Vocal fold(s)
    paralysis of, glottic obstruction in, 1066–1067
Vocal fold(s). See also Larynx; Voice; Voice therapy
    anatomy, 819–820
    benign lesions of
        epithelial, 837–838
        granuloma, 840
        midmembranous, 838–839
        Reinke edema, 840
        rheumatologic, 840
        vascular, 840
    bilateral paralysis of
        clinical presentation and evaluation, 860–862, 861f

clinical history, 860–861
direct microlaryngoscopy, 862, 862f
imaging, 861
laryngeal electromyography, 861–862, 881
neurology and internal medicine workup, 861
palpation for mobility, 862
physical examination, 861
serology, 861
common voice therapy applications for, 889t
etiology, 859–860, 860t
non-surgical, 860t
management
initial, of airway, 862–863
long-term surgical solutions, 863–864, 863f, 864f
temporizing treatments, 863
carcinoma, early treatment of, 911
hematoma of, 955f
immobility
bilateral, etiology, 859–860, 860t
congenital presentation, 1126
laryngeal trauma management and, 957t
paresis, or paralysis of, 873–874
laceration of, 955f
repair of, 955f
medialization of, in laryngeal incompetence, 1114
paradoxical motion disorder, 878–879, 878f
common voice therapy applications for, 889t
paralysis of, 873–874. See also Vocal fold(s), bilateral paralysis of; Vocal fold(s), unilateral paralysis
in children, 1058
Polytef (Teflon) injection for, 911
stridor in, 1106–1107
paroxysmal motion of, stridor in, 1108
phonation and, 700–701
phonomicrosurgery of
equipment for, 841–842
overview, 840–841
preoperative considerations, 841
procedures, techniques, and methods, 842–845, 843f, 844f
scar, 839–840
appropriate voice therapy referrals for, 890
sessile papilloma lesions involving, 1169f
unilateral paralysis of, 873–874
appropriate voice therapy referrals for, 890
common voice therapy applications for, 889t

etiology, 847, 848f, 849–850, 849t, 851f
surgical or iatrogenic, 849t
history
airway, 850–851
vocal inventory, 850
vocal quality and swallowing, 850
physical examination
general, 851–852
laryngeal, 852–854, 852f, 853f, 854f, 881
Polytef (Teflon) injection for, 911
surgery for
injection augmentation, 856–857, 857t, 858f
laryngeal framework, 857–859
treatment, 855–859
determining need for early intervention, 856
patient factors in, 856t
workup
imaging studies, 854–855
serology, 854
Vocal function exercises, in voice therapy, 888
Vogt-Koyanagi-Harada syndrome, otologic manifestations of, 2161–2162
Voice. See also Larynx; Professional voice; Vocal fold(s); Voice therapy
abnormalities of
in elderly, 239t, 240, 240t
electromyography, 881
upper airway obstruction and, 803
abuse of
laryngitis and, 830t
vocal therapy and reduction of, 884
anatomy
laryngeal changes with age, 821
laryngeal framework, 817–819
membranous vocal fold, 820–821
muscles and nerves, 819–820
evaluation
examination, 825–826
history, 824–825
neurolaryngology examination, 869t
physiology
airway protection, 821
larynx and, 822–824, 823f
respiration and, 822
Valsalva maneuver and, 822
rest, for vocal difficulties, 904
Voice prosthesis
duckbill, following laryngectomy, 1781–1782, 1782f
low-pressure, following laryngectomy, 1782, 1783f
Voice rehabilitation, after laryngectomy, 1779–1791
mechanics of, 1779–1782

Voice restoration, during laryngectomy, 1787, 1787f, 1788f
results of, 1787–1789, 1788t, 1789f
Voice therapy
approaches, 885
accent method, 885
confidential, 885–886
facilitating techniques, 886
inspiratory and expiratory pressure threshold training, 886
Lee Silverman Voice Therapy, 870–871, 871t, 886
manual circumlaryngeal techniques, 886–887
resonant voice, 887
respiratory retraining, 887–888
stretch and flow phonation, 888
vocal function exercises, 888
appropriate referrals for, 890–891
commonly associated applications to voice disorders, 889t
limitation to success, 891
model for, 883–885, 884f
common applications to voice disorders, 889t
coordinated vocal production, 884–885
interaction in, 885f
phonotrauma reduction, 884
vocal hygiene, 884
reasons for success or failure, 891t
success, connotations of, 891
Von Langenbeck technique, for cleft lip, 1328
Von Recklinghausen disease, 1382, 1382f, 2793
hearing loss in, 1310–1311

W

W-plasty, for scar camouflage, 2414, 2414f, 2415f
Waardenburg syndrome, 49, 1305t, 1311–1312, 1385–1386, 1385f, 2795–2796
Waldeyer ring lymphoma, 1621–1627. See also Lymphoma, extranodal
Wallenberg syndrome, 2796
Wardill-Kilner-Peet technique, for cleft lip, 1328
Wardill-Kilner V-Y advancement, for cleft palate, 1330, 1332f
Warfarin, 218, 219
Warthin tumor, 1516–1517, 1518f
of salivary glands, 538–540, 540f
Warts, 2739, 2739f
treatment of, 2747
Weber syndrome, 119, 2796
Webs, congenital
glottic, 1126
laryngeal stenosis and, 1135

Webster-modified Bernard cheiloplasty,
     1546–1547, 1546*f*
Wegener granulomatosis, 176–177,
     177*f*, 380–381, 407
  laryngitis and, 830*t*, 832
  otologic manifestations of,
     2159–2160
White-eyed fracture, in children, 1347
Wildervack syndrome, 2796
Wilson disease, laryngeal dysfunction
     and, 872
Winkler disease, 2014, 2796
Wound healing
  bone healing and, 210
  coagulation phase of, 199
  collagen metabolism and, 202–204
  cytokines in, 204–206, 205*t*
  delayed primary, 197, 198*f*
  dynamics of, 197–213
  epidermal growth factor in, 204–205
  factors impeding, 206–208, 206*t*
  fetal, 208–209
  fibroblast growth factors in, 205–206
  fibroplasia phase of, 199
  future of, 211
  growth hormone in, 206
  hypertrophic scars and, 211
  inflammatory phase of, 199
  keloids and, 211
  manipulation of, 208–209
     mucosal, 210
     nerve regeneration in, 209–210, 210*f*
     normal process of, 197–202
     phases of, 198, 199*f*
     platelet-derived growth factor in, 205
     primary, 197, 198*f*
     remodeling phase of, 201–202, 201*f*
     sequence of events in, 198, 200*f*
     spontaneous, 197, 198*f*
     transforming growth factors in, 204
Wounds, antimicrobial agents in, 64
Wrisberg cartilage, 2796
Wrisberg nerve, 2796

X
X-linked inheritance, 1372*f*, 1373
Xenographs, for soft-tissue
     augmentation, 2765–2766,
     2766*f*
Xeroradiography, of larynx, 92–93
Xerostomia, 557–558
     radiation-induced, 1451, 1855, 1855*f*

Y
Young's syndrome, 407

Z
Z-line, assessment of, 747, 747*f*
Z-plasty, for scar camouflage,
     2413–2414, 2413*f*, 2414*f*
Zafirlukast, 400
ZD 1839, 1431–1432
Zenker's diverticula, dysphagia in,
     728–729, 729*f*
Zidovudine, 274
Zileuton, 400
Zinc deficiency, wound healing and,
     207
Zithromax (Azithromycin), 59, 183
Zoster, 2180–2181
  otologic manifestations of,
     2155–2156
  stomatitis due to
     clinical features of, 581
     etiology of, 580–581
     treatment of, 581
  treatment of, 2180–2181, 2181*t*
Zoster sine herpete, 2180
Zygoma
  anatomy of, 976, 976*f*
  displaced, treatment of, 981–984,
     982*f*, 983*f*
Zygomaticomalar complex fractures, in
     children, 1338–1342. *See also*
     Facial fractures, in children
  surgery of, 1345–1346
Zygomaticomaxillary complex fractures,
     978–979
Zyvox (linezolid), 61